J. Javier Servat • Evan H. Black
Frank A. Nesi • Geoffrey J. Gladstone
Christopher J. Calvano
Editors

Smith and Nesi's Ophthalmic Plastic and Reconstructive Surgery

Fourth Edition

Springer

Editors
J. Javier Servat, MD
Oculofacial Plastic Surgeons of Georgia
Suwanee, GA
USA

Department of Ophthalmology
Georgia Regents University
University of Georgia
Athens, GA
USA

Frank A. Nesi, MD, FACS, FAACS
Beaumont Eye Institute
William Beaumont School of Medicine of Oakland University
Rochester, MI
USA

Kresge Eye Institute
Wayne State University School of Medicine
Detroit, MI
USA

Christopher J. Calvano, MD, PhD
San Antonio Military Medical Center/Wilford Hall Ambulatory Surgery Center
Department of Ophthalmology and Oculoplastic Surgery
San Antonio, TX
USA

Evan H. Black, MD, FACS
Consultants in Ophthalmic and Facial Plastic Surgery, P.C.
Southfield, MI
USA

Wayne State University School of Medicine/Kresge Eye Institute
Detroit, MI
USA

Oakland University/William Beaumont Hospital School of Medicine
Department of Ophthalmology
Royal Oak, MI
USA

Geoffrey J. Gladstone, MD
Consultants in Ophthalmic and Facial Plastic Surgery, P.C.
Southfield, MI
USA

Oakland University/William Beaumont Hospital School of Medicine
Department of Ophthalmology
Royal Oak, MI
USA

ISBN 978-3-030-41719-2 ISBN 978-3-030-41720-8 (eBook)
https://doi.org/10.1007/978-3-030-41720-8

This Springer imprint is published by the registered company Springer Nature Switzerland AG
The registered company address is: Gewerbestrasse 11, 6330 Cham, Switzerland

Preface

It has been 7 years since the publication of the third edition of *Smith and Nesi's Ophthalmic Plastic and Reconstructive Surgery*. The innovations in surgical technique and technology have been occurring at an astonishing pace. For half a century, our specialty has led the way in medical and surgical treatment of disease involving the eyelids, orbit, and lacrimal system, and ophthalmic plastic surgeons have become recognized experts in these areas. Over the past several decades, ophthalmic and facial plastic surgeons have created, developed, improved, and mastered techniques in forehead, brow, and facial plastic surgery.

In this fourth edition, you will find extensive updates on functional, reconstructive, aesthetic, and orbital surgery. The collaborative effort of this text includes 75 chapters by over 200 authors all well-recognized in their field. With over 1500 figures and thousands of references to peer-reviewed manuscripts, the reader can quickly locate the information they need to update their knowledge base, fill practice gaps, and improve patient medical and surgical care.

This referenced text has been the gold standard resource for oculofacial plastic surgeons, orbital surgeons, fellows, and residents since its first publication in 1987. The previous editions have also proven to be a treasured resource for comprehensive ophthalmologists, plastic surgeons, otolaryngologists, dermatologists, and many physicians in other specialties. This fourth edition promises to continue the tradition of providing an invaluable means to all who wish to stay on the cutting edge of this unique and intricate specialty.

Athens, GA, USA — J. Javier Servat
Southfield, MI, USA — Evan H. Black
Frank A. Nesi
Geoffrey J. Gladstone
Detroit, MI, USA — Christopher J. Calvano

From the Editor

"It's very easy to get mired in routine and fall into habitual patterns with your 'work'" – those were some of the last words of advice that Dr. Nesi gave me, years ago, during my time in Michigan. After an extensive phone conversation with him last spring, I knew I was embarking into no ordinary "work," by being the managing editor for the *Smith and Nesi's fourth* edition. The journey, although challenging, has been a complete privilege.

Science is an endless frontier. The horizons for ophthalmic plastic continue to evolve dramatically on several fronts prompting us to deliver this text in 11 sections. This volume, larger and with more detailed content than the previous editions, has achieved an unprecedented clinical and scientific value. The book provides an objective, comprehensive, up-to-date overview by experts of current recommendations and strategies in the field of ophthalmic plastic and reconstructive surgery.

From the beginning, a group of experts, all of them enthusiastically agreeing to function as section editors, were put together and able to finish their work in record time. More than 200 authors, with their wealth of information and expertise, have participated. Such a massive task would have been impossible without the tireless cooperation of Michael Griffin from Springer Science + Business Media, LLC.

The addition of three new chapters, including the use of image-guided orbital surgery, combat casualty ophthalmic care for the oculoplastic surgeon, and lacrimal probing and balloon dacryoplasty, cannot help but facilitate the continued astonishing progress that has characterized our dynamic field in the recent years. The edition has an additional 250+ color illustrations, which will engage the reader with text more deeply and critically. Some of the outdated material was also deleted, as we felt it was covered by other current comprehensive ophthalmic resources.

I would like to specifically thank the team of section editors who have been instrumental in supporting the book. The task of reviewing chapters is no ordinary review job, and so much more is demanded of them. They were largely up to the task. In terms of quality and promptitude, they have excelled in their delivery of reviews.

On a personal note, I am forever grateful to Drs. Bruce Shields, Brian DeBroff, Robert Bernardino, and Cesar Sierra from Yale University. I am keenly aware that I couldn't have reached this point without you. A large debt of gratitude also goes to the Fasanella-Petrelli family for your support during the past 15 years and Dr. Yuri Nakasato, who was my clinical mentor and guided me through the beginning of my career.

For all the foundation and assistance you have given me, sometimes saying thank you is not enough to express all the appreciation I feel toward my mentors, Drs. Frank Nesi, Geoffrey Gladstone, and Evan Black. To my mother Elisa, thank you infinitely for your never-ending love, support, and selfless help. Special thanks to my son, Javier, who is on a path to be a superb man; my daughters, Paloma Lucia and Almudena, who gave me a whole new enthusiastic perspective of life; and my beautiful wife, Paloma, who has stood by me for over 15 years. Thank you for allowing me time away from you to research and write; without your love and support, this would not have been possible. Finally, heartfelt thanks to my late father, Javier Servat Sr., the best father you could possibly have! Thank you for your love and all you taught me.

J. Javier Servat, MD

Acknowledgments

Dr. Byron Capleese Smith, for whom this text is named, was born in Kansas in 1908. He is considered to be one of the founders of our specialty of Ophthalmic Plastic and Reconstructive Surgery. During his over 50 years in practice, Dr. Smith trained many fellows in our specialty and in his innovative techniques. Many of these fellows are well-recognized names in ophthalmology, oculoplastic surgery, and medicine in general. Dr. Frank A. Nesi was one of those fellows in 1977 and 1978. Along with Robert C. Della Rocca and Richard D. Lisman, Frank A. Nesi was an obvious choice for developing the first edition of this one-of-a-kind oculoplastic surgery text. Dr. Nesi has trained an astonishingly large number of residents and fellows and has influenced not only their lives but also the lives of countless patients for whom they care. This next generation of fellows, some of whom have been in practice for 20–30 years, continues to carry on the tradition of compiling this information so that both the time-tested and modern techniques in our specialty can been shared with all who are interested in lifelong learning.

For this fourth edition, Juan Javier Servat, our former fellow and son of the renowned Dr. Javier Servat, has led the charge in managing this extensive project. Dr. Servat has distinguished himself as a brilliant physician and skilled surgeon as well as a prolific author. Dr. Servat has overseen this venture with superb organizational skill. Our section editors deserve special recognition for their efforts in revising the major subdivisions of this updated text. Thanks to all our authors for their outstanding work on each individual chapter, including photos, illustrations, and references.

Once again, extraordinary thanks goes to my mentors and coeditors, Drs. Frank Nesi and Geoffrey Gladstone, for all they have done professionally and personally for me and all students, residents, and fellows who have been fortunate enough to train with them. We owe gratitude always to my wife Nickole and children Liam and Mollie for being patient while we work on projects such as this on "their time!" My unending gratefulness extends to my parents Eileen and Marty Black who have continually guided the way and to my uncle Dr. Charles Weiss and aunt Teena Weiss for introducing me to medicine.

Evan H. Black, MD, FACS

Contents

Part I Anatomy
J. Javier Servat

1 **Anatomy of the Ocular Adnexa, Orbit, and Related Facial Structures** 3
J. Javier Servat, Francesca Nesi-Eloff, and Eric Baylin

Part II General Considerations
Frank A. Nesi and Richard D. Lisman

2 **Basic Principles of Ophthalmic Plastic Surgery** 65
Shani Golan, Christopher I. Zoumalan, Frank A. Nesi, and Gary J. Lelli Jr.

3 **Ophthalmic Plastic Surgery: A History in the Making** 87
Alberto G. Distefano, Emily Li, and Mahsa A. Sohrab

4 **Instrumentation in Ophthalmic Plastic Surgery** 105
Shani Golan, Christopher I. Zoumalan, Frank A. Nesi, and Gary J. Lelli Jr.

5 **Neuro-Ophthalmology Approach to Oculoplastic Disorders** 119
Tiffany L. Kent, J. Banks Shepherd III, and Gregory P. Van Stavern

6 **Traumatic Cranial Neuropathies** 145
Ann P. Murchison, Jurij R. Bilyk, and Peter J. Savino

Part III Eyelid Malpositions
John B. Holds

7 **Entropion** 181
Srinivas S. Iyengar, Eric B. Hamill, and Steven C. Dresner

8 **Trichiasis** 189
Kenneth V. Cahill

9 **Ectropion** 195
Steven M. Couch and Philip L. Custer

10 **Facial Palsy: Periocular Management** 205
John B. Holds

11 **Essential Blepharospasm and Hemifacial Spasm** 219
Leon Rafailov, Richard Lee Anderson, and Ilya Michael Leyngold

12 **Ocular Cicatricial Pemphigoid** 231
Sravanthi Vegunta and Alison V. Crum

Part IV Blepharoptosis
Geoffrey J. Gladstone

13 **Ptosis in Neurologic Disease** 243
Ann P. Murchison, Jurij R. Bilyk, and Peter J. Savino

14 **Congenital Ptosis** . . . 279
Alison V. Crum and Rebekah H. Gensure

15 **Acquired Ptosis: Classification and Evaluation** . . . 295
John D. Siddens, Jenna M. Kim, and Geoffrey J. Gladstone

16 **Management of Acquired Ptosis** . . . 307
John D. Siddens, Jenna M. Kim, and Geoffrey J. Gladstone

Part V Cosmetic Surgery
Evan H. Black

17 **Upper Eyelid Blepharoplasty** . . . 325
Mohit A. Dewan and Dale R. Meyer

18 **Lower Eyelid Blepharoplasty** . . . 333
Brett S. Kotlus

19 **Asian Blepharoplasty: Anatomy and Surgical Techniques** . . . 343
Steven Chen

20 **Forehead/Brow Ptosis** . . . 351
Evan H. Black and Dianne Marie-Boesch Schlachter

21 **Injectables and Fillers** . . . 359
Audrey E. Ahuero and Bryan S. Sires

22 **Facelift and Midface Lift** . . . 391
Richard A. Zoumalan, Christopher I. Zoumalan, and Wayne F. Larrabee Jr.

23 **Lasers and Related Technologies** . . . 397
Robert Anolik, Hao Feng, and Roy G. Geronemus

24 **Complications of Blepharoplasty** . . . 409
Helen Merritt, Margaret L. Pfeiffer, and Karina Richani

Part VI Eyelid Tumors and Reconstruction
Richard Allen

25 **Eyelid and Conjunctival Neoplasms** . . . 423
Lilly Wagner, Aaron Savar, and Bita Esmaeli

26 **Eyelid and Ocular Adnexal Reconstruction** . . . 439
Roman Shinder and Bita Esmaeli

27 **Mohs Micrographic Surgery of the Periorbital Area** . . . 459
Michael R. Migden and Sirunya Silapunt

28 **Sentinel Lymph Node Biopsy for Conjunctival and Eyelid Tumors** . . . 477
Aaron Savar and Bita Esmaeli

29 **Oculoplastic Complications of Cancer Therapy** . . . 483
Michael A. Connor and Bita Esmaeli

Part VII Lacrimal Disease and Surgery
Aaron Fay

30 **Lacrimal Sac Tumors: Diagnosis and Treatment** . . . 497
H. Jane Kim and Paul D. Langer

31 **Dysfunctional Tear Film, Etiology, Diagnosis, and Treatment in Oculoplastic Surgery** . . . 505
Mark R. Levine and Essam A. El Toukhy

32 **Congenital Causes of Nasolacrimal Duct Obstruction** 513
Christopher B. Chambers, William Rocamora Katowitz, and James A. Katowitz

33 **Acquired Causes of Lacrimal System Obstructions** 521
Jamie Lea Schaefer and Daniel P. Schaefer

34 **Clinical Evaluation and Imaging of Lacrimal System Obstruction** 545
Jonathan J. Dutton and Jeffrey J. White

35 **Surgery of the Punctum and Canaliculus** 559
Harry Marshak

36 **Primary External Dacryocystorhinostomy** 565
Natalie A. Homer and Aaron Fay

37 **Primary Endoscopic Dacryocystorhinostomy** 571
Roger A. Dailey and Jennifer Murdock

38 **Endoscopic Conjunctivodacryocystorhinostomy** 577
Geoffrey J. Gladstone and Jenna M. Kim

39 **Nasolacrimal Duct Probing, Intubation, and Balloon Dacryoplasty** 583
Peter W. MacIntosh

40 **Transcanalicular Laser-Assisted Dacryocystorhinostomy** 589
Dianne Marie-Boesch Schlachter and Evan H. Black

41 **Management of the Failed Dacryocystorhinostomy** 593
Adam J. Cohen

Part VIII Orbital Disease and Surgery
Alon Kahana

42 **Orbital Evaluation** 603
Dane H. Slentz, Brian J. Lee, and Christine C. Nelson

43 **Orbital Radiology** 615
Tabassum A. Kennedy and Lindell R. Gentry

44 **Orbital Signs of Parasellar Syndromes** 667
Christina H. Choe and Wayne T. Cornblath

45 **Methods for Obtaining and Processing Periocular Tissues for Pathologic Diagnosis** 689
Irina V. Koreen and Victor M. Elner

46 **Surgical Approaches to the Orbit and Optic Nerve** 703
Ayelet Priel, Sang-Rog Oh, Don O. Kikkawa, and Bobby S. Korn

47 **Transcranial Approach to the Orbit** 717
Alon Kahana

48 **Evaluation and Management of Lacrimal Gland Diseases** 721
David T. Tse

49 **Orbital Inflammation** 743
Shivani Gupta, Hakan Demirci, Brian J. Lee, Victor M. Elner, and Alon Kahana

50 **Ocular Adnexal Lymphoproliferative Disease** 769
Jurij R. Bilyk and Ann P. Murchison

51 **Orbital Vascular Anomalies** 817
Anaïs L. Carniciu and Alon Kahana

52 Pediatric Orbital Disease . . . 831
Mithra O. Gonzalez, Natalie A. Homer, and Vikram D. Durairaj

53 Orbital Exenteration . . . 859
Raymond I. Cho and Alon Kahana

54 Image-Guided Orbital Surgery . . . 871
Anaïs L. Carniciu and Alon Kahana

55 Silent Sinus Syndrome . . . 879
Steven E. Katz, Bryan R. Costin, and Mark R. Levine

56 Orbital Tumors . . . 883
Jonathan J. Dutton, Daniel T. Sines, and Victor M. Elner

57 Pathogenesis and Medical Management of Thyroid Eye Disease . . . 983
Anaïs L. Carniciu and Alon Kahana

58 Surgical Management of Thyroid Eye Disease . . . 1001
Anaïs L. Carniciu, Raymond I. Cho, and Alon Kahana

Part IX Socket Surgery
David R. Jordan

59 Enucleation, Evisceration, and Secondary Orbital Implantation . . . 1029
David R. Jordan and Stephen R. Klapper

60 Evaluation and Management of the Anophthalmic Socket and Socket Reconstruction . . . 1055
David R. Jordan and Stephen R. Klapper

Part X Pediatric Considerations
Ann P. Murchison

61 Considerations in Pediatric Oculoplastic Examination . . . 1103
Christopher B. Chambers, William Rocamora Katowitz, and James A. Katowitz

62 Child Abuse Concerns in Oculoplastics . . . 1113
Brian John Forbes

63 Genetics in Oculoplastics . . . 1115
Karthikeyan Arcot Sadagopan

64 Congenital Soft Tissue Deformities . . . 1145
Antonio Augusto Velasco e Cruz and John C. Mustarde

65 Specific Issues in Pediatric Periocular Trauma . . . 1165
Ann P. Murchison and Jurij R. Bilyk

66 Anesthesia and the Pediatric Oculoplastics Patient . . . 1191
Carlo Rob Bernardino

Part XI Eyelid and Orbital Trauma
Christopher J. Calvano and J. Javier Servat

67 Management of Ocular Adnexal Trauma . . . 1201
Jackson F. Lever, Anne Barmettler, and Mark R. Levine

68 Adnexal Burns . . . 1223
Wesley Lawrence Brundridge

69 General Principles of Management of Orbital Fractures 1231
Peter Timoney, Kevin Tomasko, William R. Nunery, and Hui Bae Harold Lee

70 Blowout Fractures of the Orbit 1237
David R. Jordan, Louise Mawn, and Stephen R. Klapper

71 Zygomaticomaxillary Complex Fractures 1263
Geoffrey M. Kwitko

72 Le Fort Fractures 1271
Gina M. Rogers-Hoffman and Richard C. Allen

73 Post-traumatic Enophthalmos and Three-Dimensional Imaging 1285
Michael K. Yoon and Robert C. Kersten

74 Orbital Foreign Bodies and Penetrating Orbital Injuries 1301
Alan A. McNab and Khami Satchi

75 Combat Casualty Ophthalmic Care for the Oculoplastic and Orbital Surgeon ... 1313
Donovan S. Reed, Brett W. Davies, and Christopher J. Calvano

Index 1321

Contributors

Audrey E. Ahuero, MD Ophthalmic Plastic Surgeons of Texas, Houston, TX, USA

Richard C. Allen, MD, PhD Cullen Eye Institute, Baylor College of Medicine, Department of Ophthalmology, Houston, TX, USA

Richard Lee Anderson, MD University of Utah, Salt Lake City, UT, USA

Robert Anolik, MD New York University School of Medicine, Department of Dermatology, New York, NY, USA

Laser & Skin Surgery Center of New York, New York, NY, USA

Anne Barmettler, MD Albert Einstein College of Medicine, Montefiore Medical Center, Department of Ophthalmology, Bronx, NY, USA

Eric Baylin, MD Oculofacial Plastic Surgeons of Georgia, Suwanee, GA, USA

Carlo Rob Bernardino, MD Oculoplastics and Aesthetic Surgery, Vantage Eye Center, Monterey, CA, USA

Jurij R. Bilyk, MD Attending Surgeon and Professor of Ophthalmology, Oculoplastic and Orbital Surgery Service, Wills Eye Hospital and Thomas Jefferson University Hospital, Philadelphia, PA, USA

Evan H. Black, MD, FACS Consultants in Ophthalmic and Facial Plastic Surgery, P.C., Southfield, MI, USA

Wayne State University School of Medicine/Kresge Eye Institute, Detroit, MI, USA

Oakland University/William Beaumont Hospital School of Medicine, Department of Ophthalmology, Royal Oak, MI, USA

Wesley Lawrence Brundridge, DO Aesthetic, Facial and Oculoplastic Surgery, San Antonio, TX, USA

Kenneth V. Cahill, MD The Ohio State University, Department of Ophthalmology, Columbus, OH, USA

Christopher J. Calvano, MD, PhD San Antonio Military Medical Center/Wilford Hall Ambulatory Surgery Center, Department of Ophthalmology and Oculoplastic Surgery, San Antonio, TX, USA

Anaïs L. Carniciu, MD Consultants in Ophthalmic and Facial Plastic Surgery, Southfield, MI, USA

Christopher B. Chambers, MD Division of Oculoplastic and Orbital Surgery, Department of Ophthalmology, University of Washington Harborview Medical Center, Seattle, WA, USA

Steven Chen, MD, FACS Oculoplastic Consultants of Arizona, Glendale, AZ, USA

Christina H. Choe, MD Carolina Ophthalmology, Asheville, NC, USA

Raymond I. Cho, MD Ophthalmic Plastic and Reconstructive Surgery, The Ohio State University Wexner Medical Center, Department of Ophthalmology and Visual Science, Columbus, OH, USA

Adam J. Cohen, MD Eyelid and Facial Plastic and Reconstructive Surgery, Glenview, IL, USA

Michael A. Connor, MD Oculoplastic and Orbital Consultants, P.A., Palm Beach Gardens, FL, USA

Wayne T. Cornblath, MD Department of Ophthalmology & Visual Sciences and Neurology, University of Michigan Kellogg Eye Center, Ann Arbor, MI, USA

Bryan R. Costin, MD Department of Oculoplastics, Cleveland Eye Clinic, Brecksville, OH, USA

Steven M. Couch, MD, FACS Washington University in St. Louis, Ophthalmology and Visual Sciences, St. Louis, MO, USA

Alison V. Crum, MD University of Utah Health Care, Moran Eye Center, Department of Ophthalmology, Salt Lake City, UT, USA

Antonio Augusto Velasco e Cruz, MD, PhD Hospital das Clínicas- FMRP-USP, Department of Ophthalmology, Ribeirão Preto, SP, Brazil

Philip L. Custer, MD, FACS Washington University in St. Louis, Ophthalmology and Visual Sciences, St. Louis, MO, USA

Roger A. Dailey, MD, FACS Oregon Health & Sciences University, Department of Ophthalmic Plastics, Portland, OR, USA

Brett W. Davies, MD, MS Ophthalmic Plastic and Reconstructive Surgery, Brooke Army Medical Center/Wilford Hall Eye Center, Department of Ophthalmology, Lackland, TX, USA

Hakan Demirci, MD University of Michigan, Department of Ophthalmology and Visual Sciences, Kellogg Eye Center, Ann Arbor, MI, USA

Mohit A. Dewan, MD Eye Plastic Surgery of Minnesota PLLC, Woodbury, MN, USA

Alberto G. Distefano, MD Boston University School of Medicine, Department of Ophthalmology, Boston, MA, USA

Steven C. Dresner, MD Roski Eye Institute, The University of Southern California, Department of Ophthalmology, Los Angeles, CA, USA

Eyesthetica, Los Angeles, CA, USA

Vikram D. Durairaj, MD, FACS Dell Medical School – University of Texas at Austin, TOC Eye and Face, Austin, TX, USA

Ophthalmic Plastic and Reconstructive Surgery, TOC Eye and Face, Austin, TX, USA

Jonathan J. Dutton, MD, PhD University of North Carolina, Department of Ophthalmology, Chapel Hill, NC, USA

Victor M. Elner, MD, PhD Eye Plastic and Orbital Surgery Service, Department of Ophthalmology and Visual Sciences, Kellogg Eye Center, University of Michigan, Ann Arbor, MI, USA

Essam A. El Toukhy, MD, FRCOph School of Medicine, Cairo University, Department of Ophthalmology, Dokki, Cairo, Egypt

Bita Esmaeli, MD, MA, FACS Orbital Oncology & Ophthalmic Plastic Surgery, Department of Plastic Surgery, MD Anderson Cancer Center, Houston, TX, USA

Aaron Fay, MD Harvard Medical School, Department of Ophthalmology, Boston, MA, USA

Hao Feng, MD, MHS University of Connecticut Health Center, Department of Dermatology, Farmington, CT, USA

Brian John Forbes, MD, PhD University of Pennsylvania, Department of Opthalmology, Philadelphia, PA, USA

Rebekah H. Gensure, MD, PhD University of Utah, Moran Eye Center, Department of Ophthalmology, Salt Lake City, UT, USA

Lindell R. Gentry, MD, FACR Radiology, Madison, WI, USA

Roy G. Geronemus, MD New York University School of Medicine, Department of Dermatology, New York, NY, USA

Laser & Skin Surgery Center of New York, New York, NY, USA

New York Eye and Ear Infirmary, Department of Plastic Surgery, New York, NY, USA

Geoffrey J. Gladstone, MD Consultants in Ophthalmic and Facial Plastic Surgery, P.C., Southfield, MI, USA

Oakland University/William Beaumont Hospital, School of Medicine, Department of Ophthalmology, Royal Oak, MI, USA

Shani Golan, MD Division of Ophthalmic Plastic, Reconstructive, and Orbital Surgery, Department of Ophthalmology, Weill Cornell Medical College, New York-Presbyterian Hospital, New York, NY, USA

Mithra O. Gonzalez, MD University of Rochester Department of Ophthalmology, Oral and Maxillofacial Surgery, Otolaryngology, Plastic and Reconstructive Surgery, Rochester, NY, USA

Shivani Gupta, MD, MPH Kaiser Permanente, Department of Ophthalmology, Panorama City, CA, USA

Eric B. Hamill, MD Roski Eye Institute, The University of Southern California, Department of Ophthalmology, Los Angeles, CA, USA

Eyesthetica, Los Angeles, CA, USA

John B. Holds, MD, FACS Saint Louis University School of Medicine, Departments of Ophthalmology and Otolaryngology/Head and Neck Surgery, St. Louis, MO, USA

Natalie A. Homer, MD Ophthalmic Plastic and Reconstructive Surgery, TOC Eye and Face, Austin, TX, USA

Srinivas S. Iyengar, MD, FACS San Diego Eyelid Specialists, Encinitas, CA, USA

David R. Jordan, MD, FACS, FRCSC Ottawa Hospital – General Campus, Eye Institute, Ottawa, ON, Canada

Alon Kahana, MD, PhD Consultants in Ophthalmic and Facial Plastic Surgery, Southfield, MI, USA

James A. Katowitz, MD The Children's Hospital of Philadelphia and The Edwin and Fannie Gray Hall Center for Appearance, The University of Pennsylvania Perelman School of Medicine, Department of Ophthalmology, Philadelphia, PA, USA

William Rocamora Katowitz, MD Perelman School of Medicine, The University of Pennsylvania, The Children's Hospital of Philadelphia and The Scheie Eye Institute, Division of Ophthalmology, Philadelphia, PA, USA

Steven E. Katz, MD Ocular & Orbital Traume Service, Riverside Methodist Hospital, Department of Opthalmology, Columbus, OH, USA

Tabassum A. Kennedy, MD Department of Radiology, University of Wisconsin Hospital and Clinics, Madison, WI, USA

Tiffany L. Kent, MD, PhD Oculoplastic Associates of West Michigan, Grand Rapids, MI, USA

Robert C. Kersten, MD University of California – San Francisco, Department of Ophthalmology, San Francisco, CA, USA

Don O. Kikkawa, MD Division of Oculofacial Plastic Surgery, Viterbi Family Department of Ophthalmology Shiley Eye Institute University of California San Diego School of Medicine, La Jolla, CA, USA

H. Jane Kim, MD Oculofacial Plastic Surgery, The Permanente Medical Group, Department of Ophthalmology, Union City, CA, USA

Jenna M. Kim, MD William Beaumont School of Medicine, Beaumont Eye Institute, Royal Oak, IL, USA

Stephen R. Klapper, MD, FACS Ophthalmology/Oculoplastic Surgery, Klapper Eyelid and Facial Plastic Surgery, Carmel, IN, USA

Irina V. Koreen, MD, PhD Eye Physicians of Orange County, P.C., Goshen, NY, USA

Bobby S. Korn, MD, PhD Division of Oculofacial Plastic Surgery, Viterbi Family Department of Ophthalmology Shiley Eye Institute University of California San Diego School of Medicine, La Jolla, CA, USA

Brett S. Kotlus, MD, MS, FACS Oculofacial Plastic Surgeon, Private Practice, New York, NY, USA

Geoffrey M. Kwitko, MD, FACS University of South Florida, Department of Ophthalmology, Tampa, FL, USA

Paul D. Langer, MD, FACS Division of Ophthalmic Plastic, Reconstructive, and Orbital Surgery, Institute of Ophthalmology and Visual Science, Rutgers New Jersey Medical School, Newark, NJ, USA

Wayne F. Larrabee Jr., MD, MSH Larrabee Center for Plastic Surgery, Seattle, WA, USA

Brian J. Lee, MD Maryland Oculoplastic Surgery, Ellicott City, MD, USA

Hui Bae Harold Lee, MD, FACS St. Vincent Hospital, Department of Ophthalmology, Indianapolis, IN, USA

Gary J. Lelli Jr., MD Weill Cornell Medical Center/New York-Presbyterian Hospital, Department of Ophthalmology, New York, NY, USA

Jackson F. Lever, MD Country Hills Eye Center, Ogden, UT, USA

Mark R. Levine, MD, FACS University Hospitals of Cleveland, Department of Ophthalmology, Cleveland, OH, USA

Ilya Michael Leyngold, MD Duke Eye Center, Division of Oculofacial and Orbital Surgery, Durham, NC, USA

Emily Li, MD University of Washington School of Medicine, Department of Ophthalmology, Seattle, WA, USA

Peter W. MacIntosh, MD University of Illinois, Ophthalmology and Visual Sciences, Chicago, IL, USA

Harry Marshak, MD Eisenhower Medical Center, Department of Surgery, Palm Desert, CA, USA

Louise Mawn, MD, FACS Vanderbilt University Medical Center, Department of Ophthalmology, Nashville, TN, USA

Alan A. McNab, FRANZCO, DMedSc Royal Victorian Eye and Ear Hospital, Orbital Plastic and Lacrimal Clinic, East Melbourne, VIC, Australia

Helen Merritt, MD Oculoplastics Associates of Texas, Dallas, TX, USA

Dale R. Meyer, MD Lions Eye Institute-Albany Medical Center, Department of Ophthalmic Plastic Surgery-Ophthalmology, Albany, NY, USA

Michael R. Migden, MD University of Texas M D Anderson Cancer Center, Department of Head and Neck, Division of Surgery, Houston, TX, USA

University of Texas M D Anderson Cancer Center, Department of Dermatology, Division of Internal Medicine, Houston, TX, USA

Ann P. Murchison, MD, MPH Attending Surgeon, Oculoplastic and Orbital Surgery Service and Director, Eye Emergency Department, Wills Eye Hospital and Thomas Jefferson University Hospital, Philadelphia, PA, USA

Jennifer Murdock, MD Oregon Health & Sciences University, Department of Ophthalmic Plastics, Portland, OR, USA

Christine C. Nelson, MD Eye Plastic, Orbital and Facial Cosmetic Surgery, University of Michigan Health System, Department of Ophthalmology and Visual Sciences (W.K. Kellogg Eye Center), Ann Arbor, MI, USA

Francesca Nesi-Eloff, MD William Beaumont Hospital, Department of Ophthalmology, Southfield, MI, USA

Frank A. Nesi, MD, FACS, FAACS Beaumont Eye Institute, William Beaumont School of Medicine of Oakland University, Rochester, MI, USA

Kresge Eye Institute, Wayne State University School of Medicine, Detroit, MI, USA

William R. Nunery, MD University of Louisville, Department of Ophthalmology & Visual Sciences, Louisville, KY, USA

Sang-Rog Oh, MD Division of Oculofacial Plastic and Reconstructive Surgery Department of Ophthalmology The Permanente Medical Group, Sacramento, CA, USA

Margaret L. Pfeiffer, MD Key-Whitman Eye Center, Dallas, TX, USA

Ayelet Priel, MD Division of Oculopfacial Plastic and Reconstructive Surgery, Goldschleger Eye Institute, Sheba Medical Center, Ramat Oan, Israel

Sackler School of Medicine, Tel Aviv University, Tel Aviv, Israel

Leon Rafailov, MD Duke Eye Center, Division of Oculofacial and Orbital Surgery, Durham, NC, USA

Donovan S. Reed, MD Brooke Army Medical Center, Department of Ophthalmology, Fort Sam Houston, TX, USA

Karina Richani, MD Ruiz Department of Ophthalmology, University of Texas, McGovern Medical School, Houston, TX, USA

Gina M. Rogers-Hoffman, MD Eye Physicians and Surgeons of Chicago, Chicago, IL, USA

Karthikeyan Arcot Sadagopan, DO, MBBS, MD, FRCS CMER (SHENZHEN) Dennis Lam Eye Hospital, Department of Pediatric Ophthalmology & Ocular Genetics, Futian District, Shenzhen, China

Khami Satchi, MB BChir MA FRCOphth, FRANZCO Orbital Plastic and Lacrimal Clinic, Royal Victorian Eye and Ear Hospital, Melbourne, VIC, Australia

Aaron Savar, MD Stein Eye Institute, UCLA, Department of Ophthalmology, Los Angeles, CA, USA

Peter J. Savino, MD Clinical Professor of Ophthalmology, Viterbi Famile Department of Ophthalmology, Shiley Eye Institute, University of Califormia San Diego, La Jolla, CA, USA

Daniel P. Schaefer, MD. FACS Clinical Professor of Ophthalmology, Director of Oculoplastic, Orbital, and Facial Plastic Reconstructive Surgery, Department of Otolaryngology, State University of New York at Buffalo, Buffalo, NY, USA

Jamie Lea Schaefer, MD Division of Ophthalmology, The Warren Alpert Medical School at Brown University, Providence, RI, USA

Dianne Marie-Boesch Schlachter, MD Consultants in Ophthalmic and Facial Plastic Surgery, P.C., Southfield, MI, USA

Oakland University/William Beaumont Hospital School of Medicine, Department of Ophthalmology, Royal Oak, MI, USA

J. Javier Servat, MD Oculofacial Plastic Surgeons of Georgia, Suwanee, GA, USA

Department of Ophthalmology, Georgia Regents University, University of Georgia, Athens, GA, USA

J. Banks Shepherd III, MD Washington University in St. Louis, Department of Visual Sciences (Ophthalmology), Saint Louis, MO, USA

Roman Shinder, MD SUNY Downstate Medical Center, Department of Ophthalmology, Otolaryngology, Brooklyn, NY, USA

John D. Siddens, DO Ophthalmic Plastic Surgery Service, Greenville Memorial Hospital, Prisma Health System Upstate, Division of Ophthalmology, Department of Surgery, Greenville, SC, USA

Sirunya Silapunt, MD University of Texas McGovern Medical School at Houston, Department of Dermatology, Houston, TX, USA

Daniel T. Sines, MD Boozman Hof Regional Eye Clinic, Rogers, AR, USA

Bryan S. Sires, MD, PhD Allure Laser Center and Medispa, Kirkland, WA, USA

Dane H. Slentz, MD Eye Plastic, Orbital and Facial Cosmetic Surgery, University of Michigan Health System, Department of Ophthalmology and Visual Sciences (W.K. Kellogg Eye Center), Ann Arbor, MI, USA

Mahsa A. Sohrab, MD Yale University, Department of Ophthalmology, New Haven, CT, USA

Peter Timoney, MBBCh University of Kentucky, Department of Ophthalmology, Lexington, KY, USA

Kevin Tomasko, MD University of Louisville, Department of Ophthalmology & Visual Sciences, Louisville, KY, USA

David T. Tse, MD Bascom Palmer Eye Institute, Department of Ophthalmology, Miami, FL, USA

Gregory P. Van Stavern, MD Washington University in St. Louis, Department of Ophthalmology and Visual Sciences, St. Louis, MO, USA

Sravanthi Vegunta, MD University of Utah Health Care, Moran Eye Center, Department of Ophthalmology, Salt Lake City, UT, USA

Lilly Wagner, MD Mayo Clinic, Department of Ophthalmology, Rochester, MN, USA

Jeffrey J. White, MD Carolina Eye Associates, P.A, Southern Pines, NC, USA

Michael K. Yoon, MD Mass Eye and Ear, Department of Ophthalmology, Harvard Medical School, Boston, MA, USA

Christopher I. Zoumalan, MD Department of Ophthalmology, Division of Ophthalmic Plastic and Reconstructive Surgery, Keck School of Medicine of USC, Los Angeles, CA, USA

Richard A. Zoumalan, MD UCLA, Cedars Sinai Medicine, Department of Otolaryngology, Beverly Hills, CA, USA

Part I

Anatomy

J. Javier Servat

Anatomy of the Ocular Adnexa, Orbit, and Related Facial Structures

1

J. Javier Servat, Francesca Nesi-Eloff, and Eric Baylin

Introduction

The sine qua non of corrective or cosmetic orbital and eyelid surgery is the exquisite and requisite knowledge of the anatomical structures contained in this relatively confined space. A study of the osteology of the orbit and its relationship to the surrounding cranial bone structures is correlated with the topographic anatomy and then the contents of the orbit, finally addressing the structures of the lids and periorbital area.

The anatomy of the bony structures segues into an analysis of the lacrimal system and its structures, followed by a study of the muscular superficial and deep structures that follow. An in-depth study of the vascular and neurological elements is then undertaken.

With this anatomic knowledge in one's armamentarium, the surgeon is able to embark on an organized and deliberate series of reconstructive or cosmetic procedures always aimed at restoring or enhancing anatomic integrity.

Osteology

Orbital Shape and Development

The confines and the relationships of the orbits are best understood by examining a skull (Fig. 1.1). Early in human development, the optic vesicles point in opposite directions. As facial development occurs, the angle between the optic stalks decreases as the eyes become situated more anteriorly. In the adult, the exact angle of the divergent optic nerves is determined in part by the placement of the optic chiasm on the sphenoid body, but it is usually about 68° [1].

The adult lateral orbital walls are approximately 90° from each other, or 45° anteroposterior. The medial orbital walls

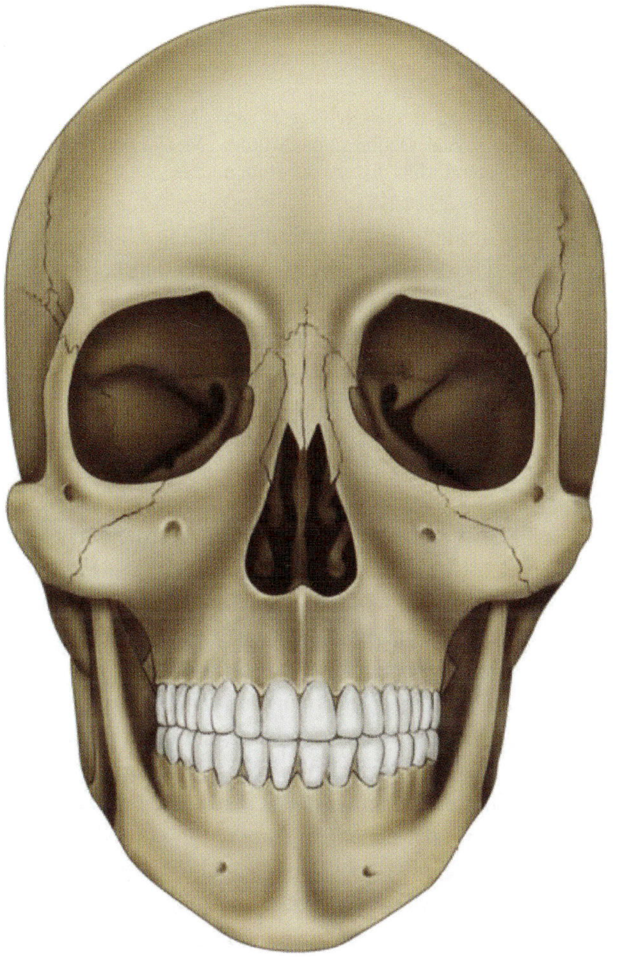

Fig. 1.1 Anteroposterior view of adult skull

J. J. Servat (✉)
Oculofacial Plastic Surgeons of Georgia, Suwanee, GA, USA

Department of Ophthalmology, Georgia Regents University, University of Georgia, Athens, GA, USA

F. Nesi-Eloff
William Beaumont Hospital, Department of Ophthalmology, Southfield, MI, USA

E. Baylin
Oculofacial Plastic Surgeons of Georgia, Suwanee, GA, USA

J. J. Servat et al. (eds.), *Smith and Nesi's Ophthalmic Plastic and Reconstructive Surgery*,
https://doi.org/10.1007/978-3-030-41720-8_1

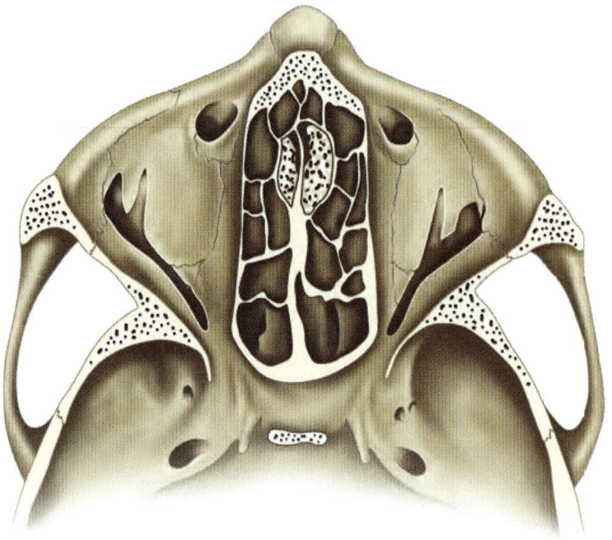

Fig. 1.2 Horizontal section through orbits. Medial walls are nearly parallel and lateral walls diverge 45° from midline

are nearly straight anteroposterior, angling slightly medial anteriorly. The divergent axis of each orbit thus becomes half of 45°, or about 23° (Fig. 1.2). The eyes tend to diverge in accordance with their bony surroundings, as is seen in individuals with acquired visual loss, under general anesthesia, or in death. It is not surprising to find the medial rectus, the thickest of the rectus muscles, because of the constant demand on it for torsion of the globe away from the orbital axis.

Facial development occurs from processes evident in the third week of development. The mandibular swellings are the most caudal and initially are separated by a midline depression. The frontonasal process is rostral with symmetric halves and is separated from the former by the median stomodeum, or primitive mouth, and laterally by the paired maxillary processes (Fig. 1.3). The frontonasal and mandibular processes form the central face and mandible, respectively, while the maxillary processes later approach the midline to form the malar eminences.

The lateral nasal process lies medial to the eye and fuses with the maxillary process situated beneath and lateral to the eye, thus forming the medial, inferior, and lateral orbital walls. The orbital roof is formed by the capsule of the developing forebrain. The enlarging globe stretches the surrounding connective tissue making it fairly dense and a relative restraint to further embryologic modeling in this area [2]. Within these condensed fibrous plates, numerous ossification centers first appear around the seventh week. Ossification of the orbital walls is completed by birth except at the orbital apex. The lesser wing of the sphenoid is initially cartilaginous, unlike the greater sphenoid wing and the other membranous orbital bones. The orbital walls are derived from cranial neural crest cells, which expand to form the frontonasal and maxillary processes.

The orbit most closely resembles a four-sided pyramid that becomes three-sided near the apex. The side lost is the floor, which is cut off by the inferior orbital fissure at two-thirds the orbital depth. The widest portion is 1 cm behind the orbital rim corresponding to the equator of the globe. The relative narrowing of the orbital rim is minimal at birth but proceeds with facial growth, especially with expansion of the frontal and maxillary sinuses. The depth of the orbit measured from the apex to the center of the orbital margin is approximately 45 mm, with substantial variation between individuals and slight differences between sides of an individual.

Orbital Margin

The adult orbital rim is a discontinuous spiral. It is roughly rectangular with a horizontal dimension of 40 mm and a vertical dimension of 32 mm. The zygomatic bone forms most of the lateral margin and the lateral half of the inferior rim (see Figs. 1.1 and 1.4). This orbital protector or "facial buttress" can withstand severe trauma before fracture which usually occurs along the suture lines. Steps may then be felt inferiorly at the zygomaticomaxillary suture and superolaterally at the zygomaticofrontal suture. The frontal bone encompasses the superior orbital margin and extends laterally and medially to form portions of these borders. The newborn superior orbital rim is sharp. It remains so in the female but becomes rounded with development in the male. Medially between the superior orbits is the smooth glabellar area below which the nasal bones arise. In most skulls, the medial superior rim is indented by a supraorbital notch formed by the supraorbital nerve and artery rising to the forehead. In some skulls, the bone covers these structures, forming a foramen.

The medial orbital margin is formed anteriorly by the maxillary bone rising to meet the maxillary process of the frontal bone. The lacrimal excretory sac complicates the medial rim by indenting the bone and forming anterior (maxillary bone) and posterior (lacrimal bone) crests (see section "Lacrimal Excretory Osteology"). Thus, the orbital rim was described by Whitnall as a single coil of an undulating spiral [3].

The infraorbital nerve and attendant artery exit 4 mm or more below the inferior rim medially. In two-thirds of skulls, a supraorbital notch can be found along the superomedial rim [4]. A foramen is seen instead of a notch in other skulls. The possibility of this variation should be considered during coronal or endoscopic brow lifting. The supraorbital ridge lies above the medial one-half of the orbit.

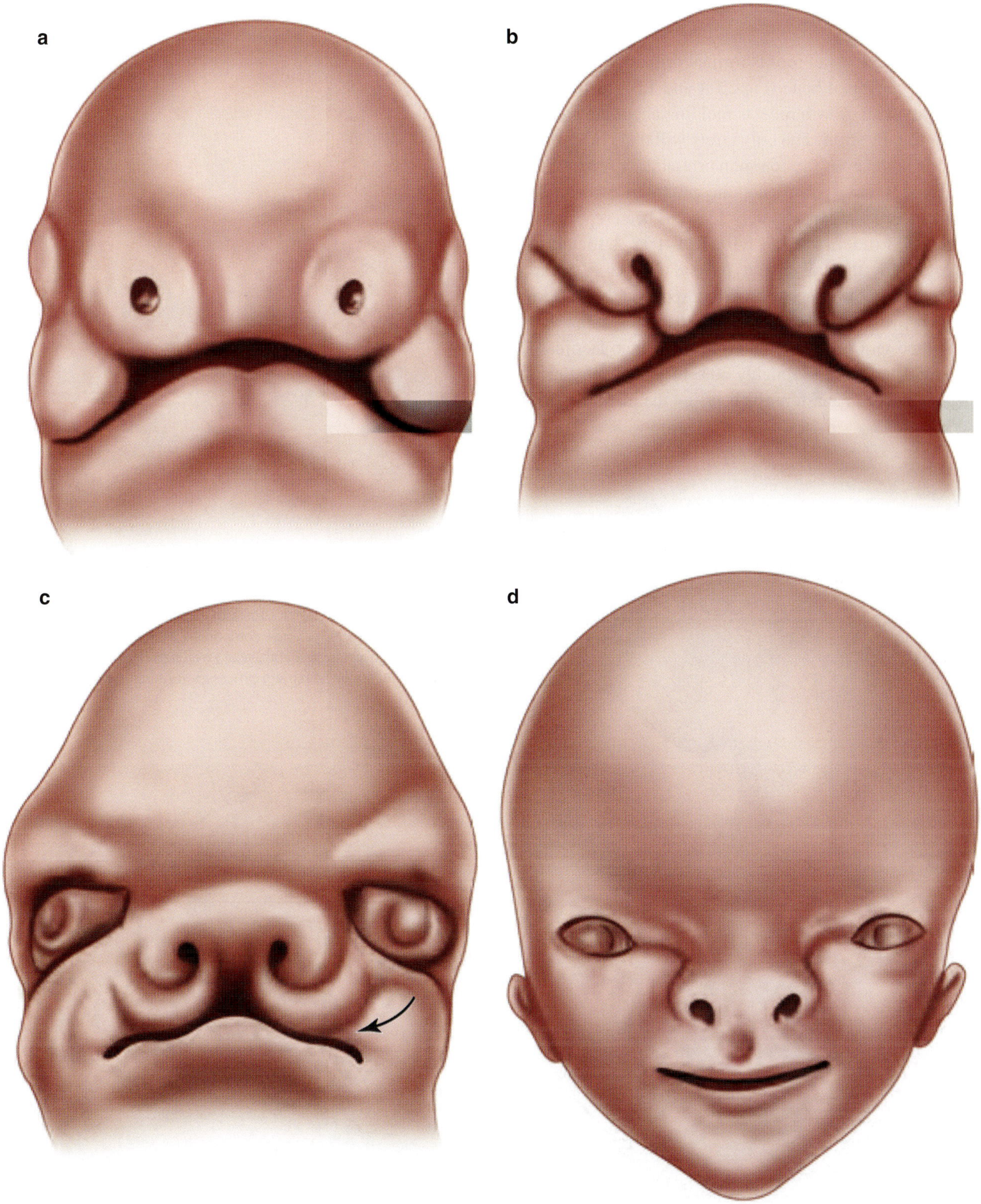

Fig. 1.3 Facial development. (**a**) Frontonasal and mandibular processes separated by maxillary processes and mouth. (**b**) Lacrimal groove develops between lateral nasal and maxillary processes. (**c**) Medial expansion of maxillary processes forming lateral wall and floor of orbit. Medial wall is formed by lateral nasal process and roof by frontal process. (**d**) Medial nasal processes fuse, forming upper lip and hard palate

Orbital Walls

The triangular orbital roof is formed primarily by the orbital plate of the frontal bone (Figs. 1.4 and 1.5). Its progressive convexity with growth reflects molding about the globe. The roof is usually strong and only rarely will blunt ocular trauma explode it, vis-a-vis the common orbital floor fracture. Small dehiscences, however, are not uncommon in the orbital roof. An incidence of approximately 15% has been reported [3, 5] (Figs. 1.5, 1.6, 1.7, 1.8, 1.9, 1.10, 1.11, 1.12, 1.13, and 1.14).

Posteriorly, the roof remains flat and receives a 1.5-cm contribution from the lesser wing of the sphenoid bone. Near the suture between the frontal and sphenoid bones, approximately 30 mm posterior to the orbital rim, a meningo-lacrimal foramen may be found. In roughly 30% of individuals, this foramen conducts an anastomosis between the middle meningeal

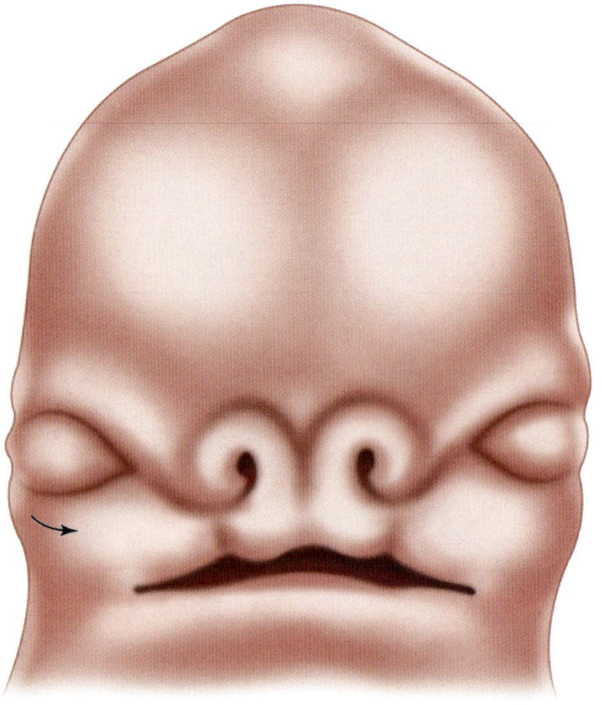

Fig. 1.6 Nasal development. Medial movement of maxillary processes compresses medial nasal swellings of frontonasal mass to form philtrum of upper lip, upper jaw component encompassing four incisor teeth, and hard palate. Lateral nasal swellings become nasal alae and medial orbital walls. Maxillary processes form nasal floor and inferior nasal wall

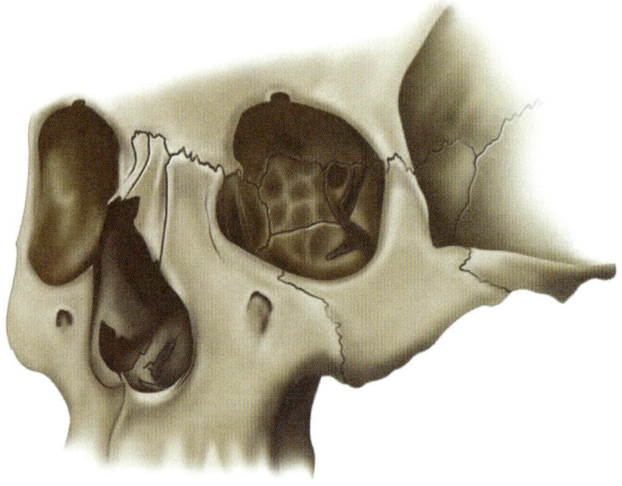

Fig. 1.4 Bones of orbit

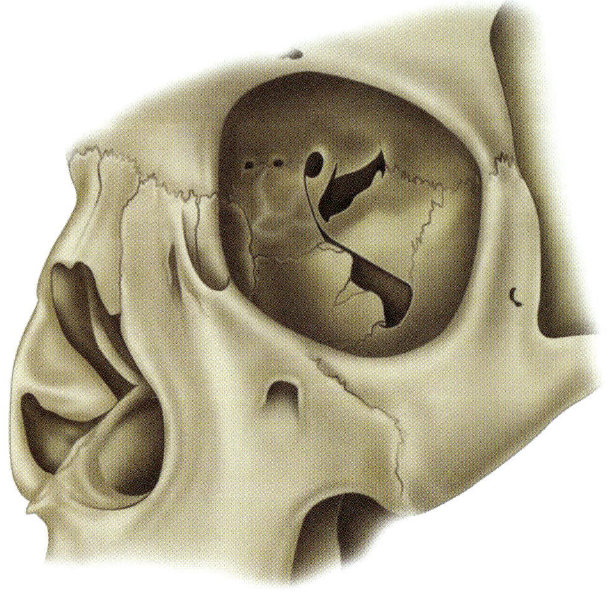

Fig. 1.5 Osteology of orbital apex

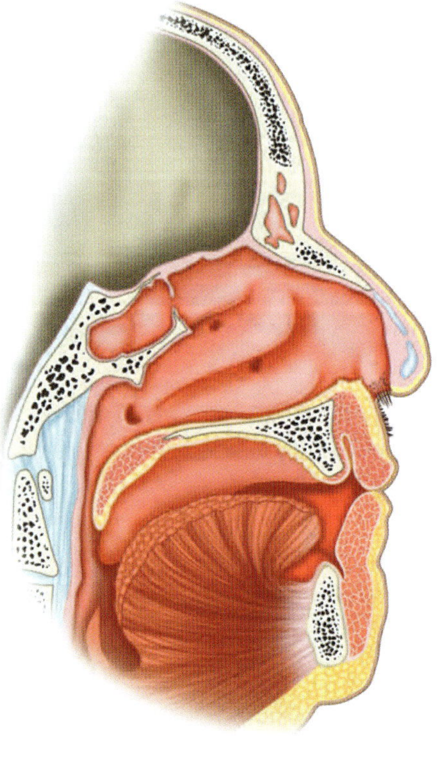

Fig. 1.7 Nasal anatomy. Each meatal space is named for turbinate that lies immediately above

artery (external carotid system) and the root of the lacrimal artery [6]. The optic nerve pierces the roof at an angle of about 35° from midline to form the optic foramen (see later). Anteromedially, the small trochlear fossa is found while the large lacrimal gland fossa is seen laterally.

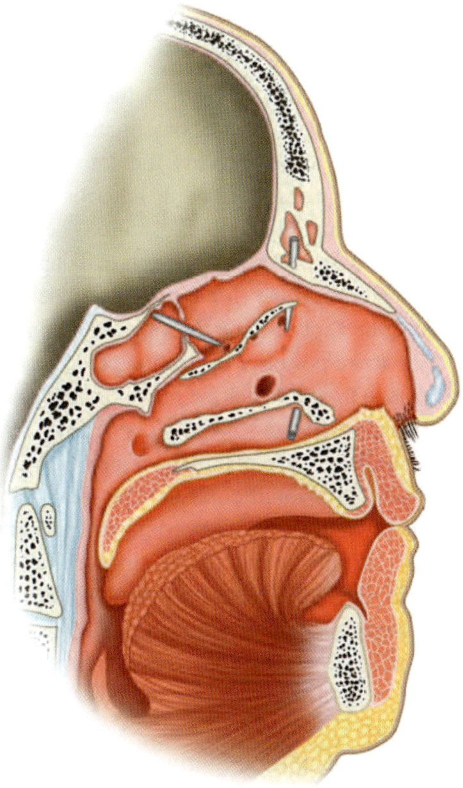

Fig. 1.8 Lateral nasal wall with middle and inferior turbinates amputated. Probes are placed in sphenoid sinus ostium and frontonasal and nasolacrimal ducts

The lateral orbital wall is bounded by the superior and inferior orbital fissures. These borders are carried anteriorly roughly by the frontosphenoidal and zygomaticomaxillary sutures. Posteriorly, the greater wing of the sphenoid forms the lateral wall. Anteriorly, the zygoma and the lateral angular (zygomatic) process of the frontal bone each contributes to the lateral orbital wall. The vertical zygomaticosphenoid suture marks the thinnest part of the lateral orbital wall and forms a convenient breaking point for bone removal during orbitotomy. Posterior and lateral to the lateral rim lies the firmly adherent temporalis muscle. The muscle has a dense superficial fascia easily harvested through a skin and superficial muscle plane incision.

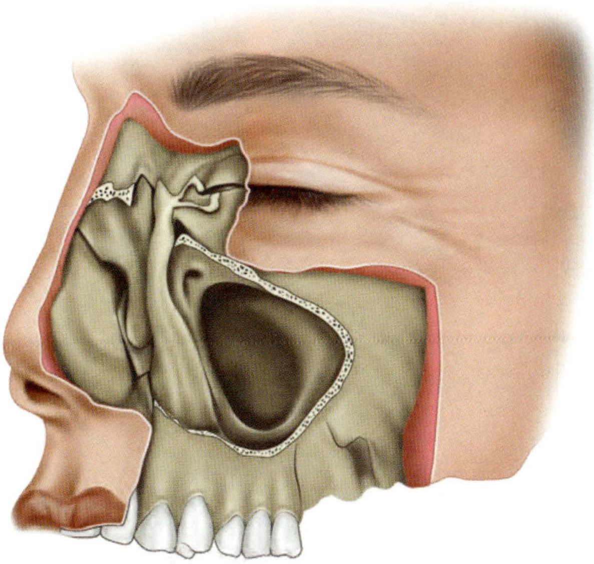

Fig. 1.10 Anterolateral view of maxillary sinus with anterior wall removed. The maxillary bone contributes the lateral two-thirds of the nasolacrimal duct

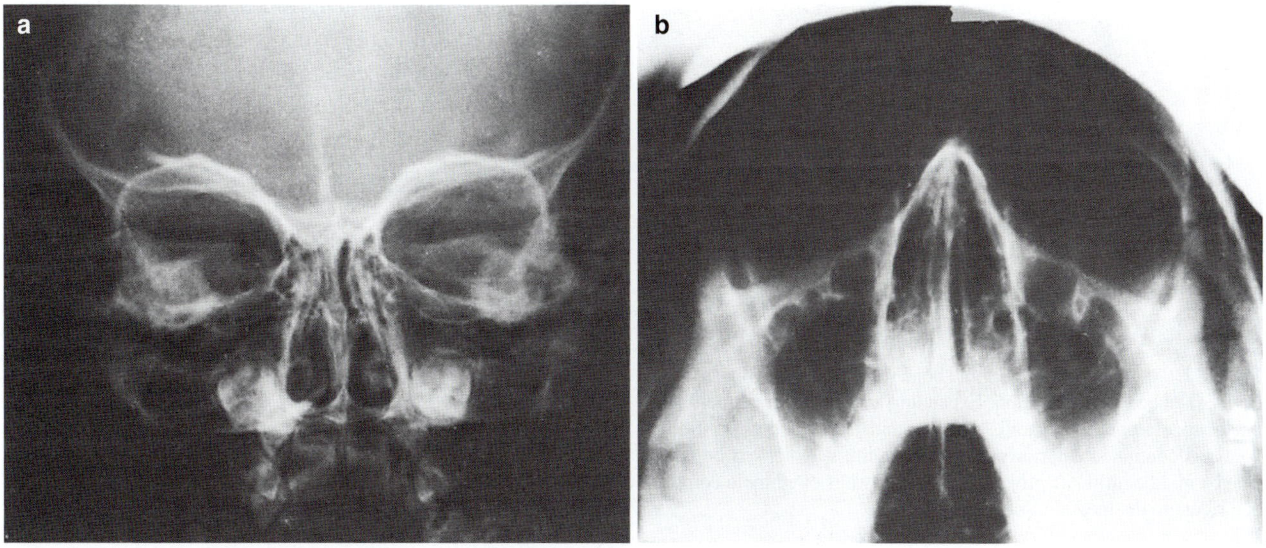

Fig. 1.9 (**a**) Radiograph of 7-year-old child shows ethmoid and maxillary sinuses. Although the ethmoid sinus is well developed, the maxillary sinus cannot complete pneumatization until secondary teeth descend. (**b**) Fully developed maxillary sinuses in adult

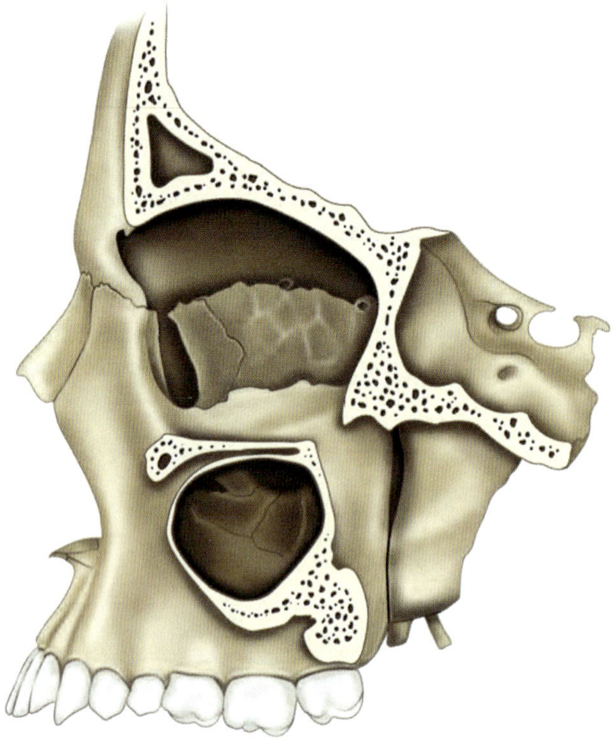

Fig. 1.11 Parasagittal view showing intimate relationship of orbit and maxillary sinus

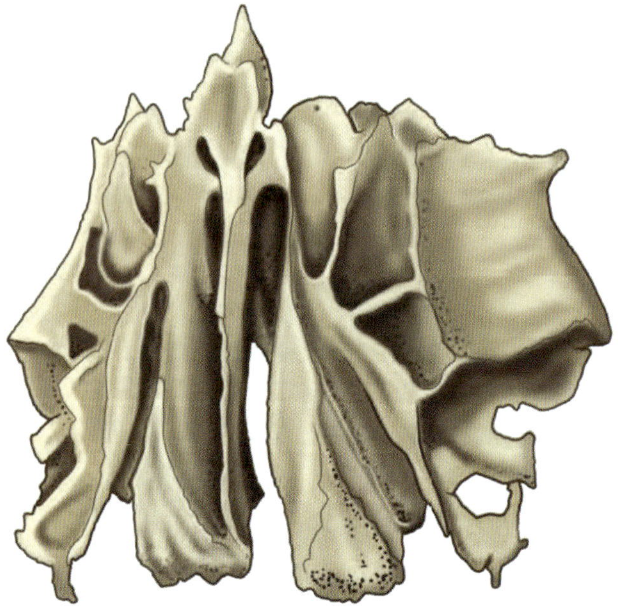

Fig. 1.12 Anterior view of ethmoid bone with left orbital rim and nasal cavity sketched for orientation. Expanding air cells from ethmoid may pneumatize frontal, sphenoid, palatine, and lacrimal bones. Midline vomer is continued anteriorly as nasal septum; it is flanked on either side by middle turbinate projections. Lateral walls of ethmoid complex contribute to the medial orbital walls

Just within the lateral orbital margin about 11 mm below the frontozygomatic suture, the lateral orbital tubercle of Whitnall is found [7]. At this important site, the lateral canthal ligament, lateral rectos check ligament, lateral horn of the levator, suspensory ligament of the eye (Lockwood's ligament), and orbital septum all attach. The zygomaticotemporal and zygomaticofacial foramina perforate the anterior lateral orbital wall and transmit neurovascular bundles.

The shortest of the orbital walls is the floor. It is shaped like an equilateral triangle. A line passing through the axis of the inferior orbital fissure forms the lateral border. The medial border can be defined with anterior and posterior extensions of the maxilloethmoidal suture. The orbital floor does not continue to the orbital apex. It ends approximately 35–40 mm posterior to the rim at the pterygopalatine fossa. This fact must be kept in mind during surgery on the orbital floor because more posterior dissection could lead to extensive hemorrhage from the internal maxillary artery located in the pterygopalatine fossa.

The orbital plate of the maxillary bone comprises nearly the entire floor, with small contributions from the palatine bone posteriorly and from the zygoma anterolaterally. The floor remains strong lateral to the infraorbital nerve but becomes thin medially with maxillary sinus expansion. This thin, unsupported dome of the maxillary sinus is where the floor usually fractures with trauma. In static loading studies, the orbital floor shows the greatest degree of deformation [8]. This location is also a convenient site for entry into the maxillary sinus during orbital decompression surgery.

The infraorbital groove is found posteriorly and centrally in the orbital floor. It carries the maxillary division of the trigeminal nerve. This groove or sulcus is converted into a canal, which ends anteriorly as the infraorbital foramen. In the embryo, the infraorbital nerve lies freely along the orbital floor, but by birth, it has been encompassed by the more rapidly growing maxillary bone. In the child, the infraorbital foramen is situated immediately below the orbital margin. In the adult, the infraorbital nerve exits approximately 6 mm inferior to the orbital rim.

The medial wall is the smallest and the thinnest of the orbital walls. It extends roughly 4.5–5 cm posterior to the anterior lacrimal crest. The ethmoid bone makes the major contribution, with extensions of its frontoethmoidal and maxilloethmoidal sutures defining the superior and inferior medial borders. The lacrimal, maxillary, and sphenoid bones also contribute to the medial wall. The medial wall becomes thicker posteriorly at the body of the sphenoid and anteriorly both at the posterior lacrimal crest of the lacrimal bone and at the anterior lacrimal crest of the maxillary

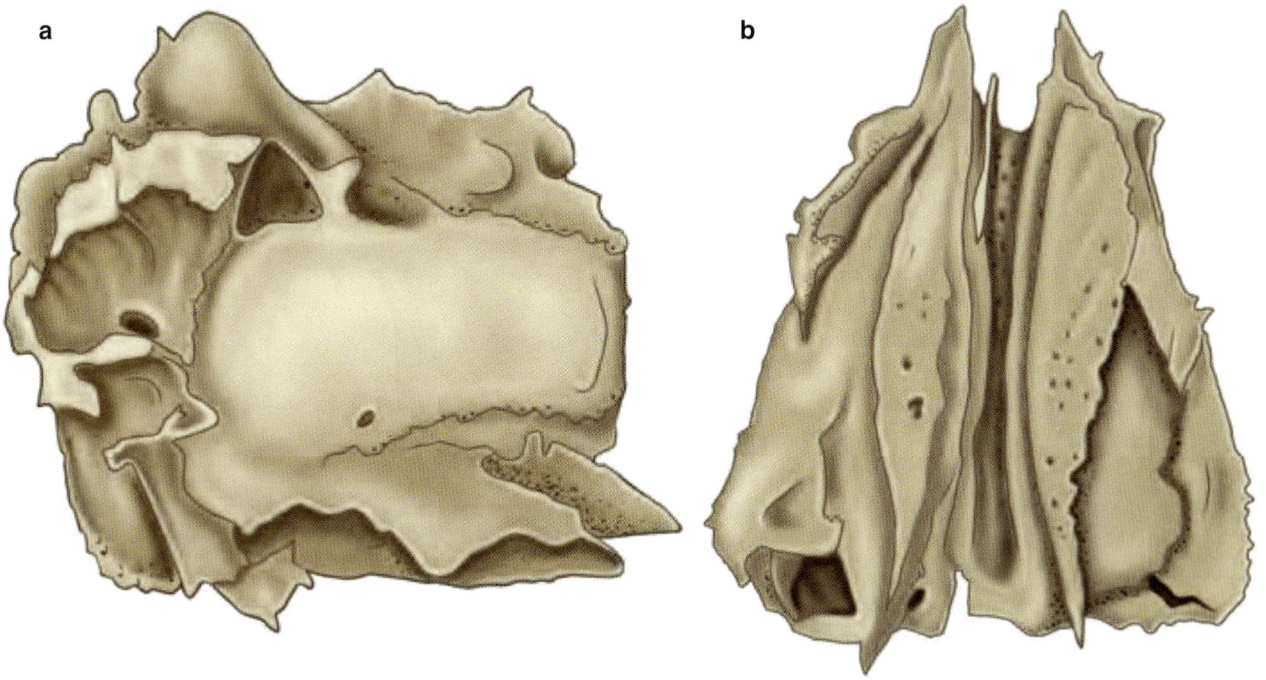

Fig. 1.13 (**a**) Left lateral view of ethmoid bone. Surface is flattened at orbital plate, where it articulates with frontal bone above, maxillary bone below, lacrimal bone anteriorly, and sphenoid bone posteriorly. (**b**) Inferior view of ethmoid bone. Note that it is slightly widened posteriorly where it articulates with sphenoid bone. Vomer projects inferiorly from center of cribriform plate. Large air cell masses project inferiorly from each of the lateral borders of cribriform plate. Middle and superior turbinates are medial projections from each air cell mass

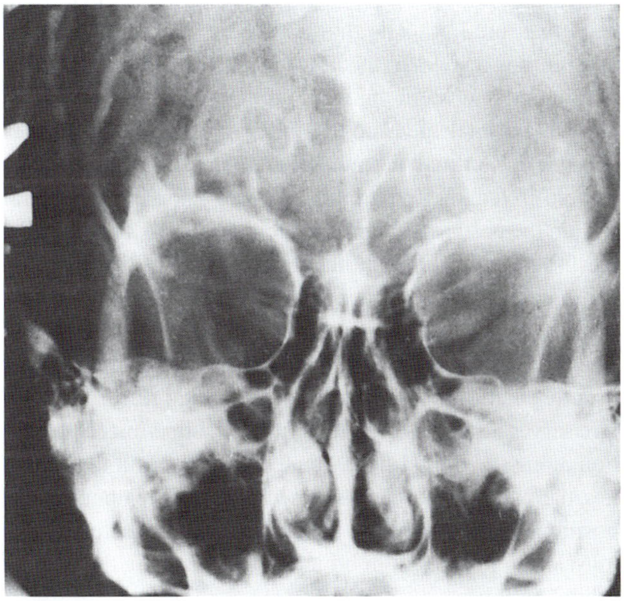

Fig. 1.14 Well-developed frontal sinus in male adult. Septum irregularly divides left and right halves

bone. The many bullae of the ethmoid pneumatization can be seen as a honeycomb pattern beneath the lamina papyracea. This supportive structure in part explains why the medial wall fractures less often than the thicker orbital floor.

Congenital dehiscences sometimes are seen at the ethmoidal suture lines, whereas age atrophy is seen centrally in the ethmoid plate. Important to the orbital surgeon are the anterior and posterior ethmoidal foramina conveying branches of the ophthalmic artery and the nasociliary nerve. They are located at the frontoethmoidal suture approximately 24 and 36 mm posterior to the anterior lacrimal crest, respectively. Additionally, the frontoethmoidal suture serves as an important guide during orbital surgery approximating the level of the floor of the anterior cranial fossa.

The position of the cribriform plate relative to the medial orbital wall is variable. At the posterior lacrimal crest, the vertical distance from the medial canthal ligament to the anterior cranial fossa ranges between 0 mm and 19 mm (mean = 6.5 mm). This distance may be 3 mm or less in 20% of individuals [9]. This variability in anatomy should be considered during dacryocystorhinostomy.

Orbital Apex

Because of its many important neural and vascular structures, the orbital apex is especially worthy of study. The orbital apex is an extremely busy area because of the narrowing of the walls associated with the exit of venous blood, the entrance of arterial blood and a large number of nerves, and the origin of six extraocular muscles.

The superior orbital fissure [10] is a transverse notch 22 mm in length between the greater and lesser wings of the sphenoid bone, which descends medially (see Fig. 1.5). There is much individual variation in the shape of the superior orbital fissure, but usually the fissure is narrower superotemporally. This fissure transmits most of the critical neurovascular structures entering the orbit. Important exceptions are the optic nerve and ophthalmic artery, which traverse the optic canal as well as the maxillary division of the trigeminal nerve, and the inferior ophthalmic vein, which courses through the inferior orbital fissure.

The lacrimal, frontal, and trochlear nerves and the superior ophthalmic vein pass through the superolateral portion of the fissure outside the annulus of Zinn. The middle meningeal artery anastomosis with the ophthalmic artery may enter here, if not through its own foramen more anteriorly in the roof. The annulus of Zinn is a fibrous ring formed by the common origin of the rectus muscles. This ring encircles the central portion of the superior orbital fissure, the oculomotor foramen, giving access to the intraconal space. Structures passing through this portion of the superior orbital fissure include the superior and inferior divisions of the third cranial nerve, the sixth cranial nerve, the nasociliary branch of the ophthalmic trigeminal nerve, and sympathetic nerve fibers. Additionally, the optic nerve and the ophthalmic artery pass through the annulus of Zinn from the optic canal.

Radiologic enlargement of the superior orbital fissure may accompany aneurysm, meningioma, chordoma, pituitary adenoma, or tumors of the orbital apex. Pathologic entities involving this region may result in superior orbital fissure syndrome manifested by total or partial ophthalmoplegia, V, anesthesia, and venous congestion.

Medial to the superior orbital fissure lies the optic foramen, which conveys the optic nerve, the ophthalmic artery, and sympathetic nerve fibers. This canal is formed by the lesser wing of the sphenoid superolaterally, the optic strut inferolaterally, and the body of the sphenoid medially. The inferior root of the lesser wing of the sphenoid, the optic strut, joins the body of the sphenoid to its lesser wing and separates the optic foramen from the superior orbital fissure (see Figs. 1.5 and 1.15). In approximately 50% of cases, the posterior ethmoid air cells are in contact with the medial aspect of the optic canal [11]. The axis of the foramen is directed downward and outward toward the lateral inferior orbital rim. Deviation away from the sagittal plane is about 35°, and descent below the horizontal plane is about 38° [12]. The optic canals measure approximately 8–10 mm in length and course posteromedially and superiorly, ending just medial and anterior to the anterior clinoid processes. This relationship is useful in differentiating the optic canals from the superior orbital fissures on neuroimaging studies. Microcryoplaning with computerized reconstruction has been performed to illustrate the anatomic relationships [13] at the orbital apex.

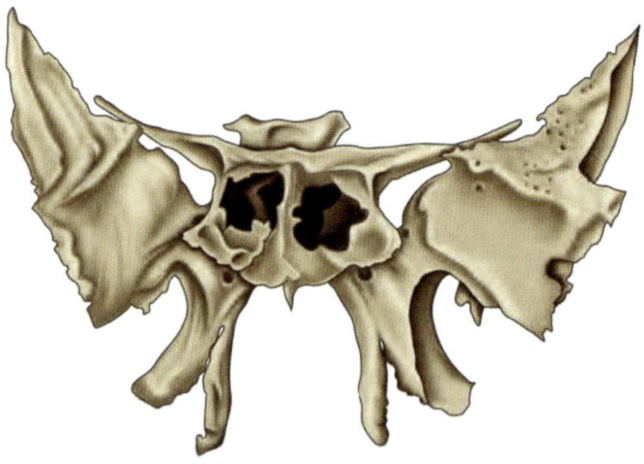

Fig. 1.15 Anterior view of disarticulated sphenoid bone. Body of sphenoid communicates anteriorly with ethmoid. Sphenoid sinus generally is divided by midline septum. The sphenoid bone is a key component of the orbital apex

The optic canal normally measures 5–6 mm in diameter. Because of a shift in the position of the ophthalmic artery relative to the optic nerve, the canal is horizontally oval posteriorly and more vertically oval anteriorly. The optic canal attains adult dimensions by age 3 years and usually exhibits symmetry within the individual. A diameter greater than 6.5 mm or a difference of more than 1 mm between sides is generally considered abnormal. Deformation of the optic canal has been demonstrated in dried skulls by direct forehead pressure [14]. The thin optic strut forming the lateral and inferior borders of the optic canal is subject to deformation in optic nerve gliomas and infraclinoid aneurysms [15].

At the orbital apex and just inferior to the optic canal lies the inferior orbital fissure. This fissure is a bony defect 20 mm in length separating the orbital floor and the lateral wall in the posterior half of the orbit (see Fig. 1.5). Laterally, the fissure is bounded by the greater wing of the sphenoid and medially by the palatine and maxillary bones. The axis of the fissure is an anterior projection of the optic foramen. The inferior fissure extends more anteriorly than the superior fissure, ending about 20 mm from the orbital rim. This structure serves as the posterolateral limit of subperiosteal dissection along the orbital floor. Immediately beneath the fissure lies the pterygopalatine fossa, with the infratemporal fossa positioned more laterally. Blunt trauma to the temporalis muscle can thus result in orbital hemorrhage via the inferior orbital fissure.

The inferior orbital fissure allows passage of the inferior ophthalmic veins to the pterygoid venous plexus. The maxillary division (V2) of the trigeminal nerve leaves the foramen rotundum to enter the orbit at the extreme superoposterior aspect of the fissure. Arriving with the maxillary nerve is a terminal branch of the internal maxillary artery, which becomes the infraorbital artery. The fissure also transmits the zygomatic nerve and accompanying postganglionic parasympathetic branches from the pterygopalatine ganglion. These parasympathetic fibers pass from the zygomaticotemporal nerve to the lacrimal nerve en route to the lacrimal gland. The inferior orbital fissure is covered by the vestigial smooth orbital muscle of Muller.

The cavernous sinus, located immediately posterior to the orbital apex, is discussed later.

Nasal and Paranasal Sinuses

The orbital roof, floor, and medial wall are intimately related to the nasal cavity. These bones are pneumatized by paranasal sinuses arising from and maintaining communication with the nasal cavity. Because of this intimate relationship, the orbital surgeon must have a solid understanding of paranasal sinus anatomy. Pathologic processes of these sinuses often create orbital effects. In addition, the lacrimal excretory system must be studied in light of these same surrounding structures.

Regional anatomy often can best be understood in terms of function. The nose, for example, filters, warms, and moistens air and collects secretions from the sinuses and nasolacrimal duct. The paranasal sinuses, however, do not enjoy a function that has been universally accepted as reason for their development. Leading theories are as follows: (1) impart resonance to the voice, (2) humidify and warm inspired air, (3) increase the area of the olfactory membrane, (4) absorb shock applied to the head for protection of sensory organs, (5) secrete mucus for keeping the nasal chambers moist, (6) thermally insulate the nervous centers, (7) aid facial growth, (8) exist as evolutionary remnants or unwanted air spaces or both, and (9) lighten the bones of the skull for maintenance of proper balance of the head [16].

Nose

The external nose is formed by the frontonasal process (Fig. 1.6). The nasal alae are cartilaginous condensations of the lateral nasal processes. The maxillary processes compress the medial nasal swellings of the frontonasal mass to form the philtrum of the upper lip, the upper jaw component encompassing the four incisors, and the anterior palate [17]. The maxillary processes contribute to the maxillary bone portion of the lateral nasal wall and the majority of the nasal floor, the posterior or secondary palate. The ethmoidal box, derived from the nasofrontal process, spans the roof of the nasal cavity, arching from the superolateral nasal walls.

The large cartilaginous anterior dilation of the nose is termed the vestibule. The space superior and posterior to the vestibule is termed the atrium. The nasal cavity is bisected anteriorly by the cartilaginous septum, which joins the vomer, a bony vertical plate of the ethmoid, posteriorly. Laterally, the nasal wall is thrown into three or more horizontal ridges termed turbinates, with a corresponding meatus below each turbinate (Fig. 1.7).

The inferior turbinate arises from the medial wall of the maxillary sinus and is the largest. The progressively smaller and more posterior middle, superior, and (variably present) supreme turbinates are outcroppings of the ethmoid. The nasolacrimal duct extends posteriorly and laterally and is formed by the maxillary bone laterally and the lacrimal and inferior turbinate bones medially. The nasolacrimal duct drains into the inferior meatus.

The posterior portion of the middle turbinate arises from the roof of the nose at the cribriform plate. More anteriorly, the middle turbinate emerges from the medial wall of the maxillary sinus. The nasolacrimal sac fossa lies anterior and lateral to the anterior tip of the middle turbinate. The middle meatus receives the drainage of the ethmoid (anterior and middle), frontal, and maxillary sinuses. Within the middle meatus lies a curvilinear ridge, the uncinate process. Superior to the uncinate process lies the bulla ethmoidalis, a prominence of the ethmoid sinus air cells. The hiatus semilunaris is a cleft that lies between these structures and receives the ostium of the maxillary sinus [18]. The anterior and middle ethmoid air cells drain into the superior aspect of the hiatus. The frontonasal duct drains the frontal sinus into the anterosuperior portion of the hiatus semilunaris.

The posterior ethmoid air cells drain into the superior meatus. The sphenoid sinus drains from an anterior ostium into the sphenoethmoidal recess. This recess is located posterior to the short superior turbinate.

When the exterior nares are dilated by a nasal speculum, the inferior turbinate and the inferior meatus can be seen by tilting the blades to look along the nasal floor. The middle turbinate and nasal atrium are seen if the blades of the speculum are directed superiorly. Because the wall of the atrium is convex medially, a dacryocystorhinostomy site located at the anterior tip of the middle turbinate is usually hidden from direct visualization without an endoscope (Fig. 1.8).

The paranasal sinuses together more than double the nasal chamber volume. Every bone housing the nasal cavity except the nasal bone is subject to pneumatization. Embryologically, the nasal ectoderm invaginates and creates tracts into the surrounding mesenchyme that persist as paranasal sinus ostia or communications with the nose in the adult. Vascular mucoperiosteum lines the sinuses. Densely populous cilia rhythmically beat mucus toward the ostia. Scarring of the mucoperiosteum can inhibit the movement of mucus and result in pathologic sequestration [19].

Maxillary Sinus

The maxillary is the largest of the paranasal sinuses (15 ml) and the first to develop (Fig. 1.9a, b). A dimple develops in the middle meatus posterior and superior to the uncinate ridge at 10–11 gestational weeks and expands to slightly more than 0.1 ml by birth. The sinus grows anteriorly and inferiorly accompanying facial growth, leaving the ostium high on the medial sinus wall. Expansion is not completed until the descent of the secondary teeth, the roots of which are seen in relief along the sinus floor in the adult. The ostium of the maxillary sinus drains into the middle meatus. In the setting of trauma, the ostium may be blocked by inferiorly displaced orbital tissue.

The sinus roof is the orbital floor. Medially it is thin and prone to fracture. It thickens laterally near the infraorbital canal. The sinus roof (orbital floor) declines from the medial wall to the lateral wall at an angle of approximately 30° (Fig. 1.10). The lateral wall of the sinus is also thin and subject to fracture with zygomatic displacement. The pterygopalatine space lies posteriorly with the internal maxillary artery intimately related to the posterior sinus wall (Fig. 1.11). The nasal cavity is medial except where the nasolacrimal canal and the inferior turbinate intervene. The position of the nasolacrimal duct must be considered during antral surgery [20].

Ethmoid Sinus

The ethmoid sinuses appear during the fifth month of gestation, and expansion continues until puberty (see Fig. 1.9a). The ethmoid air cells are the most exuberant growing sinuses and may pneumatize the frontal, sphenoid, palatine, and lacrimal bones (Fig. 1.12). Normally, 3–15 air cells expand from each lateral border of the cribriform plate. The air cell masses convolute medially to form the middle, superior, and supreme (if present) turbinates. The anterior and middle ethmoid air cells drain into the middle meatus; the posterior cells drain into the superior meatus. Anterior ethmoid air cells are smaller, have smaller ostia, and are more subject to occlusion with inflammation. Medial wall fracture and injury to the medial rectus muscle with resulting motility dysfunction may occur with intranasal or endoscopic ethmoidectomy [21]. Damage to the lacrimal duct may result from middle meatus antrostomy [22].

The ethmoid bone can best be understood as a box slightly wider posteriorly where it articulates with the sphenoid (Fig. 1.13). Medially, the floor of the anterior cranial fossa slopes inferiorly to join the superomedial aspect of the anterior ethmoid bone at a crease termed the fovea ethmoidalis. The fovea ethmoidalis lies inferior to the orbital roof and is therefore vulnerable during orbital surgery.

Frontal Sinus

The frontal sinus evaginates from the frontal recess superior to the nasal hiatus semilunaris (see Fig. 1.8). Pits are present at birth, but the frontal infundibulum is not well developed or radiographically evident until about the sixth year of life. Frontal sinus expansion continues until early adulthood and attains greater proportions in the male (Fig. 1.14). The frontal sinus is bisected inferiorly by a midline septum that meanders more superiorly. Each sinus is a single chamber appearing scalloped radiologically because of intrasinus septa. The frontonasal duct drains into the anterior middle meatus. The frontal sinus is particularly susceptible to mucocele formation.

Sphenoid Sinus

The sphenoid sinus evaginates from the most posterior portion of the nasal roof in the fourth gestational month (see Fig. 1.8). Growth continues until adulthood with varying degrees of pneumatization of the sphenoid body. A midline septum divides the sinus into two portions that are rarely equal (Fig. 1.15). They rarely are absent or may, to varying degrees, extend into the sphenoid wings or may even surround the optic nerve and extend into the pterygoid plates. Air cells from the ethmoid anteriorly articulating with sphenoid bone may pneumatize it. In the instance in which the sphenoid body is nearly completely replaced by air, only sinus mucoperiosteum, a thin layer of bone, and periosteum separate the respiratory tract from the internal carotid artery, the cavernous sinus, and the branches of the trigeminal nerve. The sphenoid sinus drains into the sphenoethmoidal recess in the posterior nasal cavity.

Lacrimal Secretory and Excretory System

Lacrimal Excretory Osteology

The osteology of the lacrimal excretory system is discussed in this section along with a description of the soft tissues. The lacrimal bony passage consists of the lacrimal sac fossa above, continuing inferiorly as the nasolacrimal canal to end under the inferior turbinate bone in the nose.

The lacrimal sac fossa is located within the widened orbital rim medially and is to be distinguished from the fossa for the lacrimal gland, which is behind the superotemporal orbital margin. The excretory fossa or groove is bounded in front by the anterior lacrimal crest of the maxillary bone frontal process and behind by the posterior lacrimal crest of the lacrimal bone (Fig. 1.16). The elevation of these crests varies considerably from skull to skull; they may be short, producing a shallow fossa, or they may be so pronounced as to create a space more like an incomplete cylinder than a groove. The fossa is about 16 mm high, 4–8 mm wide, and 2 mm deep [23]. The lacrimal fossa is narrower in women.

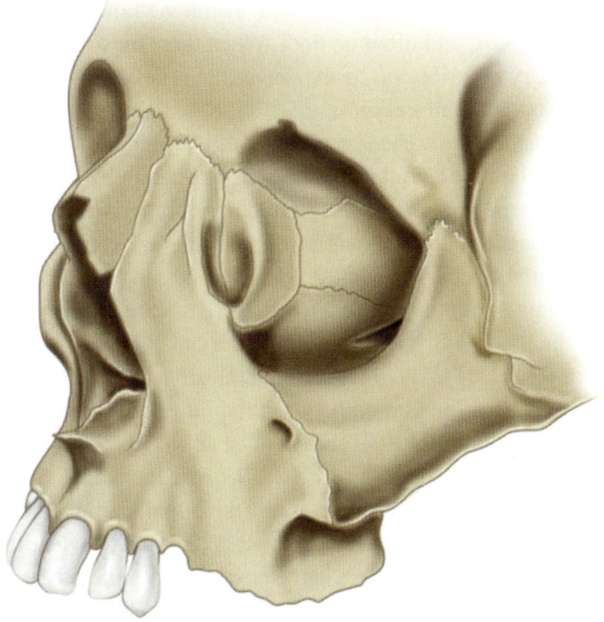

Fig. 1.16 Lacrimal excretory fossa

Perhaps, narrower osteology leads to the increased percentage of females requiring dacryocystorhinostomy. Active bone remodeling may be seen in the nasolacrimal fossa in patients with chronic dacryocystitis [24].

The anterior lacrimal crest continues as the superomedial extension of the inferior orbital rim, a relation to bear in mind when it is underdeveloped and palpated with difficulty during surgery. The medial canthal ligament attaches to the anterior lacrimal crest superiorly, where a small lacrimal tubercle sometimes is noted. Inferiorly, the orbital septum and some superficial fibers of the orbicularis attach. On its posterior aspect, the anterior lacrimal crest periorbita gives rise to the lacrimal fascia that covers the lacrimal sac.

The posterior lacrimal crest of the lacrimal bone is better defined and may sometimes curve slightly anteriorly, partially covering the sac with a bony roof. The superior portion of the posterior crest is stronger and flatter where the pretarsal deep heads of the orbicularis muscle (Horner–Duverney muscle) insert. Continuing from the arcus marginalis above, the orbital septum inserts just behind the posterior lacrimal crest.

A vertical suture generally runs centrally between the lacrimal and maxillary bones of the anterior and posterior crests. The maxillary–lacrimal union may be more posteriorly placed, however, indicating predominance of the maxillary bone, or more anteriorly placed, indicating that the lacrimal bone predominates. For the lacrimal surgeon performing an osteotomy, this variation has some importance because a fossa formed chiefly by the lacrimal bone is easily penetrated with a blunt instrument. A maxillary bone, predominant lacrimal fossa, as is frequently seen in Asian patients, has a much denser bony floor, and the surgeon must place the instrument more posteriorly and inferiorly in order to break through. The maxillary contribution to the lacrimal fossa is thought to be greater in skulls with heavy bone structure [25]. Conversely, a lacrimal predominant fossa is likely to be associated with small anterior ethmoidal air cells and is more likely to be opposed on the nasal side by the anterior tip of the middle turbinate.

The lacrimal bone is pneumatized by anterior ethmoidal cells termed agger nasi bullae, which rarely may also extend into the maxillary frontal process. The frequency with which the agger nasi cells intervene between the lacrimal fossa and the nasal cavity has been studied by Whitnall [26]. In 54% of skulls, the air cells extended anteriorly to the anterior lacrimal crest and as far as the maxillary–lacrimal suture in an additional 32% (Fig. 1.17). The middle turbinate extension of the ethmoid is also related at its anterior aspect to the superior portion of the lacrimal fossa; indeed, it sometimes must be excised during dacryocystorhinostomy to accomplish an unobstructed opening to the nasal cavity. The inferior lacrimal fossa is directly related to the middle meatus of the nose. The frontonasal duct drains into the middle meatus of the nose under the middle turbinate in a relationship analogous to the relationship the nasolacrimal duct has with the inferior turbinate. However, the frontonasal duct is situated more posteriorly in the middle meatus than the lacrimal fossa relation.

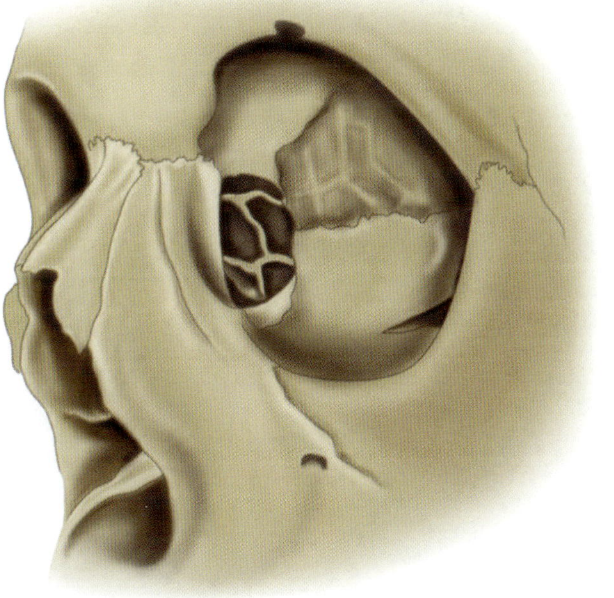

Fig. 1.17 Lacrimal bone removed to show variant of anterior ethmoidal air cells intervening between lacrimal fossa and nasal cavity

The variable position of the floor of the anterior cranial fossa relative to the lacrimal sac fossa again deserves mention. At the horizontal midpoint of the lacrimal sac fossa, the distance from the medial canthal ligament to the anterior cranial fossa averages 8.3 mm, with a range of 1–30 mm. At the posterior lacrimal crest, this distance decreases to 0–19 mm (mean = 6.5). In 20% of individuals, the distance may be 3 mm or less [9]. This relationship should be considered during dacryocystorhinostomy.

The bony nasolacrimal canal conveys the nasolacrimal excretory sac (here called the nasolacrimal duct) to the inferior meatus of the nose under the inferior turbinate. The maxillary and lacrimal bones that form the lacrimal fossa entrance are joined by the inferior turbinate bone to complete the nasolacrimal canal. The lateral two-thirds of the nasolacrimal canal are contributed by the maxillary bone. The medial aspect is formed by a descending process of the lacrimal bone joining the lacrimal or ascending process of the inferior turbinate (Fig. 1.18). In some instances, the medial nasolacrimal canal is nearly or completely formed by the maxilla, with a corresponding diminution of the lacrimal and inferior turbinate components (Figs. 1.19 and 1.20), resulting in narrowing of the nasolacrimal duct lumen [27]. The maxillary bone is the first of the orbital bones to develop (16 mm stage), whereas the lacrimal bone appears much later (75 mm stage) [28]; this interval may explain the occasional preempting of the second bone.

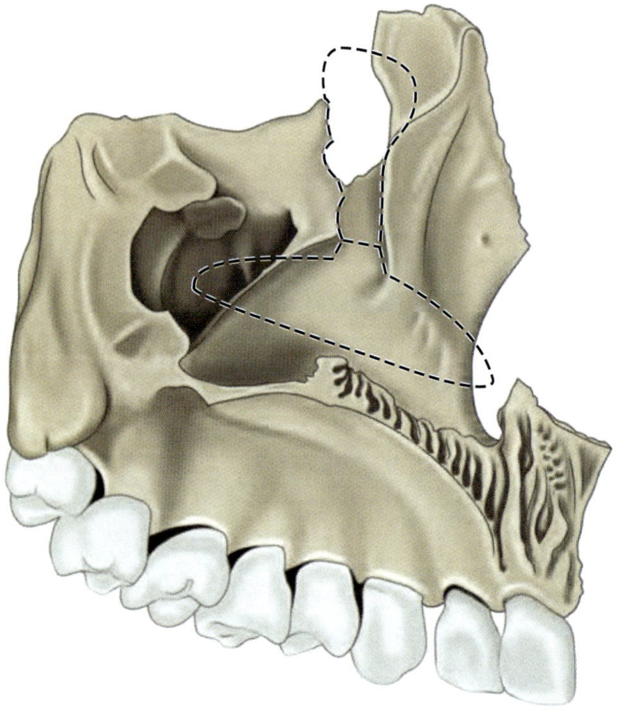

Fig. 1.18 Medial, inferior view of right maxillary bone to show nasolacrimal canal articulating lacrimal and inferior turbinate form medial aspect of canal and are represented with dotted lines

The nasolacrimal canal may appear in relief on the medial wall of the maxillary sinus, on the lateral wall of the middle nasal meatus, and often on both. When there exists a greater maxillary contribution to the canal, the relief is favored on the maxillary sinus aspect.

Considerable variation in the width, length, and angulation of the nasolacrimal canal exists, attested to by the clinician experienced in nasolacrimal duct probing. The average bony canal is slightly oval in the parasagittal plane with a width of 4.5 mm. The average length of the canal is 12.5 mm. Beginning with the lacrimal fossa, there is about a 15° posterior inclination from the vertical as the canal descends to the nose (Fig. 1.21). This inclination clinically can be estimated by imaging a line drawn between the inner canthus and the first molar tooth. The nasolacrimal canal also angles slightly laterally in its descent (Fig. 1.22). Because the course of the canal is somewhat convex laterally, the initial lateral angulation suggested in the lacrimal fossa is diminished when the probe completes its course in the nose. A good external landmark to the end of the nasolacrimal duct is the ala nasi. A line drawn between the tear sac and this structure is a good approximation of the nasolacrimal duct course. Individuals with narrow intercanthal distances or with wide noses are thus observed to exhibit greater lateral angulation of the nasolacrimal excretory system.

Lacrimal Secretors

The tear layer consists of surface oils secreted by the meibomian and Zeis glands, an aqueous component produced by the main lacrimal gland and the accessory lacrimal glands of Krause and Wolfring, and a basal mucinous layer secreted by conjunctival goblet cells. The superficial oily layer is thinner than a wavelength of light, yet it functions to slow the evaporation of tears by a factor of 15 [29]. Increased evaporation has been reported as accounting for the majority of tear insufficiency in patients with dry eye [30]. Meibomian gland dysfunction is a frequent cause of increased tear evaporation [31]. The aqueous component is uniformly about 6.5 mm(um) thick across the cornea. It is actually a salt solution that contains the bactericidal lysozyme and 13-lysin proteins [32]. The pH of tears averages 7.4 [33]. Because of considerable surface tension factors, there is little downflow of the aqueous film, provided the surface corneal epithelium is intact. The mucous layer is important for proper wetting of the corneal surface; corneal drying occurs despite adequate aqueous and oil layers in conditions that destroy the conjunctival goblet cells [34].

Jones proposed that the secretory system be divided into basic secretors and reflex secretors [35]. The basic secretors are the mucin and oil glands, as well as the accessory lacrimal glands of Krause and Wolfring. These are thought to provide

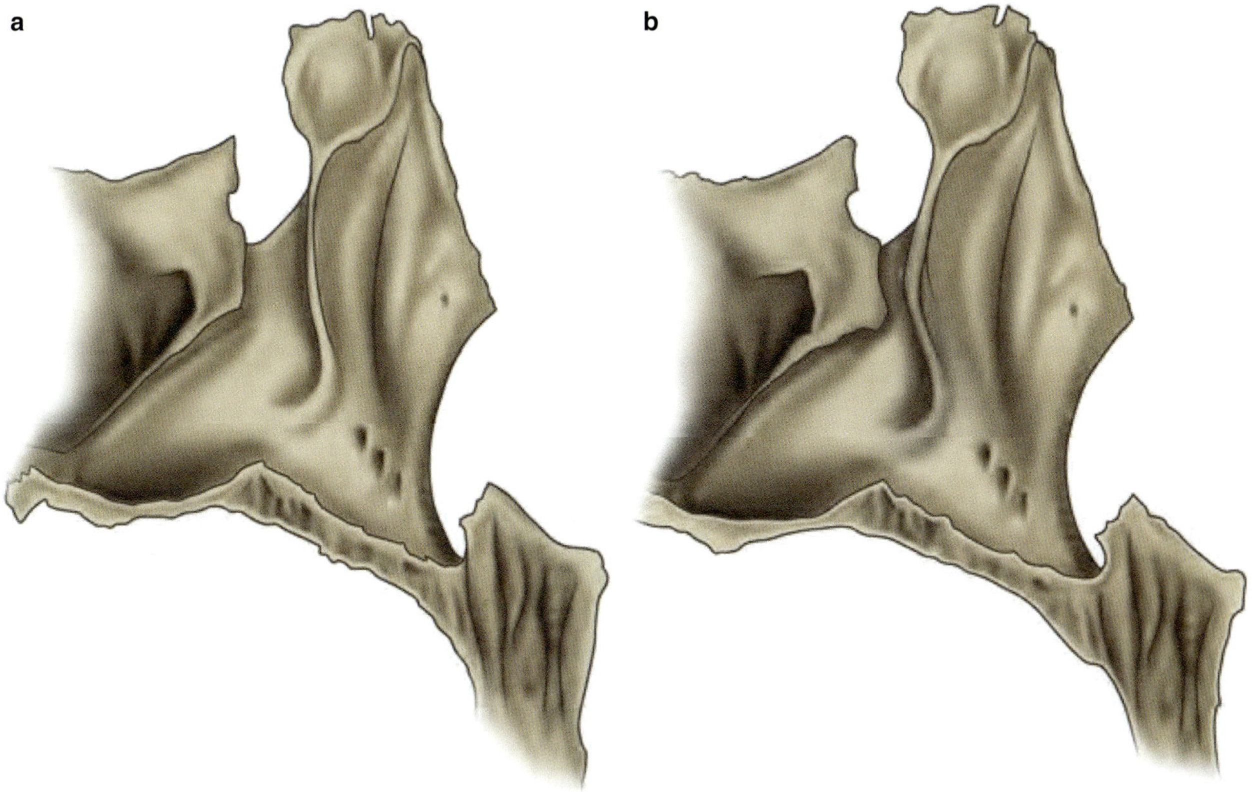

Fig. 1.19 (**a**) Lacrimal bone predominant and (**b**) maxillary bone predominant nasolacrimal canal. In latter instance, lumen of canal is narrowed

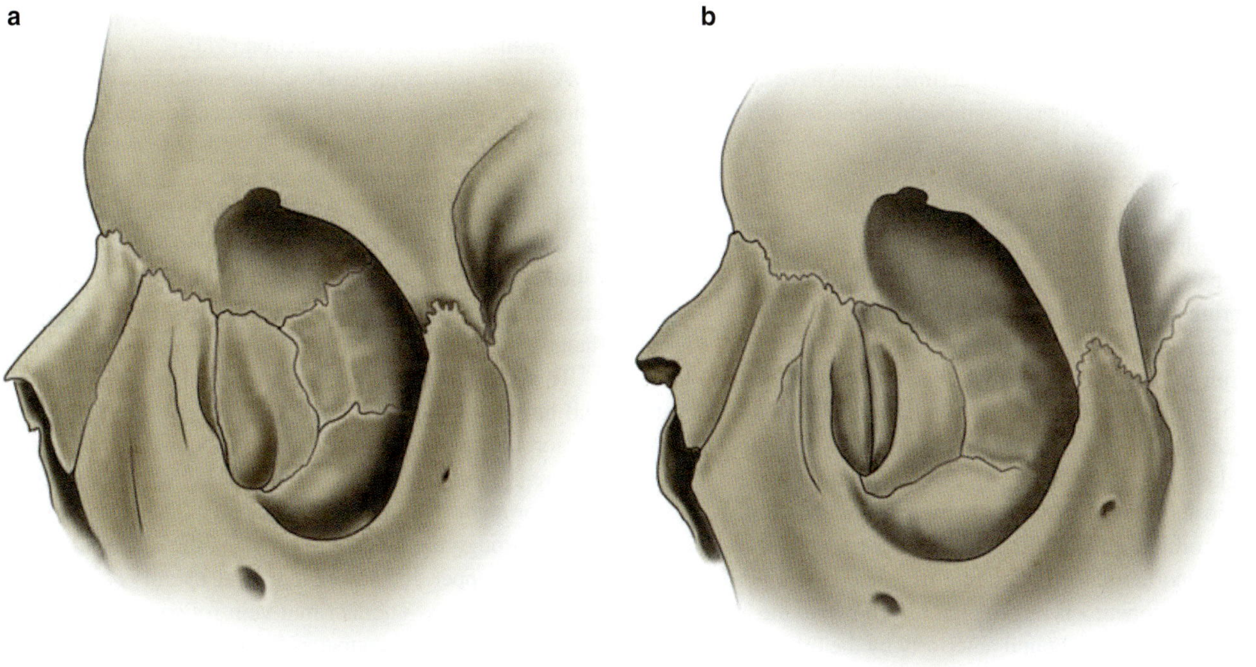

Fig. 1.20 (**a**) Lacrimal bone predominant and (**b**) maxillary bone predominant nasolacrimal canal. In the former instance, thin lacrimal bone is easily broken during dacryocystorhinostomy

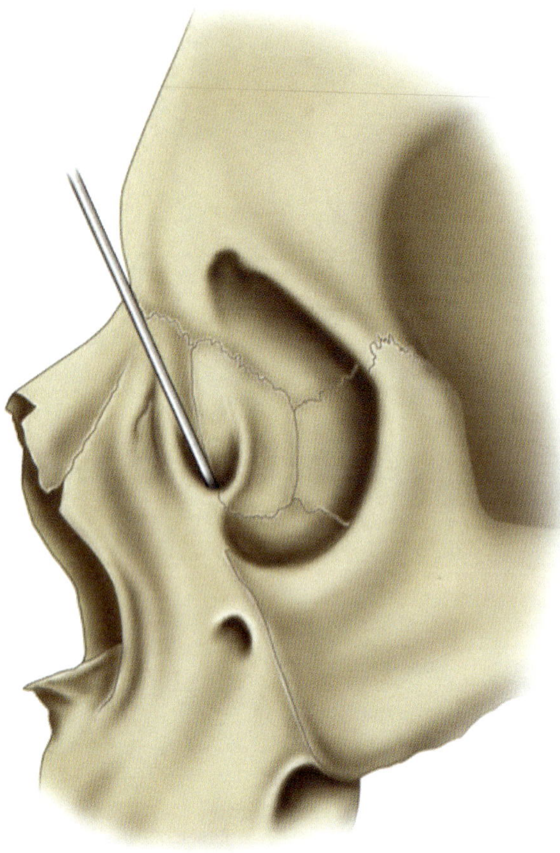

Fig. 1.21 Probe placed in nasolacrimal canal to show 15° posterior inclination

the tear film under ordinary conditions. These accessory glands may also respond to reflex stimulation [36]. The orbital and palpebral lobes of the lacrimal gland have a parasympathetic nerve supply and are thought primarily to participate in reflexive lacrimation. Removal of the lacrimal gland, however, can produce keratoconjunctivitis sicca despite normally functioning accessory lacrimal glands [37]. Clinical testing of tear film sufficiency is achieved by variations of the Schirmer test, using filter paper strips in the inferior lateral conjunctival fornix [35], and by tear breakup time [38, 39].

The main lacrimal gland resides superotemporally in the orbit in the shallow lacrimal gland fossa of the frontal bone. The gland is partially divided by the lateral horn of the levator into a larger orbital lobe above and a lesser palpebral lobe below (Figs. 1.23 and 1.24). Division is not complete because a posterior wall of parenchyma persists between the lobes. The orbital lobe conforms to the space between the orbital wall and the globe, extending from the lateral border of the levator aponeurosis on which it rests down to the frontozygomatic suture. It is bound anteriorly by the orbital septum and the preaponeurotic fat pad, posteriorly by orbital fat, medially by the intermuscular membrane between the superior and lateral recti, and laterally by bone. The orbital lobe measures approximately 20 mm long, 12 mm wide, and 5 mm thick [3].

The palpebral lobe of the lacrimal gland lies underneath the levator aponeurosis in the subaponeurotic Jones' space. It is separated from the conjunctiva only medially where the superior tarsal muscle intervenes. Early anatomists attributed various supporting ligaments to the gland, but in reality, it is secured primarily by the conjunctiva and intermuscular membranes below, by the lacrimal fascia linking it with Whitnall's ligament, and by the levator horn around which it is wrapped. Disruption of Whitnall's ligament may result in prolapse of the lacrimal gland.

The lacrimal gland lacks a true capsule. The parenchyma of the gland can be seen grossly as a pinkish-gray collection of small lobules separated by a fine mesh of connective tissue. Care must be taken during blepharoplasty and ptosis surgery to avoid inadvertent excision of lacrimal gland mistaken for preaponeurotic fat. Each lobule consists of many acini that drain into tubules, which, in turn, are tributaries of still larger ducts (Fig. 1.25). The acini are made up of a basal myoepithelial cell layer with inner columnar secretory cells. Electron microscopy has demonstrated mucopolysaccharides in secretory granules, which implies that the lacrimal gland is a modified mucus gland [40].

Secretory ducts from the palpebral lobe drain into the superotemporal conjunctival fornix, as do those from the orbital lobe. The orbital lobe secretory ducts pass through the palpebral lobe parenchyma or remain tightly bound to its capsule. Palpebral dacryoadenectomy therefore interrupts drainage from the remaining orbital portion. Surgical resection of the conjunctiva in the superolateral upper eyelid may also result in secretory dysfunction [41].

A light microscopic study of lacrimal glands removed at autopsy by Roen and associates revealed abnormalities in 80% [42]. Chronic inflammation and periductular fibrosis were the most common changes seen. In another work [43], diffuse atrophy and fibrosis of the orbital lobe were significantly correlated with advancing age and female sex. Age-related decrease in lacrimation seems to be associated with loss of gland parenchyma and closure of some of the efferent ducts.

The lacrimal gland receives arterial blood from the lacrimal branch of the ophthalmic artery, from a branch of the infraorbital artery, and often from a contribution from the recurrent meningeal artery, which may join the lacrimal artery or enter the gland independently. The lacrimal artery passes through the gland and provides the major blood supply to the upper and lower temporal eyelids as the lateral palpebral arteries. The lacrimal vein follows approximately the same intraorbital course as the artery and drains into the superior ophthalmic vein. Both artery and vein communicate with the gland on its posterior surface.

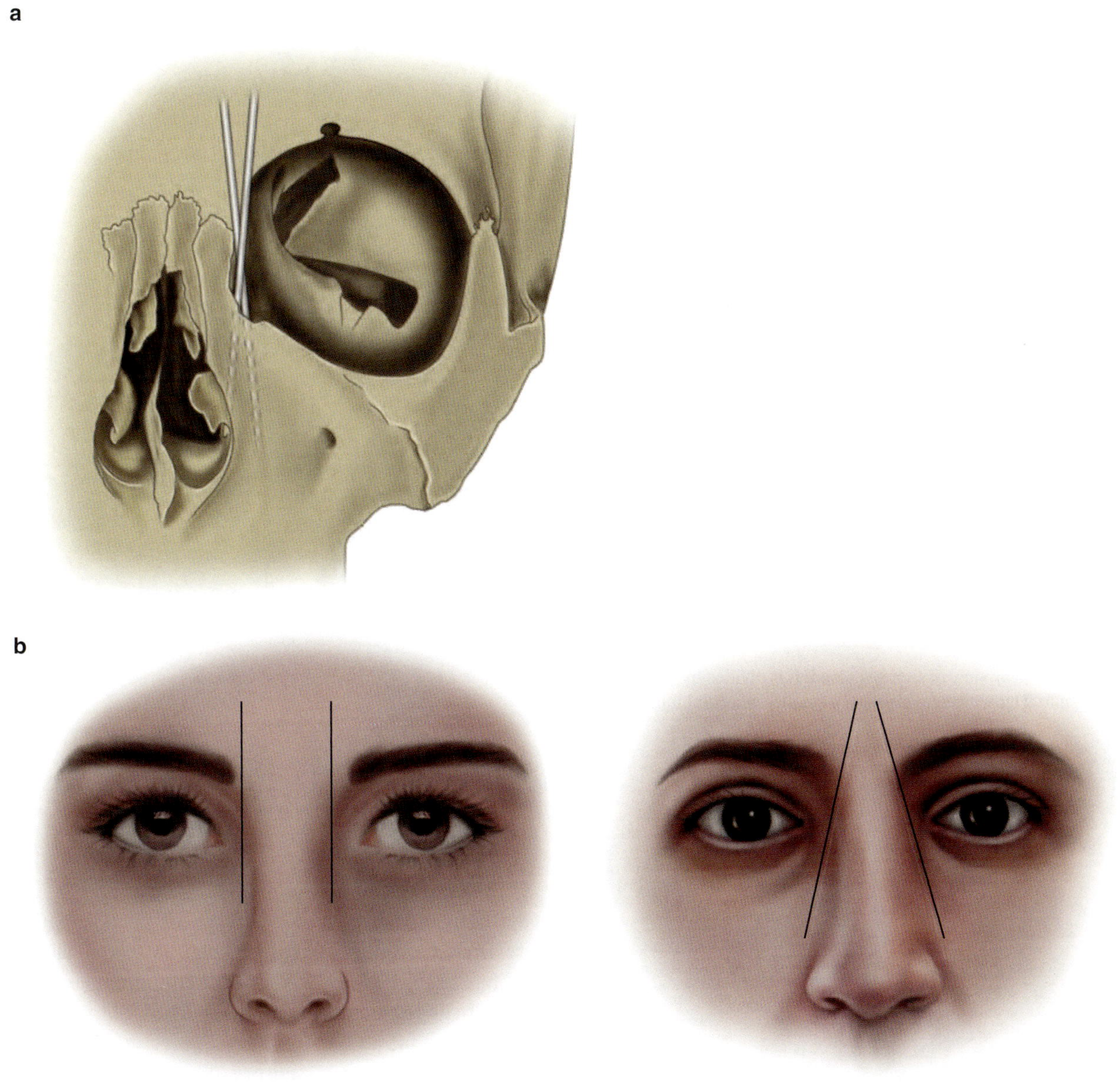

Fig. 1.22 (**a**) Probes placed in nasolacrimal canal to show variation in lateral inclination. (**b**) Individuals with narrow intercanthal distances or with wide noses are observed to exhibit greater lateral angulation of nasolacrimal canal

The lacrimal gland receives innervation from the fifth and seventh cranial nerves, as well as from the sympathetics of the superior cervical ganglion. The lacrimal nerve branch of the ophthalmic trigeminal travels superotemporally in the orbit just underneath the periorbita to enter the gland with the vessels. Like the artery, the lacrimal nerve continues through the gland to supply more superficial eyelid structures. Sympathetic nerves arrive with the lacrimal artery and along with parasympathetics in the zygomatic nerve.

The long parasympathetic path to the lacrimal gland is diagrammed in Fig. 1.26. Parasympathetic input from the facial nerve complex joins the zygomatic nerve via the sphenopalatine ganglion. The zygomatic nerve enters the orbit 5 mm behind the anterior limit of the inferior orbital fissure and may indent the zygomatic bone (zygomatic groove) on its anterior and superior course. The zygomatic nerve may give off a lacrimal branch before dividing into zygomaticotemporal and zygomaticofacial branches. This lacrimal branch anastomoses with a branch from the lacrimal nerve or travels along the periorbita to independently enter the gland at its posterior lateral aspect. Separate zygomaticofacial and zygomaticotemporal nerves may enter the orbit and exit separately, in which case the latter carries the lacrimal branch. Other parasympathetic pathways are likely

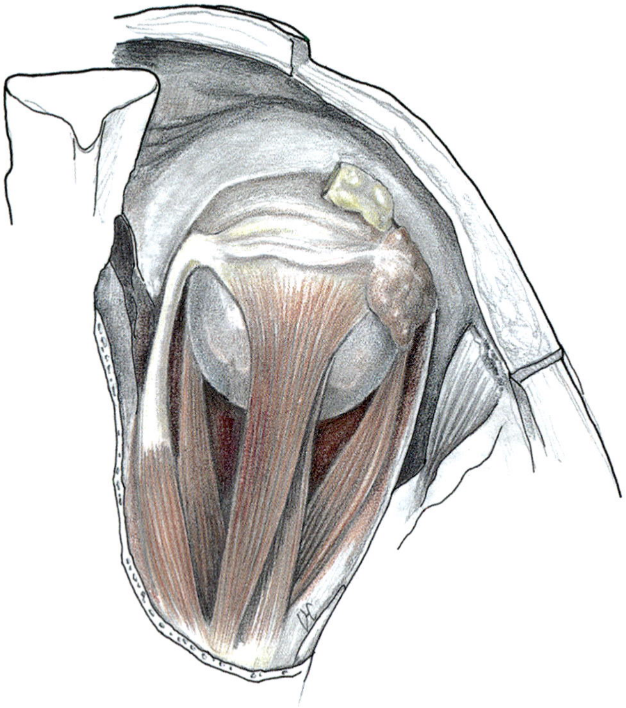

Fig. 1.23 Superior view of lacrimal gland. It is divided by lateral horn of levator into a larger orbital lobe and a smaller palpebral lobe

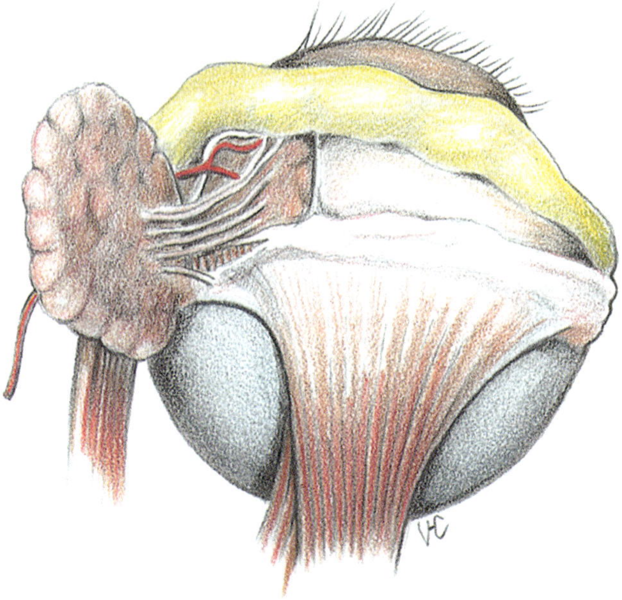

Fig. 1.24 Reflected orbital lobe of lacrimal gland with levator horn partially excised to show secretory ducts and palpebral lobe. Ducts from main lobe pass through palpebral lobe or remain tightly bound to its capsule. Damage to the palpebral lobe may thus influence secretion from the orbital lobe

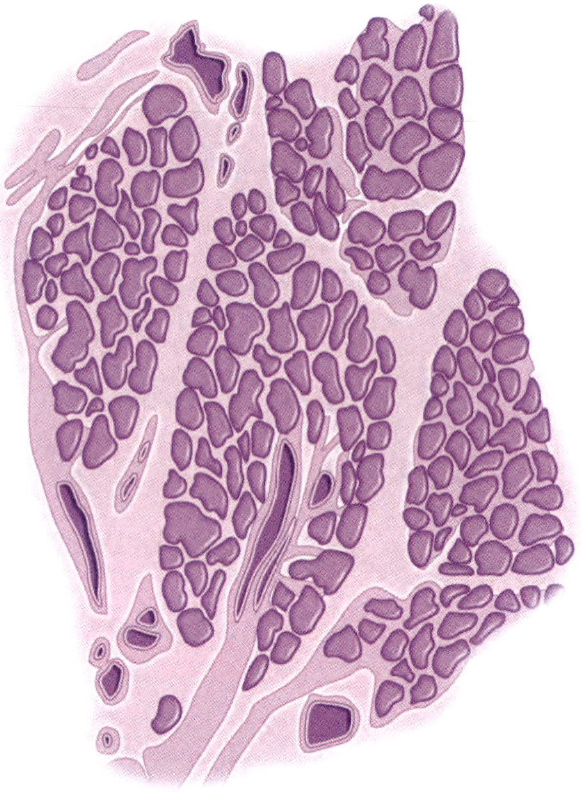

Fig. 1.25 Schematic drawings of tubuloalveolar structure of lacrimal gland. Each lobule consists of many acini that drain into tubules, which, in turn, are tributaries of still larger ducts

to exist. In monkeys, direct passage of parasympathetic fibers from the pterygopalatine ganglion to the lacrimal gland has been demonstrated [44]. Additionally, evidence in the cat suggests that secretomotor fibers run within the lacrimal nerve [45].

The lacrimal nerve is sensory (although it may carry some sympathetic fibers gained while traversing the cavernous sinus). The seventh nerve supply to the lacrimal gland (via the zygomatic) provides the main secretomotor function, whereas the sympathetics are thought to stimulate basal secretion [46]. Blocking the sphenopalatine ganglion greatly diminishes tear production but does not eliminate it entirely [47]. Lacrimal gland hyposecretion is noted in central autonomic dysfunction states such as the Riley–Day syndrome [48].

Embryologically, the lacrimal gland develops from outpouchings of the conjunctiva, those of the orbital lobe appearing earlier than the accessory lacrimal glands. In

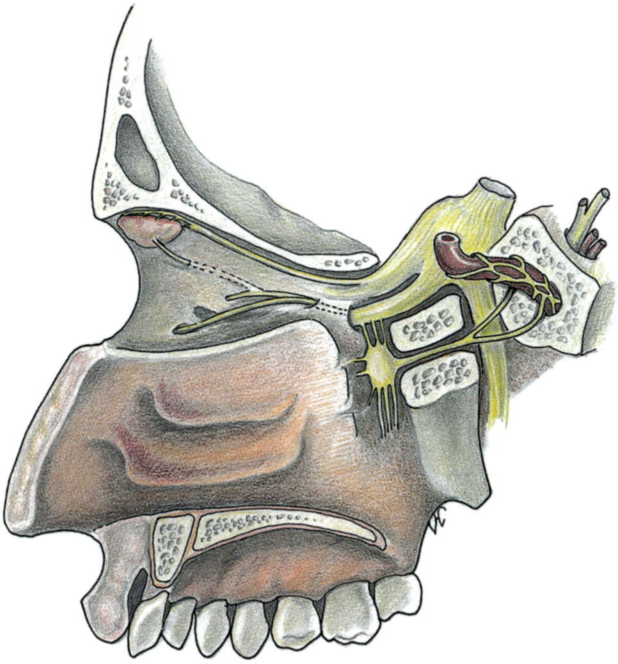

Fig. 1.26 Parasympathetic innervation of lacrimal gland. Fibers from facial nerve emerge from temporal bone as greater superficial petrosal nerve, pass through vidian canal of sphenoid bone as vidian nerve to enter sphenopalatine ganglion, communicate with maxillary nerve via sphenopalatine nerves, and leave maxillary nerve shortly thereafter as zygomatic nerve. Zygomatic branch to lacrimal gland usually joins lacrimal nerve before entering gland, but in this specimen, the zygomatic branch was seen entering separately

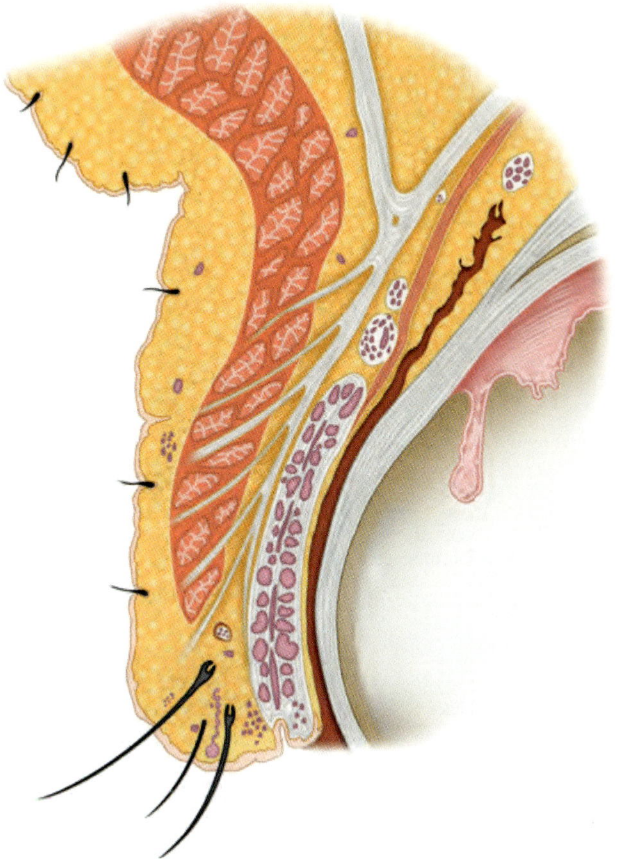

Fig. 1.27 Basal lacrimal secretors. Accessory lacrimal glands of Krause and Wolfring, mucin glands of Manz and Henle, oil glands of Meibomius and Zeis, and sweat glands of Moll

lower animals, the main gland is found in the lower eyelid; phylogenetically, it can be followed to reach the superotemporal orbit.

The accessory lacrimal glands of Krause and Wolfring structurally resemble the lacrimal gland and may develop identical types of metaplasia. They differ, however, in that they lack parasympathetic innervation. About 20 glands of Krause are located in the superior conjunctival fornix, and perhaps half that number is present in the inferior fornix. Several glands of Wolfring can be found along the upper border of the superior tarsus. Sevel [49] reported between 4 and 42 accessory lacrimal glands in the upper conjunctiva and 6 or fewer in the lower fornix. Accessory lacrimal glands may also be found in the caruncle and in the plica semilunaris (Fig. 1.27).

Mucus-secreting goblet cells are located throughout the conjunctiva but are most concentrated at the lid margins, the conjunctival fornices, the antimarginal tarsal borders, and near the corneoscleral limbus. The meibomian glands and the eyelid margin glands are discussed in the eyelid section.

Canaliculi

Lacrimal Excretory System

The proximal portion of the lacrimal drainage system is formed by the lacrimal canaliculi (Fig. 1.28). A dense fibroelastic ring, the papilla marks the beginning of the canaliculus, 10 mm from the tear sac in the lower eyelid and 8 mm distant in the upper lid (Fig. 1.29). A 0.3-mm punctum opens at the mucocutaneous junction in the center of each papilla. The lower punctum is generally larger than the upper punctum [50, 51]. The superior punctum is placed medially, and the inferior punctum is lateral to the plica semilunaris. Because of the posterior pull of the pars lacrimalis muscle of Horner–Duverney, the puncta are directed into the tear lake [52]. The tear lake occurs because the caruncle and plica intervene between the medial eyelid and the globe.

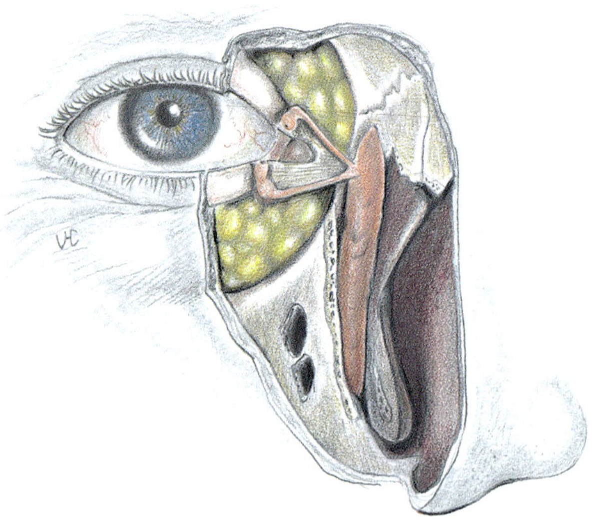

Fig. 1.28 Nasolacrimal excretory system

their walls, they can dilate considerably with instrumentation or with chronic nasolacrimal duct obstruction. The canaliculi may run immediately beneath the surface of the eyelid margin but usually are buried within orbicularis muscle.

The lacrimal canaliculi separately traverse the tissue between the anterior crus and posterior crus of the medial canthal ligament. In more than 90% of instances, the canaliculi conjoin to form a common canaliculus. The common canaliculus represents a diverticulum of the lacrimal sac (Whitnall) and, if dilated, is termed a Maier's sinus (Fig. 1.30). The valve of Rosenmuller is present at the medial end of the common canaliculus. Retrograde filling studies [53] have called into question the functional significance of this structure. The common canaliculus joins the lacrimal sac at an acute mean angle of 58°, which may have a valve effect [54]. The common internal punctum enters the posterolateral

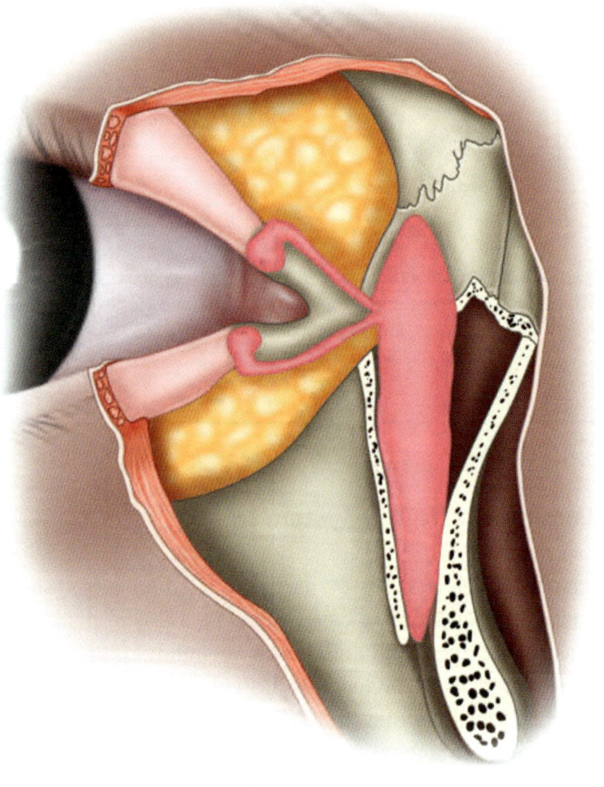

Fig. 1.29 Approximate dimensions of nasolacrimal excretory system. In the adult, the length of system is about 35 mm; in the newborn the system measures about 25 mm

The initial 2 mm of each canaliculus is vertical, turning medially at a right angle dilation termed the ampulla. The ampullae are situated on the anterior surface of the medial tarsal plates. The tubes have a diameter of 0.5–1 mm in the horizontal portion, but because of the elastic character of

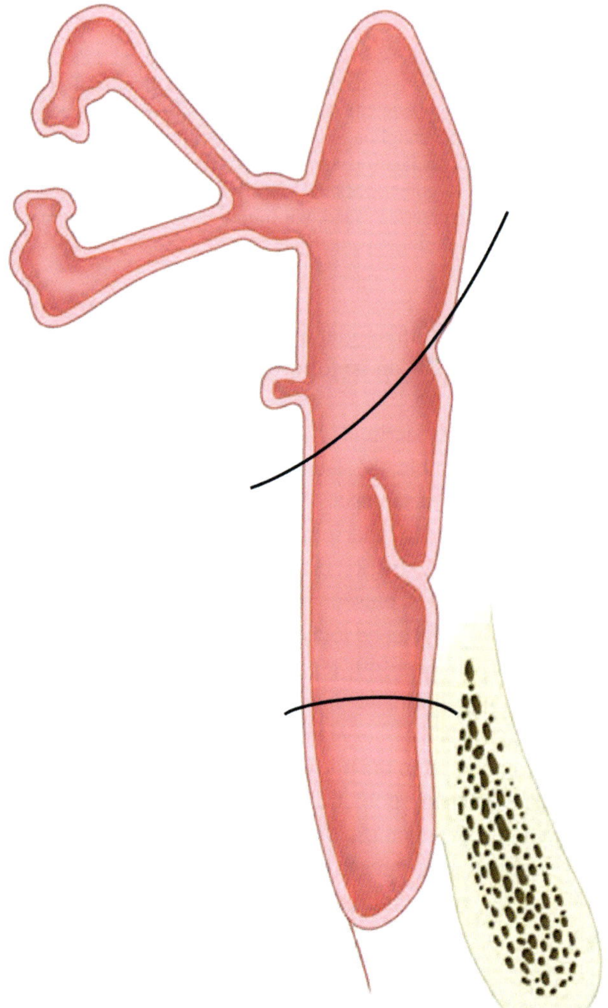

Fig. 1.30 Schematic drawing of nasolacrimal excretory system to show valves

sac 2–3 mm deep and slightly superior to the anterior crus of the medial canthal ligament.

Nasolacrimal Sac and Duct

The lacrimal sac and the nasolacrimal duct are differently named portions of the same structure, and they differ in their surrounding relationships. The lacrimal sac is bound tightly by the lacrimal fascia laterally and nestled into the bony lacrimal fossa medially. The nasolacrimal duct is entirely intraosseous until its inferior termination in the inferior meatus. The sac (Fig. 1.31) measures about 12 mm in height, with the 4-mm fundus above the medial canthal ligament. Conforming to the shape of the lacrimal fossa, the sac is 4–8 mm anteroposteriorly and several millimeters in width. The lacrimal fossa is narrower in the female, [23] thereby containing a smaller lacrimal sac. The intraosseous duct extends 12.5 mm on average and ends with a 2–5 mm extension into the inferior nasal meatus.

The anterior limb of the medial canthal ligament lies anterior to the upper lacrimal sac and inserts on the anterior lacrimal crest. The medial canthal ligament has a smaller posterior crus inserting on the lacrimal fascia and posterior lacrimal crest. This posterior limb is crucial in the maintenance of eyelid–globe apposition medially. The lacrimal muscle of Horner is a specialized extension of the pretarsal orbicularis, which inserts immediately behind, above, and below the posterior crus [55]. The deep head of the preseptal orbicularis from the upper eyelid inserts onto the superior anterior aspect of the sac. These muscles are important in the lacrimal pump mechanism [55, 56].

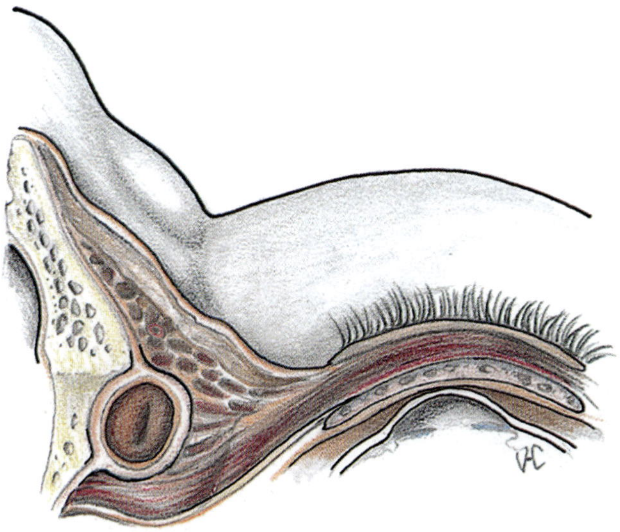

Fig. 1.31 Horizontal section through the right upper eyelid near palpebral margin to show relations of lacrimal sac. At medial commissure (slightly below this cut), fibrous medial canthal ligament replaces Horner–Duverney muscle in immediate contact with lacrimal fascia

The orbital septum extends from the inferior orbital rim to insert along the anterior lacrimal crest until the medial canthal ligament is met. The orbital septum from the superior orbital rim inserts posterior to the Horner–Duverney lacrimal muscle at the posterior lacrimal crest. Laterally, the septum fuses with the lacrimal fascia. Because of this arrangement, the lacrimal sac is a preseptal structure. Additionally, a transcaruncular incision, followed by dissection between the lacrimal muscle and the septum at the posterior lacrimal crest, may be used to obtain access to the medial orbit.

The inferior portion of the sac not bound by the medial canthal ligament is susceptible to anterior distention in acute dacryocystitis. Behind the inferior lacrimal sac and fascia lies the orbital fat unless a prominent hamular process of the lacrimal bone intervenes. Just lateral to the lacrimal sac lies the origin of the inferior oblique on the orbital floor.

The intraosseous nasolacrimal duct conforms to the bony nasolacrimal canal. The membranous nasolacrimal sac and upper nasolacrimal duct can be easily separated from the bone; farther down in the canal, the tissue becomes adherent to the bone as it assumes more of the mucoperiosteum quality of the nasal lining. This fact explains why false tracts made by probings superiorly meet greater resistance between the duct and bone more inferiorly. The histology of the nasolacrimal system shows transition from the stratified squamous epithelium and elastic support of the canaliculi to the more fibrous coat of the sac lined with a columnar epithelium and to the fibrous wall of the nasolacrimal duct with an erectile venous plexus similar to that seen in the nose. Various reports exist of cilia and mucous glands within the nasolacrimal canal. Therefore, conditions affecting the nasal mucosa are likely to involve the inferior nasolacrimal system.

The membranous portion of the nasolacrimal duct usually empties immediately beneath the inferior turbinate but may extend to the nasal floor and remain imperforate [56]. The opening of the duct into the nose may be a slit or a mucosal flap valve hinged from above (Hasner's valve) (see Fig. 1.30). The degree to which this valve is incompetent determines the extent to which the individual can inflate the tear sac with nose blowing. The numerous nasolacrimal duct diverticula noted in some individuals are presumably pneumatically induced. An incompetent valve of Rosenmuller allows nasal air to escape from the puncta.

Lacrimal Excretory Development

The developmental anatomy of the nasolacrimal duct has received considerable interest because of the frequency of congenital obstruction. Between the lateral nasal and maxillary processes in the 7-mm embryo, a depression develops termed the nasolacrimal groove (see Fig. 1.3). The ectoderm in this region thickens and becomes buried as the maxillary mesoderm moves medially overriding it. Previous literature states that a central mass of ectoderm is buried and extensions develop on either end to reach the eyelids and the nose, respectively. A work by Sevel [49], studying serial sections of embryos, suggests that a single, complete nasolacrimal ectodermal cord is buried. Accessory lacrimal fistulous tracts, termed anlage ducts by Jones and Wobig, may occur throughout the course of the nasolacrimal system [56, 57].

Canalization of the ectodermal rod begins at 32- to 36-mm stage of development [58]. Areas of imperfect disintegration result in persistent membranes or "valves" seen in the adult. Some literature states that the process of the canalization is segmented, whereas Sevel found the entire nasolacrimal system to hollow concurrently. The central cells of the cord degenerate, leaving a lumen closed on the proximal end by a thin membrane of fused conjunctival and canalicular epithelium and closed on the distal end by a similar membrane with nasolacrimal and nasal components. The nasolacrimal epithelium desquamates, and a plug of debris accumulates at the inferior end of the tube. The superior membrane is virtually always open by birth, whereas the inferior membrane is reported to persist 35–73% of the time, perhaps protected by the desquamated epithelial debris [59]. Others have reported congenital epiphora from nasolacrimal duct obstruction in 5% of newborns [60]. Hydrostatic massage of the lacrimal sac often opens the thin nasal membrane, thus avoiding later probing or silicone intubation of the nasolacrimal duct [61, 62]. Congenital absence of any portion of the nasolacrimal canal, supernumerary puncta, and lacrimal fistula demonstrates the variability of development in this area [57, 58, 63].

Eyelid Anatomy

The eyelids are complex specialized facial adaptations designed to protect, moisten, and clean the ocular surfaces. These superficial components are modified by structures arising from within the orbit, adding complexity to the function and anatomy. Consideration of eyelid anatomy as a superficial component with deep modifiers clarifies the relationships to the surrounding face.

Eyebrow and Superficial Musculoaponeurotic System

The eyebrow skin is thick with a correspondingly thick subcutaneous fibroadipose layer. Large hair follicles with attendant sweat and sebaceous glands abound, interspersed between which are the inserting fibers of the underlying muscles. Hair angulation is somewhat less than 30° downward from the vertical in the upper eyebrow and somewhat less than 30° upward in the lower eyebrow with an abrupt reversal at the center or horizontal crest of the structure (Fig. 1.32). This reversal does not occur at the medial end of the eyebrow, where the hair sweeps uninterruptedly superolaterally. The horizontal and vertical eyebrow hair angulations should be kept in mind while performing incisions in the eyebrow region [64]. Incisions adjacent to the brow should be made parallel to the cilia.

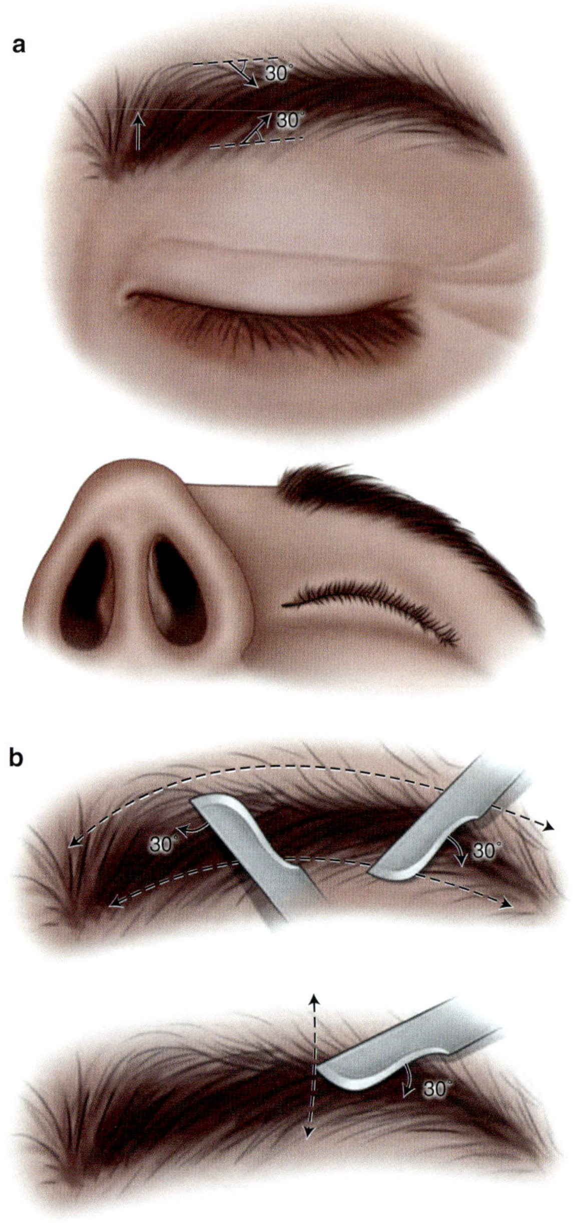

Fig. 1.32 (**a**) Hair direction in adult eyebrow. Hair angulation is about 30° downward from vertical in the upper eyebrow and about 30° upward in the lower eyebrow with an abrupt reversal at center of the eyebrow. This reversal does not occur at medial end of the eyebrow, where hair sweeps upward uninterrupted from below. (**b**) Hair also angles laterally, at least 30° from vertical

The eyebrow is a specialized area of the superficial muscle plane of the face where the frontalis and orbicularis muscles interdigitate [65]. The bilateral corrugator supercilii muscles arise from the smooth, superomedial orbital margin and extend superolaterally to insert in the muscle and skin of the medial eyebrow. The procerus muscle overlying the glabella is continuous with the frontalis and indistinguishable from it during dissection. Various authors have considered the corrugator and procerus muscles as "heads" of the frontalis, but because the corrugator muscles arise from a different superficial muscle plane lamina and are served by different branches of the facial nerve, the value of these concepts is questioned.

The superficial musculoaponeurotic system (SMAS) was described by Mitz and Peyronie [66]. Their work demonstrated a fascia dividing the subcutaneous fat in the parotid and cheek into two layers. This structure showed continuity between the posterior part of the frontalis muscle in the upper face and the platysma of the lower face (Fig. 1.33). The details and functional significance of this structure have been controversial [51, 67]. Thaller and co-workers [68] further characterized the SMAS in human and rhesus monkey specimens, reporting contiguity with the orbicularis oculi and identifying the superficial temporalis fascia (temporoparietal fascia) as part of the structure. Work by others [51] did not show continuity between the SMAS and the temporoparietal fascia.

Kikkawa and colleagues [69] detailed the orbital and eyelid relationships of the SMAS. The SMAS (Figs. 1.34 and 1.35) was shown to invest the orbicularis muscle, being continuous with the anterior and posterior orbicularis fascia. The eyebrow fat pad, the sub-SMAS fat in the malar region (malar fat pad), and the postorbicularis layer of the lower eyelid were all shown to be contiguous. Additionally, collagen and elastin attachments were found extending from the inferior orbital rim, traveling through the orbicularis, and inserting into the skin of the nasojugal and malar folds. Kikkawa termed this structure the orbitomalar ligament. Scanning electron microscopy of SMAS tissue [70] demonstrated an irregular, loose, and interwoven network of elastin and collagen.

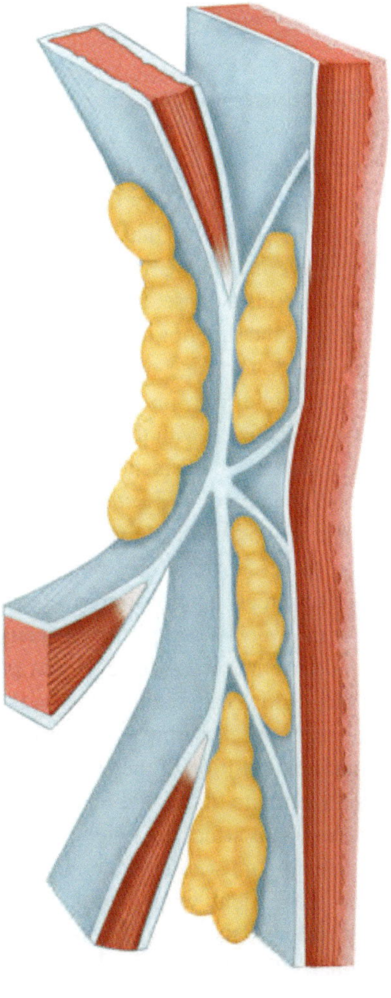

Fig. 1.33 The superficial musculoaponeurotic system (SMAS) is an important facial layer with continuity between the frontalis and the platysma

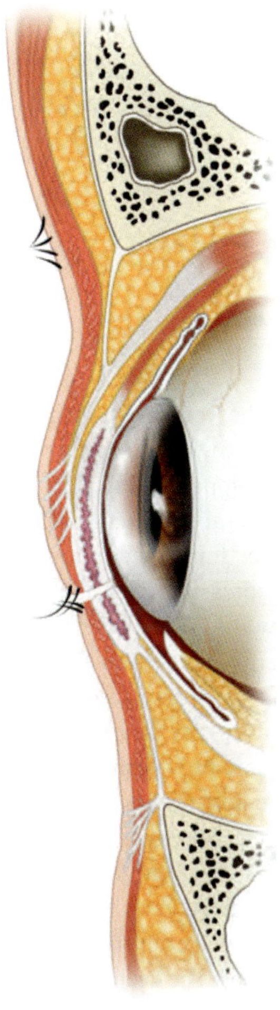

Fig. 1.34 The SMAS extends into the eyelids as the anterior and posterior fascia which envelops the orbicularis muscle. The orbitomalar ligament is an important supporting structure of the SMAS

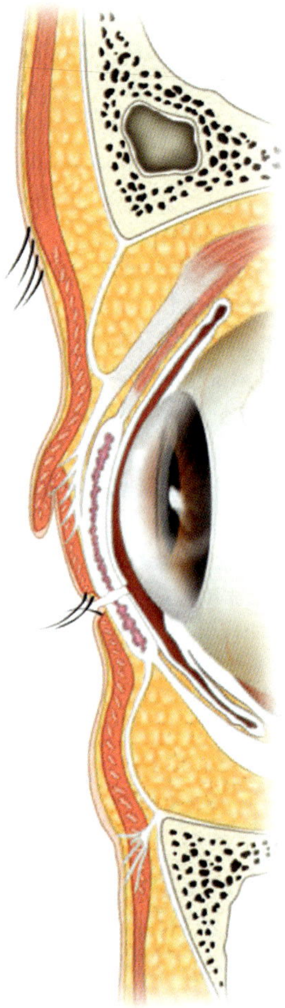

Fig. 1.35 Aging SMAS

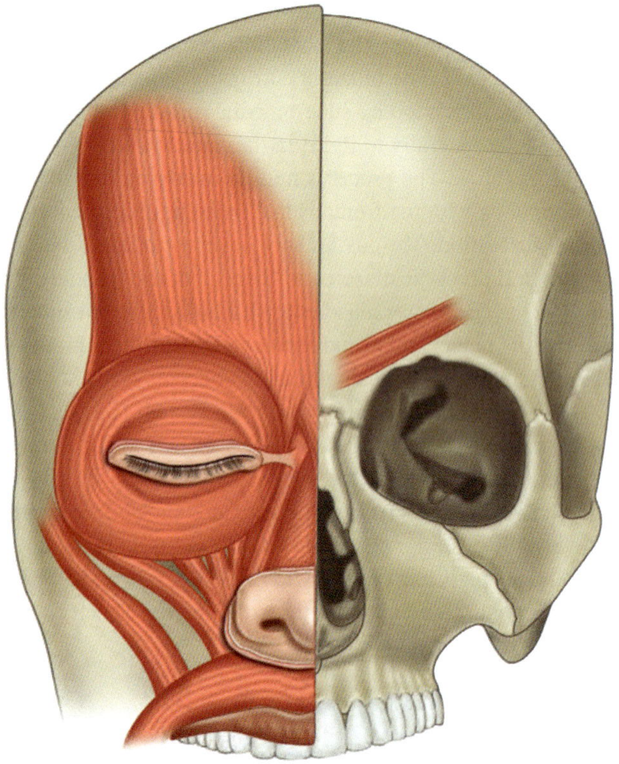

Fig. 1.36 Superficial muscle plane of the face

Contraction of the vertically oriented frontalis elevates the eyebrow (Fig. 1.36). The frontalis can serve as an accessory elevator of the upper eyelid. This function is the basis of frontalis sling operations used for the correction of ptosis with poor levator function. Contraction of the corrugator results in a depression over the medial eyebrow and draws the eyebrow inferomedially, producing vertical glabellar folds. Procerus contraction also depresses the medial eyebrow, resulting in horizontal creases. The corrugator and procerus muscles are intentionally weakened during coronal or endoscopic brow-elevating procedures.

The galea aponeurotica joins the frontalis anteriorly with the occipitalis muscle posteriorly. The galea splits about the frontalis muscle to form a superficial and deep galea (Fig. 1.37). The superficial galea is thinner and continues into the upper eyelid as the anterior muscle sheath of the frontalis and orbicularis muscles. The deep galea serves as the posterior muscle sheath of the frontalis and orbicularis muscles. The deep galea layer divides here to encompass the fat pad of the eyebrow, termed "fatty cushion" by Charpy [71]. This same layer continues into the eyelid as the posterior orbicularis fascia described by Putterman and Urist [72]. The posterior limit of the eyebrow fat pad is a dense, fibrous layer continuous in the upper eyelid with the superior orbital septum.

Occasionally, the lower edge of the brow fat pad droops inferiorly into the eyelid. The inexperienced ptosis surgeon must avoid confusing this fat with the preaponeurotic fat pad. Such a mistake could lead to misidentifying of the orbital septum as the levator aponeurosis. Dissection in the plane between the orbicularis and the posterior orbicularis fascia and continuing in the same plane superiorly between the frontalis and brow fat pad are key steps in posterior brow fixation [73, 74]. Because the lateral eyebrow is less densely attached to the bone lateral to the supraorbital ridge eyebrow, ptosis usually occurs first in this region. This segment is also the most common site for the recurrence of brow ptosis postoperatively.

The anatomic juxtaposition of the eyebrow and the upper eyelid confers an intimate functional relationship. The position of the eyebrow can affect the height and the excursion of the upper eyelid and must be considered in the evaluation and surgery of the patient with blepharoptosis [75, 76]. Likewise, the position of the eyebrow must be considered in the patient evaluated for blepharoplasty [77–81].

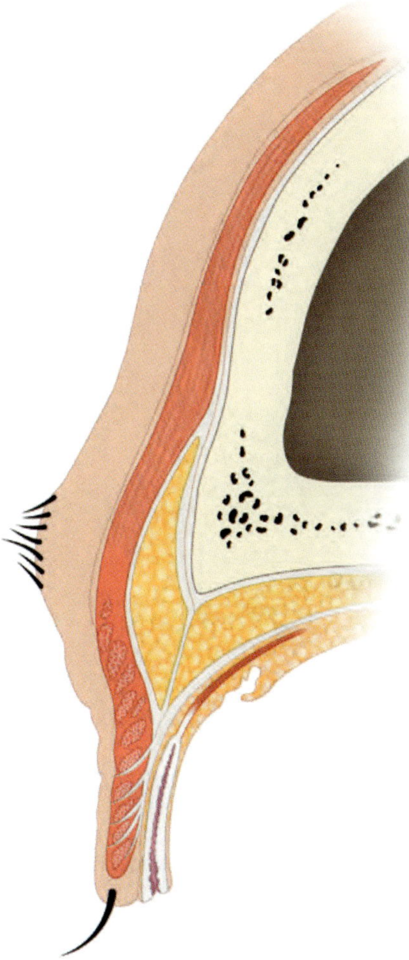

Fig. 1.37 Relationships of galea aponeurotica

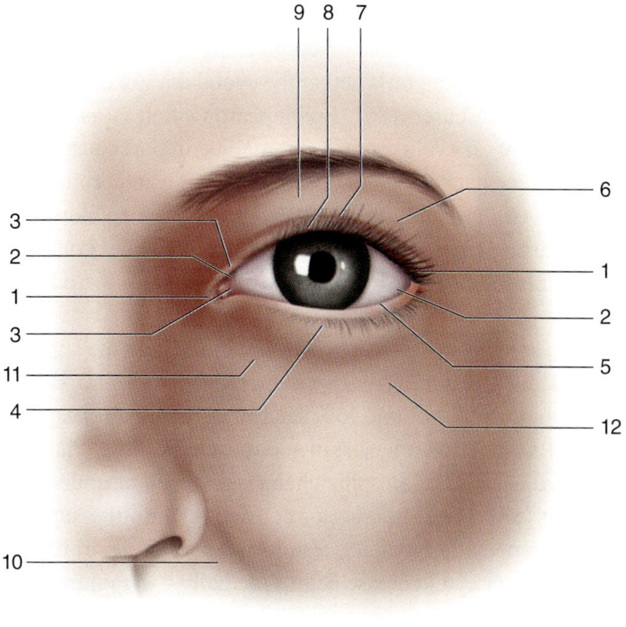

Fig. 1.38 Topographic eyelid anatomy. *1* Commissures. *2* Canthal angles, medial and lateral. *3* Puncta. *4* Inferior lid crease. *5* Lowest point of curve. *6* Superior eyelid skin fold. *7* Superior lid crease. *8* Highest point of curve. *9* Superior orbital sulcus. *10* Nasolabial fold. *11* Nasojugal fold. *12* Malar fold (see text)

Superficial Eyelid Anatomy

The topographic anatomy of the eyelids is shown in Fig. 1.38. The palpebral fissure between the eyelid margins measures vertically about 9–11 mm in the non-ptotic adult. The upper eyelid rests at the upper limbus in children and about 1.5–2 mm below in adults. The lower eyelid is generally found at the lower limbus. The highest point of the curved upper eyelid is slightly nasal to the pupil. The lowest point of the lower eyelid is slightly temporal. The contour of the closed eyelids roughly is that of the open lower eyelid [82]. The commissures are the junction points between the upper and lower eyelids where they meet medially and laterally. The horizontal distance between the commissures is about 28–30 mm. The lateral commissure rests on the globe, whereas the medial commissure is separated by the intervening caruncle and plica semilunaris. The medial and lateral canthi are the angles formed by the eyelids at these commissures. The lateral canthal angle should be about 2 mm higher than the medial canthal angle.

The upper eyelid crease results from the superficial insertion of levator fibers. The crease lies about 8–11 mm above the central lid margin, generally higher in women than in men. A recent study of healthy white subjects [83] suggested lower crease heights than traditionally reported but confirmed relatively higher lid creases in females and with advancing age. During blepharoplasty or levator surgery, the lid crease should usually be reformed by attachment of the eyelid skin and/or pretarsal orbicularis muscle to the levator aponeurosis [84] or superior tarsal margin. The eyelid crease in Asian patients is only several millimeters from the eyelid margin because the superior orbital septum inserts on the levator aponeurosis at this low level, preventing the higher cutaneous insertions of the levator seen in other patients [85]. Tissue overlapping the upper eyelid crease, the upper eyelid fold, assumes greater proportions with the loss of skin elasticity in advancing age. A less well-defined crease can be seen in the lower eyelid where the retractors superficially insert.

An excessive skin fold that may be associated with underlying orbicularis is called an epiblepharon fold or an epicanthal fold depending on whether the eyelid margin or the inner canthus is obscured [86]. Epiblepharon often is associated with loss of an eyelid crease and may be in part caused by a lack of deep anchoring of the superficial skin and orbicularis. Chronic ocular irritation may be caused by the epiblepharon fold causing the eyelashes to rub on the cornea, a condition often misdiagnosed as infectious conjunctivitis or dacryocystitis [87].

The area between the upper eyelid crease and the superior orbital margin is referred to as the superior orbital sulcus. With the orbital volume loss seen in aging or after enucleation, the superior sulcus skin and muscle become relatively concave because of atrophic changes and lack of underlying support [88]. Focal bulging or convexities into the superior sulcus, especially medially, result from herniating orbital fat.

The lower eyelid crease begins medially 4–5 mm from the eyelid margin and slopes slightly inferiorly as it moves temporally. A less well-defined oblique malar crease marks the junction between the orbicularis muscle and the malar fat. The malar crease accentuates with the rise of the cheek during a smile and forms the lower border of eyelid edema. An even more oblique nasolabial fold marks the inferior border of the malar fat pad. A dense fibrous septum anchors the nasolabial fold to the maxilla. This fold divides the levator labii superioris alaeque nasi from the orbicularis muscle above and from the levator labii superioris below. Within this fold run the angular vessels.

Wrinkling of the facial skin is predictable in pattern, although individual forms differ because of the habitual use of different muscles of expression (Fig. 1.39). The horizontal forehead furrows topographically show the lateral extent of the frontalis muscle and provide evidence for the chronic physiologic correction of eyebrow ptosis. Horizontal skin creases radiating from the lateral eyelid commissure represent the vertical shortening of orbicularis muscle throwing the relatively immobile skin of this region into folds. A horizontal fold across the glabella indicates procerus depression of the medial eyebrows. The vertical fold through the medial eyebrow represents corrugator action.

The skin of the eyelids is thin; that of the medial upper eyelid being the thinnest found in the body. Well-placed incisions within this thin skin usually result in minimal scarring. Transition to the thick skin of the eyebrow above and to the malar region below is rather abrupt. Subcutaneous fat is sparse in the preorbital and preseptal skin and is absent in the pretarsal skin. Edema of the loose subcutaneous eyelid tissues is typically well demarcated, with a specific border at the surrounding areas having a denser subcutaneous fibroadipose.

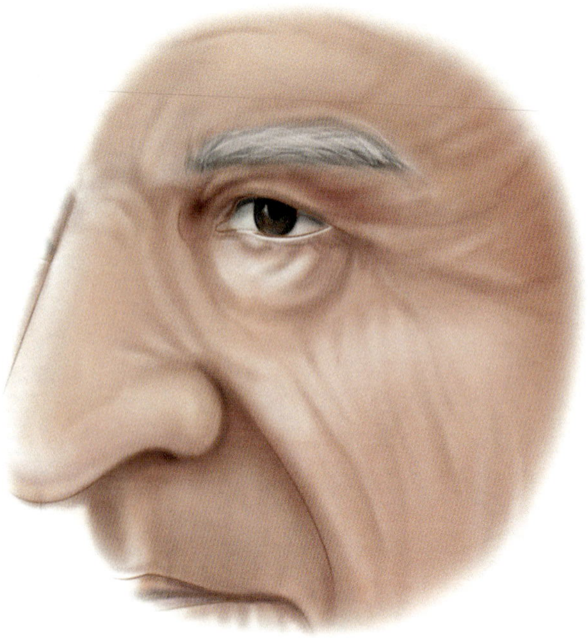

Fig. 1.39 Drawing of adult wrinkled face

Eyelid Margin

The eyelid margin is divided into a medial lacrimal portion and a lateral palpebral portion by the lacrimal punctum. Medially, the margin is rounded, without lashes, and carries the lacrimal canaliculus a variable depth beneath its surface. A cross-section through the eyelid at this point demonstrates pretarsal muscle encompassing the canaliculus. The lacrimal papilla is a fibrous ring within the medial end of the tarsus; the canaliculus dives anteriorly to the ampulla. The palpebral portion of the eyelid margin is squared off because of pressure from the opposite lid and the eyeball behind (Fig. 1.40).

The number of cilia located on the anterior eyelid margin is around 100 in the upper eyelid and 50 in the lower lid. Several sebaceous glands (Zeis glands) empty into each follicle. Between each follicle is a spiral sweat gland (Moll's gland) ending either onto the eyelid margin, a sebaceous gland, or a follicle. Centrally, the margin exhibits a fine gray line, which represents the terminal extensions of the orbicularis muscle of Riolan. This line serves as a dissection guide to split the eyelid into an anterior lamella of skin, muscle, and lashes and a posterior lamella of tarsus and conjunctiva. Such a division is only approximate; however, because fibrous elements from the tarsus splay anteriorly, follicles may extend posteriorly to embed in the tarsus, and orbicularis elements are seen even posterior to the meibomian glands (pars subtarsalis or Klodt's muscle).

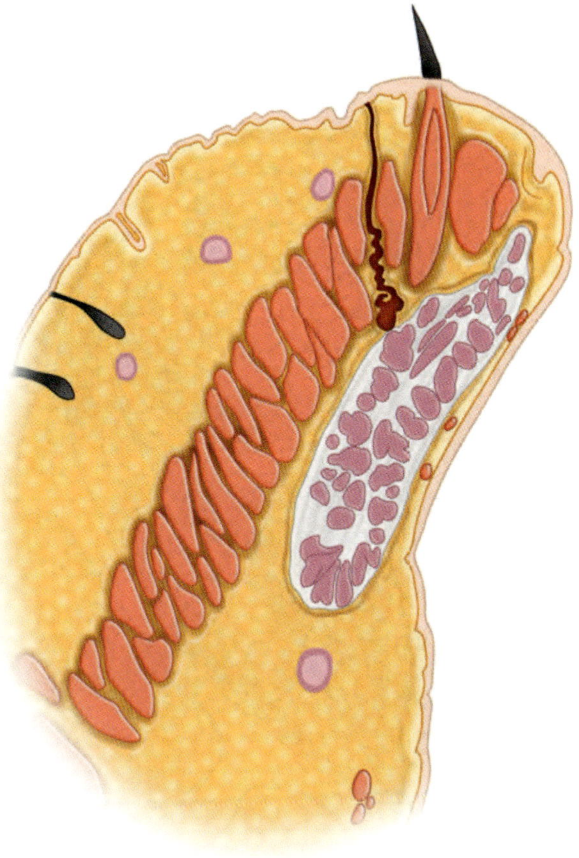

Fig. 1.40 Cross-section of lower eyelid margin

Orbicularis Oculi Muscle

The orbicularis oculi muscle is the superficial muscle plane covering of the orbit and is continuous with other facial muscles in this plane. It is separated from the dermis by a fibroadipose layer 4–6 mm thick beneath the brow tapering to less than 0.1 mm in the pretarsal eyelid [89]. Fibrous septa from the dermis interdigitate with the orbicularis fibers, keeping the skin and muscle adherent. Together, the skin and underlying orbicularis are often referred to as the anterior lamella.

The peripheral orbicularis fibers are coarse and loosely associated, whereas those close to the lid margins are fine and densely arranged. Around the palpebral fissure, the fibers are parallel and concentric. The peripheral fibers may be gently curved or may run tangential to the inner curves (Fig. 1.41). The vertical lateral fibers are important in the formation of horizontal skin wrinkles at the lateral angle of the eye [65]. Jones [90] has reemphasized the division of the orbicularis muscle into pretarsal, preseptal, and orbital components.

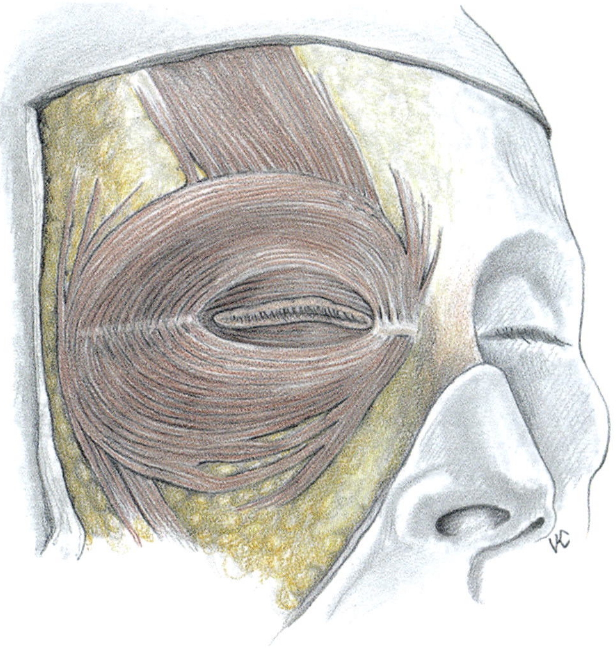

Fig. 1.41 Superficial orbicularis oculi muscle

The pretarsal orbicularis is tightly adherent to the tarsus and levator. The pretarsal component originates from the superficial and deep limbs of the medial canthal ligament. The superficial heads overlie the ampullae and surround the canaliculi. The superficial heads of the orbicularis muscle are also continuous with and overlie the superficial medial canthal ligament in the newborn (Whitnall), but they are seen to terminate along this structure in the adult (Fig. 1.42). The deep pretarsal heads (Horner–Duverney muscle) [52, 91] insert on the posterior lacrimal crest and the lacrimal fascia (Figs. 1.43 and 1.44). Thus, the superficial and deep components of the pretarsal orbicularis both contribute to the lacrimal pump mechanism [92, 93]. The deep component (Horner–Duverney muscle) is also crucial in maintaining globe–eyelid apposition. A very small component of the orbicularis, the muscle of Riolan, lies separated from the pretarsal fibers by the follicles of the eyelashes. This component forms the gray line of the eyelid margins [94].

The preseptal orbicularis lies anterior to the orbital septum, separated from it by the postorbicularis fascia. This fascia is continuous with the eyebrow fat pad. The fibers of the preseptal orbicularis originate along the upper and lower margins of the medial canthal ligament. The preseptal muscles arc around the eyelids toward the lateral canthus. At the lateral canthus, the preseptal orbicularis fibers attach to the zygoma along a horizontal line, the lateral palpebral raphe.

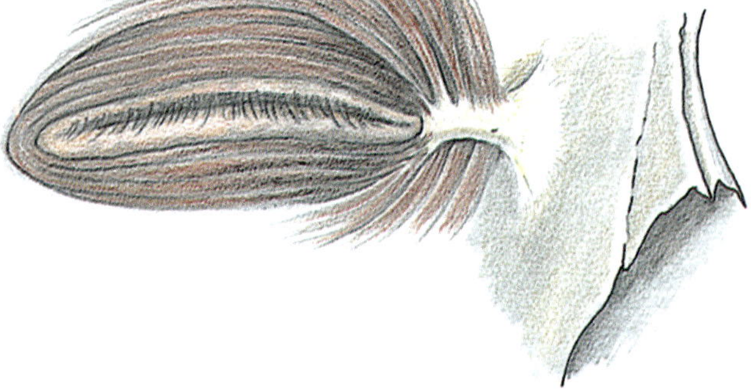

Fig. 1.42 Superficial medial canthal ligament. Superficial muscle fibers overlie this structure in the newborn but are seen to terminate along this structure in the adult

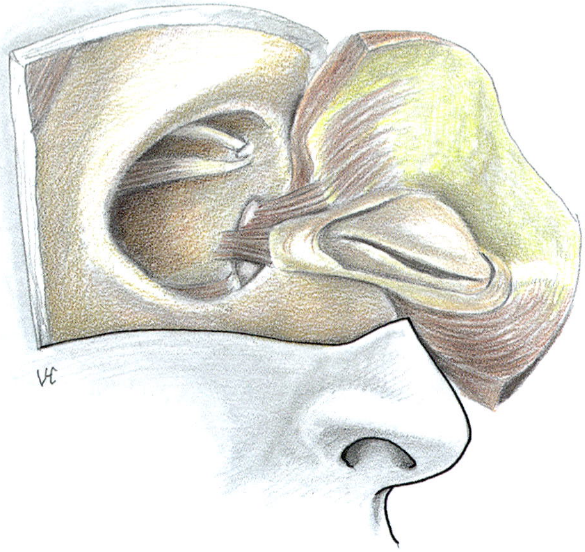

Fig. 1.43 Duplication of Homer's dissection to show pars lacrimalis muscle. Superficial muscle plane and skin has been reflected medially and orbital contents have been largely removed

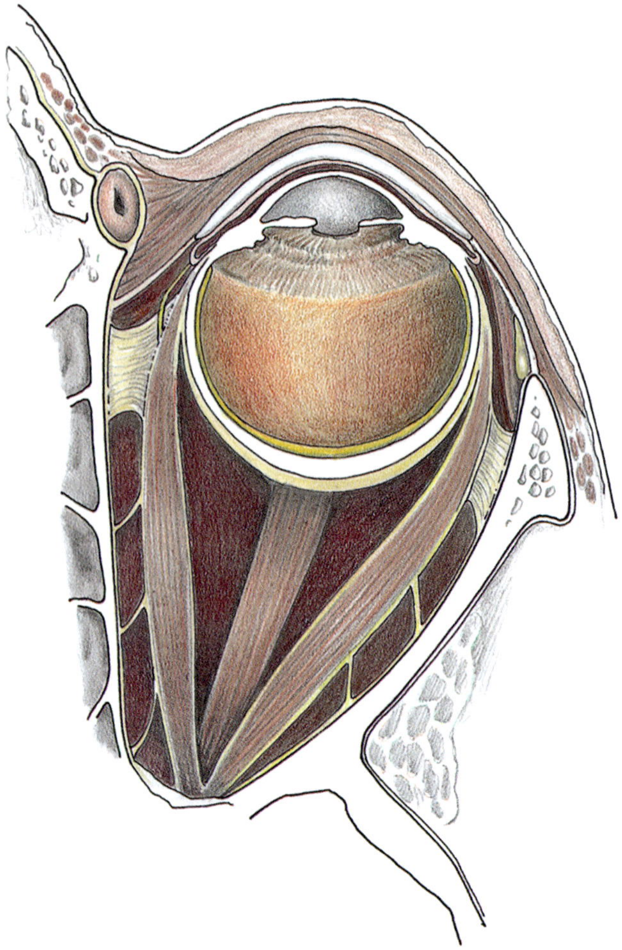

Fig. 1.44 Horizontal section through the upper eyelid near the palpebral margin. Anterior crus of medial canthal ligament is seen more inferiorly. Posterior fibers in Horner–Duverney muscle arise from pretarsal orbicularis muscle, while the more anterior fibers inserting on lacrimal fascia originate in preseptal orbicularis. Posterior crus of medial canthal ligament is seen in more inferior cuts; it replaces Horner–Duverney muscle in immediate relations to lacrimal fascia

The orbital portion of the orbicularis covers the orbital rims. It originates from insertions on the frontal process of the maxillary bone, from the orbital process of the frontal bone, and from the medial canthal ligament. Its fibers pass around the orbital rim without interruption at the lateral commissure and insert just inferior to their origin [89]. Just as the postorbicularis fascia of the upper eyelid is continuous with the brow fat pad, the malar fat pad lies directly beneath the postorbicularis fascia of the peripheral lower lid. To emphasize this anatomic relationship, the malar fat pad has been referred to as the "suborbicularis oculi fat" (SOOF) [95].

Involuntary blink and unforced eyelid closure result from pretarsal and preseptal function. Increasingly forceful eyelid closure results in centripetal overriding by the preseptal and the orbital components. Forced eyelid closure is achieved by orbital orbicularis contraction. The preseptal and orbital components move more freely except where they are attached to a bone at the lateral palpebral raphe, the supraorbital ridge, the nasoorbital valley, and the malar crease.

Medial and Lateral Canthal Ligaments

Attached to the medial and lateral orbital rims are the fibrous connections to the tarsal plates, the medial and lateral canthal ligaments. The term ligament is probably more appropriate than tendon because these structures connect fibrous tissue to the bone and serve as structural support for the orbicularis muscle. The medial canthal ligament extends anteriorly to the anterior lacrimal crest and superiorly along the frontal process of the maxilla and the frontal bone [96, 97]. Deep fibers of the medial canthal ligament pass along the lacrimal fascia to insert on the posterior lacrimal crest [55]. These deep fibers serve structurally as the anterior border of deep pretarsal muscles (Fig. 1.44). The superficial medial canthal ligament is seen more prominently through the skin in the aged and may even calcify.

The structure and function of the medial deep pretarsal muscles (pars lacrimalis, or Horner–Duverney muscle) are best appreciated by recreating the dissection (Fig. 1.43) of Horner [52]. The posterior placement of the insertion along the lacrimal fascia and posterior lacrimal crest provides a posterior anchor, allowing the eyelids to follow and cover the convex globe. Successful medial canthal reconstructive surgery depends on the reestablishment of this important posterior vector. Chronic epiphora in patients with centurion syndrome [98] (anomalous anterior displacement of the anterior crus of the medial canthal ligament) demonstrates this point.

Contraction of the orbicularis draws the eyelids (especially the lower lid) medially and posteriorly. The resulting lateral pull on the lacrimal diaphragm creates a negative pressure in the lacrimal sac that draws the tears from the canaliculi. Moreover, compression of the lacrimal ampullae by pretarsal muscle pushes fluid toward the sac. The contraction of the Horner–Duverney muscle creating these several effects is termed "lacrimal pump" by Jones [93].

Weakening of the eyelid muscles can cause epiphora through the loss of an effective lacrimal pump, despite a normally positioned punctum [99, 100]. Similarly, a lax lower eyelid can result in epiphora because of tear pump failure [99]. With more advanced eyelid laxity, frank ectropion occurs. The laxity may rarely reflect elongation of the tarsus or, more commonly, either the lateral or medial canthal ligaments or any combination of the three structures. The lateral canthal ligament is most commonly implicated in cases of lower eyelid laxity [101, 102].

The lateral canthal region is less complex than its medial counterpart. Fibrous strands continuous with the tarsi (Fig. 1.45) become the crura of the lateral canthal ligament. These crura form a common ligament 1 mm thick, 3 mm wide, and 5–7 mm long [89]. The ligament inserts at Whitnall's lateral orbital tubercle, just inside the lateral orbital rim (Fig. 1.46). The pretarsal orbicularis inserts 3–4 mm deep to the lateral palpebral raphe along with the lateral canthal ligament [103]. Appreciation of the posterior direction of the lateral canthal ligament is crucial in lower lid ectropion and reconstructive surgery.

The lateral canthal ligament is connected to the lateral rectus check ligament, resulting in slight lateral displacement of the lateral canthal angle on extreme abduction [104]. Additionally inserting on the lateral orbital tubercle are the orbital septum anteriorly, the lateral horn of the levator and the lacrimal gland fascia superiorly, and the lateral portion of

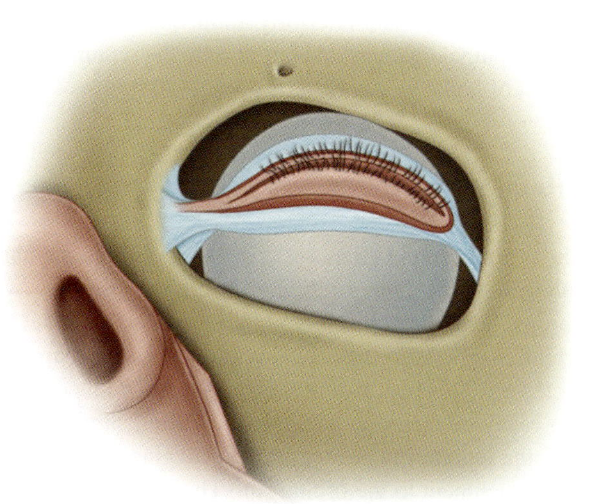

Fig. 1.45 Anteroinferior view of tarsi with canthal ligaments. Deep heads of orbicularis muscles have been removed. Medial canthal ligament inserts anteriorly to anterior lacrimal crest and fans posteriorly to lacrimal fascia and posterior lacrimal crests; it is bound superiorly, inferiorly, and posteriorly by Horner–Duverney muscle. Superficial crus of lateral canthal ligament is shown with underlying deep orbicularis heads removed. Deep crus of lateral canthal ligament, which underlies deep orbicularis head, is not shown

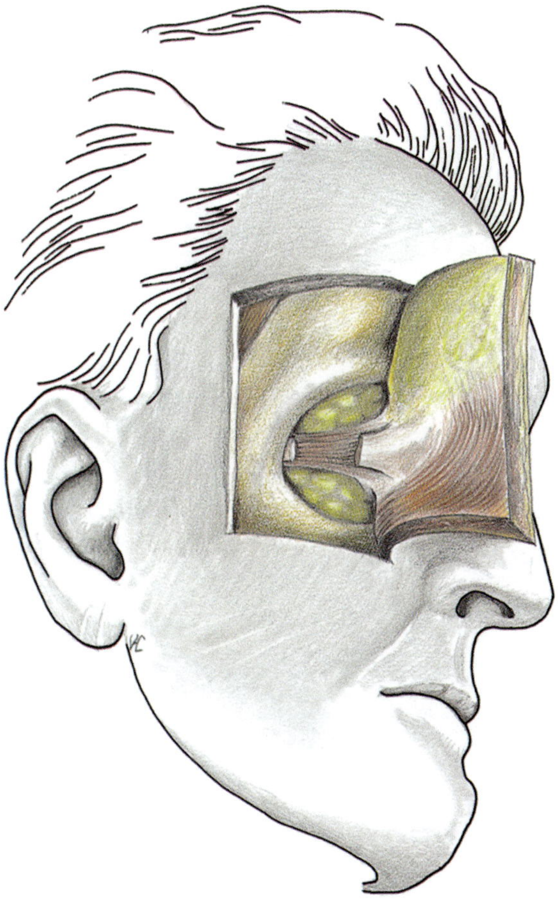

Fig. 1.46 Deep lateral canthal structures. Superficial muscle plane is partially reflected medially. Superficial head of lateral canthal ligament has been divided to show deep insertion on Whitnall's tubercle

Lockwood's ligament inferiorly. Immediately anterior to the lateral canthal ligament and posterior to the septum is a small pocket of fat known as Eisler's pocket [105].

Orbital Septum

The orbital septum (Fig. 1.47) is a thin, fibrous membrane delineating the anterior boundary of the orbit. A white fibrous line, the arcus marginalia, appears on the bony orbital margin after the orbital septum has been sharply dissected off. This fusion of the orbital septum with periosteum can easily be traced in the cadaver. During surgical dissection, the septum can be identified by tugging on it to confirm firm attachment to the orbital rim. The septum is redundant medially and laterally. Medially, the septum covers the posterior aspect of the lacrimal muscle as it inserts along the posterior lacrimal crest.

It is described by Whitnall to cross the midlacrimal fossa adherent to lacrimal fascia to reach the anterior lacrimal crest (Fig. 1.48). In this way, the lacrimal sac is isolated from the orbit and the eyelid. Laterally, the septum posterior to the superficial orbicularis inserts anterior to the lateral canthal ligament. A sheath of septum posterior to the deep orbicularis muscle inserts at Whitnall's tubercle behind the muscle.

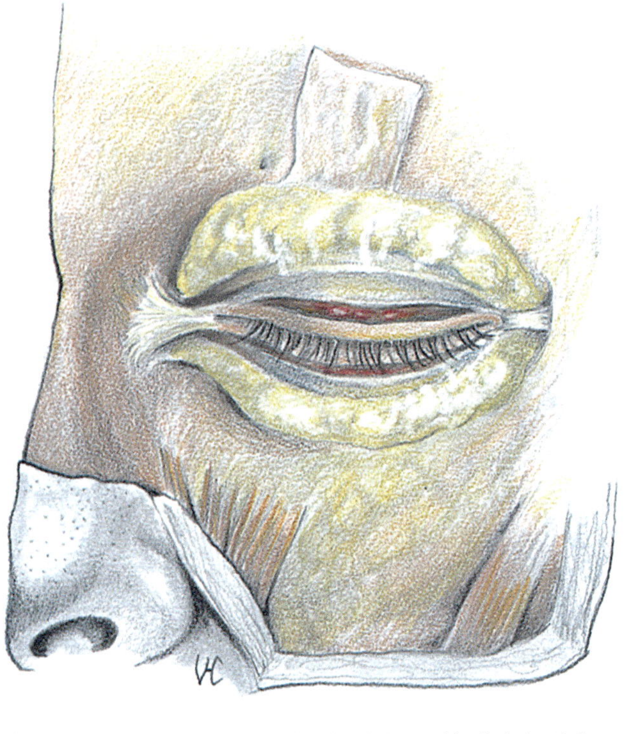

Fig. 1.47 Orbital septum. Superficial and deep orbicularis heads have been removed. Tag of deep galea, which forms posterior border of eyebrow fat pad, has been left to show its continuity with orbital septum as posterior limit of superficial muscle plane

The septum inserts on the inferior tarsal margin after joining with the lower eyelid retractors 4–5 mm below this structure. The superior orbital septum does not reach the superior tarsal plate because of the intervening aponeurosis of the levator muscle. Instead, in whites, it inserts on the aponeurosis about 2–5 mm above the superior tarsal border [106]. In Asians, the septum joins the levator at a lower level.

Directly posterior to the septum lie the preaponeurotic and the lower eyelid fat pads. Loose areolar tissue lies immediately before the septum, termed the suborbicularis fascia by Putterman and Urist [72]. This tissue shares the same plane as the eyebrow and malar fat pads further from the eyelid margins. Considerable variation in septum strength is seen between individuals, and the membrane may attenuate with age, allowing orbital fat to herniate forward.

Levator Palpebrae Superioris

The levator palpebrae superioris is the major retractor of the upper eyelid and provides excellent vertical mobility. The superior tarsal muscle complements the function of the levator and is controlled by sympathetic innervation. The lower eyelid does not require substantial vertical excursion. Accordingly, the lower eyelid retractors are much less developed and serve to depress the eyelid only several millimeters in downgaze. Despite this difference in size and function, the retractors of the eyelid exhibit structural similarities (Fig. 1.49).

The levator palpebrae superioris is composed of striated muscle. Arising from the annulus of Zinn at the lesser sphenoid wing, the levator origin is lateral to the superior oblique and above the superior rectus. The levator extends anteriorly in the superior orbit with a thin layer of fat, the supraorbital artery, the frontal nerve, and the trochlear nerve separating it from the orbital roof. The muscle is about 36 mm in length [107]. Beneath the levator lies the superior rectus, on which it rests (Fig. 1.50). These muscles are easily divided, except along their medial borders, where they are attached by a fascial sheath.

The levator and the superior rectus muscles are both innervated by the superior division of the oculomotor nerve, which enters the muscles on their undersides, about 12–13 mm from the orbital apex. The nerve to the levator usually passes around the lateral side of the superior rectus but may pass directly through it. Evidence suggests that the frequent association of superior rectus muscle underaction and levator muscle underaction stems from the development of these muscles from the same superior mesodermal complex [108]. Whether the defect lies in the common superior division of the oculomotor nerve remains unknown. Experimental development of a method to measure levator force [109] has been applied to patients with blepharoptosis.

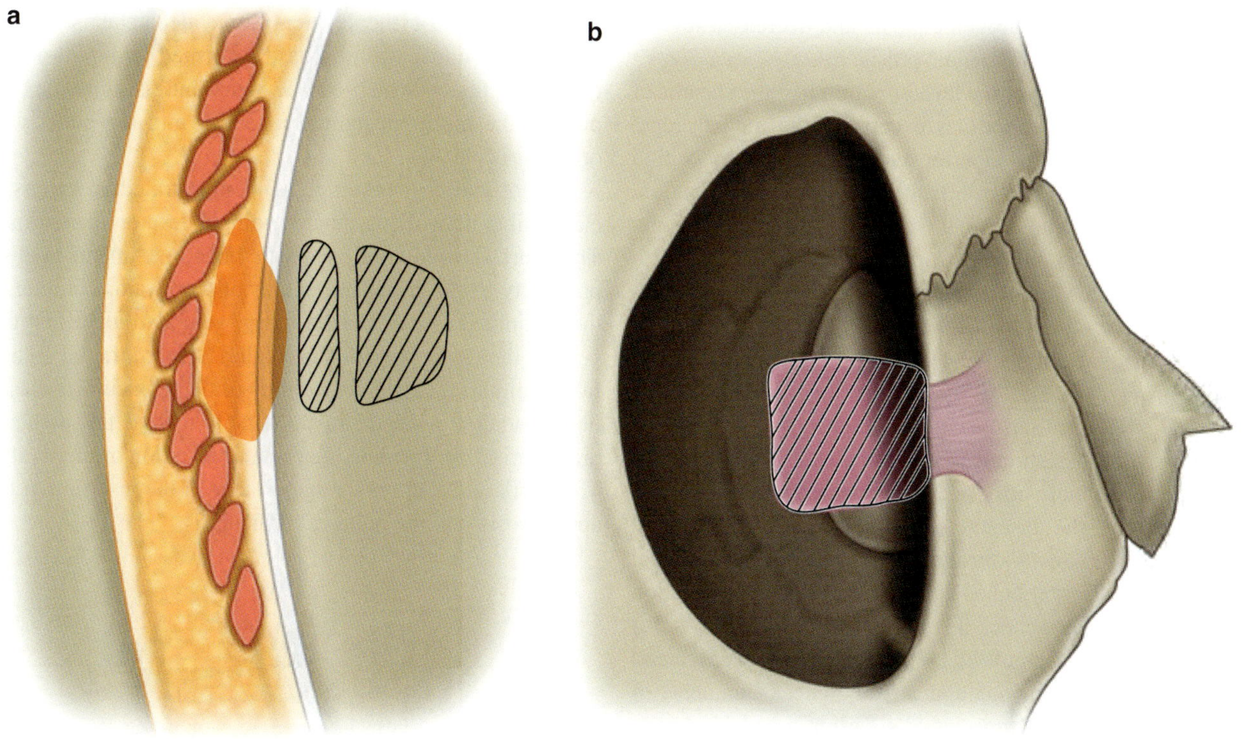

Fig. 1.48 Schematic drawings to show (**a**) lateral and (**b**) medial insertions of orbital septum represented by *dashed lines*. In both cases, deep orbicularis heads carry orbital septum behind them into orbit

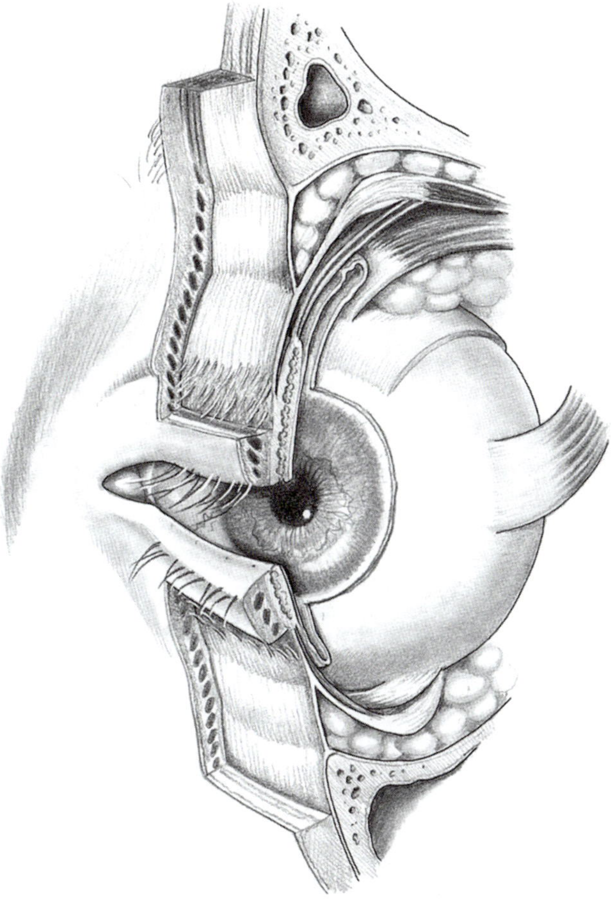

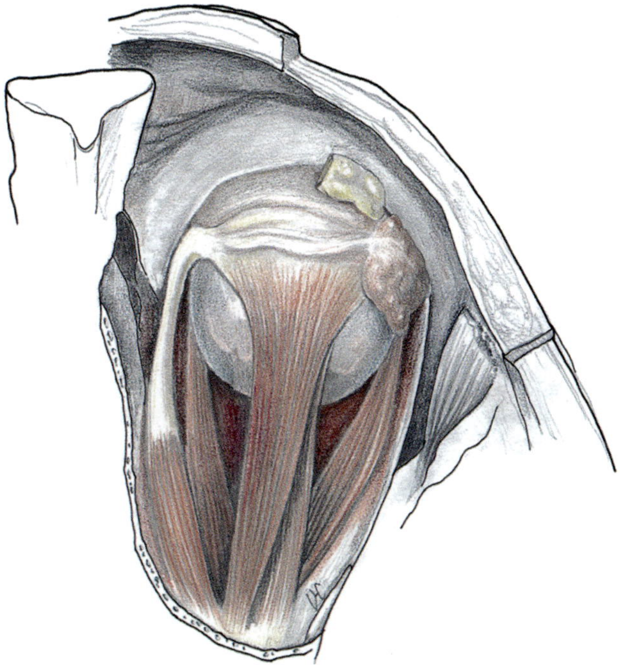

Fig. 1.50 Superior view of levator palpebrae superioris muscle and its relations. Note superior transverse Whitnall's ligament attaching medially to trochlear fascia and laterally to fascia investing the lacrimal gland. Levator is bound on its medial side to superior rectus muscle and is innervated by the same superior oculomotor nerve division

Fig. 1.49 Oblique section through upper and lower eyelids

Extension of this work [110] verified normal force generation in patients with aponeurogenic ptosis and decreased levator force in patients with myogenic ptosis.

The muscle sheath of the levator is thin like the sheaths of the other extraocular muscles except on the medial edge, where it joins with the superior rectus. Immediately behind the superior orbital rim, a transverse fibrous condensation, Whitnall's ligament, attaches superiorly to the widening levator [111]. This fibrous structure is variable in strength but always can be found in the cadaver.

Attachment of Whitnall's ligament to the levator muscle sheath is firm medially and laterally but can be partially separated from it centrally by depression of the muscle. Whitnall's ligament terminates medially in fascia about the trochlea, in fibrous strands to the bone beneath the superior oblique muscle more posteriorly, and possibly anteriorly as a blending with the fascia closing the supraorbital notch. Laterally, the ligament joins with the capsule of the lacrimal gland and the frontal bone. Whitnall described the function of this structure as a check ligament of the levator because it limited the posterior pull of the muscle in the cadaver and because its location is analogous to the check ligaments of the other extraocular muscles. As earlier noted by Jones, Anderson and Dixon stress the importance of the ligament as support for the upper eyelid [112]. They termed it a fulcrum for the levator and noted that larger levator resections are necessary if the ligament is cut. Using high-resolution magnetic resonance imaging, Goldberg and coworkers [113] documented Whitnall's function as a swinging suspender rather than a fulcrum. Shore and McCord suggested that medial ptosis of the eyelid can result from medial disinsertion of the ligament [114]. It has been emphasized that Whitnall's ligament surrounds the levator in a sleevelike fashion on both the superior and inferior surfaces of the levator complex [115]. The relationship of Whitnall's ligament to the levator is fixed; the levator does not slide through it freely as in a fulcrum.

The fibrous levator aponeurosis begins at the level of Whitnall's ligament. Anderson and Beard stated that the length of the aponeurosis is 14–20 mm from Whitnall's transverse ligament to the anterior inferior tarsus border [116], a measurement with which the authors concur. In his extensive description of the levator aponeurosis [117], Whitnall gave a length of 7 mm from the aponeurosis origin to its orbicularis and cutaneous insertions.

Whitnall [3] also noted two distinct divisions in the aponeurosis in which the upper fibers "meet and fuse with the orbital septum," whereas the lower fibers "insert into the lower third of the face of the tarsal plate." Similarly, Siegel [118] demonstrated a fusion of the levator aponeurosis, the orbital septum, and the postorbicularis fascia in this area. This union was termed the conjoined fascia. The levator aponeurosis also has extensive insertions into the pretarsal orbicularis. Figure 1.51 shows in schematic form the palpebral insertions of the levator. Some debate exists about whether the upper eyelid crease is formed by a pull on the cutaneous fibers, which can be weak and variable, or by a pull on the more substantial insertion into the underlying orbicularis [119].

Stasior and co-workers [120] demonstrated an extensive elastic fiber network associated with the levator aponeurosis. This work showed multiple elastic fiber attachments in close proximity to the collagen bundles of the levator complex at the conjoined fascia. Elastic fibers were also identified traversing the lower preseptal orbicularis toward the lid crease. In the midtarsal region, two-thirds of the aponeurotic elastic fibers radiated away from the tarsus, toward the pretarsal orbicularis, thus forming the primary insertion of the levator. This work underscores the importance of the insertion of the aponeurosis into the pretarsal orbicularis.

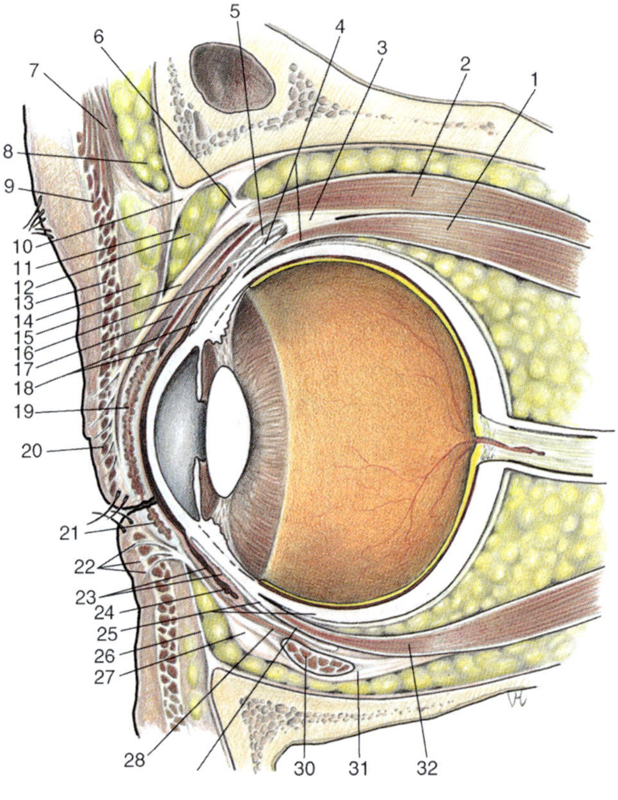

Fig. 1.51 Parasagittal section to show anterior orbital structures. *1* Superior rectus muscle. *2* Levator muscle. *3* Conjoining of SRM with levator muscle sheath. *4* Tenon's capsule. *5* Suspensory ligament of superior fornix. *6* Whitnall's ligament. *7* Frontalis muscle. *8* Brow fat pad. *9* Orbital orbicularis. *10* Arcus marginalis. *11* Orbital septum. *12* Preaponeurotic fat pad. *13* Preseptal orbicularis. *14* Postorbicularis fascia. *15* Levator aponeurosis. *16* Superior conjunctival fornix. *17* Muller's muscle. *18* Conjunctiva. *19* Superior tarsus. *20* Pretarsal orbicularis. *21* Inferior tarsus. *22* Musculocutaneous retractor insertion. *23* Conjunctiva. *24* Inferior conjunctival fornix. *25* Tenon's capsule. *26* Inferior orbital septum. *27* Lockwood's ligament. *28* Inferior tarsal muscle. *29* Suspensory ligament of inferior fornix. *30* Inferior oblique. *31* Capsulopalpebral fascia. *32* Inferior rectus muscle

In addition to the palpebral insertions, the levator aponeurosis expands into a broad, fibrous sheet to insert into the orbital margins behind the medial and lateral commissures of the eye. These insertions, termed medial and lateral "horns" of the levator, may be severed during levator resection surgery. Confusion between the levator horns below and the extremities of the transverse suspensory ligament above should be avoided. The lateral horn is a strong, fibrous band incompletely dividing the lacrimal gland into two lobes and continuing inferiorly to insert on the lateral orbital tubercle and the lateral canthal tendon. The medial horn, in contrast, becomes filmy as it passes over the reflected superior oblique tendon to reach the medial canthal tendon and the posterior lacrimal crest. This less dense attachment medially allows a greater mobility to the medial upper eyelid [116]. Dehiscence of the levator aponeurosis results in acquired involutional ptosis [121].

Müller's Muscle

The smooth superior tarsal muscle of Muller arises from the underside of the striated levator muscle about 15 mm above the superior tarsal border. Muller's muscle inserts at the upper border of the tarsus [122]. It is firmly attached to the levator near its origin but may be more easily separated inferiorly to form the post aponeurotic space described by Jones. Conversely, the attachment to the conjunctiva is firm near the upper tarsal border but looser superiorly. Interruption of sympathetic innervation from the superior cervical ganglion results in the 2 mm of Horner's blepharoptosis. The exact course/courses of sympathetic nerves to this smooth muscle is/are unknown [123, 124]. Using the cynomolgous monkey, Lyon and co-workers [125] detailed the sympathetic nerve anatomy in the cavernous sinus and orbit. All sympathetic fibers destined for the orbit entered through the superior orbital fissure. Within the orbit, the fibers were associated with the ophthalmic artery and with the sensory root to the ciliary ganglion. Muller's muscle infiltration and scarring occur in thyroid disease and contribute to excessive upper eyelid retraction [126]. Surgical excision with levator aponeurosis recession is sometimes necessary for such patients [127, 128].

Lower Eyelid Retractors

The retractors of the lower eyelid are less developed than the corresponding structures of the upper lid. Vertical excursion of the lower eyelid is linked to downgaze. Not surprisingly, the retractors for this action are palpebral extensions from the inferior rectus (see Fig. 1.51). This muscle sends off a peripheral capsulopalpebral head that splits to encompass the inferior oblique muscle [129]. The inferior portion is a thin fibrous layer, whereas the layer coursing over the inferior oblique is thicker and contains smooth muscle cells. These layers fuse again anterior to the inferior oblique muscle to form Lockwood's suspensory ligament. Jones noted that the suspensory ligament maintains the globe position in the orbit even if all bone inferior to its attachments at the medial and lateral orbital walls is removed. This support is not always dependable, however, as evidenced by the occasional development of hypoglobus in patients undergoing decompression of the orbital floor.

Anterior to Lockwood's ligament, the capsulopalpebral head has three insertions. The innermost is Tenon's fascia. The central main mass, a continuation of the inferior tarsal muscle, inserts on the inferior tarsal border. The inferior tarsal muscle is analogous to the Muller's muscle of the upper eyelid. The external head of the capsulopalpebral muscle fuses with the orbital septum 5 mm inferior to the tarsus before extending to the tarsus and sending fibers to the orbicularis and the skin. This capsulopalpebral muscle is the lower eyelid analog of the levator muscle. The physiology of the lower eyelid retractors has been investigated with high-resolution magnetic resonance imaging [130].

The conjunctiva of the inferior fornix anchors in the cleft between Tenon's fascia and the inferior tarsal muscle, the latter structure becoming mostly fibrous as the tarsus is approached. The inferior tether of the tarsus consists of the orbital septum and the capsulopalpebral heads.

Tarsal Plates

The tarsal plates are formed of dense fibrous tissue and provide structural integrity to the eyelids. The tarsal plates extend to the eyelid margins. The antimarginal edges curve in a convex direction away from the lid margins (Fig. 1.52). A tarsal height of about 10 mm is measured centrally in the upper eyelid. The height of the lower tarsus ranges from 3.2 to 5.0 mm, with an average vertical height of 3.7 mm [131]. Disparity between the upper and lower tarsal dimensions directly reflects the contribution of the respective eyelids in covering the globe. Medially and laterally, the tarsal plates taper to a height of approximately 2 mm before becoming the canthal ligaments. Pretarsal orbicularis muscle is densely adherent to the entire anterior surface of the inferior tarsal plate. An identical situation in the upper eyelid is prevented by the intervening levator aponeurosis insertion, except along the margin. Posteriorly, the tarsal plates are lined by a tightly adherent conjunctiva that continues on the eyelid margin to the gray line or mucocutaneous junction. Together, the tarsus and the palpebral conjunctiva may be considered as the posterior lamella of the eyelid.

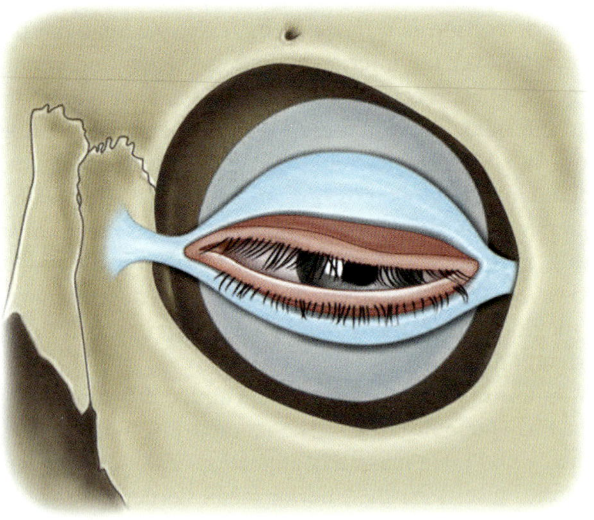

Fig. 1.52 Skeletonized tarsal plates with eyelid margins left intact. Disparity between upper and lower tarsal dimensions directly reflects contribution of their respective eyelids in covering globe anteriorly

In youth, the tarsal plates and canthal ligaments hold the eyelids firmly against the eye. With aging, the ligaments and the tarsus itself may stretch, allowing the eyelids to be distracted mechanically from the globe 6 mm or more [132]. Habitual rubbing of the eyelid likewise can cause stretching. The tarsal plates are particularly lax in patients with floppy eyelid syndrome [133]. Recent work has demonstrated a marked decrease in elastin but normal distribution of types I and III collagen in the tarsal plates of patients with floppy eyelid syndrome [134].

Meibomian Glands

Each tarsus contains many branched acinal glands with long central ducts extending nearly the vertical height of the plate. These meibomian glands (about 25 in the upper tarsus and 20 in the lower) are sebaceous, secreting the oil component of the tear film. The ducts are lined by keratinized epithelium, abnormalities of which may lead to various types of gland dysfunction states [135]. The meibomian gland orifices are located on the posterior lid margin between the mucocutaneous junction and the gray line.

Following chronic inflammation, the meibomian gland orifices may develop abnormal distichiasis hair follicles [136]. In congenital distichiasis, the abnormal cilia emerge from the meibomian orifices. This is not surprising because the glands represent primitive sebaceous vestiges of a secondary row of eyelashes that has disappeared in humans [3]. In the very young eyelid or one covering a microphthalmic globe, the meibomian gland orifices are seen very closely spaced, suggesting horizontal lengthening, perhaps by stretching, of the intervening tarsus with growth. The glands also increase in diameter and length with tarsal growth. Obstruction of the meibomian orifices may result in lipogranulomatous inflammation and chalazion.

Conjunctiva

The conjunctiva covers the tarsal plates at the posterior eyelid margins and over their posterior surfaces. In the upper eyelid, the palpebral portion of the conjunctiva continues to the superior fornix applied to the smooth superior tarsal muscle of Muller. Immediately above the tarsus, the conjunctiva and superior tarsal muscle are tightly adherent, but separation is easier more superiorly. In the lower eyelid, the conjunctiva can be elevated from the lower eyelid retractors without difficulty. The superior reflection of the conjunctiva is about 13 mm from the open eyelid margin and 20–25 mm with the eye closed [3]. Assuming the tarsal component of the palpebral conjunctiva remains constant at 10 mm, a difference of 10 mm of superior palpebral conjunctival length exists between closed and open eyelid positions, affording a large magnitude of play between the upper eyelid and the globe.

The suspensory ligament of the superior fornix consists of smooth muscle and fibrous tissue arising from the conjoined fascia of the levator and superior rectus muscles to provide elevation of the fornix in upgaze. Surgical disruption of this suspensory ligament may result in postoperative conjunctival prolapse. The inferior fornix reflection remains 8–10 mm from the lower eyelid margin because the lower eyelid does not significantly elevate with closure. The inferior suspensory ligament arises from fascia extending from Lockwood's ligament.

Bulbar conjunctiva reflected on the globe is loosely adherent to the underlying Tenon's fascia until the corneal limbus is approached, where the layers are tightly bound to the episclera. The conjunctiva consists of a nonkeratinized stratified epithelium with goblet cells overlying a loose layer of connective tissue, the lamina propria. The glands of the conjunctiva are described in the section on lacrimal secretors.

Eyelid Comparison

Comparison of the eyelids reveals many similarities, but the differences are instructive. The upper eyelid is vertically mobile with a well-developed levator muscle and aponeurosis. Vertical mobility of the lower eyelid is more limited with less-developed retractors inserting into a thicker eyelid. Congenital or acquired disinsertion of the levator aponeurosis results in ptosis of the upper eyelid. Disinsertion of the lower eyelid retractors results in instability of the lower eyelid tarsus and may result in congenital or acquired entropion [137, 138]. Because the levator aponeurosis extends to insert on the anterior inferior aspect of the upper tarsus, the superior orbital septum fails to reach the superior tarsal border, but instead, terminates on the aponeurosis. The degree of tarsal development roughly approximates the surface area of the globe, which must be anteriorly covered. The upper tarsus meibomian glands and cilia are correspondingly greater in size and number.

Eyelid Vessels

The eyelids receive arterial blood from both the external and internal carotid systems. The major contributions from the external carotid include the facial artery, the superficial temporal artery, and the infraorbital artery. The facial artery arises from the external carotid below the angle of the jaw and crosses the mandible anterior to the masseter muscle, coursing diagonally to the nasolabial fold (Fig. 1.53). Here, it travels beneath the levators of the lip, becoming more superficial to lie between the levator labii superioris and levator alae nasi muscles. It becomes the angular artery at the medial canthus, lying superficially beneath the orbicularis muscle 6–8 mm medial to the canthus and 5 mm anterior to the lacrimal sac. External dacryocystorhinostomy incisions should be positioned to avoid damage to and resultant hemorrhage from the angular artery.

At the medial canthus, the angular artery anastomoses with branches of the dorsal nasal and infraorbital arteries. The angular artery perforates the orbital septum above the medial canthal ligament to anastomose with branches of the ophthalmic artery.

The external carotid artery continues superiorly to give rise to the internal maxillary and superficial temporal arteries (Fig. 1.54). The internal maxillary artery supplies deep structures of the face. This artery and its branches are described in the section on the orbit.

The superficial temporal artery is also a terminal branch of the external carotid originating 1 cm anterior to the external auditory canal approximately 6.5 mm posterior to the lateral orbital rim [139]. After a preauricular course, it lies superficial to the temporalis muscle, separated from the skin by a varying amount of subcutaneous tissue. In patients suspected of having temporal arteritis, this vessel is easily biopsied. Three named branches serve the eyelids: the frontal, the zygomaticofacial, and the transverse facial arteries.

Other arterial supply to the eyelids is derived from the internal carotid system. The cutaneous terminations of the ophthalmic artery include the lacrimal, frontal, supraorbital, supratrochlear, and nasal arteries (Fig. 1.53).

Several deep anastomoses between the lacrimal and nasal arteries traverse the upper eyelid as the marginal and peripheral tarsal arcades. Usually, the medial vessels arise from the terminal nasal branch of the ophthalmic artery before it passes through the orbital septum, yet they originate external to the septum in the specimen shown in Fig. 1.55.

The marginal arcade lies on the anterior tarsal surface 2–4 mm superior to the eyelid margin. Tucker and Lindberg

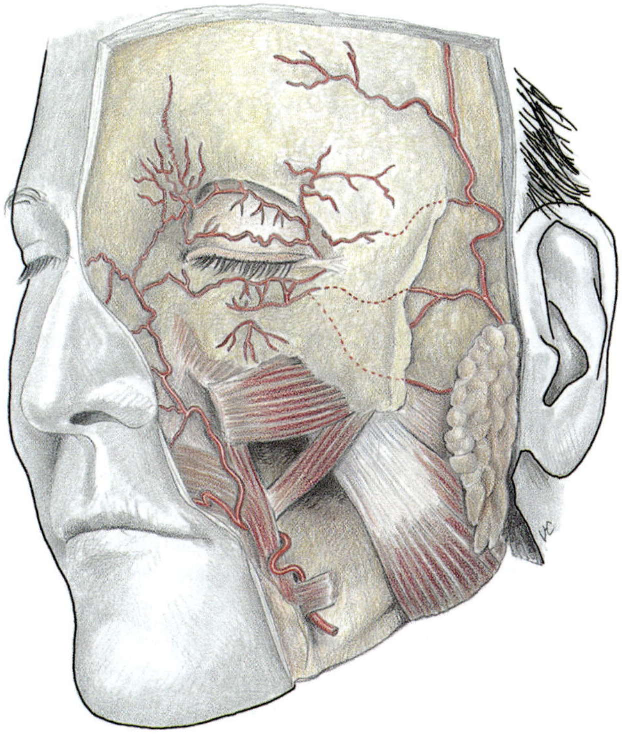

Fig. 1.53 Superficial arteries of ocular region

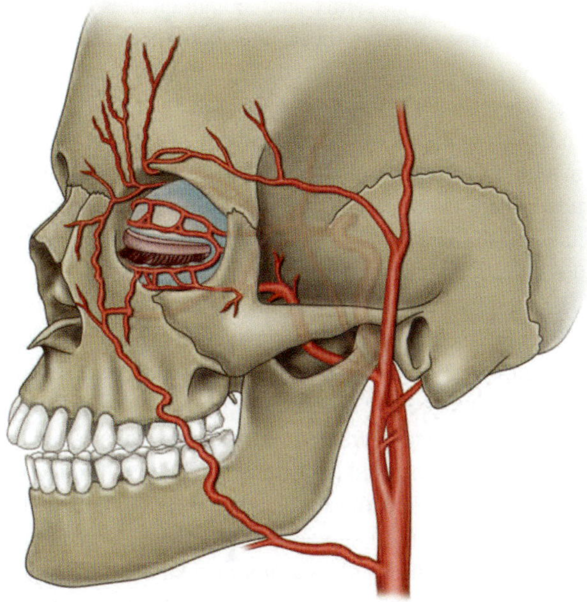

Fig. 1.54 Deep facial arteries. Note external and internal carotid contributions to orbital blood supply

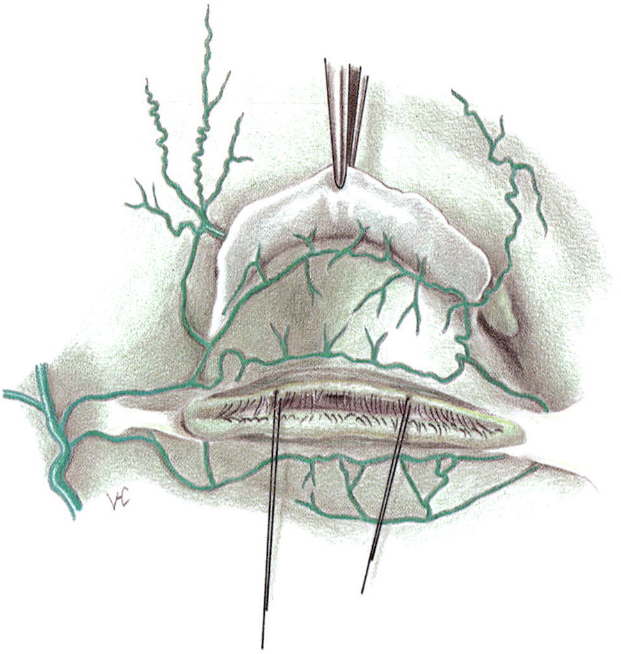

Fig. 1.55 Tarsal arterial arcades. Terminal branches of ophthalmic artery medially communicate with lacrimal artery laterally. Marginal artery is larger than peripheral artery and is located 2–3 mm from tarsal margin. Peripheral arcade in the upper eyelid is found between Muller's muscle and levator aponeurosis

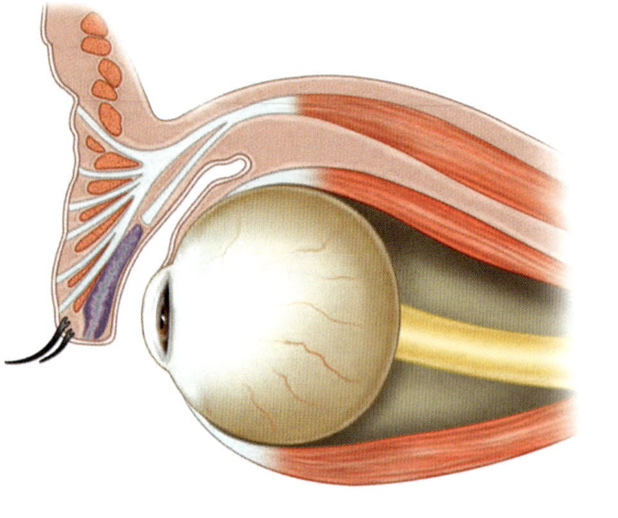

Fig. 1.56 Schematic drawing showing communication between palpebral arterial arcades and anterior ciliary arteries near corneoscleral limbus

[140] reported mean distances of 4.1, 2.2, and 1.8 mm from the eyelid margin at the medial canthus, midlid, and lateral canthus, respectively. This arcade should be respected during reconstructive tarsal-sharing techniques. The peripheral arcade lies superiorly at the tarsal border on the surface of Muller's muscle. This deeper peripheral system supplies the superior conjunctival fornix and communicates with the anterior ciliary arteries near the corneoscleral limbus (Fig. 1.56). Brisk arterial bleeding from this source often occurs when the levator horns are incised.

In the lower eyelid, a marginal arcade is also seen arising from a branch of the nasal artery. A lesser-developed double-arcade system is sometimes present. Laterally, anastomoses occur with the lacrimal artery and zygomaticofacial branch of the superficial temporal artery.

The facial vein is the main superficial venous structure, arising at the medial eyebrow as the confluence of the frontal and supraorbital veins (Fig. 1.57). The facial vein follows roughly the same course as the artery bearing the same name but is superficial and lateral to it. The facial vein is called the angular vein near the medial canthus. Often seen through the thin skin of this region, the angular vein is 6–8 mm medial to the inner canthus. The supraorbital vein runs horizontally beneath the orbicularis and does not medially surface to join the frontal vein until it communicates with the superior ophthalmic vein of the orbit. The supraorbital vein forms a deep preauricular plexus lateral to the lateral canthus underneath the orbicularis and passes posteriorly to the ear via the superficial temporal vein.

A second superficial to deep communication occurs between the facial vein and the pterygoid plexus via the deep facial vein. The pterygoid plexus communicates with the cavernous sinus directly and by sending branches through the inferior orbital fissure to the inferior ophthalmic vein.

The veins of the face do not have valves. This lack of valves and the anastomoses between the superficial and deep veins makes superficial infection in the facial region a potentially dangerous problem. A superficial facial infection may spread to the cavernous sinus via communication of the angular, supraorbital, and superior ophthalmic veins.

The lymphatic drainage of the eyelids occurs via a medial and a larger lateral system passing to the submandibular and preauricular lymph chains, respectively (Fig. 1.58). The lateral two-thirds of the upper eyelid and the lateral third of the lower eyelid drain to the preauricular nodes. Conversely, the medial third of the upper eyelid and the medial two-thirds of the lower eyelid drain to the submandibular chains.

Eyelid Nerves

The nerves serving the eyelids are the facial (motor), the oculomotor (motor), the ophthalmic and maxillary divisions of the trigeminal nerve (sensory), and the sympathetics from the superior cervical ganglion.

The facial nerve (VII) leaves the pons to enter the temporal bone at the internal acoustic meatus along with the sensory intermediate nerve and the acoustic nerve. It exits the facial canal behind the styloid process at the stylomastoid

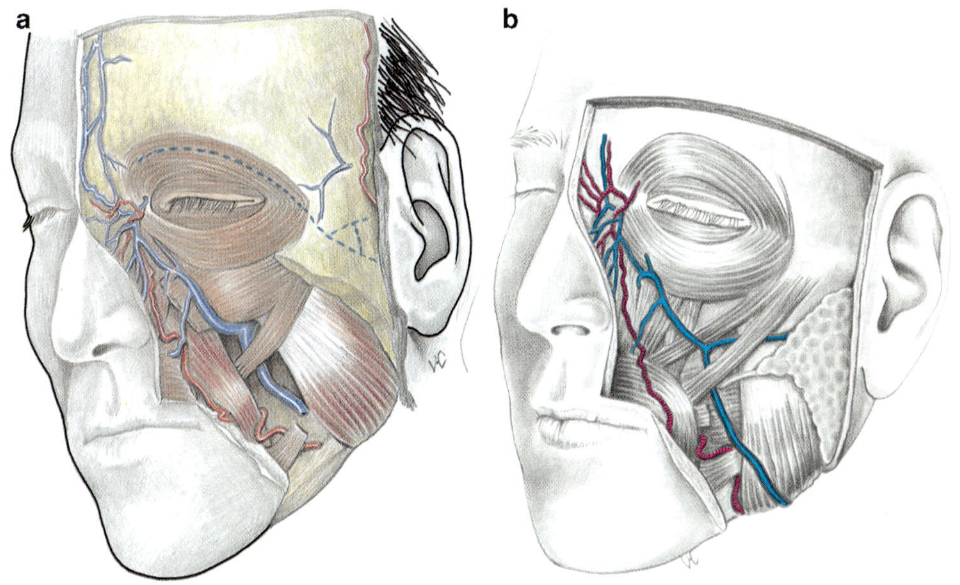

Fig. 1.57 (**a**, **b**) Superficial veins of ocular region. Angular vein lies 6–8 mm medial to inner commissure; it communicates superficially with frontal and facial veins, joins horizontal supraorbital vein beneath orbicularis, and becomes superior ophthalmic vein after piercing orbital septum

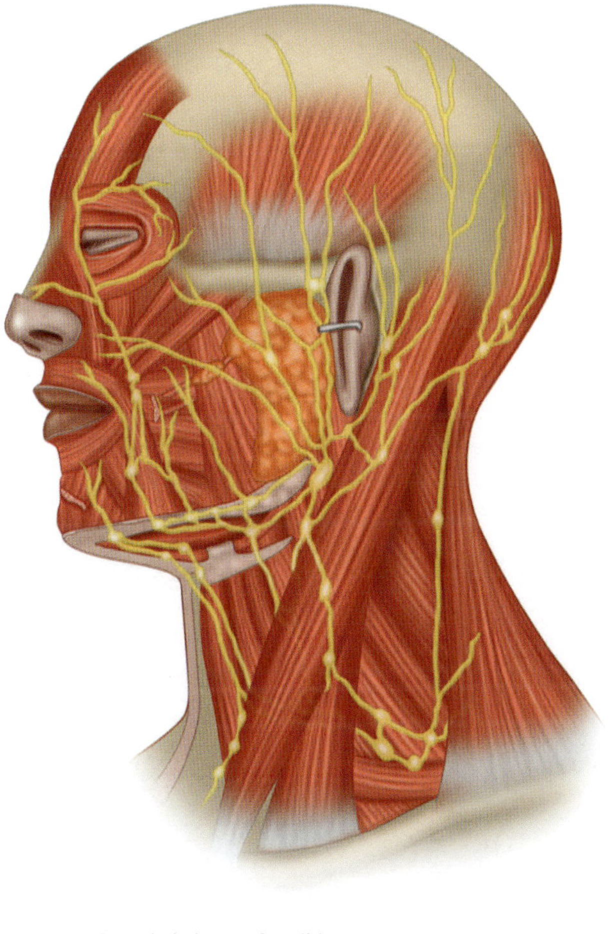

Fig. 1.58 Lymph drainage of eyelids

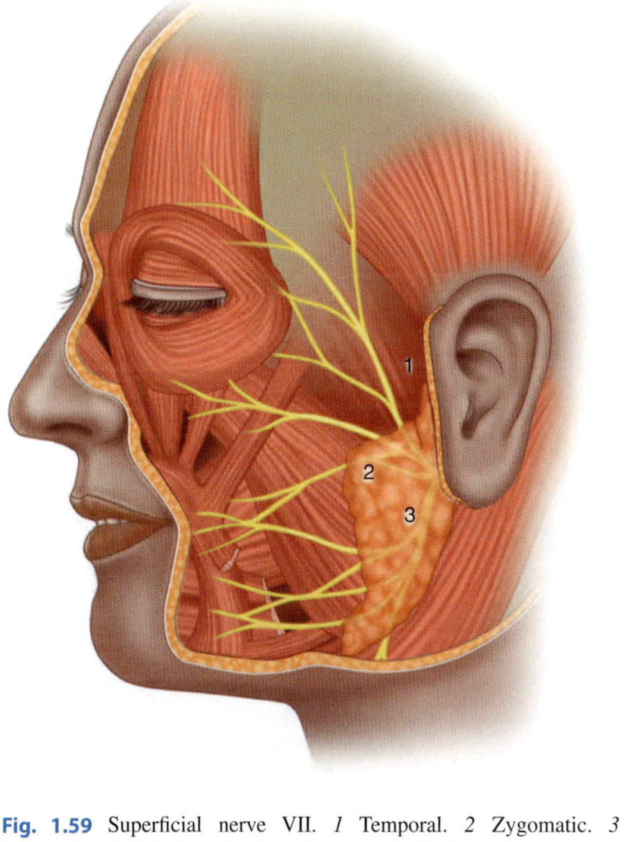

Fig. 1.59 Superficial nerve VII. *1* Temporal. *2* Zygomatic. *3* Cervicofacial with three divisions: buccal, mandibular, and cervical

foramen and passes anteriorly to the parotid gland. Within the gland, the nerve divides as shown in Fig. 1.59. The nerve lies beneath the orbicularis and the other muscles of the superficial plane that it serves. The orbicularis is served by the temporal and the zygomatic branches, and sometimes by the buccal division. Extensive interdigitation is often present between these branches. The procerus innervation passes inferior to the eye, whereas the corrugator nerve may be inferior or superior [141].

The frontal branch of the facial nerve arises from the temporal division. This branch innervates the frontalis muscle and travels within the temporoparietal (superficial temporalis) fascia [142]. Damage to this branch results in unilateral forehead paralysis. Detailed knowledge of the course of this branch of the facial nerve is essential for the surgeon performing coronal or endoscopic brow lifts. Such dissection should be performed directly on the deep temporalis fascia to avoid damage to the more superficial frontal nerve.

The superior division of the oculomotor nerve supplies the levator muscle to retract the upper eyelid. The capsulopalpebral muscle, the main retractor of the lower eyelid, is innervated by the inferior division of the oculomotor nerve.

Two sensory branches of the trigeminal nerve, the ophthalmic and the maxillary, pass through the orbit to reach the face. The cutaneous distributions of the trigeminal nerve are pictured in Fig. 1.60. Sensory input from the upper eyelid travels via the supraorbital, supratrochlear, and lacrimal nerves.

A detailed description of the surgically important supraorbital nerve has been provided by Knize [143]. At the superior orbital rim, the nerve divides into a superficial branch medially and a deep branch laterally. Branches of the superficial division penetrate the frontalis at various points from the orbital rim to the midforehead, providing sensation to the forehead skin up to the anterior margin of the scalp. The deeper lateral division travels between the periosteum and the galea aponeurotica superotemporally, coursing 0.5–1.5 cm medial to the temporal fusion line. The branches of the deep division penetrate the galea just anterior to the coronal suture to enter the frontoparietal scalp.

The lower eyelid is served centrally by the infraorbital nerve, temporally by the zygomaticofacial branch of the maxillary nerve, and medially by part of the infratrochlear branch of the ophthalmic division [89]. Note the overlap between the areas in the naso-orbital valley and at the outer canthus. The intraorbital division of these nerves is discussed more fully in the section on the orbit.

The sympathetic nerves supply the superior and inferior smooth tarsal muscles. Disruption of the superior cervical sympathetic chain results in Horner's syndrome, the eyelid

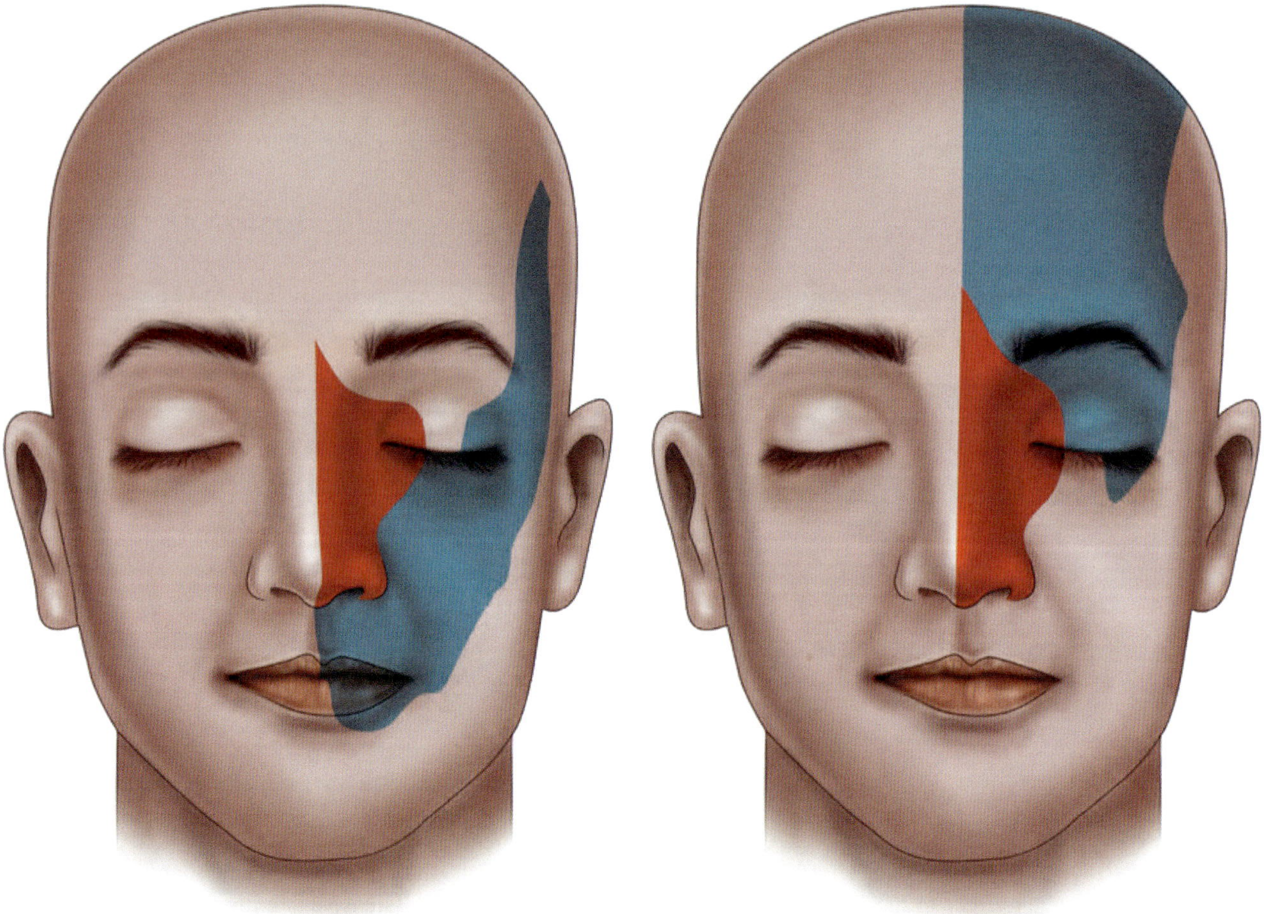

Fig. 1.60 Cutaneous distribution of nerve V

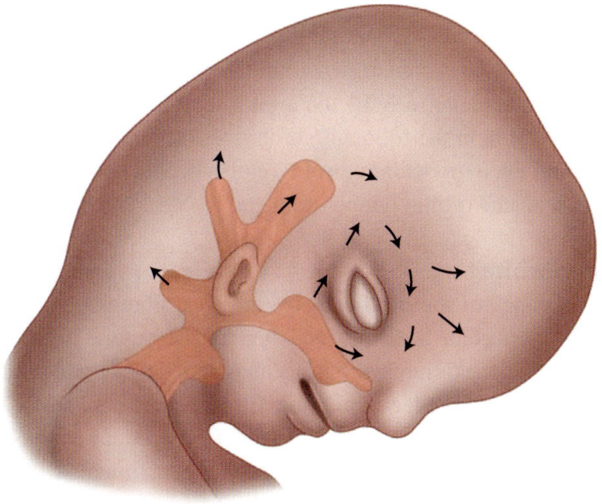

Fig. 1.61 Developing superficial muscle plane of head. Frontalis muscle arises from temporal lamina, whereas orbicularis oculi, corrugator superciliaris, and procerus muscles arise from infraorbital lamina

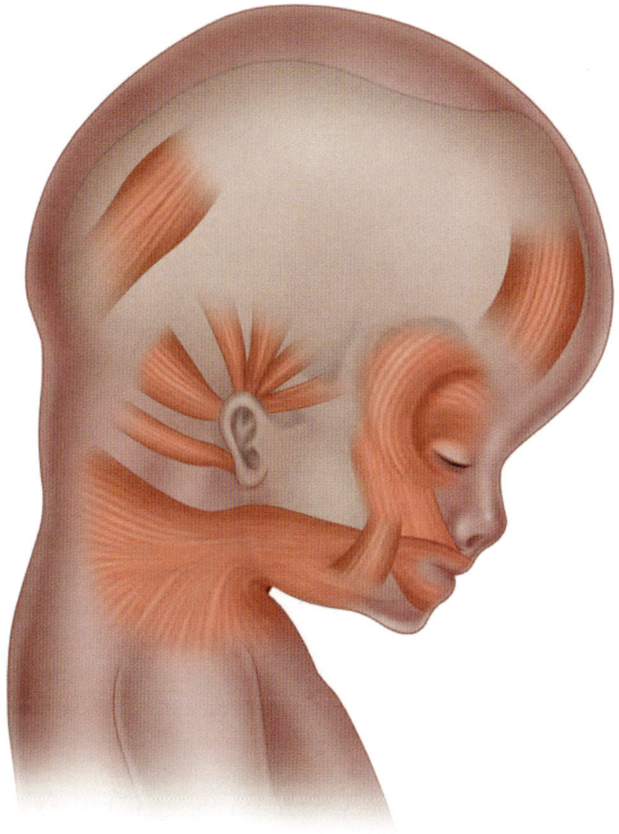

Fig. 1.62 Further stage in superficial muscle plane development

effects of which are 2 mm of upper blepharoptosis and slight elevation of the lower eyelid. The exact path of the sympathetics in the orbit remains controversial. Most investigators believe the plexus runs with cranial nerve VI in the cavernous sinus before joining the ophthalmic division of the trigeminal nerve. The cavernous sinus and orbital sympathetic nerve anatomy has been carefully studied in the cynomolgus monkey [125].

Eyelid Development

The mesenchymal structures of the head develop from the neural crest and mesodermal origin. In the embryo, a sheet of immature mesoderm immediately beneath the skin originates from the second branchial arch and spreads to cover the entire head and neck [144]. This development may actually represent successive myoblast induction rather than actual migration (Figs. 1.61 and 1.62). The frontalis muscle arises from the temporal lamina, whereas the orbicularis oculi, corrugator supercilii, and procerus muscles arise from the infraorbital lamina. The developing attendant facial nerve is seen trailing the enlarging myoblast laminae. The developed superficial muscles are continuous with intervening fibrous sheets and together form the superficial muscle plane of the head (see SMAS earlier). The nuchal ridges and the supraorbital ridges are areas of deep superficial muscle plane attachment where secondary bony hypertrophy has occurred from chronic stress.

The upper and lower eyelids develop from mesenchymal folds above (frontonasal) and below (maxillary) the optic cup during the 8- to 12-mm embryonic stage [145]. The upper eyelid is formed by medial and lateral extensions of the nasofrontal process, whereas the lower eyelid is formed from the maxillary process. By about the stage of 10 weeks, the eyelids have fused [146], with increased lengthening of the lower canaliculus relative to the upper canaliculus (Figs. 1.63 and 1.64).

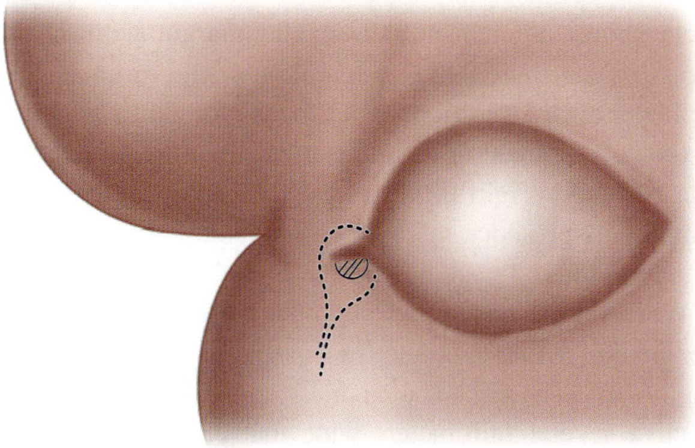

Fig. 1.63 Developing eyelids before fusion

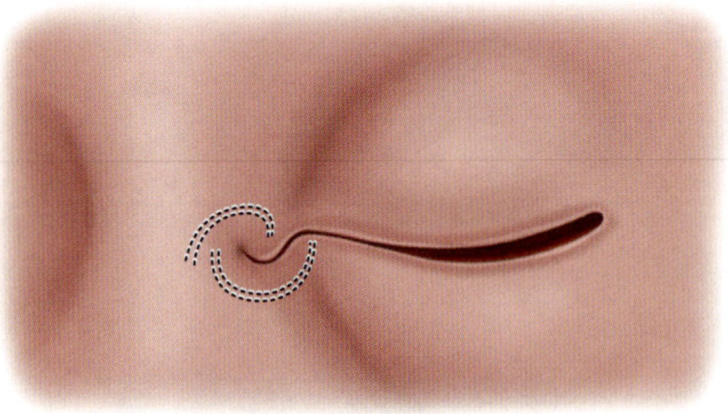

Fig. 1.64 Developing eyelids at fusion

After the eyelids fuse to cover the eye, the tissues juxtaposed to the globe are modified to become conjunctiva. The conjunctival mucous membrane is formed by a surface epithelium resting on a mesodermal substantia propria. Mucous glands and accessory lacrimal glands develop as shown in Fig. 1.27. The lacrimal gland also develops from the surface epithelium and is discussed under lacrimal secretors. Interestingly, in cases of eyelid coloboma in which surfaces of the eye are not embryologically covered by fused eyelid, dermoid growths sometimes develop.

During the period of eyelid fusion, the eyelashes and the meibomian, Zeis, and Moll glands develop. The separation of the eyelids at the end of the fifth month is thought to be effected by gland secretion breaking down the epithelial adhesion [1]. Abnormal separation results in ankyloblepharon.

The caruncle separates from the most medial segment of the lower eyelid between the medial commissure and the lacrimal papillary prominence. Histologic study of the caruncle shows elements of the eyelid margin with several accessory lacrimal glands. Separation of the caruncle from the lower eyelid traditionally has been thought to be caused by the development of the inferior canaliculus. An independent caruncle origin theory has since been postulated that explains its presence in cases of congenital absence of the canaliculi [85].

While the caruncle is developing, a neighboring fold from the medial bulbar conjunctiva enlarges to form the plica semilunaris. The plica is a medially convex crescent of conjunctiva several millimeters wide that extends toward the conjunctival fornices. It contains fat and is anchored to fibers of the medial rectus check ligament and the caruncle. The thickening of the conjunctival space caused by the plica slightly separates the medial eyelid from the globe, allowing pooling of the tears in a lacrimal lake.

Orbit

The soft tissues contained within the bony walls of the orbit and limited anteriorly by the orbital septum are discussed in this section in the following order: periorbita, orbital fascia, orbital fat, extraocular muscles, globe, orbital nerves, orbital vessels, and orbital lymph drainage.

Periorbita

The bones of the orbit are covered by a fibrous periorbita. This periorbita is firmly attached at the suture lines, the foramina, the fissures, the arcus marginalis, the lateral orbital tubercle, and the lacrimal crest. Elsewhere, it may easily be lifted from the bone by the surgeon or by accumulations of blood or pus. Anteriorly, the periorbita is continuous with the frontal, zygomatic, malar, and nasal periosteum. The periorbita is thickened along the orbital rim at the arcus marginalis where the orbital septum originates. The periorbita lines the lacrimal sac fossa, and an extension, the lacrimal fascia, covers the lacrimal sac between the anterior and posterior lacrimal crests.

Except where it is pierced by the nerves and vessels, the superior orbital fissure is bound by thickened periorbita, which is continuous with the dura mater. The optic foramen periorbita is likewise continuous with the dura mater surrounding the optic nerve. The periosteum is also continuous with the bones of the sphenopalatine and temporal fossae through the inferior orbital fissure. The inferior orbital fissure structure is covered in life by the smooth orbital muscle of Muller.

The periorbita is extensively vascularized on both its bone and soft tissue sides. These vessels are interconnected so the periorbita does not serve as a vascular border area. It is supplied by twigs from regional branches of the intraorbital trigeminal nerve.

Orbital Fascia

The orbital contents are supported by a highly developed connective tissue system. Extensive work by Koornneef has shown a highly organized complexity of the orbital fascia and muscle by means of a thick serial section technique [147, 148]. The fascia may be divided for discussion purposes into three parts: the fascia covering the globe (Tenon's fascia), the coverings of the extraocular muscles, and the check ligament extensions of the extraocular muscle fascia that reach to the surrounding bone and eyelids. Jones presented an interesting concept unifying all the fascial layers as extensions or heads of the extraocular muscle fascia [56].

Tenon's capsule, or fascia bulbi, is a fibroelastic membrane that extends anteriorly from the dural sheath of the optic nerve, where it is thinnest, to fuse with the conjunctiva immediately posterior to the corneoscleral limbus. It is loosely applied to the episclera posteriorly but adherent anterior to the rectus muscle insertions. Tenon's capsule separates the globe from the intraconal orbital fat. The rectus muscles penetrate Tenon's capsule posterior to the equator of the globe. The nerves and vessels en route to the globe (Fig. 1.65) also penetrate Tenon's capsule. The potential space between the globe and Tenon's membrane is termed Tenon's space.

Externally, Tenon's membrane is joined to the network of fibrous septa dividing the lobules of orbital fat. The globe is thus loosely related to the surrounding orbital fat, and freedom of movement is afforded by the distensibility of the elastic fibers of the surrounding fascia. Orbital implants used after enucleation are placed either within this fibrous space or posterior to it within the muscle cone. Careful closure of Tenon's layer is important to prevent extrusion of enucleation implants.

The muscular fascia ensheaths the extraocular muscles and stretches between the muscles as the intermuscular septum (Fig. 1.66). The extraocular muscle fascial coverings are thin posteriorly but become much denser anteriorly [82]. The muscular membranes are seen to connect externally to the orbital walls and internally to the fibrous septa dividing the intraconal fat lobules [149]. An extensive system of fascial septa radiates from the muscle sheaths to the posterior part of Tenon's capsule [89]. The bulbar side of the muscular sheath is thinner than the external aspect that forms the check ligaments yet is thicker than the posterior portion of Tenon's capsule [150]. Smooth muscle fibers are scattered throughout the membrane and are innervated by the sympathetic nervous system [3]. Enlargement of the tensor intermuscularis muscle (sparse circumferential striated muscle within the superolateral intermuscular septum) has been demonstrated in Graves' orbitopathy [151].

The muscles are connected to the surrounding fascia throughout the anterior one-third of their lengths, especially so where they insert onto the globe. This prevents their retraction far posteriorly in the orbit if they are lost during strabismus surgery (unless the muscle has been dissected free). These connections also explain the persistent movement of the eye socket after enucleation when the muscles have not been specially sewn to the implant.

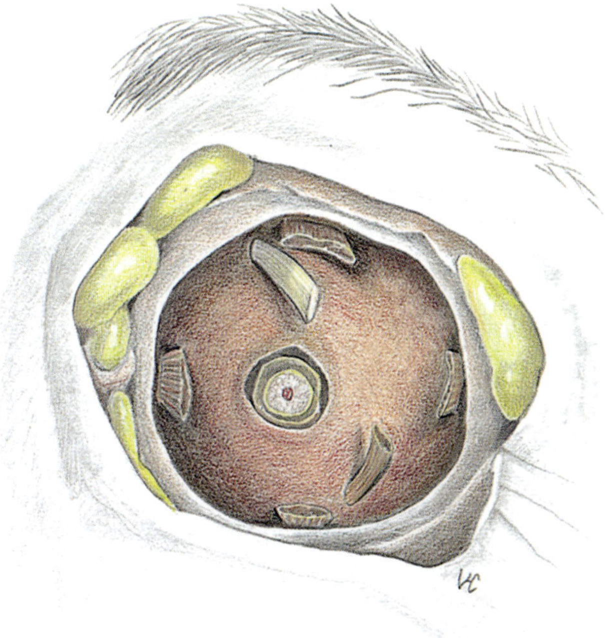

Fig. 1.65 Enucleated left socket to show internal aspect of Tenon's capsule. It is continuous with sheaths of muscles piercing it

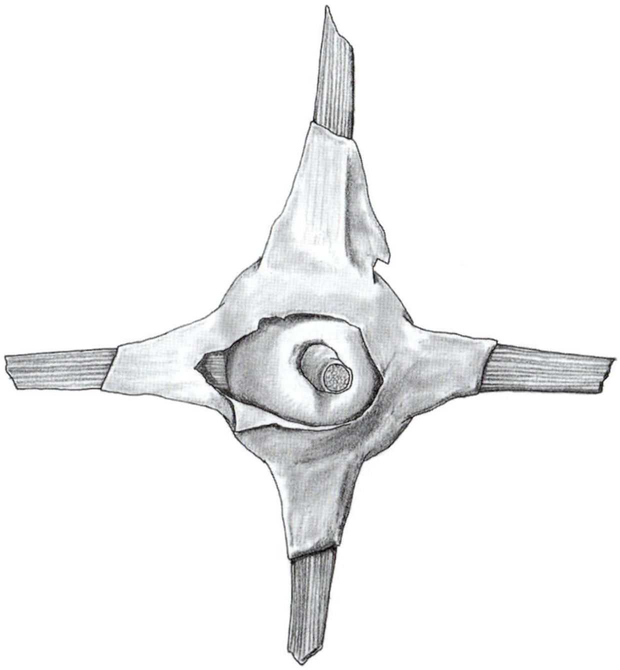

Fig. 1.66 Muscular fascia

As noted earlier, each of the extraocular muscle sheaths sends extensions to the orbital walls. Anteriorly, they become especially prominent, sufficient to deserve designation as check ligaments. The best developed check ligaments are those of the medial and lateral rectus muscles. The lateral check ligament is the strongest and inserts primarily on the posterior aspect of Whitnall's lateral orbital tubercle with lesser extensions to the lateral conjunctival fornix and to the lateral orbital septum. The medial check ligament inserts to the bone behind the posterior lacrimal crest and to the medial orbital septum, caruncle, and plica semilunaris. The superior rectus muscle sheath is joined by an intermuscular fascia anteriorly to that of the levator palpebral superioris muscle [152]. The fused inferior rectus and inferior oblique muscle sheaths send fascial connections to the inferior periorbita, which might have some checking function.

The superior transverse ligament [111] arises from the fascia of the levator in the region of its transition from muscle to aponeurosis. Whitnall's ligament is attached medially to the periorbita near the trochlea. Laterally, it travels between the lobes of the lacrimal gland to insert at the lateral orbital tubercle. An extension of Whitnall's ligament joins the medial head of Lockwood's ligament [89]. Whitnall's ligament appears to limit the posterior movement of the levator muscle [107] and may be important in achieving a vertical vector of force from the levator's mainly anteroposterior direction [112, 113]. Fine fibers from Whitnall's ligament contribute to the suspensory ligament of the superior fornix.

Lockwood described a hammock-like structure extending to the medial and lateral orbital walls from the fused fascia of the inferior rectus and inferior oblique muscles [153]. It is strongest immediately anterior to the inferior oblique muscle [129]. This suspensory ligament of the eye usually supports the globe following maxillectomy with the removal of the orbital floor as long as its attachments in the medial and lateral retinacula are not disturbed (Fig. 1.67). Globe ptosis, however, does sometimes occur following surgical removal of the orbital floor [154]. Additionally, Manson and colleagues [155] demonstrated substantial hypoglobus in autopsy specimens by removing the intraconal fat. They concluded that Lockwood's ligament alone was insufficient to maintain the position of the globe. Preservation of the maxilloethmoid strut may be helpful in preventing globe ptosis following orbital decompression [156].

Jones studied the comparative anatomy of the orbit and related human fascia and rectus anatomy to different forms [106]. He noted that all the structures in the orbit are embedded in a fatty retinaculum divided into lobes by the rectus muscles. The primitive rectus muscle has a smaller ocular head and a larger capsulopalpebral head. The capsulopalpebral head is best developed in the superior rectus complex with the formation of a distinct levator muscle. The outermost aponeurotic heads are horizontally represented as medial and lateral check ligaments. Smooth muscle fibers are found in the fascia of all the muscles, although they are best developed superiorly and inferiorly. Jones regarded the innermost capsular heads as forming the anterior Tenon's fascia.

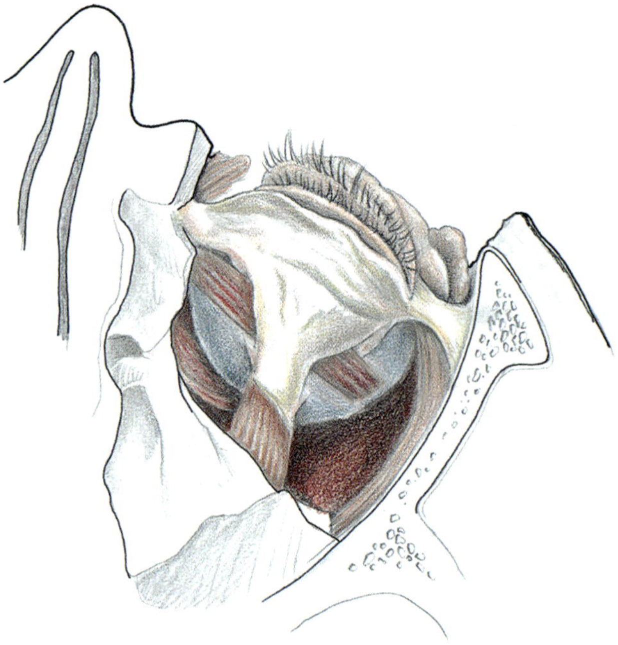

Fig. 1.67 Left orbit viewed from below to show Lockwood's ligament

Koornneef significantly improved understanding of the orbital fascia [147, 157]. He documented a consistent interrelation of all the fibrous structures within the orbit (Figs. 1.68, 1.69, and 1.70). The fascia and blood vessels are the first mesenchymal structures to differentiate in the embryo, with the adult configuration reached by the 125 mm stage. Each muscle has a fascial complex that can vary between individuals, yet it is fairly constant between the two orbits of the individual. No common muscle sheath was found in his serial section technique. A supportive hammock for the superior ophthalmic vein is described. The orbital veins are supported by the fascia, whereas the arteries course independently through it.

The complex orbital fascial system has many clinical implications. Koornneef [158] has shown that motility restriction following orbital fracture is usually the result of entrapment of connective tissue septa rather than direct muscular incarceration. In thyroid orbitopathy, hypertrophy of the fascial septa [159] may contribute to motility dysfunction. Fibrosis of the septal tissues and venous compression have been postulated as mechanisms of congestion in Graves' orbitopathy when muscular enlargement is not prominent [160].

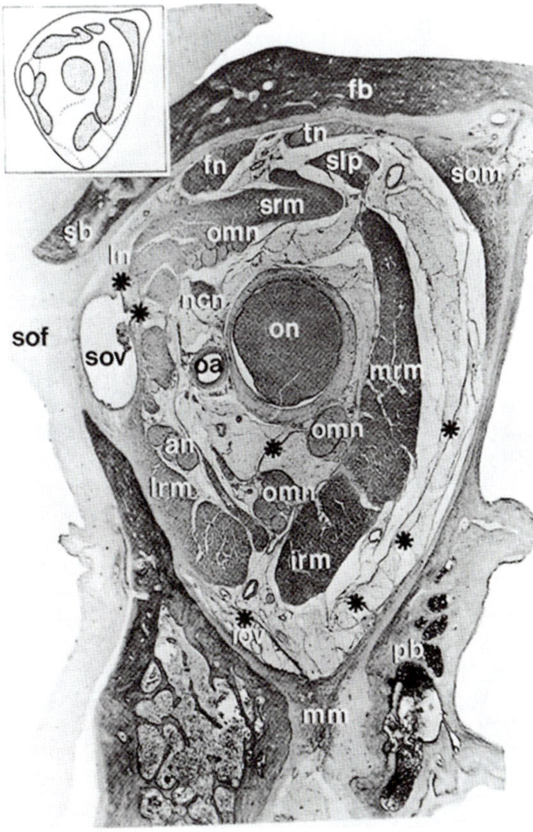

Fig. 1.68 A view 18.4 mm from back of globe. Vertical diameter 1.5 cm; transversal diameter 1.1 cm. Enlargement approximately 11 times. The following artifacts are present in this section. Inside muscle cone several holes in adipose tissue are seen. Outside the cone adipose tissue is torn off from frontal and trochlear nerves, superior levator palpebrae/superior rectus complex, medial and inferior recti muscles, and medial orbital wall; *fb* frontal bone, *sb* sphenoid bone, *sof* superior orbital fissure, *mm* Muller's muscle, *pb* palatine bone, *on* optic nerve, *fn* frontal nerve, *In* lacrimal nerve, *ncn* nasociliary nerve, *tn* trochlear nerve, *an* abducens nerve, *omn* oculomotor nerve, *oa* ophthalmic artery, *soy* superior ophthalmic vein, *My* inferior ophthalmic vein, *slp* superior levator palpebrae muscle, *srm* superior rectus muscle, *lrm* lateral rectus muscle, *irm* inferior rectus muscle, *mrm* medial rectus muscle, *som* superior oblique muscle, and *asterisks* (∗) connective tissue septa. (Reproduced from [148])

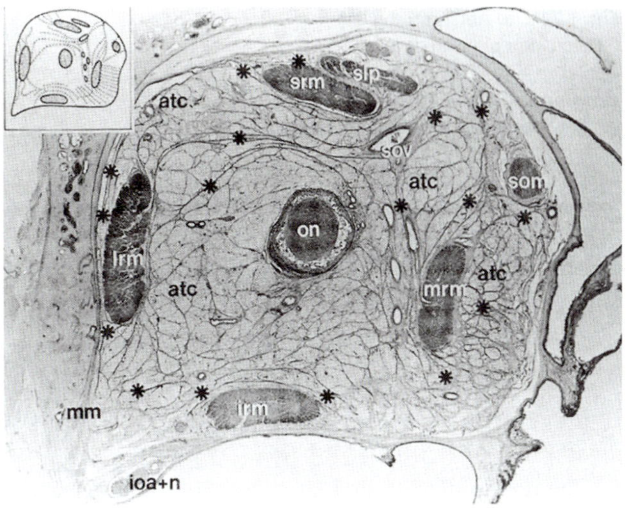

Fig. 1.69 A view 1.4 mm from hind surface of the eye. Vertical diameter, 2.4 cm; transversal diameter, 2.7 cm. Enlargement approximately 3.5 times. Note artifacts in superior, medial, and inferolateral areas; *on* optic nerve, *sov* superior ophthalmic vein, *slp* superior levator palpebrae muscle, *srm* superior rectus muscle, *lrm* lateral rectus muscle, *irm* inferior rectus muscle, *mrm* medial rectus muscle, *som* superior oblique muscle, *asterisk* (∗) connective tissue septa, *atc* adipose tissue compartment, *ioa + n* infraorbital artery and nerve, and *mm* Muller's muscle. (Reproduced from [148])

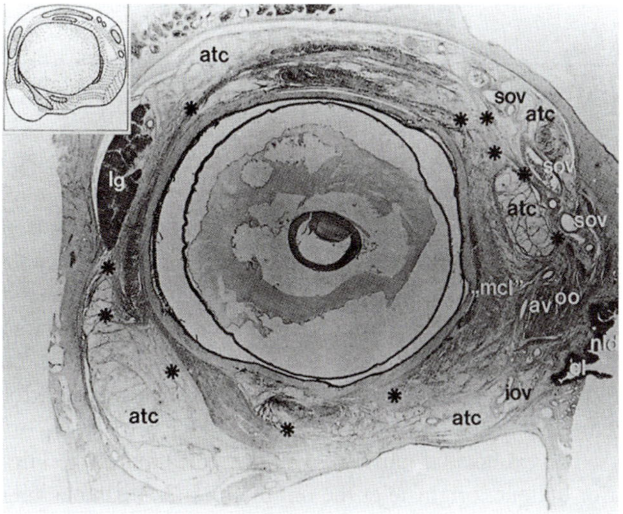

Fig. 1.70 A view 7.0 mm anteriorly to back of the eye. Vertical diameter, 3.1 cm; transversal diameter, 3.7 cm. Enlargement approximately 2.5 times. *cl* lacrimal canaliculus, *nld* nasolacrimal duct, *av* angular vein, *sov* superior ophthalmic vein, *iov* inferior ophthalmic vein, *lg* lacrimal gland, *oo* orbicularis oculi muscle, *mcl* medial check ligament, *atc* adipose tissue compartment, and *asterisk* (∗) connective tissue septa. (Reproduced from [148])

Orbital Fat

All of the orbital space not containing fascia, globe, muscle, nerves, vessels, or glandular structures is filled with fat. Anteriorly in the orbit, the fat is fibrous, whereas larger lobules are found posteriorly due to the decreased fascial structure in the posterior orbit. The fat serves as a cushion that supports and stabilizes the globe. Atrophy from aging or chronic ocular inflammation may result in enophthalmos or deepening of the superior sulcus. Acquired anophthalmia in monkeys did not result in fat atrophy [161].

Posterior to the orbital septum in the upper eyelid, a yellow preaponeurotic fat pad is seen (Fig. 1.71). This structure is a useful landmark to the ptosis surgeon. Medial and inferior to the trochlea is the medial fat pad of the upper eyelid. This fat pad is firmer, more lobulated, and lighter in color. The associated infratrochlear nerve and the medial palpebral artery explain the tendency for intraoperative pain and bleeding, respectively, in this region. Damage to the nearby trochlea or tendon of the superior oblique may result in Brown's syndrome or superior oblique palsy [162, 163].

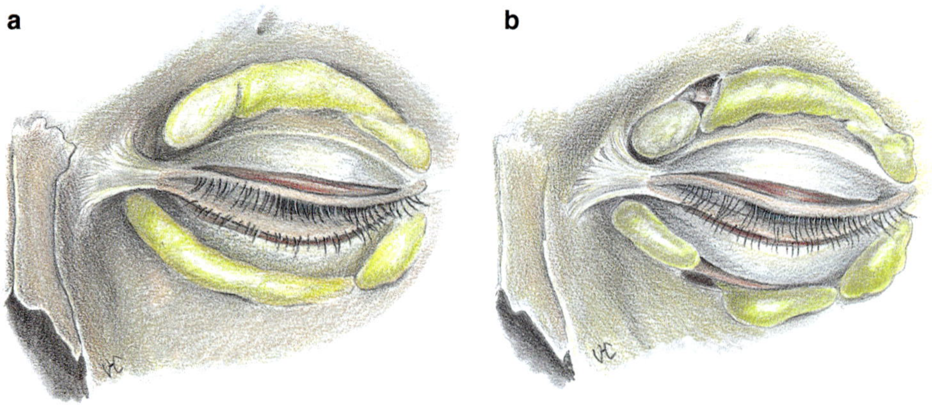

Fig. 1.71 (**a**) Anterior orbital fat seen after removal of orbital septum. (**b**) Deeper dissection of orbital fat pads to show trochlea dividing fat pads in upper eyelid. Fascial attachments from inferior oblique muscle presumably serve to divide large medial and middle fat pads in the lower eyelid

The precapsulopalpebral fat pockets of the lower eyelid are analogous to the preaponeurotic fat of the upper lid. Clinically, in the inferior anterior orbit, there are three fat pads [164]. Studies using dye in patients undergoing lower eyelid blepharoplasty have demonstrated compartmentalization [165]. The lateral fat pad is divided from the central fat by the arcuate expansion of the inferior oblique passing to the orbital floor inferotemporally. The medial fat pad is separated deeply from the central pad by the inferior oblique muscle. Dissection during lower eyelid blepharoplasty must respect the inferior oblique muscle [166].

Extraocular Muscles

The extraocular muscles are specialized striated skeletal muscles. Two fiber types have been recognized with light microscopy. Fibrillenstruktur fibers are fine, well-organized myofibrils arranged in discrete bundles. They contract briskly and are responsible for rapid saccadic and pursuit movements. Felderstruktur fibers show a more random arrangement of myofibrils [167]. These fibers contract more slowly in a graded fashion. They are probably responsible for muscle tonicity.

The extraocular muscles, with the exception of the inferior oblique, originate at the orbital apex. A tendinous ring (annulus of Zinn) spans the optic foramen and the central portion of the superior orbital fissure, where the four rectus muscles take their origin (Fig. 1.72). The levator and the superior oblique muscles arise more superiorly and medially on the lesser sphenoid wing. The annulus of Zinn is connected posteriorly to the dura and medially and laterally to the lesser and greater wings of the sphenoid, respectively. In most cases, a short spine develops at the annulus attachment on the greater wing of the sphenoid at the origin of the lateral rectus.

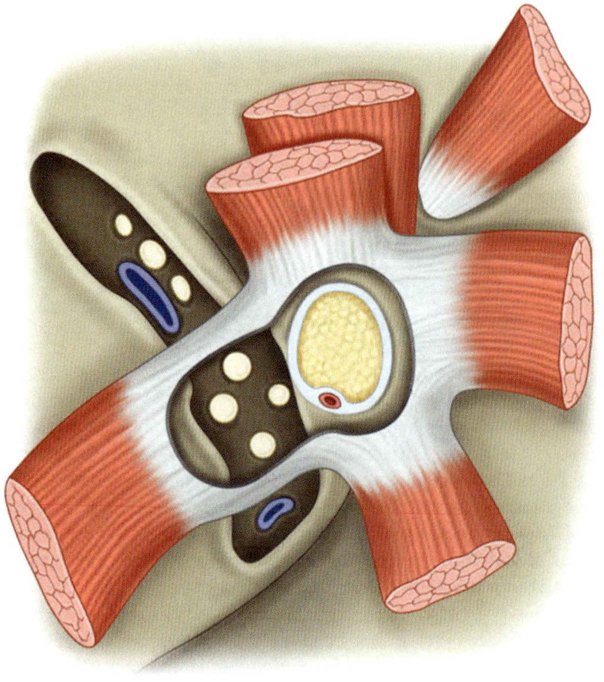

Fig. 1.72 Schematic drawing of annulus of Zinn spanning superior orbital fissure. Levator palpebrae superioris and superior oblique muscles arise from sphenoid lesser wing above and medial to anulus

The central opening of the annulus of Zinn is named the oculomotor foramen. This opening circumscribes the central portion of the superior orbital fissure and the optic foramen. Passing through the annulus are the optic nerve, the superior and inferior oculomotor nerve divisions, the nasociliary nerve, and the abducens nerves. The ophthalmic artery and sympathetic nerve fibers course through the oculomotor foramen as well.

The extraocular muscles grow in childhood as the orbit and eye enlarge yet maintain the same angular relationships

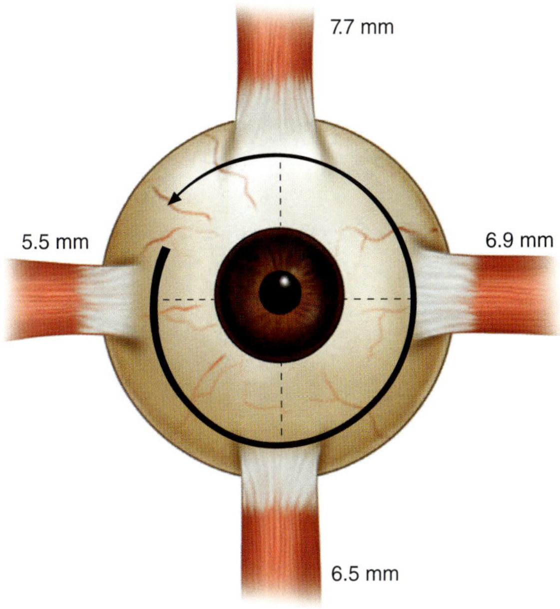

Fig. 1.73 Spiral of Tillaux O.S

to the eye [168]. The horizontal recti attain a length (excluding the tendon) of about 40.5 mm while the superior rectus is slightly longer and the inferior rectus is slightly shorter. The medial has the greatest mass of the recti and the superior the least. Insertions of the recti onto the globe are shown in Fig. 1.73. The progressively increased distance from the corneal limbus (going in a clockwise fashion on the right eye) to the medial rectus is termed the spiral of Tillaux. The location and shape of the insertions vary. In a series of eyes at autopsy measured by Apt, the distance from the corneoscleral limbus of the insertions was found to vary by over 3 mm for each rectus muscle [169].

The medial and inferior rectus muscles and the inferior oblique are supplied by the inferior division of the oculomotor nerve, the superior rectus by the superior oculomotor division, and the lateral rectus by the abducens nerve. Each enters the muscle at the junction of the posterior third with the anterior two-thirds; the nerve to the inferior oblique enters the muscle near its midpoint. The superior oblique is innervated by the trochlear nerve. Similarly, an inferior branch of the ophthalmic artery provides blood supply to the medial rectus, inferior rectus, and inferior oblique muscles. A superior branch of the ophthalmic artery supplies the remaining extraocular muscles.

The medial rectus remains close to the medial orbital wall until the anterior third of its course when it angles laterally to insert on the eye. It has the greatest mass of the recti, perhaps resulting from the constant need to maintain the eye in a primary or convergent position, in spite of an orbital axis 22° divergent. Just above the muscle lie terminal branches of the nasociliary nerve and ophthalmic artery. The sole action of the muscle is to adduct the eye.

The inferior rectus lies juxtaposed to the orbital floor posteriorly in the region of the palatine bone but elevates from it more anteriorly to be separated by fat. Koornneef has shown that a series of fibrous septa radiate to the inferior periorbita, suggesting that incarceration of this tissue alone in a floor fracture may yield restriction of the muscle [158]. The primary action of the inferior rectus is infraduction. Because the inferior rectus muscle must angle laterally from the orbital apex to reach the eye, secondary actions are excyclotorsion and adduction with the eye in primary position.

The inferior oblique muscle originates from the periosteum of the maxillary bone approximately 1.5 mm lateral to the ostium of the nasolacrimal duct just posterior to the orbital rim. The muscle travels in a course similar to that of the reflected superior oblique tendon, although somewhat more divergent from the medial wall. The 37-mm inferior oblique muscle remains muscular until its insertion on the globe, where a tendon several millimeters in length or the muscle fibers themselves may enter the sclera. The insertion is 2.2 mm inferior and lateral to the macula. It may be found 9.5 mm posterior to the lateral rectus insertion. The inferior oblique muscle travels inferior to the inferior rectus muscle. Their conjoined fascia forms Lockwood's suspensory ligament. The large inferior oculomotor nerve division to the inferior oblique muscle travels along the lateral border of the inferior rectus. The nerve enters the muscle midway along its length. The inferior oblique elevates, extorts, and abducts the eye.

The lateral rectus is separated from the optic nerve by the other nerves entering the oculomotor foramen (see Fig. 1.72). It remains separated from the nerve by the ciliary ganglion, the nasociliary nerve, and the ophthalmic artery, which are embedded in the loose intraconal orbital fat. Anteriorly, the lacrimal gland with attendant artery and nerve is just above, whereas fat intervenes laterally. The only action of the lateral rectus is abduction.

The superior rectus is the main elevator of the globe. The primary relation of the superior rectus is to the levator of the upper eyelid, which lies immediately above it. Having the same embryonic origin, the muscles remain fused at their medial borders. The nasociliary nerve and ophthalmic artery leave the lateral orbit to cross beneath the superior rectus. The insertion of the superior rectus is posterior to the ora serrata; a poorly directed bridle suture may thus result in retinal perforation. The superior rectus elevates, adducts, and intorts the eye.

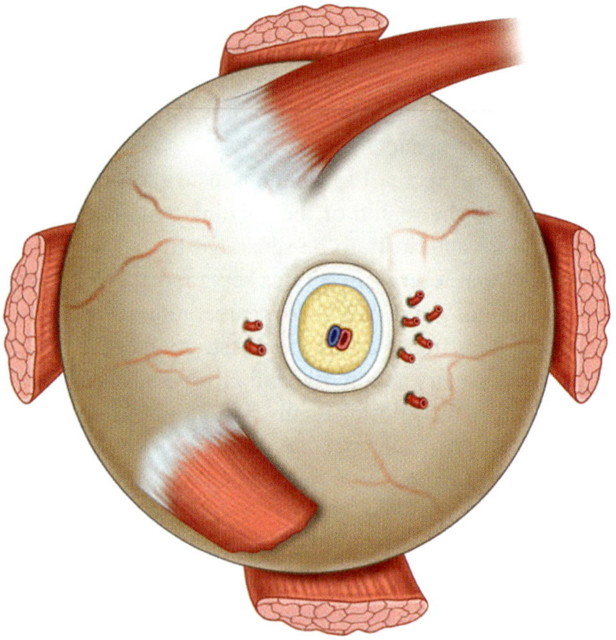

Fig. 1.74 Posterior view of left globe (which is slightly abducted) to show insertions of oblique muscles

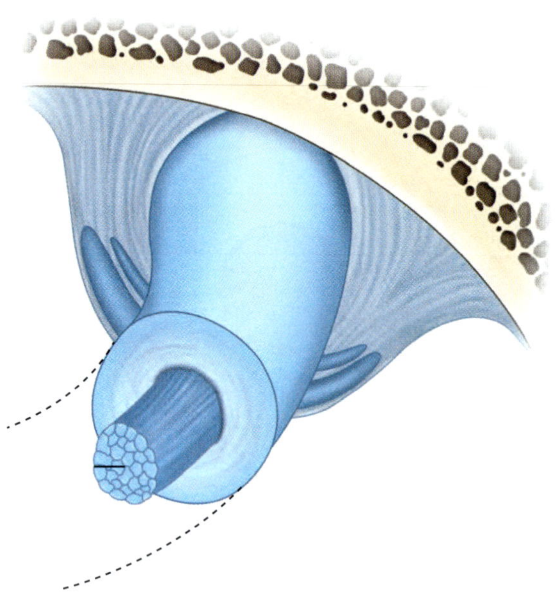

Fig. 1.75 Schematic drawing of right trochlea. Tendon is supported by layer of cartilage slung by fibrous supports from periorbita. Central fibers of tendon are strong with few attachments peripherally

The superior oblique courses anteriorly and superiorly for 40 mm from its origin (see Fig. 1.72), closely applied to the lesser wing of the sphenoid at the superomedial orbital wall. Beneath it, and separating it from the medial rectus, are the terminal branches of the nasociliary nerve and ophthalmic artery. It passes through the trochlea and makes a 54° angle to the sagittal plane to continue posteriorly, laterally, and inferiorly to the eye. The tendon begins 10 mm behind the globe and narrows to 1–2 mm as it passes through the trochlea. The 2.8-cm reflected tendon passes underneath the superior rectus and fans out to insert on the posterior lateral surface of the globe. Generally, the insertion is 10–11 mm long along a posterolateral convex line, but this insertion is the most variable of the extraocular muscles (Fig. 1.74). The distance between the temporal ends of the superior rectus and superior oblique tendons averages 4.7 mm [170]. The superior oblique depresses, intorts, and abducts the eye.

The trochlea is situated in a shallow fossa bearing its name on the anteromedial orbital roof. A crescent-shaped cartilage is suspended from the periorbita on either end by fibrous pillars (Fig. 1.75). The central fibers of the reflected tendon exhibit few adhesions to neighboring fibers, whereas those peripheral in the tendon are related in a loose fashion to the fibers of the tendon. Located between the cartilage and the tendon is a bursa-like structure, presumably to reduce friction [171]. The cartilage is a U-shaped ring with a grooved flange that supports the reflected tendon posteriorly and laterally from the front of the trochlea [172]. The periorbita to which the trochlea is attached can be elevated carefully from the bone by the surgeon and replaced with variable detriment to superior oblique function.

The levator palpebrae superioris has been discussed earlier in the section on the eyelid.

For the additional study of extraocular muscle structure and function, the reader is referred to the extensive review by Porter and colleagues [173].

Globe Topography

The eyeball occupies the anterior orbit. The superior, medial, and inferior orbital rims extend to approximately the same frontal plane as the surface of the eye. The lateral rim is recessed 1–2 cm. Attached to the eye are the six extraocular muscles, the optic nerve, the long and short posterior ciliary nerves, the anterior and posterior ciliary arteries, and the vortex veins. The globe is covered behind the corneal limbus by Tenon's fascia and is supported in the orbit by Lockwood's ligament and surrounding fat.

The average volume of the eyeball is about 6.5 ml compared with the orbital volume, which is about 29.7 ml [7]. The shape is not truly spherical; rather, it is formed by the union of two spheres (corneal and scleral) with different curvatures. The average dimensions are 24 mm anteroposteriorly, 23 mm vertically, and 23.5 mm horizontally.

At birth, the anteroposterior diameter is approximately 16 mm. By 20 months of age, the globe reaches 90% of its adult size. Changes in Hertel exophthalmometry and interpupillary distance have been studied [174]. Hertel measurements increase until age 20. Interpupillary distances increase in the elderly, possibly related to laxity and atrophy of the senescent orbital tissues.

Orbital Nerves

Five of the 12 cranial nerves innervate the orbit. These include the optic (second), the oculomotor (third), the trochlear (fourth), the abducens (sixth), and the first and second divisions of the trigeminal (fifth). The orbit also receives sympathetic and parasympathetic innervation. The nerves crowd together along with the ophthalmic artery to enter the orbit at its apex, at the point where orbital venous blood drains into the cavernous sinus. Single lesions in this complex area can result in multiple deficits. The intraorbital courses of the nerves are discussed later; the intracranial pathways are described in the section on intracranial orbital relationships.

The Optic Nerve (II)

The optic nerve is essentially an orbital extension of the brain. Unlike the other cranial nerves, the optic nerve contains supporting neuroglial cells, is bathed by cerebrospinal fluid, and is covered by meninges. The optic nerve is divided into intraocular, intraorbital, intracanalicular, and intracranial segments.

The axons of the nerve arise from the ganglion cell layer of the retina and converge at the optic disk to course through the lamina cribrosa. The optic disk is 1.5 mm in diameter, but the nerve expands to 3 mm at the junction with the globe because of an increase in supporting neuroglial cells and the onset of myelination [175]. The intraocular segment is 1 mm in length.

The intraorbital segment of the optic nerve measures 24 mm, on average, between the back of the globe and the entrance into the optic foramen, but the distance between these structures is only about 18 mm [3].

This 6 mm of slack in the optic nerve results in a gentle curve, with the convexity directed inferotemporally in the orbit (Fig. 1.76). This degree of laxity in the nerve allows free movement of the globe under physiologic conditions and affords a margin of safety in proptotic states. In very severe proptosis, this slack may be insufficient and tension on the globe results. This may be observed radiologically as "globe tenting" [176]. Excessive stretching of the nerve and compression by taut dura may result in visual loss [177].

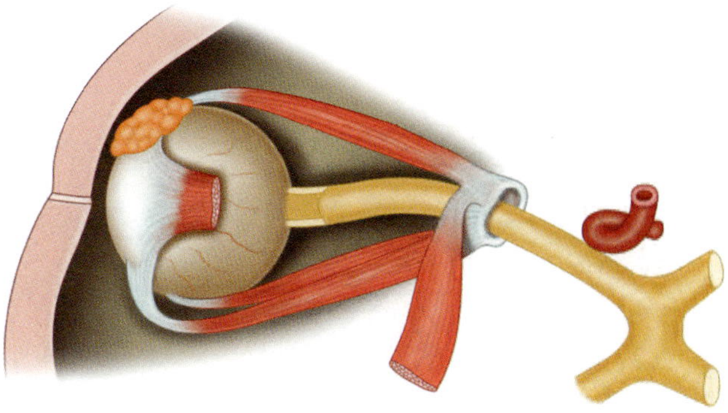

Fig. 1.76 Dissection of right orbit to show inferolateral convexity of optic nerve. Intraorbital optic nerve measures 24 mm, while posterior globe is 18 mm from optic foramen

The intraorbital optic nerve is surrounded and cushioned by large lobules of intraconal fat. The intraorbital nerve is covered by dura that is continuous with superficial scleral fibers and thickens near the optic canal. The cerebrospinal fluid communicates freely with the fluid bathing the midbrain, explaining instances of sudden respiratory arrest following retrobulbar injection [178]. Release of this cerebrospinal fluid can be seen intraoperatively during optic nerve sheath fenestration for pseudotumor cerebri.

The Oculomotor Nerve (III)

The third cranial nerve innervates the medial, superior, and inferior recti, the inferior oblique, and the levator palpebrae superioris muscles. Additionally, the oculomotor nerve provides parasympathetic innervation to the eye. The third nerve courses through the lateral roof of the cavernous sinus, slightly superior and medial to the abducens nerve. Within the anterior portion of the cavernous sinus or near the superior orbital fissure, the third nerve divides into a superior and an inferior division. The branches enter the orbit through the oculomotor foramen. The superior branch rises within the muscle cone to reach the superior rectus on its internal side, 15 mm from the orbital apex. Fibers then proceed to the levator palpebrae superioris by passing medial to the superior rectus (90%) or through it (Fig. 1.77).

The inferior branch of the oculomotor nerve travels underneath the optic nerve to innervate the medial and inferior rectus muscles. Its large terminal branch to the inferior oblique continues anteriorly along the lateral border of the inferior rectus. This latter branch gives off a parasympathetic twig to the ciliary ganglion above. The pupillomotor fibers are contained within this parasympathetic bundle. Damage to these fibers may result in postoperative mydriasis following orbital floor fracture repair [179].

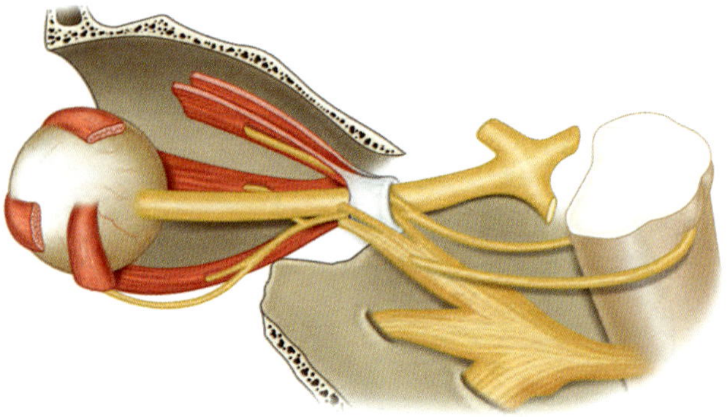

Fig. 1.77 Extraocular muscle branches of oculomotor nerve. Superior and inferior divisions are separated by nasociliary nerve within oculomotor foramen. Superior division supplies superior rectus and levator muscle. Inferior division supplies inferior and medial rectus muscles and inferior oblique muscle. Parasympathetic fibers from inferior oblique nerve to ciliary ganglion are not shown

The Trochlear Nerve (IV)

The trochlear nerve enters the orbit through the superior orbital fissure superotemporal to the annulus of Zinn and medial to the frontal nerve. It courses outside the muscle cone, attested to by the fact that the superior oblique is relatively resistant to a retrobulbar block. The trochlear nerve crosses medially over the origin of the levator and superior rectus muscles and runs anteriorly between the orbital roof and the levator muscle. The nerve enters the posterior one-third of the superior oblique. If the superior periorbita alone is removed during dissection, its entire course is visible (Fig. 1.78).

The Abducens Nerve (VI)

After leaving the cavernous sinus, the abducens nerve passes through the oculomotor foramen to enter the orbit. It travels anteriorly between the optic nerve and the lateral rectus muscle. The sixth nerve inserts into the inner surface of the muscle, where its posterior third meets the anterior two-thirds. A similar point of entry is observed as the oculomotor nerve supplies the other recti muscles.

The Trigeminal Nerve (V)

The trigeminal nerve is composed of ophthalmic, maxillary, and mandibular divisions. The nerve complex is largely sensory with a small motor component within the mandibular division. The ophthalmic and maxillary divisions of the sensory trigeminal nerve supply the superior two-thirds of the face (see Figs. 1.60 and 1.79). The deeper structures underlying the cutaneous distribution are likewise served.

The ophthalmic division enters the orbit through the superior orbital fissure as three branches – the lacrimal, frontal, and nasociliary. The lacrimal nerve is the smallest branch and is situated most laterally in the superior orbital fissure. It joins the lacrimal artery to pass superotemporally to the posterior aspect of the lacrimal gland (Fig. 1.78). Here, it forms superior and inferior branches; the former supplies the gland, nearby conjunctiva, and the lateral upper eyelid; the latter supplies the gland and anastomoses with the fibers from the zygomaticotemporal nerve. The frontal branch travels just beneath the periorbita, where it divides somewhat anteriorly in the orbit to form the supratrochlear branch and a larger, more lateral supraorbital branch (Fig. 1.78). The supratrochlear innervates the medial upper eyelid, glabellar skin, and lower forehead; the supraorbital nerve supplies the majority of the forehead and the anterior scalp (see section "Eyelid Nerves"). The nasociliary nerve of the ophthalmic division is the only branch to pass through the annulus of Zinn. It passes over the optic nerve with the ophthalmic artery to lie between the superior oblique and medial rectus muscles (Fig. 1.80). The nasociliary nerve gives off a sensory root to the ciliary ganglion, two or three long ciliary nerves to the globe, the anterior and posterior ethmoidal nerves, and a terminal infratrochlear branch. Anterior ethmoidal and infratrochlear nerve blocks are useful when performing dacryocystorhinostomy under local anesthesia.

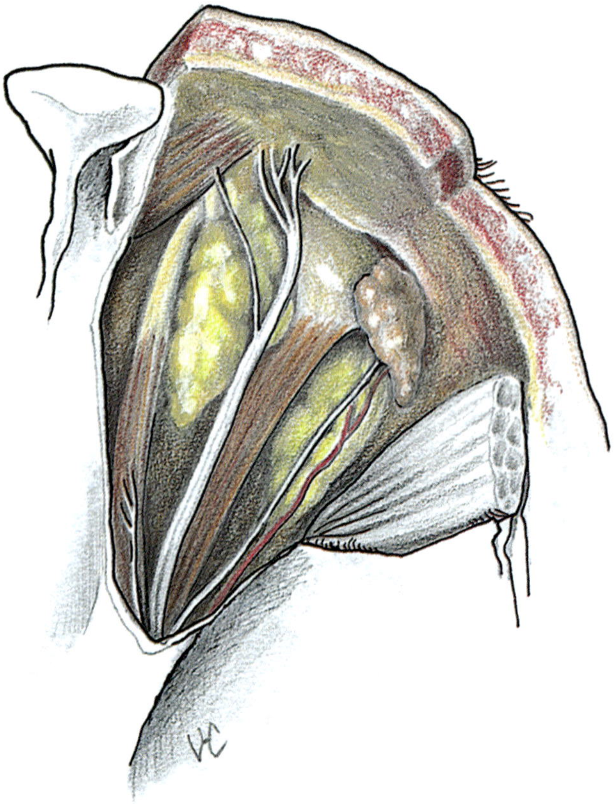

Fig. 1.78 Dissection to show superior nerves of orbit entering through superior orbital fissure outside annulus of Zinn. Trochlear nerve has the shortest intraorbital course. Frontal and lacrimal nerves are branches of trigeminal ophthalmic division

The maxillary division of the trigeminal nerve gives rise to the sphenopalatine, posterior superior alveolar, and zygo-

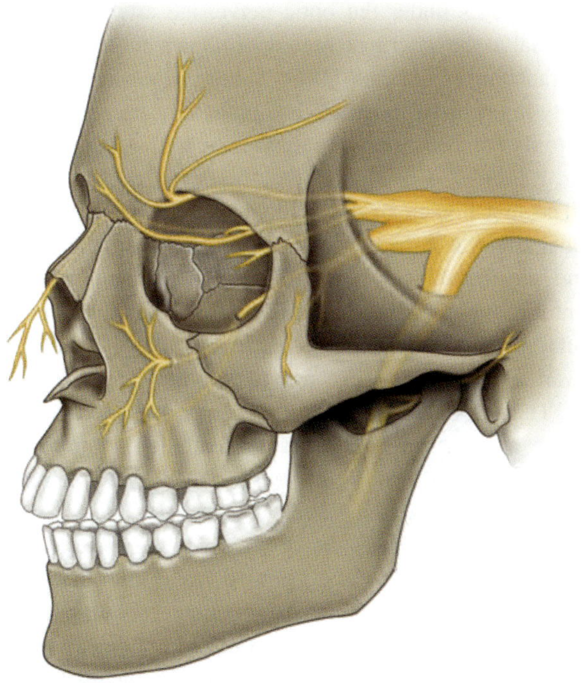

Fig. 1.79 Trigeminal nerve pathways

matic branches in the pterygopalatine fossa. The zygomatic nerve enters the orbit through the inferior orbital fissure and gives off the zygomaticotemporal and zygomaticofacial nerves, which supply the lateral brow and lateral cheek, respectively. Parasympathetic secretomotor fibers from the sphenopalatine ganglion travel with the zygomaticotemporal nerve before joining the lacrimal nerve en route to the lacrimal gland. The bulk of the maxillary nerve enters the orbit through the inferior orbital fissure and courses along the orbital floor as the infraorbital nerve. In the newborn, this course parallels the medial wall but becomes slightly convex laterally with the expansion of the maxillary sinus. The infraorbital nerve enters the infraorbital groove and emerges from the infraorbital foramen 4–6 mm inferior to the orbital rim. Middle and anterior superior alveolar branches are given off in the infraorbital canal. The terminal branches of the infraorbital nerve (inferior palpebral, lateral nasal, and superior labial) provide sensation to the lower eyelid (see Fig. 1.60) as well as to the nose, cheek, and upper lip.

The trigeminal nerve also provides proprioceptive sensory branches to the third, fourth, and sixth nerves while in the cavernous sinus and may exhibit anastomosis with the facial nerve peripherally beneath the superficial muscle plane.

The Sympathetic Nerves

The sympathetic nerve supply to the orbit allows for pupillary dilation, the function of the smooth muscles of the eyelids, and vasoconstriction. Postganglionic sympathetic

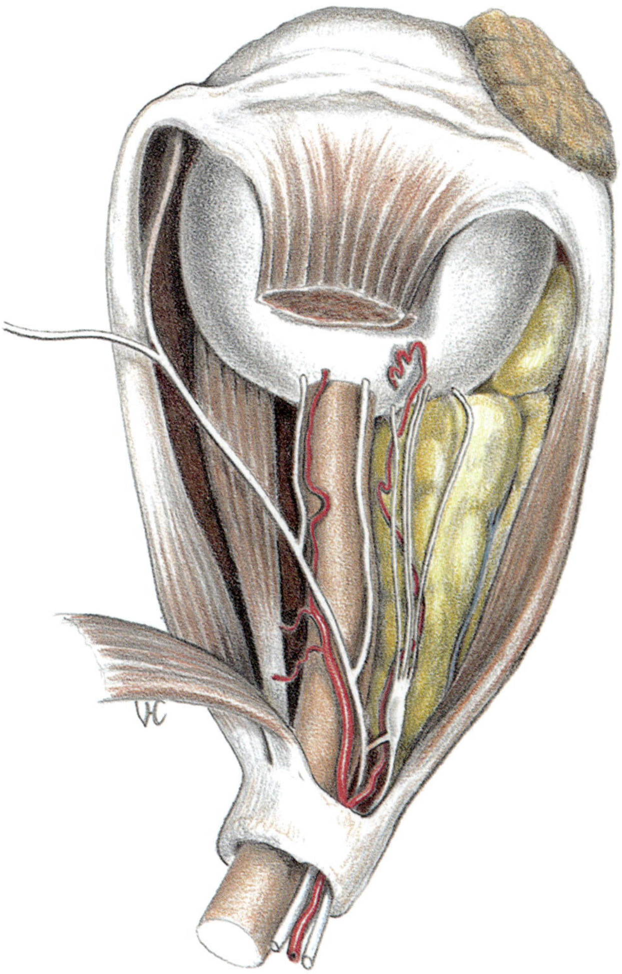

Fig. 1.80 Dissection to show intraorbital nasociliary nerve course

fibers arise in the superior cervical ganglion and enter the cavernous sinus with the internal carotid artery. Within the cavernous sinus, the exact relationships of the sympathetic pathway remain controversial. Whitnall described entry into the orbit via the optic canal, superior orbital fissure, and inferior orbital fissure [3]. Wolff states that the major dilator fibers pass through nasociliary and the long posterior ciliary nerves to the globe. Work in primates by Lyon and colleagues [125] showed that the pathway may be exclusive via the superior orbital fissure. This work also demonstrated sympathetic fibers traveling with the sixth nerve and the ophthalmic (V1) division of the fifth nerve. Most investigators agree that some of the sympathetics run a short course with the abducens nerve before entering the orbit via the ophthalmic division of the trigeminal nerve. Cases of Horner's syndrome with the sixth nerve paresis [180, 181] have been reported. Pathways to the superior and inferior tarsal muscles are not entirely understood, but evidence suggests that sympathetic nerves may travel along with the motor nerves that supply the extraocular muscles rather than with supplying arteries [158].

Ciliary Ganglion and Parasympathetic Nerves

Parasympathetic nerves to the orbit supply the pupil, ciliary muscle, and lacrimal gland. Preganglionic fibers from the Edinger–Westphal portion of the oculomotor nucleus destined for the eye travel with the inferior division of the oculomotor nerve. They synapse in the ciliary ganglion and continue to the eye via the short ciliary nerves. The majority of these fibers supply the ciliary body, and the remaining 10% innervate the pupil.

Fibers destined for the lacrimal gland originate in the superior salivatory nucleus and travel via the nervus intermedius [182] branch of the facial nerve. These fibers travel with the greater superficial petrosal nerve and then the vidian nerve, to synapse in the sphenopalatine ganglion. The remainder of the course to the lacrimal gland via the second and, then, first division of the trigeminal was described previously.

The ciliary ganglion is situated 10 mm from the orbital apex and 15 mm posterior to the globe between the lateral rectus and the optic nerve (see Fig. 1.80). The sensory root from the nasociliary nerve contributes fibers that pass through the ganglion without synapsing. These sensory fibers travel from the iris, ciliary body, and cornea via the short ciliary nerves. The sympathetic supply may arrive from a direct branch from the sympathetic plexus, from a twig from the ophthalmic artery, or both [183]. The sympathetic fibers en route to the choroidal vasculature travel through the ciliary ganglion without synapsing. The sympathetic fibers innervating the pupil, however, bypass the ciliary ganglion and travel via the long posterior ciliary nerves to the iris [89]. The short ciliary nerves leaving the ganglion usually number five or six. The majority are lateral to the optic nerve, with one or two usually crossing to enter medially.

Orbital Arteries

The orbital arteries are primarily branches of the ophthalmic artery with small contributions from the middle meningeal and internal maxillary arteries. Bergen (attributed to Henle) spatially separates the orbital arteries into three groups that radiate in three conical planes coaxial to the axis between the optic foramen and the central retinal artery: the innermost cone represents the posterior ciliary arteries, the middle cone is formed by the radiating muscular arteries, and the external cone is formed by the lacrimal, supraorbital, and ophthalmic arteries (Fig. 1.81a).

The ophthalmic artery is usually the first branch of the internal carotid and provides the primary arterial supply to the orbit and the eye in 96% of individuals. In 3%, the middle meningeal contributes equally via the recurrent meningeal branch, and in 1%, the middle meningeal is the only arterial supply to the orbit [184]. The ophthalmic artery enters the orbit inferolateral to the optic nerve and courses medially [185, 186]. In approximately 75%–80% of orbits, the ophthalmic artery crosses above the optic nerve. At this point, the artery is firmly fixed to the optic nerve sheath. If the artery crosses under the optic nerve, the arterial segment proximal to the anterior ethmoidal foramen and the order of its branching is affected [186]. There is considerable variability in the order in which the ophthalmic artery gives origin to its branches; only the most frequent pattern is shown (Fig. 1.81b).

The first branch of the ophthalmic artery is the central retinal artery. It originates at the orbital apex and pierces the dural sheath to enter the optic nerve inferomedially about 10 mm posterior to the globe in conjunction with the central retinal vein [187]. The point of entry into the optic nerve can be variable, ranging from 5 mm to 16 mm behind the globe [89]. The possibility of an unusually anterior entry should be kept in mind during optic nerve sheath fenestration. The artery then penetrates the nerve substance to run centrally within the nerve into the globe.

The ophthalmic artery then gives rise to the posterior ciliary arteries, usually as two trunks dividing into numerous branches. These divide further into about 15 twigs, which enter the sclera to supply the choroid and optic nerve head. Two branches of the posterior ciliary system, the medial and lateral long posterior ciliary arteries, travel anteriorly to the ciliary body and iris.

The muscular arteries that supply the extraocular muscles generally arise as a lateral (superior) and a medial (inferior) trunk. The former supplies the levator, superior oblique, superior rectus, and lateral rectus muscles. Each rectus muscular artery terminates into two anterior ciliary arteries, except that of the lateral rectus, which has only one. These enter the eye anterior to the muscle insertions and anastomose with the long posterior ciliary arteries.

The lacrimal artery arises from the ophthalmic artery and travels superotemporally in the orbit to reach the gland on its posterior surface. It often develops a recurrent meningeal branch to anastomose with the meningeal artery via the superior orbital fissure. The lacrimal artery also gives off the zygomaticofacial, zygomaticotemporal, and lateral palpebral branches. The lateral palpebral branch supplies the lateral aspect of the arcades of the upper and lower eyelids.

The supraorbital artery travels between the levator and the orbital roof after leaving the ophthalmic artery. It contributes small muscular branches to the levator, superior rectus, and superior oblique muscles before exiting the orbit through the supraorbital notch. The supraorbital artery supplies the eyebrow and forehead. The medial termination of the ophthalmic artery gives off a posterior and a larger anterior ethmoidal branch, each passing through its respective foramen. The posterior ethmoidal artery supplies mucosa of the posterior ethmoidal air cells. The larger anterior ethmoidal artery supplies the middle and anterior ethmoid cells, nasal septum, and mucosa, as well as the frontal sinus and dura near the cribriform plate.

The ophthalmic artery is accompanied by the nasociliary nerve, while the lacrimal and supraorbital arteries are

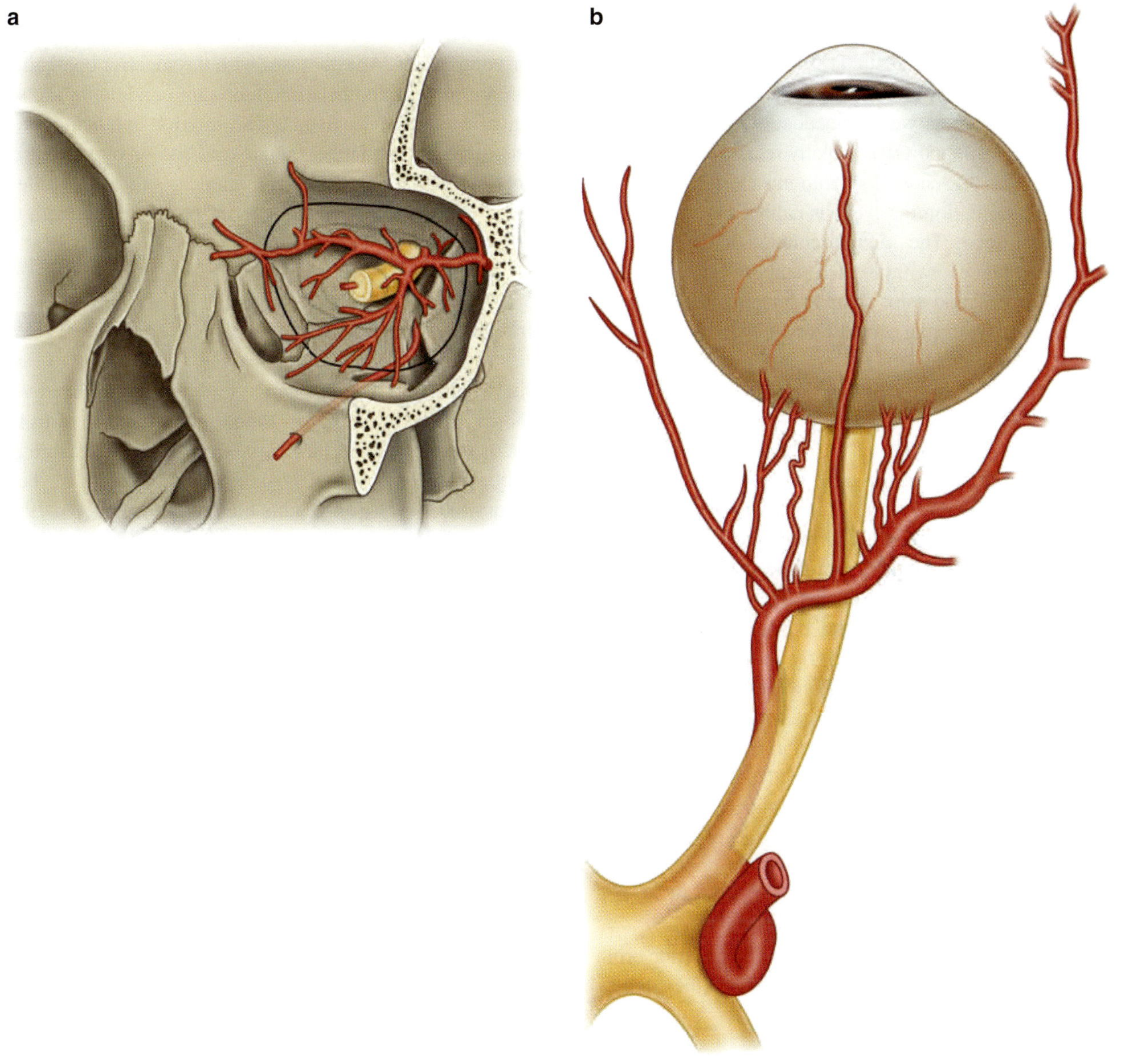

Fig. 1.81 Orbital arteries. (**a**) Bergen spatially separates orbital arteries into three groups that radiate in three conical planes coaxial to axis between optic foramen and central retinal artery; innermost cone represents posterior ciliary arteries; middle cone surface is formed by radiating muscular arteries; outermost cone is completed on its superior surface only by lacrimal, supraorbital, and ophthalmic arteries. (**b**) Most common branching pattern of ophthalmic artery in orbit

accompanied by the lacrimal and supraorbital nerves, respectively. The ophthalmic artery gives rise to the nasofrontal artery superomedially, which divides to form the supratrochlear and the medial palpebral arteries. The palpebral terminations are discussed in the section on eyelid anatomy.

The external carotid bifurcates within the parotid gland to form the superficial temporal artery and the maxillary (internal maxillary) arteries. The latter pass deep to the mandible to enter the pterygopalatine fossa via the infratemporal fossa [188]. A terminal branch of the maxillary artery, the infraorbital, enters the orbit through the inferior orbital fissure. It passes into the infraorbital sulcus and gives branches to the inferior rectus and inferior oblique muscles, lacrimal gland, and the orbital fat. Emerging from the infraorbital foramen, it terminates in eyelid, labial, and nasal branches.

The middle meningeal branch of the external carotid enters the orbit through the superior orbital fissure or its own foramen to anastomose with the lacrimal artery. The recurrent meningeal branch is usually diminutive, but rarely, it may supply the majority of orbital arterial blood in individuals with congenital atresia of the ophthalmic artery or acquired ipsilateral internal carotid stenosis.

Bergen studied the serial thick histologic sections produced by Koornneef to determine vascular relationships to the connective tissue septa [189–191]. He observed the orbital arteries to be independent of the fibrous septa. On the other hand, the veins were embedded within the septa; the degree of septal support was directly related to the caliber of the vessel. The presence of smooth muscle cells in the septa raises the speculation that venous caliber may be related to sympathetic tone. The microcirculation tended to remain compartmentalized within each adipose space. Doppler ultrasound [192] and color Doppler imaging [193] have been used to quantify normal orbital blood flow.

Orbital Veins

The venous drainage of the orbit is carried by the superior and inferior ophthalmic veins. The superior ophthalmic vein is the larger of the two and is formed anteromedially by the union of the supraorbital, supratrochlear, and angular veins (see Fig. 1.82). It is situated superiorly in the orbit, suspended from the roof periorbita by septa forming a hammock. The vessel courses posteriorly along the medial border of the superior rectus muscle. It crosses between the optic nerve and the superior rectus muscle, continuing posteriorly along the lateral aspect of the superior rectus muscle. Within the muscle cone, the superior ophthalmic vein receives branches from the ciliary veins and superior vortex veins. The superior ophthalmic vein enters the cavernous sinus through the superior orbital fissure. At the point where the vein leaves the orbit, usually above the annulus of Zinn, it is encased by fibrous tissues.

The inferior ophthalmic vein drains the inferior orbit. It begins as a diffuse venous plexus beneath the globe. Its course within the orbit is more variable. It receives venous drainage from the inferior extraocular muscles and the inferior vortex veins. Anastomoses with the superior ophthalmic vein are present and become important conduits in the setting of a dural sinus fistula. The inferior ophthalmic vein exits the orbit below the annulus of Zinn or by joining the superior ophthalmic vein. It communicates through Muller's orbital muscle [194] and the inferior orbital fissure with the pterygoid venous plexus.

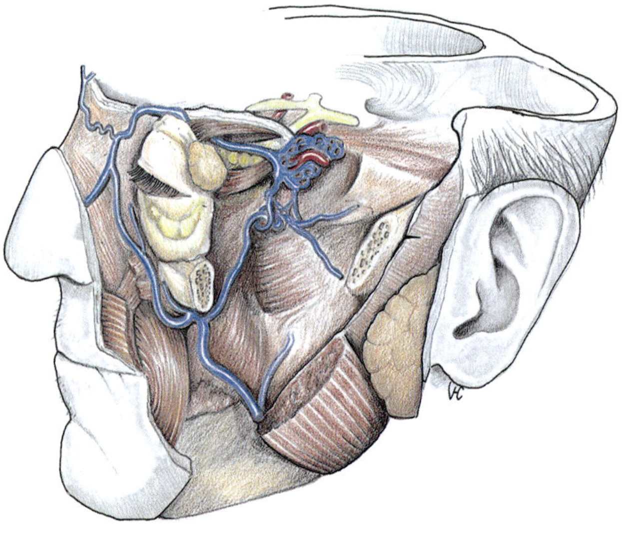

Fig. 1.82 Orbital venous drainage (see text)

Orbital Lymph Drainage

The lymphatic system is a network of endothelial-lined vessels serving to return extravasated protein and fluid to the venous system. Duke-Elder stated that "in the orbit there are no lymphatic nodes, and no lymphatic vessels have been demonstrated" [195]. From his literature review up to 1968, he concluded that the principal lymph drainage accompanies the veins in perivascular channels through "the inferior orbital fissure to the internal maxillary nodes, thence to the superior deep cervical nodes." Wolff [175] concurred about the lack of orbital lymphatics. There has since been a report of an orbital lymph node, which the authors thought was probably ectopic and congenital [196].

No true lymphatics (endothelial-lined channels) have been found in the brain, either. Millen and Woollam injected carbon colloid into the subarachnoid space of rats and recovered some of the material in reticular tissue around the blood vessels [197]. Foldi and coworkers tied off cervical lymphatics of dogs and produced cerebral edema [198]. Pathologic examination of the perivascular reticular space showed dilation with clear or eosinophilic fluid. It was postulated that the reticular tissue, derived from the pia and arachnoid layers, functions as lymph channels. The authors concluded that the spaces should be termed "pre-lymphatic," unless endothelial cells were found on electron microscopy. Endothelial cells have not been found since.

Orbital lymph drainage has been studied by injecting radioactive colloid solutions into the different orbital spaces of the rabbit and then characterizing their dispersion in the sacrificed animal [199–203]. Injection into the retrobulbar space resulted in the highest concentrations in the bilateral deep cervical lymph nodes, with minor concentrations found in ipsilateral superficial cervical and mandibular nodes. Injection into the anterior chamber or vitreous body yielded radioactivity in the retrobulbar space (especially around the optic nerve) and in the bilateral deep cervical lymph nodes. Subconjunctival injection on the right side resulted in measurable radioactivity in the bilateral deep cervical nodes, the right superficial cervical node, and the right mandibular node, as well as in the eye, in the retrobulbar space, and along the optic nerve. Drainage from the subconjunctival space took place rapidly, but the deeper injections were measured after about 1 week.

McGetrick and associates studied the lymphatic drainage from the orbit of a cynomolgus monkey using retrobulbar injections of technetium-99 (99Tc) antimony sulfide colloid and India ink [197]. Injections outside the extraocular muscle cone were removed by the conjunctival and eyelid lymphatics. Colloids injected into the intraconal orbit spread along the connective tissue septa and did not reach lymph nodes over a 24-h period. A small amount of India ink left the posterior orbit and was demonstrated entering the contralateral orbit.

A further search for orbital lymphatics in the primate has been carried out by Sherman and associates [204]. Using a 5′-nucleotidase enzyme histochemical method [205] and strict morphologic criteria, as well as electron microscopy with strict ultrastructural grading, lymphatics were consistently demonstrated in the optic nerve arachnoid and in the lacrimal gland. Lymphatics were inconsistently identified in the extraocular muscles. Lymphatics were not found within the connective tissue septa of the orbital fat.

Intracranial Orbital Relationships

Pertinent Intracranial Osteology

The anterior cranial fossa lies above the orbit, separated from it by the frontal bone. Posteriorly, the anterior cranial fossa is bounded by the lesser wing of the sphenoid. The crista galli lies in the center of the fossa. The cribriform plates lie on either side of the crista galli.

The middle cranial fossa consists of two lateral depressions that straddle the body of the sphenoid at the midline. The sphenoid bone articulates with the occipital bone behind, with the temporal bones laterally, and with the frontal and ethmoid bones anteriorly (Fig. 1.83a, b). It is of particular interest to the orbital surgeon because most structures entering or leaving the orbit pass through it.

The lesser wing of the sphenoid terminates medially at the anterior clinoid process. This process lies slightly superior, posterior, and lateral to the optic canal (Figs. 1.84 and 1.85). The anterior clinoid process is a useful marker when differentiating the optic canal from the superior orbital fissure on an axial computed tomograph. The hypophyseal fossa lies between the tuberculum sellae anteriorly and the dorsum sellae posteriorly. The hypophyseal fossa and its ridges collectively are termed the sella turcica. The projections found at the lateral aspects of the dorsum sella are the posterior clinoid processes, which anchor the tentorium cerebelli. The lateral wall of the sphenoid bone is indented by the carotid groove, which accommodates the carotid artery and the cavernous sinus. The sphenoid body pneumatizes to a variable degree, forming the sphenoid sinus over which the cavernous sinus is draped.

The optic foramen is formed within the lesser sphenoid wing. The superior orbital fissure is a defect between the greater and lesser sphenoid wings, through which pass most of the nerves entering the orbit, as well as the exiting venous blood and recurrent meningeal artery (see Fig. 1.72; also see section "Orbital Apex"). The foramen rotundum and the foramen ovale conduct the second and third divisions of the trigeminal nerves, respectively. Immediately posterolateral to the foramen ovale is the foramen spinosum, through which enters the middle meningeal branch of the maxillary artery.

Dura Mater

In humans, it is believed that the dura mater and the leptomeninges (pia and arachnoid layers) all arise from loose mesenchyme surrounding the developing nervous system, with neural crest cells contributing to the pia layer. The cranial dura mater is, at first, indistinguishable from the mesenchyme that later forms the skull and can be differentiated from it only when the blood sinuses appear [97].

The dura is separated from the arachnoid by a potential subdural space, whereas the cerebrospinal fluid separates the pia from the arachnoid in the subarachnoid space. These relationships are continued in the optic nerve sheath within the orbit. The dura mater is composed of an outer endosteal layer and an inner meningeal layer, which separate only to accommodate blood sinuses. The outer layer is especially densely attached to the bone sutures and is continuous with the periosteum lining the orbit. The inner layer covers the nerves as they exit the cranium and blends with the peripheral epineurium cover. Because of the frequent presence of atrophic orbital roof defects in the elderly [5], particular care must be taken to avoid damage to the dura and subsequent cerebrospinal fluid leak.

Cavernous Sinus

The cavernous sinus [206–208] covers the lateral aspects of the sphenoid body with a height of about 1 cm and a length of about 2 cm. Like other intracranial venous sinuses, it is formed by a split in the dura mater. Although one or two main venous channels exist in each side of the sinus, a reticulated network of endothelial-lined septa subdivide the sinus into a plexus. The nerves within the cavernous sinus may be separated from the venous blood by just an endothelial layer. It is believed that pulsations of the contained carotid arteries help pump blood from the sinus [198]. The sinus seems

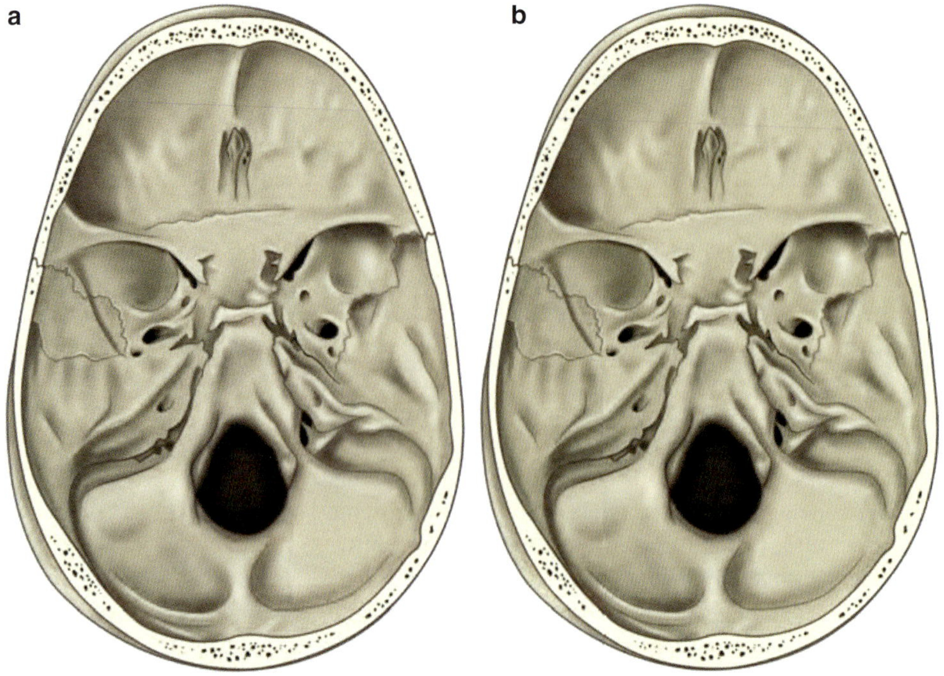

Fig. 1.83 (**a**) Cranial fossae. (**b**) Sphenoid contribution to middle cranial fossa is indicated by *shaded area*

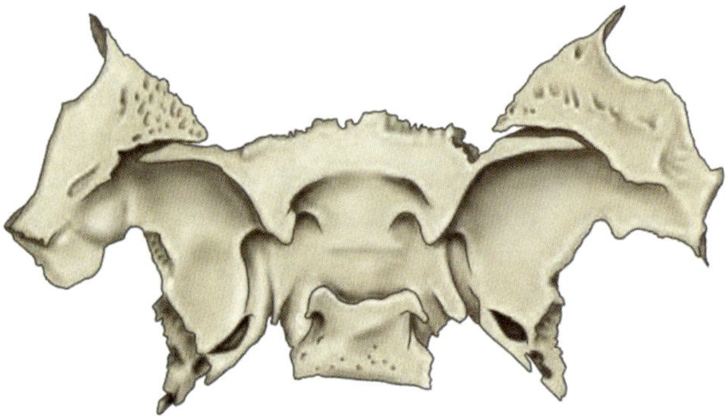

Fig. 1.84 Posterior superior view of sphenoid bone

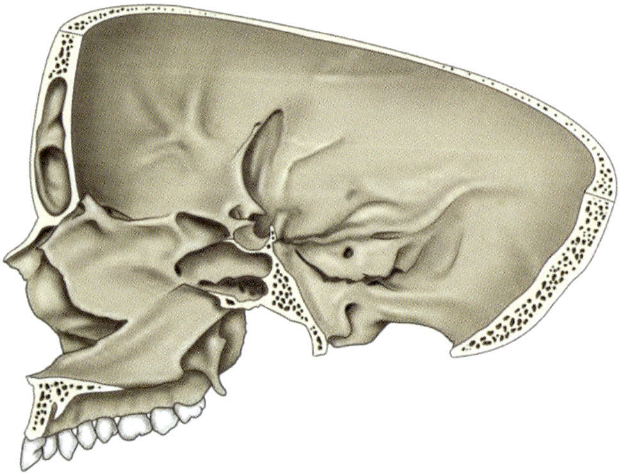

Fig. 1.85 Sagittal section through skull showing sphenoid structures

flattened against the sphenoid bone in the cadaver, yet it is inflated during life [209].

Anteriorly, the sinus receives venous blood from the superior ophthalmic vein, a branch from or the entire inferior ophthalmic vein, the sphenopalatine sinus, the middle meningeal veins, and the superficial middle cerebral veins; sometimes the central retinal vein will drain directly into it as do minor orbital veins (Fig. 1.86). The primary outflow of the cavernous sinus is to the superior and the inferior petrosal veins. The two sides of the cavernous sinuses communicate freely via the valveless anterior and posterior intercavernous sinus and the basilar plexus [210]. A unilateral orbital cellulitis that becomes bilateral is highly suggestive of septic thrombosis of the cavernous sinus.

The carotid siphon and the sixth cranial nerve lie within the sinus. The oculomotor, trochlear, and ophthalmic nerves travel within the lateral wall of the cavernous sinus [206, 207]. The maxillary nerve is outside the sinus but closely associated posteriorly. The locations of the nerves and the carotid artery within the anterior cavernous sinus are pictured schematically in Fig. 1.87.

Arteriovenous communications may involve the cavernous sinus in several ways. Spontaneous shunts may develop between small meningeal arteries and the cavernous sinus, producing signs of orbital congestion [211, 212]. A much more severe clinical picture is seen after the traumatic rupture of the intracavernous carotid artery causing a carotid-cavernous fistula with pulsatile exophthalmos [213, 214].

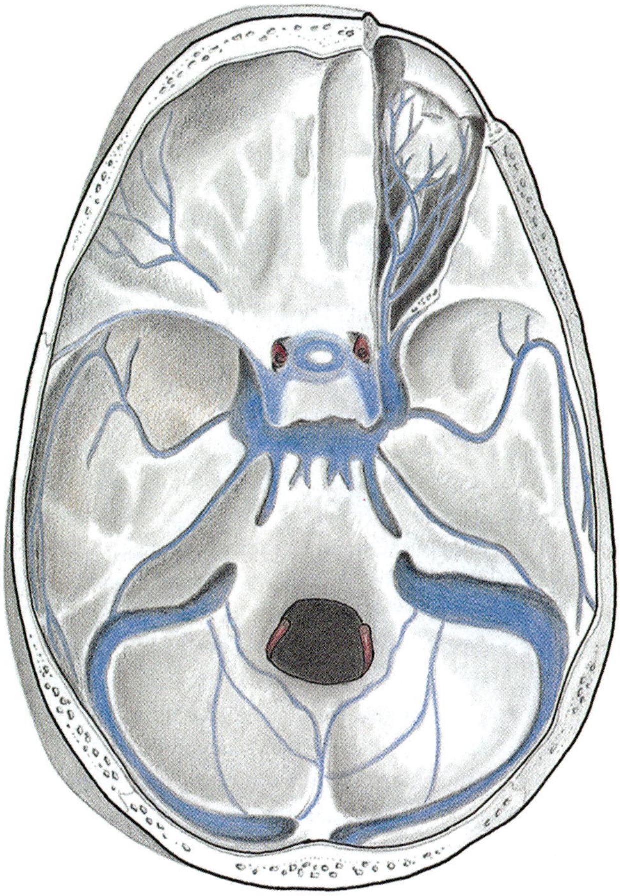

Fig. 1.86 Cavernous sinus and venous connections

Cranial Nerves

The fascicular portion of the oculomotor nerve courses through the midbrain and exits the medial surface of the cerebral peduncle (Figs. 1.88 and 1.89). The nerve gains an arachnoid covering 15–20 mm from the site of origin and a dural coat 5 mm later [215]. The oculomotor nerve travels anterolaterally to the cavernous sinus in the subarachnoid space, just lateral to the posterior communicating artery. Aneurysm at this point is a cause of third nerve palsy. At the posterior clinoid process, the oculomotor nerve enters the dura to lie temporally in the cavernous sinus. The superior and inferior divisions of the nerve separate within the sinus to enter the orbit above and below the nasociliary nerve (see Fig. 1.72).

The trochlear nerve is the smallest of the cranial nerves, has the longest course, and is the only one to arise dorsally. The rootlets of origin arise from the superior medullary velum above the fourth ventricle and travel 40 mm before dural investment. The total length of the nerve equals 85 mm. Situated in the subarachnoid space, the nerve runs between the superior cerebellar and posterior cerebral arteries. It passes to the ventral surface of the brain between the temporal lobe and the pons and enters the dura behind the posterior clinoid attachment for the tentorium cerebelli (see Figs. 1.88 and 1.89). It remains superficial within the dura to enter the cavernous sinus laterally just below the third nerve. The fourth nerve enters the orbit through the superior orbital fissure, superolateral to the annulus of Zinn.

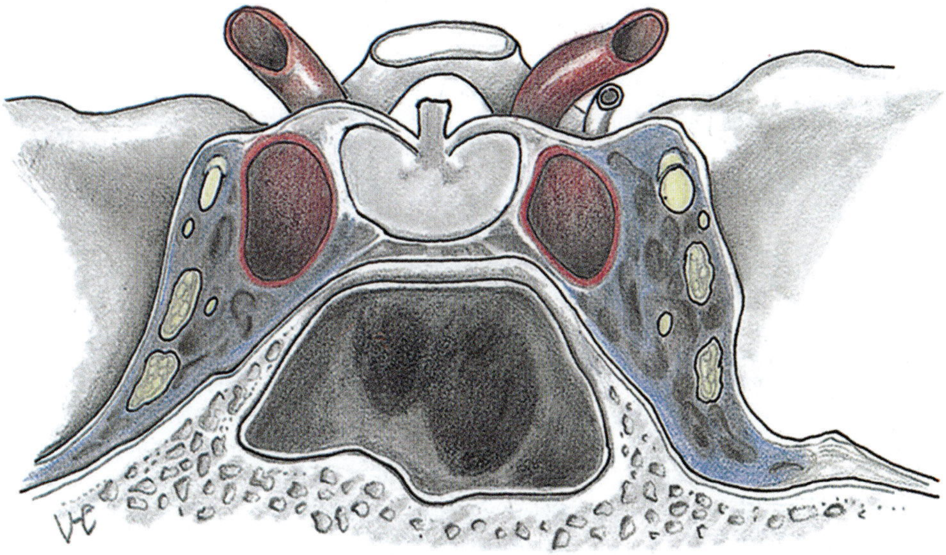

Fig. 1.87 Schematic drawing showing structures in anterior cavernous sinus. More posteriorly the abducens nerve is applied to the side of carotid artery

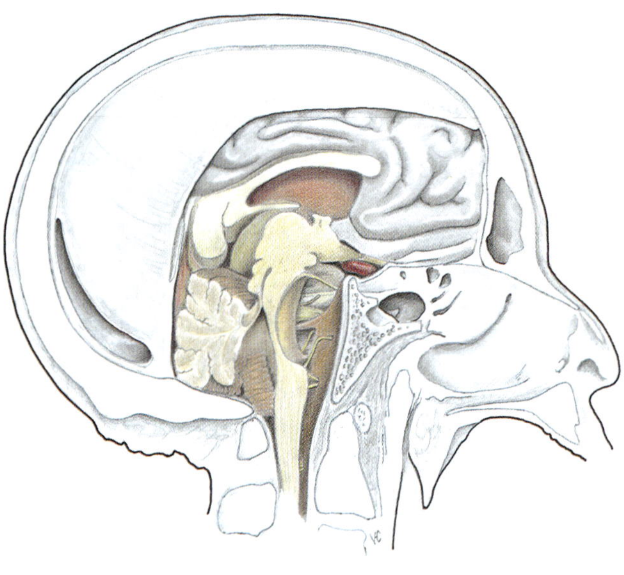

Fig. 1.88 Sagittal section of the head with basilar pons cut away to show cranial nerves, which pass anteriorly to enter orbit. (Dissection by Dr. Jesse G. Kennedy III)

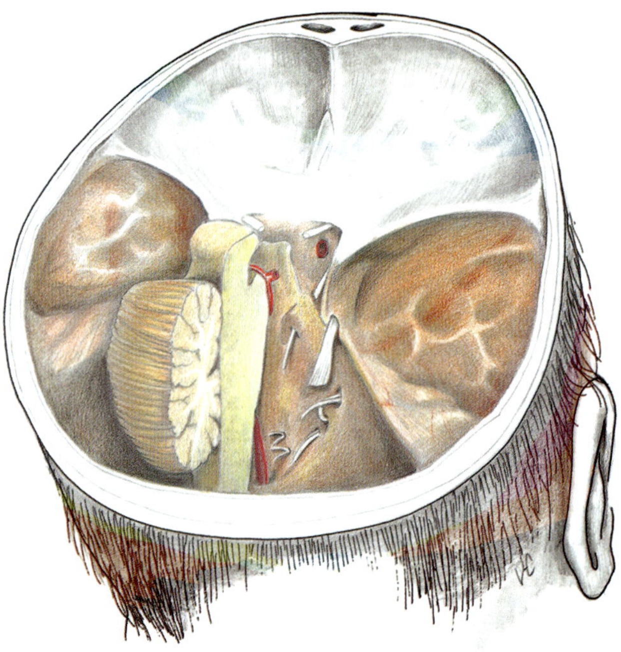

Fig. 1.89 Posterior lateral view of head with right side of brainstem removed to show cranial nerves entering dura mater. (Dissection by Dr. Jesse G. Kennedy III)

The abducens or sixth cranial nerve leaves the pons just lateral to the cerebral pyramid, and the rootlets remain attached to the pons for several millimeters. In the subarachnoid space, it travels superiorly and anteriorly to ascend the clivus, before entering the dura (Dorello's canal) below and medial to the fifth nerve. It crosses the sharp petrous ridge of the temporal bone, bending abruptly to enter the cavernous sinus under the petrosphenoidal ligament (see Figs. 1.89 and 1.90). Here, it lies temporal to the carotid artery, bound to it by the sympathetic plexus (Fig. 1.90). Unlike the oculomotor and the trochlear nerves, the abducens nerve runs within the body of the cavernous sinus rather than within the wall [206]. The sharp bend of the nerve renders it the most sensitive to damage resulting from increased intracranial pressure [216]. The close relationship of the abducens nerve with the mastoid bone is emphasized by the association of suppurative otitis media and abducens nerve paresis or paralysis (Gradenigo's syndrome) [217]. The sixth nerve enters the orbit through the annulus of Zinn.

The trigeminal nerve arises from the side of the pons with a sensory and a small motor root. The sensory root pierces the dura beneath the tentorium cerebelli and enters the middle cranial fossa to join the trigeminal ganglion, residing in Meckel's cave on the petrous ridge of the temporal bone [217]. Meckel's cave results from the doubling of dura mater because dura from the posterior cranial fossa continues to ensheath the fifth nerve structures as they pass anteriorly beneath the dura of the middle cranial fossa. The motor root emerges from the pons cephalad to the oncoming sensory root and traverses the trigeminal ganglion on its medial side, as does the greater superficial petrosal nerve. The ophthalmic division differentiates the earliest, and it maintains its identity from the maxillary and mandibular segments within the ganglion topographically, separated by a depression (Fig. 1.91).

The ophthalmic nerve traverses the cavernous sinus on its lateral side to lie between the trochlear nerve above and the maxillary nerve below. Within the cavernous sinus, the ophthalmic nerve receives a recurrent branch from the dura and proprioceptive branches from the third, fourth, and sixth motor nerves. Sympathetic nerve fibers also join the ophthalmic nerve. At the anterior end of the cavernous sinus, the nerve terminates in the lacrimal, frontal, and nasociliary nerves.

The maxillary nerve travels in close proximity to the posterior cavernous sinus before entering the foramen rotundum. It is in close association with the carotid artery, whereas the ophthalmic division is cushioned by intervening sinus venous blood spaces [218].

Carotid and Intracranial Ophthalmic Arteries

The carotid artery enters the cranial cavity through the carotid canal and passes over the foramen lacerum to lie on the lateral side of the sphenoid body (Fig. 1.92). Here, it causes a depression in the lateral wall of the sphenoid sinus as it traverses the medial cavernous sinus. Medial to the anterior clinoid process, the artery arches upward and backward (carotid siphon) to enter the middle cranial fossa. The carotid siphon lies in the cavernous sinus medial to the cranial nerves. Just before dividing into the anterior and middle cerebral branches, it gives rise to the ophthalmic artery. Whitnall notes that the caliber of the carotid artery drops from 5.4 mm at the cavernous sinus entry to 3.8 mm distal to the origin of the ophthalmic artery [3]. He postulated that the increased pressure before the constriction may aid blood flow to the important ophthalmic artery. The ophthalmic

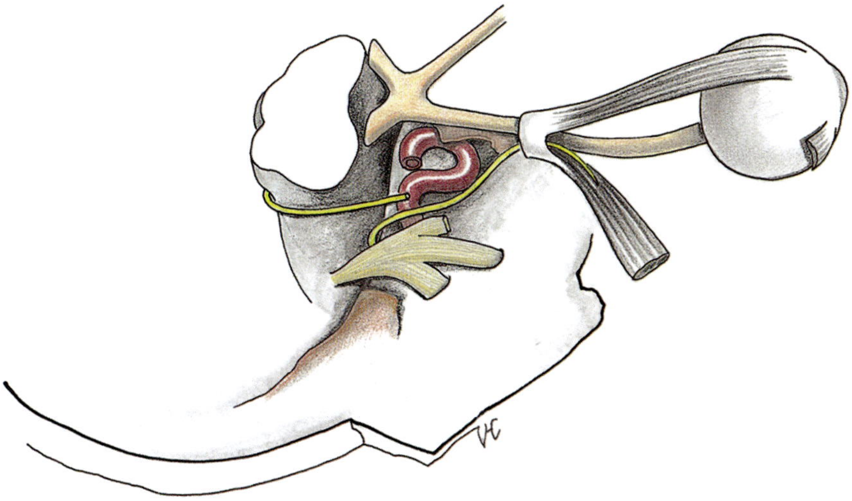

Fig. 1.90 Schematic drawing of abducens nerve course to emphasize sharp angle formed when passing under petrosphenoidal ligament. Note close association with carotid artery while abducens nerve is in posterior cavernous sinus

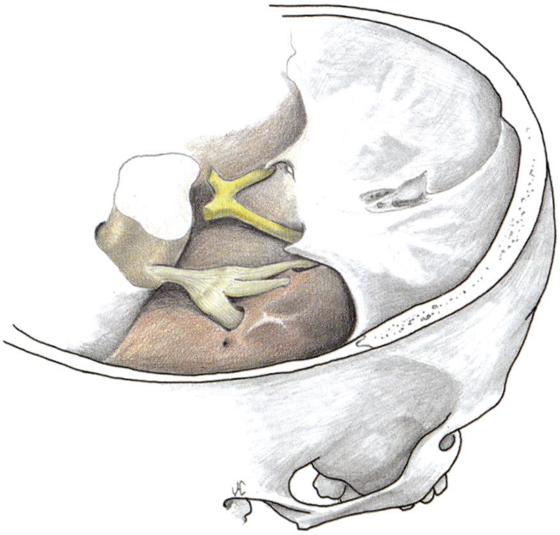

Fig. 1.91 Trigeminal ganglion. Ophthalmic division enters orbit through superior orbital fissure to form lacrimal, frontal, and nasociliary nerves. Maxillary division exits skull through foramen rotundum and enters orbit through inferior orbital fissure as infraorbital and zygomatic nerves

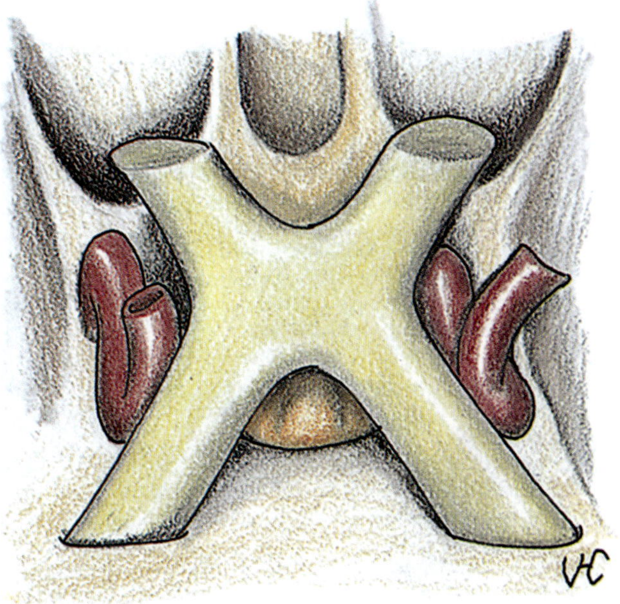

Fig. 1.93 Optic chiasm

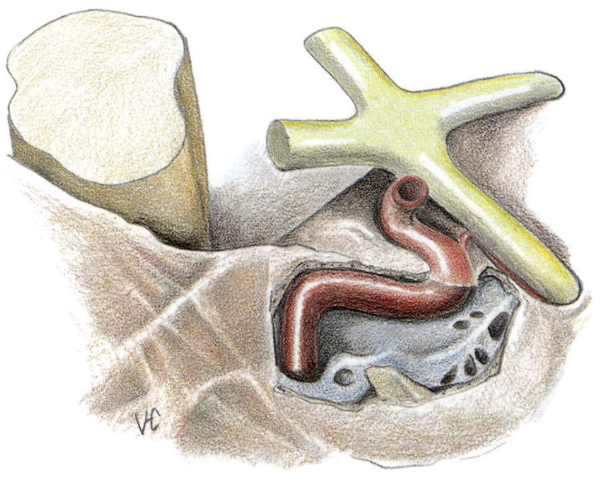

Fig. 1.92 Carotid artery. Cavernous sinus structures have been stripped away

artery passes anteriorly, entering the optic foramen below the optic nerve before exiting the canal inferolateral to the nerve.

Optic Chiasm

The optic chiasm location above the body of the sphenoid is subject to variation. It usually rests directly above the dorsum sellae but may be positioned either anterior or posterior to the dorsum sellae. This variability accounts for the different patterns of visual field loss resulting from pituitary lesions. The chiasm is separated from the diaphragm sellae by the subarachnoid basal cistern in which it resides covered by pia mater (Fig. 1.93). The third ventricle is located above the chiasm. The carotid artery rises along the lateral side of the chiasm to divide into middle and anterior cerebral arteries.

References

1. Mann I. The development of the human eye. New York: Grune & Stratton; 1950.
2. Blechschmidt E, Gasser RF. Biokinetics and biodynamics of human differentiation. Springfield: Charles C Thomas; 1978. p. 130.
3. Whitnall SE. The anatomy of the human orbit and accessory organs of vision. 2nd ed. New York: Oxford University Press; 1932.
4. Webster RC, et al. Supraorbital and supratrochlear notches and foramina: anatomical variations and surgical relevance. Laryngoscope. 1986;96:311.
5. Wulc AE, Adams JL, Dryden RM. Cerebrospinal fluid leakage complicating exenteration. Arch Ophthalmol. 1989;107:827.
6. Diamond MK. Homologies of the meningeal-orbital arteries of humans: a reappraisal. J Anat. 1991;178:223.
7. Whitnall SE. On a tubercle on the malar bone, and on the lateral attachments of the tarsal plates. J Anat Physiol. 1911; 45:426.
8. Jo A, Rizen V, Nikolic V, Banovic B. The role of orbital wall morphological properties in the etiology of "blow-out" fractures. Surg Radiol Anat. 1989;11:241.
9. Kurihashi K, Yamashita A. Anatomical consideration for dacryocystorhinostomy. Ophthalmologica. 1991;203:1.
10. Natori Y, Rhoton AL. Microsurgical anatomy of the superior orbital fissure. Neurosurgery. 1995;36:762.
11. Bansberg SF, Harner SG, Forbes G. Relationship of the optic nerve to the paranasal sinuses as shown by computed tomography. Otolaryngol Head Neck Surg. 1987;96:331.
12. Goalwin HA. One thousand optic canals. JAMA. 1927;89:1745.
13. Goldberg RA, Hannani K, Toga AW. Microanatomy of the orbital apex: computed tomography and microcryoplaning of soft and hard tissue. Ophthalmology. 1992;99:1447.
14. Rochels R. Holographic deformation analysis of the optic canal in blunt cranial trauma. Fortschr Ophthalmol. 1990;87:182.
15. Cares HL, Bakay L. The clinical significance of the optic strut. J Neurosurg. 1971;34:355.
16. Blanton PL, Biggs NL. Eighteen hundred years of controversy: the paranasal sinuses. Am J Anat. 1969;124:135.
17. Langman J. Medical embryology. 2nd ed. Baltimore: Williams & Wilkins; 1969. p. 355.
18. Bridger MWM, VanNostrand AWP. The nose and paranasal sinuses – applied surgical anatomy. J Otolaryngol. 1978;7:2.
19. Ritter FN. The paranasal sinuses, anatomy and technique. 2nd ed. CV Mosby: St. Louis; 1978.
20. Serdahl CL, Berris CE, Chole RA. Nasolacrimal duct obstruction after endoscopic sinus surgery. Arch Ophthalmol. 1990; 108:391.
21. Penne RB, et al. Ocular motility disorders secondary to sinus surgery. Ophthal Plast Reconstr Surg. 1993;9:53.
22. Bolger WE, et al. Lacrimal drainage system injury in functional endoscopic sinus surgery. Arch Otolaryngol Head Neck Surg. 1992;118:1179.
23. Bailey JH. Surgical anatomy of the lacrimal sac. Am J Ophthalmol. 1923;6:665.
24. Hinton P, Hurwitz JJ, Cruickshank B. Nasolacrimal bone changes in diseases of the lacrimal drainage system. Ophthalmic Surg. 1984;15:516.
25. Patton JM. Regional anatomy of the tear sac. Ann Otol Rhinol Laryngol. 1923;32:58.
26. Whitnall SE. The relations of the lacrimal fossa to the ethmoidal cells. Ophthalmic Rev. 1911;30:321.
27. Whitnall SE. The nasolacrimal canal: the extent to which it is influenced by the maxilla, and the influence of this upon its calibre. Ophthalmoscope. 1912;10:557.
28. deHaan AB, Willekens BL. Embryology of the orbital walls: a preliminary report. Proceedings of the 2nd international symposium on orbital disorders, Amsterdam, 1973. Mod Prob Ophthalmol. 1975;14:57.
29. Mishima S. Some physiologic aspects of the precorneal tear film. Arch Ophthalmol. 1965;73:233.
30. Mathers WD, Daley TE. Tear flow and evaporation in patients with and without dry eye. Ophthalmology. 1996;103:664.
31. Mathers WD. Ocular evaporation in meibomian gland dysfunction and dry eye. Ophthalmology. 1993;100:347.
32. Ford LC, Delange RJ, Petty RW. Identification of a nonlysozymal bactericidal factor (beta lysin) in human tears and aqueous humor. Am J Ophthalmol. 1976;81:30.
33. Hurwitz JJ. The lacrimal system. Philadelphia: Lippincott-Raven; 1996. p. 331.
34. Lemp MA, Dohlman CH, Holly FJ. Corneal desiccation despite normal tear volume. Ann Ophthalmol. 1970;2:258.
35. Jones LT. The lacrimal secretory system and its treatment. Am J Ophthalmol. 1966;62:47.
36. Jordan A, Baum J. Basic tear flow. Does it exist? Ophthalmology. 1980;87:920–30.
37. Scherz W, Dohlman CH. Is the lacrimal gland dispensable? Keratoconjunctivitis sicca after lacrimal gland removal. Arch Ophthalmol. 1975;93:281.
38. Holly FJ, Lemp MD. Tear physiology and dry eyes. Surv Ophthalmol. 1977;22:69.
39. Lemp MA, Hamill JR. Factors affecting tear film break-up in normal eyes. Arch Ophthalmol. 1973;89:103.
40. Iwamoto T, Jakobiec FA. Lacrimal glands. In: Jakobiec F, editor. Ocular anatomy, embryology, and teratology. New York: Harper & Row; 1982. p. 762.
41. Smith B, Petrelli R. Surgical repair of the prolapsed lacrimal gland. Arch Ophthalmol. 1978;96:113.
42. Roen JL, Stasior OG, Jakobiec FA. Aging changes in the human lacrimal gland: role of the ducts. CLAO J. 1985;11:237.
43. Obata H, et al. Histopathologic study of human lacrimal gland: statistical analysis with special reference to aging. Ophthalmology. 1995;102:678.
44. Ruskell GL. The distribution of autonomic post-ganglionic nerve fibers to the lacrimal gland in monkeys. J Anat. 1971;109:229.
45. Botelho SY, Hisada M, Fuenmayor N. Functional innervation of the lacrimal gland in the cat. Arch Ophthalmol. 1966;76:581.
46. Whitwell J. Denervation of the lacrimal gland. Br J Ophthalmol. 1958;42:518.
47. Ruskin SL. Control of tearing by blocking the nasal ganglion. Arch Ophthalmol. 1930;4:208.
48. Riley CM, et al. Central autonomic dysfunction with defective lacrimation. Pediatrics. 1949;3:468.
49. Sevel D. Development and congenital abnormalities of the nasolacrimal apparatus. J Pediatr Ophthalmol Strabismus. 1981;18:13.
50. Carter KD, Nelson CC, Martonyi CL. Size variation of the lacrimal punctum in adults. Ophthal Plast Reconstr Surg. 1988;4:231.
51. Gosain AK, et al. Surgical anatomy of the SMAS: a reinvestigation. Plast Reconstr Surg. 1993;92:1254.
52. Homer WE. Description of a small muscle at the internal commissure of the eyelids. J Med Phys Sci. 1824;8:70.
53. Aubaret E. The valves of the lacrymonasal passages. Arch Ophthalmol. 1908;28:211.
54. Tucker NA, Tucker SM, Linberg JV. The anatomy of the common canaliculus. Arch Ophthalmol. 1996;114:1231.
55. Ahl NC, Hill JD. Horner's muscle and the lacrimal system. Arch Ophthalmol. 1982;100:488.
56. Jones LT, Wobig JL. Surgery of the eyelids and lacrimal system. Birmingham: Aesculapius; 1976.
57. Masi AV. Congenital fistula of the lacrimal sac. Arch Ophthalmol. 1969;81:701.

58. Cassady JV. Developmental anatomy of nasolacrimal duct. Arch Ophthalmol. 1952;47:141.
59. Ffooks OO. Dacryocystitis in infancy. Br J Ophthalmol. 1962;46:422.
60. Petersen RA, Robb RM. The natural course of congenital obstruction of the nasolacrimal duct. J Pediatr Ophthalmol Strabismus. 1978;15:246.
61. Kushner BJ. Congenital nasolacrimal system obstruction. Arch Ophthalmol. 1982;100:597.
62. Robb RM. Probing and irrigation for congenital nasolacrimal duct obstruction. Arch Ophthalmol. 1986;104:378.
63. Kirk RC. Developmental anomalies of the lacrimal passages: a review of the literature and presentation of three unusual cases. Am J Ophthalmol. 1956;42:227.
64. Lemke BN, Stasior OG. Eyebrow incision making. Adv Ophthalmic Plast Reconstr Surg. 1983;2:19.
65. Lemke BN, Stasior OG. The anatomy of eyebrow ptosis. Arch Ophthalmol. 1982;100:981.
66. Mitz V, Peyronie M. The superficial musculoaponeurotic system (SMAS) in the parotid and cheek area. Plast Reconstr Surg. 1976;58:80.
67. Jost G, Levet Y. Parotid fascia and face lifting: a critical evaluation of the SMAS concept. Plast Reconstr Surg. 1984;74:42.
68. Thaller SR, et al. The submuscular aponeurotic system (SMAS): a histologic and comparative anatomy evaluation. Plast Reconstr Surg. 1990;86:690.
69. Kikkawa DO, Lemke BN, Dortzbach RK. Relations of the superficial musculoaponeurotic system to the orbit and characterization of the orbitomalar ligament. Ophthal Plast Reconstr Surg. 1996;12:77.
70. Har-Shai Y, et al. Mechanical properties and microstructure of the superficial musculoaponeurotic system. Plast Reconstr Surg. 1996;98:59.
71. Charpy A. Le coussinet adipeux du sourcil. Bibl Anat. 1909;19:47.
72. Putterman AM, Urist MJ. Surgical anatomy of the orbital septum. Ann Ophthalmol. 1974;6:290.
73. McCord CD, Doxanas MT. Browplasty and browpexy: an adjunct to blepharoplasty. Plast Reconstr Surg. 1990;86:248.
74. Stasior OG, Lemke BN. The posterior eyebrow fixation. Adv Ophthalmic Plast Reconstr Surg. 1983;2:193.
75. Knize D. An anatomically based study of the mechanism of eyebrow ptosis. Plast Reconstr Surg. 1996;97:1321.
76. Lemke BN, Stasior OG. Eyebrow considerations in blepharoptosis. Adv Ophthalmic Plast Reconstr Surg. 1982;1:55.
77. Barnes HO. Frown disfigurement and ptosis of the eyebrow. Plast Reconstr Surg. 1959;19:337.
78. Castanares S. Forehead wrinkles: glabellar frown and ptosis of the eye-brows. Plast Reconstr Surg. 1964;31:106.
79. Johnson C, Anderson J, Katz R. The brow lift, 1978. Arch Otolaryngol. 1979;105:124.
80. Spira M, Hardy S. The brow lift. In: Conley J, Dickerson J, editors. Plastic and reconstructive surgery of the face and neck: first international symposium, vol. 1. New York: Grune & Stratton; 1970. p. 17–20.
81. Vinas J. Forehead rhytidoplasty and brow lifting. Plast Reconstr Surg. 1976;57:445.
82. Hargiss JL. Surgical anatomy of the eyelids. Trans Pac Coast Otolaryngol Soc. 1963;44:193.
83. Cartwright MJ, et al. Measurements of upper eyelid and eyebrow dimensions in healthy white individuals. Am J Ophthalmol. 1994;117:231.
84. Gavaris P. Editor's note: the lid crease. Adv Ophthalmic Plast Reconstr Surg. 1982;1:89.
85. Doxanas MT, Anderson RL. Clinical orbital anatomy. William & Wilkins: Baltimore; 1984.
86. Johnson CC. Epicanthus and epiblepharon. Arch Ophthalmol. 1978;96:1030.
87. Lemke BN, Stasior OG. Epiblepharon: an important and often missed diagnosis. Clin Pediatr. 1981;20:661.
88. Spivey BE, Allen L, Stewart W. Surgical correction of superior sulcus deformity occurring after enucleation. Am J Ophthalmol. 1976;82:365.
89. Dutton JJ. Atlas of clinical and surgical orbital anatomy. Philadelphia: WB Saunders; 1994. p. 116.
90. Jones LT. An anatomical approach to the problems of the eyelids and lacrimal apparatus. Arch Ophthalmol. 1961;66:111.
91. Duverney M. Oeuvres anatomiques. Paris: Biblioteque Nationale de France; 1761. p. 130.
92. Becker BB. Tricompartment model of the lacrimal pump mechanism. Ophthalmology. 1992;99:1139.
93. Jones LT. Epiphora: its causes and new surgical procedures for its cure. Am J Ophthalmol. 1954;38:824.
94. Wulc AE, Dryden RM, Khatchaturian T. Where is the gray line? Arch Ophthalmol. 1987;105:1092.
95. Aiche AE, Ramirez OH. The suborbicularis oculi fat pads: an anatomic and clinical study. Plast Reconstr Surg. 1995;95:37.
96. Anderson RL. The medial canthal tendon branches out. Arch Ophthalmol. 1977;95:2051.
97. Williams PL, Warwick R, editors. Gray's anatomy. 36th ed. Philadelphia: WB Saunders; 1980. p. 531.
98. Sullivan TJ, Welham RAN, Collin JRO. Centurion syndrome: idiopathic anterior displacement of the medial canthus. Ophthalmology. 1993;100:328.
99. Hill JC. Treatment of epiphora owing to flaccid eyelids. Arch Ophthalmol. 1979;97:323.
100. Jacobs HB. Epiphora due to weak lid muscles. Br J Ophthalmol. 1959;43:332.
101. Hill JC. An analysis of senile changes in the palpebral fissure. Can J Ophthalmol. 1975;10:32.
102. Ousterhout DK, Weil RB. The role of the lateral canthal tendon in lower eyelid laxity. Plast Reconstr Surg. 1982;69:620.
103. Jones LT. The anatomy of the lower eyelid and its relations to the cause and cure of ectropion. Am J Ophthalmol. 1960; 49:29.
104. Gioia VM, Linberg JV, McCormick SM. The anatomy of the lateral canthal tendon. Arch Ophthalmol. 1987;105:529.
105. Kestenbaum A. Applied anatomy of the eye. New York: Grune & Stratton; 1963. p. 264.
106. Jones LT. A new concept of the orbital fascia and rectus muscle sheaths and its surgical implications. Trans Am Acad Ophthalmol Otolaryngol. 1968;72:755.
107. Lemke BN, Stasior OG, Rosenberg PN. The surgical relations of the levator palpebrae superioris muscle. Ophthal Plast Reconstr Surg. 1988;4:25.
108. Sevel D. Ptosis and underaction of the superior rectus muscle. Ophthalmology. 1984;91:1080.
109. Frueh BR, Musch DC. Levator force generation in normal subjects. Trans Am Ophthalmol Soc. 1990;88:109.
110. Frueh BR, Musch DC. Evaluation of levator muscle integrity in ptosis with levator force measurement. Ophthalmology. 1996;103:244.
111. Whitnall SE. On a ligament acting as a check to the action of the levator palpebrae superioris. J Anat Physiol. 1910;14:131.
112. Anderson RL, Dixon RS. The role of Whitnall's ligament in ptosis surgery. Arch Ophthalmol. 1979;97:705.
113. Goldberg RA, et al. Eyelid anatomy revisited. Dynamic high-resolution images of Whitnall's ligament and upper eyelid structures with the use of a surface coil. Arch Ophthalmol. 1992;110:1598.
114. Shore JW, McCord CD. Anatomic changes in involutional blepharoptosis. Am J Ophthalmol. 1984;98:21.
115. Codere F, Tucker NA, Renaldi B. The anatomy of Whitnall ligament. Ophthalmology. 1995;102:2016.

116. Anderson RL, Beard C. The levator aponeurosis attachments and their clinical significance. Arch Ophthalmol. 1977;95:1437.
117. Whitnall SE. The levator palpebrae superioris muscle: the attachments and relations of its aponeurosis. Ophthalmoscope. 1914;12:258.
118. Siegel R. Surgical anatomy of the upper eyelid fascia. Ann Plast Surg. 1984;13:263.
119. Collin JRO, Beard C, Wood I. Experimental and clinical data on the insertion of the levator palpebrae superioris muscle. Am J Ophthalmol. 1978;85:792.
120. Stasior GO, Lemke BN, Wallow IH, Dortzbach RK. Levator aponeurosis elastic fiber network. Ophthal Plast Reconstr Surg. 1993;9:1.
121. Dortzbach RK, Sutula FC. Involutional blepharoptosis: a histopathological study. Arch Ophthalmol. 1980;98:2045.
122. Kuwabara T, Cogan DG, Johnson CC. Structure of the muscles of the upper eyelid. Arch Ophthalmol. 1975;93:1189.
123. Collin JRO, Beard C, Wood I. Terminal course of nerve supply to Muller's muscle in the rhesus monkey and its clinical significance. Am J Ophthalmol. 1979;87:234.
124. Manson PN, et al. Pathways of sympathetic innervation to the superior and inferior (Muller's) tarsal muscle. Plast Reconstr Surg. 1986;78:33.
125. Lyon DB, et al. Sympathetic nerve anatomy in the cavernous sinus and retrobulbar orbit of the cynomolgous monkey. Ophthal Plast Reconstr Surg. 1992;8:1.
126. Lemke BN. Anatomic considerations in upper eyelid retraction. Ophthal Plast Reconstr Surg. 1991;7:158.
127. Chafflin J, Putterman AM. Muller's muscle excision and levator recession in retracted upper lid: treatment of thyroid-related retraction. Arch Ophthalmol. 1979;97:1487.
128. Lemke BN, Shovlin JP. Thyroid eye disease. In: Dortzbach R, editor. Ophthalmic plastic surgery: prevention and management of complications. New York: Raven Press; 1994. p. 402.
129. Hawes MJ, Dortzbach RK. The microscopic anatomy of the lower eyelid retractors. Arch Ophthalmol. 1982;100:1313.
130. Goldberg RA, et al. Physiology of the lower eyelid retractors: tight linkage of the anterior capsulopalpebral fascia demonstrated using dynamic ultrafine surface coil MRI. Ophthal Plast Reconstr Surg. 1994;10:87.
131. Wesley RE, McCord CD, Jones NA. Height of the tarsus of the lower eyelid. Am J Ophthalmol. 1980;90:102.
132. Liu D, Stasior OG. Lower eyelid laxity and ocular symptoms. Am J Ophthalmol. 1983;95:545.
133. Culbertson WW, Ostler HB. The floppy eyelid syndrome. Am J Ophthalmol. 1981;92:568.
134. Netland PA, Sugrue SP, Albert DM, Shore JW. Histopathologic features of the floppy eyelid syndrome. Involvement of tarsal elastin. Ophthalmology. 1994;101:174.
135. Jester JV, Nicolaides N, Smith RE. Meibomian gland studies: histologic and ultrastructural investigations. Invest Ophthalmol Vis Sci. 1981;20:537.
136. Scheie HG, Albert DM. Distichiasis and trichiasis: origin and management. Am J Ophthalmol. 1966;61:718.
137. Jones LT, Reeh MJ, Tsujimura JK. Senile entropion. Am J Ophthalmol. 1963;55:463.
138. Tse DT, Anderson RL, Fratkin JD. Aponeurosis disinsertion in congenital entropion. Arch Ophthalmol. 1983;101:436.
139. Stock AL, Collins HP, Davidson TM. Anatomy of the superficial temporal artery. Head Neck Surg. 1980;2:466.
140. Tucker SM, Lindberg JV. Vascular anatomy of the eyelid. Ophthalmology. 1994;101:1118.
141. Huber E. Zur morphology der supraorbital und glabellarmuskulatur des menschen. Experimentelle bestimmung der innervation des M. procerus nasi. Anatomischer Anseiger. 1926/7;62:25.
142. Stuzin JM, et al. Anatomy of the frontal branch of the facial nerve: the significance of the temporal fat pad. Plast Reconstr Surg. 1989;83:265.
143. Knize DM. A study of the supraorbital nerve. Plast Reconstr Surg. 1995;96:564.
144. Gasser RF. The development of facial muscles in man. Am J Anat. 1967;120:357.
145. Sevel D. A reappraisal of the development of the eyelids. Eye. 1988;2:123.
146. Barber AN. Embryology of the human eye. CV Mosby: St Louis; 1955.
147. Koornneef L. Spatial aspects of orbital musculo-fibrous tissue in man: a new anatomical and histological approach. Amsterdam: Swets and Zeitlinger; 1977.
148. Koornneef L. Orbital septa: anatomy and function. Ophthalmology. 1979;86:876.
149. Sutton JE. The fascia of the human orbit. Anat Rec. 1920;18:141.
150. Hosakawa H. A note on the fibrous apparatus surrounding the human eyeball. Okajimas Folia Anat Jpn. 1956;28:165.
151. Goodall KL, et al. Enlargement of the tensor intermuscularis muscle in Graves' ophthalmopathy. Arch Ophthalmol. 1995;113:1286.
152. Fink WH. An anatomical study of the check mechanism of the vertical muscles of the eyes. Am J Ophthalmol. 1957;44:800.
153. Lockwood CB. The anatomy of the muscles, ligaments, and fasciae of the orbit, including an account of the capsule of Tenon, the check ligaments of the recti, and of the suspensory ligament of the eye. J Anat Physiol. 1886;20:1.
154. Long JA, Baylis HI. Hypoglobus following orbital decompression for dysthyroid ophthalmopathy. Ophthal Plast Reconstr Surg. 1990;6:185.
155. Manson PN, et al. Mechanisms of global support and posttraumatic enophthalmos: I. The anatomy of the ligament sling and its relation to intramuscular cone orbital fat. Plast Reconstr Surg. 1986;77:193.
156. Goldberg RA, Shorr N, Cohen MS. The medial orbital strut in the prevention of postdecompression dystopia in dysthyroid ophthalmopathy. Ophthal Plast Reconstr Surg. 1992;1992(8):32.
157. Koornneef L. New insights in the human orbital connective tissue: results of a new anatomic approach. Arch Ophthalmol. 1977;95:1269.
158. Koornneef L. Eyelid and orbital fascial attachments and their clinical significance. Eye. 1988;2:130.
159. Kronish JW, et al. The pathophysiology of the anophthalmic socket. Part I. Analysis of orbital blood flow. Ophthal Plast Reconstr Surg. 1990;6:77.
160. Hudson HL, Levin L, Feldon SE. Graves' exophthalmos unrelated to extraocular muscle enlargement. Ophthalmology. 1991;98:1495.
161. Kronish JW, et al. The pathophysiology of the anophthalmic socket. Part II. Analysis of orbital fat. Ophthal Plast Reconstr Surg. 1990;6:88.
162. Neely KA, Ernest JT, Mottier M. Combined superior oblique paresis and Brown's syndrome after blepharoplasty. Am J Ophthalmol. 1990;109:347.
163. Wesley RE, Pollard SF, McCord CD. Superior oblique paresis after blepharoplasty. Plast Reconstr Surg. 1980;66:283.
164. Castanares S. Blepharoplasty for herniated intraorbital fat: anatomical basis for a new approach. Plast Reconstr Surg. 1951;8:46.
165. Barker DE. Dye injection studies of intraorbital fat components. Plast Reconstr Surg. 1977;59:82.
166. Jordan DR, Anderson RL, Thiese SM. Avoiding inferior oblique injury during lower blepharoplasty. Arch Ophthalmol. 1989;107:1382.
167. Kruger P. Die innervation der tetanischen and tonischen fasern der quergestreiften skelettmusculatur der wierbeltiere. Anat Anaz. 1949;97:169.

168. Eggers HM. Functional anatomy of the extraocular muscles. In: Jakobiec F, editor. Ocular anatomy, embryology, and teratology. New York: Harper & Row; 1982. p. 783.
169. Apt L. An anatomic reevaluation of rectus muscle insertions. Trans Am Ophthalmol Soc. 1980;78:365.
170. Fink WH. The surgical anatomy of the superior oblique muscle. Trans Am Ophthalmol Soc. 1948;46:154.
171. Helveston EM, et al. The trochlea: a study of the anatomy and physiology. Ophthalmology. 1982;89:124.
172. Sacks JG. The shape of the trochlea. Arch Ophthalmol. 1984;102:932.
173. Porter JD, et al. Extraocular muscles: basic and clinical aspects of structure and function. Surv Ophthalmol. 1995;39:451.
174. Fledelius HC, Stubgaard M. Changes in eye position during growth and adult life based on exophthalmometry, interpupillary distance, and orbital distance measurements. Acta Ophthalmol (Copenh). 1986;64:481.
175. Warwick R. Eugene Wolff s anatomy of the eye and orbit. 7th ed. Philadelphia: WB Saunders; 1976.
176. Dailey RW, Robertson WD, Rootman J. Globe tenting: a sign of increased orbital tension. Am J Neuroradiol. 1989;10:181.
177. Dolman PJ, et al. Mechanisms of visual loss in severe proptosis. Ophthal Plast Reconstr Surg. 1991;7:256.
178. Drysdale DB. Experimental subdural retrobulbar injection of anesthetic. Ann Ophthalmol. 1984;16:716.
179. Hornblass A. Pupillary dilation in fractures of the floor of the orbit. Ophthalmic Surg. 1979;10:44.
180. Abad JM, Alvarez F, Blazquez MG. An unrecognized neurological syndrome: sixth-nerve palsy and Homer's syndrome due to traumatic intracavernous carotid aneurysm. Surg Neurol. 1981;16:140.
181. Hartmann B, et al. Cavernous sinus infection manifested by Horner's syndrome and ipsilateral sixth nerve palsy. J Clin Neuroophthalmol. 1987;7:223.
182. Jordan DR. The nerves intermedius. Arch Ophthalmol. 1993;111:1691.
183. Sinnreich Z, Nathan H. The ciliary ganglion in man (anatomical observations). Anat Anz. 1981;150:287.
184. Hayreh SS, Dass R. The ophthalmic artery. I. Origin and intracranial and intracanalicular course. Br J Ophthalmol. 1962;46:65.
185. Bergen MP. A literature review of the vascular system in the human orbit. Acta Morphol Neerl Scand. 1981;19:273.
186. Hayreh SS. The ophthalmic artery. III. Branches. Br J Ophthalmol. 1962;46:212.
187. Singh S, Dass R. The central artery of the retina. Br J Ophthalmol. 1960;44:193.
188. Pearson BW, Mackenzie RG, Goodman WS. The anatomical basis of transantral ligation of the maxillary artery in severe epistaxis. Laryngoscope. 1969;79:969.
189. Bergen MP. A spatial reconstruction of the orbital vascular pattern in relation with the connective tissue system. Acta Morphol Neerl Scand. 1982;20:117.
190. Bergen MP. Relationship between arteries and veins and the connective tissue system in the human orbit, parts I, II, and III. Acta Morphol Neerl Scand. 1982;20:1.
191. Bergen MP. Microvessels in the human orbit in relation to the connective tissue system. Acta Morphol Neerl Scand. 1982; 20:139.
192. Rojanapongpun P, Drance SM. Velocity of ophthalmic arterial flow re-corded by Doppler ultrasound in normal subjects. Am J Ophthalmol. 1993;115:174.
193. Greenfield DS, Heggerick PA, Hedges TR. Color Doppler imaging of normal orbital vasculature. Ophthalmology. 1995; 102:1598.
194. Jordan DR. The orbital muscle of Muller. Arch Ophthalmol. 1992;110:1798.
195. Duke-Elder S, Wybar KC. The anatomy of the visual system. St. Louis: CV Mosby; 1961. p. 479.
196. Wolter JR, Roosenberg RJ. Ectopic lymph node of the orbit simulating a lacrimal gland tumor. Am J Ophthalmol. 1977;83:908.
197. Millen JW, Woollam DHM. The reticular perivascular tissue of the central nervous system. J Neurol Neurosurg Psychiatry. 1954;17:286.
198. Foldi M, et al. Lymphogenic haemongiopathy. Angiologica. 1968;5:250.
199. Gruntzig J, Huth F. Studien zur lymphdrainage des auges: 3 untersu-chungen zum tuscheabfluss aus dem glaskorper nach beidseitiger zer-vikaler lymphblockade. Klin Monatsbl Augenheilk. 1977;171:774.
200. Gruntzig J, et al. Abfluss der radioaktiven lymphpflichtigen substan-zen Au-198-kolloid und Tc-99 m-schwefelkolloid aus der orbita des kan-inchens. Graefes Arch Klin Exp Ophthalmol. 1977;204:161.
201. Gruntzig J, et al. Studien zur lymphdrainage des auges: 2. Abfluss lymphpflichtiger radioaktiver indicatoren aus der vorderkammer. Klin Monatsbl Augenheilk. 1977;171:571.
202. Gruntzig J, et al. Studien zur lymphdrainage des auges: 4. Abfluss lymphpflichtiger radioaktiver tracer (99mTC-mikrokolloid) nach intra-virtealar injektion. Klin Monatsbl Augenheilk. 1978;172:87.
203. Gruntzig J, et al. Studien zur lymphdrainage des auges: 5. Quantitative erfassung des lymphtransportes ans dem subkonjunctivalraum mit einem radioaktiven tracer. Klin Monatsbl Augenheilk. 1978;172:872.
204. Sherman DD, et al. Identification of orbital lymphatics: enzyme and histochemical light microscopic and electron microscopic studies. Ophthal Plast Reconstr Surg. 1993;9:153.
205. Werner JA, et al. Description and importance of lymphatics of the vocal fold. Otolaryngology. 1990;102:13.
206. Harris FS, Rhoton AL. Anatomy of the cavernous sinus: a microsurgical study. J Neurosurg. 1976;45:169.
207. Umansky F, Nathan H. The lateral wall of the cavernous sinus with special reference to the nerves related to it. J Neurosurg. 1982;56:228.
208. Umansky F, Valarezo A, Elidan J. The superior wall of the cavernous sinus: a microanatomical study. J Neurosurg. 1994;81:914.
209. Kline LB, Acker JD, Post MJD. Computed tomographic evaluation of the cavernous sinus. Ophthalmology. 1982;89:374.
210. Kaplan HA, Browder J, Krieger AJ. Intercavernous connections of the cavernous sinuses: the superior and inferior circular sinuses. J Neurosurg. 1976;45:166.
211. Goldberg RA, et al. Management of cavernous sinus – dural fistulas. Arch Ophthalmol. 1996;114:707.
212. Grove AS. The dural shunt syndrome: pathophysiology and clinical course. Ophthalmology. 1984;91:31.
213. Dandy WE, Follis RH. On the pathology of carotid-cavernous aneurysms (pulsating exophthalmos). Am J Ophthalmol. 1941;24:365.
214. Meadows SP. Intracavernous aneurysms of the internal carotid artery: their clinical features and natural history. Arch Ophthalmol. 1959;62:56.
215. Barrat JOW. Observations on the structure of the third, fourth, and sixth cranial nerves. J Anat Physiol. 1901;35:214.
216. Wolff E. A bend in the sixth cranial nerve and its probable significance. Br J Ophthalmol. 1928;12:22.
217. Meltzer PE. Gradenigo's syndrome: anatomic aspects. Arch Otolaryngol. 1931;13:87.
218. Frazier DH, Whitehead E. The morphology of the gasserian ganglion. Brain. 1925;48:458.

Part II

General Considerations

Frank A. Nesi and Richard D. Lisman

Basic Principles of Ophthalmic Plastic Surgery

2

Shani Golan, Christopher I. Zoumalan, Frank A. Nesi, and Gary J. Lelli Jr.

Introduction

Ophthalmic plastic and reconstructive surgery combines the precision of ophthalmic microsurgery with plastic and reconstructive surgical principles, allowing for subspecialized care of the eyelid, orbital, and lacrimal system. A foundation in ophthalmology grants the oculoplastic surgeon the knowledge and skills to safely and successfully protect the globe while achieving functional and aesthetic results. Certain basic ophthalmic and plastic surgical considerations form the necessary framework for the successful practice of oculoplastic surgery.

Preparation of the Patient

Consistent surgical outcomes depend on optimal preoperative preparation and patient counseling. The patient's oculoplastic, ophthalmic, psychological, and general physical condition must be evaluated and documented. The surgeon needs to understand the concerns that have caused the patient to seek consultation. Every patient deserves a discussion of the goals of treatment (medical or surgical), along with an honest appraisal of the expected outcomes and potential pitfalls that may prevent the patient from achieving the desired results.

The patient's preoperative condition must be assessed and documented in a manner consistent with the risk and complexity of the proposed procedure. This may include a general physical examination, an ocular examination, and an ophthalmic plastic examination, as indicated. A typical preoperative oculoplastic evaluation includes a problem-specific examination of the eyes, eyelids, and adnexal structures. It may include specialized testing such as lacrimal probing and irrigation, ocular photography, or orbital imaging.

Laboratory and ancillary evaluation should adequately satisfy the patient's needs and be consistent with the diagnosis and planned intervention. This may include complete blood count (CBC), electrolyte panel, prothrombin time (PT), partial thromboplastin time (PTT), chest radiograph, electrocardiography, magnetic resonance imaging (MRI), and/or orbital computed tomography (CT).

Many nonorbital oculoplastic procedures are now performed with local anesthetic and intravenous sedation as needed, with monitored anesthesia care provided by an anesthesiologist. These cases may not require any ancillary testing if the patients are under 40 years of age and without a history of diabetes, diuretic use, or coagulopathy. In some instances, a CBC and coagulation panel is performed, depending on the patient's age and comorbidities and the proposed procedure. Patients who are diabetics require measurement of their glucose level. Patients on a diuretic need measurement of their potassium level. A recent electrocardiogram is usually necessary for patients older than 40 years. The same procedure performed in the office setting with local anesthesia and oral sedation usually does not require any laboratory evaluation.

When possible, medications that decrease clotting should be stopped before oculoplastic surgery. Ideally the patient is given a list of all aspirin-containing medications, both pre-

S. Golan (✉)
Division of Ophthalmic Plastic, Reconstructive, and Orbital Surgery, Department of Ophthalmology, Weill Cornell Medical College, New York-Presbyterian Hospital, New York, NY, USA

C. I. Zoumalan
Department of Ophthalmology, Division of Ophthalmic Plastic and Reconstructive Surgery, Keck School of Medicine of USC, Los Angeles, CA, USA

F. A. Nesi
Beaumont Eye Institute, William Beaumont School of Medicine of Oakland University, Rochester, MI, USA

Kresge Eye Institute, Wayne State University School of Medicine, Detroit, MI, USA
e-mail: llion1@comcast.net

G. J. Lelli Jr.
Weill Cornell Medical Center/New York-Presbyterian Hospital, Department of Ophthalmology, New York, NY, USA
e-mail: gjl9003@med.cornell.edu

J. J. Servat et al. (eds.), *Smith and Nesi's Ophthalmic Plastic and Reconstructive Surgery*,
https://doi.org/10.1007/978-3-030-41720-8_2

scription over the counter and homeopathic, and instructed not to use these for 1 or 2 weeks before surgery. However, for patients with certain medical conditions, such as a mechanical heart valve or cardiac stent, it is not always advisable to stop anticoagulation. Working in coordination with the patient's primary-care doctor or cardiologist will allow an individualized decision based upon the cardiac history and the surgical risk of bleeding [1, 2]. When abnormal bleeding cannot be avoided during surgery, the surgeon and the patient need to reevaluate the relative necessity of the surgery and the inherent risks involved.

All patients with periocular or remote trauma need to have their tetanus immunization status evaluated. Any patient who has been previously immunized for tetanus but was last immunized over 5 years ago needs to have a booster for tetanus toxoid. Any patient with a contaminated wound and no prior tetanus immunization needs to have a tetanus immune globulin injection immediately followed by a complete tetanus vaccination sequence.

Perioperative Antibiotics

Perioperative antibiotics have limited usefulness in most oculoplastic procedures. Infection is very unlikely following oculoplastic surgery, and preoperative antibiotics have not been demonstrated to reduce the incidence of postoperative infection in most oculoplastic procedures, and as such their uses among oculoplastic surgeons are not consistent [3, 4]. Although there is no consensus, antibiotics may be useful in cases of trauma, particularly bite wounds (with anerobic coverage needed), and in cases of preoperative infection. Antibiotic selection should be directed to the most likely category of bacterial contamination, such as gram-positive organisms from the skin and anaerobes from the sinuses. When deemed appropriate and if the patient is not allergic to penicillins or cephalosporins, 1 g of cefazolin covers the most common pathogens.

Skin Markings and Local Anesthesia

Many oculoplastic procedures require meticulous skin marking as a guide to incision making. It is commonly preferable to place incisions on natural skin creases or adjacent to anatomic structures to hide the scar. The skin marking should be done before local anesthesia is injected.

Local anesthesia with epinephrine should be used for all procedures to provide some hemostasis. The most commonly used local anesthetic mixture is 2% lidocaine with 1:100,000 epinephrine in combination with 0.5% bupivacaine. The anesthesia should be injected very slowly to minimize pain.

Incisions

Incisions in and around the eyelids demand precision but offer the attentive surgeon the possibility of completely hiding well-constructed wounds in the natural skin folds and creases around the eye [5, 6]. To make successful skin incisions into the eyelids requires an understanding of their muscular, fibrous, and vascular anatomy as well as that of all of the adjacent structures. It also requires knowledge of the surgical principles involved.

Whenever possible the incisions should be placed in or parallel to skin folds and skin tension lines. These skin lines often coincide with lines of facial expression and are especially prominent around the eyes. Subtle skin tension lines can be identified by compressing the skin at 90° angle and observing the indentation pattern. Incisions in or along periocular rhytids help decrease wound tension, thereby creating thinner scars (Fig. 2.1). Cutting the skin can be achieved using several instruments – scalpels, scissors, cautery, etc. (all discussed in detail in Chap. 4) – and each is used in specific circumstances to achieve the best postoperative anesthetic goal.

Lymphatic drainage from the eyelids can be adversely affected by poor incision placement. Poor lymphatic drainage can significantly delay wound healing and can lead to a suboptimal long-term result. The normal lymphatic channels of the eyelid extend obliquely, posteriorly, and inferiorly from the lateral eyelids to the preauricular and submandibu-

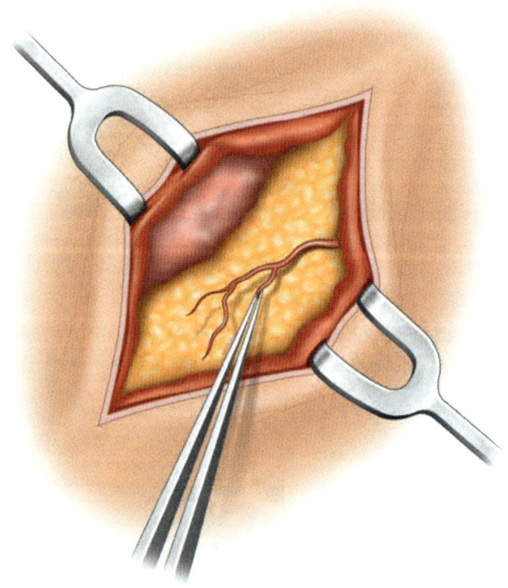

Fig. 2.1 Suggested incision sites in the periocular region

lar lymph nodes. Vertical incisions in the lateral canthus tend to disrupt the flow of lymph fluid and heal poorly. Vertical incisions in the medial canthus do not affect the lymphatics as much as those in the lateral canthus. Simultaneous vertical incisions in the medial and lateral canthal regions of the same eyelid may cause chronic eyelid lymphedema.

Retraction and Exposure

Exposure in the oculoplastic surgery is crucial in preforming the surgery and appropriate retraction is important to visualize the surgical field as the orbit is a small compartment.

It can be achieved primarily using the fingers as retractors. But other methods of retraction exist: skin hooks are available in different sizes and are used in eyelid surgery. Forceps are the most common instrument used to hold and retract tissues. Smooth forceps cause more trauma than forceps with teeth. Forceps with teeth offer better grip and less crushing of tissue.

Th majority of orbital surgery consists of separating tissue planes, rather than cutting. Meticulous learning of "pulling" techniques and separating tissues is required before preforming orbital surgery.

There are three types of retractors: self-retaining retractors, like the eyelid speculum; handheld retractors such as the Desmarres lid retractor, whose shape is perfect for a traumatically retracting tissue; and suture retractors, usually using the 4-0 silk suture.

Hemostasis

The eyelids and ocular adnexa are richly vascularized with arcades oriented in the eyelid in predictable locations. Although this generous blood supply reduces the risk of necrosis and infection, it makes perioperative hemostasis more difficult. Excessive bleeding obscures the surgical field and can prolong intraoperative time. The final surgical result may be delayed by hematoma, or the desired result may not be accomplished. Uncontrolled postoperative bleeding can lead to orbital hemorrhage and vision loss [7].

Preoperative

The possibility of abnormal bleeding always exists. Historical clues should be sought preoperatively such as easy bruising with minor trauma or excessive bleeding during prior surgery, including dental surgery. This issue must be thoroughly reviewed with the patient, who frequently may not recall this information even with specific prompting. The patient's medication list should be carefully evaluated, and nonsteroidal anti-inflammatory drugs should be stopped 3–5 days before surgery. Preoperative bleeding studies may be considered such as platelet count and a coagulation profile (PT/PTT/INR). In rare instances, a bleeding time may be beneficial.

Control of perioperative blood pressure is an important preventive measure to avoid excessive bleeding during and after surgery. This is best accomplished by having the patient take his or her usual medication with a small drink of water the morning of surgery. Of particular note, the patient should take their midday medications if they are on the afternoon surgery schedule. If necessary, the patient can be given an additional long-acting oral agent to control the blood pressure on arrival to the surgical preoperative holding area.

Additional systemic measures can decrease the chance of hemorrhage in the perioperative period. They include the use of Antitussive as needed and the use of antiemetics to prevent Valsalva during or after a procedure.

Careful attention to perioperative hemostasis is a critical element of any oculoplastic surgery. Injection of local anesthetic with a vasoconstrictor, such as epinephrine (1:100,000 or 1:200,000), is extremely helpful. It is important to pay particular attention to the time of injection, as epinephrine requires approximately 10 min for its effects to occur and has its maximal effect between 20 min and 60 min after injection. Ideally the critical part of the surgery will be completed within this time. Additionally, epinephrine significantly prolongs the action of lidocaine and other similar anesthetics. Phenylephrine is an acceptable alternative when epinephrine is contraindicated owing to cardiac or other reasons. It can be added to a local anesthetic to achieve similar hemostasis as epinephrine without as much cardiac stimulation.

Conjunctival and mucosal bleeding frequently can be minimized or prevented by proper preoperative planning. When a conjunctival incision is planned, the application of phenylephrine drops 20 min before the incision can frequently eliminate most if not all of the bleeding typically encountered from this type of incision. Likewise, the use of 0.5% phenylephrine nasal spray before a dacryocystorhinostomy can dramatically reduce the amount of nasal mucosal oozing.

Intraoperative

An easy way to control bleeding is sing a temponade with either finger, gause pad or q-tip. Compressing the bleeding tissue against bone will stop most bleedings. This is usually a temporary measure that will minimize blood loss and facilitate cautery usage.

Cautery is the mainstay of intraoperative hemostasis. It is targeted and works immediately. When used properly, it tends to cause minimal associated thermal damage while closing the bleeding vessels. There are three types of commonly used cautery: (1) hot wire, (2) high-frequency radio waves, and (3) laser. All three methods use heat to coagulate the blood vessel and adjacent tissue to stop the bleeding.

Hot-wire cautery is generally accomplished with a handheld, battery-operated instrument. They are available in low- and high-temperature varieties. Low-temperature cautery usually contains a single AA battery and reaches a temperature of 1000 °C. The wire does not glow red. It is often used for ocular and periocular surgery. The high-temperature cautery usually contains two AA batteries and reaches a temperature of 2200 °C. The wire glows orange red. The color of the tip glow indicates the temperature of the cautery; a bright orange is the maximum temperature. This temperature is helpful for dissection. Temperature and heat are different measures of the same phenomenon and should not be confused with each other. Temperature is determined by the relative speed of the molecules in an object. Heat is a product of the relative speed of the object's molecules and the object's mass. Although the two batteries in the cautery can raise the temperature of the wire to several thousand degrees, the total heat in the wire is small, even when the tip is glowing orange. Therefore it is important to apply the cautery with the tip glowing. This method allows maximum cauterization at the surface with minimal deep thermal effects. If the cautery is applied to the tissue before the wire glows orange, the cautery will be inefficient. The temperature does not rise much because the tissues absorb the extra energy and a deeper, less effective burn occurs that unnecessarily damages normal tissue.

High-frequency electrocautery is extremely useful in oculoplastic surgery. It is useful for dissecting as well as cauterizing tissue. The relative action of the instruments is controlled by the frequency and shape of the electrical wave that emanates from its tip. The power level controls the intensity of these effects. It can be used as a unipolar or bipolar instrument. In the unipolar mode, it is a very effective dissecting instrument and can coagulate vessels that are smaller than 1 mm in diameter by direct obliterative cautery. In the bipolar mode, it is a poor dissecting instrument but an unparalleled coagulator of larger vessels that are difficult to control with any other means. The bipolar mode seals larger vessels by also cauterizing and recruiting the surrounding connective tissue into the zone of coagulation and collagen shrinkage (Fig. 2.2).

Bipolar cautery is very helpful for shrinking prolapsed orbital fat. During orbital surgery, fat frequently prolapses into the surgical field. One option for managing this problem is bipolar cautery. The surface of the fat is lightly moistened with saline. The bipolar cautery power is set relatively low.

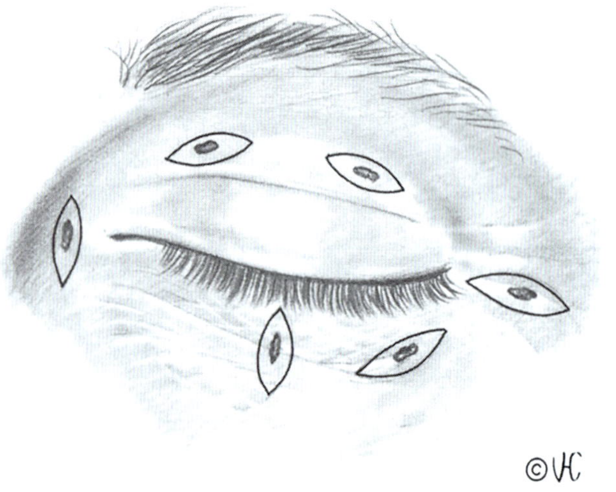

Fig. 2.2 Bipolar cautery is applied directly to a blood vessel after the forceps are placed in apposition

The tips are applied to the fat's surface in a painting motion with the power on and the waveform set to coagulate. The fat consistently contracts out of the field without the need to incise it and without the risk of causing bleeding.

The carbon dioxide laser can function as a scalpel or cautery, or both. When the laser's energy flux or density is very high, it vaporizes tissue without leaving any heat in the remaining tissue to coagulate it. In this fashion the laser makes an excellent scalpel, but there is tremendous bleeding associated with its use. Conversely, the laser can be adjusted to heat tissue without cutting it, but causing tissue necrosis from the thermal effects. Most of the time, the carbon dioxide laser is used to simultaneously cut and coagulate. The relative effects are controlled by varying the intensity and duration of the beam.

Adjuvant Agents

Some bleeding is so diffuse that cautery is impractical or unwise. This happens frequently with mucosal surface bleeding, especially when preoperative hemostasis has not been effective before a dacryocystorhinostomy. In these cases hemostasis is augmented nicely by several different materials. An excellent option is to utilize one of the charged collagen products such as Helistat or Collistat. These materials are sheets containing many ends of charged collagen simulating a cut tissue surface. These sheets strongly induce thrombogenesis. They may be left in the operative field, although some believe that a small inflammatory reaction may ensue. Other readily available materials include absorbable gelatin foam (Gelfoam), oxidized cellulose (Surgicel), and microfibrillar collagen (Avitene). Gelfoam and Avitene can be left in the surgical field. Surgicel may cause too much inflammation to be left in the eyelids or orbit.

Bleeding from bone is best controlled with direct application of bone wax into the bleeding sites. It is very difficult to control bone bleeding with cautery of any kind even with a well-defined bleeding site because the vessels do not have much surrounding connective tissue that can be incorporated into the coagulated area.

Postoperative

Suction drains can be used postoperatively to increase hemostasis. Some surgeons use active suction devices in surgeries involving large flaps. Some use passive drains like Penrose or rubber band drains routinely for orbital procedures.

Nasal packing is often used after DCR surgeries for hemostasis.

Wound Closure

Closure of incisions in the periocular area usually requires sutures. Staples and tissue adhesives are generally poor choices for the eyelids and surrounding areas owing to the great mobility of the skin and surrounding structures. Great care must be taken with suture placement and suture tension. A tight suture can cheese-wire (pull) through thin eyelid skin and can cause necrosis, especially in association with significant edema (Fig. 2.3). Attention must be paid to needle type and size, suture type and thickness, and suture placement and tension. All of these factors have a significant effect on the surgical result.

Suture Needles

The choice of needles is critical in eyelid surgery. The type of needle determines the ease with which the needle penetrates the tissue. The size and shape of the needle influence the amount of trauma induced by passing the suture. Cutting or reverse-cutting needle configurations are the most useful in ophthalmic plastic surgery. Spatulated needles are helpful for lamellar passes through tissues such as sclera and tarsus (Fig. 2.4). Round or tapered needles, often used in vascular surgery, have a limited role in ophthalmic plastic surgery, but can be used to decrease bruising in certain procedures, such as temporary eyelid closure (tarsorrhaphy).

The size and curvature of the needle are also important. Slightly curved needles are helpful for suturing eyelid skin and tarsus. Highly curved (semicircle) needles are helpful for tight spaces such as the medial or lateral canthus or deeper suture passes in dacryocystorhinostomy surgery.

Suture Placement

Sutures should be used when clearly indicated. For skin closures, correctly placed sutures slightly pucker the wound edges.

A simple, interrupted suture is a single rectangular to trapezoid-shaped loop that can approximate tissue well when there is little tension on the wound. The base of the loop should be wider than the top to ensure skin edge eversion (Fig. 2.5). A vertical mattress suture creates a U-shaped loop with the outer limits placed deep and the inner limits placed superficially through the skin alone. The vertical mattress suture is used to ensure an approximated and everted skin edge for a wound where there is significant tension (Fig. 2.6). A figure-of-eight suture is a variant of

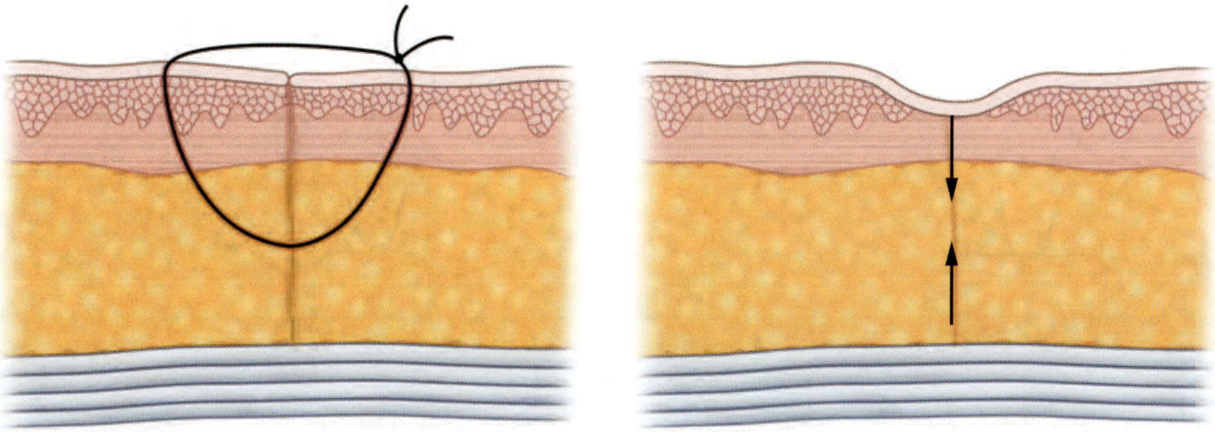

Fig. 2.3 Depressed scar caused by overly tight suture

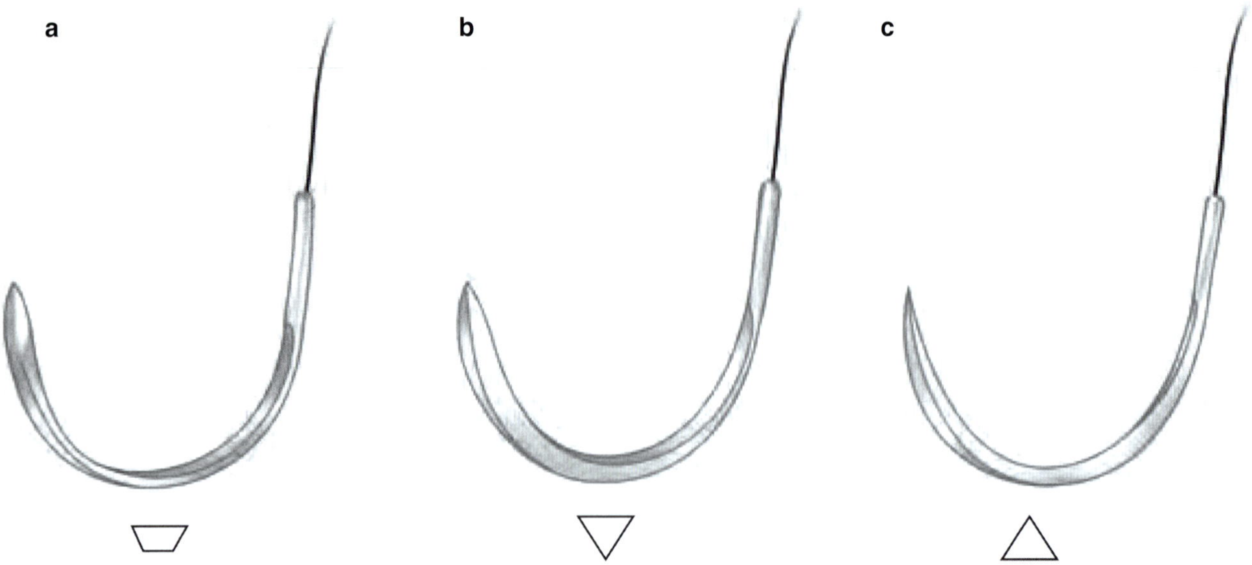

Fig. 2.4 (**a**) Spatula needle. (**b**) Cutting needle. (**c**) Reverse cutting needle

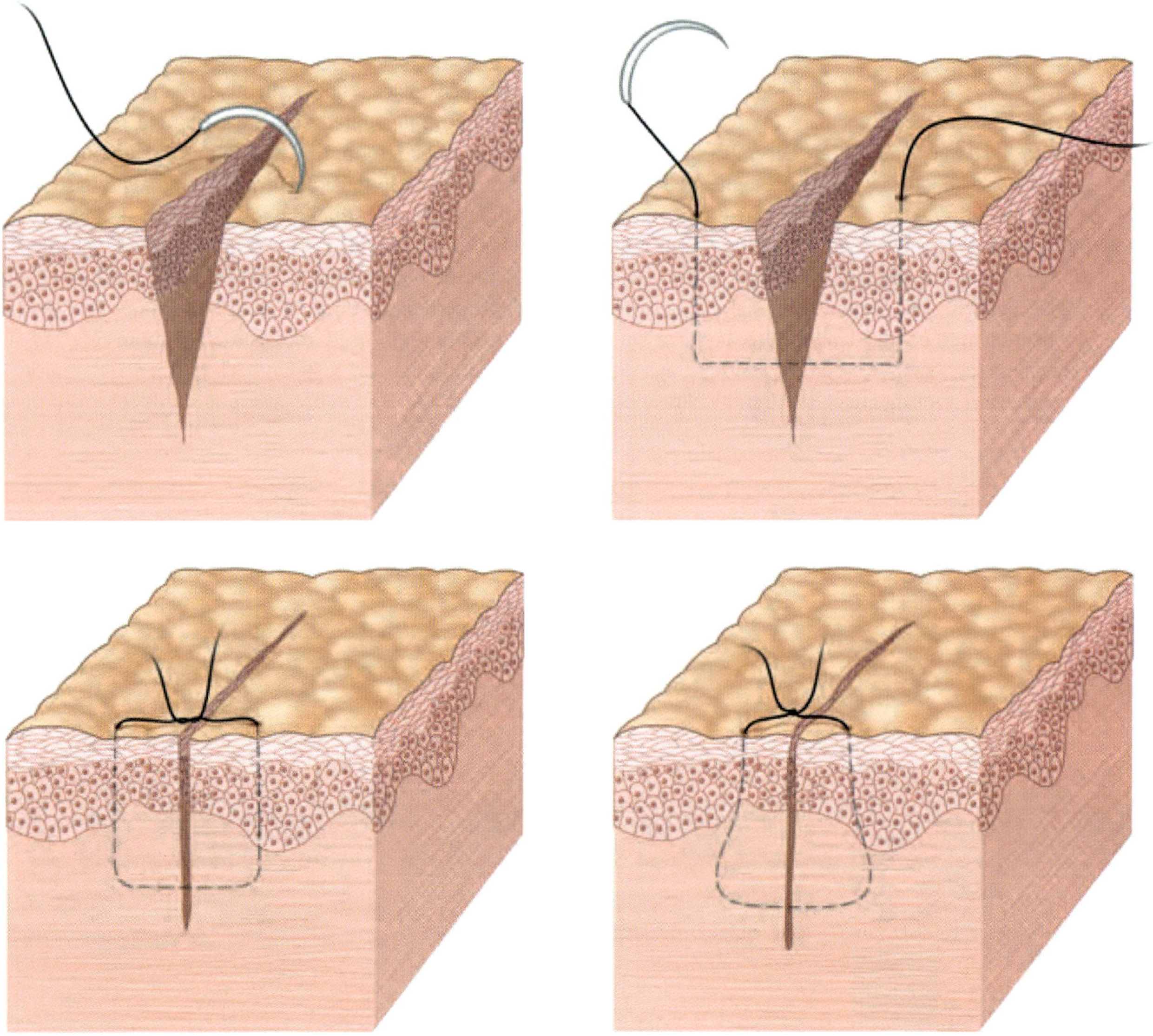

Fig. 2.5 Correctly placed interrupted superficial closure with skin edges slightly puckered after tying

the vertical mattress suture (Fig. 2.7). A horizontal mattress suture is created by tying two connected simple sutures together (Fig. 2.8). A horizontal mattress suture is commonly used to reattach the lateral canthal tendon to the inner aspect of the lateral orbital rim during lower eyelid tightening. The horizontal mattress suture, like a continuous, locking, running suture, is a means of reducing the number of knots and the time required to tie them (Fig. 2.9). Subcuticular sutures form an S-shaped chain linking the dermis. Such sutures, largely buried, suit a skin closure with little tension in which the surgeon wishes to reduce the effect of suture materials on epidermal scarring. The subcuticular sutures are exteriorized at the wound ends and left free and tied or sutured to skin at the ends (Fig. 2.10).

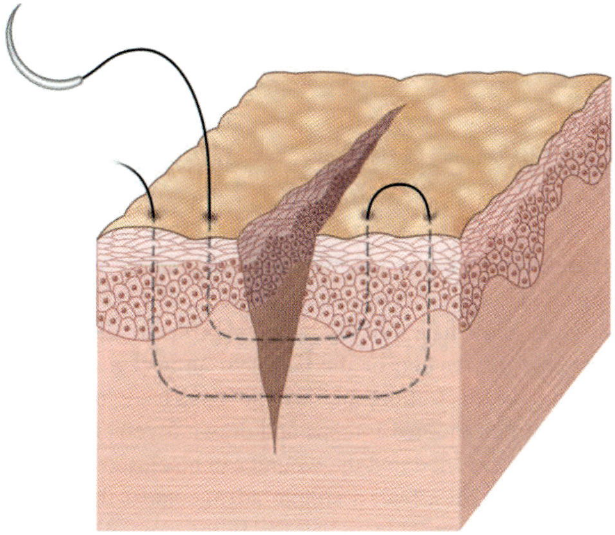

Fig. 2.6 Vertical mattress suture provides excellent deep and superficial support and helps to evert wound edges. A far-far, near-near suture pass is utilized

Suture Materials

Both absorbable and nonabsorbable sutures are useful, depending on the desired effect. The sizes for ophthalmic plastic surgery are usually between 4–0 (largest) and 8–0 (smallest). Absorbable sutures consist of naturally occurring materials such as catgut and collagen and synthetic materials. The first are usually monofilaments and are degraded by enzymatic action that is somewhat variable between individual patients (Table 2.1). Therefore the effectiveness of these suture materials is somewhat unpredictable, but they are shorter acting than the synthetic materials. The synthetic materials such as polyglactin are usually braided and are degraded by hydrolysis, which is more predictable but takes longer to complete. The braided sutures make the most effective knots but also have spaces between the braids that are too small for white cells to enter while allowing bacterial proliferation. Sutures that inhibit bacterial colonization by impregnation with triclosan are now available (Ethicon Plus Sutures, Ethicon, Somerville, NJ).

Nonabsorbable sutures usually last at least several years or longer. When externalized, they are frequently removed after several days to weeks. They tend to cause less inflammation than absorbable sutures because they are more inert and relatively ignored by the body's immune system. Silk sutures are the principal exceptions to the abovementioned guidelines. Silk causes significantly more inflammation than the synthetic monofilament sutures, but offers excellent ease of use. Supramid, polyester, and silicone are used predominantly for eyelid suspensions and canthal reconstructions. Steel wire is used for joining bones and for canthal reconstruction but is rarely used now with the wide availability of plating sets (Fig. 2.11).

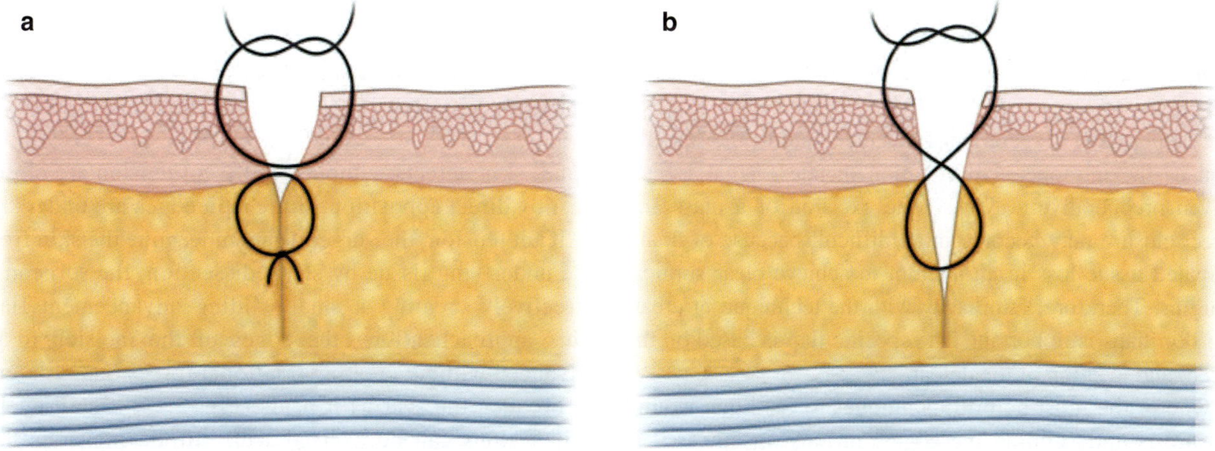

Fig. 2.7 (**a**) Buried suture used to close deeper layers. Superficial layer closed with interrupted suture. (**b**) Figure-of-eight suture used to achieve same closure

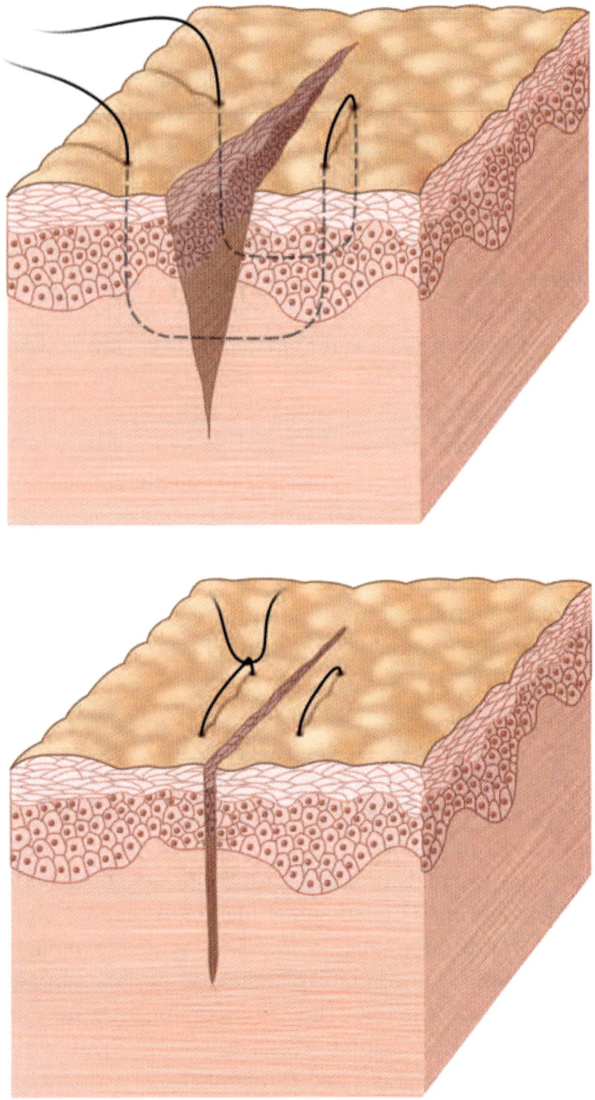

Fig. 2.8 Horizontal mattress suture allows speed of placement secondary to less tying and is useful for wounds under tension, as in reapproximation of the lateral canthal tendon during the lateral tarsal strip procedure

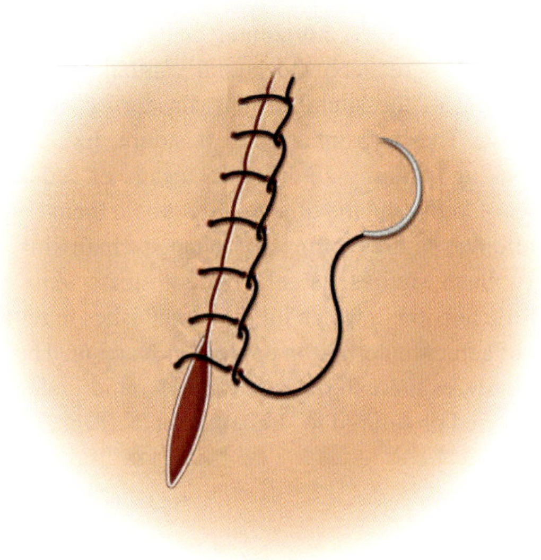

Fig. 2.9 Continuous locking suture

Skin Defects

The oculoplastic surgeon must be able to adjust the surgical plan as the intraoperative situation dictates. What is perceived preoperatively as a simple excision of a mass and direct closure may become more difficult because of unanticipated tissue loss in an attempt to achieve clear surgical margins. Therefore, familiarity with the technique of creating skin flaps is important. The specific flap is based on the extent and location of the defect.

One of the most helpful techniques to facilitate wound closure is undermining the edges. In most instances it is straightforward to undermine the adjacent tissue in the subcutaneous planes beginning at the wound margins. The surgeon may have to dissect a significant distance to decrease the tension of the tissue to an acceptable level. During the dissection, the wound edges are repeatedly grasped with toothed forceps and drawn together until the surgeon is satisfied that the wound can be closed relatively tension-free. In effect, a simple advancement flap is created without any skin incisions. If the wound is closed with significant, persistent skin tension, the scar will broaden postoperatively and will tend to either hypertrophy or atrophy. This is particularly true if the scar has repetitive stretching forces on it, such as a scar in the upper eyelid.

When undermining is insufficient to relieve incisional stress, more advanced techniques are necessary.

Primary Closure

Small skin defects without significant tension are closed best by direct apposition. If the skin edges are under significant tension, the surgeon can undermine the skin from the underlying tissue by sharp dissection; the surgeon is effectively creating a small sliding advancement flap. This approach allows the edges of the incision to be advanced without creating tractional forces that will tend to broaden the scar as it heals (Fig. 2.12). Small eyelid skin lesions can be excised with elliptic incisions that easily convert to linear closures with minimal tissue distortion (Fig. 2.13). As with all incisions, it is important to evert the wound edges as they are closed. All tissue margins are swollen during the wound closure. Detumescence occurs as the scar heals. A depressed scar is avoided by carefully and consistently everting the wound edges during the closure (Fig. 2.14). Each layer of skin should be approximated to the equivalent layer in the opposite wound edge to avoid creating a bump in the scar. If a raw edge is sutured to an epidermal surface, an elliptic abnormality in the scar will result because the two will not properly seal.

Table 2.1 Commonly used suture materials in oculoplastic surgery

Suture	Characteristics	Strength retention	Typical use
Nylon	Synthetic, monofilament	Permanent	Skin closure
Prolene	Synthetic, monofilament	Permanent	Skin closure
Silk	Natural, multifilament	2 years	Lid margin repair
Plain gut	Natural, monofilament	7–10 days	Skin and conjunctival closure
Chromic gut	Natural, monofilament	2–3 weeks	Deep buried wound closure, tarsal sutures
Polyglactin	Synthetic, multifilament	3–4 weeks	Deep buried wound closure, tarsal sutures
Polydioxanone	Synthetic, monofilament	4–6 weeks	Deep suspension sutures, tissue flap support

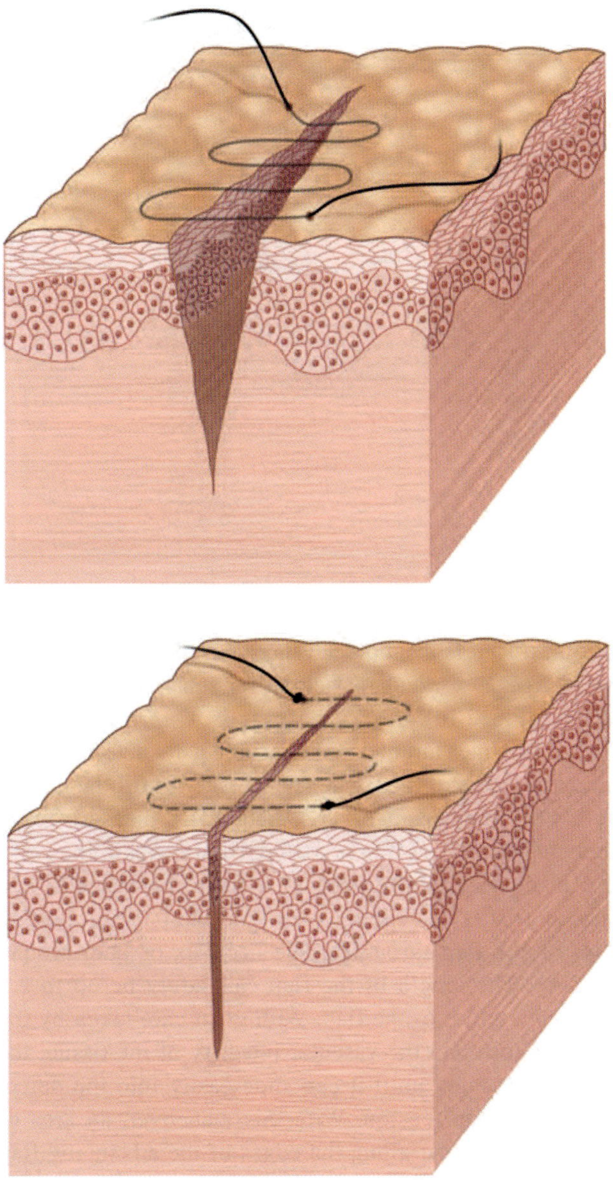

Fig. 2.10 Buried running subcuticular closure affords excellent cosmesis and ease of removal

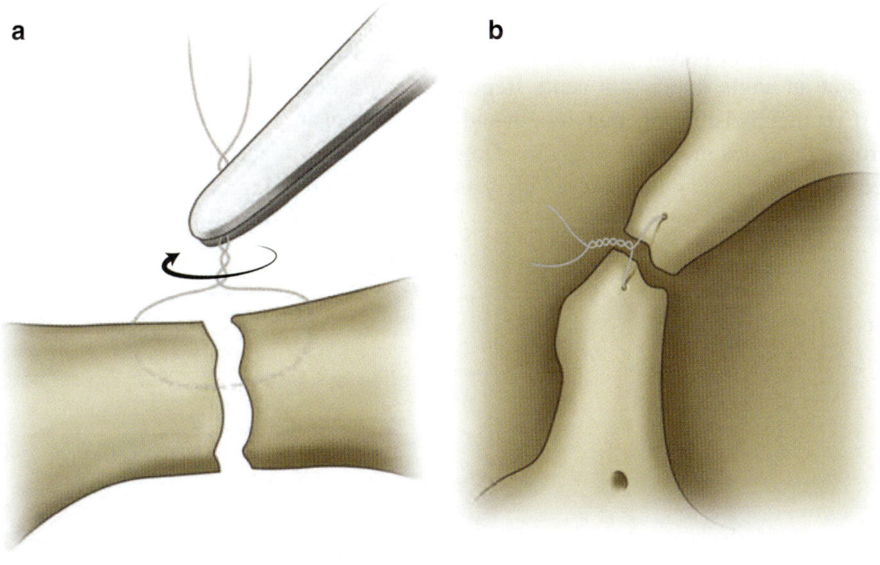

Fig. 2.11 (**a**) Wire is twisted to hold it in position; it is not tied. (**b**) After the wire is twisted, the free end is bent toward the bone and deeply buried. Wire causes very little tissue reaction if the end is well buried

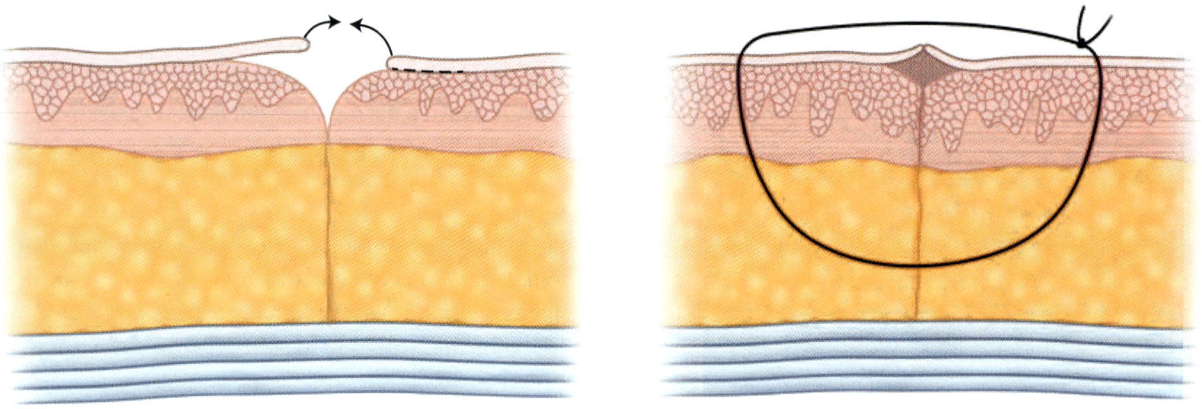

Fig. 2.12 Undermining of wound edges with slight eversion of the wound margin

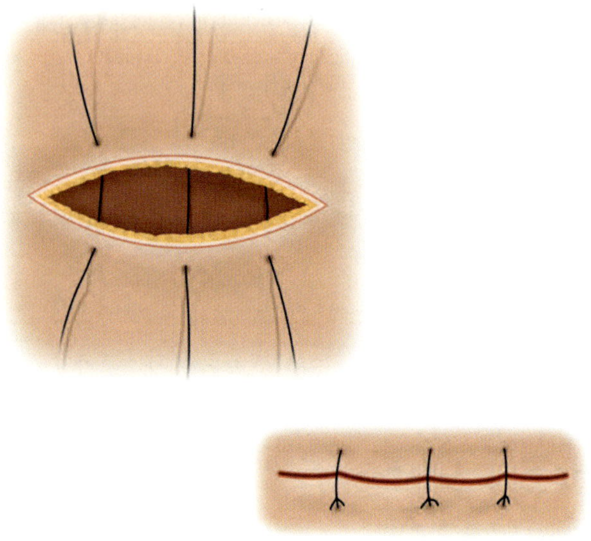

Fig. 2.13 Elliptic defect closed with interrupted sutures

Dog Ears

Dog ears are created by redundant tissue at the termination of an incision. Unequal incision lengths and incisions joined at an angle that is too acute frequently cause dog ears. Creating incisions of equal length and joining them at appropriate angles minimize dog ears. Dog ears are eliminated by creating a flat, unpuckered incision before closure (Fig. 2.15).

Flaps

The next step is a simple advancement flap with skin incisions. This is particularly helpful for square or rectangular defects (Fig. 2.16).

Careful measurement of the defect to determine the size and shape of the tissue is necessary to fill the defect, following the woodworker's dictum of "measure twice and cut once." The flap is outlined and the skin incisions are made sufficiently deep to include the vascular bed that nourishes it. Failure to include the bed can lead to loss of the flap through tissue necrosis or poor wound healing. The length of the flap can safely be up to 2.5 times the width of the flap. With great care taken by the surgeon to retain the vascular integrity of the tissue, the flap is dissected until it can slide easily into the defect with minimum tension. With this maneuver, an area of stress may appear along the edges of the advancing flap that may impede the successful advancement of the flap. The eyelids are a privileged site with great vascularity; therefore it is rare to see tissue slough. Nevertheless, these principles apply to the periorbital region as well as other sites. Small releasing triangles, called Burrow's triangles, may be made at these stress points to lessen the tension and minimize scarring (Fig. 2.17). After the flap is advanced into position and the apparent stress is acceptable, it is sutured into position. In those areas with larger flaps, buried absorbable sutures may be used to join opposing subcutaneous tissue and obliterate the sur-

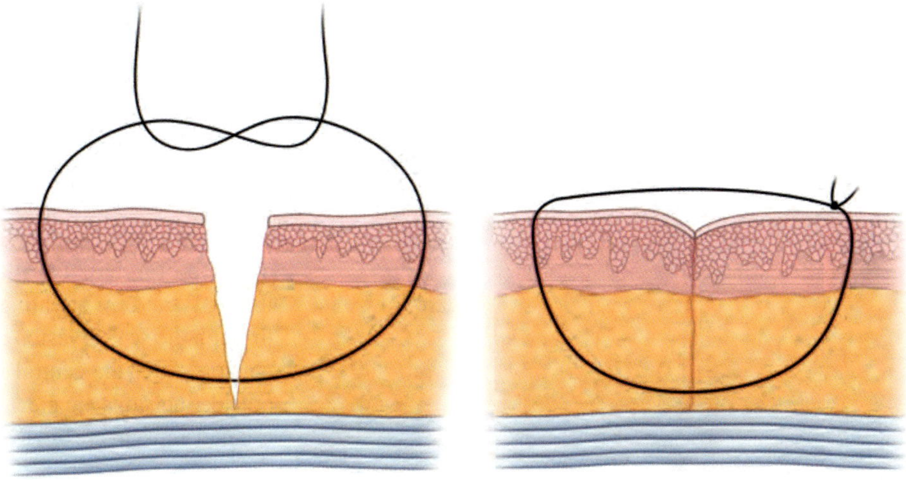

Fig. 2.14 Poorly placed suture is too far from the wound and caused inverted wound edges

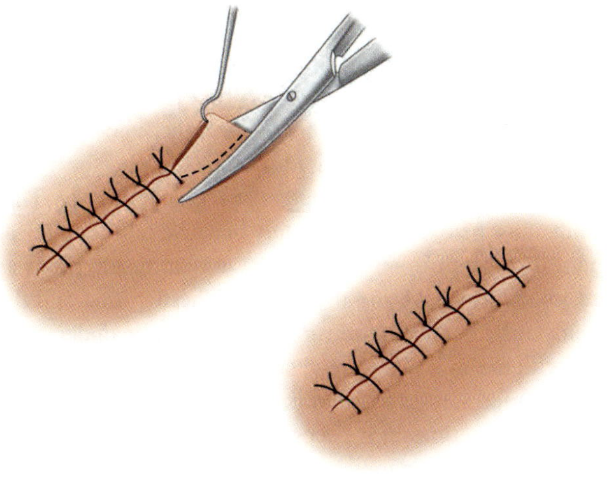

Fig. 2.15 Correction of dog ears requires stretching the redundant skin edges and excising the redundancy in the line of the incision. A single cut treats both edges simultaneously; folding the redundancy and cutting with one blade inside the fold treat each edge separately

gical dead space (Fig. 2.18). These buried sutures also decrease the tension on the skin and distribute it more evenly.

An alternative method of tension reduction is the V-Y plasty ("V to Y plasty"). Determining the force vector on the skin is critical for this flap. Once the direction of the main vector is known, a V-shaped incision is made along the meridian of the main vector bisecting the V. The area lateral to the V is undermined. This results in a release of the V in one direction, and the former base of the V lengthens. This area is then closed by suturing the former base of the V in a linear fashion. The arms of the V are automatically converted into a Y (Fig. 2.19). It is also possible to make a Y into a V by a reverse process. These techniques are most helpful in the reconstruction of the medial and lateral canthi.

A rotation flap is very helpful for rotating tissue around a fixed base to fill in a defect. A flap of tissue is dissected free of the subcutaneous tissue, as in a simple advancement flap. The flap is rotated into position, and the defect is closed by beginning at both ends to minimize undue tension (Fig. 2.20). Those areas of puckered tissue can be excised as a triangle and closed with interrupted sutures.

The Limberg or rhomboid rotational flap is a useful variation of the standard rotational flap for situations that make a less complicated flap insufficient to close the defect [8, 9]. It is particularly helpful for closing diamond-shaped incisions or elliptic incisions that have been converted to a rhomboid shape. The configuration of the flap is shown. The critical elements are the 120° and 60° angles, as indicated, so that the flap sits snugly into position (Fig. 2.21). The key to success is the orientation of the excision site. Before demarcating the lesion, the surgeon should determine in which direction the skin is most extensible. This line becomes the lateral aspect of the channel. This approach ensures minimal wound tension at the conclusion of the procedure. The guideline cannot be perpendicular to the lid margins because this position may cause abnormal tension and result in malposition of the eyelid (Fig. 2.22). The procedure lends itself well to use in the orbital adnexal areas. After creation of the defect, the flap is formed with the top extending from an imaginary line bisecting the 120° angle. It has the same length as the corresponding side of the diamond. To complete the flap, the lateral incision is formed by placing it at a 60° angle and parallel to the bottom or top side of the diamond, depend-

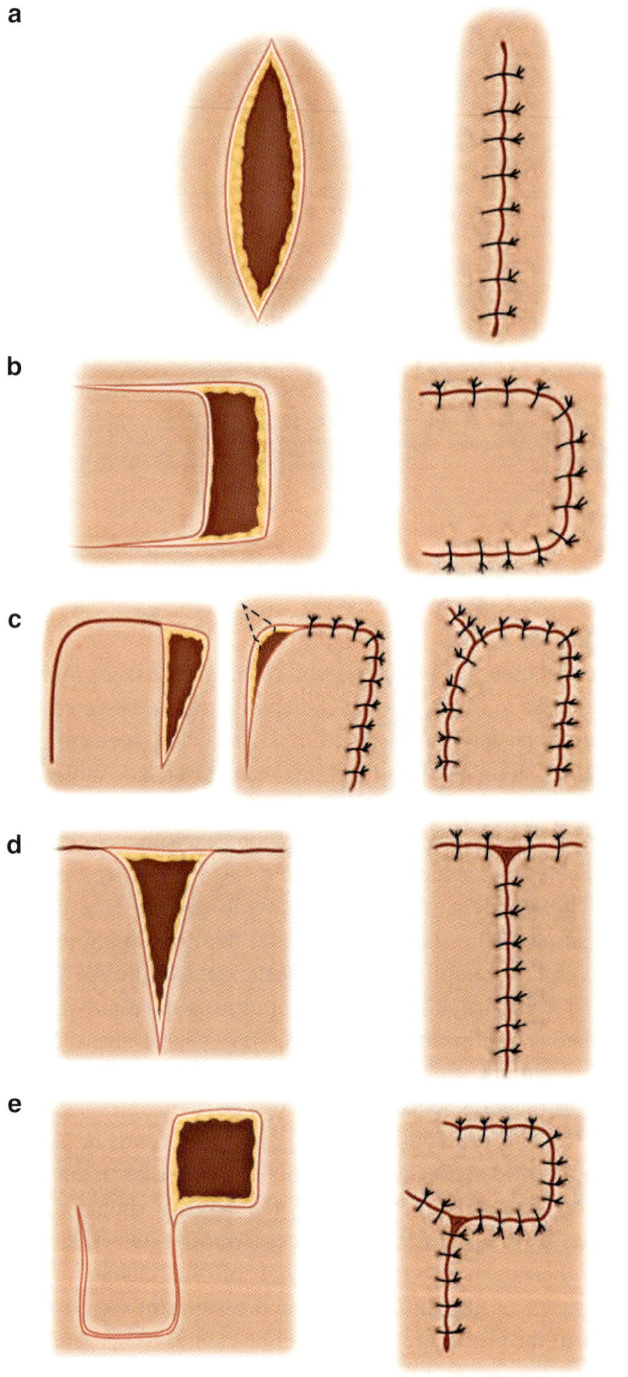

Fig. 2.16 (**a**) Wound margin is undermined in shaded region to achieve sliding flap closure. (**b**) Simple linear advancement flap. (**c**) Rotation flap with triangle removed to facilitate closure. (**d**) Combined sliding and advancement flap. (**e**) Transpositional flap used to close nonadjacent defects

ing on which way the flap will be rotated. Meticulous dissection is used to properly undermine and isolate the flap until it can be rotated into the defect. After it is rotated, near-far, far-near sutures are used to secure it.

Z-plasty

Z-plasty is an important surgical option to release a contracted scar. It is a transpositional flap, and it is used to decrease the tension on a scar. It is also possible to completely excise the scar or a mass within the central incision of the Z-plasty by enclosing it within a spindle-shaped excision. The combination of a Z-plasty with a spindle-shaped excision of a mass is called an O-Z plasty (Fig. 2.23). The flap is started by orienting the long or central arm of the Z through the scar or lesion and parallel to the principle line of tension. After the central incision is oriented and sized, the outside incisions are created with an equal length to the central incision and are angled at 60° to the central incision. This creates two flaps shaped like equilateral triangles of equal size. The flaps are undermined extensively so they can be rotated into position and joined together without significant tension (Fig. 2.24). This process is facilitated by creating flaps of equal size that are mirror images of each other across the central incision.

Once the triangular flaps are formed, the subdermal tissue is examined. Subcutaneous fibrous bands may be present that the surgeon had not appreciated preoperatively. These bands must be excised completely because failure to release them may result in an inadequate surgical result. The flaps are joined by anchoring the bases of the flap first and then evenly distributing the tension along the remainder of the flap with multiple interrupted sutures. It may be appropriate to use buried sutures to minimize the effects of late scar contracture. Sometimes it is necessary to anchor the flap apexes with vertical or horizontal mattress sutures to distribute the tension better along the flap edges. Undue stress caused by inequality of the flaps promotes poor or incorrect wound healing. Such problems may actually exacerbate the underlying condition rather than improve it. If it is not possible to make these flaps of equal angles, there should be no more than 20° of difference between them.

The use of the Z-plasty may range from apparently simple applications to extremely complex situations. It is useful for relieving vertical contracture in the eyelids after trauma. It is also helpful for long, complicated scars of the face.

To correct a vertical shortening of the upper eyelid from scar contracture, the tension-relieving incision or excision is made vertically through the cicatrized area of the lid. The two arms of the Z are made at 60° angle to the central incision to form the two equilateral triangles. The flaps are completely mobilized. All of the underlying scar tissue is excised. Any scar tissue that remains will compromise the desired surgical result. The flaps are carefully transposed. A significant lengthening of the vertical dimension of the eyelid will result. It is frequently possible to increase the vertical dimension of the eyelid by one-third of the length of the scar (Fig. 2.25). To enhance the early healing process, a traction

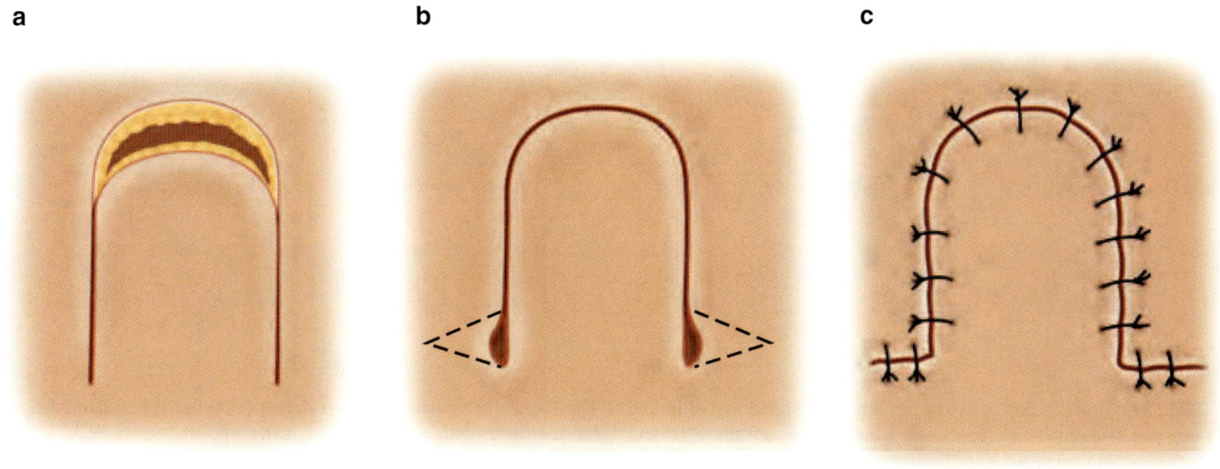

Fig. 2.17 (**a–c**) Tongue-in-groove advancement flap with Burrow's triangles excised from the end of the incision

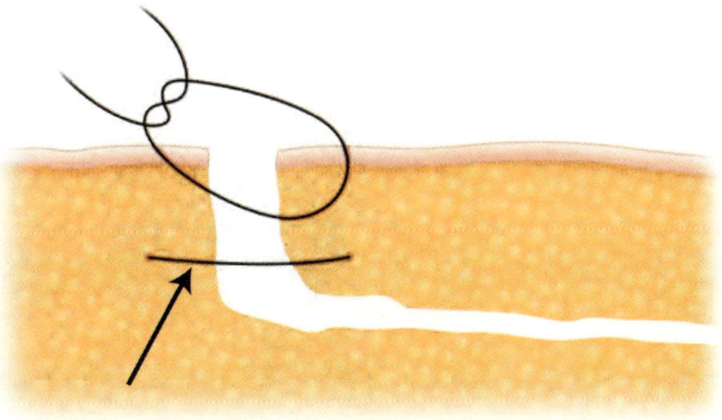

Fig. 2.18 Elimination of surgical dead space with flap advancement

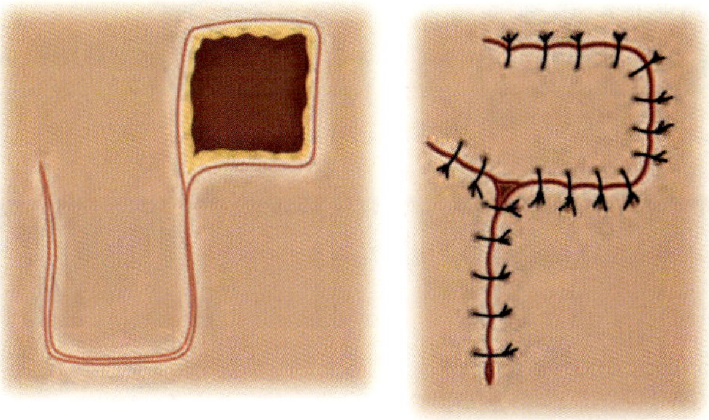

Fig. 2.20 Transposition flap from nonadjacent area

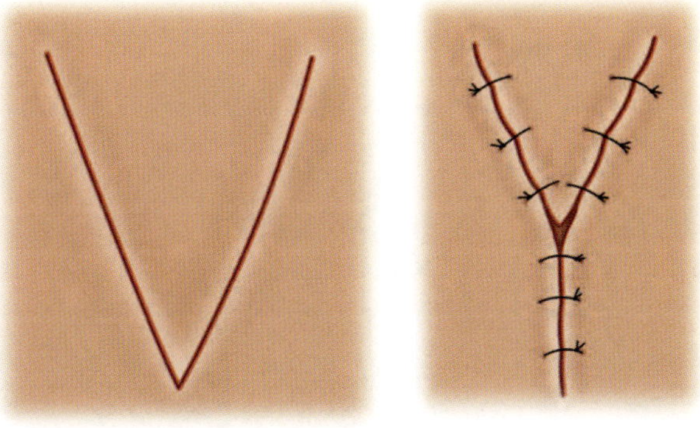

Fig. 2.19 V-Y plasty

suture should be placed through the upper eyelid margin and taped to the cheek for approximately 1 week. A double-armed 6–0 silk suture with cutting needles is placed through the eyelid margin directly below the Z-plasty, over a bolster material of the surgeon's choice (Fig. 2.26). At the surgeon's discretion, the suture may be brought through the lower eyelid margin to completely close the eyelids for the week that the suture is in place. By keeping the eyelid stretched for the first week, the initial wound contraction is controlled and the vertical elongation of the eyelid is enhanced. Gentle massage of the area can soften the subcutaneous scar.

Z-plasty can also be used for more complex types of facial scars. Multiple Z-plasties can be used for long scars that would not respond well to a single large Z-plasty. The initial, central incision is made through the center of the scar. The first two arms are created at 60° to the central incision to create the first two equilateral triangles of tissue for the flaps. Additional arms are created as necessary to completely treat the scar (Fig. 2.27). Great care must be taken to ensure that these incisions parallel the original offset incisions. It is easy to become slightly disoriented, and each mistake will result in successive mistakes in placement of the incision. The number of pairs of incisions depends on

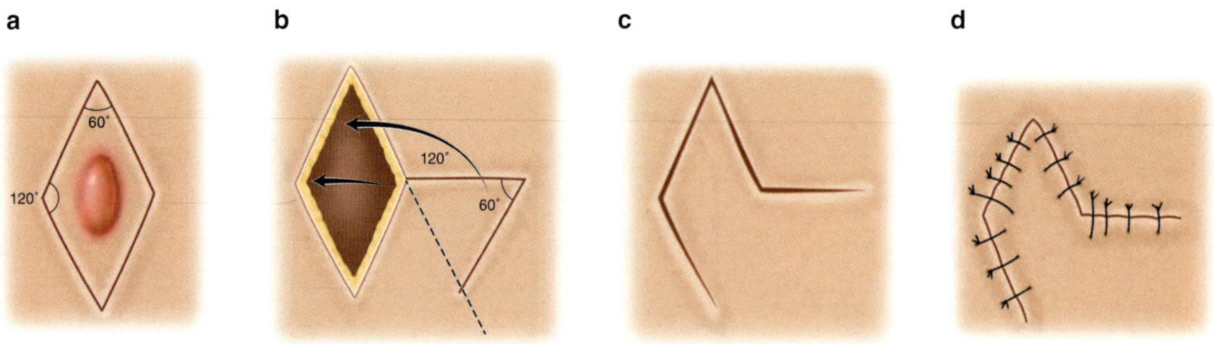

Fig. 2.21 The limberg flap is used for diamond- shaped and elliptical incisions (**a**). The critical elements of a Limberg flap are the 120° and 60° angles, as indicated, so that the flap sits snugly into position (**b**). The flap is then rotated into the defect (**c**). After it is rotated, near-far, far-near sutures are used to secure it (**d**)

Fig. 2.22 Lines of direction altered to preserve eyelid function

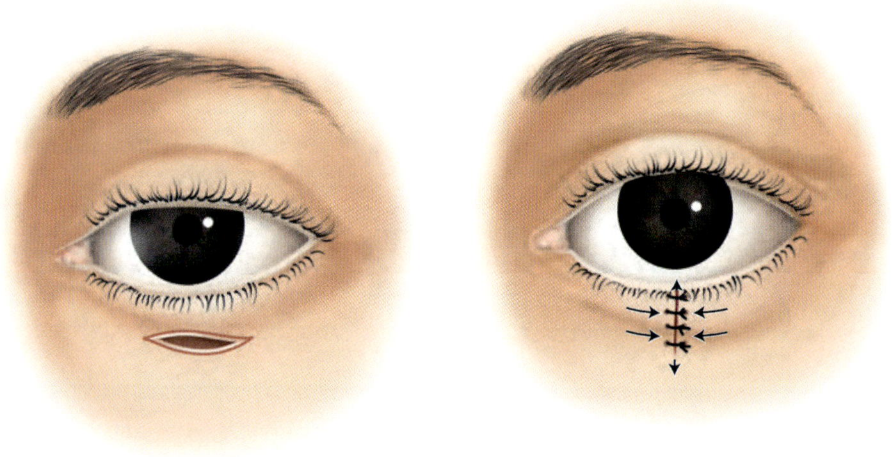

Fig. 2.23 O-Z plasty

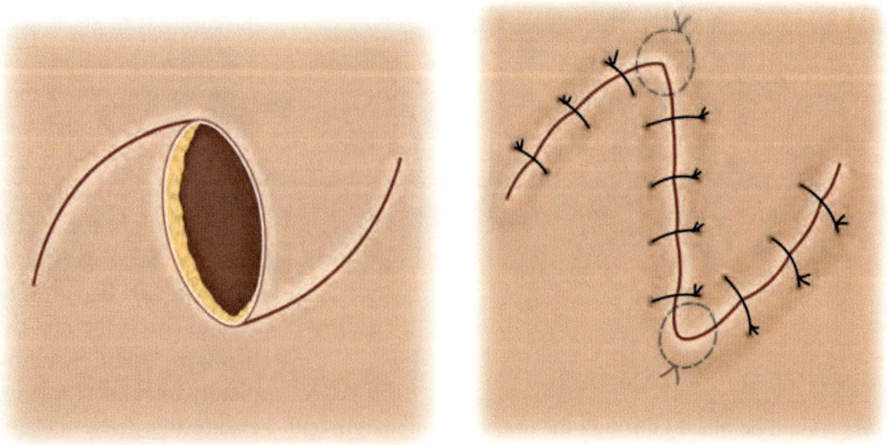

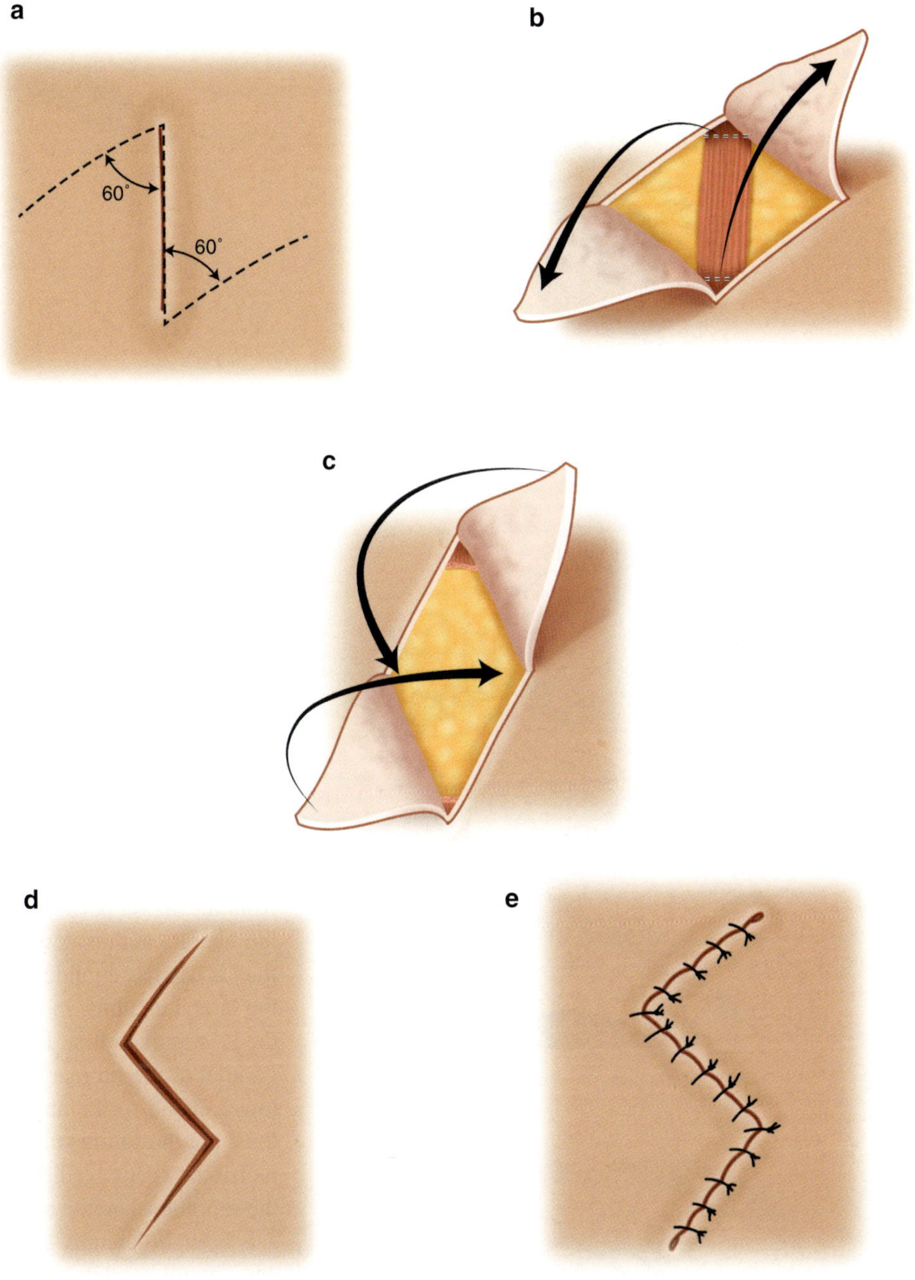

Fig. 2.24 (**a**) Central incision through line of traction with arm line offset by 60° angle. (**b**) Flaps dissected free and elevated. (**c**) Fibrotic band excised and flaps ready for transposition. (**d**) Flaps have been transposed. (**e**) Flaps sutured into position

the length of the scar and adequate distribution of the wound tension. Each pair of offset incisions that forms a Z-plasty is treated as described above.

Z-plasty is also helpful to rotate the eyelid or brow margin. In this role it can be a useful alternative to skin grafting. When caring for burn patients, there is minimal skin available for grafting, and avoiding a graft can be critical. To enhance incision placement and accuracy, the surgeon places the eyelid on stretch before the incision. This can be accomplished with a 4–0 silk suture. The incision is made through the skin 2–3 mm outside of the ciliary margin. The arms of the Z are completed on the side of the eyelid that the tissue flaps will be moved toward (Fig. 2.28). The flaps are meticulously dissected, and all fibrotic bands are excised. In cases of lateral or medial canthal transposition, the angle of the flaps may not be at 60° angle. It may be necessary to angle the flaps more acutely to allow the flaps to work within the available space. It may also be necessary to incise and reattach the lateral canthal tendon before final placement of the flaps.

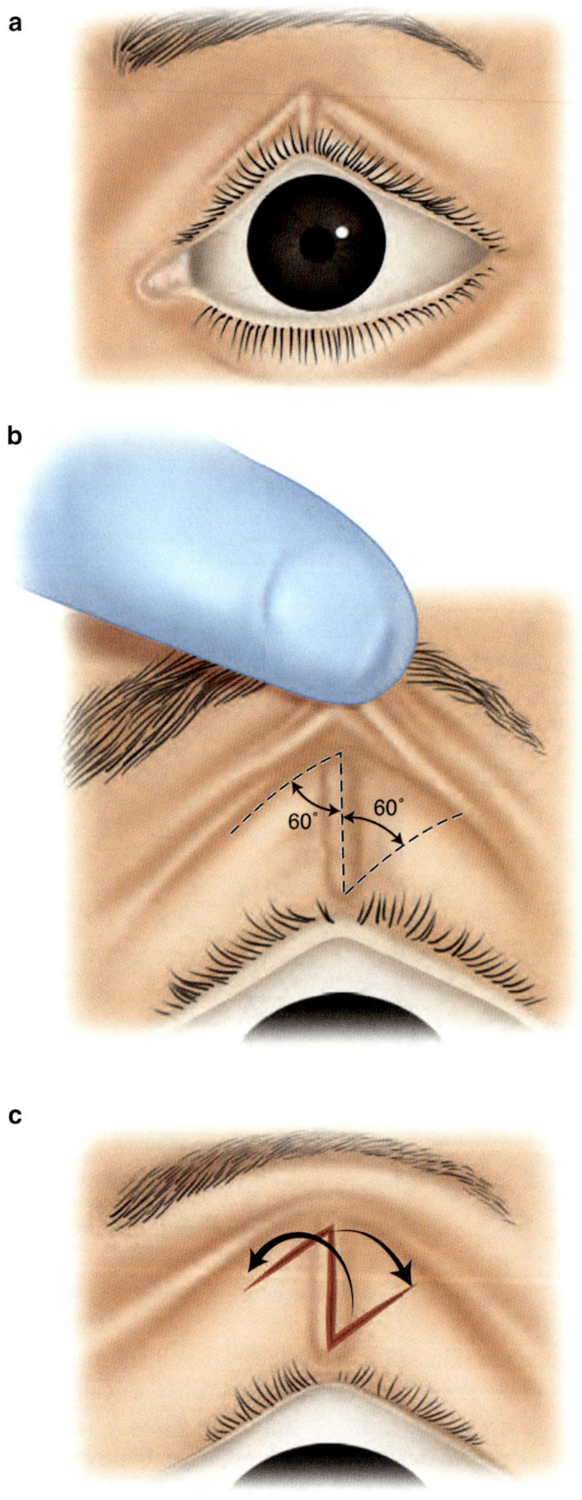

Fig. 2.25 (**a**) Cicatricial band causing vertical shortening of the upper lid. (**b**) Central line through scar with arms offset at 60° angle. (**c**) Flaps dissected free and ready to be transposed

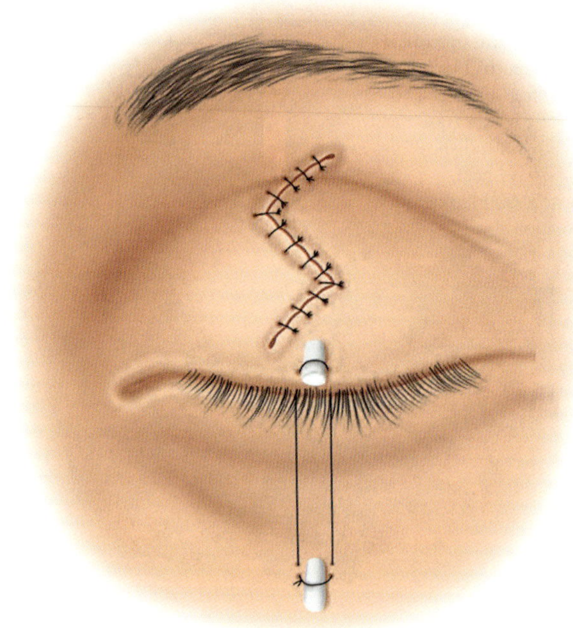

Fig. 2.26 Upper lid placed on stretch with bolsters after completion of the Z-plasty

A similar problem such as elevation of the lateral canthus can be solved by adapting this technique. The flap is taken from the lateral portion of the lower eyelid and used to rotate the lateral canthus downward. The level of the medial canthus is used as a guide to estimate the optimal placement of the lateral canthus. In this adaptation, the central portion of the Z is marked first. It is placed 3 mm below the cilia line. Parallel to the lid margin, it extends from the middle of the lower eyelid to the angle of the malpositioned lateral canthus, not the future site of the new lateral canthus. Then the incision sweeps medially, superiorly, and obliquely toward the supratarsal crease of the upper lid. The inferior arm of the Z is brought laterally and ends at the desired position of the new lateral canthus. This step is extremely important. The cicatrix creating an abnormal canthal position is excised segmentally until the lateral canthus freely drops into the desired position. The inferior angle is then transferred to fill the superior defect. Skin hooks or delicate atraumatic forceps are extremely helpful during these manipulations. The wound is then closed.

An elevated brow can also be corrected by a Z-plasty. The incisions are marked out while keeping in mind that the future position of the elevated brow will be determined by its placement in the temporal and inferior arm of the Z (Fig. 2.29). The site is estimated by comparison to both the contralateral

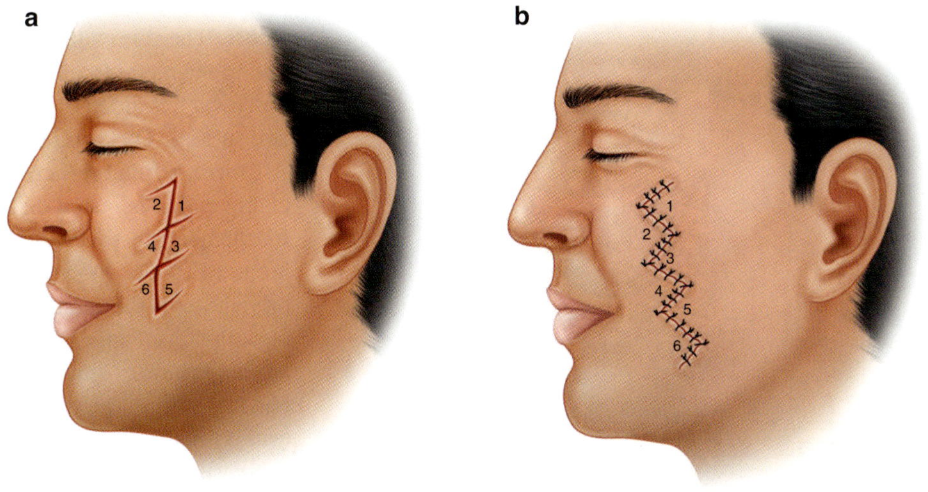

Fig. 2.27 (**a**) Multiple Z-plasty marked out and incised. (**b**) Flaps carefully transposed and sutured into position

brow and the medial aspect of the ipsilateral brow. The absence of cilia in the elevated brow or aberrant growth should be noted. If they are found, placement of the brow should be adjusted accordingly. The central portion of the Z is placed under and parallel to the arch of the affected brow. The superior arm is then offset to follow the curve of the superior orbital rim. The inferior arm of the Z is placed parallel to the superior incision. It may be necessary to extend the lateral aspect of the inferior incision slightly in order to lessen wound tension and accommodate the transposition. This frequently makes the Z resemble the number 2. The flaps are dissected carefully to minimize the risk of injury to the lash follicles. The flaps are transposed as shown and sutured into position.

Reconstruction of the Eyelid

The goals of eyelid reconstruction include structural and functional restoration with an acceptable aesthetic result. Structural restoration of the anterior and posterior lamella provides skin coverage and blood supply to the eyelid (anterior) while supporting the eyelid and a nonabrasive mucosal surface (posterior). Functional restoration of the upper eyelid allows adequate mobility to protect the cornea, and that of the lower eyelid allows it to appose the globe and have stability, aiding in the normal flow of tears.

Pentagonal Excision with Direct Closure Full-thickness defects of the lower eyelid up to 25% of its length can be converted into a pentagonal excision and closed directly in the younger patient with less eyelid laxity.

The medial wound edge is first straightened with a super-sharp knife or a No. 11 Bard-Parker scalpel (Fig. 2.30). This allows a more precise closure and removes debris from the incision. The eyelid margin is grasped with toothed forceps. While keeping the eyelid under tension, the blade is inserted through full-thickness eyelid. It is brought upward in one continuous motion to remove all of the irregular tissue while creating a smooth wound edge. The lateral wound edge is treated in a similar fashion. Attention is directed to closing the wound edge without leaving a notch in the eyelid margin. The center point of this effort is placing three 6–0 silk sutures through the eyelid margin. The sutures should be passed through the meibomian gland orifices, the gray line, and the lash line approximately 2–2.5 mm from the wound margin on either side (Fig. 2.31). The first suture passed should be through the gray line, just anterior to the mucocutaneous junction. A double throw is placed in the suture and the eyelid margin is evaluated. The eyelid margin should be well approximated with a solid mirror-image pass. If the wound edges are symmetrically joined, the suture is completed with two more throws to make square knots, and the suture is cut long and placed within a hemostat which is rested on the patient's brow and aids in retraction for the next pass. If the wound edges are not symmetrically joined, the abovementioned process needs to be repeated. The second suture is placed through the lash line by starting the needle 2–2.5 mm from the wound edge and passing it in a smooth, symmetric fashion through the opposite side of the wound at the same level. This suture is tied, cut long and placed in a hemostat, and retracted inferiorly (rested over the

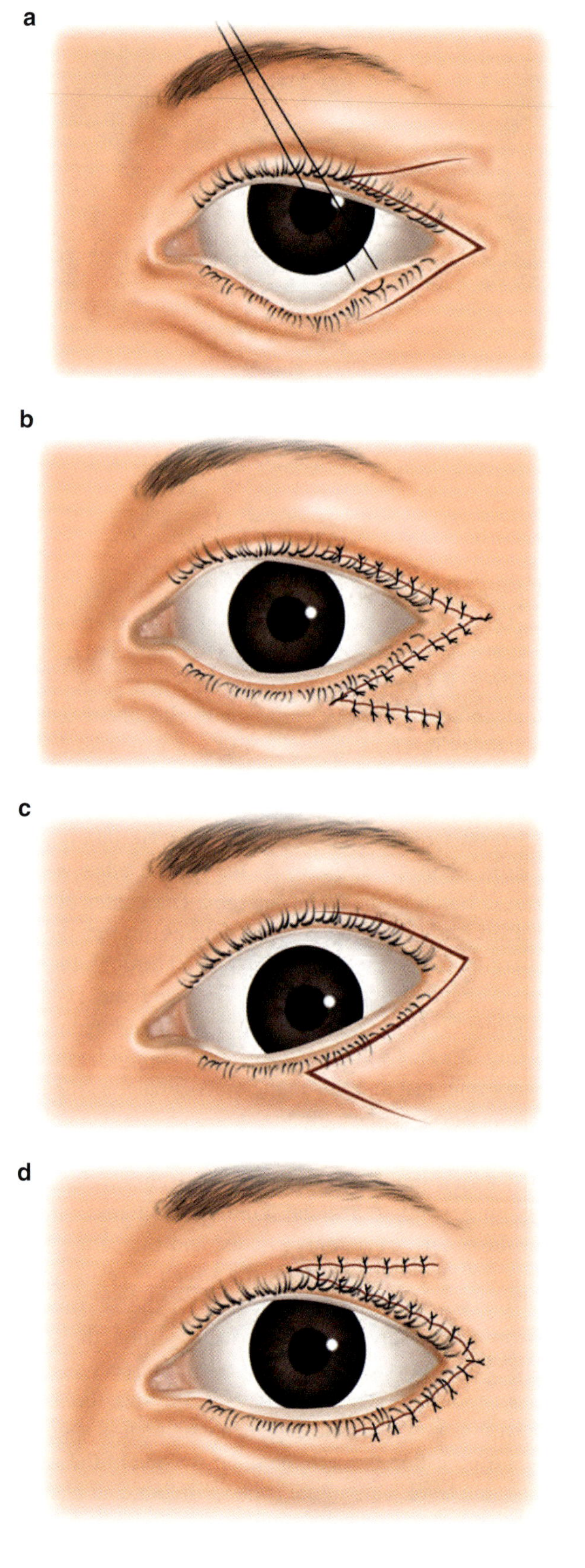

Fig. 2.28 (**a**) Z-type incision prepared to correct lower-lid deficiency. (**b**) Upper lid flap transposed to fill deficiency and sutured into place. (**c**) Central incision made along lid margin in attempt to lower lateral canthus. (**d**) Lower-lid flap transposed to upper lid and sutured in place

patient's cheek) to aid in retraction for the last lid margin suture. The third suture is passed in between the first two (along the meibomian gland orifices), usually in one single pass which is aided by the retraction provided by the initial two sutures. This suture is also cut and left long (Fig. 2.32). All three lid margin sutures are then placed in the same clamp which is rested on the brow and provides retraction for the deep, tarsal closure. Absorbable 5–0 or 6–0 sutures are used to close the tarsal plate. They are passed anteriorly through the tarsus in a lamellar fashion to approximate the tarsal edges during the healing phase and to avoid any exposure of the suture on the conjunctival side. By placing sutures in the tarsus, the wound stress is more evenly distributed, the likelihood of a dehiscence is decreased, and the risk of a lid notch is minimized (Fig. 2.33). The skin is closed with interrupted 6–0 sutures, and the lid margin sutures are tied inferiorly into one of the skin sutures to avoid corneal-suture touch. The patient is instructed not to rub the eyelid and to wear a shield whenever sleeping for the first 2 weeks after surgery to avoid inadvertently rubbing the eyelid during twilight sleep (Fig. 2.34). The lid margin sutures are left for 7–14 days. The patient is usually seen at 7 days, and a determination is made at that time regarding optimal suture removal. The decision of when to remove the lid margin sutures is greatly influenced by the surgeon's personal experience and the patient's ability to heal. Since the dense connective tissue of the tarsus requires 9–10 days to heal, removal of these sutures is most often performed at about 10 days from surgery.

After suture removal, the lid margin should be slightly everted. The eversion resolves with complete resolution of the postoperative edema. It is also acceptable to have the lid margin smooth and flat. A small depression developing at the incision site will fill in with epithelium. If a depression larger than 2 mm develops, it will probably require surgical revision.

Sometimes the defect is too large to allow direct closure. In these cases, it is necessary to obtain additional tissue to relieve the tension on the wound; otherwise, the wound will stretch and separate in the early postoperative period.

The simplest way to obtain additional tissue is through a lateral canthotomy. A straight mosquito hemostat is placed around the lateral canthus, with the blades straddling the horizontal raphe. The hemostat is advanced until the inner tip reaches the cul-de-sac at the level of the bony rim. The canthal tissue is crushed (Fig. 2.35). The area is then incised with minimal bleeding. The eyelid has now gained several millimeters of additional horizontal length. If this is sufficient, the wound is closed and the canthal incision is closed with interrupted sutures. If additional tissue is required to close the incision, the appropriate crus of the lateral canthal tendon can be partially or completely lysed. The tendon is isolated from the orbicularis anteriorly and the conjunctiva

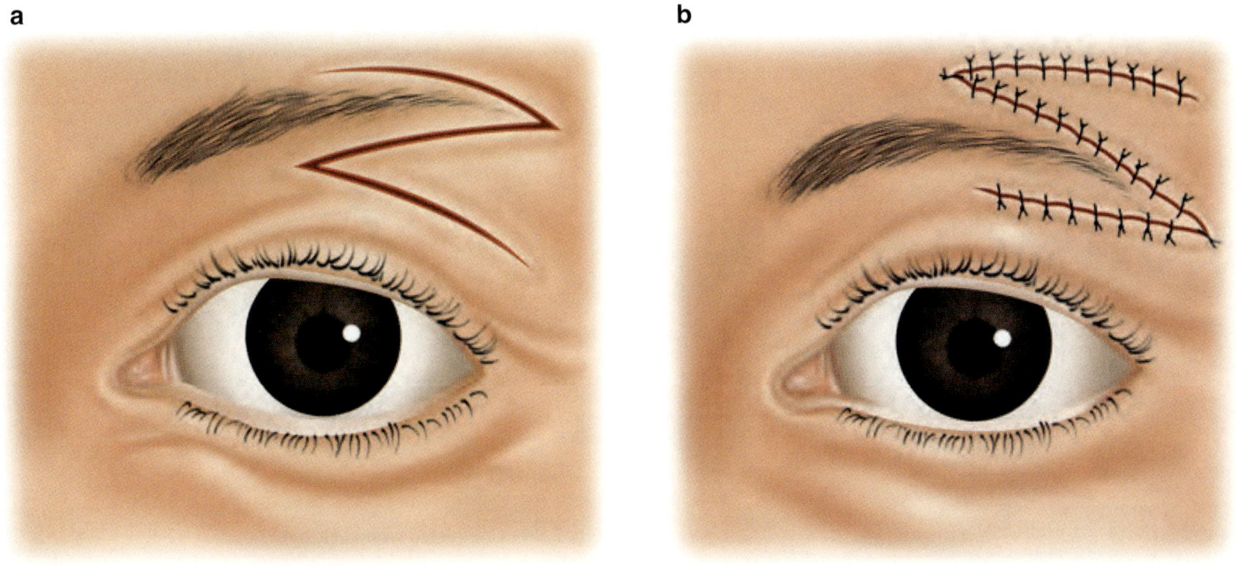

Fig. 2.29 (**a**) Correction of elevated brow by Z-type incision. (**b**) Transposed brow with placement at temporal end of lower arm

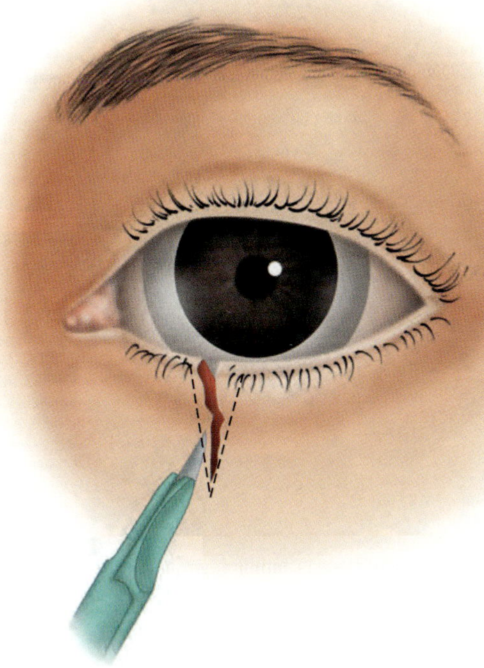

Fig. 2.30 Freshening of wound edges

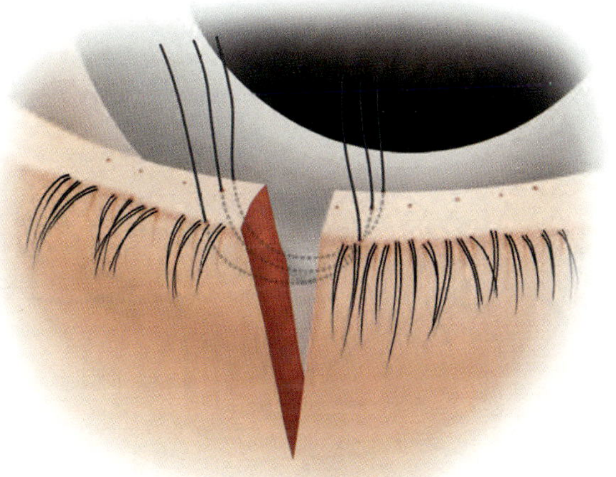

Fig. 2.31 Correct placement of sutures for full-thickness eyelid repair

posteriorly by carefully dissecting within the canthotomy incision (Fig. 2.36). The tendon can be incised in a graded fashion to provide progressively more horizontal lid tissue until the tendon is completely severed (Fig. 2.37). Complete severing of the inferior crus of the lateral canthal tendon creates approximately 8–10 mm of additional eyelid length (Fig. 2.38). When properly dissected away from the surrounding tissues, severing the tendon does not significantly affect the position or function of the eyelid. The primary wound is closed first followed by the canthal incision (Fig. 2.39). When the inferior crus of the lateral canthal tendon has been completely lysed, deep sutures are useful from the lateral aspect of the eyelid orbicularis and tarsus to the inner aspect of the lateral orbital rim, to serve as lower eyelid support and reforming sutures.

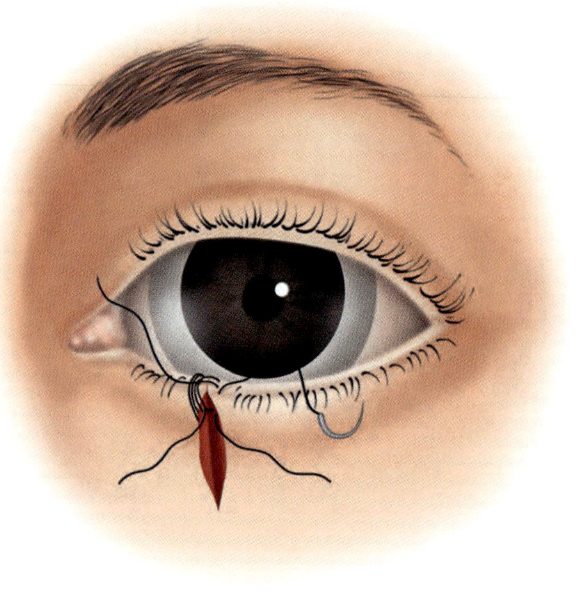

Fig. 2.32 Closure of posterior lid margin sutures away from the cornea

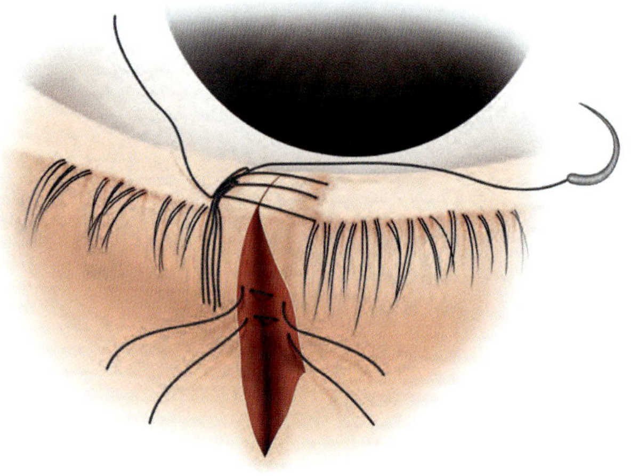

Fig. 2.33 Closure of vertical wound's subcutaneous layer which includes the tarsal layer closure

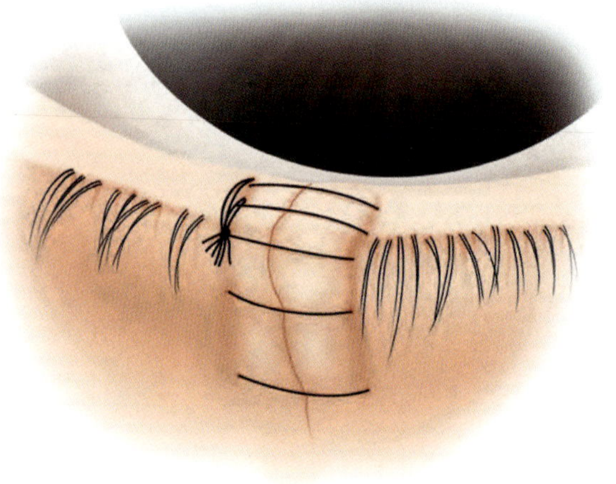

Fig. 2.34 Completed wound closure

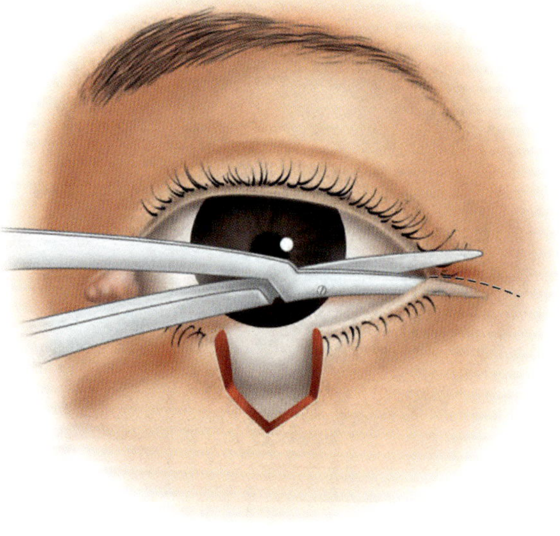

Fig. 2.35 Formation of lateral canthotomy

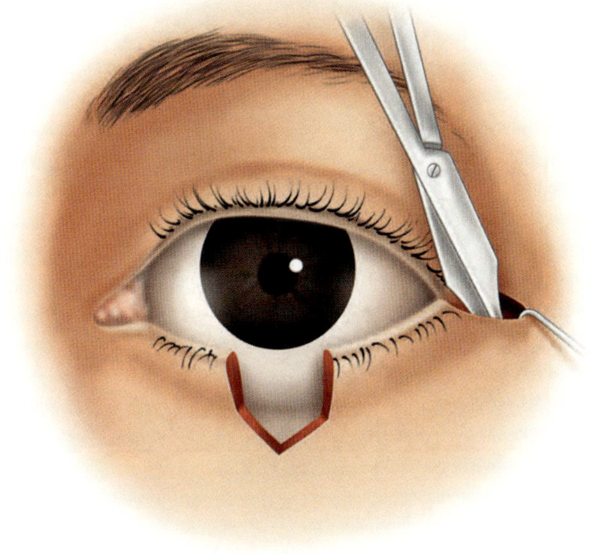

Fig. 2.36 Isolation of inferior crus of the lateral canthal tendon

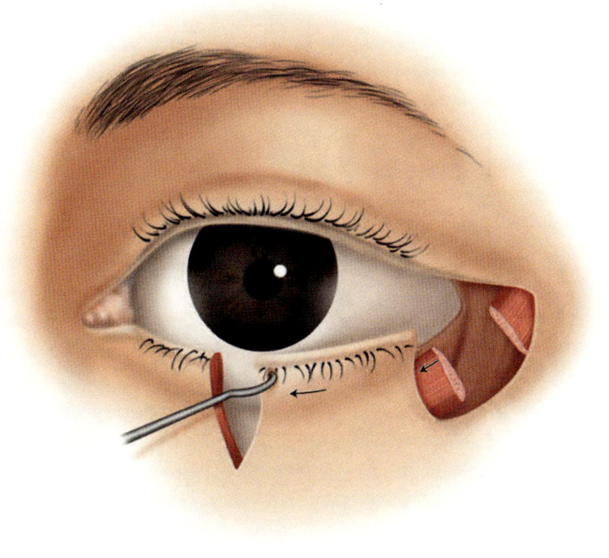

Fig. 2.38 Sliding full-thickness eyelid into place medially after lysis of the inferior crus of the lateral canthal tendon

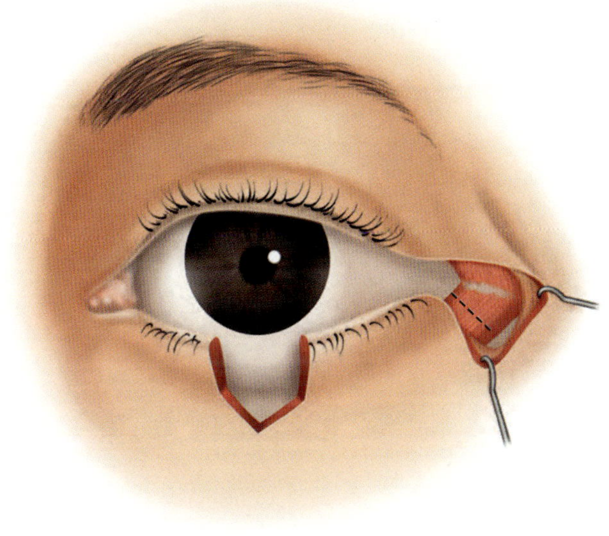

Fig. 2.37 Lysis of the inferior crus of the lateral canthal tendon

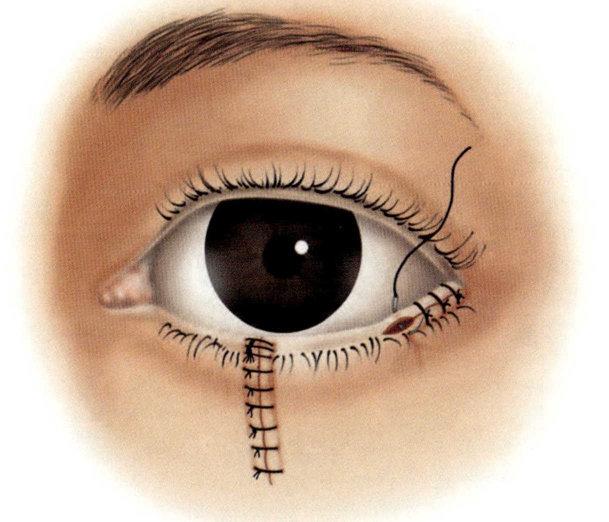

Fig. 2.39 Final closure of incisions after lateral canthotomy and inferior cantholysis for lid margin reconstruction

References

1. Esparaz ES, Sobel RK. Perioperative management of anticoagulants and antiplatelet agents in oculoplastic surgery. Curr Opin Ophthalmol. 2015 Jul;26(5):422–8.
2. Isted A, Cooper L, Colville RJ. Bleeding on the cutting edge: A systematic review of anticoagulant and antiplatelet continuation in minor cutaneous surgery. J Plast Reconstr Aesthet Surg. 2018;71(4):455–67.
3. Lee E, Holtebeck AC, Harrison AR. Infection rates in outpatient eyelid surgery. Ophthal Plast Reconstr Surg. 2009;25(2):109–10.
4. Fay A, Nallasamy N, Bernardini F, Wladis EJ, Durand ML, Devoto MH, Meyer D, Hartstein M, Honavar S, Osaki MH, Osaki TH, Santiago YM, Sales-Sanz M, Vadala G, Verity D. Multinational Comparison of Prophylactic Antibiotic Use for Eyelid Surgery. JAMA Ophthalmol. 2015;133(7):778–84.
5. Lister GD, Gibson DT. Closure of rhomboid skin defects: the flaps of Limberg and Dufourmentel. Br J Plast Surg. 1972;25:300–14.
6. Stein JD, Antonyshyn OM. Aesthetic eyelid reconstruction. Clin Plast Surg. 2009;36(3):379–97.
7. Hass AN, Penne RB, Stefanyszyn MA, Flanagan JC. Incidence of postblepharoplasty orbital hemorrhage and associated visual loss. Ophthal Plast Reconstr Surg. 2004;20(6):426–32.
8. Courtiss EH, Longacre JJ, Destefano GA, Brizio L, Homstrand K. The placement of elective skin incisions. Plast Reconstr Surg. 1963;31(1):31–44.
9. Lister GD, Gibson DT. Closure of rhomboid skin defects: the flaps of Limberg and Dufourmentel. Br J Plast Surg. 1972;25:300–14.

3 Ophthalmic Plastic Surgery: A History in the Making

Alberto G. Distefano, Emily Li, and Mahsa A. Sohrab

Introduction

The subspecialty of ophthalmic plastic surgery was born in the mid-twentieth century in the United States at the conclusion of World War II. The art of oculoplastic surgery, however, is centuries old, bearing its roots in antiquity in India, the Far East, and Europe. The principles and basic techniques that have been improved upon and refined over the years are inherent in the disciplines of ophthalmology and plastic surgery. Thus, a history of ophthalmic plastic surgery is inevitably a history of the development of both fields. The various procedures that have evolved over centuries can be divided into several general categories: reconstructive, restorative, and cosmetic. Each of these categories deals with restoring or enhancing structure as well function to damaged or malfunctioning adnexal structures. Numerous adnexal structures make up the periorbita, and throughout time, oculoplastic surgeons have perfected, refined, and pioneered new techniques of lacrimal surgery, ptosis repair and blepharoplasty, orbital surgery, lid malpositions, and flaps and grafts. Oculoplastic surgery became recognized as a unique subspecialty of ophthalmology at the end of World War II. Numerous orbital and periocular injuries were treated by general ophthalmologists without prior training or exposure to ophthalmic plastic surgery. For these surgeons, review of the existing literature, exchange of experiences with colleagues and across disciplines, and, more often than not, trial and error were keys in developing these procedures. After the war, interest in the subfield of ophthalmic surgery grew, and eventually, an organized association dedicated solely to the field of ophthalmic plastic surgery was formed. This chapter is a testament to those great minds that weaved the broad array of ophthalmic techniques into a quilt of a distinct subspecialty.

Eyelid Repair and Reconstruction

The earliest attempt at modern lid reconstruction was documented by Von Graefe in 1818. He devised a cheek flap to repair an upper eyelid deformed by erysipelas in a young girl. His cheek flap was reminiscent of the primitive sliding advancement skin flaps of Celsus [1]. Numerous flaps have been described in the literature since the time of Celsus (see Table 3.1) [2]. Another curious record of an early-nineteenth-century eyelid repair was made by Dzondi, who used the hand of one of his students as the source for the free graft [3]. Von Graefe, von Walther, Dieffenbach, and von Ammon made unsuccessful attempts at free skin grafting in the nineteenth century. Not until 1869 did Reverdin definitively demonstrate that a free piece of the epidermis could be placed in a new bed and survive if protected and allowed to maintain contact with underlying tissues long enough for union of the tissues to occur [4]. Sichel, Lawson, Bunger, and Warren reported methods for grafting free full-thickness skin grafts in the 1870s, an approach that was later popularized by Le Fort and Wolfe. The split-thickness skin graft was introduced by Ollier and Thiersch in 1874 [2].

In 1835, Dieffenbach reported what was thought to be the first account of a cheek sliding flap for total lower lid reconstruction [5]. It was later shown, however, that De Argumosa of Spain had presented "Dieffenbach's" method 3 years prior to the Faculty of Medicine in Madrid [6]. Sichel suggested a skin flap from the arm for eyelid reconstruction, which was later performed by Ray Burger of Paris in 1879 (see Fig. 3.1) [7, 8]. The Z-plasty or switch flap was first described by Horner in 1837 and then by Denonvillers in 1854 [9].

A. G. Distefano
Boston University School of Medicine, Department of Ophthalmology, Boston, MA, USA

E. Li
University of Washington School of Medicine, Department of Ophthalmology, Seattle, WA, USA

M. A. Sohrab (✉)
Yale University, Department of Ophthalmology, New Haven, CT, USA

J. J. Servat et al. (eds.), *Smith and Nesi's Ophthalmic Plastic and Reconstructive Surgery*,
https://doi.org/10.1007/978-3-030-41720-8_3

Table 3.1 Various flaps in ophthalmic plastic surgery since the time of Celsus

Advancement	Celsus	c. AD 25
(applied to eyelids)	Dzondi	1818
Upper extremity	A. Branca	c. 1460
(publication)	Taglicozzi	1597
(applied to eyelids)	Sichel	1834
Pedicle transposition	Fricke	1829
Transposition/rotation	de Argumosa y Obregón	1833
	Hysern y Molleras	1834
	Dieffenbach	1835
Z-plasty	Horner	1837
	Denonvilliers	1854
Pedicle transposition	Von Langenbeck	1874
Tarsoconjunctival	Landolt	1881
Bipedicle skin	Landolt	1885
	Tripier	1889
Skin island orbicularis (brow to lower lid)	Tripier	1889
Vascularized island pedicle	Monks	1898
Cervical (not tubed)	Snydacker	1907
	Morax	1908
Tubed pedicle from neck	Filatov	1917
Compostive eyelid transpostion	Gillies	1918
(upper to lower)	Esser	1919
Tarsoconjunctival	Dupuy-Dutemps	1921
	Hughes	1937
Nasojugal flap	Spaeth	1925
Composite bridge	Cutler and Beard	1955
Cheek rotation with or without eyelid transposition	Mustardé	1966
Semicircular myocutaneous	Tenzel	1975
Tarsoconjunctival		
(laterally based)	Hewes–Sullivan–Beard	1976

From [2]

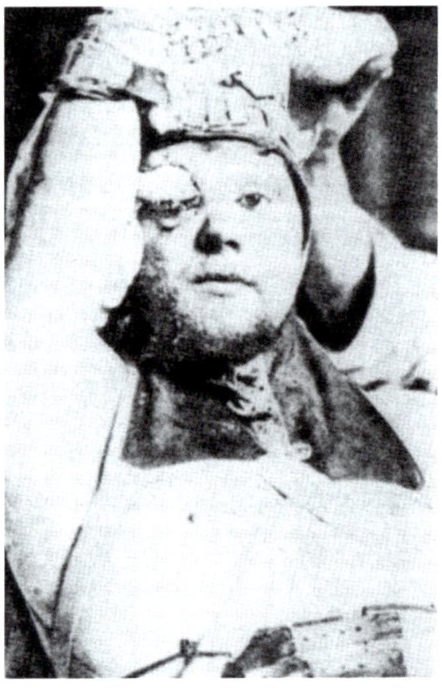

Fig. 3.1 Pedicle flap reconstruction in the nineteenth century. (This photograph probably appeared in a nineteenth-century publication De Vincentiis: Saggio di blepharoplastica)

Vascularized pedicle flaps were suggested by Dunham in 1892 and carried out by Monks in 1898. He isolated a temporal facial skin flap along with its blood supply from a branch of the temporal artery and transposed this flap to the lower lid [10]. In 1917, Filatov reported the first tubed pedicle flap in lower eyelid reconstruction [11]. In 1928, Imre of Budapest described the rotational cheek flap to the lower lid [12]. Fricke described the temporal forehead flap in 1929 [13], and Kazanjian and Roopenian devised the forehead flap in 1956 [14] for the repair of a full-thickness eyelid defect. Both of these surgical approaches require separate reconstruction of the posterior lamella.

During and after World War I, the field of ophthalmic plastic surgery blossomed especially in the area of eyelid reconstruction. Propelled by the horrific casualties of war, surgeons experimented with old methods and innovated new ones for the reparation of the periorbita. Wheeler (1879–1938) served in the Army Medical Corps in World War I and contributed many novel reparative post-traumatic operations and prostheses. His "halving lid incision" became a popular method to repair the upper lid [15]. Spaeth, like Wheeler, was instrumental to the advancement of the techniques used for eyelid reconstruction post-World War I. In 1925, he published *Newer Methods of Ophthalmic Plastic Surgery*, the first text dedicated solely to the subspecialty. In this book, Spaeth delineated numerous applications and modifications to pedicle and flap grafting along with numerous other innovations for orbital surgeries post-enucleation [16].

One of Wheeler's most renowned students was Wendell Hughes, who trained under Wheeler from 1924 to 1935 at Bellevue Hospital. Among Hughes' numerous accomplishments in ophthalmology, he became the first president of ASOPRS in 1969, was deeply involved in education at national meetings and of his fellows, and played a leading role in the development of microneedles and improved suture materials. He is well known for his method of repair of a full-thickness lower lid defect, published in 1937. The posterior lamella was reformed with a tarsoconjunctival flap from the upper eyelid, and a full-thickness skin graft was then transplanted to reform the anterior lamella (see Fig. 3.2) [17, 18]. Interestingly, the idea for this procedure had been the brainchild of Landolt as early as 1881 and the operation had previously been carried out by Dupuy-Dutemps in 1921 [2].

World War II bred a second wave of talented and motivated ophthalmologists whose advents in the field of ophthalmic plastic surgery propelled the field forward. Among them were Scheie, Smith, Stallard, and Mustarde. Smith first described and coined the term "blowout fracture" of the floor of the orbit [19]. Mustarde described the rotational cheek flap for lower eyelid repair and the lower eyelid full-thickness transposition surgery with a pedicled flap for upper eyelid repair (see Fig. 3.3) [20]. In 1955, Cutler and Beard described their bridge flap for reparation of a full-thickness central

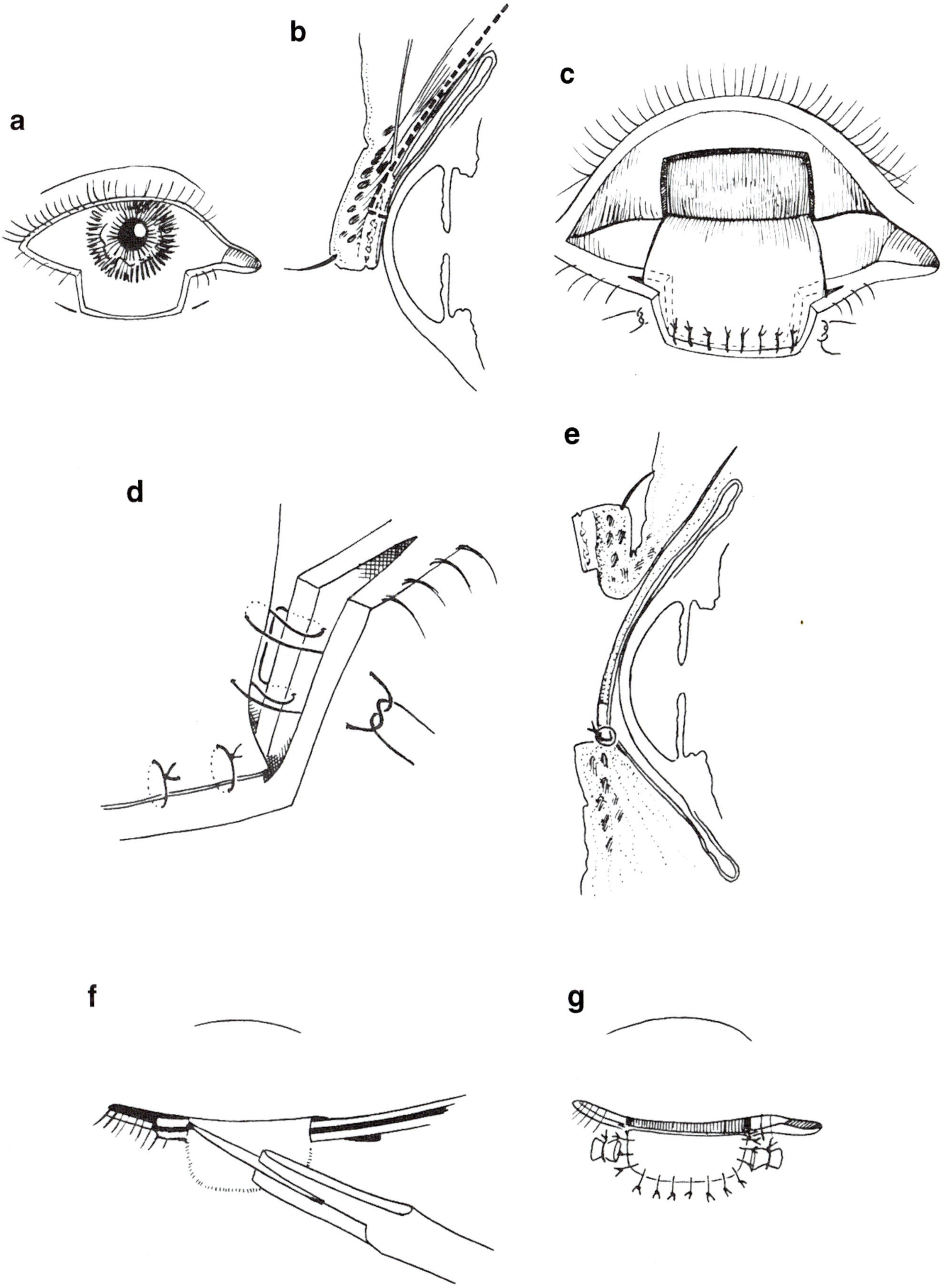

Fig. 3.2 (**a**–**g**) Kollner–Hughes procedure for lower lid reconstruction, originally described by Hughes in 1937. (From Meltzer [115]. With permission)

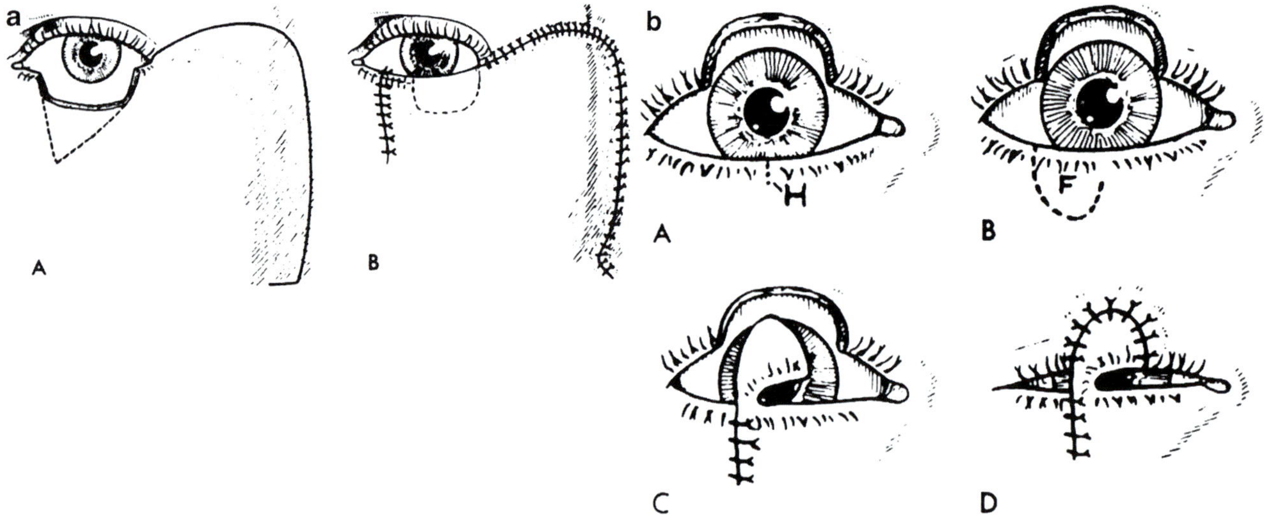

Fig. 3.3 Original diagram of Mustarde's (**a**) lower lid repair with cheek flap; (**b**) upper lid repair with pedicle flap from lower lid. (From Mustarde [116])

upper lid defect in 1955. They described the creation of a temporary full-thickness bridge flap from the lower to the upper lid (see Fig. 3.4) [18, 21]. Tenzel devised his rotational semicircular flap in 1975 for the reconstruction of upper and lower lid defects of 30–40% [22].

Ptosis

Antiquity

Ptosis and dermatochalasis were most likely considered to be the same entity by the surgeons of antiquity as they treated both conditions by simple excision of redundant skin indiscriminately. Celsus' description of the treatment of the "relaxed eyelid" written in the first century AD is surprisingly reminiscent of the modern day blepharoplasty:

> …seize a fold of skin between a finger and thumb, and so to raise it; then consider how much must be removed for the lid to be in a natural position for the future…Next where it is seen that the incision is to be made, a mark must be made first in the case of the upper lid, but the second for the lower one…the edges of the wound are to be brought into apposition by one stitch…on the fourth day the sutures are taken out and a salve for repressing inflammation is smeared on [1].

Another ingenious technique of blepharochalasis repair was the method of "controlled tissue necrosis" described by the Arabic physician Ali ibn Isa (AD 940–1010). He advocated using two wooden sticks compressing excessive skin, which would become ischemic and fall off in several days without scarring (see Fig. 3.5) [23].

Approaches to Levato

George James Guthrie (1785–1856) was the first to comment on the limitations of skin excision in the correction of the pathogenesis of ptosis [24]. Surgeons attempted various methods of improving on the simple method of skin excision to correct ptosis. Von Graefe, for example, described resection of an elliptical wedge of orbicularis in addition to simple blepharoplasty in 1863 [25]. However, it was not until 1857 that Sir William Bowman described the first true ptosis surgery that focused on the levator muscle. The procedure involved levator shortening through the excision of the tarsus and levator tendon via the transconjunctival approach [2]. In 1883, Everbusch illustrated the anterior cutaneous approach to ptosis repair where he described the folding and advancement of the levator [26]. Numerous modifications to both of these approaches were made throughout the nineteenth and twentieth centuries. De Blaskovics and Imre (1920s) reintroduced Bowman's posterior approach in Europe, and Berke (1944), Iliff (1950s–1960s), and Beard (see Fig. 3.6) popularized it in the United States. De Lapersonne modified this technique in 1903 by carrying out the first true levator resection with advancement of the muscle onto the tarsus [27]. Surgery on the levator muscle thus comprised the main surgical approach to ptosis surgery for over a century, beginning in 1857.

Tarsectomy/Mullerectomy

In 1891, Gillet de Grandmont described a cutaneous approach to ptosis correction that involved a partial tarsal and Muller's resection [28]. Grandmont utilized the external approach in

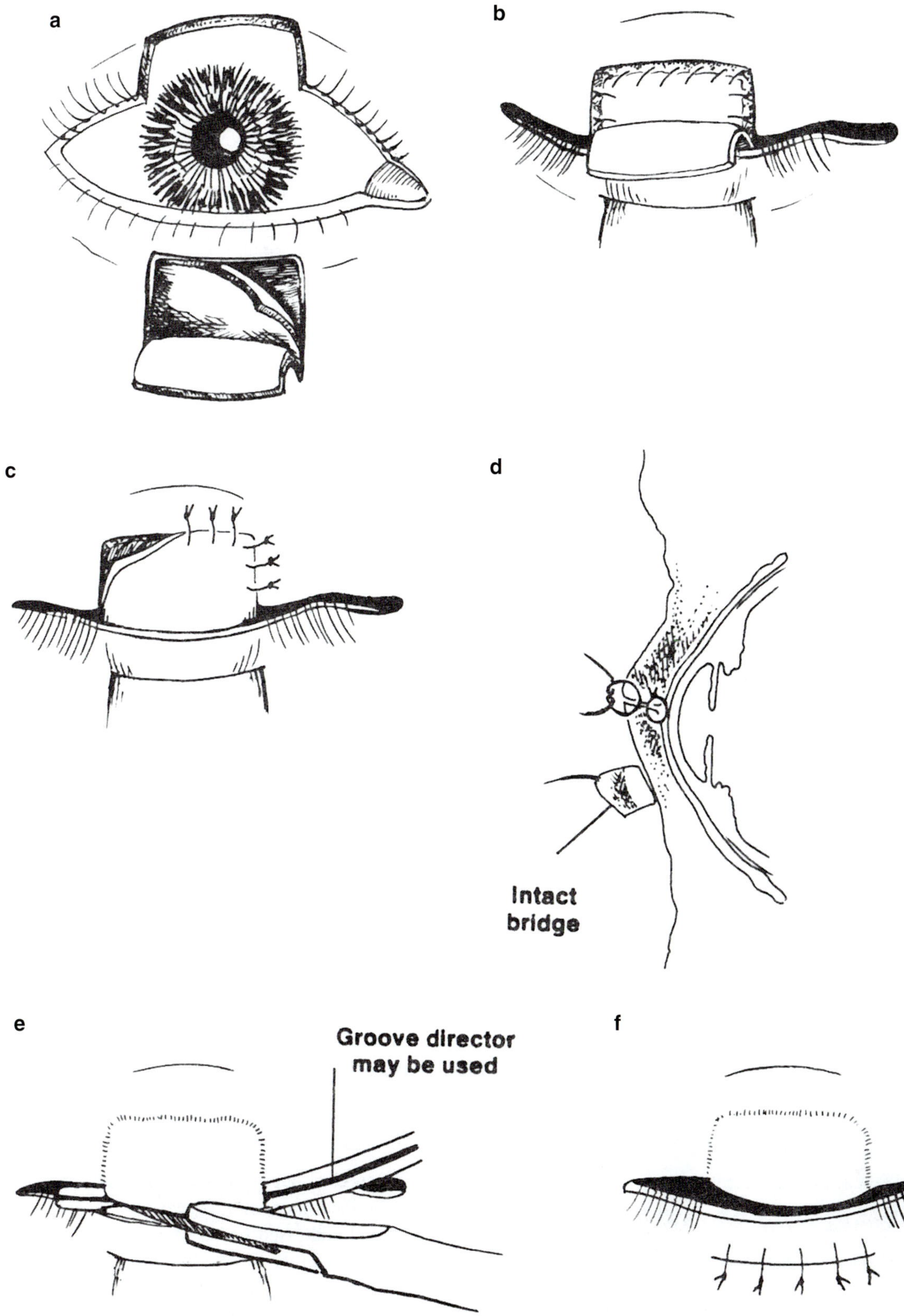

Fig. 3.4 (**a–f**) Method of Cutler and Beard for reconstruction of upper lid defects with a bridging flap from the lower lid. (From Meltzer [115]. With permission)

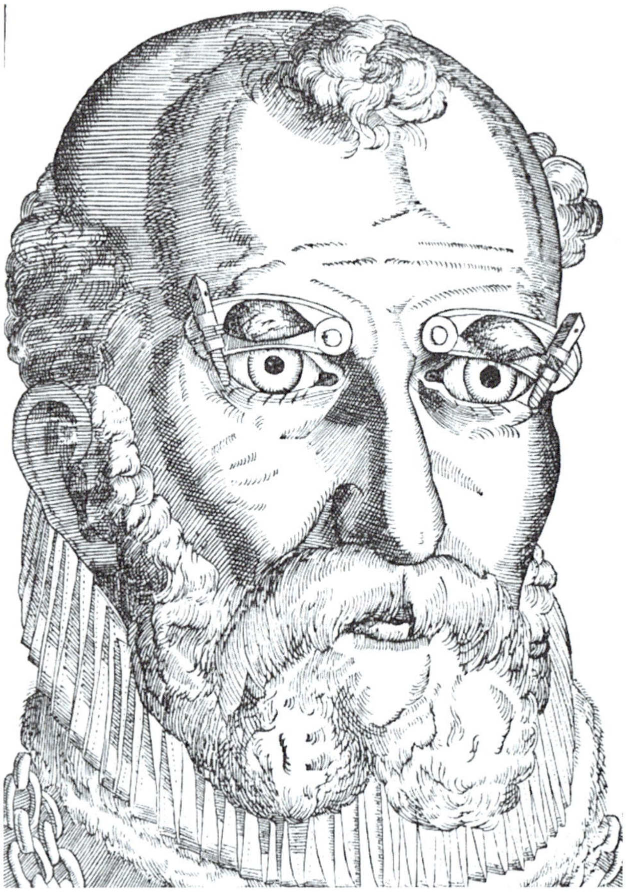

Fig. 3.5 Ali ibn Isa's method of controlled tissue necrosis

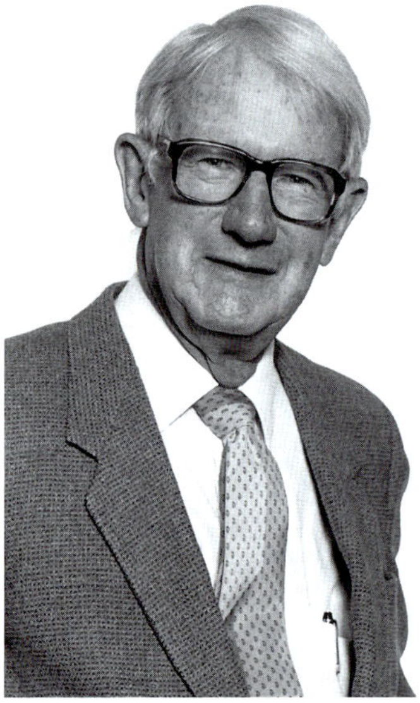

Fig. 3.6 Photograph of Crowell Beard. (This photograph appeared in transactions of the American Ophthalmological Society 139th Annual Meeting and republished with permission of the American Ophthalmological Society)

the correction of congenital ptosis, and later, it was modified and applied to cases of acquired ptosis by Emil Gruening and Wilbur Marple in the early twentieth century. Tarsectomy via the posterior approach was developed by Hervouet and Tessier [29, 30].

Modern approaches to the correction of mild ptosis via the mullerectomy are based on the methods originally described by Fasanella, Servat, Werb, and Putterman. In 1961, Fasanella and Servat described their approach to minimal ptosis surgery as a small resection of levator combined with tarsectomy. Only through pathological studies did the presence of Muller's muscle in the resection become manifest [31]. Interestingly, many texts still refer to the Fasanella–Servat procedure as a surgery on the levator. The great simplicity and predictable, reproducible outcomes of this surgery made ptosis surgery possible even for the general ophthalmologist (see Fig. 3.7) [32]. Werb advocated a method quite similar to the Fasanella–Servat procedure with resection of Muller's muscle in conjunction with tarsal resection, which resulted in some advancement of the muscle [33]. Putterman's procedure involved resection of Muller's muscle and conjunctiva with the aid of a special clamp, without tarsal resection, and is currently advocated for mild to moderate degrees of ptosis [34, 35].

Suspensions. Numerous materials have been used to suspend the ptotic lid. Dransart advocated suspension with absorbable subcutaneous sutures (1880), Panas devised an "eyelid skin sling" to the frontalis muscle (1894), and Motais and Perinaud attempted to suspend the eyelid from the superior rectus muscle (1897). Payr adapted fascia lata for suspension from the tarsal border to the brow (1909), and Wright (1922) and Derby (1928) further improved upon this technique by suggesting a double fascia lata sling and a hammock sling [36]. In 1965, Beard described the use of a bilateral frontalis sling using autologous fascia lata for severe unilateral ptosis and Marcus Gunn jaw-winking syndrome [37].

Lid Malpositions

Antiquity

A variety of surgical approaches to repair lid malpositions have been described since antiquity. No matter which method was utilized, all addressed one or more underlying pathological mechanisms of the ill-positioned eyelid (entropion or ectropion) such as horizontal tightening, repair of lid retractors, and redirecting the vector force of the orbicularis muscle. Everting sutures for the correction of entropion were described by Hippocrates as early as 380 BC. The great

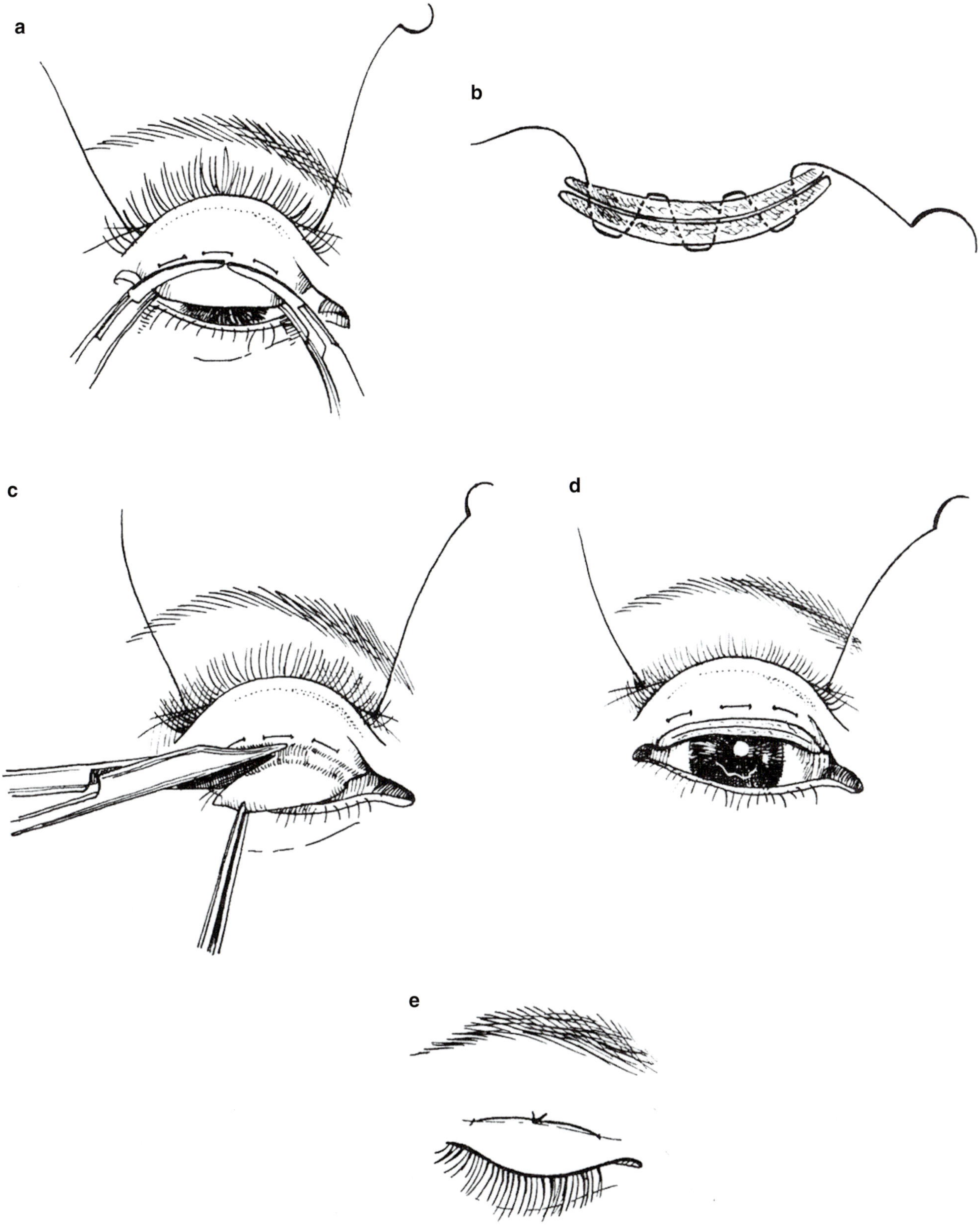

Fig. 3.7 (**a**–**e**) Fasanella–Servat procedure for the correction of mild ptosis. (From Meltzer [115]. With permission)

ancient Greek surgeons Leonidas (200 BC) and Aetius of Amida (sixth century) treated the inturned eyelid with excision of skin and full-thickness eyelid incision, followed by lid-margin everting sutures [38]. Snellen (1862) full-thickness sutures [39] and Ziegler (1909) cautery [40] were used to repair eyelid margin malpositions but were successful only in cases of mild ectropion and did not address the lateral canthal tendon or eyelid laxity. Recognizing these limitations, various procedures to shorten and tighten the lid were undertaken over the years.

Ectropion

In 1835, Dieffenbach reported a procedure of horizontal tightening of the atonic lower lid via excision of a triangle of skin distal to the lateral canthus. Dieffenbach also described modification to this procedure for the correction of cicatricial ectropion and combined it with lateral tarsorrhaphy for magnified effect. Dieffenbach is recognized for innovations of surgical technique in several important areas of ophthalmology and plastic surgery. He was one of the few physicians (along with von Graefe and von Ammon) to be a candidate for the title of "father of plastic surgery" for his innovations in graft and flap reconstructions and rhinostomy procedures, as well as "father of strabismus surgery" for popularizing this corrective method [2]. In the 1860s, Szymanowski developed a modification on Dieffenbach's technique of ectropion repair by moving the excised skin triangle superiorly as well as laterally, thus achieving lift of the lax eyelid in addition to horizontal tightening [36].

In 1812, William Adams, an English surgeon, described the first full-thickness wedge eyelid resection for ectropion repair. Unaware of Adams' work, von Ammon of Germany reported a similar procedure for ectropion repair in 1839 – first describing a central eyelid wedge and later a lateral wedge resection. Besides his contributions to the oculoplastic body of knowledge, von Ammon had many notable achievements in ophthalmology, among which was the publication of one of the first journals in history to be dedicated solely to ophthalmology, *Zeitschrift für die Ophthalmologie* [36, 41].

Building on Adams' experience with tarsal wedge excision, Kuhnt described excision of a portion of the posterior lamella of the eyelid after splitting the lid at the gray line. This approach was criticized by some due to its association with numerous complications such as lid notching, frequent inability to correct medial ectropion, and eyelash damage [36]. Despite these shortcomings, Meller (late nineteenth century) implemented Kuhnt's posterior lamellar resection in combination with Szymanowski's anterior lateral lid resection (Kuhnt–Szymanowski procedure) [41]. Despite numerous modifications of this technique, shortcomings associated with resection of the midtarsal portion of the eyelid included damage to meibomian glands and phimosis and lateralization of the punctum. Attempting to avoid these complications, Bick described a full-thickness resection of the temporal eyelid [42]. Unfortunately, this approach can also lead to deformities of the lateral canthal angle and was thus not the ideal solution to the posed problem.

Tenzel (1977) described the approach of lateral canthal suspension without excision of any portion of the eyelid by fracturing the tarsus and rotating the lid margin. While this technique worked well for mild cases of marginal ectropion, it failed to correct severe cases associated with large amounts of medial and lateral canthal laxity [43]. Imre suggested an approach to the medial portion of the eyelid in the correction of senile ectropion in 1935 [44]. Just 2 years after the elucidation of the lateral canthal suspension, Anderson and Gordy reported the lateral tarsal strip method for the correction of lid malpositions. This procedure, on its own and in combination with other previously described approaches, has become the most commonly practiced corrective surgery for various types of ectropion and some cases of entropion. In this procedure, Anderson described the severing of the inferior crus of the lateral canthal tendon, separation of the anterior and posterior lamellae at the lateral aspect of the lid, excision of a wedge of the posterior and anterior lamellae, and reinsertion of the lateral aspect of the tarsus to the inner lateral orbital wall [45]. For medial ectropion, Meltzer described a procedure combining horizontal lid shortening with vertical lengthening in [46].

Entropion

More surgical approaches to entropion correction have been described than all other procedures for lid malpositions put together. Several lid margin everting suture techniques have been illustrated by Quickert [47] and Feldstein [48] and provide good temporary relief of lid inversion. Modifications of the Bick procedure have also been adapted for the correction of involutional entropion [42]. Weis reported transverse blepharotomy combined with marginal rotation sutures for the treatment of spastic entropion [49]. Ballen later adapted the Weis procedure for upper lid entropion [50]. To fixate the orbicularis, Wheeler (1938) resected a portion of the pretarsal orbicularis and transposed it to the inferior transorbital fascia in order to evert the eyelid edge in involutional entropion [51]. Hill (1967) further modified this technique in order to reduce the incidence of recurrent overriding of the preseptal orbicularis by creating a firmer attachment between the muscle, skin, and tarsus and reattaching the shortened orbicularis muscle directly to the inferior border of the tarsus [52]. Various sources for posterior lamellar grafting for entropion repair have since been described (see Table 3.2) [53].

Table 3.2 Sources utilized for posterior lamellar grafting for entropion repair

Conchal cartilage
Nasal chondromucosa
Palatal mucoperichondrium
Buccal mucosa
Tarsoconjunctival composite graft

Adapted from [53]

In 1993, Dresner and Karesh described the tarsoconjunctival approach for repair of involutional entropion. The procedure addressed the etiological mechanisms of involutional entropion and involved horizontal eyelid shortening, lateral canthal resuspension, and reinsertion retractors of the lower eyelid [54].

Lacrimal Surgery

The earliest surviving description of an ophthalmic plastic procedure is a description of the treatment of an infected lacrimal sac by incision and drainage, in the Code of the Hammurabi (2300 BC). These laws from the King of Babylon also warned that a physician would face loss of his hands should the patient's eye be lost in an unsuccessful surgery [55]. In the first century, the great Roman philosopher Cornelius Celsus described the treatment of a lacrimal sac fistula with excision and "burning to the bone" [1], while Archigenes (second century AD) suggested the usage of caustics to destroy the infected sac in dacryocystitis and bore holes through the nose for drainage [36]. In the seventeenth century, Georg Ernst Stahl identified nasolacrimal duct stenosis as the pathophysiologic mechanism of dacryocystitis and advocated treating the entity with incision and drainage, followed by stenting – with a violin string [56]. The field of lacrimal surgery was revolutionized in 1713 by Dominique Anel who described irrigation and probing of the lacrimal system and developed the earliest probes and cannulae for this purpose [57].

The earliest and most intriguing account of an attempt at dacryocystorhinostomy (DCR) was offered in the eighteenth century by the poet Johann Wolfgang von Goethe:

> Goethe watched the operation and noted that horse hair was used as a stent and placed through the lacrimal punctum, the open lacrimal sac, the anastomosis and out through the nose. This hair was moved every day in order to ensure a free communication. Goethe stayed with Herder for a while in Strasbourg and took care of his postoperative needs. However, after a long and expensive treatment by the "fat surgeon" the anastomosis scarred down and the operation was a failure [7].

The first account of a modern version of a DCR by an external approach appeared in the early twentieth century (1904) by Italian otolaryngologist Addeo Toti and ushered in the modern era of lacrimal surgery. The procedure involved the excision of a wall of the lacrimal sac, creation of a passage within the nasal bone with a hammer and chisel, and removal of overlying nasal mucosa [58]. The external approach was popularized in the late nineteenth and early twentieth centuries by Louis Dupuy-Dutemps and Bourget who described the anastomosis of the lacrimal and nasal mucosa [59].

Dacryocystorhinostomy through the endonasal (intranasal) approach was originally described by G.W. Caldwell in 1893. Utility of this technique at the time was limited due to the inadequate visibility of endonasal structures. J.M. West, an ENT surgeon from Johns Hopkins University, revived the technique in 1910 and claimed a 90% success rate. However, this approach was not employed often during the twentieth century because it was plagued by technical difficulties that had to do with poor visualization of the operative site. Interest in endonasal DCR resurfaced in 1979 with Cohen's advent of a technique for endoscopic viewing into the lacrimal sac and coined the term "dacryoscopy" [60]. The fiberoptic scopes that were developed allowed for improved visualization of the endonasal anatomy. A modified version of the original technique, which utilized argon laser for the creation of the DCR fistula, was popularized in the 1990s by Gonnering and Massaro [61].

Various natural and synthetic materials have been used as temporary stents to correct acute and chronic lacrimal obstructions and disruptions. Canalicular obstruction has been treated by stenting as early as the 1700s. Some of the earliest attempts at preventing lacrimal system closure after canalization utilized animal or human hair, and others attempted stenting with strings of musical instruments (see above).

Henderson advocated polyethylene tubing of the canalicular system at the time of DCR in 1950 [62]. Huggert [63] used polyethylene tubing for stenting, and Werb [64, 65] conceived of the bicanalicular polyethylene intubation. The stiff polyethylene tubing was prone to causing punctual erosion, canalicular lacerations, and frequent tube kinking. For canalicular repair, Worst's spiral "pigtail" probe in 1962 provided a simpler method of canalicular intubation that avoided the surgical opening of the lacrimal sac [66]. Various malleable metal stents have been used to repair lacerated canaliculi (Veirs [67], Johnson [68]). The advent of the softer silicone tubing in the late 1960s alleviated some of these common complications of lacrimal reparative surgery. In the 1970s, Quickert and Dryden described silastic tubing fashioned with a probe for stenting the lacrimal and for canalicular repair [69]. Guibor and Crawford further adapted the instruments and the technical aspects of the procedure to facilitate passage and retrieval of the tubing [70, 71]. In 1996, Ritleng created an intubation set consisting of a silicone tube linked to a polypropylene tube and ending in a metal probe for lacrimal insertion [72].

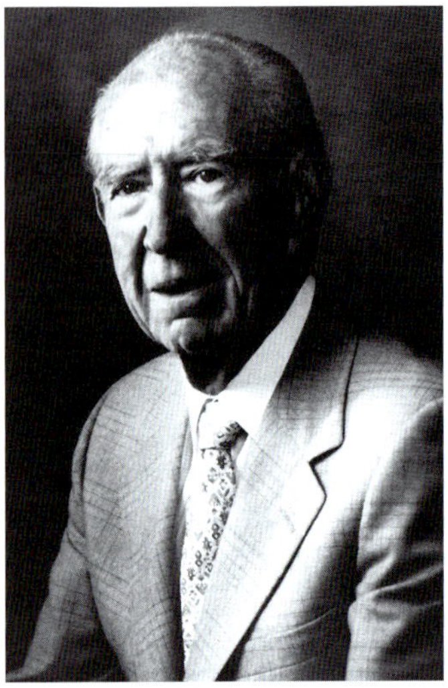

Fig. 3.8 Photograph of Lester T. Jones (1894–1983). (With permission from ASOPRS and David M. Reifler)

In 1961, another milestone in lacrimal surgery was reached when Jones (see Fig. 3.8) published his landmark paper on the first CDCR using a glass pyrex tube for treatment of epiphora in patients with upper lacrimal system dysfunction [73]. Sisler offered yet another technique for bypassing canalicular obstruction by using a minitrephine to reestablish patency of a blocked lacrimal passage, followed by intubation of the system [74].

Finally, in 1985, Werb glimpsed into the future and envisioned a definitive solution for irreparable canalicular damage – the canalicular transplant: "…dare one speak of the possibility of transplanting an intact canalicular system which will include puncta, canaliculi and an appropriate segment of the lateral wall of the lacrimal sac?" [65]. The first successful canalicular transplant was carried out by Meltzer via an en bloc full-thickness lid transplantation published in 2010 [75].

Orbital Surgery

Antiquity

The earliest records of orbital surgery date back to the sixteenth century. Bartisch's method of extirpation of the eyeball, in today's terms, would be deemed a subtotal exenteration sans anesthesia. He advocated the passing of a large tractional suture through the eyeball and then cut away portions of the globe until it was completely detached from surrounding structures (see Fig. 3.9) [76].

With a spoon-shaped knife "sharp as any razor can be, press it into a groove under the upper lid however very close to the bone and on the skull-cup to the very backmost ground, turn then quickly and dextrously the entire eye, especially so that it may be emptied out and made loose on the hinder place in all parts, very fine and close around on the skull-cap and bones in order that the corrupted material, the bad humors, veins and nerves may be brought out and away completely at all places. Yet everyone ought, who goes about this, to see to it industriously in advance that he does not injure the upper and the lower lid, so that it may not afterward heal hideously and hatefully" [76].

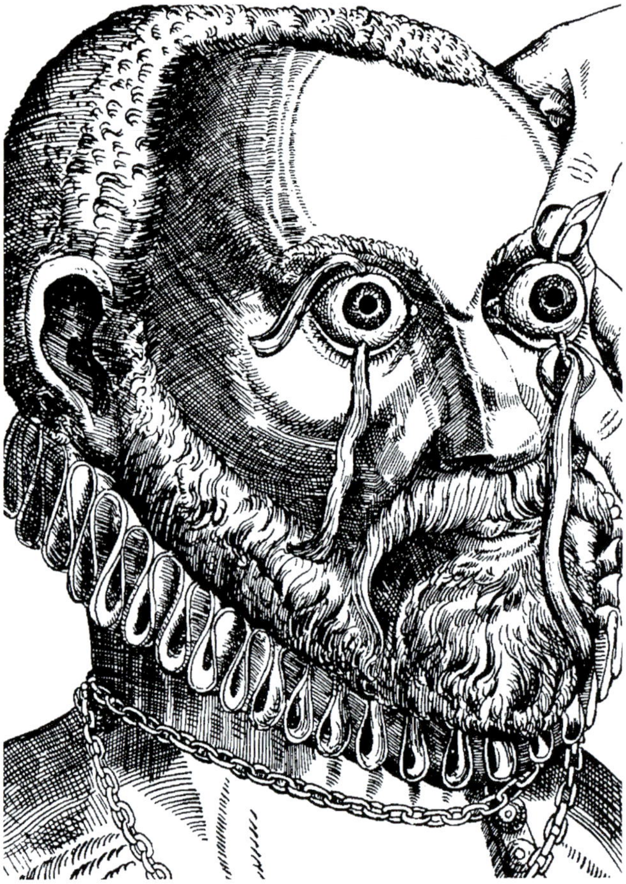

Fig. 3.9 Method of extirpation as described by Bartisch, 1535–1606

Although it was heralded as one of the most barbaric ocular surgical procedures, extirpation was the accepted method of enucleation for over a century. The modern method of enucleation was initially described by Cleobурey in 1826 and then again independently by Bonnet and O'Farrell in 1841 [77–79]. The technique required separation of the sclera from Tenon's capsule and the subsequent severing of the extraocular muscles and optic nerve. Although not present in the original descriptions of Bonnet and O'Farrell, conjunctival closure after enucleation was routinely practiced at the end of the nineteenth century [80]. Post-enucleation socket ablation was advocated by Streatfeild, Green, and Alt in the late nineteenth century and was repopularized for special cases by Rycroft in the 1960s [2]. Gooch is credited with being the first to describe an exenteration in 1767 [81]. The first modern exenteration was carried out in 1864 by Collis [82].

Ocular Prostheses

The first ocular prosthesis was a hollow glass ball that was sutured within Tenon's capsule after evisceration by Mules in 1885 [83]. The Mules implant was fragile and was plagued by complications of frequent extrusion and temperature- or trauma-induced shattering. Frost and Lang separately described glass ocular prostheses over which they sutured the rectus muscles [36, 84]. Various materials have since been used to try to improve complication rates (see Table 3.3) [85].

In the 1930s, Wheeler described a hollow-ball implant with grooves for the rectus muscles [86]. This prosthesis significantly decreased extrusion rates and also allowed for some implant mobility. Wheeler is also remembered for being the first to suggest implanting autologous fat after enucleation – an approach that was later popularized by a young student of Dr. Hughes [87].

Acrylic prostheses became widespread during the 1940s when the large number of wartime ocular casualties could not be supported with glass implants that were manufactured abroad. Ruedemann made significant contributions to the field of anophthalmic socket repair and created the first "integrated orbital implant" in 1945. This was a two-part implant that consisted of an anterior conformer and a posterior tantalum mesh that had four attachment points for the extraocular muscles [88]. Although this implant was more durable than its glass counterparts and allowed for greater globe mobility, its utility was limited by its associated complications such as socket infections and implant migration. Despite this, the Ruedmann implant opened the door to the various improved integrated implants that followed. Notably, Ruedmann was also instrumental to forging the alliance between ophthalmologists and ocularists and to the formation of the American Society of Ocularists (ASO) in 1958 [2].

Table 3.3 Various materials used for enucleation implants

Agar	Paraffin
Aluminum	Peat
Asbestos	Plastic
Bone	Platinum
Cartilage	Polymethyl methacrylate[a]
Cat gut	Polyvinyl sponge
Cellulose	Rubber
Coral (hydroxyapatite)[a]	Silk
Cork	Silver
Charred bone	Silicone (solid or inflatable)[a]
Fat[a]	Stainless steel
Fascia lata	Tantalum
Glass (single hollow ball or beads)	Vaseline
Gold	Vitallium
Ivory	Wool

From [85]. With permission
[a]Commonly in use today

One year after Ruedemann described his implant, Cutler devised a new partially buried two-piece integrated implant. Made of methyl methacrylate, the posterior portion fit into the anterior artificial eye shell via a male–female socket configuration. Several years after he designed his first implant, Cutler created a tantalum mesh "universal implant" that could be used for either enucleations or eviscerations [89]. In 1949, Troutman developed a magnetic, buried, integrated implant. Most of the integrated implants, including those of Cutler and Troutman and later modifications, were not well tolerated and tended to cause socket infections and frequently extruded. Additionally, Troutman's implant suffered from slippage between the buried and external portion that led to conjunctival erosion [90]. A variety of buried orbital implants have been described through the years (see Fig. 3.10) [91].

A major advance in orbital implants came about in 1985, when Perry introduced the hydroxyapatite orbital implant. This new material was much more compatible than glass and PMMA. However, more importantly because of the porous nature of hydroxyapatite, it allows the body to vascularize through the implant and thus improves ocular motility and minimizes implant migration. Perry also introduced the concept of post-op drilling for peg insertion to improve motility of the prosthesis [92].

Approaches to the Orbit

Parker described making a transconjunctival incision in 1841 in order to remove a cystic lesion from the lateral orbit [93]. Knapp, de Wecker, and Carter all reported using the transconjunctival orbitotomy to access pathological entities of the optic nerve [2]. Passavant is credited with performing the first lateral orbitotomy in the 1860s in order to resect an orbital aneurysm [94]. The lateral orbitotomy incision described by Kronlein in 1888 revolutionalized orbital surgery because it enabled the surgeon to access the retrobulbar compartment [95]. This incision, however, left an unsightly half-moon scar over the temple. Stallard popularized the S-shaped under-brow lateral orbitotomy incision that was initially described by Cirincione in 1901 [96, 97]. In 1907, Rollet reported the first anterior orbitotomy, which involved making an incision beneath the brow and dissecting subperiosteally in order to gain entry to the orbit. The transcranial approach was initially described by Dandy in 1922 [94].

In 1962, Smith described the vertical full-thickness lid split approach to the superomedial orbit [98]. This incision provided good access to the intraconal space with minimal morbidity. Over the last 10 years, the eyelid crease incision has become one of the standard approaches used to access the superomedial orbit [99]. Initially described by Wolfley in 1985, this incision's popularity is heralded by the large area

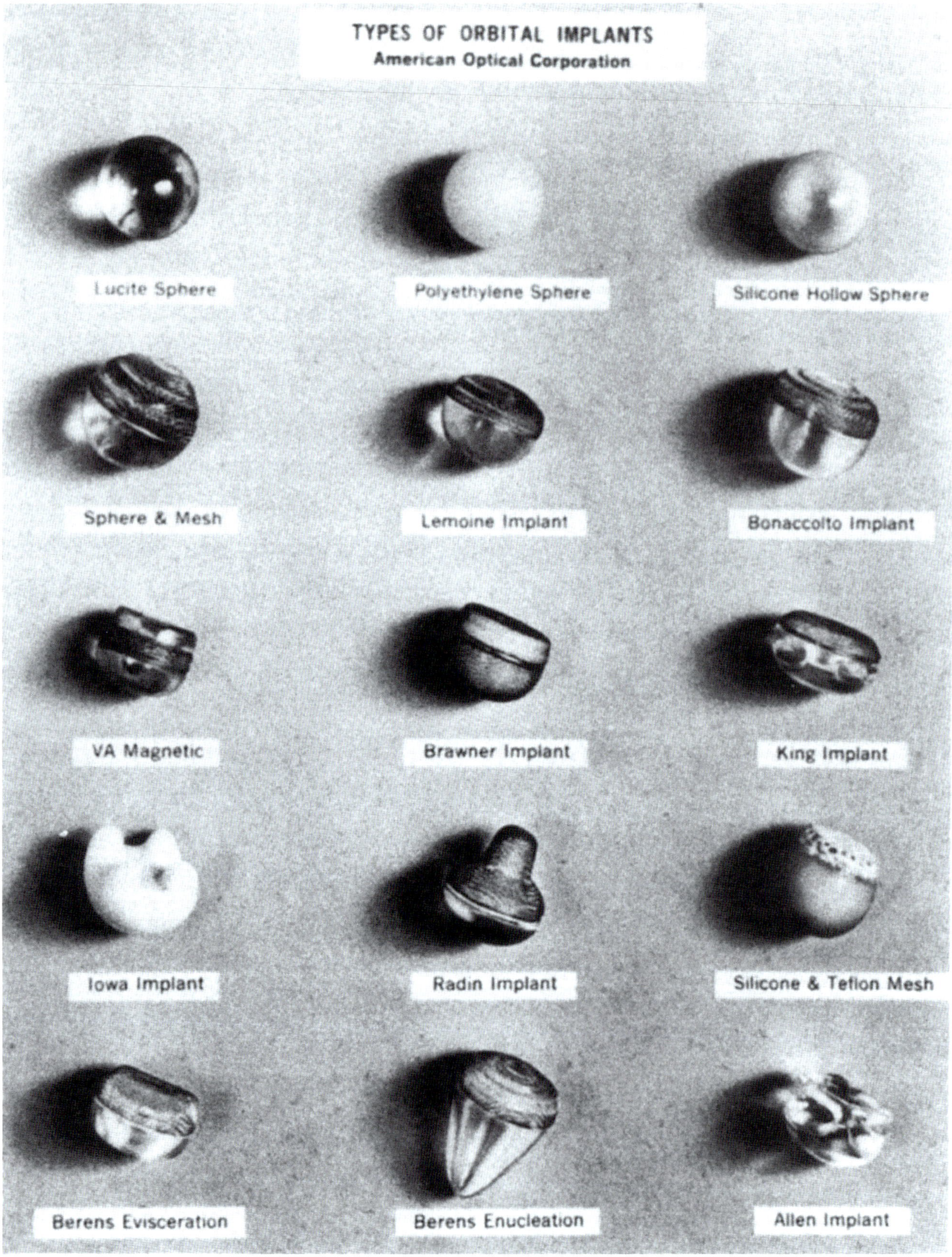

Fig. 3.10 Types of integrated orbital implants. (With permission from [91])

of exposure to the anterior orbit that it provides and the minimal scarring it leaves behind. Although both the lid crease approach and the vertical split approach were initially exclusively utilized to access the medial anterior orbit, in the past few years, both of these incisions have been used to reach the posterior orbit for various interventions such as optic nerve fenestration [100].

Several different approaches to the medial orbit are described in the literature. The Lynch transcutaneous incision was made by incising the skin over the superomedial orbital rim. This incision frequently resulted in webbing and scarring of the nasal canthal area. The transconjunctival approach (see above) decreased scarring but did not allow adequate exposure of the medial aspect of the orbit. The transcaruncular approach, devised by Balch et al. in 1998 and popularized by Goldberg, allowed for greater access to the medial orbit and orbital apex with minimal resultant scarring [101].

Orbital Decompression

Decompression of every wall of the orbit has been described in twentieth-century ophthalmic literature. The first decompression for Graves' ophthalmopathy via the Kronlein lateral orbitotomy approach was performed by Dollinger in 1911. Anterior cranial fossa decompression was described by Naffziger, a neurosurgeon, in 1931, and Sewall performed the first medial wall decompression in 1936 [2, 102]. Orbital floor decompression into the maxillary sinus was published by Hirsch in 1950 [102]. The Caldwell–Luc decompression of the medial and inferior walls, intra-orally via the maxillary sinus, was reported by Walsh and Ogura in 1957 [103]. More recently, the transnasal endoscopic decompression of the medial wall has been described by Kennedy et al. in 1990 [104]. Finally, Kazim, Trokel, and Moore innovated the fat decompression technique for Graves' orbitopathy in 1993 [105].

ASOPRS

In 1969, several of Byron Smith's fellows founded the American Society of Ophthalmic Plastic and Reconstructive Surgery (ASOPRS) [2]. Beyer, Buerger, Cherubini, Obear, Wilkins, and Pidde conceived of the idea for a society that could function as a forum for the exchange of ideas in the growing subspecialty of ophthalmic plastic surgery and to optimize the quality of the training of ophthalmic plastic surgeons in the United States. In his description of the events surrounding the society's founding, Buerger credited Margaret Obear's enthusiasm and organizing endeavors to the success of the effort. Cherubini reminisced about the atmosphere surrounding the time of the society's creation:

> The actual idea of the ASOPRS was hatched in a Third Avenue bar where we would assemble, more or fewer of us, once in a while after work for refreshment. Out of those (sometimes hilarious) meetings the idea became reality…We all [five] worked like hell on the founding [of the Society] [2].

The young ASOPRS received great support from many prominent oculoplastic surgeons and especially from Byron Smith (see Fig. 3.11) and Alston Callahan (see Fig. 3.12). The first ASOPRS meeting was held in 1969 concurrently with the American Academy of Ophthalmology (AAO) meeting. Sixty people signed up for charter membership, and Wendell Hughes (see Fig. 3.13) was elected the society's first president (see Table 3.4). He trained many of the field's leaders, including Cole and Stasior. Stasior was chosen as

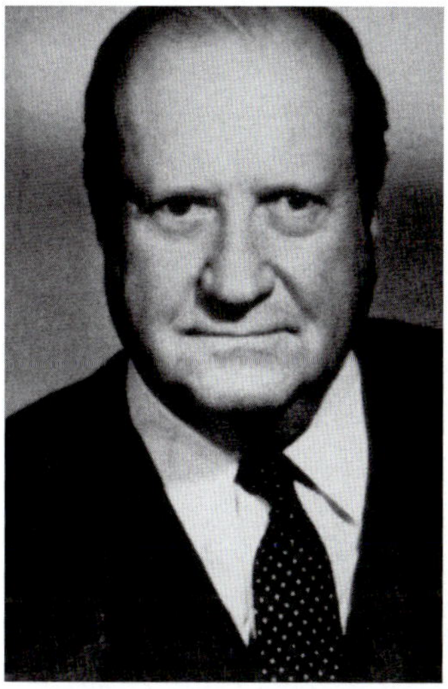

Fig. 3.11 Photograph of Byron Capleese Smith (1908–1990). (Courtesy of ASOPRS and David M. Reifler)

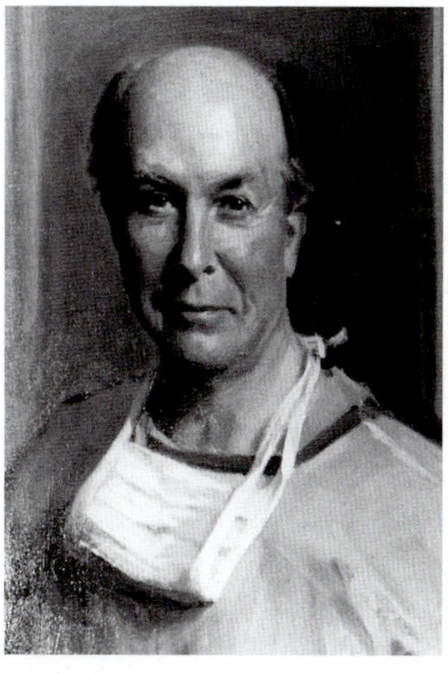

Fig. 3.12 Alston Callahan. A photograph of an oil painting displayed at the Eye Foundation Hospital in Birmingham. (Courtesy of ASOPRS and David M. Reifler)

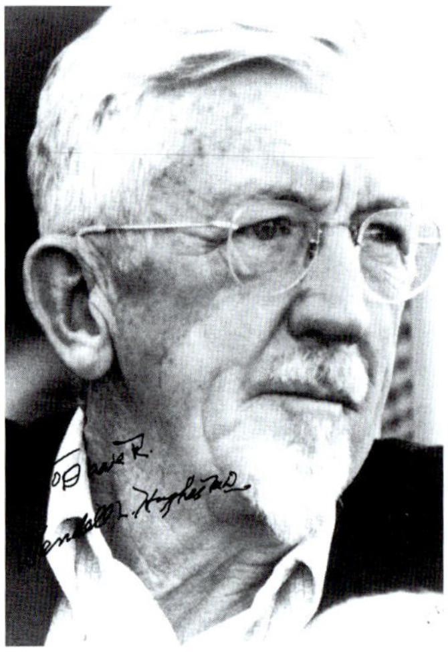

Fig. 3.13 Photograph of Wendell Hughes. (Courtesy of ASOPRS and David M. Reifler)

Table 3.4 Founding and charter members of the ASOPRS in 1969

ASOPRS founding and charter fellows	
Peter H. Ballen	Ira S. Jones
Henry I. Baylis	Lester T. Jones
Crowell Beard	Burton Krimmer
James E. Bennett	Charles R. Leone, Jr.
Raynold N. Berke	Jack V. Lisman
A. Jan Berlin	Edward L. Liva
Charles K. Beyer	Virginia Lubkin
David W. Bishop	Charles S.G. Maris
Martin Bodian	Clinton D. McCord, Jr.
Alvin H. Brackup	Murray A. Meltzer
George F. Buerger	Gordon R. Miller
Alston Callahan	Fay E. Millett
Thomas Cherubini	Margaret F. Obear
John S. Crawford	William J. Pidde
Robert D. Deitch	Marvin H. Quickert
Robert M. Dryden	Merrill J. Reeh
Rocko M. Fasanella	Albert D. Ruedemann, Sr.
Morris Feldstein	Robert A. Schimek
John R. Finlay	Gerard M. Shannon
Joseph C. Flanagan	Daniel Silva
Sidney A. Fox	Bernd Silver
James L. Hargiss	Robert A. Silver
Deane C. Hartman	Byron C. Smith
Sanford D. Hecht	David B. Soll
Joseph C. Hill	Edmund B. Spaeth
Wendell L. Hughes	Orkan George Stasior
John W. Huneke	Richard R. Tenzel
Charles E. Iliff	Robert B. Wilkins
Carl C. Johnson	

Courtesy of ASOPRS

the second president of ASOPRS in 1971 and was followed by Obear in 1972.

In 1979, the first oral exams in ophthalmic plastic surgery were given under the direction of Flanagan and in 1984 the first written exams by Sutula. By the early 1980s, ASOPRS had an official seat on the AAO council and had officially sponsored courses in ophthalmic plastics instruction at the AAO meetings. By 1985, the Ad Hoc Committee on Fellowship training headed by Grove made recommendations for fellowship training that were soon implemented by the executive committee.

The ASOPRS expanded the horizon of ocular and orbital work to encompass both reconstructive and cosmetic surgery. Currently, all ASOPRS-trained fellows are well trained in all aspects of reconstructive and aesthetic plastic surgery.

In July of 2010, Evan Black's ASOPRS fellowship (Consultants in Ophthalmic and Facial Plastic Surgery, PC/Wayne State University School of Medicine) became the first program to be accredited by the Accreditation Council for Graduate Medical Education (ACGME). The ACGME sets standards for US graduate medical education programs and confers accreditation with compliance to these standards. This voluntary process gives participating programs further recognition that they meet certain benchmarks in quality and dedication to education. Other currently ACGME-accredited programs include the University of Texas MD Anderson Cancer Center under Bita Esmaeli, the University of Louisville School of Medicine under Bill Nunnery, and West Virginia University under John Nguyen. Massachusetts Eye and Ear Infirmary voluntarily withdrew from ACGME accreditation in July of 2017.

Cosmetic Oculoplastic Surgery

Surgical techniques utilized specifically for enhancement purposes did not come about until the early twentieth century. As described before, during antiquity, the pinch technique was an early attempt at the correction of ptosis and sagging of excess upper eyelid skin. These early surgeries were conducted more for functional rather than cosmetic purposes. As the nuances of periocular and ocular anatomy became elucidated in the eighteenth century, the difference between ptosis and dermatochalasis became more apparent. In 1906, Miller published the first article dedicated solely to cosmetic blepharoplasty [106]. He then published a second manuscript that addressed surgical correction of facial wrinkles and lower lid dermatochalasis [107]. Miller faced some criticism over the years from his more functionally oriented colleagues but continued in his efforts and went on to publish several texts on cosmetic oculoplastic surgery.

Another pioneer in enhancing oculoplastic surgery was Kolle, who published a significant textbook, elucidating oculoplastic techniques for wrinkle removal in 1911 [108]. Bourgett described a transconjunctival approach for excision of fat from the lower lid in 1923, but it was abandoned until

1955 when Tessier used it to gain access to the inferior orbit for reconstruction of congenital facial defects [109, 110].

Castaneres popularized lower lid blepharoplasty with prolapsed fat resection in America in the 1950s [111]. Grafting herniated fat pads to fill the sunken infraorbital sulcus was initially described by Loeb and later popularized by Hamra [112]. Lower eyelid fat herniation was managed by both percutaneous approach described in 1988 by de La Plaza and Arroyo [113] and the transconjunctival method described by Camirand in the 1990s [114]. Numerous other surgical and medical approaches to cosmetic periocular surgery have been described since but are beyond the scope of this chapter.

Closing Remarks

Since antiquity, physicians have been performing surgery on the eye and its cradling structures. Elucidation of the ocular and adnexal anatomy as well as the advent of anesthesia and antisepsis in the mid-nineteenth century allowed surgeons to experiment and improve upon existing methods, as well as to innovate new techniques for reparation and enhancement of the eye and periorbita. Collaborations between individuals and disciplines have allowed for the blossoming of the oculoplastic subspecialty over the past two centuries. The creation of ASOPRS established a platform for the exchange of ideas and standardized the educational requirements for training in ophthalmic plastic surgery. Each year with the graduation of new trainees, we wait for the birth of new ideas and pioneering of new innovative techniques in this still young and evolving subspecialty of ophthalmology.

Although ASOPRS was the first formal organization dedicated solely to training and certifying oculoplastic surgeons, several other organizations with similar objectives arose throughout the world over the past three decades. The European Society of Ophthalmic Plastic and Reconstructive Surgery (ESOPRS) and the Canadian Society of Oculoplastic Surgery were founded in the early 1980s (88, 89), and the Asia Pacific Society of Ophthalmic Plastic and Reconstructive Surgery (APSOPRS) was founded in 2000.

References

1. Celsus AC. DE Medicina. With English translation by WG Spencer. Cambridge, MA, Harvard University Press, 1935, v3, pp338–343.
2. Reifler DM, editor. The American Society of Ophthalmic Plastic and Reconstructive Surgery (*ASOPRS*). Winter Park: ASOPRS/ Norman; 1994.
3. Katzen LB. The history of cosmetic blepharoplasty. In: Putterman A, editor. Cosmetic oculoplastic surgery. New York: Grune & Stratton; 1982. Reprinted, in part, in Advanced Ophthlamic Plastic and Reconstructive Surgery 1986; 5:80–96.
4. Reverdin JL. Greffe epidermique. Bull Soc Imperiale Chir (Paris). 1869;10:483–511.
5. Dieffenbach JF. Eininge Bemerkungen aus uber Paris. Wchnschr f d Res Heilk. 1835;4:7–11.
6. Hughes WL. Reconstructive surgery of the eyelids. St Louis, CV Mosby, 1943. Reprinted, in part, in. Adv Ophthalmic Plast Reconstr Surg. 1986;5:25–87.
7. Hirschberg J. The history of ophthalmology. (Translated in II volumes by Frederick Blodi. Originally published under the title Gescichte der Augenheilkunde Julius Hirschberg, Springer Verlag, Berlin). Bonn: JP Wayenborough, v1–11ptl; 1982–1992.
8. Sichel J. Une discussion sur la blephoroplastique. Gaz d Hop. 1834;8:276.
9. Borges AF, Gibson T. The original Z-plasty. Br J Plast Surg. 1973;26:237–46.
10. Bosniak SL. Ophthalmic and plastic reconstructive surgery in the United States: 1893–1970. Adv Plast Reconstr Surg. 1986;5:241–81.
11. Filatov VP. Plastika na kruglom stebl. Vestnik Oftamologii. 1917;34(4–5):149–58.
12. Imre J. Schetamejplastikat (Lidplastik). Budapest: Studium Kiadasa; 1928.
13. Fricke JCG. Die Bildung neuer Augenlider (Blepharoplastik) nach Zerstorungen und dadurch hervorgebrachten Auswartswendungen derselben. Perthes and Bessler: Hamburg; 1929.
14. Kazanjian VH, Roopenian A. Median forehead flaps in the repair of defects of the nose and surrounding areas. Trans Am Acad Ophthalmol Otolaryngol. 1956;60:557.
15. Wheeler JM. Halving wounds in facial plastic surgery. Proceedings of the 2nd congress Pan Pacific Surgery Association. 1936, p. 289–95.
16. Spaeth EB. Newer methods of ophthalmic plastic surgery. Philadelphia: P Blakiston's; 1925.
17. Hughes WL. A new method of rebuilding the lower lid. Arch Ophthalmol. 1937;17:1008–17.
18. Kohn R. Textbook of ophthalmic plastic and reconstructive surgery. Philadelphia: Lea & Febiger; 1988.
19. Converse JM, Smith B. Enophthalmos and diplopia in fractures of the orbital floor. Br J Plast Surg. 1957;9(4):265–74.
20. Mustarde JC. Repair and reconstruction in the orbital region. 2nd ed. Edinburgh: Churchill Livingstone; 1980.
21. Cutler N, Beard C. A method for partial and total upper lid reconstruction. Am J Ophthalmol. 1955;39:1–7.
22. Tenzel RR. Reconstruction of the central one half of an eyelid. Arch Ophthalmol. 1975;93:125.
23. Wood CA. Memorandum book of a tenth century oculist for the use of modern ophthalmologists. A translation of the TADHKIRAT of Ali ibn Isa of Baghdad. Chicago: Northwestern University; 1936.
24. Guthrie GJ. Lectures on the operative surgery of the eye. London: Burgess and Hill; 1823.
25. von Graefe A. Operation der ptosis. Arch Ophthalmol. 1863;9:57.
26. Rogers PA. Development of oculoplastic surgery in Australia. Adv Ophthal Plast Reconstr Surg. 1986;5:417–20.
27. Beard C. History of ptosis surgery. Adv Ophthalmic Plast Reconstr Surg. 1986;5:125–31.
28. de Grandmont G. Nouvelle Operation du ptosis congenital. Recueil d'Ophthalmol (Paris). 1891;13:267–70.
29. Reifler DM. The tarsectomy operation of A.P.L. Gillet de Grandmont (1837–1894) and its periodic rediscovery. Doc Ophthalmol. 1837–1894;89(1–2):153–62.
30. Hervouet F, Tessier P. Technique chirurgicale du ptosis. Bull Mem Soc Fr Ophthalmol. 1956:239–42.
31. Fasanella RM. Surgery for minimal ptosis: the Fasanella-Servat operation, 1973. Trans Ophthalmol Soc UK. 1973;93:425–38.
32. Albert DM, editor. Ophthalmic surgery: principles and techniques. Malden: Blackwell Science; 1999.

33. Werb A. Ptosis. Trans Ophthalmol Soc NZ. 1976;28:29–32.
34. Putterman AM. Müllers muscle-conjunctival resection ptosis procedure. Aust NZ J Ophthalmol. 1985;13(2):179–83.
35. Putterman AM. Mueller's muscle-conjunctival resection-ptosis procedure combined with upper blepharoplasty, Chapter. In: Putterman AM, editor. Cosmetic oculoplastic surgery. 3rd ed. Philadelphia: WB Saunders Co; 1999. p. 145.
36. Fox SA. Ophthalmic plastic surgery. 5th ed. New York: Grune & Stratton; 1976.
37. Beard C. A new treatment for severe unilateral congenital ptosis and for ptosis with jaw-winking. Am J Ophthalmol. 1965;59:252–8.
38. Montadon D. History of plastic surgery of the orbital region. In: Aston SJ, editor. Third international symposium of plastic and reconstructive surgery of the eye and adnexa. Baltimore: Williams & Wilkins; 1982. p. 2–10.
39. Snellen H. Suture for ectropion. Congr Int Opt. 1862;2:236.
40. Ziegler SL. Galvanocautery puncture ectropion and entropion. JAMA. 1909;53:183–6.
41. Smith B, Cherubini TD. Oculoplastic surgery: a compendium of principles and techniques. St Louis: CV Mosby; 1970.
42. Bick MW. Surgical management of orbital tarsal disparity. Arch Ophthalmol. 1966;75(3):386–9.
43. Tenzel RR, Buffam FV, Miller GR. The use of the "lateral canthal sling" in ectropion repair. Can J Ophthalmol. 1977;12:199–202.
44. Imre J Jr. Operation for senile ectropion. Klin Mbl Augenheilk. 1935;95:303–5.
45. Anderson RL, Gordy DD. The tarsal strip procedure. Arch Ophthalmol. 1979;97(11):2192–6.
46. Meltzer MA. Medial ectropion repair. A new procedure. Ophthal Plast Reconstr Surg. 1989;5(3):182–5.
47. Quickert MH, Rathbun E. Suture repair of entropion. Arch Ophthalmol. 1971;85(3):304–5.
48. Feldstein M. Suture correction of senile entropion by inferior lid retractor tuck. Adv Ophthalmic Plast Reconstr Surg. 1983;2:269–74.
49. Weis FA. Spastic entropion. Trans Acad Ophthalmol Otolaryngol. 1955;59:503–6.
50. Ballen PH. A simple procedure for the relief of trichiasis and entropion of the upper lid. Arch Ophthalmol. 1964;72:239–40.
51. Wheeler JM. Spastic entropion correction by orbicularis transplantation. Am J Ophthal. 1939;22:477.
52. Hill JC, Feldman F. Tissue barrier modifications of a Wheeler II operation for entropion. Arch Ophthalmol. 1967;78:621–3.
53. Stein JD, Antonyshyn OM. Aesthetic eyelid reconstruction. Clin Plast Surg. 2009;36(3):379–97.
54. Dresner SC, Karesh JW. Transconjunctival entropion repair. Arch Ophthalmol. 1993;111:1144–8.
55. Harper RF. The code of Hammurabi. Chicago: University of Chicago Press; 1904. p. P79.
56. Stahl GE. De fistula lachrymali. Halle; 1702.
57. Anel D. Observation Singuliere sur la Fistule Lacrimale. Torino. 1713.
58. Toti A. The treatment of dacryocystitis by the formation of a fresh passage from sac to nasal cavity (dacryocystorhinostomy). Ophthalmol Rev. 1909;28:287.
59. Dupuy-Dutemps L, Bourguet J. Cure de la dacryocystite cronique commune et du larmoiemet par la dacryocysto-rhinosto,ie plastique. Bull Acad de Med (Paris). 1921;86:293–5.
60. Cohen SW, Prescott R, Sherman M, Banko W, Castillejos ME. Dacryoscopy. Ophthalmic Surg. 1979;10(11):57–63.
61. Massaro BM, Gonnering RS, Harris GJ. Endonasal laser dacryocystorhinostomy. A new approach to nasolacrimal duct obstruction. Arch Ophthalmol. 1990;108:1172–6.
62. Henderson JW. Management of obstructions of the lacrimal canaliculi with polyethylene tubes: a follow-up study. Arch Ophthalmol. 1953;49:182–4.
63. Huggert A, Sandmark E. Treatment of lacrimal obstruction with temporarily applied polyethylene tubes – technique and results. Am I Ophthalmol. 1965;60:603–10.
64. Werb A. Role of polyethylene tubing in lacrimal obstructions. In proceedings of the second international symposium on plastic and reconstructive surgery of the eye and adnexa. St. Louis: C.V. Mosby Co; 1967. p. 157–70.
65. Werb A. A lacrimal perspective. Ophthal Plast Reconstr Surg. 1985;1(2):81–2.
66. Worst JGF. Method for reconstructing torn lacrimal canaliculus. Am J Ophthal. 1962;53:520–2.
67. Veirs ER. Malleable rods for immediate repair of the traumatically severed lacrimal canaliculus. Trans Am Acad Ophthalmol Otolaryngol. 1962;66:263–4.
68. Johnson CC. A canaliculus wire. Am J Ophthalmol. 1974;78(5):854–5.
69. Quickert MH, Dryden RM. Probes for intubation in lacrimal drainage. Trans Am Acad Ophthalmol Otolaryngol. 1970;74(2):431–3.
70. Guibor P. Canaliculus intubation set. Ophthalmology. 1975;79:419–20.
71. Crawford JS. Intubation of obstructions in the lacrimal system. Can J Ophthalmol. 1977;12:289–92.
72. Ritleng P. A simplified technique for lacrimal intubation. Ocul Surg News. 1996;14(7)
73. Jones LT. Wobig: surgery of the eyelids and lacrimal system. Aesculapius: Birmingham; 1976.
74. Sisler HA, Allarakhia L. A new ophthalmic microtrephine. Ophthalmic Surg. 1990;21:656–7.
75. Meltzer MA, Zatezalo CC, Zoltan S. Lacrimal canalicular transplantation with composite eyelid graft. Ophthal Plast Reconstr Surg. 2010;26(1):23–5.
76. Snyder C. An operation designated "The extirpation of the eye". Arch Ophthalmol. 1965;74:429–32.
77. Cleobury W. A review of the different operations performed on the eyes. London: T. & G. Underwood; 1826. p. 261.
78. Ferrall JM. On the anatomy and pathology of certain structures in the orbit not previously described. Dublin J M Sc. 1841;19:329.
79. Bonnet A. Nouvelles recherches sur l'anatomie des aponevroses et des muscles de l'oeil. Ann d'oculist. 1841;5:27.
80. Guyton JS. Enucleation and allied procedures: a review and description of a new operation. Trans Am Ophthalmol Soc. 1948;46:472–527.
81. Frezzotti R, Bonanni R, Nuti A, Polito E. Radical orbital resections. Adv Ophthal Plast Reconstr Surg. 1992;9:175–92.
82. Collis MH. On the diagnosis of cancer and the tumor. London: John Churchill and Sons editors; 1864. p. 68–70.
83. Mules PH. Evisceration of the globe with artificial vitreous. Trans Ophthalmol Soc UK. 1885;5:200–6.
84. Frost WA. What is the best method of dealing with a lost eye? Br Med J. 1887;1:1153–4.
85. Sami D, Young S, Petersen R. Perspective on orbital enucleation implants. Surv Ophthalmol. 2007;52(3):244–65.
86. Wheeler JM. Implantation of hollow grooved body into orbit for filling. Arch Ophthalmol. 1938;20:709–12.
87. Soll DB. Evolution and current concepts in the surgical treatment of the anophthalmic orbit. Ophthal Plast Reconstr Surg. 1988;2:163–71.
88. Ruedemann AD. Plastic eye implant. Trans Am Ophthalmol Soc. 1945;43:304–12.
89. Cutler NL. A universal type integrated implant. Am J Ophthalmol. 1949;32:253–8.
90. Troutman RC. A magnetic implant. Arch Ophthalmol. 1950;43:1123–4.

91. King JH Jr. Wadsworth JAC: an atlas of ophthalmic surgery. 3rd ed. Philadelphia: JB Lippincott; 1981.
92. Perry AC. Integrated orbital implants. Adv Ophthalmic Plast Reconstr Surg. 1990;8:75–81.
93. Khan JA, Albert DM. Willard Parker's 1841 orbital operation. Surv Ophthalmol. 1988;33:117–9.
94. Duke-Elder S, MacFaul PA. The ccular adnexa. In: Duke-Elder S, editor. System of ophthalmology, v13: pt 1 Diseases of the eyelids; pt 2 Lacrimal, orbital and para-orbital diseases. St Louis: CV Mosby; 1974.
95. Kronlein RU. Zur Pathologie und operative Bedhandlung der Dermoidcysten der Orbita. Beitr Klin Chir. 1888; 4:149–63.
96. Hughes WL. The evolution of ophthalmic sutures. Adv Ophthalmic Plast Reconstr Surg. 1986;5:177–83.
97. Stallard HB. The evolution of lateral orbitotomy. Trans Ophthalmol Soc UK. 1973;93:1–17.
98. Smith B. The anterior surgical approach to orbital tumors. Trans Am Acad Ophthalmol Otolayngol. 1966;70:607–11.
99. Wolfley DE. The lid crease approach to the superomedial orbit. Ophthalmic Surg. 1985;16(10):652–6.
100. Pelton RW. The anterior eyelid crease approach to the orbit. Curr Opin Ophthalmol. 2009;20(5):401–5.
101. Balch KC, Goldberg RA, Green JP, Shorr N. The transcaruncular approach to the medial orbit and ethmoid sinus. A cosmetically superior option to the cutaneous (Lynch) incision. Facial Plast Surg Clin North Am. 1998;6:71–7.
102. Alper MG. Pioneers in the history of orbital decompression for graves' ophthalmopathy. R.U. Kroenlein (1847–1910), O. Hirsch (1877–1965) and H.C. Naffziger (1884–1961). Doc Ophthalmol. 1995;89(1–2):163–71.
103. Walsh TE, Ogura JH. Transantral orbital decompression for malignant exophthalmos. Trans Am Laryngol Rhinol Otol Soc. 1957;59:56–81.
104. Kennedy DW, Goodstein ML, Miller NR, Zinreich J. Endoscopic transantral orbital decompression. Arch Otolaryngol Head Neck Surg. 1990;116:275–82.
105. Trokel S, Kazim M, Moore S. Orbital fat removal. Decompression for Graves orbitopathy. Ophthalmology. 1993;100(5):674–82.
106. Miller CC. The excision of bag-like folds of skin from the region about the eyes. Med Brief. 1906;34:648.
107. Miller CC, Miller FL. Folds, bags and wrinkles of the skin about the eyes and their eradication by simple surgical methods. Med Bief. 1907;35:540.
108. Kolle FS. Plastic and cosmetic surgery, vol. 54. New York: D Appleton & Co; 1911. p. 717.
109. Bourget I. La Correction esthetique des diverses deformation nasals. Rev Int de Laryngologie. 1926;Oct:133–7.
110. Katzen LB. The history of cosmetic blepharoplasty. Adv Ophthalmic Plast Recostruct Surg. 1986;5:89–96.
111. Castanares S. Blepharoplasty for herniated intraorbital fat: anatomical basis for a new approach. Plast Reconstr Surg. 1951;8:46.
112. Loeb R. Clin Plast Surg. 1981;8:757–76.
113. de la Plaza R, Arroyo JM. A new technique for the treatment of palpebral bags. Plast Reconstr Surg. 1988;81(5):677–87.
114. Camirand A. Canthopexy and transconjunctival blepharoplasty are preferable to lower blepharoplasty. Can J Plast Surg. 1993/1994;1:184.
115. Meltzer M. Ophthalmic plastic surgery for the general ophthalmologist. The Williams & Wilkins Company: Baltimore; 1979.
116. Mustarde JC. Repair and reconstruction of the orbital region. Baltimore/Edinburgh/London: E&S Livingston; 1966.

Instrumentation in Ophthalmic Plastic Surgery

4

Shani Golan, Christopher I. Zoumalan, Frank A. Nesi, and Gary J. Lelli Jr.

Introduction

The use of proper instrumentation in ophthalmic plastic surgery is an essential element to successful surgical outcomes. However, the surgeon must be aware that without proper adherence to the basic surgical principles, surgical outcomes will be suboptimal. The surgeon must have an intimate knowledge of the eyelid, orbital, and facial anatomy. Furthermore, an understanding of the anatomy and the natural tissue planes allows the surgeon to surgically dissect the tissue planes as atraumatically as possible with the aid of appropriate and adequate instrumentation.

This chapter will describe the various instruments ophthalmic plastic surgeons have at their disposal when managing their patients both in the office and in the operating room.

S. Golan (✉)
Division of Ophthalmic Plastic, Reconstructive, and Orbital Surgery, Department of Ophthalmology, Weill Cornell Medical College, New York-Presbyterian Hospital, New York, NY, USA

C. I. Zoumalan
Department of Ophthalmology, Division of Ophthalmic Plastic and Reconstructive Surgery, Keck School of Medicine of USC, Los Angeles, CA, USA

F. A. Nesi
Beaumont Eye Institute, William Beaumont School of Medicine of Oakland University, Rochester, MI, USA

Kresge Eye Institute, Wayne State University School of Medicine, Detroit, MI, USA

G. J. Lelli Jr.
Weill Cornell Medical Center/New York-Presbyterian Hospital, Department of Ophthalmology, New York, NY, USA

Photography

Photography is absolutely essential pre- and postoperatively. Although the best images are often captured by a professional, high-quality images can be taken in the physician's office after some practice. Standard digital SLR cameras offer excellent quality and greater control than point-and-shoot cameras. Polaroid cameras allow the user to instantly develop photos that can be placed in the patient's chart. The full ophthalmic plastic series typically includes photos of the entire face, both eyes isolated in up and down gaze, left and right facial profiles, and each eye individually (seven photos). Photography and videotaping through the surgical microscope are now routinely available.

Skin Marking

A surgical marking pen should be used to define the area of incision prior to infiltration with lidocaine. The mark should be placed parallel to relaxed skin tension lines and along a natural skinfold or crease if possible. Fine-pointed marking pens allow for more accurate skin marking. Intraoperatively, further markings can be made using brilliant green (4% in 95% ethyl alcohol) or Bonnie's blue (1% gentian violet and 1% brilliant green in 50% ethyl alcohol) on a fine-pointed toothpick rather than with the commercial pen.

Draping

Drapes should be organized to freely expose not only the eyelids but also the brows and cheeks, bilaterally. One must be able to mobilize surrounding tissues when remodeling

J. J. Servat et al. (eds.), *Smith and Nesi's Ophthalmic Plastic and Reconstructive Surgery*,
https://doi.org/10.1007/978-3-030-41720-8_4

lids. In order to help prevent any burn injuries, oxygen should not be placed under a drape. The surgical drape should be placed under the nose or mouth.

Surgeon Position

In order to prevent fatigue and musculoskeletal injury, the surgeon must maintain proper positioning. Furthermore, the surgeon should obtain adequate exposure of the surgical field and a proper working distance. In general, whether sitting or standing, the operating table height should be adjusted so that the surgical plane is just below the surgeon's elbow. This position allows for maximal muscle control and ideal function [1].

Visibility of Field

Although some procedures do not require magnification, many ophthalmic plastic surgeons prefer to use surgical loupes. Typical magnification is from 2.5 to 3.5 times with an adequate field of view and working distance. The operating microscope may be used in selected cases – for example, electroepilation of trichiatic cilia, conjunctival lesions, selected orbital cases, and determining margins of resection for infiltrative lesions.

Incisions

A precision grip in which the pulps of the thumb and the second finger, along with the radial portion of the distal third finger, is used to create a stable three-point fixation of the surgical instrument. Stabilizing the forearms relaxes the large muscles of the forearm and upper arm, effectively minimizing hand tremors (see Fig. 4.1). Figure 4.2 also illustrates acceptable ways to grasp scissors and needle holders.

Various scalpel blades are available for skin incisions, but the most commonly used blade is a #15 Bard–Parker. It is best for straight or gently arching incisions. The belly of the blade should be used rather than its point. The #11 scalpel blade is tapered to a fine point. This can be used for removal of a very small lesion or for making accurate stab incisions such as in chalazion excisions with the assistance of a chalazion clamp along the posterior lamellae (Fig. 4.3). Similarly, a Beaver #57 blade can be used for very accurate excisions of small lesions and is helpful for tarsal dissection (i.e., Hughes flap construction). A #10 blade has a larger belly when compared to a #15 Bard-Parker, and some surgeons prefer this blade when

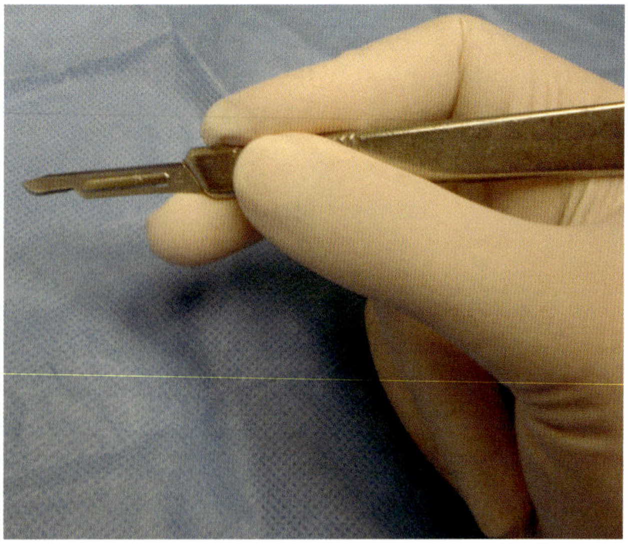

Fig. 4.1 Surgeon showing a proper three-point fixation grip when using a scalpel. The pulps of the thumb and the second finger along with the radial portion of the distal third finger create a three-point fixation

performing large facial incisions, flap formations and in harvesting of dermis fat grafts (see Fig. 4.4).

Over the last decade, other skin incision modalities have been available with variable surgeon preference. These devices allow for excellent hemostasis. Fine-needle-tipped electrocautery can be used to incise skin, but the resulting thermal damage to adjacent tissue makes it less desirable to many surgeons. Similarly, carbon dioxide (CO_2) laser uses a laser platform to incise tissue. Alternatively, the thin eyelid skin can be incised accurately with the use of sharp scissors, particularly along the lower eyelid subciliary line.

Tissue Dissection

An intimate knowledge of anatomy allows the surgeon to appropriately dissect through the eyelid and orbital soft tissue using blunt and sharp dissection. Most incisions in the soft tissue planes begin with blunt-tipped dissection using blunt-tipped Stevens or Westcott scissors. Metzenbaum scissors can be used in areas of denser tissue. Connective tissue bands can be lysed directly with the use of the above scissors (see Fig. 4.5). Refer to Fig. 4.6 for the majority of standard instruments found in an oculoplastic tray. Table 4.1 lists the complete set of standard instruments found in an oculoplastic tray.

During orbital surgery, a periosteal freer elevator is helpful for various dissection techniques (see Fig. 4.7). Its primary role is to allow the gentle release of the periosteal layer from the underlying bone in orbital fracture

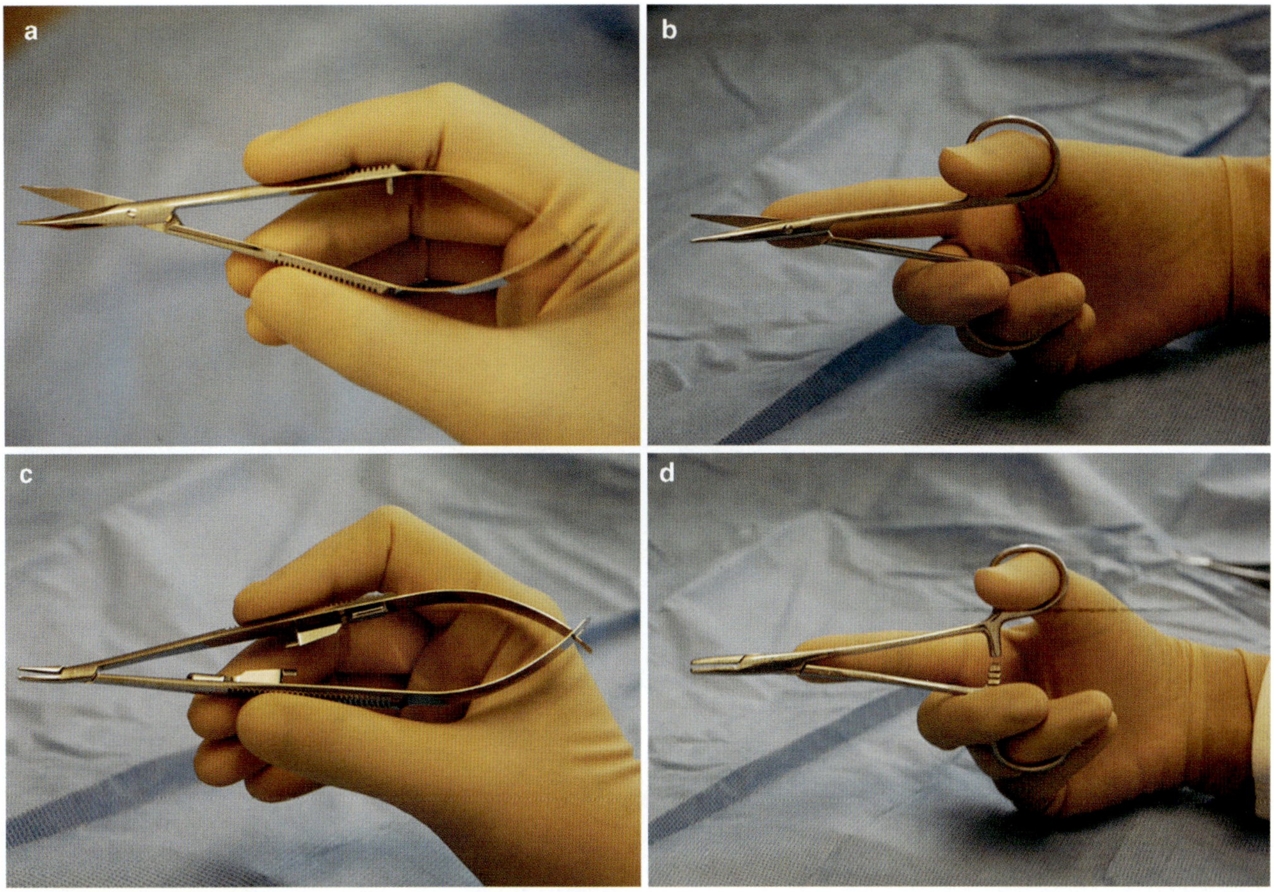

Fig. 4.2 Acceptable ways to grasp (**a**) Westcott scissors, (**b**) Stevens scissors, (**c**) Castroviejo needle holder, and (**d**) Webster needle holder

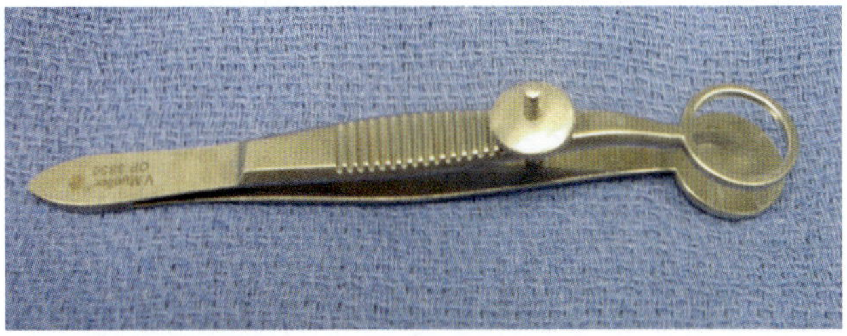

Fig. 4.3 Chalazion clamp

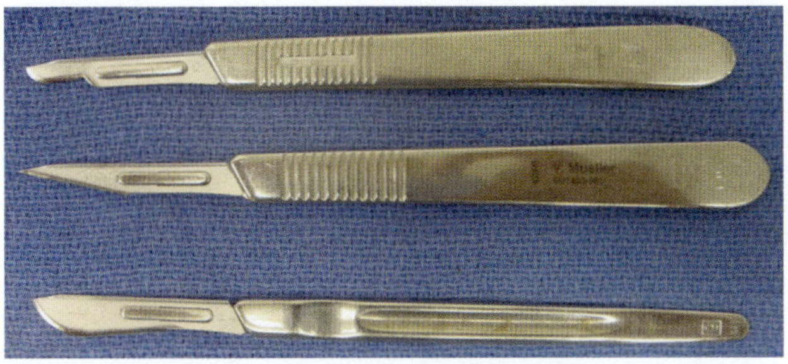

Fig. 4.4 Different surgical blades used in ophthalmic plastic surgery: #15 Bard–Parker blade (*top*), #11 blade (*center*), #10 blade (*bottom*)

repairs, orbitotomies, and dacryocystorhinostomies. The instrument allows for blunt dissection through orbital tissue with minimal trauma of the surrounding tissue. It can gently release the bands of connective tissue surrounding an orbital tumor such as a cavernous hemangioma. It can also serve as a retractor and help in repositioning orbital soft tissues that have prolapsed through a fracture site.

Blunt dissection using neurosurgical cottonoids or cotton-tipped applicators are also useful within the orbit. They allow for the gentle release of connective tissues surrounding orbital lesions for easier delivery. Additional instruments such as a cryoprobe can be used to aid in the delivery of a lesion once it is directly visualized.

Exposure of the Surgical Field

Maintaining adequate exposure of the surgical field is crucial. Lid margin sutures, Desmarres retractors, and skin hooks or rakes can sufficiently expose the surgical field in

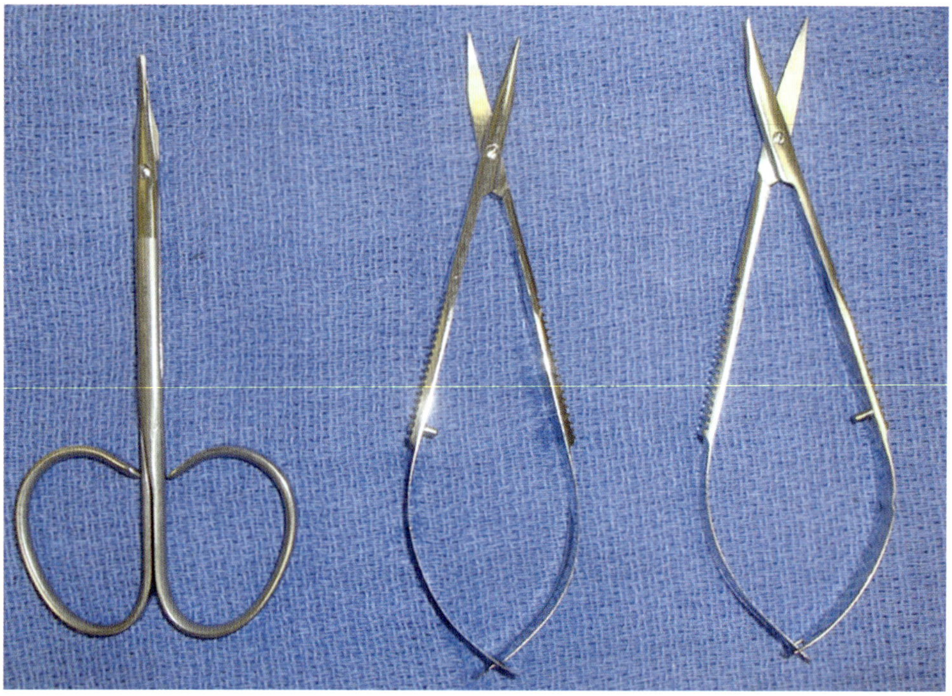

Fig. 4.5 Various scissors used in ophthalmic plastic surgery include blunt-tipped Stevens scissors (*left*), blunt-tipped Westcott scissors (*center*), and sharp-tipped Westcott scissors (*right*)

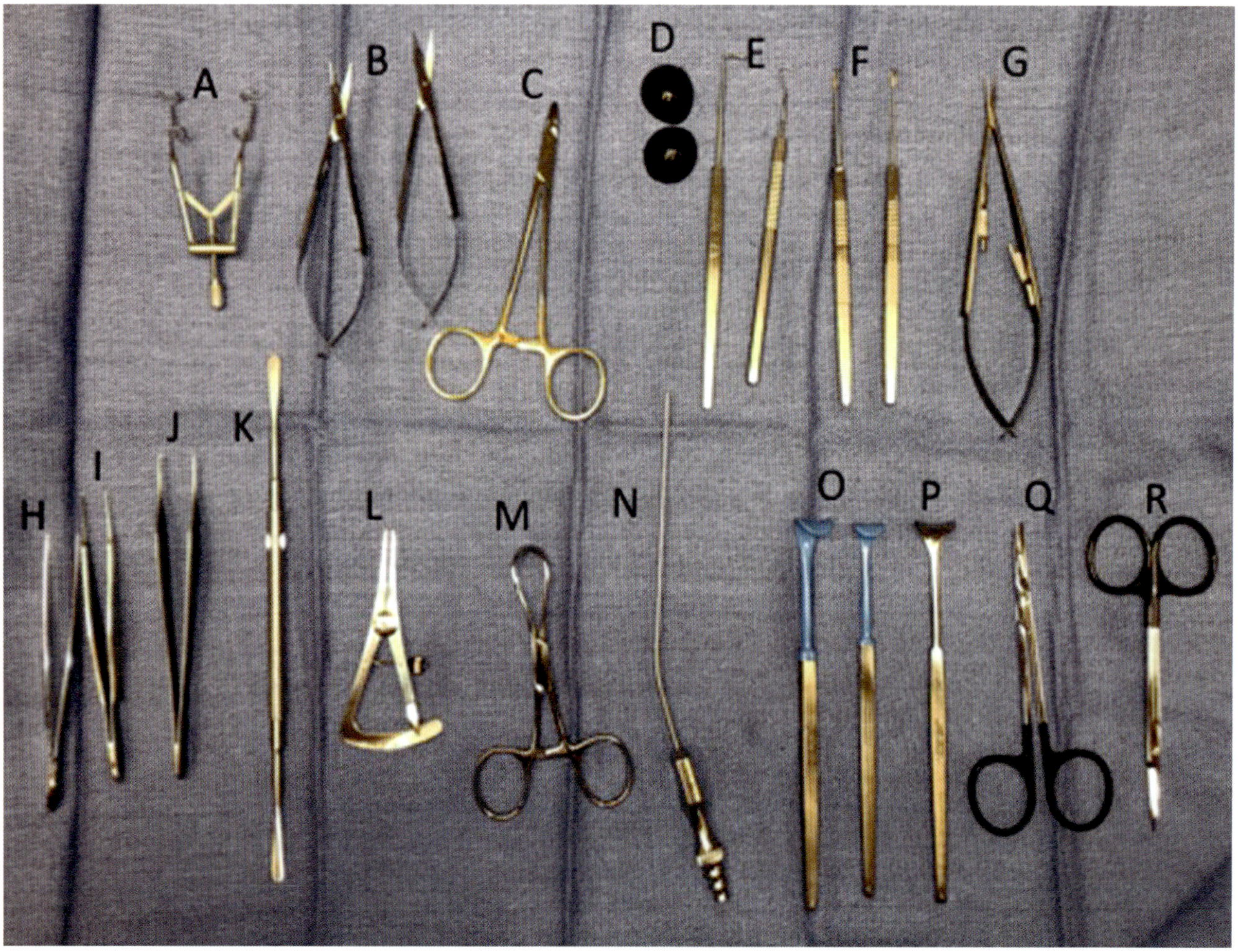

Fig. 4.6 An oculoplastic tray containing (**a**) lid speculum, (**b**) blunt and sharp Westcott scissors, (**c**) Webster needle driver, (**d**) corneal shields, (**e**) muscle hooks × 2, (**f**) Skin hooks × 2, (**g**) Castroviejo needle driver, (**h**) non-toothed forceps, (**i**) 0.5 forceps, (**j**) Adson forceps with teeth, (**k**) periosteal freer elevator, (**l**) caliper, (**m**) towel clamp, (**n**) Frazier suction, (**o**) insulated Desmarres retractors × 2, (**p**) Desmarres retractor, (**q**) straight iris scissors, (**r**) curved iris scissors

most aesthetic and reconstructive eyelid surgeries (Fig. 4.8). In orbital cases, the use of thin- or medium-sized malleables, Desmarres, Converse, or Senn retractors can aid in the visualization of deeper surgical fields.

Hemostasis

While bleeding from large vessels often requires ligation, small-vessel hemorrhages are often controlled by direct pressure. Electrocautery uses electricity to heat tissue for hemostasis. The most common mode of cautery is the Bovie type, which is monopolar and requires a reference electrode that is placed under the back or thigh of the patient. Bovie cautery provides hemostasis and also allows for cutting and fulguration of tissue. One must be aware of patients with pacemakers because they can be disabled or more likely cause the defibrillator to discharge by the monopolar current, even with the reference electrode in place. Thus, a limit of 30 s per discharge is advisable, as well as the presence of an anesthesiologist to monitor the electrocardiogram (ECG) [2].

Bipolar cautery incorporates the active and reference electrodes at the site of surgery, typically in the parallel tines of a pair of forceps. Thus, current is passed only through the tissue held between the two electrodes (this characteristic eliminates the risk to patients with pacemakers). This results in a more refined area of coagulation and minimal damage to surrounding tissue, a quality that is particularly important in orbital surgery. Although bipolar cautery has many advantages over monopolar, it may require a longer time for hemo-

Table 4.1 Standard oculoplastic tray

Oculoplastic set
Mosquito clamps curved, 4
Iris scissors (straight), 1
Iris scissors (curved), 1
Jameson muscle hook, 1
Blair retractor sharp (rake), 2
Knapp retractor blunt (rake), 2
0.3 mm forceps, 2
0.5 mm forceps, 2
Westcott scissors (sharp), 1
Westcott scissors (blunt), 2
Bayonet forceps, 1
Wire speculum
Webster needle holder, 1
Orbital retractor (small), 2
Orbital retractor (big), 2
Senn retractor (blunt), 1
Senn retractor (sharp), 1
Skin hook, 2
Mayo scissors, 1
Nasal speculum, 1
Suction tube (7FR, 8FR, 9FR)
Desmarres retractors (0,1,2,3)
Allis clamps, 1
Ruler, 1
Castroviejo needle holder, 1
Periosteal freer elevator, 2
Jewelers forceps, 1
Bard–Parker handle, 2
Adson dressing forceps, 1
Adson tissue forceps, 2
Brown–Adson forceps, 2
Steven scissors (straight), 1
Steven scissors (curved), 1
Bipolar forceps, 1

Numbers after the comma indicate the recommended quantity of each instrument

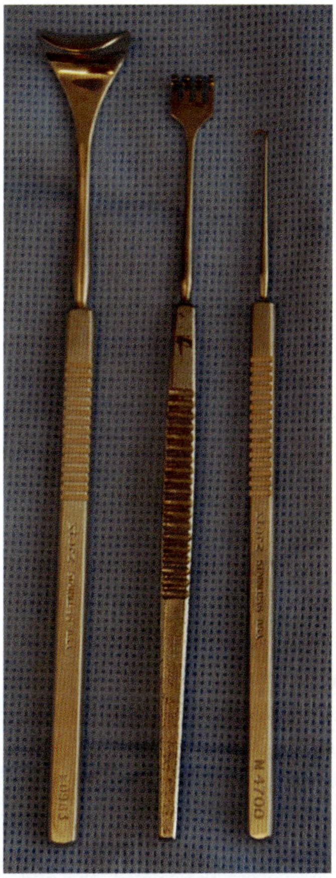

Fig. 4.8 Desmarres retractor (*left*), skin rake (*center*), and skin hook (*right*) can help in providing optimal exposure of the surgical field

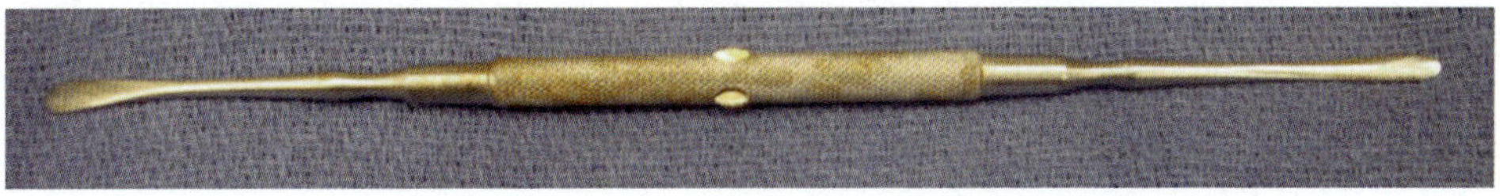

Fig. 4.7 Standard periosteal freer elevator

stasis due to lower power settings and may tear blood vessels due to stronger adherence to tissue.

When clearing the field of blood or other fluids, suction is mandatory, but it does not dry the field. Cottonoids and 4×4 gauze sponges effectively dry the field, but they need manipulation to work well.

Alternative Hemostasis Technology

Thrombin and microfibrillar collagen products may be used directly on diffusely oozing surfaces; the latter can even be effective in anticoagulated patients who are taking aspirin or heparin.

Should all hemostatic measures fail, the Hemovac drainage system, Jackson-Pratt, or even a fine Silastic tubing carried from the interior of the wound into a venipuncture vacuum test tube may be required.

Traction and Exposure

The classic traction device in surgery has always been the second assistant. The small size of the field in ophthalmic plastic surgery has encouraged the invention of mechanical assistance, such as the lacrimal speculum, the lid speculum (see Fig. 4.9). Exposure can be optimized by the use of malleables and Desmarres retractors (Fig. 4.10). Mattress sutures clamped to the surgical drape with two opposing hemostats joined by a sterile rubber band can also provide adequate retraction.

Along with the many benefits of good palpebral exposure come the hazards of corneal abrasion and *epithelial defects* during lid surgery. Adequate lubrication of the globe and corneal protectors can prevent corneal injury.

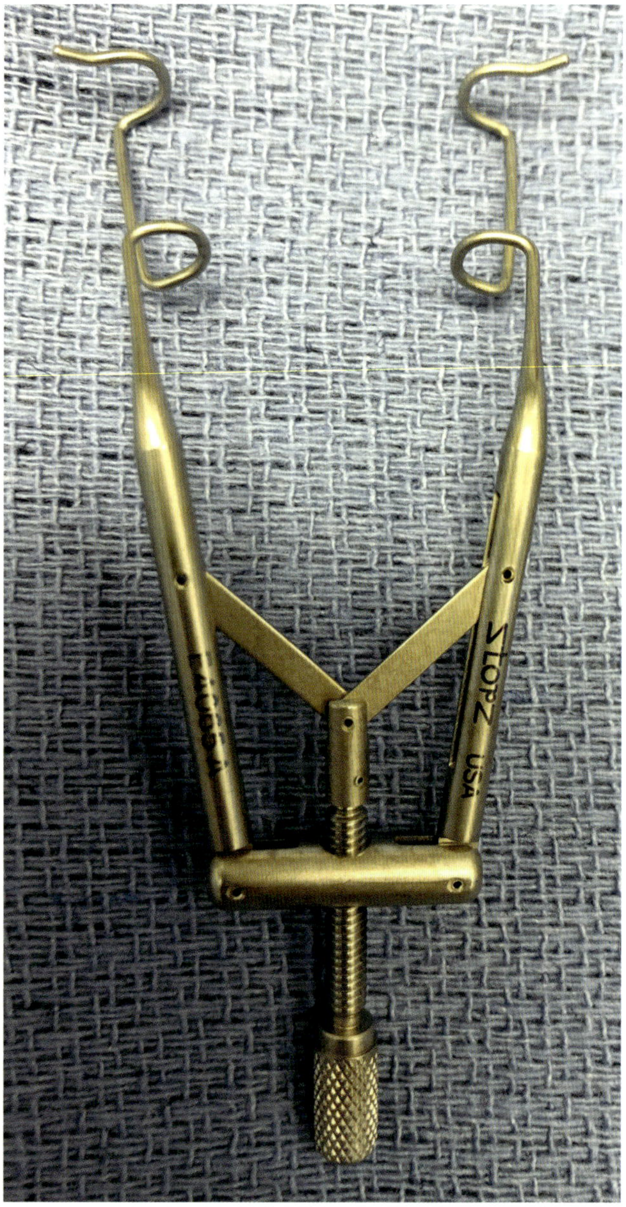

Fig. 4.9 An adjustable lid speculum with 14 mm blades. Overall length: 83 mm, 3.3 inches. Made of stainless steel. (Storz®, USA)

Soft Tissue Grafts

Amniotic membrane grafts have been widely used over the last decade for corneal and conjunctival diseases, such as in pterygium excisions. Because amnion is readily available; convenient and easy to use; and reduces inflammation, vascularization, and scarring, it has also become a useful medium for forniceal reconstruction [3].

When reconstructing the eyelid, the end goal is an aesthetically optimal restoration of anatomy and anatomic function with a minimum of surgical morbidity. Attention to reconstitution of the trilamellar eyelid structure is essential. The surgeon must create an anterior lamella of adequate and aesthetically appropriate skin, preserving dynamic orbicularis muscle function whenever possible, and create a posterior lamella replacing tarsus at the eyelid margin and providing for a smooth mucosal surface that protects and preserves the cornea.

Hand cutting for full-thickness skin grafts is still routine in eyelid surgery, but a dermatome provides larger split-thickness skin grafts when reconstructing a socket after an exenteration. Meshing instruments can expand grafts up to nine times. On a similar note, the Castroviejo mucotome is extremely useful in harvesting mucous membrane grafts. It permits regeneration of the mucosa with the opportunity to reharvest grafts repeatedly if required.

Hard palate mucosal grafts are an excellent posterior lamella substitute for select cases of eyelid malpositions such as retraction, cicatricial entropion, and trichiasis. They

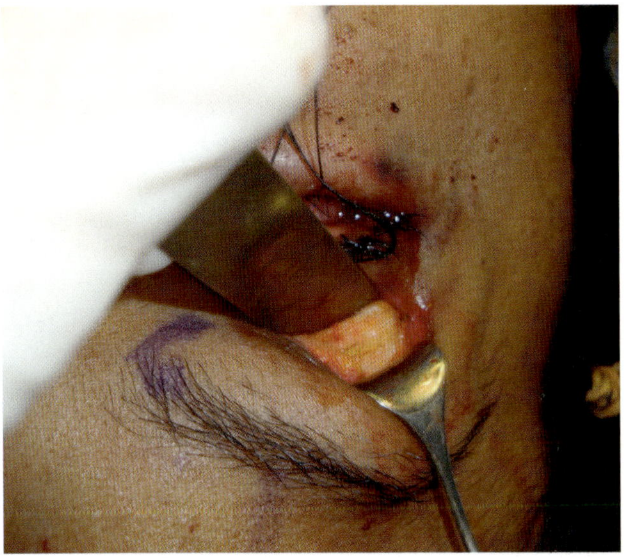

Fig. 4.10 Malleables and Desmarres retractors used to allow for optimal exposure in orbital reconstructive surgery

avoid any morbidity to the contralateral eye, such as that caused by free tarsal grafts, and provide rigidity and flexibility to the eyelid. However, the keratinized mucosa of hard palate may be irritating to the cornea, and there can be significant morbidity at the donor site [4].

Newer synthetic agents such as AlloDerm (Lifecell Corp., Woodlands, TX), a type of acellular human dermis, have become a viable alternative to autologous grafts in eyelid reconstruction. These acellular dermal matrices derived from cadaveric dermis are immunologically inert, are rigid enough to replace tarsus, and provide the necessary substrate for conjunctival epithelial migration and repopulation of the graft surface. Although synthetic agents avoid the need for harvesting from a donor site and provide adequate results, many surgeons still prefer hard palate grafts in certain cases of eyelid reconstruction, given their proven longevity in providing good lid position [5, 6].

Dry Eye Evaluation

It is important to evaluate patients who are undergoing eyelid surgery for signs and symptoms of dry eyes, as changes in eyelid position can worsen this condition. A thorough corneal examination including fluorescein staining and evaluation of meibomian gland function, with special attention to the tear film, is critical for the prevention of dry eye postoperatively. A Schirmer test with anesthesia, which consists of the insertion of paper strips into the lower fornices for a set amount of time, usually 5 min, and measuring how much moisture is absorbed by the paper can also be used to diagnose aqueous tear deficiency.

Often, artificial tears and lubricating ointments are enough to treat symptoms of postoperative dry eyes. Humidifiers and moisture shields can also be helpful. Patients with moderate to severe dry eyes may benefit from punctal occlusion. Alternatively, one can use collagen plugs. They dissolve within a few days and may be used as a trial before inserting permanent plugs.

Bone and Cartilage

Bone work involves either drilling or removing bone via osteotomies. This is integral to orbital fracture repair, orbital surgery, orbital decompression, and dacryocystorhinostomy (DCR). Periosteal freer elevators are crucial in denuding the bone of periosteum. For procedures involving controlled fractures, such as orbital decompressions and DCRs, a smaller-tipped osteotome and mallet can be used efficiently. Removal of bone is performed with biting instruments such as rongeurs. A straight rongeur, similar to a pair of pliers, allows for direct removal of bone using the biting tip on the distal end. A rongeur needs to be used carefully in a gentle side-to-side rocking motion in order to prevent inadvertent extension of fractures posteriorly. Similarly, a long-handed Kerrison rongeur can reach deep bone, as required for orbital decompressions and DCRs. Kerrison rongeurs allow for further widening of osteotomies once a bony dehiscence exists (Fig. 4.11).

Air-powered drills and saws allow for controlled osteotomies in orbital surgery. Air-powered drills (such as a 3 M drill or Hall drill) are required to create holes for the placement of screws, sutures, and wires. Figure 4.12 illustrates a standard set for placement of titanium screws and plates within the

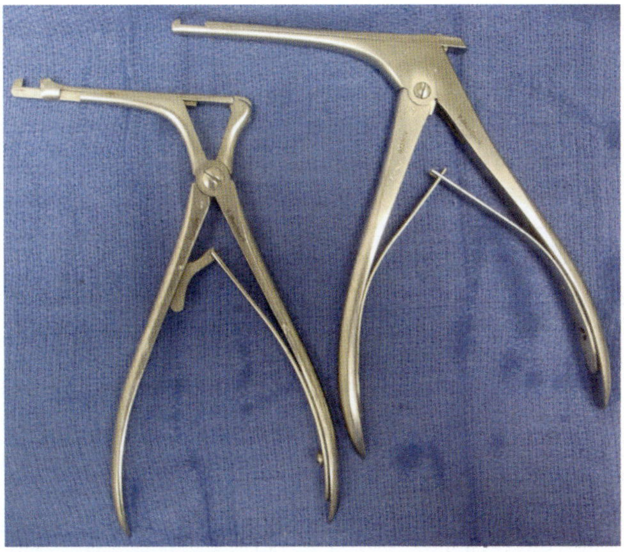

Fig. 4.11 Kerrison rongeurs

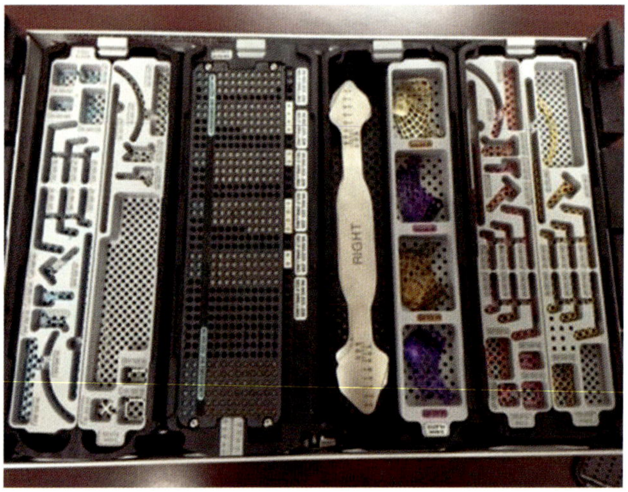

Fig. 4.12 Standard titanium plating system for orbital surgery. (MIDFACE Plating System Synthes®)

orbit. Cutting bits can be attached to these particular drills for bony contouring and sculpting, as required for certain lateral decompression cases. Various compatible plating systems are available for use with these drills, including those composed of titanium, vitallium, and stainless steel. Titanium plates are popular as they are well tolerated, lightweight, and not paramagnetic. Titanium wires or plates can also be used to repair congenital and acquired telecanthus [7]. Air-powered oscillating saws are often employed in cases of lateral orbitotomies that require a bony window for better intraoperative visualization. Typically, a sagittal saw is used for this particular approach. The blade should be in motion prior to making the initial cut, should be held firmly with the blade in constant orientation to the bone which is to be cut, and should be withdrawn from the osteotomy while still in motion when completed. During the osteotomy, the bone is irrigated with saline in order to prevent bone necrosis, and the orbital contents are protected by the assistant with malleable retractors [1].

As for cartilage grafts, sources include the nasal septum, the external ear, or the rib, and the instruments used are "cartilage knives," nasal speculums, and nasal scissors, as used in nasal surgery.

Orbital Implants

Repairing Orbital Fractures

Repair of orbital fractures often involves reconstruction of the floor, medial wall, or rarely the roof. Many different autogenous grafts and alloplastic materials are available for this purpose (see Table 4.2).

Alloplastic implants have largely replaced autogenous bone grafts, which can have variable rates of resorption. The ideal alloplastic material is chemically inert, biocompatible, noncarcinogenic, and nonallergenic and should provide structural support to recreate normal anatomy. Alloplastic implants can be grouped into two categories: nonporous and porous. Nonporous implants provide structural support, but most do not allow for vascular ingrowth, usually forming a capsule at the graft–host interface. Examples include Teflon, nylon foil (SupraFOIL), silicone (Silastic), and titanium mesh. Titanium mesh provides excellent structural support, is physiologically inert, and can undergo osseointegration. It is easy to manipulate and reshape to fit various orbital defects. In contrast, the porosity of materials such as Medpor (porous high-density polyethylene) allows for vascular and osseous ingrowth, which allows for greater biocompatibility. Medpor is manufactured to have a large pore size (100–200 μm), which is ideal for tissue ingrowth. This property prevents capsule formation, maintains the host immune response, and minimizes infection [8]. Structurally, however, Medpor has some disadvantages. It is not as malleable as titanium, has less memory, and is not visualized well on imaging studies. Porous polyethylene implants with embedded titanium mesh have recently been developed to combine the advantages of these two materials. This new material provides excellent structural support and malleability while allowing for rapid host integration and resistance to infection [6, 9, 10].

Table 4.2 This table outlines the various different types autologous and alloplastic implants used in orbital surgery

Orbital implants
Autologous tissue
Autologous bone
Autologous cartilage
Alloplastic implants
Nonporous implants
Silicone polymer (Silastic)
Polyurethane
Aluminum oxide ceramic
Teflon (polytetrafluoroethylene polymer)
Supramid (polyamide)
Nylon foil (SupraFOIL)
Titanium mesh
Vitallium mesh
Polydioxanone plates
Porous implants
Hydroxyapatite
Methyl methacrylate
Gore-Tex (expanded polytetrafluoroethylene)
Gelatin film
Polyvinyl sponge
Vicryl mesh (polyglactin)
Polylactide plates
Porous polyethylene (Medpor)

There are both nonporous and porous alloplastic orbital implants available for use

Orbit Volume Enhancement

Orbital spherical implants are also used in the orbit to replace intra-orbital volume loss and to impart motility to an ocular prosthetic after removal of the globe. Similar to implants used in fractures (as described above), alloplastic spherical implants are also classified as integrated or nonintegrated. There are advantages and disadvantages to using either one, but a recent Cochrane base review [11] did not provide sufficient evidence to assess the effect of integrated and nonintegrated material orbital implants for treating anophthalmic sockets.

Nonintegrated (Nonporous)

These implants are single spheres of inert material such as silicone, acrylic, or poly(methyl methacrylate) (PMMA). Unlike integrated implants, these implants do not provide for integration of the extraocular muscles (EOMs). When using nonintegrated implants, imbrication of the EOMs in front of the implant can impart motility to the implant and the overlying prosthesis and can also migrate within the orbit. The advantages of using this implants are the low cost and the low risk of implant exposure.

Integrated (Porous)

Porous implants, typically hydroxyapatite or porous polyethylene (Medpor), allow for fibrovascular ingrowth and incorporation of the implant within the orbit, giving them a theoretical advantage over nonintegrated implants. Other advantages of this implant are its excellent mobility, the fact that it rarely migrates and it can be pegged. However, it carries higher risks of infection and extrusion and is also more expensive than the nonintegrated implants.

Hydroxyapatite

This commonly used material is a salt of calcium phosphate which is present in human bone. Its innately rough surface can cause erosion through the overlying soft tissue after placement. Therefore, a wrapping material is commonly used to encapsulate the implant prior to placement. The EOMs are directly sutured onto the wrapping material. Hydroxyapatite is readily available from the manufacturer precovered with and without integrated openings to allow suture placement. The unwrapped implants are still available, but precovered implants eliminate the need to surgically wrap them.

Porous Polyethylene (Medpor)

This implant, approved by the Food and Drug Administration in 1985, is another commonly used porous implant. It also allows for fibrovascular ingrowth, though at a slower rate than the hydroxyapatite implant. The implant is designed to allow direct attachment of the EOMs, although many surgeons prefer wrapping Medpor implants (i.e., Vicryl mesh).

Wrapping Materials

As previously mentioned, wrapping materials can be used to encapsulate the implant prior to placement. Donor sclera is the most commonly used material; however, autologous tissues such as fascia lata and synthetic materials are also used.

Pegged Implants

A peg can be implanted into integrated implants to create mechanical fixation between the implant and prosthesis. This was thought to create more stability and enhance mobility of the prosthetic. Pegs are used less routinely today due to a relatively high complication rate [12, 13]. Pegging does allow for smaller and lighter prostheses since they are affixed to the implant and therefore do not have the weight and bulk to push a lower eyelid inferiorly with time.

Orbital Tissue Expanders

Clinical congenital anophthalmia is a condition in which some or all ocular tissues fail to develop properly, resulting in micro-orbitism and micro-blepharon. Without bony orbital growth, the entire hemiface will remain underdeveloped. Traditionally, progressively larger conformers and spherical orbital implants have been used for orbital and periocular soft tissue expansion. Hydrogel tissue expanders composed of highly hydrophilic polymers that self-expand via osmosis of surrounding water have recently been adapted for use in anophthalmia. Able to expand up to tenfold, these implants exert a constant hydrostatic pressure, theoretically stimulating normal orbital growth. More recently, an integrated orbital tissue expander model is being introduced in selected cases of anophthalmia [14–16].

Ptosis Surgery

Frontalis sling surgery. The instruments employed in frontalis sling ptosis surgery are unique and not commonly used in other ophthalmic plastic surgeries. Methods of suspension

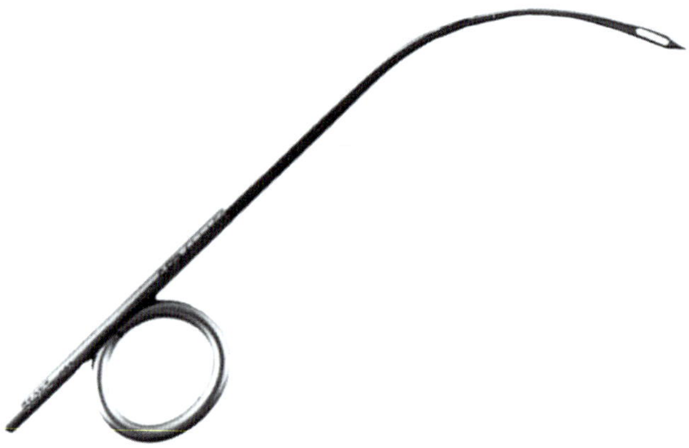

Fig. 4.13 Wright needle is used in frontalis fixation ptosis surgery. (Courtesy of Bartley R. Frueh, MD, deceased)

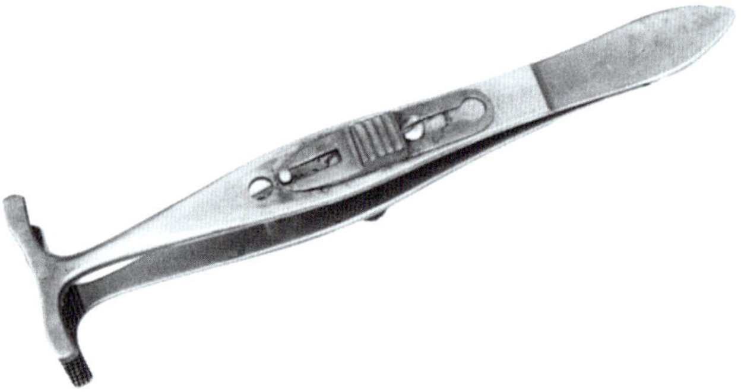

Fig. 4.14 Putterman clamp used in Müller's muscle–conjunctival resection ptosis repair

vary from a simple suture (such as 4-0 Supramid on a ski needle), to silicone bands (such as no. 240 used in scleral surgery for retinal detachment) or a 1-mm silicone rod (Dow Corning), the classic fascia lata strip, banked fascia lata or tendon transfers [17–19]. Instruments in use are the Reese ptosis knife (with the eye enlarged if the silicone band is used) or the Wright needle (see Fig. 4.13).

Müllerectomy. The Putterman clamp is commonly used in Müller's muscle–conjunctival resection ptosis repair and allows for efficient and accurate removal of the desired tissue (see Fig. 4.14). Fibrant sealant (Tisseel) has been recently reported to be a safe and effective method of wound closure in Müller's muscle–conjunctival resection ptosis repair [20].

Canalicular Laceration Repair

Any canalicular or nasolacrimal probing that may involve the need for silicone tube intubation requires perioperative nasal packing composed of neurosurgical cottonoids soaked in a vasoconstrictor (i.e., Afrin, phenylephrine, or cocaine) using a nasal speculum and bayonet instrument.

If the proximal end of the damaged canaliculus is not found on direct examination nor discovered by following the path of the probe used to explore the torn distal end, a pigtail probe may be used to intubate the intact side of the lacrimal system. The probe will pass through the intact canaliculus, curve through the common canaliculus, and enter the distal end of the torn canaliculus to exit within the wound.

Canalicular Stents

Numerous methods of stenting the canaliculi have been described in literature, including rubber, silk thread, steel, nylon sutures, and silicone. Both bicanalicular and monocanalicular silicone stents have been described and are currently the most commonly employed stents. The "Mini Monoka" is used for laceration of a single canaliculus and is properly angled to fit the ampulla, with a plug designed with a collarette to lie flush against the eyelid margin or even perforated plugs to keep the punctum open while allowing it to drain tears [21].

Balloon Catheter Dilation in Lacrimal System

Balloon dacryoplasty is a term used for a set of minimally invasive lacrimal procedures that utilizes specially designed balloons, targeted at different points in the lacrimal system for a wide range of indications. Balloon dacryoplasty and balloon-assisted primary and revision dacryocystorhinostomy are gaining ground in minimally invasive lacrimal surgeries with increasing indications for their use. This technique involves passing a lubricated, inflatable balloon (Fig. 4.15) along a guide wire into the nasolacrimal duct and through the level of obstruction [22]. The balloon is then inflated for 90 seconds to dilate the obstruction, deflated, and reinflated a second time or removed. Theoretically, this technique offers relief of epiphora with fewer complications and without the need to return to the operating room to remove inserted stents [23–24].

Endoscopic Surgery

Endoscopes have been increasing in use among ophthalmic plastic surgeons for forehead rejuvenation surgery (brow lifting), dacryocystorhinostimies (DCRs), and removal of certain orbital tumors. Endoscopes allow for adequate visualization while minimizing the use of incisions. The necessary equipment for performing endoscopic surgery includes the endoscope and video camera equipment. The rigid endoscope is typically between 18 and 23 cm in length, 4.5 mm in diameter, and consists of a 0- or 30-degree lens (see Fig. 4.16). It is equipped with a coupling device that projects the scope lens image onto a monitor. The illumination of the endoscope is provided by a halogen or xenon light source.

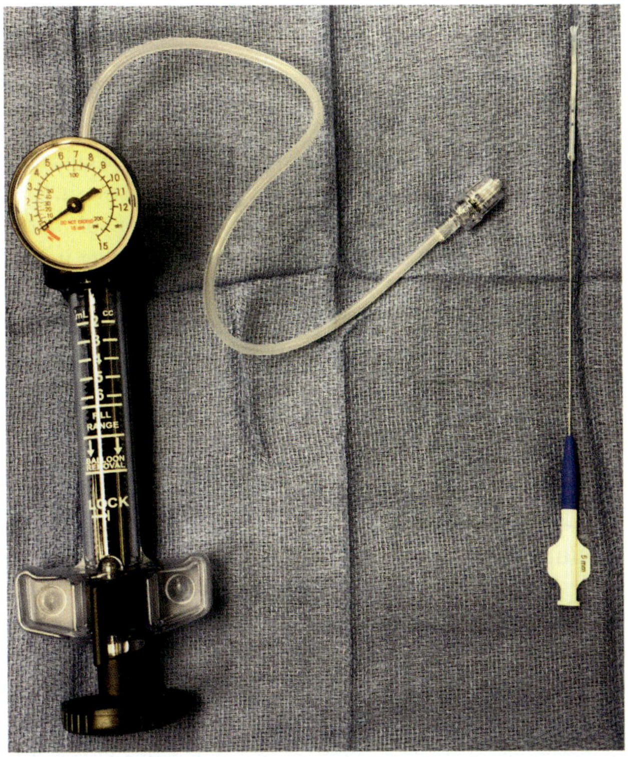

Fig. 4.15 Balloon dacryoplasty system including lacrimal duct catheter and inflation device. (LacriCATH; Quest Medical, Allen, TX, USA)

Endoscopic Brow Lifting

The endoscope can safely and effectively provide visualization while performing brow resuspension in cases of mild brow ptosis. The paramedian forehead and temporal hairline incisions are minimal so that healing times are minimized and postoperative comfort is maximized. A 30° lens provides optimal visualization.

Although most endoscopic surgical instruments are now standardized, some specialized instruments are available. Angled endoscopic sheaths extend beyond the scope tip to permit better visualization while performing bimanual dissection. The surgeon should have straight and curved periosteal elevators in anticipation of forehead anatomical variations. Sharp- and blunt-tipped elevators should be available to address periosteal adhesions.

Various methods have been described to resuspend the brow, which include bone tunnel sutures, screw fixation, Mitek 2.0-mm Quickanchor screw (Ethicon, Norwood, MA, USA), and Endotine Forehead devices (Coapt Systems, Inc., Palo Alto, CA) fixation [25, 26].

Endoscopic DCR

Endoscopes are also used in DCRs because they provide adequate visualization of the paranasal sinuses, obviating an external incision. The success rates for endoscopic DCR compare reasonably well with those of standard external DCR in the hands of experienced surgeons. In endoscopic DCRs, an ENT sinus tray is often helpful in providing equip-

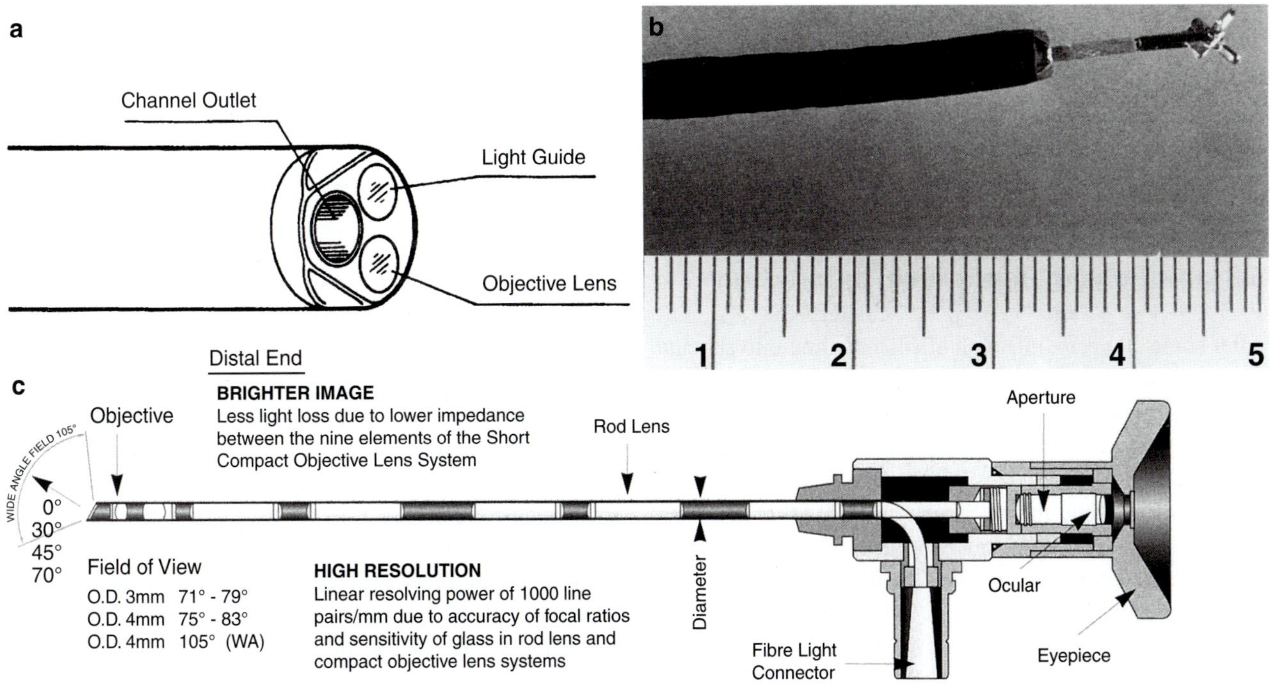

Fig. 4.16 (**a**) Diagram of endoscope tip, (**b**) biopsy forceps, and (**c**) detail of fiber-optic light

Table 4.3 Standard dacryocystorhinostomy set

Dacryocystorhinostomy (DCR) set
Periosteal elevator, 1
Kerrison rongeur (small, medium, large), 3
Mallet, 1
Osteotome 3 mm, 4 mm, 5 mm; 3
Stevenson retractor, 2
Takahashi forceps, 1
Lempert rongeur (small, medium), 2
Curette (small, medium), 2
Crawford hook, 1
Lacrimal cannula, 2
Bowman probes (0000–000, 00–0, 1–2, 3–4, 5–6)
Punctal dilator, 1

Numbers after the comma indicate the recommended quantity of each instrument

Table 4.4 Standard endoscopic dacryocystorhinostomy set

Endoscopic dacryocystorhinostomy (DCR) set
Includes standard DCR tray in addition to the following:
Storz endoscope (0° or 30°), 1
Sickle knife (blunt, sharp), 1
Rhinoforce Blakesley, 1
Rhinoforce upturn 45°,1

Numbers after the comma indicate the recommended quantity of each instrument

ment such as Takahashi and Blakesley forceps to grasp mucosa and bone fragments. A fiber-optic light pipe (20-gauge diameter) can be cannulated through the upper canaliculus to allow for transillumination of the osteotomy site [27, 28]. In addition to the standard DCR tray (Table 4.3), the following table lists the instruments usually required for an endoscopic DCR (Table 4.4).

Nonsurgical Facial Aesthetics

Botulinum toxin discussed in detail in Chapter 31

Subdermal fillers discussed in detail in Chapter 31

Silicone (Polyorganosiloxane) by Injection

After some 30 years, injection of silicone fluid into subcutaneous spaces has not yet received FDA approval. The reason for this withholding is essentially based on the errors of massive injections, of added or accidental adulterants, and of the use of nonmedical-grade silicone. The correct technique consists of multiple minute injections with 30-gauge sharp needles, each about 0.05 mL, within a few millimeters of each other, perhaps 1 mL at a session, distributed over a large facial area and repeated monthly. These deposits are gradually augmented by the patient's own collagen. Nevertheless, the safety of the use of liquid injectable silicone for cosmetic purposes is controversial and that it should not be used outside legitimately approved clinical trials.

Complementary Fat Grafting

A major contributor to facial aging is fat atrophy of the periorbital region leading to a skeletonized appearance of the orbit and midface, resulting in the classic double-convexity deformity. Autologous fat grafts have been gaining popularity since the early 1990s as a way of orbital volume enhancement for rejuvenation, as well as for processes such as hemifacial atrophy and radiation damage. Other soft tissue fillers, as described above, have problems including impermanence and allergic reaction. Autologous fat is theoretically an ideal soft tissue filler because it is readily available, inexpensive, and potentially long lasting and has no immune response. Fat is usually harvested from the periumbilical, lumbar, and trochanteric regions, refined and injected into the appropriate area [29, 30–32].

Facial Skin Rejuvenation

With the gravitational and atrophic effects of aging come changes to the skin including epidermal and dermal thinning, flattening, and loss of elasticity. Extrinsic factors such as actinic damage due to chronic ultraviolet exposure contribute to wrinkling, pigmentary changes, and skin laxity. Skin resurfacing should be considered along with blepharoplasty or soft tissue injections for many rejuvenation regimens. Skin resurfacing can be accomplished by topical therapy, as well as ablative therapies, such as chemical peels, microdermabrasion, and laser resurfacing, in which the superficial layers of the skin are wounded, thereby removing damaged tissue and stimulating collagen and fibroblast production [33].

Chemical Peel

Chemical peeling is a process by which chemicals are applied to damaged and aged skin to destroy the outer layers, causing exfoliation and stimulating new collagen production. Chemical peels can improve actinic damage, smooth wrinkles, flatten scarring, and treat acne. Chemical peels may be divided into superficial, medium, and deep peels. Superficial peels, typically made up of alpha hydroxy acids such as glycolic acid, can penetrate and damage the epithelium, leading to exfoliation and a smoother complexion. Medium-depth peels penetrate through the epidermis and superficial dermis and are usually made up of various concentrations of trichloroacetic acid (TCA). Deep peels, which are composed of different phenol compositions such as the Baker–Gordon formula (phenol, tap water, soap, and cotton oil), can penetrate the reticular dermis and stimulate new collagen production. Caution should be used for patients with cardiac, hepatic, or renal disease as phenols are cardiotoxic, metabolized in the liver, and renally excreted.

Microdermabrasion

Microdermabrasion is a technique in which a high-pressure stream of fine particles, usually aluminum oxide crystals, is sprayed onto the skin, resulting in exfoliation. Multiple sessions are required. This procedure has been shown to induce fibroblast proliferation and new collagen deposition. Clinical benefits include improvement in wrinkles, acne scars, and decrease in pore size.

Laser Resurfacing

Laser skin resurfacing has been gaining popularity primarily due to the operator's ability to control the depth of ablation during the procedure, allowing for more predictable clinical results. The two most commonly used wavelengths are pulsed carbon dioxide (CO_2) and erbium:yttrium-aluminum-garnet (Er:YAG). CO_2 is more aggressive than Er:YAG, removing 50–100 μm per pulse vs 25–30 μm. Er:YAG laser energy is absorbed more superficially than CO_2 and causes less collateral thermal damage. Newer hybrid lasers that combine the two modalities achieve the benefits of both, with the depth of CO_2 and the precision and minimal tissue necrosis of Er:YAG.

Ablative lasers, such as those described above, often are accompanied by adverse postoperative complications, such as erythema. Newer, nonablative laser modalities cause a dermal wound without epidermal ablation. Thus, new collagen formation is stimulated, without disruption to the epidermis and minimal postoperative erythema. Common modalities include pulsed dye lasers, intense pulsed light, 1320-nm Nd:YAG, 1450-nm diode laser, and Q-switched Nd:YAG laser. Fractional photothermolysis (i.e., Fraxel or Fractal) causes thermal necrosis in many microscopic areas of skin via small laser beams. The small areas of necrosis heal quickly, resulting in fewer complications. These particular laser platforms have been shown to be effective for abnormal pigmentation, wrinkles, and facial scarring.

References

1. Della Rocca RC, Bedrossian EH, Arthurs AP. Ophthalmic plastic surgery: decision making and techniques. New York: McGraw-Hill Professional; 2001.
2. Sherman DD, Dortzbach RK. Monopolar electrocautery dissection in ophthalmic plastic surgery. Ophthal Plast Reconstr Surg. 1993;9:143–7.
3. Solomon A, Espana EM, Tseng SC. Amniotic membrane transplantation for reconstruction of the conjunctival fornices. Ophthalmology. 2003;110:93–100.
4. Cohen MS, Shorr N. Eyelid reconstruction with hard palate mucosa grafts. Ophthal Plast Reconstr Surg. 1992;8:183–95.
5. Rubin PA, Fay AM, Remulla HD, Maus M. Ophthalmic plastic applications of acellular dermal allografts. Ophthalmology. 1999;106:2091–7.
6. Lee S, Maronian N, Most SP, et al. Porous high-density polyethylene for orbital reconstruction. Arch Otolaryngol Head Neck Surg. 2005;131:446–50.
7. Mauriello JA Jr, Caputo AR. Treatment of congenital forms of telecanthus with custom-designed titanium medial canthal tendon screws. Ophthal Plast Reconstr Surg. 1994;10:195–9.
8. Romano JJ, Iliff NT, Manson PN. Use of Medpor porous polyethylene implants in 140 patients with facial fractures. J Craniofac Surg. 1993;4:142–7.
9. Ellis E III, Messo E. Use of nonresorbable alloplastic implants for internal orbital reconstruction. J Oral Maxillofac Surg. 2004;62:873–81.
10. Garibaldi DC, Iliff NT, Grant MP, Merbs SL. Use of porous polyethylene with embedded titanium in orbital reconstruction: a review of 106 patients. Ophthal Plast Reconstr Surg. 2007;23:439–44.
11. Schellini S, El Dib R, Silva LR, Farat JG, Zhang Y, Jorge EC. Integrated versus non-integrated orbital implants for treating anophthalmic sockets. Cochrane Database Syst Rev. 2016;11:CD010293.
12. Moshfeghi DM, Moshfeghi AA, Finger PT. Enucleation. Surv Ophthalmol. 2000;44:277–301.
13. Stewart WB. Surgery of the eyelid, orbit, and lacrimal system. San Francisco: American Academy of Ophthalmology; 1995.
14. Mazzoli RA, Raymond WR, Ainbinder DJ, Hansen EA. Use of self-expanding, hydrophilic osmotic expanders (hydrogel) in the reconstruction of congenital clinical anophthalmos. Curr Opin Ophthalmol. 2004;15:426–31.
15. Tse DT, Pinchuk L, Davis S, et al. Evaluation of an integrated orbital tissue expander in an anophthalmic feline model. Am J Ophthalmol. 2007;143:317–27.
16. Gundlach KK, Guthoff RF, Hingst VH, Schittkowski MP, Bier UC. Expansion of the socket and orbit for congenital clinical anophthalmia. Plast Reconstr Surg. 2005;116:1214–22.
17. Park S, Shin Y. Results of long-term follow-up observations of blepharoptosis correction using the palmaris longus tendon. Aesthet Plast Surg. 2008;32:614–9.
18. Leibovitch I, Leibovitch L, Dray JP. Long-term results of frontalis suspension using autogenous fascia lata for congenital ptosis in children under 3 years of age. Am J Ophthalmol. 2003;136:866–71.
19. Esmaeli B, Chung H, Pashby RC. Long-term results of frontalis suspension using irradiated, banked fascia lata. Ophthal Plast Reconstr Surg. 1998;14:159–63.
20. Foster JA, Holck DE, Perry JD, et al. Fibrin sealant for Muller muscle-conjunctiva resection ptosis repair. Ophthal Plast Reconstr Surg. 2006;22:184–7.
21. Reifler DM. Management of canalicular laceration. Surv Ophthalmol. 1991;36:113–32.
22. Wladis EJ, Aakalu VK, Yen MT, Bilyk JR, Mawn LA. Balloon dacryoplasty for congenital nasolacrimal duct obstruction: a report by the American Academy of Ophthalmology. Ophthalmology. 2018;125(10):1654–7.
23. Zoumalan CI, Maher EA, Lelli GJ, Lisman RD. Balloon canaliculoplasty for acquired canalicular stenosis. Ophthal Plast Reconstr Surg. 2010;26:459–61.

24. Ali MJ, Naik MN, Honavar SG. Balloon dacryoplasty: ushering the new and routine era in minimally invasive lacrimal surgeries. Int Ophthalmol. 2013;33:203e210.
25. Romo T III, Zoumalan RA, Rafii BY. Current concepts in the management of the aging forehead in facial plastic surgery. Curr Opin Otolaryngol Head Neck Surg. 2010;18:272–7.
26. Chowdhury S, Malhotra R, Smith R, Arnstein P. Patient and surgeon experience with the endotine forehead device for brow and forehead lift. Ophthal Plast Reconstr Surg. 2007;23:358–62.
27. Codere F, Denton P, Corona J. Endonasal dacryocystorhinostomy: a modified technique with preservation of the nasal and lacrimal mucosa. Ophthal Plast Reconstr Surg. 2010;26:161–4.
28. Tsirbas A, Davis G, Wormald PJ. Mechanical endonasal dacryocystorhinostomy versus external dacryocystorhinostomy. Ophthal Plast Reconstr Surg. 2004;20:50–6.
29. Coleman KR, Carruthers J. Combination therapy with BOTOX and fillers: the new rejuvnation paradigm. Dermatol Ther. 2006;19:177–88.
30. Carruthers A, Carruthers J. Non-animal-based hyaluronic acid fillers: scientific and technical considerations. Plast Reconstr Surg. 2007;120:33S–40S.
31. Coleman SR. Structural fat grafting: more than a permanent filler. Plast Reconstr Surg. 2006;118:108S–20S.
32. Pu LL, Coleman SR, Cui X, Ferguson RE Jr, Vasconez HC. Autologous fat grafts harvested and refined by the Coleman technique: a comparative study. Plast Reconstr Surg. 2008;122:932–7.
33. Holck DE, Ng JD. Facial skin rejuvenation. Curr Opin Ophthalmol. 2003;14:246–52.

Neuro-Ophthalmology Approach to Oculoplastic Disorders

5

Tiffany L. Kent, J. Banks Shepherd III, and Gregory P. Van Stavern

Neuro-ophthalmologists often participate in the care of patients with oculoplastic disorders. Their role may be the initial diagnosis, with subsequent referral; managing a patient ultimately found to have a neurologic reason for the oculoplastic condition (e.g., a patient with ptosis found to be secondary to myasthenia gravis); or coordinated care of diseases which straddle both specialties (e.g., thyroid orbitopathy, chronic progressive external ophthalmoplegia, skull base tumors, and orbital inflammatory syndrome). As with all of medical practice, good communication is an essential foundation for a fruitful and successful partnership in the care of patients.

Each neuro-ophthalmologist has his or her own unique style, but in general, the approach to each patient is similar. This chapter will briefly introduce oculoplastic surgeons to the manner in which neuro-ophthalmologists approach each patient and discuss the possible roles a neuro-ophthalmologist may play in the care of oculoplastic patients. We will also discuss neuro-ophthalmic disorders which may present to the oculoplastic surgeon and those in whose care the oculoplastic surgeon may participate.

Localization in Neuro-Ophthalmology

It may appear that, with the advent of sophisticated neuroimaging, there is little value to precise clinical localization: after all, when in doubt, why not just get a scan? However, we would argue forcefully that the reverse is more often the case: more sophisticated (and necessarily more expensive and time-consuming) imaging techniques compel us to be even more precise with clinical diagnosis and rational clinical decision-making. Even when imaging is necessary, it is critical to know what image to order (CT or MRI), how to order (with or without contrast, orbital views with fat saturation), and where to image (brain, orbit, cervical spine, skull base). Extensive use of unnecessary ancillary procedures (including neuroimaging) results in discomfort for patients and wasted resources. A targeted approach, informed by clinical localization and categorization, provides a good balance between looking only for common conditions that are easy to diagnose and testing for every possible disease that can cause the patient's complaint. In general, the wider the diagnostic net is cast, the higher the chance that unrelated positive findings may surface to further muddy the waters. It should also be kept in mind that every diagnostic test, including blood work, imaging, and even histopathology, has a false positive rate, and every positive finding needs to be matched to the patient, particularly if it does not fit the clinical scenario. For example, an MRI of the brain is performed on a patient presenting with unilateral ptosis, and it shows a large ipsilateral parasellar meningioma. That is clearly a positive finding – but does it have anything to do with the ptosis? If the ptosis is ultimately due to levator dehiscence, the tumor is an incidental finding, and there may be no need for intervention upon an asymptomatic benign tumor.

Principles of Localization

Localization derives from a Latin term locus, or site [1]. This refers to the diagnostic practice of determining from the symptoms and signs that the patient is displaying what portion of the nervous system has been affected. Injury to the neurovisual system causes abnormal function, and it is the characteristics of the dysfunction which allow a topographical diagnosis.

T. L. Kent
Oculoplastic Associates of West Michigan, Grand Rapids, MI, USA

J. Banks Shepherd III
Washington University in St. Louis, Department of Visual Sciences (Ophthalmology), Saint Louis, MO, USA

G. P. Van Stavern (✉)
Washington University in St. Louis, Department of Ophthalmology and Visual Sciences, St. Louis, MO, USA
e-mail: vanstaverng@wustl.edu

J. J. Servat et al. (eds.), *Smith and Nesi's Ophthalmic Plastic and Reconstructive Surgery*,
https://doi.org/10.1007/978-3-030-41720-8_5

Localization in medicine has a rich and distinguished history. The oldest known document regarding neurologic localization was recorded in an Egyptian papyrus circa 3000–2500 B.C. [2]. Hippocrates and others in ancient Greece recognized that injury to one side of the brain resulted in contralateral symptoms [1]. Paul Broca introduced the concept of functional organization and lateralization with pioneering work in aphasic patients [3]. Neuroimaging techniques, beginning with X-ray in the early twentieth century and progressing to current state-of-the-art MRI scanners, have refined our understanding of localization even further. However, even the highest-quality brain MRI is dependent upon human interpretation, which includes fitting the results of the scan into the patient's symptom complex and examination.

Clinical localization in neuro-ophthalmology involves the following steps:

1. Recognition of impaired visual function – afferent, efferent, or both
2. Identification of what site of the neurovisual system has been affected – e.g., retina, optic nerve, and chiasm
3. Listing the most likely etiologic entities, with a prioritized differential diagnosis
4. Use of ancillary testing (imaging, bloodwork, etc.) to determine a specific diagnosis

The recognition of impaired visual function is dependent upon a careful and thorough neuro-ophthalmological examination. This is built upon a foundation of experience and knowledge including examination techniques, neuroanatomy, and the range of normal visual function. Inexperience or too rapid examination technique may result either in over-interpretation of normal findings (e.g., misinterpreting physiologic hippus for an afferent pupillary defect) or missing subtle deficits (such as a noncomitant esotropia due to partial sixth nerve palsy).

Neuroanatomy provides the roadmap for localization. This encompasses both morphology of the structure and its functional representation – that is, the function mediated by a given structure. For example, the neuroanatomy of the oculomotor nerve includes its origin in the midbrain, the various regions through which it passes in its course, the separation into superior and inferior divisions, the location of fibers controlling pupillary function, and the central representation of the muscles innervated by that nerve. With this information, the combination of unilateral ptosis and elevation defect indicates superior divisional third nerve palsy. This narrows the region of interest on the roadmap considerably, but to find a specific address requires knowledge of anatomic detail – in this case, the clinical division of the third nerve occurs in the cavernous sinus or superior orbital fissure.

When there is more than one deficit present, localization becomes both easier and harder. It becomes easier since now we can find a common element to both deficits and harder because the possible neuroanatomic locations expand.

Common Locations

This is perhaps the most useful and practical way to localize findings. This method relies upon the concept of *medical parsimony* or *Occam's razor*: with multiple findings, a common underlying cause is likely. Given an array of neuro-ophthalmic deficits, we begin looking for an anatomic intersection where all of the structures involved meet. For example, a patient presenting with unilateral third, fourth, and sixth cranial nerve palsies most likely has a lesion in the ipsilateral cavernous sinus. A combination of ipsilateral fifth, sixth, and seventh nerve palsies (Gradenigo's syndrome) suggests a lesion at the ipsilateral petrous apex.

The absence of deficits provides critical information, as well. Complete, bilateral ophthalmoplegia resulting from a brainstem process would involve a long contiguous or multifocal lesion, resulting in long-tract signs (spasticity, weakness, hemisensory loss) and possibly alteration of consciousness (if the reticular activating system was affected). The lack of such findings would suggest multiple cranial nerve palsies, neuromuscular junction disease (myasthenia gravis or botulism), or ocular myopathy.

Common Anatomy

There are situations where shared anatomic features provide clues to localization. All cranial nerves are invested by the leptomeninges, and all pass through the subarachnoid space [4]. Therefore, diffuse meningeal processes (e.g., acute or chronic meningitis, meningeal carcinomatosis, subarachnoid hemorrhage) often cause multiple, bilateral cranial nerve palsies. Similarly, all cranial nerves are supplied by microvascular branches of the large vessels in the circle of Willis. This microvasculature is preferentially affected by conditions such as diabetes mellitus and hypertension. Single, isolated cranial nerve palsies in susceptible patients have a favorable prognosis and rarely need extensive workup. Certain infectious organisms, particular herpes viruses and fungi, are basophilic and may cause an associated infectious vasculitis, resulting in multiple cranial nerve palsies.

Prioritized Differential Diagnosis

Generating a differential diagnosis is the final outcome of a comprehensive history and examination. Although the differential needs to be inclusive, it should not be exhaustive – a real value of subspecialty consultation is to help narrow the differential diagnosis and tailor any further diagnostic testing to what is most likely.

All physicians rely upon clinical reasoning skills when generating a differential diagnosis. Although the rise of subspecialized care and the advent of modern technology (particularly the twenty-first century neuroimaging techniques) have changed the landscape of medicine, the manner in which we reason through clinical cases has changed little over the past several decades. Elstein [5] described the essential components of the clinical reasoning process – the *hypothetico-deductive model.* We reduce uncertainty in a clinical case by generating one or more diagnostic hypotheses and procure additional information to confirm or exclude one or more of these hypotheses. The problem is placed in a deductive framework: if patient has X, then he must exhibit these features. This process might be simple or complex, depending upon the clinical scenario, the experience of the clinician, the urgency of the situation, and other factors.

This type of reasoning, also called *analytical reasoning*, implicitly or explicitly incorporates Bayes theorem or regression analysis [6, 7]. Briefly, these models assume that each clinician is cognizant of the a priori probability with which a particular diagnosis may present and the conditional probability associating each bit of evidence (clinical findings, presenting symptoms, diagnostic tests) with the diagnosis. This *forward flow* – reasoning from evidence to diagnosis – is the essence of analytical clinical reasoning.

However, most physicians rely upon what some have called *nonanalytic* clinical reasoning or, less technically, pattern recognition [8]. These medical heuristics, or *rules of thumb*, are derived from time spent in training and years of clinical experience. For example, an oculoplastic surgeon is generally able to make a diagnosis of levator dehiscence within a short period of time, with minimal diagnostic challenge. This occurs because he or she has seen many cases of ptosis, is familiar with the presentation of a variety of conditions which cause ptosis, and is *tuned in* to red flags in the history or exam which would suggest an alternate diagnosis. Most of us rely heavily upon these heuristics, and they serve us well. They allow us to see large numbers of patients and successfully run a busy practice.

There is a price, however, in that even the most astute diagnostician is prone to cognitive errors as a result of a too heavy reliance upon pattern recognition and experience. Diagnostic errors in medicine have become the focus of increased attention over the past decade. Graber [9] and others [10] have published strong evidence that cognitive-processing errors (or cognitive biases) are far more common than knowledge gaps. There are a large number of biases to which we as physicians and humans are prone – most such lists are overcomplete and redundant. These are the biases that seem to be the primary sources of diagnostic error [11].

1. *Availability bias:*
   the tendency to judge diagnoses as more likely if they are more easily retrievable from memory
2. *Base rate neglect:*
   the tendency to ignore the true rate of disease and pursue rare but more exotic diagnoses (*looking for zebras*)
3. *Representativeness:*
   the tendency to be guided by prototypical features of the disease and miss atypical variants
4. *Confirmation bias:*
   the tendency to seek data to confirm, not refute, the hypothesis (*we only find what we're looking for*)
5. *Premature closure:*
   the tendency to stop too soon and not order the critical test or gather the critical information

All of these biases may be in play in any clinical situation – the degree to which they compromise clinical decision-making varies from case to case and is dependent upon a number of different factors, not the least of which is the individual clinicians' awareness of these tendencies. Limited evidence suggests that awareness of the cognitive processes used to make decisions can reduce the likelihood of poor decision-making.

There is certainly nothing unique about the clinical decision-making skills possessed by neuro-ophthalmologist versus any other clinical physician. However, in some ways, subspecialists (such as neuro-ophthalmologists) may be even more prone to certain errors. For example, we often see patients already seen by a primary ophthalmologist or neurologist. There is therefore an often unconscious assumption that the patient has already been *screened* for nonneurologic conditions such as refractive error, cataract, and decompensated congenital strabismus. In many cases, this turns out not to be the case, and it becomes critical to keep common disorders in mind, even in a tertiary or quaternary referral clinic. Such clinics also tend to see rare diseases more frequently, and one can easily fall prey to base rate neglect – thinking every case is a *zebra* and spending an enormous amount of time and money to prove that it is, indeed, just a horse.

Role of Neuro-Ophthalmologist in Oculoplastics

Aside from aiding in differential diagnosis, the neuro-ophthalmologist may be a valuable resource for interpreting neuroimaging studies and the medical management of certain conditions.

Neuro-ophthalmologists may be primarily trained in either neurology or ophthalmology (or, rarely, both). Ophthalmology-trained neuro-ophthalmologists may perform strabismus surgery, some orbital surgery, or practice some general ophthalmology. Neurology-trained neuro-ophthalmologists often treat the neurologic diseases that present to their clinic, such as myasthenia gravis, multiple sclerosis, and migraine. They are also familiar with the use of immunomodulatory agents and could be a valuable resource when managing patients requiring long-term immunosuppression (recurrent orbital inflammatory syndrome, sarcoidosis, etc.). Such patients are often referred to rheumatologists, who may not be familiar with underlying disease process and lack the capacity to carefully monitor visual function.

Although oculoplastic specialists are quite familiar with interpreting orbital imaging, some are less comfortable evaluating intracranial structures. As we will discuss in detail, lesions of the intracranial visual pathways (both afferent and efferent) can present to the oculoplastic clinic. The high sensitivity of MRI is a double-edged sword: not only it can detect many small, pathologic lesions missed by CT scan but also it can identify clinically insignificant abnormalities that, when improperly interpreted, may lead to further, unnecessary testing [12]. A neuro-ophthalmologist may be helpful in reviewing the films and helping to decide whether further testing is warranted. The explosion of imaging techniques over the past decade leads to confusion – what part of the neuraxis to image (brain, orbit, cervical spine, etc.), whether to add gadolinium or not, whether to image the vascular system (MR angiogram, CT angiogram, MR venogram, etc.), and special sequences (diffusion-weighted imaging, susceptibility-weighted imaging). All of these techniques have their role but are usually only needed for particular clinical indications. We have included a more in-depth discussion of neuroimaging later in the chapter, but in general, neuro-ophthalmologists assess the intracranial visual pathways more frequently than oculoplastic surgeon, and neuroimaging can be helpful to have on hand when reviewing scans.

Neurologic Conditions with Oculoplastic Manifestations

Lesions at any level of the neuraxis above the spine can cause damage resulting in oculoplastic consultation. In general, the lower the level of the lesion, the more likely it is to present to an oculoplastic surgeon. We will review this topic anatomically, beginning at the highest level (cerebral cortex) and moving caudally. Table 5.1 reviews the hierarchical organization of eye movement control descending from the cortex to brainstem, with predicted oculomotor dysfunction and associated neurologic deficits.

Table 5.1 Localization of eye movement disorders

Brain level	Ocular motor structure	Lesions result in	Other neurologic deficits
Cerebral cortex	Cortical gaze centers (eye fields)	Ipsilateral gaze deviation Hypometric saccades Impaired smooth pursuit	Contralateral weakness Hemisensory loss
Basal ganglia	Descending gaze control pathways	Saccadic intrusions Impaired smooth pursuit Hypometric saccades	Axial rigidity Dyskinesias
Thalamus	Descending gaze control pathways Vergence pathways	Wrong way deviation Thalamic esotropia	Hemisensory loss Visual field defect
Midbrain	Vertical gaze centers (riMFL, INC) Trochlear nucleus and fascicle Oculomotor nucleus and fascicle	Vertical gaze palsy Superior oblique palsy Convergence-retraction nystagmus Third nerve palsy	Contralateral hemiparesis Light-near dissociation Contralateral tremor
Pons	Abducens nucleus and fascicle PPRF MLF	INO Horizontal gaze palsy Sixth nerve palsy Skew deviation	Facial nerve palsy Trigeminal neuropathy Hearing loss Contralateral weakness

riMLF rostral interstitial nucleus of medial longitudinal fasciculus, *INC* interstitial nucleus of Cajal, *PPRF* paramedian pontine reticular formation, *MLF* medial longitudinal fasciculus

Cerebral Gaze Deviation

Acute, unilateral hemispheric injury may cause transient gaze palsy or gaze deviation [13]. This most often occurs with parietal and right-sided lesions. The eyes are deviated ipsilateral to the lesion. The gaze deviation may be overcome with horizontal oculocephalics and usually changes within days to a gaze preference. Other localizing features, such as hemineglect, visual field defect, and anosognosia, are often present. The most common causes are stroke and tumor. The gaze deviation usually improves to a gaze preference and often resolves completely over several weeks or months, depending upon the severity of the initial insult. Such patients rarely require oculoplastic procedures.

Cerebral Ptosis

Although eyelid dysfunction was once thought to rare with cerebral hemispheric lesions, more recent reports suggest that it may be more common than suspected. Averbuch-Heller et al. [14] studied 64 consecutive patients with acute hemispheric stroke, with standardized measurement of palpebral fissures, margin reflex distance, and levator function. They found that 24/64 patients had neurogenic ptosis, 10 of whom had bilateral involvement. Only one-third of these patients had complete ptosis, and somewhat surprisingly, the ptosis was often greater ipsilateral to the lesion. The majority of patients improved spontaneously, with complete normalization of eyelid function. This suggests that even when cerebral ptosis develops, it is self-limited and will only rarely require oculoplastic consultation and intervention.

Basal Ganglia

The basal ganglia are grouped subcortical structures sharing common functional attributes. They are variably defined but are considered to include the following [1]:

1. The corpus striatum, composed of the putamen and caudate nucleus
2. The claustrum
3. The substantia nigra, consisting of the pars compacta and pars reticularis
4. The globus pallidus, with internal and external portions
5. The subthalamic nucleus

A detailed review of the neuroanatomy and neurophysiology of the basal ganglia is well beyond the scope of this chapter. Broadly, the basal ganglia help control posture and movement. They are heavily involved in learned motor activities that occur at a subconscious or preconscious level. Lesions involving the basal ganglia are often diffuse and can result in a wide range of abnormal motor function.

The basal ganglia also play a major role in eye movement control, particularly saccades [15]. The pathways through the basal ganglia maintain balance between reflexive and purposeful voluntary saccades and help prevent intrusive saccades. Basal ganglia diseases often cause impaired smooth pursuit and hypometric saccades (i.e., more than one eye movement is needed to acquire a new target). Saccadic intrusions (rapid eye movements interrupting fixation) are frequently found in these conditions. In many cases, these findings are asymptomatic or minimally symptomatic. There are several basal ganglia diseases that cause significant ocular motor and eyelid dysfunction and may result in an oculoplastic consultation. We will cover these in more detail.

Parkinson's Disease

Parkinson's disease (PD) is a primary neurodegenerative disorder characterized pathologically by loss of dopaminergic cells within the substantia nigra and clinically by resting tremor, bradykinesia, and rigidity. The precise etiology is unknown, and treatment is largely symptomatic, most commonly with dopaminergic agonists, such as levodopa.

Visual symptoms are frequently present in patients with PD but are rarely a presenting feature. The complaints may be relatively vague and direct, and specific questioning may be needed to clarify. Visual hallucinations occur in up to 25% of PD patients; this may occur as a result of dopaminergic medications or visual cortical dysfunction [16].

Eyelid disorders are common in PD. Decreased blink rate is frequent, resulting in dry eye and assorted afferent visual symptoms. Blepharospasm can occur as well, possibly due to disinhibition of the facial nucleus and spontaneous firing of orbicularis oculi muscles. Apraxia of eyelid opening (AEO) occurs less frequently; in this condition, the patient has difficulty initiating opening of the eyelids. Lepore and Duvoisin [17] reported the clinical criteria for the diagnosis of AEO as transitory inability to initiate eyelid opening; no evidence of ongoing orbicularis oculi contraction, such as lowering of the brows beneath the superior orbital margins (Charcot's eyebrow sign of blepharospasm); vigorous frontalis contraction during periods of inability to raise eyelids; and no oculomotor or ocular sympathetic nerve dysfunction and no ocular myopathy.

The supranuclear ocular motor system is affected in PD. Convergence is impaired in many patients, resulting in convergence insufficiency (CI). Indeed, CI should be a leading consideration in PD patients with diplopia [16]. Historical features supporting CI include horizontal diplopia at near, visual blurring at near after reading for a set time period (usually 5–10 min), and relief of symptoms with monocular occlusion. Examination findings confirming CI include reduced convergence amplitudes, remote near point of convergence, and exodeviation at near. Correct diagnosis in the appropriate clinically setting would obviate the need for extensive workup for alternate causes. Treatment usually involves adequate presbyopic correction and prisms.

Progressive Supranuclear Palsy

Progressive supranuclear palsy (PSP) is an uncommon neurodegenerative disorder with prominent neuro-ophthalmic findings [18]. Current diagnostic criteria include gradually progressive disorder, onset age >40 years, either vertical supranuclear palsy or both slowing of vertical saccades and postural instability with falls in the first year of onset. Patients with PSP have *parkinsonian* features such as decreased blink rate, masked facies, axial rigidity, and en bloc turns and may initially be mistakenly diagnosed with PD. However, clues to the diagnosis include greater axial and neck rigidity, marked micrographia, frequent spastic dysarthria and dysphonia, lack of resting tremor, eye movement abnormalities, and minimal response to dopaminergic therapy.

As suggested by the name of the condition, the supranuclear eye movement system is often abnormal in PSP. The ocular motor findings are often present early in the disease course and may help differentiating PSP from PD and other causes of parkinsonism.

Saccades are initially slowed. The classic abnormality is a supranuclear vertical gaze paresis, initially for vertical eye movements but ultimately affecting eye movements in all planes. Patients may progress to complete ophthalmoplegia. The vestibulo-ocular reflex remains intact until late in the disease course. Saccadic intrusions (square wave jerks) may be seen in at least 60% of patients. Frequent or continuous square wave jerks are commonly seen and are more frequent in PSP than PD. The ratio of square wave jerks to blink rate may help distinguish PSP from idiopathic PD [19].

Eyelid disorders are common in PSP, similar to PD. Decreased blink rate is common and results in dry eye, occasionally severe. Blepharospasm and apraxia of eyelid opening may occur as well.

Management of eyelid disorders in both PD and PSP is symptomatic and similar to conventional treatment. Dry eye should be treated aggressively with lubricating drops and ointments and punctal plugs for refractory patients. Dopaminergic replacement has no benefit for eyelid dysfunction. Botox is the treatment of choice for symptomatic blepharospasm and has been used successfully for AEO as well [18].

Other Basal Ganglia Diseases

Hereditary neurodegenerative diseases may selectively involve the basal ganglia. These include *Huntington's disease*, *Wilson's disease*, *Hallervorden–Spatz* disease, and others, most exceedingly rare. As a general rule, these conditions result in saccadic dysfunction to varying degrees. Eyelid disorders such as blepharospasm and AEO seem to be less common, although they may occur [15].

Tourette's syndrome has been associated with blepharospasm, although the saccadic and ocular motor system is typically normal. This should be distinguished from benign eyelid tics, which usually resolve with age. Treatment of blepharospasm in Tourette's is similar to essential blepharospasm.

Brainstem Ocular Motility Disorders

The brainstem is composed primarily of three parts: the midbrain, the pons, and the medulla. Together these structures are about the size of a thumb but contain a complex array of prenuclear, internuclear, and nuclear centers that control many of the basic functions of the body, including eye movement and image stabilization. Because of its dense and intricate anatomy, lesions of brainstem pathways can cause a wide variety of complex ocular motility deficits. Three archetypal brainstem ocular motility syndromes will be reviewed: the dorsal midbrain syndrome, internuclear ophthalmoplegia, and skew deviation. Patients with these conditions may present to the oculoplastic surgeon with complaints of ptosis, diplopia, or eyelid retraction [20]. Early recognition of these conditions will help direct appropriate workup, diagnosis, and treatment.

Internuclear Ophthalmoplegia

The medial longitudinal fasciculus (MLF) is a tract of internuclear neurons that runs the length of the brainstem whose purpose is to coordinate eye movements by yoking together the third, fourth, sixth, and eighth cranial nerve nuclei. A lesion of the MLF interrupts these connections and manifests clinically as an *internuclear ophthalmoplegia* (INO). The most noticeable clinical manifestation of an INO is incoordination of horizontal eye movements: slow and/or incomplete adduction of one or, in the case of bilateral INO, both eyes accompanied by compensatory nystagmus of the abducting fellow eye in extreme lateral gaze. Unless the lesion is high in the midbrain, convergence remains intact [21]. Patients with INO are often asymptomatic but may have diplopia, oscillopsia, or vertigo with eye and head movement. In most cases of INO, the eyes are aligned in primary gaze; however, some patients develop an exotropia (a so-called wall-eyed INO), particularly if convergence is impaired and/or if the patient has an underlying strabismus.

Unilateral INO is most often caused by small-vessel ischemia of the pons or midbrain. Bilateral INO is most commonly associated with demyelinating disease; however, small-vessel ischemia, brainstem hemorrhage, trauma, tumors, and hydrocephalus may also present with bilateral INO. As a rule, any patient with an INO should have imaging of the brain, brainstem, and skull base with MRI. Additionally, myasthenia gravis and Guillain–Barré (Fisher) syndrome should be considered in any patient with weak adduction, particularly if ptosis is present and/or if nystagmus of the abducted fellow eye is absent.

Causes of Internuclear Ophthalmoplegia
- Multiple sclerosis (typically bilateral)
- Infarction (typically unilateral)
- Brainstem and fourth ventricular tumors
- Hemorrhage
- Trauma
- Arnold–Chiari malformation
- Hydrocephalus

Dorsal Midbrain (Pretectal, Parinaud) Syndrome

Midbrain structures important for supranuclear control of vertical eye movements surround the aqueduct of Sylvius. Lesions affecting the posterior aspect of the midbrain can damage these structures and result in a cluster of neuro-ophthalmic findings known as the dorsal midbrain (pretectal, Sylvian aqueduct, or Parinaud) syndrome. Although vertical gaze paresis is a key finding of the dorsal midbrain syndrome, it is important to note that all of these findings need not be present in any given patient.

The most common causes of the dorsal midbrain syndrome are hydrocephalus and tumors near the tectum (e.g., pineal germinomas, glioma); however, trauma, multiple sclerosis, stroke, and midbrain hemorrhage may also cause the dorsal midbrain syndrome (Fig. 5.1).

Because patients with the dorsal midbrain syndrome may have clinical features similar to those with restrictive orbital myopathies (e.g., thyroid orbitopathy), any patient with bilateral upper eyelid retraction and restriction of elevation should have a careful examination of pupil function and for convergence-retraction nystagmus. Any patient with signs of dorsal midbrain syndrome should undergo cerebral imaging urgently (Table 5.2).

Table 5.2 Features of the dorsal midbrain syndrome

Limitation of upward eye movement
Convergence retraction with attempted upward saccades
Large, often asymmetric, pupils with light-near dissociation
Eyelid retraction (Collier's sign)
Slow abduction (pseudoabducens palsy) due to increased convergence tone

Skew Deviation

Skew deviation is a vertical misalignment of the eyes resulting from asymmetric impairment of vestibular inputs to the midbrain gaze centers. Interruption of these pathways causes the oculomotor centers to misperceive head position and results in a hypertropia that may either be the same in all directions of gaze (comitant) or change across gaze directions (incomitant). In its incomitant form, skew deviation may mimic isolated extraocular muscle paresis; however, unlike lesions of the oculomotor nerves or muscles, secondary deviation does not occur with skew deviation [22]. Occasionally, a skew deviation is associated with significant bilateral ocular torsion and head tilt known as the ocular tilt reaction and is more likely to be associated with vestibular disease (inner ear, vestibulocochlear nerve, or vestibular nucleus) [23].

Skew deviation can result from vestibular, brainstem, or cerebellar dysfunction and may be caused by brainstem or cerebellar stroke, tumors, or demyelination. Rarely, skew deviation may be seen with increased intracranial pressure [24].

The Ocular Motor Nerves and their Nuclei

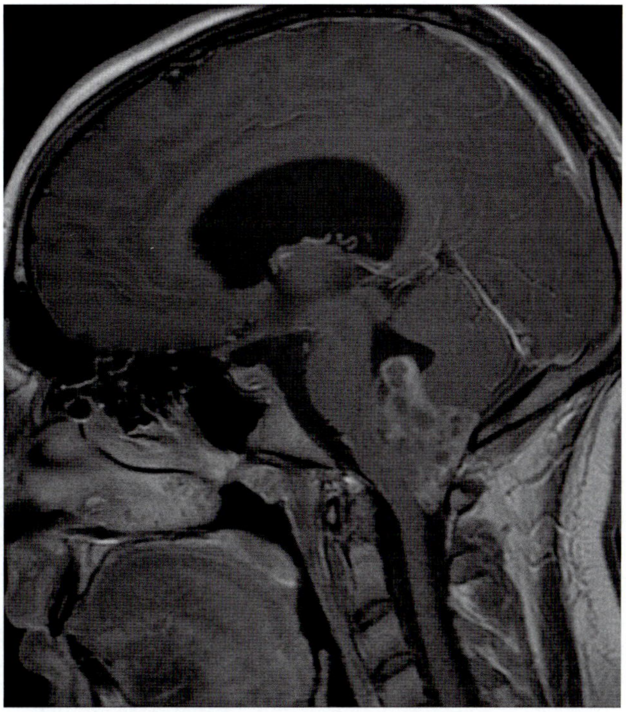

Fig. 5.1 Sagittal T1 MRI with Gadolinium. Note the enhancing mass obstructing the fourth ventricle. This was found at pathology to be an ependymoma [25–27]

The Oculomotor (Third) Nerve

The oculomotor nerve supplies the levator muscle of the upper eyelid, the superior rectus, medial rectus, inferior rectus, and inferior oblique muscles. Additionally, the oculomotor nerves supply parasympathetic input to the ciliary ganglion for accommodation and pupillary constriction. Paralysis of the oculomotor nerve results in a combination of weak elevation, adduction, depression of the globe, ptosis, poor pupillary constriction, and loss of accommodation. The two most common causes of oculomotor paresis are compression from an intracranial aneurysm and microvascular infarction [26].

Anatomy

The oculomotor nuclear complex lies within the central midbrain anterior to the aqueduct of Sylvius near the floor of the third ventricle. Motor fibers from the nucleus pass anteriorly through the MLF, red nucleus, and medial portion of the superior cerebellar peduncle before exiting the midbrain in the interpeduncular fossa. Passing between the posterior cerebral and superior cerebellar arteries in the subarachnoid space, the oculomotor nerve continues anterolaterally, crossing closely under the posterior communicating artery. The nerve then passes under the medial edge of the tentorium cerebelli before piercing the dura at the posterior clinoid process. It then travels along the lateral dural wall of the cavernous sinus in a layer of dense connective tissue before separating into superior and inferior divisions as it passes through the superior orbital fissure into the orbit.

A unique anatomical feature of the oculomotor nerve is that the parasympathetic fibers are located on the exterior surface of the nerve and derive their blood supply from pial blood vessels. By contrast, the interior of the nerve (where the somatic motor fibers are located) derives a majority of its perfusion from a central nutrient artery. As a result, microvascular infarction of the nerve tends to spare pupillary function even as it results in complete motor paresis otherwise. Conversely, compressive lesions (tumor, aneurysm, and herniation) or trauma to the nerve tends to involve pupillary fibers in addition to the ocular motor deficits (Fig. 5.2).

Pathology

Given the tight arrangement of the oculomotor nuclear complex and its fascicles, midbrain lesions typically result in bilateral ocular motility deficits with symmetrical involvement of the levator muscles. Thus, unilateral oculomotor paresis with bilateral ptosis and/or contralateral superior rectus weakness is likely midbrain in origin [28]. Similarly, if unilateral paresis is accompanied by evidence of damage to the red nucleus or cerebellar peduncle (contralateral ataxia, tremor, or hemiparesis), the site of damage is likely in the anterior midbrain. The most common midbrain lesions are infarction and hemorrhage, although demyelination and intrinsic tumors should be considered.

Because of its firm dural attachment to the sphenoid bone, the oculomotor nerve is vulnerable to shearing and compressive forces in the subarachnoid space. The most important cause of damage at this site is compression of the nerve by

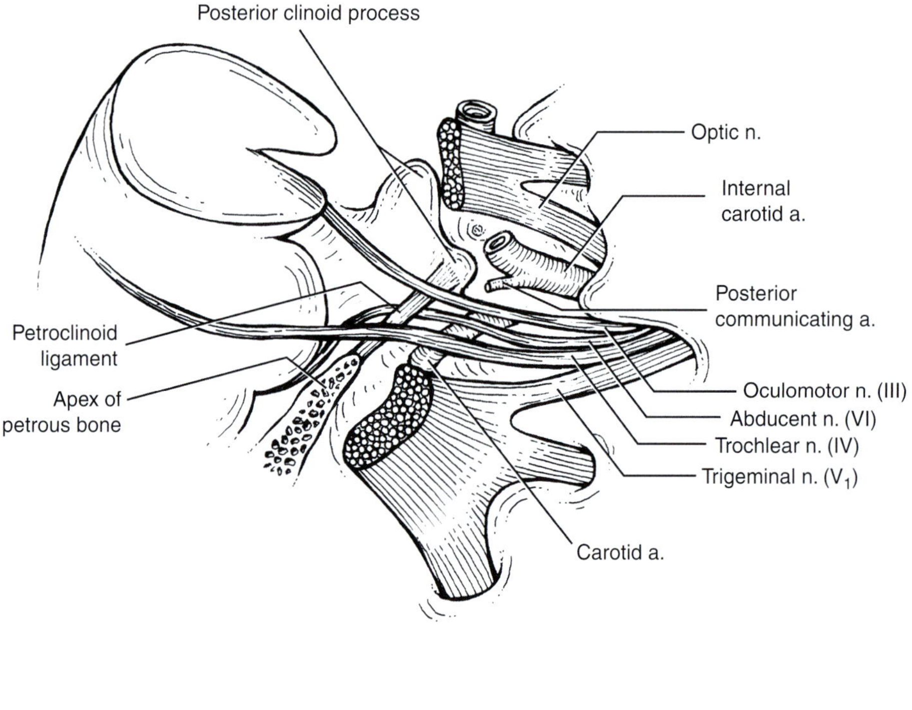

Fig. 5.2 Illustration of the posterior portion of the cavernous sinus and intracranial courses of the relevant cranial nerves and vascular structures

an expanding skull base aneurysm (Fig. 5.3a, b); however, mass lesions, head trauma, and cerebral herniation are also important causes.

Within the cavernous sinus, lesions affecting the third nerve often cause concomitant dysfunction of the trochlear, abducens, and/or upper divisions of the trigeminal nerve. The presence of oculosympathetic paresis (Horner syndrome) is highly suggestive of a cavernous sinus lesion. See *cavernous sinus syndrome* below.

Within the superior orbital fissure, the superior division innervates the levator and superior rectus muscles, while the inferior division innervates the inferior rectus, inferior oblique, and medial rectus muscles as well as transmits the parasympathetic fibers destined for the ciliary ganglion. Any patient with unilateral ptosis and reduced levator function should be evaluated for diplopia in upgaze (superior rectus weakness), whether or not a motility deficit can be appreciated clinically. Myasthenia gravis should also be carefully considered in patients with ptosis and weak elevation of the globe.

Emergent cerebral imaging with angiography (MRI/MRA or CT/CTA) is indicated in all cases of new onset third nerve paresis [29]. The only exception is if the clinical evidence overwhelmingly supports microvascular disease: complete oculomotor paresis with *sparing of pupillary function* in an older individual with no relevant systemic disease, other than vasculopathic risk factors [30]. However, should the nerve paresis not recover in 3 months or aberrant regeneration (most commonly retraction of the eyelid with downgaze or adduction) occur, cerebral and vascular imaging should be obtained.

The Trochlear (Fourth) Nerve

The trochlear (fourth) nerve innervates the superior oblique muscle and is the longest of the ocular motor nerves. Paralysis of the trochlear nerve results in vertical diplopia (hypertropia) that is most troublesome in downgaze and contralateral sidegaze. The patient may tilt his or her head toward the opposite shoulder to minimize the diplopia. The most common causes of fourth nerve palsy are congenital weakness that manifests in adulthood, microvascular infarction, and head trauma [1, 26].

Anatomy

The fourth nerve nucleus lies anterior to cerebral aqueduct directly caudal to the oculomotor nuclear complex. The fascicles of the nerve course posteriorly around the aqueduct and decussate near the roof of the fourth ventricle and exit at the level of the inferior colliculi. The trochlear nerve then courses around the brainstem in the subarachnoid space; passes along the underside of the tentorium cerebelli, under the petroclinoid ligament; and pierces the dura just inferior to the oculomotor nerve at the posterior clinoid process. Within the cavernous sinus, the fourth nerve travels along the thickened dural layer of the lateral wall inferior to the oculomotor nerve and superior to the ophthalmic division of the trigeminal nerve. It then passes through the superior orbital fissure and into the orbit.

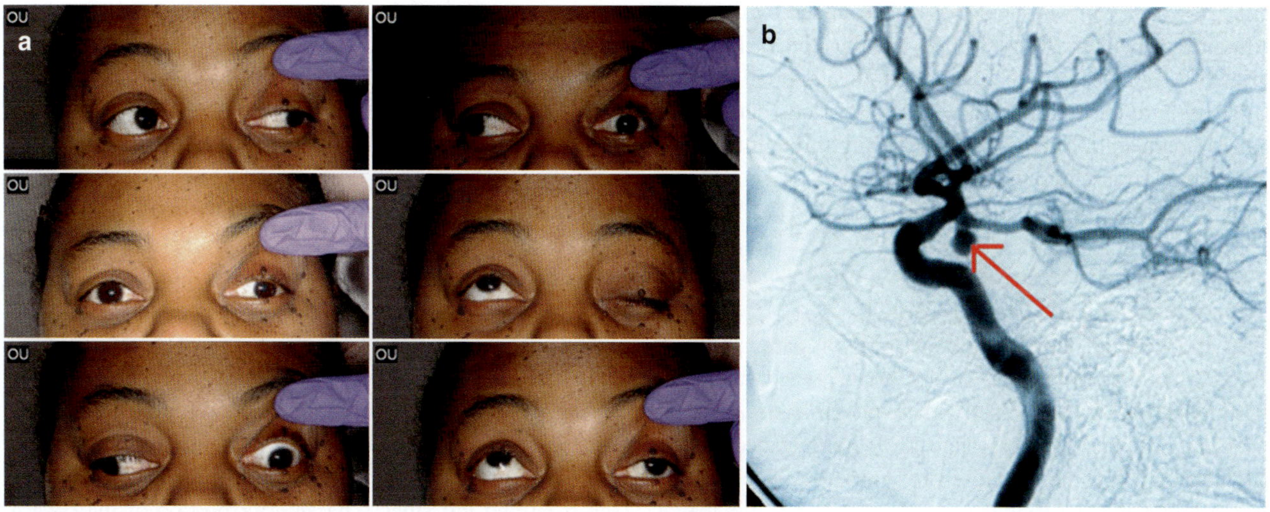

Fig. 5.3 (**a**) Motility photos of a 39-year-old woman who had presented with painful diplopia and left ptosis. Note the limited adduction, elevation, and depression, with left ptosis. Pupils are pharmacologically dilated in the photograph; she had presented with isocoric, reactive pupils. MRI and MRA were nondiagnostic. Cerebral angiography (**b**) demonstrates a left posterior communicating artery aneurysm (*arrow*)

Pathology

The most frequent causes of unilateral fourth nerve palsy are microvascular disease and decompensation of a congenital trochlear nerve paresis. The most frequent cause of bilateral fourth nerve palsy is head trauma. Compression by posterior fossa tumors and meningiopathies (neoplastic, infectious, etc.) is uncommon [31].

The Abducens (Sixth) Nerve

The abducens (sixth) nerve innervates the lateral rectus muscle. Paresis of the abducens nerve results in a monocular esotropia that worsens toward the side of the paresis with or without visible abduction paresis. The most common causes of sixth nerve paresis is microvascular infarction, head trauma, and cavernous sinus disease.

Anatomy

The nucleus of the sixth nerve is located in the central pons and contains two groups of neurons: motor neurons supplying the ipsilateral abducens nerve and interneurons projecting via the MLF to the contralateral medial rectus subnucleus in the oculomotor nucleus. Exiting nerve fibers pass anteriorly through the medial lemniscus and the lateral portion of the corticospinal tracts before exiting the ventral surface of the pons. The abducens nerve then ascends through the subarachnoid space along the slope of the clivus before passing into Dorello's canal (a small passage bounded by the petroclinoid ligament, the petrous apex, and the clivus). The nerve traverses the cavernous sinus, largely unsupported, in close apposition to the carotid artery (where it briefly carries ocular sympathetic afferents) before passing through the superior orbital fissure into the orbit.

Pathology

The abducens nucleus is the final common pathway for all horizontal eye movement except convergence; therefore, lesions of the nucleus itself result in *paralysis of conjugate gaze* to the ipsilateral side [32]. Further, because the abducens nucleus lies in close proximity to the genu of the facial nerve, nuclear lesions very commonly result in ipsilateral facial weakness. More anterior lesions of the pons may damage the fascicles of the sixth nerve and produce isolated unilateral lateral rectus weakness; however, signs of concomitant damage to surrounding midbrain structures (contralateral hemiparesis, facial weakness) betray the location of the damage.

Because the nerve is firmly tethered at Dorello's canal, the nerve is vulnerable to stretching and shearing in the subarachnoid space. Downward displacement of the brainstem due to increased intracranial pressure or head trauma can cause unilateral or bilateral sixth nerve paresis.

Within the confined space of Dorello's canal, expansile or inflammatory lesions of the clivus or petrous apex can cause abducens nerve paresis. The Gradenigo syndrome [33] of unilateral abducens nerve paresis, hemifacial pain, and variable facial weakness results from inflammation of the apex of the petrous ridge and the overlying meninges. Sometimes referred to as *petrous apicitis* [34], Gradenigo syndrome is most commonly a sequela of otitis media and mastoiditis [35], although it may also be seen with tuberculous infection of the skull base, aneurysms of the intrapetrosal carotid artery, traumatic petrous fracture, and thrombosis of the inferior petrosal sinus. Similarly, expansile lesions of the clivus can cause unilateral or bilateral sixth nerve paresis. These include chordomas, meningiomas, and bony metastases.

The overall incidence among all ages of a tumor as the etiology of a nontraumatic, isolated sixth nerve palsy is approximately 20% [36]. Microvascular disease is a more common cause in older adults. Thus, patients at risk for microvascular disease may be observed initially, as 86% of microvascular palsies spontaneously recover within 3 months [37]. If recovery does not occur, if other neurologic abnormalities are present, or for bilateral sixth nerve pareses, neuroimaging is then required. In adults younger than 50 years old, MRI is indicated initially, as the incidence of a space-occupying lesion increases with decreasing age [38].

Cavernous Sinus (Fig. 5.4)

Anatomy

The cavernous sinus is a collection of thin-walled venous channels lateral to the sella turcica. It is bounded by sphenoid bone inferomedially and by a free dural layer superiorly and laterally. The cavernous sinus receives venous inflow from the superior/inferior ophthalmic, middle cerebral, and sphenoparietal veins and drains into the inferior and superior petrosal sinuses. There are variable collaterals that connect the right and left sides. The anterior portion of the cavernous sinus lies just underneath the optic foramen and directly abuts the superior orbital fissure [25, 30].

Along its lateral wall, dense connective tissue encases the cavernous segments of the oculomotor and trochlear nerves as well as the first (ophthalmic) and second (maxillary) divisions of the trigeminal nerves. Medially, the inter-

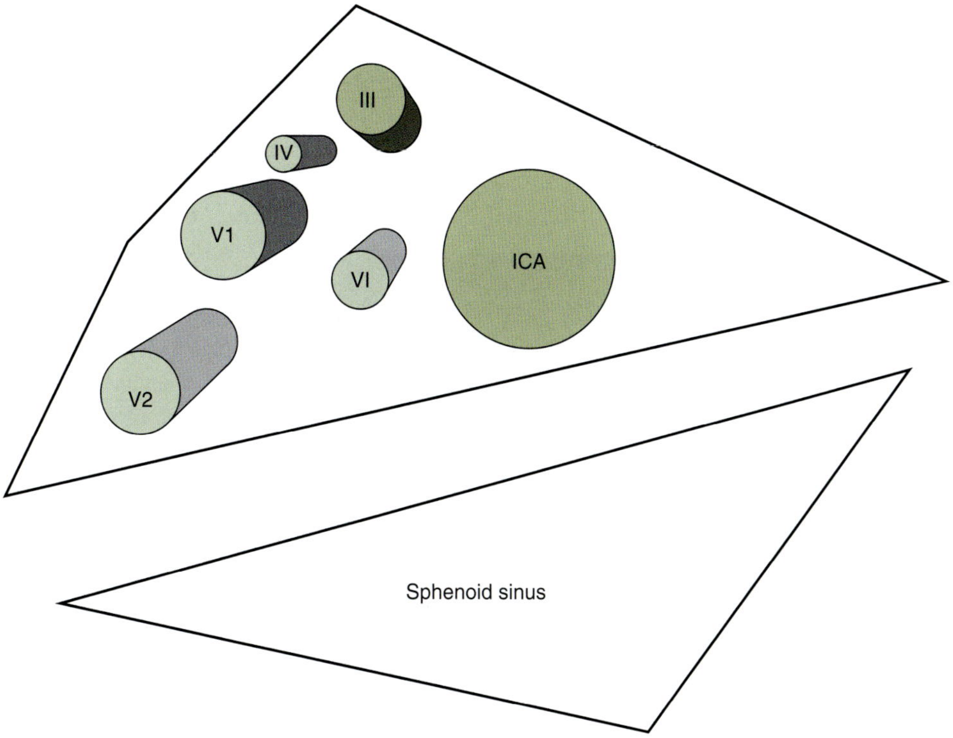

Fig. 5.4 Schematic diagram of the right cavernous sinus, with neuroanatomic relationships. *IC* internal carotid artery, III: oculomotor nerve; VI: abducens nerve; IV: trochlear nerve; *V1* ophthalmic division of trigeminal nerve, *V2* maxillary division of trigeminal nerve. Note the close proximity of the abducens nerve to the internal carotid artery

nal carotid artery courses through the cavernous sinus in close apposition to the abducens nerve, delivering postganglionic sympathetic fibers to the orbit via the abducens and trigeminal nerves.

Pathology

Cavernous sinus disease (space-occupying lesions, thrombosis, infection, fistula, etc.) typically results in varying degrees of ophthalmoplegia (ocular motility deficit attributable to more than one ipsilateral cranial nerve), oculosympathetic paresis, and/or pain in the distribution of the ophthalmic and (less commonly) maxillary branches of the trigeminal nerve [39].

Slowly expanding lesions of the cavernous sinus lead to gradually progressive ophthalmoplegia, often starting with abducens paresis (with or without oculosympathetic paresis) for medially based lesions (laterally breaking pituitary tumors, meningiomas of the greater wing of the sphenoid, and fusiform aneurysms of the carotid siphon) or oculomotor paresis for lateral lesions (meningiomas, meningeal carcinomatosis). Rapidly expanding and/or inflammatory lesions (metastases, nasopharyngeal carcinoma, lymphoma, sarcoidosis, mycosis, pituitary apoplexy) often cause rapid total or near-total ophthalmoplegia, oculosympathetic paresis (Horner syndrome), and periocular pain.

Directly apposed to the anterior cavernous sinus, the superior orbital fissure transmits the third, fourth, and sixth nerves, in addition to the ophthalmic division of the trigeminal nerve and the superior ophthalmic vein. In isolation and without the aid of neuroimaging, lesions of the superior orbital fissure (tumor, trauma, aneurysm, fungal infection, etc.) are clinically indistinguishable from those of the cavernous sinus. Although uncommon, involvement of the maxillary division of the trigeminal nerve indicates cavernous sinus disease.

Tolosa–Hunt Syndrome

The Tolosa–Hunt Syndrome (THS) of painful ophthalmoplegia is the result of idiopathic granulomatous inflammation of the orbital apex, superior orbital fissure, or cavernous sinus [40, 41]. Patients with THS respond rapidly to corticosteroids, with pain often resolving within 24 h and improvement of ophthalmoplegia within days; however, symptoms can recur during attempted taper and may require long-term steroid sparing immunosuppression. The sensitivity of MRI for detecting focal abnormalities at the anterior cavernous sinus/orbital apex is greater than 90% [42]. The strongest systemic association is with inflammatory bowel disease and systemic lupus erythematosus [43]; however, THS may be isolated.

The diagnosis of Tolosa–Hunt syndrome should be made cautiously and after a thorough search (MRI, lumber puncture, body imaging, laboratory tests) has ruled out other plausible causes of inflammatory cavernous sinus disease (lymphoma, mycosis, sarcoidosis, metastasis, etc.) (Fig. 5.5).

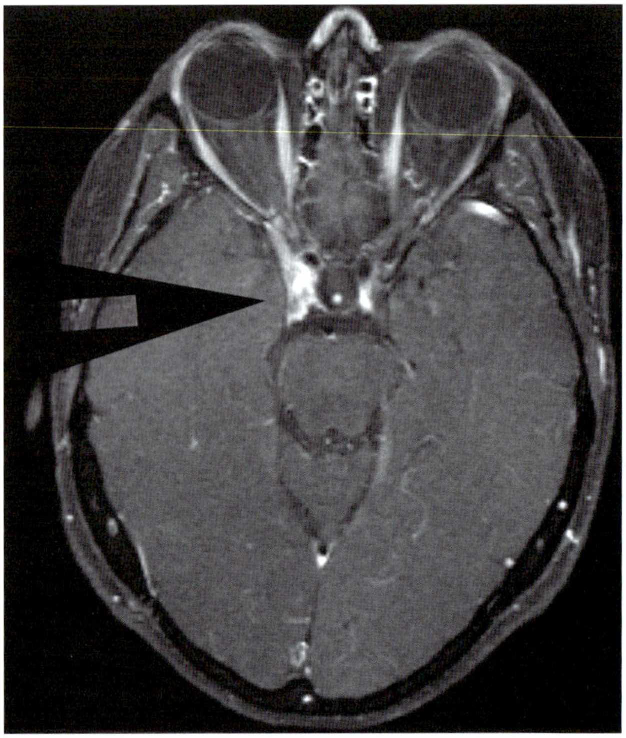

Fig. 5.5 Axial T1 MRI with gadolinium and fat saturation. Note the asymmetric, increased enhancement of the right cavernous sinus, consistent with Tolosa–Hunt syndrome (*arrow*)

Carotid-Cavernous Fistula (CCF)

The close relationship with the carotid artery and its tributaries renders the cavernous sinus prone to arterial pressurization from arteriovenous fistula formation. There are two major forms of carotid-cavernous fistula: direct and indirect [44].

Direct CCFs are high-flow, high-pressure fistulas resulting from direct communication of the internal carotid artery and the cavernous sinus. Considered an emergency, a direct CCF may result from head trauma (with or without skull base fracture), spontaneous rupture of a preexisting cavernous carotid artery aneurysm, or less commonly atherosclerosis. Because direct CCFs often drain anteriorly into the superior and inferior ophthalmic veins, they result in rapid, dramatic orbital congestion. Signs of a direct CCF are marked proptosis, ophthalmoplegia, eyelid swelling, pain, conjunctival injection/hemorrhage and chemosis, orbital bruit, severely increased intraocular pressure, and/or retinal vascular congestion (Fig. 5.6a, c). Progressive thrombosis of ipsilateral draining veins may cause shunting to the contralateral cavernous sinus and asymmetrically bilateral ocular findings. MRI or CT may reveal an enlarged superior ophthalmic vein and enlarged extraocular muscles; however, catheter angiography is often required to identify (and treat) the fistula. Following successful closure of the fistula, resolution of ocular symptoms occurs in roughly 80% of patients.

Indirect CCFs are low-flow/low-pressure fistulas and the result of rupture of small dural branches of the carotid artery into the cavernous sinus. Most commonly arising from expanded collateral vessels, they are more common in postpartum or postmenopausal women. Indirect CCFs cause much less dramatic orbital congestion and ocular

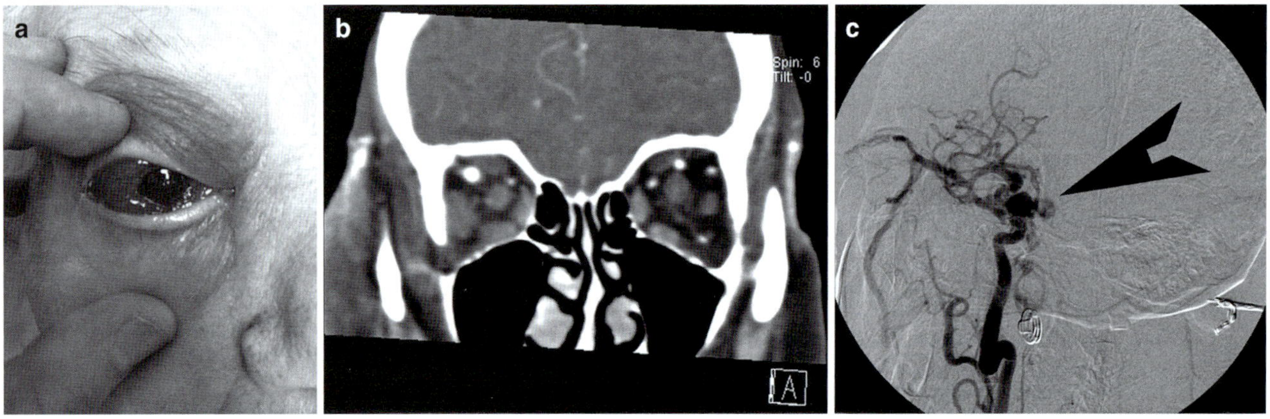

Fig. 5.6 (**a**) Right-sided direct carotid-cavernous fistula (CCF) with severe proptosis and hemorrhagic chemosis. There was complete ophthalmoplegia OD. (**b**) Orbital non-contrast CT scan demonstrating enlarged extraocular muscles and dilated right superior ophthalmic vein. These findings indicated increased orbital venous pressure. (**c**) Right-sided direct CCF visualized with digital subtraction catheter angiography (*arrow*)

hypertension than direct fistulas and may close spontaneously. Endovascular treatment of indirect fistulas is reserved for refractory ocular hypertension, diplopia, pain, or optic neuropathy.

Causes of the cavernous sinus syndrome

- Tumors
- Meningioma
- Pituitary adenoma (with or without apoplexy)
- Craniopharyngioma
- Nasopharyngeal carcinoma
- Squamous cell carcinoma
- Multiple myeloma
- Lymphoma
- Metastatic tumors (esp. breast, prostate, lung)
- Inflammatory
- Sarcoidosis
- Tolosa–Hunt Syndrome
- Infectious
- Fungal (mucormycosis, aspergillosis)
- Tuberculosis
- Vascular
- Carotid aneurysm
- Carotid-cavernous (direct) fistula
- Dural-cavernous (indirect) fistula

Orbital Apex Syndrome

Often presenting with ophthalmoplegia and vision loss, lesions of the orbital apex are often similar in nature to those that affect the anterior cavernous sinus and superior orbital fissure [45]. Oculosympathetic paresis and periocular pain may also be present; however, the absence of pain does not rule out the diagnosis. Proptosis is also a common feature of the orbital apex syndrome, resulting from both orbital venous congestion (from compression of the superior ophthalmic vein) and mass effect.

The orbital apex syndrome may be caused by tumors, infection, inflammation, trauma, or ischemia. Because of the proximity of the orbital apex to the posterior ethmoidal air cells, care should be taken in diabetic and immunosuppressed patients as rhinogenic mycosis (esp. *mucormycosis* and *aspergillosis*) spreads rapidly and has a high rate of mortality [46] (Fig. 5.7a–c).

Because lesions of the orbital apex may also involve the superior orbital fissure and cavernous sinus, MRI is preferred; however, CT scanning may be useful in cases of trauma and to evaluate bony involvement.

While centralized and peripheral nerve lesions may manifest themselves with predictable deficits of specific muscles, disorders of the neuromuscular junction or the muscles themselves present with more generalized deficits. Disorders of both the neuromuscular junction and ocular myopathies can not only result in ptosis but also lead to deficits in extraocular muscle (EOM) function. The ptosis seen in these disorders can be variable, unilateral, bilateral, and symmetrical or bilateral and asymmetrical. Similarly, disorders of the EOMs can result in variable and asymmetric involvement of specific muscles, causing diplopia, or more generalized involvement in which patients will suffer from external ophthalmoplegia, without complaints of diplopia. Understanding the physiologic causes of ptosis and motility disorders will not only provide the best treatment plan but also lead patients to other specialists, if necessary. Table 5.3 summarizes the clinical features of neuromuscular disorders which can affect the extraocular muscles.

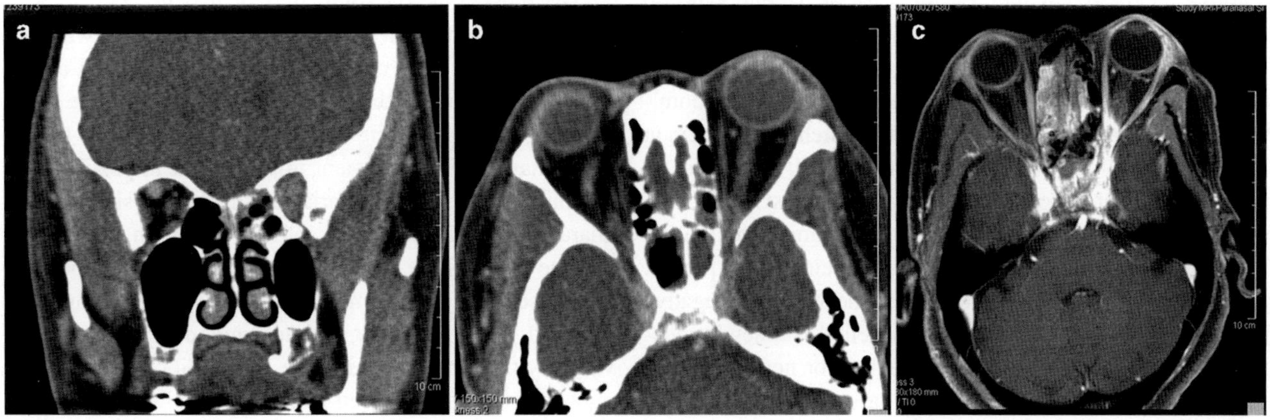

Fig. 5.7 (**a**–**c**) This is a 62-year-old woman with diabetes mellitus who presented with severe visual loss and complete ophthalmoplegia OS. (**a**) and (**b**) are axial and coronal CT scans demonstrating infiltration into the left orbital apex with extensive sphenoid sinus disease. (**c**) is an axial T1 MRI with gadolinium showing increased enhancement in the left orbital apex with normal size extraocular muscles. Biopsy showed mucormycosis

Table 5.3 Summary of the clinical features of neuromuscular disorders that can affect the extraocular muscles

Disease	Bell's phenomenon	Surgery recommendations	Muscle weakness	Intraocular findings
Myasthenia gravis	Normal	No, except refractory cases	Extraocular, bulbar, limb, and axial	None
Lambert–Eaton	Normal	No	Ascending proximal limb	None
Botulism	Normal	No	Descending	None
Mitochondrial myopathies with CPEO	Poor	Variable, proceed with caution	Generalized	±Pigmentary retinopathy
Myotonic dystrophy	Decreased	Yes, with caution	Distal limb	Pigmentary retinopathy, cataract
Oculopharyngeal dystrophy	Normal	Yes	Proximal limb, pharyngeal, ocular	None

Myasthenia Gravis

The patient with autoimmune myasthenia gravis may present to the oculoplastic surgeon with complaints of ptosis. Myasthenia gravis (MG) is a disorder in which autoantibodies block nicotinic acetylcholine receptors at the postsynaptic neuromuscular junction. Despite healthy neuronal and muscle tissue, released acetylcholine is precluded from stimulating the striated muscle, secondarily resulting in muscle weakness. As the autoantibodies are only directed against the nicotinic acetylcholine receptors, the hallmark of myasthenia gravis is fluctuating skeletal muscle weakness without associated neurologic findings, such as paresthesias. The muscle weakness in myasthenic patients is not static in that it may wax and wane throughout the day, characteristically worsening with activity.

Myasthenia gravis is a heterogeneous disease, most commonly an autoimmune disorder. However, in approximately 15% of MG patients, the disease is a paraneoplastic process, the result of a thymoma. Approximately 80–85% of patients with MG will have detectable antibodies against acetylcholine receptors (AChR). Of the 15% of patients who do not have detectable antibodies against AChR's, up to 50% will have antibodies against muscle-specific tyrosine kinase (MuSK) [47]. Patients with MuSK antibodies have predominantly bulbar and cranial involvement, which makes them at higher risk for respiratory failure. Envoli et al. found that up to half of patients who produce antibodies against MuSK may have a respiratory crisis that requires mechanical ventilation [48]. More recently, antibodies to lipoprotein-related protein 4 (LRP4) have been associated with otherwise seronegative MG [49, 50]. Lipoprotein-related protein 4 is a newly identified receptor for aging and is essential for neuromuscular junction formation. Zhang et al. [50] assessed serum sample for 120 patients with securely diagnosed MG with no detectable acetylcholine receptor or MuSK antibodies. Anti-LRP4 antibodies were detected in 11/120 patients with neither AChR or MuSK antibodies and 1/36 patients without AchR antibodies but with MuSK antibodies. It is unclear at this time whether the LRP4 antibodies are associated with a specific phenotype, and their sensitivity and specificity remains unclear. However, they likely account for a proportion of ocular myasthenics who are seronegative. These antibodies are now available commercially.

Patients suffering from autoimmune myasthenia *without* thymoma can be further subdivided. Ocular MG tends to manifest with diplopia and ptosis. Of those with ocular MG, only 50% of patients produce antibodies against AChR. Generalized MG has a bimodal distribution with characteristic features. In the early onset group, patients present prior to age 40 are predominately female and will demonstrate thymus hyperplasia. Approximately 90% of these patients will express antibodies against AChR and respond best to thymectomy. In contrast to the early-onset group, the late-onset MG patients have more diffuse muscle involvement. There is no sex predilection in this group, with males and females equally affected. The vast majority of these patients produce antibodies against AChR and have an atrophic thymus, subsequently rendering thymectomy a less effective treatment modality.

The most common complaints of patients with MG are ptosis and/or diplopia. More than half of patients with MG initially present with ocular complaints. The ptosis of MG patients is unique in that with sustained upgaze, the ptosis worsens, whereas having the patient close their eyes temporarily may result in transient improvement in ptosis. These patients may describe a variable, shifting ptosis, which is characteristic of MG, since intrinsically, both the neurons and the muscles are intact. Ocular motility should be carefully assessed. Usually, more than one extraocular muscle is involved, asymmetrically, and not limited to muscles innervated by the same cranial nerve. In addition, these patients may have weakness of their facial muscles. Detection of MG is important as it directs the treatment plan, but most importantly, there is a mortality risk associated with a myasthenic crisis.

If a patient with ptosis is suspected of having MG, further support of the diagnosis can be made in clinic using an icepack test. Patients with MG and ptosis may demonstrate an improvement in symptoms following application of an icepack to the affected muscles. In addition, diagnosis can be supported with the Tensilon (edrophonium) test, in which MG patients will demonstrate an improvement in muscle strength following administration. Alternatively, electrophysiological testing can also be employed in which muscle fibers will demonstrate a decremental response with repetitive stimulation. Most commonly, however, antibody tests are used in the diagnosis of MG.

Antibodies against the AChR are specific for MG; therefore, antibody testing can be used for confirmation of disease. It is important to note, however, that since not all MG patients express the AChR antibody, blood testing cannot rule out the disease. There are three types of AChR antibodies that are commonly tested in patients with MG: binding, blocking, and modulating. The binding antibody is the most common, while the blocking antibody is the least prevalent [49]. Of those patients who test positive for antibodies against AChR, testing for both the binding and blocking antibodies will identify 97% of patients, whereas testing for the modulating antibody only identified 93% [50]. Therefore, it is recommended that in patients suspected of MG, initial blood testing should be performed to detect the binding and blocking antibodies, and if positive, additional testing for the modulating antibody should be performed. In addition to AChR antibody testing, screening for anti-MuSK antibodies may determine which patients are at greater risk for respiratory failure and anti-striated muscle antibodies, as they have been found to be positive in many patients with thymoma. Once the diagnosis of MG has been confirmed, all patients will require additional screening tests. A chest CT is required to rule out a thymoma; in addition, as MG patients have be noted to be concomitantly affected with thyroid disease, lupus, or rheumatoid arthritis, thyroid function tests, ANA tests, and rheumatoid factor testing are suggested [51–56].

Once the diagnosis has been made, patients diagnosed with MG are treated symptomatically using acetylcholinesterase inhibitors, which prevent acetylcholine from being metabolized at the neuromuscular junction. These drugs functionally increase acetylcholine concentrations, resulting in adequate skeletal muscle stimulation. While usually well tolerated, some patients may experience side effects related to over stimulation of both muscarinic and nicotinic acetylcholine receptors, by virtue of increased systemic acetylcholine concentrations. In those patients with thymoma, thymectomy is recommended. If patients experience progression of symptoms, signifying worsening of disease, immunomodulator/suppressants are recommended [8]. The surgical management of MG only involves thymectomy. When ptosis in these patients is caused solely by MG, there is no role for surgical ptosis repair. However, if patients suffer with severe, refractory MG, who have demonstrated stable measurements for at least 1 year, modest ptosis correction with a frontalis sling procedure may provide benefit [57, 58].

Lambert–Eaton

Similar to MG, the pathophysiology of Lambert–Eaton myasthenic syndrome (LEMS) involves antibody-mediated interference of neuromuscular signaling. In contrast to MG, these antibodies are directed against the neuronal presynaptic voltage-gated calcium channels. Calcium-mediated acetylcholine release is essential in neuromuscular communication. Inhibition of voltage-gated calcium channels by antibodies prevents acetylcholine release, inhibiting the signaling cascade for muscle contraction. Subsequently, calcium channels can be downregulated at the neuromuscular junction.

Patients with LEMS commonly present with ascending proximal limb weakness, absent deep tendon reflexes, fatigability, and autonomic dysfunction. While ptosis is a less frequently observed symptom [59], it will likely be the chief complaint of patients presenting to the oculoplastic surgeon [60, 61]. In contrast to MG, patients with LEMS have been shown to demonstrate a transient improvement in their ptosis following prolonged upgaze [62]. The symptoms of LEMS will also tend to fluctuate less than those in MG patients.

The ability to both diagnose LEMS and differentiate it from MG is paramount for patient care. As many as 70% of patients with LEMS harbor an underlying malignancy, most commonly small-cell bronchogenic carcinoma. Patients may not have a diagnosis of malignancy upon presentation, as the paraneoplastic LEMS can precede the diagnosis of cancer by months to years. Therefore, any patient presenting with LEMS should have a thorough malignancy workup, including CT and PET scans [63].

Traditionally, nerve conduction studies have been used for diagnosis of LEMS. Results will demonstrate characteristic incremental responses to repetitive stimulation. However, antibodies directed against the voltage-gated calcium channels (VGCCs) have been detected in up to 85% of patients with LEMS, and even higher rates have been reported in those patients with both LEMS and small-cell lung cancer [64]. Serum screening for antibodies to VGCCs can be sent to several commercial labs. Patients with both LEMS and small-cell lung cancer have also been shown to express SOX1 antibodies in 43% of patients [65]. While those LEMS patients who were seronegative for the voltage-gated calcium channels were less likely to have small-cell lung cancer [66], all seronegative patients diagnosed with LEMS should have very close follow-up.

The management of patients with LEMS is medical. All patients with LEMS need referrals to oncologists to identify potential malignancies. In those patients with known malignancies, the primary treatment is directed toward the underlying malignancy. For symptomatic treatment, current recommendations suggest 3,4-diaminopyridine which functionally increases acetylcholine in the neuromuscular junction and/or intravenous immunoglobins [67]. If symptomatic improvement is not achieved, immunosuppressive agents (prednisone, azathioprine) can be considered provided malignancy has been ruled out. Recently, however, it has been reported that two LEMS patients with diplopia underwent strabismus surgery with successful results [68]. While two isolated cases were successful, the pathophysiology of LEMS involves the neuromuscular junction, and surgical repair of ptosis is unlikely to be long-lasting.

Botulism

The majority of disorders of the neuromuscular junction will occur as a result of antibody blockade. However, in rare instances, exogenous agents, such as botulinum toxin, may interfere with neuromuscular signaling. Botulinum toxin is a potent neurotoxin produced by the anaerobic, spore-forming bacterium *Clostridium botulinum*. This bacterium can be found in soil, water, and improperly handled foods, leading to the four major types of botulism: infant botulism, foodborne, wound inoculation, and intestinal colonization. Commonly, outbreaks occur as a result of ingested food and involve multiple patients [69–71].

As a potent neurotoxin, botulinum toxin binds presynaptically and irreversibly prevents acetylcholine release from the nerve terminal. This blockade results in a descending flaccid paralysis and autonomic dysfunction, symmetrically involving cranial nerves. Because botulism is characterized by a descending paralysis, the cranial nerves are likely involved first, and patients may initially present to their ophthalmologist. Common ocular complaints are ptosis and blurred vision. However, examination may reveal pupillary abnormalities such as sluggish light responses to fixed and dilated.

Diagnosis requires a high index of suspicion and can be performed by assaying blood, gastrointestinal secretions, and food products for the toxin [72]. Treatment of botulism is prompt medical care. Patients should be monitored closely in an ICU setting, as botulism may progress to respiratory paralysis, requiring mechanical ventilation to sustain life. In addition, antitoxin is available and will bind to circulating toxin, but not toxin that had previously bound to the nerve terminal [73]. There is no role for surgery in the treatment of ptosis from botulism.

Mitochondrial Myopathies

Chronic progressive external ophthalmoplegia (CPEO) is a common finding in mitochondrial myopathies. In general, patients develop a painless, symmetrical loss of ocular motility and generally do not complain of diplopia. However, patients do commonly present with complaints of ptosis and may not even be aware of their CPEO. Systemically, they may also have generalized muscle weakness. There are often common phenotypic features with all of these disorders, and muscle biopsy remains the definitive diagnostic test for many, showing characteristic red, ragged fibers. However, these mitochondrial myopathies are distinct entities which require variable approaches for the proper management of the patient.

The genetic mutations leading to mitochondrial myopathies with CPEO are variable. Table 5.4 provides an overview of mitochondrial myopathies which can affect the extraocular muscles. Traditionally, mitochondrial diseases are inherited in a maternally transmitted fashion, with mutations in mitochondrial DNA (mtDNA) being passed from the mother to all offspring. However, not all patients will inherit these conditions maternally, as sporadic mutations may occur in mtDNA in patients with a negative family history. In addition to defects in mtDNA, patients can also inherit these diseases in an autosomal fashion, in which the genetic mutation affects specific nuclear DNA loci, which are responsible for mitochondrial function. The genes that have been implicated in autosomal dominant CPEO include POLG [74, 75], Twinkle (PEO1) [76], and ANT1 [77]. Most patients with autosomal dominant CPEO will present with ophthalmoplegia and ptosis; however, other features may include generalized fatigue, myopathies, and cardiac abnormalities. As an alternative to muscle biopsy, current diagnostic techniques allow screening for these conditions with whole blood.

Table 5.4 Overview of mitochondrial myopathies that can affect the extraocular muscles

Mitochondrial myopathy	Inheritance	Genetic defect	Diagnosis
Sporadic CPEO	Sporadic, without family history	Single large-scale rearrangement/deletion of mtDNA	Genetic testing of mtDNA, muscle biopsy
Maternal CPEO	Maternally	Point mutations in mitochondrial tRNA	Genetic testing of mt-tRNA, muscle biopsy
Autosomal CPEO	Mendelian	Nuclear gene mutation results in multiple large-scale rearrangements/deletions of mtDNA	Genetic testing of nuclear genes, muscle biopsy

Patients with CPEO commonly present by the second decade. These patients will present with symmetric loss of ocular motility, with eyes fixed to oculocephalic stimulation (Fig. 5.8a–d). Not only will patients have weakened orbicularis function, but also they will have a very poor Bell's phenomenon. A weakened orbicularis can also cause lagophthalmos and ectropion in these patients, a combination which puts them at risk for exposure keratopathy. Mitochondrial myopathies also affect the levator, resulting in ptosis. When examining these patients, expected findings include decreased levator function, without fatigability. These symptoms experienced by these patients will slowly progress, but will not wax and wane throughout the day.

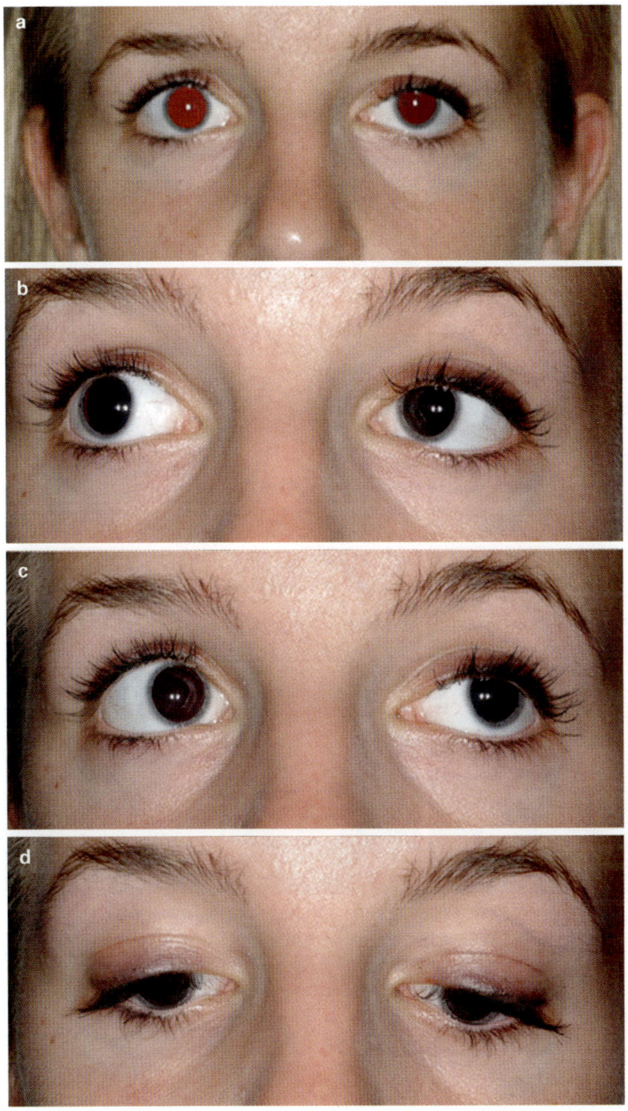

Fig. 5.8 (**a–d**) This is a 17-year-old woman with a lifelong history of progressive ophthalmoplegia and ptosis. Figure (**a–d**) shows primary gaze (**a**), right gaze (**b**), left gaze (**c**), and down gaze (**d**). Note the relatively mild and asymmetric ptosis, as well as limitation of versions in all directions. Triceps muscle biopsy showed ragged red fibers, consistent with mitochondrial myopathy

Diagnosis of CPEO can be suspected by history, physical exam, and certain laboratory findings, but for most patients, specific diagnosis requires muscle biopsy. As CPEO is a mitochondrial myopathy, biopsy results may reveal ragged red fibers. There may be false negative biopsies, however, depending on the location of the skeletal muscle biopsy. While success has been noted using proximal limb biopsies [78], taking a muscle biopsy from the orbicularis or levator muscle, especially at the time of surgery, has yielded satisfactory results [79]. Large-scale deletion and rearrangements in mtDNA have been implicated in the sporadic disease [80].

While the majority of patients who present with a mitochondrial myopathy will suffer from sporadic CPEO, there is a subset of patients who will suffer from CPEO plus syndromes. These syndromes are characterized by a CPEO *plus* other symptomatic and diagnostic features [81].

Kearns–Sayre syndrome (KSS), described by Kearns and Sayre in 1958, is a disorder which combines CPEO, a pigmentary retinopathy, and complete heart block [82]. Primary features of KSS include onset of ophthalmoplegia prior to age of 20 years, pigmentary retinopathy, and either heart block, elevated cerebrospinal fluid protein, or cerebellar ataxia (Fig. 5.9a, b). As these findings suggest, KSS is a descriptive term encompassing several mitochondrial disorders, which share overlapping phenotypic features, all resulting from deletions and rearrangements of mtDNA. It is important for the clinician to be aware of KSS as it has been reported that up to 60% of patients with KSS have cardiac conduction defects [83]. These patients require frequent monitoring with cardiologist, and some may even require permanent pacemakers.

Similar to patients with sporadic CPEO, patients with KSS have large-scale deletion mutations in mitochondrial DNA [84]. However, the deletions seen in KSS may be distinct from those in isolated CPEO, likely influencing the phenotypic differences between the two disease entities. Similar to other mitochondrial myopathies, patients with KSS will demonstrate ragged red fibers upon muscle biopsy. Since the ultimate pathologic mechanism is thought to be bioenergetic failure at a cellular level, substrates that supplement and enhance oxidative phosphorylation could potentially benefit these patients. One study demonstrated that KSS patients who were treated for 3 months with vitamin coenzyme Q10 had decreased serum levels of lactate and pyruvate and improvement in both cardiac conduction and ocular movements [85]. However, recent reviews have found no conclusive evidence to support any effective treatments [86].

Mitochondrial encephalomyopathy, lactic acidosis, and stroke-like episodes (MELAS) is a distinct syndrome seen in children and young adults. These patients experience an encephalopathy that consists of transient hemianopsia and hemiparesis with permanent neurologic damage and spon-

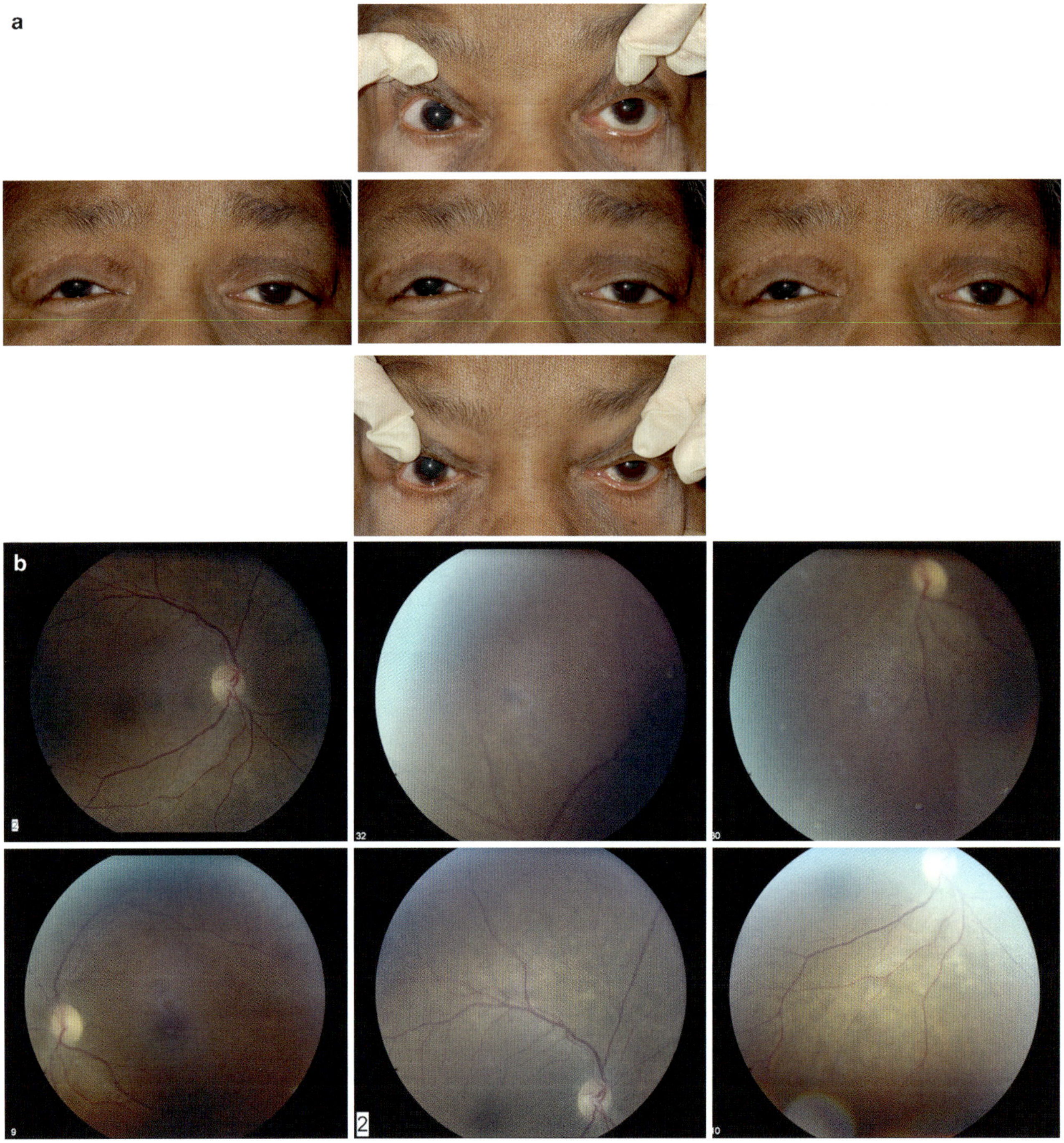

Fig. 5.9 (**a**, **b**) This is a 62-year-old woman with Kearns–Sayre syndrome. (**a**) demonstrates severe, bilateral, symmetric ptosis and marked limitation of versions in all directions, in a symmetric pattern. (**b**) shows a fundus photograph from the same patient. Note the speckled, mottled appearance of the retinal pigment epithelium in the periphery in both eyes. Also note the absence of pigment clumping and bony spicules, which are usually absent in KSS. Limb muscle biopsy showed ragged red fibers, consistent with mitochondrial myopathy. Mitochondrial genetic analysis showed large-scale deletions and rearrangements of mitochondrial DNA

giform cortical degenerations. However, in addition to the aforementioned symptoms, patients can also present with CPEO [87, 88]. Clinical criteria have been developed to aid in diagnosis, which require the presence of a stroke-like episode prior to the age of 40, encephalopathy, and the presence of lactic acidosis or ragged red fibers on muscle biopsy [89]. Point mutations in the 3243 location in mtDNA have been associated with the MELAS phenotype and can be screened for commercially. Currently, patients are managed with supportive therapy, although there is ongoing research for potential treatment options including antioxidants and vitamin supplements [90].

The treatment of CPEO syndromes is supportive and includes management of symptoms, including ptosis. Surgical management of patients with CPEO or a CPEO plus syndrome requires careful planning. It is recommended that patients be considered for surgical repair only if they are having functional difficulties and if vision is functionally impaired [3]. The consequences of surgical repair without careful consideration of the underlying disorder can result in deleterious effects on the cornea and subsequent visual potential of these patients. It has been reported that patients who underwent too aggressive of surgical repair later presented with inadequate lid closure resulting in corneal ulcers from chronic exposure [91].

Using standard levator resection techniques of an already weakened muscle may not provide enough elevation without subsequently increasing lagophthalmos in the setting of a poor Bells' phenomenon and weakened orbicularis function. Wong et al. and others suggest that if levator function is less than 8 mm, resection should not be considered [6, 92]. Therefore, employing other muscles to lift the eyelids can be considered. Frontalis sling procedures theoretically have a greater chance of success, although it should be noted that patients with CPEO also suffer from generalized muscle weakness and may have weakened frontalis function. There have successful reports of ptosis repair using frontalis sling procedures with multiple materials. Fascia, both donor and autologous, have been used [7, 94], as well as monofilament nylon [95] and silicone rods [96]. Lelli et al. recommend using silicone rods for the frontalis sling because of the ease of adjustment if optimal results are not obtained following the implantation [58]. Regardless of the type of surgical repair employed, the priority in these patients is to increase their field of view while maintaining adequate corneal coverage to minimize the risk of exposure keratopathy.

Myotonic Dystrophy

Although a rare autosomal dominant disease, myotonic dystrophy is the most common adult onset muscular dystrophy. Diagnosis can be made by a blood test to detect nucleotide repeat mutations in either chromosome 19 or 3 [97] and by electromyogram, which demonstrates myotonic discharges. Patients with myotonic dystrophy begin to experience symptoms in adolescence or early adulthood. Myotonic dystrophy manifests with weakness of the distal limb musculature, which progresses to include weakness of the oropharyngeal musculature and wasting of the temporalis and masseter muscles, which produces the characteristic *hatchet face* (Fig. 5.10). Myotonia implies failure of muscle relaxation, so traditionally, after a handshake, myotonic dystrophy patients will demonstrate difficulty releasing their grasp. Their symptoms can be worsened by excitement, cold temperatures, or fatigue. Other loosely associated features include low intelligence, frontal balding, testicular atrophy, uterine atony, insulin resistance, and cardiac conduction abnormalities. There have also been rare associations with thymoma and myasthenia gravis [98].

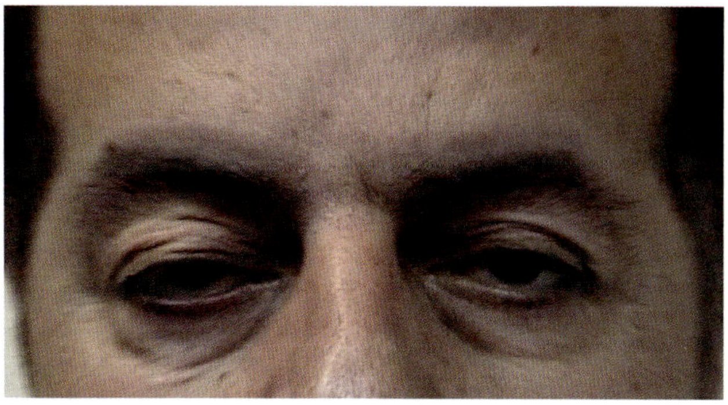

Fig. 5.10 This is a 58-year-old Iraqi man with a several decade history of progressive ptosis and some limb weakness. Similar findings were present in his brother and niece. Note the bilateral, symmetric ptosis. Also demonstrated is frontal balding, a feature often seen with myotonic dystrophy. Electromyography and subsequent genetic testing confirmed this diagnosis

Ocular findings include symmetric external ophthalmoplegia, weakness of the orbicularis muscle, myotonic lag, blepharitis, pigmentary retinopathy, enophthalmos, and polychromatic lenticular deposits (Christmas tree cataracts) [99]. Ptosis usually predominates, with ophthalmoplegia less common. Pupils may be miotic with sluggish light responses. However, most patients with myotonic dystrophy present to the oculoplastic surgeon with complaints of ptosis. Surgical repair has been described with both silicone slings and levator resection and advancement [92, 100]. However, as these patients experience decreased orbicularis tone and may have decreased Bell's phenomenon, careful consideration must be made when planning ptosis surgery since they are at risk for exposure keratopathy.

Oculopharyngeal Dystrophy

Oculopharyngeal dystrophy is a rare hereditary disorder that may present in middle age, with the average age of onset in the fifth and sixth decades. Patients develop progressive dysphagia followed by bilateral ptosis and proximal limb weakness. Eventually, patients may develop a progressive ophthalmoplegia.

The inheritance of oculopharyngeal dystrophy is most commonly autosomal dominant [101] but has also been reported as autosomal recessive [102]. Diagnosis is typically suspected in patients with a history of ptosis, dysphagia, and a positive family history. However, genetic testing can be performed to detect an increased number of trinucleotide repeats in the PABPN1 gene (formerly PABP2). Genotypically, the autosomal dominant and recessive forms of the disease differ by the number of trinucleotide repeats [103]. Muscle biopsy can be performed which reveals a vacuolar myopathy with intranuclear inclusions, but this is rarely necessary with the availability of genetic testing.

In contrast to myotonic dystrophy, OPMD patients do not experience decreased orbicularis tone [93, 104] and have a normal Bell's phenomenon, which makes them ideal candidates for surgical repair of their ptosis [105, 106]. However, because this disease is progressive, patients may need multiple repairs throughout life.

Rare Myopathies

There are other rare myopathies that may cause ocular symptoms. Facioscapulohumeral muscular dystrophy is an autosomal dominant, slowly progressive disease that usually begins in their second decade. Patients will likely complaint of muscular weakness, as the disease affects facial muscles and muscles of the scapula and dorsiflexors of the feet. These patients may also have hearing loss and retinal telangiectasias [107, 108]. Muscle biopsy and genetic testing can be used for diagnosis. Weakness of facial muscles may result in weakened orbicularis function, which puts these patients at risk for lagophthalmos and exposure keratopathy, for which aggressive corneal lubrication is recommended. It is conceivable that if the orbicularis weakness is so severe, there may be a role for insertion of eyelids weights to minimize lagophthalmos. Other muscular dystrophies that may affect facial muscles include Emery–Dreifuss muscular dystrophy [3].

Neuroophthalmic Imaging Techniques

With the advent of computerized tomography (CT) scans and magnetic resonance imaging (MRI) in the 1970s, it became possible to differentially image blood, water, bone, air, and soft tissues within the body. Both techniques have undergone significant advancement over the past 30 years, and it is now possible to create high-resolution images of soft tissue, bone, CSF, and blood vessels in two or three dimensions. Despite these advances, CT and MRI remain fundamentally different imaging methods, and each has distinct advantages and disadvantages.

Computerized Tomography (CT)

CT scans are obtained by passing thin beams of X-rays from an array of emitters on one side of the patient's body to detectors on the opposite side. The emitter/detector complex is mounted on a rotating gantry through which the body (or body part) is passed. Detectors record X-ray attenuation levels along the detector array as a function of the orientation of the gantry through its 360 rotation. Fourier calculations allow image *slices* to be constructed computationally and displayed in grayscale as a function of relative radiodensity of the tissues. Modern helical (spiral) scanners, taking advantage of advanced acquisition protocols and significant image processing power, now allow three-dimensional volumetric images to be obtained, allowing multiple-angle viewing and variable-plane reconstructions with a minimum loss of resolution [109].

CT is superior to MRI in detailing bony anatomy of the orbit, skull base, and sinuses. Additionally, CT is highly sensitive for detecting acute blood and has a very short acquisition time (single images can be obtained in less than 1 s and whole scans in 30–60 s). CT is the imaging technique of choice in cases of trauma and when bony lesions or calcium-containing masses (meningiomas, optic nerve drusen) are suspected.

Magnetic Resonance Imaging (MRI)

The principle of magnetic resonance imaging (MRI) is significantly more complex than CT scanning but is far more versatile. MRI takes advantage of the fact that magnetic atoms (those having an odd number of electrons or protons) align their axis of spin in a magnetic field [12, 26]. The patient is placed within the bore of a large magnet (0.5–3.0 T). By turning on a radiofrequency (RF) field within the magnetic field, some atoms will flip their axis of spin. When the radiofrequency field is turned off again, atoms' spin will decay (*relax*) back to their original orientation and, in so doing, emit a photon of energy in the radiofrequency range. These signals (typically from hydrogen atoms) can be reconstructed into high-resolution two- or three-dimensional images. By varying RF pulse sequences and scanning parameters, contrast between varying types of tissue or fluid can be differentially imaged. Compared with CT, MRI provides significantly greater spatial resolution, soft tissue differentiation, and avoids bony artifact. Some of the most common imaging sequences for MRI scanning are as follows:

- *T1*: Best for showing anatomy. CSF appears black, normal brain appears gray, and abnormal brain typically appears darker, owing to increased water content. Pre- and post-contrast T1 series are commonly compared to identify areas of pathology (where the blood–brain barrier has become permeable).
- *T2 and FLAIR*: Very sensitive to water content and is good for showing pathology. Since increased water content is common for pathologic processes (tumors, edema, demyelination, and infarction) within the brain, T2 images appear brighter than normal brain in these areas, even without contrast. With T2 images, CSF appears white,

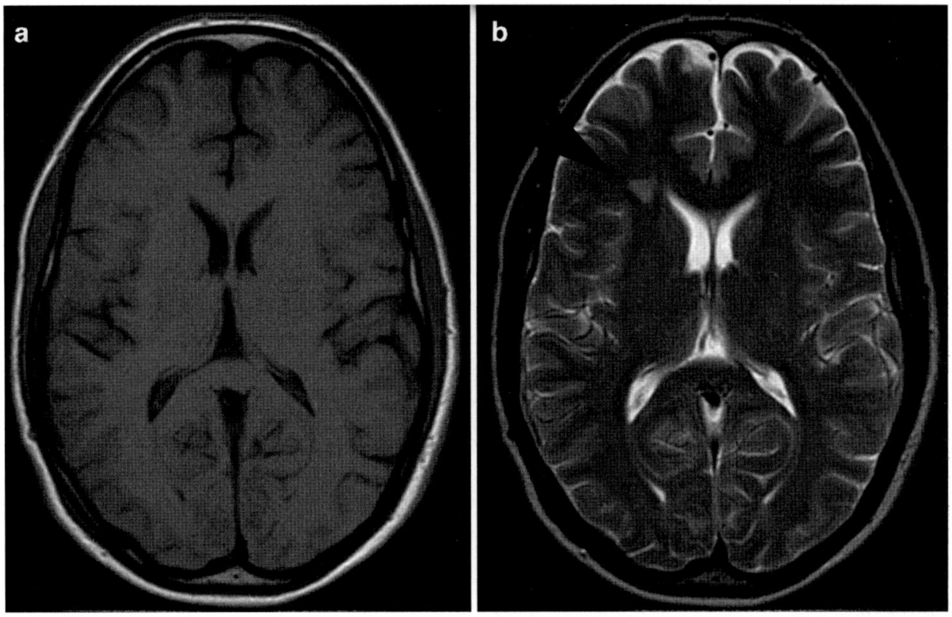

Fig. 5.11 (**a**, **b**) Non-contrasted axial T1-weighted (**a**) and (**b**) T2-weighted MRI of a patient with a right periventricular demyelinating plaque. On the T1-weighted image, the plaque is barely visible; however, due to increased water content, it is much more apparent with T2-weighted imaging (*arrowhead*)

whereas with FLAIR, CSF appears black and allows improved visualization of white matter disease near CSF (periventricular white matter, optic nerve, etc.).

- See Fig. 5.11a, b.
- *Diffusion-weighted imaging (DWI)*: A specialized form of MR imaging. DWI provides image contrast based on the molecular movement of water, which may be alerted in disease states. In standard DWI imaging, tissue in which water movement is limited (*restricted*) appears bright, as in cases of ischemic cytotoxic edema (as ion pumps fail, water enters the cell and cannot diffuse. Later as cells burst, water diffusivity actually increases above normal, and the area appears darker than the surrounding brain tissue). DWI is currently used chiefly in early identification of ischemia (diffusion restriction can be detected within minutes of an ischemic stroke) but is being increasingly used to investigate tumors as well as demyelinating and inflammatory brain pathologies.

CT Versus MRI

Because of the superiority of MRI in differentiating soft tissue and water content, MRI is superior to CT scan for intracranial disease. Because CT has superior bone imaging and is less prone to fat suppression artifact, it is generally considered superior for orbital imaging.

CT

Advantages: Lower cost, rapid acquisition, excellent imaging of bony structures, acute blood easily identified, and safe with ferromagnetic implants and indwelling electronics

Disadvantages: Poor resolution of soft tissue structures near skull base due to bony artifact, ionizing radiation exposure limits the number of scans

MRI

Advantages: High spatial resolution, excellent gray-white differentiation, no ionizing radiation exposure, not affected by bony attenuation, and able to image in any plane

Disadvantages: Slow acquisition, may exacerbate claustrophobia, movement degrades image quality, not safe with indwelling electronics or ferromagnetic materials, poor bony imaging

CT and MR Angiography

MRI and CT are both capable of acquiring high-resolution images of vascular structures. Both techniques, when interpreted by experienced radiologists, can be highly sensitive and specific compared with catheter angiography.

With CT angiography (CTA), iodinated contrast media is injected into a vein, and using high-speed CT scanning and digital tissue subtraction, high-resolution three-dimensional reconstruction of cerebral arteries can be obtained rapidly and with minimal artifact. In many academic centers, CTA is now considered the primary imaging technique for detecting important cerebral vascular abnormalities (dissection, aneurysm, etc.) in patients with normal renal function [12].

MR angiography (MRA) can be obtained using two different techniques: contrast-enhanced MRA (CE-MRA) and non-enhanced MRA (NE-MRA). Contrast-enhanced MRA provides fast acquisition of high-resolution images

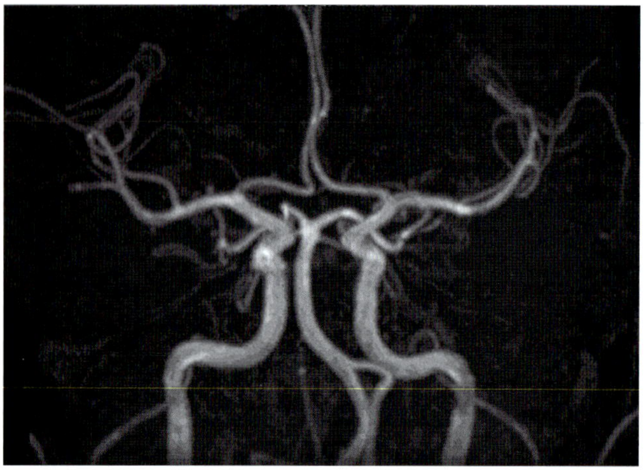

Fig. 5.12 Normal MR angiogram of the circle of Willis

but depends highly on proper technique (bolus delivery and acquisition timing) and should be used with caution in patients with renal disease (see below). NE-MRA is most useful in patients with renal disease as no contrast media is required; however, this technique is more susceptible to artifact from turbulent blood flow and is less sensitive to slow-moving blood (as in large aneurismal cavities) (Fig. 5.12).

Gadolinium and Nephrogenic Systemic Fibrosis (NSF)

Gadolinium is a rare earth element with powerful paramagnetic properties that make it an ideal contrast agent for MRI and MR angiography [110]. Gadolinium must be chelated however, as unbound gadolinium is a potent inhibitor of calcium channels and is highly cardio- and neurotoxic [111]. In the USA, seven gadolinium chelates are currently approved for use, and it was believed for many years that these agents were essentially risk-free.

Nephrogenic systemic fibrosis (NSF) is a rare condition consisting of insidious fibrosis of the skin, joints, and internal organs. Occurring exclusively in patients with renal insufficiency, the first case series was published in 2000 [112]. Although the cause of NSF was not initially known, an Austrian study published in 2006 suggested a link between gadodiamide (Omniscan®; GE Healthcare, Buckinghamshire, UK) and NSF [8]. Later that same year, additional gadodiamide-related NSF cases were reported in Denmark [9] and in the USA. The FDA first issued a black box warning in June of 2006 for all gadolinium formulations. Currently, four of the seven approved chelates have been associated with NSF, with gadodiamide having the highest risk, followed by gadoversetamide (OptiMark®), gadopentetate dimeglumine (Magnevist®), and gadobenate dimeglumine (MultiHance®). To date, the FDA is the only regulatory agency in the world to issue NSF warnings for all gadolinium formulations.

The FDA currently recommends that all gadolinium chelates be used with caution in patients whose estimated glomerular filtration rate (eGFR) is <30 mL/min/1.73 m^2 and that gadodiamide, gadoversetamide, and gadopentetate dimeglumine be avoided altogether in these patients [113]. Recent studies have suggested that modification of the use of gadolinium-based contrast agents in renally impaired patients has reduced the incidence of NSF [114].

References

1. Brazis PW. General principles. In: Brazis PW, Masdeu JC, Biller J, editors. Localization in clinical neurology. 5th ed. Philadelphia: Lippincott, Williams & Wilkins; 2006. p. 1–24.
2. Breasted J. The Edwin Smith surgical papyrus. Chicago: Chicago University Press; 1930.
3. Berker EA, Berker AH, Smith A. Translation of Broca's 1865 report. Localization of speech in the third left frontal convolution. Arch Neurol. 1986;43:1065–72.
4. Wilson-Pauwels L, Akesson EJ, Stewart PA. Sandoz course. Cranial nerve: anatomy and clinical comments. Philadelphia: B.C. Decker; 1988.
5. Elstein AS, Shulman LS, Sprafka SA. Medical problem solving: an analysis of clinical reasoning. Cambridge, MA: Harvard University Press; 1978. p. 64–6.
6. Wigton RS. Use of linear models to analyse physicians' decisions. Med Decis Mak. 1988;8:241–52.
7. Eva KW. What every teacher needs to know about clinical reasoning. Med Educ. 2004;39:98–106.
8. Norman G, Young M, Brooks L. Non-analytical models of clinical reasoning: the role of experience. Med Educ. 2007;41:1140–5.
9. Graber M, Gordon R, Franklin N. Reducing diagnostic errors in medicine: what's the goal? Acad Med. 2002;77:981–92.
10. Croskerry P. The importance of cognitive errors in diagnosis and the strategies to minimize them. Acad Med. 2003;78:775–80.
11. Norman GR, Eva KW. Diagnostic error and clinical reasoning. Med Educ. 2010;44:94–100.
12. Bose S. Neuroimaging in neuro-ophthalmology. Neurosurg Focus. 2007;23:1–9.
13. Lekwuwa GU, Barnes GR. Cerebral control of eye movements. Brain. 1996;119:473–90.
14. Averbuch-Heller L, Leigh RJ, Mermelstein V, Zagalsky L, et al. Ptosis in patients with hemispheric strokes. Neurology. 2002;58:620–4.
15. Van Stavern GP. Efferent: supranuclear motility continuum lifelong learning. Neurology. 2009;15(4):127–48.
16. Biousse V, Skibell BC, Watts RL, Loupe DN, et al. Ophthalmologic features of Parkinson's disease. Neurology. 2004;62:177–80.
17. Lepore FE, Devoisin RC. "Apraxia" of eyelid opening: an involuntary levator inhibition. Neurology. 1985;35:423–7.
18. Pelak VS, Hall DA. Neuro-ophthalmologic manifestations of neurodegenerative disease. Ophthalmol Clin N Am. 2004;17:311–20.
19. Altiparmak U, Eggenberger E, Coleman A, Condon K. The ratio of square wave jerk rates to blink rates distinguishes progressive supranuclear palsy from Parkinson's disease. J Neuroophthalmol. 2006;26:257–9.
20. Kerrison JB, Newman NJ. Five things oculoplastic surgeons should know about neuro-ophthalmology. Ophthal Plast Reconstr Surg. 1999;15(6):373–7.

21. Cogan DG. Internuclear ophthalmoplegia: typical and atypical. Arch Ophthalmol. 1970;84:583–9.
22. Keane JR. Ocular skew deviation. Analysis of 100 cases. Arch Neurol. 1975;32:185–90.
23. Dieterich M, Brandt T. Ocular torsion and tilt of subjective visual vertical are sensitive brainstem signs. Ann Neurol. 1993;33:292–9.
24. Frohman LP, Kupersmith MJ. Reversible vertical ocular deviations associated with raised intracranial pressure. J Clin Neuroophthalmol. 1985;5:158–63.
25. Haines DE, Lancon JA. Neuroanatomy, North American edition: an Atlas of structures, sections, and systems. 7th ed. Philadelphia: Lippincott, Williams & Wilkins; 2007.
26. Biousse V, Newman NJ. Neuro-ophthalmology illustrated. 1st ed. New York: Thieme Medical Publishers; 2009.
27. Miller NR, Newman NJ. Walsh and Hoyt's clinical neuro-ophthalmology. 6th ed. Philadelphia: Lippincott, Williams & Wilkins; 2004.
28. Bruce BB, Biousse V, Newman NJ. Third nerve palsies. Semin Neurol. 2007;27(3):257–68.
29. Trobe JD. Rapid diagnosis in Ophthalmology series: Neuro-Ophthalmology. 1st ed. Mosby; 2007.
30. Brazis PW. Isolated palsies of cranial nerves III, IV, and VI. Semin Neurol. 2009;29(1):14–28.
31. Brazis PW. Palsies of the trochlear nerve: diagnosis and localization–recent concepts. Mayo Clin Proc. 1993;68(5):501–9.
32. Carpenter MB, Batton RR. Abducens internuclear neurons and their role in conjugate horizontal gaze. J Comp Neurol. 1980;189:191–209.
33. Gradenigo G. A special syndrome of endocranial otitic complications (paralysis of the motor oculi externus of otitic origin). Ann Otol Rhinol Laryngol. 1904;13:637.
34. Rambo JH, Petti GH. Petrous apicitis. AMA Arch Otolaryngol. 1957;65(5):523–4.
35. DeGraaf J, Cats H, de Jager AEJ. Gradenigo's syndrome: a rare complication of otitis media. Clin Neurol Neurosurg. 1988;90:237–9.
36. Miller RW, Lee AG, Schiffman JS, et al. A practice pathway for the initial diagnostic evaluation of isolated sixth cranial nerve palsies. Med Decis Mak. 1999;19:42–8.
37. Sanders SK, Kawasaki A, Purvin VA. Long-term prognosis in patients with vasculopathic sixth nerve palsy. Am J Ophthalmol. 2002;134:81–4.
38. Lee MS, Galetta SL, Volpe NJ, Liu GT. Sixth nerve palsies in children. Pediatr Neurol. 1999;20:49–52.
39. Keane JR. Cavernous sinus syndrome. Analysis of 151 cases. Arch Neurol. 1996;53:967–71.
40. Colnaghi S, Versino M, Marchioni E, et al. ICHD-II diagnostic criteria for Tolosa-Hunt syndrome in idiopathic inflammatory syndromes of the orbit and/or the cavernous sinus. Cephalalgia. 2008;28:577.
41. Kline LB, Hoyt WF. The Tolosa-Hunt syndrome. J Neurol Neurosurg Psychiatry. 2001;71(5):577–82.
42. Areaya AA, Cerezal L, Canga A, et al. Neuroimaging diagnosis of Tolosa-Hunt syndrome: MRI contribution. Headache. 1999;39(5):321–5.
43. Evans OB, Lexow SS. Painful ophthalmoplegia in systemic lupus erythematosus. Ann Neurol. 1978;4:584–5.
44. Miller NR. Diagnosis and management of dural carotid-cavernous sinus fistulas. Neurosurg Focus. 2007;23(5):E13.
45. Yeh S, Foroozan R. Orbital apex syndrome. Curr Opin Ophthalmol. 2004;15:490–8.
46. Spellberg B, Edwards J, Ibrahim A. Novel perspectives on mucormycosis: pathophysiology, presentation, and management. Clin Microbiol Rev. 2005;18(3):556–69.
47. Hoch W, McConville J, Helms S, Newsom-Davis J, Melms A, Vincent A. Auto-antibodies to the receptor tyrosine kinase MuSK in patients with myasthenia gravis without acetylcholine receptor antibodies. Nat Med. 2001;7:365–8.
48. Evoli A, Tonali PA, Padua L, et al. Clinical correlates with anti-MuSK antibodies in generalized seronegative myasthenia gravis. Brain. 2003;126:2304–11.
49. Higuchi O, Hamuro J, Motomura, et al. Autoantibodies to LRP4 in myasthenia gravis. Ann Neurol. 2011;69:418–22.
50. Zhang B, Tzartos JS, Belimezi M, et al. Autoantibodies to LRP4 in patients with double seronegative myasthenia gravis. Arch Neurol. 2012;69:445–51.
51. Cruz AA, Akaishi PM, Vargas MA, de Paula SA. Association between thyroid autoimmune dysfunction and non-thyroid autoimmune diseases. Ophthal Plast Reconstr Surg. 2007;23:104–8.
52. Tellez-Zenteno JF, Cardenas G, Estanol B, Garcia-Ramos G, Weder-Cisneros N. Associated conditions in myasthenia gravis: response to thymectomy. Eur J Neurol. 2004;11:767–73.
53. Tellez-Zenteno JF, Remes-Troche JM, Mimenza-Alvarado A, Garcia-Ramos G, Estanol B, Vega-Boada F. The association of myasthenia gravis and connective tissue diseases. Effects of thymectomy in six cases with rheumatoid arthritis and one case with systemic lupus erythematosus. Neurologia. 2003;18:54–8.
54. Christensen PB, Jensen TS, Tsiropoulos I, et al. Associated autoimmune diseases in myasthenia gravis. A population-based study. Acta Neurol Scand. 1995;91:192–5.
55. Thorlacius S, Aarli JA, Riise T, Matre R, Johnsen HJ. Associated disorders in myasthenia gravis: autoimmune diseases and their relation to thymectomy. Acta Neurol Scand. 1989;80:290–5.
56. Monden Y, Uyama T, Nakahara K, et al. Clinical characteristics and prognosis of myasthenia gravis with other autoimmune diseases. Ann Thorac Surg. 1986;41:189–92.
57. Yu CC, Chen SG, Chen TM. Frontalis slings with palmaris tendon as an adjuvant treatment for myasthenic blepharoptosis: a case report. Ann Plast Surg. 2007;58:577–9.
58. Lelli GJ Jr, Musch DC, Frueh BR, Nelson CC. Outcomes in silicone rod frontalis suspension surgery for high-risk noncongenital blepharoptosis. Ophthal Plast Reconstr Surg. 2009;25:361–5.
59. Wirtz PW, Sotodeh M, Nijnuis M, et al. Difference in distribution of muscle weakness between myasthenia gravis and the Lambert-Eaton myasthenic syndrome. J Neurol Neurosurg Psychiatry. 2002;73:766–8.
60. Cruciger MP, Brown B, Denys EH, et al. Clinical and subclinical oculomotor findings in the Eaton-Lambert syndrome. J Clin Neuroophthalmol. 1983;3:19–22.
61. O'Neill JH, Murray NM, Newsom-Davis J. The Lambert-Eaton myasthenic syndrome. A review of 50 cases. Brain. 1988;111(Pt 3):577–96.
62. Breen LA, Gutmann L, Brick JF, Riggs JR. Paradoxical lid elevation with sustained upgaze: a sign of Lambert-Eaton syndrome. Muscle Nerve. 1991;14:863–6.
63. Titulaer MJ, Wirtz PW, Willems LN, van Kralingen KW, Smitt PA, Verschuuren JJ. Screening for small-cell lung cancer: a follow-up study of patients with Lambert-Eaton myasthenic syndrome. J Clin Oncol. 2008;26:4276–81.
64. Motomura M, Johnston I, Lang B, Vincent A, Newsom-Davis J. An improved diagnostic assay for Lambert-Eaton myasthenic syndrome. J Neurol Neurosurg Psychiatry. 1995;58:85–7.
65. Sabater L, Titulaer M, Saiz A, Verschuuren J, Gure AO, Graus F. SOX1 antibodies are markers of paraneoplastic Lambert-Eaton myasthenic syndrome. Neurology. 2008;70:924–8.
66. Nakao YK, Motomura M, Fukudome T, et al. Seronegative Lambert-Eaton myasthenic syndrome: study of 110 Japanese patients. Neurology. 2002;59:1773–5.
67. Maddison P, Newsom-Davis J. Treatment for Lambert-Eaton myasthenic syndrome. Cochrane Database Syst Rev. 2003;(2):CD003279.

68. Krieger FT, Goldchmit M. Surgical correction of strabismus in Lambert-Eaton myasthenic syndrome: case reports. Arq Bras Oftalmol. 2009;72:99–102.
69. Villar RG, Shapiro RL, Busto S, et al. Outbreak of type A botulism and development of a botulism surveillance and antitoxin release system in Argentina. JAMA. 1999;281:1334–8, 1340.
70. Townes JM, Cieslak PR, Hatheway CL, et al. An outbreak of type A botulism associated with a commercial cheese sauce. Ann Intern Med. 1996;125:558–63.
71. Kongsaengdao S, Samintarapanya K, Rusmeechan S, et al. An outbreak of botulism in Thailand: clinical manifestations and management of severe respiratory failure. Clin Infect Dis. 2006;43:1247–56.
72. Dowell VR Jr, McCroskey LM, Hatheway CL, Lombard GL, Hughes JM, Merson MH. Coproexamination for botulinal toxin and clostridium botulinum. A new procedure for laboratory diagnosis of botulism. JAMA. 1977;238:1829–32.
73. Shapiro RL, Hatheway C, Becher J, Swerdlow DL. Botulism surveillance and emergency response. A public health strategy for a global challenge. JAMA. 1997;278:433–5.
74. Lamantea E, Tiranti V, Bordoni A, et al. Mutations of mitochondrial DNA polymerase gamma are a frequent cause of autosomal dominant or recessive progressive external ophthalmoplegia. Ann Neurol. 2002;52:211–9.
75. Van Goethem G, Dermaut B, Lofgren A, Martin JJ, Van Broeckhoven C. Mutation of POLG is associated with progressive external ophthalmoplegia characterized by mtDNA deletions. Nat Genet. 2001;28:211–2.
76. Fratter C, Gorman GS, Stewart JD, et al. The clinical, histochemical, and molecular spectrum of PEO1 (Twinkle)-linked adPEO. Neurology. 2010;74:1619–26.
77. Kaukonen J, Juselius JK, Tiranti V, et al. Role of adenine nucleotide translocator 1 in mtDNA maintenance. Science. 2000;289:782–5.
78. Schoser BG, Pongratz D. Extraocular mitochondrial myopathies and their differential diagnoses. Strabismus. 2006;14:107–13.
79. Almousa R, Charlton A, Rajesh ST, Sundar G, Amrith S. Optimizing muscle biopsy for the diagnosis of mitochondrial myopathy. Ophthal Plast Reconstr Surg. 2009;25:366–70.
80. Harding AE, Hammans SR. Deletions of the mitochondrial genome. J Inherit Metab Dis. 1992;15:480–6.
81. Drachman DA. Ophthalmoplegia plus. The neurodegenerative disorders associated with progressive external ophthalmoplegia. Arch Neurol. 1968;18:654–74.
82. Kearns TP, Sayre GP. Retinitis pigmentosa, external ophthalmoplegia, and complete heart block: unusual syndrome with histologic study in one of two cases. AMA Arch Ophthalmol. 1958;60:280–9.
83. Berenberg RA, Pellock JM, DiMauro S, et al. Lumping or splitting? "Ophthalmoplegia-plus" or Kearns-Sayre syndrome? Ann Neurol. 1977;1:37–54.
84. Lopez-Gallardo E, Lopez-Perez MJ, Montoya J, Ruiz-Pesini E. CPEO and KSS differ in the percentage and location of the mtDNA deletion. Mitochondrion. 2009;9:314–7.
85. Ogasahara S, Yorifuji S, Nishikawa Y, et al. Improvement of abnormal pyruvate metabolism and cardiac conduction defect with coenzyme Q10 in Kearns-Sayre syndrome. Neurology. 1985;35:372–7.
86. Chinnery P, Majamaa K, Turnbull D, Thorburn D. Treatment for mitochondrial disorders. Cochrane Database Syst Rev. 2006;(1):CD004426.
87. Fang W, Huang CC, Lee CC, Cheng SY, Pang CY, Wei YH. Ophthalmologic manifestations in MELAS syndrome. Arch Neurol. 1993;50:977–80.
88. Hsu CC, Chuang YH, Tsai JL, et al. CPEO and carnitine deficiency overlapping in MELAS syndrome. Acta Neurol Scand. 1995;92:252–5.
89. Hirano M, Ricci E, Koenigsberger MR, et al. Melas: an original case and clinical criteria for diagnosis. Neuromuscul Disord. 1992;2:125–35.
90. Thambisetty M, Newman NJ. Diagnosis and management of MELAS. Expert Rev Mol Diagn. 2004;4:631–44.
91. Daut PM, Steinemann TL, Westfall CT. Chronic exposure keratopathy complicating surgical correction of ptosis in patients with chronic progressive external ophthalmoplegia. Am J Ophthalmol. 2000;130:519–21.
92. Wong VA, Beckingsale PS, Oley CA, Sullivan TJ. Management of myogenic ptosis. Ophthalmology. 2002;109:1023–31.
93. Johnson CC, Kuwabara T. Oculopharyngeal muscular dystrophy. Am J Ophthalmol. 1974;77:872–9.
94. Salvi SM, Currie ZI. Frontalis suspension sling using palmaris longus tendon in chronic progressive external ophthalmoplegia. Ophthal Plast Reconstr Surg. 2009;25:140–1.
95. Soejima K, Sakurai H, Nozaki M, et al. Surgical treatment of blepharoptosis caused by chronic progressive external ophthalmoplegia. Ann Plast Surg. 2006;56:439–42.
96. Bernardini FP, de Conciliis C, Devoto MH. Frontalis suspension sling using a silicone rod in patients affected by myogenic blepharoptosis. Orbit. 2002;21:195–8.
97. Brook JD, McCurrach ME, Harley HG, et al. Molecular basis of myotonic dystrophy: expansion of a trinucleotide (CTG) repeat at the 3′ end of a transcript encoding a protein kinase family member. Cell. 1992;69:385.
98. Feyma T, Carter GT, Weiss MD. Myotonic dystrophy type 1 coexisting with myasthenia gravis and thymoma. Muscle Nerve. 2008;38:916–20.
99. Burian HM, Burns CA. Ocular changes in myotonic dystrophy. Trans Am Ophthalmol Soc. 1966;64:250–73.
100. Waller RR. Management of myogenic (myopathic) ptosis. Trans Sect Ophthalmol Am Acad Ophthalmol Otolaryngol. 1975;79:697–702.
101. Fan X, Rouleau GA. Progress in understanding the pathogenesis of oculopharyngeal muscular dystrophy. Can J Neurol Sci. 2003;30:8–14.
102. Hebbar S, Webberley MJ, Lunt P, Robinson DO. Siblings with recessive oculopharyngeal muscular dystrophy. Neuromuscul Disord. 2007;17:254–7.
103. Brais B, Bouchard JP, Xie YG, et al. Short GCG expansions in the PABP2 gene cause oculopharyngeal muscular dystrophy. Nat Genet. 1998;18:164–7.
104. Molgat YM, Rodrigue D. Correction of blepharoptosis in oculopharyngeal muscular dystrophy: review of 91 cases. Can J Ophthalmol. 1993;28:11–4.
105. Jordan DR, Addison DJ. Surgical results and pathological findings in the oculopharyngeal dystrophy syndrome. Can J Ophthalmol. 1993;28:15–8.
106. Kang DH, Koo SH, Ahn DS, Park SH, Yoon ES. Correction of blepharoptosis in oculopharyngeal muscular dystrophy. Ann Plast Surg. 2002;49:419–23.
107. Tawil R, Van Der Maarel SM. Facioscapulohumeral muscular dystrophy. Muscle Nerve. 2006;34:1–15.
108. Longmuir SQ, Mathews KD, Longmuir RA, Joshi V, Olson RJ, Abramoff MD. Retinal arterial but not venous tortuosity correlates with facioscapulohumeral muscular dystrophy severity. J AAPOS. 2010;14:240–3.

109. Flohr TG, Schaller S, Stierstorfer K, Bruder H, Ohnesorge BM, Schoepf UJ. Multi-detector row CT systems and image-reconstruction techniques. Radiology. 2005;235:756–73.
110. Caille JM, et al. Gadolinium as a contrast agent for NMR. Am J Neuroradiol. 1983;4:1041–2.
111. Haley TJ, Raymond K, Komesu N, Upham HC. Toxicological and pharmacological effects of gadolinium and samarium chlorides. Br J Pharmacol Chemother. 1961;17:526–32.
112. Cowper SE, Robin HS, Steinberg SM, Su LD, Gupta S, LeBoit PE. Scleromyxoedema-like cutaneous diseases in renal-dialysis patients. Lancet. 2000;356:1000–1.
113. US Food and Drug Administration, Information for healthcare professionals gadolinium-based contrast agents for magnetic resonance imaging (marketed as Magnevist, MultiHance, Omniscan, OptiMARK, ProHance) Updated 23 May 2007. http://www.fda.gov/Drugs/DrugSafety/PostmarketDrugSafetyInformationforPatientsandProviders/ucm142884.htm. Accessed 21 Aug 2010.
114. Martin DR, Kalb B, Salman K, et al. Decreased incidence of NSF in patients on dialysis after changing gadolinium contrast-enhanced MRI protocols. J Magn Reson Imaging. 2010;31(2):440–6.

Traumatic Cranial Neuropathies

6

Ann P. Murchison, Jurij R. Bilyk, and Peter J. Savino

Introduction

Many patients who sustain head trauma may have associated orbital injuries that necessitate a thorough, systematic ophthalmic evaluation. In patients with recent cranial injury, bedside testing may be difficult and limited. At times, the pupillary examination, forced duction testing, anterior segment examination, and direct ophthalmoscopy are all that are initially feasible. This information, along with imaging studies, guides much of the early treatment of head injury patients. Motor vehicle accidents are the most common cause of head trauma, and cranial nerve injuries occur in approximately 13% of these patients [1]. This chapter will discuss the diagnosis and management of traumatic injury to the optic nerve and the motor nerves of the orbit. Discussion of trigeminal and facial nerve injury is found in other chapters.

Traumatic Optic Neuropathy

Traumatic optic neuropathy (TON) is not encountered frequently in an outpatient setting of a comprehensive ophthalmologist's office. However, TON is not at all uncommon in emergency rooms, especially in institutions dealing with a high volume of head trauma. TON has been reported to occur in 0.5–5% of cases following head trauma and in 2.5–6% of patients with zygomaticomaxillary (tripod) fractures [2–8].

Two issues need to be clarified at the outset of this discussion. First, the term "traumatic optic neuropathy" has become synonymous with a specific type of TON – posterior indirect TON. In reality, TON can occur from a variety of mechanisms. Second, with the notable exception of compressive TON from orbital hemorrhage, effective medical or surgical management of TON is for the most part extremely limited and of dubious value.

Types of TON

There are a variety of classification schema for TON, but the easiest and most practical is that proposed by Miller [9]. In this paradigm, TON is divided both anatomically and mechanistically. From the anatomic standpoint, TON is separated into an anterior and posterior form at the level of the entry point of the central retinal artery into the optic nerve, an admittedly arbitrary but practical anatomic landmark. Miller's classification includes the intracanalicular optic nerve in addition to the intraorbital and intrascleral segments. From the mechanistic standpoint, injury to the optic nerve occurs either directly or indirectly.

Direct optic nerve injury typically results in a penetrating orbital injury that contuses, lacerates, compresses, or transects the optic nerve. Typical examples include transection by a sharp object or compression by a foreign body. Indirect injury is the result of rotational or deceleration forces applied to the optic nerve secondarily, usually without significant disruption of the surrounding anatomy. Posterior indirect TON (PITON) is an example of such a mechanism. As a general rule, direct TON typically results in more severe and less reversible injury than indirect TON [9].

TON secondary to orbital hemorrhage is harder to characterize both anatomically and mechanistically, since orbital compartment syndrome usually causes diffuse intraorbital pressure spikes affecting all parts of the intraorbital

A. P. Murchison (✉)
Department of Ophthalmology, Oculoplastic and Orbital Surgery Service, Eye Emergency Room, Wills Eye Hospital and Thomas Jefferson University Hospital, Philadelphia, PA, USA
e-mail: amuchison@willseye.org

J. R. Bilyk
Attending Surgeon and Professor of Ophthalmology, Oculoplastic and Orbital Surgery Service, Wills Eye Hospital and Thomas Jefferson University Hospital, Philadelphia, PA, USA

P. J. Savino
Clinical Professor of Ophthalmology, Viterbi Famile Department of Ophthalmology, Shiley Eye Institute, University of Califormia San Diego, La Jolla, CA, USA

J. J. Servat et al. (eds.), *Smith and Nesi's Ophthalmic Plastic and Reconstructive Surgery*,
https://doi.org/10.1007/978-3-030-41720-8_6

optic nerve, and the mechanism may include both direct compression on the nerve or secondary ischemia from inadequate vascular supply. Chiasmal injury will also be discussed in this section, although from a strictly anatomic standpoint, the optic chiasm is not part of the optic nerve.

Optic Nerve Anatomy

The optic nerve is divided into four anatomic segments: intrascleral, orbital, canalicular, and prechiasmal [10, 11]. The entire optic nerve is about 50 mm in length, containing 1.5–2.0 million axons. The short intrascleral portion measures 1 mm and contains unmyelinated nerve fibers. The optic nerve head derives its arterial supply from three sources, forming the circle of Zinn-Haller: choroidal feeders, several dedicated short posterior ciliary arteries, and pial vessels from the proximal optic nerve sheath. To put it more simply, the vast majority of optic nerve head perfusion arises exclusively from the posterior ciliary arterial supply [12–15].

As the nerve exits the sclera through the lamina cribrosa, the axons become myelinated, doubling the optic nerve thickness. In addition, the orbital optic nerve becomes invested in a meningeal sheath composed of pia, arachnoid, and dura mater. The subarachnoid space of the optic nerve is contiguous with the middle cranial fossa, with a pseudocistern in the bulbous proximal optic nerve immediately behind the globe. The orbital optic nerve travels in a gentle S-shaped course toward the optic canal, with an average length of about 25 mm. The average distance between the posterior sclera and optic canal is about 18 mm, allowing for about 7 mm of excess optic nerve length within the orbit. This accommodation allows for ductions to occur without putting excessive tension on the nerve fibers and thereby avoiding ductional amaurosis. Theoretically, the excess intraorbital length provides a buffer for 5–7 mm of tolerable exophthalmos, although this should not be assumed as an absolute in all clinical presentations.

Long and short posterior ciliary arteries course over the surface of the optic nerve to supply the globe. One long posterior ciliary artery is generally found on the medial and lateral surface of the optic nerve sheath, and each pierces the posterior sclera partial thickness to supply the anterior segment as a contributor to the major arterial circle. The 15–20 short posterior ciliary arteries travel in a more haphazard fashion to supply the optic nerve head and choroid plexus in a segmental fashion. Sensory innervation to the globe travels with the ciliary arteries. The central retinal artery enters the optic nerve approximately 10–15 mm behind the globe. Interestingly, neither the overlying ciliary arteries nor the central retinal artery provide any significant supply to the orbital optic nerve; instead, perforating pial vessels are exclusively responsible for blood supply.

The optic nerve ascends toward the optic foramen in the orbital apex. The ciliary ganglion is found on the lateral aspect of the optic nerve about 10 mm anterior to the orbital apex. The optic foramen is situated in the posterior portion of the medial orbital wall and is tilted medially and superiorly, pointing toward the optic chiasm [16]. The optic nerve and ophthalmic artery travel within the optic canal along with a portion of the sympathetic supply to the globe and orbit. The optic canal typically measures 5–10 mm in length and lies superomedial to the cavernous sinus, shifting from a vertical elliptical shape within the orbit to a horizontal ellipse intracranially. The dura of the nerve fuses with the annulus of Zinn at the orbital apex and within the optic canal additional adhesions are found to the periosteum superomedially, effectively tethering the nerve into position and making it and the attendant nutrient vessels from the pia vulnerable to shearing forces. The canal also forms a natural enclosed compartment, potentially allowing for compression of the intracanalicular optic nerve in a number of pathologic processes. Two other points regarding the intracanalicular optic nerve are important clinically. First, the optic canal is formed laterally by the anterior clinoid process. On axial imaging, identification of the anterior clinoid process is critical in correctly identifying the optic canal and distinguishing it from the more laterally and inferiorly placed superior orbital fissure. Second, from the transnasal endoscopic standpoint, the optic canal is typically seen superiorly within the lateral wall of the sphenoid sinus [17]. The bulge of the intracavernous carotid siphon is noted just below the canal and may have little overlying bone in some patients [16]. These are crucial landmarks to identify during skull base surgery and specifically during attempted optic canal decompression.

As the optic nerve exits the canal, it is additionally tethered by a superior dural sheath. The intracranial portion of the nerve continues its course superiorly and medially to form the optic chiasm about 10 mm from the intracranial edge of the canal, lying adjacent to the internal carotid artery at its lateral edge. The optic chiasm forms as a midline confluence and partial crossover of both optic nerves. It is found approximately 10 mm above the pituitary fossa and gland but may have a significant variation in its anterior to posterior relationship with the pituitary fossa mainly due to normal differences in the length of the intracranial optic nerve. This feature is important clinically and explains the variety of possible perimetry patterns of enlarging pituitary lesions.

Specific TON Subtypes

Anterior Indirect

Anterior indirect TON usually occurs in the setting of a rapid rotational force applied to the globe. The rotation results in damage to the optic nerve head, ranging clinically from optic

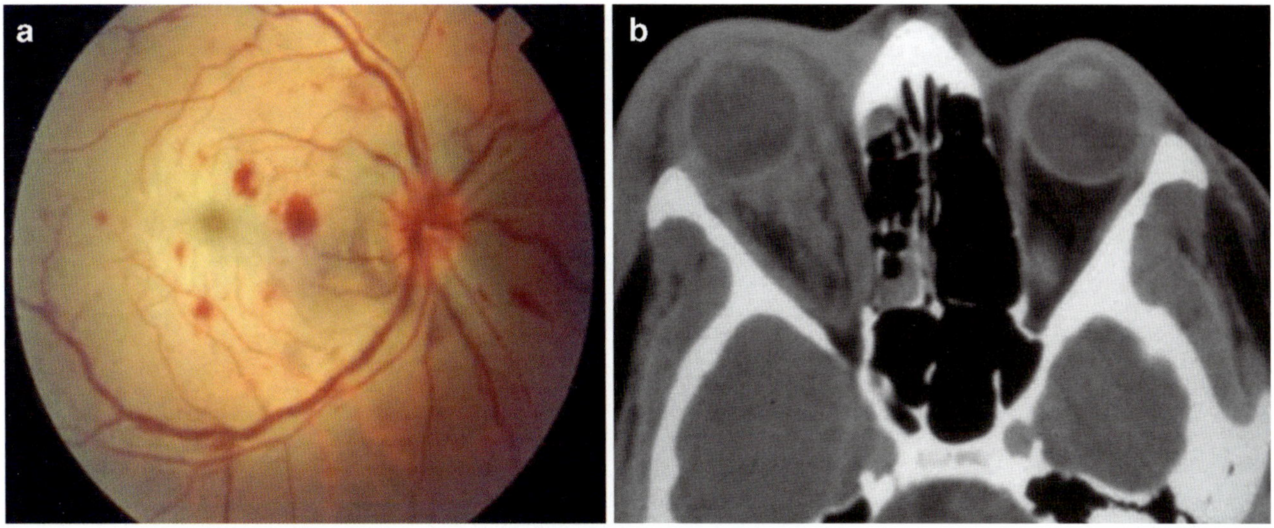

Fig. 6.1 Direct anterior TON. Fundus photo of a patient who suffered a finger poke to the right eye with immediate visual loss to the hand-motion level. A conjunctival laceration was noted on clinical exam. (**a**) On fundus exam, note the signs of combined central arterial and venous occlusion, including nerve fiber layer edema with a "cherry-red spot" and flame hemorrhages. (**b**) On axial CT, hemorrhage is noted in the orbital fat surrounding the optic nerve

nerve head edema (Fig. 6.1) with or without hemorrhage to complete avulsion of the optic nerve from the posterior sclera (Fig. 6.2) [18]. The classic history is that of a finger poke to the globe [19]. The authors have managed several such patients, and as a side note, being poked in the eye during a basketball game seems at least anecdotally to be a common mechanism [20]. Optic nerve head avulsion is rarely caused by assault, since a closed fist is unlikely to result in globe torsion; however, martial arts practitioners will on occasion purposely attempt to pluck out an eye with two fingers and in some cases successfully avulse the optic nerve head. Other mechanisms may also play a role. An acute rise in intraocular pressure has been postulated as a mechanism for optic nerve head avulsion, in effect blowing out the optic nerve posteriorly [20, 21]. An anterior displacement of the globe may also occur, acutely stretching the orbital optic nerve until avulsion occurs at the posterior sclera [22, 23]. Optic nerve head avulsion has been reported with motor vehicle accidents, bicycle accidents, and falls [18].

The severity of visual loss secondary to optic nerve head injury varies, but if partial or complete avulsion has occurred, visual loss is typically profound [18]. The initial diagnosis may be difficult to make, since the view of the optic nerve head may be obscured by vitreous hemorrhage (Fig. 6.2); definitive diagnosis may require surgical exploration [20, 21, 24]. Retinal detachment or infarction may be noted if the vitreous hemorrhage remains localized around the lamina cribrosa [18, 25]. CT imaging is usually not diagnostic, since the optic nerve sheath may still be intact (Fig. 6.2) [19, 23]. MRI may also prove inconclusive [21, 23]. B-scan ultrasonography appears to provide the best information (Fig. 6.3) [21, 26]. Early diagnosis of optic nerve head avulsion has no impact on clinical management and prognosis, since there is no known effective treatment. Corticosteroids are sometimes prescribed, but there is no evidence to support their use [20]. If external ophthalmoplegia is present, it is reasonable to explore the globe and extraocular muscles (EOMs), since the torsional mechanism of the initial injury may on occasion also avulse one or more EOMs. Reapproximation of the torn muscle back onto the globe may at least allow for better long-term extraocular motility of the injured eye. Severe globe luxation can also be present and may be dependent on the mechanism of injury (anterior globe displacement rather than torsion), number of avulsed or lacerated EOMs, and presence of orbital hemorrhage [24]. In such cases, an initial attempt to reposition the globe into the orbit is reasonable; neither sympathetic ophthalmia nor ocular ischemia has been reported in cases of optic nerve head avulsion, although the total number of reports is admittedly small [24]. Although phthisis bulbi may eventually occur, there is little reason to complete the enucleation early on, and retention of the globe may offer at least some psychological comfort to the unfortunate patient [24].

Direct TON

Direct TON is usually the result of a penetrating orbital injury, with or without concomitant globe penetration [27, 28]. Some type of missile typically directly contuses, lacerates, abuts, or lodges within the optic nerve (Fig. 6.4) [22]. In many cases, visual loss is profound, sudden, and permanent. Funduscopy varies from completely normal to findings consistent with arterial occlusion. In cases of contusion and laceration, little can be offered in terms of effective therapy. If a foreign body or bone fragment is found abutting or lodged

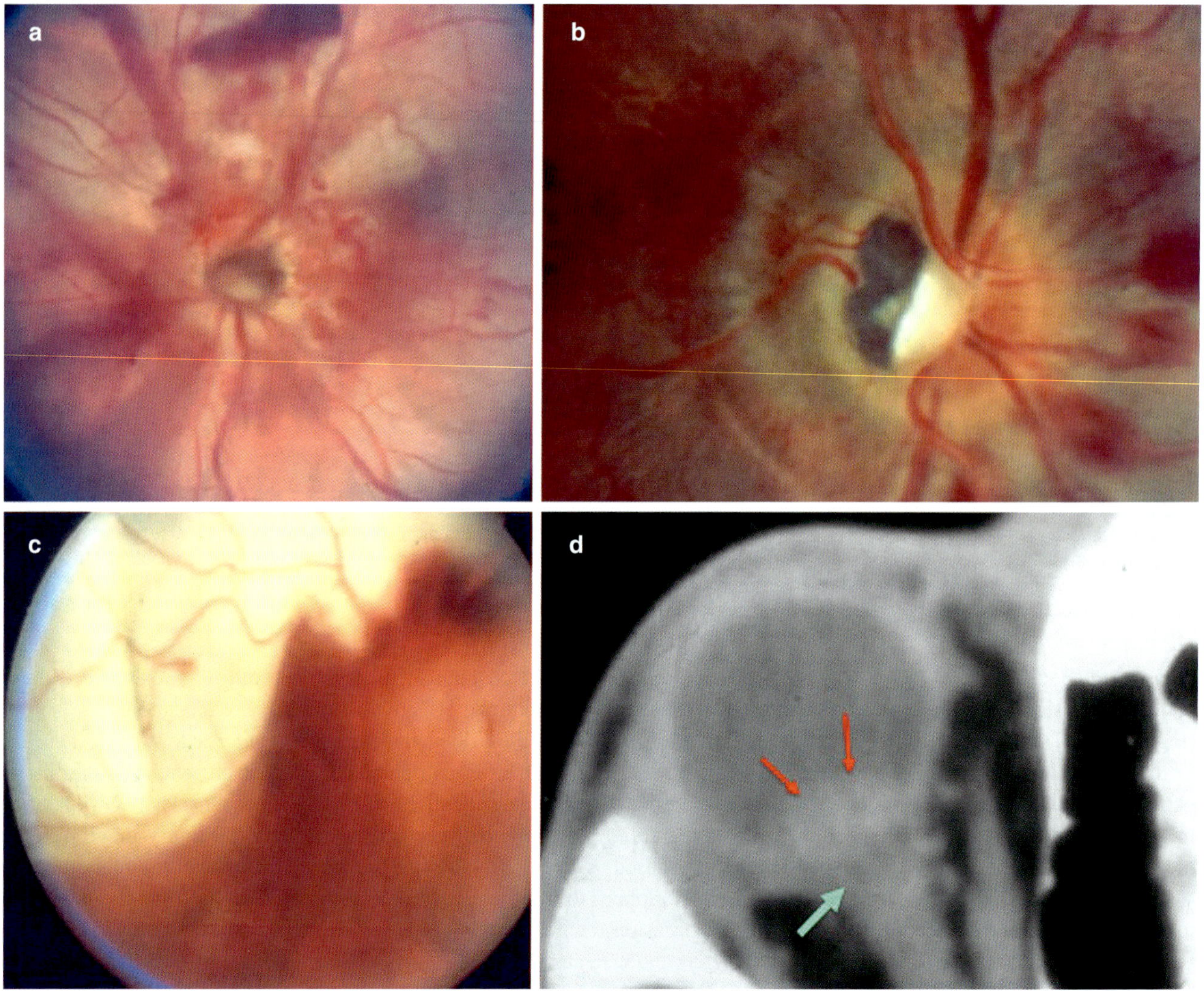

Fig. 6.2 Avulsion of the optic nerve head. (**a**) Complete optic nerve head avulsion. (**b**) Partial optic nerve head avulsion. (**c**) Typical acute fundus appearance of an optic nerve head avulsion. Note the prepapillary vitreous hemorrhage obscuring the optic nerve head. The retina is detached and infarcted. (**d**) Close-up of an axial CT image of the patient in C. The findings are nondiagnostic but suspicious for optic nerve head avulsion. There is a prepapillary vitreous hemorrhage (red arrows). The nerve sheath is still attached to the globe, but three narrow lucencies (green arrow) suggest avulsion of the optic nerve

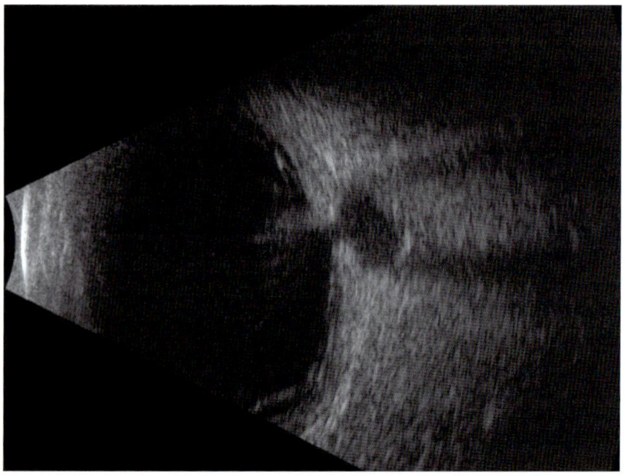

Fig. 6.3 B-scan of an optic nerve head avulsion clearly demonstrates the retracted optic nerve within its sheath, along with overlying vitreous hemorrhage

in the optic nerve on CT imaging (Fig. 6.5), consideration may be given to timely removal of the offending material. However, successful surgery may prove difficult because of the location of the foreign body, an associated posterior globe rupture that may be difficult to access, an orbital apical location, or significant orbital soft tissue edema and hemorrhage, which may limit visualization. If orbital hemorrhage is present to any significant degree, it should be managed aggressively, since it is often impossible to conclude the etiology of the visual loss in the early stages [29].

Optic nerve sheath hemorrhage represents a rare subtype of direct TON but may also occur via an indirect mechanism in the setting of subarachnoid hemorrhage (as a form of Terson syndrome) or secondary to acute spikes in intracranial pressure [30]. Retinal and vitreous hemorrhage may be present. Based on postmortem studies by Walsh and Hedges, the hemorrhage typically occurs in the subdural space

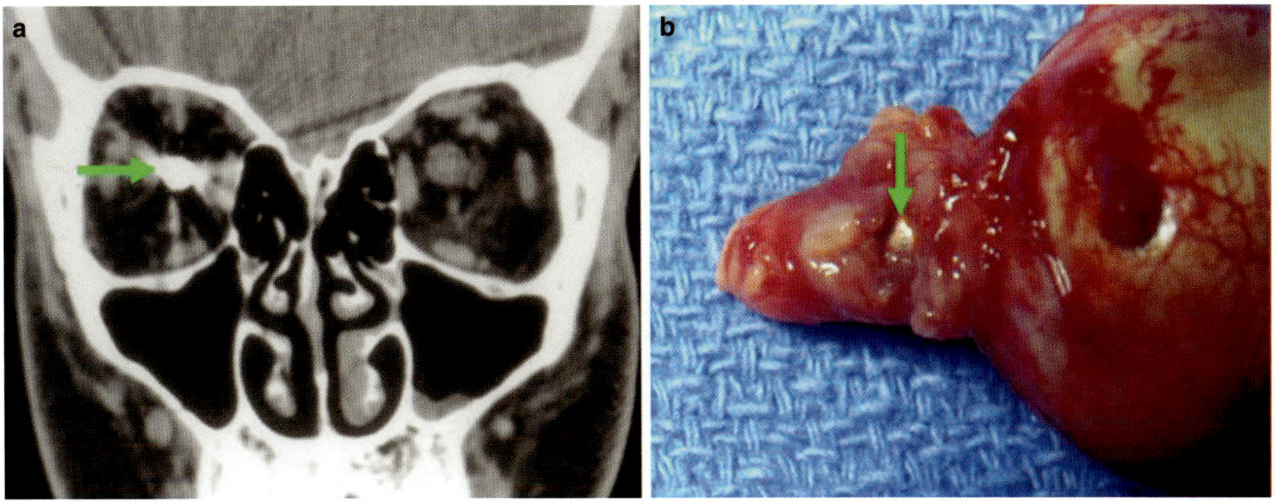

Fig. 6.4 (**a**) Direct TON from a foreign body. A coronal CT shows a radiopaque foreign body (arrow) in the area of the right optic nerve. (**b**) On subsequent enucleation, the BB pellet is seen lodged in the optic nerve (arrow). Also note the posterior globe rupture from the penetrating injury

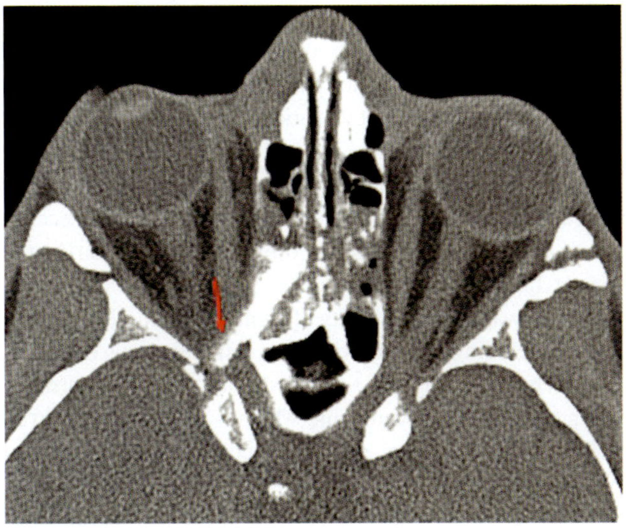

Fig. 6.5 Direct TON from a bone fragment. Bone from an orbital roof fracture (arrow) is seen either abutting or transecting the right optic nerve

(60%), with subarachnoid blood found less frequently; thus, in cases of raised intracranial pressure from subarachnoid hemorrhage, the optic nerve sheath hemorrhage is a consequence of localized bleeding rather than migrating blood into the optic nerve sheath from a intracranial location [31]. If the hemorrhage within the sheath continues to expand, a compartment syndrome may occur. Clinically, this manifests as progressive visual loss and an evolving retinal arterial and venous obstruction on serial fundus exams. Imaging may not be diagnostic. On CT, it may be difficult to distinguish true subarachnoid optic nerve sheath hemorrhage from a localized epidural hemorrhage occurring within the perineural fat compartments (Fig. 6.6). MRI may be helpful in such cases: oblique coronal views perpendicular to the long axis of the optic nerve may elucidate the exact location of the hemorrhage. In suspected cases of optic nerve sheath hemorrhage with normal visual function, observation alone is sufficient. However, if compression of the optic nerve and the attendant retinal vessels occurs, optic nerve sheath decompression is recommended to evacuate the hematoma and open the compartment formed by the optic nerve's meningeal covering. Because of the rarity of this diagnosis, it remains unclear whether surgical decompression is effective in reversing visual loss, but it remains a reasonable option in an otherwise stable patient with progressive visual loss; the decision to operate is much more difficult in an obtunded and possibly neurologically unstable patient with optic nerve sheath hemorrhage and a limited ophthalmic examination.

Orbital Hemorrhage and Orbital Compartment Syndrome

Limited orbital hemorrhage is a frequent phenomenon following craniofacial trauma and is usually inconsequential in the long term. However, because the bony orbit along with the orbital septum and the tarsoligamentous system of the eyelids effectively form a closed compartment, any excessive volume from a secondary source (blood, pus, air, edema) will eventually result in a compartment syndrome with compressive optic neuropathy [32–36]. Because of the ubiquity of orbital trauma and subsequent hemorrhage, compressive optic neuropathy from orbital hemorrhage is in all likelihood the most common form of TON.

Following orbital injury, hemorrhage can occur from a variety of sources, including bleeding from any of the myriad intraorbital arteries. There are also multiple arteries that exit the orbit either along or through bone, including the anterior and posterior ethmoidal, supratrochlear, supraorbital, infraorbital, zygomaticofacial, zygomaticotemporal, and recurrent meningeal arteries, which can be avulsed or lacerated as a result of injury. Bleeding may be facilitated by an underlying inherent or pharmacologic (aspirin, warfarin, etc.) coag-

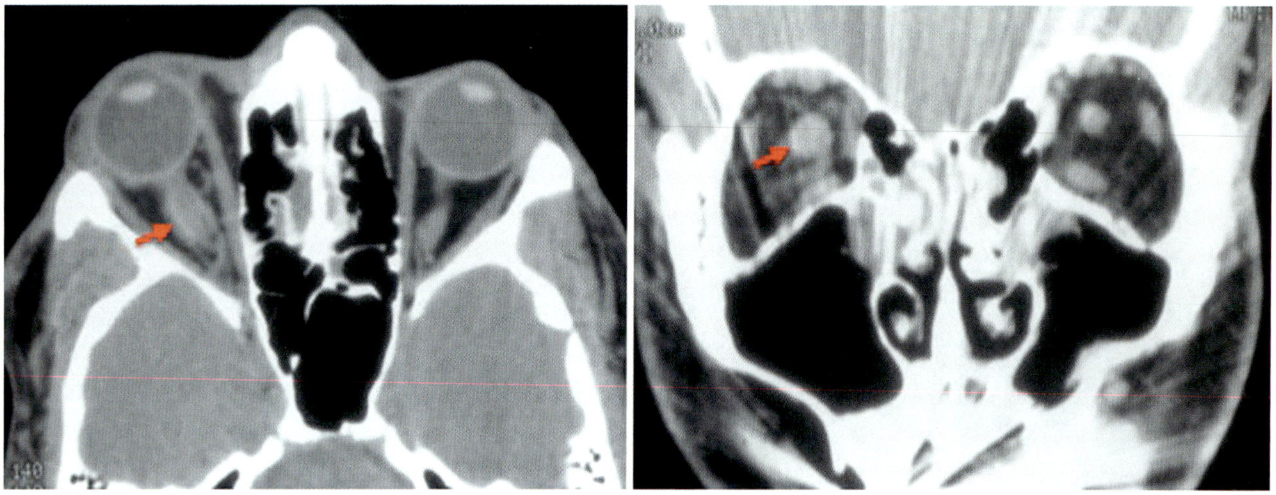

Fig. 6.6 Suspected optic nerve sheath hemorrhage following orbital penetration by an antenna. CT imaging shows an enlargement of the optic nerve sheath (arrows). However, funduscopic exam showed no evidence of vascular occlusion despite no light perception vision. Emergent orbital exploration revealed only epidural hemorrhage in the area of the optic nerve sheath. Exploration of the subarachnoid space of optic nerve sheath failed to reveal any blood

ulopathy and other systemic comorbidities (hematologic, oncologic, etc.), including uncontrolled hypertension [37]. Although an associated orbital fracture communicating with an adjacent paranasal sinus may have a decompressive effect on the orbital compartment, this is not always the case, and orbital compartment syndrome is not infrequently seen with orbital fractures communicating with the paranasal sinuses.

Visual loss from orbital hemorrhage occurs from several mechanisms, and in all likelihood, multiple mechanisms are present in a typical case of orbital compartment syndrome (OCS) [37, 38]. As intraocular pressure rapidly increases, retinal perfusion becomes compromised and central retinal artery occlusion may occur. The retina can tolerate arterial occlusion for only a limited time (~100 minutes) before permanent damage occurs [39]. Primate studies have also demonstrated permanent optic nerve damage of varying severity occurred with a sustained IOP of >50 mmHg for more than 180 minutes [40]. Increased intraorbital pressure may result in decreased venous drainage from the eye, resulting in central retinal vein occlusion or hemorrhagic choroidal detachment. High intraorbital pressure may also cause occlusion of the ophthalmic artery, as demonstrated angiographically by Wladis et al. [41]. Ischemic optic neuropathy is probable from several mechanisms: (1) direct compression on the axons, (2) direct compression of the pial vessels supplying the nerve, and (3) shearing of the pial vessels as the optic nerve is stretched from axial proptosis [32, 38, 40, 42–44].

Orbital hemorrhage is per se not a difficult diagnosis to make clinically. Accurate evaluation of optic nerve function in the face of a tight orbit, on the other hand, is often not straightforward for a variety of reasons, including difficulty in opening the eyelids, poor patient cooperation, and altered mental status. Adequate evaluation is especially difficult for a non-ophthalmologist.

The presentation of orbital hemorrhage spans a broad spectrum from mild proptosis with eyelid edema and ecchymosis to "rock hard" lids and orbit (Fig. 6.7) requiring the use of lid retractors for adequate assessment. In addition, there is always the possibility of significant underlying globe injury, including rupture, which necessitates gentle examination techniques (Fig. 6.8). Patients with orbital hemorrhage often complain of severe pain, which is not surprising given the rapid expansion of soft tissue edema. Varying degrees of eyelid ecchymosis, edema, and exophthalmos are present. On occasion, deep orbital hemorrhage may manifest as severe visual loss but only minimal eyelid signs. External ophthalmoplegia can also be present but may be difficult to assess because of poor cooperation. Depending on the degree of lid edema and visual loss, the patient may not complain of diplopia even in the face of obvious strabismus.

Measurement of intraocular pressure is important in the setting of OCS. First, it assesses the presence of unacceptably high intraocular pressure that may result in vascular occlusion. Second, it provides a baseline measure and valuable indirect evidence regarding the effectiveness of subsequent therapy: in an experimental model of orbital hemorrhage, Zoumalan and colleagues showed that IOP closely parallels intraorbital pressure and that IOP is in all likelihood a reasonably accurate predictor of pressure within the confines of the orbital compartment (Fig. 6.9) [45]. However, IOP may

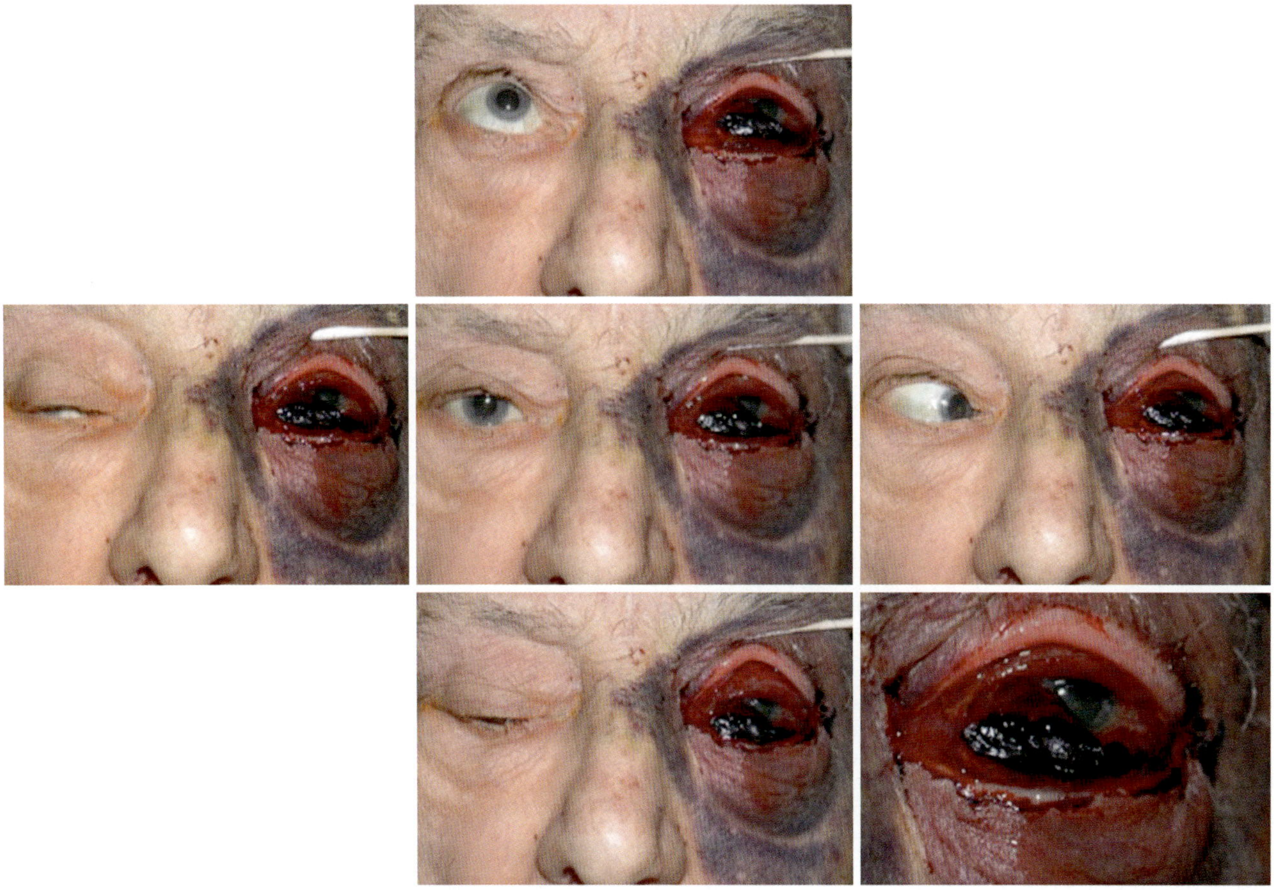

Fig. 6.7 Orbital compartment syndrome from hemorrhage. Note the proptosis, limited extraocular motility, and severe hemorrhagic chemosis. Vision was decreased to 20/100 with an afferent pupillary defect. The OCS occurred after mininal trauma, but the patient was using warfarin and had a markedly elevated international normalized ratio (INR)

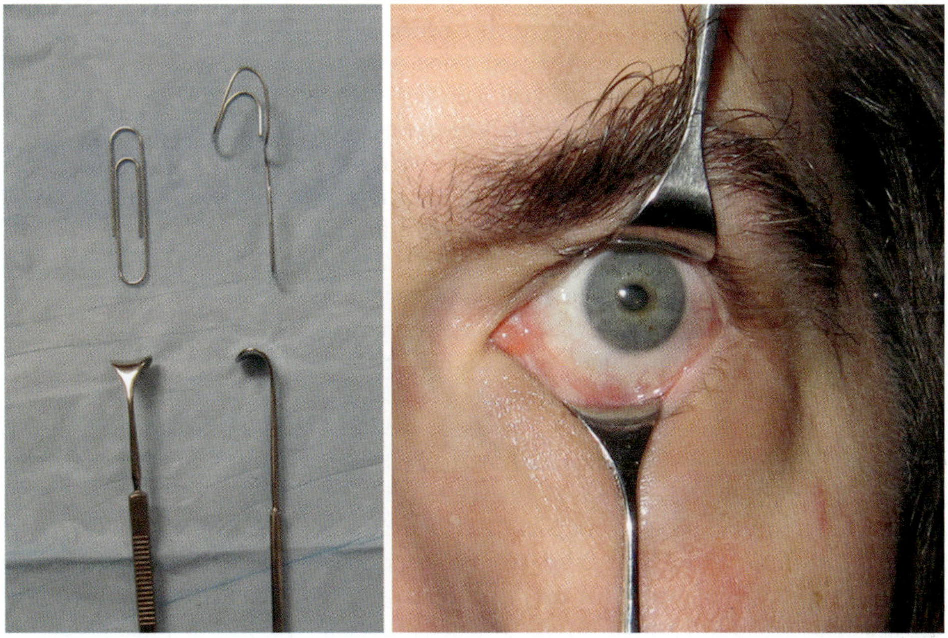

Fig. 6.8 Desmarres retractors are highly effective in opening the eyelids, even with a tight orbit. If they are not available, two bent paper clips may be improvised into the appropriate shape

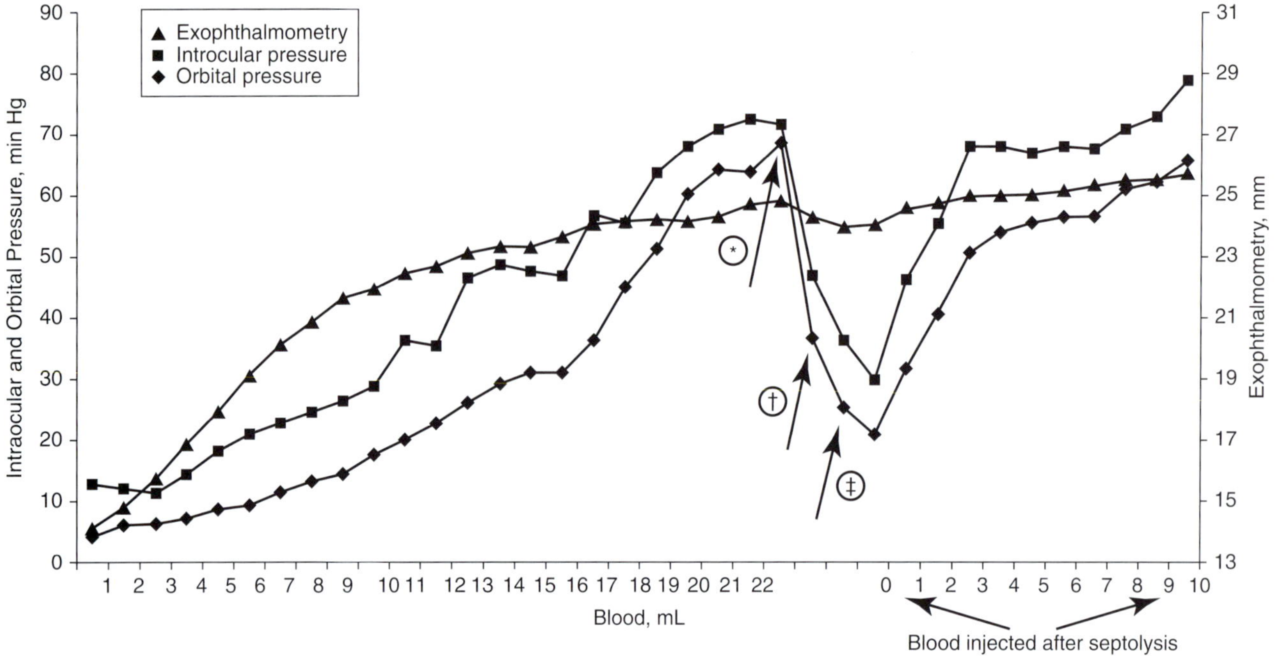

Fig. 6.9 Intraorbital and intraocular pressures in orbital hemorrhage. Note the nearly parallel rise in the two parameters with increased blood volume in the orbital compartment. • = Lateral canthotomy. † = Inferior cantholysis. ‡ = Inferior septolysis. Note that these maneuvers are effective in reducing intraorbital and, secondarily, intraocular pressures but are transient in the face of persistent bleeding. (Ref. [44]. Used with permission)

not always be elevated in cases of orbital hemorrhage, especially in cases of localized posterior orbital hemorrhage or severe ocular ischemia with ciliary body shutdown.

Clinical evaluation of orbital hemorrhage follows the same general tenets as for any ocular trauma: assess visual function, rule out intraocular injury or globe rupture, and then examine for periocular injury. In the case of orbital hemorrhage, one factor is essential: time. If a patient presents with an obviously tight orbit, decreased vision, and evidence of optic nerve dysfunction (afferent pupillary defect, dyschromatopsia), any significant delay in definitive therapy may result in permanent visual loss. Thus, it is often possible to only clear the anterior segment of the eye initially before proceeding with emergent intervention. This is also true for imaging. Orbital compartment syndrome (OCS) is a *clinical* diagnosis, and does not require radiologic confirmation. Delay in therapy while awaiting an imaging study is not recommended. Certainly, subsequent CT is indicated for a more elucidative assessment of deeper injury but should be performed after the OCS has been stabilized. The clinician should also not make any unfounded conclusions about the duration of posttraumatic visual loss and defer cantholysis because "too much time has elapsed." First, visual loss may have occurred several hours after the initial injury, and because of eyelid edema, very often, the patient cannot report an accurate timeline regarding visual function. Second, despite the aforementioned timeframes for retinal and optic nerve damage, clinical medicine does not necessarily mirror experimental models, and visual recovery in orbital hemorrhage has been reported even after delayed orbital decompression [46, 47].

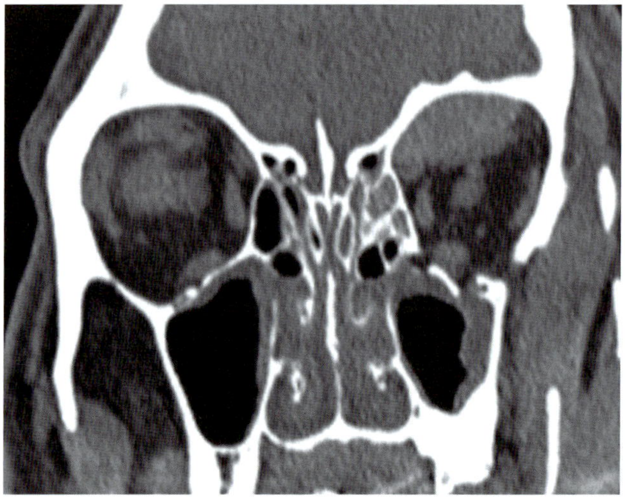

Fig. 6.10 A left superior, subperiosteal hematoma on coronal CT. An orbital floor fracture is also present

CT imaging of OCS from orbital hemorrhage is typically nonspecific. On occasion, a localized subperiosteal hematoma may be present (Fig. 6.10), but this is the exception to the rule of a nonspecific, increased reticular pattern seen in the intraconal space. Associated fracture may be present. In one study by Dailey and colleagues, the angle of the posterior

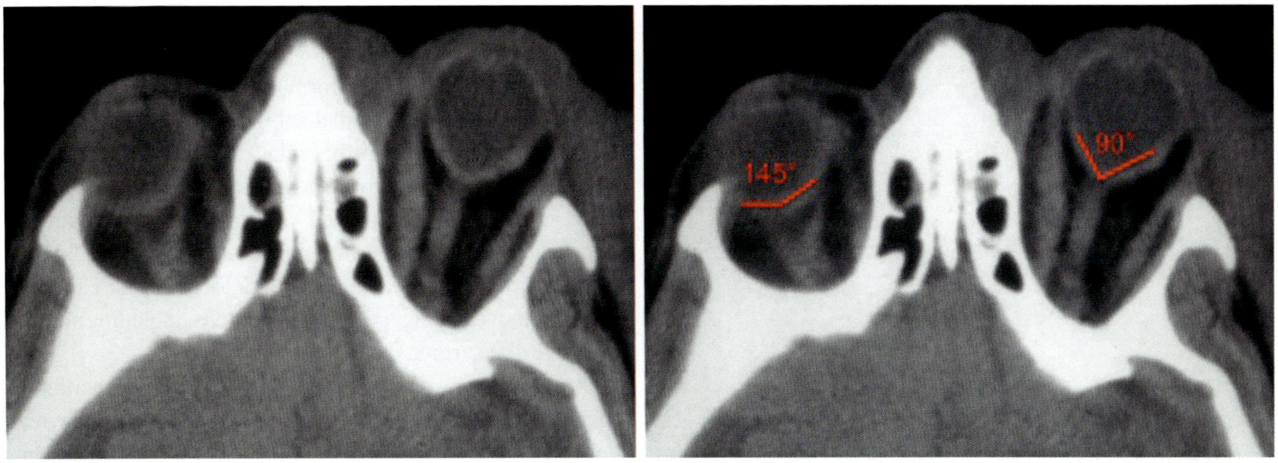

Fig. 6.11 Axial CT demonstrating globe tenting from a left orbital hemorrhage. Note the normal posterior scleral angle of about 150° on the right compared to 90° on the abnormal side

sclera correlated with the severity of the visual compromise [48]. The normal posterior scleral angle measure approximately 150°; a decreased angle to 120–130° was associated clinically with only mild visual symptoms, whereas an angle of less than 120° was ominous, indicating severe visual compromise and variable recovery. This so-called "globe tenting" or "tear-drop sign" on axial CT indicates that the intraorbital optic nerve has stretched to its maximum length and that the acute proptosis is significant enough to distort the posterior sclera (Fig. 6.11).

While medical therapy is helpful as an adjunct, the mainstay of management remains soft tissue decompression of the orbit by lateral canthotomy and inferior cantholysis. Two studies have shown the effectiveness of this procedure in decreasing both intraorbital and intraocular pressure in experimental models [45, 49]. Two points about the procedure need to be stressed. First, lateral canthotomy alone is inadequate in lowering intraorbital pressure adequately; inferior cantholysis should also be performed in all cases. Second, lateral canthotomy and inferior cantholysis are temporizing measures only [45]. In other words, if an active intraorbital process persists after cantholysis (persistent bleeding, abscess expansion, etc.), then the OCS will recur. This is best exemplified by the OCS seen following either spontaneous thrombosis of the superior ophthalmic vein or iatrogenic closure of a cavernous sinus fistula through as transvenous approach; in this situation, the orbit suddenly has no venous egress, and cantholysis may provide only temporary relief as the orbit once again refills from the arterial side but has not yet established an alternate venous route to drain [50]. Fortunately, the vast majority of OCS in trauma occurs from a hemorrhage that has tamponaded itself and is no longer active.

Additional measures, including intravenous corticosteroids (methylprednisolone 250 mg every 6 hours in adults), frequent ice compresses, acetazolamide, and intravenous mannitol may be considered if IOP remains dangerously high. Topical antiglaucoma medications may also be helpful. Of note, a recent animal study in OCS found a significant reduction in both IOP and intraorbital pressure with mannitol infusion [51]. While this reduction was transient and not considered definitive therapy, mannitol use may "buy time," while definitive therapy with cantholysis is being arranged. This may be especially helpful if there is a delay because of patient transfer or physician arrival. The use of intravenous mannitol infusion should be cleared with the primary team and, in the case of concomitant intracranial injury, with the neurosurgeon to assure there are no contraindications for its use.

If an inferior cantholysis fails to improve visual function and IOP over the span of 15–20 minutes, several scenarios need to be considered. A common cause for the lack of improvement is an incomplete cantholysis. While the technique seems quite straightforward and is not difficult in experienced hands, in the setting of trauma (tight orbit with swollen lids, uncooperative patient, poor effectiveness of injected local anesthetics, etc.), an inferior cantholysis may prove difficult. The adequacy of the inferior cantholysis is crucial to the success of the procedure [45, 49]. One useful maneuver is to check the patient at the slit lamp following the cantholysis. In the setting of a tight orbit, a disinserted lateral canthus should move medially to the level of the lateral limbus (Fig. 6.12). If any eyelid margin is still noted in the vicinity of the lateral canthus, the cantholysis is incomplete, and another attempt at disinsertion should be made.

If the inferior cantholysis is indeed adequate, then two possibilities exist. First, too much time may have elapsed between the development of OCS and the cantholysis, and no additional therapy will be effective. Second, the inferior cantholysis, although complete, has not adequately decom-

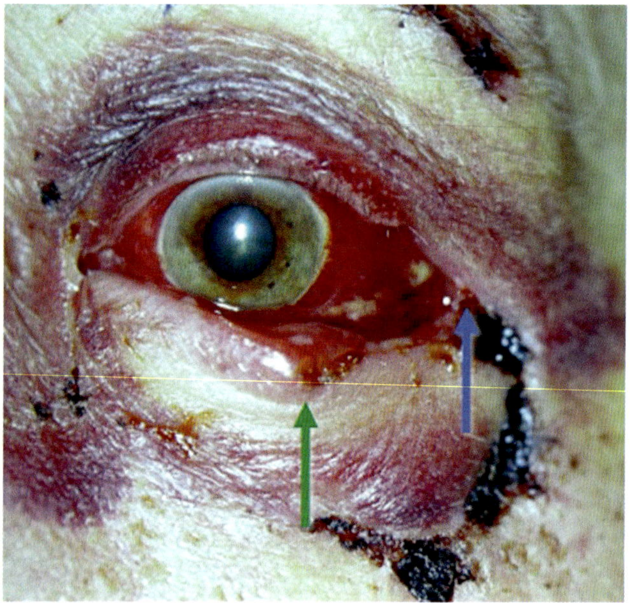

Fig. 6.12 Successful cantholysis. Note that in a tight orbit, the entire lateral eyelid (including the margin) should move from its original position at the lateral canthus (blue arrow) medially to a position near the lateral limbus (green arrow)

pressed the orbit. The differentiation between these two scenarios may be difficult, but IOP provides an important clue. As noted, Zoumalan and colleagues found that intraorbital pressure mirrored IOP fairly accurately [45]. A successful lateral canthotomy and inferior cantholysis decreased intraorbital pressure by 59% and IOP by 55%. Therefore, if visual function fails to improve in the setting of a successful inferior cantholysis and a marked reduction in IOP, in all likelihood, too much time has elapsed since the initial OCS. If the IOP remains high and additional therapy is warranted, then a superior cantholysis should be performed immediately, although this may not add any significant soft tissue release. Furthermore, because of the proximity and vascularity of the lacrimal gland, superior cantholysis usually results in significantly more bleeding than its inferior counterpart. An inferior septolysis (essentially a medial extension of the inferior cantholysis which opens the orbital septum transconjunctivally) is a simple adjunct to inferior cantholysis and is advocated by some experts [45]. Several anecdotal case reports have recommended a limited bony decompression of the orbital floor using a curved hemostat through the canthotomy incision in a blind fashion [52, 53]. The authors have never faced a clinical situation which necessitated this maneuver and caution that if performed, an operating room with anesthesia support be available in case of inadvertent laceration of the infraorbital artery either by the hemostat or the resultant bony fragments. If bony decompression is necessary, it is safest to proceed to the operating room and perform the surgery in a controlled fashion under direct visualization. In such cases, Dolman and colleagues have recommended a posterior decompression of the orbit [32]. Our preferred method (but certainly not the only method) is to perform with transnasal endoscopic decompression of the medial orbital wall posteriorly under image guidance, since this provides excellent visualization of the skull base and approaches an already tight orbital apex from an extraorbital approach, avoiding the soft tissue traction that is necessary during transorbital surgery. A large or expanding subperiosteal hematoma or loculated air collection can be removed using a variety of methods, including surgical drainage and syringe decompression [34].

Another issue of some contention is the not uncommon scenario of a patient who presents with recent injury, evidence of periocular edema and ecchymosis, and a varying amount of orbital congestion without any evidence of visual compromise. At what point does the clinician decide that the orbital process is no longer evolving and it is safe to discharge the patient? Once again, the evidence is anecdotal, and the decision is largely based on personal experience. A series by Hass et al. concluded that the highest risk for orbital hemorrhage following eyelid surgery occurred within the first 3 hours following the procedure and decreased significantly after 24 hours [54]. Other single case reports have demonstrated postoperative orbital hemorrhage days after the initial surgery [44, 54, 55]. A reasonable, though admittedly unproven, algorithm is to monitor the patient until 8 hours has elapsed from the initial injury [37]. In other words, if a patient presents 2 hours after injury and has evidence of orbital congestion, he should be followed closely for an additional 6 hours before discharge. This may be impractical for a variety of reasons. At the very least, any patient with recent trauma and periocular edema should be given detailed instruction on how to monitor visual function closely. An emergency number should also be provided so that the patient can be reevaluated immediately if increased pain, increased swelling, and/or decreased vision occur.

Lateral Canthotomy and Inferior Cantholysis: Surgical Technique

Compressive optic neuropathy from an orbital hemorrhage (OCS) is an ophthalmic emergency because of possible permanent visual loss. As already noted, the diagnosis is made clinically, and treatment should not be delayed while waiting for "confirmation" on imaging studies. The main surgical treatment of OCS is a soft tissue decompression of the orbit by lateral canthotomy and inferior cantholysis (Fig. 6.13). The procedure requires few instruments and is readily performed at the bedside.

Local anesthetic is infiltrated along the lateral canthus, with the needle always pointing away from the globe. The patient must be warned that despite anesthetic injection, a

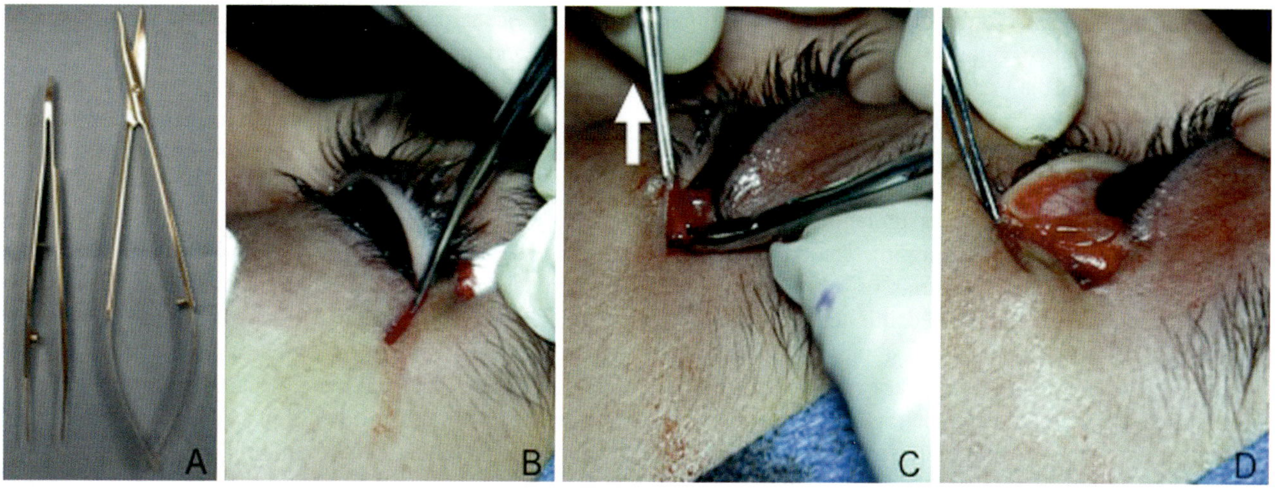

Fig. 6.13 Lateral canthotomy and inferior cantholysis. See text for details

significant amount of pain may be encountered during the procedure, since local anesthetic may not work effectively in already edematous, tense, and ischemic anatomy.

Only two instruments are needed for the procedure: a pair of *blunt*-tipped Westcott or curved Stevens scissors (Storz; #E3320 RS or E3562) and toothed 0.5 mm Castroviejo or Bishop-Harmon forceps (Storz; #E1798 or E1500) (Fig. 6.13a). With the patient in a supine position, a lateral canthotomy is performed by passing the posterior blade of the scissors along the conjunctival side of the lateral canthus and cutting across the canthus in a full-thickness fashion. No forceps are needed for this step (Fig. 6.13b). It is important to remember that a lateral canthotomy has limited decompressive effect and is performed primarily to provide access to the inferior crus of the lateral canthal tendon (LCT). The inferior cantholysis is performed next and provides definitive soft tissue decompression. Of note, the surgeon should not expect to see, palpate, or strum the inferior crus of the LCT. Instead, the surgeon will simply see and feel the lower lid release away from the globe. The cut edge of the lateral lower lid is grasped across the tarsal plate with toothed forceps, and the eyelid is pulled upward toward the ceiling (Fig. 6.13c). This upward traction is crucial to monitor the extent of the cantholysis. The scissors are then inserted into the wound, pointed toward the tip of the nose, and a subcutaneous incision across the eyelid is made just below the level of the tarsal plate (approximately 5 mm below the eyelid margin). Sharp dissection continues until a release of the eyelid away from the orbital rim is noted with the forceps (Fig. 6.13d). The release is not subtle: the eyelid should elevate markedly away from the globe (Fig. 6.14). Hemostasis is typically achieved with pressure over the lateral canthus.

Following successful inferior cantholysis, there is no rush to repair the lateral canthus. Several days may be needed to allow the orbit to soften completely, and up to one-third of patients will heal spontaneously.

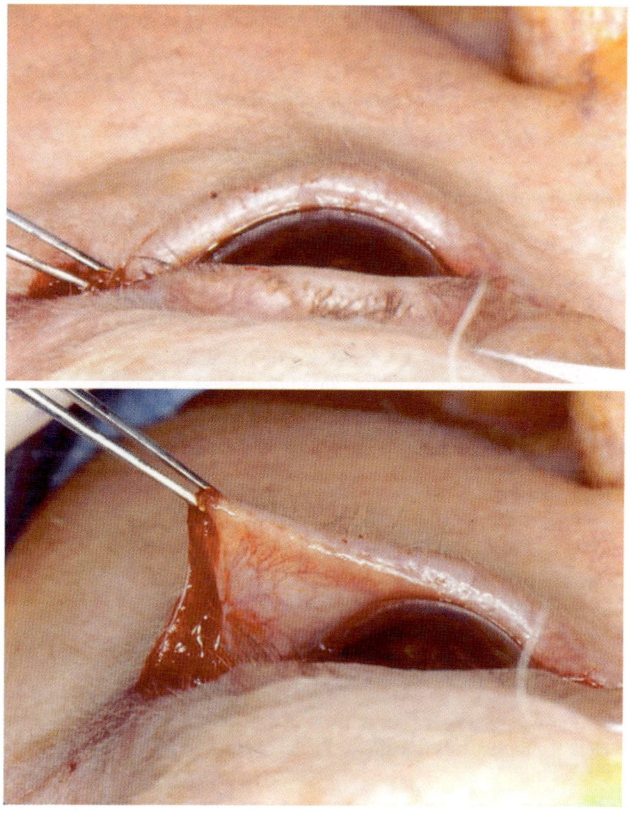

Fig. 6.14 Successful cantholysis. Top, original position of the lower eyelid as seen from above. Bottom, with successful cantholysis, the lower eyelid moves away from the lateral orbital rim dramatically

Management of Anticoagulants in the Trauma Setting

With regard to orbital hemorrhage, especially in the perioperative or peritraumatic period, three additional issues need to be considered: (1) the management of a patient's chronic anticoagulant therapy before and after periocular surgery, (2) the utility for anticoagulants in the perioperative or peritraumatic period for the prevention of deep vein thrombosis (DVT) and pulmonary embolism (PE), and (3) the increased risk of a thromboembolic (TE) event because of cessation or reduction of anticoagulant therapy [56].

The need to discontinue anticoagulants prior to periocular surgery is not clearly defined [56]. The patient and surgeon must weigh the potential risk of orbital hemorrhage and permanent visual loss with continued anticoagulation in the perioperative period against the known increased risk of TE events (stroke, pulmonary embolism, etc.) with discontinuance of anticoagulant therapy. One must also remember that surgery in general increases the potential for a TE event by 1.2% [57]. Dutton has estimated that if all anticoagulants were stopped in all patients undergoing ophthalmic or periocular surgery, a surgeon performing 1000 procedures annually should expect to encounter 1 TE event per year [57]. There is no easy answer to the common scenario of the anticoagulated patient who needs surgery, and any decision is based on stratification of risk [57, 58]. As a sweeping statement, the ophthalmologist alone should not make any decision regarding anticoagulant therapy in the perioperative period, but instead discuss this with the patient and communicate with the patient's primary care physician or cardiologist and then arrive at a consensus decision (Tables 6.1 and 6.2). There are also certain "absolutes" regarding anticoagulation that must be respected. Foremost of these is the critical need to continue low-dose aspirin *and* a $P2Y_{12}$ inhibitor (e.g., clopidogrel), also known as dual antiplatelet therapy (DAPT) therapy for at least 1 month following placement of a bare-metal coronary artery stent (BMS) and for at least 6 months following placement of a drug-eluting stent (DES) to prevent stent thrombosis [59]. Premature cessation of either drug increases the risk of myocardial infarction with a reported mortality rate of 40% [56]. Furthermore, elective noncardiac surgery should be delayed for at least 30 days follow-

Table 6.1 Properties of common anticoagulants

Agent generic name (trade name)	Mechanism of action	Anticoagulant effect (after the first dose)	Discontinue (preoperative)	Resume (postoperative)
Acetylsalicylic acid/aspirin	COX-1 and COX-2 inhibitor (decreases platelet aggregation)	Minutes	7–10 days	24–hours after hemostasis achieved
Warfarin (Coumadin)	Vitamin K antagonist	3–5 days	4–7 days (longer in older patients, higher INR)	Night of surgery for PM dosing. Morning after surgery for AM dosing
NSAID	Reversible platelet inhibition	3–5 days	Five times the specific drug's half-life	24–hours after hemostasis achieved
Clopidogrel (Plavix)	$P2Y_{12}$ inhibitor (irreversible platelet inhibition)	2 hours	5–7 days	24– hours after hemostasis achieved
Dabigatran (Pradaxa)	Factor IIa inhibitor	0.5–2 hours	2–5 days	24–hours after hemostasis achieved
Apixaban (Eliquis), edoxaban (Savaysa), rivaroxaban (Xarelto)	Factor Xa inhibitor	1–4 hours	2–4 days	24–hours after hemostasis achieved
Enoxaparin (Lovenox)	Factor Xa inhibitor	10 minutes if IV 3–5 hours if SC	1–4 hours if IV 8–12 hours if SC	12–24 hours after hemostasis achieved.
Heparin	Factor Xa inhibitor	Immediate if IV 20–60 minutes if SC	5 hours	12–24 hours after hemostasis achieved
Herbal supplements (the three Gs, vitamin E, etc.)	Platelet aggregation, among others	Variable	10–14 days	1 week after hemostasis achieved

Modified from Refs. [56, 57]. Used with permission of authors

NSAID nonsteroidal anti-inflammatory drug, *INR* international normalized ratio, *IV* intravenous, *SC* subcutaneous, *Three Gs* garlic, ginger, and *Ginkgo biloba*

Table 6.2 Relative risk of continued anticoagulation versus cessation of anticoagulation in low to moderate risk procedures

Preoperative decision	Total number of patients	Complication studied	Complication %	Permanent consequences
Continuation of anticoagulants	35,173	Excessive intraoperative or postoperative bleeding	3.0	None
Cessation of anticoagulants	29,588	Thromboembolic event	1.7 (0–9.5%)	Severe[a]

Modified from Ref. [57] Used with permission of author

[a]Includes pulmonary embolism, stroke, and death

ing placement of a BMS and at least 6 months following DES placement [59]. Note that these recommendations are also dependent on the stability of the individual patient's coronary artery disease.

Certain ophthalmic procedures (e.g., temporal artery biopsy, chalazion excision, and excision of eyelid lesion) carry little if any risk of causing an orbital compartment syndrome, and in such instances, anticoagulation may be continued, with the understanding that this may result in increased postoperative ecchymosis and prolonged postoperative blood oozing (Fig. 6.15). Eyelid surgery (e.g., ptosis repair and ectropion repair) carries a relatively low risk of OCS, but nevertheless, a risk still remains. In such cases, a clear discussion with the patient and the patient's primary care physician or cardiologist typically clarifies the relative risk and the patient's tolerance to accept the risk [56]. Orbital surgery carries the highest risk of OCS and permanent visual loss, and in most cases, anticoagulation should be discontinued if possible. If this is not feasible, then an elective procedure should be postponed, and other modalities may be offered. As an example, in an elderly, anticoagulated patient with an orbital fracture, it may be prudent for the surgeon to defer surgery, since a potential posttraumatic orbital deformity may be much more acceptable to the patient than permanent visual loss from orbital hemorrhage. In cases where deep orbitotomy and continued anticoagulation are necessary, the patient and family must understand that even with ideal surgical technique and postoperative care, OCS with permanent visual loss is possible.

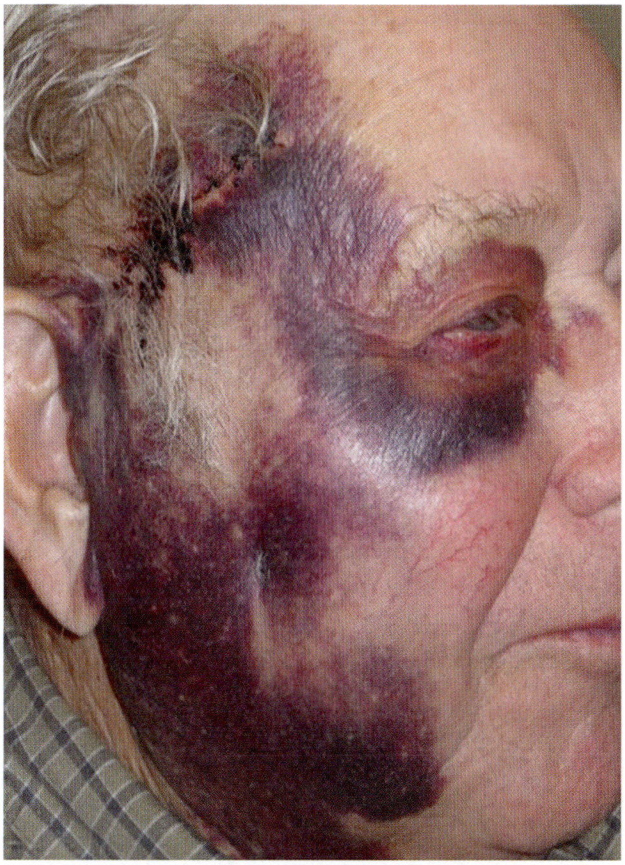

Fig. 6.15 Ecchymosis following temporal artery biopsy in a patient on warfarin therapy. Although the external appearance is dramatic, the fascial planes of the face and orbit prevent hemorrhage from extending into the orbital compartment, with essentially no risk of OCS

The role of anticoagulation for DVT/PE prevention in postoperative or posttrauma patients is still debated, but a significant pool of data exists to allow for a rational approach. Although anecdotal reports have described orbital hemorrhage in patients with orbital and midfacial fractures who were anticoagulated for prophylaxis against DVT [6], multiple large studies have also demonstrated an increased risk of DVT and PE in postoperative patients who are obtunded or cannot ambulate. As an example, in a small cohort of patients following neurosurgical procedures, Taniguchi et al. documented a DVT incidence of 13.5%, and 60% of those patients developed PE [60].

Most patients suffering from periocular trauma are young, can be ambulated immediately after repair, and are usually home within 24 hours of fracture repair, and in this group of patients, postoperative anticoagulation is a moot point. Similarly, older patients who are not on routine anticoagulation therapy and undergo outpatient periocular surgery also do not require specific DVT prophylaxis. However, this still leaves a significant group of patients who are immobile following severe head and bodily injury and may be obtunded or comatose. If concomitant orbital injury (e.g., fractures, hemorrhage, and penetrating injury) is present or if orbital surgery is being planned, the clinician is in a quandary regarding DVT prophylaxis. At the very least, all inpatients with orbital injuries involving intraorbital hemorrhage, awaiting surgery, or in the immediate postoperative period should be placed on intermittent pneumatic compression (IPC) therapy (unless a documented DVT is present in the leg) and encouraged to ambulate. Studies have shown that IPC alone decreases the incidence of DVT by two-thirds and PE by two-fifths, although these conclusions are not universal [61, 62]. Overall, oral anticoagulants appear to result in less postoperative hemorrhage than heparin and its derivatives, but they are also less effective in decreasing the risk of DVT and PE [61]. A meta-analysis by Kakkos and colleagues concluded that combination therapy (IPC plus anticoagulation) was more effective in reducing the postoperative incidence of DVT (0.65–1.6%) and PE (1.1%) than IPC alone (DVT = 4%; PE = 2.7%) or anticoagulation alone (DVT = 4.21%; PE data insufficient) [63]. Studies in the neurosurgical literature have also shown no increased risk of intracranial hemorrhage in patients who receive low molecular weight heparin (LMWH) therapy in combination with IPC and elastic stockings following craniotomy, although in many cases this therapy is delayed for 24–48 hours following surgery [64, 65]. The results of a meta-analysis by Dutton are summarized in Table 6.2. In this review, Dutton analyzed the incidence of "excessive bleeding" for procedures considered low to medium risk, including ophthalmic, dental, dermatologic, plastic surgical, gynecologic, and endoscopic (colonoscopy) surgery [57]. The analysis did not include higher risk categories such as neurosurgery and cardiothoracic surgery.

In patients at high risk for DVT, including those who are obtunded from concomitant intracranial injury or those immobilized because of other injuries, a detailed discussion with the primary team regarding anticoagulation should be documented, and the risks for and against such therapy should be discussed in detail with the patient and family. Based on the neurosurgical literature, it is reasonable to begin IPC therapy immediately and LMWH therapy in patients at high risk for DVT 24–48 hours after initial orbital trauma or orbital fracture repair if no active orbital hemorrhage is present and there is no evidence of OCS. Close clinical monitoring of visual function should be maintained in patients on LMWH in the immediate posttraumatic or postoperative period.

Posterior Indirect TON

The exact microscopic mechanism of PITON is not known with any degree of certainty, but the pattern of injury is elucidating. PITON is typically encountered in deceleration injury [66]. Simply put, the skull (usually the forehead) or, less commonly, the midface strikes a solid, immovable object. The bone absorbs the shock with two consequences. First, while the bony anatomy stops suddenly, the soft tissue anatomy of the head (including the orbit) continues to move forward until its native tensile strength tethers the tissue. As already noted, the orbital optic nerve has approximately 7 mm of excess length. Beyond this, a significant force is applied at the point of optic nerve tethering at the optic canal. As noted in the anatomy section, the meningeal optic nerve sheath is tightly bound to the annulus of Zinn and the periosteum of the optic canal, and the optic nerve is further tethered by a dural fold as it exists the canal intracranially [67]. As shearing forces are applied, the nutrient pial vessels supplying the optic nerve presumably tear, resulting in localized optic nerve infarction, leading to acute axonal loss [68]. Shearing injury may also occur directly within the optic nerve axons [2]. Subsequent optic nerve edema within the confines of the optic canal may result in a localized compartment syndrome, further ischemia, and a cascade of secondary injury by a variety of mechanisms, including free radical formation [17, 69]. Simultaneously, a shock wave from the bony impact is transmitted posteriorly [2]. Cadaver studies have shown that a blunt force applied to the forehead is transmitted toward the orbital apex and is concentrated in the area of the optic canal [70, 71]. This second mechanism may cause additional injury, including contusion to the intracanalicular optic nerve or direct injury from optic canal fracture. There is no treatment to reverse infarction to the optic nerve axons. The goal of PITON management is to decrease the expression of physiologic cascades that result in secondary injury in the hopes of diminishing progressive injury and perhaps reversing an ongoing noxious process.

Patients with PITON typically note visual loss immediately following the trauma. Progressive visual loss is distinctly uncommon in PITON, occurring in fewer than 10% of cases; when progressive visual loss is noted, other potential mechanisms should be investigated (evolving OCS, intraocular injury, etc.). Not surprisingly, PITON occurs most frequently in young males, who also have a relatively high incidence of traumatic brain injury (TBI) when compared to the general population [66, 72]. While a deceleration mechanism to the forehead is frequently encountered (motor vehicle accidents, bicycle accidents, etc.), trauma not involving deceleration injury can certainly occur (assault, etc.) [2, 73]. The diagnosis of PITON requires the absence of other intraocular or periocular injuries which could explain the visual loss. Thus, it would be difficult to make a diagnosis of PITON in a patient with a traumatic retinal detachment and an afferent pupillary defect, although both could certainly coexist. Similarly, it is essentially impossible to distinguish the degree of visual loss from direct versus indirect TON in a patient who suffered a deceleration injury that resulted in an OCS from hemorrhage [2]. Visual acuity in PITON spans the spectrum from normal to no light perception. Some degree of afferent pupillary defect and/or dyschromatopsia must be present to make the diagnosis. In acute cases, the optic nerve head appears normal on fundus examination. Many patients with PITON will have other head and neck injuries, including skull fracture, intracranial hemorrhage, and maxillofacial fractures, further complicating assessment, especially if mental status is compromised [72]. It is also important to note that 40–72% of patients with PITON have suffered loss of consciousness and may be considered as suffering from TBI; the significance of TBI will be discussed shortly [74]. Bilateral PITON may also occur, and it is important to remember that an afferent pupillary defect is a *relative* measure of optic nerve function; it is completely plausible for a patient to have an afferent pupillary defect from bilateral, asymmetric PITON or no afferent pupillary defect but significant visual loss from bilateral, symmetric PITON.

CT imaging is performed with particular attention to the skull base and optic canals [65]. In general, CT is not helpful in making the diagnosis or predicting the severity of PITON, but is performed for two reasons [2, 75, 76]: First, CT will help to rule out possible impingement on the

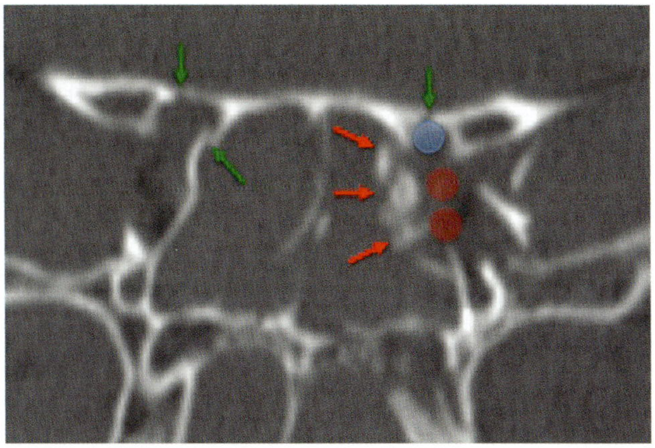

Fig. 6.16 Bilateral optic canal fractures and TON. Coronal CT (bone window) of a patient assaulted with a baseball bat. Initial ophthalmologic evaluation was limited by a comatose state, but a left afferent defect was noted. CT shows bilateral optic canal fractures (green arrows) along with comminuted fracture of the medial wall of the left cavernous sinus (red arrows). The approximate positions of the left optic nerve (blue circle) and carotid siphon (red circles) are noted. Corticosteroids were contraindicated because of the TBI. Decompressive surgery was not offered because the unstable skull base and the patient's tenuous neurologic status in the acute phase. Final vision was 20/80 OD and hand motions OS

intraorbital or intracanalicular optic nerve by bone fragments or other foreign bodies (Fig. 6.5). Second, CT provides a good assessment of the bony skull base anatomy and is helpful in diagnosing other fractures of the skull base (Fig. 6.16). MRI is not helpful in the initial diagnosis and management of PITON, but can be obtained for further assessment of the surrounding soft tissue anatomy (e.g., cavernous sinus and pituitary gland). Nonimpinging fractures of the optic canal are certainly seen in PITON, but this finding is of questionable significance: some experts argue that a nonimpinging optic canal fracture may in theory have the paradoxical benefit of decompressing the intracanalicular optic nerve.

In most cases, the diagnosis of PITON is relatively straightforward, but several caveats are worth mentioning [2]. First, as noted, care must be taken in initial trauma assessment to not prematurely exclude the possibility of contralateral optic nerve damage. Optic nerve assessment may be limited in an emergency room and inpatient setting, and subtle contralateral injury can therefore be missed. It is best not to make any conclusive, sweeping statements about the health of the contralateral optic nerve until a full assessment has been carried out at a later date. This is especially important in comatose or obtunded patients, in whom the degree of optic nerve function is impossible to assess with any certainty; the family should be informed at the outset of the limitations of the assessment and the potential for significant, permanent unilateral or bilateral visual loss. Second, it is extremely important to make the diagnosis of PITON as early as possible following trauma and to discuss this in detail with the patient and family. As already noted, it is not uncommon for concomitant injury to exist. Some patients will require urgent intracranial surgery or skull and facial fracture repair. The preoperative diagnosis and documentation of unilateral or bilateral PITON decreases the possibility of future claims of iatrogenic optic nerve injury.

Treatment of PITON

The treatment paradigm of PITON has changed significantly over the past two decades. Although this has been a contentious issue in the past, there is a growing consensus among orbital specialists that there is little, if any, effective treatment for PITON and that in the vast majority of cases, no intervention is indicated. That said, it is worthwhile to review the available evidence on this issue to allow the readers to come to their own conclusions.

Put succinctly, there are five potential management possibilities for PITON: (1) observation alone, (2) megadose intravenous corticosteroid therapy, (3) surgical decompression of the optic canal, (4) a combination of options 2 and 3, and (4) experimental modalities [2, 77].

Megadose Corticosteroids

The use of megadose intravenous corticosteroid therapy for PITON was popularized following the results of the National Acute Spinal Cord Injury Studies (NASCIS II and III), and in the past, the results were extended to the management of central nervous system injury [78, 79]. The NASCIS studies concluded that treatment of acute spinal cord injury using large amounts of intravenous methylprednisolone instituted within an 8-hour posttraumatic window resulted in a better final outcome than placebo alone. The dosages recommended were far higher than those usually used in neuro-ophthalmology: a 30 mg/kg loading dose of methylprednisolone followed by either a continuous infusion at 5.4 mg/kg/hour or a bolus dosing schedule of 15 mg/kg every 6 hours, for a total course of 48–72 hours [5]. This amounted to an average adult loading dose of 2 g of methylprednisolone followed by 1 g every 6 hours, compared to the recommended dose of 250 mg of intravenous methylprednisolone infused every 6 hours for acute optic neuritis from demyelinating disease [80]. This higher dose was justified by previous laboratory work showing an antioxidant effect that decreased free radical damage in the acute stage of central nervous system injury [69, 74, 81–86]. Megadoses also appeared to improve spinal cord microcirculation in animal models [84]. The ophthalmic community quickly embraced this potentially beneficial therapy for PITON, perhaps prematurely and erroneously extrapolating laboratory and clinical data related to spinal cord axons to the optic nerve, despite significant histopathologic differences between the two tissues [2, 77, 87, 88]. In addition, there was no known contraindication to the use of megadose corticosteroids in the setting of TBI; in fact, neurosurgeons had been using megadose corticosteroids routinely in the management of acute TBI for quite some time [89–92]. The only major downside of megadose corticosteroid therapy was the potential for significant systemic side effects, which could presumably be treated effectively if and when they occurred [66, 79, 93].

As the use of megadose corticosteroids in PITON became routine, it became painfully evident that there was little supportive clinical data on steroid efficacy in this disease [76, 94–97]. Any studies claiming efficacy were typically retrospective, non-randomized, and small. In fact, to date, no randomized, controlled study on the subject exists [2]. A valiant effort was made to better quantify efficacy in the multicenter International Optic Nerve Trauma Study (IONTS), but even this attempt was fraught with confounding factors, and no conclusive evidence could be found to support the use of corticosteroids. Other subsequent studies have also failed to find significant evidence for corticosteroid use. Although the IONTS failed to prove efficacy, it also did not show any detrimental effects on optic nerve function, and many practitioners continued to offer megadose corticosteroid therapy. However, at the turn of this century, new data emerged from several sources that effectively applied the brakes on the enthusiastic use of corticosteroids in PITON. First, an experimental study by Steinsapir and colleagues found that high-dose methylprednisolone exacerbated axonal loss in rodent optic nerves following crush injury [98]. Whether or not crush injury was a valid mechanism for studying PITON notwithstanding, the findings were disturbing for advocates of megadose corticosteroids. Second, several years prior, the NASCIS III study concluded that the institution of megadose corticosteroids after the initial 8-hour posttraumatic window in spinal cord injury was detrimental to final outcome. If a parallelism of optic nerve and spinal cord injury were to be followed, then one would have to conclude that corticosteroid therapy should not be offered to PITON patients outside of this initial 8-hour window.

Finally and perhaps most importantly, a landmark study on the use of megadose corticosteroids in TBI was published in 1997 [2, 92]. The Corticosteroid Randomization After Significant Head Injury Trial, also known as the CRASH study, followed over 10,000 patients with TBI prospectively. The study found a small but statistically significant increase in neurologic morbidity and mortality in TBI patients treated with corticosteroids when compared to placebo – a finding with enough significance that further enrollment in the study was stopped. The neurosurgical community in general embraced the findings of the study and ceased the routine use of megadose corticosteroids in TBI [99, 100].

So what stance does the oculoplastic surgeon take regarding the use of megadose corticosteroids in PITON? The evidence, although admittedly not perfect, can be summarized thusly:

1. The IONTS showed no significant benefit of corticosteroid therapy in the treatment of PITON.
2. Three sequential Cochrane meta-analyses found no conclusive evidence that megadose corticosteroids are effective in PITON [2, 101, 102].
3. The NASCIS studies concluded that megadose corticosteroid therapy outside of the initial 8-hour posttraumatic window was detrimental. There are criticisms of the NASCIS results, citing possible randomization bias [2, 74, 103].
4. The NASCIS studies found an increased risk of systemic side effects (sepsis, pneumonia) potentially related to corticosteroid therapy.
5. Animal models of optic nerve crush injuries (again, may not apply to the actual mechanism of PITON) showed a detrimental effect of high-dose corticosteroid therapy.
6. The CRASH study showed an increased long-term morbidity and mortality in patients with TBI who received megadose corticosteroids.

Based on these findings, at present, the clinician is hard pressed to recommend either high- or low-dose corticosteroids therapy to any patient presenting with PITON, especially if the initial 8-hour window has expired or the patient has concomitant TBI [74]. It appears that, regarding the medical management of PITON, we are back to the proverbial "square one" of observation alone. One might still argue that the rare patient who presents within the 8-hour window, is otherwise healthy, and has no evidence of TBI might be offered the option of megadose corticosteroids along with a detailed discussion of the limited efficacy data and potential systemic side effects of corticosteroid therapy, but for the vast majority of patients with PITON, corticosteroid therapy is no longer a valid option [2]. The results of the CRASH study also place a sobering onus on the ophthalmologist: would anyone recommend corticosteroids for PITON based on dubious data in the face of solid evidence that corticosteroids are detrimental for TBI? *Primum non nocere* comes to mind.

Optic Canal Decompression

The optic nerve is tightly encased within the optic canal, and hemorrhage or edema can potentially result in a compartment syndrome. One rationale for optic canal decompression is to open this bony compartment, presumably releasing pressure on the intracanalicular optic nerve in the hopes of limiting or reversing injury. A variety of techniques have been described for canal decompression, including an external transethmoidal approach, a transcranial approach, and most recently an endoscopic transnasal approach, with or without intraoperative image guidance. Sofferman hypothesized that three criteria were necessary for adequate optic canal decompression: removal of one-half of the optic canal diameter, removal of bone along the entire length of the canal, and incision of the optic nerve sheath [104]. Whether all three criteria are achieved intraoperatively on a routine basis is debatable.

The efficacy of this procedure remains largely unproven. No randomized controlled studies exist, and reported series are small with multiple confounding factors. One recurring feature in most series on optic canal decompression is an inherent selection bias toward more severe cases of TON [105]. Typically, optic canal decompression in the published reports is reserved for patients with poor baseline visual function, limited or no perceived response to corticosteroid therapy, or a combination of the two. Since the prognosis for visual recovery in TON is at least in part due to initial severity of visual loss, such selection bias gravitates to patients who will predictably have a poorer prognosis, making it difficult to assess the true effectiveness (or ineffectiveness) of the procedure [105]. In addition, optic canal decompression has its own set of inherent risks, many of which are significant. Because of the proximity of critical skull base structures, including the brain, cavernous sinus, pituitary gland, and carotid artery, as well as unstable posttraumatic bony anatomy, decompressive surgery may have potentially devastating consequences [106, 107]. The IONTS noted a 10% incidence of cerebrospinal fluid leakage and one case of meningitis [66]. Rare anecdotal, unpublished reports of carotid laceration and death have also circulated among the orbital community. A meta-analysis of available data concluded there was no evidence to support the efficacy of optic canal decompression in PITON [105]. In addition, the intracanalicular optic nerve may be vulnerable to injury during attempted surgical decompression because of the inherent anatomy of the optic canal. A study by Onufrey and colleagues demonstrated a tethered anatomic complex consisting of the bony optic canal, dural/periosteal adhesions, and the intracanalicular optic nerve [17]. Potential iatrogenic optic nerve compression during bony elevation and laceration of nutrient vessels or axons during incision of the neural sheath was noted in cadaver specimens, and possible thermal and vibrational injury from microdrill use was also posited by the authors [17].

A second potential indication for optic canal decompression is the removal of impinging fragments on the optic nerve. Since this type of direct trauma is not the same mechanism postulated for PITON, efficacy once again comes into question, since a grouping of surgical results for different forms of TON may be invalid [105].

Given the unproven efficacy of the procedure, the technical difficulty of the procedure (especially in the presence of a fractured, unstable skull base), and the recent report by Onufrey et al., optic canal decompression at best should be offered in only a minority of TON cases (possibly only to those patents with significant bone impingement from infracturing of the canal) and only if a skilled endoscopic surgeon or neurosurgeon with extensive skull base experience is available [17]. The potential risks of the procedure should be discussed in detail with the patient and/or family.

Experimental Modalities

Although a variety of medications and modalities have been offered for the treatment of PITON, two stand out as having gained at least a foothold: erythropoietin (EPO) and transcorneal electrical stimulation (TES).

EPO is a renally produced cytokine that promotes hematopoiesis. Numerous studies have shown a neuroprotective effect of EPO, with reduction of neuronal apoptosis, inflammation, ischemia, and oxidative stress in traumatic and ischemic models [108–114]. The drug has been studied in both cerebral and myocardial ischemia and in spinal cord injury. That said, to date, EPO is not considered standard of care in the treatment of stroke. An animal model of optic nerve transection treated with EPO has also been published [115].

In 2010, Kashkouli and colleagues published a nonrandomized, pilot study of three doses of intravenous EPO used to treat seven patients with PITON and compared the results to eight PITON patients managed with observation alone [116]. They found a statistically significant improvement in final best corrected visual acuity (BCVA) in the EPO group. However, a subsequent open-label, phase 3, multicenter study of 100 patients (69 treated with EPO at 20,000 units/day for 3 days in adults, 15 with methylprednisolone 250 mg four times daily for 3 days, and 16 with observation) found no statistically significant difference in BCVA, although the EPO group did have a statistically significant improvement in color vision (the authors noted that not all patients had documented color vision testing) [117]. As already mentioned, neither the patient nor the investigator was masked to the treatment. Randomization was attempted, but could not be achieved, resulting in the skewed treatment groups listed. Intravitreal EPO for PITON treatment has also been reported in one study [118]. The authors concluded improvement in BCVA, visually evoked response (VER) amplitude, and VER latency. However, the study was small, nonrandomized, and without a strict methodology.

At present, any definitive conclusion for the use of EPO for the treatment of PITON cannot be made, since the available evidence is limited by study design, low power, and the lack of randomization and masking; EPO should *not* be considered as standard of care for the management of PITON.

TES has been studied for a variety of optic nerve pathologies, including PITON. The exact mechanism of TES efficacy on the optic nerve is not well understood [119–122].

An upregulation after TES of insulin-like growth factor 1 may play a role [123]. In 2006, Fujikado and colleagues published limited data on the efficacy of TES in TON [119]. Four of five patients with TON showed an improvement in BCVA. However, the study had no control arm and lacked statistical power. Two of the authors (APM, JRB) have just completed a study on the use of TES in PITON and found an improvement in BCVA in the PITON patients ($p = 0.001$) but not in the sham patients ($p = 0.628$); however, the difference between the two groups was not statistically significant ($p = 0.114$). Similar to EPO, at present, TES should *not* be considered as a standard treatment for PITON.

Prognosis for PITON

The prognosis for visual recovery in PITON is highly variable and unpredictable. Overall, spontaneous recovery occurs in 40–60% of patients with PITON managed with observation alone (Fig. 6.17) [2, 124]. The IONTS found that 57% of untreated patients recovered ≥ three lines of Snellen visual acuity at 1 month and 50% at 3 months [66]. In general, patients presenting with 20/200 or better vision fare better than those with initial vision of hand motions or worse. Initial no-light-perception vision is a poor prognostic factor, as are the loss of consciousness and lack of improvement

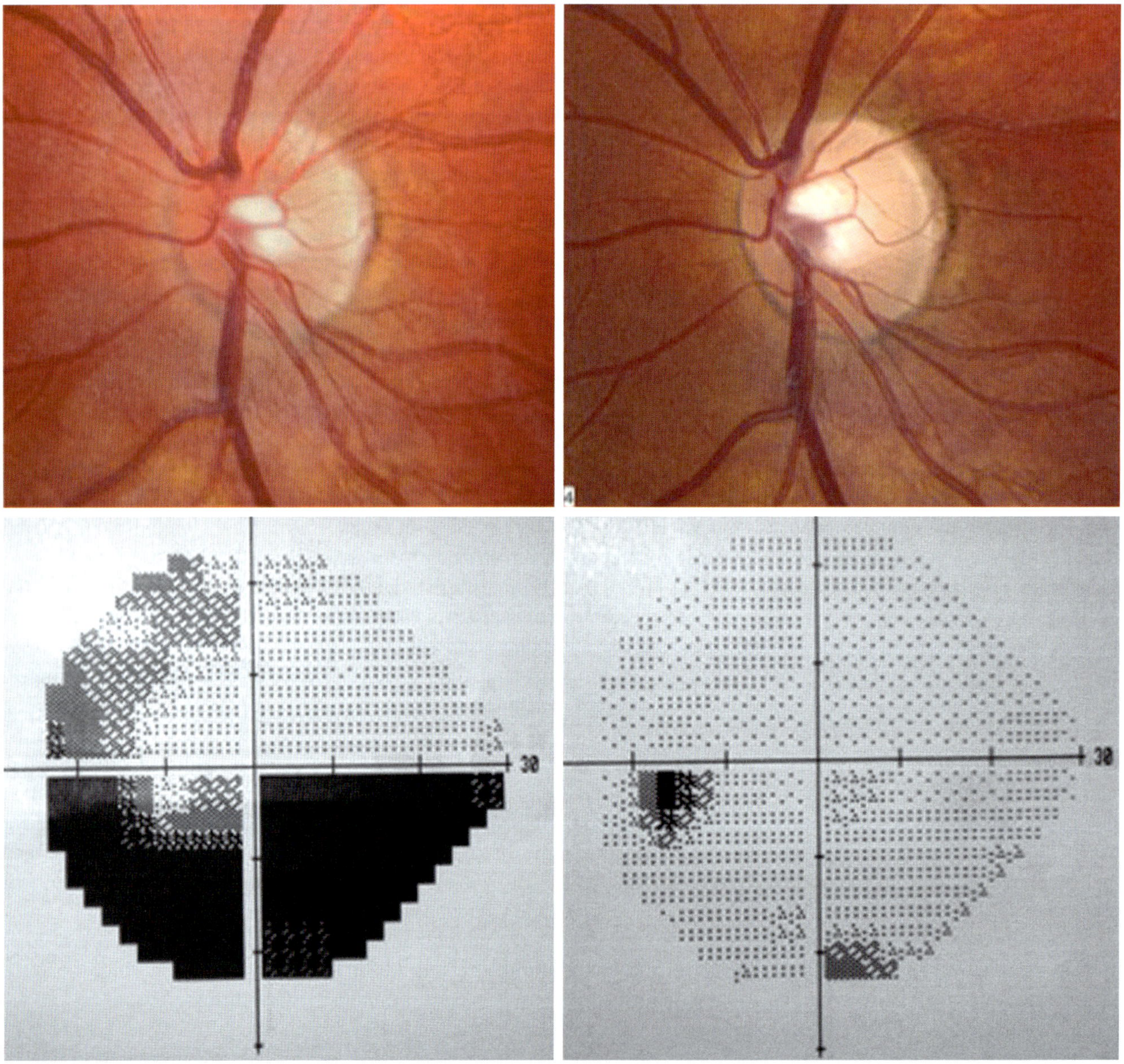

Fig. 6.17 Spontaneous visual recovery in TON. A 17-year-old female presented with counting fingers vision OS secondary to TON. Initial exam revealed a normal optic disc and a dense inferior arcuate defect (left). She was followed without treatment. On follow-up 3 months later, vision improved to 20/30, and the visual field cleared markedly, despite the development of optic nerve pallor (right)

over the initial 48 hours [2, 125]. The presence of optic canal fracture is not an accurate prognosticator.

Based on the available evidence, the authors presently do not recommend any therapeutic intervention in the vast majority of patients with PITON.

Chiasmal Injury and Posterior Optic Nerve Avulsion

Chiasmal injury is rare and may occur by a variety of mechanisms. Deceleration injury may result in chiasmal contusion, subarachnoid or pituitary bleeding may secondarily affect the chiasm, penetrating intracranial injury may lacerate portions of the chiasm, or posterior optic nerve avulsion may extend to the chiasm. Regardless of the mechanism, suspected chiasmal injury on clinical exam typically leads to neuroimaging to better assess the skull base and any associated intracranial injuries. Because of the proximity of the pituitary gland, detailed imaging of this region is warranted, and the patient should be followed closely by the primary team for the development of diabetes insipidus and Addisonian crisis.

In a related note, posterior avulsion of the optic nerve in many cases results from an identical mechanism as that seen in optic nerve head avulsion [22]. On occasion, severe TBI, as seen in high-speed motor vehicle accidents or other blunt force trauma, can result in either avulsion or laceration of the posterior optic nerve [22, 24, 126]. Gouging and biting of the eye have also resulted in optic nerve avulsion (Fig. 6.18) [28, 29]. The avulsion may occur at any point of the skull base from the orbital side of the optic canal to the chiasm itself. Because the ophthalmic artery abuts the optic nerve and is partially bound to it in this region, ophthalmic artery laceration may result in orbital hemorrhage. EOM avulsion may be found on subsequent orbital exploration. As with optic nerve head avulsions, the globe need not be enucleated if enough anterior arterial supply is present, although this may be difficult to gauge in the acute stage. Certainly, if concomitant ophthalmic artery injury is present, the risk of ocular and orbital ischemia increases. In rare cases, avulsion of the ophthalmic artery at its origin on the internal carotid artery can lead to significant subarachnoid bleeding and carotid arterial vasospasm with severe neurologic sequelae (Fig. 6.19) [126–129]. Once the patient has been stabilized, formal visual field testing should be performed to rule out the possibility of chiasmal injury and contralateral visual field deficits [130, 131].

One subtype of optic nerve avulsion is worth mentioning. Autoenucleation, also known as oedipism, typically occurs in schizophrenic patients or secondary to drug-induced psychosis [132]. The reasoning by the patient for such self-inflicted injury varies but may involve the delusion that the eyes are responsible for a variety of unwanted, evil thoughts and may include the biblical invocation found in the Book

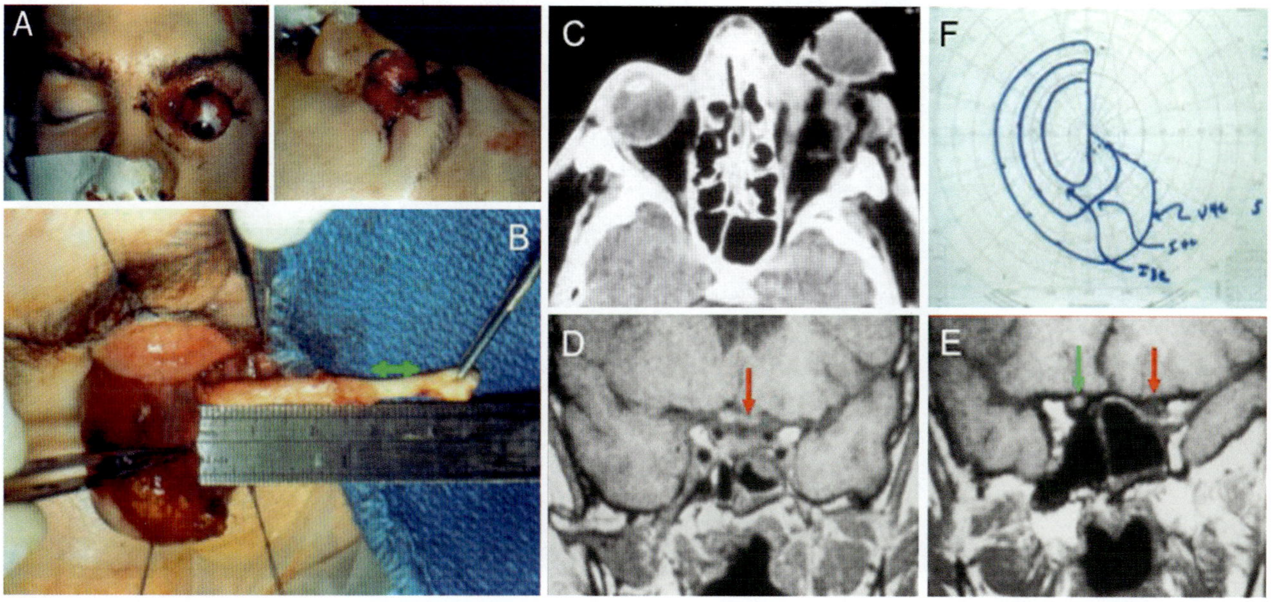

Fig. 6.18 Posterior optic nerve avulsion with chiasmal injury. (**a**) Clinical photographs. (**b**) Intraoperatively, the avulsed optic nerve was identified, measured, and reposited in the orbit. Note that the intracanalicular portion of the optic nerve (green arrow) is devoid of overlying dura, which remained tethered in the optic canal. (**c**) Initial CT demonstrating posterior avulsion of the left optic nerve. (**d**) On subsequent MRI (T-1 weighted), note the asymmetry of the anterior chiasm, with the edge of the avulsion identified by the arrow. (**e**) Coronal MRI (T-1 weighted) of the optic canals demonstrates a normal-appearing right intracanalicular optic nerve (green arrow) and an empty optic canal on the left except for a cuff of residual optic nerve sheath (red arrow). (**f**) Subsequent perimetry OD shows a chiasmal defect. (Courtesy of Peter A. D. Rubin, MD)

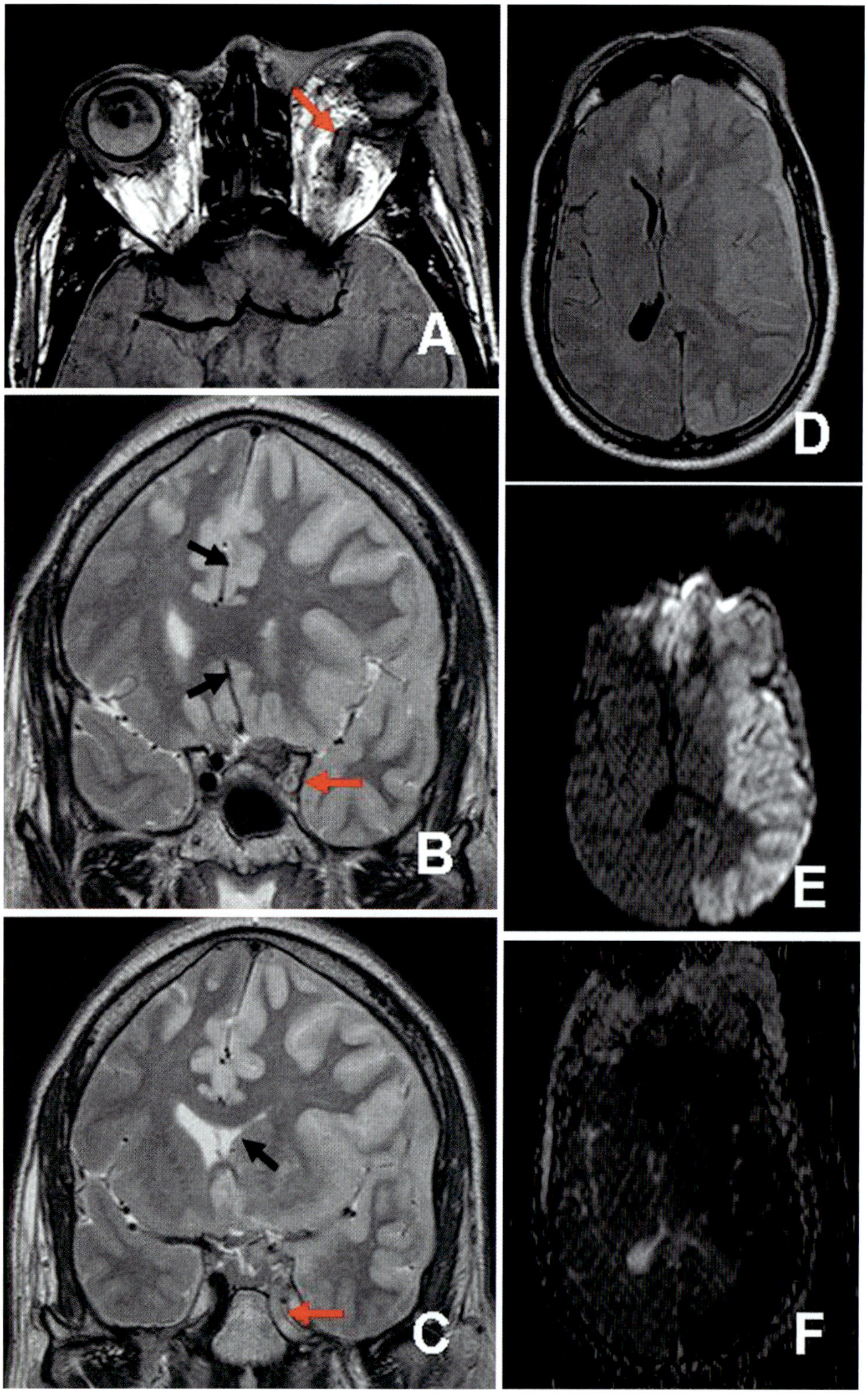

Fig. 6.19 Serial oedipism in a patient with schizoaffective disorder resulting in intracranial injury and death. (**a**) Two days after attempted autoenucleation of the right eye with resultant diffuse vitreous hemorrhage and possible optic nerve head avulsion, the patient autoenucleated the left eye and immediately became unresponsive. On T1-weighted MRI, a lax and kinked left optic nerve is noted (arrow), consistent with posterior optic nerve avulsion. (**b**) On coronal T2-weighted imaging, thrombosis and complete occlusion of the carotid siphon within the cavernous sinus is noted (red arrow). Midline shift is also obvious (black arrows). (**c**) Coronal T2-weighted image shows thrombus and no flow through the left internal carotid artery (red arrow), compared to the normal flow void of the right carotid artery. Note nearly complete effacement of the left lateral ventricle (black arrow). (**d**) Axial FLAIR image demonstrating left hemispheric infarction with involvement of the right frontal lobe. (**e**) Diffusion image of the infarcted area. (**f**) ADC map. In all likelihood, the ophthalmic artery avulsed near its root at the time of the optic nerve injury, with resultant dissection of the internal carotid artery, hemispheric stroke, cerebral edema, and brain death

of Matthew that "if thy right eye offend thee, pluck it out." [130, 132] The avulsion may occur at any point along the optic nerve course, with most occurring between 15–30 mm from the posterior sclera [130]. In such cases, it is important to remind the psychiatry team caring for the patient that there is a high risk of a contralateral autoenucleation attempt and that appropriate patient supervision should be established [132–135]: in a review of the literature, Krauss et al. noted that sequential, bilateral autoenucleation occurred in 38% of reported patients, with an additional 12% making an unsuccessful contralateral attempt [130]. Patients with oedipism also appear to be at higher risk for suicide [132, 133].

Injury to the Motor Nerves of the Orbit

Injury to the oculomotor (CN-III), trochlear (CN-IV), and abducens (CN-VI) nerves can occur at any point along their course along the skull base. As a general rule, traumatic ocular motor neuropathy is associated with relatively severe TBI (lower Glasgow Coma Score (GCS)) and may affect one or more cranial nerves either unilaterally or bilaterally. Good data on the subject comes from a retrospective study from the University of Michigan, which compared a group of TBI patients without ocular motor palsy to a group with single or multiple palsy [136]. When compared to a control group of patients with head trauma but no resultant ocular motor nerve injury, Dhaliwal and colleagues found that in the cohort with traumatic ocular motor palsies not only was the GCS lower (a lower number indicates more severe TBI), but also this group of patients had a higher rate of ocular, optic nerve, ocular adnexal, and chest injuries [136]. In addition, patients with ocular motor palsy had a much higher rate of craniofacial fractures (49% compared to 13% in controls) and radiographic findings of intracranial injury (67% vs 4% in controls) (Fig. 6.20) [136].

The findings by Dhaliwal and colleagues are supported by previous, smaller studies on the subject, and the overall findings are worth a succinct summary. First, craniofacial fractures are present in >50% of patients with ocular motor nerve injury [137–139]. Second, there appears to be little correlation between the location of TBI and craniofacial fracture on imaging and the specific ocular motor palsy, with the exception that CN-III dysfunction seems to be associated with a higher rate of temporal lobe injury. This is an important point to remember. Multiple small studies have posited various mechanisms and anatomic locations for cranial nerve injury based on neuroimaging, when in fact the injury may occur at any point or points along the course of the individual cranial nerve [1, 140–146]. Third, the rate of loss of consciousness (LOC) (>80%) was equal among patients with and without traumatic ocular motor palsy. Therefore, the presence of LOC is not a good predictor of motor palsy incidence. That said, multiple studies have shown that mild TBI, as defined by no LOC, is unlikely to result in ocular motor injury [136].

One limitation of Dhaliwal et al.'s analysis is possible selection bias, which may have skewed both patient cohorts to more severe TBI overall. Coello and colleagues have reported a large series of patients with a variety of traumatic cranial neuropathies after seemingly mild TBI (GCS 14–15) [147]. In this study, the olfactory (CN-I) and facial (CN-VII) nerves were affected more frequently (27% and 22%, respectively) than the ocular motor nerves (CN-VI 16%, CN-III 14%, CN-IV 14%). However, on further analysis of the authors' data, only 19 patients with either isolated or multiple CN-III, CN-IV, and CN-VI injury were identified out of 16,440 total patients with mild TBI. This calculates to an incidence rate of ocular motor injury in mild TBI of only

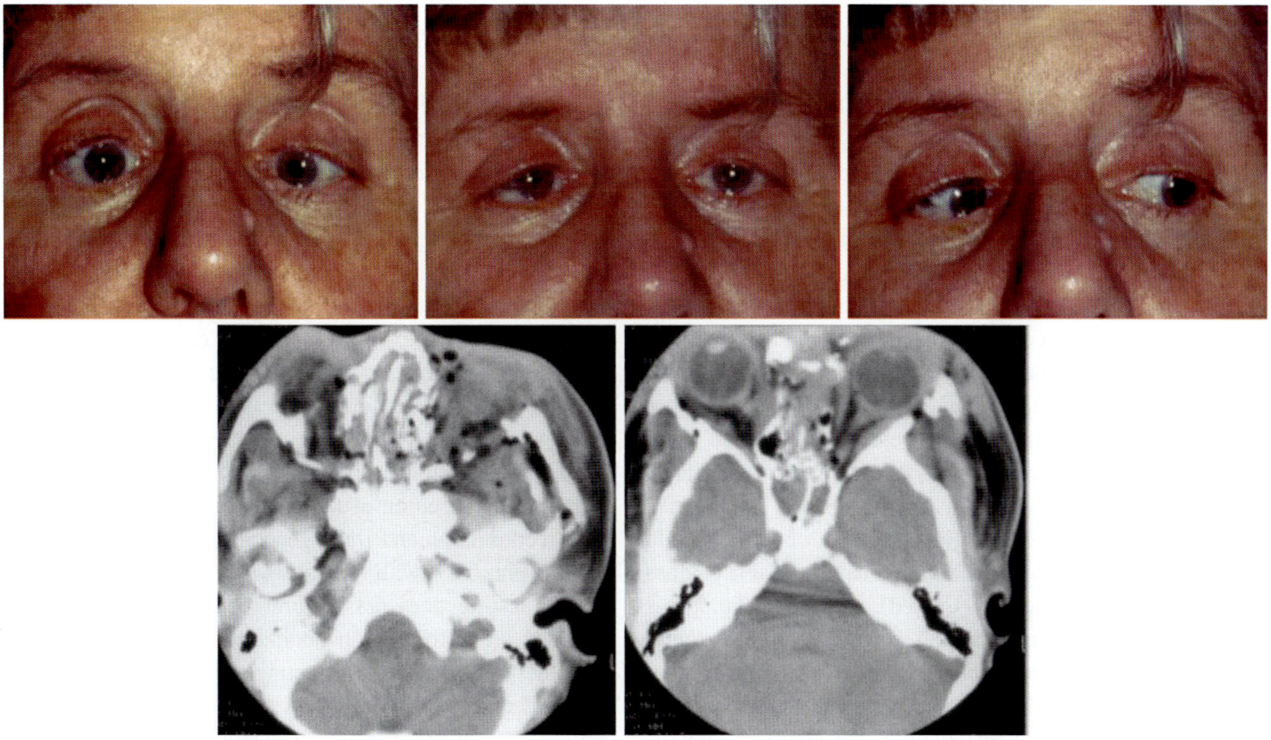

Fig. 6.20 Ocular motor palsy and craniofacial fractures. Right CN-VI palsy and left CN-VI paresis associated with LeFort III fractures (top clinical photos, bottom axial CT scans)

0.12%, consistent with Dhaliwal et al.'s conclusion that mild TBI is unlikely to result in ocular motor nerve injury. As a corollary, Dhaliwal and colleagues prudently recommend that if ocular motor injury is present in the setting of mild TBI, other etiologies (aneurysm, intracranial tumor, etc.) should be considered and appropriately investigated [136, 148–151].

Among the three ocular motor nerves, CN-III injury is associated with the lowest GCS [136]. In other words, CN-IV and CN-VI palsies overall occur with less severe TBI than CN-III dysfunction. In addition, patients with isolated CN-VI injury needed less inpatient rehabilitation than other groups, suggesting that this subgroup had the least severe injuries overall (head and body). Somewhat counterintuitively, patients with multiple traumatic cranial neuropathies had a higher GCS than those with isolated CN-III injury in Dhaliwal et al.'s analysis; although additional detailed data is not available in the manuscript, one possibility is that the cohort of multiple motor nerve palsies mainly included bilateral CN-IV and CN-VI injuries or the combination of CN-IV and CN-VI, and this supposition is somewhat supported by the authors' finding that bilateral CN-IV palsy occurred with mild TBI [136].

Diagnosis

Ideally, a definitive diagnosis of traumatic ocular motor nerve injury should be made in an awake and cooperative patient with no other confounding posttraumatic processes. Since cranial nerve injury is related to the severity of TBI, a careful history is helpful in distinguishing traumatic cranial neuropathy from that due to other etiologies where the head trauma was an incidental, noncontributory issue. Pupillary and eyelid examinations are important (see Chap. 13), since these structures may be affected and often offer a clue to the nature of the patient's posttraumatic diplopia. The circumstance related to the initial injury should also be documented carefully, especially in the more chronic phase, since patients may perceive a secondary gain based on the severity of their symptoms. Leading questions by the physicians are usually counterproductive in this regard; it is best to allow the patient to describe their diplopia symptoms and, when necessary, to fine-tune the history by asking open-ended questions. As a first order of business, the clinician should determine whether or not the diplopia is binocular (i.e., does it resolve when either eye is covered); monocular diplopia is not due to cranial neuropathy and, if present, should prompt an investigation for intraocular pathology (corneal, lenticular, macular, etc.). If binocular diplopia is indeed present, then the pattern should be elicited, and additional details of the history should be sought: Is it horizontal, vertical, or oblique? Does it change with gaze or head position? Is the pattern constant or intermittent and variable? Are there other systemic symptoms (headache, nausea/vomiting, shortness of breath, dysphagia, extremity weakness, etc.)? What is the temporal relationship between the onset of diplopia and the trauma? What was the initial workup following trauma? Was neuroimaging performed, and if so, what type (CT, MRI) and what were the findings (specifically, was orbital or skull fracture found)?

Once the history is obtained, a complete ocular and adnexal examination should be performed, including a bilateral dilated funduscopic examination. This tenet is especially important in the acute phase to not only rule out concomitant intraocular injury or globe rupture but also assess the fundus for any signs related to subarachnoid hemorrhage (Terson syndrome) or increased intracranial pressure (papilledema). Of note, initial pupillary dilation may be contraindicated in acute cases of TBI, since pupillary examination may be the only reliable initial method of following the patient neurologically; the ophthalmologist should clear the use of mydriatic agents with either the primary trauma team or the neurosurgical consultant, and the instillation of mydriatics should be clearly discussed with the nursing staff and documented in the patient's chart and details posted above the patient's bed. The extraocular motility should first be checked grossly with ductions and versions and then more precisely using prism bars in the cardinal gazes. A head tilt examination is critical in any patient complaining of vertical or oblique diplopia (see CN-IV injury below).

Isolated, unilateral CN-III and CN-VI palsy is relatively straightforward to diagnose using these techniques. CN-IV, multiple, or bilateral ocular motor nerve injury may make diagnosis more difficult. Furthermore, if the patient is obtunded or comatose, initial diagnosis may be impossible and is further confounded if there is significant concomitant orbital injury and associated hemorrhagic edema. Globe position in primary gaze and extraocular motility may be abnormal due to single cranial neuropathy, multiple cranial neuropathies, soft tissue entrapment within orbital fractures, soft tissue edema, extraocular muscle contusion or laceration, or any combination of the aforementioned factors.

Forced duction and force generation testing may be helpful in some cases, with the caveat that patient cooperation and associated clinical findings may significantly affect any accurate interpretation of these maneuvers. The techniques for forced duction and force generation testing are summarized in Fig. 6.21, with several tips listed here. First, forced duction testing does not require the patient's cooperation and may be performed on obtunded or comatose patients; conversely, force generation testing necessitates the patient's assistance. Second, the use of viscous lidocaine gel on the conjunctiva greatly reduces discomfort during testing, improving the accuracy of test. Third, although a variety of fixation points on the globe can be used to perform the test,

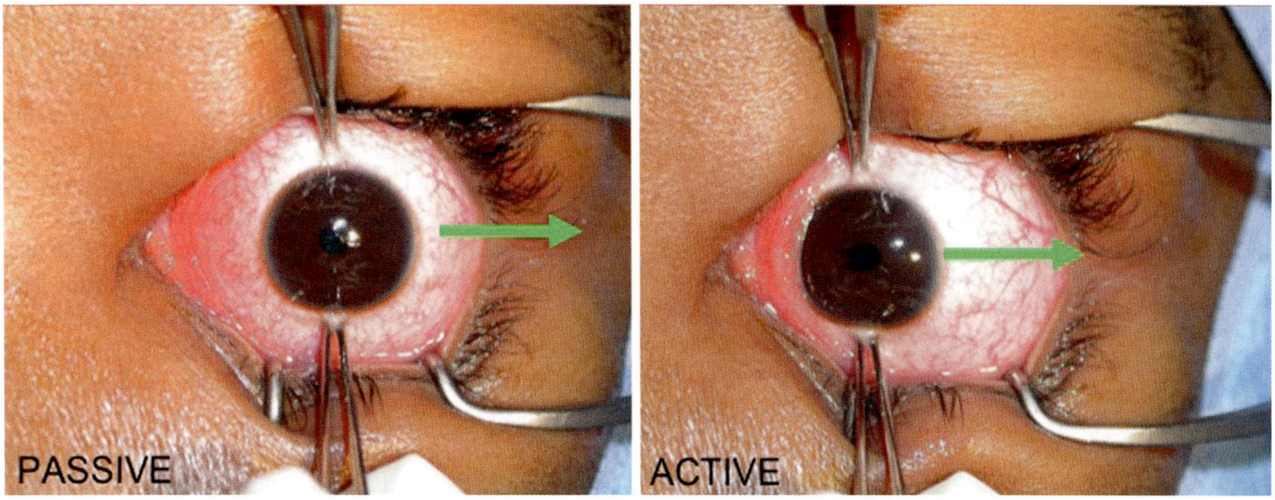

Fig. 6.21 Forced duction and force generation testing. Left, to test for medial rectus muscle restriction, the limbus is grasped at 6 and 12 o'clock, and the globe is rotated temporally. Forced duction testing is a passive test from the patient's standpoint. Right, to test for CN-VI paresis, the globe is grasped and rotated medially. The patient is then asked to actively abduct the eye while the examiner maintains resistance. Force generation testing requires patient participation. The lid speculum (shown in these intraoperative photos) is usually not necessary

the authors' preferred method is the use of two large-toothed forceps (0.5 mm Castroviejo or Bishop-Harmon) on the limbus 90° from the EOM being tested to minimize the chance of corneal abrasion. The novice tester will have a tendency to grasp minimal tissue in an effort to reduce iatrogenic injury, when in fact this technique increases the risk of corneal abrasion and conjunctiva laceration. It is best to open the forceps and, on opposites edges of the limbus, to push the globe into the orbit and then close the forceps around the limbal tissue, thereby providing a firm grasp on the globe.

In a forced duction test, the globe is moved away from the muscle and the surrounding orbital soft tissue that are potentially entrapped (e.g., abducting the eye if medial rectus muscle restriction is suspected). If resistance to movement is noted, then there is an abnormality in the orbital soft tissue, although the specific pathology cannot be determined by forced duction testing. In other words, the examiner cannot distinguish muscle entrapment from orbital fat entrapment, muscle edema, etc.

A force generation test is performed if EOM paresis is suspected, usually due to cranial nerve dysfunction. As already noted, this test requires patient cooperation. The patient is first asked to look in the direction opposite of the presumed paresis (e.g., if a CN-VI palsy is suspected, then the patient is asked to adduct the eye). The limbus is grasped 90° from the EOM being tested with two toothed forceps, and the patient is then asked to look in the direction of the paresis (in the case of CN-VI paresis, to abduct the eye) while the examiner maintains tension on the globe in the opposing direction. If the muscle and supplying nerve are normal, force is generated. If, on the other hand, paresis is present, then no or little force generation is perceived by the examiner. An abnormal force generation test indicates poor muscle function, which can be due to a variety of causes, including cranial nerve palsy, muscle paresis from contusion injury, or muscle laceration.

As already noted, because of the complex nature of craniofacial trauma, forced duction and force generation testing may not be helpful in making a definitive diagnosis of cranial neuropathy in many cases, especially in the early post-traumatic stage, when concomitant soft tissue swelling and decreased patient cooperation make interpretation difficult. Orbital computed tomography may be helpful in such cases.

Oculomotor Nerve (CN-III) Injury

The oculomotor nerve supplies three rectus muscles (medial, superior, and inferior), the inferior oblique muscle, and the levator palpebrae superioris (levator) muscle. It also carries parasympathetic nerve supply to the orbit from the Edinger-Westphal nucleus. The CN-III nucleus is located in the midbrain with a topographical distribution of subnuclei related to specific muscles. Three anatomic pearls should be remembered regarding these subnuclei: (1) Only one midline subnucleus supplies both levator muscles. (2) The supply to the superior rectus muscles is crossed, with fibers traveling through the opposite subnucleus before exiting the midbrain. Thus, if one superior rectus subnucleus is involved in pathology (hemorrhage, stroke, etc.), both superior rectus muscles will likely be affected. (3) The remaining subnuclei are paired and supply the ipsilateral muscles.

CN-III fascicles exit the cerebral peduncle and form the trunk of the oculomotor nerve, traveling between the supe-

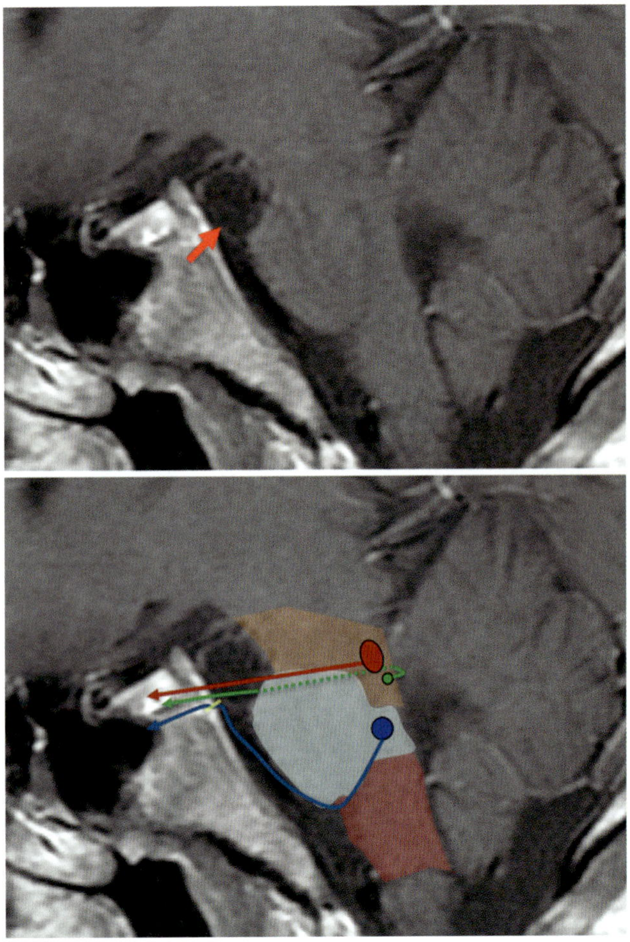

Fig. 6.22 Anatomy of CN-III, IV, and VI. Top, an arachnoid cyst abutting the ventral surface of the midbrain and resulting in partial CN-III dysfunction. Bottom, the nuclei and courses of CN-III (*red*), CN-IV (*green*), and CN-VI (*blue*). Note that CN-IV exits dorsally and travels around the dorsal aspect of the midbrain to supply the contralateral side

rior cerebellar and posterior cerebral arteries through the subarachnoid cistern (Fig. 6.22) [11]. The trunk continues forward just lateral to the posterior clinoid process at the top of the clivus in proximity to the posterior communicating artery, piercing through the dura to enter the cavernous sinus. It is bound within the lateral dural wall of the cavernous sinus along with the trochlear nerve and the first division of the trigeminal nerve. Throughout the intracranial course of CN-III, the parasympathetic fibers are located in the periphery (superomedially), making them susceptible to compression from expanding lesions, most notably posterior communicating artery aneurysms. At some point between the anterior cavernous sinus and the orbital apex, CN-III divides into a superior and inferior division, coursing through the superior orbital fissure to assume an intraconal position within the annulus of Zinn. The superior division supplies the levator and superior rectus muscles, while the inferior division supplies the inferior and medial rectus muscles and the inferior oblique muscle. Two additional anatomic pearls are worth remembering: (1) the nerve to the inferior oblique muscle travels anteriorly along the lateral border of the inferior rectus muscle, where it is susceptible to injury and (2) the parasympathetic fibers exit from the inferior division (usually associated with those fibers destined for the inferior oblique muscle) at the orbital apex to enter and synapse in the ciliary ganglion. Traction on the inferior rectus muscle could then not only cause paresis to the inferior oblique muscle but also result in a tonic (Adie) pupil due to parasympathetic fiber damage, occasionally seen after orbital fracture repair.

Trauma is the leading cause of acquired CN-III palsies in children and the second or third leading cause in adults [152]. The majority of traumatic CN-III palsies are due to motor vehicle accidents with severe TBI, and they can also be associated with intracranial hemorrhage or a ruptured aneurysm (Fig. 6.23) [136, 139, 153]. As already noted, Dhaliwal et al. reported that patients with traumatic CN-III palsy overall had a lower GCS, worse clinical outcomes, and higher rates of temporal region injury on intracranial imaging [136]. In other words, initial diagnosis may be difficult because traumatic CN-III injury is usually associated with more severe TBI and craniofacial injury, and there is therefore a higher probability that the exam is limited by poor neurologic status.

CN-III palsy may manifest in a variety of ways. Acutely, either partial or complete palsy is possible, with or without pupillary involvement (Fig. 6.23). If the pattern of CN-III injury progresses over the first few hours or days following TBI, it is prudent to reimage the patient with CT and/or MRI as well as CTA or MRA, looking for evidence of new intracranial hemorrhage, cavernous sinus fistula, or posttraumatic aneurysm. Over the course of several weeks, aberrant regeneration may manifest (Fig. 6.24). The clinical features of CN-III paresis and aberrant regeneration are summarized in Chap. 13.

Trochlear Nerve (CN-IV) Injury

The trochlear nerve nucleus is located in the midbrain just caudal to the much larger oculomotor nuclear complex [11]. As an interesting side note, embryologically, both the CN-III and CN-IV nuclei begin as one neural aggregate in the 10 mm embryo, differentiating into two separate nuclei in the 18–24 mm embryo. The CN-IV nucleus is located at the level of the inferior colliculus, with fibers exiting to supply the superior oblique muscle in a unique way: CN-IV is the only cranial nerve to cross and exit at the dorsal side of the midbrain (Fig. 6.22) [154]. It is also the smallest cranial nerve, containing approximately 1500 axons. The nerve then travels in a circuitous route around the brainstem just above the pons to pierce the dura at the posterior cavernous sinus, coursing within the lateral dural wall of the cavernous sinus just below CN-III. CN-IV enters the orbit through the superior orbital fissure extraconally, above the annulus of Zinn.

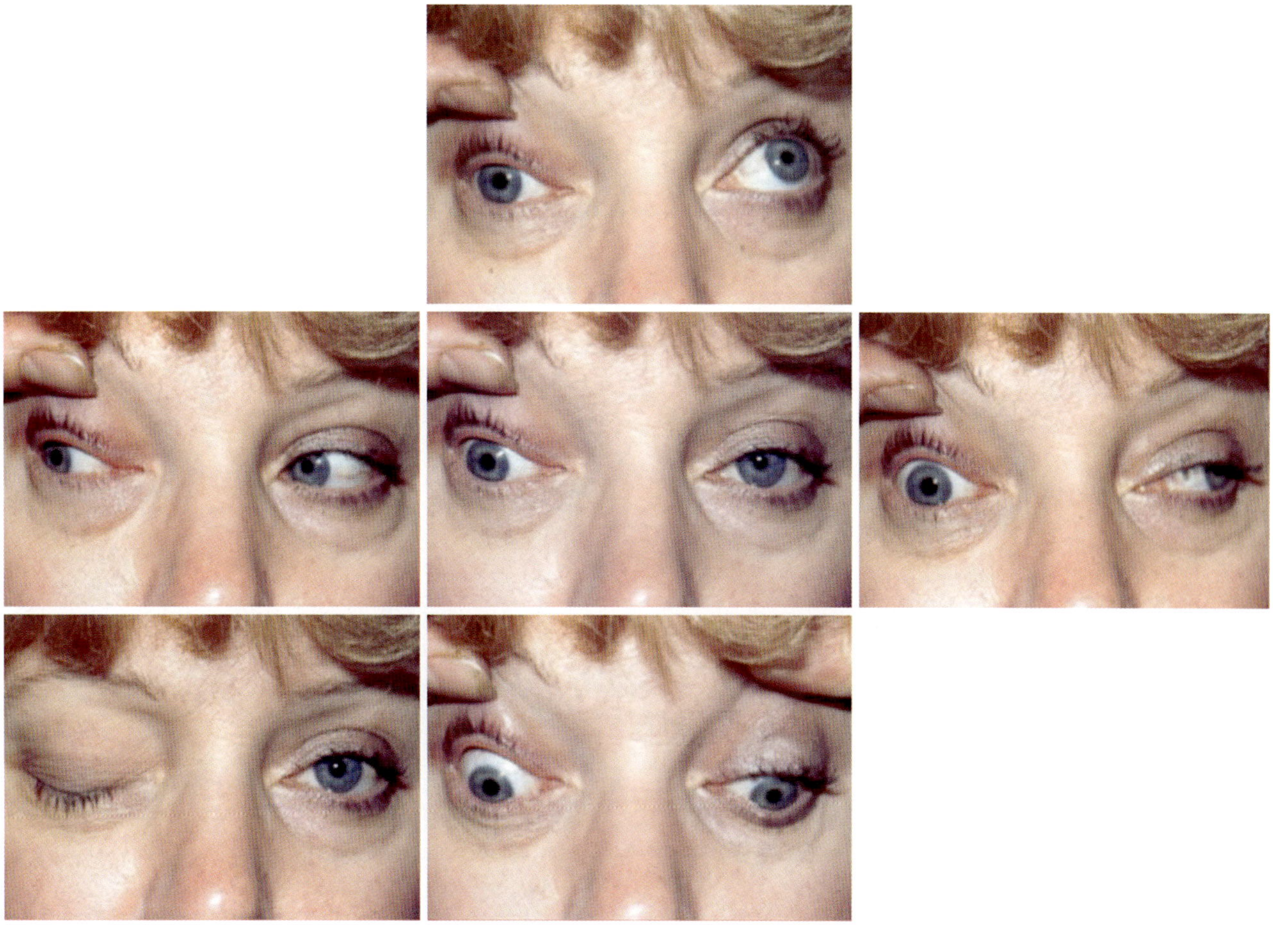

Fig. 6.23 Right third nerve palsy following motor vehicle accident

It then meanders medially, first above the superior rectus muscle and then along the medial edge of the levator muscle to enter the lateral aspect of the superior oblique muscle [11]. The long and circuitous intracranial and intraorbital course of CN-IV, coupled with its small size, makes it vulnerable to injury. The nerve can also be avulsed at its exit point from the dorsal brainstem [141, 155]. Additionally, the decussation makes bilateral traumatic trochlear palsies more likely, and this bilaterality can be difficult to initially discern [156, 157]. Unlike isolated CN-III and CN-VI palsies, which can occur from a variety of pathologic processes, isolated CN-IV is generally due to trauma [158]. CN-IV palsy can occur with even minor head trauma, though it is more common with an intermediate severity of TBI [136, 159–161].

Patients with CN-IV palsy typically complain of a vertical or oblique binocular diplopia. In cases of concomitant TBI and orbital injury (especially orbital floor fracture), careful extraocular motility examination is needed to distinguish inferior rectus muscle restriction from CN-IV injury. The patient will often notice that the diplopia resolves with a combined head turn and head tilt, and just as often not notice this but present to the physician with just such a head position. CN-IV is most accurately diagnosed with the so-called three-step (Parks-Bielschowsky) test [162]. The strabismus is measured in primary and secondary gazes with prism bars and either a red filter or red Maddox rod. In a unilateral CN-IV palsy, the incomitant hypertropia will increase in opposite horizontal gaze and ipsilateral head tilt (Fig. 6.25); thus, the mnemonic, "hypertropia worse in opposite gaze and same head tilt." Typically, unilateral CN-IV palsies are distinguished from bilateral involvement by the amount of excyclotorsion present (in addition to the presence of alternating hypertropias in bilateral involvement): unilateral palsy usually will manifest less than 10° of torsion. History, old photos, and vertical fusional amplitudes can be used to distinguish an acquired from a congenital CN-IV palsy. While some studies demonstrate no need for neuroimaging in an isolated, traumatic CN-IV palsy [1, 163], there are rare cases of CN-IV palsies after trauma associated with an underlying intracranial tumor [149, 150]. Since most TBI patients are imaged, often before an ophthalmologist is called, this is generally a moot point.

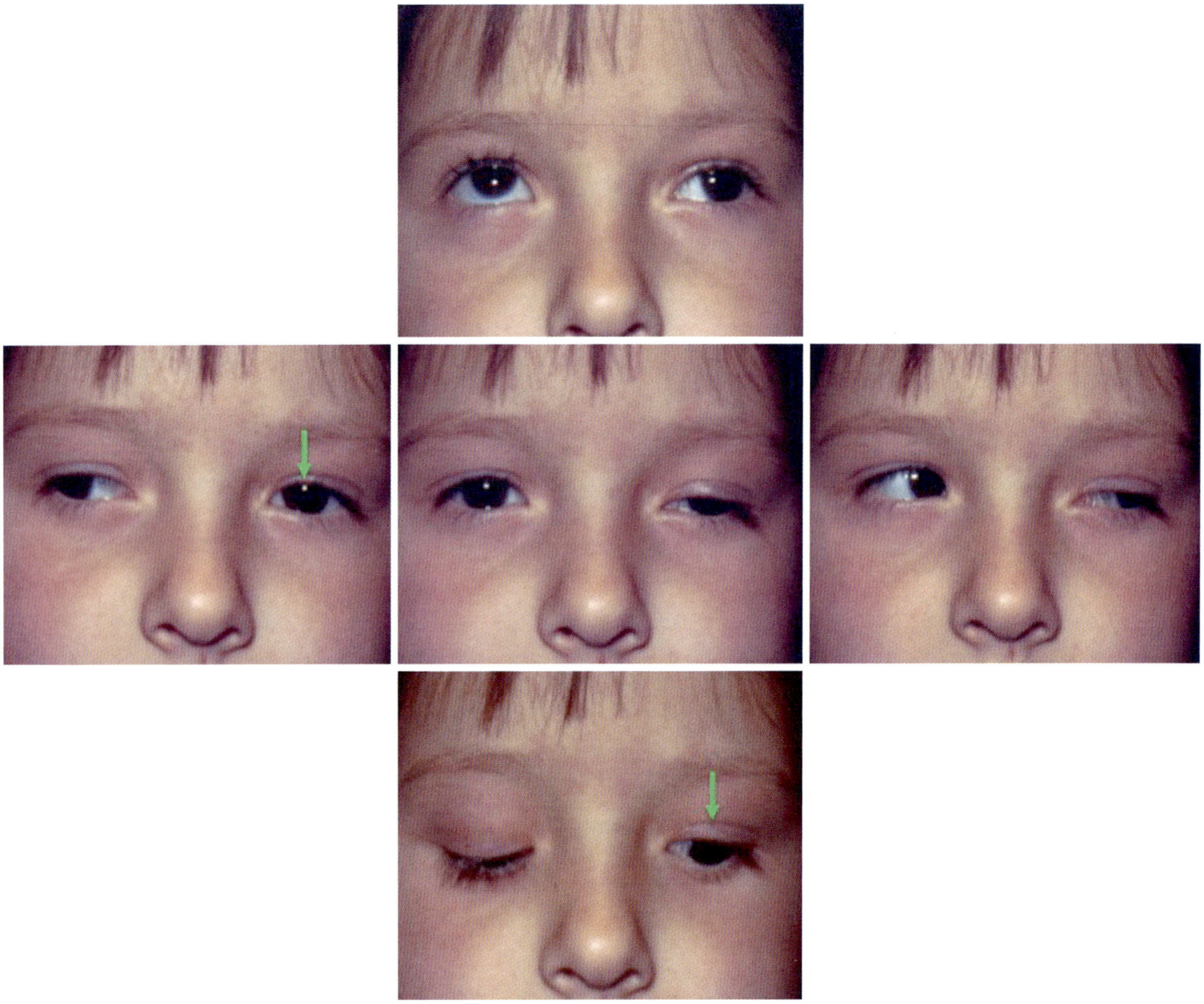

Fig. 6.24 Aberrant third nerve palsy following motor vehicle accident 3 years earlier. In addition to the left external ophthalmoplegia, note the upper eyelid retraction (pseudo-von Graefe sign) in adduction and infraduction (arrows)

Abducens Nerve (CN-VI) Injury

The paired abducens nuclei lie in the dorsal pons along the floor of the fourth ventricle adjacent to CN-VII fasicles [11]. Fibers exit the pons ventrally and then travel upward along the clivus (Fig. 6.22). After piercing the dura, CN-VI continues superiorly to the petrous apex, where it bends acutely (almost 90°) into Dorello's canal and is tethered by various trabeculae, the most notable being the petroclinoid (Gruber's) ligament. The nerve then enters the posterior cavernous sinus, but unlike CN-III and CN-IV, it does not travel through the protective stability of the lateral dural wall. Instead, it meanders through the venous spaces of the cavernous sinus in close proximity to the carotid siphon. CN-VI exits the cavernous sinus through the superior orbital fissure within the confines of the annulus of Zinn to supply the lateral rectus muscle. The long intracranial course along the petrous ridge, as well as the angulated exit from the pons and angulated tethering of the nerve at the petrous apex makes CN-VI vulnerable to traumatic injury.

Patients with CN-VI palsy typically present with an esotropia in primary gaze and may often assume a gaze position away from the involved side to minimize symptoms of diplopia. Horizontal gaze testing will reveal a defect in abduction on the affected side (Fig. 6.26). Due to the large deviation, CN-VI damage is generally easier to recognize than CN-IV palsy and is much easier to map out at the bedside without the need of prism bars. Traumatic CN-VI palsies are thought to be due to transmitted petrous bone injuries or stretch injuries from hyperextension of the neck [142, 164–166]. However, one critical point regarding CN-VI palsy must be stressed: CN-VI palsy may be the initial and only manifestation of increased intracranial pressure (Fig. 6.27). In cases of trauma, CN-VI palsy may indicate active intracranial bleeding and impending uncal herniation. Optic disc swelling (papilledema) may or may not be present. It is therefore important to urgently image all patients presenting with post-traumatic CN-VI palsy. As a side note, in cases of craniofacial trauma involving the orbit, the clinician may assume

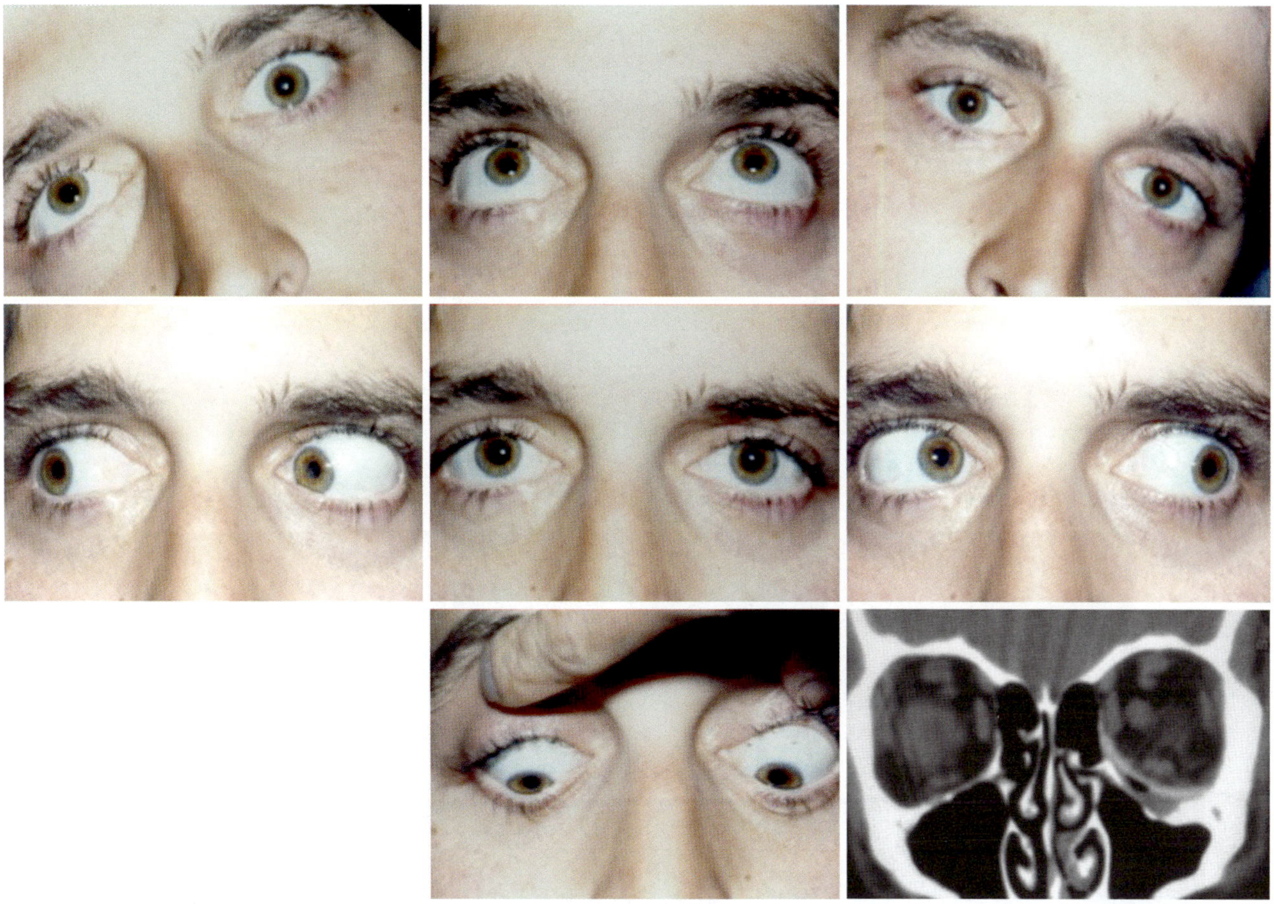

Fig. 6.25 Right CN-IV palsy. The patient was referred for persistent vertical diplopia following left orbital floor fracture repair. On coronal CT, the orbital implant appears to be in good position (lower right). The diplopia pattern was mapped with prism bars and revealed a right hypertropia increasing in left gaze and right head tilt. The diplopia resolved completely with left head tilt and right gaze

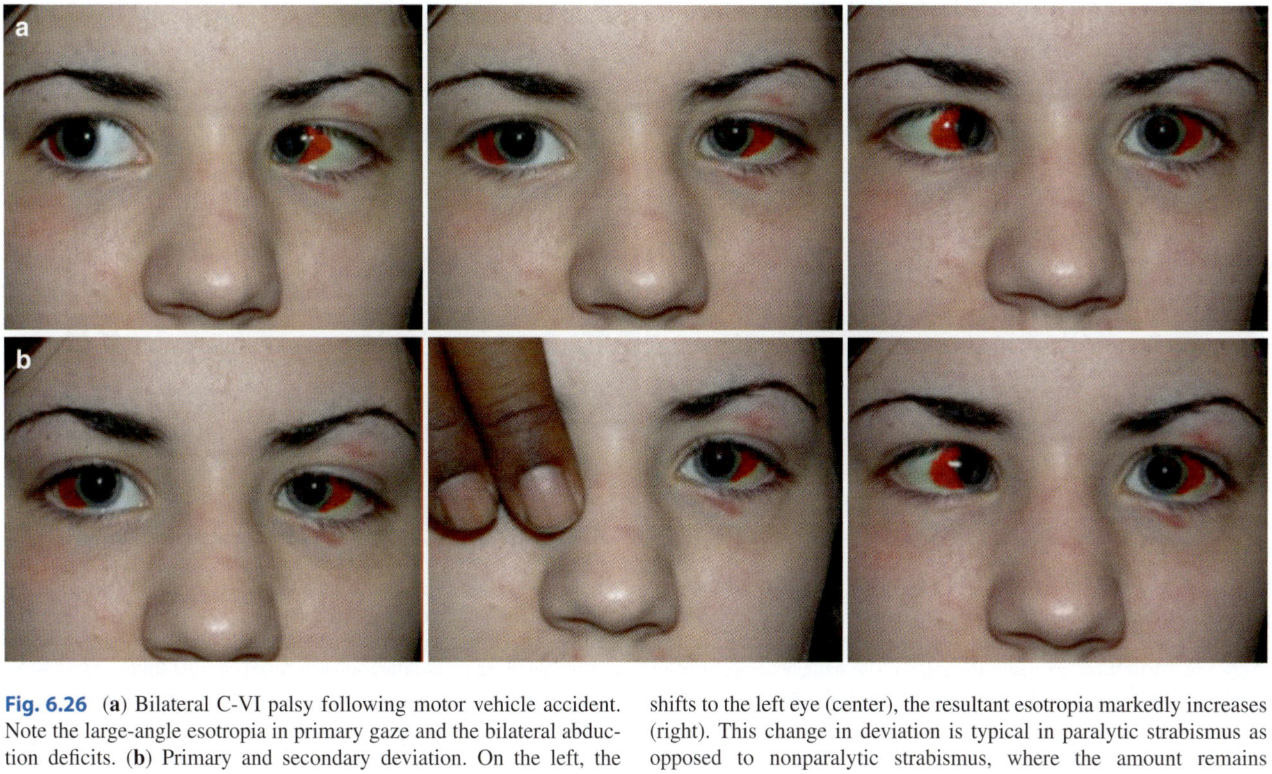

Fig. 6.26 (**a**) Bilateral C-VI palsy following motor vehicle accident. Note the large-angle esotropia in primary gaze and the bilateral abduction deficits. (**b**) Primary and secondary deviation. On the left, the patient fixates with her right eye. After the right is occluded and fixation shifts to the left eye (center), the resultant esotropia markedly increases (right). This change in deviation is typical in paralytic strabismus as opposed to nonparalytic strabismus, where the amount remains constant

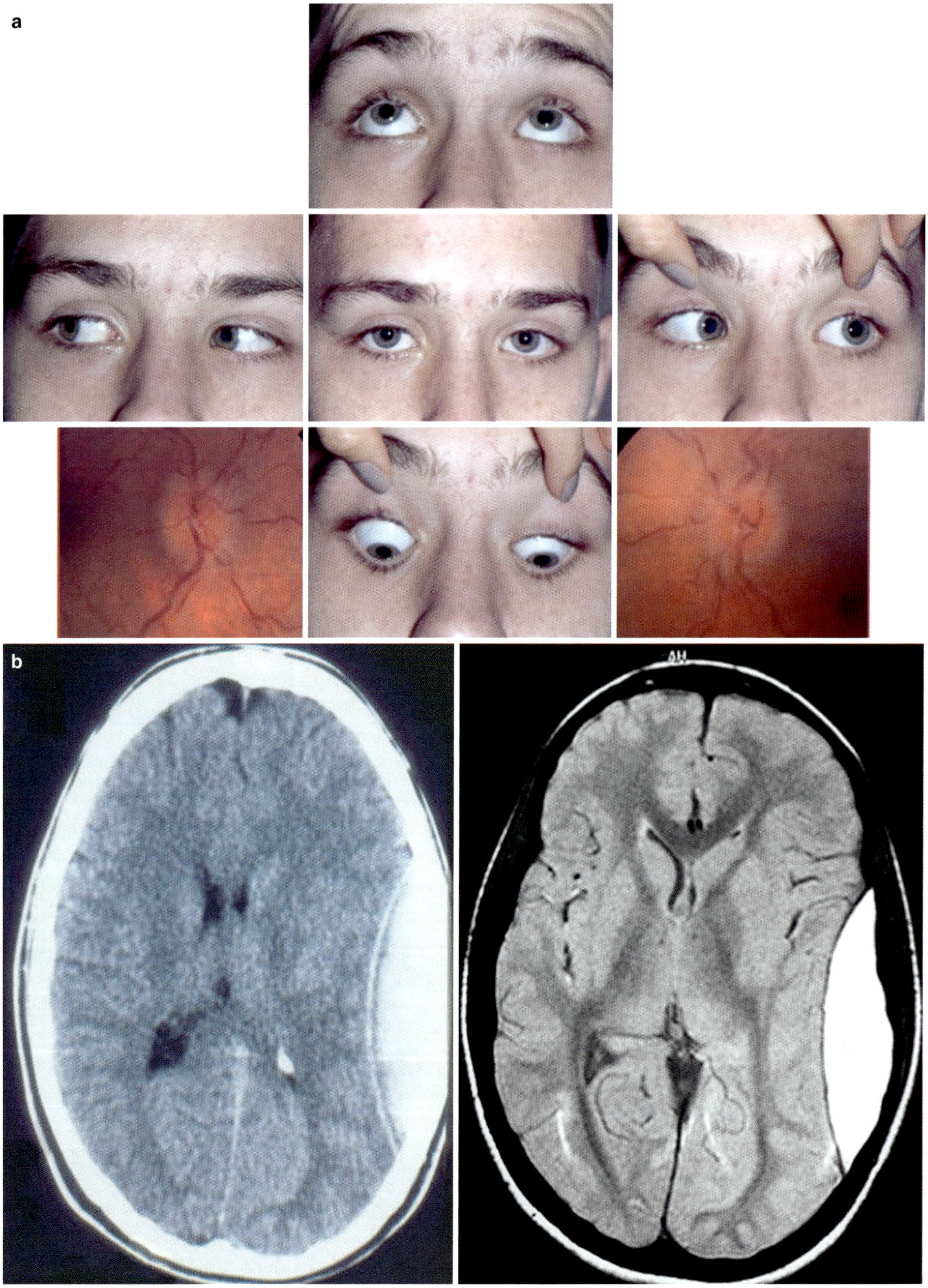

Fig. 6.27 (**a**) CN-VI palsy from increased intracranial pressure. A 17-year-old male referred for repair of left medial wall fracture 2 weeks after sustaining a poorly described head injury. No imaging or funduscopy was performed following the injury. The patient complained of headaches, and the parents noted lethargy. (**a**) External exam shows a left abduction deficit and a distinct lack of any signs of left periorbital injury. Funduscopy revealed bilateral disc swelling. (**b**) Urgent CT (left) showed a large epidural hematoma with midline shift. No intraparenchymal bleeding or infarction was noted on MRI (right). The CN-VI palsy resolved completely within 2 weeks of hematoma evacuation

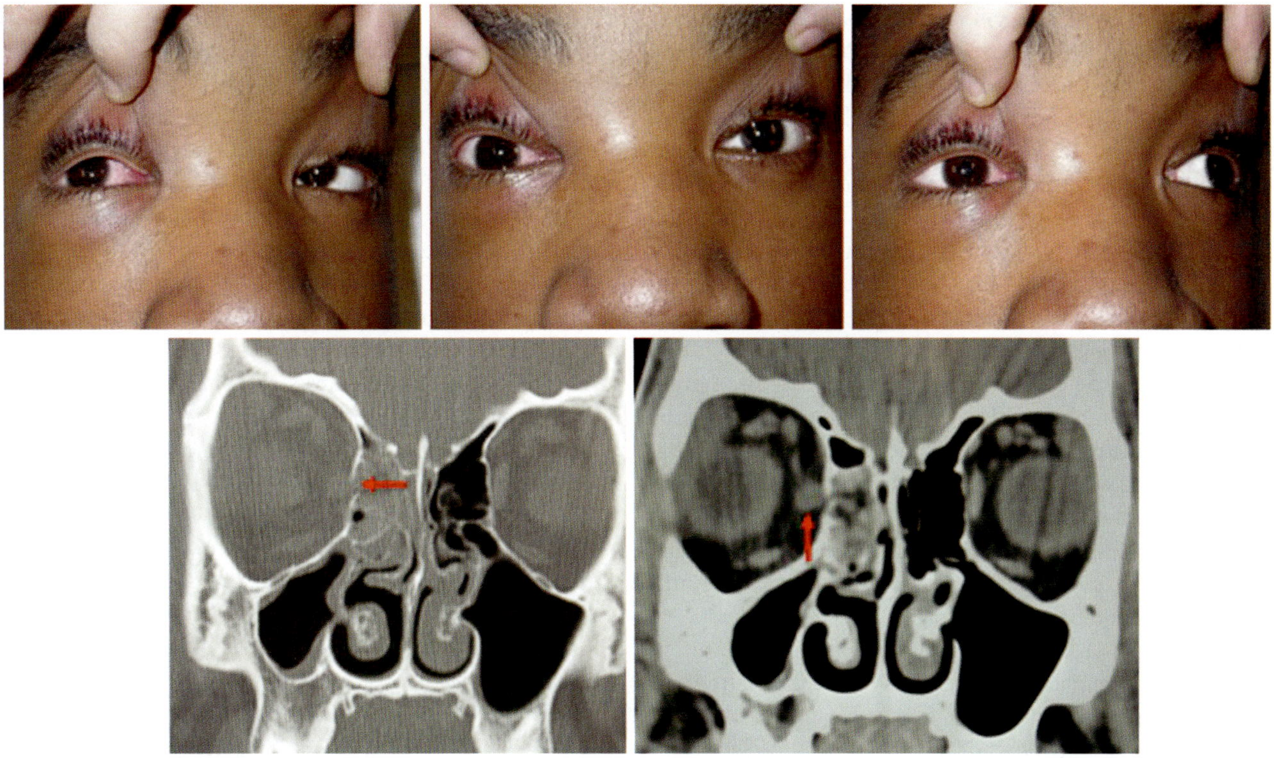

Fig. 6.28 Medial wall fracture mimicking CN-VI paresis. A 15-year-old male with a right abduction deficit secondary to a white-eyed blow-out fracture of the medial wall (arrow, bottom left) and incarceration of the medial rectus muscle. Note the distortion of the muscle (arrow, bottom right) on coronal CT. Also note the right adduction deficit, inconsistent with an isolated CN-VI injury

that an abduction deficit is secondary to medial orbital wall fracture and restriction of the medial rectus muscle. While this may indeed be the case (Fig. 6.28), as a first order of business, CN-VI palsy needs to be ruled out. Forced duction and force generation testing may be helpful in distinguishing a CN-VI injury from an entrapped medial rectus muscle. Other associated findings may be found, including an ipsilateral facial paralysis and facial pain (pseudo-Gradenigo syndrome) from a petrous bone fracture. Interestingly, in one series, patients with CN-VI palsies had lower severity of TBI than those with CN-III or IV palsies overall and, inexplicably, the highest rate of extremity injury [136].

Management

In general, traumatic ocular motor nerve palsy should be treated nonsurgically for at least 6 months following initial injury because of a high rate of spontaneous recovery or improvement. The rate of spontaneous recovery following trauma to each of the ocular motor nerves is difficult to assess with any accuracy because few studies with adequate patient cohorts have looked specifically at posttraumatic palsies. As an example, of 206 patients with CN-III, CN-IV, and/or CN-VI dysfunction from a variety of causes reported by Park and coauthors, only 44 cases were secondary to TBI [167]. In this study, the overall rate of complete recovery measured 87.5%. In a series of over 1200 patients with a variety of ocular motor cranial neuropathies, either partial or complete recovery from trauma was about 55%, compared to about 70% in patients with vascular etiologies and 57.3% from all etiologies [168]. The use of botulinum toxin during this period is controversial, and the available data is difficult to interpret, since many series include various etiologies [169–176]. In case of posttraumatic ocular motor palsy, botulinum toxin injection to the antagonist muscle(s) may decrease diplopia symptoms and theoretically decrease the possibility of fibrosis and contracture of the paretic muscle. However, botulinum toxin injection into an EOM is not without risk [169].

In children younger than 5 years, the development of amblyopia is an important issue and requires more aggressive nonsurgical therapy in the early posttraumatic stages [177]. The clinician should also remember that in cases of pediatric CN-III palsy, amblyopia may be due to occlusive ptosis in addition to strabismus.

CN-III Injury

The surgical goal in strabismic repair is to provide binocular fusion in primary position and is difficult for complete CN-III palsies. Ptosis repair should not be undertaken until any efforts to treat the diplopia are complete and with the understanding by the patient that any residual diplopia may be unmasked by ptosis correction. The overall spontaneous recovery rate for CN-III injury is about 30% [139]. Surgical management of CN-III palsy is difficult because of the paucity of remaining fully functional extraocular muscles (lateral rectus and superior oblique) coupled with potentially visually obstructive ptosis with limited levator function [178–180]. In their study of CN-III dysfunction in children, Mudgil and Repka noted that only patients who recovered fully from their CN-III regained stereopsis; no patients regained stereopsis following strabismus surgery [181]. Acquired pediatric cases of CN-III dysfunction also have a higher rate of amblyopia than their congenital counterparts, and posttraumatic cases (along with those secondary to neoplasia) had the worst prognosis when compared to other congenital or acquired etiologies [181, 182]. Elstone noted that most adults with traumatic CN-III dysfunction fail to regain sensory fusion, even after surgery, and that any strabismus correction should be aimed primarily at cosmesis [139].

In a study of 18 children with CN-III palsy from a variety of etiologies, trauma (four cases plus one case of iatrogenic surgical injury) was the most frequent cause of acquired palsy [177]. Of note, none of the posttraumatic cases went on to develop aberrant regeneration; this is not surprising, since aberrant CN-III regeneration is usually associated with slowly progressive oculomotor nerve injury (neoplasm, aneurysm) rather than acute trauma. However, the authors have seen several cases of posttraumatic aberrant CN-III regeneration. Ing and colleagues reported that six of 18 children (33%) with traumatic CN-III injury went on to develop aberrant regeneration, and Elstone noted that 19 of 20 adults developed this finding (Fig. 6.23) [139, 153]. That said, detailed neuroimaging is indicated in any patient presenting with a vague history of head trauma and aberrant CN-III regeneration to rule out nontraumatic intracranial processes [136].

CN-IV Injury

Most trochlear palsies will resolve, although the recovery following trauma is lower than the overall rate for all acquired etiologies, with less than 50% resolution and the potential for incomplete recovery [161, 183]. Myokymia of the superior oblique muscle may occur after CN-IV injury [184]. If there is no recovery or incomplete recovery leading to disabling diplopia or neck problems from a head tilt, surgery can be performed. As with all posttraumatic ocular motor palsies, stable measurements over several months should be documented before attempted repair. In addition, careful strabismus and torsional measurements should be performed to unmask bilateral palsy. The surgical options include superior oblique tuck, inferior oblique recession (ipsilateral or contralateral), superior oblique tendon advancement, and a Knapp procedure [185–187].

CN-VI Injury

The overall recovery rate of traumatic CN-VI palsy is 73% at 6 months, with a median time period of 90 days [188–190]. As with CN-III injury, the rate of recovery drops in cases of complete or bilateral CN-VI palsy: in one study, unilateral cases resolved in 84% of patients, while bilateral cases resolved in only 38% [188]. The routine use of botulinum toxin in cases of CN-VI palsy, as already mentioned for CN-III injury, is still being debated, with several studies showing essentially identical recovery rates with or without the use of the toxin [170, 191]. Surgical correction depends on the extent of the residual abducens nerve paresis and spans the gamut from horizontal muscle resection and/or recession, vertical muscle transposition, or a combination of vertical and horizontal muscle surgery (Jensen procedure) [192–194].

References

1. Baker RS, Epstein AD. Ocular motor abnormalities from head trauma. Surv Ophthalmol. 1991;35(4):245–67.
2. Yu-Wai-Man P, Griffiths PG. Steroids for traumatic optic neuropathy. Cochrane Database Syst Rev. 2007;4:CD006032.
3. Kline LB, Morawetz RB, Swaid SN. Indirect injury of the optic nerve. Neurosurgery. 1984;14(6):756–64.
4. Kallela I, Hyrkas T, Paukku P, Iizuka T, Lindqvist C. Blindness after maxillofacial blunt trauma. Evaluation of candidates for optic nerve decompression surgery. J Craniomaxillofac Surg. 1994;22(4):220–5.
5. Bilyk JR, Joseph MP. Traumatic optic neuropathy. Semin Ophthalmol. 1994;9(3):200–11.
6. Jamal BT, Diecidue RJ, Taub D, Champion A, Bilyk JR. Orbital hemorrhage and compressive optic neuropathy in patients with midfacial fractures receiving low-molecular weight heparin therapy. J Oral Maxillofac Surg. 2009;67(7):1416–9.
7. al-Qurainy IA, Stassen LF, Dutton GN, Moos KF, el-Attar A. The characteristics of midfacial fractures and the association with ocular injury: a prospective study. Br J Oral Maxillofac Surg. 1991;29(5):291–301.
8. Jamal BT, Pfahler SM, Lane KA, et al. Ophthalmic injuries in patients with zygomaticomaxillary complex fractures requiring surgical repair. J Oral Maxillofac Surg. 2009;67(5):986–9.
9. Steinsapir KD, Goldberg RA. Traumatic optic neuropathies. In: Miller NR, Newman NJ, editors. Walsh and Hoyt's clinical neuro-ophthalmology. 5th ed. Baltimore: Williams and Wilkins; 1998. p. 278–89.
10. Miller NR. Anatomy and physiology of the retina and optic nerve. In: Miller NR, Newman NJ, editors. Walsh and Hoyt's clinical neuro-ophthalmology. 5th ed. Baltimore: Williams and Wilkins; 1998. p. 77–84.
11. Dutton JJ. Clinical and surgical orbital anatomy. Philadelphia: W.B. Saunders; 1994.
12. Hayreh SS. Blood supply of the optic nerve head and its role in optic atrophy, glaucoma, and oedema of the optic disc. Br J Ophthalmol. 1969;53(11):721–48.
13. Hayreh SS, Baines JA. Occlusion of the posterior ciliary artery. I. Effects on choroidal circulation. Br J Ophthalmol. 1972;56(10):719–35.
14. Hayreh SS, Baines JA. Occlusion of the posterior ciliary artery. II Chorio-retinal lesions. Br J Ophthalmol. 1972;56(10): 736–53.

15. Hayreh SS, Baines JA. Occlusion of the posterior ciliary artery. 3. Effects on the optic nerve head. Br J Ophthalmol. 1972;56(10):754–64.
16. Dutton JJ. Orbital nerves. In: Dutton JJ, editor. Atlas of clinical and surgical orbital anatomy. 2nd ed. New York: Elsevier Saunders; 2011. p. 51–4.
17. Onofrey CB, Tse DT, Johnson TE, et al. Optic canal decompression: a cadaveric study of the effects of surgery. Ophthal Plast Reconstr Surg. 2007;23(4):261–6.
18. Sturm V, Menke MN, Bergamin O, Landau K. Longterm follow-up of children with traumatic optic nerve avulsion. Acta Ophthalmol. 2010;88(4):486–9.
19. Anand S, Harvey R, Sandramouli S. Accidental self-inflicted optic nerve head avulsion. Eye (Lond). 2003;17(5):646–7.
20. Zinn KM, Kirban EH. Partial avulsion of the optic nerve head secondary to local trauma: case report. Mt Sinai J Med. 1984;51(5):629–32.
21. Simsek T, Simsek E, Ilhan B, Ozalp S, Sekercioglu B, Zilelioglu O. Traumatic optic nerve avulsion. J Pediatr Ophthalmol Strabismus. 2006;43(6):367–9.
22. Morris WR, Osborn FD, Fleming JC. Traumatic evulsion of the globe. Ophthal Plast Reconstr Surg. 2002;18(4):261–7.
23. Killer HE, Blumer BK, Rust ON. Avulsion of the optic disc after a blow to swimming goggles. J Pediatr Ophthalmol Strabismus. 1999;36(2):92–3.
24. Lelli GJ Jr, Demirci H, Frueh BR. Avulsion of the optic nerve with luxation of the eye after motor vehicle accident. Ophthal Plast Reconstr Surg. 2007;23(2):158–60.
25. Andreou P, Clarke MP, Feeney P. A case of traumatic retinal avulsion at the optic nerve head. Br J Ophthalmol. 1996;80(6):575–6.
26. Talwar D, Kumar A, Verma L, Tewari HK, Khosla PK. Ultrasonography in optic nerve head avulsion. Acta Ophthalmol. 1991;69(1):121–3.
27. Lee MW, Lee SY, Ong SG. Optic disc laceration with combined retinal artery and vein occlusion following penetrating injury. Clin Experiment Ophthalmol. 2007;35(5):486–8.
28. Hindman HB, Srikumaran D, Halfpenny C, Hirschbein MJ. Traumatic globe luxation and enucleation caused by a human bite injury. Ophthal Plast Reconstr Surg. 2007;23(5):422–3.
29. Shneck M, Oshry T, Marcus M, Lifshitz T. Attempted bilateral manual enucleation (gouging) during a physical assault. Ophthalmology. 2003;110(3):575–7.
30. Gauntt CD, Sherry RG, Kannan C. Terson syndrome with bilateral optic nerve sheath hemorrhage. J Neuroophthalmol. 2007;27(3):193–4.
31. Walsh FB, Hedges TR Jr. Optic nerve sheath hemorrhage. Am J Ophthalmol. 1951;34(4):509–27.
32. Dolman PJ, Glazer LC, Harris GJ, Beatty RL, Massaro BM. Mechanisms of visual loss in severe proptosis. Ophthal Plast Reconstr Surg. 1991;7(4):256–60.
33. Lima V, Burt B, Leibovitch I, Prabhakaran V, Goldberg RA, Selva D. Orbital compartment syndrome: the ophthalmic surgical emergency. Surv Ophthalmol. 2009;54(4):441–9.
34. Hunts JH, Patrinely JR, Holds JB, Anderson RL. Orbital emphysema. Staging and acute management. Ophthalmology. 1994;101(5):960–6.
35. Al-Shammari L, Majithia A, Adams A, Chatrath P. Tension pneumo-orbit treated by endoscopic, endonasal decompression: case report and literature review. J Laryngol Otol. 2008;122(3):e8.
36. Key SJ, Ryba F, Holmes S, Manisali M. Orbital emphysema – the need for surgical intervention. J Craniomaxillofac Surg. 2008;36(8):473–6.
37. Callahan MA. Prevention of blindness after blepharoplasty. Ophthalmology. 1983;90(9):1047–51.
38. Anderson RL, Edwards JJ. Bilateral visual loss after blepharoplasty. Ann Plast Surg. 1980;5(4):288–92.
39. Hayreh SS, Kolder HE, Weingeist TA. Central retinal artery occlusion and retinal tolerance time. Ophthalmology. 1980;87(1):75–8.
40. Hargaden M, Goldberg SH, Cunningham D, Breton ME, Griffith JW, Lang CM. Optic neuropathy following simulation of orbital hemorrhage in the nonhuman primate. Ophthal Plast Reconstr Surg. 1996;12(4):264–72.
41. Wladis EJ, Peebles TR, Weinberg DA. Management of acute orbital hemorrhage with obstruction of the ophthalmic artery during attempted coil embolization of a dural arteriovenous fistula of the cavernous sinus. Ophthal Plast Reconstr Surg. 2007;23(1):57–9.
42. Hayreh SS. Posterior ischaemic optic neuropathy: clinical features, pathogenesis, and management. Eye (Lond). 2004;18(11):1188–206.
43. Goldberg RA, Marmor MF, Shorr N, Christenbury JD. Blindness following blepharoplasty: two case reports, and a discussion of management. Ophthalmic Surg. 1990;21(2):85–9.
44. Cruz AA, Ando A, Monteiro CA, Elias J Jr. Delayed retrobulbar hematoma after blepharoplasty. Ophthal Plast Reconstr Surg. 2001;17(2):126–30.
45. Zoumalan CI, Bullock JD, Warwar RE, Fuller B, McCulley TJ. Evaluation of intraocular and orbital pressure in the management of orbital hemorrhage: an experimental model. Arch Ophthalmol. 2008;126(9):1257–60.
46. Katz B, Herschler J, Brick DC. Orbital haemorrhage and prolonged blindness: a treatable posterior optic neuropathy. Br J Ophthalmol. 1983;67(8):549–53.
47. McCartney DL, Char DH. Return of vision following orbital decompression after 36 hours of postoperative blindness. Am J Ophthalmol. 1985;100(4):602–4.
48. Dalley RW, Robertson WD, Rootman J. Globe tenting: a sign of increased orbital tension. AJNR Am J Neuroradiol. 1989;10(1):181–6.
49. Yung CW, Moorthy RS, Lindley D, Ringle M, Nunery WR. Efficacy of lateral canthotomy and cantholysis in orbital hemorrhage. Ophthal Plast Reconstr Surg. 1994;10(2):137–41.
50. Sergott RC, Grossman RI, Savino PJ, Bosley TM, Schatz NJ. The syndrome of paradoxical worsening of dural-cavernous sinus arteriovenous malformations. Ophthalmology. 1987;94(3):205–12.
51. Johnson D, Winterborn A, Kratky V. Efficacy of intravenous mannitol in the management of orbital compartment syndrome: a nonhuman primate model. Ophthal Plast Reconstr Surg. 2016;32(3):187–90.
52. Liu D. A simplified technique of orbital decompression for severe retrobulbar hemorrhage. Am J Ophthalmol. 1993;116(1):34–7.
53. Markovits AS. A simplified technique of orbital decompression for severe retrobulbar hemorrhage. Am J Ophthalmol. 1994;117(1):124.
54. Hass AN, Penne RB, Stefanyszyn MA, Flanagan JC. Incidence of postblepharoplasty orbital hemorrhage and associated visual loss. Ophthal Plast Reconstr Surg. 2004;20(6):426–32.
55. Teng CC, Reddy S, Wong JJ, Lisman RD. Retrobulbar hemorrhage nine days after cosmetic blepharoplasty resulting in permanent visual loss. Ophthal Plast Reconstr Surg. 2006;22(5):388–9.
56. Fountain T. What about anticoagulation? In: Kersten RC, McCulley TJ, editors. Curbside consultation in oculoplastics. 1st ed. Thorofare: Slack Incorporated; 2011. p. 79–82.
57. Dutton JJ. Controversies in ophthalmic plastic and reconstructive surgery: anticoagulation. Chicago: American Academy of Ophthalmology, Subspecialty Day; 2010.
58. Enzer YR. Controversies in ophthalmic plastic and reconstructive surgery: anticoagulation. Chicago: American Academy of Ophthalmology, Subspecialty Day; 2010.
59. Levine GN, Bates ER, Bittl JA, et al. 2016 ACC/AHA guideline focused update on duration of dual antiplatelet therapy in patients with coronary artery disease: a report of the American College of Cardiology/American Heart Association Task Force on Clinical Practice Guidelines. J Am Coll Cardiol. 2016;68(10):1082–115.

60. Taniguchi S, Fukuda I, Daitoku K, et al. Prevalence of venous thromboembolism in neurosurgical patients. Heart Vessels. 2009;24(6):425–8.
61. Roderick P, Ferris G, Wilson K, et al. Towards evidence-based guidelines for the prevention of venous thromboembolism: systematic reviews of mechanical methods, oral anticoagulation, dextran and regional anaesthesia as thromboprophylaxis. Health Technol Assess. 2005;9(49):iii–iv, ix–x, 1–78.
62. Naccarato M, Chiodo Grandi F, Dennis M, Sandercock PA. Physical methods for preventing deep vein thrombosis in stroke. Cochrane Database Syst Rev. 2010;8:CD001922.
63. Kakkos SK, Caprini JA, Geroulakos G, Nicolaides AN, Stansby GP, Reddy DJ. Combined intermittent pneumatic leg compression and pharmacological prophylaxis for prevention of venous thromboembolism in high-risk patients. Cochrane Database Syst Rev. 2008;4:CD005258.
64. Collen JF, Jackson JL, Shorr AF, Moores LK. Prevention of venous thromboembolism in neurosurgery: a metaanalysis. Chest. 2008;134(2):237–49.
65. Goldhaber SZ, Dunn K, Gerhard-Herman M, Park JK, Black PM. Low rate of venous thromboembolism after craniotomy for brain tumor using multimodality prophylaxis. Chest. 2002;122(6):1933–7.
66. Levin LA, Beck RW, Joseph MP, Seiff S, Kraker R. The treatment of traumatic optic neuropathy: the International Optic Nerve Trauma Study. Ophthalmology. 1999;106(7):1268–77.
67. Crompton MR. Visual lesions in closed head injury. Brain. 1970;93(4):785–92.
68. Walsh FB. Pathological-clinical correlations. I. Indirect trauma to the optic nerves and chiasm. II. Certain cerebral involvements associated with defective blood supply. Invest Ophthalmol. 1966;5(5):433–49.
69. Flamm ES, Demopoulos HB, Seligman ML, Poser RG, Ransohoff J. Free radicals in cerebral ischemia. Stroke. 1978;9(5):445–7.
70. Anderson RL, Panje WR, Gross CE. Optic nerve blindness following blunt forehead trauma. Ophthalmology. 1982;89(5):445–55.
71. Gross CE, DeKock JR, Panje WR, Hershkowitz N, Newman J. Evidence for orbital deformation that may contribute to monocular blindness following minor frontal head trauma. J Neurosurg. 1981;55(6):963–6.
72. Lee V, Ford RL, Xing W, Bunce C, Foot B. Surveillance of traumatic optic neuropathy in the UK. Eye (Lond). 2010;24(2):240–50.
73. Steinsapir KD. Traumatic optic neuropathy. Curr Opin Ophthalmol. 1999;10(5):340–2.
74. Steinsapir KD. Treatment of traumatic optic neuropathy with high-dose corticosteroid. J Neuroophthalmol. 2006;26(1):65–7.
75. Levin LA, Joseph MP, Rizzo JF 3rd, Lessell S. Optic canal decompression in indirect optic nerve trauma. Ophthalmology. 1994;101(3):566–9.
76. Seiff SR. High dose corticosteroids for treatment of vision loss due to indirect injury to the optic nerve. Ophthalmic Surg. 1990;21(6):389–95.
77. Levin LA, Baker RS. Management of traumatic optic neuropathy. J Neuroophthalmol. 2003;23(1):72–5.
78. Bracken MB, Shepard MJ, Collins WF, et al. A randomized, controlled trial of methylprednisolone or naloxone in the treatment of acute spinal-cord injury. Results of the Second National Acute Spinal Cord Injury Study. N Engl J Med. 1990;322(20):1405–11.
79. Bracken MB, Shepard MJ, Holford TR, et al. Administration of methylprednisolone for 24 or 48 hours or tirilazad mesylate for 48 hours in the treatment of acute spinal cord injury. Results of the Third National Acute Spinal Cord Injury Randomized Controlled Trial. National Acute Spinal Cord Injury Study. JAMA. 1997;277(20):1597–604.
80. Beck RW, Gal RL. Treatment of acute optic neuritis: a summary of findings from the optic neuritis treatment trial. Arch Ophthalmol. 2008;126(7):994–5.
81. Demopoulos HB, Flamm ES, Pietronigro DD, Seligman ML. The free radical pathology and the microcirculation in the major central nervous system disorders. Acta Physiol Scand Suppl. 1980;492:91–119.
82. Demopoulos HB, Flamm ES, Seligman ML, Pietronigro DD, Tomasula J, DeCrescito V. Further studies on free-radical pathology in the major central nervous system disorders: effect of very high doses of methylprednisolone on the functional outcome, morphology, and chemistry of experimental spinal cord impact injury. Can J Physiol Pharmacol. 1982;60(11):1415–24.
83. Hall ED, Braughler JM. Glucocorticoid mechanisms in acute spinal cord injury: a review and therapeutic rationale. Surg Neurol. 1982;18(5):320–7.
84. Anderson DK, Means ED, Waters TR, Green ES. Microvascular perfusion and metabolism in injured spinal cord after methylprednisolone treatment. J Neurosurg. 1982;56(1):106–13.
85. Braughler JM, Hall ED. Effects of multi-dose methylprednisolone sodium succinate administration on injured cat spinal cord neurofilament degradation and energy metabolism. J Neurosurg. 1984;61(2):290–5.
86. Braughler JM, Hall ED, Means ED, Waters TR, Anderson DK. Evaluation of an intensive methylprednisolone sodium succinate dosing regimen in experimental spinal cord injury. J Neurosurg. 1987;67(1):102–5.
87. Steinsapir KD, Seiff SR, Goldberg RA. Traumatic optic neuropathy: where do we stand? Ophthal Plast Reconstr Surg. 2002;18(3):232–4.
88. Steinsapir KD, Goldberg RA. Traumatic optic neuropathy. Surv Ophthalmol. 1994;38(6):487–518.
89. Roberts I, Yates D, Sandercock P, et al. Effect of intravenous corticosteroids on death within 14 days in 10008 adults with clinically significant head injury (MRC CRASH trial): randomised placebo-controlled trial. Lancet. 2004;364(9442):1321–8.
90. Bracken MB. CRASH (Corticosteroid Randomization after Significant Head Injury Trial): landmark and storm warning. Neurosurgery. 2005;57(6):1300–2; discussion 1300–302.
91. Alderson P, Roberts I. Corticosteroids in acute traumatic brain injury: systematic review of randomised controlled trials. BMJ. 1997;314(7098):1855–9.
92. Edwards P, Arango M, Balica L, et al. Final results of MRC CRASH, a randomised placebo-controlled trial of intravenous corticosteroid in adults with head injury-outcomes at 6 months. Lancet. 2005;365(9475):1957–9.
93. Beck RW. Optic neuritis or anterior ischemic optic neuropathy? Arch Ophthalmol. 1992;110(10):1357.
94. Cook MW, Levin LA, Joseph MP, Pinczower EF. Traumatic optic neuropathy. A meta-analysis. Arch Otolaryngol Head Neck Surg. 1996;122(4):389–92.
95. Joseph MP, Lessell S, Rizzo J, Momose KJ. Extracranial optic nerve decompression for traumatic optic neuropathy. Arch Ophthalmol. 1990;108(8):1091–3.
96. Entezari M, Rajavi Z, Sedighi N, Daftarian N, Sanagoo M. High-dose intravenous methylprednisolone in recent traumatic optic neuropathy; a randomized double-masked placebo-controlled clinical trial. Graefes Arch Clin Exp Ophthalmol. 2007;245(9):1267–71.
97. Yip CC, Chng NW, Au Eong KG, Heng WJ, Lim TH, Lim WK. Low-dose intravenous methylprednisolone or conservative treatment in the management of traumatic optic neuropathy. Eur J Ophthalmol. 2002;12(4):309–14.
98. Steinsapir KD, Goldberg RA, Sinha S, Hovda DA. Methylprednisolone exacerbates axonal loss following optic nerve trauma in rats. Restor Neurol Neurosci. 2000;17(4):157–63.

99. Alderson P, Roberts I. Corticosteroids for acute traumatic brain injury. Cochrane Database Syst Rev. 2000;2:CD000196.
100. Alderson P, Roberts I. Corticosteroids for acute traumatic brain injury. Cochrane Database Syst Rev. 2005;1:CD000196.
101. Yu-Wai-Man P, Griffiths PG. Steroids for traumatic optic neuropathy. Cochrane Database Syst Rev. 2013;6:CD006032.
102. Yu-Wai-Man P, Griffiths PG. Steroids for traumatic optic neuropathy. Cochrane Database Syst Rev. 2011;1:CD006032.
103. Nesathurai S. Steroids and spinal cord injury: revisiting the NASCIS 2 and NASCIS 3 trials. J Trauma. 1998;45(6):1088–93.
104. Sofferman RA. Sphenoethmoid approach to the optic nerve. Laryngoscope. 1981;91(2):184–96.
105. Yu Wai Man P, Griffiths PG. Surgery for traumatic optic neuropathy. Cochrane Database Syst Rev. 2005;(4):CD005024.
106. Goldberg RA, Steinsapir KD. Extracranial optic canal decompression: indications and technique. Ophthal Plast Reconstr Surg. 1996;12(3):163–70.
107. Abuzayed B, Tanriover N, Gazioglu N, Eraslan BS, Akar Z. Endoscopic endonasal approach to the orbital apex and medial orbital wall: anatomic study and clinical applications. J Craniofac Surg. 2009;20(5):1594–600.
108. Gorio A, Gokmen N, Erbayraktar S, et al. Recombinant human erythropoietin counteracts secondary injury and markedly enhances neurological recovery from experimental spinal cord trauma. Proc Natl Acad Sci U S A. 2002;99(14):9450–5.
109. Mammis A, McIntosh TK, Maniker AH. Erythropoietin as a neuroprotective agent in traumatic brain injury review. Surg Neurol. 2009;71(5):527–31; discussion 531.
110. Brines ML, Ghezzi P, Keenan S, et al. Erythropoietin crosses the blood-brain barrier to protect against experimental brain injury. Proc Natl Acad Sci U S A. 2000;97(19):10526–31.
111. Feng Q. Beyond erythropoiesis: the anti-inflammatory effects of erythropoietin. Cardiovasc Res. 2006;71(4):615–7.
112. Sun Y, Calvert JW, Zhang JH. Neonatal hypoxia/ischemia is associated with decreased inflammatory mediators after erythropoietin administration. Stroke. 2005;36(8):1672–8.
113. Ehrenreich H, Weissenborn K, Prange H, et al. Recombinant human erythropoietin in the treatment of acute ischemic stroke. Stroke. 2009;40(12):e647–56.
114. Siren AL, Fasshauer T, Bartels C, Ehrenreich H. Therapeutic potential of erythropoietin and its structural or functional variants in the nervous system. Neurotherapeutics. 2009;6(1):108–27.
115. King CE, Rodger J, Bartlett C, Esmaili T, Dunlop SA, Beazley LD. Erythropoietin is both neuroprotective and neuroregenerative following optic nerve transection. Exp Neurol. 2007;205(1):48–55.
116. Kashkouli MB, Pakdel F, Sanjari MS, et al. Erythropoietin: a novel treatment for traumatic optic neuropathy-a pilot study. Graefes Arch Clin Exp Ophthalmol. 2011;249(5):731–6.
117. Kashkouli MB, Yousefi S, Nojomi M, et al. Traumatic optic neuropathy treatment trial (TONTT): open label, phase 3, multicenter, semi-experimental trial. Graefes Arch Clin Exp Ophthalmol. 2018;256(1):209–18.
118. Rashad MA, Abdel Latif AAM, Mostafa HA, Fawzy SM, Abdel Latif MAM. Visual-evoked-response-supported outcome of intravitreal erythropoietin in management of indirect traumatic optic neuropathy. J Ophthalmol. 2018;2018:2750632.
119. Fujikado T, Morimoto T, Matsushita K, Shimojo H, Okawa Y, Tano Y. Effect of transcorneal electrical stimulation in patients with nonarteritic ischemic optic neuropathy or traumatic optic neuropathy. Jpn J Ophthalmol. 2006;50(3):266–73.
120. Morimoto T, Fukui T, Matsushita K, et al. Evaluation of residual retinal function by pupillary constrictions and phosphenes using transcorneal electrical stimulation in patients with retinal degeneration. Graefes Arch Clin Exp Ophthalmol. 2006;244(10):1283–92.
121. Morimoto T, Miyoshi T, Fujikado T, Tano Y, Fukuda Y. Electrical stimulation enhances the survival of axotomized retinal ganglion cells in vivo. Neuroreport. 2002;13(2):227–30.
122. Franklin JL, Sanz-Rodriguez C, Juhasz A, Deckwerth TL, Johnson EM Jr. Chronic depolarization prevents programmed death of sympathetic neurons in vitro but does not support growth: requirement for Ca2+ influx but not Trk activation. J Neurosci. 1995;15(1 Pt 2):643–64.
123. Morimoto T, Miyoshi T, Matsuda S, Tano Y, Fujikado T, Fukuda Y. Transcorneal electrical stimulation rescues axotomized retinal ganglion cells by activating endogenous retinal IGF-1 system. Invest Ophthalmol Vis Sci. 2005;46(6):2147–55.
124. Steinsapir KD, Goldberg R. Traumatic optic neuropathy: a critical update. Comprehensive Ophthal Update. 2005;1:1–14.
125. Carta A, Ferrigno L, Salvo M, Bianchi-Marzoli S, Boschi A, Carta F. Visual prognosis after indirect traumatic optic neuropathy. J Neurol Neurosurg Psychiatry. 2003;74(2):246–8.
126. Limbrick DD Jr, Behdad A, Derdeyn CP, Custer PL, Zipfel GJ, Santiago P. Traumatic enucleation with avulsion of the ophthalmic artery resulting in aneurysm-like subarachnoid hemorrhage. J Neurosurg. 2009;111(4):653–7.
127. Middleton TH 3rd, Smith RR. Optic nerve avulsion secondary to traumatic enucleation. Neurosurgery. 1987;21(1):89–91.
128. Suzuki N, Fujitsu K, Tanaka N, Sekino T, Kuwabara T, Yuda K. Traumatic enucleation of the eye ball – report of a case and considerations concerning the pathogenic mechanism of intracranial complications. No Shinkei Geka. 1988;16(11):1293–7.
129. Kotlus BS, Lo MW. Subarachnoid hemorrhage and vasospastic stroke after self-enucleation. Ophthal Plast Reconstr Surg. 2007;23(5):425–7.
130. Krauss HR, Yee RD, Foos RY. Autoenucleation. Surv Ophthalmol. 1984;29(3):179–87.
131. Arkin MS, Rubin PA, Bilyk JR, Buchbinder B. Anterior chiasmal optic nerve avulsion. AJNR Am J Neuroradiol. 1996;17(9):1777–81.
132. Jones NP. Self-enucleation and psychosis. Br J Ophthalmol. 1990;74(9):571–3.
133. Khan JA, Buescher L, Ide CH, Pettigrove B. Medical management of self-enucleation. Arch Ophthalmol. 1985;103(3):386–9.
134. Field HL, Waldfogel S. Severe ocular self-injury. Gen Hosp Psychiatry. 1995;17(3):224–7.
135. Kumar AV, Geist CE. A case report of bilateral autoenucleation and its prevention. Orbit. 2007;26(4):309–13.
136. Dhaliwal A, West AL, Trobe JD, Musch DC. Third, fourth, and sixth cranial nerve palsies following closed head injury. J Neuroophthalmol. 2006;26(1):4–10.
137. Green WR, Hackett ER, Schlezinger NS. Neuro-ophthalmologic evaluation of oculomotor nerve paralysis. Arch Ophthalmol. 1964;72:154–67.
138. Memon MY, Paine KW. Direct injury of the oculomotor nerve in craniocerebral trauma. J Neurosurg. 1971;35(4):461–4.
139. Elston JS. Traumatic third nerve palsy. Br J Ophthalmol. 1984;68(8):538–43.
140. Mariak Z, Stankiewicz A. Cranial nerve II-VII injuries in fatal closed head trauma. Eur J Ophthalmol. 1997;7(1):68–72.
141. Heinze J. Cranial nerve avulsion and other neural injuries in road accidents. Med J Aust. 1969;2(25):1246–9.
142. Lindenberg R, Freytag E. Brainstem lesions characteristic of traumatic hyperextension of the head. Arch Pathol. 1970;90(6):509–15.
143. Lindenberg R. Significance of the tentorium in head injuries from blunt forces. Clin Neurosurg. 1964;12:129–42.
144. Adams JH, Graham DI, Murray LS, Scott G. Diffuse axonal injury due to nonmissile head injury in humans: an analysis of 45 cases. Ann Neurol. 1982;12(6):557–63.

145. Adams JH, Graham DI, Gennarelli TA. Head injury in man and experimental animals: neuropathology. Acta Neurochir Suppl (Wien). 1983;32:15–30.
146. Gennarelli TA. Head injury in man and experimental animals: clinical aspects. Acta Neurochir Suppl (Wien). 1983;32:1–13.
147. Coello AF, Canals AG, Gonzalez JM, Martin JJ. Cranial nerve injury after minor head trauma. J Neurosurg. 2010;113(3):547–55.
148. Eyster EF, Hoyt WF, Wilson CB. Oculomotor palsy from minor head trauma. An initial sign of basal intracranial tumor. JAMA. 1972;220(8):1083–6.
149. Neetens A, Van Aerde F. Extra-ocular muscle palsy from minor head trauma. Initial sign of intracranial tumour. Bull Soc Belge Ophtalmol. 1981;193:161–7.
150. Jacobson DM, Warner JJ, Choucair AK, Ptacek LJ. Trochlear nerve palsy following minor head trauma. A sign of structural disorder. J Clin Neuroophthalmol. 1988;8(4):263–8.
151. Walter KA, Newman NJ, Lessell S. Oculomotor palsy from minor head trauma: initial sign of intracranial aneurysm. Neurology. 1994;44(1):148–50.
152. McCann JD, Seiff S. Traumatic neuropathies of the optic nerve, optic chiasm, and ocular motor nerves. Curr Opin Ophthalmol. 1994;5(6):3–10.
153. Ing EB, Sullivan TJ, Clarke MP, Buncic JR. Oculomotor nerve palsies in children. J Pediatr Ophthalmol Strabismus. 1992;29(6):331–6.
154. Miyazaki S. Bilateral innervation of the superior oblique muscle by the trochlear nucleus. Brain Res. 1985;348(1):52–6.
155. Lavin PJ, Troost BT. Traumatic fourth nerve palsy. Clinicoanatomic correlations with computed tomographic scan. Arch Neurol. 1984;41(6):679–80.
156. Sydnor CF, Seaber JH, Buckley EG. Traumatic superior oblique palsies. Ophthalmology. 1982;89(2):134–8.
157. Hermann JS. Masked bilateral superior oblique paresis. J Pediatr Ophthalmol Strabismus. 1981;18(2):43–8.
158. Mansour AM, Reinecke RD. Central trochlear palsy. Surv Ophthalmol. 1986;30(5):279–97.
159. Younge BR, Sutula F. Analysis of trochlear nerve palsies. Diagnosis, etiology, and treatment. Mayo Clin Proc. 1977;52(1):11–8.
160. Khawam E, Scott AB, Jampolsky A. Acquired superior oblique palsy. Diagnosis and management. Arch Ophthalmol. 1967;77(6):761–8.
161. Teller J, Karmon G, Savir H. Long-term follow-up of traumatic unilateral superior oblique palsy. Ann Ophthalmol. 1988;20(11):424–5.
162. Parks MM. Isolated cyclovertical muscle palsy. AMA Arch Ophthalmol. 1958;60(6):1027–35.
163. Hoya K, Kirino T. Traumatic trochlear nerve palsy following minor occipital impact – four case reports. Neurol Med Chir (Tokyo). 2000;40(7):358–60.
164. Moster ML, Savino PJ, Sergott RC, Bosley TM, Schatz NJ. Isolated sixth-nerve palsies in younger adults. Arch Ophthalmol. 1984;102(9):1328–30.
165. Schneider RC, Johnson FD. Bilateral traumatic abducens palsy. A mechanism of injury suggested by the study of associated cervical spine fractures. J Neurosurg. 1971;34(1):33–7.
166. Rosa L, Carol M, Bellegarrigue R, Ducker TB. Multiple cranial nerve palsies due to a hyperextension injury to the cervical spine. Case report. J Neurosurg. 1984;61(1):172–3.
167. Park UC, Kim SJ, Hwang JM, Yu YS. Clinical features and natural history of acquired third, fourth, and sixth cranial nerve palsy. Eye (Lond). 2008;22(5):691–6.
168. Richards BW, Jones FR Jr, Younge BR. Causes and prognosis in 4,278 cases of paralysis of the oculomotor, trochlear, and abducens cranial nerves. Am J Ophthalmol. 1992;113(5):489–96.
169. Rowe FJ, Noonan CP. Botulinum toxin for the treatment of strabismus. Cochrane Database Syst Rev. 2009;2:CD006499.
170. Hung HL, Kao LY, Sun MH. Botulinum toxin treatment for acute traumatic complete sixth nerve palsy. Eye (Lond). 2005;19(3):337–41.
171. Metz HS, Mazow M. Botulinum toxin treatment of acute sixth and third nerve palsy. Graefes Arch Clin Exp Ophthalmol. 1988;226(2):141–4.
172. Scott AB, Kraft SP. Botulinum toxin injection in the management of lateral rectus paresis. Ophthalmology. 1985;92(5):676–83.
173. Murray AD. Early and late botulinum toxin treatment of acute sixth nerve palsy. Aust N Z J Ophthalmol. 1989;17(3):239–45.
174. Metz HS, Dickey CF. Treatment of unilateral acute sixth-nerve palsy with botulinum toxin. Am J Ophthalmol. 1991;112(4):381–4.
175. Wagner RS, Frohman LP. Long-term results: botulinum for sixth nerve palsy. J Pediatr Ophthalmol Strabismus. 1989;26(3):106–8.
176. Repka MX, Lam GC, Morrison NA. The efficacy of botulinum neurotoxin A for the treatment of complete and partially recovered chronic sixth nerve palsy. J Pediatr Ophthalmol Strabismus. 1994;31(2):79–83; discussion 84.
177. Ng YS, Lyons CJ. Oculomotor nerve palsy in childhood. Can J Ophthalmol. 2005;40(5):645–53.
178. Gottlob I, Catalano RA, Reinecke RD. Surgical management of oculomotor nerve palsy. Am J Ophthalmol. 1991;111(1):71–6.
179. Kose S, Uretmen O, Pamukcu K. An approach to the surgical management of total oculomotor nerve palsy. Strabismus. 2001;9(1):1–8.
180. Maruo T, Iwashige H, Kubota N, et al. Results of surgery for paralytic exotropia due to oculomotor palsy. Ophthalmologica. 1996;210(3):163–7.
181. Mudgil AV, Repka MX. Ophthalmologic outcome after third cranial nerve palsy or paresis in childhood. J AAPOS. 1999;3(1):2–8.
182. Schumacher-Feero LA, Yoo KW, Solari FM, Biglan AW. Results following treatment of third cranial nerve palsy in children. Trans Am Ophthalmol Soc. 1998;96:455–72; discussion 472–4.
183. Rush JA, Younge BR. Paralysis of cranial nerves III, IV, and VI. Cause and prognosis in 1,000 cases. Arch Ophthalmol. 1981;99(1):76–9.
184. Brazis PW, Miller NR, Henderer JD, Lee AG. The natural history and results of treatment of superior oblique myokymia. Arch Ophthalmol. 1994;112(8):1063–7.
185. Kushner BJ. Vertical rectus surgery for Knapp class II superior oblique muscle paresis. Arch Ophthalmol. 2010;128(5):585–8.
186. Helveston EM, Mora JS, Lipsky SN, et al. Surgical treatment of superior oblique palsy. Trans Am Ophthalmol Soc. 1996;94:315–28; discussion 328–34.
187. von Noorden GK, Murray E, Wong SY. Superior oblique paralysis. A review of 270 cases. Arch Ophthalmol. 1986;104(12):1771–6.
188. Holmes JM, Beck RW, Kip KE, Droste PJ, Leske DA. Predictors of nonrecovery in acute traumatic sixth nerve palsy and paresis. Ophthalmology. 2001;108(8):1457–60.
189. Holmes JM, Droste PJ, Beck RW. The natural history of acute traumatic sixth nerve palsy or paresis. J AAPOS. 1998;2(5):265–8.
190. Mutyala S, Holmes JM, Hodge DO, Younge BR. Spontaneous recovery rate in traumatic sixth-nerve palsy. Am J Ophthalmol. 1996;122(6):898–9.
191. Holmes JM, Beck RW, Kip KE, Droste PJ, Leske DA. Botulinum toxin treatment versus conservative management in acute traumatic sixth nerve palsy or paresis. J AAPOS. 2000;4(3):145–9.
192. Nowakowska O, Loba P, Broniarczyk-Loba A. The efficacy of vertical rectus transposition and its modalities in patients with abducens nerve palsy. Eur J Ophthalmol. 2011;(21):223–7.
193. Selezinka W, Sandall GS, Henderson JW. Rectus muscle union in sixth nerve paralysis. Jensen rectus muscle union. Arch Ophthalmol. 1974;92(5):382–6.
194. Jensen CD. Rectus muscle union: a new operation for paralysis of the rectus muscles. Trans Pac Coast Otoophthalmol Soc Annu Meet. 1964;45:359–87.

Part III

Eyelid Malpositions

John B. Holds

Entropion

7

Srinivas S. Iyengar, Eric B. Hamill, and Steven C. Dresner

Introduction

Entropion is the inversion of the eyelid margin. It may be classified as congenital, involutional, or cicatricial. Correction of entropion is aimed at the underlying mechanism for eyelid margin inversion. The most common mechanism is destabilization of the anatomic components of the eyelid, such as horizontal eyelid laxity or disinsertion of the eyelid retractions, but may also be related to scarring or congenital abnormalities. As such, therapeutic surgical interventions must be modified to the type of entropion.

Classification

Congenital Entropion

True congenital entropion is rare. These patients have a history of eyelid margin inversion since birth, most commonly involving the lower eyelid, and this is typically caused by disinsertion of the lower-eyelid retractors [1]. Surgical repair is aimed at reinsertion of the retractors. Less commonly, congenital entropion may be caused by a tarsal kink in which a structural abnormality in the tarsal plate turns the eyelid inward; this type of congenital entropion occurs more commonly in the upper eyelid.

Some children have lower-eyelid pretarsal orbicularis and skin that override the eyelid margin and may cause rotation of the cilia toward the cornea (Fig. 7.1). This condition is called *epiblepharon* and, though not a true entropion, exists along the same continuum. Epiblepharon is more commonly seen in Asian infants and may be associated with an elevated body mass index [2]. Epiblepharon is generally asymptomatic and tends to resolve as the child gets older, but when corneal irritation and injury are eminent, surgical intervention is warranted.

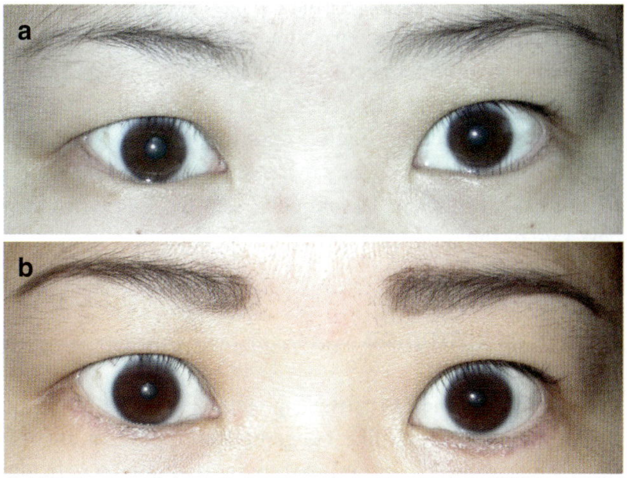

Fig. 7.1 (**a**) Child with epiblepharon of both lower eyelids and symptomatic trichiasis. (**b**) Following small pinch excision of lower-eyelid skin and minimal orbicularis oculi resection

Involutional Entropion

Involutional entropion is the most common type of entropion (Fig. 7.2) and almost exclusively occurs in the lower eyelid. Classically, the causes of involutional entropion include lower-eyelid laxity, an overriding orbicularis oculi muscle, and disinsertion, or attenuation, of the lower-eyelid retractors [3]. Clinically, lower-eyelid laxity is identified by the eyelid distraction or snapback test. In cases of involution entropion, the eyelid can be pulled more than 6 mm from the globe. The overriding or superior migration of the preseptal orbicularis oculi is seen during forceful eyelid closure. The

S. S. Iyengar
San Diego Eyelid Specialists, Encinitas, CA, USA

E. B. Hamill (✉) · S. C. Dresner
Roski Eye Institute, The University of Southern California, Department of Ophthalmology, Los Angeles, CA, USA

Eyesthetica, Los Angeles, CA, USA

J. J. Servat et al. (eds.), *Smith and Nesi's Ophthalmic Plastic and Reconstructive Surgery*,
https://doi.org/10.1007/978-3-030-41720-8_7

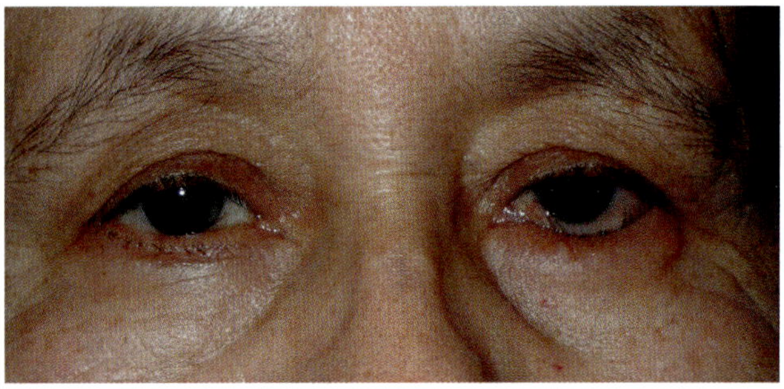

Fig. 7.2 Involutional entropion of the left lower eyelid. Note the comparison between the position of the inverted left lower eyelid and normal right lower eyelid

disinserted lower-eyelid retractors may occasionally be seen as a white band of connective tissue fibers inferior to the tarsal plate. The inferior fornix may also be deeper than normal. With each of these three factors contributing to the destabilization of eyelid position, any therapeutic procedure that fails to address all of these factors decreases the long-term success rate of the procedure.

Cicatricial Entropion

Cicatricial entropion is caused by vertical contracture of the posterior lamellae. Unlike congenital entropion or involutional entropion, cicatricial entropion is often seen in the upper eyelid as well. Causes of cicatricial entropion include ocular cicatricial pemphigoid, Stevens–Johnson syndrome, trachoma, herpetic infection or other chronic inflammatory diseases, trauma, or iatrogenic causes from previous surgery or topical glaucoma and other medications. Clinically, evaluation of the tarsus and conjunctiva of the eyelid in cases of cicatricial entropion shows scarring and difficulty with digital eversion of the eyelid.

Therapy

Treatment of Epiblepharon

There are various methods described to treat epiblepharon. The highest success rate and lowest rate of overcorrection are achieved by the following method. The lower-eyelid skin is gently pinched with a forceps, assessing the minimal amount of skin excision needed to position the eyelashes away from the cornea. This skin is then excised with Westcott scissors. A small strip of orbicularis is excised, and the skin is closed with 6-0 plain or fast-absorbing gut suture (Fig. 7.1a, b). There are other methods [2] described that involve manipulation of the lower-eyelid retractors; this is unnecessary in the surgical correction of true epiblepharon. Some surgeons have injected hyaluronic acid gel to mechanically fill the eyelid and expand the eyelid fold in epiblepharon [4], although the duration of effect may be limited.

Treatment of Involutional Entropion

Involutional lower-eyelid entropion has three underlying correctable causes: eyelid laxity, overriding of the orbicularis oculi muscle, and attenuation of the lower-eyelid retractors. Historically, some procedures described for the correction of involutional entropion failed to address all three of these causes, with suboptimal surgical outcomes.

Wies [5] attempted to create a more permanent scar between the anterior and posterior lamellae of the eyelid with a full-thickness transverse blepharotomy combined with rotation sutures. This technique prevented overriding of the preseptal orbicularis oculi muscle but did not address eyelid laxity or the lower-eyelid retractors. The Wies procedure is helpful in certain cases of cicatricial entropion, although overcorrections and poor cosmesis limit its usefulness. To prevent overriding of the preseptal orbicularis oculi muscle, Wheeler [6] transposed a strap of this muscle from the pretarsal area inferiorly. This corrected the problem with orbicularis oculi muscle override; it did not address horizontal eyelid laxity or abnormalities of the lower-eyelid retractors.

Quickert and Rathbun [7] described a suture technique to create a rotational vector and, hopefully, scarring similar to that created by the Wies procedure. This was modified by Rainin [8] to include deeper cul-de-sac sutures to imbricate the lower-eyelid retractors. Both of these techniques can temporize before a definitive procedure is performed. Neither achieves a high degree of permanence. To correct horizontal laxity, Bick [9] described a technique of full-thickness eyelid shortening. While correcting one underlying cause of entropion, it left the orbicularis oculi muscle and eyelid retractors untouched.

Leone [10] described a technique of transconjunctival tarsectomy and orbiculectomy to correct involutional entropion. This technique excised central tarsus instead of correcting the eyelid laxity at the lateral canthus, where it is most effectively and permanently tightened. In addition, it did not correct attenuation of the lower-eyelid retractors. Jones et al. [11] described dysfunction of the lower-eyelid retractors in involutional entropion and advocated tucking or resecting the abnormal retractors. Dryden et al. [12] described similarly reattaching the retractors directly to the inferior tarsus.

Carroll and Allen [13] have described a combined technique of retractor reinsertion and eyelid shortening that requires a full-thickness blepharotomy. Wesley and Collins [14] have also presented a combined technique of lower-eyelid retractor repair with horizontal eyelid shortening. A modification of this technique has also been described by Nowinski [15]. These later techniques provide long-term success and address the three important elements causing entropion (lower-eyelid laxity, retractor attenuation, and overriding orbicularis oculi muscle) but require a subciliary incision. Overcorrection and postoperative eyelid retraction with the anterior subciliary approach are problematic and may yield less than satisfactory cosmetic results.

The ideal procedure would address all causative factors and avoid a subciliary incision. The approach described by Karesh and Dresner [16] utilizes a transconjunctival approach to address both the lower-eyelid retractors and the orbicularis oculi. Combining this technique with lateral canthal resuspension anatomically corrects the entropion. Long-term studies have shown good functional outcome with minimal complications [17].

Transconjunctival Entropion Repair

The lower eyelid is anesthetized with a transconjunctival injection of 2 mL of 1% xylocaine hydrochloride with a 1:100,000 dilution of epinephrine or other preferred anesthetic solution [16]. One milliliter of anesthetic is injected into the lateral canthus down to the periosteum. A protective eye shield is placed.

A no. 15 blade is used to make a horizontal incision at the lateral canthus. A lateral canthotomy is performed with a straight tenotomy scissors (Fig. 7.3a). The inferior crus of the lateral canthal tendon is released (Fig. 7.3b). A small retractor is placed in the lateral canthal incision. Beginning at the lateral canthus and extending to just lateral to the punctum, an incision is made with a cutting unipolar cautery through the conjunctiva and lower-eyelid retractors just below the lower tarsal border (Fig. 7.3c). Little bleeding is usually encountered as this is a relatively bloodless plane. The orbital septum and the orbicularis oculi muscle are left undisturbed. The conjunctiva and lower-eyelid retractors are elevated and separated from the anterior eyelid lamella and orbicularis muscle. The surgical plane is carried inferiorly 4–5 mm between the lower-eyelid retractors and the fat pads (Fig. 7.3d). Downward traction on the lower eyelid with either a rake or a small Desmarres retractor is used for improving exposure.

Once the fat pads are identified, a transconjunctival blepharoplasty is performed when desired. Gentle pressure on the globe or upward traction on the lower-eyelid retractors is helpful for demonstrating the three lower-eyelid fat compartments. The fine connective tissues covering the fat pads are incised with the cutting cautery. Each fat pad is excised with the needle tip of the cutting cautery without clamping. Small vessels in the fat are cauterized. When the entropion is unilateral, a limited fat excision or none at all is performed to ensure symmetry with the other eyelid. One may perform fat repositioning if desired.

The lower tarsal border is then pulled upward, everting the eyelid. Cutting cautery is used to excise a strip of orbicularis oculi muscle below the tarsus along the full length of the incision (Fig. 7.3e). Since the orbital septum fuses with the lower-eyelid retractors approximately 5 mm below the tarsal border, excision of the orbicularis oculi in this area is performed without violating the orbital septum. The lower-eyelid retractors are firmly adherent to the conjunctiva and immediately posterior to the fat compartments. If there is any uncertainty about their location, the patient can be asked to look upward and downward to identify the edge of the retractors.

The retractors are separated from the conjunctiva with the cutting cautery to create a free edge (Fig. 7.4a). Sharp dissection is then performed at the inferior tarsal border to expose the anterior surface. The free retractor edge is then reinserted into the inferior and anterior tarsal border with two buried 6-0 Vicryl (polygalactin 910) sutures (Fig. 7.4b, c). Reattaching the retractors to the anterior surface of the tarsus appreciably everts the eyelid margin. No closure of the conjunctiva is necessary since the conjunctiva readily reattaches to the inferior tarsal border.

The eyelid is then horizontally shortened to correct all eyelid laxity, and a tarsal strip is performed (Fig. 7.4d). The mucocutaneous junction is excised, and a no. 15 blade is used to scrape the epithelium from the posterior surface of the lateral tarsus. Shortening of the strip before its reattachment to the lateral orbital rim periosteum prevents the formation of a lateral subcutaneous lump after closure of the skin. The tarsal strip is reinserted into the lateral orbital rim with two 4-0 Vicryl sutures. The canthotomy incision can then be closed in standard fashion.

This approach is successful in 96.7% of cases [17]; it circumvents the risk of lower-eyelid retraction and overcorrection that may occur with the transcutaneous approach. An external approach is preferred in cases where lid laxity is minimal or absent, significant festoons are present, or prominent lower-eyelid dermatochalasis is present.

Treatment of Cicatricial Entropion

Often the causes of cicatricial entropion are systemic and progressive. Medical control of the underlying cause is optimized before surgical correction of the eyelid malposition. Methods used in the surgical repair include anterior lamellar resection, partial or complete tarsal infracture, mucous membrane grafting, and lash follicle excision. The decision on which of these procedures to employ depends on the severity, age, and etiology of cicatricial entropion. Skin resection

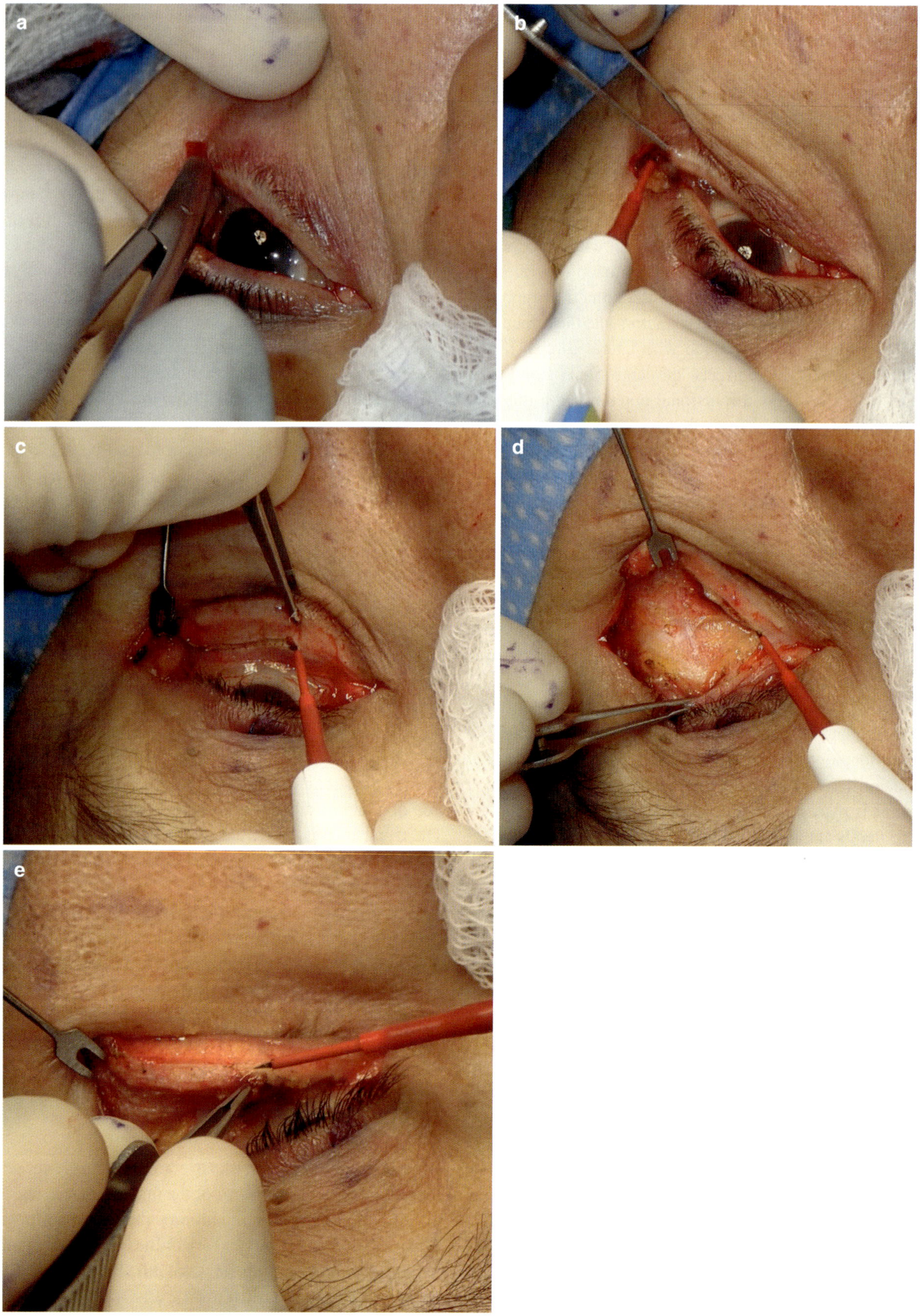

Fig. 7.3 (**a**) A lateral canthotomy is performed with a straight tenotomy scissors "view inverted". (**b**) The inferior crus of the lateral canthal tendon is released. (**c**) An incision is made with a unipolar cutting cautery immediately below the tarsal border through the conjunctiva and lower-eyelid retractors. (**d**) Dissection is carried out inferiorly 4–5 mm between the eyelid retractors and fat pads. (**e**) A cutting cautery is used to excise a strip of orbicularis muscle along the full length of the incision

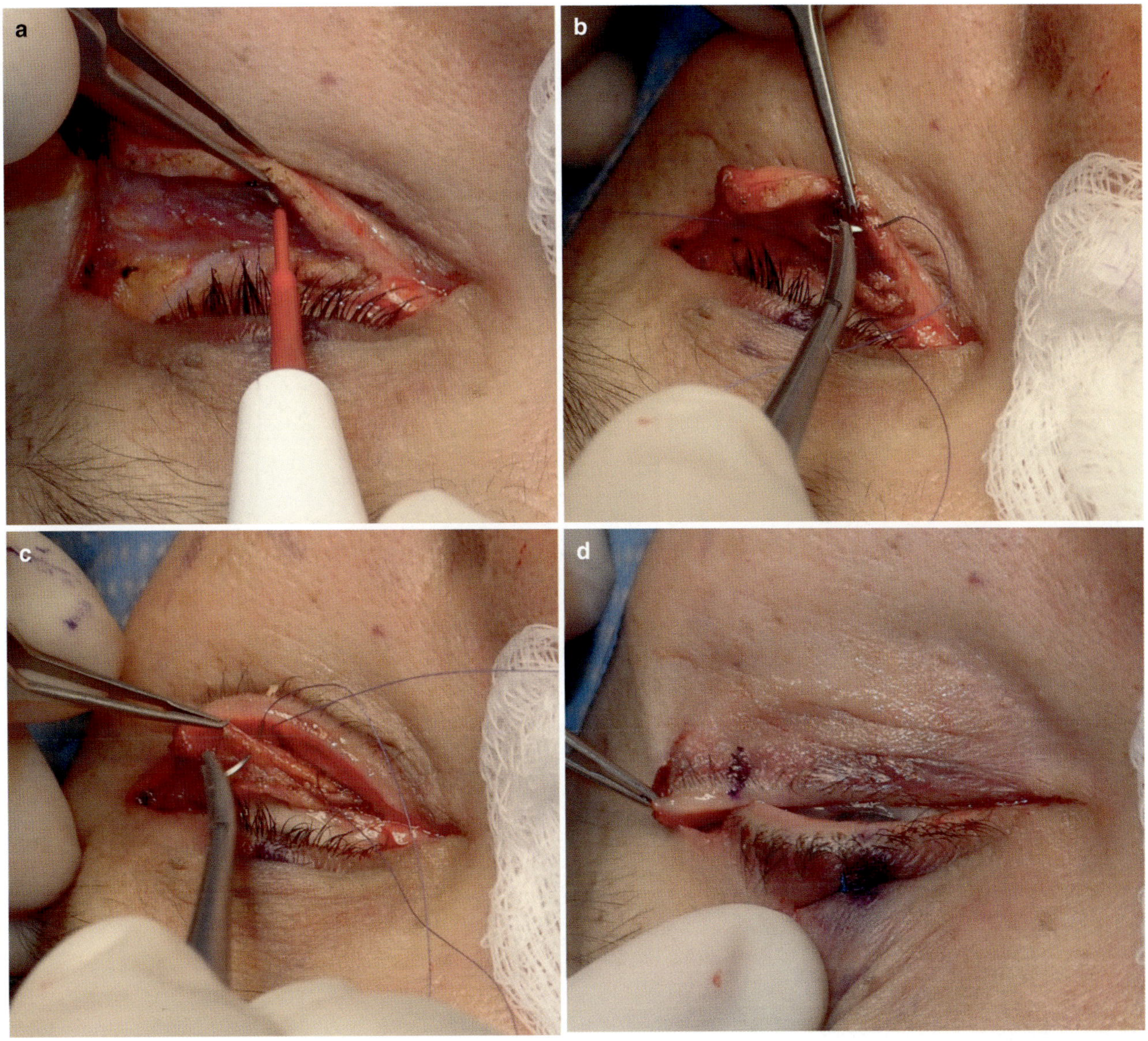

Fig. 7.4 (**a**) A cutting cautery is used to create a potential space anterior to the tarsal plate. (**b**) A suture is placed in the inferior anterior surface of the tarsal plate. (**c**) The same 6-0 Vicryl suture is passed through the lower-eyelid retractors to reapproximate the retractors with the tarsus. (**d**) A horizontal eyelid shortening and eyelid resuspension through tarsal strip formation are then performed to tighten the eyelids

or blepharoplasty alone may rotate the eyelid margin sufficiently away from the cornea in mild cases.

In moderate cases, in which lash preservation is not as much of a concern, lash follicle excision may be performed. In this procedure, a no. 11 blade is used to make a horizontal lamellar-splitting incision posterior to the lashes, and Westcott scissors are used to excise the lashes. Electrocautery is then applied for hemostasis and at the base of excised lash follicles. Cryotherapy may also suffice when there are limited sectoral areas of lash-corneal touch (see Chap. 8 regarding treatment of trichiasis).

In cases of significant cicatricial entropion, when lash preservation is desired, tarsal infracture, partial or complete, is considered. For the upper eyelid, after local anesthesia, placement of a corneal shield, and skin incision with or without blepharoplasty, the tarsal plate is exposed. Partial tarsotomy is then performed and extended with Stevens scissors. Double-armed everting 6-0 Vicryl sutures are then placed through partial-thickness tarsus and externalized. The lid margin is then reassessed and full-thickness transverse tarsotomy performed. Everting sutures are replaced, rotating the lid margin away from the cornea. Standard skin closure is performed.

More severe cicatricial entropion in the lower eyelid may warrant the placement of a hard palate mucosal graft or other mucous membrane graft to lengthen and support the posterior lamella after releasing all scar tissue (Fig. 7.5a–e). Graft choice is particularly important in the upper eyelid as the graft directly contacts the cornea. Free tarsoconjunctival grafts are particularly useful here, especially if the patient is undergoing simultaneous posterior approach ptosis surgery. In the lower eyelid, we prefer the use of hard palate mucosa over the currently available synthetic tarsal substitutes.

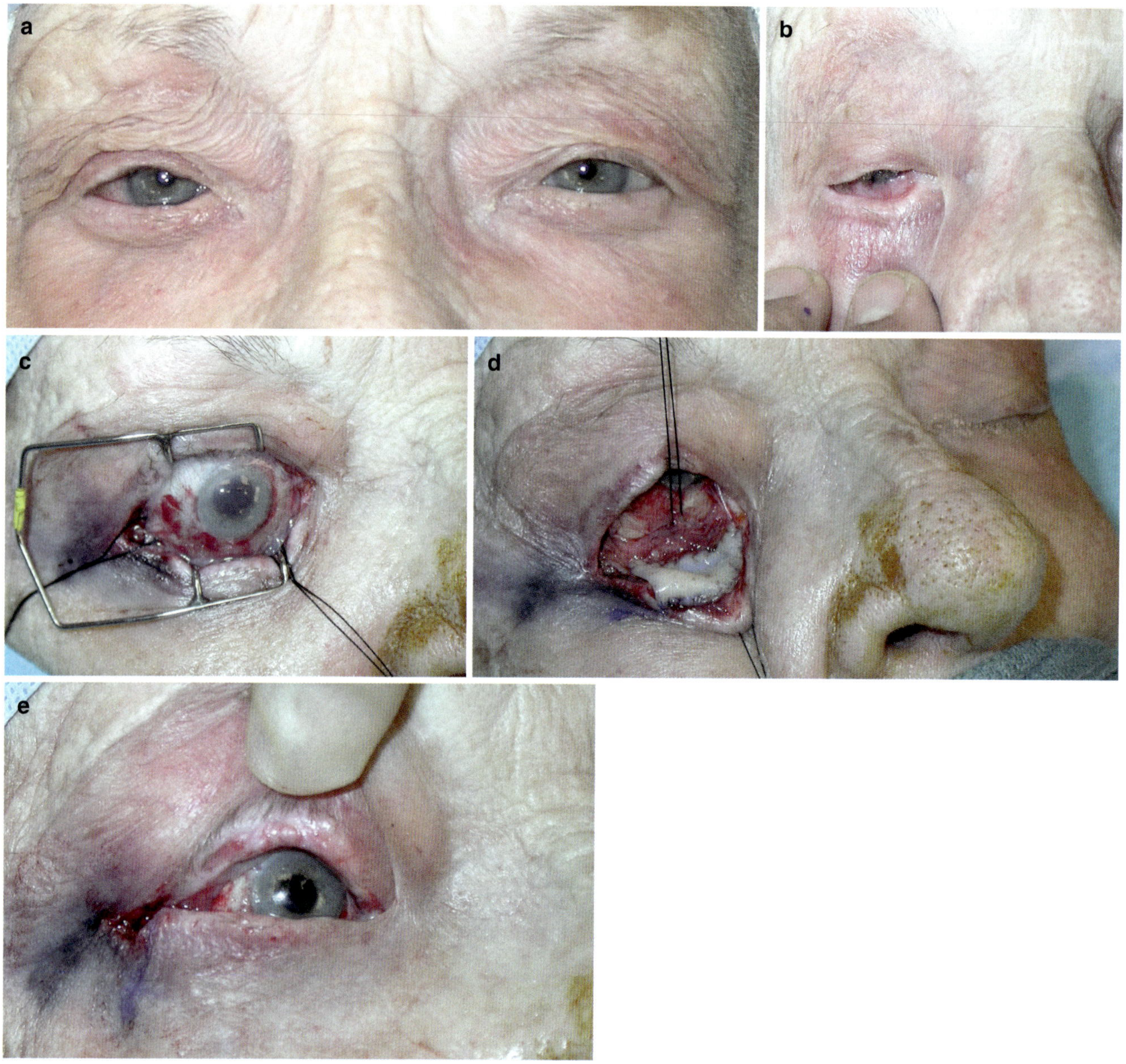

Fig. 7.5 (**a**) Patient with a cicatricial entropion of the right lower eyelid. (**b**) Manual inferior traction on the right lower eyelid shows extensive symblepharon causing posterior lamellar shortening. (**c**) Intraoperative photograph showing the first stage of cicatricial entropion repair, which in this case is lysis of symblepharon of the right lower eyelid. (**d**) Intraoperative photograph showing placement of hard palate graft to lengthen the posterior lamella of the right lower eyelid. (**e**) Right lower eyelid after horizontal lid shortening and eyelid resuspension via lateral tarsal strip in the correction of cicatricial entropion

Conclusion

The structures of the eyelid, including the orbicularis muscle, canthal tendons, conjunctiva, and lower-eyelid retractors, contribute to the stability of the lower-eyelid margin position. Treatment for the cause of entropion, namely, congenital entropion, epiblepharon, and involutional or cicatricial entropion, is directed at addressing those specific anatomical factors directly responsible for the eyelid margin instability, so as to maximize success and minimize recurrence while maintaining an optimal aesthetic result.

References

1. Tse DT, Anderson RL, Frakker JD. Aponeurosis disinsertion in congenital entropion. Arch Ophthalmol. 1983;101:436.
2. Ahn HB, Seo JW, Yoo JH, Jeong WJ, Park WC, Rho SH. Epiblepharon related to high body mass index in Korean children. J Pediatr Ophthalmol Strabismus. 2010;30:1–4.
3. Collin JRO, Rathbun JE. Involutional entropion: a review with evaluation of a procedure. Arch Ophthalmol. 1978;96:1058–64.
4. Naik MN, Ali MJ, Das S, Honavar SG. Nonsurgical management of epiblepharon using hyaluronic acid gel. Ophthal Plast Reconstr Surg. 2010;26(3):215–7.
5. Wies FA. Spastic entropion. Trans Am Acad Ophthalmol Otolaryngol. 1955;59:503–6.

6. Wheeler JM. Spastic entropion corrected by orbicularis transplantation. Trans Am Ophthalmol Soc. 1938;36:157–62.
7. Quickert MH, Rathbun E. Suture repair of entropion. Arch Ophthalmol. 1971;85:304–5.
8. Rainin EA. Senile entropion. Arch Ophthalmol. 1979;97:928–30.
9. Bick MW. Surgical management of orbital tarsal disparity. Arch Ophthalmol. 1966;75:386–9.
10. Leone CR. Internal tarsus-orbicularis resection for senile spastic entropion. Ann Ophthalmol. 1975;7:1004–6.
11. Jones LT, Reeh MJ, Wobig JL. Senile entropion: a new concept for correction. Am J Ophthalmol. 1972;74:327–9.
12. Dryden RM, Leibsohn J, Wobig JL. Senile entropion: pathogenesis and treatment. Arch Ophthalmol. 1978;96:1883–5.
13. Carroll RP, Allen SE. Combined procedure for repair of involutional entropion. Ophthal Plast Reconstr Surg. 1991;7:123–7.
14. Wesley RE, Collins JW. Combined procedure for senile entropion. Ophthalmic Surg. 1983;14:401–5.
15. Nowinski TS. Orbicularis oculi muscle extirpation in a combined procedure for involutional entropion. Ophthalmology. 1991;98:1250–6.
16. Dresner SC, Karesh JW. Transconjunctival entropion repair. Arch Ophthalmol. 1993;111(8):1144–8.
17. Erb MH, Uzcategui N, Dresner SC. Efficacy and complications of the transconjunctival entropion repair for lower eyelid involutional entropion. Ophthalmology. 2006;113(12):2351–6.

8 Trichiasis

Kenneth V. Cahill

Introduction

Eyelashes play a protective role in keeping foreign material out of the eye. They emanate from the anterior edge of the rectangular lid margin. Each lash has a gently tapering shaft that arches anteriorly and away from the eyelid fissure. The lash follicles are approximately 2 mm deep in the upper lid and 1.75 in the lower lid. If a follicle becomes distorted in shape and/or orientation, the lash will grow with abnormal curvature or direction, defined as trichiasis. Lashes that touch the ocular surface can cause irritation, reflex epiphora, and abrasions which can lead to ocular surface infections, erosions, and scarring with temporary or permanent visual loss.

A number of eyelid abnormalities cause abnormal eyelash position. These may or may not occur in conjunction with trichiasis. Entropion is an inward rotation of the lid margin and tarsus. Since the lid margin is rotated inward, the lashes rub against the ocular surface. In epiblepharon, a fold of redundant lower lid subciliary anterior lamellar tissue consisting of the skin, subcutaneous connective tissue, and orbicularis oculi muscle presses the lashes toward the globe where they can rub the ocular surface. In the upper lid, an excessive lid fold forming above the lid crease (dermatochalasis) can hang down over the lashes. In some cases, the lashes are not able to support this extra weight and are pressed down against the globe. Sometimes lash ptosis develops in which the upper lid lashes sag downward due to anterior lamellar laxity in the pretarsal area including the lash follicles.

In distichiasis, lashes grow out of the meibomian gland orifices in the posterior lid lamella near the posterior lid margin. Meibomian glands arise from embryologic structures with the potential to be a pilosebaceous unit. Distichiasis can occur as a congenital anomaly or as an acquired defect following eyelid inflammation. These lashes are usually straight and touch the ocular surface. Occasionally, a loose eyelash will become lodged in a meibomian gland or a vertical canaliculus and cause temporary irritation until it comes out or is removed.

Trichiasis results from many causes and may be associated with other eyelid abnormalities. It is important to try to identify the cause so that the optimal treatment is chosen and so that future problems can be averted or at least minimized.

In general, the treatment of trichiasis involves medical treatment of underlying infections and cicatricial disorders, epilation, electrolysis, and surgical repair of the lid margin and adjacent lid abnormalities.

Occasionally, an eyelash will become ingrown, with its shaft visible under the thin lid skin. This is termed cilia incarnata [1]. It is a variation of pili incarnata, which refers to any ingrown hair. If the shaft of the lash is not buried adjacent to its follicle, it can usually be teased out at this exposed site using the rounded side of a hypodermic needle. If there is no exposure of the lash shaft, an opening can be made with a blade after application of topical or local anesthetic. Ingrown lashes are rarely recurrent and usually do not cause problems unless the site of lash ingrowth becomes infected.

Sometimes a solitary lash will grow aberrantly and cause ocular irritation. If there is no prior history of this and no structural abnormality of the lid is evident, then epilation (pulling) of the lash is appropriate. If the lash epilates with minimal resistance, it is possible that the lash was about to fall out, and its abnormal direction was due to being loose in the follicle. If the lash regrows, which can begin in as little as 2 weeks, and causes recurrent irritation, then permanent eradication by selective electrolysis is reasonable. Sometimes a patient or their relatives are able to epilate the lash and prefer repeated epilation to electrolysis. Such efforts often result in numerous "innocent bystander" lashes being epilated without relief, while the offending lash(es) are too fine or too short to be accurately identified and removed by the patient or their family.

Focal trichiasis may occur due to the distortion caused by a lid margin lesion, such as a nevus, benign squamous papil-

K. V. Cahill (✉)
The Ohio State University, Department of Ophthalmology, Columbus, OH, USA

J. J. Servat et al. (eds.), *Smith and Nesi's Ophthalmic Plastic and Reconstructive Surgery*,
https://doi.org/10.1007/978-3-030-41720-8_8

loma, glandular cyst (sebaceous or serous), or a chalazion. Seborrheic keratoses are frequent lid margin lesions but rarely cause lash follicle distortion. Treatment of the offending lesion is a good first step. For most of the benign growths, a lid margin shave excision with light superficial cautery clinically eliminates the growth even though "clear" margins are not necessarily achieved. Full-thickness wedge excisions of eyelid margin benign lesions are rarely necessary. Lid margin cysts are usually controlled by excising the exposed half of their cyst wall, evacuating their contents, and lightly cauterizing the remaining deep half of their wall. In the unusual instance that a symptomatic notch remains in the eyelid, a wedge excision and repair can be performed. Chalazia are also treated and resolved before definitive lash treatment is undertaken. We epilate the offending lashes at the time of treatment of the lid margin lesion. Any symptomatic trichiasis which persists when the margin is fully healed can be eliminated by electrolysis. In the unusual circumstance that a full-thickness pentagonal wedge excision is required, this will usually also remove the eyelid segment with the trichiasis.

Accidental or surgical lid margin trauma can result in trichiasis. If it is a focal problem such as trichiasis at the site of an otherwise well-healed marginal full-thickness lid laceration, electrolysis is used. If there is a traumatic notch along with trichiasis, then a pentagonal wedge excision and repair is used (Fig. 8.1). If the damage is not focal, such as from thermal or chemical injury, then more extensive lid reconstruction is required, as discussed in other chapters.

Trichiasis can occur in conjunction with entropion and ectropion. One of the most common forms of combined involutional entropion and trichiasis we see is an acquired lower lid margin thinning and distortion that is most prominent centrally (Fig. 8.2). This was described by Mills and Meyer [2]. Chronic blepharitis is a suspected etiology. The irritation caused by the lid margin thinning and trichiasis may lead to increased forceful blinking, resulting in a spastic or involutional entropion. If only a few lashes are misdirected, selective electrolysis may suffice, although the problem can continue to progress. In extreme cases, a lid splitting procedure may be necessary. This is technically challenging in these patients since the tarsal plate is thin and weakened.

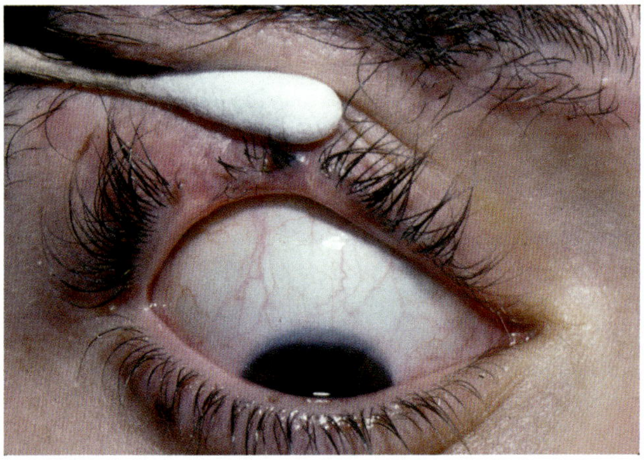

Fig. 8.1 Full-thickness lid margin trichiasis following a complex full-thickness upper lid laceration. If selective electrolysis is not successful, a pentagonal wedge resection and repair is used

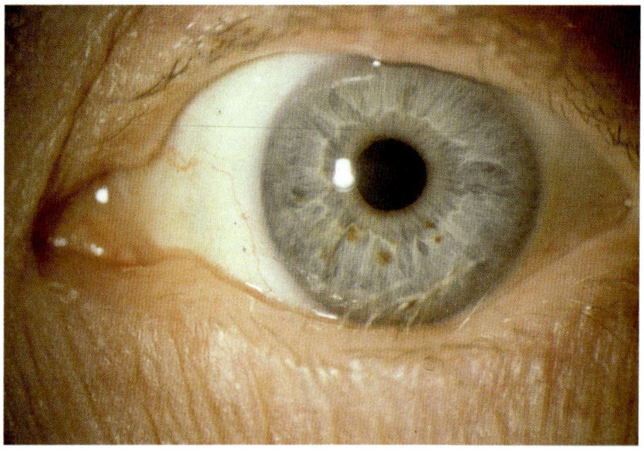

Fig. 8.2 Involutional lower lid margin thinning, entropion, and trichiasis. This example is too extensive to be treated with a wedge resection. Selective electrolysis of the most posterior trichiasis may provide a satisfactory solution. If not, a lid splitting procedure can be utilized

Chronic involutional entropion and ectropion may be associated with a rounding deformity of the lid margin with secondary trichiasis. Suspicious lashes are epilated at the time of the surgical lid margin position repair. If trichiasis remains a problem after the patient has recovered from surgery, selective electrolysis is usually sufficient treatment.

Cicatricial entropion is frequently accompanied by trichiasis. The scarring process that alters the position of the tarsus and lid margin usually distorts the lash follicles as well. Sometimes this entropion and trichiasis is due to a single event, such as scarring from a lower cul-de-sac surgical incision. Many causes of cicatricial entropion are chronic and progressive. A diagnosis is sought and medical therapy provided for treatable disorders.

Trachoma, ocular cicatricial pemphigoid, linear IgG, graft versus host disease, and Stevens–Johnson syndrome are conditions which should be medically stabilized before surgical repair. Periodic epilation and selective electrolysis provide temporary ocular protection. Surgical repair should avoid incising the conjunctiva. If the conjunctival surface must be increased, this may be performed in combination with trichiasis treatment or in separate staged procedures, depending on the specific techniques required. This is generally deferred until the underlying cicatricial disease is medically controlled.

Upper lid lash ptosis can be a component of floppy eyelid syndrome, involutional lateral upper lid entropion described by Camara et al. [3] (Fig. 8.3), various forms of ptosis, and as an isolated occurrence. Ordinarily, fibers of the levator aponeurosis extend into the orbicularis oculi muscle and terminate at the dermal layer of the skin, contributing to the formation of the upper lid crease and maintaining the orientation of the lash follicles. Laxity or disruption of this support can lead to anterior lamellar descent and lash ptosis. Various

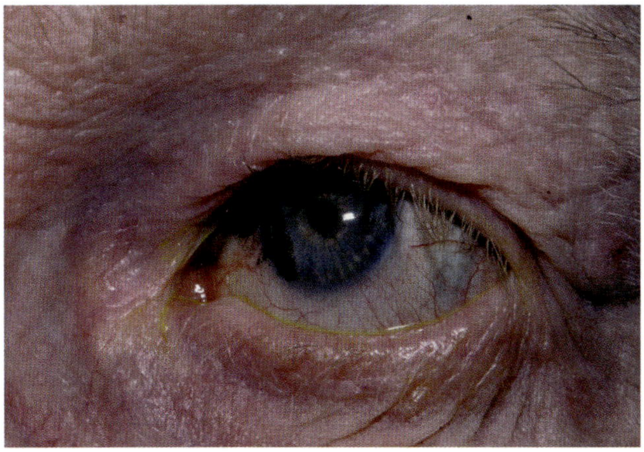

Fig. 8.3 Involutional lateral upper lid entropion can occur in all races. This patient had too much of the lid involved to make electrolysis appropriate, and surgical repair was utilized

authors have described a skin resection to correct this problem. We have found that undermining the anterior lamella along the anterior tarsal surface from the crease incision down to the lash follicles with attachment of this lamella to the levator aponeurosis provides a more predictable and lasting repair.

Lower lid trichiasis, entropion, and retraction are sometimes seen following transconjunctival approaches to repair extensive trauma to the inferior orbital rim and/or floor. If this begins to appear, steroid (Kenalog 10 mg/mL) injections, 5% 5-FU injections, or other means of preventing scar tissue contracture may avert more serious problems. If the contracture is already extensive, an infratarsal spacer graft usually corrects the problem. A graft of autogenous tarsus, split thickness dermis, or hard palate mucosa which can be left uncovered is usually best. Some allo- and xenografts such as preserved sclera, AlloDerm®, Enduragen®, or Tarsys® may be placed to serve as temporary spacers. Additional conjunctival surface area is usually needed in addition to lengthening the lower lid retractors, scarred septum, etc.

Electrolysis Technique

For electrolysis, we use the Ellman Surgitron FFPF EMC radiosurgery unit (Ellman International, Inc., Oceanside, NY) [4]. The affected area of the lid is infiltrated with local anesthetic and given time to reach full anesthesia.

The electrolysis needle which we use is a very fine wire in which only the tip is not insulated (Ellman sterile needle H137 handpiece XH136). The procedure is best performed at the slit lamp. We have used the operating microscope for visualization but do not feel it offers the same accuracy and depth perception.

The needle is advanced into the follicle at least 2 mm. For full-sized eyelash cilia, the needle should pass without any resistance so that it slides into the follicle alongside the eyelash. The current is applied for 1–2 s using the partially rectified mode at a power level of 2. This cauterizes the follicle. Very mild blanching is seen on the surface of the lid margin. The lash will oftentimes slide out of the follicle with the needle when it is withdrawn. If the lash does not slide out with the needle and if there is any resistance when forceps removal is attempted, it has not been adequately treated. The lash should have no adhesion to the follicle after proper treatment. It is sometimes difficult to align an eyelid so that the needle can be passed directly into the follicles in cases where the lashes are highly distorted. No posttreatment care or analgesics are necessary.

The success rate for permanent elimination of aberrant cilia is approximately 80% with this technique. It is only used if the offending lashes are present, so epilation should be avoided for 3–6 weeks before a treatment. A second treatment session is often necessary 6–8 weeks after the first treatment to eliminate the 20% of lashes for which treatment failed and any aberrant lashes that were not actively growing at the time of the first treatment. If a higher power level is used to try to increase the success rate above 80%, there is a greater risk of causing thermal injury to the adjacent lid tissues.

There is not an absolute limit to the number of aberrant lash cilia that can be treated in one lid with electrolysis. As a rough guideline, if more 20 lashes are symptomatic in a lid, a surgical approach may be a better option.

Since distichiasis lashes emanate from a meibomian gland pilosebaceous follicle, they are quite amenable to treatment with electrolysis. Procedures with resection of the involved tarsal plate and replacement with a mucous membrane graft have been described. This may leave a red posterior lid margin. We have not found this approach to be necessary.

Cryotherapy Technique

Many surgeons have abandoned cryotherapy for treating trichiasis. Cryotherapy may damage the adjacent structures, including normal lashes, the tarsal plate, and the posterior lid margin, and alter skin pigmentation. Performing cryotherapy selectively to the anterior lid lamella during lid splitting surgery avoids some of this damage. Cryotherapy may be an unnecessary adjunct to lid splitting surgery. If trichiasis is treated with cryotherapy utilizing a nitrous oxide gas retinal cryoprobe, the following techniques will successfully destroy eyelash cilia with the noted shortcomings:

Local infiltration with a 50:50 lidocaine/bupivacaine mixture provides patient comfort for the procedure and for several hours afterward. A topical anesthetic is instilled, and a protective eye shield is placed. A nitrous oxide cryotherapy unit fitted with a 1.5 mm retinal tip can be used. The freezing tip should be positioned on the conjunctiva surface of the lid adjacent to the lid margin where abnormal lashes are present. If a thermocouple is available, its needle-point probe should be positioned among the lash cilia follicles to be treated. A freeze, thaw, and freeze cycle achieving −25 °C on the thermocouple meter for 45 seconds during each freeze is usually sufficient. If no thermocouple is available, the end point for the freeze cycle can be

45 seconds of freezing after the ice ball reaches the anterior lid surface. The temperature of the retinal tip should register −60 °C or lower during each 45 seconds freeze cycle.

The protective scleral shell is removed, and an antibiotic ophthalmic ointment is instilled. Analgesics, such as acetaminophen with codeine or oxycodone, and a bedtime sedative are usually indicated for the first few days after treatment. The lid margin area forms bullae followed by a scab. The patient continues to use antibiotic ointment several times daily until this scab is shed. One week after treatment, the lashes should pull out with no resistance. Resistance to epilation at this time suggests that inadequate cryotherapy was administered. Some skin depigmentation may result from properly performed eyelid cryotherapy. This must be considered before recommending cryotherapy in darkly pigmented patients.

Laser Techniques

An argon or diode 532 mm ophthalmic laser can be used to treat trichiasis. The hair shaft needs to be pigmented for this to work well. Local anesthesia and eye protection are necessary. A narrow laser beam of 50 μm diameter in continuous mode with high energy (1 W plus) is used to ablate the entire follicular portion of the shaft which extends approximately 2 mm below the lid margin surface. It can be a challenge to orient and immobilize the lid so that the lash follicle to be treated is precisely aligned with the laser beam for the duration of treatment. We find electrolysis to be easier and to have a higher success rate.

Lid Splitting Technique

A lid splitting technique is used when there is extensive trichiasis that occurred as a result of cicatricial entropion which is inactive. It is generally performed under local anesthesia. The affected lid margin is stabilized with a very wide chalazion clamp, bone plate, or other means. A sharp blade is used to initiate the lamellar split immediately posterior to the lashes and anterior to the remaining meibomian orifices, posterior lid margin, and tarsus. It is of utmost importance to preserve whatever is left of these posterior lid margin structures or lid margin defects will result with a functional failure. The dissection is carried along the entire anterior surface of the tarsus, which may be curved or irregular due to the cicatricial process. The recessed anterior lamella is fixated to the posterior lamella with 5-0 chromic sutures or with 5-0 silk, nylon, or polypropylene sutures which are removed 3 weeks later. A spatulated needle works best to make a partial-thickness pass through the posterior lamella. In the lower lid, 2–3 mm of vertical tarsal height is left bare. Three to 4 mm is left bare in the upper lid (Fig. 8.4a). The appearance of the lid does not change for 2 weeks. Then from the second to the third postoperative week, there is granulation that forms a new anterior lid margin. The appearance is mildly erythematous at first, but with time, it forms a remarkably aesthetic lid margin plateau (Fig. 8.4b, c). We find the appearance and patient satisfaction of this technique to be better than mucous membrane grafts (Fig. 8.5). If there has

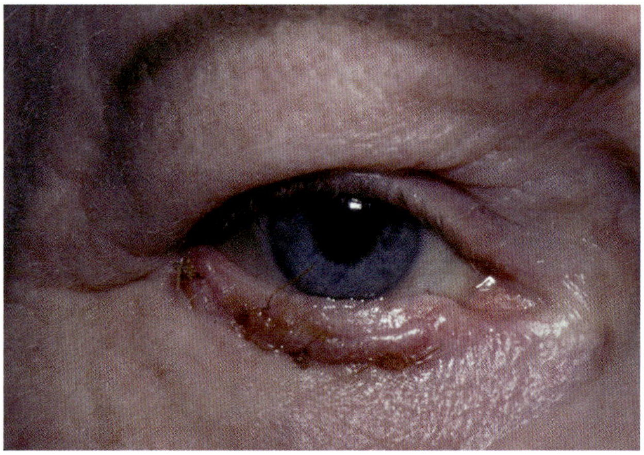

Fig. 8.5 Lower lid splitting at 3 weeks showing the absence of erythema typically seen in mucous membrane grafts

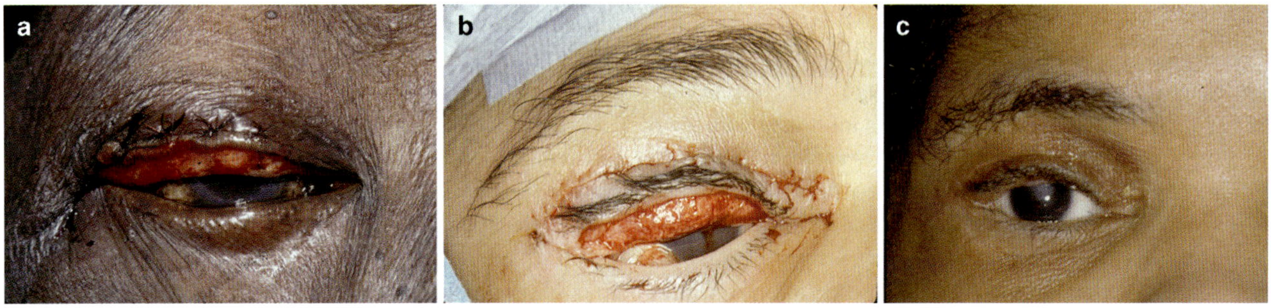

Fig. 8.4 (**a**) Upper lid splitting procedure for trichiasis due to cicatricial entropion. The anterior lamella was recessed 4 mm and secured in this position with sutures. (**b**) Upper lid splitting procedure in a patient with uncontrolled corneal abrasion unable to tolerate a bandage contact lens. (**c**) Postoperatively, the patient was comfortable, the corneal epithelium was intact, corneal stromal opacification partially regressed, and a lid margin plateau was present

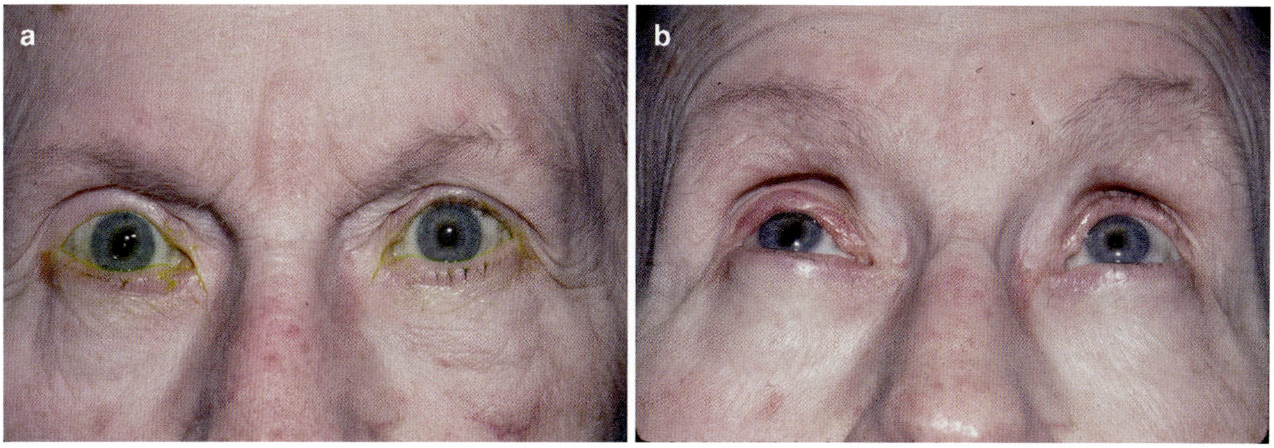

Fig. 8.6 (a) Preoperatively, the right upper lid margin was rounded with loss of all lashes from previous cryotherapy. Keratinized skin continued to cause right ocular surface abrasions. (b) Both upper lids have healed from a splitting procedure. With no lashes, the right upper lid still looks "bald." Both eyes became comfortable, and corneal abrasions were eliminated

been extensive lash loss, this procedure will still work, but the resultant new margin will have a rounded, "bald" appearance (Fig. 8.6a, b).

Conclusion

Trichiasis may occur due to a number of mechanisms related to trauma, surgery, chronic cicatrizing disease, and other causes. Epilation followed by focal electrocautery and treatment of any underlying instigating cause are important initial treatments. Cryotherapy has fallen into disfavor in many surgeons' hands but still has a role in the treatment of some patients. Lid splitting and excision techniques are also valuable for recalcitrant patients. A careful assessment and appropriate choice of treatment improve comfort for most patients with trichiasis.

References

1. Lowry JC, Bartley GB. Cilia incarnata. Arch Ophthalmol. 1995;113:110.
2. Mills DM, Meyers DR. Central lower eyelid thinning with trichiasis: characterization and management of a unique subset of entropion in elderly patients. Ophthal Plast Reconstr Surg. 2009;25(6):445.
3. Camara JG, et al. Involutional lateral entropion of the upper eyelids. Arch Ophthalmol. 2002;120:1682.
4. Ferreira IS, Bernardes TF, Bonfioli AA. Trichiasis. Semin Ophthalmol. 2010;25(3):66–71.

Ectropion

9

Steven M. Couch and Philip L. Custer

Introduction

Eyelid ectropion is present when the lid margin is displaced outward from the ocular surface. This eyelid malposition is commonly encountered in clinical practice and generally affects the lower eyelid. The etiologies of eyelid ectropion include involutional, cicatricial, paralytic, mechanical, and congenital disorders; however, multifactorial causes are frequently present.

Eyelid retraction describes inferior displacement of the eyelid margin with the development of inferior scleral show. While ectropion and retraction can both be present, retraction differs from ectropion in that the lid margin remains approximated to the globe.

Etiology

Normally, the posterior surface of the lower eyelid is closely apposed to the globe, with the edge of the lid margin positioned slightly above the inferior corneal limbus. The eyelid margin is square-shaped with the mucocutaneous junction occurring just posterior to the meibomian gland orifices. The marginal orbicularis muscle (muscle of Riolan) is responsible for tight apposition of the eyelid margin to the ocular surface. A relative shortage of skin, horizontal eyelid laxity, orbicularis muscle weakness, thinning of the normal square-shaped eyelid margin, and disinsertion of the lower eyelid retractors may all contribute to the development of ectropion.

Clinical Presentation

Patients with lower eyelid ectropion present with symptoms related to ocular or conjunctival exposure, cosmetic deformity, or lacrimal dysfunction. Ocular surface irritation secondary to exposure is common secondary to incomplete palpebral closure and poor blink. When the lower eyelid is ectropic, the palpebral conjunctiva can become irritated, erythematous, and keratinized leading to ocular irritation, discharge, and cosmetic deformity. Ectropion-related tearing is frequently multifactorial [1]. Reflex lacrimation may be present secondary to superficial keratitis and exposure. Punctal malposition inhibits lacrimal outflow [2]. Coexisting punctal stenosis often develops in patients with chronic ectropion. The lacrimal pump may be inadequate in patients with significant horizontal laxity.

While the symptoms are commonly the same among the different types of ectropion, historical clues may provide value in determining the predominant cause of ectropion. Involutional ectropion is generally gradual but progressive in onset. Commonly, involutional changes follow a specific pattern of development by starting as punctal eversion and progressing to medial ectropion and then diffuse ectropion. It is important to elicit any history of trauma, chemical exposure or systemic cicatrizing disease, extensive sun exposure, or history of skin cancer if concerned about cicatricial ectropion. Cicatricial ectropion may be gradual in development or sometimes has a sudden onset, especially if related to a specific precipitating event such as trauma, surgery, or acute blepharitis. Long-standing involutional ectropion can cause cicatricial anterior lamellar changes secondary to skin contraction. Paralytic ectropion may be present in patients with previous history of facial palsy.

S. M. Couch (✉) · P. L. Custer
Washington University in St. Louis, Ophthalmology and Visual Sciences, St. Louis, MO, USA
e-mail: couchs@wustl.edu

J. J. Servat et al. (eds.), *Smith and Nesi's Ophthalmic Plastic and Reconstructive Surgery*,
https://doi.org/10.1007/978-3-030-41720-8_9

Evaluation of the Patient with Ectropion

The defining cause of ectropion may be ascertained through historical clues, but the most important indication is found with careful physical examination. Specific attention should be paid to the eyelid margin, character of anterior and posterior lamella, horizontal laxity of lower eyelid, horizontal extent of the ectropion across the eyelid margin, and canthal position [3].

Eyelid Margin

The transition between nonkeratinized conjunctival epithelium and keratinized eyelid margin epithelium is abrupt and should occur just behind the orifices of the meibomian glands. Posterior migration of the mucocutaneous junction occurs in long-standing ectropion, and the level of keratinization can be assessed using rose bengal or lissamine green if it is not easily visualized. The normal square eyelid margin takes on a rounded appearance in chronic ectropion. When severe, this marginal cicatrization can cause posterior rotation of the eyelash line, resulting in trichiasis after the ectropion is corrected surgically.

Eyelid Puncta

Evaluation of the punctal position and aperture is important. When observing the eyelid in its natural resting position, the punctum should not be visible; if the punctum is perceptible, eversion may be present. Chronic malposition can lead to stenosis or obliteration of the lower puncta, and surgical repair of the puncta may be required.

Eyelid Distraction Test

Horizontal eyelid laxity can be assessed with vertical distraction testing of the lower eyelid. Normal values are 6 mm or less. While laxity tends to increase with age, excessive laxity may need to be addressed with horizontal eyelid tightening techniques.

Snapback Test

Another method of assessing horizontal eyelid laxity and eyelid tone is performing a snapback test. When the normal lower eyelid is downwardly distracted from the globe and released, it returns to position abutting the globe without blinking (Fig. 9.1). The eyelid tone can be graded from 1 to 4+ based on the amount of time or number of blinks required for the eyelid to return to its normal position, normal being immediately without blinking. This test is most helpful in mild cases of ectropion and does not rule out paralytic or cicatricial ectropion.

Character of Anterior Lamella

Anterior lamellar shortening is the hallmark of cicatricial ectropion. Mild cases of cicatrization can be easily overlooked; vertical rhytids in the medial lid are an early sign of skin shortage (Fig. 9.2). Limitation of superior migration of the lid margin in upgaze and eversion of the margin when opening the mouth widely also indicate inadequacy of the anterior lamella. In severe cases of cicatricial ectropion, it can be impossible to manually reposition the lid because of tethering from the tight skin.

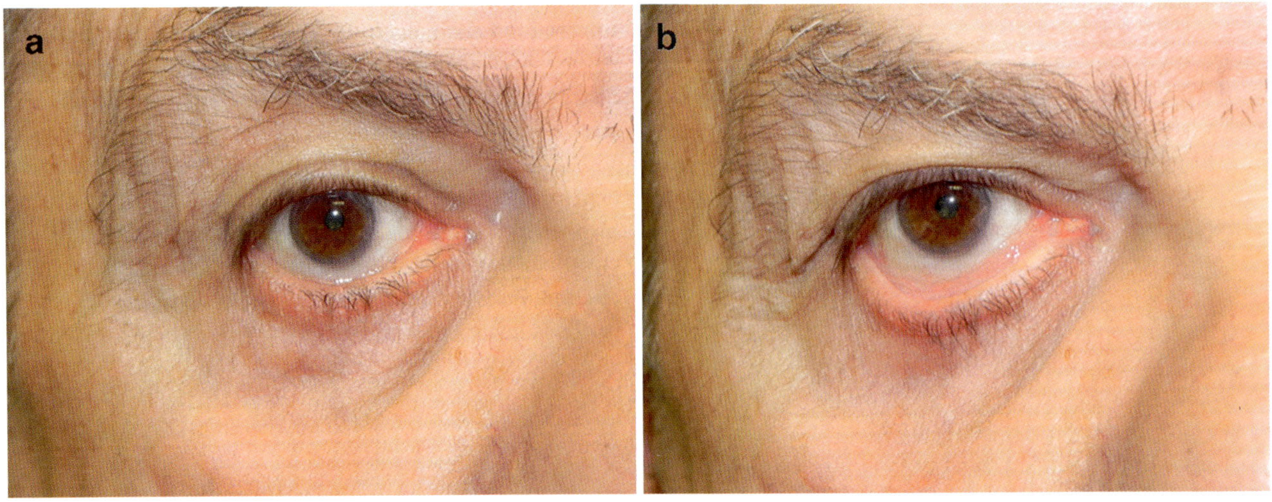

Fig. 9.1 Before (**a**) and after (**b**) inferior distraction of the lower eyelid. The amount of time required for the eyelid to return to normal resting position may indicate degree of laxity

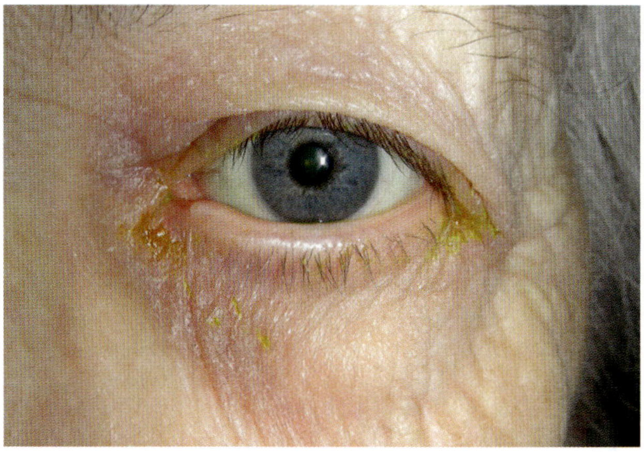

Fig. 9.2 Vertically oriented anterior lamella striae may be a subtle sign of early cicatricial ectropion

Orbicularis Oculi Muscle Tone

At rest the orbicularis oculi muscle in the lower eyelid functions to keep the eyelid margin in normal position, and good muscle tone is required to keep the tarsal plate apposed to the ocular surface. In addition, normal muscle tone is required for the tear pump to function correctly. Passive and active orbicularis contracture can be assessed by asking the patient to squeeze their eyes and release.

Lateral Canthus Evaluation

Lengthening and poor fixation of the lateral canthal tendon is one of the most common mechanisms for horizontal eyelid laxity and can be observed in many cases of ectropion. At times, the entire canthus is dehiscent. Repair of horizontal laxity or canthal instability is mandatory for the long-term success of ectropion surgery.

Medial Canthus Evaluation

Poor fixation of the medial canthus can be evaluated by horizontal distraction testing. The degree of punctal displacement is evaluated while pulling the eyelid temporally. Excessive distraction may signify medial canthal tendon laxity. When mild, medial canthal tendon laxity can often be observed. In patients with marked dehiscence, surgeons may attempt to repair the tendon, a procedure that is difficult because of the close proximity of the tendon to the lacrimal drainage system.

Posterior Eyelid Inspection

Inspection of the conjunctival surface of the lower eyelids allows visualization of the relationship between the tarsal plate and the lower eyelid retractors. Occasionally, ectropion can be caused by excessive eyelid retractor laxity or dehiscence. If the lower eyelid retractors are dehiscent, this may require surgical repair [4–6].

Treatment [6] (See Fig. 9.3)

Involutional Ectropion

Involutional ectropion typically progresses from mild punctal eversion secondary to medial retractor laxity to more diffuse ectropion with associated horizontal lid laxity. The degree of laxity and horizontal extent of the ectropion dictate the surgical procedure(s) required [7]. Mild cases can frequently be corrected with some variation of the medial spindle procedure [8]. Unless there is an isolated area of lid margin pathology, horizontal tightening of the lower eyelid is usually best performed at the lateral canthus. A small wedge excision is appropriate when minimal laxity is present. Significant laxity or canthal instability is best corrected with a tarsal strip procedure. Medial canthal laxity is only corrected when severe. Plication or shortening of the anterior limb of the medial canthal tendon often displaces the punctum away from the globe and tear film. Repair of the posterior limb of the medial canthal tendon can be effective but is difficult because of the close proximity of the lacrimal drainage system and the attenuated tissue.

Lateral Tarsal Strip

Advantages of the lateral tarsal strip procedure over other horizontal eyelid shortening techniques include minimal visible scarring, less symptomatic trichiasis, preservation of tarsus, creation or maintenance of a sharp lateral canthal angle, and reestablishing lateral canthal fixation and position. This operation involves recreation and repositioning the inferior crus of the lateral canthal tendon to the periosteum of the lateral orbital rim. The tarsal strip is fashioned by laterally separating the anterior and posterior lamella, freeing the lower eyelid retractors, and removing the mucocutaneous junction. The tarsal strip is then secured to the periosteum of the lateral orbital rim [9].

Local anesthesia is infiltrated in the lower eyelid and lateral canthus. Care must be taken to achieve proper anesthesia of the lateral orbital rim as the periosteal exposure and suturing can be a source of discomfort for the patient. A horizontal canthotomy and inferior cantholysis are performed (Fig. 9.4). The lower crus of the canthal tendon is recognized visually or identified by performing a strumming motion to locate firm attachments to the lateral orbital rim. After cantholysis is achieved, the lower eyelid margin should be completely free of any lateral attachments. The upper arm of the

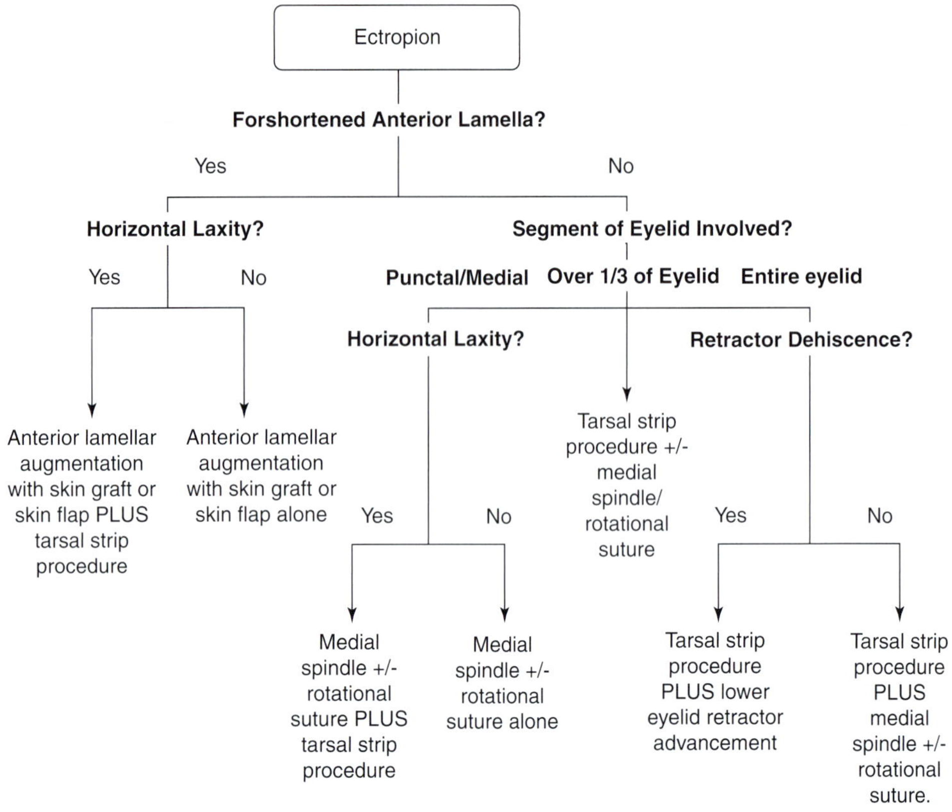

Fig. 9.3 Ectropion therapy flowchart

canthal tendon is preserved as the inner and outer surfaces of the periosteum are exposed. Cautery will be necessary for hemostasis through the dissection. The amount of horizontal shortening is determined by drawing the lid laterally until the desired tension is achieved. The point where the canthal angle intersects the lower lid margin is marked. Care is taken not to shorten the lower eyelid excessively so as to avoid disparity between the length of the upper and lower eyelids. The tarsal strip is fashioned from the redundant lid by separating the anterior and posterior lamella, freeing the lower eyelid retractors, and removing the mucocutaneous junction. A sharp horizontal incision at the base of the lashes is performed, and a small skin-muscle flap is raised. The gray line is then split and lash follicles are removed. The lower eyelid retractors and conjunctiva are divided at the tarsal base, and the mucosa of the remaining lid margin is removed. While the conjunctiva on the posterior lamella can be scraped with a scalpel, it is easier to ablate the epithelium with bipolar cautery. An excessively long tarsal strip may need to be slightly shortened by transecting its distal end. A pocket to receive the tarsal strip is fashioned posterior to the orbital rim, medial to the upper limb of the lateral canthal tendon. The strip is then secured to the periosteum along the inside of the lateral orbital rim with double-armed 5-0 Prolene (polypropylene) suture in a mattress fashion. Care is taken to direct the sutures under the upper crus of the canthal tendon so that the strip is directed into the pocket previously created. Some surgeons use Vicryl (polyglactin 910), Mersilene (braided polyester), or PDS (polydioxanone) sutures for tarsal strip anchoring. The strip is secured with moderate tightness and in a slightly superior location, carefully assessing both the lid contour and canthal position. An excessively tight eyelid may be drawn underneath the globe in patients with prominent eyes. The tarsal suture should be adjusted or replaced if the location of the lid or canthus is not appropriate. Polyglactin (6-0 Vicryl) sutures are used to reform the lateral canthal angle and close the orbicularis muscle. The overlying skin is rearranged and sutured with 6-0 plain gut suture.

Medial Spindle with Rotational Suture

Many times complete repair of an ectropion cannot be achieved with a tarsal strip procedure alone. A medial spindle operation can be used as an adjunctive technique with tarsal strip (Fig. 9.5). In cases where horizontal eyelid shortening is not necessary, the medial spindle procedure can

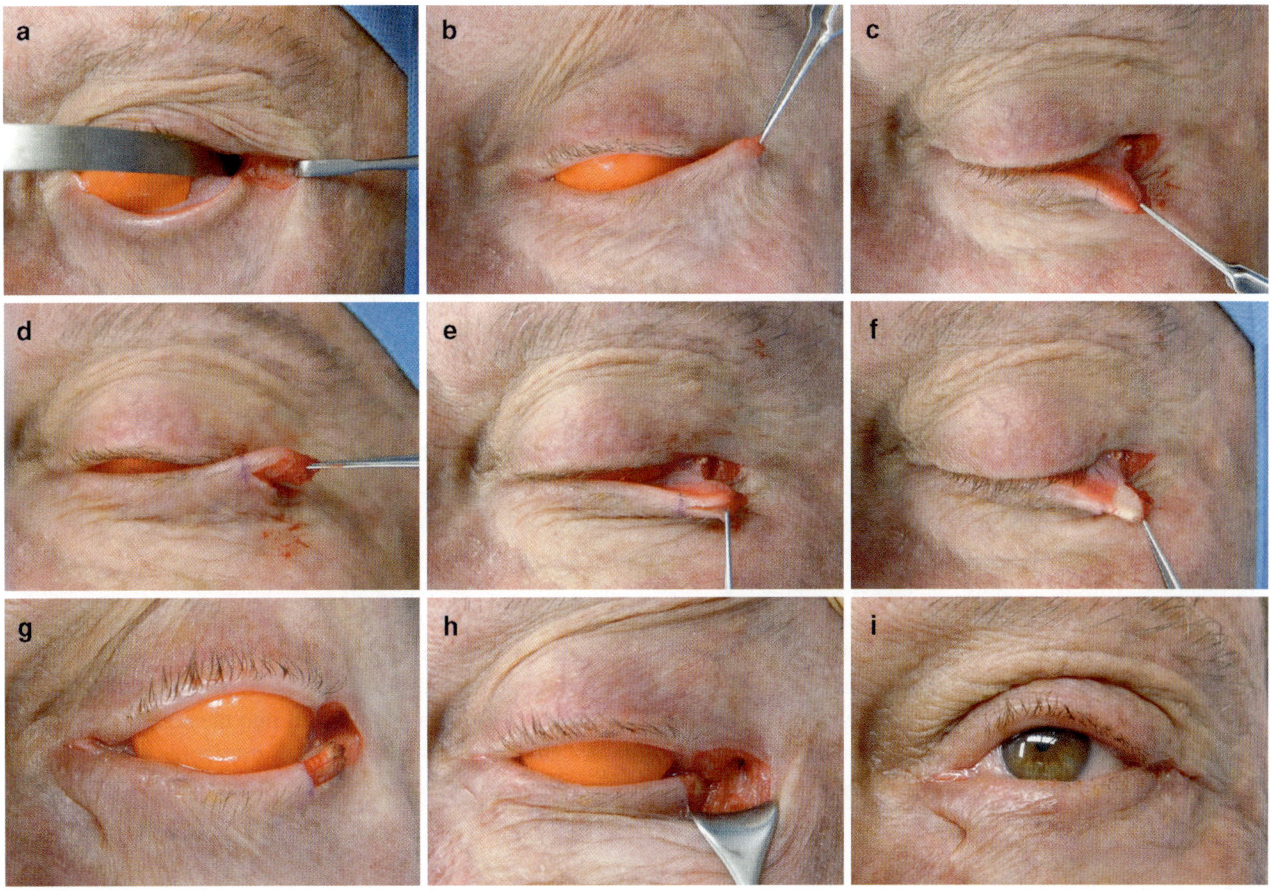

Fig. 9.4 Lateral tarsal strip procedure. Lateral canthotomy (**a**) and inferior cantholysis (**b**) performed. The lower eyelid is marked at the proposed new lateral canthal angle and the lower eyelid retractors released (**c**). An incision is made at the base of the lashes and a skin-muscle flap dissected (**d**). The eyelid is then split in the gray line and the lash follicles are removed (**e**). The conjunctival epithelium is denuded (**f**). A pocket is created medial to the upper limb of the lateral canthal tendon, posterior to the orbital rim (**g**). Note that a medial spindle procedure (if required) should be performed prior to suturing the tarsal strip into place. The tarsal strip is then sutured into position within the newly created pocket (**h**). The lateral canthal angle may be reformed and the overlying skin rearranged and sutured in position (**i**)

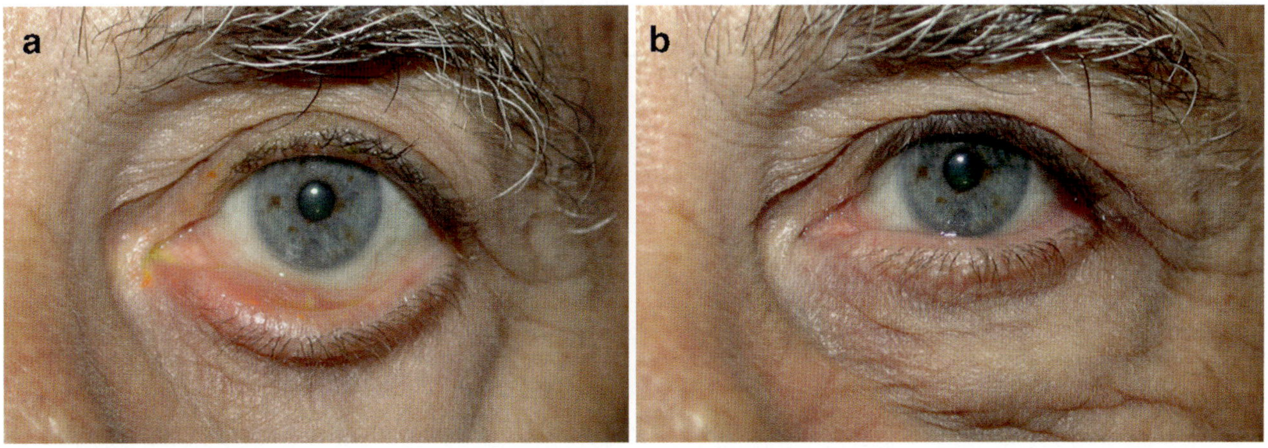

Fig. 9.5 Involutional ectropion before (**a**) and after (**b**) treatment with lateral tarsal strip and medial spindle with rotational suture

be performed alone. This procedure involves making a defect in the posterior lamellae at the medial eyelid, advancement of lower eyelid retractors in the small area, and mechanical eversion of the eyelid with full-thickness mattress sutures.

Local anesthesia is infiltrated in the anterior and posterior lamella of the medial lower eyelid. If needed, a Bowman probe can be placed in the lower canaliculus to both protect the canaliculus and evert the lower eyelid as an elliptical resection of redundant conjunctiva and subconjunctival tissue is performed just below the inferior tarsal border (Fig. 9.6). A mattressed double-armed 5-0 chromic gut suture is used for segmental advancement of the retractors to the tarsal border. Each arm of the 5-0 chromic gut suture is placed sequentially through the inferior edge of the tarsus, upper edge of the lower eyelid retractors, exiting the skin. The exit point for the rotational sutures must be inferior to the entrance point to provide additive rotational effect. The externalized sutures are then tied. Multiple sutures or longer conjunctival resection can be performed in more severe cases. It is important to avoid excessive conjunctival resection to avoid cicatricial entropion development. If the eyelid does not rotate inward adequately, then consider replacement of sutures or other factors, especially cicatricial anterior lamellar changes.

Lazy-T Procedure

Some techniques of ectropion repair, such as the Kuhnt-Szymanowski [10, 11] procedure, have fallen out of favor as surgical techniques have improved. The lazy-T technique of medial ectropion repair originally favored by Byron Smith [12] combines a medial wedge resection with a medial spindle-type conjunctival resection (Fig. 9.7). It sometimes proves useful in the treatment of medial ectropion associated with some eyelid laxity. Oftentimes medial ectropion with a cicatricial component is successfully treated with this technique.

Retractor Advancement

Severe ectropion that involves the entire length of the lower eyelid can be caused by dehiscence of the lower eyelid retractors. Total tarsal ectropion is a common obvious endpoint. Resection of redundant posterior lamella with retractor reattachment is performed across the entire length of the lid. This is commonly included with the tarsal strip procedure.

Local anesthesia is infiltrated into the anterior and posterior lamella of the lower eyelid. A transconjunctival incision

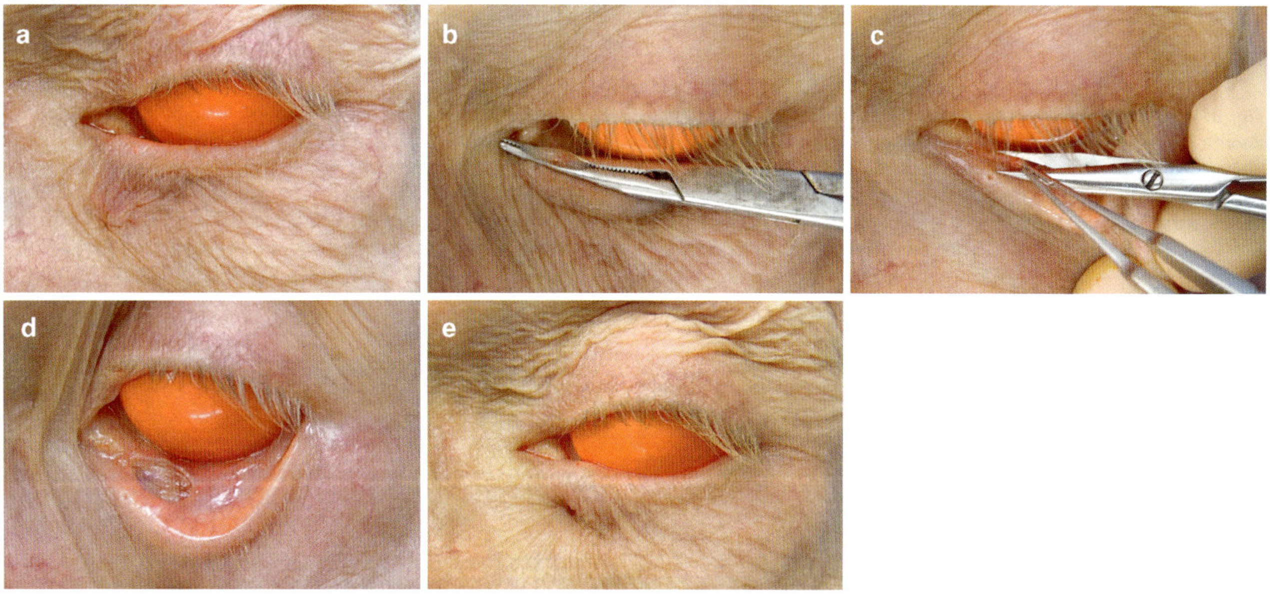

Fig. 9.6 Medial spindle procedure with rotational suture. Medial ectropion with no horizontal laxity (**a**). Following administration of local anesthesia to the medial lower eyelid, a hemostat is placed over the redundant conjunctiva just inferior to the puncta (**b**). Following release of the hemostat, redundant conjunctiva is excised (**c**) exposing the lower eyelid retractors (**d**). Double-armed 5-0 chromic sutures are placed in a mattress fashion and externalized. Each arm of the suture is placed sequentially through the inferior edge of the tarsus, the upper edge of the lower eyelid retractors, and the anterior eyelid lamella. This suture functions to both advance the lower eyelid retractors and close the conjunctival defect (**e**)

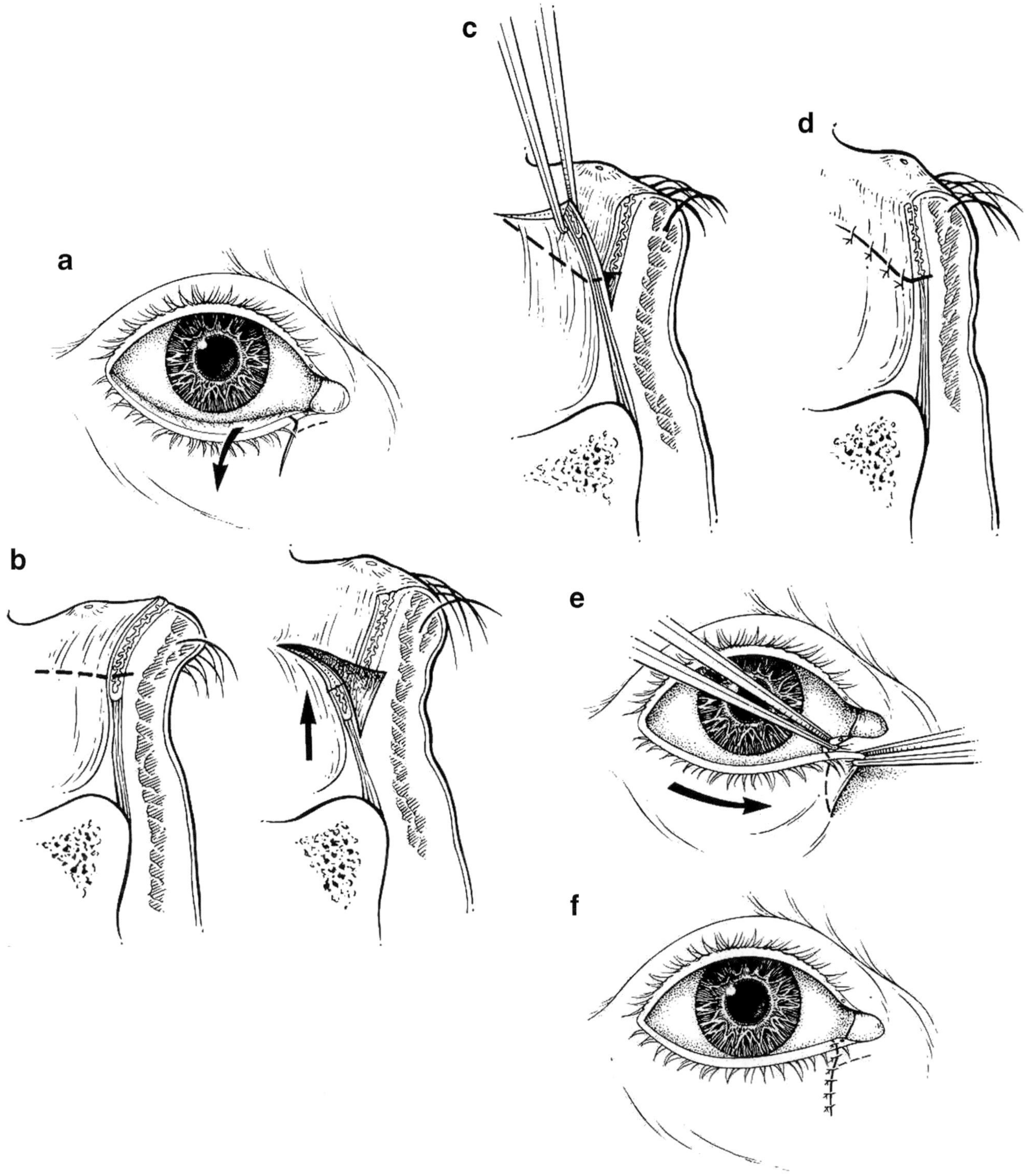

Fig. 9.7 (**a**–**f**) Lazy-T procedure for medial ectropion

is made at the inferior tarsal border along the length of the eyelid [13].Dissection is carried out to the lower eyelid retractor plane, and redundant conjunctiva is excised. Advancement of the retractors is carried out with buried 6-0 Vicryl sutures or 5-0 chromic gut sutures tied similar to the medial spindle procedure.

Cicatricial Ectropion

Cicatrization of the anterior lamella in the lower eyelid can occur following trauma, after lower eyelid blepharoplasty, due to facial actinic changes and with other dermatologic conditions. Detailed evaluation and determination of the cause are necessary as occasionally acute causes such as allergic blepharitis can be reversed with discontinuation of the offending agent or a trial of topical steroids. Cutaneous fibrosis and infiltration can be seen with certain malignancies and infiltrative processes. Suspicious lesions should be biopsied prior to eyelid surgery. Epidermal contraction can also be seen following long-standing involutional or paralytic ectropion. Cicatricial disorders can be segmental or involve the entire lower eyelid, and the treatment depends on the cause, extent, and location of the changes.

Skin Flaps

Localized cicatricial changes are occasionally treated by redirecting the resting skin tension lines and lengthening the anterior lamella through Z-plasty or other types of skin flaps. Mild, diffuse cicatricial ectropion in patients with some degree of cheek ptosis may respond to elevation of cheek with vertical mobilization of the eyelid skin through midface or SOOF lifting procedures. Some regression of surgical effect is common with these procedures, and long-term results may be disappointing.

Anterior Lamellar Skin Graft

Full-thickness skin grafts lengthen the anterior lamella and commonly return the eyelid to a normal position. The color and thickness of the surrounding skin are considered when choosing an appropriate skin graft donor site. Options include the upper eyelid, retroauricular, preauricular, supraclavicular, and upper arm areas. Attempts are made to find the thinnest, most color-compatible tissue possible. Commonly, skin grafting is combined with a lateral tarsal strip operation.

Local anesthesia is infiltrated into the anterior lamella of the lower eyelid and into the donor site. In patients with isolated scarring, a horizontal incision is usually created at the upper border of the fibrosed tissue. In patients with diffuse skin shortage, a subciliary skin incision is often used. Sharp dissection is carried into the lower eyelid to release any deep cicatricial bands while attempting to maintain a viable recipient bed. Once all cicatrized areas are released, the lid margin should be easily elevated to normal position. With the eyelid margin elevated to its normal position, the remaining anterior lamellar defect is measured. An appropriate-sized graft is marked and harvested from the donor site. It is generally helpful to harvest a graft 1–2 mm larger in each dimension than the defect. Care is taken to ensure that a full-thickness graft is harvested, separating dermis from the underlying subcutaneous fat. The donor site is closed appropriately, dependent on the location. The graft is thinned and remaining subcutaneous tissue removed. The skin graft is then placed into position, appropriately trimmed, and secured at the edges with absorbable suture such as 6-0 plain gut. When possible, a gauze bolster is secured over the graft with mattress sutures to prevent dislocation or fluid collecting under the graft, helping successful graft healing (Fig. 9.8).

Paralytic Ectropion

Strong orbicularis oculi tone is required for correct function and position of the lower eyelid; however, without horizontal eyelid laxity, facial nerve paralysis seldom leads to ectropion. Surgical management of paralytic ectropion commonly requires techniques described above for horizontal eyelid shortening in addition to other techniques, including medial canthoplasty and tarsorrhaphy [14]. Periocular management of facial nerve palsy is discussed in Chap. 10 and includes the management of paralytic ectropion.

Mechanical Ectropion

Classically, eyelid margin neoplasms can physically displace the lower eyelid margin or, through gravitational forces, weigh the eyelid margin down and away from the globe. Commonly, patients with marginal eyelid tumors have other mechanisms that lead to ectropion including cicatricial and involutional changes. In addition to removal of the offending neoplasm and surgical management of any carcinomatous spread, the other factors causing the ectropion must be addressed with the above surgical techniques.

Congenital Ectropion

Rarely, neonates can present with congenital ectropion secondary to anterior lamella deficiency or inadequate eyelid retractor insertion. Management of patients with congenital ectropion depends on severity of ocular complications.

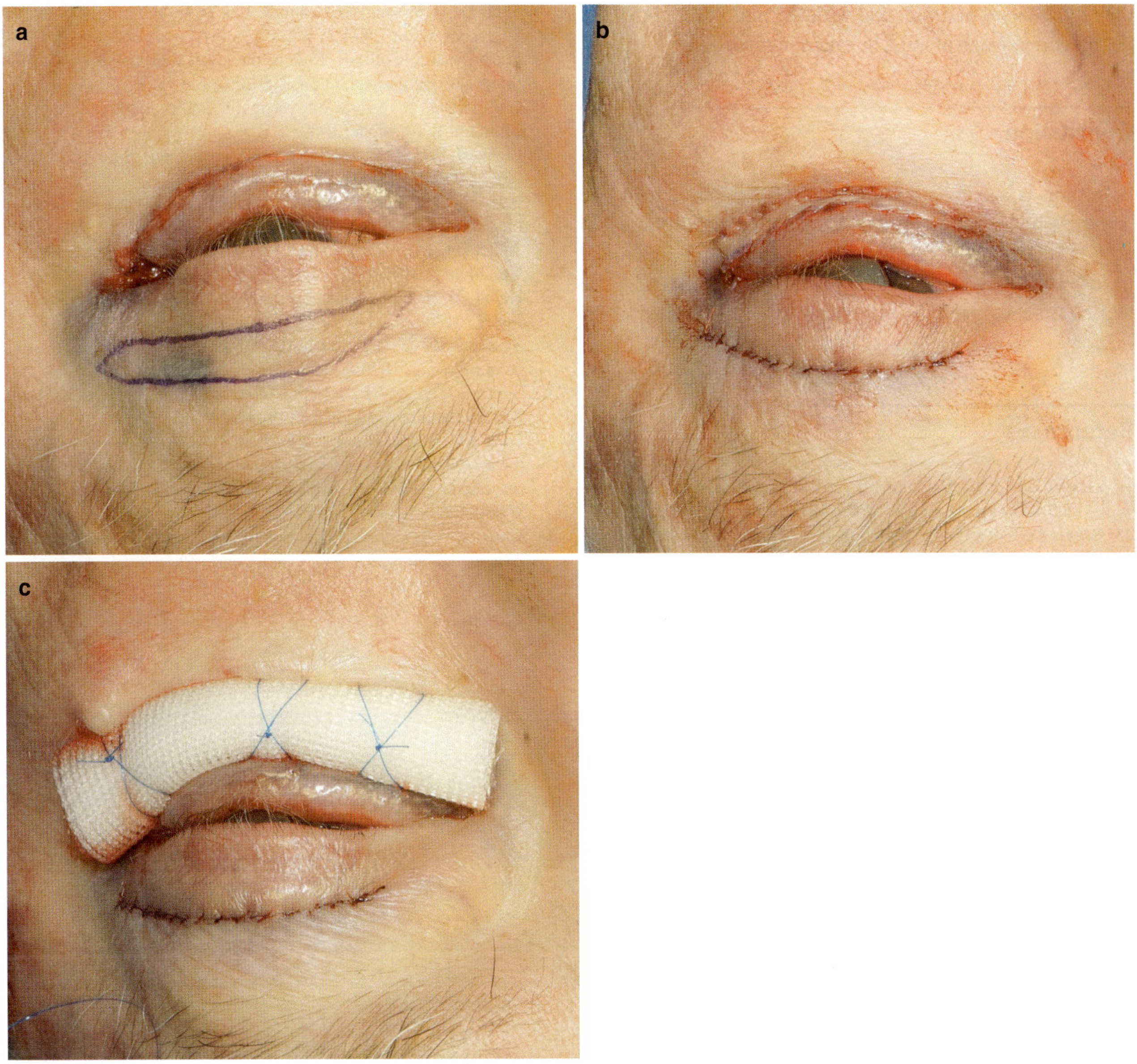

Fig. 9.8 Cicatricial ectropion repair with tarsal strip and full thickness skin graft (**a**), intraoperative following cicatricial release and upper eyelid donor site marking (**b**), intraoperative following skin graft suturing and donor site closure (**c**), intraoperative following bolster placement with Vaseline gauze

Mixed Mechanism Ectropion

One definitive cause for lower eyelid ectropion cannot be delineated in many patients. Sometimes one mechanism induces the ectropion, with worsening through other mechanisms. For example, chronic involutional ectropion commonly leads to anterior lamellar cicatrization. Careful physical exam allows the clinician to isolate the causes and surgically correct the predominant causes of the ectropion through combining techniques described previously. Cases of operative failure or recurrent ectropion should be reevaluated, attempting to determine the disorders contributing to the present malposition. Additional surgery is then directed to correct those factors.

Upper Eyelid Ectropion

Ectropion of the upper eyelid is considerably less common than in the lower eyelid. The same factors can play a role in upper eyelid ectropion, but cicatricial mechanisms predominate in causing upper lid ectropion. Similar mechanistic treatment paradigms would apply in the upper eyelid as described in the lower eyelid. Differences in anatomy with the higher tarsus and function with the importance of eyelid height and movement must be taken into account.

Conclusion

Ectropion is a common eyelid malposition, usually in the lower eyelid. A variety of approaches to treatment take into account the mechanism of the ectropion and the functional needs of the patient. Careful application of these diagnostic and treatment principles generally results in a satisfactory outcome.

References

1. Vick VL, Holds JB, Hartstein ME, et al. Tarsal strip procedure for the correction of tearing. Ophthal Plast Reconstr Surg. 2004;20:37–9.
2. Adenis JP, Grivet D. Ectropion of the lacrimal point: the shoelace technique. Eur J Ophthalmol. 2005;15:267–70.
3. Frueh BR, Schoengarth LD. Evaluation and treatment of the patient with ectropion. Ophthalmology. 1982;89:1049–54.
4. Shah-Desai S, Sandy C, Collin R. Lax eyelid or "progeria" of eyelid tissues. Orbit. 2004;23:3–12.
5. Shah-Desai S, Collin R. Role of the lower lid retractors in involutional ectropion repair. Orbit. 2001;20:81–6.
6. Collin JRO. A manual of systematic eyelid surgery. Edinburgh: Churchill Livingstone; 1989.
7. Liebau J, Schultz A, Arens A, et al. Management of lower lid ectropion. Dermatol Surg. 2006;32:1050–6.
8. Nowinski TS, Anderson RL. The medial spindle procedure for involutional medial ectropion. Arch Ophthalmol. 1985;103:1750–17553.
9. Anderson RL, Gordy DD. The tarsal strip procedure. Arch Ophthalmol. 1979;97:2192–6.
10. Kuhnt H. Beitrage zur Operationen augenheikunder. Jena: G Fischer; 1883. p. 44–55.
11. Symanowski J. Handbuch der Operationen chirurgie. Berlin: Braunschweig; 1870. p. 243.
12. Smith B. The lazy-T correction of ectropion of the lower punctum. Arch Ophthalmol. 1976;94:1149–50.
13. Fong KC, Mavrikakis I, Sagili S, et al. Correction of involutional lower eyelid ectropion with transconjunctival approach retractor plication and lateral tarsal strip. Acta Ophthalmol Scand. 2006;84:246–9.
14. Crawford GJ, Collin JRO, Moriarty PAJ. The correction of paralytic medial ectropion. Br J Ophthalmol. 1984;68:639–41.

Facial Palsy: Periocular Management

10

John B. Holds

Introduction

The eye and periocular structures are central to the evaluation and treatment of conditions of facial paralysis and associated conditions of seventh cranial (facial) nerve dysfunction. As a result of the complex course and innervation of the facial nerve, physicians from multiple specialties including neurologists, neurosurgeons, otolaryngologists, ophthalmologists, and plastic surgeons have a role in the evaluation and treatment of facial paralysis.

Abnormalities of the seventh nerve produce significant issues impacting ocular and facial comfort, protection, function, and appearance. Rehabilitation must routinely balance concerns of corneal exposure and ocular protection, eyelid malposition and dysfunction, facial deformity, and secondary symptoms such as tearing. The variability of clinical signs and symptoms necessitates a carefully tailored approach to each patient's findings.

Anatomy

The functions of the facial nerve include innervation of the muscles of facial expression including the orbicularis and frontalis muscles, which are particularly relevant to the eye, and the innervation of lacrimal and salivary secretion. The sensory innervation of the external ear and taste fibers on the anterior two-thirds of the tongue provided by the seventh nerve are less relevant to the eye but provide diagnostic clues in patient evaluation [1].

The facial nerve exits the brainstem at the cerebellopontine angle and with the eighth cranial nerve enters the internal auditory canal. The 30 mm intraosseous course of the facial nerve makes it vulnerable to edema and injury. The motor portion of the nerve bends posteriorly at the geniculate ganglion; the fibers for lacrimal secretory function branch off via the greater superficial petrosal nerve, passing to the lacrimal gland via the pterygopalatine ganglion and infraorbital and frontozygomatic nerves to the lacrimal gland.

The main motor portion of the facial nerve runs from the geniculate ganglion into the labyrinthine segment, its narrowest part, before exiting the skull at the stylomastoid foramen and dividing into five major branches: temporal (frontal), zygomatic, buccal, marginal mandibular, and cervical. The main branches divide deep in the parotid gland (Fig. 10.1) and branch further to innervate the muscles of facial expression (Fig. 10.2).

Forehead dissection lateral to the temporal line for browlift and related surgical exposures is carried out in a plane deep to the (superficial) temporoparietal fascia, which is continuous with the galea aponeurotica over the forehead and the superficial musculoaponeurotic system (SMAS) over the lower face. This elevates the forehead tissues in a plane deep to the temporal branch of the facial nerve but superficial to the deep temporal fascia which overlies the temporalis muscle (Fig. 10.3). Below the zygomatic arch, the facial nerve branches run deep to the SMAS, so dissection superficial to the SMAS avoids injury to the facial nerve branches [2].

Clinical Syndromes

The clinical syndromes associated with facial nerve dysfunction can be divided into problems of partial or complete paralysis, aberrant regeneration symptoms, disorders of hyperactivity, and other facial dyskinesias (movement disorders). The most frequent cause of decreased facial movement (especially unilateral weakness) is facial palsy. Facial palsy may be a result of surgical or other trauma to the facial nerve, facial (e.g., parotid) or brain (e.g., acoustic neuroma) tumor, or inflammatory and infiltrative processes that may affect the facial nerve.

J. B. Holds (✉)
Saint Louis University School of Medicine, Departments of Ophthalmology and Otolaryngology/Head and Neck Surgery, St. Louis, MO, USA

J. J. Servat et al. (eds.), *Smith and Nesi's Ophthalmic Plastic and Reconstructive Surgery*,
https://doi.org/10.1007/978-3-030-41720-8_10

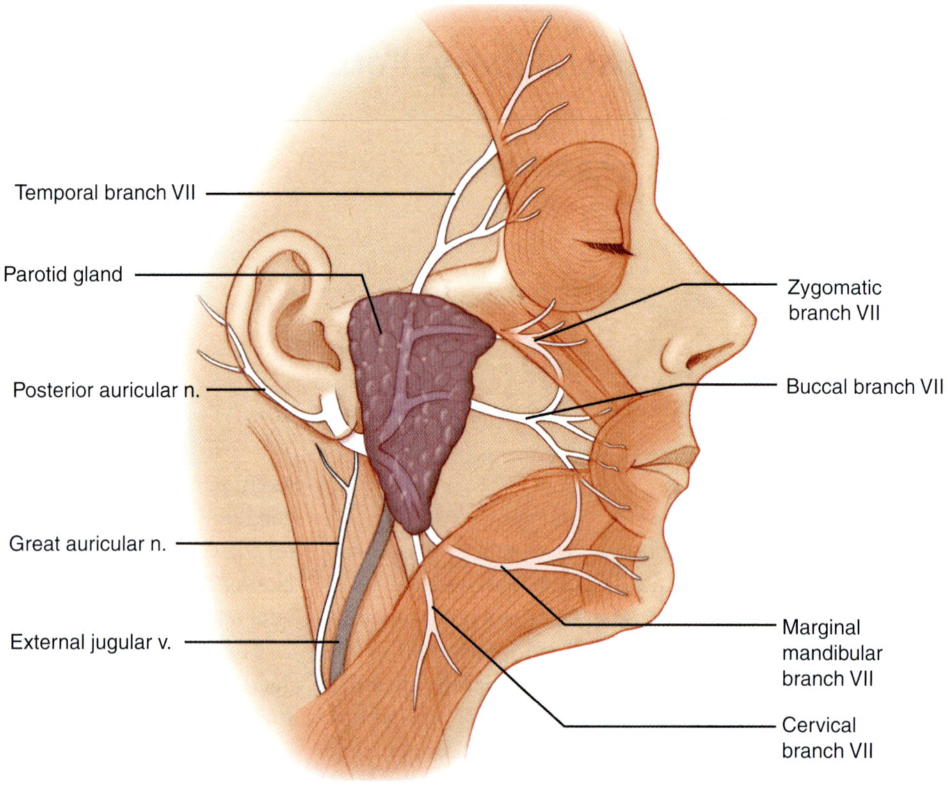

Fig. 10.1 Five major external branches of the facial nerve. (Reproduced with permission [2], Fig. Hyperlink "https://doi.org/10.1007/978-1-4614-0971-7_9"\h9.3)

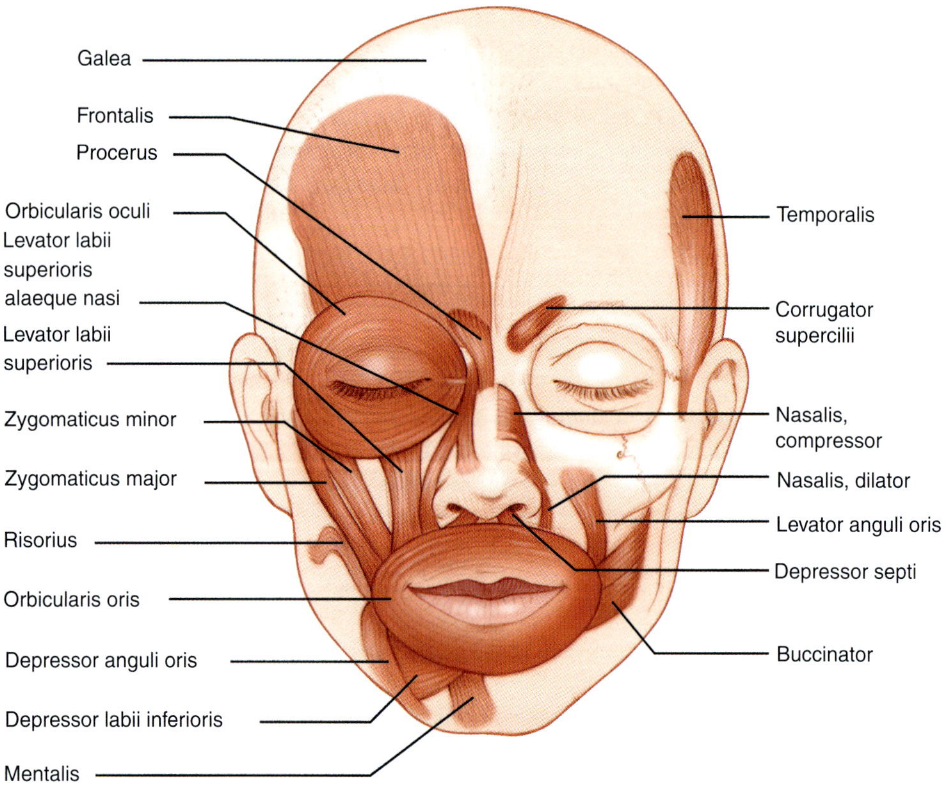

Fig. 10.2 Muscles of facial expression. (Reproduced with permission [2])

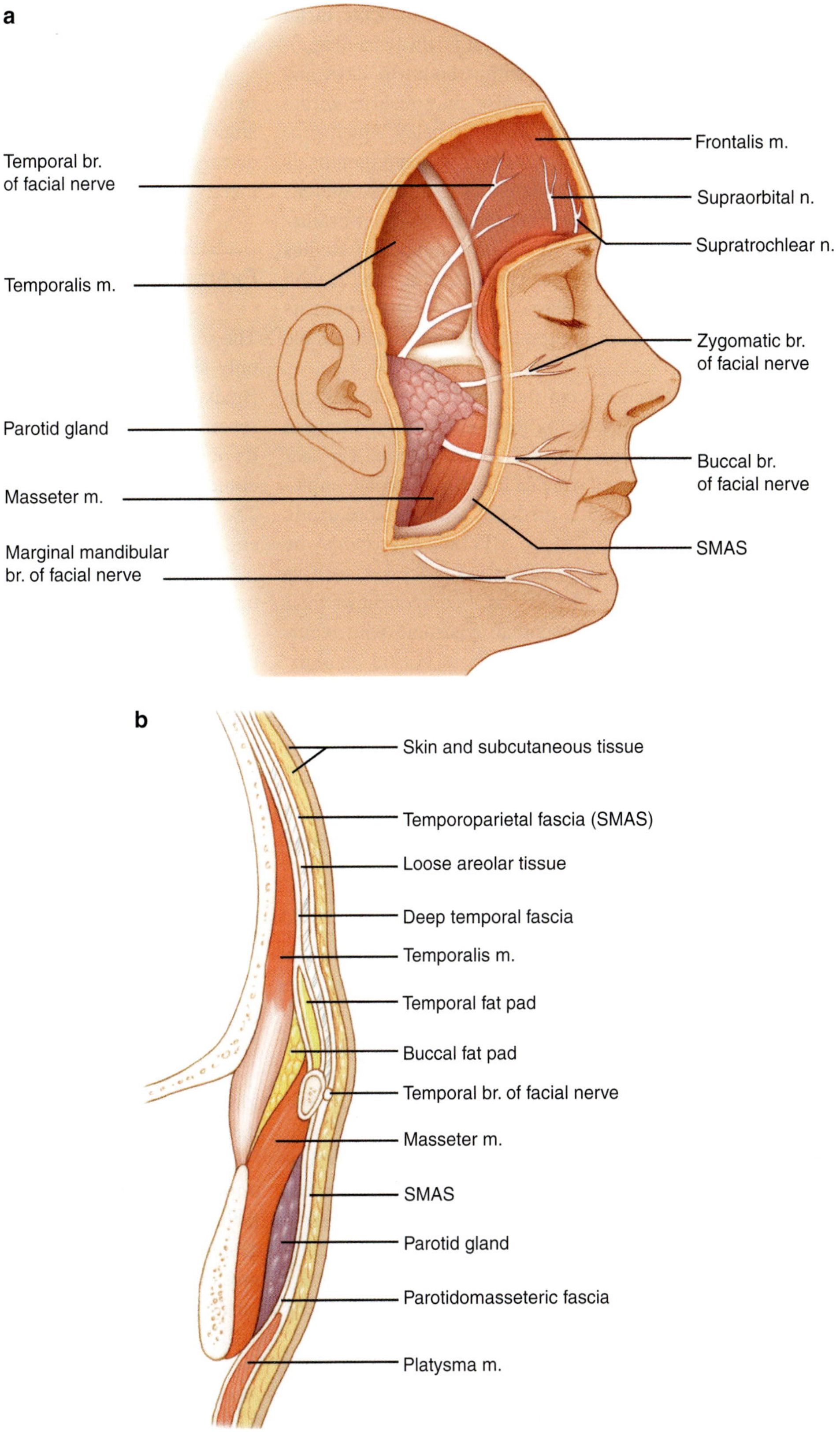

Fig. 10.3 Relationship of the facial nerve to the facial tissue planes. (**a**) Above the zygomatic arch, the frontal branch of the facial nerve lies in the temporoparietal (superficial temporal) fascia, which is continuous inferiorly with the SMAS. (**b**) Inferior to the arch, the facial nerve branches lie deep to the SMAS. (Reproduced with permission [2], Fig. Hyperlink "https://doi.org/10.1007/978-1-4614-0971-7_9"\h9.1)

Bell's palsy is the most common cause of acute facial paralysis. As an idiopathic diagnosis, it is always a diagnosis of exclusion. Onset occurs within hours to days and peaks within 2 weeks, and the palsy may resolve within weeks or slowly over months. A Bell's palsy which progresses beyond 3 weeks, fails to recover within 6 months, is of bilateral onset, or recurs unilaterally is more suspicious for tumor or other process and may prompt further evaluation. Although considered idiopathic, a number of studies point to a reactivation of herpes simplex virus type 1, with the theory being that the inflamed nerve swells within its tightly encased course in the temporal bone, causing acute dysfunction.

A variety of infectious and inflammatory processes can affect the facial nerve including Ramsay Hunt syndrome in which typical herpes zoster lesions of the external ear near the external auditory canal provide the clue to initiate immediate antiviral therapy. Otitis media as well as more exotic infections including Lyme disease, HIV, and leprosy may be associated with facial palsy. Infiltrative processes such as sarcoidosis may have facial palsy as a component of their presentation. Melkersson–Rosenthal syndrome with recurrent alternating facial palsy, recurrent facial edema, cheilitis, and a fissured tongue should be excluded. Bilateral simultaneous palsy may represent Bell's palsy, but workup is essential, with Guillain–Barre syndrome and infiltrative processes being more likely causes.

Clinical Presentation

History is important both diagnostically and in determining the patient's course, symptoms, prior therapy, and ability to provide care to the eye. The longitudinal course of the patient's symptoms is of considerable importance in deciding when to intervene surgically. A patient who has managed well with medical therapy of the eye for 2 months and is believed to have a reversible injury might appropriately wait a full 6 months before planning surgical rehabilitation. Conversely, a patient whose nerve was resected at surgery will not be expected to show recovery, and long-term rehabilitation of the eye and face may be planned immediately [3]. It is frequently helpful to speak with colleagues who may have operated on or examined the patient, both in determining course to the present and the likelihood of recovery of the facial nerve.

Specific ophthalmic symptoms to elicit include complaints of visual obstruction, visual disturbance, dry eye versus tearing complaints, and the patient's current topical medication regimen. Tearing symptoms may be largely reflexive secondary to corneal exposure, primary epiphora related to eyelid malposition and failure of the lacrimal pump system, or gustatory (crocodile tears) due to aberrant reinnervation of the autonomic fibers of the nerve.

Likewise, aberrant reinnervation may lead to involuntary twitching or closure of the eyelids on the affected eye with attempts at other facial movements (facial synkinesis). These disconcerting issues should be noted in planning subsequent therapy.

Examination

The severity of facial paresis may vary from very mild with only slight noticeable weakness to complete. The House–Brackmann [4] scale (Fig. 10.4) may be used to grade the severity of facial palsy. Careful notation regarding the severity of involvement in specific segments of the face along with clinical photographs can be helpful in following patients. The longer lasting and more severe the facial palsy, the generally worse the prognosis.

In the periocular area, facial palsy causes a number of troublesome signs. A weakened blink, lax lower eyelid, and lagophthalmos contribute to the frequent finding of corneal exposure in the setting of facial palsy. In addition to a careful slit lamp examination, one should document corneal sensation. Often diminished after acoustic neuroma surgery, and sometimes in other situations, corneal anesthesia will be synergistic with the facial palsy in producing keratopathy. The acronym "BAD" denoting poor *B*ell's phenomenon, *a*nesthesia, and *d*ryness may be used to help one remember the aggravating factors, threatening the eye in the presence of facial palsy [3]. More aggressive treatment and careful follow-up are warranted in such patients. Patients with a sensory and motor (CN 5 and 7) palsy are much more likely to develop a severe neurotrophic keratitis and require more aggressive treatment including the corneal neurotization procedure discussed later [5].

Eyebrow position, associated dermatochalasis, upper and lower eyelid position and the blink, and amount of lagophthalmos must all be carefully noted. A tendency to upper eyelid closure with lower facial animation is a potentially important finding, suggesting aberrant regeneration of the facial nerve. This finding is observed only months after true acute-onset palsy. The finding of aberrant regeneration at the presentation of a reportedly acute palsy implies a chronic onset. A complete workup with neuroimaging is indicated to rule out a tumor or other cause of the palsy [6].

As previously noted, tearing symptoms require careful evaluation and oftentimes diagnostic trials of treatments. Reflex tearing from exposure requires treatment of the exposure. Tearing due to punctal or lower eyelid malposition requires treatment of the eyelid malposition. Gustatory tearing is a difficult and troublesome symptom to treat because of the aberrant nerve reinnervation causing it. The evaluation

Grade	Characteristics
I. Normal	Normal facial function in all areas
II. Mild dysfunction	Gross Slight weakness noticeable on close inspection May have slight synkinesis At rest, normal symmetry and tone Motion Forehead - Moderate-to-good function Eye - Complete closure with minimal effort Mouth - Slight asymmetry
III. Moderate dysfunction	Gross Obvious but not disfiguring difference between sides Noticeable but not severe synkinesis, contracture, or hemifacial spasm At rest, normal symmetry and tone Motion Forehead - Slight-to-moderate movement Eye - Complete closure with effort Mouth - Slightly weak with maximum effort
IV. Moderately severe dysfunction	Gross Obvious weakness and/or disfiguring asymmetry At rest, normal symmetry and tone Motion Forehead - None Eye - Incomplete closure Mouth - Asymmetric with maximum effort
V. Severe dysfunction	Gross Only barely perceptible motion At rest, asymmetry Motion Forehead - None Eye - Incomplete closure Mouth - Slight movement
VI. Total paralysis	No movement

Fig. 10.4 House–Brackmann scale for grading facial paralysis. (Adapted from [4])

of best vision may require an initial vigorous rinse of the eye with saline to remove ointment. The combination of topical lubricants and a poor blink often severely decreases recorded visual acuity.

Therapy

Medical

The patient's age, physical and mental capabilities, nature and expected duration of the palsy, and physical findings will all dictate the intensity of treatment and timetable for consideration of surgical options. Lubrication with tear drops and ophthalmic ointment is a cornerstone of treatment for most patients. The patient should be encouraged to use lubricants at a frequency that avoids rather than reacts to ocular irritation. Ointment is generally applied at night to minimize prolonged exposure while sleeping. Patients with corneal anesthesia are at special risk. Preservative-free lubricants are preferred and necessary for some patients.

Additional measures may include wearing a patch or moisture chamber, shrouding the lens of the patient's spectacles to create a moisture chamber, and placing tape from the lower lid past the lateral canthus to support a grossly ectropic lower eyelid. Taping the eye shut at night is difficult to perform properly and repeatedly and may result in damage to the eye from the tape slipping. The placement of an external weight on the pretarsal skin of the upper eyelid will provide a mechanical load that will decrease lagophthalmos and protect the eye in the same fashion as an implanted weight [7]. This provides a means to test the effectiveness of the weight and may be used short or long term in protecting the eye.

Another alternative for temporary eye protection is to induce a protective ptosis with botulinum toxin injection. Although various techniques are reported, the usual technique entails the placement of 5–7.5 u of onabotulinumtoxinA (Botox®) in the mid-superior orbit at a depth of 12 mm, in a fashion similar to the placement of a frontal nerve block. An attempt to inject in an intramuscular fashion increases the risk for superior rectus underaction posttreatment. Ptosis lasts for approximately 6 weeks, which may allow time for the recovery of facial nerve function or to evaluate other treatment options [8].

Surgical

Tarsorrhaphy

The creation of an adhesion between the upper and lower eyelids may be done on a temporary or permanent (but reversible) basis. This approach narrows the eyelid fissure in a graded fashion, both horizontally and vertically, and thus diminishes lagophthalmos, the area of exposure, and the surface area exposed to evaporation.

The simplest tarsorrhaphy will be performed on a temporary basis with a suture passed through the gray line, as described in the technique of lateral tarsorrhaphy below, and no incision of the eyelid. The advantage is the simple and readily reversible nature of such a suture tarsorrhaphy. The disadvantage of such an approach is the inability to leave a suture in place longer than 3 weeks.

Lateral Tarsorrhaphy

A basic procedure of considerable utility in the treatment of facial palsy and corneal disease, lateral tarsorrhaphy is best approached as a graded and possibly adjunctive procedure combined with other surgical approaches or as a semipermanent temporizing measure. It is best to utilize a technique which allows the adhesion to be partially or completely divided at a later date without apparent distortion of the eyelid margin or other sequelae.

Local anesthesia should be achieved with topical proparacaine followed by local anesthetic given subcutaneously adjacent to the lid margin and a posterior transconjunctival injection for complete anesthesia. The author favors a variation of the technique described by Stamler and Tse [9] and others with denuding of the mucocutaneous junction of the upper and lower eyelid, splitting of the anterior and posterior lamellae to a depth of 1.5 mm, and suturing designed to achieve adhesion of the anterior and posterior lamellae (Fig. 10.5). Suturing may be accomplished using the technique of an externalized suture tied over foam bolsters or a layered closure with an absorbable 5-0 polyglactin 910 (Vicryl®) suture adhering the posterior lamellae and a 6-0 plain gut suture to the anterior lamellae. Sutures are removed in 12–14 days. The externalized suture tied over foam bolsters is used in the placement of a temporary tarsorrhaphy, allowing a bow knot which can be undone to examine the eye, if needed.

Medial Tarsorrhaphy

A medial adhesion can be created lateral to the punctum with a small adhesion as described for lateral tarsorrhaphy. As this will often encroach on the papillary axis and allow only a narrow lid opening (when combined with a lateral tarsorrhaphy), it is generally an appropriate technique only to temporize in following a healing compromised cornea or in extreme cases of exposure. Alternative techniques to use medially are the tarsal pillar tarsorrhaphy technique [10], which allows for some opening of the eye, or a modified technique of medial tarsorrhaphy which preserves the canalicular system.

The modified technique of medial tarsorrhaphy incises the eyelid anterior to the puncta and canalicular system, avoiding damage to these structures [11]. The technique requires a local anesthetic injection, the possible placement of a lacrimal probe (if desired to ensure against damage to the canalicular system), the incision into the anterior lamella tissues, and a layered closure to create an adhesion (Fig. 10.6).

The cosmesis of tarsorrhaphy surgery and resultant patient acceptance is always an issue. These procedures are performed in a graded fashion and may be combined with other reanimation procedures including lower lid tightening and gold weight implant placement of the upper eyelid to give a balanced approach to ocular protection while minimizing the cosmetic consequences of surgery.

Ectropion Repair

The ectropion of many patients with facial paralysis can be treated with a standard tarsal strip type [12], with or without a medial spindle operation [13] to improve punctal ectropion. The principal differences between this procedure in the setting of facial paralysis and in the routine involutional ectropion are the possible need for a greater shortening of the eyelid and the frequent need for adjunctive procedures such as a posterior lamella spacer graft, midface lift, or full-thickness skin graft to augment the repair.

Lower eyelid retraction, in addition to ectropion, is frequent in the setting of facial palsy. In patients with adequate anterior lamella, division of the conjunctiva and lower eyelid retractors inferior to the lower tarsus and the placement of a

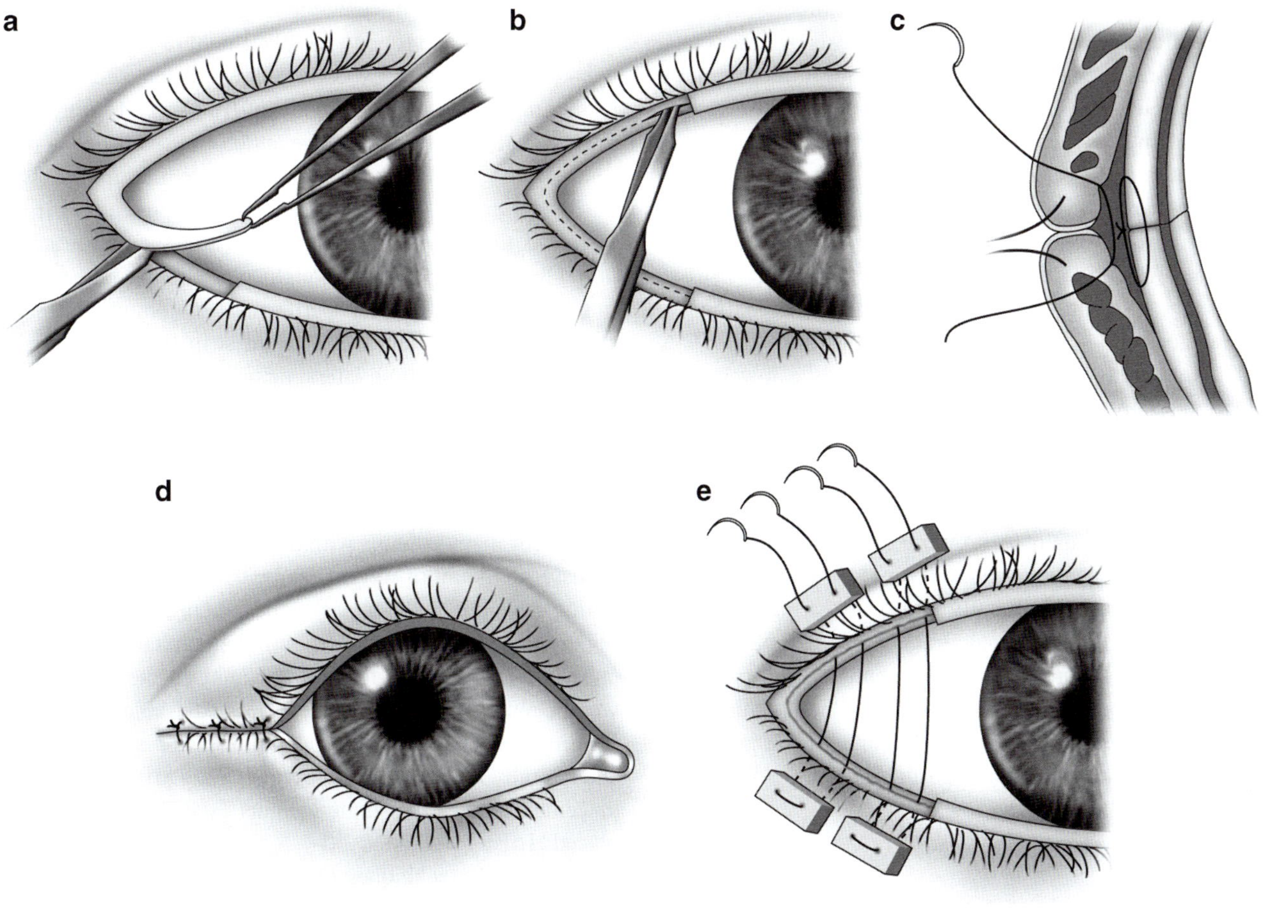

Fig. 10.5 Technique of lateral tarsorrhaphy showing (**a**) denuding of the lid margin at the mucocutaneous junction; (**b**) splitting of the anterior and posterior lamella to a depth of 1.5 mm; (**c**) suturing with a layered suture technique, 5-0 polyglactin 910 suture deep; (**d**) external appearance after skin closure with 6-0 plain gut suture; and (**e**) alternate suturing technique using a bolstered externalized suture

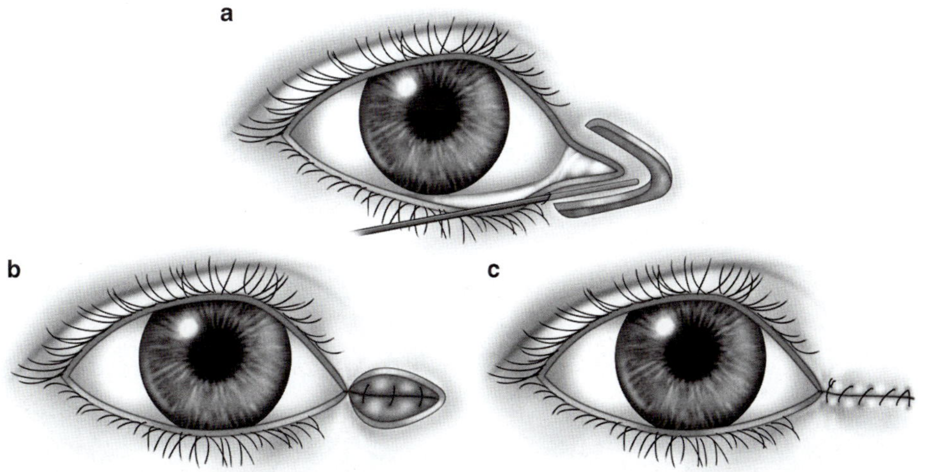

Fig. 10.6 Technique of medial tarsorrhaphy with incision anterior to canalicular system and a layered closure. (**a**) With a Bowman probe in place for canalicular protection, an incision is made in the skin using a scalpel blade or scissors. (**b**) Deep closure of 5-0 polyglactin 910 (Vicryl) suture is placed, avoiding the lacrimal canalicular system. (**c**) The skin is closed anterior to the canalicular system with 6-0 plain gut suture. (Adapted from Nerad [11])

subtarsal spacer graft will often help to raise the lower eyelid margin relative to the cornea, reducing exposure keratitis. Effective allograft spacers include preserved sclera, other preserved collagen allografts (Alloderm, Allergan PLC, Dublin, Ireland; Enduragen, Stryker CMF, Kalamazoo, MI, USA) are frequently effective spacers. Autogenous cartilage may be placed as a splint to vertically support the eyelid. Hard palate mucosal grafts [14] are the best lower lid spacers but carry the downside of the need for a graft harvest with donor site discomfort and healing time.

Patients with a shortage of anterior lamella, resulting from a shortage of skin due to facial ptosis or other cause, may require additional treatment including techniques of midface elevation (described below) or full-thickness skin grafting of the eyelid. Although it appears elegant and anatomically appropriate to lift the midface rather than grafting skin, long-term results are seldom as impressive as those obtained early on with midface elevation, and full-thickness skin grafting sometimes proves necessary if the anterior lamella is tight and causing eyelid retraction.

The correction of ectropion improves the lower eyelid position relative to the cornea, decreasing exposure keratitis and resultant ocular irritation. Improved punctal position and eyelid tone may help the lacrimal pump system in patients with an incomplete paralysis so that tearing is markedly improved. Most patients with more complete paralysis have an incompetent lacrimal pump. Nonetheless, improvement in corneal exposure frequently improves tearing complaints to a significant degree. Recalcitrant cases of epiphora due to lacrimal pump failure necessitate a conjunctivodacryocystorhinostomy (Jones tube) procedure to allow lacrimal drainage. This procedure should only be undertaken in suitable patients at minimal risk for exposure keratitis as it may significantly dry the eye.

Gold Weight Implantation

As previously noted, an external weight can be placed to test whether a mechanical load in the upper eyelid will adequately diminish lagophthalmos [7]. The usual technique of placement is to suture the weight directly to the tarsus in the central eyelid [15]. An alternate surgical approach is to place the weight supratarsal, sutured to the levator aponeurosis laterally and/or medially. Tower and Dailey [16] have described a series of 59 patients treated with a 2.2 g weight placed in a supratarsal position.

The basic surgical technique (Fig. 10.7) entails systemic antibiotic coverage (due to the placement of an implant), an eyelid crease incision, exposure of the recipient site, suturing of the implant with 5-0 polyglactin 910 (Vicryl) suture, and a layered closure. Postoperative antibiotic coverage is a routine. Additional surgical options include multiple weight placement and/or recession of the levator aponeurosis if the patient is thought to have a degree of true eyelid retraction not fully relieved by gold weight placement. Gold weight implantation is routinely performed in conjunction with other procedures including a tarsal strip tightening of the lower eyelid (Fig. 10.8), lateral tarsorrhaphy, or browlift.

Weights are available in 0.2 g increments from 0.6 to 2.8 g (Meddev Co., Palo Alto, CA). Platinum weights are also available in the rare case or suspicion of gold allergy. Most patients require at least 1.2 g of weight, with 1.4 g needed for many patients with only one weight in place. The necessary amount of weight can be determined by taping or gluing a weight to the upper eyelid preoperatively. The end point will be a marked reduction in lagophthalmos with the patient upright and up to 1 mm of induced ptosis from the weight. With pretarsal placement, it is advisable to consider splitting the load into two separate weights placed medially and laterally if the total mass exceeds 1.2 g [10]. Supratarsal placement allows for single weights exceeding 2.0 g to be placed [16].

Many other techniques of eyelid rehabilitation in facial palsy have been devised over the years. The Arion sling is a technique of periocular cerclage using a silicone rod or fascia. This sling is anchored under the medial and lateral canthal tendons and runs near the upper and lower eyelid margins in hopes of narrowing the eyelid fissure and lessening lagophthalmos. Problems with loosening, breakage, infection, and extrusion have kept this procedure from ever gaining widespread acceptance. Palpebral spring placement is another much talked-about but seldom performed procedure. In theory, this will provide a dynamic rehabilitation of the upper eyelid with a custom-formed piece of orthodontic wire

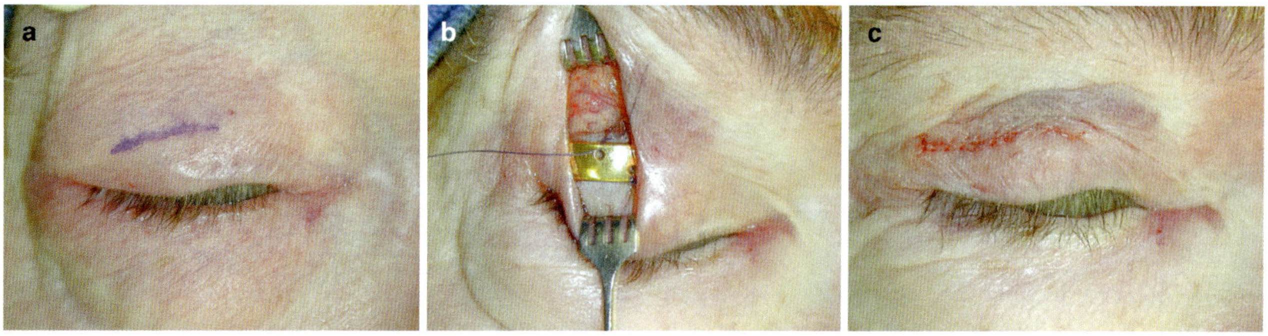

Fig. 10.7 Modified technique of supratarsal gold weight placement showing (**a**) lateral eyelid incision; (**b**) suturing of the gold weight to the levator aponeurosis just above the upper edge of tarsus with 5-0 polyglactin 910 (Vicryl) suture; (**c**) following layered closure of the orbicularis muscle and skin with 6-0 plain gut suture

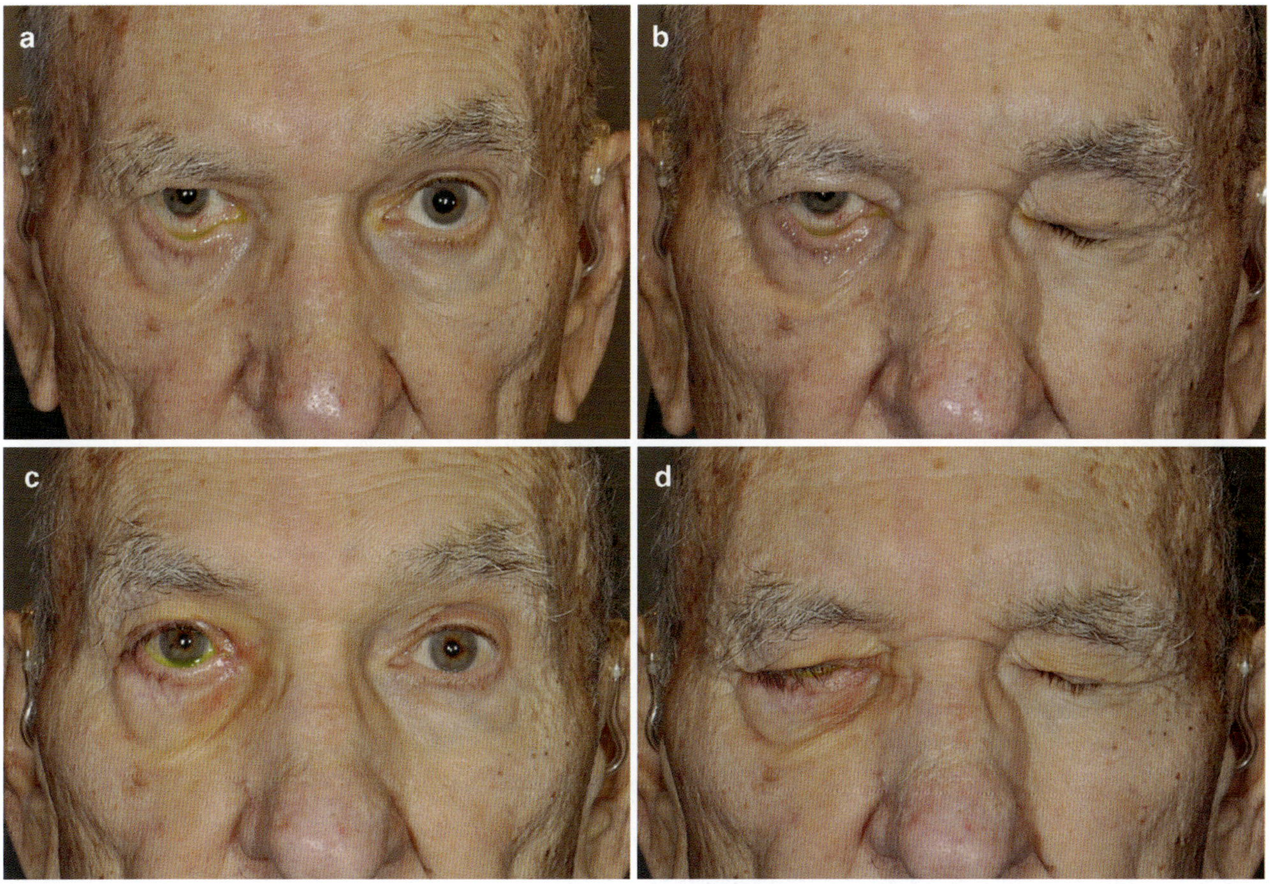

Fig. 10.8 Patient before (**a**, **b**) and after (**c**, **d**) tarsal strip ectropion repair and gold weight placement. Lagophthalmos is minimized, ectropion corrected, and eyelid position improved. Despite the persistent increased tear lake, tearing symptoms are minimal postoperatively

implanted between the upper lid and the brow. In practice, this technique is generally fraught with problems with appropriate adjustment, migration, infection, and extrusion.

Periocular Adjuncts

Browlift

The loss of frontalis tone which accompanies facial paresis generally causes a profound brow ptosis. All of the techniques of browlift otherwise employed and described in chapter 20 may be used to address the brow ptosis associated with facial paresis, although more powerful techniques of direct, mid-forehead, and pretrichial browlift are probably most applicable to the generally severe and asymmetric brow ptosis associated with facial paralysis.

In general, the closer the incision to the eyebrow, the more efficient and permanent the lift induced. The direct browlift is a common and time-honored technique which may be used to correct brow ptosis. The downside to a direct lift is the prominence of the scar and the difficulty in blending the contour across the entire brow. For this reason, a mid-forehead or pretrichial lift [17] has the advantage of lifting across the entire side of the forehead with the potential for a more natural-looking brow and forehead contour. The primary disadvantages are the longer incision, the potential prominence of the scar, and the greater chance of prolonged forehead numbness. Despite these concerns, mid-forehead browlift is particularly applicable in the facial palsy patient.

Facial Suspension

A variety of techniques of cheek, midface, and perioral suspension exist. Although limited and less invasive than full-face suspensions, eyelid incision-only techniques of cheek, midface, or SOOF (suborbicularis oculi fat) lift are of limited long-term benefit, especially in the presence of facial paralysis. The lift achieved with all of these techniques relaxes somewhat with time, and techniques of limited scope generally have little long-term effect on a ptotic cheek and midface.

Temporalis muscle transfer is used to reanimate the mouth [18]. This technique offers the advantage of long-term rehabilitation of the perioral area with limitations of extensive surgery which may leave a temporal defect with poor rehabilitation of other facial areas.

The orbital rim and suture suspension are used to lift and stabilize a subperiosteal cheek and midface lift passing into the nasolabial fold [19]. A complete subperiosteal midface release is followed by the placement of three mattress sutures from the nasolabial fold to the orbital rim. There, the sutures are stabilized to bone tunnels or Mitek anchors (Fig. 10.9). This technique helps to functionally and aesthetically rehabilitate the patient (Fig. 10.10) and is readily performed at the time of eyelid rehabilitation surgery.

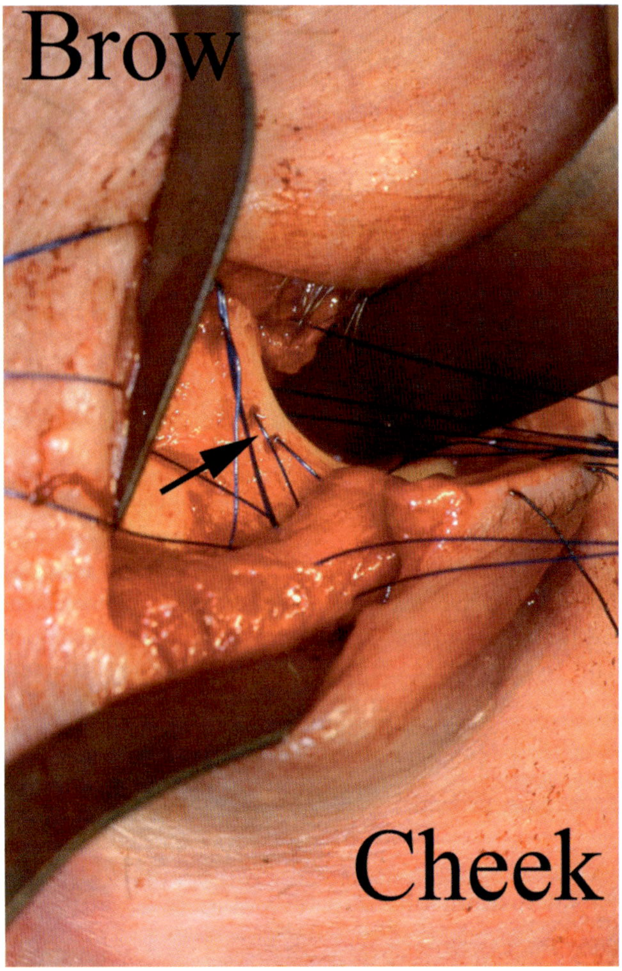

Fig. 10.9 Lateral intraoperative view of subperiosteal midface release and suture midface suspension. *Arrow* shows bone tunnels at lateral orbital rim with Tevdek suspension sutures passed. Three such sutures pass from the orbital rim to the nasolabial fold and are anchored by bone tunnels or Mitek® anchors. (Images courtesy of Roberta Gausas, MD)

Other Treatments

Surgeons will always attempt to preserve and repair the facial nerve after surgical or other trauma. Nonetheless, these repairs are fraught with failures and complications. Decompression of the facial nerve in severe cases of Bell's palsy has had proponents over the years, but the procedure carries significant risks and questionable benefits, making it an uncommon recommendation at this time. In patients who have a clear permanent loss of facial nerve integrity, completion of a hypoglossal nerve transfer in the first few months after definitive injury may provide some reinnervation of the face which maintains tone and some animation [20].

Other techniques of nerve grafting including cross-cable grafting of the face are seldom attempted or effective. Similarly, a microvascular functional muscle transfer is a technical tour de force with few indications in routine facial palsy.

Aberrant Regeneration

Aberrant regeneration is a result of severe injuries to the facial nerve and a cause of facial synkinesis. This finding is typically associated with the degeneration of over 95% of fibers and the crossover of axonal sprouts between different muscle units. Gustatory tearing or "crocodile tears" occur when a damaged facial nerve has fibers which should innervate the salivary glands that cross over to innervate the lacrimal gland.

Narrowing of the eyelid fissure with lower facial movement is the most commonly bothersome facial movement associated with facial synkinesis (Fig. 10.11a). This finding is often treated with the local injection of small amounts of onabotulinumtoxinA (Botox®) (Fig. 10.11b) [21]. Because of the damaged facial nerve and frequent finding of weakness despite the observed hyperactivity, it is prudent to begin with very small doses of 0–1 unit Botox in the medial eyelid and 2–3 units laterally. Interestingly, the clinical effect of the toxin in these patients sometimes exceeds 12 months.

Botulinum toxin may also be used to treat gustatory tearing by the direct injection of 5 units of onabotulinumtoxinA (Botox®) into the palpebral lobe of the lacrimal gland. This author has had variable success with this approach, with failure and mild temporary ptosis the most frequent complications. Nonetheless, this off-label use of botulinum toxin may be considered in the symptomatic patient who has failed other therapy.

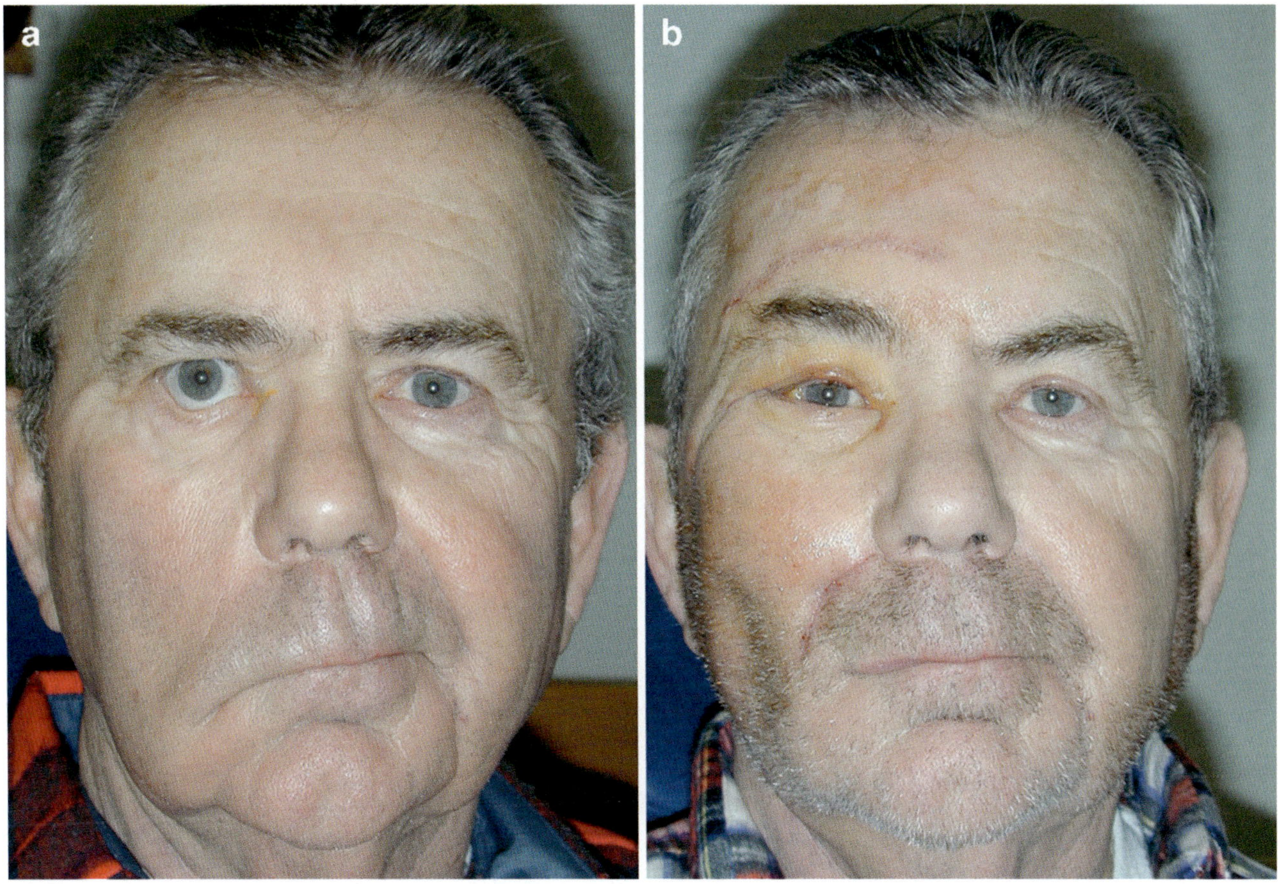

Fig. 10.10 (**a**) Patient preoperatively before undergoing mid-forehead browlift, upper eyelid gold weight implant, subperiosteal midface suspension, and lateral canthoplasty; (**b**) the same patient postoperatively showing improved position of the eyelid, cheek, and lip. (Images courtesy of Roberta Gausas, MD)

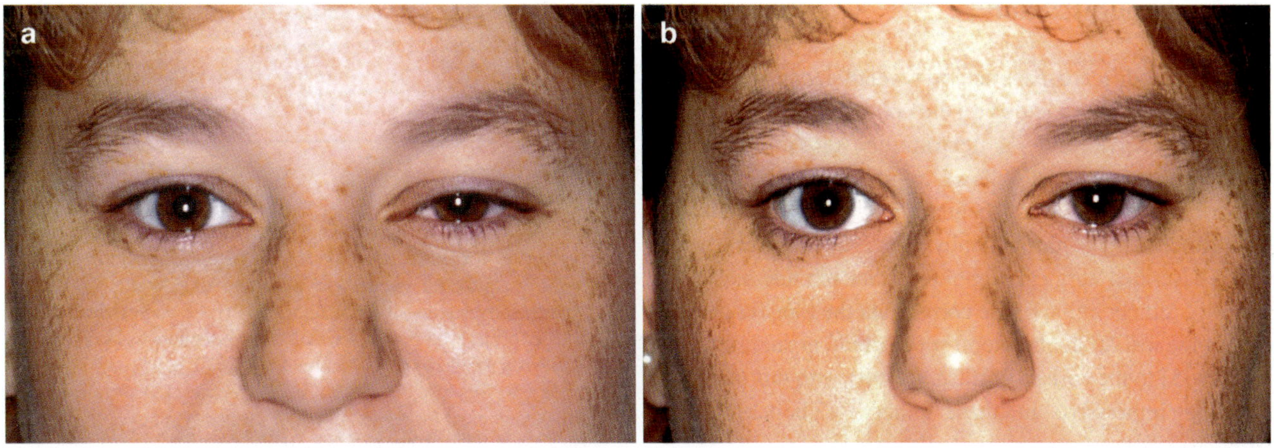

Fig. 10.11 (**a**) Patient with history of facial palsy, left synkinesis, and facial contracture. Note: left ptosis prior to onabotulinumtoxinA (Botox) treatment. (**b**) The same patient after botulinum toxin treatment to the left periocular area showing relaxation of the orbicularis muscle and improvement in the left ptosis

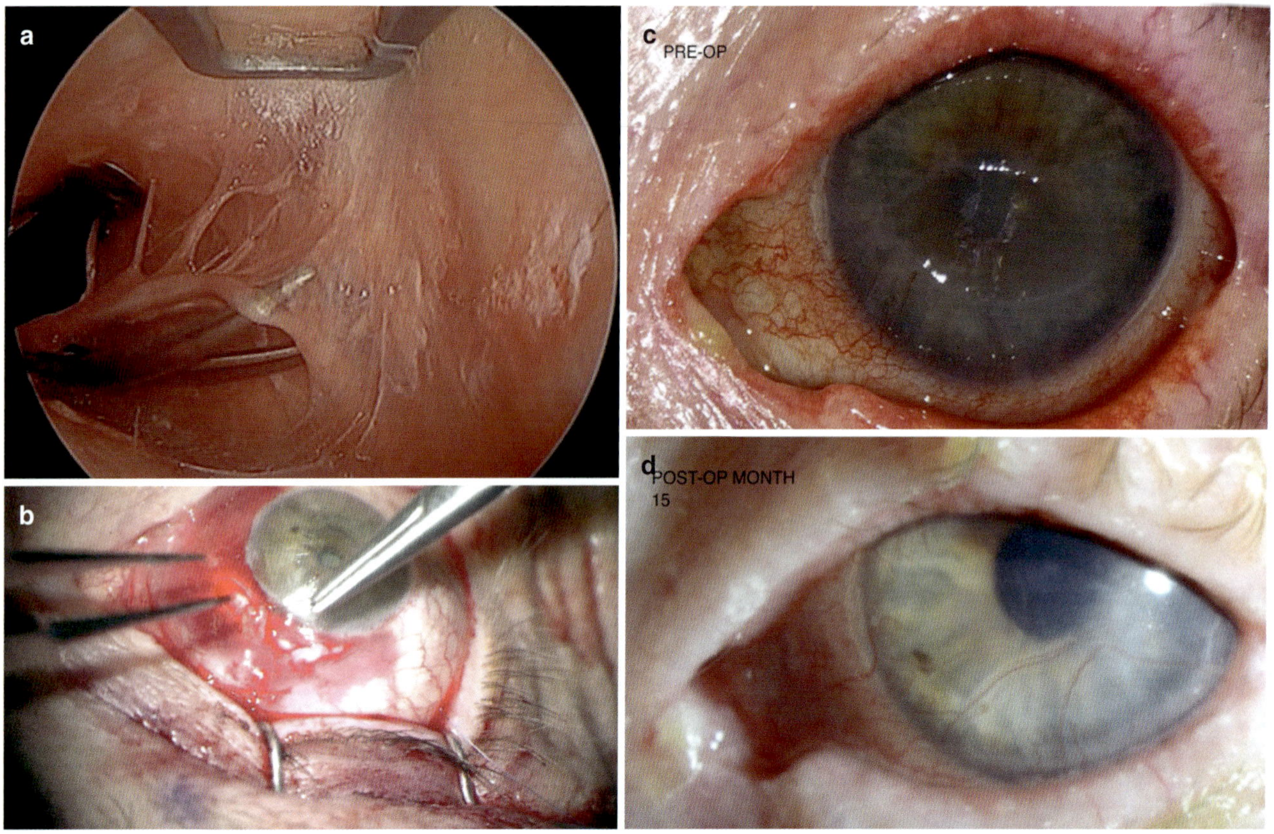

Fig. 10.12 (**a**) Isolation of the right supratrochlear nerve in preparation for nerve grafting to the left cornea. (**b**) Left cornea showing tunneling of the nerve graft and insertion of the nerve fascicles onto the corneal limbus. (**c**) Surgical patient's left neurotrophic cornea following maximal medical therapy with nonhealing central neurotrophic ulcer and peripheral corneal vasculatization. (**d**) The same patient's cornea 15 months postoperatively with healed ulcer and significant resolution of neurotrophic corneal changes. (Images courtesy of Ilya Leyngold, MD)

Corneal Neurotization

Sometimes an accompaniment to seventh nerve palsy, loss of corneal sensation provided by the ophthalmic division of the trigeminal nerve results in neurotrophic keratitis. Treatment of corneal breakdown follows a similar paradigm to that described for facial palsy, beginning with ocular lubrication and proceeding to tarsorrhaphy. Since 2014 several teams have described surgical techniques that provide successful sensory reinnervation of the cornea, via the transfer or grafting of the ipsi- or contralateral supraorbital or supratrochlear nerves [5] to the corneal surface. Results with this technique can be impressive in these otherwise hopeless cases (Fig. 10.12).

Conclusion

Numerous face and especially eye problems result from facial palsy. Psychological issues with self-image and social handicaps add to the physical disabilities. A careful history, examination, medical therapy, and, at an appropriate interval, surgical therapy can successfully manage many of the problems associated with facial palsy.

References

1. Gausas RE. Facial nerve paralysis: diagnosis and treatment. In: Guthoff R, Katowitz JA, editors. Essentials in ophthalmology – oculoplastics and orbit. Heidelberg: Springer; 2005. p. 191–204.
2. American Academy of Ophthalmology. Basic and clinical science course: orbit, eyelids and lacrimal system, section 7. San Francisco: American Academy of Ophthalmology; 2010. p. 131–4.
3. Maas CS, Benecke JE, Holds JB, Schoenrock LD. Primary surgical management for rehabilitation of the paralyzed eye. Otolaryngol Head Neck Surg. 1994;110:288–95.
4. House JW, Brackmann DE. Facial nerve grading system. Otolaryngol Head Neck Surg. 1985;93:146–7.
5. Leyngold IM, Yen MT, Tian J, Leyngold MM, Vora GK, Weller C. Minimally invasive corneal neurotization with acellular nerve allograft: surgical technique and clinical outcomes. Ophthalmic Plast Reconstr Surg. 2018. [Epub ahead of print].
6. Kumar A, Mafee MF, Mason T. Value of imaging in disorders of the facial nerve. Top Magn Reson Imaging. 2000;11:38–51.
7. Seiff SR, Boerner M, Carter SR. Treatment of facial palsies with external eyelid weights. Am J Ophthalmol. 1995;120:652–7.

8. Kirkness CM, Adams GG, Dilly PN, Lee JP. Botulinum toxin A-induced protective ptosis in corneal disease. Ophthalmology. 1988;95:473–80.
9. Stamler JF, Tse DT. A simple and reliable technique for permanent lateral tarsorrhaphy. Arch Ophthalmol. 1990;108:125–7.
10. Tanenbaum M, Gossman MD, Bergin DJ, Friedman HI, Lett D, Haines P, McCord CD Jr. The tarsal pillar technique for narrowing and maintenance of the interpalpebral fissure. Ophthalmic Surg. 1992;23:418–25.
11. Nerad JA. Ch 9. Abnormal facial movements. Techniques in ophthalmic plastic surgery: a personal tutorial. Philadelphia: Saunders Elsevier; 2010. p. 237–60.
12. Jordan DR, Anderson RL. The lateral tarsal strip revisited. The enhanced tarsal strip. Arch Ophthalmol. 1989;107:604–6.
13. Nowinski TS, Anderson RL. The medial spindle procedure for involutional medial ectropion. Arch Ophthalmol. 1985;103:1750–3.
14. Kersten RC, Kulwin DR, Levartovsky S, Tiradellis H, Tse DT. Management of lower-lid retraction with hard-palate mucosa grafting. Arch Ophthalmol. 1990;108:1339–43.
15. Rofagha S, Seiff SR. Long-term results for the use of gold eyelid load weights in the management of facial paralysis. Plast Reconstr Surg. 2010;125:142–9.
16. Tower RN, Dailey RA. Gold weight implantation: a better way? Ophthal Plast Reconstr Surg. 2004;20:202–6.
17. Cook TA, Brownrigg PJ, Wang TD, Quatela VC. The versatile midforehead browlift. Arch Otolaryngol Head Neck Surg. 1989;115:163–8.
18. May M, Drucker C. Temporalis muscle for facial reanimation. A 13-year experience with 224 procedures. Arch Otolaryngol Head Neck Surg. 1993;119:378–82.
19. Douglas RS, Gausas RE. A systematic comprehensive approach to management of irreversible facial paralysis. Facial Plast Surg. 2003;19:107–12.
20. May M, Sobol SM, Mester SJ. Hypoglossal-facial nerve interpositional-jump graft for facial reanimation without tongue atrophy. Otolaryngol Head Neck Surg. 1991;104:818–25.
21. Putterman AM. Botulinum toxin injections in the treatment of seventh nerve misdirection. Am J Ophthalmol. 1990;110:205–6.

11 Essential Blepharospasm and Hemifacial Spasm

Leon Rafailov, Richard Lee Anderson, and Ilya Michael Leyngold

Introduction

Benign essential blepharospasm (henceforth "blepharospasm") and hemifacial spasm are conditions which are linked in the final manifestation of facial spasm and are similar in regard to basic approaches to treatment. Both these diseases are movement disorders but have completely different pathophysiology. For this reason, this chapter is divided into two sections, the first on blepharospasm and the second on hemifacial spasm.

Blepharospasm

Blepharospasm is a debilitating condition of unknown cause characterized by bilateral, involuntary, and persistent closure of the eyelids:

- Presents with persistent and involuntary eyelid closure commonly with mid- and lower facial dystonia.
- Blepharospasm is a clinical diagnosis.
- Benign essential blepharospasm is by definition idiopathic and without identifiable structural changes.
- Blepharospasm is likely a result of "defective circuitry."
- Botulinum-A toxin injection is the mainstay of treatment.
- Myectomy is reserved for botulinum-A toxin failures.
- Support groups, counseling, oral medication, and surgery are important adjuncts to treatment.

Only very few advances were made in understanding and treating blepharospasm and facial dystonia for many centuries, and until the mid-1900s, most patients were still regarded as having a mental disorder or having voluntary eyelid squeezing. The first report of blepharospasm in the medical literature was in 1870, when Wood and Talkow [1] described patients with facial and eyelid squeezing disorders. In 1907, Meige [2] described a similar patient, and this dystonia has become known as Meige syndrome [3]. In the beginning of the twentieth century, the treatments for blepharospasm, such as alcohol injection of the facial nerve, neurotomy, neurectomy, and selective facial nerve avulsion, began to evolve [4–6].

Early interventions were directed at destroying the facial nerve, and patients suffered from a high recurrence rate and severe side effects such as loss of facial expression and sequelae of facial paralysis. In addition, the functional and cosmetic deformities associated with blepharospasm, such as brow ptosis, eyelid ptosis, dermatochalasis, and eyelid malpositions, were aggravated by facial nerve operations, so that the treatment was nearly as bad as the disease [7].

Treatments such as myectomy surgery, botulinum-A toxin therapy, psychosocial counseling and support groups, and oral medications were not codified until the last quarter of the twentieth century.

Classification

Blepharospasm describes what is frequently a more extensive facial dystonia. If patients with blepharospasm are followed clinically, only approximately 20% remain with isolated eyelid spasms. Most either present with or progress to more extensive facial dystonias. Patients with blepharospasm have been classified into several categories to aid in treatment decisions including (1) blepharospasm, spasms only in eyelids (Fig. 11.1); (2) Meige syndrome, spasms in eyelids and midface (Fig. 11.2); (3) Brueghel syndrome (oro-mandibular dystonia), spasms in eyelids associated with marked spasms in the lower face and neck (Fig. 11.3); (4) segmental cranial dys-

L. Rafailov (✉) · I. M. Leyngold
Duke Eye Center, Division of Oculofacial and Orbital Surgery, Durham, NC, USA

R. L. Anderson
University of Utah, Salt Lake City, UT, USA

J. J. Servat et al. (eds.), *Smith and Nesi's Ophthalmic Plastic and Reconstructive Surgery*,
https://doi.org/10.1007/978-3-030-41720-8_11

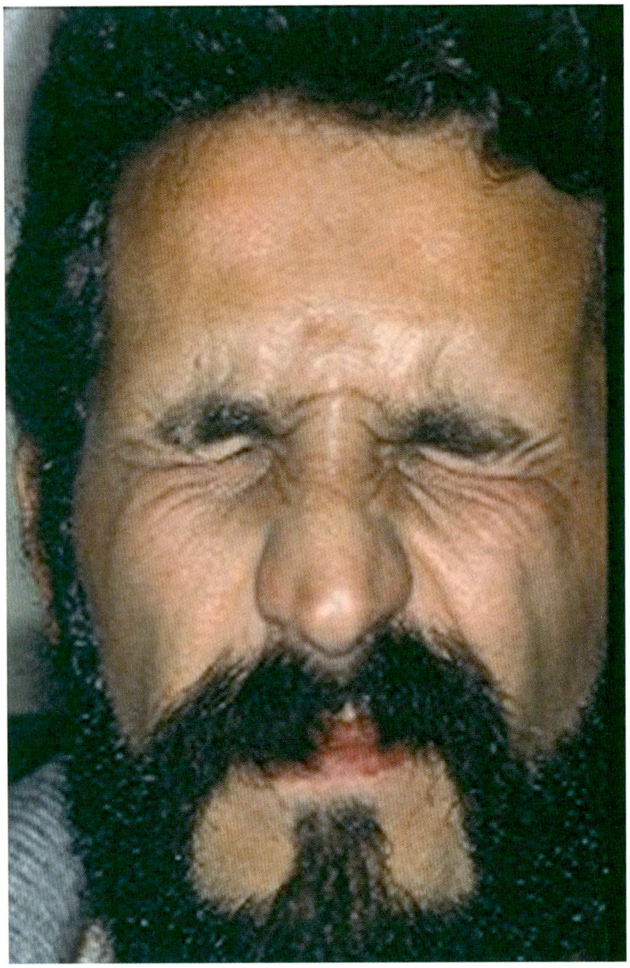

Fig. 11.1 A patient with benign essential blepharospasm without pronounced lower facial dystonia

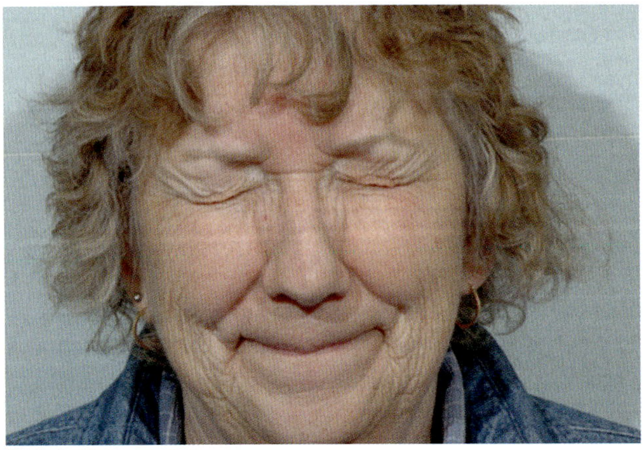

Fig. 11.2 Patient with Meige syndrome with spasms of the eyelids and midface

tonia, eyelid and facial spasms associated with spasms in cranial nerve distributions in addition to the seventh nerve; and (5) generalized dystonia, eyelid and facial spasms associated with spasms in additional body sites.

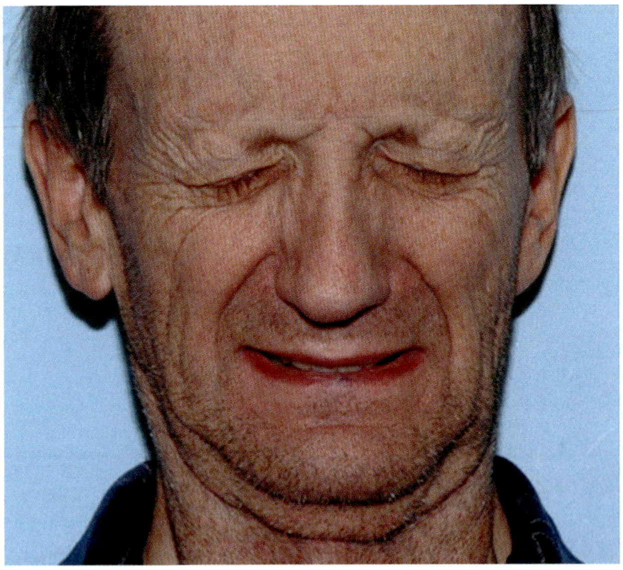

Fig. 11.3 Patient with Brueghel syndrome demonstrating spasms of the eyelids, lower face, and neck

Clinical Presentation

The typical age at presentation is in the 60s; however, it is not uncommon for patients to present in their 50s or even earlier. Frequently, early signs of the disease include increased blink rate progressing to more forceful eyelid closure. Often, the spasms appear to decrease with activities such as doctor's visits or hobbies. This phenomenon may result in an underestimate or misdiagnosis of the condition by less experienced practitioners. Control of eyelid spasm with whistling, singing, or humming is an almost pathognomic sign found in perhaps 20% of patients. On the other hand, symptoms may worsen in severity and frequency during activities such as reading or driving. In severe cases, the affected individuals are disabled to the point where they are incapable of performing the most basic activities of daily living such as cooking, reading, etc. Patients often complain of dry and irritated eyes and photophobia, especially to fluorescent lights. Although the condition is bilateral, initially, patients may notice mostly one affected side due to asymmetrical involvement.

On examination, the physician should notice increased blink frequency in early stages and forceful eyelid squeezing in more advanced cases. During eyelid spasms, simultaneous with orbicularis contraction, the eyebrows are pulled down toward the midline through the action of corrugator and depressor superciliaris muscles (Charcot's sign). Mid- and lower facial dystonias are frequently associated with blepharospasm characterized by abnormal facial movements such as lip pursing.

When the patient has difficulty opening his or her eyes after the spasm despite a lack of apparent eyelid squeezing,

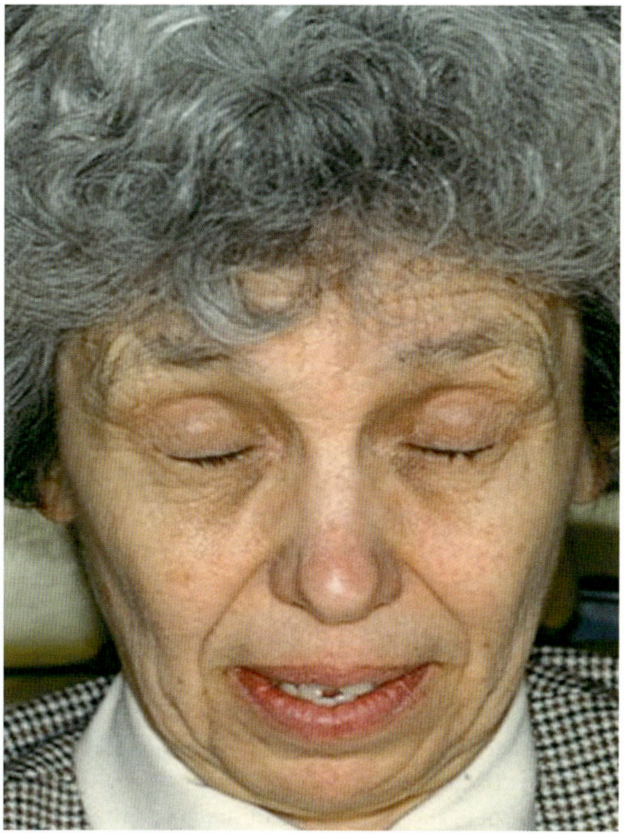

Fig. 11.4 Apparent apraxia of eyelid opening in a patient with blepharospasm

apraxia of eyelid opening (ALO) may be present (Fig. 11.4). Although strict neurophysiologic requirements for the diagnosis of ALO exist, it is clinically useful to refer to the inability of otherwise normal eyelids to open in the absence of apparent orbicularis spasm as ALO associated with blepharospasm [8, 9]. Commonly, patients with this condition are misdiagnosed as botulinum toxin treatment failures since they continue to be functionally impaired despite increasing dose of the botulinum toxin. The incidence of ALO is around 7% in the general population of patients with blepharospasm and almost 50% in patients who are "failures" of botulinum-A toxin therapy [10]. We currently believe that there is an 88% prevalence of ALO in patients refractory to botulinum-A injections who present for myectomy operation [11].

Etiologic Factors

A specific cause for blepharospasm and its central control remains elusive. From years of clinical experience, research and patient population studies [12] suggest that blepharospasm is multifactorial in origin and manifestation. Genetic predisposition may be a factor as 21% of patients report having a first- or second-degree relative with blepharospasm [13]. Some authors view blepharospasm as a defective circuit rather than a single defective locus. An as yet unidentified central defect appears to exist in the region of the basal ganglia and mid-brain [14–18]. This control center fails to modulate the blinking in blepharospasm, but it is only a part of an overloaded circuit [14].

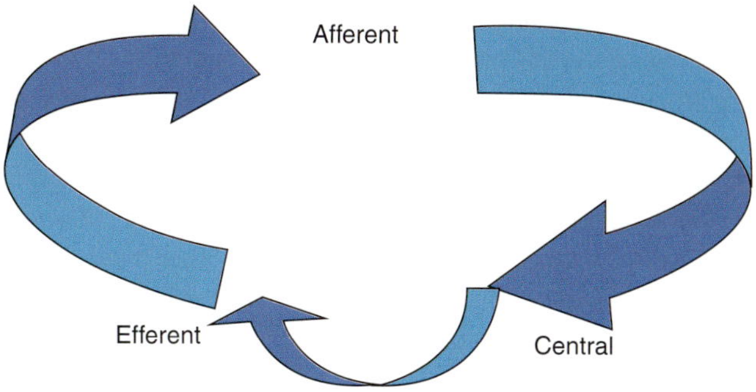

Fig. 11.5 Theoretical vicious cycle in blepharospasm

Anderson et al. [12] simplify the complex circuitry in blepharospasm into a three-component loop, with an afferent or input limb, a central control, and an efferent or response limb (Fig. 11.5). The afferent limb receives multiple stimuli, including light, corneal or eyelid irritation, pain, emotion, stress, psychic issues, and virtually any trigeminal nerve stimulation or outside irritation. These stimuli are transmitted to a central control, probably in or near the basal ganglia. The efferent pathway is transmitted via the facial nucleus, facial nerve, orbicularis oculi, corrugator, and procerus muscles. In more extensive dystonias, virtually all of the muscles supplied by the facial nerve, and even other remote nerves in the body, are involved in the efferent squeezing response. This circuit can become self-stimulating, with afferent stimuli causing efferent spasm and vice versa. The central control may be defective or weakened by anything from a genetic predisposition to injury and thereby unable to modulate this overloaded circuit. Many patients relate one stressful event, injury, or irritation as the cause of the blepharospasm, although this was probably just the final event which made the process obvious.

Therapy

Therapy is designed to interrupt the vicious cycle discussed previously. There are four major therapies directed at the treatment of blepharospasm. These are supportive therapies, oral medications, botulinum-A toxin, and myectomy surgery.

Supportive Therapies

Patients with blepharospasm suffer the same ocular irritants of any individual, with the addition of the abnormal activation of the afferent arc of their disease by these irritants.

Occasional patients with early or mild blepharospasm will experience a near-complete remission of symptoms with the treatment of other irritating factors. All patients who experience painful light sensitivity (oculophotodynia) are encouraged to wear tinted glasses with ultraviolet block. Ocular hygiene helps decrease blepharitis symptoms and irritation, and artificial tears, punctal occlusion, and other treatment of dry eye provide symptomatic relief. Supportive therapy to help manage other irritations, emotional upset, and stress is also extremely important [12].

Oral Drug Therapy

Anticholinergic class drugs are the most commonly used and effective, with GABA-ergic drugs generally the second most effective group [12]. Sedative drugs are sometimes helpful but generally decrease blepharospasm at approximately the same rate that they slow down the patient in general. Recently, due to the connection of blepharospasm with dopamine depletion, studies have shown some promise with methylphenidate [19, 20]. Methylphenidate provides an appealing alternative as it does not have the same sedative effect as traditional medications. Tachyphylaxis is common with all oral medications, with the degree of improvement and length of improvement generally limited. At present, oral medications are used more as an adjunctive therapy to botulinum-A toxin or myectomy rather than a primary long-term treatment for eyelid spasms. However, drugs may be the most useful treatment in lower facial dystonia and generalized dystonia, where botulinum-A toxin and surgery provide little relief. In another study, researchers found that of 1653 patients with blepharospasm, 1162 (70%) had tried oral therapy [12]. Forty-three percent of the patients trying drug therapy noted improvement. Outside of oral drug therapy, topical therapy with apraclonidine has also been tried due to its effect on Muller's muscle but has been limited by a small and transient improvement in symptoms [21].

Botulinum Toxin Therapy

Botulinum-A toxin, a neurotoxin produced by *Clostridium botulinum* bacteria, temporarily induces paralysis by blocking the release of acetylcholine at the nerve terminal in the neuromuscular junction. The effect is overcome in about 3 months via sprouting of new terminal axons to the motor endplate [22].

In the early 1980s, Scott described botulinum-A toxin treatment for strabismus, and soon after, clinicians began using it in blepharospasm [23, 24]. Since its approval in 1989, botulinum-A toxin became the first-line therapy for essential blepharospasm. Different brands of botulinum-A toxin have been developed and successfully used including onabotulinumtoxinA (Botox, Allergan Pharmaceuticals), abobotulinumtoxinA (Dysport, Ipsen Pharmaceuticals), and incobotulinumtoxinA (Xeomin, Merz Pharmaceuticals). It should be noted that because they are made using different processes, their dosages are not interchangeable. To date, there are no large studies which demonstrate any significant difference in efficacy, durability, or adverse events between the three types of botulinum-A toxin available for blepharospasm [25]. Subjective preferences among those who have tried both onabotulinumtoxinA (Botox) and incobotulinumtoxinA (Xeomin) indicate those who preferred onabotulinumtoxinA believed it was "more effective," whereas those who preferred incobotulinumtoxinA felt that it had had a "longer duration" [26]. We generally use a 2 mL dilution of a 100 unit vial of onabotulinumtoxinA (Botox) with a resultant concentration of 5 units/0.1 mL. Manufacturer's instructions specify the use of non-preserved saline for mixing the botulinum toxins, but most practitioners use a preserved or bacteriostatic saline to mix the drug. This considerably decreases the discomfort as the drug is injected due to the mild anesthetic properties of the bacteriostatic saline and increases the safety margin if the drug is refrigerated for several days. Using the botulinum toxins more than 6 h after mixing them again goes outside of the manufacturer's recommendations, and the "safe and effective" interval for which it may be kept is controversial. Nonetheless, keeping it refrigerated after mixing with bacteriostatic saline for up to 1 week appears to be safe.

At the initial session, the corrugator, depressor supercilii aris, and the orbicularis muscles are injected as shown in Fig. 11.6. Usually, 4–8 units per injection site are given into the corrugator muscles and 3–6 units per injection site into the orbicularis muscle. The central portion of the upper eyelid and the medial portion of the lower eyelid are avoided given the proximity of the levator and inferior oblique muscles, respectively. Some of the mid- and lower facial muscles are injected in more involved cases. The low volume of injections minimizes the potential complications of blepharoptosis and diplopia by limiting toxin spread while provid-

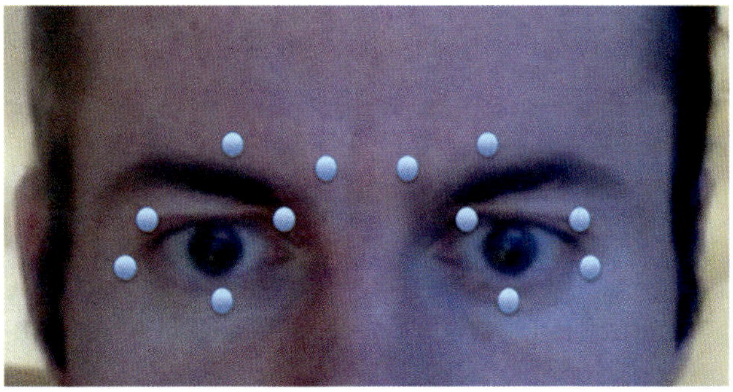

Fig. 11.6 Initial pattern of periocular injections for blepharospasm

ing maximum relief of spasms. Approximately 10% of patients receiving botulinum toxin for blepharospasm develop dose-dependent antibodies to the toxin over 10 years, which may decrease its efficacy over time [27]. One should attempt to use the maximum interval between injections since higher frequency of neurotoxin protein exposure has been positively correlated with development of immunity [28]. In cases of progressive immunity, changing the brand of botulinum toxin may allow the patient to regain the efficacy of the toxin. While there has been one study showing increased duration and subjective effect of botulinum toxin treatment with dietary zinc and phytase supplementation [29], there remain questions as to whether this can be replicated due to limits in study design [30]. Multiple studies show an 86–95% success rate with botulinum-A toxin injection alone for the treatment of blepharospasm [12, 14]. Many patients noting limited improvement with neurotoxin therapy have associated ALO and/or acquired eyelid malpositions such as ptosis which interfere with the therapeutic effect. In cases of ALO, injection of the pretarsal central upper eyelid can be an effective treatment with low rate of resulting ptosis [31, 32].

Botulinum-B neurotoxin (Myobloc, Elan Pharmaceuticals) has been available on an FDA-approved basis since 2000. Once thought to be the possible solution for the "Botox-resistant" patient, results of treatment are generally disappointing. Drug doses are generally 75–100 times those administered with Botox due to interspecies variability in the potency of the toxin serotypes, and the duration of effect and efficacy are generally considerably less for patients previously treated with a botulinum-A toxin, lasting an average of 7.3 weeks [33]. This drug now has a small ancillary role in patient treatment in most practices.

Myectomy Surgery

Given the significant morbidity and recurrence following neurectomy surgery (Fig. 11.7), one of the authors (R.L.A.) developed what has been termed the "full myectomy." Previously, blepharoplasty with removal of the orbicularis muscle was described as useful in blepharospasm, but these cases recurred with time [5]. In our early operations beginning in 1974, only the upper eyelid orbicularis muscle was removed, similar to what we now refer to as a "very limited myectomy," and all of these patients experienced recurrence of blepharospasm with time. The operation evolved into a more aggressive procedure, removing virtually all of the orbicularis muscle as well as the corrugators, procerus, and depressor superciliaris muscles. Since the myectomy operation removes all the orbicularis muscle in the extended lateral raphe, it also removes the peripheral branches of the facial nerve. The long-lasting effect of surgery comes largely

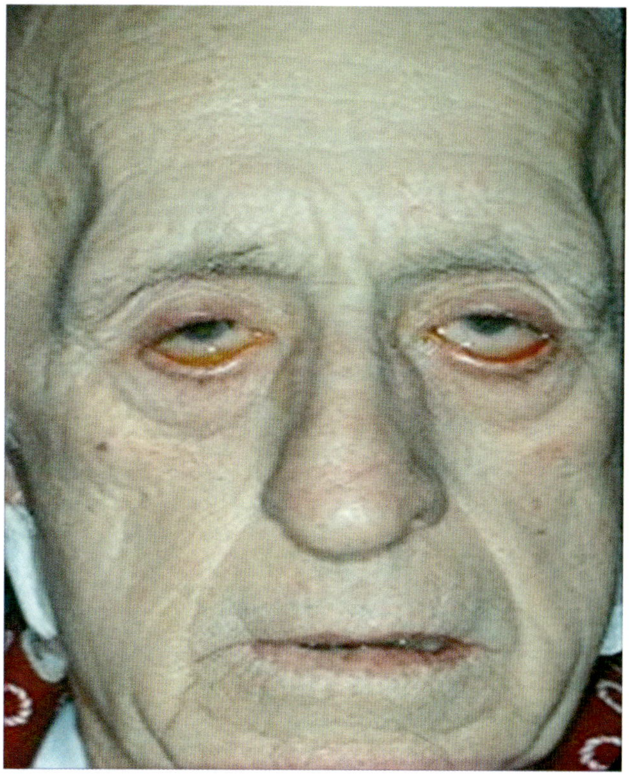

Fig. 11.7 Peripheral bilateral facial nerve paralysis following neurectomy operation for blepharospasm

from the myectomy as peripheral nerves regenerate. Since the first description of this operation in 1981, a number of subsequent papers describing our and other surgeons' experiences have been published [34–38]. The myectomy procedure is a difficult and technically demanding eyelid operation requiring experience and anatomical and surgical expertise. Results are directly related to the meticulous and complete removal of squeezing muscles. The muscles must be removed en bloc rather than piecemeal to ensure complete removal, to protect normal anatomy and vascular supply, and to decrease blood loss.

After botulinum-A toxin (onabotulinumtoxinA) approval by the Food and Drug Administration in 1989, the full myectomy operation is reserved for true botulinum-A toxin failures or patients who refuse to receive botulinum-A toxin. A "limited myectomy," removal of the entire upper, lateral, and inferotemporal orbicularis fibers, corrugator, and depressor superciliaris with sparing of most of the lower orbicularis muscle (Fig. 11.8), is used for patients who are inadequate botulinum-A toxin responders or botulinum-A toxin responders who have a poor clinical response to botulinum toxin due to ALO and/or functional deformities associated with blepharospasm. Many patients considered botulinum-A toxin "failures" are found post treatment to have a greatly weakened orbicularis on evaluating their ability to forcibly close the eyelids. Thus, the botulinum-A toxin is working but is

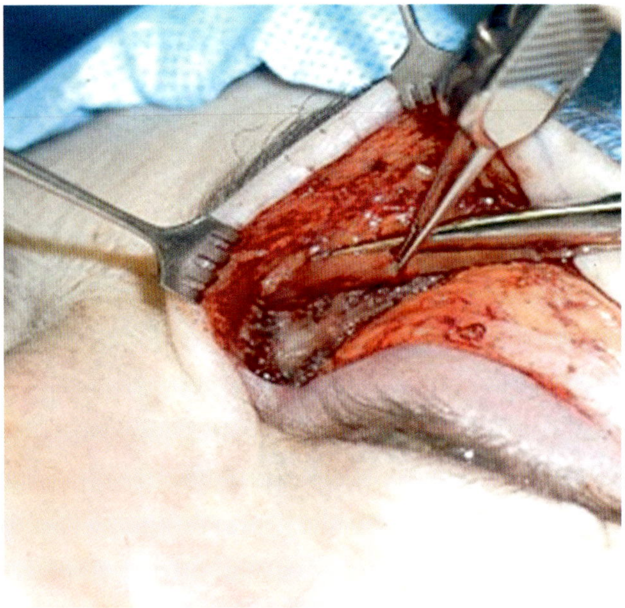

Fig. 11.8 En bloc removal of the corrugator muscle during limited myectomy surgery

not providing functional relief. Most patients presenting for myectomy, who feel that the botulinum-A toxin is not working, have ALO and/or a suboptimal response related to acquired ptosis or other functional eyelid issues. Significantly increasing the dose of the botulinum toxin in these patients often worsens the symptoms by weakening the levator muscle. In addition, the underlying deformities such as ptosis, dermatochalasis, brow ptosis, entropion, canthal tendon laxity, phimosis, and other eyelid malpositions aggravate the blepharospasm and may be a greater problem after botulinum toxin treatment than the residual blepharospasm. In cases where there is a question regarding botulinum toxin resistance, one may inject 6–8 units above a forehead rhytid in one spot and follow the effect.

At present, virtually all patients presenting for myectomy have "failed" botulinum-A toxin and drug therapy, creating a more surgically challenging group. Of the patients undergoing a myectomy operation, close to 90% note improvement.

However, there is a range in the degree of improvement achieved with myectomy. Our own study found that 27% note less than 50% improvement, 21% noted 50–75% improvement, 29% noted 75–90% improvement, and 23% noted more than 90% improvement [12]. To maximize the success of myectomy in patients with ALO, it is imperative to remove every orbicularis fiber down to the lash follicles.

Most patients continue to require botulinum-A toxin after the myectomy operation, but at lower doses and decreased frequency [39]. In true botulinum-A toxin failures, a lower myectomy may be necessary, performed 6 months following the "limited" myectomy operation. Simultaneous upper and lower myectomy, or full myectomy, is to be advised against. The tissue disruption after a myectomy procedure is marked, and considerable lymphedema generally follows the surgery. It usually requires months for complete healing after myectomy. Patients continue to improve functionally and cosmetically for 6 months to 1 year after myectomy surgery.

Over the years, modifications have been introduced to optimize the functional and cosmetic outcomes following myectomy. The "integrated upper myectomy," or "limited myectomy" with additional functional and cosmetic procedures, commonly performed today includes external aponeurotic ptosis repair, upper blepharoplasty, internal brow fat sculpting, and lateral canthopexy. To elevate and support the lower eyelid and prevent postoperative tissue depression and retraction, midface lift and orbicularis muscle grafts are now performed in many patients [40]. The orbicularis muscle grafts provide an excellent filler effect in the lateral raphe, retaining approximately 50% of their volume on long-term follow-up [40]. The effect of integrated surgery on the daily functioning of blepharospasm patients with ALO is dramatic and consistent with our previously reported study [12].

In most cases, cosmesis is improved because of decreased wrinkles and excess tissues as well as correction of brow and eyelid ptosis. Subsequent minor surgery is necessary in many patients to improve cosmesis; however, our study found an 82% satisfaction rate in appearance at 1 year following the operation [12]. The "integrated upper myectomy" gives a more predictable cosmetic improvement. However, it only provides adequate relief in patients who are also responding to botulinum-A toxin.

There are several negative side effects of myectomy. They are predictable and occur to some degree in all patients. The main concern is lymphedema, which may be present for days, months, or, rarely, even years in some patients. Lymphedema is much worse when an upper and lower myectomy is performed at the same setting (Fig. 11.9).

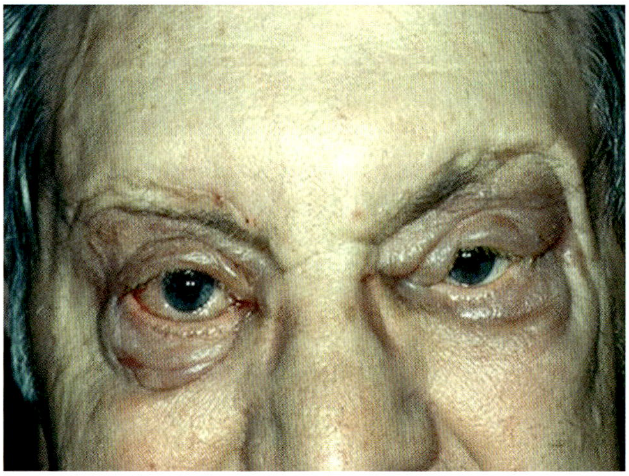

Fig. 11.9 Lymphedema following upper and lower eyelid myectomy performed at the same surgical setting

Another negative side effect of full myectomy is supraorbital anesthesia or hypoesthesia. It is impossible to completely remove the corrugator and depressor superciliaris muscles without damage to the supraorbital nerve. Supraorbital anesthesia improves over months in most patients.

Decreased orbicularis function and lagophthalmos are necessary negative side effects but may result in corneal exposure and increased dry eyes, necessitating more lubricants. This is temporary in most patients. It is surprising that a permanent severe dry eye and exposure does not always occur with myectomy and botulinum-A toxin. The eyelids may act as better "windshield wipers" or resurfacing agents for the cornea after relieving the spasms and may open and close in a more physiologic fashion after healing. The lacrimal pump is weakened, which increases the tear lake and may help dry eyes. Punctal occlusion is very useful in those experiencing dry eye in addition to blepharospasm.

One of the authors (RLA) has performed over 2000 myectomy operations. A review of complications experienced in over 500 myectomy operations included infection, hematoma or hemorrhage, brow hair loss, skin loss requiring skin graft, ptosis, upper lid retraction, lower lid retraction, trichiasis, and canthal deformity. Fortunately, except for some permanent cosmetic disfigurement, most of these complications were minor or correctable with additional surgery. There was no occurrence of permanent visual loss, and despite the extensive nature of a myectomy operation in an older patient population, there was no occurrence of death or permanent disability from surgery.

Current Therapeutic Protocol

Referral to a patient support group such as the Benign Essential Blepharospasm Research Foundation (BEBRF) for education regarding their disease and support is recommended for all patients. If blepharospasm or torticollis (not discussed in this chapter) is the main problem, then botulinum-A toxin is the primary treatment. If lower facial or body spasm is the main problem and eyelid spasm is a minor or secondary component, then oral therapy should be tried first. If a patient has both eyelid and lower facial components, then botulinum-A toxin as well as oral therapy may be required. If a patient with blepharospasm is a rare but true nonresponder to botulinum-A toxin, then a full myectomy operation is required. Patients with blepharospasm who are true botulinum-A toxin nonresponders will generally require an upper as well as lower myectomy, but at least 6 months between operations is advised. Some patients who are considered botulinum-A toxin nonresponders may be converted to botulinum-A toxin responders in their lower eyelids after a limited myectomy. If a patient is only a functional "failure" of botulinum-A toxin or is obtaining inadequate relief, but the toxin is providing orbicularis weakening, then the patient usually has associated ALO and functional lid deformities. In this case, a limited myectomy is recommended.

Patient Support

Patient support groups such as the BEBRF, founded by Mattie Lou Koster in 1981, have provided the great support for blepharospasm sufferers worldwide. These groups brought blepharospasm "out of the closet" and to the attention of patients, physicians, and the public. Newly diagnosed patients with blepharospasm may wish to be placed in touch with the BEBRF or similar groups such as the Dystonia Foundation to provide education and support, helping them to cope with their disease and providing a forum for patients to share experiences.

In summary, blepharospasm is a challenging disorder with dysfunctional circuitry rather than a specific abnormal locus. In addition to disabling eyelid squeezing, most of the affected patients also have significant involutional periorbital changes contributing to their symptoms. Although no cure is available for blepharospasm, its treatment had evolved over the years with botulinum-A toxin becoming the mainstay of therapy. Currently, most patients obtain relief from neurotoxin injections alone, but myectomy remains a viable option for nonresponders. Oral drug therapy is less effective for blepharospasm but may be more successful for lower facial dystonias. Finally, all of the blepharospasm patients should join BEBRF for psychological support, education, and counseling.

Hemifacial Spasm

Hemifacial spasm, first described in 1884 by Gowes, is characterized by a segmental typically unilateral myoclonus of facial musculature innervated by cranial nerve VII:

- Presents with unilateral fasciculations of periocular and/or facial muscles.
- Possible etiologies include idiopathic, ectatic cranial vasculature and intracranial mass.
- Evaluation includes careful history, clinical exam, and imaging.
- Treatment includes botulinum toxin, oral medications, surgical decompression, and myectomy.

They were a few meters apart when the left side of the man's face was suddenly contorted by a sort of spasm. It happened again just as they were passing one another. It was only a twitch, a quiver, rapid as the clicking of a camera shutter, but obviously habitual.

George Orwell, *1984*.

Hemifacial spasm is an uncommon disorder with an annual incidence of 0.78/100,000, most often presenting between the fourth and sixth decade of life. The largest study conducted to date suggests it is about two times more prevalent among women (14.5/100,000) than men (7.4/100,000). While rare reports of familial cases exist, most cases are sporadic [41].

Etiologic Factors

The most common identifiable cause of hemifacial spasm is compression of the facial nerve root by an ectatic blood vessel (most often anterior inferior cerebellar artery, posterior inferior cerebellar artery, or vertebral artery) as it exits from the brainstem [29, 42–44].

Compression of the facial nerve root leads to nerve damage with demyelination, resulting in aberrant signal conduction in response to nerve irritation, and thereby involuntary contraction of the innervated facial musculature. This mechanism has been supported by electrophysiological studies [45, 46]. In addition, studies have shown resolution of the aberrant nerve signaling following surgical decompression [34, 47]. Some researchers have implicated hypertension in the pathophysiology of hemifacial spasm (HFS) by suggesting that hypertension-induced vascular thickening may produce ectasia of the offending vessel, but data have not proven conclusive [48]. Intracranial mass lesions (e.g., meningioma, lipoma, epidermoid) have also been identified as etiologic in rare cases of hemifacial spasm [42, 44]. The remainder of hemifacial spasm cases are classified as idiopathic, with as many as 62% having no identifiable underlying cause of facial nerve dysfunction [49]. Hemifacial spasm must also be distinguished from aberrant reinnervation after facial nerve palsy with facial synkinesis in which movement in one part of the face triggers movement in other areas or hemifacial contracture with a tonic contracture of facial musculature. History and examination generally make it easy to discriminate these processes.

Clinical Presentation

The initial presentation of hemifacial spasm is typified by unilateral fasciculations and clonic contracture of periocular orbicularis oculi musculature. The contractions are often exacerbated by stress, anxiety, fatigue, voluntary facial movements, or a combination thereof [50, 51]. With time, the involuntary contractures tend to migrate to a larger area of the ipsilateral midface and lower facial muscles, often developing a component of tonic contracture (Fig. 11.10). Spontaneous resolution has been reported but is exceedingly rare [42, 51]. Some patients report experiencing low-pitched tinnitus, presumably secondary to contracture of the stapedius muscle, which is also innervated by cranial nerve VII. In contrast to benign essential blepharospasm, hemifacial spasm symptoms tend to persist during sleep. As hemifacial spasm becomes chronic in nature, most patients will demonstrate some degree of ipsilateral facial weakness [50]. Bilateral hemifacial spasm has been reported but is exceedingly rare [52]. In bilateral cases, the facial contractions are asynchronous and cause ipsilateral brow elevation during contracture ("Babinski sign"), differentiating them from bilaterally symmetric contractions that depress the brows ("Charcot's sign") characteristic of blepharospasm.

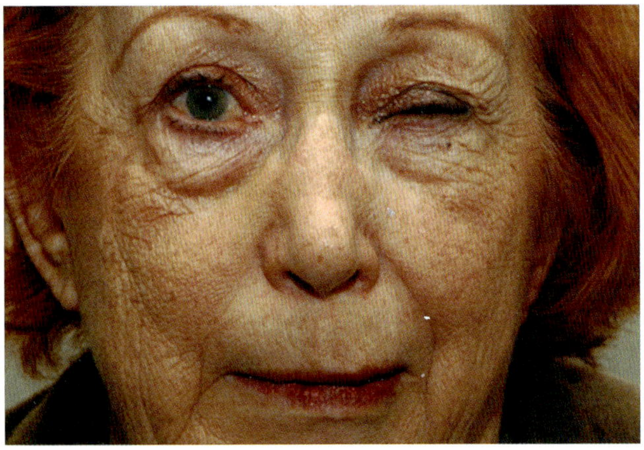

Fig. 11.10 A patient with hemifacial spasm demonstrating left-sided facial contracture

Diagnosis/Work-Up

Hemifacial spasm is largely a clinical diagnosis based upon a compatible patient history and observation of facial contractures. In straightforward cases presenting with classic features, many clinicians perform no additional work-up. However, if any question of the diagnosis exists, or atypical features such as numbness, weakness, or additional neurological abnormalities exist, further work-up is warranted to rule out an atypical etiology of facial contractures. The most common diagnostic modality employed is a combination of MRI and MRA of the head and neck [41]. Three-dimensional MRI and MRA scans are increasingly being employed, particularly if surgical intervention is desired [43], as these can assist in surgical planning. This approach looks for a possible mass lesion and may demonstrate the etiologic dolichoectatic vessel impinging on the facial nerve root. Electrophysiologic studies may also be used in the work-up to demonstrate features unique to hemifacial spasm. Facial electromyographic studies demonstrate high-frequency bursts (150–400 Hz) of motor unit action potentials during periods of clinically observed facial contracture.

Therapy

Hemifacial spasm treatment can be divided into surgical and nonsurgical options.

Medical

In cases demonstrating vascular compression of the facial nerve on neuroimaging, treatment is tailored to patient preference. Most patients wish to avoid surgery, and therefore, botulinum toxin injection is the mainstay of treatment. Botulinum toxin functions via chemodenervation of neuromuscular junctions in the area of injection. Symptomatic improvement with botulinum toxin is achieved in greater than 95% of patients [53] with hemifacial spasm while maintaining a low rate of complications once the patient is outside of his or her early titration phase [54]. Following injection into the involved facial musculature, symptoms typically improve within 3–5 days, with maximal improvement 10–14 days post-injection (Fig. 11.11). Average duration of clinical effect is approximately 3 months, with reports varying from 3 to 6+ months [53, 55]. In general, the duration of clinical efficacy of botulinum toxin is slightly longer among hemifacial spasm patients when compared with patients with blepharospasm.

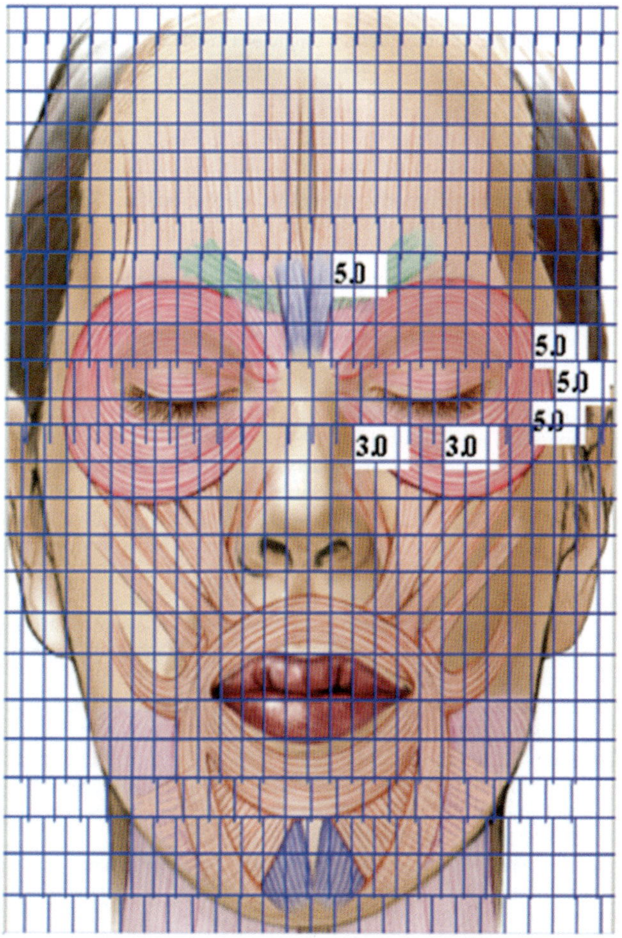

Fig. 11.11 Typical initial injection pattern for hemifacial spasm in our practice with corresponding units of Botox®

One may inject botulinum toxin in the contralateral facial musculature (e.g., crow's feet) to avoid facial asymmetry and improve cosmesis. Long-term results with repeated botulinum toxin injections are favorable with low rates of side effects [53, 56]. The most common side effects include dry eye, ipsilateral ptosis, lower facial weakness, and diplopia, all of which can be minimized with proper dosing, careful injection technique, and knowledge of periocular anatomy [53, 57].

Oral medications offer another nonsurgical treatment option for hemifacial spasm. Carbamazepine, baclofen, and benzodiazepines are among the most commonly employed oral medications in hemifacial spasm [42]. In most patients, oral medications are much less effective at ameliorating involuntary facial contractions compared with botulinum toxin therapy, and the side effects of oral medications tend to outweigh the symptomatic relief achieved [44, 58, 59].

Surgical Treatment Options

Should botulinum toxin injections prove inadequate to control symptoms of hemifacial spasm, orbicularis myectomy is an available replacement or adjunct therapy. A study of hemifacial spasm patients undergoing unilateral myectomy suggested improvement in 94% of those treated [11]. Contralateral blepharoplasty will provide a cosmetic outcome by improving symmetry. Following myectomy, patients may continue to require botulinum toxin injections; however, fewer units are required, and the symptom-free interval between injections is typically increased [11, 60].

In patients with radiographically demonstrable vascular compression of the facial nerve, surgical decompression of the facial nerve at the cerebellopontine angle is a therapeutic option. Microvascular decompression of the facial nerve is reported to alleviate symptoms of hemifacial spasm in greater than 90% of patients [61, 62]. Risks of the surgery include permanent facial nerve injury and hearing loss [63], in addition to the risks of craniotomy; 9–10% rates of recurrence are reported after successful surgical decompression [62, 64]. Given the surgical morbidity and risks involved, patient selection for microvascular decompressive surgery is paramount. Ideal candidates are young, otherwise healthy patients, or older patients with associated pain unrelieved by botulinum toxin, in whom an identifiable etiology exists on neuroimaging [65].

Summary

In summary, hemifacial spasm is a physically, psychologically, and socially debilitating disorder that frequently goes unrecognized and therefore untreated. With appropriate treatment, the vast majority of patients achieve long-term improvement in quality-of-life measures, with few if any signs or symptoms of the disorder. Given these facts, increased awareness of hemifacial spasm among treating physicians holds great potential to reduce the impact of this disorder on the lives of affected individuals.

References

1. Talkow J. Klonische krampfe der angelinder: neurotomie der supraorbitalnerven. Klin Montasbl Augenheilkd. 1870;8:129–45.
2. Meige H. Les convulsion de la face une form clinique de convulsion faciale, bilateral et mediane. Rev Neurol (Paris). 1907;10:437–43.
3. Jankovic JJ. Etiology and differential diagnosis of blepharospasm and oromandibular dystonia. Adv Neurol. 1988;49:103–16.
4. Reynolds DH, Smith JL, Walsh TJ. Differential section of the facial nerve for blepharospasm. Trans Am Acad Ophthalmol Otolaryngol. 1967;71:656–64.
5. Callahan A. Surgical correction of intractable blepharospasm: technical improvements. Am J Ophthalmol. 1965;60:788–91.
6. Weingarten CZ, Putterman AM. Management of patients with essential blepharospasm. Eye Ear Nose Throat Mon. 1976;55:8–24.
7. Henderson JW. Essential blepharospasm. Trans Am Ophthalmol Soc. 1956;54:453–520.
8. Goldstein JE, Cogan DG. Apraxia of lid opening. Arch Ophthalmol. 1965;73:155–9.
9. Lepore FE, Devoisin RC. 'Apraxia' of eyelid opening: an involuntary levator inhibition. Neurology. 1985;35:423–7.
10. Jordan DR, Anderson RL, Digre KB. Apraxia of lid opening in blepharospasm. Ophthalmic Surg. 1990;21:331–4.
11. Georgescu D, Vagefi MR, McMullan TF, McCann JD, Anderson RL. Upper eyelid myectomy in blepharospasm with associated apraxia of lid opening. Am J Ophthalmol. 2008;145(3):541–7.
12. Anderson RL, Patel BC, Holds JB, Jordan DR. Blepharospasm: past, present, and future. Ophthal Plast Reconstr Surg. 1998;14:305–17.
13. Peckham EL, Lopez G, Shamim EA, et al. Clinical features of patients with blepharospasm: a report of 240 patients. Eur J Neurol. 2011;18(3):382–6.
14. Jankovic JJ, Patel SC. Blepharospasm associated with brainstem lesions. Neurology. 1983;33:1237–40.
15. Aramideh M, Bour LJ, Koelman JH, et al. Abnormal eye movements in blepharospasm and involuntary levator palpebrae inhibition. Brain. 1994;117:1457–74.
16. Hotson JR, Boman DR. Memory-contingent saccades and the substantia nigra postulate for essential blepharospasm. Brain. 1991;114:295–307.
17. Jankovic JJ. Clinical features, differential diagnosis and pathogenesis of blepharospasm and cranial-cervical dystonia. In: Bosniak SL, Smith BC, editors. Advances in ophthalmic plastic and reconstructive surgery, vol. 4. New York: Pergamon Press; 1985. p. 67–82.
18. Creel DJ, Holds JB, Anderson RL. Auditory brain-stem responses in blepharospasm. Electroencephalogr Clin Neurophysiol. 1993;86:138–40.
19. Eftekhari K, Choe CH, Vagefi MR, et al. Oral methylphenidate for the treatment of refractory facial dystonias. Ophthalmic Plast Reconstr Surg. 2015;31(3):e65–6.
20. Price KM, Ramey NA, Richard MJ, et al. Can methylphenidate objectively provide relief in patients with uncontrolled blepharospasm? A pilot study using surface electromyography. Ophthalmic Plast Reconstr Surg. 2010;26(5):353–6.
21. Vijayakumar D, Wijemanne S, Jankovic J. Treatment of blepharospasm with apraclonidine. J Neurol Sci. 2017;372:57–9.
22. Alderson K, Holds JB, Anderson RL. Botulinum-induced alterations of nerve-muscle interactions in the human orbicularis oculi following treatment for blepharospasm. Neurology. 1991;41:1800–5.
23. Scott AB. Botulinum toxin injection of eye muscles to correct strabismus. Trans Am Ophthalmol Soc. 1981;79:734–70.
24. Kennedy RA, Stubbs HA. Botulinum-A toxin injection as a treatment for blepharospasm. Arch Ophthalmol. 1985;103:347–50.
25. Kollewe K, Mohammadi B, Kohler S, et al. Blepharospasm: long-term treatment with either Botox(R), Xeomin(R) or Dysport(R). J Neural Transm (Vienna). 2015;122(3):427–31.
26. Chundury RV, Couch SM, Holds JB. Comparison of preferences between onabotulinumtoxinA (Botox) and incobotulinumtoxinA (Xeomin) in the treatment of benign essential blepharospasm. Ophthalmic Plast Reconstr Surg. 2013;29(3):205–7.
27. Albrecht P, Jansen A, Lee JI, et al. High prevalence of neutralizing antibodies after long-term botulinum neurotoxin therapy. Neurology. 2019;92(1):e48–54.
28. Adler CH, Factor SA, Brin M, Sethi KD. Secondary nonresponsiveness to botulinum toxin type A in patients with oromandibular dystonia. Mov Disord. 2002;17(1):158–61.
29. Koshy JC, Sharabi SE, Feldman EM, et al. Effect of dietary zinc and phytase supplementation on botulinum toxin treatments. J Drugs Dermatol. 2012;11(4):507–12.
30. Cohen JL. Scientific skepticism and new discoveries: an analysis of a report of zinc/phytase supplementation and the efficacy of botulinum toxins in treating cosmetic facial rhytides, hemifacial spasm and benign essential blepharospasm. J Cosmet Laser Ther. 2014;16(5):258–62.
31. Esposito M, Fasano A, Crisci C, et al. The combined treatment with orbital and pretarsal botulinum toxin injections in the management of poorly responsive blepharospasm. Neurol Sci. 2014;35(3):397–400.
32. Huang L, Costin BR, Sakolsatayadorn N, Perry JD. Safety of onabotulinum toxin a injection to the central upper eyelid and eyebrow regions. Ophthalmic Plast Reconstr Surg. 2014;30(5):377–80.
33. Dutton JJ, White JJ, Richard MJ. Myobloc for the treatment of benign essential blepharospasm in patients refractory to botox. Ophthalmic Plast Reconstr Surg. 2006;22(3):173–7.
34. Gillum WN, Anderson RL. Blepharospasm surgery: anatomic approach. Arch Ophthalmol. 1981;99:1056–62.
35. Jordan DR, Patrinely JR, Anderson RL, et al. Essential blepharospasm and related dystonias. Surv Ophthalmol. 1989;34:123–32.
36. McCord CD, Coles WH, Shore JW, et al. Treatment of essential blepharospasm. I. Comparison of facial nerve avulsion and eyebrow-eyelid muscle stripping procedure. Arch Ophthalmol. 1984;102:266–8.
37. Frueh BR, Musch DC, Bersani TA. Effects of eyelid protractor excision for the treatment of benign essential blepharospasm. Am J Ophthalmol. 1992;113:681–6.
38. Patel BCK, Anderson RL. Blepharospasm and related facial movement disorders. Curr Opin Ophthalmol. 1995;5:86–99.
39. Kent TL, Petris CK, Holds JB. Effect of upper eyelid myectomy on subsequent chemodenervation in the management of benign essential blepharospasm. Ophthalmic Plast Reconstr Surg. 2015;31(3):222–6.
40. Yen MT, Anderson RL, Small RG. Orbicularis oculi muscle graft augmentation after protractor myectomy in blepharospasm. Ophthal Plast Reconstr Surg. 2003;19:287–96.
41. Adler CH, Zimmerman RA, Savino PJ, et al. Hemifacial spasm: evaluation by magnetic resonance imaging and magnetic resonance tomographic angiography. Ann Neurol. 1992;32(4):502–6.
42. Digre K, Corbett JJ. Hemifacial spasm: differential diagnosis, mechanism, and treatment. Adv Neurol. 1988;49:151–76.

43. Girard N, Poncet M, Caces F, et al. Three-dimensional MRI of hemifacial spasm with surgical correlation. Neuroradiology. 1997;39(1):46–51.
44. Jannetta PJ, Abbasy M, Maroon JC, Ramos FM, Albin MS. Etiology and definitive microsurgical treatment of hemifacial spasm. Operative techniques and results in 47 patients. J Neurosurg. 1977;47(3):321–8.
45. Nielsen VK. Pathophysiology of hemifacial spasm: I. Ephaptic transmission and ectopic excitation. Neurology. 1984;34(4):418–26.
46. Nielsen VK. Pathophysiology of hemifacial spasm: II. Lateral spread of the supraorbital nerve reflex. Neurology. 1984;34(4):427–31.
47. Nielsen VK, Jannetta PJ. Pathophysiology of hemifacial spasm: III. Effects of facial nerve decompression. Neurology. 1984;34(7):891–7.
48. Tan EK, Jankovic J. Hemifacial spasm and hypertension: how strong is the association? Mov Disord. 2000;15(2):363–5.
49. Yaltho TC, Jankovic J. The many faces of hemifacial spasm: differential diagnosis of unilateral facial spasms. Mov Disord. 2011;26(9):1582–92.
50. Wang A, Jankovic J. Hemifacial spasm: clinical findings and treatment. Muscle Nerve. 1998;21(12):1740–7.
51. Ehni G, Woltman HW. Hemifacial spasm: review of one hundred and six cases. Arch Neurol Psychiatr. 1945;53(3):205–11.
52. Tan EK, Jankovic J. Bilateral hemifacial spasm: a report of five cases and a literature review. Mov Disord. 1999;14(2):345–9.
53. Defazio G, Abbruzzese G, Girlanda P, et al. Botulinum toxin A treatment for primary hemifacial spasm: a 10-year multicenter study. Arch Neurol. 2002;59(3):418–20.
54. Czyz CN, Burns JA, Petrie TP, et al. Long-term botulinum toxin treatment of benign essential blepharospasm, hemifacial spasm, and Meige syndrome. Am J Ophthalmol. 2013;156(1):173–7. e2
55. Schellini SA, Matai O, Igami TZ, Padovani CR, Padovani CP. Essential blepharospasm and hemifacial spasm: characteristic of the patient, botulinum toxin A treatment and literature review. Arq Bras Oftalmol. 2006;69(1):23–6.
56. Calace P, Cortese G, Piscopo R, et al. Treatment of blepharospasm with botulinum neurotoxin type A: long-term results. Eur J Ophthalmol. 2003;13(4):331–6.
57. Vartanian AJ, Dayan SH. Complications of botulinum toxin a use in facial rejuvenation. Facial Plast Surg Clin North Am. 2005;13(1):1–10.
58. Eckman PB, Kramer RA, Altrocchi PH. Hemifacial spasm. Arch Neurol. 1971;25(1):81–7.
59. Savino PJ, Sergott RC, Bosley TM, Schatz NJ. Hemifacial spasm treated with botulinum A toxin injection. Arch Ophthalmol. 1985;103(9):1305–6.
60. Garland PE, Patrinely JR, Anderson RL. Hemifacial spasm. Results of unilateral myectomy. Ophthalmology. 1987;94(3):288–94.
61. Tan N, Chan L, Tan E. Hemifacial spasm and involuntary facial movements. QJM. 2002;95(8):493–500.
62. Miller LE, Miller VM. Safety and effectiveness of microvascular decompression for treatment of hemifacial spasm: a systematic review. Br J Neurosurg. 2012;26(4):438–44.
63. Sindou M, Fobé JL, Ciriano D, Fischer C. Hearing prognosis and intraoperative guidance of brainstem auditory evoked potential in microvascular decompression. Laryngoscope. 1992;102(6):678–82.
64. Payner TD, Tew JM. Recurrence of hemifacial spasm after microvascular decompression. Neurosurgery. 1996;38(4):686–90; discussion 690–1
65. Han I, Chang JH, Chang JW, Huh R, Chung SS. Unusual causes and presentations of hemifacial spasm. Neurosurgery. 2009;65(1):130–7; discussion 137

Ocular Cicatricial Pemphigoid

12

Sravanthi Vegunta and Alison V. Crum

Introduction

Mucous membrane pemphigoid is a chronic autoimmune disease that mainly affects mucous membranes. Skin lesions occur in 10–43% of patients [1]. The conjunctiva is involved in about 70% of patients [2]. The component of the disease that affects the conjunctiva, regardless of involvement of nonocular sites, is commonly called ocular cicatricial pemphigoid. It is a bilateral, asymmetric, sight-threatening disease characterized by progressive conjunctival cicatrization associated with trichiasis, eyelid entropion, symblepharon, secondary corneal neovascularization, and scarring. It is characterized by IgG, IgA, or C3 (complement component) deposition in a linear fashion along the epithelial basement membrane zone. The disease usually presents between the ages of 30 and 90 years; it affects males twice as often as females [3, 4].

Mucous membrane pemphigoid (MMP) is the most common cause of cicatrizing conjunctivitis in developed countries. It is a chronic autoimmune disease that mainly affects the subepidermal tissue of mucous membranes. Oral mucosae have the highest rate of involvement followed by ocular, nasal, nasopharyngeal, anogenital, skin, laryngeal, and esophageal mucosae [5]. Conjunctiva is involved in about 70% of cases and skin lesions occur in 10–43% [3]. It is a bilateral, asymmetric, sight-threatening disease characterized by progressive conjunctival cicatrization associated with trichiasis, eyelid entropion, symblepharon, and secondary corneal neovascularization and scarring. The disease usually presents between the ages of 30 and 90 years, and it affects males twice as often as females [3, 4]. It is characterized by IgG, IgA, or C3 (complement component) deposition in a linear fashion along the epithelial basement membrane zone (BMZ) [5].

The nomenclature of the disease itself has undergone changes and is sometimes confused with other bullous diseases. According to the 2002 International Consensus Statement on Mucous Membrane Pemphigoid, the most appropriate term to characterize this group of diseases is mucous membrane pemphigoid rather than ocular MMP, as more than one site is commonly involved. Additionally, the term *cicatricial* incorrectly eliminates patients who have ocular disease without scarring [6].

MMP should be distinguished from two other bullous diseases that mainly affect nonocular sites, pemphigus vulgaris and bullous pemphigoid. Pemphigus vulgaris is an acute or chronic intraepidermal bullous autoimmune disease that starts with erosion of mucous membranes of the mouth and nose, followed by involvement of the skin in a localized or generalized form [7]. Bullous pemphigoid is a subepidermal blistering dermatosis that mainly affects the skin with limited mucosal and conjunctival involvement. In contrast to MMP, bullous pemphigoid is a non-scarring disease. It resembles MMP in the localization of the immunoreactants to the subepidermal BMZ, which is found with a high prevalence in the conjunctiva. However, clinical changes of the conjunctiva are typically absent [1, 8].

Clinical Presentation

MMP systemically creates a bullous rash of skin and inflammatory lesions of mucosal subepidermal tissue. This leads to irreversible scarring of mucosal surfaces. In extreme cases, death may occur from esophageal and/or tracheal strictures resulting in asphyxiation [9]. The eye is the first site of involvement in about one-third of patients [10]. Subclinical ocular MMP can become active and be diagnosed after ocular trauma, eyelid surgery, or strabismus surgery.

S. Vegunta · A. V. Crum (✉)
University of Utah Health Care, Moran Eye Center, Department of Ophthalmology, Salt Lake City, UT, USA
e-mail: Alison.crum@hsc.utah.edu

J. J. Servat et al. (eds.), *Smith and Nesi's Ophthalmic Plastic and Reconstructive Surgery*,
https://doi.org/10.1007/978-3-030-41720-8_12

Ocular MMP, which is usually asymmetric, can ultimately destroy all three layers of the tear film—goblet cells, accessory lacrimal glands of Wolfring and Krause, and meibomian gland orifices. Trichiasis and cicatricial entropion cause microabrasions and ocular surface irritation. Symblepharon or contracted posterior lamellae can lead to lagophthalmos, impairment of Bell's phenomenon, and restricted extraocular motility. Local inflammation can result in punctal or lacrimal apparatus obstruction [11]. Tear spread and renewal are thus compromised (Figs. 12.1 and 12.2) [5].

Pathology of the eyelids, ocular surface, and lacrimal apparatus combine to generate keratoconjunctivitis sicca, conjunctival keratinization, pseudopterygium, infectious keratitis, corneal ulceration, corneal neovascularization, corneal scarring, corneal perforation, subconjunctival fibrosis, forniceal shortening, symblepharon, and lagophthalmos. The end stage of the disease is characterized by severe limbal stem cell deficiency, ankyloblepharon, frozen globe, and blindness.

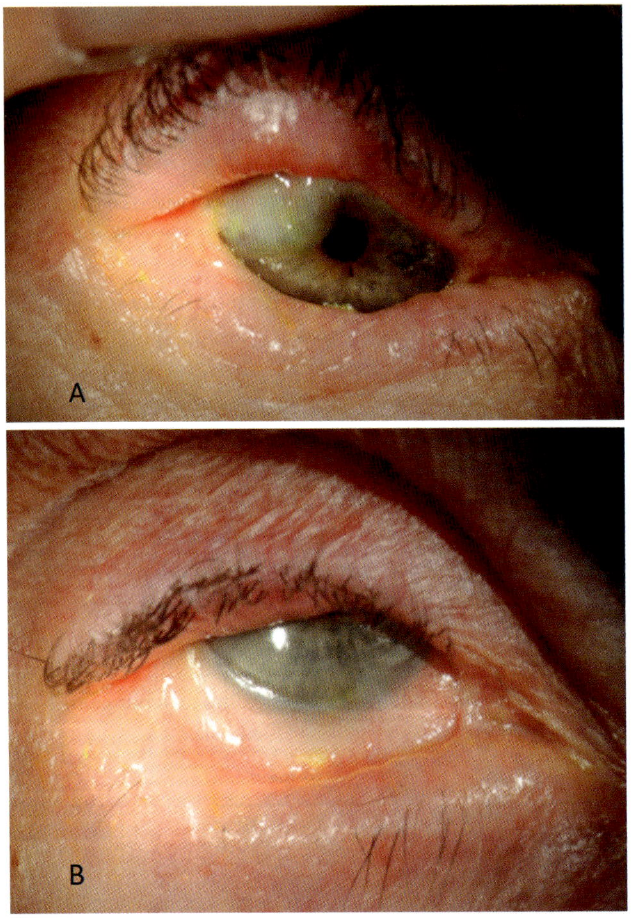

Fig. 12.1 Slit lamp photographs of the right eye of Foster stage III direct immunofluorescence microscopy-confirmed mucous membrane pemphigoid with fluorescein staining. Note upper and lower eyelid margin thickening and keratinization, lower eyelid madarosis after treatment of trichiasis with electrolysis, conjunctivalization of the cornea and pseudopterygium, and limbal stem cell deficiency. Visual acuity is 20/40 in the right eye. (**a**) Lower eyelid entropion is seen, lack of eyelashes (madarosis) noted. (**b**) Lower eyelid is retracted to show conjunctival scarring, shortened inferior fornix, and nasal and temporal symblephara. (Images courtesy of Moran Eye Center Photography, Department of Ophthalmology, University of Utah, Salt Lake City, Utah)

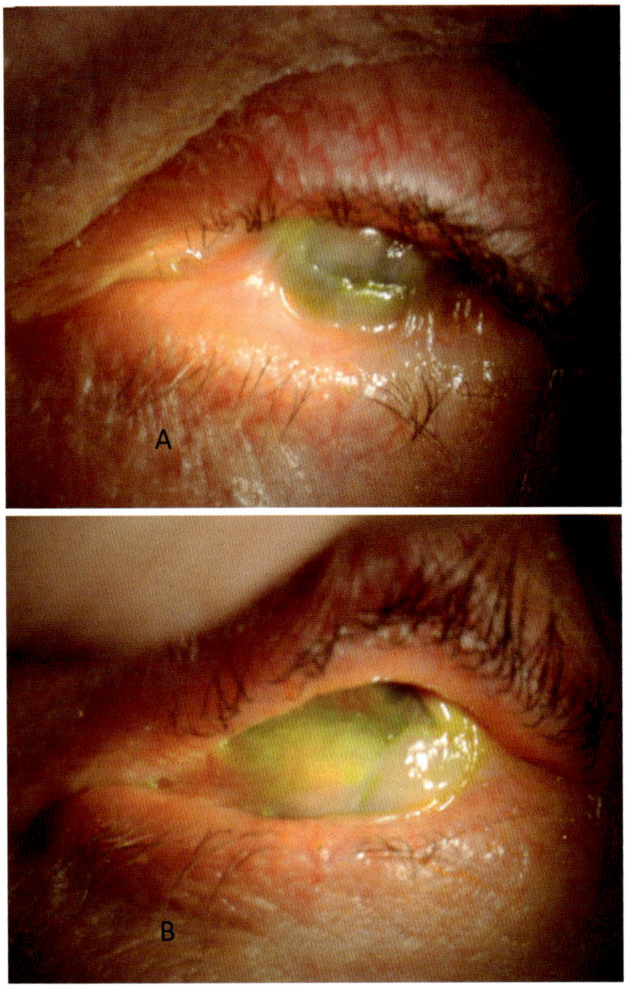

Fig. 12.2 Slit lamp photographs of the left eye of Foster stage III direct immunofluorescence microscopy-confirmed mucous membrane pemphigoid with fluorescein staining. (Photos of the same patient as in Fig. 12.1.) Note greater disease severity of the left eye. Patient has upper and lower eyelid thickening, lower eyelid symblepharon, obliteration of upper and lower fornices, severe bulbar conjunctival thickening and keratinization, minimal superior clear cornea, severe limbal stem cell deficiency, and corneal vascularization, conjunctivalization, and keratinization. Visual acuity is hand motion in the left eye. The patient is currently treated with rituximab and intravenous immunoglobulin. (**a**) Symblepharon medially and laterally. (**b**) Upper eyelid is retracted. (Image courtesy of Moran Eye Center Photography, Department of Ophthalmology, University of Utah, Salt Lake City, Utah)

Staging

Grading systems are used to stage the severity of disease and follow progression and treatment response. The four most common grading systems, Foster, Mondino and Brown, Tauber, and Rowsey, are listed in Table 12.1.

Table 12.1 Grading systems of ocular mucous membrane pemphigoid

Foster stages [13]	
I	Subconjunctival scarring and fibrosis
II	Fornix foreshortening of any degree
III	Presence of symblepharon and degree
IV	Ankyloblepharon, frozen globe
Mondino and Brown stages [14]	
I	0–25% loss of inferior fornix depth
II	25–50% loss of inferior fornix depth
III	50–75% loss of inferior fornix depth
IV	75–100% loss of inferior fornix depth
Tauber stages based on Foster stages with subdivisions within stages II and III (a–d corresponding to Mondino and Brown stages) [15]	
II	% loss of inferior fornix depth
III (n)	% loss of horizontal involvement by symblephara (number of symblephara)
Rowsey stages mm/45 (100%): total of three measurements of the distance from the inferior limbus to the posterior edge of the retracted lower eyelid (at 5, 6, and 7 o'clock) [16]	
35–45 mm	<25% of conjunctival loss
24–34 mm	25–50% of conjunctival loss
12–23 mm	50–75% of conjunctival loss
0–11 mm	>75% of conjunctival loss

Modified from Sobolewska et al. [12]

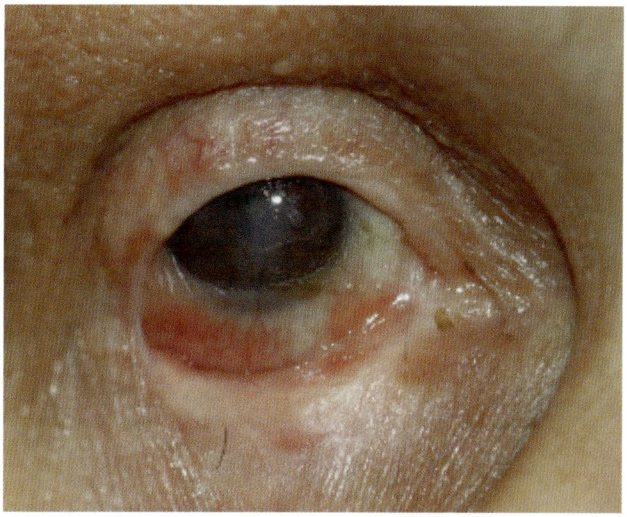

Fig. 12.3 External photograph of the right eye of Foster stage III direct immunofluorescence microscopy-confirmed ocular mucous membrane pemphigoid with upper and lower forniceal shortening, multiple trichiatic lashes of the lower eyelid, keratinization of the conjunctiva, lateral symblepharon, keratinization of inferior cornea, stromal neovascularization, and 50% corneal thinning. This patient has 3+ nuclear sclerotic cataract and light perception vision. (Image courtesy of Moran Eye Center Photography, Department of Ophthalmology, University of Utah, Salt Lake City, Utah)

Pathophysiology

MMP is characterized by IgA, IgG, and C3 complement deposition on the BMZ of the conjunctival subepithelium, igniting inflammation and cicatricial changes through a type II hypersensitivity reaction [17]. Mouse models of the passive transfer of basement membrane antibodies to newborn mice show induced skin blister formation, indicating that these antibodies are likely pathogenic in vivo [18–20]. Various epithelial basement membrane components have been identified as potential targets of MMP. These include bullous pemphigoid antigens 1 and 2, type VII collagen, laminin-5 and laminin-6, α-6 and β-4 integrin subunits, and a 120 kDa undefined epithelial antigen. A striking association between MMP and major histocompatibility class II gene DQB1*0301 has been observed. The role of these alleles is unclear in antigen presentation to T cells [21].

A putative pathophysiological cause of MMP may be "epitope spreading," where a prior inflammatory event might expose epithelial basement membrane components that were previously "hidden" from autoreactive T and B cells, leading to a secondary autoimmune phenomenon and the eventual development of MMP [22]. Chan et al. reported on ocular MMP that subsequently developed in several patients who had suffered an episode of Stevens-Johnson syndrome affecting the ocular mucosae [23]. This mechanism could also explain how true MMP is triggered after use of topical drops (see "Differential Diagnosis" section to distinguish from pseudopemphigoid).

Diagnosis

Diagnosis is made by clinical, histological, and immunohistopathological findings of conjunctival, oral, other mucosal, or skin biopsy. Conjunctival biopsy in the setting of inflammation can result in further scarring. If a skin site is involved, biopsy should be taken from there first. If a nonocular mucosal site is involved, it would be the second choice for skin biopsy. Conjunctival biopsy should be reserved for cases in which only conjunctiva is involved [6]. Biopsy of tissue adjacent to inflamed bulbar conjunctiva is submitted for direct immunofluorescent studies [17, 24]. Biopsy should not be taken from the bulla because the BMZ in this area may be destroyed. In MMP, direct immunofluorescent (DIF) staining with linear deposits of IgG and/or of C3 along the BMZ is the most common finding and generally considered sufficient for diagnosis [25–27]. Occasionally findings of an IgA band along the BMZ may be present (Figs. 12.3, 12.4, 12.5, and 12.6) [21, 28].

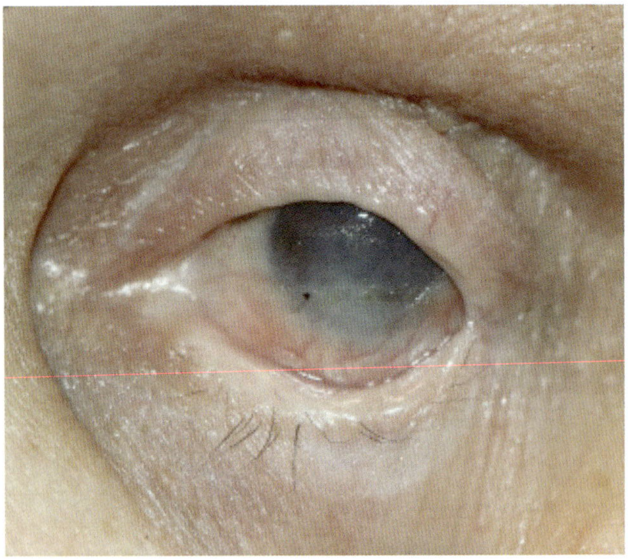

Fig. 12.4 External photographs of the left eye of the same patient as in Fig. 12.3 with Foster stage III direct immunofluorescence microscopy-confirmed ocular mucous membrane pemphigoid with near obliteration of the lower fornix, multiple trichiatic lashes of the lower eyelid, keratinization of the conjunctiva, near-complete keratinization of entire cornea, neovascularization of the inferior and superior cornea, and nasal corneal thinning. The patient has 3+ nuclear sclerotic cataract and light perception vision. The patient has had multiple eyelid procedures to treat entropion and exposure keratopathy. Due to severe limbal stem cell deficiency, corneal transplantation would likely not be successful. Treatment with oral dapsone has stabilized the condition. The next step is to consider type II keratoprosthesis. (Image courtesy of Moran Eye Center Photography, Department of Ophthalmology, University of Utah, Salt Lake City, Utah)

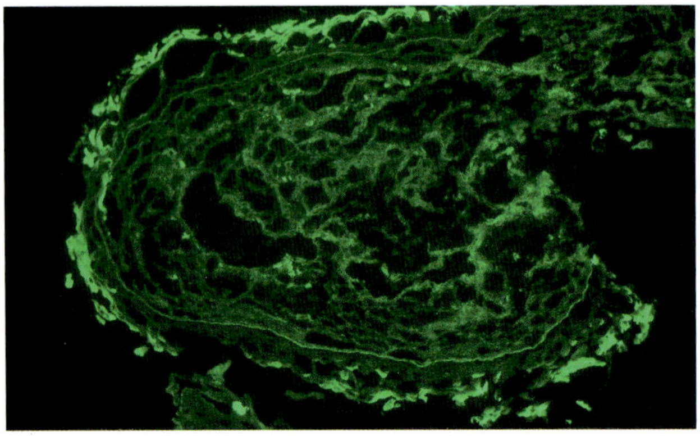

Fig. 12.5 Direct immunofluorescence microscopy image of a conjunctival mucosal specimen from a patient with mucous membrane pemphigoid - this demonstrates linear IgA basement membrane zone staining, original magnification 100×. Note positive staining of scattered subepithelial inflammatory cells (likely eosinophils and/or plasma cells), epithelial cells (likely constitutive and/or nonspecific), and expression of IgA in mucosa

A considerable proportion of patients (3–80%) with clinically diagnosed MMP have a negative DIF result regardless of site of biopsy [17, 29–31]. Labowsky et al. found, in a retrospective review of 55 patients treated for ocular MMP at a tertiary care center, that a higher proportion of patients with ocular disease alone (46.2%) had negative conjunctival biopsies compared to those with both ocular and extraocular diseases (6.9%; Fisher exact test, $P < 0.001$) [32]. *Biopsy site strongly influences the sensitivity of DIF.* Power et al. propose the routine use of an immunoperoxidase technique in immunofluorescent-negative biopsies, which in their study increased the diagnostic yields to 80% [7]. Other times, it may be beneficial to repeat biopsies in different locations (oropharynx) to maximize the yield. Mehra et al., in a retrospective review of 54 patients with suspected ocular MMP in Germany, found higher sensitivity and negative predictive value for DIF of cutaneous samples compared to conjunctival samples [33]. A negative biopsy, however, does not exclude the diagnosis of pemphigoid.

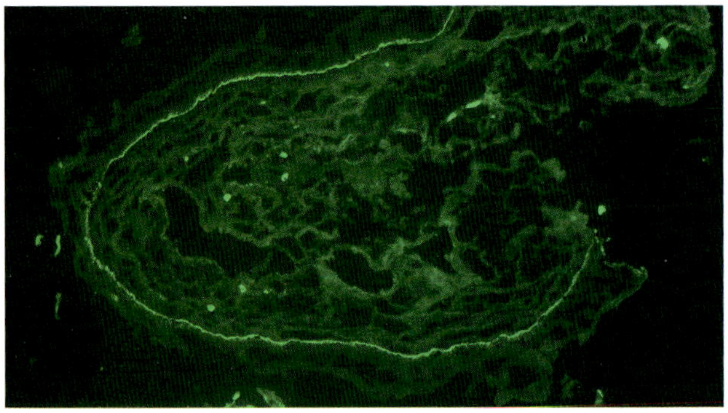

Fig. 12.6 Direct immunofluorescence microscopy image of conjunctival mucosal specimen from a patient with mucous membrane demonstrates linear IgG4 basement membrane zone staining, original magnification 100×. Note positive staining of scattered subepithelial inflammatory cells (likely eosinophils and/or plasma cells). (Images courtesy of Immunodermatology Laboratory, Department of Dermatology, University of Utah, Salt Lake City, Utah)

Patients with negative biopsies and clinical signs of MMP are still considered to have MMP, if alternative diagnoses for cicatrizing conjunctivitis have been excluded. Due to its reported high sensitivity, indirect immunofluorescence testing for circulating serum basement membrane autoantibodies to BP-180 and BP-230 to screen for pemphigoid diseases is recommended [34]. Positive serum autoantibodies, however, are not considered a criterion for diagnosis [6, 35–37].

Differential Diagnosis

The differential diagnosis of eyelid cicatrizing diseases is extensive and includes infections, medications, trauma, and other immunologic disorders (Table 12.2).

It is imperative to know that there are drugs that can induce a clinical picture similar to idiopathic MMP. Implicated medicines include pilocarpine, epinephrine, timolol, idoxuridine, echothiophate iodide, demecarium bromide, and

Table 12.2 Differential diagnosis of ocular mucous membrane pemphigoid

Infection	Herpes simplex virus
	Adenovirus
	Chlamydia trachomatis
	Corynebacterium diphtheriae
	Chronic mucocutaneous candidiasis
Mucocutaneous and immunobullous disorders	Pemphigus vulgaris
	Bullous pemphigoid
	Dermatitis herpetiformis/linear immunoglobulin A disease
	Erythema multiforme
	Stevens-Johnson syndrome
	Toxic epidermal necrolysis
	Systemic lupus erythematosus
	Chronic atopic keratoconjunctivitis
	Conjunctival lichen planus
	Ectodermal dysplasia
	Porphyria cutanea tarda
	Congenital ichthyosiform erythroderma
Neoplasia	Ocular surface neoplasia
	Sebaceous cell carcinoma
	Lymphoma
Systemic diseases	Ocular rosacea
	Sjögren syndrome
	Sarcoidosis
	Inflammatory bowel disease
	Chronic graft-versus-host disease
	Immune complex disease
Trauma	Eyelid surgeries
	Radiation injury
	Chemical injuries

Modified from Saw et al. and Dart et al. [5, 38]

latanoprost [39]. These medications can mimic, promote, or even trigger cicatricial pemphigoid. Drug-induced pseudopemphigoid is a self-limited reaction to the medication itself without any systemic features [40]. In contrast, drugs can trigger true MMP. In this case, inflammation and cicatrization continue despite stopping the medication. The cause is thought to be epitope spreading (see "Pathophysiology" section). Pseudopemphigoid is a term used to describe conditions that mimic MMP. In a retrospective review of 280 patients who presented with suspected MMP, Thorne et al. found the most frequent presumed causes of pseudopemphigoid were topical glaucoma medications (28.3%), rosacea blepharoconjunctivitis (20.0%), atopic keratoconjunctivitis (8.3%), and conjunctival lichen planus (8.3%) [30].

Drug-induced pseudopemphigoid may be caused by the toxicity of the drug itself or preservatives in solution. Benzalkonium chloride (BAK) has a disruptive effect on the tear film by exerting a detergent effect on the lipid layer and predisposes the eye to inflammation and conjunctival metaplasia. In addition, BAK has a destructive effect on mucus-secreting cells reducing the number of goblet cells, inciting inflammation of the substantia propria, and leading to subconjunctival fibrosis [41].

Treatment

According to the First International Consensus on MMP, ocular involvement is defined as "high risk" and is an indication for systemic immunomodulatory treatment [6]. Hence, therapy should be started when Foster stage II disease is diagnosed. The goal of the treatment is to control the inflammation and stop the cicatrizing process. Immunomodulatory agents are selected in a stepwise approach depending on disease severity, incidence of adverse reactions, and tolerability of side effects. Therapy should be started in conjunction with all consultants involved in the patients' care—ophthalmologist, otolaryngologist, dermatologist, and rheumatologist—to ensure all disease areas are monitored and treated. If mild inflammatory activity continues during therapy, providers should consider increased dosage of the drug, addition of systemic corticosteroid (1 mg/kg/day tapered gradually), and/or replacing the immunomodulatory therapy. Signs of clinical progression of disease are conjunctival inflammatory activity, but more importantly, conjunctival shrinkage and symblepharon formation. Inflammation may be influenced by other compounding factors such as dry eyes, trichiasis, entropion, and irritation from keratinized tissue in contact with the corneal surface. Furthermore, conjunctival shrinkage can still progress in a quiet eye [24, 42].

First-Line Therapy

Mycophenolate mofetil is considered a first-line therapy for non-vision-threatening ocular MMP. Mycophenolate mofetil is more successful in controlling inflammation than the sulfa derivatives—dapsone, sulfasalazine, and sulfapyridine—and has a lower rate of discontinuation [12]. Saw et al. found that mycophenolate had the lowest rate of side effects (15%) of all first-line immunomodulatory therapies [43]. Methotrexate is a good alternative to mycophenolate mofetil in patients with mild, non-vision-threatening disease. The main concern with methotrexate is the risk of irreversible hepatic and pulmonary fibrosis in patients receiving therapy long term [12].

Sulfa-derivative medications are also considered first line. Dapsone has more side effects (hemolytic anemia, skin rash, malaise, and gastrointestinal problems) and poorer compliance compared to sulfasalazine and sulfapyridine. Dapsone is contraindicated in patients with sulfa allergy and deficiency of erythrocytic *glucose-6-phosphate dehydrogenase.* Azathioprine has similar success rate to the sulfa derivatives but higher frequency of side effects such as gastrointestinal problems, headache, malaise, dizziness, elevated liver function tests, and myelosuppression [12, 40].

Second-Line Therapy

Cyclophosphamide is the next line option for patients who fail the above options or have more severe disease. However, cyclophosphamide also has more severe side effects. Among 44 MMP patients treated with cyclophosphamide, Thorne et al. reported infection (48.6%), pneumonia (5.8%), hematuria (45.5%), hematuria leading to temporary/permanent discontinuation of treatment (24.2%), anemia (38.8%), severe leukopenia (16.2%), and cancer including bladder cancer (13%) [44]. Patients should be monitored with complete blood counts and platelet levels.

Third-Line Therapy

Intravenous immunoglobulin therapy (*IVIg*) is employed if the above options are not effective [45, 46]. It should be considered for patients who are resistant to conventional therapy, have significant adverse effects, or have uncontrolled, rapidly progressive disease. Cycles are repeated every 2–4 weeks for months to years depending on disease severity. Adverse effects are very rare [47].

Few case reports and one study by El Darouti et al. have been published about adding biologics to cyclophosphamide or IVIg therapy in patients who do not have adequate response to any of the above treatments. Adding etanercept and infliximab results in stable or improved disease. Foster et al. reported that rituximab combined with IVIg in six patients with persistent inflammation and blindness in one eye resulted in stable disease and visual acuity [48, 49]. Patients need to be monitored for infection, anemia, pancytopenia, and malignancy among other adverse effects. High-dose steroids can be used to treat acute flare-ups at any disease stage. Steroids should be tapered as disease improves or remains stable. See Fig. 12.7 for a summary of treatment recommendations.

Therapy can last months or years before the disease is subdued. You et al. studied 34 patients (66 eyes) with biopsy-proven OCP (Ocular Cicatricial Pemphigoid) who were able to stay in long-term remission off IMT after finishing a 2-year IMT regimen without active disease. Patients had mean sustained remission time of 36 months. Patients were in various Foster stages at the time treatment was started: stage I 22.7%, stage II 28.8%, stage III 40.9%, and stage IV 7.6%. During a mean follow-up time of 63.4 months, two patients had mild flare-up over 2 years after stopping therapy. One patient had reactivation of disease 5 years after stopping therapy [50].

Because of the systemic toxicity of these medications, several papers have been presented on subconjunctival mitomycin-C for the treatment of cicatricial pemphigoid. Mitomycin-C is an alkylating agent that acts by inhibiting DNA synthesis. In these studies, it appears to inhibit fibroblast proliferation at the level of the episclera. In a limited case series by Donnenfeld et al., eight of nine patients showed quiescence of their MMP after mitomycin-C use. Patients were given a 0.25 mL injection of 0.2 mg/mL of mitomycin-C to both the inferior and superior cul-de-sacs for a total dose of 0.5 mL [51]. Patients were followed for a mean of 23.5 months. Secchi et al. described a method of intraoperative symblepharon surgical lysis and treatment with mitomycin-C. Conjunctival adhesions were surgically lysed, and then sponges soaked in 0.4 mg/mL of mitomycin-C were applied to the dissected conjunctiva for 3–5 minutes.

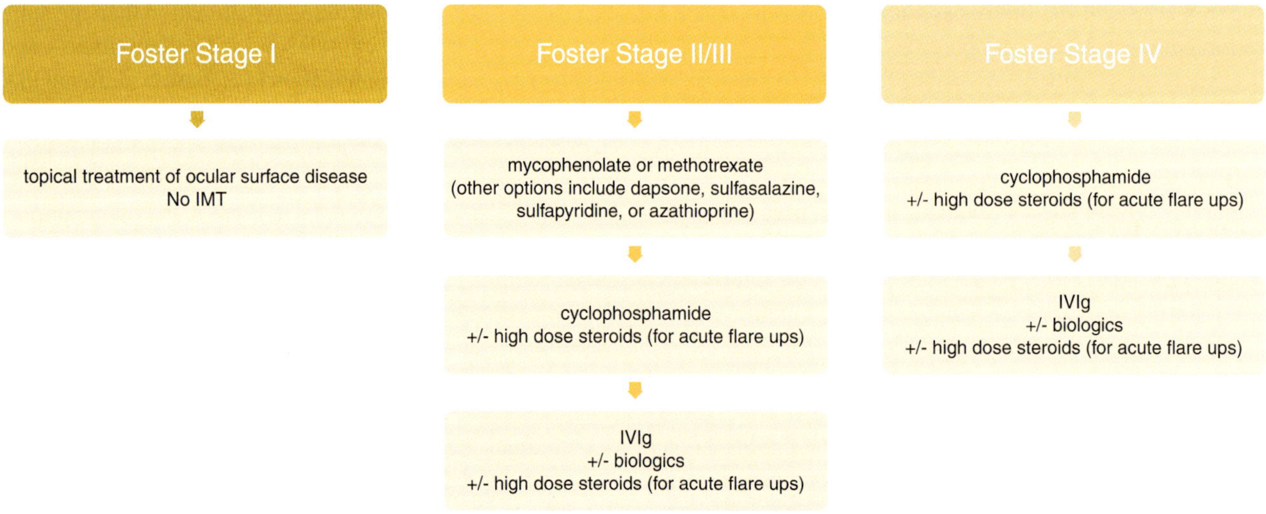

Fig. 12.7 Summary of the stepwise treatment regimens by stage of MMP. IMT, immunomodulatory therapy. IVIg, intravenous immunoglobulin. (Modified from Saw et al. and Sobolewska et al. [12, 43])

This method showed promise in five patients during the follow-up period of 12–19 months. Unfortunately, mitomycin-C is also associated with significant complications, including infectious keratitis, corneal melting, endophthalmitis, choroidal effusion, and hypotony [52].

Systemic treatment must be accompanied by local aggressive lubrication, punctal occlusion, tarsorrhaphy, soft contact lenses, and gas-permeable lenses as needed. Trichiasis can be managed with cryoablation, argon laser thermoablation, electrolysis, or excision of lash follicle complexes. Care should be taken to avoid scarring.

Because OCP is a systemic disease, topical medications are used only as a temporary measure to relieve symptoms before systemic therapy has time to take effect [13]. Topical corticosteroids, calcineurin inhibitors, cyclosporine A, and tacrolimus have been used to treat ocular MMP.

Surgical Therapies

Surgical intervention during active disease can be problematic and complicated by increased scarring. It is imperative that any surgical intervention in these patients be preceded by complete control of the disease, as the failure rate may be quite high [53]. Heiligenhaus et al. suggest at least a 6-week period of disease control prior to surgical intervention. Manipulation of the conjunctival surface during the active course of the disease can promote progression of cicatrization. Patients should continue their immunosuppressive therapy perioperatively, and a perioperative oral steroid taper can be considered to help reduce risk of disease activation [53].

Amniotic membrane transplantation (AMT) can be used to prevent symblepharon formation and treat ocular surface disease. As the membrane is absorbed, effectiveness deteriorates over months. Barabino et al. reported nine eyes of nine patients treated with AMT had conjunctival surfaces free from symblepharon for the first 16 weeks [54]. At the week 28 examination, a small area of symblepharon was present in four eyes (44.4%). The depth of the fornix was significantly (P <0.0001, analysis of variance) improved at weeks 4, 16, and 28.

Oral mucosal grafts, sutured to cover the keratinized eyelid margin, can add height to the tarsus to treat lagophthalmos and treat blink-related microtrauma of the cornea caused by keratinization of the eyelid margin. Fu et al. found among 39 eyelids (22 eyes of 19 patients) lagophthalmos persisted in 12 (54.5%) eyes, was completely corrected in 9 eyes, and was much improved in the remaining 3 eyes [55]. During a mean follow-up of 16.2 months, reports of foreign body sensation, photophobia, pain, burning, tearing, and discharge were relieved significantly in 17 of 22 eyes (77.3%). Corneal epithelial defects and superficial punctate keratopathy were healed rapidly or improved in 14 eyes (63.6%).

The most common eyelid procedures performed are entropion repair and symblepharon repair. For mild to moderate entropion without lagophthalmos, another option is gray line eyelid splitting procedure and anterior lamellar excision or repositioning. Fornix reconstruction can be performed with grafts from labial or buccal mucous membranes. Posterior lamellae can be reconstructed with hard palate or nasal mucosal grafts. Graft sites should be carefully examined to ensure they do not have pemphigoid changes. Gibbons et al. report successful surgical outcomes without recurrence in entropion repair of 11 eyes of 7 patients followed for a mean of 20.8 months [56]. Tarsotomies were performed on upper eyelids, and the Weis procedure was performed on the lower eyelids. Elder et al. reported entropion repair of 16 eyelids of 11 patients through gray line splitting procedure and anterior lamellar repositioning, which resulted in 72% anatomic success rate at 4 years [57]. Rosser and Collins reported on lower eyelid retractor plication of seven eyelids with lower eyelid entropion. Their technique avoided surgery on the conjunctiva. The patients had successful outcomes without acute exacerbation of disease [58]. Nonsurgical management of entropion and trichiasis is possible with repeat manual epilation and contact lens use.

Treatment of Corneal and Surface Disease

Corneal scarring can result in irregular corneal astigmatism that may require rigid gas-permeable contact lenses to correct vision. Scleral lenses can be considered for patients who have adequate forniceal depth. Patients must be monitored for worsening corneal neovascularization while using these contact lenses [5].

Corneal complications can result in the need for keratoplasty and keratoprosthesis. Tugan-Tutkal et al. studied the efficacy of penetrating keratoplasty in eyes with end-stage cicatrizing conjunctival diseases including MMP, Stevens-Johnson syndrome, and toxic epidermal necrolysis [59]. Visual improvement was limited. After a mean follow-up period of 4.6 years, eight eyes (50%) had clear grafts, and three eyes (18.7%) had 20/200 or better visual acuity. Causes of graft failure included epithelial defects, ulceration, perforation, and graft rejection. Destruction of limbal stem cells is an important cause of keratoplasty failure.

Stem cell transplantation does not have good long-term efficacy in MMP patients. Tsubota et al. reported successful visual improvement at 5 months in all nine eyes of nine patients with MMP treated with limbal allografts and AMT in conjunction with systemic dapsone and cyclosporine [60]. Penetrating keratoplasty was also performed in five of nine eyes. However, these improvements were not sustained with prolonged follow-up.

Summary

MMP is an immune inflammatory disorder that may result in major morbidity due to conjunctival scarring and obliterative surface changes. Diagnosis is made by clinical presentation and biopsy with direct immunofluorescence assay. Patients can experience significant ocular surface and eyelid disease that can result in frozen globe and blindness. Immunosuppressive treatment and stabilization of disease must precede surgical repair to avoid worsening the disease.

References

1. Michel B, Thomas CI, Levine M, Waisman M, Bean SF. Cicatricial pemphigoid and its relationship to ocular pemphigus and essential shrinkage of the conjunctiva. Ann Ophthalmol. 1975;7(1):11–20.
2. Queisi MM, Zein M, Lamba N, Meese H, Foster CS. Update on ocular cicatricial pemphigoid and emerging treatments. Surv Ophthalmol. 2016;61(3):314–7.
3. Rauz S, Maddison PG, Dart JKG. Evaluation of mucous membrane pemphigoid with ocular involvement in young patients. Ophthalmology. 2005;112(7):1268–74.
4. Xu H-H, Werth VP, Parisi E, Sollecito TP. Mucous membrane pemphigoid. Dent Clin N Am. 2013;57(4):611–30.
5. Saw VPJ, Dart JKG. Ocular mucous membrane pemphigoid: diagnosis and management strategies. Ocul Surf. 2008;6(3):128–42.
6. Chan LS, Ahmed AR, Anhalt GJ, Bernauer W, Cooper KD, Elder MJ, et al. The first international consensus on mucous membrane pemphigoid: definition, diagnostic criteria, pathogenic factors, medical treatment, and prognostic indicators. Arch Dermatol. 2002;138(3):370–9.
7. Buhac J, Bhol K, Padilla T, Foster CS, Ahmed AR. Coexistence of pemphigus vulgaris and ocular cicatricial pemphigoid. J Am Acad Dermatol. 1996;34(5 Pt 2):884–6.
8. Frith PA, Venning VA, Wojnarowska F, Millard PR, Bron AJ. Conjunctival involvement in cicatricial and bullous pemphigoid: a clinical and immunopathological study. Br J Ophthalmol. 1989;73(1):52–6.
9. Neumann R, Tauber J, Foster CS. Remission and recurrence after withdrawal of therapy for ocular cicatricial pemphigoid. Ophthalmology. 1991;98(6):858–62.
10. Hardy KM, Perry HO, Pingree GC, Kirby TJ. Benign mucous membrane pemphigoid. Arch Dermatol. 1971;104(5):467–75.
11. Satchi K, McNab AA. Conjunctival cicatrizing disease presenting with lacrimal obstruction. Orbit. 2016;35(6):321–3.
12. Sobolewska B, Deuter C, Zierhut M. Current medical treatment of ocular mucous membrane pemphigoid. Ocul Surf. 2013;11(4):259–66.
13. Foster CS. Cicatricial pemphigoid. Trans Am Ophthalmol Soc. 1986;84:527–663.
14. Mondino BJ, Brown SI. Ocular cicatricial pemphigoid. Ophthalmology. 1981;88(2):95–100.
15. Tauber J, Jabbur N, Foster CS. Improved detection of disease progression in ocular cicatricial pemphigoid. Cornea. 1992;11(5):446–51.
16. Rowsey JJ, Macias-Rodriguez Y, Cukrowski C. A new method for measuring progression in patients with ocular cicatricial pemphigoid. Arch Ophthalmol (Chicago, Ill 1960). 2004;122(2):179–84.
17. Power WJ, Neves RA, Rodriguez A, Dutt JE, Foster CS. Increasing the diagnostic yield of conjunctival biopsy in patients with suspected ocular cicatricial pemphigoid. Ophthalmology. 1995;102(8):1158–63.
18. Liu Z, Giudice GJ, Swartz SJ, Fairley JA, Till GO, Troy JL, et al. The role of complement in experimental bullous pemphigoid. J Clin Invest. 1995;95(4):1539–44.
19. Liu Z, Diaz LA, Troy JL, Taylor AF, Emery DJ, Fairley JA, et al. A passive transfer model of the organ-specific autoimmune disease, bullous pemphigoid, using antibodies generated against the hemidesmosomal antigen, BP180. J Clin Invest. 1993;92(5):2480–8.
20. Lazarova Z, Yee C, Darling T, Briggaman RA, Yancey KB. Passive transfer of anti-laminin 5 antibodies induces subepidermal blisters in neonatal mice. J Clin Invest. 1996;98(7):1509–18.
21. Chan LS. Ocular and oral mucous membrane pemphigoid (cicatricial pemphigoid). Clin Dermatol. 2012;30(1):34–7.
22. Chan LS, Vanderlugt CJ, Hashimoto T, Nishikawa T, Zone JJ, Black MM, et al. Epitope spreading: lessons from autoimmune skin diseases. J Invest Dermatol. 1998;110(2):103–9.
23. Chan LS, Soong HK, Foster CS, Hammerberg C, Cooper KD. Ocular cicatricial pemphigoid occurring as a sequela of Stevens-Johnson syndrome. JAMA. 1991;266(11):1543–6.
24. Foster CS, Wilson LA, Ekins MB. Immunosuppressive therapy for progressive ocular cicatricial pemphigoid. Ophthalmology. 1982;89(4):340–53.
25. Mutasim DF, Adams BB. Immunofluorescence in dermatology. J Am Acad Dermatol. 2001;45(6):803–24.
26. Morrison LH. Direct immunofluorescence microscopy in the diagnosis of autoimmune bullous dermatoses. Clin Dermatol. 2001;19(5):607–13.
27. Leonard JN, Hobday CM, Haffenden GP, Griffiths CE, Powles AV, Wright P, et al. Immunofluorescent studies in ocular cicatricial pemphigoid. Br J Dermatol. 1988;118(2):209–17.
28. Bruch-Gerharz D, Hertl M, Ruzicka T. Mucous membrane pemphigoid: clinical aspects, immunopathological features and therapy. Eur J Dermatol. 2007;17(3):191–200.
29. Kirzhner M, Jakobiec FA. Ocular cicatricial pemphigoid: a review of clinical features, immunopathology, differential diagnosis, and current management. Semin Ophthalmol. 2011;26(4–5):270–7.
30. Thorne JE, Anhalt GJ, Jabs DA. Mucous membrane pemphigoid and pseudopemphigoid. Ophthalmology 2004;111(1):45–52.
31. Goldich Y, Ziai S, Artornsombudh P, Avni-Zauberman N, Elbaz U, Rootman DS, et al. Characteristics of patients with ocular cicatricial pemphigoid referred to major tertiary hospital. Can J Ophthalmol. 2015;50(2):137–42.
32. Labowsky MT, Stinnett SS, Liss J, Daluvoy M, Hall RP, Shieh C. Clinical implications of direct immunofluorescence findings in patients with ocular mucous membrane pemphigoid. Am J Ophthalmol. 2017;183:48–55.
33. Mehra T, Guenova E, Dechent F, Würth F, Zierhut M, Röcken M, et al. Diagnostic relevance of direct immunofluorescence in ocular mucous membrane pemphigoid. J Dtsch Dermatol Ges. 2015;13(12):1268–74.
34. Thoma-Uszynski S, Uter W, Schwietzke S, Hofmann SC, Hunziker T, Bernard P, et al. BP230- and BP180-specific auto-antibodies in bullous pemphigoid. J Invest Dermatol. 2004;122(6):1413–22.
35. Setterfield J, Shirlaw PJ, Kerr-Muir M, Neill S, Bhogal BS, Morgan P, et al. Mucous membrane pemphigoid: a dual circulating antibody response with IgG and IgA signifies a more severe and persistent disease. Br J Dermatol. 1998;138(4):602–10.
36. Setterfield J, Shirlaw PJ, Bhogal BS, Tilling K, Challacombe SJ, Black MM. Cicatricial pemphigoid: serial titres of circulating IgG and IgA antibasement membrane antibodies correlate with disease activity. Br J Dermatol. 1999;140(4):645–50.
37. Leiferman K, Tebo A. Pemphigoid [Internet]. [cited 2019 Feb 13]. Available from: https://arupconsult.com/content/pemphigoid.

38. Dart JK. The 2016 Bowman Lecture Conjunctival curses: scarring conjunctivitis 30 years on. Eye (Lond). 2017;31(2):301–32.
39. Fiore PM, Jacobs IH, Goldberg DB. Drug-induced pemphigoid. A spectrum of diseases. Arch Ophthalmol (Chicago, Ill 1960). 1987;105(12):1660–3.
40. Huang LC. Pseudopemphigoid as caused by topical drugs and pemphigus disease. World J Ophthalmol. 2015;5(1):1.
41. Petr I. Drops show long term effects [Internet]. [cited 2010 Jan 15]. Available from www.Ophthalmologytimes.com.
42. Rosenthal P, Cotter JM. Surgical reconstruction of the ocular surface in advanced ocular cicatricial pemphigoid and Stevens-Johnson syndrome. Am J Ophthalmol. 1996;122(6):914–5.
43. Saw VPJ, Dart JKG, Rauz S, Ramsay A, Bunce C, Xing W, et al. Immunosuppressive therapy for ocular mucous membrane pemphigoid. Ophthalmology. 2008;115(2):253–261.e1.
44. Thorne JE, Woreta FA, Jabs DA, Anhalt GJ. Treatment of ocular mucous membrane pemphigoid with immunosuppressive drug therapy. Ophthalmology. 2008;115(12):2146–2152.e1.
45. Houssiau FA, Vasconcelos C, D'Cruz D, Sebastiani GD, de Ramon GE, Danieli MG, et al. The 10-year follow-up data of the Euro-Lupus Nephritis Trial comparing low-dose and high-dose intravenous cyclophosphamide. Ann Rheum Dis. 2010;69(1):61–4.
46. Houssiau FA, Vasconcelos C, D'Cruz D, Sebastiani GD, Garrido Ed Ede R, Danieli MG, et al. Immunosuppressive therapy in lupus nephritis: The Euro-Lupus Nephritis Trial, a randomized trial of low-dose versus high-dose intravenous cyclophosphamide. Arthritis Rheum. 2002;46(8):2121–31.
47. Ahmed AR, Dahl MV. Consensus statement on the use of intravenous immunoglobulin therapy in the treatment of autoimmune mucocutaneous blistering diseases. Arch Dermatol. 2003;139(8):1051–9.
48. You C, Lamba N, Lasave AF, Ma L, Diaz MH, Foster CS. Rituximab in the treatment of ocular cicatricial pemphigoid: a retrospective cohort study. Graefes Arch Clin Exp Ophthalmol. 2017;255(6):1221–8.
49. Foster CS, Chang PY, Ahmed AR. Combination of rituximab and intravenous immunoglobulin for recalcitrant ocular cicatricial pemphigoid: a preliminary report. Ophthalmology. 2010;117(5):861–9.
50. You C, Ma L, Anesi SD, Stephen FC. Long-term remission of ocular cicatricial pemphigoid off immunomodulatory therapy. Eur J Ophthalmol. 2018;28(2):157–62.
51. Donnenfeld ED, Perry HD, Wallerstein A, Caronia RM, Kanellopoulos AJ, Sforza PD, et al. Subconjunctival mitomycin C for the treatment of ocular cicatricial pemphigoid. Ophthalmology. 1999;106(1):72–8; discussion 79
52. Secchi AG, Tognon MS. Intraoperative mitomycin C in the treatment of cicatricial obliterations of conjunctival fornices. Am J Ophthalmol. 1996;122(5):728–30.
53. Heiligenhaus A, Shore JW, Rubin PA, Foster CS. Long-term results of mucous membrane grafting in ocular cicatricial pemphigoid. Implications for patient selection and surgical considerations. Ophthalmology. 1993;100(9):1283–8.
54. Barabino S, Rolando M, Bentivoglio G, Mingari C, Zanardi S, Bellomo R, et al. Role of amniotic membrane transplantation for conjunctival reconstruction in ocular-cicatricial pemphigoid. Ophthalmology. 2003;110(3):474–80.
55. Fu Y, Liu J, Tseng SCG. Oral mucosal graft to correct lid margin pathologic features in cicatricial ocular surface diseases. Am J Ophthalmol. 2011;152(4):600–608.e1.
56. Gibbons A, Johnson TE, Wester ST, Gonzalez AE, Farias CC, Betancurt C, et al. Management of patients with confirmed and presumed mucous membrane pemphigoid undergoing entropion repair. Am J Ophthalmol. 2015;159(5):846–52.e2.
57. Elder MJ, Collin R. Anterior lamellar repositioning and grey line split for upper lid entropion in ocular cicatricial pemphigoid. Eye (Lond). 1996;10(Pt 4)(4):439–42.
58. Rosser PM, Collin JR. Retractor plication for lower lid entropion in ocular cicatricial pemphigoid. Aust N Z J Ophthalmol. 1993;21(2):93–7.
59. Tugal-Tutkun I, Akova YA, Foster CS. Penetrating keratoplasty in cicatrizing conjunctival diseases. Ophthalmology. 1995;102(4):576–85.
60. Tsubota K, Satake Y, Ohyama M, Toda I, Takano Y, Ono M, et al. Surgical reconstruction of the ocular surface in advanced ocular cicatricial pemphigoid and Stevens-Johnson syndrome. Am J Ophthalmol. 1996;122(1):38–52.

Part IV

Blepharoptosis

Geoffrey J. Gladstone

Ptosis in Neurologic Disease

13

Ann P. Murchison, Jurij R. Bilyk, and Peter J. Savino

Introduction

"Ptosis," derived from the Greek word "fall," is the abnormal lowering or prolapse of a structure; blepharoptosis refers to a lowering of the upper eyelid [1]. The normal position of the upper eyelid is dependent on the gender and ethnicity of each individual [2, 3]. The true frequency of ptosis and its particular subtypes is not known. A recent review of 251 patients across all ages in a tertiary care center reported aponeurotic ptosis as the most frequent subtype (60%), followed by a relatively similar distribution of traumatic, congenital, and mechanical (9–11%). Neurogenic etiologies made up a minority of cases (6%), with 38% due to oculomotor palsy, 29% from myasthenia gravis, and 7% from Horner syndrome [4].

The surgical techniques and nuances of blepharoptosis correction are covered elsewhere in this text. The purpose of this chapter is to familiarize the clinician with the neurogenic causes of ptosis. Of the myriad categories, neurogenic ptosis is the most worrisome to the oculoplastic surgeon because of potential systemic morbidity and mortality. The clinician must be aware of this possibility and follow a standard algorithm in the evaluation of *all* ptosis patients to assure that neurologic disease is not overlooked.

A. P. Murchison (✉)
Attending Surgeon, Oculoplastic and Orbital Surgery Service and Director, Eye Emergency Department, Wills Eye Hospital and Thomas Jefferson University Hospital, Philadelphia, PA, USA
e-mail: amuchison@willseye.org

J. R. Bilyk
Attending Surgeon and Professor of Ophthalmology, Oculoplastic and Orbital Surgery Service, Wills Eye Hospital and Thomas Jefferson University Hospital, Philadelphia, PA, USA

P. J. Savino
Clinical Professor of Ophthalmology, Viterbi Famile Department of Ophthalmology, Shiley Eye Institute, University of Califormia San Diego, La Jolla, CA, USA

Examination Pearls

A patient with ptosis most commonly presents complaining of heaviness of the eyelids, the appearance of droopy lids, or difficulty with a visual activity, such as in driving [5, 6]. Other information that should be noted and may not be volunteered by the patient includes headache, variation in the eyelid position during the day, vision changes, timing of onset, duration, and history of previous trauma or surgery. In most cases, "neurologic ptosis" presents with associated findings and symptoms. However, if these factors are not actively sought out and documented, the true nature of the droopy lid may be missed. A complete history is important and should always include a detailed review of systems. As an example, a patient with bilateral eyelid droop may not bother to mention to an ophthalmologist that he/she has had a gastrointestinal work-up for dysphagia and has had recent difficulty in climbing stairs, but these could be important clues to the presence of myasthenia gravis.

Specific factors to explore include the presence of diplopia, variability of ptosis throughout the day or from day to day, acuity of onset, and systemic symptoms as noted throughout this chapter. Of note, a complaint of worsening of ptosis in the evening is not a helpful symptom; essentially all ptosis, regardless of etiology, worsens toward the end of the day as the patient becomes tired of using the frontalis muscle to raise the eyelid secondarily (Fig. 13.1).

In addition to a detailed history with targeted questions, examination must be complete and clearly documented in all patients presenting with ptosis. A simple tetrad of clinical documentation is essential and represents a basic tenet of neuro-ophthalmology: always document eyelid position, pupillary examination, extraocular motility, and globe position in detail, especially if one of the four is abnormal. Thus, in any patient presenting with ptosis, it is critical to carefully check *and* document size and reactivity of pupils and any diplopia or external ophthalmoplegia, along with any globe dystopia (e.g., enophthalmos, hyperglobus, etc.). It is safest to be

J. J. Servat et al. (eds.), *Smith and Nesi's Ophthalmic Plastic and Reconstructive Surgery*,
https://doi.org/10.1007/978-3-030-41720-8_13

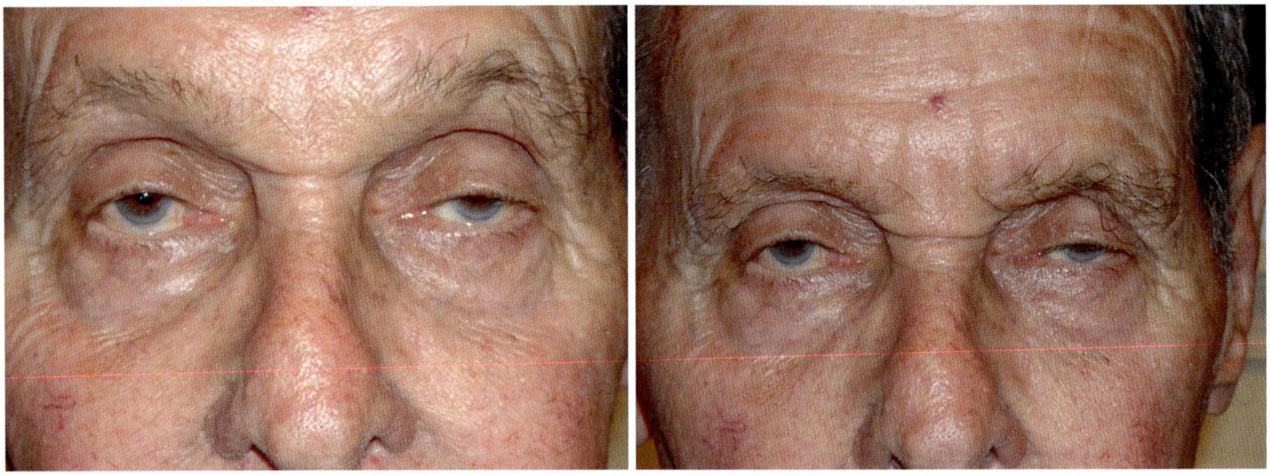

Fig. 13.1 Sustained frontalis use in ptosis. On the left, note the recruitment of the frontalis muscles in an effort to clear the visual axes. Right, with frontalis relaxation, both visual axes are effectively blocked. Patients with ptosis often complain of worsening eyelid droop at the end of the day secondary to frontalis fatigue

specific about pupillary, extraocular motility (EOM), and orbital examinations. In other words, it is much better to document the pupils as "equal, briskly reactive, without afferent pupillarydefect (APD)" than to simply state "pupils normal." Although this point seems somewhat pedestrian, the mantra of "ptosis, pupils, EOMs and globe position – if one is abnormal check the other three" cannot be overemphasized.

The concept of physiologic anisocoria must also be clearly understood by the oculoplastic surgeon because it occurs so commonly in the general population. Depending on the measureable amount of pupillary disparity, physiologic anisocoria is present in up to 21% of the general population and increases with age [7, 8]. It is obvious that, because of the ubiquity of levator dehiscence and physiologic anisocoria, the majority of patients with ptosis and unequal pupils will simply have two benign conditions. However, a minority will have real neurologic disease.

By definition, in physiologic anisocoria, the amount of pupillary disparity remains constant in light and dark conditions. This finding, when present, should be documented in any patient presenting with unilateral ptosis. Any patient presenting with ptosis whose anisocoria cannot be clearly documented as physiologic needs additional investigation.

Pseudoptosis

Pseudoptosis is an apparent blepharoptosis without true decreased margin-to-reflex distance (MRD) or a ptosis secondary to underlying globe malposition. As mentioned elsewhere, the margin-to-reflex distance is defined as the distance from the corneal light reflex to the upper eyelid margin (not to overhanging skin) measured in primary gaze. Multiple causes for pseudoptosis exist and are outlined below. The conditions should be differentiated from true ptosis to guide patient care and the approach to possible surgical correction. Given the spectrum of pathology that can present as pseudoptosis, it is difficult to determine the true prevalence. Within the broad unilateral pseudoptosis category and excluding dermatiochalasis, contralateral upper lid retraction is thought to be the most frequent cause [6].

Dermatochalasis

Dermatochalasis may exist with ptosis or be mistaken for ptosis. The eyelid skin should be gently lifted off the pretarsal eyelid to reveal the eyelid margin and to allow correct measurement of the MRD. This allows the differentiation of true ptosis from pseudoptosis due to dermatochalasis (Fig. 13.2).

Contralateral Lid Retraction

Contralateral upper eyelid retraction may be the most common cause of *unilateral* pseudoptosis (Fig. 13.3). By far the leading etiology of unilateral eyelid retraction is thyroid eye disease (TED), which is found in up to 90% of patients with thyroid dysfunction at some point during their clinical course [9]. A classification of non-TED etiologies of unilateral eyelid retraction into neurogenic, myogenic, and mechanical has been proposed [10]. If thyroid disease is ruled out, the differential diagnosis is quite diverse and beyond the scope of this chapter [11]. That said, it is important to note that patients with lid retraction and a euthyroid state may still go on to develop thyroid function abnormalities and progressive TED if monitored carefully over the ensuing 48 months, with over 80% developing thyroid dysfunction within 12 months [12].

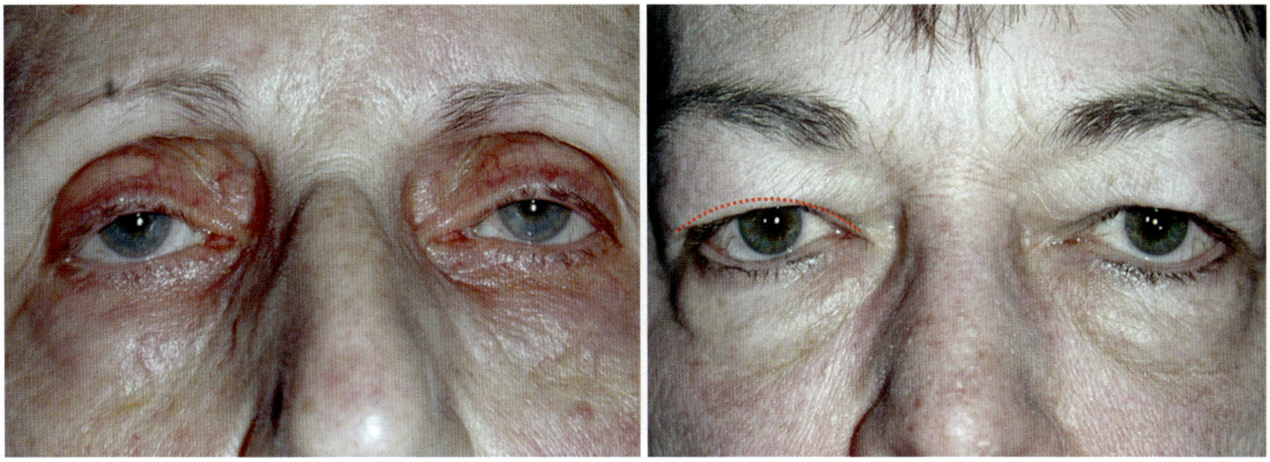

Fig. 13.2 True ptosis versus pseudoptosis. On the left, the patient's MRDs are clearly decreased, with high lid creases and deep superior sulci consistent with levator dehiscence. On the right, pseudoptosis from dermatochalasis is evident. The true eyelid margin position (dotted line) is masked by overhanging skin

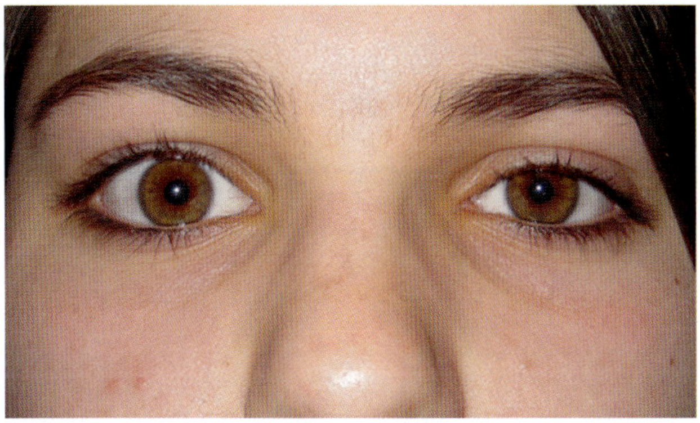

Fig. 13.3 Contralateral eyelid retraction. A 14-year-old female referred for correction of left upper lid ptosis. Note the superior scleral show and lid retraction on the right side. Subsequent serologies revealed a markedly elevated thyroid-stimulating immunoglobulin level, with eventual development of hyperthyroidism

Both levator muscles are supplied by the superior division of the oculomotor nerve and are uniquely subserved by one midline subnucleus located on the superior surface of the oculomotor nuclei. On occasion, unilateral ptosis can result in contralateral lid retraction due to Hering's law (Fig. 13.4). This typically requires occlusion or near occlusion of one visual axis by the ptotic lid and may be seen more frequently if the contralateral eye has poorer vision.

Enophthalmos

Enophthalmos, or the relative posterior displacement of the globe in relation to the orbital rim, is not always clinically evident. An initial misdiagnosis of enophthalmos as ptosis is not uncommon as most cases are associated with some degree of ptosis secondary to abnormal globe position and a deep superior sulcus [13, 14].

Three mechanisms can be used to categorize enophthalmos: structural abnormality, fat atrophy, and traction [14]. Structural abnormalities can result in an increase in bony orbital volume. The most common cause is trauma, though silent sinus syndrome (maxillary sinus atelectasis) and congenital abnormalities can also lead to enophthalmos and secondary ptosis or pseudoptosis. Fat atrophy leads to a reduction in orbital content volume and thus a relatively larger orbit. This is most common with age-related fat atrophy but can be the result of lipodystrophy (e.g., from topical prostaglandin analogs used in glaucoma), traumatic contusion injury, or other orbital pathologies. Interestingly, weight loss does not lead to a decrease in orbital fat [15]. Posterior traction, due to fibrosis within the orbit, can lead to enophthalmos and is generally associated with extraocular motility problems. The majority of enophthalmos is secondary to trauma and orbital floor fracture (Fig. 13.5).

Though much less common, non-traumatic causes of enophthalmos resulting in ptosis or pseudoptosis must also be considered due to the potential for an underlying systemic process and/or morbidity [16]. There are two additional etiologies that are important for the clinician to remember. First, metastatic scirrhous breast carcinoma, which typically also presents with restrictive external ophthalmoplegia, may present as a progressive ptosis and enophthalmos over several months' duration, with or without a previous history of breast carcinoma (Fig. 13.6) [17, 18]. Diagnosis may be difficult because orbital imaging (CT or MRI) may reveal a paucity of findings, including an increased reticular pattern to the intraconal orbital fat (Fig. 13.6). Ptosis and enophthalmos secondary to maxillary sinus atelectasis, the so-called silent sinus syndrome, present in a similar fashion, but with

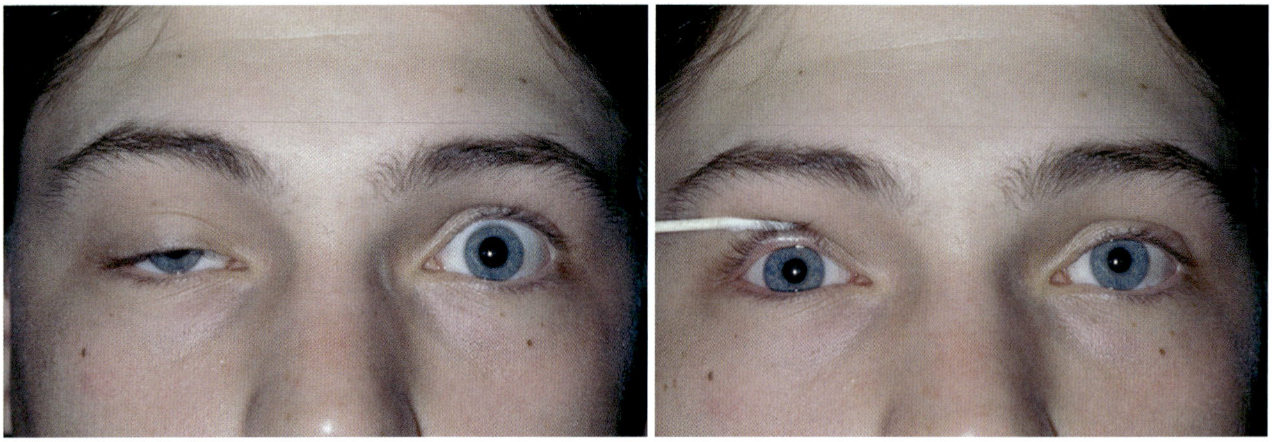

Fig. 13.4 Ptosis with secondary contralateral lid retraction. A patient with left monofixation syndrome and right upper lid ptosis. Left, there is left upper lid retraction as the patient tries to clear the right visual axis. Right, with elevation of the right upper lid, the left upper lid position normalizes

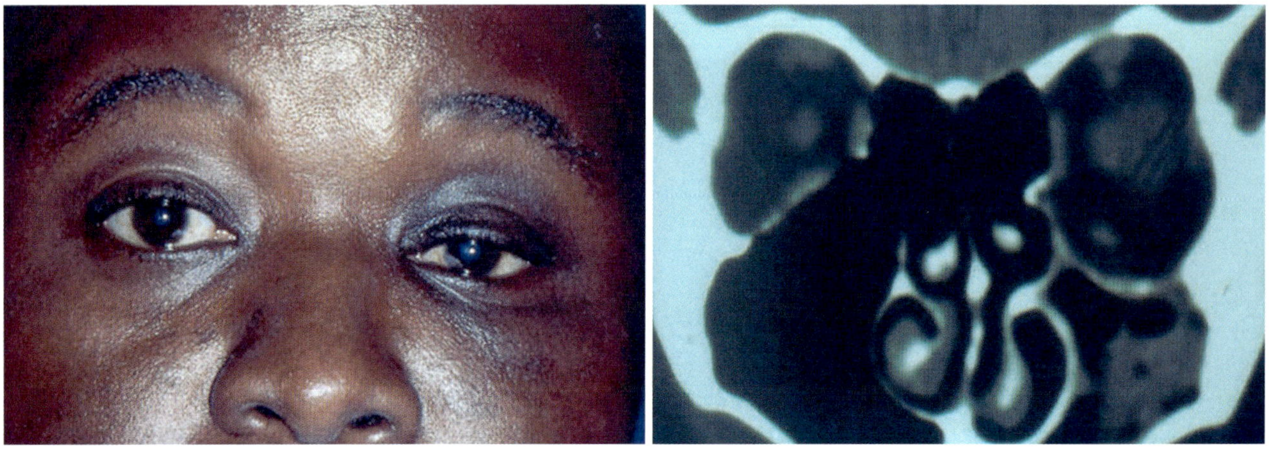

Fig. 13.5 Ptosis secondary to posttraumatic enophthalmos. The left upper lid is ptotic secondary to enophthalmos (left) from a large old orbital floor fracture seen on CT (right). Note that left hypoglobus is also present

a notable lack of significant diplopia or external ophthalmoplegia (Fig. 13.7) [19]. Many patients will have either a minimal or no history of significant paranasal sinus disease. CT will typically reveal complete opacification of the affected maxillary sinus with an inward bowing of all of the sinus walls, secondarily expanding the orbital cavity (Fig. 13.7).

Globe Asymmetry

Decreased orbital volume, from decreased volume of the globe or the orbital fat, can lead to pseudoptosis. Unilateral myopia may result in asymmetry of eyelid position, with a perceived contralateral lid droop; pseudoptosis is more common with conditions such as microphthalmia or phthisis bulbi.

Ocular Misalignment

A patient with vertical strabismus may have a component of pseudoptosis, as the lid will follow the hypotropic eye. On occasion, a patient with hypertropia or hyperglobus will also present with pseudoptosis. Evaluating each eye independently in the primary position through cross-cover testing should unmask this pseudoptosis secondary to strabismus [20]. Hyperglobus may be more difficult to assess and requires clinical comparison to the contralateral eye (Fig. 13.8). Relative globe position is an important concept to remember when evaluating any ptotic lid. On occasion, a localized process in the superior orbit may result in ptosis and hypoglobus without axial proptosis (Fig. 13.9). In older individuals, ocular adnexal lymphoproliferative disease (including lymphoma) molding to the superior orbit or cul-de-sac may

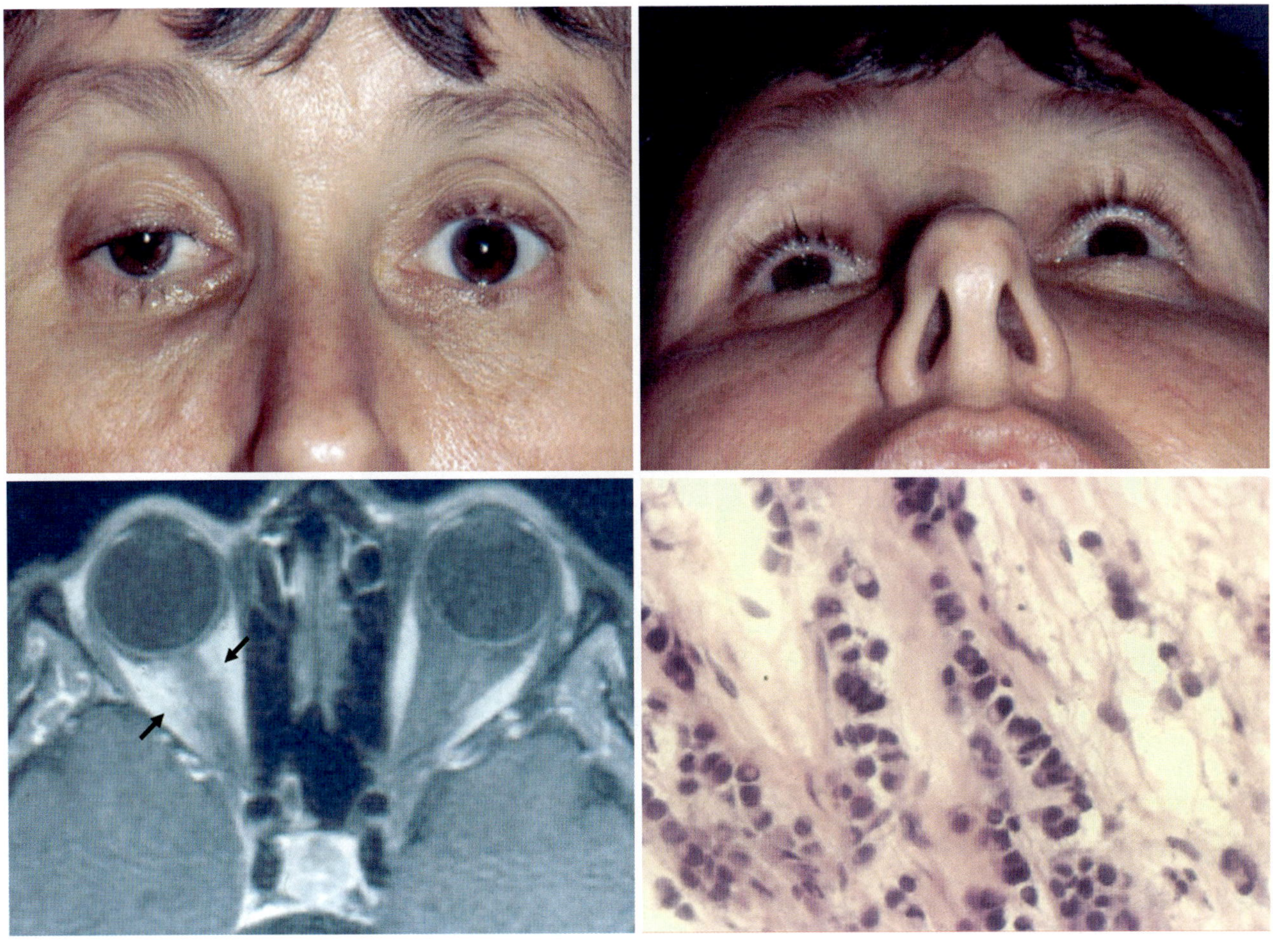

Fig. 13.6 Ptosis and enophthalmos from metastatic scirrhous breast carcinoma. Top, clinical photographs. External ophthalmoplegia without diplopia was also present. Bottom left, MRI (T-1, post-contrast with fat suppression) showing an ill-defined infiltration of the right intraconal space (arrows). Bottom right, histopathology showing an "Indian file" carcinomatous infiltration of the orbit with an intense fibrous reaction

present as simple ptosis. Palpation of the superior orbit and examination of the superior cul-de-sac are essential in all patients presenting with ptosis.

Spastic Disorders

Focal dystonias, including benign essential blepharospasm (BEB), apraxia of eyelid opening (AEO), hemifacial spasm (HFS), and spastic paretic facial contracture, can present with a pseudoptosis.

BEB is an idiopathic disorder of bilateral, involuntary contractions of the eyelids that disappears during sleep (Fig. 13.10). The terminology is deeply ingrained despite the criticism of the dystonia rarely being "benign" and never being "essential." [21] One hypothesis on the etiology is basal ganglia dysfunction leading to the hyperexcitability of brainstem neurons [22]. As imaging technology has improved, other studies evaluating morphometry and white matter integrity on MRI in patients with dystonias have begun, and this may shed some light on the etiology of blepharospasm in the future [23–25]. Additionally, PET studies looking at increased areas of activity have begun on patients with BEB, which may demonstrate the area(s) of abnormality, but to date, no reproducible abnormalities have been identified [26, 27]. Of note, there is no indication for routine neuroimaging in patients presenting with classic BEB. Secondary blepharospasm clinically appears similar to BEB but is due to an underlying cause such as local ocular irritation or dry eye syndrome.

The prevalence of BEB varies in reports from 12 to 133 per million by region, although it is unclear if there is a true geographic variance or simply a disparity in clinical definition and reporting [28–30]. Risk factors for BEB include increasing age and female gender, with women being 2.3 times more likely to be effected than men [30, 31]. Additionally, family history of a dystonia is a factor, and epidemiologic studies suggest that BEB is an autosomal domi-

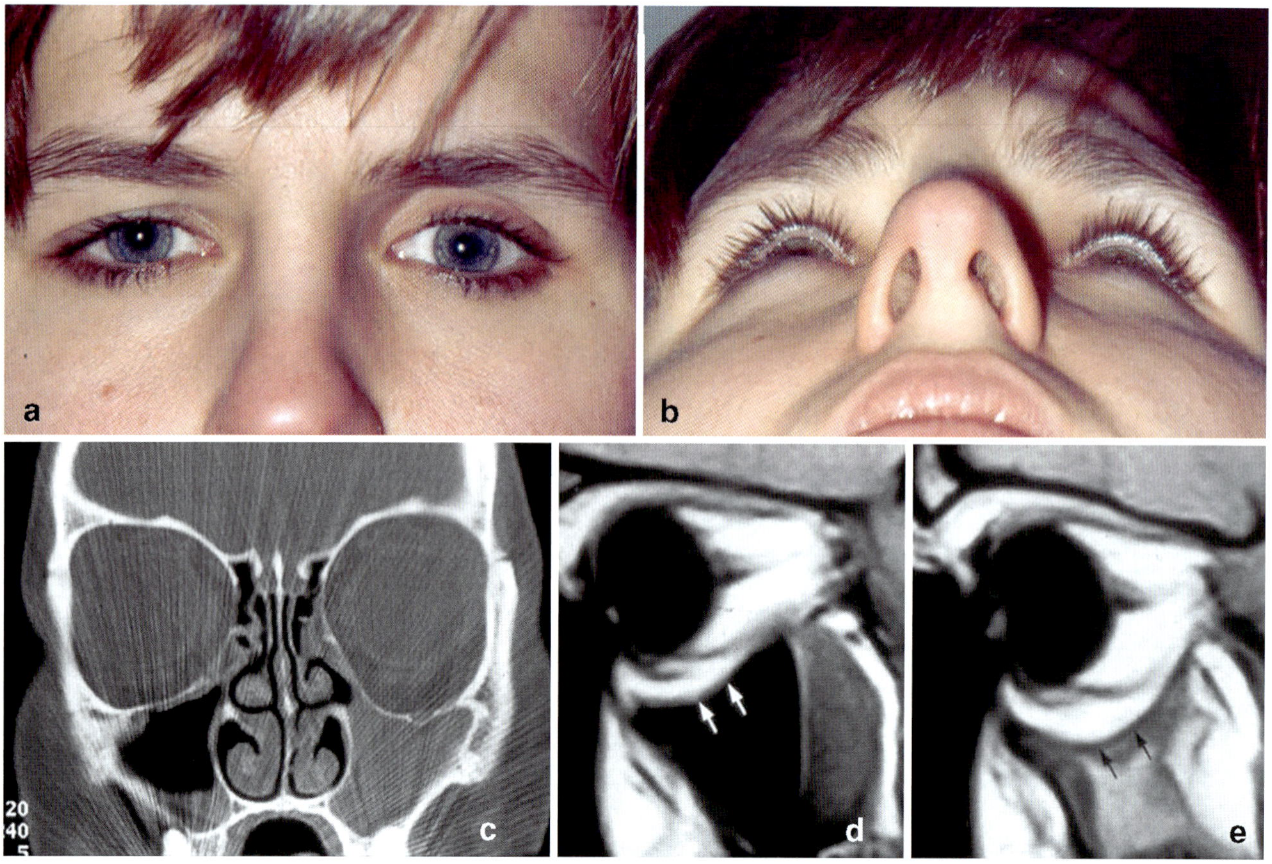

Fig. 13.7 Silent sinus syndrome. A 35-year-old woman referred for eyelid asymmetry and progressive inability to wear a left contact lens. (**a**) External examination shows a deep left superior sulcus deformity suggestive of levator dehiscence. There is a suggestion of left hypoglobus. (**b**) Left enophthalmos. (**c**) Coronal CT (bone window) shows atelectasis and opacification of the left maxillary, resulting in a downward bowing of the orbital floor and secondary expansion of the left orbit. (**d**) Parasagittal MRI (T-1) of the uninvolved right orbit with a normal orbital floor contour (arrows). (**e**) Parasagittal MRI (T-1) of the involved left orbit showing obvious bowing of the orbital floor (arrows) along with an inward collapse of the anterior and posterior maxillary sinus walls

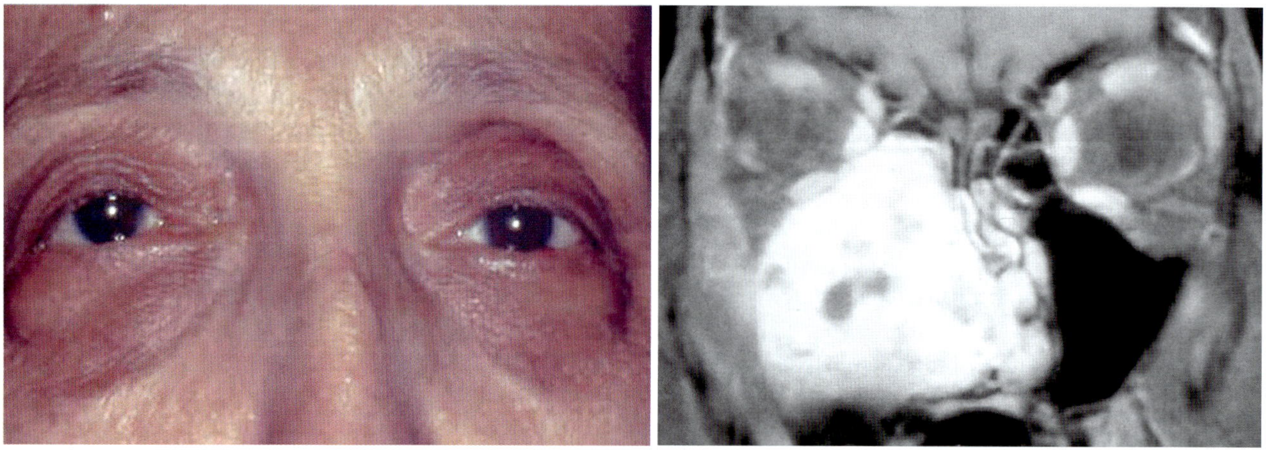

Fig. 13.8 Eyelid asymmetry secondary to hyperglobus. Left, clinical view of a patient seeking an opinion regarding her lids after being told by members of her bridge club that her "eyes and lids look funny." Ptosis is present bilaterally. The asymmetric dermatochalasis on the right is secondary to hyperglobus. Right, coronal MRI (T-1, post-contrast with fat suppression) shows a mass filling the right maxillary sinus and nasal cavity with secondary extension into the orbit. Extirpation of the sinus pleomorphic adenoma was curative and the globe/lid malpositions resolved

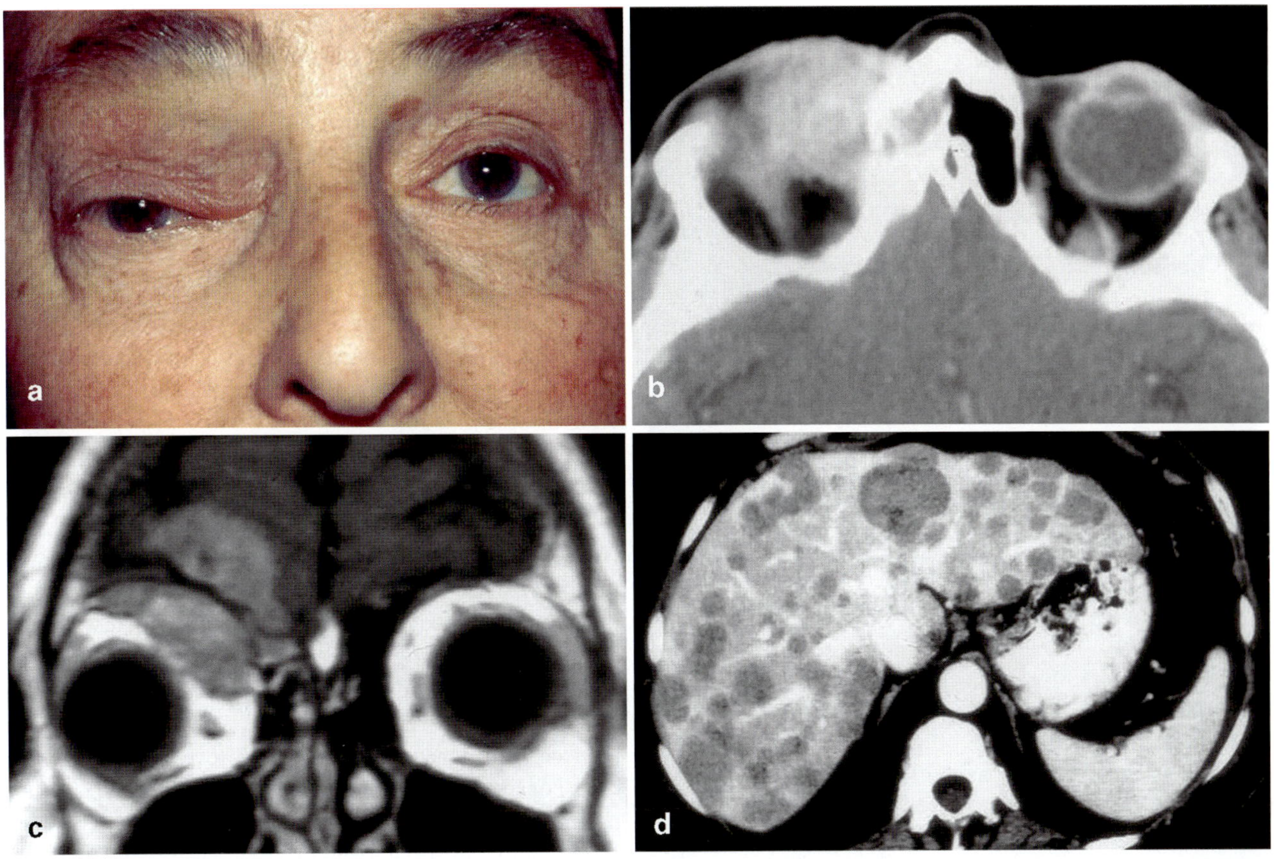

Fig. 13.9 Ptosis secondary to a superior orbital mass. (**a**) Clinical photograph of a patient presenting with ptosis 6 months after an automobile accident. A fixed, rubbery mass was palpated along the superior orbital rim and a possible posttraumatic frontoethmoidal mucocele was suspected. (**b**) Axial CT views of the lesion. Bony erosion and possible intracranial extension were noted on other images. (**c**) MRI (T-1, post-contrast) delineated the intracranial extent. Biopsy showed metastatic lung carcinoma. (**d**) On systemic work-up, diffuse hepatic metastases were noted

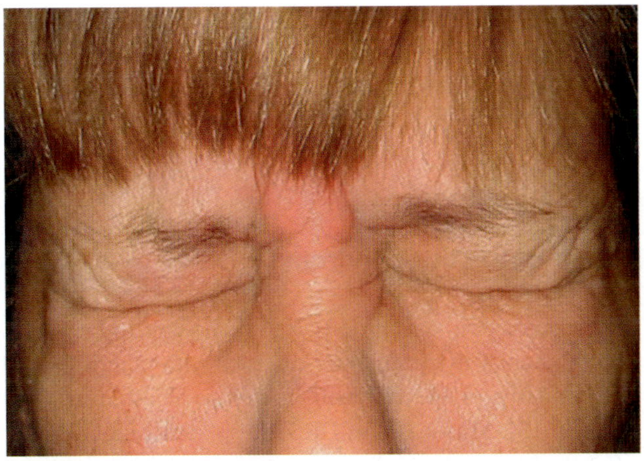

Fig. 13.10 Benign essential blepharospasm. Note the bilateral forced closure of the eyelids secondary to uncontrolled spasm of the orbicularis oculi muscles

nant disorder with reduced penetrance, though specific genetic markers have not been found [32–34]. This disorder can extend to other areas of the face or neck, as a forme fruste of Meige syndrome and oromandibular dystonia [35]. Additionally there can be spread to other areas of the body [36]. True eyelid position is often difficult to ascertain in BEB patients because of the variable degree of blepharospasm at any given moment, as well as the effect of any ongoing treatment (e.g., botulinum toxin injection). Ptosis in BEB is in all likelihood secondary to orbicularis contraction (pseudoptosis) early in the course of the disease. However, over time, true levator dehiscence or attenuation occurs; this is due at least in part by patients' understandable habit of frequently trying to digitally force the eyelids open against the spasm.

Apraxia of eyelid opening (AEO) is an uncommon disorder, usually occurring with another spastic disorder but rarely manifesting as an isolated entity [37, 38]. Clinically, the patient presents with an apparent inability to raise the eyelids voluntarily, despite normal levator function (Fig. 13.11). The apraxia is typically intermittent and, in cases of pure AEO, is not associated with orbicularis spasm. AEO has been reported in patients with neurodegenerative diseases, such as Parkinson disease and spinocerebellar ataxia, but can also be idiopathic or drug-induced [39–41]. This is generally a bilateral phenomenon, with limited reports of unilateral cases [42]. As AEO is thought to be due to prolonged levator palpebrae superioris inhibition, it

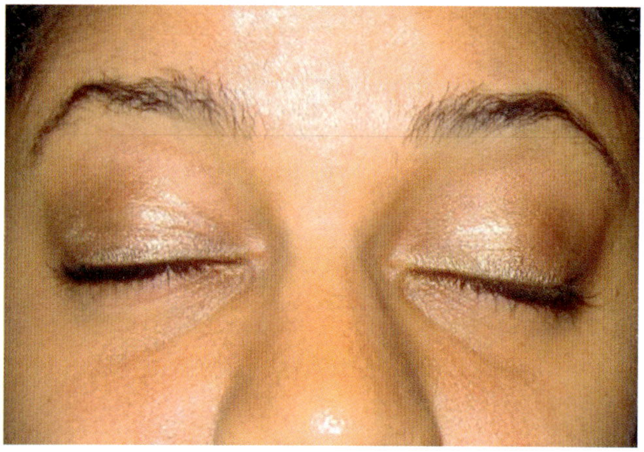

Fig. 13.11 Apraxia of lid opening. Note the inability to open the eyelids despite contraction of the frontalis muscles and relaxation of the orbicularis oculi muscles. The phenomenon is usually transient and often occurs during stressful situations, such as attempted examination of the eyes

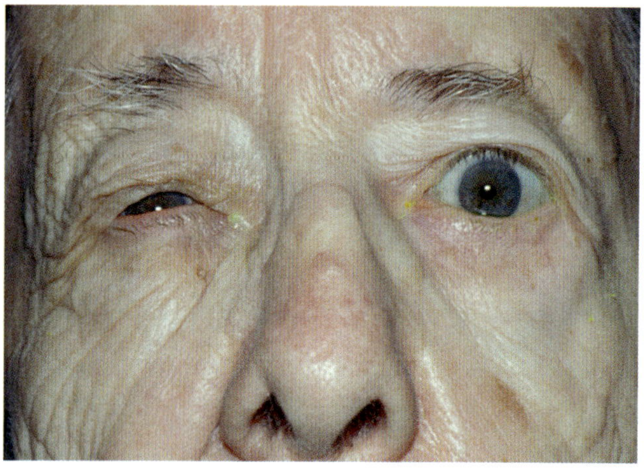

Fig. 13.12 Hemifacial spasm. Note contraction of the right facial muscles which results in uncontrolled unilateral eyelid closure and distortion of the lower face

is included in the spectrum of dystonias [39, 43]. Reports suggest a higher prevalence of AEO in patients with BEB [43, 44].

Unlike BEB, HFS is nearly always unilateral, persists during sleep, and generally has an identifiable underlying condition (Fig. 13.12) [45]. Many patients with HFS will also present with subtle weakness of the ipsilateral facial musculature, suggestive of mild facial nerve paresis. The incidence of HFS increases with age and is more common in women [46]. The majority of patients have either a normal or aberrant artery in contact with the root of the facial nerve, but it is unclear if this leads to focal demyelination or some other underlying pathophysiology [47–51]. While HFS is a clinical diagnosis, baseline MRI with attention to the course of the facial nerve is worthwhile to exclude rare cases associated with a vascular malformation or tumor [52–54]. HFS can range in severity from slight unilateral lid twitching to intense spasm of one side of the face and neck and on occasion presents initially as an isolated eyelid myokymia which progresses over months to years to manifest as obvious HFS [54]. While it is generally a benign condition, HFS can cause severe functional disability and spontaneous recovery is rare.

Spastic paretic hemifacial contracture (SPHC) is an uncommon condition with unilateral contraction of the facial muscles and an evolving ipsilateral facial paresis. Unlike HFS, this is a chronic, persistent contracture. The anatomic localization is pontine, usually due to neoplasia or demyelinating disease [55, 56].

The mainstay of treatment for facial dystonias is botulinum toxin injections and supportive therapies. Botulinum toxin has high efficacy and low risk [57–59]. Patients with BEB are generally very photophobic, and tinted lenses, most notably FL-41, may be useful [60]. Anticholinergic and dopaminergic medications benefit some patients, though usually not alleviating the need for concomitant treatment(s). Orbicularis oculi myectomies (with or without levator advancement) and neurectomy of selected facial nerve branches are generally reserved for severe cases of BEB unresponsive to medical treatments [61–64]. It appears that patients with a higher level of disability from BEB benefit most from surgical intervention [61]. Even with successful myectomy, about 50% of patients will eventually require additional botulinum toxin therapy [61]. Studies on deep brain stimulation are ongoing, showing some effect in other forms of dystonia, and may prove useful in the future for BEB [21].

Microvascular decompression of the facial nerve at the pons is a surgical approach for HFS [65]. This surgery requires a small craniectomy with the associated risks and complications. More recently, an endoscopic approach has been used with a high success rate and fewer potential complications [66].

Duane Retraction Syndrome

Duane retraction syndrome (DRS) is thought to be a congenital cranial dysinnervation disorder with embryological cranial nerve maldevelopment and anomalous innervation (Fig. 13.13). Most cases of DRS are sporadic, though up to 5% may be autosomal dominant [67]. There is a slight predominance of females, and the majority of cases are unilateral, with the left eye being involved more frequently [68, 69]. The classification of DRS can be difficult, and several systems have been reported. The most commonly used classification system is based on electromyographic (EMG) data and distinguishes three types of DRS (Table 13.1) [70]. The degree of ptosis associated with DRS typically varies with

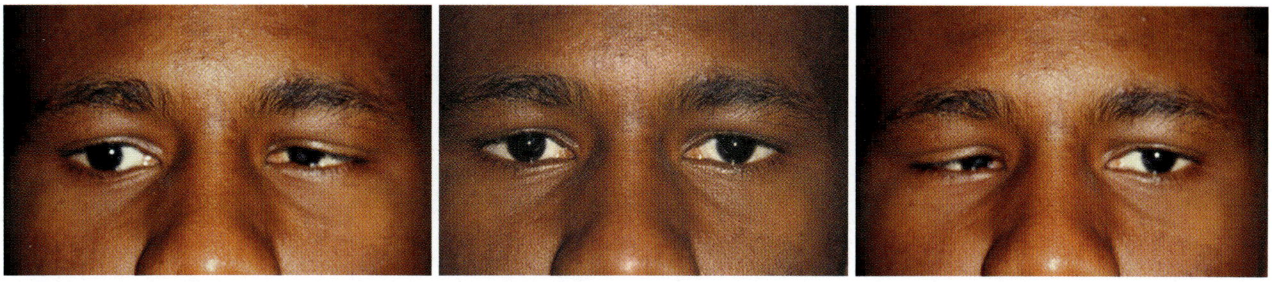

Fig. 13.13 Duane retraction syndrome. A patient with Type III DRS. Note the bilateral limitation of horizontal gaze with globe retraction and narrowing of the palpebral fissure on attempted adduction of each eye

Table 13.1 Characteristics of Duane retraction syndrome (DRS). Lateral rectus msucel = LR. Medial rectus muscle = MR

DRS type	Prevalence	Primary gaze	Adduction	Abduction	Palpebral fissure narrowing	EMG activity
I	85%	Generally esotropic	Normal	Limited (improves with elevation or depression)	Adduction	LR and MR on adduction
II	14%	Exodeviation	Limited/absent	Normal	Adduction	LR with adduction and abduction
III	1%	Varies	Limited/absent	Limited/absent	Adduction	LR and MR with primary gaze, adduction, or abduction

horizontal gaze. The horizontal gaze restriction usually alerts the clinician that the lid droop is not simply a typical case of congenital ptosis. While most patients with DRS are otherwise healthy, there are associated systemic and conditions including Goldenhar syndrome, iris dysplasia, and colobomas [71]. Treatment is difficult and is generally primarily performed to address strabismus.

Parinaud Syndrome

Parinaud, or dorsal midbrain, syndrome consists of supranuclear impaired superior gaze and convergence retraction nystagmus. Generally bilateral upper lid retraction is seen, but ptosis can occur and pseudoptosis with retraction may be evident. Given the other findings with this syndrome, the ptosis is generally not mistaken as a benign, isolated condition.

Floppy Eyelid Syndrome

Floppy eyelid syndrome (FES), a subgroup of eyelid laxity, is a rubbery eyelid laxity with papillary conjunctivitis seen in obese individuals (Fig. 13.14) [72]. The etiology of FES is likely multifactorial, with evidence of elastin depletion and upregulation of matrix metalloproteinases [73, 74]. FES is associated with a variety of disorders including obstructive sleep apnea (OSA), blepharoptosis, eyelash ptosis, keratoconus and dermatochalasis [75–78]. While the relationship between OSA and FES may be an epiphenomenon related to obesity, it is important to consider referral for OSA screening due to the associated morbidity and mortality of OSA [72]. Ophthalmic treatment can include conservative therapy, with lubrication and patching, and surgical horizontal lid shortening [75, 79]. Levator advancement alone will fail to resolve ptosis in floppy eyelid syndrome. Some form of horizontal lid tightening is recommended. Surgical repair of eyelids in patients with FES is complicated by an increased incidence of wound dehiscence, most likely secondary to impaired healing from the underlying condition. Not infrequently, successful management of OSA with continuous positive airway pressure (CPAP) therapy improves the ocular symptoms, presumably because the patient sleeps more peacefully in a supine position, with less mechanical irritation to the eyelid and tarsal conjunctiva against the pillowcase.

Aberrant Facial Nerve Regeneration

The majority of unilateral peripheral facial palsies are idiopathic or Bell palsies. The incidence rate is approximately 25 per 100,000 [80]. Generally this palsy resolves without sequelae. However, about 20% of patients will develop synkinesis. Wallerian degeneration of axons with resultant abnormal branching during axonal regeneration is the most commonly proposed mechanism, though nuclear hyperexcitability and/or central cortex reorganization may play roles [81–85]. Regardless of the mechanism, synkinetic movements can begin 3 months after the onset of the palsy and range from subclinical to massive hemifacial contractures [86]. Commonly patients will have intermittent ptosis with

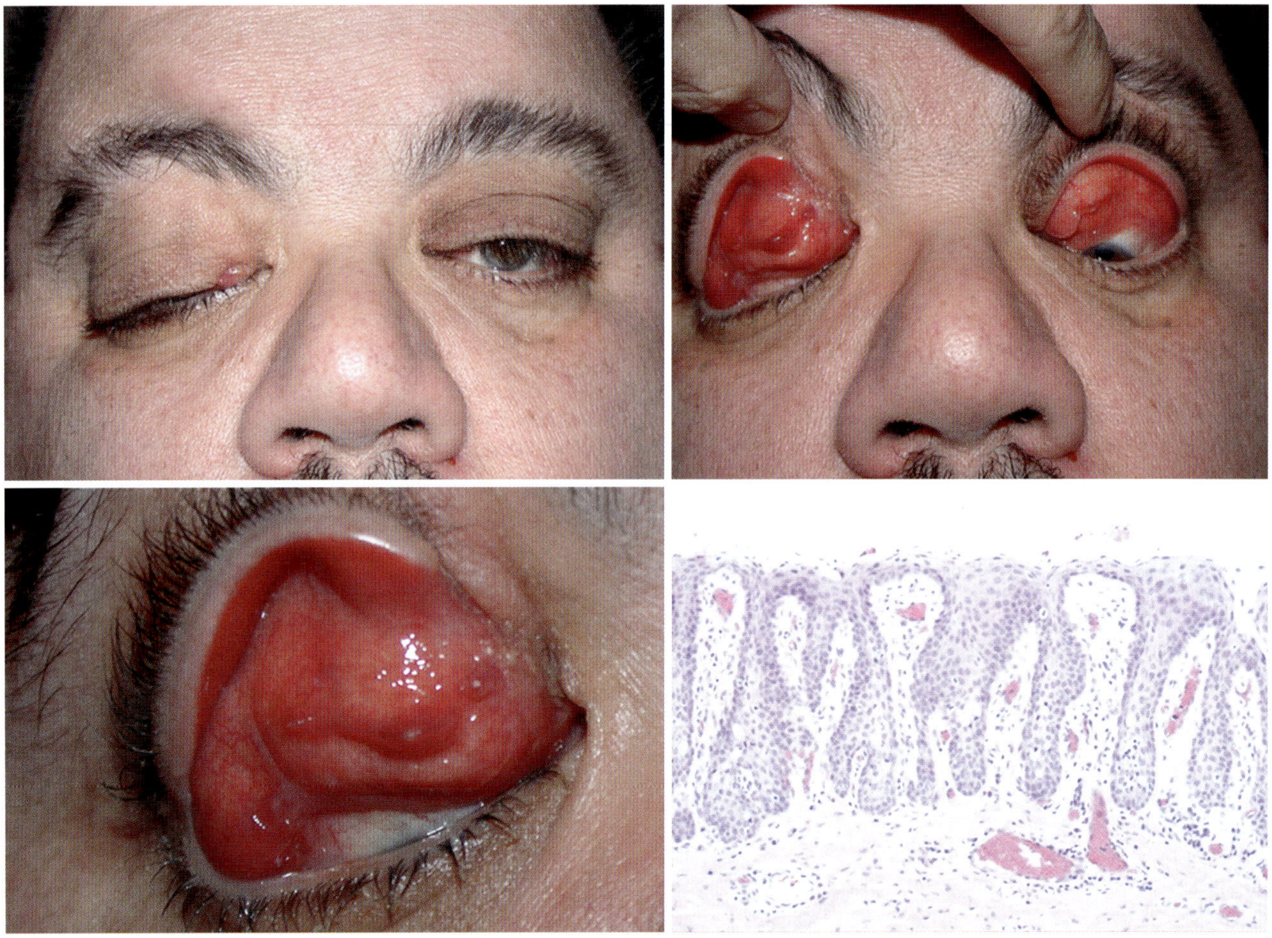

Fig. 13.14 Floppy eyelid syndrome. An obese patient with a history of obstructive sleep apnea presents for ptosis evaluation. On further questioning, a history of chronic mucous discharge and daily "sticky eyelids" on awakening is elicited. Top, external appearance. Note eversion of the eyelids with minimal effort. Marked laxity was noted, along with conjunctival thickening suggestive of a "salmon patch." Lower left, marked papillary conjunctivitis noted on slit lamp examination, which was confirmed on wedge resection (bottom right)

mouth closure from co-contraction of orbicularis oris and oculi and may develop gustatory lacrimation or "crocodile tearing." [84] However, any pattern of facial synkinesis can develop. The hypersecretion and synkinetic movements can generally be successfully treated with botulinum toxin injections, making surgical intervention rare [87, 88]. Facial physical therapy with biofeedback using a mirror or surface EMG may also have some benefit [89, 90].

True Ptosis: Neurologic Etiologies

Myogenic Ptosis

Congenital Fibrosis of the Extraocular Muscles

Congenital fibrosis of the extraocular muscles (CFEOM) is a disorder with congenital, non-progressive, restrictive ophthalmoparesis and bilateral ptosis (Fig. 13.15). Nystagmus and Marcus Gunn jaw-winking are variably present. In the past, this was considered a primary myopathy. However, more recent data suggests aberrant oculomotor and/or trochlear muscle innervation, which would classify CFEOM as a congenital cranial dysinnervation disorder [91–93]. The pathophysiology is unknown, and the categorization between

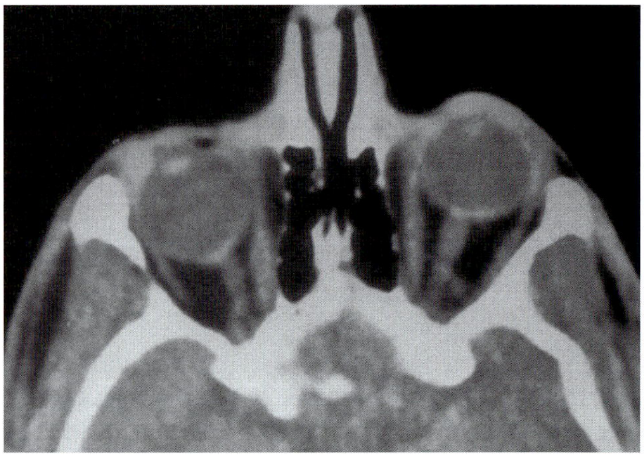

Fig. 13.15 Congenital fibrosis of the extraocular muscles

myogenic and neurogenic is unclear [94]. Three familial types have been found, CFEOM1, CFEOM2, and CFEOM3, and may be either autosomal dominant or autosomal recessive [95–99]. Interestingly, the phenotype also varies between the familial types [100]. Treatment is aimed primarily at the strabismus. If ptosis surgery is later needed, a frontalis sling is generally the procedure of choice, with a goal of just clearing the pupillary axis [101].

Muscular Dystrophy

Myotonic dystrophy (MD) is the most common form of muscular dystrophy in adults. These autosomal dominantly inherited disorders have been found to have two different loci and distinct phenotypes. Muscle dysfunction, the most common presenting complaint, and myotonia, or involuntary muscle contraction and delayed relaxation, are found with each form [102, 103]. The periocular findings of iridescent cataracts, facial weakness, temporalis wasting, frontal hair loss, and bilateral ptosis create a characteristic facial appearance (Fig. 13.16). Systemic findings are seen as well, including cardiac and endocrine abnormalities [104]. The progression of the disease is slow, but life expectancy is reduced due to cardiac disease, neoplasms, and respiratory disease [105].

Oculopharyngeal Muscular Dystrophy

Oculopharyngeal muscular dystrophy (OPMD) is an uncommon disorder. The prevalence of OPMD varies by ethnic population, from a high of 1:600 among Bukharan Jews in Israel to 1:1000 in French Canadians in Quebec and 1:100,000 in France. The majority of OPMD-affected individuals in the United States have a French-Canadian background, though more recently populations of Hispanic Americans with Spanish ancestry in Texas, New Mexico, Arizona, and California have also been recognized [106–110].

Patients with OPMD generally present with an insidious, progressive, late-onset ptosis, dysphagia, and positive family history (Fig. 13.17). The ptosis begins at a mean age of 48 years but can occur as late as 65 years. Development of dysphagia may lag a bit behind the ptosis, with a mean age of onset of 51 years, but specific questioning may be suggestive, including avoidance of dry foods and increased time to complete a meal [111]. External ophthalmoplegia is a less typical sign, though some reports note motility limitation in up to 50% of patients at the time of presentation [112–114]. The severity of the disease is variable, and the life span appears unchanged. However, more severe cases tend to be

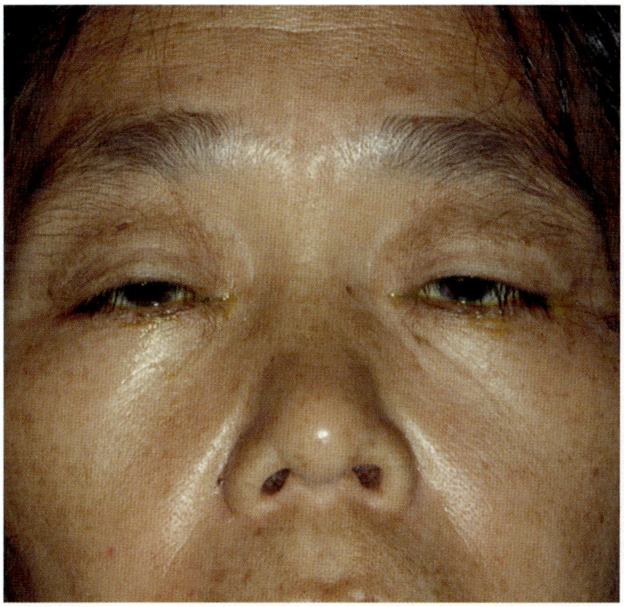

Fig. 13.16 Myotonic dystrophy. Severe bilateral ptosis with poor levator function is present bilaterally. Note the wasting of the facial muscles, resulting in a mask-like facies

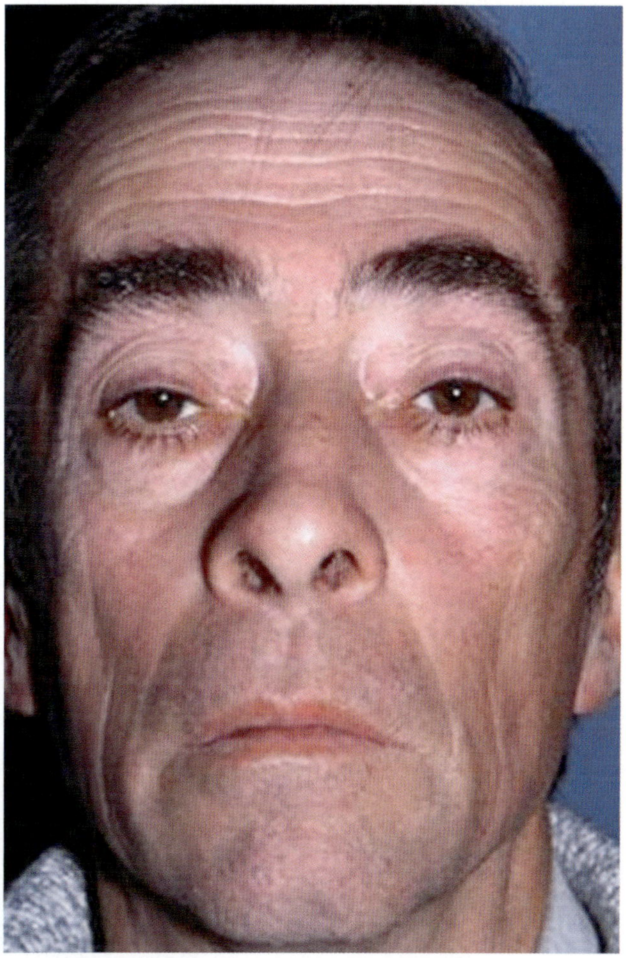

Fig. 13.17 Oculopharyngeal muscular dystrophy. A patient of French-Canadian heritage with severe ptosis, dysphagia, and a strong family history of oculopharyngeal dystrophy. Note the diffuse facial muscle wasting with hollowing of the temporalis fossae. (Courtesy of Isabelle Hardy, MD)

autosomal dominant and generally have an earlier onset of ptosis and dysphagia [115, 116].

The disease can be autosomal dominant or autosomal recessive. First-line testing for diagnosis is generally non-invasive genetic probing for expansions of trinucleotide repeats. Invasive testing with muscle biopsy or electromyography (EMG) is generally reserved for patients with clinical findings and non-diagnostic genetic tests or an unclear clinical presentation. Muscle biopsy with the presence of intranuclear inclusions, specific tubulofilamentous characteristics on electron microscopy, small angulated fibers, and rimmed vacuoles is generally diagnostic [117]. EMG may reveal a myopathic pattern and help rule out other conditions, such as myasthenia gravis (MG).

Levator resection or frontalis suspension can be utilized when ptosis surgery is warranted. When levator surgery is performed, the patients should be counseled that frequently this will need to be repeated [118]. Frontalis suspension should certainly be used in patients with severe ptosis and poor levator function (<4 mm) and may be used in less severe cases as well [119]. Some patients with OPMD have atypical responses to anesthetics, but general anesthesia is not contraindicated in this population [120]. Patients should be referred for swallowing studies and genetic counseling.

Chronic Progressive External Ophthalmoplegia

Chronic progressive external ophthalmoplegia (CPEO) describes a collection of syndromes caused by an underlying mitochondrial myopathy [121]. The true prevalence is unknown but estimated as at least 1 in 5000 [121]. The extraocular muscles appear to be preferentially affected when compared to other skeletal muscles, possibly due to a lower mutational threshold and a resultant more pronounced mitochondrial defect [122]. It is also possible that structures with high baseline metabolic rates (extraocular muscles, retinal pigment epithelium, photoreceptors, heart) requiring high mitochondrial activity show preferential involvement.

Ptosis may be the first manifestation of CPEO; external ophthalmoplegia may be absent or minimally present in the early stages (Fig. 13.18). Ptosis is eventually bilateral but may present initially as a unilateral phenomenon. Ptosis from CPEO has two characteristics that distinguish it from other forms of blepharoptosis. First, unlike the normal or near-normal levator function of acquired ptosis from levator dehiscence, poor levator function is the hallmark of CPEO-associated ptosis. Second, ptosis from CPEO is fixed and does not vary throughout the day, in contradistinction to myasthenic ptosis; that said, on occasion, it may be difficult

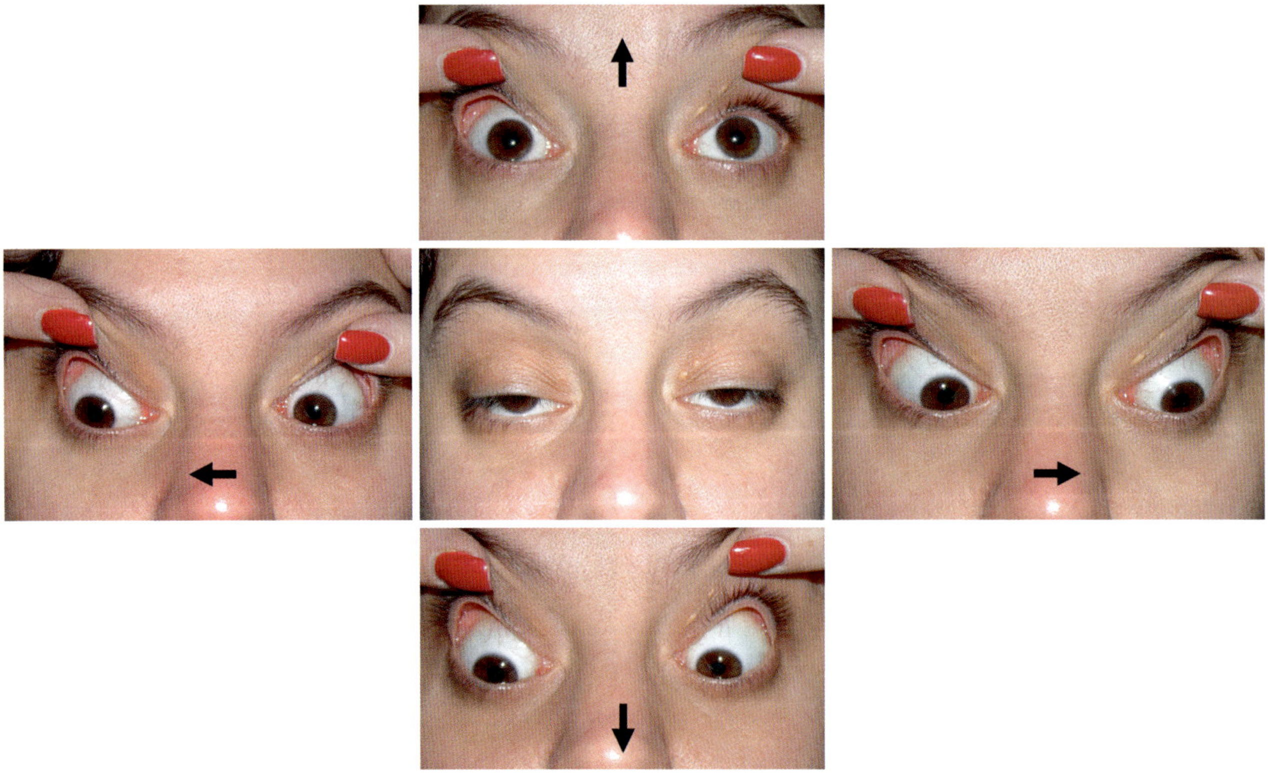

Fig. 13.18 Chronic progressive external ophthalmoplegia: ophthalmoplegia plus syndrome. A 31-year-old woman presented with progressive ptosis over the past 5 years. Pigmentary retinopathy had been noted several years prior. She denied diplopia or any history of cardiac disease. Severe ptosis with absent levator function is noted, along with obvious external ophthalmoplegia (arrows indicate attempted direction of gaze). As a precaution, she was referred to a cardiologist for long-term follow-up

to distinguish CPEO from ocular myasthenia [123]. As ptosis from CPEO worsens, patients develop a classic chin-up position. Importantly, most patients with CPEO develop a symmetric external ophthalmoplegia and do not complain of diplopia. If EOMs are not checked carefully, the true diagnosis may be missed. Many patients with CPEO also have orbicularis oculi weakness and lagophthalmos. This is an important consideration when planning ptosis repair [124].

The diagnosis of CPEO is typically made by examining the skeletal muscle for the so-called ragged-red fibers, caused by abnormal accumulations of mitochondria within muscle fibers. Electron microscopy may be very helpful but requires that the skeletal muscle specimen be fixed in glutaraldehyde. If CPEO is suspected, a strip of orbicularis oculi muscle may be excised either as a separate procedure or during ptosis repair and sent for analysis in three sections: formalin-fixed, frozen for cryostat and mitochondrial studies, and in glutaraldehyde for electron microscopy [125].

The most dangerous form of CPEO is Kearns-Sayre syndrome (KSS). It is important to remember that at least clinically, KSS represents a specific subtype of CPEO. Thus, all KSS is CPEO, but not all CPEO is KSS; however, recent studies on mitochondrial defects in a variety of mitochondrial disorders suggest that, in fact, KSS may be secondary to distinct mitochondrial genetic deletions not seen in CPEO [126]. KSS is typified by the triad of CPEO, retinopathy (with or without pigmentation), and young age of presentation (<20 years) (Fig. 13.19). Patients presenting with this triad after the age of 20 years are diagnosed with "ophthalmoplegia plus" syndrome (Fig. 13.18) [121]. Any patient presenting with a pattern suggestive of KSS must undergo urgent cardiac work-up, since many patients will have a high-degree heart block, which could prove fatal. If initial cardiac work-up is normal, the patient must be followed over the long term, as cardiac conduction defects may occur several years after the ocular manifestations. Early implantation of cardiac pacemakers is recommended, but conduction defects may be progressive [127]. Patients with KSS may also manifest other signs, including deafness, cerebral ataxia, and abnormal facies. Endocrine problems may also occur and warrant close endocrinologic follow-up.

The retinopathy of KSS is variable and in early stages is easily missed. In general, KSS retinopathy has a predilection for the posterior pole and, although often described as mimicking retinitis pigmentosa, does not usually affect the peripheral retina or form "bone spicules." Instead, a depigmentation of the retina is more typical of KSS in the early stages, with increased pigmentation and atrophy occurring over time (Fig. 13.19) [128]. Despite pronounced fundus abnormalities, visual loss is mild in most cases [121].

Correction of ptosis in CPEO mimics that of ptosis repair in MG, with the exception that bilateral ptosis repair can be performed in CPEO with a much lower risk of postoperative diplopia.

Guillain-Barré Syndrome

Guillain-Barré syndrome (GBS) is an idiopathic, acute, progressive paralyzing illness. Cranial nerve involvement, generally bilateral facial weakness, can be a component. It is thought to be an autoimmune response triggered by an infection and targeting peripheral nerve antigens. The Miller Fisher variant of GBS (MFS) is more limited, with no systemic weakness. MFS is described by the clinical triad of ataxia, areflexia, and external ophthalmoplegia, with ophthalmoplegia being the most prevalent and consistent finding [129]. One to two per 100,000 people are affected, and it is more common in the elderly and in men [130, 131]. Cerbrospinal fluid examinations generally show increased protein concentration in 90% of patients after 2 weeks, and the concentrations of haptoglobin, alpha-1 antitrypsin, neurofilaments, and apolipoprotein are also increased. EMG can also be helpful in the diagnosis and subclassification of GBS [132, 133].

Plasma exchange and intravenous immunoglobulin treatments have both been found to be beneficial in GBS [134, 135]. Corticosteroids alone do not significantly alter the outcome and have known risk factors [131].

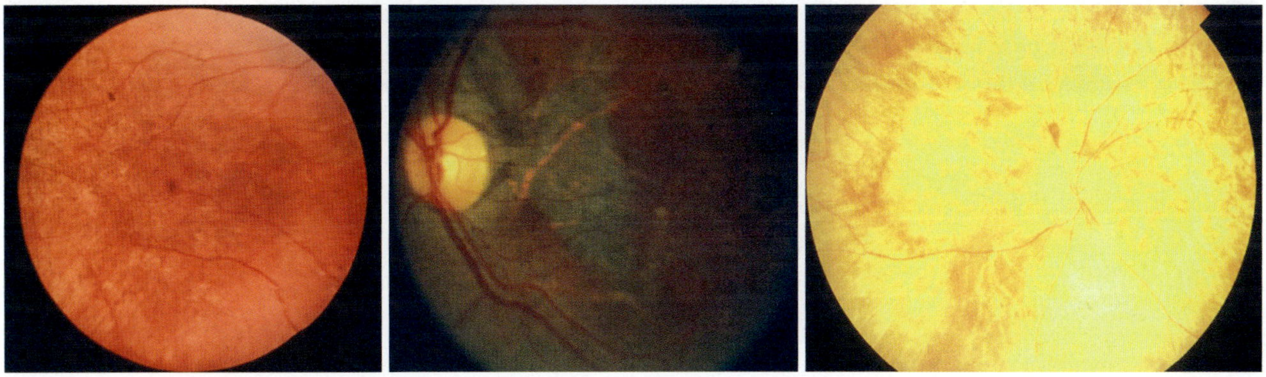

Fig. 13.19 Retinopathy in Kearns-Sayre syndrome. Note that the abnormalities mainly affect the posterior fundus. Left, early dropout of the retinal pigment epithelium (RPE) with no secondary pigmentation. Center, placoid atrophy. Right, diffuse RPE dropout and chorioretinal atrophy. Note the absence of the typical bone spicules characteristic of retinitis pigmentosa

Neurogenic Ptosis

Oculomotor Nerve Dysfunction

Abnormalities of the oculomotor nerve may occur anywhere along its course from the midbrain nucleus through its intracranial course up to its division into superior and inferior branches as it exits the skull base into the orbit. Nuclear and perinuclear lesions will not be discussed in this chapter. Acquired abnormalities of CN-III are relatively common and may have a variety of etiologies, including vascular (aneurysmal), ischemic (including giant cell arteritis), neoplastic, demyelinating, inflammatory, and traumatic [136–140].

Oculomotor nerve dysfunction may present as unilateral ptosis with or without complaints of diplopia or pupillary abnormality; some degree of external ophthalmoplegia is always present. Several patterns may manifest clinically [140]. First, complete third nerve palsy with or without pupillary involvement may occur (Fig. 13.20). This diagnosis is typically straightforward clinically, with findings of complete ptosis and absence of adduction, infraduction, and supraduction. The involved globe is typically "down and out." Because of the complete, visually obstructive ptosis, the patient may not notice diplopia unless the eyelid is elevated above the visual axis. Two issues are important in complete third nerve palsy: pupillary involvement and patient age. Any significant anisocoria (>2 mm) requires urgent neuroimaging with either MRI/MRA (magnetic resonance arteriography) or CT (computed tomography)/CTA (computed tomographic arteriogra-

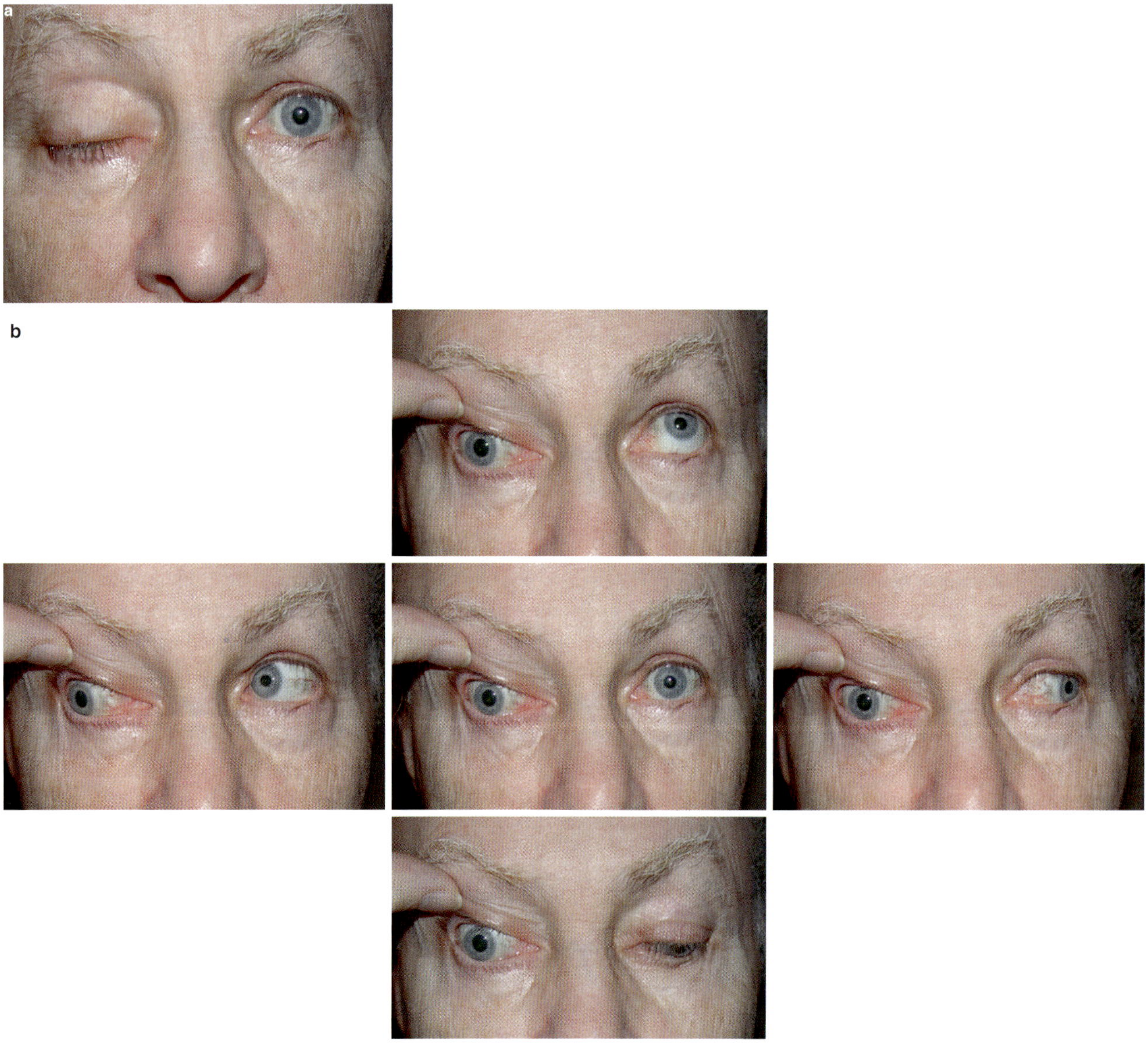

Fig. 13.20 Oculomotor nerve palsy. (**a**) A patient presenting with a sudden onset of right upper eyelid ptosis and pain. Because the eyelid is completely obstructing the visual axis, the patient does not perceive diplopia. (**b**) With the patient's eyelid elevated, obvious right internal and external ophthalmoplegia are evident. Urgent neuroimaging confirmed an intracranial aneurysm

phy) to rule out a posterior communicating artery aneurysm, regardless of patient age, although aneurysm under age 10 is a rare cause of CN-III dysfunction [140–142]. Although subtle anisocoria may occur in microvascular ischemic CN-III palsies, it is usually less than 1 mm [140, 143, 144].

The previous protocol for the work-up of oculomotor nerve dysfunction depended on several clinical findings. If the pupil was "not involved" (<2 mm of anisocoria), then patient age and medical history came into play. Patients younger than 50 years also required neuroimaging to rule out a vascular, inflammatory, or neoplastic intracranial processes [145, 146]. For those older than 50 years with a vasculopathic history, some clinicians followed the patient over the first week to assure that no anisocoria developed and then rechecked the patient several weeks later, assuming a microvascular ischemic etiology for the palsy and eventual recovery. (As mentioned, in patients over the age of 55 years, giant cell arteritis must be ruled out by history and, when necessary, serology or temporal artery biopsy is performed.) Neuroimaging was performed only if the patient fails to improve over the ensuing 12 weeks or develops additional cranial neuropathies [140]. The aforementioned recommendations should be considered outdated. *All patients presenting with oculomotor nerve dysfunction, regardless of age, vasculopathic risk factors, or pupillary involvement should undergo neuroimaging, including MRA and/or CTA* [147]. Pain and headache are not accurate predictors of the etiology of the palsy: most patients (77%) with a microvascular ischemic CN-III dysfunction will complain of pain or headache that is indistinguishable from that of aneurysm [146, 148, 149]. Similarly, a history of ischemic risk factors (diabetes mellitus, smoking, hypertension) does not help distinguish microvascular CN-III palsy, since these entities also predispose to weakening of arterial walls and aneurysm formation [146].

A partial CN-III palsy is often more difficult to diagnose because of a variety of subtle presentations (Fig. 13.21). Varying degrees of ptosis, external ophthalmoplegia, and anisocoria are possible. The most important rule for the clinician to remember regarding partial CN-III palsy is that all patients suspected of having this diagnosis, regardless of age, pupillary involvement, and vasculopathic risk factors, must be treated as if they have a complete and pupil-involving CN-III palsy; in other words, all patients with partial CN-III palsy must undergo urgent neuroimaging to rule out an actively expanding aneurysm [140].

Aberrant oculomotor nerve regeneration (AONR) may also present as a clinical conundrum. Often patients will

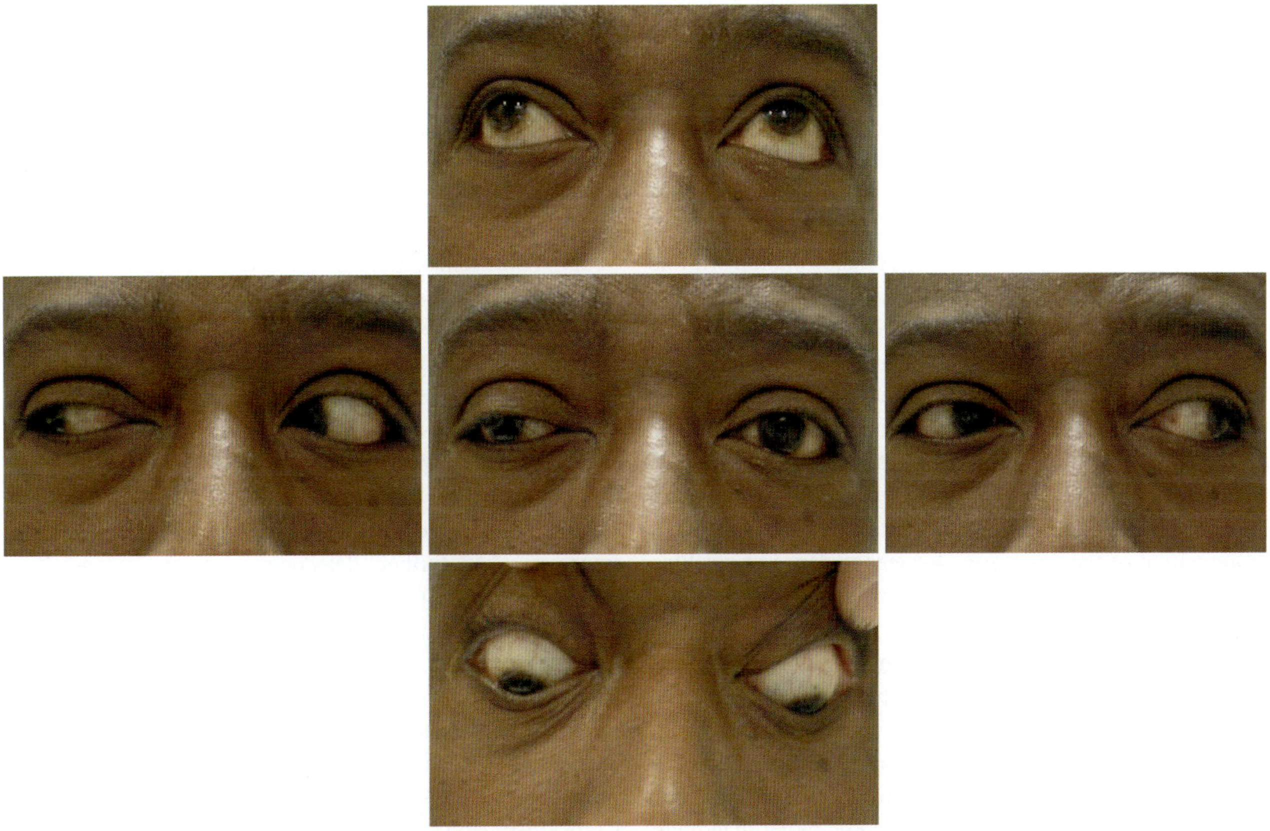

Fig. 13.21 Partial (incomplete) CN-III palsy. Note the right ptosis in primary gaze with a small-angle exotropia. Ductions reveal a subtle deficit in right upgaze and adduction. Neuroimaging showed a right cavernous sinus mass. (Courtesy of Scott Uretsky, MD)

report a history of CN-III palsy from a variety of etiologies, but on occasion, a slowly progressive intracranial process may affect the oculomotor nerve in a subtle fashion. Of note, aberrant regeneration from a microvascular ischemic oculomotor nerve palsy is so rare that the clinician should never assume AONR is due to ischemia [140]. Cavernous sinus meningiomas, aneurysms, pituitary tumors, and other intracranial pathologies have been reported in AONR [150–152].

Most patients with aberrant AONR will have some degree of ptosis in primary gaze (Fig. 13.22). A head tilt may also be present if the patient has learned to turn his/her head to avoid diplopia. External ophthalmoplegia and anisocoria may be noted. The key to diagnosis for AONR is the position of the upper eyelid and size of the pupil during ductions. Many cases of AONR will manifest lid retraction in attempted adduction and/or infraduction (pseudo-von Graefe sign). Ipsilateral miosis may also occur in these ductions. Unless there is a complete history and documentation of clearly defined pathology that resulted in CN-III dysfunction (e.g., well-documented previous head injury, including radiographic examination), all cases of AONR require neuroimaging to rule out intracranial pathology. Repair of ptosis in AONR can be frustrating, since upper lid position will change with ductions. If the patient has a significant head tilt, it is prudent to have the patient evaluated by a strabismologist first to assess whether extraocular muscle surgery is indicated to resolve the head tilt. Ptosis repair can then be performed as a second stage. If the patient refuses strabismus surgery, then eyelid height should be evaluated with the head tilt, and not in primary gaze. As with all forms of ptosis, the technique of eyelid repair is dependent on levator function.

On rare occasions, an isolated pupillary dilation with no external ophthalmoplegia can be caused by basilar artery aneurysms [153, 154]. That said, a CN-III etiology for a truly isolated, dilated, nonreactive pupil in an awake patient is exceedingly rare, and the isolated pupillary abnormality is most likely due to ciliary ganglion damage or pharmacologic blockade. The clinician should always remember that an isolated, dilated pupil may be the first sign of increased intracranial pressure (this is especially important in trauma settings); examination of the optic discs for any evidence of swelling should be documented, and neuroimaging should be performed.

Congenital oculomotor palsies may mimic congenital ptosis with varying degrees of external ophthalmoplegia. Anisocoria is a common feature of congenital oculomotor nerve palsy and is a helpful distinguishing feature from typical congenital ptosis. Counterintuitively, most congenital oculomotor paresis presents with a miotic, rather than mydriatic, pupil, possibly due to secondary aberrant regeneration. All infants with suspected congenital oculomotor nerve palsy should undergo neuroimaging to rule out intracranial pathology. Of note, computed tomographic arteriography (CTA) should be avoided in infants and young children because of the low incidence of aneurysm in this age group and the significant radiation exposure inherent to CTA; magnetic resonance arteriography (MRA) is preferable in these cases.

A brief discussion on imaging of CN-III palsy will be presented here. For additional details, the reader is referred to other excellent reviews, such as by Chaudhary et al. and Lee et al. [155, 156]

The vast majority of aneurysms causing oculomotor nerve dysfunction are at least 4 mm in diameter [156, 157]; this number is an important one to remember when considering imaging modalities. In other words, the sensitivity of the modality is not the only issue to consider when ordering a study. The clinician must also consider other extremely important issues: availability of the technology, morbidity of the modality, correct use of the technology, and correct interpretation of the study [155, 156]. As an example, it may be prudent to image a patient with a suspected aneurysmal cause for CN-III palsy on immediately available but older technology that has an adequate resolution, rather than delaying initial imaging until the optimum modality is available. Similarly, it may be perfectly reasonable to obtain an MRA to effectively rule out an aneurysm >4 mm in size rather than subject an at-risk patient to the morbidities of conventional angiography [140].

There are essentially three choices in imaging of CN-III palsy, catheter cerebral angiography (CCA), MRI/MRA, and CT/CTA, and each modality has particular advantages and disadvantages (Fig. 13.23).

CCA still remains the gold standard for identification of aneurysms, but does carry a 5% risk of catheter complications and a 0.3–1.0% risk of neurologic injury, which appears to increase with age [155, 156]. In addition, classic CCA provides images in only two dimensions, which may miss smaller aneurysms; in one study, two-dimensional CCA missed 29% of aneurysms between 0.5 and 4.0 mm [158]. With the use of newer three-dimensional rotational angiography (3DRA) with post-processing of images, sensitivity improves even further, detecting aneurysms as small as 1–2 mm [155, 156].

CTA, especially when used with multi-detector scanners and the newest reconstruction algorithms, has an excellent spatial resolution, with the ability to detect aneurysms as small as 1 mm. In a study by Mathew and colleagues, all aneurysms in a cohort of patients were detected by CTA, and no new aneurysms were found on subsequent therapeutic CCA [159]. However, because of the proximity of the skull base to aneurysms causing CN-III dysfunction, care must be taken to separate signal from the bone that may mimic aneu-

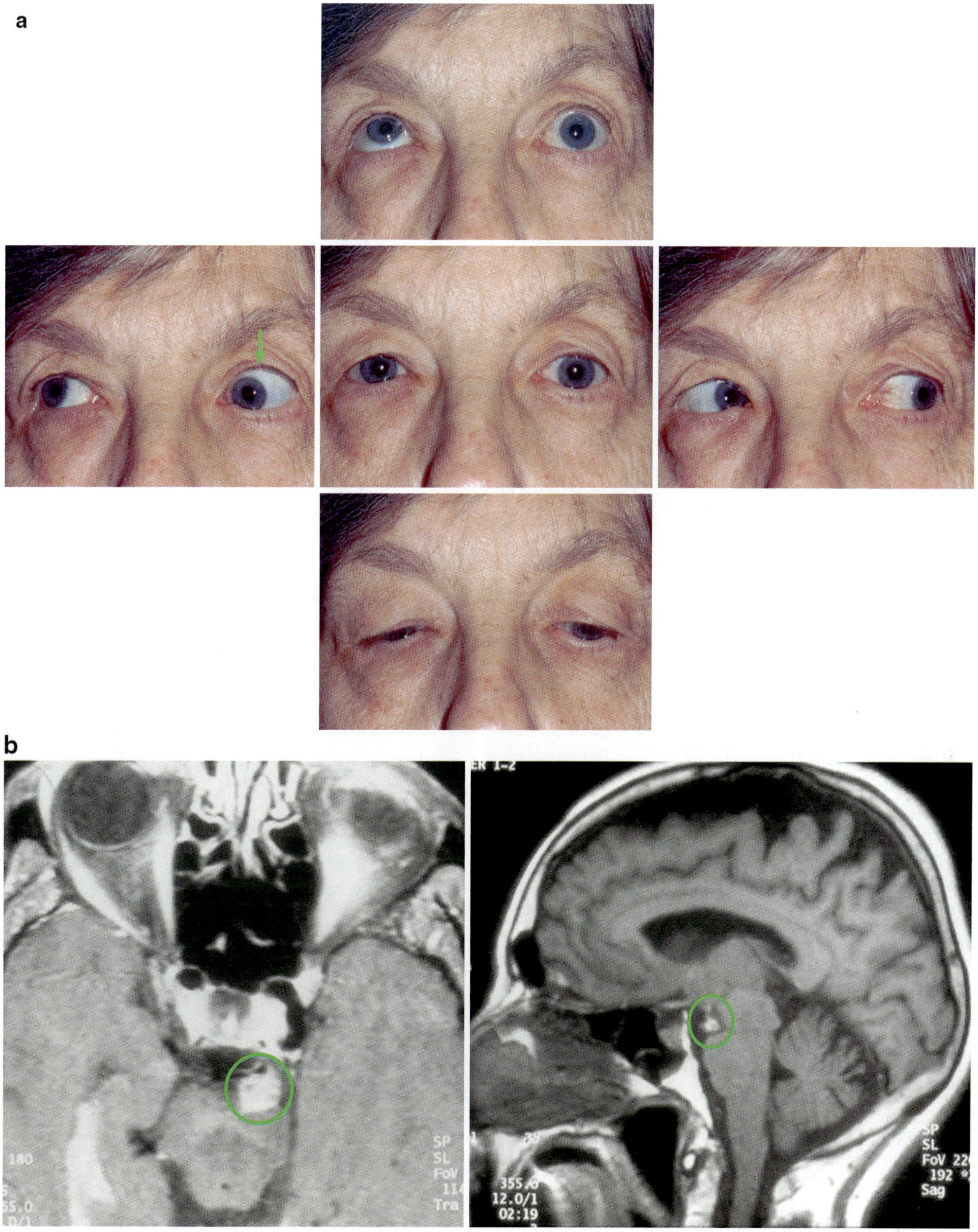

Fig. 13.22 Aberrant CN-III regeneration. (**a**) The patient presented with a complaint of right upper eyelid ptosis. She denied diplopia. On external exam, a chin-up position (not shown) was noted. Note the limitation in upgaze and adduction on the left, contralateral to her perceived ptotic lid. In primary gaze, there is a suggestion of left upper lid retraction, which increases in adduction (arrow). Subtle lid retraction is also present in downgaze (pseudo-von Graefe sign). (**b**) Neuroimaging showed an inoperable, partially thrombosed brainstem aneurysm (green circles)

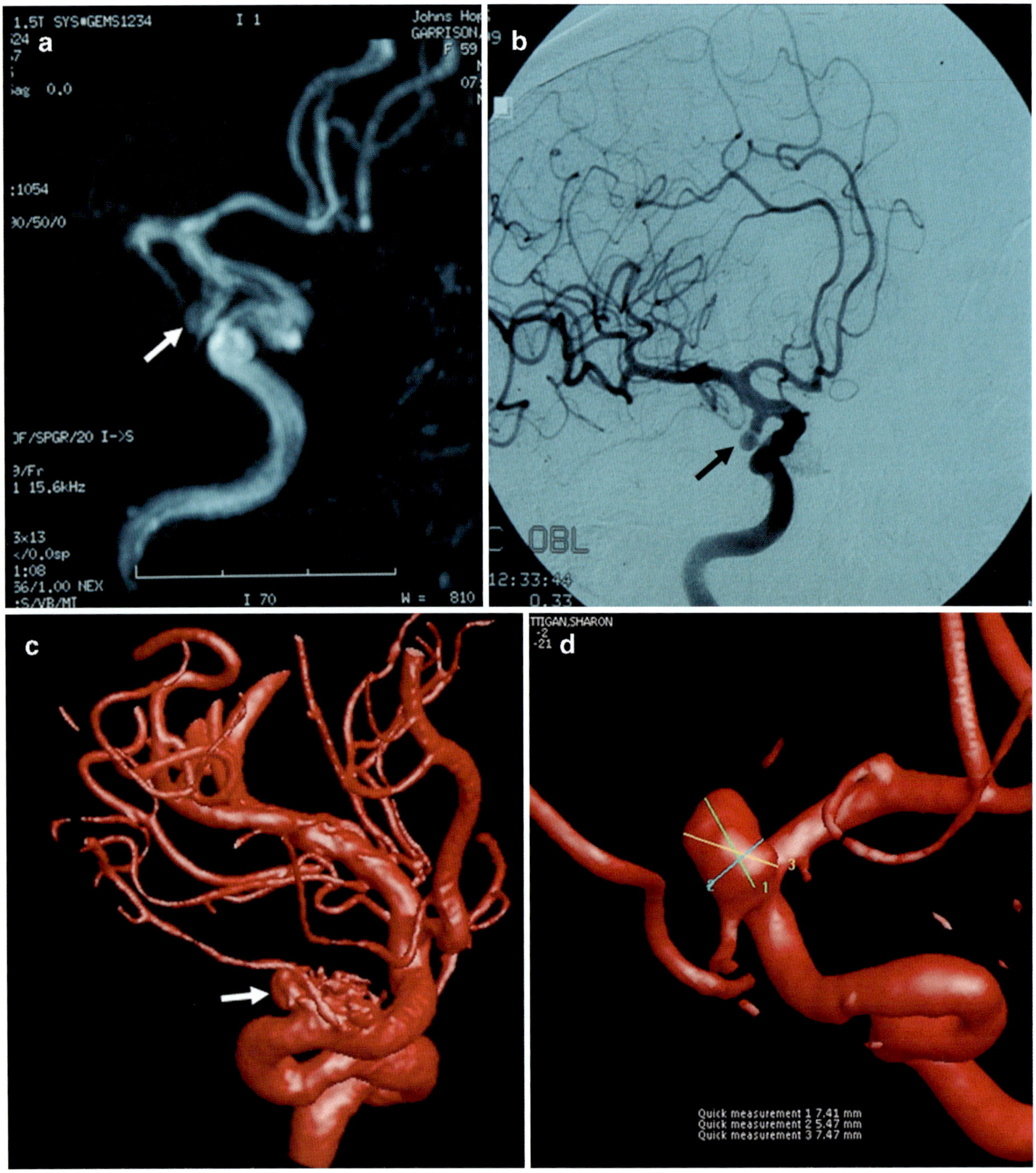

Fig. 13.23 Imaging modalities in CN-III palsy. (**a**) MRA of a posterior communicating artery aneurysm (arrow). (**b**) The same lesion on conventional angiography. (**c**) CTA of two aneurysms (arrow) with three-dimensional reconstruction. (**a** and **b** courtesy of Neil Miller, MD)

rysm and vice versa. CTA also requires the use of a large amount of intravenous contrast and radiation, which limits the use of this modality in children, in pregnant patients, and in those with limited renal function [155].

MRA is based on two differing technologies: time-of-flight (TOF-MRA) and phase-contrast MRA (PC-MRA). Under ideal circumstances, PC-MRA may be superior to TOF-MRA, but because of longer acquisition times, image degradation from patient motion is more of a concern with PC-MRA and may limit interpretation. As a broad statement, a higher-field strength (i.e., a stronger magnet) will improve the resolution of MRA. In addition, one advantage of MRI/MRA over CT/CTA is the superiority of MRI in identifying non-aneurysmal causes of CN-III dysfunction (Fig. 13.24)

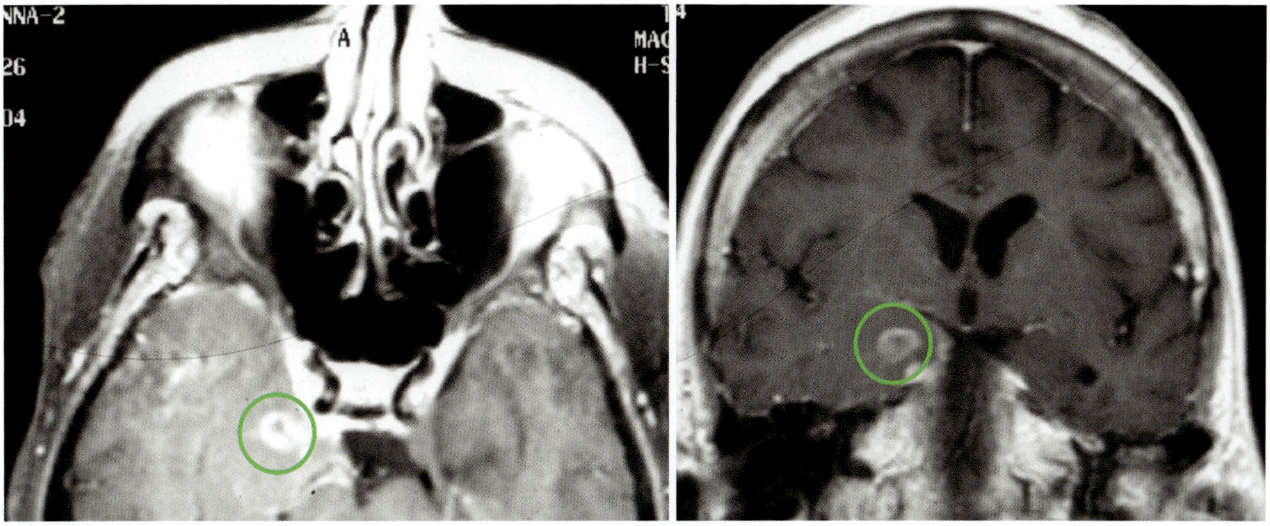

Fig. 13.24 CN-III palsy secondary to intracranial mass. A patient presented with a pupil-involving CN-III palsy. No aneurysm was noted on MRA, but MRI showed a ring-enhancing lesion. Biopsy confirmed glioblastoma

[156]. Of note, intravenous contrast (gadolinium) is not used in MRA; MRA can therefore be performed safely in patients with poor renal function.

Finally, as noted previously, no technology supersedes the ability of study interpretation. The availability of an experienced neuroradiologist is imperative in obtaining an optimum reading. Studies have shown that neuroradiologists in general are more adept at identifying both aneurysmal and non-aneurysmal pathologies in the head and neck when compared to comprehensive radiologists [160, 161]. It is also important for the clinician to clearly point the neuroradiologist toward the suspected location of the intracranial abnormality based on the clinical exam [162]. Thus, a request form that states "right CN-III palsy, rule out posterior communicating artery aneurysm" will result in a better diagnostic yield than one which states "diplopia, rule out aneurysm."

What, then, is the optimum protocol for a clinician faced with a patient with a possible aneurysmal CN-III dysfunction? Assuming the availability of the newest imaging modalities, most experts would recommend CTA over MRA as long as radiation and contrast injection are not contraindicated. If clinical suspicion for aneurysm or soft tissue mass is still high, MRI/MRA would be a reasonable next step. CCA is reserved for those patients in whom small aneurysms must be ruled out, or for the therapeutic management of aneurysm found with other modalities [155].

Marcus Gunn Jaw-Winking Synkinesis

Ptosis with synkinetic winking motion of the lid with jaw movement is termed Marcus Gunn jaw-winking (MGJW) (Fig. 13.25). This phenomenon is commonly thought to be due to an aberrant connection between motor branches of the trigeminal nerve and the superior division of the oculomotor nerve [163, 164]. The incidence of MGJW in congenital ptosis is about 5% [165]. More than half of the cases are associated with strabismus, and it is generally noted at birth when the infant is feeding [165]. Once any strabismus is addressed, ptosis correction can be considered. If the ptosis is treated, the approach varies based on the severity of the ptosis. When the jaw-wink is significant, the levator must be ablated and either unilateral or bilateral frontalis suspension performed [166]. The technique for eliminating levator function varies from complete excision of the muscle to the orbital apex to excising a portion of the muscle [167, 168]. Patients with MGJW ptosis are at greater risk of developing arrhythmias during surgery and should be monitored.

Myasthenia Gravis

Myasthenia gravis (MG) is an autoimmune disease that results in a depletion of acetylcholine (ACH) by secondary autoantibodies [169–171]. This results in clinical manifestations of muscle weakness and easy fatigability. As an oversimplification, myasthenia gravis (MG) typically occurs in two flavors. Early-onset MG, defined as onset younger than the age of 50 years, is classically a disease of females with a high incidence of thymic hyperplasia; of note, the female predilection disappears with onset between 40 and 50 years [172, 173]. Late-onset MG, which occurs after 50 years old, is more common in males [174]. Symptom severity usually peaks within 3 years of onset [175]. About 10% to 15% of all MG remains limited to the extraocular muscles and is called ocular MG (OM). External ophthalmoplegia (with or without diplopia) is the presenting sign in approximately 75% to 85% of patients with MG [170]. Interestingly, pediatric MG

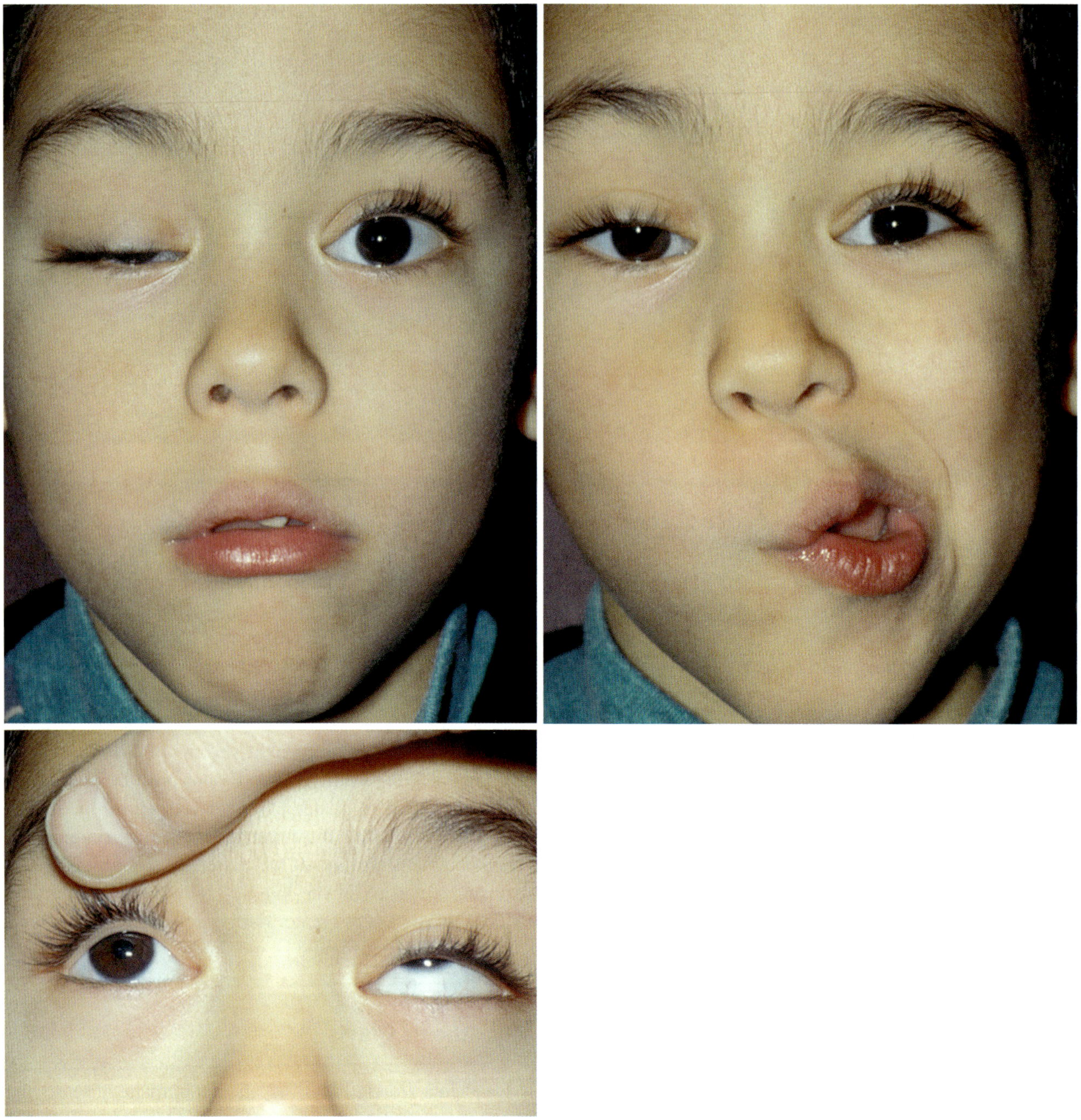

Fig. 13.25 Marcus Gunn jaw-winking synkinesis. Right ptosis improves with jaw movement. A right double elevator palsy was also present

is uncommon in North America and Europe, comprising about 10% to 15% of all MG cases, but this number increases to almost 50% in Asia [176, 177]. Familial disease is very rare [173]. A more extensive list of MG variants is found in Table 13.2.

MG has an estimated incidence of 4–11/1 million persons and a prevalence of 5–15/100,000 persons in the United States [170]. Of note, MG may be underdiagnosed in the elderly population and occur with a higher frequency of bulbar symptoms (shortness of breath, slurred speech, etc.), possibly because of confusion with other diseases seen frequently in older individuals [178]; this is an important consideration for the oculoplastic surgeon, who frequently evaluates older patients for ptosis.

Periocular symptoms and signs are extremely common in MG (eventually occurring in 90% of patients and as an initial manifestation in 75%) because the levator, extraocular, and orbicularis oculi muscles are the most commonly affected [170]. About 40% of patients will have signs and symptoms limited to the periocular region and are termed to have

Table 13.2 Characteristic features of myasthenia gravis by subtype

MG subtype	Characteristic features
Early-onset MG	Age of onset <50 years, predominantly females (60–70%) Thymic follicular hyperplasia common Probable influence of sex hormones Other autoimmune disease is common, including thyroiditis IgG1 and IgG3 antibody isotypes
Late-onset MG	Age of onset 50–60 years, no gender predominance Thymoma common Typically manifests as severe, generalized MG with significant bulbar symptoms IgG1 and IgG3 antibody isotypes Thymoma-associated MG occurs in 10–15% of all cases
Late late-onset MG	Age of onset >60 years Clear male predominance Thymic atrophy
Ocular MG	Limited to the extraocular muscles and eyelids Diagnosis is made if no generalized symptoms occur after 2 years 50% have negative AChR and MuSK antibodies
MG with MuSK antibodies	Early age of onset, typically in females Clinical presentation is usually more severe, with significant respiratory and other bulbar signs. Muscular atrophy is common, but ocular symptoms are rare Antibody titer correlates with disease severity Therapeutic management is difficult Thymus is usually normal IgG4 antibody isotypes
MG with LRP4 antibodies ("double seronegative MG")	Typically occurs in younger females (similar to MuSK+ MG) MG symptoms are usually mild IgG1 antibody isotypes
Seronegative MG	MG symptoms are usually mild Includes both generalized and purely ocular MG and clinically indistinguishable from AChR+ MG May have mild thymic follicular hyperplasia Testing for clustered AChR antibodies recommended

AChR acetylcholine receptor, *MuSK* muscle-specific receptor tyrosine kinase, *IgG* immunoglobulin G

OM. Overall, about 50–80% of patients with OM will eventually develop generalized myasthenia [179–181]. A reasonable, but by no means absolute, rule is that patients with OM who do not develop generalized signs within 2 years will in all likelihood remain localized [169, 170, 182, 183]. Patients >50 years of age who present with OM are at higher risk for developing generalized symptoms, including respiratory problems.

Variability of signs and symptoms is the hallmark of MG. While essentially all ptosis, regardless of etiology, appears to worsen toward the end of the day, the ptosis of MG is variable throughout the day and may alternate sides. Unilateral ptosis may occur. Diplopia may not be a presenting complaint if ptosis is severe enough to block one visual axis (Fig. 13.26). Of note, the combination of ptosis and orbicularis oculi weakness is highly suspicious for MG. Additional clinical findings are also suggestive of MG. Upgaze fatigue may be seen with sustained upgaze, manifesting as worsening of ptosis [170]. Enhanced ptosis is also an important sign to document and is relatively specific for MG: when one eyelid is manually elevated by the examiner, the contralateral lid should drop significantly based on Hering's law (Fig. 13.27) [184, 185]. A Cogan lid twitch may also be observed in patients with MG [186]. After looking down for several seconds, the patient is asked to make a saccade to primary gaze. The upper lids may overshoot and then either become ptotic or twitch several times before settling into a stable position.

The pattern of strabismus in MG is so myriad, often mimicking cranial nerve palsies or internuclear ophthalmoplegia, that for all intents and purposes, MG should be included in the differential diagnosis of any patient presenting with external ophthalmoplegia. Of note, MG affects striated muscles and, for practical purposes, can never cause an internal ophthalmoplegia; therefore, MG should not be considered as the only etiology in the setting of external ophthalmoplegia and nonphysiologic anisocoria. A detailed history and review of systems should be performed in any patient suspected of having MG and, for that matter, in all patients presenting with acquired ptosis. Frequently, patients will not volunteer information regarding muscle weakness, dysphagia, or shortness of breath to their ophthalmologist. Prompt referral for treatment is crucial in any patient who presents with so-called bulbar symptoms (dysphagia or respiratory difficulties) to avoid a myasthenic crisis.

The diagnosis of MG can be made in a variety of ways, including clinical, pharmacologic, serologic, and electrophysiologic testing (Table 13.3). Several caveats will be mentioned here.

Ice testing is highly specific for MG, with a sensitivity of 80–90% [187–189]. However, these numbers are typically derived from studies that include patients with possible myasthenic ptosis. A recent study which performed an ice test on all patients presenting with ptosis found a sensitivity of 92% and specificity of only 79% (positive and negative likelihood ratios of 4.35 and 0.11, respectively), casting doubt on the specificity of the test [190]. The ice test is performed by measuring the MRD, followed by placing an ice pack over the closed eyelids for 2 minutes and remeasuring the palpebral fissure. An improvement of 2 mm or more in the patient's ptosis is considered positive (Fig. 13.28) [188, 189]. A portion of this improvement is attributing to resting the lid [187]. Diplopia may also improve, but not resolve, with the ice applied for 5 minutes [191].

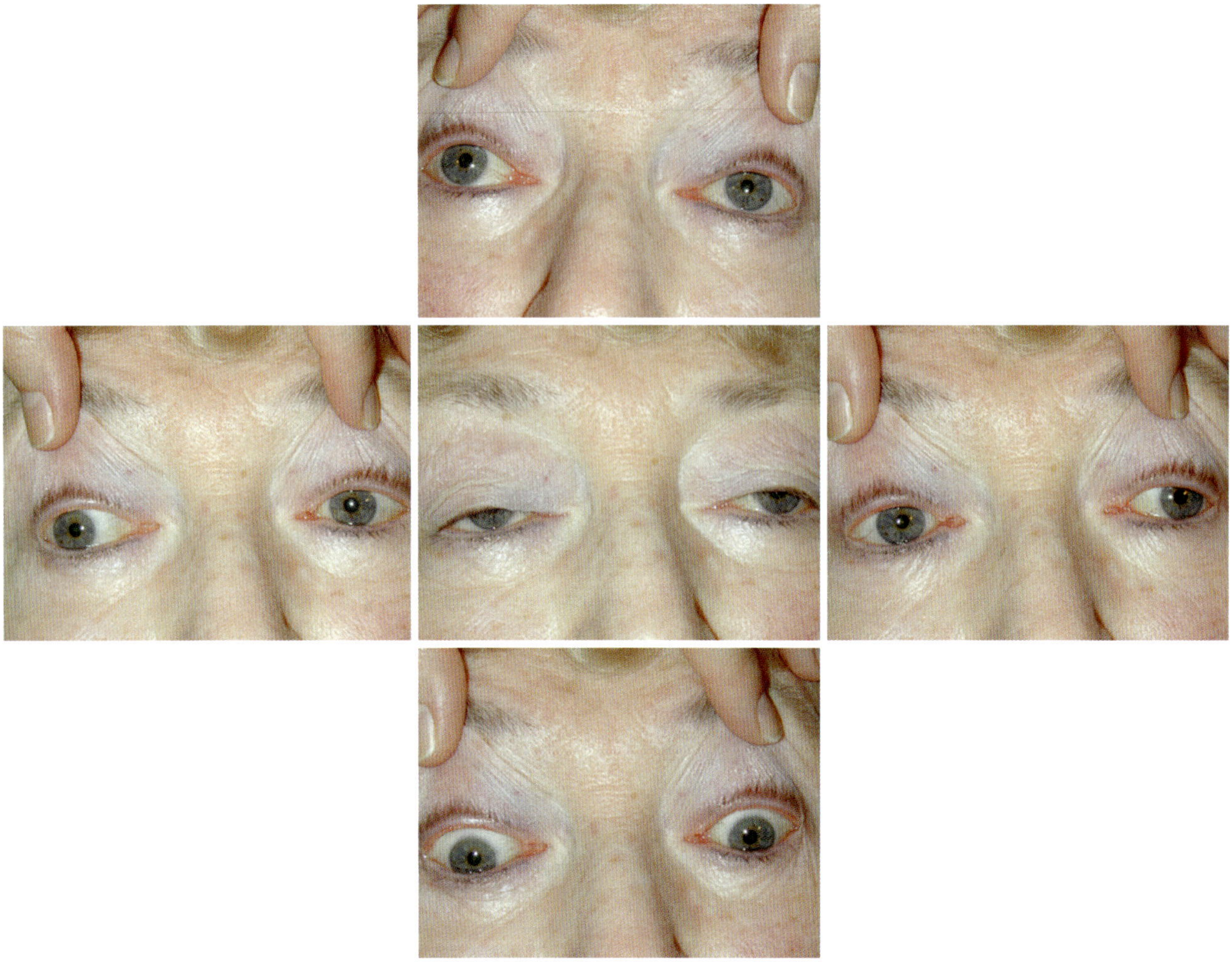

Fig. 13.26 Myasthenia gravis. Severe ptosis is noted in primary gaze, along with diffuse external ophthalmoplegia. Orbicularis oculi weakness is also present

Edrophonium (Tensilon) testing is still performed in many centers; the authors have abandoned this test in favor of other modalities. Although helpful if positive, a negative edrophonium test does not rule out MG. Furthermore, rare but significant cardiac side effects may occur, including bradycardia and asystole; the test should not be performed without careful cardiac monitoring in older patients with a history of cardiac disease [192, 193].

Testing for acetylcholine receptor (AChR) antibodies is highly specific if positive, but negative tests may be seen in up to 20% of patients with MG and in about one-half of patients (40–77%) with OM [169, 170, 194, 195]. In those patients with thymoma, positive AChR antibodies are the rule. However, patients diagnosed with MG early in their disease may initially lack AChR antibodies; the majority of such patients will develop antibodies within 1 year, and retesting in suspected cases over several months is therefore prudent [196–198]. Although AChR antibodies are highly specific for MG, occasionally other disease states (lupus, rheumatoid arthritis, paraneoplastic disease [Lambert-Eaton syndrome, usually associated with small cell lung cancer], etc.) may also manifest positive AChR antibodies on testing [196–198]. Of the three available antibody assays – binding, modulating, and blocking, the binding antibody has the highest sensitivity for both MG and OM. The combination of binding and blocking AChR antibody testing (the "reflex panel") has a very high sensitivity and specificity for generalized MG. The chance of a positive modulating antibody in the face of negative blocking and binding antibodies is very low (0.4%); the modulating antibody is therefore typically used as a confirmatory test in cases of positive binding and blocking antibody titers.

If the AChR antibody test is negative, then a muscle-specific receptor tyrosine kinase (MuSK) assay may be helpful [170, 199]. Of the 15% to 20% of MG patients with negative AChR antibodies, 40% will be positive to MuSK antibody testing [174, 200]. Overall, MuSK antibodies are found in about 5% of MG patients [201]. Myasthenia gravis

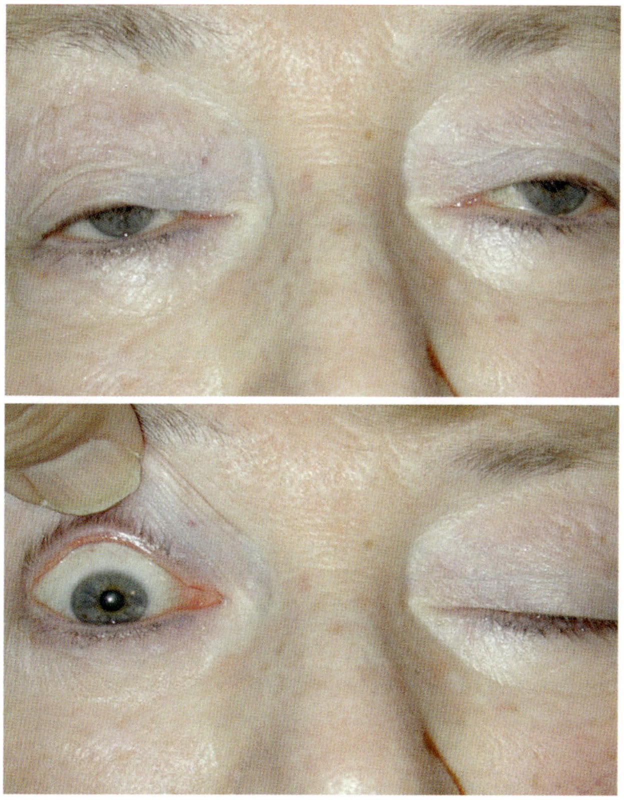

Fig. 13.27 Enhanced ptosis

Table 13.3 Sensitivity and specificity of testing for ocular myasthenia

Test	Sensitivity (%)	Specificity (%)	References
Rest	50[a]	100[a]	A
Ice	80–92[a]	79–100[a]	A, E
Edrophonium (Tensilon)	86–97	83	B, C
ACH receptor antibody (all types)	25–77	100	A, D
ACH receptor antibody (binding)	71	100	D
MuSK	50–70[b]		D
Single-fiber EMG	62–92		A, D
Chest CT	Up to 65–70[c]	89[d]	D

Refs: A [182], *B* [188], C [180], *D* [189], E [190]

[a]For ptosis

[b]Of ACH receptor antibody-negative patients with generalized myasthenia

[c]With generalized myasthenia and younger age

[d]For generalized myasthenia

with MuSK antibodies is distinctly more severe than typical AChR-positive MG, as noted in Table 13.2 [202, 203]. Of note, ocular symptoms are uncommon in this subgroup of MG.

Electromyography (EMG) is also useful in MG but must be ordered appropriately, especially in patients with OM. In general, single-fiber EMG (SFEMG) is preferable to conventional EMG. In cases of suspected OM, SFEMG of the deltoid will not suffice; instead, testing of either the frontalis or orbicularis oculi muscle must be performed. The authors have found that the combination of ice test, AChR antibody

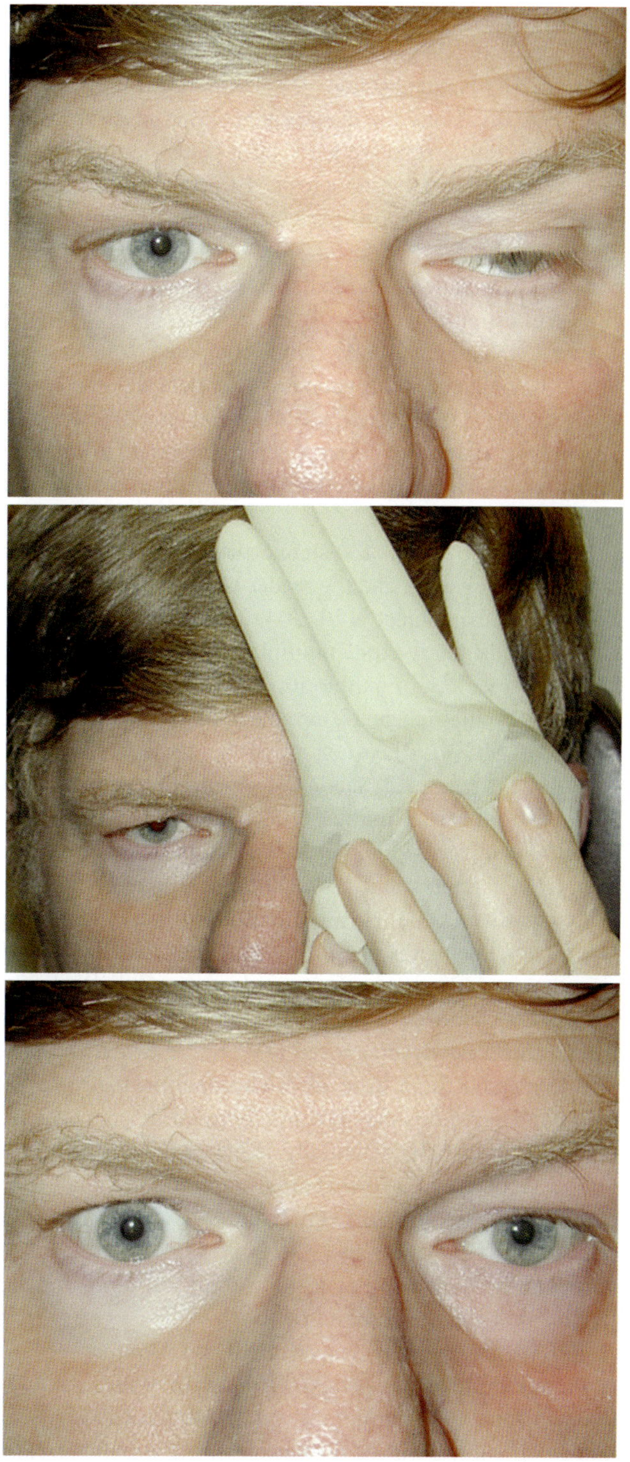

Fig. 13.28 Positive ice test. Top, initial clinical presentation. Middle, ice is applied to the eyelid, crushed for better contouring around the orbit. Bottom, 2 minutes later, a marked improvement in upper eyelid position is evident

titers, and SFEMG of the orbicularis oculi muscle has a high sensitivity in the diagnosis of even OM, although admittedly the sensitivity is not absolute.

On rare occasions, the diagnosis of OM is suspected even in patients with a negative work-up, usually because of the severity of the presenting ptosis. In such patients, some experts advocate a trial of pyridostigmine (Mestinon) prior to offering surgery. Pyridostigmine should be used with caution in elderly patients and in those with a history of cardiac disease or asthma.

Chest imaging, usually with computed tomography, should be obtained in all patients to rule out thymic hyperplasia or thymoma, which occurs in about 10% of MG patients overall [169]. This is especially important in younger patients, who have a higher incidence of thymic mass as a cause for MG [170].

The various forms of systemic therapy are beyond the scope of this chapter, and the reader is referred to other discussions on the subject [170, 204, 205]. Only three points will be made here. First, multiple systemic medications, including a variety of antibiotics, anticonvulsants, and cardiac and psychiatric agents, have been implicated in exacerbation of MG [170]; when possible, these medications should be discontinued. Second, it appears that patients who are diagnosed earlier in their clinical course (within 1 year of initial symptoms) fare better than those who are treated later. This connotes that earlier treatment may be helpful. With regard to OM, early corticosteroid therapy may be helpful in reducing the possibility of developing generalized myasthenia [179–181]. That said, the ophthalmologist should be cautious when prescribing corticosteroids for patients with newly diagnosed OM. Some experts recommend an initial high dose of prednisone, on the order of 60–80 mg daily; this may potentially result in a myasthenic crisis, a serious and potentially lethal development [206]. Others recommend a lower initial dose of 5–15 mg every other day, titrated upward slowly until the patient notes an improvement in symptoms [170, 206]. Corticosteroids also appear to be beneficial, at least in the short term, for the treatment of generalized MG [205].

Ptosis correction in patients with MG is frustrating because of the variability of the ptosis, the presence of external ophthalmoplegia, and poor corneal protective mechanisms secondary to orbicularis oculi weakness. As a general rule, systemic therapy should be tried first. If this fails, either a unilateral or bilateral ptosis crutch is often an adequate therapy, which has a great advantage of being instantly reversible if excessive keratopathy occurs. In cases where surgical repair is warranted, unilateral ptosis correction is often preferable, since this may minimize postoperative diplopia. The specific form of ptosis repair is controversial, although many experts will typically offer a frontalis sling using easily reversible material, including sutures or silicone rods [124, 207]. One possible surgical technique relies on simply moving the palpebral fissure to a higher level, theoretically minimizing any postoperative exacerbation of lagophthalmos [208]. The technique involves excision of a free tarsoconjunctival graft from the upper lid with internal levator advancement, with suturing of the free graft into the recipient bed of the lower lid after recession of the conjunctiva and lower lid retractors. In essence, both the upper and lower eyelids are raised the same height. Finally, the anesthesia team should be warned in advance of the patient's MG, as this may affect the amount and specific type of intravenous agents used. In some cases, it may be prudent to perform surgery in a hospital setting rather than in an ambulatory care center in case postoperative respiratory support is necessary.

Horner Syndrome (Oculosympathetic Paresis)

A patient with Horner syndrome (HS) will typically present with complaints of unilateral ptosis; bilateral HS occurs in only a small minority of patients. HS is the result of injury at some point along the oculosympathetic pathway which begins at the skull base (hypothalamus), travels down the neck in the cervical spine to the lung apex, and then reverses course to travel back up the neck as a neural net wrapped around the common and internal carotid arteries to reenter the skull base and the orbit via the cavernous sinus and optic canal [143, 209, 210].

An injury to the nerve fibers anywhere along this pathway will produce a paresis of the sympathetically innervated secondary eyelid retractors in the upper and lower eyelids and miosis of the ipsilateral pupil (Fig. 13.29) [209]. Anhydrosis and other more subtle findings, such as transient conjunctival injection, are less commonly encountered in clinical practice (Fig. 13.30) [209, 210]. If the iris is light in color, miosis may be noticed by the patient, but is otherwise uniformly missed in dark-colored irides. The anisocoria is visually asymptomatic in essentially all patients with HS.

Clinically, the ptosis in HS is not severe, with a disparity in the MRD1 of only 1–3 mm, consistent with the function of the Müller muscle. The finding of the awkwardly named "reverse ptosis" of the lower lid, when present, is extremely helpful and is due to paresis of the inferior tarsal muscle (Fig. 13.29) [209]. The anisocoria of HS is worse in dim than in ambient lighting, since the paretic iris dilator muscle cannot react as quickly as the uninvolved pupil. A so-called dilation lag is also a typical feature of HS [209]. Note that pupillary measurements in dim lighting should be performed efficiently, since the paretic pupil of HS will eventually dilate.

In many cases, clinical examination alone is sufficient to raise or rule out the possibility of HS, especially if reverse ptosis and nonphysiologic anisocoria are present. However, in some cases, clinical findings may be equivocal; this is

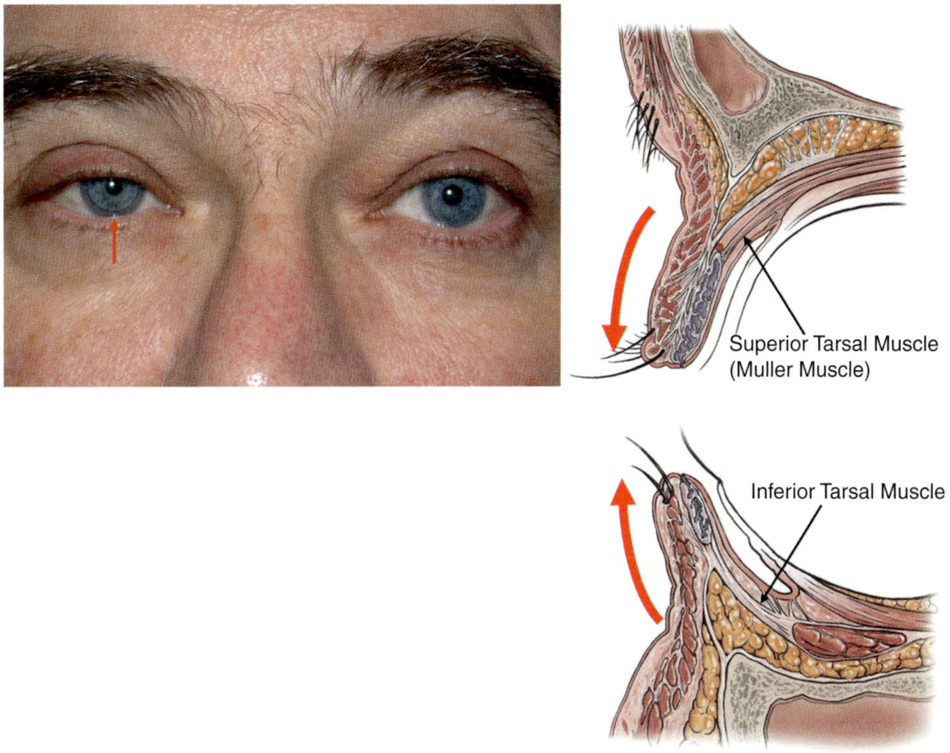

Fig. 13.29 Horner syndrome. Right upper eyelid ptosis and miosis are present. Ptosis of the lower eyelid (arrow), when present, is helpful in confirming the diagnosis clinically. Right, the anatomy of the sympathetically innervated superior and inferior tarsal muscles is shown. Paresis results in movement of both lids to narrow the palpebral fissure (arrows)

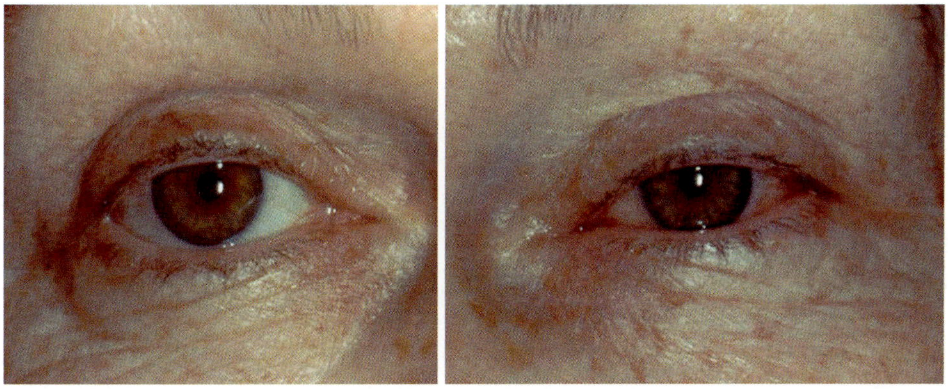

Fig. 13.30 Conjunctival hyperemia in acute left Horner syndrome. Conjunctival hyperemia on the affected side is an uncommon and transient manifestation of HS, usually disappearing in days to weeks. Hyperemia occurs because of the lack of baseline sympathetic tone on the conjunctival vessels, allowing them to dilate. Also note the presence of lower lid "reverse ptosis"

especially true in patients with dark irides, in whom accurate pupillary testing in dim and ambient lighting may be difficult. A variety of pharmacologic tests are available to confirm the diagnosis of HS and offer clues as to the etiology and duration, but many of these agents are difficult to obtain and maintain in an oculoplastic surgery office setting [210]. Four topical pharmacologic agents have been used for the diagnosis of HS: cocaine (10%), hydroxyamphetamine, diluted phenylephrine (1%), and apraclonidine (0.5%). Of these, two are impractical: hydroxyamphetamine is very difficult to obtain and cannot be used on the same day as cocaine, prompting Trobe to comment that hydroxyamphetamine testing is "a waste of time" [143, 209]; diluted phenylephrine must be mixed properly to give reasonably reliable results and requires an unspecified time lag for the development of denervation supersensitivity before it works [143]. The remaining two agents, cocaine and apraclonidine, still have a place in the diagnosis of HS [143].

Cocaine dilates the normal pupil by blocking the reuptake of norepinephrine at the neuromuscular junction of the pupil. If the oculosympathetic pathway is intact, norepinephrine is normally secreted. Blocked reuptake will result in pupillary dilation. Two drops of 10% solution are placed in each eye, and the patient is reassessed 20 minutes to 1 hour later [209].

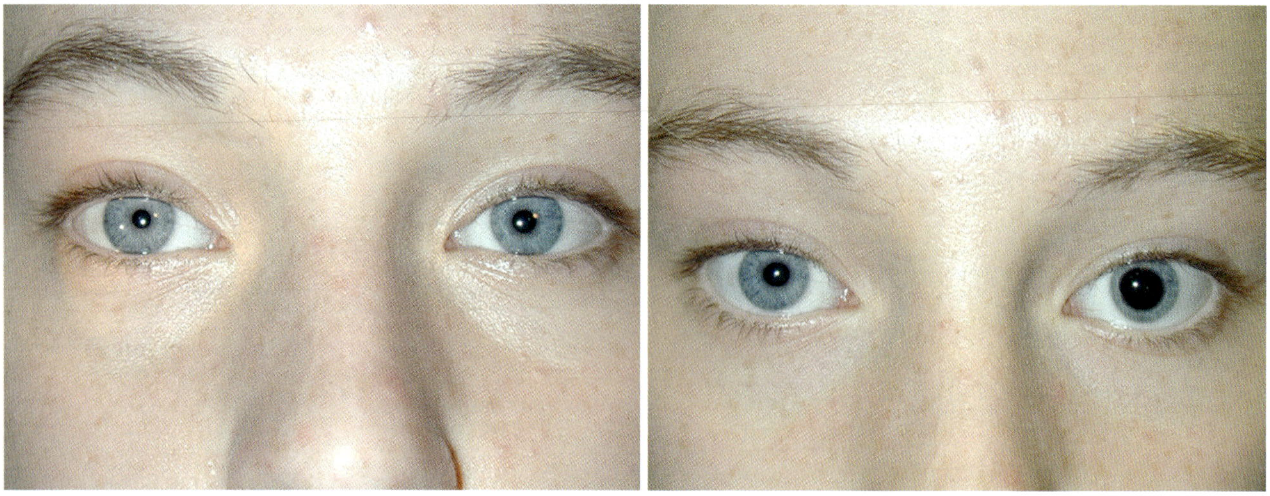

Fig. 13.31 Cocaine test. Left, initial clinical appearance. Right, after instillation of cocaine drops in both eyes, the affected right pupil fails to dilate

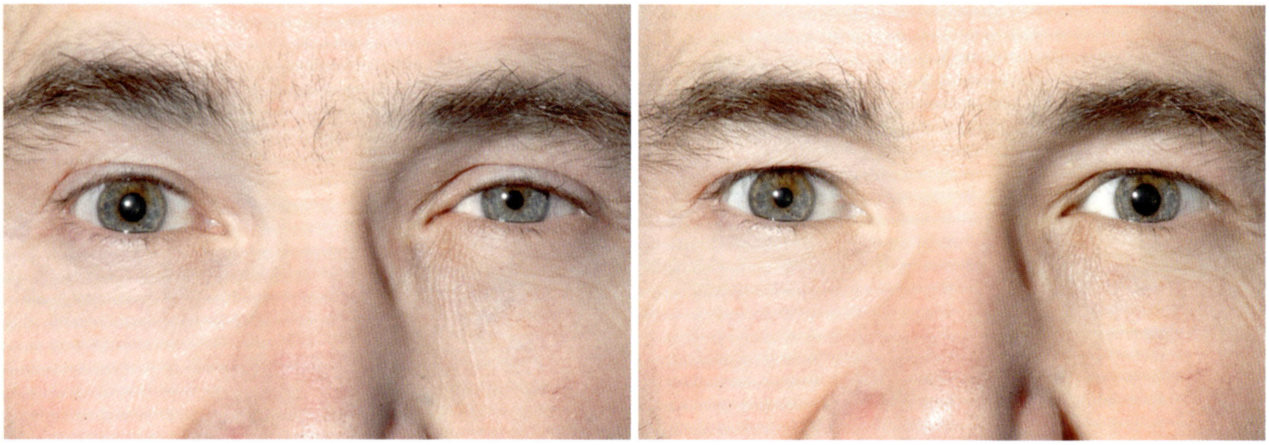

Fig. 13.32 Apraclonidine test. Left, initial clinical appearance 3 months after excision of a left cervical schwannoma. Right, instillation of apraclonidine drops in both eyes results in a reversal of anisocoria. Bilateral lid retraction, as noted here, does not always manifest

In a case of HS, the affected pupil will fail to dilate, while the normal pupil does (Fig. 13.31). The great advantage of cocaine testing is that it does not require denervation hypersensitivity to work. In other words, a positive cocaine test should be seen in even an acute HS. The disadvantages of topical cocaine include difficulty in obtaining and maintaining the medication (Schedule II drug with a shelf life of about 2 weeks), corneal toxicity, and the possibility of positive urine drug screening following the test [209–211].

Apraclonidine 0.5% (AC) is a relatively ubiquitous agent in an ophthalmologist's office and is easily available. It is an α-2 adrenergic agonist with weak α-1 action used in glaucoma treatment or as prophylaxis against intraocular pressure spikes following anterior segment laser procedures. In physiologic conditions, instillation will result in a slight miosis of the pupil and in some patients a mild upper lid retraction. In cases of HS with denervation hypersensitivity, the weak α-1 agonist property of AC will act to dilate the affected pupil. Thus, in a case of HS, the unaffected pupil will become miotic, and the affected pupil will dilate, causing a reversal of anisocoria (Fig. 13.32). Both upper eyelids may also elevate. The advantage of AC, in addition to its easy availability, is that it provides a positive finding (pupillary dilation) on the affected side. The disadvantage is that AC relies on the presence of denervation hypersensitivity, which may take days to weeks to develop, although some experts posit that AC is a relaible test 4-5 days after the onset of HS [212]. However, the sensitivity of AC in the diagnosis of acute or subacute HS is at present simply not known, and a negative AC test in such situations may not effectively rule out the possibility of HS [212, 213]. However, the sensitivity of AC in chronic HS reportedly equals (and in one study exceeds) that of cocaine [212, 214].

In most cases of HS, the etiology can be ascertained with a reasonable degree of certainty at the time of initial presentation. In a recent study of 52 patients with HS, 62% of patients had a known etiology on presentation, and an additional 21% had enough clinical clues to allow for targeted imaging [215]. That said, a selection bias based on referral patterns might have been present in this series, since most patients with a known etiology of HS were referred after head and neck surgery. It is important to obtain a detailed history that may confirm the diagnosis as well as the eiology of HS. A history of smoking, lung or breast cancer, and scapular pain suggest a lesion at the lung apex. Previous neck surgery (including thyroid, parathyroid, spine, or carotid artery procedures) points to a neck etiology.

Trobe has published practical guidelines for the initial work-up of HS, and it is useful to review these tenets here [143].

First, all patients with HS will require imaging with two exceptions. First, any patient presenting with HS following neck, cervical spine, or thoracic apex surgery does not require further work-up; the iatrogenic cause for the HS is obvious. Second, any *teenager* or *adult* presenting with classic congenital HS, which would include iris heterochromia, needs no further work-up (Fig. 13.33). All other patients with HS should be imaged.

Second, the correct imaging should be ordered in all patients. A common clinical reflex with HS is to order imaging of the brain, which in fact is one area of the head and neck that does not require radiologic examination. As already mentioned, the anatomic routing of the oculosympathetic system spans the skull base to the lung apex, and does *not* include the majority of the central nervous system. Similarly, an orbital or cavernous sinus process rarely, if ever, causes an *isolated* HS. Within the compact and richly innervated cavernous sinus, HS without other cranial neuropathy in the setting of a mass is highly unlikely. In the orbit, sympathetic fibers travel with arterial and sensory nerve branches, arborizing into a diffuse and complex system immediately in the orbital apex [216]. Isolated HS from an orbital process is anatomically untenable. Thus, dedicated orbital and cavernous sinus imaging is also not necessary in *isolated* HS. Finally, because the oculosympathetic pathway is closely aligned to the common and internal carotid arteries, a dedicated radiologic examination of these structures is indicated. Therefore, conventional MRI or CT of the neck is inadequate; MRA or CTA should be obtained as well in all cases. Imaging of the lung apex, either with a conventional X-ray techniques or with chest CT, should be performed if no definitive pathology is noted on head and neck imaging, or performed as the initial study if clinical clues suggest this anatomic area (Fig. 13.34).

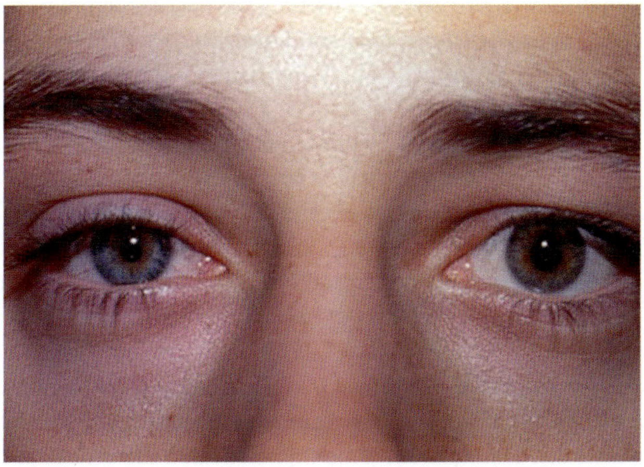

Fig. 13.33 Congenital Horner syndrome. A teenager presents with iris heterochromia and right ptosis with miosis present since birth. No further work-up is indicated

Third, timing of imaging is critical in patients with new-onset HS to rule out the possibility of acute carotid artery dissection. If the droopy lid has been present for more than 4 weeks, then routine imaging can be scheduled. In more acute or subacute cases, it is important to document whether or not head or neck pain, periorbital tingling, or other dysesthesia is present. If so, then urgent imaging is warranted to rule out carotid artery dissection (Fig. 13.35). A history of trauma may not be elicited, as even trivial trauma has been linked to carotid dissection [217, 218]. The clinician should avoid attributing painful HS to such poorly understood entities as cluster headache or Raeder's trigeminal neuralgia, which often mimic symptoms of carotid dissection [219]. HS is seen in 44–82% of patients with carotid dissection, either in isolation or with other ophthalmologic signs [218, 220]. Patients with carotid dissection are at risk for hemispheric stroke, with 88% of ocular or cerebral infarctions occurring during the first 14 days [220]. Whether the sensitivity and specificity for diagnosis of dissection are better with MRI/MRA or CT/CTA is debatable [143, 209]. At present, many experts lean toward CTA as the most sensitive modality [221], but certainly MRI/MRA is an acceptable alternative, and MRI may show thrombus within the wall of the artery better than CT; as already noted, when possible, CTA should be avoided in neonates and children because of the high radiation exposure. The final decision of what modality to order depends on the availability of each modality and the preference of the neuroradiologist. Conventional arteriography should be avoided in cases of suspected carotid dissection, since the procedure may propagate the dissection into the CNS. Whether or not anticoagulation is effective in the treatment of carotid dissection is also debatable, but most experts would at least offer antiplatelet therapy or anticoagulation to the patient [143, 218, 220, 222].

Fourth is the issue of HS in children. Not all HS in young children is necessarily congenital, and not all congenital HS in young children is benign. A recent study of pediatric HS found that no cases of malignancy were found in 20 patients presenting with congenital or acquired HS; the most frequent etiologies were traumatic (including iatrogenic) or idiopathic [223]. That said, other researchers have found significant pathology in 21–55% of pediatric HS cases [224, 225]. Acquired pediatric HS appears to have a higher incidence of a serious underlying disease (55%) than congenital HS (3%) [224]. Young children (less than 2 years of age) with classic

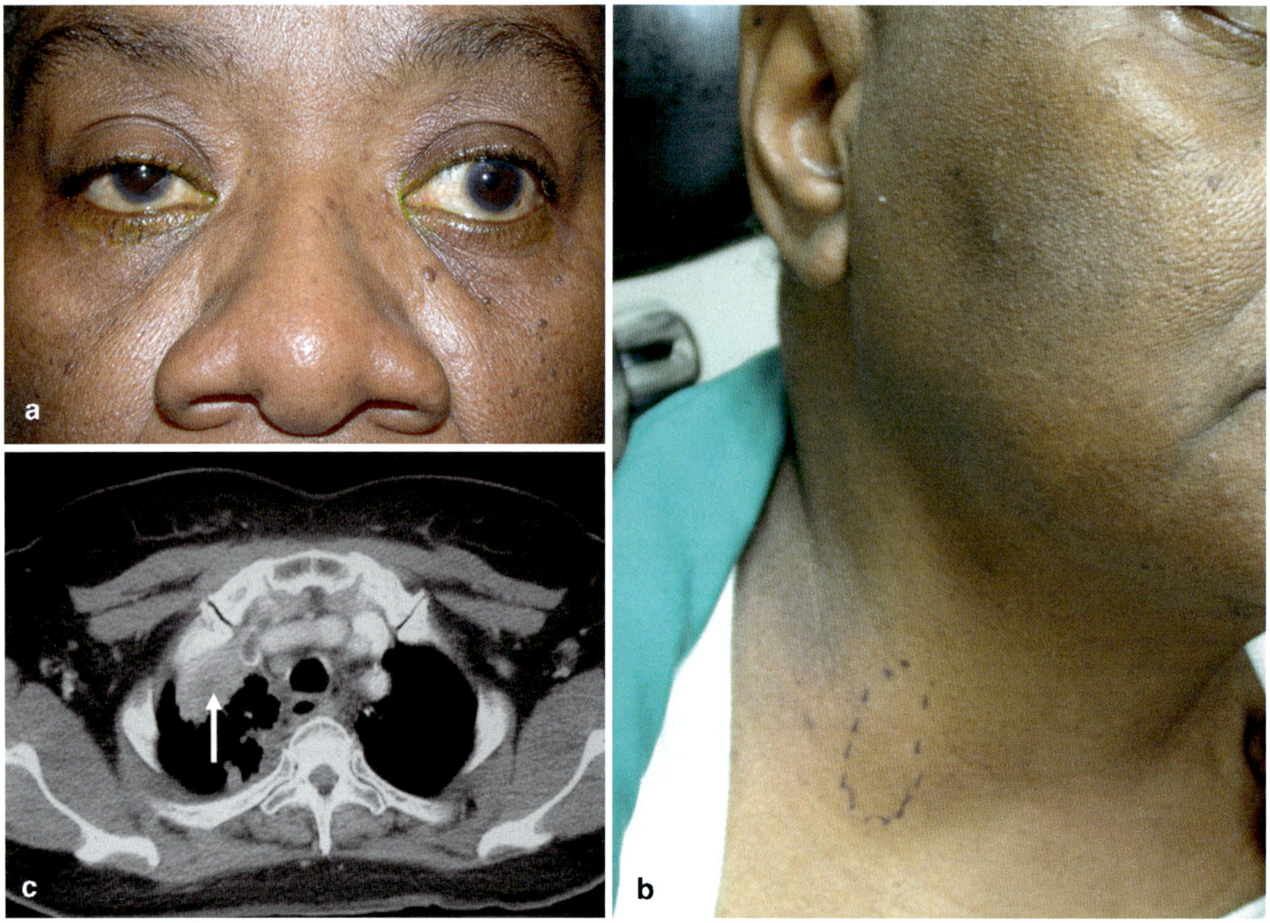

Fig. 13.34 Horner syndrome from an apical lung mass. Top left, a patient diagnosed with HS by her neurologist was referred for right ptosis repair. She had a previous history of unrelated left amblyopia and exotropia. Brain imaging was normal. Right, during initial ophthalmologic consultation, a 60-pack-year tobacco history was obtained, and fixed (**a**), rubbery lymph node was palpated just above the clavicle (**b**). Bottom left, chest CT showed an infiltrating mass extending into the right lung apex (*arrow*). Carcinoma was confirmed on bronchoscopic biopsy (**c**)

congenital HS should still undergo neuroimaging to rule out skull base or neck pathology [224–226]. Acquired HS in children must also be worked up with neuroimaging and urine catecholamine metabolite studies (homovanillic acid and vanillylmandelic acid) to rule out the possibility of malignancy, most commonly metastatic neuroblastoma (Fig. 13.36) [224]. One additional point about pediatric HS is important: avoid apraclonidine testing in children less than 1 year old unless cardiac and respiratory monitoring is available for 2 hours following eye drop instillation [143, 210]. Infants have an incomplete blood-brain barrier, and apraclonidine may cause an acute dysautonomia (cardiovascular depression).

Correction of the paralytic ptosis of HS typically requires surgery. Topical therapy with phenylephrine, apraclonidine, or brimonidine is typically not feasible over the long term because of symptomatic mydriasis. In most cases, ptosis from HS responds well to conjunctivomüllerectomy.

Botulism

Botulism is a rare disease caused by the neurotoxin produced by the anaerobe *Clostridium botulinum*. The action of the subtypes of toxins, primarily A, B and E, all result in a failure of ACH release [227]. The mode of exposure determines the types of botulism: foodborne, wound, infant, and iatrogenic botulism. Typically the presentation begins with ophthalmic signs of ptosis and ophthalmoplegia and progresses with a descending paralysis and autonomic involvement [169]. Treatment consists of antitoxin administration and supportive care in a hospital setting. The overall mortality with treatment has decreased from 79% to 3–5% [169, 228]. If a botulism outbreak is suspected, public health authorities should be informed.

Of note, the authors have seen multiple cases of paralytic ptosis due to botulinum toxin injections into the eyelids and forehead for functional or cosmetic reasons. In one case, the patient presented with ptosis and external ophthalmoplegia

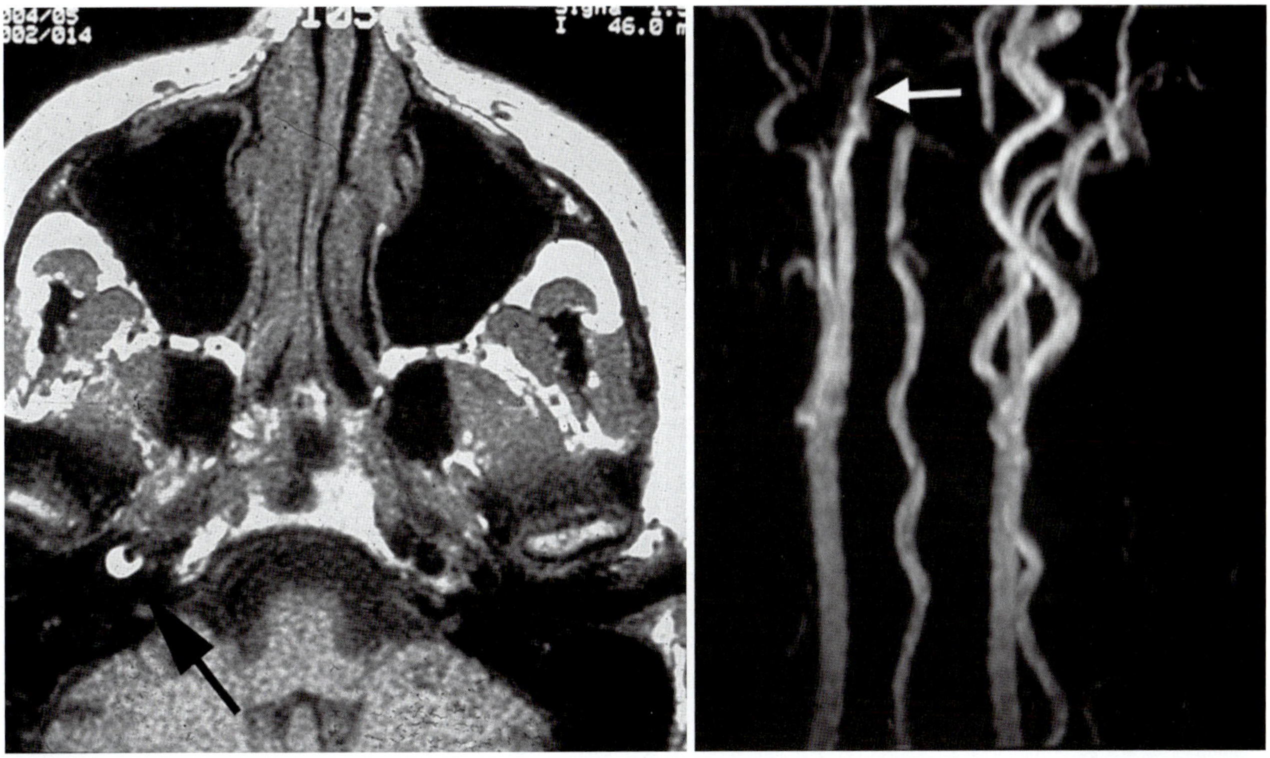

Fig. 13.35 Carotid artery dissection. Left, MRI shows a bright, crescent-shaped thrombus within the wall of the right internal carotid artery (arrow), with marked narrowing of the lumen (compare the normal left carotid flow void with the abnormally narrow right flow void). Right, MRA shows a markedly narrowed internal carotid lumen (arrow) in the area of the dissection

and underwent extensive neuroimaging for a possible oculomotor paresis despite having had cosmetic botulinum toxin injected into the forehead 1 week prior; her symptoms resolved within 2 weeks. A previous injection of botulinum toxin for either functional or cosmetic reasons should be sought in all patients presenting with an acute onset of ptosis. Very frequently patients will not disclose the injection as part of the history because they do not realize its importance.

Cluster Headache

Cluster headache (CH) is a benign neurologic disease with a series of intense, generally unilateral headaches occurring periodically [229]. CH may be associated with dietary triggers, including red wine or other alchohol consumption. Unlike migraines, CH occurs four to seven times more commonly in males than females [230]. Generally one or more autonomic symptoms occur ipsilateral to the headache, including ptosis, miosis, lacrimation, and conjunctival injection (Fig. 13.37). It is important to distinguish such cases from acute HS. The etiology of CH is not clear, though one widely accepted theory posits a hypothalamic abnormality [231]. There appears to be a genetic component to CH as well as environmental triggers for some people, including alcohol or nicotine [232, 233]. Treatments are generally categorized as either prophylactic, such as calcium channel blockers, or abortive [234]. Abortive treatments to break CH include 100% inhaled oxygen and triptans.

Recurrent Ophthalmoplegic Cranial Neuropathy

Recurrent ophthalmoplegic cranial neuropathy (previously called "ophthalmoplegic migraine") begins with migraine symptoms and progresses to include oculomotor, abducens, or trochlear neuropathies that may persist for days or weeks. This condition is usually seen in boys under the age of 10 years with an incidence of about 0.7 per million [235]. Previously this rare condition was thought of as a migraine variant. It has been recently reclassified as a neuralgia [236]. Vital in the diagnosis is the exclusion of other etiologies of painful ophthalmoplegia, such as an aneurysm [237]. MRI may show enhancement of the involved cranial nerve, generally CN-III, which disappears as the symptoms resolve [238]. Corticosteroids are generally recommended to resolve an acute episode [239].

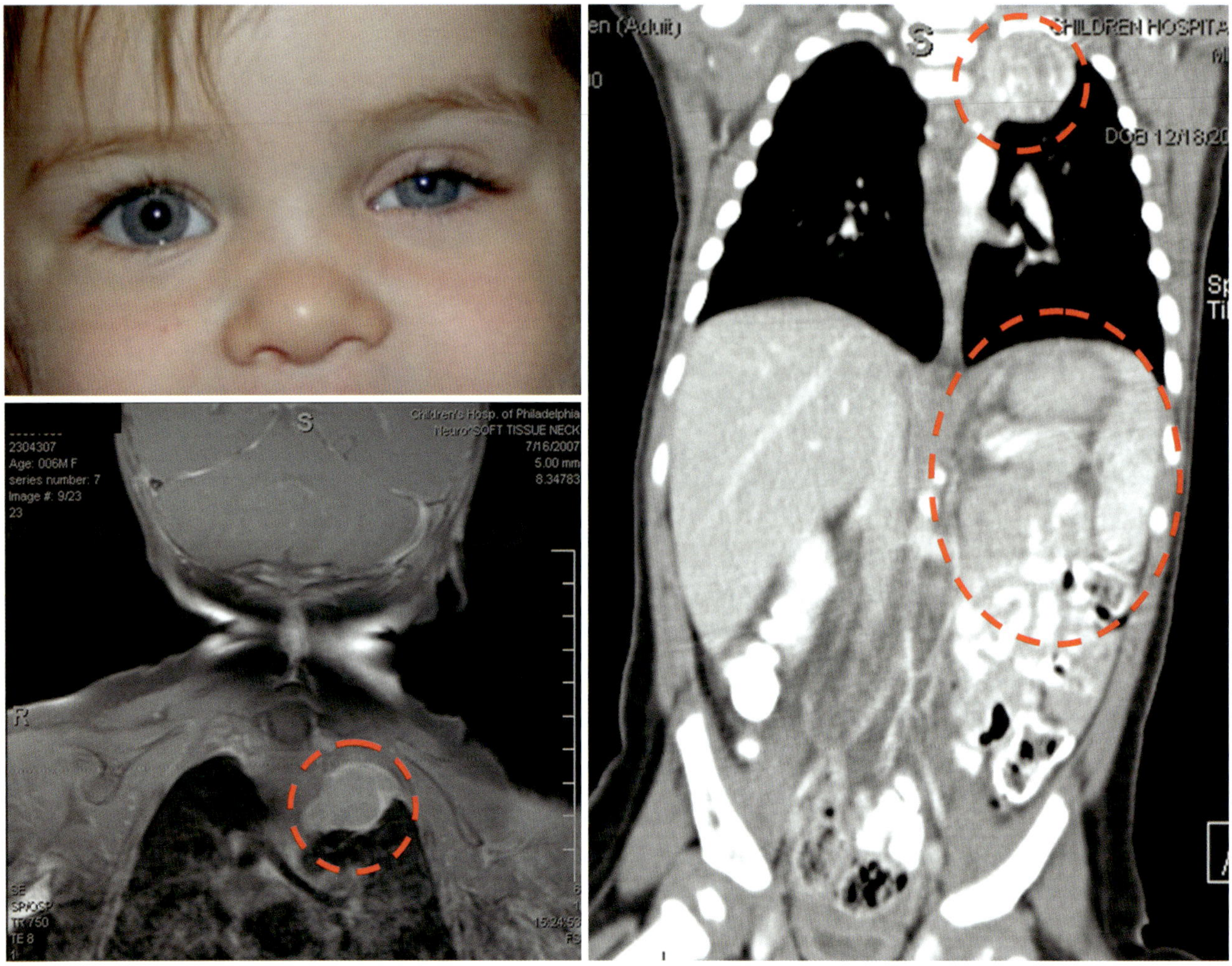

Fig. 13.36 Pediatric Horner syndrome. Top left, A 3-year-old child presents with left upper lid ptosis for 2 months. Bottom left, MRI (T-1) shows a mass at the left lung apex. Right, CT demonstrates the left lung mass and abdominal mass. Histopathology showed neuroblastoma. (Courtesy of James A. Katowitz, MD)

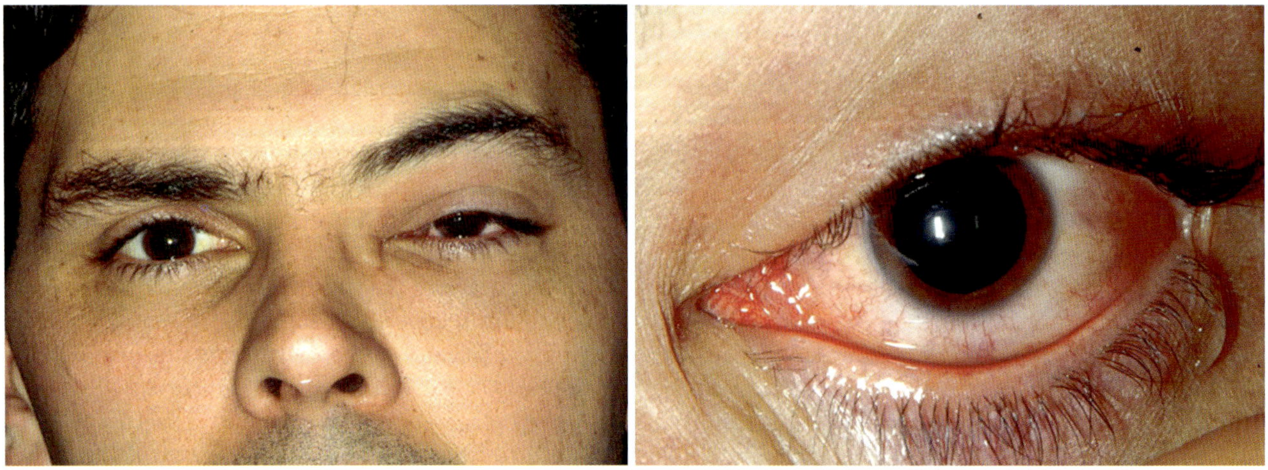

Fig. 13.37 Cluster headache. A 36-year-old man was referred for evaluation of episodes of intense left headache associated with left ptosis. He returned for evaluation during an episode. On clinical exam, note the facial grimacing, ptosis, and conjunctival hyperemia. Diffuse nasal discharge also occurred during the attacks. On detailed history, the symptoms typically occurred after alcohol use. Neuroimaging failed to reveal any intracranial abnormalities

References

1. Houghton Mifflin Harcourt Publishing Company. The American Heritage dictionary of the English language. 4th ed. Boston: Houghton Mifflin; 2000.
2. Murchison AP, Sires BA, Jian-Amadi A. Margin reflex distance in different ethnic groups. Arch Facial Plast Surg. 2009;11(5):303–5.
3. Price KM, Gupta PK, Woodward JA, Stinnett SS, Murchison AP. Eyebrow and eyelid dimensions: an anthropometric analysis of African Americans and Caucasians. Plast Reconstr Surg. 2009;124(2):615–23.
4. Lim JM, Hou JH, Singa RM, Aakalu VK, Setabutr P. Relative incidence of blepharoptosis subtypes in an oculoplastics practice at a tertiary care center. Orbit. 2013;32(4):231–4.
5. Nerad J. Evaluation and treatment of the patient with ptosis. In: Nerad JA, editor. Oculoplastic surgery the requisites in ophthalmology. St. Louis: Mosby Inc; 2001. p. 157–92.
6. Putman JRNW, Tanenbaum M, McCord CD Jr. Blepharoptosis. In: McCord Jr CD, Tannenbaum M, Nunery WR, editors. Oculoplastic surgery. New York: Raven Press; 1995. p. 175–220.
7. Lam BL, Thompson HS, Corbett JJ. The prevalence of simple anisocoria. Am J Ophthalmol. 1987;104(1):69–73.
8. Moeller JJ, Maxner CE. The dilated pupil: an update. Curr Neurol Neurosci Rep. 2007;7(5):417–22.
9. Bartley GB. The epidemiologic characteristics and clinical course of ophthalmopathy associated with autoimmune thyroid disease in Olmsted County, Minnesota. Trans Am Ophthalmol Soc. 1994;92:477–588.
10. Bartley GB. The differential diagnosis and classification of eyelid retraction. Ophthalmology. 1996;103(1):168–76.
11. Chang EL, Rubin PA. Upper and lower eyelid retraction. Int Ophthalmol Clin. 2002;42(2):45–59.
12. Bartley GB, Fatourechi V, Kadrmas EF, et al. Chronology of Graves' ophthalmopathy in an incidence cohort. Am J Ophthalmol. 1996;121(4):426–34.
13. Rubin PA, Rumelt S. Functional indications for enophthalmos repair. Ophthal Plast Reconstr Surg. 1999;15(4):284–92.
14. Cline RA, Rootman J. Enophthalmos: a clinical review. Ophthalmology. 1984;91(3):229–37.
15. Mattacks CA, Pond CM. The effects of dietary restriction and exercise on the volume of adipocytes in two intra-orbital depots in the guinea-pig. Br J Nutr. 1985;53(2):207–13.
16. Athanasiov PA, Prabhakaran VC, Selva D. Non-traumatic enophthalmos: a review. Acta Ophthalmol. 2008;86(4):356–64.
17. Shields CL, Stopyra GA, Marr BP, Moster ML, Shields JA. Enophthalmos as initial manifestation of occult, mammogram-negative carcinoma of the breast. Ophthalmic Surg Lasers Imaging. 2004;35(1):56–7.
18. Goldberg RA, Rootman J. Clinical characteristics of metastatic orbital tumors. Ophthalmology. 1990;97(5):620–4.
19. Soparkar CN, Patrinely JR, Cuaycong MJ, et al. The silent sinus syndrome. A cause of spontaneous enophthalmos. Ophthalmology. 1994;101(4):772–8.
20. Ficker LA, Collin JR, Lee JP. Management of ipsilateral ptosis with hypotropia. Br J Ophthalmol. 1986;70(10):732–6.
21. Hallett M, Evinger C, Jankovic J, Stacy M. Update on blepharospasm: report from the BEBRF international workshop. Neurology. 2008;71(16):1275–82.
22. Frueh BR, Musch DC. Treatment of facial spasm with botulinum toxin. An interim report. Ophthalmology. 1986;93(7):917–23.
23. Etgen T, Muhlau M, Gaser C, Sander D. Bilateral grey-matter increase in the putamen in primary blepharospasm. J Neurol Neurosurg Psychiatry. 2006;77(9):1017–20.
24. Obermann M, Yaldizli O, De Greiff A, et al. Morphometric changes of sensorimotor structures in focal dystonia. Mov Disord. 2007;22(8):1117–23.
25. Colosimo C, Pantano P, Calistri V, Totaro P, Fabbrini G, Berardelli A. Diffusion tensor imaging in primary cervical dystonia. J Neurol Neurosurg Psychiatry. 2005;76(11):1591–3.
26. Kerrison JB, Lancaster JL, Zamarripa FE, et al. Positron emission tomography scanning in essential blepharospasm. Am J Ophthalmol. 2003;136(5):846–52.
27. Suzuki Y, Mizoguchi S, Kiyosawa M, et al. Glucose hypermetabolism in the thalamus of patients with essential blepharospasm. J Neurol. 2007;254(7):890–6.
28. Nakashima K, Kusumi M, Inoue Y, Takahashi K. Prevalence of focal dystonias in the western area of Tottori Prefecture in Japan. Mov Disord. 1995;10(4):440–3.
29. Nutt JG, Muenter MD, Aronson A, Kurland LT, Melton LJ 3rd. Epidemiology of focal and generalized dystonia in Rochester, Minnesota. Mov Disord. 1988;3(3):188–94.
30. Epidemiological Study of Dystonia in Europe (ESDE) Collaborative Group. A prevalence study of primary dystonia in eight European countries. J Neurol. 2000;247(10):787–92.
31. Epidemiologic Study of Dystonia in Europe (ESDE) Collaborative Group. Sex-related influences on the frequency and age of onset of primary dystonia. Neurology. 1999;53(8):1871–3.
32. Defazio G, Berardelli A, Abbruzzese G, et al. Possible risk factors for primary adult onset dystonia: a case-control investigation by the Italian Movement Disorders Study Group. J Neurol Neurosurg Psychiatry. 1998;64(1):25–32.
33. Hallett M, Daroff RB. Blepharospasm: report of a workshop. Neurology. 1996;46(5):1213–8.
34. Defazio G, Martino D, Aniello MS, et al. A family study on primary blepharospasm. J Neurol Neurosurg Psychiatry. 2006;77(2):252–4.
35. Seiff SR, Zwick OM. Botulinum toxin management of upper facial rhytidosis and blepharospasm. Otolaryngol Clin N Am. 2005;38(5):887–902.
36. Defazio G, Berardelli A, Abbruzzese G, et al. Risk factors for spread of primary adult onset blepharospasm: a multicentre investigation of the Italian movement disorders study group. J Neurol Neurosurg Psychiatry. 1999;67(5):613–9.
37. Kanazawa M, Shimohata T, Sato M, Onodera O, Tanaka K, Nishizawa M. Botulinum toxin A injections improve apraxia of eyelid opening without overt blepharospasm associated with neurodegenerative diseases. Mov Disord. 2007;22(4):597–8.
38. Lamberti P, De Mari M, Zenzola A, Aniello MS, Defazio G. Frequency of apraxia of eyelid opening in the general population and in patients with extrapyramidal disorders. Neurol Sci. 2002;23(Suppl 2):S81–2.
39. Krack P, Marion MH. "Apraxia of lid opening," a focal eyelid dystonia: clinical study of 32 patients. Mov Disord. 1994;9(6):610–5.
40. Boghen D. Apraxia of lid opening: a review. Neurology. 1997;48(6):1491–4.
41. Defazio G, Livrea P, Lamberti P, et al. Isolated so-called apraxia of eyelid opening: report of 10 cases and a review of the literature. Eur Neurol. 1998;39(4):204–10.
42. Cherian V, Foroozan R. Benign unilateral apraxia of eyelid opening. Ophthalmology. 2010;117(6):1265–8.
43. Jordan DR, Anderson RL, Digre KB. Apraxia of lid opening in blepharospasm. Ophthalmic Surg. 1990;21(5):331–4.
44. Kerty E, Eidal K. Apraxia of eyelid opening: clinical features and therapy. Eur J Ophthalmol. 2006;16(2):204–8.
45. Holds JB, Anderson RL, Jordan DR, Patrinely JR. Bilateral hemifacial spasm. J Clin Neuroophthalmol. 1990;10(2):153–4.
46. Auger RG, Whisnant JP. Hemifacial spasm in Rochester and Olmsted County, Minnesota, 1960 to 1984. Arch Neurol. 1990;47(11):1233–4.
47. Bernardi B, Zimmerman RA, Savino PJ, Adler C. Magnetic resonance tomographic angiography in the investigation of hemifacial spasm. Neuroradiology. 1993;35(8):606–11.

48. Hosoya T, Watanabe N, Yamaguchi K, Saito S, Nakai O. Three-dimensional-MRI of neurovascular compression in patients with hemifacial spasm. Neuroradiology. 1995;37(5):350–2.
49. Nielsen VK, Jannetta PJ. Pathophysiology of hemifacial spasm: III. Effects of facial nerve decompression. Neurology. 1984;34(7):891–7.
50. Nielsen VK. Pathophysiology of hemifacial spasm: II. Lateral spread of the supraorbital nerve reflex. Neurology. 1984;34(4):427–31.
51. Nielsen VK. Pathophysiology of hemifacial spasm: I. Ephaptic transmission and ectopic excitation. Neurology. 1984;34(4):418–26.
52. Matsuura N, Kondo A. Trigeminal neuralgia and hemifacial spasm as false localizing signs in patients with a contralateral mass of the posterior cranial fossa. Report of three cases. J Neurosurg. 1996;84(6):1067–71.
53. Nagata S, Matsushima T, Fujii K, Fukui M, Kuromatsu C. Hemifacial spasm due to tumor, aneurysm, or arteriovenous malformation. Surg Neurol. 1992;38(3):204–9.
54. Wang A, Jankovic J. Hemifacial spasm: clinical findings and treatment. Muscle Nerve. 1998;21(12):1740–7.
55. Koutsis G, Kokotis P, Sarrigiannis P, Anagnostouli M, Sfagos C, Karandreas N. Spastic paretic hemifacial contracture in multiple sclerosis: a neglected clinical and EMG entity. Mult Scler. 2008;14(7):927–32.
56. Krauss JK, Wakhloo AK, Scheremet R, Seeger W. Facial myokymia and spastic paretic facial contracture as the result of anaplastic pontocerebellar glioma. Neurosurgery. 1993;32(6):1031–4.
57. Savino PJ, Maus M. Botulinum toxin therapy. Neurol Clin. 1991;9(1):205–24.
58. Simpson DM, Blitzer A, Brashear A, et al. Assessment: botulinum neurotoxin for the treatment of movement disorders (an evidence-based review): report of the Therapeutics and Technology Assessment Subcommittee of the American Academy of Neurology. Neurology. 2008;70(19):1699–706.
59. Bilyk JR, Yen MT, Bradley EA, Wladis EJ, Mawn LA. Chemodenervation for the treatment of facial dystonia: a report by the American Academy of Ophthalmology. Ophthalmology. 2018;125(9):1459–67.
60. Blackburn MK, Lamb RD, Digre KB, et al. FL-41 tint improves blink frequency, light sensitivity, and functional limitations in patients with benign essential blepharospasm. Ophthalmology. 2009;116(5):997–1001.
61. Chapman KL, Bartley GB, Waller RR, Hodge DO. Follow-up of patients with essential blepharospasm who underwent eyelid protractor myectomy at the Mayo Clinic from 1980 through 1995. Ophthal Plast Reconstr Surg. 1999;15(2):106–10.
62. Grivet D, Robert PY, Thuret G, et al. Assessment of blepharospasm surgery using an improved disability scale: study of 138 patients. Ophthal Plast Reconstr Surg. 2005;21(3):230–4.
63. Nicoletti AG, Pereira IC, Matayoshi S. Browlifting as an alternative procedure for apraxia of eyelid opening. Ophthal Plast Reconstr Surg. 2009;25(1):46–7.
64. Fante RG, Frueh BR. Differential section of the seventh nerve as a tertiary procedure for the treatment of benign essential blepharospasm. Ophthal Plast Reconstr Surg. 2001;17(4):276–80.
65. Barker FG 2nd, Jannetta PJ, Bissonette DJ, Shields PT, Larkins MV, Jho HD. Microvascular decompression for hemifacial spasm. J Neurosurg. 1995;82(2):201–10.
66. Artz GJ, Hux FJ, Larouere MJ, Bojrab DI, Babu S, Pieper DR. Endoscopic vascular decompression. Otol Neurotol. 2008;29(7):995–1000.
67. Pfaffenbach DD, Cross HE, Kearns TP. Congenital anomalies in Duane's retraction syndrome. Arch Ophthalmol. 1972;88(6):635–9.
68. DeRespinis PA, Caputo AR, Wagner RS, Guo S. Duane's retraction syndrome. Surv Ophthalmol. 1993;38(3):257–88.
69. Raab EL. Clinical features of Duane's syndrome. J Pediatr Ophthalmol Strabismus. 1986;23(2):64–8.
70. Huber A. Electrophysiology of the retraction syndromes. Br J Ophthalmol. 1974;58(3):293–300.
71. Alexandrakis G, Saunders RA. Duane retraction syndrome. Ophthalmol Clin N Am. 2001;14(3):407–17.
72. Fowler AM, Dutton JJ. Floppy eyelid syndrome as a subset of lax eyelid conditions: relationships and clinical relevance (an ASOPRS thesis). Ophthal Plast Reconstr Surg. 2010;26(3):195–204.
73. Taban M, Perry JD. Plasma leptin levels in patients with floppy eyelid syndrome. Ophthal Plast Reconstr Surg. 2006;22(5):375–7.
74. Schlotzer-Schrehardt U, Stojkovic M, Hofmann-Rummelt C, Cursiefen C, Kruse FE, Holbach LM. The pathogenesis of floppy eyelid syndrome: involvement of matrix metalloproteinases in elastic fiber degradation. Ophthalmology. 2005;112(4):694–704.
75. Goldberg R, Seiff S, McFarland J, Simons K, Shorr N. Floppy eyelid syndrome and blepharochalasis. Am J Ophthalmol. 1986;102(3):376–81.
76. McNab AA. Floppy eyelid syndrome and obstructive sleep apnea. Ophthal Plast Reconstr Surg. 1997;13(2):98–114.
77. Langford JD, Linberg JV. A new physical finding in floppy eyelid syndrome. Ophthalmology. 1998;105(1):165–9.
78. Culbertson WW, Tseng SC. Corneal disorders in floppy eyelid syndrome. Cornea. 1994;13(1):33–42.
79. Dutton JJ. Surgical management of floppy eyelid syndrome. Am J Ophthalmol. 1985;99(5):557–60.
80. Katusic SK, Beard CM, Wiederholt WC, Bergstralh EJ, Kurland LT. Incidence, clinical features, and prognosis in Bell's palsy, Rochester, Minnesota, 1968-1982. Ann Neurol. 1986;20(5):622–7.
81. Kimura J, Rodnitzky RL, Okawara SH. Electrophysiologic analysis of aberrant regeneration after facial nerve paralysis. Neurology. 1975;25(10):989–93.
82. Celik M, Forta H, Vural C. The development of synkinesis after facial nerve paralysis. Eur Neurol. 2000;43(3):147–51.
83. Yamamoto E, Nishimura H, Hirono Y. Occurrence of sequelae in Bell's palsy. Acta Otolaryngol Suppl. 1988;446:93–6.
84. Moran CJ, Neely JG. Patterns of facial nerve synkinesis. Laryngoscope. 1996;106(12 Pt 1):1491–6.
85. Rijntjes M, Tegenthoff M, Liepert J, et al. Cortical reorganization in patients with facial palsy. Ann Neurol. 1997;41(5):621–30.
86. Valls-Sole J, Montero J. Movement disorders in patients with peripheral facial palsy. Mov Disord. 2003;18(12):1424–35.
87. Keegan DJ, Geerling G, Lee JP, Blake G, Collin JR, Plant GT. Botulinum toxin treatment for hyperlacrimation secondary to aberrant regenerated seventh nerve palsy or salivary gland transplantation. Br J Ophthalmol. 2002;86(1):43–6.
88. Lee V, Currie Z, Collin JR. Ophthalmic management of facial nerve palsy. Eye (Lond). 2004;18(12):1225–34.
89. VanSwearingen JM, Brach JS. Changes in facial movement and synkinesis with facial neuromuscular reeducation. Plast Reconstr Surg. 2003;111(7):2370–5.
90. Cronin GW, Steenerson RL. The effectiveness of neuromuscular facial retraining combined with electromyography in facial paralysis rehabilitation. Otolaryngol Head Neck Surg. 2003;128(4):534–8.
91. Demer JL, Clark RA, Engle EC. Magnetic resonance imaging evidence for widespread orbital dysinnervation in congenital fibrosis of extraocular muscles due to mutations in KIF21A. Invest Ophthalmol Vis Sci. 2005;46(2):530–9.
92. Engle EC, Goumnerov BC, McKeown CA, et al. Oculomotor nerve and muscle abnormalities in congenital fibrosis of the extraocular muscles. Ann Neurol. 1997;41(3):314–25.
93. Engle EC. The genetic basis of complex strabismus. Pediatr Res. 2006;59(3):343–8.
94. Egan RA, Kerrison JB. Survey of genetic neuro-ophthalmic disorders. Ophthalmol Clin N Am. 2003;16(4):595–605, vii.

95. Engle EC, Kunkel LM, Specht LA, Beggs AH. Mapping a gene for congenital fibrosis of the extraocular muscles to the centromeric region of chromosome 12. Nat Genet. 1994;7(1):69–73.
96. Wang SM, Zwaan J, Mullaney PB, et al. Congenital fibrosis of the extraocular muscles type 2, an inherited exotropic strabismus fixus, maps to distal 11q13. Am J Hum Genet. 1998;63(2):517–25.
97. Engle EC, Marondel I, Houtman WA, et al. Congenital fibrosis of the extraocular muscles (autosomal dominant congenital external ophthalmoplegia): genetic homogeneity, linkage refinement, and physical mapping on chromosome 12. Am J Hum Genet. 1995;57(5):1086–94.
98. Aubourg P, Krahn M, Bernard R, et al. Assignment of a new congenital fibrosis of extraocular muscles type 3 (CFEOM3) locus, FEOM4, based on a balanced translocation t(2;13) (q37.3;q12.11) and identification of candidate genes. J Med Genet. 2005;42(3):253–9.
99. Doherty EJ, Macy ME, Wang SM, Dykeman CP, Melanson MT, Engle EC. CFEOM3: a new extraocular congenital fibrosis syndrome that maps to 16q24.2-q24.3. Invest Ophthalmol Vis Sci. 1999;40(8):1687–94.
100. Heidary G, Engle EC, Hunter DG. Congenital fibrosis of the extraocular muscles. Semin Ophthalmol. 2008;23(1):3–8.
101. Harley RD, Rodrigues MM, Crawford JS. Congenital fibrosis of the extraocular muscles. J Pediatr Ophthalmol Strabismus. 1978;15(6):346–58.
102. MOxley RT 3rd. Proximal myotonic myopathy: mini-review of a recently delineated clinical disorder. Neuromuscul Disord. 1996;6(2):87–93.
103. Day JW, Ricker K, Jacobsen JF, et al. Myotonic dystrophy type 2: molecular, diagnostic and clinical spectrum. Neurology. 2003;60(4):657–64.
104. Ranum LP, Day JW. Myotonic dystrophy: RNA pathogenesis comes into focus. Am J Hum Genet. 2004;74(5):793–804.
105. Mathieu J, Allard P, Potvin L, Prevost C, Begin P. A 10-year study of mortality in a cohort of patients with myotonic dystrophy. Neurology. 1999;52(8):1658–62.
106. Brais B, Xie YG, Sanson M, et al. The oculopharyngeal muscular dystrophy locus maps to the region of the cardiac alpha and beta myosin heavy chain genes on chromosome 14q11.2-q13. Hum Mol Genet. 1995;4(3):429–34.
107. Blumen SC, Nisipeanu P, Sadeh M, et al. Epidemiology and inheritance of oculopharyngeal muscular dystrophy in Israel. Neuromuscul Disord. 1997;7(Suppl 1):S38–40.
108. Brunet G, Tome FM, Eymard B, Robert JM, Fardeau M. Genealogical study of oculopharyngeal muscular dystrophy in France. Neuromuscul Disord. 1997;7(Suppl 1):S34–7.
109. Grewal RP, Karkera JD, Grewal RK, Detera-Wadleigh SD. Mutation analysis of oculopharyngeal muscular dystrophy in Hispanic American families. Arch Neurol. 1999;56(11):1378–81.
110. Becher MW, Morrison L, Davis LE, et al. Oculopharyngeal muscular dystrophy in Hispanic New Mexicans. JAMA. 2001;286(19):2437–40.
111. Bouchard JP, Brais B, Brunet D, Gould PV, Rouleau GA. Recent studies on oculopharyngeal muscular dystrophy in Quebec. Neuromuscul Disord. 1997;7(Suppl 1):S22–9.
112. Victor M, Hayes R, Adams RD. Oculopharyngeal muscular dystrophy. A familial disease of late life characterized by dysphagia and progressive ptosis of the eyelids. N Engl J Med. 1962;267:1267–72.
113. Murphy SF, Drachman DB. The oculopharyngeal syndrome. JAMA. 1968;203(12):1003–8.
114. Hill ME, Creed GA, McMullan TF, et al. Oculopharyngeal muscular dystrophy: phenotypic and genotypic studies in a UK population. Brain. 2001;124(Pt 3):522–6.
115. Brais B, Bouchard JP, Xie YG, et al. Short GCG expansions in the PABP2 gene cause oculopharyngeal muscular dystrophy. Nat Genet. 1998;18(2):164–7.
116. Blumen SC, Brais B, Korczyn AD, et al. Homozygotes for oculopharyngeal muscular dystrophy have a severe form of the disease. Ann Neurol. 1999;46(1):115–8.
117. Ruegg S, Lehky Hagen M, Hohl U, et al. Oculopharyngeal muscular dystrophy - an under-diagnosed disorder? Swiss Med Wkly. 2005;135(39–40):574–86.
118. Rodrigue D, Molgat YM. Surgical correction of blepharoptosis in oculopharyngeal muscular dystrophy. Neuromuscul Disord. 1997;7(Suppl 1):S82–4.
119. Codere F. Oculopharyngeal muscular dystrophy. Can J Ophthalmol. 1993;28(1):1–2.
120. Caron MJ, Girard F, Girard DC, et al. Cisatracurium pharmacodynamics in patients with oculopharyngeal muscular dystrophy. Anesth Analg. 2005;100(2):393–7.
121. Edmond JC. Mitochondrial disorders. Int Ophthalmol Clin. 2009;49(3):27–33.
122. Greaves LC, Yu-Wai-Man P, Blakely EL, et al. Mitochondrial DNA defects and selective extraocular muscle involvement in CPEO. Invest Ophthalmol Vis Sci. 2010;51(7):3340–6.
123. Finsterer J. Mitochondrial disorder mimicking ocular myasthenia. Acta Neurol Belg. 2010;110(1):110–2.
124. Lelli GJ Jr, Musch DC, Frueh BR, Nelson CC. Outcomes in silicone rod frontalis suspension surgery for high-risk noncongenital blepharoptosis. Ophthal Plast Reconstr Surg. 2009;25(5):361–5.
125. Almousa R, Charlton A, Rajesh ST, Sundar G, Amrith S. Optimizing muscle biopsy for the diagnosis of mitochondrial myopathy. Ophthal Plast Reconstr Surg. 2009;25(5):366–70.
126. Lopez-Gallardo E, Lopez-Perez MJ, Montoya J, Ruiz-Pesini E. CPEO and KSS differ in the percentage and location of the mtDNA deletion. Mitochondrion. 2009;9(5):314–7.
127. Yesil M, Bayata S, Postaci N, Arikan E. Progression of conduction system disease in a paced patient with Kearns-Sayre syndrome. Clin Cardiol. 2009;32(6):E65–7.
128. Gronlund MA, Honarvar AK, Andersson S, et al. Ophthalmological findings in children and young adults with genetically verified mitochondrial disease. Br J Ophthalmol. 2010;94(1):121–7.
129. Snyder LA, Rismondo V, Miller NR. The Fisher variant of Guillain-Barre syndrome (Fisher syndrome). J Neuroophthalmol. 2009;29(4):312–24.
130. Hughes RA, Cornblath DR. Guillain-Barre syndrome. Lancet. 2005;366(9497):1653–66.
131. Hughes RA, Swan AV, van Doorn PA. Corticosteroids for Guillain-Barre syndrome. Cochrane Database Syst Rev. 2010;2:CD001446.
132. van der Meche FG, van Doorn PA. Guillain-Barre syndrome and chronic inflammatory demyelinating polyneuropathy: immune mechanisms and update on current therapies. Ann Neurol. 1995;37(Suppl 1):S14–31.
133. Yang YR, Liu SL, Qin ZY, et al. Comparative proteomics analysis of cerebrospinal fluid of patients with Guillain-Barre syndrome. Cell Mol Neurobiol. 2008;28(5):737–44.
134. Raphael JC, Chevret S, Hughes RA, Annane D. Plasma exchange for Guillain-Barre syndrome. Cochrane Database Syst Rev. 2002;2:CD001798.
135. Hughes RA, Raphael JC, Swan AV, van Doorn PA. Intravenous immunoglobulin for Guillain-Barre syndrome. Cochrane Database Syst Rev. 2006;1:CD002063.
136. Tan H. Bilateral oculomotor palsy secondary to pseudotumor cerebri. Pediatr Neurol. 2010;42(2):141–2.
137. Bahmani Kashkouli M, Khalatbari MR, Yahyavi ST, Borghei-Razavi H, Soltan-Sanjari M. Pituitary apoplexy presenting as acute painful isolated unilateral third cranial nerve palsy. Arch Iran Med. 2008;11(4):466–8.

138. Beckmann YY, Deniz B, Gelal F, Secil Y. Third cranial nerve palsy as the presenting neuro-ophthalmic feature of nasopharyngeal carcinoma. J Neuroophthalmol. 2010;30(1):102–3.
139. Beleza P, Machado A, Soares-Fernandes J, et al. Isolated oculomotor nerve paresis as the presenting sign of multiple sclerosis. Arq Neuropsiquiatr. 2008;66(2A):254–5.
140. Brazis PW. Isolated palsies of cranial nerves III, IV, and VI. Semin Neurol. 2009;29(1):14–28.
141. Akagi T, Miyamoto K, Kashii S, Yoshimura N. Cause and prognosis of neurologically isolated third, fourth, or sixth cranial nerve dysfunction in cases of oculomotor palsy. Jpn J Ophthalmol. 2008;52(1):32–5.
142. Cullom ME, Savino PJ, Sergott RC, Bosley TM. Relative pupillary sparing third nerve palsies. To arteriogram or not? J Neuroophthalmol. 1995;15(3):136–40; discussion 140–131.
143. Trobe JD. The evaluation of horner syndrome. J Neuroophthalmol. 2010;30(1):1–2.
144. Jacobson DM. Pupil involvement in patients with diabetes-associated oculomotor nerve palsy. Arch Ophthalmol. 1998;116(6):723–7.
145. Jacobson DM, Trobe JD. The emerging role of magnetic resonance angiography in the management of patients with third cranial nerve palsy. Am J Ophthalmol. 1999;128(1):94–6.
146. Trobe JD. Searching for brain aneurysm in third cranial nerve palsy. J Neuroophthalmol. 2009;29(3):171–3.
147. Tamhankar MA, Biousse V, Ying GS, et al. Isolated third, fourth, and sixth cranial nerve palsies from presumed microvascular versus other causes: a prospective study. Ophthalmology. 2013;120(11):2264–9.
148. Wilker SC, Rucker JC, Newman NJ, Biousse V, Tomsak RL. Pain in ischaemic ocular motor cranial nerve palsies. Br J Ophthalmol. 2009;93(12):1657–9.
149. Cogan DG, Lincoff HA. Unilateral headache and oculomotor paralysis not caused by aneurysm. AMA Arch Ophthalmol. 1957;57(2):181–9.
150. Landau K. Discovering a dys-covering lid. Surv Ophthalmol. 1997;42(1):87–91.
151. Carrasco JR, Savino PJ, Bilyk JR. Primary aberrant oculomotor nerve regeneration from a posterior communicating artery aneurysm. Arch Ophthalmol. 2002;120(5):663–5.
152. Varma R, Miller NR. Primary oculomotor nerve synkinesis caused by an extracavernous intradural aneurysm. Am J Ophthalmol. 1994;118(1):83–7.
153. Bartleson JD, Trautmann JC, Sundt TM Jr. Minimal oculomotor nerve paresis secondary to unruptured intracranial aneurysm. Arch Neurol. 1986;43(10):1015–20.
154. Payne JW, Adamkiewicz J Jr. Unilateral internal ophthalmoplegia with intracranial aneurysm. Am J Ophthalmol. 1969;68(2):349–52.
155. Chaudhary N, Davagnanam I, Ansari SA, Pandey A, Thompson BG, Gemmete JJ. Imaging of intracranial aneurysms causing isolated third cranial nerve palsy. J Neuroophthalmol. 2009;29(3):238–44.
156. Lee AG, Johnson MC, Policeni BA, Smoker WR. Imaging for neuro-ophthalmic and orbital disease – a review. Clin Exp Ophthalmol. 2009;37(1):30–53.
157. Lee AG, Hayman LA, Brazis PW. The evaluation of isolated third nerve palsy revisited: an update on the evolving role of magnetic resonance, computed tomography, and catheter angiography. Surv Ophthalmol. 2002;47(2):137–57.
158. van Rooij WJ, Sprengers ME, de Gast AN, Peluso JP, Sluzewski M. 3D rotational angiography: the new gold standard in the detection of additional intracranial aneurysms. AJNR Am J Neuroradiol. 2008;29(5):976–9.
159. Mathew MR, Teasdale E, McFadzean RM. Multidetector computed tomographic angiography in isolated third nerve palsy. Ophthalmology. 2008;115(8):1411–5.
160. White PM, Wardlaw JM, Lindsay KW, Sloss S, Patel DK, Teasdale EM. The non-invasive detection of intracranial aneurysms: are neuroradiologists any better than other observers? Eur Radiol. 2003;13(2):389–96.
161. Loevner LA, Sonners AI, Schulman BJ, et al. Reinterpretation of cross-sectional images in patients with head and neck cancer in the setting of a multidisciplinary cancer center. AJNR Am J Neuroradiol. 2002;23(10):1622–6.
162. Elmalem VI, Hudgins PA, Bruce BB, Newman NJ, Biousse V. Underdiagnosis of posterior communicating artery aneurysm in noninvasive brain vascular studies. J Neuroophthalmol. 2011;31(2):103–9.
163. Beard C. Ptosis. 3rd ed. St. Louis: Mosby; 1981.
164. Duke-Elder S. System of ophthalmology. London: Kimpton; 1976.
165. Pratt SG, Beyer CK, Johnson CC. The Marcus Gunn phenomenon. A review of 71 cases. Ophthalmology. 1984;91(1):27–30.
166. Demirci H, Frueh BR, Nelson CC. Marcus Gunn jaw-winking synkinesis: clinical features and management. Ophthalmology. 2010;117(7):1447–52.
167. Bowyer JD, Sullivan TJ. Management of Marcus Gunn jaw winking synkinesis. Ophthal Plast Reconstr Surg. 2004;20(2):92–8.
168. Dillman DB, Anderson RL. Levator myectomy in synkinetic ptosis. Arch Ophthalmol. 1984;102(3):422–3.
169. Spillane J, Beeson DJ, Kullmann DM. Myasthenia and related disorders of the neuromuscular junction. J Neurol Neurosurg Psychiatry. 2010;81(8):850–7.
170. Elrod RD, Weinberg DA. Ocular myasthenia gravis. Ophthalmol Clin N Am. 2004;17(3):275–309; v.
171. Seybold ME. Myasthenia gravis. A clinical and basic science review. JAMA. 1983;250(18):2516–21.
172. Berrih-Aknin S, Frenkian-Cuvelier M, Eymard B. Diagnostic and clinical classification of autoimmune myasthenia gravis. J Autoimmun. 2014;48–49:143–8.
173. Punga T, Le Panse R, Andersson M, Truffault F, Berrih-Aknin S, Punga AR. Circulating miRNAs in myasthenia gravis: miR-150-5p as a new potential biomarker. Ann Clin Transl Neurol. 2014;1(1):49–58.
174. Jayam Trouth A, Dabi A, Solieman N, Kurukumbi M, Kalyanam J. Myasthenia gravis: a review. Autoimmune Dis. 2012;2012:874680.
175. Grob D, Brunner NG, Namba T. The natural course of myasthenia gravis and effect of therapeutic measures. Ann N Y Acad Sci. 1981;377:652–69.
176. Zhang X, Yang M, Xu J, et al. Clinical and serological study of myasthenia gravis in HuBei Province, China. J Neurol Neurosurg Psychiatry. 2007;78(4):386–90.
177. Eymard B, Vernet-der Garabedian B, Berrih-Aknin S, Pannier C, Bach JF, Morel E. Anti-acetylcholine receptor antibodies in neonatal myasthenia gravis: heterogeneity and pathogenic significance. J Autoimmun. 1991;4(2):185–95.
178. Vincent A, Clover L, Buckley C, Grimley Evans J, Rothwell PM. Evidence of underdiagnosis of myasthenia gravis in older people. J Neurol Neurosurg Psychiatry. 2003;74(8):1105–8.
179. Sommer N, Sigg B, Melms A, et al. Ocular myasthenia gravis: response to long-term immunosuppressive treatment. J Neurol Neurosurg Psychiatry. 1997;62(2):156–62.
180. Monsul NT, Patwa HS, Knorr AM, Lesser RL, Goldstein JM. The effect of prednisone on the progression from ocular to generalized myasthenia gravis. J Neurol Sci. 2004;217(2):131–3.
181. Kupersmith MJ, Latkany R, Homel P. Development of generalized disease at 2 years in patients with ocular myasthenia gravis. Arch Neurol. 2003;60(2):243–8.
182. Grob D, Brunner N, Namba T, Pagala M. Lifetime course of myasthenia gravis. Muscle Nerve. 2008;37(2):141–9.

183. Bever CT Jr, Aquino AV, Penn AS, Lovelace RE, Rowland LP. Prognosis of ocular myasthenia. Ann Neurol. 1983;14(5):516–9.
184. Gorelick PB, Rosenberg M, Pagano RJ. Enhanced ptosis in myasthenia gravis. Arch Neurol. 1981;38(8):531.
185. Gay AJ, Salmon ML, Windsor CE. Hering's law, the levators, and their relationship in disease states. Arch Ophthalmol. 1967;77(2):157–60.
186. Cogan DG. Myasthenia gravis: a review of the disease and a description of lid twitch as a characteristic sign. Arch Ophthalmol. 1965;74:217–21.
187. Kubis KC, Danesh-Meyer HV, Savino PJ, Sergott RC. The ice test versus the rest test in myasthenia gravis. Ophthalmology. 2000;107(11):1995–8.
188. Sethi KD, Rivner MH, Swift TR. Ice pack test for myasthenia gravis. Neurology. 1987;37(8):1383–5.
189. Golnik KC, Pena R, Lee AG, Eggenberger ER. An ice test for the diagnosis of myasthenia gravis. Ophthalmology. 1999;106(7):1282–6.
190. Fakiri MO, Tavy DL, Hama-Amin AD, Wirtz PW. Accuracy of the ice test in the diagnosis of myasthenia gravis in patients with ptosis. Muscle Nerve. 2013;48(6):902–4.
191. Chatzistefanou KI, Kouris T, Iliakis E, et al. The ice pack test in the differential diagnosis of myasthenic diplopia. Ophthalmology. 2009;116(11):2236–43.
192. Seybold ME. The office Tensilon test for ocular myasthenia gravis. Arch Neurol. 1986;43(8):842–3.
193. Barton JJ, Fouladvand M. Ocular aspects of myasthenia gravis. Semin Neurol. 2000;20(1):7–20.
194. Vincent A, Newsom-Davis J. Acetylcholine receptor antibody as a diagnostic test for myasthenia gravis: results in 153 validated cases and 2967 diagnostic assays. J Neurol Neurosurg Psychiatry. 1985;48(12):1246–52.
195. Srinivasan A, Kleinberg TT, Murchison AP, Bilyk JR. Laboratory investigations for diagnosis of autoimmune and inflammatory periocular disease: part I. Ophthal Plast Reconstr Surg. 2016;32(5):321–8.
196. Bindu PS, Nirmala M, Patil SA, Taly AB. Myasthenia gravis and acetylcholine receptor antibodies: a clinico immunological correlative study on South Indian patients. Ann Indian Acad Neurol. 2008;11(4):242–4.
197. Fulpius BW, Miskin R, Reich E. Antibodies from myasthenic patients that compete with cholinergic agents for binding to nicotinic receptors. Proc Natl Acad Sci U S A. 1980;77(7):4326–30.
198. Keesey JC. Clinical evaluation and management of myasthenia gravis. Muscle Nerve. 2004;29(4):484–505.
199. Vrolix K, Fraussen J, Molenaar PC, et al. The auto-antigen repertoire in myasthenia gravis. Autoimmunity. 2010;43(5–6):380–400.
200. Berrih-Aknin S, Le Panse R. Myasthenia gravis: a comprehensive review of immune dysregulation and etiological mechanisms. J Autoimmun. 2014;52:90–100.
201. Hoch W, McConville J, Helms S, Newsom-Davis J, Melms A, Vincent A. Auto-antibodies to the receptor tyrosine kinase MuSK in patients with myasthenia gravis without acetylcholine receptor antibodies. Nat Med. 2001;7(3):365–8.
202. Evoli A, Tonali PA, Padua L, et al. Clinical correlates with anti-MuSK antibodies in generalized seronegative myasthenia gravis. Brain. 2003;126(Pt 10):2304–11.
203. Leite MI, Strobel P, Jones M, et al. Fewer thymic changes in MuSK antibody-positive than in MuSK antibody-negative MG. Ann Neurol. 2005;57(3):444–8.
204. Drachman DB. Myasthenia gravis. N Engl J Med. 1994;330(25):1797–810.
205. Benatar M, Kaminski H. Medical and surgical treatment for ocular myasthenia. Cochrane Database Syst Rev. 2006;2:CD005081.
206. Seybold ME, Drachman DB. Gradually increasing doses of prednisone in myasthenia gravis. Reducing the hazards of treatment. N Engl J Med. 1974;290(2):81–4.
207. Wong VA, Beckingsale PS, Oley CA, Sullivan TJ. Management of myogenic ptosis. Ophthalmology. 2002;109(5):1023–31.
208. Demartelaere SL, Blaydon SM, Shore JW. Tarsal switch levator resection for the treatment of blepharoptosis in patients with poor eye protective mechanisms. Ophthalmology. 2006;113(12):2357–63.
209. Walton KA, Buono LM. Horner syndrome. Curr Opin Ophthalmol. 2003;14(6):357–63.
210. Mughal M, Longmuir R. Current pharmacologic testing for Horner syndrome. Curr Neurol Neurosci Rep. 2009;9(5):384–9.
211. Jacobson DM, Berg R, Grinstead GF, Kruse JR. Duration of positive urine for cocaine metabolite after ophthalmic administration: implications for testing patients with suspected Horner syndrome using ophthalmic cocaine. Am J Ophthalmol. 2001;131(6):742–7.
212. Dewan MA, Harrison AR, Lee MS. False-negative apraclonidine testing in acute Horner syndrome. Can J Ophthalmol. 2009;44(1):109–10.
213. Kawasaki A, Borruat FX. False negative apraclonidine test in two patients with Horner syndrome. Klin Monatsbl Augenheilkd. 2008;225(5):520–2.
214. Bremner F. Apraclonidine is better than cocaine for detection of Horner syndrome. Front Neurol. 2019;10:55.
215. Almog Y, Gepstein R, Kesler A. Diagnostic value of imaging in horner syndrome in adults. J Neuroophthalmol. 2010;30(1):7–11.
216. Thakker MM, Huang J, Possin DE, et al. Human orbital sympathetic nerve pathways. Ophthal Plast Reconstr Surg. 2008;24(5):360–6.
217. Demetriades AM, Miller NR, Garibaldi DC. Bilateral internal carotid artery dissection presenting as isolated unilateral Horner syndrome. Ophthal Plast Reconstr Surg. 2009;25(6):485–6.
218. Kerty E. The ophthalmology of internal carotid artery dissection. Acta Ophthalmol Scand. 1999;77(4):418–21.
219. Rigamonti A, Iurlaro S, Reganati P, Zilioli A, Agostoni E. Cluster headache and internal carotid artery dissection: two cases and review of the literature. Headache. 2008;48(3):467–70.
220. Biousse V, Touboul PJ, D'Anglejan-Chatillon J, Levy C, Schaison M, Bousser MG. Ophthalmologic manifestations of internal carotid artery dissection. Am J Ophthalmol. 1998;126(4):565–77.
221. Reede DL, Garcon E, Smoker WR, Kardon R. Horner's syndrome: clinical and radiographic evaluation. Neuroimaging Clin N Am. 2008;18(2):369–85, xi.
222. Menon R, Kerry S, Norris JW, Markus HS. Treatment of cervical artery dissection: a systematic review and meta-analysis. J Neurol Neurosurg Psychiatry. 2008;79(10):1122–7.
223. Smith SJ, Diehl N, Leavitt JA, Mohney BG. Incidence of pediatric Horner syndrome and the risk of neuroblastoma: a population-based study. Arch Ophthalmol. 2010;128(3):324–9.
224. Jeffery AR, Ellis FJ, Repka MX, Buncic JR. Pediatric Horner syndrome. J AAPOS. 1998;2(3):159–67.
225. Mahoney NR, Liu GT, Menacker SJ, Wilson MC, Hogarty MD, Maris JM. Pediatric horner syndrome: etiologies and roles of imaging and urine studies to detect neuroblastoma and other responsible mass lesions. Am J Ophthalmol. 2006;142(4):651–9.
226. Pirouzian A, Holz HA, Ip KC, Sudesh R. Acquired infantile Horner syndrome and spontaneous internal carotid artery dissection: a case report and review of literature. J AAPOS. 2010;14(2):172–4.
227. Sobel J. Botulism. Clin Infect Dis. 2005;41(8):1167–73.
228. Caya JG. Clostridium botulinum and the ophthalmologist: a review of botulism, including biological warfare ramifications of botulinum toxin. Surv Ophthalmol. 2001;46(1):25–34.
229. Capobianco DJ, Dodick DW. Diagnosis and treatment of cluster headache. Semin Neurol. 2006;26(2):242–59.

230. Silberstein SD, Lipton RB, Dodick D, Wolff HG. In: Silberstein SD, Lipton RB, Dodick DW, editors. Wolff's headache and other head pain. 8th ed. Oxford/New York: Oxford University Press; 2008.
231. DaSilva AF, Goadsby PJ, Borsook D. Cluster headache: a review of neuroimaging findings. Curr Pain Headache Rep. 2007;11(2):131–6.
232. Pinessi L, Rainero I, Rivoiro C, Rubino E, Gallone S. Genetics of cluster headache: an update. J Headache Pain. 2005;6(4):234–6.
233. Schurks M, Diener HC. Cluster headache and lifestyle habits. Curr Pain Headache Rep. 2008;12(2):115–21.
234. May A, Leone M, Afra J, et al. EFNS guidelines on the treatment of cluster headache and other trigeminal-autonomic cephalalgias. Eur J Neurol. 2006;13(10):1066–77.
235. Hansen SL, Borelli-Moller L, Strange P, Nielsen BM, Olesen J. Ophthalmoplegic migraine: diagnostic criteria, incidence of hospitalization and possible etiology. Acta Neurol Scand. 1990;81(1):54–60.
236. Levin M, Ward TN. Ophthalmoplegic migraine. Curr Pain Headache Rep. 2004;8(4):306–9.
237. Headache Classification Committee of the International Headache Society. Classification and diagnostic criteria for headache disorders, cranial neuralgias and facial pain. Cephalalgia. 1988;8(Suppl 7):1–96.
238. Bek S, Genc G, Demirkaya S, Eroglu E, Odabasi Z. Ophthalmoplegic migraine. Neurologist. 2009;15(3):147–9.
239. Carlow TJ. Oculomotor ophthalmoplegic migraine: is it really migraine? J Neuroophthalmol. 2002;22(3):215–21.

Congenital Ptosis

14

Alison V. Crum and Rebekah H. Gensure

Introduction

Congenital ptosis is a malposition of one or both upper eyelids present at birth due to abnormal development of the levator palpebrae superioris muscle, the primary elevator of the eyelid. The condition can occur in isolation or may be associated with other ocular or systemic conditions. This chapter discusses important surgical considerations including the pathophysiology, evaluation, and management of congenital ptosis, as well as timing of surgery, surgical techniques, and materials studied for repair. Appropriate pre- and postoperative management of congenital ptosis are essential to avoid complications and to achieve the goal of normal visual development.

Pathology and Epidemiology

The pathophysiologic basis of congenital ptosis is a deficiency of striated muscle fibers in the levator palpebrae superioris muscle, with the severity of the ptosis proportional to the extent of the muscle deficiency [1, 2]. This decrease in muscle size and number of fibers causes an inability of the muscle both to contract sufficiently to elevate the eyelid to its normal level in primary gaze and also to relax inadequately, resulting in eyelid lag on downgaze. In a classic study, Berke and Wadsworth found Müller's superior tarsal muscle to be histologically normal in all congenital ptosis specimens in contrast to the levator muscle [1]. Of note, although the size of the muscle itself and number of fibers is reduced, a small case series found that the size of each muscle fiber was not significantly smaller in congenital ptosis patients compared to normal controls [3]. Other more rare etiologies of congenital ptosis : include levator palpebrae superioris muscle defect due to fibrosis or levator disinsertion due to birth trauma [4].

Congenital ptosis often occurs in isolation but can also exist as part of a syndrome with other ocular or systemic components. Systemic disorders have been reported in up to 35% of patients with congenital ptosis, most commonly genetic/chromosomal, craniofacial, or neurologic disorders [5]. Ptosis may be the presenting sign in these cases. Careful evaluation of the face and a careful history including birth history, prior eye trauma, and family ocular history may help clue in the oculoplastic surgeon to other potential syndromic findings.

Genetic Associations

With the advances in genetic research in recent years, we have gained additional understanding about genetic associations with congenital ptosis, although the published studies are typically limited in application given high degrees of genetic variability across ethnic groups. A Chinese epidemiologic study found 0.18% prevalence of congenital ptosis, with the majority coming from sporadic cases (67.1%), 18.4% autosomal dominant (8.3% BPES (blepharophimosis-ptosis-epicanthus inversus syndrome)), and 14.5% autosomal recessive. Several of the genome association studies have begun to implicate specific genes. Gene mutations, such as mutations of PAX6, have been studied in congenital aniridia and have also recently been proposed to be indicated in congenital ptosis [6]. The National Institutes of Health (NIH) identified a zinc finger protein of unknown function (ZNF462) in a ptosis-related condition by sequencing families in which they identified a phenotype of ptosis, craniosynostosis, metopic ridge (triangular-shaped forehead), corpus callosum dysgenesis, and developmental delay [7]. Other researchers have identified associations with RYR1, the skeletal muscle ryanodine receptor which is implicated in malignant hyperthermia [8].

A. V. Crum (✉) · R. H. Gensure
University of Utah, Moran Eye Center, Department of Ophthalmology, Salt Lake City, UT, USA
e-mail: Alison.crum@hsc.utah.edu

J. J. Servat et al. (eds.), *Smith and Nesi's Ophthalmic Plastic and Reconstructive Surgery*,
https://doi.org/10.1007/978-3-030-41720-8_14

The association between heart disease and congenital ptosis has been demonstrated in two larger case series [9, 10]. Larned studied a series of 156 patients with congenital ptosis and found congenital heart disease in 7/156 (4.5%). A case series by Mansour and colleagues found congenital ptosis in 12 of 240 subjects (5%) with congenital heart disease [9]. Given the low prevalence of congenital ptosis in the general population (0.18%) compared to the congenital heart disease population (5%), the association between congenital heart disease and congenital ptosis appears likely.

Coexisting eye abnormalities are more common in population with congenital ptosis than in the general population. About 75% of congenital ptosis cases are unilateral. Amblyopia is found in about 20% of patients, often secondary to convergent strabismus, high astigmatism, or anisometropia. Anderson and Baumgartner initially proposed that the instances of amblyopia they observed were due to the ptotic occlusion of the pupil [11]. A recent systematic review by Wang and colleagues included 24 studies and estimated the pooled prevalence of amblyopia at 22%, strabismus 19.6%, and refractive error 30.2% [12]. Complications from these comorbid eye conditions can be reduced by timely surgical repair of congenital ptosis.

Special Categories and Subtypes

Superior Rectus Weakness (Double Elevator Palsy)

A deficiency in elevation of the ipsilateral eye is present in approximately 5% of patients with congenital ptosis. This condition is referred to as double elevator palsy or monocular elevation deficiency (given its usual unilateral presentation). Many of these cases of hypotropia appear to be due to superior rectus weakness, but the inferior oblique may also be implicated. The levator and the superior rectus muscles arise from the same mesodermal bud, which is one theory regarding the pathophysiologic basis of this condition. Histologic studies of the superior rectus muscles of patients in this category have not been reported; however, a small case study of magnetic resonance imaging in these patients confirms decreased volume of the superior rectus [13]. Some of these patients have fusion in the primary position, masking the condition with a compensatory chin elevation. With an elevation deficit and ptosis, the hypotropia needs to be corrected before the ptosis can be addressed [14]. Surgery must be individualized according to forced duction testing and preoperative assessment of Bell's reflex. Further details regarding the background, subtypes, and management of this condition have been documented by Bagheri and colleagues over their 10-year experience [15].

Blepharophimosis-Ptosis-Epicanthus Inversus Syndrome (BPES)

First described by Komoto in 1921, blepharophimosis-ptosis-epicanthus inversus syndrome (BPES) is a condition involving a narrowed horizontal palpebral fissure, telecanthus, severe bilateral ptosis (usually with associated chin lift), and an extra skin fold arising from the lower eyelid [16]. It can occur sporadically or can be inherited in autosomal dominant fashion. Mutations in FOXL2 have been identified in patients with BPES. Sporadic cases may also have associated mental retardation. The two subtypes are categorized according to gonadal status: Type I has premature ovarian failure and infertility, whereas Type II does not.

Anatomy, Evaluation, and Preoperative Considerations

Anatomy

For surgical planning purposes in the repair of congenital ptosis, we will briefly review the relevant anatomy and physiology that allows for normal eyelid elevation. The levator palpebrae superioris (LPS) is the primary elevator of the upper eyelid and is composed of skeletal (striated) muscle that is innervated by the superior division of CN III, the oculomotor nerve. The LPS originates on the lesser wing of sphenoid at the annulus of Zinn and extends about 40 mm in total length between its origin and where it inserts into the skin and the anterior tarsus. Whitnall's ligament is a transition point for the LPS muscle, changing its force vector from anterior-posterior to inferior-superior; this also marks the transition to the levator aponeurosis. The secondary elevator of the upper eyelid is the Müller muscle, which is composed of smooth rather than striated muscle and is innervated by the autonomic nervous system. Müller's muscle contributes to approximately 2–3 mm of elevation. Overall contributions from both the LPS and Müller's muscle maintain the upper eyelid height 1–2 mm below the superior limbus at rest.

Evaluation

Two authors have shaped the historical approach to levator resection for congenital ptosis: Berke and Beard. The early method described by Berke in 1961 employed only measurement of preoperative levator function, disregarding lid height and instead anticipating a lid fall after surgery if levator function was less than 8 mm or a lid rise if levator function was greater than 8 mm [17]. Several years later, Beard, whose approach is still commonly used, recommended a quantitative approach to resection of a predetermined amount of levator muscle based on two critical pieces of preoperative data: the degree of levator function as well as the height of the palpebral fissure in the primary position of gaze [18]. Hardy and colleagues published their experience using a method largely based on Beard's, which yielded a high success rate (86%) [19]. Although implementation of technique may vary, most modern oculoplastic surgeons agree on the levator function and lid height as essential components in their surgical planning.

It is usually preferable to examine children on two or three occasions before surgery in order to confirm and refine these critical measurements. Surgery based on false assumptions or inaccurate measurements is bound to fail. If the child is a toddler when first seen, and an examination is performed every 6–12 months, a reliable body of data can be generated by the summer that precedes starting elementary school. This is usually the most convenient time for elective surgery. An important exception occurs when the pupillary axis is partially or completely covered by the eyelid. Here, the eyelid should be elevated on an urgent if not an emergent basis to prevent the development of deprivation amblyopia.

Formal visual fields with and without lid elevation, such as those performed for insurance purposes in adult patients with ptosis, are not a part of the preoperative evaluation in congenital ptosis. Children do not perform well with visual field testing. The results would likely confirm obstruction of the upper visual field proportional to the degree of pupillary encroachment by the upper eyelid margin. Oculoplastic surgeons can take advantage of modern electronic medical record systems that allow the surgeon to easily record sequential anatomical and functional measurements, which is usually sufficient for surgical planning as well as any necessary insurance documentation.

Any child being evaluated for congenital ptosis should be followed closely with a careful ocular motility examination and vision assessment at frequent intervals. If amblyopia or refractive error is diagnosed, it should be treated with appropriate occlusion therapy and spectacles. Amblyopia may develop postoperatively even if it is absent preoperatively; Merriam, Ellis, and Helveston reported the increase of astigmatism postoperatively in 10 of 65 patients (15%) undergoing ptosis surgery; 6 of these 10 patients (60%) later developed amblyopia in the operated eye [20]. These early studies led to the theory that delaying surgery until the age of 5 years may allow time for the visual system to mature.

Monitoring of congenital ptosis does not stop once surgery is complete. Postoperative congenital ptosis patients may have refractive error and amblyopia and thus may still need glasses, patching, or other therapy. Additional studies have confirmed refractive error changes after surgery, most commonly a shift in astigmatism toward the oblique axis, which can be amblyogenic and needs appropriate evaluation and treatment [21]. Paik and colleagues found postoperative oblique astigmatism rates of 73% (19/26 eyes) compared to 38% (10/26) preoperatively [21]. A recent study by Savino and colleagues took a quantitative approach and evaluated corneal topography before and after congenital ptosis repair; they found that the steep corneal curvature attributed to the presence of ptosis flattened after surgery [22]. Ptosis repair surgery in this retrospective group resulted in reduced astigmatism, improved best-corrected visual acuity, and improved corneal symmetry.

Informed Consent for Surgery

During the informed consent process, a thorough discussion with parents of children with ptosis will help set up a framework for what to expect from surgery. There is an art to maintaining a positive and realistic attitude toward surgery while also reviewing all the possible complications. Much of this art can be gleaned from experience, but there is at least one excellent reference to help the young oculoplastic surgeon begin to learn how to effectively communicate with their patients [23]. It is best to point out that perfect eyelid symmetry is not guaranteed, although in some patients may be achievable. Secondary operations are occasionally required. Generally, the functional result is proportional to the amount of preoperative levator function: patients with mild (2 mm) ptosis and good (8–12 mm) or excellent (13 mm or more) levator function often have better results than those with more severe pathology. In patients with poor (4 mm or less) levator function and severe (4 mm or more) ptosis, the primary surgical goal is to aim for equal eyelid fissure heights when the eyes are directed in the primary position. Eyelid lag and lagophthalmos must be accepted as potential side effects of the procedure. The surgeon can assure parents that these problems often improve with the passage of time.

Now more than ever before, in the setting of rapidly accessible information via the Internet, the public is better informed concerning medical issues, and their appetite for such information appears insatiable. Many patients (and parents) desire to know the surgical details of how the operation is performed in addition to explicit descriptions of what specific complications are most likely to be encountered. It is not unusual for surgical prospects to request the surgeon to show them illustrations or videos of the steps in the proposed operation. Patients may request to see preoperative and postoperative photographs of other patients undergoing similar surgery. Such requests should be respectfully welcomed and fulfilled to the extent possible, because prospective parents and patients who are familiar with the potential problems that confront the surgeon are far easier to communicate with than those who are uninformed, especially if complications unexpectedly arise.

The following dialogue, which was developed for the prior version of this text, may be useful in preoperative consultation with parents of children with congenital ptosis [24]: “The muscle that lifts the eyelid is somewhat like an elastic band. When your child was born, that muscle was not fully developed. Instead of being strong and functional, it is now weak and not functioning well. To raise the eyelid, we must tighten the muscle by surgically removing a very small piece of it. We determine the amount to adjust according to the muscle’s strength and the severity of the droop. Even though the operations we use are time-tested and reliable, there is some variability in the result. Muscle is living tissue (rather than a block of wood or piece of steel that can be measured and cut to exact specifications). You are probably aware that no matter how detailed the set of plans, construction of a house from such plans may sometimes not turn out as desired. Unfortunately, eyelid reconstructive surgery sometimes suffers from the same drawbacks. I will do all that is humanly possible to have a successful outcome. My goal is equal and symmetric opening of the eyelids when the child is looking straight ahead. Additionally, our goal in lifting the eyelid(s) is to facilitate normal development of vision in both eyes.”

Anesthesia

General anesthesia is required for ptosis surgery on infants and children. A thorough history and physical examination should always be performed preoperatively, because the rate of congenital heart disease is five times greater in patients with ptosis than in the general pediatric population [9, 10, 25]. A family history of malignant hyperthermia should be specifically examined, because this congenital anesthetic-induced muscular abnormality, which has an incidence of 1/15,000 in children and a significant mortality rate, may be transmitted as an autosomal dominant trait [26, 27]. Sometimes teenagers need general anesthesia, too, unless they are unusually stoic. The final decision as to the selection of the optimal general anesthetic agent should be left in the hands of a pediatric anesthesiologist.

Surgery for Congenital Ptosis

Most cases of congenital ptosis can be corrected by one of three operative procedures:

- Levator resection by skin approach
- Levator resection by conjunctival approach
- Eyebrow suspension of the eyelids

The quantitative approach to levator resection by either the conjunctival or skin approach is strongly recommended for repair of ptosis when the levator has adequate function (5 mm or more). Its basic premise is that, depending on the severity of ptosis and, in particular, the amount of levator function, excising a predetermined amount of levator muscle should be expected to raise the eyelid to a certain height. Many authorities agree that this technique yields more predictable results than a qualitative system for the determination of levator resection to elevate the eyelid [18, 19, 28, 29]. In the past, a qualitative system has been taught by using such vagaries as “just the right amount of levator is resected” or “the amount resected is judged by the experience of the operation.” However, the results can be variable and challenging to reproduce. The quantitative approach is also preferred to another method advocated by some authors who advise intraoperative determination of levator resection by the relation of the eyelid margin to the upper corneoscleral limbus [30–33]. This approach does not apply to patients with poor levator function (4 mm or less) in whom eyebrow suspension is indicated.

Even though the levator muscle is the best source of power for elevating a ptotic eyelid, there are patients with severely ptotic eyelids with weak levator muscles that are incapable of lifting them. In these cases of severe ptosis with poor levator function, an alternate muscular source must be employed. This second choice almost always is the frontalis muscle.

The old rule of thumb was that 2 mm of levator should be resected for each 1 mm of ptosis [34]. In congenital ptosis, this usually led to undercorrection; in fact, resection of 8 mm (or less) of levator aponeurosis in an eyelid with mild (2 mm or less) ptosis would yield no elevation even when the levator function is good (8–12 mm). Perhaps this is because Müller’s muscle is also affected, which results in loss of a significant amount of lifting power. Other algorithms of varying complexity have been employed, such as simple ones (4 mm resection per 1 mm of ptosis [35]) or more complex ones [36].

With careful preoperative examination, a surgeon can make an educated assessment regarding which eyelids can be raised by levator resection, which cannot, and how much levator to resect in appropriate cases. The definitions for the various parameters for ptosis, levator function, and levator resection are presented in Tables 14.1, 14.2, and 14.3, respectively, as a guide rather than absolute rule for surgical planning. Table 14.4 correlates levator function and degree of ptosis to aid the surgeon in choosing a suggested operation for correction of congenital ptosis. For optimal results, surgeons should ideally be familiar with multiple methods to determine the best option for each patient.

Table 14.1 Definitions of the degree of ptosis

Ptosis severity	Reduction in lid height from normal level (mm)
Mild	≤2
Moderate	3
Severe	≥4

Table 14.2 Definitions of levator function

Category	Eyelid excursion (mm)
Excellent	≥13
Good	8–12
Fair	5–7
Poor	≤4

Table 14.3 Definitions of levator resection

Type of resection	Amount of levator excised (mm)
Small	10–13
Moderate	14–17
Large	18–22
Maximum	23–26
Supermaximal	27–30

Table 14.4 Recommended amount of levator resection for congenital ptosis

Degree of ptosis	Levator function	Choice of procedure, amount of levator resection
Mild (≤2 mm)	Good (8–12 mm)	Small levator resection (10–13 mm)
Moderate (3 mm)	Fair (5–7 mm) Good (8–12 mm) Fair (5–7 mm) Poor (≤4 mm)	Moderate levator resection (14–17 mm) Moderate levator resection (14–17 mm) Large levator resection (18–22 mm) Maximum levator resection (23–27 mm)
Severe (4 mm or more)	Fair (5–7 mm)	Maximum levator resection (23–27 mm)
	Poor (≤4 mm)	Callahan procedure Beard procedure Supermaximal levator resection (27 mm) Unilateral sling

It is noted in Table 14.4 that the amount of indicated levator resection sometimes may vary by as much as 3 mm, depending on the amount of levator function. For instance, when a patient needs a moderate levator resection, one might resect 17 mm of levator (if the levator function is 8 mm) or 14 mm (if the levator function is 11 mm). Larger resections are preferred over smaller resections, as the natural tendency of these surgeries leans toward undercorrection rather than overcorrection, and undercorrections are infinitely easier to treat.

Additional elevation of the eyelid margin can be gained by either advancing the levator down the anterior tarsal surface or resecting the superior 2–3 mm of the tarsus. These supplemental techniques should usually be reserved for cases of severe (4 mm or more) ptosis with poor (4 mm or less) to fair (5–6 mm) levator function. Because the tarsus is the eyelid's skeleton, one should never resect more than one half its vertical height due to the possibility of peaking or ectropion.

Methods

Levator Resection

Levator resection can be accomplished through either skin or conjunctival incisions and is the operation of choice with good levator function (at least 5 mm). The advantages of the skin incision approach include (1) the anatomy is easier to follow because the eyelid is not altered by eversion; (2) important structures in the upper orbit are exposed (Whitnall's ligament and the medial and lateral horns), allowing a greater length of levator to be dissected and resected more easily; (3) sutures can be advanced lower on the tarsus, enhancing the elevating effect; (4) the location of the eyelid crease can be altered; (5) excess skin can be excised simultaneously; and (6) bleeding can be controlled more easily [31].

The skin approach has been described in detail in prior editions [24] and is summarized elaborately in several other references [4, 37] (Fig. 14.1a, b). Briefly, the skin is incised at the desired site of the eyelid crease (with the exact location depending on age and eyelid size). Dissection is carried through the orbicularis and preaponeurotic fat pad down to the levator aponeurosis, which is then reattached to the upper tarsus at the desired location. The levator can either be resected or plicated, each of which has advantages and disadvantages. Maximum resections performed for moderate (3 mm) and severe (4 mm) ptosis should result in an eyelid margin at or near the upper limbus, assuming the globe is approximately in the primary position. The resultant eyelid height is dependent on the accuracy of the careful preoperative and intraoperative measurements. When the patient is under general anesthesia, remember that it is not unusual for the tarsus to be slightly lifted off of the cornea in resections greater than 18–20 mm. At the conclusion of surgery, copious ointment should be applied to the cornea.

A conjunctival approach to levator resection is much less common but may be preferred for small (10–13 mm) resections or for reoperations on undercorrected congenital ptosis in children in which overcorrection is a true hazard (Fig. 14.2a, b). The primary advantage of the conjunctival approach is that the exteriorized mattress sutures, which are used to join the levator to the tarsus, can be removed in 4–7 days if an overcorrection occurs. With the conjunctival approach to levator resection, there is also less edema than with the skin approach, because the full thickness of the eyelid is not transected, and there is no external scar. Moreover, without external scarring, operative time is shortened [38]. Historically, Blaskovics published his procedure in 1923, and this may have been the first approach to levator surgery, even before the external skin approach [39]. Prior editions of this text provide a detailed description of a modification of the Blaskovics operation [24], which was reported by Agatson in 1942 [40, 41].

Complications of Levator Resection (Table 14.5)

Severe unilateral congenital ptosis (4 mm or more) is always accompanied by levator function that is less than good; the majority of such patients have poor (4 or less) function, and the rest have fair (5–7 mm) function.

The ptotic eyelid with fair (5–7 mm) function can be elevated by levator resection (23–26 mm) combined with advancement of the levator (2–3 mm) inferiorly on the tarsus and excision of a 4–5 mm crescent of the skin superior to the eyelid crease. If the levator function is poor (4 mm or less), a supermaximal levator resection (27–30 mm) can be performed [44], with advancement of the levator down on the inferior aspect of the tarsus and superior 3 mm tarsectomy with crescentic (4–5 mm) skin resection. These cases result in slight undercorrection with moderate to severe accompanying eyelid lag and akinetic appearance to the eyelid in everyday life with bizarre asymmetry in upgaze, downgaze, and blinking.

Several alternative procedures have been suggested in cases of poor levator function. The first was proposed in 1965 by Beard; it consists of levator disinsertion on the normal side, creating bilateral severe (4 mm or more) ptosis and then performing bilateral eyebrow suspension with autogenous fascia. The levator disinsertion and bilateral slings are all performed during the same operation [45]. This procedure obtained results similar to fascia lata sling for bilateral severe ptosis. Alternatively, suspension of the tarsus to Whitnall's ligament (an internal sling, sometimes referred to as Whitnall's sling) has also been proposed. The Whitnall's sling yields a similar postoperative eyelid position to a supermaximal (27–30 mm) resection [46]. Alston Callahan suggested another procedure, which involves insertion of eyebrow suspension slings in both eyelids without excising

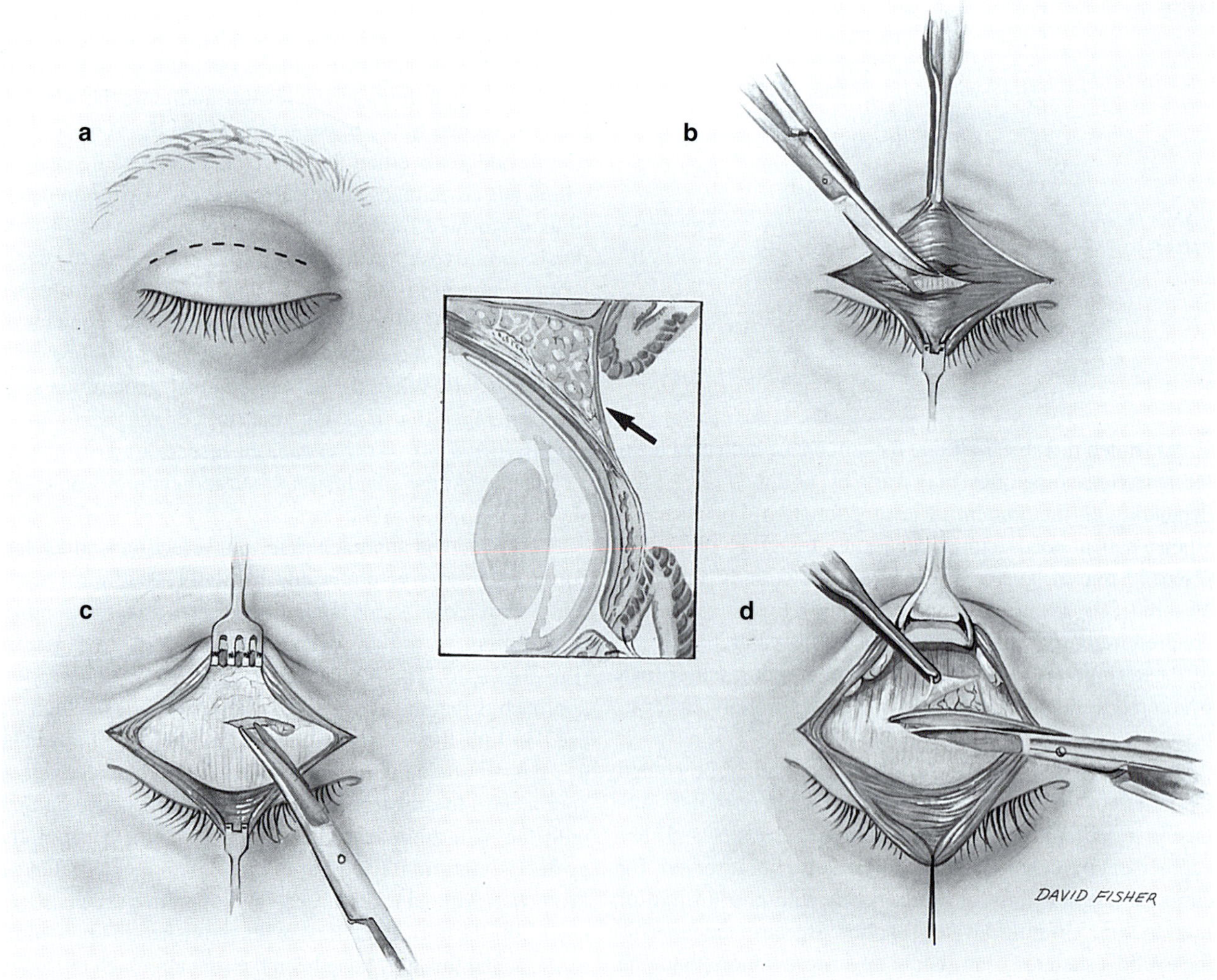

Fig. 14.1 Technique of levator resection, skin approach

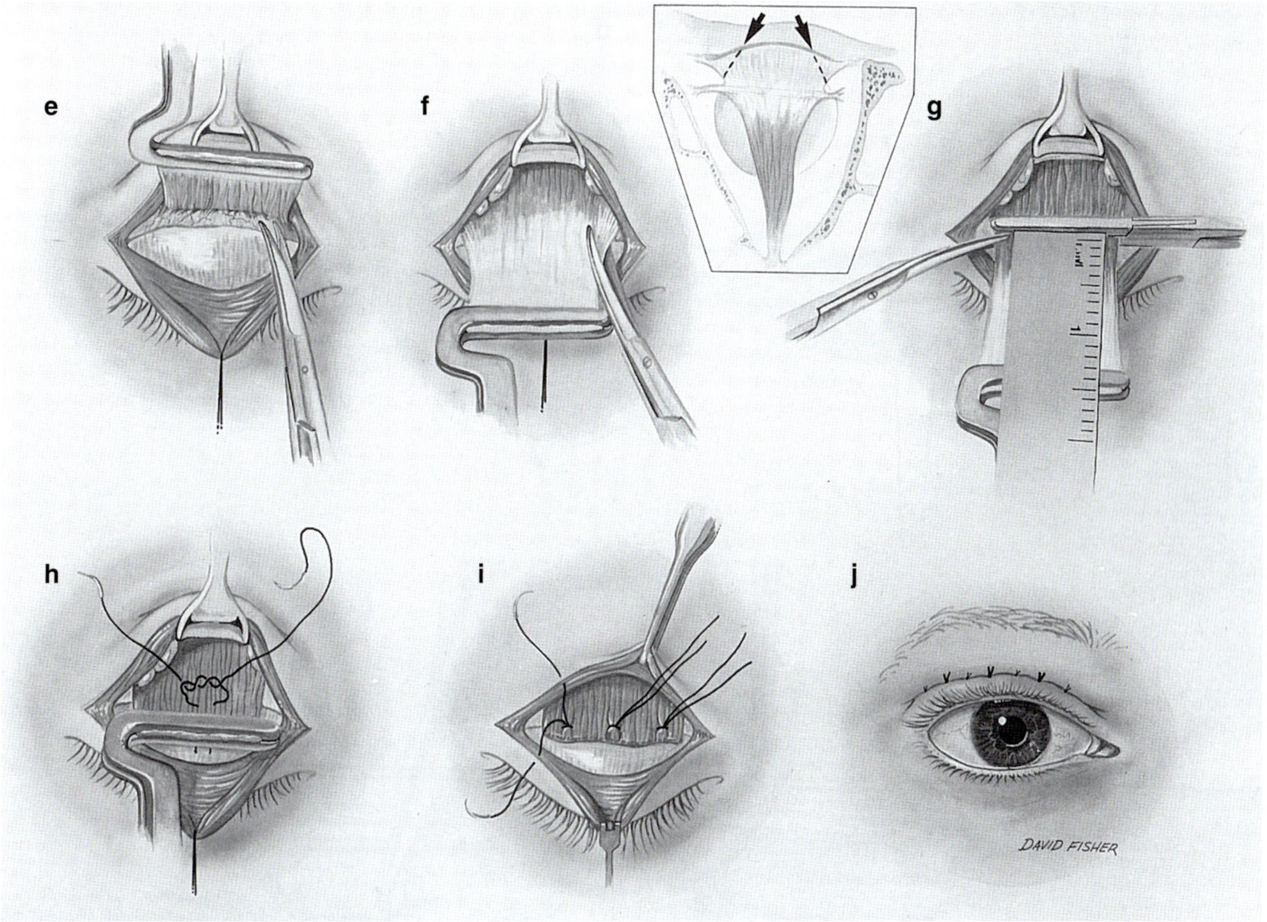

Fig. 14.1 (continued)

the levator on the normal side, using either silicone rods or autogenous fascia lata [47]. The tension of the sling is somewhat loose on the normal side so that the normal levator is not restricted in the primary position of gaze or in upgaze; the tension of the sling in the ptotic eyelid is tighter, so it is symmetric with the normal eyelid in the primary position of gaze. On downgaze, the slings suspend both eyelids at approximately the same level, thus achieving symmetric eyelid lag.

Frontalis Suspension or Sling

For blepharoptosis with poor levator function, a frontalis sling had been proposed to elevate the eyelid by attaching the frontalis muscle to the upper eyelid tarsal plate, bypassing the need of elevation of the eyelid by the levator palpebrae superioris muscle. The "frontalis muscle suspension" treatment was first described with use of fascia lata in 1909 by Payr and Wright in 1922 [48].

Materials for Frontalis Sling

There are various materials that have been used in the past decades to create a frontalis sling:

Common materials for frontalis sling
Autologous fascia lata
Preserved fascia lata
Fascia temporalis
Umbilical vein
Autologous palmaris longus tendon
Silicone rod
(Mersilene) Polyester fiber mesh
(Supramid) Monofilament nylon
(Prolene) Polypropylene
(Gore-Tex) Expanded polytetrafluoroethylene

Many surgeons feel that AFL (autologous fascia lata) has good long-term outcomes and remains the principal material used. The argument for AFL is that it integrates with the patient's tissues, providing better vascularization and long-term functionality. No perfect material has been found [49].

Techniques for Frontalis Sling

The frontalis sling has also been modified over the years and different techniques have surfaced (Figs. 14.3 and 14.4):

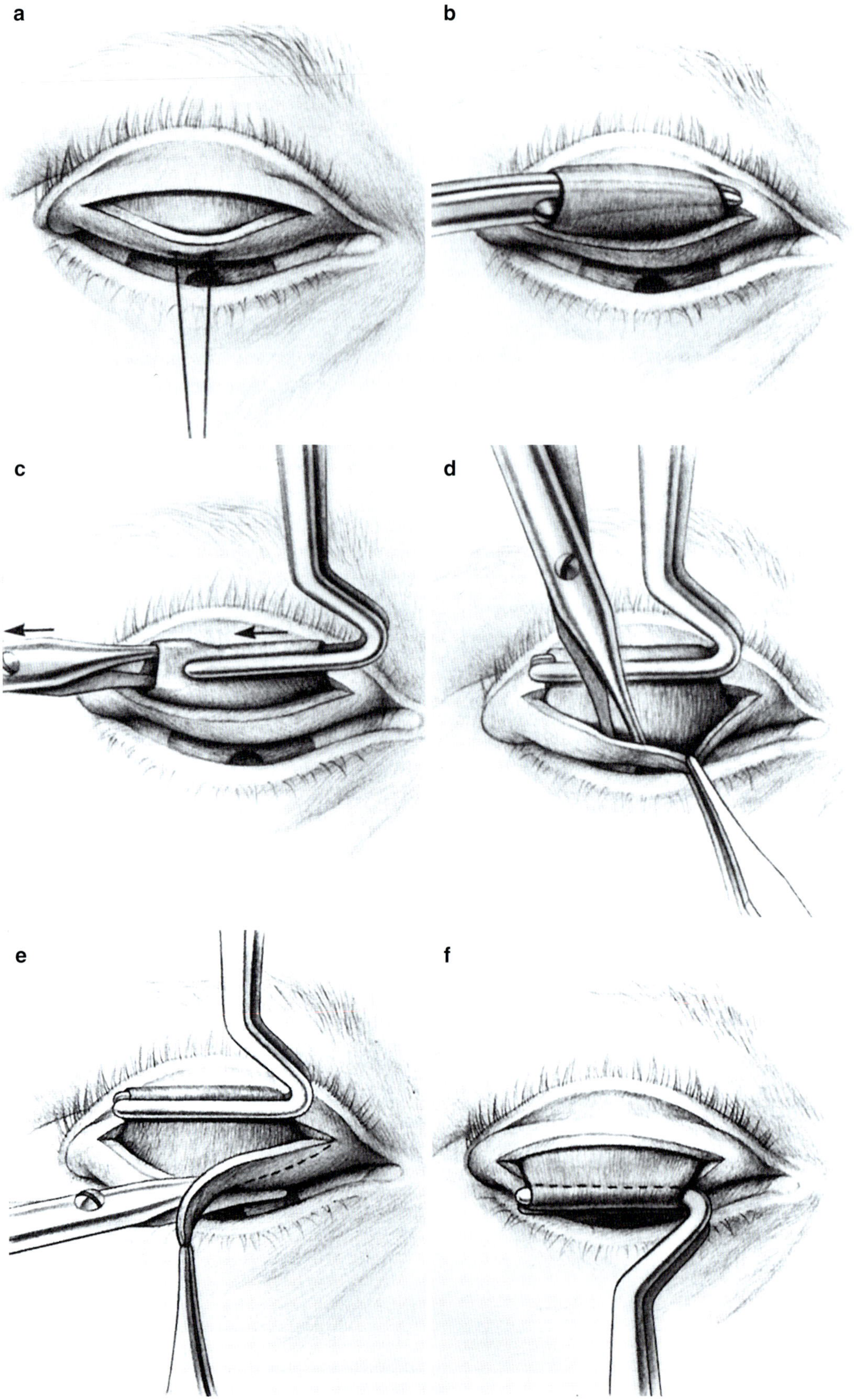

Fig. 14.2 Technique of levator resection, conjunctival approach

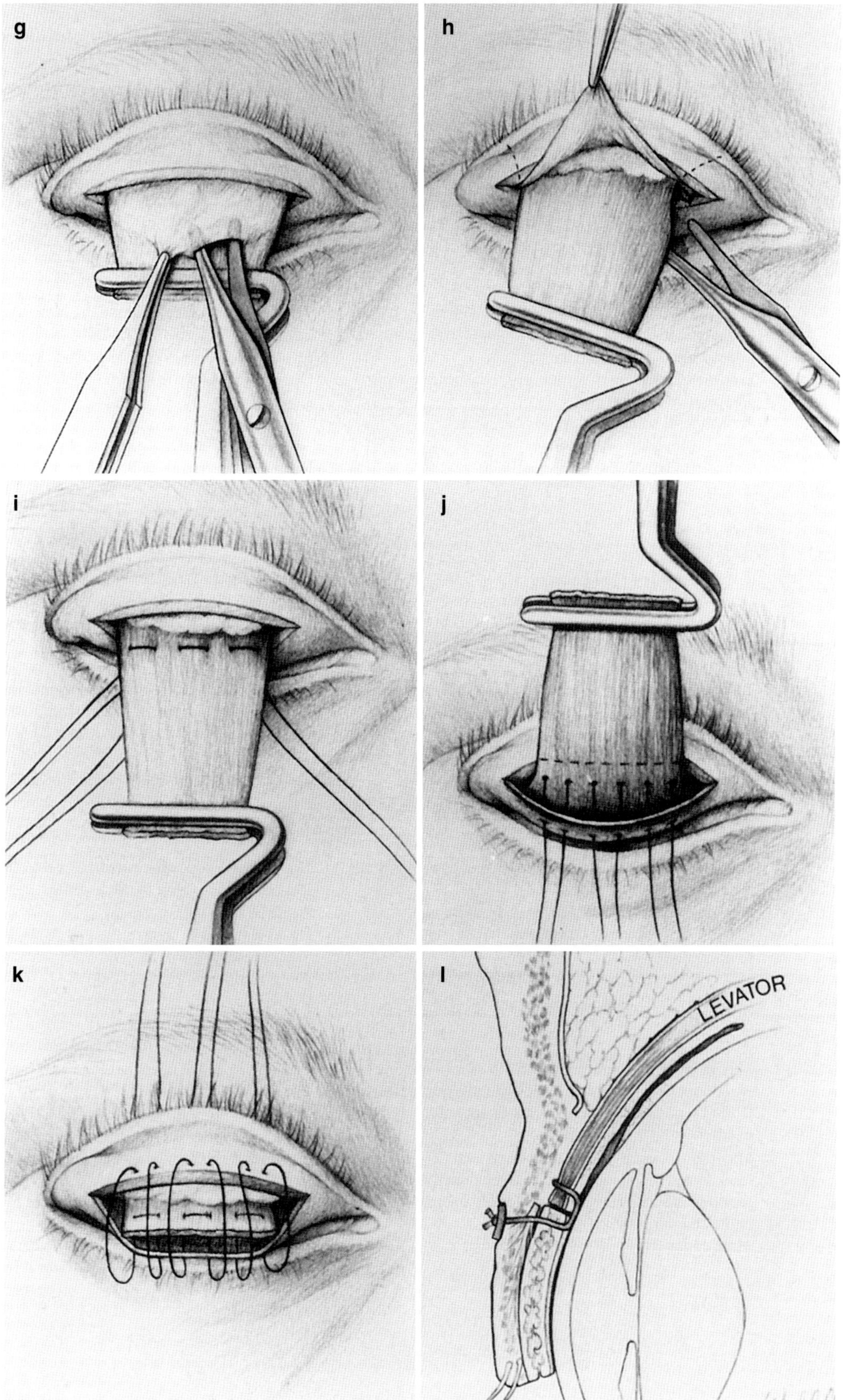

Fig. 14.2 (continued)

Table 14.5 Complications of levator resection congenital ptosis repair and treatment

Complication	Description/cause	Treatment/repair
Small overcorrection (0–1.5 mm)		Observation (often lid will lower after 2–3 months) Downward eyelid massage (5 min, 3 times a day for 1–2 weeks) Forcible downward traction on eyelashes
Large overcorrection (>1.5 mm)	Rare after congenital ptosis surgery	Removal of mattress suture for conjunctival approach Transconjunctival or transcutaneous levator recession; skin approach preferred with spacer between levator and tarsus [42]
Pseudo-overcorrection	Measurable drop in the contralateral eyelid postoperatively gives the operated eyelid the appearance of an overcorrection May be due to Hering's law as well as underlying phoria/tropia/monofixational syndrome in ptotic eye	Prevent with preoperative testing: Manually elevate the ptotic eye while the patient fixates on a distant object Temporarily occlude vision in the ptotic eye
Small undercorrection (0.5–1 mm)	Improper choice of procedure Inadequate resection of levator due to inaccurate preoperative measurements Premature dissolution of absorbable sutures Large postoperative hematomas	Ensuring hemostasis prior to wound closure Observation (likely to improve somewhat as edema subsides)
Large undercorrection (>1 mm)	Unlikely to improve as edema subsides	Reoperation excising additional levator, usually by the skin approach Segmental Fasanella-Servat procedure or Müllerectomy Segmental full-thickness eyelid resection procedure
Abnormal eyelid contour: nasal notching	More common with superior tarsectomy due to destabilization of eyelid margin Occurs when medial horn of levator has not been severed completely in maximum levator resections or when the superior oblique or its fascia has been unintentionally caught in the levator tarsus sutures	Minor: massage and observation Major: extraocular muscle imbalance and diplopia may necessitate immediate opening of the wound and removing the nasal sutures before fibrous adhesions form
Abnormal eyelid contour: central peaking	Too far apart spacing of levator-tarsus sutures in the central position of the tarsus Too close spacing of sutures to the eyelid margin Taking too long a bite of tarsus	If the angle of the notch is acute, resuture the levator to the tarsus over a broader area or replace the sutures further away from the margin
Abnormal eyelid contour: temporal notching/flare	Levator is sutured too far temporally on the tarsus Lateral horn is not severed in large (18–22 mm) levator resections	Suture replacement as in nasal notching
Eyelid lag	Severity increases in proportion to the amount of levator resected	Not a true complication but rather a side effect; becomes less conspicuous with passage of time
Exposure keratitis	Due to incomplete blink amplitude from lid lag Usually mild, resulting in minimal burning and foreign body sensation Milder in cases with normal Bell's phenomenon	Artificial tears during the day Bland ointment at night Treat any abrasion or ulceration with therapeutic soft contact lens or collagen shield
Lagophthalmos	Lack of eyelid closure during sleep	Frequent artificial tears during the day Bland ointment at night Tape eyelids closed at night (if severe)
Intractable lagophthalmos	May indicate erroneous inclusion of superior oblique tendon (would see vertical diplopia + ipsilateral hypotropia) Orbital septum included in levator-tarsus sutures (use forced traction eyelid testing to diagnose)	If severe – need to open incision and remove troublesome suture(s)
Entropion	May follow large (18–22 mm) or maximal (23–26 mm) resections when too much tarsus or conjunctiva is removed, resulting in shortening of the posterior lamella with respect to the anterior lamella More common with conjunctival approach	Watchful waiting and massage (mild) Free levator adhesions to tarsus and resuture it down to anterior surface of tarsus 4–5 mm above eyelashes (severe) Resect additional levator if undercorrected Add spacer between tarsus and levator if overcorrected [42]

Table 14.5 (continued)

Complication	Description/cause	Treatment/repair
Ectropion	May follow large (18–22 mm) or maximal (23–26 mm) resections via skin approach when skin incision is too low and crease is fixed too high, rotating the margin outward May occur in conjunctival approach – due to mattress sutures being brought out too close to the eyelashes and tied too tightly	Reverse of above for entropion but do not excise skin
Eyelid crease deformity (too high or too low)	Can occur with faulty marking of incisions preoperatively or inaccurate tarsal fixation	Prevent by proper preoperative marking
Conjunctival prolapse	Occurs in large (18–22 mm), maximum (23–26 mm), or supermaximal (27–30 mm) levator resections when the suspensory ligament between the conjunctival fornix and levator-superior rectus complex is severed	Avoid by examining the position of the conjunctiva before the skin is closed and tacking redundant conjunctiva to the levator with two or three well-placed mattress sutures (Wolfley 1987) Avoid by excising a 5–6 mm ellipse of it and then suturing the edges together with a fine absorbable suture (chromic 7-0) If mild, treat with topical steroid-antibiotic drops QID for 2–3 weeks Inject hyaluronidase (150 TBU/1 mL saline solution) directly Can treat with simple excision or placement of double-armed mattress sutures (chromic 6-0) through full thickness of eyelid
Loss of eyelashes	Rare; caused by surgical dissection and cauterization within 2 mm of cilia follicles at marginal artery or tying sutures too tightly near the eyelashes Traumatic alopecia can be idiosyncratic reaction to general anesthesia	Passage of time (2–3 months) for regrowth of eyelids If severe and permanent, can treat with surgical wedge resection or eyelash autografts (tedious)
Diplopia	Often temporary	Passage of time (weeks to months)
Eyelid cysts	Rare [43] Burying of conjunctival epithelium Obstruction of gland of Krause Injury to main lacrimal gland or duct Accessory lacrimal gland fistula	Avoid by careful dissection and suturing

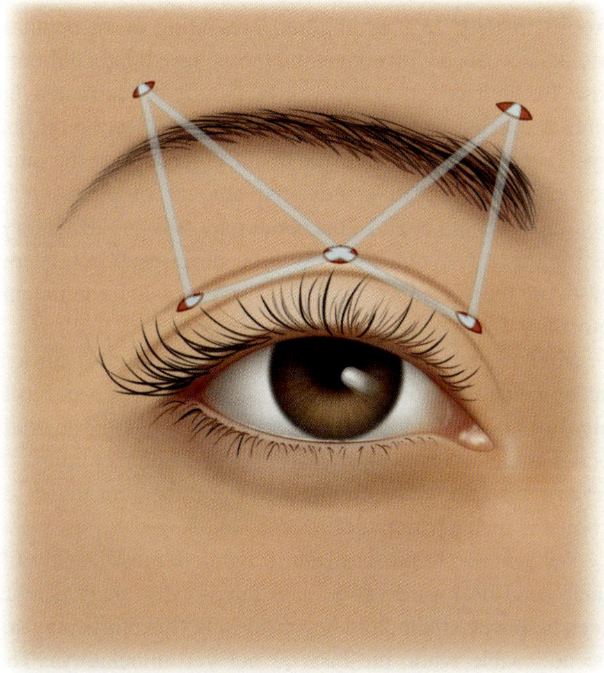

Fig. 14.3 Double triangle technique

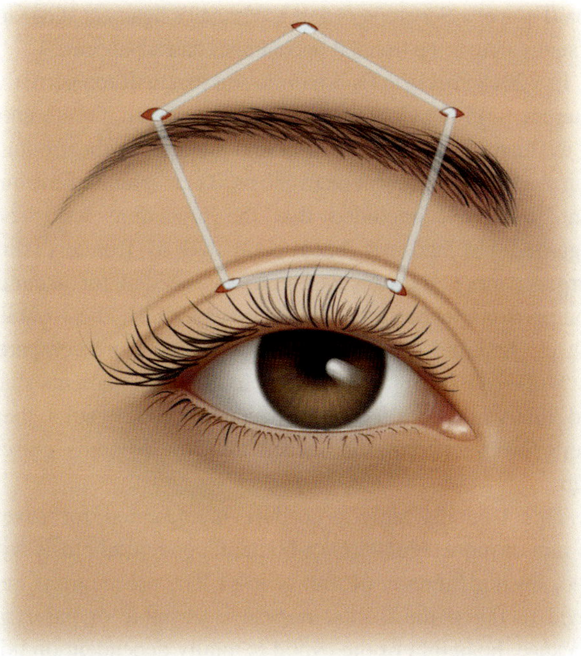

Fig. 14.4 Single pentagon technique

Techniques for frontalis sling
Single triangle/double triangle
Single rhomboid/double rhomboid
Double trapezoid
Single pentagon/double pentagon

The two most commonly used are the Fox pentagon and the modified Crawford double triangle. The reader is referred to additional references for more about these techniques and modifications upon them:

1. Fox SA. Congenital ptosis frontal sling. J Pediatr Ophthalmol. 1966:325–8.
2. Fox SA. Complications of frontalis sling surgery. Am J Ophthalmol. 1967;63:758–62.
3. Crawford JS. Correction of unilateral blepharoptosis with bilateral eyelid suspension. Am J Ophthalmol. 1972;74:321–6.
4. Friedenwald JS, Guyton JS. A simple ptosis operation: utilization of the frontalis by means of a single rhomboid-shaped suture. Am J Ophthalmol. 1948;31:411–14.
5. Iliff CE. Surgical management of ptosis. Somerville: Ethicon; 1963. p. 9–12.
6. Goldberger S, Conn H, Lemor M. Double rhomboid silicone rod frontalis suspension. Ophthal Plast Reconstr Surg. 1991;7:48–53.

Alternative Procedures for Severe Ptosis with Poor Levator Function

Another method beyond maximal levator resection, Mueller's muscle surgery, conjunctivo-tarso-Muller's muscle-levator resection (Fasanella-Servat procedure), Whitnall's ligament sling, and frontalis sling is the frontalis aponeurosis flap advancement.

In a 2018 article in Ophthalmic and Plastic Reconstructive Surgery (OPRS), Cruz and Akaishi researched the literature to evaluate the standardization and success of the frontalis flap as correction for blepharoptosis. Their search of the current literature concluded that the procedure was well-regarded but had not been compared to frontalis sling surgery; more vigorous research was needed for accurate comparisons to be drawn [50]. In one study, the frontalis muscle flap and maximal levator resection were compared by Wolley-Dod [51]. The authors found, in 58 patients studied, that while both techniques achieved good results, there were fewer reoperations needed with the frontalis muscle flap.

This frontalis sling procedure is indicated for severe (4 mm or more) unilateral or bilateral congenital ptosis with poor levator function (4 mm or less). The procedure is destined to fail if the frontal muscle is atrophic or paralytic, because the height of the eyelid is totally dependent on how tight the surgeon ties the fascial strips and also on how much force the frontal muscle can transmit to the eyelid through the strips.

Retrieval of Autogenous Fascia Lata from the Thigh

With its low rate of complication and recurrence, autogenous fascia lata has become the gold standard material of choice for eyebrow suspension [52–54]. It is usually not sufficiently developed as donor material until the child is 3–4 years of age. If surgery must be performed because of amblyopia before the child attains this age, preserved fascia lata or other sling materials can be used, although there is an increased risk of recurrence and infection transmission with preserved fascia lata [24] (Fig. 14.5).

Frontalis Suspension Method

The approach to the frontalis suspension is similar whether the Crawford (triangle) [55] or Fox (pentagon) [56] approaches are used. Again, the procedure has been documented extensively in the academic literature as well as in prior editions of this text [24]. Briefly, equidistant 4 mm skin incisions are made in the eyelid and eyebrow, and then strips are threaded and passed superficially (anterior to the tarsus) from the eyelid incisions to the eyebrow incisions. Of note, the fascia should be tied with almost maximum tension at the time of operation for a successful outcome.

Complications of Eyebrow Suspension (Table 14.6)

Bilateral Congenital Ptosis

Approximately 25% of children presenting to an ophthalmologist's office with congenital ptosis have bilateral drooping. In such cases, both eyelids should be corrected by similar operations (i.e., do not use levator resection on one eyelid and frontalis suspension on the other) during the same session. If less than the desired amount of elevation is obtained on both eyelids, the result may still be satisfactory, as long as it is symmetric. The procedures used in bilateral cases are the same ones as previously described for unilateral ptosis.

Mild (2 mm or less) bilateral ptosis is almost always accompanied by good (8–12 mm) levator function and usually does not present a difficult surgical problem. The bilateral Fasanella-Servat operation, 8 mm Müllerectomies, or levator resection (10–13mm) would be the procedures of choice if such a patient desires correction.

With moderate ptosis (3 mm), toddlers must usually tilt their head backward to see, and this is why many parents seek help when their child begins to walk (the ptosis may not be noticeable while the baby is not yet ambulatory). The quantitative rules for levator resection are similar to those for

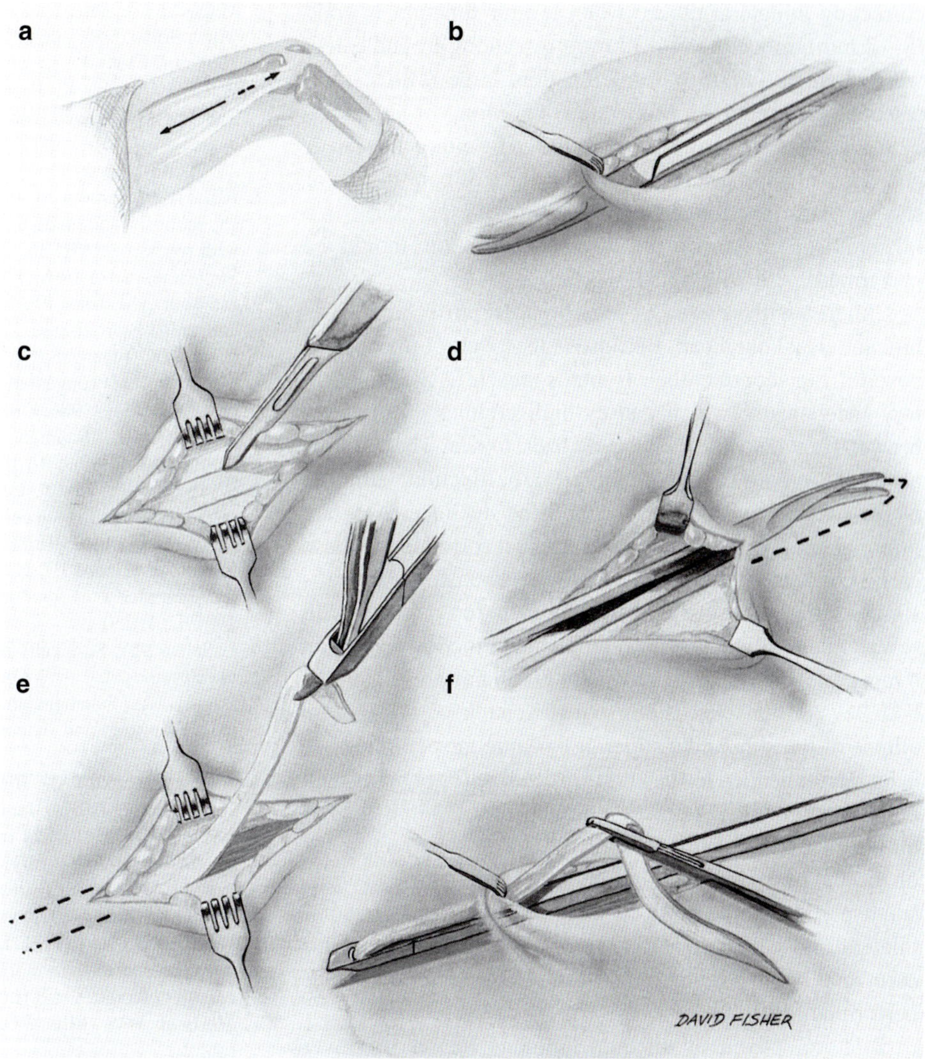

Fig. 14.5 Technique of removing autogenous fascia lata

Table 14.6 Complications of eyebrow suspension

Complication	Description/cause	Treatment/repair
Small overcorrection (0–1.5 mm)	Rare	Fascia can be tied as tightly as its strength will bear If corneal exposure is bothersome, knots can be untied during the first 10–14 postoperative days
Undercorrection	Slippage of the fascial knot (most common) Mechanical restriction of eyelid due to intraoperative hemorrhage	Open eyebrow incision and retie knot
Infection	Can have small incisional abscesses above eyebrow due to wound contamination	Broad-spectrum antibiotics If abscesses do not drain spontaneously or resolve with warm compresses, can be opened in office
Poor eyelid contour	Like with levator resection, can have nasal, central, or temporal peaking due to improper spacing of incisions or placement too close to eyelid margin	Correct intraoperatively before skin incisions are closed
Lagophthalmos	Usually occurs transiently	Patient can protect cornea by voluntary orbicularis muscle contraction (over time, this becomes involuntary)
Exposure keratopathy	May result in photophobia on waking in the morning	Artificial tears during the day Bland ointment at nighttime Ulceration is rare Treat persistent corneal breakdown with nightly eyelid taping or with moisture chamber goggles

correcting unilateral ptosis; when levator function is good (8–12 mm), moderate (14–17 mm) resections are indicated; when there is fair (5–7 mm) function, large (18–22 mm) resections are required. Moderate (14–17 mm) or large (18–22 mm) resections may be accomplished by either the skin or conjunctival approach. In the rare instance of poor (4 mm or less) levator function, bilateral eyebrow suspensions or a bilateral supermaximal (27–30 mm) resection should be performed.

Children with severe (≥4 mm) bilateral ptosis have a significant visual handicap. Because at least half of the pupil is covered, they contract their frontalis muscle as a compensatory mechanism, which causes high arching of the eyebrows. They also tilt their heads back to see. They almost always have poor (4 mm or more) levator function with little or no striated muscle present, and the eyelid creases are minimal or absent. The preferred surgical correction in these cases consists of bilateral eyebrow suspension. Frontalis sling is the current preferred approach for patients with severe bilateral ptosis with poor levator function (less than 4 mm). In the past, supermaximal (27–30 mm) resections of both levator muscles, along with excision of a 3–4 mm ellipse of the skin and a superior 3–4 mm tarsectomy, have been recommended as the "first" procedure for patients with poor (4 mm or more) function because it was more "physiologic." However, such patients are apt to have recurrence of the ptosis years later and need eyebrow suspension. A small percentage of patients with severe (4 mm or more) bilateral ptosis have fair (5–7 mm) levator function; in this case, maximum (23–26 mm) levator resection should be performed.

Bilateral ptosis of unequal amounts in the two eyes occurs frequently. Each eyelid must be considered separately to determine the amount of levator to be resected according to the quantitative rules. Bilateral levator resections (with a varying amount of muscle resected for each eye depending on the preoperative measurements) or frontalis muscle suspension would be the best procedure in these cases.

References

1. Berke RN, Wadsworth JA. Histology of levator muscle in congenital and acquired ptosis. Arch Ophthalmol. 1955;53(3):413–28.
2. Isaksson I, Mellgren J. Pathological-anatomical changes in the levator palpebrae sup. muscle in congenital blepharoptosis. Acta Pathol Microbiol Scand Suppl. 1961;51(Suppl 1):157–60.
3. Edmunds B, Manners RM, Weller RO, Steart P, Collin JRO. Levator palpebrae superioris fibre size in normals and patients with congenital ptosis. Eye. 1998;12(1):47–50.
4. Jubbal KT, Kania K, Braun TL, Katowitz WR, Marx DP. Pediatric blepharoptosis. Semin Plast Surg. 2017;31(1):58–64.
5. Stein A, Kelly JP, Weiss AH. Congenital eyelid ptosis: Onset and prevalence of amblyopia, associations with systemic disorders, and treatment outcomes. J Pediatr. 2014;165(4):820–824.e2.
6. Malandrini A, Mari F, Palmeri S, et al. PAX6 mutation in a family with aniridia, congenital ptosis, and mental retardation. Clin Genet. 2008;60(2):151–4.
7. Weiss K, Wigby K, Fannemel M, et al. Haploinsufficiency of ZNF462 is associated with craniofacial anomalies, corpus callosum dysgenesis, ptosis, and developmental delay. Eur J Hum Genet. 2017;25(8):946–51.
8. AlBakri A, Karaoui M, Alkuraya FS, Khan AO. Congenital ptosis, scoliosis, and malignant hyperthermia susceptibility in siblings with recessive RYR1 mutations. J Am Assoc Pediatr Ophthalmol Strabismus. 2015;19(6):577–9.
9. Mansour AM, Bitar FF, Traboulsi EI, et al. Ocular pathology in congenital heart disease. Eye (Lond). 2005;19(1):29–34.
10. Larned DC, Flanagan JC, Nelson LE, Harley RD, Wilson TW. The association of congenital ptosis and congenital heart disease. Ophthalmology. 1986;93(4):492–4.
11. Anderson RL, Baumgartner SA. Amblyopia in ptosis. Arch Ophthalmol. 1980;98(6):1068–9.
12. Wang Y, Xu Y, Liu X, Lou L, Ye J. Amblyopia, strabismus and refractive errors in congenital ptosis: a systematic review and meta-analysis. Sci Rep. 2018;8(1):1–9.
13. Cadera W, Bloom JN, Karlik S, Viirre E. A magnetic resonance imaging study of double elevator palsy. Can J Ophthalmol. 1997;32(4):250–3.
14. Callahan MA. Surgically mismanaged ptosis associated with double elevator palsy. Arch Ophthalmol. 1981;99(1):108–12.
15. Bagheri A, Sahebghalam R, Abrishami M. Double elevator palsy, subtypes and outcomes of surgery. J Ophthalmic Vis Res. 2008;3(2):108–13.
16. Allen CE, Rubin PAD. Blepharophimosis-ptosis-epicanthus inversus syndrome (BPES). Int Ophthalmol Clin. 2008;48(2):15–23.
17. Berke RN. The surgical treatment of congenital ptosis. Trans Pa Acad Ophthalmol Otolaryngol. 1961;14:57–61.
18. Beard C. The surgical treatment of blepharoptosis: a quantitative approach. Trans Am Ophthalmol Soc. 1966;64:401–87.
19. Nguyen CT, Hardy TG. Levator resection for congenital ptosis: does pre-operative levator function or degree of ptosis affect successful outcome? Orbit (London). 2017;36(5):325–30.
20. Merriam WW, Ellis RD, Helveston EM. Congenital blepharoptosis, anisometropia, and amblyopia. Am J Ophthalmol. 1980;89(3):401–7.
21. Paik JS, Kim SA, Park SH, Yang SW. Refractive error characteristics in patients with congenital blepharoptosis before and after ptosis repair surgery. BMC Ophthalmol. 2016;16(1):1–7.
22. Savino G, Battendieri R, Riso M, et al. Corneal topographic changes after eyelid ptosis surgery. Cornea. 2016;35(4):501–5.
23. Goldwyn RM. The patient and the plastic surgeon. Little, Brown & Company: Boston; 1981.
24. Black EH, Nesi FA, Calvano CJ, Gladstone GJ, Levine MR. Smith and Nesi's ophthalmic plastic and reconstructive surgery. New York: Springer; 2012.
25. Sonoda T, Ohdo S, Ohba K, Okishima T, Hayakawa K. Association of congenital heart disease, blepharoptosis, and short stature. Jpn J Hum Genet. 1989;34(4):291–6.
26. Marmor M. Malignant hyperthermia. Surv Ophthalmol. 1983;28(2):117–27.
27. Salazar JH, Yang J, Shen L, Abdullah F, Kim TW. Pediatric malignant hyperthermia: risk factors, morbidity, and mortality identified from the Nationwide Inpatient Sample and Kids' Inpatient Database. Paediatr Anaesth. 2014;24(12):1212–6.
28. Fox SA. A modified Fasanella-Servat procedure for ptosis. Arch Ophthalmol. 1975;93(8):639–40.
29. Fox SA. Surgery in ptosis. Arch Ophthalmol. 1980;98(1):186.
30. Berke RN. Blepharoptosis. Arch Ophthalmol. 1945;34:434–50.
31. Berke RN. Results of resection of the levator muscle through a skin incision in congenital ptosis. Trans Am Ophthalmol Soc. 1958;56:288–322; discussion 323–6.

32. Johnson CC. Blepharoptosis: a general consideration of surgical methods: with the results in 162 operations. Am J Ophthalmol. 1954;38(2):129–62.
33. Jones LT. The anatomy of the upper eyelid and its relation to ptosis surgery. Am J Ophthalmol. 1964;57(6):943–59.
34. Katowitz JA. Frontalis suspension in congenital ptosis using a polyfilament, cable-type suture. Arch Ophthalmol. 1979;97(9):1659–63.
35. Carraway JH, Vincent MP. Levator advancement technique for eyelid ptosis. Plast Reconstr Surg. 1986;77(3):394–403.
36. Harvey DJ, Iamphongsai S, Gosain AK. Unilateral congenital blepharoptosis repair by anterior levator advancement and resection: an educational review. Plast Reconstr Surg. 2010;126(4):1325–31.
37. SooHoo JR, Davies BW, Allard FD, Durairaj VD. Congenital ptosis. Surv Ophthalmol. 2014;59(5):483–92.
38. Ichinose A, Leibovitch I. Transconjunctival levator aponeurosis advancement without resection of Müller's muscle in aponeurotic ptosis repair. Open Ophthalmol J. 2010;4:85–90.
39. Blaskovicz L. A new operation for ptosis with shortening of the levator and tarsus. Arch Ophthalmol. 1923;52:563–73.
40. Agatson SA. Resection of levator palpebrae muscle by the conjunctival route for ptosis. Arch Ophthalmol. 1942;27(5):994.
41. Patel V, Malhotra R. Transconjunctival blepharoptosis surgery: a review of posterior approach ptosis surgery and posterior approach white-line advancement. Open Ophthalmol J. 2010;4:81–4.
42. Schwarz GS, Spinelli HM. Correction of upper eyelid retraction using deep temporal fascia spacer grafts. Plast Reconstr Surg. 2008;122(3):765–74.
43. Gonnering RS, Carroll RP. Cystic lesions of the eyelid following ptosis repair. Ophthal Plast Reconstr Surg. 1986;2(2):89–93.
44. Epstein GA, Putterman AM. Super-maximum levator resection for severe unilateral congenital blepharoptosis. Ophthalmic Surg. 1984;15(12):971–9.
45. Beard C. A new treatment for severe unilateral congenital ptosis and for ptosis with jaw-winking. Am J Ophthalmol. 1965;59(2):252–8.
46. Holds JB, McLeish WM, Anderson RL. Whitnall's sling with superior tarsectomy for the correction of severe unilateral blepharoptosis. Arch Ophthalmol. 1993;111(9):1285.
47. Callahan A. Correction of unilateral Blepharoptosis with bilateral eyelid suspension. Am J Ophthalmol. 1972;74(2):321–6.
48. Wasserman BN, Sprunger DT, Helveston EM. Comparison of materials used in frontalis suspension. Arch Ophthalmol. 2001;119(5):687.
49. Ben Simon GJ, Macedo AA, Schwarcz RM, Wang DY, McCann JD, Goldberg RA. Frontalis suspension for upper eyelid ptosis: evaluation of different surgical designs and suture material. Am J Ophthalmol. 2005;140(5):877–85.
50. Cruz AAV, Akaishi APMS. Frontalis-orbicularis muscle advancement for correction of upper eyelid ptosis: a systematic literature review. Ophthal Plast Reconstr Surg. 2018;34(6):510–5.
51. Medel R, Molina S, Vasquez LM, Visa J, Wert A, Wolley-Dod C. Frontalis muscle flap versus maximal anterior levator resection as first option for patients with severe congenital ptosis. Ophthal Plast Reconstr Surg. 2018;34(6):565–9.
52. Lee MJ, Oh JY, Choung H-K, Kim NJ, Sung MS, Khwarg SI. Frontalis sling operation using silicone rod compared with preserved fascia lata for congenital ptosis: a three-year follow-up study. Ophthalmology. 2009;116(1):123–9.
53. Bernardini FP, Cetinkaya A, Zambelli A. Treatment of unilateral congenital ptosis: putting the debate to rest. Curr Opin Ophthalmol. 2013;24(5):484–7.
54. Lee J, Lee H, Chang M, Park M, Baek S. Clinical results of modified frontalis suspension technique using preserved fascia lata for congenital ptosis. J Craniofac Surg. 2016;27(5):e477–81.
55. Crawford JS. Repair of ptosis using frontalis muscle and fascia lata. Trans Am Acad Ophthalmol Otolaryngol. 1956;60:672–82.
56. Fox SA. A new frontalis skin sling for ptosis. Am J Ophthalmol. 1968;65(3):359–62.

Acquired Ptosis: Classification and Evaluation

15

John D. Siddens, Jenna M. Kim, and Geoffrey J. Gladstone

Introduction

Blepharoptosis, or ptosis, is a unilateral or bilateral droop of the upper eyelid with the patient's head in the fully upright position and eyes in primary gaze. Patients often seek medical attention because of visual obstruction or cosmetic deformity caused by ptotic lids. Ptosis is often recognized by friends or family but some cases may be seen only by a physician. Ptosis may be an isolated condition, or it may occur from a number of different causes.

Anatomy and Physiology

A detailed description of the anatomy of the eyelid and levator complex may be found elsewhere in this text. Knowledge of this anatomy is paramount for appropriate surgical reconstruction of ptotic eyelids. Early authors described in great detail the relationship of the levator palpebrae superioris muscle with its insertion into the tarsus, orbicularis muscle, and skin [1, 2]. Recent investigators have improved our understanding of the relationship of the levator aponeurosis with the tarsal plate and anterior skin structures [3, 4].

The origin of the levator muscle is at the apex of the orbit, just above the annulus of Zinn. The length of the levator is approximately 60 mm, 40 mm of which is muscular and the distal 15–20 mm of which is fibrous aponeurosis. The superior transverse ligament, also known as Whitnall's ligament, is a condensation of the anterior sheath of the levator muscle. This ligament is found at the approximate area of transition from levator muscle to levator aponeurosis. Whitnall's ligament functions as a suspensory support for the upper eyelid and orbital tissue along with acting as a fulcrum and suspensory component for the levator complex. Whitnall's ligament attaches to the connective tissue around the trochlea medially, and it courses through the lacrimal gland laterally to attach to the inner aspect of the lateral orbital wall approximately 10 mm above the orbital tubercle.

The transition from muscular levator to fibrous aponeurosis is gradual but tends to occur 10–12 mm above the tarsal plate. At this level, the sympathetically innervated smooth muscle fibers of Müller's muscle arise from the undersurface of the levator aponeurosis. This muscle runs along the posterior surface of the aponeurosis to insert on the superior tarsal border. Müller's muscle is adherent to the conjunctiva posteriorly but is much less firmly attached to the aponeurosis. This superior tarsal muscle may provide approximately 2 mm of lift for the upper eyelid and accounts for 2 mm of vertical palpebral fissure height in a fully awake individual. The peripheral marginal arterial arcade is found between the aponeurosis and Müller's muscle just above the superior tarsal border.

As the levator courses forward, fibers from the orbital septum fuse with the aponeurosis 3–5 mm above the superior tarsal border. Just beneath this fusion, fibers frm the aponeurosis course forward to insert into the subcutaneous fibers of the skin. The insertion helps to form the natural eyelid crease. The remaining levator fibers then run along the anterior surface of the tarsal plate. The fibers are loosely attached to the upper 2–3 mm of tarsus and are most firmly attached 3 mm above the eyelid margin.

The medial and lateral fibers of the levator form horns, which are much stronger than the middle aspects of the levator complex. The lateral horn is a broad, strong band about 4 mm in width, which divides the lacrimal gland into a palpebral and an orbital lobe. The lateral horn then attaches to

J. D. Siddens
Ophthalmic Plastic Surgery Service, Greenville Memorial Hospital, Prisma Health System Upstate, Division of Ophthalmology, Department of Surgery, Greenville, SC, USA

J. M. Kim
William Beaumont School of Medicine, Beaumont Eye Institute, Royal Oak, IL, USA

G. J. Gladstone (✉)
Consultants in Ophthalmic and Facial Plastic Surgery, P.C., Southfield, MI, USA

Oakland University/William Beaumont Hospital, School of Medicine, Department of Ophthalmology, Royal Oak, MI, USA

J. J. Servat et al. (eds.), *Smith and Nesi's Ophthalmic Plastic and Reconstructive Surgery*,
https://doi.org/10.1007/978-3-030-41720-8_15

the periorbita at the lateral orbital tubercle, along with the lateral canthal tendon. The medial horn is much thinner and more delicate, and as it passes nasally, it inserts loosely to portions of the medial canthal tendon and an area at the posterior lacrimal crest [5].

Classification

Acquired ptoses account for approximately 60% of all ptosis cases. The most useful classification of acquired ptoses was proposed by Beard [6]. Later authors have added subclassifications [7, 8].

It is perhaps most useful to classify the acquired ptoses according to the underlying cause. These include aponeurotic, myogenic, neurogenic, traumatic, and mechanical. The clinical presentation of patients with ptosis often involves one or more categories, and management is based on the etiology. Pseudoptosis may be an additional category and includes patients with dermatochalasis, enophthalmos, hypotropia, or phthisis bulbi.

Aponeurotic Ptosis

Aponeurotic ptosis is considered the most frequent form of acquired ptosis. This condition may occur as the result of a localized or generalized disinsertion or dehiscence of the aponeurosis from the tarsal plate. Clinical features of this type of ptosis may include a high or absent lid crease, good levator function, and thin eyelid tissue (Fig. 15.1). Typically, aponeurotic ptosis occurs as a result of aging changes, including microinfarction of collagen bundles and other tissue within the aponeurosis [9]. Occasionally, levator fibers may be replaced with bundles of adipose tissue, leading to fatty infiltration of the levator.

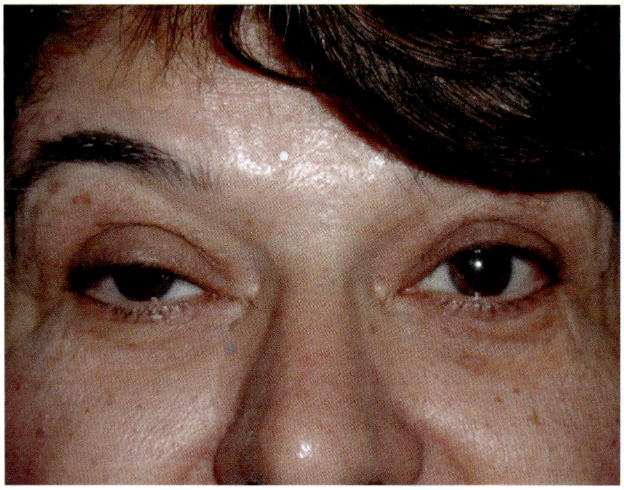

Fig. 15.1 Ptosis of the left upper eyelid due to aponeurotic disinsertion

This type of ptosis typically is found in elderly patients and is referred to as involutional ptosis in some text; however, younger patients may have aponeurotic ptosis due to previous trauma [10], postsurgical changes [11], contact lens wear [12], long-standing Graves'-related lid retraction [13] that has eventually led to levator dehiscence, or pregnancy.

Myogenic Ptosis

Ptosis in this category often overlaps with ptosis of neurogenic etiology. Conditions that result in ptosis include myasthenia gravis, chronic progressive external ophthalmoplegia, and myotonic dystrophy.

Myasthenia Gravis

Myasthenia gravis (MG) is an autoimmune disease in which antibodies to acetylcholine receptor sites of neuromotor end plates impair the transfer of acetylcholine from the neuron to the muscle. In this situation, muscle fatigue and weakness occur. MG is more common in women, although it affects all races, ages, and both sexes [14, 15]. Approximately 85–90% of patients with MG present with localized ocular signs, although the disease may be generalized. Ptosis is the most frequent clinical manifestation (Figs. 15.2 a, b and 15.3), and it may be unilateral or bilateral and is variable in nature [16]. Ptosis may worsen as the day progresses and is usually more pronounced with a sustained upgaze. (Refer to Chap. 13 for discussion of diagnosis and treatment of myasthenia gravis.)

Chronic Progressive External Ophthalmoplegia

This disorder occurs due to a defect in mitochondrial function in which a slowly progressive weakness of the extraocular and periocular muscles occurs. Although autosomal-dominant inheritance has been described, sporadic cases may occur. Chronic progressive external ophthalmoplegia (CPEO) is called external because the extraocular and periocular muscles are involved, whereas the iris and ciliary body muscles are not. CPEO typically begins in childhood or adolescence and progresses very slowly over the next 40–50 years. Almost any of the body's muscles may be affected, but usually, bilateral ptosis is the first symptom noted (Fig. 15.4a, b). At an advanced stage, the eyes may be totally immobile, and if the face is involved, a myopathic (Hutchinson's) facies occurs. A multitude of associated neurodegenerative disease may occur with CPEO. These

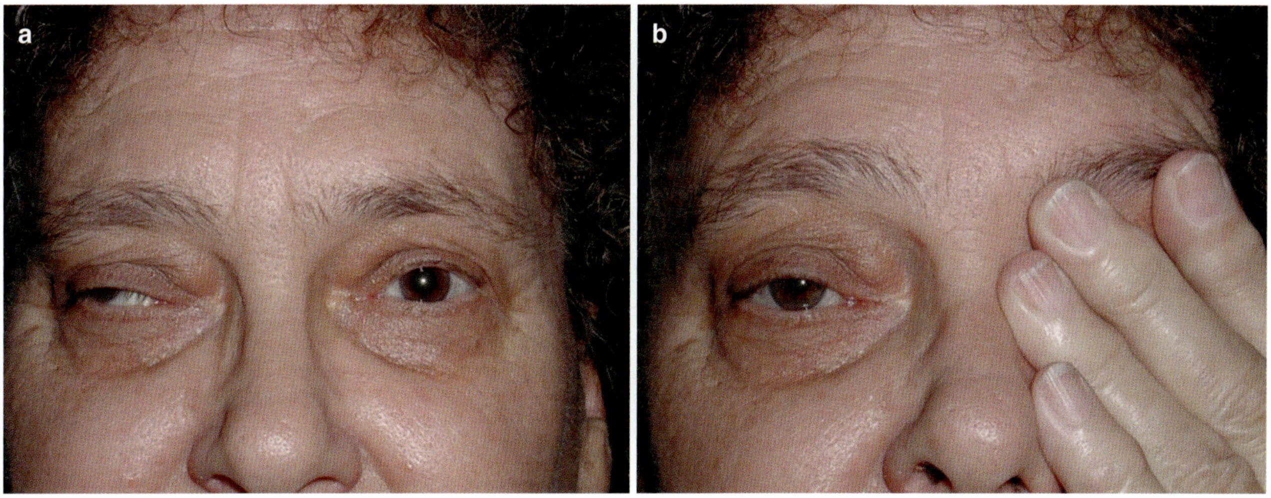

Fig. 15.2 (**a**) and (**b**) Ptosis in both upper eyelids caused by myasthenia gravis

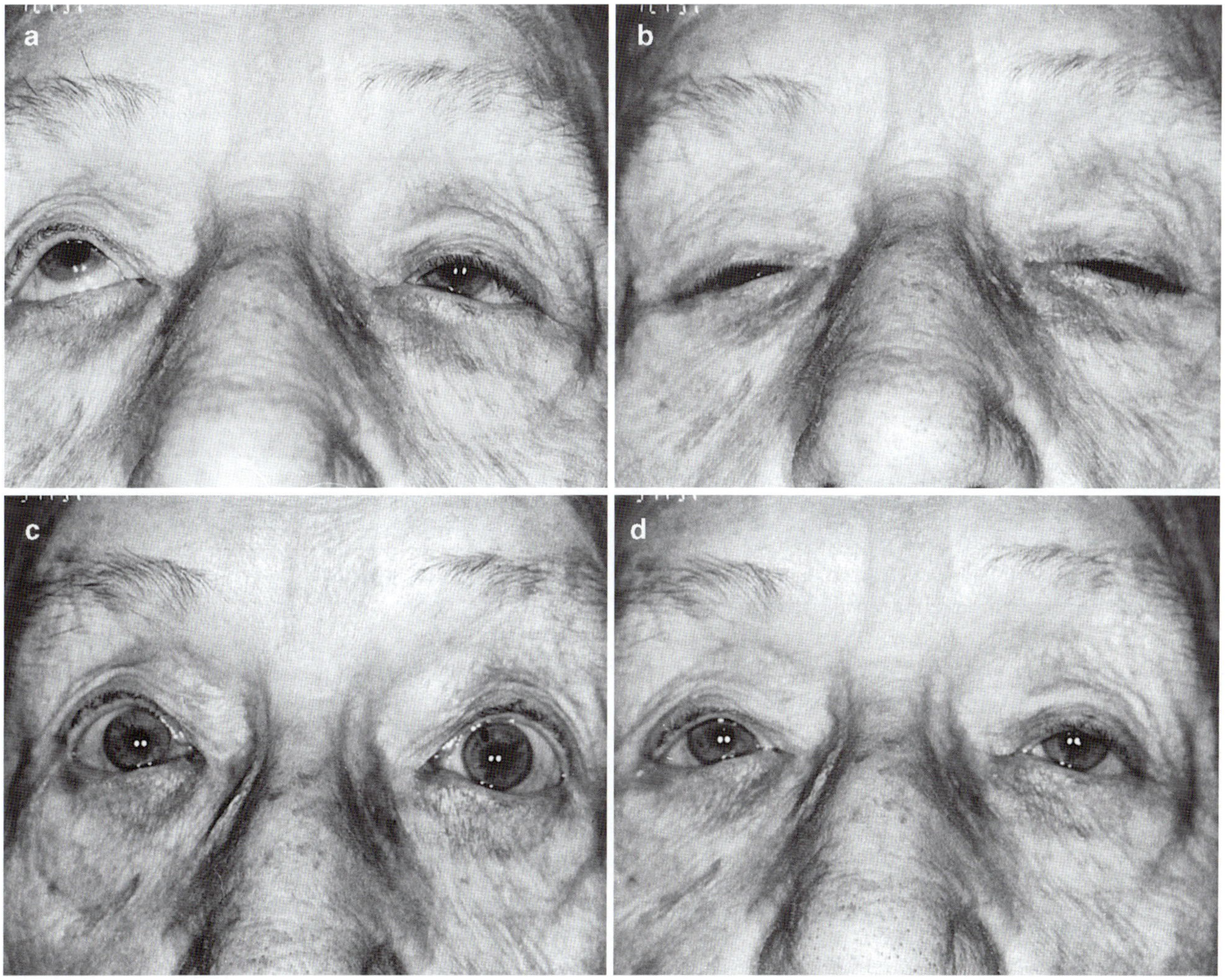

Fig. 15.3 (**a**) Patient with myasthenia gravis in upgaze. (**b**) Same patient in downgaze. (**c**) Patient 90 s after administration of Tensilon. (**d**) Patient 5 min after administration of Tensilon

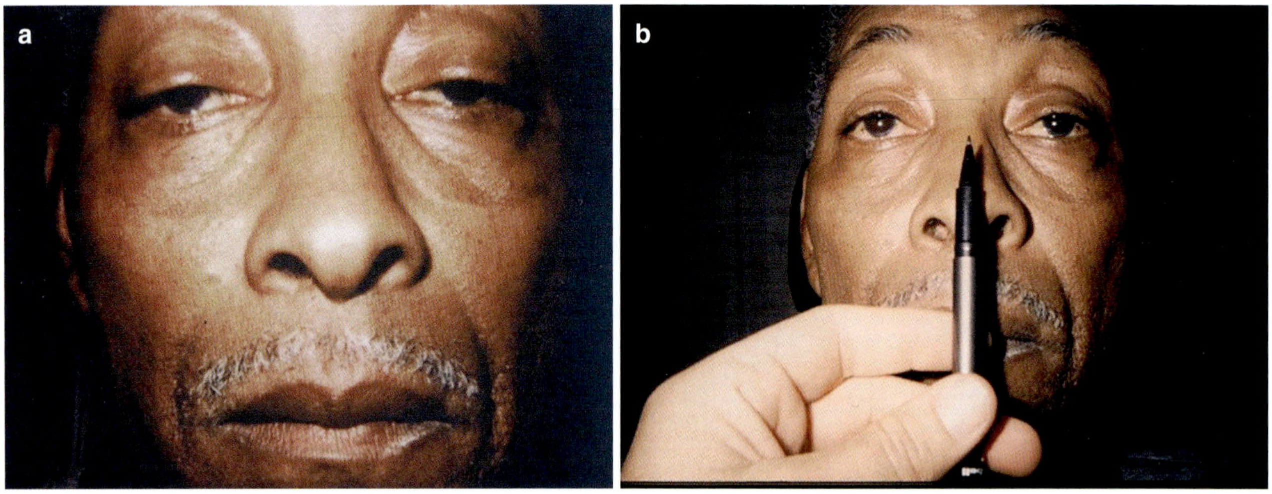

Fig. 15.4 (**a**) Marked ptosis of both upper eyelids caused by chronic progressive external ophthalmoplegia: primary gaze. (**b**) Same patient in upgaze

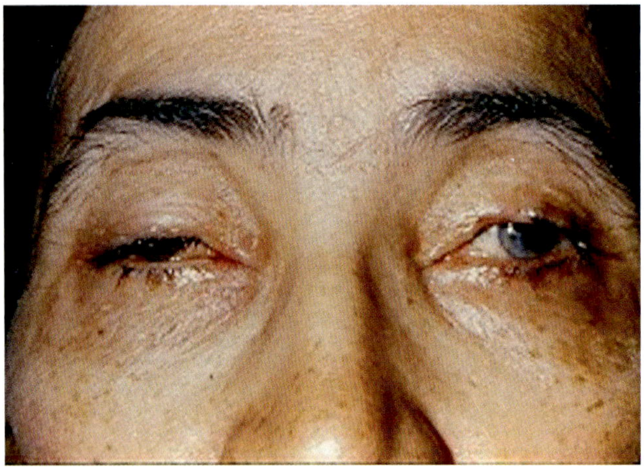

Fig. 15.5 Marked ptosis in both upper eyelids caused by chronic oculopharyngeal dystrophy

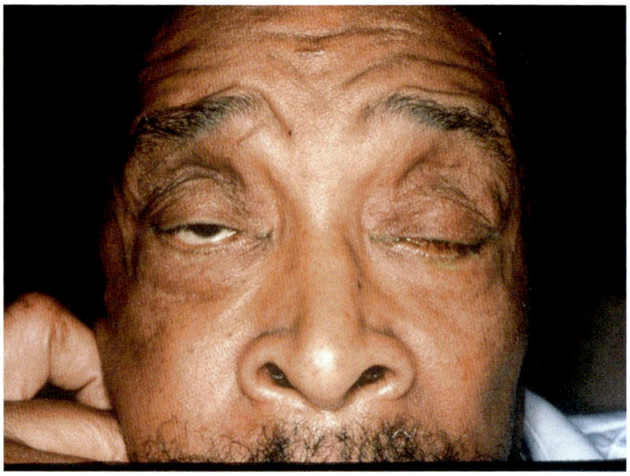

Fig. 15.6 Ptosis in both upper eyelids caused by myotonic dystrophy

include thyroid orbitopathy, myasthenia gravis, myotonic dystrophy, Refsum's disease, and oculopharyngeal dystrophy, among others.

Kearns and Sayre described a form of CPEO in which retinitis pigmentosa, CPEO, and complete heart block occurred typically by the age of 20 years. Other manifestations include short stature, ataxia, neuropathy, and endocrine dysfunction. Ragged red fibers in muscle biopsies are suggestive of mitochondrial disease, as is the presence of spongy degeneration of the central nervous system. Patients with Kearns–Sayre syndrome require serial electrocardiograms to monitor for heart block.

Oculopharyngeal dystrophy is a myopathic form of CPEO that begins after age 40 and consists of slowly progressive ptosis with dysphagia and dysarthria. This results from pharyngeal dystrophy, and in some patients, the extraocular muscles, shoulder muscles, and pelvic girdle muscles may be involved. Inheritance is autosomal dominant, and many have French-Canadian ancestry (Fig. 15.5) [17].

Myotonic Dystrophy

Myotonic dystrophy is a genetic disease with an autosomal-dominant inheritance, and it may be associated with varying degrees of bilateral ptosis (Fig. 15.6), orbicularis weakness, poor lid closure, ophthalmoparesis, and poor blinking. Additional findings may include chromatic cataracts, testicular atrophy, diabetes mellitus, first-degree heart block, and frontal alopecia [18].

Neurogenic Ptosis

Neurogenic ptosis may result from a multitude of neurologic disorders. The author presents the most likely ptosis seen by an ophthalmologist. Conditions that are listed in this category include third nerve palsy, Horner's syndrome, ophthalmoplegic migraine, multiple sclerosis, Marcus Gunn syndrome, and Guillain–Barré syndrome.

Third Cranial Nerve Palsy

Lesions of the oculomotor (CN III) nerve cause ptosis along with deficits of adduction, elevation, and depression of the eye (Fig. 15.7). The pupil may be normal or dilated. Lesions of the superior division of the third nerve involve only the superior rectus and levator muscles, with resultant ptosis and decreased upgaze. Congenital third nerve palsy usually presents with ptosis and ophthalmoparesis, as well as a miotic pupil (as a result of misdirected third nerve regeneration). Acquired third nerve palsy may be a neurosurgical emergency if the pupil is involved typically due to a compressive lesion, such as a posterior communicating artery aneurysm. Other causes of neurosurgical third nerve palsy include infection, cavernous sinus thrombosis, fistulas, tumors, and contiguous paranasal sinus disease [19]. (Refer to Chap. 34 for detailed discussion of third cranial nerve palsy.)

Horner's Syndrome (Ocular Sympathetic Paresis)

Horner's syndrome consists of mild ptosis, pupillary miosis, and at times facial anhidrosis. Pseudoenophthalmos may be apparent and is the result of a decreased palpebral fissure size. Ptosis is due to decreased sympathetic tone in Müller's muscle (Fig. 15.8). Loss of sympathetic innervation to the lower lid retractors may cause elevation of the lower eyelid, the so-called upside-down ptosis.

Horner's syndrome may be caused by lesions in any of the three levels of neurons that carry sympathetic impulses to the eye. The first-order neuron begins at the hypothalamus and

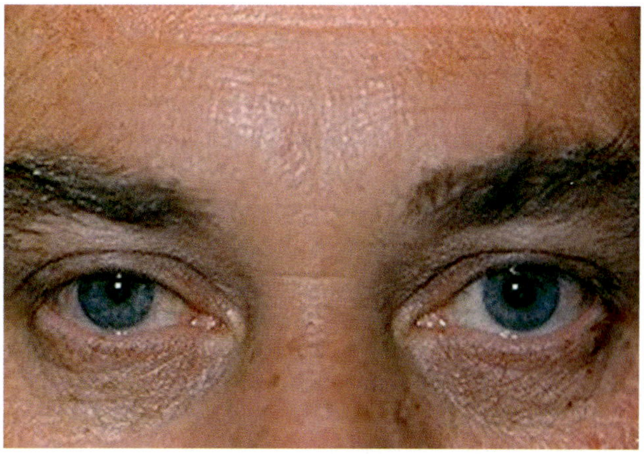

Fig. 15.8 Minimal ptosis in right upper eyelid caused by Horner's syndrome following excision of tumor in the neck. Miotic left pupil is also present

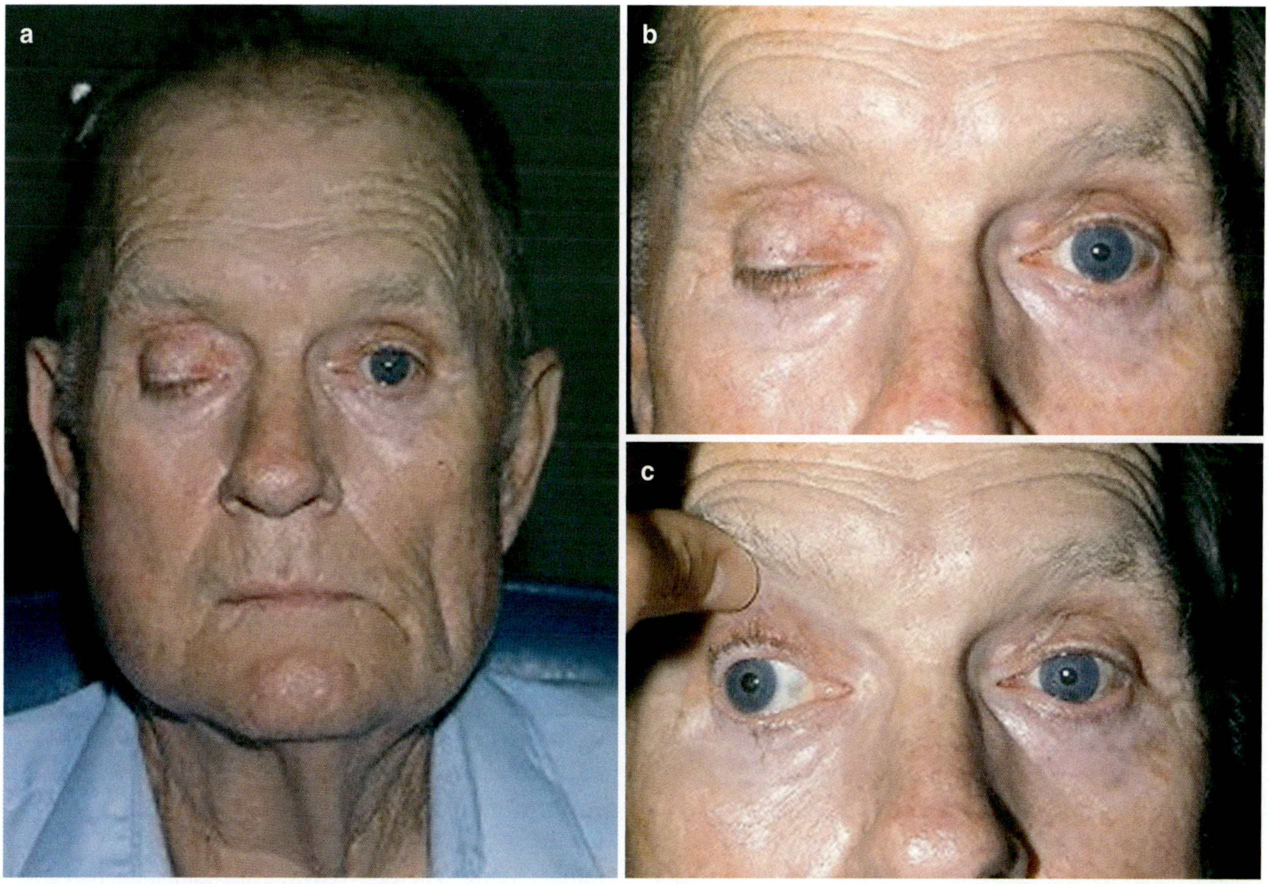

Fig. 15.7 (**a**) Complete right upper eyelid ptosis caused by third cranial nerve palsy. (**b**) and (**c**) Typical position of globe with exotropia and hypotropia associated with dilated pupil

terminates in the intermediolateral cell column of the spinal cord at the level of C8–T2 (ciliospinal center of Budge). The second-order preganglïotic neuron begins here, ascends through the sympathetic chain in close proximity to the pulmonary apex and subclavian artery, and synapses at the superior cervical ganglion. The third-order postganglionic neuron in this chain then travels along the internal carotid artery to terminate at the tarsal muscles and pupillary dilator muscles. Patients with congenital Horner's syndrome may show iris hypochromia due to lack of sympathetic stimulation interferes with melanin pigmentation of melanocytes in the superficial iris stroma. These cases are typically due to brachial plexus injury during birth. Occasionally, other lesions, including tumors, may be responsible for congenital Horner's syndrome [20, 21].

Differentiation of the involved neuron in Horner's syndrome is important. Testing with cocaine and hydroxyamphetamine (Paredrine) eye drops may be performed to confirm the diagnosis of Horner's syndrome and to localize the lesion to the first-, second-, or third-order neuron in the chain. Four percent cocaine solution, which blocks the reuptake of norepinephrine, may be given as one drop in each eye, followed by one additional drop 5 min later, and the pupils are measured after 30 min. If the suspect pupil does not dilate and the presumed normal pupil does, then Horner's syndrome is confirmed. In situations where obtaining cocaine for testing is difficult, alpha-agonist apraclonidine can be used. Apraclonidine leads to a reversal of miosis on the side affected with Horner's syndrome. Testing cannot differentiate between the first- and second-order neurons, but the Paredrine test may demonstrate a third-order neuron lesion. One percent Paredrine ophthalmic solution is administered as one drop in each eye, followed by one drop in each eye 5 min later. If the suspect pupil fails to dilate and the normal pupil does dilate, this confirms Horner's syndrome as a third-order neuron. The cocaine and Paredrine test must be separated by at least 24 hours. Pharmacologic testing is important to localize the lesion because the third-order neuron lesion is typically benign, whereas first- and second-order Horner's syndrome may often be caused by malignancy, and further investigation may be warranted.

Ophthalmoplegic Migraine

Ophthalmoplegic migraine is a rare cause of third nerve palsy. Patients are typically young adults or children, often with a history of migraine headaches. Fifty percent of these patients have a family history of migraines. The mechanism of ophthalmoplegic migraine is unclear; however, it is believed that dilation of the carotid artery may play a factor. Compression of the third nerve usually occurs as the patient begins to complain of severe headaches, followed by ptosis and extraocular muscle paralysis [22, 23]. The pupil is involved in the majority of patients. Ophthalmoplegic migraine usually responds dramatically to oral steroids, and recovery is usually complete after the initial attack. However, if repeated episodes occur, permanent ophthalmoparesis may occur.

Multiple Sclerosis

Multiple sclerosis (MS) is an idiopathic autoimmune disease that occurs when multifocal demyelination occurs within the white matter of the central nervous system. MS occurs most often in young adults with a female predominance and an average age of 30 years. The most common presenting symptoms are weakness, numbness, and paresthesias of the extremities.

Involvement of the visual system usually takes the form of ocular inflammation or an eye movement disorder. Optic neuritis occurs in about 50% of patients with MS, and in about 20% of patients, it is the presenting sign. Rapid onset of unilateral decrease in visual acuity is the most frequent manifestation, followed by pain with eye movement, afferent pupillary defect, and eye movement disorders, including ptosis [24]. Recurrent attacks are frequent, and symptoms follow a pattern of exacerbation and remission lasting weeks to months. Evaluation includes brain magnetic resonance imaging studies, cerebrospinal fluid (CSF) studies, and histocompatibility antigen studies. The Optic Neuritis Treatment Trial suggests that the use of oral corticosteroids alone is ineffective in the treatment of optic neuritis and that this approach may actually increase the risk of developing new episodes [25]. In more severe cases, high-dose intravenous steroids, followed by an 11-day course of oral steroids, have been shown to speed recovery in the first few weeks, but no long-term beneficial effect for vision persists. Immunomodulatory drugs, such as interferon beta-1a, interferon beta-1b, and glatiramer, are proven to reduce morbidity in the relapsing–remitting form of MS. At present, treatment needs to be individualized for the patient [26, 27].

Jaw-Winking (Marcus Gunn Syndrome)

Some patients display an unusual synkinetic movement of elevation of the unilateral ptotic eyelid with jaw movements. This Marcus Gunn jaw-winking phenomenon is caused by aberrant connections between the motor division of cranial nerve V and the levator muscle. When the jaw opens widely or is deviated to the contralateral side, the pterygoid muscles are stimulated. The resultant impulse is sent through abnormal fibers to the levator muscle, causing the eyelid to open and close repeatedly [28].

Guillain–Barré Syndrome

Guillain–Barré syndrome (GBS; acute idiopathic polyneuritis) is a motor neuropathy which often occurs following a viral illness. The lower extremities often exhibit weakness and numbness, and these problems typically progress in an ascending fashion. Ptosis is a frequent manifestation of GBS. The Fisher variant, a limited form of GBS, consists of bilateral ophthalmoplegia and ptosis. Ataxia and areflexia occur as well, but there is no systemic weakness. The CSF contains an elevated amount of protein with relatively few cells (albuminocytologic dissociation) [29].

Traumatic Ptosis

Ptosis may occur from stress or trauma to the levator aponeurosis both from external and iatrogenic causes. Blunt or sharp injury may cause local damage to the levator muscle or aponeurosis or both. Injury to the periocular tissues may cause edema, hemorrhage, or infection, which may also cause ptosis (Fig. 15.9). Orbital fractures and foreign bodies may impair levator function either directly or subsequently.

Ptosis has also been shown to occur from injury to the levator aponeurosis as a result of surgery. Cataract and trabeculectomy surgery have been shown to cause ptosis in up to 10–20% of cases [30].

Mechanical Ptosis

Mechanical ptosis may be caused by lid tumors, scarring, or blepharochalasis. Lid tumors may cause ptosis as a result of increased weight on the upper eyelid or cause disinsertion by stretching the levator (Fig. 15.10). Cicatricial ptosis may be caused as a result of trauma or diseases that involve the conjunctiva or levator complex. Blepharochalasis is a rare condition of unknown etiology. This is typically inherited and is more common in young women. This condition is manifested by intermittent transient episodes of periocular edema and erythema. As the inflammatory episodes become more frequent, the upper eyelid tissues are stretched and may cause disinsertion of the levator complex. The orbital septum may become thinned and atrophic with prolapse of periorbital adipose tissue into the eyelid as well as thinning and discoloration of the eyelid skin. Reoperation is often necessary owing to the recurrent nature of this syndrome [31].

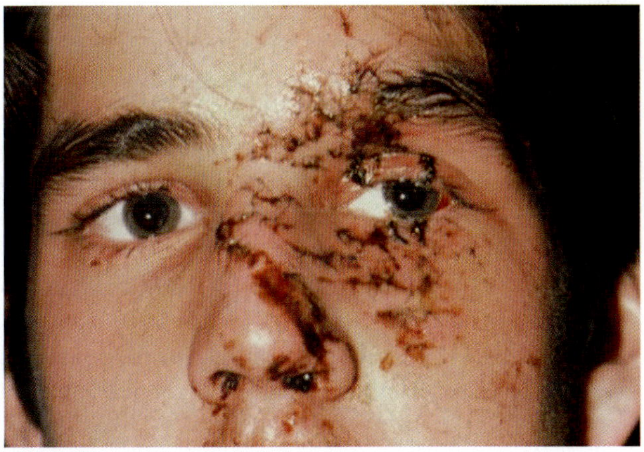

Fig. 15.9 Multiple facial lacerations sustained during a fall while skiing. Lacerations involved full-thickness tissue of eyelid and the levator aponeurosis

Pseudoptosis

A patient may appear with apparent ptosis when true eyelid ptosis is not actually present. There are several reasons that may cause this type of confusing picture. Inflammatory conditions of the eye, including keratitis, photophobia, or functional complaints that cause squinting or guarding, may cause an apparent ptosis. Lack of posterior lid support, such as in an anophthalmic eye, a posttraumatic eye (Fig. 15.11), or the presence of an orbital prosthesis, may result in ptosis. A hypotropic eye may appear to have a droopy eyelid, although this normalizes when the patient is asked to fix on an object with the hypotropic eye. Dermatochalasis

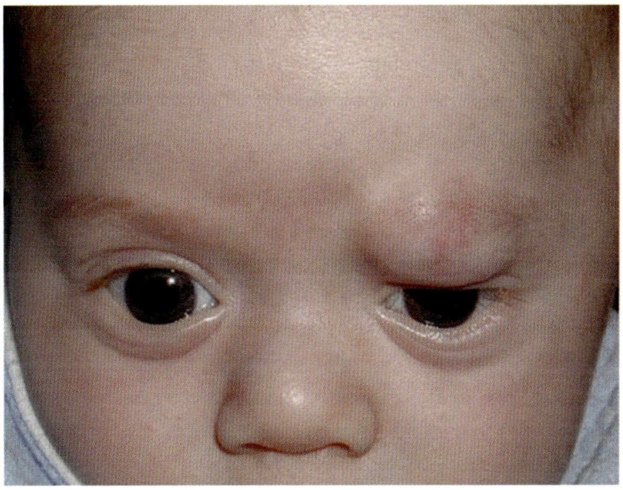

Fig. 15.10 Hemangioma resulting in mechanical ptosis

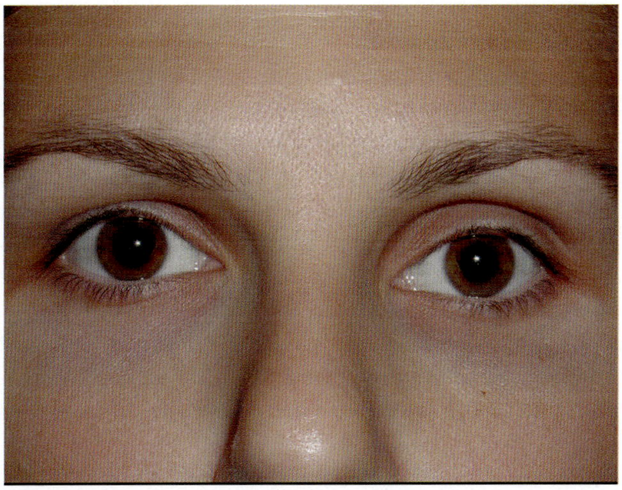

Fig. 15.11 Pseudoptosis in left upper eyelid due to posttraumatic enophthalmos

(redundant upper eyelid skin) may also cause the appearance of a droopy eyelid, although when lifting the skin off of the eyelid, the margin typically returns to normal position. Retraction of one eye may often cause the appearance of ptosis of the fellow eye. This occurs commonly in thyroid eye disease and in cases of cicatricial eyelid retraction.

Evaluation

History

A careful history helps identify the etiology of ptosis. The history should include the approximate time of onset of ptosis and an indication as to whether or not the condition is improving, worsening, or remaining unchanged. Related symptoms should be reviewed, including the loss of peripheral vision, the use of eyebrows or fingers to open the eyelids, and the possibility of previous trauma. Often, the history must be obtained from the family, and birth injuries or a neonatal illness may be important. Eyelid or globe surgery and contact lens use are important, as is a family history of eye abnormalities. Old photographs of the patient and family members may help determine the time of onset and type of ptosis. An estimation of the mental status of the patient can usually be obtained at this time.

A thorough review of the patient's systemic history may lead to clues for the cause of ptosis. Questions regarding childhood health and development, general health, and systemic illnesses should be asked and recorded. Medications and dosages, as well as allergic reactions to medications, should also be documented. Any regular use of aspirin or other blood thinners should be specifically covered as well as bleeding tendencies. Questions about previous surgeries, including the patient's reaction to anesthesia, should be asked.

Usually, the questions and answers lead to a specific direction and provide a very clear picture of the patient's background and type of ptosis.

Physical Examination

The examination of a patient with ptosis is probably the single most important factor in determining the type of surgical approach. If not previously performed, a complete eye examination is necessary. However, topical medications should be avoided until all baseline eyelid measurements have been obtained. Visual acuity must be documented with and without correction. The refraction status of the patient should be known.

Careful inspection and palpation of the eyelids and orbits help determine the extent of asymmetry and proptosis, if present. Exophthalmometry is helpful to assess for globe position and the possible presence of orbital masses or enophthalmos. The presence or absence of an eyelid crease and its distance from the eyelid margin are noted and recorded. The amount of brow effort may be estimated by the presence of deep forehead creases. The amount of redundant eyelid skin is also noted, and eversion of the eyelids helps determine the presence of foreign bodies or inflammatory conjunctivitis. Head position is noted because the presence of ptosis may cause a compensatory chin-up head posture.

The size and reaction of pupils should be measured both in light and in dark. A slit lamp examination and fundus evaluation help determine the presence of ocular disease, surgery, or previous trauma to the eyes. An evaluation of ocular motility is important even if the patient is not complaining of diplopia. Motility disturbances along with ptosis may be noted in conditions, such as orbital masses, myasthenia gravis, CPEO, or other neurogenic causes. The strength of the orbicularis muscle is also noted.

The presence of Bell's phenomenon, Schirmer testing, and corneal reflex testing may be checked preoperatively to determine the potential for exposure keratitis following ptosis repair. Two simple tests may be performed in the office to determine the amount of lacrimal secretion. The basic secretion test is performed by placing one or two drops of topical anesthesia in the conjunctiva. The inferior cul-de-sac is then blotted dry, and a Schirmer strip is placed in the inferior cul-de-sac for 5 min. Ten millimeters or more of moisture should be present on the filter paper strip. The Schirmer I test measures both reflex and basic secretion. A strip of filter paper is placed in the inferior cul-de-sac for 5 min with no topical anesthesia. Normal wetting should be at least 12–15 mm.

Eyelid Measurements

Eyelid measurements provide objective information that helps determine the type of procedure that will best correct ptosis. The amount of eyelid droop is measured in millimeters and can easily be measured with most vision cards or millimeter rulers. If a patient is unable or unwilling to allow accurate eyelid measurements, measurements can be estimated by noting the relationship of the eyelid margin to the upper limbus and the upper pupillary border. The most accurate measurement of eyelid function is determined by the location of the corneal light reflex (from a handheld penlight or other small light source) in relation to the position of the eyelid margins.

A variety of measurements of eyelid position and excursion have been made a part of ptosis evaluation by many surgeons (Box 15.1) [32–34]. Although each of these methods may have a place in determining the type of surgical approach

Box 15.1. Eyelid Measurements

PF (PRIMARY FISSURE) The distance between the upper eyelid and lower eyelid margins. Variable, depending upon globe position. Fixate brow to measure.

MRD1 (UPPER EYELID MARGIN–CORNEAL LIGHT REFLEX IN PRIMARY GAZE) The distance from the upper eyelid margin to the corneal light reflex in primary gaze. Best measure of true ptosis. Normal, 3.0–4.5 mm.

MRD2 (LOWER EYELID MARGIN–CORNEAL LIGHT REFLEX IN PRIMARY GAZE) The distance from lower eyelid margin to corneal light reflex in primary gaze. Aids in comparing true eyelid position. Normal, 4.0–5.0 mm.

LF (LEVATOR FUNCTION) The amount of upper eyelid excursion from maximum upgaze to maximum downgaze. Normal, 12.0–18.0 mm.

PFD (PALPEBRAL FISSURE IN DOWNGAZE) Distance from upper eyelid to lower eyelid margins in maximum downgaze. Smaller on ptotic side in acquired ptosis. Larger in congenital ptosis and thyroid eyelid retraction.

LAG (LAGOPHTHALMOS) PF with *gentle* eyelid closure. Normally less than 1.0 mm.

for ptosis repair, several are indispensable. The margin to reflex distance in primary gaze (MRD1) is the distance between the upper lid margin and the corneal light reflex. This is the best measurement of true ptosis and is measured with the ipsilateral frontalis muscle suppressed, and contralateral eyelid is elevated if ptotic to avoid Herring's law effects. MRD1 usually measures 3.0–5.0 mm, but negative values are possible. The levator function (LF) indicates the distance of the total excursion of the upper eyelid margin from maximum upgaze to maximum downgaze. Normal LF is 12–18 mm. Frontalis muscle effort may alter this measurement and is negated by applying brow fixation, with the thumb above the brow. The LF is the most important measurement, and an operative procedure cannot be well planned without a precise LF. The measurement should be repeated several times until it is believed to be accurate. The primary fissure in downgaze (PFD) is an indication of the ability of the levator muscle to relax. In congenital ptosis, the upper lid will lag and allow more of the eye to be seen in downgaze compared to the normal eye. If the ptotic eyelid is at a lower level on downgaze compared to the normal lid, acquired ptosis is usually present. Lagophthalmos (LAG) indicates the width of the palpebral fissure with gentle eyelid closure. The presence of lagophthalmos is an indication of potential corneal exposure following ptosis repair.

The amount of redundant eyelid skin should also be measured as well as the position and appearance of the eyelid crease. The normal position of the eyelid crease is 7–10 mm above the eyelid margin, and this measurement is often increased in aponeurotic ptosis. Previous evidence of surgical or accidental trauma should be determined, and eyelashes should be examined and abnormalities be documented. The patient should be asked to chew or move the jaw sideways to rule out Marcus Gunn (jaw-winking) type of ptosis.

In patients with good levator function, a phenylephrine test can be employed. As originally described by Putterman, two drops of 10% phenylephrine are instilled into the upper fornix of the ptotic eye to elicit the response of sympathetically innervated Müller's muscle. Some advocate the use of 2.5% phenylephrine for this testing to minimize adverse systemic effects. It is reported that the 10% dosage of phenylephrine resulted in a statistically significantly, 0.2-mm-higher, upper eyelid elevation compared to the 2.5% dosage [35]. The maximum height of the eyelid takes approximately 3–5 min to occur and is measured as an MRD1. If a significantly increased eyelid height after phenylephrine is observed, this is an indication that a conjunctival–Müller's muscle resection may be useful. The Müller's muscle–conjunctival resection provides up to 2 or 3 mm of lid lift. If ptosis exceeds 4 mm, this test is not an accurate predictor of surgical success [36].

The amount of Müller's muscle–conjunctival resection performed can vary from 6.5 to 9.5 mm. If the eyelid achieves the desired height after phenylephrine testing, a resection of 8.0 mm is performed. If the lid responds to phenylephrine but not to the desired height, the amount of resection is increased up to a maximum of 9.5 mm. If the eyelid over-responds to the phenylephrine, the amount of resection is decreased to a minimum of 6.5 mm. The Müller's muscle–conjunctival resection provides any amount of lift as indicated by the preoperative testing. Typically, this procedure is avoided in patients with glaucoma filtration surgery due to theoretical bleb-related complications [37] and those with conjunctival deficiency, such as ocular cicatricial pemphigoid.

Photography

Photographic documentation of the preoperative and postoperative eyelid appearance is important for the surgeon performing ptosis repair. Photographs allow documentation of the eyelid position before and after surgery and may also help demonstrate medical necessity for insurance purposes

[38]. Photographs also allow patients to see improvements in eyelid position following surgery, especially when patients forget what they looked like before surgery. Photographs may also help a surgeon explain the approach needed to repair ptosis and also help provide information in medicolegal disputes.

The technique for photographing eyelid position needs to be consistent to yield best results [33]. The type of lens, camera, and lighting used in eyelid photography depends on the surgeon's preference but needs to remain consistent. Taking photographs under different conditions with different cameras limits the usefulness in comparing preoperative and postoperative photographs.

Eyelid photographs are usually taken with a digital camera. These digital cameras produce instant results, which make patient education and surgical planning easier. Digital photos may be stored for reference, before and after differentiation, and insurance needs. Photographic prints may be easily made and are an excellent method for record keeping. Digital photos may be submitted to insurance companies, patients, or other persons as necessary.

Documenting eyelid position in ptosis surgery usually involves several photographic views. It is often beneficial to have full-face photographs as well as the eyelids framed along, side views, and one in downgaze. The patient should be photographed with the head in an upright position. Additionally, the eyes can be photographed closed or one eye at a time [39, 40]. The background should be nondistracting, with no headrest, slit lamps, or other equipment in view. The use of heavy makeup should be discouraged.

Visual Fields

Ptosis is known to produce defects in the superior visual field. This superior field impairment is a very important functional consideration in the presurgical evaluation of ptosis patients and also is an important factor in documenting medical necessity. Upper eyelid ptosis has been shown to cause a reduction in both the central and peripheral superior visual fields [41–43]. Some patients with acquired ptosis also exhibit difficulty with reading owing to the decreased palpebral fissure in the ptotic eyelid when the patient looks down to read [40, 44, 45].

Visual field testing may be performed by a number of different methods, including confrontation, tangent screen, Goldmann, and automated static perimetry. Increasing requirements by insurance companies [46, 47] to document visual field loss has led to several makers of automated perimetry machines to produce special programs for ptosis fields.

Our preference is for the Zeiss Humphrey HFA II-i 750i visual field analyzer (Humphrey Instruments, Inc., Carl Zeiss Group, San Leandro, California). Visual field testing in a primary gaze may be performed using a threshold-related screening strategy using a 10° resolution grid. The custom ptosis screening test is a modification of the blepharoplasty screening test and may be programmed either by a Humphrey representative or by the surgeon or his/her staff. Stimuli are placed in a grid pattern beginning 10° below the midline and extended upward in 10° increments to 60° or 70° above midline. The patient's refractive status is corrected in the usual method for visual field testing.

In most cases, patients are tested in primary gaze. This should demonstrate a significant decrease in the superior visual field of a patient with ptosis (Fig. 15.12a, b), but to demonstrate the potential benefit of ptosis surgery, the eyelids are taped open. Retesting the patient with taped eyelids should demonstrate an improvement in the superior visual field, consistent with results expected from ptosis surgery (Fig. 15.12c, d). Most modern visual field machines are digital and, as in the case of photographs, may be stored digitally and then be sent to insurance companies digitally for review.

Psychological Aspects

Various authors have identified psychological issues in cosmetic surgery [48, 49]. These issues are complex in nature; however, most surgeons will want to take them into account when planning surgery, including ptosis surgery. It is reasonable to assess the patient during the history for potential problems, including psychiatric illness or emotional instability. A history of multiple surgeries may indicate self-dissatisfaction or the psychological need for surgery.

In most situations, the patient with ptosis seeks surgery for legitimate reasons, usually to improve vision. Occasionally, a patient may have other expectations or considerations, and these need to be determined before surgery. The patient must be made aware of the most likely outcome of surgery as well as what to expect visually. In most cases, central visual acuity will not change, but a patient should expect an improvement in the peripheral visual field. Although complications are unusual in ptosis surgery, these should be explained in detail to the patient, with documentation made that the patient has heard and understood these potential problems.

Several factors can improve patient satisfaction with ptosis surgery, including honest, open communication between the surgeon and patient; realistic expectations of what will occur before, during, and after surgery [50]; and clear patient understanding of the goals involved in ptosis repair.

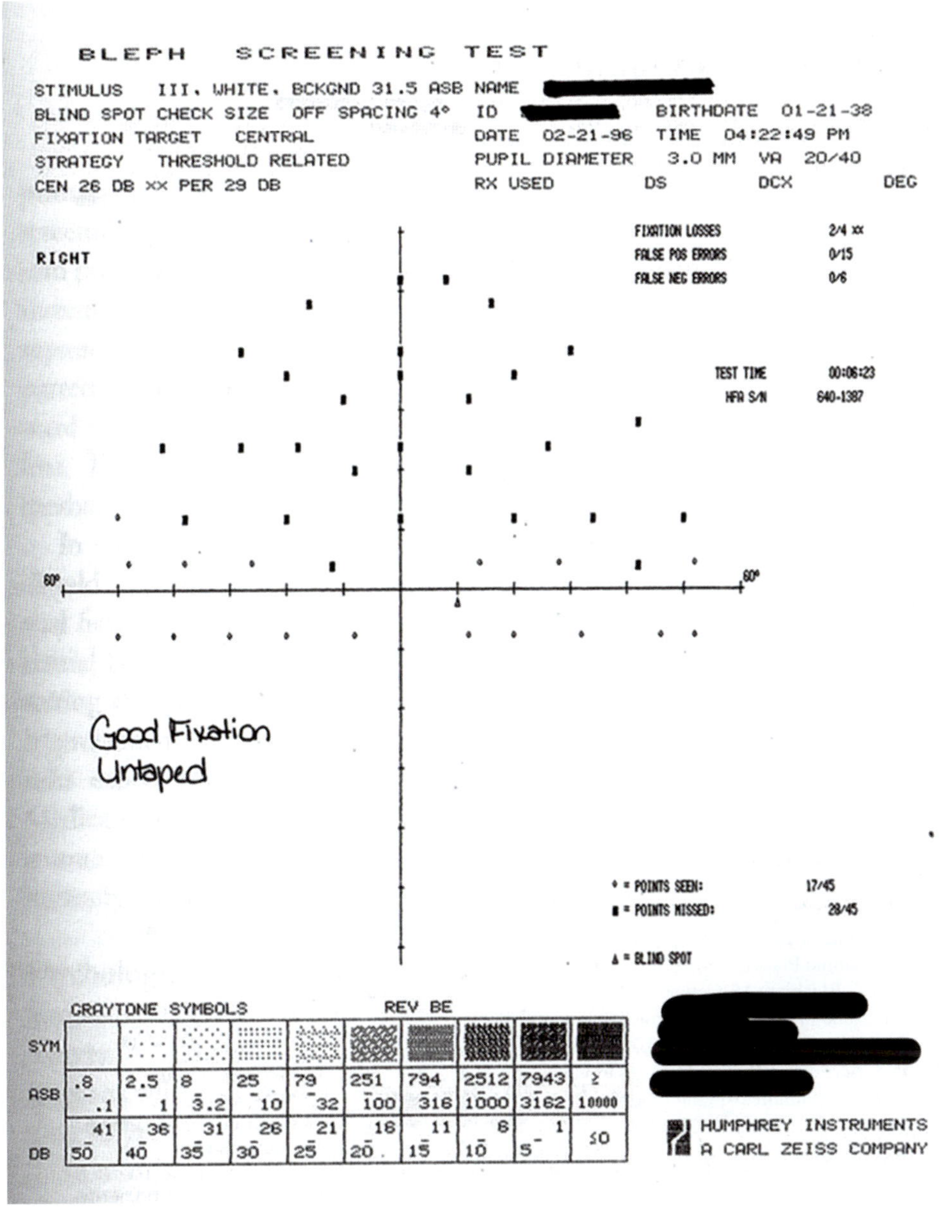

Fig. 15.12 Ptosis visual field with eyelid taped

References

1. Anderson RL, Beard C. The levator aponeurosis. Attachments and their clinical significance. Arch Ophthalmol. 1977;95(8):1437–41.
2. Berke RN, Wadsworth JA. Histology of levator muscle in congenital and acquired ptosis. AMA Arch Ophthalmol. 1955;53(3):413–28.
3. Kakizaki H, Leibovitch I, Selva D, et al. Orbital septum attachment on the levator aponeurosis in Asians: in vivo and cadaver study. Ophthalmology. 2009;116(10):2031–5.
4. Kakizaki H, Zako M, Nakano T, et al. The levator aponeurosis consists of two layers that include smooth muscle. Ophthalmic Plast Reconstr Surg. 2005;21(4):281–4.
5. Kang H, Takahashi Y, Nakano T, et al. Medial canthal support structures: the medial retinaculum: a review. Ann Plast Surg. 2015;74(4):508–14.
6. Beard C. Ptosis surgery: past, present, and future. Ophthalmic Plast Reconstr Surg. 1985;1(1):69–72.
7. Frueh BR. The mechanistic classification of ptosis. Ophthalmology. 1980;87(10):1019–21.
8. De Sanctis U, Alovisi C, Actis AG, et al. Blepharoptosis. Minerva Chir. 2013;68(6 Suppl 1):37–47.
9. Latting MW, Huggins AB, Marx DP, Giacometti JN. Clinical evaluation of blepharoptosis: distinguishing age-related ptosis from masquerade conditions. Semin Plast Surg. 2017;31(1):5–16.
10. Rasiah S, Hardy TG, Elder JE, et al. Etiology of pediatric acquired blepharoptosis. J AAPOS. 2017;21(6):485–7.
11. Mehat MS, Sood V, Madge S. Blepharoptosis following anterior segment surgery: a new theory for an old problem. Orbit. 2012;31(4):274–8.
12. Hwang K, Kim JH. The risk of blepharoptosis in contact lens wearers. J Craniofac Surg. 2015;26(5):e373–4.
13. Selvan C, Dutta D, Maisnam I, et al. Thyroid associated orbitopathy with ocular myasthenia in primary hypothyroidism: keep those eyes open. Indian J Endocrinol Metab. 2013;17(Suppl 3):S657–9.

14. Fortin E, Cestari DM, Weinberg DH. Ocular myasthenia gravis: an update on diagnosis and treatment. Curr Opin Ophthalmol. 2018;29(6):477–84.
15. Pasnoor M, Dimachkie MM, Farmakidis C, Barohn RJ. Diagnosis of myasthenia gravis. Neurol Clin. 2018;36(2):261–74.
16. Al-Haidar M, Benatar M, Kaminski HJ. Ocular myasthenia. Neurol Clin. 2018;36(2):241–51.
17. Feinstein E, Chen J, Setabutr P. Recent onset of bilateral ptosis. JAMA Ophthalmol. 2017;135(4):397–8.
18. Turner C, Hilton-Jones D. Myotonic dystrophy: diagnosis, management and new therapies. Curr Opin Neurol. 2014;27(5):599–606.
19. Singh A, Bahuguna C, Nagpal R, Kumar B. Surgical management of third nerve palsy. Oman J Ophthalmol. 2016;9(2):80–6.
20. Xu X, Li X, Ren F, et al. Primary chondroma of posterior mediastinum with Horner's syndrome: a case report. World J Surg Oncol. 2018;16(1):209.
21. Nabavizadeh SA, Zimmerman RA, Mattei P, Liu GT. Infantile myofibroma of the carotid space presenting as horner syndrome. J Neuroophthalmol. 2017;37(4):459–60.
22. Gulkilik G, Cagatay HH, Oba EM, Uslu C. Ophthalmoplegic migraine associated with recurrent isolated ptosis. Ann Ophthalmol (Skokie). 2009;41(3–4):206–7.
23. Bek S, Genc G, Demirkaya S, et al. Ophthalmoplegic migraine. Neurologist. 2009;15(3):147–9.
24. Yetimalar Y, Secil Y, Inceoglu AK, et al. Unusual primary manifestations of multiple sclerosis. N Z Med J. 2008;121(1277):47–59.
25. Beck RW. The optic neuritis treatment trial. Arch Ophthalmol. 1988;106(8):1051–3.
26. Feinstein A, Freeman J, Lo AC. Treatment of progressive multiple sclerosis: what works, what does not, and what is needed. Lancet Neurol. 2015;14(2):194–207.
27. Fernandez O, Delvecchio M, Edan G, et al. Survey of diagnostic and treatment practices for multiple sclerosis in Europe. Eur J Neurol. 2017;24(3):516–22.
28. Pearce FC, McNab AA, Hardy TG. Marcus Gunn jaw-winking syndrome: a comprehensive review and report of four novel cases. Ophthalmic Plast Reconstr Surg. 2017;33(5):325–8.
29. Illes Z, Blaabjerg M. Cerebrospinal fluid findings in Guillain-Barre syndrome and chronic inflammatory demyelinating polyneuropathies. Handb Clin Neurol. 2017;146:125–38.
30. Park AJ, Eliassi-Rad B, Desai MA. Ptosis after glaucoma surgery. Clin Ophthalmol. 2017;11:1483–9.
31. Takahashi Y, Zheng X, Mito H, et al. Recurrent ptosis in a patient with blepharochalasis: clinical and histopathologic findings. J Craniofac Surg. 2015;26(1):e52–3.
32. Danesh J, Ugradar S, Goldberg R, Rootman DB. A novel technique for the measurement of eyelid contour to compare outcomes following Muller's muscle-conjunctival resection and external levator resection surgery. Eye (Lond). 2018;32(9):1493–7.
33. Choi CJ, Chou JC, Lefebvre DR, Yoon MK. Margin reflex distance: differences based on camera and flash positions. Ophthalmic Plast Reconstr Surg. 2016;32(3):199–203.
34. Small RG, Sabates NR, Burrows D. The measurement and definition of ptosis. Ophthalmic Plast Reconstr Surg. 1989;5(3):171–5.
35. Glatt HJ, Fett DR, Putterman AM. Comparison of 2.5% and 10% phenylephrine in the elevation of upper eyelids with ptosis. Ophthalmic Surg. 1990;21(3):173–6.
36. Wee SW, Lee JK. Clinical outcomes of conjunctiva-Muller muscle resection: association with phenylephrine test-negative blepharoptosis and dry eye syndrome. J Craniofac Surg. 2014;25(3):898–901.
37. Michels KS, Vagefi MR, Steele E, et al. Muller muscle-conjunctiva resection to correct ptosis in high-risk patients. Ophthalmic Plast Reconstr Surg. 2007;23(5):363–6.
38. Guterman EL, Botelho JV, Horton JC. Diagnosis of tensilon-negative ocular myasthenia gravis by daily selfie. J Neuroophthalmol. 2016;36(3):292–3.
39. Wojno TH. Downgaze ptosis. Ophthalmic Plast Reconstr Surg. 1993;9(2):83–8; discussion 8–9.
40. Dryden RM, Kahanic DA. Worsening of blepharoptosis in downgaze. Ophthalmic Plast Reconstr Surg. 1992;8(2):126–9.
41. Cahill KV, Burns JA, Weber PA. The effect of blepharoptosis on the field of vision. Ophthalmic Plast Reconstr Surg. 1987;3(3):121–5.
42. Meyer DR, Linberg JV, Powell SR, Odom JV. Quantitating the superior visual field loss associated with ptosis. Arch Ophthalmol. 1989;107(6):840–3.
43. Alniemi ST, Pang NK, Woog JJ, Bradley EA. Comparison of automated and manual perimetry in patients with blepharoptosis. Ophthalmic Plast Reconstr Surg. 2013;29(5):361–3.
44. Patipa M. Visual field loss in primary gaze and reading gaze due to acquired blepharoptosis and visual field improvement following ptosis surgery. Arch Ophthalmol. 1992;110(1):63–7.
45. Olson JJ, Putterman A. Loss of vertical palpebral fissure height on downgaze in acquired blepharoptosis. Arch Ophthalmol. 1995;113(10):1293–7.
46. Local coverage determination (lcd): blepharoplasty, blepharoptosis and brow lift centers for medicare & medicaid services, 2018; v. 2018.
47. Aetna. Eyelid Surgery Clinical Policy Bulletins Policy for acquired ptosis 2018; v. 2018.
48. Berros P, Armstrong BK, Foti P, Mancini R. Cosmetic adolescent filler: an innovative treatment of the "selfie" complex. Ophthalmic Plast Reconstr Surg. 2018;34(4):366–8.
49. Joseph AW, Ishii L, Joseph SS, et al. Prevalence of body dysmorphic disorder and surgeon diagnostic accuracy in facial plastic and oculoplastic surgery clinics. JAMA Facial Plast Surg. 2017;19(4):269–74.
50. Putterman AM. Patient satisfaction in oculoplastic surgery. Ophthalmic Surg. 1990;21(1):15–21.

Management of Acquired Ptosis

16

John D. Siddens, Jenna M. Kim, and Geoffrey J. Gladstone

Introduction

Ptosis repair is one of the most challenging problems faced by oculoplastic surgeons. There is no single procedure that will suffice for every case, and there is a considerable difference of opinion as to which procedure is the best. Many different techniques have been discussed and tried, and it appears that the procedure of choice rests with the experience of the surgeon and the needs of the patient. In this chapter, the four most common surgical methods of approaching ptosis—frontalis suspension, levator advancement, the Fasanella-Servat operation, and Müller's muscle-conjunctival resection—are discussed.

Anesthesia

Ptosis surgery may be performed alone or in conjunction with other oculoplastic procedures. Ptosis surgery may be performed under general anesthesia, but paralysis of the eyelid muscles makes postoperative prediction of the final eyelid position extremely difficult and postoperative success less predictable [1]. Local anesthesia is the standard delivery method because it is associated with decreased bleeding, decreased patient cost, decreased stress on the airway and cardiovascular system, and a shortened recovery time [2, 3]. The use of short-acting intravenous anesthesia and local anesthetic has allowed ptosis surgery to become much more accurate because the process is performed on dynamic tissue, and anatomic structures are much more easily identified [3]. In this situation, the action of the levator muscle is not impaired, and the effect of the aponeurotic repair may be assessed during surgery.

All types of ptosis surgery may be performed under local anesthesia with intravenous sedation, provided that the patient is emotionally stable and of sufficient age to provide intraoperative cooperation. This technique may be performed on adults and adolescents as young as 10 or 11 years of age. In some cases, ptosis surgery may be performed using only local anesthesia. Patient selection is the most important factor in this situation. When the procedure is performed in the office or without an anesthetist, oral premedication can be very effective. A benzodiazepine may be given orally 30 min before surgery, and this relieves patient anxiety in most situations.

The routine preoperative evaluation of a patient for outpatient surgery includes an interview and evaluation by an anesthesiologist. The medical history is reviewed, along with information on any previous surgery and anesthesia. Any previous adverse reactions by the patient or family members to anesthetic agents are reviewed. This information allows appropriate individualization of anesthesia for the patient's benefit.

In conjunction with intravenous sedation, preoperative medication may include narcotics, barbiturates, and tranquilizers. Narcotics such as morphine sulfate and fentanyl must be used with caution owing to their tendency to cause respiratory depression. Barbiturates and tranquilizers are typically avoided because of their long-acting properties, which negates the ability to open or close eyelids during surgery.

Topical anesthetics are useful preoperatively to provide corneal comfort during surgery. In situations where corneoscleral protective shells are necessary, topical anesthetics provide for comfort. Lidocaine 2.5% and prilocaine 2.5% cream (Emla, Astra Pharmaceuticals, Westborough, MA) has been shown to provide significant anesthesia of the

J. D. Siddens
Ophthalmic Plastic Surgery Service, Greenville Memorial Hospital, Prisma Health System Upstate, Division of Ophthalmology, Department of Surgery, Greenville, SC, USA

J. M. Kim
William Beaumont School of Medicine, Beaumont Eye Institute, Royal Oak, IL, USA

G. J. Gladstone (✉)
Consultants in Ophthalmic and Facial Plastic Surgery, P.C., Southfield, MI, USA

Oakland University/William Beaumont Hospital, School of Medicine, Department of Ophthalmology, Royal Oak, MI, USA

J. J. Servat et al. (eds.), *Smith and Nesi's Ophthalmic Plastic and Reconstructive Surgery*,
https://doi.org/10.1007/978-3-030-41720-8_16

skin surface. Application of this cream for 45 min or longer before incision helps provide significant comfort during the actual injection of local anesthesia. Infiltration anesthesia is the most widely used form of preventing patient discomfort during ptosis surgery. Toxic reactions to these agents include convulsions, respiratory arrest, and cardiovascular collapse. Judicious use of infiltration anesthesia should prevent the need for cardiopulmonary resuscitation should severe reactions to these drugs occur.

Lidocaine is the most commonly used agent because it diffuses well through tissue and produces little irritation. It is available in solutions of 0.5–2.0%, with and without epinephrine. The maximum dose is 4–7 mg/kg. The onset of effect is typically within 5 min, and the duration of lidocaine averages 2–3 h.

Bupivacaine (0.25%, 0.5%, and 0.75%) is a solution in which the effect of anesthesia lasts 4–12 h. The time of onset for action is typically 10–12 min.

Some patients have true allergy to Xylocaine or bupivacaine as a result of an amide chemical linkage in the local anesthesia molecule. Procaine is a local anesthetic with an ester chemical linkage and may be used in patients with true allergy to Xylocaine.

Epinephrine is a potent vasoconstrictor, and in solutions of 1:100,000 or less, it provides an excellent prolongation of anesthetic effect and also helps provide hemostasis. Epinephrine should be avoided in patients with thyrotoxicosis and severe coronary artery disease.

Hyaluronidase is an enzyme that degrades hyaluronic acid, which helps increase tissue permeability and enhances the diffusion of local anesthesia agents. Hyaluronidase also helps obtain adequate deep orbital fat anesthesia.

Sodium bicarbonate has been shown to reduce discomfort associated with infiltration by changing the pH of the anesthetic agent solution [3, 4]. Injection of local anesthesia slowly also helps decrease the discomfort during injection.

Patient sedation, analgesia, and amnesia may be obtained using intravenous medications. While the patient is sedated, the local anesthesia may be administered with minimal patient discomfort, and the patient's memory of the event is essentially nonexistent. This allows adequate anesthesia of the surgical field while preventing deleterious changes in the cardiovascular or pulmonary functions. The level of intravenous sedation has become more or less an art form, depending significantly on communication between the surgeon, the anesthetist or anesthesiologist, and the patient.

Several agents are effective in inducing this level of sedation. Thiopental sodium is a short-acting sedative with no analgesic effects. This agent is useful when the patient is extremely anxious or when other forms of premedication have minimal effect. Full alertness is typically regained within 5–10 min. Methohexital sodium is a rapid ultrashort-acting barbiturate. It is twice as potent as thiopental, and its duration of action is half as long. Propofol is a sedative and hypnotic agent and allows rapid induction of anesthesia. Its onset of action is typically within 1 min, and its effect lasts usually 3–6 min. Titration of propofol provides an excellent plan of anesthesia for longer procedures.

Other agents, including narcotics, midazolam, ketamine, and diazepam, are also useful in maintaining anesthesia during a procedure. By using the anesthetic agents in appropriate dosages, ptosis surgery may be carried out in a predictable and reproducible fashion while maintaining patient comfort.

Management of Acquired Ptosis

Principles

Repair of patients with ptosis may be traced back to ancient Arabian surgeons, who resected crescents of skin in an attempt to lift eyelids [5]. The literature is filled with a vast amount of data concerning attempts to repair ptosis. It is most advantageous to base the treatment of ptosis on an accurate assessment of its cause. If an incorrect diagnosis is made, even the most accurate and well-executed procedure may be unsuccessful. The surgeon must very carefully determine the needs of each patient and direct management to meet those specific needs.

A variety of procedures have been described to repair ptosis, and most fall under three categories. The first is an attachment of the eyelid to the frontalis muscle complex, and this works well in patients with little or no levator function. An anterior approach provides the second means of ptosis correction, in which an incision is made through the skin, and an external repair of the levator complex is carried out. The third method involves a posterior approach, in which an incision is made through the palpebral conjunctiva, with attention given to repair of the tarsus, conjunctiva, Müller's muscle, and even the levator complex at times. There is often intense discussion as to which method is the best. Whether the approach for repair is anterior, posterior, or suspensory, the end result most often depends on the surgeon's comfort level with his or her skills, dissecting technique, and knowledge of eyelid anatomy.

Nonsurgical Management

There are some patients in whom surgical repair of ptosis may be unnecessary or unwarranted. If there is a poor prognosis for a good functional or cosmetic result from surgery, observation of the patient may be an appropriate means to treat the condition. An example would be a patient in whom a neurogenic ptosis is present, along with poor levator function and poor Bell's phenomenon. In this situation, ptosis repair may increase the chances for exposure keratopathy or diplopia.

If the ptosis has an identifiable cause that would respond to medical treatment, such as myasthenia gravis, surgery should be deferred until the patient is medically stable. Ptosis that results from blunt trauma is another situation in which surgical intervention may not be necessary. Traumatic ptosis often resolves spontaneously within the first 4–6 months after injury. If resolution is incomplete after this time, surgical repair may be effective.

Another method for treating acquired ptosis involves the use of crutch glass (Fig. 16.1). These are spectacles in which a metal bar (crutch) extends posteriorly from the superior one-third of the lens frame. This bar inserts into the eyelid crease, helping to mechanically elevate the lid margin. Crutch glasses are usually most helpful on a trial basis, and this is very helpful to determine if an underlying strabismus or diplopia will be debilitating. These glasses are seldom useful over a long period of time due to decreased blinking and exposure keratopathy.

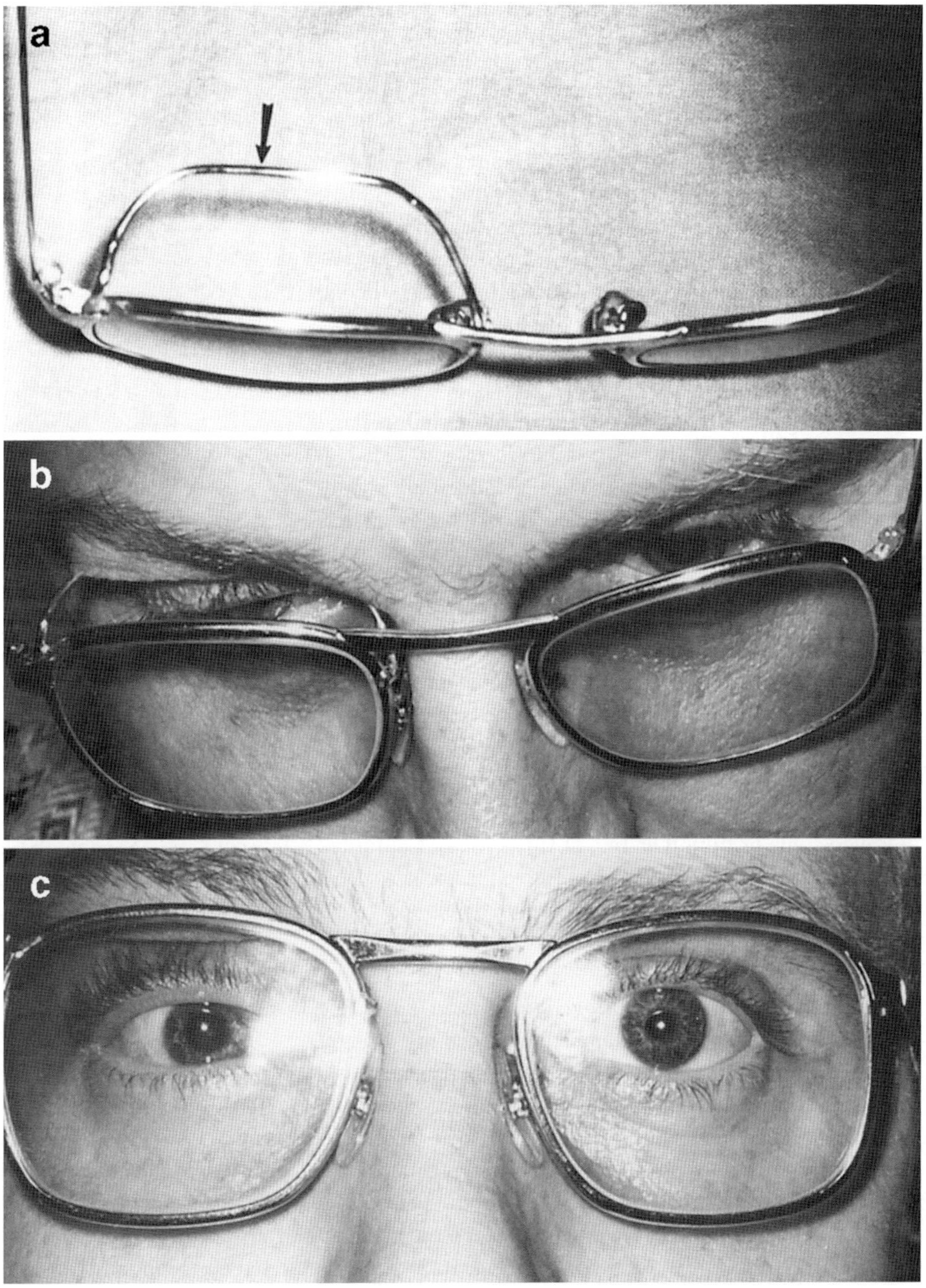

Fig. 16.1 (**a**) Crutch glasses with metal crutch (*arrow*) extending posteriorly from superior part of glasses frame. (**b**) Superior view showing crutch holding up right upper eyelid in patient with third cranial nerve palsy. (**c**) Frontal view showing position of right upper eyelid and camouflage of crutch by glasses frame

Surgical Management

The Anterior Approach to Ptosis Repair

Frontalis Suspension Surgery At present, suspension of the upper eyelid to the frontalis muscle complex is the standard technique for the correction of severe ptosis with poor or no levator muscle function. Dransart is generally given credit as the first to utilize this technique in the 1880s [6]. He used non-buried sutures to attach the eyelid to the brow. In 1899, Koster [7] modified this technique and buried the sutures. Later, surgeons used strips of skin that were buried; however, this technique has the obvious disadvantage of causing subcutaneous cysts from residual epithelial cells. Reese fashioned a suspensory system based on strips of orbicularis muscle [8]. Crawford modified the use of fascia lata suspensory slings in 1956 [9]. This approach was modified further by Fox in 1966 [10]. Other authors have modified the placement and position of the fascia lata, and in 1977, Crawford provided a 20-year review of this technique [11]. In 1966, Tillett used silicone rods in an effort to prove elasticity to the eyelid [12]. This effectively allowed an adequate blink reflex and closure but still provided lift.

Other surgeons have provided a variety of techniques and materials used in brow suspension ptosis surgery [12–16]. Current materials other than fascia lata include suture (nylon, Prolene, Supramid, Mersilene) [17], silicone bands or rods [18], expanded polytetrafluoroethylene (ePTFE) commonly known as Gore-Tex, and palmaris longus tendon or temporalis fasica [19].

Despite numerous modifications in both technique and materials, fascia lata appears to remain the most popular material of choice in frontalis suspension surgery. Fascia lata is used in either of two forms, autogenous or preserved [20]. Preserved fascia lata may be obtained from various sources, including the Eye Bank at the Wills Eye Hospital in Philadelphia or from IOP, Inc. of Costa Mesa, California. The choice of autogenous versus preserved fascia lata seems to depend on the training and experience of the individual surgeon.

Technique for Harvesting Autogenous Fascia Lata The patient may be placed supine, and leg is placed in a straight position with the toes rotated mediallyGeneral anesthesia may be administered, but this technique may be performed with monitored intravenous sedation and local anesthesiaTwo reference points are marked: the lateral femoral condyle and a point just anterior to the anterior superior iliac crest. The fibers of the iliotibial tract in general run along an imaginary line between these two points (Fig. 16.2). A marking pen is used to outline a vertical incision site 2 cm long,

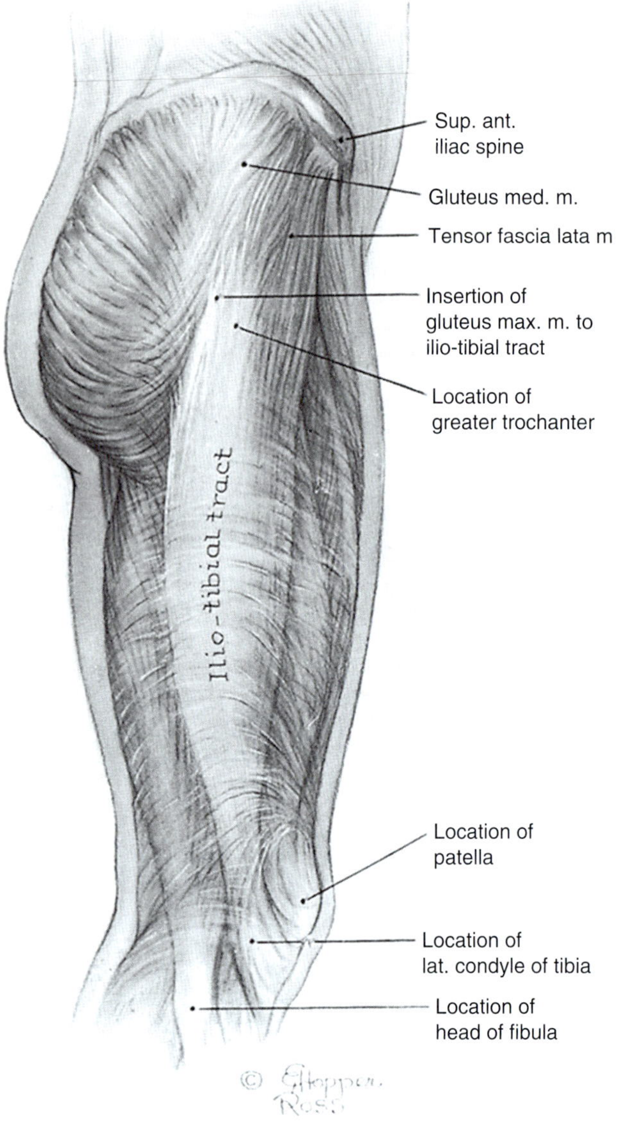

Fig. 16.2 Diagram of muscles of leg demonstrating position of fascia lata

located 6 cm above the lateral femoral condyle. The author prefers to inject a solution with a 1:1 ratio of 1.0% lidocaine with 1:100,000 epinephrine and 0.5% bupivacaine with 1:200,000 epinephrine in the subcutaneous area.

The skin is incised with a scalpel blade along a 2-cm segment, and dissection is carried through the subcutaneous fat to the level of the glistening fascia lata fibers. The subcutaneous tissues are spread, and the fascia lata fibers are carefully exposed. Metzenbaum scissors are used to bluntly dissect a plane between fascia lata and overlying subcutaneous fat for a distance of 12–15 cm along the surgical site toward the reference point anterior to the iliac crest. With the scissors removed, two parallel incisions are made along the distal end of the fascia lata 1 cm apart, each incision being 2 cm long. The scissors are then placed beneath the fascia lata, and another surgical plane is dissected superiorly between the fascia lata fibers and the tensor fascia lata muscle for a distance of 12–15 cm. The distal ends of the two incisions are joined, creating a stump of fascia lata (Fig. 16.3a–e).

A Crawford or Masson fascia stripper is used to then harvest the fascia lata (Fig. 16.4). The end of the Crawford separator is placed over the stump of the fascia lata strip and is very carefully passed along the superior path of the fascia lata fiber tract. This effectively cuts a 1-cm-wide strip of fascia lata. In some cases, scissors may be necessary to place the lateral cuts of the fascia lata strip; however, care must be used due to the blind nature of the procedure. Once the separator is removed, the stump of the fascia lata strip is passed through the cutting port of a Crawford stripper. The stripper is then passed upward for 12–15 cm, and the cutting blade lock is released, severing the superior end. The fascia lata strip is then removed. Pressure is placed for approximately 5 min to avoid subcutaneous bleeding. The subcutaneous tissues are closed with deep inverted interrupted 4-0 Vicryl or chromic sutures. Vertical mattress sutures of 5-0 silk or nylon are then used to close the skin. A non-encircling pressure dressing is then applied for 48 h. Antibiotic ointment must be placed on the suture line for at least 7 days, after which the skin sutures may be removed.

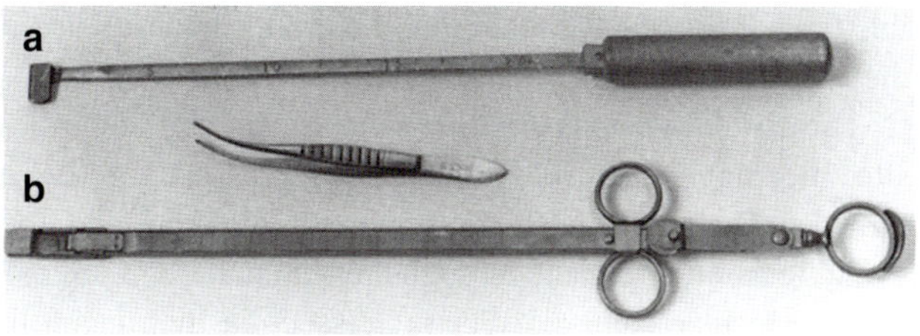

Fig. 16.4 (**a**) Crawford separator. (**b**) Crawford stripper and curved forceps for pulling fascia through end of stripper

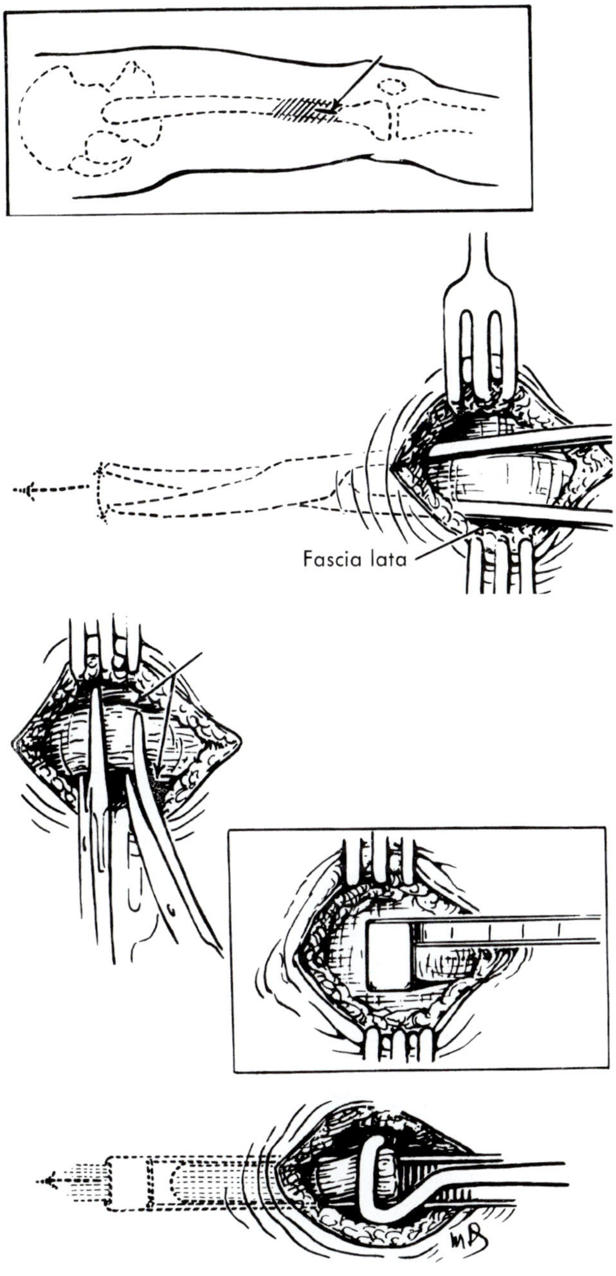

Fig. 16.3 Method of taking fascia lata from the thigh

The fascia lata is then prepared for implantation by trimming any adherent fat or areolar tissue. The fascia is then very carefully cut into 2-mm-wide strips, with care being taken to ensure the cuts are parallel to the collagen bundles.

Preserved fascia lata is prepared for implantation by following the reconstitution instructions in the product packaging.

Surgical Technique for Frontalis Suspension

General anesthesia may be used for young children or noncooperative adults; however, local anesthesia with intravenous sedation is preferable in adults and cooperative children. With the patient in a sitting position, two incision sites are marked on the eyelid with a marking pen. The eyelid incisions are placed above the position where the corneoscleral limbus intersects with the lid margin. Three brow incision sites are marked symmetrically above the brow to provide a pentagonal shape for the fascia lata. The central brow incision should be 2–3 mm above the level of the lateral brow incisions. The patient is then placed in the supine position, and after topical anesthesia is applied, corneoscleral protectors are put into position. After intravenous sedation is administered, a 1:1 ratio of 1.0% lidocaine with 1:100,000 epinephrine and 0.5% bupivacaine with 1:200,000 epinephrine is injected. Pressure is applied to this area for several minutes. If bilateral surgery will take place, the other lid is injected at this time. The patient should then be prepped and draped in the usual fashion for sterile technique.

Three stab incisions are then made in each brow incision site. Bleeding is controlled by applying pressure for several minutes. Then, with adequate protection for the globe, two eyelid incisions are made through the skin to the level of pretarsal orbicularis muscle. Scissor dissection then carefully exposes the tarsal plate (Fig. 16.5a).

A Jaeger lid plate is placed under the eyelid and brought into contact with the orbital rim. A Wright fascia needle is then passed through the temporal brow incision and brought out through the lateral upper incision (Fig. 16.5b). It is extremely important in this situation to maintain visual and palpable contact with the tip of the Wright needle. The needle should be passed in a direction to remain beneath the orbicularis muscle but anterior to the orbital septum, levator aponeurosis, and tarsal plate. Fascia lata is then loaded into the eye of the Wright needle, which is then withdrawn through the tissues. A 2-cm segment of fascia lata is pulled out of the temporal brow incision. The Wright needle is then passed from the nasal lid incision to the temporal lid incision, and the free end of the fascia lata is pulled along the surface of the tarsal plate and out of the nasal eyelid incision (Fig. 16.5c). The Wright needle is then similarly passed from the nasal brow wound along the suborbicularis surgical plane and out through the nasal eyelid incision (Fig. 16.5d). The fascia lata is then loaded and withdrawn from the eyelid out the brow incision. The Wright needle is then passed from the central brow incision to both the central and nasal brow incisions (Fig. 16.5e), which will allow the fascia lata to be brought out of the central brow incision. This maneuver completes the pentagon shape of the fascia lata (Fig. 16.5f).

The patient is then assisted into a sitting position, and the fascia lata is elevated until the eyelid contour is appropriate. The eyelid margin is elevated to a position of 1–3 mm of overcorrection. The ends of the fascial strips is tied with a square knot, and the knot is secured with a 6–0 Vicryl suture. The knot is then placed deep within the central brow incision, allowing the lid to drop approximately 1 mm. The brow incisions are closed with one or two 6–0 mild chromic sutures; the eyelid incisions may not require suturing (Fig. 16.5g). Alternative methods of placing fascia lata include the use of three or four incisions on the upper eyelid. The eyelid may be opened with a single incision to facilitate suturing the fascia lata to the tarsal plate. The fascia lata strips may be interlocked to avoid "cheese-wiring" of the bands. Silicone rods, Supramid sutures, and other materials have also been shown to be useful for frontalis suspension surgery (Fig. 16.6a, b) [18, 21–23].

Postoperative care includes the use of ice compresses for the first 24–48 h. Intensive ocular lubrication, including ophthalmic antibiotic ointment, is used two to four times a day and at bedtime for at least 7 days. Nonabsorbable sutures are removed after 5–7 days. Bland ophthalmic ointment should be used at bedtime in the eye for a period of 2–3 weeks following frontalis suspension surgery.

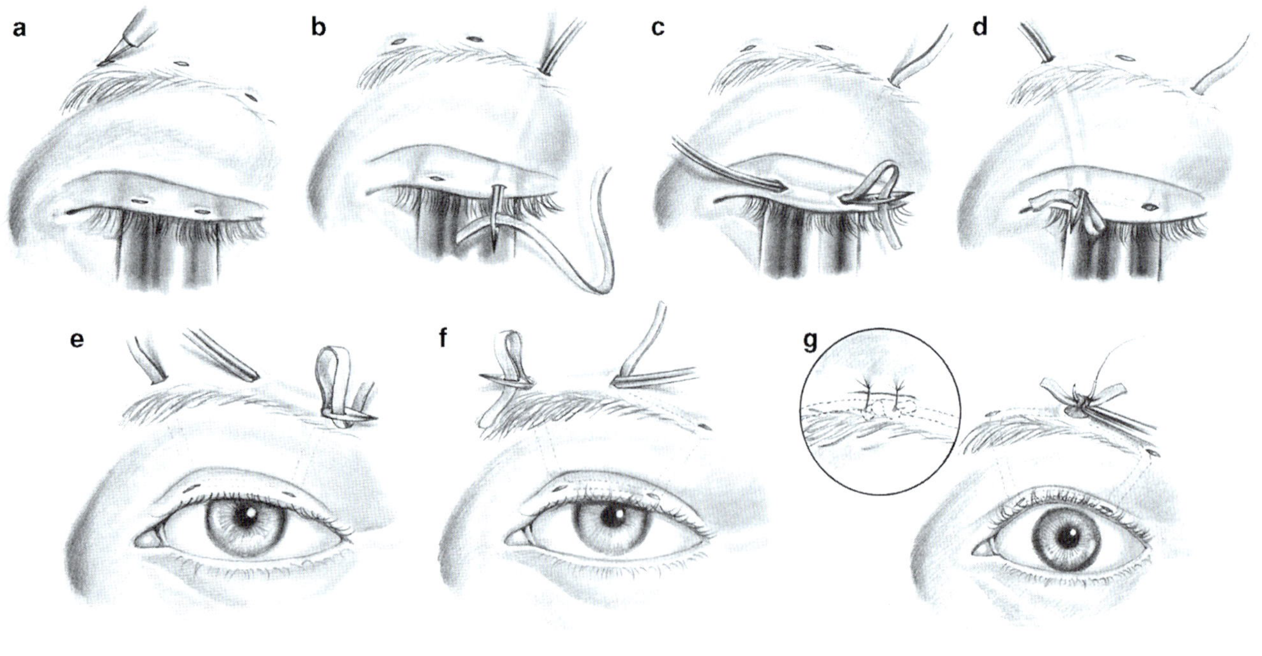

Fig. 16.5 Frontalis suspension surgery. (**a**) Brow and eyelid stab incisions are made. (**b**) Wright needle passed and fascia lata threaded into it. (**c**) Fascia lata threaded through the lid. (**d**) Fascia lata brought through brow incision. (**e**) Fascia lata passed from temporal to central brow incisions. (**f**) Fascia lata passed from nasal brow incision to central brow incision. (**g**) Lid elevated and fascia lata secured. (From Nesi et al.; reproduced with permission of Elsevier)

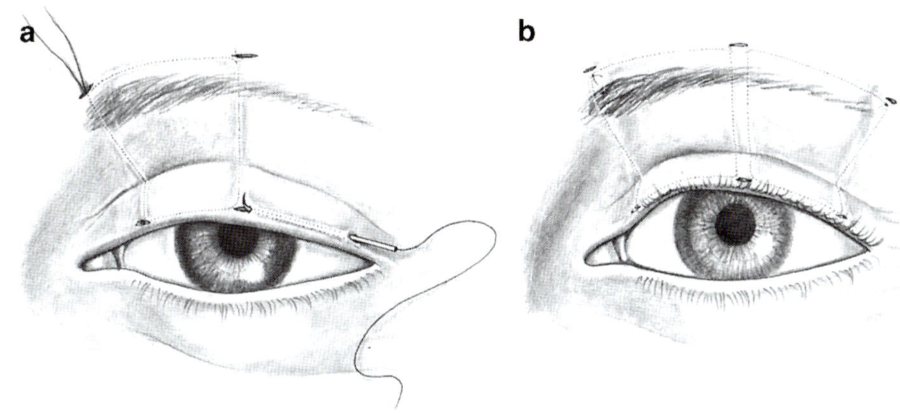

Fig. 16.6 (**a**) Ski needle used to carry Supramid suture through stab incisions. (**b**) Completion of double rhomboid-type fixation. (From Nesi et al.; reproduced with permission of Elsevier)

Levator Aponeurosis Surgery

Eversbusch is generally credited with the first anterior approach in using the levator muscle for ptosis repair [24]. He performed a tuck of the levator by an external approach. Wolf further modified this approach in 1896 by resecting the levator aponeurosis [25]. Ptosis surgery has been repeatedly changed, modified, and improved. The works of Jones, Quikert, Wobig, and others have demonstrated that repair of the levator aponeurosis is one of the best means for repairing ptosis [26–30]. Various techniques have been described, including the tarsoaponeurotomy [31], the anterior tarsectomy [32], and a multilevel, full-thickness eyelid resection. Later work has turned its attention to treatment of ptosis by levator surgery along with adjustable sutures [33–35].

It is important to understand that despite the apparent simple problem, ptosis surgery may be difficult. To get superior results consistently, each surgeon must use an approach with which the results are consistent and reproducible. As our knowledge of ptosis and the multiple physiologic changes that occur with this defect grow, the results from ptosis surgery should improve.

Surgical Technique Ptosis surgery is more accurate when performed on an awake patient. A cooperative patient enables the surgeon to move the eyelid margin accurately in position as well as reform the normal eyelid contour. Ptosis surgery may be performed in the office under straight local anesthesia, whereas others may require intravenous sedation. Regional blocks are unnecessary. If it is used, intravenous sedation must not interfere with the patient's ability to cooperate with the surgeon when patients are asked to open and close their eyes. In an upright position, the proposed eyelid crease or incision sites are marked with a marking pen. If bilateral surgery is performed and the proposed eyelid crease is not apparent, the incision line is drawn 8–10 mm above the eyelid margin centrally. The proposed lid crease should taper to approximately 4–6 mm medially and 5–6 mm laterally. Once the proposed surgical site is marked, the patient is placed in a supine position.

The closed eyelids of both eyes are scrubbed and prepped in the usual fashion for ophthalmic surgery. The author prefers povidone-iodine (Betadine) prep applied with folded sterile gauze. Topical anesthesia is instilled into the conjunctival sac of both eyes. The operative field is then draped leaving both eyes uncovered. Corneoscleral protectors may be used to protect the eye. If they are used, these must be removed before final positioning of the eyelid margin.

If the procedure is performed in the office, it is often helpful to augment oral sedative agents with topical Emla cream. The cream is applied thickly to the eyelids 45 min before the procedure and is then removed with a moistened cloth before injection, prepping, and draping. If this procedure is performed in an ambulatory surgical setting, Emla cream is not usually necessary since intravenous sedation is given. The eyelid is infiltrated with a 1:1 ratio of 1.0% lidocaine with 1:100,000 epinephrine and 0.5% bupivacaine with 1:200,000 epinephrine. The injection is made just below the skin. This will prevent any anesthetic effect on the levator or Müller's muscles. Usually, a 1–1.5 mL of local anesthetic is all that is necessary for ptosis repair (Fig. 16.7a). Adequate time is allowed for the anesthetic to take effect, as well as to maximize hemostasis. The skin is held taut to prevent buckling, and a scalpel blade is used to make an incision along the course of the marked eyelid crease line. The orbicularis muscle fibers should be visible through the incision. Radio frequency or laser incisions are now becoming accepted as means of replacing cold steel incision surgery.

Hemostasis is maintained using a hot-tip, handheld cautery. Occasionally, bipolar cautery or a Bovie cautery may be necessary. Excessive cautery is avoided to prevent complications associated with thermal damage.

The skin edges are then tented with forceps, and Westcott scissors are used to cut through the orbicularis muscle. The angle of the scissors should be approximately 45°, angling along the anatomic plane of the levator aponeurosis. The orbicularis is opened both nasally and temporally, forming superior and inferior skin-orbicularis flaps. The orbital septum should become visible along with the underlying preaponeurotic orbital fat. Blunt dissection using a cotton-tipped applicator is often helpful in accurately identifying the septum, which inserts onto the aponeurosis 3–5 mm above the tarsal plate (Fig. 16.7b).

The septum is then positively identified by grasping the tissue believed to be septum with forceps. Traction on this tissue takes place while the surgeon palpates the superior orbital rim. The septum is firmly attached to the orbital rim,

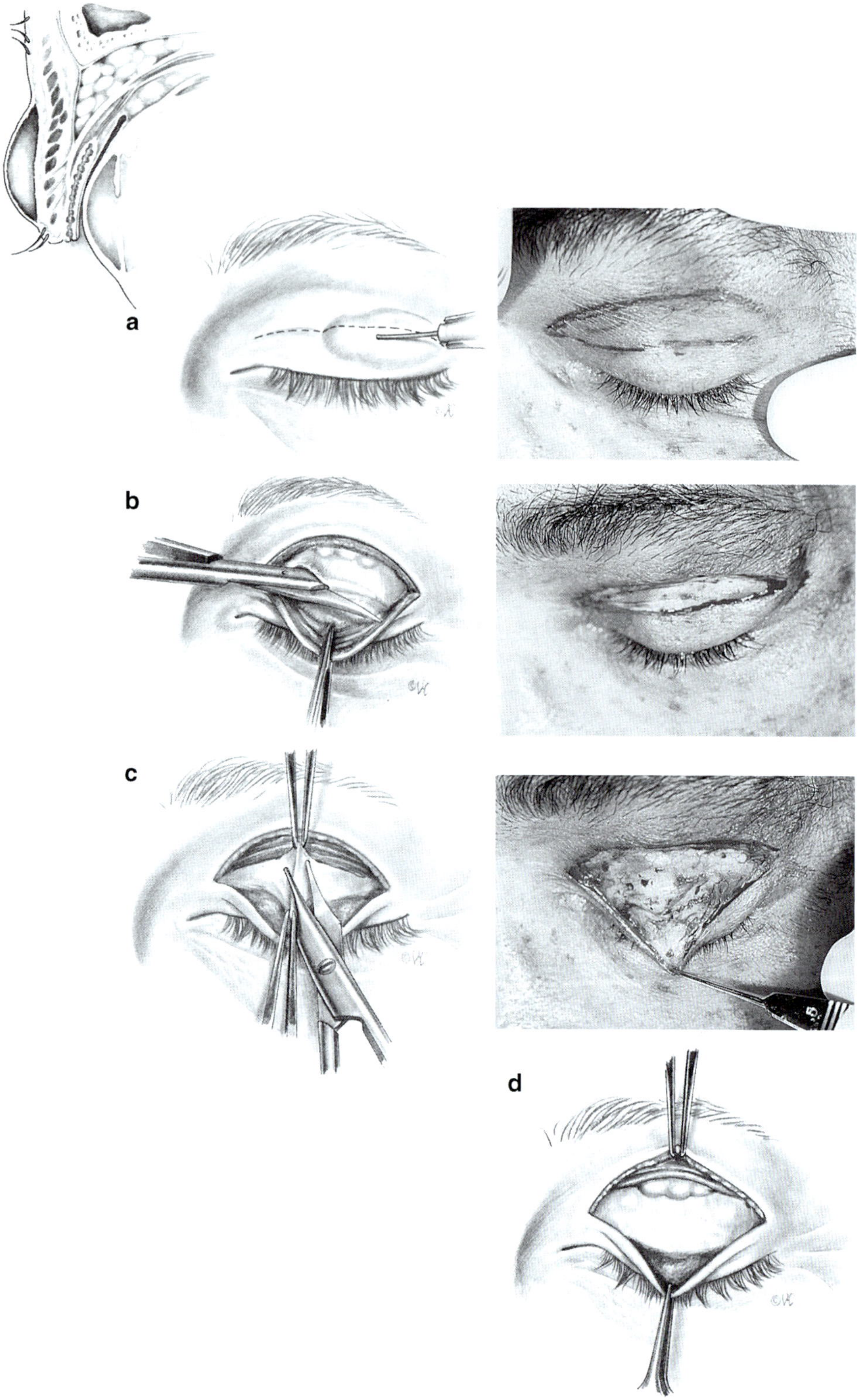

Fig. 16.7 Levator aponeurosis surgery. (**a**) Incision site outlined and lid infiltrated with anesthetic solution. (**b**) Orbital septum opened. (**c**) Orbital septum is tented upward and incised. (**d**) Levator exposed, with preaponeurotic fat anterior to it. (From Nesi et al.; reproduced with permission of Elsevier)

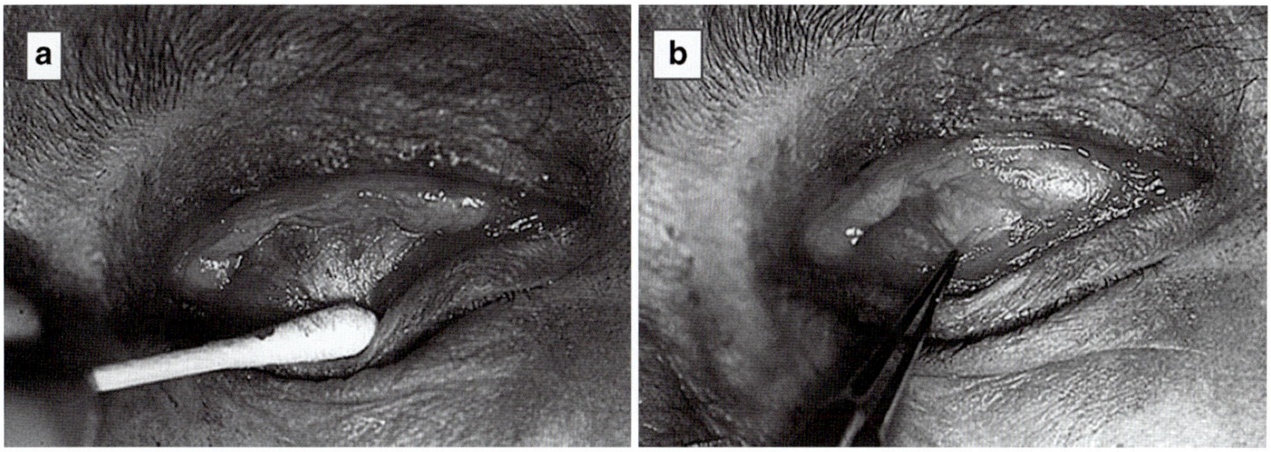

Fig. 16.8 (**a**) Dark iris visible beneath the conjunctiva. (**b**) Disinserted levator visible in grasp of forceps

and the surgeon will feel this tautness as the septum is pulled. The levator aponeurosis may be tested in the same way; however, there will be no feeling of tightness because there is no attachment of the levator to the orbital rim. The levator can also be identified positively by asking the patient to look upward, which will cause the tip of the grasping forceps to be pulled along with it.

The orbital septum is opened by placing a small buttonhole in the center and extending this hole both laterally and nasally (Fig. 16.7c). Preaponeurotic fat then bulges into the surgical wound, and this fat may be brushed upward using gentle retraction with the cotton-tipped applicator. The levator is revealed as a glistening white structure with vertical fibers extending from the tarsal plate upward, becoming muscular fibers approximately 20 mm from the eyelid margin (Fig. 16.7d). The status of the aponeurosis may be evaluated at this time. Redundant or disinserted aponeurosis must be repaired. If the levator is disinserted, Müller's muscle will be visible beneath the lower edge of the aponeurosis, and the peripheral vascular arcade will be seen running horizontally just above the superior tarsal border (Fig. 16.8a, b).

The levator aponeurosis is then gently dissected free from Müller's muscle and conjunctiva with either scissors or cotton-tipped applicators. Carrying this dissection 5–8 mm superiorly is usually enough to mobilize the levator aponeurosis adequately (Fig. 16.9a). Postoperative conjunctival prolapse may occur if excessive separation of Müller's muscle from the levator aponeurosis occurs. If levator disinsertion has occurred, reattachment is necessary. If the levator is still attached but stretched thin, resection may be necessary. A small strip of pretarsal orbicularis muscle is removed from above the inferior wound edge, revealing the tarsal plate (Fig. 16.9b).

Reattaching the aponeurosis to the tarsal plate is accomplished by placing one or more sutures through partial thickness of the tarsus, approximately 3 mm from its upper border. The central suture should be placed in a position to achieve the appropriate eyelid height and contour (Fig. 16.9c). An additional suture may be placed 5–7 mm nasal and lateral to the central suture, if necessary, to adjust the lid contour. Each time the suture is passed, it is important to avoid full-thickness penetration of the tarsal plate and conjunctiva. Eversion of the tarsal plate demonstrates the presence of suture through the tarsus. Sutures placed in this method can cause severe corneal abrasions and their sequelae. The author prefers to use 5–0 Mersilene suture on an S-24 needle, but other absorbable or nonabsorbable sutures may be used [36]. The author favors a technique in which the central suture is broad-based, with the tarsal bite being 5–5.5 mm in width. A more narrow bite may cause peaking of the eyelid margin, whereas a bite larger than 6 mm may cause a flattened contour. Using a double-armed suture, both needles are passed through the levator aponeurosis in an appropriate distance from the inferior levator edge to elevate the eyelid margin (Fig. 16.9d). A temporary knot is thrown, and the patient is assisted into a sitting position and asked to open the eyes. The height and contour of the eyelid margin may be adjusted by tightening the suture or by adjusting either side. Once the appropriate lid height and contour have been obtained, the suture is tied and the tails are cut (Fig. 16.9e). If other sutures are necessary, these are placed at this time. Each time a suture is passed, the lid is everted to examine for inadvertent penetration of the conjunctiva.

At this time, excision of preaponeurotic orbital fat may be achieved using handheld cautery or clamp-cut cauterized methods. If necessary, excessive or redundant skin may be removed at this point as well. A small amount of orbicularis muscle may be excised from the superior lid incision, preventing excessive skin overhang. The skin is closed using running or interrupted 6–0 mild chromic, plain gut, or Prolene sutures [37]. The eyelid crease is reformed by three cardinal sutures, which are placed laterally, centrally, and

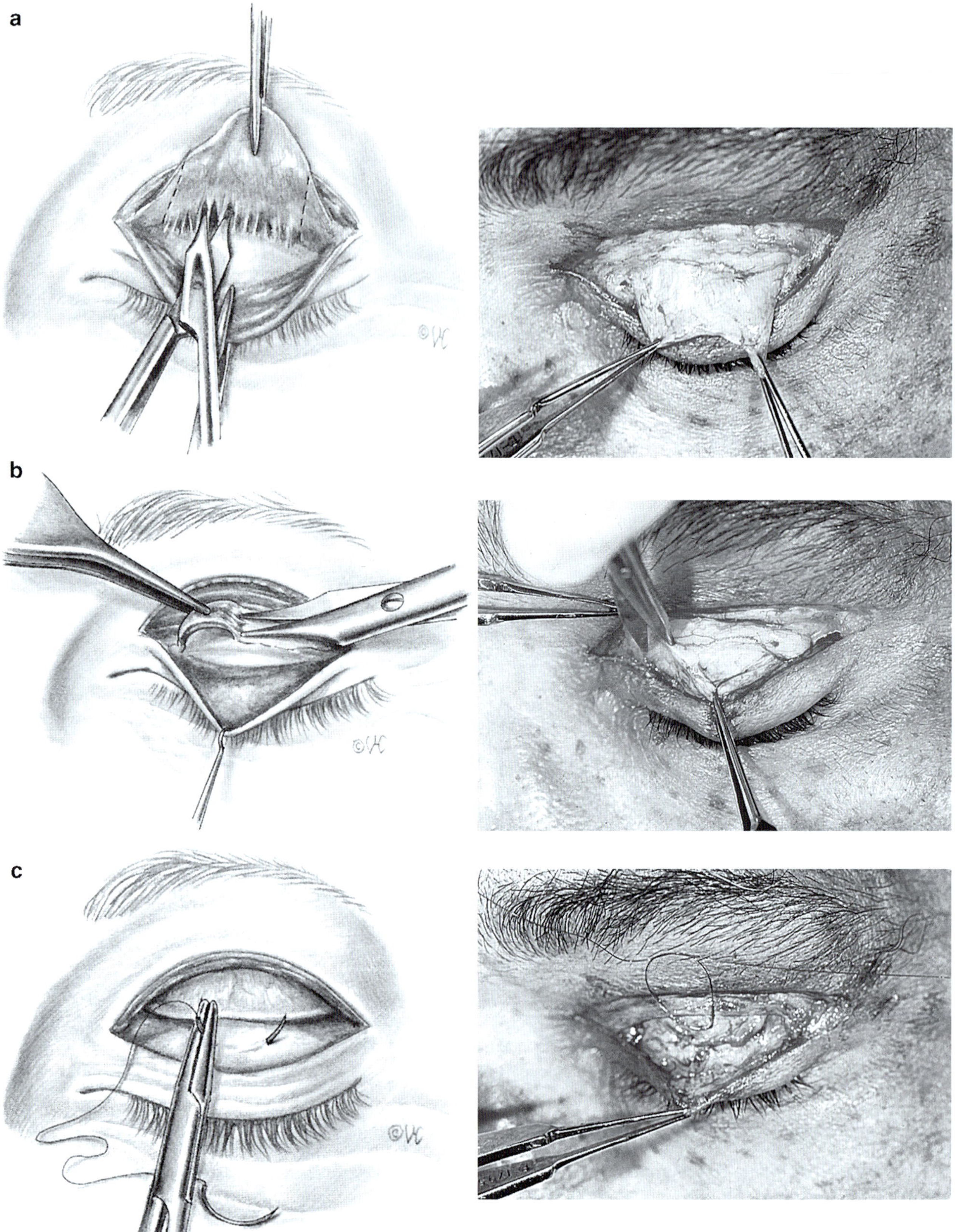

Fig. 16.9 Levator aponeurosis surgery. (**a**) Levator grasped and Müller's muscle dissected free from the conjunctiva. (**b**) Superior third of pretarsal orbicularis is removed. (**c**) Suture is placed with a 5-mm horizontal bite. (From Nesi et al.; reproduced with permission of Elsevier). (**d**) Suture brought through levator and Müller's muscle. (**e**) Suture tied and lid level evaluated. (**f**) Incision site closed with 6–0 mild chromic suture

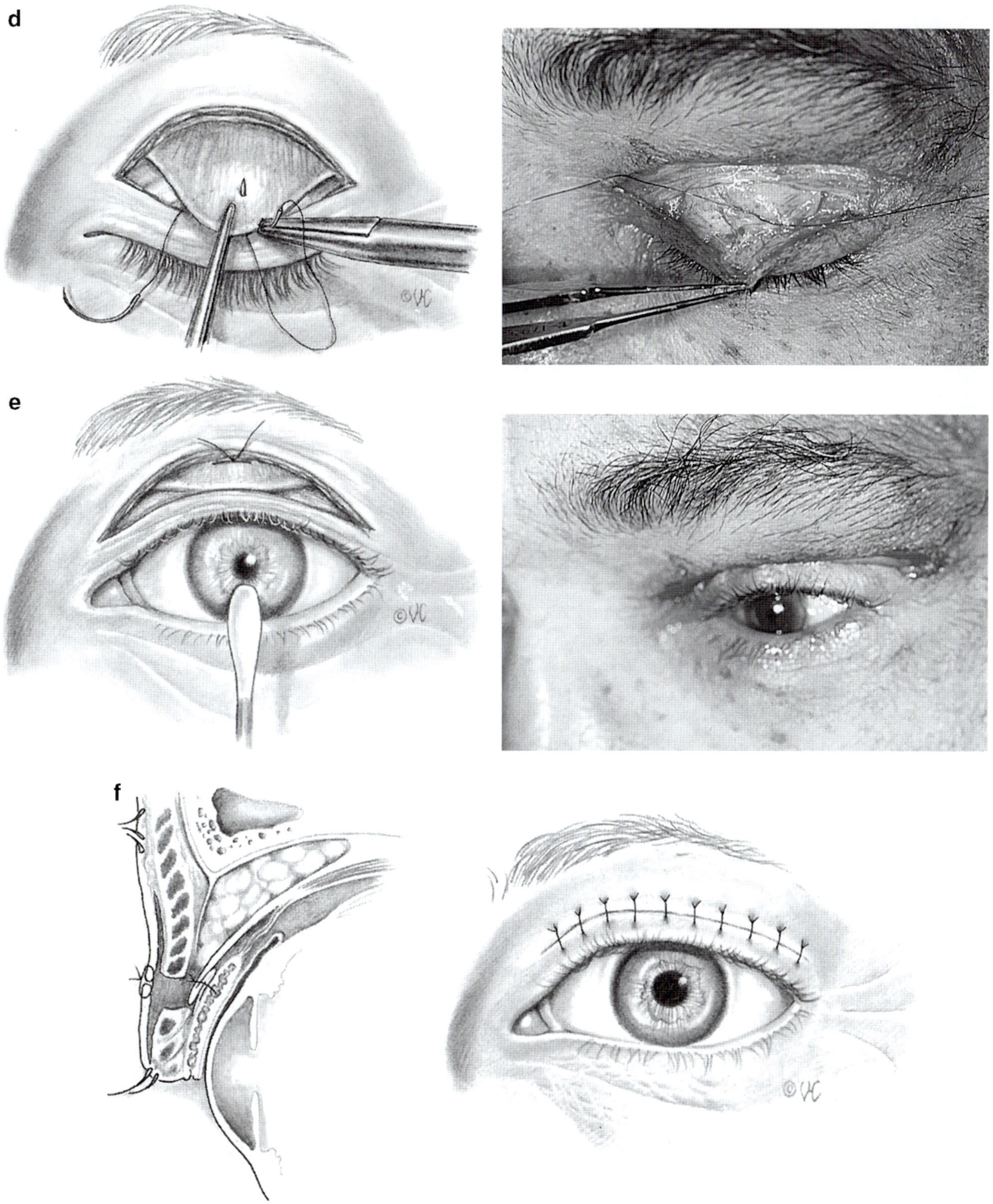

Fig. 16.9 (continued)

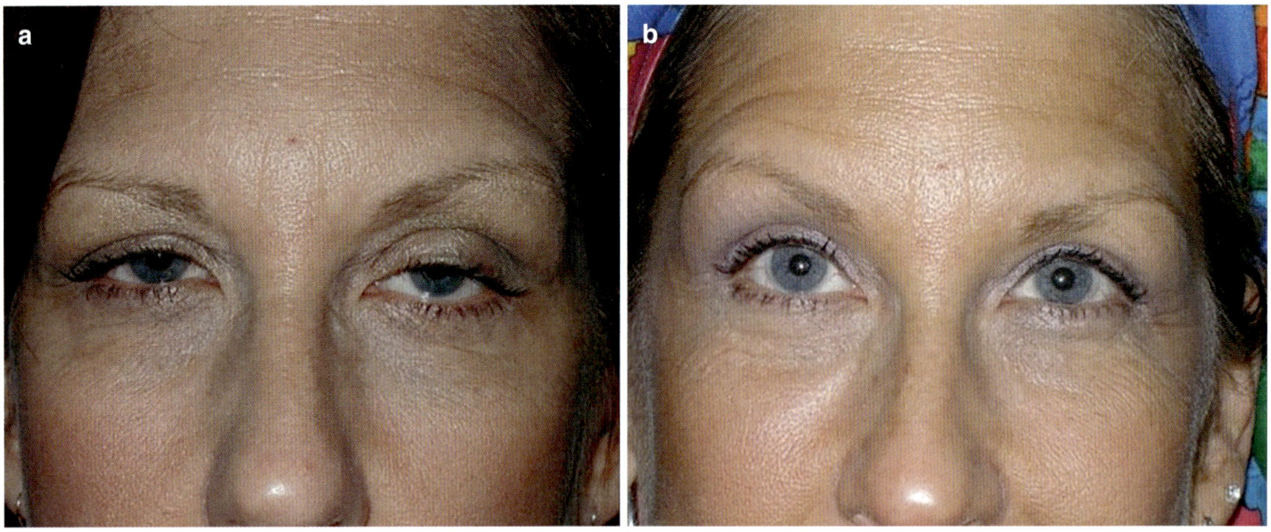

Fig. 16.10 (**a**) Preoperative views. (**b**) Postoperative view 1 month after surgery

medially (Fig. 16.9f). Each is passed through the skin along the inferior incision, through a small edge of aponeurosis, and through the superior skin edge. This step is omitted when an Asian lid crease is to be maintained.

At the conclusion of every ptosis procedure, the surgeon should pull the upper eyelid margin down to see if any restriction of lid closure occurs. This would indicate inadvertent suturing of the orbital septum to the tarsal plate, with subsequent check ligament effect. A Steri-Strip dressing may be placed on the wound, along with antibiotic ointment. The author prefers not to use eye patches, but cold compresses are applied for 15–20 min every hour for the first postoperative day (Fig. 16.10a, b).

The Steri-Strip may be removed on the second day, and nonabsorbable sutures should be removed by the fourth or fifth postoperative day. Any absorbable suture remnants should be removed by the tenth day. A shield may be placed over the eye at bedtime if there is suspicion of potential rubbing by the patient during sleep. If the lid position needs to be corrected, reoperation may be performed within a few days to weeks with the same technique.

The Posterior Approach to Ptosis Repair

Tarsal-Conjunctival-Müller's Muscle Resection (Fasanella-Servat Operation)

The Fasanella-Servat operation (FSO) [38] is a procedure used mainly in mild to moderate blepharoptosis with good levator function (above 8 mm). It can correct up to 2 mm of congenital ptosis and 2.5–4 mm of acquired ptosis. It is particularly useful in treating patients with Horner's syndrome. Other common indications are steroid-induced ptosis and myasthenia gravis. It is a quick, reliable, and predictable procedure. Proper patient selection, adequate patient evaluation, and meticulous surgical technique are essential in this procedure.

In the FSO, the ratio of tarsectomy to eyelid elevation is approximately 2:1 [39]. Phenylephrine hydrochloride 2.5% can be used preoperatively to ascertain whether the ptotic eyelid will rise with the FSO. If after the installation of phenylephrine the eyelid in question is not within 1 mm of the desired level, other procedures such as levator advancement should be considered. If the lid is within 1 mm, incorporation of more conjunctiva-Müller's muscle in the resection is recommended (up to 8 mm). If overcorrection is present, the surgeon should double check for the presence of a Hering's law (equal innervation). If no Hering's law is present, a less aggressive tarsectomy should be performed (for every 1 mm of overcorrection, 2 mm less of tarsus).

In cases of 1–1.5 mm of ptosis, the FSO with the modification by Lauring (sutureless) is indicated [40]. In cases between 1.5 and 4 mm of ptosis, the original FSO or any of its modifications by Iliff [41] (pressure on skin) or Stasior [42] (maximal tarsal resection) could be used.

Local anesthesia should be used with or without sedation by infiltrating 2% lidocaine with epinephrine subcutaneously, approximately 10 mm superior to the eyelid margin. A modified frontal block can also be used. Some surgeons infiltrate along the border of the tarsus subconjunctivally, with the eyelid everted. We find this tends to distort the tissues and the measurement. Several drops of 0.5% proparacaine are instilled in the eye. An Adson forceps is used to fixate the upper eyelid margin. A 5–0 nylon suture (alternatively 5–0 chromic gut/original FSO suture) on a P1 or FS-2 needle is passed at the superior palpebral crease temporally from the skin surface to the conjunctival surface just above the tarsus (Fig. 16.11). A plastic corneoscleral protector should be used to protect the globe. The upper eyelid is everted by a Desmarres retractor. Two equally curved hemostats are

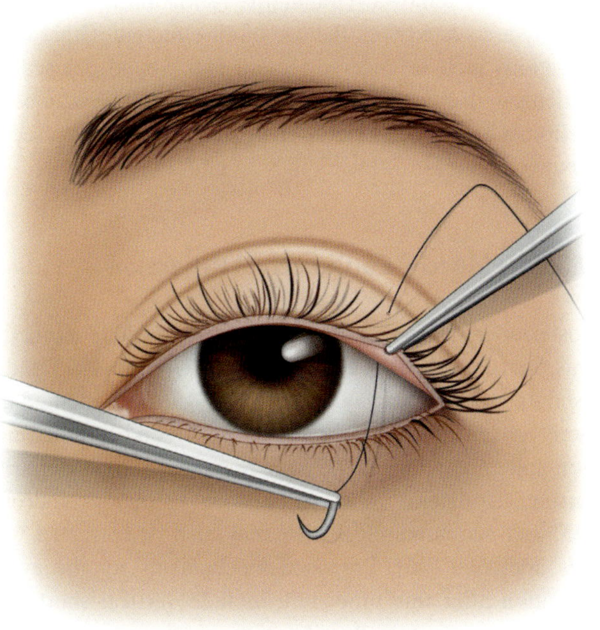

Fig. 16.11 A 5–0 suture is passed at the superior palpebral crease temporally

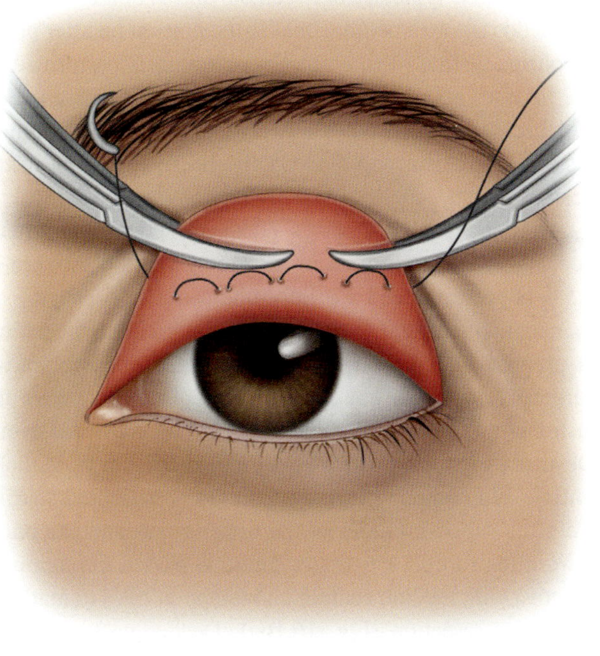

Fig. 16.12 Two equally curved hemostats are placed at about 3 mm from the superior tarsal margin

placed at about 3 mm from the superior tarsal margin. The clamp will incorporate tarsus, Müller's muscle, and conjunctiva. Care must be taken to clamp no more tarsus centrally. This central placement of the clamp will lead to central eyelid peaking. Alternatively, a Putterman clamp 6 can be used. If more than 3 mm of ptosis is present, an additional 4–6 mm

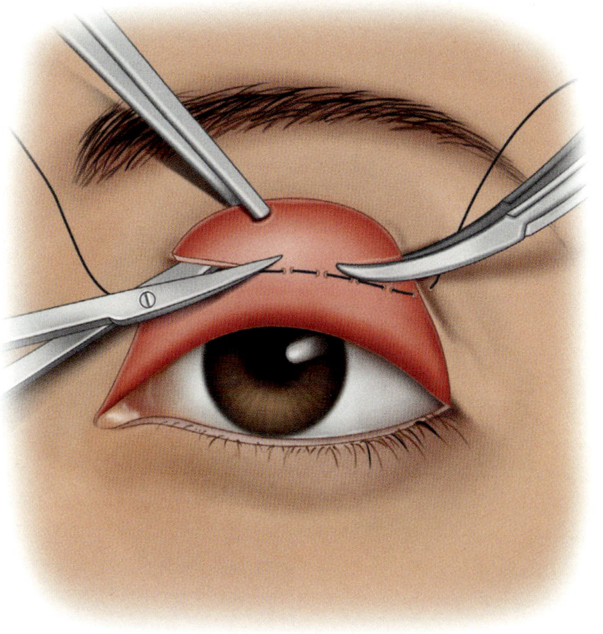

Fig. 16.13 Westcott scissors are then used to cut the conjunctiva-tarsus-Müller's muscle above the suture line and against the clamps

of conjunctival/Müller's muscle may be incorporated into the clamps (Fig. 16.12).

The suture is placed below the clamps from the temporal to the nasal side. The suture should pass approximately 2 mm below the clamp (toward the fornix). An effort is made to pass the needle at the same level and to tighten the suture on each pass. This will bring the suture under the conjunctiva and avoid corneal abrasions. After the needle is passed the whole length of the clamps, it is further passed nasally, from the conjunctiva through the full thickness of the eyelid and out the skin, at the superior palpebral crease. A 15-blade or Westcott scissors are then used to cut the conjunctiva-tarsus-Müllers muscle above the suture line and against the hemostats or clamp (Fig. 16.13).

In case of concomitant lower eyelid retraction, the excised tissue could be used as a graft to elevate the lower eyelid or in other reconstructive procedures (Fig. 16.14). Any rough irregularities on the inner surface of the eyelid is removed. Each end of the suture is then tied to itself (Fig. 16.15). The plastic corneoscleral shield is removed, and an antibiotic is placed on the eye.

Postoperative Management

Ice compresses are used for the first 24 h. This procedure is usually done on an ambulatory basis, and the patient goes home the same day of surgery. Systemic antibiotics and a short course of steroids may be used prophylactically. The suture is removed in 10 days. If there is overcorrection, the suture should be removed earlier than 10 days, and gentle traction should be placed on the eyelid to separate the wound adhesion to the desired level. Final results are usually obtained after 21 days.

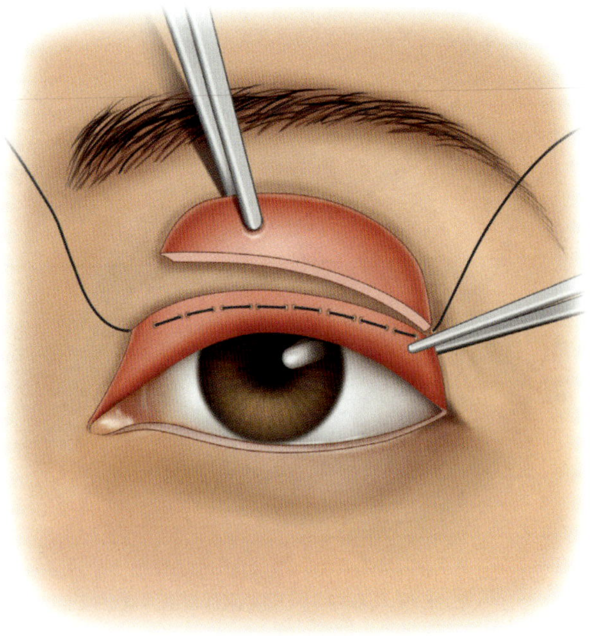

Fig. 16.14 In case of concomitant lower eyelid retraction, the excised tissue could be used as a graft

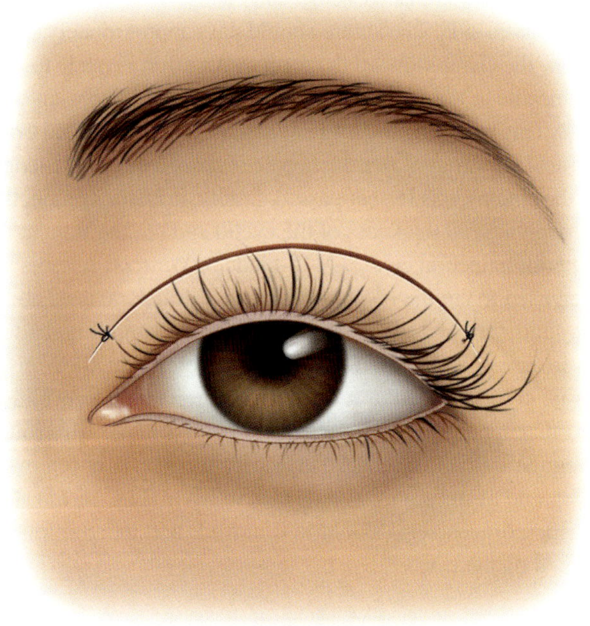

Fig. 16.15 Each end of the suture is then tied to itself

Complications

Possible complications include a peaked eyelid or segmental ptosis because of a misapplication of the hemostats, corneal abrasion from too much exposed suture material on the tarsus, and occasional duplication of the eyelid crease secondary to tarsus removal. Granuloma formation is rare and is usually associated with the use of chromic gut. Other complications include undercorrection and wound dehiscence. Patients with concomitant lower eyelid retraction may benefit from a lower eyelid elevation procedure using the resected tarsus-conjunctiva-Müller's muscle graft [43].

Müller's Muscle-Conjunctival Resection

Posterior resection of Müller's muscle and conjunctiva was first described by Putterman and Urist in 1975 and is used to treat mild to moderate ptosis [44]. This method has been proven effective in patients with good levator function and an appropriate positive response to phenylephrine testing. Unilateral ptosis related to Horner's syndrome [45] and anophthalmic socket may also be corrected with this approach [46]. Proposed mechanisms for the eyelid elevation after this procedure include vertical shortening of the posterior lamella, plication or advancement of the Müller's muscle and levator aponeurosis, and cicatricial changes. Careful preoperative measurements and planning are essential since intraoperative adjustments are not possible, unlike levator advancement surgery [47]. The range of resection is typically between 6.5 and 9.5 mm. When the ptotic lid rises to a height equal to the normal lid after phenylephrine testing [48], an 8-mm resection is performed. If the lid rises above the normal lid, the amount of resection is decreased as low as 6.5 mm. A maximum of 9.5 mm of resection is performed if the ptotic lid rises but not to the desired height.

After the patient receives adequate sedation, a frontal nerve block is performed by injecting a 50:50 mixture of 0.5% bupivacaine and 2% lidocaine using a 25 gauge, 1.5-in. needle just lateral to the supraorbital groove. The patient is prepped and draped as previously described for ptosis surgery. A 6–0 silk traction suture is place just above the lash margin centrally, and the upper eyelid is everted over a Desmarres retractor. The predetermined amount of Müller's muscle and conjunctiva to be resected is measured starting from the superior border of the upper tarsus and extending toward the fornix. A 6–0 silk suture is passed through conjunctiva with medial, central, and temporal bites to mark the tissue for resection (Fig. 16.16a). Deeper passes through the vascularized Müller's muscle may elicit bleeding. The conjunctiva and Müller's muscle are loosened from the overlying levator aponeurosis by grasping and elevating with forceps. A Putterman clamp designed for Müller's muscle resection is placed between the 6–0 marking suture and the superior tarsal border. The clamp is closed around the conjunctiva and Müller's muscle (Fig. 16.16b). A 6–0 double-armed plain gut suture is passed 1.5 mm below the clamp as a running horizontal mattress suture (Fig. 16.16c). A #15

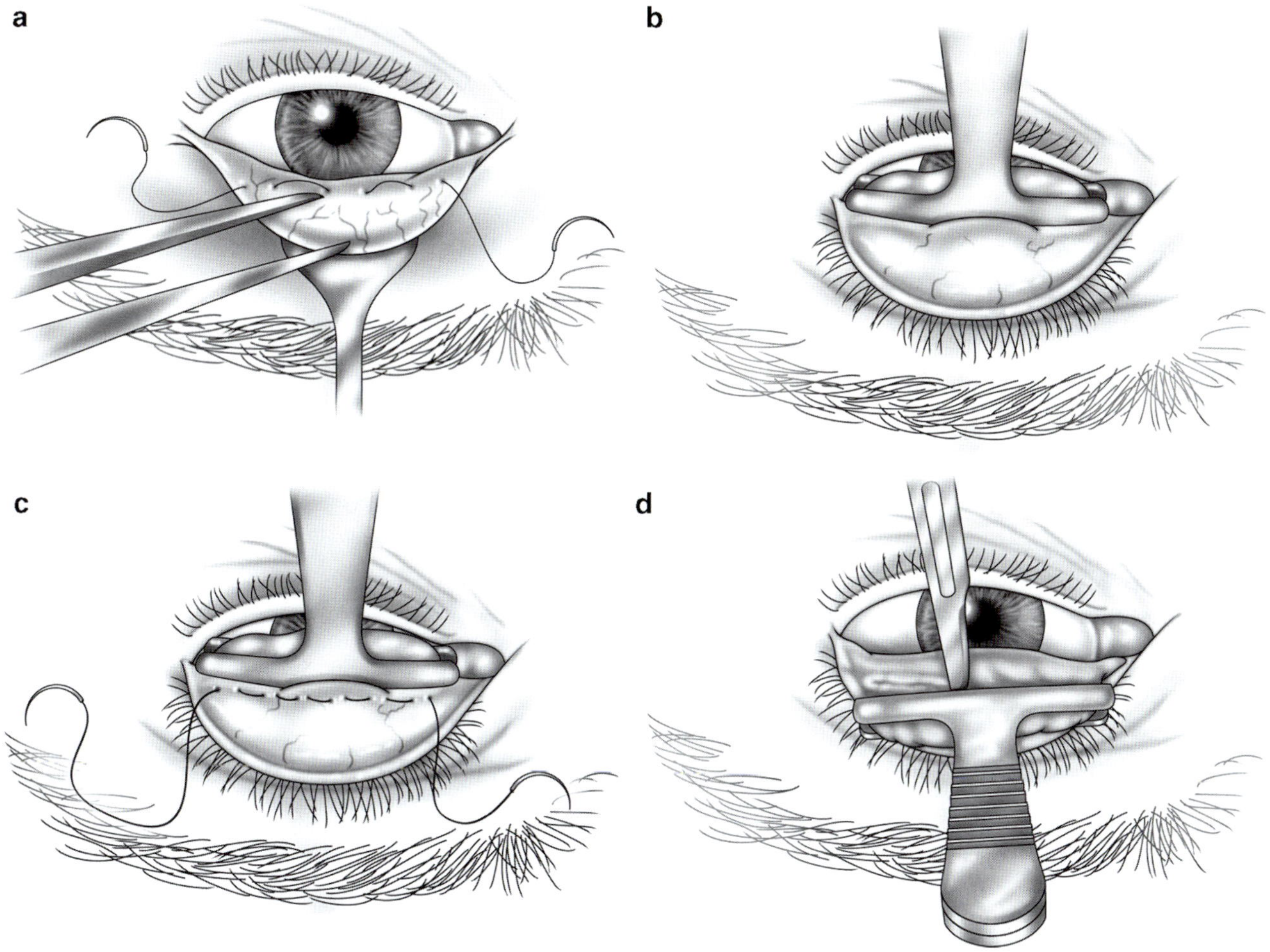

Fig. 16.16 (**a**) A marking suture is placed in a predetermined distance from the superior tarsal border. (**b**) A clamp is placed which now contains conjunctiva and Müller's muscle. (**c**) A 6–0 plain gut suture is placed superior to the clamp in a running mattress fashion. (**d**) The tissue within the clamp is removed with the blade, maintaining a metal-on-metal feel to minimize the chances of cutting the suture

blade is used to remove the tissue secured within the clamp. Maintaining a metal-on-metal contact between the blade and the Putterman clamp during resection helps to avoid cutting the suture (Fig. 16.16d). Both needles are passed full thickness through the eyelid and are secured on the skin surface with a small piece of surgical tape which can be removed in 1 week.

Advantages of this procedure are maintaining eyelid contour by avoiding tarsus resection and low reoperation rate. Putterman and others have shown that 90% of eyelids achieve satisfactory symmetry compared to the fellow eye [38, 43]. Most commonly encountered postoperative complications include eyelid retraction and mild lagophthalmos. Concerns have been raised that excision of conjunctival goblet cells and accessory lacrimal glands of Wolfring situated at the upper tarsal border may aggravate dry eyes, although evidence against such concerns has also been published [49, 50]. An open-sky technique for Müller's muscle and conjunctival resection without the use of a clamp has been described [50], and further modification of this technique in order to preserve conjunctiva has been published [51, 52]. Sutureless mullerectomy as an adjunct to blepharoplasty has also been described [53, 54].

References

1. Beard C. The surgical treatment of blepharoptosis: a quantitative approach. Trans Am Ophthalmol Soc. 1966;64:401–87.
2. Linberg JV, Vasquez RJ, Chao GM. Aponeurotic ptosis repair under local anesthesia. Prediction of results from operative lid height. Ophthalmology. 1988;95(8):1046–52.
3. Metzinger SE, Rigby PL, Bailey DJ, Brousse RG. Local anesthesia in blepharoplasty: a new look? South Med J. 1994;87(2):225–7.
4. Vasan A, Baker JA, Shelby RA, Soo MSC. Impact of sodium bicarbonate-buffered lidocaine on patient pain during image-guided breast biopsy. J Am Coll Radiol. 2017;14(9):1194–201.
5. Beard C. Ptosis. 2nd ed. St. Louis: Mosby; 1976.
6. Dransart H. Un cas de blépharoptose opéré par un procédé spécial à l'auteur. Analectes ophtalmologiques. 1880;84:88.

7. Koster WG. De verhouding van den musculus tarsalis superior Mülleri bij ptosis congenita. Ned Tijdschr Geneeskd. 1899;35:412.
8. Reese RG. An operation for Blepharoptosis, with the formation of a fold in the lid. Trans Am Ophthalmol Soc. 1923;21:71–8.
9. Crawford JS. Repair of ptosis using frontalis muscle and fascia lata. Trans Am Acad Ophthalmol Otolaryngol. 1956;60(5):672–8.
10. Fox SA. Congenital ptosis: II. Frontalis sling. J Pediatr Ophthalmol Strabismus. 1966;3(2):25–8.
11. Crawford JS. Repair of ptosis using frontalis muscle and fascia lata: a 20-year review. Ophthalmic Surg. 1977;8(4):31–40.
12. Tillett CW, Tillett GM. Silicone sling in the correction of ptosis. Am J Ophthalmol. 1966;62(3):521–3.
13. Downes RN, Collin JR. The Mersilene mesh sling--a new concept in ptosis surgery. Br J Ophthalmol. 1989;73(7):498–501.
14. Ruban JM, Mallem M, Tabone E, Donne C. A new biomaterial in surgery of ptosis with frontalis suspension: wide pore PTFE. J Fr Ophtalmol. 1995;18(3):207–19.
15. Bach A, Sanchez-Gonzalez M, Warman R. Double rhomboid suture technique for congenital ptosis. J Pediatr Ophthalmol Strabismus. 2018;55(2):117–21.
16. Beyer CK, Albert DM. The use and fate of fascia lata and sclera in ophthalmic plastic and reconstructive surgery. Ophthalmology. 1981;88(9):869–86.
17. Wasserman BN, Sprunger DT, Helveston EM. Comparison of materials used in frontalis suspension. Arch Ophthalmol. 2001;119(5):687–91.
18. Ben Simon GJ, Macedo AA, Schwarcz RM, et al. Frontalis suspension for upper eyelid ptosis: evaluation of different surgical designs and suture material. Am J Ophthalmol. 2005;140(5):877–85.
19. Bernardini FP, Devoto MH, Priolo E. Treatment of unilateral congenital ptosis. Ophthalmology. 2007;114(3):622–3.
20. Suh JY, Ahn HB. Ptosis repair using preserved fascia lata with the modified direct tarsal fixation technique. Korean J Ophthalmol. 2013;27(5):311–5.
21. Spoor TC, Kwitko GM. Blepharoptosis repair by fascia lata suspension with direct tarsal and frontalis fixation. Am J Ophthalmol. 1990;109(3):314–7.
22. Antoszyk JH, Tucker N, Ling C, Codere F. Interlocking Crawford triangles in frontalis suspension. Arch Ophthalmol. 1993;111(6):875–8.
23. Wagner RS. Comparing suture materials used in frontalis suspension procedures. J Pediatr Ophthalmol Strabismus. 2015;52(2):76.
24. Eversbusch O. Zur operation der congenitalen blepharoptosis. Klin Monatsbl Augenheilkd 1883;21:100–7.
25. Wolff H. Die vorlagerung des Musc. Levator pal. Superioris mit Plurchtrengnung der Insertion. Zwei neue Methoden gegen Ptosis congenita. Arch Augenheilkd 1896(33).
26. Anderson RL, Beard C. The levator aponeurosis. Attachments and their clinical significance. Arch Ophthalmol. 1977;95(8):1437–41.
27. Anderson RL, Dixon RS. Aponeurotic ptosis surgery. Arch Ophthalmol. 1979;97(6):1123–8.
28. Berke RN. A simplified Blaskovics operation for blepharoptosis; results in ninety-one operations. AMA Arch Ophthalmol. 1952;48(4):460–95.
29. Jones LT, Quickert MH, Wobig JL. The cure of ptosis by aponeurotic repair. Arch Ophthalmol. 1975;93(8):629–34.
30. Older JJ. Levator aponeurosis surgery for the correction of acquired ptosis. Analysis of 113 procedures. Ophthalmology. 1983;90(9):1056–9.
31. McCord CD Jr. An external minimal ptosis procedure – external tarsoaponeurectomy. Trans Sect Ophthalmol Am Acad Ophthalmol Otolaryngol. 1975;79(5):683–6.
32. Baylis HI, Shorr N. Anterior tarsectomy reoperation for upper eyelid blepharoptosis or contour abnormalities. Am J Ophthalmol. 1977;84(1):67–71.
33. Collin JR, O'Donnell BA. Adjustable sutures in eyelid surgery for ptosis and lid retraction. Br J Ophthalmol. 1994;78(3):167–74.
34. Hylkema HA, Koornneef L. Treatment of ptosis by levator resection with adjustable sutures via the anterior approach. Br J Ophthalmol. 1989;73(6):416–8.
35. Karesh JW. Multilevel full-thickness eyelid resection for the correction of severe acquired ptosis in the poorly functioning eyelid. Ophthalmic Surg. 1991;22(7):399–405.
36. Linberg JV, Mangano LM, Odom JV. Comparison of nonabsorbable and absorbable sutures for use in oculoplastic surgery. Ophthalmic Plast Reconstr Surg. 1991;7(1):1–7.
37. Jaggi R, Hart R, Taylor SM. Absorbable suture compared with nonabsorbable suture in upper eyelid blepharoplasty closure. Arch Facial Plast Surg. 2009;11(5):349–52.
38. Fasanella R, Servat J. Levator resection for minimal ptosis: another simplified operation. Arch Ophthalmol. 1961;65:493–6.
39. Samimi DB, Erb MH, Lane CJ, Dresner SC. The modified fasanella-servat procedure: description and quantified analysis. Ophthal Plast Reconstr Surg. 2013;29(1):30–4.
40. Lauring L. Blepharoptosis correction with the sutureless Fasanella-Servat operation. Arch Ophthalmol. 1977;95(4):671–4.
41. As cited: Fasanella RM. Surgery for minimal ptosis: the Fasanella-Servat operation, 1973. Trans Ophthalmol Soc U K. 1973;93(0):425–38.
42. As cited: Callahan A. Ptosis associated with congenital defects; blepharophimosis, epicanthus and other syndromes. In: Symposium on surgery of the orbit and adnexa. Transactions New Orleans Academy of Ophthalmology. St. Louis, C. V. Mosby Company, 1974.
43. Putterman AM. A clamp for strengthening Müller's muscle in the treatment of ptosis. Modification, theory, and clamp for the Fasanella-Servat ptosis operation. Arch Ophthalmol. 1972;87(6):665–7.
44. Putterman AM, Urist MJ. Muller muscle-conjunctiva resection. Technique for treatment of blepharoptosis. Arch Ophthalmol. 1975;93(8):619–23.
45. Glatt HJ, Putterman AM, Fett DR. Muller's muscle-conjunctival resection procedure in the treatment of ptosis in Horner's syndrome. Ophthalmic Surg. 1990;21(2):93–6.
46. Ha SW, Lee JM, Jeung WJ, Ahn HB. Clinical effects of conjunctiva-Muller muscle resection in anophthalmic ptosis. Korean J Ophthalmol. 2007;21(2):65–9.
47. Ben Simon GJ, Lee S, Schwarcz RM, et al. External levator advancement vs Muller's muscle-conjunctival resection for correction of upper eyelid involutional ptosis. Am J Ophthalmol. 2005;140(3):426–32.
48. Ramesh S, Mancini R. Dynamic analysis of Muller's muscle response to phenylephrine. Ophthalmic Plast Reconstr Surg. 2016;32(1):46–8.
49. Saonanon P, Sithanon S. External levator advancement versus Muller muscle-conjunctival resection for aponeurotic blepharoptosis: a randomized clinical trial. Plast Reconstr Surg. 2018;141(2):213e–9e.
50. Lake S, Mohammad-Ali FH, Khooshabeh R. Open sky Muller's muscle-conjunctiva resection for ptosis surgery. Eye (Lond). 2003;17(9):1008–12.
51. Bautista SA, Wladis EJ, Schultze RL. Quantitative assessment of dry eye parameters after Muller's muscle-conjunctival resection. Ophthalmic Plast Reconstr Surg. 2018;34(6):562–4.
52. Peter NM, Khooshabeh R. Open-sky isolated subtotal Muller's muscle resection for ptosis surgery: a review of over 300 cases and assessment of long-term outcome. Eye (Lond). 2013;27(4):519–24.
53. Baldwin HC, Bhagey J, Khooshabeh R. Open sky Muller muscle-conjunctival resection in phenylephrine test-negative blepharoptosis patients. Ophthalmic Plast Reconstr Surg. 2005;21(4):276–80.
54. Gildener-Leapman JR, Sheps I, Stein R, et al. The sutureless Mullerectomy. Ophthalmic Plast Reconstr Surg. 2019;35(3):290–3.

Part V

Cosmetic Surgery

Evan H. Black

Upper Eyelid Blepharoplasty

17

Mohit A. Dewan and Dale R. Meyer

Introduction

Studies on facial recognition and aesthetic beauty indicate that the upper and lower eyelids, eyebrows, and midface all play a vital role in the overall aesthetic and memorability of the face. Concepts of beauty, however, are widely variable and constantly evolving throughout the world, with certain facial contours more desirable than others depending upon the societal norms. These contours can be altered surgically during upper eyelid blepharoplasty. Each patient has individual desires and concerns which the surgeon can take into consideration in attempting to achieve the desired aesthetic outcome. This patient-centered approach to blepharoplasty requires a healthy patient-physician relationship that can ultimately be both rewarding and challenging.

Evolution of Beauty

Beauty is the perception of attractiveness as appreciated by the observer, that is, "the eye of the beholder." It is influenced by the combination of innate physical attributes and the presentation of these attributes in society. Importantly, the desirability of certain attributes changes over time, creating an ever-evolving scale of attractiveness. For instance, clothing, hairstyle, and makeup fads change constantly as our perceptions of their relative beauty are fluid. Facial beauty, as it relates to desirability of certain anatomic characteristics, is also evolving. Of note, in the early 1980s, blepharoplasty included the removal of large amounts of fat as the trend was to create a very deep superior sulcus. Studies now indicate that orbital fat atrophies as time passes, creating a natural hollowing around the eyes. As a result, modern techniques of facial rejuvenation recommend very little or no fat removal, and some patients may even benefit from additional transfer of fat (or other agents) to "volumize" the lid and/or immediately adjacent region (e.g., brows for upper lids). The customizability of this surgery has resulted in it being among the most performed plastic surgery procedures in the world, with over 300,000 surgical cases in the US in 2017 alone (Fig. 17.1).

Because the eyelids are a single aesthetic unit often influenced by the facial features around them, the surgeon must also evaluate the entirety of the face when considering blepharoplasty. While the most common presenting concern for patients is "excess eyelid skin," concomitant upper eyelid ptosis (i.e., droop of the true eyelid margin) or brow ptosis is often present. As Fig. 17.2 shows, upper eyelid blepharoplasty is not always the solution. In this case, only brow ptosis was present, and a brow lift achieved a good aesthetic outcome.

Surgical Planning and Applied Eyelid Anatomy

Successful surgery of the upper eyelid requires thorough knowledge of the associated anatomy. A detailed description of eyelid anatomy can be found in Chap. 1. It is important to gain an understanding of how each anatomical structure of the eyelid influences the overall appearance of the patient and subsequently apply surgical principles to address each of these areas.

For instance, the orbital septum and levator aponeurosis of an Asian upper eyelid typically insert more inferiorly than an occidental lid, creating a fuller appearance and a lower or absent eyelid crease. In Asians, the sub-brow fat layer also extends more inferiorly into the lid adding yet more fullness. To preserve these Asian characteristics during blepharoplasty,

M. A. Dewan (✉)
Eye Plastic Surgery of Minnesota PLLC, Woodbury, MN, USA
e-mail: mohit.dewan@eyeplasticsmn.com

D. R. Meyer
Lions Eye Institute-Albany Medical Center, Department of Ophthalmic Plastic Surgery-Ophthalmology, Albany, NY, USA

J. J. Servat et al. (eds.), *Smith and Nesi's Ophthalmic Plastic and Reconstructive Surgery*,
https://doi.org/10.1007/978-3-030-41720-8_17

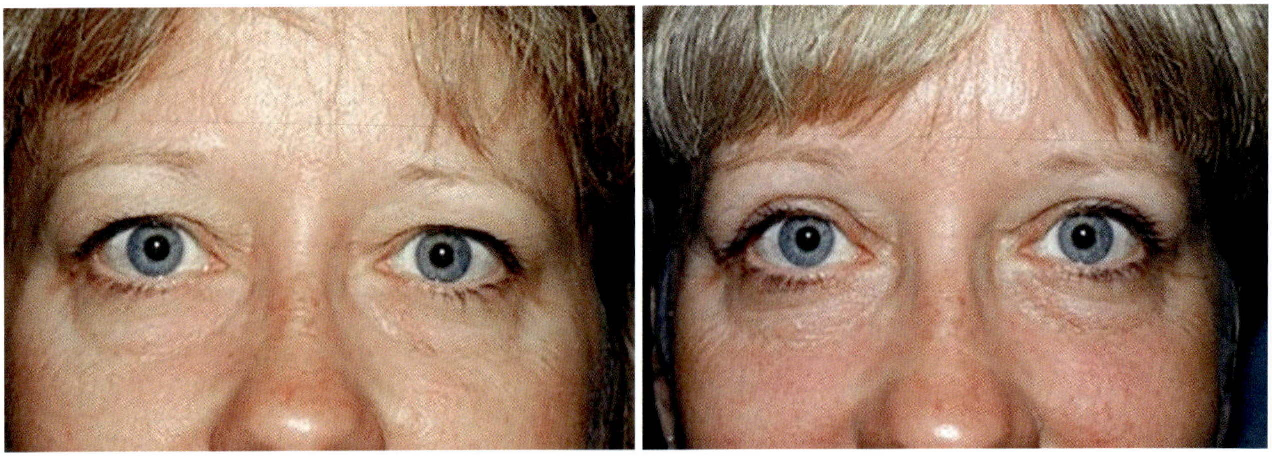

Fig. 17.1 Pre- and postoperative results with no fat removal. This patient underwent upper lid blepharoplasty with no fat removal. The excess skin has been removed, creating a new platform for the application of eyelid makeup. Note the youthful fullness in the lateral brow

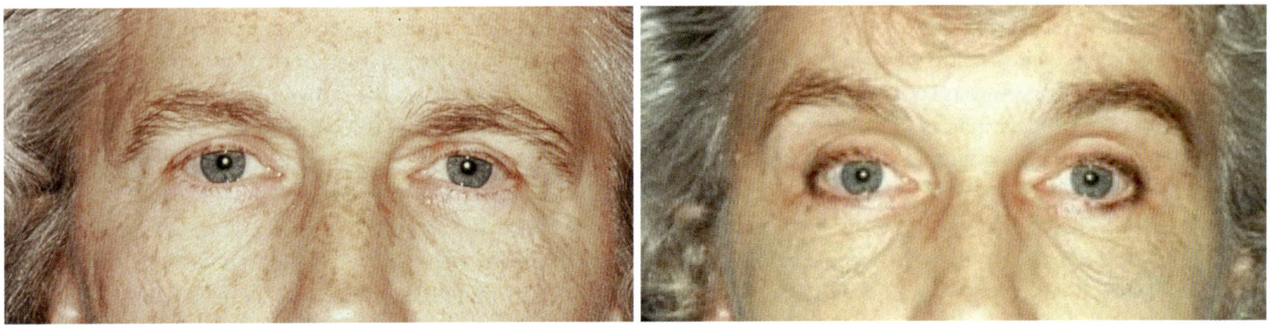

Fig. 17.2 Preoperative and postoperative brow lift photos. This patient presented to the office with "too much skin on the upper eyelids." Elevation of the brows without upper eyelid blepharoplasty corrected this complaint, as evidenced in the postoperative photo on the right

a minimum of skin and fat removal, with definition of the more subtle eyelid crease, is necessary.

African-American eyelids often have a greater amount of fat and more prominent-appearing eyes. To avoid an exophthalmic postoperative appearance, careful removal of orbital fat and skin is necessary, allowing the natural fullness of the lid to hide the proptosis of the eyes.

The retro-orbicularis oculi fat ("ROOF"), sits deep to the eyebrow, and this submuscular fibroadipose layer can be of variable thickness in the eyelids and eyebrows. This can create a fuller-appearing upper eyelid but should not be mistaken for preaponeurotic fat when performing surgical dissection. Erroneously excising the ROOF in this case may lead to a hollowed, aged appearance of the upper eyelid.

Attention should also be directed to the eyelid crease and its position. For many women, a well-defined eyelid crease provides the perception of a more youthful appearance, and the area of skin anterior to the tarsal plate creates a "platform" for the application of makeup. As a patient ages and the orbital fat atrophies, deepening the superior sulcus, this eyelid platform may extend superiorly (and posteriorly) to Whitnall's ligament, indicating the need for crease fixation at the time of blepharoplasty. Often, the incision is made further superiorly in these patients to allow the incision to hide in the deeper sulcus. Conversely, a similar approach in a male patient may feminize the eyelids and should be avoided. The male eyelid crease is typically lower than the female, and surgical planning should account for this.

The medial canthal region should generally be avoided with a blepharoplasty incision, with most surgeons suggesting the incision stay lateral to the punctum as this region is a confluence of different skin types—thin upper eyelid skin and the thicker nose and glabellar skin. Furthermore, the concave shape of this area, along with these different types of tissues, can lead to postoperative webbing and poor cosmesis. If extreme redundancy is present in this area, lifting the medial eyebrow tissue may be a more effective solution than blepharoplasty alone.

Surgical Technique

Anesthesia

Upper eyelid blepharoplasty is typically performed under local anesthesia or with monitored care anesthesia with adjunctive local anesthetic. Under MAC, the local anesthetic is typically injected after the administration of sedation for maximum patient comfort. The preferred local anesthetic is 2% lidocaine with 1:100,000 epinephrine which provides for sufficient anesthetic time and vasoconstriction to limit intraoperative bleeding. Surgeons may also elect to add sodium bicarbonate in a 1:10 concentration (e.g., 2 ml of buffer in 20 ml of local anesthetic) to aid patient comfort. This is particularly useful in surgery performed solely with local anesthesia. Additionally, surgeons may add hyaluronic acid to the local anesthetic to facilitate spread of the injection. This is generally avoided in patients undergoing concomitant ptosis repair to allow for intraoperative adjustments.

Local anesthetic is injected after incision marking is complete. We prefer to use a 27 g needle for administration of local anesthetic as it allows for good patient comfort and controlled injection, and approximately 1–2 ml of anesthetic is generally sufficient. Additional injections can be given as necessary intraoperatively if the patient feels discomfort during portions of the surgery.

Incision Marking

Incision marking is, perhaps, the most important part of blepharoplasty surgery as it, in many ways, determines the overall results of the surgery. Marking, in fact, is responsible for the two most important factors of the surgery: the position of the eyelid crease and how much skin is removed from the eyelid.

The eyelid can be marked for surgery in many ways. One method is to place the lower marking along the natural eyelid crease of the patient. This affords a natural appearance and, for most patients, a desirable outcome. The incision should be marked starting just lateral to the lower punctum, along the eyelid crease, and ending at the lateral canthus. The incision can be carried further laterally in a slightly upward oblique fashion if there is a significant amount of lateral skin excess. Alternatively, the eyelid "crease" marking can be placed using measurements based on standard lid crease height. In most women, the lid crease is typically between 7 and 10 mm above the lid margin centrally, while in men, the crease is 5–8 mm above the margin. In Asian patients, the crease is lower, typically 3–6 mm in height (Fig. 17.3).

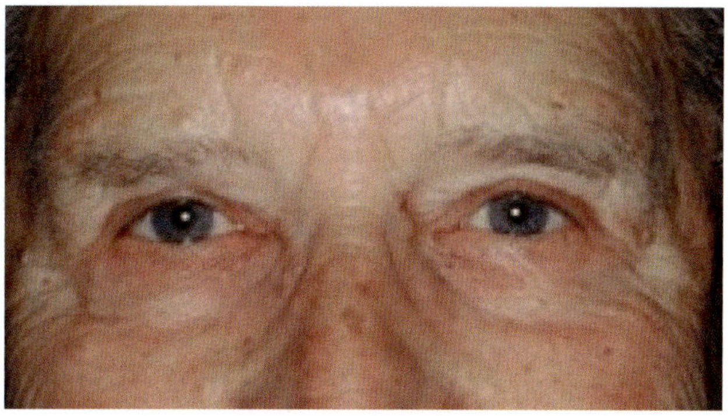

Fig. 17.3 Lid crease height in men. This patient has had upper eyelid blepharoplasty. Note the position of the eyelid crease is lower than on women. No crease fixation is used in this patient to avoid a feminine appearance

The upper marking can be placed using a variety of techniques. Many surgeons prefer the "skin pinch" method of marking. This is accomplished by using forceps to elevate the skin from the lower lid crease until the amount of skin in the forceps is maximized without causing lagophthalmos. The superior marking is then placed at the position of the superior tine of the forceps. Alternatively, Flowers' rule suggests that the eyelid should have 20 mm of skin present between the brow and lashes to prevent postoperative lagophthalmos. The authors prefer a combination of these techniques. We mark the eyelid using the natural eyelid crease, then perform a skin pinch to ensure no lagophthalmos, and place the more superior marking at this point (which will typically be about 8–9 mm above the crease). We generally prefer to leave at least 10 mm (1 cm) of skin below the brows. This conservative approach leads to a more natural postoperative appearance with little risk of lagophthalmos and coincident corneal exposure (Fig. 17.4).

Surgical Technique

After the incision is marked, sedation induced, and anesthesia injected, incision can begin. Many instruments are available to perform the skin incision, including the scalpel, scissors, radio frequency devices, and carbon dioxide laser. Each instrument has advantages and disadvantages related to cost, safety, and healing. Scalpel techniques and scissor dissection are the most familiar to surgeons and are also the least costly. The laser is advantageous because of the ease and precision of incision, relatively bloodless field, and easy tissue dissection. However, the laser dissection is entirely visual, which takes experience to master, and has a significantly higher cost associated with the equipment. Additionally, laser safety precautions must be taken in the

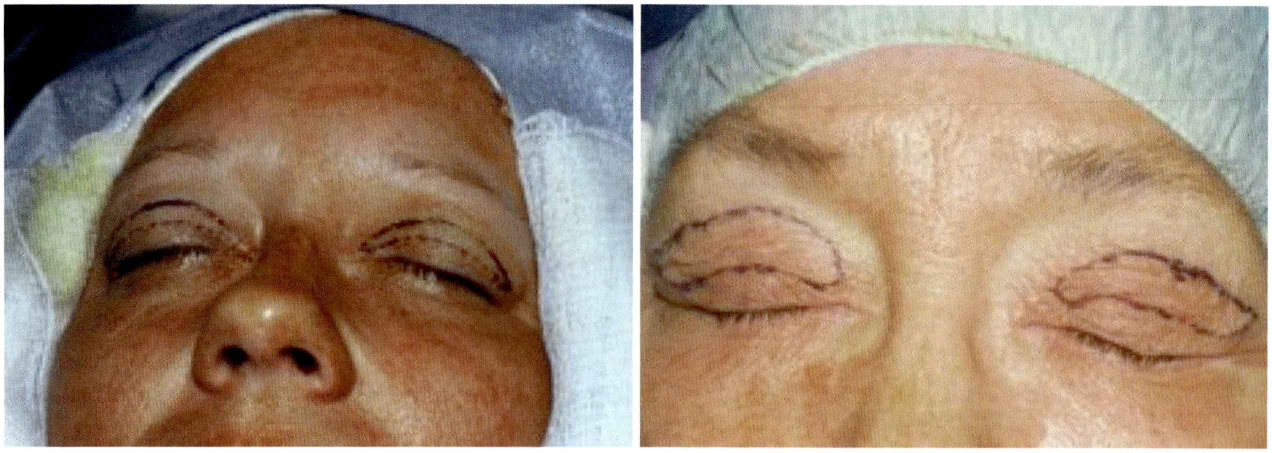

Fig. 17.4 Skin marking. The lower incision is marked using the natural lid crease. The superior incision is marked by following the orbital rim contour, taking care to leave enough superior skin to allow lid closure. Of note, the markings are of different style: The left photo, a younger patient with minimal skin excess, is marked with a tapered point on the medial and lateral ends. The right photo, an older patient with marked skin excess, shows a boat-shaped marking. Either is acceptable, with the boat shape allowing for more skin removal medially and laterally. A skin pinch is performed prior to incision to ensure no postoperative lagophthalmos is present

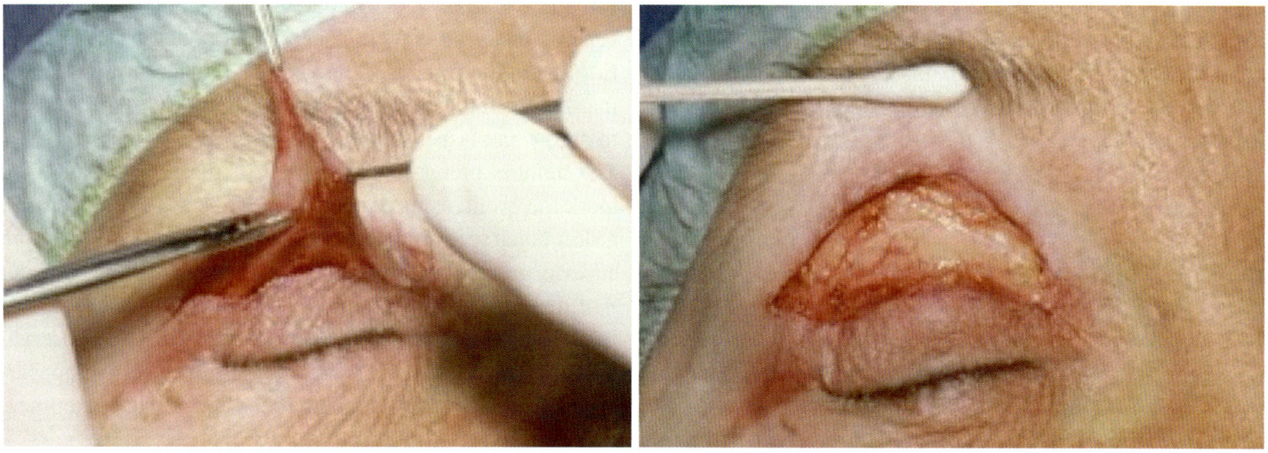

Fig. 17.5 Skin excision and musculocutaneous flap removal. The skin is incised with the scissors and the musculocutaneous flap removed in the suborbicularis plane. On the right, the intact orbital septum is visible with a small cuff of pretarsal orbicularis remaining

operating room, making the laser logistically more complex than traditional instrumentation.

After the initial incision is made, the musculocutaneous flap is removed—taking both the skin and orbicularis muscle. The scissors, laser, radio frequency devices, monopolar cautery, or handheld high-temperature cautery can be employed for this step. Care must be taken to avoid a deeper-than-intended dissection which may be associated with postoperative complications (Fig. 17.5).

Upon removal of the musculocutaneous flap, the orbital septum is visualized. If no orbital fat is to be sculpted or removed, the surgeon can proceed to closure at this time. If orbital fat is to be addressed, the septum should be opened horizontally above the fat pads, providing access to the preaponeurotic fat pads.

The upper eyelid consists of two major fat pads, the medial and central. The medial fat pad is often the primary target of facial rejuvenation, with a youthful face having a concavity near the nasal bridge. To restore this concavity, excess fat can be sculpted with monopolar or high-temperature cautery, the traditional "clamp-cut-cautery" method utilizing the scissors, or with the laser. Traction on the fat often produces a deep discomfort for patients, as intertwined nerves and blood vessels are present within the pad. Prior to excision, additional local anesthetic may be injected into the base of the fat to alleviate this discomfort. Our technique of fat removal requires a small opening being made in the fat pad capsule, applying light downward pressure on the globe, and using a forceps to gently elevate the fat out of its capsule where it can be excised. As discussed earlier, the amount of fat removal should be customized to the patient's ethnic and gender features to achieve the desired aesthetic goal (Figs. 17.6 and 17.7).

Lateral upper eyelid bulging can be caused by lacrimal gland prolapse. There is no lateral fat pad to be removed, but the preaponeurotic space can be filled by a prolapsed lacrimal gland. The lacrimal gland can be identified by its paler color, generally light pinkish-gray, lateral location, and its firmer texture. The bulging of the gland can be addressed by repositing it in the lacrimal gland fossa utilizing sutures plicating the gland to the underlying periosteum.

If fat pad bulging is a minimal concern, application of laser or monopolar cautery to the orbital septum or directly to the fat pads will tighten and shrink these structures and may be sufficient to achieve the desired effect. This can address a mild bulge in the lid without creating a hollow effect postoperatively.

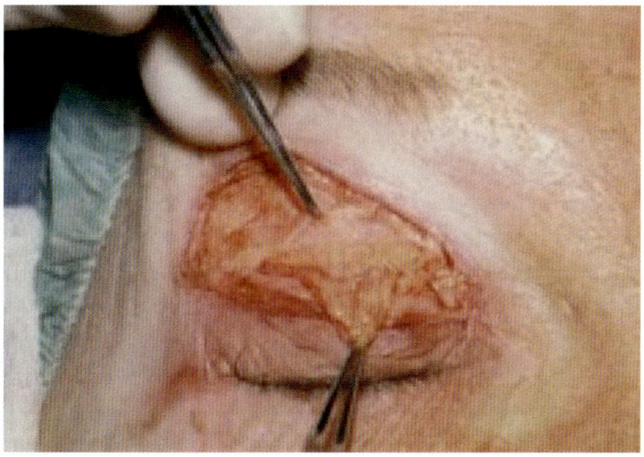

Fig. 17.6 Central fat pad exposed. The orbital septum has been incised (held by superior forceps), exposing the central fat pad. The levator is visible underneath the fat pad. Excision or sculpting of the fat pad can be accomplished at this time

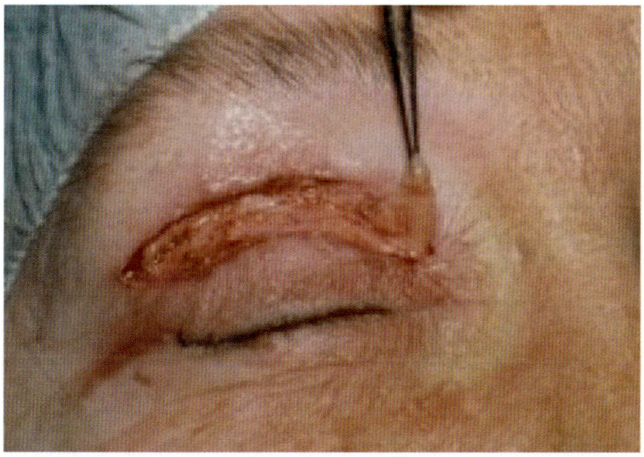

Fig. 17.7 Medial fat pad exposure. The medial fat pad is slightly whiter in color than the central fat pad. Exposure is accomplished by making a small "window" in the fat pad capsule and applying gentle pressure on the globe. The medial fat pad will prolapse through the window and can be excised or sculpted

Crease Fixation and Closure

Crease fixation is an option step in the closure of the blepharoplasty incision. The authors use crease fixation in cases that require firm definition of the eyelid crease. This is more commonly preferred among woman patients as a defined crease provides a youthful, feminine appearance. Crease fixation is also utilized in those patients with thinner lids and higher creases to establish the new crease at the desired height. Unless specifically requested, or to address crease asymmetry, we typically avoid crease fixation in most men as it may give a more feminine appearance to the eyelids (Fig. 17.8).

Crease fixation is performed by passing a needle through the pretarsal skin, capturing the edge of the levator aponeurosis, and through the superior incision edge in a single interrupted pass. The authors typically use a single 6–0 fast-absorbing plain gut, or similar absorbable, suture in the middle eyelid at the level of the medial limbus for crease fixation. Additional sutures can be placed laterally through the lid for more lateral definition of the crease. Another technique involves capturing the levator on each pass of a running suture to close the incision.

Incision closure is then performed using a running 6–0 absorbable or nonabsorbable suture. The authors prefer a 6–0 fast-absorbing plain gut suture. Care must be taken to avoid overtightening the suture as the skin edges need only touch for healing to occur. This "loose running" stitch provides excellent cosmesis without excess tension on the tissue and also provides an avenue for blood to escape the wound, preventing hematoma formation (Fig. 17.9).

Postoperative Management

Patients are asked to apply ice compresses for the first 48 h postoperatively, followed by warm compresses thereafter for the next 48 h. The application of ice and heat helps with resolution of edema and ecchymosis. Preliminary studies of arnica ointment are nondefinitive as to their effectivity in resolving postoperative blepharoplasty edema and ecchymosis. Postoperative infections of the eyelids are exceedingly rare, and the authors do not utilize systemic antibiotics, and only antibiotic ophthalmic ointment is placed on the incisions four times daily.

Postoperative pain is managed typically with acetaminophen, and only rarely are narcotics considered necessary. Patient complaints of excessive pain should be evaluated

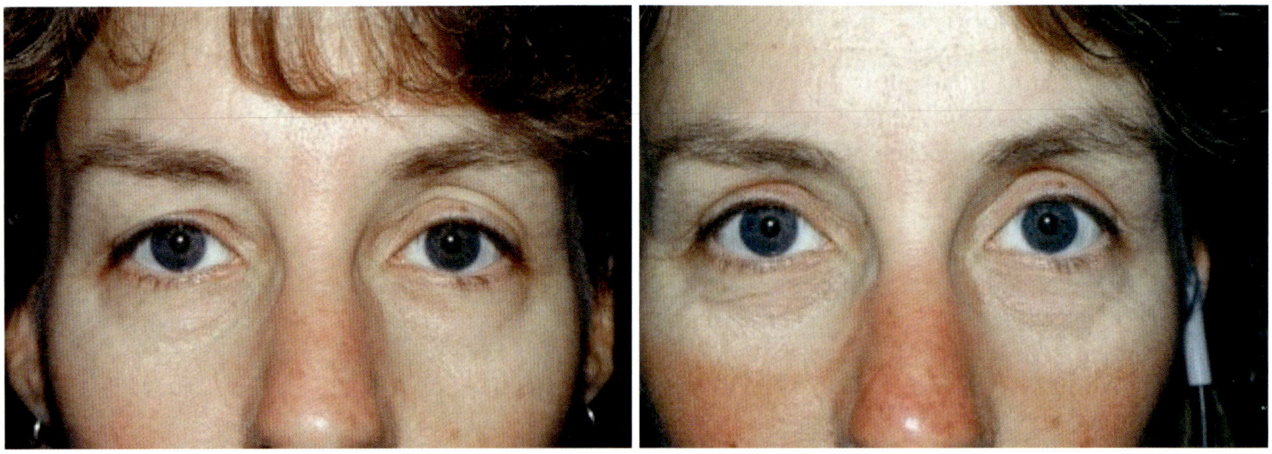

Fig. 17.8 Crease fixation used to adjust height of lid crease. This patient presented with an asymmetric lid crease, with the left upper eyelid having a higher lid crease than the right. The height of the lid crease created a "double-fold" appearance to the lid. The second photo (postoperative) shows correction by excision of the excess skin on each side and crease fixation sutures to provide a higher lid crease on the right and further definition of the crease on the left

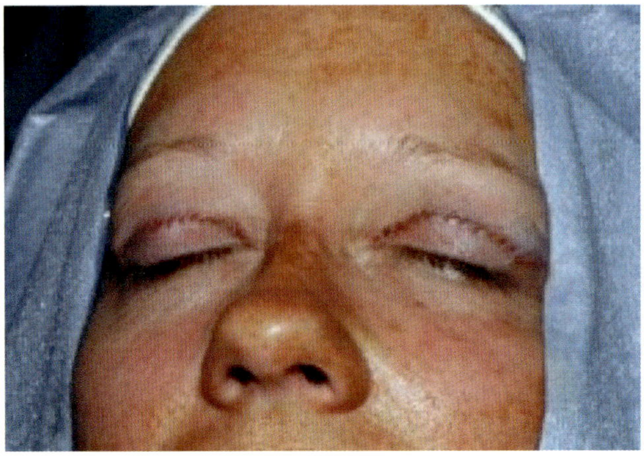

Fig. 17.9 Skin closure. A running 6–0 fast-absorbing suture is used to close the skin incision. This suture is placed in a "loose running" fashion as the skin edges need only to just come together to ensure wound closure with minimal scarring. A nonabsorbable suture can be used if preferred

thoroughly, with the concern for orbital hemorrhage at the forefront of concern for the surgeon. Hemorrhage should be ruled out immediately, with opening and evacuation of the wound performed should hemorrhage with ocular compromise be present. Further discussion of blepharoplasty complications and management can be found in Chap. 24.

The authors typically call patients on postoperative day 1 to ensure everything is progressing as expected. This reassures patients and provides them a chance to ask any questions they may have. A postoperative examination is performed approximately 1 week after surgery. If used, nonabsorbable sutures are removed at this time.

Subtle asymmetries and contour irregularities can be noted after edema and ecchymosis have resolved—typically 2 weeks after surgery. It is important for patients to understand that healing continues over the first 6 weeks and even up to 6 months after surgery and many subtle irregularities will resolve with time. Thus, any decision for further surgery would typically be postponed until after healing has had a chance to occur, unless a more marked problem, such as significant lagophthalmos, is noted.

Conclusion

Success in upper eyelid blepharoplasty is achievable with a thorough understanding of the anatomy of the eyelids and eyebrows and, specifically, the application of this anatomical knowledge to the patient's concerns and facial features. A comprehensive discussion including a discussion of the nature, risks, and limitations of surgery with the patient and formulation of an appropriate operative plan provides the highest chance of achieving the desired outcomes.

Suggested Readings

Chen WP. Asian blepharoplasty. J Ophthalmic Plast Reconstr Surg. 1987;3:135–40.
Dailey RA. Upper eyelid blepharoplasty. Focal Points: Clinical Modules for Ophthalmologists. 1995;13:8.
Dailey RA, Jones LT. Rejuvenation of the aging face. Focal Points: Clinical Modules for Ophthalmologists. 2003;21:11.
Fagien S. Advanced rejuvenative upper blepharoplasty. Enhancing aesthetics of the upper periorbita. Plast Reconstr Surg. 2002;110:278.
Flowers RS. Periorbital aesthetic surgery for men. Eyelids and related structures. Clin Plast Surg. 1991;18:689.
Flowers RS. Optimal procedure in secondary blepharoplasty. Clin Plast Surg. 1993;20:225.

Flowers RS, Flowers SS. Precision planning in blepharoplasty. The importance of preoperative mapping. Clin Plast Surg. 1993;20:303.

Goldbaum AM, Woog JJ. The CO2 laser in oculoplastic surgery. Surv Ophthalmol. 1997;42:255–67.

Jelks GW, Jelks EB. Preoperative evaluation of the blepharoplasty patient. Bypassing the pitfalls. Clin Plast Surg. 1993; 20:213.

Kerth JD, Toriumi DM. Management of the aging forehead. Arch Otolaryngol Head Neck Surg. 1990;116:1137–42.

Levine MR, et al. Complications of blepharoplasty. Ophthalmic Surg. 1975;6:53.

Lowry JC, Bartley GB. Complications of blepharoplasty. Surv Ophthalmol. 1994;38:327–50.

May JW Jr, Fearon J, Zingarelli P. Retro-orbicularis oculus fat (ROOF) resection in aesthetic blepharoplasry: a 6-year study in 63 patients. Plast Reconstr Surg. 1990;86:682.

McCord CD, Doxanas MT. Browplasty and browpexy: an adjunct to blepharoplasty. Plast Reconstr Surg. 1990;86:248–54.

Meyer DR, Linber JV, Wobig JL, McCormick SA. Anatomy of the orbital septum and associated eyelid connective tissues. Ophthalmol Plast Reconstr Surg. 1991;7:104–13.

Neuhaus RW. Complications of blepharoplasty. Focal Points: Clinical Modules for Ophthalmologists. 1990;8:3.

Parkes M, Fein W, Brennan HG. Pinch technique for repair of cosmetic eyelid deformities. Arch Ophthalmol. 1973;89:324.

Perman KI. Upper eyelid blepharoplasty. J Dermatol Surg Oncol. 1992;18:1096.

Lower Eyelid Blepharoplasty

18

Brett S. Kotlus

Introduction

Lower blepharoplasty is a procedure that encompasses a constellation of strategies and techniques that aim to improve the appearance of the lower eyelids. Depending on the perspectives of the surgeon and the patient, aesthetic improvement of the lower eyelids may have different directives. For example, one's goal may be to improve the effects of skin surface photoaging or the topographic contour as influenced by prominent underlying fat, or both may be targeted concerns. Ultimately, the specific approach chosen by the surgeon in discussion with a patient takes a multitude of factors into consideration and is largely driven by the results of a thorough oculofacial evaluation.

Lower Eyelid Aging

While some prospective lower blepharoplasty candidates are young individuals with unwanted lower eyelid fat prominences (Fig. 18.1), a significant proportion of individuals seeking this procedure are interested in lower eyelid rejuvenation after noticing senescent changes. These externally visible changes with age reflect the anatomic aging changes that occur within the orbit, the eyelids, and the midface.

The bony orbit tends to enlarge over time which may contribute to under-eye concavities and the visibility of lower eyelid fat [1]. At the same time, the orbital fat tends to expand with age [2], further accentuating the appearance of lower eye bags [3] which are visible at the anterior face of the lower orbital fat. The maxillary bone, suborbicularis oculi fat, and malar fat lose volume with age [4] and are associated with progression of tear trough depth and diminished lower eyelid structural support [5].

On the more superficial level, photoaging leads to thinning of the skin and the subcutaneous adipose layer [5] which exposes contours that are influenced by the underlying ligamentous attachments including the orbital retaining ligaments along the tear trough and lateral orbital rim and the zygomatic retaining ligaments along the transverse malar (palpebromalar) crease [6] (Fig. 18.2). These atrophic changes that occur at all tissue layers lead to the appearance of gravitationally influenced tissue descent [7], and current rejuvenation techniques aim to preserve or enhance volume in the aging patient to offer an anatomically based treatment strategy.

Evaluation

A comprehensive evaluation for lower blepharoplasty includes an examination of the eyelid structure and function along with a broader examination of facial balance, symmetry, and the relationships between the facial subunits. This physical examination influences the selection of specific techniques during surgical planning.

Skin evaluation using the Glogau Photoaging Classification [8] documents the degree of wrinkles, dyschromia, telangiectasias, and overall sun damage. The skin is also graded using the Fitzpatrick phototype scale [9] to rate their response to sun exposure and expected response to energy-based or chemical skin treatments.

Lower eyelid skin is examined to identify and grade the degree of redundancy (dermatochalasis) or anterior lamella insufficiency, rhytidosis, dyschromia and hyperpigmentation, lesions, visibility of dermal glands, and scars. It should be noted that photoaging can be present with or without lower eyelid skin redundancy, and the latter can often be identified or ruled out by asking the patient to gaze upward and open their mouth while observing the lower eyelid skin

B. S. Kotlus (✉)
Oculofacial Plastic Surgeon, Private Practice, New York, NY, USA
e-mail: drkotlus@drkotlus.com

J. J. Servat et al. (eds.), *Smith and Nesi's Ophthalmic Plastic and Reconstructive Surgery*,
https://doi.org/10.1007/978-3-030-41720-8_18

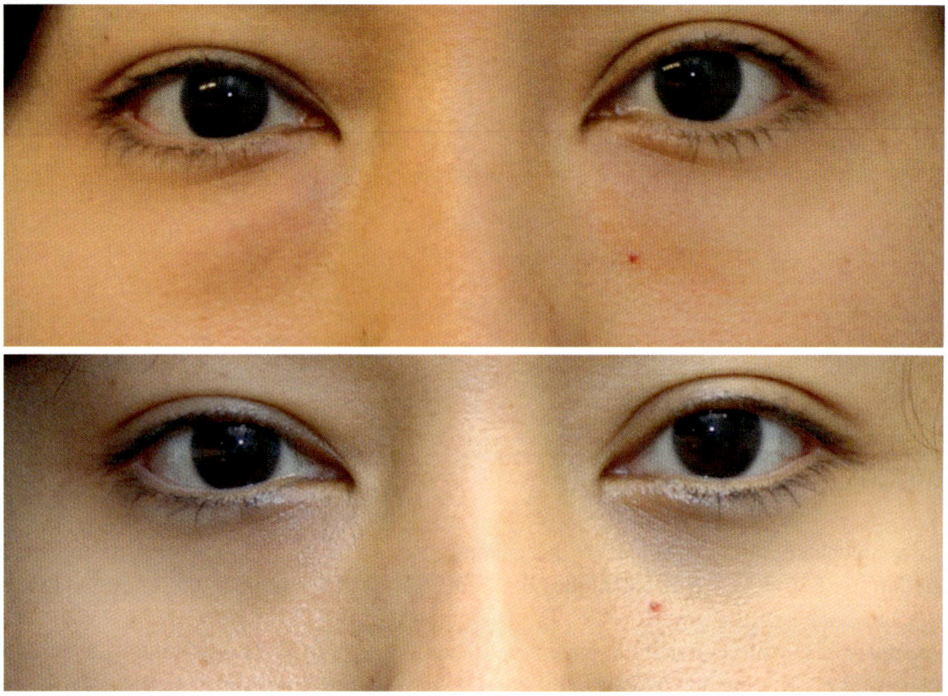

Fig. 18.1 Prominent lower eyelid fat in a young woman (above) and after transconjunctival blepharoplasty (below)

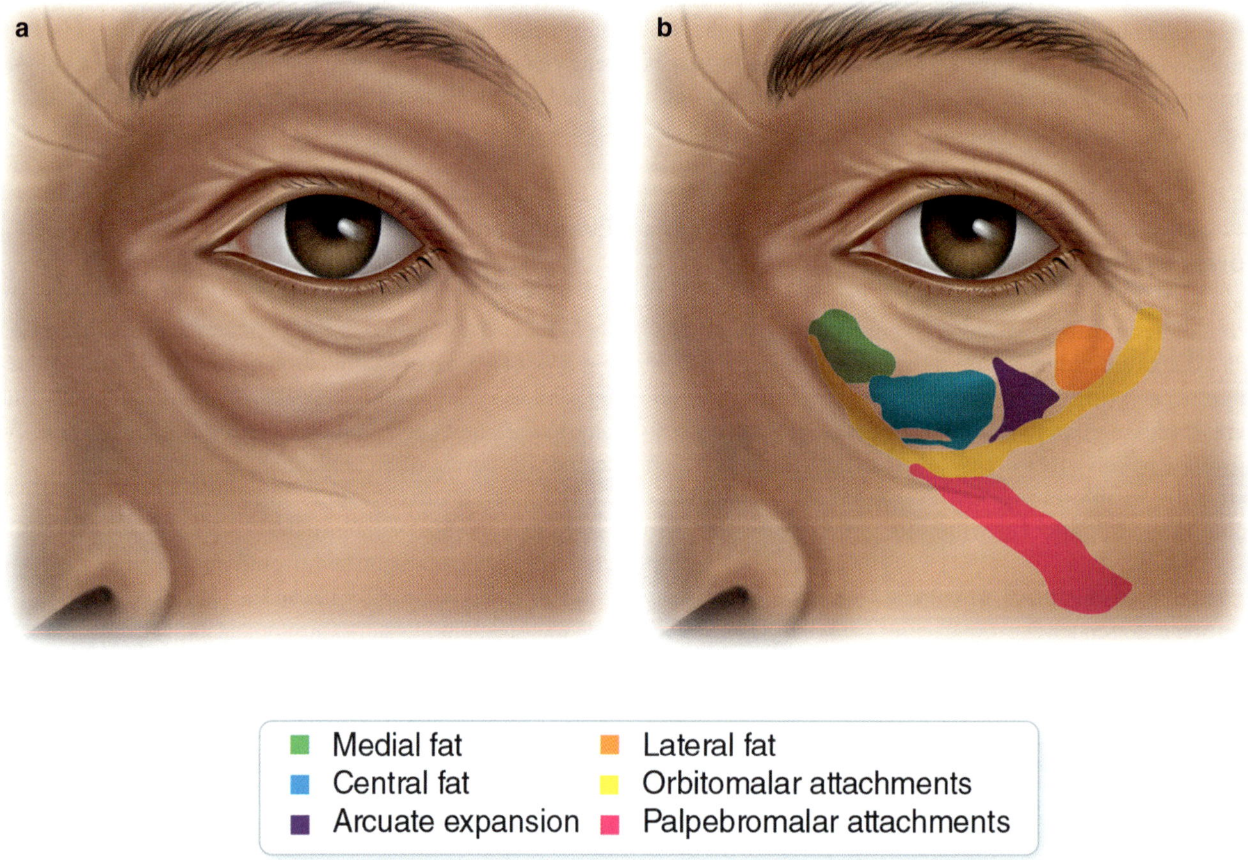

Fig. 18.2 (**a**) Periorbital aging signs with photoaging, protruding lower eyelid fat, infraorbital hollowing, and palpebromalar crease formation. (**b**) Green, medial fat; blue, central fat; purple, arcuate expansion; orange, lateral fat; yellow, orbitomalar attachments; magenta, palpebromalar attachments

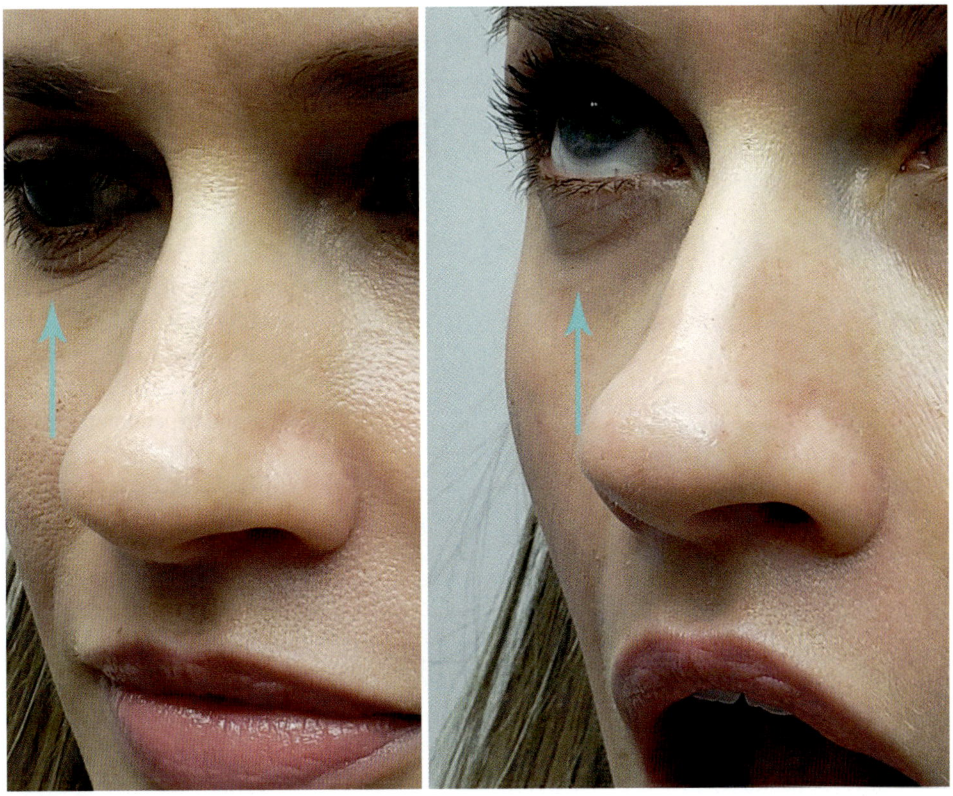

Fig. 18.3 Evaluation of lower eyelid redundancy in slight downgaze followed by upgaze with mouth open

appearance (Fig. 18.3). The presence of an infraciliary crease can be congenital or acquired and should be noted if a skin incision is planned so as to align the resultant scar with a preexisting landmark.

The eyelid position is evaluated to determine if ectropion or entropion exists and to determine if additional support may be required to prevent post-blepharoplasty downward traction. The lateral canthal angle is examined to identify medialization and shortening of the horizontal aperture which may be associated with lateral canthal rounding and possible lower eyelid laxity. Dehiscence of the lateral canthal attachments can also impact the upper eyelid position which should also be evaluated. The lateral canthal angle position and its relationship to the medial canthus can also influence the decision to modify the eyelid tilt with lateral canthoplasty during blepharoplasty.

The surface contour as influenced by the subsurface lower eyelid structures is evaluated including the presence of prominent lower eyelid fat pads. These common bulges that contribute to the appearance of "eye bags" are the anterior projection of the inferior orbital fat and frequently contribute to the shadows termed under-eye "dark circles." The lower eyelid fat is generally described as three contiguous pouches: medial, central, and lateral. These may appear as a single, elongated mound that sits above and spans the horizontal length of the inferior orbital rim, or they may present as discrete pouches of varying size and shape with the medial and central fat separated by the inferior oblique muscle and the central and lateral fat separated by the fascia known as the arcuate expansion. The appearance of the lower eyelid fat compartments can be accentuated by asking the patient to gaze upward or by gently applying posterior pressure (ballottement) to the globe with the eye closed.

A recess or concavity is typically seen inferior to the lower eyelid fat prominences. The depth of the nasojugal groove (or tear trough) and lateral infraorbital recess is evaluated as well as the degree of condensation of layers where the orbitomalar attachments reside. The overall malar and zygomatic volume status is assessed along with the presence and severity of a transverse malar groove and malar mounds or festoons as bound superiorly by the orbitomalar attachments and inferiorly by the zygomatico-cutaneous attachments.

The relationship between the eyelids, globe, orbital rim, and orbital volume with its contents is considered. A prominent globe may be associated with a wider vertical palpebral aperture, and if present along with a so-called negative vector or anterior globe position in relationship to the eyelid/orbital rim complex, there is a predisposition for downward displacement of the lower eyelid or retraction after blepharoplasty due to insufficient structural support [10]. Asymmetry of the internal dimensions of the orbital space and three-dimensional position will often be represented externally as an eye asymmetry with globe dystopia, asymmetry of infraorbital concavities, and asymmetry in the appearance or severity of "eye bags" and "dark circles" (Fig. 18.4).

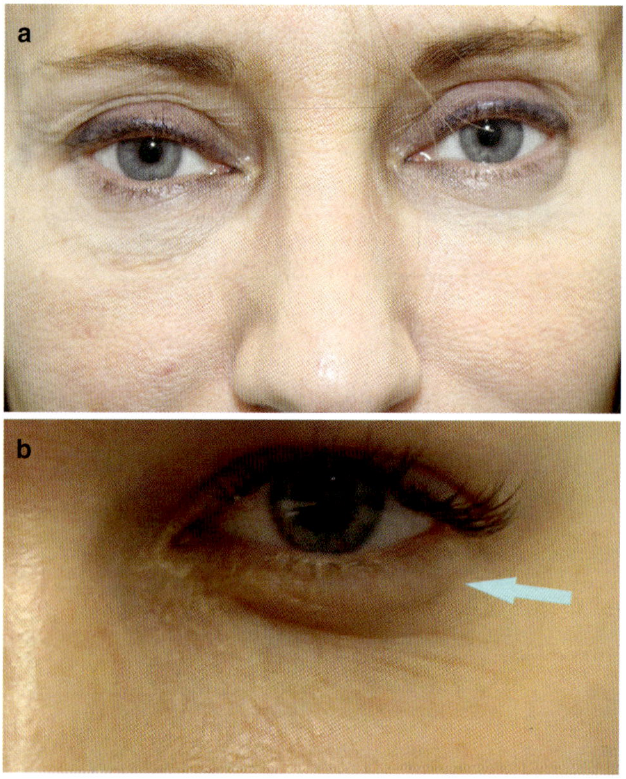

Fig. 18.4 (**a**) Orbital volume asymmetry (with vertical orbital dystopia) manifesting as asymmetric infraorbital hollows, (**b**) Lower eyelid orbicularis roll evident with muscle contraction

Dynamic eyelid movements are observed for signs of dysfunction, asymmetry, and aesthetic concerns related to facial expression. An infraciliary muscle roll may appear or become more pronounced with orbicularis muscle contraction (Fig. 18.4b), and some patients may desire a reduction of the muscle roll or, alternatively, a more pronounced roll (Aegyo Sal in South Korea) [11]. The patient is asked to smile, and as the cheek elevates and projects, the lower eyelids may exhibit apparent skin redundancy and folding which is also influenced by skin thickness, quality, and infraorbital/cheek volume status in all structural layers. It should be considered that injectable neuromodulators will alter the muscular contraction and possibly the upper and lower eyelid position [12]. Incomplete closure with either forced or relaxed blinking should be noted as should blink rate, quality, and asymmetry [13].

Documentation of the pre-procedural evaluation includes photography with standardized lighting and patient positioning. The patient is asked to maintain a straight gaze, unless the provider wishes to obtain additional upgaze angles that cause enhanced protrusion of the lower eyelid fat. The head should be positioned so that the auriculo-orbital plane (from the external auditory meatus to the inferior orbital rim) is parallel to the floor. Photographs are obtained in frontal view, 45-degree angle oblique views, and lateral views. Images taken separately with direct and indirect light (without a flash or a light bounced from the ceiling) can aid in representing the lower eyelid contours which may be "washed out" when using a direct flash alone. Three-dimensional imaging may offer a higher quality representation of the surface shape, but the quality is also dependent on the choice of lighting technique.

In the case of patients who are seeking a rejuvenative procedure, the use of a "retroscope" by means of previous photographs, preferably with the subject not smiling, can be a useful tool to determine how the patient has changed over time and to establish a starting point for the discussion about what the expectations are after a proposed procedure.

Techniques

Anesthesia

The lower eyelids are anesthetized with local anesthetic such as lidocaine using a combination of local infiltration and nerve blocks. Epinephrine is included to induce vasoconstriction, reduce bleeding, and prolong the anesthetic effect. A waiting period of at least 7 min after injection of anesthetic with epinephrine ensures a maximum vasoconstrictive effect [14]. The procedure can be performed with local anesthesia alone or paired with systemic analgesia, sedation, and/or general anesthesia.

Lower Eyelid Fat Modification

The lower eyelid fat can be accessed from an anterior approach (transcutaneous) or a posterior approach (transconjunctival) [15]. Many surgeons advocate the posterior approach which has been shown to reduce the risk of post-blepharoplasty retraction resulting from middle lamellar scarring [16], likely along the orbicularis oculus muscle, suborbicularis fascia, and septal continuum. The lateral lower eyelid fat which is often the most challenging to access due to the posterior curvature of the lateral eyelid and tight lateral canthal attachments can also be approached from a lateral upper eyelid incision. If there is a forwardly located globe or relative orbital congestion and a transconjunctival approach does not afford adequate exposure, a lateral canthotomy and inferior cantholysis (swinging eyelid approach) allow for wider access.

In some cases, simple removal of prominent lower eyelid fat is performed. A Desmarres retractor with its anatomic curvature affords visualization of the posterior aspect of the eyelid and the lower eyelid fornix. An incision is created between the lower edge of the tarsus and the fornix through the conjunctiva and lower eyelid retractors (Fig. 18.5a). Depending

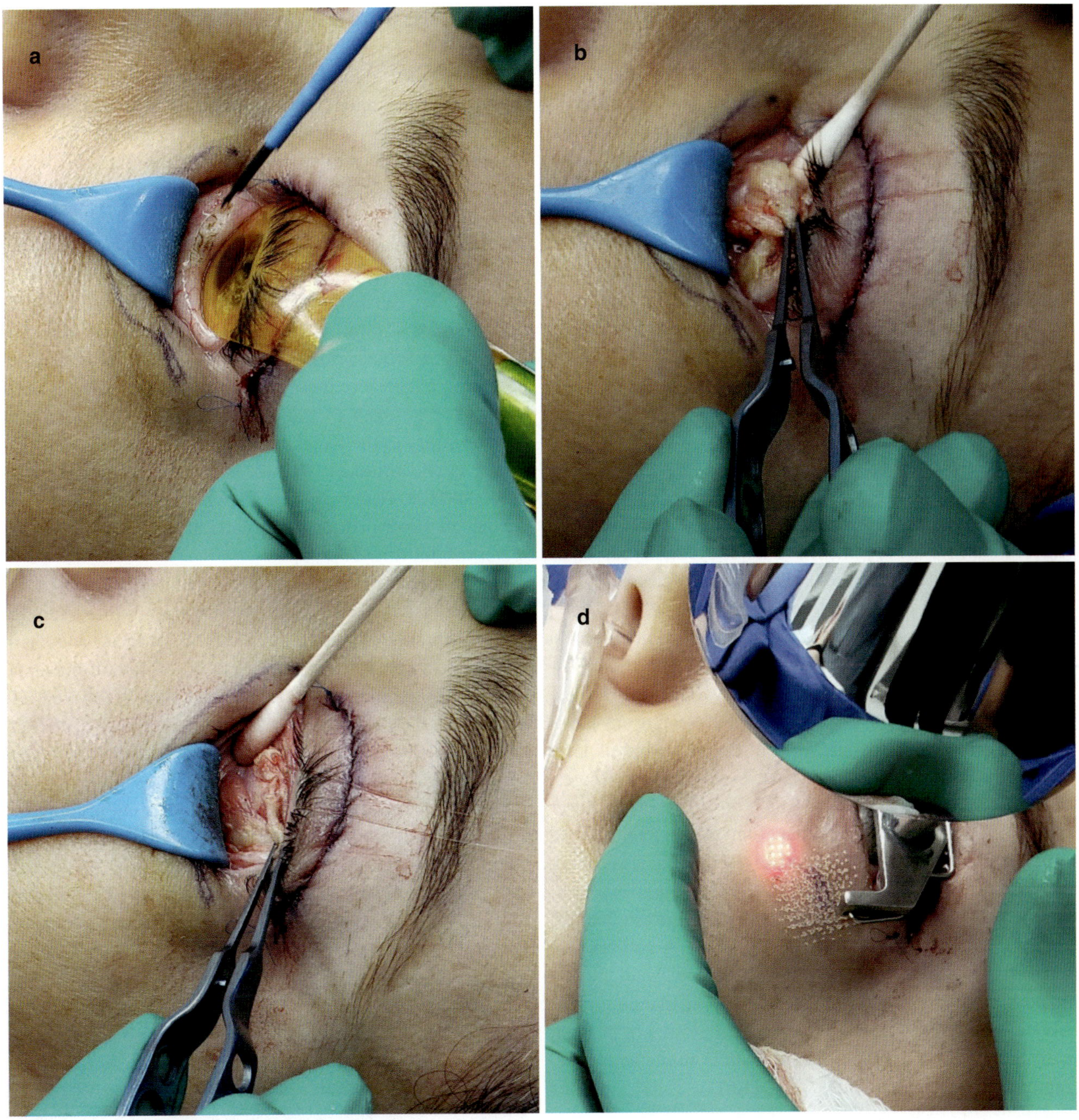

Fig. 18.5 (**a–d**) Clockwise. (**a**) Transconjunctival incision with coated Desmarres retractor and Jaeger plate. (**b**) Medial fat pedicle in forceps, traction sutures placed in lower eyelid retractors. (**c**) Inferior oblique muscle visible lateral to cotton-tipped applicator. (**d**) Fractional erbium lower eyelid skin resurfacing with nonreflective, steel corneal protector in place

on the incision location, dissection may proceed in the preseptal plane or enter directly into the orbital fat compartment [17]. Once orbital fat is encountered, it is dissected from the connective tissue attachments and, if necessary, the inferior oblique muscle (Fig. 18.5b, c). Each of the three lower eyelid fat subdivisions can be debulked so the most anterior extent of the fat prominence projects no further than the anterior face of the lower orbital rim. Hemostasis is meticulously maintained using monopolar or bipolar cautery to reduce the risk of post-septal hemorrhage and vision-threatening compartment syndrome. Disruption of the ligamentous attachments along the orbital rim has not been shown to improve the aesthetic outcome [18]. The conjunctival incision may be left to heal by opposition, or fine absorbable sutures may be loosely placed to align the conjunctival edges without creating a watertight seal so as to allow for the efflux of anesthetic and blood.

The transconjunctival approach can also be used to modify the infraorbital hollows with lower eyelid fat repositioning via a redraping technique [19] or free fat placement [20]. After isolating the relevant lower eyelid fat compartments but before excising fat, a subperiosteal or suborbicularis muscle pocket is created along the areas of externally visible concavities, typically underlying the middle and central fat pads and corresponding with the nasojugal depression. For repositioning, a pedicle is created and temporarily sutured transcutaneously to maintain its position during early healing. Alternatively, after excising redundant fat, 1–2 mm in diameter parcels of fat can be placed in the infraorbital pockets as free grafts which can act as a spacer to prevent reattachment.

Skin Excision

If redundant skin is present or if it is deemed that skin redraping will improve the appearance of lower eyelid rhytidosis, an infraciliary incision is created along an existing crease or wrinkle, typically 1–2 mm inferior to the eyelash line. The lateral extent of the incision often extends lateral to the outer canthal angle within a natural expression line; the length of the incision depends on the degree of skin removal planned with the aim of minimizing the overall length while avoiding any pleating. Dissection proceeds inferiorly in the subcutaneous level beyond the lower limit of planned skin excision. In some cases, undermining extends inferiorly to the boundary of the lower orbital rim as an extended skin flap. Skin is then redraped in a superotemporal direction. Alternatively, if the goal is to simply excise a strip of skin, a "pinch" technique can be used by crushing the skin with a fine hemostat inferior the eyelash line and excising the skin roll with Westcott scissors. A conservative removal of skin is often warranted to avoid downward traction on the eyelid margin. A canthal or lateral eyelid margin support technique may be performed prior to final closure or in some cases prior to skin excision. The incision is closed with interrupted and running fine sutures (Fig. 18.6).

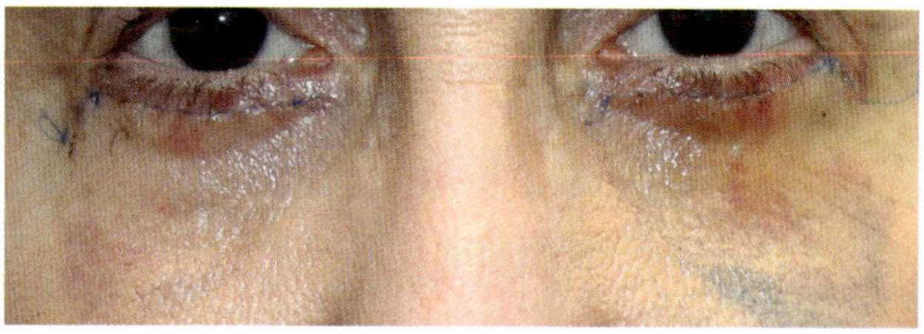

Fig. 18.6 Seven days after skin pinch lower blepharoplasty with monofilament sutures in place, the incision is 2 mm inferior to the eyelash line

Orbicularis Suspension

The orbicularis oculi muscle is continuous with the superficial muscular aponeurotic system and can act as a support and "lifting" structure for the lower eyelid. There are several approaches to suspension of the orbicularis which in turn can aid in effacing a pronounced nasojugal recess or fold.

An infraciliary incision provides anterior access to the orbicularis muscle. From this incision, a composite skin/muscle flap can be initiated or a skin-only flap may be initiated for several millimeters, and dissection is transitioned to a suborbicularis flap at the preseptal portion of the muscle therefore preserving the pre-tarsal muscle function. Care is taken to avoid sharp dissection to minimize risk of injury to the facial nerve branches that innervate the lower eyelid orbicularis oculi, entering the muscle on its undersurface. Excess muscle may be trimmed. The flap is advanced superiorly or superolaterally and sutured to the outer orbital rim [21].

The orbicularis oculi may be suspended without extensive submuscular dissection by creating a limited superolateral orbicularis muscle flap (Fig. 18.7). Blunt and sharp dissection is used to initiate a flap at the lateral preseptal or orbital orbicularis muscle, and this flap is elevated and sutured to the periosteum at the external aspect of the lateral orbital rim.

The inferior portion of the orbicularis muscle may also be suspended utilizing the muscle condensation along the inferolateral orbital rim often termed the orbitomalar ligament or orbicularis retaining ligament [22]. The dissection proceeds after creating a subciliary incision. The condensation is identified in the suborbicularis plane along the

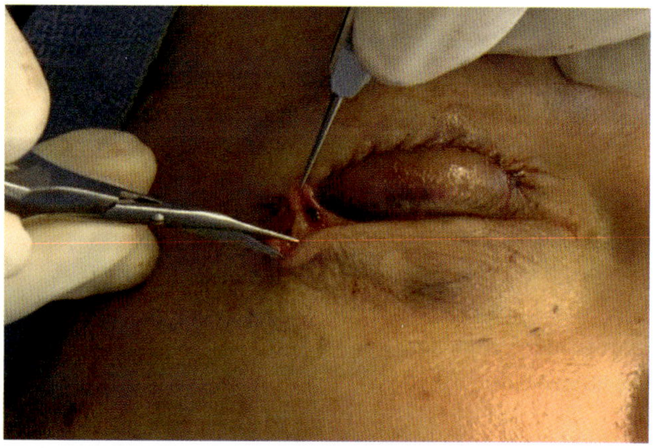

Fig. 18.7 Orbicularis muscle flap initiated from an infraciliary incision. The flap is anchored to the periosteum at the external aspect of the lateral orbital rim to elevate and support the lower eyelid

inferolateral orbital rim or in the subperiosteal plane in the same location. The ligamentous attachment is released with sharp dissection and anchored superiorly to the periosteum on the external face of the lateral orbital rim. If dissection is in the subperiosteal space, a lower periosteal relaxing incision is created to allow for upward shift of the periosteal/muscular flap.

Orbicularis muscle imbrication is a technique that employs interrupted absorbable sutures to infold a lax orbicularis oculus without incising or disrupting the muscle fibers [23].

Canthoplasty/Canthopexy

A lower eyelid tightening procedure is performed as part of an aesthetic lower blepharoplasty if warranted due to preexisting lower eyelid laxity, eyelid malposition, or a predisposing factor that could cause the eyelid to become lax or inferiorly displaced as a result of blepharoplasty [24]. The pre-procedure evaluation informs this decision based on the lower eyelid distraction and snap-back tests.

A canthoplasty is the more robust option as it entirely dislocates and reconstructs the lateral lower eyelid attachments. A method of canthoplasty is the lateral tarsal strip procedure which offers an effective means of lower eyelid and lateral canthal tightening. Canthopexy may be less powerful but also less invasive and can be done in an open or semi-closed manner using a suture plication or suspension [25] to tighten the lateral lower eyelid at the lateral canthal tendinous condensation or the lateral tarsus from an incision in the lateral lower eyelid, lateral canthus (sparing the canthal angle) , or the lateral upper eyelid.

Eyelid Skin Resurfacing

The surface skin quality, rhytidosis, dyspigmentation, and general photoaging can be improved during blepharoplasty with skin resurfacing using laser/energy or chemical agents. The most commonly used ablative laser devices are carbon dioxide [26] or erbium:YAG which targets water molecules in the skin to produce a photothermal effect (Fig. 18.5d). Fractional laser devices create noncontiguous zones of injury which leads to a shorter recovery compared to full-field ablation. Chemical resurfacing agents including trichloroacetic acid and phenol [27] which are available at varying strengths (which reach varying skin depths) cause coagulation and protein denaturation in the outer skin layers [28]. Whether energy or chemical is used, a skin injury induces a healing response with the desired effect of smoother, more even, and in some cases tighter skin after a recovery period.

If resurfacing is performed, the pre-procedural evaluation determines if the patient is an appropriate candidate for the selected modality based on a multitude of factors including skin type. Laser settings or acid strength is tailored to the patient's characteristics, the desired effect, and the patient's tolerance for downtime.

Fat Grafting

Autogenous fat cells can be used to enhance infraorbital volume as an alternative to lower eyelid fat repositioning techniques [29–31]. Fat is harvested from a suitable donor site which may include the abdomen, flanks, thighs, or medial arms. Tumescent anesthesia including diluted lidocaine and epinephrine [32] is infiltrated to the subcutaneous compartment at the donor site. After a waiting period to allow for the anesthetic and vasoconstrictive effects, a blunt-tipped suction cannula is used to harvest fat under low suction pressures. The fat is separated from the infranatant consisting of anesthetic fluid and red blood cells and the supranatant consisting of oil by gravity, centrifugation, manual drainage on sterile nonwoven gauze, or with a commercial filtering system [33] (Fig. 18.8). Fat is then deposited in small aliquots (less than 0.01 mL per droplet or channel) with a blunt-

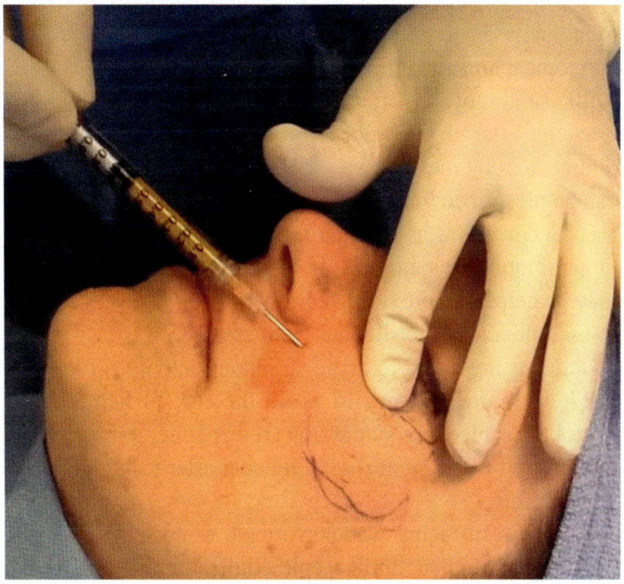

Fig. 18.8 Autologous fat grafting performed with a blunt-tipped, disposable cannula to enhance the infraorbital and malar volume after transconjunctival fat removal. The nondominant hand touches the edge of the orbital rim to palpate the location of the cannula tip

tipped injection cannula attached to a 1 mL syringe in a plane deep to the orbicularis oculi. Fat may be added along the tear trough, lateral infraorbital hollows, and blended into an atrophic malar fat compartment. The survival rate of injected fat is variable and has been reported from 30% to 70% of the original injected volume due to reabsorption or non-survival with subsequent cell replacement [34, 35]. It has been suggested yet not entirely accepted that platelet-rich plasma [36] and mesenchymal adipose cells known as stromal vascular fraction (also known as SVT or nanofat) [37, 38] can each be added to grafted fat to enhance the adipocyte survival rate.

Injectable Fillers

If infraorbital volume enhancement is indicated, injectable fillers may be used as an adjunct or alternative to lower eyelid fat redraping or fat grafting. Injectable, stabilized, cross-linked hyaluronic acid gel fillers are reversible implants that can be introduced in the subdermal or suborbicularis plane in the infraorbital hollows and tear trough as an off-label application. These products degrade over time and require maintenance treatments for continual volume augmentation.

Aftercare and Recovery

Edema and ecchymosis are typical in the postsurgical period and are often marked in the first 1–2 weeks. Ice or cold compression has not been shown to reduce edema but is commonly advised and may reduce postoperative pain [39]. Oral and topical homeopathics such as Arnica montana have been studied and shown to offer no benefit in reducing ecchymosis or edema after blepharoplasty [40, 41]. Topical antibiotics as ointment along incision lines or eye drops instilled in the eye can be prescribed with or without a steroid additive. There is no true consensus as whether topical and/or oral prophylactic antibiotics are beneficial in all cases [42]. Artificial tears may be helpful in providing comfort during recovery when a transconjunctival incision has been created.

Patients are asked to avoid strenuous activity for the first 7–14 days after surgery to avoid the risk of hemorrhage. Retrobulbar bleeding symptoms are explained to the patient in the case of this event should it occur after leaving the surgical facility.

If skin resurfacing was performed, a moist or occlusive dressing is applied until reepithelialization. Dilute acetic acid soaks may aid in recovery.

After the initial recovery phase, it can take several months for swelling to fully resolve and for external incisions to mature (Fig. 18.9). It is recommended to avoid sun exposure [43]. Hypertrophic scars may be injected with corticosteroids and/or 5-fluorouracil [44].

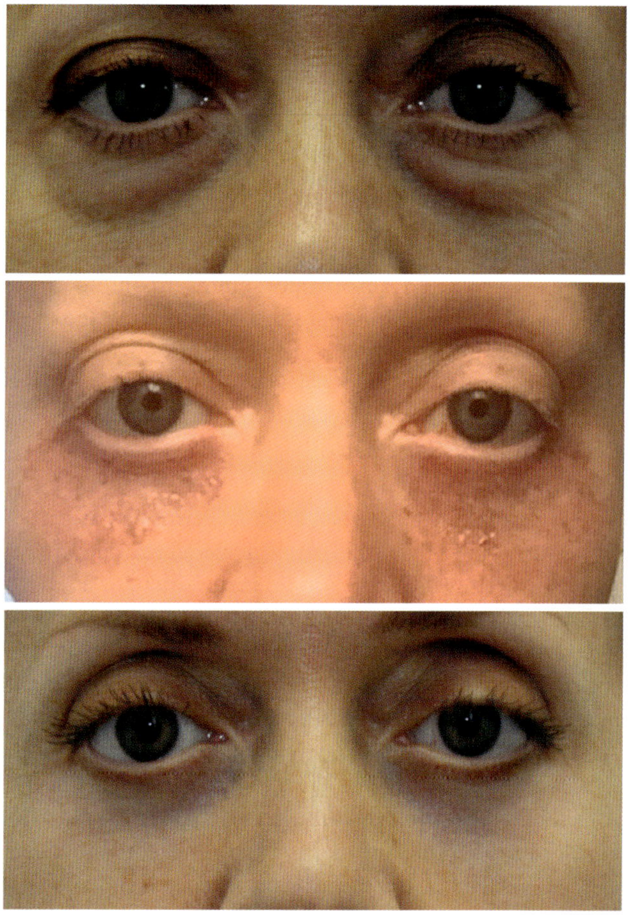

Fig. 18.9 Before lower blepharoplasty (top), 5 days after lower blepharoplasty with fractional CO_2 laser resurfacing and infraorbital fat grafting (middle), and 4 months after blepharoplasty (bottom)

References

1. Kahn DM, Shaw RB Jr. Aging of the bony orbit: a three-dimensional computed tomographic study. Aesthet Surg J. 2008;28(3):258–64.
2. Darcy SJ, Miller TA, Goldberg RA, Villablanca JP, Demer JL, Rudkin GH. Magnetic resonance imaging characterization of orbital changes with age and associated contributions to lower eyelid prominence. Plast Reconstr Surg. 2008;122(3):921–9; discussion 930–1
3. Kim J, Park SW, Choi J, Jeong W, Lee S. Ageing of the bony orbit is a major cause of age-related intraorbital fat herniation. J Plast Reconstr Aesthet Surg. 2018;71(5):658–64.
4. Kahn DM, Shaw RB. Overview of current thoughts on facial volume and aging. Facial Plast Surg. 2010;26(5):350–5.
5. Glaser A, Lambros V, Kolodziejczyk J, Magyar A, Dorries K, Gallagher CJ. Relationship between midface volume deficits and the appearance of tear troughs and nasolabial folds. Dermatol Surg. 2018;44(12):1547–54.
6. Han A, Chien AL, Kang S. Photoaging. Dermatol Clin. 2014;32(3):291–9.
7. Yang C, Zhang P, Xing X. Tear trough and palpebromalar groove in young versus elderly adults: a sectional anatomy study. Plast Reconstr Surg. 2013;132(4):796–808.

8. Mally P, Czyz CN, Wulc AE. The role of gravity in periorbital and midfacial aging. Aesthet Surg J. 2014;34(6):809–22.
9. Glogau RG. Physiologic and structural changes associated with aging skin. Dermatol Clin. 1997;15(4):555–9.
10. Fitzpatrick RE. Laser resurfacing. Adv Dermatol. 1997;13:463–501.
11. Hirmand H, Codner MA, McCord CD, Hester TR Jr, Nahai F. Prominent eye: operative management in lower lid and midfacial rejuvenation and the morphologic classification system. Plast Reconstr Surg. 2002;110(2):620–8; discussion 629–34
12. Jeon YR, Rah DK, Lew DH, Roh TS, Kim YS, Choi HL. Pretarsal augmented lower blepharoplasty. Plast Reconstr Surg. 2016;138(1):74–82.
13. Fagien S. Temporary management of upper lid ptosis, lid malposition, and eyelid fissure asymmetry with botulinum toxin type A. Plast Reconstr Surg. 2004;114(7):1892–902.
14. Hult J, Sheikh R, Nguyen CD, Tenland K, Dahlstrand U, Malmsjö M. A waiting time of 7 min is sufficient to reduce bleeding in oculoplastic surgery following the administration of epinephrine together with local anaesthesia. Acta Ophthalmol. 2018;96(5):499–502.
15. Weinberg DA, Baylis HI. Transconjunctival lower eyelid blepharoplasty. Dermatol Surg. 1995;21(5):407–10.
16. Mullins JB, Holds JB, Branham GH, Thomas JR. Complications of the transconjunctival approach. A review of 400 cases. Arch Otolaryngol Head Neck Surg. 1997;123(4):385–8.
17. Undavia S, Briceño CA, Massry GG. Quantified incision placement for postseptal approach transconjunctival blepharoplasty. Ophthalmic Plast Reconstr Surg. 2016;32(3):191–4.
18. Chan NJ, Nazemzadeh M, Hartstein ME, Holds JB, Massry GG, Wulc AE. Orbicularis retaining ligament release in lower blepharoplasty: assessing efficacy and complications. Ophthalmic Plast Reconstr Surg. 2018;34(2):155–61.
19. Goldberg RA, Edelstein C, Balch K, Shorr N. Fat repositioning in lower eyelid blepharoplasty. Semin Ophthalmol. 1998;13(3):103–6.
20. Miranda SG, Codner MA. Micro free orbital fat grafts to the tear trough deformity during lower blepharoplasty. Plast Reconstr Surg. 2017;139(6):1335–43.
21. Mladick RA. The muscle-suspension lower blepharoplasty. Plast Reconstr Surg. 1979;64(2):171–5.
22. Korn BS, Kikkawa DO, Cohen SR. Transcutaneous lower eyelid blepharoplasty with orbitomalar suspension: retrospective review of 212 consecutive cases. Plast Reconstr Surg. 2010;125(1):315–23.
23. Nakra T. Biplanar contour-oriented approach to lower eyelid and midface rejuvenation. JAMA Facial Plast Surg. 2015;17(5):374–81.
24. Goldberg RA. Review of prophylactic lateral canthopexy in lower blepharoplasties. Arch Facial Plast Surg. 2003;5(3):272–5.
25. Gladstone HB, Moy RL. Suspension suture canthopexy: a minimally invasive procedure for correcting mild to moderate ectropion. J Cosmet Dermatol. 2009;8(4):289–94.
26. Kotlus BS. Dual-depth fractional carbon dioxide laser resurfacing for periocular rhytidosis. Dermatol Surg. 2010;36(5):623–8.
27. Gatti JE. Eyelid phenol peel: an important adjunct to blepharoplasty. Ann Plast Surg. 2008;60(1):14–8; discussion 19–20
28. Manaloto RM, Alster TS. Periorbital rejuvenation: a review of dermatologic treatments. Dermatol Surg. 1999;25(1):1–9.
29. Kranendonk S, Obagi S. Autologous fat transfer for periorbital rejuvenation: indications, technique, and complications. Dermatol Surg. 2007;33(5):572–8.
30. Massry GG, Azizzadeh B. Periorbital fat grafting. Facial Plast Surg. 2013;29(1):46–57.
31. Tonnard PL, Verpaele AM, Zeltzer AA. Augmentation blepharoplasty: a review of 500 consecutive patients. Aesthet Surg J. 2013;33(3):341–52.
32. Klein JA. Anesthetic formulation of tumescent solutions. Dermatol Clin. 1999;17(4):751–9.
33. Cleveland EC, Albano NJ, Hazen A. Roll, spin, wash, or filter? Processing of lipoaspirate for autologous fat grafting: an updated, evidence-based review of the literature. Plast Reconstr Surg. 2015;136(4):706–13.
34. Harrison BL, Malafa M, Davis K, Rohrich RJ. The discordant histology of grafted fat: a systematic review of the literature. Plast Reconstr Surg. 2015;135(3):542e–55e.
35. Coleman SR, Katzel EB. Fat grafting for facial filling and regeneration. Clin Plast Surg. 2015;42(3):289–300.
36. Luck J, Smith OJ, Mosahebi A. A systematic review of autologous platelet-rich plasma and fat graft preparation methods. Plast Reconstr Surg Glob Open. 2017;5(12):e1596.
37. James IB, Coleman SR, Rubin JP. Fat, stem cells, and platelet-rich plasma. Clin Plast Surg. 2016;43(3):473–88.
38. Laloze J, Varin A, Gilhodes J, et al. Cell-assisted lipotransfer: friend or foe in fat grafting? Systematic review and meta-analysis. J Tissue Eng Regen Med. 2018;12(2):e1237–50.
39. Pool SM, van Exsel DC, Melenhorst WB, Cromheecke M, van der Lei B. The effect of eyelid cooling on pain, edema, erythema, and hematoma after upper blepharoplasty: a randomized, controlled, observer-blinded evaluation study. Plast Reconstr Surg. 2015;135(2):277e–81e.
40. Kotlus BS, Heringer DM, Dryden RM. Evaluation of homeopathic Arnica montana for ecchymosis after upper blepharoplasty: a placebo-controlled, randomized, double-blind study. Ophthalmic Plast Reconstr Surg. 2010;26(6):395–7.
41. Kahana A, Kotlus B, Black E. Re: Assessing the effectiveness of Arnica montana and Rhododendron tomentosum (Ledum palustre) in the reduction of ecchymosis and edema after oculofacial surgery: preliminary results. Ophthalmic Plast Reconstr Surg. 2017;33(1):74.
42. Ferneini EM, Halepas S. Aronin SI antibiotic prophylaxis in blepharoplasty: review of the current literature. J Oral Maxillofac Surg. 2017;75(7):1477–81.
43. Meaume S, Le Pillouer-Prost A, Richert B, Roseeuw D, Vadoud J. Management of scars: updated practical guidelines and use of silicones. Eur J Dermatol. 2014;24(4):435–43.
44. Ren Y, Zhou X, Wei Z, Lin W, Fan B, Feng S. Efficacy and safety of triamcinolone acetonide alone and in combination with 5-fluorouracil for treating hypertrophic scars and keloids: a systematic review and meta-analysis. Int Wound J. 2017;14(3):480–7.

Asian Blepharoplasty: Anatomy and Surgical Techniques

19

Steven Chen

There is a keen interest in aesthetic eyelid surgery within the Asian population. In the past several decades, with the increasing number of affluent Asians, especially from China, the demand for aesthetic surgery has grown steadily in the Eastern Hemisphere [32]. Upper eyelid blepharoplasty is the most commonly performed aesthetic procedure among affluent Asians [1, 2, 31]. The vast majority of patients desire the formation of an upper lid crease, or a "double eyelid." This procedure has been given various names such as "double eyelid procedure," "oriental blepharoplasty," "lid crease procedure," and "Asian blepharoplasty." The term "Asian blepharoplasty" is utilized because this includes the various ethnic groups inhabiting the Eastern Hemisphere.

The terms "single" and "double" eyelid are used frequently by both the general public and the medical profession. A single eyelid lacks a crease, which is accompanied by a fullness of the pretarsal tissues. In contrast, a double eyelid possesses a crease, which is created by a folding of the eyelid skin (Fig. 19.1). Approximately 50% of Asians have an upper lid crease, which can be complete, partial, or intermittent. Many patients requesting blepharoplasty desire the formation of a crease, or a double eyelid. A common misconception is that the endpoint of Asian blepharoplasty is the creation of a more "Westernized" appearance [4, 6]. To the contrary, the majority of these patients do not desire a more Westernized appearance but rather an enhancement of their Asian features; they desire to have an eyelid crease like other Asians [3]. In the Asian patient, the anatomy of the upper eyelid, aesthetic goals, and surgical techniques are vastly different from that of Caucasian patients. The surgeon must be cognizant of these differences in order to be proficient in Asian blepharoplasty.

S. Chen (✉)
Oculoplastic Consultants of Arizona, Glendale, AZ, USA

Anatomy

Doxonas and Anderson demonstrated important anatomic differences in the upper eyelids of Caucasian and Asian patients, which arise from the relationship of the orbital septum to the levator aponeurosis. Other authors have further clarified these anatomic differences through cadaver dissection and magnetic resonance imaging [8–12]. The levator palpebrae superioris originates from the orbital apex and courses anteriorly in the superior orbit. As it passes through the superior transverse ligament (Whitnall's ligament), the transition from levator muscle to levator aponeurosis occurs. The levator aponeurosis then fuses with the lower anterior surface of the tarsal plate, fusing to a distinct pretarsal fascial layer [10, 11]. These distal aponeurotic fibers also interdigitate with the pretarsal orbicularis muscle to produce an eyelid crease. The largest concentration of these interdigitations is along the superior tarsal border. The extent to which the levator aponeurosis interdigitates with the pretarsal orbicularis determines whether the crease will be complete, partial, or intermittent. Among Asians, approximately 50% lack these interdigitations that are responsible for the crease. In Caucasians, the orbital septum fuses to the levator aponeurosis above the superior tarsal border. The intact septum prevents the anterior prolapse of orbital fat. In Asians, however, the orbital septum fuses with the levator aponeurosis well below the superior tarsal border (Fig. 19.2). The primary insertion of the levator aponeurosis also tends to be closer to the lid margin in Asians. This lower insertion results in two important differences from the Caucasian eyelid. First, the preaponeurotic fat pad extends more anteriorly and inferiorly, giving the upper eyelid a "fuller" appearance and making the crease, if present, less discernible. Second, the inferior extension of the orbital septum may prevent the terminal fibers of the levator aponeurosis from forming interdigitations with the pretarsal orbicularis muscle. As a result, the upper eyelid crease in Asians may

J. J. Servat et al. (eds.), *Smith and Nesi's Ophthalmic Plastic and Reconstructive Surgery*,
https://doi.org/10.1007/978-3-030-41720-8_19

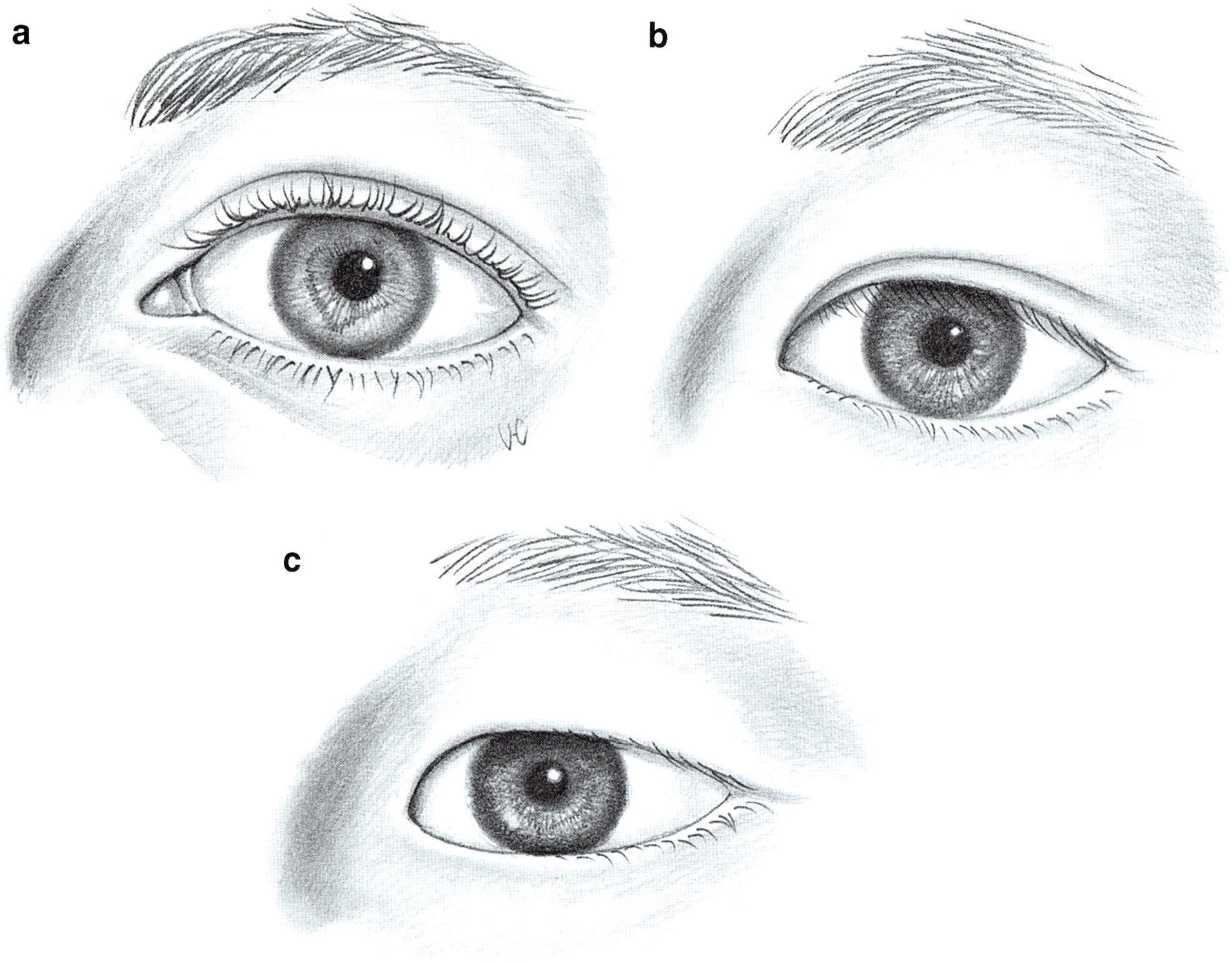

Fig. 19.1 (**a**) Caucasian eyelid crease. (**b**) Asian eyelid crease. (**c**) Asian eyelid, no crease

be absent or poorly developed. The increased "fullness" of the Asian eyelid is also attributable to the presence of a pretarsal fat pad.

In the lower eyelid, the anatomic differences are more subtle, owing to the more rudimentary development of the lower eyelid structure in both Caucasians and Asians. In Asians, the orbital septum fuses with the lower lid retractors in a slightly higher position than in Caucasians. This allows the preaponeurotic fat to prolapse anteriorly, producing the appearance of a fuller lid. In addition, the higher septal insertion may block the subcutaneous insertion of the distal fibers of the lower lid retractors, allowing the preaponeurotic fat to project more superiorly. In some cases, this may allow the preseptal skin to override the tarsus, producing an epiblepharon with secondary trichiasis [12].

The height of the crease differs significantly among Caucasians and Asians, notably due to the differences in the height of the tarsal plate. The tarsal height is 10–12 mm in Caucasians compared with 6–8 mm in Asians. As a result, the Asian crease is somewhat lower. The goal of Asian blepharoplasty should be to create an eyelid crease that is consistent with the patient's ethnic appearance. Therefore, creating a Western crease on an Asian patient may result in an unusually high eyelid crease, resulting in an unnatural appearance.

The epicanthal fold presents a difficult set of challenges. Some patients request reduction or elimination of the epicanthal fold. Numerous procedures to eliminate or reduce the epicanthal fold have been described, most involving some variation of a Y-V plasty [5]. While these techniques may work well for the experienced surgeon with a high number of Asian patients, the author does not recommend this procedure for the novice surgeon. In general, it is best not to alter the epicanthal fold in Asian patients. Rather, the author recommends blending the lid fold into the epicanthal fold. For those who do desire removal of the epicanthal fold, such a procedure should be discouraged, because the epicanthal skin is thicker and has a higher propensity toward scarring and keloid formation.

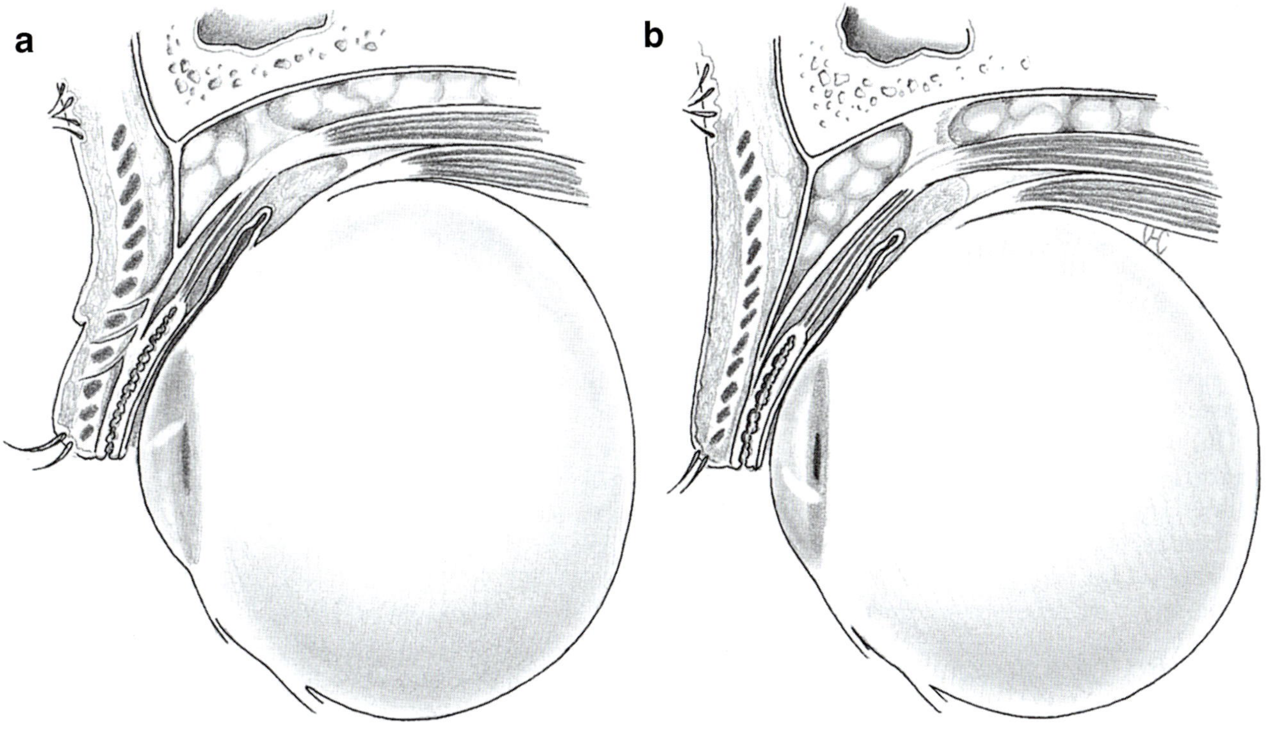

Fig. 19.2 (**a**) Caucasian upper lid. (**b**) Asian upper lid

Preoperative Evaluation

As with any type of aesthetic surgery, it is important for the surgeon to determine what the patient hopes to achieve with surgery. There must be clear communication between the surgeon and the patient regarding the shape and height of the crease desired. Sometimes, the patient has an idea regarding the desired result but is unable to articulate this to the patients, while at other times, the patient does not know what he or she wants and looks to the surgeon for guidance. Therefore, a thorough examination and discussion are vital so that the patient and surgeon can share the same common vision for the final surgical outcome [15]. Some patients have been known to wear clear plastic adhesive strips, commercially sold in Asian catalogs, for the purpose of creating an eyelid crease. The patient should be examined with and without these adhesive strips to determine the preoperative anatomy and the desired result. As with any type of aesthetic surgery, the patient may have unrealistic expectations about what surgery can accomplish, such as promotion in a career or improvement of a relationship. It must be made clear as to what surgery realistically can be achieved. In addition, common patient misconceptions must be addressed: Some patients expect no swelling, and some patients expect no incision and no sutures [4]. The use of a hand mirror and a cotton-tipped applicator (or similar device) to simulate the lid fold is often useful in the preoperative evaluation and discussion. Visual aids, such as pre- and postoperative photographs of representative patients, are often helpful in the discussion.

As with any surgical procedure, a comprehensive ophthalmic examination is mandatory before surgery. It is important to document preexisting ocular pathology, such as dry eye, and eyelid malpositions, such as entropion, ectropion, and eyelid retraction. A basic secretor test and slit lamp examination should be performed on all patients to determine the presence of dry eyes. In addition, lid height, levator function, margin fold distance, and margin crease distance all should be measured. If blepharoptosis is present, its etiology must be determined and then managed appropriately. This may require simultaneous surgery on the levator aponeurosis at the time of blepharoplasty" [9, 25].

Surgical Techniques

Numerous surgical techniques have been devised to create a double eyelid. These techniques fall into one of two broad categories: suture techniques or external incision approach. Suture techniques involve the use of full-thickness sutures to create a scar tract between the skin and conjunctiva at the desired height, thus creating an eyelid crease. Mikamo published the first description of the suture technique in 1896 [19]. Numerous variations of the suture technique have been described [2, 20, 26], all with one common goal—creating adhesions along the superior tarsal border between the levator aponeurosis and the overlying skin and orbicularis muscle (Fig. 19.3). Over the years, the popularity of suture techniques has waxed and waned, compared to external incision techniques. Recently, there has been renewed interest in the suture techniques, especially in Asia [5, 13, 14, 16, 22]. Various types of suture materials have been advocated, some absorbable and some permanent. Suture techniques have the advantage of being relatively less invasive and are generally easier to perform. However, there are relative disadvantages associated with this technique. Over time, the crease has a greater tendency to fade or disappear, compared to the external incision approach. Because the suture techniques do not require a large skin incision, they are not recommended in patients requiring skin or fat removal.

After anesthetizing the eyelid with local anesthetic, the lid is everted and the superior tarsal border identified. Three double-armed sutures are passed from the conjunctival side toward the skin surface. The sutures then can be brought out onto the skin surface and tied or buried beneath small stab incisions. An alternate method employs a threaded needle that may be passed through the pretarsal tissues along the superior tarsal border through several stab incisions. A 4–0 silk suture is then passed in a continuous fashion along the defect. A section of rubber catheter is sutured externally, and the compressive effect of the catheter combined with the scarring from the needle tract produces an eyelid crease [27, 28]. In these techniques, the sutures are left in place for as brief as 2–3 days or as long as 8–10 days, depending on the technique and the surgeon's assessment of postoperative crease formation.

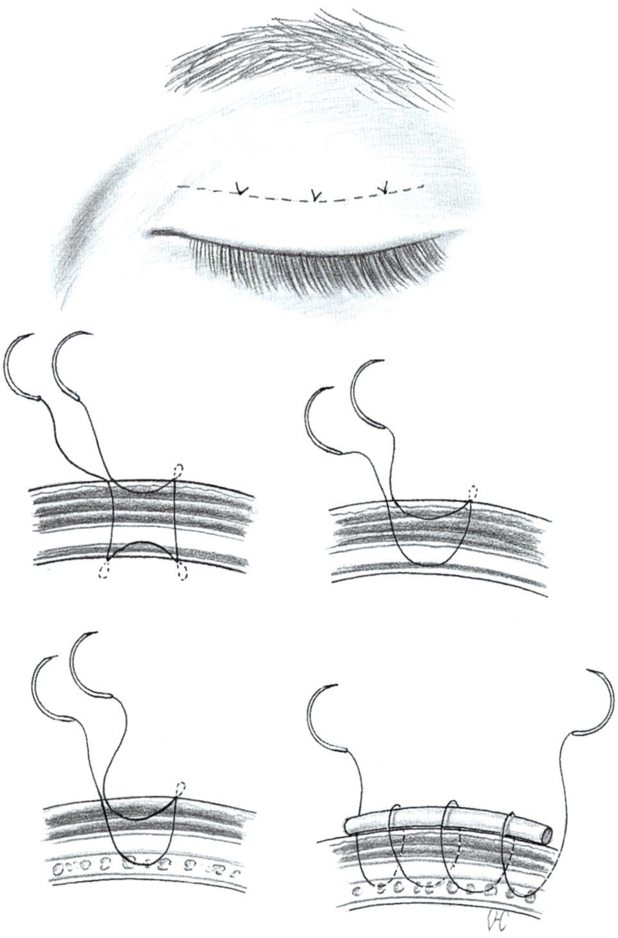

Fig. 19.3 Suture techniques to create a double eyelid

The earliest description of an external incision approach dates to 1929, when Maruo published both his suturing and incision techniques [18]. Asian blepharoplasty via an external incision is the author's preferred surgical approach. The technique is more technically difficult and more time consuming but, when performed properly, yields superior results. The crease is more likely to be permanent, and excess upper lid skin and herniated orbital fat can be debulked if desired. When performed properly, formation of an eyelid crease using an external skin incision produces a crease that is more physiologic or "dynamic" in appearance. This dynamic effect is achieved by fixing the superior and inferior edges of the skin incision to the levator aponeurosis, approximately at the height of the superior tarsal border. The slight redundancy of skin superiorly is allowed to drape over the incision, producing the fold or "double eyelid." The eyelid crease is most visible when the eyes are open and tends to disappear during downgaze or eyelid closure [7, 8]. In contrast, suture techniques produce a "static" crease, which tends to remain visible even with eyelid closure.

To determine the height of the crease, the lid is everted and the height of the tarsus is then measured. The incision is then outlined with a tapering toward the epicanthal fold, if present. The surgeon may use the same local anesthetic mixture that he or she uses for other types of blepharoplasty. The author prefers 2% lidocaine with epinephrine (1:100,000) mixed equally with 0.5% bupivacaine with epinephrine (1:200,000). One milliliter of sodium bicarbonate may be added to 9 ml of the above mixture to raise the pH and thereby reduce the pain associated with injection. Preoperative ice compresses and topical anesthetics may also be used at the surgeon's discretion. The choice of office surgery versus intravenous sedation in an outpatient surgery center will depend upon the health and cooperation of the patient.

After excision of skin and orbicularis muscle, the orbital septum can be opened and the preaponeurotic fat removed, if desired (Fig. 19.4). Younger patients generally require a small skin excision, whereas older patients may require greater skin removal. The amount of skin removal will determine the margin fold distance. The amount of fat removal required in an Asian patient is generally less than that in a

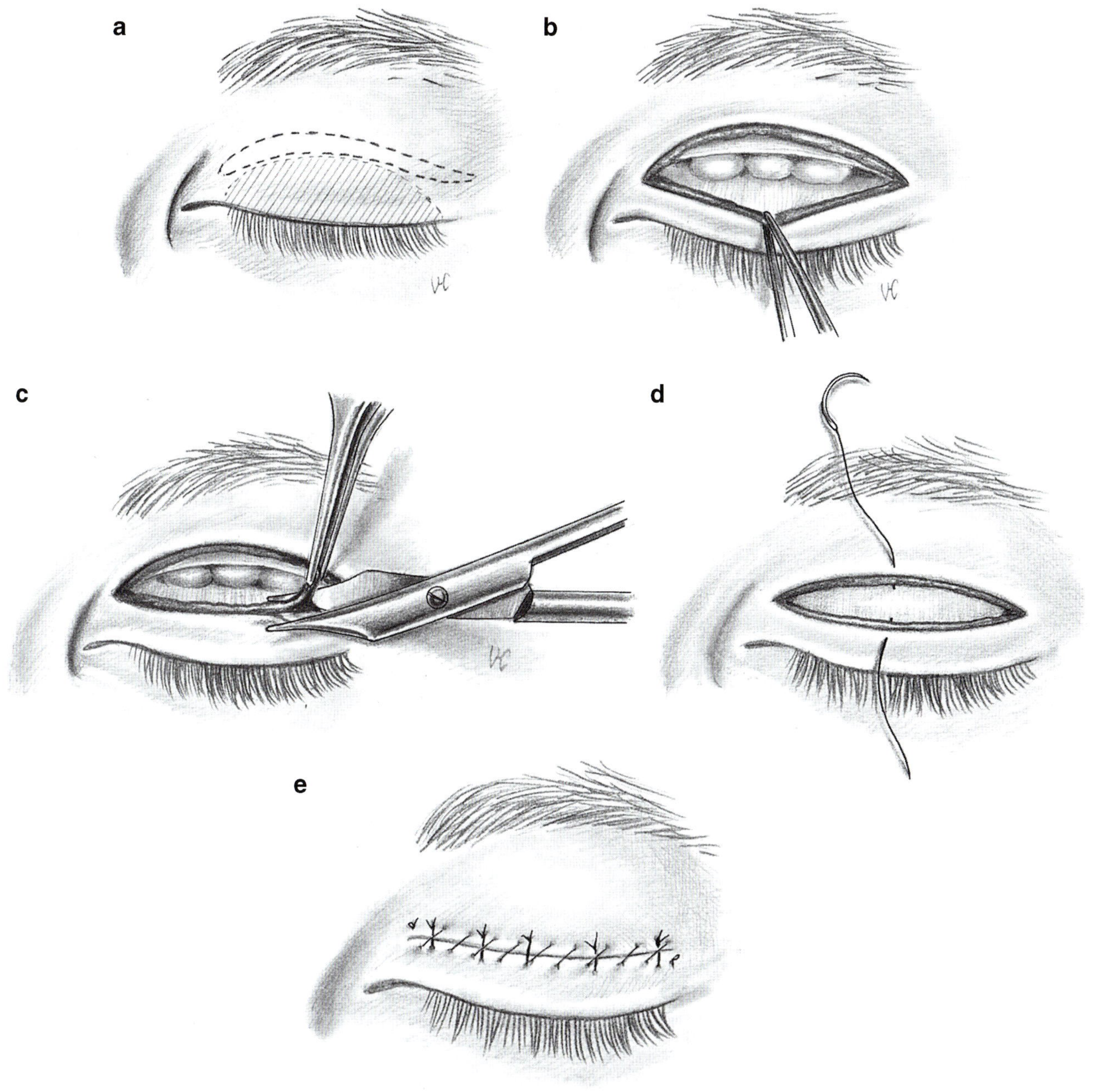

Fig. 19.4 (**a**) Skin marked at approximate edge of superior tarsal border. (**b**) Opening for removal of preaponeurotic fat. (**c**) Trimming edge of pretarsal orbicularis to provide exposure to tarsus. (**d**) Crease sutures of levator aponeurosis. (**e**) Five crease sutures placed. Remainder of skin closed with running suture

Caucasian but may be important if the eyelid has a full or bulky appearance. The amount of fat removed should be conservative so as to avoid hollowing of the superior sulcus. The patient's perception of a successful result is dependent upon symmetry and height of the eyelid fold, as well as a reduction in the bulk of the upper eyelid. Therefore, the appropriate amount of skin and fat excision requires both experience and artistic judgment [29, 30].

As with all surgical procedures, thorough knowledge of eyelid anatomy is important. Iatrogenic damage to the levator aponeurosis, which lies beneath the orbital septum and fat, can result in ptosis and is difficult to repair. As with any form of surgery, meticulous hemostasis must be maintained in order to avoid the dreaded complication of retrobulbar hemorrhage. The lid crease then can be formed using one of several methods. Five or six interrupted sutures incorporating skin, levator aponeurosis, and skin in each bite may be used to form the lid crease. Alternatively, these sutures may incorporate skin, tarsus, and skin with each bite (Fig. 19.5) [1]. A third method employs buried sutures incorporating tar-

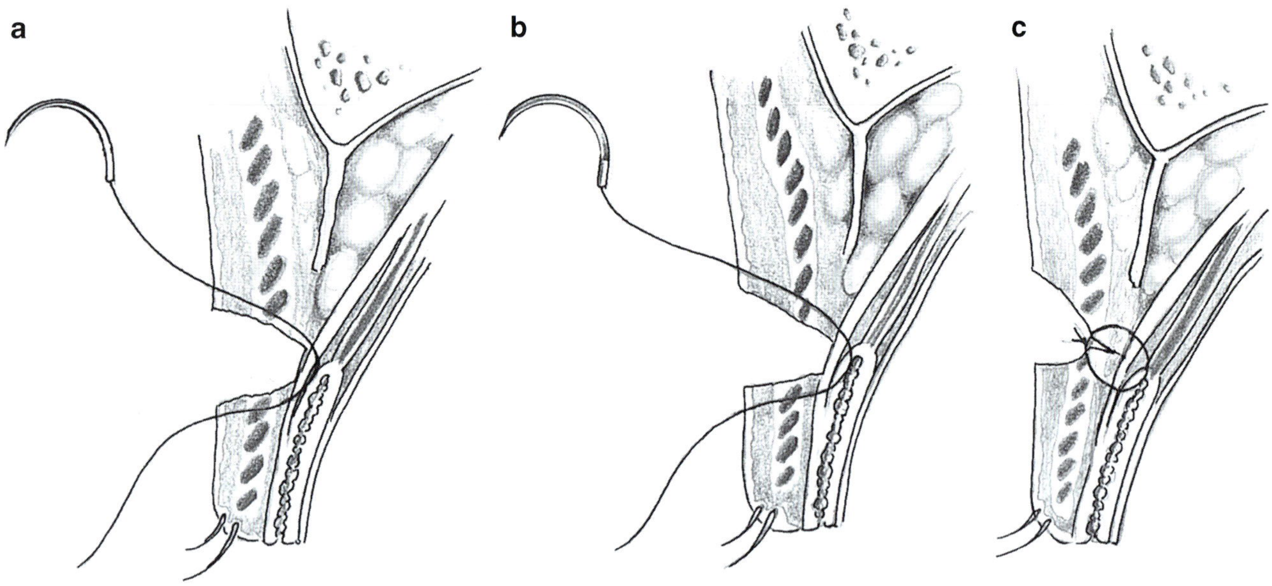

Fig. 19.5 Wound closure. (**a**) Skin, levator, and skin sutures. (**b**) Skin, tarsus, and skin sutures. (**c**) Subcuticular tissue, tarsus, and subcuticular tissue sutures

sus and subcutaneous tissue with each bite [21, 23, 24, 27]. The remainder of the skin incision then can be closed with either running or interrupted sutures. Permanent or absorbable sutures may be used. The author prefers 6–0 nylon, which is removed approximately 1 week postoperatively. Representative preoperative and postoperative photographs are presented for review.

Postoperative Care

The postoperative care of these patients is similar to that of any blepharoplasty patient. They are instructed to avoid strenuous exercise, sun exposure, and aspirin or other anticoagulants. An antibiotic ointment is used on the wounds three to four times daily, and ice compresses are applied for the first 48–72 h. Acetaminophen is helpful for postoperative analgesia.

If nonabsorbing sutures are used, they may be removed approximately 5–7 days after surgery. Interrupted sutures used to form the eyelid crease may be left longer if the crease formation appears to be delayed. The patient should expect a moderate amount of edema and ecchymosis. It is normal for the crease to appear somewhat high initially due to postoperative edema. As the edema resolves, the crease will then appear to be lower. As with all blepharoplasty patients, the surgeon should counsel the patient about the possibility of minor postoperative revisions, which usually can be performed with local anesthesia in an office setting. One should wait a minimum of 1 month after surgery to determine the final height and contour of the upper eyelid fold. Pretarsal edema can especially influence the perceived height of the upper lid fold.

Complications

Numerous complications may be associated with blepharoplasty of any type. They can include common problems such as excessive or insufficient skin or fat removal, abnormalities of the lid crease, ptosis, lagophthalmos, lid retraction, exposure keratopathy, and lacrimal gland prolapse. Rare but serious problems such as infection, orbital hemorrhage, and blindness also may occur [7, 17]. These complications are discussed in greater detail elsewhere in the text.

The problems most commonly seen in Asian blepharoplasty patients are related to the height, shape, and permanence of the eyelid crease. An abnormality of the crease height most often results from excessively high placement of the crease. This usually results from the surgeon's failure to recognize the differences in tarsal height among Asians or from an error in marking the crease height preoperatively. An overzealous removal of eyelid skin or the preaponeurotic fat pads may result in superior sulcus hollowing and may further accentuate the crease height. Asymmetric skin removal may alter the margin fold distance, giving the illusion that the crease is higher on one side compared with that of the other side. The surgeon should consider the possibility of an undetected ptosis when the crease of one eyelid appears higher than the other [23].

If the skin is inadequately fixated to the underlying levator aponeurosis, disappearance of all or part of the crease may

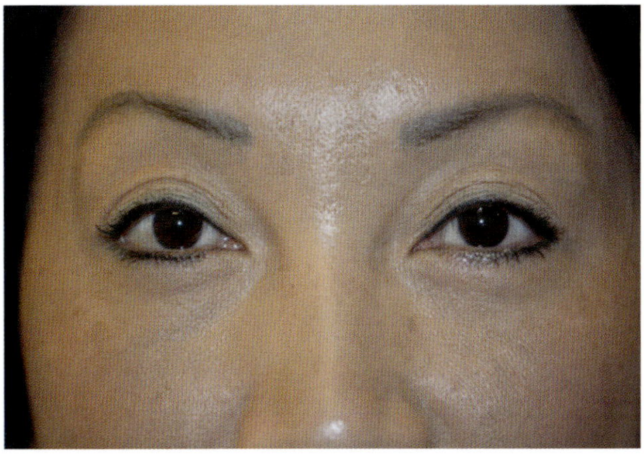

Fig. 19.6 An Asian female presented for consultation after having a bilateral upper lid blepharoplasty performed elsewhere. Her complaint was that the eyelid folds did not look "clean." On examination, she was found to have two high creases and multiple pretarsal creases

occur (Fig. 19.5). The resulting appearance is a crease that is shallow, discontinuous, or obliterated. Multiple creases may arise after unpredictable scar formation after reoperations (Fig. 19.6). Occasionally, the patient may desire reversal of the lid crease procedure [3, 4].

Conclusion

Blepharoplasty in the Asian patient represents a unique set of challenges. The eyelid anatomy, aesthetic goals, and surgical techniques are vastly different from that of Caucasian patients. In Caucasians, upper eyelid blepharoplasty is largely a procedure to debulk skin and preaponeurotic fat. In Asians, the primary goal is to create an eyelid crease. Debulking of skin and preaponeurotic fat is secondary and mainly to enhance the appearance of the crease. The common mistake made by surgeons is to apply Western concepts of anatomy, aesthetics, and surgical techniques to Asian patients. The majority of Asian patients desire the formation of an eyelid crease to enhance their natural Asian features. Ophthalmic surgeons who have gained familiarity with the anatomy and surgical techniques involved are most able to help the patient achieve his or her desired outcome.

References

1. Amrith S. Oriental eyelids—anatomical and surgical considerations. Singap Med J. 1991;32:316.
2. Chashi K. The double eyelid operation using electrocautery. Jpn Rev Clin Ophthalmol. 1951;46:723.
3. Chen WPD. Upper blepharoplasty in the Asian patient. In: Fagien S, editor. Putterman's cosmetic oculoplastic surgery. 3rd ed. Philadelphia: WB Saunders Co.; 2008.
4. Chen WPD. Asian blepharoplasty and the eyelid crease. Philadelphia: Butterworth-Heinemann; 2006.
5. Park J, Toriumi D. Asian facial cosmetic surgery. Philadelphia: WB Saunders Co.; 2008.
6. Harahap M. Blepharoplasty for orientals. J Dermatol Surg Oncol. 1981;7(4):334–9. (ISSN: 0148-0812).
7. Dortzbach RK, editor. Ophthalmic plastic surgery: prevention and management of complications. New York: Raven Press; 1994.
8. Doxonas MT, Anderson RL. Oriental eyelids: anatomic studies. Arch Ophthalmol. 1984;102:1232.
9. Jeong S, Lemke BN, Dortzbach RK, Park YG, Kang HK. The Asian upper eyelid: an anatomical study with comparison to the Caucasian eyelid. Arch Ophthalmol. 1999;117(7):907–12. (ISSN: 0003-9950).
10. Haramoto U, Kubo T, Tamatani M, Hosokawa MK. Anatomic study of the insertions of the levator aponeurosis and Müller's muscle in oriental eyelids. Ann Plast Surg. 2001;47(5):528–33. (ISSN: 0148-7043).
11. Siegel R. Surgical anatomy of the upper eyelid fascia. Ann Plast Surg. 1984;13(4):263–73. (ISSN: 0148-7043).
12. Carter SR, Seiff SR, Grant PE, Vigneron DB. The Asian lower eyelid: a comparative anatomic study using high-resolution magnetic resonance imaging. Ophthal Plast Reconstr Surg. 1998;14(4):227–34. (ISSN: 0740-9303).
13. Fernandez LR. Double eyelid operation in the oriental in Hawaii. Plast Reconstr Surg. 1960;25:257.
14. Fernandez LR. The east Asian eyelid—open technique. Clin Plast Surg. 1993;20(2):247.
15. Jelks GW, Jelks EB. Preoperative evaluation of the blepharoplasty patient. Bypassing the pitfalls. Clin Plast Surg. 1993;20(2):213.
16. Khoo BC. Some aspects of plastic (cosmetic) surgery in orientals. Br J Plast Surg. 1969;22:60.
17. Lowry JC, Bartley GB. Complications of blepharoplasty. Surv Ophthalmol. 1994;38(4):327.
18. Maruo M. Plastic construction of a double-eyelid. Jpn Rev Clin Ophthalmol. 1929;24:393.
19. Mikamo K. A technique in the double eyelid operation. J Chugaishinpo. 1896;396:9.
20. Pang HG. Surgical formation of upper lid fold. Arch Ophthalmol. 1961;65:783.
21. Putterman AM, Urist MJ. Reconstruction of the upper eyelid crease and fold. Arch Ophthalmol. 1976;94:1941.
22. Sayoc BT. Plastic construction of the superior palpebral fold. Am J Ophthalmol. 1954;38:556.
23. Sheen JH. Supratarsal fixation in upper blepharoplasty. Plast Reconstr Surg. 1974;54:424.
24. Sheen JH. A change in the technique of supratarsal fixation in upper blepharoplasty. Plast Reconstr Surg. 1977;59:831.
25. Stasior OG, Ballitch HA. Ptosis repair in aesthetic blepharoplasty. Clin Plast Surg. 1993;20(2):247.
26. Uchida K. The Uchida method for the double-eyelid operation in 1,523 cases. Jpn J Ophthalmol. 1926;30:593.
27. Weingarten CZ. Blepharoplasty in the oriental eye. Trans Am Acad Ophthalmol Otol. 1976;82:442.
28. Yang PY. Double eyelid operation by the twisted needle and compressive suturing technique. Clin J Plast Surg Burn. 1987;3:191.
29. Kim DW, Bhatki AM. Upper blepharoplasty in the Asian eyelid. Facial Plast Surg Clin North Am. 2007;15(3):327–35, vi (ISSN: 1064-7406).
30. Ichinose A, Tahara S. Extended preseptal fat resection in Asian blepharoplasty. Ann Plast Surg. 2008;60(2):121–6. (ISSN: 0148-7043).
31. 2009 AAFPRS Membership Study, http://www.aafprs.org/media/stats_polls/m_stats.html. Accessed 19 July 2010.
32. LaFraniere, S. For many Chinese, New Wealth and a Fresh Face, New York Times, April 23, 2011.

Forehead/Brow Ptosis

20

Evan H. Black and Dianne Marie-Boesch Schlachter

Introduction

Descent of the upper face and brow area occurs frequently with age. With brow ptosis in particular, many patients complain of appearing tired, angry, or sad. Returning the brow, sub-brow fat, and forehead to an improved anatomic position is important to achieve an aesthetically pleasing appearance of the upper face and periorbital area. Numerous techniques exist to elevate the forehead and brow area, so a thorough evaluation and discussion will help determine which technique is appropriate for each patient.

Clinical Evaluation

Understanding the changes which occur in the upper face with age is prerequisite when evaluating a patient for eyelid surgery. Brow ptosis should be suspected in every patient who has redundant upper eyelid skin even if the eyebrow initially appears to be in a normal position. Patients typically lift up the eyebrow with their finger when they want eyelid surgery (Flower's sign). This action should be a cue to the surgeon to evaluate the patient's brow and forehead position as they may be better served with a brow lift in addition to, or instead of, eyelid surgery. Upper eyelid skin extending over the eyelid margin in the lateral periorbital area (Connell's sign) is a hallmark of brow ptosis. Patients with deep transverse forehead creases, from prolonged contraction of the frontalis muscle, also commonly suffer from brow ptosis and may give the false impression of a normal brow position. By having the patient gently close their eyes while placing a hand above the brow to fixate the forehead position in the relaxed state, the true level of brow ptosis can be measured when the patient opens their eyes gently. It is also important to note many individuals (women more so than men) epilate their lateral or inferior brow cilia to create an illusion of a normal brow position. Patients may also attempt to correct a low brow appearance by tattooing above the location of the natural brow to correct the appearance of brow ptosis. The frequent nonanatomic position and permanent nature of eyebrow tattoos present unique challenges with brow and forehead lifting and should be discussed with these patients prior to surgery.

The goal of brow-lifting surgery is to elevate the brow and sub-brow fat, decrease forehead rhytides, decrease vertical glabellar rhytides, improve lateral canthal hooding and rhytides, and decrease infrabrow skin. During the exam, patients should be given a handheld mirror. The mirror will provide patients the opportunity to specifically identify areas of concern and describe their goals. The mirror will also allow the surgeon an opportunity to point out the correct position of the brow, the possible contribution of eyelid skin and blepharoptosis, and possible realistic surgical outcomes. The position of the hairline, forehead rhytides, brow position, and upper eyelids should all be evaluated and discussed with the patient. The upper eyelid crease height should also be noted as a low crease can contribute to significant eyelid crowding with minimal brow descent. It is often helpful to demonstrate to the patient how the appearance of the eyelids is changed by correcting the forehead and brow position. A cotton tip applicator or lid creasing instrument can also be used to simulate removal

E. H. Black (✉)
Consultants in Ophthalmic and Facial Plastic Surgery, P.C., Southfield, MI, USA

Wayne State University School of Medicine/Kresge Eye Institute, Detroit, MI, USA

Oakland University/William Beaumont Hospital School of Medicine, Department of Ophthalmology, Royal Oak, MI, USA

D. M.-B. Schlachter
Consultants in Ophthalmic and Facial Plastic Surgery, P.C., Southfield, MI, USA

Oakland University/William Beaumont Hospital School of Medicine, Department of Ophthalmology, Royal Oak, MI, USA

J. J. Servat et al. (eds.), *Smith and Nesi's Ophthalmic Plastic and Reconstructive Surgery*,
https://doi.org/10.1007/978-3-030-41720-8_20

of eyelid skin with the brow in the relaxed and elevated position. This maneuver is especially important to illustrate to the patient possible surgical outcomes when the patient is deciding between brow and lid surgery. All discussions should be documented in writing and by preoperative photographs.

Anatomic Considerations

The position of the eyebrow is affected by brow elevator and depressor muscles, genetics, gravity, and the patient's expressivity. All or some of these factors can affect the position of the brow. Although each eyebrow has its own shape, position, and contour, the female eyebrow should lie approximately at or slightly above the superior orbital rim in the relaxed state. The tail of brow should be positioned higher than the head of the brow with a gently arched shape. The peak of the arch should be at the junction of the medial two-thirds and the lateral third. In contrast, the male eyebrow should be at the level of the superior orbital rim with a flatter configuration. When planning brow surgery, the function of the frontalis, orbicularis oculi, depressor supercilii, corrugator, and procerus muscles must be specifically addressed. Their individual actions influence the position of the eyebrows and the presence or absence of rhytides.

The frontalis muscle originates at the galea aponeurotica and inserts into the eyebrow skin and the superficial fascia of the orbicularis oculi muscle. The main function of the frontalis muscle is to elevate the eyebrows, and it is responsible for transverse rhytides in the forehead. The corrugator muscle originates from the medial orbital rim and inserts into the frontalis muscle and skin of the eyebrow. It primarily shortens the glabellar space between the heads of the brows and secondarily causes descent of the brow tail. It is responsible for vertical glabellar frown lines. The orbicularis oculi muscle originates at the medial orbital rim and medial canthal tendon and inserts on the lateral aspect of the bony orbit. It depresses the brow and is responsible for vertical and horizontal rhytides. The depressor supercilii muscle also originates at the medial orbital rim and medial canthal tendon and inserts on the medial aspect of the bony orbit. It is responsible for depressing the head of the brow. The procerus muscle originates at the nasal bone fascia and inserts onto the skin of the medial lower forehead. Like the depressor supercilii, the procerus depresses the head of the brow and is responsible for horizontal rhytides at the radix of the nose. The surgeon must be thoroughly familiar with these muscles in order to adequately evaluate and treat brow ptosis.

Motor innervation of the forehead musculature is provided by the frontal branch of the facial nerve. As this nerve branch traverses the zygomatic arch from the lower face, it assumes a superficial course running within the substance of the superficial musculoaponeurotic system (SMAS) on the deep surface of the temporoparietal fascia. The superficial nature of this nerve branch is in contrast to the facial nerve branches in the lower face which run deep to the facial fascial layers. Distally, the frontal branch pierces the temporoparietal fascia to innervate the frontalis muscle on its deep surface (1). With undermining of the tissues of the lateral forehead during endoscopic brow lifting, extreme care must be taken to protect the nerve as damage can cause prolonged paresis or permanent paralysis of the eyebrow.

Sensory innervation of the forehead is supplied by the supraorbital and supratrochlear branches of the ophthalmic division of the trigeminal nerve. The supraorbital nerve exits the skull by either a supraorbital foramen or supraorbital notch and continues superiorly. When present, the foramen is located just above the superior orbital rim approximately 2–3 cm from the midline. The notch is located in the superior orbital rim between the medial one-third and lateral two-thirds of the orbit. Approximately 50% of skulls have bilateral supraorbital notches, 25% have bilateral supraorbital foramina, and 25% have a foramen on one side and a notch on the other (2). The supraorbital nerve branches near its exit into a deep and superficial branch. The deep branch runs superolaterally to pierce the galea near the coronal suture and supplies sensation to the frontoparietal region. The superficial branch pierces the frontalis muscle and provides sensory innervation to the forehead and anterior scalp. The supratrochlear nerve also exits the orbit at a foramen or notch located above the trochlea and medial to the supraorbital nerve. Similar to the supraorbital nerve, variation exists between skulls with 97% having bilateral notches, 1% having bilateral foramina, and 2% having a notch on one side and a foramen on the other (2). The nerve penetrates the corrugator muscle and frontalis muscle to supply cutaneous sensation to the forehead and medial upper eyelid. Whether the surgeon is directly removing tissue in the brow area, or undermining tissue during endoscopic brow lifting, extreme care must be taken to protect these nerves as damage can cause prolonged hypoesthesia of the forehead and scalp.

Medical Management

Medical management for brow ptosis is limited. In mild cases, botulinum toxin can be used for eyebrow elevation. This effect is temporary, lasting approximately 3–4 months. By injecting the superolateral portion of the orbicularis oculi muscle below the lateral third of the brow, a noticeable eyebrow lift can be achieved in some patients (3). Injection of the central portion of orbicularis muscle below the brow has also been shown to produce some lifting effect in female patients (4). In contrast, selective inhibition of the central portion of the frontalis muscle with sparing of the lateral aspect can also give moderate elevation of the lateral brows. However, care must be taken to adequately paralyze the frontalis muscle past the central brow on each side to avoid an aesthetically unpleasing medially displaced arch. One must also titrate the dose when using this technique to prevent an unnaturally high arch which is also aesthetically unpleasant. Another common mistake in patients with significant horizontal forehead rhytides from severe brow ptosis is to use botulinum toxin to paralyze the entire frontalis muscle. This action weakens the brow elevators and worsens the brow ptosis (though the rhytides will usually resolve). In a severely low brow, paralysis of the brow depressor muscles and/or selective inhibition of the medial frontalis muscle is unlikely to make a noticeable improvement.

Chemical peels, laser skin resurfacing, and other techniques have been used to accomplish mild brow elevation. Several of these measures rely on skin tightening above the brow and are dependent on the amount of correction of skin laxity that can be attained. The use of silicone tape can also be applied to the temporal skin to temporarily lift the lateral brows; however, these tapes must be able to be hidden by hair. The use of filler or fat injections to replace volume in the temple area can also give a mild amount of lateral brow lift. However, all of these techniques are relatively temporary and are of minimal benefit in a severely low brow.

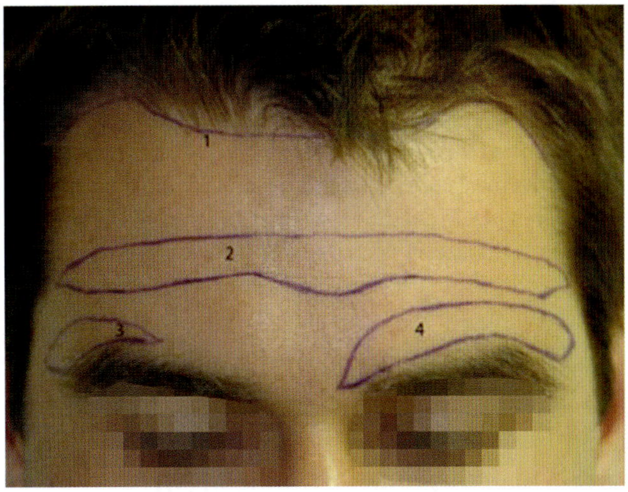

Fig. 20.1 Forehead incisions. 1. Pretrichial /Trichophytic forehead lift. 2. Midforehead lift. 3. Temporal direct brow lift. 4.Direct brow lift

Surgical Management

A variety of surgical procedures are available to lift the forehead and brow area, and choosing one depends largely on both the desired surgical outcome and patient preference. During the initial consultation, it is important to discuss patients' expectations, note the position of the brow and hairline, and determine if the patient is interested in brow lifting primarily to improve visual function or cosmetic appearance. A thorough discussion regarding possible postsurgical scarring is also imperative as certain procedures may leave a noticeable scar.

Direct and Temporal Direct Brow Lift

If the patient is interested in lifting the brow primarily to improve visual function, a direct brow lift can provide a good functional result. The procedure lifts the entire brow, and the contour of the brow can be altered by varying the amount and location of skin excised. An ellipse of tissue is removed directly above each brow while attempting to hide the incisions in a forehead furrow if possible (see Fig. 20.1, 4). The lateral edge of each ellipse should not extend more than 1 cm lateral to the tail of the brow to avoid damage to the frontal branch of the facial nerve, and medial dissection should be maintained in a superficial, subcutaneous plane to avoid damage to the supraorbital nerve. The superior-most brow hair follicles are protected by beveling the incision 30 degrees away from the brow. To decrease postoperative scarring, the superior incision should be beveled in the *same* (italics) direction by 45 degrees. This beveling technique will create an everted wound edge with closure to minimize the appearance of the scar. The skin is then closed with deep tissue and skin sutures. For patients with temporal brow ptosis, a temporal direct brow lift can be considered as well. In this technique, the incisions are placed laterally over the temporal brow (see Fig. 20.1, 3). The lateral nature of this incision tends to hide better than the full direct brow lift; however, it is important to keep in mind these techniques are not recommended for patients desiring a cosmetic outcome as noticeable scars will occur.

Midforehead Lift

A midforehead lift is a brow-lifting option for patients with deep forehead rhytides. An incision line is marked along a forehead furrow 2–4 cm above the brows along the length of the forehead. An ellipse is drawn above or below the initial incision line, and skin and subcutaneous tissue are excised (see Fig. 20.1, 2). The frontalis muscle should be spared to prevent forehead weakness. The wound is then closed with a layered closure. Alternatively, a skin flap may be created by making an initial incision along a forehead furrow. The tissue is then dissected in a plane above the frontalis muscle to the level of the brow. Sutures are used to suspend the brow, and the excess skin at the incision line is trimmed and closed in a layered fashion. Similar to the direct and temporal brow lift, this procedure can cause significant scarring and should be avoided in a cosmetic patient.

Transblepharoplasty Brow Lift

The transblepharoplasty brow lift is performed through an upper lid skin crease incision. This procedure is commonly accomplished with upper lid blepharoplasty in patients with mild brow ptosis or temporal brow ptosis who do not desire a full forehead lift. At the superior edge of the blepharoplasty incision, a dissection is carried out superiorly to a predetermined point above the superior orbital rim. The brow is then fixated to this location with sutures or an implantable fixation device. The medial brow should not be lifted with this procedure to avoid damage to the supraorbital nerve.

Pretrichial/Trichophytic Forehead Lift

The pretrichial forehead lift is useful for patients with a high forehead. The trichophytic incision, placed just anterior to the hairline, effectively raises the brows while lowering the hairline (see Fig. 20.1, 1). The incision may also be wavy or "zig-zag" to help hide the scar. The lateral extent of the incision can be placed behind or at the edge of the temporal hairline. Centrally, a dissection is carried out down to the loose areolar tissue between the galea and periosteum. Along this subgaleal plane, blunt dissection is carried out inferiorly until just above the superior orbital rim. Some surgeons prefer to dissect the central forehead in the subperiosteal plane. Near the superior orbital rims, care is taken to avoid the supraorbital vessels and nerves. Laterally, the incision is deepened until the deep temporalis fascia is visible. Along the surface of the deep temporalis fascia, the dissection is carried forward until the conjoined tendon is reached at the temporal line. Maintaining the correct plane of dissection in this area is important to avoid damage to the frontal branch of the facial nerve. Using sharp dissection, the conjoined tendon is released inferiorly to the lateral brow, joining the two planes of dissection. Once the forehead is released, the corrugators are released from their deep attachments. The forehead is elevated to the correct position, and excess skin is trimmed along the incision line. The wound is then closed in a layered fashion. The same procedure performed just behind the hairline is known as a trichophytic forehead lift.

Coronal Forehead Lift

The coronal forehead lift raises the forehead through an elliptical scalp incision extending from ear to ear anterior to the coronal suture. The hair is often shaved in the area of tissue to be removed. The skin is incised to the level of the subgaleal plane centrally and the deep temporalis fascia laterally. A dissection is then carried forward under direct visualization similar to the pretrichial forehead lift, taking care to avoid the frontal branch of the facial nerve and the supraorbital nerve. Careful hemostasis is also achieved while avoiding damage to the hair follicles. Similar to the pretrichial forehead lift, some surgeons prefer to use a subperiosteal plane of dissection in the central forehead area. Once the entire forehead is released, the forehead is elevated to the proper position and the excess skin is trimmed. Skin resection should be conservative as wound closure under tension can cause secondary alopecia within the scar. The scalp wound is closed with a layered closure, and the use of surgical staples for skin closure is helpful to prevent strangulation of the wound margin and severe alopecia. Permanent hypoesthesia of the scalp and incisional alopecia are common with this older technique.

Endoscopic Forehead Lift

Advances in endoscopic surgery have allowed surgeons to modify the forehead lifting procedure in such a way as to minimize postoperative scarring and tissue disruption. The endoscopic forehead lift is an elegant alternative to offer the cosmetic patient, and many patients are pleased with the less invasive approach.

Marking is critical when planning for surgery. The right and left temporal crescents, denoting the fusion of periosteum, deep temporal fascia, and temporoparietal fascia at the conjoined tendon, are palpated and marked. This ridge is more pronounced when the patient clenches the jaw. A marking is then placed at the right and left lateral orbital rims at the level of the lateral canthal angle. This mark denotes the area of the zygomaticotemporal (sentinel) vein and should be the extent of the lateral dissection for this procedure to avoid damage to the frontal branch of the facial nerve. The supraorbital notch is then palpated on each side, and a "safety zone" of approximately 2 cm is drawn around these areas to protect the supraorbital and supratrochlear nerves during later dissection. Blind subperiosteal dissection can be done safely up to these markings. One central vertical and two paramedian vertical incision sites are then marked just posterior to the hairline. The central incision is marked at or 1 cm behind the hairline, extending 1.0–1.5 cm in length. The paramedial incisions are marked approximately 4.5 cm lateral to the central incision site. Alternatively, in males, a single central elliptical incision can be placed in a coronal orientation at or approximately 1 cm behind the hairline. This ellipse will help maintain the natural flattened contour of the male brow and replaces the three vertical incisions. The size and shape of the ellipse are determined by preoperative measurements. Two paramedian incisions can also be placed horizontally in males rather than using an ellipse or three vertical incisions (see Fig. 20.2). These parame-

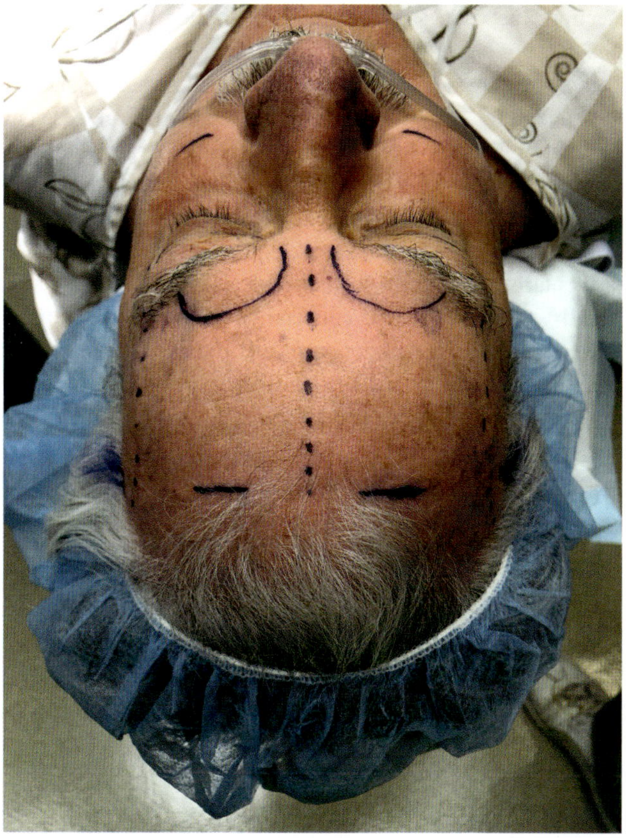

Fig. 20.2 Representative male endoscopic forehead lift markings with two paramedian incisions

dian incisions are useful when a central ellipse would be visible without adequate hair coverage. The approximate placement of the fixation devices should then be drawn just anterior and lateral to the paramedian incision sites. Careful scrutiny of preoperative photographs is important intraoperatively to determine the correct placement of the fixation devices. Any asymmetry between the brows should be noted, and corrected if possible, by varying the position of the fixation devices. In a female patient, the placement of the fixation devices should be at the location of maximum desired lift, or arch, of the brow. Moving the fixation devices slighly lower will give more lift to the brows. However, care should be taken to remain above the level of the midforehead to avoid too much inferior traction on the devices during healing. More lift of the head of the brow will also be attained by moving the devices medially. In male patients, a more medial placement will also help ensure the preferred "T-shaped" brow contour. Bilateral simple or elliptical incisions are then marked in the temporal areas. If an ellipse is used, the size of each ellipse is determined by the preoperative evaluation. The orientation of these incisions is perpendicular to a line drawn from the lateral nasal ala to the lateral canthal angle on each side. These incisions are responsible for lifting the

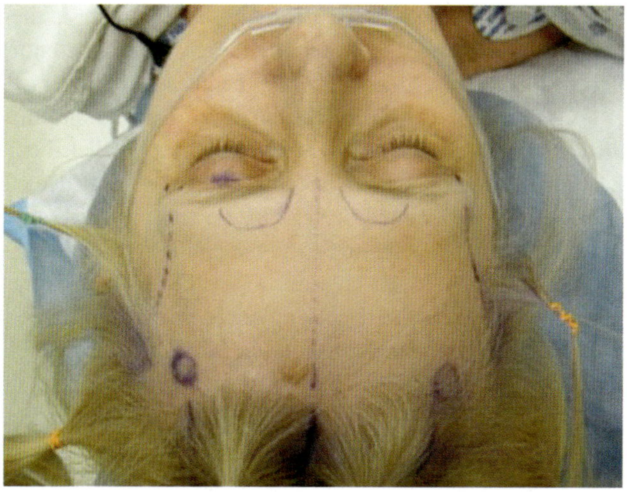

Fig. 20.3 Representative female endoscopic forehead lift markings

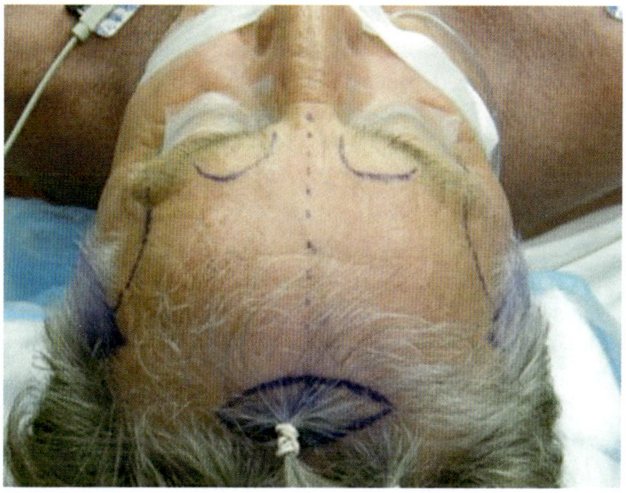

Fig. 20.4 Representative male endoscopic forehead lift markings with central ellipse

lateral canthal area and temporal brow, and ellipses add to the effectiveness of the procedure. The proper angle of these incisions is critical to a good cosmetic outcome. By tilting the inferior most aspect of these incisions posteriorly, more lift in the lateral canthal areas can be attained. In the presence of male pattern baldness, these incisions can be made behind the fringe line. The hair should not be shaved but can be twisted with rubber bands to maximize visualization during surgery (see Figs. 20.3 and 20.4).

Endoscopic forehead lifting can be performed under local anesthesia with sedation or general anesthesia. A bilateral, supraorbital nerve block is given using a 50/50 mixture of 2% lidocaine with 1:100,000 epinephrine and 0.5% bupivacaine with 1:100,000 epinephrine. If ptosis repair is scheduled with the forehead lift, this block should be done after the ptosis repair as it may impair levator function.

Additional local anesthesia using the same mixture is then administered along the surgical markings, across the entire forehead and brow area, and along the lateral orbital rims.

A scalpel is used to incise the temporal skin over the elliptical marking on each side. These incisions are beveled outward with increasing depth from the ellipse on both edges to create an everted wound during closure and minimize scarring. The skin flap is removed and the temporoparietal fascia is exposed. This fascial layer moves with the skin. Further dissection exposes the deep temporalis fascia immediately superficial to the temporalis muscle. This fascial layer is firmly attached to the surface of the temporalis muscle and will not move with the skin. The superficial layer of the deep temporalis fascia lies immediately superficial to this fascial layer. The plane of dissection is between the superficial and deep temporalis fascia. The frontal branch of the facial nerve lies within the temporoparietal fascia and is superficial to the surgical plane. Maintaining the correct plane of dissection in this area is important to avoid damage to the nerve. The temporal artery is often encountered during dissection and should be avoided, cauterized, or tied off with ligature suture as necessary.

The endoscope is introduced through the temporal incision above the deep temporalis fascia. Continuing in each temporal pocket, dissection is carried out toward the lateral canthal angle with direct endoscopic visualization. It is important to stay on the surface of the deep temporalis fascia to avoid damage to the facial nerve branches. At the lateral orbit, the orbicularis-temporal ligament is visible as a tough ligament joining the lateral orbicularis to the deep temporalis fascia. Careful dissection beyond this point reveals the zygomaticotemporal (sentinel) vein. This vein is typically 5 mm temporal to the zygomaticofrontal suture line, and dissection should be minimal in this location to protect branches of the facial nerve. The lateral canthal ligament is then detached under endoscopic visualization.

At the central and paramedian incisions, a scalpel is used to incise the skin, scalp, and periosteum to bone. A periosteal elevator is then used to blindly release the periosteum across the forehead in a subperiosteal plane until the markings are reached above the supraorbital nerves on each side. Subperiosteal dissection is also accomplished 5–10 centimeters posterior to the incision lines. The endoscope is then introduced into one of the vertical incisions in order to accomplish the remaining dissection in the vicinity of the supraorbital nerves. Under direct visualization, the supraorbital nerve is located and avoided. A supraperiosteal pocket is then formed above the bridge of the nose to address the depressor muscles (procerus, corrugators, depressor supercilii, and orbicularis oculi). Using blunt dissection, the tissues are moved side to side to separate the muscles for better visualization. The corrugators are avulsed, rather than cut, to prevent injury to the supratrochlear nerve and unnatural spreading of the brow heads. This release can be accomplished with endoscopic scissors. Branches of the supratrochlear nerve are sometimes seen within the corrugators and should be avoided. The procerus and depressor supercilii muscles are addressed in a similar fashion. The orbicularis oculi muscle can also be visualized laterally, and small vertically oriented cuts can be made with scissors to weaken the downward action of this muscle temporally. To eliminate the glabellar lines, vertical incisions can be made in the periosteum centrally up to the dermis. When cutting the orbicularis laterally or periosteum centrally, care should be taken to maintain a deep plane as skin irregularities can be seen if the cuts are too superficial. Using blunt and sharp dissection, the temporal crescents are released on each side joining the subperiosteal and deep temporalis fascial planes. This maneuver releases the entire forehead from its deep attachments. The key to a successful and lasting endoscopic forehead procedure centers on meticulous release of the periosteum and brow depressor muscles. Skin hooks can then be used to grasp to posterior edges of the vertical incisions and pull the forehead superiorly. If the release is adequate, the entire forehead and brows will move easily into an elevated position.

Following release of the periosteum, attention is given to fixation. Many methods are available to fixate the scalp. Anchor or screw techniques include the use of a screw or plate, internal screw/anchor device (Mitek™), external screw, and k-wire. Further options include galea-frontalis-occipitalis release, use of lateral suspension sutures or bolster fixation sutures, anterior scalp port excision, galea-frontalis advancement, creation of a cortical tunnel, and use of tissue adhesives. The Endotine™ forehead fixation device (MicroAire, Charlottesville, VA) was introduced in 2003. This anchoring device utilizes a biodegradable, polylactic acid implant on a triangular platform with 5 tines and a bone peg for attachment to the skull. In 2006, a modification of the Endotine was introduced called the Ultratine™ forehead fixation device. This device used a similar platform and attachment peg and was developed by combining polyglycolic acid and polylactic acid for quicker resorption. Unfortunately, this modification resulted in a high rate of cyst formation at the implant site, so these devices are not recommended (5). Regardless of the technique, the fixation method must be safe and reproducible and have long-term results. Fixation devices should be placed according to the manufacturer's instructions.

The superficial temporalis fascia is closed with deep, buried absorbable or nylon sutures, and the skin is closed with surgical staples. A firm dressing is placed around the forehead to prevent postoperative swelling and left in place for 24–48 h. Postoperative antibiotics, analgesia, and anti-inflammatory medication are provided at the surgeon's discretion. The staples are removed in 7–10 days. Patients can usually return to work in 3–5 days, although bending and heavy lifting should be avoided for at least 1 week. Patients should also avoid any hair dye near the scalp incisions for at least 4–6 weeks. Patients are warned preoperatively of expected V_1 hypoesthesia, transient (and rarely permanent) facial neuropraxia, and possible alopecia near the incision sites. Preoperative discussion regarding the type of fixation device is also important as patients may palpate the anchors.

The endoscopic forehead lift procedure is an effective, long-lasting procedure available to patients interested in forehead and brow lifting. With a higher patient acceptance rate than the traditional coronal lift, the endoscopic lift is a nice addition to the surgeon's armamentarium (6–8).

References

1. Stuzin JM, Wagstrom L, Kawamoto HK, et al. Anatomy of the frontal branch of the facial nerve: the significance of the temporal fat pad. Plast Reconstr Surg. 1989;83(2):265–71.
2. Webster RC, Gaunt JM, Hamdan US, et al. Supraorbital and supratrochlear notches and foramina: anatomical variations and surgical relevance. Laryngoscope. 1986;96(3):311–5.
3. Ahn MS, Catten M, Maas CS. Temporal brow lift using botulinum toxin A. Plast Reconstr Surg. 2000;105(3):1129–35.
4. Huang W, Rogachefsky AS, Foster JA. Browlift with botulinum toxin. Dermatol Surg. 2000;26:55–60.
5. Servat JJ, Black EH. A comparison of surgical outcomes with the use of two different biodegradable multipoint fixation devices for endoscopic forehead lift. Ophthal Plast Reconstr Surg. 2012;28(6):401–4. PMID: 23138199.
6. Nesi FA, Gladstone GJ, Brazzo BG, Myint S, Black EH. Ophthalmic and facial plastic surgery: a compendium of reconstructive and aesthetic techniques. Thorofare: Slack Inc; 2001. p. 219–25.
7. Gladstone GJ, Black EH, Myint S, Brazzo BG, Nesi FA. Gladstone and Nesi's oculoplastic surgery atlas: cosmetic facial surgery. New York: Springer New York, Inc; 2005. p. 25–42.
8. Nerad JA. Techniques in ophthalmic plastic surgery: a personal tutorial. Oxford: Saunders Elsevier, Inc; 2010. p. 129–86.

Injectables and Fillers

21

Audrey E. Ahuero and Bryan S. Sires

Introduction

Facial aging involves volumetric change, alteration of tissue quality, and the effects of long-standing facial muscular animation [1]. These factors lead to soft tissue ptosis and static and dynamic rhytids [1]. The traditional concept of beauty involves the "triangle of beauty" with high cheekbones and a defined jaw, whereas the "reverse triangle" or pyramid with flattened cheeks, drooping eyes, and jowling is considered unattractive [2]. Facial rhytids can be classified as dynamic or static. Dynamic rhytids occur with muscle action and are best treated by specifically targeting facial muscles with botulinum toxin [2]. Facial expression not only contributes to the development of facial lines but also influences atrophy of soft tissue and malposition [3]. More facially animated individuals typically demonstrate increased lines and furrows relative to their less animated counterparts [3]. Static rhytids result from the natural aging process with collagen loss and photodamage [4]. They are visible at rest and are addressed with volume replacement or combination therapy. Sun exposure and smoking additionally contribute to facial aging [3]. The trend in facial rejuvenation has increasingly emphasized the three-dimensional aspects of facial aging [5]. The three critical components of facial augmentation involve control of movement, improvement of contour, and restoration of volume [5]. The volume loss in the aging face involves atrophy of subcutaneous fat, which is variable between race and gender [5]. Bone loss plays a minor role as well [5]. Characteristics of the aesthetic ideal differ between men and women and need to be considered when developing a treatment plan [5].

A. E. Ahuero
Ophthalmic Plastic Surgeons of Texas, Houston, TX, USA

B. S. Sires (✉)
Allure Laser Center and Medispa, Kirkland, WA, USA

Botulinum Toxin

Botulinum neurotoxin type A (BoNTA) is a key component in facial rejuvenation and has become the mainstay of therapy for dynamic rhytids. It is also used for soft tissue malposition and adjunctively for static rhytids. Also, it has applications for facial aesthetic surgery and has additional uses [1]. BoNTA injections are the most popular nonsurgical cosmetic procedures in the United States [2, 6, 7]. The worldwide sales of Botox reached 2.3 billion in 2017 [8], and according to the ASPS survey in 2016, sales continue to grow [9].

Pathophysiology

Pierard and Lapiere first described the role of muscle action in formation of facial lines. They used postmortem microanatomic studies [10, 11]. The utility of botulinum neurotoxin stems from its role in chemodenervation. Botulinum neurotoxin is derived from *Clostridium botulinum.* This anaerobic, spore-forming bacterium produces eight exotoxins, five of which can affect the human nervous system [1, 12]. Type A was the first toxin purified and is the one most easily grown in culture [1]. Types A, B, and E are the subtypes associated with botulism [12]. Botulinum toxin is a protein composed of a heavy chain and light chain connected by a fragile disulfide bond [7]. This toxin induces muscle paralysis by inhibiting the release of acetylcholine at the presynaptic terminal of the neuromuscular junction [1]. The different exotoxins act on different proteins at the presynaptic terminal. BoNTA and botulinum toxin type E cleave SNAP-25, and BoNTB cleaves synaptobrevin [13]. The effect of the toxin is dose-related and at very high doses can affect autonomic cholinergic ganglia [1]. The toxin rapidly and irreversibly binds, but the effect is not permanent due to turnover of neuromuscular junctions [4, 12] and axonal nerve sprouting [1]. Muscle biopsies from treated

J. J. Servat et al. (eds.), *Smith and Nesi's Ophthalmic Plastic and Reconstructive Surgery*,
https://doi.org/10.1007/978-3-030-41720-8_21

patients in a study did not demonstrate evidence of permanent degeneration or atrophy [12]. One study suggests that facial muscles have different distribution and quantity of motor endplates compared to skeletal muscles [14]. The toxin does not have any reported central nervous system effects because it does not cross the blood-brain barrier [1]. One unit of botulinum toxin is described as the amount of toxin required to kill 50% of mice when injected intraperitoneally [7]. The toxic dose in humans is thought to be around 3000 units based on animal models [7]. The suspected lethal dose has been far exceeded in a few patients injected with unlicensed, highly concentrated botulinum toxin, and these patients survived [7, 15]. Systemic spread is a possible adverse effect but not commonly reported [16].

History

Justinus Kerner first described botulism, a foodborne illness, following the ingestion of contaminated sausage in the early 1800s [7, 17]. The Latin word for sausage is *botulus*. He subsequently studied the disease and observed that the toxin disrupted the autonomic and somatic nervous system [7]. The concept of chemodenervation with botulinum toxin originated in the 1920s [10]. Prior to chemodenervation, surgical resection of facial muscles was attempted as a means of facial enhancement [3, 18]. The therapeutic use of botulinum toxin type A began in the late 1970s when Dr. Alan Scott and Dr. Edward Schantz produced BoNTA for therapeutic use [10]. He published his results of injecting BoNTA into extraocular muscles for treatment of strabismus in 1981 [19–21].

The use of botulinum toxin in the treatment of blepharospasm began the following year [19] and expanded to include treatment of hemifacial spasm and lower eyelid entropion [19] as well as for numerous other disorders such as focal dystonias and hyperhidrosis [22, 23], bruxism, muscle spasm, tremor, tics, spastic bladder, rigidity [1, 10, 24], Frey's syndrome, excessive perspiration, anal fissures, esophageal motility disorders [4], tension headaches, and migraines [1, 10, 24]. Expanded ocular and periocular uses include treatment of nystagmus, aberrant regeneration, corneal disease, and amblyopia [1, 10]. It has also been found to be useful in facial reconstructive surgery [25]. The original Botox was reformulated in 1997 and now has approximately 20% of the protein load of the original formulation, which reduces its antigenicity [1]. The FDA approved one BoNTA formulation, Botox, in 1989 for use in blepharospasm, strabismus, and hemifacial spasm [7, 12].

The initial insight that BoNTA may be a viable modality for facial rejuvenation resulted from the observation that glabellar rhytids were improved in patients treated for facial spastic disorders [1, 26]. Its use for cosmetic purposes began in 1987, and studies demonstrated excellent efficacy and safety [22, 23, 26, 27]. In particular, Carruthers and Carruthers began using the toxin for cosmetic purposes in 1987 [7] and described the positive effects on glabellar furrows in patients treated for benign essential blepharospasm in 1992 [4, 26]. In 1989, Botox was used to correct facial asymmetry resulting from facial nerve paralysis after rhytidectomy [4, 28]. Glabellar furrows, horizontal forehead furrows, and lateral canthal lines were the most emphasized areas for cosmetic Botox treatment initially [3]. The efficacy and longevity of BoNTA for cosmetic purposes were also found to be dose-dependent [29].

BoNTA officially entered the US cosmetic market on April 15, 2002 with initial FDA approval of Botox Cosmetic (onabotulinumtoxinA; Allergan, Inc., Irvine, CA, USA) for the treatment of moderate to severe glabellar rhytids [4, 30]. In 2013, Botox was approved for the temporary improvement of moderate to severe crow's feet lines and in 2017 gained FDA approval for the temporary improvement of moderate to severe forehead lines associated with frontalis muscle activity in adults. In 2009, a second formulation of botulinum toxin type A, Dysport (abobotulinumtoxin A; Galderma, Lausanne, Switzerland) [13, 30] was FDA approved in the United States. Product labeling has been modified to clearly distinguish between the two BoNTA products [31]. Dysport is thought to have increased diffusion compared to Botox [2, 5], but data may suggest a longer duration of action compared to Botox [13, 32]. The BoNTA formulations also differ in molecular weight, dosing, and units per vial [5]. There is not a single conversion ratio between the BoNTA formulations; thus, they are not interchangeable [13]. For most procedures, 1 U of Botox is equivalent to 3–4 U of Dysport [7, 33]. A third botulinum toxin type A formulation, Xeomin (incobotulinum toxin A; Merz Aesthetics, Frankfurt, Germany), was granted FDA approval in 2011 for the temporary improvement in moderate to severe glabellar lines in adult patients. The newest formulation, Jeuveau (prabotulinumtoxinA-xvfs; Evolus, Inc., Santa Barbara, California), was approved by the FDA on February 1, 2019 for the temporary improvement in the appearance of moderate to severe glabellar lines in adult patients. Botulinum toxin type B (rimabotulinumtoxin B; Myobloc/Neurobloc; Solstice Neurosciences, Inc., South San Francisco, California) is the first botulinum toxin type B FDA approved for human use in the United States [13]. It is not favored for cosmetic use due to discomfort upon injection due to its acidic pH and the short duration of treatment effect [5, 13], though it does have faster onset [13]. Worldwide, there are several other BoNTA formulations known as PurTox, Neuronox, and BTX-A [13]. A topical formulation of BoNTA, RT001 by Revance Therapeutics, Inc. (Newark, CA), was under investigation for treatment of lateral canthal rhytids (crow's feet) and axillary hyperhidrosis [34], but in phase 3 trials, it did not achieve its endpoints and development was discontinued [35]. Since there is more information available and greater US experience with

Botox, all of the dosages and recommendations are based on Botox within this chapter.

Technique

The muscles targeted for BoNTA treatment lie at different depths; thus, a thorough understanding of facial anatomy is crucial [2] (Fig. 21.1). The treatment should be customized for each individual patient, and it is necessary to assess the patient's muscle tone, mass, activity, and strength in order to determine the proper dosage and placement [2]. The face should be observed at rest and with facial expression, and the muscles palpated prior to treatment [2].

A thorough history is important to ensure that the patient is not pregnant or breastfeeding. They should not have any neuromuscular disorders like Lambert-Eaton syndrome or allergy to human albumin. Botox is classified as a pregnancy category C drug as formal human studies in pregnancy have not been performed; however, reports indicate that women inadvertently treated during pregnancy have not experienced any sequelae [12]. A review of the patient's medications is necessary as aminoglycoside antibiotics can potentiate the effect of the toxin [1]. Aminoquinolones, calcium channel blockers, cyclosporine, and D-penicillamine can impact the effect of the toxin as well [1, 4]. Proper informed consent is imperative. It is important to elicit the patient expectations. In addition, proper education about the expected effects of treatment should be stressed along with the expected time of onset, maximum effect, and duration of results. The inability to fully treat static rhytids should be discussed as well [4].

Lidocaine can prolong the half-life of botulinum toxin; thus, co-administration is not recommended [7, 36]. Patients who have a history of botulism may have a reduced treatment effect due to antibody formation [1]. Patients with diabetes and alcoholism and those being treated with chemotherapy or immunosuppression are at increased risk of infection following any procedure [7]. Cleansing the skin prior to injection is important in every patient. In addition, injections should not be performed in any area of active infection [7]. It is also essential to carefully document the treatment in order to refer to later for future duplication or modification [2].

The vial of BoNTA can be reconstituted with different volumes of saline, but it is important to be consistent so that the concentration of the product is standardized. BoNTA is quite fragile because of the disulfide bond. It comes in a vial

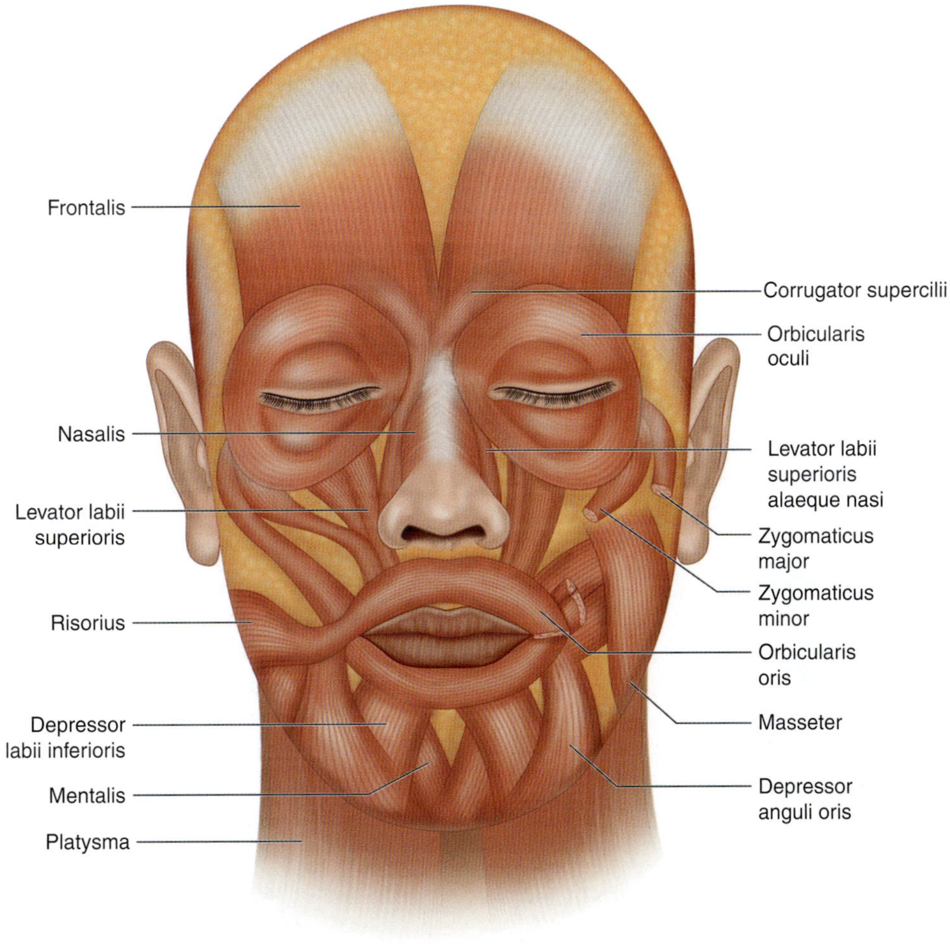

Fig. 21.1 Diagram of facial muscles, many of which are targets of BoNTA treatment

containing 50 or 100 units of freeze-dried toxin in a crystalline complex that should be immediately frozen (−20 °C) [1, 7]. It can be stored up to 24 months [7]. The Botox package insert advises that it be reconstituted with nonpreserved normal saline, but one study demonstrated that preserved saline was less painful [7, 37]. Preservatives also have subtle local anesthetic effects. In addition, microbial contamination may be reduced with preserved saline [7, 38]. On average, each point of injection is thought to denervate a 2.5–3-cm area [12]. One implication of a more dilute concentration is that due to the increased volume of the injected product, increased diffusion may occur [7, 39, 40]. Double-blinded studies have not demonstrated any statistically significant difference in safety or efficacy between concentrations [7, 41]. In addition, more dilute formulations with increased diffusion usually have a shorter duration of effect [12]. During reconstitution, it is important to allow alcohol to dry and to avoid turbulence when injecting saline in order to prevent denaturing the toxin [1]. If the vacuum in the vial does not draw in the dilutant, indicating loss of the negative pressure seal, the vial should not be used [7]. The toxin should be drawn using an 18-gauge needle and placed into either a tuberculin syringe or an insulin syringe. Recommendations on type of syringe and gauge of needle vary depending on injector preference; however, smaller gauge needles, i.e., 30 and 32 gauge, will reduce pain and risk of bruising [4] (Fig. 21.2). It is important to refrigerate the vial following reconstitution [1], but it should not be frozen because that will decrease the efficacy of the toxin [4]. Xeomin does not require refrigeration. There is no clear consensus regarding the appropriate length of time that a vial may be used following reconstitution; however, most practitioners have observed efficacy for at least 1 week post-reconstitution, and one study demonstrated equal efficacy up to 6 weeks later [7, 42].

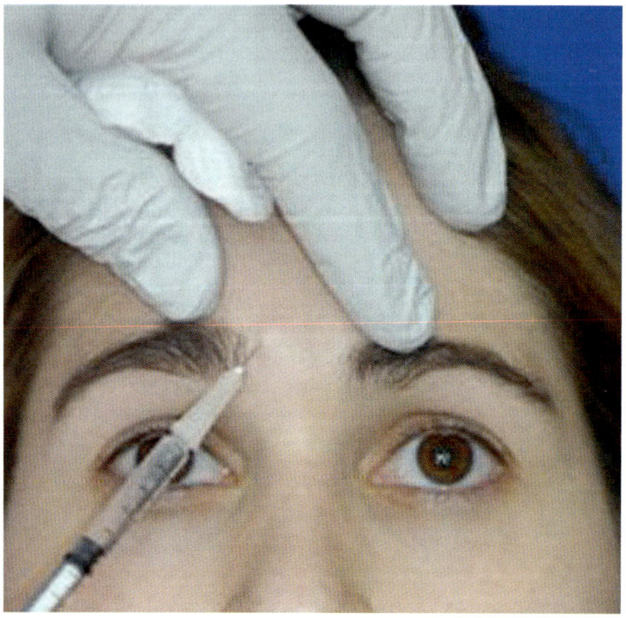

Fig. 21.2 Injection technique for BoNTA with standard needle and syringe combination

In order to minimize risk of bruising, the patient should hold aspirin and blood-thinning medications for 14 days if possible prior to treatment [1]. Patients may elect to take two herbal supplements, Arnica montana and bromelain, which may reduce the risk of bruising. Manual pressure is often applied to the injection site to help prevent bruising [33]. Anesthesia can be obtained by using ice or topical lidocaine preparations, but as previously mentioned, injected local anesthesia is contraindicated [1]. Some practitioners use pressure or vibration anesthesia as a means of improving patient comfort based on the gate-control theory [5].

In certain areas, the injection must be placed intramuscularly, i.e., corrugator, but in other areas, i.e., orbicularis oculi, subcutaneous injection is optimal [1]. EMG guidance is not usually necessary [1]. Many practitioners instruct patients to stay upright and avoid deep massage, saunas, or exercise for several hours following injections in order to minimize unwanted spread of the toxin [4, 7]. EMG studies have indicated the potential for spread to distant muscles, thus emphasizing the importance of precise placement and appropriate dosing [1, 4]. It is theorized that contraction of treated muscles may increase the uptake of the toxin and limit diffusion [1, 7, 12]. The onset of noticeable effect of the toxin is usually 3–7 days postinjection, but some patients notice improvement even earlier [1]. The peak of action is typically at 2–3 weeks, and the duration of effect ranges from 3 to 6 months [1] depending on the dosage used, area treated, and patient-dependent factors. It is not advisable to use both Botox and Dysport or Xeomin in the same treatment session as it would be difficult to discern which product was involved if there was a problem with the treatment [2]. In addition, the maximum Botox dose given in a procedure should not exceed 400 U [33].

Treatment Areas

The use of BoNTA in the upper face is well established, particularly for treatment of the glabella, forehead, and crow's feet [2]. In the upper face, dynamic wrinkling is the major sign of aging as the upper face is more muscular with less fat than the lower face [2]. In addition, treatment of the upper face is relatively predictable and safe [2], and higher treatment doses are tolerated in the upper face, as precise movement is not as essential as it is in the lower face. Higher doses are typically used in the upper face than in the lower face to achieve the amount of paralysis required to achieve optimal cosmetic results [43].

The agonist/antagonist relationship is crucial to facial augmentation with BoNTA [39]. In certain regions, injection of the antagonist allows the agonist to work unopposed, thus achieving the desired effect by altering the position of the overlying soft tissue [39]. While treatments should be individualized, consensus recommendations provide a reasonable guideline [2, 44]. The mass of the muscle, gender of the patient, prior exposure, and time interval since prior injection all influence the amount of toxin necessary for adequate treatment [4].

Upper Face

Important anatomic considerations in the upper face include the varying depth of the muscles and the presence of the frontal branches of the facial nerve, the supratrochlear and supraorbital complexes, and the lacrimal gland [2] in addition to the eye and orbit.

A placebo-controlled, double-blind study demonstrated what practitioners had previously observed that multiple areas of the upper face could be safely and effectively treated in a single session [5]. Treatment of the glabella targets the superficial procerus and deeper corrugator supercilii muscles [2] (Fig. 21.3). The procerus is a fan-shaped muscle originating from the nasal bones and inserting into the skin between the brows [7] which functions to draw the medial head of the eyebrows inferiorly, producing rhytids over the bridge of the nose [1]. The corrugator supercilii are paired muscles that originate near the junction of the frontal and nasal bones and pass through the orbicularis oculi and frontalis as they course laterally to insert in the skin in the midbrow [7]. The corrugator supercilii also draws the medial head of the eyebrows inferiorly but also medially, thus creating the vertical frown lines in the glabella [1]. Dosages for women range from 10 to 30 units and 20 to 40 units in men over one to ten sites [2, 5]. Several authors have described the glabellar injection technique [2, 7]. The glabellar area is particularly amenable to treatment as facial expressions involving these lines typically have negative connotations such as anger [26]. Rarely, upper eyelid ptosis has been described resulting from glabellar treatment [12]. This effect typically lasts for only a few weeks as it is due to distant diffusion through the septum affecting the levator muscle [4, 45]. Iatrogenic ptosis can be temporarily improved by the use of topical antihistamine or adrenergic eye drops [4, 45]. Apraclonidine 0.5% TID to the affected eye can accomplish the desired improvement [7].

The frontalis muscle is responsible for horizontal forehead rhytids (Fig. 21.4). The frontalis is a thin muscle that originates from the galea aponeurotica and inserts into the skin of the brow [7]. The frontalis elevates the brow and opposes the action of the brow depressors [7]. The frontalis does not extend as far laterally as the lateral brow retractors, the orbital portion of the orbicularis oculi [7]. The treatment of horizontal forehead rhytids is particularly variable. The target is the frontalis muscle in each case, but the height of the forehead and pattern of the rhytids merit evaluation. In general, a dose of 6–15 units distributed over four to eight sites is used [5]. The previous recommendations were for higher doses in this area, but it has since been modified [5]. It is recommended to remain 1.5–2 cm above the brow margin to minimize brow droop [2]. Some choose to extend the injections lateral enough to avoid an excessively peaked brow contour [2]; however, particular care should be taken when injecting lateral to the midpupil to

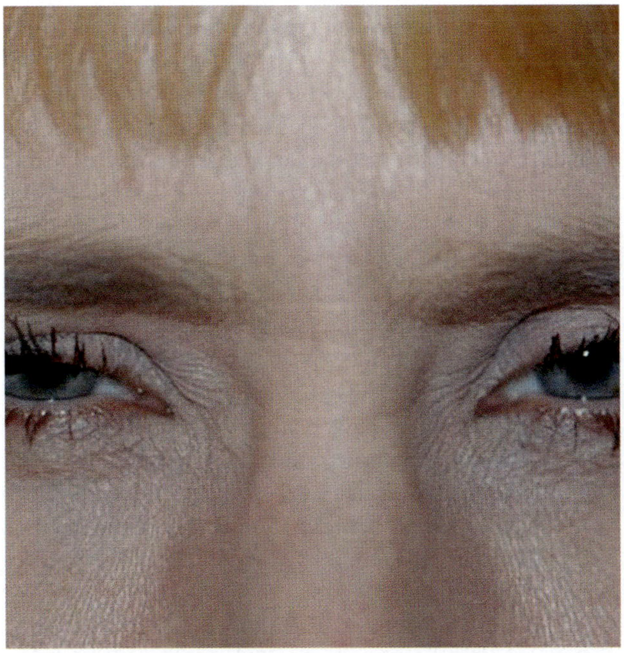

Fig. 21.3 The photo demonstrates glabellar frown lines. This is the original FDA-approved treatment area for cosmetic BoNTA

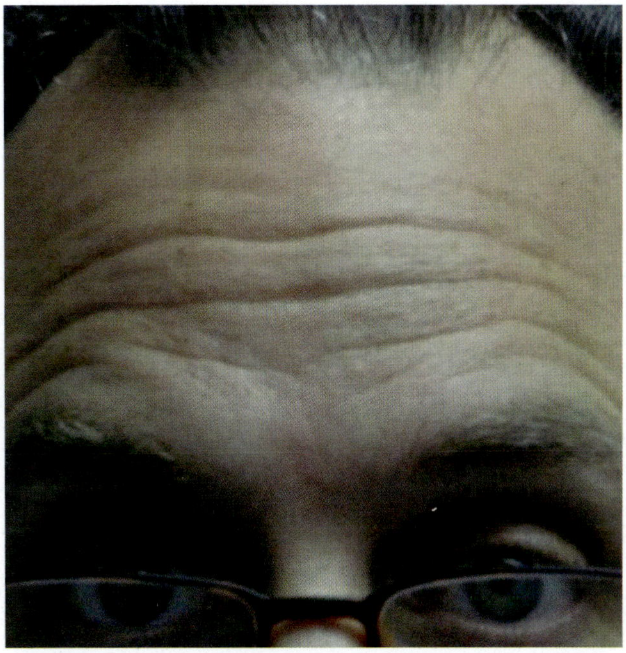

Fig. 21.4 Horizontal forehead rhytids

avoid lateral brow ptosis. Superficial injection as opposed to deeper injections near the periosteum may reduce the risk of brow ptosis [4]. Treatment of the frontalis should be avoided in patients with severe preexisting brow ptosis [3]. Occasionally, treatment of the frontalis may unmask upper eyelid ptosis as patients often compensate for ptosis by raising their brows; thus, pretreatment assessment needs to be attentive to this possibility [4]. Older patients should be treated with a decreased number of units in this area relative to a younger patient [5]. In addition, most injectors prefer not to overtreat the frontalis which can lead to a "frozen" look [5]. In general, doses greater than 20 units in this area lead to a less-than-optimal outcome [5]. One technique used to weaken but not paralyze the frontalis is to inject very small doses subcutaneously rather than into the muscle at 1–2-cm intervals across the forehead [12, 46]. Intradermal injection of small doses of BoNTA is also used to improve skin texture and pore size [47].

Lateral canthal rhytids (crow's feet) occur due to the action of the orbicularis oculi muscle, which is circumferential surrounding the eye and divided into three parts [2] (Fig. 21.5). Contraction of the orbital component is usually the underlying source of lateral canthal rhytids [1]. In addition to formation of lateral canthal rhytids, repeated contraction of the orbicularis oculi, as with squinting and smiling, contributes to lower eyelid orbicularis oculi hypertrophy, lateral brow ptosis, and the development of lateral canthal disinsertion [3]. For adequate chemodenervation of the orbicularis oculi, typically 10–30+ units spread among two to five plus sites are used [2, 5]. The injections should be placed tangentially at or outside the orbital rim to minimize diffusion [2]. Also, the lateral portion of the orbital component should be targeted as this area pulls down the tail of the eyebrow with forced contraction [2]. Injection should be performed 1.5 cm from the lateral canthus to avoid a ridge extending laterally [2]. The periocular area has numerous vessels, so it is particularly prone to bruising [2, 48]. Magnification with loupes can help visually identify vessels and help avoid puncturing them. Subcutaneous rather than intramuscular injection can minimize the risk of ecchymosis by enabling treatment of a larger area with a fewer number of punctures [4]. Generally, it is best not to inject too far medially on the lower lid to avoid scleral show, retraction, ectropion, lagophthalmos, and epiphora [4]. In addition, injecting too far inferiorly can affect the zygomaticus major muscle and lead to lip ptosis, drooling, and an asymmetric smile [4] as this muscle is located deep to the inferior fibers of orbicularis [7]. Patients who have severe dry eyes or lower eyelid malposition are not good candidates for botulinum toxin treatment for lateral canthal rhytids.

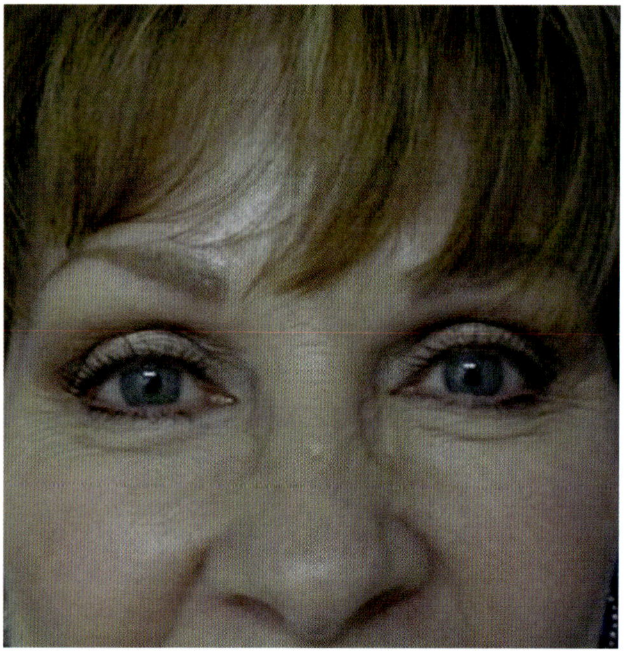

Fig. 21.5 Lateral canthal rhytids or "crow's feet"

Brow ptosis is influenced by repeated action of the lateral orbicularis oculi muscle that weakens the lateral brow-retaining ligaments [3]. The lateral brow is more affected than the medial brow, as the frontalis does not extend laterally past the arcuate line; thus, the action of the orbicularis oculi on the tail of the brow is unopposed [3]. The procerus and corrugator supercilii and to a small degree the medial portion of the orbicularis oculi act as depressors of the medial brow, while the lateral orbital portion of the orbicularis oculi depresses the lateral brow. A lift of 1–2 mm can be accomplished by chemodenervation of the brow depressors [4, 27]. For patients with mild brow ptosis or asymmetry, this may be sufficient. For patients with more substantial brow ptosis, a surgical brow lift is necessary to accomplish appropriate correction [27]. The ideal contour of the brow in women is thought to consist of an arch with maximal height at the level of the lateral canthus and the medial and lateral portions located at the same horizontal level [49]. Brow contouring to attain a proper arch can be achieved by chemodenervation of both the frontalis centrally over the medial portion of the brow and the lateral orbicularis oculi (brow retractors) [3] or the procerus and corrugator for selective brow elevation. In particular, careful placement of the injections in the frontalis muscle can achieve the desired brow peak at the lateral limbus by injecting the frontalis 2–3 cm higher in that location than the other injections [49]. The risk of blepharoptosis is higher in this particular region as well [48] but can be minimized by careful placement and by using a high toxin concentration of 1 U/0.01 cc (i.e., reconstitution of Botox with 1 cc of saline) [50]. Treatment of the glabella alone can raise the medial portion of the brow, which many find to be aesthetically displeasing [49].

However, treatment of the adjacent frontalis neutralizes this effect [48]. If an overly peaked brow appearance results, this can be easily corrected by placing 1–3 units in the untreated frontalis fibers above the peaked area [5, 48]. For patients in the entertainment industry who need to maintain animated expression, lower doses with placement of 7–10 units in the glabella and only up to 2.5 units in the supralateral brow for a total of 10–14 units can provide aesthetic improvement and still permit movement [50]. Studies demonstrate that nonsurgical brow lifting is more effective in younger patients than in older patients likely due to the diminished action of the frontalis muscle on the brow associated with soft tissue ptosis [49].

Palpebral fissure asymmetry can also be improved with BoNTA treatment. The modification of the agonist (orbicularis oculi) or antagonist (upper lid elevators or lower lid retractors) can influence lid height [45]. Injection of low doses (1–2 units) of BoNTA into the lateral aspect of the lower eyelid and in the pretarsal orbicularis at midpupil can improve orbicularis hypertrophy with associated lower lid elevation or confer greater symmetry in cases of unilateral lower eyelid retraction by treating the non-retracted lid [45]. It has been described that upper eyelid retraction can be improved by injection of low doses of BoNTA transconjunctivally into Mueller's muscle, though this application risks substantial ptosis. In addition, the observation has been made that in a certain subset of patients with upper eyelid retraction, treatment of the brow lowers the retracted upper lid [45]. These patients are typically contact lens wearers [45]. BoNTA treatment has also been demonstrated to be effective in treating mild upper eyelid ptosis by placing 1-unit doses in the lateral and medial pretarsal orbicularis oculi [45]. In this situation, Hering's law applies typically as one would expect [45]. Particular care must be taken when using BoNTA for palpebral fissure asymmetry. There is greater risk of lagophthalmos, exposure, worsening ptosis, and epiphora with this technique [45].

Treatment of lower eyelid rhytids should target the preseptal orbicularis rather than the pretarsal as it is more effective in treating the peripheral portions of the rhytids and has less risk of unwanted side effects [45]. The technique is well described [51]. The hypertrophic orbicularis, however, has been reportedly improved by injection of 2 U of Botox into the lower pretarsal orbicularis [33]. Patients with a history of poor snap test, prior lower eyelid blepharoplasty, or lower eyelid resurfacing are not good candidates for this treatment unless they had canthopexy to support the lower eyelid position [33, 45].

Midface

Facial rejuvenation of the mid- and lower face and neck is more complex than the upper face as volumetric changes predominate here as opposed to the dynamic muscle effects of the upper face [2]. Much lower doses are used in order to preserve proper function and appearance of the mouth. Some of the feared side effects of treatment in this area include an asymmetric smile, drooling from an incompetent mouth, and problems with biting a flaccid cheek [12].

The nasalis muscle originates from the dorsal portion of the nose and inserts onto the maxilla and the skin of the nose above the ala [7]. Contraction of this muscle leads to rhytids along the lateral nasal wall commonly referred to as "bunny lines" (Fig. 21.6). Treating bunny lines is a nice complement to treatment of the glabella and involves placement of 2–5 units between two sites into the nasalis [2]. Treatment of the glabella alone can accentuate bunny lines [3] as recruitment of the nasalis occurs with attempts to contract the glabella [7]. Care should be taken to place the injections above the nasofacial groove to avoid affecting the levator labii superioris and subsequent upper lip ptosis [27, 33]. Optimal placement is into the belly of the upper nasalis as it crosses the nasal bone [33]. The injections should be placed high on the lateral nasal wall inferior to the angular vein in order to avoid substantial bruising [33].

Zygomaticus smile lines often connect to the lower lateral canthal rhytids, and if the orbicularis alone is treated, these lines can worsen because of descent of redundant cheek skin [27]. The zygomaticus can be carefully weakened to improve the midfacial contour in this situation, though this is a very advanced application with a high risk of unwanted side effects [27]. Treatment should be placed in the origin of the zygomaticus major [3]. Typically, only 1–2 units are injected per side [33]. Lip ptosis and increased prominence of a malar bag may result from this despite careful placement and low doses used [3].

The nasolabial fold is affected by the levator labii superioris alaeque nasi along the medial aspect of the fold and the levator labii superioris on the middle of the fold [4]. The zygomaticus muscles additionally influence the nasolabial fold [3, 4]. Improvement in the nasolabial fold with che-

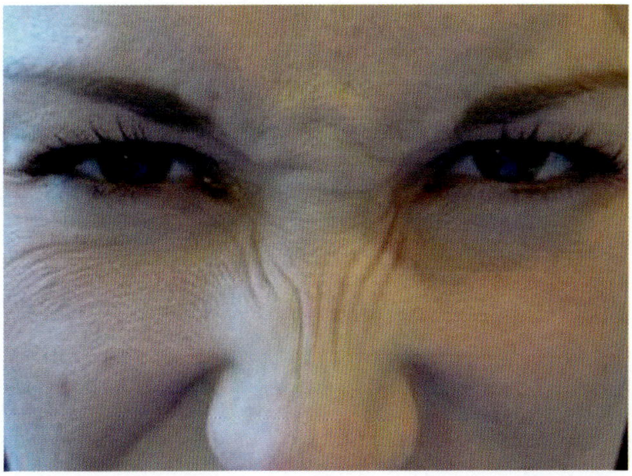

Fig. 21.6 Bunny lines (nasalis muscle)

modenervation has been attempted; however, most of the results were unsatisfactory [4], and other modalities may be preferable for rejuvenation of this area [4]. Two to three units can be injected under EMG guidance into the levator labii superioris alaeque nasi [33]. Injection directly into the nasolabial fold can cause upper lip ptosis and an asymmetric smile [33].

Alteration of the nose can also be achieved with BoNTA. Excessive involuntary nostril flaring can be ameliorated with injection of five units on each side of the nostril in the nasalis where the lower nasalis fibers pass over the lateral nasal ala in the area of maximal muscle contraction [4, 33]. This treatment can, however, lead to elongation of the upper lip, which in many patients is undesirable. Nasal tip droop is caused by the action of the depressor septi and can be improved with injection of 2–3 units at the base of the columella [33]. This will slightly elevate the nasal tip, but there is a risk of lip ptosis with this procedure [33].

Patients concerned about a "gummy smile" may observe some improvement with targeting of the levator labii superioris alaeque nasi and zygomaticus major [2]. Approximately 5–7.5 units can be injected 5 mm lateral to the inferior aspect of the nostril to weaken the levator labii superioris alaeque nasi and 1–3 units in the zygomaticus major [2].

Lower Face

Vertical lip lines result from repeated animation (i.e., smoking) and volume loss [3] (Fig. 21.7). The orbicularis oris originates from the mandible and maxilla and runs circumferentially around the mouth with superficial fibers inserting into the skin and deep fibers inserting into the lip mucosa [7]. Multiple modalities have been utilized for perioral rejuvenation including injectable fillers and laser or microdermabrasion [3]. The vertical lines are softened using 4–5 [5, 27] units in 2–11 sites placed carefully and symmetrically in the orbicularis oris [2]. Low doses of BoNTA should be placed at the vermillion border and only for deeper lines [27] to soften the lip sphincter. In addition, do not inject the philtrum or Cupid's bow as flattening of these areas is not attractive [33]. The corners of the lips should be avoided to prevent drooping of the corner of the mouth [33]. No more than 2 units per lip quadrant should be placed [33]. In addition to softening the lines, eversion of the vermilion border occurs creating more upper lip show [3]. An alternative injection technique is to thread the injection evenly across the upper lip on each side sparing the philtrum, which is thought to provide a more natural result [7, 52]. Treatment of the orbicularis oris should not be performed in people who play wind instruments, professional singers, or speakers [33].

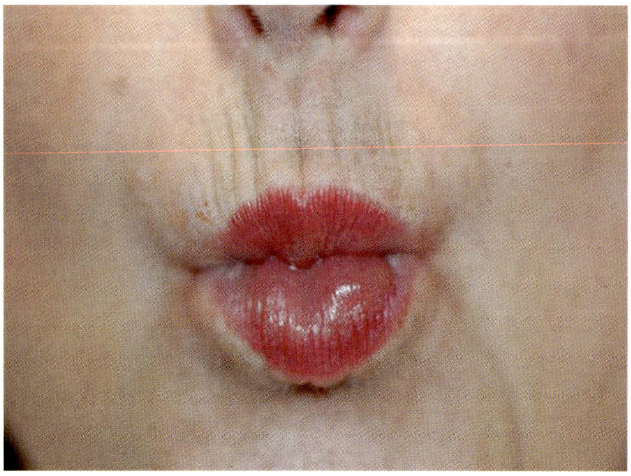

Fig. 21.7 Perioral rhytids or "lipstick lines" or "smoker's lines"

The depressor anguli oris originates on the mandible and inserts at the modiolus [7]. This muscle helps control the resting position of the oral commissures and upon contraction turns the corners of the mouth downward [7]. Over time, this muscle contributes to the development of rhytids extending inferiorly from the mouth resembling a marionette mouth; thus, they are referred to as marionette lines or labiomandibular fold. Marionette lines can be improved by weakening the depressor anguli oris with a total of 4–6 units over two sites [2], one on each side anterior to the masseter near the mandible to avoid diffusion into the depressor labii inferioris and an asymmetric smile. In particular, the injection should be placed quite inferior and lateral to the mouth, specifically more than 1 cm lateral to the oral commissure and near the inferior border of the mandible [7]. Care should be taken to avoid the marginal mandibular branch of the facial artery which courses along the edge of the mandible at the anterior part of the masseter and can be palpated [2].

The mentalis elevates the soft tissue of the chin [7]. It originates from the anterior mandible, interdigitates with fibers from the platysma, and inserts into the skin of the chin [7]. A hyperactive mentalis can lead to a deep transverse mental crease and a peau d'orange appearance of the chin as the mentalis fibers insert on the skin [7]. The appearance of a pebbly chin can be remedied by placing 4–10 units in one to two sites in the mentalis by injecting along the inferior aspect of the chin in a perpendicular fashion [5]. Alternatively, a total of 10 units in several injections can be placed subcutaneously at least 1 centimeter inferior to the mental sulcus to avoid unwanted effects on the mouth [4]. Other authors recommend 5–10 units into the mentalis at the prominence of the chin [33]. For horizontal mentalis creases, injection of 3–5 units into the mentalis at the bony mentum can soften the crease and avoid unwanted weakening of the orbicularis oris [33].

The use of botulinum toxin for treatment of masseter muscle hypertrophy was first reported in 1994 [53]. It can improve facial contour by smoothing a square jaw [53]. It has become quite popular among the Asian population. An initial dose of 10–20 units per masseter is recommended divided among two to four injections along the inferior edge of the masseter, deep within the muscle [5, 7, 54]. This treatment is associated with local side effects that affect form and function [53]. Difficulty in chewing foods and a sunken appearance of the cheeks have been described [7, 55]. Avoid injecting the masseter too far superiorly or anteriorly to minimize side effects [7]. For patients with asymmetric jaw movement, intraoral injection of 10–15 units into the internal pterygoid can relax the jaw, which eases discomfort with chewing [33].

Botulinum toxin injection will not improve lipodystrophy or static rhytids, but it can improve the effects of a hyperkinetic platysma [4]. The platysma is a wide, thin muscle that depresses the skin of the lower face and neck [7]. It originates from the fascia overlying the pectoralis and deltoid muscles and inserts into the skin of the lower face and neck and superficial musculoaponeurotic system (SMAS) [7]. Horizontal necklines can be improved with injections of 1–2 units in the deep intradermal plane placed 1 cm apart for 10–15 units total [4, 33]. The appearance of vertical platysmal bands can be treated with careful injection of 10–30 units in women and up to 40 units in men distributed in 2–12 sites [2]. Typically less than 10 units per band or up to 40–60 units per treatment session is effective [5]. It is important to grasp the band and inject into the muscle and limit the dose in order to avoid deeper laryngeal and pharyngeal side effects [2, 33]. It is important to avoid injecting the sternocleidomastoid, which can lead to neck weakness [12]. Botox can be used to create a nonsurgical jaw lift by placing 2–3 units superficially 1–1.5 cm apart along the mandibular jaw line lateral to the nasolabial folds, along the mandibular ramus and down any platysmal bands [7]. A dose of 30 units should not be exceeded [7].

Adjuvant Use

BoNTA is also a useful adjunct to other facial cosmetic procedures. BoNTA can effectively complement and enhance soft tissue augmentation with fillers and fat. This combination achieves more optimal correction than either product alone. In addition, the longevity of correction is improved [1, 10, 39]. The mechanism of the collaborative benefit is thought to be reduced extrusion of the product and stress due to adjacent muscle action [39].

BoNTA treatment of the brow depressors is a particularly useful adjunct to surgical brow lifting. This reduces the resistance to brow repositioning, thus enabling more secure healing of the brow in the elevated position [1, 10, 27, 39].

Pretreatment of lateral canthal rhytids can improve the aesthetic outcome of cosmetic blepharoplasty by eliminating the need to extend the incision past the orbital rim in order to soften the crow's feet [27]. In addition, chemodenervation enables more accurate estimation of the amount of skin to be removed [27]. With brow asymmetry, pretreatment of the relatively ptotic brow will enhance symmetry and prevent over-excision of upper eyelid skin [27].

Lower lid tightening can be aided by chemodenervation of the lateral orbital orbicularis fibers which place medial traction on lateral canthal wounds as part of the lacrimal pump, which would help improve wound security and reduce wound dehiscence [1, 27, 39].

Laser resurfacing yields initial improvement, but if the underlying hyperdynamic muscle action is not appropriately addressed, new folds may emerge that are more evident than prior to treatment [1, 10, 27]. The most common areas of recurrent post-laser rhytids are glabellar furrows and periocular and perioral rhytids [39]. Botox pretreatment should occur approximately 1 week prior to laser resurfacing [39]. Care should be taken to avoid injecting close to the lower eyelid margin to prevent subsequent lower lid retraction or ectropion [39]. Interestingly, in patients pretreated with BoNTA prior to laser resurfacing, the duration of Botox effect is somewhat shortened for unknown reasons [39].

BoNTA can also be useful in rhytidectomy procedures because despite plication of the platysma, banding can recur, which can be treated with BoNTA [27]. In addition, post-facelift synkinesis resulting from damage to the buccal branch of the facial nerve can be improved by injection of 1–2 units of BoNTA into the levator labii superioris after careful localization with EMG [27].

BoNTA has also been a useful adjunct for facial reconstruction, particularly in the forehead. It functions to provide immobilization of the wound in order to limit tractional forces, which reduces hypertrophy, width, and pigmentation of a wound [7]. A double-blind study demonstrated that a single treatment of Botox following simple closure of forehead wounds improved the cosmetic outcome at 6 months [7, 56]. BoNTA is also being studied as a possible treatment option for improvement of rosacea as well as hair loss [57, 58].

Complications

Lack of effect is the most common adverse reaction. This is usually due to an inadequate number of units injected in a given area. Reported adverse reactions with the use of BoNTA for all approved conditions include globe perforation, retrobulbar hemorrhage, Adie's pupil, lagophthalmos, dry eye, exposure keratitis, epiphora, ectropion, ptosis, and diplopia. Other undesirable effects with cosmetic use include bruising, brow abnormalities (ptosis, asymmetry, exaggerated peaking), eyelid retraction, asymmetric smile, lip dysfunction, and mouth droop [1]. Oral use of 60-mg pyridostigmine has been described to counteract some of the side effects of BoNTA [5]. Due to the high side effect profile of this medication, however, routine use is discouraged [5]. Headache is a well-described occurrence following BoNTA treatment; however, this is usually temporary. It is thought to be due to initial muscle spasm, which subsequently relaxes [12]. BoNTA has demonstrated a role in reducing migraine frequency, severity, and abortive medication use [7, 59]. OnabotulinumtoxinA received FDA approval for treatment of chronic migraine in 2010 [60]. Neutralizing antibodies have not been described with cosmetic use [7], and antibodies against one serotype are not thought to block the biologic activity of another serotype [12]. Antibody formation relates to protein load, and the newer formulation has an exceedingly low rate of antibody formation at 1–2% [1, 12] which is thought to be more likely related to overall dose exceeding 300 units and less to treatment interval [12]. Only a few reports of acute type I reactions to BoNTA exist [12].

The discovery and development of BoNTA have revolutionized the aesthetic realm. There are countless applications for BoNTA treatment. It is overall safe and well tolerated with very high degree of patient satisfaction.

Dermal Fillers

History

The concept of manufactured fillers began in 1899 when the first use of paraffin was described by Gersuny who reported injection of paraffin into the scrotum of a young man to replace resected testicles [61]. Subsequently, paraffin was described for use in the face in 1907 [61]. Unfortunately, this practice resulted in numerous granulomas, emboli, infection, and yellowish skin plaques and was ultimately found to be unacceptable [62–64]. In the following years, mineral oil, lanolin, beeswax, and vegetable oil were used for cosmetic injections but were also found to have too many undesirable side effects [64]. In the 1920s, rubber and purified latex were used as filling agents [61]. In the 1960s, medical-grade liquid silicone began being used off-label for facial augmentation [62]. For the next 30 years, silicone in various forms continued to be used [63]. The first approved facial filler was bovine collagen, which was granted FDA approval in 1981 [62]. Dermal fillers are approved for correction of moderate to severe wrinkles and folds (i.e., nasolabial folds) with product placement in the mid- to deep dermis [65]. Various approved cosmetic uses include treatment of moderate to severe facial wrinkles and folds, such as the nasolabial folds, for most products. Several products have other approved indications such as Radiesse for volume loss on the back of the hand, Juvederm Voluma for volume loss of the cheek, Belotero Balance for wrinkles and folds especially around the nose and mouth, and Sculptra for shallow to deep folds and other facial wrinkles [66]. Filler products have been used and approved for non-cosmetic purposes such as improvement of cutaneous defects, HIV-associated lipodystrophy, anophthalmic orbit, unilateral paralysis of the vocal cords, augmentation of the lip and palate in cleft palate patients, and as a bulking agent for the esophageal sphincter in GERD and the anus and bladder neck for incontinence [67]. The ideal filler is safe, stable, long-lasting, volumizing, natural looking [68], and pliable, will not migrate, does not induce a foreign body reaction, does not require skin testing, is painless, and will not cause granulomas [67–69]. Filler products may be derived from a patient's own tissue (autogenic), another human (allogenic), animal, or bioengineering of bacteria (xenogenic) or synthetic [62].

Treatment Areas

Upper Face

Dynamic lines are best treated initially with BoNTA; however, residual static furrows may be corrected with dermal fillers [65]. A study demonstrated that a combination of BoNTA and hyaluronic acid filler treatment of glabellar rhytids resulted in improved outcomes compared to hyaluronic acid filler alone in both overall improvement and duration of improvement [5]. Historically, intradermal injection of a hyaluronic acid filler corrected superficial rhytids, but deeper furrows were better addressed with thicker products [65]; however, with the advent of thicker, more versatile hyaluronic acid products, that is no longer the case. Treatment of the glabella typically involves very low volume of filler (<0.25 cc most often) with placement of the product in the superficial to mid-dermis [5]. Care should be taken to aspirate prior to injecting in order to prevent intravascular injection and avoid compressing vessels [5]. Dermal fillers may be used in the forehead for filling of various defects, but softer products are optimal to avoid beading [5]. Fluid, non-particulate hyaluronic acids are the most suitable products to place in the forehead [70]. Bunny lines may be softened with a soft filler product [5], but special care should be taken to avoid the angular vessels.

The crow's feet may be treated with a small amount of a soft filler product. Usually, 0.25 cc or less is injected, and hyaluronic acid fillers should be placed deeply to avoid the Tyndall effect [5]. The Tyndall effect is a blue-gray discoloration that occurs particularly in the eyelid area as the eyelid skin is the thinnest in the body, approximately 400–500 microns on average [71]. The Tyndall effect is specific to hyaluronic acid fillers and occurs due to the fact that blue is the shortest wavelength of light, and it is more easily scattered and reflected than the longer red wavelengths that penetrate deeper in tissue [72].

In addition to brow contouring with BoNTA, the vast majority of practitioners use filler to replace volume in the brow area [5]. Filler can be placed in the temple and under the lateral brow to enhance brow contour and provide a lateral brow elevation. This can be combined with BoNTA at the tail of the brow to achieve a very pleasing result [5]. Hyaluronic acid fillers should be placed superficially in the immediate subcutaneous plane [71], while fat and other permanent fillers should be injected between the galea aponeurosis and the periosteum [71]. Care should be taken to place the products lateral to the supraorbital complex to avoid intravascular injection or damage to the nerves [71].

Another application is correction of age-related volume loss in the temples [5]. With aging, the temporal fossa becomes increasingly hollow due to a combination of increased concavity of the temporal bone, temporalis muscle atrophy, and reduction in the volume of the temporal fat pad [71]. There are three possible planes for soft tissue augmentation in the temple area. Subcutaneous injection of dermal fillers in a cross-hatched fashion adequately restores volume in this area and is best suited for hyaluronic acid fillers [65, 71]. In addition, injection just deep to the temporoparietal fascia is another option for hyaluronic acid fillers [71]. Placement of autologous fat or permanent fillers should be done in the plane deep to the temporalis muscle to avoid migration or clumping of the product [71].

A nonsurgical lower eyelid lift can be accomplished by careful placement of filler injected in small amounts (typically 0.2–0.3 cc) in the tear trough [5]. It is important to avoid the inferior oblique muscle, infraorbital nerve, and periorbital blood vessels [5]. Hyaluronic acids and autologous fat are most suitable in this dangerous and difficult area [70].

Midface

Restoration of volume is the key principle in rejuvenation of the midface. In general, malar contour is restored first followed by the orbital-malar groove and nasojugal fold [5]. Placement in this order helps lift the cheeks, thus minimizing the nasolabial fold and often eliminating the need to treat the tear trough, which is a more challenging technique [5]. The infraorbital hollow, malar smile lines, nasolabial fold, and nasal dorsum and tip can also be addressed with filler agents [5]. Care should be taken to avoid the globe, infraorbital nerve, and numerous blood vessels [5]. Knowledge of the anatomy of the sub-orbicularis oculi fat pads (medial and lateral) and their relationship to the deep cheek fat is important for successful volume augmentation in this area [73]. For restoring malar projection, several bulkier products work well. Injection may be submuscular or subdermal [5]. Malar smile lines are nicely corrected with 0.2–0.4 cc per side. Deep dermal or subdermal placement is optimal in this region [5].

The product should be placed deeply, particularly in the nasojugal fold and tear trough deformity where the Tyndall effect is problematic. This area can be difficult to achieve a good result [65]. The patient should be seated upright in order to determine proper product placement as the contour can be different when supine due to the fat pad changes with gravity [65]. The product should be placed pre-periosteal along the orbital rim in order to avoid worsening the fat pad pseudo-herniation that creates the original uneven contour [65]. Tangential placement should be used as direct penetration with bolus placement can lead to extrusion of the material and nodule formation. A small volume of product is placed in multiple passes for the tear trough with a typical range of 0.1–0.2 cc per eyelid [5]. Undercorrection is preferred, and many routinely see the patient again in 2–4 weeks to determine if additional product is needed [5]. Correction of several years may be achieved since this area is relatively immobile [65]. The infraorbital hollow is generally treated using 0.2–0.5 cc injected per side, and care should be taken to avoid injecting deep to the orbital septum [5].

The nasolabial fold is one of the most satisfying areas for dermal filler placement (Fig. 21.8). It is the main region that is FDA approved for treatment. On average, 0.5–1.0 cc/side is placed in a layered fashion. Massage is particularly helpful in this area [5]. Linear threading is the technique of choice, and care should be taken when withdrawing the needle to avoid superficial placement of the product, which can lead to a nodular texture [65].

Contouring of the nasal dorsum or tip can be accomplished with a variety of filler agents. Specifically, fillers can recontour the saddlenose and nasal tip through careful placement and help elevate the nasal tip by injecting at the base of the columella [5]. Some believe that injection of filler at the bridge of

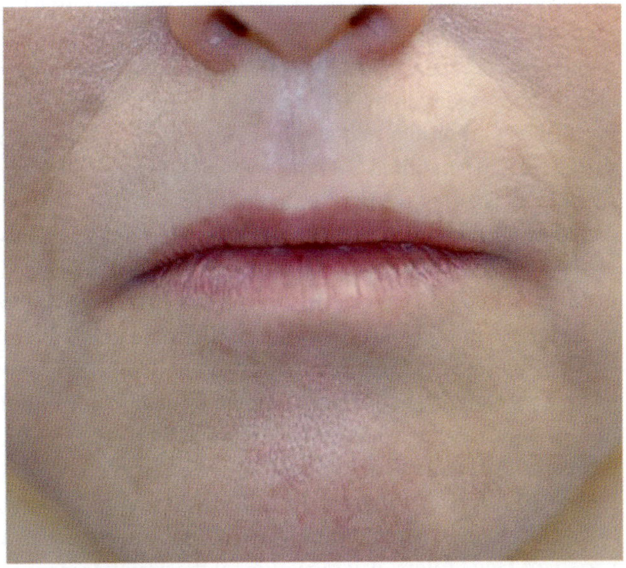

Fig. 21.8 Nasolabial folds

the nose can help soften the appearance of epicanthal folds in Asian patients. Care should be taken to avoid injecting deeply in the nasal septum, and practitioners should exercise caution in order to avoid overfilling this area. Most injectors place less than 0.5 cc in the nasal dorsum and tip. This procedure can be used after rhinoplasty to refine the results [5]. There are notable risks which will be described later.

Lower Face

The lower face is the area most commonly treated with facial fillers [65]. The lower face is particularly susceptible to aging changes. The development of perioral rhytids (lipstick lines), wrinkled lips, downturned oral commissures, marionette lines, and irregular chin lines is particularly distressing to patients [5]. Descent of the malar fat pad worsens nasolabial folds and the prejowl sulcus [65].

The orbicularis oris muscle largely influences the development of perioral rhytids. The marionette lines result from the actions of the depressor anguli oris on the oral commissures. Lip changes can consist of overall volume loss, flattening of the Cupid's bow, reduced vermillion border, and overall vertical elongation [5]. Loss of the deep fat below the orbicularis oris muscle and the mentalis muscle contributes to the deflated lip appearance and must be adequately restored by careful placement of fillers [74]. Rejuvenation of the lower face must restore volume and control muscle movement to a tolerable degree [5]. Large volumes of fillers are typically not used in the lower face, as it is such a mobile, active area.

As the lips are the focal point of the lower face, restoring volume in the lips can greatly enhance one's appearance. Treatment of this area is painful; thus, many practitioners used to block the infraorbital and mental nerves [65], however many filler products now include lidocaine which has reduced the need for an anesthetic block. The majority of practitioners use 1.0 cc to fill the vermillion border and restore volume within the lip itself [5]. Retrograde linear threading is used to fill the vermillion border. The Cupid's bow and lateral commissures may also be improved with the addition of filler. Serial puncture or linear threading in the mid-dermis is used to fill the perioral rhytids [65]. The philtral columns may be filled as well. Care should be taken not to overfill the lips, and attention to detail regarding the proportion and contour of the upper and lower lips is important [5]. Hyaluronic acid products are the best tolerated in this area. Radiesse has been associated with nodule formation in the lips, so it is no longer recommended for use in this area.

The marionette lines are nicely filled using a cross-hatching technique, and many different products can be used in this area to achieve a satisfactory effect (Fig. 21.9). Concurrent treatment of the lateral commissures complements the effect of the marionette line correction. In addition, chin and jaw contouring may be performed using a variety of facial fillers. Augmentation of the prejowl sulcus is quite effective, but avoid overcorrection.

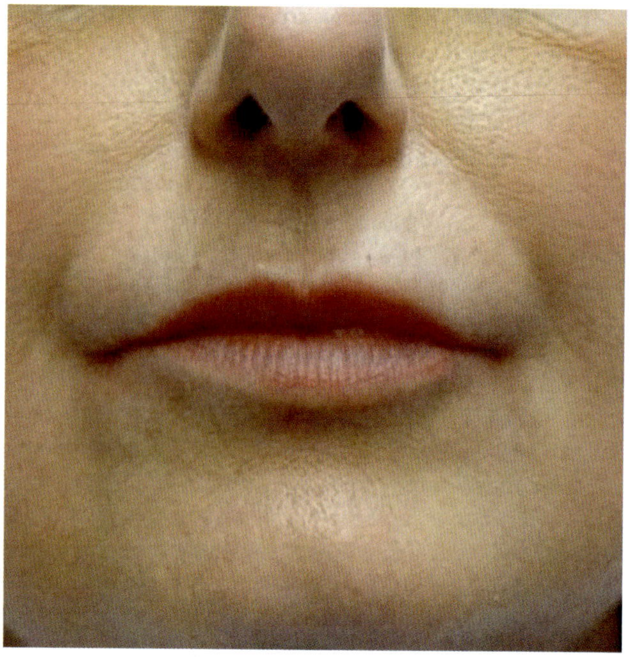

Fig. 21.9 Marionette lines

There are several other applications of fillers in the lower face. The appearance of chin implants may be softened by placement of hyaluronic acid fillers adjacent to the implant to soften the transition to native tissue. There may be some benefit for treating acne scars by using hyaluronic acid fillers, particularly to restore volume in atrophic scars. Textural changes are best addressed by laser resurfacing or chemical peels. The effects of which can be enhanced by the use of sunblock and cosmeceuticals. Fillers should not be used in actively inflamed or infected areas [5].

Technique

Pretreatment recommendations include cessation of blood-thinning agents for 14 days prior to treatment in order to minimize bruising [75]. Arnica montana [76] and bromelain are herbal supplements that may be used in patients without coagulopathy or heart disease in order to minimize bruising. Careful documentation of any allergies is important. Product selection must take into account the patient goals and medical history [70]. If lower face, especially lip, augmentation with facial fillers is planned, antiviral prophylaxis against HSV must be provided if the patient has a history of cold sores. Informed consent must be obtained with each treatment. The face should be cleansed with an antiseptic such as isopropyl alcohol or Betadine. Pretreatment photos must be taken to adequately document appearance before and after treatment [75].

Anesthesia may be obtained using several different methods. EMLA cream (lidocaine 2.5% and prilocaine 2.5% in an emulsion base) (AstraZeneca Canada, Inc., Mississauga, Ontario) or betacaine/lidocaine/tetracaine should be applied for 30 minutes prior to treatment [77]. Ice or blown freezing air provides anesthesia and minimizes bruising by constricting blood vessels [65, 75]. A 0.2 cc of 1% lidocaine with 1:100,000 epinephrine may be mixed with a filler product not already containing lidocaine to facilitate anesthesia. Occasionally, dental blocks of 2% lidocaine are used to block the infraorbital and mental nerves for lip augmentation or if a patient is very pain intolerant for nasolabial fold augmentation, but beware that tissue distortion may occur with the dental block. Ice packs may be applied throughout the procedure to improve comfort and minimize swelling [75]. Some practitioners also use vibration or pressure anesthesia to improve patient comfort [5].

Administration of the filler product is typically done using 28- to 32-gauge needles half-inch to 1 ¼ inch on prefilled syringes. It is helpful to minimize the number of needlesticks [75]. In addition, many practitioners are using blunt cannulas to place filler products. One of the most crucial factors in safe and successful facial augmentation is slow injection rate [75]. Inject slowly (<0.3 cc per minute) and apply gentle pressure to the syringe to avoid traumatizing the tissue [5]. In addition, slow injection speed is less painful [75]. The filler should be massaged or molded to distribute it evenly and carefully assess the effect [5]. Vigorous massage should be avoided in order to minimize swelling [75].

Depth of placement is dependent on the viscosity of the product [62, 69]. Deeper defects should be treated with more viscous filler, which should be placed in deep dermis or subdermis. More superficial defects need shallow correction, and less viscous fillers work better for this and should be placed in the upper dermis, which may cause blanching at the time of the filler placement [65]. Product selection is influenced by many factors. The desire to maintain a youthful appearance has been influenced by the need to remain competitive in the workforce, increased life expectancy, and the psychological and social consequences associated with aging. Aging is a dynamic process, and needs may change over time; thus, semipermanent fillers serve an optimal role for soft tissue augmentation [78].

The main techniques used are serial puncture, linear threading, fanning, and cross-hatching. With the serial puncture technique, the skin is pulled taut and multiple injections are given with small boluses of material in a close enough proximity to create a continuous product placement. If there are small gaps, this may be remedied with massage. This technique works well for acne scarring and treatment of the glabella, among other uses. Larger, separate boluses may be used to place product deeply in order to augment the cheeks. The linear threading technique involves advancing the needle for its full length along the wrinkle. Anterograde or retrograde injection may be used with this technique. This technique is well suited for treatment of the nasolabial folds and augmentation of the vermillion border of the lips. Both the cross-hatching and fanning techniques are variations of linear threading. Larger defects may be more adequately corrected with these particular techniques. Cross-hatching involves placement of multiple linear threads perpendicularly in a grid pattern using numerous punctures. The fanning technique minimizes the number of needle insertions so that one insertion site is used to place multiple threads emanating from that point [65]. This technique is useful for marionette lines.

There is some debate about whether anterograde injection or retrograde injection is better. The majority of experts who inject in an anterograde fashion do so in order to minimize tissue trauma and mechanically move blood vessels out of the course of the needle. Practitioners who advocate retrograde injection do so as they feel slow injection as the needle is being withdrawn helps prevent intravascular injection. It is also possibly beneficial in the malar region or below the eyes, which are soft, thin, or vascular areas [5].

At the conclusion of the treatment, topical Arnica montana gel or vitamin K cream may be applied [79]. Some practitioners send patients home with a sample of the cream to apply to bruised areas to speed resorption [75]. Typed post-treatment instructions should be given to the patient.

Products

There are currently over 150 injectable fillers on the market worldwide; however, in the past decade, more have FDA approval [65] but are still the minority [66]. Only FDA-approved fillers should be used, as complications of non-FDA-approved fillers will not be covered by malpractice insurance [75]. It is also important that the products be purchased from a US distributor [75].

The behavior of the various filler products is influenced by the particle shape, size, degree of cross-linking, and concentration [80]. The longevity of facial fillers relates to phagocytosis, which is the body's natural reaction to a foreign body in the tissue. In general, macrophages can ingest particles smaller than 15–20 microns; larger particles persist [80]. Increased cross-linking and increased concentration improve resistance to phagocytosis. Also, hydrophilic particles are not phagocytosed as early. In addition, particle shape influences phagocytosis and encapsulation [80]. Irregularly shaped particles are more likely to induce active granulomas, and smooth particles are more safely encapsulated [80]. In fact, irregular particles may be induced to form active granulomas decades after placement particularly with trauma, repeat injection, or surgery [80].

Collagen

The first collagen products were Zyderm and Zyplast (Inamed Corp., Toronto, Ontario; now distributed by Allergan, Inc.) [63, 65]. Zyderm was approved in 1981 following 6 years of rigorous testing [64]. These products required skin testing due to the possibility of allergic reactions. Allergic reactions to skin testing occur in 3–5% of patients [80, 81]. Many practitioners advocate double skin testing [80, 82]. The tests should be 1 month apart with treatment at least 2 weeks following the second test [80], thus delaying treatment by 4–6 weeks [69]. Double skin testing reduces the allergy risk to 0.5% [81, 83]. Collagen should not be injected in patients with autoimmune disease [80]. The bovine collagen source was a closed herd of cattle to prevent the transmission of bovine encephalopathy virus [64]. Collagen products are overall effective and safe, but the duration of effect was limited [63]. Since that time, several different collagen formulations entered the market including Fibrel (Serono Laboratories, Darmstadt, Germany). In addition, Autologen (Collagenesis, Inc., Beverly, MA) was developed from surgically excised human skin, and Dermalogen, a less expensive version, was derived from cadaver skin; however, the company filed for bankruptcy in 2001, and the products are no longer produced [63]. Isolagen (Isolagen, Inc., Houston, TX) used the patient's own tissue from a 3-mm punch from which the collagen is harvested and grown [63]. Subsequently, CosmoDerm and CosmoPlast (Inamed 2003, acquired by Allergan, Inc., Irvine, CA 2006) began production from human genetically engineered dermal tissue and do not require skin testing [63, 80]. These products are not being actively marketed by Allergan, which reflects the trend toward hyaluronic acid products [65]. Evolence (Ortho Dermatologics, Los Angeles, CA), a porcine collagen product, was introduced in June 2008, but distribution of this product was stopped in November 2009 [65]. The collagen dermal fillers in general are particularly good for filling perioral rhytids given their consistency and ability to be placed superficially but are used less often now. The duration of correction with these products was relatively short, and the incidence of beading was fairly common [69].

Hyaluronic Acid

Hyaluronic acid fillers were FDA approved in 2003 (Restylane) and were quickly embraced due to the improved longevity over collagen and the fact that no skin testing is required [66]. A 2017 data from the American Society of Aesthetic Plastic Surgeons revealed that the hyaluronic acid fillers were the most popular with approximately 722,000 treatments, followed by Radiesse and Sculptra [84]. Hyaluronic acid is a naturally occurring glycosaminoglycan in living organisms that is part of the extracellular matrix [5, 85, 86]. It is one of the basic components of the dermis and all connective tissue [63]. Fifty percent of hyaluronic acid in the body is found in the skin [87]. Interestingly, it has impressively high biologic compatibility and demonstrates no species specificity; thus, there is no risk of immunologic reaction in humans [63, 68]. In the skin, the molecules have a substantial ability to bind water and create volume [63, 68] in part due to its highly charged nature [87]. Hyaluronic acid was first discovered in the vitreous of the cow eye in 1934 [65, 75]. Hyaluronic acid substances were originally used in cataract surgery and for injections into joints [5]. They have become incredibly popular dermal filling agents.

Naturally occurring hyaluronic acid has a very short half-life, which product manufacturers have increased by cross-linking, which also results in larger molecules that are more stable and less water-soluble [5]. The characteristics of hyaluronic acid that affect the product performance include cross-linking, concentration of hyaluronic acid, molecular weight, and gel hardness or consistency of the product [5, 68]. The optimum degree of cross-linking has not yet been determined [80]. There are several different chemicals used for cross-linking of injectables [65]. Butanediol diglycidyl ether (BDDE) is used in Restylane, Juvederm, and Belotero, while divinyl sulfone (DVS) was used in Prevelle Silk, Captique, Hylaform [65]. Different cross-linkers were used for Elevess and products not yet available in the United States [87]. The cross-linkers may be toxic to the skin; thus, residual stabilizer must be removed [75]. Newer cross-linking technology has been introduced recently with Vycross used in some Juvederm products and XpresHAn used in some Restylane products [88]. Juvederm's Vycross technology combines some longer HA chains with a high molecular weight and shorter chains with a lower molecular weight. The earlier generation of fillers by Allergan used cross-linked HA chains of uniform molecular weight [88]. While older Restylane products relied on higher G Prime and particle size to achieve higher lift, based on HA particle dimension, which is established through a sizing process during the division of the gel, the newest Restylane products Restylane Defyne and Restylane Refyne use XpresHAn technology of cross-linking which creates a smooth gel that allows maintaining natural movement and expression [88]. Merz patented technology known as CPM (Cohesive Polydensified Matrix) to cross-link their Belotero balance product [89].

The cross-linking process may be used to create a particulate or nonparticulate form of hyaluronic acid [75]. Particulate hyaluronic acid products achieve a greater filling power based on particle size, while nonparticulate hyaluronic acid fillers rely on greater cross-linking to enable greater filling power. The degree of cross-linking may be affected by the fact that a cross-linker may sometimes bond only at one end of a hyaluronic acid strand instead of connecting two strands, which leaves the other end pendant [87]. Overall, increasing the cross-linking density results in a harder product, but if the majority of the hyaluronic acid has pendant modification, a low cross-link density product occurs which leads to a softer gel formulation [87]. Rheology describes the consistency and flow of a gel [75]. Rheology is influenced by particle size, concentration of hyaluronic acid, and gel hardness [75]. Elastic modulus or G is a characteristic that describes a material's resistance to deformation for both the viscous and elastic components [87]. Hard gels require more syringe pressure to inject [75]. They also may disrupt tissue more and incite more discomfort and swelling [75]. Soft gels do not resist deformation as much and inject under less pressure, feel softer under the skin, and are better suited to areas of thin skin [75]. Particle size is important for the ability of the product to pass through a needle, typically 27–32 gauge [87]. This relates to the extrusion force. The extrusion force of a filler can be reduced by reducing the particle size [87]. For hyaluronic acid fillers, larger particle size does not appear to extend the duration of the product as the particle size does not vary substantially [87]. Hyaluronic acid concentration does influence product duration but mainly indirectly by the amount of cross-linking [87]. The rheologic characteristics influence the different behavior of various HA fillers [90].

Originally, rooster combs, umbilical cord, vitreous humor, tendons, skin, and bacterial cultures were used as sources of hyaluronic acid [68]. Hylaform (Allergan, Inc., Irvine, CA), the first hyaluronic acid developed for dermal filling, was originally used in Europe in 1996 and FDA approved in 2004 [75]. It was derived from rooster combs [68] and had a low concentration but high molecular weight and a less viscous consistency [68]. It provided excellent results but did not seem to last as long as the bacterial-fermented products [64]. Allergy to avian proteins may occur with this product [75]. Hylaform, Hylaform Plus, and Captique were manufactured by Genzyme (Ridgefield, NJ) and were initially distributed by Inamed but are now owned by Allergan, Inc. (Irvine, CA) [75]. All of these three products have been phased out of production, and Captique was reformulated with lidocaine and FDA approved as Prevelle Silk (Mentor) in 2008 [91].

The most popular current products are biosynthetically produced by fermentation of *Streptococcus equi* bacterium and vary in consistency [5, 63, 75, 80]. The main products on the US market are the Restylane product line (Galderma, Lausanne, Switzerland), Juvederm product line (Allergan, Inc., Irvine, CA), and Belotero Balance (Merz Aesthetics, Frankfurt, Germany). More recently, Revanesse (Prollenium Medical Technologies, Canada) received FDA approval in 2017 [88]. Many of these filler products have added lidocaine to the original formulation. Restylane products (Restylane, Restylane Silk, Restylane Lyft, Restylane-L, Restylane Refyne, and Restylane Defyne) have a hyaluronic acid concentration of 20 mg/cc, while Juvederm Ultra XC and Ultra Plus XC have a higher concentration of 24 mg/cc and are more cross-linked with a smoother consistency [5, 80], but their newer products Juvederm Volbella XC, Juvederm Vollure XC, and Juvederm Voluma XC have HA concentrations of 15 mg/mL, 17.5 mg/mL, and 20 mg/mL, respectively [88]. Belotero Balance has a hyaluronic acid concentration of 22.5 mg/mL, and Revanesse Versa has a hyaluronic acid concentration of 25 mg/mL [88]. Restylane was available in Europe in 1996 and approved by the FDA in December 2003 [75]. Studies demonstrated its superiority to bovine collagen in a randomized, double-blinded, split-face study [75]. Perlane was approved in 2007 with a larger particle size. Lidocaine was added to Restylane to make Restylane-L in 2012. Particle size is the only difference between Restylane-L, Restylane Lyft (Perlane relabeled in 2015), and Restylane Silk (2014). Restylane Refyne and Defyne were granted FDA approval in 2016 [66] and use different cross-linking technology previously described. All of the Restylane products are approved for treatment of moderate to severe facial folds and wrinkles in patients over the age of 21; however, Restylane, Restylane-L, and Restylane Silk are also indicated for use in lip volume augmentation. Restylane Lyft recently received specific FDA approval for midface injection via cannula [92] as well as for rejuvenation of the hands [66].

Juvederm Ultra and Juvederm Ultra Plus were FDA approved in 2006 [75]. They are created using a patented Hylacross technology, which is responsible for the homogeneous, nonparticulate smooth consistency and approximately 20% thicker viscosity [75]. Both of these products demonstrated superiority over collagen in initial and sustained correction [75]. Juvederm Ultra Plus is double cross-linked [69]. The XC designation was used after 0.3% lidocaine was added to the products in 2010 [66]. Juvederm Voluma XC (2013), Juvederm Volbella XC (2016), and Juvederm Vollure XC (2017) are more recent additions to the product line and use different cross-linking technology as previously described. The Juvederm products are indicated for correction of moderate to severe facial wrinkles and folds; however, Juvederm Voluma XC is also indicated for deep injection for cheek augmentation, and Juvederm Volbella is indicated for injection into the lips for lip augmentation [66]. Belotero Balance (Merz Aesthetics, Frankfurt, Germany) was approved in 2011 for injection into facial tissue to smooth wrinkles and folds, especially around the nose and mouth [66]. Revanesse (Prollenium Medical Technologies, Canada) was approved in 2017 and is indicated for injection into the mid- to deep dermis for correction of moderate to severe facial wrinkles and folds, such as nasolabial folds, in adults 22 years of age or more [66].

Several new dermal hyaluronic acid fillers are being produced and have not yet obtained FDA approval. The various gels have very low levels of impurities, i.e., fermentation by-products [68].

Hyaluronic acid fillers are temporary, which enables satisfactory correction without the risks associated with permanent fillers [5]. They are becoming increasingly long-lasting [5]. The different commercially available hyaluronic acid products have different properties, which provide tailoring product selection to patient need [5]. The various properties make the different products suitable for injection at different layers in the skin [63]. In general, most practitioners use softer gels for more superficial use and stiffer, more robust product for deeper use [5].

Local reactions may include erythema, pain, itching, and tenderness [63]. Hyaluronic acid is theorized to have a mild, local, heparin-like effect that can result in increased bruising relative to other fillers [80]. The Tyndall effect is specific to hyaluronic acid fillers and appears as a blue-gray hue in the area of the injected filler. It can be related to injection in areas of thin, pale skin or superficial placement of product. The blue color results from the fact that blue is the shortest wavelength of light, and it is more easily scattered and reflected than the longer red wavelengths that penetrate deeper in tissue [72]. Q-switch laser treatment may be used to correct the Tyndall effect as well [72].

One benefit to hyaluronic acid filling agents is that overcorrection, visible lumps, Tyndall effect, or inflammatory reactions can be ameliorated with the off-label use of hyaluronidase [93]. Hyaluronidase is an enzyme that degrades hyaluronic acid. It has been used as a dispersive agent for retrobulbar anesthesia for many years [93]. Soparkar et al. [94] and Lambros [72, 95] both first reported the use of hyaluronidase to dissolve hyaluronic acid in 2004, and it has since been used by many practitioners for this purpose [72]. The onset is rapid and it is generally well tolerated [93]. Dissolution of hyaluronic acid typically occurs within 24 hours [93]. It has also been used in cases of impending skin necrosis due to inadvertent intravascular injection of filler and embolic complications [93]. Preliminary skin testing for hypersensitivity is recommended due to the theoretical risk of allergy [93]. There are no reported anaphylactic reactions following subepidermal injection [93]. It is postulated that injection of high concentrations of hyaluronidase could destroy the native hyaluronic acid and possibly lead to atrophy, though this specific occurrence has not been reported [93]. There has been speculation that collagenase may be used to reverse the effect of unwanted collagen filler akin to the use of hyaluronidase for hyaluronic acid.

Biosynthetic Polymers

Calcium hydroxylapatite, Radiesse (BioForm Medical, San Mateo, CA, 2006) is a volumizing filler found to incite collagen neogenesis. Radiesse was granted FDA approval for treatment of moderate to severe lines and wrinkles such as nasolabial folds as well as HIV-associated facial lipoatrophy in late 2006 [65, 96]. It is opaque and has the consistency of wet toothpaste [77]. It must be placed subdermally [80]. It consists of 30% calcium hydroxylapatite spheres 25–45 microns in size suspended in a methylcellulose carrier gel (70%) [80]. It is minimally immunogenic [80]. In 2015, Radiesse was granted FDA approval for subdermal implantation for hand augmentation to correct volume loss on the dorsum of the hands [66]. Due to the composition, the product is visible on CT scans and less on plain films; thus, it is also used as a radiological tissue marker [77, 80]. It has not been reported to obscure CT studies or radiographic findings [77]. It promotes collagen formation in the deep dermis and subdermis [80] but does not induce osteogenesis [77]. Over time, the microspheres degrade into calcium and phosphate ions [77]. It has impressive longevity of up to 12 months according to the FDA [66]. The duration of Radiesse has been reported from 9 to 36 months, though studies demonstrate reduction in degree of correction following 12–14 months [96]. Due to the relatively high viscosity of the product, it is better suited for correction of deeper rhytids and volume loss as opposed to fine lines and wrinkles [69]. This product should be injected in the subdermal and, in some cases, supraperiosteal plane [77]. Care should be taken to stop injecting prior to withdrawal from the skin and avoid dermal placement as a visible white lump can result [77]. Radiesse has a shelf life of 3 years and does not need to be refrigerated [77]. Discomfort with injection of this product has been ameliorated following the mid-2009 FDA approval of lidocaine addition to this product immediately prior to injection [96]. A 0.2 cc of plain 2% lidocaine was mixed with 1.3 cc of Radiesse via a Luer-lock connector and mixed [96]. Now, the product is formulated as Radiesse (+) and includes 0.3% integral lidocaine. The addition of lidocaine to Radiesse has decreased the extrusion force of the product [96].

Studies have demonstrated favorable results with Radiesse compared to collagen and Radiesse compared to several hyaluronic acid fillers [77]. A recent study demonstrated safety of Radiesse for soft tissue augmentation in persons of color [77, 96, 97]. A special 28-gauge needle with an interior equivalent to a 27 gauge is included and is less traumatic to the tissues [96]. Radiesse should not be used for lip augmentation due to the propensity for nodule formation in this area [77, 80, 96]. The supraperiosteal approach has been advocated with the use of this product for the zygoma and temporal fossa [96]. Some practitioners use an intraoral route to augment the midface, though concern has been raised about the potential for biofilm formation [96]. Radiesse produces the least amount of tissue reactivity compared to poly-L-lactic acid and polymethyl methacrylate, which all have fibroblast-stimulating properties [96].

Poly-L-lactic acid (PLLA), Sculptra (Sanofi-Aventis, Dermik Laboratories, Bridgewater, NJ 2004), stimulates collagen neogenesis by granulomatous inflammation [65, 80]. Like Radiesse, it is marketed for semipermanent augmentation [80]. It is the same synthetic material found in absorbable suture material [80]. It is an inert polymer from the alpha hydroxy acid family and contains microparticles measuring 40–63 microns [98]. Poly-L-lactic acid has been used in medical products for over 30 years [99]. It does not require allergy testing [98]. The initial volumizing is very transient. The stimulation of fibroblasts to produce collagen is the only effect of this product; thus, it is a dermal stimulating volumizer or augmentation product as opposed to a filler like the other products [80]. It is important to undercorrect initially [98]. Correction is observed initially, but the carrier is absorbed over the following weeks, and 2 or more months elapse before correction is achieved by stimulation of collagen and fibrous tissue in response to the degradation of the product [69]. This product is not a good option for patients who want instant results but is well suited for individuals desiring gradual, long-lasting correction [100]. This product must be injected subdermally [80]. Multiple treatments may be necessary to build up to the desired correction [65]. Typically, at least three treatment sessions over 3 months are needed with results occurring over 4–6 months [100]. Correction has been reported to last up to 30–40 months according to one study [101, 102], though most data demonstrates continued improvement at 2 years [101]. It was originally used in Europe since 1999 [99] and was FDA approved for HIV-associated facial lipoatrophy in 2004. Sculptra gained approval for volumizing and facial augmentation of facial rhytids such as nasolabial folds on July 28, 2009 [101, 103, 104]. Sculptra is used off-label for other cosmetic purposes [80]. The majority of data is available in the HIV population, but their characteristics are different from the cosmetic patient such as gender being mostly male as opposed to the female cosmetic patient, and the degree of correction needed is much worse in the HIV population [101]. The studies involve a varying number of treatment sessions as well [101]. Sculptra is initially in a freeze-dried preparation and is best reconstituted the night before use with 3–5 cc of sterile water [80]. Lidocaine may be added to the preparation [80]. Massage of the treated area for 3–7 days following injection helps to evenly distribute the particles [80]. Sculptra should not be used to fill lines; it is intended to augment deep rhytids and restore volume [100]. Nodule formation is the most common adverse effect and typically is seen in the periorbital area and oral commissures [80]. Subcutaneous papules formerly occurred in approximately 5–44% of patients treated for HIV lipoatrophy [105]. Evolution in the use of Sculptra has reduced this incidence to less than 1% by placing emphasis on thorough mixing, avoiding injection in the thin periorbital skin, use of a 5 cc or more dilution, and thorough massage after product placement [105]. In addition, patients are instructed to massage the treated areas for 10 days [100]. The incidence of granuloma formation is reported to range from 0.2% to 12%. Various treatment modalities attempted for granulomas include steroid injections, oral steroids, subcision, and injection of 5-FU [80].

ArteFill (Artes Medical, Inc., San Diego, CA) consists of PMMA microspheres suspended in a 3.5% solution of bovine collagen [63] and lidocaine hydrochloride 0.3% [63]. It is the first "permanent" facial filler approved by the FDA in October 2006 [69, 80]. There are approximately six million PMMA microspheres per cubic centimeter of ArteFill [76]. PMMA is biocompatible and was originally used as a hip prosthesis in 1947, and its use as tissue cement expanded to many fields [80]. The collagen is degraded in 1–3 months with the remaining PMMA microspheres becoming encapsulated as they are too large to be taken up by the vasculature or degraded by phagocytosis [63]; thus, the result is long-lasting. Patients should be extensively counseled regarding the permanent nature of this product and the possibility of late adverse reactions [76]. This product is thought to stimulate collagen neogenesis [80]. It is important to avoid overcorrection with this product because it is permanent [63]. Contour irregularities such as beading, ridging, and nodules have been reported and are associated with superficial product placement. Care should be taken to inject the product into the deep dermis. Double skin testing is recommended for the collagen component [63, 80]. The bovine collagen comes from a restricted, closed herd [76]. Prior to product injection, the ArteFill should be allowed to thaw for 30–45 min [76]. Granuloma formation has a reported incidence of 1/1000 [63]. Late granuloma formation is not infrequent [80]. The prior version of the product, Artecoll, available in Europe, had a much higher rate, which was attributed to the gelatin carrier and inconsistent particle size [80]. It is helpful to perform a biopsy to achieve a histologic diagnosis in the case of a suspected granuloma [76]. Intralesional steroids, oral steroids, or intralesional 5-fluorouracil may be used to correct granulomas [76]. The microspheres are poorly phagocytosed and becomes surrounded by a fibrous capsule, which accounts for the augmentation [80]. Nodules may also be a problem with this product, particularly in the lips. Biofilm formation has been reported with orthopedic implants bonded with PMMA cement [80]. ArteFill was rebranded as Bellafill (Suneva Medical, Inc., San Diego, CA) and received FDA approval in 2015 for moderate to severe, atrophic, distensible facial acne scars on the cheek in patients over the age of 21 years [106].

Silicone is a generic name used to refer to a family of polymers derived from the element silicon (atomic number 14) [107]. Silicone compounds can exist as solids, foams, gels, and liquids [108]. It has a wide variety of industrial and medical applications [108]. The medical-grade silicone is polydimethylsiloxane [107]. Liquid silicone has been used for over 40 years for soft tissue augmentation [108]. It originally was used in the 1960 as a cosmetic treatment though it had been previously used for breast augmentation in Japan in the 1940s [64]. Silicone use has been extremely controversial. Following reports of disastrous local and systemic complications resulting from injectable liquid silicone, the FDA and AMA condemned its use in 1970 [64]. In 2017, the FDA issued a specific warning against injectable silicone for body contouring and enhancement [66]. There are two medical-grade liquid silicone products produced since 1994 that may be legally used for soft tissue augmentation in the United States based on the FDA Modernization Act from 1997 that allows any FDA-approved device to be prescribed or administered for any condition or disease within a doctor-patient relationship [108]. AdatoSil (Bausch & Lomb, Claremont, CA, USA) and Silikon (Alcon Labs, Fort Worth, TX, USA) are both approved for retinal tamponade; therefore, their use has extended to soft tissue augmentation [108] which remains off-label use. The cosmetic use of liquid silicone is considered illegal in Nevada, California, and Colorado, however [64, 80]. The use of impure products or large volumes leads to many complications [63, 107]. Disfigurement has occurred due to patients' self-injecting or unlicensed practitioners injecting other forms of silicone and oil. In addition, misuse of the product with injection into unsuitable areas such as the breasts has caused major problems [107].

It has been reported that delayed nodules may still occur in patients treated with pure medical-grade silicone by experienced injectors, which may implicate the host response as a crucial factor [109]. Injection of small volumes (i.e., microdroplet technique) elicits a local fibroblastic reaction, whereas larger volumes could create an inflammatory granulomatous reaction [107]. Inflammatory reactions associated with liquid silicone may be treated with intralesional corticosteroids [107]. There is some debate about whether late granulomatous reactions may represent a reaction to biofilm contamination as opposed to the product itself [79].

Two other permanent synthetic polymers are Bio-alcamid (Ascente Medical) and Aquamid (Contura International), which are 4% polyalkylimide and polyacrylamide hydrogel, respectively [65]. They have not been granted FDA approval at this time [65]. There are numerous other products available internationally that are not used in the United States at this time.

Complications

Complications from dermal fillers may be categorized as immediate, early, late, and permanent [65, 110].

A 2008 report by the FDA found 823 adverse events with 638 (78%) that responded to medication, 94 (11%) requiring surgical intervention, and 19 (2%) that required emergency admission due to problems with hypersensitivity [65]. Fortunately, no deaths have been reported [111]. Complications occur more commonly with permanent fillers [65]. Permanent fillers do not age in a similar fashion to the rest of the face, which may lead to undesirable long-term outcomes [5]. Complications occur more frequently with inexperienced injectors. States vary widely regarding who is allowed to inject fillers and how much training is required [111].

Immediate side effects include bruising, swelling, needle marks, pruritus, erythema, and bumps or contour irregularity [75]. All of these should be discussed prior to the filler treatment. They are not true complications but are simply expected to occur initially with treatment. They typically resolve in approximately 1 week [75]. Significant lip edema is occasionally treated with ice or oral prednisone [69]. Underreporting by patients of herbal supplement use or alcohol use often occurs in the screening process, which contributes to increased bruising in some patients [72]. In addition, though the fanning technique involves fewer needlesticks, it may increase the likelihood of bleeding [72]. Persistent erythema may require intense pulsed light treatments or steroid injections [111].

Actual complications include intravascular injection, tissue necrosis, granuloma formation, infection, allergic reaction, and a visible blue hue with hyaluronic acid fillers (Tyndall effect). Postinjection telangiectasias occur most commonly in the area of the nasolabial fold [79]. Laser therapy, sclerotherapy, or electrodesiccation may be needed to treat the telangiectasias [79]. Postinjection hyperpigmentation is typically post-inflammatory and may be improved with the use of topical hydroquinones, retinoids, or corticosteroids [79]. Migration of the product has been reported and may be difficult to treat [72]. Hypersensitivity to hyaluronic acid occurs in 1 in 5000 patients and is typically self-limited [72]. Facial lipoatrophy has been reported with the filler Profill, which is not used in the United States [112].

Other complications include visible product such as with incorrect placement, beading, clumping, or overcorrection [5]. In order to prevent this occurrence, use a smaller-gauge needle and a serial puncture technique [5]. Massage in the area can also help distribute clumped or excess filler [5] by combining the warmth of the fingertips and consistent pressure.

Nodules posttreatment may be divided into early appearing, intermediate, and late appearing [79]. Early appearing nodules typically represent misplacement of the product, but some may indicate hypersensitivity [79]. Early nodules may be treated with antibiotics, massage, or hyaluronidase injection depending on the degree of inflammation [79]. Intermediate nodules are rare and are usually best treated with antibiotics [79]. Late-appearing nodules are usually granulomas and must be diagnosed histologically [79]. First-line treatment is antibiotics and intralesional steroids or 5-FU has been described [79]. Incising, squeezing, and surgical excision of nodules is sometimes necessary [111].

Granuloma formation is theoretically possible with all of the different filler materials [80] and has been reported recently [113].

Biofilm formation is an additional concern [80]. Biofilms are collections of microorganisms in an encapsulated environment with nutrients and bacterial waste products that can sustain the microorganisms for an extended duration [80]. This is thought to be the mechanism behind indolent, low-grade infection in some patients with a history of facial fillers [80]. Minocycline has been reported to be beneficial in the treatment of silicon granulomas [72] alone or in combination with celecoxib [114]. Intralesional injections of bleomycin or allopurinol have been attempted, as well, for granulomas [72]. Other treatment regimens involving antibiotics, corticosteroids, and 5-FU have been described [115]. Allergic granuloma formation has been described with hyaluronic acid fillers and may require surgical correction [116–118]. Allergy or hypersensitivity to hyaluronic acid can be tested for, and double skin tests should be performed in this situation [119, 120].

Scarring following filler treatment is rare; however, hypertrophic scarring and keloid formation have been reported [111]. Treatment includes IPL, pulsed dye laser, intralesional steroid, and pressure [111].

The most feared complication from dermal filler injection is necrosis, which occurs when filler is inadvertently injected intravascularly or externally compresses an artery. Certain locations are more prone to this complication such as the glabella; thus, a thorough understanding of the anatomy and injecting experience is crucial when treating this area [5]. The major danger zones are the supratrochlear arteries near the glabella, facial artery at the alar-facial angle and the dorsal nasal arteries located at the nasal dorsum [65]. Intravascular injection presents with sudden pain, blanching [5], and development of livedo reticularis. If blanching occurs, the injection should be immediately ceased, and the plunger should be pulled back in an attempt to elicit a flash of blood to confirm intravascular placement [79]. Hyaluronidase, aspirin, warm compresses, and nitropaste should be available in every office in order to provide immediate treatment in situations of possible vascular compromise [75, 121]. More recently, treatment of skin necrosis with platelet-rich plasma has been described [122].

Decreasing the rate of injection (<0.3 cc/min) and using smaller-gauge needles (i.e., 30 g) no longer than 1 inch decrease the complication rate [5, 79]. Use of a cannula as opposed to a needle is thought to reduce the risk of vascular injection as well [123]. In vascular areas such as the glabella, it is important to avoid placing stiffer products superficially where the capillary bed can be occluded leading to necrosis [5]. If this serious situation occurs, it is important to inject hyaluronidase immediately. Various different dosage protocols have been described [124, 125]. Use of a vasodilator such as nitropaste on the affected area has become more controversial. In addition, applying a warm compress, massage, and oral aspirin can be beneficial [124]. The patient should be examined daily.

Vision loss has also been reported following injection of filler in the glabella [81]. It has also occurred following injections of other particulate substances in the mouth, nose, and face [126]. It is thought to result from inadvertent injection into one of the peripheral branches of the ophthalmic artery [126]. This can occur even with typical placement of product since individual anatomy is variable [126]. Slow injection with minimal force and use of a small-diameter needle can help minimize this risk [126].

Abscess formation is rare but has been reported following bovine collagen injection and can be a late occurrence [81]. Fluctuance is the hallmark in this situation [81]. Cultures most often demonstrate *Staphylococcus epidermidis* [81]. Abscesses may be treated with incision and drainage and can be improved with intralesional steroids [81]. The development of a lesion more than 2 weeks after treatment may indicate an atypical infection such as mycobacteria [72, 127]. The activation of herpes simplex labialis is well known, which is why prophylaxis is provided; however, reactivation of herpes zoster following facial filler injection has also been described [128] (Fig. 21.10).

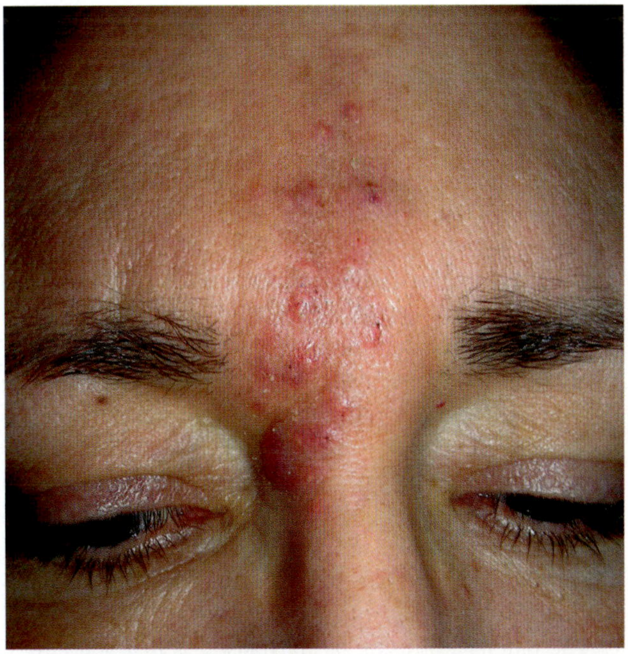

Fig. 21.10 Herpes zoster following filler placement in the glabella. (Reprinted with permission from [128])

Dermal fillers provide overall effective and safe facial augmentation. There are numerous off-label applications. Many different products are available that enable treatment to be customized. Complications are rare.

Fat Transfer

Facial aging is associated with loss of elasticity, descent, and deflation of the soft tissues. Fillers including the transfer of fat to facial regions are advocated to address the issue of deflation. Reinflation also has a secondary effect to help elevate the soft tissues. Over the past decades, much of the emphasis has been on lifting and draping procedures such as blepharoplasty and rhytidectomy. This alone has been shown to be inadequate to address the issues of facial aging. In fact, it has been shown with careful photographic analysis in patients that as they age, the primary cause of visible aging is the concentric contraction of facial volume rather than tissue descent [129]. This would be akin to a plump juicy grape that becomes deflated and wrinkled with dehydration as it becomes a raisin. Fat transfer adds an additional dimension to address the changes of facial aging alone or in conjunction with other surgical techniques. This section of the chapter will provide an emphasis on periorbital and facial fat transfer techniques with the many varied approaches including their pros and cons. This will allow the surgeon to decide what may work best, as an ongoing debate exists in regard to clinical outcome and fat graft survival and longevity. This chapter also provides a basis for research to modify and refine the technique for the optimal clinical outcome in the future.

History and Rationale

Fat was first used as whole grafts for a filler material in 1893 [130]. A variety of alloplastic materials like paraffin [131, 132], gold, silver, filigree wire, hard rubber [133], sponge rubber, silk, gutta-percha, ivory [134], and latex were used later but fell out of favor due to complications. However, Miller revisited fat use as a filler material in 1926 when he described his technique and outcomes with infiltration of fatty tissue through cannulas [135]. Its use never became popular due to the difficulty of preparing and placing en bloc fat through cannulas. It was not until the 1980s when tumescent liposuction techniques were described that widespread use of fat transfer could be utilized [136, 137]. The liposuction techniques allowed the production of "fat pearls" which could easily be harvested and then could pass through narrow cannulas to the site of interest [138].

The rationale of using fat for transfer is that you have a living autologous tissue graft that could potentially provide a lasting effect without repetitive injections. If the fat survives the transfer to the intended site, then you have a basis for a permanent treatment. The fat is also readily accepted by the body as it is the patient's own autologous tissue. One advantage over other facial fillers is the absence of both early and late hypersensitivity reactions and granuloma formation with autologous fat [139]. There is also usually an ample supply of fat. It is unclear what cells survive. It is known that preadipocytes and adipocytes are both transferred as evidenced by the expression of adiponectin [140] and CD 34 [141]. Do the actual adipocytes or the preadipocytes or both survive? Both may be true, but the latter would then confer that regeneration of new cells plays a role in the transfer. It is becoming apparent that the long-term volumizing effect is more likely the result from fat regeneration rather than fat transfer. Transfer and differentiation of stem cells or preadipocytes enable fat regeneration [141].

It has been shown that volume retention will often dip in the first 3–4 months with resolving edema and as vascularization occurs. A rebound with improved facial volume at 1 year or later follows this. The delayed volumetric effect is either the uptake of fatty acids into the cytoplasm of the surviving adipocytes or the differentiation of the stem cells becoming fat cells that mature and grow. It is also unclear what percent of the transferred cells survive. Studies have reported widely variable retention results ranging from 13% to 68%, objective measurements are challenging, and the variability may be related to the importance of the location for long-term retention of the reinjected fat [139]. This is important in deciding how much fat to place considering the anticipated loss. Access of the fat pearls to the surrounding blood supply plays a critical role. Most surgeons are overcorrecting due to the anticipated loss. An unknown critical maximum volume exists whereby additional fat pearl volume will lack adequate exposure to blood supply nourishment. This will lead to cell death and atrophy due to inadequate oxygenation and nutrition. This notion is supported by the placement of optimal volumes of fat rather than overfilling to get the desired effect [142]. The goal is to place a total of 30–50 cc of fat into the facial regions compared with the 100–150 cc some authors advocate. This helps retention and avoids contour issues as well. If further research can enhance fat pearl survival, then overcorrection will become less important. Overcorrection has been found to be not as necessary in the pediatric population with fat transfer performed for functional reasons [143]. Also, most patients have an extensive source of fat for harvesting, which could be utilized for repeat injections if needed. However, ideally, it would be best to avoid additional harvesting of fat. Potentially extra fat that is initially harvested could be preserved for future use to fill undercorrections or modify small regions of unevenness. This would be akin to touch-ups with off-the-shelf fillers. Extra harvested fat has been frozen for later use, but the best conditions to do this have not entirely been elucidated [144]. It is known that the fat must be cryoprotected and frozen and stored in a controlled fashion [145].

Preoperative Exam

Facial Exam

Understanding the patients' unbiased goals and expectations of the procedure is the first step of the exam. These should align with the anatomic changes on the physical exam and, if so, then a customized treatment plan can be formulated. Standardized photography should be used including full-face AP and oblique and side views when relaxed as well as in positions of facial expression like smiling and grimacing. The patient should have a good understanding of the financial commitment and the recuperation process. The latter issue may take longer than some patients willing to tolerate due to the time for edema resolution. Patients with significant past medical history should be eliminated from consideration of having this technique.

The key to planning where to inject the fat pearls is based on a thorough understanding of the patient's expectations. In addition, the exam findings and careful study of photographs influence final decision-making. There are well-defined and agreed-upon facial changes that occur from decade to decade. Briefly, from teenage years to the early or mid-30s, individuals typically lose their baby fat. Most woman like this change as it gives them a supported full face without age-related volume loss. Over the next 10–15 years, gravitational forces (descent) and volumetric contraction (deflation) occur which lead to predictable aging changes. There is a squaring off of the face from the youthful heart shape. Changes include variable amounts of brow ptosis/deflation, formation of the tear trough deformity, malar fat descent/deflation, buccal soft tissue deflation, nasolabial fold development, jowl formation, lip atrophy, marionette lines, and platysmal banding. Think of a topographical map where there are peaks and valleys. The same is true for the aging deflated face. Drawing the topographical lines of isometric elevation can help direct the surgeon's eye to areas of deflation during the assessment (Fig. 21.11). Sharp transitions from peaks to valleys will be seen with closely bunched isometric lines indicative of what we would see with aging.

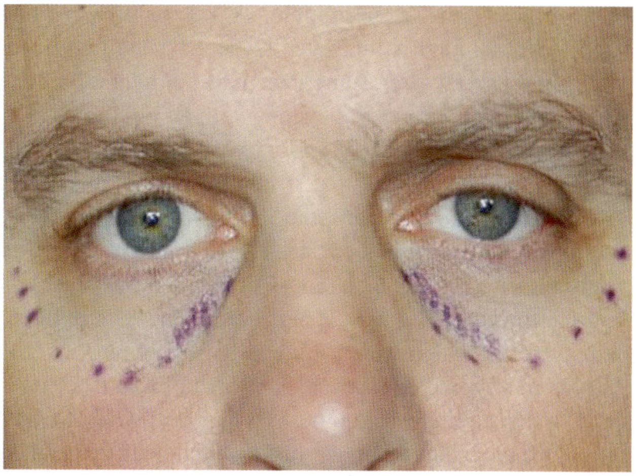

Fig. 21.11 A surgical marking pen is used to delineate facial hollows and areas to be treated with fat transfer

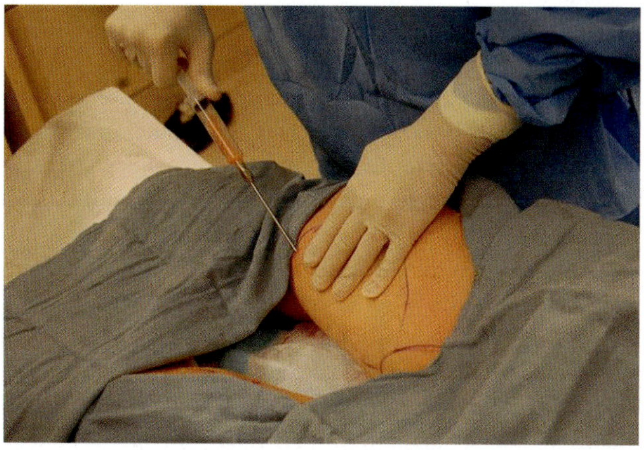

Fig. 21.12 Fat harvesting technique. Following infusion of tumescent anesthesia, a cannula is used to harvest fat from the donor site

Procedural Technique

Body Harvest Site

The most important concept of fat pearl harvest is to determine optimal donor location. The rationale is that this fat would be most resistant to atrophy, cell death, and weight change after transfer. Also, it is known that different fat regions of the body have biochemical differences [146, 147]. It is unclear if this makes a difference in survival or effect when deciding what area to use for fat harvest. A simple question you can ask the patient is what region of their body is most resistant to weight loss or body contouring with diet and exercise. Most patients will say their abdomen or outer thighs. The abdomen has more saturated fat than the unsaturated fat around the eye. This makes sense as the region of the eye experiences much more movement than does the abdomen. There are many possible harvest sites. These sites include the abdomen, outer thigh, anterior thigh, knee, hip, buttock, waist roll, and triceps [148]. It is important to perform an exam of the harvest site prior to the day of the procedure. This is particularly true if one is harvesting from the abdomen. You must be aware of a history or the finding on exam of a ventral abdominal or umbilical hernia. If there has been a history of a hernia, then you should be aware if this has been repaired or not and determine if another harvest location should be found.

Harvest is performed using standard tumescent liposuction technique [136, 137] (Fig. 21.12). A full discussion is beyond the scope of this chapter, but suffice it to say that all surgeons who contemplate fat transfer should be fully skilled at standard tumescent liposuction. Briefly, this technique utilizes dilute solutions of buffered (10 cc of 8.4% of sodium bicarbonate) lidocaine (100 cc of 1% lidocaine) and epinephrine (1 mg or an ampule) in 1 L of 0.9% normal saline. The solution is infiltrated throughout the fatty layer within the harvest site. Tumescent infiltration can be done with either a pump or syringe along with an infiltration cannula. Ample time should pass prior to harvesting. The advantage of this technique is that it minimizes bleeding while providing a long-lasting anesthetic effect. Harvest starts by creating a wheal with local anesthetic at the small entry point. Either a 2-mm punch biopsy device or a #11 blade can be used for entry through the skin. Both devices require no suture to close and provide a minimally perceptible scar. The entry points should be inferior to the area of harvest. This is done so that any serosanguinous discharge after the completion of the procedure can drain in a gravitationally dependent fashion.

The harvest technique is similar to standard therapeutic liposuction with two exceptions. Those differences first include aspiration of the fat with handheld syringes rather than mechanical pumps. Also, the ideal size syringes to use are 10-cc syringes [149]. This effort is made to decrease barotrauma injury to harvested fat cells. This is done best by using handheld 10-cc syringes with the aspiration cannulas rather than a pump to harvest fat [150]. If pumps are used, then the lowest pressure possible should be used. Also, fat harvest with a 10-cc syringe can be facilitated with a fine needle aspiration gun. This avoids fatigue to the surgeon's hand and provides a more even pressure during harvest. Secondly, the volume of tumescent anesthetic and aspirated fat is much less compared to therapeutic liposuction. The margin of safety is much greater as there is less chance of lidocaine toxicity and physiologic fluid shifts in the patient. However, equal amounts of fat should be harvested from the two sides of the region of interest to attain body symmetry in case any change is produced. Patients need to be told that the amount of fat removed from the harvest site will do little to nothing to improve their body contour unless they want to have therapeutic liposuction involving much greater amounts of tumescent infiltration and fat aspiration. The amount of irrigation used for just fat transfer compared to therapeutic liposuction is significantly below the toxic dose for lidocaine. Never exceed 50 mg/kg of lidocaine.

Fat Transfer

Fat transfer can be performed with facial regional blocks, local anesthetic infiltration with either oral or IV sedation, or general anesthesia especially if done in conjunction with other facial surgeries. Anesthetic infiltration into the recipient site needs to be minimized as this can distort the tissue volume and can affect the accuracy of estimating fat transfer needs. The local anesthetics from the harvest and the placement of the fat into the recipient region should be minimized as well. It is known that they reduce functionality and viability of the preadipocytes and adipocytes [140, 150]. Also, it is known that different local anesthetics have variable effects on these cells [140]. Local anesthetics markedly impair the differentiation to adipocytes. The ideal local anesthetic is not known. Removal of the anesthetic before transfer is imperative. This is done with a separation technique. There are several separation techniques, but the optimal one has not been determined.

Also, systemic antibiotics should be given at the start of the procedure. One can use either 2 g of oral amoxicillin 1 hour before treatment or 1 g of IV cefazolin at the time of treatment. Intraoperative and postoperative steroids can also be considered to minimize the early postoperative edema. Oral bromelain and arnica may also help ecchymosis turnover.

There are three basic methods to separate, clean, and prepare the fat pearls for transfer to the facial region. They include passive sedimentation, filtering, and centrifugation. All are done under sterile conditions. Sedimentation is the passive separation of the components based on their inherent densities. This was generally not a well-utilized technique due to the duration (approximately 10 minutes) the fat spends at room temperature separating. However, quantitative histological comparison of these three techniques shows that sedimentation appears to yield a higher proportion of viable adipocytes than does filtering or centrifugation [151]. Adipocyte viability in air is somewhat controversial. Brief exposure to air has been reported to induce cytoplasmic lysis of up to 50% of fatty tissue [152, 153]. However, another study demonstrated comparable or superior results of fat grafting in terms of volume persistence when fat grafts were dried in the open air with a towel [153, 154]. Filtering is performed by placing the harvested material into stainless steel screened cups and then rinsing with saline (Figure 21.13a). This eliminates blood, tumescent solution, and oil. This likely does a poorer job on removing oil since the oil is not soluble in saline. Blotting the fat is then performed to remove any free oil. However, this is the only technique that uses a solution like saline to rinse the fat, which eliminates the lidocaine. Filtration and irrigation in vitro have been shown to return adipocyte function to normal [150]. Centrifugation is typically performed at 2000–4000 rpm for 2–3 min. The result is three layers in the syringe (Fig. 21.13b). The top layer or supernatant is least dense and contains oil from ruptured fat cells. This can be decanted and wicked off with gauze. Removal of as much oil as possible is important as it can incite inflammation and lead to loss or atrophy of the fat pearls. The middle layer contains the usable fat and connective tissue. And the dense bottom layer contains blood and the tumescent solution and is drained. Regardless of the separation technique, the fat is then transferred from 10-cc syringes into 1-cc syringes with a double

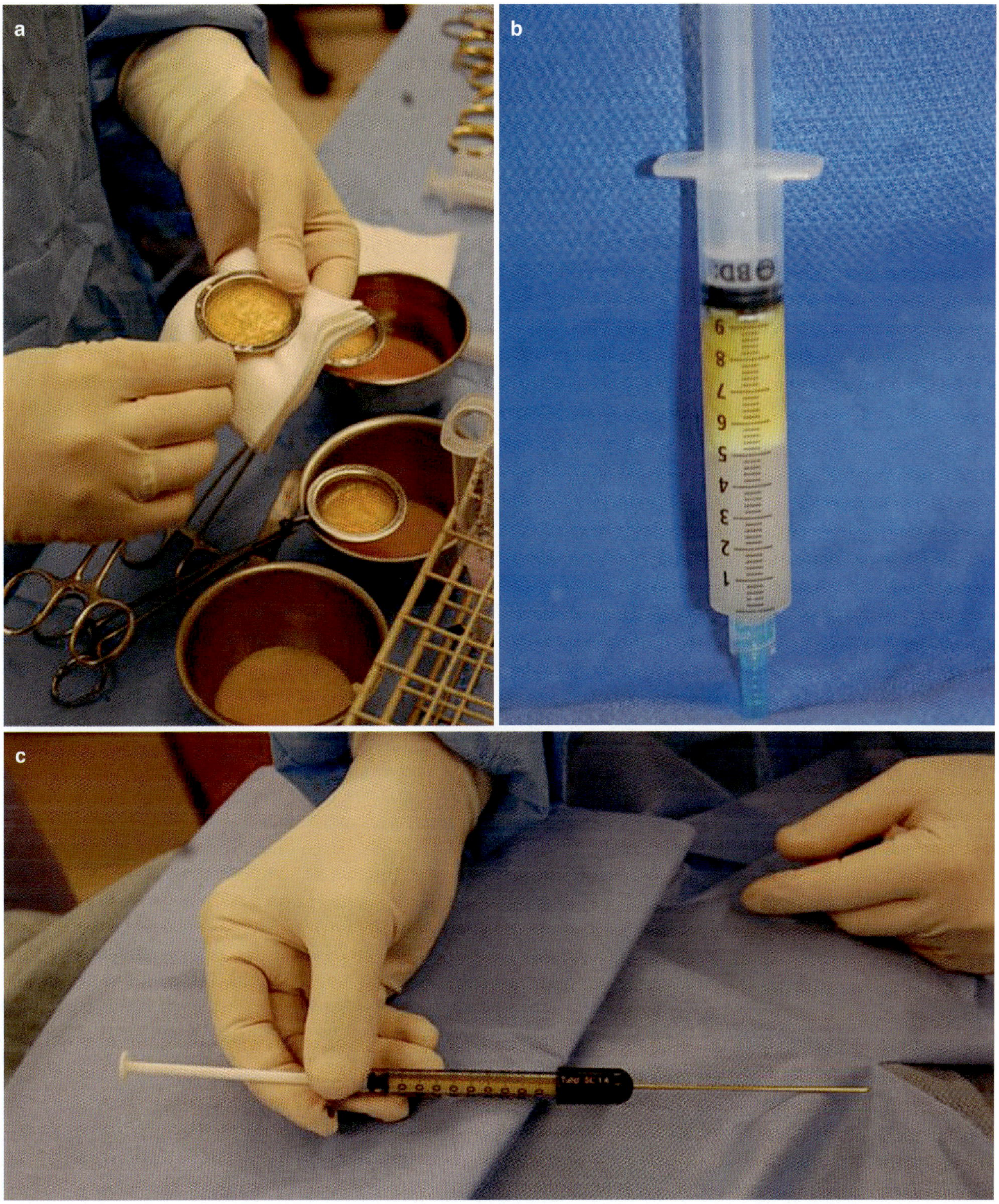

Fig. 21.13 Fat isolation techniques. (**a**) Filtering is performed by placing the harvested material into stainless steel screened cups and rinsing with saline. (**b**) Passive sedimentation results in three layers in the syringe. The dense water layer is discarded. (**c**) The fat is transferred to 1-cc syringes to be used for fat placement with special blunt-tipped cannulas

female Luer-lock connector. Injection control is best with small-volume syringes. Special blunt-tipped injection cannulas are then placed on the 1-cc syringes (Fig. 21.13c). The blunt-tipped injection cannulas are designed to avoid disrupting underlying neurovascular structures, which could lead to temporary or permanent neuropraxia or hematomas. Hematoma or ecchymosis leads to alterations in nutrition availability for the transferred fat cells and decreases their viability.

Once the fat has been harvested, there are many potential tissue engineering manipulations to enhance preadipocyte and adipocyte survival and functionality. Studies involving autologous substances added to the fat to improve retention have also been performed [139, 155–157]. They are worth mentioning as they may play a more pivotal role in the technique of fat transfer over the next decade [158]. The tissue engineering manipulations come in three forms. They are the addition of various growth factors like bFGF, IGF-1, VEGF, PDGF-BB, and insulin to the fat pearls [159, 160], placement on uniform extracellular matrix scaffolds like collagen and fibrin [161, 162], and the cotransplantation with other helper cells [163, 164]. A combination of 20% plasma-rich platelets to 80% fat pearls has been employed.

The goal is to transfer the fat pearls to within 1.5 mm of living vascularized tissue for optimal survival [165]. Fat within a thicker bolus may not have access to nutrients leading to cell death. Another advantage of having fat in close proximity to living vascularized tissue is that it is more likely to adhere to the living tissue with a fibrovascular bond, thereby minimizing migration. This leads to a more predictable result.

Fat transfer has been found to be an excellent complement to other facial rejuvenation procedures [166]. If fat transfer is being done in conjunction with other facial surgeries like blepharoplasty and rhytidectomy, it was originally thought best to do the fat transfer first followed by the incisional surgery. The rationale is that the transferred fat is situated within the tissue and migration of this fat is minimized when crossing the two-dimensional plane of dissection, as it is a smaller amount of exposed fat. If the fat transfer follows the incisional surgery, the fat during injection can overaccumulate in a dissection plane because it will follow the path of least resistance. This fat would accumulate in a three-dimensional space and would not likely fulfill the 1.5-mm goal for viability mentioned above. Also, the transferred fat could migrate out of the wound as it follows the pathway of least resistance. This could have deleterious effect on the healing of the incisional surgery outcome. More recently, surgeons are using fat transfer as a complement to blepharoplasty, and the fat is placed after the lower eyelid fat pads have been addressed [167]. The main facial regions that can be addressed by fat transfer include the temporalis fossa, the lateral eyebrow, the upper eyelid, the lower eyelid, the zygomatic region, the nasojugal fold, the buccal area, the nasolabial fold, the labiomandibular (marionette) folds, the labiomental sulcus, the prejowl sulcus, and the lateral mandible [168].

An 18-gauge needle stabs in different locations on the face provide access to these facial regions. The infiltration cannulas to place the fat in the face fit nicely through these stab wounds. These stab wounds also heal well without a suture. The stabs can be placed strategically in order to minimize the number of wounds. Multiple facial areas can be accessed by one stab wound if they are placed properly. The three most commonly used locations include the lateral canthal area, the central malar region horizontal to the ala, and the anterior jowl along the mandible. The lateral canthal stab can be used to fill the temporalis fossa, the lateral eyebrow, the lateral upper and lower eyelids, and the zygomatic region. The central malar stab can be used to fill the lower eyelid, the malar region, the nasojugal fold, the buccal area, and the nasolabial fold. The anterior jowl stab can be used to fill the buccal area, the labiomandibular fold, the labiomental sulcus, the prejowl sulcus, and the lateral mandible. Many of the regions can be filled from two stabs which allows for cross-hatching of the fat and the creation of a three-dimensional matrix for even volumetric filling. Again, these three locations are only suggestions, and additional stabs can be made to enhance the placement of the fat.

There are many considerations when injecting the fat after deciding where to place it. First, blunt-tipped cannulas should be used. They are manufactured by many companies and come in straight and curved models. They minimize injury to the surrounding tissues. They tend to slide through the tissue without lacerating vital structures like nerves and blood vessels. When injecting the fat, the material is expressed from a side port near the tip. The cannula should be advanced to the start of the injection location without expressing any fat. Fat injection should occur only upon withdrawing the cannula (i.e., retrograde). Minimal force should be used to inject the fat. If there is any difficulty or resistance encountered, then the cannula should be removed without any force on the plunger. This will avoid an inadvertent over bolus of the fat. The cannula opening can get obstructed with connective tissue and should be cleaned. This may be prevented by manually removing large strands of connective tissue following separation. Recall that fat normally resides within a connective tissue matrix that supports it. Both fat and connective tissue are typically harvested together.

Next, the depth of injection is variable depending on the specific location. The three levels from superficial to deep include the subcutaneous plane (superficial), the musculofascial plane (intermediate), and the supraperiosteal plane (deep). The following are the preferred depths of injection according to the region of interest. The brow is filled in the intermediate to deep planes. The lateral canthus is filled in the deep plane only. The inferior orbital rim requires a deep foundation followed by intermediate-level refinement. This is best performed from the inferior injection site as opposed to the lateral injection site to avoid either a lump or bulge of fat. The other areas are more amenable to cross-hatching the fat. The nasojugal fold should be filled in the deep plane. The lateral cheek should be filled in all three levels. The buccal area should be filled in the deep superficial plane. The prejowl sulcus is filled in all three planes.

The volume of fat to be placed in each region along with the amount per individual injection has been well described by many authors [61, 148, 169]. The range per region is anywhere from 0.3 cc in the upper eyelid to 5 cc in the buccal area. The volume of each injection is at most 0.1 cc. The periorbital region is treated using approximately 1 cc total with three to five passes per 0.1 cc for the medial inferior orbital rim in the deep plane [148]. The same parameters apply to the lateral aspect of the inferior orbital rim and the superior orbital rim [148]. The lateral canthal region does not require as much volume, and generally, 0.5 cc total is placed deeply using three to five passes per 0.1 cc. This area has denser connective tissue adhesions and many blood vessels. The tear trough is filled with 1 cc of fat placed at intermediate depth with three to five passes per 0.1 cc, whereas the nasojugal groove is filled deeply with 1 cc total in ten passes of 0.1 cc. A combination of fat repositioning and fat transfer has been described particularly for Ristow's space. Fat repositioning involves a fat pedicle flap as opposed to fat pearl grafts [170]. Fat grafting to the central upper eyelid is an advanced technique [148]. Midfacial filling can be very effective. Volume restoration of the anterior cheek typically involves 4–5 cc total with multiple deep, intermediate, and superficial passes of 0.1 cc each from two different entry points. Care should be taken when injecting from the lateral direction, as this is more predisposed to irregular contour. The lateral cheek may require up to 4–6 cc placed in the same fashion. The nasolabial fold can be augmented with 1–2 cc placed superficially using three to five passes per 0.1 cc. There are several possible targets for volume enhancement in the lower face. There is a reduced longevity of fat grafts in this region owing to the increased movement with chewing and speech. The marionette lines may be treated with 1–2-cc fat grafting placed superficially with 0.1 cc per pass. The prejowl sulcus requires around 3 cc placed in all three planes with 0.1 cc per pass. The lateral jawline may be refined with 1 cc of fat placed in all three planes with 0.1 cc per pass [148]. Fat grafting to the chin has also been described [171]. A strategic sequence of injections is helpful. Care should be taken to monitor the volume of fat injected per side to ensure symmetry.

Tissue motion stabilization is performed at the completion of the fat transfer to the different facial regions. This is done with a casting technique that allows the fat to integrate into the desired location with less risk for migration. The casting tape technique utilizes micropore tape with Mastisol. Taping is done in a cross-hatched fashion over the desired area after applying Mastisol. This performs two functions. First, it reminds patients to not touch or manipulate the area of the fat transfer while holding the region relatively still for a 48–96-hour period. This increases the chances the fat will stay in the desired location. This taping cannot be done if the patient undergoes concomitant skin resurfacing.

Postoperative Evaluations

The key to accurately evaluate postoperative results is to correlate the subjective patient response with the physical exam findings, photography, and a quantitative measurement of volume or topography. Of late, more work has been done in the quantification of results, and surgeons are becoming more critical of their results and are introducing objective evaluation techniques such as digital profilometry analysis [172]. Humans have inherent visual abilities to identify what is a good outcome and how it improves one's aging. It is easy to see with the eye and describe, but this does not quantitatively measure the differences before and after treatment (Fig. 21.14a–d). It does not allow rigid comparison for research purposes. Until standardization of results is performed, there will be no basis to study the many remaining questions about the optimization of this technique. Fortunately, studies have been undertaken to measure the results of fat transfer over time. This includes the use of MRI and three-dimensional imaging [173, 174]. Both techniques show about 50% and about 33% volumetric retention at 1 and 1.5 years, respectively, but some more recent studies depict improved retention [155].

Complications

Complications range from serious loss of function to easily managed situations. Anticipation of these issues will allow the surgeon to quickly and rapidly deal with the presenting situation. The most devastating complication is death and blindness following injection. This likely occurs by fat injection into the vascular system akin to fat emboli. The fat likely traverses the external carotid system and occludes the cerebrovascular system [175] leading to stroke. Blindness results from central retinal artery occlusion [176]. Standard treatment for central retinal artery occlusion should be attempted. These include lowering the eye pressure with drops, oral medications, and massage along with carbogen inhalation and anterior chamber paracentesis. The mechanism of fat emboli can also lead to the possibility of regional facial skin

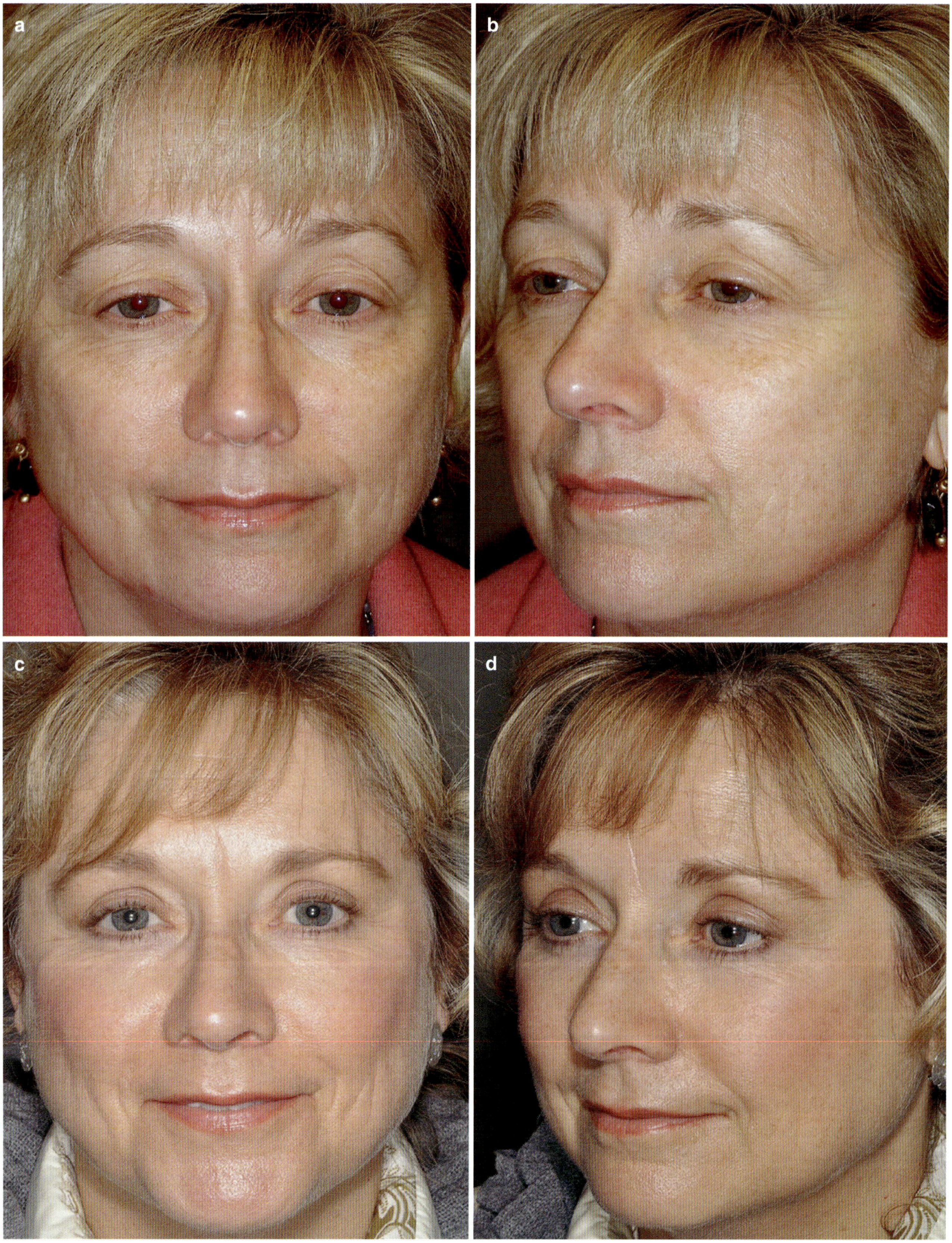

Fig. 21.14 (**a**, **b**) Before photos of a patient who underwent fat transfer to the tear trough and nasojugal fold bilaterally. (**c**, **d**) After photos of the patient following fat transfer to the tear troughs and nasojugal folds, four-lid blepharoplasty, and laser resurfacing. Note the substantially improved lid-cheek interface contour. (Courtesy of John B. Holds, M.D.)

ischemia and necrosis. This has been seen with the use of industry-manufactured fillers in the glabellar furrows and nasolabial folds near the ala of the nose [177, 178]. Treatment of ischemia and necrosis should include aspirin, application of nitroglycerin paste, and warm compresses to the affected area. Hyperbaric oxygen may also provide a beneficial role [179, 180]. All of the above treatments work at reestablishing flow to the area and increasing oxygenation.

More easily managed complications are related to uneven, inadequate, or excess placement of the fat at the time of transfer [142, 148]. This would include lumps, bulges, over- or undercorrection, and depressions at the injection site. Persistent edema can also be problematic. This is especially true in area of the malar bag. Carefully check patients to determine if they may be predisposed to having this occur and, if so, have an informed discussion with them. A lump of fat usually occurs in the inferior periorbital region where the skin is thin and there is minimal subcutaneous tissue. Overapplication of fat or placement too superficially is the etiology of a lump. Treatment can be either local steroid injection or actual excision of the excess fat. The best way to avoid a lump that occurs along the inferior orbital rim is to inject from the malar area superiorly in a perpendicular fashion. Avoid injecting parallel to the inferior orbital rim from the lateral canthal region. A bulge is a larger area of elevation of a recipient site. The three causes include fibrosis, edema, or excess fat. Induration of the area can be determined with palpation. If indurated from fibrosis, then intralesional steroids can be used. Diluted, low-dose steroid is suggested to avoid surrounding tissue atrophy and hypopigmentation of the overlying skin. Excessive fat can be removed with liposuction once time has passed to determine that edema is no longer present. Excess fat overcorrection needs to be distinguished from edema. At least 6 months should pass before a determination is made to intervene. Reduction of overcorrection is performed with a fine-gauge liposuction cannula. Undercorrection is simply treated with the addition of more fat. Also, be aware that smokers and avid exercisers can have more atrophy. Some surgeons store frozen fat for this purpose of treating undercorrection. The best temperature and cryopreservation conditions to store fat for viability have not been determined, and reports regarding the viability of cryopreserved fat vary widely [144, 181, 182]. Storage of fat may present an increased infection risk as well [183]. Others simply harvest fresh fat and refill the undercorrected areas. Lifting procedures tend to have a slight overcorrection as the goal in order to overcome the effects of gravity as the edema resolves. Fat transfer on the other hand has the goal of proper correction or to err on the side of undercorrection. The addition of more fat is simpler than trying to remove fat in the complex anatomical facial region by liposuction techniques.

Summary

Fat transfer offers an alternative to biosynthetic materials for the volume replenishment of the face. It is easily combined with traditional incisional surgery. It appears that with technique refinement, there is a long-lasting effect. It is well tolerated with typically mild complications. Further investigation will elucidate the optimal technique for enhanced and persistent results. Rejuvenation medicine is a field of interest which is growing [184].

References

1. Fagien S, Brandt FS. Primary and adjunctive use of botulinum toxin type A (Botox) in facial aesthetic surgery: beyond the glabella. Clin Plast Surg. 2001;28(1):127–48.
2. Fagien S, Raspaldo H. Facial rejuvenation with botulinum neurotoxin: an anatomical and experiential perspective. J Cosmet Laser Ther. 2007;9(Suppl 1):23–31.
3. Fagien S. Botulinum toxin type A for facial aesthetic enhancement: role in facial shaping. Plast Reconstr Surg. 2003;112(5 Suppl):6S–18S; discussion 19S–20S.
4. Rohrich RJ, et al. The cosmetic use of botulinum toxin. Plast Reconstr Surg. 2003;112(5 Suppl):177S–88S; quiz 188S, 192S; discussion 189S–91S.
5. Carruthers JD, Glogau RG, Blitzer A. Advances in facial rejuvenation: botulinum toxin type a, hyaluronic acid dermal fillers, and combination therapies–consensus recommendations. Plast Reconstr Surg. 2008;121(5 Suppl):5S–30S; quiz 31S–6S
6. Carruthers A, Carruthers J. History of the cosmetic use of botulinum a exotoxin. Dermatol Surg. 1998;24(11):1168–70.
7. Walgama EAR, Gilmore J. Botulinum toxin for the facial cosmetic surgeon. Am J Cosmet Surg. 2010;27(2):49–61.
8. Statista.com. Global revenue of allergan botox. 2017. Available from: https://www.statista.com/statistics/737487/global-revenue-of-allergan-botox-by-region/.
9. ASPS. Plastic surgery statistics report. 2017. Available from: https://www.plasticsurgery.org/documents/News/Statistics/2017/plastic-surgery-statistics-full-report-2017.pdf.
10. Fagien S. Botox for the treatment of dynamic and hyperkinetic facial lines and furrows: adjunctive use in facial aesthetic surgery. Plast Reconstr Surg. 1999;103(2):701–13.
11. Pierard GE, Lapiere CM. The microanatomical basis of facial frown lines. Arch Dermatol. 1989;125(8):1090–2.
12. Klein AW. Contraindications and complications with the use of botulinum toxin. Clin Dermatol. 2004;22(1):66–75.
13. Flynn TC. Botulinum toxin: examining duration of effect in facial aesthetic applications. Am J Clin Dermatol. 2010;11(3):183–99.
14. Happak W, et al. Human facial muscles: dimensions, motor endplate distribution, and presence of muscle fibers with multiple motor endplates. Anat Rec. 1997;249(2):276–84.
15. Chertow DS, et al. Botulism in 4 adults following cosmetic injections with an unlicensed, highly concentrated botulinum preparation. JAMA. 2006;296(20):2476–9.
16. Chang MA. Possible adverse effects of repeated botulinum toxin a injections to decrease post-stroke spasticity in adults undergoing rehabilitation: a review of the literature. J Allied Health. 2015;44(3):140–4.
17. Erbguth FJ, Naumann M. Historical aspects of botulinum toxin: Justinus Kerner (1786–1862) and the "sausage poison". Neurology. 1999;53(8):1850–3.

18. Pessa JE. Improving the acute nasolabial angle and medial nasolabial fold by levator alae muscle resection. Ann Plast Surg. 1992;29(1):23–30.
19. Carruthers J, Stubbs HA. Botulinum toxin for benign essential blepharospasm, hemifacial spasm and age-related lower eyelid entropion. Can J Neurol Sci. 1987;14(1):42–5.
20. Scott AB. Botulinum toxin injection into extraocular muscles as an alternative to strabismus surgery. Ophthalmology. 1980;87(10):1044–9.
21. Scott AB. Botulinum toxin injection into extraocular muscles as an alternative to strabismus surgery. J Pediatr Ophthalmol Strabismus. 1980;17(1):21–5.
22. Carruthers JA, et al. A multicenter, double-blind, randomized, placebo-controlled study of the efficacy and safety of botulinum toxin type A in the treatment of glabellar lines. J Am Acad Dermatol. 2002;46(6):840–9.
23. Carruthers JD, et al. Double-blind, placebo-controlled study of the safety and efficacy of botulinum toxin type A for patients with glabellar lines. Plast Reconstr Surg. 2003;112(4):1089–98.
24. Jankovic J. Botulinum toxin in movement disorders. Curr Opin Neurol. 1994;7(4):358–66.
25. Choi JC, Lucarelli MJ, Shore JW. Use of botulinum A toxin in patients at risk of wound complications following eyelid reconstruction. Ophthal Plast Reconstr Surg. 1997;13(4):259–64.
26. Carruthers JD, Carruthers JA. Treatment of glabellar frown lines with C. botulinum-A exotoxin. J Dermatol Surg Oncol. 1992;18(1):17–21.
27. Carruthers J, Carruthers A. The adjunctive usage of botulinum toxin. Dermatol Surg. 1998;24(11):1244–7.
28. Clark RP, Berris CE. Botulinum toxin: a treatment for facial asymmetry caused by facial nerve paralysis. Plast Reconstr Surg. 1989;84(2):353–5.
29. Carruthers A, Carruthers J, Cohen J. A prospective, double-blind, randomized, parallel- group, dose-ranging study of botulinum toxin type a in female subjects with horizontal forehead rhytides. Dermatol Surg. 2003;29(5):461–7.
30. Rohrich RJ, et al. Botulinum toxin: expanding role in medicine. Plast Reconstr Surg. 2003;112(5 Suppl):1S–3S.
31. Safety warnings for botulinum toxin. J Drugs Dermatol. 2009;8(10):959.
32. Kassir R, Kolluru A, Kassir M. Triple-blind, prospective, internally controlled comparative study between abobotulinumtoxinA and onabotulinumtoxinA for the treatment of facial rhytids. Dermatol Ther (Heidelb). 2013;3(2):179–89.
33. Carruthers J, Carruthers A. Aesthetic botulinum A toxin in the mid and lower face and neck. Dermatol Surg. 2003;29(5):468–76.
34. Kane M. RT001 by revance shows promise for topical delivery of botulinum toxin type A. Plastic Surgery Pulse News. 2010;2(1):20.
35. Revance. Available from: https://investors.revance.com/news-releases/news-release-details/revance-reports-results-rt001-topical-phase-3-trial-lateral.
36. Wollina U, Konrad H. Managing adverse events associated with botulinum toxin type A: a focus on cosmetic procedures. Am J Clin Dermatol. 2005;6(3):141–50.
37. Alam M, Dover JS, Arndt KA. Pain associated with injection of botulinum A exotoxin reconstituted using isotonic sodium chloride with and without preservative: a double-blind, randomized controlled trial. Arch Dermatol. 2002;138(4):510–4.
38. Alam M, et al. Sterility assessment of multiple use botulinum A exotoxin vials: a prospective simulation. J Am Acad Dermatol. 2006;55(2):272–5.
39. Fagien S. Extended use of botulinum toxin type a in facial aesthetic surgery. Aesthet Surg J. 1998;18(3):215–9.
40. Hsu TS, Dover JS, Arndt KA. Effect of volume and concentration on the diffusion of botulinum exotoxin a. Arch Dermatol. 2004;140(11):1351–4.
41. Carruthers A, Carruthers J, Cohen J. Dilution volume of botulinum toxin type A for the treatment of glabellar rhytides: does it matter?. Dermatol Surg. 2007;33(1 Spec No):S97–104.
42. Hexsel DM, et al. Multicenter, double-blind study of the efficacy of injections with botulinum toxin type a reconstituted up to six consecutive weeks before application. Dermatol Surg. 2003;29(5):523–9; discussion 529
43. Winn BJ, Sires BS. Electromyographic differences between normal upper and lower facial muscles and the influence of onabotulinum toxin a. JAMA Facial Plast Surg. 2013;15(3):211–7.
44. Carruthers J, Fagien S, Matarasso SL. Consensus recommendations on the use of botulinum toxin type a in facial aesthetics. Plast Reconstr Surg. 2004;114(6 Suppl):1S–22S.
45. Fagien S. Temporary management of upper lid ptosis, lid malposition, and eyelid fissure asymmetry with botulinum toxin type a. Plast Reconstr Surg. 2004;114(7):1892–902.
46. Carruthers A, Kiene K, Carruthers J. Botulinum A exotoxin use in clinical dermatology. J Am Acad Dermatol. 1996;34(5 Pt 1):788–97.
47. Shah AR. Use of intradermal botulinum toxin to reduce sebum production and facial pore size. J Drugs Dermatol. 2008;7(9):847–50.
48. Fagien S. Temporal brow lift using botulinum toxin A. Plast Reconstr Surg. 2003;112(S5):105S–7S.
49. Maas CS, Kim EJ. Temporal brow lift using botulinum toxin A: an update. Plast Reconstr Surg. 2003;112(5 Suppl):109S–12S; discussion 113S–4S.
50. Huilgol SC, Carruthers A, Carruthers JD. Raising eyebrows with botulinum toxin. Dermatol Surg. 1999;25(5):373–5; discussion 376
51. Flynn TC, Carruthers JA, Carruthers JA. Botulinum-A toxin treatment of the lower eyelid improves infraorbital rhytides and widens the eye. Dermatol Surg. 2001;27(8):703–8.
52. Kane MA. The functional anatomy of the lower face as it applies to rejuvenation via chemodenervation. Facial Plast Surg. 2005;21(1):55–64.
53. Park MY, Ahn KY, Jung DS. Botulinum toxin type A treatment for contouring of the lower face. Dermatol Surg. 2003;29(5):477–83; discussion 483
54. Choe SW, et al. Effects of botulinum toxin type a on contouring of the lower face. Dermatol Surg. 2005;31(5):502–7; discussion 507–8
55. Yu CC, Chen PK, Chen YR. Botulinum toxin a for lower facial contouring: a prospective study. Aesthet Plast Surg. 2007;31(5):445–51; discussion 452–3
56. Gassner HG, et al. Botulinum toxin to improve facial wound healing: a prospective, blinded, placebo-controlled study. Mayo Clin Proc. 2006;81(8):1023–8.
57. Park KY, et al. Botulinum toxin for the treatment of refractory erythema and flushing of rosacea. Dermatology. 2015;230(4):299–301.
58. Cutrer FM, Pittelkow MR. Cephalalgic alopecia areata: a syndrome of neuralgiform head pain and hair loss responsive to botulinum A toxin injection. Cephalalgia. 2006;26(6):747–51.
59. Gobel H. Botulinum toxin in migraine prophylaxis. J Neurol. 2004;251(Suppl 1):I8–11.
60. Singer N. In New York Times. 2010.
61. Coleman SR. Structural fat grafts: the ideal filler? Clin Plast Surg. 2001;28(1):111–9.
62. Murray CA, Zloty D, Warshawski L. The evolution of soft tissue fillers in clinical practice. Dermatol Clin. 2005;23(2):343–63.
63. Jordan DR. Soft-tissue fillers for wrinkles, folds and volume augmentation. Can J Ophthalmol. 2003;38(4):285–8.
64. Kontis TC, Rivkin A. The history of injectable facial fillers. Facial Plast Surg. 2009;25(2):67–72.

65. Bray D, Hopkins C, Roberts DN. A review of dermal fillers in facial plastic surgery. Curr Opin Otolaryngol Head Neck Surg. 2010;18(4):295–302.
66. FDA. Available from: https://www.fda.gov/MedicalDevices/ProductsandMedicalProcedures/DeviceApprovalsandClearances/Recently-ApprovedDevices/ucm589391.htm.
67. Lemperle G, Morhenn V, Charrier U. Human histology and persistence of various injectable filler substances for soft tissue augmentation. Aesthet Plast Surg. 2003;27(5):354–66; discussion 367
68. Duranti F, et al. Injectable hyaluronic acid gel for soft tissue augmentation. A clinical and histological study. Dermatol Surg. 1998;24(12):1317–25.
69. Wesley NO, Dover JS. The filler revolution: a six-year retrospective. J Drugs Dermatol. 2009;8(10):903–7.
70. Bergeret-Galley C. Choosing injectable implants according to treatment area: the European experience. Facial Plast Surg. 2009;25(2):135–42.
71. Sykes JM. Applied anatomy of the temporal region and forehead for injectable fillers. J Drugs Dermatol. 2009;8(10 Suppl):s24–7.
72. Hirsch RJ, Stier M. Complications of soft tissue augmentation. J Drugs Dermatol. 2008;7(9):841–5.
73. Rohrich RJ, et al. The anatomy of suborbicularis fat: implications for periorbital rejuvenation. Plast Reconstr Surg. 2009;124(3):946–51.
74. Rohrich RJ, Pessa JE. The anatomy and clinical implications of perioral submuscular fat. Plast Reconstr Surg. 2009;124(1):266–71.
75. Beasley KL, Weiss MA, Weiss RA. Hyaluronic acid fillers: a comprehensive review. Facial Plast Surg. 2009;25(2):86–94.
76. Hilinski JM, Cohen SR. Soft tissue augmentation with ArteFill. Facial Plast Surg. 2009;25(2):114–9.
77. Ridenour B, Kontis TC. Injectable calcium hydroxylapatite microspheres (Radiesse). Facial Plast Surg. 2009;25(2):100–5.
78. Lupo MP. Natural look in volume restoration. J Drugs Dermatol. 2008;7(9):833–9.
79. Carruthers J, et al. The science and art of dermal fillers for soft-tissue augmentation. J Drugs Dermatol. 2009;8(4):335–50.
80. Bentkover SH. The biology of facial fillers. Facial Plast Surg. 2009;25(2):73–85.
81. Cockerham K, Hsu VJ. Collagen-based dermal fillers: past, present, future. Facial Plast Surg. 2009;25(2):106–13.
82. Klein AW. In favor of double testing. J Dermatol Surg Oncol. 1989;15(3):263.
83. Elson ML. The role of skin testing in the use of collagen injectable materials. J Dermatol Surg Oncol. 1989;15(3):301–3.
84. Surgeons, A.S.o.A.P. Available from: https://www.surgery.org/sites/default/files/ASAPS-Stats2017.pdf.
85. Hirsch RJ, Cohen JL. Soft tissue augmentation. Cutis. 2006;78(3):165–72.
86. Monheit GD, Coleman KM. Hyaluronic acid fillers. Dermatol Ther. 2006;19(3):141–50.
87. Kablik J, et al. Comparative physical properties of hyaluronic acid dermal fillers. Dermatol Surg. 2009;35(Suppl 1):302–12.
88. MAIPS. Medical Aesthetics Information Platform and Solutions. Available from: http://www.maips.com/all_facial_injectable_fillers.html.
89. MERZ. Available from: https://www.belotero.com/how-it-works/.
90. Sundaram H, Cassuto D. Biophysical characteristics of hyaluronic acid soft-tissue fillers and their relevance to aesthetic applications. Plast Reconstr Surg. 2013;132(4 Suppl 2):5S–21S.
91. Sundaram H. Going with the flow: an overview of soft tissue filler rheology and its potential clinical applications. Pract Dermatol. 2011;2:23–8.
92. Galderma. Galderma announces FDA approval of restylane lyft for midface injection via cannula. Available from: https://www.prnewswire.com/news-releases/galderma-announces-fda-approval-of-restylane-lyft-for-midface-injection-via-cannula-300743490.html.
93. Lee A, et al. Hyaluronidase. Dermatol Surg. 2010;36(7):1071–7.
94. Soparkar CN, Patrinely JR, Tschen J. Erasing restylane. Ophthal Plast Reconstr Surg. 2004;20(4):317–8.
95. Lambros V. The use of hyaluronidase to reverse the effects of hyaluronic acid filler. Plast Reconstr Surg. 2004;114(1):277.
96. Busso M. Calcium hydroxylapatite (Radiesse): safety, techniques and pain reduction. J Drugs Dermatol. 2009;8(10 Suppl):s21–3.
97. Marmur ES, et al. Six-month safety results of calcium hydroxylapatite for treatment of nasolabial folds in Fitzpatrick skin types IV to VI. Dermatol Surg. 2009;35(Suppl 2):1641–5.
98. Vleggaar D. Facial volumetric correction with injectable poly-L-lactic acid. Dermatol Surg. 2005;31(11 Pt 2):1511–7; discussion 1517–8
99. Vleggaar D, Bauer U. Facial enhancement and the European experience with Sculptra (poly-l-lactic acid). J Drugs Dermatol. 2004;3(5):542–7.
100. Lacombe V. Sculptra: a stimulatory filler. Facial Plast Surg. 2009;25(2):95–9.
101. Palm MD, Goldman MP. Patient satisfaction and duration of effect with PLLA: a review of the literature. J Drugs Dermatol. 2009;8(10 Suppl):s15–20.
102. Vleggaar D. Soft-tissue augmentation and the role of poly-L-lactic acid. Plast Reconstr Surg. 2006;118(3 Suppl):46S–54S.
103. Jones D. HIV facial lipoatrophy: causes and treatment options. Dermatol Surg. 2005;31(11 Pt 2):1519–29; discussion 1529
104. FDA approves poly-L-lactic acid for nasolabial folds. J Drugs Dermatol. 2009:8(10):959.
105. Physicians' Coalition for Injectable Safety. Current concepts in utilization of collagen stimulators. Release date: October 1, 2009. J Drugs Dermatol. 2009;8(10 Suppl):s3–4.
106. Medical S. Available from: http://www.sunevamedical.com/bellafill-receives-fda-approval-for-treatment-of-acne-scars-2/.
107. Naoum C, et al. A histological and immunohistochemical study of medical-grade fluid silicone. Dermatol Surg. 1998;24(8):867–70.
108. Duffy DM. Liquid silicone for soft tissue augmentation. Dermatol Surg. 2005;31(11 Pt 2):1530–41.
109. Rapaport MJ, Vinnik C, Zarem H. Injectable silicone: cause of facial nodules, cellulitis, ulceration, and migration. Aesthet Plast Surg. 1996;20(3):267–76.
110. Urdiales-Galvez F, et al. Treatment of soft tissue filler complications: expert consensus recommendations. Aesthet Plast Surg. 2018;42(2):498–510.
111. Winslow CP. The management of dermal filler complications. Facial Plast Surg. 2009;25(2):124–8.
112. Andre P, Wechsler J, Revuz J. Facial lipoatrophy: report of five cases after injection of synthetic filler into naso-labial folds. J Cosmet Dermatol. 2002;1(3):120–3.
113. Gandy J, Bierman D, Zachary C. Granulomatous reaction to Belotero balance: a case study. J Cosmet Laser Ther. 2017;19(5):307–9.
114. Beer K. Delayed onset nodules from liquid injectable silicone: report of a case, evaluation of associated histopathology and results of treatment with minocycline and celecoxib. J Drugs Dermatol. 2009;8(10):952–4.
115. Dumitrascu DI, Georgescu AV. The management of biofilm formation after hyaluronic acid gel filler injections: a review. Clujul Med. 2013;86(3):192–5.
116. Gelfer A, et al. The natural history of polymethylmethacrylate microspheres granulomas. Dermatol Surg. 2007;33(5):614–20.
117. Shafir R, Amir A, Gur E. Long-term complications of facial injections with Restylane (injectable hyaluronic acid). Plast Reconstr Surg. 2000;106(5):1215–6.
118. Honig JF, Brink U, Korabiowska M. Severe granulomatous allergic tissue reaction after hyaluronic acid injection in the treat-

ment of facial lines and its surgical correction. J Craniofac Surg. 2003;14(2):197–200.
119. Lowe NJ, et al. Hyaluronic acid skin fillers: adverse reactions and skin testing. J Am Acad Dermatol. 2001;45(6):930–3.
120. Lupton JR, Alster TS. Cutaneous hypersensitivity reaction to injectable hyaluronic acid gel. Dermatol Surg. 2000;26(2):135–7.
121. Kim JH, et al. Treatment algorithm of complications after filler injection: based on wound healing process. J Korean Med Sci. 2014;29(Suppl 3):S176–82.
122. Kang BK, et al. Treatment of glabella skin necrosis following injection of hyaluronic acid filler using platelet-rich plasma. J Cosmet Laser Ther. 2016;18(2):111–2.
123. Andre P, Haneke E. Nicolau syndrome due to hyaluronic acid injections. J Cosmet Laser Ther. 2016;18(4):239–44.
124. DeLorenzi C. Complications of injectable fillers, part 2: vascular complications. Aesthet Surg J. 2014;34(4):584–600.
125. Cohen JL, et al. Treatment of hyaluronic acid filler-induced impending necrosis with hyaluronidase: consensus recommendations. Aesthet Surg J. 2015;35(7):844–9.
126. McCleve DE, Goldstein JC. Blindness secondary to injections in the nose, mouth, and face: cause and prevention. Ear Nose Throat J. 1995;74(3):182–8.
127. Weinberg MJ, Solish N. Complications of hyaluronic acid fillers. Facial Plast Surg. 2009;25(5):324–8.
128. Sires B, Laukaitis S, Whitehouse P. Radiesse-induced herpes zoster. Ophthal Plast Reconstr Surg. 2008;24(3):218–9.
129. Lambros V. The dynamics of facial aging. In American Academy of Facial Plastic and Reconstructive Surgery, winter meeting, 2009, Telluride.
130. Neuber F. Bericht uber die Verhandlungen der Dt Ges f Chir. Zentalbl Chir. 1893;22:66.
131. Miller C. The limitations and use of paraffin in cosmetic surgery. Wis Med Recorder. 1908;11:277.
132. Kolle F. Plastic and cosmetic surgery, vol. 209-338. New York: Appleton and Company; 1911.
133. Beck J. Implantation method: plastic surgery of the nose and ear. In: Loeb H, editor. Operative surgery of the nose, throat and ear. St. Louis: CV Mosby; 1917. p. 3.
134. Rogers BO. A chronologic history of cosmetic surgery. Bull N Y Acad Med. 1971;47(3):265–302.
135. Miller C. Cannula implants and review of implantation techniques in esthetic surgery. Chicago: Oak Press; 1926. p. 15.
136. Klein JA. Tumescent technique for regional anesthesia permits lidocaine doses of 35 mg/kg for liposuction. J Dermatol Surg Oncol. 1990;16(3):248–63.
137. Coleman WP 3rd, Badame A, Phillips JH 3rd. A new technique for injection of tumescent anesthetic mixtures. J Dermatol Surg Oncol. 1991;17(6):535–7.
138. Chajchir A, Benzaquen I. Liposuction fat grafts in face wrinkles and hemifacial atrophy. Aesthet Plast Surg. 1986;10(2):115–7.
139. Groen JW, et al. Autologous fat transfer for facial rejuvenation: a systematic review on technique, efficacy, and satisfaction. Plast Reconstr Surg Glob Open. 2017;5(12):e1606.
140. Keck M, et al. Local anesthetics have a major impact on viability of preadipocytes and their differentiation to adipocytes. Plast Reconstr Surg. 2010;126:1500.
141. Stashower M, et al. Stromal progenitor cells present within liposuction and reduction abdominoplasty fat for autologous transfer to aged skin. Dermatol Surg. 1999;25(12):945–9.
142. Glasgold RA, Lam SM, Glasgold MJ. Facial fat grafting: the new paradigm. Arch Facial Plast Surg. 2008;10(6):417–8.
143. Tringale KR, et al. Sustained overcorrection after autologous facial fat grafting in the pediatric population: a case series. Ann Plast Surg. 2017;78(5 Suppl 4):S217–21.
144. Erol OO, Agaoglu G. Facial rejuvenation with staged injections of cryopreserved fat and tissue cocktail: clinical outcomes in the past 10 years. Aesthet Surg J. 2013;33(5):639–53.
145. Moscatello DK, et al. Cryopreservation of human fat for soft tissue augmentation: viability requires use of cryoprotectant and controlled freezing and storage. Dermatol Surg. 2005;31(11 Pt 2):1506–10.
146. Sadick NS, Hudgins LC. Fatty acid analysis of transplanted adipose tissue. Arch Dermatol. 2001;137(6):723–7.
147. Sires BS, et al. Characterization of human orbital fat and connective tissue. Ophthal Plast Reconstr Surg. 1998;14(6):403–14.
148. Lam SM, Glasgold MJ, Glasgold RA. Operative technique. In: Complementary fat grafting. Philadelphia: Wolters Kluwer-Lippincott Williams & Wilkins; 2007. p. 32–82.
149. Gonzalez AM, et al. An alternative method for harvest and processing fat grafts: an in vitro study of cell viability and survival. Plast Reconstr Surg. 2007;120(1):285–94.
150. Moore JH Jr, et al. Viability of fat obtained by syringe suction lipectomy: effects of local anesthesia with lidocaine. Aesthet Plast Surg. 1995;19(4):335–9.
151. Rose JG Jr, et al. Histologic comparison of autologous fat processing methods. Ophthal Plast Reconstr Surg. 2006;22(3):195–200.
152. Aboudib Junior JH, de Castro CC, Gradel J. Hand rejuvenescence by fat filling. Ann Plast Surg. 1992;28(6):559–64.
153. Kaufman MR, et al. Autologous fat transfer for facial recontouring: is there science behind the art? Plast Reconstr Surg. 2007;119(7):2287–96.
154. Ramon Y, et al. Enhancing the take of injected adipose tissue by a simple method for concentrating fat cells. Plast Reconstr Surg. 2005;115(1):197–201; discussion 202–3
155. Gontijo-de-Amorim NF, Charles-de-Sa L, Rigotti G. Mechanical supplementation with the stromal vascular fraction yields improved volume retention in facial lipotransfer: a 1-year comparative study. Aesthet Surg J. 2017;37(9):975–85.
156. Sasaki GH. The safety and efficacy of cell-assisted fat grafting to traditional fat grafting in the anterior mid-face: an indirect assessment by 3D imaging. Aesthet Plast Surg. 2015;39(6):833–46.
157. Mailey B, et al. A comparison of cell-enriched fat transfer to conventional fat grafting after aesthetic procedures using a patient satisfaction survey. Ann Plast Surg. 2013;70(4):410–5.
158. Wan DC, Lim AT, Longaker MT. Craniofacial autologous fat transfer. J Craniofac Surg. 2009;20(2):273–4.
159. Hong SJ, et al. Enhancing the viability of fat grafts using new transfer medium containing insulin and beta-fibroblast growth factor in autologous fat transplantation. J Plast Reconstr Aesthet Surg. 2010;63(7):1202–8.
160. Pallua N, et al. Content of the growth factors bFGF, IGF-1, VEGF, and PDGF-BB in freshly harvested lipoaspirate after centrifugation and incubation. Plast Reconstr Surg. 2009;123(3):826–33.
161. Rubin JP, et al. Collagenous microbeads as a scaffold for tissue engineering with adipose-derived stem cells. Plast Reconstr Surg. 2007;120(2):414–24.
162. Torio-Padron N, et al. Engineering of adipose tissue by injection of human preadipocytes in fibrin. Aesthet Plast Surg. 2007;31(3):285–93.
163. Matsumoto D, et al. Cell-assisted lipotransfer: supportive use of human adipose-derived cells for soft tissue augmentation with lipoinjection. Tissue Eng. 2006;12(12):3375–82.
164. Zhu M, et al. Supplementation of fat grafts with adipose-derived regenerative cells improves long-term graft retention. Ann Plast Surg. 2012;64(2):222–8.
165. Carpaneda CA, Ribeiro MT. Study of the histologic alterations and viability of the adipose graft in humans. Aesthet Plast Surg. 1993;17(1):43–7.

166. Rohrich RJ, et al. Lift-and-fill face lift: integrating the fat compartments. Plast Reconstr Surg. 2014;133(6):756e–67e.
167. Stein R, et al. Phi, fat, and the mathematics of a beautiful midface. Ophthalmic Plast Reconstr Surg. 2018;34(5):491–6.
168. Shue S, Kurlander DE, Guyuron B. Fat injection: a systematic review of injection volumes by facial subunit. Aesthet Plast Surg. 2018;42(5):1261–70.
169. Ellenbogen R. Fat transfer: current use in practice. Clin Plast Surg. 2000;27(4):545–56.
170. Einan-Lifshitz A, et al. Volumetric rejuvenation of the tear trough with repo and Ristow. Ophthalmic Plast Reconstr Surg. 2013;29(6):481–5.
171. Rohrich RJ, Sanniec K, Afrooz PN. Autologous fat grafting to the Chin: a useful adjunct in complete aesthetic facial rejuvenation. Plast Reconstr Surg. 2018;142(4):921–5.
172. Trivisonno A, et al. Facial skin rejuvenation by autologous dermal microfat transfer in photoaged patients: clinical evaluation and skin surface digital profilometry analysis. J Plast Reconstr Aesthet Surg. 2017;70(8):1118–28.
173. Horl HW, Feller AM, Biemer E. Technique for liposuction fat reimplantation and long-term volume evaluation by magnetic resonance imaging. Ann Plast Surg. 1991;26(3):248–58.
174. Meier JD, Glasgold RA, Glasgold MJ. Autologous fat grafting: long-term evidence of its efficacy in midfacial rejuvenation. Arch Facial Plast Surg. 2009;11(1):24–8.
175. Yoon SS, Chang DI, Chung KC. Acute fatal stroke immediately following autologous fat injection into the face. Neurology. 2003;61(8):1151–2.
176. Dreizen NG, Framm L. Sudden unilateral visual loss after autologous fat injection into the glabellar area. Am J Ophthalmol. 1989;107(1):85–7.
177. Glaich AS, Cohen JL, Goldberg LH. Injection necrosis of the glabella: protocol for prevention and treatment after use of dermal fillers. Dermatol Surg. 2006;32(2):276–81.
178. Grunebaum LD, et al. The risk of alar necrosis associated with dermal filler injection. Dermatol Surg. 2009;35(Suppl 2):1635–40.
179. Henderson R, Reilly DA, Cooper JS. Hyperbaric oxygen for ischemia due to injection of cosmetic fillers: case report and issues. Plast Reconstr Surg Glob Open. 2018;6(1):e1618.
180. Darling MD, Peterson JD, Fabi SG. Impending necrosis after injection of hyaluronic acid and calcium hydroxylapatite fillers: report of 2 cases treated with hyperbaric oxygen therapy. Dermatol Surg. 2014;40(9):1049–52.
181. Mashiko T, et al. Biological properties and therapeutic value of cryopreserved fat tissue. Plast Reconstr Surg. 2018;141(1):104–15.
182. Li BW, et al. Cryopreservation of fat tissue and application in autologous fat graft: in vitro and in vivo study. Aesthet Plast Surg. 2012;36(3):714–22.
183. Kim SK, Kim HJ, Hwang K. Mixed infection of an atypical Mycobacterium and Aspergillus following a cryopreserved fat graft to a face. J Craniofac Surg. 2013;24(5):1676–8.
184. James IB, Coleman SR, Rubin JP. Fat, stem cells, and platelet-rich plasma. Clin Plast Surg. 2016;43(3):473–88.

Facelift and Midface Lift

22

Richard A. Zoumalan, Christopher I. Zoumalan, and Wayne F. Larrabee Jr.

Introduction

Facelift and midface lifts are performed to give a more youthful appearance to the face. While this type of surgery is mostly performed on the aging face, it can also be used for patients with facial paralysis. Overall, aging involves gradual thinning of the epidermis, flattening of the epidermal-dermal border, loss of collagen and thickness in the dermis, decrease in collagen type I to type III ratio, and reduction in the skin cellular and protein components. Sun damage can worsen and accelerate this process. Lax skin with decreased collagen manifests through sagging and increased propensity to be wrinkled and furrowed. In addition, muscle laxity and atrophy can add to sagging tissues and lack of face, mandibular, and neck definition. This can be seen in the increase in the cervicomental angle of the neck and jowling, which is sagging of tissues along the mandibular line. These particular effects of aging can be amenable to a facelift or midface lift [5].

Until the 1970s, much of facelift surgery involved a superficial skin dissection with the excision of excess skin. While there are some who still perform this, skin excision did not provide a long-term benefit, nor did this procedure affect the midface. In the 1970s, dissection and manipulation of the superficial muscular aponeurotic system (SMAS) began to take place. This began an era of different strategies to attain optimal vector pull fat pad repositioning. Since then, the field has seen the implementation of endoscopic techniques, cable sutures, and blepharoplasty incision approaches as ways to improve previous techniques. We will discuss the most commonly used techniques [6].

R. A. Zoumalan
UCLA, Cedars Sinai Medicine, Department of Otolaryngology, Beverly Hills, CA, USA

C. I. Zoumalan (✉)
Department of Ophthalmology, Division of Ophthalmic Plastic and Reconstructive Surgery, Keck School of Medicine of USC, Los Angeles, CA, USA

W. F. Larrabee Jr.
Larrabee Center for Plastic Surgery, Seattle, WA, USA

Anatomy

Superficial Muscular Aponeurotic System (SMAS)

The key to understanding facelift surgery is the concept of the SMAS. The SMAS is a fibromuscular fascial layer which invests and interlinks the muscles of facial expression. It maintains consistent relationships with the vessels and nerves. Inferiorly, it is contiguous with the platysma. Superiorly, it is contiguous with the temporoparietal fascia. Medially, it has attachments to the zygomaticus major and minor as well as the dermis of the upper lip. The SMAS also has fascial condensations which are adherent to the overlying dermis and underlying muscle and bone. While not true ligaments, they are termed as such and act as supportfor the soft tissues of the cheek [3].

Platysma

The platysma is a thin layer of muscle in the neck which is deep to the dermis. It is contiguous with the SMAS and is innervated by the cervical branch of the facial nerve, which is deep to the muscle. Medially, at the level of the thyroid cartilage, the platysma fibers interdigitate, forming an inverted "V." The apex can be at the level of the chin or slightly below at the level of the thyroid cartilage. Because of this, the submental area may or may not be covered by the muscle fibers. If there is laxity or dehiscence of the anterior borders of the muscle, it creates banding in the midline, which occurs with age. Patients may then also have a chin droop, as the submental area lacks tissue. Laxity of the platysma can lead to "turkey gobbler" deformity and an increased cervicomental

J. J. Servat et al. (eds.), *Smith and Nesi's Ophthalmic Plastic and Reconstructive Surgery*,
https://doi.org/10.1007/978-3-030-41720-8_22

angle. The flaccidity of the superolateral fibers of the platysma muscle may be a contributing factor to chin droop and jowling [7, 12].

Facial Nerve

The facial nerveexits the stylomastoid foramen and courses through the parotid gland. It branches into five branches: temporal (or frontal), zygomatic, buccal (marginal), mandibular, and cervical rami. Within the parotid gland, the main trunk usually divides a superior (temporofacial) and inferior (cervicofacial) branches. From there, the branching pattern becomes variable. After exiting the parotid gland in the face, the nerve branches are just deep to the parotideomasseteric fascia, which is a barely appreciable thin facial layer just deep to the SMAS. The frontal and marginal branches are the most commonly injured branches in facelift [11]. The frontal branch runs within the temporoparietal fascia and is superficial to the superficial layer of the deep temporal fascia. It crosses the zygoma midway between the tragus and lateral canthus of the eye. The marginal mandibular branch runs just deep to the platysma and can be found as low as the level of the hyoid bone, usually two fingerbreadths below the mandibular line [4].

Greater Auricular Nerve

The greater auricular nerve provides sensation to the upper lateral neck and ear lobule. Derived from second and third cervical nerves (C2 and C3), it emerges at the posterior border of the sternocleidomastoid muscle 6 cm inferior to the external auditory canal, wraps around this border, and ascends in the neck on the surface of the SCM. Eventually, it gives off a small postauricular branch and then pierces the parotid gland to provide its sensory innervation [10].

Patient Evaluation

Each patient is entirely different and requires a different approach. Some patients require a more extensive dissection. The surgeon must inquire on and understand the most pressing concerns of the patient. In addition to the patient's desires, the inclusion of various procedures depends on the age and overall health of the patient and their medical history. Patients are counseled on expected outcomes which may include the limitations of the surgery. They are informed of the areas of incisions and reasoning behind placement of these incisions. Patients should also be counseled on all the risks of the surgery, which are discussed later in this chapter.

Surgical Techniques

Skin Excision

While this type of excision is less commonly used today, subcutaneous rhytidectomy has the lowest complication rate of nerve injury. The flap is elevated just superficial to the SMAS and platysma. Superiorly, it avoids injury to the frontal branch by dissecting superficial to the temporalis fascia. In the parotid region, injury is increased as the dissection continues beyond the parotid gland, but it is still low due to having an SMAS layer between the dissection and the facial nerve branches. Inferiorly, there is risk to the greater auricular nerve. A shorter flap may be used in patients with comorbidities which have propensity toward flap ischemia. Figure 22.1 shows skin elevation which can be used for both skin excision technique as well as other types of rhytidectomy. This type of lift has the least ability to rejuvenate and lasts the least amount of time. This type of lift also tends to have higher chance of telltale signs of surgery such as a lateral sweep. In addition, because there is tension on the skin and suture line, and not deeper tissues, incisions do not heal as well [9].

Sub-SMAS Rhytidectomy

Techniques which address the SMAS-platysma complex have longer-lasting and more favorable results than skin excision. The SMAS can be addressed in a variety of ways. One way is to suture plicate, or infold, the SMAS. This allows the surgeon to mobilize the SMAS without exposing

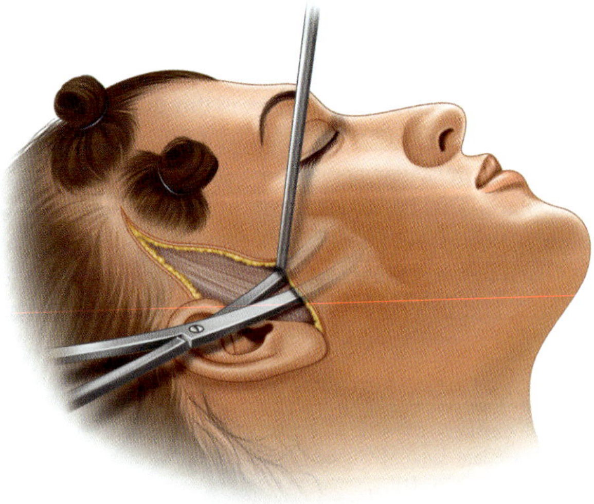

Fig. 22.1 Skin elevation which can be used for both skin excision technique as well as other types of rhytidectomy

the facial nerve to potential injury. However, it does not free up the SMAS or platysma to allow it to mobilize as freely as elevating a sub-SMAS flap. In this flap, incision is made into the SMAS just anterior to the ear and carried anteriorly in the plane just immediately deep to the SMAS [8]. Figure 22.2 shows a variation of an incision that can be used to enter the sub-SMAS plane. This dissection is stopped just inferior to the zygomatic arch, and while it can be carried anterior to the parotid gland and inferior to the mandibular angle, facial nerve branches lie here. Excess tissue is excised and flaps are sutured posterosuperiorly. A posterosuperior vector rejuvenates not only the mandibular line but also the neck. In addition, it can move descended cheek in more superior and lateral position which can even volumize the cheek. The inferior part of the flap is sutured to the mastoid periosteum. The superior portion of the flap is sutured to the temporalis fascia. In the temporalis fascia, a horizontally placed suture is a stronger fixation point than a vertically placed suture due to fibers of the fascia being vertical. Figure 22.3 shows a variation of resuspension of the SMAS flap performed before skin closure [6].

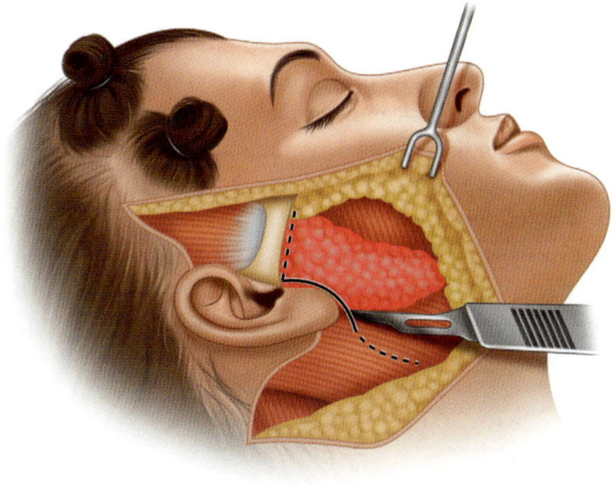

Fig. 22.2 Variation of an incision which can be used to enter the sub-SMAS plane

Composite rhytidectomy is a variation of deep plane technique. It targets the melolabial fold and malar area more precisely. A composite flap is created, which begins with a subcutaneous dissection to a line from the malar eminence to mandibular angle. Then the surgeon performs subplatysmal dissection in the neck, suborbicularis oculi dissection, and separation of the zygomaticus from the SMAS-platysma complex to release the melolabial fold. The zygomaticocutaneous and madibulocutaneous ligaments are released to allow for more mobilization. The flap which not consists of both the SMAS and platysma is then sutured in a posterior and supe-

Fig. 22.3 Variation of resuspension of the SMAS flap performed before skin closure

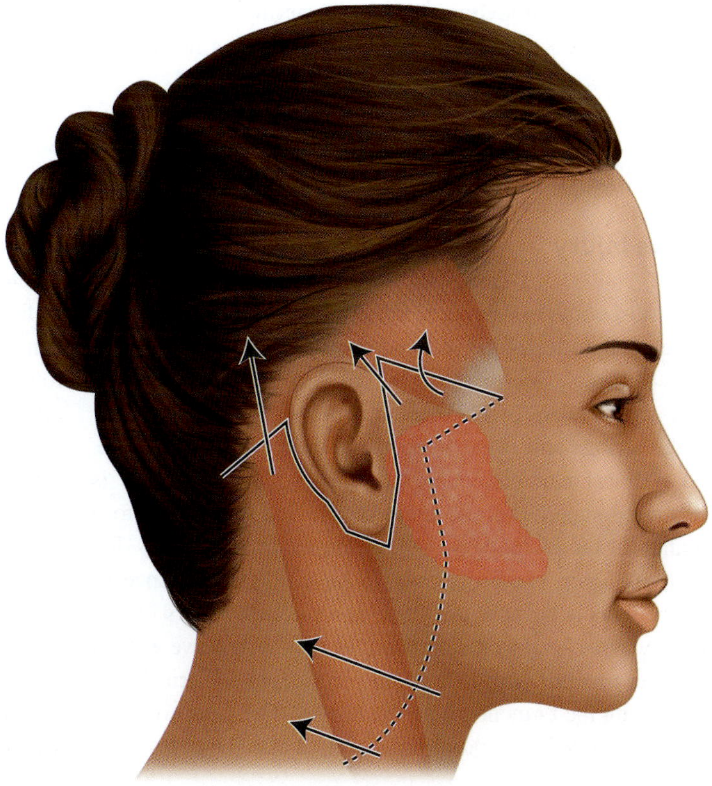

rior direction which tightens the submental area, tightens the mandibular line, improves jowls, and also volumizes the midface. Tension is all placed on this flap so skin incisions have little to no tension, and this leads to more favorable healing. The sub-SMAS-platysma complex is sutured posterosuperiorly in one unit [2].

The Mini-lift and Short Scar Lift

Originally, these operations involved minimal subcutaneous skin undermining and limited skin excision with subsequently minimal improvement and short-lived results (Fig. 22.3). However, the mini-facelift, or mini-lift, and short scar lift have evolved to describe a variety of facelifts which utilize minimal incisions, decreasing the need for postauricular and scalp incisions. Typically, candidates who are excellent fits for a mini-lift are younger patients with limited skin laxity and patients requiring "tuck-ups." One can tell if a patient is a good candidate for this by pulling tissue superiorly and laterally with hands and seeing if the submental tissue easily flattens out. The advantages of these lifts are limited incisions, shorter surgical time, better potential of sedation, risk minimization, and quicker recovery. The disadvantages are limited access to the neck, limited access and improvement in the midface, and difficulty for visualization which is required for suture placement and hemostasis. Also, if too much movement of tissue is performed, the lateral aspect of the lift will have pleats. This does not occur with patients with mild laxity, so the power of this procedure lies in patient evaluation and experience in knowing how much laxity can be well treated with limited incisions [16].

Complications

Nerve Injury

The most commonly injured nerve during facelift surgery is the greater auricular nerve, occurring in up to 7% of patients. This can cause anesthesia of the earlobe. For some patients, this is permanent and bothersome as they have a hard time with earrings and using a telephone on that particular side. As postauricular dissection has thinner skin, the nerve is relatively superficial and must be avoided. An injury to a branch of the facial nerve is less common. Sub-SMAS dissections (deep plane dissections) have a higher chance of injury. This is because the plane of dissection occurs immediately superficial to the branches of the facial nerve as they exit the parotid, with just a thin parotideomasseteric fascia separating the branches from the SMAS. The most common injuries are to the temporal and marginal branches. However, the likelihood of a branch being injured depends on surgical technique and areas of dissection [13].

Hematoma

Hematoma formationis the most common major complication after facelift. Hematomas can lead to tissue ischemia, prolonged facial edema, hyperpigmentation, reoperation, and patient dissatisfaction. If dissection occurs into the neck, airway obstruction can occur, which can be life threatening. Large expanding hematomas require immediate evacuation. The incidence of hematoma ranges from 0.2% to 8.1%, and it is much more common in males. These hematomas must be evacuated as soon as possible. What is more common is to have smaller seromas after surgery, and simple needle drainage and compression dressing solve these smaller fluid collections [14].

Infection

Surgical site infectionoccurs in facelifts in less than 1% of cases (18–65%). Involved areas are usually at the incisions, with possible collections that need to be opened and drained. Early culture and treatment is important, and there is an increasing incidence of methicillin-resistant *Staphylococcus aureus* (MRSA). Protocols to reduce this include the use of chlorhexidine washes before surgery, intranasal mupirocin before surgery, and aggressive culture and antibiotic-directed treatment for any erythema or suspicious collections [15].

Scars

Patientsmust be counseled on the fact that they may have visible scars long-term which are either hyper- or hypopigmented. As with any surgery, scarring is an expected outcome of facelift. In addition, hypertrophic scarring may occur and can be seen as early as 2 weeks after surgery. This is due to excess tension on the incision. With well-closed incisions which are not under tension (tension should be placed on the deep plane), incisionscan heal imperceptibly.

Alopecia

Hair loss is a minor complication or rhytidectomy, and it may be temporary or permanent. It is especially noticeable in the temporal area. The three reasons why alopecia occurs are compromised hair follicles from trauma, an expanding scar which cannot grow hair, and posterior placement of temporal incisions leading to elevation of hairline. Using an incision at the temporal tuft can preclude this [1].

Earlobe Deformity

A pixie or Satyr's ear (devil's ear) deformity can occur due to excessive skin tension at the inferior aspect of the lobe. During the healing period, the lobe is drawn inferiorly. It is caused by the earlobe not being tucked up properly during closure. This is a telltale sign of facelift surgery, and repair can be difficult. This can be prevented by not excessively removing tissue under the earlobe.

Rejuvenation of the Midface

While many think of rejuvenationof the aging face as rhytidectomy, the face ages in other areas that are not addressed by facelift alone. Over time, the midface also descends. If the facelift has a sufficient pull of the SMAS in the posterior and superior direction, the midface will also be pulled and can volumize the lateral midface. In some patients, there is need with further volumization either with fat at the same time of surgery or with fillers at a later date if there is hollowing. In some patients who only want to have midface volumization, a midface lift can help. However, the increased use of facial filler and the use of fat grafting to the face have decreased the use and demand for midface lifts.

Midface Lift

Midface Anatomy

The malar prominence is the upper lateral mound of the cheek. It is composed of a subcutaneous malar fat pad with underlying orbicularis oculi. Deep to the orbicularis oculi is the suborbicularis orbital fat (SOOF). Motor supply is from the zygomatic and buccal branches, and sensation is by V2 from the infraorbital foramen and the zygomaticotemporal branch of the trigeminal nerve laterally. During aging, the cheek prominence descends inferomedially and consequently deepens the nasolabial crease. Midface lifts serve to both decrease the depth of the nasolabial crease as well as to elevate and recreate the prominence of the cheek.

There are two basic planes via which the midface can be dissected in order to place suspension sutures which will elevate the cheek. One is to approach the midface superficial to the investing fascia of the zygomaticus major muscle. The other is to approach it via a subperiosteal dissection. Choice of dissection plane depends on the patient's anatomy and desires. Once the appropriate dissection plane is chosen, there are four different means to access the midface: via facelift incision, blepharoplasty incision, transoral, and endoscopic temporal approach (similar to endoscopic brow).

In an endoscopic midface lift, the midface is approached via the temporal or forehead area. Endoscopic forehead approach with midface suspension can be performed without a browlift. However, some lower eyelid procedure usually has to be performed because elevation of the midface causes bunching of skin under the eye. Dissection is carried in a subperiosteal plane from the temporal line to the superior orbital rim. Dissection in the temporal region is over the deep temporal fascia to zygomatic arch bone. Tissue over the arch is released, and the midface tissues are released in a subperiosteal plane. Dissection is carried out all the way to the nasal bones and piriform aperture. As with the brow, there are many ways to suspend the midface/SOOF, including suture and absorbable suspension systems.

Patients often experience edema and distortion that may not resolve for 6 weeks. They may experience masticatory tenderness for a week due to release of masseter muscle and suturing in the temporalis muscle.

Conclusion

In the right patients, these procedures are effective tools to give patients a more youthful appearance. The approach must be tailored for each patient individually, and communication with the patient to understand their goals and desires is an essential element in achieving an optimal result in aging face surgery.

References

1. Brennan HG, Toft KM, Dunham BP, Goode RL, Koch RJ. Prevention and correction of temporal hair loss in rhytidectomy. Plast Reconstr Surg. 1999;104(7):2219–25; discussion 2226–8
2. Carron MA, Zoumalan RA, Miller PJ, Shah AR. Biomechanical analysis of anchoring points in rhytidectomy. Arch Facial Plast Surg. 2010;12(1):37–9; Hamra.
3. Furnas DW. The retaining ligaments of the cheek. Plast Reconstr Surg. 1989;83(1):11–6; Matarasso
4. Gassner HG, Rafii A, Young A, Murakami C, Moe KS, Larrabee WF Jr. Surgical anatomy of the face: implications for modern face-lift techniques. Arch Facial Plast Surg. 2008;10(1):9–19.
5. Gonzales-Ulloa M. Facial wrinkles: integral elimination. Plast Reconstr Surg. 1962;29:658.
6. Hamra ST. The deep-plane rhytidectomy. Plast Reconstr Surg. 1990;86:53.
7. Hunt H. Plastic surgery of the head, face and neck. Philadelphia: Lea & Febiger; 1926.

8. Larrabee WF Jr, Henderson JL. Face lift: the anatomic basis for a safe, long-lasting procedure. Facial Plast Surg. 2000;16(3):239–53.
9. Larrabee WF Jr, Ridenour BD. Rhytidectomy: technique and complications. Am J Otolaryngol. 1992;13(1):1–15.
10. Larrabee WF, Makielski KH, Henderson JL. Surgical anatomy of the face. 2nd ed. Philadelphia: Lippincott Williams & Wilkins; 2004.
11. Salinas NL, Jackson O, Dunham B, Bartlett SP. Anatomical dissection and modified Sihler stain of the lower branches of the facial nerve. Plast Reconstr Surg. 2009;124(6):1905–15.
12. Shah AR, Rosenberg D. Defining the facial extent of the platysma muscle: a review of 71 consecutive face-lifts. Arch Facial Plast Surg. 2009;11(6):405–8.
13. Sherris DA, Larrabee WF Jr. Anatomic considerations in rhytidectomy. Facial Plast Surg. 1996;12(3):215–22.
14. Zoumalan R, Rizk SS. Hematoma rates in drainless deep-plane face-lift surgery with and without the use of fibrin glue. Arch Facial Plast Surg. 2008;10(2):103–7.
15. Zoumalan RA, Rosenberg DB. Methicillin-resistant Staphylococcus aureus-positive surgical site infections in face-lift surgery. Arch Facial Plast Surg. 2008;10(2):116–23.
16. Zoumalan RA, Shah AR, Westine J. Chapter 38: Short incision or mini-lift. In: Thomas JR, editor. Advanced therapy in facial plastic and reconstructive surgery. Shelton: People's Medical Publishing House; 2009. p. 429–36.

Lasers and Related Technologies

23

Robert Anolik, Hao Feng, and Roy G. Geronemus

Introduction

When Albert Einstein first developed the concept of laser radiation in *The Quantum Theory of Radiation*, none could have predicted all its future roles in the applied sciences [1]. Since that time, physicians have used lasers along with other components of the electromagnetic spectrum in a variety of medical and cosmetic applications. In part because of accessibility, many of these developments have involved the skin and eyes.

Appreciation of the physics behind lasers provides a foundation for understanding its applications. The electromagnetic spectrum comprises radiation energy spanning short gamma waves to long radio waves and includes X-rays, ultraviolet radiation, visible light, infrared light, and microwaves in between. If sufficient electromagnetic radiation is absorbed by resting atoms, their electrons are stimulated to excited states. When these electrons eventually return to resting states, the atom releases the same absorbed energy at its same wavelength in a process known as "spontaneous emission."

Spontaneous emission may be hastened, or stimulated, when an excited atom is irradiated a second time with the same wavelength used to excite it originally. The second hit may come from a new source of energy or from spontaneous emissions of nearby atoms. As a result, if atoms are concentrated in a particular medium and confined within a reflective charged cavity, emissions may become markedly amplified because of the interaction of the spontaneous emissions and surrounding stimulated atoms.

Maiman was first to demonstrate Einstein's theories of stimulated emission using visible light [2]. This led to his coining the now familiar acronym LASER, which stands for Light Amplification by Stimulated Emission of Radiation. Although light technically refers to the visible spectrum, all laser emissions, whether in the visible spectrum or not, are generally referred to as laser light. The wavelength of the laser light is dependent on the medium of the reflective charged cavity. In the Maiman study, ruby crystal made up the medium, but since that time, several other mediums, such as alexandrite, potassium-titanyl-phosphate (KTP), and others, have been used to generate other wavelengths in medicine.

Laser light is monochromatic, coherent, and collimated. Monochromicity results from its consisting of one wavelength. Coherence refers to light waves that travel in phase, both in time and space, and collimation relates to the parallel nature and lack of divergence of the light waves.

Use of lasers by physicians was revolutionized by the concept of selective photothermolysis [3]. Essentially, selective photothermolysis takes advantage of the heterogeneous absorption spectra of anatomic structures, particularly melanin, hemoglobin, and water. The preferential absorption of these structures for different wavelengths permits their controlled ablation, coagulation, or thermal damage and preservation of surrounding structures.

Successful laser use, however, relies on more than wavelength and target. Training, experience, and management of settings such as fluence, spot size, and pulse width are critical to clinical outcome. Fluence is a measure of the laser's joules (i.e., energy) per centimeter squared. Spot size is clinically important since larger spots may cause peripheral dam-

R. Anolik
New York University School of Medicine,
Department of Dermatology, New York, NY, USA

Laser & Skin Surgery Center of New York, New York, NY, USA

H. Feng
University of Connecticut Health Center,
Department of Dermatology, Farmington, CT, USA

R. G. Geronemus (✉)
New York University School of Medicine,
Department of Dermatology, New York, NY, USA

Laser & Skin Surgery Center of New York, New York, NY, USA

New York Eye and Ear Infirmary, Department of Plastic Surgery,
New York, NY, USA
e-mail: rgeronemus@laserskinsurgery.com

J. J. Servat et al. (eds.), *Smith and Nesi's Ophthalmic Plastic and Reconstructive Surgery*,
https://doi.org/10.1007/978-3-030-41720-8_23

age around a small target. It also results in deeper penetration of the laser's effects but with more scatter. Pulse width is a measure of laser exposure time and is clinically relevant because of its relationship to thermal relaxation time (TRT). For a given tissue target, TRT is the time required to lose half of its heat. If pulse width is longer than the TRT, less ablation and more surrounding reversible and irreversible (coagulative necrosis) damage occur.

The objective of this chapter is to review common applications of lasers and related technologies for the treatment of periorbital concerns. These applications are broad and include resurfacing as well as the elimination of unwanted vascular and pigmented lesions. Although some of the technologies discussed in this chapter now serve as novel tools in traditional surgery, such as lasers in place of scalpels for making incisions, the following discussion will primarily concentrate on the role of the technologies when employed as the primary therapeutic strategy.

Vascular Concerns of the Periorbital Skin

Numerous vascular concerns of the periorbital skin are effectively treated with lasers, commonly the pulsed dye laser (PDL) or potassium-titanyl-phosphate (KTP), as their wavelengths can target hemoglobin. Examples include superficial infantile hemangiomas, capillary vascular malformations, venous malformations, spider angiomas, cherry angiomas, telangiectasias, reticular veins, pyogenic granulomas, and purpura.

Hemangiomas are benign proliferative vascular tumors of endothelial tissue that affect 2–3% of newborns and up to 10% of infants within the first year [4, 5]. The majority affect the head and neck, with 16% of facial hemangiomas involving the eyelid [6, 7]. They may present as superficial, deep, or compound (superficial and deep) and display many months of a proliferative phase followed by spontaneous involution at rates of about 10% per year [6]. Particular attention must be paid to deep and compound hemangiomas around the eye because of potential for amblyopia from anisometropia, strabismus, and obstruction, all of which can be exacerbated during the hemangioma's proliferative phase [8]. Despite involution, residual cosmetically upsetting effects are not uncommon in any form of hemangioma. Some report textural changes in up to 50% of hemangiomas after involution [9]. Long-term residua from hemangiomas are more common when involution occurs over a longer period of time, and unfortunately, no methods of identifying rate of involution presently exist [6]. The hemangioma and potential residua are recognized as causing psychological strain in children and family members. In general, laser therapy is not the ideal choice for deep hemangiomas because of their limited depth of penetration. However, for superficial hemangiomas, the pulsed dye laser (PDL) is an excellent treatment option as it is safe and effective and minimizes extent of proliferation and residua if treated early [10].

A report of 22 patients highlights the value of early treatment of superficial eyelid hemangiomas with the 595-nm pulsed dye laser (PDL) [10]. These patients underwent 2–14 treatments, initiating therapy at 5–28 weeks of age. Of these patients, 77.3% received an improvement rating of excellent (76–100% improvement), and 36% demonstrated complete clearance. No scarring, atrophy, hypopigmentation, infections, or ulcerations occurred during the study period, with the only side effect being hyperpigmentation in two subjects. Catalyzing its resolution and presumably limiting the proliferative phase likely contributed to the patients having no hemangioma residua. This report is in contrast to historical reports that resulted in side effects, particularly atrophy and hypopigmentation, but these side effects are attributable to use of higher fluences, smaller spot sizes, absence of epidermal cooling, and different PDL wavelengths [11].

Vascular malformations are localized defects of vascular morphogenesis, which is in contrast to the neoplastic nature of hemangiomas. They are categorized by their anomalous vessels (e.g., capillary, venous, arterial, lymphatic) and by whether they are fast or slow flow (i.e., arterial vs. other).

Capillary vascular malformations (CVM), often referred to as port-wine stains, are observed in 0.03% of the population [4]. Facial CVMs classically course along the distribution of trigeminal nerve sensory branches, namely, V1 (ophthalmic), V2 (maxillary), and V3 (mandibular) branches. When present, especially around the eye, risks of coincident glaucoma and choroidal vascular malformations exist, as do concerns for syndromic capillary venous malformations such as Sturge–Weber syndrome, von Hippel–Lindau syndrome, and Bonnet–Dechaume syndrome [12]. Over years and without treatment, CVMs typically develop vessel ectasia, which corresponds to the thickening, darkening, and cobblestoning appearance in aged lesions [13, 14]. Exuberant overgrowth can potentially lead to visual field obstruction of the eye or airway depending on location [12]. The PDL is an important therapy in the treatment of periorbital CVMs and should be considered a treatment of choice for flat or mildly hypertrophic lesions [12]. Other technologies are helpful, however, as intense pulsed light and the alexandrite laser, among others, have demonstrated efficacy and even advantage in some situations [15, 16]. Early treatment has been shown to be safe and more effective [17]. Although anatomic differences do exist in terms of response to laser and light treatments, periorbital CVMs tend to respond well [18].

Venous malformations are examples of defective venous morphogenesis. While sclerotherapy with or without surgical excision is an important therapeutic option, relatively long wavelength lasers that penetrate more deeply into cutaneous veins may serve as a therapeutic option as well [19]. When faced with appropriate candidates in our practice, the authors of this chapter often utilize a long pulsed 532- or 1064-nm KTP laser with effective results.

Other collections of superficial vessels, including spider angiomas, cherry angiomas, telangiectasias, reticular veins, and pyogenic granulomas, also respond to laser therapy [20–24].

A relatively new use of laser is for the treatment of purpura, which is a common occurrence following periorbital surgical procedures [25]. Most patients requiring medically necessary surgical interventions generally expect and accept purpura. However, purpura from a cosmetic procedure is often more frustrating for patients as many of these patients demand little downtime or choose to have the procedure before important social events. Whatever the cause of purpura, the PDL can effectively accelerate purpura resolution. This was demonstrated in a study of ten adults with far more rapid resolution in the days after treatment with a 595-nm PDL at a spot size of 10 mm, fluence of 7.5 J/cm^2, and pulse duration of 6 ms [25].

Pigmented Concerns of the Periorbital Skin

Several pigmented concerns of the periorbital skin respond to laser therapy. Commonly used lasers for pigment include the ruby laser, alexandrite, diode, and the neodymium-doped yttrium aluminum garnet (Nd:YAG) as their wavelengths can target melanin. These lasers effectively treat periorbital lesions such as ephelis, lentigo, café au lait spot, nevus spilus, Nevus of Ota, congenital melanocytic nevus, and tattoo.

Ephelides, also known as freckles, arise on sun-exposed areas as well-defined circular or oval hyperpigmented macules of just a few millimeters. While not precancerous themselves, high concentrations on the face have been associated with melanoma development [26]. On pathology, an ephelis demonstrates normal epidermal configuration but tends to have larger melanocytes in the basal layer with additional dendritic branching.

Lentigines may be characterized as simple or solar and may involve mucosal surfaces, unlike ephelides. Simple lentigines arise earlier and in any location when compared to solar lentigines, which arise in adulthood and in sun-exposed areas. Like ephelides, lentigines are well-defined circular or oval hyperpigmented macules but tend to be slightly darker and larger. Lentigines display elongated rete ridges on pathology, with more numerous melanocytes than typical skin. The solar lentigo rete ridges are more uniform and clubbed in appearance when compared to simple lentigo rete ridges. Lentigines are associated with several genetic syndromes, including LEOPARD, which also demonstrates ocular hypertelorism, and Peutz–Jeghers syndrome, which often includes periorbital and conjunctival lentigines.

Ephelides and lentigines are treated similarly and effectively with lasers targeting pigment. A study of 34 pigmented lesions, including lentigines, was performed using the Q-switched ruby laser at settings of 694 nm, 40 ns pulse duration, and 4.5 and/or 7.5 J/cm^2 [27]. Substantial clearing was appreciated in the lentigines with just one treatment at either fluence. Even mucosal lentigines are effectively treated with these strategies [28]. Long-term follow-up reveals efficacy in the majority of patients with lentigines. In another study of ten patients with solar lentigines treated once or twice with the Q-switched ruby laser, 77% demonstrated continued response at 10–21 months follow-up [29].

Café au lait spots are larger brown patches in the ranges of 2–5 cm. These are not uncommon, usually arise in infancy or childhood, and may be found periorbitally. Although unusual syndromes are associated with numerous café au lait spots, the vast majority of café au lait spots are isolated and harmless, without evidence of malignant transformation. Pathology demonstrates a normal-appearing epidermis with slightly increased melanin in the basal layer. Removal is often a challenge with these lesions. Hydroquinone and sun protection have little to no effect. Laser treatments can improve or even resolve the appearance, but recurrence rates are high. A study of 12 patients with café au lait spots treated one to six times with the Q-switched ruby laser showed a response rate of just 33% at 10–21 months follow-up [29]. Similar responses of café au lait spots were shown in a retrospective analysis of the Q-switched alexandrite laser [30]. Another study of 22 café au lait spots using the Q-switched Nd:YAG also showed discouraging results but found certain features, such as irregular borders, as a predictor of a better outcome [31].

The nevus spilus, or speckled lentiginous nevus, comprises a café au lait-like patch with more darkly pigmented melanocytic nevi within it. Like the café au lait, the nevus spilus is a challenge to treat. This has been highlighted in retrospective reviews evaluating efficacy of the Q-switched ruby and alexandrite, among other strategies [27, 30]. Few reports of nonlaser light sources, such as the intense pulsed light, have shown some success, but long-term follow-up is not available in these cases [32].

A Nevus of Ota is a blue-brown patch that usually arises in infancy or around puberty. A favored site is the periorbital skin. Often, the ipsilateral sclera shows blue-brown hyperpigmentation as well. Less commonly, other components of the eye can be affected, and, importantly, glaucoma may be seen in 10% of those affected with Nevus of Ota [33]. The pathology explains the blue hue to the skin, namely, a higher than normal concentration of melanocytes in the dermis. Laser treatment is effective against the cutaneous periorbital features of Nevus of Ota and has been demonstrated with numerous lasers, including the alexandrite, ruby, and Nd:YAG [34–36]. Notably, these same laser measures are

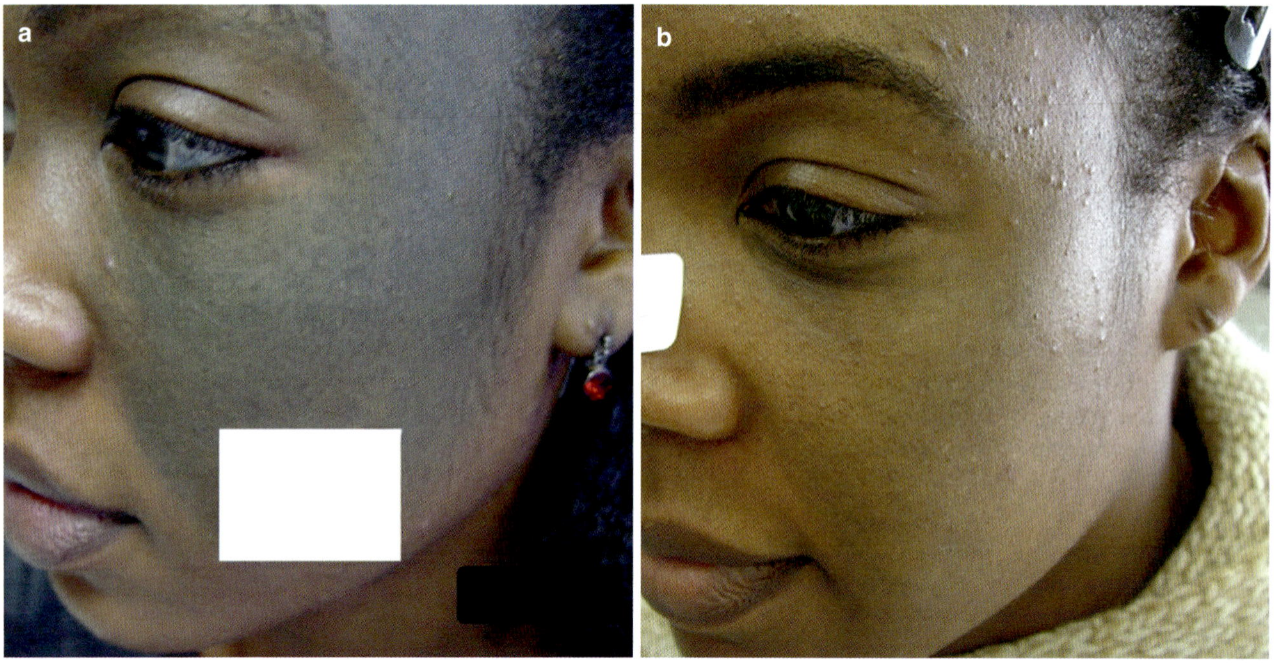

Fig. 23.1 A 19-year-old woman with Nevus of Ota before (**a**) and after (**b**) eight treatments using either the Q-switched Nd:YAG, Q-switched ruby, or Q-switched alexandrite laser at each session over 3 years

not safe as therapy for scleral involvement of the pigment. An example of the potential cutaneous improvement is demonstrated in Fig. 23.1. One study comprised of 602 Chinese Nevus of Ota patients found benefits with each additional treatment using a Q-switched alexandrite laser [37]. The study also found poorer response on the eyelid skin, which is referred to by some as the "panda sign." Another study of 119 Nevus of Ota patients found periorbital under-response [38]. They recommend discounting the traditional Tanino classification of Nevus of Ota, which is based on clinical distribution, and instead adopting a system based on response to laser treatment.

Congenital melanocytic nevi are collections of melanocytes presenting as flat or raised blue-brown lesions, with or without excess and course hair, and with an increased risk of melanoma when giant [39, 40]. Intervention depends on risk of progression to melanoma, cosmetic disfigurement of the lesion, and complexity of removal. Laser therapy is helpful but is also controversial based on questions of dysplastic effects of lasers on nevi and an increased risk of melanoma in some congenital nevi [40, 41]. In addition, recurrence of lesion and color is not uncommon. One strategy for treatment is laser ablation. In a study of 13 patients with medium-sized congenital nevi, as much tissue as possible was excised, followed by erbium:YAG ablation of residua [42]. Eighty-three percent of the patients were rated as having good to excellent results by the physicians global assessment scale. Seventy-seven percent of the patients reported good to excellent results at 4 months after treatment. Ablative lasers have also been successful in dark skin types [43]. Another approach involves pigment-specific lasers. In a study of nine patients with medium-sized congenital nevi on the face or upper limbs, the patients were treated on average 9.6 times with a Q-switched ruby laser [44]. After treatment, 0–20% of the lesions' color remained. However, eight demonstrated slight repigmentation that responded to additional treatment. One lesion returned to its original color within a month of its final treatment and therefore was simply excised.

In addition to the endogenous pigment concerns cited above, exogenous pigments in the form of tattoos are commonly found around the eyes. However, along with the rise in use of tattooed makeup, there has been a rise in patients seeking periorbital tattoo removal. Common challenges to periorbital tattoo removal are preservation of hair follicles, since these tattoos are typically placed along the eyelash and eyebrow, as well as avoidance of red, white, and beige/brown tattoo pigment since these paradoxically darken with Q-switched laser treatment [45]. Picosecond laser can be efficacious and possess similar efficacy and safety as Q-switched lasers. The phenomenon of paradoxical darkening is generally attributed to the reduction of ferric oxide (Fe^{3+}) to ferrous oxide (Fe^{2+}) in the pigment. Because of both challenges, periorbital tattoo removal is often accomplished with the careful use of a Q-switched Nd:YAG and/or an ablative laser, particularly a fractionated carbon dioxide laser. The Q-switched Nd:YAG allows for small spot sizes that better target fine eyelid tattoos and lessen risk of adjacent follicle damage [46]. Ablative lasers are incorporated when red, white, and beige/brown pigments are present since these lasers do not cause paradoxical darkening [47]. They effectively clear tattoos via superficial tissue vaporization with subsequent transepidermal elimination of unwanted tattoo pigment.

Periorbital Photodamage and Rejuvenation

Noninvasive and minimally invasive treatments for periorbital photodamage and rejuvenation have grown markedly in recent years. Today's strategies commonly employ resurfacing lasers in addition to the related technology of radio frequency. These technologies have shown effectiveness against laxity, rhytides, scars, and more recently premalignant changes of the skin, namely, actinic keratoses.

Originally, resurfacing lasers were nonfractional and fully ablative carbon dioxide lasers. Though they delivered impressive results, they came with substantial risks, particularly for scarring and hypopigmentation. With regard to periorbital treatments, scarring could further lead to ectropion, entropion, and epiphora. Nonfractional, nonablative laser alternatives followed, which were safer but delivered less impressive results. With the advent of fractional lasers, meaningful rejuvenation became achievable with far less risk [48]. The seminal concept of fractional laser delivery was first described in 2004 and has since been applied to nonablative and ablative devices [49]. In essence, a fractional system delivers laser in a pixilated pattern, creating zones of injury surrounded by areas of unaffected skin. Evidence for the efficacy and safety of these systems for periorbital treatment is now supported throughout the literature.

A study of 45 patients demonstrated that café au lait with jagged or ill-defined borders of the coast of Maine subtype tend to respond well to laser treatment, whereas those with smooth and well-defined borders of the coast of California subtype tend to have poor response. Several studies have demonstrated clinical efficacy of picosecond lasers. A retrospective study of 31 patients treated with a nonablative fractional resurfacing laser to the upper and lower eyelids was evaluated for changes in eyelid tightening and eyelid aperture [50, 51]. The laser consisted of a fractionated 1550-nm erbium-doped fiber laser and was delivered over three to seven treatment sessions. All patients achieved eyelid tightening, without any concerning adverse effects or downtime. Just over half, specifically 55.9%, also achieved increase in eyelid aperture.

Ablative systems have also been formally evaluated around the eye. A prospective study of 15 patients evaluated the effect of an ablative fractional carbon dioxide laser resurfacing treatment for laxity of the eyelid and periorbital skin [52]. Investigators found a 53.1% improvement in rhytidosis and 42.0% improvement in skin redundancy. No unusual adverse effects occurred in the study, although two patients did experience postinflammatory hyperpigmentation for 3 months that resolved with hydroquinone and sunscreen.

Surgeons should notably be aware of the value of these rejuvenating laser systems for the improvement of surgical scars since their efficacy has been shown for a variety of scar types [53, 54]. One study objectively and quantifiably examined the effect of ablative fractional carbon dioxide laser resurfacing of 19 atrophic scars resulting from surgery or trauma [55]. Subjects were treated three times and followed for 6 months. Subjective assessment of treated scars both by investigators and patients found improvement in skin texture. These findings were confirmed by optical tomographic analysis that quantifiably demonstrated a 38.0% mean reduction of volume and 35.6% mean reduction of scar depth.

In addition to laser resurfacing, radio frequency allows for periorbital rejuvenation. Radio frequency effects result from a uniformly distributed three-dimensional heat referred to as volumetric bulk heating. The heat is generated from resistance to the flow of electrical current through tissue. The uniform heat is thought to have two effects. First, the collagen fibrils have some degree of denaturation, which then recover with shortening in length. Second, the inflammatory cascade leads to production of new collagen synthesis. It is these changes that are thought to result in the clinically evident cosmetic enhancement of tightening [56].

An early study of nine patients addressed the effect of radio frequency on the lower eyelid [57]. After one treatment to the temporal and/or zygomatic periorbital skin, the investigators claim to have achieved cosmetic improvement. A larger multicenter study followed involving 72 patients undergoing one session of radio frequency therapy [58]. The investigators demonstrated upper eyelid tightening in 88%, reduction of hooding in 86%, and lower eyelid tightening in 71–74%. Since these studies, several others have emerged, similarly showing mild to modest periorbital tightening benefits along with a good safety profile [59, 60].

Treatment with newer picosecond alexandrite and Nd:YAG lasers has demonstrated significant clinical improvement in congenital melanocytic nevi, including treatment-recalcitrant lesions, with potential fewer side effects. In addition to the cosmetic enhancements achievable with these technologies, the medical value should not be underestimated. Periorbital skin cancers commonly challenge ophthalmic and dermatologic surgeons. Laser resurfacing has recently proven itself to be valuable against premalignant changes, namely, actinic keratoses, which may serve as precursors to squamous cell carcinoma [61]. The mechanism of therapy is not yet understood, but the clinical response is evident, as in Fig. 23.2. The authors of this

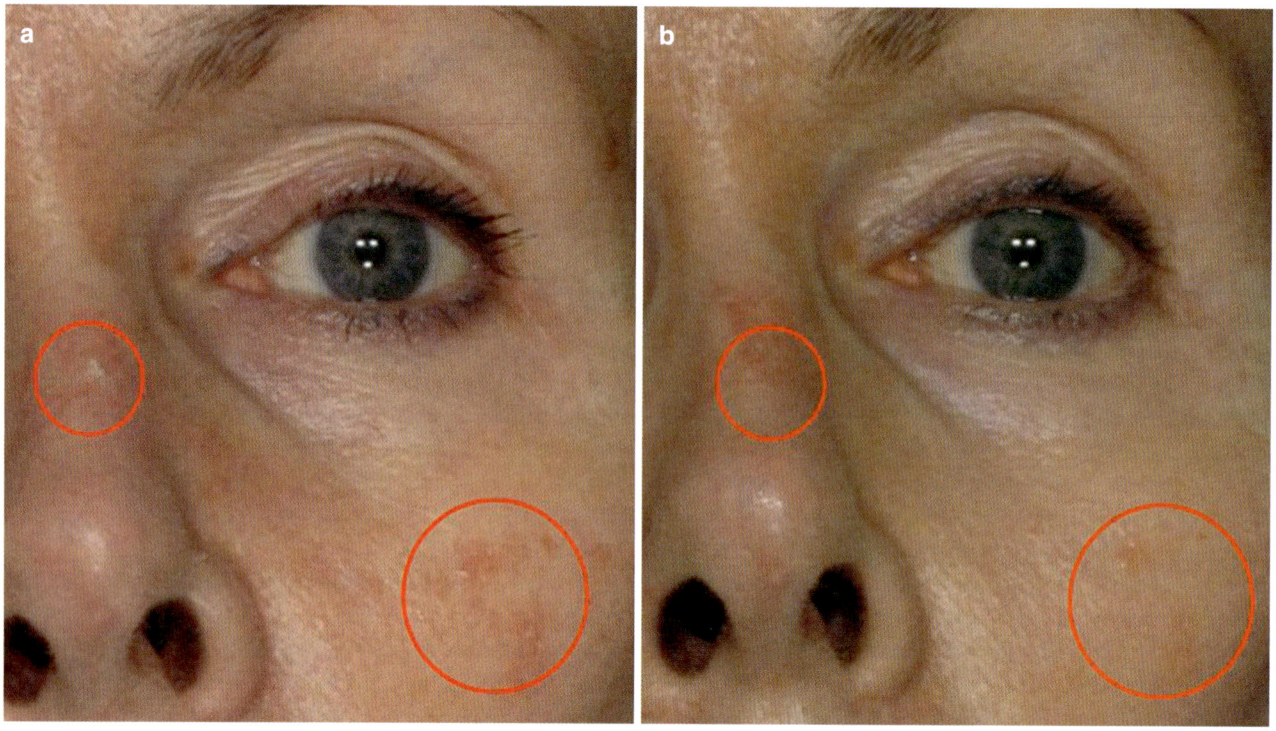

Fig. 23.2 A 63-year-old woman with widespread actinic keratoses, including those periorbital lesions shown here, before (**a**) and after (**b**) four treatments using a 1927-nm thulium nonablative fractional laser over 10 weeks demonstrating marked resolution

chapter commonly employ a nonablative fractional thulium 1927-nm laser as field treatment to reduce actinic keratoses over the face, including periorbital skin.

Infraorbital Dark Circles

Infraorbital dark circles do not stem from a single pathology but rather are a shared endpoint. The clinical appearance may result from hyperpigmentation, relatively translucent skin overlying muscle and vessels, or shadowing because of skin laxity and/or pronounced tear troughs from festooning or pseudoherniation of fat pads. To achieve a cosmetic improvement, the cause or causes should be identified in order to choose the correct treatment approach. Fortunately, laser technologies offer several options for the treatment of these concerns.

Traction on the infraorbital cheek assists in deciphering the cause. If the pigmented area grows proportionally with the stretching without blanching or change in color, dermal melanocytosis is likely [62]. If traction causes spread of pigment, yet the area develops a deeper violaceous hue, then thin and translucent skin is likely the cause [63]. In other words, as the skin is stretched thin, the underlying violaceous structures are more visible. Finally, if traction on the cheek diminishes the pigmentation, especially in a brightly lit room, shadowing is likely the driver.

Because of the diversity of causes, a variety of treatment modalities exist for dark circles. Surgery and filler certainly have their role, as do the slow improvement topical bleaching agents might bring, such as hydroquinone and retinoids. Fortunately, newer technologies exist which might contribute to therapy. Pigment lasers, such as the Q-switched ruby, alexandrite, and Nd:YAG, have demonstrated efficacy [64–66]. The 1064-nm Q-switched Nd:YAG shows particular value, as it appears to ably treat both melanocytic and vascular components of dark circles [63].

Transparency, thin skin, laxity, fat pseudoherniation, and festooning may be improved with the strategies for rejuvenation discussed earlier in this chapter. These tactics include ablative and nonablative fractional resurfacing and radio frequency. With these treatments, dermal collagen remodeling may contribute to a thicker dermis and thereby diminish visibility of vessels and musculature. Additionally, subsequent tightening contributes to minimized shadowing. Picosecond laser may be helpful in treating paradoxical darkening, although additional studies are needed.

Xanthelasma

Xanthelasma, or xanthelasma palpebrarum, are soft, yellow-hued papules and plaques involving the periorbital skin. Histologically, the lesions consist of foamy, lipid-filled histiocytes. For some, xanthelasma is a sign of systemic disease, such as hyperlipidemia, although half of patients are normolipidemic and only a minority have familial hypercholesterolemia [67]. Benefits of diet or medical therapy are unconvincing, leaving most patients to rely on surgical or laser intervention if removal is desired [68]. Traditionally destructive methods, such as cryotherapy, chemical peeling, scalpel surgery, and electrosurgery, have not delivered sustained results and bring substantial risks for scar, dyspigmentation, ectropion, and eyelid asymmetry [68].

Interestingly, several types of lasers have shown efficacy against xanthelasma, including those traditionally used for pigment, blood vessels, and resurfacing [69–73]. Ablative lasers were studied initially. One study of 23 patients with a cumulative total of 52 xanthelasma lesions assessed efficacy of an ultrapulsed carbon dioxide laser with a follow-up period of 10 months [73]. One treatment cleared all lesions, although three patients developed recurrence and dyspigmentation was found in 17%. Importantly, no scarring was reported. Another study investigated the use of the erbium:YAG laser in 15 patients with 33 xanthelasma lesions [70]. With one treatment, the authors report complete clearance without dyspigmentation or scarring.

Despite success with ablative lasers, nonablative alternatives are desirable to minimize risks even further as well as to bypass the need for wounding, pain from injection of local anesthetic, and downtime. Some claim benefits of the 1064-nm Nd:YAG [74]. However, a subsequent report of 37 patients with 76 lesions found both the 1064- and 532-nm Nd:YAG ineffective, even with more aggressive parameters [72]. However, another nonablative alternative, specifically the PDL, has shown greater promise. In a study of 20 patients with 38 lesions, patients underwent five treatments with the 585-nm PDL at 2- to 3-week intervals. About two-thirds demonstrated greater than 50% improvement, and one-quarter demonstrated greater than 75% improvement.

More recently, evidence supports nonablative fractional resurfacing as a means to remedy xanthelasma. A report of a 52-year-old woman with 4 years of xanthelasma was treated with the 1550-nm-wavelength, erbium-doped fractional laser [69, 75]. After seven treatments at 4- to 11-week intervals, the patient achieved near total improvement.

Adnexal Structures of Periorbital Skin

Periorbital adnexal structures, both normal and abnormal, can be removed with success using lasers. These structures include unwanted normal hair, trichiasis, syringomas, and hidrocystomas.

Laser hair removal has become a practical and often permanent means to remove unwanted hair [76]. Removal generally relies on pigment-specific lasers that target melanin in the hair follicle, although intense pulsed light devices are sometimes used with good response [77]. Hair follicle elimination and destruction are observed clinically and histologically following laser treatment [76]. Because pigment serves as the target chromophore, fair-colored or white hairs are not responsive to treatment.

Abnormal hair may also be targeted, so long as it is still pigmented. One report demonstrated efficacy of periorbital laser hair removal in ten patients with eyelid trichiasis after treatment with the ruby laser [78]. At settings of 3 J and a 3.5-mm spot size, the ruby laser completely eliminated eyelid trichiasis in six patients after one to three sessions. Another three patients achieved a partial response. The tenth patient was lost to follow-up. Importantly, there were no reported complications and the procedure was well tolerated. Picosecond laser with a diffractive lens array represents a new technologic advancement in the treatment of rejuvenation, striae, and scars. A series of six treatment sessions of facial acne scars in 20 adult patients with the 755-nm picosecond laser with diffractive lens array produced improvement in appearance and texture at 3 months after the last treatment, with objective findings similar to those published for a series of fractional ablative laser treatments. In contrast to other nonablative and ablative laser modalities, this system has shown to be safe in darker phototype individuals with no serious adverse events and only transient hyperpigmentation that self-resolved.

Abnormal tumors of the adnexae, most commonly syringomas and hidrocystomas, are also treatable with lasers. Syringomas and hidrocystomas are benign adnexal neoplasms that may be solitary, multiple, or eruptive lesions [79, 80]. Essentially, effective treatment involves lesion destruction. This could be achieved using excision, electrodesiccation with curettage, and dermabrasion, among other destructive methods, but these come with risks for scarring and dyspigmentation. The benefit of laser resurfacing as a means of lesion destruction is the minimization of complications in tandem with efficacy. In a study using an ablative nonfractional carbon dioxide laser, ten patients with multiple periorbital syringomas were treated at 5 W, 0.2-s scan time, and 3-mm spot size [81]. Two to four passes over one to four treatment sessions were performed resulting in elimination of syringomas in all patients over a median follow-up period of 16 months. Adverse effects included transient erythema lasting 6–12 weeks in all patients and hyperpigmentation in a patient with type IV skin that resolved over 8–12 weeks. Erbium laser ablation has also shown efficacy against syringomas. In a study of 104 patients with a variety of skin lesions, some with syringomas, the erbium:YAG system successfully eliminated the lesions using a 0.350 ms pulse duration and 0.1–1.7 J [82]. The syringomas were successfully vaporized with minimal peripheral thermal damage and good to excellent cosmetic outcome.

Hidrocystomas have also been treated effectively with lasers. Surprisingly, some report successful treatment of hidrocystomas using the pulsed dye laser (PDL). This is unexpected since the PDL's target chromophore in a hidrocystoma is not known. In one report, a 585-nm pulsed dye laser was used at fluences of 7.0–7.5 J/cm^2 over 6–8 weeks intervals [83]. After four treatments, there was near total resolution of the lesions. Other reports, however, have not had such success with the PDL, raising questions about the real effectiveness of this strategy [84]. As would be predicted, however, hidrocystomas can be successfully treated using ablative lasers, such as the carbon dioxide laser [85]. Conceptually, this makes sense as destruction of the cyst wall itself could lead to resolution of the lesion.

Relatively inventive strategies have also been developed for these adnexal structures. One paper studied the effectiveness of a so-called multiple-drilling carbon dioxide laser method [86]. Rather than resurfacing or cutting the skin, the clinicians created several relatively deep holes with the ablative laser into the targeted lesions. This strategy was taken in an attempt to reach the deep components of the adnexal structures. Eleven patients were treated, ten with periorbital lesions and one with vulvar, over one to four treatment sessions. All patients were found to achieve good to excellent clinical responses. No serious complications were noted.

Another group cleverly integrated temporary tattooing into the treatment of patients' syringomas [87]. In this report, multiple periorbital syringomas had their surface epithelium removed with a carbon dioxide laser. Afterward, droplets of black ink were laid on the syringomas, and iontophoresis was performed to create a tattooed lesion. Finally, the Q-switched alexandrite laser was applied to the lesion. The majority of syringomas disappeared by the 1-week follow-up evaluation. The only significant adverse effect was hyperpigmentation lasting more than 2 months in a patient with type V skin.

Despite success with lasers for these adnexal lesions, some groups still rely and endorse electrosurgery and excision [88, 89]. Certainly, these options are successful in some circumstances, such as cases of giant histiocytomas, and are relatively more accessible in clinicians' offices. However, the authors of this chapter encourage clinicians not to choose these alternatives simply because laser systems may not be available in their immediate practice.

Microneedle radio frequency technology has additionally shown to improve and possibly resolve festoons and offers patients a simple, noninvasive, and nonsurgical treatment method that additionally rejuvenates the lower eyelid complex.

Microfocused ultrasound can tighten and elevate skin with minimal downtime via collagen denaturation and neocollagenesis. Unlike radio frequency, microfocused ultrasound allows direct visualization and is able to heat the tissue up to between 60 and 70 degrees Celsius via targeted heat generation in the dermis and subcutaneous tissue without affecting more superficial tissue or the need for surface cooling. In a prospective rater-blinded study of 35 subjects, 30 individuals had clinically significant improvement in brow elevation with a mean of 1.7 mm 90 days after a single treatment and no adverse events. Microfocused ultrasound may also be useful for lower eyelid rejuvenation. In a prospective study of 15 Korean patients who received 1–2 treatments to bilateral lower eyelids for infraorbital laxity, 2 (13.33%) were much improved, 11 (73.33%) were improved, and 2 (13.33%) were unchanged 6 months posttreatment. In a case series of seven Korean patients, both qualitative and quantitative improvements were observed via targeting of orbital septum, intraseptal fat, and orbicularis oculi.

Safety and Complications (Including Contraindications)

The use of lasers around the eyes raises a number of safety concerns. Physicians must be fluent in these concerns and know the appropriate measures to protect themselves, their staff, and the patients.

Ocular damage from inadvertent exposure is always a risk with lasers. Ocular melanin and vasculature are at particular risk when using pigment and vascular lasers, respectively. Cornea and sclera are at particular risk when using resurfacing lasers because of the high water content of these structures.

In practice, if any reasonable risk exists to the eyes, everyone must have protective eyewear. For the physician and staff, wraparound goggles should be worn that are rated as having an optical density (OD) of 4 or greater. OD is calculated as log (1/T) where T is the transmittance of light through the eyewear. A particular pair of goggle's OD differs based on wavelength and should be specified on the glasses themselves. One shouldn't simply rely on the color of the protective goggles as a determinant of which pair to wear.

For patients, external or internal eye shields may be used. When the laser is not in or directed at the immediate eyelid vicinity, external opaque shields should be adequate. When internal shields are required, nonreflective metal shields should be used. Internal plastic shields used by some surgeons during nonlaser procedures do not adequately protect against some lasers, such as the carbon dioxide laser, since they may penetrate the shield. Eye shields are generally well tolerated. Pretreatment with ophthalmic anesthetic drops may alleviate patient discomfort.

Despite available safety protocols, complications from periorbital laser use are reported, especially when the appropriate precautions are not met [90–93]. Complications include iris atrophy, posterior synechiae, iris pigment dispersion, anterior uveitis, and blindness. In most reports of these cases, the patient simply closed their eyes, covered their eyes with their own fingers, or inadequately covered the eyes with displaced external shields. Several of the reports stem from laser hair removal of the lower aspect of the eyebrow. Often, external eye shields were displaced or removed to allow a bulky laser tip to treat the target area. The laser's proximity in combination with Bell's phenomenon puts the patient's eyes at substantial risk when lasing the lower eyebrow.

Despite proper shielding, patients may still appreciate a flash of light concurrent with each periorbital laser pulse. The pulse is thought to somehow trigger the retinal photoreceptors. Safety concerns have been raised, but the evidence does not show any harmful effects. In one study, five patients undergoing diode laser hair removal for severe trichiasis were evaluated with pre- and posttreatment ophthalmic exams [94]. These exams included slit-lamp, pupillary, fundoscopic, and objective retinal electroretinogram studies. Although three of the five patients experienced the sensation of flashing lights during treatment, there was no detectable change in any of the listed exams after treatment.

Aside from ophthalmic risks, lasers bring safety concerns for fires and burns, particularly when flammable materials such as paper drapes, alcohol, or supplied oxygen are used in settings of carbon dioxide and erbium lasers. PDL and other lasers may pose risks as well [95]. Therefore, flammable material should be removed from the treatment area. Additionally, when a sedated patient requires concentrated oxygen and/or nitrous oxygen, use of a laryngeal mask or endotracheal intubation limits release of the flammable gas. Moist surgical drapes contribute to fire hazard safety and may even be wrapped around the portion of a laryngeal mask or endotracheal tube exiting the mouth. Aerosolization of infectious agents, like viruses, and tissue particles is also a concern with laser treatment. These risks are still being clarified, but appropriate ventilation, vacuum use, gloves, and masks may assist in preventing consequences from these risks.

Conclusion

Lasers and related technologies are invaluable for medical and cosmetic concerns around the eyes. Rejuvenation and the elimination of pigment, vascular lesions, dark circles, adnexal tumors, and xanthelasma are all possible. With advances of existing technologies and the development of newer technologies on the horizon, periorbital concerns will be more effectively and more safely treated.

References

1. Einstein A. Zur quantentheorie der strahlung. Physiol Z. 1917;18:121–8.
2. Maiman TH. Stimulated optical radiation in ruby. Nature. 1960;187:493–4.
3. Anderson RR, Parrish JA. Selective photothermolysis: precise microsurgery by selective absorption of pulsed radiation. Science. 1983;220(4596):524–7.
4. Jacobs AH, Walton RG. The incidence of birthmarks in the neonate. Pediatrics. 1976;58(2):218–22.
5. Jacobs AH. Strawberry hemangiomas; the natural history of the untreated lesion. Calif Med. 1957;86(1):8–10.
6. Finn MC, Glowacki J, Mulliken JB. Congenital vascular lesions: clinical application of a new classification. J Pediatr Surg. 1983;18(6):894–900.
7. Waner M, North PE, Scherer KA, Frieden IJ, Waner A, Mihm MC Jr. The nonrandom distribution of facial hemangiomas. Arch Dermatol. 2003;139(7):869–75.
8. Ceisler E, Blei F. Ophthalmic issues in hemangiomas of infancy. Lymphat Res Biol. 2003;1(4):321–30.
9. Mulliken JB, Fishman SJ, Burrows PE. Vascular anomalies. Curr Probl Surg. 2000;37(8):517–84.
10. Hunzeker CM, Geronemus RG. Treatment of superficial infantile hemangiomas of the eyelid using the 595-nm pulsed dye laser. Dermatol Surg. 2010;36(5):590–7.
11. Batta K, Goodyear HM, Moss C, Williams HC, Hiller L, Waters R. Randomised controlled study of early pulsed dye laser treatment of uncomplicated childhood haemangiomas: results of a 1-year analysis. Lancet. 2002;360(9332):521–7.
12. Holy A, Geronemus RG. Treatment of periorbital port-wine stains with the flashlamp-pumped pulsed dye laser. Arch Ophthalmol. 1992;110(6):793–7.
13. Barsky SH, Rosen S, Geer DE, Noe JM. The nature and evolution of port wine stains: a computer-assisted study. J Invest Dermatol. 1980;74(3):154–7.
14. Geronemus RG, Ashinoff R. The medical necessity of evaluation and treatment of port-wine stains. J Dermatol Surg Oncol. 1991;17(1):76–9.
15. Faurschou A, Togsverd-Bo K, Zachariae C, Haedersdal M. Pulsed dye laser vs. intense pulsed light for port-wine stains: a randomized side-by-side trial with blinded response evaluation. Br J Dermatol. 2009;160(2):359–64.
16. Izikson L, Nelson JS, Anderson RR. Treatment of hypertrophic and resistant port wine stains with a 755 nm laser: a case series of 20 patients. Lasers Surg Med. 2009;41(6):427–32.
17. Chapas AM, Eickhorst K, Geronemus RG. Efficacy of early treatment of facial port wine stains in newborns: a review of 49 cases. Lasers Surg Med. 2007;39(7):563–8.
18. Renfro L, Geronemus RG. Anatomical differences of port-wine stains in response to treatment with the pulsed dye laser. Arch Dermatol. 1993;129(2):182–8.
19. Bagazgoitia L, Boixeda P, Lopez-Caballero C, Bea S, Santiago JL, Jaen P. Venous malformation of the eyelid treated with pulsed-dye-1064-nm neodymium yttrium aluminum garnet sequential laser: an effective and safe treatment. Ophthal Plast Reconstr Surg. 2008;24(6):488–90.
20. Hare McCoppin HH, Goldberg DJ. Laser treatment of facial telangiectases: an update. Dermatol Surg. 2010;36(8):1221–30.
21. Dawn G, Gupta G. Comparison of potassium titanyl phosphate vascular laser and hyfrecator in the treatment of vascular spiders and cherry angiomas. Clin Exp Dermatol. 2003;28(6):581–3.
22. Lai SW, Goldman MP. Treatment of facial reticular veins with dynamically cooled, variable spot-sized 1064 nm Nd:YAG laser. J Cosmet Dermatol. 2007;6(1):6–8.
23. Clark C, Cameron H, Moseley H, Ferguson J, Ibbotson SH. Treatment of superficial cutaneous vascular lesions: experience with the KTP 532 nm laser. Lasers Med Sci. 2004;19(1):1–5.
24. Sud AR, Tan ST. Pyogenic granuloma-treatment by shave-excision and/or pulsed-dye laser. J Plast Reconstr Aesthet Surg. 2010;63(8):1364–8.
25. Karen JK, Hale EK, Geronemus RG. A simple solution to the common problem of ecchymosis. Arch Dermatol. 2010;146(1):94–5.

26. Rhodes AR, Albert LS, Barnhill RL, Weinstock MA. Sun-induced freckles in children and young adults. A correlation of clinical and histopathologic features. Cancer. 1991;67(7):1990–2001.
27. Taylor CR, Anderson RR. Treatment of benign pigmented epidermal lesions by Q-switched ruby laser. Int J Dermatol. 1993;32(12):908–12.
28. Ashinoff R, Geronemus RG. Q-switched ruby laser treatment of labial lentigos. J Am Acad Dermatol. 1992;27(5 Pt 2):809–11.
29. Shimbashi T, Kamide R, Hashimoto T. Long-term follow-up in treatment of solar lentigo and cafe-au-lait macules with Q-switched ruby laser. Aesthet Plast Surg. 1997;21(6):445–8.
30. Kagami S, Asahina A, Watanabe R, et al. Treatment of 153 Japanese patients with Q-switched alexandrite laser. Lasers Med Sci. 2007;22(3):159–63.
31. Levy JL, Mordon S, Pizzi-Anselme M. Treatment of individual cafe au lait macules with the Q-switched Nd:YAG: a clinicopathologic correlation. J Cutan Laser Ther. 1999;1(4):217–23.
32. Gold MH, Foster TD, Bell MW. Nevus spilus successfully treated with an intense pulsed light source. Dermatol Surg. 1999;25(3):254–5.
33. Teekhasaenee C, Ritch R, Rutnin U, Leelawongs N. Ocular findings in oculodermal melanocytosis. Arch Ophthalmol. 1990;108(8):1114–20.
34. Lowe NJ, Wieder JM, Sawcer D, Burrows P, Chalet M. Nevus of Ota: treatment with high energy fluences of the Q-switched ruby laser. J Am Acad Dermatol. 1993;29(6):997–1001.
35. Chan HH, Ying SY, Ho WS, Kono T, King WW. An in vivo trial comparing the clinical efficacy and complications of Q-switched 755 nm alexandrite and Q-switched 1064 nm Nd:YAG lasers in the treatment of nevus of Ota. Dermatol Surg. 2000;26(10):919–22.
36. Tse Y, Levine VJ, McClain SA, Ashinoff R. The removal of cutaneous pigmented lesions with the Q-switched ruby laser and the Q-switched neodymium: yttrium-aluminum-garnet laser. A comparative study. J Dermatol Surg Oncol. 1994;20(12):795–800.
37. Wang HW, Liu YH, Zhang GK, et al. Analysis of 602 Chinese cases of nevus of Ota and the treatment results treated by Q-switched alexandrite laser. Dermatol Surg. 2007;33(4):455–60.
38. Chan HH, Lam LK, Wong DS, et al. Nevus of Ota: a new classification based on the response to laser treatment. Lasers Surg Med. 2001;28(3):267–72.
39. Dohil MA, Baugh WP, Eichenfield LF. Vascular and pigmented birthmarks. Pediatr Clin N Am. 2000;47(4):783–812. v–vi
40. Swerdlow AJ, English JS, Qiao Z. The risk of melanoma in patients with congenital nevi: a cohort study. J Am Acad Dermatol. 1995;32(4):595–9.
41. Soden CE, Smith K, Skelton H. Histologic features seen in changing nevi after therapy with an 810 nm pulsed diode laser for hair removal in patients with dysplastic nevi. Int J Dermatol. 2001;40(8):500–4.
42. Lim JY, Jeong Y, Whang KK. A combination of dual-mode 2,940 nm Er:YAG laser ablation with surgical excision for treating medium-sized congenital melanocytic nevus. Ann Dermatol. 2009;21(2):120–4.
43. Rajpar SF, Abdullah A, Lanigan SW. Er:YAG laser resurfacing for inoperable medium-sized facial congenital melanocytic naevi in children. Clin Exp Dermatol. 2007;32(2):159–61.
44. Kishi K, Okabe K, Ninomiya R, et al. Early serial Q-switched ruby laser therapy for medium-sized to giant congenital melanocytic naevi. Br J Dermatol. 2009;161(2):345–52.
45. Anderson RR, Geronemus R, Kilmer SL, Farinelli W, Fitzpatrick RE. Cosmetic tattoo ink darkening. A complication of Q-switched and pulsed-laser treatment. Arch Dermatol. 1993;129(8):1010–4.
46. Geronemus RG. Surgical pearl: Q-switched Nd:YAG laser removal of eyeliner tattoo. J Am Acad Dermatol. 1996;35(1):101–2.
47. Mafong EA, Kauvar AN, Geronemus RG. Surgical pearl: removal of cosmetic lip-liner tattoo with the pulsed carbon dioxide laser. J Am Acad Dermatol. 2003;48(2):271–2.
48. Brightman LA, Brauer JA, Anolik R, et al. Ablative and fractional ablative lasers. Dermatol Clin. 2009;27(4):479–89. vi–vii
49. Manstein D, Herron GS, Sink RK, Tanner H, Anderson RR. Fractional photothermolysis: a new concept for cutaneous remodeling using microscopic patterns of thermal injury. Lasers Surg Med. 2004;34(5):426–38.
50. Sukal SA, Chapas AM, Bernstein LJ, Hale EK, Kim KH, Geronemus RG. Eyelid tightening and improved eyelid aperture through nonablative fractional resurfacing. Dermatol Surg. 2008;34(11):1454–8.
51. Geronemus RG. Fractional photothermolysis: current and future applications. Lasers Surg Med. 2006;38(3):169–76.
52. Kotlus BS. Dual-depth fractional carbon dioxide laser resurfacing for periocular rhytidosis. Dermatol Surg. 2010;36(5):623–8.
53. Kunishige JH, Katz TM, Goldberg LH, Friedman PM. Fractional photothermolysis for the treatment of surgical scars. Dermatol Surg. 2010;36(4):538–41.
54. Behroozan DS, Goldberg LH, Dai T, Geronemus RG, Friedman PM. Fractional photothermolysis for the treatment of surgical scars: a case report. J Cosmet Laser Ther. 2006;8(1):35–8.
55. Weiss ET, Chapas A, Brightman L, et al. Successful treatment of atrophic postoperative and traumatic scarring with carbon dioxide ablative fractional resurfacing: quantitative volumetric scar improvement. Arch Dermatol. 2010;146(2):133–40.
56. Fitzpatrick R, Geronemus R, Goldberg D, Kaminer M, Kilmer S, Ruiz-Esparza J. Multicenter study of noninvasive radiofrequency for periorbital tissue tightening. Lasers Surg Med. 2003;33(4):232–42.
57. Ruiz-Esparza J. Noninvasive lower eyelid blepharoplasty: a new technique using nonablative radiofrequency on periorbital skin. Dermatol Surg. 2004;30(2 Pt 1):125–9.
58. Biesman BS, Baker SS, Carruthers J, Silva HL, Holloman EL. Monopolar radiofrequency treatment of human eyelids: a prospective, multicenter, efficacy trial. Lasers Surg Med. 2006;38(10):890–8.
59. Friedman DJ, Gilead LT. The use of hybrid radiofrequency device for the treatment of rhytides and lax skin. Dermatol Surg. 2007;33(5):543–51.
60. Biesman BS, Pope K. Monopolar radiofrequency treatment of the eyelids: a safety evaluation. Dermatol Surg. 2007;33(7):794–801.
61. Geronemus RG, Chapas AM, Desai S, Brightman L, Hale EK, Karen JK, Bernstein LJ. Finally! A well-tolerated and effective treatment for actinic keratoses on the face. American Society for Laser Medicine and Surgery 30th Annual Conference. Phoenix, 2010.
62. Epstein JS. Management of infraorbital dark circles. A significant cosmetic concern. Arch Facial Plast Surg. 1999;1(4):303–7.
63. Roh MR, Chung KY. Infraorbital dark circles: definition, causes, and treatment options. Dermatol Surg. 2009;35(8):1163–71.
64. Watanabe S, Nakai K, Ohnishi T. Condition known as "dark rings under the eyes" in the Japanese population is a kind of dermal melanocytosis which can be successfully treated by Q-switched ruby laser. Dermatol Surg. 2006;32(6):785–9; discussion 789
65. Momosawa A, Kurita M, Ozaki M, et al. Combined therapy using Q-switched ruby laser and bleaching treatment with tretinoin and hydroquinone for periorbital skin hyperpigmentation in Asians. Plast Reconstr Surg. 2008;121(1):282–8.
66. West TB, Alster TS. Improvement of infraorbital hyperpigmentation following carbon dioxide laser resurfacing. Dermatol Surg. 1998;24(6):615–6.
67. Bergman R. The pathogenesis and clinical significance of xanthelasma palpebrarum. J Am Acad Dermatol. 1994;30(2 Pt 1):236–42.
68. Rohrich RJ, Janis JE, Pownell PH. Xanthelasma palpebrarum: a review and current management principles. Plast Reconstr Surg. 2002;110(5):1310–4.

69. Alster TS, West TB. Ultrapulse CO_2 laser ablation of xanthelasma. J Am Acad Dermatol. 1996;34(5 Pt 1):848–9.
70. Borelli C, Kaudewitz P. Xanthelasma palpebrarum: treatment with the erbium:YAG laser. Lasers Surg Med. 2001;29(3):260–4.
71. Karsai S, Czarnecka A, Raulin C. Treatment of xanthelasma palpebrarum using a pulsed dye laser: a prospective clinical trial in 38 cases. Dermatol Surg. 2010;36(5):610–7.
72. Karsai S, Schmitt L, Raulin C. Is Q-switched neodymium-doped yttrium aluminium garnet laser an effective approach to treat xanthelasma palpebrarum? Results from a clinical study of 76 cases. Dermatol Surg. 2009;35(12):1962–9.
73. Raulin C, Schoenermark MP, Werner S, Greve B. Xanthelasma palpebrarum: treatment with the ultrapulsed CO_2 laser. Lasers Surg Med. 1999;24(2):122–7.
74. Fusade T. Treatment of xanthelasma palpebrarum by 1064-nm Q-switched Nd:YAG laser: a study of 11 cases. Br J Dermatol. 2008;158(1):84–7.
75. Katz TM, Goldberg LH, Friedman PM. Fractional photothermolysis: a new therapeutic modality for xanthelasma. Arch Dermatol. 2009;145(10):1091–4.
76. Grossman MC, Dierickx C, Farinelli W, Flotte T, Anderson RR. Damage to hair follicles by normal-mode ruby laser pulses. J Am Acad Dermatol. 1996;35(6):889–94.
77. Toosi P, Sadighha A, Sharifian A, Razavi GM. A comparison study of the efficacy and side effects of different light sources in hair removal. Lasers Med Sci. 2006;21(1):1–4.
78. Moore J, De Silva SR, O'Hare K, Humphry RC. Ruby laser for the treatment of trichiasis. Lasers Med Sci. 2009;24(2):137–9.
79. Patrizi A, Neri I, Marzaduri S, Varotti E, Passarini B. Syringoma: a review of twenty-nine cases. Acta Derm Venereol. 1998;78(6):460–2.
80. Smith JD, Chernosky ME. Hidrocystomas. Arch Dermatol. 1973;108(5):676–9.
81. Wang JI, Roenigk HH Jr. Treatment of multiple facial syringomas with the carbon dioxide (CO_2) laser. Dermatol Surg. 1999;25(2):136–9.
82. Riedel F, Windberger J, Stein E, Hormann K. Treatment of periocular skin lesions with the erbium:YAG laser. Ophthalmologe. 1998;95(11):771–5.
83. Tanzi E, Alster TS. Pulsed dye laser treatment of multiple eccrine hidrocystomas: a novel approach. Dermatol Surg. 2001;27(10):898–900.
84. Choi JE, Ko NY, Son SW. Lack of effect of the pulsed-dye laser in the treatment of multiple eccrine hidrocystomas: a report of two cases. Dermatol Surg. 2007;33(12):1513–5.
85. Madan V, August PJ, Ferguson J. Multiple eccrine hidrocystomas – response to treatment with carbon dioxide and pulsed dye lasers. Dermatol Surg. 2009;35(6):1015–7.
86. Park HJ, Lee DY, Lee JH, Yang JM, Lee ES, Kim WS. The treatment of syringomas by $CO_{(2)}$ laser using a multiple-drilling method. Dermatol Surg. 2007;33(3):310–3.
87. Park HJ, Lim SH, Kang HA, Byun DG, Houh D. Temporary tattooing followed by Q-switched alexandrite laser for treatment of syringomas. Dermatol Surg. 2001;27(1):28–30.
88. Gupta S, Handa U, Handa S, Mohan H. The efficacy of electrosurgery and excision in treating patients with multiple apocrine hidrocystomas. Dermatol Surg. 2001;27(4):382–4.
89. Al Aradi IK. Periorbital syringoma: a pilot study of the efficacy of low-voltage electrocoagulation. Dermatol Surg. 2006;32(10):1244–50.
90. Hammes S, Augustin A, Raulin C, Ockenfels HM, Fischer E. Pupil damage after periorbital laser treatment of a port-wine stain. Arch Dermatol. 2007;143(3):392–4.
91. Halkiadakis I, Skouriotis S, Stefanaki C, et al. Iris atrophy and posterior synechiae as a complication of eyebrow laser epilation. J Am Acad Dermatol. 2007;57(2 Suppl):S4–5.
92. Le Jeune M, Autie M, Monnet D, Brezin AP. Ocular complications after laser epilation of eyebrows. Eur J Dermatol. 2007;17(6):553–4.
93. Shulman S, Bichler I. Ocular complications of laser-assisted eyebrow epilation. Eye (Lond). 2009;23(4):982–3.
94. Pham RT, Tzekov RT, Biesman BS, Marmor MF. Retinal evaluation after 810 nm Dioderm laser removal of eyelashes. Dermatol Surg. 2002;28(9):836–40.
95. Fretzin S, Beeson WH, Hanke CW. Ignition potential of the 585-nm pulsed-dye laser. Review of the literature and safety recommendations. Dermatol Surg. 1996;22(8):699–702.

Complications of Blepharoplasty

24

Helen Merritt, Margaret L. Pfeiffer, and Karina Richani

Introduction

Blepharoplasty, like any other surgical procedure, may be associated with postoperative complications that are upsetting to both the surgeon and the patient [1–3]. Many postoperative complications can be avoided by vigilant presurgical planning and meticulous surgical technique [2]. The indications and benefits of surgery as well as the possible complications should be discussed carefully with the patient before surgery, both to build rapport with the patient and to set realistic expectations [4, 5]. The surgeon should encourage the cosmetic blepharoplasty patient to speak openly in the preoperative assessment about his or her aesthetic desires [6]. A handheld mirror is useful to help patients point out eyelid features that are bothersome. In doing so, the surgeon minimizes the risk of misunderstanding the patient's requests. The surgeon should be cautious of patients who believe that a complication is unacceptable under any circumstance because this patient is not suitable for surgery. Finally, photographic documentation is valuable as an objective record for the patient who may question the surgical result.

A complete preoperative evaluation of the blepharoplasty patient is mandatory. The evaluation should include a complete history (including use of topical and systemic medications and drug sensitivities), a physical evaluation, and a thorough ocular evaluation. The complete ophthalmic examination is performed with particular attention to conditions that could adversely affect the outcome of blepharoplasty including dry eye, lagophthalmos, meibomian gland dysfunction, keratitis, and corneal dystrophies [6].

H. Merritt · M. L. Pfeiffer
Oculoplastics Associates of Texas, Dallas, TX, USA

M. L. Pfeiffer
Key-Whitman Eye Center, Dallas, TX, USA

K. Richani (✉)
Ruiz Department of Ophthalmology, University of Texas, McGovern Medical School, Houston, TX, USA
e-mail: KarinaRichani@cizikeye.org

The oculoplastic surgeon should pay close attention to concomitant brow ptosis, which may accentuate dermatochalasis and lead to poor cosmetic results if it is uncorrected. The physician should also carefully measure the upper lid margin reflex distance (MRD-1) to detect the preoperative presence of blepharoptosis in the blepharoplasty patient so that both may be treated simultaneously. In addition, preoperative documentation noting the amount and position of redundant skin and prolapsed orbital fat should be performed to aid in surgical decisions. Prolapse of the lateral tissue of the upper lids should alert the surgeon to possible lacrimal gland prolapse, a prominent sub-brow fat pad, or unrecognized brow ptosis [1]. Lower lid laxity should be assessed with either the "distraction" or "snap" test. The ability to distract a lid from the globe by gentle pinching for a distance of 6 mm or greater represents a positive distraction test for laxity [7]. A positive snap test is demonstrated by a distracted lid that fails to return promptly to its normal position after release, except with blinking or manipulation. The tendency to lower lid entropion should also be elicited by having the patient forcefully close the eyelids. It is important to correct documented laxity or entropion before or at the time of blepharoplasty surgery. Finally, neuromuscular disease affecting the eyes, such as myasthenia gravis or myotonic dystrophy, should be ruled out.

Complications of Upper Lid Blepharoplasty

The complications of upper lid blepharoplasty range from the relatively innocuous and easily treated, such as incisional milia, to the most devastating outcome of blindness. These complications may be divided into those caused by errors in preoperative assessment, intraoperative complications, and postoperative complications. (Box 24.1).

J. J. Servat et al. (eds.), *Smith and Nesi's Ophthalmic Plastic and Reconstructive Surgery*,
https://doi.org/10.1007/978-3-030-41720-8_24

Box 24.1: Upper eyelid blepharoplasty complications

Errors in Preoperative Planning or Surgical Judgment

- Undercorrected redundant skin
- Lid or crease asymmetry
- Canthal webbing
- Superior sulcus deformity
- Failure to recognize concomitant ptosis or brow ptosis
- Dry eye/Exposure keratopathy and lagophthalmos
- Ptosis
- Lacrimal gland injury

Operative Complications

- Orbital hemorrhage
- Ocular injury
- Fire and facial burns

Postoperative Complications

- Incision irregularities
- Hypertrophic scar
- Wound dehiscence
- Infection
- Diplopia
- Numbness or hypesthesia
- Blindness

Complications Arising from Preoperative Planning or Surgical Judgment

As previously discussed, preoperative assessment and careful surgical decision-making are essential to minimize complications. Errors of judgment regarding wound placement or extent or those resulting in undercorrection or overcorrection can lead to asymmetry, undesirable appearance, need for wound modulation or revision, and ocular exposure.

Undercorrected Redundant Skin or Fat

Insufficient lid skin removal, while considered in this chapter of blepharoplasty complications, is an expected occasional outcome of the prudent surgeon. The surgeon must ensure that postoperative edema has resolved prior to deciding to remove additional skin, as early edema may give the illusion of excess skin. If a revision is to be performed and the lid crease is desirable, the surgeon should maintain the same crease and remove excess skin only as necessary. This may be easily performed in an office setting under local anesthesia.

As with skin, undercorrection of herniated fat removal is less problematic than overcorrection. However, it tends to be much more common. In the preoperative evaluation, it is prudent to assess the patient for the presence and amount of herniated orbital fat in each compartment to guide surgical decision-making. In the upper lid, the medial fat pad tends to be underexcised far more commonly than the preaponeurotic fat pad. Retropulsion of the globe during surgery can help to reveal herniating fat.

Surgical revision to remove excess skin or fat should be performed once postoperative edema has completely resolved, typically at least 3 months after surgery.

Lid or Crease Asymmetry

The differences between the male and female eyelid crease have been well described [1]. The eyelid crease in women should be well demarcated and run at least 7–8 mm above the lash line. This nicely demonstrates the lashes and provides a pretarsal platform for makeup placement. The typical male crease is usually lower (5–6 mm above the lash line) and more subtle. Careful preanesthetic skin marking and proper incision placement help minimize eyelid crease asymmetry. Removing a strip of orbicularis muscle beneath the inferior skin edge is useful to reform a firmer crease when this is desired, often in Asian patients. Supratarsal fixation of the wound edges may also be performed to establish a new lid crease.

Cases of early postoperative asymmetry can frequently be adequately managed with massage and observation over time. Persistent lid crease problems may require a secondary operation utilizing supratarsal fixation. In cases of lid asymmetry, it is important to realize that lowering an eyelid crease is more difficult than raising it.

If there is undesirable erythema, prominence to the eyelid crease, or hypertrophic scar, intralesional triamcinolone or 5-fluorouracil may be injected to modulate wound healing and soften the scar.

Canthal Webbing

When canthal webbing occurs, it is almost always at the medial canthus (pseudoepicanthus), although cases of lateral canthal webbing may occur. Medial canthal webbing results most frequently from carrying the skin incision too far medially and near the upper eyelid margin or aggressive excision.

Massage tends to have little value in treatment of medial canthal webbing. Intralesional triamcinolone or 5-fluorouracil may be helpful to modulate wound healing, but patients often require surgical revision. One can repair this condition with a V-Y plasty, a Y-V plasty, a diamond plasty, a Z-plasty, or a series of Z-plasties [8, 9]. The surgeon must decide, based on his or her experience and evaluation of the patient's physical condition, which procedure is best for the patient.

Lateral canthal webbing may occur when the incisions of upper and lower lid blepharoplasties are made too close together. It has been suggested that incisions should not be placed closer together than 5 mm [1]. Similar advancement flaps used for the treatment of medial canthal webbing may be used for management of this problem.

Superior Sulcus Deformity

Excessive removal of fat during blepharoplasty may result in hollowing of the superior sulcus and A-frame deformity. Whereas traditional upper blepharoplasty was subtractive, our knowledge of volume loss and its contribution to the aging face has led surgeons to value volume preservation. This has led to a trend in lower blepharoplasty of fat repositioning rather than resection, and this same principle has been applied to upper blepharoplasty. There are a variety of techniques for repositioning of the nasal and central upper eyelid fat compartments for volumization in patients with preoperative hollowing [10, 11].

If aggressive fat removal does lead to bothersome superior sulcus deformity, volume may be added using hyaluronic acid fillers or autologous fat transfer [12, 13]. The effect of the filler is temporary, so maintenance injections are required. Another option involves the removal of additional fat on the opposite side in order to achieve a symmetric appearance [4]. Finally, cosmetics may be used to mask the area of concern. It is best to err on the side of conservative excision because additional removal of fat may be accomplished, whereas adding fat is more challenging.

Dry Eye and Exposure Keratopathy

In addition to providing mechanical protection of the globe, the eyelids help lubricate the cornea by spreading the tear film during the spontaneous blink. Disruption or surgical excision of the orbicularis oculi, the muscle of eyelid closure, may compromise the muscle's function and may result in exposure keratopathy. As with many upper lid blepharoplasty complications, preoperative evaluation is a crucial step in avoiding this result. Every patient should be routinely checked for the presence of preoperative dry eye with inspection for corneal staining, basal secretion test, tear break-up time, and assessment of Bell's phenomenon. With timely detection of an abnormality, the surgeon can modify the approach. Preoperative counseling regarding potential worsening dry eye after blepharoplasty is crucial.

Frequently, postoperative poor blink, dry eye, and exposure symptoms are transient in nature. A small amount of postoperative lagophthalmos usually resolves in several days to weeks or the patient becomes accustomed to the new post-surgical amount of ocular exposure. A variety of different over-the-counter artificial tears and lubricating ointments, as well as lid taping or patching or punctal plugs, may be used in the interim to assist the patient's comfort during this period.

Lagophthalmos

Occasionally, lagophthalmos from aggressive skin and/or orbicularis oculi resection may persist permanently postoperatively (Fig. 24.1A, B). Preoperative assessment of the amount of excess skin and brow position and careful skin markings are crucial to avoid excess skin removal. There often is a subtle internal and external bias to remove more rather than less skin from the upper lids during blepharoplasty to improve a patient's postoperative cosmetic appearance. However, the surgeon should always keep one thing in mind: insufficient skin removal may lead to an unhappy patient, but excessive excision can cause a plethora of clinical problems that are much more difficult to treat. Flowers has stated that 20 mm of anterior lamellar tissue is required for normal functioning of the upper eyelid [14]. In cases of purposefully uncorrected brow ptosis, the surgeon may wish to remove a few millimeters more of skin. Conversely, a more conservative excision may be desirable if brow ptosis is being surgically addressed at the same time. Approximately 10–12 mm of anterior lamella should be left between the inferior brow and the superior incision line [15].

For cases of aggressive anterior lamellar resection and marked lagophthalmos, early suture removal and lid massage

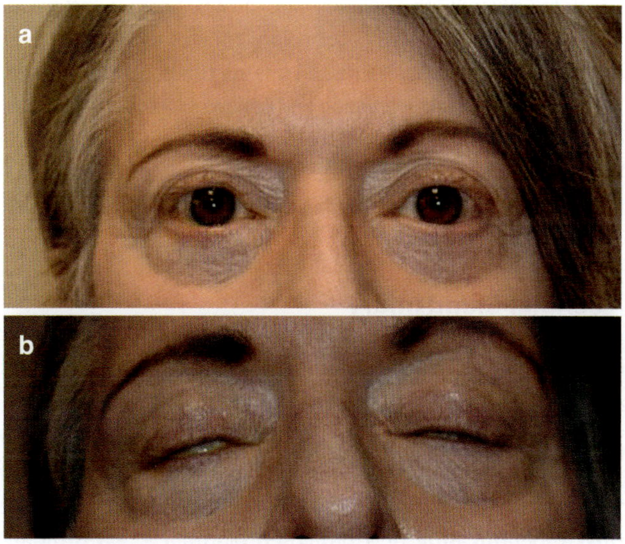

Fig. 24.1 (**a** and **b**) Bilateral postoperative lagophthalmos, in which the right eye is worse than the left

can be beneficial. The lid massage is downward in nature and should be started no sooner that 1 week after surgery to avoid wound dehiscence.

If conservative therapies do not remedy this problem, full-thickness skin grafting may be necessary. Although the degree of exposure symptoms may necessitate earlier intervention, it is probably prudent to wait at least 3 months and more desirably 6 months before proceeding to this step. This will allow postoperative healing to occur and lid scarring to "soften," enabling an easier dissection. Contralateral upper eyelid skin is the best match for a skin graft, but the frequent bilateral nature of blepharoplasty renders this solution impossible. Retroauricular, preauricular, or supraclavicular skin also provides reasonably good matches. The scar release and graft placement should take place above the lid crease, thus hiding the graft in the superior sulcus in primary gaze [4]. If the lid crease was made too low originally, one may want to consider creating a new, higher lid crease at the inferior border of the graft. The graft size should be slightly larger than the defect to allow for healing contracture [1]. Finally, a Frost suture may be applied to help ensure correction.

Often the patient with multiple prior eyelid surgeries has poor orbicularis function and poor blink contributing to lagophthalmos. This may not improve and is best managed with topical lubricants rather than repeat surgery, as each successive surgery has the potential to cause more trauma to the orbicularis.

If the orbital septum is traumatized during blepharoplasty, there may be middle lamellar scarring that contributes to persistent lagophthalmos, and this may be assessed at the time of surgical revision, if necessary.

Ptosis

As noted earlier in this chapter, care must be taken in the preoperative evaluation to rule out concomitant ptosis before a blepharoplasty, so as not to "unmask" this condition postoperatively to the surprise of both surgeon and patient. However, if the ptosis is a new finding after blepharoplasty, it should be treated as a traumatic ptosis and observed for up to 6 months for improvement. Ptosis remaining after this time may be treated surgically.

Lacrimal Gland Injury

Preoperative evaluation should include inspection of the lacrimal gland for prolapse, so as not to confuse this condition with herniated orbital fat. Typically, there is no temporal fat pad in the upper lid although, on occasion, the central preaponeurotic pad will have a lateral component that may make identification of a prolapsed lacrimal gland difficult. Intraoperatively, fat may be distinguished from lacrimal gland by color and texture. Fat tends to be yellow, soft, and billowy, whereas the lacrimal gland appears pinkish gray and contained within a tough, diaphanous membrane. Frequently, the two structures abut one another.

Care should be taken not to excise the lacrimal gland because this may lead to debilitating dry eye. A prolapsed lacrimal gland may be reattached to the periosteum of the lacrimal gland fossa by a mattress suture with 5-0 Prolene or other comparable suture [16].

Operative Complications

While more rare than complications arising from preoperative planning and judgment, unexpected errors or adverse events during upper blepharoplasty can be devastating and sight-threatening. An acute awareness of the possibilities of injury to the eye, orbital hemorrhage, and intraoperative fire is necessary to take preventative measures.

Ocular Injury

All surgeries carry inherent risk of damage to surrounding structures, therefore ocular injury may be a rare but devastating occurrence. Injury can range from mild corneal abrasions to globe perforation. Corneal shields are easily obtained and can protect the globes from intraoperative desiccation of the ocular surface and other trauma. Care must be taken to remove these protectors prior to the end of the case.

Hemorrhage

Significant hemorrhage after upper lid blepharoplasty is uncommon. Orbital hemorrhage may lead to compartment syndrome and vision loss and thus should be managed emergently. This topic is covered under the "Complications of Lower Lid Blepharoplasty" section.

Fire and Facial Burns

Surgery such as upper or lower eyelid blepharoplasty carries a rare but serious risk of intraoperative fire, especially with the common use of handheld or electrosurgical cautery devices and in the setting of supplemental oxygen. Risk of fire and subsequent eyelid or facial burns can be reduced by increased awareness of this risk, judicious use of supplemental oxygen, avoidance of flammable drapes or skin preparations, and placement of ignition sources (i.e. electrocautery, fiber-optic illumination light sources, or lasers) in a designated area away from the patient (e.g. in a holster or a safety cover) and not directly on the patient or surgical drapes [17].

Postoperative Complications

Complications arising after surgery range in severity and may occur even in the most routine of cases and with the most experienced of surgeons. Careful and timely follow-up, early recognition, and appropriate management can often prevent long-term sequelae.

Incision Irregularities

Incision irregularities may consist of inclusion cysts (milia), granulomas, microabscesses, and epithelial suture tunnels (Fig. 24.2). Each has slightly varying etiologies and treatments.

Milia are inclusion cysts that result from the occlusion of glandular ducts or the trapping of epithelial debris in the operative wound. They generally occur 1–2 months after blepharoplasty and usually enlarge, rupture, and atrophy within the next few months. The use of hot, wet compresses or the unroofing of these milia with a blade or needle will hasten their resolution.

Granulomas result from a foreign-body reaction to debris trapped in the wound, including eyelashes and retained suture, and they appear as nodular thickenings in the suture line or underneath the nearby skin. Treatment options include excision or injection with corticosteroids.

Epithelial suture tunnels arise along suture penetration tracts and can be lessened by the use of monofilament sutures, a subcuticular wound closure, as well as the early removal of sutures [1]. A needle, blade, or light cautery may be used to unroof suture tunnels should they occur.

Wound Dehiscence

Meticulous closure with careful reapproximation of the wound edges is an important preventative step to avoid dehiscence. Additionally, patient factors such as smoking, immunocompromise, and rubbing may increase the risk, and appropriate counseling should be performed.

A small wound dehiscence may be observed without intervention, but a larger dehiscence may be repaired by resuturing, use of glue, or tissue adhesive and tape (Fig. 24.3). If there has been a significant time period between wound dehiscence and repair, it is essential that the wound edges be "freshened" using a blade in order to allow the wound to heal properly.

Infection

Infection after blepharoplasty is rare, with a reported incidence of 0.2% in patients undergoing a combination of upper and lower blepharoplasties [18]. A majority of infections are easily treated, yet severe infectious complications have been reported after upper blepharoplasty including blindness from orbital cellulitis [19] and necrotizing fasciitis [20, 21].

Acute postoperative preseptal infection presents with worsening lid edema, erythema, and warmth. The patient should be assessed for orbital involvement by examining vision, relative afferent pupillary defect, extraocular motility, chemosis, and proptosis. Management of such infections is essentially identical to management in the

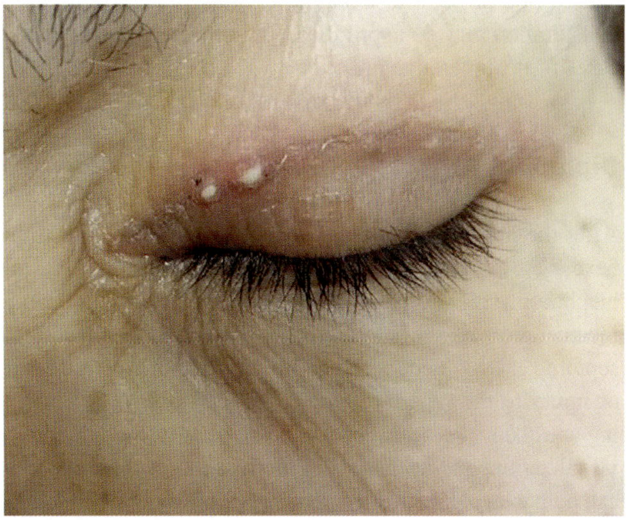

Fig. 24.2 Incisional microabscesses after upper blepharoplasty

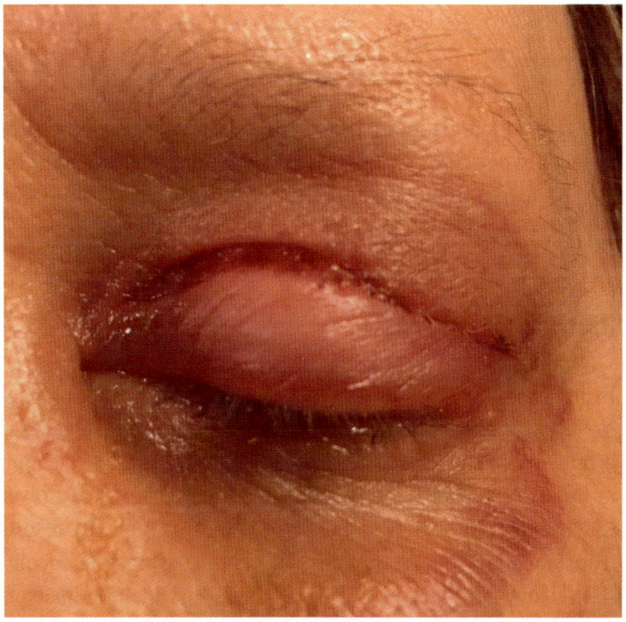

Fig. 24.3 Wound dehiscence after upper blepharoplasty

unoperated patient. Gram stain and culture should be performed on any open wound or drainage. A complete blood count and blood cultures should be strongly considered for severe cases of preseptal and orbital cellulitis or for febrile or toxic patients.

Preseptal cellulitis may be managed with oral antibiotics. Orbital cellulitis or severe preseptal cellulitis requires hospitalization and careful monitoring. A computed tomography (CT) scan of the orbits should be obtained, and any abscess should be drained. Although such infections would be suspected to be Gram-positive, broad coverage is important. Additionally, chronic cutaneous infection with atypical *Mycobacterium* species may also occur after eyelid surgery and can be difficult to treat [22, 23]. An infectious disease consultation may be appropriate for severe or nonresponsive cases of postoperative infection.

Diplopia

After the inferior oblique muscle, the superior oblique is the next most common extraocular muscle to be injured during blepharoplasty [1]. Causes of this condition may include incarceration of the superior oblique tendon in the orbital septum, excess electrocautery in the superonasal quadrant, or injury to the superior oblique while excising fat or injecting anesthetic. Fat resection should be performed under direct visualization, and awareness of the location of these muscles can help to avoid inadvertent damage [2]. If diplopia develops, observation for 3 to 6 months is usually recommended, with patching or Fresnel prisms as temporary treatment. If diplopia in primary gaze persist, strabismus surgery may be necessary.

Numbness

The occasional patient will complain of postoperative numbness between the lid crease incision and the lid margin. No good treatment exists for this condition, but it tends to resolve over several months.

Blindness

Blindness is an occasional devastating complication of blepharoplasty [5, 19]. The feature common to most reported cases is orbital hemorrhage, which is discussed ahead at greater length in the "Hemorrhage" section under "Complications of Lower Lid Blepharoplasty." Blindness in these cases typically results from ischemic optic neuropathy and central retinal artery occlusion. Three other lesser causes of visual loss include inadvertent globe perforation, severe postoperative infection, and the use of monopolar cautery with channeling into the orbital apex.

Complications of Lower Lid Blepharoplasty

As with upper lid blepharoplasty, complications can arise from lower lid blepharoplasty. These range from mild and easily corrected to severe complications with irreversible outcomes (Box 24.2).

Box 24.2: Lower eyelid blepharoplasty complications

Errors in Preoperative Assessment or Surgical Judgment
- Ectropion and eyelid retraction
- Over or undercorrected excess skin
- Over or undercorrected herniated fat
- Asymmetry

Operative Complications
- Fire and/facial burns
- Hemorrhage
- Ocular injury

Postoperative Complications
- Incision irregularities
- Nonaesthetic incision
- Canthal webbing
- Diplopia
- Conjunctival chemosis
- Canalicular laceration and epiphora
- Infection
- Inflammation
- Blindness

Complications Arising from Preoperative Planning or Surgical Judgment

Ectropion and Eyelid Retraction

One of the most common postoperative complications from lower eyelid blepharoplasty is ectropion and eyelid retraction with subsequent lagophthalmos (Figs. 24.4 and 24.5). The major causative factors are excessive anterior lamella removal, unrecognized laxity of the lower eyelid or canthal tendons, orbicularis weakness, and negative-vector topography [24]. Scarring at the level of the orbital septum has also been implicated but may be a less common factor [24, 25].

Laxity of the lower eyelid and weakened canthal tendons should be addressed together. Careful preoperative attention should be paid to preexisting lower lid laxity by the distraction and snap tests. The medial and lateral canthal tendons should similarly be assessed for laxity by

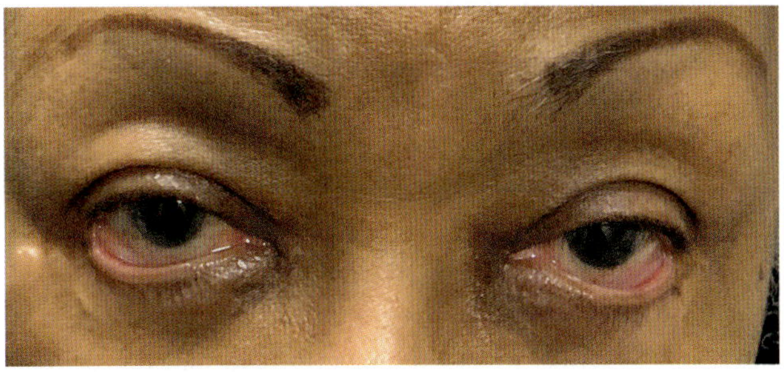

Fig. 24.4 Frank ectropion of the lower lid following lower lid blepharoplasty

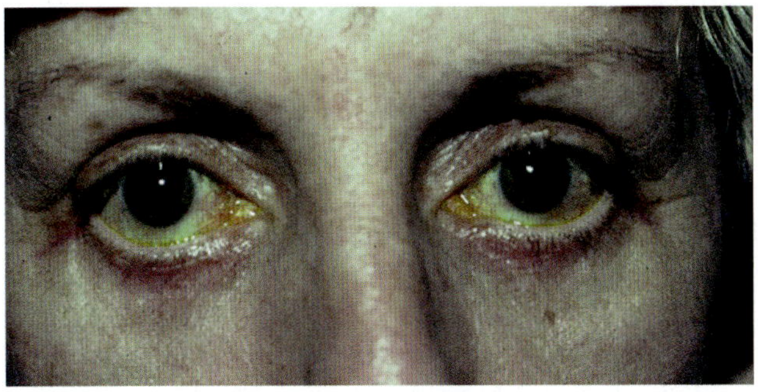

Fig. 24.5 Lower lid retraction after blepharoplasty

"medializing" the lateral canthal tendon and vice versa to check for significant excess motion. A medial canthal tendon tightening may be warranted for significant laxity present in this structure. For general laxity, however, attention may be given to the lateral canthal tendon. A simple plication of the inferior crus of this tendon with 5-0 Prolene or comparable suture works well for mild-to-moderate lid laxity and generally is easily integrated with the standard external blepharoplasty incision. A full tarsal strip procedure may be indicated for severe laxity. These similar procedures may be used for correction of eyelid malpositions that occur postoperatively secondary to horizontal laxity that does not improve spontaneously with resolving edema.

Removing excess skin causing anterior lamellar shortening is a common cause of lower lid retraction after blepharoplasty. This condition can be avoided or minimized by careful assessment of the amount of dermatochalasis and conservative excision during surgery. Preservation of the orbicularis oculi muscle is crucial during skin excision. If the procedure is performed under sedation, the patient should be instructed to look up and open the mouth to place the periocular skin on maximal stretch while the surgeon is assessing skin redundancy. If the patient is under general anesthesia, the surgeon may manually open the mouth. Skin excision should err on the conservative side.

If mild ectropion or retraction secondary to an anterior lamella shortage is noted early in the postoperative period, an attempt may be made to loosen the vertical tension through suture removal and careful opening of the wound, leaving a 2–3 mm area below the lashes bare of skin [26]. This area is allowed to heal by secondary intention. Wound modulation with injection of 5-fluorouracil or triamcinolone may be considered. Aggressive, upward massage for several weeks is recommended in mild cases. The surgeon may consider placement of Frost/traction sutures in the lower lid to put the lid in moderate upward traction for 7–10 days [27].

Persistent lower lid retraction not improved by conservative measures will require repeat surgical intervention. Surgical options include canthoplasty, recession of the lower lid retractors, midfacial or suborbicularis oculi fat (SOOF) lifting, and posterior lamellar spacer grafting such as ear cartilage, hard palate, or allografts [28, 29] Often, a combination of these procedures is necessary and must be determined based on the severity of eyelid retraction. Care should be taken to identify and lyse any focal scarring or adhesions, which may be in the septal plane.

Often these measures can help avoid the need for skin grafting, although this may be reserved for severe, refractory cases. If necessary, a subciliary incision is made, and a full-thickness skin graft is placed into the lower lid, similar to the treatment of a cicatricial ectropion [26]. It is important to thin the graft carefully of its subdermal elements to promote the best healing and ultimate cosmetic result.

Overcorrected or Undercorrected Redundant Skin

Overcorrection of redundant skin can lead to eyelid retraction, which is discussed in the previous section. If redundant skin persist after initial lower eyelid blepharoplasty, additional skin removal can be performed with a skin pinch under local anesthesia in an office or procedure room setting (Fig. 24.6) [30]. As with upper blepharoplasty, it is prudent to wait 3 months after surgery prior to revision to allow for adequate healing and resolution of edema. Again,

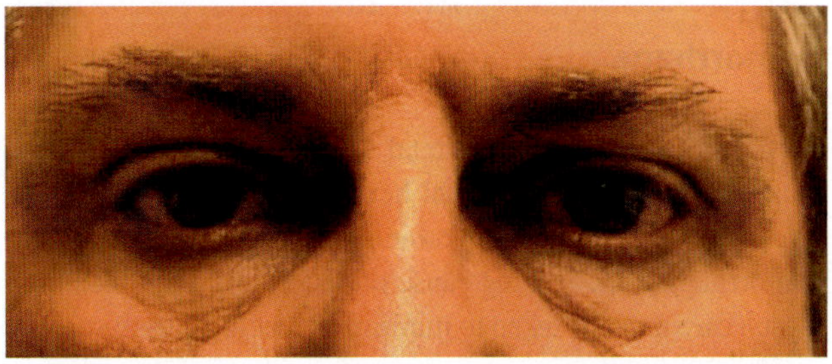

Fig. 24.6 Residual left lower lid skin following lower blepharoplasty

care should be taken to preserve the orbicularis muscle and to ensure that additional skin removal will not cause eyelid retraction. Applications of fractional carbon dioxide laser to the lower lids can be used alternatively in particular patient with residual excess skin.

Overcorrected or Undercorrected Herniated Orbital Fat

The principles of removal or preservation of the orbital fat pads are essentially identical to those mentioned in the "Complications of Upper Lid Blepharoplasty" section. The main difference between the two lids is the presence of three, rather than two, fat pads in the lower lid that need to be addressed surgically. It is once again important to grade the fat pads preoperatively to appropriately estimate the amount of fat to be removed during surgery. It is noteworthy that the lateral fat pad is the compartment most often undercorrected during lower blepharoplasty secondary to its more numerous fibrous adhesions and less billowing nature. Also, access to the lateral fat pad can be more difficult if canthotomy and cantholysis are not performed, leading to undercorrection.

Operative Complications

Ocular Injuries

Ocular complications during surgery vary from corneal abrasion to severe ocular injuries such as globe perforation or laceration, which are extremely rare during lower lid blepharoplasty. The use of lubricating ointments and corneal protectors is recommended during this procedure.

Fire/Facial Burns

The cause and management of this complication have been addressed in "Complications of Upper Lid Blepharoplasty" section above.

Hemorrhage

Persistent bleeding from orbital fat or the orbicularis oculi muscle can lead to superficial hematoma formation, progressive ecchymosis, or deep orbital hemorrhage [2]. Because hemorrhage is the leading cause of vision loss from blepharoplasty, care must be taken to minimize bleeding during surgery.

This caution begins preoperatively with careful scrutiny of preoperative medications. It is recommended that the patients be off aspirin 7–10 days before surgery. Other anticoagulants like warfarin should be discontinued 5 days before surgery. The oral antithrombin anticoagulants should be stopped 2 days prior to surgery. Over-the-counter supplements and nonsteroidal anti-inflammatory drugs should be stopped as well.

During the operation, bleeding must be controlled meticulously by pressure, hemostats, sutures, or cautery as necessary. Of particular importance are the careful dissection of the orbital septum when this is performed and the delicate manipulation of orbital fat. One technique to remove orbital fat is the "3-C," or clamp, cut, and cauterize, approach. The fat is first gently clamped with a hemostat, taking care not to exert upward traction. Next, the fat is excised with a pair of scissors, leaving a small stump. Finally, the fat is cauterized thoroughly with a cautery unit of choice. As also described by others, we suggest that before removing the clamp, the fat should be gently grasped and lightly stretched with forceps to ensure direct visualization of the tissue by the surgeon. This allows the physician to verify that complete hemostasis has occurred before allowing the fat to retract back into the orbit [31].

Intraoperatively or postoperatively, iced compresses and head elevation may be used to suppress bleeding and edema. Occlusive dressings are not recommended after blepharoplasty, and the patients should be instructed to monitor their vision at home and report any changes to the surgeon. The patient should be reexamined immediately by the surgeon if he/she develops acute eye or periorbital pain, significant swelling or proptosis, chemosis, ophthalmoplegia, or vision changes. Vision and intraocular pressure should be assessed, and a direct ophthalmoscope may be used to visualize the optic nerve. The surgeon should intervene if retrobulbar hemorrhage is causing an orbital compartment syndrome with increased intraocular pressure or optic nerve or vision compromise. An immediate and often effective treatment is to open up the surgical wound and to evacuate the free blood and clots. Simultaneously, intravenous acetazolamide or mannitol may be given unless it is contraindicated by the patient's medical status. More aggressive actions may be considered if the abovementioned treatment fails. This includes the creation of a lateral canthotomy and cantholysis, or orbital exploration and bone decompression for refractory orbital hemorrhage.

Postoperative Complications

Nonaesthetic Incision and Incision Irregularities

Causes of a noticeable lower lid blepharoplasty scar are generally threefold: early wound dehiscence, an inferiorly placed incision away from the lash line, and extension of the incision past the canthus. Wound dehiscence should be reclosed in a timely fashion, if possible. If this is impractical or if significant scarring persists, 3–6 months should be allowed to pass before additional surgery is undertaken. This allows complete wound healing, resolution of edema, relaxation of the skin tension, and time to reevaluate the cosmetic condition. A similar waiting period should be allotted for noticeable scars secondary to the other two etiologies. Hypertrophic scars may be injected with a small amount of triamcinolone or 5-fluorouracil. Topical steroids, silicone, or growth factors can also be used to treat and prevent hypertrophic scars.

Scars inferior to the lash line may be corrected through careful excision with a strip of skin taken as necessary above the wound to raise and bury the incision. This procedure should be performed judiciously because it may lead to ectropion and retraction. Noticeable lateral incisions and webbing may be treated with scar revisions such as the Z- or W-plasty to change the tension or direction of the scar or to irregularize the scar, respectively. Dermabrasion, carbon dioxide laser, and microneedling may also be advantageous as nonincisional approaches to resurfacing and remodeling the offending tissue, leading to a smoother transition between scarred and normal tissues [29, 32, 33]. Noticeable lateral canthal webbing may be treated with scar revisions such as the Z- or W-plasty as discussed in the Complications of Upper lid Blepharoplasty section.

Diplopia

Double vision after blepharoplasty occasionally is caused by a periorbital or retrobulbar hemorrhage or edema, which should resolve with resolution of the blood or fluid. Mechanisms of extraocular muscle injury include intramuscular hemorrhage and edema, cicatricial changes within the muscle, and accidental incorporation of extraocular muscle in closure of orbital septum [34, 35].

The inferior oblique is the extraocular muscle most often injured during blepharoplasty. It arises from the orbital floor and can be found between the medial and central fat pads traveling superiorly, laterally, and posteriorly. It is prudent for the surgeon to locate and identify this structure so that it can be avoided with fat excision. Careful dissection of the medial and central fat pads from the inferior oblique is recommended during orbital fat repositioning to prevent excess tension on the muscle. If there is inadvertent severing of the inferior oblique during the surgery, primary repair can be attempted. For most cases of lesser trauma to the muscle, double vision will resolve with time.

For diplopia that persists, the surgeon may consider transconjunctival exploration of the inferior oblique for mechanical restriction. If strabismus surgery is necessary, it is recommended to wait 3 months prior to intervention.

Canalicular Laceration and Epiphora

The inferior canaliculus may be injured during either an external or transconjunctival blepharoplasty with extension of the incision too medially or too close to the eyelid margin. Realization of a severed canaliculus during the surgery should prompt the surgeon to attempt a primary repair with intubation.

Eyelid swelling and ecchymosis in the early postoperative period decrease eyelid motility and interfere with the mechanics of blinking. It is common to have tearing and ocular discomfort during this period. Treatment consisting of lubricating drops can be used, especially if lagophthalmos is present. Persistent tearing detected after surgery should undergo a full epiphora workup including a search for lagophthalmos or exposure, punctal ectropion, severed canaliculi, or outflow obstruction.

Conjunctival Chemosis

Transient chemosis after lower blepharoplasty is common and may occur after transconjunctival or transcutaneous blepharoplasty. However, chronic chemosis that persists for several months is uncommon [36]. The cause is multifactorial: manipulation of the conjunctiva, ocular surface exposure, disruption of the orbital lymphatic channels, and corneal injury or infection. Fortunately, most cases resolve spontaneously with time and reassurance. Symptomatic palliation such as topical lubricants and steroids are used to treat this condition. In cases of persistent chemosis, high-frequency radiowave electrosurgery has been reported to produce significant reduction in the chemosis [37]. In this procedure, subconjunctival coagulation of the edematous conjunctiva with a fine-needle electrode is performed using a high-frequency radiowave electrosurgical unit in coagulation mode. This is followed by subconjunctival fluid drainage by application of gentle pressure. Other treatments have been described to treat chronic bulbar chemosis such as conjunctivotomy and the injection of 2% tetracycline [38].

Infection

Preseptal and orbital cellulitis can rarely occur after a lower lid blepharoplasty. The management is similar to that described earlier in the "Complications of Upper Lid Blepharoplasty" section.

Inflammation

Persistent postoperative lower eyelid inflammation or edema can occur after lower lid blepharoplasty. When this occurs, time should be allowed for spontaneous resolution. In cases where there is no improvement, off-label intralesional injections of triamcinolone, tetracycline, or doxycycline have been used with variable success.

Blindness

Rarely permanent vision loss can occur from a lower lid blepharoplasty and can result from orbital hemorrhage, orbital cellulitis, or globe perforation.

References

1. Lowry JC, Bartley GB. Complications of blepharoplasty. Surv Ophthalmol. 1994;38(4):327–50. PubMed PMID: 8160107.
2. Mauriello JA. Unfavorable results of eyelid and lacrimal surgery: prevention and management. Boston: Butterworth-Heinemann; 2000. p. 3–25.
3. Iliff CE, Iliff WJ, Iliff NT. Oculoplastic surgery. Boston: WB Saunders; 1979.
4. Kulwin DR, Kersten RC. Blepharoplasty and brow elevation. In: Dortzbach RK, editor. Ophthalmic plastic surgery—prevention and management of complications. New York: Raven; 1984.
5. Stasior OG. The Wendell L. Hughes lecture. Complications of ophthalmic plastic surgery and their prevention. Trans Sect Ophthalmol Am Acad Ophthalmol Otolaryngol. 1976;81(4 Pt 1):OP543–52. PubMed PMID: 960377.
6. Gladstone GJ, Black EH, Myint S, et al. Gladstone and Nesi's oculoplastic surgery atlas. New York: Springer; 2005. p. 63–78.
7. Shagets FW, Shore JW. The management of eyelid laxity during lower eyelid blepharoplasty. Arch Otolaryngol Head Neck Surg. 1986;112(7):729–32. PubMed PMID: 3707734.
8. Massry GG. Cicatricial canthal webs. Ophthalmic Plast Reconstr Surg. 2011;27(6):426–30. https://doi.org/10.1097/IOP.0b013e318222f4a1. PubMed PMID: 21862949.
9. Field LM. Repair of a cicatricial epicanthal fold by a double Z-plasty (Spaeth). J Dermatol Surg Oncol. 1982;8(3):215–7. PubMed PMID: 7040520.
10. Massry GG. Nasal fat preservation in upper eyelid blepharoplasty. Ophthalmic Plast Reconstr Surg. 2011;27(5):352–5. https://doi.org/10.1097/IOP.0b013e31821524c3. PubMed PMID: 21904172.
11. Chen CC, Chen SN, Huang CL. Correction of sunken upper-eyelid deformity in young Asians by minimally-invasive double-eyelid procedure and simultaneous orbital fat pad repositioning: a one-year follow-up study of 250 cases. Aesthet Surg J. 2015;35(4):359–66. https://doi.org/10.1093/asj/sju083. Epub 2015/03/24. PubMed PMID: 25804503.
12. Holck DE, Lopez MA. Periocular autologous fat transfer. Facial Plast Surg Clin North Am 2008;16(4):417–27, vi. https://doi.org/10.1016/j.fsc.2008.06.001. PubMed PMID: 19056054.
13. Goldberg RA, Fiaschetti D. Filling the periorbital hollows with hyaluronic acid gel: initial experience with 244 injections. Ophthalmic Plast Reconstr Surg 2006;22(5):335–41; discussion 41–3. doi: https://doi.org/10.1097/01.iop.0000235820.00633.61. PubMed PMID: 16985414.
14. Flowers RS. Blepharoplasty. In: Courtiss EH, editor. Male aesthetic surgery. St. Louis: C.V. Mosby; 1982.
15. Seiff SR. Eyebrow ptosis and blepharoplasty. In: Stewart WB, editor. Surgery of the eyelid, orbit, and lacrimal system, vol. 2. San Francisco: American Academy of Ophthalmology; 1994.
16. Nesi FN, Waltz KL. Smith's practical techniques in ophthalmic plastic surgery. C.V. Mosby: St. Louis; 1994.
17. Lucarelli MJ, Lemke BN. Monopolar electrosurgical flash fire. Ophthalmic Surg Lasers. 1998;29(3):249–50. PubMed PMID: 9547782.
18. Carter SR, Stewart JM, Khan J, Archer KF, Holds JB, Seiff SR, et al. Infection after blepharoplasty with and without carbon dioxide laser resurfacing. Ophthalmology. 2003;110(7):1430–2. https://doi.org/10.1016/S0161-6420(03)00447-0. PubMed PMID: 12867404.
19. Morgan SC. Orbital cellulitis and blindness following a blepharoplasty. Plast Reconstr Surg. 1979;64(6):823–6. PubMed PMID: 515236.
20. Suñer IJ, Meldrum ML, Johnson TE, Tse DT. Necrotizing fasciitis after cosmetic blepharoplasty. Am J Ophthalmol. 1999;128(3):367–8. PubMed PMID: 10511038.
21. Jordan DR, Mawn L, Marshall DH. Necrotizing fasciitis caused by group A streptococcus infection after laser blepharoplasty. Am J Ophthalmol. 1998;125(2):265–6. PubMed PMID: 9467463.
22. Crosswell EG, Leyngold IM. Atypical mycobacterial infection following upper eyelid blepharoplasty. Ophthalmic Plast Reconstr Surg. 2016;32(5):e116–8. https://doi.org/10.1097/IOP.0000000000000285. PubMed PMID: 25210873.
23. Mauriello JA, Group AMS. Atypical mycobacterial infection of the periocular region after periocular and facial surgery. Ophthalmic Plast Reconstr Surg. 2003;19(3):182–8. PubMed PMID: 12918551.
24. Griffin G, Azizzadeh B, Massry GG. New insights into physical findings associated with postblepharoplasty lower eyelid retraction. Aesthet Surg J. 2014;34(7):995–1004. https://doi.org/10.1177/1090820X14544306. PubMed PMID: 25168805.
25. Schwarcz R, Fezza JP, Jacono A, Massry GG. Stop blaming the septum. Ophthalmic Plast Reconstr Surg. 2016;32(1):49–52. https://doi.org/10.1097/IOP.0000000000000420. PubMed PMID: 25719376.
26. Dortzbach RK. Ophthalmic plastic surgery: prevention and management of complications. New York: Raven; 1994. p. 91–111.
27. Baylis HI, Wilson MC, Groth MJ. Complications of lower blepharoplasty. In: Putterman AM, editor. Cosmetic oculoplastic surgery. 2nd ed. Philadelphia: W.B. Saunders; 1993.
28. Marshak H, Morrow DM, Dresner SC. Small incision preperiosteal midface lift for correction of lower eyelid retraction. Ophthalmic Plast Reconstr Surg. 2010;26(3):176–81. https://doi.org/10.1097/IOP.0b013e3181b8c00a. PubMed PMID: 20489542.
29. Kotlus B, Schwarcz RM. Management of postblepharoplasty lower eyelid retraction. Clin Plast Surg. 2015;42(1):73–7. https://doi.org/10.1016/j.cps.2014.09.006. Epub 2014/10/11. PubMed PMID: 25440743.
30. Taban M, Perry JD. Lower eyelid position after transconjunctival lower blepharoplasty with versus without a skin pinch. Ophthalmic Plast Reconstr Surg. 2008;24(1):7–9. https://doi.org/10.1097/IOP.0b013e318160f3a0. PubMed PMID: 18209632.
31. Wilkins RB, Hunter GJ. Blepharoplasty: cosmetic and functional. In: McCord CD, editor. Oculoplastic surgery. New York: Raven; 1981.
32. Ramaut L, Hoeksema H, Pirayesh A, Stillaert F, Monstrey S. Microneedling: where do we stand now? A systematic review of the literature. J Plast Reconstr Aesthet Surg. 2018;71(1):1–14. https://doi.org/10.1016/j.bjps.2017.06.006. Epub 2017/06/17. PubMed PMID: 28690124.

33. Zduńska K, Kołodziejczak A, Rotsztejn H. Is skin microneedling a good alternative method of various skin defects removal. Dermatol Ther. 2018;31(6):e12714. https://doi.org/10.1111/dth.12714. Epub 2018/09/24. PubMed PMID: 30246914.
34. Ghabrial R, Lisman RD, Kane MA, Milite J, Richards R. Diplopia following transconjunctival blepharoplasty. Plast Reconstr Surg. 1998;102(4):1219–25. PubMed PMID: 9734448.
35. Syniuta LA, Goldberg RA, Thacker NM, Rosenbaum AL. Acquired strabismus following cosmetic blepharoplasty. Plast Reconstr Surg. 2003;111(6):2053–9. https://doi.org/10.1097/01.PRS.0000056840.61348.35. PubMed PMID: 12711971.
36. Weinfeld AB, Burke R, Codner MA. The comprehensive management of chemosis following cosmetic lower blepharoplasty. Plast Reconstr Surg. 2008;122(2):579–86. https://doi.org/10.1097/PRS.0b013e31818001d0. PubMed PMID: 18626377.
37. Woo KI, Choi CY. High-frequency radiowave electrosurgery for persistent conjunctival chemosis following cosmetic blepharoplasty. Plast Reconstr Surg. 2014;133(6):1336–42. https://doi.org/10.1097/PRS.0000000000000175. PubMed PMID: 24867715.
38. Moesen I, Mombaerts I. Subconjunctival injection of tetracycline 2% for chronic bulbar chemosis after transcutaneous four-eyelid blepharoplasty. Ophthalmic Plast Reconstr Surg. 2008;24(3):219–20. https://doi.org/10.1097/IOP.0b013e31816e2f27. PubMed PMID: 18520839.

Part VI

Eyelid Tumors and Reconstruction

Richard Allen

Eyelid and Conjunctival Neoplasms

25

Lilly Wagner, Aaron Savar, and Bita Esmaeli

Introduction

There are numerous neoplastic lesions that can affect the eyelids and conjunctiva. These most commonly arise from the epithelial layer, but can also arise from any cell type, including connective tissue and lymphoid tissue. Some neoplastic lesions primarily affect the bulbar conjunctiva, some primarily affect the eyelid skin or palpebral conjunctiva, and some neoplastic lesions involve all these structures to various extents. In the following chapter, we will discuss the more common malignant lesions of the eyelid and conjunctiva, covering epidemiology, clinical and pathologic features, and treatments.

Eyelid Neoplasms

Basal Cell Carcinoma

Basal cell carcinoma (BCC) is the most common malignant neoplasm of the eyelid, accounting for 86–91% of cases [1, 2]. BCC is also the most common malignancy in humans worldwide. A study from Spain found a population-based incidence of 253 cases per 100,000 individuals per year, and in Australia, the incidence was as high as 7067 cases per 100,000 men per year and 3379 cases per 100,000 women per year [3, 4]. Most patients are in their seventh decade at the time of diagnosis, and men are affected more frequently than women [5, 6].

Exposure to ultraviolet light and fair skin type are the most notable risk factors for BCC [7]. Several other extrinsic and intrinsic factors have been reported to promote development of BCC, including radiation, arsenic exposure, and immunosuppression. Furthermore, BCC can arise from scars and ulcers, and individuals with xeroderma pigmentosum and Gorlin–Goltz syndrome are predisposed to develop multiple BCCs at a young age [8, 9]. BCC rarely metastasizes, and mortality rates are low; however, destruction of periocular structures and orbital invasion can cause extensive functional and cosmetic impairment.

Pathologic Features

BCC originates from the basal cell layer of the epidermis. The neoplastic cells have large hyperchromatic nuclei and scant cytoplasm. Aggregates of tumor cells form basophilic cords and nests in the dermis. The neoplastic foci show characteristic peripheral palisading of nuclei (Fig. 25.1) and a retraction artifact that appears as a cleft between the tumor nests and the surrounding stroma.

Currently, there is no uniform histologic classification for BCC. However, certain architectural growth patterns have been found to predict subclinical spread, which is associated with increased risk of incomplete excision and local recurrence [6, 10]. The various subtypes of BCC are divided into more and less aggressive forms. The aggressive subtypes include infiltrative (also referred to as morpheaform or sclerosing) BCC, micronodular BCC, and basosquamous carcinoma. Nodular BCC is a well-circumscribed form of BCC that exhibits less aggressive biologic behavior. The aggressiveness of superficial BCC is controversial.

Nodular BCC, the most common subtype, is composed of multiple round nests of various size that show the characteristics described in the first paragraph of this section. In infiltrative BCC, the second most common subtype, tumor cells form irregularly shaped thin cords and nests (Fig. 25.2) with

L. Wagner
Mayo Clinic, Department of Ophthalmology, Rochester, MN, USA

A. Savar
Stein Eye Institute, UCLA, Department of Ophthalmology, Los Angeles, CA, USA

B. Esmaeli (✉)
Orbital Oncology & Ophthalmic Plastic Surgery, Department of Plastic Surgery, MD Anderson Cancer Center, Houston, TX, USA
e-mail: besmaeli@mdanderson.org

J. J. Servat et al. (eds.), *Smith and Nesi's Ophthalmic Plastic and Reconstructive Surgery*,
https://doi.org/10.1007/978-3-030-41720-8_25

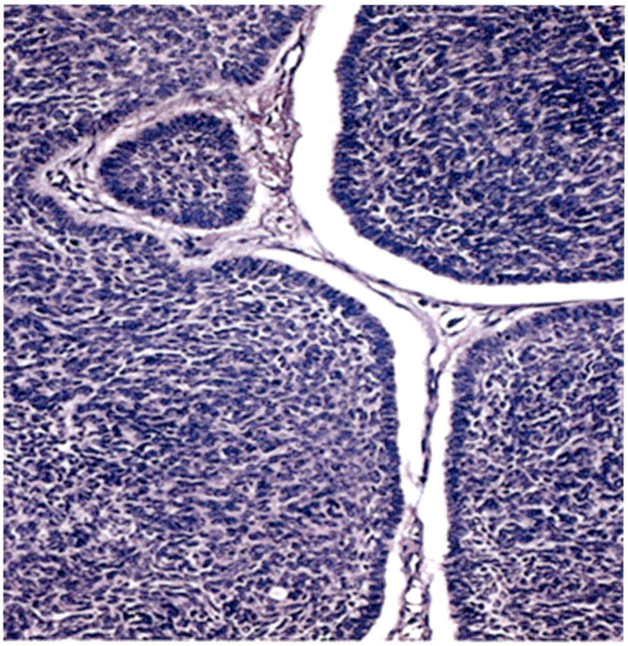

Fig. 25.1 Histologic section of a nodular basal cell carcinoma demonstrating peripheral palisading

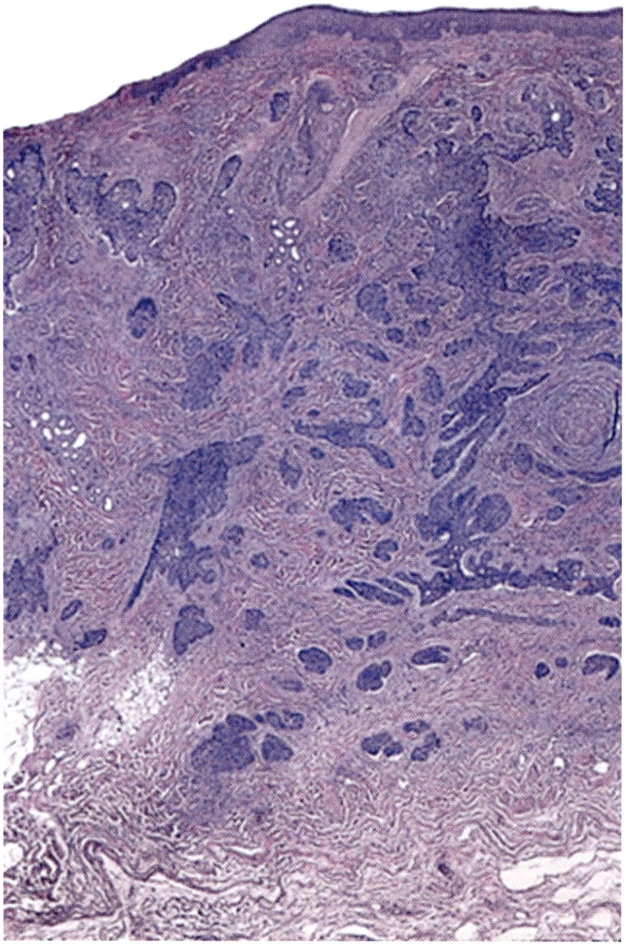

Fig. 25.2 Histologic section of an infiltrative (morpheaform) basal cell carcinoma

jagged contours, and the surrounding stroma is frequently fibrotic and intensely collagenized. Various degrees of differentiation into follicular, eccrine, apocrine, and sebaceous structures can be observed in all subtypes of BCC. However, the grade of differentiation has not been found to be prognostically significant.

Recurrence rates of periocular BCC after complete surgical excision range from 0% to 17%. Higher rates were found with tumor-free margins <2 mm, recurrent lesions, medial canthus location, and aggressive histologic subtype [6, 11, 12]. Perineural invasion has been reported in 1–3% of patients with periocular BCC and is associated with increased risk of subclinical extension, a higher recurrence rate, and a high rate of orbital invasion [13, 14].

The incidence of metastasis is very low—several large studies have reported a metastasis rate of 0.1% among all patients with BCC [15, 16]. In contrast, in a case series including 28 patients with basosquamous carcinoma, 14% of patients developed metastases, a finding that highlights the malignant potential of this particular subtype [17]. Reported sites of metastasis include lymph nodes, lung, bones, and liver [16, 18].

Clinical Presentation

Periocular BCC is most frequently located on the lower lid, followed by the medial canthus, upper lid, and lateral canthus [6, 14]. The classic lesion is of the nodular histologic subtype and is a slowly growing, painless, skin-colored or pinkish papule with well-defined pearly margins and telangiectasias (Fig. 25.3), sometimes accompanied by crusting and bleeding. As the tumor progresses, central ulceration occurs, and the edges appear rolled.

In contrast, infiltrative (morpheaform) BCC usually presents clinically as a pale-white, yellowish, or reddish scar-like plaque with irregular, indurated edges and a waxy, scaly

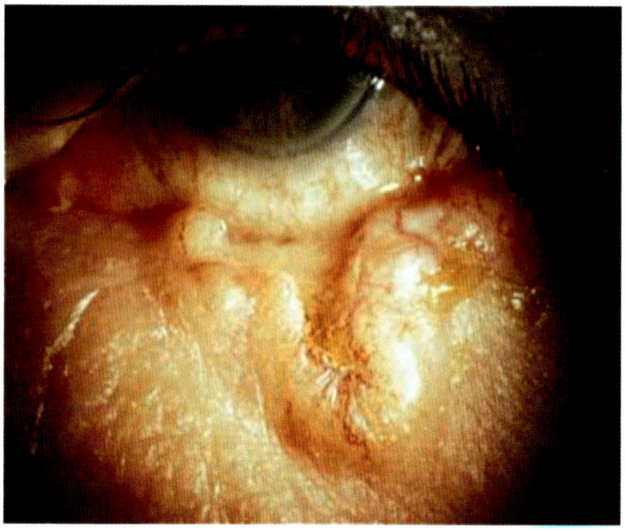

Fig. 25.3 Clinical photograph of basal cell carcinoma of the eyelid with telangiectasia and "pearly gray" borders

surface. In superficial BCC, single or multiple erythematous plaques with slightly raised margins create an eczema-like image. Pigmented BCC is usually of the nodular histologic subtype and can be mistaken for melanoma.

Although the biologic behavior of BCC is usually benign, clinicians must be alert to the possibility of perineural invasion or orbital invasion. Patients with perineural invasion can experience paresthesia, motor function loss, pain, or anesthesia [19]. Signs of orbital invasion include a visible or palpable mass with or without bone fixation, limitation of ocular motility, globe displacement, epiphora, and ptosis [20].

Management

Surgical excision is the treatment of choice for periocular BCC. A large retrospective study documented an incomplete excision rate of 25% after excision with 3 mm clinical margins [6]. Another study found local recurrence in 27% of patients with positive histologic margins [11]. These data show that BCC has a high potential for subclinical spread and that histologic margin control is essential for successful surgical treatment.

Both frozen section control and Mohs micrographic surgery achieve very good local control; 5-year recurrence rates with these approaches are 0–2.4% [13, 14, 21]. In cases with perineural invasion, however, the recurrence rate has been reported to be as high as 7.7% [13].

Radiation therapy has been suggested for tumors that are very large, recurrent, or involve the lacrimal apparatus and for patients who are not good surgical candidates. Radiation therapy has been shown to yield local control rates of 94% and 67% for primary and recurrent tumors, respectively [22]. Adjuvant radiation therapy after surgical resection of BCC may be indicated if there are high-risk histologic features in the surgical specimen, such as microscopic perineural invasion.

Promising results have been observed with other nonsurgical treatments, including photodynamic therapy and topical treatment with imiquimod [23, 24]. However, large studies and long-term follow-up data are needed to establish these modalities as valuable alternatives to surgical treatment.

The hedgehog inhibitors vismodegib and sonidegib have shown great promise in the treatment of lesions that had previously been considered unresectable or resectable only with exenteration [25–28]. Vismodegib is approved for treatment of locally advanced basal cell carcinomas, and sonidegib is approved for treatment of metastatic basal cell carcinomas. Side effects (alopecia, dysgeusia, dysosmia, diarrhea, constipation) have been significant enough in some patients to warrant discontinuation of the therapy. These agents have also shown success in treatment of basal cell nevus syndrome [29].

Squamous Cell Carcinoma

Squamous cell carcinoma (SCC) is the second most common cancer of the eyelids. The incidence of SCC of the eyelid has been reported to be approximately 10% that of BCC, with 1.37 cases per 100,000 individuals per year [1, 2]. In patients with SCC of the eyelid, aggressive tumor growth and the proximity of the tumor to multiple sensitive structures can cause significant morbidity. The capacity of SCC for lymphatic, perineural, and hematogenous spread makes SCC a potentially lethal disease.

While exposure to ultraviolet light and a fair complexion are the most commonly identified risk factors [30], several other conditions have also been shown to increase the risk of development of SCC, including chronic ulcers, scars, human papillomavirus infection, radiation, and various chemical agents. Furthermore, immunocompromised individuals and patients with genetic skin disorders, including xeroderma pigmentosum and albinism, exhibit an increased incidence of SCC as well as more aggressive growth of SCC [31–33].

Pathologic Features

In most cases, SCC develops from preexisting intraepidermal lesions characterized as SCC in situ or actinic keratosis. The distinction between these premalignant lesions is not highly reproducible among different dermatopathologists, and some authors propose considering SCC in situ and actinic keratosis as one entity [34]. SCC can also develop de novo in previously normal skin; this variety of SCC has been found to be associated with increased risk of regional and distant metastases [35].

Invasive SCC is an SCC in which there is invasion of atypical keratinocytes into the dermis. They form fingerlike extensions that appear on tissue sections as distinct nests and cords. In the most common histopathologic subtype, simplex (also referred to as generic) SCC, tumor cells present with eosinophilic cytoplasm; enlarged, hyperchromatic nuclei with high mitotic activity; and formation of keratin pearls (Fig. 25.4). The typical features of keratinization decrease in less differentiated subtypes, like spindle-cell or small-cell SCC. In these variants, immunostaining for cytokeratins shows a positive signal with diffuse cytoplasmic distribution and can be a helpful tool in making a diagnosis [36].

The most common sites of metastasis of SCC are regional lymph nodes, predominantly the parotid/preauricular and submental/submandibular nodes [37]. Less frequently, hematogenous spread to distant sites, such as lung, can be seen.

Several features have been identified that help predict the likelihood of local recurrence and metastasis. Tumor size >2 cm doubles the risk of local recurrence (7.4% versus 15.2%) and triples the risk of metastasis (9.1% versus 30.3%). Other indicators of increased malignant potential

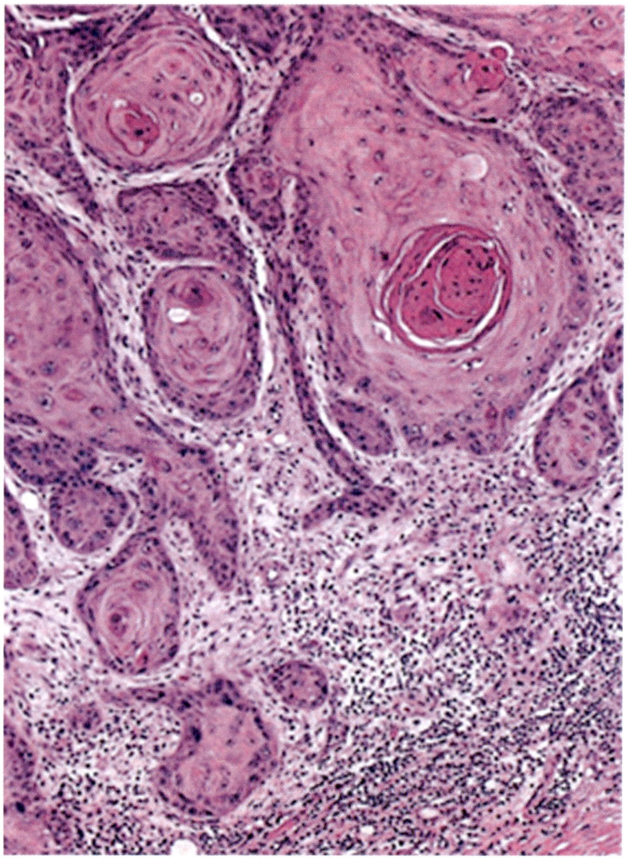

Fig. 25.4 Histologic section of squamous cell carcinoma with typical keratin pearls

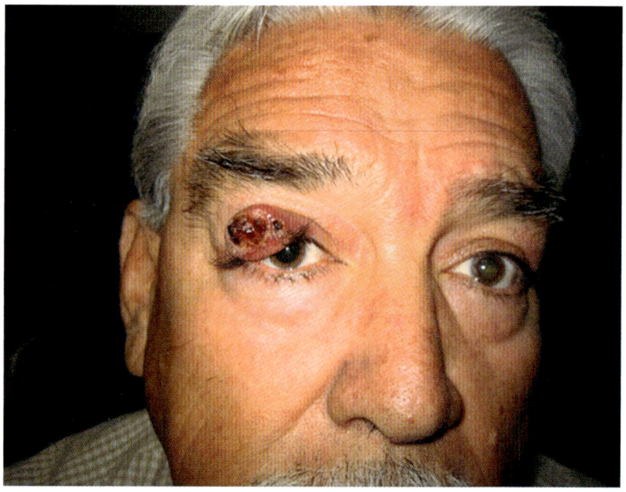

Fig. 25.5 Clinical photograph of squamous cell carcinoma of the eyelid

include depth of invasion >4 mm, poor differentiation, desmoplastic or adenosquamous subtype, occurrence in scar tissue, and recurrent disease. The most significant predictor of aggressiveness of SCC, however, is perineural invasion: 47.2% of lesions with perineural invasion show local recurrence and 47.3% of lesions with perineural invasion show metastasis [38]. Perineural invasion has been observed in 4.3–8.1% of cases of periocular SCC [37, 39], and identification of these cases by meticulous histologic analysis is mandatory for the development of an adequate treatment strategy.

Clinical Presentation

The most common location of periocular SCC is the lower eyelid, followed by the medial canthus, upper eyelid (Fig. 25.5), and lateral canthus [37, 40]. The clinical diagnosis can be challenging because of a broad variety of morphologic presentations. Typically, SCC initially appears as a painless plaque or nodule with chronic erythema, scaling, and fissuring that gradually enlarges and develops ulceration, bleeding, and discomfort. The lesion can be well circumscribed or poorly defined. It can present as a large fungating mass, mimicking keratoacanthoma, cutaneous horn, or BCC with pearly edges and telangiectasias.

Invasion of the orbit through direct or perineural spread can cause globe fixation, proptosis, dystopia, and symptoms and signs of cranial nerve involvement, including pain, numbness, ophthalmoplegia, ptosis, and facial nerve palsy. A series of 17 cases of SCC with perineural spread to the ocular adnexa found that the affected cranial nerves, in order of decreasing frequency, were the ophthalmic and maxillary divisions of the trigeminal nerve (V1, V2), the extraocular motor nerves (III, IV, VI), the facial nerve (VII), and the optic nerve (II) [41].

Management

Complete surgical excision is the primary treatment for most periocular SCCs. Lesions for which an initial treatment attempt has failed are associated with a higher risk of local recurrence and metastasis following subsequent treatments [38]; therefore, complete resection during the initial procedure should be the goal. A review of 68 cases found that the rate of incomplete excision was 25% when 5 mm clinically clear margins were used to determine the area of resection, showing the potential for extensive subclinical spread [6]. In contrast, surgical resection with histologic margin control and immediate reconstruction is associated with a cure rate of over 95% and is the standard modality in the management of periocular SCC [39, 40, 42].

The local control rate in cases with high-risk features, such as positive or close margins or perineural invasion, can be improved by postoperative adjuvant radiation therapy [43]. Patients with lymph node metastasis should undergo lymphadenectomy and possibly adjuvant irradiation of the affected area [44]. Distant metastasis necessitates treatment with systemic chemotherapy [45, 46]. Orbital invasion usually necessitates exenteration as the only potentially curative treatment [47]; however, targeted therapy (see below) shows some promise in treating these patients.

Primary radiation therapy is a reasonable alternative in cases in which surgical treatment is contraindicated because of comorbidities or concerns regarding the functional and cosmetic results and has been shown to achieve local control rates of 89–93% [43, 48]. Because of the potential ocular side effects of radiation therapy, surgical excision remains the first-line therapy.

Other treatment modalities have been used in selected cases, including cryotherapy, intralesional chemotherapy, and photodynamic therapy [49, 50]; however, large studies and long-term results are lacking. These modalities should be employed only when the aforementioned options are not available or are contraindicated.

Targeted therapy inhibiting the fibroblast growth factor/fibroblast growth factor receptor pathway with cetuximab, gefitinib, and erlotinib has been described for the treatment of extensive disease [51]. In addition, successful treatment of advanced squamous cell carcinoma with immunotherapy has been reported [52].

Sebaceous Carcinoma

Sebaceous carcinoma (SC) usually arises from the sebaceous glands of the ocular adnexa, including the meibomian glands, the glands of Zeis, the glands of the eyebrows, the caruncle, and the glands of the fine hair follicles on the cutaneous surface of the eyelid. The periocular region is the most common location for SC; this fact is thought to be due to the abundance of sebaceous glands in this area. Rarely, SC occurs at extraocular sites, and extraocular SC has been shown to exhibit a relatively benign biologic behavior [53].

The mean age at diagnosis of SC is 64–72 years, and 59–73% of affected patients are female [54–56]. In the United States and Europe, SC has been reported to account for approximately 1–3% of all eyelid malignancies [1, 57]. In contrast, several studies from Asia have reported that SC accounts for up to 30% of malignant eyelid neoplasms [58] suggesting an increased relative frequency of SC in the Asian population compared to individuals of Western European descent. However, the reasons for these apparent racial differences remain to be investigated, and a large retrospective study could not confirm the previous findings [59].

The hallmark of eyelid SC is its propensity to masquerade as various benign conditions or other eyelid malignancies. This unique behavior of SC often leads to a delay in diagnosis and treatment; therefore, SC is associated with an unfavorable prognosis, including mortality rates of up to 22% [54]. More recent studies, however, indicate that early detection and treatment can lead to a significantly improved outcome [55, 60].

There are no reports of an association between SC and exposure to ultraviolet light; however, there are case reports suggesting that radiation therapy promotes the development of SC. Several patients have been reported to have developed SC of the eyelid after exposure to radiation therapy for treatment of acne or for treatment of various cancers [56, 61, 62]. Furthermore, SC occurs frequently in patients with Muir–Torre syndrome, a rare autosomal-dominant disorder characterized by neoplasms of the sebaceous glands and visceral malignancies that is caused by mutation of DNA mismatch repair genes [63]. Because of this association, patients with SC should be queried about signs and symptoms of gynecologic and gastrointestinal malignancies, and referral for work-up should be considered.

Pathologic Features

The light microscopic analysis of SC is often challenging because of poor differentiation or expression of features characteristic of BCC or SCC; therefore, in a high proportion of cases of SC, the initial histopathologic diagnosis is incorrect [56]. Lipid stains such as Oil Red O can be helpful to establish a diagnosis (Fig. 25.6).

SCs can be classified histopathologically on the basis of grade of differentiation (well, moderately, or poorly differentiated) and growth pattern (e.g., lobular, comedocarcinoma, papillary, or mixed type) [54, 56, 64]. Well-differentiated SC can mimic the architecture of normal sebaceous glands and contains mainly large polygonal cells with vacuolated cytoplasm and prominent nucleoli. With loss of differentiation, the cytoplasm becomes scant and appears more basophilic, the nuclei are hyperchromatic and pleomorphic, and mitotic activity is increased [65, 66].

In addition to foci of abnormal cells in the dermis, SC can exhibit intraepithelial spread to the eyelid skin and conjunctiva in a pagetoid or bowenoid (carcinoma in situ-like) pattern [54]. Pagetoid spread (also referred to as intraepithelial

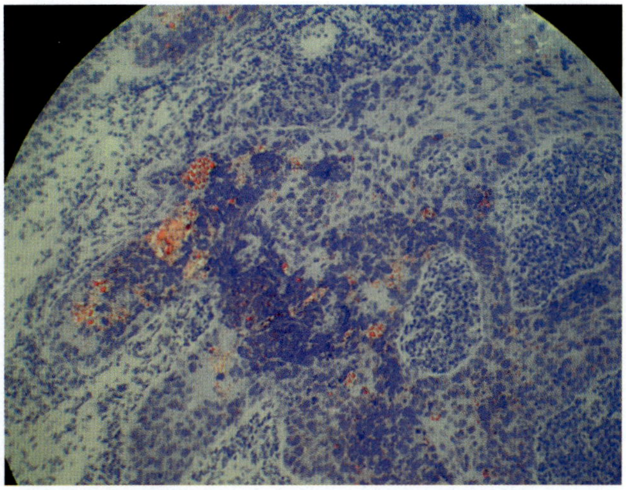

Fig. 25.6 Histologic section of sebaceous carcinoma of eyelid stained with the fat stain Oil Red O

neoplasia) is found in approximately 50% of patients with SC [56, 65], and conflicting reports exist regarding the prognostic relevance of this distinct feature [54, 65]. However, most authorities agree that the presence of pagetoid spread is associated with a higher risk of local recurrence. Features that have been linked to increased mortality are large tumor size; vascular, lymphatic, or orbital invasion; longer duration of symptoms; poor differentiation; and multicentric origin [54, 55]. In a recent review of 44 patients with SC, tumors ≥T2b according to the seventh edition of *the AJCC Cancer Staging Manual* were associated with increased risk of lymph node metastasis, and tumors ≥T3b were associated with distant metastasis and death [67]. Periocular SC most commonly metastasizes to regional lymph nodes; regional lymph node metastasis occurs in 8–20% of patients [56, 68]. Sites of distant metastasis of SC include lung, liver, bones, and brain [69].

Clinical Presentation

In contrast to periocular BCC and SCC, the most common location for periocular SC is the upper eyelid, followed by the lower eyelid and caruncle [56, 65]. The majority of cases present as either a painless yellow solitary nodule (Fig. 25.7a) or diffuse erythema and thickening of the eyelid margin (Fig. 25.7b). The latter variant has been associated with intraepithelial invasion (pagetoid spread) [70]. Patients usually complain of an eyelid mass, irritation, redness, or discharge. Less frequent presentations include ulceration and a pedunculated mass.

The aforementioned propensity of SC to mimic benign conditions has been termed a "masquerade syndrome" and is associated with a high proportion of cases being initially misdiagnosed. Common misdiagnoses include chalazion, blepharoconjunctivitis, benign tumor, BCC, SCC, trichiasis, ectropion, and entropion [54, 65]. Clinical observations that should raise high suspicion for SC are a recurrent "chalazion," chronic unilateral blepharitis, and conjunctivitis and madarosis (loss of cilia).

Management

Surgical excision is the treatment of choice for SC of the eyelid. Complete removal can be complicated because of the high propensity of SC for intraepithelial spread. Intraepithelial neoplasia can occur in normal-appearing skin or conjunctiva in the form of so-called skip lesions that are not contiguous with the primary lesion. Therefore, the reliability of techniques that aim at ensuring clear margins—such as Mohs micrographic surgery and simple frozen section control—may be limited. Several studies have shown that these two techniques yield similar rates of local control, ranging from 82% to 90% [56, 70], but some older reports found a much higher recurrence rate after Mohs micrographic surgery [71, 72]. However, large case series and standardized treatment regiments for eyelid SC are lacking. The largest published series to date included 60 patients with eyelid SC and reported a local recurrence rate of 18% following surgical excision with frozen section control of margins [56].

Intraoperative map biopsies allow assessment of the degree of conjunctival involvement and help determine whether adjuvant therapies are needed [73]. Adjuvant therapies, such as postexcisional cryotherapy and topical use of mitomycin C, have been advocated to improve outcome of patients with SC and evidence of intraepithelial neoplasia on map biopsies [74]. Even though SC has traditionally been thought to exhibit little radiosensitivity, radiation therapy has been described to be effective in single cases as an alternative to surgical treatment in patients who may be poor surgical candidates [74, 75]. Invasion of orbital structures usually necessitates an orbital exenteration. Regional lymph node metastasis is treated with neck dissection and radiation, and

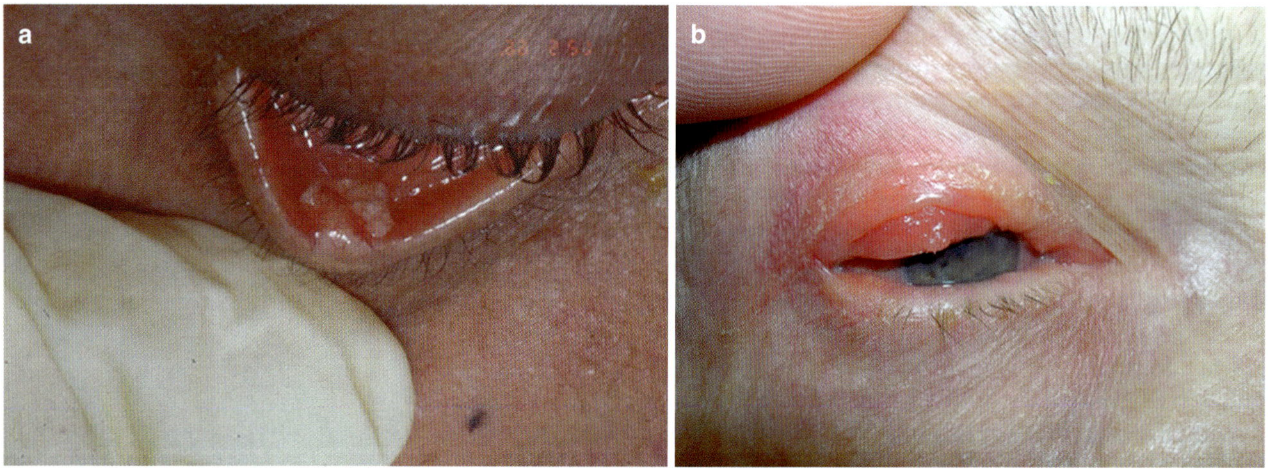

Fig. 25.7 (**a**) Example of a solitary sebaceous carcinoma of the lower eyelid. (**b**) Example of a more diffuse variety of sebaceous carcinoma with diffuse erythema and thickening of the eyelid margin

distant metastasis is treated with systemic chemotherapy. However, the prognosis for patients with SC who develop distant metastasis remains extremely poor [69].

Malignant Melanoma

Malignant transformation of melanocytes in the skin gives rise to cutaneous malignant melanoma (MM). Periocular MM is relatively rare, accounting for less than 1% of malignant eyelid neoplasms [2], and few reports exist describing the specific epidemiology and clinicopathologic features of eyelid MM. A large retrospective study showed that facial MM was relatively overrepresented compared to MM at other anatomic sites but that overall survival rates of patients with MM of the head and neck and those with MM at other anatomic regions were not significantly different [76]. According to estimates of the National Cancer Institute, MM accounted for slightly less than 7% of skin cancer cases but caused nearly 90% of skin cancer-related deaths in the USA in 2009. Five-year survival rates of patients with MM are 98.1%, 61.9%, and 15% for patients with local, regional, and distant disease, respectively [77]. These data underscore the importance of early detection of MM. Targeted therapy and immunotherapy have proven to offer better prognosis for patients with metastatic disease [78, 79].

The majority of patients with MM present in their sixth or seventh decade, and the incidence of MM is similar in males and females. Phenotypic characteristics associated with a markedly increased risk of developing MM are high density of freckles and melanocytic nevi, light complexion, and reaction to sun exposure with burn and no subsequent tanning [80]. The number of painful sunburns appears to be more significant than lifetime sun exposure [81]. Shorter distance from the equator has been linked to increased incidence of eyelid MM [82], and incidence differs significantly by race and ethnicity: Whites are at much greater risk than Blacks and Hispanics [83]. During the last few decades, the incidence of MM has increased considerably, although the rate of increase has slowed in recent years [84]. The increase in the incidence of MM is thought to be due to increased recreational exposure to sunlight. Use of tanning beds has likewise been shown to increase the risk of MM, especially in young women [85]. Furthermore, individuals with xeroderma pigmentosum are predisposed to the development of multiple MMs [86], and single cases of MM after radiation exposure and exposure to pesticides have been documented [87, 88].

Pathologic Features

MM of the eyelid can be divided into three subtypes with distinct histologic and clinical features [89]. The most common type in the periocular area is lentigo maligna melanoma, followed by superficial spreading melanoma and nodular melanoma. In lentigo maligna melanoma and superficial spreading melanoma, a phase of radial growth confined to the epidermis precedes the invasion of subepidermal structures. In contrast, nodular melanoma enters the vertical growth phase without prior intraepidermal spread. Lentigo maligna, the precursor lesion of lentigo maligna melanoma, is considered a melanoma in situ and shows proliferation of atypical melanocytes in the basal epidermal layer; periadnexal involvement is frequently evident. Foci of invasion of the substantia propria mark the progression to lentigo maligna melanoma. In the epidermal component of superficial spreading melanoma, atypical melanocytes are found in all layers, demonstrating a pattern of pagetoid spread. The depth of invasion can be documented in terms of Clark level (I–IV) using anatomic structures as landmarks or in terms of Breslow thickness, with the largest tumor thickness measured in millimeter.

The neoplastic cells in all three types of MM can be spindle-shaped, epithelioid, or nevus-like, and many tumors show a mixture of these cell types. The degree of cytoplasmic pigmentation is highly variable. Further features of atypical melanocytes are large pleomorphic and hyperchromatic nuclei, prominent nucleoli, and high mitotic activity.

Factors that have been found to be associated with a worse prognosis are deeper invasion, presence of vascular invasion, microscopic satellitosis, ulceration, and higher mitotic rate. The relevance of histologic type, patient age, and sex is controversial [90–92].

A retrospective study showed that in 30 patients with MM of the eyelid and conjunctiva with thickness >1 mm, Clark level IV, or presence of ulceration, 33% developed regional and distant metastases [68]. Mapping of sentinel lymph nodes reveals that intraparotid, preauricular, submandibular, and cervical nodes drain the eyelid skin [93]. Sites of distant metastasis from periocular MM include lung, brain, and liver. For a further discussion of sentinel lymph node biopsy for melanomas and other eyelid or conjunctival tumors, please see Chap. 10.

Clinical Presentation

Patients with MM most commonly present with a morphologic change in a preexisting pigmented lesion. Increase in size and color changes appear in early lesions, whereas elevation, tenderness, itching, bleeding, and ulceration are indicators of more advanced tumors [94, 95]. However, MM can also arise de novo. Application of the ABCDE criteria (asymmetry, border, color, diameter, evolutionary change) has proven to be a useful tool for differentiating benign from malignant pigmented lesions [96].

Eyelid MM is most frequently located on the lower eyelid, followed by the upper lid, lateral canthus, and medial canthus [90, 97]. Lentigo maligna melanoma presents as a

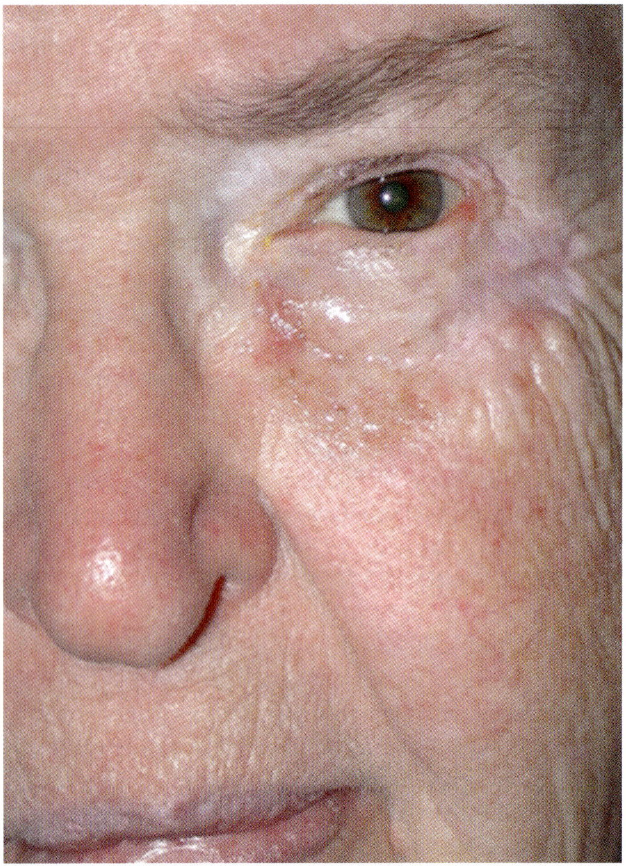

Fig. 25.8 Clinical photograph of lentigo maligna of the lower eyelid

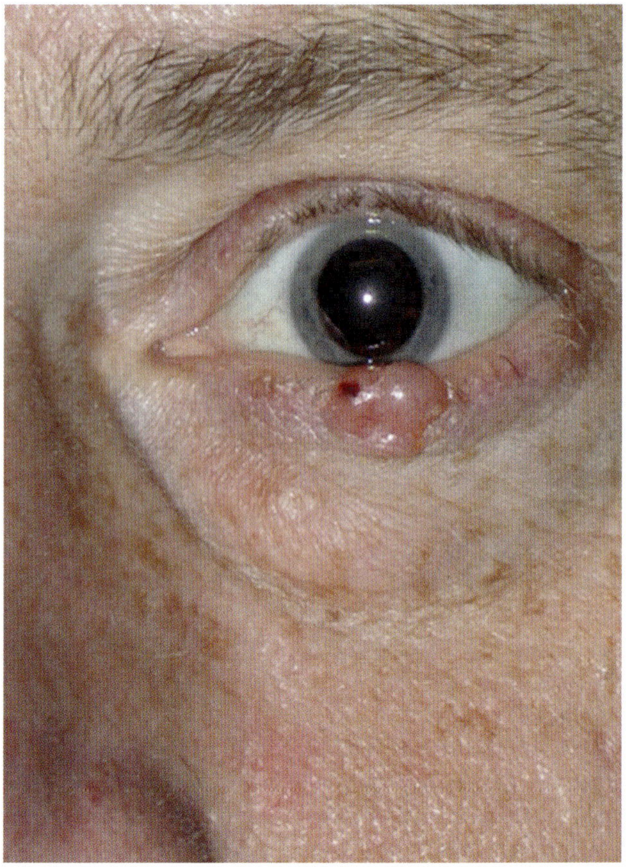

Fig. 25.9 Clinical photograph of a nodular melanoma of the lower eyelid. This lesion is relatively amelanotic

slowly growing pale-brown to black macular lesion with an ill-defined geographic outline and patchy pigmentation (Fig. 25.8); areas of spontaneous regression appear bluish gray. The occurrence of palpable areas marks the transformation to invasive growth. Superficial spreading melanoma tends to be slightly more circumscribed, showing scattered palpable areas and irregular coloration. Nodular melanoma appears as a nodular blue-black, reddish, or brown lesion without pigmentation of the surrounding epidermis (Fig. 25.9). Amelanotic MMs are exceedingly rare and pose a particular diagnostic challenge. They have been shown to be associated with advanced stage at diagnosis and unfavorable outcome compared to that of pigmented lesions [96, 97]. Other unusual presentations of periocular MM include cases of MM arising from a blue nevus and in association with oculodermal melanosis (nevus of Ota) [98–101].

Management

Wide local excision is the treatment of choice for MM. The general guidelines for primary cutaneous melanoma advise 1 cm clinical excision margins for lesions <2 mm thick and 2 cm clinical excision margins for lesions >2 mm thick [102]. However, these guidelines are difficult to follow in the periocular area without causing extensive functional impairment and cosmetic disfigurement. A retrospective study analyzing 44 cases of eyelid MM found that Breslow thickness was the only statistically significant predictor of local recurrence and regional and distant metastases. Rates of recurrence and metastasis differ significantly between patients with margins of excision <5 mm and those with margins >5 mm. These findings suggest that 5 mm margins may be adequate for thin MM of the eyelid skin; however, larger case numbers will be necessary for a definitive recommendation [103]. The postsurgical defect after histologic clearance of margins is often considerably greater than the clinically apparent lesion, showing that periocular MM has a propensity for subclinical spread [94, 104]. A retrospective study found a local recurrence rate of 77.8% in patients with positive histologic margins, underscoring that histologic confirmation of complete excision is essential for successful treatment [97]. However, standard frozen section control was shown to be unreliable for MM [105]. Instead, evaluation of paraffin-embedded sections with delayed repair after confirmation of negative margins is advocated. For modified Mohs micrographic surgery with rush permanent paraffin-embedded sections, local control rates of 82.8–85.7%

have been reported [104, 106]. Furthermore, the use of immunostains has been practiced for improved accuracy in frozen section interpretation [107].

In selected cases of MM with extensive or recurrent local disease, radiation therapy has been suggested as a reasonable alternative to surgical excision [108]. Numerous chemotherapy regimens are employed in the management of metastatic disease. The prognosis for patients with metastatic MM was traditionally poor; however, the advent of targeted therapy and immunotherapy has shown great advances in survival.

Rare Eyelid Neoplasms

Sweat Gland Tumors

Malignant neoplasms arising from the sweat glands of the eyelid can be divided into apocrine and eccrine carcinomas. Apocrine carcinomas originate from the glands of Moll at the base of cilia and usually present as a painless nodule near the eyelid margin. In cases with conjunctival involvement, patients may complain of discomfort and excessive lacrimation [109]. Eccrine carcinomas include mucinous, signet ring cell, and sclerosing sweat duct carcinomas. The clinical presentation varies in terms of location, contour (plaque, nodule, pedunculated, or fungating mass), color (translucent, bluish, or red), texture (firm or cystic), and surface characteristics (smooth, crusty, telangiectasias, ulcerated, or bleeding) [110–112].

Sweat gland carcinomas have a high rate of local recurrence [113]. They can exhibit extensive local infiltration and metastasize to lymph nodes and distant sites [109, 114]. Sweat gland carcinomas are diagnosed on the basis of histopathologic analysis and immunohistochemical markers. Treatment consists primarily of wide local excision with histologic margin control [115]. Radiation therapy has been advocated as an adjuvant treatment or as an alternative modality when surgical therapy is contraindicated [110, 113, 116].

Merkel Cell Carcinoma

Merkel cells are receptors located in the basal layer of the epidermis that mediate fine touch sensation. They give rise to Merkel cell carcinoma, also referred to as cutaneous neuroendocrine carcinoma. Merkel cell carcinoma is very rare: the incidence is <0.5 cases per 100,000 person-years, and only 0.8% of cases are located on the eyelid [117, 118]. Ultraviolet light and immunosuppressive therapy after organ transplantation have been found to increase the risk of development of Merkel cell carcinoma [118, 119].

Merkel cell carcinoma presents clinically as a painless reddish-blue nonulcerated nodule that grows rapidly; Merkel cell carcinoma is frequently misdiagnosed as chalazion [120]. In a large case series that included patients with Merkel cell carcinoma of all anatomic regions, lymph node metastasis was present in 23% and distant metastasis in 6% of cases. The overall 5-year survival rate was 67.5%. Several histopathologic parameters were found to be associated with worse prognosis, including greater tumor thickness, greater tumor size, infiltrative growth pattern, lymphovascular invasion, and presence of tumor-infiltrating lymphocytes [121]. Postoperative radiation therapy has been found to improve locoregional control as well as overall survival compared to complete surgical excision alone [122–124]. Given the high rate of recurrence in regional lymph nodes, elective adjuvant irradiation of regional lymph node basins has been suggested [125, 126]. More recently, consideration has been given to sentinel lymph node biopsy for Merkel cell carcinoma of the eyelid to better evaluate which nodal basins may harbor microscopic metastasis and need further treatment [127].

Vascular Tumors

Cutaneous angiosarcoma is a malignant neoplasm originating from lymphatic or vascular endothelial cells. It carries a poor prognosis: the 5-year survival rate is 13–50% [128, 129]. Risk factors for the development of angiosarcoma are prior radiation therapy and chronic lymphedema [130, 131]. The clinical diagnosis of angiosarcoma is frequently delayed because of this neoplasm's variable and often benign appearance. The most commonly reported clinical picture is a reddish or purple maculopapular lesion, but cases presenting as recurrent edema, cellulitis, and yellowish plaques resembling xanthelasma have been described as well [132, 133]. Management of angiosarcoma is complicated by its predilection for diffuse and multifocal growth [134]. A combination of surgical excision and radiation therapy and, more recently, neoadjuvant chemotherapy has been found to be the most effective approach [129, 135].

Kaposi sarcoma is an endothelial cell malignancy associated with HHV-6 infection. The incidence of Kaposi sarcoma is highly increased in HIV-positive patients, and Kaposi sarcoma is considered an AIDS-defining illness. The classic form, which typically occurs in HIV-negative patients, follows a less aggressive course [136]. Lesions present as erythematous, bluish, brown, or black plaques or nodules with a smooth, scaly, or ulcerated surface. Single lesions are treated with complete excision or intralesional chemotherapy, whereas multiple lesions in HIV-positive patients are usually treated with palliative radiation therapy [137, 138].

Lymphoma

Primary eyelid lymphomas are rare; lymphoma is more commonly found in the orbit. B-cell lymphoma usually appears as a painless subcutaneous mass but can also present with inflammation, recurrent swelling, and discoloration [139]. In cutaneous T-cell lymphoma (mycosis fungoides), involvement of skin and cutaneous appendages in the form of ulceration, induration, and madarosis has been reported and can cause an eczematoid rash and sometimes secondary cicatricial ectropion (Fig. 25.10) [140, 141]. Localized lesions can be controlled with radiation therapy, whereas disseminated disease is treated with chemotherapy.

Metastatic Lesions

Isolated metastasis to the eyelid occurs less frequently than isolated metastasis to the orbit or the uvea. Isolated eyelid metastasis usually presents as a painless nodule or diffuse swelling, sometimes accompanied by erythema, and can be misdiagnosed as blepharitis or chalazion [142–144]. Primary malignancies that have been reported to metastasize to the eyelid include melanoma, breast cancer, renal cell carcinoma, prostate and lung cancers, leiomyosarcoma, salivary gland carcinoma, and hepatocellular carcinoma [144–146]. Prognosis and treatment depend on the nature and stage of the primary malignancy.

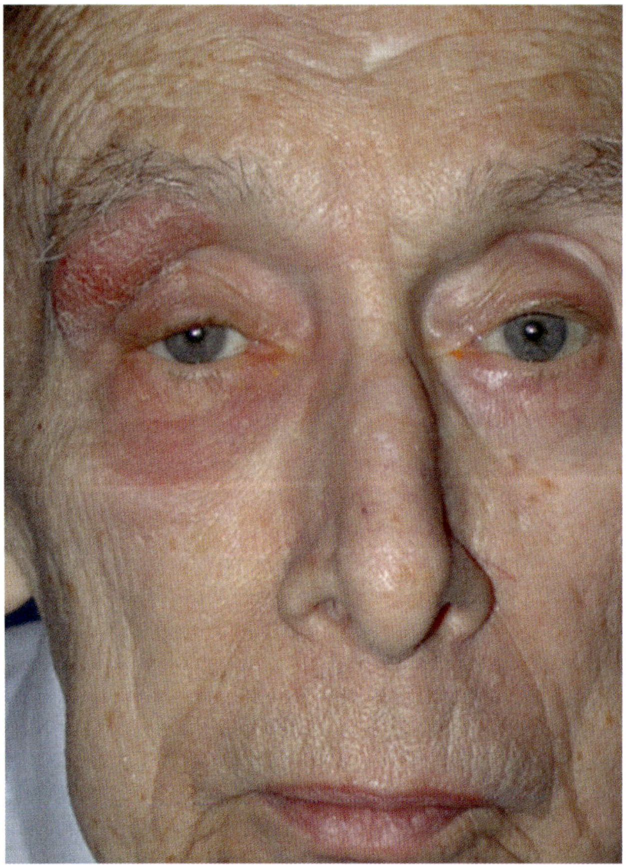

Fig. 25.10 Clinical photograph of mycosis fungoides with involvement of the periocular skin

Conjunctival Neoplasms

Melanocytic Tumors

Conjunctival melanoma is rare. After analyzing data from the North American Association of Central Cancer Registries collected between 1996 and 2000, McLaughlin et al. reported that conjunctival melanoma accounted for 4.8% of noncutaneous melanomas and 0.2% of melanomas overall [147]. As with cutaneous melanoma, fair complexion is a risk factor for conjunctival melanoma [148].

Pathologic Features

Conjunctival melanoma can arise from primary acquired melanosis (PAM) with atypia, from nevi, or de novo. There has been considerable debate in the literature between dermatopathologists and ophthalmic pathologists over the appropriate terminology for premalignant melanocytic lesions of the conjunctiva [149, 150]. "Primary acquired melanosis" has traditionally been used by ophthalmic pathologists, while melanoma in situ is preferred by dermatopathologists. Melanoma in situ and PAM with severe atypia may be equivalent, though this concept has been contested. In a study of 311 eyes with PAM, progression to invasive melanoma was seen in none of the eyes with PAM without atypia, none of the eyes with PAM with mild atypia, and 13% of the eyes with PAM with severe atypia [151]. Variability among ophthalmic pathologists in the grading of mild versus moderate versus severe atypia complicates the problem of determining whether PAM with severe atypia and melanoma in situ are equivalent. Nevertheless, most authorities agree that conjunctival PAM with severe atypia has the potential for spread to wide areas of the ocular surface as well as the potential for transformation to invasive melanoma; thus, it should be treated with this potential in mind.

Most conjunctival melanomas are of the acral (mucosal) subtype. Histopathologically, conjunctival melanoma is characterized by anaplastic melanocytes, though the diagnosis is not always straightforward. When diagnosis is difficult, immunohistochemical studies for HMB-45 and Ki-67 can be helpful. S-100 and MART-1 have also been used, though they may also be positive in benign melanocytic lesions [152].

Factors associated with worse prognosis include increased tumor thickness, nonlimbal location, positive excision margins [148, 153], and nodal metastasis. Ulceration is known to indicate a worse prognosis for cutaneous melanoma [153, 154] and may indicate a worse prognosis for conjunctival melanoma [93, 155].

Clinical Presentation

The presenting complaint in patients with conjunctival melanoma is most commonly a visible pigmented lesion (Fig. 25.11). The lesion is usually brown and elevated, often with a visible feeder vessel, though amelanotic lesions are possible. The majority of lesions are present on the bulbar conjunctiva with involvement of the limbus. There is a high risk of local recurrence—26–36% at 5 years according to two large recent studies [148, 153]. Mortality rates at 10 years in these two studies were 13% [148] and 38% [153].

Meticulous attention to margin status and judicious use of adjuvant treatments, such as cryotherapy, topical chemotherapy, and radiation therapy, can yield local control rates of close to 90% [155].

Management

Wide local excision is the mainstay of treatment for conjunctival melanoma. More radical surgery, such as enucleation or orbital exenteration, has not been shown to increase survival [148, 156] and is therefore reserved for cases in which there is orbital extension of the tumor. Margins of 4 mm have been suggested. In addition, treatment of the corneal epithelium with alcohol and treatment of the surgical margins with cryotherapy are thought to be beneficial [148]; however, there have not been any prospective randomized trials to evaluate these techniques. Topical mitomycin C is a useful adjuvant for cases in which there has been incomplete excision. Mitomycin C is an alkylating agent and is typically administered at a concentration of 0.02% or 0.04% [157]. Various regimens have been reported, but a typical regimen is one drop to the affected eye four times per day in four cycles of 4 days on and 10 days off. Mitomycin C can cause conjunctivitis as well as pannus formation and corneal haze [157]. Radiation therapy may be appropriate for some tumors [155, 158].

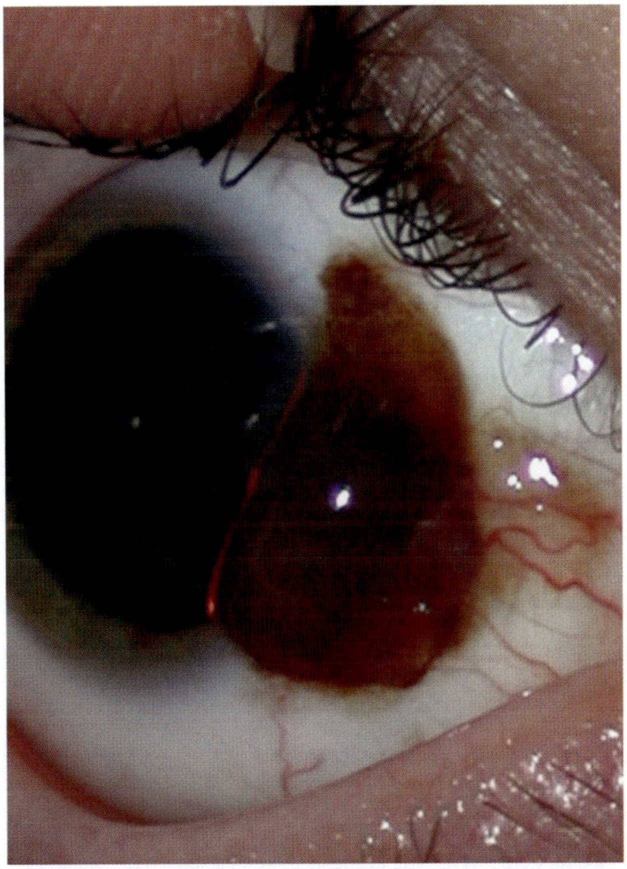

Fig. 25.11 Example of conjunctival melanoma involving the bulbar conjunctiva

Squamous Neoplasia

Squamous neoplasia includes a spectrum of lesions from conjunctival intraepithelial neoplasia to conjunctival SCC. Several factors have been shown to increase the risk of conjunctival SCC, including sun exposure, older age, and immunosuppression. Infections can also increase the risk. Human papillomavirus infection, most commonly with serotypes 5 and 8 [159], and HIV infection have been associated with conjunctival SCC [160]. In a study of conjunctival malignancy in patients with AIDS, SCC was the most common subtype and was the first presenting sign of HIV in 50% of the patients [161].

Pathologic Features

Conjunctival intraepithelial neoplasia is a precursor to SCC in which the basement membrane has not been violated by dysplastic cells. Typical conjunctival SCC is characterized by sheets of atypical epithelial cells. Several variants of conjunctival SCC have been identified, including mucoepidermoid carcinoma, spindle-cell carcinoma, lymphoepithelioma-like SCC [162], and acantholytic/adenoid SCC [163]. These are all uncommon but appear to be more aggressive than typical SCC. Recent studies have shown that tumor-associated lymphangiogenesis may indicate a higher risk of recurrence in SCC [164].

Clinical Presentation

Presenting symptoms of conjunctival SCC often include symptoms of ocular surface irritation, such as conjunctival injection and foreign body sensation. Conjunctival SCC is most commonly seen on the bulbar conjunctiva in the interpalpebral zone [165] (Fig. 25.12). The clinical appearance of conjunctival SCC is quite variable; these lesions can present as both pedunculated and sessile lesions that can be

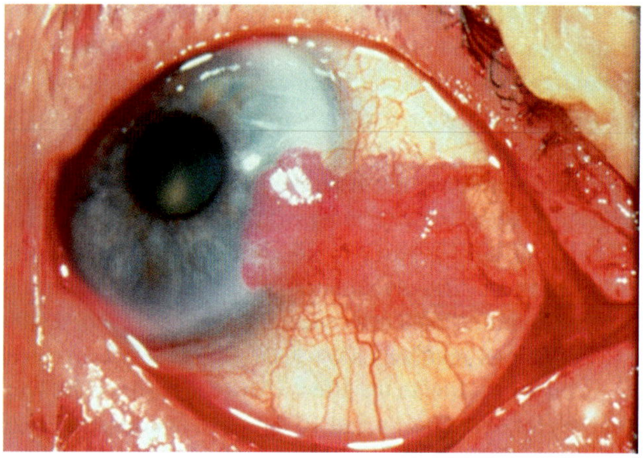

Fig. 25.12 Example of conjunctival squamous cell carcinoma

pink, white, or, rarely, pigmented. Historically, regional and distant metastases have been thought to be uncommon with conjunctival SCC. In a study including 286 patients with conjunctival SCC, only 2 (0.7%) had nodal metastasis [162]. The rates may be higher in immunocompromised individuals.

Management

Wide local excision is the primary treatment in most cases of conjunctival SCC [162]. Application of alcohol and cryotherapy are often used after excision. Fluorouracil, an antimetabolite used in the treatment of many cancers elsewhere in the body, has also been used topically to treat SCC of the conjunctiva. Fluorouracil is typically given in a 1% solution and administered four times daily [166, 167]. Intralesional interferon alpha-2b has also been used with success for the treatment of conjunctival SCC. Karp et al. reported resolution of disease in 13 of 15 eyes treated with subconjunctival injections of interferon alpha-2b [168]. Orbital exenteration and radiation therapy have also been used in locally advanced cases [163]. A study of the immunohistochemical profile of conjunctival SCC showed high levels of expression of epidermal growth factor receptor [169]. This receptor has served as a target for several targeted chemotherapeutic agents. It is possible that such targeted therapies may have a role in the treatment of conjunctival SCC in the future.

Other Conjunctival Malignancies

A number of other, less common tumors can involve the conjunctiva, including Kaposi sarcoma [161], rhabdomyosarcoma [170], and many others that have been described only in case reports. Metastasis to the conjunctiva is extremely rare. In a series of eleven such cases, four were from breast cancer; two each were from lung cancer, laryngeal cancer, and melanoma; and one was from an unknown site [171].

References

1. Deprez M, Uffer S. Clinicopathological features of eyelid skin tumors. A retrospective study of 5504 cases and review of literature. Am J Dermatopathol. 2009;31(3):256–62. https://doi.org/10.1097/DAD.1090b1013e3181961861.
2. Cook BE Jr, Bartley GB. Epidemiologic characteristics and clinical course of patients with malignant eyelid tumors in an incidence cohort in Olmsted County, Minnesota. Ophthalmology. 1999;106(4):746–50.
3. Bielsa I, Soria X, Esteve M, Ferrandiz C. Population-based incidence of basal cell carcinoma in a Spanish Mediterranean area. Br J Dermatol. 2009;161(6):1341–6.
4. Dallas RE, Anne K, Peter JH, Peter LR, Michael GW, Bruce KA. Incidence of non-melanocytic skin cancer in Geraldton, Western Australia. Int J Cancer. 1997;73(5):629–33.
5. Malhotra R, Huilgol SC, Huynh NT, Selva D. The Australian Mohs database, part I: periocular basal cell carcinoma experience over 7 years. Ophthalmology. 2004;111(4):624–30.
6. Nemet AY, Deckel Y, Martin PA, Kourt G, Chilov M, Sharma V, et al. Management of periocular basal and squamous cell carcinoma: a series of 485 cases. Am J Ophthalmol. 2006;142(2):293–7.
7. Zanetti R, Rosso S, Martinez C, Navarro C, Schraub S, Sancho-Garnier H, et al. The multicentre south European Study 'Helios'. I: skin characteristics and sunburns in basal cell and squamous cell carcinomas of the skin. Br J Cancer. 1996;73(11):1440–6.
8. Honavar SG, Shields JA, Shields CL, Eagle RC Jr, Demirci H, Mahmood EZ. Basal cell carcinoma of the eyelid associated with Gorlin-Goltz syndrome. Ophthalmology. 2001;108(6):1115–23.
9. Malhotra AK, Somesh G, Binod KK, Kaushal KV. Multiple basal cell carcinomas in xeroderma pigmentosum treated with imiquimod 5% cream. Pediatr Dermatol. 2008;25(4):488–91.
10. Batra RS, Larisa CK. A risk scale for predicting extensive subclinical spread of nonmelanoma skin cancer. Dermatol Surg. 2002;28(2):107–12.
11. Auw-Haedrich C, Frick S, Boehringer D, Mittelviefhaus H. Histologic safety margin in basal cell carcinoma of the eyelid: correlation with recurrence rate. Ophthalmology. 2009;116(4):802–6.
12. Smeets NWJ, Kuijpers DIM, Nelemans P, Ostertag JU, Verhaegh MEJM, Krekels GAM, et al. Mohs' micrographic surgery for treatment of basal cell carcinoma of the face–results of a retrospective study and review of the literature. Br J Dermatol. 2004;151(1):141–7.
13. Leibovitch I, Huilgol SC, Selva D, Richards S, Paver R. Basal cell carcinoma treated with Mohs surgery in Australia III. Perineural invasion. J Am Acad Dermatol. 2005;53(3):458–63.
14. Wong VA, Marshall JA, Whitehead KJ, Williamson RM, Sullivan TJ. Management of periocular basal cell carcinoma with modified En face frozen section controlled excision. Ophthal Plast Reconstr Surg. 2002;18(6):430–5.
15. Ramzi SC. Metastasizing basal cell carcinomas. Cancer. 1961;14(5):1036–40.
16. von Domarus H, Stevens PJ. Metastatic basal cell carcinoma. Report of five cases and review of 170 cases in the literature. J Am Acad Dermatol. 1984;10(6):1043–60.
17. Robert CGM II, Michael JE, Thomas GC, Catherine LS, Kelly MM. Basosquamous carcinoma. Cancer. 2000;88(6):1365–9.
18. Evan RF, Elson BH. Metastatic basal cell carcinoma: a clinicopathologic study of seventeen cases. Cancer. 1980;46(4):748–57.
19. McCord MW, Mendenhall WM, Parsons JT, Amdur RJ, Stringer SP, Cassisi NJ, et al. Skin cancer of the head and neck with clinical perineural invasion. Int J Radiat Oncol Biol Phys. 2000;47(1):89–93.

20. Leibovitch I, McNab A, Sullivan T, Davis G, Selva D. Orbital invasion by periocular basal cell carcinoma. Ophthalmology. 2005;112(4):717–23.
21. Conway RM, Themel S, Holbach LM. Surgery for primary basal cell carcinoma including the eyelid margins with intraoperative frozen section control: comparative interventional study with a minimum clinical follow up of 5 years. Br J Ophthalmol. 2004;88(2):236–8.
22. Erika LS, Robert JA, William MM, Christopher GM, Jessica MK, Franklin F. Radiotherapy for basal cell carcinoma of the medial canthus region. Laryngoscope. 2009;119(12):2366–8.
23. Rhodes LE, de Rie MA, Leifsdottir R, Yu RC, Bachmann I, Goulden V, et al. Five-year follow-up of a randomized, prospective trial of topical methyl aminolevulinate photodynamic therapy vs surgery for nodular basal cell carcinoma. Arch Dermatol. 2007;143(9):1131–6.
24. Ll J, Kai K, Hannu U, Matti K. Imiquimod in the treatment of eyelid basal cell carcinoma. Acta Ophthalmol Scand. 2007;85(5):566–8.
25. Demirci H, Worden F, Nelson CC, Elner VM, Kahana A. Efficacy of Vismodegib (Erivedge) for basal cell carcinoma involving the orbit and periocular area. Ophthal Plast Reconstr Surg. 2015;31(6):463–6.
26. Gills HS, Moscato EE, Chang AL, Soon S, Silkiss RZ. Vismodegib for periocular and orbital basal cell carcinoma. JAMA Ophthalmol. 2013;131(12):1591–4.
27. Kahana A, Worden FP, Elner VM. Vismodegib as eye-sparing adjuvant treatment for orbital basal cell carcinoma. JAMA Ophthalmol. 2013;131(10):1364–6.
28. Yin VT, Pfeiffer ML, Esmaeli B. Targeted therapy for orbital and periocular basal cell carcinoma and squamous cell carcinoma. Ophthal Plast Reconstr Surg. 2013;29(2):87–92.
29. Tang JY, Mackay-Wiggan JM, Aszterbaum M, et al. Inhibiting the hedgehog pathway in patients with basal-cell nevus syndrome. N Engl J Med. 2012;366(23):2180–8.
30. Gallagher RP, Hill GB, Bajdik CD, Coldman AJ, Fincham S, McLean DI, et al. Sunlight exposure, pigmentation factors, and risk of nonmelanocytic skin cancer. II. Squamous cell carcinoma. Arch Dermatol. 1995;131(2):164–9.
31. Maurice EA, Ogbu N, Godwin E, Ekpo EB. Skin cancers amongst four Nigerian albinos. Int J Dermatol. 2009;48(6):636–8.
32. Herman S, Rogers HD, Ratner D. Immunosuppression and squamous cell carcinoma: a focus on solid organ transplant. Skinmed. 2007;6(5):234–8.
33. Perry JD, Polito SC, Chundury RV, et al. Periocular skin cancer in solid organ transplant recipients. Ophthalmology. 2016;123(1):203–8.
34. Röwert-Huber J, Patel MJ, Forschner T, Ulrich C, Eberle J, Kerl H, et al. Actinic keratosis is an early in situ squamous cell carcinoma: a proposal for reclassification. Br J Dermatol. 2007;156(Suppl3):8–12.
35. Cassarino DS, Derienzo DP, Barr RJ. Cutaneous squamous cell carcinoma: a comprehensive clinicopathologic classification–part two. J Cutan Pathol. 2006;33(4):261–79.
36. Lohmann CM, Solomon AR. Clinicopathologic variants of cutaneous squamous cell carcinoma. Adv Anat Pathol. 2001;8(1):27–36.
37. Faustina M, Diba R, Ahmadi MA, Esmaeli B. Patterns of regional and distant metastasis in patients with eyelid and periocular squamous cell carcinoma. Ophthalmology. 2004;111(10):1930–2.
38. Rowe DE, Carroll RJ, Day CL Jr. Prognostic factors for local recurrence, metastasis, and survival rates in squamous cell carcinoma of the skin, ear, and lip. Implications for treatment modality selection. J Am Acad Dermatol. 1992;26(6):976–90.
39. Malhotra R, Huilgol SC, Huynh NT, Selva D. The Australian Mohs database: periocular squamous cell carcinoma. Ophthalmology. 2004;111(4):617–23.
40. Donaldson MJ, Sullivan TJ, Whitehead KJ, Williamson RM. Squamous cell carcinoma of the eyelids. Br J Ophthalmol. 2002;86(10):1161–5.
41. Bowyer JD, Sullivan TJ, Whitehead KJ, Kelly LE, Allison RW. The management of perineural spread of squamous cell carcinoma to the ocular adnexae. Ophthal Plast Reconstr Surg. 2003;19(4):275–81.
42. Cook BE Jr, Bartley GB. Treatment options and future prospects for the management of eyelid malignancies: an evidence-based update. Ophthalmology. 2001;108(11):2099–100.
43. Petsuksiri J, Frank SJ, Garden AS, Ang KK, Morrison WH, Chao KSC, et al. Outcomes after radiotherapy for squamous cell carcinoma of the eyelid. Cancer. 2008;112(1):111–8.
44. Russell WH, Daniel JI, Robert JA, Christopher GM, John WW, Mikhail V, et al. Cutaneous squamous cell carcinoma metastatic to parotid-area lymph nodes. Laryngoscope. 2008;118(11):1989–96.
45. Phan R, Phan L, Ginsberg LE, Blumenschein G, Williams MD, Esmaeli B. Durable response to chemotherapy for recurrent squamous cell carcinoma of the cheek with perineural spread. Arch Ophthalmol. 2009;127(8):1074–5.
46. Shin DM, Glisson BS, Khuri FR, Ginsberg L, Papadimitrakopoulou V, Lee JJ, et al. Phase II trial of paclitaxel, ifosfamide, and cisplatin in patients with recurrent head and neck squamous cell carcinoma. J Clin Oncol. 1998;16(4):1325–30.
47. Rahman I, Maino A, Cook AE, Leatherbarrow B. Mortality following exenteration for malignant tumours of the orbit. Br J Ophthalmol. 2005;89(11):1445–8.
48. Fitzpatrick PJ, Thompson GA, Easterbrook WM, Gallie BL, Payne DG. Basal and squamous cell carcinoma of the eyelids and their treatment by radiotherapy. Int J Radiat Oncol Biol Phys. 1984;10(4):449–54.
49. Calista D, Riccioni L, Coccia L. Successful treatment of squamous cell carcinoma of the lower eyelid with intralesional cidofovir. Br J Ophthalmol. 2002;86(8):932–3.
50. Calzavara-Pinton PG, Venturini M, Sala R, Capezzera R, Parrinello G, Specchia C, et al. Methylaminolaevulinate-based photodynamic therapy of Bowen's disease and squamous cell carcinoma. Br J Dermatol. 2008;159(1):137–44.
51. Yin VT, Merritt H, Esmaeli B. Targeting EGFR and sonic hedgehog pathways for locally advanced eyelid and periocular carcinomas. World J Clin Cases. 2014;16(9):432–8.
52. Migden MR, Rischin D, Schmults CD, et al. PD-1 blockade with cemiplimab in advanced cutaneous squamous-cell carcinoma. N Engl J Med. 2018;379:341–51.
53. David BR, Elson BH. Cutaneous sebaceous neoplasms. Cancer. 1974;33(1):82–102.
54. Rao NA, Hidayat AA, McLean IW, Zimmerman LE. Sebaceous carcinomas of the ocular adnexa: a clinicopathologic study of 104 cases, with five-year follow-up data. Hum Pathol. 1982;13(2):113–22.
55. Song A, Carter KD, Syed NA, Song J, Nerad JA. Sebaceous cell carcinoma of the ocular adnexa: clinical presentations, histopathology, and outcomes. Ophthal Plast Reconstr Surg. 2008;24(3):194–200.
56. Shields JA, Demirci H, Marr BP, Eagle RC Jr, Shields CL. Sebaceous carcinoma of the eyelids: personal experience with 60 cases. Ophthalmology. 2004;111(12):2151–7.
57. Boniuk M, Zimmermann LE. Sebaceous carcinoma of the eyelid, eyebrow, caruncle and orbit. Int Ophthalmol Clin. 1972;12(1):225–57.
58. Takamura H, Yamashita H. Clinicopathological analysis of malignant eyelid tumor cases at Yamagata university hospital: statistical comparison of tumor incidence in Japan and in other countries. Jpn J Ophthalmol. 2005;49(5):349–54.
59. Tina D, Lynn DW, James BY. A retrospective review of 1349 cases of sebaceous carcinoma. Cancer. 2009;115(1):158–65.

60. Muqit MM, Roberts F, Lee WR, Kemp E. Improved survival rates in sebaceous carcinoma of the eyelid. Eye (Lond). 2004;18(1):49–53.
61. Richard PH, William JL, William HS, Edward GB, Jonathan JD, Gordon KK, et al. Sebaceous gland carcinoma: a subtle second malignancy following radiation therapy in patients with bilateral retinoblastoma. Cancer. 1998;83(4):767–71.
62. Rumelt S, Hogan NR, Rubin PA, Jakobiec FA. Four-eyelid sebaceous cell carcinoma following irradiation. Arch Ophthalmol. 1998;116(12):1670–2.
63. Rishi K, Font RL. Sebaceous gland tumors of the eyelids and conjunctiva in the Muir-Torre syndrome: a clinicopathologic study of five cases and literature review. Ophthal Plast Reconstr Surg. 2004;20(1):31–6.
64. Tan KC, Lee ST, Cheah ST. Surgical treatment of sebaceous carcinoma of eyelids with clinico-pathological correlation. Br J Plast Surg. 1991;44(2):117–21.
65. Doxanas MT, Green WR. Sebaceous gland carcinoma: review of 40 cases. Arch Ophthalmol. 1984;102(2):245–9.
66. Miki I, Kiyoshi M, Takeshi N, Jun M, Keiichi I, Cheng-Sheng C, et al. Sebaceous carcinoma of the eyelids: thirty cases from Japan. Pathol Int. 2008;58(8):483–8.
67. Esmaeli B, Nasser QJ, Cruz H, Fellman M, Warneke CL, Ivan D. American Joint Committee on Cancer T category for eyelid sebaceous carcinoma correlates with nodal metastasis and survival. Ophthalmology. 2012;119(5):1078–82.
68. Ho VH, Ross MI, Prieto VG, Khaleeq A, Kim S, Esmaeli B. Sentinel lymph node biopsy for sebaceous cell carcinoma and melanoma of the ocular adnexa. Arch Otolaryngol Head Neck Surg. 2007;133(8):820–6.
69. Husain A, Blumenschein G, Esmaeli B. Treatment and outcomes for metastatic sebaceous cell carcinoma of the eyelid. Int J Dermatol. 2008;47(3):276–9.
70. Chao AN, Shields CL, Krema H, Shields JA. Outcome of patients with periocular sebaceous gland carcinoma with and without conjunctival intraepithelial invasion. Ophthalmology. 2001;108(10):1877–83.
71. Spencer JM, Nossa R, Tse DT, Sequeira M. Sebaceous carcinoma of the eyelid treated with Mohs micrographic surgery. J Am Acad Dermatol. 2001;44(6):1004–9.
72. Folberg R, Whitaker DC, Tse DT, Nerad JA. Recurrent and residual sebaceous carcinoma after Mohs' excision of the primary lesion. Am J Ophthalmol. 1987;103(6):817–23.
73. Shields JA, Demirci H, Marr BP, Eagle RC Jr, Stefanyszyn M, Shields CL. Conjunctival epithelial involvement by eyelid sebaceous carcinoma. The 2003 J. Howard stokes lecture. Ophthal Plast Reconstr Surg. 2005;21(2):92–6.
74. Adam KR, James SM. Mitomycin-C as adjuvant therapy in the treatment of sebaceous gland carcinoma in high-risk locations. Clin Exp Ophthalmol. 2009;37(4):352–6.
75. Yen MT, Tse DT, Wu X, Wolfson AH. Radiation therapy for local control of eyelid sebaceous cell carcinoma: report of two cases and review of the literature. Ophthal Plast Reconstr Surg. 2000;16(3):211–5.
76. Hoersch B, Leiter U, Garbe C. Is head and neck melanoma a distinct entity? A clinical registry-based comparative study in 5702 patients with melanoma. Br J Dermatol. 2006;155(4):771–7.
77. Horner MJ, Ries LAG, Krapcho M, Neyman N, Aminou R, Howlader N, Altekruse SF, Feuer EJ, Huang L, Mariotto A, Miller BA, Lewis DR, Eisner MP, Stinchcomb DG, Edwards BK (eds). Seer cancer statistics review. Bethesda, 2010. http://seer.cancer.gov/csr/1975_2006/. Accessed 25 Feb 2010 based on November 2008 SEER data submission, posted to the SEER web site (2009).
78. Flaherty KT, Robert C, Hersey P, et al. Improved survival with MEK inhibition in BRAF-mutated melanoma. N Engl J Med. 2012;367(2):107–14.
79. Atkins M. Immunotherapy combinations with checkpoint inhibitors in metastatic melanoma: current approaches and future directions. Semin Oncol. 2015;42(Suppl 3):s12–9.
80. Marrett LD, King WD, Walter SD, From L. Use of host factors to identify people at high risk for cutaneous malignant melanoma. CMAJ. 1992;147(4):445–53.
81. Kennedy C, Bajdik CD, Willemze R, De Gruijl FR, Bouwes Bavinck JN. The influence of painful sunburns and lifetime sun exposure on the risk of actinic keratoses, seborrheic warts, melanocytic nevi, atypical nevi, and skin cancer. J Invest Dermatol. 2003;120(6):1087–93.
82. Yu GP, Hu DM, McCormick SA. Latitude and incidence of ocular melanoma. Photochem Photobiol. 2006;82(6):1621–6.
83. Tsai T, Vu C, Henson DE. Cutaneous, ocular and visceral melanoma in African Americans and Caucasians. Melanoma Res. 2005;15(3):213–7.
84. Newnham A, Moller H. Trends in the incidence of cutaneous malignant melanomas in the south east of England, 1960–1998. J Public Health. 2002;24(4):268–75.
85. William T, Kara S, Natalie NC, Michael P, Hobart WW. Tanning Bed exposure increases the risk of malignant melanoma. Int J Dermatol. 2007;46(12):1253–7.
86. Wang Y, Digiovanna JJ, Stern JB, Hornyak TJ, Raffeld M, Khan SG, et al. Evidence of ultraviolet type mutations in xeroderma pigmentosum melanomas. Proc Natl Acad Sci U S A. 2009;106(15):6279–84.
87. Margo CE, Duncan WC, Rich A, Garcia E, Stricker J. Periocular cutaneous melanoma arising in a radiotherapy field. Ophthal Plast Reconstr Surg. 2004;20(4):319–20.
88. Fortes C, Mastroeni S, Melchi F, Pilla MA, Alotto M, Antonelli G, et al. The association between residential pesticide use and cutaneous melanoma. Eur J Cancer. 2007;43(6):1066–75.
89. Sanchez R, Ivan D, Esmaeli B. Eyelid and periorbital cutaneous malignant melanoma. Int Ophthalmol Clin. 2009;49(4):25–43.
90. Esmaeli B, Wang B, Deavers M, Gillenwater A, Goepfert H, Diaz E, et al. Prognostic factors for survival in malignant melanoma of the eyelid skin. Ophthal Plast Reconstr Surg. 2000;16(4):250–7.
91. Golger A, Young DS, Ghazarian D, Neligan PC. Epidemiological features and prognostic factors of cutaneous head and neck melanoma: a population-based study. Arch Otolaryngol Head Neck Surg. 2007;133(5):442–7.
92. Nagore E, Oliver V, Botella-Estrada R, Moreno-Picot S, Insa A, Fortea JM. Prognostic factors in localized invasive cutaneous melanoma: high value of mitotic rate, vascular invasion and microscopic satellitosis. Melanoma Res. 2005;15(3):169–77.
93. Savar A, Ross MI, Prieto VG, Ivan D, Kim S, Esmaeli B. Sentinel lymph node biopsy for ocular adnexal melanoma: experience in 30 patients. Ophthalmology. 2009;116(11):2217–23.
94. Chan FM, O'Donnel BA, Whitehead K, Ryman W, Sullivan TJ. Treatment and outcomes of malignant melanoma of the eyelid: a review of 29 cases in Australia. Ophthalmology. 2007;114(1):187–92.
95. Michael MW, Arthur JS, Thomas BF, Martin CM, Alfred WK, Wallace HC, et al. Clinical characteristics of early cutaneous melanoma. Cancer. 1980;45(10):2684–6.
96. Kittler H, Seltenheim M, Dawid M, Pehamberger H, Wolff K, Binder M. Morphologic changes of pigmented skin lesions: a useful extension of the ABCD rule for dermatoscopy. J Am Acad Dermatol. 1999;40(4):558–62.
97. Vaziri M, Buffam FV, Martinka M, Oryschak A, Dhaliwal H, White VA. Clinicopathologic features and behavior of cutaneous eyelid melanoma. Ophthalmology. 2002;109(5):901–8.
98. Lessner A, Sexton M, Margo CE. Amelanotic malignant melanoma of the eyelid. Arch Ophthalmol. 1991;109(8):1166–7.
99. Gualandri L, Betti R, Crosti C. Clinical features of 36 cases of amelanotic melanomas and considerations about the relationship

between histologic subtypes and diagnostic delay. J Eur Acad Dermatol Venereol. 2009;23(3):283–7.
100. Gündüz K, Shields JA, Shields CL, Eagle RC Jr. Periorbital cellular blue nevus leading to orbitopalpebral and intracranial melanoma. Ophthalmology. 1998;105(11):2046–50.
101. Patel BC, Egan CA, Lucius RW, Gerwels JW, Mamalis N, Anderson RL. Cutaneous malignant melanoma and oculodermal melanocytosis (nevus of Ota): report of a case and review of the literature. J Am Acad Dermatol. 1998;38(5 Pt 2):862–5.
102. Sober AJ, Chuang TY, Duvic M, Farmer ER, Grichnik JM, Halpern AC, et al. Guidelines/outcomes committee: guidelines of care for primary cutaneous melanoma. J Am Acad Dermatol. 2001;45(4):579–86.
103. Esmaeli B, Youssef A, Naderi A, Ahmadi MA, Meyer DR, McNab A. Margins of excision for cutaneous melanoma of the eyelid skin: the collaborative eyelid skin melanoma group report. Ophthal Plast Reconstr Surg. 2003;19(2):96–101.
104. Then SY, Malhotra R, Barlow R, Kurwa H, Huilgol S, Joshi N, et al. Early cure rates with narrow-margin slow-mohs surgery for periocular malignant melanoma. Dermatol Surg. 2009;35(1):17–23.
105. Prieto VG, Argenyi ZB, Barnhill RL, Duray PH, Elenitsas R, From L, et al. Are En face frozen sections accurate for diagnosing margin status in melanocytic lesions? Am J Clin Pathol. 2003;120(2):203–8.
106. Shumaker PR, Kelley B, Swann MH, Greenway HT. Modified Mohs micrographic surgery for periocular melanoma and melanoma in situ: long-term experience at Scripps clinic. Dermatol Surg. 2009;35(8):1263–70.
107. Menaker GM, Chiang JK, Tabila B, Moy RL. Rapid Hmb-45 staining in Mohs micrographic surgery for melanoma in situ and invasive melanoma. J Am Acad Dermatol. 2001;44(5):833–6.
108. Stannard CE, Sealy GR, Hering ER, Pereira SB, Knowles R, Hill JC. Malignant melanoma of the eyelid and palpebral conjunctiva treated with iodine-125 brachytherapy. Ophthalmology. 2000;107(5):951–8.
109. Masayuki S, Kohji T, Hidehiko Y, Airo T, Yasuaki N, Kazuo N. Apocrine adenocarcinoma of the eyelid with aggressive biological behavior: report of a case. Pathol Int. 2002;52(2):169–73.
110. Hoppenreijs VPT, Reuser TTQ, Mooy CM, de Keizer RJW, Mourits MP. Syringomatous carcinoma of the eyelid and orbit: a clinical and histopathological challenge. Br J Ophthalmol. 1997;81(8):668–72.
111. John DW, Ramon LF. Mucinous sweat gland adenocarcinoma of eyelid. A clinicopathologic study of 21 cases with histochemical and electron microscopic observations. Cancer. 1979;44(5):1757–68.
112. Duffy MT, Harrison W, Sassoon J, Hornblass A. Sclerosing sweat duct carcinoma of the eyelid margin: unusual presentation of a rare tumor. Ophthalmology. 1999;106(4):751–6.
113. Durairaj VD, Hink EM, Kahook MY, Hawes MJ, Paniker PU, Esmaeli B. Mucinous eccrine adenocarcinoma of the periocular region. Ophthal Plast Reconstr Surg. 2006;22(1):30–5.
114. Wollensak G, Witschel H, Böhm N. Signet ring cell carcinoma of the eccrine sweat glands in the eyelid. Ophthalmology. 1996;103(11):1788–93.
115. Baker MS, Yin VT, Ivan D, Allen RC, Carter KD, Esmaeli B, Shriver EM. Epidemiology and prognosis of primary periocular sweat gland carcinomas. Ophthalmic Plast Reconstr Surg. 2017;33(2):101–5.
116. Auw-Haedrich C, Boehm N, Weissenberger C. Signet ring carcinoma of the eccrine sweat gland in the eyelid, treated by radiotherapy alone. Br J Ophthalmol. 2001;85(1):112–3.
117. Agelli M, Clegg LX. Epidemiology of primary Merkel cell carcinoma in the United States. J Am Acad Dermatol. 2003;49(5):832–41.
118. Miller RW, Rabkin CS. Merkel cell carcinoma and melanoma: etiological similarities and differences. Cancer Epidemiol Biomark Prev. 1999;8(2):153–8.
119. Buell JF, Trofe J, Hanaway MJ, Beebe TM, Gross TG, Alloway RR, et al. Immunosuppression and Merkel cell cancer. Transplant Proc. 2002;34(5):1780–1.
120. Rawlings NG, Brownstein S, Jordan DR. Merkel cell carcinoma masquerading as chalazion. Can J Ophthalmol. 2007;24(3):469–70.
121. Andea AA, Coit DG, Amin B, Busam KJ. Merkel cell carcinoma: histopathologic features and prognosis. Cancer. 2008;113(9):2549–58.
122. Gillenwater AM, Hessel AC, Morrison WH, Burgess MA, Silva EG, Roberts D, et al. Merkel cell carcinoma of the head and neck: effect of surgical excision and radiation on recurrence and survival. Arch Otolaryngol Head Neck Surg. 2001;127(2):149–54.
123. Jonathan RC, Michael JV, Ralph G, Christopher JOB, Patrick JG. Merkel cell carcinoma of the head and neck: is adjuvant radiotherapy necessary? Head Neck. 2007;29(3):249–57.
124. Medina-Franco H, Urist MM, Fiveash J, Heslin MJ, Bland KI, Beenken SW. Multimodality treatment of Merkel cell carcinoma: case series and literature review of 1024 cases. Ann Surg Oncol. 2001;8(3):204–8.
125. Eich HT, Eich D, Staar S, Mauch C, Stützer H, Groth W, et al. Role of postoperative radiotherapy in the management of Merkel cell carcinoma. Am J Clin Oncol. 2002;25(1):50–6.
126. Michael JV, Gary JM, Val G. Adjuvant locoregional radiotherapy as best practice in patients with Merkel cell carcinoma of the head and neck. Head Neck. 2005;27(3):208–16.
127. Esmaeli B, Naderi A, Hidaji L, Blumenschein G, Prieto VG. Merkel cell carcinoma of the eyelid with a positive sentinel node. Arch Ophthalmol. 2002;120(5):646–8.
128. Luir MT, Rufus M, Robert M, Thomas CC, Robert GP. Sarcomas of the head and neck. Prognostic factors and treatment strategies. Cancer. 1992;70(1):169–77.
129. William HM, Robert MB, Adam SG, Harry LE, Ang KK, Lester JP. Cutaneous angiosarcoma of the head and neck. A therapeutic dilemma. Cancer. 1995;76(2):319–27.
130. Billings SD, McKenney JK, Folpe AL, Hardacre MC, Weiss SW. Cutaneous angiosarcoma following breast-conserving surgery and radiation: an analysis of 27 cases. Am J Surg Pathol. 2004;28(6):781–8.
131. Mauricio G-Y. Cutaneous angiosarcoma arising on the radiation site of a congenital facial hemangioma. Int J Dermatol. 1998;37(8):638–9.
132. Lapidus CS, Sutula FC, Stadecker MJ, Vine JE, Grande DJ. Angiosarcoma of the eyelid: yellow plaques causing ptosis. J Am Acad Dermatol. 1996;34(2 Pt 1):308–10.
133. Ettl T, Kleinheinz J, Mehrotra R, Schwarz S, Reichert T, Driemel O. Infraorbital cutaneous angiosarcoma: a diagnostic and therapeutic dilemma. Head Face Med. 2008;4(1):18.
134. Rosai J, Sumner HW, Kostianovsky M, Perez-Mesa C. Angiosarcoma of the skin. A clinicopathologic and fine structural study. Hum Pathol. 1976;7(1):83–109.
135. DeMartelaere SL, Roberts D, Burgess MA, Morrison WH, Pisters PW, Sturgis EM, et al. Neoadjuvant chemotherapy-specific and overall treatment outcomes in patients with cutaneous angiosarcoma of the face with periorbital involvement. Head Neck. 2008;30(5):639–46.
136. Reiser BJ, Mok A, Kukes G, Kim JW. Non-AIDS-related Kaposi sarcoma involving the tarsal conjunctiva and eyelid margin. Arch Ophthalmol. 2007;125(6):838–40.
137. Qureshi YA, Karp CL, Dubovy SR. Intralesional interferon alpha-2b therapy for adnexal Kaposi sarcoma. Cornea. 2009;28(8):941–3. https://doi.org/10.1097/ICO.1090b1013e3181967338.

138. Kirova YM, Belembaogo E, Frikha H, Haddad E, Calitchi E, Levy E, et al. Radiotherapy in the management of epidemic Kaposi's sarcoma: a retrospective study of 643 cases. Radiother Oncol. 1998;46(1):19–22.
139. Vivek BP, Conway RM, Simon FT. Primary cutaneous B cell lymphoma presenting as recurrent eyelid swelling. Clin Exp Ophthalmol. 2008;36(7):672–4.
140. Justin AG, Rodger D. Mycosis fungoides causing severe lower eyelid ulceration. Clin Exp Ophthalmol. 2002;30(5):369–71.
141. Lker GL, SeÁil S, Erkan A, Zeliha Y, Murat DRZ. Uncommon presentation of mycosis fungoides: eyelid margin involvement. J Dermatol. 2008;35(9):581–4.
142. Fonseca NL Jr, Lucci LMD, Cha SB, Rossetti C, Rehder JRCL. Metastatic eyelid disease associated with primary breast carcinoma: case report. Arq Bras Oftalmol. 2009;72:390–3.
143. Douglas RS, Goldstein SM, Einhorn E, Ibarra MS, Gausas RE. Metastatic breast cancer to 4 eyelids: a clinicopathologic report. Cutis. 2002;70(5):291–5.
144. Yeung SN, Blicker JA, Buffam FV, Chung SW, White VA. Metastatic eyelid disease associated with hepatocellular carcinoma. Can J Ophthalmol. 2007;42(5):752–4.
145. Bianciotto C, Demirci H, Shields CL, Eagle RC Jr, Shields JA. Metastatic tumors to the eyelid: report of 20 cases and review of the literature. Arch Ophthalmol. 2009;127(8):999–1005.
146. Esmaeli B, Cleary KL, Ho L, Safar S, Prieto VG. Leiomyosarcoma of the esophagus metastatic to the eyelid: a clinicopathologic report. Ophthal Plast Reconstr Surg. 2002;18(2):159–61.
147. McLaughlin CC, Wu XC, Jemal A, Martin HJ, Roche LM, Chen VW. Incidence of noncutaneous melanomas in the US. Cancer. 2005;103(5):1000 7.
148. Shields CL, Shields JA, Gunduz K, Cater J, Mercado GV, Gross N, et al. Conjunctival melanoma: risk factors for recurrence, exenteration, metastasis, and death in 150 consecutive patients. Arch Ophthalmol. 2000;118(11):1497–507.
149. Ackerman AB, Sood R, Koenig M. Primary acquired melanosis of the conjunctiva is melanoma in situ. Mod Pathol. 1991;4(2):253–63.
150. Folberg R, Jakobiec FA, McLean IW, Zimmerman LE. Is primary acquired melanosis of the conjunctiva equivalent to melanoma in situ? Mod Pathol. 1992;5(1):2–5. discussion 6–8.
151. Shields JA, Shields CL, Mashayekhi A, Marr BP, Benavides R, Thangappan A, et al. Primary acquired melanosis of the conjunctiva: experience with 311 eyes. Trans Am Ophthalmol Soc. 2007;105:61–71. discussion 71–62.
152. Jakobiec FA, Bhat P, Colby KA. Immunohistochemical studies of conjunctival nevi and melanomas. Arch Ophthalmol. 2010;128(2):174–83.
153. Tuomaala S, Eskelin S, Tarkkanen A, Kivela T. Population-based assessment of clinical characteristics predicting outcome of conjunctival melanoma in whites. Invest Ophthalmol Vis Sci. 2002;43(11):3399–408.
154. Balch CM, Wilkerson JA, Murad TM, Soong SJ, Ingalls AL, Maddox WA. The prognostic significance of ulceration of cutaneous melanoma. Cancer. 1980;45(12):3012–7.
155. Savar A, Esmaeli B, Ho H, Liu S, Prieto VG. Conjunctival melanoma: localregional control rates, and impact of high-risk histologic features. J Cutan Patho. 2011;38(1):18–24.
156. Norregaard JC, Gerner N, Jensen OA, Prause JU. Malignant melanoma of the conjunctiva: occurrence and survival following surgery and radiotherapy in a Danish population. Graefes Arch Clin Exp Ophthalmol. 1996;234(9):569–72.
157. Kurli M, Finger PT. Topical mitomycin chemotherapy for conjunctival malignant melanoma and primary acquired melanosis with atypia: 12 years' experience. Graefes Arch Clin Exp Ophthalmol. 2005;243(11):1108–14.
158. Hsu A, Frank SJ, Ballo MT, Garden AS, Morrison WH, Rosenthal DI, et al. Post-operative adjuvant external-beam radiation therapy for cancers of the eyelid and conjunctiva. Ophthal Plast Reconstr Surg. 2008;24(6):444–9.
159. Ateenyi-Agaba C, Franceschi S, Wabwire-Mangen F, Arslan A, Othieno E, Binta-Kahwa J, et al. Human papillomavirus infection and squamous cell carcinoma of the conjunctiva. Br J Cancer. 2010;102(2):262–7.
160. Guech-Ongey M, Engels EA, Goedert JJ, Biggar RJ, Mbulaiteye SM. Elevated risk for squamous cell carcinoma of the conjunctiva among adults with AIDS in the United States. Int J Cancer. 2008;122(11):2590–3.
161. Porges Y, Groisman GM. Prevalence of HIV with conjunctival squamous cell neoplasia in an African provincial hospital. Cornea. 2003;22(1):1–4.
162. Cervantes G, Rodriguez AA Jr, Leal AG. Squamous cell carcinoma of the conjunctiva: clinicopathological features in 287 cases. Can J Ophthalmol. 2002;37(1):14–9. discussion 19–20.
163. Mauriello JA Jr, Abdelsalam A, McLean IW. Adenoid squamous carcinoma of the conjunctiva-a clinicopathological study of 14 cases. Br J Ophthalmol. 1997;81(11):1001–5.
164. Heindl LM, Hofmann-Rummelt C, Adler W, Holbach LM, Naumann GO, Kruse FE, et al. Tumor-associated lymphangiogenesis in the development of conjunctival squamous cell carcinoma. Ophthalmology. 2010;117(4):649–58.
165. Cha SB, Shields JA, Shields CL, Wang MX. Squamous cell carcinoma of the conjunctiva. Int Ophthalmol Clin. 1993;33(3):19–24.
166. Midena E, Angeli CD, Valenti M, de Belvis V, Boccato P. Treatment of conjunctival squamous cell carcinoma with topical 5-fluorouracil. Br J Ophthalmol. 2000;84(3):268–72.
167. Kim JW, Abramson DH. Topical treatment options for conjunctival neoplasms. Clin Ophthalmol. 2008;2(3):503–15.
168. Karp CL, Galor A, Chhabra S, Barnes SD, Alfonso EC. Subconjunctival/perilesional recombinant interferon alpha2b for ocular surface squamous neoplasia a 10-year review. Ophthalmology. 2010;117(12):2241–6. [epub ahead of print].
169. Shepler TR, Prieto VG, Diba R, Neuhaus RW, Shore JW, Esmaeli B. Expression of the epidermal growth factor receptor in conjunctival squamous cell carcinoma. Ophthal Plast Reconstr Surg. 2006;22(2):113–5.
170. Shields CL, Shields JA, Honavar SG, Demirci H. Primary ophthalmic rhabdomyosarcoma in 33 patients. Trans Am Ophthalmol Soc. 2001;99:133–42. discussion 142–133
171. Kiratli H, Shields CL, Shields JA, DePotter P. Metastatic tumours to the conjunctiva: report of 10 cases. Br J Ophthalmol. 1996;80(1):5–8.

26 Eyelid and Ocular Adnexal Reconstruction

Roman Shinder and Bita Esmaeli

Introduction

Reconstruction of an acquired defect following ocular adnexal cancer excision is a common challenge to ophthalmic plastic surgeons, and various surgical techniques may be employed during repair. With a depleting ozone layer and increasing ultraviolet radiation exposure, the incidence of eyelid cancers is on the rise, and we can expect a growing need for eyelid reconstruction. Several reconstructive techniques may be appropriate for a particular eyelid defect. The choice of procedure by the surgeon depends on the patient's age, the degree of eyelid laxity and quality of eyelid skin, the location and size of the defect, and the surgeon's preference. Regardless of the surgical procedure chosen, the goals of the procedure should be restoration of both the anatomy and the dynamic function of the eyelid, creation of a stable eyelid margin, acceptable vertical eyelid height, adequate eyelid closure, smooth posterior epithelial surface, canthal fixation, and maximum cosmesis and symmetry. Surgeons must have a repertoire of procedures that can be used either singly or in combination to reconstruct ocular adnexal defects.

General Principles

The goals of reconstructive procedures in the periocular region should be restoration of both the anatomy and the dynamic function of the eyelid, creation of a stable eyelid margin, acceptable vertical eyelid height, adequate eyelid closure, smooth posterior epithelial surface, and maximum cosmesis and symmetry. The reconstructive technique chosen for eyelid defects largely depends on the extent of full-thickness horizontal lid resection. The surgeon may be surprised at the final size of a lid defect following tumor excision. Frozen-section histopathologic examination or Mohs surgery may prove the tumor to be more extensive than clinically estimated. Therefore, the patient should be counseled about the potential extent of the eyelid defect based on the anatomic location and type of cancer.

For the purposes of repair, the eyelids can be thought of as consisting of anterior and posterior lamellae. The anterior lamella consists of the skin and orbicularis muscle, while the posterior lamella is made up of the tarsus and conjunctiva. It is important to reconstruct both the anterior and posterior lamellae. Reconstruction of either the anterior or posterior lamella may be accomplished with a graft but grafts should not be used to reconstruct both lamellae since one of the layers must provide the blood supply. Prior or future radiation therapy to the reconstructive site must be considered when choosing a graft or a flap for reconstruction. Grafts may not take as well in irradiated areas, and surgeons may instead choose a flap to prevent shrinkage or sloughing of tissue.

Horizontal tension should be maximized at the expense of vertical tension to avoid postoperative lid malposition. In so doing, the surgeon must evaluate for horizontal lid laxity. Eyelid tissue may have different flexibility in different individuals. In the older age group, tissues are more lax, and larger defects may be reduced to a smaller size by simple stretching. In other individuals, especially in the younger age group, the eyelid is not as lax and the defect cannot be reduced as much in size by stretching. Particularly severe examples of stiff eyelids are those that have been damaged by irradiation, burns, surgery, or fibrosing conditions such as scleroderma. In general, the defect can be reduced by 15% or more in an older patient with lax tissue than in a younger patient.

Another factor that is important to consider is the availability of tissue for reconstruction. One source of tissue for repair

R. Shinder
SUNY Downstate Medical Center, Department of Ophthalmology, Otolaryngology, Brooklyn, NY, USA

B. Esmaeli (✉)
Orbital Oncology & Ophthalmic Plastic Surgery, Department of Plastic Surgery, MD Anderson Cancer Center, Houston, TX, USA
e-mail: besmaeli@mdanderson.org

J. J. Servat et al. (eds.), *Smith and Nesi's Ophthalmic Plastic and Reconstructive Surgery*,
https://doi.org/10.1007/978-3-030-41720-8_26

is adjacent tissue, which can be advanced directly or with undermining and incision. Direct closure, advancement, and rotational flaps are examples of this. In many cases, the opposing eyelid is used for donor material to repair the damaged eyelid—this is the underlying principle of the Cutler–Beard and Hughes tarsoconjunctival flap procedures. The availability of the free graft tissue, whether full-thickness skin, autogenous cartilage, or mucous membrane, is important.

Medial and lateral canthal fixation should always be optimized, and an attempt should be made to match like tissue to like tissue in each lamella. Before any graft is sized, the anatomical defect should be narrowed as much as possible. The surgeon should avoid, whenever feasible, creating a defect that cannot be closed. When presented with alternatives, choosing the simplest technique is often wise. Finally, for complex and large defects encompassing more than the immediate periorbital soft tissues, it may be necessary to engage specialists from other disciplines, such as facial plastic surgery, to collaborate with the oculoplastic surgeon in surgical planning and reconstruction.

Eyelid Defects Not Involving the Eyelid Margin

Partial-thickness eyelid defects not involving the eyelid margin frequently result from Mohs surgery for skin cancers. Defects that do not involve the eyelid margin can be repaired by direct closure as long as the procedure does not distort the eyelid margin. Undermining of superficial tissues may sometimes be necessary to avoid undue wound tension. Tension of wound closure should be directed horizontally to avoid lower eyelid ectropion, eyelid retraction, and lagophthalmos. Avoiding vertical tension requires the placement of vertically oriented incision lines.

When undermining does not allow direct approximation, advancement or transposition procedures utilizing local skin flaps may be undertaken. The most commonly used flaps are advancement flaps, including sliding and rotation flaps, and transposition flaps, including z-plasty and rhomboid flaps [1]. The simplest skin-and-muscle flap is a sliding flap. It requires wide undermining to allow it to "slide" into the defect. The second simplest flap is the advancement flap, which requires wide undermining followed by relaxing incisions to allow the flap to "advance" into the defect (Fig. 26.1). The resultant excess tissue adjacent to the flap can be trimmed by removing Burrow's triangles of skin on either side of the flap. Semicircular and rotational flaps are types of advancement flaps that are rotated into the defect. Z-plasty and rhomboid flaps are transposition flaps, entailing transfer of the flap from a nonadjacent area into the defect by lifting the flap over normal tissue [2]. Transposition flaps are often helpful in the repair of larger defects. These different flaps are often used in combination to work around facial contours. Flaps typically provide the best tissue match and cosmetic result but necessitate planning to limit secondary deformities. Although skin graft procedures are usually less challenging to perform, the final contour, texture, and aesthetic results are generally better with flaps.

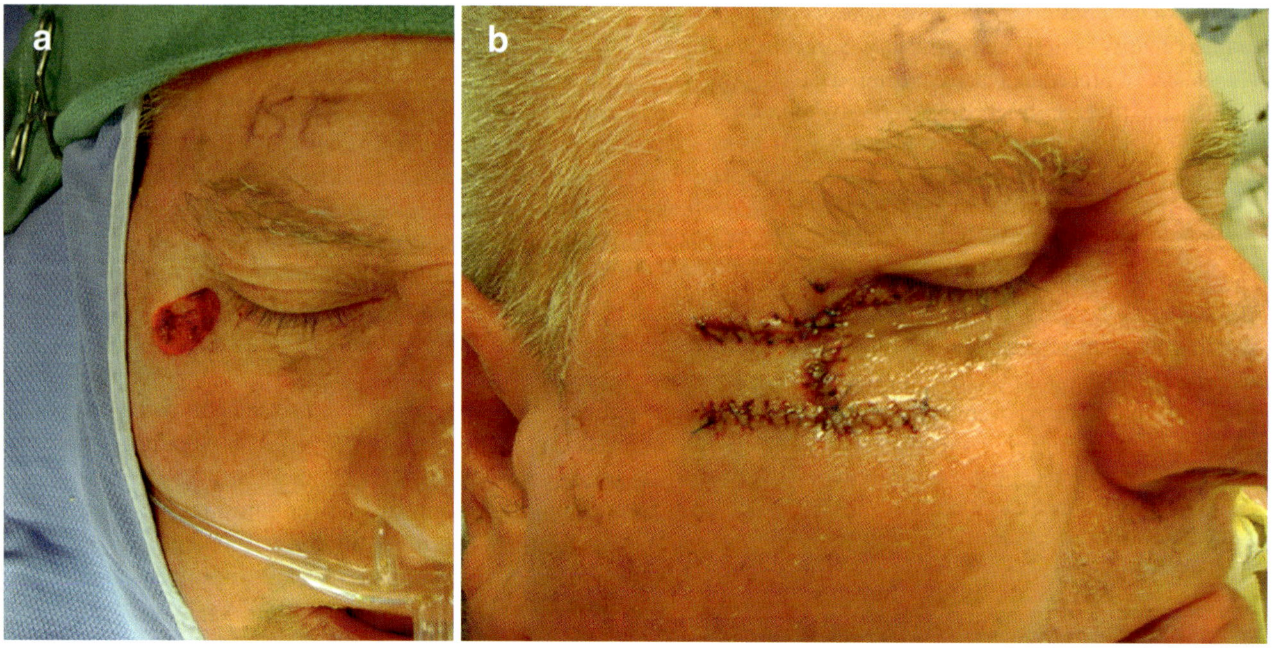

Fig. 26.1 Shallow right lateral periocular defect repaired with local medial and laterally based advancement myocutaneous flaps. (**a**) Defect. (**b**) Intraoperative appearance after flap placement

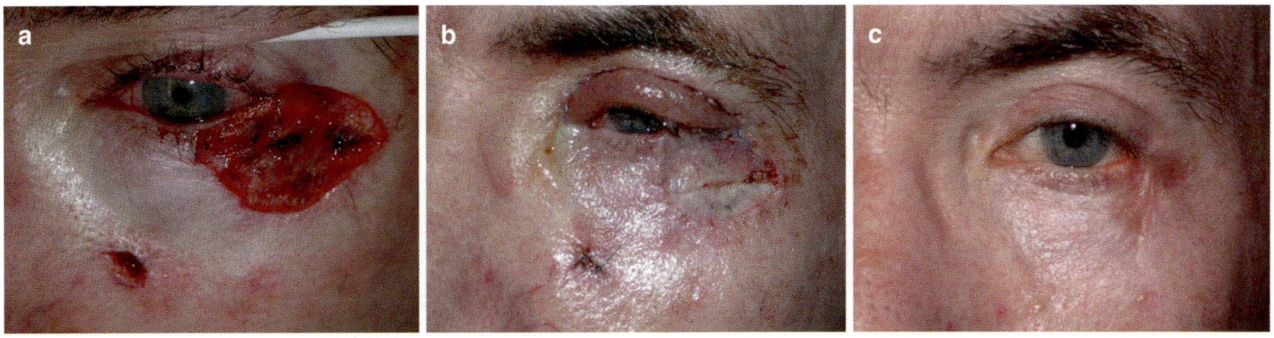

Fig. 26.2 Shallow left lower eyelid and lateral canthal defect repaired with full-thickness skin graft harvested from left upper eyelid. (**a**) Defect. (**b**) Postoperative appearance 1 week after repair showing well vascularized graft. (**c**) Postoperative appearance 3 months after repair

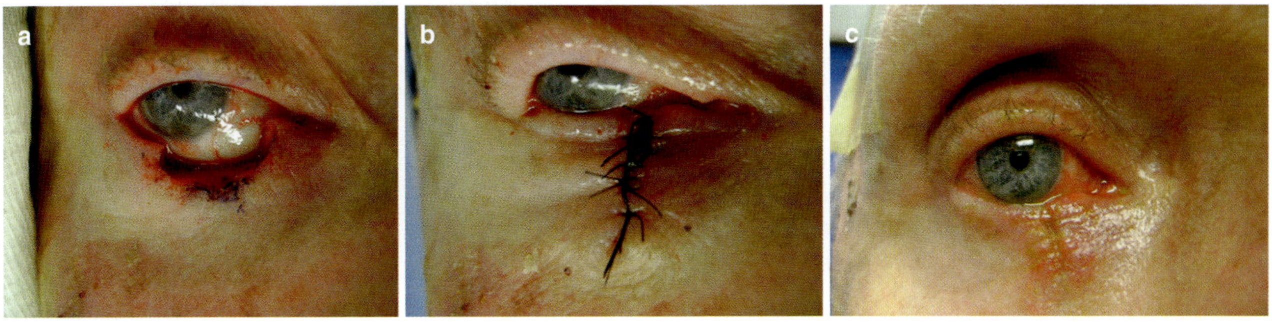

Fig. 26.3 Small right lower eyelid margin defect closed directly (pentagonal wedge). (**a**) Defect. (**b**, **c**) Postoperative appearance 1 week after repair

Upper eyelid defects involving the anterior lamella are best repaired with full-thickness skin grafts from the contralateral upper lid. Preauricular or retroauricular grafts may also be utilized, but their greater thickness may hinder upper lid mobility and cosmesis. Lower eyelid defects not involving the margin and without significant soft tissue depth can be repaired using a skin graft from the upper eyelid or preauricular or retroauricular skin (Fig. 26.2). When tissue is not available from the upper lid or periauricular locations, full-thickness grafts may be harvested from the supraclavicular fossa or the inner upper arm. It should be remembered that skin grafts will shrink, somewhat, and produce some traction on the eyelid in the direction of the graft. Surgeons must be vigilant not to place hair-bearing skin grafts near the eyelid margin as this may lead to future corneal irritation.

Split-thickness grafts should be avoided in periocular reconstructions as the cosmetic result is inferior to full-thickness grafts. They are only recommended in the surgical care of severe facial burns when adequate full-thickness skin is unavailable.

Small Defects Involving the Lower Eyelid Margin

Small defects that involve the lower eyelid margin can be repaired by direct closure assuming the surrounding tissue is sufficiently lax so that undue tension is not placed on the wound. Primary closure is typically carried out when less than 33% (25% in young patients) of the lid margin is involved (Fig. 26.3). Increased laxity of tissue in older patients may allow direct closure of defects involving up to 40% of the eyelid or more. If a larger defect is present, adjacent tissue advancement or grafting of distant tissue may be needed. During primary closure, an additional 3–5 mm of medial mobilization may be obtained from the remaining lateral lid margin by severing the inferior limb of the lateral canthal tendon via canthotomy and cantholysis (Figs. 26.4 and 26.5). If the eyelid tension is excessive during trial approximation, an inferior cantholysis should be performed. To perform a lateral canthotomy and inferior cantholysis, an incision is made horizontally at the lateral canthus down to the orbital rim. Scissors are then used to detach the lower limb of the lateral canthal tendon from the bony orbital rim. Alternatively, an internal cantholysis can be performed. The cantholysis is performed in a piecemeal manner until the desired amount of laxity is obtained. Direct closure of eyelid defects is preferred as it allows a continuity of the lash line.

When excising the tumor, parallel wound edges are created perpendicular to the lid margin and should encompass the entire vertical length of the tarsus. During closure, the lid margin should be repaired with interrupted 6–0 silk sutures, which are left long, draped anteriorly over the eyelid surface, and incorporated into subsequent skin sutures to ensure that they do not rub against the cornea. Three margin sutures should be placed—through the tarsus, the lash line, and the gray line. The suture bites should be equally distant from the wound on each side of the defect. The vertical cut edges of the tarsus should be repaired with interrupted 5–0 absorbable polyglactin suture. These sutures should be partial thickness through the tarsus so that the knots are buried on the anterior surface of the tarsus, so as not to abrade the cornea. The most important part of direct closure is proper approximation of the tarsal plate, in as exact a manner as possible, as it acts as the framework of the eyelid. Finally, the skin and orbicularis layer is closed with interrupted 6–0 silk sutures. Postoperatively, where the eyelid tissue has been stretched, the eyelid may appear tight but over the following few weeks the eyelid will undergo relaxation and provide a normal appearance and position. Sutures can be removed after 7 days of normal wound healing. In many cases, the eyelid appears tight after repair, but the patient can be reassured that over the next several weeks the tissue will relax and the eyelid will develop good motility and cosmetic appearance.

Lower medial eyelid and canalicular system defects can be repaired by reattaching the tarsal plate with a nonabsorbable suture to the residual medial canthal tendon or periosteum of the posterior lacrimal crest. The suture is placed in a vertical direction through the tarsal remnant. The conjunctival defect is repaired with fine absorbable sutures before the permanent

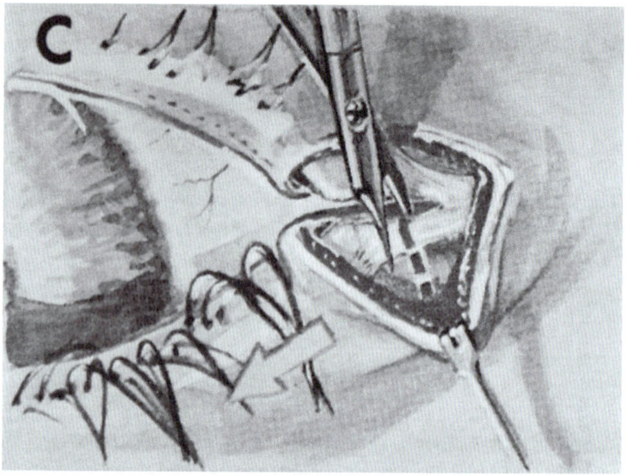

Fig. 26.4 Inferior crus of lateral canthal tendon being cut to allow eyelid to shift medially

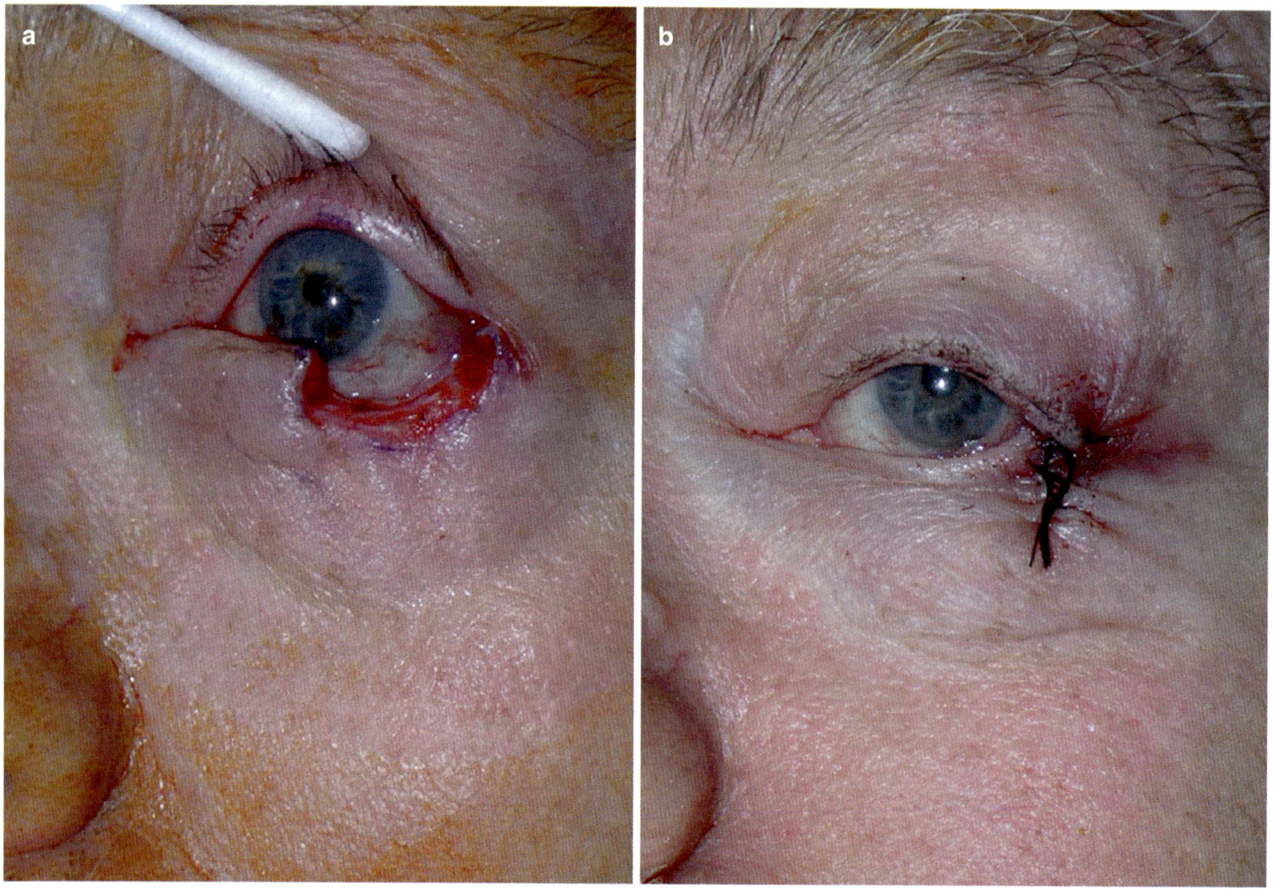

Fig. 26.5 Moderate left lower eyelid margin defect repaired with primary closure after lateral canthotomy and inferior cantholysis. (**a**) Defect. (**b**) Intraoperative appearance after repair

suture is tied. Even when the tear drainage system cannot be reestablished during primary surgery, many patients have no epiphora after resection of one or both canaliculi as long as the eyelids are in apposition to the globe; one should delay lacrimal bypass surgery (dacryocystorhinostomy) until the newly reconstructed eyelid position is final and the patient can be assessed for degree of epiphora. Timing for establishing lacrimal outflow in the patient with epiphora through a dacryocystorhinostomy (DCR) or conjunctivodacryocystorhinostomy (cDCR) is controversial. There is the potential to create a tract for spread of any residual tumor or recurrence through a bony defect into the nasal passages or sinuses. Most surgeons would recommend waiting at least a year and performing imaging prior to DCR or cDCR.

Possible complications resulting from direct closure include a notch at the eyelid margin and wound dehiscence. A notch at the eyelid margin can be prevented by ensuring precise approximation of the tarsal margin and placing additional silk sutures at the eyelid margin. During tumor excision, the full vertical height of the tarsus should be excised in parallel incisions to aid in tarsal approximation during reconstruction. Hesitation on the part of the surgeon to create a full vertical excision of the tarsal plate to its inferior border will result in notching of the eyelid margin or buckling of the eyelid with an abnormal contour. Occasionally, wound dehiscence may occur. This tends to happen when there is excess tension on the wound or when the tissues are chronically inflamed. If the wound is too tight, thought should be given to performing a cantholysis to relieve the tension. Additionally, well-placed tarsal sutures at the lid margin and tarsal base help prevent dehiscence.

Moderate Defects Involving the Lower Eyelid Margin

Moderate defects are defined as those involving 33–50% of the margin. They are repaired by advancement of the lateral portion of the eyelid using semicircular advancement or rotation flaps. The most common repair technique utilizes a modified superior Tenzel semicircular rotation flap in conjunction with an inferior cantholysis. This is simply an extension of the direct closure technique to include a local advancement flap. The arching incision line is marked beginning at the lateral canthus arching superiorly and rotating inferiorly. The diameter of the flap should be approximately 20 mm. The flap should not extend as far as the brow superiorly, nor should it extend beyond the lateral orbital rim laterally.

The skin flap incision is then made, together with a lateral canthotomy. Dissection is carried to the lateral orbital rim, where the ramus of the lateral canthal tendon is severed and detached completely from the rim so that the lateral aspect of the eyelid can be mobilized nasally. The semicircular flap is thoroughly undermined and rotated nasally. Care should be taken to avoid damage to the lacrimal gland. The lateral eyelid tissue containing some tarsal remnant is advanced to the medial edge of the defect and fixated in a similar manner to direct closure. The deep tissue of the flap must be securely fixed to the periorbita on the inner aspect of the lateral orbital rim, since ectropion and lateral canthal dystopia may result from poor fixation. The lateral incision is then closed directly with interrupted 6–0 silk sutures as in primary closure.

Additional complications resulting from the use of the semicircular flap are usually caused by poor placement of the flap at the lateral canthus. Also, the semicircular rotation flap may result in a rounded lateral canthus, making secondary revisions necessary. Another potential pitfall is encountered if the flap is used to correct the defect it cannot encompass; some difficulty may occur in reforming the lateral eyelid tissues.

Tarsoconjunctival flaps are very useful for larger lower eyelid defects. These flaps are taken from the undersurface of the upper eyelid and mobilized into the lower lid defect to reconstruct the posterior lamella. The next section provides more details.

Large Defects Involving the Lower Eyelid Margin

Lower eyelid defects—those involving greater than 50% of the lid margin—require adjacent tissue advancement for repair (Fig. 26.6a). One such approach involves the use of a modified tarsoconjunctival flap (Hughes flap) taken from the undersurface of the upper eyelid. During tumor excision, the wound margins of the lower eyelid are made perpendicular with respect to the eyelid margin, and their vertical extent should go below the level of the inferior tarsal margin. The base of the wound is fashioned so that the wound itself is rectangular. Once the lower eyelid wound is properly prepared, the upper eyelid is everted and a horizontal line parallel to the upper eyelid margin on the tarsal plate is marked with a sterile surgical pen at least 3–4 mm from the upper eyelid margin. The length of the line should approximate the size of the lower eyelid defect. Care should be taken when the tarsal flap is harvested to preserve the marginal 3–4 mm tarsal height in the upper eyelid to prevent donor-lid margin distortion. Two vertical lines are then delineated at the medial and lateral edge of the horizontal line and extend toward the superior fornix. The outlined flap is then incised going through both conjunctiva and tarsus and separating the tarsus from the levator aponeurosis. Dissection is continued superiorly in a plane between Muller's muscle and the levator aponeurosis, taking care not to violate Muller's muscle. The flap is then advanced from the upper lid into the posterior lamellar defect of the lower lid (Fig. 26.6b) [3]. The inferior tarsal

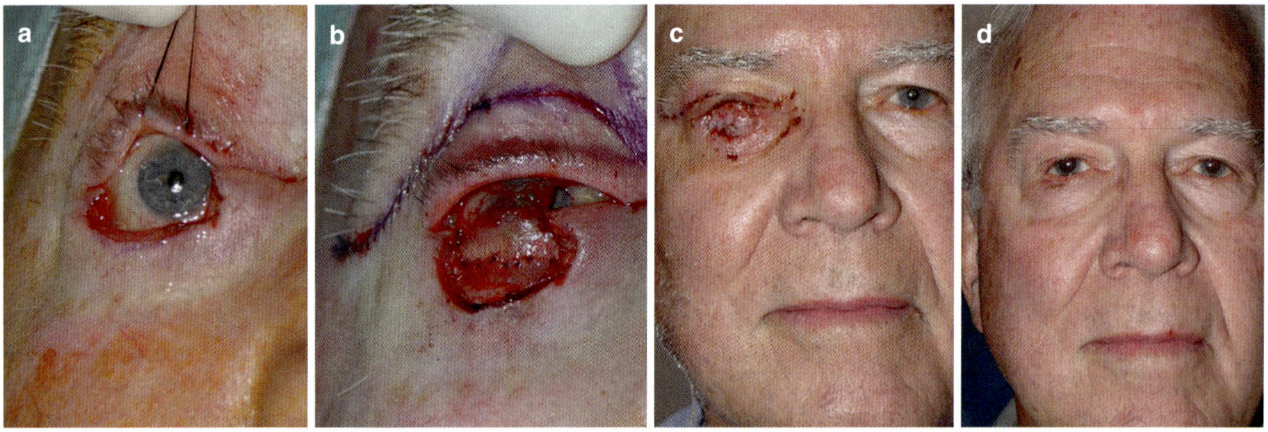

Fig. 26.6 Large right lower eyelid defect closed with a Hughes flap. (**a**) Defect. (**b**) Intraoperative appearance after tarsoconjunctival flap harvested from upper eyelid has been sutured to lower eyelid. (**c**) Postoperative appearance 1 week after repair utilizing full-thickness skin graft harvested from upper eyelid to reconstruct anterior lamella over tarsoconjunctival flap. (**d**) Postoperative appearance 3 months after second stage

border of the flap is sutured to the conjunctival edge of the lower eyelid defect with 6–0 absorbable polyglactin suture. The lateral superior edge of the tarsal flap is sutured to the lateral lower eyelid superior tarsal wound edge, if available, or the periosteum of the orbital rim if no lateral tarsus remains. The medial superior edge of the tarsal flap is sutured to the medial lower eyelid superior tarsal wound edge, if available, or the periosteum that lines the posterior lacrimal crest if no medial tarsus remains.

Once the reconstructed posterior lamella is securely in place, the tarsoconjunctival flap can be covered with various types of skin flaps, including advancing a myocutaneous flap superiorly from the remaining lower eyelid tissue into the defect if enough lax skin exists, or a full-thickness skin graft [4, 5]. A skin graft can be harvested from the upper eyelid using a blepharoplasty-type incision, usually from the same side, or it can be harvested from the retroauricular area (Fig. 26.6c). Once the skin graft is harvested, all subcutaneous tissue is dissected off and the graft is sutured into the defect with interrupted 6–0 silk sutures. The superior edge of the graft is sutured to the conjunctival flap 2 mm superior to the future lower eyelid margin. A bolster is then placed over the flap and left in place for 5 days.

The modified Hughes procedure thus results in a bridge of conjunctiva from the upper lid across the visual axis. The vascularized pedicle of conjunctiva is subsequently released in a staged, second procedure once vascularization of the lower lid flap is achieved (Fig. 26.6d). The timing of the second stage of the modified Hughes procedure (when the pedicle of the flap is severed) depends on many factors. From the standpoint of vascular supply, studies have shown that a Hughes flap with good blood supply can be separated as early as 2 weeks after the first stage. However, there is a higher likelihood of lower eyelid ectropion and retraction after early separation of the flap. When postoperative adjuvant radiation therapy is planned for cutaneous cancers of the lower eyelid, it is necessary to separate the Hughes flap within 4–6 weeks after the first stage to allow for shielding of the globe and to allow radiation therapy to begin in a timely fashion (within 4 6 weeks after ablative surgery). The technique for the second stage begins with local anesthesia infiltrated into the conjunctival flap, and a grooved director is placed under the conjunctival flap for globe protection. The conjunctiva is pulled away from the globe and incised parallel to the eyelid margin as close to the origin of the flap under the superior eyelid as possible. Once the upper eyelid is released, dissection is carried out in the upper eyelid between Muller's muscle and the levator aponeurosis superiorly into the superior fornix to prevent upper eyelid retraction. Excess skin and conjunctiva from the reconstructed lower eyelid are then excised at the level of the lower eyelid margin. The conjunctiva is then sutured to the new lower eyelid margin with a mild amount of eversion using 6–0 plain gut suture to avoid entropion and keratopathy.

Because it is an eyelid sharing technique and may result in complications, the modified Hughes procedure should be avoided in certain patient groups whenever possible. Children under age 7 should not undergo this procedure as it may precipitate occlusion amblyopia. This procedure should also be avoided in the seeing eye of a monocular patient. Several complications may result following a modified Hughes procedure. For instance, the patient may develop an eyelid malposition. If the lower eyelid margin skin rotates inward, the patient is likely to develop keratitis, either from the keratinized skin surface or from the fine lanugo hairs arising from the skin. The risk of this complication can be reduced during the second stage of the procedure, when the surgeon transects the advancement flap. Specifically, care should be taken to angle the incision to create a longer posterior lamella with more conjunctiva than skin. The conjunctiva can then be advanced over the lid margin, leaving it nonkeratinized. Another complication that may occur following the modified Hughes procedure is upper lid retraction. To reduce this risk, the Muller's muscle should be dissected away from conjunctiva and not advanced with the tarsoconjunctival flap during the first stage of the procedure. During the second stage of the procedure, the conjunctiva of the upper lid is left unsutured, and Muller's muscle and the levator aponeurosis are recessed to decrease the likelihood of postoperative upper eyelid retraction. Sloughing of the skin graft may also occur following the Hughes procedure, but this is an uncommon occurrence. If blood or fluid collect beneath the donor skin graft, poor donor–host apposition will occur, resulting in graft failure. Drainage holes in the skin graft will prevent any fluid accumulation under the graft. A bolster suture that is placed over the graft will keep it firmly apposed to the underlying vascular bed. Necrosis of the tarsoconjunctival flap is another rare complication and results from a poorly vascularized flap.

Alternative procedures include full-thickness pedicled flaps [6, 7] and a free tarsoconjunctival graft from the contralateral upper lid with an overlying vascularized bipedicled skin-and-muscle flap [8]. Another useful technique is the tarsal transposition flap, as described by Hewes et al. [9]. The advantage of these procedures is that only one surgical stage is needed and visual axis occlusion is avoided, but in our experience, the outcomes are not as predictable as those of a modified Hughes procedure for large defects of the lower eyelid.

A large rotating cheek flap (Mustardé flap) works well for repair of a large anterior lamellar defect, but for posterior lamellar replacement, it must be coupled with a tarsal substitute, such as a free tarsoconjunctival autograft, hard palate mucosa, nasal septum cartilage and mucosa, full-thickness buccal mucous membrane, Hughes flap, free periosteal graft, or homologous tarsus [9–15].

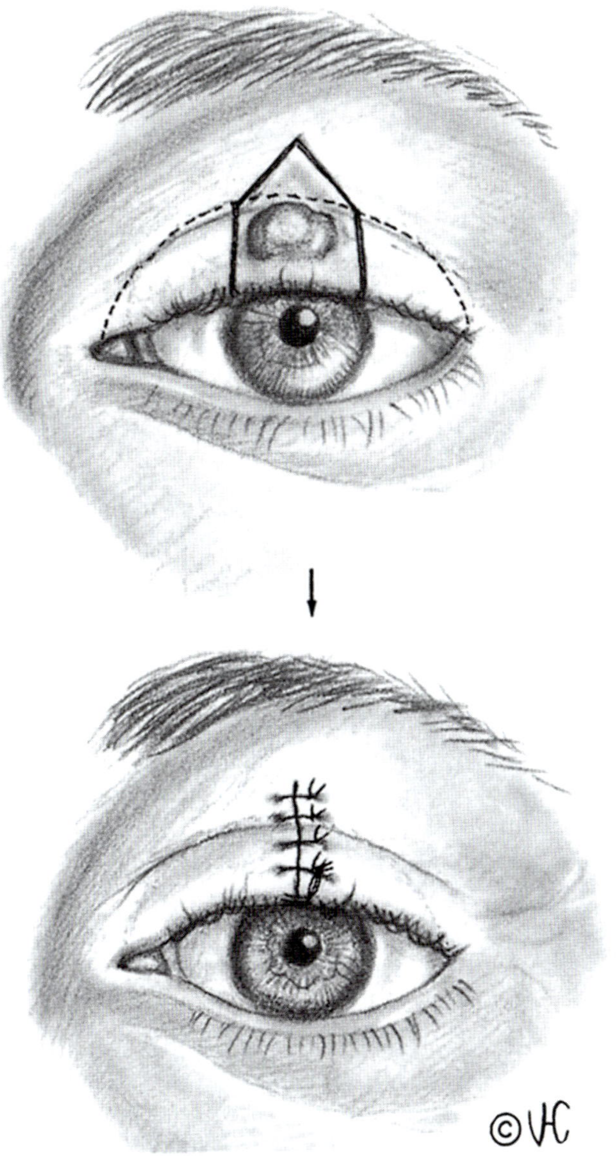

Fig. 26.7 Closure of upper lid defects. Upper lid defects should have parallel-sided edges and should encompass entire vertical width of tarsus as shown in Fig. 26.9a

Small Defects Involving the Upper Eyelid Margin

Upper eyelid defects involving less than 33% of the lid margin can be repaired by primary closure (Figs. 26.7, 26.8, and 26.9). Mirroring what is possible with the lower lid, the superior crus of the lateral canthal tendon can be lysed to obtain an additional 3–5 mm of medial mobilization of the remaining lateral lid margin. Although a relatively tight lower eyelid is preferred after reconstruction, a tight upper eyelid may result in ptosis.

Moderate Defects Involving the Upper Eyelid Margin

Moderate defects involving 33–50% of the upper eyelid margin are repaired by advancement of the lateral portion of the lid. A lateral canthotomy and superior cantholysis are performed, and a reverse Tenzel semicircular skin flap is created inferior to the lateral brow and canthus to allow additional mobilization of the lid [16–18]. The arching incision line is marked beginning at the lateral canthus arching inferiorly and rotating superiorly (Fig. 26.10).

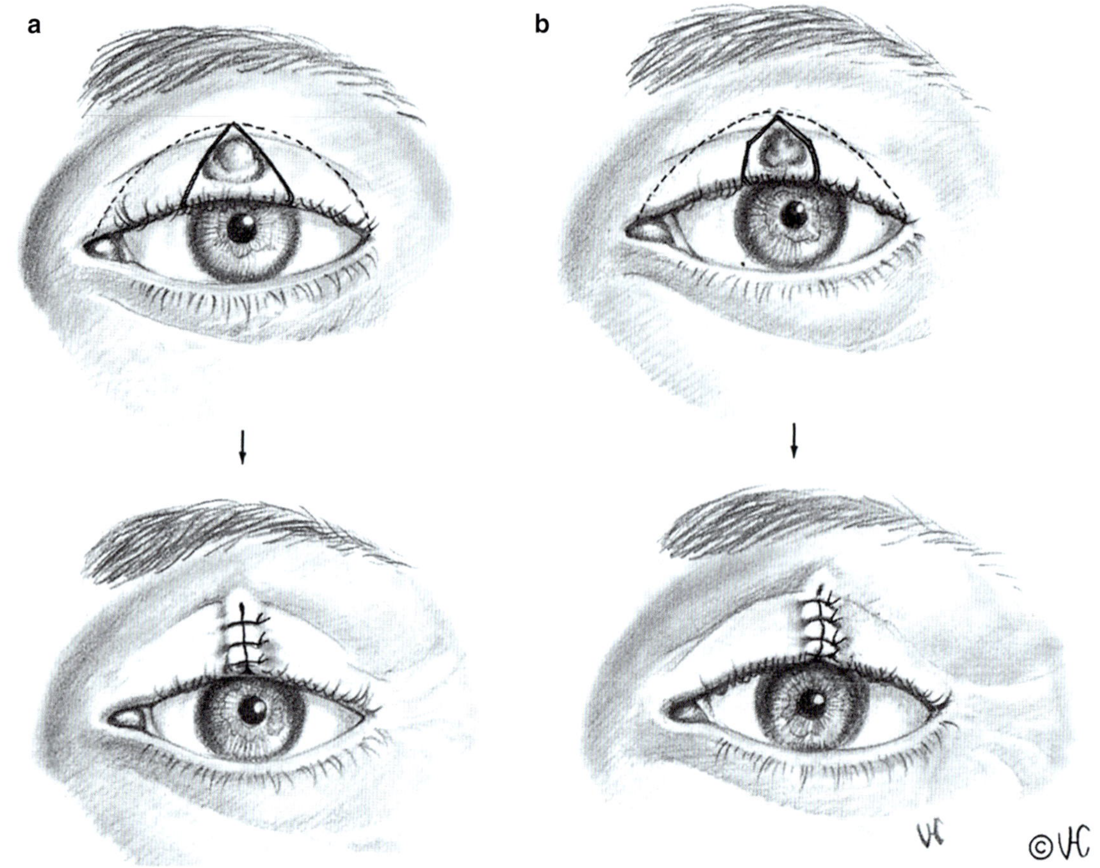

Fig. 26.8 Pitfalls in closure of upper lid defects. (**a**) Nonparallel-sided "pie-shaped" wedge, when removed, will ultimately result in lid notch. (**b**) Parallel-sided defect that does not extend through full vertical width of tarsus. Closure of this defect results in buckling of superior tarsus and notching

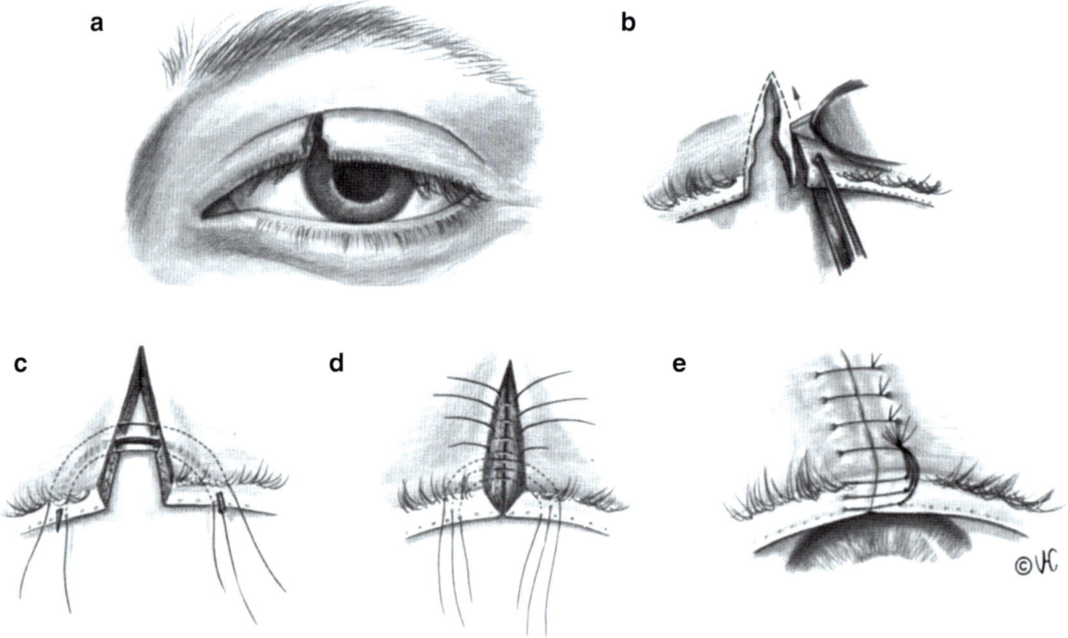

Fig. 26.9 (**a**) Eyelid margin laceration. (**b**) Edges are minimally debrided to convert them to straight surgical wound. (**c**) Eyelid margin is repaired by three-suture technique. First suture goes through meibomian glands, second at posterior lash line, and third through gray line. (**d**) Tarsus is approximated using several 5–0 absorbable sutures. (**e**) Skin is closed using 6–0 silk sutures. The three eyelid margin sutures are tied anteriorly under skin suture to keep them from rubbing cornea

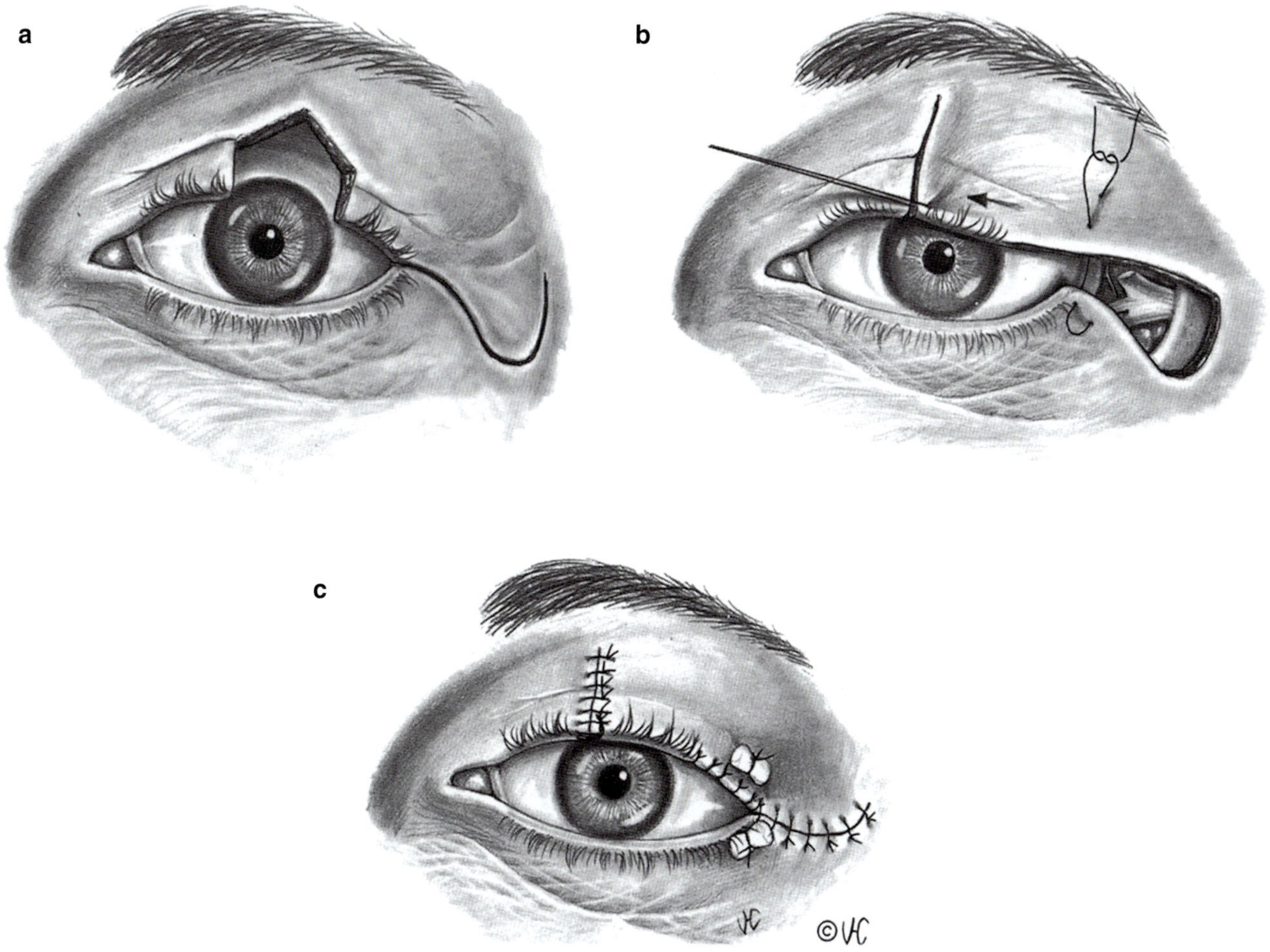

Fig. 26.10 Tenzel semicircular flap for closure of upper lid defect. (**a**) Upper lid defects, with outline of lateral semicircular advancement flap to be developed. (**b**) Advancement of skin muscle flap, which fills upper lid defect, from lateral canthal area. Flap should be fixated at lateral canthus at lateral orbital tubercle with mattress suture that encompasses lower ramus of lateral canthal tendon. (**c**) Final closure of Tenzel semicircular flap to correct upper lid. Lateral canthal area has been reformed, and conjunctiva has been stretched and sutured to new lid margin

Tarsal sharing procedures, which consist of an adjacent sliding tarsoconjunctival flap from the remaining part of the upper lid covered by either a skin–orbicularis advancement flap or a full-thickness skin graft, have also been described for repair of the upper lid [19–21]. This technique is best when used in the canthal angles and should be used when the defect is slightly larger than can be repaired with an advancement flap, but the surgeon does not want to resort to a Cutler–Beard bridge flap. It is best when used on isolated medial or lateral defects of the upper eyelid (Figs 26.11a and 26.12a).

To reconstruct the defect in the area described, the eyelid remnant is everted over a Desmarres retractor (Fig. 26.11b). The horizontal incision is then made in the tarsal plate in the residual eyelid remnant, 3–4 mm above the eyelid margin. The horizontal width should be approximately the width of the defect to be corrected. One should reduce the size of the defect somewhat by stretching the edges of the defect before developing the tarsal flap. A second relaxing incision is then made vertically through the tarsus to the superior border and up into the superior fornix. The tarsoconjunctival flap is then attached to the periosteum in the canthal area—or to remnants of the canthal tendon, if it is still present—inside the orbital rim with permanent suture on a half-circle needle (Fig. 26.11c). It is imperative that medial or lateral canthal fixation be accomplished properly to ensure that the eyelid position and contour are adequate (Fig. 26.11d, e). The superior border of the tarsal flap is then sutured to the cut edge of the defect. The edge of the tarsal flap next to the remaining upper eyelid margin is anchored to the margin with a 6–0 polyglactin suture. The suture is then placed through partial tarsal thickness so as not to extend underneath the eyelid and abrade the cornea (Fig. 26.11f). A full-thickness skin graft can then be harvested from the contralateral upper eyelid or retroauricular area and placed over the tarsoconjunctival flap and sutured into place in an appropriate manner. If there is lax tissue available, a myocutaneous advancement flap can also be advanced over the tarsoconjunctival flap (Figs. 26.11g, h and 26.12b). If a graft is used, the bolster dressing of the

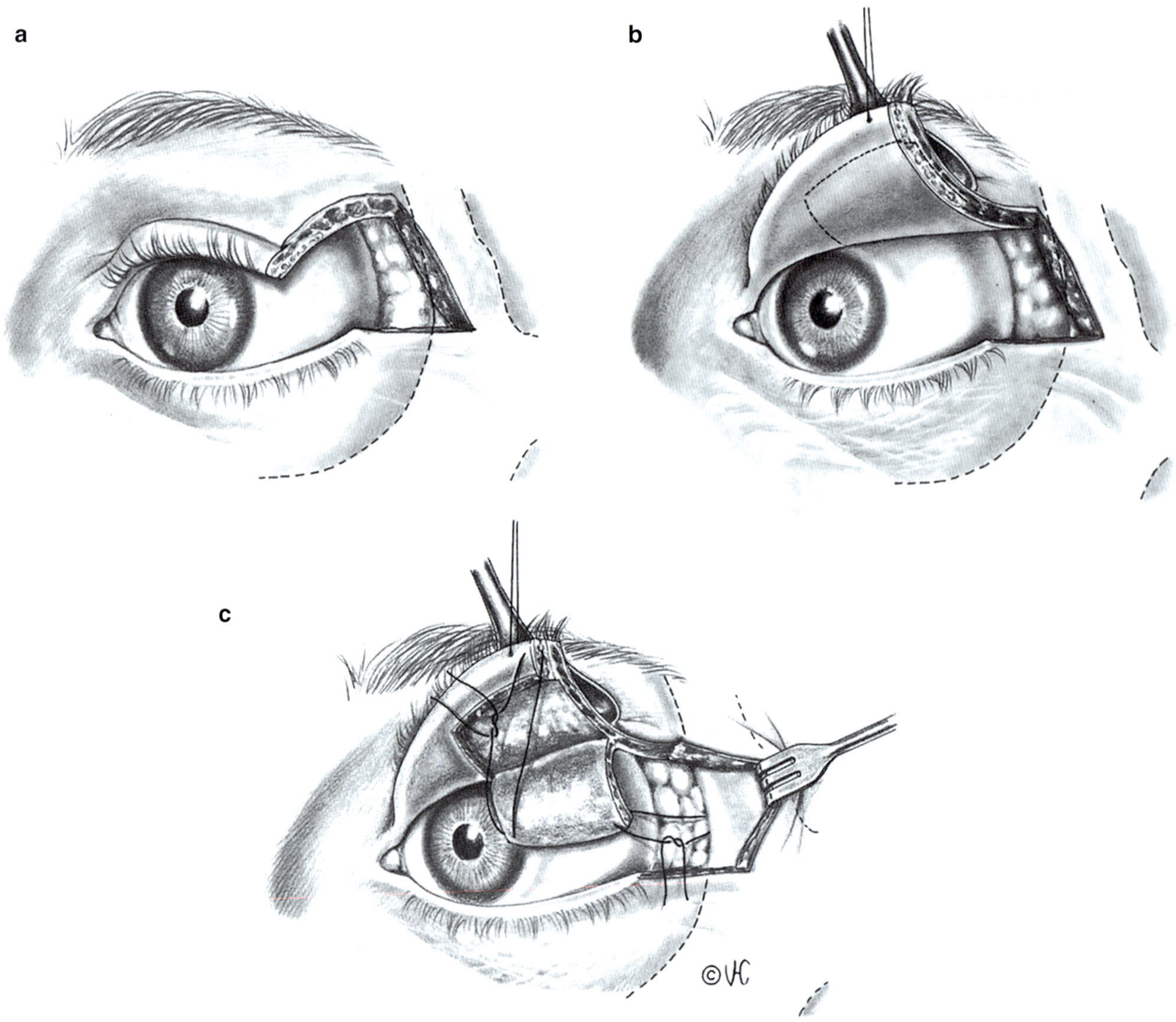

Fig. 26.11 Sliding tarsal flap—upper lid reconstruction. (**a**) Lateral upper lid full-thickness defect, including temporal portion of lid and portion of canthus. (**b**) Eversion of upper lid and outline of tarsoconjunctival flap to be developed from inner surface of residual upper lid. Margin of 4 mm should be spared to ensure stability of residual upper lid. Vertical incision in lid is made into upper fornix. (**c**) Mobilization of tarsoconjunctival flap to be slid horizontally into lateral canthal angle. Lateral canthal fixation of flap is carried out with suture inside lateral orbital rim at lateral orbital tubercle. Residual lid edge is then sutured to advanced edge of tarsoconjunctival flap. (**d**) Direction of fixation of flap with nasally placed defect. Proper direction of pull of any flap in inner canthal area is toward posterior lacrimal crest, posterior reflection of medial canthal tendon. (**e**) Fixation of advanced tarsoconjunctival flap to margin of upper lid remnant with suture placed in a position to stabilize flap and yet not abrade cornea. (**f**) Coverage of advanced tarsoconjunctival flap with full-thickness skin graft. (**g**) Coverage of advanced tarsoconjunctival flap with advance of musculocutaneous flap

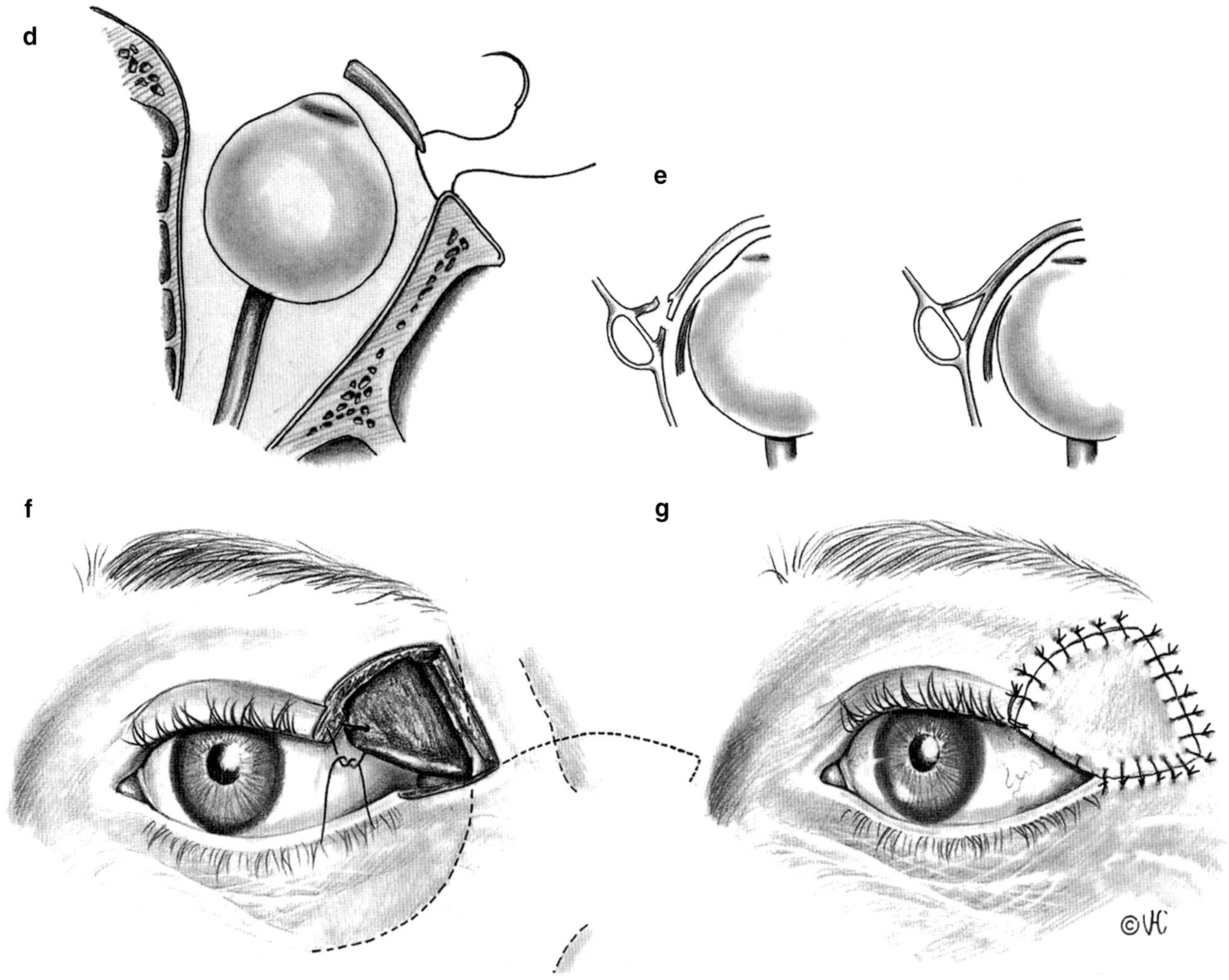

Fig. 26.11 (continued)

graft is important to ensure an adequate take of the graft without contracture. A moderate-pressure patch should be placed over the wound.

This procedure can be used successfully with medial and lateral canthal defects, but it is important that fixation of the sliding tarsal flap in the canthal area be made properly. If the flap is fixed too anteriorly, the resultant eyelid will not coat or follow the contour of the globe, and separation of the eyelid from the globe with exposure keratopathy and conjunctivitis will occur. The skin graft or flap should not override the eyelid margin because the keratinized epithelium will result in keratopathy. If an overlying skin graft is used, a 6–0 silk Frost traction suture should be placed at the juncture of the flap and eyelid margin for 5 days. Failure to do so can result in shrinkage and notching of the eyelid in area of repair.

Large Defects Involving the Upper Eyelid Margin

Upper eyelid defects involving greater than 50% of the lid margin are most commonly repaired utilizing a Cutler–Beard procedure (Fig. 26.13a). This technique involves advancing a composite full-thickness lower eyelid flap into the upper eyelid defect by passing it posterior to the remaining lower lid margin (Fig. 26.13b) [22]. Because the advanced flap lacks tarsus to maintain stability and prevent shrinkage, a relatively thick and immobile reconstructed upper eyelid results. Upper eyelid stability is enhanced by placing a spacer tarsal substitute graft, such as donor sclera, autogenous cartilage, or AlloDerm, in the upper eyelid between the myocutaneous layer and conjunctiva [20, 23–25]. We do not prefer donor sclera as it has been associated with significant lid sloughing.

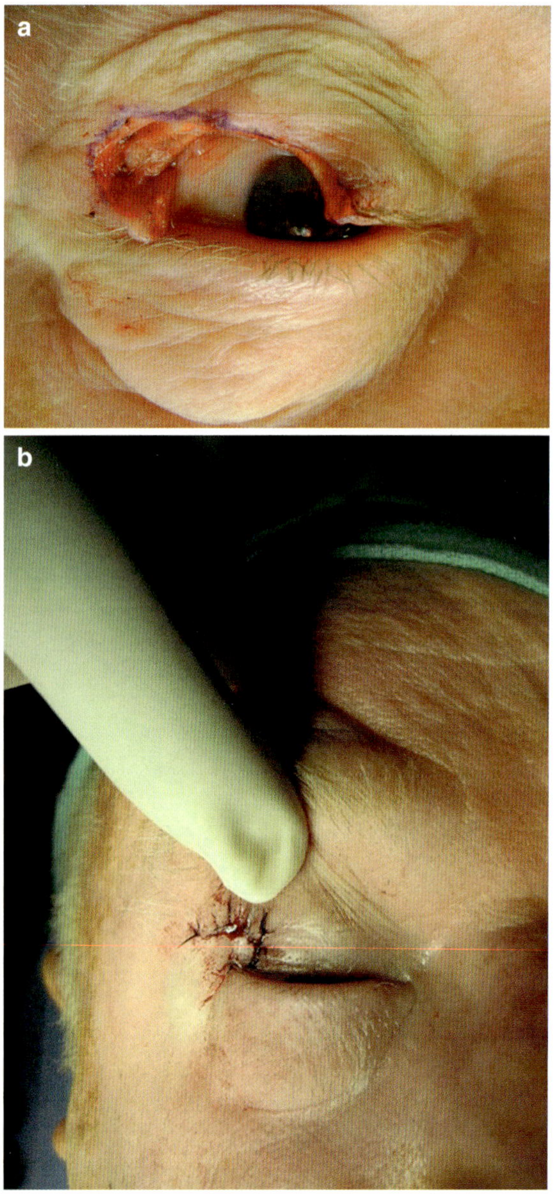

Fig. 26.12 Moderate right upper eyelid margin defect repaired with a sliding tarsoconjunctival flap harvested from the medial right upper eyelid remnant and a local advancement flap to reconstruct the anterior lamella. (**a**) Defect. (**b**) Intraoperative appearance after repair

The surgery begins with the creation of a rectangular upper eyelid defect during tumor excision (Fig. 26.14a). The flap of tissue from the lower eyelid should be approximately the same width as the upper eyelid defect. However, in very lax upper eyelids the flap of tissue from the lower eyelid can be narrower because the upper eyelid edges can be stretched somewhat to reduce the size of the defect.

A horizontal full-thickness incision is made in the lower eyelid 4–5 mm below the eyelid margin, which is just below the base of the tarsus and the inferior marginal arcade. During this incision, a corneal protector or lid plate should be used to protect the globe. At the edges of the horizontal incisions, full-thickness incisions are then carried vertically down to the lowest aspect of the inferior fornix on the conjunctival side. In younger patients with very elastic tissue, the flap may appear contracted so that the horizontal dimension is shorter than needed; however, this will stretch to fill the defect created if it has been measured properly initially. The flap is then separated into a conjunctivocapsulopalpebral fascia layer and a skin muscle layer. Both flaps are then advanced underneath the remaining bridge of the lower eyelid; however, some relaxing incisions in the capsulopalpebral fascia may be needed to advance the conjunctiva. The conjunctival layer, after being advanced under the bridge, is secured to the conjunctiva of the upper eyelid defect with 6–0 polyglactin suture (Fig. 26.14b). The tarsal substitute spacer graft chosen is then fashioned to fit the defect (Fig. 26.14c). If alloderm is chosen, it is cut to shape and secured with interrupted 6–0 polyglactin suture medially and laterally to the tarsal remnants of the upper eyelid, or to the medial and lateral canthal tendons if the tarsus has been excised, and superiorly to the cut edge of the levator aponeurosis. If the aponeurosis has been excised completely, then the graft should be sutured directly to the levator palpebrae superioris muscle. If autogenous cartilage is chosen, an ideal harvest site location is the flat scaphoid part of the ear. The skin muscle portion of the flap from the lower eyelid is then advanced under the bridge of the lower eyelid margin and sutured to the skin edges of the upper eyelid with interrupted 6–0 silk suture (Fig. 26.14d). Additional undermining of the

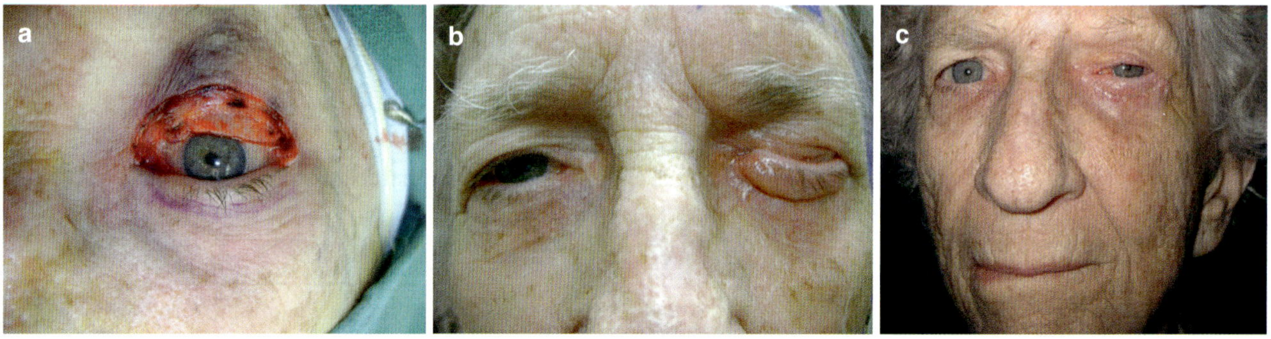

Fig. 26.13 Large left upper eyelid defect closed with a Cutler–Beard flap. (**a**) Defect. (**b**) Postoperative appearance following first stage of procedure showing the full-thickness lower eyelid flap sutured into the upper eyelid defect, coursing posterior to the intact lower eyelid margin. (**c**) Postoperative appearance of reconstructed left upper eyelid after second stage of procedure

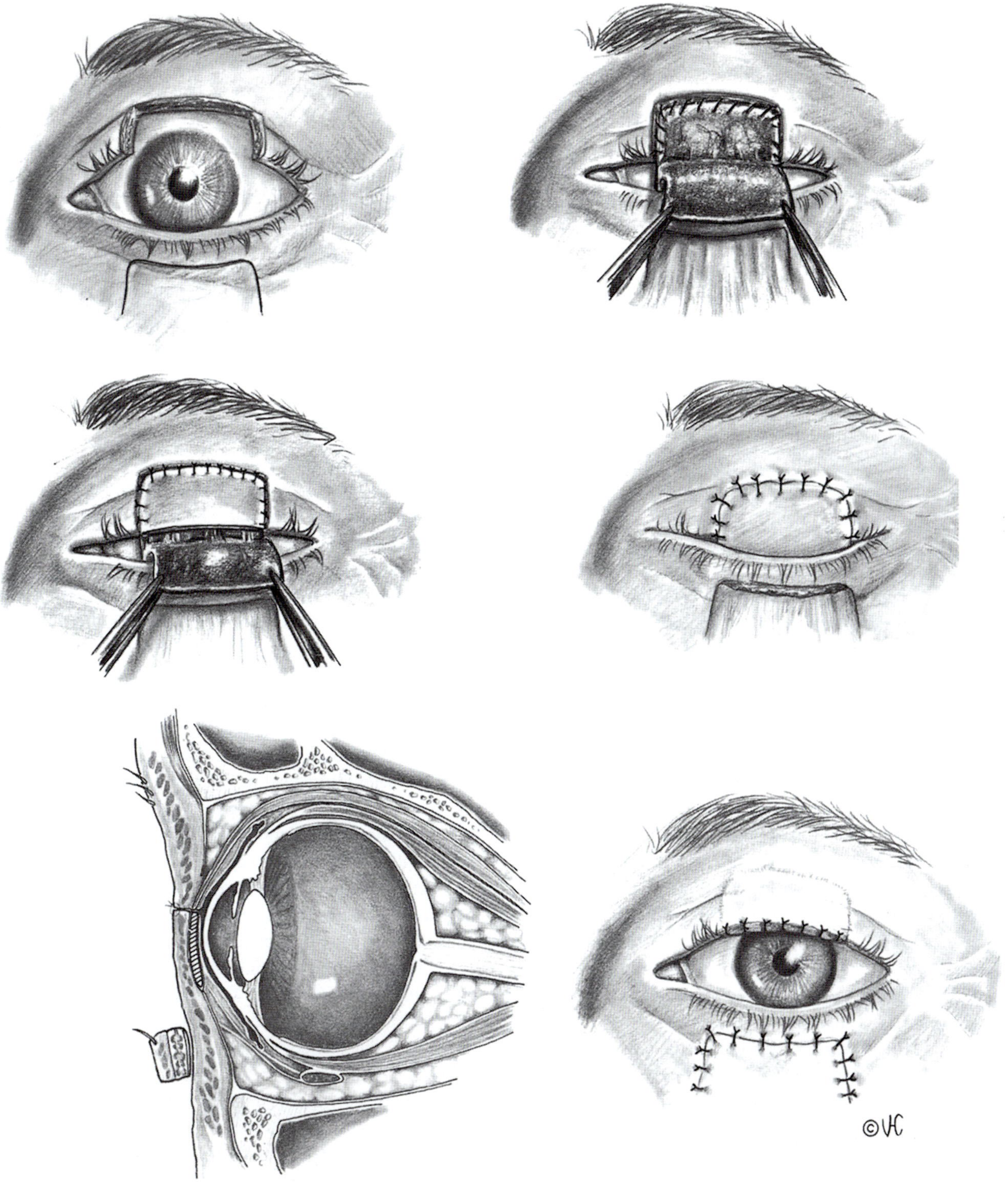

Fig. 26.14 Cutler–Beard bridge flap technique. (**a**) Rectangular upper lid defect that can be reduced by stretching horizontally so that proper width of lower lid advancement flap can be determined. Lower lid skin muscle conjunctival flap should be developed with horizontal incision not closer than 5 mm to lid margin. (**b**) Advancement of full-thickness lid flap from lower lid into upper lid defect. Inner layer of conjunctiva and capsulopalpebral fascia has been sutured to conjunctiva of upper lid. (**c**) Autogenous cartilage has been sutured in position attached to remnants of tarsal edge and levator muscle. This step is often unnecessary. Occasionally materials introduced into advancement flap can cause lid slough. (**d**) Skin muscle flap is then sutured into skin muscle defect in upper lid. (**e**) Sagittal view of lower lid flap in place. Autogenous cartilage graft is shown sandwiched between conjunctiva from lower lid and skin muscle flap. (**f**) Patient after separation of flap 6 weeks later. It is important in separating flap to ensure that there is extra conjunctiva to evert around upper lid margin, as shown here. Small traction folds must be excised for lower lid to close properly

skin flap over the malar eminence may be necessary to allow this flap to advance properly. The orbicularis muscle of the flap will fit the shape of the defect without undue tension as the skin is closed. The spacer graft has now been interposed in a sandwich manner between the flap of conjunctiva and the skin muscle layer from the lower eyelid (Fig. 26.14e).

Lysis of the flap is the second stage of the procedure and typically is performed 6–8 weeks after the first stage (Fig. 26.13c). At the time of flap separation, a surgical marking pen is used to mark the incision 2 mm below the desired position of the upper eyelid margin. As the assistant provides downward traction on the bridge, a grooved director is inserted under the flap so that a scalpel can be used to make the incision full thickness. Then 1–2 mm of the skin muscle is trimmed, leaving a 2 mm extra fold of conjunctiva that can be draped forward over the eyelid margin so that the lid margin will be mucous membrane rather than keratinized epithelium (Fig. 26.14f). This will decrease the likelihood of postoperative keratopathy from keratinized epithelium or fine lanugo hairs abrading the cornea.

The lower eyelid must be reformed after the inferior margin of the bridge is freshened. The lower eyelid conjunctiva can simply be left open and will heal by secondary intention. The lower eyelid skin edges are closed with 6–0 silk sutures, but the lower aspects of the cheek incisions may need to be undermined with excision of traction folds to promote smooth closure and to prevent lower eyelid malposition. An upper eyelid crease can be ensured by placing sutures through the eyelid fold at the desired location. All sutures are removed 1 week after separation of the flap. There is usually some edema in the upper eyelid for about 4–6 weeks, after which the eyelid achieves a more normal appearance, with a stable margin and vertical motility.

Other potential complications of a Cutler–Beard procedure besides keratopathy include blepharoptosis, lagophthalmos, and even lid retraction. Upper eyelid retraction can be avoided by waiting a minimum of 6 weeks before performing the second-stage procedure and by transecting the flap approximately 2 mm below the level of the upper lid. Necrosis of the bridge in the lower lid may result if the vascular supply is compromised. In creating the bridge during the first-stage procedure, the marginal arterial arcade should be avoided by making the incision 4–5 mm below the lid margin to preserve the vascular supply. Another shortcoming of the procedure is that it requires two stages and occlusion of the eye for a period of weeks. It should therefore be avoided if possible in monocular patients and children in whom occlusion amblyopia may develop. Additionally, there are no cilia present in the reconstructed upper eyelid. Hair-bearing grafts have been attempted at the desired location before separation of the flap; however, these grafts do not have the appearance of normal eyelashes. A shorter-than-desired reconstructed upper eyelid can be prevented by suturing the upper lid remnants as far down as possible on the advanced flap, so that the greatest amount of skin muscle and new tissue is included in the reconstructed lid.

A potential alternative to a Cutler–Beard procedure for large upper lid defects is placement of a free tarsoconjunctival graft from the contralateral upper lid and coverage of this graft with a skin–muscle flap if the amount of redundant upper lid skin is adequate. However, for deep defects of the upper eyelid with loss of tissue extending into the conjunctival fornix and anterior orbit, a free tarsoconjunctival graft is not adequate, and a Cutler–Beard flap would be more appropriate.

If the upper lid defect is wide but shallow, involving only the lid margin, a tarsoconjunctival flap from the area just superior to the defect can be advanced inferiorly to replace the posterior lamella. This flap must be well dissected toward the fornix. The levator aponeurosis is dissected away from the anterior face of the tarsus to prevent upper lid retraction during the postoperative period. It may then be covered by either a full-thickness skin graft or a skin–orbicularis flap.

In many cases of massive tissue loss of the upper eyelid, tissue cannot be borrowed from the opposing lower eyelid or adjacent areas for reconstruction of the defect. Flaps that contain their own blood supply must be brought in from more remote areas (usually the forehead) [26]. The forehead flap can be based nasally, using a median forehead flap, or based temporally, using the superficial temporal artery as its vascular supply. These techniques are used to reconstruct the upper eyelid when no other techniques are available.

In the median forehead flap, a flap of vertically oriented skin is outlined with a marking pen in the midforehead area; ideally, the flap should not exceed five times the width. The width of the flap should be sufficient to give adequate vertical length to the reconstructed upper eyelid. The flap is then incised and elevated from the midforehead area, retaining as much deep tissue and vascularization at the base as possible (Fig. 26.15a). The surrounding tissue in the forehead is undermined to allow the flap to rotate into the defect and to allow closure of the donor site. The vertical donor site is closed with subcutaneous interrupted 5–0 polyglactin suture and 6–0 silk skin closure. The undersurface of this flap, which opposes the globe, must be lined with mucous membrane to prevent shrinkage and to provide a proper surface to oppose the cornea (Fig. 26.15b). This lining may be gained from remnants of the conjunctiva that can be advanced from the superior or inferior fornix, or, if necessary, free buccal mucous membrane grafts. The free grafts in most cases "take" on a well-vascularized flap. The ideal lining of the flap is conjunctiva from either the superior or inferior fornix, if available. The flap is then attached to the levator aponeurosis or remnants of the levator palpebrae superioris muscle with 6–0 silk mattress sutures through the flap to give appropriate motility to the upper eyelid. Laterally, the tip of the

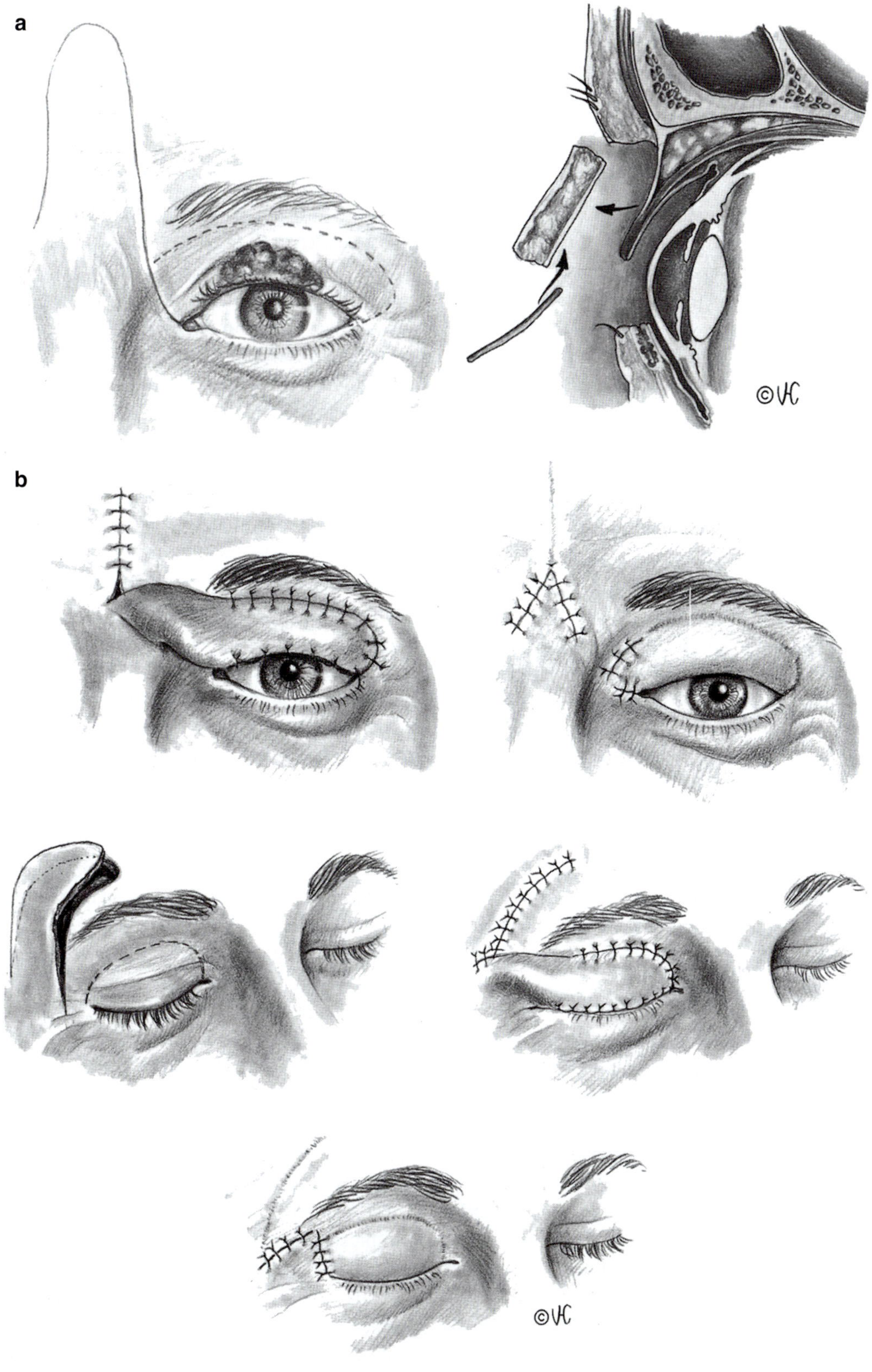

Fig. 26.15 Reconstruction of upper lid with forehead flaps: median forehead and temporal forehead flaps. (**a**) Upper lid to be excised for large eyelid tumor and development of median forehead flap. (**b**) Lining of flap tissue with alternative sources of mucous membrane. Free mucous membrane graft may be applied to flap, or conjunctiva can be advanced from upper or lower lid to undersurface of flaps. (**c**) Transposition of forehead flap to upper lid with pedicle intact. (**d**) Separation of pedicle of median forehead flap with replacement of tissue to glabellar area and trimming of flap. (**e**) Development of temporal forehead flap based on superficial temporal artery and intended area of excision of upper lid. (**f**) Placement of flap into upper lid donor area, with closure of donor site. (**g**) There is some buckling of tissue temporally, and pedicle must be separated and replaced later, as with median forehead flap

flap is attached with Prolene suture to the remnants of the lateral canthal tendon. The graft of mucous membrane or conjunctival flap is carefully rotated around the flap margin—which will become the new upper eyelid margin—and sutured in place with 7–0 silk to ensure that mucous membrane rather than keratinized epithelium will be in future contact with the cornea (Fig. 26.15c). If the undersurface of the forehead flap has been lined with advanced conjunctiva from the lower eyelid, it can be separated in 2 weeks, leaving enough conjunctiva to cover the lower edge of the flap, which becomes the new upper eyelid margin.

Eight weeks later, the flap is separated, and the base of the pedicle is replaced in the donor (glabellar) area (Fig. 26.15d). The remaining donor incisions are closed with interrupted 6–0 silk sutures. Some contracture will occur in the postoperative period. Vertical shortening generally is more of a problem than excessive length of the upper eyelid. Excess tissue can be trimmed later, if necessary. The upper eyelid will appear tight for many weeks until the levator palpebrae superioris muscle begins to provide vertical motility. The resultant eyelid skin is abnormally thick and may be cautiously thinned down at a later time.

A temporal forehead transposition flap based in the lateral temporal area can be used to reconstruct the upper eyelid when there are no other alternatives. This flap is based on the superficial temporal artery, which travels along the lateral orbital rim and above the brow in that area. One should palpate the artery by tracing its pulsations or by using Doppler ultrasound and mark the location of the artery on the skin so that it can be included in the flap (Fig. 26.15e). The full-thickness skin from the brow area is then outlined to include the artery at its base. Care should be taken that the flap is long enough to rotate and cover the desired area for the upper eyelid. The tip of the flap is dissected free from the thick forehead skin above the brow, generally including some subcutaneous fat, which can be dissected from the dermis. The flap is then developed down to its base in the temporal area; care should be taken to avoid cutting the superficial temporal artery. Some undermining may be necessary to allow the flap to be turned onto the lid. There will be some buckling at the base of the flap, as there was in the forehead flap, although not as severe (Fig. 26.15f). The flap should then be anchored medially, either to the eyelid remnant or to the posterior reflection of the medial canthal tendon. However, before being sutured into position, it should be lined with mucous membrane and either an advancement conjunctival flap from the superior fornix or lower eyelid, or a free buccal mucous membrane graft (Fig. 26.15g). If possible, the levator aponeurosis should be attached to the undersurface or the edge of the flap. The forehead defect must be undermined for closure; vertical mattress sutures can be used to take tension off the edges in the forehead. At the temporal portion of the brow, there may be some difficulty in closure. This area can be left open during the 3–4 week interval before the base of the flap is separated. The base of the flap, after being separated from the eyelid, can be repositioned, avoiding displacement of the brow temporally. The disadvantages of this flap are the same as those of the forehead flap: The skin is very thick and not as soft and mobile as normal upper eyelid skin should be. However, this is a valuable technique when there is no other alternative.

Lateral Canthal Defects

A key element of reconstruction in the lateral canthus is maintenance of the lower eyelid position and avoidance of lower eyelid ectropion. This is usually achieved by a lower eyelid tightening procedure that involves attaching the lower eyelid to the lateral orbital rim. If the periorbita is of poor quality or absent, drill holes can be placed in the lateral orbital rim near Whitnall's tubercle (the lateral orbital tubercle). In most individuals, the vertical position of the lateral canthus is approximately 2 mm higher than the vertical position of the medial canthus. Following extensive lower lid surgery, the lateral canthus tends to retract inferiorly. Thus, the lateral canthus should be positioned superiorly enough that the lower lid and canthus maintain good anatomic orientation.

Laterally based transposition flaps or an upper eyelid Hughes tarsoconjunctival flap can be utilized for large lower lid defects that extend to the lateral canthus [27]. Free skin grafts can be used to cover these flaps. Semicircular advancement skin flaps may also be used for defects extending to the lateral canthus. Occasionally, strips of periosteum and temporalis fascia still attached at the lateral orbital rim can be used to attach the remaining lateral lid margins to the lateral orbital rim, when the eyelid remnant cannot reach the orbital rim periosteum [27–29]. To create the periosteal flap, cut a 5-mm-high strip of periosteum angled superiorly, starting slightly above where the lateral canthal tendon should be. The strip is then sutured to the lateral tarsal eyelid remnant.

Medial Canthal Defects

The medial canthal area is the second most common site for basal cell carcinoma of the eyelids. The size and depth of the defect determine the method of reconstruction—direct closure, full-thickness skin graft, local myocutaneous flap, or spontaneous granulation. The medial canthal region represents a complex anatomic area. Maintaining the posterior displacement of the medial canthal tendon is paramount in obtaining the normal configuration of the medial commissure. A functional and cosmetic result is based on sound anatomic knowledge and appropriate surgical reconstruction. It must be remembered that tumors of the medial canthus are notorious for their deep penetration. Complete tumor removal is the first priority. Lacrimal drainage can be established as a secondary procedure.

Full-thickness skin grafts are ideal for small, shallow defects of the medial canthus (Figs. 26.16 and 26.17). Eyelid, postauricular, supraclavicular, and upper underarm are good donor sites, with acceptable color matches in descending order. An imprint of the defect is made on sterile paper and placed on the donor site. The donor tissue is excised, and the defect is closed. The graft is usually thinned and sutured into the defect with interrupted 6–0 silk sutures. The graft is kept taut.

Pie crusting of the graft with multiple stab incisions may be carried out to prevent elevation of the graft resulting from postoperative oozing of the recipient site (Fig. 26.18). Contact between the graft and its bed is maintained with a bolster (Fig. 26.19). The sutures are removed in 5–10 days.

Larger medial canthal defects require good fixation of the residual upper and lower eyelid remnants to the medial canthal tendon insertion area. The fixation suture should be posterior enough and with solid attachment to the bone to achieve good apposition of the eyelid against the globe to restore the natural direction and shape of the medial canthal angle (Figs. 26.20 and 26.21). The attachment of the eyelids to the deep periosteum facilitates the placement, when necessary, of a silicone stent tube. Fixation may be carried out with heavy 4–0 permanent suture, wire, or titanium miniplates [30]. In the majority of cases, the lid can be fixated by suturing its medial aspect to the deep tissues in the region of the posterior lacrimal crest, where the posterior limb of the medial canthal tendon normally inserts. Once the edges of the eyelid remnants are in their proper position, the superficial defect can either heal by spontaneous granulation or be covered with a full-thickness skin graft.

For deep defects, various forms of transposition flaps are more appropriate. Deep nonmarginal canthal lesions requiring excision of muscle, periosteum, and bone should not be allowed to heal by granulation. Also, free skin grafts are unacceptable if bone is exposed. A very useful flap for this location is a glabellar flap (Figs. 26.22 and 26.23) [31–33].

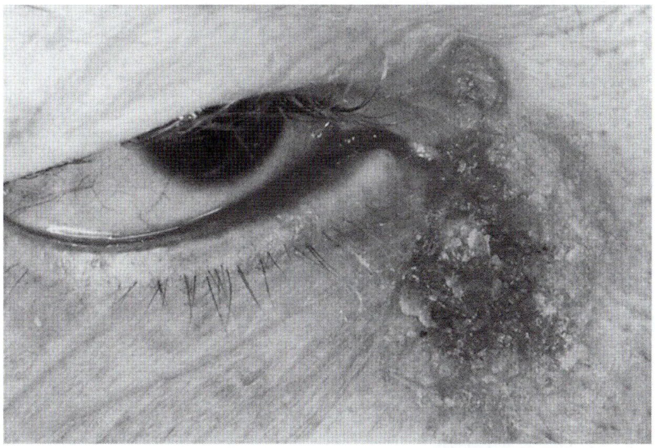

Fig. 26.16 Basal cell carcinoma with only superficial involvement of medial canthus

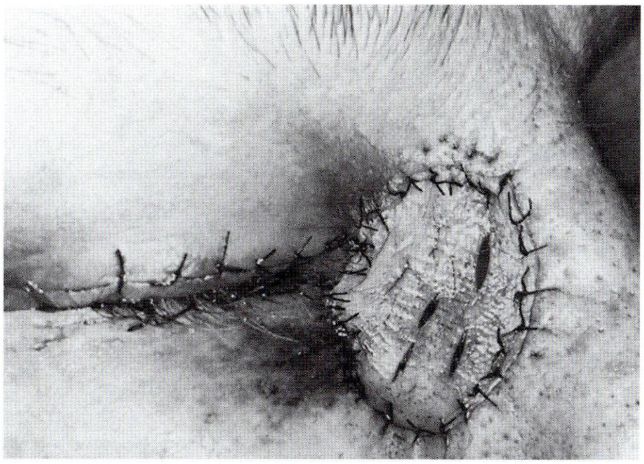

Fig. 26.18 Defect in Fig. 26.11 covered with postauricular full-thickness skin graft. Defect was made smaller by sliding skin flaps from the upper and lower eyelids. Pie crusting is clearly evident in graft

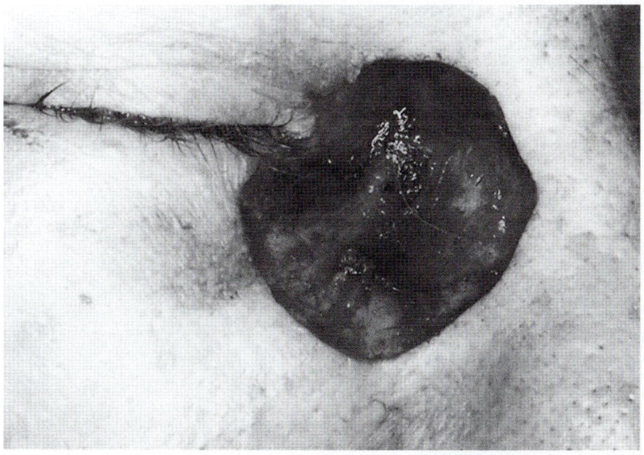

Fig. 26.17 Extent of defect after frozen section excision of tumor seen in Fig. 26.10. Note that margins of eyelids are undisturbed, as is medial canthal tendon

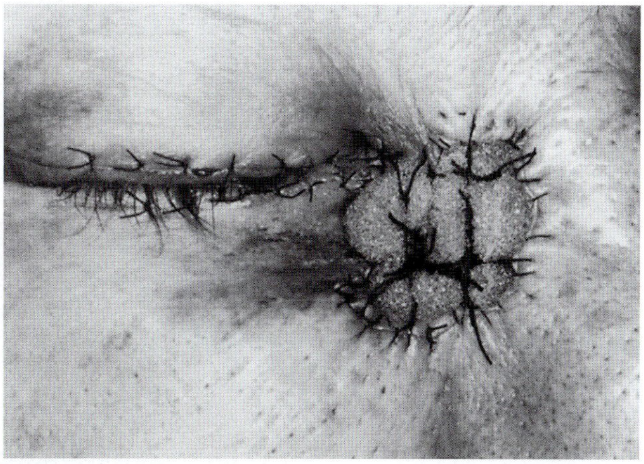

Fig. 26.19 Foam rubber bolster used to maintain contact between graft and its bed to increase chances of graft survival

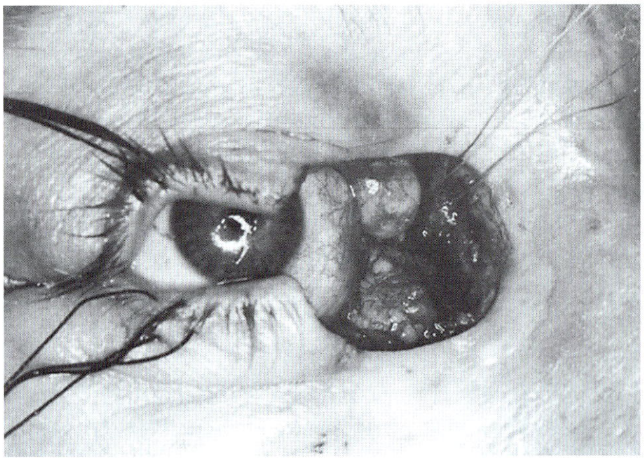

Fig. 26.20 Central medial canthal defect after removal of basal cell carcinoma

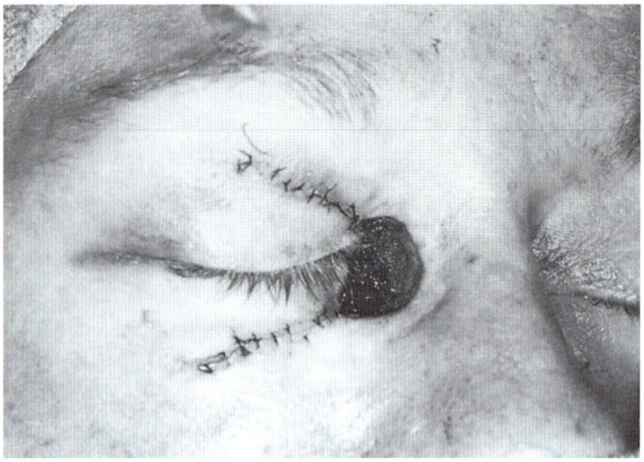

Fig. 26.21 Same patient as in Fig. 26.20 after attachment of lid margins to periosteum of posterior lacrimal crest and reapproximation of conjunctiva. This defect was allowed to heal by granulation

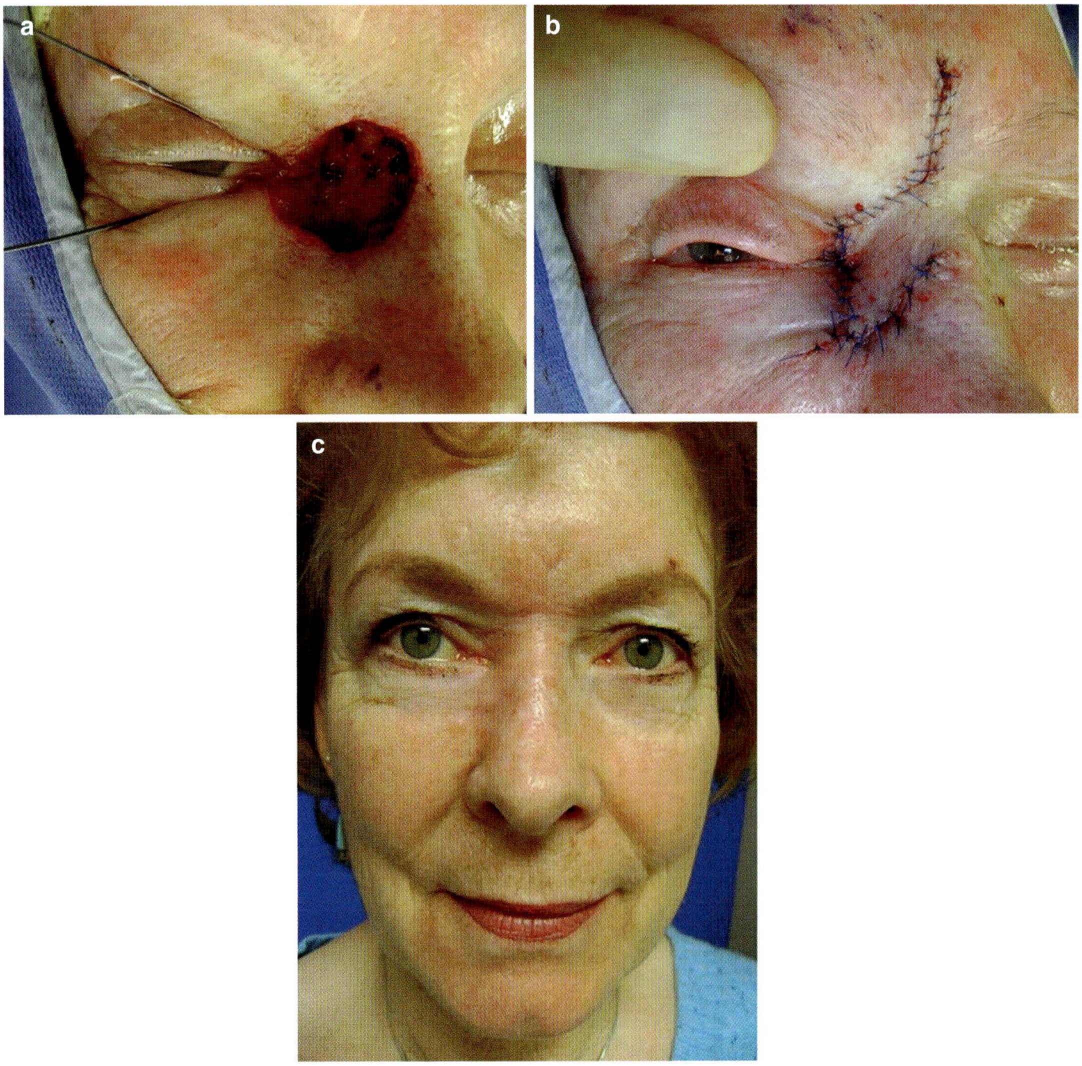

Fig. 26.22 Large and deep right medial canthal defect repaired with a glabellar myocutaneous flap. (**a**) Defect showing lacrimal probes in the canaliculi with disruption of the superior canaliculus. (**b**) Intraoperative appearance after flap placement. (**c**) Postoperative appearance 5 months after repair

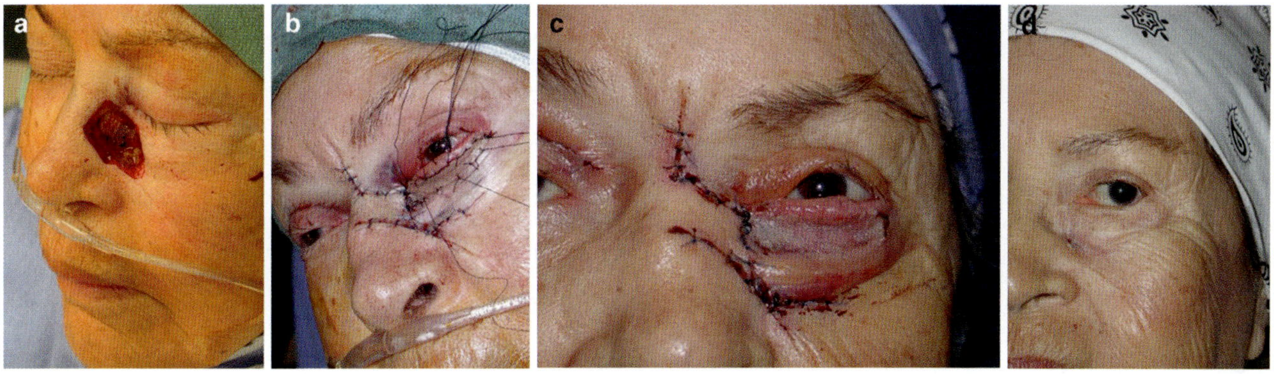

Fig. 26.23 Large left medial canthal defect closed with a combination of a glabellar flap, full-thickness skin graft harvested from the right upper eyelid, and a local advancement myocutaneous flap. (**a**) Defect. (**b**) Intraoperative appearance showing skin graft superior to advancement flap. (**c**) Postoperative appearance 1 week after repair showing well-vascularized graft and flaps. (**d**) Postoperative appearance 3 months after repair

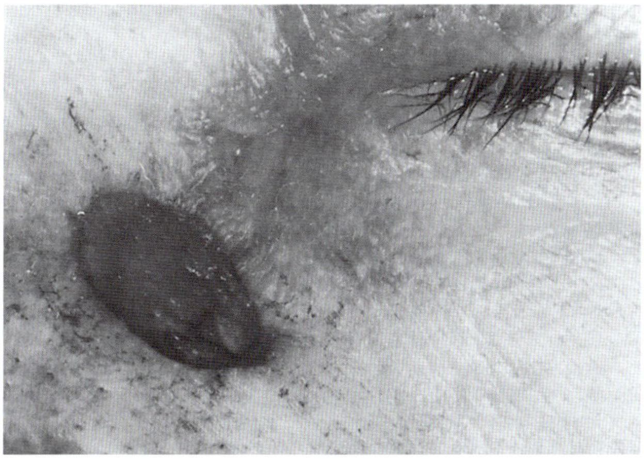

Fig. 26.24 Defect of medial canthus after tumor excision. Note that eyelid margins are intact

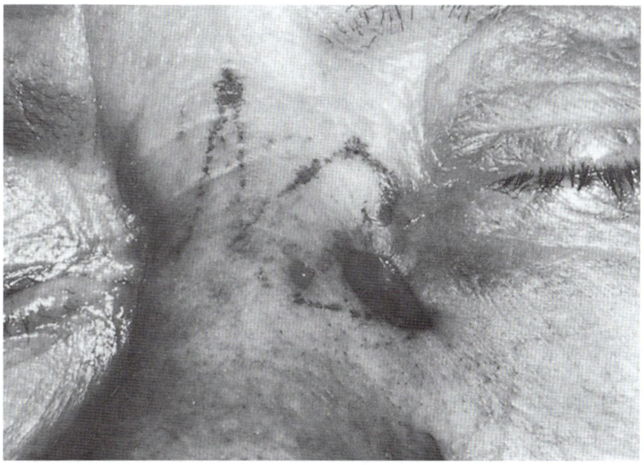

Fig. 26.25 Outline of proposed bilobed flap. Skin of entire area is undermined, and flaps are transposed

The flap and adjacent area are undermined to allow the flap to rotate into the defect without tension. Midline or oblique forehead flaps can be used for longer defects (Figs. 26.24, 26.25, 26.26, and 26.27). Flaps can withstand postoperative adjuvant radiation therapy, if it is needed [32].

Loss of the lacrimal drainage apparatus, including the canaliculi, is common after removal of medial canthal cancers. We typically do primary repair of canaliculi with silicone stenting only for defects that involve up to 5 mm of canalicular loss; otherwise, we prefer to perform lacrimal bypass surgery, including placement of a Pyrex glass tube ("Jones tube"), after the soft tissue reconstruction in the medial canthal angle has stabilized and only if the patient has symptomatic epiphora. Most surgeons would wait at least one year prior to fistulization into the nasal passages with

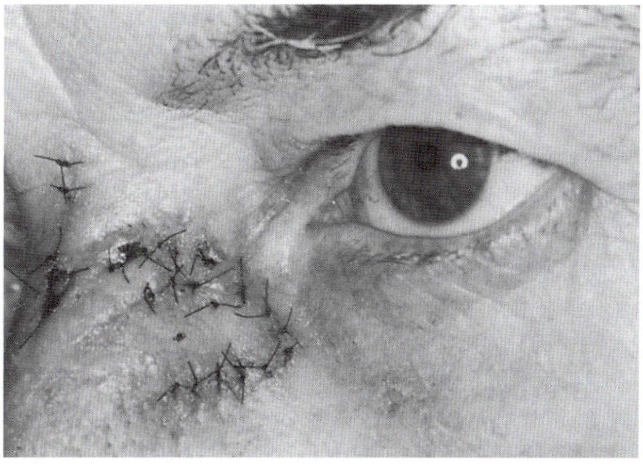

Fig. 26.26 Flaps sutured in place

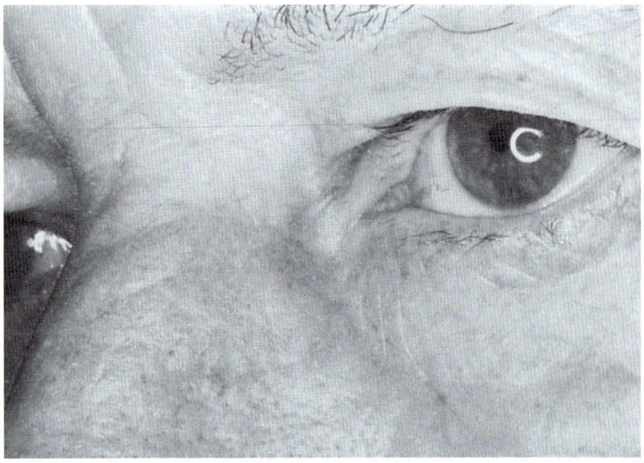

Fig. 26.27 Postoperative appearance. Note that scars are well hidden by skin tension lines

either a DCR or cDCR and perform preoperative imaging to ensure no recurrence of tumor.

Spontaneous granulation ("laissez faire" granulation) of anterior lamellar defects has been used with varying success because of cicatrix formation [34]. This is best used when the defect straddles the medial canthal tendon with approximately equal areas above and below the tendon. In such cases, tissue shrinkage that occurs postoperatively should be symmetrical, minimizing the risk of displacement of the canthus or of lower eyelid ectropion. Superior or inferior defects allowed to spontaneously granulate can result in cicatricial contraction and ectropion. During medial reconstruction of the upper and lower eyelid margins, the cut ends of the conjunctiva are sutured together to form a new medial cul-de-sac. The lid margins are sutured together and attached to the periosteum of the posterior lacrimal crest with a nonabsorbable suture. The remaining defect is left to heal by granulation. Of note, healing takes much longer with a laissez faire strategy than with grafts and flaps and requires daily care to avoid infection and prominent scars. The weeping open wound requires frequent dressing changes for 6–8 weeks.

References

1. Patrinely JR, Marines HM, Anderson RL. Skin flaps in periorbital reconstruction. Surv Ophthalmol. 1987;31:249–61.
2. Harvey J. Modified "double Z-plasty" in the closure of medial canthal defects. Ophthalmic Surg. 1987;18:120–2.
3. Hughes WL, editor. Reconstructive surgery of the eyelids. 2nd ed. St. Louis: Mosby; 1954.
4. Smith B, Lisman R. Preparation of split thickness auricular cartilage for use in ophthalmic plastic surgery. Ophthalmic Surg. 1982;13:1018–21.
5. Baylis HI, Rosen N, Neuhaus RW. Obtaining auricular cartilage for reconstructive surgery. Am J Ophthalmol. 1982;93:709–12.
6. Anderson RL, Weinstein GS. Full thickness bipedicle flap for total lower eyelid reconstruction. Arch Ophthalmol. 1987;105:570–6.
7. Anderson RL, Jordan DR, Beard C. Full-thickness unipedicle flap for lower eyelid reconstruction. Arch Ophthalmol. 1988;106:122–5.
8. Leone CR, Van Gemert JV. Lower lid reconstruction using tarsoconjunctival grafts and bipedicle skin-muscle flap. Arch Ophthalmol. 1989;107:758–60.
9. Hewes EH, Sullivan JH, Beard C. Lower eyelid reconstruction by tarsal transposition. Am J Ophthalmol. 1976;81:512–4.
10. Putterman AM. Viable composite grafting in eyelid reconstruction. Am J Ophthalmol. 1978;85:237–41.
11. Cohen MS, Shorr N. Eyelid reconstruction with hard palate mucosa grafts. Ophthal Plast Reconstr Surg. 1992;8:183–95.
12. Siegel RJ. Palatal grafts for eyelid reconstruction. Plast Reconstr Surg. 1985;76:411–4.
13. Brown BZ. The use of homologous tarsus as a donor graft in lid surgery. Ophthal Plast Reconstr Surg. 1985;1:91–5.
14. Hurwitz JJ, Corin SM, Tucker SM. The use of free periosteal grafts in extensive lower lid reconstruction. Ophthalmic Surg. 1989;20:415–9.
15. Jordan DR, Tse DT, Anderson RL, et al. Irradiated homologous tarsal plate banking: a new alternative in eyelid reconstruction: part II. Human data Ophthal Plast Reconstr Surg. 1990;6:168–76.
16. Tenzel RR. Reconstruction of the central one-half of an eyelid. Arch Ophthalmol. 1975;93:125–6.
17. Tenzel RR, Stewart WB. Eyelid reconstruction by the semicircle flap technique. Ophthalmology. 1978;85:1164–9.
18. Levine MR, Buckman G. Semicircular flap revisited. Arch Ophthalmol. 1986;104:915.
19. Anderson RL, Edwards JJ. Reconstruction by myocutaneous eyelid flaps. Arch Ophthalmol. 1979;97:2358.
20. Leone CR. Tarsal conjunctival advancement flaps for upper eyelid reconstruction. Ophthalmic Surg. 1973;4:68.
21. Smith B. A technique for extirpation and replacement of the lateral canthus. Trans Am Acad Ophthalmol Otolaryngol. 1953;50:738.
22. Cutler NL, Beard C. A method for partial and total upper eyelid reconstruction. Am J Ophthalmol. 1955;39:1.
23. Wesley RE, McCord CD. Transplantation of eyebank sclera in the cutler–beard method of upper eyelid reconstruction. Ophthalmology. 1980;87:1022.
24. Baylis HI, Rosen N, Neuhaus RW. Obtaining auricular cartilage for reconstructive surgery. Am J Ophthalmol. 1981;93:709.
25. Smith B, Obear MF. Bridge flap technique for reconstruction of large upper lid defects. Plast Reconstr Surg. 1966;38:45.
26. Kazanjian VH, Roopenian J. Median forehead flaps and the repair of defects of the nose and surrounding areas. Trans Am Acad Ophthalmol Otolaryngol. 1956;60:557.
27. Leone CR. Lateral canthal reconstruction. Ophthalmology. 1987;94:238–41.
28. Holt JE, Holt GR, Van Kirk M. Use of temporalis fascia in eyelid reconstruction. Ophthalmology. 1984;91:89–93.
29. Weinstein GS, Anderson RL, Tse DT, et al. The use of a periosteal strip for eyelid reconstruction. Arch Ophthalmol. 1985;103:357–9.
30. Howard GR, Nerad JA, Kersten RC. Medial canthoplasty with microplate fixation. Arch Ophthalmol. 1992;110:1793–7.
31. Dortzbach RK, Hawes MJ. Midline forehead flap in reconstructive procedures of the eyelids and exenterated socket. Ophthalmic Surg. 1981;12:257–68.
32. Teske SA, Kersten RC, Devoto MH, et al. The modified rhomboid transposition flap in periocular reconstruction. Ophthal Plast Reconstr Surg. 1998;14:360–6.
33. Spinelli HM, Jelks GW. Periocular reconstruction: a systematic approach. Plast Reconstr Surg. 1993;91:1017–24.
34. Lowry JC, Bartley GB, Garrity JA. The role of second-intention healing in periocular reconstruction. Ophthal Plast Reconstr Surg. 1997;13:174–88.

Mohs Micrographic Surgery of the Periorbital Area

27

Michael R. Migden and Sirunya Silapunt

Introduction

Mohs micrographic surgery (MMS) has been advocated as an effective method of dealing with periorbital skin malignancy especially basal cell carcinoma (BCC) and squamous cell carcinoma (SCC). It has been shown to have high rates of tumor clearance with minimal loss of normal tissue, thus making oculoplastic reconstruction easier and functional preservation better. Mohs [1] reported a 99% and 98% 5-year cure rate for BCC and SCC of the eyelids, respectively. Menn et al. [2] reported that 47% of recurrent lesions recurred a second time when treated with other methods, excluding Mohs surgery. Recurrent periorbital lesions are more difficult to eradicate because of earlier invasion, possible histological transformation, or local tissue alteration due to previous surgery. Complete removal at first diagnosis of periorbital tumors should be the main aim of treatment. MMS is the most effective method for achieving this.

Treatment Goals for Periorbital Malignancy

- Eliminate tumor while preserving normal tissue
- Preserve function whenever possible
- Restore structural form and cosmesis

Preservation of healthy tissue has been highlighted by Kumar et al. in 1997 [3]. They reviewed 24 cases of primary ($n = 18$) and recurrent ($n = 6$) periorbital basal and squamous cell carcinomas managed by MMS excision and oculoplastic reconstruction. They found that in 12 of 24 cases (50%), the posterior lamella was preserved. Posterior lamella preservation makes reconstruction of the defect easier and helps maintain function, particularly in elderly patients in whom the ocular surface is already compromised by reduced tear function. In some cases where the tumor clinically appeared fixed to underlying bone, MMS facilitated complete resection without resorting to exenteration.

History of Mohs Micrographic Surgery

In 1933, Dr. Frederick Mohs began his pioneering work in microscopic chemosurgery as a research assistant at the University of Wisconsin in the Department of Zoology [4]. Working under the head of the department, he assessed the effects of injecting platinum and other chemicals into cancers implanted in rats. The effects of the various chemicals injected were evaluated by shaving a specimen from the injected implanted tumors parallel to the skin surface and examining them in the horizontal excision plane. When the chemical injected was zinc chloride solution, an unexpected observation was that excellent histologic structural features were preserved. This led to the concept of "micrographic" observation of a tumor's surgical margins following zinc chloride in vivo "fixation" in order to confirm complete tumor removal. The term micrographic was created to recognize the components of microscopic examination and mapping of the surgical resection plane.

In 1936, when Dr. Mohs began using his micrographic chemosurgery method to treat patients, the method was considered controversial. This was due to the pain and tissue morbidity associated with in vivo zinc chloride tissue fixation as well as the long-since-debunked theory that prevailed at the time that cutting through malignancies would cause them to spread locally or metastasize. As a consequence of

M. R. Migden (✉)
University of Texas M D Anderson Cancer Center, Department of Head and Neck, Division of Surgery, Houston, TX, USA

University of Texas M D Anderson Cancer Center, Department of Dermatology, Division of Internal Medicine, Houston, TX, USA
e-mail: mrmigden@mdanderson.org

S. Silapunt
University of Texas McGovern Medical School at Houston, Department of Dermatology, Houston, TX, USA

J. J. Servat et al. (eds.), *Smith and Nesi's Ophthalmic Plastic and Reconstructive Surgery*,
https://doi.org/10.1007/978-3-030-41720-8_27

this controversy, his early patients were restricted to those with extremely advanced cancers who were considered to be incurable. Dr. Mohs kept meticulous records as he treated these extensive tumors. Although his data first reported in 1941 showed the technique to be very effective in the most difficult of tumors, suspicion of the micrographic chemosurgery approach continued.

Use of the zinc chloride fixative caused this process to be a very complex and time-consuming process. It often required several days to complete because the fixative paste had to remain in place for up to 24 h between each surgical procedure. During the process of fixation of tissue by the paste, patients usually experienced severe pain and occasionally systemic fever secondarily to marked inflammation within tissues. Some normal tissues would slough when the last layer of fixed tissue separated from its underlying bed of unfixed tissue. This additional loss of normal tissue would be undesirable in the treatment of cancers located on the eyelids, nasal ala, and the helix of the ears. Baylis and Cies discussed problems concerning wound healing, such as cicatricial distortion of the eyelids that occurred secondarily to the use of the zinc chloride fixative [5].

In the periorbital area, there was a concern that the zinc chloride paste, which would occasionally migrate beyond the intended site of application, would damage the ocular surface. Because of the complexities of using the paste in the periorbital area, most Mohs surgeons ultimately omitted the fixative when treating cancers occurring within this anatomic region. In several cases in which the tumor invaded eyelids and the cancer cells approached the globe, Dr. Mohs applied the fixative for only a few minutes in order not to damage that important ocular structure [6]. Clearly, these disadvantages of the fixative precluded its use for most periorbital skin cancers.

Evolution of the technique to replace the chemosurgery fixation with fresh frozen sections was a creative modification borne out of necessity. In 1953, while making an instructional film demonstrating the Mohs technique, Dr. Mohs needed to complete a multistage excision of the eyelid basal carcinoma within a single day. The camera crew and equipment were available only for 1 day. Replacing the chemosurgical in vivo fixation with frozen sections prepared from fresh tissue allowed the filming to be completed on schedule. The decreased inflammation noted on microscopic evaluation using this modification led Dr. Mohs to use the fresh tissue technique for removal of eyelid cancers from that date forward.

Adopting the micrographic fresh frozen section approach over traditional chemosurgery was based on the obvious benefits of changing from a multi-day process to that of a single-day procedure performed without the significant inflammatory effects of zinc chloride paste.

Originally, this procedure was referred to as chemosurgery, then microscopically controlled surgical excision. In 1987, the term Mohs micrographic surgery was becoming more common and is presently accepted as the preferred descriptor of the procedure originally attributed to Dr. Mohs.

Margin Control: Methods and Considerations

The goal of cancer surgery is complete removal of the tumor while sparing as much normal tissue as possible. The most optimal approach for achieving this goal is early cancer screening and early detection of the smallest possible primary lesion before it becomes more locally destructive, has greater subclinical extension, or develops in transit or distant metastasis. The key concept is that early complete excision of a naïve primary tumor affords the best protection against developing a larger, more locally destructive, recurrent, or metastatic skin cancer.

One might argue, the more high risk the tumor, the larger the margin should be in order to decrease the likelihood of incomplete removal, local extension, or metastasis. Recommended wide local excision margins are based on tumor type, subtype, grade, and stage, as well as other features such as depth of invasion, ulceration, and perineural involvement. These margins recommend the amount of additional tissue beyond the clinical tumor which should be taken in order to include and thereby contain the irregular subclinical extension of tumors which often occur but may not be detected in standard bread-loafed sections. In the absence of any local metastasis, substantially increasing margins beyond what will completely clear the primary tumor has not been demonstrated to provide benefit in decreasing recurrence rate or increasing long-term survival.

Wide Local Excision (WLE)

Most wide local excisions are evaluated by transverse sectioning of tissue in "bread loaf" orientation, providing a survey of excision margins. These parallel cross-sectional sections are performed in series from one end of the specimen to the other. Although each section from a "bread-loafed" specimen contains a component of peripheral margin, the sum of all of the peripheral margins from these sections may total 1–2% or less of the complete peripheral margin available in the excision specimen (Fig. 27.1a).

This method is appropriate for evaluating the margins of tumors having less subclinical extension and those where the edges of the tumor are less irregular. For tumors with a high degree of irregular subclinical extension, a root or vein of the

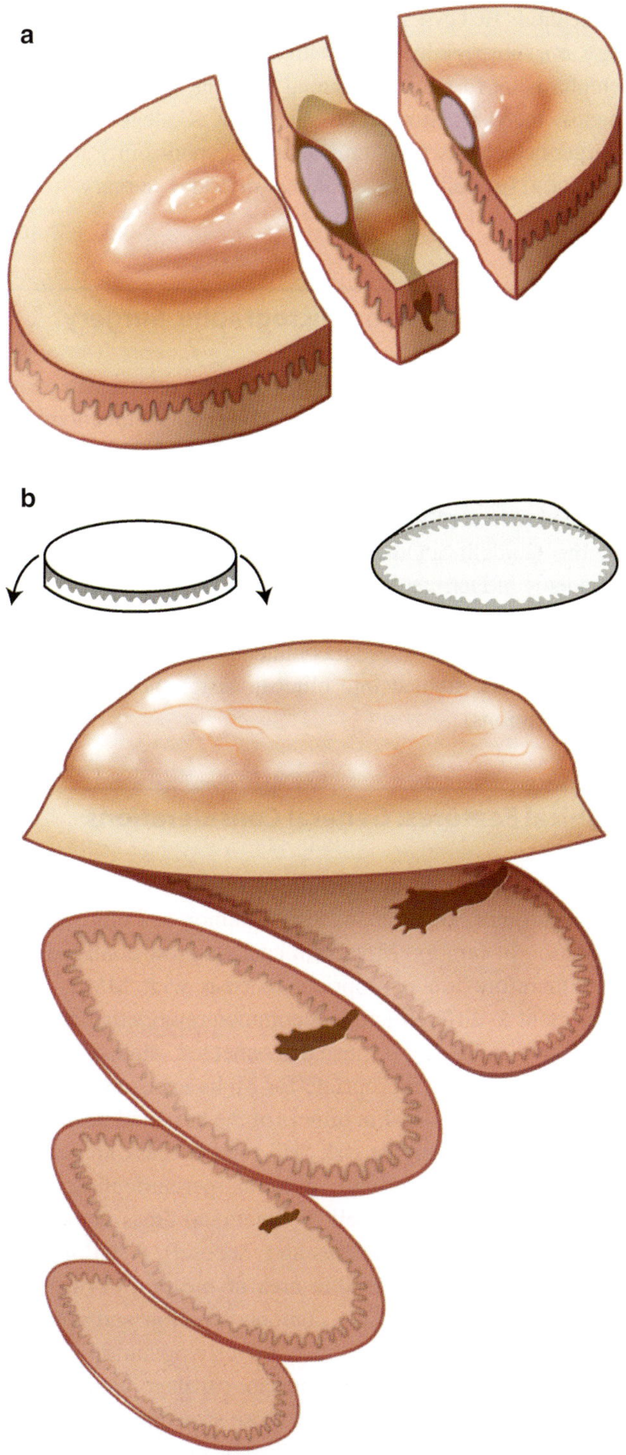

Fig. 27.1 (**a**) Standard bread loafed sectioning visualizes that portion of the margin where the specimen is divided transversely. Margin located between the sections is not evaluable. In this case, unidentifiable tumor is present along the peripheral margin between the areas of sectioning. (**b**) Mohs stage with 100% en face evaluation of both the deep and contiguous peripheral margins. All marginal tumor at contact area with patient is evaluable in the sections prepared

malignancy may fall between transverse sections prepared, and in this case, a negative margin may be erroneously reported. When performing wide local resection, adhering to the recommended margins appropriate for tumor type and subtype may compensate for some of the subclinical irregular extension. Attempts to narrow standard margins using wide local excision may result in incomplete excision. For timely and more detailed scrutiny of selected areas, intraoperative en face frozen sections may also be performed. This may be combined with intraoperative mapping of the areas selected. The challenge with most intraoperative frozen sections is to predict which portion of the total margin should be excised and evaluated. Oculoplastic surgeons advocate treating small-size cutaneous lesions that involve the eyelid and periocular region with intraoperative frozen section evaluation of en face margins. They consider this approach practical for surgeons who have access to expert dermatopathology support for immediate evaluation of en face margins for the entire specimen.

Wide local excision also has an important role in cutaneous malignancies that are not appropriate for MMS such as (1) tumors that are not contiguous, (2) cutaneous malignancies so deep or extensive that they are unlikely to be completely removed with Mohs resection, (3) tumors in patients who are not willing to have surgery under local anesthesia, and (4) tumors that do not meet the indication criteria for MMS and therefore can be treated by other means including standard excision.

Mohs Micrographic Surgery (MMS)

Mohs surgery specimens are not cross-sectioned. They are instead processed in order to examine 100% of the contact area between the Mohs specimen obtained and the wound bed from which it came. This “complete view” is similar to compiling a mosaic of all possible adjacent contiguous en face sections, with each face parallel to a specific portion of the total contact area (Fig. 27.1b).

If the Mohs excision specimen were to be thought of as a freshly baked pie and the wound bed from where it was excised a pie pan, the Mohs frozen sections would examine all of the pie crust contact area where it contacts the pie pan: the sides of the crust as well as the bottom. By evaluating 100% of the margin of excision as is the case in MMS, there is substantially decreased chance of missing a root of malignancy.

One primary advantage of MMS is the single physician continuity across all aspects of the Mohs process. One Mohs surgeon meticulously performs all steps of the Mohs micrographic process. This includes resection of Mohs layer specimens while maintaining strict anatomical orientation, laboratory processing with or without relaxing incisions, specimen annotation with tissue dye, specimen mapping, interpretation of frozen section slides, and precisely marking the Mohs map with any tumor identified to guide any additional resection indicated. It is this single physician continuity approach to margin assessment that provides the most complete margin control for excising most cutaneous and mucosal tumors.

Precisely mapped 100% margin evaluation with Mohs frozen sections provides the Mohs surgeon with the information necessary to continue surgical excision, tracking irregular extension of the tumor beyond that clinically apparent on the surface. Performed while the wound bed is "fresh," resection is completed prior to extensive inflammation and early granulation tissue formation. Returning to a surgical site for additional margins days after the original excision may produce specimens with significant inflammation and other postsurgical changes that can make histologic interpretation more challenging. Standard staged excisions with paraffin sections are also subject to postsurgical wound distortion and contraction that can alter the surgical site's contour, making accurate determination of orientation at surgical site markings more difficult.

Mohs Surgery Training

Mohs surgeons function in the capacity of both surgeon and pathologist, so that he or she can make critical judgments using ongoing clinicopathologic correlation throughout the surgical case. The key training components for MMS are precise Mohs excision, processing, and mapping of an appropriate excision specimen. Substantial training beyond residency prepares the Mohs surgeon for the multiple roles of cutaneous oncologic surgeon, frozen section dermatopathologist with emphasis on cutaneous malignancy, and cutaneous restorative surgeon. Dermatology is the only specialty other than pathology where diagnostic histopathology training in relevant diseases—dermatopathology—comprises a substantial portion of the overall training during residency. Dermatologists are qualified to read and generate reports on the skin biopsies they perform.

Training in MMS began in the early days when Dr. Mohs, as well as a small number of physicians he trained, provided informal training for physicians who rotated in their clinics for variable periods of time in order to learn the process. In 1966, Dr. Perry Robbins became the first Mohs surgeon to establish a 1-year fellowship training program at NYU [4]. In 1983, formalized 1–2-year fellowships following dermatology residency were developed under the direction of the American College of Chemosurgery. In 1985, the name was changed to American College of Mohs Micrographic Surgery and Cutaneous Oncology (ACMMSCO), and in 2007, it became the American College of Mohs Surgery (ACMS). In 2002, the Accreditation Counsel for Graduate Medical Education (ACGME) began support of procedural dermatology as a subspecialty of dermatology that included a primary emphasis on formalized training in Mohs surgery and cutaneous reconstruction. The American College of Mohs Surgery elected to transfer oversight, responsibility, and certification for fellowship training in Mohs surgery to the ACGME.

Indications for Mohs Micrographic Surgery

Although MMS has been shown to be very effective in treating a wide range of skin cancers, and specific indications are described in many publications, there is no multidisciplinary consensus that requires its use to treat these malignancies. A detailed review of indications for its use has been published in the Guidelines/Outcomes Committee of the American Academy of Dermatology [7]. A variety of more recent publications including several articles from other specialties continue to support these recommendations [8]. Indications for MMS are divided into clinical, histologic, and patient considerations.

Clinical Features: General Considerations

Clinical features to be considered for MMS include contiguous tumor, location and size of tumor, and clinical presentation of tumors. Most skin cancers grow contiguously and therefore are appropriate to treat with MMS. It is important to differentiate less common tumors that are significantly multifocal or have disconnected satellite components that are not appropriate for Mohs excision. MMS is appropriate for most skin tumors of the head and neck. This encompasses the higher risk "H" zone or mask area of the face including periorbital, perioral, periauricular, nasal, and glabellar units as well as functional areas contained: eyelids, ears, lips (cutaneous and mucosal), distal intranasal vestibule, and accessible area of the oral cavity. The central face has extensive contour variation and is often comprised of thin skin or mucosa overlying multiple tissue types and planes including muscle, cartilage, and glands. Skin cancers frequently invade these structures and planes and can cause substantial destruction. In these areas, contour variation and proximity to vital structures can make resection of recommended standard excision margins while avoiding anatomic distortion and functional compromise much more difficult. Other locations where Mohs surgery is indicated include hands, feet, digits, anogenital, and pretibial lower extremity skin. These areas share a common theme of having limited tissue reservoir available for reconstruction, and functional anatomic structures may lie more superficially below the skin.

Increased tumor size may qualify a skin malignancy for treatment with MMS because it is associated with higher risk. Increased tumor size correlates with increased risk for deeper invasion and wider subclinical extension. Based on size alone, BCC and SCC lesions greater than 2 cm in any location are appropriate to consider for treatment with MMS.

Tumors that are recurrent, ill-defined, rapidly growing, ulcerated, or associated with significant pain or paresthesia are appropriate to treat with MMS. Marjolin's ulcer, a particularly aggressive SCC forming in an area of trauma, chronic inflammation, or scar often associated with burn may also be suitable for MMS if size and degree of local extension are clinically appropriate. When very large or extending deeply, Marjolin tumors may be better managed using a multidisciplinary approach.

Clinical Features: Periorbital Considerations

Given the high-risk anatomic location, appropriate periorbital skin cancers should be considered for treatment with MMS even in tumors less than 5 mm in size. Larger appropriate tumors including those with substantial depth of soft tissue involvement or those known to approach periosteum may be effectively treated by MMS. Treatment for these tumors may be enhanced by comanagement with an oculoplastic surgeon. Periorbital tumors with bone invasion or those that have infiltrated beyond the orbital septum, which can be recognized by presence of ocular motility restriction, proptosis or computed tomography (CT) and magnetic resonance imaging (MRI) evidence of involvement of retrobulbar fat or post-septal structures, are unsuitable for MMS.

Histologic Features

MMS is suitable for tumor type that is identifiable on frozen section histology. It is most frequently used for periorbital basal cell carcinoma and squamous cell carcinoma. It has also been demonstrated to be an effective treatment for a variety of other periorbital cutaneous malignancies such as sebaceous carcinoma, microcystic adnexal carcinoma, and Merkel cell carcinoma. MMS for specific cutaneous malignancies of the periorbital area is discussed later in the chapter.

Patient Considerations

There are many patient specific variables that are valid when considering treatment with Mohs surgery. MMS is appropriate in individuals forming a larger number of skin cancers due to any cause or in those where the tumors are frequently more aggressive, placing them at increased risk for substantial tissue destruction, functional loss, and/or metastasis. Extreme environmental exposure such as overwhelmingly sun-damaged patients who continuously develop a large number of tumors are best treated with MMS. They need tissue sparing of their cutaneous "real estate" in order to facilitate resection and reconstruction at sites of their future lesions. Other environmental exposures including arsenic exposure and high non-ultraviolet radiation exposure may predispose patients to an ongoing substantial incidence of tumor formation. Chronic immunosuppression such as that medically induced in patients who have had solid organ transplants, immunosuppression resulting as a consequence of decreased native immune function notable in chronic lymphocytic leukemia and other leukemia/lymphoma, and immunosuppression were both factors may play a role such as graft-versus-host disease are appropriate to treat with MMS. Patients having genetic conditions producing a large number of skin cancers such as basal cell nevus syndrome, albinism, and xeroderma pigmentosa, qualify for treatment with MMS.

Elderly patients are more likely to have significant medical comorbidities that may place them at "high risk" for complications from general anesthesia, but they may be suitable for treatment with MMS using local anesthesia. They should be evaluated preoperatively to make sure that they are stable enough even for MMS performed in an outpatient setting. MMS is appropriate in individuals who are found to have skin cancers at a young age due to early increased ultraviolet exposure, increasing risk for more aggressive lesions such as sclerosing basal cell carcinoma and/or invasive squamous cell carcinomas as well as for forming a significantly increased number of skin cancers over their lifetimes.

Relative Contraindications to Mohs Surgery

1. Tumor that is not contiguous.
2. Tumor that is not readily identifiable in Mohs frozen sections.
3. Anatomical access is limited such as tumor locale deep beyond orbital rim.
4. Location having substantial risk for tissue fragmentation such as lacrimal crest.
5. Structure is not amenable to resection in the outpatient environment, such as tumors involving the bone or tumor within the globe.
6. Limitations of local anesthesia such as extensive tumor in low-threshold pain-sensitive patient.
7. Patient has strong psychological aversion to procedure performed under local anesthesia.
8. Advanced age or significant medical comorbidities.

Mohs Micrographic Surgery Technique

Safe and effective Mohs resection begins with a thorough preoperative patient evaluation. Vital signs, medical history including comorbidities, relevant cancer history, medications, and allergies are reviewed. Inquiry should be made about symptoms such as paresthesia, burning, numbing, and pain. Physical examination should note surface features such as ulceration or proximity to vital structures. Palpation of "Z" axis is performed, assessing for apparent depth and whether the tumor is freely mobile. The Mohs surgeon must evaluate the tumor while considering whether it is likely to be cleared with MMS in the outpatient operatory setting under local anesthesia. If there is a question of potential in transit metastasis, lymph node involvement, or involvement of deep structures, CT scan or MRI imaging is performed and additional scouting biopsies may be considered. If the periorbital lesion is extensively fixed and bound down, with a seemingly low probability for clearing with MMS, imaging is ordered and the patient is sent for consultation with an oculoplastic surgeon. When the skin tumor is extraordinarily large, fixed, and bound down to periosteum or very deep structures, or there are features that otherwise indicate it to be beyond the reach of surgery in the outpatient setting, Mohs surgery may be used to obtain a peripheral clear margin under local anesthesia and combined with subsequent oculoplastic or head and neck surgical en bloc central resection performed under general anesthesia. If the Mohs defect is anticipated to be extensive and/or the patient is deemed inappropriate for reconstruction in the outpatient setting under local anesthesia, preoperative consultation with an oculoplastic surgeon is appropriate. Mohs surgical resection can easily be coordinated with delayed oculoplastic surgery reconstruction.

If the patient and tumor are deemed appropriate for MMS following preoperative assessment, a detailed explanation of the procedure is provided. The patient is made aware of the logistics for surgical stages and reconstruction after tumor clearance. The consent is explained and signed. Preoperative prescriptions, as appropriate, are prescribed.

Correct identification of the biopsy site is essential. It is made with the patient using preoperative biopsy site photos if available. While viewing the general area in a mirror, the patient is asked to verify the proposed treatment site as correct. The clinical lesion is assessed for precise tumor marking using optimal lighting with or without wood's lamp, polarized magnification, or surgical loops. A surgical marker or gentian violet liquid is used to accurately mark the outer edge of the lesion. A 1–5-mm uninvolved margin is also precisely marked outside of the clinical tumor marking, depending on tumor type, subtype, grade, recurrence, and other features such as perineural involvement. The Mohs surgeon may choose a round, oval, or angulated geometric pattern for outer margin, depending on the size and shape of the tumor. Choice of an appropriate size, shape, and thickness of a Mohs layer that can be prepared in the Mohs frozen section histology lab can be complex, depending on the size, tumor grade, tissue involved (e.g., cartilage, mucosa, muscle, and periosteum), anatomic location, and perceived depth of tumor.

Preoperative markings may include short orientation "hash marks" that traverse the Mohs margin outlined with skin marker. The confirmed surgical site is anesthetized with local anesthesia and the patient prepped and draped in a sterile fashion.

Depending on the technique of the surgeon, the first stage of resection is performed with a varying degree of peripheral bevel ranging from 30° to 90°. The latter produces a "no bevel" Mohs layer. The outer margin "hash marks" may be scored with short superficial transverse nicks placed lightly for accurate specimen orientation. Prior to resecting the first stage, the central non-margin portion of the lesion may be surgically debulked, curetted, or treated with intraoperative relaxing incisions. These techniques assist in processing the specimen by allowing the peripheral skin edge to more freely rotate down to the level of the deep tissue plane for contiguous 100% evaluation of both the deep and peripheral margins. When performed properly, these central specimen maneuvers do not violate any of the external margins of the specimen (the key portion of the Mohs layer).

The first Mohs stage is placed on the transfer medium with appropriate annotation placed for precise specimen orientation. The transfer medium may include a photograph or drawing of the surgical anatomic location that corresponds with the same design on the Mohs map.

The transfer medium is taken to the Mohs laboratory for processing. It may be submitted as a single piece of tissue or divided into smaller sections; the sum of which will be analyzed to evaluate the complete margin. Processing is performed to allow viewing of both the entire bottom and all of the sides of the specimen. Processing may be simple or very complex, depending on the technique of the Mohs surgeon and the individual case. The advanced techniques required to process more difficult specimens are a vital part of Mohs surgery training. Improper processing of the specimen can lead to frozen sections that are impossible to evaluate or that contain substantial artifact, limiting assessment for tumor. The specimen is precisely marked with colored tissue dye to accurately maintain orientation. A precisely oriented representation of the Mohs layer is drawn on the Mohs map with the same color markings used on the specimen.

The specimen is embedded in optimal cutting temperature compound (OCT), and frozen sections are prepared. The glass slides are then stained in hematoxylin and eosin or toluidine blue. After cover slips are placed, the frozen section slides are ready for evaluation by the Mohs surgeon. Immunohistochemical frozen section staining can provide additional information in selected cases and specific tumor types.

The corresponding Mohs map for the slides evaluated is placed next to the microscope. If tumor is identified, it is precisely marked on the Mohs map and annotated for subtype and tissue depth. The patient is then anesthetized, prepped, and draped for an additional layer to resect the areas found to be positive in stage I. If, after stage I, 100% of the margin is found to be clear of tumor, the patient is notified, and reconstruction can be performed or a dressing can be placed if delayed reconstruction was planned. In our practice, each stage takes approximately 30 min.

If a second stage is required, a new transfer medium is used to transfer the second stage of resection to the laboratory. The second stage is also processed and marked with colored tissue dye. A second stage is drawn on the Mohs map to accurately document additional tissue taken in relationship to tumor-positive areas marked on stage I. Again, the identical color orientation that was applied to the second stage specimen is annotated (Fig. 27.2).

The process of evaluation of additional stages and obtaining an additional Mohs layer if the prior stage is found to be positive is repeated until all of the margins are clear of tumor. Once the site is clear of all tumors, the patient is prepared for reconstruction, delayed reconstruction, or second-intention healing. Delayed reconstruction could be in a form of patients returning on the following days or undergoing planned reconstruction by an oculoplastic surgeon. When proper patient selection and the defect size permit, Mohs surgeons commonly repair acquired defects resulting from the tumors they resect. By doing so, they provide their patients expertise in cutaneous reconstruction, efficiency of care, and the convenience of having the wound closure completed soon after tumor clearance. Identification of precancerous changes surrounding the surgical site can provide the Mohs surgeon indispensable information when selecting appropriate tissue reservoir for cutaneous restoration. When the extent of the defect is significant and beyond the scope of individual Mohs surgeon's training, referral to oculoplastic surgery is advised.

MMS and Periorbital Cutaneous Malignancy

Basal Cell Carcinoma

Basal cell carcinoma is the most common cutaneous malignancy of the periorbital area.

They occur more frequently on the lower eyelid and at the medial canthus. BCCs arising in the medial canthal region are at particular high risk for intraorbital and intracranial extension. Although smaller lesions are common, larger tumors when encountered are well suited for treatment by the Mohs technique (Fig. 27.3a–c).

A prospective series of 1295 patients with periocular BCCs showed the tumor locations were 615 (47.5%) lower eyelid, 626 (48.3%) medial canthus, and 51 (3.9%) upper eyelid. The most common histologic subtypes were nodulocystic (39.5%) and infiltrating (34.8%). Sixty-eight percent were primary and 32% were recurrent tumors. Recurrent BCCs were larger, with larger defects than primary BCCs, and had more subclinical extension. Perineural invasion was found in 1% of cases, with greater subclinical tumor extension noted [9].

For the treatment of periorbital BCCs, several different modalities have been reported. These include excision, cryotherapy, radiotherapy, and photodynamic therapy. For appropriate tumors, Mohs micrographic surgery is considered to be the most optimal treatment because MMS provides the best assurance of complete removal of the tumor and preserves the maximal amount of normal tissue. MMS is indicated as a treatment for periorbital BCC due to the increased recurrence risk at this anatomic location. Higher-risk basal cell carcinoma histologic subtypes include infiltrative, morpheaform or sclerosing, basosquamous, and micronodular. These subtypes are appropriate for treatment with MMS independent of their size and location. Perineural BCC may be a harbinger of aggressive behavior that is well-suited for treatment with MMS. When significant perineural invasion is encountered, consultation with radiation oncologist is appropriate.

Although commonly found to be less aggressive than recurrent basal cell carcinoma, ill-defined superficial BCCs of the periorbital area are also appropriate for treatment with MMS. This subtype's subclinical extension is unpredictable, and it may develop into a virtually contiguous "multifocal" pattern. Periocular basal cell carcinomas occurring in basal cell carcinoma nevus syndrome (nevoid basal cell carcinoma syndrome, Gorlin's syndrome) are another indication for Mohs surgery. These tumors commonly invade beyond clinical margins. Recurrent BCC after radiation therapy is particularly difficult to treat.

The recurrence rate for primary BCCs treated with MMS is very low, ranging from 0% to 2% [6, 10, 11]. Following the removal of periorbital tumor, the defects should be reconstructed by standard oculoplastic procedures and should be performed expeditiously. Cryotherapy might be a reasonable choice for the treatment of periocular nodular or noduloulcerative BCC in patients who are poor candidates for surgery.

Mohs in 1978 [6] reported a 5-year cure rate of 98.7% in 699 patients using the technique with zinc chloride paste fixative. The site of origin of the basal cell carcinoma was a factor in prognosis. The 5-year cure rates for upper and lower eyelids, medial and lateral canthus were 99.3%, 99.1%, 98.1%, and 92.2%, respectively. The role of previous treatments was a factor in reducing cure rates to 93.2% for 162 patients who had received previous surgical or radiation treatments versus cure rates of 99.8% in 537 patients who received no previous treatment. Dr. Mohs also showed that the cure rates decreased as the tumors increased in size. The 5-year cure rate of 31 BCCs which were 3 cm or greater in size was 81%. Later, Mohs [1] in 1986 reported 5-year cure rates of 99.4% for 1124 primary BCCs and 92.4% for 290 recurrent BCCs.

Robins et al. in 1985 [11] reported 5-year cure rates of 98.1% from 318 primary (previously untreated) lesions and

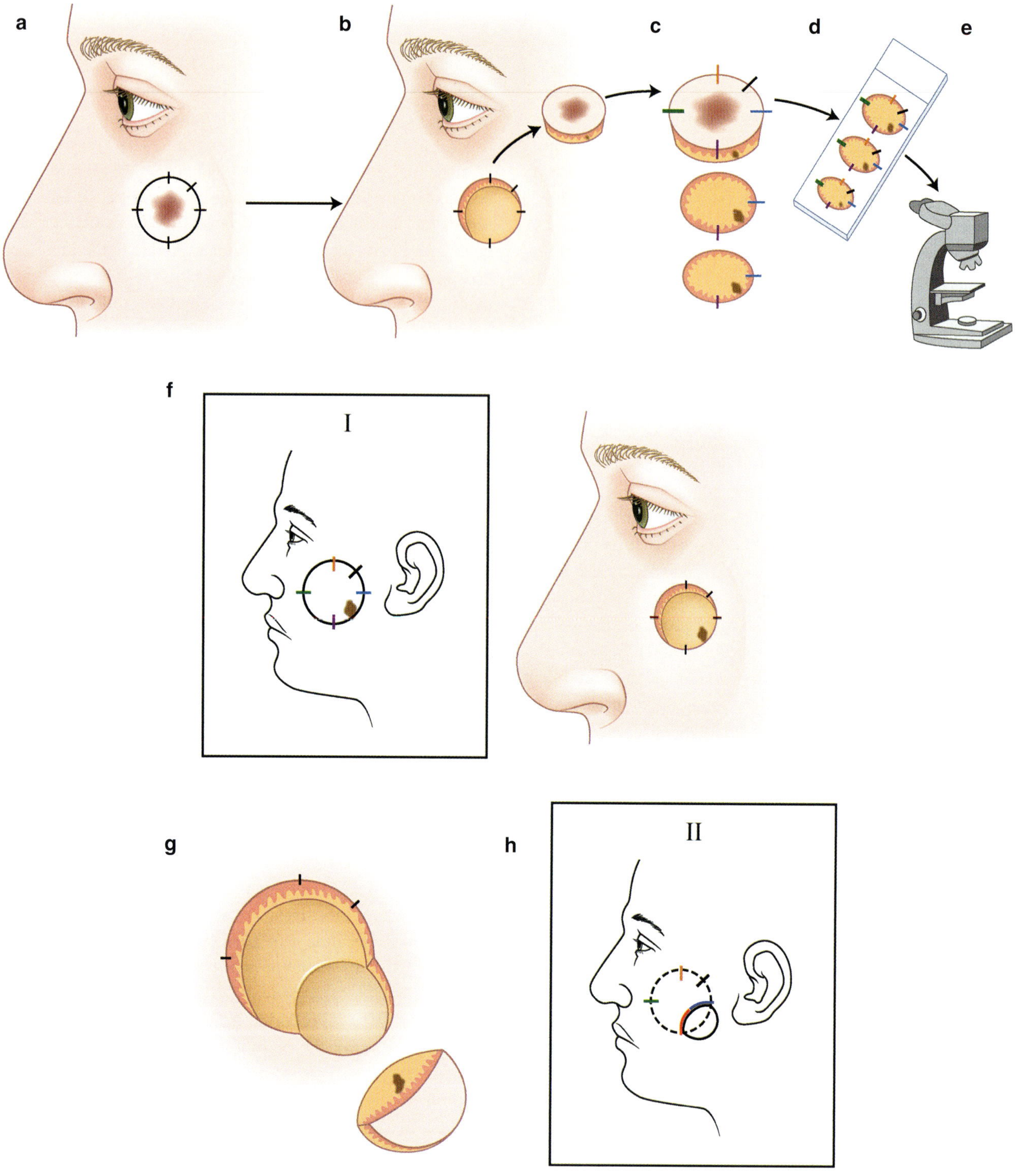

Fig. 27.2 (**a**) Plan for stage I of Mohs resection with orientation hash lines marked on patient. (**b**) Resection of Mohs stage contains both peripheral and contiguous deep margins. (**c**) The layer is "processed" in the Mohs laboratory and frozen for sectioning of both peripheral and deep margin visualized in a single view. Colored tissue dye landmarks are placed for precise specimen orientation. (**d**) Hundred percent margin evaluation sections are transferred to glass slides. (**e**) Microscopic review of frozen sections confirms tumor between colored tissue dye orientation markings. (**f**) Tumor location and depth (deep versus peripheral margins) marked on the corresponding color annotated Mohs map for stage I. (**g**) Returning to the patient with the annotated stage I Mohs map allows for precise resection of stage II tissue only in the areas of positivity. (**h**) Stage II is marked on the Mohs map with corresponding colored orientation markings. The process is repeated until all margins reported clear

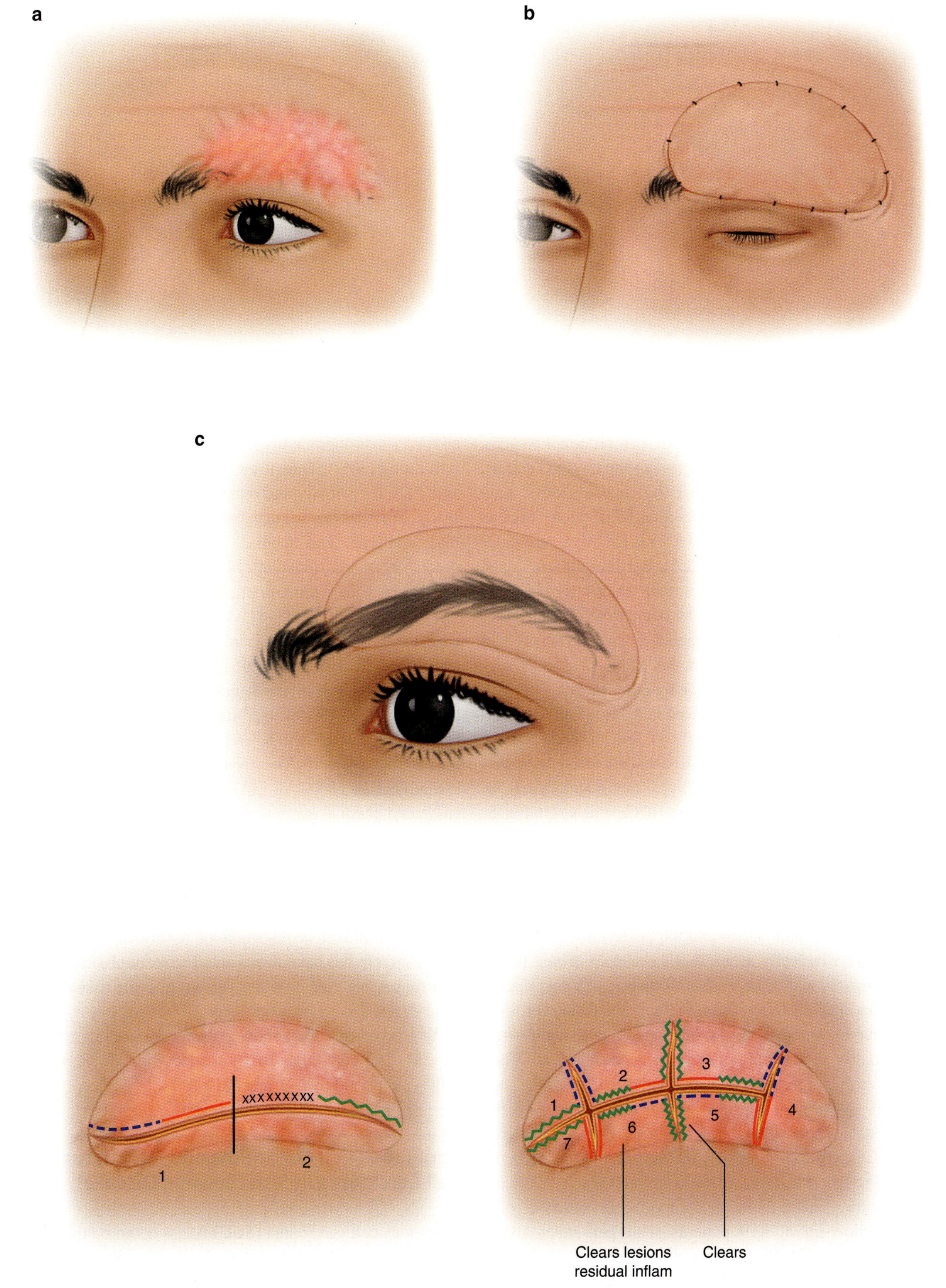

Fig. 27.3 Large, long-standing BCC. (**a**) Preop. (**b**) Mohs surgical tumor clearance in two stages, nine sections. (**c**) Mohs map with clear stage shown on the left. Patient referred for oculoplastic reconstruction

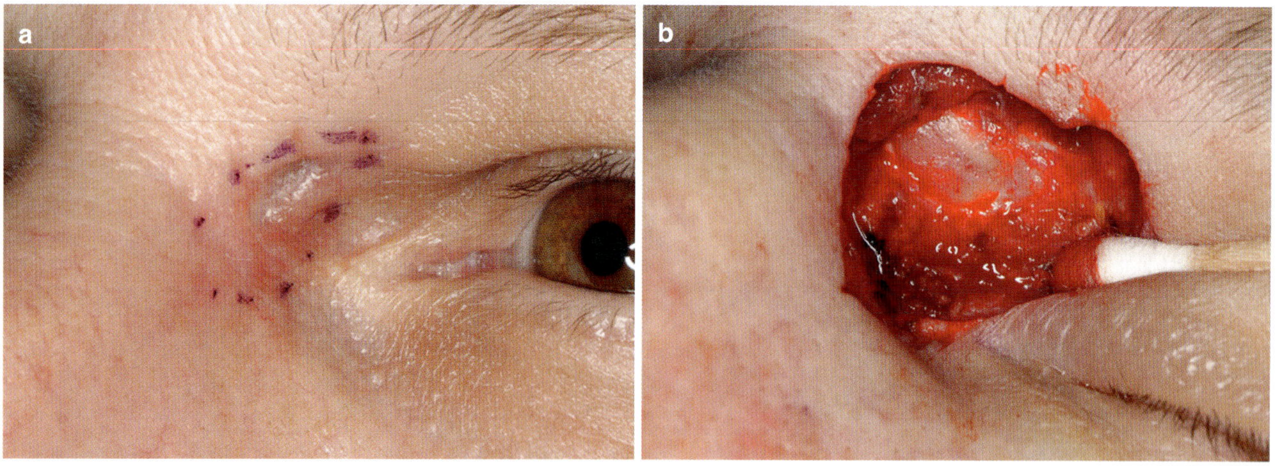

Fig. 27.4 Recurrent infiltrative BCC following multiple prior wide local excisions. (**a**) Preop. (**b**) Closeup photo showing Mohs surgical clearance after two stages, three sections with periosteal resection, and preserved medial canthal ligament. Patient referred for oculoplastic reconstruction

93.6% from 313 recurrent lesions. All recurrences of primary lesions treated by MMS were located in the medial canthus. Among lesions previously treated by methods other than Mohs surgery, the recurrence rates after MMS were twice as high for medial canthal lesions (9.5%) as for other periocular basal cell carcinomas (4.5%). There was a threefold increased risk of recurrence for medial canthal lesions (post-MMS) previously treated by radiation as compared with all other treatment modalities. This high rate of recurrence may reflect past practices of treating large medial canthal basal cell carcinomas with radiation rather than by other means.

Monheit et al. in 1989 [10] treated 283 basal cell carcinomas with a 5-year recurrence rate of less than 2%. Those cases included complex recurrent basal cell carcinomas that had previously undergone multiple treatments, such as surgical excision and radiation, and BCCs with orbital invasion. It is important to note that they point out that tumors with certain degrees of orbital invasion can be successfully resected. They reported that the globe can be salvaged even after tumors have invaded into periorbital fat, extraocular muscles, bulbar conjunctiva, and the posterior medial orbit. The authors are clearly aware that these deep orbital resections ultimately lead to peribulbar fibrosis involving muscles and fascia, and thus, compromise function. However, they argued that in such patients, limited binocular vision is a better alternative than having one eye or no vision at all. They emphasize the importance of evaluating the status of the contralateral eye when considering an exenteration. These authors stated that orbital exenteration should be considered when BCCs extends well past the equator of the globe or involves fat, muscle, bone, or walls of the globe.

Malhotra et al. [12] in 2004 reported an outcome of a 5-year follow-up of 819 patients with periocular BCCs treated with MMS. The most common locations were 257 (54%) lower eyelid and 195 (41%) medial canthus. The most common histologic subtypes were nodulocystic (43%) and infiltrating (30%). They found 5-year recurrence rates of 0% and 7.8% for primary and recurrent periocular BCC, respectively. Previous recurrence, infiltrating or superficial histologic subtype, and medial canthal site were the main predictors of recurrence after MMS. This study emphasized that MMS is the treatment of choice for periocular BCC.

Nemet et al. in 2006 [13] reviewed medical records of 469 patients with confirmed eyelid cancer treated with surgical excision with 3–5-mm clinically clear margins and histologic confirmation of the surgical margins. Frozen section histology or MMS was used for incompletely excised cases and those located in the medial canthus or close to the lacrimal drainage system. They found that excision was initially incomplete in 25.4% of all tumors. Morpheaform type of BCC and medial canthus location BCCs were associated with a higher incomplete resection rate. Twenty-seven patients (5.6%) had a recurrent tumor. After initial incomplete excision, there was no recurrence following subsequent treatment with MMS. Although the best opportunity for complete removal is resection of a surgical naive lesion, Mohs surgery has been found an effective approach to recurrent tumor and still provides opportunity for tissue sparing (Fig. 27.4a, b).

Several other studies showed the recurrence rates of 0–2% for 231–282 periocular BCCs treated with MMS, with the follow-up period of 1–9 years [14–16].

Squamous Cell Carcinoma and Squamous Cell Carcinoma In Situ (Bowen's Disease)

Squamous cell carcinoma (SCC) is less common than BCC; however, it is well known to be a generally higher-risk cutaneous malignancy when compared to BCC. It can arise de

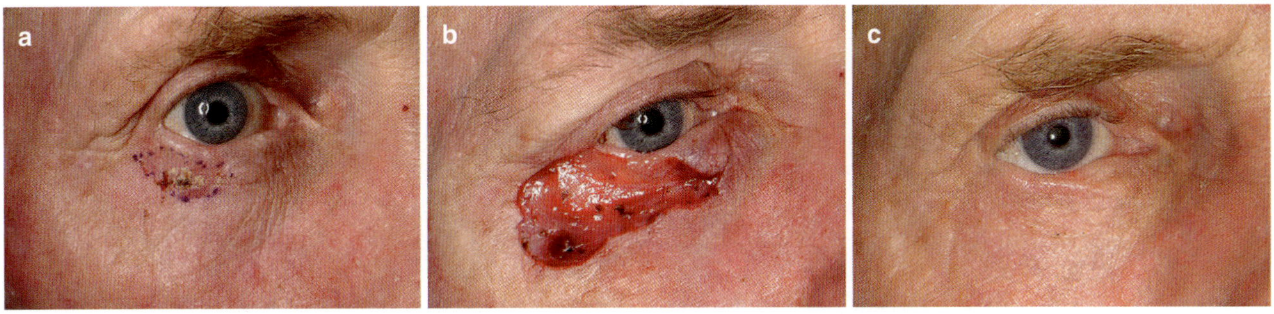

Fig. 27.5 Invasive squamous cell carcinoma. (**a**) Preop. (**b**) Clearance after three stages, six sections. (**c**) Follow-up after Mohs reconstruction, consisting of partial wound narrowing and full-thickness skin graft (Courtesy of Tri H. Nguyen, MD)

novo or from areas of actinic keratosis or Bowen's disease (squamous cell carcinoma in situ). Unlike BCC, squamous cell carcinoma has a substantial potential for metastatic spread through direct extension or indirectly via lymphatic and hematogenous routes. SCC also has a greater tendency than BCC to recur locally. MMS may be considered the treatment of choice for SCCs of the periorbital area, given this high-risk anatomic location (Fig.27.5a–c).

Keratoacanthoma is a form of well-differentiated SCC. It appears initially as a flesh-colored papule on the lower eyelid and rapidly develops into a dome-shaped nodule with elevated margins and a central crater filled with keratin. Although some clinicians believe they often resolve spontaneously, they can be very locally destructive and are appropriate for complete surgical extirpation. The preferred treatment of keratoacanthoma in the periorbital area remains MMS [17]. Although squamous cell carcinoma in situ also known as Bowen's disease may be treated with superficial destruction or topical 5-FU, in larger lesions, tumors having significant adnexal involvement or lesions involving the eyelid margin, MMS is appropriate.

Mohs [1] in 1986 reported the 5-year cure rates of 98.1% in 213 cases of squamous cell carcinoma of the eyelids. Malhotra et al. [9] in 2004 reported the prospective series of 79 periocular SCCs managed by MMS, with a median follow-up of over 7 years. The tumor locations were lower eyelid (68%), medial canthus (24%), and upper eyelid (7.6%). The most common histologic subtypes were well differentiated (48.7%) and moderately differentiated (35.1%). Seventy-three percent were primary tumors, and 27% were recurrent tumors. Three (4.3%) cases had histologically confirmed perineural invasion. A median follow-up of 73 months was available in 56 (71%) cases, of which two (3.64%) recurred. Both cases were primary, moderately differentiated SCCs. There were no recurrences for cases with perineural invasion after treatment with MMS. They demonstrated that MMS has the lowest reported recurrence rate (3.64%) of any treatment modality for periocular SCC.

Perineural infiltration facilitates spreading of SCC into the orbit, intracranial cavity, and periorbital structures along the branches of the trigeminal nerve, the facial nerve, and the ocular motor nerves [18]. Faustina et al. [19] retrospectively reviewed 111 patients with SCCs of eyelids and periocular skin. They reported an incidence of regional lymph node metastasis of 24.3%, a 6.2% risk of distant metastasis, and an 8.1% risk of perineural invasion. Postoperative adjuvant radiation therapy is recommended for lesions with perineural invasion to decrease the risk of local recurrence.

In addition to clinical features of large size, recurrent tumor and high-risk location, characteristics of SCC that increase risk for metastasis include moderately and poorly differentiated tumor, deeply invasive lesion, perineural or perivascular involvement, acantholytic subtype, desmoplastic tumor, and tumor with spindle cell features.

The most common site for squamous cell carcinoma in situ (SCC in situ) was the lower eyelid (51%), followed by the medial canthus [20, 21]. Periocular SCC in situ seems to carry a high risk of incomplete excision and recurrence due to the anatomy of the eyelid, with numerous eyelash follicles and pilosebaceous structures extending into deeper structures including the tarsal plate. The role of MMS for SCC in situ is supported by the significant subclinical tumor extension seen in 25% of cases in one series [21]. This study found a recurrence rate of 5.3% (1 of 19) for primary periocular SCC in situ and 11.8% (2 of 17) for recurrent periocular SCC in situ treated with MMS [21]. Recurrent SCC in situ may represent a greater likelihood of skip lesions being present within the tumor. These skip areas are commonly seen and may remain undetected even with treatment by MMS technique [22].

Sebaceous Carcinoma

Sebaceous carcinoma (SC) is a relatively rare and aggressive tumor found most commonly on the eyelids of patients with advanced age [23]. Other areas of the head and neck can also be involved (Fig. 27.6a–f). Sebaceous carcinoma commonly arises from the meibomian glands of the eyelids and other sebaceous glands of the ocular adnexa. It can

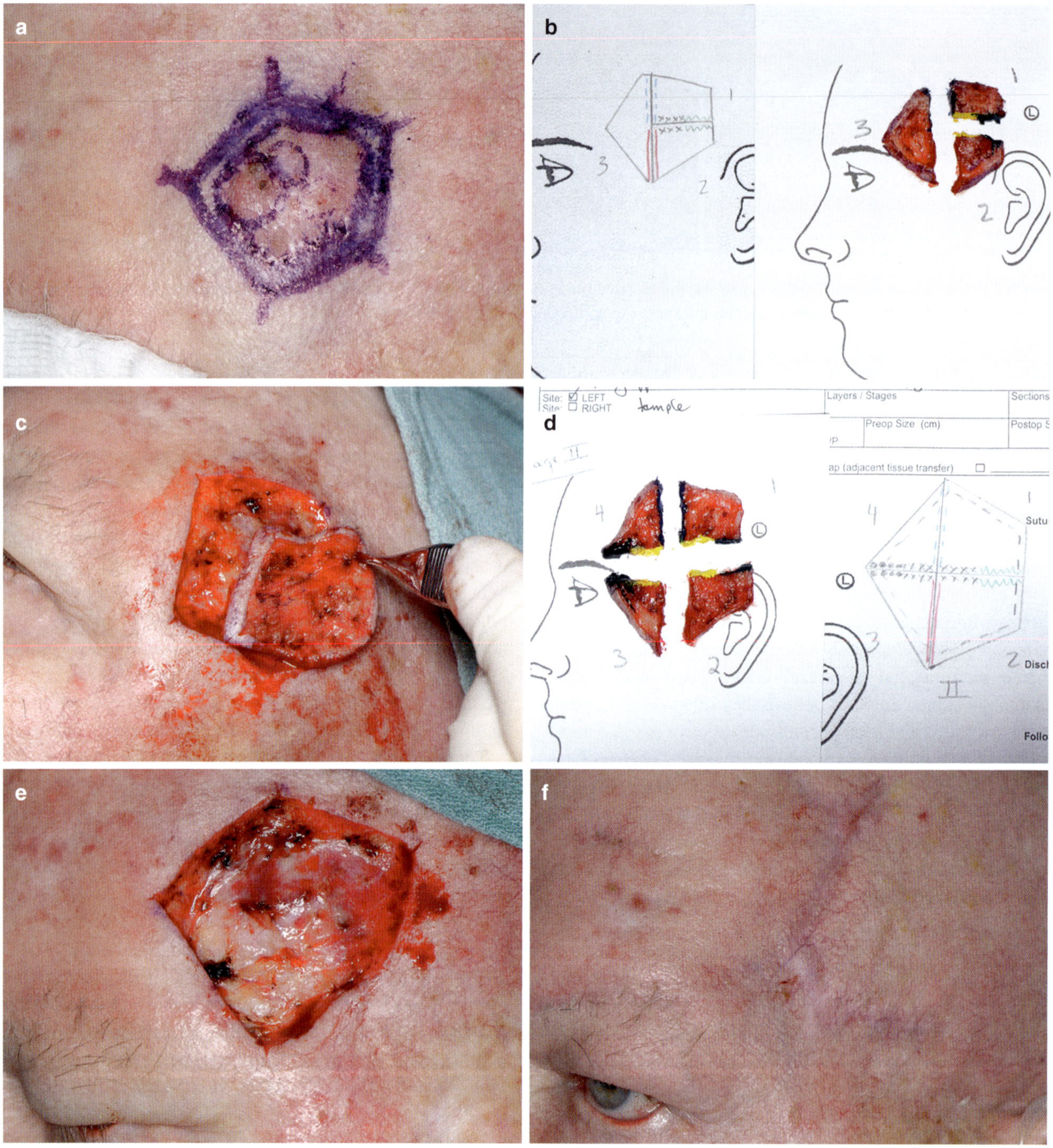

Fig. 27.6 Sebaceous carcinoma. (**a**) Angulated plan for Mohs stage I. (**b**) Sectioned and inked Mohs stage I on tissue transfer card annotated on matching Mohs map. (**c**) Mohs stage II resection. (**d**) Mohs stage II sectioned for processing and inked on transfer card with corresponding map. (**e**) Mohs surgical clearance after three stages, eight sections. (**f**) Three months following Mohs reconstruction

present initially as a painless yellowish to pink papule or nodule that may be mistaken for chalazion, blepharitis, or conjunctivitis. Muir–Torre syndrome should be considered in patients with this finding. SC may be basaloid or squamous and therefore can be misdiagnosed as BCC or SCC. Regional lymph node metastasis is estimated to be 17–30% [24, 25], and when lymph node metastasis is present, the 5-year survival rate is estimated to be 50% [26]. Distant metastasis to muscle, liver, spleen, viscera, and the brain is less frequent and has a dismal 5-year survival rate [27]. Correct early diagnosis with complete surgical extirpation within the first 6 months correlates with a much more favorable prognosis. Sebaceous carcinomas tend to have an intraepithelial growth phase (pagetoid spread), which may extend over the palpebral and bulbar conjunctiva. Intraepithelial conjunctival extension has been reported to be present in 44–80% of patients with sebaceous gland carcinoma, and the epithelium of the conjunctiva can display multifocal involvement with skip areas [28]. Chao et al. evaluated outcomes of 25 patients with eyelid sebaceous gland carcinoma with and without conjunctival intraepithelial (pagetoid) invasion. Local recurrences and distant metastases of the tumor have been reported to be similar in both groups. Orbital invasion was found in 36% of tumors with intraepithelial invasion compared with 7% of tumors without invasion, suggesting that when it is present, intraepithelial involvement is a risk factor for more invasive behavior of the tumor and subsequent orbital exenteration [29].

Although the most common location of sebaceous carcinoma is the upper eyelid, this tumor has a potential for multifocal organization, making any method of surgical resection more challenging. One report found multifocal disease in 6% of cases reviewed [30]. Intraepithelial (pagetoid) spread was found in 50% of the cases (24 of 48) reviewed [30]. Some authors advocate combining conjunctival map biopsies with MMS to track pagetoid conjunctival spread, that an additional layer of MMS be performed beyond the stage appearing to clear the tumor, and/or that tissue be submitted for paraffin sections as confirmation of negative margins [24, 31–34]. Recurrence rates with MMS have been reported to be approximately 11–12% [25, 30, 33, 35, 36]. Close collaboration with oculoplastic and head and neck surgeons can be key in coordinating a multidisciplinary approach to treatment. Adjuvant-controlled cryotherapy to treat conjunctival extension, radiotherapy, chemotherapy, and lymph node dissection has been used in conjunction with MMS as well as WLE. Radiotherapy and treatment with electron beam may be ineffective [24, 37]. Topical mitomycin-C treatment of intraepithelial neoplasia involving the conjunctiva may play a role in temporizing local recurrence from pagetoid intraepithelial spread of sebaceous carcinoma [38–40]. Meticulous and frequent postsurgical patient follow-up is essential to identify local recurrences early. Recent reports have suggested that sentinel lymph node biopsy may be effective at identifying early microscopic nodal metastasis in patients with sebaceous carcinoma of the eyelid [41].

Merkel Cell Carcinoma

Merkel cell carcinoma (MC) is a rare and highly malignant tumor which frequently forms in sun-exposed areas. In MC patients having periorbital tumors, the upper eyelids are more commonly involved. The tumor shows a rapid growth pattern to a significant size (>10 mm) within 2–3 months. It tends to recur locally and develop regional nodal metastasis in 30–50% of patients. Location on the head and neck is associated with a worse prognosis, and local recurrence after surgery is high [42, 43]. A review of 86 patients by O'Connor et al. [44] reported the marginal persistent rate in 12 patients who underwent MMS to be 8.3% and 31.7% in 41 patients who had WLE. Regional lymph node metastasis in 45 patients who had MMS followed for 27.8 months was 15.6%. In 102 patients who underwent WLE followed for 35 months, metastasis to regional lymph node was 39.2%. Management of MC may be enhanced by a multidisciplinary approach. MMS or WLE may be combined with sentinel lymph node biopsy (SLNB) with complete lymph node dissection (CLND) if positive, chemotherapy, and postoperative radiation.

In a study of 122 patients with no nodal disease found by physical examination, sentinel lymph node biopsy revealed occult nodal involvement in 32% of cases. The recurrence rate for patients with a positive lymph node biopsy proved to be three times higher, and for these patients, adjuvant nodal therapy significantly improved the prognosis [45]. The authors conclude that SLNB is important for both prognosis and therapy and should be performed routinely for patients with MC. Even though use of SLNB/CLND has been reported in combination with MMS, it has not been found consistently beneficial. At our center, patients with Merkel cell carcinoma of eyelid are recommended to have postoperative adjuvant radiation therapy to the local surgical site and either prophylactic radiation therapy to the regional lymph nodes or sentinel lymph node biopsy to map out which regional nodal basins to treat with radiation therapy. For lesions greater than 2 cm in size, consideration is also given to adjuvant systemic chemotherapy.

A literature review on 1254 patients with Merkel cell carcinomas affecting the head and neck region indicated that surgery plus local adjuvant irradiation was associated with significantly lower rates of local and regional recurrence of MC than surgery alone even in presence of free surgical margins [46]. Lawenda et al. reviewed effect of radiation therapy for the control of Merkel cell carcinoma of the head and neck based on 36 cases [47]. They reported that there is no long-term evidence of increased survival rates with postoperative radiation even though it seems to be helpful in improving local control.

Microcystic Adnexal Carcinoma

Microcystic adnexal carcinoma (MAC) also called sclerosing sweat duct carcinoma is a less frequently encountered, very invasive facial malignancy that clinically is often poorly defined and may be difficult to diagnose. The subclinical extent of the tumor is frequently found to be far beyond that of initial impression and may be the cause of the higher rate of recurrence with wide local excision (Fig. 27.7a–d). One

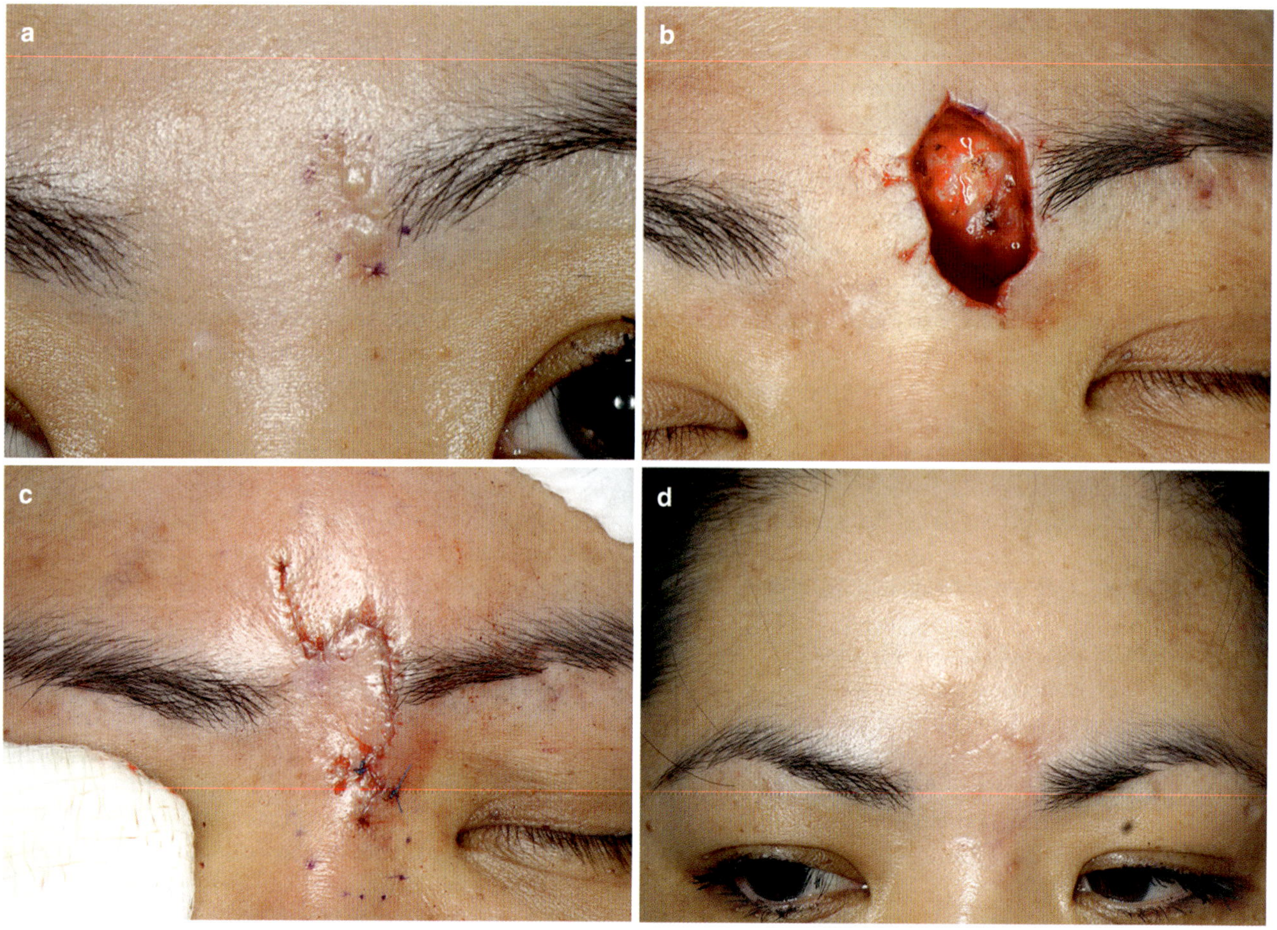

Fig. 27.7 Microcystic adnexal carcinoma. (**a**) Preop. (**b**) Mohs surgical clearance after two stages, three sections. (**c**) Immediate Mohs reconstruction. (**d**) Four months postoperatively (Courtesy of Tri H. Nguyen, MD)

study found it is misdiagnosed in 30% of cases and that treating these skin cancers with MMS to track tumor extension resulted in a mean defect four times the size of the initial lesion measurement [48]. Perineural invasion is often encountered. This locally aggressive but usually slow-growing tumor has a predilection for perioral, periocular, perinasal, or scalp tissue. Metastasis is rare. Local excision has an approximately 50% recurrence rate, and MMS has been reported to have an approximately 5–10% recurrence rate [48, 49]. Due to the poorly defined nature of this disease, mapped scouting biopsies prior to treatment may provide a better starting point for the first stage of MMS. Mohs surgery is a treatment of choice. Tumor with deep subcutaneous extension beyond the reach of Mohs surgery is appropriate for additional wide local excision. Confirmatory paraffin sections or immunohistochemistry may enhance the Mohs surgical outcome. Some have advocated subsequent wider excision followed with delay repair when paraffin sections and immunohistochemistry confirm clearance of tumor because of the aggressive infiltrative nature of MAC. When MAC infiltrates in the orbital fat or when perineural orbital involvement is detected, orbital exenteration may be required. Radiotherapy may be considered in cases with multiple recurrences and presence of perineural invasion.

Melanoma In Situ and Invasive Malignant Melanoma

Although the topic remains controversial, treatment of invasive malignant melanoma (MM) and melanoma in situ (MIS) with MMS has been reported to be effective in multiple published case series. These include a 15-year pivotal study by Zitelli et al. that compared treatment of 553 primary stage I melanomas including 369 invasive tumors with MMS to historical data of 15,798 melanomas treated by WLE [50]. The first stage of MMS was taken with a 6-mm margin. In this study, treatment with MMS had a very low 0.5% overall local recurrence rate and a 1.2% local recurrence rate on the head, neck, hands, and feet. After stratification by Breslow depth into five groups, the metastasis and 5-year survival rates of the MMS groups were either equivalent to or better than those in the WLE group. The majority of melanomas were completely excised using 6-mm margins (83%) and 95% with margins less than 1 cm regardless of Breslow thickness identified on skin biopsy. A significant finding was that most of the cases requiring greater than 1-cm margins for clearance were with melanoma found on the head, neck, hands, and feet (5%). A compelling argument made by the authors is that standard margins do not account for unpredictable subclinical extension of tumor and in many cases are either too large or too small. Their conviction in using MMS to treat melanoma is based on confidence that complete removal of the primary lesion provides the highest cure rate together with the greatest tissue sparing as reported in their study. They do not agree that adding additional margin to include possible local micrometastasis in the excision provides benefit because the presence of micrometastasis is associated with a worse prognosis that is not improved by performing a larger local resection. If it did, they reason that their study would not have shown a lower 5-year recurrence rate with MMS than with WLE. The authors acknowledge that the results are dependent on the Mohs surgeon's experience as well as maintaining the highest standards of tissue processing in the Mohs histology laboratory. This study was followed by a 2006 case series of 202 melanomas including 69 invasive tumors reported in the Journal of Surgical Oncology by Temple and Arlett [51]. This 9-year review of melanoma treated with MMS using an initial 5-mm margin supported the conclusions of the prior larger study. The authors found zero recurrences over a mean follow-up of 29.8 months. Studies have reported that lentigo maligna (LM, melanoma in situ occurring in sun-damaged skin), which is notorious for frequently having ill-defined clinical margins and higher local recurrence rates, may be better suited for treatment with MMS, particularly in anatomically sensitive locations [52–54].

Surgical excision with margin control has been employed for melanoma of the head and neck, including periocular melanoma, in order to maximize the cure rate and minimize postoperative morbidity by sparing normal tissue [55–63]. Margin-control options include traditional MMS with frozen sections with or without immunostains, and MMS with paraffin-embedded tissue sections. These variations of MMS techniques are to accommodate better visualization of melanocytes. Published reports using these MMS with or without modifications have shown lower recurrence rates than with standard surgical excision. Margin-control surgery uniformly offers lower local recurrence rates for head and neck MM and MIS, ranging from 0% to 5% after 2–5 years [51, 53, 55, 64, 65].

One surgical excision technique that may be appropriate for eyelid melanomas is the use of overnight, "rush," permanent paraffin-embedded tissue sections combined with traditional Mohs mapping and en face mounting to achieve both better visualization of melanocytes and 100% margin control [52, 66, 67]. In one study [61], 29 patients with periocular MM and MIS were followed after they were treated with a staged, modified Mohs excision technique with rush permanent, paraffin-embedded tissue sections. The recurrence rate for primary tumors was 5%, with the follow-up period of greater than 5 years. Still others prefer the "square technique" of staged excision with en face permanent section evaluation of the margins prior to delayed resection of the central portion of the lesion once the margins are proven clear over either MMS or standard WLE for treating LM [24, 68]. Demirci et al. [69] in 2008 evaluated the outcome of the "square procedure," a multidisciplinary, staged excision technique using standard formalin-fixed, vertically oriented sections for 40 patients with periocular MM and MIS. The recurrence was observed in 2.5% of patients at 8 months after the square procedure, and a Kaplan–Meier survival curve estimated a local recurrence rate of 2.5% at 8 years.

Mapped serial excision uses vertical sections obtained through "bread loafing," with serial sections at 1–2-mm intervals or radial sections at 1-mm intervals. Although greater attention is given to tumor margins with mapped serial excision, the main disadvantage is that it fails to evaluate 100% of the margin.

The use of MMS with frozen sections is controversial because of the difficulty in distinguishing residual MIS from background atypical melanocytic hyperplasia at tumor margins on sun-damaged skin. Physicians who do not recommend MMS for treating melanoma argue that there are no prospective studies showing its efficacy, that MM and MIS are not easy to visualize on frozen sections, and that current standard margins for WLE appear to provide effective treatment in most cases. Some argue that in MM and MIS, the tumor architecture is best visualized in cross-sectioned tissue like in the case of WLE. Proponents of MMS treatment for MM and MIS argue that the highest-quality thin Mohs frozen sections provide better histology than commonly produced with standard frozen sections. They believe that together with the addition of MART-1 and other immunostains, there is excellent frozen section visualization of MM/MIS. Rapid immunostaining on frozen section can be achieved in 16–20 min [70, 71]. Although immunostains may help identify melanocytes at tumor margins, no test can reliably distinguish benign from malignant melanocytes. The identification of positive or negative margins is still subject to some degree of interpretation.

Though the American Academy of Dermatology and the National Institutes of Health have acknowledged the potential benefits of MMS in treating melanoma [50, 72, 73], additional studies including prospective trials with more than 5-year follow-up period may help address the ongoing controversy over its use in these diagnoses. To provide optimal treatment, treatment of malignant melanoma of the eyelids and periocular region should be pursued using a multidisciplinary approach. Sentinel lymph node biopsy as well as work-up for systemic disease should be considered. For locally advanced disease with orbital involvement, an orbital exenteration may be indicated.

Summary

MMS has become a preferred treatment for many skin cancers of periorbital area such as BCC and SCC. The role of MMS for melanomas is controversial, and its use in Merkel cell carcinomas is less well-established. MMS adheres to the three core treatment goals, because it has the highest 5-year cure rate. Keeping the margins appropriately narrow when 100% of the excisional contact area is meticulously evaluated provides two additional key benefits. MMS preserves more normal tissue, lowering risk of functional loss, and decreasing postoperative surgical morbidity. With a smaller resulting defect, there is less extensive reconstruction required, improving the opportunity for optimal functional and aesthetic restoration. The periorbital area contains a number of vital structures which are adjacent to each other, such as skin, conjunctiva, eyelash, sebaceous glands, lacrimal ducts, and glands. Preservation of adjacent normal tissue to the tumor in this area is vital in order to maintain function and cosmesis of orbital structures.

MMS is a detailed time-consuming process that is indicated for appropriate higher-risk cutaneous malignancies. These higher-risk skin cancers include those where Mohs surgery can access the entire contiguous tumor and the tumor threatens extensive tissue loss or functional impairment, disfigurement, recurrence, or development of metastatic extension. If indicated, MMS may be followed with other treatment modalities such as radiation, chemotherapy, and targeted biologic therapy.

The team efforts of the Mohs surgeon working in conjunction with oculoplastic surgeons and other medical and surgical specialists have greatly enhanced the complete cycle of the patient's care by optimizing cure rates, functionality, and cosmetic appearance.

References

1. Mohs FE. Micrographic surgery for the microscopically controlled excision of eyelid cancers. Arch Ophthalmol. 1986;104(6):901–9.
2. Menn H, Robins P, Kopf AW, Bart RS. The recurrent basal cell epithelioma. A study of 100 cases of recurrent, re-treated basal cell epitheliomas. Arch Dermatol. 1971;103(6):628–31.
3. Kumar B, Roden D, Vinciullo C, Elliott T. A review of 24 cases of Mohs surgery and ophthalmic plastic reconstruction. Aust N Z J Ophthalmol. 1997;25(4):289–93.
4. Brodland DG, Amonette R, Hanke CW, Robins P. The history and evolution of Mohs micrographic surgery. Dermatol Surg. 2000;26(4):303–7.
5. Baylis HI, Cies WA. Complications of Mohs' chemosurgical excision of eyelid and canthal tumors. Am J Ophthalmol. 1975;80(1):116–22.
6. Mohs F. Chemosurgery: microscopically controlled surgery for skin cancer. Thomas: Springfield; 1978.
7. Drake LA, Dinehart SM, Goltz RW, et al. Guidelines of care for Mohs micrographic surgery. American Academy of Dermatology. J Am Acad Dermatol. 1995;33(2 Pt 1):271–8.
8. Minton TJ. Contemporary Mohs surgery applications. Curr Opin Otolaryngol Head Neck Surg. 2008;16(4):376–80.
9. Malhotra R, Huilgol SC, Huynh NT, Selva D. The Australian Mohs database, part I: periocular basal cell carcinoma experience over 7 years. Ophthalmology. 2004;111(4):624–30.
10. Monheit GD, Callahan MA, Callahan A. Mohs micrographic surgery for periorbital skin cancer. Dermatol Clin. 1989;7(4):677–97.
11. Robins P, Rodriguez-Sains R, Rabinovitz H, Rigel D. Mohs surgery for periocular basal cell carcinomas. J Dermatol Surg Oncol. 1985;11(12):1203–7.
12. Malhotra R, Huilgol SC, Huynh NT, Selva D. The Australian Mohs database, part II: periocular basal cell carcinoma outcome at 5-year follow-up. Ophthalmology. 2004;111(4):631–6.
13. Nemet AY, Deckel Y, Martin PA, et al. Management of periocular basal and squamous cell carcinoma: a series of 485 cases. Am J Ophthalmol. 2006;142(2):293–7.
14. Miller PK, Roenigk RK, Brodland DG, Randle HW. Cutaneous micrographic surgery: Mohs procedure. Mayo Clin Proc. 1992;67(10):971–80.
15. Arlette JP, Carruthers A, Threlfall WJ, Warshawski LM. Basal cell carcinoma of the periocular region. J Cutan Med Surg. 1998;2(4):205–8.
16. Callahan A, Monheit GD, Callahan MA. Cancer excision from eyelids and ocular adnexa: the Mohs fresh tissue technique and reconstruction. CA Cancer J Clin. 1982;32(6):322–9.
17. Donaldson MJ, Sullivan TJ, Whitehead KJ, Williamson RM. Periocular keratoacanthoma: clinical features, pathology, and management. Ophthalmology. 2003;110(7):1403–7.
18. Cottel WI. Perineural invasion by squamous-cell carcinoma. J Dermatol Surg Oncol. 1982;8(7):589–600.
19. Faustina M, Diba R, Ahmadi MA, Esmaeli B. Patterns of regional and distant metastasis in patients with eyelid and periocular squamous cell carcinoma. Ophthalmology. 2004;111(10):1930–2.
20. Sullivan TJ, Boulton JE, Whitehead KJ. Intraepidermal carcinoma of the eyelid. Clin Exp Ophthalmol. 2002;30(1):23–7.
21. Malhotra R, James CL, Selva D, Huynh N, Huilgol SC. The Australian Mohs database: periocular squamous intraepidermal carcinoma. Ophthalmology. 2004;111(10):1925–9.
22. Smith KJ, Skelton HG, Holland TT. Recent advances and controversies concerning adnexal neoplasms. Dermatol Clin. 1992;10(1):117–60.
23. Dasgupta T, Wilson LD, Yu JB. A retrospective review of 1349 cases of sebaceous carcinoma. Cancer. 2009;115(1):158–65.
24. Cook BE Jr, Bartley GB. Treatment options and future prospects for the management of eyelid malignancies: an evidence-based update. Ophthalmology. 2001;108(11):2088–98; quiz 2099–2100, 2121.
25. Ratz JL, Luu-Duong S, Kulwin DR. Sebaceous carcinoma of the eyelid treated with Mohs' surgery. J Am Acad Dermatol. 1986;14(4):668–73.
26. O'Neal ML, Brunson A, Spadafora J. Ocular sebaceous carcinoma: case report and review of the literature. Compr Ther. 2001;27(2):144–7.

27. Husain A, Blumenschein G, Esmaeli B. Treatment and outcomes for metastatic sebaceous cell carcinoma of the eyelid. Int J Dermatol. 2008;47(3):276–9.
28. Rao NA, Hidayat AA, McLean IW, Zimmerman LE. Sebaceous carcinomas of the ocular adnexa: a clinicopathologic study of 104 cases, with five-year follow-up data. Hum Pathol. 1982;13(2): 113–22.
29. Chao AN, Shields CL, Krema H, Shields JA. Outcome of patients with periocular sebaceous gland carcinoma with and without conjunctival intraepithelial invasion. Ophthalmology. 2001;108(10):1877–83.
30. Snow SN, Larson PO, Lucarelli MJ, Lemke BN, Madjar DD. Sebaceous carcinoma of the eyelids treated by Mohs micrographic surgery: report of nine cases with review of the literature. Dermatol Surg. 2002;28(7):623–31.
31. Arora A, Barlow RJ, Williamson JM, Olver JM. Eyelid sebaceous gland carcinoma (SGC) treated with 'slow' Mohs' micrographic surgery. Eye (Lond). 2004;18(8):854–5.
32. Yount AB, Bylund D, Pratt SG, Greenway HT. Mohs micrographic excision of sebaceous carcinoma of the eyelids. J Dermatol Surg Oncol. 1994;20(8):523–9.
33. Dzubow LM. Sebaceous carcinoma of the eyelid: treatment with Mohs surgery. J Dermatol Surg Oncol. 1985;11(1):40–4.
34. Putterman AM. Conjunctival map biopsy to determine pagetoid spread. Am J Ophthalmol. 1986;102(1):87–90.
35. Spencer JM, Nossa R, Tse DT, Sequeira M. Sebaceous carcinoma of the eyelid treated with Mohs micrographic surgery. J Am Acad Dermatol. 2001;44(6):1004–9.
36. Dixon RS, Mikhail GR, Slater HC. Sebaceous carcinoma of the eyelid. J Am Acad Dermatol. 1980;3(3):241–3.
37. Rigel DS. Cancer of the skin. Philadelphia: Elsevier Saunders; 2005. p. 277–88.
38. Rudkin AK, Muecke JS. Mitomycin-C as adjuvant therapy in the treatment of sebaceous gland carcinoma in high-risk locations. Clin Exp Ophthalmol. 2009;37(4):352–6.
39. Tumuluri K, Kourt G, Martin P. Mitomycin C in sebaceous gland carcinoma with pagetoid spread. Br J Ophthalmol. 2004;88(5): 718–9.
40. Shields CL, Naseripour M, Shields JA, Eagle RC Jr. Topical mitomycin-C for pagetoid invasion of the conjunctiva by eyelid sebaceous gland carcinoma. Ophthalmology. 2002;109(11):2129–33.
41. Savar A, Oellers P, Myers J, et al. Positive sentinel node in sebaceous carcinoma of the eyelid. Ophthal Plast Reconstr Surg. 2011;27(1):e4–6.
42. Kivela T, Tarkkanen A. The Merkel cell and associated neoplasms in the eyelids and periocular region. Surv Ophthalmol. 1990;35(3):171–87.
43. Rubsamen PE, Tanenbaum M, Grove AS, Gould E. Merkel cell carcinoma of the eyelid and periocular tissues. Am J Ophthalmol. 1992;113(6):674–80.
44. O'Connor WJ, Roenigk RK, Brodland DG. Merkel cell carcinoma. Comparison of Mohs micrographic surgery and wide excision in eighty-six patients. Dermatol Surg. 1997;23(10):929–33.
45. Gupta SG, Wang LC, Penas PF, Gellenthin M, Lee SJ, Nghiem P. Sentinel lymph node biopsy for evaluation and treatment of patients with Merkel cell carcinoma: the Dana-Farber experience and meta-analysis of the literature. Arch Dermatol. 2006;142(6):685–90.
46. Lewis KG, Weinstock MA, Weaver AL, Otley CC. Adjuvant local irradiation for Merkel cell carcinoma. Arch Dermatol. 2006;142(6):693–700.
47. Lawenda BD, Arnold MG, Tokarz VA, et al. Analysis of radiation therapy for the control of Merkel cell carcinoma of the head and neck based on 36 cases and a literature review. Ear Nose Throat J. 2008;87(11):634–43.
48. Chiller K, Passaro D, Scheuller M, Singer M, McCalmont T, Grekin RC. Microcystic adnexal carcinoma: forty-eight cases, their treatment, and their outcome. Arch Dermatol. 2000;136(11):1355–9.
49. Snow S, Madjar DD, Hardy S, et al. Microcystic adnexal carcinoma: report of 13 cases and review of the literature. Dermatol Surg. 2001;27(4):401–8.
50. Zitelli JA, Brown C, Hanusa BH. Mohs micrographic surgery for the treatment of primary cutaneous melanoma. J Am Acad Dermatol. 1997;37(2 Pt 1):236–45.
51. Temple CL, Arlette JP. Mohs micrographic surgery in the treatment of lentigo maligna and melanoma. J Surg Oncol. 2006;94(4):287–92.
52. Cohen LM, McCall MW, Zax RH. Mohs micrographic surgery for lentigo maligna and lentigo maligna melanoma. A follow-up study. Dermatol Surg. 1998;24(6):673–7.
53. Cohen LM, McCall MW, Hodge SJ, Freedman JD, Callen JP, Zax RH. Successful treatment of lentigo maligna and lentigo maligna melanoma with Mohs' micrographic surgery aided by rush permanent sections. Cancer. 1994;73(12):2964–70.
54. Zitelli JA. Mohs surgery for lentigo maligna. Arch Dermatol. 1991;127(11):1729–30.
55. McKenna JK, Florell SR, Goldman GD, Bowen GM. Lentigo maligna/lentigo maligna melanoma: current state of diagnosis and treatment. Dermatol Surg. 2006;32(4):493–504.
56. Vaziri M, Buffam FV, Martinka M, Oryschak A, Dhaliwal H, White VA. Clinicopathologic features and behavior of cutaneous eyelid melanoma. Ophthalmology. 2002;109(5):901–8.
57. Tahery DP, Goldberg R, Moy RL. Malignant melanoma of the eyelid. A report of eight cases and a review of the literature. J Am Acad Dermatol. 1992;27(1):17–21.
58. Garner A, Koornneef L, Levene A, Collin JR. Malignant melanoma of the eyelid skin: histopathology and behaviour. Br J Ophthalmol. 1985;69(3):180–6.
59. Esmaeli B, Wang B, Deavers M, et al. Prognostic factors for survival in malignant melanoma of the eyelid skin. Ophthal Plast Reconstr Surg. 2000;16(4):250–7.
60. Agarwal-Antal N, Bowen GM, Gerwels JW. Histologic evaluation of lentigo maligna with permanent sections: implications regarding current guidelines. J Am Acad Dermatol. 2002;47(5):743–8.
61. Shumaker PR, Kelley B, Swann MH, Greenway HT Jr. Modified Mohs micrographic surgery for periocular melanoma and melanoma in situ: long-term experience at Scripps Clinic. Dermatol Surg. 2009;35(8):1263–70.
62. Malhotra R, Chen C, Huilgol SC, Hill DC, Selva D. Mapped serial excision for periocular lentigo maligna and lentigo maligna melanoma. Ophthalmology. 2003;110(10):2011–8.
63. Kimyai-Asadi A, Katz T, Goldberg LH, et al. Margin involvement after the excision of melanoma in situ: the need for complete en face examination of the surgical margins. Dermatol Surg. 2007;33(12):1434–9; discussion 1439–1441.
64. Bub JL, Berg D, Slee A, Odland PB. Management of lentigo maligna and lentigo maligna melanoma with staged excision: a 5-year follow-up. Arch Dermatol. 2004;140(5):552–8.
65. Zitelli JA, Moy RL, Abell E. The reliability of frozen sections in the evaluation of surgical margins for melanoma. J Am Acad Dermatol. 1991;24(1):102–6.
66. Dhawan SS, Wolf DJ, Rabinovitz HS, Poulos E. Lentigo maligna. The use of rush permanent sections in therapy. Arch Dermatol. 1990;126(7):928–30.
67. Zalla MJ, Lim KK, Dicaudo DJ, Gagnot MM. Mohs micrographic excision of melanoma using immunostains. Dermatol Surg. 2000;26(8):771–84.
68. Johnson TM, Headington JT, Baker SR, Lowe L. Usefulness of the staged excision for lentigo maligna and lentigo maligna melanoma: the "square" procedure. J Am Acad Dermatol. 1997;37(5 Pt 1):758–64.

69. Demirci H, Johnson TM, Frueh BR, Musch DC, Fullen DR, Nelson CC. Management of periocular cutaneous melanoma with a staged excision technique and permanent sections the square procedure. Ophthalmology. 2008;115(12):2295–300. e2293
70. Chang KH, Finn DT, Lee D, Bhawan J, Dallal GE, Rogers GS. Novel 16-minute technique for evaluating melanoma resection margins during Mohs surgery. J Am Acad Dermatol. 2011;64(1): 107–12.
71. Kimyai-Asadi A, Ayala GB, Goldberg LH, Vujevich J, Jih MH. The 20-minute rapid MART-1 immunostain for malignant melanoma frozen sections. Dermatol Surg. 2008;34(4):498–500.
72. Committee on Guidelines of Care. Task Force on Malignant Melanoma. Guidelines of care for malignant melanoma. J Am Acad Dermatol. 1993;28(4):638–41.
73. NIH Consensus conference. Diagnosis and treatment of early melanoma. JAMA. 1992;268(10):1314–9.

Sentinel Lymph Node Biopsy for Conjunctival and Eyelid Tumors

28

Aaron Savar and Bita Esmaeli

Introduction

For conjunctival and eyelid tumors, as for solid tumors at other anatomic sites, the status of the regional lymph nodes is an important prognostic factor. Elective regional lymph node dissection is not normally performed for ocular tumors and has not proven to be beneficial for other head and neck skin cancers. Sentinel lymph node biopsy (SLNB) offers a minimally invasive way to get information about the regional lymph nodes without having to do a standard complete lymph node dissection. In this chapter, we discuss the rationale for and history of SLNB and then turn to the use of SLNB in the management of conjunctival and eyelid tumors.

Sentinel Lymph Node Biopsy

Cancers can metastasize via both blood vessels and lymphatics. In certain cancers, lymphatic spread is observed before hematogenous spread. Sentinel lymph node biopsy (SLNB) is a procedure to identify and remove the first draining lymph node, or sentinel lymph node (SLN), for a tumor in a patient without clinical evidence of regional lymph node metastasis. SLNB is performed by injecting a tracer into the tissue surrounding a tumor, detecting uptake of the tracer in the regional lymph nodes, and then removing the first draining lymph node along each lymphatic pathway leading away from the tumor. The tracer is either a dye, which allows visual identification of the first draining lymph node, or a radiolabeled molecule such as technetium-labeled sulfur colloid, which is taken up by lymph nodes and can be detected using a gamma probe.

The histologic status of the SLN provides important prognostic information and can guide treatment. If the SLN is histologically negative, there is a low likelihood of disease being present in that nodal basin. If the SLN is positive, the patient has microscopic regional lymph node metastasis and further treatment is needed. Ideally, SLNB can allow for identification of microscopic disease within the lymph nodes that develops before hematogenous seeding develops. SLNB allows for early detection of microscopic metastases that would otherwise be detected by clinical or radiologic examination much later, perhaps after the development of distant metastases, or at a stage when many additional lymph nodes may also be involved increasing the risk of recurrence and death. SLNB also allows for better selection of patients who would benefit from more invasive procedures, such as more extensive lymphadenectomy, or additional treatment of regional lymph nodes with radiation.

SLNB was first described by Morton et al. for use in patients with skin melanoma [1] and then by Krag et al. for use in patients with breast cancer [2]. It has become a standard part of the management of these cancers and has also been used in a variety of other malignancies, including Merkel cell carcinoma, squamous cell carcinoma, thyroid cancer, gastrointestinal cancers, and gynecologic cancers. In 2008, the International Sentinel Node Society issued a consensus statement on the use of SLNB for cutaneous melanoma [3]. They recommended SLNB in patients with a greater than 10% risk of nodal metastasis if the procedure could provide useful prognostic information or the results would be helpful in planning further treatment [3].

There are opponents of SLNB who believe that microscopic metastases detected by SLNB are not clinically significant and may never progress to advanced disease [4]. Indeed, whether or not micrometastases would progress to advanced disease may be difficult to prove in a prospective trial, but clinical experience suggests that microscopic

A. Savar
Stein Eye Institute, UCLA, Department of Ophthalmology, Los Angeles, CA, USA

B. Esmaeli (✉)
Orbital Oncology & Ophthalmic Plastic Surgery, Department of Plastic Surgery, MD Anderson Cancer Center, Houston, TX, USA
e-mail: besmaeli@mdanderson.org

J. J. Servat et al. (eds.), *Smith and Nesi's Ophthalmic Plastic and Reconstructive Surgery*,
https://doi.org/10.1007/978-3-030-41720-8_28

metastasis, if untreated, likely will lead to overt extensive clinically detectable metastatic disease eventually. A growing body of data supports the concept that SLNB provides important prognostic information and facilitates decision-making about treatment [3, 5]. A randomized prospective trial of SLNB in patients with intermediate-thickness melanoma, the Multicenter Selective Lymphadenectomy Trial, compared wide local excision plus observation to wide local excision plus SLNB [5]. Patients in the observation group underwent complete lymph node dissection if nodal disease became clinically apparent. Patients in the SLNB group without a positive SLN received no further surgery; those with a positive SLN underwent immediate complete lymph node dissection. Although this trial did not show an overall survival benefit in the SLNB group, it did provide strong evidence that SLNB can provide useful prognostic information and guide treatment. It also showed a survival benefit for the subset of patients who had a positive SLN and underwent immediate complete lymph node dissection compared to the subset of patients in the observation arm who were found to have lymph node metastases by traditional methods (clinical examination) (hazard ratio for death, 0.51; P = 0.004) [5].

SLNB for Conjunctival and Eyelid Tumors

The use of SLNB in the periocular region was first reported in 2001 [6, 7]. We have since studied SLNB for tumors of the conjunctiva and eyelid as part of prospective Institutional Review Board approved trials at The University of Texas MD Anderson Cancer Center [8–16]. Additional reviews and studies have supported the use of SLNB for selected conjunctival and eyelid conditions [17–20].

Our Experience to Date: Feasibility, Safety, and False-Negative Rate

We have demonstrated that SLNB is feasible for conjunctival and eyelid tumors with only minor adaptation of the technique used for skin or breast tumors [7–10]. We have further demonstrated that SLNB is associated with minimal risk (discussed in more detail in the section Risks below) [15, 16]. We have also provided proof of the principle that microscopically positive SLNs can be identified in patients with conjunctival melanoma (both bulbar and palpebral conjunctival tumors) [7, 11, 12], eyelid melanoma [12], eyelid Merkel cell carcinoma [13], and eyelid sebaceous carcinoma [11, 14]. In 2009, we published results of a prospective nonrandomized trial in which 30 patients with conjunctival or eyelid melanoma underwent SLNB and were then followed up clinically for a median of 24 months [12]. An SLN was identified in all 30 patients (100% identification rate). In many patients, more than one SLN was identified (median 2, range 1–5). Five patients had SLNs that were positive (16% positivity rate). There were two false-negative events (6%). The overall SLN positivity rate in our report was similar to the reported positivity rates for intermediate-thickness cutaneous melanomas. The false-negative event rate was slightly higher than the rate reported for cutaneous melanoma of the extremities in the Multicenter Selective Lymphadenectomy Trial (3.3%) [5] and rates previously reported for head and neck melanomas (2–5.9%) [21, 22].

In appropriately selected patients, a negative SLNB result should provide reassurance that the tumor has not metastasized to the lymph nodes. However, because false-negative events do occur, ongoing surveillance is necessary.

If microscopic metastases are found in an SLN, additional treatment is recommended. Usually this consists of additional lymphadenectomy, including parotidectomy and complete neck dissection. In some patients, including those with multiple positive nodes or with extracapsular extension based on evaluation of the lymphadenectomy specimens, irradiation of the nodal basin may also be appropriate. Furthermore, in patients with melanoma or Merkel cell carcinoma of the conjunctiva or eyelid who have lymph node metastases identified, systemic treatments can be considered – e.g., chemotherapy, immunotherapy, and vaccine trials.

Technique

Lymphatics of the periocular region can drain to the preauricular, submandibular, and cervical regions, all of which are potential sites for regional lymph node metastasis [23]. Therefore, before SLNB for a conjunctival or eyelid tumor, lymphoscintigraphy is performed to identify the location of the SLN [22]. A radioactive tracer is injected in the subconjunctival space for conjunctival tumors (Fig. 28.1) and intradermally in the eyelid skin for eyelid tumors. In some centers,

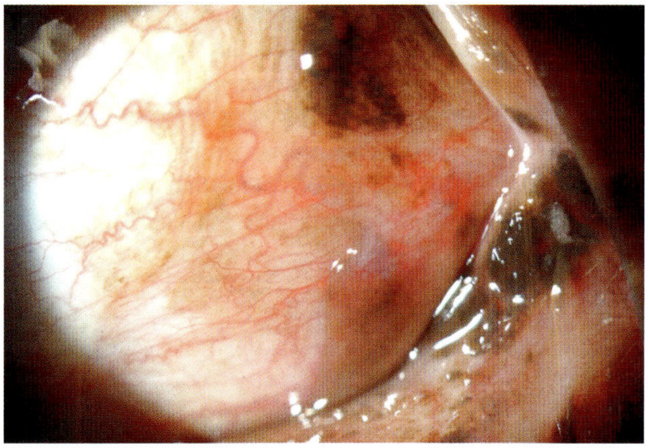

Fig. 28.1 Conjunctival melanoma involving the caruncle, with histologic tumor thickness of 5 mm and evidence of ulceration. This patient underwent SLNB at the time of surgical resection of his conjunctival melanoma and had a histologically positive sentinel node

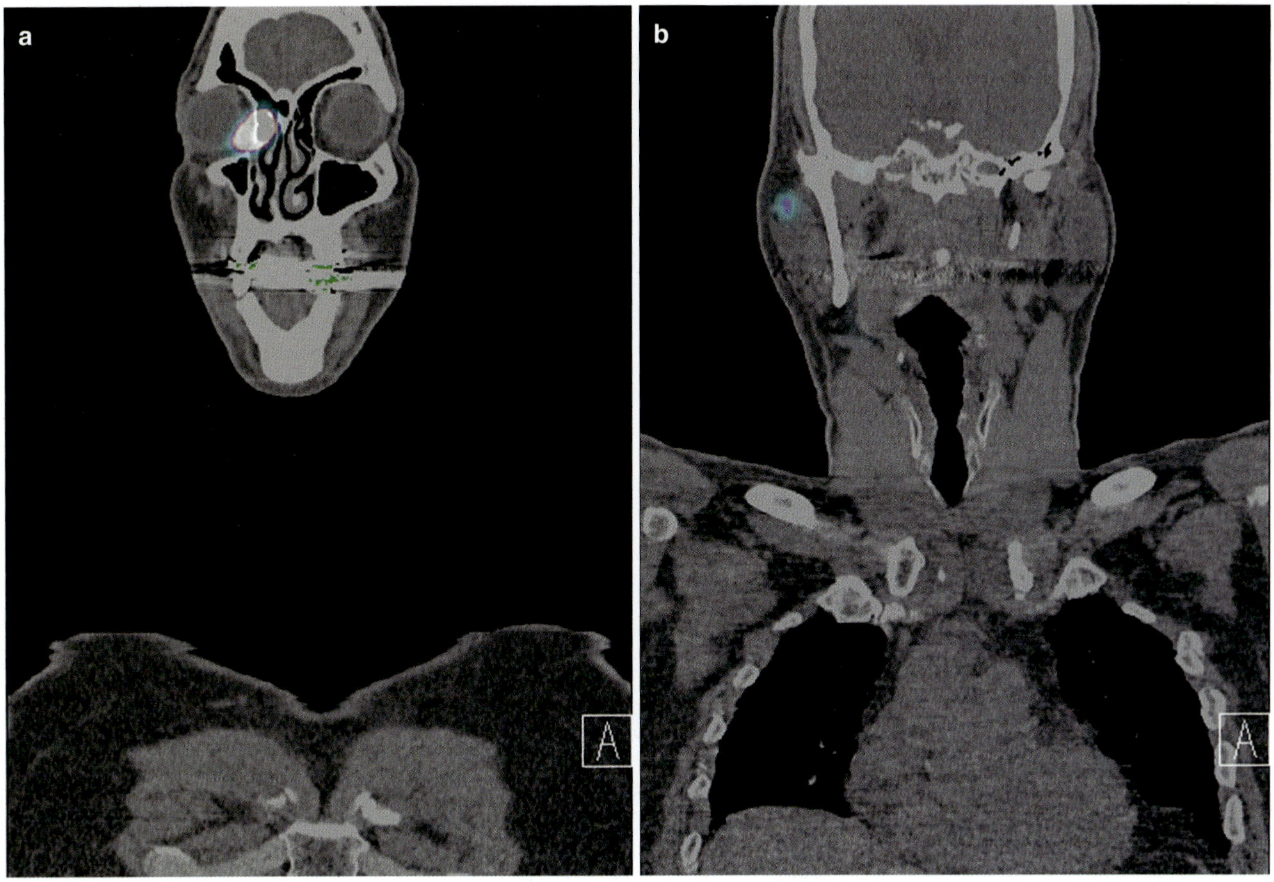

Fig. 28.2 SPECT/CT scan of the patient in Fig. 28.1 demonstrates the area of injection of tracer in the caruncle (**a**) and nodal uptake of tracer in the parotid region (**b**)

in addition to standard lymphoscintigraphy, single photon emission computed tomography/computed tomography (SPECT/CT) is being performed. SPECT/CT can offer higher resolution and better localization of the SLN (Fig. 28.2). As part of the multidisciplinary team required for SLNB, a nuclear medicine physician familiar with SLNB is needed to help with interpretation of preoperative lymphoscintigraphy.

The timing of SLNB varies, but the procedure is ideally done at the time of tumor excision or as soon as possible afterward. Roughly 1 h prior to surgery, the tumor bed is infiltrated with 0.2 ml (0.3 mCi) of technetium-99 m sulfur colloid, which is injected in the subconjunctival space for conjunctival tumors and intradermally in the eyelid skin for eyelid tumors. Lymph nodes in which the radiotracer has accumulated are identified transcutaneously using a hand-held gamma probe [7, 9, 10]. In the first 16 patients with conjunctival or eyelid tumors who had SLNB at MD Anderson, we also injected blue dye in the tumor bed. However, in these 16 patients, none of the SLNs identified on the basis of technetium uptake and use of a gamma probe were blue, even though some of these SLNs were microscopically positive [16]. We concluded that addition of the blue dye as a tracer is probably not necessary and does not improve detection capabilities over and above those with technetium alone. Thus, we stopped using blue dye after these first 16 patients. Likely explanations for the SLNs not being blue include the small volume of dye that was injected in the subconjunctival space or eyelid skin and rapid rate of transit of the blue dye in the head and neck region. In these 16 patients in whom blue dye was used, we did not encounter any cases of permanent discoloration of the conjunctiva or eyelid skin or any cases of anaphylactic shock in reaction to the blue dye [7, 11, 16].

For conjunctival and eyelid tumors, it is best for the technetium to be injected by an ophthalmologist familiar with subconjunctival injection techniques or intradermal injection close to the globe. This is an important modification of the standard procedure for SLNB for tumors at other anatomic sites, which often involves injection of the tracer by a nurse or technician in the Nuclear Medicine Department. For the safety reasons discussed later in this chapter, special training in handling of radioactive tracers is necessary for all health-care professionals who are involved in injection or handling of radiotracers.

During the SLN biopsy procedure, through a small incision in the overlying skin, the SLNs are removed and handed off to the pathologist to be processed, as described in the next section. In our hands, SLNB adds approximately 30–90 min of surgical time. It is best done at the time of surgical excision of the primary conjunctival or eyelid tumor, but we have shown that it can also successfully identify a positive SLN even if the primary tumor has previously been removed [24]. We prefer to perform SLNB with a multidisciplinary surgical team that includes the ophthalmic surgeon and either a surgical oncologist or a head and neck surgeon with extensive experience with SLNB and knowledge of the lymphatic anatomy in the head and neck region.

Evaluation of SLNs

Evaluation of SLNs requires an experienced pathologist familiar with bread-loafing and special histologic evaluation of SLNs and analyzing such specimens. Prieto and Clark described the technique used at MD Anderson in assessing SLNs for melanoma [25]. This involves cutting the nodes perpendicularly to the long axis into slices 1–2 mm thick ("bread-loafing") and then placing the resulting slices into tissue cassettes. A hematoxylin-eosin (H&E)-stained section is reviewed from each of these cassettes. This initial review of H&E-stained sections identifies metastatic cells in 15% of SLN specimens for intermediate-thickness cutaneous melanomas and in about the same percentage of SLN specimens for ocular adnexal melanomas. If no melanoma is identified on review of a first H&E-stained section, additional sections are reviewed, both with H&E staining and for immunohistochemical markers, including HMB-45, anti-MART1, and anti-tyrosinase. The addition of this step identifies nodal metastases in 3% to 5% of patients in whom nodal metastases were not initially identified on H&E [25]. For carcinomas, such as eyelid sebaceous carcinoma or Merkel cell carcinoma, if the H&E-stained sections are negative, immunohistochemical staining with cytokeratin is done to further identify lymph node metastasis.

Risks

Although SLNB is performed via a small incision overlying the SLN, injury to nerves or vessels is a risk. For conjunctival and eyelid tumors, the facial nerve is at risk given that the majority of tumors drain to the parotid region. In our experience, however, the risk of damage to the facial nerve is negligible when the procedure is done by experienced surgeons. In over 50 patients with conjunctival or eyelid tumors who underwent SLNB at MD Anderson, only two patients developed temporary weakness of the marginal mandibular branch of the facial nerve. Both cases resolved spontaneously and did not require any additional intervention [11, 12].

There is also a theoretical risk of harm from exposure to radiation during lymphatic mapping. Both the patient and members of the health-care team, including operating room and pathology staff, could be at risk. We specifically estimated radiation exposure for patients with conjunctival and eyelid tumors and found the amount of radiation to be well below the dose that may cause cataracts [23, 26] and less than one-tenth the dose that would cause more serious ocular damage, such as radiation retinopathy or optic neuropathy. Exposure to radiation during lymphatic mapping and SLNB has also been examined for breast cancer. Law et al. found that the effective radiation dose for the patient was roughly equal to that from one to five chest radiographs, depending on the protocol followed [27]. Law et al. also examined the radiation exposure of health-care workers and found that a surgeon would have to perform 2000 SLNB procedures to reach the recommended limit for occupational radiation exposure in a year [27].

Indications

The indications for SLNB in patients with ocular adnexal tumors are in evolution. Patients with clinical or radiographic evidence of metastasis should not undergo SLNB as the presence of metastatic nodal disease is already known. In all patients with conjunctival and eyelid tumors who are being considered for SLNB, we advocate computed tomography and ultrasonography of the regional lymph nodes, and only if these imaging tests are negative do we consider performing SLNB.

Among patients with eyelid or conjunctival melanoma, performing SLNB in a patient with in situ disease would have a very low yield and would put the patient at risk for complications related to facial or neck surgery. The melanoma patients most likely to benefit from SLNB are those with eyelid melanomas of intermediate-thickness tumors (greater than 1.5 mm Breslow thickness), or high-risk histologic features, such as ulceration. For conjunctival melanomas, several studies suggest a cutoff point of 2 mm tumor thickness as a reasonable criterion for selecting patients for SLNB [12, 28]. In addition, we have found that histologic ulceration is a risk factor associated with more aggressive tumors and SLN positivity [12, 29]; thus, patients with conjunctival melanoma who have ulceration identified on evaluation of the surgical specimen should also be considered for SLNB [12, 28].

SLNB has been advocated for Merkel cell carcinoma at various anatomic sites, including the eyelid [13, 30–32]. The overall lymph node positivity rate for Merkel cell carcinomas in various locations is greater than 30%, which provides a compelling argument for SLNB for Merkel cell carcinoma. However, some authorities advocate prophylactic irradiation of the regional lymph nodes at risk instead of SLNB in patients with Merkel cell carcinoma because of the high risk of nodal metastasis and because Merkel cell carcinoma is thought to be particularly radiosensitive. Radiation therapy is also used as adjuvant therapy for the primary tumor bed at most centers, even in light of negative surgical resection margins.

SLNB for other eyelid tumors, such as sebaceous carcinoma, is still considered investigational. At MD Anderson, we have been able to successfully identify microscopically positive SLNs in patients with eyelid sebaceous carcinoma [14]. In a cohort of 50 patients with eyelid sebaceous carcinoma treated at MD Anderson, our observations suggested that eyelid sebaceous carcinomas that are T2b or greater according to the seventh edition of the American Joint Committee on Cancer staging system are more likely to be associated with regional lymph node metastasis [33].

Future Directions

There is a need to more clearly define which histologic features correlate with positive SLNs in patients with tumors of the conjunctiva and eyelid. Future studies should focus on analyzing such features in large cohorts of patients. More widespread use of SLNB for ocular adnexal tumors through multi-institutional collaborations will most likely lead to better patient selection and higher yields and possibly lower false-negative rates through improved techniques and greater surgeon experience.

Tracers used for identifying SLNs have evolved over time, and new targeted tracers are becoming available. ^{99}mTc-diethylenetriaminepentaacetic acid-mannosyl-dextran (^{99}mTc-DTPA-mannosyl-dextran; Lymphoseek) is a new tracer designed for rapid clearance from the injection site. It contains a mannose moiety that is bound selectively by lymphoid tissue. Because of this feature, ^{99}mTc-DTPA-mannosyl-dextran is more likely than ^{99}mTc sulfur colloid to stay in the first draining node and not accumulate in distal nodes [34]. ^{99}mTc-DTPA-mannosyl-dextran has been evaluated for use in SLNB for melanoma and breast cancer [35, 36].

Conclusion

SLNB for tumors of the conjunctiva and eyelid is feasible and relatively safe. It can successfully identify regional lymph nodes that harbor microscopic disease that would otherwise go undetected. It makes treatment of lymph node metastases possible earlier in the course of disease. SLNB should be considered for the following ocular adnexal tumors: conjunctival melanomas with greater than 2 mm tumor thickness and/or histologic evidence of ulceration, for eyelid melanomas of intermediate thickness (>1.5 mm Breslow thickness) or evidence of ulceration, for eyelid Merkel cell carcinoma, and for sebaceous carcinomas of the eyelid that are greater than T2b according to the seventh edition of the American Joint Commission on Cancer staging system. SLNB requires a multidisciplinary team including an ophthalmic surgeon, a surgical oncologist or head and neck surgeon with extensive experience with SLNB and familiarity with lymphatics in the head and neck region, an experienced pathologist familiar with bread-loafing and special histologic evaluation of SLNs, and a nuclear medicine physician to help with interpretation of preoperative lymphoscintigraphy and administration of the radioactive tracers. As experience with SLNB for ocular adnexal tumors grows, this procedure is likely to become part of the management of patients with tumors of the ocular adnexa that have high-risk clinical and histologic features predictive of a positive SLN.

References

1. Morton DL, Wen DR, Wong JH, et al. Technical details of intraoperative lymphatic mapping for early stage melanoma. Arch Surg. 1992;127(4):392–29.
2. Krag DN, Weaver DL, Alex JC, Fairbank JT. Surgical resection and radiolocalization of the sentinel lymph node in breast cancer using a gamma probe. Surg Oncol. 1993;2(6):335–9.
3. Balch CM, Morton DL, Gershenwald JE, et al. Sentinel node biopsy and standard of care for melanoma. J Am Acad Dermatol. 2009;60(5):872–5.
4. Thomas JM. Prognostic false-positivity of the sentinel node in melanoma. Nat Clin Pract Oncol. 2008;5(1):18–23.
5. Morton DL, Thompson JF, Cochran AJ, et al. Sentinel-node biopsy or nodal observation in melanoma. N Engl J Med. 2006;355(13):1307–17.
6. Wilson MW, Fleming JC, Fleming RM, Haik BG. Sentinel node biopsy for orbital and ocular adnexal tumors. Ophthal Plast Reconstr Surg. 2001;17(5):338–44.
7. Esmaeli B, Eicher S, Popp J, et al. Sentinel lymph node biopsy for conjunctival melanoma. Ophthal Plast Reconstr Surg. 2001;17(6):436–42.
8. Esmaeli B. Sentinel lymph node mapping for patients with cutaneous and conjunctival malignant melanoma. Ophthal Plast Reconstr Surg. 2000;16(3):170–2.
9. Esmaeli B. Sentinel node biopsy as a tool for accurate staging of eyelid and conjunctival malignancies. Curr Opin Ophthalmol. 2002;13(5):317–23.
10. Esmaeli B. Advances in the management of malignant eyelid tumors: the role of sentinel node biopsy. Int Ophthalmol Clin. 2002;42(2):151–62.
11. Ho VH, Ross MI, Prieto VG, et al. Sentinel lymph node biopsy for sebaceous cell carcinoma and melanoma of the ocular adnexa. Arch Otolaryngol Head Neck Surg. 2007;133(8):820–6.
12. Savar A, Ross MI, Prieto VG, et al. Sentinel lymph node biopsy for ocular adnexal melanoma: experience in 30 patients. Ophthalmology. 2009;116(11):2217–23.
13. Esmaeli B, Naderi A, Hidaji L, et al. Merkel cell carcinoma of the eyelid with a positive sentinel node. Arch Ophthalmol. 2002;120(5):646–8.

14. Savar A, Oellers P, Myers J, Prieto VG, Torres-Cabala C, Frank SJ, Ivan D, Esmaeli B. Positive sentinel node in sebaceous carcinoma of the eyelid. Ophthal Plast Reconstr Surg. 2011;27(1):e4–6.
15. Amato M, Esmaeli B, Ahmadi MA, et al. Feasibility of preoperative lymphoscintigraphy for identification of sentinel lymph nodes in patients with conjunctival and periocular skin malignancies. Ophthal Plast Reconstr Surg. 2003;19:102–6.
16. Nijhawan N, Ross MI, Diba R, Ahmadi MA, Esmaeli B. Experience with sentinel lymph node biopsy for eyelid and conjunctival malignancies at a cancer center. Ophthal Plast Reconstr Surg. 2004;20(4):291–5.
17. Ling J, Tauscher R, Mehta V, Zhang M, Daniels A, Kohanim S. The role of sentinel lymph node biopsy in the management of conjunctival melanoma. Int Ophthalmol Clin. 2017;57(1):87–101.
18. Pfeiffer ML, Ozgur OK, Myers JN, et al. Sentinel lymph node biopsy for ocular adnexal melanoma. Acta Ophthalmol. 2017;95(4):e323–8.
19. Vora GK, Demirci H, Marr B, Mruthyunjaya P. Advances in the management of conjunctival melanoma. Surv Ophthalmol. 2017;62(1):26–42.
20. Campbell AA, Grob SR, Freitag SK. Controversies in sentinel lymph node biopsy for ocular neoplasms. Int Ophthalmol Clin. 2015;55(4):73–9.
21. Agnese DM, Maupin R, Tillman B, Pozderac RD, Magro C, Walker MJ. Head and neck melanoma in the sentinel lymph node era. Arch Otolaryngol Head Neck Surg. 2007;133(11):1121–4.
22. Gomez-Rivera F, Santillan A, McMurphey AB, Paraskevopoulos G, Roberts DB, Prieto VG, et al. Sentinel node biopsy in patients with cutaneous melanoma of the head and neck: recurrence and survival study. Head Neck. 2008;30(10):1284–94.
23. Esmaeli B, Wang X, Youssef A, Gershenwald JE. Patterns of regional and distant metastasis in patients with conjunctival melanoma: experience at a cancer center over four decades. Ophthalmology. 2001;108(11):2101–5.
24. Esmaeli B, Reifler D, Prieto VG, et al. Conjunctival melanoma with a positive sentinel lymph node. Arch Ophthalmol. 2003;121(12):1779–83.
25. Prieto VG, Clark SH. Processing of sentinel lymph nodes for detection of metastatic melanoma. Ann Diagn Pathol. 2002;6(4):257–64.
26. Henk JM, Whitelocke RA, Warrington AP, et al. Radiation dose to the lens and cataract formation. Int J Radiat Oncol Biol Phys. 1993;25:815–20.
27. Law M, Chow LW, Kwong A, Lam CK. Sentinel lymph node technique for breast cancer: radiation safety issues. Semin Oncol. 2004;31(3):298–303.
28. Tuomaala S, Kivelä T. Metastatic pattern and survival in disseminated conjunctival melanoma: implications for sentinel lymph node biopsy. Ophthalmology. 2004;111(4):816–21.
29. Savar A, Esmaeli B, Ho H, Liu S, Prieto VG. Conjunctival melanoma: local-regional control rates, and impact of high-risk histopathologic features. J Cutan Pathol. 2011;38:18–24.
30. Mehrany K, Otley CC, Weenig RH, et al. A meta-analysis of the prognostic significance of sentinel lymph node status in Merkel cell carcinoma. Dermatol Surg. 2002;28(2):113–7.
31. Ruan JH, Reeves M. A Merkel cell carcinoma treatment algorithm. Arch Surg. 2009;144(6):582–5.
32. Herbert HM, Sun MT, Selva D, et al. Merkel cell carcinoma of the eyelid: management and prognosis. JAMA Ophthalmol. 2014 Feb;132(2):197–204.
33. Esmaeli B, Nasser QJ, Cruz H, Fellman M, Warneki CL, Ivan D. American Joint Committee on Cancer T category for eyelid sebaceous carcinoma correlates with nodal metastasis and survival. Ophthalmology. 2012 May;119(5):1078–82.
34. Vera DR, Wallace AM, Hoh CK, Mattrey RF. A synthetic macromolecule for sentinel node detection: (99 m)Tc-DTPA-mannosyl-dextran. J Nucl Med. 2001;42(6):951–9.
35. Wallace AM, Hoh CK, Ellner SJ, et al. Lymphoseek: a molecular imaging agent for melanoma sentinel lymph node mapping. Ann Surg Oncol. 2007;14(2):913–21.
36. Wallace AM, Hoh CK, Darrah DD, et al. Sentinel lymph node mapping of breast cancer via intradermal administration of Lymphoseek. Nucl Med Biol. 2007;34(7):849–53.

Oculoplastic Complications of Cancer Therapy

29

Michael A. Connor and Bita Esmaeli

Introduction

Many modalities exist for cancer therapy, and like most medical interventions, cancer therapies can produce side effects and complications. Ultimately, the goal in treating cancer is to prolong survival, and side effects are often unavoidable. Careful individualized planning is required to limit the risks and side effects of cancer treatment. The incidence and severity of side effects depend on the treatment method and on individual patient characteristics; for a given treatment, the incidence and severity of side effects can vary widely among patients [1].

Localized treatments, such as surgical excision and radiation therapy, as well as systemic treatments, such as chemotherapy, can all lead to ocular and oculoplastic complications. Oculoplastic complications of cancer therapy may be a result of direct cellular damage, as from radiation therapy, or a result of biochemical changes, as occur with systemic treatment. The structures most commonly involved in oculoplastic complications of cancer therapy are the eyelids, eyelashes, lacrimal gland, lacrimal drainage system, skin, orbital soft tissue, and cranial nerves. Ocular morbidity from cancer therapy is also well described in the literature but is beyond the scope of this chapter.

M. A. Connor
Oculoplastic and Orbital Consultants, P.A., Palm Beach Gardens, FL, USA

B. Esmaeli (✉)
Orbital Oncology & Ophthalmic Plastic Surgery, Department of Plastic Surgery, MD Anderson Cancer Center, Houston, TX, USA
e-mail: besmaeli@mdanderson.org

Oculoplastic Complications of Radiation Therapy

Radiation therapy in the periocular region has long been used in the management of cutaneous eyelid cancers, intraocular cancers, and orbital processes such as tumors or inflammatory conditions. Radiation therapy has both curative and palliative indications. The dose of radiation is limited by the radiation tolerance of the surrounding healthy tissue as the field of radiation extends well beyond the target tissue (Fig. 29.1). Radiation therapy for an ocular or periocular process may damage periorbital tissue; radiation therapy for nearby intracranial and paranasal lesions may also damage periorbital tissue [2].

Radiation therapy in the periocular region requires careful planning because of the vital and radiosensitive orbital and ocular structures. Specialized treatment and shielding techniques are used to minimize irradiation of surrounding tissues while delivering the appropriate dose to the target tissue. In order to reduce the effects on nearby healthy tissue, radiation is delivered in multiple doses—an approach known as fractionated radiation therapy. This approach effectively allows time for healthy surrounding tissue to repair damage induced by the energy of radiation; cancer cells lack this intrinsic repair capability and undergo apoptosis. Cytokine-mediated and inflammatory responses in the surrounding tissues exacerbate the damage induced by the radiation itself [3]. Even with the use of fractionated radiation therapy, however, healthy tissue frequently sustains permanent damage. This damage can become apparent weeks, months, or even years later. Clinical sequelae may result from cell death and the wound healing cascade initiated within irradiated tissue [3].

Many radiation therapy modalities exist. In external beam radiation therapy, photons, protons, or electrons are used to directly damage DNA or interact with nearby molecules to form free radicals resulting in cell death. Stereotactic

J. J. Servat et al. (eds.), *Smith and Nesi's Ophthalmic Plastic and Reconstructive Surgery*,
https://doi.org/10.1007/978-3-030-41720-8_29

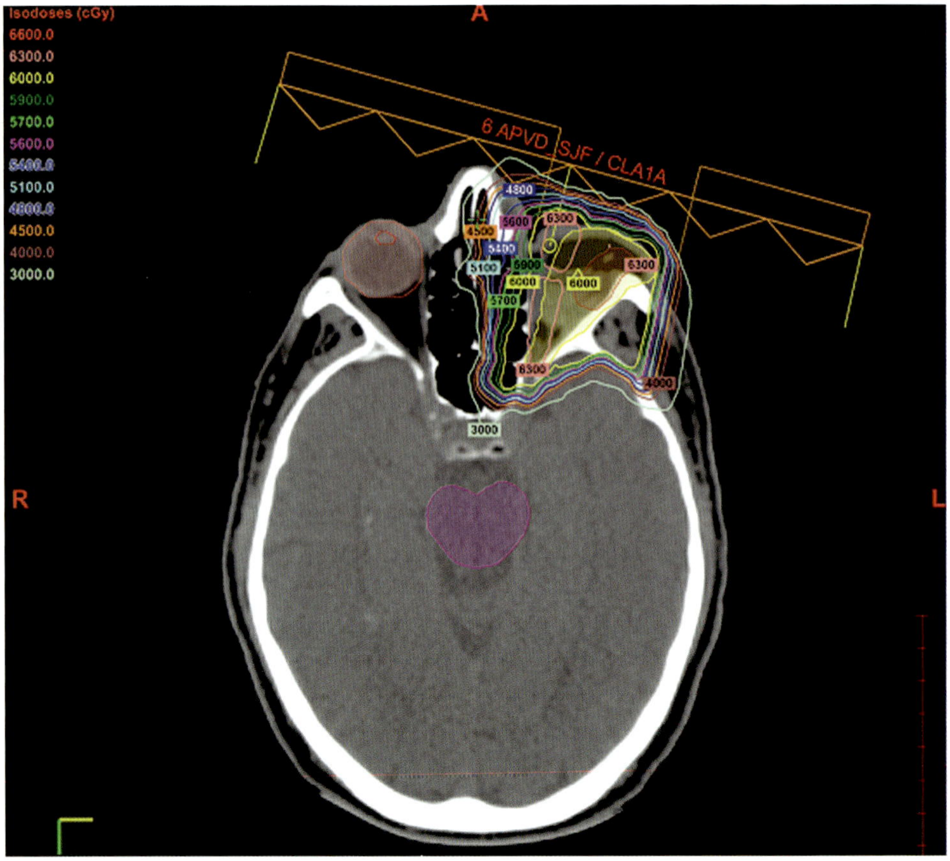

Fig. 29.1 A 76-year-old man with invasive squamous cell carcinoma with perineural invasion of the left lacrimal gland underwent orbital exenteration with free-flap reconstruction. Above is a map of the postoperative proton beam radiation plan for cobalt 60 60-Gy equivalents in 30 fractions to improve local control and survival. Careful mapping was done to minimize the dose to the optic chiasm, contralateral eye, and brain

radiosurgery (gamma knife) is used to deliver fixed fields of radiation to well-defined tumors while sparing the surrounding normal tissue. Plaque brachytherapy is a way of delivering radiation to a localized area with short-range-emitting radioactive particles such as iodine 125, palladium 103, ruthenium 106, and strontium 90. Plaque brachytherapy is commonly used for treating intraocular tumors.

Early and late side effects of radiation therapy differ [1, 3]. Early side effects, those occurring during or within weeks after radiation therapy, include skin erythema, dry or moist desquamation of the skin, mucositis, and nausea. Acute damage is most prominent in tissues with rapidly proliferating cells, such as epithelial surfaces [3]. All periocular tissue that has been irradiated demonstrates edema, vascular congestion, and diffuse neutrophil infiltration [4]. Late side effects, those occurring months to years after radiation therapy, include fibrosis, scarring, atrophy, vascular and neural damage, and secondary malignancies [1, 3]. These side effects manifest in different ways depending on the tissue type affected in the periocular region. The exact etiology of late side effects of radiation therapy is not well understood; however, the etiology is thought to be related to depletion of slowly proliferating stem cells and vascular damage [5]. The use of concurrent chemotherapy can exacerbate radiation side effects by limiting normal repair mechanisms in healthy tissue [6, 7].

Normal Tissue Damage

Skin and Conjunctiva

Although radiation therapy is a fairly targeted treatment option, in most cases, radiation must unavoidably pass through the skin. Skin cells are derived from rapidly reproducing differentiated stem cells and are therefore radiosensitive [5]. Skin damage is one of the earliest and most noticeable side effects of radiation. The onset of skin damage usually occurs within 2 weeks of initiation of treatment [5], and management of skin injury can be challenging. Radiation factors directly proportional to the degree of injury include field size, total dose, and dose per fraction [5]. Although skin reactions are dose dependent [5, 8], there is significant interpatient variation in response [9]. Other factors also contribute to the degree of skin damage after irradiation, including age, gender, skin type, systemic diseases such as diabetes mellitus or collagen vascular disease, and prior sun exposure [5, 9]. For instance, heavily solar damaged skin with chronic vasodilatory changes will frequently develop significant erythema following radiation therapy [9].

The skin exhibits acute-phase reactions (dermatitis, madarosis) and late-phase reactions (photosensitivity, telangiectasias, skin atrophy, fibrosis, and depigmentation) to radiation therapy [5, 10] (Fig. 29.2). In the acute phase,

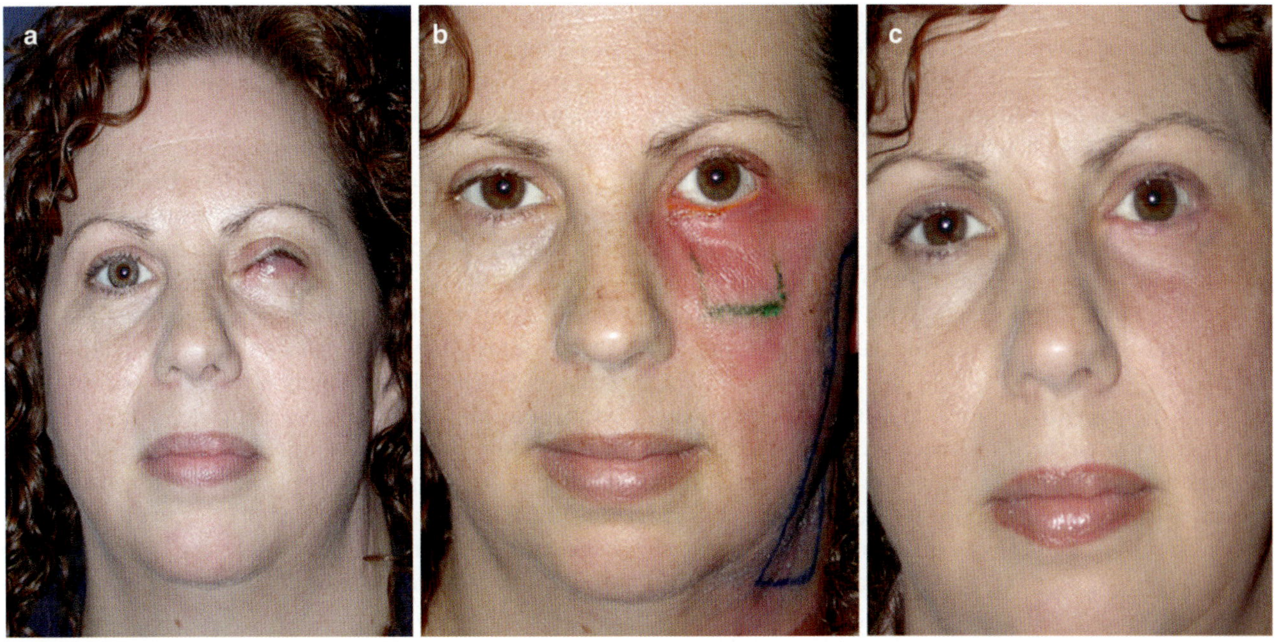

Fig. 29.2 (**a**) Newly reconstructed lower eyelid after excision of a squamous cell carcinoma of the eyelid and reconstruction using a Hughes tarsoconjunctival flap and a full-thickness skin graft. (**b**) The patient had postoperative radiation therapy. Note the radiation-induced burn immediately after radiation therapy. (**c**) Appearance of eyelid 6 months after opening of the Hughes flap (second stage of the tarsoconjunctival flap procedure) and completion of postoperative adjuvant radiation therapy. There is slight discoloration of the skin of the lower eyelid, but overall there is a very nice outcome both functionally and cosmetically. The patient had some symptoms of dry eye syndrome and mild ocular surface irritation relieved with topical lubrication

primary erythema occurs within 24 h of treatment initiation and subsides within a week [11]. The skin and conjunctiva become hyperemic secondary to vascular congestion, vasodilation, and plasma leakage [3]. Inflammatory signals released by cells damaged but not killed by radiation also play a role in the mediation of skin erythema [11]. The late-phase damage is mediated by the release of long-acting vasodilatory substances such as prostaglandin E2 as well as additional inflammatory mediators released days later by necrotic cells actually killed by radiation [11]. Radiation directly induces a premature terminal differentiation of fibroblasts, leading to a significant increase in collagen deposition over the course of months, resulting in cicatricial changes [12, 13].

In severe dermatitis reactions, loss of the epithelium overlying a bed of inflammation predisposes the patient to infectious processes, which can acutely lead to cellulitis and bacteremia and chronically cause unsightly scarring. Cicatricial changes in the thin preseptal periocular skin and in the thicker premaxillary skin can lead to downward traction on the lower eyelid resulting in a cicatricial ectropion. In the upper eyelid, severe anterior lamellar tightening can result in lagophthalmos.

The palpebral and bulbar conjunctiva is composed of nonkeratinized squamous epithelium with goblet cells overlying a thin substantia propria and can undergo changes similar to those observed in the periocular skin in response to radiation therapy [2]. Radiation-induced side effects of the conjunctiva mimic other processes that lead to chronic irritation and inflammation of the ocular surface and clinically present as injection, dry eye, mucus stranding, and keratinization [2]. In the acute phase, days to weeks after treatment initiation, injection and chemosis are most prominent. Chronic keratoconjunctivitis sicca occurs secondary to loss of the accessory lacrimal glands (the Krause glands and glands of Wolfring), resulting in a reduction in basal tear secretion. Focal loss of epithelial cells, squamous metaplasia, conjunctival keratinization, and forniceal shortening has also been reported [2, 14].

Eyelid

The eyelid margin is composed of skin, hair follicles, sebaceous glands, and mucous membrane. Each component can be damaged by radiation therapy. Eyelid alopecia or trichiasis frequently occurs when the eyelid is within or near the field of radiation. When the eyelashes are completely lost, regrowth is determined by the viability of the lash pilosebaceous unit. When the hair follicle is viable, the eyelashes may grow in aberrant directions and lead to recurrent trichiasis or distichiasis.

The sebaceous glands (meibomian glands and glands of Zeis) exhibit an acute inflammatory response to radiation therapy [4]. Karp et al. [15] demonstrated diffuse involutional atrophy of the meibomian glands of eight specimens removed 5–16 days after irradiation. In three eyes, there was a complete loss of meibomian glands and ducts [16]. Long-term effects of irradiation of the eyelid can include loss of meibomian glands and ducts, dilated ducts filled with keratin and squamous metaplasia [2]. Radiation therapy causes chronic meibomian gland dysfunction, which predisposes a patient to dry eye, chalazia, meibomitis, and blepharitis.

Positional changes of the eyelid margin following radiation therapy to the head and neck are not uncommon. In patients with lower eyelid laxity, entropion can result from cicatricial changes occurring in the posterior lamella, and ectropion can result from cicatricial changes occurring in the anterior lamella. Surgical repair consists of lower eyelid tightening and, depending on the severity of cicatrix present, may require the use of conjunctival grafts or full-thickness skin grafts.

Lacrimal System

The lacrimal gland is irradiated in the treatment of lacrimal gland tumors, orbital tumors, and orbital inflammatory processes such as orbital pseudotumor, myositis, and Graves ophthalmopathy and in wide-field radiation therapy for lesions adjacent to the lacrimal gland in the lateral canthus, temple, or scalp. Similar to radiation-induced damage to the salivary glands, radiation-induced damage to the lacrimal glands usually occurs in the parenchyma secondary to inflammation, vascular changes, and edema [4, 17]. Swelling and tenderness can occur after the first dose of radiation but usually subside in a few days [3]. Within 48 h after the first dose of radiation, extensive necrosis and serous acinar cell damage have been demonstrated. Clinically, this manifests as pain and discomfort in the lacrimal gland region and is described as necrotizing dacryoadenitis [4]. Accessory lacrimal glands, such as the Krause glands and glands of Wolfring in the conjunctiva, also exhibit pathologic changes after irradiation [4].

Dry eye is one of the most common complaints in patients who have undergone irradiation of periocular structures [14]. Parsons et al. reported that among 33 patients who underwent external beam radiation treatment of the orbit for extracranial tumors, 30% of patients who received less than 45 Gy and 100% of those who received 57 Gy or more developed severe dry eye [18]. In another study, Parsons et al. found that a patient's risk of developing severe dry eye following irradiation of the orbit significantly increased at doses greater than 40 Gy [19].

The lacrimal drainage apparatus can also be damaged if it lies within the field of radiation. Radiation passing through the medial canthal region can cause canalicular stenosis from intraluminal adhesions and scarring. Prophylactically stenting the canalicular system prior to treatment may reduce the risk of this complication [16]. However, because it is not known exactly how often canalicular stenosis occurs with various fields of radiation, the exact indications for silicone stenting of the lacrimal drainage apparatus are not well established in the literature. Bothersome epiphora and canalicular stenosis following radiation therapy are difficult to manage. Silicone intubation is not always possible, and attempts to place silicone tubes can create a false passage that will scar down following removal of the tube. Even when the tube is appropriately placed in the canalicular system, inflammation and fibrosis often occur while the tube is in place. Patients who have canalicular stenosis secondary to radiation therapy may ultimately require a conjunctivodacryocystorhinostomy with placement of a Pyrex glass tube to relieve their symptoms of excessive tearing [20].

Orbital Bone

Radiation therapy leads to loss of bone vitality secondary to osteocyte, osteoblast, and osteoclast injury as well as surrounding tissue hypoxia from vascular damage [5]. This can predispose periorbital and facial bones to osteoradionecrosis [21]. The incidence of osteoradionecrosis in the head and neck region ranges widely, from 0.4% to 56% [22]; osteoradionecrosis in the head and neck typically occurs in the maxilla and mandible. For extensive bony reconstruction of the orbit following tumor resection, bone grafts should be used with caution in patients who will require postoperative irradiation of this region. Rates of survival of osseointegrated implants in irradiated sites within the orbit have been reported to be as low as 27% [23].

In the pediatric population, radiation therapy can alter the growth of the orbit. The facial skeleton is most susceptible to radiation before the age of 6 years [24, 25]. All bone cell populations are affected, including osteoblasts and osteoclasts [26]. Osteoclasts regain function faster than osteoblasts, which leads to bone resorption [27]. Long-term sequelae result from intraosseous vascular damage [26, 27]. The Intergroup Rhabdomyosarcoma Study reported orbital hypoplasia in approximately 60% of 131 pediatric patients treated with radiation therapy for orbital rhabdomyosarcoma [25, 28]. In pediatric patients with head and neck cancer treated with radiation therapy, 60–100% of long-term survivors developed profound disturbances in craniofacial bone growth [27]. Management of orbital hypoplasia secondary to radiation therapy can be extremely difficult, especially in patients with an anophthalmic socket. Reconstructive efforts to improve symmetry in patients with orbital hypoplasia usually involve cooperation among multiple subspecialists, including oral maxillofacial surgeons, otolaryngologists, and ophthalmic plastic surgeons.

Delayed Wound Healing

Wound healing is a complex process mediated by proinflammatory cytokines and angiogenesis signals released immediately following tissue damage [29]. Several factors influence this process, including age; nutritional status; smoking; comorbidities such as diabetes, anemia, and cancer; and immune status [29, 30]. Radiation therapy given in fractional doses over consecutive days causes repeated insults to tissue. Chronic inflammation and damage to the microvasculature can delay angiogenesis and potentiate tissue hypoxia, leading to a delay in wound healing and possibly wound necrosis. This is especially important for surgical planning in patients requiring adjuvant radiation therapy.

For example, following a lid-sharing procedure for upper or lower eyelid defects, an appropriate period of healing should be allowed before postoperative adjuvant radiation therapy is started to permit stabilization of the pedicle; however, radiation therapy needs to be started within the usual 4- to 6-week window after surgery to ensure the greatest potential effectiveness against any residual microscopic cancer [14]. Full-thickness skin grafts survive well in the periocular region because of the rich vascular blood supply; however, if adjuvant radiation therapy is required in the early postoperative period, vascularized sliding or rotational flaps that maintain their own blood supply should be considered whenever possible. In patients undergoing orbital exenteration, preoperative and postoperative radiation therapy are considered contraindications to full-thickness skin grafting because of the increased risk of poor graft take and graft failure [31]. Other options for socket reconstruction in patients undergoing orbital exenteration who require radiation therapy include an eyelid-sparing exenteration technique [32] when the orbital defect is shallow and limited to the orbit or a microvascularized free flap harvested from a site such as the anterolateral thigh or radial forearm when the orbital defect is deep and there is possible involvement of adjacent periorbital structures such as paranasal sinuses or the intracranial structures (Fig. 29.3).

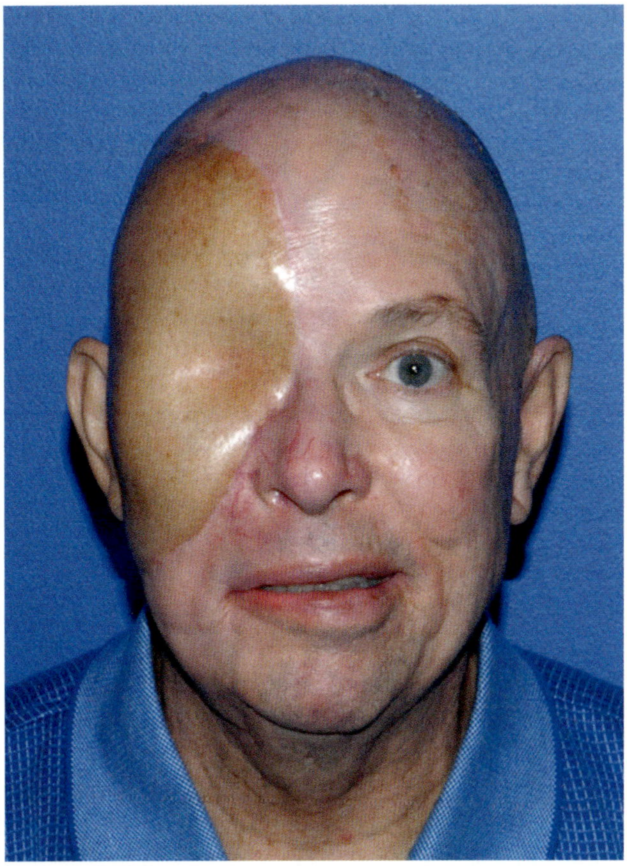

Fig. 29.3 Postoperative appearance after placement of an anterior lateral-thigh free flap to cover the orbital exenteration cavity and paranasal sinuses

Secondary Neoplasms

A secondary malignancy is one that is distinct from the original cancer; secondary malignancies often affect long-term morbidity as well as mortality [33]. Compared to individuals in the general population, patients who undergo the treatment of cancer with radiation have an increased risk of developing a secondary malignancy [33, 34]. However, a cause-and-effect relationship between radiation therapy and secondary malignancies has not been established. The estimated incidence of secondary malignancy in patients who undergo radiation therapy is 0.4–1.0% [35, 36]. The risk is higher in pediatric cancer patients and patients who have been treated with both radiation and chemotherapy or who have other carcinogenic exposures such as exposure to tobacco [33]. The probability of developing a new malignancy in pediatric cancer patients treated with radiation therapy has been reported to be as high as 17% [37]. Both solid tumor and hematologic secondary malignancies have been described [38]. Despite attempts to localize the radiation field as much as possible, certain delivery techniques can expose larger fields to radiation. Thus, radiation therapy for head and neck malignancies has been associated with secondary neoplasms not only in the periocular region but also elsewhere in the body [39].

Therapy-induced carcinogenesis is multifactorial and usually does not manifest until at least 5 years after treatment [40]. The absolute risk of developing a secondary malignancy after radiation therapy for head and neck cancer is difficult to assess because of the multitude of delivery modalities, variety of adjuvant multiple-agent chemotherapy regimens, specific patient risk factors, and range of survival times after cancer treatment. However, the risk appears to increase with increased total dose of radiation, concurrent or adjuvant chemotherapy, and increased survival time [25, 40]. Patients who are germline-mutation retinoblastoma survivors, especially those who have received radiation to the orbit, are at an increased risk of orbital sarcomas [41].

Solid tumors such as sarcoma and carcinoma as well as hematologic malignancies such as leukemia, lymphoma, and multiple myeloma have all been described as secondary malignancies following radiation therapy [38, 42–44]. In the head and neck, squamous-cell carcinoma is the most common secondary malignancy [38, 42–44]. The latency period between irradiation and diagnosis of secondary malignancy ranges from 3 to 40 years and appears to be related to the dose of radiation received as well as the type of secondary malignancy [42, 44]. Sarcomas consistently have shorter latency periods, on average about 22 years, whereas squamous-cell carcinomas occur within an average of 31–36.5 years [35, 44–46].

The treatment of secondary malignancies following radiation therapy is generally surgical resection because radiation-induced malignancies do not respond well to further radiation therapy or adjuvant chemotherapy [42, 45]. The prognosis is usually poor; 5-year survival rates have been reported to be 10–30% [47]. Despite the low incidence of secondary malignancies following radiation therapy, heightened awareness is essential for early detection. The poor prognosis and variability in latency period necessitate lifelong follow-up and close monitoring of the field of radiation.

Summary of Oculoplastic Complications of Radiation Therapy

The risks associated with radiation therapy can be significant and depend on the location of the target tissue, the amount of radiation delivered, and individual patient factors. Some side effects are self-limited, while others lead to complications requiring surgical intervention. A thorough understanding of the complications associated with radiation therapy is critical in scheduling appropriate follow-up and planning appropriate treatment of cancer.

Oculoplastic Complications of Chemotherapy

Side effects of chemotherapy are systemic, and many chemotherapeutic agents are associated with ocular and oculoplastic side effects [48]. Ocular side effects of chemotherapy are beyond the scope of this chapter; however, they can be referenced at the National Registry of Drug-Induced Ocular Side Effects website (www.eyedrugregistry.com) [49]. In this section, we focus on the chemotherapy-associated side effects most commonly encountered by oculoplastic surgeons.

Epiphora, Canalicular Stenosis, and Nasolacrimal Duct Blockage

Tearing in a cancer patient receiving chemotherapy is common, and a clinical distinction should be made between excessive tearing, a symptom, and tear outflow blockage, an anatomic finding on probing and irrigation. Many chemotherapeutic agents have been associated with ocular surface irritation causing pseudoepiphora; however, only five drugs, docetaxel (Taxotere), 5-fluorouracil, S-1, iodine-131, and topical mitomycin C, have been reported to date to cause functional blockage of the lacrimal outflow system.

Docetaxel is a potent taxane used in the treatment of breast and prostate cancer [50]. A common adverse effect of docetaxel is canalicular stenosis [51–54]. A small fraction of the unbound plasma docetaxel is secreted in the tears; this is thought to be the mechanism for induction of canalicular inflammation ultimately leading to fibrosis [55]. In a prospective study by Esmaeli et al., 64% of patients receiving weekly docetaxel injections and 39% of patients receiving docetaxel injections every 3 weeks reported epiphora [53]. One-third of the patients receiving weekly docetaxel developed moderate to severe canalicular stenosis, whereas patients on the every-3-week schedule had epiphora but no evidence of canalicular stenosis. Prospective, frequent in-office probing and irrigation with subsequent topical steroid administration may prevent permanent canalicular scarring, particularly in patients who are receiving docetaxel every 3 weeks or those who are exposed to docetaxel for a short period of time (<6–8 weeks) [53, 56]. When recurrent or progressive canalicular stenosis is observed on probing and irrigation, early bilateral silicone tube intubation of the canalicular system should be strongly considered and may prevent permanent canalicular scarring and the need for further invasive surgery [56]. The silicone tubes should be left in place for at least 4–6 weeks after cessation of docetaxel [56]. In severe cases of canalicular scarring secondary to docetaxel, a conjunctivodacryocystorhinostomy with permanent placement of a Pyrex glass tube (Jones tube) may be the only option for symptomatic resolution of epiphora.

Secretion of 5-fluorouracil has also been demonstrated in the tears of patients who receive this drug and report epiphora [57]. 5-Fluorouracil is a fluorinated pyrimidine used in the treatment of colon, breast, rectal, stomach, and pancreatic cancer and is known to cause mucosal inflammation as it has its greatest effect on rapidly dividing cells [48]. Systemic 5-fluorouracil is thought to be secreted by the lacrimal gland, causing ocular surface irritation and excess lacrimation, which usually resolve following discontinuation of the drug [58]. Eiseman et al. found that in 52 patients receiving systemic 5-fluorouracil over a period of at least 3 months, 14 (26.9%) complained of tearing, while only four (5.8%) demonstrated punctal-canalicular stenosis [59]. Obstruction of the canaliculi, scarring of the lacrimal sac, and fibrosis of the punctum and adjacent tissue have all been reported in patients with dacryostenosis receiving long-term therapy with 5-fluorouracil [60]. This risk appears to be related to the total dose given and duration of treatment [61]. Epiphora is reversible with discontinuation of 5-fluorouracil if dacryostenosis is not present. Surgical intervention usually involves a dacryocystorhinostomy with placement of silicone tubes; however, Fezza et al. reported that 26.7% of patients with 5-fluorouracil-induced dacryostenosis required a conjunctivodacryocystorhinostomy and placement of a Pyrex glass tube due to the severity of canalicular scarring [62]. 5-Fluorouracil has also been associated with dermatitis, cicatricial ectropion, keratinization of the eyelid margin, madarosis, and ankyloblepharon [63].

S-1, an oral prodrug of 5-fluorouracil, is an antineoplastic agent with fewer reported side effects than 5-fluorouracil used in the treatment of gastrointestinal cancer as well as other solid tumors [64]. S-1 is approved for treatment of gastrointestinal cancers in Japan but is not yet approved by the US Food and Drug Administration. S-1 has recently been reported to cause epiphora, and some reported cases resulted from canalicular stenosis or nasolacrimal duct blockage [65]. The etiology of canalicular stenosis in patients receiving S-1 has not been studied; however, given that S-1 is a prodrug of 5-fluorouracil, most likely the mechanism of canalicular stenosis is the same as for 5-fluorouracil. The management of canalicular stenosis caused by S-1 should be similar to the management of canalicular stenosis caused by docetaxel or 5-fluorouracil.

Punctal and canalicular stenosis have also been reported with topical use of mitomycin C [66, 67]. The underlying pathophysiology is unknown. A retrospective study of 100 eyes treated with topical mitomycin C (0.04%) four times a day for one to three 7-day cycles showed a 14% incidence of epiphora secondary to punctal stenosis [68].

Treatment of thyroid carcinoma with radioactive iodine, iodine 131 (^{131}I), has also been associated with nasolacrimal duct obstruction [69–71]. The same iodine symporter found in the thyroid gland that is responsible for uptake of ^{131}I has also been found in the epithelium of the lacrimal sac and nasolacrimal duct but not in the canaliculi. Systemic treatment with ^{131}I can cause inflammation and fibrosis of the lacrimal sac and nasolacrimal duct resulting in nasolacrimal obstruction [72]; canalicular fibrosis is not as much of a problem with ^{131}I. Patients with nasolacrimal duct blockage associated with ^{131}I do very well after a standard dacryocystorhinostomy. Silicone tubes may have to be left in place for the duration of anticipated treatment with ^{131}I if repeated treatments are expected.

Trichomegaly

Trichomegaly, excessive and aberrant eyelash growth, has been associated with inhibitors of epidermal growth factor receptor (EGFR), including cetuximab (Erbitux) and erlotinib (Tarceva) [73, 74]. EGFR is expressed in the epidermis and the outer root sheath of the hair follicles [75]. Extensive eyelash growth can occur within 2 months of the start of treatment with an EGFR inhibitor (Fig. 29.4). Long misdirected eyelashes are associated with ocular surface irritation and can cause mechanical breakdown of the corneal epithelium. Patients may require frequent eyelash trimming and epilation while receiving EGFR inhibitors.

Chalazia

Bortezomib is a boronic acid-derived proteasome inhibitor used in the treatment of patients with multiple myeloma. There have been a number of reports of persistent chalazia in patients treated with bortezomib, which resolved with discontinuation of the medication [76–78].

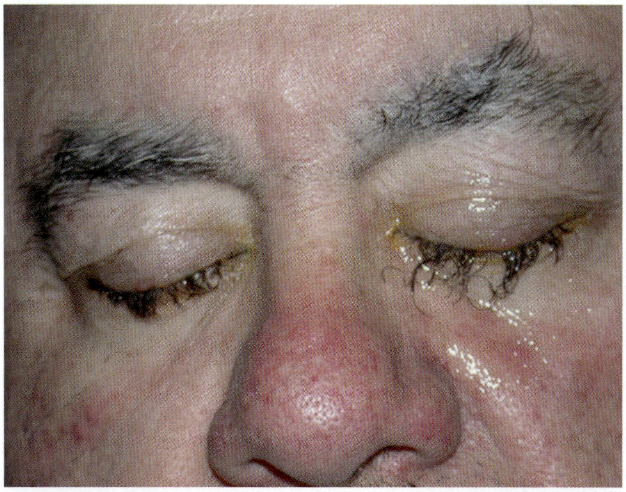

Fig. 29.4 Trichomegaly in a patient treated with erlotinib for non-small cell lung cancer

Orbital and Periorbital Edema

Orbital and periorbital edema have been reported to be side effects of many chemotherapy agents. The edema is usually transient and does not lead to long-term sequelae. Edema typically resolves within days of when the inciting drug is stopped. Chemotherapy-induced orbital edema is a rare side effect, so the literature on this condition consists mostly of case reports. Orbital or periorbital edema has been reported to be associated with methotrexate, imatinib mesylate (Gleevec) [79–82], busulfan, cyclophosphamide, doxorubicin, interleukin, etoposide, and thiotepa.

The drug associated with the most dramatic cases of periorbital edema is imatinib mesylate [79–82]. The exact etiology of periorbital edema associated with imatinib mesylate is unknown; however, histologically there is evidence of local acute and chronic inflammation [82]. Conservative management is ideal. Severe cases have been treated with a low-salt diet, topical corticosteroids, topical phenylephrine, and oral diuretics; in severe and refractory cases, surgical excision of large festoons has been successful (Fig. 29.5) [82].

Oculoplastic Complications of Ablative Surgery in Patients with Head and Neck Cancer

Despite significant advances in chemotherapy agents and radiation therapy techniques, surgical resection remains the primary treatment for head and neck cancers amenable to surgery. Surgical resection of tumors around the orbit leads to oculoplastic complications in 2–8% of patients depending on the location of the primary tumor and the extent of resection [83, 84].

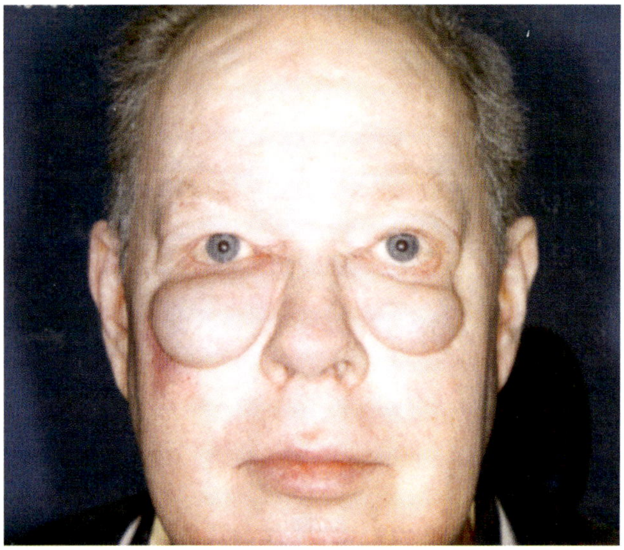

Fig. 29.5 Severe periorbital edema associated with imatinib mesylate. This patient had to have surgical resection of his large lower eyelid festoons to be able to see to read in downgaze

Orbital invasion occurs in approximately 60–80% of tumors in the maxillary and ethmoidal sinuses [73, 85]. Clear surgical margins are the goal of surgical resection, and attaining this goal can require dissection well into the orbit. When the globe and orbital soft tissues are preserved despite aggressive debulking, sequelae can include globe dystopia, entrapped orbital contents, proptosis, enophthalmos, epiphora, dacryocystitis, eyelid malposition, extraocular muscle damage, and restrictive myopathy (Fig. 29.6). Patients who have had disruption of the bony barrier between the orbit and sinus cavities are also at risk of developing a mucocele encroaching on the orbit. Exposure to the bacterial flora of the sinus can predispose a patient to orbital cellulitis. Orbital repair with synthetic implants or bone grafts at the time of resection can greatly reduce the risk of these complications [86]; however, the use of synthetic material is discouraged in most head and neck cancer patients who are expected to undergo postoperative radiation therapy because of fears of infection and extrusion of synthetic implants in this setting.

Local recurrence is also a risk following surgical resection of a tumor anywhere in the body. The reported incidence of local orbital recurrence following surgical resection of sinonasal malignancies invading the orbit is 7.8–29% [86–88]. Thus, patients who have undergone resection of a sinonasal malignancy require lifelong follow-up even when tumor clearance was achieved at the time of surgery.

Endoscopic resection of sinonasal tumors is not without risk. Complications associated with this approach include retrobulbar hematoma, extraocular muscle injury or entrapment, ocular dysmotility, orbital emphysema, nasolacrimal duct injury, and optic nerve damage [89]. Iatrogenic orbital bleeding during endoscopic sinus surgery can result from damage to the anterior or posterior ethmoidal arteries, which can retract into the orbit. Clinically, orbital bleeding presents with acute proptosis and can lead to loss of vision. Subacute proptosis, change in vision, and pain following endoscopic sinus surgery can occur from venous damage or damage to the lamina papyracea [89]. Both presentations are oculoplastic emergencies. Management includes close observation of visual acuity, intraocular pressure, and pupil function. A lateral canthotomy and cantholysis can be performed to relieve orbital pressure; if bleeding persists, surgical exploration for active bleeding may be necessary.

Surgical resection of sinonasal tumors, lacrimal sac tumors, and invasive skin cancers of the medial canthus may result in damage to or complete loss of the lacrimal drainage apparatus [20]. Chronic dacryocystitis and/or epiphora may result. Management depends on the status of the canalicular system, lacrimal sac, and nasolacrimal duct. Surgical options include dacryocystorhinostomy with silicone tube placement or conjunctivodacryocystorhinostomy with placement of a

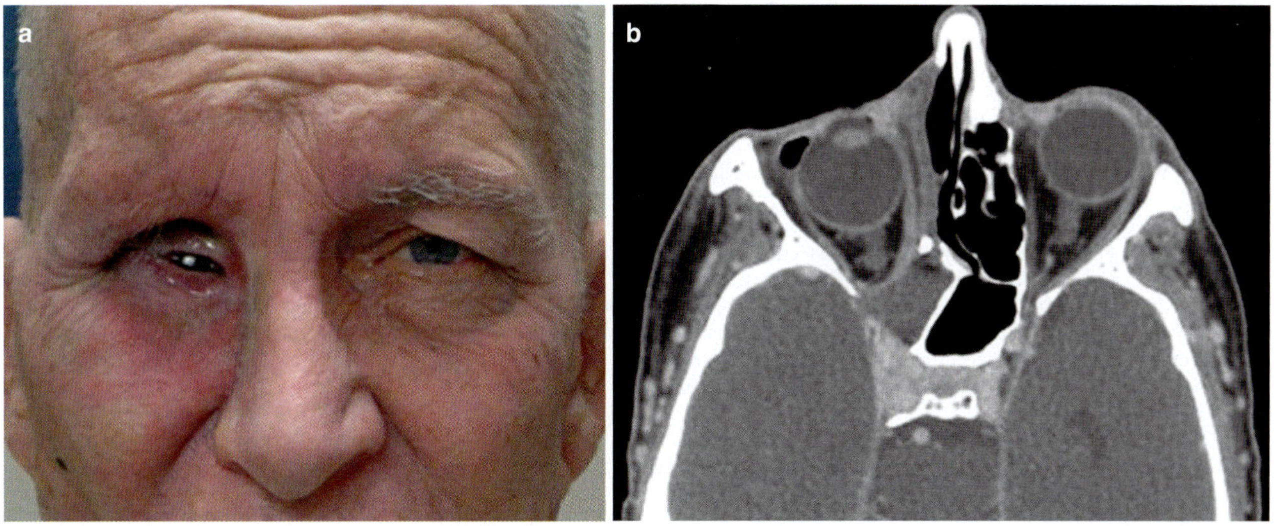

Fig. 29.6 (**a**) A 65-year-old man with right enophthalmos, hypoglobus, and medial and lateral canthal dystopia following a maxillectomy and ethmoidectomy. (**b**) Axial computed tomography image demonstrating enophthalmos

Pyrex glass tube. Placement of a silicone tube at the time of initial surgical resection of the tumor does not always prevent nasolacrimal obstruction and can lead to canalicular erosion [20]. The failure rate for dacryocystorhinostomy in patients with head and neck cancer is 17%, versus only 2–5% in patients with idiopathic nasolacrimal obstruction [20, 90, 91].

Patients with head and neck cancers may present for oculoplastic consultation with lagophthalmos, exposure keratopathy, eyebrow ptosis, and paralytic ectropion secondary to a facial palsy due to cancer directly involving the parotid gland or due to iatrogenic damage to the facial nerve. Strict ophthalmic lubrication may be sufficient for some patients with minor corneal exposure. In most patients, however, surgical intervention is required to reduce the palpebral fissure and ultimately the surface area of exposure. Such surgery may include all or a combination of the following: lower eyelid tightening, insertion of an upper eyelid gold weight, and a tarsorrhaphy. A midface cheek lift may also help support the paralytic lower eyelid. If the superior visual field is affected by the eyebrow ptosis, surgical elevation of the eyebrow can be added.

Primary wide local surgical excision with surgical margin control and Mohs micrographic surgery are the two gold-standard treatments for most malignant eyelid neoplasms [92]. In the head and neck region, Mohs micrographic surgery can create a defect that is challenging to repair, especially when the defect involves multiple neighboring aesthetic units such as the cheek, eyelid, or eyebrow. Both functional and aesthetic complications can result.

Surgical defects in the periocular region are commonly repaired using skin-muscle flaps and, when possible, direct skin closure. Reconstruction efforts resulting in vertical traction on the upper or lower eyelid may cause cicatricial eyelid malpositions such as entropion, ectropion, and lagophthalmos.

A detailed discussion of eyelid reconstruction after ablative surgery for eyelid and periocular cancers can be found in Chap. 10. Full-thickness eyelid defects can be closed directly if the defect involves less than 50% of the length of the eyelid. Upper eyelid ptosis can occur if direct closure of the upper eyelid results in a tight upper eyelid in which the levator muscle is not able to actively elevate the overly tightened eyelid. An overly tightened lower eyelid can cause the eyelid to slip below the globe, resulting in inferior scleral show and lagophthalmos. Reconstruction of eyelid defects involving greater than 50% of the eyelid is more complex and involves lid-sharing procedures and free grafts, which are described in Chap. 10.

Surgical excision and repair of surgical defects in the temporal fossa can damage the superficial temporal branch of the facial nerve, resulting in irreversible paralysis of the forehead and eyebrow. Other nerves commonly damaged in repairing periocular defects include the supraorbital and infraorbital sensory nerves; damage of these nerves can lead to numbness in the forehead/scalp and the cheek/upper lip, respectively. Understanding of the anatomy as well as the functional and aesthetic units in the periocular region is of paramount importance in successful reconstruction of skin defects resulting from surgical excision of cutaneous malignancies around the eye.

References

1. Bentzen SM. Preventing or reducing late side effects of radiation therapy: radiobiology meets molecular pathology. Nat Rev Cancer. 2006;6(9):702–13.
2. Gordon KB, Char DH, Sagerman RH. Late effects of radiation on the eye and ocular adnexa. Int J Radiat Oncol Biol Phys. 1995;31(5):1123–39.

3. Stone HB, Coleman CN, Anscher MS, McBride WH. Effects of radiation on normal tissue: consequences and mechanisms. Lancet Oncol. 2003;4(9):529–36.
4. Stephens LC, Schultheiss TE, Peters LJ, Ang KK, Gray KN. Acute radiation injury of ocular adnexa. Arch Ophthalmol. 1988;106(3):389–91.
5. Small W, Woloschak G. Radiation toxicity: a practical guide. New York: Springer; 2006.
6. Giro C, Berger B, Bokle E, et al. High rate of severe radiation dermatitis during radiation therapy with concurrent cetuximab in head and neck cancer: results of a survey in EORTC institutes. Radiother Oncol. 2009;90(2):166–71.
7. Koutcher LD, Wolden S, Lee N. Severe radiation dermatitis in patients with locally advanced head and neck cancer treated with concurrent radiation and cetuximab. Am J Clin Oncol. 2009;32(5):472–6.
8. Archambeau J. Relative radiation sensitivity of the integumentary system dose response of the epidermal, microvascular, and dermal populations, vol. 12. San Diego: Academic; 1987.
9. Denham JW, Hamilton CS, Simpson SA, et al. Factors influencing the degree of erythematous skin reactions in humans. Radiother Oncol. 1995;36:107–20.
10. Durkin SR, Roos D, Higgs B, Casson RJ, Selva D. Ophthalmic and adnexal complications of radiotherapy. Acta Ophthalmol Scand. 2007;85:240–50.
11. Simonen P, Hamilton C, Ferguson S, Ostwald P, O'Brien M, O'Brien P, et al. Do inflammatory processes contribute to radiation induced erythema observed in the skin of humans? Radiother Oncol. 1998;46:73–82.
12. Burger A, Loffler H, Bamberg M, Rodemann HP. Molecular and cellular basis of radiation fibrosis. Int J Radiat Biol. 1998;73(4):401–8.
13. Rodemann HP, Bamberg M. Cellular basis of radiation-induced fibrosis. Radiother Oncol. 1995;35(2):83–90.
14. Hsu A, Frank S, Ballo M, et al. Postoperative adjuvant external-beam radiation therapy for cancers of the eyelid and conjunctiva. Ophthal Plast Reconstr Surg. 2008;24(6):444–9.
15. Karp LA, Streeten BW, Cogan DG. Radiation-induced atrophy of the meibomian glands. Arch Ophthalmol. 1979;97(2):303–5.
16. Berman A, Rengan R, Tripuraneni P. Radiotherapy for eyelid, periocular and periorbital skin cancers. Int Ophthalmol Clin. 2009;49(4):129–42.
17. Cooper JS, Fu K, Marks J, Silverman S. Late effects of radiation therapy in the head and neck region. Int J Radiat Oncol Biol Phys. 1995;31:1141–64.
18. Parsons JT, Bova FJ, Fitzgerald CR, Mendenhall WM, Million RR. Severe dry-eye syndrome following external beam irradiation. Int J Radiat Oncol Biol Phys. 1994;30(4):775–80.
19. Parsons J, Bova F, Mendenhall W, Million R, Fitzgerald C. Response of the normal eye to high dose radiotherapy. Oncology. 1996;6(10):847–8.
20. Diba R, Saadati H, Esmaeli B. Outcomes of dacryocystorhinostomy in patients with head and neck tumors. Head Neck. 2005;27(1):72–5.
21. Katz TS, Mendenhall WM, Morris CG, Amdur RJ, Hinerman RW, Villaret DB. Malignant tumors of the nasal cavity and paranasal sinuses. Head Neck. 2002;24(9):821–9.
22. Jereczeck-Fossa B, Orecchia R. Radiotherapy-induced mandibular bone complications. Cancer Treat Rev. 2002;28:65–74.
23. Roumanas E, Chang T, Beumer J. Use of osseointegrated implants in the restoration of head and neck defects. J Calif Dent Assoc. 2006;34(9):711–8.
24. Probert J, Parker B. The effect of radiation on bone growth. Radiology. 1975;114:155–62.
25. Raney RB, James RA, Jeffrey K, et al. Late effects of therapy in 94 patients with localized rhabdomyosarcoma of the orbit: report from the Intergroup Rhabdomyosarcoma Study (IRS)-III, 1984–1991. Med Pediatr Oncol. 2000;34(6):413–20.
26. El-Naggar AM, Hanna IRA, Chanana AD, Arland LC, Cronkite EP. Bone marrow changes after localized acute and fractionated X irradiation. Radiat Res. 1980;84(1):46–52.
27. Gevorgyan A, La Scala GC, Neligan PC, Pang CY, Forrest CR. Radiation-induced craniofacial bone growth disturbances. J Craniofac Surg. 2007;18(5):1001–7.
28. Heyn R, Ragab A, Raney R, et al. Late effects of therapy in orbital rhabdomyosarcoma in children. A report from the Intergroup Rhabdomyosarcoma Study. Cancer. 1986;57(9):1738–43.
29. Cohen I, Diegelmann R, Lindbald W. Wound healing: biochemical and clinical aspects. Philadelphia: Saunders; 1992.
30. Porock D, Nikoletti S, Cameron F. The relationship between factors that impair wound healing and the severity of acute radiation skin and mucosal toxicities in head and neck cancer. Cancer Nurs. 2004;27(1):71–8.
31. Hanasono MMMD, Lee JCBA, Yang JSBS, Skoracki RJMD, Reece GPMD, Esmaeli BMD. An algorithmic approach to reconstructive surgery and prosthetic rehabilitation after orbital exenteration. Plast Reconstr Surg. 2009;123(1):98–105.
32. Shields JAMD, Shields CLMD, Demirci HMD, Honavar SGMD, Singh ADMD. Experience with eyelid-sparing orbital exenteration: the 2000 Tullos O Coston Lecture. Ophthal Plast Reconstr Surg. 2001;17(5):355–61.
33. Allan JM, Travis LB. Mechanisms of therapy-related carcinogenesis. Nat Rev Cancer. 2005;5(12):943–55.
34. Little J. Radiation carcinogenesis. Carcinogenesis. 2000;21:397–404.
35. Sale K, Wallace D, Girod D, Tsue T. Radiation-induced malignancy of the head and neck. Otolaryngol Head Neck Surg. 2004;131:643–5.
36. Lustig L, Jackler R, Lanser M. Radiation induced tumors of the temporal bone. Am J Otol. 1997;18:230–5.
37. Li F, Cassady J, Jaffe N. Risk of second tumors in survivors of childhood cancer. Cancer. 1975;35:1230–5.
38. Toda K, Shibuya H, Hayashi K, Aukawa F. Radiation-induced cancer after radiotherapy for non-Hodgkin's lymphoma of the head and neck: a retrospective study. Radiat Oncol. 2009;4:21–8.
39. Verellen D, Banhavere F. Risk assessment of radiation-induced malignancies based on whole-body equivalent dose estimates for IMRT treatment in the head and neck region. Radiother Oncol. 1999;53:199–203.
40. Kry SF, Salehpour M, Followill DS, et al. The calculated risk of fatal secondary malignancies from intensity-modulated radiation therapy. Int J Radiat Oncol Biol Phys. 2005;62(4):1195–203.
41. Baker MS, McConnell LK, Kleinberg TT, Shriver EM, Bilyk JR, Allen RC. Orbital sarcomas in retinoblastoma patients: recommendations for screening and treatment guidelines. Curr Opin Ophthalmol. 2016;27:443–8.
42. Miyahara H, Sato T, Yoshino K. Radiation-induced cancer of the head and neck region. Acta Otolaryngol. 1998;533:60–4.
43. Umatani K, Satoh T, Yoshino K, et al. Radiation-induced cancers of the head and neck (III). Nihon Kikan Shokudoka Gakkai Kaiho. 1989;4(40):313–9.
44. van der Laan BF, Baris G, Gregor R, et al. Radiation-induced tumours of the head and neck. J Laryngol Otol. 1995;109:346–9.
45. King A, Ahuja A, Teo P, Tse G, Kew J. Radiation induced sarcomas of the head and neck following radiotherapy for nasopharyngeal carcinoma. Clin Radiol. 2000;55:684–9.
46. Robinson E, Neugut A, Wylie P. Clinical aspects of postirradiation sarcomas. J Natl Cancer Inst. 1988;80:233–40.
47. Mark R, Poen J, Tran L, Selch Y, Parker R. Postirradiation sarcomas. A single-institution study and review of the literature. Cancer. 1994;73:2653–62.
48. Schmid KE, Kornek GV, Scheithauer W, Binder S. Update on ocular complications of systemic cancer chemotherapy. Surv Ophthalmol. 2006;51(1):19–40.
49. National registry of drug-induced ocular side effects. http://www.eyedrugregistry.com/. Accessed June 2010.

50. Valero V. Primary chemotherapy with docetaxel for the management of breast cancer. Oncology. 2002;16:35–43.
51. Esmaeli B, Valero V, Ahmadi MA, Booser D. Canalicular stenosis secondary to docetaxel (taxotere): a newly recognized side effect. Ophthalmology. 2001;108(5):994–5.
52. Esmaeli B, Hidaji L, Adinin RB, et al. Blockage of the lacrimal drainage apparatus as a side effect of docetaxel therapy. Cancer. 2003;98(3):504–7.
53. Esmaeli B, Amin S, Valero V, et al. Prospective study of incidence and severity of epiphora and canalicular stenosis in patients with metastatic breast cancer receiving docetaxel. J Clin Oncol. 2006;24(22):3619–22.
54. Esmaeli BMD, Burnstine MAMD, Ahmadi MAMD, Prieto VGMDP. Docetaxel-induced histologic changes in the lacrimal sac and the nasal mucosa. Ophthal Plast Reconstr Surg. 2003;19(4):305–8.
55. Esmaeli B, Ahmadi MA, Rivera E, et al. Docetaxel secretion in tears: association with lacrimal drainage obstruction. Arch Ophthalmol. 2002;120(9):1180–2.
56. Ahmadi MA, Esmaeli B. Surgical treatment of canalicular stenosis in patients receiving docetaxel weekly. Arch Ophthalmol. 2001;119(12):1802–4.
57. Christophidis N, Vajda F, Lucas I, Louis W. Ocular side effects with 5-fluorouracil. Aust NZ J Med. 1979;9(2):143–4.
58. Prasad S, Kamath GG, Phillips RP. Lacrimal canalicular stenosis associated with systemic 5-fluorouracil therapy. Acta Ophthalmol Scand. 2000;78(1):110–3.
59. Eiseman ASMD, Flanagan JCMD, Brooks ABMD, Mitchell EPMD, Pemberton CHMD. Ocular surface, ocular adnexal, and lacrimal complications associated with the use of systemic 5-fluorouracil. Ophthal Plast Reconstr Surg. 2003;19(3):216–24.
60. Haidak DJ, Hurwitz BS, Yeung KY. Tear–duct fibrosis (dacryostenosis) due to 5–fluorouracil. Ann Intern Med. 1978;88(5):657.
61. Hassan A, Hurwitz J, Burkes R. Epiphora in patients receiving systemic 5-fluorouracil therapy. Can J Ophthalmol. 1998;33(1):14–9.
62. Fezza J, Wesley R, Klippenstein K. The treatment of punctal and canalicular stenosis in patients on systemic 5-FU. Ophthalmic Surg Lasers. 1999;30(2):105–8.
63. Ng J. Orbital and periorbital side effects of chemotherapy. In: Esmaeli B, editor. Ophthalmic oncology. New York: Springer; 2011. p. 327–38.
64. Pa S. The modulated oral fluoropyrimidine prodrug S-1, and its use in gastrointestinal cancer and other solid tumors. Anti-Cancer Drugs. 2004;15(2):85–106.
65. Esmaeli B, Golio D, Lubecki L, Ajani J. Canalicular and nasolacrimal duct blockage: an ocular side effect associated with the antineoplastic drug S-1. Am J Ophthalmol. 2005;140(2):325–7.
66. Kopp E, Seregard S. Epiphora as a side effect of topical mitomycin C. Br J Ophthalmol. 2004;88(11):1422–4.
67. Billing K, Karagiannis A, Selva D. Punctal-canalicular stenosis associated with mitomycin-C for corneal epithelial dysplasia. Am J Ophthalmol. 2003;136(4):746–7.
68. Khong JJ, Muecke J. Complications of mitomycin C therapy in 100 eyes with ocular surface neoplasia. Br J Ophthalmol. 2006;90(7):819–22.
69. Kloos R, Duvuuri V, Jhaing S, Cahill K, Foster J, Burns J. Nasolacrimal drainage system obstruction from radioactive iodine therapy for thyroid carcinoma. J Clin Endocrinol Metab. 2002;87:5817–20.
70. Shepler T, Sherman S, Faustina M, Busaidy N, Ahmadi M, Esmaeli B. Nasolacrimal duct obstruction associated with radioactive iodine therapy for thyroid carcinoma. Ophthal Plast Reconstr Surg. 2003;19(6):479–81.
71. Burns J, Morgenstern K, Cahill K, Foster J, Jhiang S, Kloos R. Nasolacrimal obstruction secondary to I(131) therapy. Ophthal Plast Reconstr Surg. 2004;20(2):126–9.
72. Morgenstern K, Vadysirisack D, Zhang Z, et al. Expression of sodium iodide symporter in the lacrimal drainage system: implication for the mechanism underlying nasolacrimal duct obstruction in I(131)-treated patients. Ophthal Plast Reconstr Surg. 2005;21(5):337–44.
73. Vaccaro M, Pollicino A, Barbuzza O, Guarneri B. Trichomegaly of the eyelashes following treatment with cetuximab. Clin Exp Dermatol. 2009;34(3):402–3.
74. Papadopoulos R, Chasapi V, Bachariou A. Trichomegaly induced by erlotinib. Orbit. 2008;27(4):329–30.
75. Bouche O, Brixi-Benmansour H, Bertin A, Perceau G, Lagarde S. Trichomegaly of the eyelashes following treatment with cetuximab. Ann Oncol. 2005;16(10):1711–2.
76. Grob SR, Jakobiec FA, Rashid A, Yoon MK. Chalazia associated with bortezomib therapy for multiple myeloma. Ophthalmology. 2014;121(9):1845–7.
77. Yun C, Mukhi N, Kremer V, Shinder R, Verma V, Olcay B. Chalazia development in multiple myeloma: a new complication associated with bortezomib therapy. Hematol Rep. 2015;7(2):5729.
78. Fraunfelder FW, Yang HK. Association between bortezomib therapy and eyelid chalazia. JAMA Ophthalmol. 2016;134:88–90.
79. Esmaeli B, Diba R, Ahmadi M, et al. Periorbital edema and epiphora as ocular side effects of imatinib mesylate (Gleevec). Eye (London). 2004;10:760–2.
80. Fraunfelder F, Solomon J, Druker B, Esmaeli B, Kuyl J. Ocular side-effects associated with imatinib mesylate (Gleevec). J Ocul Pharmacol Ther. 2003;19:371–5.
81. Esmaeli B, Prieto V, Butler C, et al. Severe periorbital edema secondary to STI571 (Gleevec). Cancer. 2002;95:881–7.
82. McClelland C, Harocopos G, Custer P. Periorbital edema secondary to imatinib mesylate. Clin Ophthalmol. 2010;4:427–31.
83. Ganly I, Patel SG, Singh B, et al. Craniofacial resection for malignant paranasal sinus tumors: report of an international collaborative study. Head Neck. 2005;27(7):575–84.
84. Akinsola F, Somefun A, Oguntoyinbo O. Ophthalmological complications of nasal, paranasal sinus diseases and head and neck tumours. East Afr Med J. 2006;12(83):674–8.
85. Iannetti G, Valentini V, Rinna C, Ventucci E, Marianetti TM. Ethmoido-orbital tumors: our experience. J Craniofac Surg. 2005;16(6):1085–91.
86. Imola MJ, Schramm J, Victor L. Orbital preservation in surgical management of sinonasal malignancy. Laryngoscope. 2002;112(8):1357–65.
87. Carrau R, Segas J, Nuss D, et al. Squamous cell carcinoma of the sinonasal tract invading the orbit. Laryngoscope. 1999;109:230–5.
88. Nazar G, Rodrigo J, Llorente J, Baragano L, Suarez C. Prognostic factors of maxillary sinus malignancies. Am J Rhinol. 2004;18(4):233–8.
89. Han JK, Higgins TS. Management of orbital complications in endoscopic sinus surgery. Curr Opin Otolaryngol Head Neck Surg. 2010;18(1):32–6.
90. Hurwitz J. Dacryocystorhinostomy. Philadelphia: Lippincott-Raven; 1996.
91. Part X. Lacrimal disease and surgery. In: Nesi F, Levine M, Lisman R, editors. Smith's ophthalmic plastic and reconstructive surgery. 2nd ed. St. Louis: Mosby-Year Book, Inc.; 1998. p. 639–78.
92. Cook B, Bartley G. Epidemiologic characteristics and clinical course of patients with malignant eyelid tumors in an incidence cohort in Olmstead County. Minnesota Ophthalmol. 1999;106:746–50.

Part VII

Lacrimal Disease and Surgery

Aaron Fay

30 Lacrimal Sac Tumors: Diagnosis and Treatment

H. Jane Kim and Paul D. Langer

Introduction

Lacrimal sac tumors are uncommon, but noteworthy as they are frequently locally invasive and can result in death. Approximately 850 cases have been reported in the literature over the last century, of which over 50% were malignant [1–15]. The benign tumors include squamous papilloma, transitional papilloma, fibrous histiocytoma, oncocytoma, and hemangiopericytoma. The malignant tumors include squamous cell carcinoma, lymphoma, melanoma, transitional carcinoma, mucoepidermoid carcinoma, and adenocarcinoma in order of frequency. The most serious malignancies of the lacrimal sac are melanoma and transitional cell carcinoma, where the latter is associated with a 100% mortality rate [2]. The recurrence rate can be particularly high for some lacrimal sac malignancies as they can be invasive, multifocal, and located in vital nasopharyngeal regions. For example, the recurrence rate for invasive squamous cell carcinoma is approximately 50%, with 50% of those being fatal [1, 16]. Clinically, lacrimal sac tumors commonly masquerade as chronic dacryocystitis and often are unknowingly monitored conservatively until far advanced. Therefore, a high index of suspicion, awareness of the clinical presentation, and judicious examination of the lacrimal sac with imaging preoperatively and inspection at the time of surgery are necessary to confirm the diagnosis and to provide proper management.

H. J. Kim (✉)
Oculofacial Plastic Surgery, The Permanente Medical Group, Department of Ophthalmology, Union City, CA, USA

P. D. Langer
Division of Ophthalmic Plastic, Reconstructive, and Orbital Surgery, Institute of Ophthalmology and Visual Science, Rutgers New Jersey Medical School, Newark, NJ, USA

Clinical Features

Lacrimal sac tumors usually affect adults in the fifth decade with a reported range from 14 to 94 years of age, although benign epithelial tumors and mesenchymal tumors are diagnosed earlier in the third or fourth decades [1–20]. There is no sex predilection for lacrimal sac tumors, in contrast to dacryocystitis that is more common in women [1, 15]. Patients can present with epiphora and signs of inflammation as seen in chronic dacryocystitis, but there are some distinguishing features. The triad of signs suspicious for malignancy include: (1) mass above the medial canthal tendon (Fig. 30.1), (2) chronic dacryocystitis that irrigates freely, and (3) sanguinous reflux on irrigation [17]. Other signs include an immobile, noncompressible mass and epistaxis. Telangiectasia or ulceration overlying the mass and preauricular, submandibular, or cervical lymphadenopathy also suggests malignancy.

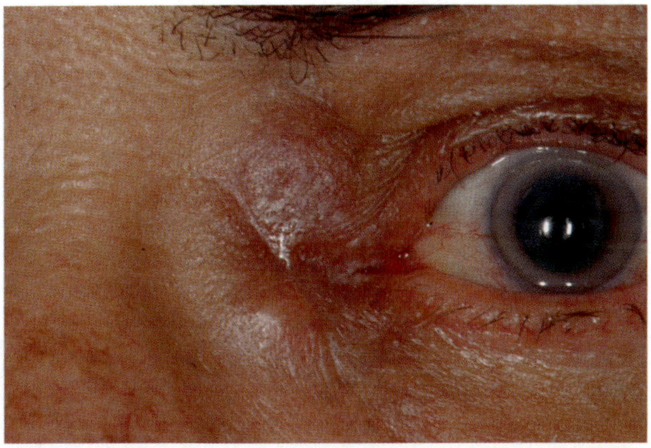

Fig. 30.1 A 74-year-old man presenting with a mass that reaches above the medial canthal tendon. Biopsy revealed squamous cell carcinoma of the lacrimal sac

J. J. Servat et al. (eds.), *Smith and Nesi's Ophthalmic Plastic and Reconstructive Surgery*,
https://doi.org/10.1007/978-3-030-41720-8_30

Diagnostic Evaluation

Preoperative imaging studies are essential in the evaluation of a lacrimal sac tumor. Computed tomography (CT) images reveal a lacrimal sac mass with possible erosion of the lacrimal fossa and, in advanced cases, invasion into neighboring structures (Fig. 30.2). Magnetic resonance imaging (MRI) can provide superior tumor definition delineating the cystic or solid nature of the mass [18] (Fig. 30.3). Dacryocystography (DCG) might reveal a filling defect due to a space-occupying lesion or a delay in contrast disappearance; however, a negative result does not rule out a tumor.

Pathology

The lacrimal sac and nasolacrimal duct are lined by stratified transitional epithelium containing mucous cells. Epithelial tumors constitute 62–94% of lacrimal sac tumors [1–3, 13, 15]. The remaining nonepithelial tumors can be further classified as mesenchymal, lymphoproliferative, melanocytic, and neural [1, 2, 8, 19, 20] (Tables 30.1a and 30.1b).

Epithelial tumors Over 70% of all lacrimal sac tumors are of epithelial origin (Tables 30.1a and 30.2). Epithelial papillomas are either squamous or transitional in type or a mixture of both types [6]. They can grow toward the lumen of the sac (exophytic) or toward the stroma of the sac wall (endophytic). Inverted papilloma displays endophytic growth often preventing complete excision and leading to frequent recurrence and malignant degeneration. Other epithelial tumors arise from oncocytes (oncocytoma, oncocytic adenocarcinoma), glandular epithelium (adenocarcinoma, adenoid cystic carcinoma) [19], or from a hybrid differentiation between mucous cells and squamous epithelial cells (mucoepidermoid). Human papillomavirus (HPV) has been associated with the majority of papillomas and about 40% of carcinomas. HPV types 6 and 11 have been associated with

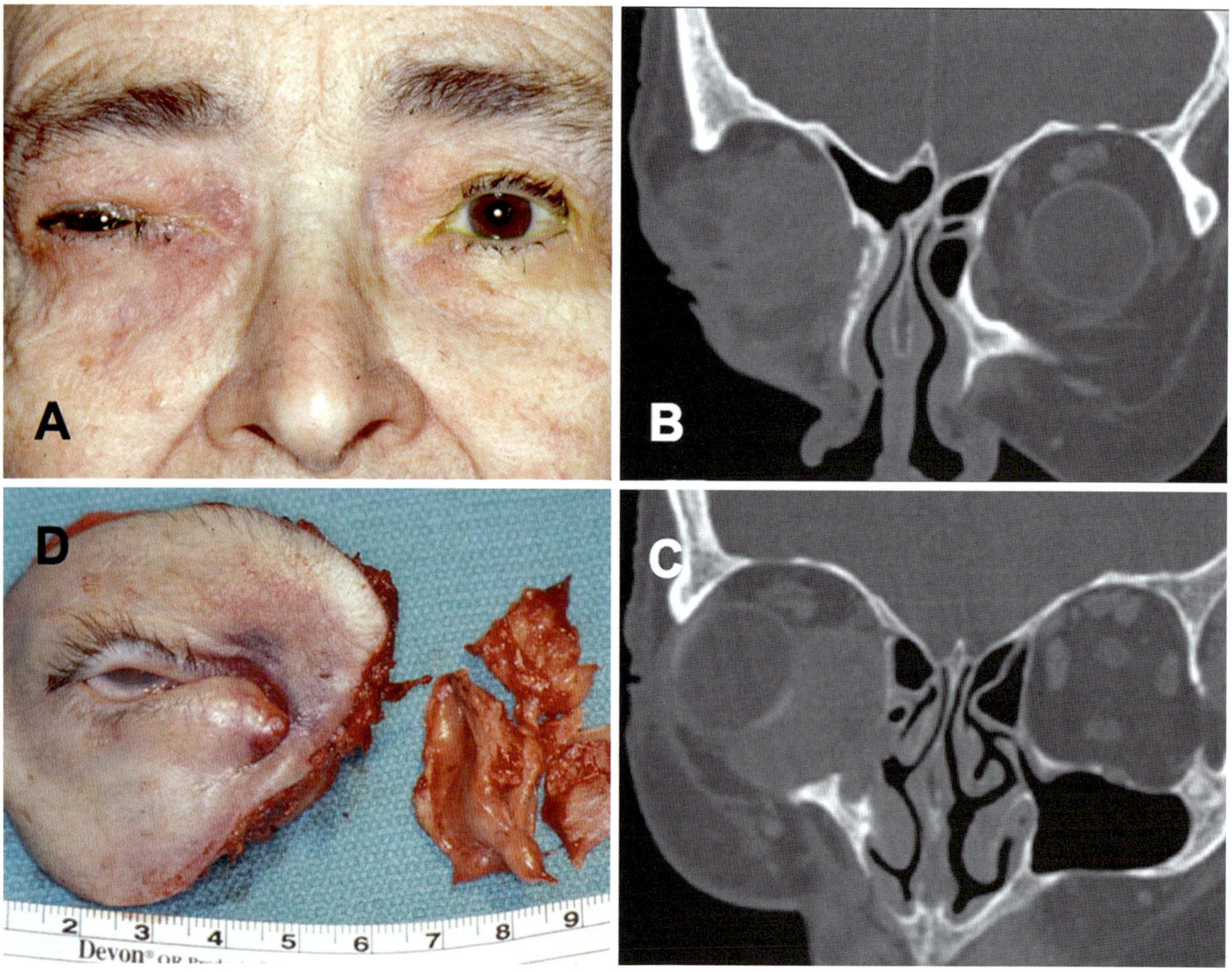

Fig. 30.2 (Clockwise) (**a**) A 89-year-old woman with nodular, nonreducible mass in the right medial canthus and inferonasal orbit displacing the globe laterally. (**b**, **c**) Noncontrast *CT demonstrates a heterogeneous, irregular mass in the right nasolacrimal system with extension* into the orbit and erosion of the lacrimal and maxillary bones medially. (**d**) Exenteration and medial maxillectomy specimen with attached lacrimal drainage system. Pathology evaluation revealed squamous cell carcinoma

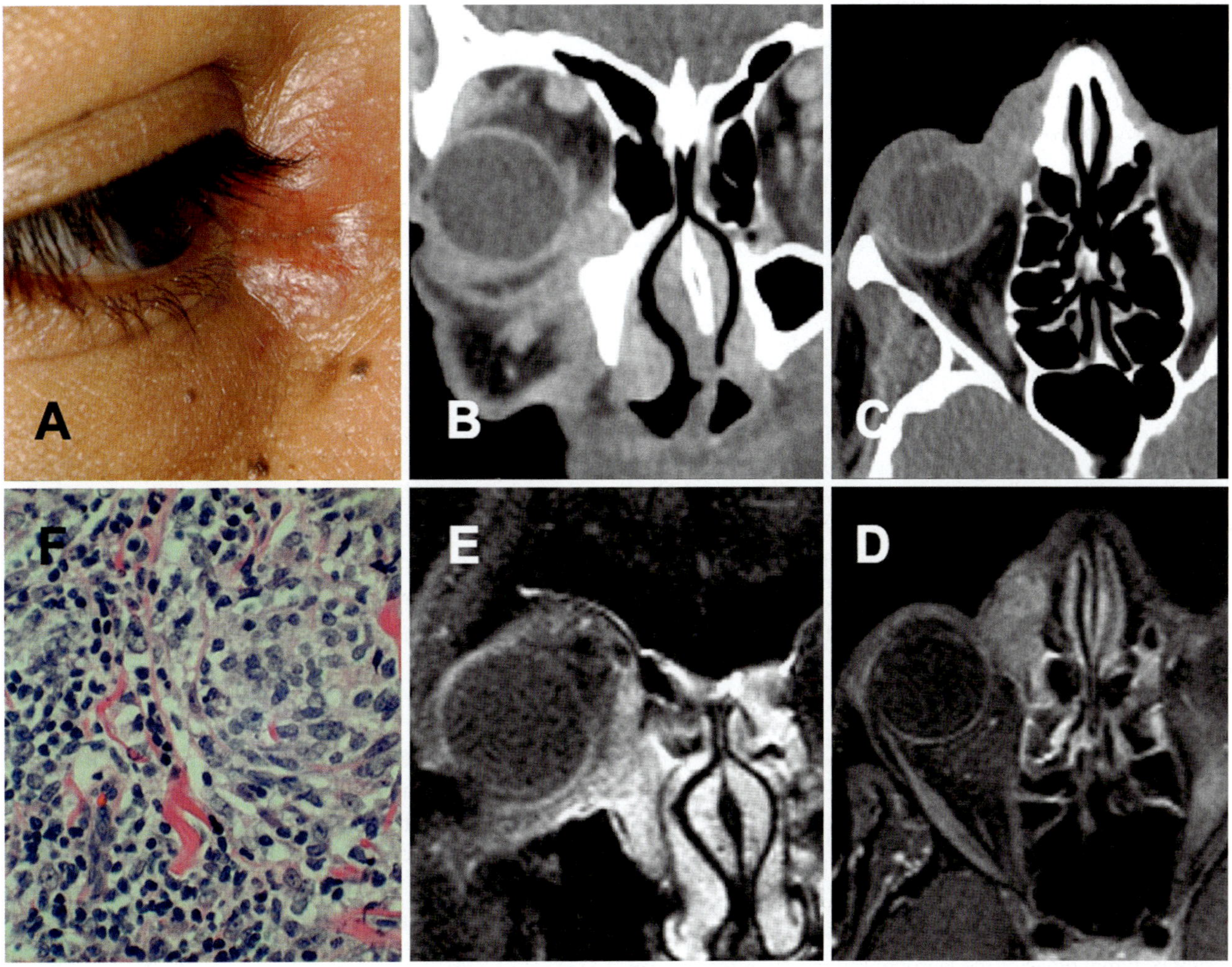

Fig. 30.3 (Clockwise) (**a**) A 54-year-old man with a firm, nodular, nonmobile subcutaneous mass located in the right medial canthus and on the side of the nose. Note the skin changes with telangiectatic vessels overlying the tumor. (**b**, **c**) Axial and coronal CT scan images reveal a homogenously enhancing mass in the right lacrimal fossa without obvious bony erosion. (**d**, **e**) Axial and coronal T1-weighted MRI images with fat suppression reveal a right lacrimal sac infiltrating mass with heterogeneous enhancement, partially occluding the right nasolacrimal duct. (**f**) Hematoxylin and eosin stain, 40X, reveals small and large lymphoid cells. Final diagnosis after immunohistochemical evaluation was low-grade B-cell lymphoma with transformation into diffuse large B-cell lymphoma

Table 30.1a Broad classification of the lacrimal sac tumors: epithelial tumors

Epithelial tumors
Benign
Squamous papilloma
Inverted papilloma
Transitional cell papilloma
Mixed cell papilloma
Oncocytoma
Pleomorphic adenoma
Cylindroma
Malignant
Squamous cell carcinoma
Transitional cell carcinoma
Mixed cell carcinoma
Oncocytic adenocarcinoma
Mucoepidermoid carcinoma
Adenoid cystic carcinoma
Adenocarcinoma

Table 30.1b Broad classification of the lacrimal sac tumors: nonepithelial tumors

Mesenchymal	Lymphoproliferative	Neural
Benign	*Benign*	*Benign*
Solitary fibrous tumor	Benign reactive lymphoid hyperplasia	Neurofibroma
Juvenile xanthogranuloma	Lymphoplasmacytic infiltrate	Schwannoma
Hemangioma		
Lipoma	*Malignant*	**Melanocytic**
Leiomyoma	Lymphoma	*Benign*
Osteoma	Leukemic infiltrate ("granulocytic sarcoma")	Nevus
	Plasmacytoma	
Malignant		*Malignant*
Kaposi's sarcoma		Melanoma

Table 30.2 Review of large (more than ten) case series of primary lacrimal sac tumors

	Epithelial benign	Epithelial malignant	Mesenchymal benign	Mesenchymal malignant	Lymphoid benign	Lymphoid malignant	Melanocytic benign	Melanocytic malignant	Neural	Total (% malignant)
Radnot and Gall [3]	22	64	5	26	1	14	1	5	0	138 (79%)
Harry and Ashton [4]	5	3	0	1	0	2	0	2	0	13 (62%)
Schenck et al. [5]	4	14	1	2	0	0	0	3	1	25 (76%)
Ryan and Font [6]	11	16	0	0	0	0	0	0	0	27 (59%)
Ni et al. [2]	6	71	1	2	0	1	0	0	1	82 (90%)
Stefanyszyn et al. [1]	38	44	15	0	2	9	0	6	1	115 (51%)
Yip et al. [7]	0	0	0	0	0	11[a]	0	0	0	11 (100%)
Anderson et al. [8]	4	4	0	0	4	10	0	0	0	22 (64%)
Parmar and Rose [9]	1	8	1	0	0	5	0	0	0	15 (87%)
Jordan [10]	6	4	0	0	4	9	0	0	0	23 (57%)
Marthin et al. [11]	11	7	0	0	0	7	0	0	0	25 (56%)
Sjo et al. [12]	0	0	0	0	0	15[b]	0	0	0	15 (100%)
Bi et al. [13]	0	83	3	0	0	5	0	3	2	96 (95%)
Sjo et al. [14]	5	6	0	0	0	0	0	0	0	11[c] (56%)
Song et al. [15]	0	79	0	1	0	7[d]	0	2	1	90 (100%)
Total	113	403	26	32	11	95	1	21	6	708

[a]Ten of 11 patients had known leukemia or lymphoma
[b]Lymphomas arising in the lacrimal sac were predominantly diffuse large B-cell lymphomas
[c]100% positive for either HPV type 6 or 11 or both
[d]Three were diffuse large B-cell lymphoma and four were extranodal marginal zone B-cell lymphoma of the mucosa-associated lymphoid tissue

squamous papillomas, whereas HPV types 16 and 18 are associated with squamous carcinoma, similar to neoplasia of the genital tract [14, 21].

Nonepithelial tumors Lymphomas and lymphocytic infiltrates are the most common nonepithelial tumors, accounting for 50% of all nonepithelial lesions of the lacrimal sac (Tables 30.1b and 30.2). Sjo and associates reported a series of 15 primary lymphomas of the lacrimal sac in which the median age of the patients was 71 years [12]. Diffuse large B-cell [12, 15], chronic lymphocytic leukemia [7] and marginal zone B-cell lymphomas [13, 15] have been described. Mesenchymal tumors constitute about 30% of nonepithelial tumors of the lacrimal sac (Table 30.2). Based on the largest report of 35 nonepithelial tumors by Pe'er and associates, the mean age of the patients with mesenchymal tumors was 34 years and fibrous histiocytoma was the most common type [20]. About 15% of nonepithelial tumors were of melanocytic origin. Fifty melanomas of the lacrimal sac have been reported in the literature [1, 3–5, 13, 15, 22–26]. Melanomas of the lacrimal sac are similar to those of the mucosal membranes of the nose and paranasal sinuses. The treatment plan is similar to mucosal melanomas, with a similar poor prognosis. Aggressive measures including wide surgical excision and radiation may delay recurrence but do little to prevent fatality in the presence of metastatic disease [1, 26].

Management

In the case of an unsuspected lacrimal sac tumor during a routine dacryocystorhinostomy (DCR), where the sac appears enlarged and hardened, a deep incisional biopsy is necessary to obtain a tumor sample and not just the peripheral inflammatory response to the tumor. If the frozen section confirms the presence of a tumor, then a dacryocystectomy should be done without disturbing the lacrimal fossa to prevent the contiguous spread of tumor into the nose or sinuses [27] (Fig. 30.4).

If a lacrimal sac tumor other than lymphoma is suspected, the patient should be informed that a dacryocystectomy will be performed with reconstruction to follow at a later date. Intraoperative frozen section analysis is recommended to verify the diagnosis and evaluate for tumor-free margins. Postoperative radiotherapy or systemic chemotherapy can be delivered in an attempt to obtain complete tumor control and minimize recurrence.

Once a tumor other than lymphoma has been confirmed, an en bloc excision is planned. If there is radiologic evidence of extension beyond the lacrimal drainage system, exenteration, lateral rhinotomy, and cervical lymph node dissection with collaboration from an otolaryngologist can offer a chance of cure (Fig. 30.2). The necessity for complete resection of tumor cannot be overemphasized. Radiotherapy is indicated when bone or lymphatic invasion is evident, or when neoplastic cells are present in the resection margins. Radiotherapy alone is not considered a treatment of choice, but only a palliative option in selected cases.

After a confirmatory biopsy, primary treatment of lymphoma with surgery, irradiation, and chemotherapy alone or in combination confers good tumor remission [12]. Treatment of lymphoma depends on the type and the extent of the lesion, the age, and clinical symptoms of the patient [20]. Close observation can be considered for a localized, low-grade histologic type lymphoid tumor in elderly patients. Irradiation (35–40 Gy) is generally indicated for

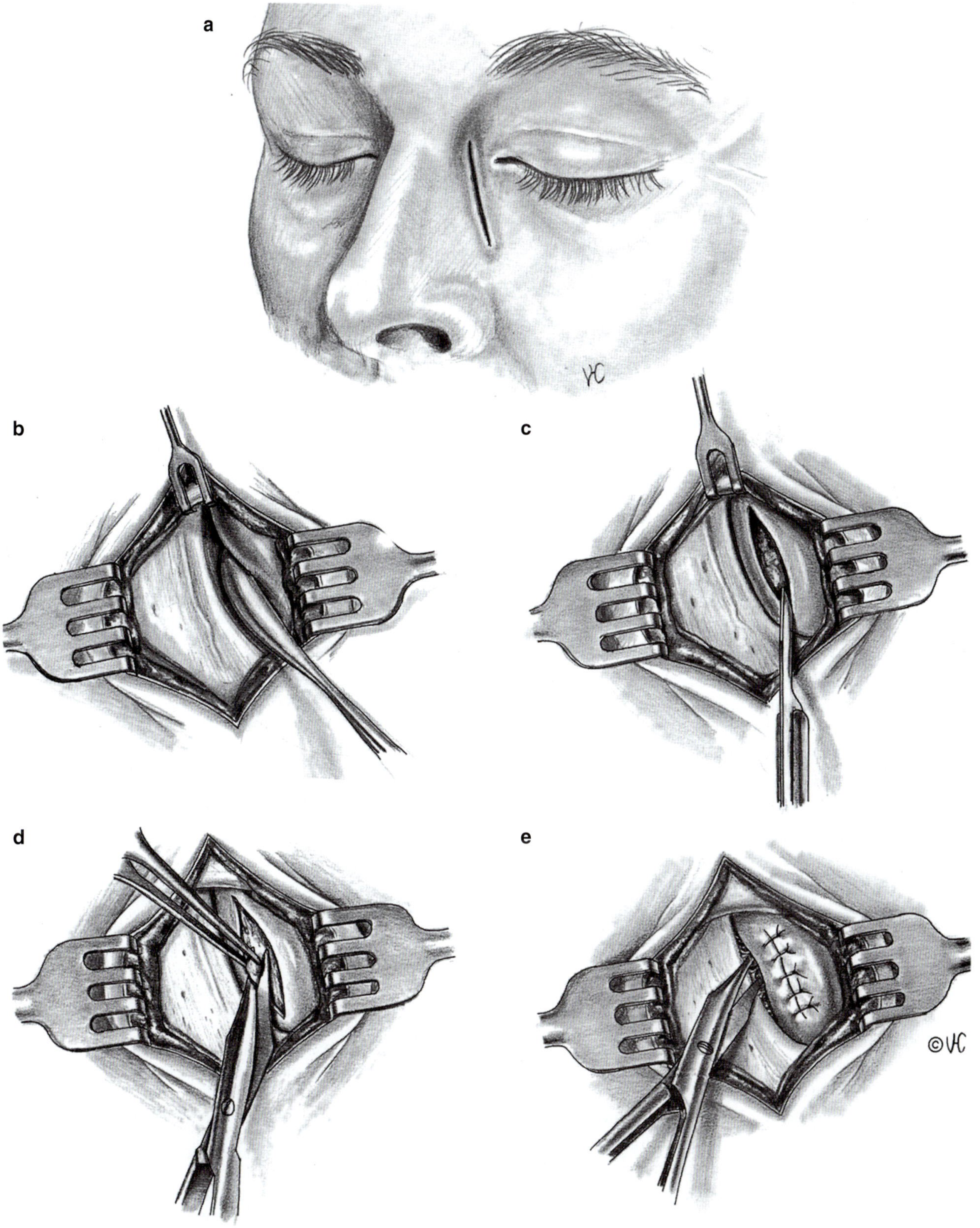

Fig. 30.4 Dacryocystectomy. (**a**) Incision for dacryocystectomy. (**b**) Skin, orbicularis, and medial canthal tendon are elevated and reflected laterally. Lacrimal sac is elevated and reflected out of lacrimal fossa. (**c**) Lacrimal sac is opened with Bard-Parker blade for inspection of interior sac. (**d**) Suspicious tissue in lacrimal sac is incised and submitted for frozen sections. (**e**) If tumor is diagnosed, sac is sutured closed and excised in its entirety with other surrounding structures as needed

solitary lymphomas. Systemic lymphoma should initially be treated with chemotherapy, such as rituximab.

Prognosis

The outcome of epithelial lacrimal sac tumors depends on the extent of the tumor and the appropriateness of treatment [2]. For malignant tumors confined to the lacrimal sac treated by dacryocystectomy and irradiation, the reported 5-year mortality rate is 44%, in contrast to those supplemented by lateral rhinotomy, with associated mortality rate of only 13% [2]. Tumor type on pathology and tumor growth pattern are major determinants of prognosis and mortality rate. Papillary squamous carcinoma has a more favorable prognosis (mortality 14%), while transitional cell carcinoma has a poor prognosis with mortality reaching 100%. Patients with exophytic growth of squamous carcinoma have shown mortality of 14%, as compared to endophytic squamous carcinoma infiltrating the sac wall that carries a higher mortality of 50%.

Of the 82 lacrimal sac tumors that Ni and colleagues reported, 74 were malignant. Among this group, direct extension to the adjacent structures was the most common mode of tumor spread (89%), but 27% developed lymphatic metastases to the preauricular, submandibular, or cervical lymph nodes, and 9% developed hematogenous dissemination mainly to the lung and less commonly to the esophagus [2].

Recurrence and mortality rates for nonepithelial lacrimal sac tumors other than lymphoma vary greatly and cannot be generalized due to the rarity of each individual subtype. Five-year survival for patients with lymphoma is 65% or higher [12]. Melanoma of the lacrimal sac is often fatal despite aggressive treatment [1]. Parma and Rose reported disease-free survival (DFS) of 60% with a median of 30 months follow-up of patients with lacrimal sac malignancy [9]. Song and colleagues reported a study of 90 malignant lacrimal sac tumors, in which DFS improved to 78% with a median of 50 months follow-up. The authors attributed higher survival to aggressive radiotherapy either as an adjuvant to surgery or as definitive treatment for those who refuse surgery or have unresectable tumors [15].

Successful management of lacrimal sac tumors requires a high index of suspicion as well as aggressive and early intervention. Although some authors advocate a routine sac biopsy in all dacryocystorhinostomy [8], what is more important is a careful intraoperative inspection of the lacrimal sac to prevent the surgeon from overlooking a lacrimal sac neoplasm [28]. For all malignant lacrimal sac tumors, patients need systemic workup including a physical exam, complete blood count (CBC), chemistry profile, lactate dehydrogenase (LDH), CT scan of chest and abdomen, and positron emission tomography (PET) scan. Bone marrow biopsy may be indicated in the presence of symptoms or abnormal blood work suspicious for systemic lymphoma.

References

1. Stefanyszyn MA, Hidayat AA, Pe'er JJ, Flanagan JC. Lacrimal sac tumors. Ophthal Plast Reconstr Surg. 1994;10:169–84.
2. Ni C, D'Amico DJ, Fan CQ, Kuo PK. Tumors of the lacrimal sac: a clinicopathological analysis of 82 cases. Int Ophthalmol Clin. 1982;22:121–40.
3. Radnot M, Gall J. Tumors of the lacrimal sac. Ophthalmologica. 1966;151:2–22.
4. Harry J, Ashton N. The pathology of tumours of the lacrimal sac. Trans Ophthalmol Soc UK. 1969;88:19–35.
5. Schenck NL, Ogura JH, Pratt LL. Cancer of the lacrimal sac. Presentation of five cases and review of the literature. Ann Otol Rhinol Laryngol. 1973;82:153–61.
6. Ryan SJ, Font RL. Primary epithelial neoplasms of the lacrimal sac. Am J Ophthalmol. 1973;76:73–88.
7. Yip CC, Bartley GB, Habermann TM, Garrity JA. Involvement of the lacrimal drainage system by leukemia or lymphoma. Ophthal Plast Reconstr Surg. 2002;18:242–6.
8. Anderson NG, Wojno TH, Grossniklaus HE. Clinicopathologic findings from lacrimal sac biopsy specimens obtained during dacryocystorhinostomy. Ophthal Plast Reconstr Surg. 2003;19:173–6.
9. Parmar DN, Rose GE. Management of lacrimal sac tumours. Eye (London). 2003;17:599–606.
10. Jordan DR. Re: "Clinicopathologic findings from lacrimal sac biopsy specimens obtained during dacryocystorhinostomy". Ophthal Plast Reconstr Surg. 2004;20:176–7.
11. Marthin JK, Lindegaard J, Prause JU, Heegaard S. Lesions of the lacrimal drainage system: a clinicopathological study of 643 biopsy specimens of the lacrimal drainage system in Denmark 1910–1999. Acta Ophthalmol Scand. 2005;83:94–9.
12. Sjo LD, Ralfkiaer E, Juhl BR, et al. Primary lymphoma of the lacrimal sac: an EORTC ophthalmic oncology task force study. Br J Ophthalmol. 2006;90:1004–9.
13. Bi YW, Chen RJ, Li XP. Clinical and pathological analysis of primary lacrimal sac tumors. Zhonghua Yan Ke Za Zhi. 2007;43:499–504.
14. Sjo NC, von Buchwald C, Cassonnet P, et al. Human papillomavirus: cause of epithelial lacrimal sac neoplasia? Acta Ophthalmol Scand. 2007;85:551–6.
15. Song X, Wang J, Wang S, Wang W, Wang S, Zhu W. Clinical analysis of 90 cases of malignant lacrimal sac tumor. Graefe's Arch Clin Exp Ophthal. 2018;256:1333–8.
16. Spaeth EB. A surgical technique for lacrimal sac malignancy. Trans Ophthalmol Soc UK. 1970;89:351–4.
17. Flanagan JC, Stokes DP. Lacrimal sac tumors. Ophthalmology. 1978;85:1282–7.
18. Schefler AC, Shields CL, Shields JA, Demirci H, Maus M, Eagle RC Jr. Lacrimal sac lymphoma in a child. Arch Ophthalmol. 2003;121:1330–3.
19. Pe'er J, Hidayat AA, Ilsar M, Landau L, Stefanyszyn MA. Glandular tumors of the lacrimal sac. Their histopathologic patterns and possible origins. Ophthalmology. 1996;103:1601–5.

20. Pe'er JJ, Stefanyszyn M, Hidayat AA. Nonepithelial tumors of the lacrimal sac. Am J Ophthalmol. 1994;118:650–8.
21. Madreperla SA, Green WR, Daniel R, Shah KV. Human papillomavirus in primary epithelial tumors of the lacrimal sac. Ophthalmology. 1993;100:569–73.
22. Gleizal A, Nimeskern N, Kodjikian L, Beziat JL. Lacrimal sac melanoma. Rev. Stomatol Chir Maxillofac. 2005;106:103–5.
23. Lee HM, Kang HJ, Choi G, et al. Two cases of primary malignant melanoma of the lacrimal sac. Head Neck. 2001;23:809–13.
24. Eide N, Refsum SB, Bakke S. Primary malignant melanoma of the lacrimal sac. Acta Ophthalmol (Copenh). 1993;71:273–6.
25. Malik TY, Sanders R, Young JD, Brennand E, Evans AT. Malignant melanoma of the lacrimal sac. Eye (Lond). 1997;11:935–7.
26. Sitole S, Zender CA, Ahmad AZ, Hammadeh R, Petruzzelli GJ. Lacrimal sac melanoma. Ophthal Plast Reconstr Surg. 2007;23:417–9.
27. Stokes DP, Flanagan JC. Dacryocystectomy for tumors of the lacrimal sac. Ophthalmic Surg. 1977;8:85–90.
28. Hurwitz JJ. Re: "Clinicopathologic findings from lacrimal sac biopsies obtained during dacryocystorhinostomy". Ophthal Plast Reconstr Surg. 2003;19:412; author reply 412–3

Dysfunctional Tear Film, Etiology, Diagnosis, and Treatment in Oculoplastic Surgery

31

Mark R. Levine and Essam A. El Toukhy

Dry eye syndrome (DES) is a complex and very prevalent disease that affects more than 10 million people, primarily women, in the United States alone. When you consider the number of contact lens wearers, computer users, patients who live and/or work in dirty environments, and patients with autoimmune disease, the number is certainly higher [1].

Why is a discussion of this problem germane in an oculoplastic surgery section? It is simply that failure to appreciate the complexity of a stable tear film (be it a decrease in aqueous tear production or meibomian gland dysfunction) may lead to an unhappy patient following ptosis or blepharoplasty surgery *as the lid position and eyelid dynamics have changed.* This can occur from unmasking a borderline condition or exacerbation of a preexisting one. Preoperatively, appreciation of the dry eye and meibomian gland dysfunction (dysfunctional tear film) with appropriate preoperative treatment may circumvent potential postoperative problems.

In addition, many patients who are referred for epiphora secondary to possible nasolacrimal duct obstruction after evaluation of the lacrimal system are found to have pseudo-epiphora (dysfunctional tear film) and not nasolacrimal duct obstruction. Finally, the concept of a dysfunctional tear film is not only a decrease in aqueous volume and increase in tear osmolarity but changes in the meibomian gland function and increase in tear evaporation. Both of these entities change a stable tear film. McCulley et al. found that 100% of patients with meibomianitis had signs of dry eye syndrome [2].

A stable tear film is composed of compositional factors (lipid, aqueous, and mucin) and hydrodynamic factors (eyelid blinking and eyelid closure). In the compositional arm, the hydrophobic lipid layer (0.4 μm thick outer layer of the tear film) is secreted by the meibomian glands and functions to prevent evaporation and maintain structural integrity of the tear film [3]. The primary component is meibom that is typically clear and free-flowing, consisting of nonpolar wax esters, cholesterol esters, and low concentration of polar triglycerides and free fatty esters. The meibomian glands make meibom from essential fatty acids. Accumulation of the meibom within the meibomian glands can lead to inflammation of the gland and bacterial colonization. The bacteria have lipases that break down wax and cholesterol esters to triglycerides and free fatty acids. The polar lipids diffuse through the aqueous layer and contaminate the mucin layer making it hydrophobic. This leads to tear film instability and a nonwetting corneal surface, and consequently a decreased tear breakup time and superficial punctate keratopathy [4–6]. In aging, there is an increase in eyelid erythema, telangiectasis, keratinization, irregular posterior lid margins, orifice metaplasia, and opaque secretions.

The middle aqueous layer is 7 μm thick [7]. The normal secretion is 1–2 μL/min with a pH of 6.5–7.6. The aqueous layer is produced by the main and accessory lacrimal glands. It hydrates the ocular surface and gives a smooth refractive surface. A healthy tear film contains, in addition to water, a complex mixture of proteins, mucins, and electrolytes. Proteins such as lysozymes and lactoferrin have antimicrobial properties, while immunoglobulins such as IgA, IgG, and IgM have protective functions. Other components of the tear include epidermal growth factor (which regulates the process for replacing epithelial cells and is necessary for healing) and electrolytes (sodium chloride, potassium, and calcium). In dry eyes, these beneficial components are reduced [8–10].

The mucus layer (0.2 μm) is produced by the goblet cells in the conjunctiva. Its lipophilic properties allow it to spread evenly over the epithelial membranes of the ocular surface, and its hydrophilic properties allow the aqueous layer to spread evenly over the corneal surface. Soluble mucin is

M. R. Levine (✉)
University Hospitals of Cleveland, Department of Ophthalmology, Cleveland, OH, USA
e-mail: mlevine@eye-lids.com

E. A. El Toukhy
School of Medicine, Cairo University, Department of Ophthalmology, Dokki, Cairo, Egypt

J. J. Servat et al. (eds.), *Smith and Nesi's Ophthalmic Plastic and Reconstructive Surgery*,
https://doi.org/10.1007/978-3-030-41720-8_31

secreted by the conjunctival goblet cells and is reduced in chronic dry eyes with loss of goblet cells.

An important concept for ocular surface health is that of the neural reflex arc. The maintenance of a normal ocular surface requires an intact neural sensory loop that connects the ocular surface to the brain, then to the lacrimal gland. Disruption of this loop will compromise the system. Without proper functioning of the lacrimal gland and its tear components, inflammatory mediators such as cytokines and proteases are released into the tear film compromising the ocular surface. Moreover, the main and accessory lacrimal glands may be susceptible to inflammation due to degenerative processes resulting from a decrease in neural or androgen support. The degenerative processes trigger chemically mediated inflammation that leads to activation of key lymphocytes. This leads to T-cell-mediated inflammation, cytokine production, the presence of cytokines in tears (interleukin 1 and tumor necrosis factor-alpha), and acinar cell apoptosis. Research has shown that cytokines in tears trigger T-cell-mediated inflammation on the ocular surface, disrupt epithelial cell function, interfere with mucin production, and decrease corneal sensitivity and thickening of the ocular surface epithelium [11, 12].

Up until this point, the compositional stability of the precorneal tear film has been discussed. From a hydrodynamic standpoint, the precorneal tear film needs to be mechanically spread to cover the entire ocular surface. Meibom needs to be expressed from the meibomian glands, and tear clearance is necessary to eliminate aqueous fluids into the nasolacrimal excretory system. This is indispensable to maintain ocular health as retention of the inflammatory mediators will only aggravate the ocular surface.

The functions of the eyelid and ocular adnexa are integrated by two reflexes, both mediated on the afferent side by the first division of the trigeminal nerve (V1). The efferent pathways are mediated by the facial nerve (CN7). The arm that is involved in the composition of the tear film is mediated by the parasympathetics of CN7, whereas the arm that involves the hydrodynamic elements is run by the motor division. We can see how in Figs. 31.1 and 31.2; these are integrated to promote a healthy ocular surface.

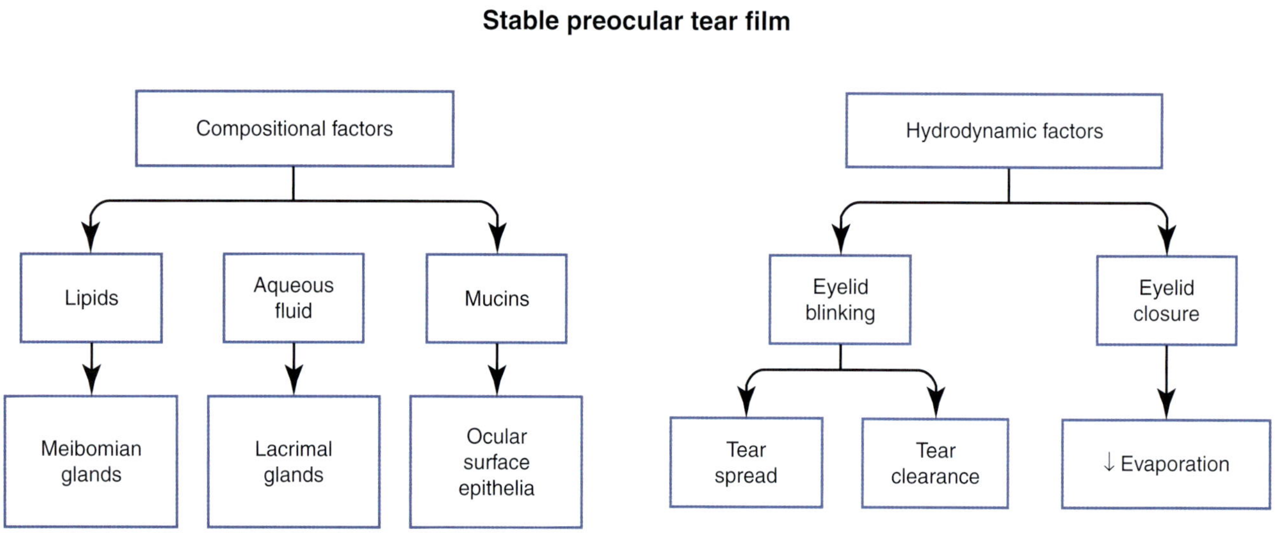

Fig. 31.1 The integration of the elements necessary to maintain a normal functioning ocular surface. (Modified from Parrish [3])

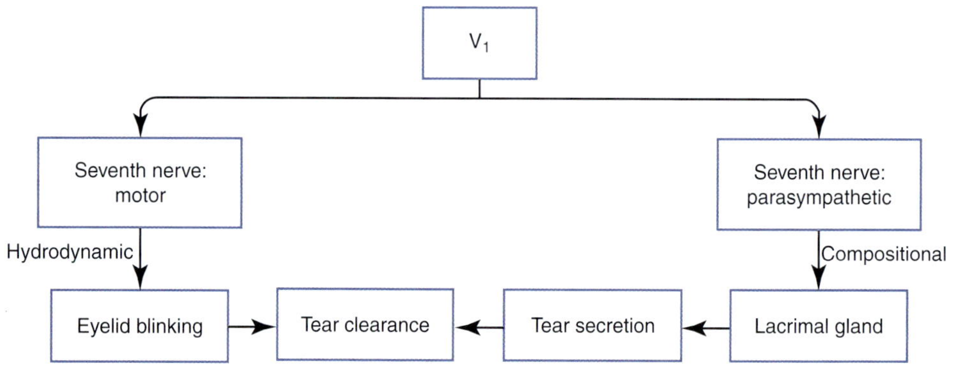

Fig. 31.2 The neural integrated arm. (Modified from Parrish [3])

When evaluating a patient with suspected dry eye syndrome (DES), there are a number of points in the history and physical examination that will help in establishing the diagnosis:

1. *Good history taking:* Particular attention should be paid to when the patient's symptoms are worse. Early morning irritation, pain, burning, and crusting that improve as the day progresses are complaints more common in patients with blepharitis and meibomian gland disease. Patients with a complaint of foreign body sensation, pain, irritation, and fluctuation in vision that gets progressively worse throughout the day, or with increased visual acuity (reading, watching TV, or working on a computer), are more indicative of dry eye syndrome. Patients with tearing down their face (gross epiphora) suggest nasolacrimal duct obstruction. Patients complain of eyes feeling wet and are about to tear but do not suggest dry eye syndrome. Patients may also complain of decreased visual acuity due to instability of the tear film. It is to be remembered that one of the functions of tear film–air interface in the cornea is its contribution to refraction. This contributes approximately 40 diopters of the total 60-diopter refractive ability of the eye (the remaining 20 diopters being in the crystalline lens). Since the tear–air interface is of paramount importance, it is easy to see how a disruption of tear film will cause significant symptoms of blurred vision.
2. *Review the patient medication list:* There are a number of medications that can exacerbate dry eye syndrome including antidepressants, decongestants, antihistamines, blood pressure medications, diuretics, ulcer medication, tranquilizers, beta blockers, oral contraceptive, and eye medications, such as antihistamine drops and glaucoma medications. Glaucoma medications have benzalkonium chloride (BAK) as a preservative (0.004–0.025% concentration). BAK has been shown to have a disruptive effect on the tear film by exerting a detergent effect on the lipid layer that predisposes the ocular surface to inflammation, as well as reducing the number of goblet cells and mucin secretion. In addition, it reduces tear production and decreases epithelial and conjunctival thickness, resulting in a decreased tear film breakup time (TBUT) [13, 14].
3. *Evaluate the patient's medical and dietary history:* Does the patient have acne rosacea? Do they eat cheese, nuts, or chocolate, or drink tea, coffee, or wine? This is most indicative of meibomian gland dysfunction.
4. *Physical examination:* Ocular rosacea is an often overlooked cause of meibomian gland dysfunction but represents an important facet in management. Look for signs of ocular or facial rosacea including rhinophyma, malar flushing, and facial telangiectasis:
   (a) Look at the patient while interviewing them and look for signs of gross epiphora versus the patient's sensation of wetness without gross epiphora.
   (b) Inspect the tear meniscus and tear breakup time. Begin by examining the tear meniscus (normal should be 1.0 mm and convex). Next, instill fluorescein in the inferior cul-de-sac and evaluate the stability of the tear film. This must be done prior to the instillation of any drops and before any manipulation of the lids. To achieve this, moisten a fluorescein strip with sterile saline and touch it to the inferior tarsal conjunctiva. Place the cobalt blue filter on and after several blinks; have the patient keep their eyes open. Look for any randomly appearing dry spots. Any spot appearing in less than 10 s is abnormal. This is indicative of an unstable tear film. Another test that correlates well with the abnormal tear breakup time is inability to hold eyes open for 10 s without burning or stinging.
   (c) Schirmer testing. This is a test of aqueous tear production. Schirmer testing is performed by placing a thin strip of filter paper in the inferior cul-de-sac (Fig. 31.3). Care must be used to place this laterally so as to minimize the effect of corneal irritation. The patient is also asked to keep the eyes closed to minimize the effect of blinking. This test can be done in several ways to measure a different secretion. This is measured following anesthetic instillation and drying out the fornix with a cotton-tipped applicator. This allows the effect of reflex tearing to be excluded in the measurement of tear production. The strips are left in for 5 min, and although normal measurements can be quite variable, a result of less than 10 mm in 5 min is highly suggestive of aqueous tear deficiency (ATD). Another more practical way to get a similar

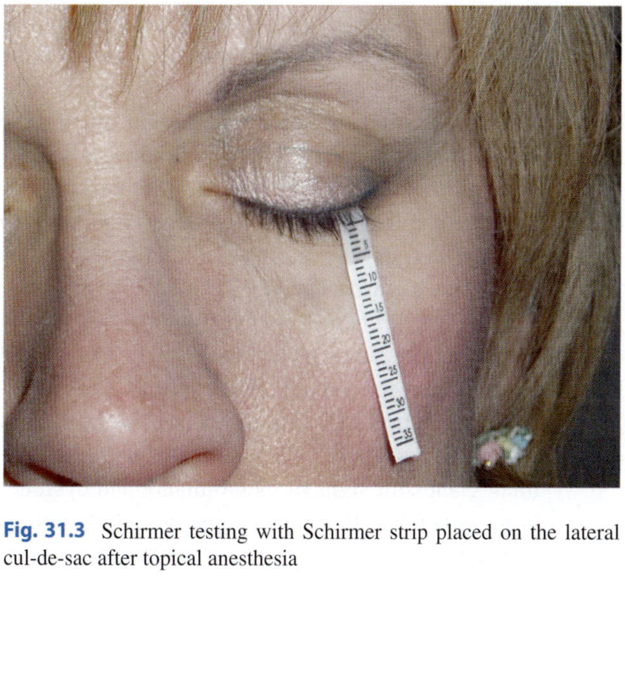

Fig. 31.3 Schirmer testing with Schirmer strip placed on the lateral cul-de-sac after topical anesthesia

(although not identical) result is to do the Schirmer test for 1 min and multiply the result by 3. This is a great way to identify those patients who have moderate to severe dry eyes as well as those who are normal. However, it may require repeated measurements in those who fall in between.

The other tests (Schirmer I and II) are more specific for evaluation of reflex tearing and are not routinely used. Most recently, tear osmolarity testing may replace a lot of these tests. If tears osmolarity testing is normal (less than 308 mOsms/L), the patient does not have dry eyes [15]. *Several devices are available for measuring tear osmolarity. Lacripen, a hand-held diagnostic tool, is one of these.*

(d) Fluorescein, rose bengal, and lissamine green staining. The pattern of staining is more important than the simple presence or absence of stain. Inferior corneal staining with fluorescein suggests probable lid etiology such as lagophthalmos, meibomianitis, and blepharitis. Using rose bengal staining (or the equally effective and less irritating lissamine green) is useful in that it can detect early changes in the progression of dry eye syndrome (DES). We know that either rose bengal or lissamine green stains the conjunctiva once goblet cell loss becomes quite significant. Again, the pattern of staining is more useful than merely the presence or absence of stain. The nasal conjunctiva stains more than the temporal conjunctiva, and the resilient cornea stains less than the conjunctiva, and later in the disease process.

(e) Gross examination of the lids. Look for the eyelid malposition and blink rate (Parkinson's). It is important to look for punctal ectropion and punctal stenosis (which may be primary or secondary to chronic meibomianitis, blepharitis, or rosacea). Pay attention to whether the patient has gross epiphora. If present, this usually points to a structural problem (lid position and lacrimal system). Remember to irrigate the lacrimal system in any patient with gross epiphora.

(f) Slit lamp examination of the lid margin. Inspect the lids for the presence of any blepharitis with scaling or lash inflammation. Bacterial lipases can directly cause destabilization of the tear film in addition to a toxic effect on the surface epithelium. Chronic blepharitis has associated meibomian abnormalities. The bacteria produce toxins that inflame the lid and cause keratinization of the meibomian glands and their subsequent stenosis. This, in turn, may result in unstable tear film that often is associated with evaporative dry eye. When looking at the meibomian glands for signs of meibomian gland dysfunction, remember that meibomian gland secretions should be clear or slightly yellow and express easily.

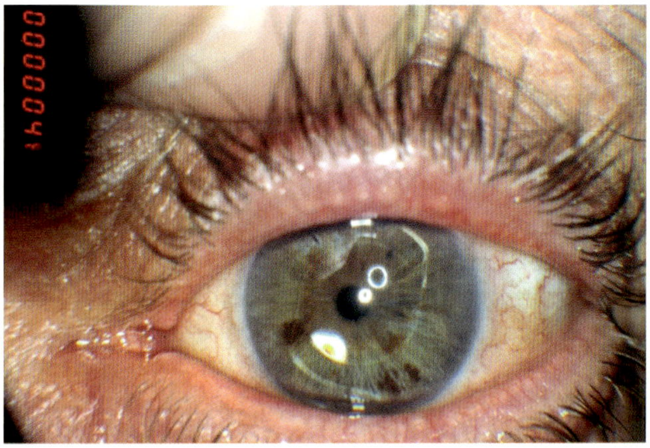

Fig. 31.4 Telangiectasia of the lid margin in an aging patient

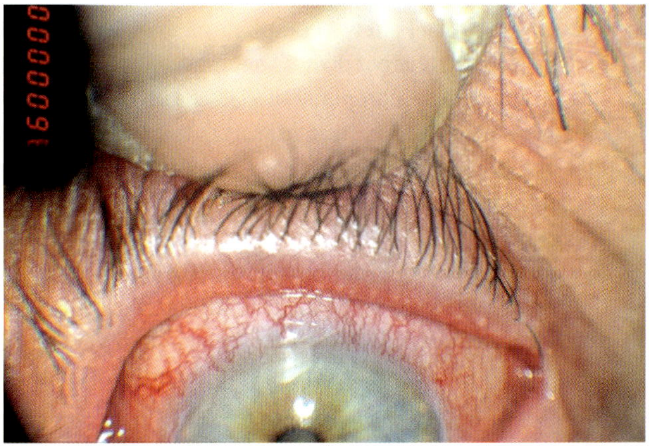

Fig. 31.5 Meibomian glands with turbid secretions

The natural progression of meibomian gland disease is as follows:

- Lid margin vascular engorgement and telangiectasis of the lid margin overlying the meibomian glands (Fig. 31.4).
- Stenosis of the meibomian gland orifices. When pressure is applied to the lid margin, oil secretion can be expressed through the stenosed orifices. These secretions are often turbid and/or have an appearance that is similar to toothpaste (Figs. 31.5 and 31.6).
- Chronic meibomianitis may lead to thickening and blunting of the lid margin that causes gland orifice obliteration (Fig. 31.7).

  Meibography can be used to grade and document meibomian gland function (Fig. 31.8).

5. *Treatment:* Treatment of DES and MGD (DTF) is multifactorial. There is no single correct treatment regimen or hierarchy of treatment protocols. The treatment must be aimed at the underlying cause, and what works for one patient may not necessarily work for another

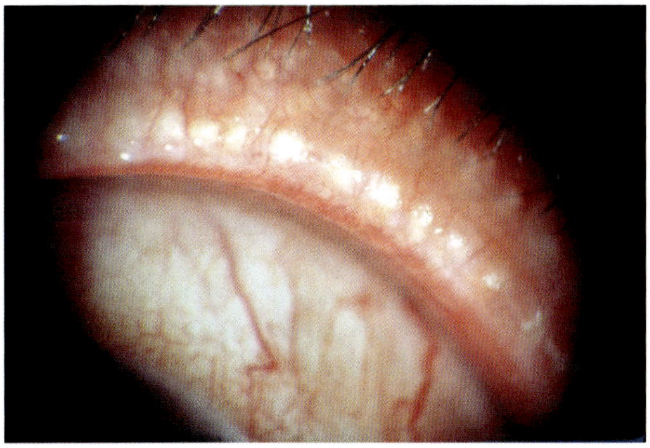

Fig. 31.6 Meibomian glands with turbid secretions

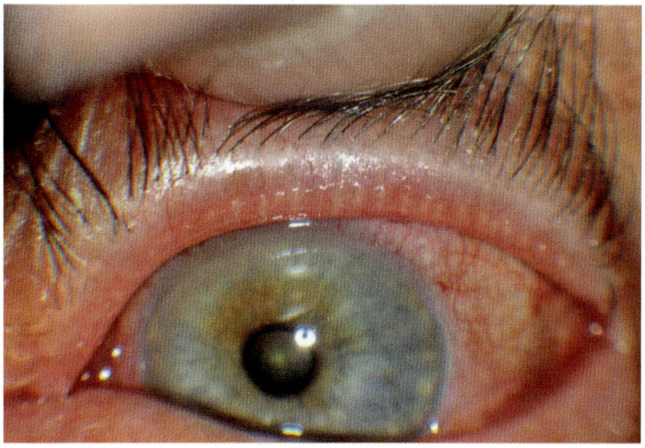

Fig. 31.7 The mucocutaneous junction of the upper lid with turbid secretions and rounding of the posterior lid border

Fig. 31.8 Meibography can be used to grade and document meibomian gland function. (Modified from Arita et al. [25])

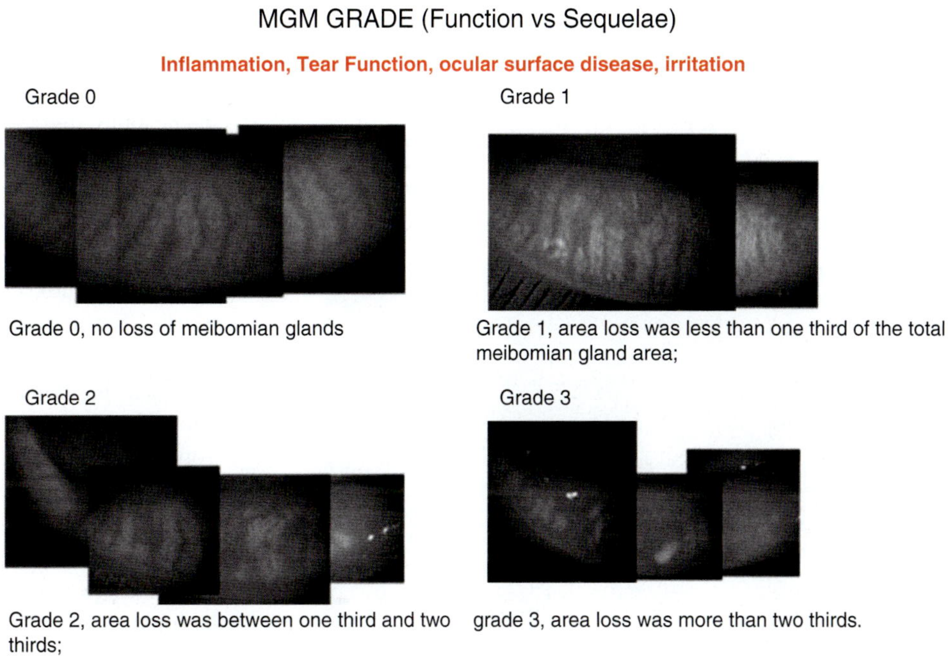

(a) Lid hygiene: Warm compresses applied to the eyelid margin can help to liquify the thick meibomian gland secretions and thus facilitate their expression. Mild nonirritating cleansing solutions such as dilute baby shampoo or commercially prepared eyelid scrubs also can be applied to the eyelids to remove clogging debris. Additionally, light pressure applied to the eyelids can aid in gland expression after application of warm compresses. *If pressure is ineffective to express meibomian gland secretions because of its thickness the Lipiflow Thermal Pulsation may be advantageous. The devise applies heat to the conjunctival surface of the lids while applying pulsatile pressure to the outer eyelid surface. This allows removal of old tenacious secretions and replacement with new more healthy effective meibom. Other thermal devices have been introduced e.g. Miboflow* [16].

(b) Punctal occlusion: Punctal occlusion is indicated when a diagnosis of aqueous tear deficiency (ATD) has been made. It should never be used when the patient has delayed clearance of tears or in meibomian gland dysfunction (MGD). If the outflow system is blocked in a patient with increased inflammatory mediators, then the ocular condition will worsen as the inflammatory components are unable to be cleared. It is, therefore, essential to have the correct diagnosis before undergoing punctal occlusion.

(c) Artificial tears: There are a number of different tears available ranging from those with preservatives (Visine Tears and HypoTears) to those with disappearing preservatives (Refresh and GenTeal) to those with no preservatives (Bion and TheraTears). Because of the frequency of application, nonpreserved artificial tears are recommended for use. Tears should be applied liberally throughout the day and, if necessary, a lubricating ointment may be used at night. This ointment may contain an antibiotic preparation.

(d) *Tear stimulation: Most recently, the Food and Drug Administration (FDA) has approved "True Tears", a hand-held device utilizing the concept of neurostimulation, to electrically stimulate the nasal mucosa resulting in reflex tear secretion from the lacrimal gland, thereby reducing the need for artificial tears* (Fig. 31.9).

(e) Topical steroids: These are useful as a temporary measure when the patient is very symptomatic and the eye and/or eyelids show moderate to severe signs of inflammation. Severe cases in which the ocular surface is filled with inflammatory mediators will likely benefit from low-dose steroids. Topical corticosteroids have a beneficial effect on the subjective and objective clinical parameters in moderate to severe dry eyes. These effects are associated with a reduction of inflammatory markers of conjunctival epithelial cells, increase goblet cell density, and smooth the corneal surface [17]. They should not be used for longer than a couple of weeks to decrease any adverse effects (steroid-induced glaucoma). Surface steroids like loteprednol have a lower risk of inducing glaucoma.

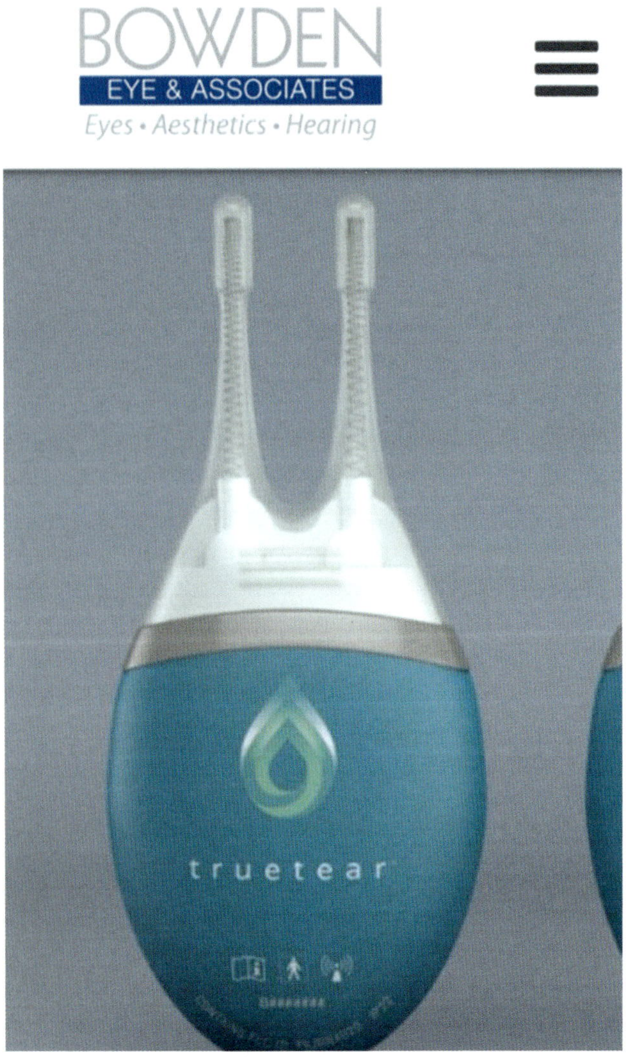

Fig. 31.9 True Tear

(f) Oral antibiotics (tetracycline): Tetracyclines represent the most common and most effective treatment regimen for rosacea. Tetracyclines have antibacterial and anti-inflammatory properties [18]. These drugs are believed to be effective, not primarily as antibiotics but rather through a secondary effect they exert on the meibomian glands. Tetracycline decreases bacteria lipase, thereby altering the fatty acid composition of meibomian gland secretions and improving their solubility. These medications are also effective in protecting the cornea from inflammatory responses by inhibiting collagenase. Among this class of medications, tetracycline and doxycycline are the most commonly used. They are both similar in their mechanisms of action, side effect profile, and efficacy, but slight differences do exist. Tetracycline, having a shorter half-life, is dosed four times per day as opposed to doxycycline that is given once or twice per day. The side effects profile is slightly more favorable for doxycycline. *Common adverse reactions are GI upset, photosensitivity, and permanent* discoloration of teeth in newborns and younger patients.

(g) Topical immunosuppressants: One immunomodulator specifically approved for dry eyes is Restasis (Cyclosporin A, Allergan). The mechanism of action is not clearly understood, although it is believed to be related to inhibition of T-cell production in the lacrimal gland. This emulsion has been shown to improve tear production that leads to improvement in tear film stability, which, in turn, resolves dry eye symptoms and returns the ocular surface to a more healthy state. In addition, it has been shown to increase goblet cell numbers and improve meibomian gland secretions as well [19]. It takes 3–4 months to achieve a clinically significant effect, and about 6 months before it achieves the full therapeutic potential. This is due to the life cycle of the T-cells (approximately 120 days).

(h) *Most recently, a new product Xiidra (lifitegrast ophthalmic solution 5%) is being used to inhibit inflammation by inhibiting the recruitment of previous and new recruited T cells blocking the release of cytokines—hopefully a helpful addition* [20].

(i) Omega-3 fatty acids: It is thought that a dysfunction in the meibomian glands leads to a defect in the lipid layer of the tear film. This, in turn, allows the aqueous to evaporate, more easily allowing for corneal surface exposure and symptoms. In recent years, the essential omega-3 fatty acids such as eicosapentaenoic (EPA) and docosahexaenoic acid (DHA) found in fish oil and alpha-linolenic acid (ALA) in flax seed oil have been found to be most helpful. Carol F. Boerner wrote one of the first articles on dry eyes being successfully treated with oral flax seed oil (1000 mg b.i.d.) [21]. The major components of flax seed oil are omega-3 (57%), omega-6 (15%), and omega-9 (18%) fatty acids. These act as precursors to different prostaglandins that affect inflammation. According to Jeffrey P. Gilbard, omega-6 fatty acids are ubiquitous in milk, ice cream, pizza, steak, fried foods, etc. These things are commonplace in the American diet, but in contrast, we are omega-3 starved (found in salmon, herring, sardines, etc.). While omega-6 fatty acids are proinflammatory, omega-3 fatty acids counterbalance them and reduce the proinflammatory mediators such as interleukin 1 and tumor necrosis factor-alpha [22, 23].

By using flax seed oil (1000 mg capsules b.i.d.) or fish oil (1200 mg capsules), not only are the inflammatory mediators lessened (similar to using doxycycline for its anti-inflammatory effects), but the secretions of the meibomian glands are also improved. This is continued indefinitely in addition to an antibiotic ointment at night (to decrease any bacteria causing inflammatory toxins). *Most recently, an article in the **New England Journal of Medicine** questioned the effectiveness of omega 3 fatty acids showing no material objective improvement in dry eye patients vs. placebo. Our experience found improved patient-subjective comfort with dry eyes however* [24].

(j) Topical antibiotics: These are used in conjunction with oral flax seed oil to reduce staphylococcal load at the eyelid margin. This is an effective adjunct when treating blepharitis. Erythromycin is a good first-line antibiotic because of its antibacterial and anti-inflammatory properties. It should be used at night for a month and reassessed. Other antibiotics such as bacitracin and tobramycin are also effective. If the patient is still symptomatic after a month, an antibiotic–steroid combination may be helpful.

The Oculoplastic Approach

Prior to ptosis or blepharoplasty surgery and after a patient has been found to have aqueous tear deficiency, they should be counseled about the risk of postoperative dry eye, and treatment should be instituted. This should include frequent application of preservative-free artificial tears and lubricating ointment at bedtime with or without the use of punctal plugs. This will help prepare the cornea adequately following more exposure from eyelid elevation. In the case of moderate-to-severe dry eyes, Restasis or **Xiidra** is started, and steroids are added as needed for comfort.

If there is a mild case of meibomian gland dysfunction, add flax seed oil 1000 mg p.o. b.i.d., or fish oil 1200 mg p.o. b.i.d. If there is more significant meibomian gland dysfunction, then a regimen of flax seed oil 1000 mg p.o. b.i.d., erythromycin ointment at bedtime, warm compresses b.i.d., and preservative-free tears (to dilute the bacterial inflammatory by-products) is instituted. Tetracycline is added as a backup as needed. It may take several months to change the dryness of the tear–lipid interface. **Lipiflow should be considered if needed to improve quality of meibom.** However, this added precaution may make the difference in achieving an uncomplicated postoperative course.

References

1. Rachid S, Jin Y, et al. Topical omega-3 and omega-6 fatty acids for treatment of dry eye. Arch Ophthalmol. 2008;126(2):219–24.
2. Mc Culley JP, Sciallis GF. Meibomian keratoconjunctivitis. Am J Ophthalmol. 1977;84(6):788–93.
3. Tseng SCG. Important concepts for ocular surface health. In: Parrish II RK, editor. Atlas of ophthalmology. Philadelphia: Butterworth-Heinemann; 2000. p. 117–20.
4. Sullivan BD, Evans JE, et al. Influence of aging on the polar and neutral lipid profiles in human meibomian gland secretions. Arch Ophthalmol. 2006;124:1286–92.
5. McCulley JP, Shine WE. The lipid layer of tears: dependent on meibomian gland function. Exp Eye Res. 2004;18:361–5.
6. McCulley JP, Shine WE. Meibomain gland function an the tear lipid layer. Ocul Surf. 2003;1(3):97–106.
7. Graham RH. There's nothing fishy about omega-3 fatty acids for dry syndrome. www.medscape.com/viewarticle/707984_print. Accessed Sep 2009. pp. 1–3.
8. Pflugfelder SC, Tsubota K, et al. Dry eye disorders involving external adnexa. In: Parrish II RK, editor. Atlas of ophthalmology. Philadelphia: Butterworth-Heinemann; 2000. p. 129–34.
9. Van Haeringen NJ. Clinical biochemistry of tears. Surv Ophthalmol. 1981;26(2):84–96.
10. Sheppard JD. Advanced therapeutic management of ocular surface disease. Ocular Surgery News. 2009. pp. 7–9.
11. Stern ME, Beuermann RW, et al. The pathology of dry eye: the interaction between the ocular surface and lacrimal glands. Cornea. 1998;17(6):584–9.
12. Tseng SCG, Pflugfelder SC, et al. Diagnostic strategies for ocular surface and tear disorders. In: Parrish II RK, editor. Atlas of ophthalmology. Philadelphia: Betterworth-Heinemann; 2000. p. 120–8.
13. Xiong C, Che D, et al. A rabbit dry eye model induced by topical medication of a preservative benzalkonium chloride. Invest Ophthalmol Vis Sci. 2008;49(5):1850–6.
14. Badouin C, de Lunardo C. Short term comparative study of topical 2% carteolol with and without benzalkonium chloride in healthy volunteers. Br J Ophthalmol. 1998;82(1):39–42.
15. Review of ophthalmology; 2011. pp. 3–10.

16. Greiner JV. A Single Lipoflow Thermal Pulsation System treatment improves meibomium gland function and reduces dry eye symptoms for nine months. J Curr Eye Res. 2012;37(4):272–8.
17. Avunduk AM, Avunduk MC, et al. The comparison of efficacies of topical corticosteroids and non steroidal anti inflammatory drops on dry eye patients; a clinical ad immunocytochemical study. Am J Ophthalmol. 2003;136(4):593–602.
18. Management and therapy of dry eye disease. Report of the management and therapy subcommittee of the international dry eye workshop. Ocul Surf. 2007;5(2):163–78.
19. Kunert KS, Tisdale AS, et al. Goblet cell numbers and epithelial proliferation in the conjunctiva of patients with dry eye syndrome treated with cyclosporin. Arch Ophthalmol. 2002;120(3):330–7.
20. Xiiadra Official Site www.xiidra.com.
21. Boerner C. Dry eye successfully treated with flaxseed oil. Ocular Surgery News. 2000. p. 14.
22. Gilbard JP. Enriched flaxseed oil no fishtail for dry eye, meibomanitis. www.ophthalmologytimes.com. Accessed Apr 2003. pp. 16–17.
23. Endes S, Ghorbani R, et al. The effect of dietary supplement with n-3 polyunsaturated fatty acids on the synthesis of interlukin-1 and tumor necrosis by mononuclear cells. N Engl J Med. 1989;320(5):265–71.
24. Asbell PA, et al. N-3 fatty acid supplement for the treatment of dry eye disease. N Engl J Med. 2018;378:1681–90.
25. Arita R, et al. Noncontact infrared meibography to document age-related changes of the meibomian glands in a normal population. Ophthalmology. 2008;115:911–5.

Congenital Causes of Nasolacrimal Duct Obstruction

32

Christopher B. Chambers, William Rocamora Katowitz, and James A. Katowitz

Introduction

This chapter discusses the anatomy and embryology of the nasolacrimal system and also describes the symptoms and various congenital causes of nasolacrimal duct obstruction (NLDO). Ninety percent of congenital nasolacrimal duct obstructions will resolve spontaneously by 1 year of age. Most commonly, the source of obstruction is due to persistence of a membrane, usually inferiorly at the valve of Hasner. The nasolacrimal system develops from a solid cord of surface ectodermal origin. Abnormal migration and canalization of this cord can lead to various types of nasolacrimal duct obstruction. Anatomic variations and mechanical pressure on the tear drainage system can lead also to nasolacrimal duct obstructions. Clefting and amniotic banding can cause nasolacrimal system abnormalities. Symptoms of nasolacrimal duct obstruction include epiphora, mattering of the lashes, and the presence of a medial canthal mass.

Anatomy and Embryology

The nasolacrimal duct arises from invagination of the surface ectoderm that starts as a solid epithelial cord. The lacrimal drainage system develops in the naso-optic groove located in a cleft between the lateral nasal process and the maxillary process [1]. This solid epithelial cord begins to develop a lumen at 12 weeks of gestation [2]. Accessory canaliculi or fistula of the nasolacrimal sac can develop if more than two cords stem from the embryologic lacrimal sac [2]. Canalization is usually complete at the puncta when the lids separate at about 7 months of gestation; however, some authors state that patency can be present at 4 months [3]. It is uncommon to have total maldevelopment of the entire nasolacrimal system; however, this can occur in patients with facial clefts, cyclops, and other rare abnormalities [4].

The nasolacrimal system begins at the punctum located 6 mm lateral to the inner canthus with the superior punctum positioned slightly temporal to the inferior punctum. The punctal opening is 0.2–0.3 mm in diameter, and the canalicular system begins at the punctum. The canaliculi are lined with stratified squamous epithelium surrounded by elastic tissue. Each canaliculus, the superior and inferior, begins with a 2 mm vertical section that turns around 90° toward the medial canthus. The internal diameter is around 1 mm and at the termination of the vertical portion where there is a dilatation called the ampulla that is about 1.5 mm in size. It is at the ampulla where the system begins its 8-mm-long horizontal course.

In approximately 90% of normal individuals, a common canaliculus is formed by the fusion of the upper and lower canaliculi. The common canaliculus travels medially to join the lacrimal sac. However, prior to joining the sac, there is a dilation of the canaliculus called the sinus of Maier. Following this dilation, there is a valve formed by folding of tissue that prevents the regurgitation of fluid called the valve of Rosenmuller. The common canaliculus typically enters the nasolacrimal sac between the upper third and lower two thirds of the sac near the medial canthal tendon. It is at this point where the canaliculus enters the nasolacrimal sac and where the upper system terminates and the lower system begins [5]. This distinction will be important in describing the different types of nasolacrimal duct obstructions (NLDO).

C. B. Chambers
Division of Oculoplastic and Orbital Surgery, Department of Ophthalmology, University of Washington Harborview Medical Center, Seattle, WA, USA

W. R. Katowitz (✉)
Perelman School of Medicine, The University of Pennsylvania, The Children's Hospital of Philadelphia and The Scheie Eye Institute, Division of Ophthalmology, Philadelphia, PA, USA

J. A. Katowitz
The Children's Hospital of Philadelphia and The Edwin and Fannie Gray Hall Center for Appearance, The University of Pennsylvania Perelman School of Medicine, Department of Ophthalmology, Philadelphia, PA, USA

J. J. Servat et al. (eds.), *Smith and Nesi's Ophthalmic Plastic and Reconstructive Surgery*,
https://doi.org/10.1007/978-3-030-41720-8_32

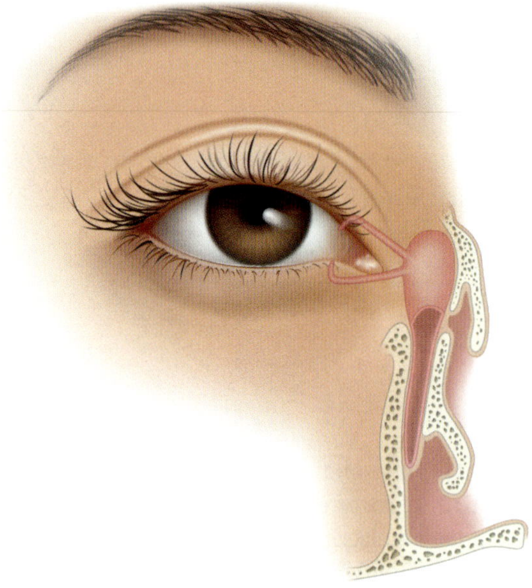

Fig. 32.1 Anatomy of nasolacrimal duct

The nasolacrimal sac is divided into two sections: the fundus, which is located above the entrance of the canaliculus, and the body, which is located below this entrance. The fundus is around 4 mm in length, while the body is around 10 mm (Fig. 32.1). The epithelial lining of the sac includes a superficial columnar layer and a deep layer of flattened cells in addition to a high concentration of mucus-secreting goblet cells [6]. The nasolacrimal sac sits in the lacrimal fossa formed anteriorly by the frontal process of the maxillary bone and posteriorly by the lacrimal bone.

The nasolacrimal duct begins as the system enters the nasolacrimal canal located in the frontal portion of the maxillary bone. The nasolacrimal duct extends in an inferior, lateral, and posterior direction to enter the nose below the inferior turbinate at the valve of Hasner [6]. The distance from the canaliculus to the nasal floor is approximately 20 mm during the first year of life, increasing to 30–40 mm in an adult. In children, the inferior meatus is flat, and there is typically crowding between the floor of the nose, the lateral nasal wall, and the inferior turbinate [5].

The inferior turbinate begins against the lateral wall of the nose. With time, the turbinate moves inferiorly and medially allowing space for opening of the nasolacrimal duct at the inferior meatus. Fusion of the inferior meatus to the lateral nose may cause a bony obstruction that can inhibit a patent system inferiorly at the valve of Hasner [2]. A detailed understanding of normal nasolacrimal system anatomy and embryology is important in diagnosing, classifying, and treating congenital NLDO.

Symptoms

Epiphora

Epiphora and the presence of an increased tear lake signify an imbalance between tear production and drainage. The presence of epiphora may represent a nasolacrimal duct obstruction; however, this symptom must be investigated to rule out nonobstructive functional abnormalities. A normal nasolacrimal pump mechanism requires good apposition of the punctae to the globe and various congenital lid abnormalities such as entropion, ectropion, telecanthus, hypertelorism, and colobomas can disrupt the anatomical position of the punctae.

Proper orbicularis function is also integral in the pump system; therefore, congenital seventh nerve palsies can lead to epiphora as well. Tearing may also occur secondary to external disease including tear film, cornea, or lash abnormalities [7]. Overproduction of tears secondary to diseases such as crocodile tears or conjunctivitis can further confound diagnosis.

Evaluation of epiphora in children can be challenging and it is important to determine if the cause of tearing is secondary to overproduction of tears or decreased drainage as this can help direct treatment for the epiphora. There are many tests oculoplastic surgeons use in clinic such as the Jones dye test and probing and irrigation of the nasolacrimal system to determine if there is an anatomic abnormality of the outflow apparatus. Though these in-clinic tests can be useful for adults, they are not typically possible in children secondary to cooperation. The dye disappearance test (DDT) in an outstanding qualitative test of tear outflow that can be used on the most uncooperative child. The DDT is performed by placing fluorescein into the inferior fornix of each eye. The excess dye is wiped from the lids and cheek immediately after application. The family is instructed to avoid rubbing the eye. After 5 minutes, the tear meniscus is examined with a cobalt blue light. At the 5-minute mark, the dye will have cleared from the fornix in a patient with normal outflow. If there is impeded flow, there will be residual fluorescein visible in the tear lake. A patient with overproduction of tears and normal outflow will have cleared the dye as well. The test is positive if there is fluorescein visible and the test is graded from trace to 3+. A rating of trace will be given when a thin strip of fluorescein is left at 5 minutes and 3+ indicates the fluorescein has dripped down the patient's face. This test is invaluable for the pediatric patient and a negative test is a good indicator that the system is patent. A positive test, on the other hand, only indicates poor outflow and does not specifically localize the problem. Further investigation of the lid function, lid position, and punctal anatomy can help direct the clinician to the probable pathology. Probing and irrigation of the nasolacrimal system in the operating room may be indicated to evaluate nasolacrimal duct obstruction.

Mattering of Lashes and Mucopurulent Discharge

Symptoms regarding the nature of tearing including the presence of mucopurulent discharge or mattering can be useful to aid diagnosis. Retrograde discharge mucoid material upon firm palpation of the lacrimal sac can help confirm the presence of nasolacrimal obstruction or stenosis [7].

Periocular Mass

The presence of a periocular mass at the medial canthal area can suggest a NLDO or may represent a periocular tumor such as a capillary hemangioma or dermoid cyst. As described above, two-thirds of the nasolacrimal sac lie below the medial canthal tendon, and a tumor above the tendon may indicate an intraorbital tumor, a nasofrontal encephalocele, or an anterior ethmoidal mucocele [7].

Diagnostic Studies

Diagnostic studies such as computed tomography (CT) scan or magnetic resonance imaging (MRI) to rule out the presence of a periocular tumor or an encephalocele can be helpful in directing treatment options. Other studies such as the dye disappearance test (DDT), Jones dye test, basal tear secretion test (BTST), Schirmer's test, irrigation of the canaliculus, dacrocystography (DCG), and lacrimal scintigraphy can be used to diagnose NLDO. These studies are described in detail in other parts of this text and will not be discussed here.

Imaging studies such as CT and DCG and lacrimal scintigraphy can be expensive, can be difficult to perform, can expose children to unnecessary radiation, and may not be necessary in many cases. Other tests such as the BTST and Jones dye test can be difficult to perform in children. The DDT (Fig. 32.2) can be safely and easily conducted on a child. This study in combination with a careful history and adnexal examination may be sufficient for diagnosis.

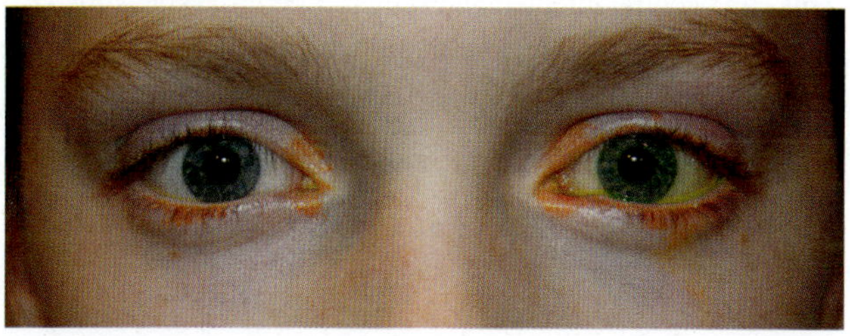

Fig. 32.2 Dye disappearance test showing retention of fluorescein in the tear lake in a NLDO on the left side and normal flow with fluorescein clearance on the right side

Congenital Etiology of Lacrimal System Obstructions

Congenital nasolacrimal duct obstruction can conveniently be grouped into upper system blockage and lower system blockage. As described above, the upper system is anatomically defined as everything before the canalicular-lacrimal sac junction (punctae, canaliculi, and common canaliculus), and the lower system includes everything after this junction (lacrimal sac and nasolacrimal duct). The causes of the obstruction can be secondary to abnormal embryogenesis with the failure of canalization of the solid epithelial cord or from retained membranous veils along the system. It may also result from tumors or strictures that hinder the normal development of the lacrimal apparatus.

It is commonly accepted that the most common site of NLDO is at the opening of the nasolacrimal duct into the inferior meatus at the valve of Hasner. Studies by Sevel substantiate this belief in that 60–70% of fetuses in his series had a membranous obstruction between the nasolacrimal duct and the inferior meatus [8]. This membranous obstruction commonly opens within a month after birth. Duke-Elder described a complete absence of the nasolacrimal passage secondary to clefting of the nasal and maxillary process during embryogenesis that occurs in rare anomalies such as cyclopia, cryptopthalmos, or from pressure of amniotic bands [9].

Upper System Obstructions

Obstruction of the upper system typically leads to epiphora with the absence of mucus discharge or mucus mattering of the lashes, as there is no connection with the mucus-secreting goblet cells located in the nasolacrimal sac.

Punctal Abnormalities

Atresia or agenesis of the punctae can occur and was documented in 1846 by Blanchet. During embryogenesis, canalization of the solid ectodermal cord, as discussed previously, progresses laterally terminating at the superior and inferior punctum. Disruption in this process can lead to punctal atresia or punctal agenesis.

Congenital Punctal Atresia

Failure of the epithelial bud to open at the punctum results in an imperforate punctum. There is commonly a thin membranous veil over the punctum that may appear as a small depression in the lid margin around 6 mm lateral to the medial canthus and, as previously discussed, the inferior punctum is typically located lateral to the superior punctum. During development of the canaliculi and punctum, the orbicularis muscle is also developing from local mesenchyme. The orbicularis covers the surface of the lids, while the lids are fused [2]. The membranous veil found overlying the punctum may have its origin from the orbicularis muscle or may be secondary to failure of the conjunctiva to properly perforate. This veil may be lysed with a safety pin or with a sharp punctal dilator. Inferior punctal atresia is more common than upper punctal atresia, and typically, only one punctum demonstrates atresia [10]. During embryogenesis, the frontal nasal process gives rise to the upper lid bud, while the lower lid bud originates from the maxillary process [2]. The distinct embryologic origin of the upper lid and lower lid may be the reason for only one punctum being affected more often than both.

Congenital Punctal Agenesis

Congenital absence of the punctum is less common than atresia; however, it can also be attributed to abnormal canalization of the ectodermal cord during embryogenesis (Fig. 32.3). Canalicular agenesis may be found in cases of punctal agenesis. Duke-Elder cited examples of autosomal-dominant inheritance patterns of punctal atresia [11]. The ectrodactyly-ectodermal dysplasia-clefting syndrome (EEC), as an addition to the Levy-Hollister syndrome, has been associated with punctal agenesis [12].

Canalicular Abnormalities

Canalicular Atresia and Agenesis

If the surface ectoderm cord migration during embryogenesis is retarded before reaching the eyelid margin or if incomplete canalization of the cord occurs, canalicular atresia or agenesis will occur. The atresia can be classified as proximal, mid-canalicular, or distal. Depending on the extent and location of canalicular abnormality, the patient may or may not be symptomatic. With total agenesis of the canalicular system, a Jones-type bypass tube will usually be indicated.

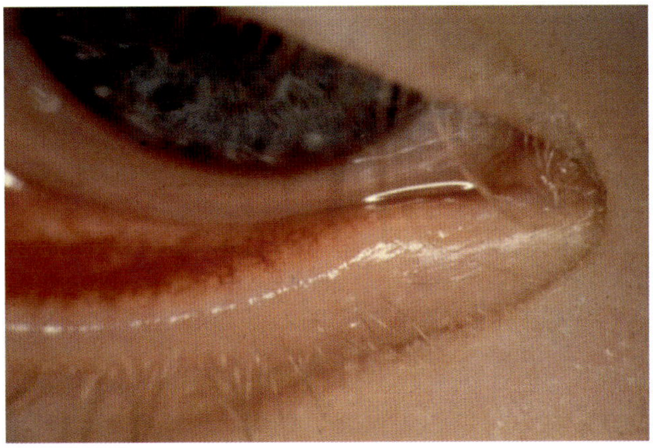

Fig. 32.3 Congenital punctal agenesis in the lower eyelid

Accessory Canaliculi and Accessory Canalicular Channels

As described earlier, if more than two cords of surface ectoderm from the canalicular system are directed toward the lid margin, accessory canaliculi may develop. If these cords terminate below the lid margin on the cutaneous surface of the lid, accessory channels can form.

Lower System Obstructions

Dacryostenosis

Obstruction of the lower nasolacrimal duct will cause tear drainage problems. The various etiologies of this obstruction will be discussed in detail. If there is a lower abnormality with a one-way valve allowing entrance of fluid via a patent upper system without egress of the fluid amniotocele, and if this becomes infected, dacryocystitis can occur.

Amniotocele and Dacryocystitis

Congenital lacrimal amniocele was described by Jones and Wobig. As previously discussed, the canalicular system ends in the sinus of Maier. The canaliculus enters the nasolacrimal sac at an acute angle at the valve of Rosenmuller, a one-way valve. Fluid is able to enter the nasolacrimal sac and retrograde flow is limited. In the presence of a lower blockage, fluid will collect in the nasolacrimal sac. At birth, a firm palpable mass may be observed below the medial canthal tendon secondary to the fluid buildup. The sac is filled with amniotic fluid and is termed an amniotocele. This fluid is sterile; however, with time, the lacrimal pump system may force unsterile fluid into the sac. This can become infected and is then called dacryocystitis [12] (Fig. 32.4). The fluid may be expressed by firm pressure on the nasolacrimal sac overcoming the one-way valve of Rosenmuller.

Anatomical Variation Causing Lower System Obstruction

Jones and Wobig described eight anatomical variations that can be observed causing obstructions of the lower nasolacrimal duct system [12].

1. The duct that ends at or near the vault of the anterior end of the inferior nasal meatus and fails to perforate the nasal mucosa. This is the most common form of lower system blockage observed and can often be cured by probing of the nasolacrimal duct system (Fig. 32.5a).
2. The duct that extends clear to the floor of the nose lateral to the nasal mucosa. It may be beneficial to infracture the inferior turbinate in addition to probing and irrigation to treat this abnormality (Fig. 32.5b).
3. The duct that extends several millimeters down lateral to the nasal mucosa without an opening (Fig. 32.5c).
4. An almost complete absence of a duct due to failure of the osseous nasolacrimal canal to form. This is frequently seen in children with cleft palate (Fig. 32.5d).
5. A blockage of the lower end of the duct due to an impacted anterior end of the inferior turbinate (Fig. 32.6a).
6. The duct that ends blindly in the anterior end of the inferior turbinate (Fig. 32.6b).
7. The duct that ends blindly in the medial wall of the maxillary sinus (Fig. 32.6c).
8. A bony nasolacrimal canal may extend to the floor of the nose without an opening (Fig. 32.6d).

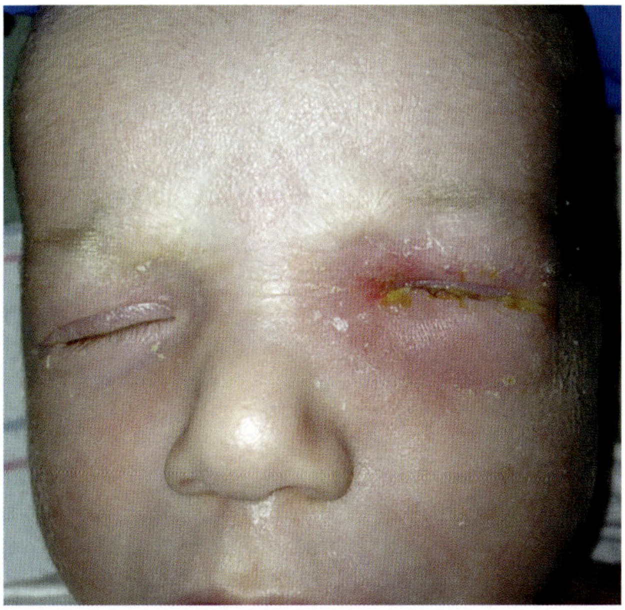

Fig. 32.4 Dacryocystitis

Supernumerary (Anlage) Ducts

Similar to the accessory canaliculi and accessory canalicular channels described above, congenital fistulas of the lacrimal sac can be observed. Jones and Wobig have named these supernumerary ducts lacrimal anlage ducts. These anlage ducts likely result from the canalization of a strand of epithelial cords originating from the lacrimal sac or lacrimal duct that terminates on the skin [12] (Fig. 32.7). Typically, normal development of the nasolacrimal system is present in these individuals.

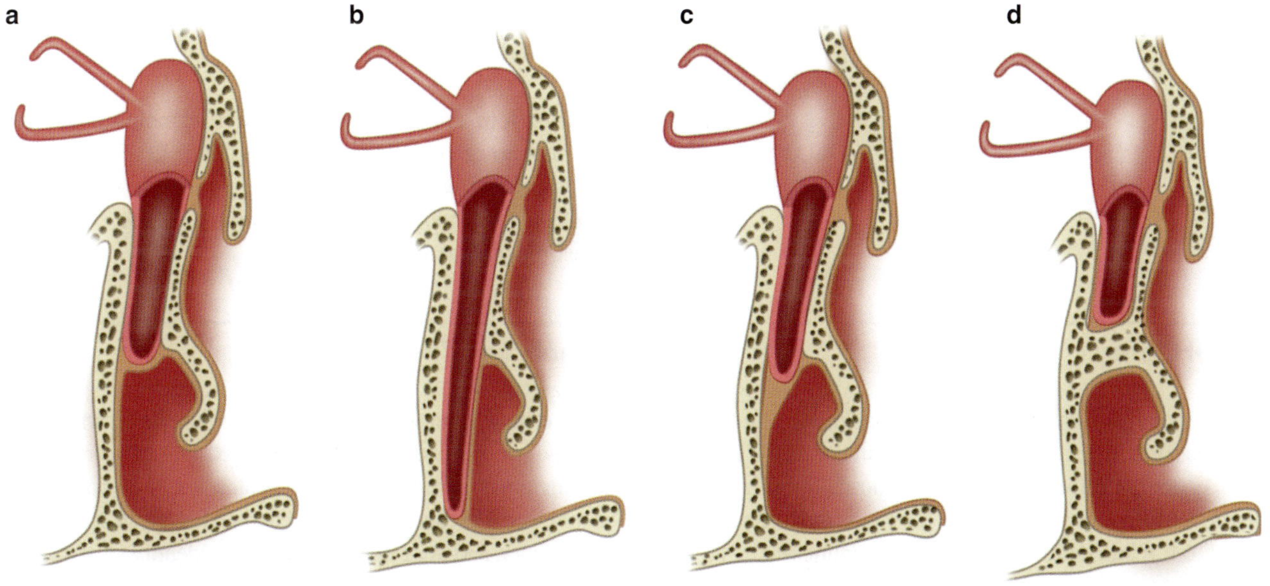

Fig. 32.5 (**a**) The duct that ends at or near the vault of the anterior end of the inferior nasal meatus and fails to perforate the nasal mucosa. (**b**) The duct that extends clear to the floor of the nose lateral to the nasal mucosa. (**c**) The duct that extends several millimeters down lateral to the nasal mucosa without an opening. (**d**) An almost complete absence of a duct due to failure of the osseous nasolacrimal canal to form

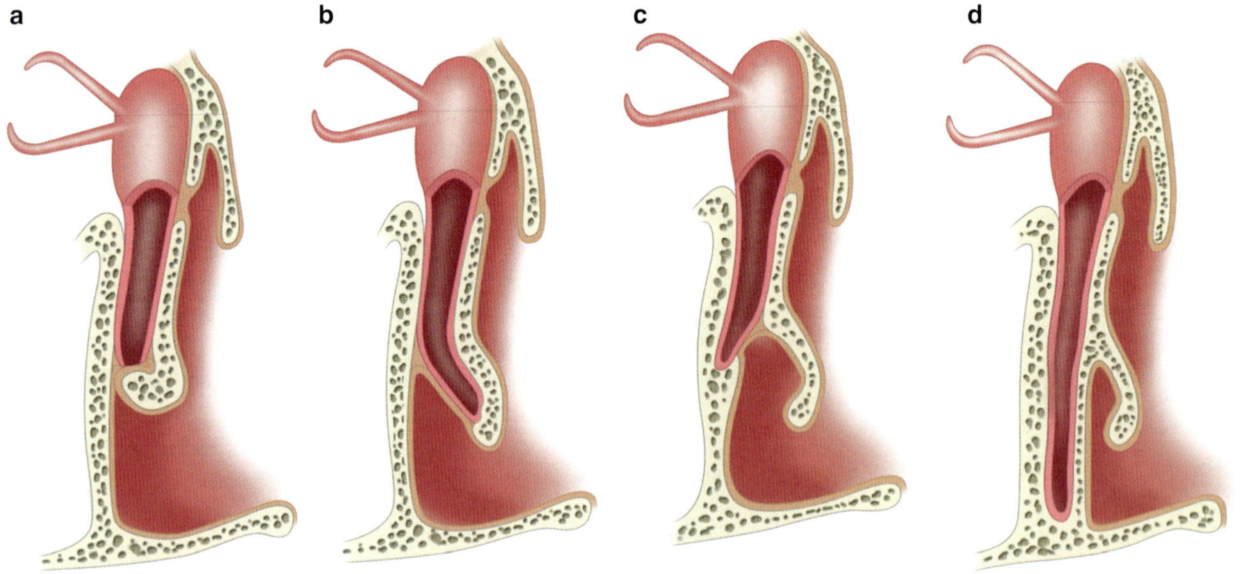

Fig. 32.6 (**a**) A blockage of the lower end of the duct due to an impacted anterior end of the inferior turbinate. (**b**) The duct that ends blindly in the anterior end of the inferior turbinate. (**c**) The duct that ends blindly in the medial wall of the maxillary sinus. (**d**) A bony nasolacrimal canal may extend to the floor of the nose without an opening

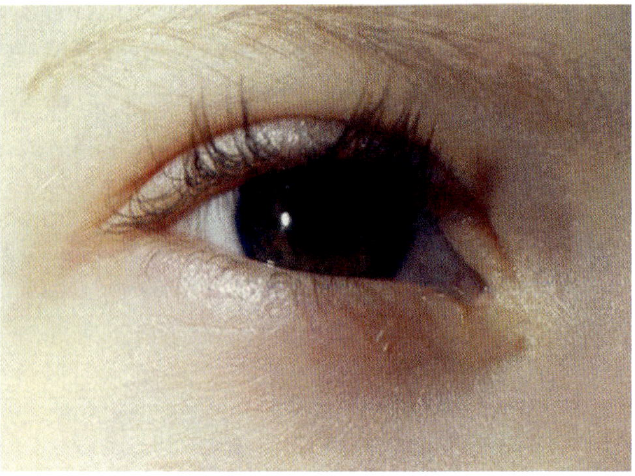

Fig. 32.7 Supernumerary (anlage) duct

Facial Clefts

Craniofacial deformities such as congenital clefting syndromes can disrupt the normal development of the nasolacrimal system. Clefting can cause abnormalities in the soft tissue and the bony structures; for more details, please see Chap. 64: (Congenital Soft Tissue deformities).

The etiology of facial clefting is not well understood. Genetic inheritance may play a role in some craniofacial clefts. Radiation has been implicated as well as exposure to various intrauterine infections or pharmacologic agents [13]. Clefting may be attributed to fusional failures during embryonic development. Some authors have implicated either the failure of neural crest cell migration or degeneration of the cells prior to migration causing clefts [14].

Amniotic Bands

Clefting from amniotic bands formed from amniotic sac rupture in utero can place physical stress on the developing fetus causing strictures and tissue necrosis. Amniotic bands can be swallowed in utero and can constrict causing congenital developmental abnormalities [13].

Tumors and Their Mass Effect

The mechanical pressure from congenital tumors on any part of the nasolacrimal duct system can cause NLDO. Tumors such as hemangiomas, dermoid cysts, encephaloceles, or mucoceles can be implicated in causing an obstruction. Good physical examination, history, and imaging studies can help identify such causes.

References

1. Tan AD, Rubin PAD, Sutula FC, Remulla HD. Congenital nasolacrimal duct obstruction. Int Ophthalmol Clin. 2001;41(4):57–69.
2. Hurwitz JJ. Embryology of the lacrimal drainage system. In: Hurwitz JJ, editor. The lacrimal system. Philadelphia: Lippincott-Raven; 1996. p. 9–13.
3. Adenis JP, Lebraud P, Leboutet MJ, Loubet R, Loubet A. Etude embryologique des vois lacrymales chez l'homme. J Fr Ophthalmol. 1983;6:351–7.
4. Mann I. Developmental abnormalities of the eye. 2nd ed. Philadelphia: Lippincott; 1957. p. 371.
5. Dei Cas RE. Evaluation of tearing in children. In: Katowitz JA, editor. Pediatric oculoplastic surgery. New York: Springer; 2002. p. 301–8.
6. Simon JW, Aaby AA, Drack AV, et al. The lacrimal drainage system. In: Cantor LB, editor. Basic and clinical science course section 6. San Francisco: American Academy of Ophthalmology; 2006. p. 239–47.
7. Katowitz JA, Goldstein SM, Kherani F, Low J. Lacrimal drainage surgery. In: Tasman W, Jaeger EA, editors. Duanes ophthalmology, vol. 5. Philadelphia: Lippincott Williams & Wilkins; 2005.
8. Sevel D. Developmental and congenital abnormalities of the nasolacrimal apparatus. J Pediatr Ophthal Strab. 1981;18(5):13–9.
9. Duke-Elder S. Congenital deformities part 2. In: Duke-Elder S, editor. System of ophthalmology, vol. 3. St. Louis: CV Mosby; 1964. p. 923–40.
10. Viers ER. Disorders of the nasolacrimal apparatus in infants and children. J Pediatr Ophthalmol. 1966;3:32.
11. Low JE, Johnson MA, Katowitz JA. Management of pediatric upper system problems: punctal and canalicular surgery. In: Katowitz JA, editor. Pediatric oculoplastic surgery. New York: Springer; 2002. p. 337–46.
12. Jones JT, Wobig JL. Congenital anomalies of the lacrimal system. In: Jones JT, Wobig JL, editors. Surgery of the eyelids and lacrimal system. Birmingham: Aesculapius; 1976. p. 157–63.
13. Fries PD, Katowitz JA. Congenital craniofacial anomalies of ophthalmic importance. Surv Ophthalmol. 1990;35(2):87–117.
14. Johnston MC. The neural crest in abnormalities of the face and brain. Birth Defects. 1975;11:416–40.

Acquired Causes of Lacrimal System Obstructions

33

Jamie Lea Schaefer and Daniel P. Schaefer

The lacrimal drainage system is composed of the puncta, canaliculi, lacrimal sac, and the nasolacrimal duct that facilitates the drainage of the tears produced by the lacrimal glands, accessory lacrimal glands, and the glands of Krause and Wolfring, along with the suspended debris in the tears. This unique physiologic system is simple and elegant in design, yet it is elaborate in the function of tear drainage, with the lacrimal pump and its anatomical construction. Tears drain through the superior and inferior puncta, canaliculi, lacrimal sac, and the nasolacrimal duct to finally empty into the inferior meatus of the nasal cavity to be absorbed by the nasal mucosa and/or be disposed of through the digestive system. The canaliculi are lined by a nonkeratinized stratified squamous epithelium surrounded by the orbicularis muscle, and the lacrimal sac and nasolacrimal duct are similarly lined with pseudostratified columnar epithelial cells with a ciliated surface. The sac contains scattered goblet cells, mucus secretors, and serous glands. The common internal punctum is the transition from the canaliculi to the lacrimal sac and shares histologic features of both [1]. Epiphora may result when there is an excessive production or hypersecretion of tears, inadequate evaporation and drainage of tears, impairment of the lacrimal pump, stenosis, or obstruction at any section of the lacrimal drainage system, or a consequence of any pathologic process that interferes with the physiology or continuity of the lacrimal drainage apparatus. It can be an isolated disorder or may involve multiple levels, at any level of the lacrimal drainage system. Our understanding and knowledge of the anatomy and pathophysiology of the lacrimal drainage system have been increased through the advancements in radiology, microbiology, and clinical studies.

Epiphora is determined by a balance between tear production and tear drainage and not by the absolute function or dysfunction of either. Symptomatic tearing can result when a normal lacrimal drainage system is overwhelmed by hypersecretion or when a drainage system is anatomically compromised and unable to handle normal tear production.

History

Tearing is a common complaint, and the evaluation of the tearing patient and lacrimal disorders requires a complete workup that is multifaceted and organized, including a detailed history as well as a comprehensive ophthalmic examination with special emphasis on the eyelids, the anterior segment, lacrimal system, and nasal cavity. This will help correctly localize the area of involvement, diagnosis, the etiology, and the development of a treatment plan.

The cause of tearing is multiple and can be secondary to hypersecretion or impairment of drainage. Patients with intranasal disease, neoplasms, corneal ulcers, and foreign bodies may develop an overproduction of tears. These conditions may cause a reflex stimulation of the ophthalmic division of the trigeminal nerve. The patient should be questioned regarding the following: unilateral versus bilateral; subjective symptoms of foreign body sensation, burning; constant versus intermittent; medications or environmental allergies; prior probings; sinus disease and/or surgeries; prior trauma, midfacial trauma, nasal fractures; radiation treatment to the periocular or paranasal sinuses area; radioiodine ablation, I^{131} therapy for thyroid carcinoma; ocular diseases; systemic or topical chemotherapy, ocular or periocular surgeries; prior episodes of lacrimal sac inflammation or infection; clear or mucous discharge or bloody tears; and present and prior topical and systemic medications.

J. L. Schaefer (✉)
Division of Ophthalmology, The Warren Alpert Medical School at Brown University, Providence, RI, USA

D. P. Schaefer
Clinical Professor of Ophthalmology, Director of Oculoplastic, Orbital, and Facial Plastic Reconstructive Surgery, Department of Otolaryngology, State University of New York at Buffalo, Buffalo, NY, USA

J. J. Servat et al. (eds.), *Smith and Nesi's Ophthalmic Plastic and Reconstructive Surgery*,
https://doi.org/10.1007/978-3-030-41720-8_33

Unilateral tearing is suggestive of a lacrimal outflow problem because of either obstruction or poor function of the tear pump due to weakness of the orbicularis muscle, seventh cranial nerve palsy, or lower lid laxity. Also to be considered in unilateral tearing is the possibility of intracranial processes or lesions that can compress the lacrimal innervation pathway in the brain and result in decreased tear production and unilateral dry eye symptoms, resulting in epiphora. Lymphoma, adenoid cystic carcinoma, or other tumors of the lacrimal gland can infiltrate the gland and/or its innervation causing decreased tear production on one side, with reflex epiphora. However, bilateral outflow abnormalities can also occur and result in bilateral tearing in these patients.

Patients with Down syndrome have been noted to develop a dacryostenosis, more frequently caused by anatomic abnormalities, canalicular stenosis, and atresia. Punctual atresia and canalicular obstruction are also more common in patients with midface abnormalities.

Examination

The evaluation of the tearing patient can usually be adequately performed with a complete ophthalmologic examination: external examination of the eyelids, periorbital area, and ocular surface; slit-lamp biomicroscopy; fluorescein and rose bengal staining; and simple office tests – the fluorescein dye disappearance test, Jones I and Jones II dye test, and diagnostic lacrimal probing and irrigation.

Inspection of the eyelids and lashes may find signs of blepharitis, concretions, cysts, molluscum contagiosum, chalazion, ectropion, entropion, trichiasis, lid laxity, lagophthalmos, meibomian gland dysfunction, squamous metaplasia of the conjunctiva, tarsal papillary or follicular reaction, floppy eyelid syndrome, poor blinking mechanism, overriding of the upper and lower lids, and seventh cranial nerve paralysis, which results in a poor lacrimal pump function. A notch on the lid margin secondary to prior trauma or surgery may allow tears to flow out of the tear pool onto the face. The punctum should be evaluated for size, stenosis or occlusion, swelling or an inflammatory pouting of the puncta as seen with canaliculitis, its position, movement with eyelid function, and for possible obstruction by the conjunctiva, conjunctivochalasis or hyperplasia, the plica semilunaris, or an enlarged caruncle. A badly slit punctum or canaliculus may also be a source of chronic epiphora. Palpation with pressure over the lacrimal sac may produce a reflux of mucoid or mucopurulent material through the canalicular system and punctum if the common canaliculus and valve of Rosenmüller are patent and there is a blockage of the nasolacrimal duct.

Disorders of the facial skin, such as psoriasis, acne rosacea, atopic dermatitis, allergies, and blepharitis, may affect the eyelids and cause ectropions, tearing and should be noted.

Examination of the nose should be performed to rule out the possibility of intranasal tumors, allergic rhinitis, polyposis, turbinate impaction, or other possible obstructions of the distal end of the nasolacrimal duct.

Lacrimal endoscopes have been developed that enable direct visualization of the lacrimal passages. Their use enables diagnostic localization of the various types of lacrimal disease, such as mucosal changes, condition of the canaliculi and lacrimal sac, inflammatory membranes, strictures, and location of the stenosis or blockage, and differentiates between partial and complete obstruction and scar tissue.

Acquired obstructions of the lacrimal excretory outflow system will produce a vicious cycle of symptoms that can include epiphora, mucopurulent discharge, discomfort, pain, dacryocystitis, cellulitis, visual disturbances, chronic eczematous inflammation of the eyelids, and even excoriation of the skin. Obstruction may lead to a visual or an eye-threatening ophthalmic process that can affect patients of all ages. The tears can well up and flood down their cheeks; the patients have to frequently dab their tears, which results in a very annoying disability and causes difficulties with reading, difficulty driving due to the difficulty seeing through the tear lake, as well as the constant questions about their emotional well-being, some or all of which will prompt the patient to seek an ophthalmologist for evaluation and treatment.

Impaired tear outflow may be functional, structural, or both. The cause may be primary, those resulting from inflammation of unknown causes that lead to occlusive fibrosis, or secondary, resulting from infections, inflammation, trauma, malignancies, toxicity, or mechanical causes. Secondary acquired dacryostenosis and obstruction may result from many causes, both common and obscure. When the obstruction is distal, below the lacrimal sac, this converts the lacrimal sac into a stagnant reservoir, leading to chronic epiphora, or may become infected causing a dacryocystitis with purulent discharge. Occasionally, the precise pathogenesis of nasolacrimal duct obstruction, in spite of years of investigations, will be elusive.

In order to properly evaluate and appropriately treat the patient, the ophthalmologist must have a comprehensive knowledge of the lacrimal anatomy, the lacrimal apparatus, pathophysiology, ocular and nasal relationships, diagnostic techniques, ophthalmic and systemic disease process, as well as the topical and systemic medications that can affect the nasolacrimal duct system. One must be able to assess if the cause is secondary to outflow anomalies, hypersecretion or reflex secretion, pseudoepiphora, eyelid malposition abnormalities, trichiasis, foreign bodies and conjunctival concretions, conjunctivochalasis, keratitis, tear film deficiencies or instability, dry eye syndromes, ocular surface abnormalities, irritation or tumors affecting the trigeminal nerve, neurotrophic keratopathy, allergy, medications, or environmental factors. Patients with hyperlacrimation frequently have the common complaints of ocular discomfort; sandy, gritty, foreign-body sensation; and/or burning due to keratitis sicca.

There is a group of patients with epiphora but have patent lacrimal systems on irrigation or syringing, a status termed functional nasolacrimal duct obstruction. In the evaluation of these patients, the primary and secondary dye tests demonstrate a functional block if the primary dye test is negative but the secondary dye test is positive. Dacryocystography, which demonstrates the anatomy of the lacrimal system, and lacrimal scintigraphy, which demonstrates the physiologic system, are useful tests in the evaluation of these patients.

Primary acquired dacryostenosis results from a fibrous obstruction secondary to chronic inflammation, but the pathophysiology of functional dacryostenosis, patients with epiphora but a patent lacrimal systemic to syringing, is not always fully understood. These patients may have an incomplete anatomic obstruction or nonfunctional segments of the lacrimal passage from prior episodes of dacryocystitis, or an anatomically normal nasolacrimal duct system, but a physiologic dysfunction of the eyelids, punctum, lacrimal pump, or a lacrimal sac that drains poorly.

Symptoms of epiphora can reflect excess tearing, or hypersecretion of tears, due to the reflex arcs initiated by such processes as keratoconjunctivitis sicca, keratitis, allergies or uveitis, etc. In some patients, the clinical examination is unremarkable and the cause of epiphora remains unclear, a functional block.

The tear film is composed of lipids, electrolyte, protein, aqueous fluid, and mucins. Tears are spread over the entire ocular surface by blinking and then drain from the eye through the superior and inferior puncta, canaliculi, and lacrimal sac and duct into the inferior meatus of the nasal cavity. Tear function is influenced by the tear components and also on this hydrodynamic system that depends on the tear secretion, tear volume, tear flow, the mucosa surface, the underlying cavernous body of the nasolacrimal drainage system, mucosal microvilli, mucins, and then drainage. Tear drainage depends on blinking to generate a pumping effect to draw tears into the lacrimal sac. Infrequent and ineffective blinking, eyelid laxity, and floppy lids contribute to the development of epiphora. Corneal sensitivity decreases with age and various eye diseases are causes of decreased blinking. Physical factors, including capillary attraction, gravity, respiration, evaporation, and reabsorption of tears through the epithelium, can affect tear drainage.

Delayed tear clearance may be associated with ocular surface inflammation. Common complaints in these patients are of an inflammatory nature with itching, redness, mucous discharge, sticking of the lids together, episodic tearing, burning, foreign body sensation, and fluctuating blurred vision, frequently resulting from an unstable tear film, which triggers the reflex tearing. Drainage also depends on the tear pump. Blinking controls tear clearance, and infrequent and ineffective blinking leads to a delayed tear clearance.

The nasolacrimal drainage system produces a broad spectrum of mucins, which may enhance tear transport as well as provide antimicrobial defenses. The nasolacrimal drainage system contains microvilli, seromucous glands, intraepithelial lipids, and a specific mucus layer like the three-layer tear film. The mucus layer is mainly synthesized by the goblet cells and intraepithelial mucus glands.

In patients with functional dacryostenosis, it has been noted that the epithelia of the nasolacrimal drainage system are characterized by squamous metaplasia with loss of goblet cells and a marked reduction of messaging for goblet-cell-associated mucins MUC2, -5 AC, and -5B. There were no changes in MUC7, which is antimicrobial and may explain the low incidence of dacryocystitis in patients with functional dacryostenosis. Mucins, a highly glycosylated, hydrophilic glycoprotein, may enhance tear transport and provide antimicrobial defenses for the nasolacrimal drainage system. Reduced level of mucin mRNA in patients with epiphora secondary to a nonfunctioning segment of the nasolacrimal drainage system, but still patent to irrigation, suggest that mucins may reduce drag and enhance tear flow through the nasolacrimal drainage system [2].

Lacrimal Pump

The lacrimal pump is the mechanism that assists the tears in their travels from the tear pool through the nasolacrimal duct system into the interior meatus of the nose. The lacrimal pump is an active, dynamic pumping mechanism. The action of the pretarsal and preseptal orbicularis oculi produces the forces that drive the lacrimal pump. Before a blink, the eyelids are open, and the canaliculi are already filled with tears. During lid closure, the puncta and medial portion of the eyelid elevates, then the superior and inferior puncta come into contact, occluding the puncta, causing the canaliculi to become compressed, creating a positive pressure, and the superior half of the lacrimal sac develops lower pressure, while the inferior half of the lacrimal sac and the nasolacrimal duct develop a positive pressure. When the eyelids open, the pressures are reversed [3]. This forces the tears into the nasolacrimal duct and nasal cavity. Also, before the eyelids open, the puncta are still opposed and occluded, creating a vacuum as the eyelids begin to open. The puncta open into the tear pool, and with the vacuum effect, tears rapidly flow into the puncta and canaliculi. The valves within the sac and duct prevent retrograde flow of the tears.

Abnormalities of lacrimal pump function can result from involutional changes, eyelid laxity, facial nerve paralysis, and floppy eyelid syndrome. All of these conditions displace the punctum from the lacrimal lake and/or cause a decrease in blinking.

Imaging Studies

Dacryocystography, dacryoscintigraphy, digital subtraction dacryocystography, echography, computed tomography (CT) and magnetic resonance imaging (MRI) scans, small-gauge fiber-optic endoscopy of the nasolacrimal drainage system, and nasal endoscopy can add further assistance when the diagnosis is in question or further confirmation is needed.

Dacryocystography will evaluate the nasolacrimal system to determine the level and degree of obstruction as well as evaluate the lacrimal sac and the presence of lacrimal mass lesions. Contrast dye is passed through the canaliculus and imagining can also be performed using computed tomography (CT) to delineate the lacrimal drainage system (see Figs. 33.1 and 33.2). This CT can better differentiate bony from soft tissue obstructions [4].

MRI can diagnose neoplasms, mucoceles, and abscesses in the lacrimal sac and can better image the surrounding soft tissue and nasal sinuses, as well as distinguish soft tissue from bony obstructions. T2-weighted fat saturation allows the contrast dye to stand out more brightly. Magnetic resonance (MR) also avoids ionizing radiation, producing high-resolution images to identify sites of obstruction. MRI with Gd-DTPA eyedrops provides a detailed morphologic and functional assessment of the nasolacrimal drainage system and surrounding structures.

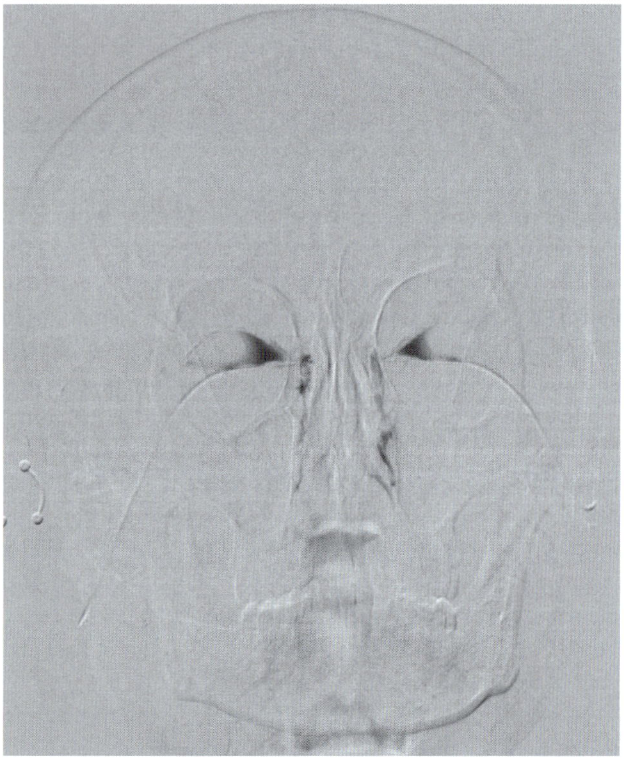

Fig. 33.1 Bilateral dacryocystogram. Right patchy filling of the lacrimal sac and nasolacrimal duct with less contrast seen exiting the inferior meatus – partial obstruction. Left with good filling of the lacrimal sac and nasolacrimal duct. (Photo courtesy of Dr. John Nguyen)

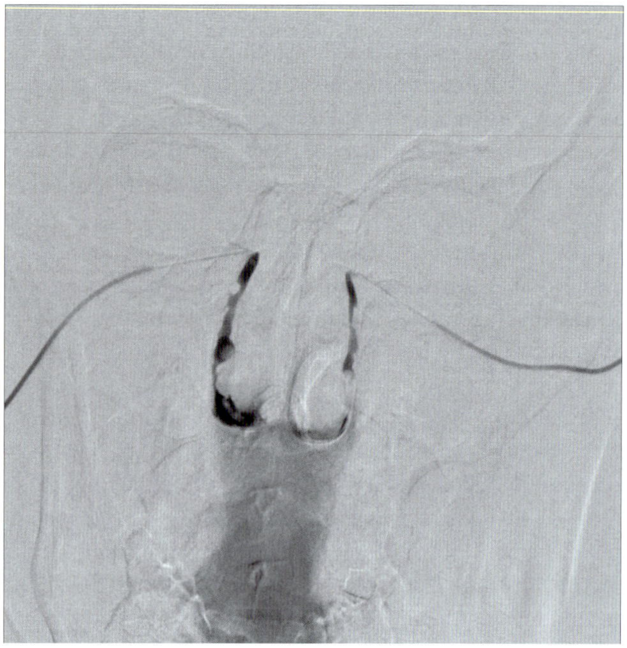

Fig. 33.2 Bilateral dacryocystogram. Right with good filling of the lacrimal sac and nasolacrimal duct. Left with stricture of the upper nasolacrimal system – partial obstruction. (Photo courtesy of Dr. John Nguyen)

These techniques, radiographic, lacrimal, and nasal endoscopy, enable one to make the proper diagnosis and allow one to select the proper surgical procedure knowing the precise cause and location of the nasolacrimal obstruction. Image-guided or stereotactic navigation systems can be a useful adjunctive tool for dacryolocalization intraoperatively, especially for the management of traumatic or otherwise challenging obstructions [5].

Bartley modified Linberg and McCormick etiologic classification system for "primary acquired nasolacrimal duct obstruction" (PANDO) and published an expanded classification for "secondary acquired lacrimal drainage obstruction" (SALDO). The etiologic causes of SALDO were divided into five categories: infectious, inflammatory, neoplastic, traumatic, and mechanical [6] (see Table 33.1).

We will first discuss the areas of the nasolacrimal system and the various processes that affect each area. Then we will review the etiologic causes.

Location of Stenosis or Occlusion

Punctum and/or Ampulla

Isolated stenosis of the lacrimal punctum is a frequent cause of epiphora, accounting for 8% of all tertiary cases with the diagnosis of epiphora, and is more obvious since it is easily visible [7]. Acquired stenosis or occlusion of the punctum and canaliculi may be caused by a variety of conditions,

Table 33.1 Causes of secondary acquired nasolacrimal duct obstruction

Neoplastic
1. *Primary neoplasms*
(a) Adenoid cystic carcinoma
(b) Adenocarcinoma
(c) Angiofibroma
(d) Angiosarcoma
(e) Cavernous hemangioma
(f) Cyst
(g) Dermoid cyst
(h) Fibroma
(i) Fibrous histiocytoma
(j) Granular cell tumors
(k) Glomus tumor
(l) Hemangioendothelioma
(m) Hemangiopericytoma
(n) Leukemia
(o) Lymphoma
(p) Lymphoplasmacytic infiltrate
(q) Lymphoproliferative diseases
(r) Melanoma
(s) Mucoepidermoid carcinoma
(t) Neurofibroma
(u) Neurilemmoma
(v) Oncocytic adenoma
(w) Oncocytic adenocarcinoma
(x) Oncocytoma
(y) Papilloma and inverted papillomas
(z) Plasmacytoma
(aa) Pleomorphic adenoma
(bb) Pyogenic granuloma
(cc) Squamous cell carcinoma
(dd) Transitional cell carcinoma
2. *Secondary involvement by neoplasm*
(a) Adenoid cystic carcinoma
(b) Amyloid
(c) Basal cell carcinoma
(d) Capillary hemangioma
(e) Dermatofibrosarcoma protuberans
(f) Esthesioneuroblastoma
(g) Fibrous dysplasia
(h) Fibrosarcoma
(i) Intraosseous cavernous hemangioma
(j) Kaposi's sarcoma
(k) Leukemia
(l) Lymphoma
(m) Maxillary and ethmoid sinus tumors
(n) Midline granuloma
(o) Mucoepidermoid carcinoma
(p) Mycosis fungoides
(q) Neurofibroma
(r) Osteoma
(s) Papilloma
(i) Conjunctival
(ii) Inverted (Schneiderian)
(t) Rhabdomyosarcoma
(u) Schwannoma
(v) Sebaceous gland carcinoma

Table 33.1 (continued)

(w) Squamous cell carcinoma
3. *Metastatic*
(a) Breast carcinoma
(b) Melanoma
(c) Prostate carcinoma
(d) Bladder carcinoma
(e) Colorectal carcinoma
(f) Esophageal carcinoma
(g) Gastric carcinoma
(h) Pharyngeal carcinoma
(i) Pulmonary carcinoma
(j) Ovarian carcinoma
(k) Thyroid carcinoma
(l) Uterine carcinoma
Inflammatory
1. *Endogenous*
(a) Wegener's granulomatosis and other forms of vasculitis
(b) Sarcoidosis and sarcoid granuloma
(c) Cicatricial pemphigoid
(d) Stevens–Johnson syndrome (erythema multiforme)
(e) Blepharitis
(f) Sinus histiocytosis
(g) Lethal midline granuloma
(h) Orbital inflammatory syndrome (pseudotumor)
(i) Linear immunoglobulin A disease
(j) Kawasaki's disease (mucocutaneous lymph node syndrome)
(k) Porphyria cutanea tarda
(l) Epidermodysplasia verruciformis, ichthyosis, scleroderma
(m) Idiopathic punctal stenosis
(n) Benign squamous metaplasia
(o) Thyroid disease
(p) Sjögren syndrome
(q) Lichen planus
(r) Nicolas–Favre lymphogranulomatosis
2. *Exogenous*
(a) Eyedrops
(i) Antiviral agents
Idoxuridine
Vidarabine
Trifluridine
Acyclovir
(ii) Antiglaucoma medications
Betaxolol
Demecarium
Echothiophate
Isoflurophate
Furmethide
Neostigmine
Physostigmine
Epinephrine
Prostaglandin analogs
Timolol
(iii) Silver nitrate, silver protein, colloidal silver
(iv) Thiotepa
(v) Cyclopentolate hydrochloride
(vi) Topical chemotherapeutic medications
Fluorouracil

(continued)

Table 33.1 (continued)

Neoplastic

Mitomycin
- (b) External radiation therapy
- (c) Cobalt and iridium brachytherapy
- (d) Radioiodine ablation, I^{131} therapy for thyroid carcinoma
- (e) Systemic chemotherapeutic medications
  - (i) Fluorouracil (systemic)
  - (ii) Docetaxel
  - (iii) Paclitaxel
  - (iv) S-1
  - (v) Capecitabine
  - (vi) Imatinib
- (f) Graft-versus-host disease
  - (i) Bone marrow transplantation
- (g) Pyogenic granuloma
- (h) Foreign body granuloma
- (i) Allergy
  - (i) Ocular
  - (ii) Nasal
- (j) Burns
  - (i) Thermal
  - (ii) Chemical
- (k) Chronic sinus disease

Infectious

1. Bacterial
- (a) *Actinomyces* sp.
  - (i) *A. israelii*
  - (ii) *A. meyeri*
- (b) *Propionibacterium propionicus* (*Arachnia propionica*)
- (c) *Fusobacterium* sp.
- (d) *Bacteroides* sp.
- (e) *Mycobacterium* sp.
  - (i) *M. fortuitum*
  - (ii) *M. leprae*
  - (iii) *M. tuberculosis*
- (f) *Chlamydia trachomatis*
- (g) *Nocardia asteroides*
- (h) *Enterobacter cloacae*
- (i) *Aeromonas hydrophila*
- (j) *Treponema pallidum*
- (k) *Staphylococcus aureus*
  - (i) Methicillin-resistant *Staphylococcus aureus* (MRSA)
  - (ii) Community-acquired MRSA (CA-MRSA)
- (l) *Staphylococcus epidermidis*
- (m) *Pseudomonas aeruginosa*
- (n) *Proteus mirabilis*
- (o) *Haemophilus influenzae*
- (p) *Peptostreptococcus*
- (q) *Streptococcus viridans*
- (r) Gamma *streptococcus*
- (s) *Diphtheroids*
- (t) *Klebsiella*
- (u) *Moraxella*
- (v) *Mononucleosis*
- (w) *Streptococcus pneumoniae*
- (x) *Moraxella*
- (y) *Escherichia coli*
- (z) *Neisseria gonorrhea*
- (aa) *Neisseria catarrhalis*
- (bb) Trachoma
- (cc) Leprosy
- (dd) Tuberculosis

2. Viral
- (a) *Herpes simplex virus*
- (b) *Herpes zoster virus*
  - (i) Varicella
- (c) Smallpox
- (d) *Adenovirus*
- (e) *Vaccinia virus*
- (f) *Epstein–Barr virus*
- (g) *Human papillomavirus*
- (h) *Mumps virus*
- (i) Epidemic keratoconjunctivitis

3. Fungal
- (a) *Aspergillus* sp.
  - (i) *A. fumigatus*
  - (ii) *A. niger*
- (b) *Candida* sp.
  - (i) *C. albicans*
  - (ii) *C. parapsilosis*
- (c) *Pityrosporon* sp.
  - (i) *P. orbiculare*
  - (ii) *P. pachydermatis*
- (d) *Rhinosporidium seeberi*
- (e) *Sporothrix schenckii*
- (f) *Streptomyces somaliensis*
- (g) *Trichophyton rubrum*
- (h) Cephalosporiosis
- (i) Blastomycosis
- (j) Cryptococcosis
- (k) *Conidiobolus coronatus* (class Zygomycetes)

4. Parasitic
- (a) *Ascaris lumbricoides*
- (b) *Distoma felineum*
- (c) Myiasis
- (d) Leishmaniasis

5. Systemic infections
- (a) Influenza
- (b) Scarlet fever
- (c) Diphtheria
- (d) Chickenpox
- (e) Smallpox
- (f) Tuberculosis

Traumatic

1. Iatrogenic
- (a) Punctal occlusion for dry eyes
- (b) After nasolacrimal duct probing with or without silicone intubation
- (c) After canalicular repair with pigtail probe
- (d) Punctoplasty – one snip, two snip, three snip, or punch
- (e) After dacryocystorhinostomy
- (f) After conjunctivodacryocystorhinostomy
- (g) After orbital fracture repair
- (h) After transantral orbital decompression
- (i) After sinus surgery (conventional or endoscopic)

Table 33.1 (continued)

(j) After rhinoplasty, rhinotomy, or other nasal surgery
(k) After craniofacial surgery
2. *Noniatrogenic*
(a) Laceration of canaliculus
(b) Laceration of lacrimal sac
(c) Avulsion of eyelid and canaliculus secondary to blunt trauma
(d) Fractures involving nasolacrimal duct nasoethmoid fractures, midfacial trauma
(e) Chemical or thermal burns
Mechanical
1. *Internal*
(a) Dacryolith
(i) Idiopathic
(ii) Eyelash nidus
(iii) Epinephrine cast
(iv) Quinacrine deposits
(v) Argyrosis
(b) Migrated or retained medical device
(i) Punctal plug
(ii) Veirs rod
(iii) Fragment of nasolacrimal probe
(vi) Modified myringotomy tube
(vii) Remnants of silicone tubing
(c) Pellet (BB)
(d) Canalicular cysts
(e) Blood
(f) Dacryops
2. *External*
(a) Kissing puncta
(b) Conjunctivochalasis; enlargement of the plica semilunaris and/ or caruncle
(c) Mucocele and mucopyoceles
(d) Migrated or malpositioned orbital floor or medial wall implants after repair of orbital floor or medial wall fractures
(e) Paget's disease
(f) Osteopetrosis
(g) Rhinolith or other nasal foreign bodies
(h) Suture stent after esophagocolostomy
(i) Exudative rhinitis
(j) Acute intranasal inflammation
(k) Nasal mucosal edema
(l) Lymphoid hyperplasia of the nasal cavity
(m) Nasal malformations
(n) Nasal polyps or polyposis
(o) Systemic syndromes or dysmorphism that involve abnormalities of facial development (clefting or malposition of the orbits or midface)
(p) Intranasal tumors
(q) Impacted or hypertrophy of the turbinate
(r) Intranasal tumors; benign and malignant
(s) Nasal packing
(t) Intranasal scaring secondary to trauma, radiation therapy, surgery, or allergic

Source: Modified table from Schaefer [57], Linberg and McCormick [58], and Bartley [6, 47]

including inflammatory conditions; infections; allergic; trachoma; cicatrizing diseases of the conjunctiva, secondary to the toxic effect of topical or systemic medications, especially systemic chemotherapeutic medications; masses in the area of the punctum; surgery; burns; trauma; long-standing ectropion or lid malposition; aging changes; blepharitis; trauma; tumors; or iatrogenic. Inferior punctal involvement is more prevalent, as expected if a medication-mediated process is suspected, as there is greater exposure of the medication-laden tear lake to the inferior puncta [8].

Punctal stenosis is more common in postmenopausal female, probably secondary to hormonal changes. Chronic blepharitis causes inflammatory and cicatricial changes resulting in inflammatory membrane formation, conjunctival epithelial overgrowth, and keratinization of the walls of the punctum. Involutional changes of these tissues, atrophy, and dense fibrous stricture of the punctum cause it to be less resilient and stenotic and the orbicularis muscle fibers to become atonic.

Even the treatment for punctal stenosis may result in punctal stenosis or occlusion. Surgical opening by punctoplasty, one snip, two snip, three snip, or punch punctoplasty, which sections the fibrous ring of the punctum, may result in the risk of cicatricial reaction and stenosis or occlusion, and may affect the lacrimal pump, by rupture of the sphincter. Many of these procedures for the management of acquired punctal stenosis include incisional techniques that disrupt the fibrous ring of the punctum and ampulla, and restenosis or occlusion may occur secondary to scar tissue formation during wound healing. Preservation of the punctal fibrous ring during these procedures should always be maintained.

Conjunctivochalasis, excess conjunctiva, can occlude the inferior punctum and is often overlooked. In mild cases, it may cause tearing due to tear film instability, and in moderate cases, it may cause obstruction of the puncta, and in severe cases, due to foreign body sensation and irritation that results from the chronic exposure of the conjunctival surface, not being covered by the eyelids (see Fig. 33.3).

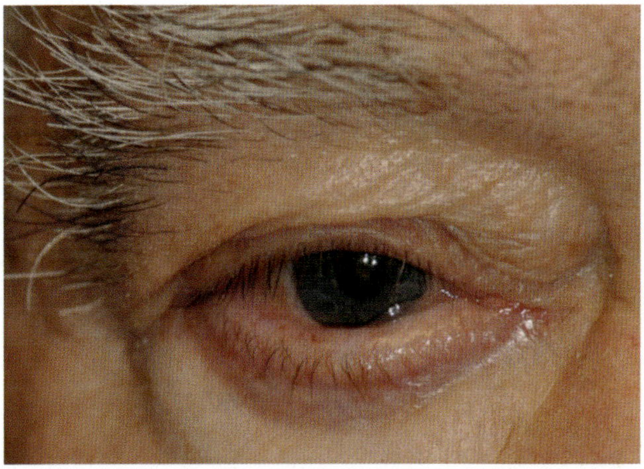

Fig. 33.3 Right eye conjunctivochalasis especially over the inferior nasal cornea to the inferior puncta

Canaliculus

Canalicular obstructions may involve the proximal segment, the first 2–3 mm, the midcanalicular segment, 3–8 mm from the puncta, and/or the distal segment, at the opening of the common canaliculus into the lacrimal sac. The predominance of canalicular obstructions has been found to involve the common canaliculus, secondary to physiologic narrowing in this area [9, 10].

Traumatic causes include chemical or thermal burns, dog bites, and lacerations after sharp penetrating wounds or blunt trauma resulting in a shearing or ripping wound of the eyelid caused by hook-like objects, teeth, fingers, etc.

Inflammatory conditions such as Stevens–Johnson syndrome, ocular cicatricial pemphigoid, chronic blepharitis, and infections such as herpes simplex, herpes zoster, infectious mononucleosis, trachoma, and dacryocystitis may cause obstruction of the canaliculi. Lichen planus, an idiopathic mucocutaneous inflammatory disease, can also cause canalicular obstruction [11].

Obstruction may occur either within the upper or lower canaliculus or in the common canaliculus. Membranous stenosis at the internal common punctum is one of the most common locations for canalicular stenosis. Causes of acquired canalicular obstruction include trauma, toxicity due to medications [5-fluorouracil, idoxuridine, phospholine iodide (echothiophate), topical cytotoxic medications, antimetabolites, eserine, etc.], infections, chlamydial infections (trachoma), viruses (herpes zoster, herpes simplex, chicken pox, and smallpox), bacteria, or cicatrizing diseases (lichen planus, Stevens–Johnson syndrome, or pemphigoid).

Canalicular cyst presents as a bluish lump or a cyst-like swelling. These cysts may arise after an episode of canaliculitis with an ecstatic canalicular diverticulum, an encysted abscess, or chronic canaliculitis.

Intrinsic canalicular tumors such as papillomas and pyogenic granulomas may occlude the canaliculi and produce a secondary inflammation and stenosis. Skin cancer may invade the puncta and canaliculi. Irradiation of tumors in the area may cause an occlusion of the canaliculi, but the placement of canalicular tubes may prevent this complication.

Punctal plugs may be associated with punctal and canalicular complications: punctal sphincter rupture during insertion, pyogenic granuloma, migration, local inflammatory reaction, canaliculitis, which may lead to stenosis or occlusion [12, 13]. Repeated probing, especially when not performed correctly, may lead to canalicular stenosis.

Lacrimal Sac

The nasolacrimal drainage system produces a broad spectrum of antimicrobial peptides that have a therapeutic potential in infections and also accelerate epithelial healing. These peptides also promote fibrin formation and cell proliferation that may also cause scarring and the resultant dacryostenosis.

The antimicrobial peptides IgA and immunocompetent cells, lymphocytes and macrophages, provide a defense mechanism. Studies indicate that the surface of the nasolacrimal duct system is also an integral part of the specific mucosal immune system and belongs to the mucosa-associated lymphoid tissue (MALT) [14]. This is an organized lymphoid tissue that has cytomorphologic and immunophenotypic characteristics of mucosa-associated lymphoid tissue.

The wall of the lacrimal sac and duct are made up of a helical system of different connective tissue fibers. The mucosal lining of the nasolacrimal sac and duct is a pseudostratified columnar epithelium and excretes a range of mucin materials, which may aid in the flow of tears and provide a defense against microbes. Researchers have identified mRNA for a variety of mucins in human lacrimal sacs and ducts [15]. Mucins play a role in nonspecific immune defense by producing a mucus layer containing different carbohydrates, TFT-peptides, and antimicrobial peptides [16, 17].

The lamina propria, beneath the epithelium, is composed of two strata: a loose connective tissue with scattered lymphocytes or groups of lymphocytes and a rich venous plexus under the loose connective tissue [18]. There is a wide luminal vascular plexus in the helical system and is connected inferior to the inferior turbinate and mucosa of the inferior meatus. This venous plexus is similar to a cavernous body and may facilitate opening and closure of the lumen of the nasolacrimal system by engorgement and shrinkage of the cavernous body, regulating the outflow of tears [19]. Factors that affect this cavernous body and its innervation may cause disturbances in the tear flow, stenosis, or total occlusion of the lacrimal drainage system. Inflammation or infections may cause swelling of the mucous membrane of the nasolacrimal duct and sac, and if this continues, will affect the helical arrangement of the connective tissue, lead to malfunctions of the subepithelial cavernous body and the resultant temporary occlusion. Repeated episodes lead to structural epithelial and subepithelial changes, which can cause a nonfunctional segment or a total fibrous closure of the lumen.

The lacrimal sac can be involved by inflammation, secondary to nongranulomatous inflammation, extraorbital manifestations of idiopathic orbital inflammatory syndrome (pseudotumor), granulomatous inflammation, granulation tissue, lymphocytic infiltrate, inflammation and ulcerations, and sarcoidosis with the most common histopathologic diagnosis on biopsy being nongranulomatous inflammation [20]. The epithelial lesions that involved the lacrimal sac are inverted papilloma, papilloma, transitional cell carcinoma, oncocytoma, granular cell tumor, carcinoma, and adenocarcinoma. The nonepithelial lesions are lymphoma, lymphoplasmacytic infiltrate, plasmacytoma, and chronic lymphocytic leukemia. Infections that involve the lacrimal sac can be secondary to fungus, viruses, and bacteria. The lacrimal sac can also be effected by dacryolith, scarring, foreign bodies, pyogenic granuloma, amyloid, orbital and midfacial fractures, blood, trauma, and papillary hyperplasia.

Several valves are present in the nasolacrimal duct system to prevent the retrograde flow of tears. The most important valve clinically is the valve of Hasner, located at the entrance of the nasolacrimal duct into the inferior meatus and frequently responsible for congenital nasolacrimal duct obstruction. The valve of Rosenmüller is found at the junction of the common canaliculus into the lacrimal sac, is not a true valve, but an angulated entrance of the common canaliculus into the sac functioning as a valve. This valve prevents retrograde flow of fluid from the sac into the canaliculi and fornix. In episodes of dacryocystitis, this valve may swell and close even more tightly. Tears and the infection cannot drain out of the sac into the nose or to the fornix. Enlargement of the lacrimal sac secondary to nasolacrimal duct obstruction changes the anatomic orientation of the common canaliculus, with an acute, inferior angulation from the superior to inferior direction in its entrance into the lacrimal sac, thus causing a functional blockage. Fibrous condensation or the development of a membrane in this location, the internal puncta, which is often adherent to the sac mucosa, is due to chronic inflammation and/or infections. This soft tissue obstruction may vary from a thin membrane to a dense fibrous condensation. If this occlusion is not identified and excised, this may compromise the results or cause failure of a dacryocystorhinostomy procedure. The common canalicular opening must be carefully examined with direct inspection and the placement of a Bowman's probe through both the superior and inferior canaliculi during surgery to ensure their patency.

Lacrimal diverticula, outpouchings of the canaliculi or the lacrimal sac, are rare but may cause intermittent or permanent swelling near the lacrimal sac. Most arise from the lateral sac wall since this area is covered only by the periorbita, offering little resistance to distention of the sac. They may be congenital, inflammatory, prior dacryocystitis, or traumatic in origin. This communication may be open or act as a one-way valve, may become symptomatic, and may cause epiphora, swelling, and/or dacryocystitis-like symptoms. Dacryoliths may form inside the diverticulum.

A retrospective study of 377 DCR specimens demonstrated nongranulomatous inflammation (321; 85.1%), granulomatous inflammation consistent with sarcoidosis (8; 2.1%), lymphoma (7; 1.9%), papilloma (4; 1.11%), lymphoplasmacytic infiltrate (4; 1.1%), transitional cell carcinoma (2; 0.5%), and single cases of adenocarcinoma, undifferentiated carcinoma, granular cell tumor, plasmacytoma, and leukemic infiltrate. Neoplasms resulting in chronic nasolacrimal duct obstruction occurred in 4.6% of cases and were unsuspected before surgery in 2.1% of patients [21].

Duct

The nasolacrimal canal is a bony conduit from the nasolacrimal fossa that enters the inferior meatus adjacent to the attachment of the inferior turbinate. This transmits the nasolacrimal duct and is formed by the three facial bones, the maxilla, the lacrimal bone, and the inferior turbinate. The nasolacrimal canal is variable and differs in size with age, gender, and race. A smaller diameter of the bony nasolacrimal duct has been noted in patients with primary acquired nasolacrimal duct obstruction by axial CT studies. Women were also noted to have a smaller diameter of the nasolacrimal canal than men, with a mean minimum diameter of 3.35 mm, versus 3.70 mm for men, which may account for the increased incidence of nasolacrimal duct obstruction in women over men [22, 23].

Nasolacrimal duct occlusion is more common in the middle-age female, is often of unknown etiology, and may present with or without dacryocystitis. This higher prevalence of primary acquired nasolacrimal duct obstruction in females may be secondary to their narrower nasolacrimal ducts or/and the possible hormonal effects on its mucosa leading to obstruction. There is an increased incidence of dacryocystitis in females (71.3%) [24].

If the cause is secondary to obstruction of the nasolacrimal duct system, the ophthalmologist must be able to determine where the anomaly is and what the cause is, in order to provide the best treatment possible for the patients.

Inflammation, trauma, or congenital defect in the drainage system may cause epiphora, dacryostenosis, and dacryocystitis. Inflammation originating at the eye, conjunctival sac, diverticula of the lacrimal system, or from the nose, and infections or diseases of the nasal mucous membrane or sinuses can induce swelling of the lacrimal system's mucous membranes, resulting in narrowing or occlusion of the nasolacrimal system from the epithelial changes and fibrosis of the lamina propria [25]. The various mechanisms that cause inflammation results in a secondary fibrosis that causes a narrowing of the nasolacrimal duct system and eventually its occlusion by scar tissue. The lacrimal sac and duct undergo similar changes: the pseudostratified, ciliated, columnar epithelium undergoes squamous metaplasia and hyperplasia with loss of goblet cells and ulceration. The underlying mucosa develops a secondary fibrosis. Basement membrane thickening may develop in the nasal mucosa but not in the lacrimal sac. The inflammation may cause a fibrosis of the lacrimal sac and the internal common punctum, which may result in obstruction, and in postoperative dacryocystorhinostomies cases may cause their failure [26].

Cicatricial nasolacrimal duct drainage obstruction has been reported to result from various medical therapies, both topical and systemic medications, radiation, radioiodine ablation, I^{131} therapy for thyroid carcinoma, systemic chemotherapy, and bone marrow transplantation.

Obstruction of the intraosseous segment of the nasolacrimal duct may be secondary to trauma, chronic sinus disease, granulomatous disease (Wegener's granulomatosis, sarcoidosis, and lethal midline granuloma), dacryocystitis, or involutional stenosis. Involutional stenosis is probably the most common cause, seen more frequently in older females.

Descending inflammation from the eye or ascending inflammation from the nasal cavity may initiate swelling of the mucous membranes of the nasolacrimal duct system, remodeling of the helical arrangement of connective tissue fibers, malfunctions in the subepithelial cavernous body with reactive hyperemia, and temporary occlusion of the nasolacrimal duct system. The submucosa is very vascular, cavernous in structure, and rich in lymphatics. The cicatricial constriction of the tissue within the bony canal makes it more likely that any swelling will lead to blockage. The submucosa of the nasolacrimal duct system surrounded by bone contains arterioles with sphincters and cavernous vessel complexes, which can cause swelling and approximation of the lumen according to the blood flow. Repeated episodes of dacryocystitis will result in permanent changes of the epithelial and subepithelial tissues, loss of goblet and epithelial cells that are important in the tear outflow mechanism, fibrosis of the helical system of connective tissue fibers, and reduction and destruction of the vascular plexus, leading to a malfunction of the tear flow mechanism, all of which result in a vicious circle [27]. These structural epithelial and subepithelial changes may cause total fibrous closure of the lumen of the nasolacrimal duct system. The changes can also develop into a nonfunctional segment that may cause chronic epiphora and discharge, but be patent to irrigation.

Obstruction of the Nasal Portion of the Nasolacrimal Duct

The orifice of the nasolacrimal canal opens 1.5 cm above the nasal floor, located on the roof of the inferior meatus, covered by the mucosal membrane termed Hasner's valve [23]. Mechanical obstruction is frequently found with enlargement, inflammation, or swelling of the inferior turbinate that may almost obliterate the anterior part of the inferior meatus and may be caused by the various nasal pathologies. A deviated septum may compress the inferior turbinate against the lateral nasal wall or even a narrow angle between the maxillary sinus medial wall and the inferior turbinate may be implicated as a causative factor [23] (see Fig. 33.4).

Inflammatory conditions, chronic nasal catarrh, and acute and suppurative infections may spread into the inferior portion of the nasolacrimal duct, resulting in obstruction. Atrophic and destructive conditions of the nasal mucosa may create an open ostium that is permitting extension of the disease process upward and allowing the direct entrance of infective secretion into the duct on blowing the nose.

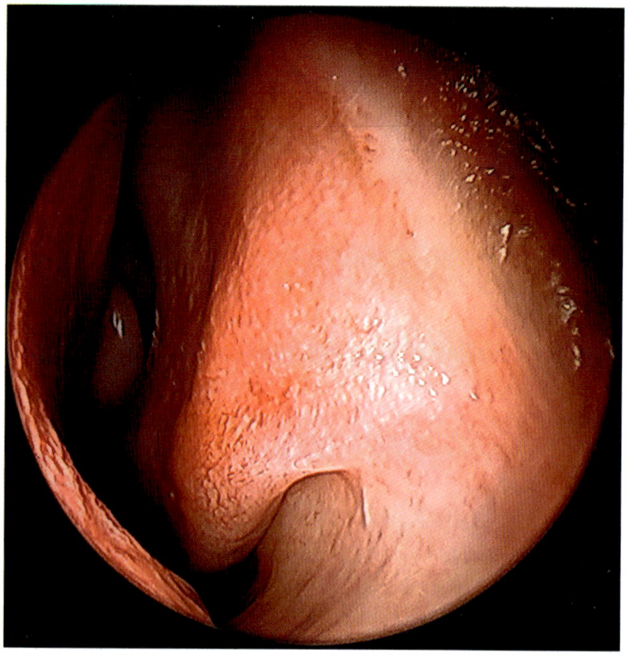

Fig. 33.4 Endoscopic view of left nasal cavity picturing the inferior turbinate and narrow inferior meatus. (Photo courtesy of Dr. John Nguyen)

Congestive and hypertrophic conditions of the nasal mucosa, vasomotor or inflammatory, may cause obstruction at or in the inferior portion of the nasolacrimal duct, as well as a nasal polyp or neoplasm. Dacryocystitis has also been reported following packing of the nose.

Intranasal pathology may affect the nasolacrimal duct. Intranasal scarring with inferior turbinate adhesions that occur from trauma, radiation therapy, surgical procedures, or nasal mucosal hypertrophy from allergic rhinitis may cause obstruction of the duct.

Dacryocystitis has various causes, but the common end result is complete obstruction of the nasolacrimal duct, resulting in stasis of tear flow, leading to secondary infections, which may progress to mucocele, pyocele–mucocele, chronic conjunctivitis, preseptal and orbital cellulitis, and abscess formation if left untreated or inadequately treated. Gram-positive bacteria are the most common cause, but gram-negative organisms should be suspected in patients with diabetes or who are immunocompromised [28].

Dacryocystitis has been reported after punctal occlusion for dry eye patients. In these patients, the nasolacrimal duct obstruction is often difficult to diagnose, since they have a decrease in tear production, and epiphora is not evident. Permanent occlusion of the canaliculi creates a closed space in the lacrimal sac, thus potentiating the development of an acute dacryocystitis [29].

Etiologic Causes

Infectious

The infectious causes of PANDO may be secondary to bacteria, viruses, fungi, and parasites. Generalized systemic infections are occasionally responsible for the onset of dacryocystitis, as seen with the occurrence of inflammation during the course of influenza, scarlet fever, diphtheria, chickenpox, smallpox, and tuberculosis.

Pathogens can enter the nasolacrimal system from the conjunctival sac, from diverticula of the lacrimal system, from the nasal cavity, or infections of the nasal mucous membranes or sinuses. The occurrence of acute dacryocystitis is dependent on the entry of a virulent strain of an organism into the stagnant contents of a lacrimal sac where the nasolacrimal duct is obstructed (see Fig. 33.5). Chronic dacryocystitis may be primary or secondary to an anatomical abnormality that has led to tear flow stasis (see Fig. 33.6). Obstructed lacrimal duct systems are colonized by increased numbers of pathogenic microorganisms. Some cases of PANDO may be secondary to unrecognized low-grade dacryocystitis. The organisms in the lacrimal sac may contribute to inflammation and scarring and therefore to the obstruction and then dacryocystitis. The microbiology of acute dacryocystitis has been reported to be frequently secondary to species of *Staphylococcus*, *Streptococcus*, *Pneumococcus*, and *Streptococcus Pyogenes*, with mixed infections being common. The most commonly

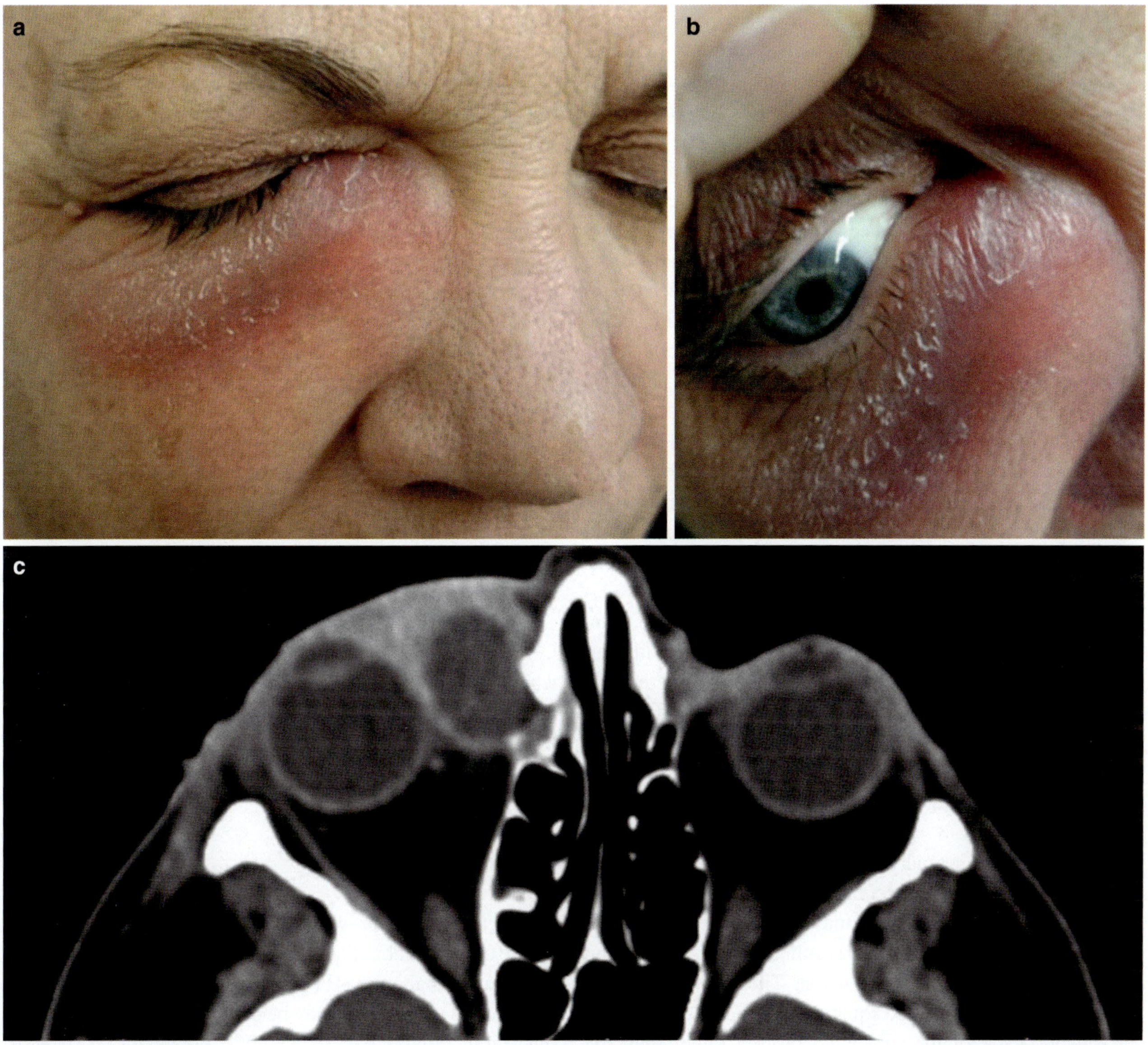

Fig. 33.5 Acute dacryocystitis, right, with enlargement of the nasolacrimal sac and surrounding preseptal cellulitis. (**a**, **b**) External photographs and (**c**) axial CT imaging

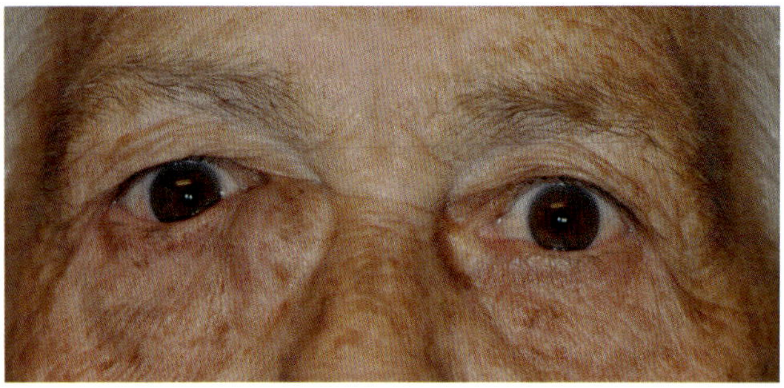

Fig. 33.6 Chronic dacryocystitis, right, with enlargement of the nasolacrimal sac

cultured organisms were *Staphylococcus epidermidis* and *Streptococcus aureus*. The common gram-negative rods include *Pseudomonas aeruginosa*, *Proteus mirabilis*, *Enterobacter cloacae*, and *Haemophilus influenzae*. Anaerobic bacteria were seen less commonly, mostly including *Propionibacterium* species. Infectious mononucleosis, mumps, and trachoma may cause dacryostenosis. The normal flora of the conjunctiva consists of gram-positive bacteria. Frequently, studies of the organisms that cause dacryocystitis are from cultures interpreted from the conjunctival cul-de-sac or are from cases of chronic dacryocystitis and therefore may not accurately identify the causative organism. Studies have shown that there is not a significant correlation between organisms cultured from the lacrimal sac to those obtained from the conjunctiva and/or nose; therefore, the preoperative conjunctival and/or nose cultures do not accurately predict the causative organism of the dacryocystitis [30].

Methicillin-resistant *Staphylococcus aureus* (MRSA) and community-acquired MRSA (CA-MRSA) are becoming increasingly prevalent as causes of ophthalmic infections, including dacryocystitis. Empiric antibiotic therapy should include coverage for MRSA especially in endemic areas until the cultures and sensitivity results are available.

Microbiologic analyses of the lacrimal sac tissue from 114 consecutive patients undergoing DCR, both with and without a history of dacryocystitis or mucocele, were positive in 44.7% of patients. Gram-positive organisms were found in 78.5% of cases, and 21.5% were gram-negative bacteria. It was suggested that an inflammatory response was caused by the initial infection resulting in fibrosis and obstruction [31].

The viruses of primary herpes simplex, herpes zoster, chicken pox, smallpox, vaccinia, epidemic keratoconjunctivitis, and Epstein–Barr viruses may cause inflammatory and cicatricial changes of the canaliculi resulting in varying degrees of obstruction or occlusion. These infections can extend beyond the stratified squamous epithelium to involve the elastic tissue of the substantia propria rather than the canalicular epithelium alone, and may also cause an adherence of the raw surfaces of the epithelium, caused by the inflammatory ulceration of the mucous membranes, resulting in stenosis and/or occlusion. Bacterial infections do not frequently affect the elastic layer. During the first few weeks of these viral infections, the mucosal epithelium is edematous, causing a functional stenosis that will still be able to be probed through. The cicatrization that occurs over the next several weeks to months generally causes an obstruction that involves the midzone or distal portions of the superior and inferior canaliculi, but occasionally may cause punctal occlusion. Early recognition, probing, and intubation, when indicated, can prevent permanent canalicular obstruction and the need for a conjunctivodacryocystorhinostomy.

Dacryocystitis has been reported to result from infections with several species of mycobacteria: *Mycobacterium fortuitum*, *M. leprae*, and *M. tuberculosis*.

Chlamydia trachomatis has been reported to cause punctual occlusion, canalicular scarring, and nasolacrimal duct obstruction.

Other bacteria associated with lacrimal drainage obstruction include *Nocardia asteroides*, *Enterobacter cloacae*, *Aeromonas hydrophila*, *Treponema pallidum*, and *S. aureus.*

Fungi generally occlude the lacrimal drainage system by the formation of stone or cast. *Aspergillus fumigatus*, *Aspergillus niger*, *Candida albicans*, *Candida parapsilosis*, *Pityrosporum orbiculare*, *Pityrosporon pachydermatis*, *Streptomyces somaliensis*, and *Trichophyton rubrum* may cause lacrimal stones or casts.

Parasitic obstruction is unusual, but has been reported with *Distoma felineum*, *Myiasis*, and the nematode *Ascaris lumbricoides*. The *Ascaris lumbricoides* worm gains entrance to the nasolacrimal system through the valve of Hasner and then emerges from the punctum. The protozoan parasite, Leishmaniasis, has been reported to cause chronic dacryocystitis [32].

Verruca vulgaris and other viruses may cause a bloody epiphora when they involve the punctum or canaliculus.

Nocardia; *Sporotrichosis*; *Rhinosporidiosis*; *Cephalosporiosis*; *Pseudomonas*; *Candida*; *Aspergillus*, which is commonly associated with other bacteria; *H. influenzae*; *Treponema vincentii*; *Rhinosporidium seeberi*; *Sporothrix fungus*; as well as *Treponema* and tuberculosis, have been reported to cause dacryocystitis.

Canaliculitis

Canaliculitis often presents as a painful, localized swelling of one of the canaliculi and may be divided into primary and secondary canaliculitis. Primary canaliculitis often refers to an infective process and may be caused by a variety of bacterial, viral, chlamydial, or mycotic organisms [33]. Most cases of canaliculitis are unilateral. *Actinomyces israelii* is reported as one of the most common causes. *Actinomyces*, previously named *Streptothrix israelii*, an obligate parasite whose only host is humans, causes a canalicular obstruction and inflammation. *A. israeli* is a gram-positive aerotolerant filamentous rod with true branching, which causes inflammation rather than a blockage of the lacrimal duct. *Actinomyces* organisms are sensitive to penicillin, but topical antibiotic therapy is usually ineffective without mechanical expression or surgical removal of the canalicular stones. *Propionibacterium propionicus*, formerly *Arachnia propionica*, is gram-positive and has a branching, rod-shape morphology. It is facultatively anaerobic; carbon dioxide is not necessary for growth, unlike *Actinomyces*. *Fusobacterium* and *Bacteroides* have also been cultured from cases of canaliculitis.

Actinomyces meyeri is principally found in the periodontal sulcus, is an uncommon pathogen, is nonfilamentous, branching, may be difficult to demonstrate, and can cause canaliculitis.

Smears and cultures will help to select the appropriate antibiotics, but expression or a surgical removal is usually required (see Fig. 33.7).

Rarely canaliculitis can be classified as idiopathic canalicular inflammatory disease (ICID) once traumatic history, cultures, collagen vascular panel, and autoimmune workup return negative. With its female preponderance presenting at a mean age of 57 years, this canaliculitis with unilateral onset often affects the other eye and punctum within 6 months. The relentless course of inflammation often ends with end-stage disease and progressive scarring despite optimal management with topical and systemic immunosuppression and with system intubation.

Secondary canaliculitis results from chemotherapy, radiotherapy, secondary to punctal plugs, or even from specific inflammations like Stevens–Johnson syndrome.

Dacryoliths

Dacryoliths are typically yellow or white "sulfur granules" and are frequently secondary to *Actinomyces* organisms but may occasionally be seen in infections secondary to *Nocardia*, *Streptomyces*, and *Staphylococcus* (see Fig. 33.8).

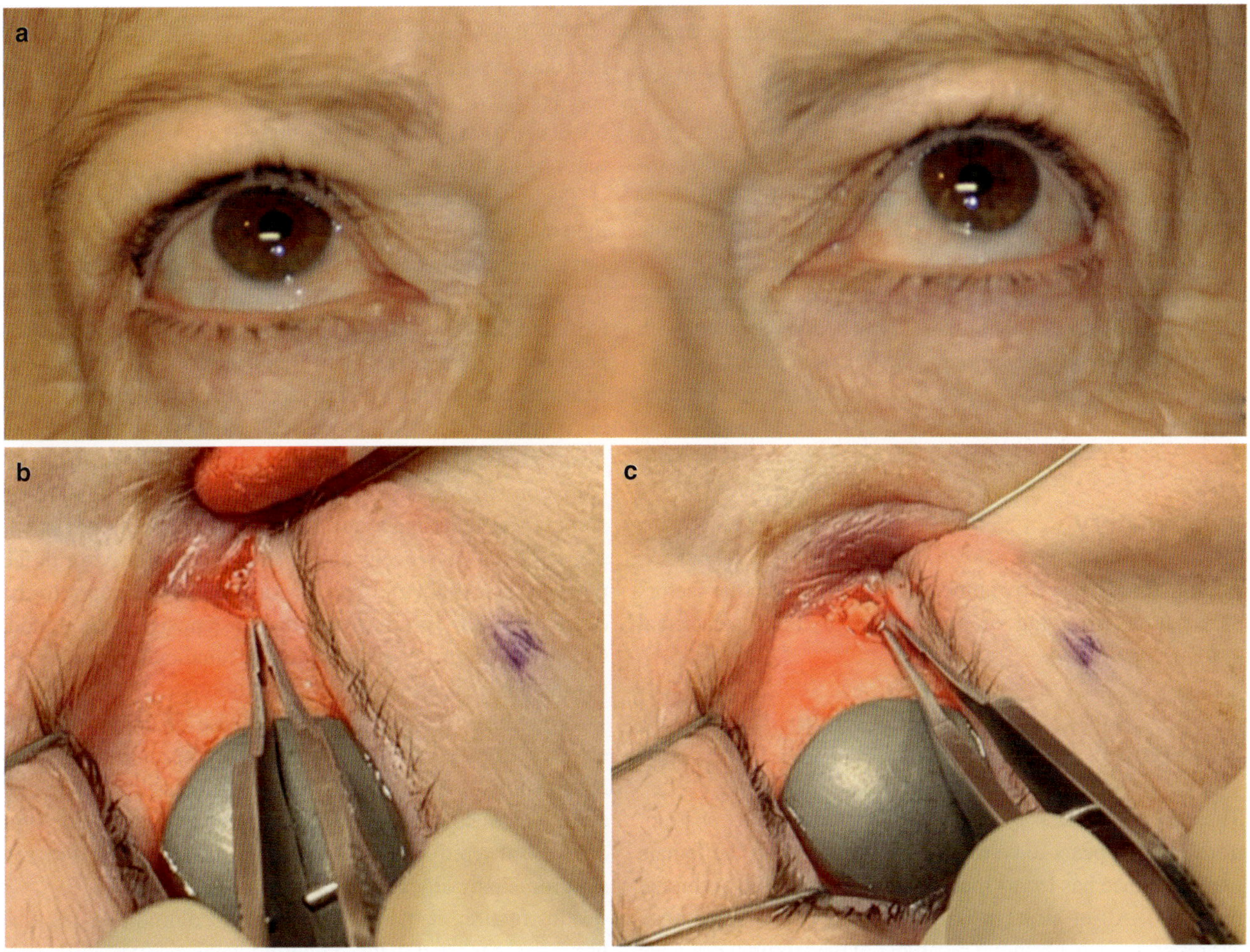

Fig. 33.7 Chronic canaliculitis presenting with (**a**) right inferior canalicular enlargement. Surgical excision (**b**, **c**) through transcanalicular incision with expression of contents. (Photos courtesy of Dr. John Nguyen)

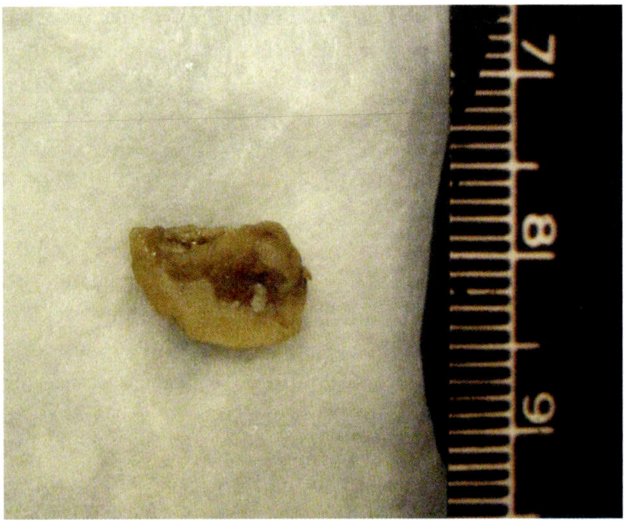

Fig. 33.8 Dacryolith. (Photo courtesy of Dr. John Nguyen)

Shed epithelial cells, amorphous debris, and lipids with or without calcium can form cast within the lacrimal sac, which can lead to obstruction. In addition to the aforementioned text, the long-term topical use of epinephrine has been reported to form casts from its oxidation products. These patients may present with the history of intermittent pain and epiphora due to the ball-valve-like behavior.

Dacryoliths may develop from foreign bodies. Cilia may act as the initial nidus for their formation. Some have postulated that metabolic factors such as high calcium and phosphate levels in the obstructed lacrimal system may contribute to their formation.

Fungi generally occlude the lacrimal drainage system by the formation of stone or cast, which can be seen with *Aspergillus fumigatus*, *A. niger*, *Candida albicans*, *C. parapsilosis*, *Pityrosporum orbiculare*, *P. pachydermatis*, *Streptomyces somaliensis*, and *Trichophyton rubrum*.

Inflammatory

Inflammation caused by numerous diseases and other factors may cause narrowing or obstruction of the nasolacrimal system.

Endogenous Origin

The etiopathogenesis of acquired nasolacrimal duct obstructions often appears to be multifactorial; however, the female predominance has led to speculations of a possible hormonal base [34]. Ali et al. have found that there is a widespread expression of sex hormone receptors in the lacrimal drainage system of cadaveric and clinical samples. The expression and distribution patterns differed between the genders and with the diseased tissues. Diseased samples showed a reduction or absence of estrogens, testosterone, progesterone, oxytocin, and oxytocin receptor expression pattern.

Granulomatous diseases can occasionally produce a mass within the lacrimal sac, as seen with extraorbital manifestations of idiopathic orbital inflammatory syndrome (idiopathic inflammatory pseudotumor), lethal midline granuloma, and sarcoidosis. In patients with sarcoidosis and the other inflammatory diseases, initially successful dacryocystorhinostomy has an increased incidence of late failure due to the reoccurrence or exacerbation of the inflammatory process in the nasal and lacrimal sac mucosa.

Wegener's granulomatosis, a vasculitis that classically involves the triad of the upper respiratory tract, the lung, and the kidneys, may cause obstruction of the nasolacrimal system. Nasolacrimal obstruction is typically associated with advanced nasal disease, late in the disease process, and has been reported in 7% of patients [35]. This obstruction is frequently secondary to contiguous nasal disease but may also be secondary to a vasculitis of the lacrimal sac mucosa. Treatment of the nasolacrimal obstruction should be deferred until the inflammation is quiescent, if possible. Other forms of vasculitis may cause similar obstruction of the nasolacrimal duct system.

Cicatricial pemphigoid, Stevens–Johnson syndrome, and Nicolas–Favre lymphogranulomatosis may cause nasolacrimal obstruction with advanced disease.

Dacryocystoceles result from mucous accumulation and the enlargement of the lacrimal sac and potentially the nasolacrimal duct. This may develop when there is obstruction of the nasolacrimal duct with either an inactive valve of Rosenmüller, punctal, or canalicular obstruction, which has been noted in patients with Steven–Johnson syndrome, a diffuse mucocutaneous inflammatory disease, as well as with dacryoliths, infectious processes, and topical or systemic medications. Dacryocystoceles in adults tend to be firmer to palpation when compared to the fluctuant congenital cases, and in these older individuals, a diminishment of the Tyndall phenomenon may occur due to the thicker overlying tissue planes [36]. Although often asymptomatic secondary to the decreased tear production, dacryostenosis is common. Cicatricial occlusion of the puncta or canaliculi may develop, as well as nasolacrimal duct obstruction.

Sinus histiocytosis (a benign disease of unknown etiology, which may be related to an allergy or an immunologic abnormality of histiocytes), linear immunoglobulin A disease, Kawasaki's disease (mucocutaneous lymph node syndrome), thyroid disease, ulcerative colitis, and Sjögren syndrome may all cause nasolacrimal obstruction.

Obstruction of the proximal sac or common canaliculus has been reported with epidermodysplasia verruciformis, ichthyosis, scleroderma, and the sclerodermoid variant of porphyria cutanea tarda. Lower lid ectropion, which often has an inflammatory or cicatricial component, which may be associated with systemic diseases, has been reported occasionally to be associated with dacryostenosis [37].

Lichen planus, an immune-mediated skin and mucosal disease similar to pemphigoid, may cause lacrimal stenosis and obstruction. There is a cell-mediated reaction at the level of the epithelial basement membrane. This may also cause a cicatrizing conjunctivitis with shortening of the fornices, symblepharon formation, and keratitis.

Exogenous Factors

Ocular and periocular disorders, such as atopic disease, sinus and nasal inflammations, exudative rhinitis, and allergies, may develop nasolacrimal stenosis and obstruction.

Epiphora may be a manifestation of ocular surface disease such as ocular allergy or ocular rosacea. Rosacea is an inflammatory condition of the facial skin. Ocular changes are present in more than 50% of patients and include meibomian gland dysfunction, telangiectasia and erythema of the eyelid margins, conjunctivitis, blepharitis, the formation of hordeolum and chalazia, keratitis, iritis, and episcleritis. Swollen and slit-like punctal openings are noted in patients with allergy, rosacea, and inflammatory meibomian gland dysfunction. This compromise in the tear drainage system leads to chronic epiphora. Conjunctivochalasis secondary to inflammatory diseases can lead to a pseudoblockage of the puncta from the overhanging conjunctiva.

Allergic conjunctivitis in patients who chronically rub their eyes can cause an intermittent allergic obstruction at the level of the puncta, canaliculus, or lacrimal sac, which may progress to a permanent occlusion.

Tumors (Neoplastic)

The signs and symptoms of tumors of the lacrimal sac are nonspecific and can easily allow the clinician to misdiagnose the various causes of primary acquired nasolacrimal duct obstruction with functional nasolacrimal duct obstruction. The insidious nature of lacrimal sac tumors may present as dacryostenosis or dacryocystitis. The mass is usually above the medial canthal tendon. The position of the medial canthal tendon does not frequently allow distention of the sac by fluid or distention from dacryocystitis superior to the tendon. A tumor within the sac can create a mass effect above the tendon that cannot be reduced on palpation or compression. Therefore, any distention of the lacrimal sac superior to the medial canthal tendon should be considered to be a tumor until proven otherwise. The nonspecific symptoms of epiphora, swelling in the lacrimal sac region, and dacryocystitis are the most frequent presenting symptoms but are shared between lymphomas, epithelial tumors, and other malignant lesions. The dacryocystitis symptoms produced may differ from other causes of dacryocystitis, in that the epiphora and dacryocystitis symptoms may be intermittent, irrigation fluid may pass into the nose, blood may reflux from the punctum, and telangiectasia may be present, as well as regional lymphadenopathy. Intermittent epiphora, sanguineous discharge, or an irreducible mass should always lead one to suspect a lacrimal sac tumor. Even imagining modalities of the nasal lacrimal system may not distinguish between lesions of the sac and functional obstruction. The clinician should always be aware that simple dacryostenosis and dacryocystitis may not always be the correct diagnosis. The symptom of bloody epiphora should always strongly indicate the need for preoperative evaluation.

Primary tumors of the nasolacrimal duct system are uncommon but can arise from within the puncta, canaliculi, lacrimal sac, nasolacrimal duct, or about its entrance into the nasal cavity, at the valve of Hasner. The epithelial tumors account for 75% of the lacrimal sac tumors, and the nonepithelial tumors for 25%, which include mesenchymal tumors, malignant melanoma and lymphomas, and leukemia, particularly in older patients with chronic lymphocytic leukemia.

Approximately 45% of lacrimal sac tumors are benign and 55% are malignant. There have been cases reported in which the initial symptoms of epiphora or dacryocystitis were found at surgery to be secondary to tumors. Squamous cell papillomas and carcinomas are the most common. Pyogenic granulomas, composed of well-vascularized friable tissue, containing an infiltration of lymphocytes, plasma cells, and a few eosinophils, may often involve the lacrimal sac. Many papillomas initially grow in an inverted pattern into the lacrimal sac wall and therefore are often incompletely excised, with recurrence, and malignant degeneration can occur. Lipoid proteinosis, Urbach–Wiethe, or hyalinosis cutis et mucosae syndrome may be associated with nasolacrimal duct obstruction.

The most common primary tumors of the nasolacrimal system of epithelial origin are papillomas and squamous cell carcinomas. Less frequently are adenoid cystic carcinoma, angiofibroma, angiosarcoma, cavernous hemangioma, dermoid cyst, fibroma, fibrous histiocytoma, hemangioendothelioma, hemangiopericytoma, lacrimal sac cyst, lymphoma, malignant melanoma, mucoepidermoid carcinoma, neurofibroma, oncocytic adenoma, oncocytic adenocarcinoma, pleomorphic adenoma, dermatofibrosarcoma protuberans, rhinoscleroma, neurilemmoma, and adenoacanthoma, and more commonly involve the lacrimal sac. Schwannoma, fibrous histiocytoma, leukemia, and granulocytic sarcoma may infiltrate the lacrimal sac. The papillomas are histologically classified as squamous cell, transitional cell, and mixed cell that are resistant to radiation therapy.

The most common neoplasms of the lacrimal sac are epithelial tumors. The most common benign epithelial tumor is a papilloma. Papillomas exhibit epithelial papillomatosis and acanthosis, and an inflammatory papilloma exhibits granulomatous tissue. Inverted papillomas can arise de novo in the lacrimal sac or more commonly from an extension from the lateral aspect of the nasal cavity or maxillary sinus. When these lesions arise from the lacrimal system, the patient presents with epiphora and a medial canthal mass. They may cause bony destruction and orbital and intracranial extension. The lesion is not malignant but has a high recurrence rate, reported to be 27–71%. Metaplastic transformation to squamous cell carcinoma occurs in 10–15% of cases and therefore should be treated as a malignant lesion. DNA viruses, human papillomavirus types 6 and 11, and the Epstein–Barr virus have been identified in these lesions. The other forms of lacrimal sac epithelial carcinomas are less common. These include adenocarcinoma and epidermoid carcinoma. Mucoepidermoid carcinoma is a very rare but aggressive cancer.

Secondary tumors and metastatic lesions can infiltrate or compress the nasolacrimal system resulting in symptoms of dacryostenosis and dacryocystitis that are much more common than primary tumors. The secondary tumors include adenoid cystic carcinoma, basal cell carcinoma, capillary hemangioma, esthesioneuroblastoma, fibrous dysplasia, fibrosarcoma, Kaposi's sarcoma, intraosseous cavernous hemangioma, leukemia, lymphoma, lymphomatous diseases, mucoepidermoid carcinoma, osteomas, breast carcinoma, bladder carcinoma, uterine carcinoma, colorectal carcinoma, esophageal carcinoma, gastric carcinoma, pulmonary carcinoma, ovarian carcinoma, pharyngeal carcinoma, prostatic carcinoma, thyroid carcinoma, conjunctival papillomas, inverted papillomas, sebaceous gland carcinoma, squamous cell carcinoma, and rhabdomyosarcoma.

The nasolacrimal drainage system has a surrounding vascular plexus that is in a system of collagen bundles, with elastic and reticular fibers arranged in a helical pattern. The mucosa of the nasolacrimal duct system may be an area where leukemic or lymphomatous tumors may form primarily or metastatically from hematologic spread due to its mucosal-associated lymphoid tissue (MALT), and occur more frequently in the middle-aged or elderly. Epiphora will often be the first complaint, before a mass develops or dacryocystitis occurs, and the system may remain patent to probing and irrigation. These lesions usually respond to local irradiation and/or chemotherapy, and stenting of the nasolacrimal duct system to prevent stenosis secondary to the radiation therapy.

Lymphoproliferative diseases may involve the nasolacrimal system leading to epiphora, and acute or chronic dacryocystitis. They are the second most common type of tumor causing nasolacrimal obstruction. Lymphomas are more frequent than benign lymphoproliferative lesions. Lymphosarcomas, reticulum cell carcinomas, and Hodgkin's disease have been reported to occur in the lacrimal sac, as well as the mesenchymal tumors: capillary and cavernous hemangiomas, hemangiopericytomas, melanomas, neurilemmoma, plexiform neuroma, osteoma, fibromas, Kaposi's sarcoma, and other sarcomas.

The presentation of bloody epiphora, a mass above the medial canthal tendon, and chronic dacryocystitis should always alert the physician to the possibility of a nasolacrimal tumor. Bleeding from the puncta may also be secondary to squamous papillomas vascular fronds, epithelial tumors, oncocytomas, melanoma, lymphoid lesions, and lymphoid hyperplasia.

The most frequent extrinsic secondary tumors are eyelid lesions, particularly basal cell carcinoma, then squamous cell carcinoma, and less frequently sebaceous cell carcinoma, which can involve the medial canthal region and the nasolacrimal duct system or cause pressure and compression, and the resultant dacryostenosis and dacryocystitis (see Fig. 33.9).

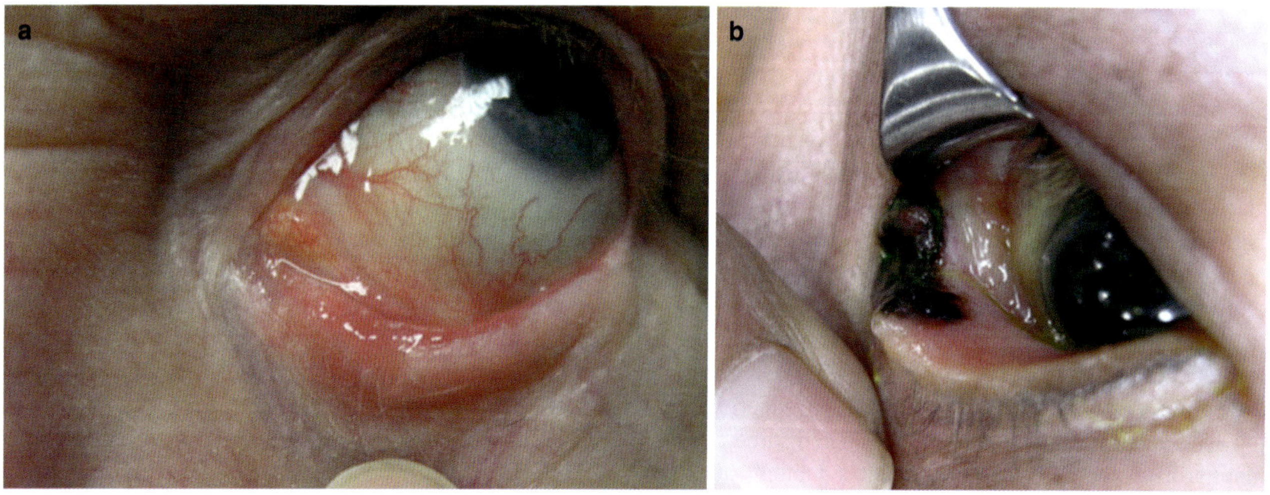

Fig. 33.9 Upper lacrimal system obstruction secondary to neoplastic eyelid tumors: (**a**) squamous cell and (**b**) melanoma. (Photos courtesy of Dr. John Nguyen)

When neoplasms are excised in the medial canthal area, complete resection must be performed with histopathologic control (frozen borders or Mohs technique), including any portion of the nasolacrimal system involved. The canaliculi may be marsupialized, but a DCR or CDCR should be delayed for 5 or more years to ensure that there are no recurrences. This preserves the natural bony barrier that helps to prevent or decreases the incidence of tumor spread into the nasal cavity, decreasing the morbidity and mortality.

The most frequent maxillary sinus lesion is squamous cell carcinoma. The most common lesions arising from the nasopharynx are lymphomatous and squamous cell carcinomas.

Sinus tumors invade the orbit and nasolacrimal duct system and can be benign or malignant. The benign lesions include inverted papillomas, osteomas, juvenile angiofibroma, and neuroectodermal tumors. Inverted papilloma is the second most common lesion that invades the orbit after squamous cell carcinoma. Inverted papillomas can arise from the lateral nasal wall or the mucosa of the ethmoidal sinus. Mucocele of the paranasal sinuses can invade the orbit and cause nasolacrimal obstruction. Squamous cell carcinoma, adenocarcinoma, adenoid cystic carcinoma, esthesioneuroblastoma, lymphoma, and melanoma can occur in the paranasal sinus. Rarer tumors are the odontogenic tumors, ameloblastoma and ameloblastic fibrosarcoma, as well as fibrosarcoma, chondrosarcoma, sinus glioblastomas multiforme, and mucoepidermoid carcinoma, and may cause dacryostenosis. The most frequent sinus tumor is squamous cell carcinoma of the maxillary sinus, then lymphomas, adenocarcinoma, adenoid cystic carcinoma, transitional cell carcinoma, olfactory neuroblastoma, osteoblastoma, and malignant histiocytosis.

The clinician must always remain vigilant in assessing any patient with dacryostenosis, considering the need for preoperative radiologic studies and inspecting the anatomy of the interior of the lacrimal sac at the time of surgery. Routine biopsy of the lacrimal sac is unnecessary if inspection does not reveal atypical pathology [38]. When taken routinely, histopathologic reports found 94.15% to have nonspecific chronic inflammation with or without fibrosis. 5.85% had lacrimal sac specific pathology, of which 24.34% were unsuspected.

Metastatic disease as a cause of dacryostenosis and/or dacryocystitis is very rare; lymphoma is the most common, but cases secondary to prostate carcinoma, breast carcinoma, and malignant melanoma have been reported [39].

Both benign and malignant tumors of mesenchymal elements, capillary and cavernous hemangiomas, and hemangiopericytomas have been reported to involve the lacrimal sac. Melanomas, neurilemmoma, plexiform neuroma, and osteoma can involve the lacrimal sac both intrinsically and extrinsically. Fibromas, Kaposi's sarcoma, and other sarcomas can rarely involve the lacrimal sac.

Traumatic

Burns are a major cause of traumatic injury and may be caused by fire, chemicals, electricity, scalding agents, and radiation. Thermal or chemical burns may cause inflammation, dacryostenosis, and obstruction.

Blunt trauma or lacerations usually damage the canaliculus, the lacrimal sac, or the nasolacrimal duct. Lacerations of the punctum are rare. The dense fibrous tissue of the tarsus is much stronger than the medial canalicular portion of the eyelid; therefore, any tractional force along the eyelid margin can result in avulsion of the medial eyelid with canalicular involvement, its weakest portion. All canalicular lacerations should be repaired within 1 day of the injury to prevent scarring and epithelialization of the wound. If there is a laceration medial to the puncta, one must always assume that there is also a laceration of the canaliculus.

Fractures

Midfacial trauma and the resultant facial fractures frequently involve the bone about the lacrimal sac fossa and/or nasolacrimal ducts, leading to obstruction of the nasolacrimal system [40]. Lacrimal system integrity in the setting of trauma or tumor extirpation may be difficult to assess initially, especially in the absence of direct or obvious disruption of the lacrimal drainage system. The nasolacrimal duct is confined by the lateral nasal wall [40]. Fractures involving portions of the nasolacrimal duct include the midface fractures of naso-orbital, LeFort II, and LeFort III fractures, frequently resulting in extensive damage to the lacrimal drainage system, including the medial canthal tendon and/or its insertion. It is always important to consider and evaluate for involvement of the nasolacrimal duct with these types of fractures rather than waiting for the patient to present with epiphora and/or dacryocystitis. The incidence of NLDO following naso-orbital-ethmoidal fractures was reported to be 68.4% by Uraloglu et al. [41]. The patients who were not treated for their fractures were more likely to present with symptoms of obstruction, concluding that early fracture repair likely reduces the incidence of posttraumatic obstruction. The diagnostic evaluation and examination, with the manipulation of the lacrimal system at the time of the initial repair, have been reported to be difficult and unreliable, and that exploratory probing may damage an intact system or exacerbate the degree of damage already present, thus discouraging early intervention. This may be true for some, but a skilled surgeon who understands and knows the anatomy, with gentle technique, not forcing the probe, should be able to perform this. Delayed assessment of the nasolacrimal system without intubation or repair may result in late cicatricial obstruction, rendering the system nonfunctional, requiring a secondary surgical repair, which is generally more difficult to perform. Even if lacrimal irrigation is easy and disappearance of fluorescein dye normal, only lacrimal duct probing can identify and define the extent of injury in these cases since the fluid may pass into the nose through boney and membranous defects caused by the trauma. The traumatic edema that develops in these cases may cause a compression of the lacrimal system and a temporary dysfunction. Detachment of the medial canthal tendon may cause compression of the lacrimal sac and may compromise the lacrimal pump function. Direct repair of these injuries is not always possible, but stent placement will help to promote patency. Prophylactic intubation with silicone tubing should be considered to prevent this occlusion when indicated. Bony fractures may also initiate an inflammatory and cicatrizing reaction that may result in nasolacrimal duct obstructions shortly after or years after the injury.

The surgical repair of these midface fractures may also damage and cause obstruction of the nasolacrimal system such as when transnasal wiring is performed incorrectly or with the improper placement of plates and/or screws.

Iatrogenic Obstruction

Dacryostenosis and obstruction may result from many procedures, such as repeated and traumatic probing of the canalicular system. Poor technique in the probing of the nasolacrimal ducts may cause the creation of a false passage and subsequent scarring of the lacrimal drainage system.

The exact risk and incidences of complications of probing have not been fully evaluated. Probing, if not performed correctly, may result in damage to the lacrimal epithelium, leading to stenosis, and may prevent the success of later treatment. There has been reported a 44% incidence of canalicular stenosis after failed probing. Bleeding from the punctum, which may be a sign of damage of the lacrimal epithelium, has been reported in 20% of 60 probings causing an iatrogenic stenosis [42, 43].

The pigtail probe has frequently been reported to cause iatrogenic damage to the nasolacrimal duct system, and many consider it to be a potentially harmful device. There have been reported cases of the treatment of a single canalicular laceration or congenital agenesis of only one puncta/canaliculus with the pigtail probe that resulted in obstruction of both canaliculi, which will then commit the patient to a conjunctivodacryocystorhinostomy and the required presence of a Jones tube and its required maintenance for life.

Cheese wiring of silicone intubation tubes through the puncta and canaliculus, as well as migrating nasally with complete healing of the eroded puncta and canaliculus, can occur. The canalicular slitting more commonly involves the inferior canaliculus. The erosion of the punctocanaliculi may also be due to chronic irritation by the tubes or tubes that were placed under tension. Rubbing of the eyelids and the horizontal movement of the puncta with orbicularis function may also be responsible for the tube pressure against the puncta causing a cheese wiring or slitting effect. The tubes may be colonized with bacteria, including atypical *Mycobacterium*. Granulation tissue formation may develop in reaction to the stent that can lead to early recurrence of dacryostenosis after the stent is removed, especially if the stent has been in place for a long period of time. The diameter of the nasolacrimal duct is small so that even a small amount of granulation tissue can occlude the passages. The stents may incite a chronic inflammatory reaction that can cause irreversible changes in the nasolacrimal system.

It is important to remove all remnants of silicone tubing from the lacrimal system to prevent secondary obstruction due to inflammatory tissue. The mucosal surfaces are prone for the development of granulation tissue, pyogenic granuloma, and true granulomas, and nongranulomatous reactions to the silicone tube may occasionally occur.

Punctoplasty, the one-, two-, three-snip, or punch procedure, may potentially cause damage to the canaliculus and its function. If too much is cut, the canaliculus may not function properly or scarring may occur in the canaliculus, and the normal anatomy and physiology of the canalicular system is not maintained. If the canaliculus is slit open, it may not be able to develop the pressure gradient that is required for the tear pump to function properly. Therefore, punctoplasties should be avoided or performed very carefully.

Punctal occlusion, which is frequently performed for the treatment of dry eye syndrome, keratoconjunctivitis sicca, may, in a few patients, cause subsequently epiphora, and, less frequently, dacryocystitis. Punctal plugs include the absorbable plugs, collagen, gelatin, catgut, and hydroxypropyl cellulose, and the nonabsorbable plugs, silicone, polymethylmethacrylate, polyethylene, and *N*-butyl cyanoacrylate plugs. Partial or complete dacryostenosis, pyogenic granulomas, intracanalicular migration, and canaliculitis have been reported after the placement of permanent punctal plugs. Distal migration of the plugs may require complicated canalicular surgery, dacryocystorhinostomy, or even a conjunctivodacryocystorhinostomy.

Collared punctal plugs are designed to be removable, but rarely there have been cases of these plugs breaking during removal, with migration of the remainder of the plug into the lacrimal system.

Intracanalicular plugs used for the treatment of dry eye syndrome are placed in the horizontal canaliculus where the plugs cannot be seen and are designed to be removed by irrigating them through the nasolacrimal system, which is not always easily accomplished in a considerable number of cases. Irrigation does not reliably flush these intracanalicular plugs from the nasolacrimal system. The collarless intracanalicular plugs theoretically can be flushed through the nasolacrimal system, but is not recovered from the nose. Therefore, successful removal cannot be objectively documented. The intracanalicular plugs have been associated with significant lacrimal complications. They have been noted to cause a higher rate of pyogenic granulomas, indicating that they may initiate an inflammatory process that disrupts the normal cellular functions, can cause a fibrosis and reactive mass, may act as a nidus for infection and inflammation, and may result in epiphora, canaliculitis, and eventually obstruction and/or dacryocystitis. Major reconstructive surgery may be required, and despite this reconstructive surgery, the symptoms may not resolve. They have also been hypothesized to facilitate the overgrowth of bacteria, and a chronic canaliculitis that can result in canalicular obstruction may erode through the canalicular mucosa, resulting in synechia, symptomatic lacrimal stenosis, or even the formation of fistula [44]. This increased incidence of complications seen with intracanalicular plugs suggests that collared punctal plugs offer a safer alternative.

Herrick plugs, an intracanalicular plug, may cause irreversible chronic adverse reactions with persistent inflammation and epiphora. They may cause destruction of the normal canalicular architecture, proliferative tissue reaction, pericanalicular fibrosis, granulomatous tissue, pyogenic granuloma, giant cell reaction, canaliculitis, dacryocystitis, and lymphocytic infiltration. The plug prevents normal tear flow and permits tear stagnation proximal to the obstruction, which serves as a nidus for inflammation and infections. Persistent inflammation and/or infection may result in chronic changes, fibrosis, and stenosis of the canaliculus. This reaction may cause chronic epiphora, canaliculitis, and/or dacryostenosis. If a patient presents with tenderness and chronic discharge, and the plug cannot be visualized, one must not assume that the plug has extruded, but must assume that the plug has migrated into the canaliculi. Removal of these plugs is the treatment of choice. Palpation of the plug may locate the plug, and probing should be performed carefully to prevent deeper migration of the plug. Forceful probing and irrigation may cause deeper migration of the plug and create greater difficulties for their removal. If the plug is located in the proximal portion of the canaliculus, it may be removed by expression, which is performed by the use of two cotton tip applicators placed medially to the plug in the canaliculi and milking it temporally out of the puncta. If this fails, a canaliculotomy and curettage may be required to remove the plug, and then repair of the damaged canaliculus and stent placement. Early removal of the plug is recommended to decrease the inflammation and possibility of secondary infections.

Cautery has also been used to occlude the puncta, but is not as easily reversible as removing punctal plugs are. The smaller sized punctal plugs were designed to facilitate their insertion, but this design increases the incidence of migration irritation, corneal erosions, canalicular stenosis after removal of the plug, foreign body sensation, epiphora, pruritus, pyogenic granuloma, fragmentation of the plug, and the possible sequelae of canaliculitis and dacryocystitis. Forceful insertion of the plug may result in the placement of the plug into the canaliculus.

Dacryostenosis may occur after a dacryocystorhinostomy due to new or persistent stenosis at the internal common punctum or to an improperly fashioned osteotomy. DCR failure may also be due to retained stenting material. Dacryostenosis and obstruction have been reported as a complication of nasal operations, paranasal sinus surgery, both endoscopic and conventional external procedures, and craniofacial procedures.

Nasoantral window procedures are generally placed at the most anterior–inferior portion of the maxillary sinus. If they are placed too high or too posterior, or if the nasolacrimal duct is in an anomalous position, damage to the duct may occur. Transantral orbital decompression that removes the medial wall and floor of the orbital, through an antrostomy, may also cause damage to the lacrimal duct, possibly secondary to delayed scarring around the nasoantral window.

The various endoscopic nasal and sinus surgeries may cause damage to the nasolacrimal drainage system. Dacryostenosis has been reported after cosmetic rhinoplasty procedures, probably secondary to damage to the membranous nasolacrimal duct during the lateral osteotomy.

Migration of orbital floor implants after orbital fracture repair into the lacrimal sac has also been reported [45]. These implants may have been improperly placed or poorly secured, and their migration may cause an external compression or occlusion of the nasolacrimal sac and/or duct.

Mechanical

Mechanical compression or blockage of the nasolacrimal duct system can result from external compression or occlusion of the system from an intraluminal foreign body, hematoma, or stone. Direct occlusion or external compression may impede or block the canaliculi or nasolacrimal duct.

Dacryoliths

The most common cause of internal mechanical obstructions is dacryoliths. Some are secondary to fungal infections, organized blood clots, and inspissated mucous plugs, but frequently, the cause is indeterminate. Foreign bodies in the lacrimal sac can be surrounded by epithelial debris and inflammatory tissue to produce a dacryolith. There are cases reported where an eyelash served as a nidus for formation of the dacryoliths, and also from the breakdown products from argyrosis. Others have postulated that metabolic factors such as high calcium and phosphate levels within an obstructed lacrimal system may contribute to the formation of dacryoliths. Various medications, including epinephrine and quinacrine, have been reported to contribute to the formation of cast of the nasolacrimal ducts. A black adrenodacryolith has been reported in a patient who was treated with topical adrenaline for chronic glaucoma. The dark color of the dacryolith was probably secondary to stimulated melanin deposition [46]. Dacryoliths occur more frequently in younger patients, under age 50 years, and in heavy smokers. These patients generally present with intermittent dacryocystitis and localized tenderness.

The foreign bodies that may cause internal mechanical obstruction are generally migrated or retained medical devices, such as punctal plugs, or incompletely removed plugs and silicone tubing. Rarely, intranasal bleeding can cause a hematoma of the lacrimal sac and duct.

External factors may cause a mechanical obstruction of the lacrimal system. Opposing superior and inferior puncta may cause a proximal obstruction, as in ptosis. Redundancy of the bulbar conjunctiva, or conjunctivochalasis, is frequently overlooked as a cause of mechanical obstruction. This condition contributes to epiphora, foreign body sensation, and disruption of the inferior tear meniscus. These symptoms tend to increase in downgaze. Excision of an ellipse of the redundant conjunctiva is often curative. Enlargement of the caruncle, megalocaruncle, may extend laterally to block the punctum or displace the puncta away from the globe and tear pool.

Orbital tumors, such as dermoid cyst, orbital lymphangioma, and osteomas, may compress the nasolacrimal system externally.

Masses arising from the paranasal sinuses, nasal polyps, mucoceles, mucopyoceles, nasal mucosal edema, lymphoid hyperplasia of the nasal cavity, exudative rhinitis, cavernous hemangioma, hypertrophy of the inferior turbinate, or tumors may cause an external compression of the lacrimal sac or duct. Nasal mucosal edema and mucopurulent exudates may lead to obstruction of the nasolacrimal duct at the intranasal ostium, the valve of Hasner. Allergic, viral, or bacterial pharyngitis and rhinitis can produce sufficient nasal mucosal edema, lymphoid hyperplasia, and exudates to result in obstruction of the nasolacrimal duct and progression to a dacryocystitis.

Lacrimal sac cysts, dacryops, are congenital or traumatic in origin. They grow slowly and may present as a painless epiphora or dacryocystitis.

Maxillary sinus cysts, antral mucoceles, retention cysts, pseudocysts, dentigerous cysts and keratocysts, ameloblastoma, ossifying fibroma, giant cell granuloma and cholesteatoma, and nasolacrimal duct orifice cysts may block the inferior meatus and cause nasolacrimal obstruction. Routine examination should be performed, direct or endoscopically, of the inferior meatus and nasal cavity to rule out or rule in these pathologies, and if found, their treatment may require a less invasive procedure that would resolve the patient's epiphora and avoid a DCR.

Nasal malformations, systemic syndromes, or dysmorphism that involves abnormalities of facial development, such as clefting or malposition of the orbits or midface, can be associated with maldevelopment of the nasolacrimal duct system. Patients with the centurion syndrome have an anterior displacement of the medial canthal tendon, a prominent nasal bridge, and displacement of the punctum away from the tear pool, resulting in epiphora.

Paget's disease and osteopetrosis have been reported as causes of acquired nasolacrimal obstruction [47]. Sarcoid granuloma, oncocytoma, rhinoliths, and nasal foreign bodies in the inferior meatus can cause a mechanical obstruction of the nasolacrimal duct system at the valve of Hasner.

Punctal eversion or ectropion may be involutional, secondary to horizontal laxity of the eyelid, medial and lateral canthal laxity, cicatricial ectropion, burns, after blepharoplasty, or the mechanical effects of tumors. The horizontal laxity will also affect the lacrimal pump and/or can cause an exposure keratitis that will stimulate the reflex tearing mechanism.

Trichiasis and distichiasis will cause a reflex tearing and will require epilation, cryosurgery, or the various eyelid margin procedures. Entropion also will cause a reflex tearing secondary to irritation from the lashes or skin.

Punctual stenosis may occasionally occur spontaneously. The punctum may become stenotic with cicatricial diseases affecting the eyelid margin. Chronic punctal eversion may also result in stenosis of the puncta.

Paralysis of the seventh cranial nerve will impair the lacrimal pump action and not drain tears properly. Horizontal shortening, as with a lateral tarsal strip procedure, Terson's spindle, and/or medical canthoplasty procedures may help, but frequently, a Jones tube is required. Any condition that impairs the contractility and elasticity of the lacrimal pump mechanism can cause epiphora, such as burns, trauma, scleroderma, and radiation fibrosis.

Medications

Acquired dacryostenosis may result from the use of antiviral, antiglaucoma, or systemic and topical chemotherapeutic medications. Cells with rapid turnover, such as those lining the nasolacrimal drainage system and the mucous membranes, are more susceptible to the cytotoxic effects of chemotherapy.

The most common cause of iatrogenic punctual or canalicular stenosis and occlusion is ophthalmic medications.

Idoxuridine, vidarabine, trifluridine, acyclovir, demecarium, echothiophate, isoflurophate, adenine arabinoside, furmethide, floxuridine, fluorouracil, neostigmine, physostigmine, epinephrine, cyclopentolate hydrochloride, pilocarpine, quinacrine, dipivefrin, timolol, betaxolol, latanoprost and the prostaglandin analogs, dorzolamide, silver preparations, and thiotepa have been most frequently associated with dacryostenosis and occlusion.

Idoxuridine, trifluridine, and adenine arabinoside generally cause occlusion of the punctum, rather than the midzone of the canaliculi as seen from viral infections. The punctal stenosis that occurs from antiviral toxicity will frequently reverse on discontinuation of the medication early on. The antiglaucoma medication may cause a cicatricial conjunctivitis that may be similar to, and indistinguishable from, cicatricial pemphigoid.

Chronic topical epinephrine may affect the vascular plexus of the nasolacrimal duct system. This specialized vascular system permits opening and closing of the lumen of the lacrimal passage, affected by the engorgement and shrinkage of the vascular system that regulate tear outflow [48]. Frequent topical cyclopentolate hydrochloride has been reported to cause dacryostenosis.

The systemic uses of some antineoplastic agents, such as 5-fluorouracil, a pyrimidine analog that blocks the enzyme thymidylate synthetase, docetaxel, and paclitaxel and similar medications have been reported to cause punctal and canalicular stenosis and occlusion with epiphora [49]. Docetaxel and paclitaxel have been demonstrated to cause keratinization of the nasal mucosa by affecting the rapidly dividing cells.

5-fluorouracil may also cause lacrimation, conjunctivitis, blepharitis, keratitis, blurred vision, pain, ankyloblepharon, and cicatricial ectropion. It may cause an inflammatory response in mucosal membranes, as evident by conjunctivitis, as well as oral and gastrointestinal inflammation. This inflammation and fibrosis of the lacrimal drainage system may cause extensive and permanent damage to the lacrimal system, with fibrous adhesions that obstruct the canaliculi and lacrimal sac [50, 51].

Docetaxel is an effective chemotherapeutic agent for advanced breast cancer and other common malignancies in the antineoplastic class of taxanes. Epiphora and permanent canalicular stenosis can occur in up to 50% of patients receiving weekly docetaxel and to a lesser percent in patients receiving docetaxel every 3 weeks. Chronic inflammation and extensive fibrotic changes have been demonstrated in the stroma of the lacrimal sac and the nasal mucosa, and probably chronic changes in the mucosal lining of the entire lacrimal drainage system. In advanced cases, this occlusion is not reversible. The mechanism of canalicular stenosis may be secondary to the secretion of docetaxel in the tear film and fibrosis of the canaliculi from direct contact, or the mucous membrane lining of the puncta and canaliculi develop a fibrosis secondary to the systemic effects of the drug similar to the widespread edema and fibrosis seen elsewhere in the body. Patients receiving docetaxel should be screened for epiphora and canalicular stenosis, and treatment in the form of silicone intubation to prevent the need for a conjunctivodacryocystorhinostomy [52]. With the newer regimens that use lower doses of the drug for shorter periods than in the past, lacrimal stenosis and occlusion should be less frequent. These patients should receive frequent monitoring and examinations, including probing and irrigation in the office to detect early involvement and, if present, treat these patients with topical steroids to decrease mucosal inflammation, as well as the use of frequent artificial tears after each infusion of docetaxel to dilute the concentration of the drug in the tear film. Moderate or progressive dacryostenosis require silicone intubation of the lacrimal drainage system to hopefully prevent the development of irreversible damage and the need for a DCR or CDCR.

Medicamentosa not only can develop from the medication but also may be secondary to the preservatives in topical drops. Patients taking topical antiglaucoma medications demonstrated an increased incidence of developing lacrimal drainage system obstruction. Routine postoperative antibiotic and steroids after intraocular surgery have also been implicated in the development of punctal occlusion. This may be associated with the medications themselves, the preservatives, and/or the duration of topical treatment. Conjunctival metaplasia, a decrease in goblet cells, an increase in macrophages, and lymphocytes in the epithelium, and an increase in fibroblasts, macrophages, mast cells, and lymphocytes in the substantia propria have been noted on histologic examination. Dacryostenosis may also occur as part of a cicatrizing process, a drug-induced pemphigoid condition, which may occur after the long-term use of antiglaucoma medications. The inflammation causes a decrease in the clearance of the medication and preservatives, and their continued use will result in more inflammation and stenosis, and therefore a longer clearance time resulting in a higher concentration and longer transit time, leading to a vicious cycle.

Topical mitomycin C is used for the treatment of corneal–conjunctival intraepithelial neoplasia, primary acquired melanosis with atypia, conjunctival malignant melanoma, and pagetoid sebaceous carcinoma, and epiphora secondary to punctal–canalicular stenosis has been reported in up to 14% [53] to 43% [54] of patients.

Radiation

External radiation in the treatment of neoplasia can cause inflammation of the lacrimal drainage system, stenosis, and occlusion. The reported required dose in the literature varies greatly, but it has been reported to occur in cases receiving as little as 1800 rad (cGy). Other reports state that the lacrimal passages are relatively immune to radiation therapy until significantly higher doses are delivered. It is hypothesized that the epiphora probably results from a combination of anatomic lacrimal obstruction, conjunctival epithelial alterations, damage to conjunctival epithelial cells, and damage to conjunctival goblet cells and glands. It is recommended that intubation should be considered in patients undergoing radiation for medical canthal tumors. Topical corticosteroid may also be useful in preventing punctal and canalicular stenosis [55].

Cobalt and iridium brachytherapy have been reported to cause severe dermatitis and lacrimal drainage stenosis. Lovato et al., in a prospective study, reported that 11 out of 12 patients who had prophylactic nasolacrimal intubation with silicone tubing maintained lacrimal duct patency, whereas 10 out of 12 patients who did not receive prophylactic silicone intubation developed punctal occlusion after helium ion therapy for uveal melanoma.

Radioiodine ablation, I^{131} therapy for thyroid carcinoma at cumulative activities of 150 mCi of I^{131} or higher, may produce clinically significant nasolacrimal drainage system obstructions in 4.6% of patients and is probably dose-related. Radioiodine has been recovered from the lacrimal gland and in the tears of patients receiving radioactive iodine therapy. The most common side effects are xerophthalmia and chronic and recurrent conjunctivitis. Sodium/iodide symporter, the ion transporter that has the ability to take up iodine, is present in the pseudostratified columnar epithelial cells of the lacrimal sac and nasolacrimal ducts. The sodium/iodide symporter is a membrane glycoprotein that mediates active iodide uptake in the thyroid gland, and in the periocular area, is located in the ciliary body, the nasolacrimal duct, and lacrimal gland. The areas of obstruction involve the nasolacrimal duct, common canaliculus, and rarely, the superior and inferior canaliculi. The mechanism of the dacryostenosis may be a contribution of local toxicity from direct radiation injury from the passive flow of radioactive tears and/or active uptake and concentration of I^{131} in the nasolacrimal drainage tissues from the blood by the sodium/iodide symporter, the same iodine uptake mechanism used by the thyroid gland. The inflammatory reaction is probably induced by radioiodine, causing a swelling and fibrosis and finally an obstruction or occlusion of the lumen. This increased incidence of dacryostenosis and obstruction is likely to be dose-related. Symptomatic patients should receive early evaluation and treatment with possible silicone tube placement since once complete obstruction has developed, it has proven to be difficult to manage [56].

Hopefully, these classification systems will be useful in the evaluation and treatment of nasolacrimal disorders. The location of the stenosis or occlusion and the etiologic classification system presented earlier provide a useful mechanism in the formulation of a differential diagnosis and help to develop the appropriate evaluation and treatment plan for each individual patient. These divisions may not be completely isolated, there will be cases that overlap, and there are some diseases and/or clinical situations that have not been included in this chapter.

References

1. McCormick SA, Linberg JV. Pathology of the nasolacrimal duct obstruction. Contemp Issues Ophthalmol Lacrimal Surg. 1988;5:169–202.
2. Paulsen FP, Corfield AP, Hinz M, et al. Characterization of mucins in human lacrimal sac and nasolacrimal duct. IOVS. 2003;44:1807–13.
3. Becher BB. Tricompartment model of the lacrimal pump mechanism. Ophthalmology. 1992;99:1139–45.
4. Ali MJ, Singh S, Naik MN, Kaliki S, Dave TV. Interactive navigation-guided ophthalmic plastic surgery: the utility of 3D CT-DCG-guided dacryolocalization in secondary acquired lacrimal duct obstruction. Clin Ophthalmol. 2017;11:127–33.
5. Ali MJ, Naik MN. Image-guided dacryolocalization (IGDL) in traumatic secondary acquired lacrimal drainage obstructions (SALDO). Ophthal Plast Reconstr Surg. 2015;31:406–9.
6. Bartley GB. Acquired lacrimal obstruction: an etiologic classification system, case report, and a review of the literature. Part 1. Ophthal Plast Reconstr Surg. 1992;8(4):237–42.
7. Mainville N, Jordan DR. Etiology of tearing: a retrospective analysis of referrals to a tertiary care oculoplastics practice. Ophthal Plast Reconstr Surg. 2011;27:155–7.
8. Starks VS, Yoon MK. Acquired obliteration of the proximal lacrimal drainage system. Ophthal Plast Reconstr Surg. 2018;35:342. https://doi.org/10.1097/IOP.0000000000001244. [Epub ahead of print].
9. Konuk O, Ilgit E, Erdinc A, Onal B, Unal M. Long-term results of balloon dacryoplasty: success rates according to the site and severity of the obstruction. Eye. 2008;22:1483–7.
10. Ohtomo K, Ueta T. Factors associated with the efficacy of probing for adult patients with lacrimal duct obstruction. Ophthal Plast Reconstr Surg. 2017;33:136–8.
11. Durrani OM, Verity DH, Meligonis G, et al. Bicanalicular obstruction in lichen planus: a characteristic pattern of disease. Ophthalmology. 2008;115:386–9.
12. Maguire LJ, Bartley GB. Complications associated with the new smaller size freeman punctal plug. Arch Ophthalmol. 1989;107:961–2.
13. Nelson C. Complications of freeman plug. Arch Ophthalmol. 1991;101:923–4.
14. Knop E, Knop N. Lacrimal drainage-associated lymphoid tissue (LDALT): a part of the human mucosal immune system. Invest Ophthalmol Vis Sci. 2001;42:566–74.
15. Paulsen F, Corfield AP, Hinz M, et al. Characterization of mucins in human lacrimal sac and nasolacrimal duct. Invest Ophthalmol Vis Sci. 2003;44(5):1807–13.
16. Paulsen F, Hinz M, Schaudig U, et al. TFF-peptides in the human efferent tear ducts. Invest Ophthalmol Vis Sci. 2002;43:3359–64.
17. Paulsen F, Pufe T, Schaudig U, et al. Detection of natural peptide antibiotics in human nasolacrimal ducts. Invest Ophthalmol Vis Sci. 2001;42:2157–63.
18. Duke-Elder S, Wybar KC. System of ophthalmology vol II. The anatomy of the visual system. St. Louis: Mosby; 1961. p. 559–81.

19. Paulsen F, Hallmann U, Paulsen J, Thale A. Innervation of the cavernous body of the human efferent tear ducts and function in tear outflow mechanism. J Anat. 2000;196:177–87.
20. Amin RM, Hussein FA, Idriss HF, Hanafy NF, Abdallah DM. Pathological, immunohistochemical and microbiological analysis of lacrimal sac biopsies in patients with chronic dacryocystitis. Int J Ophthalmol. 2013;6(6):817–26.
21. Anderson NG, Wojno TH, Grossniklaus HE. Clinicopathologic findings from lacrimal sac biopsy specimens obtained during dacryocystorhinostomy. Ophthal Plast Reconstr Surg. 2003;19:173–6.
22. Janssen AG, Mansour K, Bos JJ, et al. Diameter of the bony lacrimal canal: normal values and values related to nasolacrimal duct obstruction: assessment with CT. AJNR Am J Neuroradiol. 2001;22:845–50.
23. Gul A, Aslan K, Karli R, Ariturk N, Can E. A possible cause of nasolacrimal duct obstruction: narrow angle between inferior turbinate and upper part of the medial wall of the maxillary sinus. Curr Eye Res. 2016;41(6):729–33.
24. Burns JA, Cahill KV. Modified Kinosian dacryocystorhinostomy: a review of 122 cases. Ophthalmic Surg. 1985;16:710–6.
25. Paulsen FP, Thale AB, Maune S, Tillman BN. New insights into the pathophysiology of primary acquired dacryostenosis. Ophthalmology. 2001;108(12):2329–36.
26. Mauriello JA, Palydowycz S, DeLuca J. Clinicopathologic study of lacrimal sac and nasal mucosa in 44 patients with complete acquired nasolacrimal duct obstruction. Ophthal Plast Reconstr Surg. 1992;8(1):13–21.
27. Paulsen FP, Thale AB, Maune S, Tillman BN. New insights into the pathophysiology of primary acquired dacryostenosis. Ophthalmology. 2001;108(12):2329–36.
28. Wladis EJ, Shinder R, LeFabvre DR, Sokol JA, Boyce M. Clinical and microbiologic features of dacryocystitis-related orbital cellulitis. Orbit. 2016;35(5):258–61.
29. Glah HJ. Acute dacryocystitis after punctal occlusion for keratoconjunctivitis. Am J Ophthalmol. 1991;111:137–40.
30. Blicker JA, Buffam FV. Lacrimal sac, conjunctival, and nasal culture results in dacryocystorhinostomy patients. Ophthal Plast Reconstr Surg. 1993;9(1):43–6.
31. DeAngelis D, Hurwitz J, Mazzulli T. The role of bacteriologic infection in the etiology of nasolacrimal duct obstruction. Can J Ophthalmol. 2001;36:134–9.
32. Baddini-Caramelli C, Matayoshe S, Moura EM, et al. Chronic dacryocystitis in American mucocutaneous leishmaniasis. Ophthal Plast Reconstr Surg. 2001;17:48–52.
33. Ali MJ. Idiopathic canalicular inflammatory disease: new disease description of clinical patterns, investigations, management, and outcomes. Ophthal Plast Reconstr Surg. 2018;34:528–32.
34. Ali MJ, Schicht M, Paulsen F. Qualitative hormonal profiling of the lacrimal drainage system: potential insights into the Etiopathogenesis of primary acquired nasolacrimal duct obstruction. Ophthal Plast Reconstr Surg. 2017;33:381–8.
35. Bullen CL, Liesegang TJ, McDonald TJ, et al. Ocular complications of Wegener's granulomatosis. Ophthalmology. 1983;90:279–90, Article Linker Bibliographic Links.
36. Perry LJP, Jakobiec FA, Zakka FR, Rubin PAD. Giant dacryocystomucopyocele in an adult: a review of lacrimal sac enlargements with clinical and histopathologic differential diagnoses. Surv Ophthalmol. 2012;57(5):474–85.
37. Bartley GB. Acquired lacrimal drainage obstruction: an etiologic classification system, case reports, and a review of the literature. Part 2. Ophthal Plast Reconstr Surg. 1992;8(4):243–9.
38. Koturovic Z, Knezevic M, Rasic DM. Clinical significance of routine lacrimal sac biopsy during dacryocystorhinostomy: a comprehensive review of literature. Bosn J Basic Med Sci. 2017;17(1):1–8.
39. Bartley GB. Acquired lacrimal drainage obstruction: an etiologic classification system, case report, and a review of the literature. Part 3. Ophthal Plast Reconstr Surg. 1993;9(1):11–26.
40. Ali MJ, Gupta H, Honavar SG, Naik MN. Acquired nasolacrimal duct obstructions secondary to Naso-orbito-ethmoidal fractures: patterns and outcomes. Ophthal Plast Reconstr Surg. 2012;28:242–5.
41. Uraloglu M, Erkin Unlu R, Ortak T, Sensoz O. Delayed assessment of the nasolacrimal system at naso-orbito-ethmoid fractures and a modified technique of dacryocystorhinostomy. J Craniofac Surg. 2006;17:184–9.
42. Lyon DB, Dortzbach RK, Lemke BN, Gonnering RS. Canalicular stenosis following probing for congenital nasolacrimal duct obstruction. Ophthalmic Surg. 1991;22:228–32.
43. Young JDH, MacEwen CJ, Ogston SA. Congenital nasolacrimal duct obstruction in the second year of life, a multicentre trial of management. Eye. 1996;10:484–91.
44. White WL, Bartley GB, Hawes MJ, et al. Iatrogenic complications related to the use of Herrick lacrimal plugs. Ophthalmology. 2001;10:1835–7.
45. Jordan DR, St. Onge P, Anderson RL, Patrinelly JR, Nerad JA. Complications associated with alloplastic implants used in orbital fracture repair. Ophthalmology. 1992;99:1600–8.
46. Daxecker F. Adrenodakryolith. Klin Monatsbl Augenbeilkd. 1992;200:140–1.
47. Bartley GB. Acquired lacrimal drainage obstruction: an etiologic classification system, case report, and a review of the literature. Part 3. Ophthal Plast Reconstr Surg. 1993;9(1):11–26.
48. Paulsen FP, Thale AB, Maune S, Tillman BN. New insights into the pathophysiology of primary acquired dacryostenosis. Ophthalmology. 2001;108(12):2329–36.
49. Esmaeli B, Valero V, Ahmadi MA, Booser D. Canalicular stenosis secondary to docetaxel (taxotere): a newly recognized side effect. Ophthalmology. 2001;108:994–5.
50. Esmaeli B, Burnstine MA, Ahmadi MA, Prieto VG. Docetaxel-induced histologic changes in the lacrimal sac and nasal mucosa. Ophthal Plast Reconstr Surg. 2003;19(4):305–8.
51. Masur C, Pfeiffer ML, Esmaeli B. Evaluation and management of chemotherapy-induced epiphora, punctal and canalicular stenosis, and nasolacrimal duct obstruction. Ophthal Plast Reconstr Surg. 2017;33:9–12.
52. Esmaeli B, Valero V, Ahmadi MA, Booser D. Canalicular stenosis secondary to docetaxel (taxotere): a newly recognized side effect. Ophthalmology. 2001;108:994–5.
53. Khong JJ, Muecke J. Complications of mitomycin C therapy in 100 eyes with ocular surface neoplasia. Br J Ophthalmol. 2006;90:819–22.
54. Koop ED, Seregard A, Selva D. Punctal-canalicular stenosis associated with mitomycin-C for corneal epithelial dysplasia. Am J Ophthalmol. 2003;136:746–7.
55. Lovato AA, Char DH, Castro JR, Kroll SM. The effect of silicone nasolacrimal intubation on epiphora after helium ion irradiation of uveal melanomas. Am J Ophthalmol. 1989;108:431–4.
56. Burns JA, Morgenstern KE, Cahill KV, et al. Nasolacrimal obstruction secondary to I^{131} therapy. Ophthal Plast Reconstr Surg. 2004;20:126–9.
57. Schaefer DP. Acquired etiologies of lacrimal system obstruction. In: Cohen AJ, Mercandetti M, Brazzo BG, editors. The lacrimal system. New York: Springer; 2006. p. 46–9.
58. Linberg JV, McCormick SA. Primary acquired nasolacrimal duct obstruction: a clinicopathologic report and biopsy technique. Ophthalmology. 1986;93:1055–62.

34 Clinical Evaluation and Imaging of Lacrimal System Obstruction

Jonathan J. Dutton and Jeffrey J. White

The lacrimal drainage apparatus is an intricate mucous membrane-lined conduit, the function of which depends on a complex interplay of anatomy and physiology. Appropriate drainage of tears depends on several factors, including the volume of tear production, eyelid position, normal pump mechanisms, anatomic status of the drainage passages, gravity, and nasal air convection currents. The patient with symptomatic epiphora may have a normal anatomic system overwhelmed by an oversecretion syndrome, or a drainage system that is anatomically compromised and is therefore unable to handle normal tear production. Conversely, patients may have partial or complete blockage of the nasolacrimal system but experience no symptoms or have symptoms of dry eye if tear production is significantly reduced. The clinical picture of bothersome epiphora thus depends on the balance of tear production and tear drainage, not on the absolute function of either one.

The etiologies of lacrimal drainage dysfunction can be divided into two categories: anatomic and physiologic. Anatomic obstruction refers to a gross structural abnormality of the nasolacrimal system. This can be a complete obstruction, such as punctal occlusion, canalicular blockage, or nasolacrimal duct fibrosis. The causes of partial obstruction include punctal or canalicular stenosis, inflammatory narrowing of the duct, and mechanical obstruction within the lacrimal sac, such as tumors or stones. Physiologic etiologies result from failure of functional mechanisms despite normal anatomy. These types of dysfunction may result from anatomic deformity, such as punctal eversion or other eyelid malposition, or from lacrimal pump inadequacy from poor orbicularis tone or eyelid laxity. Determining the type of dysfunction and the exact location of the anatomic blockage with physical exam and ancillary testing is essential if appropriate therapy is to be offered.

The clinical evaluation of gross lacrimal function is usually not difficult, and the diagnosis of epiphora can oftentimes be made largely on history alone. However, determination of the etiology of epiphora may be more difficult and often requires a variety of diagnostic procedures. There is no single test that will pinpoint the anatomic site or physiologic basis for an imbalance between tear production and tear drainage. A host of clinical tests have been described, many of which must be used together to diagnose specific disease processes correctly. In this chapter, we briefly describe the most important tests and imaging techniques and discuss the clinical significance of each.

Clinical Diagnosis

The following diagnostic tests have been devised to evaluate the tear production and lacrimal drainage systems. These tests include some simple clinical procedures that should be a routine part of every evaluation, as well as more complex radiographic and echographic examinations that are used in selected patients. In most cases of epiphora, a number of tests must be employed to determine the specific etiology and to plan appropriate therapy.

Clinical History

Clinical history is one of the most important aspects in the evaluation of the patient with symptomatic epiphora, yet it is frequently glossed over or completely overlooked. Taking an adequate history can occasionally localize the site of obstruction and in most cases will allow the surgeon to decide which tests are appropriate. Epiphora in a child with a history of tearing since birth is almost always the result of a blockage at Hasner's membrane, whereas acquired epiphora in a child

J. J. Dutton (✉)
University of North Carolina, Department of Ophthalmology, Chapel Hill, NC, USA
e-mail: jonathan_dutton@med.unc.edu

J. J. White
Carolina Eye Associates, P.A, Southern Pines, NC, USA

J. J. Servat et al. (eds.), *Smith and Nesi's Ophthalmic Plastic and Reconstructive Surgery*,
https://doi.org/10.1007/978-3-030-41720-8_34

may have a very different etiology such as canalicular obstruction. It is important to elicit a history of prior facial trauma or intranasal cautery, as this should prompt evaluation of the bony nasolacrimal canal. Prior use of ophthalmic medications (i.e., phospholine iodide), certain systemic chemotherapeutic agents, or orbital irradiation should lead the clinician to suspect canalicular obstruction. Previous sinus surgery, particularly intranasal antrostomy or ethmoidectomy should alert the surgeon to potential direct duct injury. History of a rapidly growing mass or bleeding from the puncta should raise the suspicion for the presence of malignancy. Intermittent epiphora can be related to early inflammation of the membranous duct or from allergic rhinitis. Recurrent episodes of dacryocystitis may suggest lower nasolacrimal duct obstruction but may lead to stenosis of the proximal system as well. Taking a thorough history as part of the routine evaluation will make further investigation considerably more efficient.

External Examination

Evaluation of epiphora begins with a careful examination of the external ocular surface and eyelid structures for causes of hypersecretion or for mechanical obstruction of drainage. Conjunctival or corneal irritation, either inflammatory or mechanical, may cause hypersecretion with resultant epiphora, even in the presence of a normally functioning drainage system. Blepharitis and allergic conjunctivitis will often trigger increased lacrimation. Occlusion of the puncta or a narrow medial palpebral fissure with resulting punctal opposition and mechanical occlusion will block tear drainage. Conjunctivochalasis is seen with increasing frequency with advancing age, and it has been shown that contact lens wear is an additional risk factor [1, 2]. When severe, the redundant conjunctiva can cover and mechanically occlude punctal drainage [3]. Mass lesions in the medial canthal region may also mechanically obstruct tear drainage. Careful palpation of the lacrimal sac will reveal the presence of a sac mucocele, and pressure behind the anterior lacrimal crest may produce reflux of mucopurulent material suggestive of lower system obstruction. Examination of the nasal vestibule must be made, as hypertrophic mucosa or nasal polyps can obstruct the nasolacrimal ostium. Such findings during external examination will direct the clinician toward further specific diagnostic tests. Eyelid malpositions such as entropion, with or without trichiasis, can produce corneal irritation and secondary reflex tearing. Ectropion from lid laxity or facial nerve palsy may lead to exposure keratopathy and reflex epiphora. Medial ectropion causes the punctum to rotate away from the tear lake, impairing tear drainage.

Eyelid laxity from aging or other causes may result in a functional acquired epiphora from a weakened orbicularis muscle pump mechanism [4–6]. In such cases, the patient may complain of epiphora and dye drainage is delayed, but there is no evidence of mechanical punctal or canalicular stenosis or obstruction, and the nasolacrimal duct (NLD) is patent to irrigation without reflux. Quantitative scintigraphy studies have shown a positive correlation between delayed drainage and eyelid or medial canthal laxity [7]. Punctal stenosis is a common finding, reported in more than 50% of normal individuals. The prevalence increases with advancing age, and it is often related to chronic blepharitis [8]. Punctal stenosis and canalicular stenosis are also common complications of chemotherapy such as systemic 5-fluorouracil and docetaxel, or topical mitomycin-C [9–11]. Since punctal stenosis can be seen without accompanying eyelid laxity, any epiphora evaluation should specifically look for this condition.

Schirmer Tests

In 1903, Schirmer described this technique for evaluation of tear production. Since that time, the Schirmer tests have become an important clinical tool for the diagnosis of dry eye and hypersecretion syndromes. The Schirmer I test is used to evaluate gross tear production. It is usually performed without topical anesthetic. A strip of #41 Whatman filter paper, 50 mm long and 5 mm wide, is folded 5 mm from one end, and the small folded end is placed into the inferior conjunctival fornix at the junction of the lateral and middle thirds of the lower eyelid. The amount of wetting on the filter paper is measured at 5 min [12]. The test should be performed in subdued lighting, and both eyes must be tested simultaneously. This test measures the aqueous component of the tear film and does not distinguish between basic and reflex tear production. It gives only a very crude estimate of true tear flow. The paper itself may stimulate reflex lacrimation. If the investigator is not careful to wipe the tear lake from the conjunctiva prior to inserting the paper strips, an excessive degree of wetting will be recorded. If the tear drainage system is functioning, a significant volume of tear flow passes into the puncta without being recorded. The fractional volume lost is in proportion to the adequacy of the drainage system and may be significantly more than the volume recorded. Normal values for the Schirmer I test range from 10 to 30 mm at 5 min, with values over 25 mm typical of patients under age 30 and values 10 mm or less in those over age 60.

If the Schirmer I test is abnormal, the test may be modified to separate the reflex component from basic secretion. A drop of topical anesthetic is instilled into the eye and the test is repeated. This test must be performed in the dark, as light can stimulate reflex tearing. Any combination of basic and reflex tearing may be found in patients with symptomatic dry eye or epiphora, and the volume of aqueous flow alone is not a complete indication of tear function.

When the Schirmer I test results are below normal, the Schirmer II test will give some indication of stressed reflex capability. Topical anesthetic is used in the eye, and the nasal mucosa is stimulated mechanically with a cotton swab or chemically with ammonium chloride. The amount by which the Schirmer II test exceeds basic production represents stressed reflex secretion.

The 5-min testing interval used in the standard Schirmer test can cause discomfort to some patients and may cause hypersecretion that can produce a falsely high test result. Karampatakis et al. [13]. showed that a 2-min test gave acceptable results that correlated well with the 5-min results in 94.5% of cases, where most normal individuals will show wetting equal to or greater than 10 mm.

Rose Bengal Staining

Rose Bengal is a chloride-substituted iodinated fluorescein dye that stains devitalized epithelial cells. Increased conjunctival staining is a sensitive indicator of inadequate tear function, regardless of gross aqueous tear flow determined by the Schirmer test. In the patient with epiphora and significant staining, reflex hypersecretion and inadequacy of tear physiology should be suspected.

Tear Break-Up Time

Stability of the normal tear film depends upon its basal mucin layer, which increases the hydrophilic quality of epithelial cells, allowing uniform wetting of the corneal surface. When this mucin component is reduced, the tear film will bead up on the relatively more hydrophobic corneal surface. The tear break-up time is a simple clinical test for evaluation of this component of tear function. One drop of fluorescein is placed in the eye and the patient is instructed to blink once. Observing the corneal surface under slit-lamp magnification with cobalt blue illumination, the observer notes at what time dry spots appear in the tear film. Normal tear break-up time is between 15 and 30 s. A tear break-up time of less than 10 s indicates a probable mucin deficiency, which may result not only in the symptoms of dry eye syndrome but in reflex hypersecretion of the aqueous component and in epiphora.

Dye Disappearance Test

The dye disappearance test is usually performed as part of the primary Jones dye test (Jones I test). It is a rudimentary measurement of the rate of tear flow out of the conjunctival sac. One drop of 2% fluorescein is placed in the lower conjunctival fornix, and the amount remaining at 5 min is graded on a 0 to 4+ scale, with 0 representing no dye remaining and 4+ representing all the dye remaining. The test is most meaningful when both sides are compared simultaneously. Little or no fluorescein remaining in the conjunctival sac (a positive test) indicates probable normal drainage outflow, whereas most or all of the dye remaining (negative test) indicates partial or complete obstruction, or pump failure. Care must be taken to note any lid overflow. Also, a significant amount of dye may disappear in the presence of a large dilated sac mucocele and distal obstruction. The test cannot distinguish between physiologic and anatomic causes of drainage dysfunction, nor can it localize the site of mechanical blockage. The dye disappearance test has been shown to be positive in 95% of asymptomatic normal individuals and may be more sensitive than the primary Jones test [14]. Unlike the latter, it does not appear to be dependent upon gross tear flow as measured by the Schirmer test.

Primary Jones Dye Test

In 1961, Jones described a simple test of lacrimal drainage function that has become one of the most used procedures in the evaluation of epiphora. The primary Jones dye test (Jones I) is a true functional test and should be carried out in as nearly physiologic conditions as possible. The patient should be in an upright position and should blink normally. Topical anesthetic is not used, although the clinician may anesthetize the nasal mucosa for comfort. Two percent fluorescein solution is instilled into the conjunctival sac, and a fine cotton-tipped applicator is passed beneath the inferior turbinate to the level of the nasolacrimal ostium after 2 min and again after 5 min. The test is positive if dye is recovered and indicates patent anatomy and adequate physiological function. However, the dye may be very difficult to retrieve, and therefore, there is a high false-negative rate with this test. Transit time for the dye to reach the nose is quite variable and shows a significant correlation with the Schirmer test. Even in eyes without epiphora, passage of dye into the nose may take considerably longer than the 5 min allowed for the test. A 10-min interval will result in a greater number of positive tests (dye being recovered in the nose). Testing conditions may alter results since transit time is influenced by factors such as blink rate, gravity, and fluorescein volume. Also, experience in placing the dye (drops vs strips) and recovery from the nose may also influence the recovery rate. Although a positive test strongly suggests a normal system, it does not completely rule out physiological dysfunction or mild anatomic obstruction. More significantly, a negative test alone does not necessarily indicate abnormal drainage, and even in asymptomatic normal patients, the overall positive recovery rate is typically in the range of 85% [15].

The fluorescein appearance test, described by Flach, is a modification of the primary Jones dye test [16]. It is designed to avoid the difficulty and variability involved in recovering dye from the inferior nasal meatus. Two percent fluorescein is placed in the conjunctival sac, and the oropharynx is examined with ultraviolet light, beginning at 5 min and continuing up to 1 h if necessary. With this technique, 90% of normal individuals are said to show oropharyngeal fluorescence within 30 min, and 100% within 60 min. This procedure is best used as a supplement to a negative primary Jones test and can be performed 20–30 min later. Because of the persistence of fluorescence, only one eye can be tested by this technique during a single office visit.

In 1973, Hornblass elaborated on a variation of the primary Jones dye test originally mentioned by Lipsius [17]. In this version, 0.4 mL of 1% sterile solution of sodium saccharin is instilled into the conjunctival sac, and the patient is asked to report when he or she tastes the solution. Hornblass found a mean transit time to the nose of 3.5 min, with 65% of normal individuals reporting a positive test within 6 min and 90% reporting positive results within 15 min [18]. Transit times in excess of 15 min suggest partial nasolacrimal duct obstruction. The test depends on a subjective response from the patient, and before the solution can be tasted, it must pass into the pharynx, where threshold taste sensitivity is quite variable. Lipsius noted that 3% of normal individuals were incapable of tasting saccharin.

Secondary Jones Dye Test

A negative primary Jones dye test suggests delayed transit time through the lacrimal drainage system, but it does not differentiate physiologic dysfunction from anatomic obstruction. The secondary Jones dye test (Jones II) evaluates anatomic patency of the system in such cases. Residual fluorescein is flushed from the conjunctival sac, and a topical anesthetic is instilled. The patient sits with head tilted forward while clear saline is irrigated into one canaliculus through a cannula. The patient is instructed to blow or spit any fluid that passes into the nose or pharynx onto a clean tissue. The presence of any fluid in the nose indicates gross anatomic patency of the nasolacrimal passages. In this situation, complete obstruction is not present since saline did traverse the system under pressure. Recovery of dye-stained saline demonstrates normal punctal and canalicular anatomy, since the dye must have passed freely into the sac during the previous Jones I test. Such a result is compatible with a partial anatomic block at the level of the lower sac or duct. Recovery of clear saline without fluorescein suggests punctal or canalicular stenosis, with failure of dye from the primary Jones test to enter the lacrimal sac. If fluid does not reach the nose at all but regurgitates from the opposite punctum, a high-grade obstruction is likely. Regurgitation of dye-stained fluid suggests blockage at the level of the lower sac or duct, with residual dye in the sac being flushed out by the irrigation. Very rarely, a dilated canalicular mucocele may retain sufficient dye to produce similar results. Regurgitation of clear saline from the opposite punctum suggests obstruction at the level of the distal common canaliculus or upper sac with no residual dye from the primary Jones test. When clear saline regurgitates from the same punctum that is being irrigated without flow from the opposite punctum, a proximal obstruction in that canaliculus is likely.

During the irrigation of saline, distension of the lacrimal sac to palpation is highly suggestive of lower nasolacrimal duct obstruction. Under such conditions, a palpable sac without fluid passing into the nose suggests complete nasolacrimal duct blockage, whereas a palpable sac with fluid passing into the nose implies a partial obstruction. However, a sac that is contracted and fibrotic because of chronic inflammation may not dilate under these conditions.

The secondary Jones dye test evaluates anatomic patency under increased hydrostatic pressure. When positive, it does not differentiate between epiphora caused by physiological dysfunction and epiphora resulting from partial anatomic obstruction. When a primary Jones test is positive, the secondary Jones test should always be positive and is therefore unnecessary. With a negative primary test, a positive secondary test would be consistent with physiologic or partial anatomic dysfunction, but would rule out complete blockage. Negative results (no dye recovered) on both the primary and secondary tests confirm high-grade obstruction.

False-positive results are not uncommon when a diagnosis of NLD obstruction is based on the irrigation test alone. Beigi et al. [19] noted a high rate of false tests where reexamination showed canalicular stenosis, punctal abnormalities, or hypersecretion.

Probing

When the secondary Jones test indicates canalicular obstruction, the canaliculus in question should be probed gently to the lacrimal sac with a small Bowman probe. The punctum may first be dilated by pulling the lid laterally to prevent canalicular kinking and inserting a pointed dilator. The distance of the stenosis or blockage from the punctum is noted in millimeters by measuring directly on the probe. In most individuals, a short common canaliculus is present 6–9 mm from the puncta. The canalicular system should not be probed without prior indication of possible obstruction because of the risk of inadvertent injury and subsequent fibrosis.

Diagnostic Imaging Techniques

Diagnostic Ultrasonography

The techniques of A- and B-mode ultrasonography provide a simple, noninvasive method of evaluating gross anatomic abnormalities of the lacrimal drainage system (Fig. 34.1) [20, 21]. Physiological dysfunction cannot be evaluated, nor can the precise site of anatomic obstruction be localized. However, a dilated lacrimal sac can easily be distinguished from one of normal dimensions (Fig. 34.2). It is also possible to differentiate air from mucus or solid masses, making the identification of lacrimal sac neoplasms possible [22]. Tost et al. [23] reported visualization of the canaliculi, but this requires intracanalicular injection of sodium hyaluronate.

With the B-mode probe oriented vertically, placed in the medial canthus, and aimed toward the lacrimal sac fossa, an oblique longitudinal cross section of the lacrimal sac and upper duct is obtained. The canaliculi cannot usually be visualized unless they are dilated. The diameter of the sac and upper duct may be evaluated, and the thickness of the walls can often be appreciated [24]. Diverticuli may also be identified, and a variety of echogenic densities within the system such as inflammatory membranes, tumors, and stones can be detected. The position and size of a surgically created ostium may also be imaged with this technique (Fig. 34.3), although its patency cannot easily be evaluated.

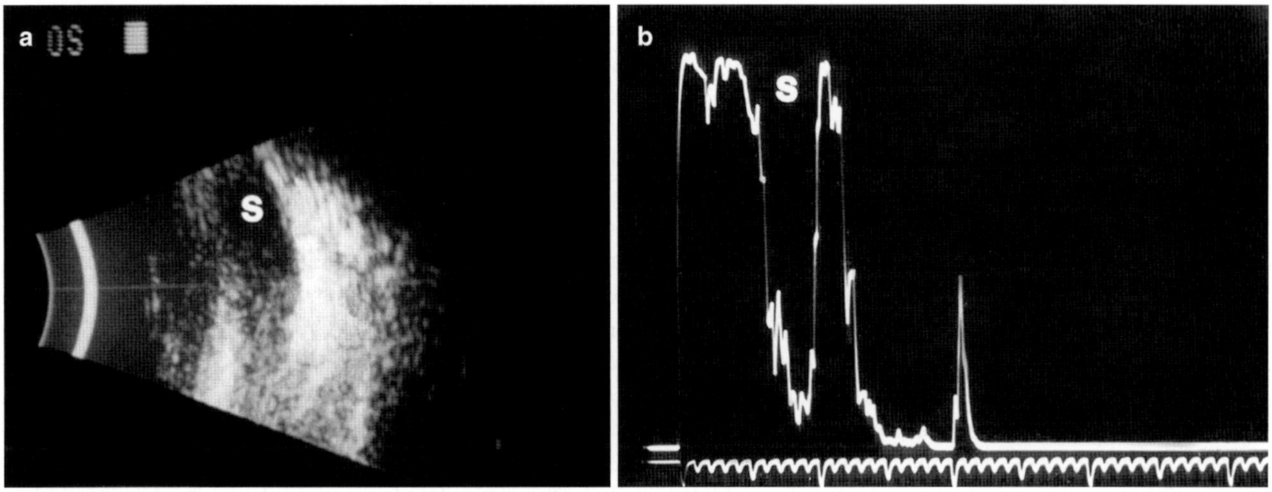

Fig. 34.1 (**a**) B-scan ultrasound of a nasolacrimal system with a normal nasolacrimal sac (S). The anterior lacrimal crest can be visualized anteriorly and inferiorly, and the lacrimal bone is seen posteriorly. (**b**) A-scan ultrasound of a normal nasolacrimal system. Nasolacrimal sac with low reflectivity (S) and sharply defined anterior and posterior walls. The smaller peak represents lacrimal bone

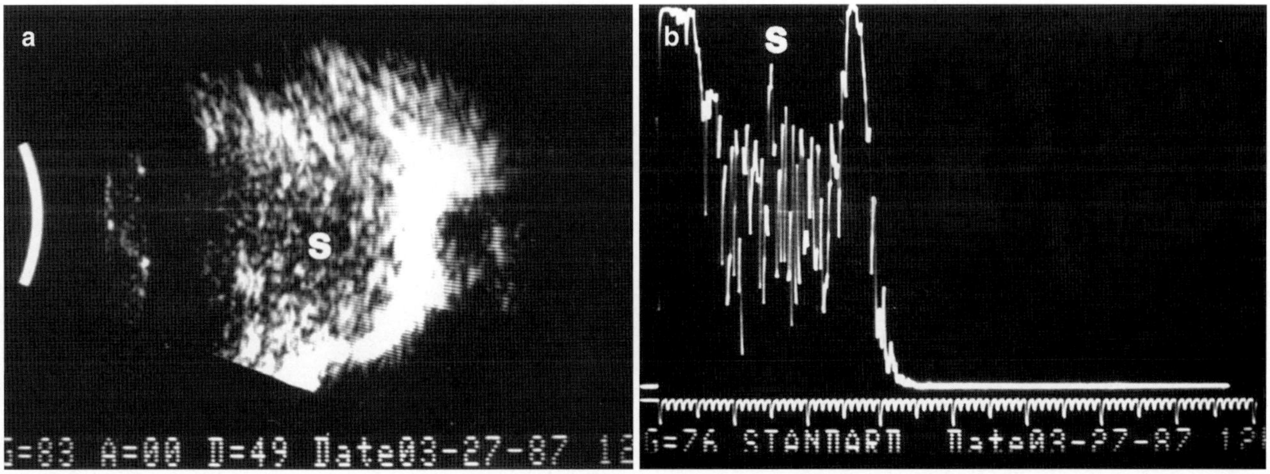

Fig. 34.2 (**a**) B-scan ultrasound of a patient with acute dacryocystitis demonstrating a massively enlarged nasolacrimal sac (S) and thickened anterior and posterior walls. (**b**) A-scan ultrasound of the same patient as Fig. 34.2a showing dilated nasolacrimal sac (S) with irregular, medium reflectivity indicating the presence of mucopurulent exudates

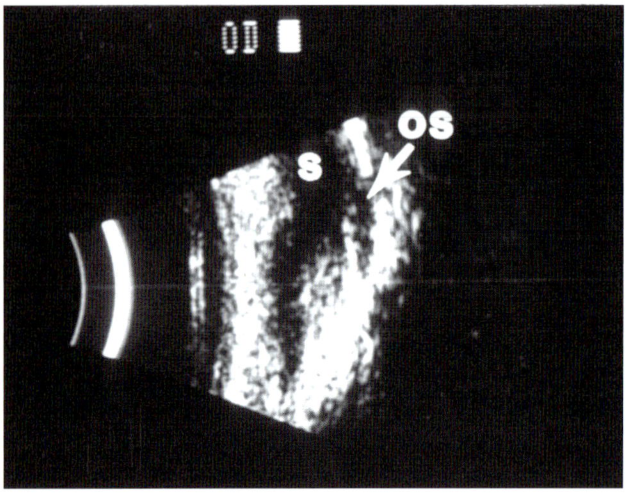

Fig. 34.3 Post-dacryocystorhinostomy B-scan ultrasonography showing the surgically created lacrimal-nasal ostium (OS). The lacrimal sac (S) is somewhat dilated because of soft tissue closure of the ostium

For precise measurements of the sac and evaluation of the internal reflectivity of sac contents, A-mode scanning must be used. The probe is first oriented as for a periocular orbital study, but with the beam aimed just behind the anterior lacrimal crest toward the sac fossa. An oblique anterolateral-posteromedial cut of the sac is thus obtained. If the sac is filled with air, it appears as an echolucent defect bounded by sharply defined vertical anterior and posterior sac walls. Often, the presence of dilated diverticula can be detected. Mucus in the sac produces uniform, homogeneous, low-density internal echoes, and inflammatory exudates and membranes show stronger, more irregular echoes. Multiple high-density, irregular echoes with infiltration of the sac walls suggest a sac tumor. A transocular A-mode image of the sac is obtained with the probe held above the lateral canthus and directed toward the lacrimal sac fossa. This technique gives an approximate horizontal cross section of the sac. The average dimensions of the sac in normal individuals are 2.5 mm (SD = 0.95 mm) in horizontal diameter and 4.0 mm (SD = 1.49 mm) in anteroposterior extent. A sac more than 4.5 mm wide or 7.0 mm deep should be considered abnormally dilated.

Contrast Dacryocystography

The first attempt to visualize the lacrimal drainage system radiographically was made by Ewing in 1909. He used bismuth paste for retrograde filling of the nasolacrimal duct. Such early attempts proved unsatisfactory, and the technique was used infrequently until the introduction of better aqueous contrast media such as Sinografin and Angiografin and especially the low-viscosity iodized oils such as Pantopaque, Ethiodol, and ultrafluid Lipiodol. In a standard dacryocystography (DCG) study, the canaliculi are intubated with intravenous catheters and contrast material is injected into the lower canaliculus on each side and films are taken immediately in Caldwell's posteroanterior frontal projection and in both lateral projections. Repeat films are obtained at 5 and 15 min, and upright films may be taken to evaluate the effects of gravity on lacrimal drainage. DCG can also be combined with computed tomography (CT) or magnetic resonance (MR) imaging to give further information on the nasolacrimal system.

In 1968, Iba and Hanafee described the technique of distension dacryocystography, first used by Barrie Jones in 1959 [25]. Here, films are taken during injection of 0.5–1.0 mL of contrast material so that the lacrimal system is imaged in the distended state. Both sides are studied simultaneously, and injection is accomplished through the placement of canalicular indwelling tapered Teflon catheters or IV catheter tubing. This method provides maximum visualization of the anatomic structure of the system and, because of the back pressure, gives good filling of the canaliculi. It is the best technique for demonstration of fistulae, diverticula, supernumerary canaliculi, and the presence of stones and sac tumors. However, it does not reveal sac and duct dimensions under normal physiologic conditions. This test also requires either the ophthalmologist or a skilled technician to be in the radiology suite to inject the material and can lead to some patient discomfort.

Improved imaging can be obtained with a technique adopted from subtraction angiography that eliminates confusing bony shadows (Fig. 34.4) [26]. A scout film is taken before injecting contrast material and is used to produce bone-free images of the dacryocystogram. More sophisticated computer-assisted digital subtraction images can be

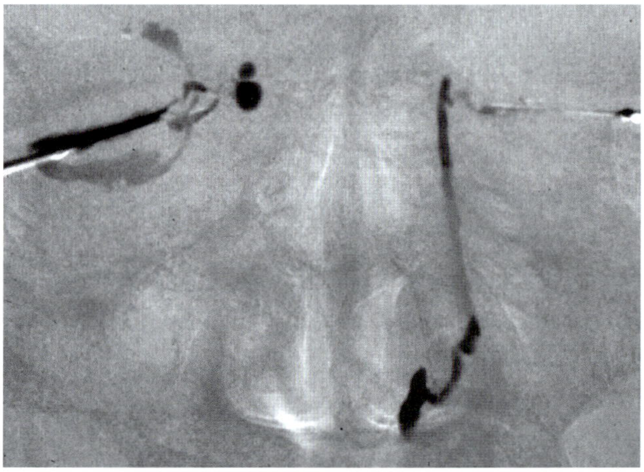

Fig. 34.4 Digital subtraction contrast dacryocystogram. Pt with normal passage of contrast through the left nasolacrimal system and complete blockage of the right proximal nasolacrimal duct and mild dilation of the right nasolacrimal sac

produced using fluoroscopically controlled angiographic equipment and an image intensifier.

The dacryocystogram of a normal lacrimal drainage system will usually show the canaliculi when less viscous aqueous contrast media are used [27]. The sac appears as a smooth, straight, or gently curved passage with the concavity facing laterally. The anteroposterior dimension is wider than the transverse. There is usually a constriction at the sac-duct junction caused by the split fascia of the orbicularis muscle as it passes around the system. The duct widens at the level of the bony rim, and its inner surface becomes more irregular because of the presence of mucosal folds. Such folds may be exceptionally well developed in younger children. Further constrictions are seen in the duct's mid-portion in the region of Hytle's and Taillefers' valves. Finally, in its lower third, the duct widens again. Visualization by DCG reveals considerable variations in the structure of the sac and duct among normal individuals. Atypical narrowing and widening of the sac and duct, as well as unusual angulations and diverticula, may all be seen in the absence of clinical symptoms.

A combination of subtraction, distension, and macrodacryocystography provides the best visualization of the anatomic structure of the lacrimal drainage system. This approach will provide accurate localization of any anatomic obstruction in the majority of cases. Imaging of the canaliculi with dye failing to pass into the sac or duct implies obstruction at the common canaliculus. Obstruction at the sac-duct junction usually results in a dilated sac with no dye reaching the duct or nose, even on late films. Obstruction at the level of the nasolacrimal duct will show dilatation of the sac, with dye in the duct, but not reaching the nose. A patent dacryocystorhinostomy ostium is easily demonstrated by passage of contrast into the nose at the level of the middle meatus. Demonstration of patent lacrimal passages by DCG in the face of epiphora suggests physiological dysfunction or a mild incomplete anatomic block.

DCG is considered the gold standard for imaging of the nasolacrimal system, but it does not allow for imaging of the soft tissue or bony structures surrounding the nasolacrimal sac or duct. DCG can be combined with CT and MR studies to better evaluate to get a complete picture of the nasolacrimal system and the surrounding anatomy.

Computed Tomography

In selected cases, computed tomography (CT) of the lacrimal system can be extremely useful in the evaluation of epiphora [28]. Axial scans through the lower orbit will show the lacrimal sac fossa as a depression in the anteromedial orbital wall. In successively lower sections, the duct appears as a round to oval defect in the frontal process of the maxillary bone at the anteromedial corner of the antrum. The duct may be filled with air or fluid. As the duct is traced inferiorly, it can be seen to open beneath the inferior turbinate. Cross sections of the system are seen in coronal reformatted images since the line of section is oriented downward and obliquely backward. Parasagittal reformatted images will reveal the entire length of the system in longitudinal section.

Dilatation of the lacrimal sac from dacryocystitis can easily be seen on CT. The modality is also useful in detecting lacrimal sac mucoceles and can sometimes show stones and tumors within the sac and duct. Extrinsic lesions such as nasosinus tumors, sinusitis, and nasal polyps that can cause tear drainage dysfunction can also often be visualized [29]. When epiphora follows trauma and subsequent clinical studies indicate nasolacrimal duct obstruction, CT dacryocystography may reveal facial fractures compressing the sac or duct [30]. CT imaging can distinguish a dacryocystocele from recurrent tumor following resection of sinonasal cancer [31]. In cases of congenital lacrimal amniocele, CT will reveal the dilated duct, often associated with bony changes. It is essential to differentiate this soft, near-midline dilated sac from a meningocele. In most cases of suspected malignancy, especially if there is a history of bloody epiphora or pain, a CT scan may demonstrate soft tissue masses of the sac or adjacent paranasal sinuses. MRI is more sensitive for soft tissue abnormalities but does not image the bony structures well.

When combined with dacryocystography, CT scan is excellent at identifying bony structures around the nasolacrimal system (Fig. 34.5). By using modern spiral CT techniques with topical or injected contrast material, the surgeon can identify accurately obstructions in the nasolacrimal system [32, 33]. This can be especially useful in patients that have had facial trauma, prior sinus or lacrimal surgery, or tumors of the medial canthus [34]. Newer techniques

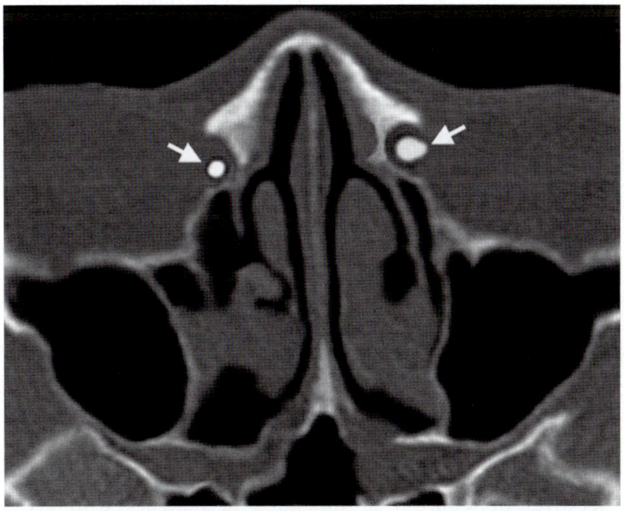

Fig. 34.5 Axial CT-DCG showing contrast-filled lacrimal sacs (*arrows*). The left lacrimal sac (*right side of the figure*) is dilated compared with the normal sac on the right

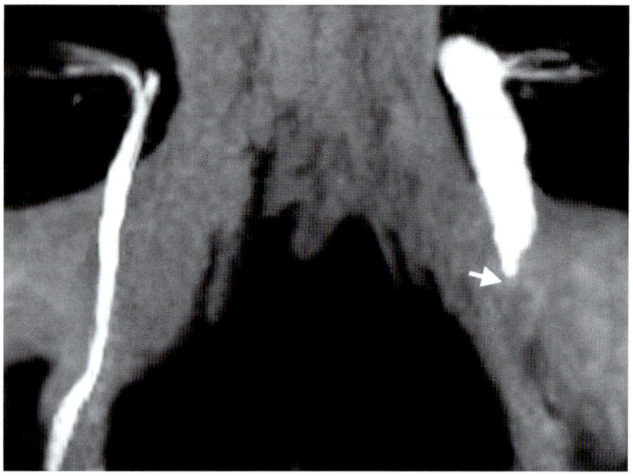

Fig. 34.6 Coronal CT-DCG reconstruction showing a normal right lacrimal drainage system. The left lacrimal sac is dilated due to a complete nasolacrimal duct obstruction (*arrow*)

utilizing spiral CT and 3D reconstruction technology have improved the diagnostic accuracy of patients with partial obstructions of the nasolacrimal system by allowing the surgeon to view a 3D image of the entire system from multiple projections (Fig. 34.6) [35].

Cone-beam computed tomography is a new technology that utilizes a C-arm angiography system that rotates around the patient to produce high-resolution 3D images with computer reconstructions in axial, coronal, and sagittal planes. The technique allows the simultaneous assessment of the nasolacrimal duct together with its surrounding soft tissue and bony structures [36].

There are some disadvantages to CT scan. As mentioned previously, it is not the best study for evaluating soft tissue masses of the nasolacrimal system. Also, in standard CT, the images are presented as a series of axial images and make identification of small obstructions difficult. Longitudinal and oblique images can be created, but this reconstruction results in decreased spatial resolution in the reformatted images. The exposure to ionizing radiation is also more than for standard DCG.

Magnetic Resonance Dacryocystography

Since 1990, dynamic magnetic resonance imaging dacryocystography (dMRI-DCG) has been used as an adjunctive diagnostic test in the evaluation of lacrimal system pathology that allows for excellent resolution of the nasolacrimal system [37–39] and minimally invasive imaging to identify the level of stenosis or blockage in patients with NLD obstruction [40]. When combined with a contrast agent, 3D MRI offers several advantages over other imaging studies [36]. Gadolinium can be given as a topical solution (Magnevist) diluted from 1:10 to 1:100 with normal saline, one drop to each eye per minute for 5 min. The patient should stay in an upright position until just prior to image acquisition. Because the lacrimal system is not cannulated, and therefore not under increased hydrostatic pressure, this study gives a picture of the functional status of the nasolacrimal system. There have been no reports of ocular complications from the administration of topical gadolinium, and this obviates the need to risk damage to puncta from the direct instillation of contrast agents. Exposure to ionizing radiation is also avoided with this technique.

MRI allows high-resolution evaluation of soft tissue structures within and surrounding the nasolacrimal drainage system, comparable to dacryoscintigraphy, dacryocystography, and computed tomography [41–45]. The superficial location of the nasolacrimal system facilitates imaging with small surface coils, which can give a spatial resolution of $0.3 \times 0.3 \times 3$ mm or better [39]. Manipulation of signal intensities, repetition times, and tip angles, as well as the use of fat suppression algorithms, can oftentimes allow for differentiation of mucous or blood from solid neoplasms. Also, because of volumetric acquisition, MRI images can be viewed in any plane without degradation of the quality of images. This is a key advantage over CT-DCG which requires reformatting of images that are out of plane and results in degradation of image resolution. Coronal images are superior for determining the distal extent of contrast transit, and axial images are excellent for examining the lumen of the nasolacrimal duct and intraductal pathology.

Although MRI can be a useful diagnostic study, it is an expensive study and therefore should not be used routinely. Other drawbacks include poor ability to image bony structures, and there can be artifact from the nearby ethmoid air cells. MRI is also susceptible to movement artifact because of the relatively long acquisition times required.

Radionuclide Dacryoscintigraphy

The first use of radionuclide tracer to image the lacrimal drainage system was by Bozoky and Korchmaros, who used radioactive ^{198}Au and measured the buildup of activity over the sac and duct. Rossomondo et al. [35] introduced the first modern nuclear imaging technique for the lacrimal drainage system. They instilled a drop of saline with [99mTc] sodium pertechnetate and imaged the system with a gamma camera. In the first clinical evaluation of the technique, Carlton et al. [46] demonstrated its value in visualizing the lacrimal system and in measuring some physiological parameters of tear flow. In their study of 28 asymptomatic volunteers, they recorded a transit time for the nuclide of 4–43 s to the sac and 4–323 s to the nose. There is a high degree of correlation between dacryoscintigraphy and contrast dacryocystography;

however, the former is more sensitive to incomplete blocks, especially in the upper system. Since dacryoscintigraphy is a physiologic test, it is also very sensitive in finding abnormalities in patients with physiologic nasolacrimal duct obstruction and can often localize the site of blockage [47, 48]. Moreover, since it does not rely on forced injection of saline or a contrast agent that can overcome a partial obstruction or stenosis, it mimics normal physiological lacrimal outflow and is therefore more suitable for the evaluation of functional epiphora [49].

The technique commonly employed today uses [99mTc] pertechnetate in saline or technetium sulfur colloid delivered as a 10 μL drop to the lateral conjunctival sac by micropipette. The patient is advised to blink normally, and the nasolacrimal system is imaged every 10 s for the first 2–3 min, and then late images are taken every 5 min for a total of 20 min. The specific activity of this dose is in the range of 50–150 μCi, and results in radiation exposure to the lens of less than 2% of that is for a complete contrast dacryocystogram.

Dacryoscintigraphy does not provide the detailed anatomic visualization available with contrast DCG. In standard nuclear studies, the proximal canalicular system is usually poorly imaged unless dilated. The sac and duct are usually well outlined (Fig. 34.7) [50]. Complete or partial obstructions of the sac or duct can be detected, with a sensitivity of better than 90% [51]. Although the precise site of obstruction is difficult to determine with scintigraphy alone, the approximate level, such as presac, preduct, and intraduct, can often be determined [52]. Generation of dynamic activity curves for specific regions of interest will demonstrate incomplete anatomic obstructions as well as rather subtle degrees of functional impairment [50, 53]. This technique is most accurate and reproducible for the upper lacrimal system. Transit times become quite variable for the lower system, with 25–32% of asymptomatic individuals showing no tracer in the nose after 12 min. This is consistent with findings on the primary Jones dye test. By using more sophisticated rapid sequence display and computer interfacing for image optimization by contrast enhancement, background subtraction, and frame arithmetic, quantitative evaluation of tracer movement provides the most revealing interpretation of lacrimal function and tear flow dynamics currently available.

A more recent "after washing" modification was introduced to improve the sensitivity and specificity of the technique. With this approach, dynamic images are obtained followed by a washing test by applying a 10-μL drop of normal saline with external massage as a secondary dynamic phase. Massoudi et al. showed that the washout technique improved sensitivity (93%) and increased specificity from 23% to 75%, with 68% of 203 obstructions at the sac-duct junction [54]. However, like previous scintigraphy methods, special resolution is low and precise anatomic evaluation is not possible.

Other Diagnostic Techniques

Percutaneous Contrast Dacryocystography

The common canaliculus is a common site of obstruction seen on radiographic imaging in patients with epiphora. When such blockages are complete, routine DCG is not possible, and the concomitant presence of lower sac or duct

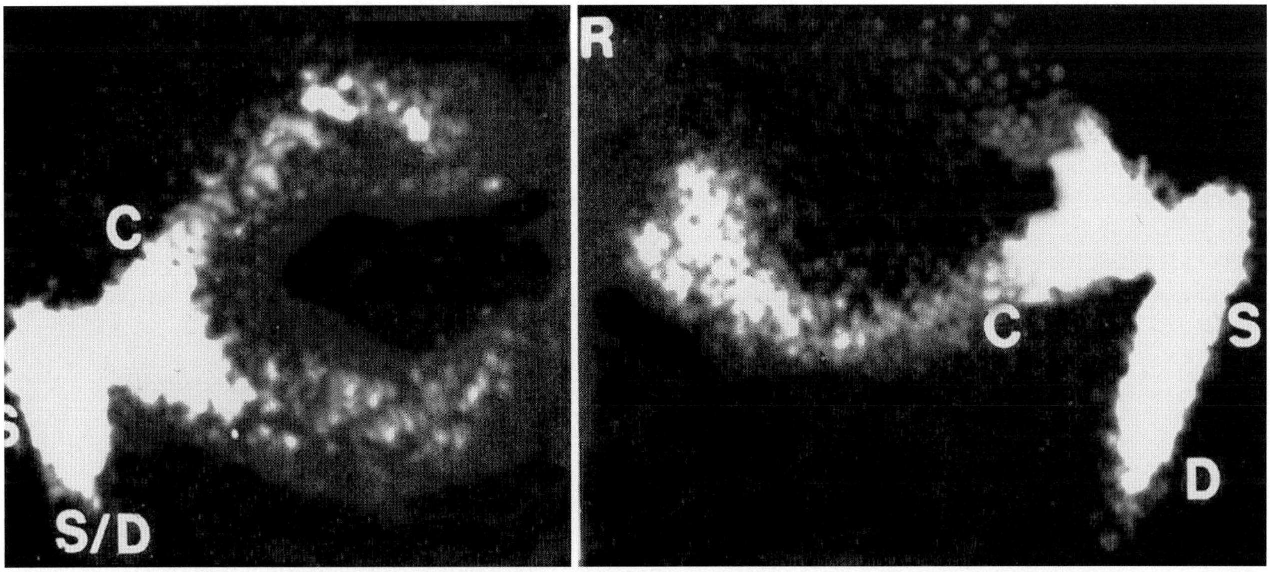

Fig. 34.7 Dacryoscintigraphy in a patient with unilateral epiphora on the left side. The right lacrimal drainage system fills normally, with tracer concentrated in the canaliculi (C), sac (S), and duct (D). The left system shows no tracer below the sac-duct junction (S/D)

pathology cannot be easily demonstrated unless echography is used to detect a dilated sac. In 1972, Putterman [55] described a technique of percutaneous injection of aqueous contrast material directly into the lacrimal sac to bypass the occluded common canaliculus. In his small series of four patients, there were no complications and results were good.

Chemiluminescence

Chemiluminescent materials are a nonradiologic technique for demonstrating the outline of the lacrimal drainage system and verifying its patency. The luminescent agents are dimethyl phthalate and tertiary butyl alcohol activated by dibutyl phthalate, which produce an intense cold light. This product is commercially used as a safety light. When these agents are injected into the lacrimal system, the glow is visible through the skin and clearly outlines the upper system. The lower duct is not readily demonstrated. The compounds are safe and nontoxic if confined within the lacrimal system, but extravasation into tissues or onto the globe can produce severe complications of corneal scarring and vascularization, purulent infection, granuloma formation, and fibrosis [56]. Chemiluminescence has not yet been used extensively enough to evaluate its clinical effectiveness as an alternative or adjunct to other procedures.

Lacrimal Thermography

Thermography is a diagnostic technique that images the heat emitted as infrared radiation from the body surface. A thermographic camera captures the radiation patterns and translates them into information encrypted in colors [57]. Unlike dacryocystography, contrast material is not injected and the patient is not touched. It allows assessment of inflammation.

The canaliculi and lacrimal sac have been visualized by thermography, using an infrared scanner and color monitor with a resolution of 0.5 °C [58]. The lacrimal system is easily differentiated from surrounding tissues by irrigation with cold water, and decreased temperature in the nose demonstrates patency. A large dilated sac can be visualized, and persistent inflammation will produce increased temperature within the sac. The duct is not demonstrated with this method.

In a related technique, a mini-thermocouple probe has been used to detect temperature differences with the lacrimal sac [59]. Increased temperatures are seen with vascularity and inflammation, and decreased temperatures with hemorrhage and mucocele formation. Nasolacrimal duct obstruction without associated inflammation shows no difference in temperature compared with the contralateral uninvolved side.

Nasolacrimal Endoscopy

High-resolution dacryoendoscopy can provide clear visualization of the lumen of the lacrimal drainage system and provide detailed information about lacrimal duct obstructions [60, 61]. It has been used successfully for the diagnosis of complex congenital nasolacrimal duct obstruction (CNLDO) in children [62] and for direct endoscopic-guided probing [63]. Takahashi et al. demonstrated its value in observing the site of fibrous obstruction in 20 cases of failed dacryocystorhinostomy [64]. Sasaki et al. introduced a pressure-controlled air-insufflation technique that provides significant improvement in image quality compared with saline-irrigated techniques [65].

Interpretation of Diagnostic Tests

Like many diagnostic tests in medicine, most of those described above required some subjective interpretation in order to determine the probable etiology of epiphora (Tables 34.1 and 34.2). Some knowledge of the variability in patient

Table 34.1 Interpretation of clinical tests in the evaluation of epiphora

Dye disappearance test	Jones I	Jones II	Probing	Palpation	Diagnosis
Rapid	+	+	Normal	Normal	Probable oversecretion
+	+	+	Normal	Normal	Normal vs. functional
+	–	+	Normal	Normal	Normal vs. functional vs. mild NLD obstruction
+	–	+	Normal	Abnormal	Partial NLD obstruction with dilated sac
Slow	–	+	Normal	Normal	Mild NLD obstruction vs. functional
Slow or –	–	+	Normal	Abnormal	Partial NLD obstruction
–	–	–	Normal	Abnormal	Complete NLD obstruction
–	–	+	Stenotic	Normal	Partial canalicular obstruction
–	–	–	Stenotic	Abnormal	Combined NLD obstruction with canalicular obstruction
–	–	–	Blocked	Normal	Complete canalicular obstruction

NLD nasolacrimal duct

Table 34.2 Results of primary and secondary Jones tests and probable sites of lacrimal system obstruction

Jones I	Jones II	Probable site of obstruction
+	+, Dye in nose	Patent system: normal vs. low-grade partial obstruction vs. functional (non-localizing)
–	+, Dye in nose	Partial NLD obstruction vs. functional
–	+, Saline in nose	Partial canalicular obstruction vs. functional
–	–, Regurgitation of dye from opposite punctum	Complete NLD obstruction
–	–, Regurgitation of saline from opposite punctum	Complete common canaliculus obstruction
–	–, Regurgitation of dye from same punctum	Complete opposite canalicular obstruction with NLD obstruction
–	–, Regurgitation of saline from same punctum	Complete canalicular obstruction

NLD nasolacrimal duct

response, as well as of the reliability of the specific tests in suggesting pathology, is needed before meaningful conclusions can be drawn. The mere demonstration of lacrimal system pathology, either anatomic or physiological, does not indicate lacrimal dysfunction. Patients with significant degrees of partial or even complete obstruction may be entirely asymptomatic as long as tear production and drainage balance is maintained.

Not every test mentioned here must be performed on each patient with epiphora. In most cases, a relatively simple clinical evaluation in the office will adequately demonstrate the cause of tearing and allow appropriate therapeutic decisions. Some cases, however, will present more difficult diagnostic challenges, particularly those with proximal system anatomic stenosis and physiologic dysfunctions. Here, more elaborate procedures, including radiographic studies, may be required.

In the face of a normal Schirmer test of basic and reflex tear response, the dye disappearance test can be a sensitive, though subjective, indicator of gross drainage. With a normally draining system, fluorescein should be almost gone within 5 min. Epiphora due to physiologic dysfunction or partial anatomic obstruction will show prolonged presence of dye in the conjunctival sac, whereas epiphora resulting from oversecretion syndrome with normal drainage should yield normal or even rapid disappearance of dye. It is important to realize that the rate of dye clearance through the lacrimal system is strongly influenced by the pressure head from above. Even in the presence of decreased drainage function, a large volume of fluorescein augmented by increased reflex tear secretion from conjunctival irritation may result in an artifactually rapid dye disappearance. It is therefore important to administer this test under conditions as nearly physiologic as possible, with the patient in an upright position, blinking normally, and receiving only one drop of fluorescein.

When the dye disappearance test is abnormal or the history strongly suggests inadequate drainage, the primary Jones dye test is usually performed next. In interpreting the results of this test, it is essential to keep in mind that in up to one-third of asymptomatic individuals, dye will not be recovered in the nose after 5 min. It is also important to remember that this test correlates well with the results of the Schirmer test and therefore with the volume of fluorescein placed into the conjunctival sac. Like the dye disappearance test, an artifactually positive Jones I test may result from volume overload even when epiphora is present under normal physiological conditions. To be meaningful, the test must be conducted under as close to normal physiological function as possible. Only a small volume of dye should be used, the patient should be in an upright position, and blinking should be normal. Variants of the Jones I test, such as the saccharin taste test, add little, and are difficult to interpret. When the primary Jones dye test is positive, one may conclude that the system is grossly patent, although minor stenoses and physiological dysfunctions cannot be ruled out. When the test is negative, it is likely that significant anatomic or physiological pathology exists, but this test alone is not sufficient to document this conclusion.

When both the dye disappearance test is prolonged and the primary Jones dye test is negative, the probability of drainage dysfunction is greater than would be indicated by a negative primary Jones dye test alone. The secondary Jones dye test is then performed and, if negative, will demonstrate complete obstruction in the system. The results of the test will indicate the location of the block. When the secondary test is negative and saline irrigated through one punctum causes dye to regurgitate from the opposite punctum, then the dye must be left over from the primary Jones test. If only clear saline regurgitates from the opposite punctum, the block is probably at the common canaliculus. Probing should encounter an obstruction at the distal canaliculus 6–9 mm from the puncta. If an obstruction or stenosis is not found, the test should be repeated with care. However, if there is a lengthy delay between the primary and secondary tests, there may be too little dye remaining in the sac to stain the regurgitating fluid.

When the secondary Jones test is positive, a low-grade partial obstruction or stenosis may be present that can be overcome by increased hydrostatic pressure, or failure of the lacrimal pump mechanism may be responsible for the negative primary Jones test and delayed dye disappearance test. Recovery of clear saline alone in the nose suggests partial canalicular obstruction since no dye entered the sac during the primary test. Appearance of dye-stained saline in the nose demonstrates free flow of fluorescein to the sac during the primary test and therefore an open canalicular system. The partial block is probably present in the distal system at the lower sac or duct. Retrograde flow out of the canaliculi may be seen even with a partially open duct if injection pressures are above 100 mmHg. A negative primary Jones test and positive secondary test could also be compatible with intact canalicular capillary action, but with pump failure in propulsion through the lower system.

When hypersecretion syndrome has been ruled out and the dye disappearance test and primary and secondary Jones tests are all negative, a complete anatomic blockage is present somewhere along the nasolacrimal system. The results of the secondary Jones test will usually indicate if the block is proximal, requiring canalicular repair or bypass, or distal enough to be corrected with a dacryocystorhinostomy. If the results are equivocal, or there is either a history of trauma, suspicion of tumor, recurrent epiphora following surgery, or persistent chronic dacryocystitis, then radiographic evaluation may be indicated to image the anatomic structure of the system and to pinpoint the site of obstruction. Dacryocystography clearly outlines the patent conduit of the lacrimal drainage system but may not demonstrate low-grade stenoses that are easily opened when the distension technique is employed. Variations in normal anatomy include widened or narrowed sac or duct, diverticulum, angulations of the system, or occlusions of one canaliculus, all of which may give false-positive indications of pathology. The test does not easily visualize the canalicular system without intubation distension and subtraction and gives no information concerning physiological function. Nevertheless, DCG gives the most reliable anatomic information of the sac and duct. In certain cases, the addition of CT or MRI in conjunction with DCG will add useful information on soft tissue and bony abnormalities within and surrounding the nasolacrimal system that can affect management and help to plan surgical approach.

When the primary Jones test is negative and the secondary test positive, the surgeon must distinguish between physiological dysfunction and partial anatomic obstruction. In the absence of obvious eyelid or punctal deformity or atonic orbicularis muscle, the problem is most likely anatomic, and the secondary Jones test should indicate whether it is proximal or distal. Nevertheless, minor degrees of stenosis and functional failure due to eyelid laxity, a dilated sac, a diverticulum, or a calculus cannot be differentiated with the above tests. Dacryocystography will usually demonstrate the presence of a stenotic segment.

If clinical and radiographic evaluations fail to show an anatomic blockage, physiological dysfunction is probably responsible for the epiphora. Radionuclide dacryoscintigraphy is indicated here, especially when used with computer interfacing for qualitative evaluation of function. Subtle functional abnormalities may be uncovered, particularly in the proximal system. However, the physiology of lacrimal drainage is poorly understood. The function of Rosenmuller's and Hasner's valves is complex, their competency varies with age, and their patency is influenced by hydrostatic pressure and volume. The results of dacryoscintigraphy are influenced by head position, blinking, and volume overload. A significant number of asymptomatic individuals will show some dysfunction with this test, making interpretation in patients with epiphora more difficult.

In summary, most patients with epiphora can be evaluated adequately with a few relatively simple office procedures. A small number of cases will require more sophisticated studies to confirm the site of anatomic block or region of physiological dysfunction. With the range of test available, appropriate medical or surgical management can be determined in the vast majority of patients with tear production and drainage imbalance.

References

1. Mimura T, Usul T, Yamamoto H, et al. Conjunctivochalasis and contact lenses. Am J Ophthalmol. 2009;148:20–2.
2. Mimura T, Yamagami S, Usul T, et al. Changes of conjunctivochalasis with age in a hospital-based study. Am J Ophthalmol. 2009;147:171–7.
3. Li QS, Zhang XR, Zou HD, et al. Epidemiologic study of conjunctivochalasis in populations equal or over 60 years old in Caoyangxincun community of Shanghai. Zhonghua Yan Ke Za Zhi. 2009;45:793–8.
4. Knijnik D. Tearing and eyelid laxity with no ectropion: is tarsal strip always effective? Arq Bras Oftalmol. 2006;69:37–9.
5. Narayanan K, Barnes EA. Epiphora with eyelid laxity. Orbit. 2005;24:201–3.
6. Vick VL, Holds JB, Hartstein ME, Massry GG. Tarsal strip procedure for the correction of tearing. Ophthal Plast Reconstr Surg. 2004;20:37–9.
7. Detorakis ET, Zissimopoulos A, Katernellis G, et al. Lower eyelid laxity in functional acquired epiphora: evaluation with quantitative scintigraphy. Ophthal Plast Reconstr Surg. 2006;22:25–9.
8. Bukhari A. Prevalence of punctal stenosis among ophthalmology patients. Middle East Afr J Ophthalmol. 2009;16:85–7.
9. Billing K, Karagiannis A, Selva D. Punctal-canalicular stenosis associated with mitomycin-C for corneal epithelial dysplasia. Am J Ophthalmol. 2003;136:746–7.
10. Eiseman AS, Flanagan JC, Brooks AB, et al. Ocular surface, ocular adnexal, and lacrimal complications associated with the use of systemic 5-fluorouracil. Ophthal Plast Reconstr Surg. 2003;19:216–24.
11. Esmaeli B, Valero V, Ahmani MA, Booser D. Canalicular stenosis secondary to docetaxel (taxotere): a newly recognized side effect. Ophthalmology. 2001;108:994–5.
12. Schirmer O. Studien zur physiology und pathology der tranenabsonderung und tranenabfuhr. Graefes Arch Clin Exp Ophthalmol. 1903;56:197–291.
13. Karampatakis V, Karamitsos A, Skriapa A, Pastiadis G. Comparison between normal values of 2- and 5-minutes Schirmer test without anesthesia. Cornea. 2010;29:497–501.
14. Zappia RJ, Milder B. Lacrimal drainage function. 2. The fluorescein dye disappearance test. Am J Ophthalmol. 1972;74:160–2.
15. Wright MM, Bersani TA, Frueh BR, Musch DC. Efficacy of the primary dye test. Ophthalmology. 1989;96:481–3.

16. Flach A. The fluorescein appearance test for lacrimal obstruction. Ann Ophthalmol. 1979;11:237–42.
17. Lipsius EI. Sodium saccharin for testing the patency of the lacrimal passages. Am J Ophthalmol. 1957;43:114–5.
18. Hornblass A. A simple taste test for lacrimal obstruction. Arch Ophthalmol. 1973;90:435–6.
19. Beigi B, Uddin JM, McMillan TF, Linardos E. Inaccuracy of diagnosis in a cohort of patients on the waiting list for dacryocystorhinostomy when the diagnosis was made by only syringing the lacrimal system. Eur J Ophthalmol. 2007;17:485–9.
20. Dutton JJ. Standardized echography in the diagnosis of lacrimal drainage dysfunction. Arch Ophthalmol. 1989;107:1010–2.
21. Rochels R, Lieb W, Nover A. Echographic diagnosis in diseases of the efferent tear ducts. Klin Monatsbl Augenheilkd. 1984;185:243–9.
22. Montanara A, Mannino G, Contestabile M. Macrodacryocystography and echography in diagnosis of disorders of the lacrimal pathways. Surv Ophthalmol. 1983;28:33–41.
23. Tost F, Bruder R, Clemens S. 20-MHz ultrasound of presaccular lacrimal ducts. Ophthalmologe. 2002;99:25–8.
24. Tobias S, Pavlidis M, Busse H, Thanos S. Presurgical and postsurgical assessment of lacrimal drainage dysfunction. Am J Ophthalmol. 2004;138:764–71.
25. Iba GB, Hanafee WN. Distention dacryocystography. Radiology. 1968;90:1020–2.
26. Galloway JE, Kavic TA, Raflo GT. Digital subtraction macrodacryocystography. Ophthalmology. 1984;91:956–62.
27. Malik SRK, Gupta AK, Chaterjee S, et al. Dacryocystography of normal and pathological lacrimal passages. Br J Ophthalmol. 1969;53:174–9.
28. Freitag S, Woog JJ, Kousoubris PD, Curtin HD. Helical computed tomography dacryocystography with three-dimensional reconstruction. Ophthal Plast Reconstr Surg. 2002;18:121–32.
29. Frances IC, Kappagoda MB, Cole IE, Bank L, Dunn GD. Computed tomography of the lacrimal drainage system: retrospective study of 107 cases of dacryostenosis. Ophthal Plast Reconstr Surg. 1999;15:217–26.
30. Glatt HJ. Evaluation of lacrimal obstruction secondary to facial fractures using computed tomography or computed tomographic dacryocystography. Ophthal Plast Reconstr Surg. 1996;12:284–93.
31. Debnam JM, Esmaeli B, Ginsberg LE. Imaging characteristics of dacryocystocele diagnosed after surgery for sinonasal cancer. Am J Neuroradiol. 2007;28:1872–5.
32. Bonnet F, Ducasse A, Marcus C, Hoeffel C. CT dacryocystography: normal findings and pathology. J Radiol. 2009;90:1685–93.
33. Udhay P, Noronha OV, Mohan RE. Helical computed tomographic dacryocystography and its role in the diagnosis and management of lacrimal drainage system blocks and medial canthal masses. Indian J Ophthalmol. 2008;56:31–7.
34. Ashenhurst M, Jaffer N, Hurwitz JJ, et al. Combined computed tomography and dacryocystography for complex lacrimal problems. Can J Ophthalmol. 1991;26:27–31.
35. Rossomondo RM, Carlton WH, Trueblood JH, et al. A new method of evaluating lacrimal drainage. Arch Ophthalmol. 1972;88:523–5.
36. Wilhelm KE, Rudorf H, Greschus S, et al. Cone-beam computed tomography (CBCT) dacryocystography for imaging of the nasolacrimal duct system. Clin Neuroradiol. 2009;19:283–91.
37. Goldberg RA, Heinz GW, Chiu L. Gadolinium magnetic resonance imaging dacryocystography. Am J Ophthalmol. 1993;115:738–41.
38. Karagulle T, Erden A, Erden I, et al. Nasolacrimal system: evaluation with gadolinium-enhanced MR dacryocystography with a three-dimensional fast spoiled gradient recalled technique. Eur Radiol. 2002;12:2343–8.
39. Rubin PA, Bilyk JR, Shore JW, et al. Magnetic resonance imaging of the lacrimal drainage system. Ophthalmology. 1994;101:235–43.
40. Higashi H, Tamada T, Mizukawa K, Katsuyoshi I. MR dacryocystography: comparison with dacryoendoscopy in positional diagnosis of nasolacrimal duct obstruction. Radiol Med. 2016;121:580–7.
41. Cubuk R, Tasali N, Aydin S, Saydam B, Sengor T. Dynamic MR dacryocystography in patients with epiphora. Eur J Radiol. 2010;73:230–3.
42. Hoffmann KT, Anders N, Hosten N, et al. High resolution functional magnetic resonance tomography with Gd-DTPA eye drops in diagnosis of lacrimal apparatus diseases. Ophthalmologe. 1998;95:542–8.
43. Kirchhof K, Hähnel S, Jansen O, et al. Gadolinium-enhanced magnetic resonance dacryocystography in patients with epiphora. J Comput Assist Tomogr. 2000;24:327–31.
44. Manfrè L, de Maria M, Todaro E, et al. MR dacryocystography: comparison with dacryocystography and CT dacryocystography. Am J Neuroradiol. 2000;21:1145–50.
45. Weber AL, Rodrigues-De Velasquez A, Lucarelli MJ, Cheng HM. Normal anatomy of the lacrimal sac and duct: evaluated by dacryocystography, computed tomography and MR imaging. Neuroimaging Clin North Am. 1996;6:199–217.
46. Carlton WH, Trueblood JH, Rossomondo RM. Clinical evaluation of microscintigraphy of the lacrimal drainage apparatus. J Nucl Med. 1973;14:89–92.
47. Jager PL, Mansour K, Vrakkink-de Zoete H, et al. Clinical value of dacryoscintigraphy using a simplified analysis. Graefes Arch Clin Exp Ophthalmol. 2005;243:1134–40.
48. Wearne MJ, Pitts J, Frank J, et al. Comparison of dacryocystography and lacrimal scintigraphy in the diagnosis of functional nasolacrimal duct obstruction. Br J Ophthalmol. 1999;83:1032–5.
49. Detorakis E, Zissimopoulos A, Ionnakis K, Kozobolis VP. Lacrimal outflow mechanisms and the role of scintigraphy: current trends. World J Nucl Med. 2014;13:16–21.
50. Amanat LA, Hilditch TE, Kwok CS, et al. Lacrimal scintigraphy II. Its role in the diagnosis of epiphora. Br J Ophthalmol. 1983;67:720–8.
51. Fard-Esfahani A, Tari AS, Saghari M, et al. Assessment of the accuracy of lacrimal scintigraphy based on a prospective analysis of patients'symptomatology. Orbit. 2008;27:237–41.
52. Jabbour J, Van der Wall H, Katelaris L, et al. Quantitative lacrimal scintigraphy in the assessment of epiphora. Clin Nucl Med. 2008;33:535–41.
53. Hilditch TE, Kwok CS, Amanat LA. Lacrimal scintigraphy I. compartmental analysis of data. Br J Ophthalmol. 1983;67:713–9.
54. Massoudi T, Shayegani H, Sedeghi R. The role of "after washing imaging" in evaluation of tear drainage system by dacryoscintigraphy. Nucl Med Rev. 2018;21:75–8.
55. Putterman AM. Dacryocystography with occluded common canaliculus. Am J Ophthalmol. 1973;76:1010–2.
56. Vettese T, Hurwitz JJ. Toxicity of the chemiluminescent material Cyalume in anatomic assessment of the nasolacrimal system. Can J Ophthalmol. 1983;18:131–5.
57. Machado MA, Silva JA, Brioschi ML, Allemann N. Using thermography for an obstruction of the lower lacrimal system. Arq Bras Oftalmol. 2016;79:46–7.
58. Raflo GT, Chart P, Hurwitz JJ. Thermographic evaluation of the human lacrimal drainage system. Ophthalmic Surg. 1982;13:119–24.
59. Billington BM, Hurwitz JJ, Galbraith DJ, Gentles W. Miniprobe for lacrimal sac temperature measurement. Ophthalmic Surg. 1984;15:680–3.
60. Matsumura N, Goto S, Yamane S, et al. High-resolution dacryoendoscopy for observation for pediatric lacrimal duct obstruction. Am J Ophthalmol Case Rep. 2016;21:23–5.
61. Singh S, Mittal V, Vashist U, et al. Utility of intraocular endoscope for lacrimal canaliculi and sac examination. Into Ophthalmol. 2019;39(8):1879–83.

62. Heichel J, Struck HG, Fiorentzis M, et al. A case series of dacryoendoscopy in childhood: a diagnostic and therapeutic alternative for complex congenital nasolacrimal duct obstruction even in the first year of life. Adv There. 2017;34:1221–32.
63. Fujimoto M, Ogino K, Matsuyama H, Miyazaki C. Success rates of dacryoendoscopy-guided probing for recalcitrant congenital nasolacrimal duct obstruction. Jon J Ophthalmol. 2016;60:274–9.
64. Takahasi Y, Nakamura Y, Kakizaki H. Dacryoendoscopic findings in the lacrimal passage in failed dacryocystorhinostomy. Ophthal Plast Reconstr Surg. 2013;29:373–5.
65. Sasaki T, Sounou T, Tsuji H, Suguyama K. Air-insufflated high-definition dacryoendoscopy yields significantly better image quality than conventional dacryoendoscopy. Clin Ophthalmol. 2017;11:1385–91.

Surgery of the Punctum and Canaliculus

35

Harry Marshak

Punctoplasty

Punctal stenosis can result from aging changes or from a history of chronic inflammation, such as blepharitis and canaliculitis, or from idiopathic causes [1]. Certain chemotherapeutic agents, such as docetaxel (Tamoxifen) and 5-fluorouracil, can cause punctal as well as canalicular stenosis [2, 3].

In order to widen the punctal opening, a three-snip punctoplasty is performed to cut the punctal sphincter [4]. Local anesthesia, 2% lidocaine with epinephrine, is injected to the medial aspect of the lid. The punctum is dilated with a punctal dilator. Small Westcott scissors are used. The first cut is made through the posterior punctal sphincter and extending approximately 2 mm down the vertical canaliculus. The second cut is made through the central punctal sphincter and extending 3–4 mm through the horizontal canaliculus. The third cut is made on the posterior aspect of the lid to connect the first two cut edges. A triangle of posterior lamellar tissue and posterior canaliculus is thus excised (Fig. 35.1). The patient is placed on a topical antibiotic-steroid drop for 1 or 2 weeks. In cases of inflammatory stenosis, stent tubes should be placed in conjunction with the punctoplasty to prevent re-scarring.

One-snip and two-snip punctoplasty procedures tend to have a high recurrence rate, as the punctum can easily scar closed [4]. In cases of recurrence, the punctoplasty should be performed in conjunction with insertion of stent tubes.

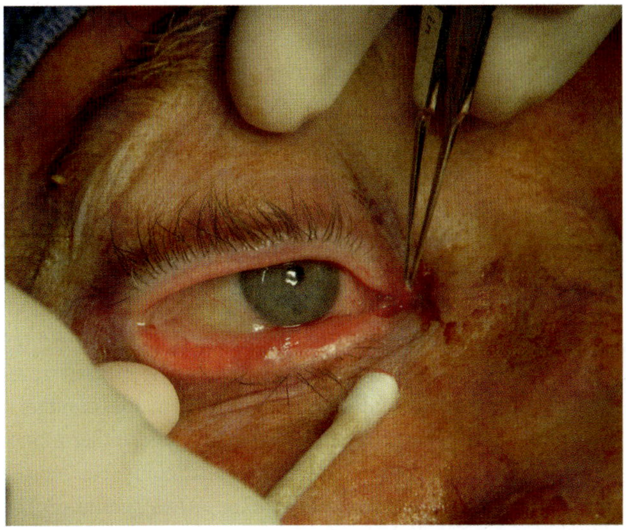

Fig. 35.1 Three-snip punctoplasty. Forceps holding triangle of posterior lamellar tissue and posterior canaliculus to be excised

Canaliculitis

The most common organism responsible for canaliculitis is *Actinomyces israelii*; however, other bacteria as well as fungi and herpesviruses have been reported [5, 6]. Medical treatment can be attempted using topical and/or oral antibiotics. However, due to the formation of concretions within the canaliculus, most patients will require surgical intervention in the form of canalicular curettage. In this procedure, a 2-mm curette is passed through a dilated punctum to access and remove the concretions. If the punctum is too small for the curette to pass, a small snip incision with scissors is made at the punctal sphincter to allow the curette to pass [7].

Large concretions or stones may require canaliculotomy. This is performed by inserting a Bowman probe into the canaliculus up to the area of concretion. The canaliculus overlying the metal probe is unroofed with a #11 blade 2 mm medial to the punctum. The punctal sphincter is left intact if possible. The roof of the canaliculus is marsupialized, and the concretions and/or stones are removed with a curette [8]. The canaliculus is irrigated, and a stent tube, either mono- or bicanalicular, is placed. The canaliculus is sutured closed over the tube with 6-0 or 7-0 vicryl suture. The patient is placed on a topical antibiotic-steroid drop for 2 weeks. The stent tube should remain in place for at least 6 weeks.

H. Marshak (✉)
Eisenhower Medical Center, Department of Surgery, Palm Desert, CA, USA
e-mail: drmarshak@drmarshak.com

J. J. Servat et al. (eds.), *Smith and Nesi's Ophthalmic Plastic and Reconstructive Surgery*, https://doi.org/10.1007/978-3-030-41720-8_35

Intracanalicular Plugs

Recent years have seen the rise in use of intracanalicular plugs for the treatment of dry eyes. The advantages of these types of plugs are that they have no external surface which may cause discomfort. They are designed to be able to be flushed out of the lacrimal duct when no longer needed. However, in practice, these plugs often become lodged within the canaliculus and can elicit an inflammatory response in the lumen of the canaliculus. Irrigation may cause the plug to become lodged in the distal canaliculus or at the common canaliculus and resist further irrigation. These plugs may create a blind pouch in the proximal canaliculus, allowing bacteria to grow, leading to canaliculitis [9].

If the plug requires removal, due to epiphora, inflammation, or infection, and cannot be dislodged with irrigation or retrograde massage, the patient may require either canaliculotomy or dacryocystorhinostomy. If the plug can be felt in the canaliculus, either by external palpation or lacrimal probing, a canaliculotomy may be attempted. A cut is made with a #11 blade over the involved portion of the canaliculus. The canaliculus is marsupialized to locate the plug. The plug will usually extrude itself easily. The canaliculus should be examined for surrounding scar tissue and the scar tissue excised (Fig. 35.2). A plug that is lodged in the common canaliculus can be excised transcutaneously by performing a cutdown in the medial canthus if the plug can be palpated externally. A stent tube, either mono- or bicanalicular, is then placed into the canaliculus. The incised area is sutured over the stent with 6-0 or 7-0 vicryl suture. The tube should remain in place for at least 6 weeks.

Lacrimal Trauma

Canalicular lacerations are commonly seen in blunt trauma due to the fact that the tarsal plate ends at the punctum, leaving only soft tissue for support in the medial canthal area. The eyelid medial to the punctum, thus, is the weakest portion of the eyelid. The laceration is most likely due to lateral traction of the eyelid during blunt trauma [10]. Canalicular lacerations are also commonly seen in association with dog bites due to the position of the dog's jaw around the victim's orbit.

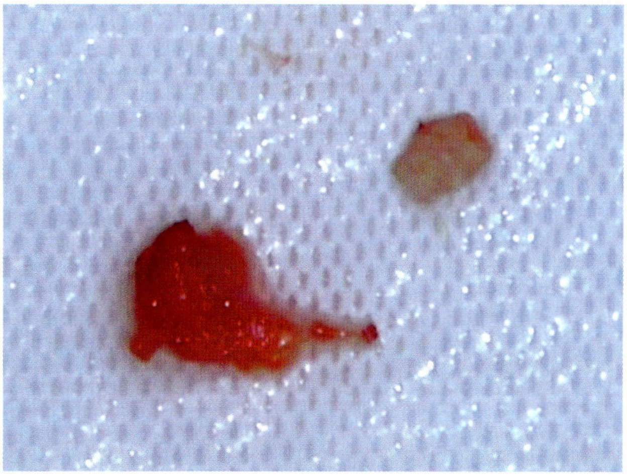

Fig. 35.2 Intracanalicular plug and surrounding scar tissue following surgical removal

Fist punches tend to be the most common mechanism for canalicular laceration (23%) [11]. Nineteen percent of canalicular lacerations occur in relation to a dog bite injury [12]. Dog bite injury is the most common cause of canalicular laceration in children [11]. These are often associated with avulsion of the medial canthal tendon.

Canalicular lacerations require repair within 24–48 h in order to ensure proper tear drainage. If a medial lid laceration is repaired without placing a stent in the canaliculus, the cut canaliculus will scar closed, committing the patient to a lifetime of tearing. Late repair is difficult, with patients often requiring conjunctivo-dacryocystorhinostomy.

Lacerations of the inferior canaliculus occur more common than superior canalicular lacerations. Meta-analysis has shown that inferior lacerations occurred in 72% of cases, superior in 16%, and 12% had both superior and inferior canalicular lacerations [12]. Medial canthal tendon avulsion has been reported to occur in 36% of canalicular lacerations [13].

Dog Bites

Dog bites to the face have a propensity to involve the medial canthus and canalicular system compared to other forms of eyelid trauma [14]. The patient should be treated with broad-spectrum systemic antibiotics, such as IV ampicillin/sulbactam, and the wound irrigated profusely. There are often associated deep facial lacerations. Generally, there is no loss of tissue [15]; however, the wound edges tend to be irregular.

Examination

After ruptured globe and other trauma have been addressed, the eyelid should be examined for laceration. If the laceration is medial to the punctum, a canalicular laceration must be suspected. After punctal dilation, a #0 Bowman probe is passed through the canaliculus until a soft stop is felt at the nose. If this is not felt, the suspicion for laceration should be high. The laceration is examined to see if the probe is visible within the wound. If this is not the case, the probe should be removed and an irrigating cannula passed into the canaliculus. The presence of a laceration will be determined by the flow of irrigation out of the eyelid in the involved area. The same procedure should be performed for the upper and lower canaliculi.

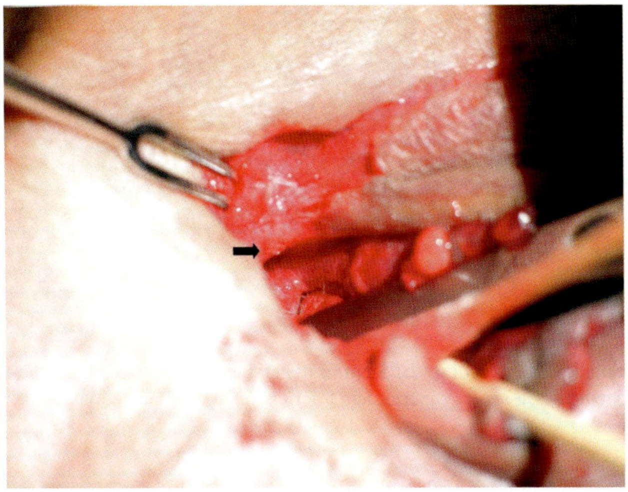

Fig. 35.3 Canalicular laceration. Medial cut edge is visible (*arrow*)

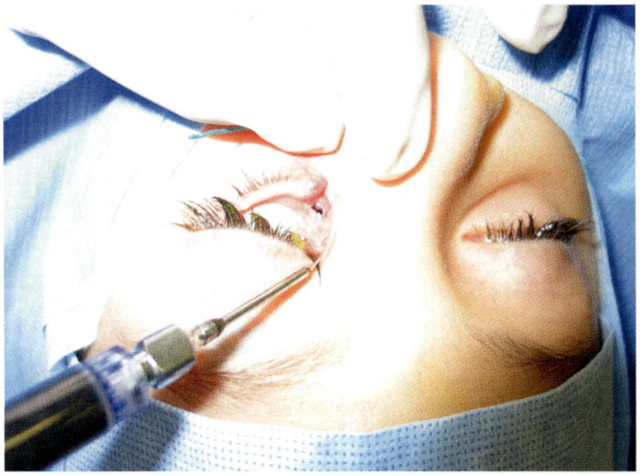

Fig. 35.4 Technique for finding cut edge of canaliculus. Viscous lidocaine with methylene blue is injected through superior canaliculus. *Blue dye* shows medial cut edge inferior canaliculus

Repair

The traditional method of repair of either mono- or bicanalicular lacerations has been with suturing over a bicanalicular stent. More recently, monocanalicular stents have become useful in the repair of simple monocanalicular lacerations that do not involve the punctum [16].

The most difficult part of canalicular repair is locating the medial cut end of the canaliculus. Under magnification with high-powered loupes or microscope, the cut edge of the canaliculus will appear as a white, glistening ring amidst the medial canthal tissue (Fig. 35.3). It is usually found posterior to the canthus. The more medial the laceration, the more posterior the cut edge will be, and the closer the two cut canaliculi will be to each other. In a monocanalicular laceration, if the cut edge cannot be found, the surgeon may be aided by slowly injecting viscous lidocaine mixed with methylene blue through the intact canaliculus and observing for reflux from the medial cut end (Fig. 35.4).

Choice of Stent

Bicanalicular intubation is the gold standard for mono- or bicanalicular lacerations. This is due to the fact that it provides a "closed loop" system which is unlikely to fall out. It does, however, require general anesthesia and nasal manipulation. Bicanalicular intubation also aids in traumatic reconstruction of the medial canthus, as the stent tubes can be clamped with mild traction at the nasal opening. This allows the cut medial canthal tissues to be drawn medially, aiding proper tissue placement prior to tissue suturing.

Monocanalicular stents can usually be inserted under local anesthesia in an office setting or monitored anesthesia care. They do not require nasal manipulation [17]. However, they are less secure and can be dislodged by a child rubbing his eye. They also cannot be used if there has been damage to the punctum, as the proximal end of the tube will not "seat" properly in a damaged or reconstructed punctum.

Bicanalicular Repair

The bicanalicular stent is passed through each punctum and proximal canaliculus and brought out through the wound. Each end is then passed into the cut edge distally and passed until a soft stop is felt at the nose. The stent is then rotated vertically and passed into the nasolacrimal duct and into the nose (Fig. 35.5). A Crawford hook is used to retrieve the tubes from under the inferior turbinate.

The preferred stent is a Crawford tube with internal suture. This allows the tubes to be tied together using the suture, allowing the tube to be cut and removed through the punctum, if necessary, without causing trauma to the punctum. This is especially useful in children who will not cooperate with tubes being removed via the nose.

Once both ends of the stent are brought out through the nose, the tubes may be clamped at the level of the nostril. This allows the tubes to provide traction on the canthal wound to aid in anatomical re-approximation. If the medial canthal tendon has been avulsed, it is closed by passing a 5-0 vicryl suture, preferably on a P-2 needle, through the periosteum of the medial wall and then through the canthal tendon, superior and inferior to the canaliculi. The pericanalicular orbicularis muscle is re-approximated using a single 7-0 vicryl mattress suture [18, 19]. The medial canthal sutures are then tied. The wound is closed with 6-0 vicryl deep sutures. The skin is closed as desired. The stents are tied to each other in the nose and sutured to the lateral wall of the nose at the

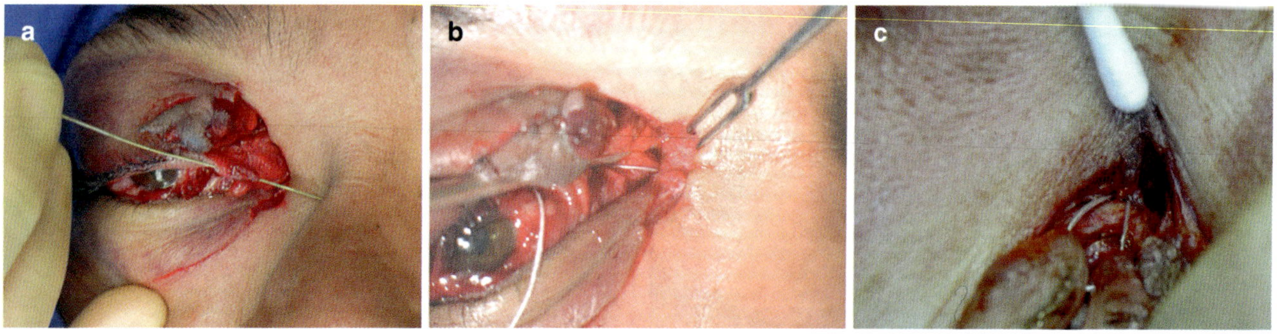

Fig. 35.5 (**a**) Probe passed through superior punctum and out through canalicular laceration. (**b**) Stent has been passed across the laceration, through the medial cut edge, and into the nasolacrimal duct into nose. (**c**) Stent passed across superior and inferior canalicular lacerations

Fig. 35.6 Monocanalicular stent. Mini Monoka. (FCI Ophthalmics Inc.©)

mucocutaneous junction with a 5-0 vicryl suture in adults and 6-0 vicryl in children. This suture will dissolve by the time the tubes are removed in approximately 6 weeks.

If the punctum is lacerated, it is sutured closed around the stent with 7-0 vicryl sutures. The stent tubes are generally left in for at least 6 weeks.

Monocanalicular Repair

The monocanalicular stent is a short silicone stent with a punctal plug at the end (Fig. 35.6). The most common is the Mini Monoka (FCI Ophthalmics). The end of the stent is passed through the punctum and brought out through the wound. The end is pulled so that the punctal plug snaps into place in the punctum (Fig. 35.7). The end of the stent is then cut to the appropriate length to reach the nasal wall. It does not need to pass into the bony nasolacrimal duct. It should be cut at an angle to aid in passage. The beveled end is passed through the cut distal canaliculus [20].

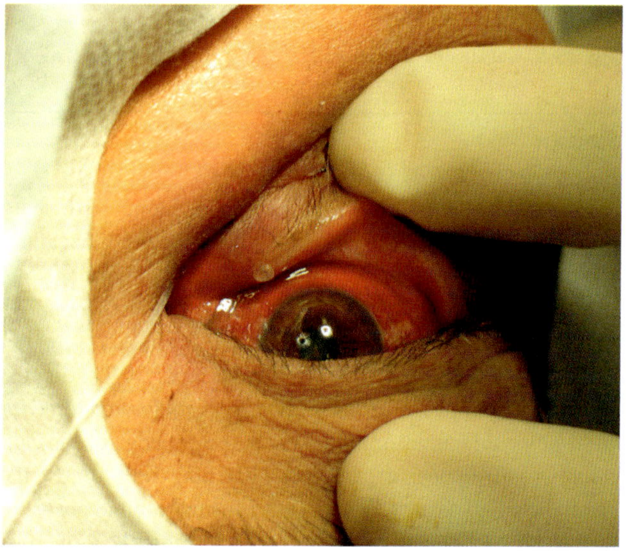

Fig. 35.7 Monocanalicular stent seated in punctum

The monocanalicular stent cannot be used if there is laceration to the punctum, as the proximal end will not seat. It also should not be used if there has been medial canthal avulsion as it cannot provide the adequate inferior and posterior traction to the wound as a bicanalicular stent tied in the nose.

Pigtail Probe

Canalicular intubation with the pigtail probe is a method of last resort when the cut end of a canaliculus cannot be located. This is because passing a curved probe around the tight turn of the common canaliculus can inadvertently cause iatrogenic trauma to the patent canaliculus, the common canaliculus, or the lacrimal sac. However, it is important to use a blunt-tipped pigtail probe in order to minimize trauma to the lacrimal system [21].

The probe is passed through the intact canaliculus with the probe handle maintained in a vertical position. It is gently

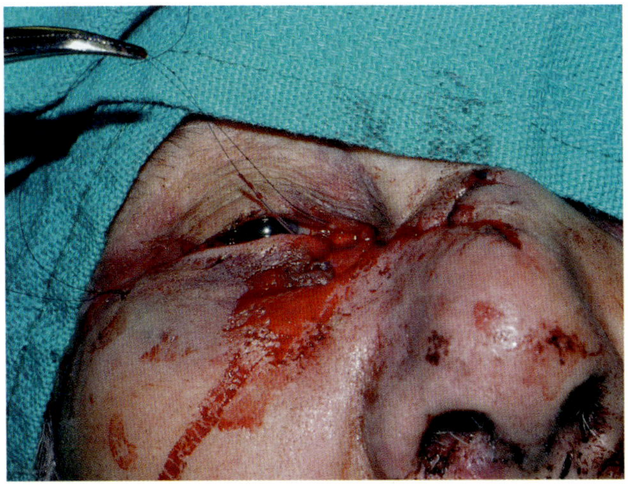

Fig. 35.8 Both ends of stent after being passed using a pigtail probe

rotated until the end of the probe is seen exiting the cut edge of the other canaliculus. A 5-0 nylon suture is passed through the eyelet of the probe. The probe is rotated out of the canaliculi, bringing the nylon with it. The opposite end of the pigtail probe is passed through the other punctum and into the wound. The nylon is threaded into the probe and the probe is withdrawn. The nylon suture is threaded into a stent tube, and a clamp is placed across the tube and suture (Fig. 35.8). The other end of the suture is pulled so that the stent tube passes through both canaliculi. The nylon suture is left in place. The cut canaliculus is sutured over the stent, and the laceration is closed. The stent is then trimmed appropriately, and the suture is tied to itself, creating a circle in the stent tube. The closed edges of the stent are rotated into the canaliculus.

Stent Removal

Canalicular stents can usually be removed approximately 6 weeks after repair. They are preferably removed from the nose after the loop between the puncta is cut. An endoscope can be used to aid in finding the nasal end of the stent. If this is not possible, as in a small child, the stent may be removed by cutting the loop between the puncta and pulling the stent out through one of the puncta. Placement of the Crawford stent tube that has an internal suture aids in removal, as there is only a small knot in the silk suture that must pass through the punctum, thus avoiding damage to the punctum.

Cutting the stent without removing it with the assumption that the patient will blow it out of the nose is not recommended as the stent may remain lodged in the lacrimal duct and lead to granuloma formation [22].

Punctal Ectropion

Anatomically, the inferior punctum should have good apposition against the globe. This allows tears to enter the canaliculus through gravity and with the normal lacrimal pump mechanism during blinking. Laxity of the medial canthal tendon can cause isolated ectropion of the medial lower eyelid and punctum, preventing the tears from entering the canaliculus and leading to chronic epiphora.

Correction of medial ectropion can be accomplished with a medial spindle procedure. A horizontal ellipse or rhombic section of tarso-conjunctiva is excised from the posterior aspect of the involved portion of the eyelid inferior to the punctum (Fig. 35.9). The lower eyelid retractors and cut edge of conjunctiva are sutured to the inferior edge of tarsus with 6-0 vicryl buried sutures (Fig. 35.10). This allows shortening

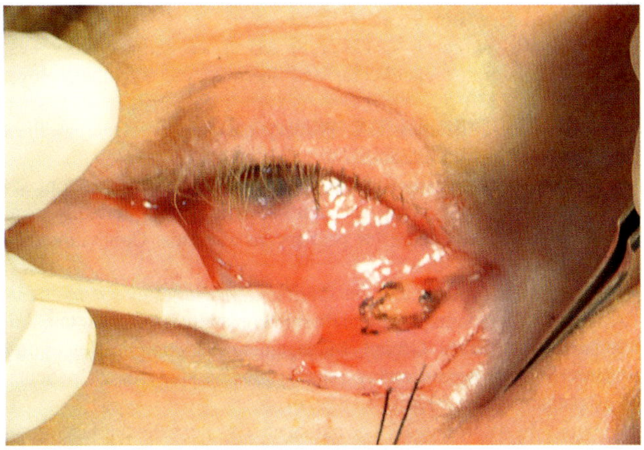

Fig. 35.9 An ellipse of tarsus and conjunctiva is excised from the posterior aspect of the medial eyelid

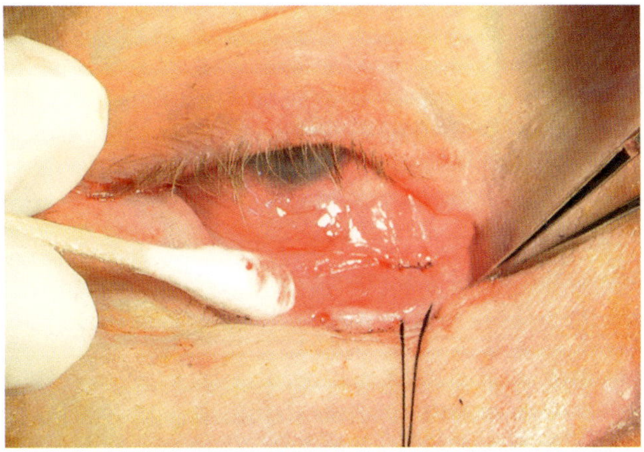

Fig. 35.10 The lower eyelid retractors and conjunctiva are sutured to the inferior edge of tarsus with 6-0 vicryl buried sutures

of the medial aspect of the posterior lamella to induce inward rotation [23]. Alternate procedures include cautery of the medial conjunctiva, medial canthoplasty, and Smith's lazy-T procedure [24–26]. If significant horizontal laxity of the lower eyelid is present, a lateral tarsal strip procedure can be added.

References

1. Kashkouli MB, Beigi B, Murthy R, Astbury N. Acquired external punctal stenosis: etiology and associated findings. Am J Ophthalmol. 2003;136:1079–84.
2. Esmaeli B, Valero V, Ahmadi MA, Booser D. Canalicular stenosis secondary to docetaxel (taxotere): a newly recognized side effect. Ophthalmology. 2001;108:994–5.
3. Lee V, Bentley CR, Olver JM. Sclerosing canaliculitis after 5-fluorouracil breast cancer chemotherapy. Eye (London). 1998;12(Pt 3a):343–9.
4. Caesar RH, McNab AA. A brief history of punctoplasty: the 3-snip revisited. Eye (London). 2005;19:16–8.
5. Repp DJ, Burkat CN, Lucarelli MJ. Lacrimal excretory system concretions: canalicular and lacrimal sac. Ophthalmology. 2009;116:2230–5.
6. Zaldivar RA, Bradley EA. Primary canaliculitis. Ophthal Plast Reconstr Surg. 2009;25:481–4.
7. Lee MJ, Choung HK, Kim NJ, Khwarg SI. One-snip punctoplasty and canalicular curettage through the punctum: a minimally invasive surgical procedure for primary canaliculitis. Ophthalmology. 2009;116:2027–30. e2
8. Khu J, Mancini R. Punctum-sparing canaliculotomy for the treatment of canaliculitis. Ophthal Plast Reconstr Surg. 2012;28(1):63–5.
9. SmartPlug Study Group. Management of complications after insertion of the SmartPlug punctal plug: a study of 28 patients. Ophthalmology. 2006;113:1859, e1–6.
10. Wulc AE, Arterberry JF. The pathogenesis of canalicular laceration. Ophthalmology. 1991;98:1243–9.
11. Kennedy RH, May J, Dailey J, Flanagan JC. Canalicular laceration. An 11-year epidemiologic and clinical study. Ophthal Plast Reconstr Surg. 1990;6:46–53.
12. Reifler DM. Management of canalicular laceration. Surv Ophthalmol. 1991;36:113–32.
13. Dortzbach RK, Angrist RA. Silicone intubation for lacerated lacrimal canaliculi. Ophthalmic Surg. 1985;16:639–42.
14. Savar A, Kirszrot J, Rubin PA. Canalicular involvement in dog bite related eyelid lacerations. Ophthal Plast Reconstr Surg. 2008;24:296–8.
15. Slonim CB. Dog bite-induced canalicular lacerations: a review of 17 cases. Ophthal Plast Reconstr Surg. 1996;12:218–22.
16. Murchison AP, Bilyk JR. Canalicular laceration repair: an analysis of variables affecting success. Ophthal Plast Reconstr Surg. 2014;30(5):410–4.
17. Naik MN, Kelapure A, Rath S, Honavar SG. Management of canalicular lacerations: epidemiological aspects and experience with Mini-Monoka monocanalicular stent. Am J Ophthalmol. 2008;145:375–80.
18. Kersten RC, Kulwin DR. "One-stitch" canalicular repair. A simplified approach for repair of canalicular laceration. Ophthalmology. 1996;103:785–9.
19. Baum JL. Canalicular function after "one-stitch" repair. Ophthalmology. 1997;104:2–3.
20. Chowdhury HR, Rose GE, Ezra DG. Long-term outcomes of monocanalicular repair of canalicular lacerations. Ophthalmology. 2014;121(8):1665–1666.e1.
21. Jordan DR, Nerad JA, Tse DT. The pigtail probe, revisited. Ophthalmology. 1990;97(4):512–9.
22. Dresner SC, Codere F, Brownstein S, Jouve P. Lacrimal drainage system inflammatory masses from retained silicone tubing. Am J Ophthalmol. 1984;98:609–13.
23. Nowinski TS, Anderson RL. The medial spindle procedure for involutional medial ectropion. Arch Ophthalmol. 1985;103:1750–3.
24. O'Donnell BA, Anderson RL, Collin JR, et al. Repair of the lax medial canthal tendon. Br J Ophthalmol. 2003;87:220–4.
25. Anderson RL, Jordan DR, Thiese SM. The medial tarsal strip. Arch Ophthalmol. 1990;108:120–4.
26. Smith B. The "lazy-T" correction of ectropion of the lower punctum. Arch Ophthalmol. 1976;94(7):1149–50.

Primary External Dacryocystorhinostomy

36

Natalie A. Homer and Aaron Fay

Nasolacrimal duct (NLD) obstruction can produce epiphora or dacryocystitis. In either case, traditional external dacryocystorhinostomy (DCR) may be performed to anastomose the nasolacrimal sac to the lateral nasal cavity. The goals of surgery are to resolve tear stasis and to prevent lacrimal sac enlargement. Specific indications for the procedure include:

- Primary acquired nasolacrimal duct obstruction (NLDO)
- Functional NLDO due to lacrimal drainage system stenosis or lacrimal pump failure
- Secondary (acquired) NLDO, resulting from sinus or nasal disease, prior midfacial and orbital trauma, dacryolithiasis, or iatrogenic injury
- Dacryocystitis, after acute infection temporization with oral antibiotic treatment
- Congenital NLDO, persisting after initial attempts at probe and intubation

Surgical Principles

External DCR establishes a low resistance pathway for tears to drain from the ocular surface to the nasal cavity. This is accomplished by suturing a fistula between the lacrimal sac mucosa and the lateral nasal mucosa. Advantages of the external DCR approach include:

1. Direct visualization of lacrimal sac pathology, including tumors, stones, and foreign bodies
2. Opportunity to suture nasolacrimal sac and nasal mucosal flaps
3. Surgical access for management of canalicular disease
4. Improved ability to maintain good hemostasis

Anesthesia

External DCR may be performed under general or local anesthesia. The decision will depend upon the preference of the patient, surgeon, and anesthesiologist. Under most conditions, general anesthesia is performed, particularly in cases of secondary obstruction or revision surgery.

Procedure

The planned surgical incision is marked halfway between the nasal dorsum and the medial caruncle, starting at level of the medial canthal tendon and extending inferiorly for a length of approximately 12 mm. When available, a natural skin crease or skin tension line is utilized (Fig. 36.1).

The local anesthesia infiltrate is prepared consisting of an equal mixture of 2% lidocaine with epinephrine and 0.5% bupivacaine. Using a 25-gauge 1.5-in. needle, approximately 5 cc of anesthetic solution is infiltrated subcutaneously and subperiosteally along the incision line and into the medial upper and lower eyelids in proximity to the lacrimal puncta and canaliculi.

An additional 5 cc of anesthetic solution is infiltrated submucosally into the lateral nasal wall in the area of the anterior middle turbinate and uncinate process, under direct visualization using a nasal speculum. Mild mucosal bleeding following injection is common and may induce a cough reflex in patients under local and intravenous sedation.

The lateral nasal wall is then packed with nasal gauze. Bayonet forceps are used to precisely place the packing under direct visualization. The author prefers to use 0.5 × 3 inch neurosurgical sponges imbibed in a topical anesthesia

N. A. Homer
Ophthalmic Plastic and Reconstructive Surgery, TOC Eye and Face, Austin, TX, USA

A. Fay (✉)
Harvard Medical School, Department of Ophthalmology, Boston, MA, USA

J. J. Servat et al. (eds.), *Smith and Nesi's Ophthalmic Plastic and Reconstructive Surgery*, https://doi.org/10.1007/978-3-030-41720-8_36

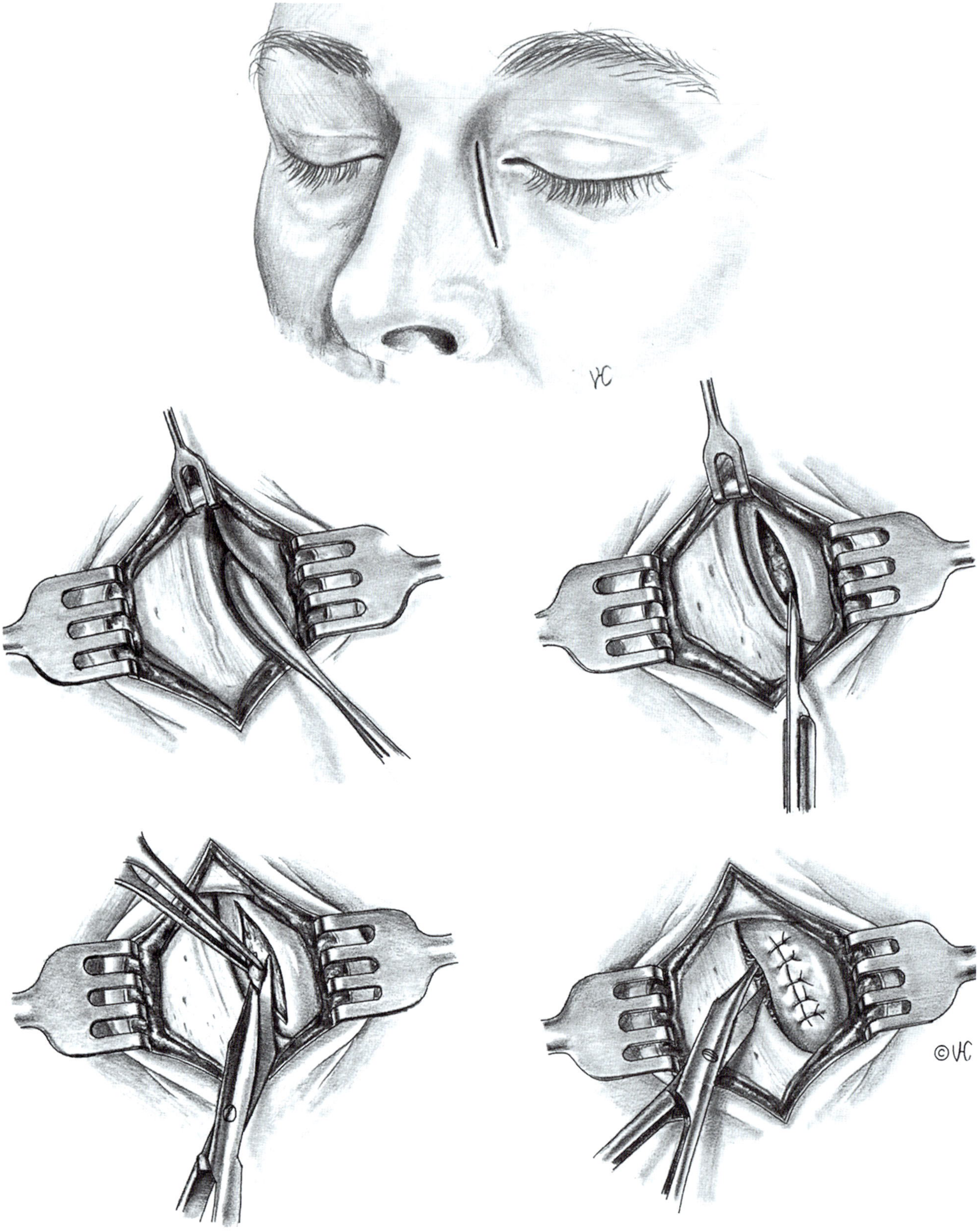

Fig. 36.1 Curvilinear incision along natural rhytid or skin tension line

solution. Sponge ribbons are left long to aid in their eventual removal. The sponges may be soaked in 2% lidocaine with epinephrine, 0.05% oxymetazoline (Afrin), or a 4% cocaine solution. The surgeon grasps one end of the nasal gauze with the Bayonet forceps and guides the sponge along the lateral nasal wall to seat it under the middle turbinate. Typically, three sponges are sufficient for unilateral packing. Precise packing allows for tamponade of post-anesthetic mucosal bleeding and reduces surgical bleeding by inducing vasoconstriction.

The patient may now be prepped and draped according to the surgeon's preference. The draping may allow the full face to be open.

The surgical marking is identified, and an incision with the appropriate instrument is made through the skin and orbicularis muscle. The incision may be performed with a #15 Bard-Parker blade or monopolar cautery on a pure-cut setting. Further dissection through the deeper tissue using a combination of monopolar cautery on a blended setting and blunt spreading with the use of a hemostat or a Freer periosteal elevator may be performed (Fig. 36.2). The dissection should continue until the periosteum of the anterior lacrimal fossa is encountered.

During this dissection, skin retractors may assist in visualization. An Alm retractor is a self-retaining skin hook which provides excellent visualization through the small incision. Two four-prong rakes, held by an assistant, may also be used to splay the wound edges. Retractors may need to be repositioned as the dissection is carried deeper.

At all times, a continuous suction device should be available to maintain a dry field and assist in viewing the deep subcutaneous tissues. Caution should be taken to avoid injury to the angular artery, located approximately 6–8 mm from the medial canthus [1]. A thoughtfully positioned incision, careful blunt dissection, and maintenance of good visualization by hemostasis and retraction help to avoid vessel injury. If arterial puncture occurs, bipolar cautery and/or vessel suture ligation may be necessitated.

Once the periosteum is adequately exposed, a vertical periosteal incision may be performed using a #11 blade or monopolar cautery. In some instances, particularly in cases of a chronic dacryocystitis, the periosteum may be significantly thinned. In such cases, the periosteum may be easily mobilized with the Freer elevator. More typically the periosteum will need to be incised with a scalpel or Bovie cautery. If this is performed, the surgeon should be careful to incise only the periosteum and not carry the incision deeper into the bone. Following incision of the periosteum, a periosteal elevator is used to elevate the lacrimal fossa periosteum and overlying lacrimal sac.

The lacrimal fossa can then be fully visualized. A small osteotomy should be initiated through the thin lacrimal bone. In most cases, a curved hemostat or periosteal elevator may be used to create an initial bony opening (Fig. 36.3). The preferred instrument is placed on the lacrimal bone, and moderate pressure is applied, directed toward the middle turbinate. The surgeon can often detect a small natural depression in the lacrimal bone which corresponds with its thinnest point. Unusually thick lacrimal bone may require initial entry with an osteotome, trephine, or drill. When a small opening is made through thick bone, the hemostat should be slowly advanced and rotated in order to achieve a larger bone window, one through which a small rongeur can fit.

Kerrison rongeurs are used to enlarge the osteotomy (Fig. 36.4). The smallest rongeur is inserted through the osteotomy, and a bite of tissue, consisting of bone and often nasal mucosa, is removed. After approximately two or three bites with this rongeur, the surgeon may elect to use a larger rongeur

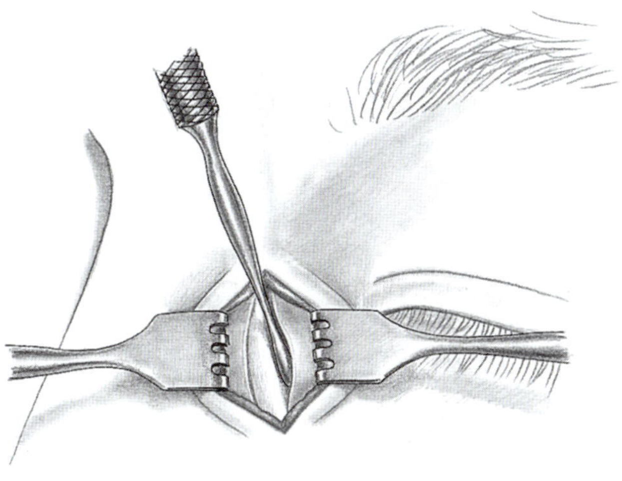

Fig. 36.2 Periosteum is incised and reflected laterally and superiorly, to expose frontal process of maxillary bone, anterior lacrimal crest, and lacrimal sac fossa

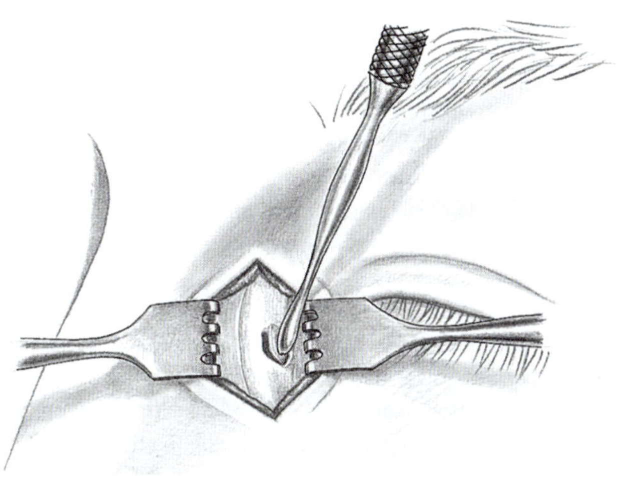

Fig. 36.3 Creation of osteotomy with periosteal elevator, just anterior to the posterior lacrimal crest

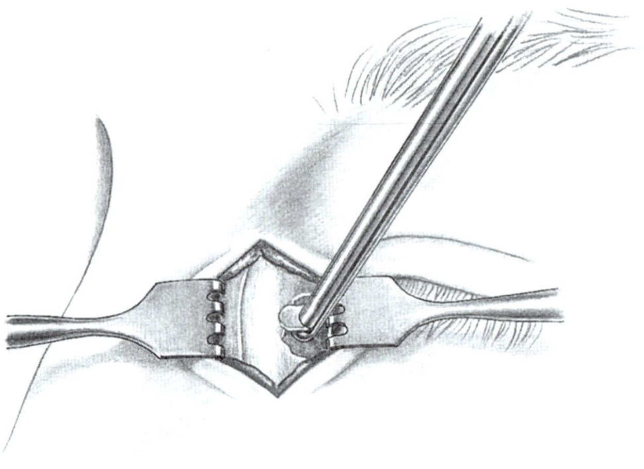

Fig. 36.4 Rongeur used to enlarge osteotomy

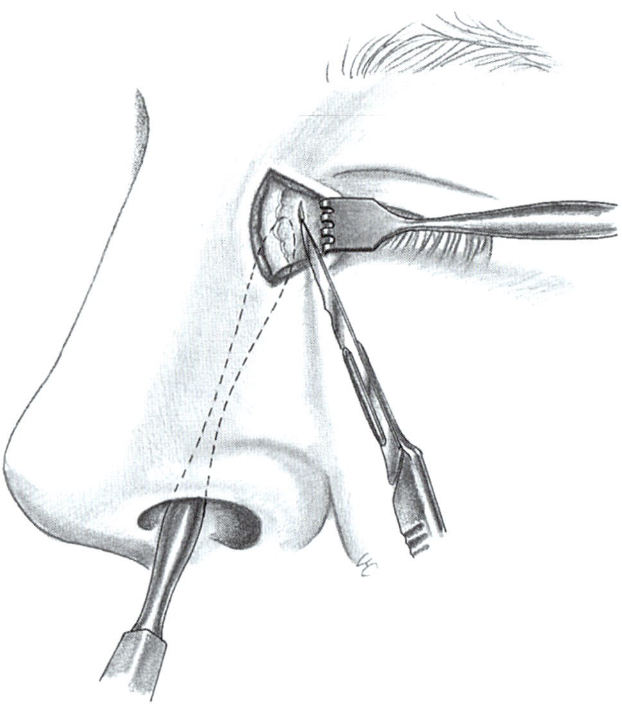

Fig. 36.5 Periosteal elevator is placed in nasal cavity and tents the nasal mucosa outward. An incision is made in the nasal mucosa. The residual mucosa may be removed or secured as a flap to the lacrimal sac

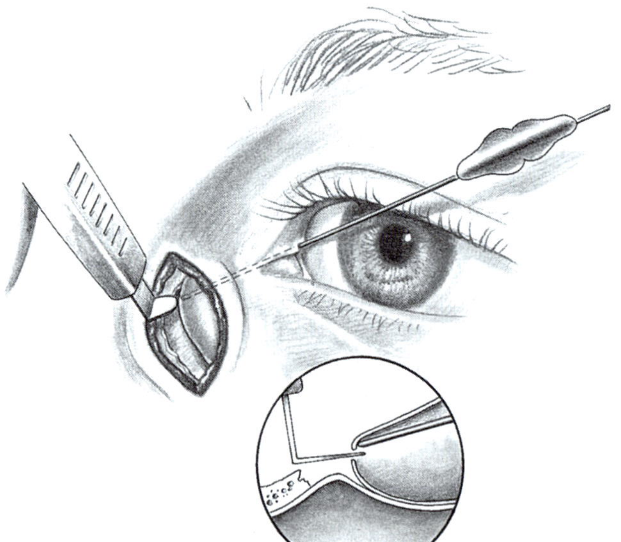

Fig. 36.6 Bowman probe passed through upper canaliculus into lacrimal sac. The tip of the probe is tenting the medial lacrimal sac. An incision is made along the medial sac to create anterior and posterior flaps. An ellipse may be excised and sent to pathology

to expedite bone removal. The osteotomy is enlarged to approximately 15 mm in diameter. This generally encompasses removal of the entire lacrimal bone. The superior-most extent of the osteotomy is up to 2 mm superior to the medial canthal tendon. At this level, the surgeon is generally more than 15 mm from the cribriform plate, which forms the base of the frontal process. It is important to avoid rotational sheering of bone at this superior osteotomy location, as this may inadvertently fracture to the overlying cribriform plate and induce a cerebrospinal fluid leak [2]. The bony opening should be carried inferiorly until the nasolacrimal canal is partially unroofed.

After completion of the osteotomy, attention is drawn to the underlying nasal mucosa. It is often the case that the nasal mucosa is incidentally entered and excised during bone removal. This can be seen by inserting a blunt instrument or periosteal elevator into the nose and directing superiorly along the lateral nasal cavity. If the nasal mucosa was entered, the instrument may be viewed easily by the surgeon through the external incision. If the nasal mucosa remains intact, the instrument may be tented toward the external opening, and the mucosa may be incised using a #11 blade (Fig. 36.5). Rongeurs may then be used to excise the remaining nasal mucosal flaps within the area of the osteotomy. The Freer elevator should at this point be fully visualized within the nasal without obstruction by the nasal mucosa. Mucosal bleeding may be encountered and temporized using careful cautery and temporary packing with the Afrin-soaked neurosurgical sponges.

After appropriate osteotomy and ethmoidectomy, attention is then directed to the lacrimal puncta and canaliculi. The upper and lower puncta should be dilated with a punctum dilator. A Bowman lacrimal probe (usually size 0 or 1) is passed through the upper and lower canaliculi in sequence, through the common canaliculus and into the lacrimal sac (Fig. 36.6), tenting it nasally. It is crucial to confirm that the osteotomy opening encompasses the entirety of the nasolacrimal sac. With the sac tented nasally, the surgeon should make a 1-cm "I"-shaped incision through the lacrimal sac near the tip of the probe. Back-cuts along the superior and inferior edges of the wound are made to create anterior and

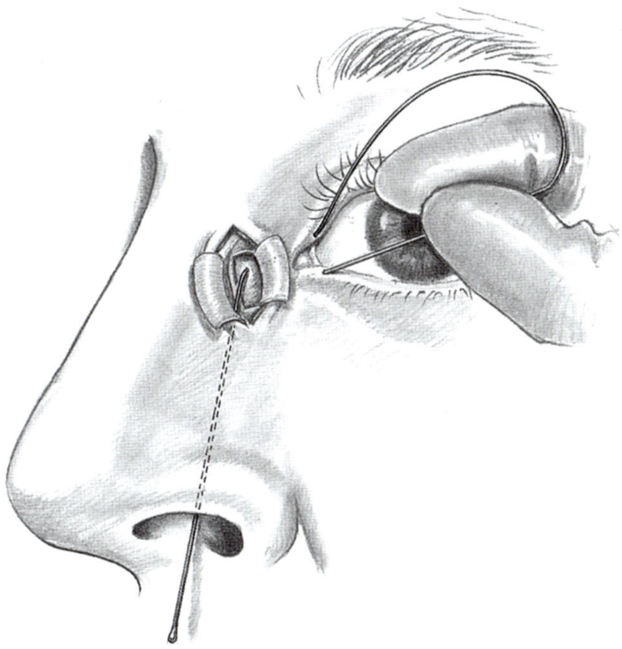

Fig. 36.7 Silicone tube with probes passed through upper and lower canaliculi into lacrimal sac area

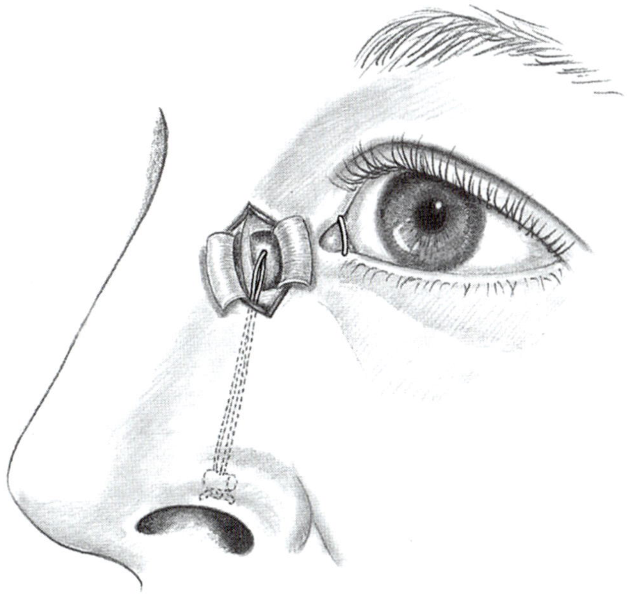

Fig. 36.8 Silicone tube ends are tied in square knot and trimmed. The knot retracts into the nose, remaining below the level of the osteotomy

posterior flaps. Avoidance of accidental skin injury can be ensured by mindful retraction.

A small ellipse of tissue can be removed from the lacrimal sac, and many surgeons prefer to send this specimen to pathology for further evaluation. If a pathological process is suspected, then it is necessary to have this tissue further evaluated. The lacrimal sac should be opened with forceps and thoroughly examined visually. If the sac appears to be free of tumor, the Bowman probe may be removed, and intubation performed.

The author prefers to intubate the lacrimal system with a standard Crawford silicone tube (Fig. 36.7). The upper and lower canalicular systems are intubated in sequence, and the tip of the probe is visualized through the incision site. A Crawford hook is placed through the nasal cavity and visualized through the osteotomy. The surgeon then grasps the end of the silicone tube with the hook and retrieves the tube through the nasal vestibule. After the upper and lower canaliculi are intubated in this fashion, the surgeon may remove both metal ends, leaving both silicone ends of the tube extruded through the nose.

A hemostat is then used to bring the tubes together and stabilize them at the base of the nose. Prior to clamping the silicone tubes, mild pressure is used to retract the tubes at the opening of the nose. The hemostat stabilizes the ends of the tube, and forceps are used to tie the ends in a simple square knot. Scissors are used to cut the ends of the tube, with attention to leave approximately 5 mm of tubing at the end of the knot to reduce the likelihood of the knot coming undone. The hemostat is opened, and the knot allowed to gently retract into the nasal cavity (Fig. 36.8). The surgeon should be able to view the ends of the silicone tube as they exit the osteotomy and rest in the lateral nasal wall.

Some advocate suture anastomosis of the respective anterior and posterior lacrimal sac and nasal mucosal flaps over the silicone tubing. While not too technically burdensome, this approach has not been shown to improve outcomes [3, 4]. This author prefers to either excise the posterior nasolacrimal duct flap or position it into the nasal cavity against the lateral nasal sidewall. The anterior sac flap may then be secured in an open position by direct apposition to the overlying orbicularis tissue using a single interrupted 5-0 Monocryl suture.

After the surgeon ensures meticulous hemostasis, the wound may be closed. The author prefers to close the wound in a layered fashion. The deep dermis is closed using 5-0 Monocryl suture in a buried interrupted fashion. The skin is then closed with a running 6-0 fast-absorbing gut suture. The wound may be dressed with Mastisol-enforced steri-strips.

Postoperative Care

Cold compresses are applied to the wound for several hours, at 15-min intervals. Once the steri-strips have spontaneously dislodged during the first postoperative week, an antibiotic ointment may be applied to the sutures three to four times a day. Ophthalmic antibiotic/steroid drops usually provide comfort and improve healing when applied four times per day for 1 week. The author routinely removes the stent tubes at 6 weeks, but surgeon preferences range from 1 to 6 months [5]. The author will often reinitiate the ophthalmic antibiotic/steroid drop for an additional 1 week following tube removal.

References

1. Chapter 6: Orbit\Lids\Adnexa. In: Friedman NJ, Kaiser PK, Trattler WB, editors. Review of ophthalmology. Saunders: Elsevier; 2018, p. 161–96.
2. Neuhaus RW, Baylis HI. Cerebrospinal fluid leakage after dacryocystorhinostomy. Ophthalmology. 1983;90(9):1091–5.
3. Kaçaniku G, Begolli I. External dacryocystorhinostomy with and without suturing the posterior mucosal flaps. Med Arch. 2014;68(1):54–6.
4. Turkcu FM, Oner V, Tas M, Alakus F, Iscan Y. Anastomosis of both posterior and anterior flaps or only anterior flaps in external dacryocystorhinostomy. Orbit. 2012;31(6):383–5.
5. Anderson RL, Edwards JJ. Indications, complications and results with silicone stents. Ophthalmology. 1979;86:1474.

Primary Endoscopic Dacryocystorhinostomy

37

Roger A. Dailey and Jennifer Murdock

Many patients present to the oculofacial specialist complaining of tearing. Although a variety of etiologies have been associated with epiphora, nasolacrimal duct obstruction is the most common. Blockage of the nasolacrimal system can be associated with chronic tearing, discharge, irritation, and recurrent infection which are often quite debilitating. A dacryocystorhinostomy (DCR) creates an alternate passageway between the lacrimal sac and nasal cavity, thus bypassing the obstructed nasolacrimal duct. DCR can be performed either by an external approach that utilizes a cutaneous incision or through an endoscopic approach, which includes an incision in the nasal cavity. An endonasal approach was initially described by Caldwell in 1893 [1]. Shortly thereafter, Toti described an external approach in 1904 [1].

A number of studies comparing the success rates of external DCR and endoscopic DCR have been performed, and the results vary. Many larger studies, however, have reported similar success rates with both procedures [2–4]. In experienced hands, endonasal surgical time can be significant less than that of an external DCR [5, 6]. Although both procedures have been shown to improve tearing in patients with distal nasolacrimal duct obstructions, each has different potential benefits and adverse outcomes.

Patient Selection

Unlike external DCR, endoscopic DCR has no external incision (Tables 37.1 and 37.2). Although the majority of these incisions heal well following surgery, some people can be unhappy with the resultant scar. An endoscopic approach is often a good option in young patients where camouflaging a cutaneous scar can be difficult [7]. Likewise, patients with a history of hypertrophic scarring or keloid formation can benefit from the endoscopic approach. Unfortunately, patients with narrow nasal passageways can pose a significant challenge to the endonasal approach, unless managed simultaneously with nasal septal surgery. Since starting performing endoscopic DCR surgeries in 1990, we now do nearly all of our DCRs endoscopically.

If underlying conditions associated with chronic epiphora such as dry eye are identified, they should be treated prior to DCR. Furthermore, all patients with chronic epiphora or chronic dacryocystitis should undergo formal Jones testing. Any systemic conditions associated with increased bleeding, inflammation, or scarring should be identified. Medications associated with nasolacrimal duct obstructions, such as Taxotere, should be noted, and their duration of use should be clearly recognized. A nasal exam should also be performed to identify a deviated septum, narrow nasal passageway, or nasal pathology. Prior to endoscopic DCR, each patient should be cleared by a primary care physician for surgery with cessation of all anticoagulants.

Table 37.1 Indications for endoscopic dacryocystorhinostomy

Indications for endoscopic dacryocystorhinostomy
The patient wants to avoid any external scars
Jones testing is consistent with a nasolacrimal duct obstruction in the setting of chronic epiphora or chronic dacryocystitis

Table 37.2 Preoperative evaluation and considerations

Preoperative evaluation
Systemic conditions (Wegener's granulomatosis) and medications (Taxotere) associated with nasolacrimal dysfunction should be identified
Predisposing bleeding conditions should be identified and addressed
Jones dye testing consistent with above indications
Nasal exam to rule out tumors, other causes for obstruction, and nasal septal deviation
Clearance by primary care physician in appropriate cases
All anticoagulants should be discontinued prior to surgery if possible

R. A. Dailey (✉) · J. Murdock
Oregon Health & Sciences University, Department of Ophthalmic Plastics, Portland, OR, USA
e-mail: daileyr@ohsu.edu

J. J. Servat et al. (eds.), *Smith and Nesi's Ophthalmic Plastic and Reconstructive Surgery*,
https://doi.org/10.1007/978-3-030-41720-8_37

Surgical Equipment

The importance of the proper equipment cannot be overemphasized. A 4-mm, 0-degree endoscope is the preferred instrument because it provides excellent visualization. In young pediatric patients, a 2.7 mm, 0-degree endoscope is recommended. A bright light source, such as Xenon, is critical to successful outcomes. Likewise, a high-resolution monitor should be placed at the eye level of the primary surgeon near the head of the patient. Recently, a microdebrider (Medtronic) has been implemented in removal of the nasal mucosa, lacrimal sac flap, and even enlargement of the osteotomy with reduced injury to adjacent tissue and an improved view with simultaneous suction of perioperative bleeding [8].

Endoscopic Dacryocystorhinostomy

Oxymetazoline HCl is sprayed into the nasal passageways of each patient prior to surgery if no contraindications exist. The nasal mucosa and middle turbinate are injected with a 50:50 mixture of 1% lidocaine with 1:100,000 epinephrine and 0.5% bupivacaine. The nasal passageway is then packed with cotton pledgets soaked in 4% cocaine solution. The above interventions provide long-acting vasoconstriction and decongestion of the nasal mucosa, decreasing the risk of intraoperative and postoperative bleeding and providing optimal visualization during the procedure.

A 4-mm endoscope, or 2.7-mm endoscope in young pediatric patients, with a zero-degree angle is then introduced into the nose. The scope should be oriented to allow for clear visualization of the nasal mucosa anterior and inferior to the middle turbinate (Fig. 37.1). A Freer elevator can be used to displace the middle turbinate gently toward the septum. If the patient has a narrow nasal passageway, a self-retaining Killian nasal speculum can be used to provide a greater view.

A keratome or sickle blade is used to create an incision into the lateral nasal mucosa anterior and inferior to the middle turbinate (Figs. 37.2 and 37.3). A caudal elevator is then used to elevate the incised mucosa from the underlying bone. The mucosal flap is then removed using Weil-Blakesley forceps (Fig. 37.4). Alternatively, a microdebrider can also be used to create and remove the mucosa over the bone. Removal of the mucosal flap allows for visualization of the underlying frontal process of the maxillary bone (Fig. 37.5).

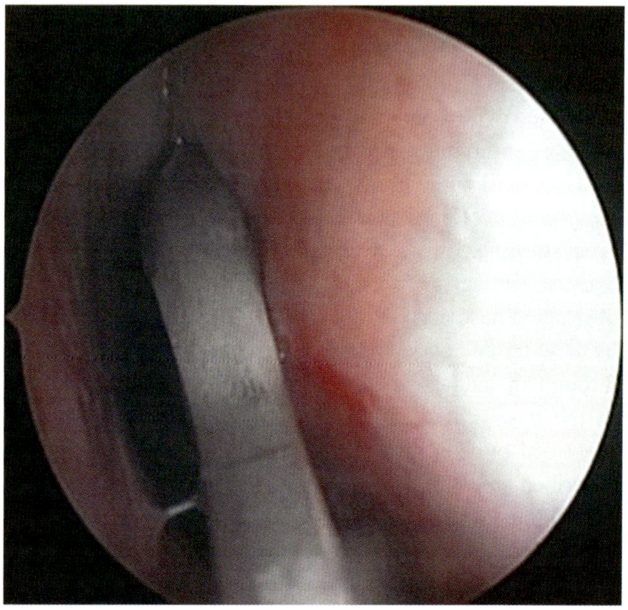

Fig. 37.2 Incision into the lateral nasal mucosa

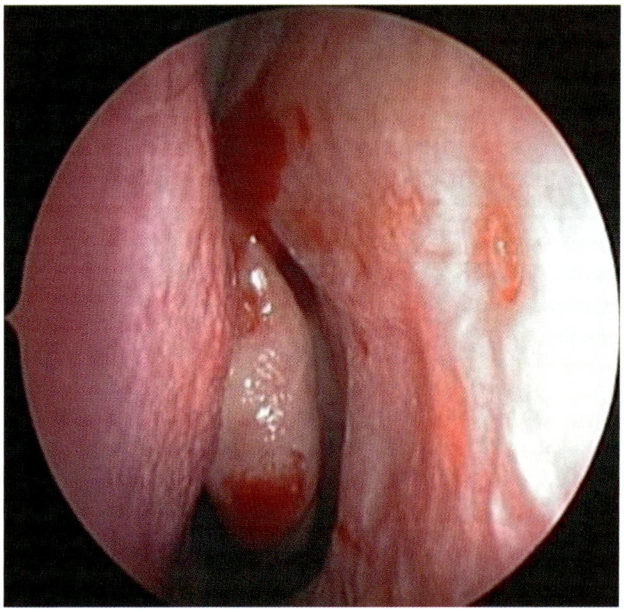

Fig. 37.1 Endoscopic view of nasal passageway

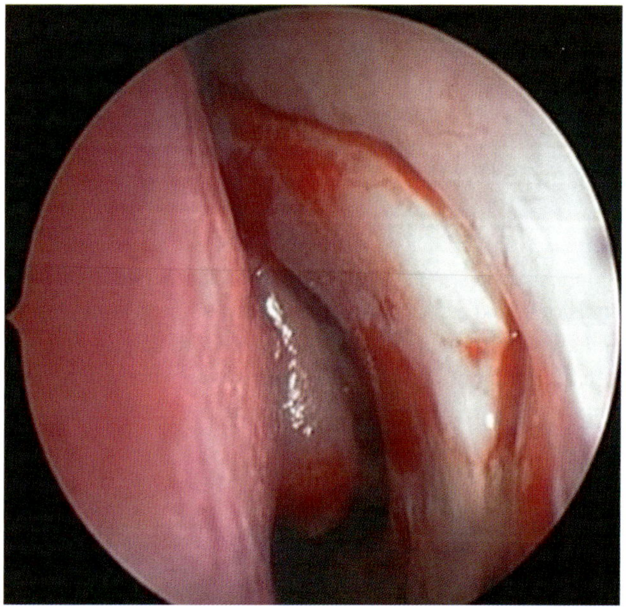

Fig. 37.3 Creation of nasal mucosal flap

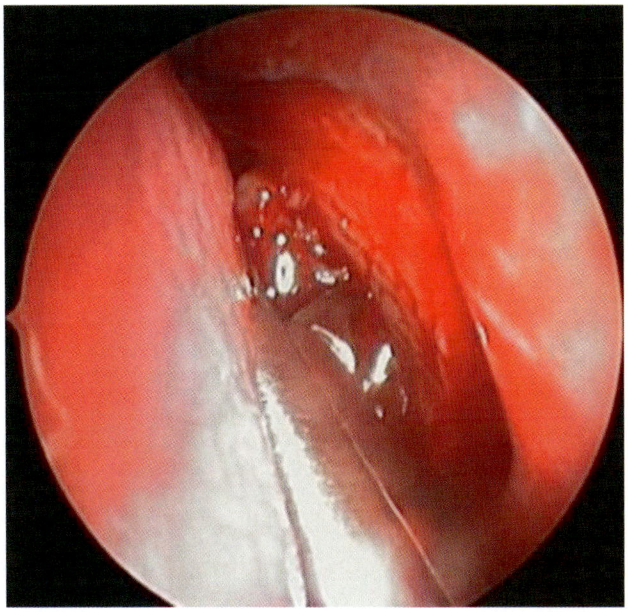

Fig. 37.4 Removal of mucosal flap with Weil-Blakesley forceps

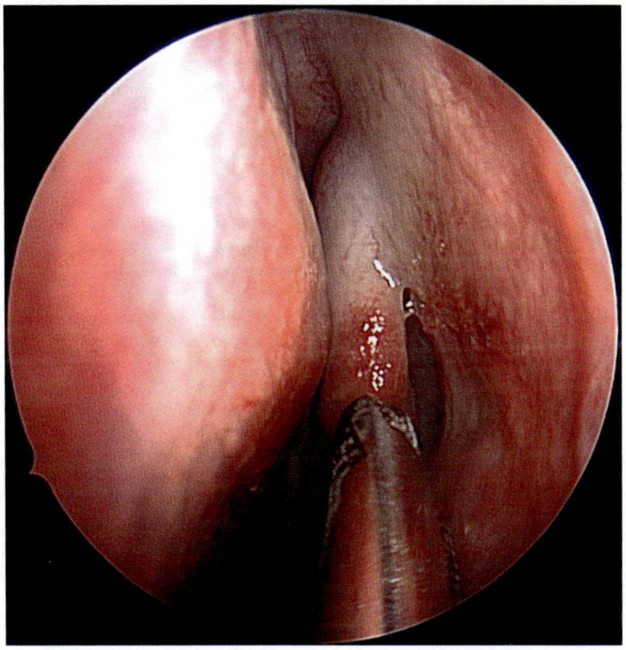

Fig. 37.5 Approach to removal of mucosa with microdebrider

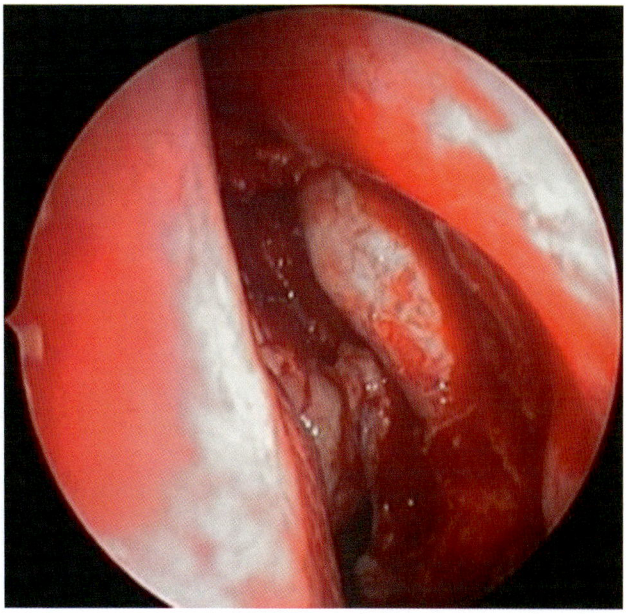

Fig. 37.6 Removal of bone to expose lacrimal sac

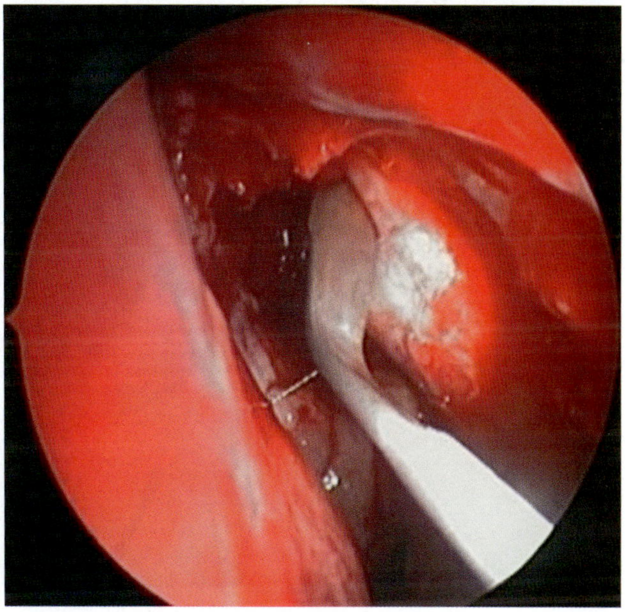

Fig. 37.7 "Tenting" of lacrimal sac with Bowman probe

A 90° Kerrison rongeur (Fig. 37.6) is then used to remove the frontal process of the maxilla and some lacrimal bone until the lacrimal sac is exposed. A high-speed diamond burr (Medtronic Xomed) can also be used to increase the osteotomy if necessary. This instrument is particularly useful superiorly where it can be difficult to remove an adequate amount of bone with the rongeur alone. The burr can also be helpful in pediatric patients [4, 9]. However, if the diamond burr is used, great care should be taken to avoid damage to the lacrimal sac or intraorbital contents. Following removal of the overlying bone, the lacrimal sac is exposed (Fig. 37.7). Ideally, the osteotomy should be large enough to expose the entire lacrimal sac.

A Jones dilator is used to dilate the upper and lower puncta. A 0 Bowman probe is then inserted into one of the canaliculi and advanced into the lacrimal sac. The lacrimal sac is then "tented" by the Bowman probe, and a keratome blade is used to open the lacrimal sac (Fig. 37.8) into anterior and posterior flaps (Fig. 37.9). The posterior portion of the

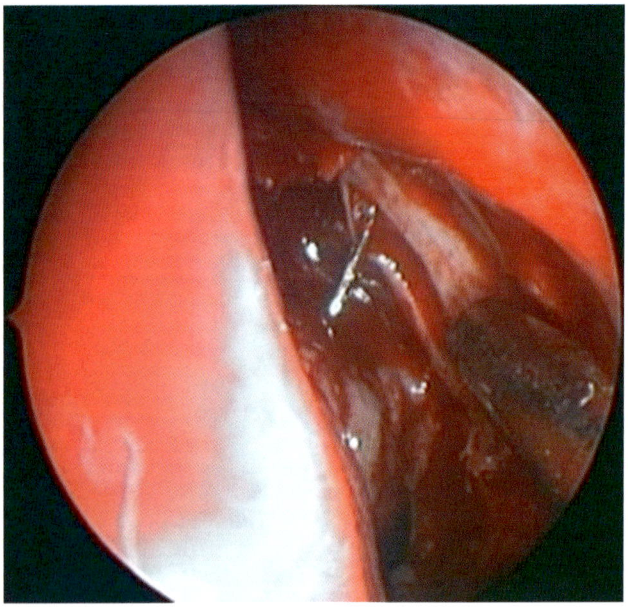

Fig. 37.8 Incision of lacrimal sac

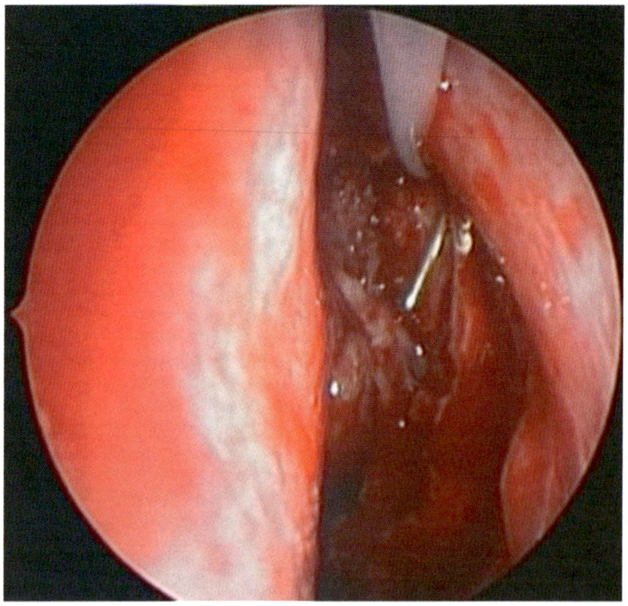

Fig. 37.10 Removal of posterior lacrimal sac flap

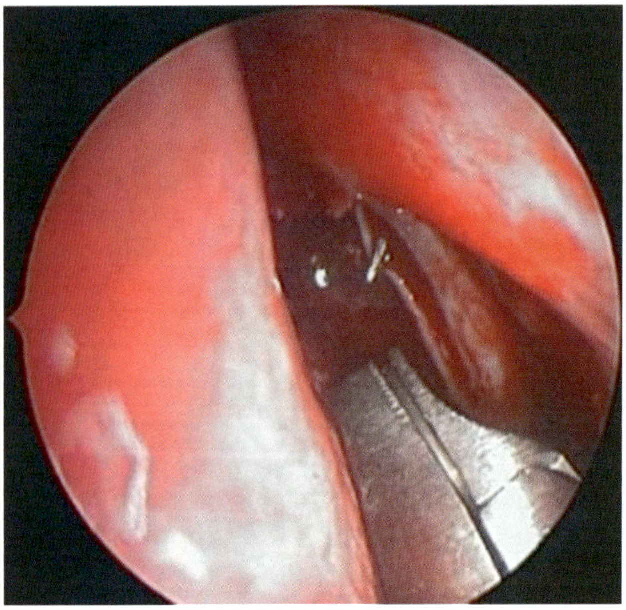

Fig. 37.9 Creation of anterior and posterior lacrimal sac flaps

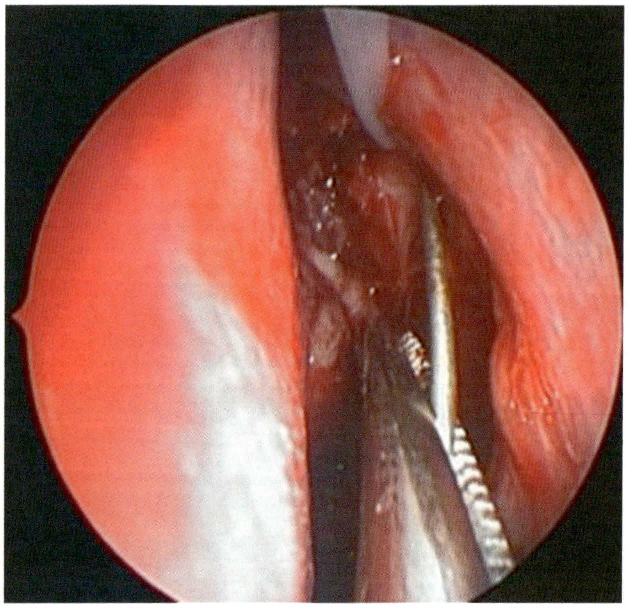

Fig. 37.11 Introduction of the silicone stents

flap is removed with "through biting" Blakesley forceps (Fig. 37.10) or microdebrider.

Silicone tubing attached to metal probes is then introduced through the upper and lower canaliculi and into the opened lacrimal sac (Fig. 37.11). The probes are retrieved through the nose with a straight hemostat or Takahashi nasal forceps individually (Fig. 37.12).

A small piece of PosiSep®, a chitosan-based hemostatic dressing and intranasal (Hemostasis LLC, Saint Paul, MN), is then inserted with bayonet forceps and placed against the osteotomy site. Local anesthetic is then injected into the body of the PosiSep to expand the dressing to provide hemostasis and prevent postoperative adhesions [10, 11] (Fig. 37.12a, b). If any significant bleeding is noted following placement of the PosiSep, Bactroban-covered Vaseline gauze should be considered for placement as an anterior nasal pack.

The metal probes are then removed from the silicone tubing. The silicone is tied in a square knot, the excess cut, and the silicone loop is allowed to recess into the nasal passageway, in a position near the inferior turbinate for easy retrieval later in a clinic setting. Following placement of the

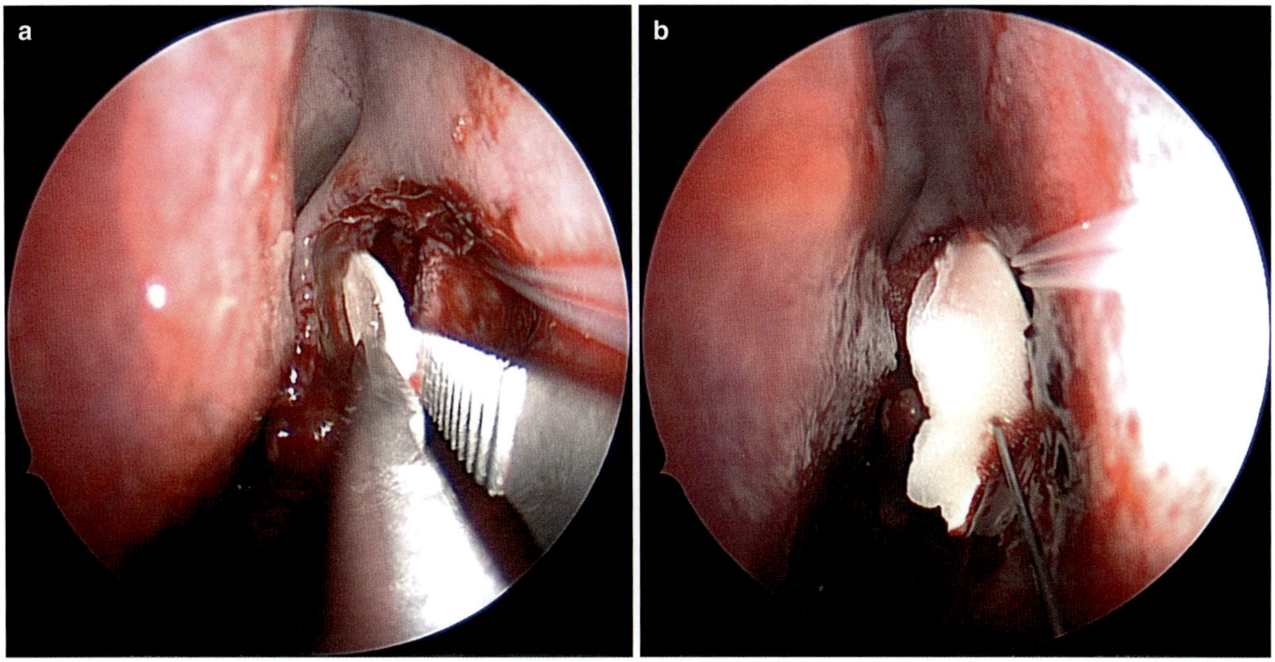

Fig. 37.12 (**a**) Retrieval of silicone stents with a straight hemostat. (**b**) Placement of PosiSep against osteotomy site for hemostasis

silicone, no significant tension should be noted at the upper and lower lid puncta. If tension is noted, the eyelids should be spread apart medially, providing some laxity of the silicone tubing in the medial canthal region. If the tension is not relieved, cheese-wiring of the silicone tubing is more likely to occur.

Postoperative Care

Following the procedure, patients are advised not to blow their nose for at least 1 week to avoid activating epistaxis. Each patient is given a narcotic for pain and asked to avoid any anticoagulants such as ibuprofen. If, however, the patient normally takes aspirin for cardiac disease, the patient is asked to coordinate continuation with their primary care physician. Furthermore, each patient is instructed to avoid bending down or lifting anything above 25 pounds for approximately 3 weeks. Postoperative antibiotics are generally only given if nasal packing other than PosiSep was utilized. Antibiotics are also used if cellulitis is present.

Complications

One of the most common complications associated with endoscopic DCR is excessive bleeding. The best management for bleeding is to prevent it from occurring in the first place. The importance of preoperative vasoconstriction, therefore, cannot be overemphasized. Likewise, cessation of anticoagulants prior to surgery is paramount. If bleeding does still occur, a Frazier suction tip allows for good visualization of the offending region. Generally, minimal bleeding will resolve on its own. Cautery is generally avoided as it tends to produce areas of loss of mucosa and intranasal adhesions for patients in the long term. When bleeding does not resolve, nasal pledgets soaked in the aforementioned local anesthetic, adrenaline, or cocaine will often control the bleeding. PosiSep can be utilized to provide excellent hemostasis in most instances. If hemostasis is still not accomplished, nasal packing can be of great value. When employed, the packing should be placed under direct visualization to ensure packing directly over the bleeding regions.

In addition to bleeding, invading adjacent structures can occur during an endoscopic DCR. Temporally, extensive dissection can result in damage to orbital tissues such as the medial rectus muscle [6]. This complication is best avoided by continually orienting oneself and cessation of dissection if any fat or muscle is identified. In order to identify these structures appropriately, excellent hemostasis is essential. Aggressive superior dissection can result in skull base injuries. This can be avoided by limiting the superior bony removal to only the region overlying the lacrimal sac. When the superior border of the lacrimal sac is in question, a light source or Bowman probe can be introduced through one of the puncta into the superior portion of the lacrimal sac. Despite careful dissection superiorly, a cerebrospinal fluid leak can still occur. In such instances, the dissection should be stopped and neurosurgical consultation should be sought.

In rare instances, extensive synechiae can occur. In patients with a history of exuberant scarring or inflammatory conditions such as Wegener's granulomatosis, mitomycin-C 0.5 mg/mL can be very beneficial [12]. Likewise, a Doyle spacer splint (Micromedics Inc., Eagan, MN) can be considered in cases that require a combined septoplasty and dacryocystorhinostomy to prevent adhesions between the two surgical surfaces.

Conclusion

Endoscopic DCR has recently been shown to have success rates comparable to external DCR. It has the advantage of no external scarring with potentially reduced surgical time. The surgical approach is often technically more challenging, especially early in the surgeon's experience, and is more difficult in patients with narrow nasal passageways [1–3, 13].

References

1. Anijeet D, Dolan L, Macewen CJ. Endonasal versus external dacryocystorhinostomy for nasolacrimal duct obstruction. Cochrane Database Syst Rev. 2011;1:CD007097.
2. Eichhorn K, Harrison AR. External vs. endonasal dacryocystorhinostomy: six of one, a half dozen of the other? Curr Opin Ophthalmol. 2010;21(5):396–403.
3. Lee DW, Chai CH, Loon SC. Primary external dacryocystorhinostomy versus primary endonasal dacryocystorhinostomy: a review. Clin Exp Ophthalmol. 2010;38(4):418–26.
4. Ali MJ, Psaltis AJ, Murphy J, Wormald PJ. Powered endoscopic dacryocystorhinostomy: a decade of experience. Ophthal Plast Reconstr Surg. 2015;31:219–21.
5. Malhotra R, Wright M, Olver JM. A consideration of the time taken to do dacryo-cystorhinostomy (DCR) surgery. Eye (London). 2003;17(6):691–6.
6. Dolman PJ. Comparison of external dacryocystorhinostomy with nonlaser endonasal dacryocystorhinostomy. Ophthalmology. 2003;110(1):78–84.
7. Caesar RH, et al. Scarring in external dacryocystorhinostomy: fact or fiction? Orbit. 2005;24(2):83–6.
8. Yoon SW, Yoon YS, Lee SH. Clinical results of endoscopic dacryocystorhinostomy using a microdebrider. Korean J Ophthalmol. 2006;20(1):1–6.
9. Pradhan P, Bhardwaj A, Mandal S, Majhi S. Double posterior based flap technique in primary endoscopic dacryocystorhinostomy with and without using powered instrument. Ind J Otolaryngol Head Neck Surg. 2017;69(4):474–9.
10. Dailey RA, Chavez MR, Choi D. Use of a chitosan-based hemostatic dressing in dacryocystorhinostomy. Ophthal Plast Reconstr Surg. 2009;25(5):350–3.
11. Hsu K, Eriksen M, Catalano P. Effect of a chitosan-based biodegradable middle meatal dressing after endoscopic sinus surgery: a prospective randomized comparative study. Dermatol Sin. 2015;1:3–12.
12. Dolmetsch AM. Nonlaser endoscopic endonasal dacryocystorhinostomy with adjunctive mitomycin C in nasolacrimal duct obstruction in adults. Ophthalmology. 2010;117(5):1037–40.
13. Huang J, Malek J, Chin D, et al. Systematic review and meta-analysis on outcomes for endoscopic versus external dacryocystorhinostomy. Orbit. 2014;33:81–90.

Endoscopic Conjunctivodacryocystorhinostomy

38

Geoffrey J. Gladstone and Jenna M. Kim

Introduction

The evaluation of a patient with excess tears involves investigating causes of excess lacrimation as well as lacrimal outflow obstruction. There are many causes of excess lacrimation, including dry eye syndrome, entropion, trichiasis, and other causes of ocular irritation. Idiopathic hypersecretion, although a diagnosis of exclusion, is an important consideration.

Preoperative Evaluation

The evaluation of a patient with excess tears involves investigating causes of excess lacrimation as well as lacrimal outflow obstruction. There are many causes of excess lacrimation, including dry eye syndrome, entropion, trichiasis, and other causes of ocular irritation [1, 2]. Idiopathic hypersecretion, although a diagnosis of exclusion, is an important consideration [3, 4].

A careful slit-lamp examination and an evaluation of the conjunctiva for signs of inflammation, symblepharon, or infection are performed. The surgeon should inspect for entropion, ectropion, trichiasis, and eyelid notching [2].

Evaluation of the outflow pathway involves probing and irrigation. Traditional Jones 1 and Jones 2 testing [5] is rarely performed. A 25-gauge lacrimal irrigating needle is used to probe the upper and lower canaliculi. Stenosis or blockage of the canaliculi is noted. Gentle irrigation of the system is attempted through the lacrimal sac. The ease of irrigation into the nasopharynx and the amount of reflux of irrigant back to the eyes are noted. Significant blockage of a canaliculus is an indication for an endoscopic conjunctivodacryocystorhinostomy (CDCR).

When considering whether to perform endoscopic CDCR, evaluation of the caruncle and medial canthus is important. There must be an appropriate place for the proximal end of the tube to rest. A previously placed medial tarsorrhaphy or other abnormality of the eyelids secondary to trauma or resection of tissue can require correction prior to the placement of the tube [6].

Nasal endoscopy must be performed to evaluate the amount of room between the septum and lateral nasal wall and the presence or absence of intranasal lesions [7]. Intranasal tumors can cause an outflow obstruction and should be treated appropriately. Benign intranasal tumors can impinge on the distal end of the tube following surgery [8]. A deviated nasal septum can make endoscopic surgery difficult or impossible [9, 10]. Additionally, the distal end of the tube must rest between the septum and the lateral nasal wall. If insufficient space is available, a septoplasty needs to be performed prior to endoscopic CDCR [9].

Gladstone–Putterman Modified Jones Tube

The original Jones tube is susceptible to internal or external migration and to ejection with nose blowing, sneezing, or coughing [11]. To alleviate these problems, an additional flange can be added to the Jones tube. This internal flange is 4 mm distal to the external flange. It acts similar to an arrowhead, locking the tube in position. This modified tube, known as the Gladstone–Putterman tube, is inserted in a similar manner as the original Jones tube [11, 12].

G. J. Gladstone (✉)
Consultants in Ophthalmic and Facial Plastic Surgery, P.C., Southfield, MI, USA

Oakland University/William Beaumont Hospital, School of Medicine, Department of Ophthalmology, Royal Oak, MI, USA

J. M. Kim
William Beaumont School of Medicine, Beaumont Eye Institute, Royal Oak, IL, USA

J. J. Servat et al. (eds.), *Smith and Nesi's Ophthalmic Plastic and Reconstructive Surgery*,
https://doi.org/10.1007/978-3-030-41720-8_38

Indications for Endoscopic CDCR

The most common indication for endoscopic CDCR is canalicular blockage [13, 14], which may be secondary to trauma [15], prior surgery, topical medications [16], or systemic chemotherapeutic agents such as 5-FU or Taxotere [17–20]. A unicanalicular or bicanalicular blockage can cause epiphora as can a significant common canalicular stenosis.

When canalicular stenosis is present, silastic intubation can be attempted. If this fails to eliminate the epiphora, then an endoscopic CDCR is indicated. With canalicular blockage, a dacryocystorhinostomy (DCR) will not be effective because the tears cannot progress to the lacrimal sac, necessitating complete bypass of the lacrimal outflow tract.

Lacrimal pump failure frequently occurs following Bell's palsy and other causes of facial paralysis [21, 22], which are common after removal of acoustic neuromas and squamous cell carcinomas. A normal probing and irrigation of the lacrimal system can be performed, but a dye retention test may be quite abnormal, with a great deal of dye remaining in the enlarged tear meniscus. Some degree of lagophthalmos, ectropion, and corneal staining is usually present [22]. It is important to consider these causes of epiphora and consider repairing or treating them before proceeding with endoscopic CDCR.

In normal patients, the lower eyelid punctum moves medially with each blink [23, 24]. This is seen most easily if the upper lid is held open and the patient is asked to blink. The absence of this movement can be an indication that an old facial paralysis is not completely resolved and that a lacrimal pump failure may be present.

The final indication for endoscopic CDCR is idiopathic hypersecretion [4]. This diagnosis of exclusion is made when the outflow tract is normal and there are no identifiable factors causing increased lacrimal gland secretion. Results from the Schirmer 1 test will be much higher than normal [25]. Referral for an external disease consultation should be considered prior to proceeding with surgery. In these cases, the modified Jones tube provides an additional and larger outflow tract to accommodate the increased tear production.

Advantages of Endoscopic Technique

Endoscopic CDCR offers a number of advantages over external CDCR. These advantages include absence of scarring, absence of ecchymosis and edema, less surgical manipulation of medial canthal tissues, and better visualization of the modified Jones tube and adjacent structures once it has been placed [26, 27]. Since no external incision is made, no external scar is created. With minimal external tissue manipulation, ecchymosis or medial canthal edema is rarely present.

With endoscopic technique, no medial canthal skin incision is necessary and no dissection of deeper tissue performed. This lack of tissue manipulation is important in the healing process, improving the chance that a properly placed modified Jones tube remains in position. With the external technique, there is a greater chance of tube displacement during healing. This change can lead to malposition of the proximal end of the tube, or the angle of the tube can be altered. It is important that the tube maintain an approximately 45° downward angle. If this angle decreases, tear drainage can also diminish.

Once the modified Jones tube is placed, endoscopic intranasal inspection of the distal end of the tube is performed. This process allows an accurate assessment of potential problems. A tube that is too short does not protrude far enough from the lateral nasal wall and is at risk for being covered by mucosa. A tube that is too long will touch the nasal septum, causing pain and leading to external tube extrusion or poor tear drainage [28]. Either of these problems is easily correctable at the time of surgery if recognized.

The relationship of the distal end of the tube to the middle turbinate is also evaluated endoscopically. The middle turbinate is often infractured at the onset of surgery to provide easier access to the uncinate process. Postoperatively, the turbinate will often assume its preoperative position and may touch the distal end of the modified Jones tube. If the surgeon believes that the shift will result in blockage of the tube, a partial turbinectomy should be performed at that time.

Surgical Technique

Thirty minutes prior to the procedure, the patient is asked to blow the nose and is then given two sprays of 0.05% oxymetazoline in the nasal cavity ipsilateral to the planned procedure. This process is repeated in 5 minutes. The majority of cases are performed under monitored intravenous sedation and local anesthesia, although some patients required general anesthesia. The nasal cavity is packed with 18 in. of 0.5 in. plain gauze soaked in 4% cocaine solution. The packing is removed after 5 minutes.

Under direct visualization with a 0° rigid endoscope, local injection of 2% lidocaine with 1:100,000 epinephrine mixed 50:50 with bupivacaine 0.75% with 1:200,000 epinephrine is administered to the submucosa of the anterior middle turbinate, uncinate process, and area anterior and superior to the uncinate. Approximately 3 cc infiltrate is applied with a 1.5-in. 25-gauge needle. The nasal cavity is repacked, carefully filling the space between the middle turbinate and the lateral nasal wall with 4% cocaine-soaked gauze for another 5 minutes. This regimen of packing is necessary to obtain adequate hemostasis. The face is draped in an appropriate fashion, but a sterile field is not required.

Under endoscopic visualization, the middle turbinate and its relationship to the lateral nasal wall are inspected. If the turbinate is obstructing the view of the uncinate process, or if the turbinate may obstruct the osteotomy site postoperatively, it may be gently infractured with a blunt periosteal elevator. The same instrument may be used to make an incision at the border of the bony lateral nasal wall and the uncinate process. The uncinate is the first protrusion of the lateral nasal wall encountered under the middle turbinate.

The mucosa overlying the lacrimal fossa is cauterized with monopolar cautery set in the coagulation mode. This area extends approximately 10 mm anterior to the uncinate process and from the level of the root of the middle turbinate superiorly and 10 mm inferiorly. The mucosa is scraped from the underlying bone with a periosteal elevator and is removed with Blakesley forceps. Thorough removal of the mucosa is important to prevent bleeding during the next step of the procedure. A medium size Kerrison bone rongeur creates an osteotomy to correspond to the area from which the mucosa was removed. The rongeur is placed onto the bony edge that was exposed following the incision of the junction between the uncinate process and the lateral nasal wall. Further bone removal proceeds superiorly and anteriorly. Usually four or five bites are needed to obtain an adequate osteotomy. At this point, the lacrimal sac can be identified.

A track for the glass tube is now created. No excision of caruncle is performed as this promotes inward migration of the modified Jones tube. A 10- or 12-gauge shielded intravenous catheter (Angiocath, BD, Franklin Lakes, NJ) is bent approximately 30° at its midpoint. A smaller 14-gauge catheter can also be used, but the passage of the Jones tube will be more difficult. Bending the catheter is intended to keep the distal end of the tube relatively anterior in the nose. The Angiocath enters the middle of the caruncle (Fig. 38.1). The shaft of the Angiocath is kept close to the eye as the catheter is advanced in a medial and inferior direction. A downward angle of 45° is attempted. The needle is visualized with the endoscope as it enters the nasal cavity. It can be redirected if necessary so it exits through the osteotomy. The metal needle is removed, leaving only the plastic sheath in position.

A 9-in.-long piece of 20-gauge wire is passed through the plastic sheath, and the sheath is removed, leaving only the wire in position (Figs. 38.2 and 38.3). The wire acts as a guide for the glass tube placement. A 4-mm by 19-mm tube is placed over the wire and pushed into proper position. When the extra flange encounters the medial canthal tissue, increased resistance will be felt. Both of the surgeon's thumbnails are place on the proximal end of the tube and used to push it firmly into position. The internal flange will lock the tube in position.

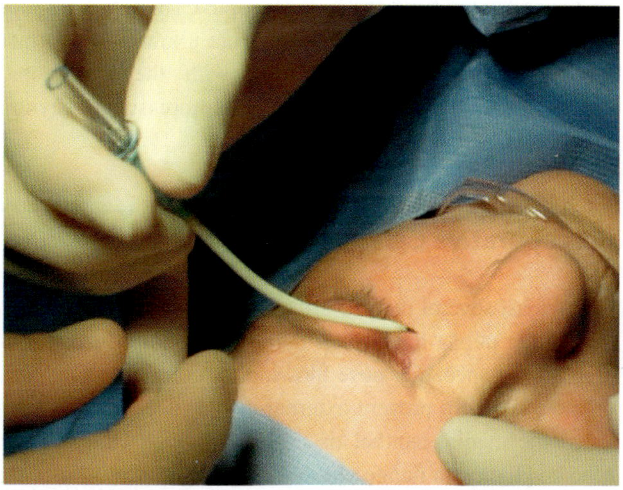

Fig. 38.1 A 12-gauge shielded intravenous catheter (Angiocath) is bent approximately 30° at its midpoint and advanced through the middle of the caruncle at a 45° angle. The catheter can be visualized entering the nasal cavity with an endoscope. (Javier Servat, MD)

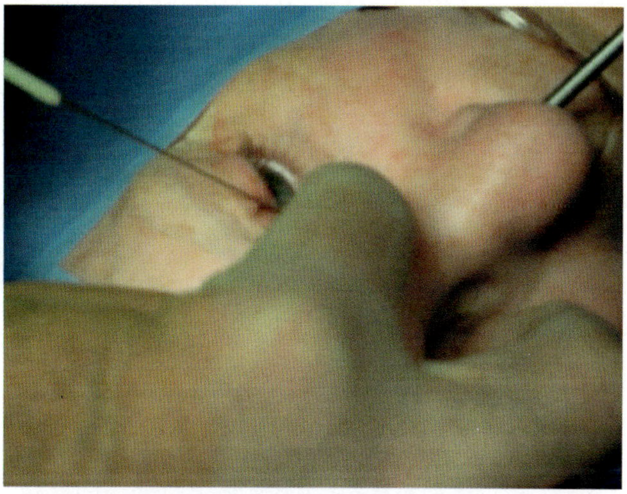

Fig. 38.2 The position of the plastic sheath is visualized inside the nose with an endoscope. (Javier Servat, MD)

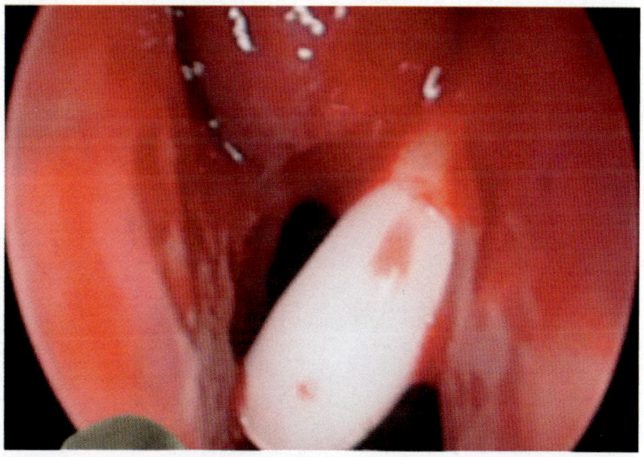

Fig. 38.3 A 9-in.-long piece of 20-gauge wire is passed through the plastic sheath, and the sheath is removed, leaving only the wire in position. The wire acts as a guide for the glass tube placement. (Javier Servat, MD)

The length and position of the tube are checked with the endoscope. The tube ideally sits halfway between the lateral nasal wall and the nasal septum (Fig. 38.4).

If the position is not appropriate, the proximal end of the tube is gently grasped with toothed forceps, and the tube is removed, leaving the guide wire in place (Fig. 38.5).

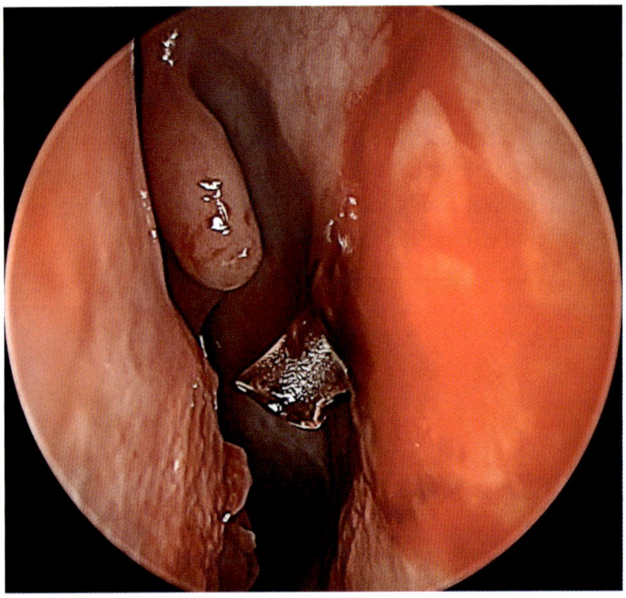

Fig. 38.4 A properly placed Gladstone-Putterman Jones tube sitting halfway between the nasal septum and the lateral nasal wall

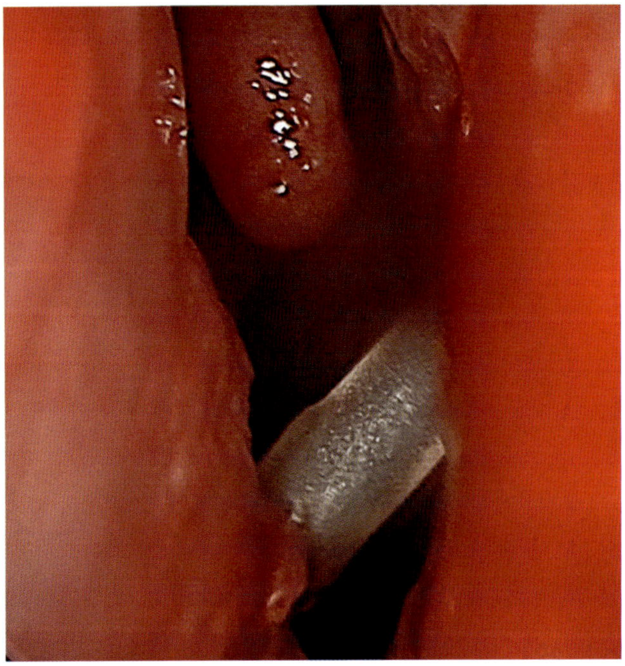

Fig. 38.5 A too long Gladstone-Putterman Jones tube that rests on the nasal septum

A tube of different lengths is inserted over the guide wire. Once an acceptable tube is placed, the guide wire is removed.

A 6-0 double-armed silk suture is wrapped twice around the proximal end of the tube. Both needles are brought from the medial side of the tube through the skin. The needles are passed through a small piece of sterile rubber band and are tied with mild tightness. This rubber band bolster and suture are removed after 1 week.

Special Surgical Considerations

After placement of the modified Jones tube, the distal end of the tube must be inspected endoscopically and its relationship to the middle turbinate appraised. If the distal end of the modified Jones tube touches the middle turbinate, this could result in external tube displacement or poor drainage of tears. To reduce the chance of this complication, a partial middle turbinectomy is performed. An additional injection of the local anesthetic mixture is given directly into the turbinate. A small curved hemostat is applied to the turbinate at the inferior border of the area to be removed. The curve of the hemostat is reversed and the instrument applied to the superior border. Care is exercised to avoid crushing the Jones tube. Ideally, the tips of the crushed areas will meet. Right and left angled endoscopic turbinate scissors are used to incise the tissue along the crushed areas. Blakesley forceps are used to gently twist and remove the section of turbinate.

An important part of the preoperative evaluation is the intranasal endoscopic examination. If a significant septal deviation is present, it will make endoscopic surgery difficult and allow insufficient room for the modified Jones tube [10]. In these situations, a septoplasty should be performed prior to the endoscopic CDCR [9]. This procedure can be performed at the time of the endoscopic CDCR, but the septum medializes better if the tissues are allowed to contract for a month before proceeding with the endoscopic CDCR. Techniques for performing a septoplasty are beyond the scope of this chapter.

Postoperative Care

For at least several months after surgery, it is important that the patient puts a finger over the tube in the medial canthal area during sneezing, nose blowing, or coughing. This precaution will help prevent external displacement of the tube. Once the medial canthal tissue has contracted around the tube and the extra flange, there exists less chance of external displacement. At a minimum, patients should be reminded to tightly close their eyes whenever they perform the above maneuvers. Nose blowing is discouraged for the first postoperative week as this may cause intranasal bleeding. After

1 week, a nasal saline rinse is used as much as desired to help cleanse the nasal cavity.

Postoperative Evaluation and Management of Complications

One of the most important aspects of postoperative evaluation is the patient's subjective evaluation of how much their epiphora has improved. This subjective evaluation is what patients consider when determining their satisfaction with the procedure.

An objective evaluation of tube function has been devised. The drainage is classified as Class I through IV. Several drops of water are place in the medial canthal area with the head tipped backward. In Class I drainage, the water drains spontaneously. In Class II drainage, the water drains with exaggerated nasal respiration. Class III drainage is present when the water will not drain with respiration, but the tube can be irrigated. Class IV drainage is present when no irrigation is possible through the tube.

When Class I or II drainage is present, the patient typically has a significant improvement in their epiphora and is usually satisfied. Class III and IV drainage problems need to be investigated and corrected; otherwise, epiphora will continue. Poor drainage can be due to many factors including displacement of the tube in an anterior or posterior direction, displacement in an internal or external direction, and blockage of the tube either externally or internally.

A tube whose proximal end is anteriorly displaced is not in position to allow entry of tears into the tube. This tube must be removed and replaced in a more posterior position. It is necessary to utilize the Angiocath and enter the caruncular tissue more posterior than the original placement. Removing the modified Jones tube can be difficult since the medial canthal tissues contract and hold the tube in position. Tying a 2-0 silk suture around the neck of the tube allows the tube to be pulled out of position without risking breaking it. Occasionally, it is necessary to use Westcott scissors to cut down to the area of the extra flange to free the tube.

A posteriorly placed tube can irritate the eye or can become blocked at its proximal end by conjunctiva. Removal of the tube and placement more anteriorly will typically be curative.

An internally migrated tube is seen more commonly when a portion of the caruncle is removed, but can occasionally occur without caruncular removal. Usually, the tube can be palpated with forceps through the overlying tissue. Westcott scissors are used to cut down to the proximal end of the tube and a 2-0 silk suture is tied around the proximal flange. This suture is used to pull the tube free. If extensive tissue manipulation is necessary to remove the tube, the canthal tissues should be allowed to heal prior to implanting another tube. Otherwise, another internal migration is likely.

External displacement of the tube places the proximal end of the tube in a position where tears cannot enter. The tube may also irritate the eye. Simple manual pressure on the proximal end of the tube may force it back into position allowing the distal flange to lock in position in the medial canthal tissue. If simple manual pressure is not adequate, endoscopic examination of the distal end of the tube is indicated. A tube that is too long can abut the nasal septum. This tube must be replaced with a tube several millimeters shorter. A tube that is too short may not be seen intranasally and should be replaced by a tube of appropriate length. If the tube abuts the middle turbinate and is obstructed, a partial middle turbinectomy should be performed. Tubes that become internally or externally displaced may benefit from the placement of a frosted Gladstone-Putterman Jones tube [26] (Fig. 38.6).

The frosting results in a rougher surface which allows the medial canthal tissues to hold the tube more securely.

A normally placed tube may have its proximal end occluded by redundant conjunctiva. An injection of the tissue with a depo steroid may be curative. If not, excision of the excess tissue can be easily performed.

Blockage of the distal end of the tube can be caused by the lateral nasal wall, the nasal septum, or the middle tur-

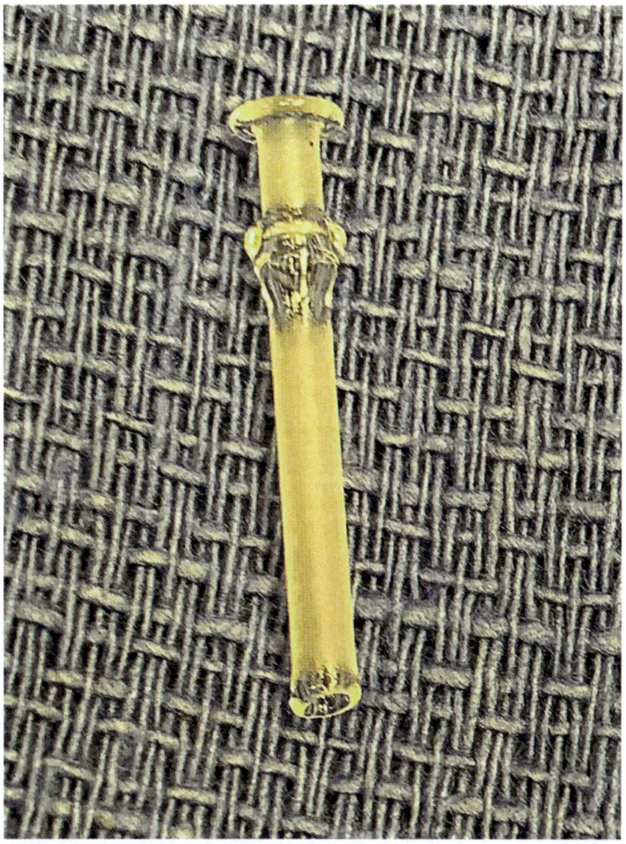

Fig. 38.6 A frosted Gladstone-Putterman Jones tube. The frosting helps prevent tube migration

binate. The treatment of these problems has been previously covered.

Occasionally, a perfectly placed and functioning tube may cause irritation of the medial canthal tissues. Topical steroid drops may resolve this condition. If not, an injection of a depo steroid can be utilized.

References

1. Boyce GH. Review of lacrymal disorders. Eye Ear Nose Throat Mon. 1946;25(11):562.
2. Tse DT, Erickson BP, Tse BC. The BLICK mnemonic for clinical-anatomical assessment of patients with epiphora. Ophthalmic Plast Reconstr Surg. 2014;30(6):450–8.
3. Clarke WN, Bastianelli F, Noel LP. Lacrimal hypersecretion in children. J Pediatr Ophthalmol Strabismus. 1987;24(4):204–6.
4. Mainville N, Jordan DR. Etiology of tearing: a retrospective analysis of referrals to a tertiary care oculoplastics practice. Ophthalmic Plast Reconstr Surg. 2011;27(3):155–7.
5. Zappia RJ, Milder B. Lacrimal drainage function. 1. The Jones fluorescein test. Am J Ophthalmol. 1972;74(1):154–9.
6. Spinelli HM, Shapiro MD, Wei LL, et al. The role of lacrimal intubation in the management of facial trauma and tumor resection. Plast Reconstr Surg. 2005;115(7):1871–6.
7. Metson R. Endoscopic surgery for lacrimal obstruction. Otolaryngol Head Neck Surg. 1991;104(4):473–9.
8. Zodpe P, Chung SW, Kang HJ, et al. Endoscopic treatment of nasolacrimal sac obstruction secondary to fibrous dysplasia of paranasal sinuses. Eur Arch Otorhinolaryngol. 2007;264(5):495–8.
9. Singh S, Alam MS, Ali MJ, Naik MN. Endoscopic intranasal findings in unilateral primary acquired nasolacrimal duct obstruction. Saudi J Ophthalmol. 2017;31(3):128–30.
10. Lee JS, Lee H, Kim JW, et al. Association of facial asymmetry and nasal septal deviation in acquired nasolacrimal duct obstruction in East Asians. J Craniofac Surg. 2013;24(5):1544–8.
11. Gladstone GJ, Putterman AM. A modified glass tube for conjunctivodacryocystorhinostomy. Arch Ophthalmol. 1985;103(8):1229–30.
12. Migliori ME, Putterman AM. Recurrent Jones tube extrusions successfully treated with a modified glass tube. Ophthalmic Plast Reconstr Surg. 1989;5(3):189–91.
13. Jones LT. Conjunctivodacryocystorhinostomy. Am J Ophthalmol. 1965;59:773–83.
14. Doucet TW, Hurwitz JJ. Canaliculodacryocystorhinostomy in the treatment of canalicular obstruction. Arch Ophthalmol. 1982;100(2):306–9.
15. Meyer DR, Kersten RC, Kulwin DR, et al. Management of canalicular injury associated with eyelid burns. Arch Ophthalmol. 1995;113(7):900–3.
16. Starks VS, Yoon MK. Acquired obliteration of the proximal lacrimal drainage system. Ophthalmic Plast Reconstr Surg. 2018;35(4):342–5.
17. Mansur C, Pfeiffer ML, Esmaeli B. Evaluation and management of chemotherapy-induced epiphora, punctal and canalicular stenosis, and nasolacrimal duct obstruction. Ophthalmic Plast Reconstr Surg. 2017;33(1):9–12.
18. Esmaeli B. Management of excessive tearing as a side effect of docetaxel. Clin Breast Cancer. 2005;5(6):455–7.
19. Esmaeli B, Hortobagyi GN, Esteva FJ, et al. Canalicular stenosis secondary to weekly versus every-3-weeks docetaxel in patients with metastatic breast cancer. Ophthalmology. 2002;109(6):1188–91.
20. Esmaeli B, Hidaji L, Adinin RB, et al. Blockage of the lacrimal drainage apparatus as a side effect of docetaxel therapy. Cancer. 2003;98(3):504–7.
21. Madge SN, Malhotra R, Desousa J, et al. The lacrimal bypass tube for lacrimal pump failure attributable to facial palsy. Am J Ophthalmol. 2010;149(1):155–9.
22. Patipa M. Ophthalmic surgical management of facial paralysis. J Fla Med Assoc. 1990;77(9):839–42.
23. Arrigg P, Miller D. A new lid sign in seventh nerve palsy. Ann Ophthalmol. 1985;17(1):43–5.
24. Shams PN, Verdick RE, Allen RC. In vivo demonstration of the lacrimal pump. Ophthalmic Plast Reconstr Surg. 2016;32(1):e25.
25. Senchyna M, Wax MB. Quantitative assessment of tear production: a review of methods and utility in dry eye drug discovery. J Ocular Biol Dis Inform. 2008;1(1):1–6.
26. Ahn ES, Dailey RA, Radmall B. The effectiveness and long-term outcome of conjunctivodacryocystorhinostomy with frosted Jones tubes. Ophthalmic Plast Reconstr Surg. 2017;33(4):294–9.
27. Trotter WL, Meyer DR. Endoscopic conjunctivodacryocystorhinostomy with Jones tube placement. Ophthalmology. 2000;107(6):1206–9.
28. Chang M, Lee H, Park M, Baek S. Long-term outcomes of endoscopic endonasal conjunctivodacryocystorhinostomy with Jones tube placement: a thirteen-year experience. J Craniomaxillofac Surg. 2015;43(1):7–10.

Nasolacrimal Duct Probing, Intubation, and Balloon Dacryoplasty

39

Peter W. MacIntosh

Introduction

Intubation of the lacrimal outflow apparatus can help maintain patency after surgical repair or in cases of partial nasolacrimal duct obstruction (NLDO). The tubing acts as a temporary stent in the canaliculi and duct, maintaining patency while the tissues around the stent heal, thereby preventing cicatricial closure. Stent placement may also be combined with dacryocystorhinostomy surgery to maintain patency of the newly created ostium.

Probing and Nasolacrimal Duct Intubation in Children

The evaluation of tearing in infants can be challenging due to lack of cooperation. Furthermore, the vast majority of congenital nasolacrimal duct obstructions resolve spontaneously by approximately 1 year of age [1–3]. As a result, there is controversy in the literature as to the optimal timing for intervention. Some studies have shown that success with nasolacrimal duct probing declines after 12–15 months of age [1], but more recent studies indicate that probing success remains high up to 4 years of age [4]. Further controversy exists regarding how to go about probing in children.

One option in infants is to probe before 6 months of age when the child is small enough to undergo probing in an office setting without general anesthesia. Advantages of early probing include avoiding general anesthesia, earlier resolution of symptoms, and reduced procedural costs. The disadvantages of early probing are the difficulty of probing an awake and uncooperative infant and performing a procedure that may have been unnecessary (due to future spontaneous resolution).

P. W. MacIntosh (✉)
University of Illinois, Ophthalmology and Visual Sciences, Chicago, IL, USA
e-mail: pmacint1@uic.edu

The other option in infants is to manage the obstruction conservatively with Crigler massage and topical antibiotics while anticipating spontaneous resolution near 12 months of age. However, if unresolved at this age, a 1-year-old is likely to require general anesthesia in an operating room with its attendant detriments and risks. The main advantages of this approach are a more controlled environment for a more successful procedure and more certainty that the procedure is indeed necessary. More confusing still, starting at 1 year of age, evidence indicates higher failure rates of probing alone in the absence of concomitant silicone intubation [1–3]; this requires a second, albeit very small, procedure to remove the tube after several months. Whether this finding is related to age itself or that these failures are related to more complicated obstruction problems than simply an imperforate valve of Hasner is not known [5]. Given the uncertainty, the best approach for each patient depends largely on the preferences and comfort level of the patient, parent, and treating physician.

Initial probing is successful in over 90% of pediatric cases if done before age 12–13 months [1–3]. If initial probing alone fails, secondary probing with silicone intubation yields a success rate of 80–90% [6, 7]. However, if during initial probing, bleeding is encountered, this may suggest injury and possible scarring of the canaliculus and/or nasolacrimal duct. In this case, silicone intubation should be considered primarily [8].

Probing and Nasolacrimal Duct Intubation in Adults

Though very successful in children with epiphora, the success of probing and silicone intubation in adults is less favorable. One study evaluated the outcome in patients with a mean age of 54.7 years and found complete resolution in 54.3%, partial improvement in 14.3%, transient improvement in 10%, and no improvement in 21.4%. However, only

J. J. Servat et al. (eds.), *Smith and Nesi's Ophthalmic Plastic and Reconstructive Surgery*,
https://doi.org/10.1007/978-3-030-41720-8_39

17% went on to elect subsequent dacryocystorhinostomy [9]. The authors further noted that their results were particularly good in patients with canalicular obstructions, which makes it difficult to interpret the data, since canalicular obstruction and NLDO are not usually grouped together and represent very different processes. Most sources conclude that nasolacrimal duct intubation (NLDI) for adult NLDO, whether partial or complete, does not yield a high success rate. Nevertheless, given the simplicity of the procedure in comparison with NLD bypass surgery (dacryocystorhinostomy), it may still be worthwhile including adult NLDI in a clinical paradigm.

Probing Technique

Probing can be done under purely local anesthesia, monitored intravenous anesthesia, or general anesthesia. Local anesthesia may consist simply of topical anesthetic eye drops or of an anterior ethmoidal block medial to the caruncle at a depth of about 1.5 cm [10]. Regardless of whether or not systemic anesthesia is administered, nasal speculum examination or nasal endoscopy should be performed to evaluate for mass lesion, nasal turbinate lateralization, or in pediatric cases intranasal dacryocystocele. Local anesthesia and vasoconstriction of the nasal mucosa are achieved by packing neurosurgical cottonoids soaked in 5% cocaine or oxymetazoline into the inferior meatus.

The puncta are first evaluated. If stenotic, they may first be gently dilated with a punctal dilator. Punctoplasty can be considered as described in Chap. 45: Surgery of the Punctum and Canaliculus. The nasal packing should now be removed.

Typically using a 00 Bowman probe, the probe is passed through the upper canaliculus starting vertically for 2 mm, then moving medially with the eyelid on lateral traction. The upper canaliculus is preferred because the angle from the horizontal canaliculus to the vertical nasolacrimal duct is less acute [11], and it avoids the risk of lower canalicular injury. Careful attention should be paid to the skin over the canaliculus for evidence of a "soft stop" which is bunching or nasalization of the skin that could indicate a stricture or stenosis of the canaliculus. If that is encountered, it is best to abort the upper canaliculus in favor of lower canalicular probing. If no "soft stop" is encountered, keep passing the probe nasally into the lacrimal sac until a "hard stop" is encountered against the lacrimal sac fossa bone. Generally, in adults, probing stops here, since probing of the nasolacrimal duct in the clinic setting is painful, and in adults less successful at achieving long-term success than in children [9, 12].

In infants, probing may continue by maintaining pressure of the probe against the lacrimal sac fossa bone as it is turned inferiorly to enter the nasolacrimal duct. There should be little resistance during this maneuver, and a sense of "crunching" or "scraping" may suggest a false passage. The probe should pass into the duct smoothly, which travels inferiorly, laterally, and posteriorly until it exits via the valve of Hasner into the inferior meatus of the nose. There may be a small amount of resistance at this valve. The probe will traverse the inferior meatus and ultimately make contact with the floor of the nose, which will create significant resistance similar to the "hard stop" in the lacrimal sac. At this point, the probe can be pulled back a few millimeters, so it is not embedded in the nasal floor mucosa. Using the other hand, the presence of the probe can be confirmed intranasally with another Bowman probe introduced via the naris until "metal on metal" contact is felt. Alternatively, a nasal endoscope can be used to visualize the instruments in the nose and reduce the risk of trauma to the nasal mucosa [13].

The process may be repeated with one or two larger sized Bowman probes. The tear outflow system should then be irrigated with balanced salt solution (BSS) to ensure patency. The BSS can be combined with fluorescein to aid visualization and then aspirated from the nose with a soft suction tip catheter to confirm patency.

Rarely, the inferior turbinate may need to be medialized if the inferior meatus is narrow or if the turbinate is fused to the lateral wall of the nose. Infracture can be accomplished using a small Freer elevator temporal and inferior to the inferior turbinate under direct visualization with a speculum and headlight. Using gentle nasal pressure, the turbinate can then be moved away from the lateral nasal wall [13, 14].

Nasolacrimal Duct Intubation Technique

Crawford

The Crawford lacrimal intubation system utilizes two flexible stainless steel wires attached to medical grade silicone tubing and a specially designed retrieval hook (Fig. 39.1a, b). Each wire has a stainless steel, olive-shaped tip that ensures atraumatic passage through the canaliculus and nasolacrimal duct and facilitates retrieval in the nose with the specialized hook.

Passage of the wires proceeds as described above for probing, starting with one wire and passing it through the upper canalicular system and into the nasolacrimal duct. The Crawford stent retrieval hook is inserted into the nose parallel to the floor of the nose and against the lateral nasal wall until "metal on metal" contact is felt. The hook should be oriented so that it can engage the olive tip of the wire. Repeated gentle pulling motion on the wire and hook will eventually engage them, and the hook can then be pulled from the nose with the wire engaged. Some surgeons prefer

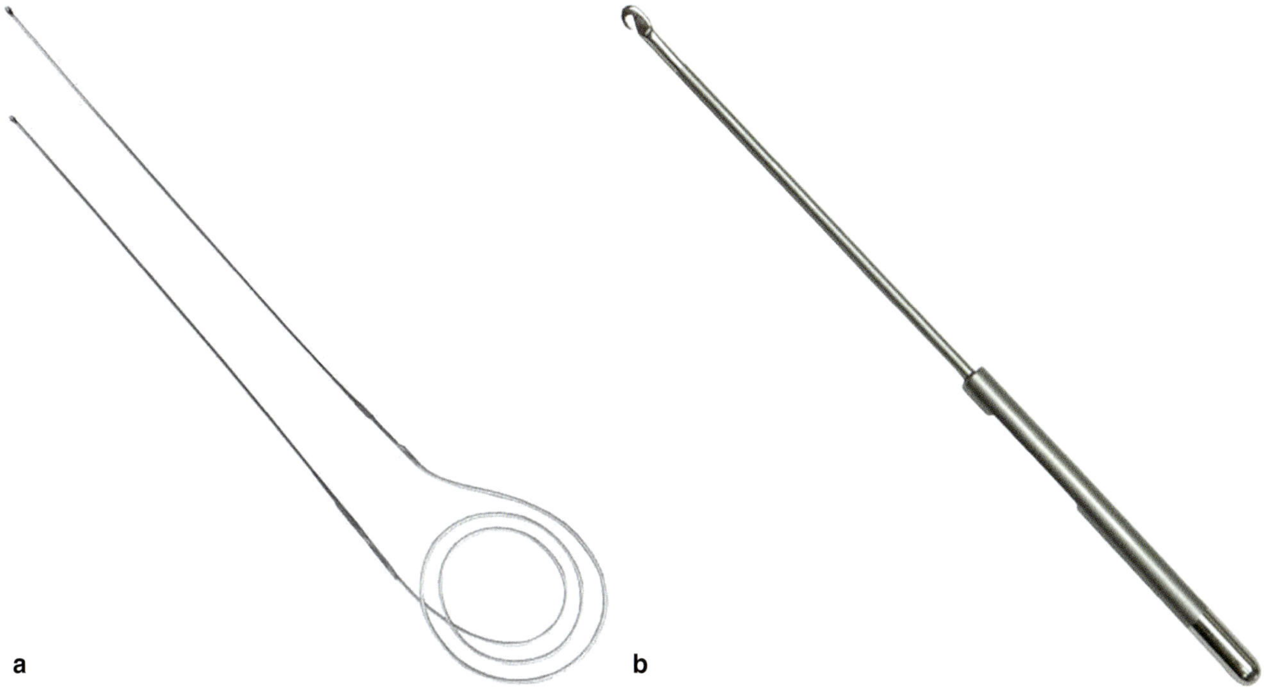

Fig. 39.1 (**a**) Crawford stent. (Image reproduced from jedmed.com). (**b**) Crawford retrieval hook. (Image reproduced from jedmed.com)

using endoscopy to visualize the instruments in the nose and reduce the risk of trauma to the nasal mucosa [13].

The same process is repeated with the other wire of the Crawford tube through the lower canaliculus. Once both ends of the tubing are retrieved from the nose, the ends should be tied together. There are several methods for anchoring the stent in the nose including suturing the stent to the lateral nasal wall, creating a hefty knot, or tying over a sleeve. One method calls for a simple square knot. This can be achieved by clamping the two silicone tubes just inside the nose with a needle driver. The flat surfaces of the needle driver prevent the silicone from inadvertently being cut by sharper-edged tools such as forceps. The knot can then be tied against the needle driver, after which the needle driver may be released to allow the knot to retract into the nose. The long tails of the silicone tubing can then be trimmed inside the nose.

The Crawford tube comes in two varieties: one bare silicone stent, which can be secured as described above, and one with a 6-0 silk suture running inside the stent. In the variety with the internal 6-0 silk suture, the silicone stent can be stripped from the suture, and the suture tied together to secure it. This knot is small enough to allow rotation of the tubing until the knot is visible between the puncta to cut and remove it. This suture was designed to allow easy removal of the Crawford tube in the office.

Postoperatively, the patient should use a steroid/antibiotic eye drop for 1 week. Generally, it is thought that the tubing should stay in longer for younger patients [8]. Under 24 months, the tube is left in for 3–6 months. Over 24 months, the tube is left in place for 6–12 months. The tubes may be left in place longer if needed. In some cases, an inflammatory response to the silicone may be seen. This can usually be quelled sufficiently with dexamethasone drops so as not to remove the stent prematurely.

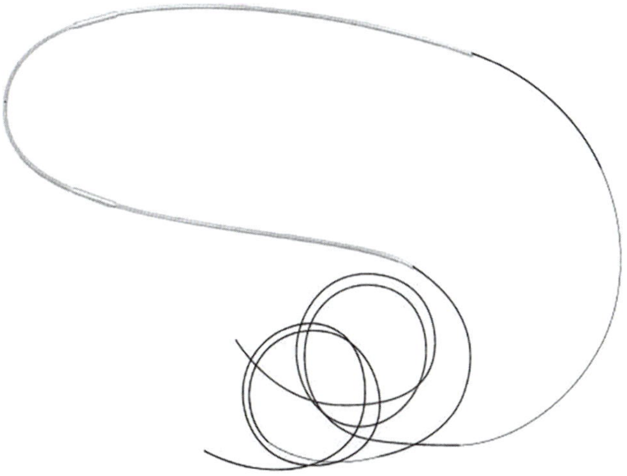

Fig. 39.2 Ritleng stent. (Image reproduced from FCI)

Ritleng

The Ritleng NLD intubation system is a novel design introduced c. 1999. Rather than passing a steel wire through the duct and nose, it employs a polypropylene leader (Fig. 39.2).

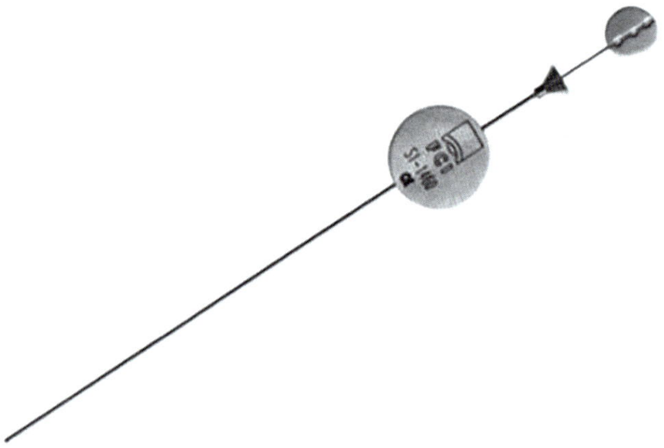

Fig. 39.3 Ritleng inserter. (Image reproduced from FCI)

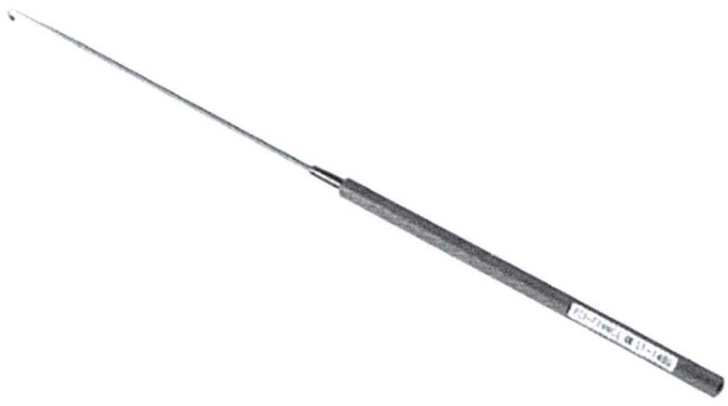

Fig. 39.4 Ritleng hook. (Image reproduced from FCI)

The stainless steel inserter contains a central groove that allows the polypropylene to escape so that the inserter can be retracted through the punctum (Fig. 39.3). The inserter is passed into the canaliculus and nasolacrimal duct in the same fashion as the Crawford stent. Once the inserter has been passed through the duct into the inferior meatus, the polypropylene leader is threaded through the introducer until several centimeters of it are looped inside the nose or exit the naris spontaneously. A special retrieving hook (Fig. 39.4) is inserted into the nose to retrieve the polypropylene fiber, which can then be pulled out of the nose pulling the silicone tubing into place. The advantage of this device is that it reduces the risk of trauma to the nasal mucosa and it is technically easier to retrieve the polypropylene thread than it is to retrieve the Crawford wire. The Ritleng comes in a bicanalicular as well as a monocanalicular variety. The latter has a special foot plate flange that sits in the punctum. The nasal end of the tubing is trimmed just inside the nose, and no knot tying is required. This tubing is easy to remove by grasping the foot plate with forceps and simply pulling it out of the punctum. There is a small risk of corneal abrasion from the large foot plate.

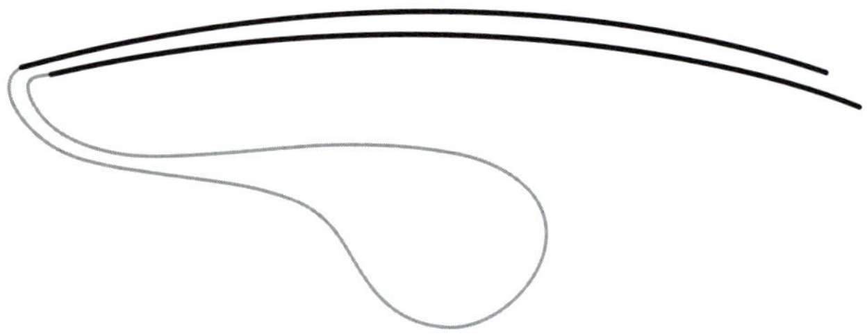

Fig. 39.5 Guibor stent. (Image reproduced from http://www.beaver-visitec.com/upload/BVI_SellSheet_Lacrimal_Duct.pdf)

Guibor and Jackson Stents

The Guibor and Jackson stents are additional stenting systems that use a stainless steel wire with a blunt end (Fig. 39.5). These are passed as described for Crawford but cannot be retrieved with a hook since it has a smooth, blunt end. Herein lies the disadvantage, as this tubing would need to be retrieved with direct visualization using nasal forceps or a grooved director. Generally, this method is less favorable than the others due to the much larger risk of trauma to the nasal mucosa and difficult retrieval technique. Guibor and Jackson stents are well suited to intubation of a dacryocystorhinostomy when indicated.

C-Line CIS

The C-Line CIS is yet another nasolacrimal system that consists of a malleable stainless steel stylet encased in a low friction nylon sheath. The stylet handles are designed to ease insertion and retraction.

Complications

Occasionally, the tubing may extrude spontaneously and present as a large loop between the puncta. Patients should be warned of this possibility in advance. Should this occur, the patient should be instructed to tape it to the side of the nose and come to the clinic as soon as possible. Unfortunately, the tubing is nearly impossible to push back down the nasolacrimal duct since the duct diameter is too small and the tubing too flexible to permit it to slide down easily. The tubing generally must be removed. However, the tubing can often be identified under nasal endoscopy, grasped, and pulled down into position. This complication can be mitigated by fixating the tubing to the lateral nasal mucosa with a loosely tied 4-0 vicryl suture on a P-2 needle [8]. The tubing can still be removed via the punctum, since the vicryl will dissolve by the time for removal, or the tubing will simply rotate out of the loosely tied vicryl suture if it is not yet dissolved. If the tubing is tied too tight in the nose, it may cause stretching or laceration of the puncta.

Tube Removal

The advantage of the single square knot to tie the tubing together inside the nose is that this knot is small enough to be pulled out via the punctum. When it is time to remove the tubing, the tube should be grasped between the puncta with fingers or a needle driver to rotate the knot into view via the upper canaliculus between the two puncta. Once the knot is visualized, the tubing can be cut and removed. If the tubing is cut before the knot is visualized, there is a risk it could break off in the nasolacrimal duct or lacrimal sac and be irretrievable and a source of obstruction in the future. Tube removal can often be done in the office with topical anesthesia, even in young children. Alternatively, the stent can be removed transnasally with endoscopic guidance. Rarely, a trip to the operating room with general anesthesia may be required if the patient is uncooperative and the tubing cannot safely be removed in the office.

Balloon Dacryoplasty

Balloon catheter dilatation of the lacrimal drainage system offers an alternative to silicone intubation and can be considered after failure of simple probing and irrigation with or without prior intubation of congenital nasolacrimal duct obstruction [15]. It can also be considered in adult patients with partial nasolacrimal duct obstruction. The system consists of a catheter with an inflatable polyurethane balloon near the tip (Fig. 39.6). Two black markings proximally on the catheter, one at 10 mm and another at 15 mm, indicate how far to insert the catheter into the nasolacrimal system (Fig. 39.7). The catheter balloon comes in two sizes: 2 mm and 3 mm. Generally, 2 mm is recommended for younger patients under 2 years of age, while the lager 3 mm is for older patients and adults.

The procedure starts similar to silicone intubation with packing of the inferior meatus with cocaine or oxymetazoline-soaked neurosurgical cottonoids and evaluation and dilation of the puncta. The cottonoids are removed and the upper and lower canaliculi should be probed as described above in order to evaluate the canaliculi and nasolacrimal duct and to break open the presumably closed valve of Hasner.

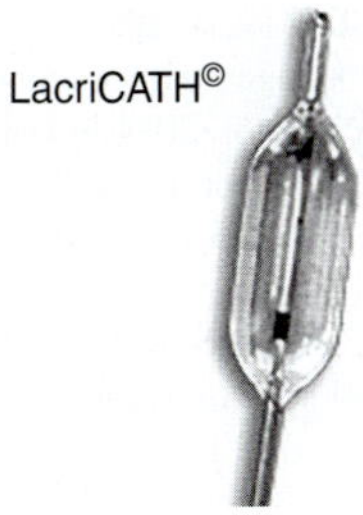

Fig. 39.6 Balloon catheter tip. (Image reproduced from Quest Medical)

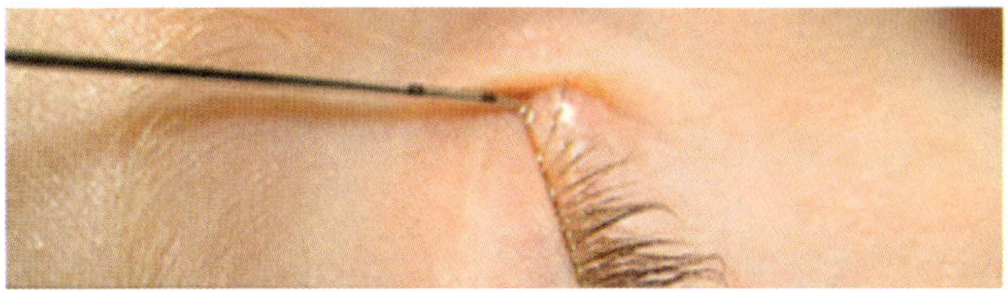

Fig. 39.7 Balloon inserted to the 10-mm mark. (Image reproduced from AAO website)

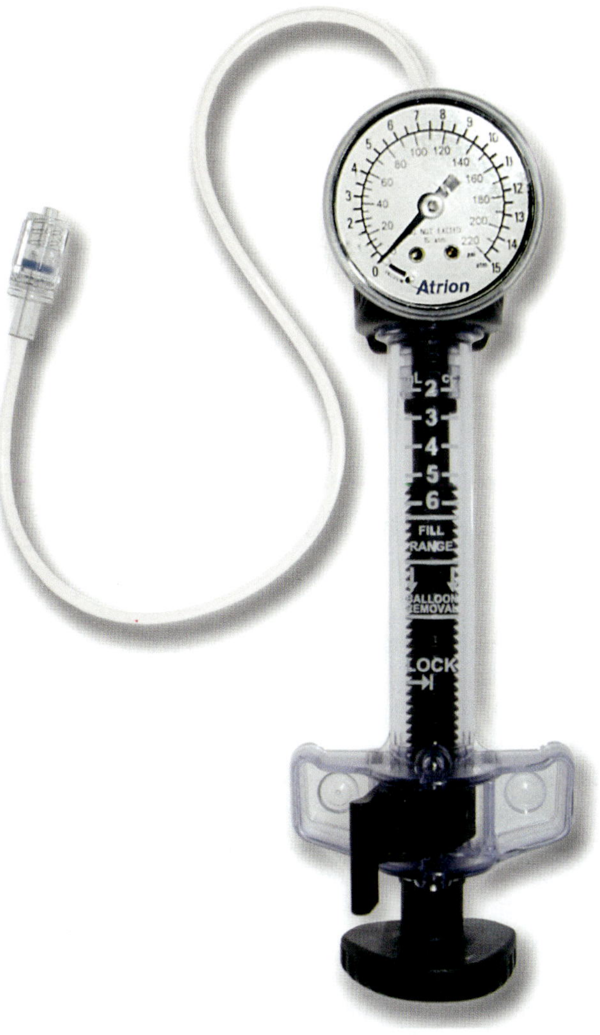

Fig. 39.8 Balloon catheter system. (Image reproduced from Quest Medical)

Once probing is complete, the balloon catheter can be prepared. It is first primed with balanced salt solution (BSS). It should then be connected to the inflator (Fig. 39.8) to confirm it inflates correctly to 8 atmospheres (atm) of pressure. Once confirmed, it is deflated and disconnected from the inflator. Next, the catheter is lubricated with lacrimal lubricant. Ensuring the balloon is completely deflated, it is inserted into the upper canaliculus and advanced into the nasolacrimal duct in a method similar to standard probing

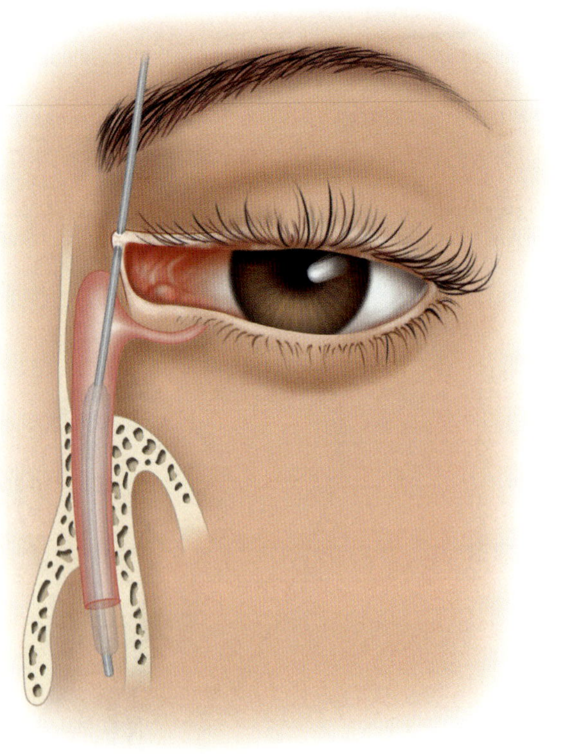

Fig. 39.9 Balloon at valve of Hasner. (Image reproduced from Quest Medical)

described above. The catheter is advanced to the 15-mm mark, which places the balloon at the valve of Hasner (Fig. 39.9). The catheter is then connected to the inflator and is inflated to 8 atm for 90 seconds. Gentle traction on the catheter ensures it is in position. Inadequate pressure or slippage of the catheter suggests malfunction, and it should be replaced. After 90 seconds, the balloon is deflated and then reinflated to 8 atm for another 60 seconds and then deflated again [15].

Next, the catheter is retracted to the 10-mm mark. This position aligns the balloon to the level of the nasolacrimal duct. The same steps of inflation and deflation are repeated as described above: 8 atm for 90 seconds, deflation, then 8 atm for 60 seconds, then deflate. Once the last deflation is completed, the catheter can be removed with a gentle twisting motion to prevent trauma to the duct and canaliculus. Once removed, the tear drain system is irrigated with BSS [15]. Silicone intubation at this point is optional, but one of the advantages of balloon dacryoplasty is that it has a high success rate in older children, even without tube placement, so it can eliminate the risk of accidental tube dislodgement and subsequent tube removal.

Postoperative steroid eye drops should be given three times daily for a week. The procedure is typically very well tolerated, without the need for special postoperative analgesics.

The success of balloon dacryoplasty has been evaluated in adults and is not as encouraging as in children. One study on patients with a mean age of 47 years found epiphora decreased at 7 days postoperative in 56% of patients but at 2 months another 45% of those were no longer patent [16]. Some authors have suggested the use of balloon dacryoplasty to treat a stenotic dacryocystorhinostomy.

References

1. Katowitz JA, Welsh MG. Timing of initial probing and irrigation in congenital nasolacrimal duct obstruction. Ophthalmology. 1987;94(6):698–705.
2. Koke MP. Treatment of occluded nasolacrimal ducts in infants. Arch Ophthalmol. 1950;43:750–4.
3. Robb RM. Probing and irrigation for congenital nasolacrimal duct obstruction. Arch Ophthalmol. 1986;104:378–789.
4. Robb RM. Success rates of nasolacrimal duct probing at time intervals after 1 year of age. Ophthalmology. 1998;105(7):1307–9.
5. Kushner BJ. Correspondence: balloon catheter dilatation for treatment of congenital nasolacrimal duct obstruction. Am J Ohpthalmol. 1996;122(4):598–9.
6. Dortzbach RK, France TD, Kushner BJ, Gonnering RS. Silicone intubation for obstruction of the nasolacrimal duct in children. Am J Ophthalmol. 1982;94(5):585–90.
7. Goldstein SM, Goldstein NB, Katowitz, JA. Monocanalicular stenting and balloon dacryoplasty following failed probing for congenital nasolacrimal duct obstruction. ASOPRS Annual Meeting, 2001.
8. Kherani F, Katowitz JA, Goldstein SM. Update on congenital nasolacrimal duct obstruction. Tech Ophthalmol. 2003;1(2):114–8.
9. Fulcher T, O-Connor M, Moriarty P. Nasolacrimal intubation in adults. Br J Ophthalmol. 1998;82:1039–41.
10. Robinson R, Turner N, Brettle P, Chell RP, Chavda SV, Murray PI. The treatment of epiphora with balloon dacryocystoplasty. Eye. 1993;7:687–90.
11. Hakim OM. A novel management for congenital nasolacrimal duct obstruction. Tech Ophthalmol. 2005;3(4):188–94.
12. Katowitz JA. Lacrimal drainage surgery, Ch 11. In: Duane TD, editor. Clinical ophthalmology, vol. 5. Philadelphia: Lipincott Co; 1983. p. 1–32.
13. Silbert DI. Evaluation and treatment of the pediatric tearing patient. Tech Ophthalmol. 2008;6(1):24–30.
14. Hakim OM. A novel management for congenital nasolacrimal duct obstruction. Tech Ophthalmol. 2011;9(4):175–80.
15. Becker BB, Berry FD, Koller H. Balloon catheter dilatation for treatment of congenital nasolacrimal duct obstruction. Am J Ophthalmol. 1996;121:304–9.
16. Song H, Ahn H, Park C, Kwon S, Kim C, Choi K. Complete obstruction of the nasolacrimal system. Radiology. 1993;186:367–71.

Transcanalicular Laser-Assisted Dacryocystorhinostomy

40

Dianne Marie-Boesch Schlachter and Evan H. Black

Introduction

Advances in endoscopic and fiberoptic technology have led to the development of innovative, minimally invasive approaches for lacrimal surgery. Lacrimal endoscopy, endocanalicular drilling, trephination, electrocauterization, and endocanalicular laser-assisted dacryocystorhinostomy (ELADCR) are techniques being used to treat nasolacrimal duct obstruction. In the endocanalicular laser-assisted DCR, a laser fiberoptic probe (Fig. 40.1) is inserted in the punctum and advanced along the canaliculus to the nasolacrimal sac. Once in the sac, the laser is used to make the osteotomy between the sac and middle meatus. Advantages of the ELADCR approach include avoidance of an external scar, improved hemostasis, limited intranasal instrumentation and tissue dissection, decreased operative time, and presumably faster recovery. A variety of lasers have been used in this method, including the argon laser, the holmium (HO):YAG laser, the potassium titanyl phosphate (KTP):YAG laser, the neodymium (Nd):YAG laser, the erbium (Er):YAG laser, and more recently, the diode laser [1–7]. The diode laser, with a 600-micron fiberoptic probe, is a portable, semiconductor contact laser of 810 nm wavelength that achieves efficient tissue dissection and instant vaporization. The laser coagulates blood vessels with minimal damage to adjacent structures, giving surgeons an alternative method for DCR surgery.

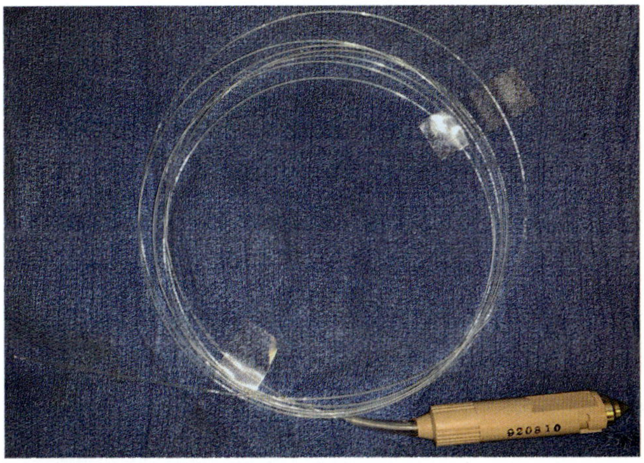

Fig. 40.1 Laser fiberoptic probe. (Courtesy of John Nguyen)

Selection of Patients

The endocanalicular approach is ideal for patients who are concerned about external scarring, as well as those with blood dyscrasias or cannot be taken off anticoagulating/antiplatelet agents. As with other endoscopic DCR techniques, a careful preoperative evaluation with intranasal endoscopy should be performed to assess the intranasal anatomy and exclude nasal pathologies such as polyps or a deviated septum that could make surgery challenging. Relative contraindications to ELADCR include suspected dacryolith, canalicular or common canalicular obstruction, canaliculitis, lacrimal sac tumor, and intranasal mass.

Description of Procedure

Thirty minutes prior to arriving in the operating room, two doses of oxymetazoline 0.05% nasal spray are administered to the ipsilateral nostril. The procedure is performed under

D. M.-B. Schlachter
Consultants in Ophthalmic and Facial Plastic Surgery, P.C., Southfield, MI, USA

Oakland University/William Beaumont Hospital School of Medicine, Department of Ophthalmology, Royal Oak, MI, USA

E. H. Black (✉)
Consultants in Ophthalmic and Facial Plastic Surgery, P.C., Southfield, MI, USA

Wayne State University School of Medicine/Kresge Eye Institute, Detroit, MI, USA

Oakland University/William Beaumont Hospital School of Medicine, Department of Ophthalmology, Royal Oak, MI, USA

J. J. Servat et al. (eds.), *Smith and Nesi's Ophthalmic Plastic and Reconstructive Surgery*,
https://doi.org/10.1007/978-3-030-41720-8_40

local anesthesia with intravenous sedation or general anesthesia. The operative side of the nose is packed with neuropaddies soaked in 4% cocaine solution placed in the middle meatus. This packing is left in place for 5 minutes and removed. A 0- or 30-degree rigid 4-mm nasal endoscope is then inserted into the nasal cavity. The middle turbinate, uncinate process, and lateral nasal wall anterior to the middle turbinate are injected with a 50/50 mixture of 2% lidocaine with epinephrine 1:100,000 and 0.5% bupivacaine with epinephrine 1:100,000. The area is repacked with cocaine-soaked neuropaddies for an additional 5 minutes. Laser-protective corneoscleral shields are inserted over both eyes.

After the packing is removed, infracture of the middle turbinate can be performed with a periosteal elevator in cases of an unusually narrow middle meatus. Infracture of the middle turbinate can improve exposure and protect the turbinate from the laser probe. The superior and inferior punctae are dilated with a punctal dilator. The 600-micron Multidiode™ fiber optic (Multidiode Endo Laser™) is then passed through the inferior punctum and fed through the canalicular system until a hard stop is felt at the medial wall of the lacrimal sac. The nasal endoscope, attached to a video monitor, is then placed into the nasal cavity. The light on the nasal endoscope is turned down in order to visualize the aiming beam of the laser as it illuminates the lateral nasal wall. Once the light appears to be in adequate position, the laser is placed on a continuous wave/pulse setting at 10 watts of power to create an osteotomy (Fig. 40.2). The power is then decreased to 5–8 watts, and the osteotomy is enlarged to prevent sump effect and stenosis of the osteotomy (Fig. 40.3). The laser is then carefully withdrawn after verifying that laser power is deactivated. Silicone tubes are then passed through the inferior

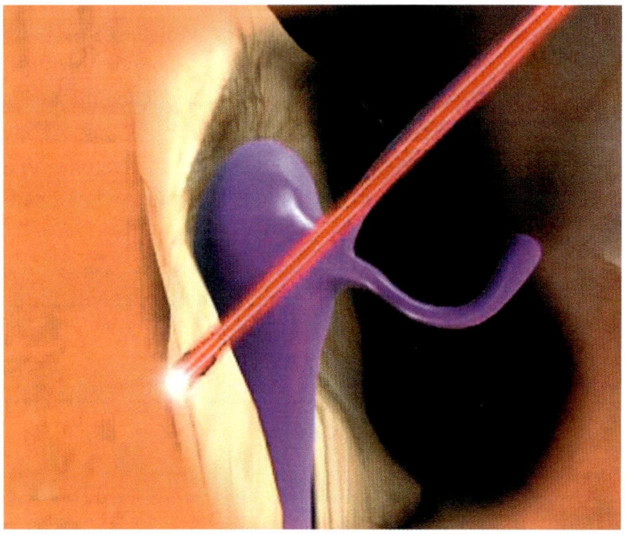

Fig. 40.2 Diagram of the laser probe placed on a continuous wave/pulse to create an osteotomy

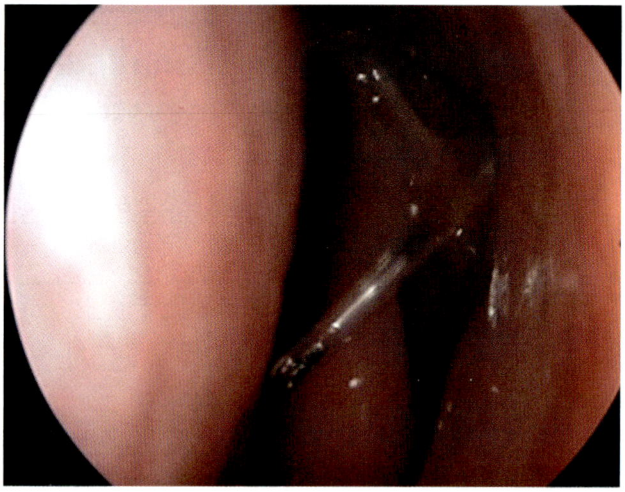

Fig. 40.3 Intranasal visualization of the laser probe. (Courtesy of John Nguyen)

and superior canaliculi and retrieved within the nose. The tubes may be tied as a single square knot and sutured to the lateral nasal wall with 6-0 vicryl.

Postoperative Care

A combined solution of topical antibiotic and steroid eye drops are used four times a day in the operative eye for 2 weeks. If nasal bleeding is present, 0.05% oxymetazoline nasal spray is recommended twice a day during the first 24–48 hours. The patient is examined at routine follow-up appointments, and the silicone tubes are typically removed in the office after approximately 3 months, when ostium contraction has presumably stabilized.

Outcomes

The success rates of surgical procedures to correct nasolacrimal duct obstruction vary depending on the technique used. The procedure thought to be associated with the highest success remains the external DCR, with success rates in the literature between 80% and 100% (majority around 90%) [8–10]. The success rates for the ELADCR are also variable, with efficacy rates in the literature between 60% and 90% [1, 2, 4, 5, 7, 11–13]. With the recent prospective study [13] indicating a 1-year success rate of 74%, the procedure in its current state is generally not used for primary DCR. Studies have suggested that there may be a role for intraoperative use of mitomycin C during endocanalicular laser-assisted DCR; however, there is not enough clinical evidence to support its continued use at this time [4, 6]. The endocanalicular laser-assisted DCR can be used for revision DCR or as a primary DCR technique for patients who are unable to discontinue antiplatelet and/or anticoagulant medications.

References

1. Cintra PP, Anselmo-Lima WT. Endocanalicular diode laser-assisted dacryocystorhinostomy. Otolaryngol Head Neck Surg. 2008;139(1):159–61.
2. Drnovsek-Olup B, Beltram M. Transcanalicular diode laser-assisted dacryocystorhinostomy. Indian J Ophthalmol. 2010;58(3):213–7.
3. Eloy P, Trussart C, Jouzdani E, Collet S, Rombaux P, Bertrand B. Transcanalicular diode laser assisted dacryocystorhinostomy. Acta Otorhinolaryngol Belg. 2000;54(2):157–63.
4. Henson RD, Henson RG Jr, Cruz HL Jr, Camara JG. Use of the diode laser with intraoperative mitomycin C in endocanalicular laser dacryocystorhinostomy. Ophthal Plast Reconstr Surg. 2007;23(2):134–7.
5. Hong JE, Hatton MP, Leib ML, Fay AM. Endocanalicular laser dacryocystorhinostomy analysis of 118 consecutive surgeries. Ophthalmology. 2005;112(9):1629–33.
6. Maeso RJ, Sellares Fabres MT. Trans-canalicular diode laser dacryocystorhinostomy: technical variations and results. Acta Otorrinolaringol Esp. 2007;58(1):10–5.
7. Plaza G, Betere F, Nogueira A. Transcanalicular dacryocystorhinostomy with diode laser: long-term results. Ophthal Plast Reconstr Surg. 2007;23(3):179–82.
8. Shun-Shin GA, Thurairajan G. External dacryocystorhinostomy--an end of an era? Br J Ophthalmol. 1997;81(9):716–7.
9. Tarbet KJ, Custer PL. External dacryocystorhinostomy. Surgical success, patient satisfaction, and economic cost. Ophthalmology. 1995;102(7):1065–70.
10. Warren JF, Seiff SR, Kavanagh MC. Long-term results of external dacryocystorhinostomy. Ophthalmic Surg Lasers Imaging. 2005;36(6):446–50.
11. Alanon Fernandez FJ, Alanon Fernandez MA, Martinez FA, Cardenas LM. Transcanalicular dacryocystorhinostomy technique using diode laser. Arch Soc Esp Oftalmol. 2004;79(7):325–30.
12. Narioka J, Ohashi Y. Transcanalicular-endonasal semiconductor diode laser-assisted revision surgery for failed external dacryocystorhinostomy. Am J Ophthalmol. 2008;146(1):60–8.
13. Schlachter DM, Richani K, Black EH. Diode laser-assisted endocanalicular dacryocystorhinostomy: a prospective study. Ophthal Plast Reconstr Surg. 2016;32(3):183–6.

Management of the Failed Dacryocystorhinostomy

41

Adam J. Cohen

Introduction

Symptomatic tearing or dacryocystitis following lacrimal bypass fistula creation (dacryocystorhinostomy (DCR)) can stem from multiple causes. Careful and thoughtful evaluation will help eliminate more obvious surgical related issues or point toward a secondary etiology that may or may not have existed prior to DCR.

Cicatricial closure of the ostium, poorly sized osteotomy, and incomplete opening of the lacrimal sac are the most common causes of DCR failure. Additionally, common canalicular obstruction, intranasal synechiae, incomplete opening of the lacrimal sac (sump syndrome), and DCR fistula malposition can also contribute to failed surgical outcomes.

A multifactorial tearing process may exist in some instances in patients who have underwent DCR but have persistent symptoms.

A nasolacrimal duct obstruction (NLDO) coupled with decreased tear pump function or hypersecretory state may exist. Although a patent fistula may exist, lower eyelid laxity or malposition, or decreased orbicularis oculi function all may contribute to tear pump insufficiency resulting in functional failure of a patent ostium. In these cases, a thorough eyelid examination prior to surgery may find eyelid signs consistent with tear pump dysfunction warranting lower eyelid tightening and/or repositioning during DCR.

Tear production testing and observing the patient for signs of dry eye prior to surgery may find a dry eye syndrome, ocular surface disorders, or gustatory tearing resulting in a secondary hypersecretory state and the need for treatment with ocular lubricants and the latter with botulinum toxin.

In some cases, patients are misdiagnosed with NLDO and the tearing is secondary to punctal or canalicular abnormalities such as canaliculitis or abnormal punctal apertures.

A. J. Cohen (✉)
Eyelid and Facial Plastic and Reconstructive Surgery, Glenview, IL, USA
e-mail: acohen@theaertofeyes.com

External versus endoscopic approaches to DCR have reported similar success rates. Of note is the lack of support against or for mucosal flaps during surgery. Given that most endoscopic approaches do not create flaps for primary intention, one could argue that flaps have limited value during fistula creation.

Also, certain autoimmune processes and lymphoma can increase surgical failure secondary to robust inflammation and scarring. Medical treatment should be maximized for quiescence of Wegener's granulomatosis, sarcoidosis, IgG4, and vasculitides prior to surgery to reduce DCR failure rates and intraoperative hemorrhage.

Surgical success in DCR is typically defined as resolution of symptoms (tearing, infection) and signs (increased tear lake, delayed dye disappearance, obstructed lacrimal irrigation). For *primary* external and endoscopic DCR, failure rates have been reported to be 5–10% or less [1, 2] and 20–40% [1, 2], respectively. Not surprisingly, the failure rate is somewhat higher with reoperation by any surgical approach. Several authors have reported lower failure rates for primary endoscopic DCR [3], but most studies have shown endonasal DCR, utilizing a variety of techniques, to carry a higher failure rate than external DCR, particularly when laser assisted. The success rate in DCR via the transcanalicular approach has been reported to be 81–83% [4, 5].

The most common causes of DCR failure are occlusion of the rhinostomy site by fibrosis, canalicular obstruction (especially at the common canaliculus) [6], cicatricial closure of the bony ostium, formation of synechiae between the ostium and the middle turbinate or the nasal septum, incomplete opening of the lacrimal sac at the time of surgery ("sump syndrome"), misdirected tear drainage into the ethmoid sinus (malpositioned DCR fistula), and granuloma formation at the ostium [6, 7].

Since flaps have not been proven to increase surgical success rate in external DCR [8], it is unclear whether or not the absence of mucosal flaps predisposes the patient to rhinos-

J. J. Servat et al. (eds.), *Smith and Nesi's Ophthalmic Plastic and Reconstructive Surgery*,
https://doi.org/10.1007/978-3-030-41720-8_41

tomy closure. Nevertheless, it has been suggested that the lack of flaps might be one reason for higher failure rates in endonasal DCR. Higher than average anatomic and functional success rates (91–98%) have been reported with the endonasal technique when a larger ostium and mucosal flaps were employed [9, 10]. The creation of mucosal flaps allows juxtaposition of the nasal and lacrimal sac mucosa, permitting primary intention rather than secondary intention healing, with theoretically less wound contracture at the site of the DCR fistula.

Prolonged postoperative silicone stent placement has been purported to increase the risk of surgical failure [11], although others have found silicone intubation during DCR to have no positive or negative impact on the surgical success rate [12, 13]. Hence, the benefits of silicone intubation in routine DCR are debated [14].

In general, there are several categories of patients who have undergone DCR and have persistent or recurrent tearing postoperatively. The first category includes those who were misdiagnosed with nasolacrimal duct obstruction (NLDO) preoperatively and instead have a different etiology of their tearing, such as canalicular occlusion or hyperlacrimation. Hyperlacrimation can rarely be primary in etiology – usually secondary to ocular surface disease, dry eye, or uncommonly to gustatory epiphora ("crocodile tears") due to aberrant regeneration of the facial nerve. The second category is comprised of patients with failure of the surgical procedure, typically secondary to scarring in or around the DCR fistula, despite a correct diagnosis of NLDO.

Finally, there are patients with NLDO plus another potential cause of tearing ("NLDO plus"), i.e., mixed-mechanism tearing. In those patients, the other cause(s) of tearing may continue to cause symptoms even after the NLDO has been successfully addressed with DCR. A patient with significant eyelid laxity or orbicularis oculi muscle weakness may have lacrimal pump failure in addition to the NLDO. In such a patient, the physiologic impairment of tear drainage may only become more obvious once the anatomic obstruction is eliminated via DCR. Therefore, one should consider tightening a very lax lower eyelid at the same time as the DCR to prevent persistent tearing due to lacrimal pump failure. Punctal ectropion, punctal stenosis, or conjunctivochalasis may also be corrected concurrently with the DCR procedure. However, if a silicone tube is placed during DCR, then snip punctoplasty for punctal stenosis is usually unnecessary and increases the risk of canalicular laceration due to cheesewiring of the tube.

It is important to keep in mind that NLDO is only one of many possible causes of tearing or lacrimal discharge. Persistent purulent discharge from the lacrimal drainage system postoperatively may indicate an initial misdiagnosis. Expression of pus from the punctum with medial canthal palpation may herald dacryocystitis associated with a NLDO, but it may also indicate canaliculitis. Clinically, it is usually easy to differentiate dacryocystitis from canaliculitis, and this is essential before undertaking any surgical intervention. While dacryocystitis displays swelling and tenderness centered at the inferior medial canthus, medial to the canthal angle, the focus of canaliculitis is along the medial upper or lower eyelid, generally between the punctum and the medial canthal angle. Lacrimal irrigation will distinguish the two conditions; in NLDO, there will be reflux from the *opposite* punctum, while canaliculitis (and any other type of canalicular occlusion) will show reflux from the *same* punctum. Therefore, it is critical to observe exactly where the irrigant refluxes.

Certain medical conditions, including lymphoma, sarcoidosis, and vasculitides, such as Wegener's granulomatosis, can cause NLDO and increase the likelihood of DCR failure. Sarcoidosis and Wegener's granulomatosis may require prolonged and intense immunosuppression to produce a patent and functioning DCR fistula [15, 16]. Many surgeons believe that the optimal timing for surgery coincides with disease remission in cases of Wegener's granulomatosis [16, 17]. While wound necrosis and nasocutaneous fistulas have been reported [18], others have found DCR to be generally quite effective in treating patients with Wegener's granulomatosis [16, 17, 19, 20].

Clinical Evaluation and Diagnostic Testing of the Symptomatic Patient After DCR

Along with a detailed general medical and ocular history, careful examination to establish the etiology of DCR failure is critical in determining the proper course of action. Close inspection of the tear lakes may reveal disparity between the eyes. In general, an increased tear lake is consistent with impairment of lacrimal drainage, while a very small tear lake suggests the possibility of reflex tearing due to low tear production. However, this can be misleading at times, particularly in patients with mixed-mechanism tearing, e.g., NLDO in a patient with low tear production who may be more symptomatic at times when there is reflex tearing. The 5-min basal tear secretion test and dye disappearance test may help differentiate between reflex tearing and impaired lacrimal drainage. In cases in which the etiology of the tearing is unclear, a trial of ocular lubricants in the dry eye may render the patient with reflex tearing asymptomatic, thereby avoiding unnecessary surgery in such a patient. Delayed dye disappearance will not differentiate an anatomic obstruction from a physiologic outflow defect (lacrimal pump failure), which may be accomplished with lacrimal irrigation or dacryoscintigraphy.

Nasal endoscopy can be performed in the office. An important diagnostic modality, endoscopy may be helpful in evaluating the size, location, and patency of the DCR fistula and for visualization of how much fluorescein dye reaches the nasal passage. Endoscopy can help detect the presence of intranasal adhesions or the middle turbinate overlying the fistula.

Preoperative nasal endoscopy is very helpful in establishing whether there is an evident nasal cause for the tearing, e.g., a mass lesion or turbinate hypertrophy. Preoperative endoscopy can help identify anatomic issues that might need to be addressed prior to or concurrent with DCR, such as a deviated nasal septum. The nose may be anesthetized with Cetacaine spray (Cetylite Industries, Pennsauken, NJ, USA) or 4–10% topical lidocaine spray. Phenylephrine 0.5% or oxymetazoline spray will provide mucosal vasoconstriction and decongestion. Certain medications, such as cocaine solution or a prepared mixture of lignocaine/phenylephrine, provide both topical anesthesia and vasoconstriction.

A modification of the Jones dye tests, originally described for evaluation of the unoperated lacrimal drainage system, can be performed. After instilling fluorescein into the inferior fornix and waiting several minutes, the rhinostomy site and nasal vault are endoscopically inspected for the appearance of fluorescein dye. If dye is present, DCR fistula patency is confirmed. A minimal amount of dye reaching the inside of the nose suggests stenosis of the canaliculi or rhinostomy. If no dye is seen with a regular light source, it may be appreciated with a cobalt blue light source, i.e., the Jones 1E test [21]. If no dye is detected, irrigation with a fluorescein solution under gentle pressure may result in the presence of dye in the nose. A quantitative assessment of the dye present in the nasal vault will help determine the patency and size of the fistula. If sparse fluorescein is found in the nose, this is likely due to a highly stenotic fistula, which can be easily overwhelmed by normal tear production or reflex tear production, resulting in symptomatic tearing at times. If dye is not visualized in the nose until after irrigation, then the problem is likely a dysfunctional lacrimal pump or perhaps still a highly stenotic DCR fistula.

In addition to the office examination, which includes the dye disappearance test, lacrimal irrigation, and nasal endoscopy, one may opt for ancillary diagnostic testing to assist in clinical evaluation. Although these diagnostic tools exist, many oculofacial surgeons do not routinely use them since most of the information necessary to effectively treat most patients can be obtained on examination in the office. Nonetheless, these special tests may be particularly helpful in selected cases.

Dacryoscintigraphy, or dacryoscintillography, is a technetium scan that provides information on physiologic tear drainage since the radioactive tracer is drawn into the lacrimal drainage system via the lacrimal pump rather than being injected into the canaliculi, as in traditional dacryocystography. It is particularly useful in cases of functional obstruction, i.e., lacrimal pump failure, or partial obstruction, either of which can present as intermittent epiphora with normal syringing or minimal reflux of the irrigant.

Dacryocystography involves imaging of the lacrimal drainage system via computed tomography (CT) or magnetic resonance imaging (MRI). When CT is used, a radiopaque agent is administered; for MRI, either a chemical contrast medium (such as gadolinium) or saline may be used [22]. When the contrast substance or saline is injected into the cannulated canaliculus, dacryocystography may discern an anatomic impairment of the lacrimal outflow system, such as canalicular stricture or the "sump syndrome," where a collection of dye can be seen pooling in the residual nasolacrimal sac that was not opened at the time of the DCR [23]. Many centers will administrate the contrast agent topically into the conjunctival fornix, in which case a more physiologic study of lacrimal drainage can be obtained, as in dacryoscintigraphy.

CT has been utilized by some to delineate the relationship between the surgical ostium and the surrounding soft tissues, as well as the size of the ostium. CT may detect obstruction of the fistula by soft tissue, scarring, neoplasia, bone, or turbinate [24], although office nasal endoscopy provides much of the same information without the expense, exposure to ionizing radiation, and risk of an IV dye reaction associated with CT scanning [6].

Management of the Failed DCR

The course of management hinges upon the basis of the surgical failure. If there is another identifiable cause for the tearing, such as punctal ectropion, or discharge, such as canaliculitis, then treatment should be directed accordingly. If the lacrimal drainage system is anatomically patent on irrigation, but dye is not reaching the nose, then one should strongly consider the possibility of lacrimal pump failure due to horizontal eyelid laxity or orbicularis oculi muscle weakness, and an eyelid tightening procedure should be considered. When there is tearing in the presence of a small tear lake or evident ocular surface disease, the possibility of reflex tearing should be entertained. Treatment for dry eye syndrome, including warm compresses, eyelid scrubs, artificial tear, and oral flax seed and fish oil supplements, may alleviate the tearing.

Patients displaying tearing or infection after DCR, an enlarged tear lake, delayed dye disappearance, the presence of little or no dye in the nose, and reflux through the opposite punctum on irrigation likely have compromise of their DCR fistula. An almost identical scenario is encountered in the patient with canalicular occlusion, except reflux presents from the same rather than the opposite punctum on lacrimal irrigation. The surgical approach is dependent upon the location of the canalicular obstruction and whether one or both canaliculi are affected. Upper and lower canalicular obstruction may necessitate conjunctivodacryocystorhinostomy (CDCR) with placement of a Jones tube or Putterman–Gladstone tube. A single patent canaliculus may be sufficient for tear drainage if the DCR is adequately sized and well-positioned. If there is a focal canalicular obstruction, which may result from an eyelid laceration, then that portion of the canaliculus may either be excised and repaired or bypassed by marsupializing the patent segment of canaliculus to the eyelid margin [25]. Diffuse canalicular occlusion proximal to the lacrimal sac, with at least 6–8 mm of patent canaliculus, can be addressed with canaliculodacryocystorhinostomy, i.e., DCR with canalicular reconstruction and silicone intubation in which the occluded portion of the canaliculus is excised and the patent segment of canaliculus is directly anastomosed to the lacrimal sac. Protracted canalicular intubation, with or without canalicular trephination, has been described, but it tends to fail if the region of canalicular occlusion is diffuse rather than focal.

When examination points toward compromise of the DCR fistula, it is important to know if there are any intranasal contributing anatomic factors, e.g., a markedly deviated septum, severe intranasal scarring, nasal polyp, or other mass lesion. If so, then those issues should be addressed before or concurrently with any further surgical attempts to reestablish lacrimal drainage.

Once it has been established that the DCR was unsuccessful and the patient is symptomatic, some form of surgical intervention will likely be necessary. Prior to surgery, one should be cognizant of the possibility that the patient may only be intermittently symptomatic due to reflex tearing. This increased tear production can overwhelm the lacrimal drainage system, typically when the patient is in windy or cold weather. In that case, one could consider botulinum toxin injection to the lacrimal gland [26], although ptosis may result and periodic reinjection is necessary. Lacrimal pump failure due to eyelid laxity may result in tearing and should be managed with horizontal lower eyelid tightening, which carries a very high success rate. Significant nasal septal deviation causing marked narrowing of the nasal passage or encroachment of the middle turbinate on the DCR fistula or intranasal scarring should be corrected to improve the likelihood of success of the revision surgery.

Balloon Dilatation [27]

The stenotic or occluded DCR fistula can often be managed successfully with balloon dilatation, using the 5-mm or 9-mm Lacricath balloon catheter (Quest Medical, Inc., Allen, TX, USA). The punctum is widely dilated to accommodate the balloon catheter, which is inserted through the upper or lower canaliculus (the superior canaliculus may be preferable, in order to avoid damage to the inferior canaliculus, which is believed by some to be functionally more important). Under endoscopic guidance, the balloon is positioned within the DCR fistula. If the DCR fistula is completely occluded, then a new opening must be created from the lacrimal sac into the nose. This may be accomplished with a trephine or large Bowman's probe. Protocols may vary for the balloon dilatation, but the authors have routinely inflated the balloon to eight atmospheres for 90 s, followed by reinflation for 60 s. As it is inflated, the balloon tends to migrate one way or the other, so it must be held in position. After dilating the fistula, the authors suggest silicone intubation. Some colleagues have advised using larger diameter tubing such as the LacriCath® STENTube (Quest Medical, Inc., Allen, TX, USA) which may serve to more effectively stent the stenotic or occluded DCR fistula. However, many have commented on the greater likelihood of the STENTube to lacerate the canaliculus and have recommended employing the usual diameter silicone tubing, e.g., the Jackson or Crawford silicone intubation set. The stent may be left in place as briefly as 4–6 weeks, but longer duration stent retention, perhaps a few months, may possibly confer more protection to the fistula. The optimal duration of silicone intubation following balloon dilatation has not yet been established, and it is unclear whether silicone intubation increases the success rate after balloon dacryoplasty for a failed DCR. Techniques for silicone intubation and fixation of the silicone tube are discussed elsewhere in this text. The authors have found balloon dilatation with silicone intubation to be highly successful in patients with stenosis of the DCR fistula.

Repeat Dacryocystorhinostomy

Should DCR fail, the procedure may occasionally need to be repeated, either from an external or internal (transnasal) approach, particularly if the DCR fistula is completely occluded. This will also permit obtaining a histopathologic specimen if deemed appropriate. The external approach may be undertaken via a transcutaneous (inferior Lynch incision), transcaruncular, or transcanalicular approach. Repeat DCR may be performed via the transnasal route, either laser assisted or not. As stated previously, the laser-assisted methods have almost universally been associated with a lower success rate. Therefore, most colleagues have abandoned the use of the laser for revision DCR. Probing of the occluded DCR fistula concurrent with nasal video endoscopy may demonstrate the site of the osteotomy and intranasal fistula by visualizing the tenting lateral nasal mucosa over the probe.

External Approach Via Skin Incision

The nose is packed with strip gauze or neurosurgical patties lightly soaked with cocaine or phenylephrine/lidocaine solution. The medial canthal region is infiltrated with local anesthetic solution containing epinephrine. An inferior Lynch (or other) skin incision is made with a scalpel. This may be placed directly over the scar from the previous surgery if an external DCR was previously employed. If the prior surgery was an endoscopic DCR, then the skin incision may be placed based on the surgeon's preference. Some asurgeons regularly use an inferomedial lower eyelid incision for DCR, which tends to camouflage very well and almost always avoids the angular vessels.

The initial portion of the DCR reoperation is the same as a primary DCR, including blunt dissection down to the inferomedial orbital rim, incising periosteum, and developing a subperiosteal plane anterior and medial to the lacrimal sac with a periosteal elevator. As the dissection proceeds medially and posteriorly, scar tissue from the prior surgery will be encountered, particularly at the site of stenosis or occlusion of the DCR fistula, i.e., in and around the osteotomy. The cicatrix will make reoperation more challenging since the surgeon will often encounter more bleeding, less effective local anesthesia, and obliteration of natural tissue planes which increases the difficulty of tissue dissection. It may be helpful to place a Bowman's probe into the lacrimal sac to help demonstrate where the osteotomy and previous fistula are located. The surgeon can make a vertical incision onto the Bowman's probe through the wall of the fistula, while staying close to the medial orbital wall to prevent inadvertent injury to the canaliculi.

If the osteotomy location is known in advance, an incision can be made through periosteum and soft tissue several millimeters anterior to the osteotomy, and subperiosteal dissection can be performed posteriorly toward the osteotomy. The osteotomy should be examined for adequacy, although the optimal osteotomy size is unclear, perhaps at least 15 mm in diameter. If it is too small or poorly positioned, the osteotomy can be enlarged, in the appropriate directions, with a Kerrison rongeur or with a burr on a high-speed drill, after lifting the soft tissue away from the bone with a periosteal elevator. The superior margin of the osteotomy should be at least a few millimeters above the level of the common internal punctum, if possible, depending on the position of the cribriform plate. Particularly with the superior edge of the osteotomy, one should avoid twisting the rongeur, which could extend a crack into the cribriform plate and produce a cerebrospinal fluid leak.

If there is obstruction at the common internal punctum, where the common canaliculus enters the lacrimal sac, then any soft tissue obstructing the opening into the nose should be resected, while saving anterior mucosal flaps on the nasal and lacrimal sac sides to create an anastomosis once a satisfactory channel into the nose has been created. If the middle turbinate encroaches on the osteotomy, then the portion of the turbinate obstructing the osteotomy is resected after infiltrating it with local anesthetic solution for analgesia and hemostasis. Light cautery may be applied to any visible bleeding vessels within the turbinate and nasal mucosa, and Surgicel (Johnson and Johnson, Inc., Piscataway, NJ, USA) may be placed, if desired, to address low-flow diffuse oozing of blood without any focal source.

Bleeding is always a potential challenge during DCR, and other maneuvers to control bleeding include placing a cottonoid, gauze, or Gelfoam® (Pharmacia and Upjohn, Kalamazoo, MI, USA) soaked in local anesthetic with epinephrine or thrombin, or the application of Avitene® (C.R. Bard, Inc., Murray Hill, NJ, USA). If there is vigorous bleeding, an active attempt should be made to find the source since such bleeding may not stop spontaneously or with pressure. It may be necessary to place a Merocel® sponge (Medtronic Xomed, Jacksonville, FL, USA), or some other form of nasal packing, soaked in antibiotic solution in the nose at the end of the case to tamponade persistent venous bleeding, but this will likely be insufficient to address active arterial bleeding.

The surgeon should avoid unnecessary trauma to the nasal mucosa, including excessive cautery, in order to limit postoperative scarring that may impact the success of the surgery. Care should be taken to protect the nasal and lacrimal sac mucosal flaps while working within the DCR fistula and nose.

Silicone tubing is commonly used to stent the reopened fistula, although some surgeons have recommended placement of a larger stent in the fistula. The two ends of the tubing may be sutured together with a slowly dissolving suture, such as poliglecaprone 25 (Monocryl®) or polyglactin 910 (Vicryl®, Ethicon, Inc. Somerville, NJ, USA), placed just medial to the common internal punctum. This tube fixation technique facilitates tube removal and helps prevent lateral tube prolapse postoperatively, which can necessitate premature removal of the tubing. The tension of the tubing at the medial canthus should be tight enough to avoid lateral prolapse and corneal irritation, but loose enough to prevent canalicular laceration from cheesewiring. The authors advocate suturing the anterior lacrimal sac and nasal mucosal flaps together since there is less tissue contraction associated with primary intention healing, as opposed to secondary intention healing (without a mucosal anastomosis). There should be little laxity in the anastomosed flaps to avoid their being drawn into the fistula and contributing to obstruction of the osteotomy.

If the sutured flaps are loose, allowing the anterior flaps to sag posteriorly toward the center of the osteotomy, this can be addressed by anchoring the flaps to overlying periosteum anterior to the fistula. In addition, if the nasal mucosal flap is too thin to retain a suture or is accidentally removed during creation of the osteotomy, then one may either extend the osteotomy further anteriorly to recruit more anterior nasal mucosa or just suture the anterior lacrimal sac flap up to periosteum along the anterior edge of the osteotomy. However, it is always preferable to juxtapose the lacrimal sac and nasal mucosa to allow for primary intention healing. The cutaneous incision is closed in a layered fashion. A "mustache" dressing may be placed below the nose at the end of the case, particularly if there is visible oozing of blood in the nose intraoperatively. In addition to intraoperative antibiotics, intraoperative and/or postoperative systemic corticosteroids may help temper the cicatricial response to surgery, especially for reoperation, where the fibroblasts may be "geared up" for a more emphatic response.

Endoscopic-Assisted Endonasal and Transcanalicular Approaches

Endoscopic-assisted approaches to failed DCR have allowed the surgeon to directly visualize intranasal anatomy as it relates to the previously formed surgical ostium without incising the skin. Two modalities are used today: the more common endonasal approach and the transcanalicular approach.

The endoscopic endonasal, or transnasal, approach to primary lacrimal bypass surgery has been described previously. The authors have found the endonasal approach coupled with balloon dilatation, and often silicone intubation, to be highly effective in treating the failed DCR.

Direct visualization of a lacrimal probe passed anterograde from a canaliculus through the previously created ostium allows for enhanced understanding of why the prior DCR failed. Initially, the surgeon should evaluate the fistula for stenosis or complete obstruction. If this is the case, the lacrimal probe may be passed through the stenotic or obstructed ostium at several points. These defects may be coalesced to form a larger defect with a Dandy nerve hook, or Blakesley forceps can be used to strip away the tissue. If the nasolacrimal sac was incompletely opened, which can produce a sump syndrome, an angled scalpel blade can be used to fillet the sac open, or Blakesley forceps can be employed to remove the portion of the medial sac wall that was not completely opened previously.

The middle turbinate is easily identified with nasal endoscopy and may contribute to DCR failure. If the middle turbinate appears to be abutting the DCR fistula, a periosteal elevator can be employed to gently infracture this bone. The surgeon should remain cognizant that overzealous manipulation of the middle turbinate may result in cerebrospinal fluid rhinorrhea due to fracture of the cribriform plate. If the lacrimal sac lies beneath, i.e., lateral to, the middle turbinate, then it may be necessary to resect the anterior portion of the turbinate to increase the chances of surgical success.

The nasal septum is easily inspected with nasal endoscopy. Deviation and scarring of the septum may result in adhesions between the fistula and the septum and possible failure of DCR. If a deviated septum is identified, septoplasty and lysis of any adhesions should be undertaken. Straightening of the septum will allow for easier endoscopic intranasal manipulations and debriding of the ostium. Following intranasal revision, balloon dacryoplasty may be performed, as described earlier.

Zeldovich et al. reported an 89% success rate of revision endoscopic DCR when betamethasone was injected into the lacrimal sac and scar tissue around the ostium at the time of surgery [28]. Tsirbas et al. reported 76.5% and 84.6% success rates for endoscopic and external DCR, respectively [29]. The transcanalicular laser-assisted approach to DCR has been described in exemplary fashion. Advantages include avoidance of a skin incision, short operative time, and lower risk of hemorrhage. When dealing with a stenotic or occluded DCR fistula or a common canalicular obstruction, this modality is ideal for revisional surgery since direct visualization is possible with the endoscope. In addition, dealing with a stenosis or completely obstructed ostium is possible, given the approach and endoscopic visualization.

Mitomycin C

Topical application of mitomycin C to the DCR fistula at the time of reoperation has been advocated by some surgeons, who have noted enhanced success compared to DCR performed without mitomycin C [3, 30–36]. Nevertheless, not all investigators have found an improved surgical success rate with the use of mitomycin C [34].

Mitomycin C is an antineoplastic antibiotic, isolated from *Streptomyces caespitosus*, that inhibits DNA and RNA replication, cell division, protein synthesis, and fibroblast proliferation. This agent has a long history of ophthalmic usage in glaucoma filtering surgery. It produces in looser, hypocellular subepithelial connective tissue. Various protocols have been utilized in dacryocystorhinostomy, including concentrations of mitomycin C ranging from 0.2 to 1 mg/ml and exposure times of 2.5–30 min (usually 5 min or less). No major complications have been reported relative to the usage of mitomycin C in DCR surgery, and it does not substantially increase the cost of surgery. One should be very careful to avoid placing the mitomycin C into direct contact with the skin edges of the wound, or this may result in impaired wound healing and possible postoperative wound dehiscence, as noted by Liao et al. [32].

Silicone Intubation

Although many surgeons incorporate silicone intubation into primary and secondary (revision) DCR procedures, this remains somewhat controversial. Not only is it unclear whether silicone intubation improves the success rate of surgery but silicone intubation has been associated with certain surgical complications, including peripunctal granulation tissue, chronic infection, canalicular laceration (slitting of the punctum), stent prolapse, discomfort, and corneal abrasions. In fact, Allen and Berlin reported an increased failure rate in DCR patients whom a silicone tube was placed at the time of surgery [11]. Some authors have suggested silicone intubation in selected patients, e.g., in those with common canalicular scarring, in patients with a small, contracted, and scarred lacrimal sac, or when the lacrimal sac–nasal mucosal flap anastomosis is suboptimal, such as when there is inadequate lacrimal sac or nasal mucosa remaining [35]. Whether or not silicone intubation is more helpful in DCR reoperations remains unproven. A variety of DCR fistula stents have been used, and it is uncertain if a larger diameter silicone tube (or other stent) makes any difference.

Summary

Post-DCR tearing patients can be challenging. A systematic history and evaluation will allow for appropriate treatment whether it is medical or surgical. At times, no clear-cut etiologies may be found prompting the surgeon to take a multifaceted approach to management. With a careful approach to the tearing patient following DCR, appropriate management usually eliminates the epiphora. It is extremely important to identify all etiologic factors contributing to the DCR failure so that they can be properly addressed. Nasal endoscopy is essential since it may reveal a deviated septum, intranasal adhesions, or a middle turbinate blocking the DCR fistula. If the DCR fistula is stenotic or occluded, then the fistula can be reopened via an external, transcanalicular, or transnasal approach, either with or without the assistance of a laser. Often, simple balloon dilatation, with or without silicone intubation, is successful. Occasionally, repeat DCR is necessary, and mitomycin C can be used in order to enhance the likelihood of surgical success. Given the fact that subsequent revisions are unlikely to be successful if the first revision fails [37], it is all the more critical that the first revision succeed. Success can usually be assured once the etiology of the DCR failure is correctly established and appropriately treated.

References

1. Hartikainen J, Antila J, Varpula M, Puuka P, Seppa H, Grenman R. Prospective randomized comparison of endonasal endoscopic dacryocystorhinostomy and external dacryocystorhinostomy. Laryngoscope. 1998;108:1861–6.
2. Hartikainen J, Grenman R, Puukka P, Seppa H. Prospective randomized comparison of endonasal endoscopic dacryocystorhinostomy and external dacryocystorhinostomy. Ophthalmology. 1998;105:1106–13.
3. Camara JG, Bengzon AU, Henson RD. The safety and efficacy of Mitomycin C in endonasal endoscopic laser-assisted dacryocystorhinostomy. Ophthal Plast Reconstr Surg. 2000;16:114–8.
4. Hong JE, Hatton MP, Leib ML, Fay AM. Endocanalicular laser dacryocystorhinostomy analysis of 118 consecutive surgeries. Ophthalmology. 2005;112:1629–33.
5. Drnovsek-Olup B, Beltram M. Transcanalicular diode laser-assisted dacryocystorhinostomy. Indian J Ophthalmol. 2010;58:213–7.
6. Allen KM, Berlin AJ, Levine HL. Intranasal endoscopic analysis of dacryocystorhinostomy failure. Ophthal Plast Reconstr Surg. 1988;4:143.
7. Woog JJ, Kennedy RH, Custer PL, Kaltreider SA, Meyer DR, Camara JG. Endonasal dacryocystorhinostomy. A report by the American Academy of Ophthalmology. Ophthalmology. 2001;108:2369–77.
8. Schepler TR, Davenport OR, Neuhaus RW, Shore JW. Dacryocystorhinostomy: flap versus no flap. Presented at the ASOPRS fall meeting, New Orleans, October 2004.
9. Tsirbas A, Wormald PJ. Endonasal dacryocystorhinostomy with mucosal flaps. Am J Ophthalmol. 2003;135:76–83.
10. Codere F, Denton P, Corona J. Endonasal dacryocystorhinostomy: a modified technique with preservation of the nasal and lacrimal mucosa. Ophthal Plast Reconstr Surg. 2010;26:161–4.
11. Allen K, Berlin AJ. Dacryocystorhinostomy failure: association with nasolacrimal silicone intubation. Ophthalmic Surg. 1989;20:486–9.
12. Walland MJ, Rose GE. The effect of silicone intubation on failure and infection rates after dacryocystorhinostomy. Ophthalmic Surg. 1994;25:597–600.
13. Saiju R, Morse LJ, Weinberg D, Shrestha MK, Ruit S. Prospective randomized comparison of external dacryocystorhinostomy with and without silicone intubation. Br J Ophthalmol. 2009;93:1220–2.
14. Madge SN, Selva D. Intubation in routine dacryocystorhinostomy: why we do what we do. Clin Exp Ophthalmol. 2009;37:620–3.
15. Chapman KL, Bartley GB, Garrity JA, Gonnering RS. Lacrimal bypass surgery in patients with sarcoidosis. Am J Ophthalmol. 1999;127(4):443–6.
16. Hardwig PW, Bartley GB, Garrity JA. Surgical management of nasolacrimal duct obstruction in patients with Wegener's granulomatosis. Ophthalmology. 1992;99(1):133–9.
17. Kwan AS, Rose GE. Lacrimal drainage surgery in Wegener's granulomatosis. Br J Ophthalmol. 2000;84(3):329–31.
18. Jordan DR, Miller D, Anderson RL. Wound necrosis following dacryocystorhinostomy in patients with Wegener's granulomatosis. Ophthalmic Surg. 1987;18:800–3.
19. Glatt JH, Putterman AM. Dacryocystorhinostomy in Wegener's granulomatosis. Ophthal Plast Reconstr Surg. 1990;6:207–10.
20. Wong RJ, Gliklich RE, Rubin PA, Goodman M. Bilateral nasolacrimal duct obstruction managed with endoscopic techniques. Arch Otolaryngol Head Neck Surg. 1998;124(6):703–6.
21. Enzer YR, Shorr N. The Jones IE test: cobalt blue endoscopic primary dye test of lacrimal excretory function. Ophthal Plast Reconstr Surg. 1997;13:204–9.

22. Goldberg RA, Heinz GW, Chiu L. Gadolinium magnetic resonance imaging dacryocystography. Am J Ophthalmol. 1993;115:738–41.
23. Welham RAN, Wulc AE. Management of unsuccessful lacrimal surgery. Br J Ophthalmol. 1987;71(2):152–7.
24. Mauriello JA, Vadehra V, Fleckner M, Shah C. Correlation of orbital computed tomographic findings with office probing and irrigation in 17 patients after successful and failed dacryocystorhinostomy. Ophthal Plast Reconstr Surg. 1999;15(2):116–20.
25. McCord CD Jr. Canalicular resection and reconstruction by canaliculostomy. Ophthalmic Surg. 1980;11:440–5.
26. Whittaker KW, Matthews BN, Fitt AW, Sandramouli S. The use of botulinum toxin A in the treatment of functional epiphora. Orbit. 2003;22(3):193–8.
27. Becker BB, Berry FD. Balloon catheter dilatation in lacrimal surgery. Ophthalmic Surg. 1989;20:193–8.
28. Selig YK, Biesman BS, Rebeiz EE. Topical application of mitomycin C in endoscopic dacryocystorhinostomy. Am J Rhinol. 2000;14:205–7.
29. Zeldovich A, Ghabrial R. Revision endoscopic dacryocystorhinostomy with betamethasone injection under assisted local anesthetic. Orbit. 2009;28(6):328–31.
30. Tsirbas A, Davis G, Wormald PJ. Revision dacryocystorhinostomy: a comparison of endoscopic and external techniques. Am J Rhinol. 2010;19(3):332–5.
31. Yeatts RP, Neves RB. Use of mitomycin C in repeat dacryocystorhinostomy. Ophthal Plast Reconstr Surg. 1999;15:19–22.
32. Liao SL, Kao SCS, Tseng JHS, Chen MS, Hou PK. Results of intraoperative mitomycin C application in dacryocystorhinostomy. Br J Ophthalmol. 2000;84:903–6.
33. You Y, Fang C. Intraoperative mitomycin C in dacryocystorhinostomy. Ophthal Plast Reconstr Surg. 2001;17:115–9.
34. Ugurbas SH, Zilelioglu G, Sargon MF, Anadolu Y, Akiner M, Akturk T. Histopathologic effects of mitomycin C on endoscopic transnasal dacryocystorhinostomy. Ophthalmic Surg Lasers. 1997;28:300–4.
35. Yalaz M, Firinciogullari E, Zeren H. Use of mitomycin C and 5-fluorouracil in external dacryocystorhinostomy. Orbit. 1999;18:239–45.
36. Zilelioglu G, Ugurbas SH, Anadolu Y, Akiner M, Akturk T. Adjunctive use of mitomycin C on endoscopic lacrimal surgery. Br J Ophthalmol. 1998;82:63–6.
37. Ben Simon GJ, Joseph J, Lee S, Schwarcz RM, McCann JD, Goldberg RA. External versus endoscopic dacryocystorhinostomy for acquired nasolacrimal duct obstruction in a tertiary referral center. Ophthalmology. 2005;112:1463–8.

Part VIII

Orbital Disease and Surgery

Alon Kahana

Orbital Evaluation

42

Dane H. Slentz, Brian J. Lee, and Christine C. Nelson

Introduction

The orbit protects and supports the eye and its adnexal structures including the optic nerve, vasculature, extraocular muscles, and lacrimal gland. Orbital disease can be benign or malignant and often fits into the categories of inflammatory, vascular, structural, or neoplastic disease. The evaluation of all patients with possible orbital pathology should be complete and systematic because even benign disease can have significant ophthalmic morbidity. The goal of the orbital evaluation is to identify the nature of the orbital disease and its location by combining elements of the patient history, examination findings, laboratory test, and imaging techniques. This knowledge guides medical and surgical treatment.

Patient History

An accurate orbital evaluation begins with a thorough history. Patients with orbital pathology often present with eyelid swelling or ptosis. More worrisome symptoms include decreased vision, diplopia, and orbital pain. Visual symptoms may also include dyschromatopsia, metamorphopsia, and visual field deficits. During history taking, it is important to elicit modifying characteristics such as waxing and waning of symptoms as well as duration and time course.

When the patient complains of diplopia, the physician must determine if the double vision is monocular or binocular, intermittent or constant, worse in a certain gaze, and identify the position of the displaced images (horizontal, vertical, or oblique). Patients with unilateral low vision or amblyopia may not report diplopia despite ocular misalignment.

Orbital pain may manifest as painful eye movements, localized tenderness, or diffuse retrobulbar pressure. Orbital pain should be clearly distinguished from corneal irritation, which tends to resolve with eyelid closure or topical anesthetic. Neuropathic pain or paresthesias in specific dermatomes of the periorbital region can give clues in localizing intraorbital pathology based on the branches of the ophthalmic and maxillary divisions of the trigeminal nerve.

A review of pertinent past medical history, surgical history, and prior treatments can also help guide the orbital evaluation. For example, orbital pathology is well known to occur in Graves' disease [1–5], inflammatory conditions such as granulomatosis with polyangiitis [6–8], sarcoidosis [9, 10], IgG4 [11], and immunosuppression due to diabetes, pharmacologics, or malignancy [12–15]. Pertinent symptoms in orbital inflammatory diseases are summarized in Table 42.1. A history of external radiation to the head or neck may lead to periorbital/orbital tissue scarring and increase the susceptibility for secondary malignancies [16–18]. Recurrence of previously treated tumors in these regions can invade the orbit by local or perineural spread [19]. Previous facial surgery can cause orbital volume changes, infections, and vascular or structural changes. If prior orbital bony reconstruction has involved alloplastic material, autologous bone, or soft tissue grafts, it is important to ascertain details from operative reports [20]. Knowledge of prior ophthalmic surgery can guide the orbital examination as well. For example, exposed scleral buckles may present with orbital findings [21].

Family history should focus on inherited diseases, such as neurofibromatosis or amyloidosis. The former is associated with optic nerve gliomas and orbital bony abnormalities and may occur in an autosomal dominant inheritance pattern [22–24], whereas the latter can also be familial and result in accumulation of amyloid deposits in the orbit [25, 26].

D. H. Slentz (✉) · C. C. Nelson
Eye Plastic, Orbital and Facial Cosmetic Surgery, University of Michigan Health System, Department of Ophthalmology and Visual Sciences (W.K. Kellogg Eye Center), Ann Arbor, MI, USA
e-mail: dslentz@umich.edu; cnelson@med.umich.edu

B. J. Lee
Maryland Oculoplastic Surgery, Ellicott City, MD, USA

J. J. Servat et al. (eds.), *Smith and Nesi's Ophthalmic Plastic and Reconstructive Surgery*,
https://doi.org/10.1007/978-3-030-41720-8_42

Table 42.1 Common orbital inflammatory diseases

Disorder	Systemic findings	Orbital and eye findings	Initial investigations
Thyroid eye disease	Tachycardia	Bilateral or unilateral	Thyroid-stimulating hormone
	Anxiety	Proptosis	Free T4
	Tremor	Eyelid retraction	Free T3
	Weight loss	Exposure keratopathy	Thyroid-stimulating immunoglobulin
	Diarrhea	Strabismus	
		Compressive optic neuropathy	
Sarcoidosis	Respiratory symptoms	Inflammation of any orbital tissues	Angiotensin converting enzyme
	Erythema nodosum		Lysozyme
		Uveitis	Chest X-ray
		Optic neuritis	Orbital biopsy
Wegener's granulomatosis	Respiratory symptoms	Inflammation of any orbital tissues	c-ANCA
	Sinusitis		CRP
	Epistaxis	Scleritis	Orbital biopsy
		Uveitis	
		Optic neuritis	
Tolosa-Hunt	Typically absent	Painful ophthalmoplegia	MRI brain and orbit
			Lumbar puncture
Lymphoproliferative disease	Lymphadenopathy	Infiltrative orbital disease	Orbital biopsy
	Fever	Subconjunctival involvement with salmon-patch appearance	Complete blood count
	Weight loss		
	Night sweats		
Metastatic disease	Variable	Extraocular muscle involvement commonly	Systemic oncology evaluation
			Orbital biopsy if primary unknown
Orbital cellulitis	Fever	Pain	Emergent orbital CT
	Sinusitis	Eyelid cellulitis	Complete blood count
	Immunosuppression	Proptosis	
		Restricted mobility	
Idiopathic orbital inflammation	Variable	Unilateral focal inflammation	Orbital biopsy
			Rapid response to corticosteroids

A complete social history contributes to the orbital evaluation. Smoking increases the incidence of head and neck cancers, which may involve the orbit [27–29]. Additionally, smoking has clearly been associated with more severe orbitopathy in thyroid eye disease [30–33]. Prior work history may provide clues for orbital foreign bodies or increased risk for sinonasal cancers [34–36].

Examination

Visual Acuity

The orbital examination begins with testing of visual acuity. This is performed using a Snellen eye chart at distance with the patient's corrective lenses. Each eye should be tested independently. In patients with significant proptosis or pathology in the medial canthus that precludes glasses wear, the examiner can use the pinhole test to approximate best-corrected visual acuity. When at the bedside for inpatient consultations, visual acuity can be tested with a handheld near card. In presbyopes, a loose +2.50 diopter lens can assist when testing near vision. For vision testing of children, "Tumbing E's" or the "HOTV" methods are useful.

Pupils

Assessment of pupillary function is important in evaluating for optic neuropathy, the most vision threatening complication of orbital pathology. It begins with measuring pupil size in ambient light. The examiner should ask the patient to fixate on a distance target to prevent accommodative pupillary constriction. Then, with the room lights dimmed, the reactivity of each pupil is assessed independently. Both a direct and consensual light response should be seen with each pupil. Typical descriptors of reactivity include brisk, sluggish, and nonreactive. The swinging light test can detect

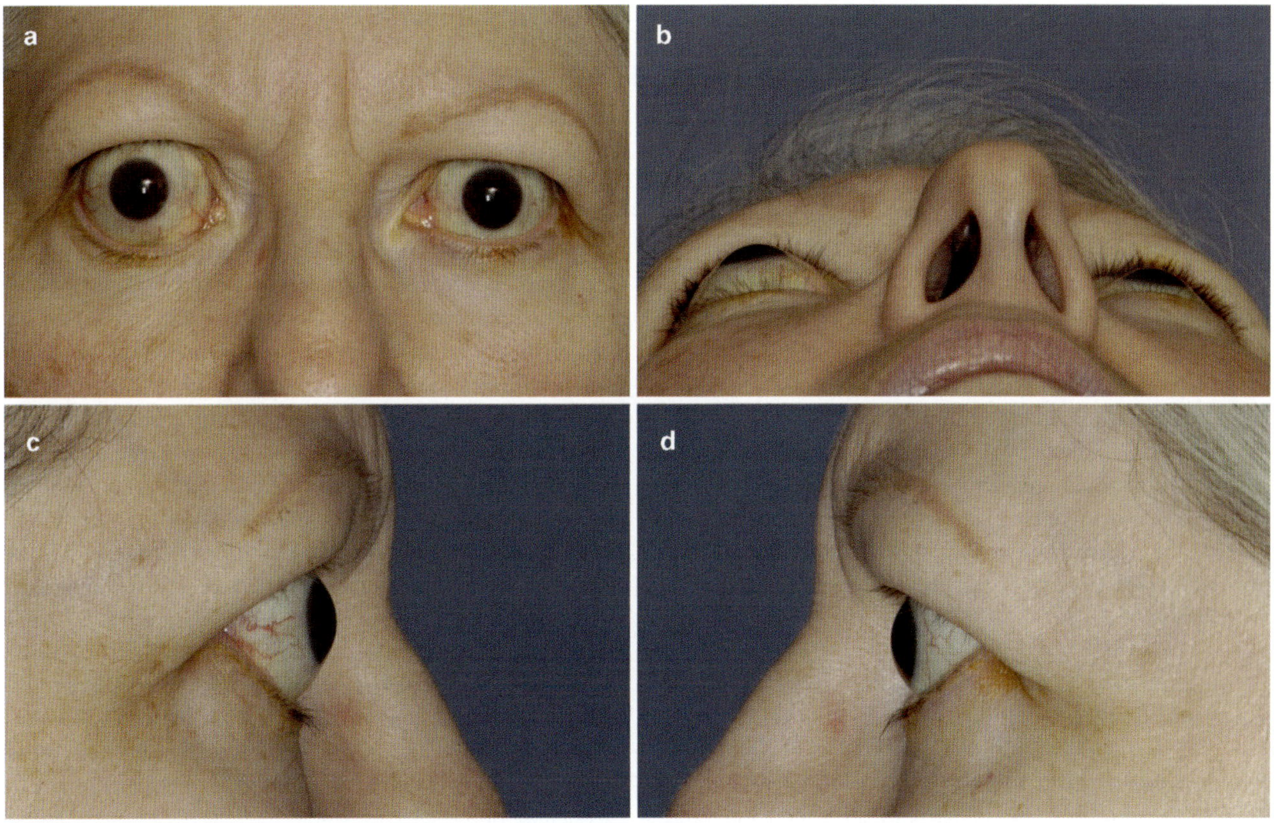

Fig. 42.1 Characteristic findings of thyroid eye disease: eyelid retraction (**a**) and proptosis (**b**, **c**, **d**)

a relative afferent pupillary defect and is graded on a 4-point scale. Such a defect localizes pathology to the ipsilateral optic nerve [37]. Optic neuropathy from orbital disease is often due to compressive or vascular abnormalities.

External Examination

External examination begins with inspection of the periocular skin. Erythema and edema are nonspecific but may suggest underlying inflammation, infection, or neoplasia. Ecchymoses or color changes of the skin may reflect deeper vascular tumors or malformations. Careful inspection also includes evaluation for possible cutaneous neoplasms that can lead to significant orbital pathology, particularly when located in the medial canthus. Typical characteristics of skin neoplasms include irregular shape, irregular borders, central ulceration, and bleeding. Skin lesions and masses should be tested for mobility over underlying bone as this may help determine the need for imaging as well as surgical planning. At the eyelid margins, skin cancers are often characterized by destruction of the normal architecture including eyelash follicles. Peripheral skin examination can reveal café-au-lait spots associated with neurofibromatosis. While we do not routinely do a whole body skin examination, we do ask the patient about suspicious lesions and examine them specifically.

Next, eyelid positions should be measured. The palpebral fissure is the distance between the upper and lower lid margins. Widening of the palpebral fissure can be associated with proptosis or eyelid retraction, while narrowing can be due to enophthalmos, eyelid edema, or eyelid ptosis. Upper eyelid position can be measured as the margin to reflex distance. Upper eyelid ptosis in orbital disease can be associated with eyelid edema or from superior orbital pathology affecting the levator palpebrae muscle. In contrast, eyelid retraction is characteristic of thyroid-associated orbitopathy (Fig. 42.1).

Complete external examination also requires palpation, which may reveal orbital rim abnormalities, masses, or lymphadenopathy. If a mass is palpated, the examiner should try to identify its location and the affected tissues. Localized tenderness on palpation can denote focal inflammatory processes such as dacryoadenitis, dacryocystitis, and trochleitis. Fluctuance suggests a fluid collection from an abscess or cyst. Increased resistance to retropulsion is a hallmark of many orbital processes. In a unilateral process such as orbital cellulitis, this finding can be compared to the uninvolved side. Orbital vascular lesions, postoperative bony defects of the frontal bone, or sphenoid wing hypoplasia may cause palpable pulsations. Auscultation with a stethoscope can reveal bruits associated with high-flow vascular lesions, such as carotid cavernous fistulas. Arterial pulsations in very anterior orbital lesions may be palpable. Additionally, Doppler ultrasound can be used to assess flow.

Lymph Node Examination

Orbital processes drain to the preauricular and submandibular lymph nodes. Palpation of these lymph nodes should be performed in patients with suspected orbital and ocular adnexal tumors. Conjunctival and eyelid melanoma, sebaceous cell carcinoma, and lacrimal gland adenoid cystic carcinoma are examples of tumors known to metastasize to the regional lymph nodes. If palpable, nodes with metastasis are usually nontender.

Lacrimal Gland

The lacrimal gland is located in the lacrimal fossa of the superotemporal orbit and consists of an orbital lobe and a smaller palpebral lobe. Lacrimal gland pathology includes prolapse, inflammation, infection, or tumor infiltration. Lacrimal gland prolapse is characterized by a palpable, soft, nontender mass in the superolateral quadrant. Distraction or eversion of the upper eyelid often allows for visualization of the prolapsed gland. Dacryoadenitis is characterized by enlargement and tenderness of the lacrimal gland with accompanying eyelid erythema and edema. Lacrimal gland tumors may or may not present with tenderness and are typically firm on palpation [38].

Nasolacrimal System

The nasolacrimal system begins in the inferomedial orbit with the canaliculi and nasolacrimal sac and extends inferiorly into the nose as the nasolacrimal duct. Benign processes include dacryocystitis and canaliculitis. Dacryocystitis is characterized by swelling and fluctuance over the nasolacrimal sac in the medial canthus. With pressure, purulence can often be expressed retrograde through the lacrimal puncta. Findings more worrisome for neoplastic processes include bloody tears and extension of masses superior to the medial canthal tendon, both of which have been associated with lacrimal sac tumors. Additionally, the nasolacrimal duct extends inferiorly from the sac and provides a potential conduit for extension of orbital tumors into the nose as well as the reverse.

Axial Displacement

Axial proptosis is often characteristic of intraconal orbital pathology. However, posterior extraconal lesions can cause axial proptosis as well. Proptosis should be measured with an exophthalmometer. The more commonly used exophthalmometers include the Hertel, Mourits, and Naugle variants (Fig. 42.2). In contrast to the Hertel and Mourits exophthalmometers, which rest on the lateral orbital rims, the Naugle exophthalmometer rests on the superior and inferior orbital rims and may be useful in patients with pathology of the lateral orbital rim such as zygomaticomaxillary complex fractures. Using the same exophthalmometry method over time with the same base allows for standardized measurements over multiple clinical visits. When exophthalmometers are not available, the bird's-eye view or worm's-eye view can be used to grossly assess for proptosis (Figs. 42.1b, 42.3b, and 42.4b). Patients with significant proptosis often demonstrate widening of the vertical palpebral fissure and eyelid retraction.

In contrast to proptosis, enophthalmos may be seen with orbital volume expansion after trauma or with sclerosing processes such as the scirrhous variant of metastatic breast cancer [39, 40]. Additional signs of enophthalmos include deepening of the superior sulcus and narrowing of the palpebral fissure (Fig. 42.3).

Nonaxial Displacement

Nonaxial globe displacement may occur due to extraconal lesions that cause mass effect. Globe displacement in this context can be measured relative to the unaffected eye. Space-occupying inflammatory, neoplastic, and vascular lesions can all cause globe displacement. Infiltrative lesions causing focal enlargement of orbital structures or localized edema can displace the globe as well.

In the superior orbit, disease involving the levator palpebrae, superior rectus muscle, or frontal nerve can cause downward displacement of the globe (Fig. 42.4). Also, bony lesions of the frontal bone or the frontal sinus can exert mass effect on the globe which may secondarily lead to refractive error (often hyperopia). In the superolateral quadrant, tumors in the lacrimal fossa, lesions of the lacrimal gland, and dermoid cysts associated with the frontozygomatic suture are common. Enlargement of the lateral rectus muscle laterally can displace the globe medially. The inferior orbit contains the inferior oblique muscle and the inferior rectus muscle with its closely associated ciliary ganglion. Lesions of the orbital floor, maxillary sinus, or nasolacrimal duct may result in superior displacement of the globe. The medial orbit is separated from the ethmoid sinuses by the thin lamina papyracea and extension of ethmoidal processes into the medial

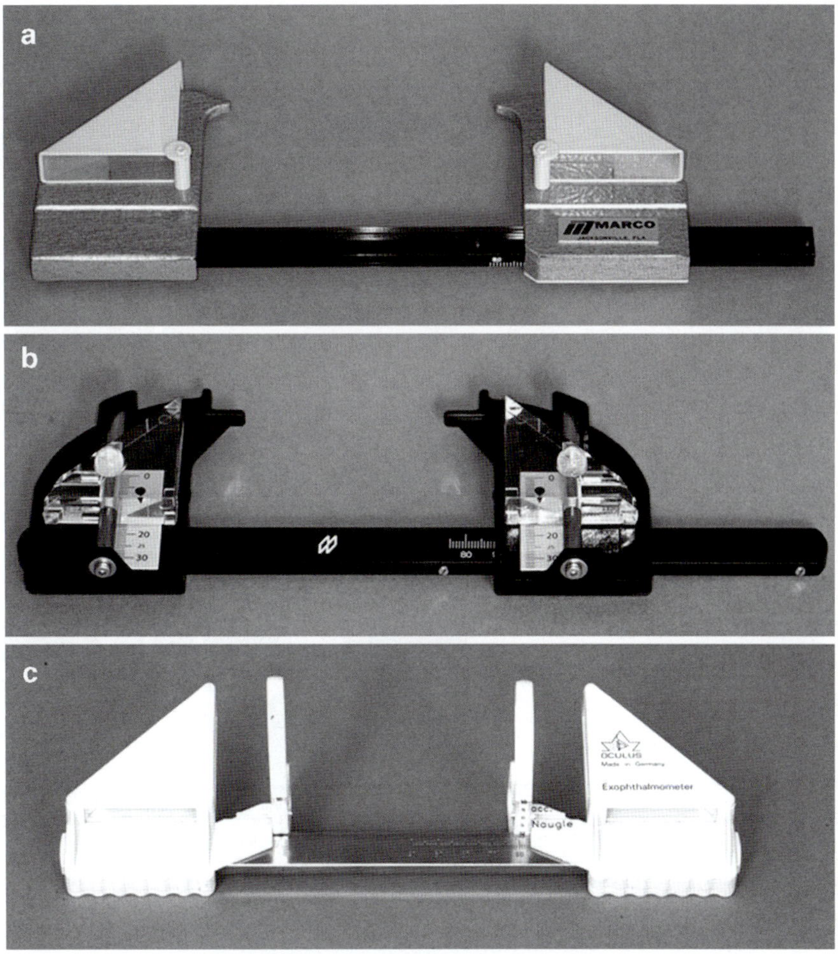

Fig. 42.2 Exophthalmometers: Hertel (**a**), Mourits (**b**), and Naugle (**c**)

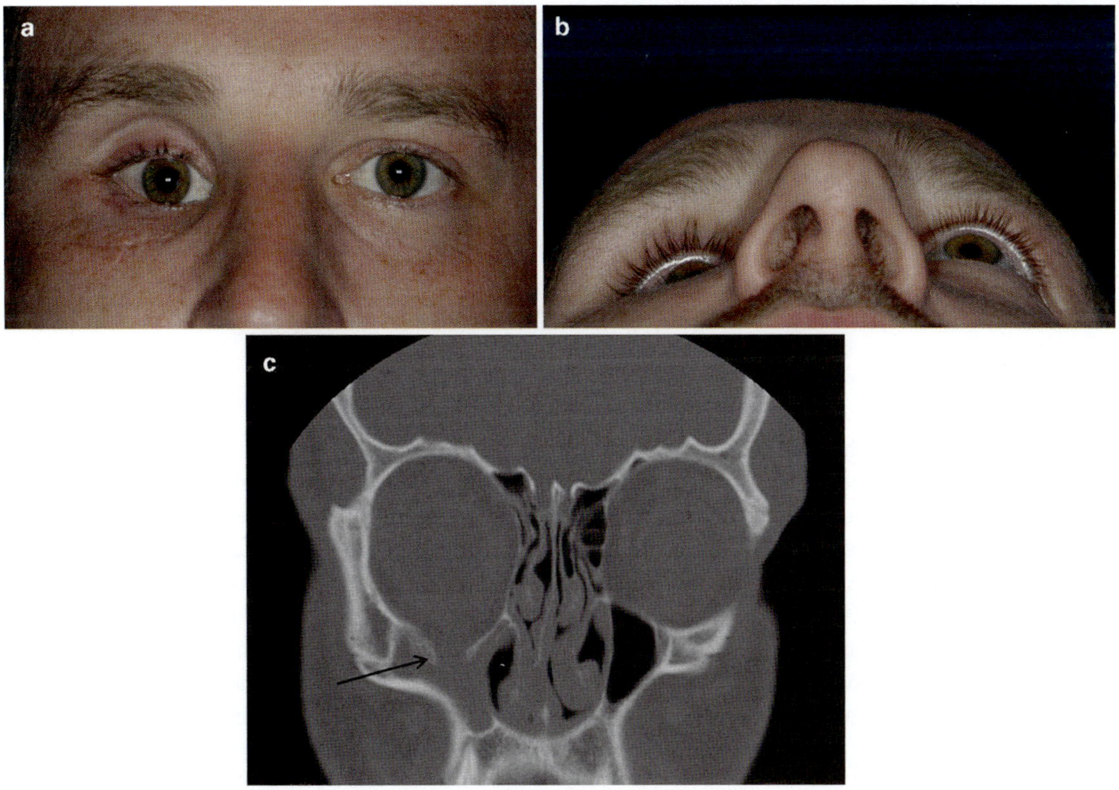

Fig. 42.3 Right inferior globe displacement (**a**) and enophthalmos (**b**) due to large orbital floor fracture. CT scan showing fracture (**c**, arrow)

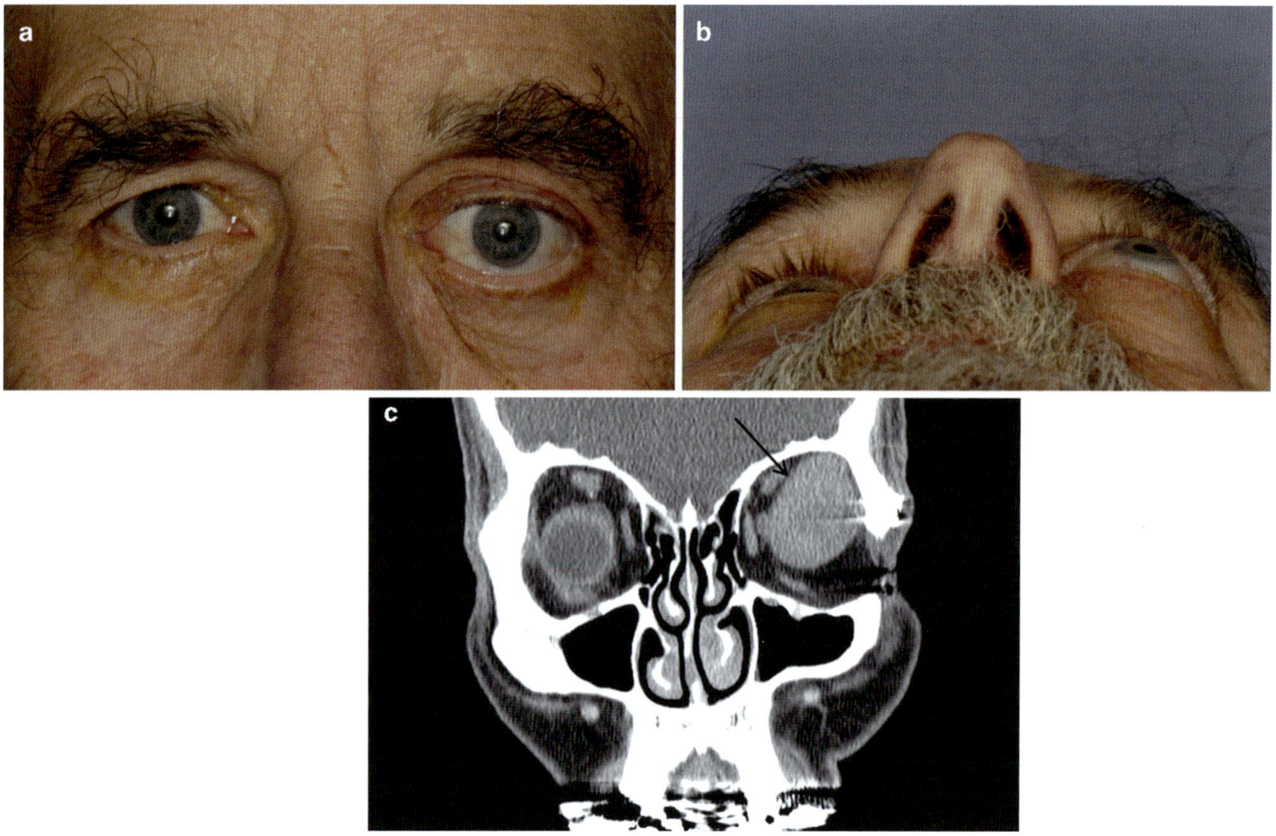

Fig. 42.4 Inferior left globe displacement (**a**) and proptosis (**b**) due to a large superolateral orbital solitary fibrous tumor. CT scan showing tumor (**c**, arrow)

orbit and lesions of this area often cause lateral globe displacement.

Inferior globe displacement can also result from bony volume expansion of the orbit after facial trauma and significant orbital fractures. Additionally, patients who have undergone prior orbital decompression or bony orbitotomy for lesion biopsy/excision may demonstrate globe dystopia.

Extraocular Motility

Binocular diplopia may occur secondary to mass effect, tumor infiltration, or inflammation of the extraocular muscles. To test the voluntary eye movements, versions are assessed with both eyes open (which allows for comparison with the unaffected side in unilateral disease), while ductions are tested with the opposing eye covered to assess for maximal motility. When motility is decreased, forced ductions can be performed to differentiate paralytic strabismus from restrictive strabismus. To perform forced duction testing, first, instill a topical anesthetic drop into the eye and then use a cotton-tipped applicator or toothed forceps to assess the mobility of the globe. In the acute trauma setting, orbital edema limits the usefulness of this test. However, after orbital and periocular swelling has decreased, it can be useful in preoperative counseling and planning and should be performed at the start and end of surgery.

Orbital processes typically cause incomitant strabismus, and diplopia fields are useful for assessing range of single vision. To quantify strabismus, cover testing with prisms should be performed. The amount of deviation can then be followed over time to assess for worsening, improvement, or stability. Consultation with pediatric ophthalmologists is particularly useful for complex patients.

Eye: Anterior Segment

The ocular examination not only can provide clues to the etiology of disease but can also reveal sequelae of orbital pathology. Examination of the anterior segment should proceed methodically and include the conjunctiva and sclera, the cornea, the anterior chamber, the iris, and the lens. In the office, this is most commonly performed at the slit lamp. When consultations are performed at the bedside, a penlight is sometimes sufficient for an initial anterior segment evaluation.

Examination of the conjunctiva can reveal inflammation or vascular changes such as venous engorgement, sentinel vessels, or corkscrew vessels. The presence of scleritis can help to narrow the differential diagnosis for orbital inflammatory disease. Examination of the cornea should focus on the epithelial integrity. Fluorescein stains exposed basement membranes and fluoresces green when illuminated with a cobalt blue light. This is useful for seeing corneal epithelial defects due to exposure keratopathy associated with proptosis and lagophthalmos. Cell and flare in the anterior chamber can reflect intraocular inflammation related to orbital inflammation. Lens opacities including subcapsular cataracts may be noted in patients who have been on steroids. Traumatic cataracts can occur from blunt trauma or from penetrating intraocular foreign bodies. Similarly, iris atrophy and disinsertion can be sequelae of blunt trauma.

Intraocular pressure is most accurately measured by applanation tonometry and is normally symmetric. A unilateral orbital vascular process may cause secondary glaucoma, and intraocular pressure may be increased on the affected side. Examples include carotid cavernous fistula, cavernous sinus thrombosis, and vascular lesions of the orbit. Additionally, steroid-responsive patients may have acute intraocular pressure increases with either topical or oral steroids. In contrast, ciliary body function may be decreased acutely after blunt trauma causing a unilateral decrease in intraocular pressure.

Eye: Posterior Segment

The posterior segment examination can be performed at the slit lamp with a fundus lens or with an indirect ophthalmoscope. It begins with examination of the optic nerve to assess its color and sharpness of the borders. Optic nerve edema is often characterized by blurring of the optic disc margin, obscuration of the peripapillary retinal vessels, peripapillary hemorrhages, or Paton's folds (peripapillary wrinkles). Optic nerve pallor usually signifies a long-standing injury. Both optic nerve edema and pallor in orbital disease can result from compression, infiltration, direct trauma, or optic neuritis. Fundus examination should then assess the retinal vasculature, macula, and periphery. With orbital masses causing indentation of the globe, choroidal folds can be observed. These can be appreciated with red-free light. Infectious processes of the posterior segment including endophthalmitis or panophthalmitis can present with orbital findings of inflammation, proptosis, and pain. Similar findings can be seen with necrosis within posterior segment tumors such as retinoblastoma or choroidal melanoma [41]. When visualization is difficult due to opaque media, B mode ultrasound is critical for evaluation of the posterior segment and can allow for identification of tumors or endophthalmitis.

Accessory Tests When Suspecting Optic Neuropathy

Decreased color vision, or dyschromatopsia, is suggestive of optic neuropathy. When the patient views a red object with each eye independently, a subjective discrepancy can be noted if disease is unilateral. Ishihara pseudoisochromatic color plates as well as the Farnsworth D-15 panel test or Farnsworth–Munsell 100-hue test can provide further characterization of color vision deficits. We typically use the Ishihara color plates to screen our patients with orbital disease for possible optic neuropathy [37].

Visual field testing is necessary for a complete orbital evaluation. Confrontational visual field testing of each eye separately can provide the clinician with a clue of gross visual field deficits such as a hemianopsia or an inferior or superior visual field deficit. However, compressive optic neuropathy often causes arcuate scotomas or paracentral scotomas that are better assessed with computerized threshold perimetry or Goldmann kinetic perimetry. These methods are more standardized and objective and allow for better comparison of visual field deficits over time.

Laboratory Evaluation

After a complete orbital examination, selected laboratory evaluation may be appropriate (Table 42.1). A complete blood count with differential can show leukocytosis or thrombocytosis reflecting infection or inflammation. Leukopenia suggests immunosuppression that can predispose patients to invasive fungal diseases such as mucormycosis and aspergillosis. In the setting of orbital infections such as cellulitis or abscess, blood cultures are invaluable for identifying causative organisms and targeting antibiotic treatment.

In patients with a constellation of proptosis, eyelid retraction, and diplopia, abnormalities of thyroid function associated with Graves' disease should be investigated. Thyroid-stimulating hormone (TSH), free T3, and free T4 should be measured. Also, stimulating antibodies to the TSH receptor can be tested [42].

Laboratory testing is most often performed in the setting of orbital inflammatory diseases looking for associated systemic diseases. Erythrocyte sedimentation rate and C-reactive protein are often elevated but are nonspecific systemic inflammatory markers. Sarcoidosis is a systemic inflammatory disorder which commonly involves the lungs but also can involve the orbital structures and the eyes [9, 10]. Angiotensin-converting enzyme and lysozyme are typically elevated in these patients, and a chest X-ray can assess for mediastinal lymphadenopathy [43].

Another cause of orbital inflammation is granulomatosis with polyangiitis (formally called Wegener's disease), a systemic necrotizing vasculitis classically involving the pulmonary parenchyma, sinuses, and kidneys [6–8, 44]. Antineutrophil cytoplasmic antibodies are elevated in this disease [44].

IgG4 disease is an inflammatory condition characterized by the development of fibroinflammatory lesions rich in IgG4+ plasma cells. In the orbit, IgG4 typically involves the lacrimal gland and causes painless lacrimal gland enlargement and inferomedial globe displacement. Diagnosis is made through a combination of histopathologic criteria, physical examination findings, elevated serum IgG4, and characteristic imaging findings. Treatment is often managed with steroids or other immunosuppressants such as rituximab [11, 45].

Less common systemic inflammatory diseases with orbital involvement include Crohn's disease, Langerhans cell histiocytosis, xanthogranuloma, and systemic lupus erythematosus [46–55]. Consultation with rheumatology specialists can help with diagnosing and treating these systemic autoimmune diseases [56–58].

Imaging

Three of the most commonly used modalities used to characterize the structures of the orbit include ultrasound, computed tomography (CT), and magnetic resonance imaging (MRI). Depending on the patient's findings, one or more are often indispensable for an accurate orbital evaluation [59].

B mode ultrasound can be used to evaluate extraocular muscle thickening seen in thyroid eye disease or orbital myositis. Other diseases with specific ultrasound findings include scleritis, choroidal melanoma, and choroidal metastases. Ultrasound can also characterize the intraocular contents when the ocular media is opaque as in endophthalmitis or vitritis.

CT imaging has become integral in the evaluation of the patient with orbital disease. Images are created based on the differential absorption of X-rays by different tissues [60]. Coronal, sagittal, and axial imaging allow for the specific localization of orbital pathology. Because CT scans delineate bone very well, they are preferable for identifying bony changes that can help characterize orbital lesions. Additionally, CT scans can characterize orbital pathology as heterogeneous or homogeneous, cystic or solid, infiltrative or encapsulated, or calcified. Intravenous contrast dye is often helpful in defining enhancement characteristics of lesions. In the trauma patient, CT scans are invaluable in identifying orbital fractures [20, 60, 61]. Thoughtful and judicious use of CT imaging in the pediatric population is important because of the deleterious effects of radiation [62–64].

MRI provides good contrast between soft tissues. This is less of an advantage in the orbit because the orbital fat naturally provides a contrast to orbital tissues or tumors and can be appreciated well on CT. Also, MRI does not show bony anatomy as well as CT. However, MRI is more sensitive than CT for detecting perineural spread of tumors and is preferable in the pediatric population to avoid radiation exposure. Because of the force of the magnet used to generate the MR image, patients with suspected metallic foreign bodies should not receive an MRI [34, 35, 65].

Patient Management

For an accurate orbital evaluation, the clinician must combine elements of the history and physical examination to recommend judicious laboratory investigations or imaging as appropriate. If a specific diagnosis can be made and medical treatment is recommended, patients should be followed carefully. However, surgical intervention is often necessary for a precise diagnosis. Table 42.2 describes the key orbital structures to preserve when considering surgery in the various orbital regions.

Table 42.2 Orbital anatomic considerations in the various orbital regions

Superomedial	*Superior*	*Superolateral*
Superior oblique muscle, trochlea, anterior and posterior ethmoidal neurovascular bundles, trochlear nerve	Superior rectus muscle, levator palpebrae muscle, frontal nerve	Lacrimal gland, lacrimal neurovascular bundle, lateral horn of the levator palpebrae
Medial	*Intraconal*	*Lateral*
Medial rectus muscle, medial canthal tendon, ethmoid sinus	Globe, ophthalmic artery, optic nerve, nerves to the recti muscles, long and short posterior ciliary arteries, nasociliary nerve, superior ophthalmic vein	Lateral rectus muscle, lateral canthal tendon, meningolacrimal artery
Inferomedial	*Inferior*	*Inferolateral*
Nasolacrimal sac, inferior oblique muscle, medial orbital strut	Infraorbital neurovascular bundle, inferior oblique, inferior rectus muscle, ciliary ganglion, capsulopalpebral fascia, maxiallary sinus	Zygomaticofacial and zygomatictemporal neurovascular bundles

When orbital surgery is required, the surgical approach is guided by the goal of the surgery, the location of the disease process, and the size of the lesion. If the suspected disease process is treatable with adjuvant therapy such as antibiotics, immunosuppression, chemotherapy, and radiation, then a less invasive orbitotomy for biopsy may be adequate. This can be achieved through upper eyelid crease, inferior fornix, or transcaruncular approaches.

In contrast, more invasive approaches are sometimes needed. For example, a large malignant lesion of the superior orbit requiring a surgical cure may demand a craniotomy with orbital roof excision. Similarly, exposure and access to large lesions of the lateral orbit may require removal of the lateral orbital wall. For medial or inferior lesions involving the paranasal sinuses, an orbitotomy combined with maxillectomy or rhinotomy may be required. Lastly, orbital exenteration is sometimes needed for aggressive orbital tumors. We recommend consultation with and assistance from neurosurgical, skull base, craniofacial, and otolaryngology colleagues if more extensive surgical planning and access are necessary.

Because of the many vital structures within the orbit and the frequent need for orbital surgery with potential complications, the clinician must perform a systematic and thorough evaluation of every patient with orbital disease to make appropriate recommendations for each patient.

References

1. Dolman PJ. Grading severity and activity in thyroid eye disease. Ophthalmic Plast Reconstr Surg. 2018;34(4S Suppl 1):S34–40. https://doi.org/10.1097/IOP.0000000000001150. PubMed PMID: 29952931.
2. Siakallis LC, Uddin JM, Miszkiel KA. Imaging investigation of thyroid eye disease. Ophthalmic Plast Reconstr Surg. 2018;34(4S Suppl 1):S41–51. https://doi.org/10.1097/IOP.0000000000001139. PubMed PMID: 29905640.
3. Dik WA, Virakul S, van Steensel L. Current perspectives on the role of orbital fibroblasts in the pathogenesis of Graves' ophthalmopathy. Exp Eye Res. 2016;142:83–91. https://doi.org/10.1016/j.exer.2015.02.007. Review. PubMed PMID: 26675405.
4. Uddin JM, Rubinstein T, Hamed-Azzam S. Phenotypes of thyroid eye disease. Ophthalmic Plast Reconstr Surg. 2018;34(4S Suppl 1):S28–33. https://doi.org/10.1097/IOP.0000000000001147. Review. PubMed PMID: 29905636.
5. Menconi F, Marcocci C, Marinò M. Diagnosis and classification of Graves' disease. Autoimmun Rev. 2014;13(4–5):398–402. https://doi.org/10.1016/j.autrev.2014.01.013. Epub 2014 Jan 12. Review. PubMed PMID: 24424182.
6. Tarabishy AB, Schulte M, Papaliodis GN, Hoffman GS. Wegener's granulomatosis: clinical manifestations, differential diagnosis, and management of ocular and systemic disease. Surv Ophthalmol. 2010;55(5):429–44. https://doi.org/10.1016/j.survophthal.2009.12.003. Epub 2010 Jul 17. Review. PubMed PMID:20638092.
7. Yang B, Yin Z, Chen S, Yuan F, Zhao W, Yang Y. Imaging diagnosis of orbital Wegener granulomatosis: a rare case report. Medicine (Baltimore). 2017;96(23):e6904. https://doi.org/10.1097/MD.0000000000006904. PubMed PMID: 28591026; PubMed Central PMCID: PMC5466204.
8. Sfiniadaki E, Tsiara I, Theodossiadis P, Chatziralli I. Ocular manifestations of granulomatosis with polyangiitis: a review of the literature. Ophthalmol Ther. 2019;8:227. https://doi.org/10.1007/s40123-019-0176-8. [Epub ahead of print] Review. PubMed PMID: 30875067.
9. Demirci H, Christianson MD. Orbital and adnexal involvement in sarcoidosis: analysis of clinical features and systemic disease in 30 cases. Am J Ophthalmol. 2011;151(6):1074–1080.e1. https://doi.org/10.1016/j.ajo.2010.12.011. Epub 2011 Mar 31. PubMed PMID: 21457924.
10. Gutman J, Shinder R. Orbital and adnexal involvement in sarcoidosis: analysis of clinical features and systemic disease in 30 cases. Am J Ophthalmol. 2011;152(5):883. https://doi.org/10.1016/j.ajo.2011.07.024. PubMed PMID: 22017852.
11. Chwalisz BK, Stone JH. Neuro-ophthalmic complications of IgG4-related disease. Curr Opin Ophthalmol. 2018;29(6):485–94. https://doi.org/10.1097/ICU.0000000000000523. Review. PubMed PMID: 30199519.
12. Neems L, Echalier EL, Subramanian PS. Orbital tumors and inflammatory disorders: diagnosis and management. Int Ophthalmol Clin. 2018;58(2):181–95. https://doi.org/10.1097/IIO.0000000000000217. Review. PubMed PMID: 29517650.
13. Pakdaman MN, Sepahdari AR, Elkhamary SM. Orbital inflammatory disease: pictorial review and differential diagnosis. World J Radiol. 2014;6(4):106–15. https://doi.org/10.4329/wjr.v6.i4.106. Review. PubMed PMID: 24778772; PubMed Central PMCID: PMC4000606.
14. Chaudhry IA, Alaraj AM, Alkatan HM. Unilateral eyelid swelling, proptosis and diplopia as initial manifestation of acute myeloid leukemia. Saudi J Ophthalmol. 2012;26(2):241–4. https://doi.org/10.1016/j.sjopt.2012.03.004. Epub 2012 Mar 19. PubMed PMID: 23960999; PubMed Central PMCID: PMC3729485.
15. Huang YC, Wang SC, Chen SN, Jou JR. Bilateral acute proptosis as initial manifestation of acute myeloid leukemia. Orbit. 2015;34(5):248–52. https://doi.org/10.3109/01676830.2015.1049371. Epub 2015 Jul 17. PubMed PMID: 26186043.
16. Neel GS, Nagel TH, Hoxworth JM, Lal D. Management of orbital involvement in sinonasal and ventral skull base malignancies. Otolaryngol Clin N Am. 2017;50(2):347–64. https://doi.org/10.1016/j.otc.2016.12.010. Review. PubMed PMID: 28314402.
17. Lisan Q, Kolb F, Temam S, Tao Y, Janot F, Moya-Plana A. Management of orbital invasion in sinonasal malignancies. Head Neck. 2016;38(11):1650–6. https://doi.org/10.1002/hed.24490. Epub 2016 Apr 30. PubMed PMID: 271313
18. Marwaha G, Macklis R, Singh AD. Radiation therapy: orbital tumors. Dev Ophthalmol. 2013;52:94–101. https://doi.org/10.1159/000351084. Epub 2013 Aug 26. Review. PubMed PMID: 23989130.
19. Suarez C, Ferlito A, Lund VJ, et al. Management of the orbit in malignant sinonasal tumors. Head Neck. 2008;30(2):242–50.
20. Holck DEE. Evaluation and treatment of orbital fractures: a multidisciplinary approach. Philadelphia: Elsevier Saunders; 2006.
21. Le Rouic JF, Bettembourg O, D'Hermies F, et al. Late swelling and removal of Miragel buckles: a comparison with silicone indentations. Retina. 2003;23(5):641–6.
22. Campen CJ, Gutmann DH. Optic pathway gliomas in neurofibromatosis type 1. J Child Neurol. 2018;33(1):73–81. https://doi.org/10.1177/0883073817739509. Review. PubMed PMID: 29246098; PubMed Central PMCID: PMC5739070.
23. de Blank PMK, Fisher MJ, Liu GT, Gutmann DH, Listernick R, Ferner RE, Avery RA. Optic pathway gliomas in neurofibromatosis type 1: an update: surveillance, treatment indications, and biomarkers of vision. J Neuroophthalmol. 2017;37(Suppl 1):S23–

32. https://doi.org/10.1097/WNO.0000000000000550. Review. PubMed PMID: 28806346
24. Friedrich RE, Stelljes C, Hagel C, et al. Dysplasia of the orbit and adjacent bone associated with plexiform neurofibroma and ocular disease in 42 NF-1 patients. Anticancer Res. 2010;30(5):1751–64.
25. Medel Jiménez R, Sánchez España JC, Vasquez LM, Tapia Bahamondes A, Rondón M, Francesc T, Ayala BE. Orbital and peri-orbital amyloidosis: a report of four cases. Orbit. 2018;22:1–6. https://doi.org/10.1080/01676830.2018.1449868. [Epub ahead of print]. PubMed PMID: 29565698.
26. Singh M, Rao KR, Das A. Primary orbital amyloidosis. JAMA Ophthalmol. 2018;136(1):e175727. https://doi.org/10.1001/jamaophthalmol.2017.5727. Epub 2018 Jan 11. PubMed PMID: 29327051.
27. Wang LE, Hu Z, Sturgis EM, et al. Reduced DNA repair capacity for removing tobacco carcinogen-induced DNA adducts contributes to risk of head and neck cancer but not tumor characteristics. Clin Cancer Res. 2010;16(2):764–74.
28. Lubin JH, Purdue M, Kelsey K, et al. Total exposure and exposure rate effects for alcohol and smoking and risk of head and neck cancer: a pooled analysis of case-control studies. Am J Epidemiol. 2009;170(8):937–47.
29. Lubin JH, Alavanja MC, Caporaso N, et al. Cigarette smoking and cancer risk: modeling total exposure and intensity. Am J Epidemiol. 2007;166(4):479–89.
30. Nita M, Grzybowski A. Smoking and eye pathologies. A Systemic review. Part II. Retina diseases, uveitis, optic neuropathies, thyroid-associated orbitopathy. Curr Pharm Des. 2017;23(4):639–54. https://doi.org/10.2174/1381612823666170111095723. Review. PubMed PMID: 28078992.
31. Sadeghi-Tari A, Jamshidian-Tehrani M, Nabavi A, Sharif-Kashani S, Elhami E, Hassanpour N, Ameli ZK. Effect of smoking on retrobulbar blood flow in thyroid eye disease. Eye (Lond). 2016;30(12):1573–8. https://doi.org/10.1038/eye.2016.184. Epub 2016 Aug 19. PubMed PMID: 27540833; PubMed Central PMCID: PMC5177752.
32. Bartalena L, Marcocci C, Tanda ML, et al. Cigarette smoking and treatment outcomes in graves ophthalmopathy. Ann Intern Med. 1998;129(8):632–5.
33. Thornton J, Kelly SP, Harrison RA, Edwards R. Cigarette smoking and thyroid eye disease: a systematic review. Eye (Lond). 2007;21(9):1135–45.
34. Finkelstein M, Legmann A, Rubin PA. Projectile metallic foreign bodies in the orbit: a retrospective study of epidemiologic factors, management, and outcomes. Ophthalmology. 1997;104(1):96–103.
35. Fulcher TP, McNab AA, Sullivan TJ. Clinical features and management of intraorbital foreign bodies. Ophthalmology. 2002;109(3):494–500.
36. Baker RS, Wilson RM, Flowers CW Jr, et al. A population-based survey of hospitalized work-related ocular injury: diagnoses, cause of injury, resource utilization, and hospitalization outcome. Ophthalmic Epidemiol. 1999;6(3):159–69.
37. Liu GT, Galetta SL. Neuro-ophthalmology. 3rd ed. Philadelphia: Elsevier; 2019.
38. Bernardini FP, Devoto MH, Croxatto JO. Epithelial tumors of the lacrimal gland: an update. Curr Opin Ophthalmol. 2008;19(5):409–13.
39. Orr CK, Cochran E, Shinder R. Metastatic scirrhous breast carcinoma to orbit causing enophthalmos. Ophthalmology. 2016;123(7):1529. https://doi.org/10.1016/j.ophtha.2016.04.012. PubMed PMID: 27342331.
40. Novitskaya E, Rene C. Enophthalmos as a sign of metastatic breast carcinoma. CMAJ. 2013;185(13):1159. https://doi.org/10.1503/cmaj.120726. Epub 2013 Mar 4. PubMed PMID: 23460637; PubMed Central PMCID: PMC3778478.
41. Blanco G. Diagnosis and treatment of orbital invasion in uveal melanoma. Can J Ophthalmol. 2004;39(4):388–96.
42. Lehmann GM, Feldon SE, Smith TJ, Phipps RP. Immune mechanisms in thyroid eye disease. Thyroid. 2008;18(9):959–65.
43. Llanos O, Hamzeh N. Sarcoidosis. Med Clin North Am. 2019;103(3):527–34. https://doi.org/10.1016/j.mcna.2018.12.011. Epub 2019 Feb 21. Review. PubMed PMID: 30955519.
44. Ungprasert P, Crowson CS, Cartin-Ceba R, Garrity JA, Smith WM, Specks U, Matteson EL, Makol A. Clinical characteristics of inflammatory ocular disease in anti-neutrophil cytoplasmic antibody associated vasculitis: a retrospective cohort study. Rheumatology (Oxford). 2017;56(10):1763–70. https://doi.org/10.1093/rheumatology/kex261. PubMed PMID: 28957561.
45. Umehara H, Okazaki K, Nakamura T, et al. Current approach to the diagnosis of IgG4-related disease – combination of comprehensive diagnostic and organ-specific criteria. Mod Rheumatol. 2017;27(3):381–91.
46. Vargason CW, Mawn LA. Orbital myositis as both a presenting and associated extraintestinal sign of crohn's disease. Ophthalmic Plast Reconstr Surg. 2017;33(3S Suppl 1):S158–60. https://doi.org/10.1097/IOP.0000000000000475. PubMed PMID: 26154590.
47. Troncoso LL, Biancardi AL, de Moraes HV Jr, Zaltman C. Ophthalmic manifestations in patients with inflammatory bowel disease: a review. World J Gastroenterol. 2017;23(32):5836–48. https://doi.org/10.3748/wjg.v23.i32.5836. Review. PubMed PMID: 28932076; PubMed Central PMCID: PMC5583569.
48. Margo CE, Goldman DR. Langerhans cell histiocytosis. Surv Ophthalmol. 2008;53(4):332–58.
49. Merritt H, Pfeiffer ML, Richani K, Phillips ME. Erdheim-Chester disease with orbital involvement: case report and ophthalmic literature review. Orbit. 2016;35(4):221–6. https://doi.org/10.1080/01676830.2016.1176211. Epub 2016 Jun 20. Review. PubMed PMID: 27322549.
50. Vosoghi H, Rodriguez-Galindo C, Wilson MW. Orbital involvement in langerhans cell histiocytosis. Ophthal Plast Reconstr Surg. 2009;25(6):430–3.
51. Elner VM, Mintz R, Demirci H, Hassan AS. Local corticosteroid treatment of eyelid and orbital xanthogranuloma. Ophthal Plast Reconstr Surg. 2006;22(1):36–40.
52. Karcioglu ZA, Sharara N, Boles TL, Nasr AM. Orbital xanthogranuloma: clinical and morphologic features in eight patients. Ophthal Plast Reconstr Surg. 2003;19(5):372–81.
53. Arthurs BP, Khalil MK, Chagnon F, et al. Orbital infarction and melting in a patient with systemic lupus erythematosus. Ophthalmology. 1999;106(12):2387–90.
54. Serop S, Vianna RN, Claeys M, De Laey JJ. Orbital myositis secondary to systemic lupus erythematosus. Acta Ophthalmol. 1994;72(4):520–3.
55. Stavrou P, Murray PI, Batta K, Gordon C. Acute ocular ischaemia and orbital inflammation associated with systemic lupus erythematosus. Br J Ophthalmol. 2002;86(4):474–5.
56. Kurz PA, Suhler EB, Choi D, Rosenbaum JT. Rituximab for treatment of ocular inflammatory disease: a series of four cases. Br J Ophthalmol. 2009;93(4):546–8.
57. Lutt JR, Lim LL, Phal PM, Rosenbaum JT. Orbital inflammatory disease. Semin Arthritis Rheum. 2008;37(4):207–22.
58. Swamy BN, McCluskey P, Nemet A, et al. Idiopathic orbital inflammatory syndrome: clinical features and treatment outcomes. Br J Ophthalmol. 2007;91(12):1667–70.
59. Dutton JJ. Atlas of clinical and surgical orbital anatomy. 2nd ed. Philadelphia: Elsevier Saunders; 2011.
60. Chen CT, Chen YR. Update on orbital reconstruction. Curr Opin Otolaryngol Head Neck Surg. 2010;18(4):311–6.

61. Bevans SE, Moe KS. Advances in the reconstruction of orbital fractures. Facial Plast Surg Clin North Am. 2017;25(4):513–35. https://doi.org/10.1016/j.fsc.2017.06.014. Review. PubMed PMID: 28941505.
62. Cohen MD. Pediatric CT radiation dose: how low can you go? AJR Am J Roentgenol. 2009;192(5):1292–303.
63. Frush DP. CT dose and risk estimates in children. Pediatr Radiol. 2011;41(Suppl 2):483–7. https://doi.org/10.1007/s00247-011-2098-z. Epub 2011 Aug 17. Review. PubMed PMID: 21847726.
64. Jeganathan VS, Wirth A, MacManus MP. Ocular risks from orbital and periorbital radiation therapy: a critical review. Int J Radiat Oncol Biol Phys. 2011;79(3):650–9. https://doi.org/10.1016/j.ijrobp.2010.09.056. Review. PubMed PMID: 21281895.
65. Pinto A, Brunese L, Daniele S, Faggian A, Guarnieri G, Muto M, Romano L. Role of computed tomography in the assessment of intraorbital foreign bodies. Semin Ultrasound CT MR. 2012;33(5):392–5. https://doi.org/10.1053/j.sult.2012.06.004. Review. PubMed PMID: 22964405.

Orbital Radiology

43

Tabassum A. Kennedy and Lindell R. Gentry

Imaging Techniques

Advances in medical imaging with computed tomography (CT) and magnetic resonance imaging (MRI) have markedly improved our ability to visualize orbital anatomy and pathology. The following section discusses the indications for orbital CT and MRI, the utility of intravenous contrast, and dynamic vascular imaging.

CT Imaging

A standard CT protocol for orbital imaging includes 0.625–1.25-mm axial images that extend from the mid-maxillary sinuses through the top of the orbits (Fig. 43.1). Two reconstruction algorithms are used to generate axial images that accentuate both soft tissue contrast and bone detail. Two-dimensional sagittal, coronal, and sagittal oblique reconstructions are then produced from the axial data set. CT imaging is usually indicated as the initial imaging study for emergent evaluation of orbital trauma and infection. CT can also be performed to assess for foreign bodies, calcifications, orbital masses, extraocular muscle pathology, and lesions involving the bony orbit [1]. CT imaging of the orbit may be performed without or with intravenous contrast. The use of contrast is always indicated for evaluation of orbital masses, vascular malformations, and infections. However, in the setting of trauma or foreign body evaluation, contrast is usually not necessary.

T. A. Kennedy (✉)
Department of Radiology, University of Wisconsin Hospital and Clinics, Madison, WI, USA
e-mail: Tkennedy@uwhealth.org

L. R. Gentry
Radiology, Madison, WI, USA

MR Imaging

There are many indications for imaging the orbit with MRI. MRI provides excellent delineation of the globe, extraocular muscles, and adjacent structures (Fig. 43.2). Orbital MR images can be obtained using a surface coil or phased array head coil. Surface coils can improve the signal-to-noise ratio (SNR) [2, 3] of MR images, but the depth of view is usually limited to one-half the radius of the coil. The SNR produced by surface coils is not homogeneous as they provide excellent signal near the coil and poor signal away from the coil, toward the orbital apex. Phased array head coils (8, 16, and 32 channels) are currently used for orbital imaging in most institutions. Phased array coils are constructed from 8 to 32 small surface coils making up the head coil. The MR signals received from each of the local surface coils are electronically integrated to make up the final MR image. Phased array coils provide many of the benefits of surface coils and avoid many of the disadvantages. In many cases, it is also important to image the brain using T1-W, T2-W, diffusion-weighted (DWI), and T2-FLAIR (fluid-attenuated inversion recovery) pulse sequences. Postcontrast images of the brain are especially helpful in patients suspected of having infectious, inflammatory, neoplastic, ischemic, or demyelinating diseases.

The ability to perform fat saturation is important when evaluating the orbit with MRI. Fat is inherently bright on both T1-weighted (T1-W) and T2-weighted (T2-W) images and therefore may mask edema on T2-W scans and hide enhancing lesions on postcontrast T1-W images. This is especially true of lesions that are adjacent to or embedded within orbital fat.

Suggested MR protocol for orbital and brain pathology includes:

A. Precontrast orbit images
   Axial T1-W
   Axial T2-W
   Oblique sagittal T1-W (parallel to the optic nerves)

J. J. Servat et al. (eds.), *Smith and Nesi's Ophthalmic Plastic and Reconstructive Surgery*,
https://doi.org/10.1007/978-3-030-41720-8_43

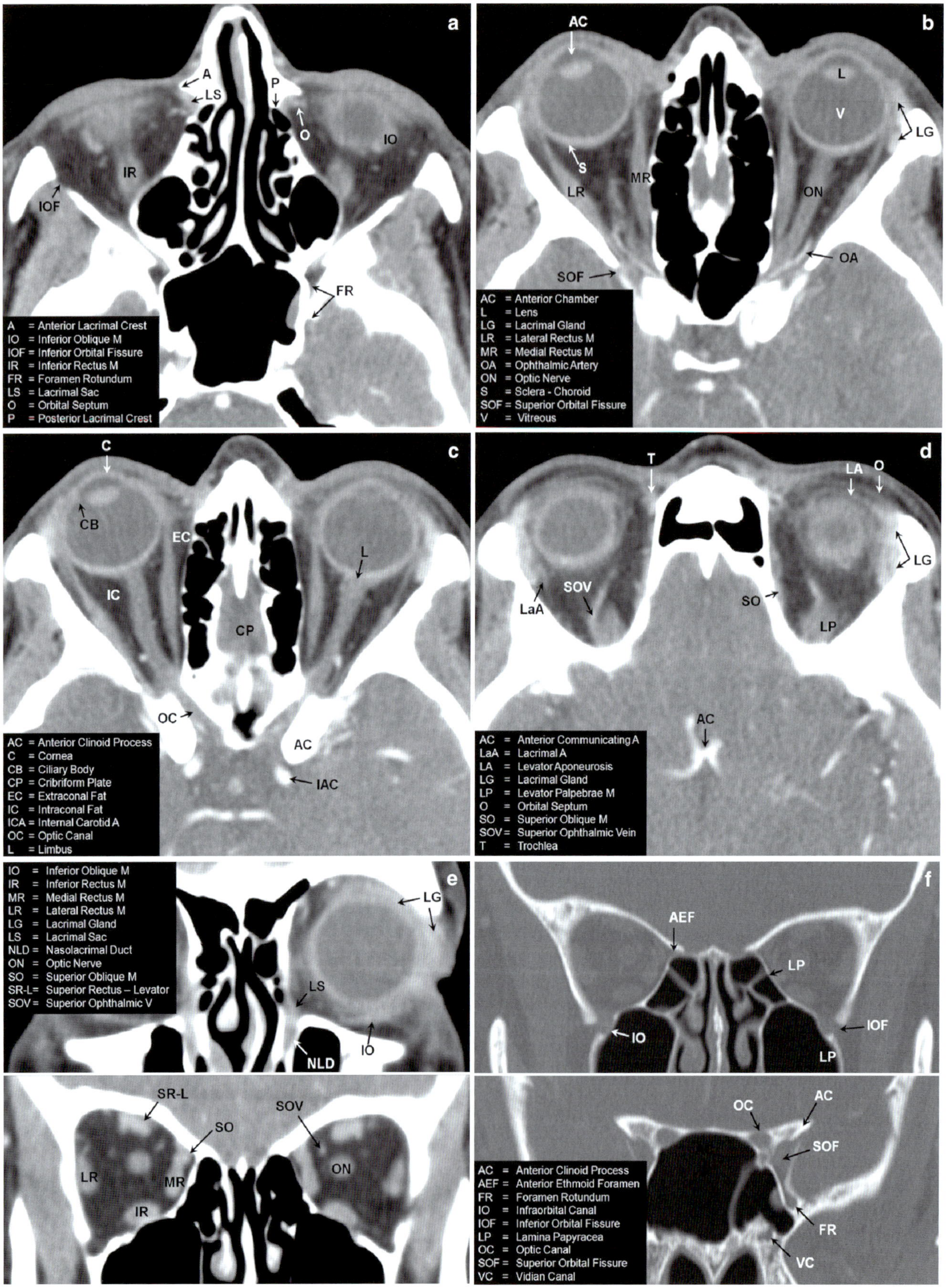

Fig. 43.1 Normal orbit CT scan: axial (**a–d**) and coronal (**e**, **f**) CT scans

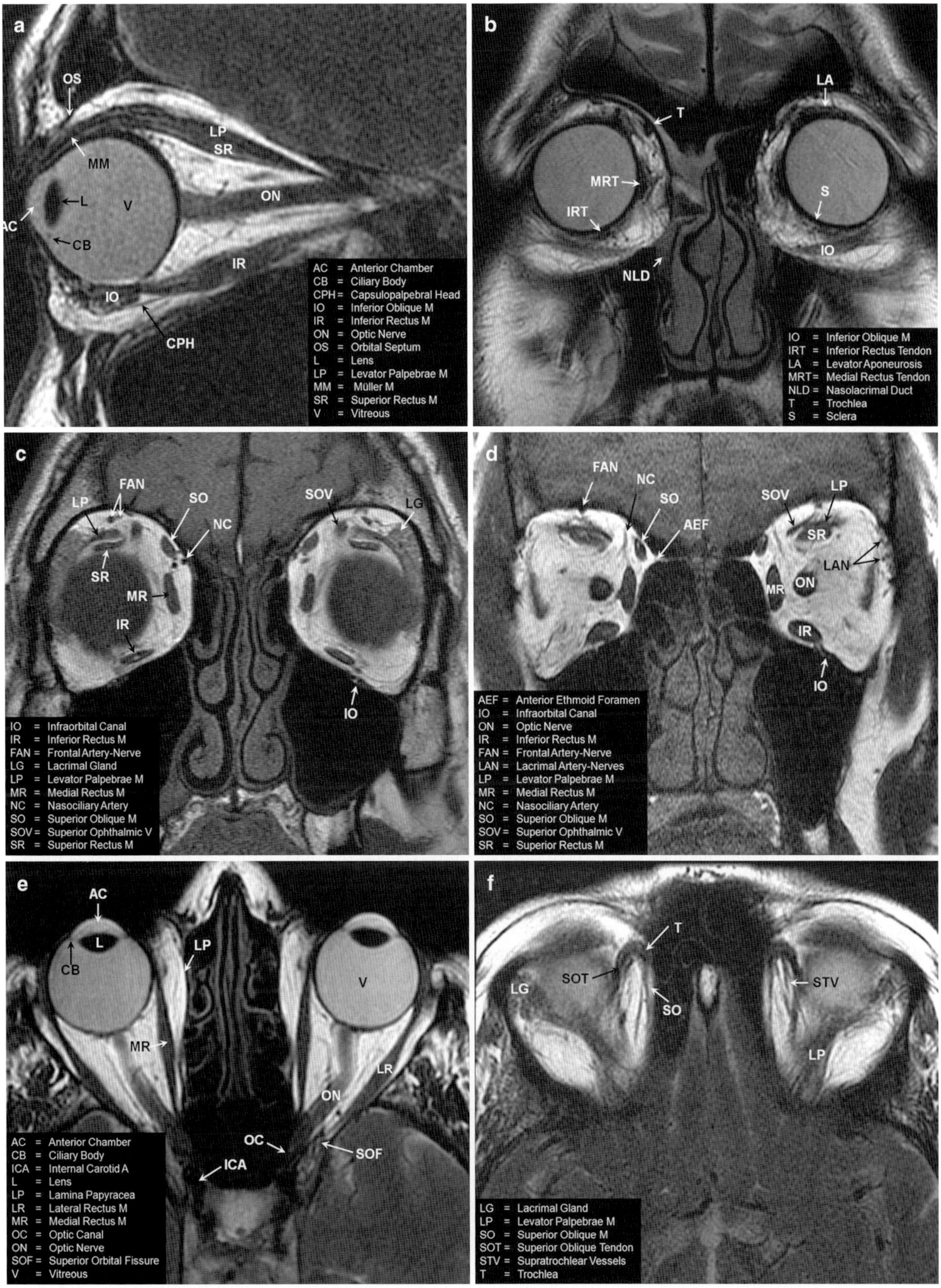

Fig. 43.2 Normal orbit MRI scan: sagittal T2-W (**a**), coronal T2-W (**b**), coronal T1-W (**c**, **d**), and axial T2-W (**e**, **f**) MR scans

Coronal T1-W (optional)
Coronal T2-W (optional)

B. Postcontrast orbit images
Axial T1-W (with fat suppression)
Coronal T1-W (with fat suppression)
Oblique sagittal T1-W (with fat suppression) (optional)

C. Precontrast brain images
Sagittal T1-W
Axial T2-W
Axial DWI

D. Postcontrast brain images
Axial T1-W
Coronal T2-FLAIR

Dynamic Vascular and Positional Imaging

There are several instances where dynamic imaging of orbital vascularity is indicated [4–14]. Both CT and MR dynamic imaging techniques are available for providing this information. Dynamic CT angiography (CTA) and MR angiographic (MRA) imaging of the orbit are especially helpful for evaluating suspected vascular orbital masses. Following a bolus injection of contrast medium, either CT or MR images can be rapidly acquired during the arterial, parenchymal, and venous phases of passage of contrast through the lesion. This will provide unique information to allow characterization of the vascularity and pattern of contrast enhancement of a particular lesion [6]. Dynamic MRA is especially beneficial since it does not require the use of ionizing radiation. In addition, pre- and post-Valsalva maneuvers may be performed to assess whether a suspected orbital lesion such as a varix changes in size after the Valsalva maneuver [11–14].

Dynamic CT or MR imaging may also be performed to assess effective contraction of the extraocular muscles with provocative maneuvers [15]. Having the patient abduct, adduct, look up, and look down during image acquisition may depict pathologic muscle contraction between normal and abnormal extraocular muscles.

Anatomy of the Orbit

The orbit is one of the most complex anatomical structures of the human body. Its small size, differing densities, complex enervation, extensive vascularity, and dynamic capability make evaluating the orbit challenging. Ophthalmoscopic evaluation can provide important information about the interior of the globe although the majority of deep orbital structures cannot be visualized by funduscopy. Imaging by CT or MR is, therefore, essential for evaluating pathologic conditions that involve the orbit. This section reviews the normal imaging anatomy of the orbit both on CT and MRI. The structures of the orbit can be grouped in several different anatomical areas including the bony orbit, the globe and optic nerve, the extraocular muscles, the lid retractor system, the lacrimal system, the vascular system, the neural structures, and orbital fat [16].

Bony Orbit

The bony orbit consists of seven separate bones that together make up four walls, four rims, and an apex. The medial wall is made up of the ethmoid bone centrally, the lacrimal bone anteriorly, sphenoid bone posteriorly, the frontal bone superiorly, and the maxillary bone inferiorly. The ethmoid bone makes up the majority of the medial wall and is paper-thin which is why some have referred to this bone as the lamina papyracea (Fig. 43.1).

The posterior two-thirds of the lateral wall of the orbit is made up of the greater wing of the sphenoid bone [16]. The zygomatic and frontal bones make up the remaining anterior and anterosuperior lateral walls, respectively.

The frontal bone composes the majority of the orbital roof with a small contribution from the lesser wing of the sphenoid bone posteriorly. The orbital floor consists primarily of the maxillary bone; however, the anterolateral aspect is partially formed by the maxillary process of the zygomatic bone.

The anterior margin of the bony orbit is divided into four rims: medial, lateral, superior, and inferior. The nasal process of the frontal bone forms the superior margin of the medial rim, and the frontal process of the maxillary bone makes up the inferior margin of the medial rim. The lateral rim is formed by the zygomatic process of the frontal bone superiorly and by the frontal process of the zygomatic bone inferiorly. The superior rim is formed by the frontal bone, whereas the inferior rim is made up of the maxillary bone medially and the zygomatic bone laterally.

The orbital apex is the posterior converging point of the four walls of the orbit. The orbital apex is made up of the lesser wing of the sphenoid medially and the greater wing of the sphenoid laterally. The strut of bone separating the superior orbital fissure from the foramen rotundum defines the inferior margin of the orbital apex, whereas the superior margin is bound by the superior portion of the lesser wing of the sphenoid. A small piece of bone called the optic strut separates the optic canal and superior orbital fissure at the orbital apex.

There are three major bony openings within the orbital apex: the optic canal, the superior orbital fissure, and the inferior orbital fissure. The optic canal transmits the optic nerve and is formed by the lesser wing of the sphenoid bone. The optic strut separates the optic nerve from the superior orbital fissure. The superior orbital fissure is formed by the lesser wing of the sphenoid medially and the greater wing of the sphenoid bone laterally. The superior orbital fissure has both horizontal and vertical components. The horizontal component which is situated lateral to the annulus of Zinn contains the trochlear nerve as well as the frontal and lacrimal branches of the ophthalmic nerve (V1). The vertical, more medial component transmits the oculomotor nerve, abducens nerve, and the nasociliary branch of V1. The margins of the inferior orbital fissure are formed by the greater wing of the sphenoid bone, palatine bone, and maxillary bone. There is communication between the inferior orbital fissure and the pterygopalatine fossa. The infraorbital fissure contains the infraorbital (V2), zygomaticotemporal, and zygomaticofacial nerves.

The anterior and posterior ethmoid nerves and arteries traverse their respective foramina within the superior aspect of the medial orbital wall.

The Globe and Optic Nerve

The globe is a spherical structure housed within the bony orbit. The lens divides the small anterior segment filled with aqueous humor from the large posterior segment filled with vitreous humor. The anterior segment is further subdivided into the anterior and posterior chambers by the iris (Fig. 43.2). The lens, located within the posterior chamber, is attached to the ciliary muscles by the zonular fibers. The ciliary body, also located within the posterior chamber, is responsible for producing the aqueous humor.

There are three primary layers of the globe: the sclera, the uvea, and the retina [3]. The sclera and cornea are the outermost layers of the globe and are primarily composed of fibrous tissue. The cornea is noted along the anterior margin of the globe and is optically clear. The posterior most part of the external surface of the globe is the sclera. The sclera and cornea are fused at the corneal limbus which is located lateral to the junction of the anterior and posterior chambers. The uvea is the highly vascularized middle layer of the globe which also has both anterior and posterior components. The iris is located anteriorly, and the highly vascular choroid is located posteriorly. These structures are separated by the ciliary muscle. The innermost layer of the globe is the retina. The retinal layer is further subdivided into the outer pigmented layer and the inner neural layer made up of rods and cones.

The globe is encompassed by a fascial sheath called Tenon's capsule, which separates the globe from the adjacent intraorbital fat [17]. Anteriorly, Tenon's capsule fuses with the conjunctiva. The posterior margin of the capsule is perforated, which allows the passage of the optic nerve, the ciliary nerves, and blood vessels. The sheath also fuses with the dural covering of the intraorbital segment of the optic nerve. The tendons of the extraocular muscles traverse the sheath to reach the underlying scleral layer. The fascial layer reflects back at the site of each tendinous insertion forming a fascial sleeve [18]. Unlike other cranial nerves, the optic nerve is not a true cranial nerve and is myelinated by oligodendrocytes and not by Schwann cells [3]. The optic nerve is formed by ganglion cells from the retina which grow posteriorly toward the diencephalon. There are four major divisions of the optic nerve: the intraocular, intraorbital, intracanalicular, and intracranial segments. The optic nerve measures approximately 50 mm in length from the optic disk to the optic chiasm [16]. The shortest segment is the intraocular component which measures only 1 mm in length [16]. The retinal ganglion cells join together along the posterior aspect of the globe at the optic disk. These unmyelinated axons course through the numerous perforations of the posterior sclera (lamina cribrosa) to form the intraorbital portion of the optic nerve. The remaining segments of the optic nerve are myelinated by oligodendrocytes. The intraorbital optic nerve is surrounded by a layer of leptomeninges (pia-arachnoid) and dura. Subarachnoid space lies in between the dura and pia-arachnoid layers and is contiguous with the intracranial subarachnoid space. The segment of optic nerve that courses through the optic canal is the intracanalicular segment. The optic nerve loses its dural layer at the level of the optic canal as it merges with the surrounding bony periosteum. The optic chiasm is located within the suprasellar cistern and is formed by the junction of the intracranial portions of both optic nerves. The nasal fibers cross at the optic chiasm and proceed into the contralateral optic tract, whereas the temporal fibers continue along the ipsilateral optic tract [3, 19, 20]. The optic tracts then terminate at the lateral geniculate nucleus of the thalamus.

The Extraocular Muscles

There are six extraocular muscles: four rectus muscles (medial, lateral, superior, and inferior) and two oblique muscles (superior and inferior) (Fig. 43.1 and 43.2). The extraocular muscles are responsible for ocular motility [15, 18, 21]. The four rectus muscles begin posteriorly at the annulus of Zinn and extend anteriorly to insert on the sclera. The tendinous insertion of the rectus muscles on the sclera has been termed the *spiral of Tillaux*, which approximates the anterior margin of the sensory retina, the ora serrata [16].

The oblique muscles originate external to the annulus of Zinn. The superior oblique muscle originates medial to the annulus of Zinn from the lesser wing of the sphenoid bone. The superior oblique muscle then extends anteriorly along the superomedial aspect of the orbit to the trochlea. The trochlea is a small cartilaginous structure that anchors the superior oblique tendon and allows it to freely move. This tendon extends laterally beneath the anterior aspect of the superior rectus muscle and inserts on the sclera posterolateral to the equator.

The inferior oblique muscle arises from the anteromedial aspect of the inferior orbit near the lacrimal sac [16]. The inferior oblique muscle runs inferior and lateral to the inferior rectus muscles. The muscle then inserts along the lateral aspect of the globe posterior to the equator. Unlike the other extraocular muscles, the inferior oblique muscle does not have a tendinous insertion but instead inserts directly to the sclera via two to six slips of muscle [16]. During contraction, the capsulopalpebral head of the inferior rectus muscle and Lockwood's ligaments help to stabilize the inferior oblique muscle [16].

The main function of the extraocular muscles is to position the eye in various directions of gaze. The superior rectus muscle elevates, whereas the inferior rectus depresses the globe in primary gaze. The lateral rectus abducts the eye and the medial rectus adducts the eye. The inferior oblique muscle elevates the globe during adduction and rotates the globe upward during primary gaze. In primary gaze, the superior oblique muscle rotates the eye downward and laterally; however, when the eye is adducted, the superior oblique acts to depress the eye.

Lid Retractor System

The upper lid retractor system begins with the levator palpebrae superioris muscle, which originates from the annulus of Zinn and the lesser wing of the sphenoid bone. The levator palpebrae superioris extends anteriorly, running superior and parallel to the superior rectus muscle. These two muscles are separated by a strong intermuscular fascia [22]. The muscle then divides into two major slips: the levator aponeurosis and Müller's muscle. The levator aponeurosis serves as the primary lid retractor and extends in a fan-like fashion to insert along the upper eye lid. Müller's muscle is innervated by sympathetic fibers and functions as an accessory retractor. This muscle may be affected in patients with Horner's syndrome.

The lower lid retractor system is complex, arising primarily from the capsulopalpebral head (CPH) [23]. The CPH extends as a fibromuscular extension from the inferior rectus muscle. At the level of the inferior oblique muscle, the CPH divides into two slips: the inferior tarsal muscle and the capsulopalpebral fascia (CPF). The inferior tarsal muscle attaches to the inferior tarsal plate and functions as the primary lower lid retractor. The CPF attaches to the orbital septum helping to form the lower lid crease. The CPF is also attached to Lockwood's ligament which serves to redirect the forces of the inferior tarsal muscle.

Vascular Supply of the Orbit

The ophthalmic artery is the major arterial supply of the adult orbit [24, 25]. The ophthalmic artery arises from the paraclinoid segment of the internal carotid artery. The artery then travels inferolateral to the optic nerve and enters the orbit through the annulus of Zinn. The central retinal artery is the first branch, and this artery supplies the optic nerve. The central retinal artery travels with the retinal vein to the level of the optic nerve head and then onto the retina. Additional smaller branches arise from the ophthalmic artery to supply the outer aspect of the optic nerve. The second portion of the ophthalmic artery gives rise to two to five short ciliary arteries which subsequently divide into up to 20 smaller braches which ultimately traverse the sclera to supply the optic nerve head and choroid [16].

The three other major terminal branches of the ophthalmic artery are the lacrimal, frontal, and nasociliary arteries (Fig. 43.1). There is some variability of the branching of these vessels. The lacrimal artery is the most constant, whereas the frontal branch is the least constant.

The lacrimal artery primarily supplies the structures within the lateral orbit including the lateral rectus muscle and lacrimal gland. The zygomaticomaxillary and zygomaticofacial arteries are branches of the lacrimal artery. These branches anastomose with branches of the external carotid artery via their respective foramina and provide an important collateral supply between the internal and external carotid arteries. The middle meningeal artery and a recurrent meningeal branch may also arise from the lacrimal artery and serve as potential external/internal carotid artery anastomoses.

The nasociliary artery supplies the medial rectus, superior rectus, and superior oblique muscles and in some instances the inferior muscle groups. Anterior and posterior ethmoid arteries arise from the nasociliary artery, which traverse their respective named foramina. The anterior ethmoid artery supplies the cribriform plate and adjacent meninges after traveling through the orbit and its named foramen. The anterior artery of the falx arises from the anterior ethmoid artery at the level of the crista galli and supplies the meninges of the anterior falx. A second external nasal branch of the anterior ethmoid artery turns inferiorly to supply the upper nasal cavity and nasal septum. The posterior ethmoid artery supplies the meninges along the posterior cribriform plate and planum sphenoidale. The infratrochlear, supratrochlear, dorsal nasal, and medial palpebral arteries are the terminal branches of the nasociliary artery.

The frontal branch may arise as a branch from the ophthalmic artery or as branch from the nasociliary or lacrimal artery. The frontal artery typically supplies the superior muscle group. The terminal branch of the frontal artery is the supraorbital artery which exits the orbit at the supraorbital notch.

The venous drainage of the orbit is typically more variable than the arterial supply and consists of valveless channels [16]. The two major draining veins of the orbit are the superior and inferior ophthalmic veins (Figs. 43.1 and 43.2). The variability is seen with the smaller tributary veins which are typically paired with their respective artery. These smaller veins will drain into one of the two major channels. The superior ophthalmic vein originates anteriorly in the superomedial orbit. It travels posterolaterally between the optic nerve and superior oblique muscle and then between the superior rectus muscle and optic nerve to exit the orbit through the superior orbital fissure. It eventually drains into the cavernous sinus. The inferior ophthalmic vein drains the inferior orbital contents and exits the orbit by way of the inferior orbital fissure to drain into the cavernous sinus and pterygoid plexus of veins. The central retinal vein drains the optic nerve and retina and eventually drains into the cavernous sinus.

Neural Structures

There are a number of different types of nerve fibers that are found within the orbit. These include both motor and sensory fibers as well as sympathetic and parasympathetic tracts. Cranial nerve VI, the abducens nerve, provides motor enervation to the lateral rectus muscle. After the nerve exits the cavernous sinus, it passes through the annulus of Zinn along with cranial nerve III to enter the orbit. The nerve passes along the lateral aspect of the intraconal space and enervates the lateral rectus muscle just beyond its midportion. Sympathetic fibers from the cavernous sinus also follow the abducens nerve to the ciliary ganglion at the orbital apex. These fibers then follow branches of the ophthalmic nerve to their various points of enervation including Müller's muscle, the inferior tarsal muscle, dilator muscle of the iris, and intraorbital blood vessels [16].

The superior oblique muscle is enervated by cranial nerve IV, the trochlear nerve. The trochlear nerve exits the cavernous sinus and enters the orbit via the superior orbital fissure, outside of the annulus of Zinn. This nerve travels in close proximity to the frontal and lacrimal branches of V1 and enervates the superior oblique muscle beyond its midsection.

Cranial nerve III, the oculomotor nerve, provides motor enervation to the remaining extraocular muscles including the medial rectus, superior rectus, inferior rectus, as well as the inferior oblique muscle and levator palpebrae superioris muscle. The oculomotor nerve traverses the superior orbital fissure to enter the orbit. The nerve then divides into superior and inferior divisions, which enter the intraconal space via the annulus of Zinn. The inferior rectus, medial rectus, and inferior oblique muscles are enervated by the inferior division, whereas the superior rectus and levator muscles are enervated by the superior division. There are also parasympathetic fibers from CN III that supply the muscles of the eye which control pupillary reaction, convergence, and accommodation [16]. Sensory fibers in the extraocular muscles provide proprioception to the brain stem.

The main sensory input of the orbit and eyelids is via the first division of cranial nerve V, the ophthalmic nerve. The frontal, lacrimal, and nasociliary nerves are the three major branches of the ophthalmic nerve. These branches all traverse the superior orbital fissure. The frontal and lacrimal branches lie outside the annulus of Zinn, whereas the nasociliary branch extends through the annulus of Zinn.

Lacrimal System

The lacrimal system consists of the lacrimal gland, lacrimal canaliculi, lacrimal sac, nasolacrimal duct, and various supporting structures (Figs. 43.1 and 43.2) [26]. The tendon of the levator palpebrae partially divides the lacrimal gland into two portions (orbital and palpebral) connected by a small isthmus. The larger orbital portion comprises two-thirds of the gland and is located within the lacrimal fossa of the frontal bone along the superolateral aspect of the orbit. The smaller palpebral segment comprises one-third of the gland, is located anterior to the orbital septum, and projects onto the upper eye lid.

There are three major constituents that make up lacrimal fluid. The primary aqueous component of tears is produced by serous secreting cells that make up the majority of the lacrimal gland. A smaller mucinous component is produced by goblet cells within the conjunctiva. The small lipid component is produced by the Meibomian glands within the eyelids [26]. This component is primarily responsible for preventing evaporation of lacrimal fluid. Lacrimal fluid is spread from the upper outer quadrant of the eye over the conjunctival surfaces of the eye during closure of the eyelids. Contraction of orbicularis oculi muscle fibers propels the lacrimal fluid toward the nasal aspect of the eye where it enters the lacrimal drainage system. Tears then drain through orifices of the superior and inferior puncta into the superior and inferior canaliculi, respectively [26]. These merge into a common canaliculus which then drains into the lacrimal sac and nasolacrimal duct. The medial canthal tendons and muscles of Riolan provide structural support to the canaliculi and lacrimal sac [26]. The nasolacrimal duct drains into the nasal cavity within the inferior meatus, inferior to the inferior nasal concha.

Orbital Fat

The majority of orbital fat is located in the retrobulbar intraconal space posterior to the globe. Orbital fat provides support to the various structures within the orbit, including the globe, optic nerve, and extraocular muscles. The soft, pliable fat allows these structures to freely move within the orbit. Interconnecting fascia courses through the orbital fat and assists in structural support. Infiltration and displacement of orbital fat can be an indirect sign of significant pathology.

Ocular, Optic Nerve, and Orbital Pathology

The following two sections cover the various pathologic processes that affect the globe and orbital contents. Ocular pathology and optic nerve pathology are discussed in the first section. Orbital pathology is covered in the second section. Within these sections, the discussion is organized based on pathologic process.

Ocular Pathology

Abnormal Globe and Optic Disk Abnormalities

Staphyloma and coloboma can appear similarly on cross-sectional imaging. However, staphyloma is an acquired anomaly, whereas colobomas arise from a developmental process. Buphthalmos is a condition where the eye may be abnormally large.

Coloboma

A coloboma is a developmental defect of the globe [27, 28]. These may occur anywhere within the globe including the iris, lens, ciliary body, retina, choroid, sclera, and optic nerve (Fig. 43.3) [27]. Three different types have been described including an optic nerve coloboma, a retinochoroidal coloboma, and a Fuchs' coloboma [28]. The typical location involves the inferior nasal portion of the globe that is caused by incomplete closure of the embryonic fissure [28]. This results in an elongated, cone-shaped globe. Colobomas can also involve the optic nerve, potentially resulting in an ocular cyst at the site of incomplete closure of the optic fissure. Colobomas can arise sporadically. Coloboma, however, is a feature of multiple systemic syndromes including CHARGE syndrome, Meckel's syndrome, trisomy 13, Aicardi syndrome, PAX2 genetic mutation, and several others [29].

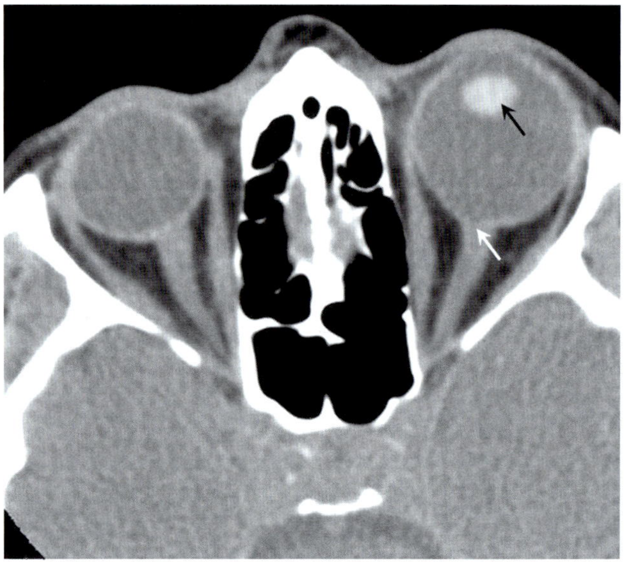

Fig. 43.3 Buphthalmos – coloboma: axial CT scan in a patient with a history of congenital glaucoma demonstrates a markedly enlarged left globe with a congenital cataract (*black arrow*) and a coloboma involving the optic nerve head (*white arrow*)

Staphyloma

Staphyloma is acquired abnormal thinning of the uvea-scleral wall which results in focal ectasia. This thinning often results in an elongated globe with a focal bulge on the temporal side of the posterior globe. Staphylomas may occur in the setting of prior infection, trauma, glaucoma, and radiation.

Buphthalmos

Prenatal or early perinatal enlargement of the globe (buphthalmos) may be seen in the eyes of a newborn with congenital glaucoma (Fig. 43.3). It is usually an autosomal recessive trait that typically appears at birth or in newborns or within the first 2–3 months of life. Early-onset congenital glaucoma with increased intraocular pressure can enlarge the globe during this early, more "plastic" stage of eye development.

Papilledema

Papilledema occurs when increased intracranial pressure is transmitted along the subarachnoid space that lies between the optic sheath and the optic nerve. Since the subarachnoid space extends anteriorly as far as the scleral limbus, the pressure is transmitted to the optic nerve head, displacing it anteriorly (Fig. 43.4). The findings are usually bilateral and symmetric unless the subarachnoid space of one nerve is selectively obstructed, in which case the findings can be unilateral.

Ocular Detachments

Retinal Detachment

The retina contains two layers: the superficial sensory retina and the deeper retinal pigment epithelium. Damage to the pigment epithelium allows fluid to accumulate within the potential subretinal space [3, 30–32]. The posterior margin of the retina is tethered at the level of the optic nerve. Therefore, retinal detachments result in a "V" shape configuration with folding of the sensory layer of the retina (Figs. 43.5, 43.6, and 43.7). Retinal detachments can occur from a variety of causes, including tumor, infection, and hemorrhage.

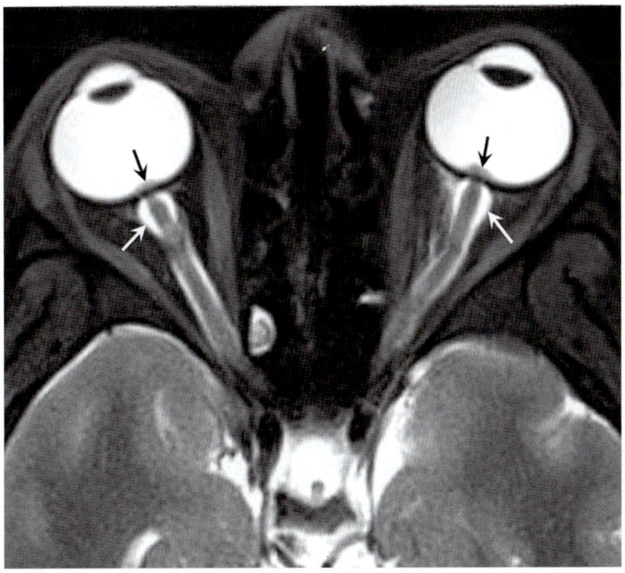

Fig. 43.4 Papilledema: axial T2-W MR image demonstrates marked bilateral elevation of the optic disks (*black arrows*) and enlargement of the subarachnoid space (*white arrows*) around the optic nerves

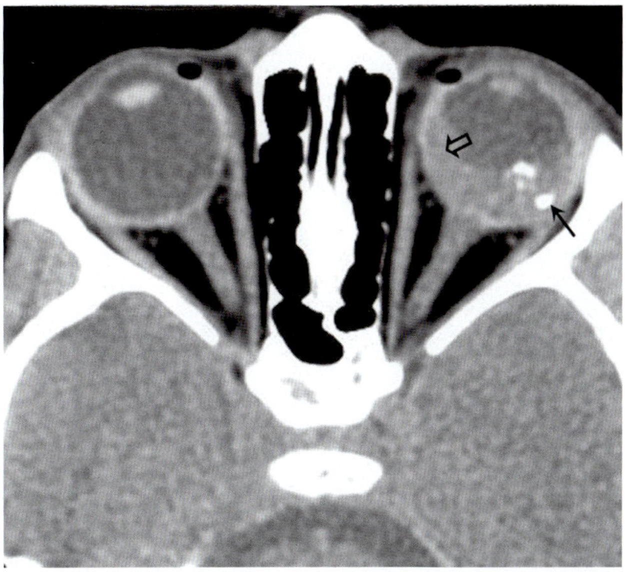

Fig. 43.5 Retinoblastoma: axial CT scan demonstrates a heterogeneously calcified retinoblastoma within the left globe (*arrow*). Also present is a concomitant retinal detachment (*open arrow*) that makes it difficult to identify the exact tumor margins

Choroidal Detachment

Choroidal detachments occur when fluid accumulates within the subchoroidal space in between the choroid and sclera [3, 30, 32–34]. This fluid can be either serous or hemorrhagic. Hemorrhagic choroidal detachments may be posttraumatic or related to complications from ocular surgery [35]. Ocular hypotony, low pressure within the globe, is associated with serous choroidal detachments [30]. Potential causes include infection, traumatic perforation, glaucoma therapy, and ocular surgery [30]. The choroid is anchored by the posterior ciliary arteries and vortex veins. Therefore, detachments that involve the subchoroidal space do not typically extend posteriorly to the level of the optic nerve, as they do with retinal detachments. This is an important differentiating feature between choroidal and retinal detachments.

The imaging appearance of choroidal detachments is variable depending on the type of fluid. Hemorrhagic detachments typically have an irregular margin, demonstrate high attenuation on CT [36], and have variable T1-W and T2-W MR signal characteristics depending on the age of the hematoma [30]. The CT attenuation and MR signal characteristics of serous choroidal effusions depend on the contents of the fluid. The greater the protein or inflammatory cells within the fluid, the higher the CT attenuation, the higher the T1-W signal intensity, and the lower the T2-W signal intensity.

Leukocoria and Its Causes

Leukocoria is defined as a white pupillary reflex occurring from the inability of light to reflect from the retina. Leukocoria can be caused by any process that prevents the passage of light through the globe. There are many causes of leukocoria including retinoblastoma, persistent hyperplastic primary vitreous, congenital cataract, retrolental fibroplasia, Coats' disease, and toxocariasis [37–60].

Retinoblastoma

Retinoblastoma is the most common intraocular tumor in children [40–42]. It is a common cause of leukocoria in infants. The most common presenting sign of retinoblastoma is leukocoria; therefore, children with this physical exam finding warrant further evaluation with imaging. Retinoblastoma will be discussed later in the chapter.

Persistent Hyperplastic Primary Vitreous (PHPV)

PHPV is the second most common cause of leukocoria in children [38]. Clinically, PHPV presents as unilateral leukocoria in a full-term baby with a small eye [40]. The con-

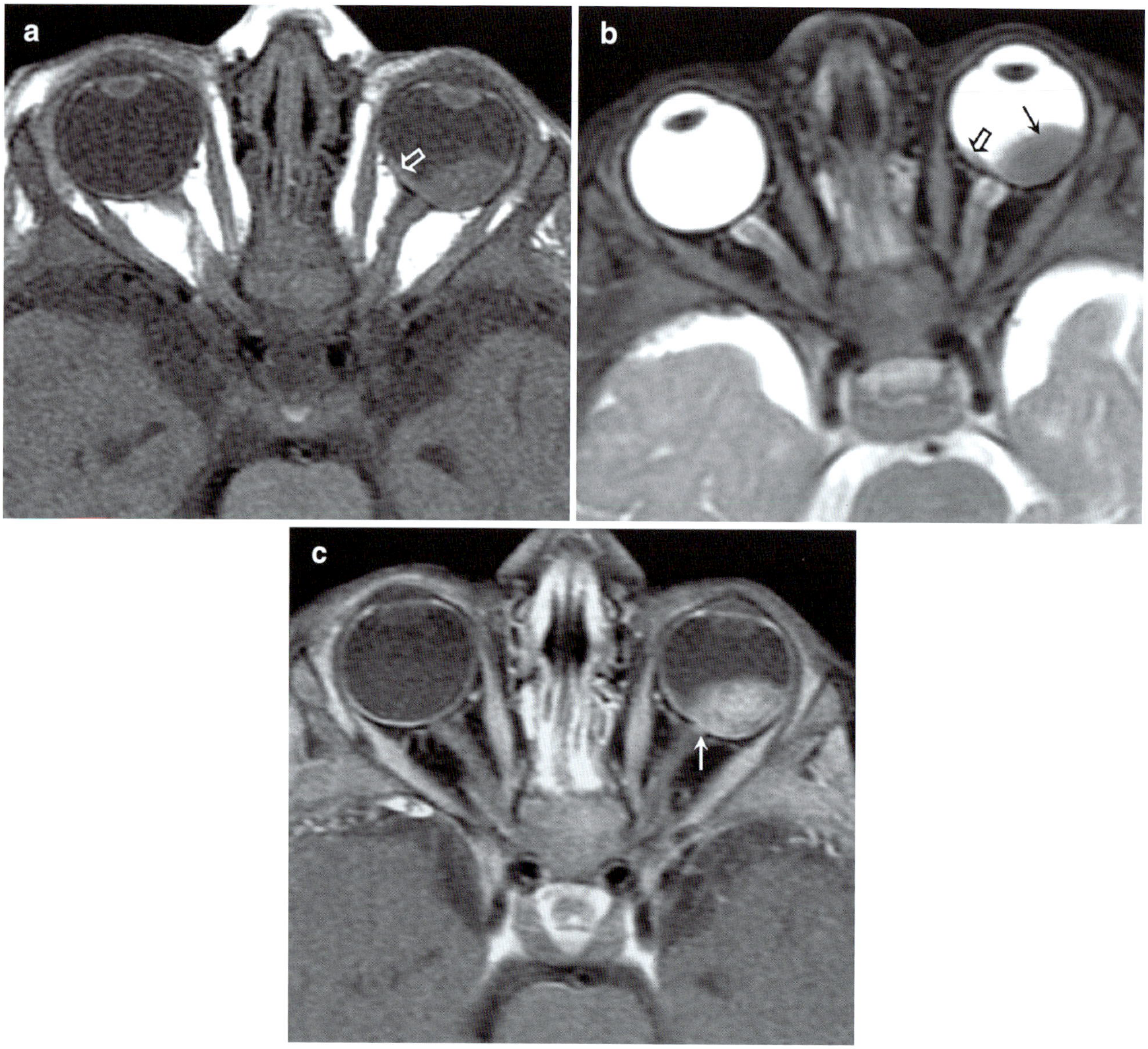

Fig. 43.6 Retinoblastoma: noncontrast axial T1-W (**a**), noncontrast axial T2-W (**b**), and postcontrast fat-suppressed axial T1-W (**c**) MR scans. The lesion is seen to be very hypointense on the T2-W image (*black arrow*) and demonstrates significant contrast enhancement. There is subtle invasion of the optic nerve (*white arrow*). A small retinal detachment (*open arrows*) is also present. Calcified areas that were seen on CT are not well seen on MRI

dition is caused by failure of the hyaloid vascular system to regress with resultant persistence of the primary vitreous [40, 53–55]. Because direct visualization with ophthalmoscopy can be challenging in some cases, CT and MRI can be useful to make the correct diagnosis (Fig. 43.7). A small eye, no associated calcifications, and normal to increased density within the vitreous are common findings on CT. MRI demonstrates microphthalmos and marked hyperintensity of the affected vitreous on T1-W and T2-W images. Retinal detachments and subretinal blood may also be seen. The diagnosis is made by visualization of Cloquet's canal on CT or MRI, which is seen as a band of fetal tissue that extends from the optic disk to the lens. The lens is often thickened in the anterior-posterior direction. Norrie disease is an inherited genetic cause of blindness associated with PHPV [49].

Coats' Disease

Coats' disease is another cause of leukocoria occurring in young boys typically before the age of 20 [29, 38]. The peak

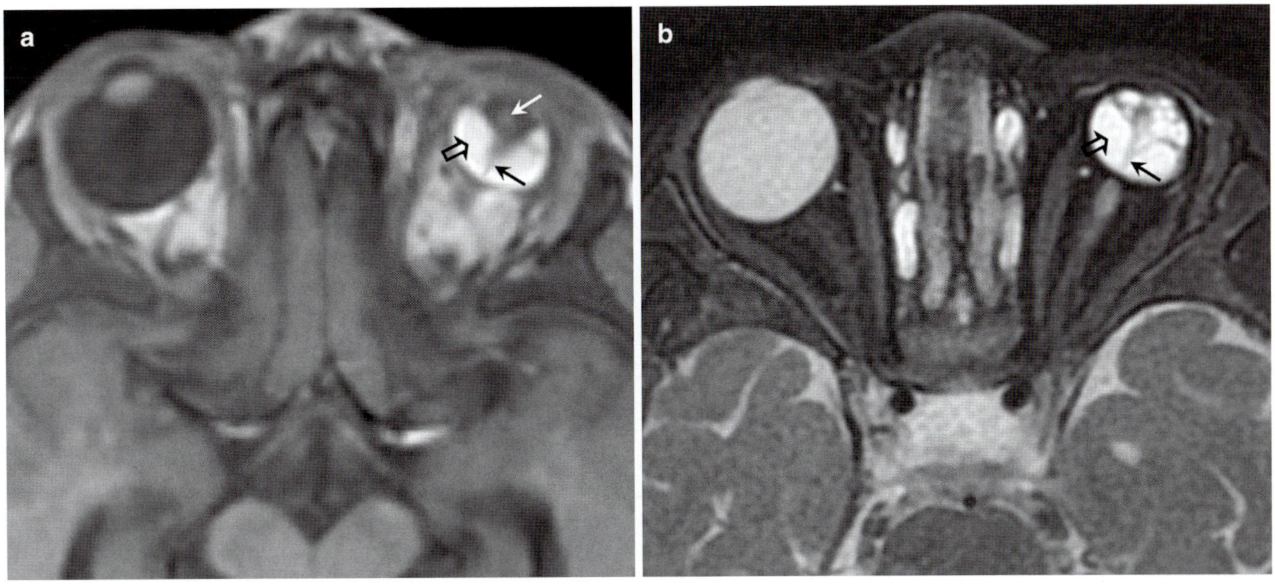

Fig. 43.7 Persistent hyperplastic primary vitreous: axial T1-W (**a**) and axial T2-W (**b**) MR images demonstrate microphthalmia of the left globe, persistence of an enlarged hyaloid (Cloquet's) canal (*black arrows*), abnormally developed lens (*white arrow*), and retinal detachment (*open arrows*)

incidence is 6–8 years of age [54]. It is a primary vascular anomaly of the retina which results in leaky telangiectatic vessels [40, 54, 56]. Serum and lipid leak into the subretinal space, resulting in lipoproteinaceous subretinal effusions [38, 49]. There may be associated retinal detachments. On CT, the globe is normal in size with high attenuation noted within the vitreous. Calcifications are not typically seen. On MRI, the vitreous is characteristically hyperintense on both T1-W and T2-W scans. This differs from the normal appearance of retinoblastoma which is typically hyperintense on T1-W images and hypointense on T2-W images. Although there is some enhancement associated with Coats' disease, the enhancement pattern differs from that seen in retinoblastoma. In Coats' disease, the enhancement is noted along the margins of the detached retina and at the attachment sites of the retina [57], whereas retinoblastomas enhance in a mass-like fashion.

Retinopathy of Prematurity

Retinopathy of prematurity (ROP), previously known as retrolental fibroplasia, is a condition seen in premature infants exposed to prolonged oxygen therapy [38, 58–60]. The severity of ROP is dependent on the degree of prematurity, the amount of oxygen exposure, and the birth weight of the infant [49]. The disease can resolve on its own or in severe cases can result in blindness. ROP is felt to result from abnormal disorganized growth of retinal blood vessels associated with scarring. This condition is often bilateral. Retinal detachments are often an associated finding. On CT, there is increased attenuation within the posterior margin of the globe. Calcifications may be seen as well.

Toxocara canis Infection

Ocular infection from *Toxocara canis* typically results in chorioretinitis and is another cause of leukocoria. *Toxocara canis* is a nematode parasite that infects dogs. Infection from *T. canis* occurs following ingestion of soil containing dog feces infested with *T. canis* ova. After the ova hatch in the gastrointestinal tract, the larvae migrate throughout the body and eventually find their way to the eye [38]. The larvae die within the globe and incite an inflammatory response. This process ultimately results in opacification of the vitreous and associated retinal detachment. Peripheral granulomas involving the retina may also be seen [38, 40]. On CT, the vitreous is high in attenuation without calcification. On MRI, the vitreous is hyperintense on both T1-W and T2-W images. Associated hemorrhage within the vitreous, subretinal, and retinal spaces can also occur.

Intraocular Masses

Retinoblastoma

Retinoblastoma is the most common intraocular tumor in children [40–42]. It is a common cause of leukocoria in infants [38]. The majority of cases occur in children less than 5 years of age [39, 43]. The most common presenting signs include leukocoria, strabismus, decreased vision, ocular pain, glaucoma, and retinal detachment [44]. The majority of retinoblastomas occur sporadically; however, 10% of cases are familial. In all cases, both Rb1 genes located on chromosome 13q14 are inactivated [3]. Sporadic cases are typically unilateral, whereas the heritable form has a propensity for bilateral and multifocal tumors [44]. Familial retinoblastoma is inherited as an autosomal dominant trait associated with chromosome 13q14 [38, 40].

Retinoblastomas most often arise from the sensory retina. These tumors can grow endophytically into the vitreous or exophytically into the subretinal space [42]. A rare diffuse infiltrating form may occur within the anterior segment of the globe and is plaque-like in morphology [40]. Individuals with the diffuse form may present with glaucoma secondary to the neovascularization of the iris [45]. Unlike the focal form, the diffuse form more often occurs in older children without calcification [42, 45]. The main differential for this infiltrating form is medulloepithelioma, which is a malignant nonhereditary tumor that arises from the ciliary body [45, 46]. These tumors are indistinguishable on imaging [45, 46].

Diagnostic imaging with both CT and MR are complimentary and crucial in making the correct diagnosis of retinoblastoma. Calcifications are a characteristic feature of retinoblastoma occurring in 95% of cases and are easily detected by CT (Fig. 43.5) [40]. The presence of calcification within the globe in a child less than 3 years of age is highly suggestive of retinoblastoma [39]. MRI is an important diagnostic tool used to differentiate between retinoblastoma (Fig. 43.6) and other causes of leukocoria [42, 47–49]. MRI is primarily used to assess the size and extent of the tumor and, in particular, involvement of the optic nerve [50]. On MRI, the tumor is hyperintense on T1-W images and hypointense on T2-W images and demonstrates intense contrast enhancement. Calcification on MRI is more challenging to visualize but usually demonstrates hyperintense signal on T1-W images and hypointense signal on T2-W images. Focal areas of hyperintense signal on T1-W images, however, may be related to calcification, tumor protein, or hemorrhagic areas within the mass. Retinal detachments may also be associated with retinoblastoma, and the fluid may have variable signal intensity.

Patients with familial retinoblastoma have a higher propensity for the development of pineoblastomas within the pineal gland and tumors within the parasellar region [51, 52]. When evaluating patients with retinoblastoma with MRI, it is important to include the entire brain to assess the parasellar and pineal regions for tumor involvement. It has been hypothesized that these tumors are not metastatic foci but rather are a manifestation of multicentric malignancy [38].

Ocular Melanoma

In adults, the most common ocular malignancy is melanoma [1]. Ocular melanoma can affect the choroid, ciliary body, and iris. Ocular melanoma is seen more often in Caucasians and is unusual in African-Americans. The liver is the most common site of metastasis from primary ocular melanoma [29]. Flat or plaque-like lesions may be difficult to identify with cross-sectional imaging and may be better evaluated with ultrasonography. Lesions that measure greater than 2–3 mm can be reliably seen with MRI [29].

On CT, uveal melanomas present as an elevated mass that is lentiform or mushroom shaped, inherently hyperdense, and enhances after contrast (Fig. 43.8) [61]. On MRI, melanotic melanomas are hyperintense on T1-W images and hypointense on T2-W images with respect to the adjacent vitreous [62]. Amelanotic melanomas, on the other hand, are similar in signal characteristics to other ocular tumors which are often hypo- to isointense on T1-W images and hyperintense on T2-W images. This difference is related to the amount of melanin within the tumor. Free radicals in melanin are known to shorten the T1 relaxation time of melanomas and may be responsible for their T1-W hyperintensity [2]. It is important to assess for extraocular extension, which will be best appreciated on the T1-W postcontrast MR images performed with fat suppression. Retinal detachments with proteinaceous effusions may also be present.

Other benign and malignant processes of the globe may mimic ocular melanoma [63, 64]. Metastasis, choroidal hemangioma, choroidal detachment, retinal detachment, macular degeneration, neurofibroma, schwannoma, choroidal lymphoma, and leiomyoma are conditions that may be confused with melanoma. Metastatic mucinous adenocarcinomas may be indistinguishable from ocular melanoma because the proteinaceous material within the tumor is typically hyperintense on T1-W images and hypointense on T2-W images.

Ocular Metastasis

The choroid is the most vascular component of the globe and is the most common location for secondary ocular malignancies (Fig. 43.9). Metastasis can also involve the retina. The most common malignancies to metastasize to the globe are from lymphoma, leukemia, lung cancer, and breast cancer. Metastasis may be bilateral, whereas ocular melanoma is typically unilateral. Retinal or choroidal detachment can be

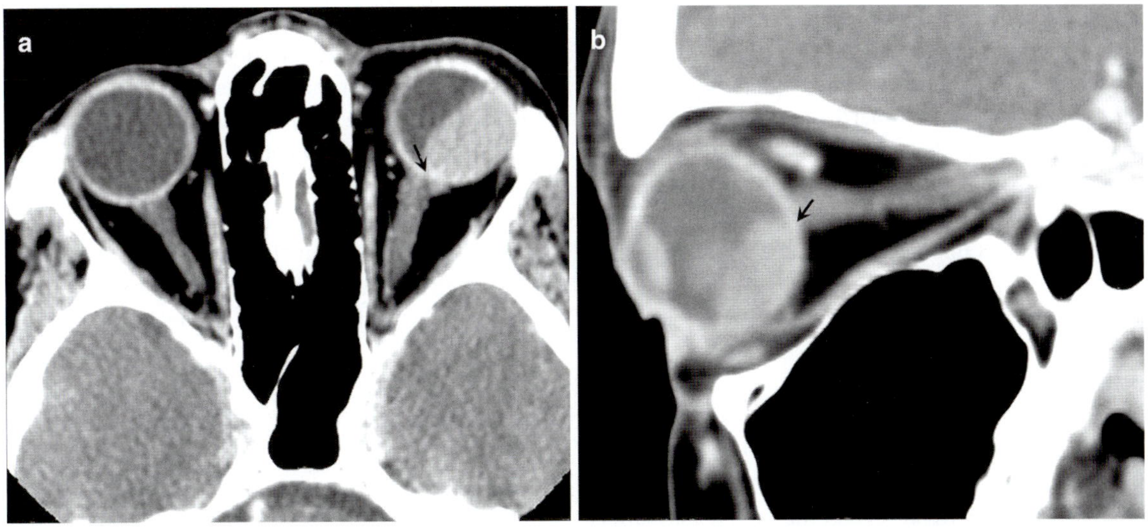

Fig. 43.8 Choroidal melanoma: axial (**a**) and oblique sagittal (**b**) postcontrast CT images reveal a well-demarcated, homogeneously enhancing choroidal melanoma that invades the optic disk (*arrows*) and sclera but does not penetrate the globe

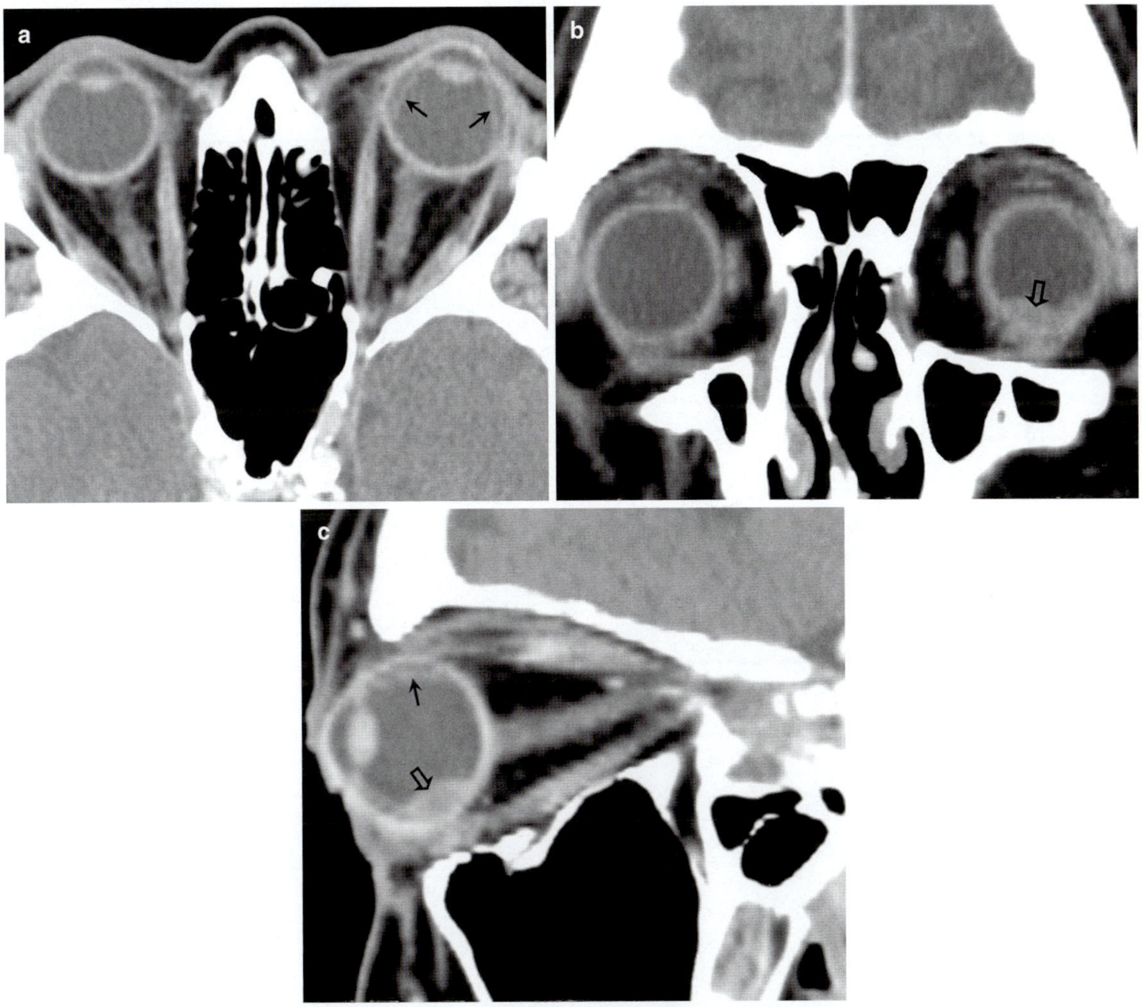

Fig. 43.9 Ocular metastasis (lung carcinoma): axial (**a**), coronal (**b**), and oblique sagittal (**c**) postcontrast CT scans demonstrate an enhancing left ocular choroidal metastasis (*open arrows*) with an associated choroidal detachment (*black arrows*). Note that the choroidal detachment does not extend back to the optic disk

an associated finding. MRI is more sensitive than CT for evaluating ocular metastasis.

The incidence of primary ocular lymphoma is rare. Systemic lymphoma, on the other hand, involves the globe more frequently. The tumor most often affects the uvea and is often bilateral. Although the signal characteristics of lymphoma resemble that of melanoma, bilateral lesions are rare in melanoma, and this finding may be used as a distinguishing feature.

Choroidal Hemangioma

Choroidal hemangiomas are vascular hamartomas. Two types have been described. They can present as a diffuse angioma associated with Sturge-Weber syndrome which may affect multiple layers of the globe [65, 66]. The second form occurs in adults as a well-circumscribed solitary lesion that is not associated with other malformations. The focal form is typically isolated to the choroid and is often located near the macula of the fundus. On both CT and MRI, the hemangioma enhances briskly after contrast (Fig. 43.10). There is some overlap between the MR appearance of a solitary choroidal hemangioma and uveal melanoma [63]. In some cases, choroidal hemangiomas are slightly hyperintense on T1-W images, similar to the appearance of melanoma [63, 64].

Retinal Angioma

Retinal angiomas are seen in association with von Hippel-Lindau disease [67]. These lesions are characterized based

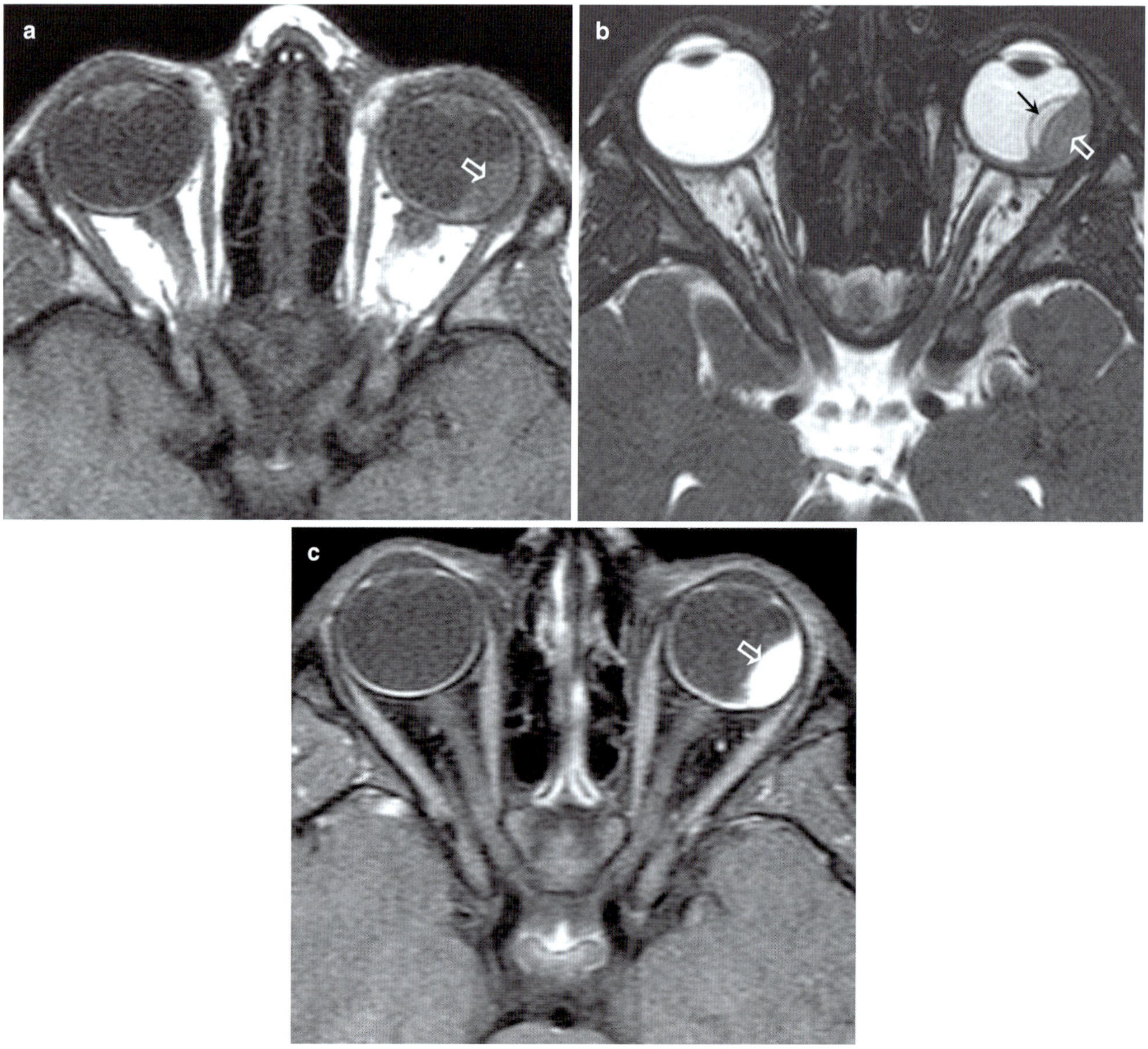

Fig. 43.10 Choroidal hemangioma: axial noncontrast T1-W (**a**), axial noncontrast T2-W (**b**), and axial postcontrast fat-suppressed T1-W (**c**) MR images reveal an intensely enhancing choroidal hemangioma (*open arrows*) with an associated choroidal detachment (*arrow*)

on their ophthalmoscopic appearance and are not typically seen on cross-sectional imaging.

Ocular Calcification

There are multiple processes that result in ocular calcification [68]. Calcifications of the globe are often seen incidentally, and it is therefore important to distinguish benign from pathologic calcification. Calcification of the globe can result from degenerative processes, trauma, neoplasm, infection/inflammatory conditions, or hypercalcemic states. Degenerative calcification is typically benign and includes cataracts, optic nerve drusen, senescent calcification (sclera plaques) of the tendinous insertions on the globe, retinal detachment, and retinopathy of prematurity [59, 69]. Tumoral calcification is seen in retinoblastoma, astrocytic hamartomas, and choroidal osteomas [42, 44, 47, 48]. Calcified congenital vascular lesions associated with Sturge-Weber syndrome and von Hippel-Lindau disease can also be seen [65, 66]. Infection from cytomegalovirus is also associated with ocular calcification [70]. Finally, calcification is also seen in the setting of hypercalcemic states such as chronic renal failure, sarcoidosis, and hyperparathyroidism.

Calcifications are best appreciated on unenhanced CT scans and are often more occult on MRI. The pattern of calcification is often pathognomonic for a specific entity. Scleral plaques occur at the tendinous insertion of the extraocular muscles along the anterior aspect of the globe and can be seen both medially and laterally [32]. Drusen are spherical acellular deposits that occur within the optic nerve near the optic nerve head (Fig. 43.11). They typically calcify later in life and are often bilateral. Drusen can be clinically misinterpreted as papilledema. Calcification is also characteristically seen in retinoblastoma and often appears as dysmorphic calcification within a mass lesion in the globe (Fig. 43.5). Phthisis bulbi is a small shrunken globe with dystrophic calcification seen in the setting of prior ocular injury such as from prior trauma or infection. Choroidal osteomas are benign tumors of the choroid that appear as a peripapillary calcified mass. These are typically unilateral occurring in young Caucasian females.

Ocular Inflammation

Inflammation of the globe can result from an infectious process, arise from a systemic illness, or may be idiopathic. Any layer of the globe may be involved. Episcleritis is inflammation of the layer of the globe external to the sclera and cornea and is usually self-limited and idiopathic. Evaluation with imaging is not typically indicated.

Imaging becomes particularly useful in evaluating for involvement of the sclera [71]. Scleritis may occur from an infectious source including viral, bacterial, or fungal organisms. There are multiple noninfectious processes that can also result in scleritis such as from collagen vascular disorders, metabolic diseases, or granulomatous diseases. Although there are multiple possible etiologies of scleritis, there are times when no underlying cause is identified. Thickening of the sclera and uvea can be either smooth and diffuse or nodular and focal. The focal type of scleritis is often secondary to granulomatous infiltrates which may resemble a focal mass and may potentially be confused with

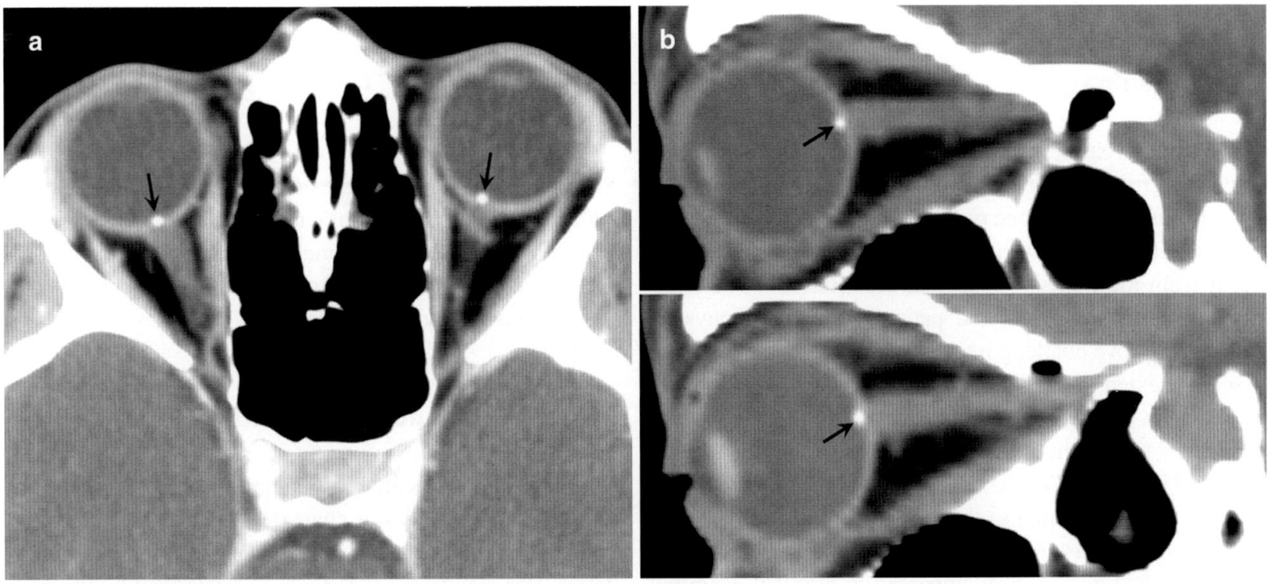

Fig. 43.11 Optic nerve head drusen: axial (**a**) and bilateral oblique sagittal (**b**) contrast-enhanced CT scans demonstrate dense focal calcifications (*arrows*) in the optic nerve heads that are pathognomonic of drusen

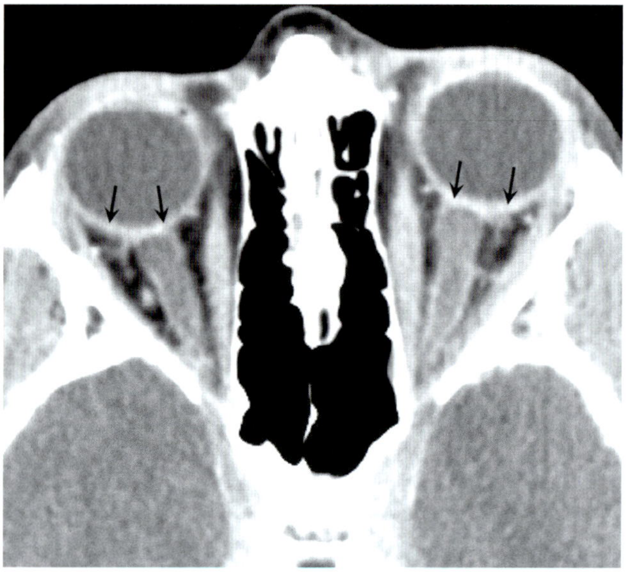

Fig. 43.12 Posterior scleritis: axial contrast-enhanced CT scan demonstrates abnormal thickening and enhancement of the posterior sclera of both globes (*arrows*) consistent with scleritis

melanoma. Diffuse scleritis, on the other hand, results in smooth thickening of the sclera which will often demonstrate enhancement on postcontrast CT and MR scans (Fig. 43.12). Concomitant choroidal detachments may be seen.

Inflammation of the uvea or retina can also result from infectious causes or may be idiopathic. *Toxoplasma gondii* and cytomegaloviruses (CMV) are two organisms that commonly cause uveitis and retinitis. CMV-induced retinitis occurs in one-third of the AIDS population not receiving highly active antiretroviral therapy (HAART) [32, 70]. Immunocompromised hosts are also at higher risk of developing ocular toxoplasmosis.

Ocular Trauma

Ocular trauma can result from direct penetrating injury, blunt trauma, or from compressive forces. Ocular injuries including lens dislocation, globe rupture, corneal tear, ocular hemorrhage, choroidal detachment, and retinal detachment can occur from these mechanisms and are often assessed clinically. In the severely injured patient, however, a physical exam may prove challenging, and imaging may be useful to assess the extent of ocular injury. CT is the imaging modality of choice in evaluating patients in the setting of trauma. CT is superior to MRI in the assessment of fractures and foreign bodies (Fig. 43.13) [72].

Hemorrhage isolated to the anterior chamber (hyphema) is the result of vascular injury in the iris and ciliary body [72]. This finding is readily apparent on physical exam but can be a subtle finding on cross-sectional imaging. CT may show high attenuation within the anterior chamber. The goal of imaging in this setting, however, is to evaluate for associated injuries.

Blunt trauma to the eye results in distortion of the globe which ultimately results in stretching of the zonular fibers that hold the lens in position [72]. These fibers may tear completely or partially resulting in lens subluxation or dislocation. The lens will most often dislocate posteriorly into the vitreous chamber. In addition, the lens may be perforated from direct penetrating injury. The lens normally is high in attenuation on CT, related to its high protein and predominant macromolecule content. Perforation of the lens results in edema with dilution of the high-density protein making it lower in attenuation on CT.

Traumatic globe rupture is a cause of blindness and should be assessed in patients with orbital trauma. The thinnest segment of the globe is at the insertion site of the extraocular muscles and, as a result, is the most common location for globe ruptures to occur [72]. A globe rupture should be suspected on CT if the globe demonstrates an abnormal contour or deflated appearance.

Surgical Change

Findings related to ocular surgery are often identifiable on cross-sectional imaging [73]. The most common surgical change is related to lens replacement for cataract surgery as well as surgery for retinal detachment [32, 73]. The replaced lens appears as a dense line seen on CT and a hypointense band on T2-W MR images. Other commonly seen devices are related to retinal detachment. The scleral buckle is seen as a circumferential band along the equator of the globe and can be seen both on CT and MRI. Intraocular gas or silicone may be seen in patients with prior retinopexy (Fig. 43.14) [73].

The Optic Nerve

Since the optic nerve is an extension of the central nervous system, many of the pathologic conditions that involve the brain can also involve the optic nerve. These include primary glial tumors, meningiomas, infections, inflammatory conditions, and demyelinating disease [3, 74].

Optic Neuritis and Demyelinating Disease

Multiple sclerosis is the most common cause of optic neuritis, which is a condition characterized by pain, decreased vision, abnormal color perception, and an afferent pupillary defect [75]. Multiple sclerosis is characterized by the presence of demyelinating plaques occurring within the white

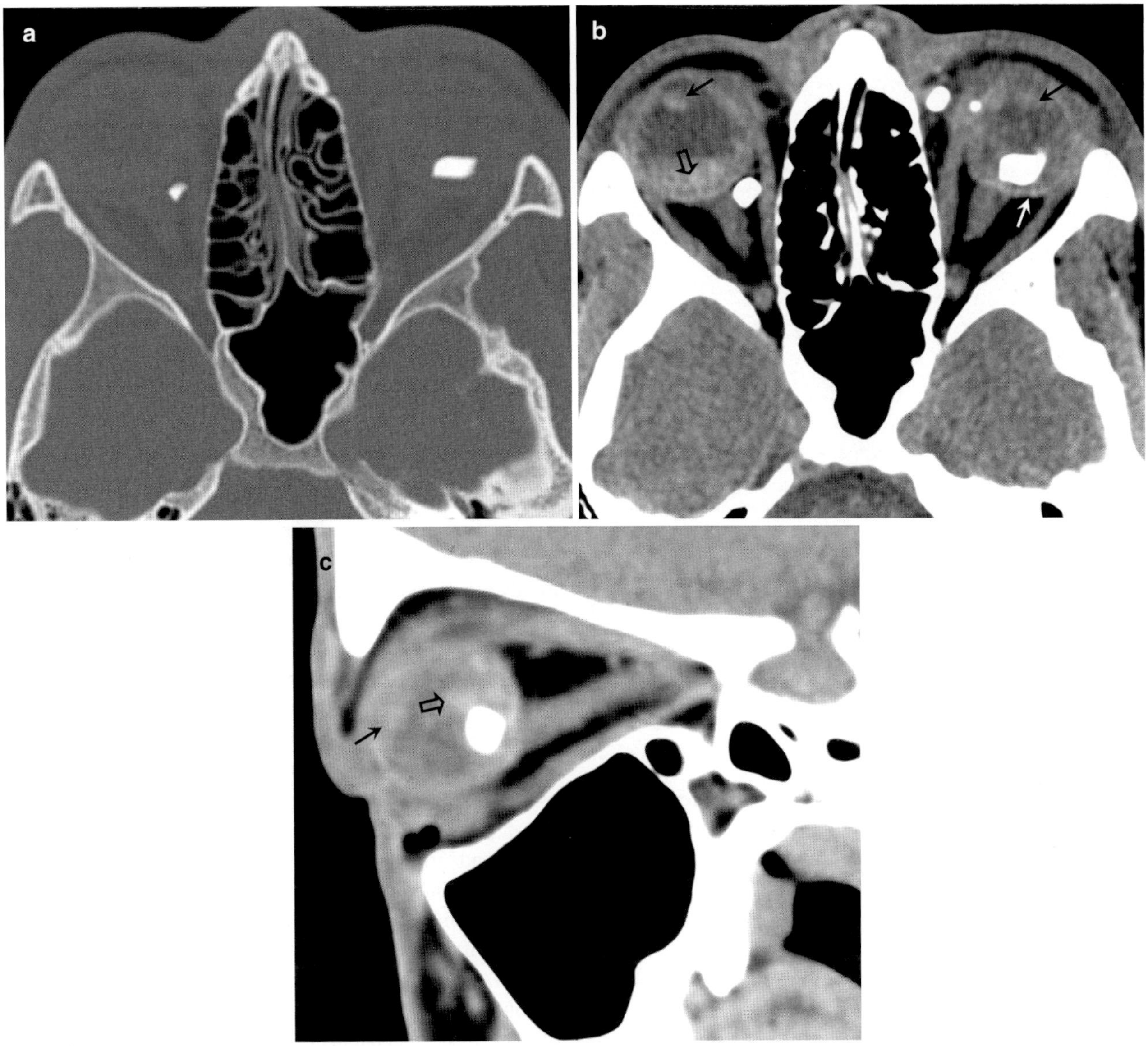

Fig. 43.13 Multiple orbital foreign bodies – ruptured globe: axial (**a**, **b**) and left oblique sagittal (**c**) CT scans in a patient who was ejected through the windshield during a motor vehicle accident. There are multiple penetrating intraocular and intraorbital foreign bodies. Note the extensive intravitreal hemorrhage (*open arrows*), bilateral lens disruption (*black arrows*), and signs of left ocular hypotony with a crenated appearance of the left globe (*white arrow*)

matter of the central nervous system that are disseminated in space and time. The optic nerves are often the first site of involvement; however, intracranial lesions are often present at the time of diagnosis (Fig. 43.15) [75]. Devic's disease (neuromyelitis optica) is another demyelinating condition that is characterized by optic neuritis and spinal cord involvement without intracranial involvement. Some of the patients will ultimately be diagnosed with multiple sclerosis, whereas others will never develop intracranial lesions [76]. Other conditions that may present with optic neuritis include various infectious agents, post-viral neuritis (Fig. 43.16), granulomatous disease (Fig. 43.17), ischemia, autoimmune conditions, metabolic-toxic demyelination, chemotherapeutic toxicity, and postradiation effects [3, 74, 76].

An MR of the orbits and brain is the imaging modality of choice when evaluating a patient with clinical symptoms suggestive of optic neuritis (Figs. 43.15, 43.16, and 43.17). The typical imaging findings of acute optic neuritis include high T2-W signal and variable contrast enhancement within a normal to minimally enlarged optic nerve [3, 23, 32, 74, 76]. In the chronic setting, the nerve may be hyperintense on T2-W images and atrophic in size. The coronal plane and images with fat saturation are particularly useful in demonstrating this finding.

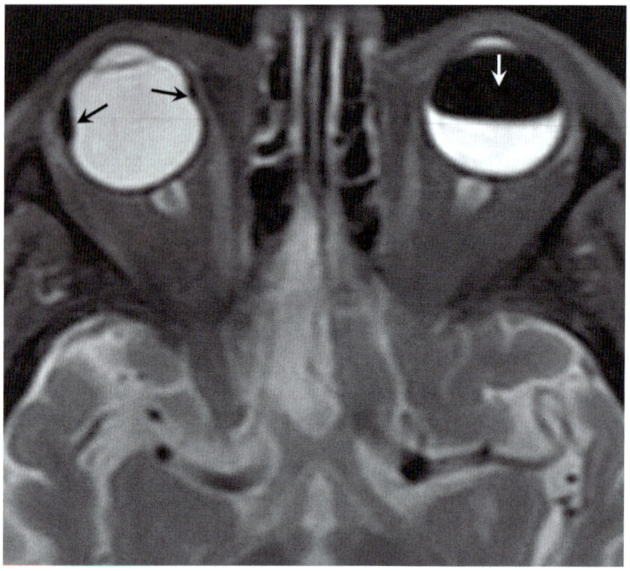

Fig. 43.14 Pneumatic retinopexy – scleral banding: axial T2-W MR scan demonstrates evidence of prior scleral banding (*black arrows*) and sulfur hexafluoride (SF_6) pneumatic retinopexy (*white arrow*) for treatment of bilateral retinal detachments. The signal intensity of the hexafluoride gas and the scleral buccal material is quite low on both T1-W and T2-W images due to the low mobile hydrogen content

Optic Perineuritis

Optic perineuritis is inflammation of the optic nerve sheath and can be confused clinically with optic neuritis [3, 77]. Patients may present with visual loss and eye pain. The differential diagnosis for optic perineuritis includes idiopathic inflammatory disease of the orbit (refer to this section later in the chapter), infection, granulomatous disease, as well as tumor including lymphoma, leukemia, subarachnoid carcinomatosis, and meningioma [74].

An MRI of the orbit demonstrates enhancement of the intraorbital optic nerve sheath rather than of the optic nerve itself (Fig. 43.18). Imaging of the brain is often normal. These patients have a dramatic improvement to corticosteroid therapy [77].

Optic Nerve Glioma

Optic nerve gliomas are the most common primary tumor of the optic nerve [3]. Optic pathway gliomas can involve any segment of the optic nerve and are classically characterized by fusiform enlargement of the optic nerve [78]. They are slow-growing tumors and classified as grade I astrocytomas according to the WHO pathologic grading system. They occur most commonly in the pediatric age group with 90% occurring in patients younger than 20 years of age [79]. Gliomas can affect one or both optic nerves. Bilateral involvement is indicative of neurofibromatosis type I. Clinically, gliomas involving the intraorbital optic nerve present with painless proptosis and decreased vision. Gliomas involving the intracranial segment of the optic nerve or chiasm may present with decreased vision in addition to symptoms related to regional mass effect on neighboring structures.

On CT and MRI, these lesions classically demonstrate fusiform enlargement of the optic nerve (Fig. 43.19) [80]. As the nerve outgrows its space, the tumor may result in kinking or bending of the nerve. Expansion of the optic canal may be seen when the intracanalicular segment of the optic nerve is involved. MRI is superior to CT in delineating the extent of tumor involvement. The tumor is typically isointense to gray matter on T1-W images and hyperintense to gray matter on T2-W images. Gliomas demonstrate variable contrast enhancement. These tumors are often managed conservatively because of their indolent course [79].

Occasionally, more aggressive primary tumors of the optic nerve (glioblastoma) may occur. These are more commonly seen in adult patients.

Optic Nerve Sheath Meningioma

In the orbit, meningiomas may arise from the meninges of the optic nerve sheath or develop from meninges near the orbital apex or superior orbital fissure, unrelated to the optic nerve [80–83]. Meningiomas occur typically within the fourth and fifth decades of life and are more common in females. Meningiomas arising from the optic nerve sheath present with proptosis and decreased vision. A central scotoma is often seen in patients with meningiomas involving the intracanalicular segment of the optic nerve. The tumors are often unilateral but may be bilateral in a small percentage of cases [84]. Management is typically conservative [84].

CT and MR imaging demonstrate circumferential thickening of the optic nerve sheath (Figs. 43.20 and 43.21). "Tram-track" calcification may be seen along the optic sheath on CT as well as adjacent osseous hyperostosis. There is low signal within the tumor on both T1-W and T2-W images relative to the optic nerve. Robust contrast enhancement is an expected feature on both CT and MRI.

The Orbit

Infection

Infections of the orbit most often result from spread of infections of the paranasal sinuses, skin, and lacrimal drainage system [32, 85]. The most common cause of orbital cellulitis is from adjacent ethmoid sinusitis. Orbital cellulitis is classified based on anatomic location and the relationship to the

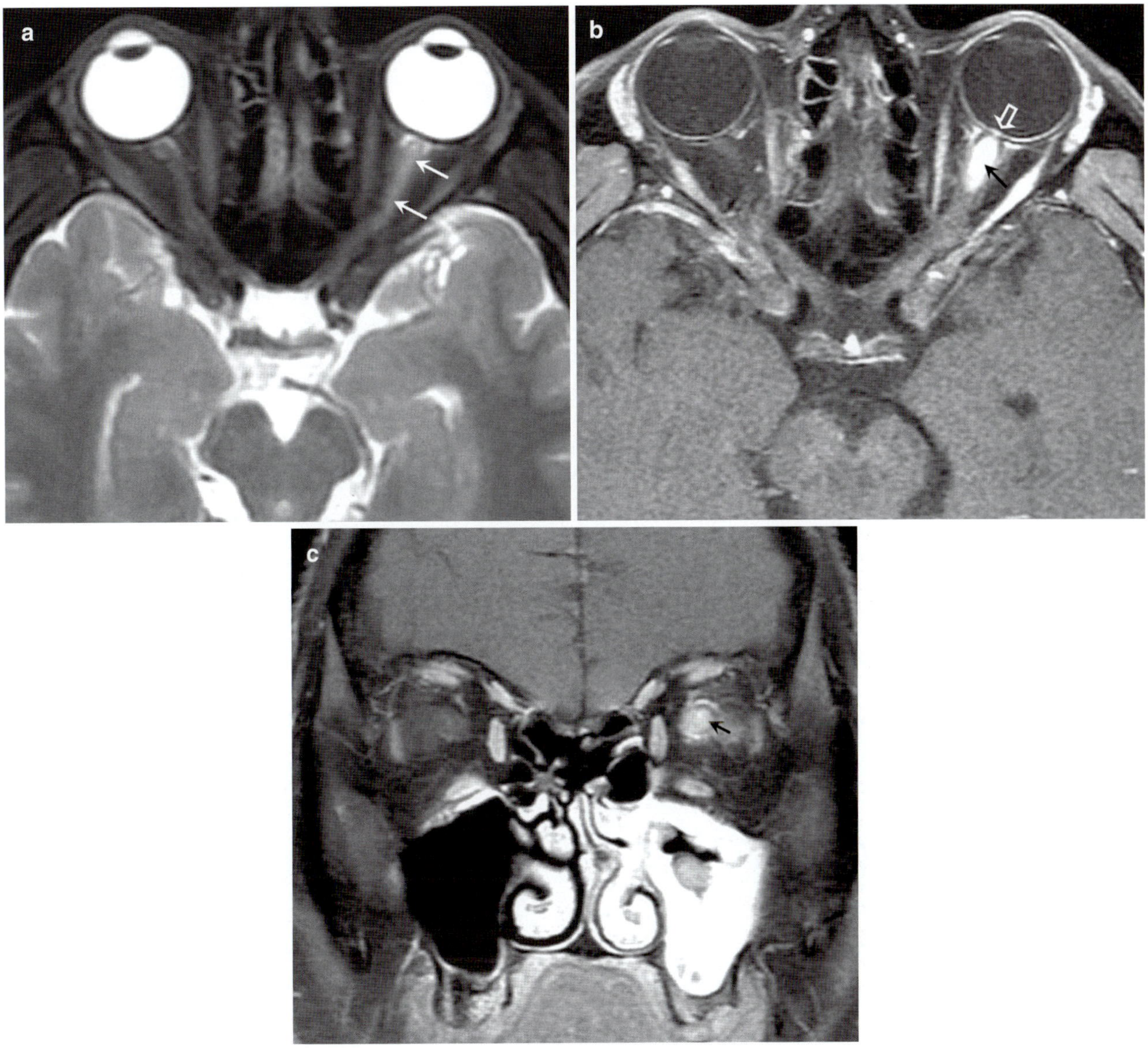

Fig. 43.15 Idiopathic optic neuritis: noncontrast axial T2-W (**a**) and axial (**b**) and coronal (**c**) postcontrast fat-suppressed T1-W MR images. There is extensive swelling and edema of the left optic nerve (*white arrows*) as well as intense enhancement of the intraorbital (*black arrows*) and papillary (*open arrow*) portions of the left optic nerve

orbital septum [32]. The orbital septum is a fibrous band that incompletely subdivides the orbit into pre- and postseptal spaces [86]. It extends from the tarsal plates to attach to the anterior aspects of the orbital walls. The orbital septum acts as an incomplete barrier preventing the initial spread of infection. Infection that involves the soft tissues including the skin and eye lid superficial to the orbital septum is termed preseptal cellulitis (Fig. 43.22). Typically, there is no associated ocular dysmotility, proptosis, or chemosis, and it is often treated medically with antibiotics.

Infection can also involve the adnexal structures of the orbit such as the lacrimal sac (Fig. 43.23), lacrimal gland (Fig. 43.24), bony orbit, and adjacent paranasal sinuses. The appearance will be dependent on the type of infection and the specific structures that are involved. Postseptal cellulitis, as the name implies, involves the soft tissues posterior to the orbital septum occurring within the orbit itself. Postseptal cellulitis may range from inflammatory edema to frank abscess formation. Clinically, these patients are more symptomatic presenting with proptosis, chemosis, decreased visual acuity, and painful ophthalmoplegia. A subperiosteal abscess results when inflammatory cells and fluid from the sinus infection collect between the orbital wall and the periorbita (Fig. 43.25) [87]. This, in turn, may lead to an abscess within the extraconal or intraconal spaces of the orbit and extraocular muscles (Figs. 43.25 and

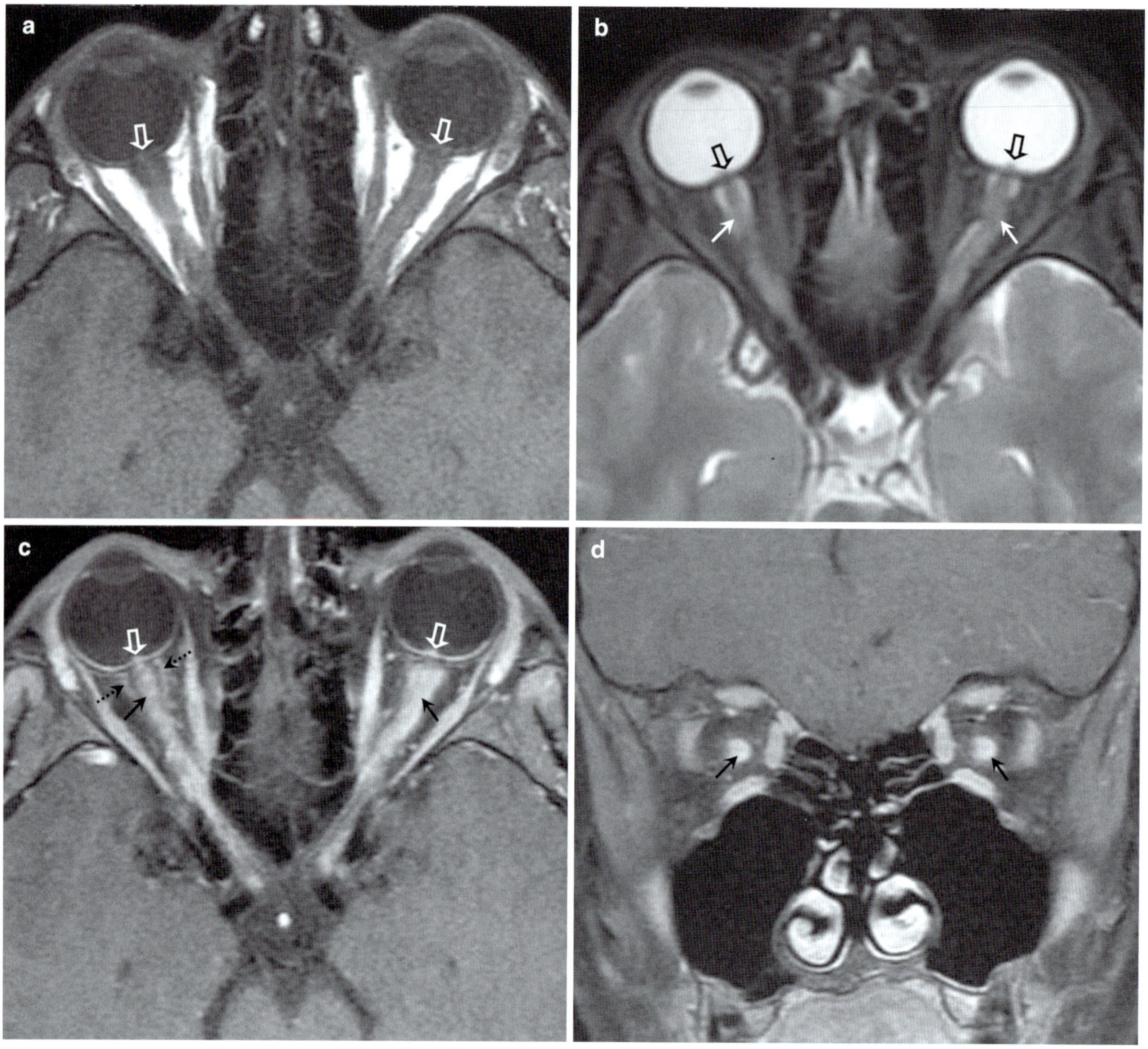

Fig. 43.16 Post-viral optic neuritis: noncontrast axial T1-W (**a**) and T2-W (**b**) as well as axial (**c**) and coronal (**d**) contrast-enhanced fat-suppressed T1-W MR images demonstrate bilateral swelling of the optic disk (*open arrows*). There is edema of the optic nerves that is best seen on the T2-W image (*white arrows*). There is diffuse intense contrast enhancement of the optic nerves (*black arrows*) as well as subtle perineuritis around the right optic nerve (*dashed arrows*)

43.26). It is not unusual to see concurrent postseptal orbital cellulitis and a subperiosteal abscess. Occasionally, preseptal cellulitis may extend posteriorly into the postseptal region to involve the retrobulbar orbital fat or extraocular muscles (Fig. 43.27). One important complication of orbital cellulitis is septic thrombophlebitis affecting the ophthalmic veins. This venous occlusion may propagate posteriorly to involve the cavernous sinus (Fig. 43.28). Cavernous sinus thrombosis should be suspected clinically if patients are extremely ill, exhibit signs of meningitis, and demonstrate multiple cranial nerve palsies including cranial nerves III, IV, V, and VI.

Contrast-enhanced CT or MR can be extremely useful to characterize the extent of disease in patients with orbital cellulitis. It is important to assess whether there is preseptal or postseptal involvement, to assess for the presence of a subperiosteal abscess, and to assess for the patency of the venous channels including the cavernous sinus. A peripherally enhancing subperiosteal collection within the orbit suggests the diagnosis of an abscess and may require surgical debridement. The cavernous sinus should enhance uniformly. The adjacent carotid artery should also enhance. In patients that have thrombosis of the cavernous sinus, there will be a lack of or incomplete contrast enhancement of the cavernous

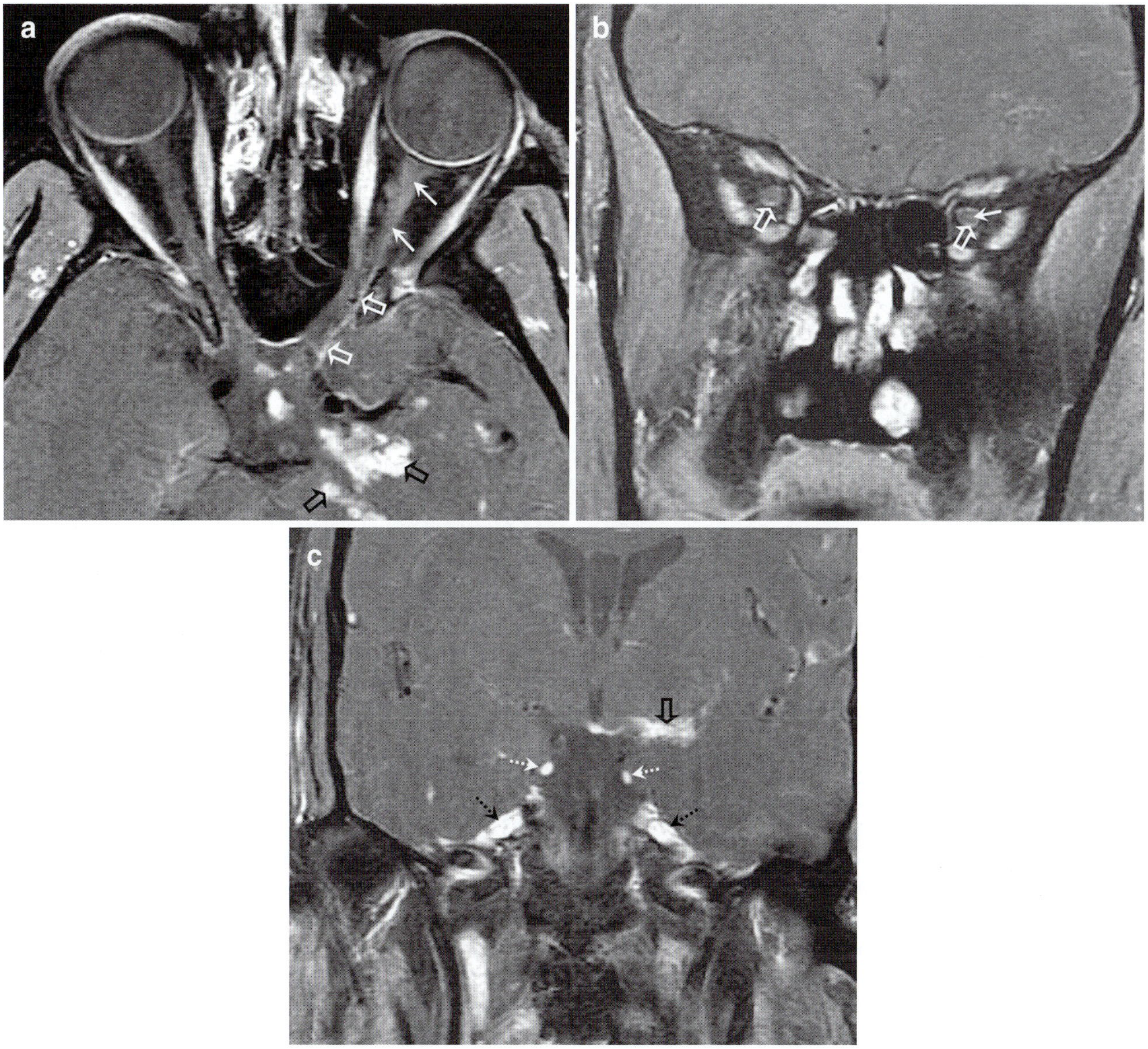

Fig. 43.17 Central nervous system neurosarcoidosis: axial (**a**) and coronal (**b**, **c**) contrast-enhanced fat-suppressed T1-W MR images reveal subtle diffuse enhancement of the left optic nerve (*white arrows*). Sarcoid granulomas also involve the optic sheaths (*open white arrows*), brain parenchyma (*open black arrows*), oculomotor nerves (*white dashed arrows*), and trigeminal nerves (*black dashed arrows*)

sinus. In addition, the superior ophthalmic veins are often enlarged and may be thrombosed [32]. Engorgement of the extraocular muscles due to vascular congestion from the absence of appropriate venous drainage and venous back pressure is often seen. This "congestive orbitopathy" may superficially resemble Graves' disease [88].

Intracranial abscesses are also a potential complication of orbital cellulitis. Contrast-enhanced MR is the most useful examination to assess for the presence of intracranial involvement. MRI may demonstrate a peripherally enhancing collection within the anterior cranial fossa subjacent to the frontal or sphenoid sinus indicative of an intracranial epidural abscess. Intracranial abscesses may be hyperintense on diffusion-weighted scans and mimic cerebral infarction. T2-FLAIR weighted sequences are extremely useful for detecting meningitis, demonstrating high signal along the cerebral sulci of the adjacent frontal lobes indicative of purulent material along the meninges. Contrast-enhanced T1-W images are more helpful than CT for detecting meningeal inflammation and infection.

Bacterial organisms are the most common source of orbital infection. However, infection from fungal organisms such as from *Mucor* and *Aspergillus* occurs in patients who are relatively immunocompromised. On MRI, fungal infection is characteristically hypointense on T2-W images and may suggest the diagnosis (Fig. 43.28). Mucormycosis and

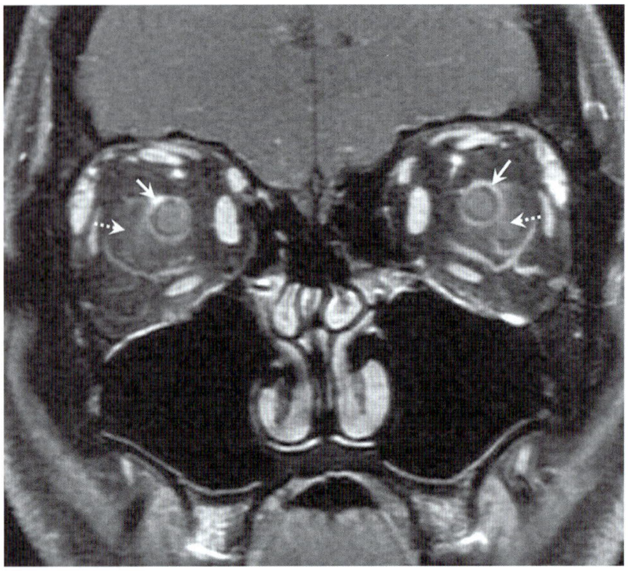

Fig. 43.18 Idiopathic perineuritis: coronal fat-suppressed T1-W contrast-enhanced MR scan reveals abnormal enhancement and thickening of the optic sheaths (*white arrows*) with minimal abnormal enhancement of the adjacent intraconal orbital fat (*dashed white arrows*)

invasive fungal *Aspergillus* may have similar imaging features.

Inflammatory Conditions

Idiopathic Orbital Inflammatory Disease

Idiopathic orbital inflammatory disease (IOID), previously known as orbital pseudotumor, occurs from the accumulation of inflammatory cells, fibrosis, and granulation tissue without an identifiable underlying cause [89]. The disease process is most commonly limited to the orbit. However, if patients also have multiple cranial neuropathies and ophthalmoplegia, a diagnosis of Tolosa-Hunt syndrome should be suspected [89, 90]. The condition is often bilateral but may be unilateral. The process may occur acutely, subacutely, or chronically. These disorders can resemble tumors, granulomatous disease, and infection [91, 92]. Clinically, the patients often present with pain, limited eye mobility, decreased visual acuity, and proptosis [89]. Idiopathic inflammatory disease of the orbit is a diagnosis of exclusion, and therefore, it is important to exclude other potentially treatable diagnoses.

Idiopathic orbital inflammatory disease can be focal or diffuse (Figs. 43.29 and 43.30). The focal form may involve the lacrimal gland, extraocular muscles, Tenon's capsule, sclera, and optic nerve sheath. The diffuse form can be transspatial, involving both the intraconal and extraconal compartments. Despite the infiltrative nature of this process, osseous erosion and globe distortion are not features of IOID as they are with orbital neoplasms [92]. The lesions of IOID tend to have low signal on T2-W and T1-W images, whereas neoplasms typically are usually higher in intensity on T2-W images (Fig. 43.30).

The extraocular muscles most commonly involved in IOID are the superior muscle group and the medial rectus muscles. The tendinous insertions are often involved producing not only a myositis but a tendinitis as well. This process can be bilateral or unilateral. On CT and MRI, there is enlargement and enhancement of the muscle bellies with extension to involve the tendinous insertions. In addition, there is often infiltration of the adjacent extraconal fat giving rise to an indistinct margin of the muscles. The main differential diagnosis is Graves' orbitopathy.

Idiopathic inflammation of the optic nerve sheath often presents with papilledema, orbital pain, painful eye mobility, and decreased visual acuity. The main differential diagnosis is that of optic neuritis which may be associated with multiple sclerosis. Infectious optic neuritis must also be considered in the differential diagnosis. On MRI, there is thickening and enhancement of the optic nerve sheath with infiltration of the adjacent retrobulbar fat.

Pain involving the upper outer quadrant of the orbit suggests a process involving the lacrimal gland. Idiopathic orbital inflammatory syndrome (IOIS) can cause enlargement and enhancement of the lacrimal gland. Other etiologies, however, including bacterial dacryoadenitis, granulomatous diseases, and tumor must be considered since many of these processes have overlapping features. Biopsy is often warranted for appropriate diagnosis.

Thyroid Orbitopathy

Thyroid orbitopathy, also known as Graves' disease, is an autoimmune disorder that typically occurs in hyperthyroid individuals, although this phenomenon can occur in euthyroid people [93]. Thyroid eye disease occurs more commonly in women, is typically bilateral, and often has a subacute onset. Clinically, individuals present with exophthalmos, eyelid edema, and limited ocular mobility [93–95]. Patients with thyroid eye disease may also develop strabismus requiring surgical intervention [93]. The primary differential diagnosis includes idiopathic inflammatory disease of the orbit, infection, metastatic disease, granulomatous disease, as well as congestive orbitopathy from dural arteriovenous fistula or orbital venous thrombosis.

CT and MRI demonstrate proptosis, increased volume of orbital fat, eyelid edema, stretching of the optic nerve, and enlargement of the bellies of the affected extraocular muscles with relative sparing of the tendinous insertion (Figs. 43.31, 43.32, and 43.33) [96]. The most frequently

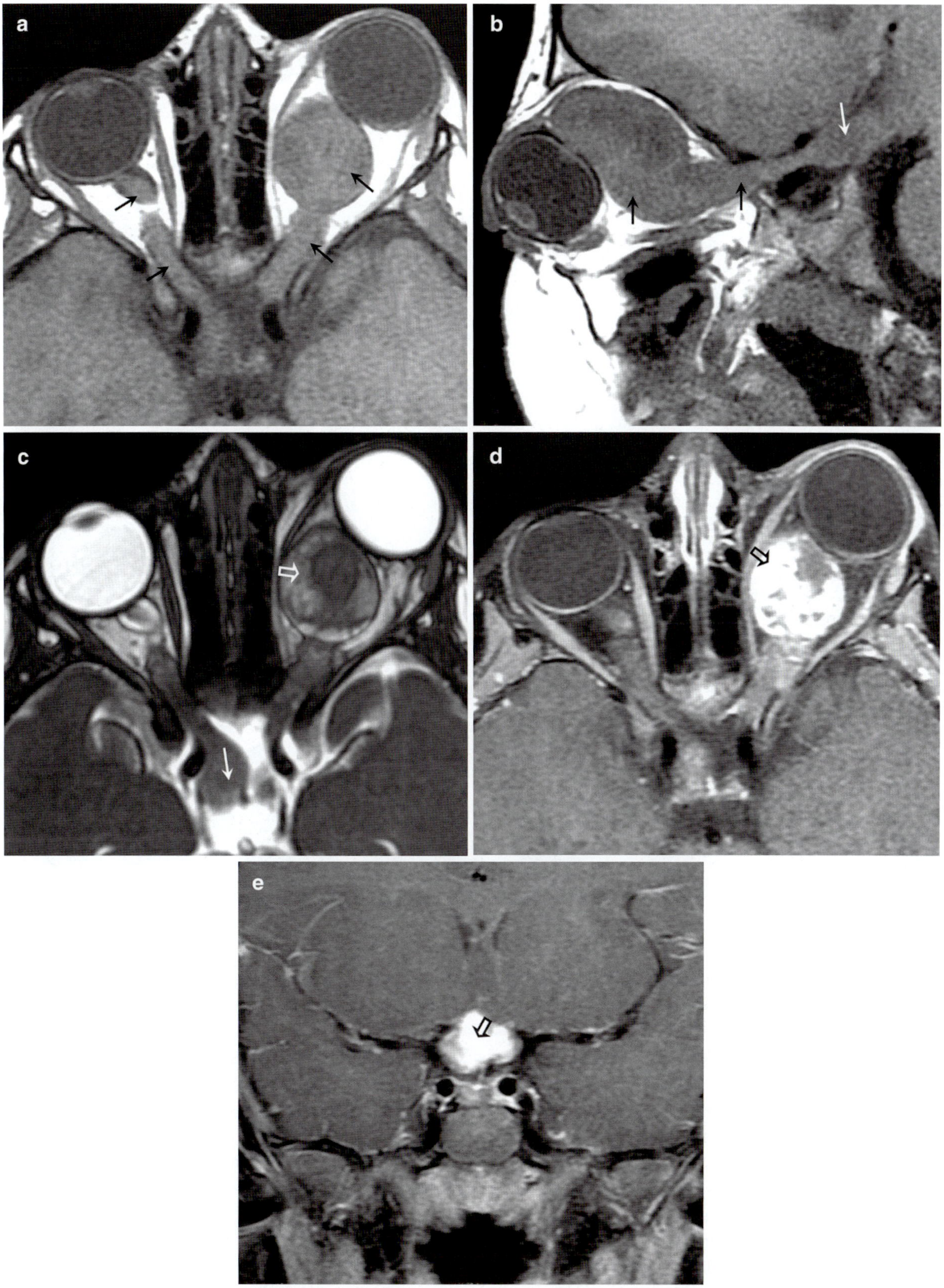

Fig. 43.19 Bilateral optic glioma – neurofibromatosis type 1: noncontrast T1-W (**a**, **b**), T2-W (**c**), and contrast-enhanced fat-suppressed T1-W (**d**, **e**) MR images reveal diffuse expansion of the orbital and intracranial portions of both optic nerves (*black arrows*) with secondary enlargement of the optic canals. There is a more focal mass of the left optic nerve with areas of intralesional edema seen on the T2-W image (*white open arrow*). The optic chiasm (*white arrows*) is also involved. There is patchy enhancement of portions of the mass (*black open arrows*) and little enhancement of other regions of the neoplasm

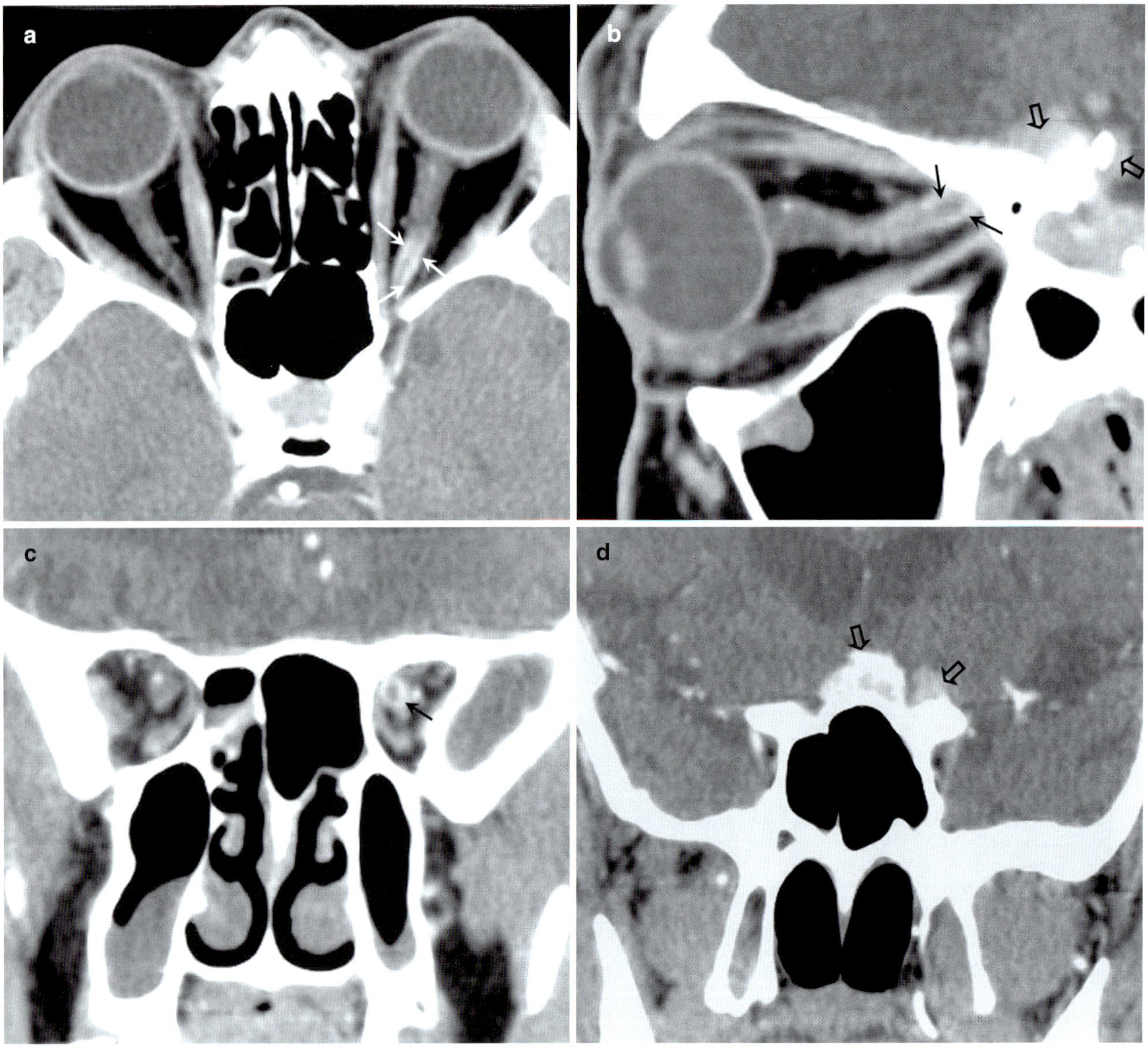

Fig. 43.20 Optic sheath meningioma: axial (**a**), oblique sagittal (**b**), and coronal (**c**, **d**) contrast-enhanced CT scans reveal focal "tram track" calcifications (*white arrows*) and abnormal enhancement along the intraorbital portion of the left optic sheath. There is extension of the meningioma through the optic canal to involve the dura (*black open arrows*) adjacent to the intracranial portion of the optic nerve. Coronal images reveal complete encasement and compression of the optic nerve by the meningioma (*black arrows*)

affected muscles are the inferior rectus and medial rectus muscles, although all of the muscles can be involved [94]. The lateral rectus muscle is not typically affected in isolation. The coronal view is the most useful imaging plane to assess relative thickness of the extraocular muscles. In the acute phase of the disease, muscle enlargement and muscle edema are the primary imaging features. There may be inflammation of the retrobulbar fat producing a "dirty fat" appearance (Fig. 43.33). In the later phase of the disease, the acute inflammation is replaced with fibrosis and fatty atrophy of the extraocular muscles (Fig. 43.32). Significant edema may be seen on T2-W MR images in the involved muscles during the acute inflammatory phase of the disease (Fig. 43.33).

Optic neuropathy can also be seen with Graves' disease. The optic nerve may be compressed or crowded at the orbital apex resulting in a compressive optic neuropathy. This can be appreciated on either axial CT or MR images [97]. Decompressive surgery may be indicated to relieve optic nerve compression [93].

Sarcoidosis

Sarcoidosis is a multisystem granulomatous disease that most often affects the pulmonary system. The orbit is also a common site of involvement, affecting 25% of patients [88]. The lacrimal gland, optic nerve, optic sheath, optic chiasm,

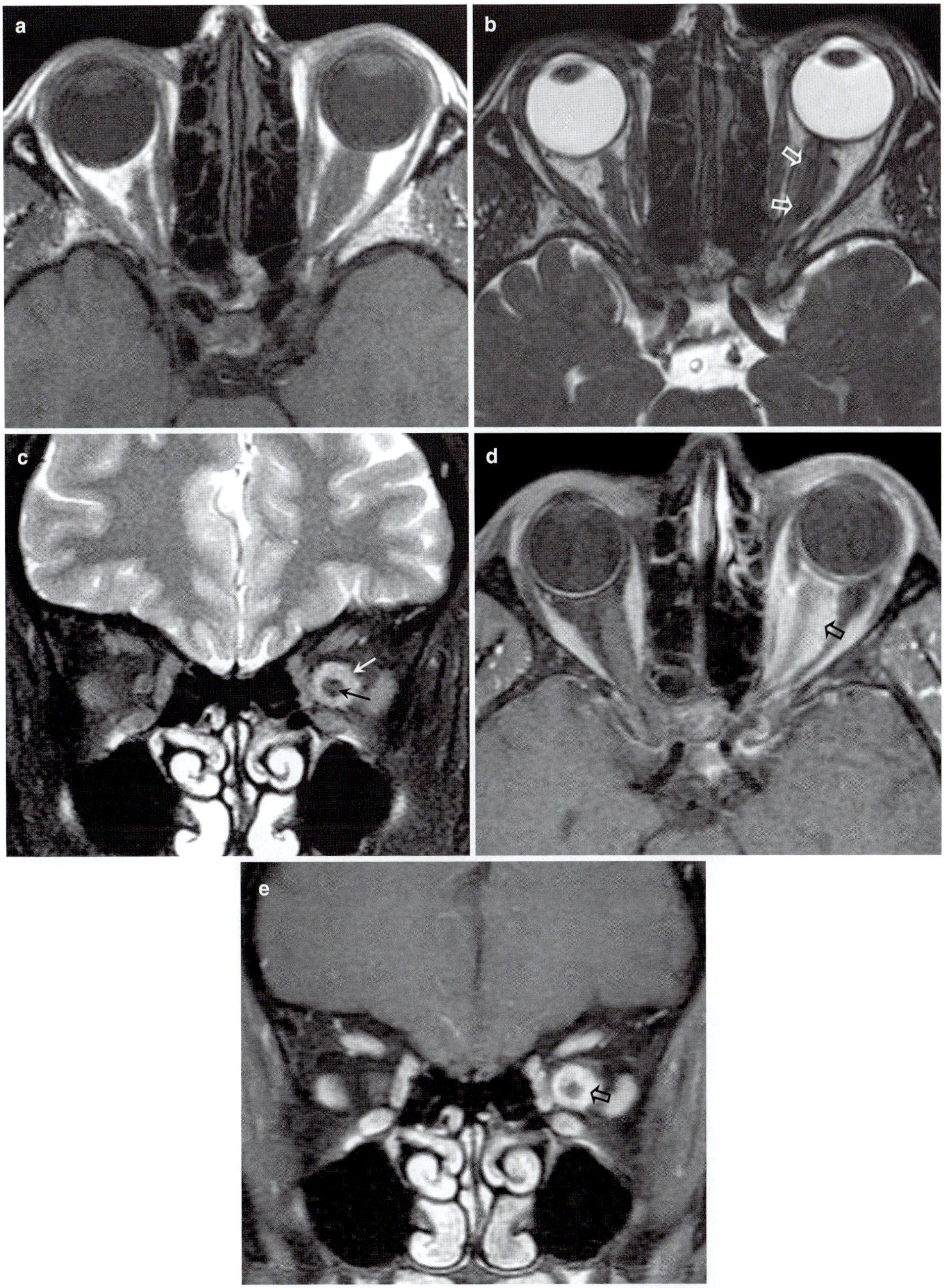

Fig. 43.21 Optic sheath meningioma: noncontrast axial T1-W (**a**), axial T2-W (**b**), and fat-suppressed STIR (**c**) MR scans demonstrate a fusiform mass of the left optic nerve extending from the globe to the optic canal. The lesion is extremely hypointense on the T2-W image (*white open arrows*) characteristic of meningioma. The neoplasm (*white arrow*) is seen to circumferentially encase the optic nerve (*black arrow*) on the fat-suppressed STIR image. Contrast-enhanced fat-suppressed T1-W MR images (**d**, **e**) reveal homogeneous intense enhancement of the lesion (*open black arrows*) typical of an optic sheath meningioma

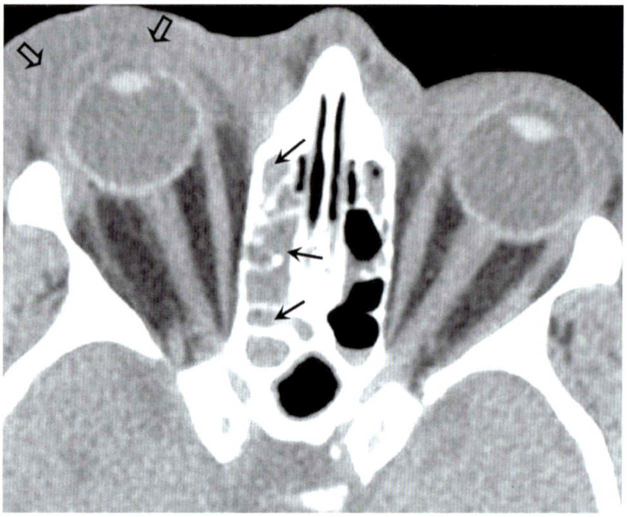

Fig. 43.22 Preseptal orbital cellulitis: axial CT scan reveals extensive soft tissue swelling of the soft tissues anterior to the right globe (*open arrows*) as well as extensive right ethmoid sinusitis (*arrows*). The post-septal orbital fat, however, is not involved

extraocular muscles, uvea, retina, and conjunctiva are the sites that may be affected [74, 98]. The disease is often accompanied by abnormal elevations of angiotensin-converting enzyme (ACE) levels. MRI is superior to CT for evaluation of the ocular and orbital manifestations of sarcoidosis. The disease process may be limited to the orbit but may also involve the brain and meninges. It is important, therefore, to simultaneously evaluate the brain as well as the orbit with imaging. On MRI, one may see nodular enhancement of the optic nerve, optic sheath, orbital adnexal structures, meninges, or brain (Fig. 43.17).

Granulomatosis with Polyangiitis

Granulomatosis with Polyangiitis (GPA, formerley called Wegener's Granulomatosis) is also a multisystem disease characterized by multi-organ small vessel vasculitis and granulomatous inflammation involving the respiratory tract [99].

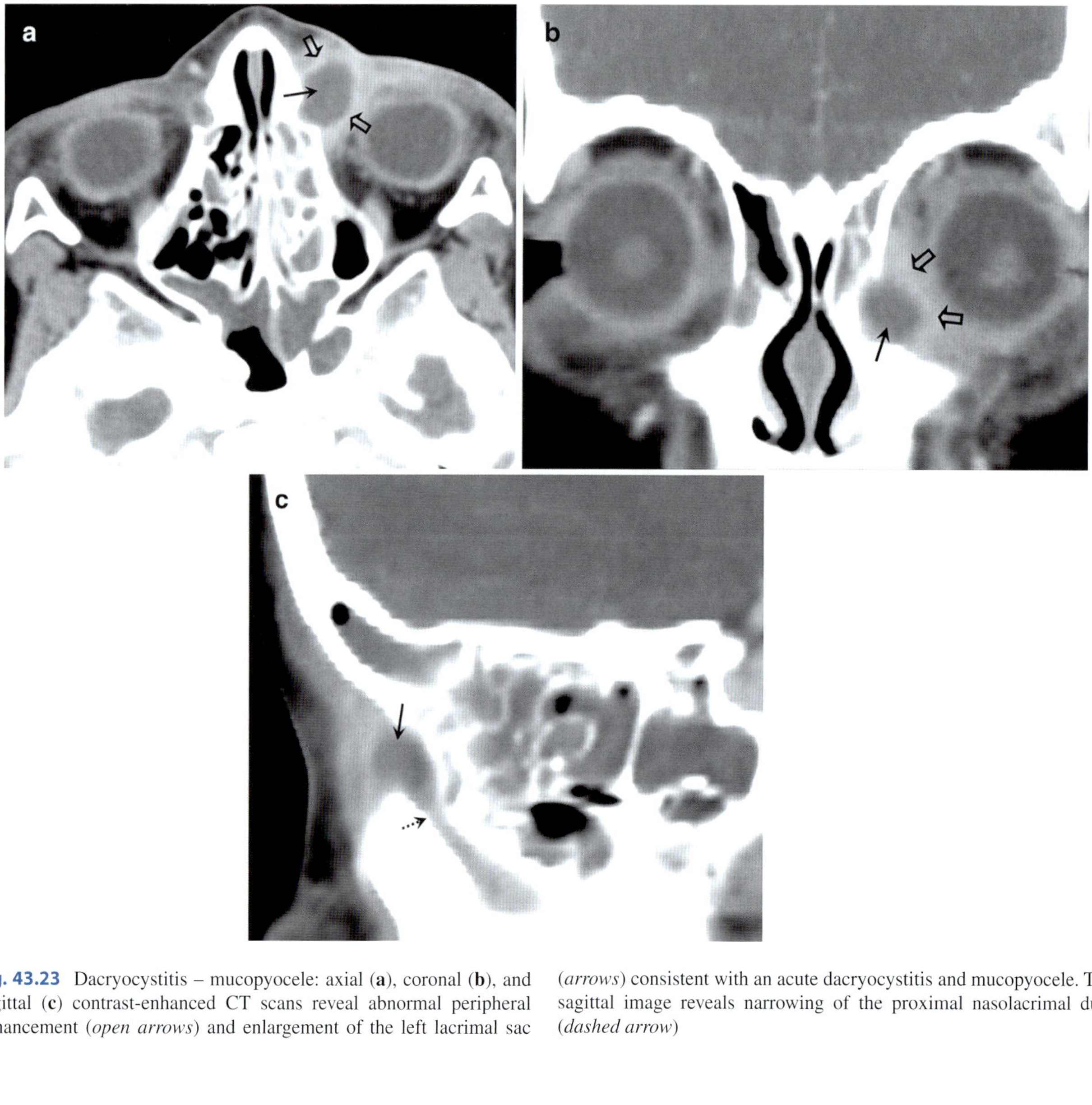

Fig. 43.23 Dacryocystitis – mucopyocele: axial (**a**), coronal (**b**), and sagittal (**c**) contrast-enhanced CT scans reveal abnormal peripheral enhancement (*open arrows*) and enlargement of the left lacrimal sac (*arrows*) consistent with an acute dacryocystitis and mucopyocele. The sagittal image reveals narrowing of the proximal nasolacrimal duct (*dashed arrow*)

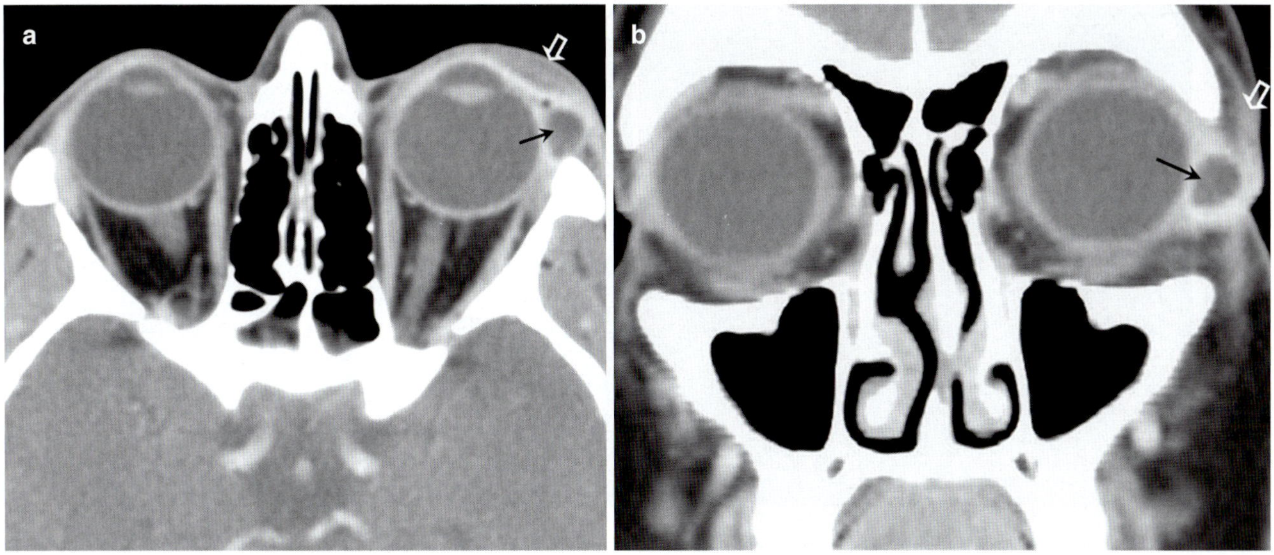

Fig. 43.24 Dacryoadenitis – lacrimal gland abscess: axial (**a**) and coronal (**b**) contrast-enhanced CT scans show evidence of preseptal cellulitis along the lateral aspect of the left eye (*open arrows*) as well as a rounded peripherally enhancing abscess (*black arrows*) within the palpebral portion of the lacrimal gland. The abscess was found to be secondary to an infected dermoid cyst

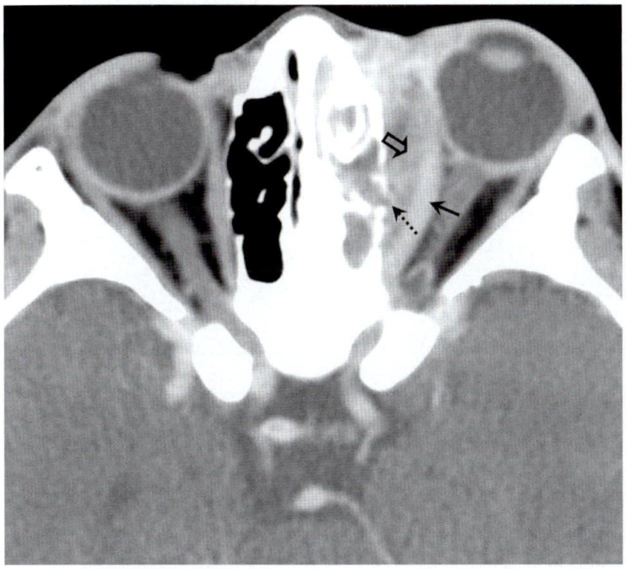

Fig. 43.25 Subperiosteal orbital abscess: axial contrast-enhanced CT scan demonstrates extensive left ethmoid sinusitis with focal erosion of the lamina papyracea (*dashed arrow*). There is a large subperiosteal abscess (*open arrow*) that displaces the extraconal orbital fat, medial rectus muscle, and globe laterally. There is mild enlargement and abnormal enhancement of the medial rectus muscle (*arrow*) consistent with associated myositis

Typically, this disease process affects the kidneys, lungs, and sinuses, although the orbit may be affected in up to 50% of patients [99]. The disease often spreads from the sinuses to the adjacent orbit, although isolated orbital disease without sinus involvement has also been described [100]. Typical clinical symptoms include proptosis, pain, eyelid edema, and limited ocular mobility. A high serum antineutrophil cytoplasmic antibody (ANCA) test is suggestive of the diagnosis, although biopsy is often warranted to exclude other diagnoses such as lymphoma, pseudotumor, sarcoidosis, and other neoplasms. GPA granulomatosis may involve both the intraconal and extraconal spaces [100]. The conjunctiva and sclera are the most common sites of orbital involvement at the time of presentation [100]. The imaging features of GPA granulomatosis are relatively nonspecific (Fig. 43.34). The MR features of GPA granulomatosis are similar to sarcoidosis, lymphoma, and pseudotumor. GPA infiltrates are typically hypointense relative to orbital fat on T2-W images and demonstrate enhancement after contrast.

Sjögren's Syndrome

Sjögren's syndrome is an autoimmune disease characterized by lymphocyte infiltration of the lacrimal and salivary glands. Clinically, the disease is characterized by dry mouth and dry eyes. This syndrome often occurs secondarily in association with other autoimmune diseases such as rheumatoid arthritis, systemic lupus erythematosus, scleroderma, and vasculitis [88]. The diagnosis of Sjögren's syndrome is often made based on a combination of clinical history and laboratory values including measuring the lacrimal flow rate, Schirmer's test. A lacrimal gland biopsy may be needed for definitive diagnosis. Patients with Sjögren's syndrome affecting the lacrimal gland will often initially have a normal size gland. As the disease progresses, the gland may hypertrophy as it becomes infiltrated with lymphocytes. The gland then eventually develops fatty atrophy with a heterogeneous stippled appearance on T1-W images that demonstrates signal dropout on fat-suppressed sequences. In the late stages of the disease, the

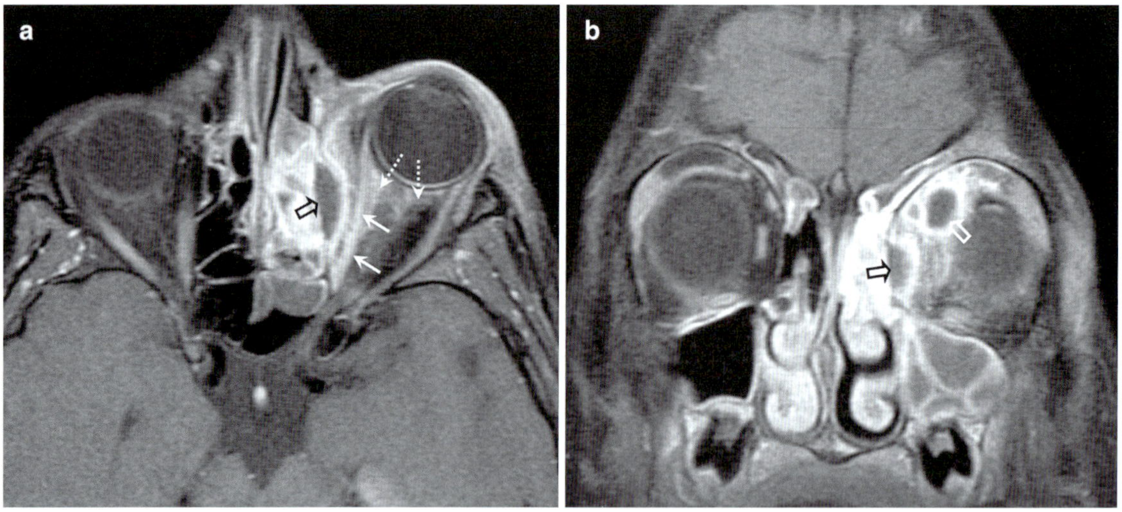

Fig. 43.26 Subperiosteal and orbital abscesses – orbital cellulitis and myositis: postcontrast fat-suppressed axial (**a**) and coronal (**b**) MR scans demonstrate several complications of left ethmoid sinusitis. There is evidence of a large subperiosteal (*open black arrows*) and retroseptal (*open white arrow*) abscesses as well as retrobulbar orbital cellulitis (*dashed white arrows*) and medial rectus myositis (*white arrows*)

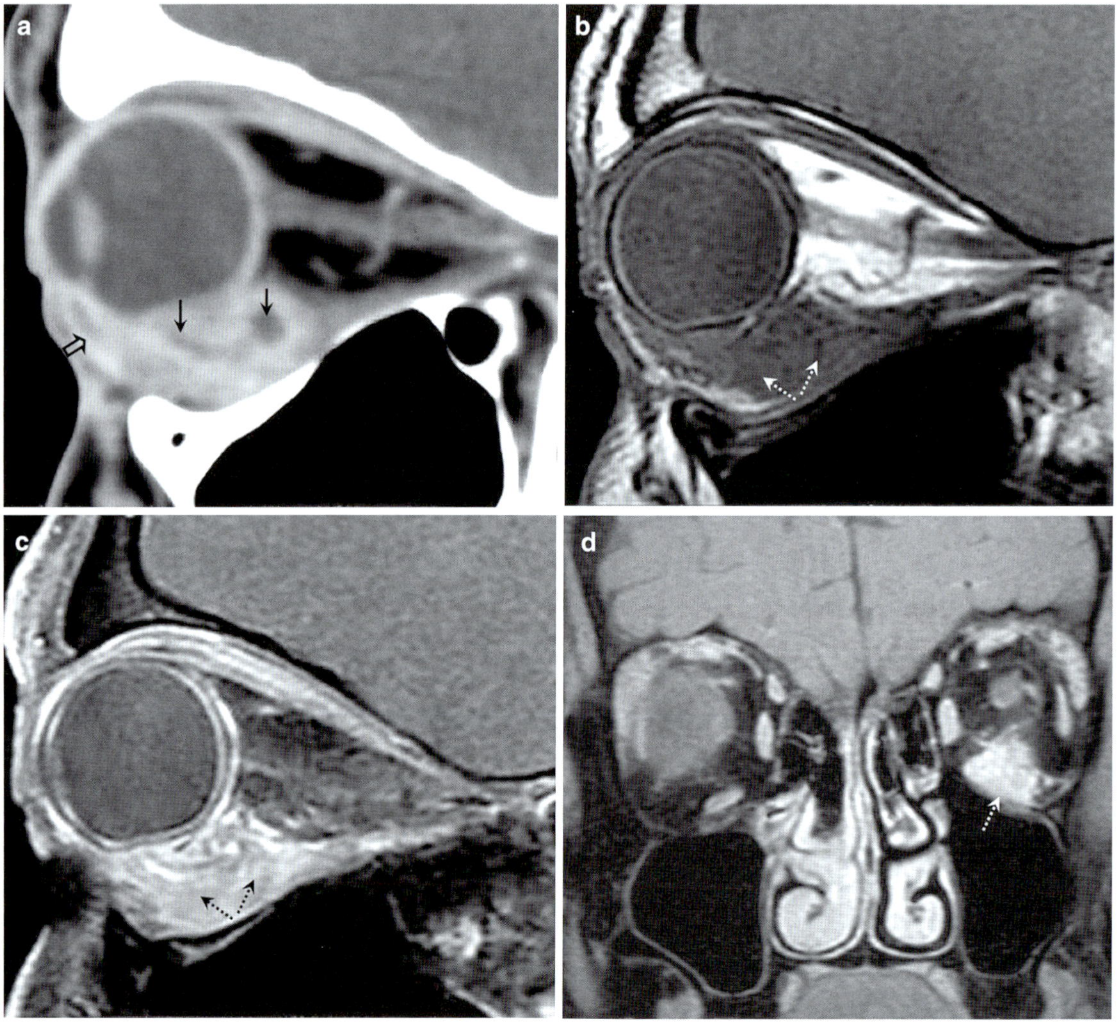

Fig. 43.27 Inferior rectus and inferior oblique muscle abscess: oblique sagittal contrast-enhanced CT scan (**a**), noncontrast oblique sagittal T1-W (**b**) scan, and fat-suppressed contrast-enhanced oblique sagittal (**c**) and coronal (**d**) MR scans demonstrate an extensive inflammatory process (*dashed arrows*) encasing the inferior oblique and inferior rectus muscles with extension into the lower eyelid (*open black arrow*). There is a focal non-enhancing abscess collection (*black arrows*) within the center of the mass. Cultures of the lesion were negative, but the patient showed dramatic improvement with intravenous ceftriaxone

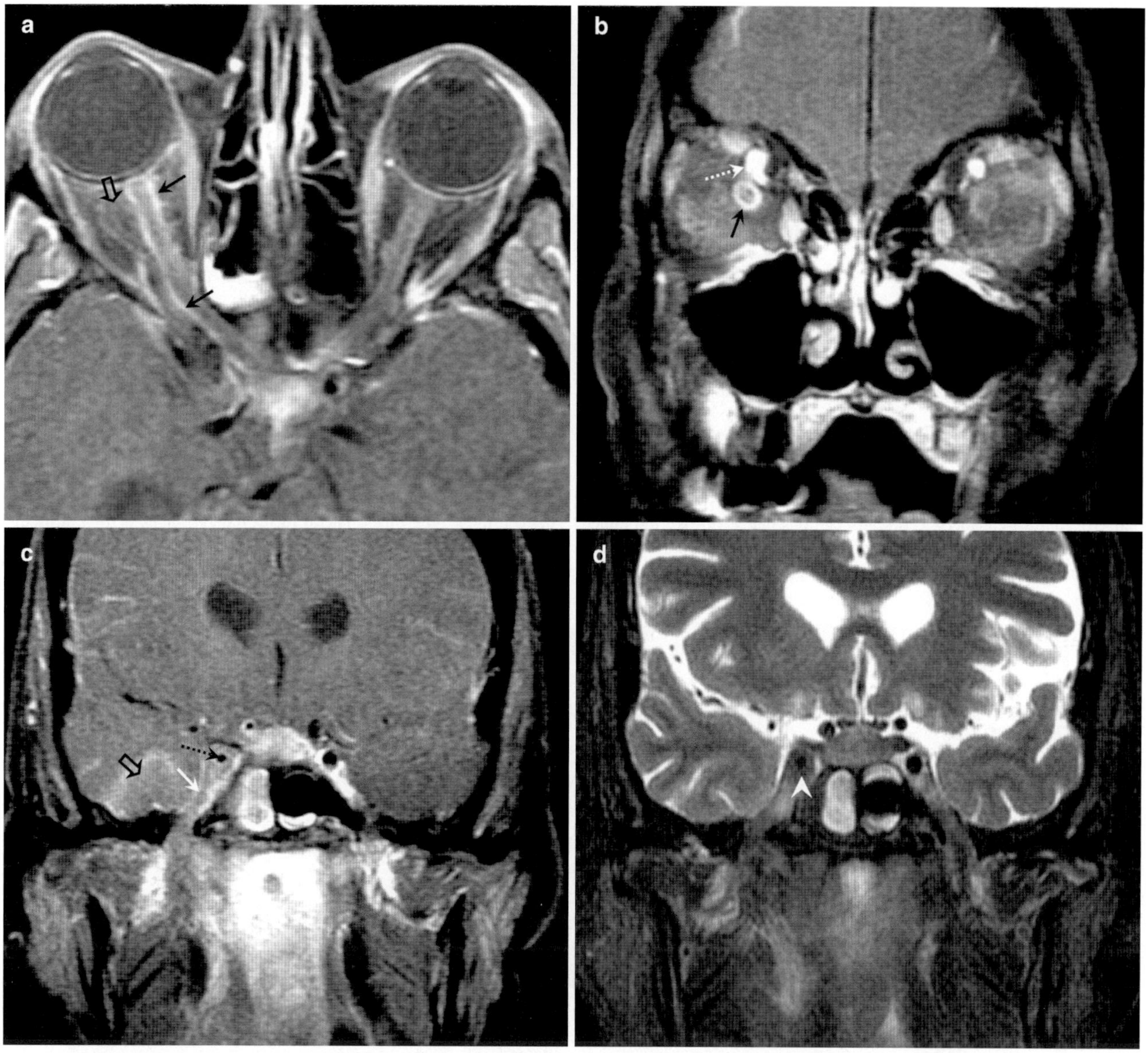

Fig. 43.28 Orbital mucormycosis – cavernous sinus thrombosis: axial (**a**) and coronal (**b**, **c**) fat-suppressed T1-W MR scans demonstrate changes of proptosis due to acute rapidly progressive right orbital cellulitis in this immunocompromised individual. There is diffuse abnormal enhancement of the retro-ocular fat (*open black arrow*), diffuse thickening and enhancement of the optic sheath (*black arrows*), and dilatation of the superior ophthalmic veins (*dashed white arrow*). The infection has extended posteriorly to involve Meckel's cave (*white arrow*), right temporal lobe (*open black arrow*), and the cavernous sinus with encasement and narrowing of the right internal carotid artery (*dashed black arrow*). A coronal T2-W MR scan (**d**) reveals that the right internal carotid artery is encased by very hypointense material (*white arrowhead*) highly suggestive of fungal infection

gland ultimately becomes completely atrophic and slit-like in appearance. The lacrimal function parallels the imaging features.

Tumors and Tumorlike Lesions

A number of developmental, benign, and malignant neoplasms occur in and around the orbit. These may occur within or adjacent to the bony orbit [2, 17, 27, 49, 85, 89, 92].

Fibro-Osseous Lesions

Fibrous dysplasia is a relatively common benign bone tumor that may present as a single lesion (monostotic), may involve more than one bone (polyostotic), or may be associated with pituitary insufficiency and endocrine abnormalities (McCune-Albright syndrome). The sphenoid and ethmoid bones of the face are the most commonly involved bones. Fibrous dysplasia typically involves the cancellous bone and causes expansion of the involved bone by an amorphous hyperdense type

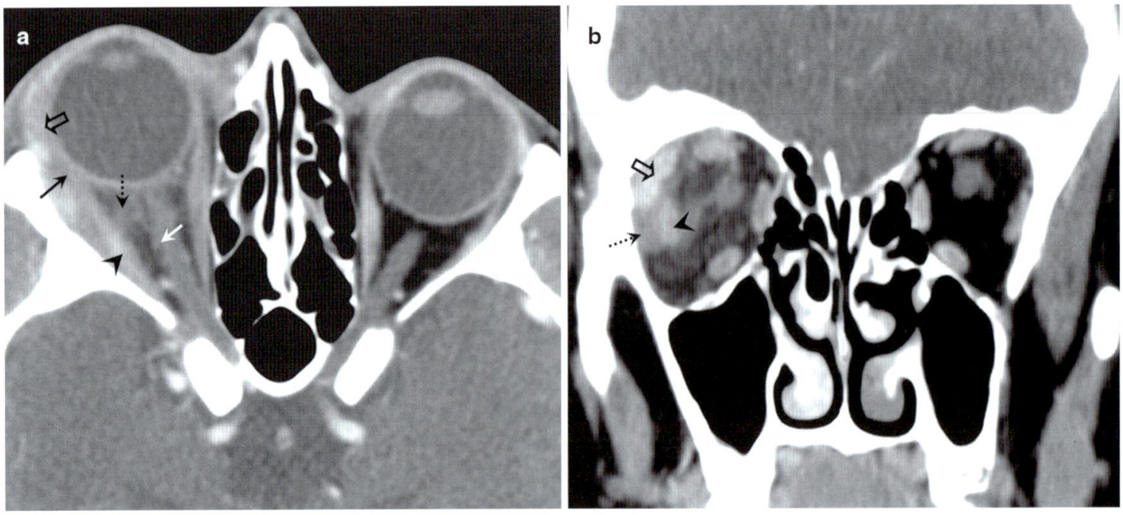

Fig. 43.29 Idiopathic orbital inflammatory disease: axial (**a**) and coronal (**b**) contrast-enhanced CT scans demonstrate a diffuse ill-defined inflammatory process involving the lacrimal gland (*open black arrows*), intraconal and extraconal spaces (*dashed black arrows*), lateral rectus muscle (*black arrowheads*), and optic sheath (*white arrow*). There is ill-defined thickening of the lateral rectus tendon (*black arrow*), a finding that is common in orbital pseudotumor. Despite the extensive abnormality, there is only mild proptosis making a neoplastic process very unlikely

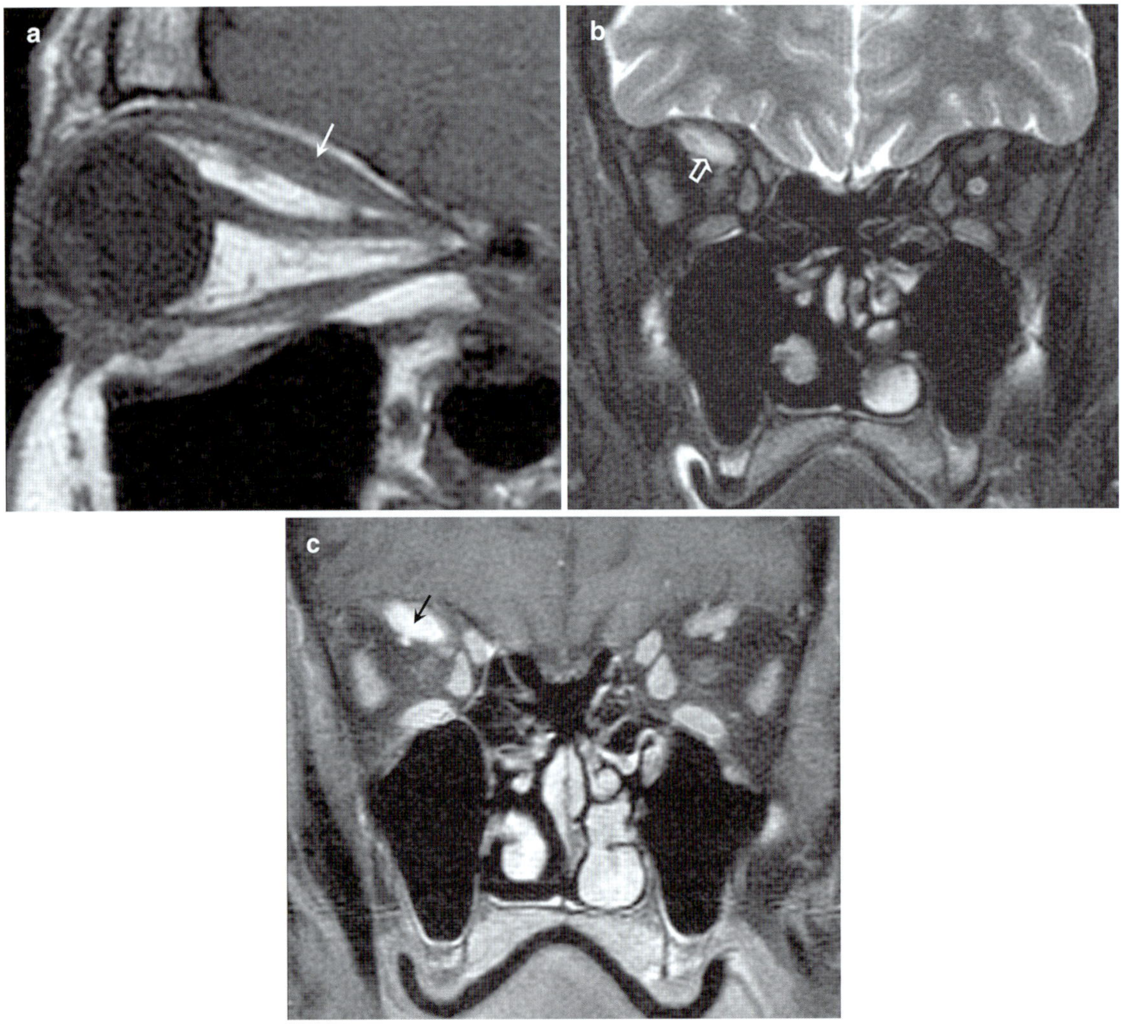

Fig. 43.30 Idiopathic orbital myositis: noncontrast oblique sagittal T1-W (**a**), noncontrast coronal T2-W (**b**), and contrast-enhanced fat-suppressed T1-W (**c**) MR scans obtained in a patient with painful right extraocular muscle movements. The right superior rectus and levator muscles show mild enlargement (*white arrow*), moderate edema (*open white arrow*), and diffuse enhancement (*black arrow*) consistent with acute idiopathic orbital myositis

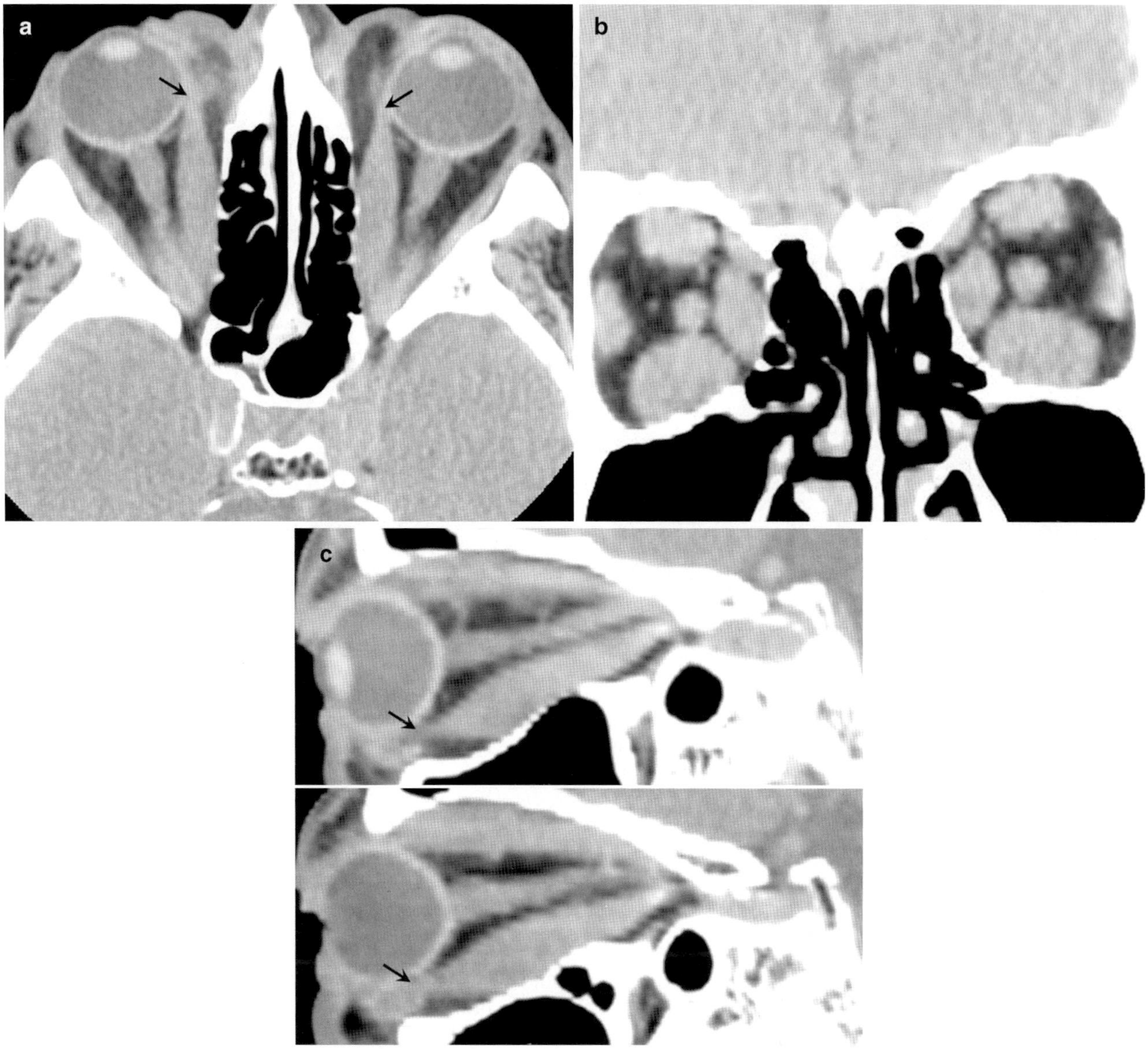

Fig. 43.31 Graves' disease (CT): axial (**a**), coronal (**b**), and sagittal (**c**) noncontrast CT scans demonstrate diffuse bilateral spindle-shaped enlargement of the extraocular muscles. The outer margins of the muscles are well circumscribed, and there is relative sparing of the tendinous insertions (*arrows*) which are differentiating features from orbital pseudotumor. Note the crowding of the optic nerve at the orbital apex

of bone that has a "ground-glass" appearance. The optic nerves and cranial nerves III–VI may be compressed if the fibrous dysplasia narrows the optic canal or skull base foramina. Osteomas are common hyperdense bone lesions that occur around the frontal and ethmoid sinus. These lesions may extend into the orbit or cause obstruction of the paranasal sinuses and produce orbital involvement by mucocele formation.

Dermoid, Epidermoid, and Lipoma

One of the most common orbital neoplasms of children occurs in the region around the lacrimal gland [27, 49, 85]. Inclusion of mesodermal elements in the tissues around the developing lacrimal gland may produce lipomas, epidermoid tumors, and dermoid tumors (Fig. 43.35). These lesions usually contain a varying amount of fat and soft tissue and are fairly easy to detect on either CT or MRI. Dermoid or epidermoid lesions may also be found near the sites of orbital suture fusion. This is especially common along the lateral wall of the orbit (Fig. 43.36).

Histiocytosis: Eosinophilic Granuloma

Histiocytosis is an idiopathic immune-related nonneoplastic disease that occurs in children. Multiple organ systems may be affected by collections of abnormal histiocytes including the calvarium and bony orbit. The soft tissue masses may

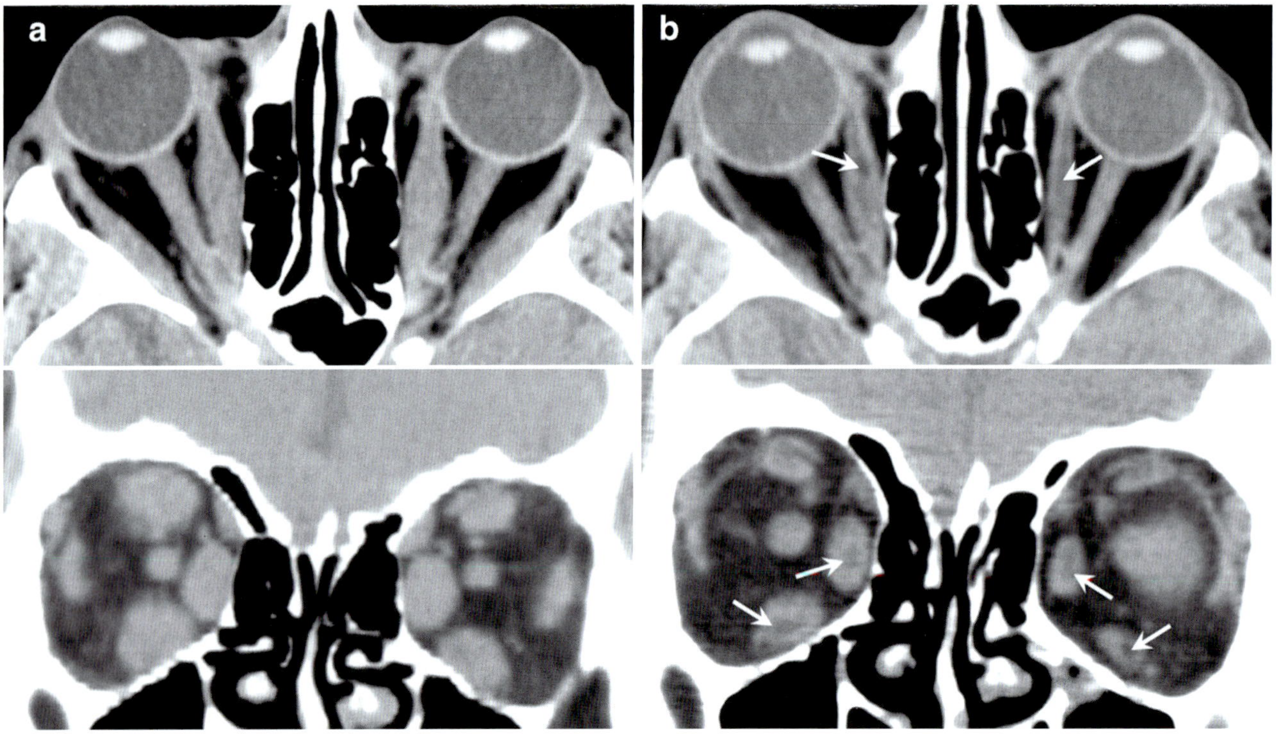

Fig. 43.32 Evolving Graves' disease: axial and coronal noncontrast CT in the acute inflammatory (**a**) and chronic (**b**) stage of the disease 3 years later. The patient has classic diffuse spindle-shaped enlargement of multiple bilateral extraocular muscles in the acute setting (**a**). There is significant decrease in the size of the extraocular muscles and significant fatty infiltration (*white arrows*) of the muscles on the follow-up scan

erode the bones of the orbit and skull producing lytic lesions that classically have irregular beveled edges (Fig. 43.37) [27, 49, 85].

Lacrimal Gland Neoplasms

Benign and malignant neoplasms may occur in the lacrimal gland [2, 17, 27, 49, 85, 89, 92]. The lacrimal gland is an exocrine secretory gland, which is situated in the superotemporal orbit. The specific neoplasms that involve the lacrimal gland are quite similar to those seen in the major salivary glands. Benign lesions include pleomorphic adenomas (Fig. 43.38), monomorphic adenomas, benign reactive lymphoid hyperplasia, and oncocytomas. These lesions are slowly growing masses more commonly found in adults in their forth to fifth decades of life. Benign lesions may cause significant bony remodeling of the lacrimal fossa of the orbit. Malignant tumors of the lacrimal gland include adenoid cystic carcinoma (Fig. 43.39), adenocarcinoma, squamous cell carcinoma, mucoepidermoid carcinoma, and malignant lymphomas. Adenoid cystic carcinoma is the most common malignant lacrimal gland tumor. Most cases are seen in the third decade of life with a second bimodal peak in the teenage years.

Orbital Lymphoma

Lymphoproliferative disorders of the orbit range from reactive lymphoid hyperplasia to malignant neoplasms which may be associated with systemic disease or may be primary to the orbit [2, 17, 49, 85, 89, 92]. Clinically, lymphoma involving the orbit occurs in the older population and presents as painless proptosis with decreased motility of the extraocular muscles and possible concomitant lacrimal gland enlargement (Figs. 43.40 and 43.41). These tumors tend to be bilateral and arise in the areas of the orbit that contain normal lymphoid tissue (lacrimal glands, conjunctiva, eyelids). Mucosa-associated lymphoid tumors (MALT), in particular, may be confined to the conjunctiva and eyelids. The imaging features of lymphoma are entirely nonspecific and may mimic other neoplasms, pseudotumor, infection, and granulomatous disease. Lymphoma will present as a soft tissue mass that is often hyperdense on CT because of high cellularity and high nuclear to cytoplasmic ratio within the tumor. The tumor is typically "plastic" in nature, insinuating itself around and molding to various structures within the orbit. Bony erosion is not a typical feature but may occasionally be present. On MRI, lymphoma is often hypointense on T1-W images and usually much darker than other tumors on T2-W images due to the marked cellularity of the lesion.

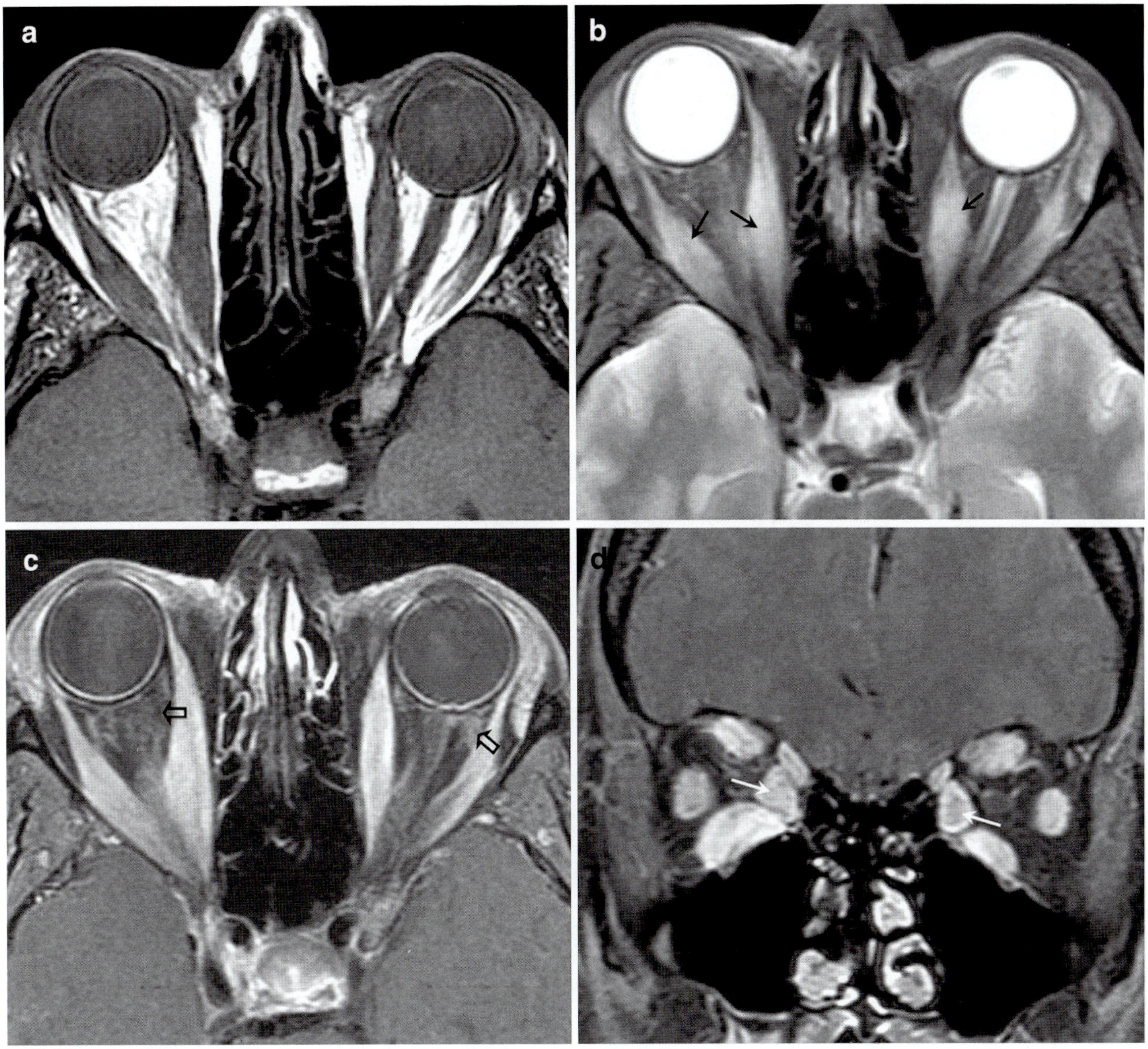

Fig. 43.33 Graves' disease (MRI): noncontrast axial T1-W (**a**), noncontrast fat-suppressed T2-W (**b**), and axial (**c**) and coronal (**d**) postcontrast fat-suppressed T1-W MR scans demonstrate diffuse bilateral spindle-shaped enlargement of the extraocular muscles with relative sparing of the tendinous insertions. The T2-W image demonstrates markedly hyperintense signal in the muscles (*black arrows*) due to acute edema. There is a "dirty fat" appearance of the retrobulbar fat (*open black arrow*) due to inflammatory infiltration and edema. The muscles enhance relatively homogeneously although there are some relatively hypovascular areas in the center of the muscles (*white arrows*) due to poor tissue perfusion of the acutely inflamed muscles

Orbital Leukemia

Unlike lymphoma, leukemia is a disease of childhood [49, 85]. Orbital involvement by leukemia occurs commonly and may in fact be the first site of involvement. Acute lymphoblastic leukemia (ALL) and acute myelogenous leukemia (AML) are the two most common subtypes that affect children (Fig. 43.42) [88]. The orbit often becomes involved by extension from leukemic infiltrates affecting the bones of the orbit typically occurring within the subperiosteal space [88]. There may be intracranial spread in addition to orbital involvement. The main differential diagnosis includes eosinophilic granuloma, rhabdomyosarcoma, neuroblastoma metastasis, infection, hematoma, and pseudotumor.

Rhabdomyosarcoma

Rhabdomyosarcoma, a malignant soft tissue tumor of skeletal muscle origin, accounts for approximately 6% of the

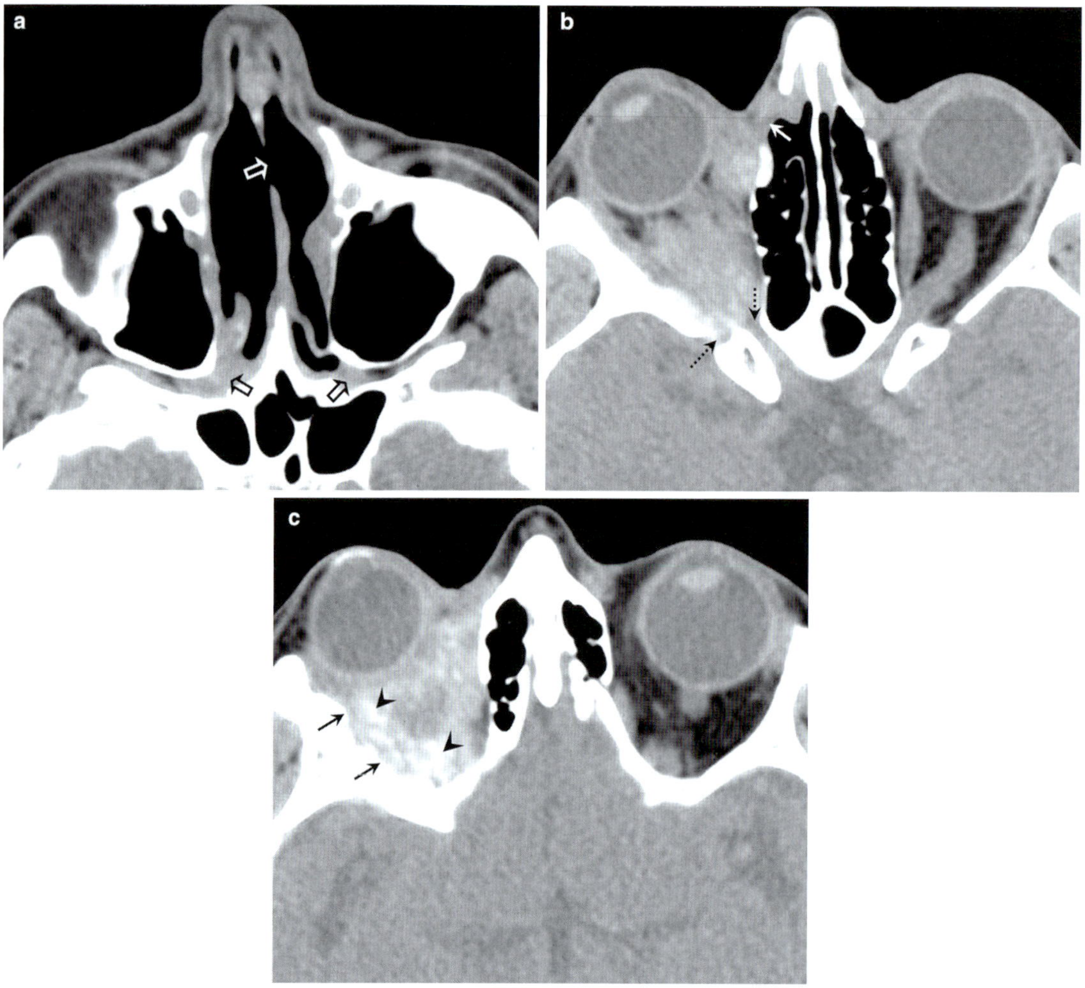

Fig. 43.34 GPA granulomatosis: axial CT scans (**a**–**c**) demonstrate classic findings of sinonasal and orbital GPA granulomatosis. There is a large area of necrosis of the nasal septum (*open white arrow*), inflammatory tissue in the pterygopalatine fossa bilaterally (*open black arrows*), and erosion of bone in the right lacrimal fossa (*white arrow*). There is an extensive area of soft tissue infiltration of the entire intraconal and extraconal orbital fat but no significant orbital proptosis. This is a distinguishing feature from infiltrating orbital neoplasms such as lymphoma. The inflammatory process is seen to involve both the superior orbital fissure and the orbital apex (*dashed black arrows*). The upper portion of the mass shows dystrophic areas of calcification (*black arrowhead*) and irregular sclerosis of the lateral orbital wall (*black arrows*), both of which would be unusual in lymphoma

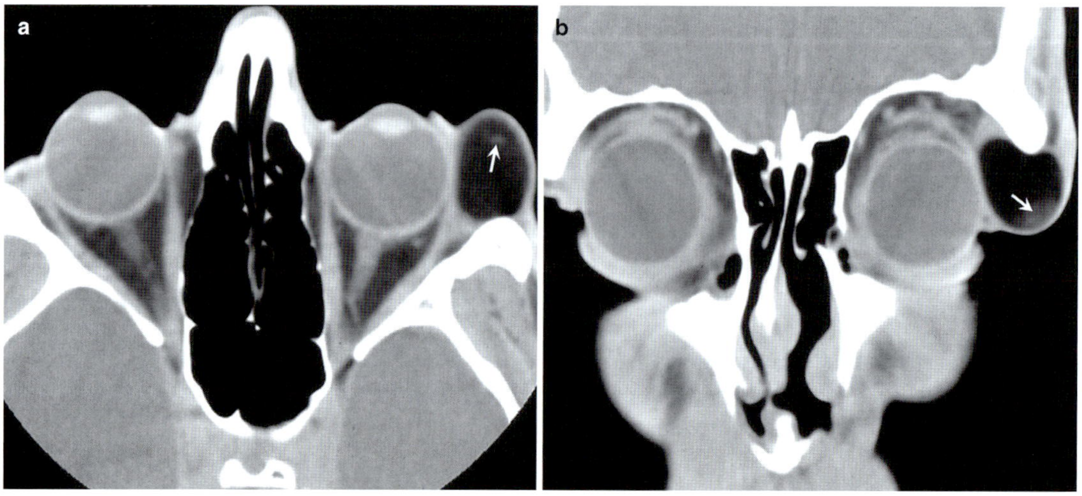

Fig. 43.35 Lipodermoid of lacrimal gland: axial (**a**) and coronal (**b**) CT scans demonstrate a well-circumscribed mass lesion primarily of fat attenuation involving the palpebral portion of the lacrimal gland. There is a small portion of the lesion that is of soft tissue attenuation (*arrows*) suggesting a dermoid tumor

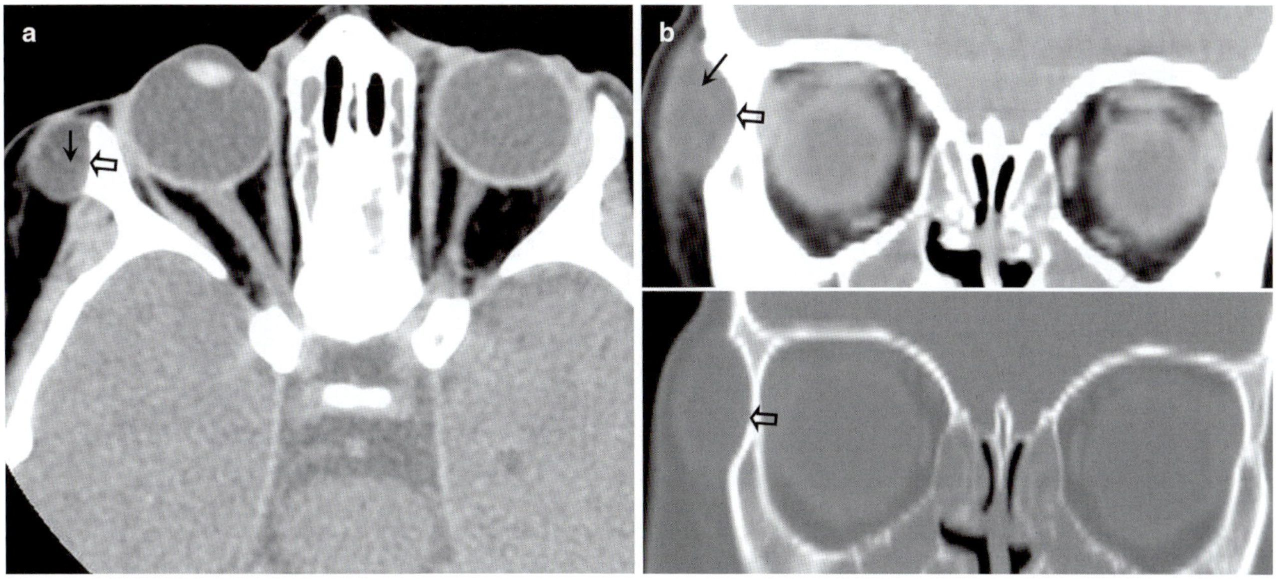

Fig. 43.36 Orbital wall epidermoid: there is a well-circumscribed mass arising from the lateral wall of the right orbit (*black arrows*) that is causing smooth scalloping of the adjacent bone (*open black arrows*). Most epidermoid tumors arise near the junction of bony sutures with this lesion beginning near the zygomaticomaxillary suture

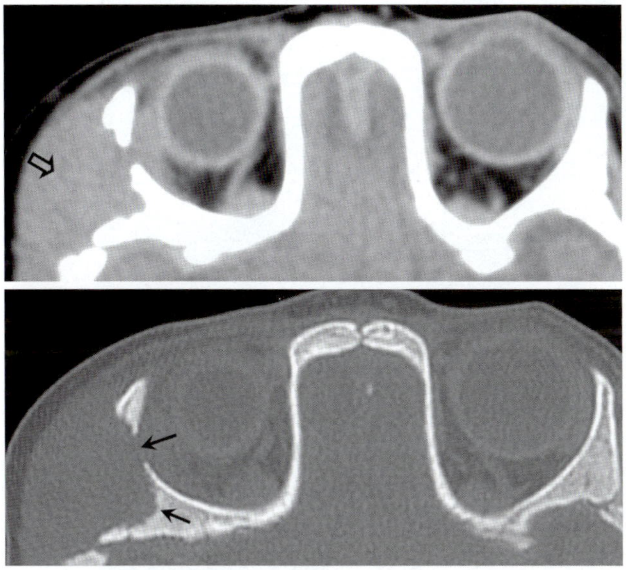

Fig. 43.37 Histiocytosis – eosinophilic granuloma: axial CT scans reveal a large soft tissue mass (*open arrow*) that is associated with irregular, ragged destruction (*arrows*) of the lateral wall of the orbit with classic beveled edges. The imaging findings in this 3-year-old child who had additional skeletal and calvarial lesions are not specific although most consistent with eosinophilic granuloma

cases of cancer among children less than 15 years of age [88]. Fifty percent of cases are seen in the first decade of life. The most common primary sites for rhabdomyosarcoma are the head, the genitourinary tract, and the extremities [88]. Two common subtypes are present (embryonal and alveolar). The embryonal type occurs more commonly in younger children, and the alveolar type is more common in older children and teenagers. Most cases of rhabdomyosarcoma occur sporadically, with no recognized predisposing factor or risk factor, although several genetic conditions may predispose to the disease. The orbit, temporal fossa, and temporal bone are common sites of head and neck rhabdomyosarcoma [49, 85].

Metastasis

Metastases to the globe, extraocular muscles, and bony orbit are fairly common in the adult to elderly patient group. Breast, lung, renal cell, thyroid, and prostate carcinomas are some of the most common cell types to involve the orbit. It is not uncommon for metastasis to spread bilaterally to the globe and extraocular muscles. Metastasis must be considered when there is enlargement of one or more extraocular muscles (Figs. 43.43 and 43.44) [2, 17, 27, 49, 85, 89, 92].

Neural Tumors

As was covered in the anatomy section of this chapter, there are multiple peripheral nerves that traverse the orbit which include cranial nerves III, IV, V, and VI. Schwannomas and neurofibromas are tumors that can arise from these nerves [101]. As the optic nerve is not a peripheral nerve, schwannomas and neurofibromas do not arise from the optic nerve. Schwannomas are slow-growing encapsulated tumors that originate from Schwann cells, which occur most commonly within the intraconal space [17]. Schwannomas affecting the nerves of the orbit share similar imaging features to schwannomas in other locations. They are characterized by fusiform enlargement of the nerve with intense homogeneous

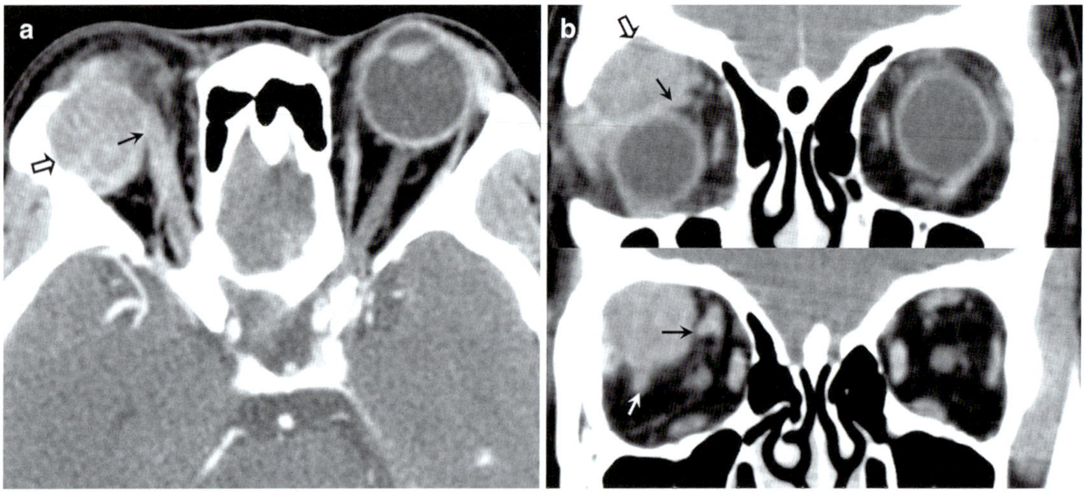

Fig. 43.38 Pleomorphic adenoma lacrimal gland: axial (**a**) and coronal (**b**) contrast-enhanced CT scans demonstrate a large, mildly enhancing, but well-circumscribed mass arising from the orbital portion of the right lacrimal gland. The well-defined shape and evidence of smooth remodeling of the bone of the lacrimal fossa (*open arrows*) suggest a nonaggressive lesion. There are medial deviation of the superior muscle group (*black arrows*) and inferior displacement of the lateral rectus muscle (*white arrow*)

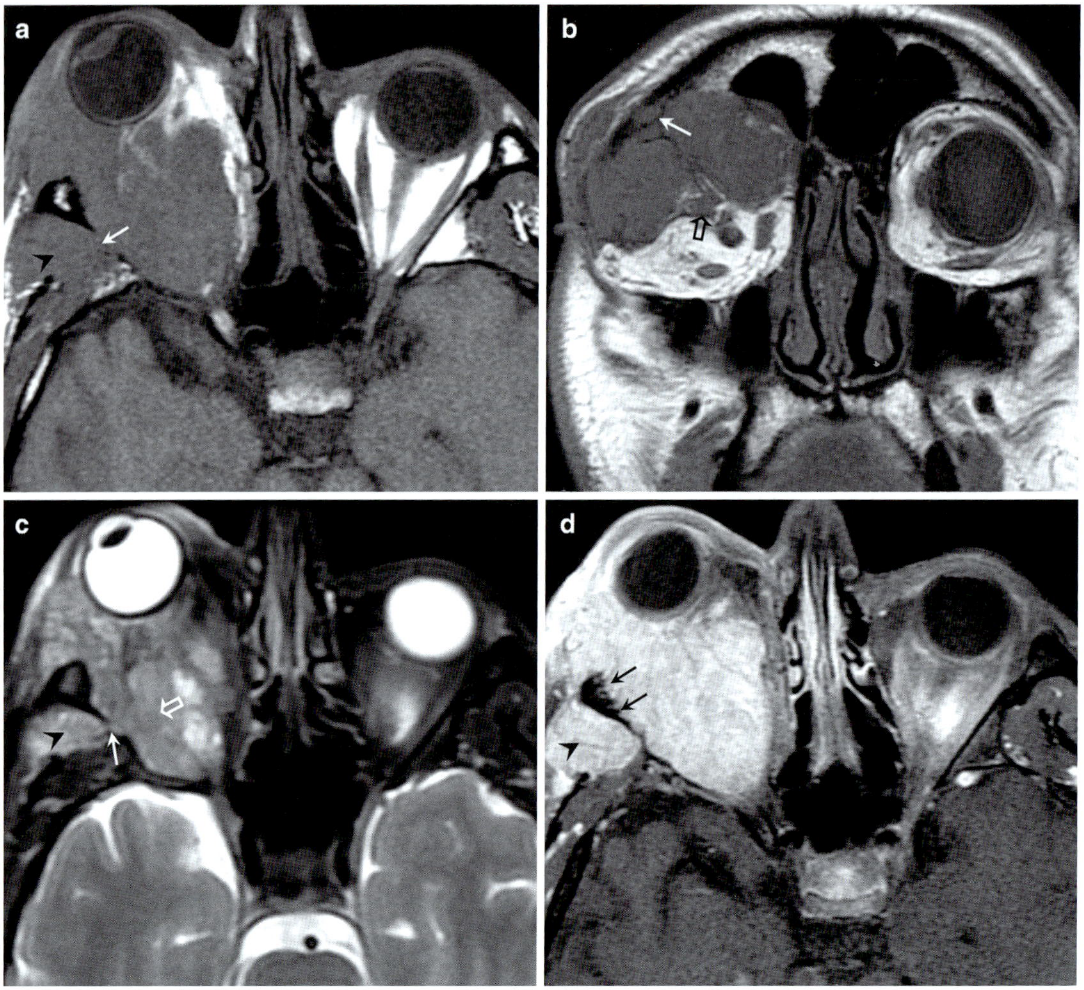

Fig. 43.39 Adenoid cystic carcinoma lacrimal gland: axial (**a**) and coronal (**b**) noncontrast T1-W, axial noncontrast T2-W (**c**), and contrast-enhanced fat-suppressed T1-W (**d**) MR images reveal a huge mass centered in the upper outer aspect of the right orbit arising near the lacrimal gland but extending laterally into the temporal fossa (*black arrowheads*). The lesion demonstrates aggressive features with focal destruction of the lateral orbital wall (*white arrows*) with areas of irregular erosion (*black arrows*). The lesion is relatively hypodense on the T2-W scan (*open white arrow*) suggestive of a highly cellular neoplasm. The mass significantly displaces the superior muscle group (*open black arrow*)

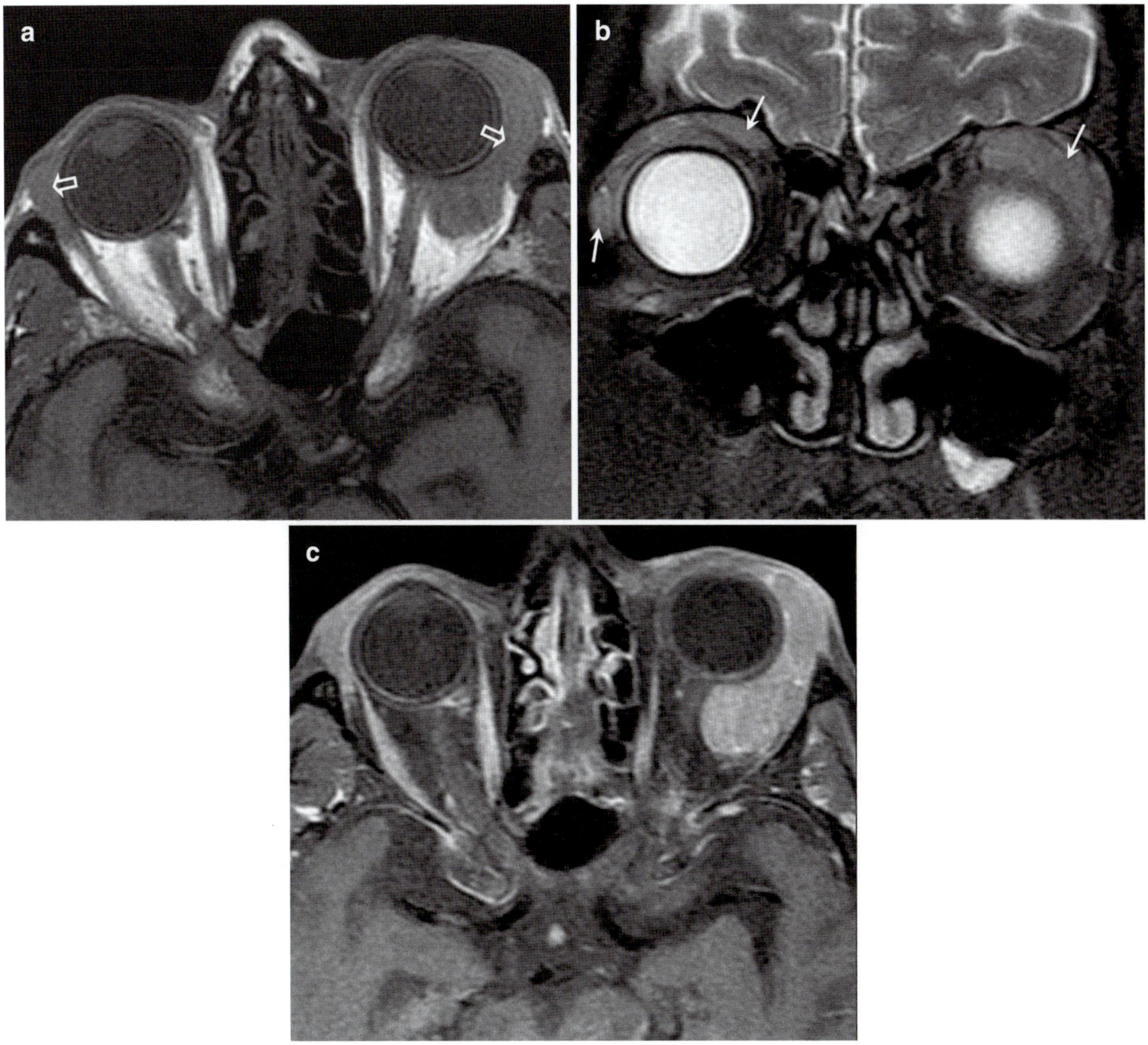

Fig. 43.40 Bilateral MALT lymphoma: noncontrast axial T1-W (**a**), noncontrast coronal T2-W (**b**), and axial contrast-enhanced fat-suppressed T1-W (**c**) MR images reveal bilateral orbital masses arising from the lacrimal glands (*open white arrows*) that "mold" to the contour of the globes. The lesions are relatively hypointense on T2-W images (*white arrows*), indicating a highly cellular neoplasm such as lymphoma. The left-sided lesion is noted to push the globe medially making lymphoma more likely than orbital pseudotumor. There is diffuse intense contrast enhancement also favoring a neoplasm

enhancement after contrast administration (Fig. 43.45). Larger lesions may show non-enhancing cystic components and focal calcifications.

Neurofibromas are also slow-growing tumors that arise from Schwann cells; however, unlike schwannomas, neurofibromas are not encapsulated tumors [17]. Neurofibromas are often associated with neurofibromatosis and may be plexiform, localized, or diffuse. Plexiform neurofibromas are characterized by fusiform enlargement of an entire peripheral nerve segment which most commonly affects the eyelids (Fig. 43.46). The diffuse subtype not only affects the nerves but may also involve the adjacent soft tissues including the extraocular muscles and orbital fat. Plexiform neurofibromas demonstrate increased vascularity and, because of this feature, demonstrate significant contrast enhancement. Differential diagnosis of peripheral nerve sheath tumor including both schwannoma and neurofibroma includes capillary hemangioma, meningioma, hemangiopericytoma, and metastasis.

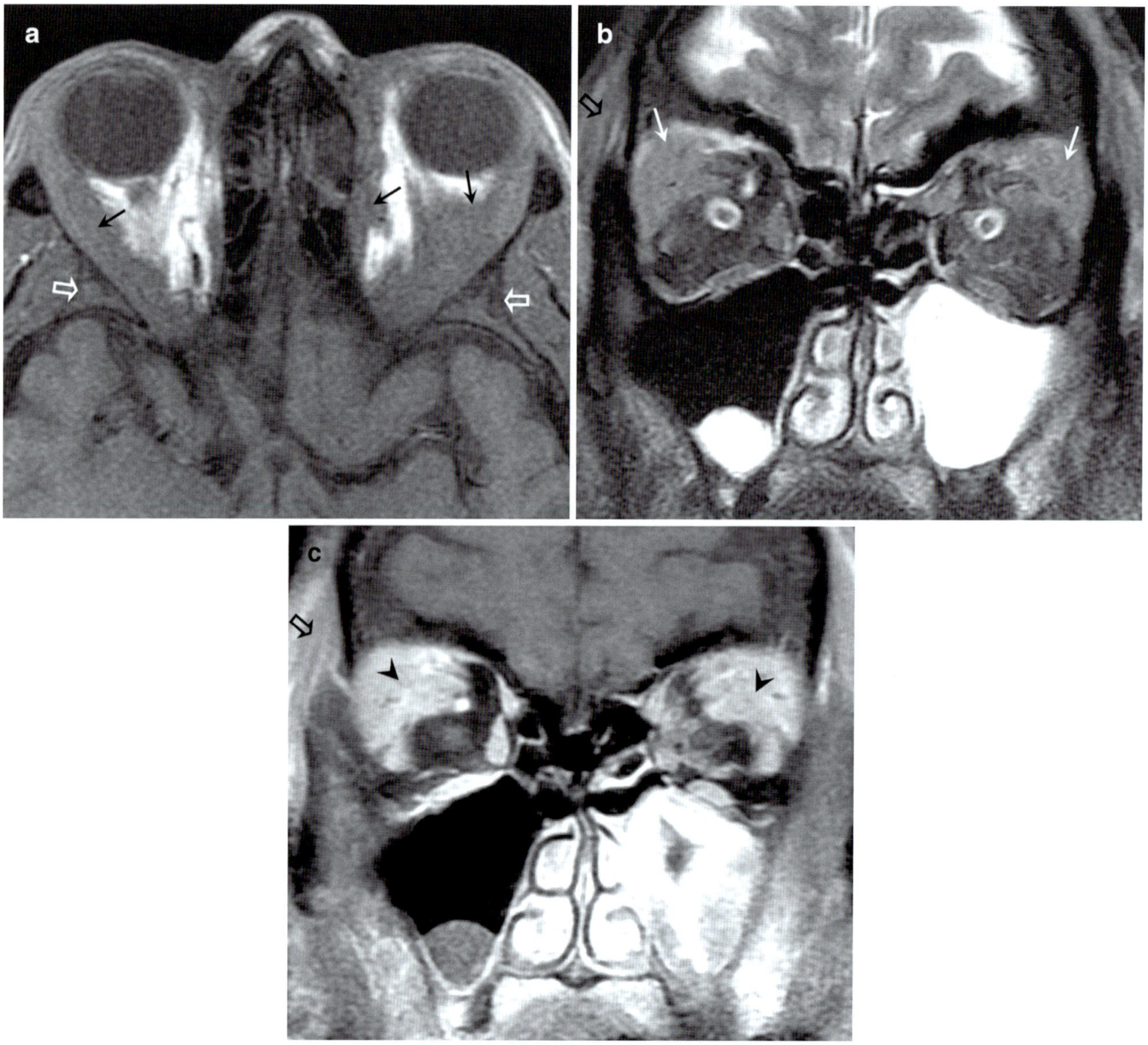

Fig. 43.41 Bilateral follicular lymphoma: noncontrast axial T1-W (**a**), noncontrast coronal T2-W (**b**), and coronal contrast-enhanced fat-suppressed T1-W (**c**) MR images reveal bilateral multi-compartmental masses arising in the superolateral aspect of the orbits. There is involvement of the bone marrow (*open white arrows*) and extension outside the right orbit (*open black arrow*). The lesions are relatively hypointense on T2-W images (*white arrows*), indicating a highly cellular neoplasm. The lesion diffusely enhances with contrast (*black arrowheads*) and infiltrates around numerous extraocular muscles

Trauma

The walls of the orbit may be fractured by a number of types of fractures [72, 102]. These fractures include orbital wall blowout, zygomaticomaxillary complex, nasomaxillary buttress, nasofrontoethmoid (nasoorbitoethmoid), and Le Fort II–III fractures. Complications of orbital trauma include ocular injury, lens dislocation, intraocular and intraorbital hemorrhage, entrapment of extraocular muscles (inferior, medial), intraocular or intraorbital foreign bodies, subperiosteal hemorrhage, traumatic optic neuropathy, and enophthalmos (Figs. 43.47, 43.48, and 43.49) [72, 102]. CT is the study of choice for initial evaluation of the vast majority of these patients because of the speed and availability of CT imaging. MRI and/or MRA may be helpful for better evaluation of the traumatized optic nerve and for diagnosis of suspected traumatic carotid-cavernous fistula.

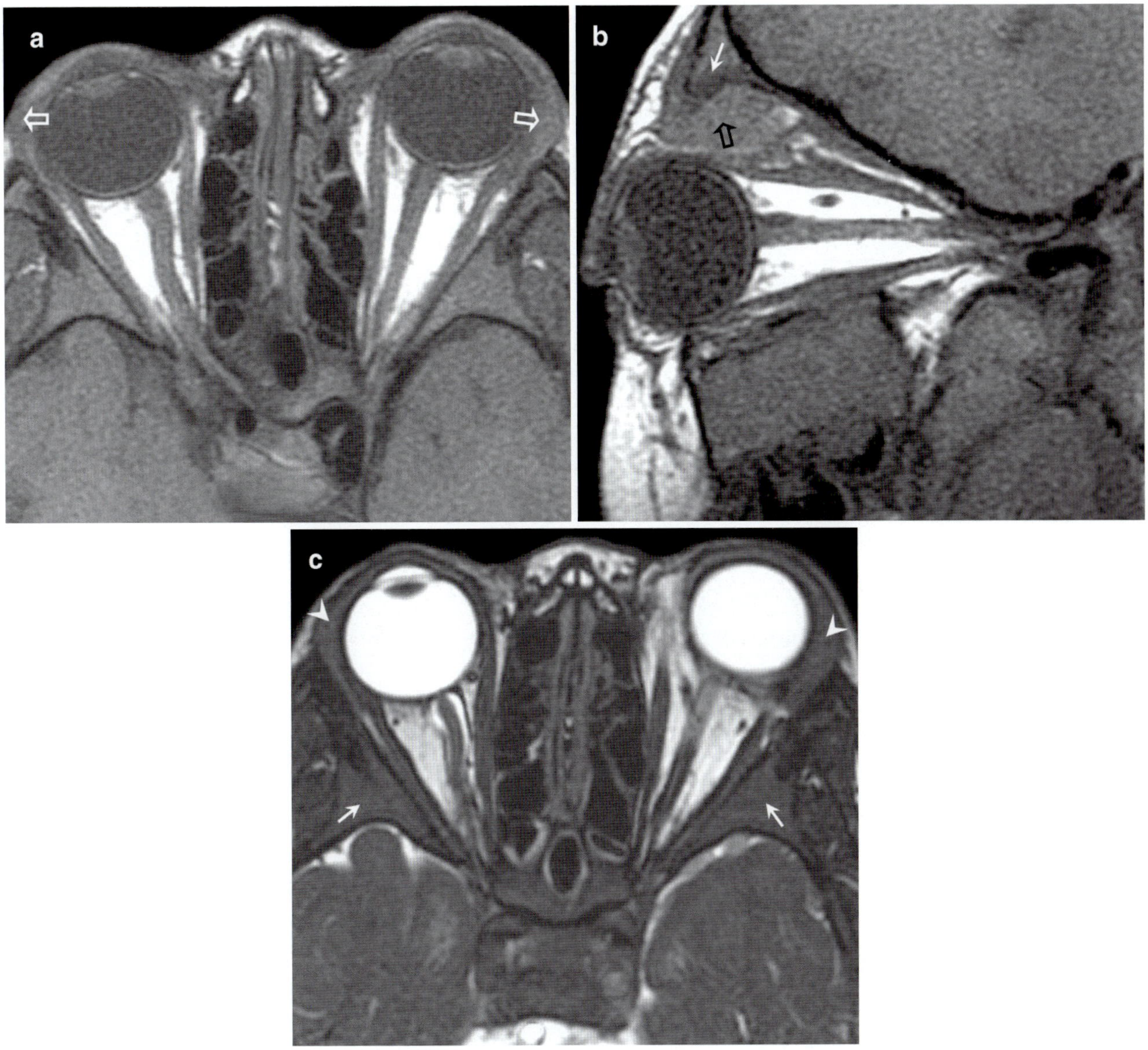

Fig. 43.42 Acute myelogenous leukemia: noncontrast T1-W axial (**a**), noncontrast oblique sagittal T1-W (**b**), and T2-W (**c**) MR images demonstrate mild enlargement of the bilateral lacrimal glands (*open white arrows*) and an infiltrating postseptal mass (*open black arrow*) in this child with known AML. There is diffuse bone marrow replacement (*white arrows*). The lacrimal gland lesions are very hypointense on T2-W scans (*white arrowheads*), indicating a highly cellular neoplasm

Vascular Masses of the Orbit

A number of classification schemes have been proposed to categorize vascular masses of the head and neck [103]. The most commonly accepted scheme proposed by Mulliken and Glowacki organizes lesions based on histology and natural history [104].

Capillary Hemangioma

The most common vascular orbital tumor in children is the capillary hemangioma [12]. Congenital and infantile forms may occur. Congenital hemangiomas are uncommon, are initially present at birth, and may have either a rapidly involuting or non-involuting course. Infantile hemangiomas, the

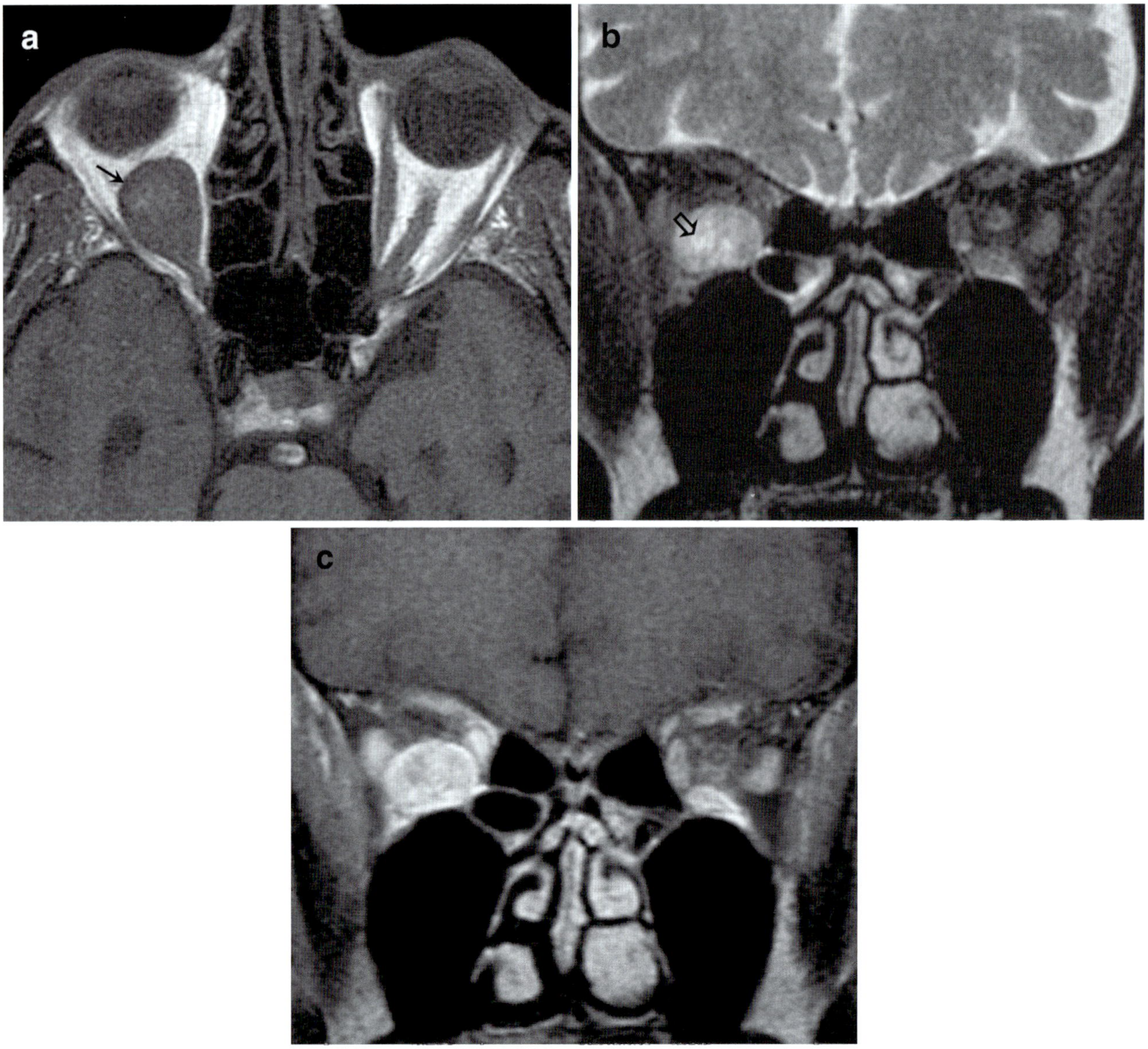

Fig. 43.43 Extraocular muscle metastasis (lung carcinoma): noncontrast axial T1-W (**a**), noncontrast coronal T2-W (**b**), and contrast-enhanced fat-suppressed T1-W (**c**) MR images reveal focal enlargement of the inferior rectus muscle (*black arrow*). There is considerable edema in the lesion as evidenced by a hyperintense appearance on the T2-W image (*black open arrow*). There is intense enhancement of the lesion following contrast administration. A metastasis would be favored over thyroid orbitopathy because of the non-spindle shape and favored over orbital myositis because of the lack of indistinct margins around the muscle

most common type of capillary hemangioma, are not usually present or are minimally present at birth but demonstrate significant subsequent growth (Fig. 43.50) [12]. This lesion often has an initial growth phase during the first year of life and subsequently gradually involutes over time [105, 106]. Histologically, capillary hemangiomas are nonencapsulated tumors that consist of vascular spaces that are surrounded by proliferating endothelial cells [12]. These masses tend to be trans-spatial but are predominately found in the extraconal space of the orbit [105, 106]. They may involve the lacrimal gland or extraocular muscles, may envelop the globe or optic nerve, and rarely may extend intracranially. Complications, although rare, include optic nerve compression, hemorrhage, and thrombosis. Conservative management is favored when possible as the natural history of these tumors is involution. In life-threatening situations, surgery, intralesional steroid administration, laser therapy, or interferon therapy may be used for treatment [12].

Capillary hemangiomas are heterogeneous in attenuation on CT and are best characterized as lobulated multispatial masses. They demonstrate avid enhancement after contrast administration. MRI is the modality of choice for the initial evaluation of these tumors due to its better multiplanar imaging capabilities, better tissue characterization, and lack of ionizing radiation when compared to CT. These masses are typically isointense on T1-W images and hyperintense on T2-W images with respect to muscle. They demonstrate avid contrast enhancement. Vascular flow voids may be seen within and adjacent to the tumor. Contrast-enhanced dynamic MRA (CED-MRA) can be useful for confirming early to midarterial phase tumor blush and demonstrating the vascular nature of these lesions (Fig. 43.51). On imaging, it is important to assess for intracranial spread and evaluate for potential complications of the mass, such as optic nerve compression.

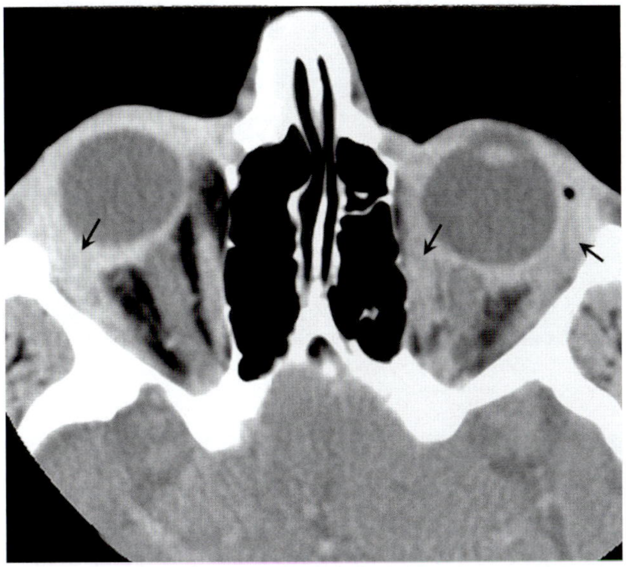

Fig. 43.44 Bilateral scirrhous breast metastasis: axial contrast-enhanced CT scan demonstrates bilateral soft tissue masses involving the lacrimal glands and extraocular muscles (*arrows*). The diagnosis of scirrhous breast metastasis can be made in this case because of mild enophthalmos due to retraction of the left globe. Most other neoplasms will cause at least some proptosis

Cavernous Malformations

Cavernous malformations, also known as cavernous hemangiomas, are the most common adult vascular lesion of the orbit [12]. These masses occur more often in women between the ages of 18 and 72 [107]. There is some controversy on the underlying etiology of cavernous malformations. Some believe that they are a slow-flow arteriovenous malformation, whereas others argue that they are an underlying anomaly primarily of venous origin. Unlike capillary hemangiomas, these masses do not involute but often slowly and progressively enlarge. Clinically, they present with painless proptosis. Unlike capillary hemangiomas, cavernous malformations have a fibrous pseudocapsule and are well-circumscribed lesions [12, 107]. They are often located within the lateral aspect of the intraconal retrobulbar space (Fig. 43.52) [12].

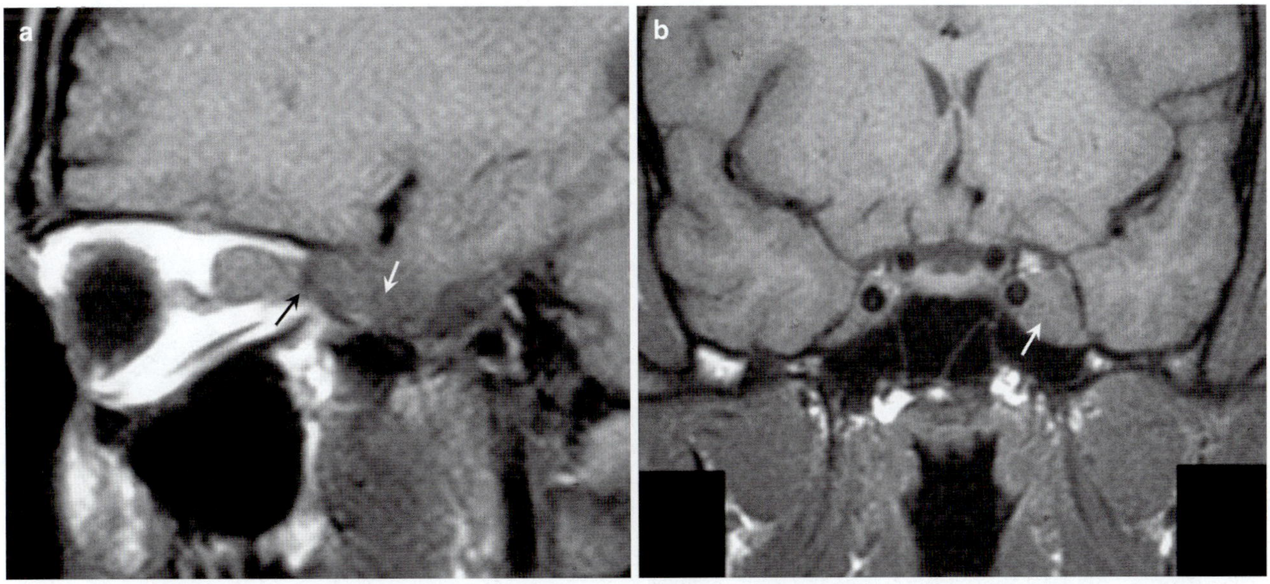

Fig. 43.45 Ophthalmic nerve schwannoma: noncontrast T1-W (**a**, **b**) and fat-suppressed contrast-enhanced T1-W (**c**, **d**) MR scans reveal an elongated, intensely enhancing, well-circumscribed mass that extends through the lateral limb of the superior orbital fissure (*black arrows*) into the cavernous sinus (*white arrows*). The lesion displaces the optic nerve inferomedially (*open black arrows*)

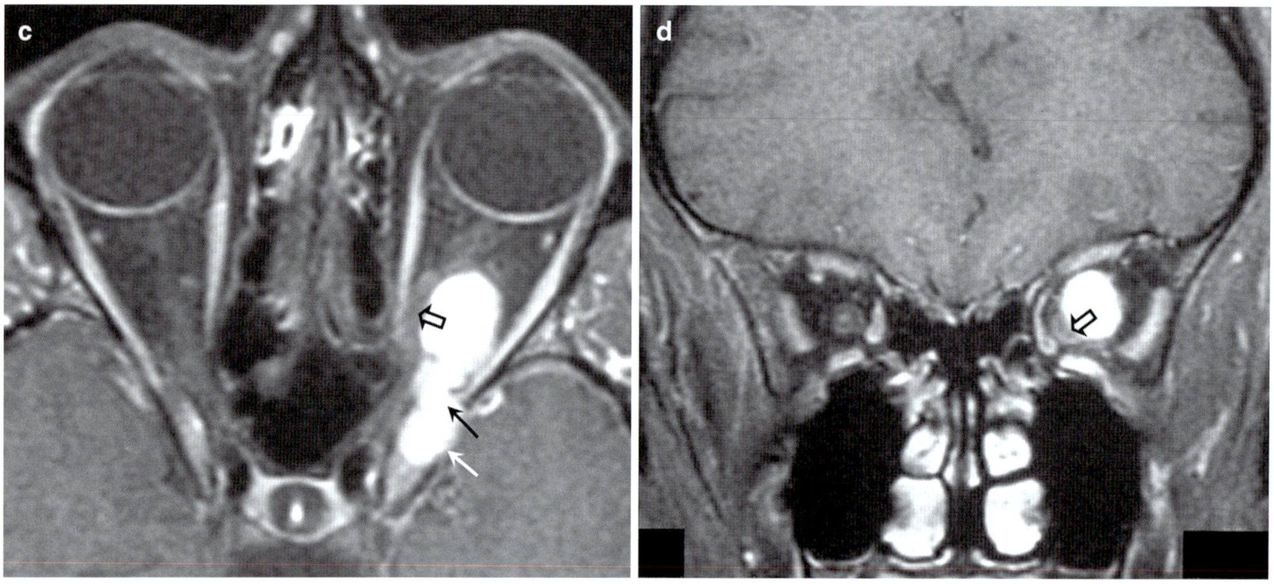

Fig. 43.45 (continued)

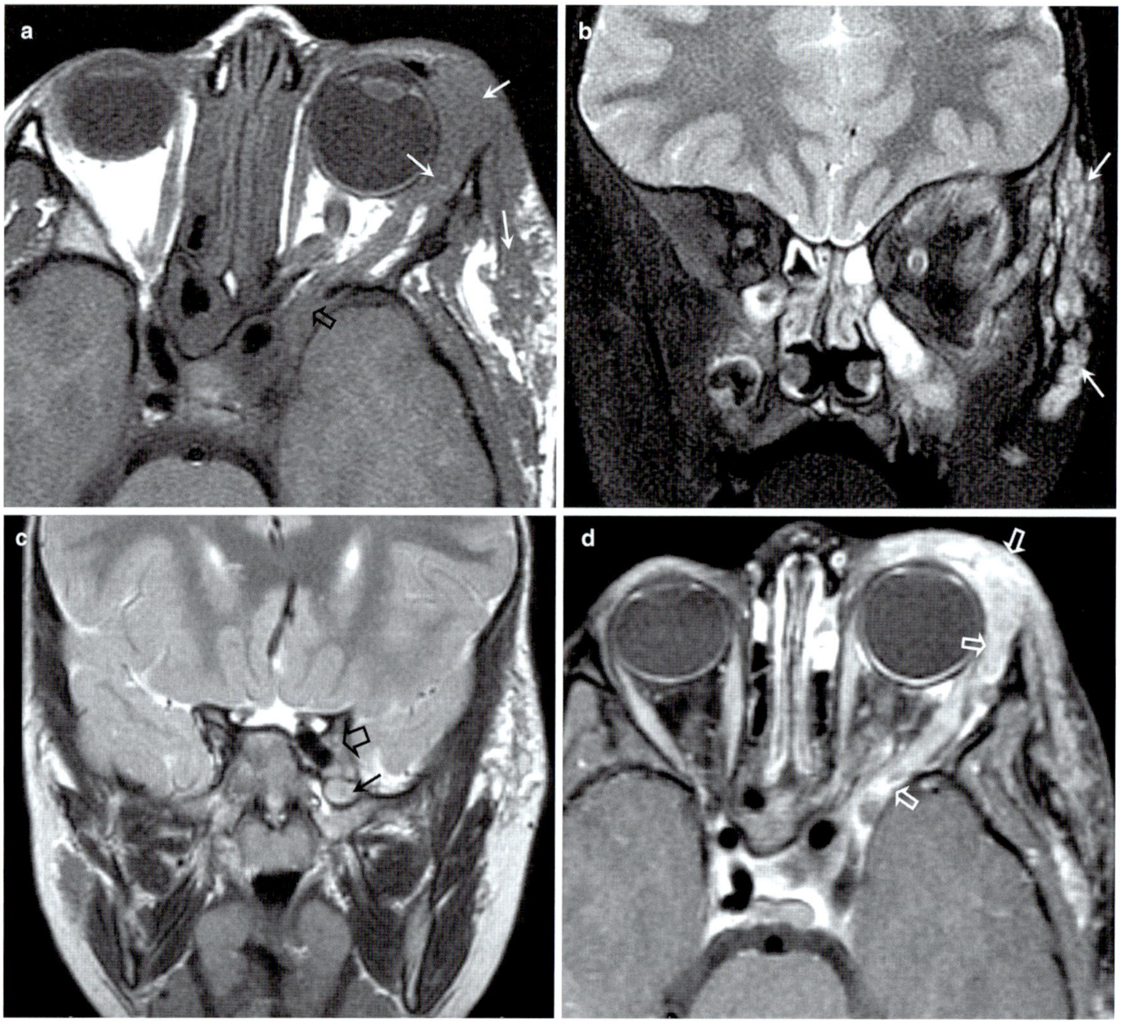

Fig. 43.46 V1 and V2 plexiform neurofibroma: axial noncontrast T1-W (**a**), noncontrast coronal T2-W (**b**, **c**), and postcontrast fat-suppressed T1-W (**d**) MR scans demonstrate a poorly marginated multilobulated mass involving the superolateral orbit, preseptal soft tissues, and overlying skin (*white arrows*). The lesion is noted to expand foramen rotundum (*black arrow*) and the superior orbital fissure (*open black arrows*), indicating the lesion is likely neural in origin. There are complex areas of abnormal contrast enhancement throughout the lesion (*white open arrow*)

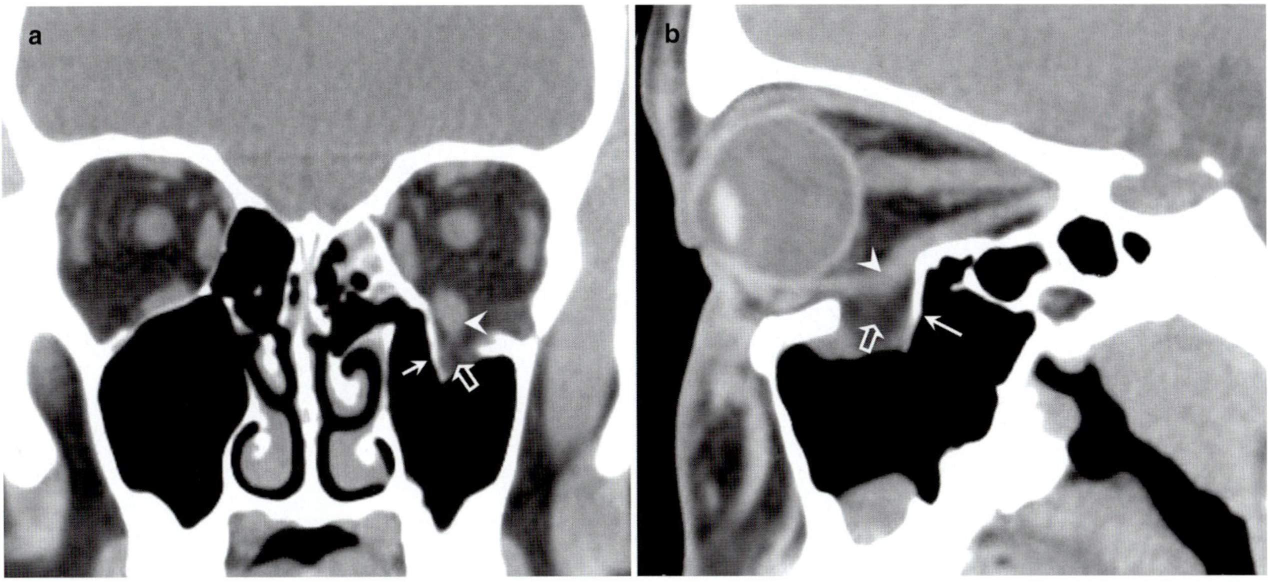

Fig. 43.47 Orbital floor fracture – inferior rectus entrapment: coronal (**a**) and oblique sagittal (**b**) CT scans reveal a trap-door "blowout" fracture of the left orbital floor (*white arrows*) with inferior displacement of orbital fat (*white open arrows*) and entrapment of the inferior rectus muscle (*white arrowhead*)

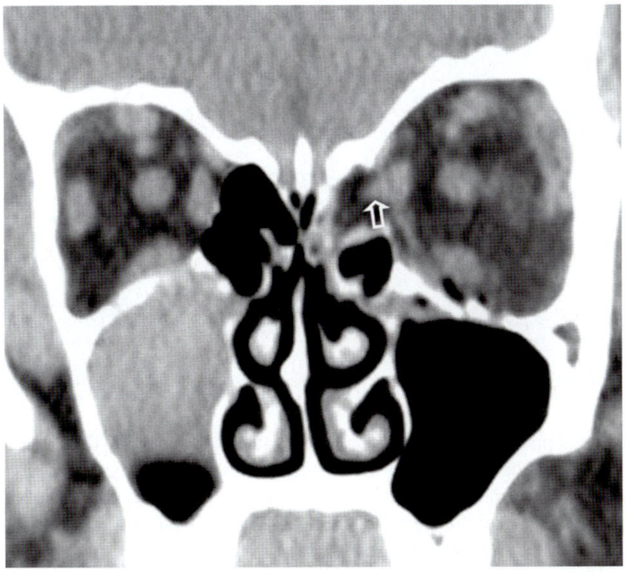

Fig. 43.48 Medial orbital wall fracture – medial rectus entrapment: coronal CT scan demonstrates fractures of the orbital floor and medial orbital wall with evidence of displacement of orbital fat and the medial rectus muscle (*open arrow*) into the ethmoid sinus. Note the "tenting" of the muscle indicating a high likelihood of entrapment

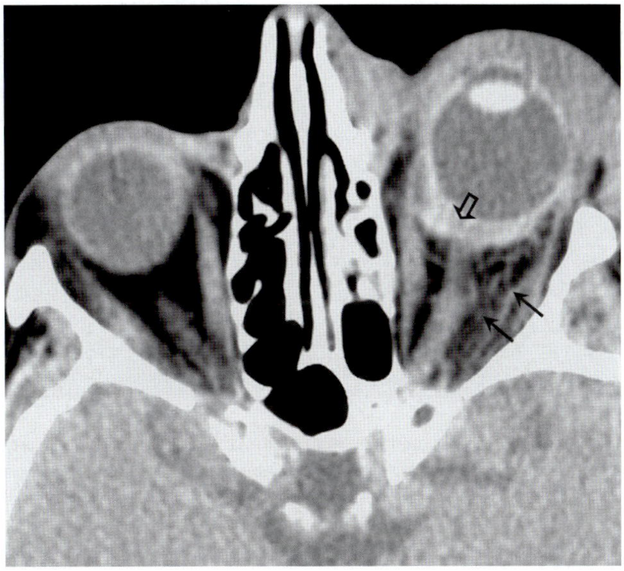

Fig. 43.49 Retrobulbar hematoma: axial CT scan following blunt left orbital trauma reveals extensive hemorrhage involving Tenon's space (*open arrow*) and the retrobulbar fat (*arrows*). A subtle medial orbital wall blowout fracture was also present on bone windows

Conservative management is favored in asymptomatic patients.

On CT, cavernous malformations are hyperdense, well-circumscribed, round masses. These malformations often displace adjacent structures without invasion. Large lesions may also cause bony remodeling of the orbital wall. These masses demonstrate little arterial phase blush on dynamic contrast CT but characteristically will demonstrate progressive enhancement during the venous phase of the scan. CED-MRA combined with early and delayed postcontrast fat-suppressed MRI is the best method for evaluation of these lesions [6].

On MRI, cavernous malformations are isointense to muscle on T1-W images and hyperintense to muscle on T2-W images. As on CT, these lesions demonstrate progressive contrast enhancement during the late venous phase.

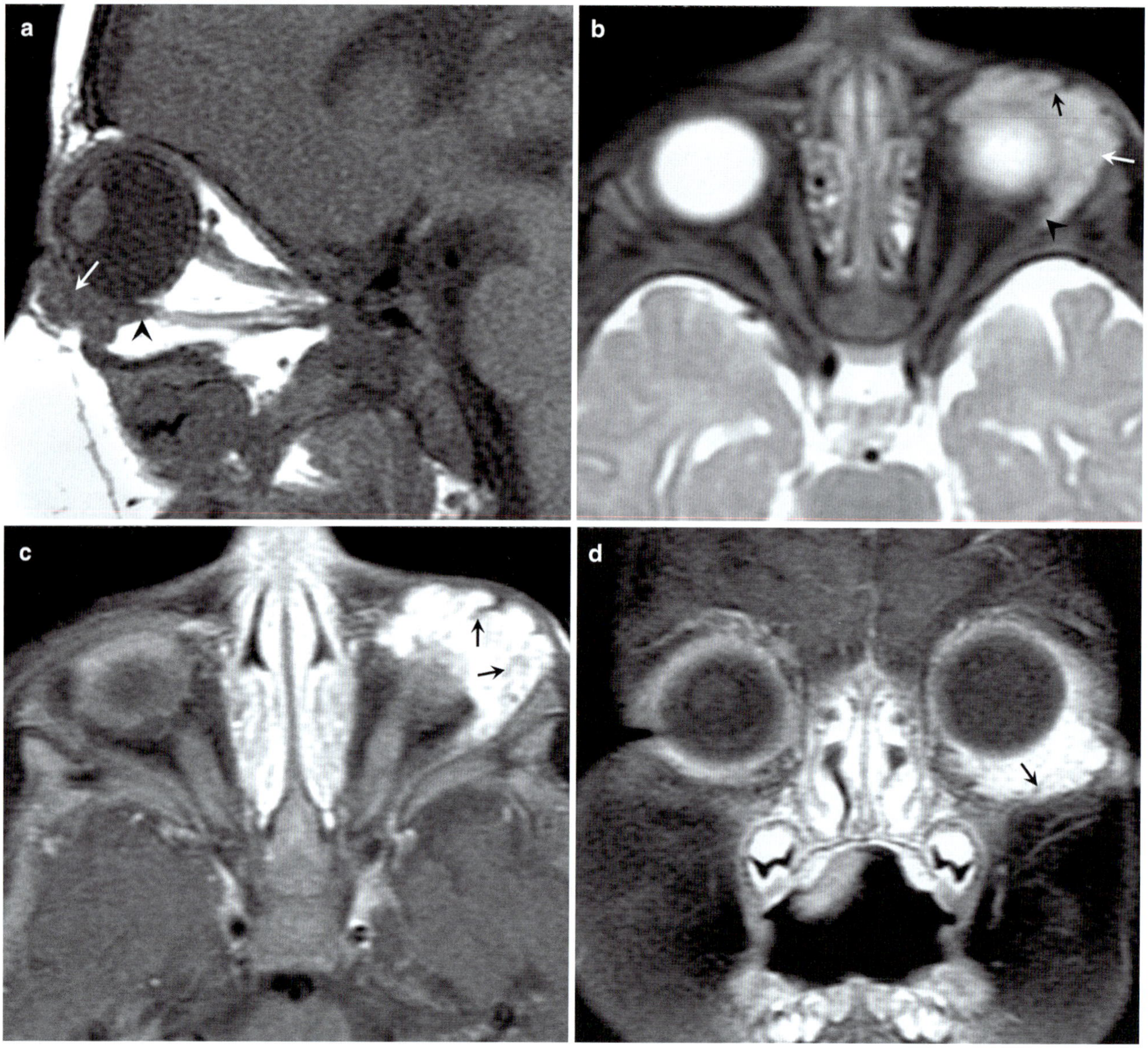

Fig. 43.50 Infantile capillary hemangioma: a 3-year-old female presenting with slowly enlarging, vascular-appearing mass along the lower eyelid that developed after birth. Noncontrast T1-W (**a**), noncontrast T2-W (**b**), and postcontrast fat-suppressed T1-W (**c**, **d**) MR images depict a poorly demarcated multi-compartmental mass along the lower lid and preseptal space (*white arrows*) with extension along the anterior aspect of the inferior and lateral rectus muscles (*black arrowheads*). There are numerous intralesional septa (*black arrows*) within the mass that are typical for capillary hemangioma as well as intense fairly homogeneous contrast enhancement

Orbital Varix

An orbital varix is an abnormally dilated valveless orbital vein that results from an underlying congenital weakness in the wall of the vessel (Fig. 43.53) [11]. Orbital varices often communicate with adjacent orbital veins and become larger during states of increased pressure including Valsalva, coughing, and bending. Clinically, patients present with pressure-induced (stress) proptosis that is relieved when the stimulus is removed. Patients with orbital varices may also present with hemorrhage or venous thrombosis which is often painful [12].

A dynamic CT, CED-MRA, or MRI performed before and during a maneuver that increases pressure, such as Valsalva or prone positioning, is often required to demonstrate the distensibility of an orbital varix [13, 14]. Thrombosed varices may not demonstrate the characteristic distensibility and enhancement. Varices have a variable appearance on imaging and may be ovoid, round, conical, or tubular in shape or may occasionally resemble a tangle of vessels. On MRI, varices range from hypointense to hyperintense on T1-W images and are typically hyperintense on T2-W scans. These lesions usually demonstrate avid contrast enhancement.

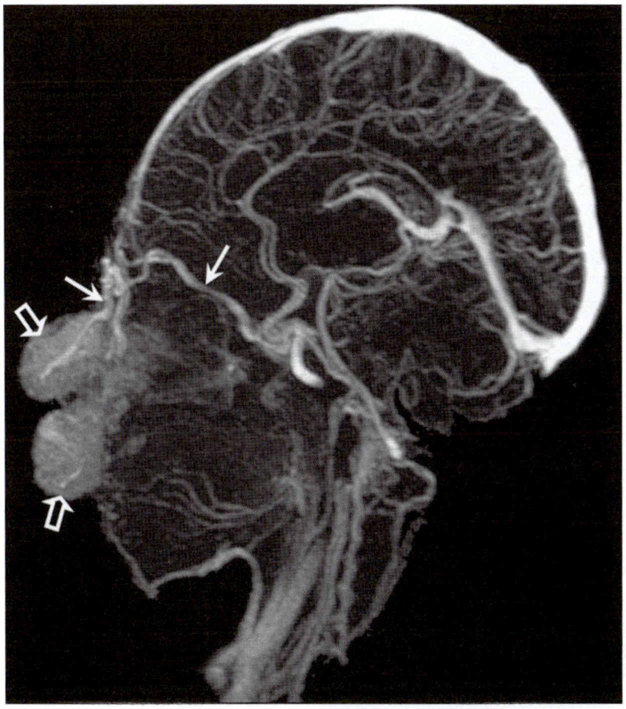

Fig. 43.51 Infantile capillary hemangioma: CED-MRA reveals intense midarterial phase blush of an infantile capillary hemangioma (*open arrows*) fed by enlarged branched of the ophthalmic artery (*white arrows*)

Lymphatic and Venolymphatic Malformations

Lymphatic malformations, also known as lymphangiomas, often manifest in early childhood [11, 14]. Like capillary hemangiomas, these masses are nonencapsulated and therefore are typically trans-spatial masses. Histologically, these lesions are composed of bloodless vascular channels lined with endothelium that are filled with lymph [12]. Loose connective tissue courses through the mass that contains small fragile blood vessels and lymphocytes. These vessels are very fragile and highly susceptible to hemorrhage [12]. Because of the lymphatic component within the lesion, they may enlarge with upper respiratory infections. Clinically, patients with lymphatic malformations present with proptosis, which is often precipitated by a hemorrhagic event. The natural history of lymphatic malformations is variable, and therefore, treatment is also variable [12, 108]. Conservative management is often favored; however, surgery may be necessary in those instances where the optic nerve, cornea, and vision are compromised. Associated noncontiguous intracranial vascular anomalies have also been described [109].

MR is superior to CT in evaluating patients with lymphatic and venolymphatic malformations (Fig. 43.54). On MRI, the lesions are often trans-spatial masses which demonstrate characteristic fluid-fluid or fluid-blood levels. These

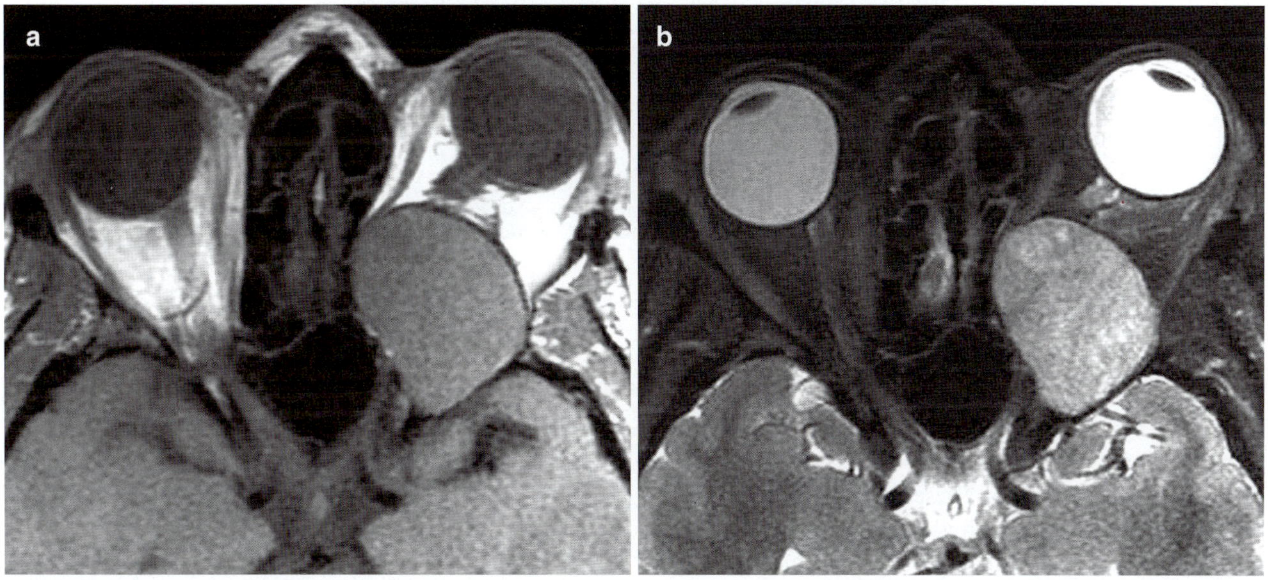

Fig. 43.52 Cavernous hemangioma: noncontrast T1-W (**a**), noncontrast T2-W (**b**), immediate postcontrast fat-suppressed T1-W (**c**), delayed fat-suppressed T1-W (**d**), and CED-MRA (**e**) reveal a large intraconal mass that is moderately hyperintense on T2-W scans. The lesion shows progressive enhancement between the immediate and delayed postcontrast scans characteristic of cavernous hemangioma. CED-MRA demonstrates a characteristic sinusoidal pattern of filling of intralesional vascular spaces within the lesion during the venous phase (*white arrows*)

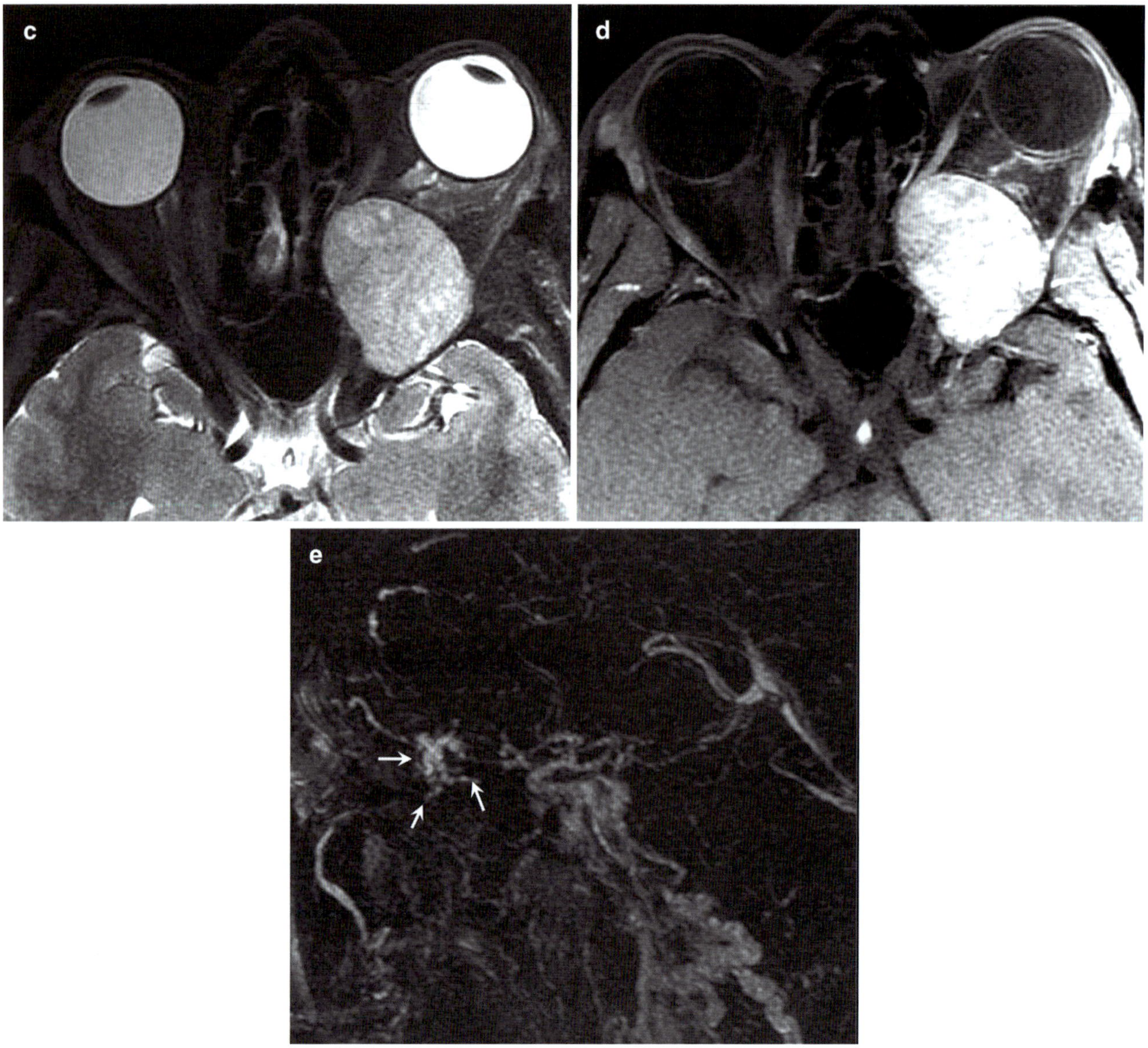

Fig. 43.52 (continued)

levels reflect various stages of hemorrhage along with proteinaceous fluid within the lesion. T1-W and T2-W images demonstrate varying amounts of proteinaceous fluid, simple fluid, and blood products. These masses do not typically enhance after contrast, which is an important distinguishing feature from hemangiomas or venous malformations. Occasionally, there may be peripheral enhancement at the very periphery of the lesion.

Arteriovenous Malformations

An arteriovenous malformation is a collection of blood vessels with an abnormal communication between the arteries and veins. No intervening capillary bed is present. Arteriovenous malformations of the orbit are rare. Clinically, these patients may present with signs of mass effect including proptosis and periorbital swelling. Other features include an audible bruit, dilated retinal veins, and palpable thrill [12].

CT and MRI using standard and dynamic vascular imaging protocols can diagnose an arteriovenous malformation. CED-MRA may often be helpful in differentiating these lesions from other vascular malformations. Conventional catheter-based angiography, however, is often indicated for accurate characterization of these complex lesions. These lesions may be treated surgically or with endovascular embolization. CT and MRI demonstrate an abnormal tangle of dilated arteries and veins within the orbit. The venous

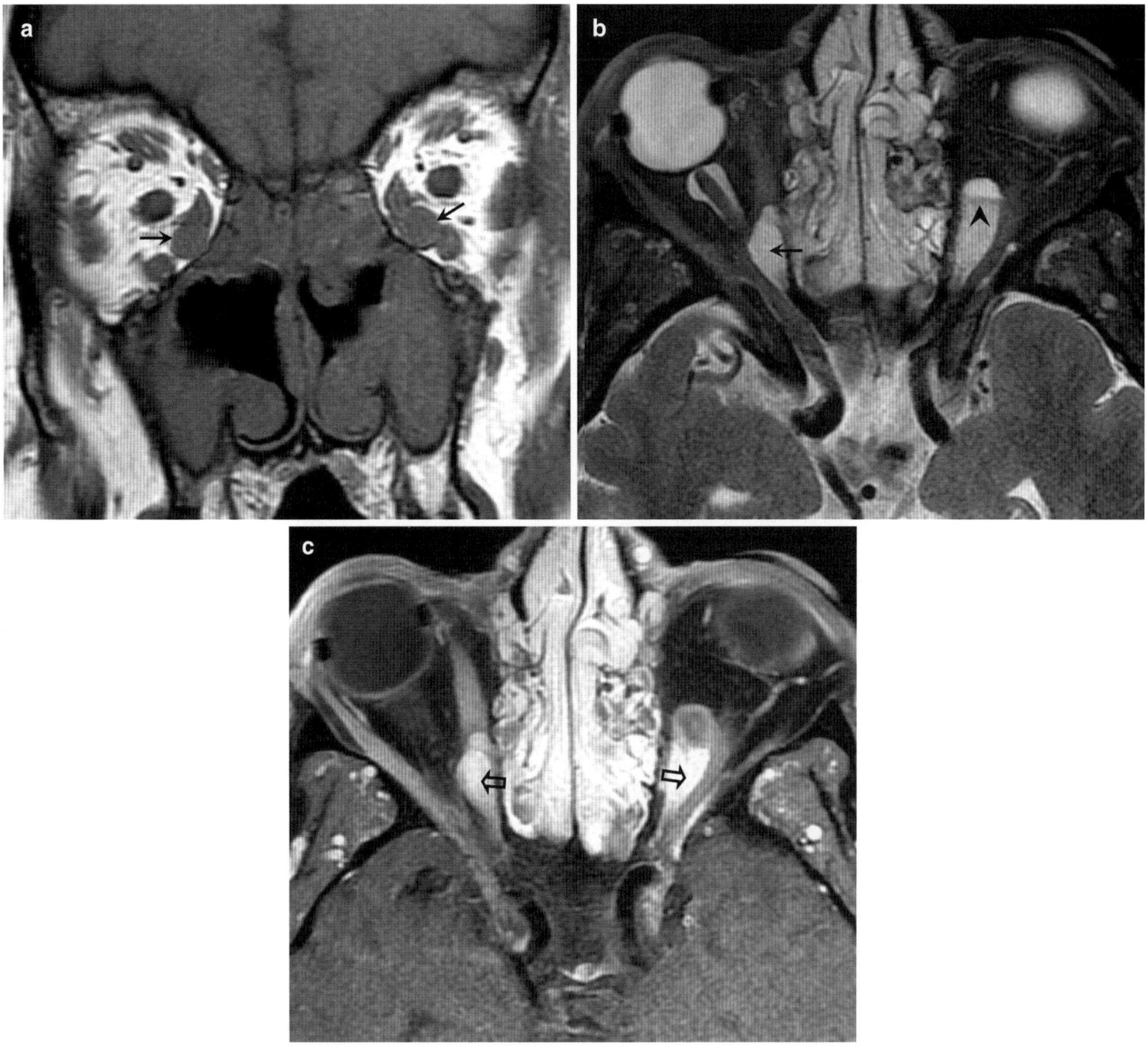

Fig. 43.53 Bilateral orbital varices: noncontrast T1-W (**a**), noncontrast T2-W (**b**), and postcontrast fat-suppressed T1-W (**c**) MR images reveal bilateral extraconal masses (*black arrows*) that lie between the medial and inferior rectus muscles. A sedimentation level (*black arrowhead*) is seen in left lesion. Postcontrast enhancement is seen within both lesions (*open black arrows*)

component is often more noticeable because the highly compliant veins are more easily distended when compared to the arteries. These lesions are often trans-spatial and poorly circumscribed. Arterial supply is most often via the ophthalmic artery. There may be intracranial or extracranial venous drainage.

Carotid Cavernous Fistulas

A carotid cavernous fistula is an abnormal connection between branches of either the internal carotid or external carotid artery and the cavernous sinus [12, 110]. The fistulous communication may be either high flow (direct) or low flow (indirect), depending on the nature of the arteriovenous shunt. Fistulas occur most commonly as a result of trauma but may also be seen in the setting of surgery, venous sinus thrombosis, and atherosclerosis or occur spontaneously. Clinically, patients may present with chemosis, pulsatile exophthalmos, congestive orbitopathy, and a bruit [12]. Palsies affecting cranial nerves III, IV, V, and VI may also be seen [111].

CT angiography and CED-MRA are useful in establishing the diagnosis of a carotid cavernous fistula. The imaging features include dilatation of the superior ophthalmic vein, extraocular muscle enlargement, proptosis, distention, and early filling of the cavernous sinus.

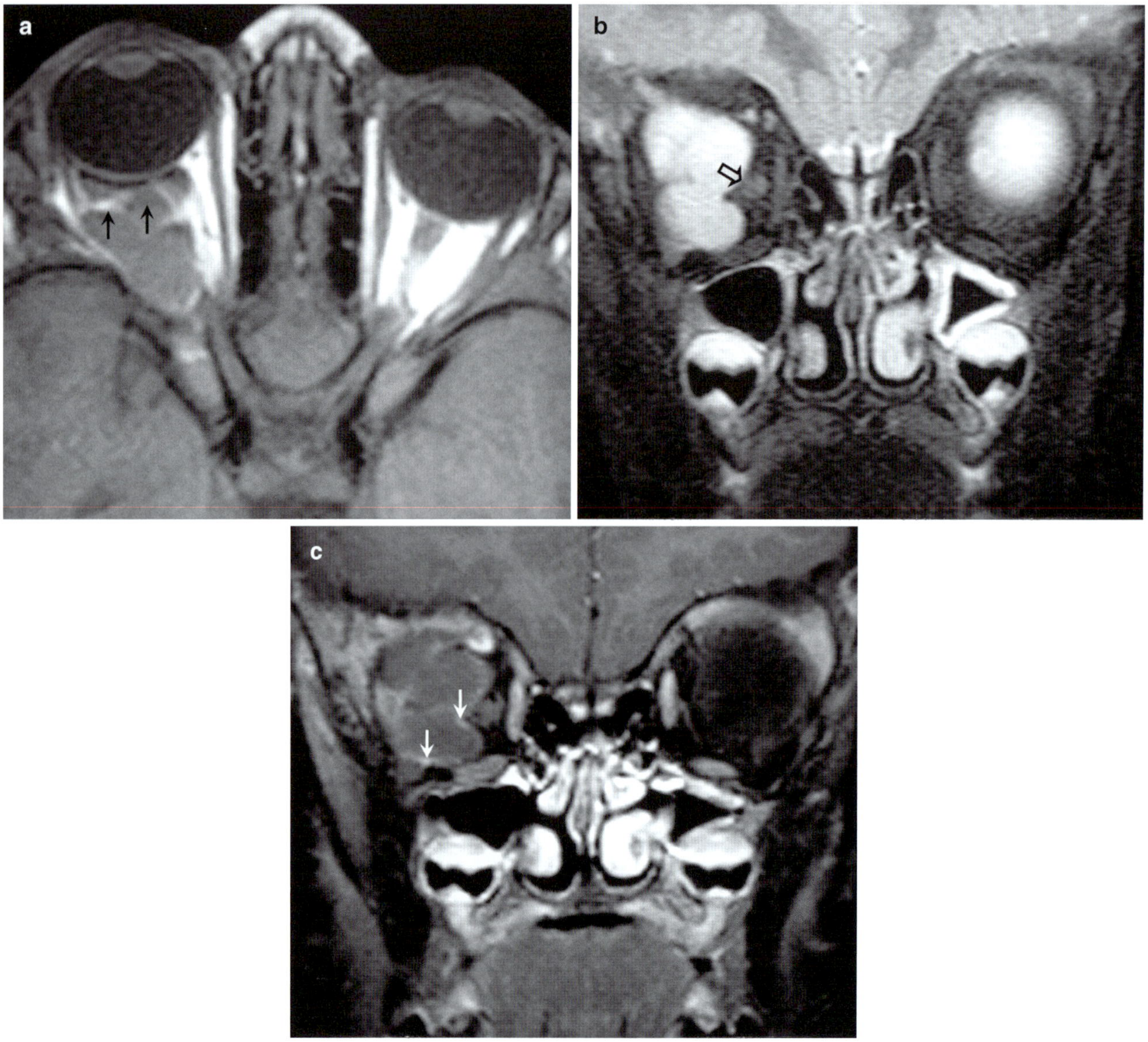

Fig. 43.54 Lymphangioma: noncontrast axial T1 (**a**), coronal T2-W (**b**), and contrast-enhanced fat-suppressed T1-W (**c**) MR images demonstrate a multilobulated mass with multiple fluid-fluid levels (*black arrows*). The lesion is very hyperintense on the T2-W image and displaces the optic nerve medially (*open black arrow*). Typical of lymphangiomas, the majority of the lesions do not enhance but only show minimal peripheral enhancement (*white arrows*)

References

1. Weber AL, Mafee MF. Evaluation of the globe using computed tomography and magnetic resonance imaging. Isr J Med Sci. 1992;28:145–52.
2. Bilaniuk LT, Atlas SW, Zimmerman RA. Magnetic resonance imaging of the orbit. Radiol Clin N Am. 1987;25:509–28.
3. Belden CJ. MR imaging of the globe and optic nerve. Magn Reson Imaging Clin N Am. 2002;10:663–78.
4. Hill JH, Mafee MF, Chow JM, Applebaum EL. Dynamic computerized tomography in the assessment of hemangioma. Am J Otolaryngol. 1985;6:23–8.
5. Hill JH, Mafee MF, Lygizos NA, Soboroff BJ. Dynamic computed tomography. Its use in the assessment of vascular malformations and angiofibroma. Arch Otolaryngol. 1985;111:62–5.
6. Kahana A, Lucarelli MJ, Grayev AM, Van Buren JJ, Burkat CN, Gentry LR. Noninvasive dynamic magnetic resonance angiography with Time-Resolved Imaging of Contrast KineticS (TRICKS) in the evaluation of orbital vascular lesions. Arch Ophthalmol. 2007;125:1635–42.
7. Forbes G. Vascular lesions in the orbit. Neuroimaging Clin N Am. 1996;6:113–22.
8. Michael AS, Mafee MF, Valvassori GE, Tan WS. Dynamic computed tomography of the head and neck: differential diagnostic value. Radiology. 1985;154:413–9.

9. Miller MT, Mafee MF. Computed tomography scanning in the evaluation of ocular motility disorders. Radiol Clin N Am. 1987;25:733–52.
10. Rootman J. Vascular malformations of the orbit: hemodynamic concepts. Orbit. 2003;22:103–20.
11. Rubin PA, Remulla HD. Orbital venous anomalies demonstrated by spiral computed tomography. Ophthalmology. 1997;104:1463–70.
12. Smoker WR, Gentry LR, Yee NK, Reede DL, Nerad JA. Vascular lesions of the orbit: more than meets the eye. Radiographics. 2008;28:185–204.
13. Winter J, Centeno RS, Bentson JR. Maneuver to aid diagnosis of orbital varix by computed tomography. AJNR Am J Neuroradiol. 1982;3:39–40.
14. Wright JE, Sullivan TJ, Garner A, Wulc AE, Moseley IF. Orbital venous anomalies. Ophthalmology. 1997;104:905–13.
15. Sa HS, Kyung SE, Oh SY. Extraocular muscle imaging in complex strabismus. Ophthalmic Surg Lasers Imaging. 2005;36:487–93.
16. Gentry LR. Anatomy of the orbit. Neuroimaging Clin N Am. 1998;8:171–94.
17. Mafee MF, Putterman A, Valvassori GE, Campos M, Capek V. Orbital space-occupying lesions: role of computed tomography and magnetic resonance imaging. An analysis of 145 cases. Radiol Clin N Am. 1987;25:529–59.
18. Demer JL, Miller JM, Poukens V, Vinters HV, Glasgow BJ. Evidence for fibromuscular pulleys of the recti extraocular muscles. Invest Ophthalmol Vis Sci. 1995;36:1125–36.
19. Langer BG, Charletta DA, Mafee MF, Spigos DG. MRI of the normal optic pathway. Semin Ultrasound CT MR. 1988;9:401–12.
20. Langer BG, Mafee MF, Pollack S, Spigos DG, Gyi B. MRI of the normal orbit and optic pathway. Radiol Clin N Am. 1987;25:429–46.
21. Porter JD, Baker RS, Ragusa RJ, Brueckner JK. Extraocular muscles: basic and clinical aspects of structure and function. Surv Ophthalmol. 1995;39:451–84.
22. Lemke BN, Stasior OG, Rosenberg PN. The surgical relations of the levator palpebrae superioris muscle. Ophthal Plast Reconstr Surg. 1988;4:25–30.
23. Hawes MJ, Dortzbach RK. The microscopic anatomy of the lower eyelid retractors. Arch Ophthalmol. 1982;100:1313–8.
24. Lang J, Kageyama I. The ophthalmic artery and its branches, measurements and clinical importance. Surg Radiol Anat. 1990;12:83–90.
25. Weinstein MA, Modic MT, Risius B, Duchesneau PM, Berlin AJ. Visualization of the arteries, veins, and nerves of the orbit by sector computed tomography. Radiology. 1981;138:83–7.
26. Ansari SA, Pak J, Shields M. Pathology and imaging of the lacrimal drainage system. Neuroimaging Clin N Am. 2005;15:221–37.
27. Kaufman LM, Villablanca JP, Mafee MF. Diagnostic imaging of cystic lesions in the child's orbit. Radiol Clin N Am. 1998;36:1149–63. xi
28. Mafee MF, Jampol LM, Langer BG, Tso M. Computed tomography of optic nerve colobomas, morning glory anomaly, and colobomatous cyst. Radiol Clin N Am. 1987;25:693–9.
29. Mafee M. The eye. In: Som PM, Curtin HD, editors. Head and neck imaging. St. Louis: Mosby; 2003. p. 441–528.
30. Mafee MF, Peyman GA. Retinal and choroidal detachments: role of magnetic resonance imaging and computed tomography. Radiol Clin N Am. 1987;25:487–507.
31. Haik BG, Saint Louis L, Smith ME, Abramson DH, Ellsworth RM. Computed tomography of the nonrhegmatogenous retinal detachment in the pediatric patient. Ophthalmology. 1985;92:1133–42.
32. LeBedis CA, Sakai O. Nontraumatic orbital conditions: diagnosis with CT and MR imaging in the emergent setting. Radiographics. 2008;28:1741–53.
33. Peyman GA, Mafee M, Schulman J. Computed tomography in choroidal detachment. Ophthalmology. 1984;91:156–62.
34. Wing GL, Schepens CL, Trempe CL, Weiter JJ. Serous choroidal detachment and the thickened-choroid sign detected by ultrasonography. Am J Ophthalmol. 1982;94:499–505.
35. Mafee MF, Linder B, Peyman GA, Langer BG, Choi KH, Capek V. Choroidal hematoma and effusion: evaluation with MR imaging. Radiology. 1988;168:781–6.
36. Mafee MF, Peyman GA. Choroidal detachment and ocular hypotony: CT evaluation. Radiology. 1984;153:697–703.
37. Howard GM, Ellsworth RM. Differential diagnosis of retinoblastoma. A statistical survey of 500 children. I. Relative frequency of the lesions which simulate retinoblastoma. Am J Ophthalmol. 1965;60:610–8.
38. Smirniotopoulos JG, Bargallo N, Mafee MF. Differential diagnosis of leukocoria: radiologic-pathologic correlation. Radiographics. 1994;14:1059–79. quiz 81–2
39. Mafee MF, Goldberg MF, Cohen SB, et al. Magnetic resonance imaging versus computed tomography of leukocoric eyes and use of in vitro proton magnetic resonance spectroscopy of retinoblastoma. Ophthalmology. 1989;96:965–75, discussion 75–6.
40. Chung EM, Specht CS, Schroeder JW. From the archives of the AFIP: pediatric orbit tumors and tumorlike lesions: neuroepithelial lesions of the ocular globe and optic nerve. Radiographics. 2007;27:1159–86.
41. Jensen RD, Miller RW. Retinoblastoma: epidemiologic characteristics. N Engl J Med. 1971;285:307–11.
42. Mafee MF, Goldberg MF, Greenwald MJ, Schulman J, Malmed A, Flanders AE. Retinoblastoma and simulating lesions: role of CT and MR imaging. Radiol Clin N Am. 1987;25:667–82.
43. Pendergrass TW, Davis S. Incidence of retinoblastoma in the United States. Arch Ophthalmol. 1980;98:1204–10.
44. Abramson DH. Retinoblastoma: diagnosis and management. CA Cancer J Clin. 1982;32:130–40.
45. Saket RR, Mafee MF. Anterior-segment retinoblastoma mimicking pseudoinflammatory angle-closure glaucoma: review of the literature and the important role of imaging. AJNR Am J Neuroradiol. 2009;30:1607–9.
46. Vajaranant TS, Mafee MF, Kapur R, Rapoport M, Edward DP. Medulloepithelioma of the ciliary body and optic nerve: clinicopathologic, CT, and MR imaging features. Neuroimaging Clin N Am. 2005;15:69–83.
47. Apushkin MA, Shapiro MJ, Mafee MF. Retinoblastoma and simulating lesions: role of imaging. Neuroimaging Clin N Am. 2005;15:49–67.
48. Kaufman LM, Mafee MF, Song CD. Retinoblastoma and simulating lesions. Role of CT, MR imaging and use of Gd-DTPA contrast enhancement. Radiol Clin N Am. 1998;36:1101–17.
49. Hopper KD, Sherman JL, Boal DK, Eggli KD. CT and MR imaging of the pediatric orbit. Radiographics. 1992;12:485–503.
50. Schulman JA, Peyman GA, Mafee MF, et al. The use of magnetic resonance imaging in the evaluation of retinoblastoma. J Pediatr Ophthalmol Strabismus. 1986;23:144–7.
51. Bader JL, Miller RW, Meadows AT, Zimmerman LE, Champion LA, Voute PA. Trilateral retinoblastoma. Lancet. 1980;2:582–3.
52. Finelli DA, Shurin SB, Bardenstein DS. Trilateral retinoblastoma: two variations. AJNR Am J Neuroradiol. 1995;16:166–70.
53. Mafee MF, Goldberg MF. Persistent hyperplastic primary vitreous (PHPV): role of computed tomography and magnetic resonance. Radiol Clin N Am. 1987;25:683–92.
54. Edward DP, Mafee MF, Garcia-Valenzuela E, Weiss RA. Coats' disease and persistent hyperplastic primary vitreous. Role of MR imaging and CT. Radiol Clin N Am. 1998;36:1119–31. x
55. Mafee MF, Goldberg MF, Valvassori GE, Capek V. Computed tomography in the evaluation of patients with persistent hyperplastic primary vitreous (PHPV). Radiology. 1982;145:713–7.

56. Chang MM, McLean IW, Merritt JC. Coats' disease: a study of 62 histologically confirmed cases. J Pediatr Ophthalmol Strabismus. 1984;21:163–8.
57. Lai WW, Edward DP, Weiss RA, Mafee MF, Tso MO. Magnetic resonance imaging findings in a case of advanced Coats' disease. Ophthalmic Surg Lasers. 1996;27:234–8.
58. Eller AW, Jabbour NM, Hirose T, Schepens CL. Retinopathy of prematurity. The association of a persistent hyaloid artery. Ophthalmology. 1987;94:444–8.
59. Tayebi H. Ocular calcification and retrolental fibroplasia. Am J Roentgenol Radium Therapy, Nucl Med. 1956;76:583–93.
60. Jabbour NM, Eller AE, Hirose T, Schepens CL, Liberfarb R. Stage 5 retinopathy of prematurity. Prognostic value of morphologic findings. Ophthalmology. 1987;94:1640–6.
61. Mafee MF, Peyman GA, McKusick MA. Malignant uveal melanoma and similar lesions studied by computed tomography. Radiology. 1985;156:403–8.
62. Mafee MF, Peyman GA, Grisolano JE, et al. Malignant uveal melanoma and simulating lesions: MR imaging evaluation. Radiology. 1986;160:773–80.
63. Mafee MF. Uveal melanoma, choroidal hemangioma, and simulating lesions. Role of MR imaging. Radiol Clin N Am. 1998;36:1083–99. x
64. Peyman GA, Mafee MF. Uveal melanoma and similar lesions: the role of magnetic resonance imaging and computed tomography. Radiol Clin N Am. 1987;25:471–86.
65. Pascual-Castroviejo I, Diaz-Gonzalez C, Garcia-Melian RM, Gonzalez-Casado I, Munoz-Hiraldo E. Sturge-Weber syndrome: study of 40 patients. Pediatr Neurol. 1993;9:283–8.
66. Wasenko JJ, Rosenbloom SA, Duchesneau PM, Lanzieri CF, Weinstein MA. The Sturge-Weber syndrome: comparison of MR and CT characteristics. AJNR Am J Neuroradiol. 1990;11:131–4.
67. Wittebol-Post D, Hes FJ, Lips CJ. The eye in von Hippel-Lindau disease. Long-term follow-up of screening and treatment: recommendations. J Intern Med. 1998;243:555–61.
68. Sudheim JL, Lapayowker MS. Calcification and ossification within the orbit. Radiology. 1976;121:391–7.
69. Rougier MB, Delyfer MN, Korobelnik JF. Imaging of optic disc drusen. J Fr Ophtalmol. 2009;32:695–6.
70. Pecorella I, Ciardi A, Garner A, McCartney AC, Lucas S. Postmortem histological survey of the ocular lesions in a British population of AIDS patients. Br J Ophthalmol. 2000;84:1275–81.
71. Chaques VJ, Lam S, Tessler HH, Mafee MF. Computed tomography and magnetic resonance imaging in the diagnosis of posterior scleritis. Ann Ophthalmol. 1993;25:89–94.
72. Kubal WS. Imaging of orbital trauma. Radiographics. 2008;28:1729–39.
73. Girardot C, Hazebroucq VG, Fery-Lemonnier E, et al. MR imaging and CT of surgical materials currently used in ophthalmology: in vitro and in vivo studies. Radiology. 1994;191:433–9.
74. Carmody RF, Mafee MF, Goodwin JA, Small K, Haery C. Orbital and optic pathway sarcoidosis: MR findings. AJNR Am J Neuroradiol. 1994;15:775–83.
75. Germann CA, Baumann MR, Hamzavi S. Ophthalmic diagnoses in the ED: optic neuritis. Am J Emerg Med. 2007;25:834–7.
76. Eggenberger ER. Inflammatory optic neuropathies. Ophthalmol Clin N Am. 2001;14:73–82.
77. Purvin V, Kawasaki A, Jacobson DM. Optic perineuritis: clinical and radiographic features. Arch Ophthalmol. 2001;119:1299–306.
78. Hollander MD, FitzPatrick M, O'Connor SG, Flanders AE, Tartaglino LM. Optic gliomas. Radiol Clin N Am. 1999;37:59–71. ix
79. Dutton JJ. Gliomas of the anterior visual pathway. Surv Ophthalmol. 1994;38:427–52.
80. Azar-Kia B, Naheedy MH, Elias DA, Mafee MF, Fine M. Optic nerve tumors: role of magnetic resonance imaging and computed tomography. Radiol Clin N Am. 1987;25:561–81.
81. Mafee MF, Goodwin J, Dorodi S. Optic nerve sheath meningiomas. Role of MR imaging. Radiol Clin N Am. 1999;37:37–58.
82. Saeed P, Rootman J, Nugent RA, White VA, Mackenzie IR, Koornneef L. Optic nerve sheath meningiomas. Ophthalmology. 2003;110:2019–30.
83. Azar-Kia B, Mafee MF, Horowitz SW, Fine M, Raofi B. CT and MRI of the optic nerve and sheath. Semin Ultrasound CT MR. 1988;9:443–54.
84. Dutton JJ. Optic nerve sheath meningiomas. Surv Ophthalmol. 1992;37:167–83.
85. Wells RG, Sty JR, Gonnering RS. Imaging of the pediatric eye and orbit. Radiographics. 1989;9:1023–44.
86. Koornneef L. Orbital septa: anatomy and function. Ophthalmology. 1979;86:876–80.
87. Dobben GD, Philip B, Mafee MF, Choi K, Belmont H, Dorodi S. Orbital subperiosteal hematoma, cholesterol granuloma, and infection. Evaluation with MR imaging and CT. Radiol Clin N Am. 1998;36:1185–200.
88. Mafee M. Orbit: embryology, anatomy, and pathology. In: Som PM, Curtin HD, editors. Head and neck imaging. St. Louis: Mosby; 2003. p. 529–654.
89. Weber AL, Romo LV, Sabates NR. Pseudotumor of the orbit. Clinical, pathologic, and radiologic evaluation. Radiol Clin N Am. 1999;37:151–68.
90. Kline LB, Hoyt WF. The Tolosa-Hunt syndrome. J Neurol Neurosurg Psychiatry. 2001;71:577–82.
91. Kapur R, Sepahdari AR, Mafee MF, et al. MR imaging of orbital inflammatory syndrome, orbital cellulitis, and orbital lymphoid lesions: the role of diffusion-weighted imaging. AJNR Am J Neuroradiol. 2009;30:64–70.
92. Flanders AE, Mafee MF, Rao VM, Choi KH. CT characteristics of orbital pseudotumors and other orbital inflammatory processes. J Comput Assist Tomogr. 1989;13:40–7.
93. Bothun ED, Scheurer RA, Harrison AR, Lee MS. Update on thyroid eye disease and management. Clin Ophthalmol. 2009;3:543–51.
94. Wiersinga WM, Smit T, van der Gaag R, Mourits M, Koornneef L. Clinical presentation of Graves' ophthalmopathy. Ophthalmic Res. 1989;21:73–82.
95. de Waard R, Koornneef L, Verbeeten B Jr. Motility disturbances in Graves' ophthalmopathy. Doc Ophthalmol. 1983;56:41–7.
96. McKinnon SG, Gentry LR. Systemic diseases involving the orbit. Semin Ultrasound CT MR. 1998;19:292–308.
97. Chan LL, Tan HE, Fook-Chong S, Teo TH, Lim LH, Seah LL. Graves ophthalmopathy: the bony orbit in optic neuropathy, its apical angular capacity, and impact on prediction of risk. AJNR Am J Neuroradiol. 2009;30:597–602.
98. Mafee MF, Dorodi S, Pai E. Sarcoidosis of the eye, orbit, and central nervous system. Role of MR imaging. Radiol Clin N Am. 1999;37:73–87.
99. Wolff SM, Fauci AS, Horn RG, Dale DC. Wegener's granulomatosis. Ann Intern Med. 1974;81:513–25.
100. Provenzale JM, Mukherji S, Allen NB, Castillo M, Weber AW. Orbital involvement by Wegener's granulomatosis: imaging findings. AJR Am J Roentgenol. 1996;166:929–34.
101. Carroll GS, Haik BG, Fleming JC, Weiss RA, Mafee MF. Peripheral nerve tumors of the orbit. Radiol Clin N Am. 1999;37:195–202. xi–xii
102. Levine LM, Sires BS, Gentry LR, Dortzbach RK. Rounding of the inferior rectus muscle: a helpful radiologic findings in the management of orbital floor fractures. Ophthal Plast Reconstr Surg. 1998;14(2):141–3.

103. Harris GJ. Orbital vascular malformations: a consensus statement on terminology and its clinical implications. Orbital Society. Am J Ophthalmol. 1999;127:453–5.
104. Mulliken JB, Glowacki J. Hemangiomas and vascular malformations in infants and children: a classification based on endothelial characteristics. Plast Reconstr Surg. 1982;69:412–22.
105. Bilaniuk LT. Orbital vascular lesions. Role of imaging. Radiol Clin N Am. 1999;37:169–83.
106. Bilaniuk LT. Vascular lesions of the orbit in children. Neuroimaging Clin N Am. 2005;15:107–20.
107. Ansari SA, Mafee MF. Orbital cavernous hemangioma: role of imaging. Neuroimaging Clin N Am. 2005;15:137–58.
108. Burrows PE, Mason KP. Percutaneous treatment of low flow vascular malformations. J Vasc Interv Radiol. 2004;15:431–45.
109. Katz SE, Rootman J, Vangveeravong S, Graeb D. Combined venous lymphatic malformations of the orbit (so-called lymphangiomas). Association with noncontiguous intracranial vascular anomalies. Ophthalmology. 1998;105:176–84.
110. Barrow DL, Spector RH, Braun IF, Landman JA, Tindall SC, Tindall GT. Classification and treatment of spontaneous carotid-cavernous sinus fistulas. J Neurosurg. 1985;62:248–56.
111. Kurata A, Takano M, Tokiwa K, Miyasaka Y, Yada K, Kan S. Spontaneous carotid cavernous fistula presenting only with cranial nerve palsies. AJNR Am J Neuroradiol. 1993;14:1097–101.

Orbital Signs of Parasellar Syndromes

44

Christina H. Choe and Wayne T. Cornblath

Introduction

Retro-orbital pathology involving the parasellar region can cause signs and symptoms that can be mistaken for orbital disease. Patients can present with a combination of proptosis, eyelid edema and erythema, chemosis, vision loss, numbness, and ophthalmoplegia with or without pain. A retro-orbital process should be considered when ophthalmoplegia is more consistent with a cranial neuropathy affecting the oculomotor nerve (CN 3), trochlear nerve (CN 4), or abducens nerve (CN 6) rather than extraocular muscle limitation. They have been divided anatomically into superior orbital fissure syndrome (SOFS), orbital apex syndrome (OAS), or cavernous sinus syndrome (CSS).

Classically, these syndromes present with multiple cranial neuropathies involving a combination of CN 2, 3, 4, 5 (first and second divisions), and 6. Bilateral involvement and dysesthesia involving the ophthalmic and maxillary divisions of the trigeminal nerve (CN V1 and V2) suggest CSS. OAS and SOFS typically are unilateral and do not involve the trigeminal nerves. Meanwhile, optic nerve involvement points to the orbital apex, which is defined as pathology involving structures passing through both the superior orbital fissure and optic canal. Vision loss should not be present in the pure definition of SOFS, which is limited to pathology affecting CN 3, 4, and 6 and branches of V1.

Despite these strict anatomic definitions, in practice, the clinical presentations represent a continuum as pathology easily progresses to involve adjacent structures. As such, the exact anatomic location is not easily pinpointed with signs and symptoms alone, and they have been inconsistently labeled in the literature. In addition, since the superior orbital fissure is the gateway between the orbit and the intracranial cavity, OAS and SOFS can be caused by both orbital and retro-orbital processes, and orbital processes can easily spread retro-orbitally and vice versa. Given these challenges, in this chapter, we will address these syndromes as a single clinical unit under the umbrella term parasellar syndromes. The differential diagnosis of parasellar syndrome is important for orbital surgeons to be familiar with.

Anatomy

The parasella is anatomically defined by the sella turcica, the depression of the sphenoid bone that contains the pituitary gland. It is situated above the sphenoid sinus and is surrounded by the cavernous sinuses, which contain a high concentration of important structures. The parasellar region contains CN 2–6, the sympathetic plexus, and the intracavernous portion of the internal carotid artery (ICA) (Fig. 44.1). Pathology affecting this eloquent region presents with many localizing signs and has the potential to cause significant morbidity and mortality.

The Orbital Apex

Anteriorly, the superior orbital fissure (SOF) and optic canal transmit many of the vital structures that pass through the parasella. The optic canal lies within the lesser wing of the sphenoid bone. It transmits the optic nerve and the ophthalmic artery. It is approximately 5–6 mm in diameter and 10–12 mm in length.

The SOF lies just lateral and inferior to the optic canal and is bounded by the lesser and greater wings of the sphenoid. It represents the largest entry point from the orbit to the middle cranial fossa. It is approximately 22 mm long, and within the orbit, it is divided by the origin of the lateral rectus

C. H. Choe
Carolina Ophthalmology, Asheville, NC, USA

W. T. Cornblath (✉)
Department of Ophthalmology & Visual Sciences and Neurology, University of Michigan Kellogg Eye Center, Ann Arbor, MI, USA
e-mail: wtc@med.umich.edu

J. J. Servat et al. (eds.), *Smith and Nesi's Ophthalmic Plastic and Reconstructive Surgery*,
https://doi.org/10.1007/978-3-030-41720-8_44

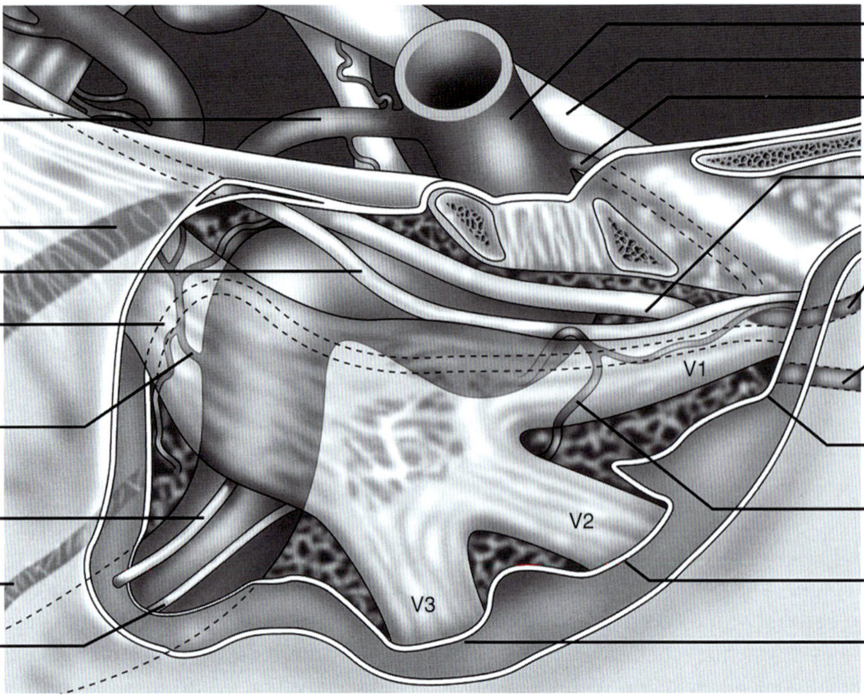

Fig. 44.1 This sagittal depiction of the parasella with the dural sheath reflected shows how intimately associated the structures in this region are. Note the S-shaped curve of the carotid artery as it traverses the cavernous sinuses

muscle in the annulus of Zinn. Inferior to the lateral rectus origin (intraconally), it transmits the superior and inferior divisions of CN 3, the nasociliary branch from CN V1, CN 6, the superior ophthalmic vein, and the pupillomotor sympathetics. Superior to the lateral rectus origin (extraconally), it transmits CN 4 and the lacrimal and frontal divisions of CN V1 (Fig. 44.2).

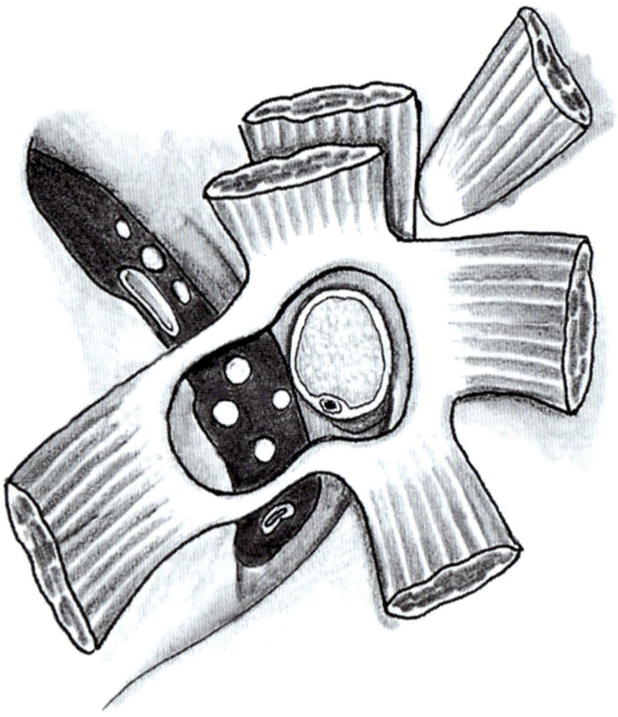

Fig. 44.2 This diagram of the orbital apex demonstrates the intra- and extraconal structures entering through the superior ophthalmic fissure

Cavernous Sinuses

Extending posteriorly from the SOF to the petrous apex are the paired cavernous sinuses. The cavernous sinuses are part of the cerebral dural venous system (Fig. 44.3). They are trabeculated venous sinuses located on the lateral aspect of the sella turcica. They communicate with each other via the anterior and posterior intracavernous sinuses. The blood supply of the orbit and eye is drained by the superior and inferior ophthalmic veins into the cavernous sinuses. The cavernous sinuses also receive drainage from the superior and inferior cerebral veins and the middle meningeal veins. They are in turn drained by the superior and inferior petrosal sinuses to the transverse sinus and inferiorly through the pterygoid plexus to the internal jugular vein.

The cerebral venous sinus system is a valveless system that is continuous with the vertebral venous plexus and the sacral plexus. It has a large capacity and is important in regulating intracranial pressure. Because they are valveless, normal venous flow can be reversed, and they may be involved in either retrograde or anterograde spread of tumors, infection, or emboli.

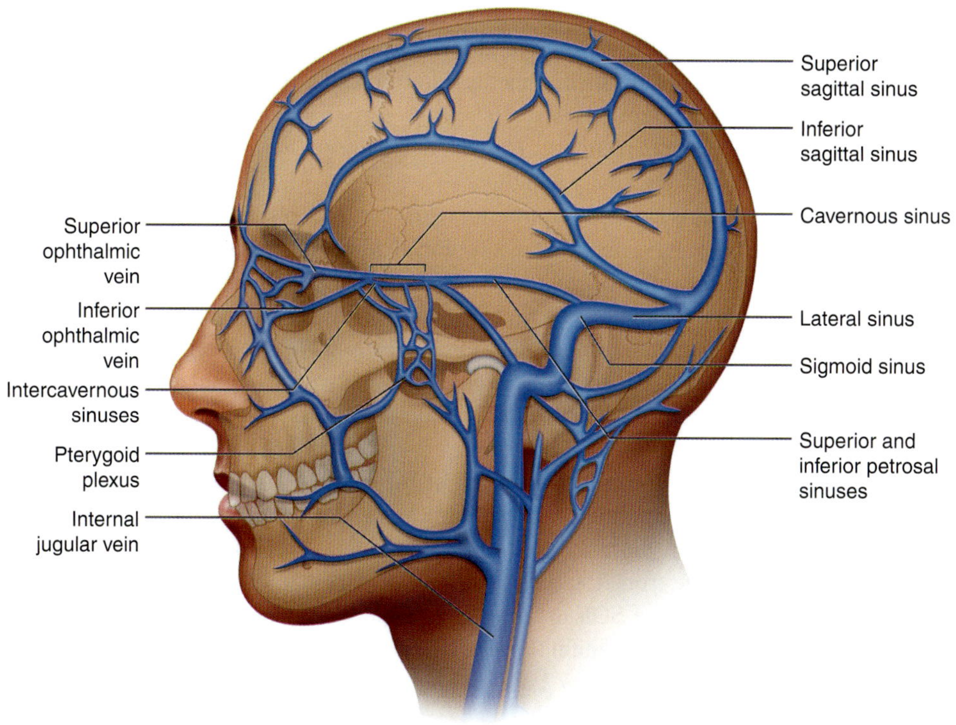

Fig. 44.3 The cerebral dural venous plexus is a valveless, high capacitance system that communicates with the vertebral and sacral venous plexuses. The cavernous sinuses are highly trabeculated and centrally located within cerebral venous system. (Modified from *Archives of Internal Medicine* 161(22): 2671–2676, 2001. Copyright 2001 American Medical Association)

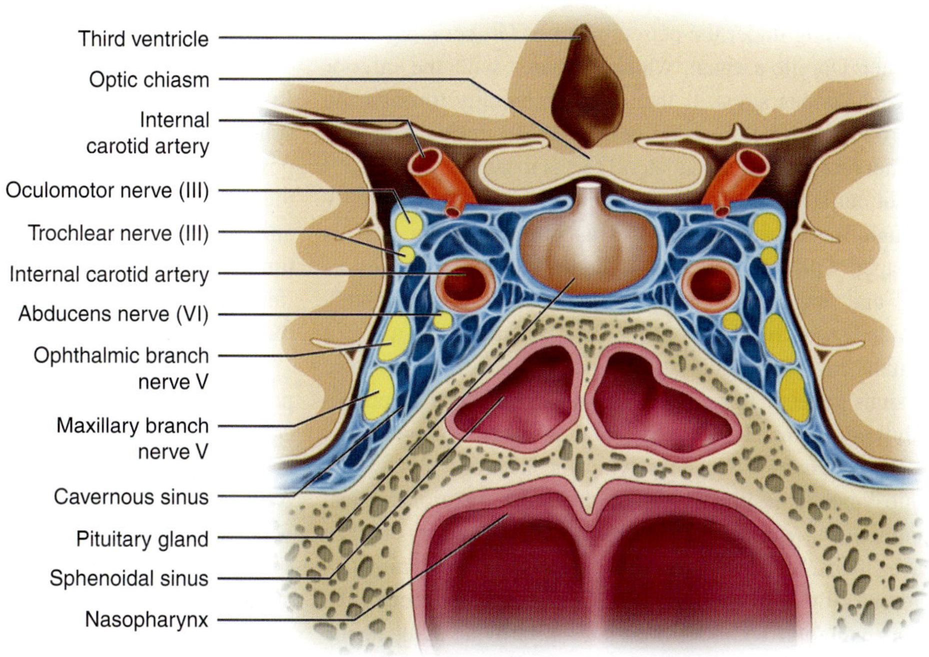

Fig. 44.4 This coronal cross-section of the cavernous sinuses provides an alternate view demonstrating the relationship of these vital structures in the cavernous sinuses. Note the relatively central position of the abducens nerve in comparison to the rest of the nerves, which traverse enveloped in the lateral dural fold. Also note the intimate relationship shared by the optic nerve, pituitary, and sphenoid sinuses. (Modified from *Archives of Internal Medicine* 161(22): 2671–2676, 2001. Copyright 2001 American Medical Association)

The cavernous sinuses are home to many important structures (Fig. 44.4). Within the cavernous sinuses pass CN 3, 4, 6, and V1 and the cavernous portion of the ICA. The oculomotor nerve lies most superiorly within the dural fold that makes up the lateral wall of the cavernous sinus. This is followed sequentially by CN 4 and CN V1. Whether CN V2 is intracavernous or extracavernous is a source of debate [1], but its close proximity results in its involvement in many parasellar pathologies.

The oculomotor nucleus originates in the midbrain at the level of the superior colliculus. It emerges between the posterior cerebral and superior cerebellar arteries and courses anteriorly to run superiorly within the lateral dural reflection of the cavernous sinus. It then splits into the superior and inferior divisions before entering the orbit intraconally through the SOF. It innervates the ipsilateral levator palpebrae superioris, superior rectus, medial rectus, inferior rectus, and inferior oblique muscles. It also carries parasympathetic supply to the papillary sphincter and ciliary body after synapsing with the ciliary ganglion.

The trochlear nucleus is situated just inferior to the oculomotor nucleus, and the nerve exits from the dorsal lower midbrain just below the inferior colliculus. It decussates before wrapping around the midbrain to course anteriorly. It enters the cavernous sinus and runs in the dural reflection just inferior to the CN 3. It then enters the orbit extraconally through the SOF. It innervates the superior oblique muscle contralateral to its nucleus.

The ophthalmic root of the trigeminal nerve is the most inferior of the nerves running through the lateral wall of the cavernous sinuses. Sensory information from the face and orbit is transmitted by the frontal, lacrimal, and nasociliary nerve, which exit through the SOF to form the ophthalmic nerve. CN V1 travels inferiorly within the lateral wall of the cavernous sinus before joining CN V2 and CN V3 to form the Gasserian ganglion in Meckel's cave.

Unlike CN 3, 4, and V1, CN 6 does not run within the wall but rather centrally within the cavernous sinus. The abducens nerve originates in the lower pons and ascends over the clivus before passing under the petroclinoid, or Gruber's, ligament to enter Dorello's canal, which it shares with the inferior petrosal venous sinus. It then passes centrally through the cavernous sinus before entering intraconally through the SOF to innervate the ipsilateral lateral rectus muscle.

The intracavernous portion of the ICA also runs centrally through the cavernous sinus. This portion of the ICA is S-shaped with a posterior ascending portion, horizontal portion, and anterior ascending portion and is approximately 2 cm in length. It is firmly anchored at its entrance to and exit from the cavernous sinus but is otherwise freely mobile within the sinus trabeculations. Involvement of the ICA by cavernous pathology can result in cerebral infarcts or hemorrhage.

The ICA carries with it the sympathetic carotid plexus. The oculosympathetic fibers originate from the superior cervical ganglion and runs along the internal carotid artery. It then leaves the ICA sheath to travel along CN 6 before joining CN 3 to enter the orbit through the SOF. They pass through the ciliary ganglion without synapsing and provide sympathetic innervation to the iris, eyelids, and lacrimal gland.

Pituitary Gland

Nestled within the sella turcica is the pituitary gland. The pituitary is a vital endocrine organ that is covered by a dural reflection known as the diaphragma sellae. The pituitary is connected to the hypothalamus by the pituitary stalk, and they form an important neuroendocrine axis that regulates systemic endocrine function. The hypothalamus produces releasing factors that act upon the pituitary to stimulate the release of pituitary hormones, including adrenocorticotropic hormone (ACTH), thyroid-stimulating hormone (TSH), prolactin (PRL), growth hormone (GH), follicle-stimulating hormone (FSH), and luteinizing hormone (LH).

It is separated into the anterior pituitary (adenohypophysis) and the posterior pituitary (neurohypophysis). The anterior pituitary is divided anatomically into the pars tuberalis, pars intermedia, and pars distalis, which is the principal, functional region of the anterior pituitary. The posterior pituitary stores and releases oxytocin and antidiuretic hormone (ADH), which is also known as arginine vasopressin (AVP). These are produced in the supraoptic and paraventricular nuclei of the hypothalamus.

Due to its location, the pituitary can become secondarily involved in parasellar pathologies. Symptoms suggestive of pituitary dysfunction include weight loss, cold or hot flashes, decreased libido and potency, anorexia, galactorrhea, and oligomenorrhea. The most concerning manifestation is adrenal crisis, which can cause systemic cardiovascular collapse, hypotension, shock, and death.

Paranasal Sinuses

Just inferior to the sella turcica is the sphenoid sinus. The sphenoid sinus and posterior ethmoid air cells comprise the posterior system of paranasal sinuses, which drain through the superior meatus into the sphenoethmoid recess. It is deep and centrally located with the nasopharynx below, the sella turcica above, and the pons dorsally. It thus can serve as an important portal for surgeons. Unfortunately, it can also be the entryway for tumors and infections.

The ethmoid sinuses are also clinically important in pathology involving this region. They are paired sinuses composed of the anterior, middle, and posterior ethmoid air cells. They share a common wall with the medial wall of the orbit. The medial wall of the orbit, or lamina papyracea, is very thin and in some patients may be dehiscent. The posterior ethmoid air cells lie just medial to the optic canal and communicate with the sphenoid sinus. Thus, they can be considered functionally as a single unit (the sphenoethmoid sinuses), and they play a vital role in the pathogenesis of parasellar syndromes.

Differential Diagnosis

Due to the multiple structures within this region, parasellar syndromes can present with variable combinations of multiple cranial neuropathies, proptosis, retro-orbital pain,

Table 44.1 Differential diagnosis of parasellar syndromes

Trauma
Neoplasm
Primary: pituitary adenoma, meningioma, craniopharyngioma, epidermoid, chordoma, chondrosarcoma, cavernous angioma
Metastatic: lymphoma, squamous cell cancer, nasopharyngeal tumors, breast, prostate, melanoma, other solid organ tumors
Secondary mass effect: sinus mucocele, adenoid cystic carcinoma
Inflammation
Secondary: sarcoidosis, Churg-Strauss syndrome, Wegener's granulomatosis, systemic lupus erythematosus
Idiopathic: Tolosa-Hunt syndrome
Vascular
Carotid artery aneurysm
Carotid artery dissection
Carotid-cavernous fistula
Carotid-cavernous thrombosis
Infectious
Fungal (mucormycosis, actinomycosis)
Mycobacterial (tuberculosis, leprae)
Spirochetes (treponema pallidum)
Viral (herpes zoster)
Bacterial (sinusitis, cellulitis, otitis, mastoiditis, dental infection)

chemosis, eyelid erythema, pupillary abnormalities, and dysesthesia involving the trigeminal nerve. However, a single cranial neuropathy is possible in up to 42% of patients, so parasellar syndromes are also considered part of the differential of painful ophthalmoplegia [2, 3].

Hirschfeld described the first case of a parasellar syndrome in 1858 [4]. This case was secondary to closed head trauma, and postmortem autopsy revealed a hematoma at the SOF. Subsequent cases were noted to improve with anti-syphilitic medications, and syphilitic periostitis was empirically presumed to be the cause of most parasellar syndromes. This became known as Rochon-Duvigneaud syndrome.

However, subsequent studies quickly recognized that tumors, trauma, other infections, and causes of inflammatory periostitis were also important etiologies of this presentation. Today, in the antibiotic era, syphilis is a rare cause of parasellar syndromes. Trauma is currently the most common cause secondary to basilar skull fractures and trauma to the vascular structures in the parasella (Table 44.1). Outside of trauma, tumors are the most common underlying etiology, followed by vascular causes and inflammation [2, 5–8]. Infection is now a rare but still important consideration.

Trauma

Trauma to the parasella, both iatrogenic and accidental, is one of the most common causes of parasellar syndrome. As previously described, the original description of parasellar syndrome was due to closed head trauma resulting in a hematoma at the SOF. It usually can be differentiated from other causes of parasellar syndrome by the history of antecedent head trauma or surgery. Basilar skull fractures can result in hematomas and foreign bodies, which cause parasellar syndrome secondary to compression. It can also cause parasellar syndrome indirectly by introducing an infection or causing vascular anomalies due to shear trauma.

Damage to the cavernous ICA can result in a carotid-cavernous fistula (CCF), which is discussed in further detail later in this chapter. Shear trauma is one of the primary causes of CCFs, but iatrogenic damage resulting in CCF is also a known complication of endovascular intervention. Iatrogenic parasellar syndrome has also been reported secondary to neurosurgical and sometimes endoscopic sinus surgeries. As such, questioning the patient regarding any recent trauma or surgeries can point the physician to the diagnosis.

Tumors

Neoplasms are one of the most common causes of a parasellar syndrome. The absence of pain increases the suspicion for tumors. However, the presence of pain does not rule out neoplasia. Tumors can be primary tumors of the parasella, originate in nearby structures including the sphenoethmoid sinuses or nasopharynx and cause secondary mass effect, or be metastatic lesions from a distant source. Nasopharyngeal carcinoma, pituitary adenomas, cavernous meningiomas, lymphomas, and metastatic lesions are common neoplastic causes of parasellar syndrome [2, 5, 6, 8]. Management is tailored to the specific neoplasm. However, surgical intervention is inherently difficult given the potential for iatrogenic damage to the cavernous sinus structures. Below is a non-comprehensive introduction to some tumors common in the parasellar region.

Nasopharyngeal Carcinoma

Nasopharyngeal carcinomas are rare, malignant tumors that arise from the roof or lateral walls of the nasopharynx. They can invade the cavernous sinuses directly by eroding through the skull base or by perineural spread along the trigeminal nerve. They may occur at any age but most commonly occur between 40 and 60 years of age with a male predilection. Ophthalmoplegia is common and can be present in up to 65% of nasopharyngeal carcinoma cases [9]. The abducens nerve is the most commonly involved ocular motor nerve.

Pituitary Adenoma

Pituitary adenomas are benign tumors of the pituitary gland and are divided into microadenomas (<10 mm) and macroadenomas (>10 mm). They can cause symptoms due to mass effect or due to secreting supranormal amounts of pituitary hormones. The clinical manifestations vary by which, if any, pituitary hormone is secreted. Adenomas commonly cause chiasmal compression and classically result in a bitemporal hemianopsia. They can also grow laterally and invade the cavernous sinuses resulting in parasellar syndrome. Pituitary adenomas are also the most common underlying cause of a potentially fatal condition called pituitary apoplexy.

Pituitary apoplexy is a fortunately rare condition consisting of hemorrhage and infarction of the pituitary gland. It usually presents with the sudden onset of headache, visual disturbance, and sometimes altered consciousness with concurrent hyponatremia and other signs of hypopituitarism. The oculomotor nerve is the most common ocular motor nerve involved resulting in ophthalmoplegia. This occurs either in isolation or as part of multiple cranial neuropathies [10]. Prompt recognition of this complication is important as close monitoring of fluid and electrolyte status with replacement of deficient hormones is vital.

Meningioma

Meningiomas involving the cavernous sinuses or sphenoid wing are benign but can cause significant neurologic morbidity. They are difficult to manage due to their proximity to many vital structures, especially if they become enmeshed around the cavernous ICA. Thus, complete surgical resection is often not possible. Observation is preferred in many cases, but in cases of symptomatic diplopia in primary gaze, pain, visual compromise, and cosmetically deforming proptosis, the combination of surgical debulking followed by radiation surgery for residual tumor is often employed for the best outcomes and decreased rates of tumor recurrence.

Lymphoma

Non-Hodgkin's, large B-cell, T-cell, and Burkitt's lymphoma have all been described in the cavernous sinuses [11, 12]. Lymphomas can be primary lesions affecting the cavernous sinuses or can be secondary, occurring through direct extension of an adjacent lesion or hematogenous spread of distant metastases. Lymphomas are classically very responsive to steroids and are an important differential in inflammatory lesions that appear to improve with corticosteroid administration.

Metastases

Metastases to the cavernous sinuses can occur with other malignancies as well. Metastases can develop hematogenously or through perineural spread along the trigeminal nerve. Solid organ tumors such as lung, prostate, and breast cancer can metastasize hematogenously to the cavernous sinuses, while perineural spread is common among head and neck cancers and cutaneous malignancies.

Adenoid cystic and squamous cell carcinomas have a particularly high propensity for perineural infiltration. CN V and CN VII are the most commonly involved nerves, and CN V1 is the typical access point to the cavernous sinuses, orbital apex, and SOF. Tumor cells invade the perineurium or endoneurium and grow concentrically. It can be asymptomatic in the early stages but eventually causes local pressure degeneration and pain. Nerve enlargement occurs with secondary foraminal enlargement. Pathologic specimens can demonstrate skip areas, so careful evaluation of nerve biopsy specimens is required. Unfortunately, perineural spread is associated with a very poor prognosis.

Miscellaneous

Other possible tumors include neural tumors such as schwannomas, plexiform neurofibromas, and malignant neurilemmoma that can affect the cavernous sinuses when they occur on CN V. Chordomas are malignant tumors originating from the notochord that tend to grow slowly with local skeletal destruction and may extend into the cavernous sinuses. Chondrosarcomas are bone tumors that can originate in the petroclival synchondrosis to secondarily infiltrate the cavernous sinuses.

Mucoceles and mucopyoceles are benign masses that can occur if the outlet of an accessory sinus is blocked, causing the accumulation of secretions and expansion and thinning of the sinus walls. They are usually sterile and known as mucoceles. If they become secondarily infected, they are known as pyoceles or mucopyoceles. Arachnoid, epidermoid, and dermoid cysts are also benign lesions that have all been documented to involve the cavernous sinuses.

The tumors that can involve the parasella are numerous. Because of the vital structures in the parasella, one of the parasellar syndromes may be the initial presentation of neoplasias that has more diffuse intracranial involvement. In addition, since neoplasia is the most common etiology of parasellar pathology, neuroimaging should be one of the first steps in the evaluation of these syndromes.

Vascular

Pathology involving the cavernous carotid artery represents the third most common cause of parasellar syndrome after neoplasia and trauma. This includes carotid-cavernous fistulas and cavernous carotid artery aneurysms.

Carotid-Cavernous Fistula

Carotid-cavernous fistulas (CCFs) are abnormal arteriovenous communications between the venous cavernous sinuses and the cavernous ICA. CCFs have a unique presentation that makes them more easily distinguished from other etiologies of parasellar syndrome. The classic presentation of CCFs involves prominent conjunctival injection with corkscrew vessels, proptosis, painful ophthalmoplegia, and an audible bruit. These manifestations are due to arterialization of the venous system and diversion of orbital blood flow. This can result in hypoxia and secondary edema of the ocular tissues. While its presentation is unique among the parasellar syndromes, it can be difficult to differentiate from other etiologies of a red eye. Familiarity with its diagnosis and management is thus important for all ophthalmologists.

Classification

CCFs are described by their flow rate on angiography (high flow or low flow) and the source of their arterial feeders (direct or indirect). The most commonly used classification system is Barrow's angiographic classification (Table 44.2) [13]. Type A CCFs are direct communications between the ICA and cavernous sinus. They are typically high-flow fistulas that occur secondary to trauma or to rupture of preexisting cavernous carotid artery aneurysm.

In contrast to direct fistulas, indirect CCFs receive their arterial supply from dural branches of the external and/or the internal carotid artery and are usually low flow. Barrow types B thru D are indirect fistulas. They are more commonly spontaneous fistulas occurring in middle aged women. Type B fistulas receive their arterial supply from dural branches of the ICA and are rare. Type C fistulas receive their arterial supply from the dural branches of the external carotid artery. Type D fistulas are supplied by dural branches of both the internal and external carotid arteries. They represent the most common CCF subtype [14–16].

Table 44.2 Barrow's angiographic subtypes

Type A: direct fistula between ICA and cavernous sinuses
Type B: arterial supply via meningeal branch of ICA
Type C: arterial supply via meningeal branch of ECA
Type D: arterial supply via meningeal branch of ICA and ECA

ICA internal carotid artery, *ECA* external carotid artery

Pathogenesis

As previously mentioned, CCFs can be secondary to shear trauma affecting the cavernous carotid artery or can be idiopathic. Traumatic CCFs and CCFs secondary to cavernous ICA aneurysm rupture tend to be high-flow, direct fistulas, while idiopathic CCFs are commonly low flow and indirect. Traumatic CCFs occur more commonly in young men, and spontaneous CCFs typically occur in postmenopausal women over 50 years old. In this population, hypertension, atherosclerosis, and diabetes may play a role. Spontaneous CCFs have also been documented during pregnancy, in young patients as a congenital lesion, and in patients with underlying connective tissue disorders like Ehlers-Danlos syndrome (EDS), fibromuscular dysplasia, and pseudoxanthoma elasticum. In these cases, it is thought that relatively minor trauma can cause intimal tears due to weak and defective arterial walls.

Spontaneous CCFs are especially common in type IV EDS, which is characterized by multiple arterial aneurysms, dissections, and fistulas. Diagnosis of the underlying condition can be missed because this subtype lacks the joint laxity typical of EDS. If suspected, it can be confirmed by looking for the *COL3A1* gene mutation. Visceral angiography is recommended in these patients due to the high incidence of systemic aneurysms. In cases where these connective tissue disorders are suspected, care needs to be taken to avoid excessive arterial manipulation, and transvenous accessto the fistula is recommended.

Venous Drainage

Although the arterial supply is important for classification and management of CCFs, the venous drainage of CCFs is equally important in determining clinical manifestations and prognosis. Anterior drainage through the superior and/or inferior ophthalmic veins occurs in up to 88% of CCFs and is the most common drainage pattern [14, 17]. This results in the classic ocular signs of CCFs that are reviewed below.

If there is drainage through the intercavernous sinuses, the clinical presentation can be bilateral or contralateral to the fistula. In addition, drainage posteriorly through the superior and inferior petrosal sinus can sometimes be present in the absence of anterior drainage. Cases such as these result in minimal ocular signs and can cause periorbital pain or ophthalmoplegia despite a normal appearing eye.

The most important venous drainage pattern to look out for is superior drainage through the sphenoparietal sinus into the cortical veins. This can be present in up to 55% of patients with CCFs [1, 17, 18]. CCFs with cortical drainage have an increased risk for intracranial complications including elevated intracranial venous pressure, intracranial and subarachnoid hemorrhage, and cerebral venous infarctions. This can lead to neurologic deficits, seizures, and strokes and can be potentially fatal. Evidence of cortical drainage would decrease the threshold for proceeding with intervention.

Clinical Presentation

The classic presentation of CCFs is a unilateral, red eye with dilated, tortuous episcleral vessels, chemosis, pulsatile proptosis, painful ophthalmoplegia, and an ocular bruit. The presentation tends to be dramatic with direct CCFs but can be indolent in cases of spontaneous, indirect CCFs. These indolent cases are often initially misdiagnosed and can be mistaken for episcleritis, conjunctivitis, or thyroid eye disease.

The almost universal sign of CCFs is tortuous conjunctival and episcleral vessels with a sharp turn at the limbus (aka "limbus loops") (Fig. 44.5). Funduscopically, this is echoed as dilated, tortuous retinal veins. Chemosis, proptosis, and diplopia are also common. Diplopia can result from a cranial neuropathy or from diffuse ophthalmoplegia secondary to orbital congestion and extraocular muscle edema [19]. If a cranial neuropathy is present, the abducens nerve is the particularly vulnerable and isolated CN 6 palsy is common. This may be due to mechanical compression and stretching of the nerve within the cavernous sinus or due to its shared course through Dorello's canal with the inferior petrosal sinus. Ophthalmoplegia secondary to orbital congestion usually recovers rapidly, while cranial neuropathy can take over 3 months to resolve. Pain and ocular bruits are less common and only seen in approximately half of CCF cases [15, 18].

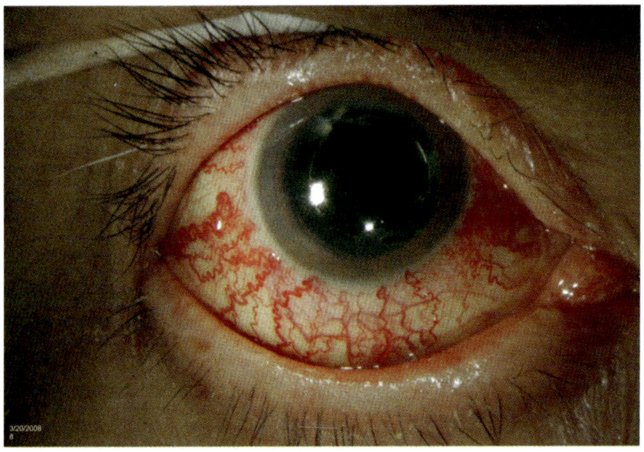

Fig. 44.5 This picture of a patient with a carotid-cavernous fistula demonstrates the classic pattern of episcleral vessel dilation ("limbal loops" with a hairpin-like turn)

Evaluation

When a CCF is suspected, bilateral selective digital subtraction angiography (DSA) of the internal and external carotid arteries remains the gold standard for diagnosis. However, angiography is invasive and has associated risks. Thus, CT angiography (CTA) is often the preferred initial diagnostic imaging modality. CTA has been shown to have similar diagnostic value to DSA and is superior to magnetic resonance angiography (MRA) in the diagnosis of CCFs [20]. Findings include a dilated superior ophthalmic vein, diffusely enlarged muscles, and convex bulging of the lateral cavernous sinus wall.

Other noninvasive diagnostic modalities including orbital and color Doppler ultrasonography play a lesser role but can have diagnostic utility. Orbital ultrasonography can be helpful because it can demonstrate a dilated superior ophthalmic vein and diffusely congested and thickened extraocular muscles. This can help differentiate a CCF from thyroid orbitopathy, which affects certain muscles selectively. Color Doppler ultrasonography can demonstrate flow reversal through the superior ophthalmic vein. Despite the availability of these noninvasive imaging techniques, DSA is recommended if surgical intervention is planned in order to fully map out feeding arteries, draining veins, and the presence of pseudoaneurysms or thrombosis.

Outcomes and Prognosis

As previously mentioned, CCFs can cause intracranial and systemic complications including elevated intracranial venous pressure, intracranial and subarachnoid hemorrhage, and cerebral venous infarctions. These complications are potentially fatal. Fortunately, these complications are rare and estimated to occur in only 15% of cases with a 3% fatality rate [21]. Thus, the overall prognosis of CCFs is systemically benign especially if cortical venous drainage is not present. However, the eye represents the organ suffering the greatest damage, and CCFs can result in significant visual morbidity.

Decreased vision has been cited to be as high as 32% [18, 22]. The eye is particularly vulnerable to the altered hemodynamics of CCFs as decreased arterial pressure is compounded by elevated intraocular pressure to reduce ocular perfusion.

Table 44.3 Goldmann's equation

Goldmann's equation: IOP = F/C + EVP
F = rate of aqueous production
C = outflow facility
EVP = episcleral venous pressure

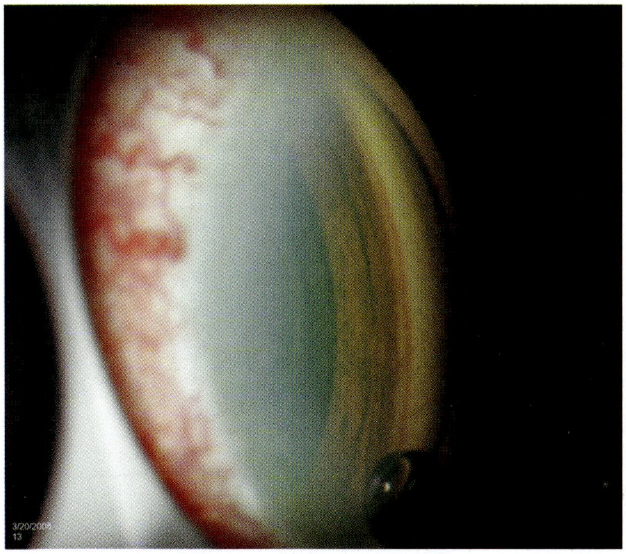

Fig. 44.6 Blood in Schlemm's canal is evidence of elevated episcleral venous pressure, a common cause of glaucoma in patients with carotid-cavernous fistulas

Vision loss can occur due to retinal vein occlusion, glaucoma, anterior segment ischemia, exposure keratitis, and ocular ischemia with secondary proliferative retinopathy and risk for vitreous hemorrhage.

Secondary glaucoma is common and occurs in up to 60% of CCFs [14, 15, 17, 18]. The majority is due to elevated episcleral venous pressure (EVP) in accordance with Goldmann's equation (Table 44.3). Blood in Schlemm's canal on gonioscopy is a classic finding (Fig. 44.6). This secondary glaucoma can be resistant to standard treatment and has an increased risk for suprachoroidal hemorrhage if incisional surgery is performed. Fortunately, the majority resolve with treatment of the underlying CCF. However, in some prolonged cases of CCF, permanent alterations in the outflow resistance are believed to be the cause of chronic unilateral glaucoma. In addition to this open angle mechanism of glaucoma, patients who develop retinal vein occlusion or ocular ischemia are at risk for neovascular glaucoma, which can be difficult to treat.

Treatment: Observation

Indirect CCFs have been documented to resolve spontaneously. This may occur in up to 30–70% of cases [16, 17]. Given the generally benign course, observation can be considered for low-flow fistulas not causing significant symptoms and without evidence of high-risk drainage patterns. If observation is elected, periodic manual compression of the ipsilateral carotid artery and jugular vein can be attempted. Alterations in vascular flow, such as air travel and angiography, have been associated with spontaneous CCF closure. For this reason, manual compression of the ipsilateral carotid artery has been advocated as a mechanism to diminish antegrade flow, elevate venous pressure, and thus promote thrombosis of the fistula [22, 23].

Manual compression is recommended only if the patient does not experience signs and symptoms of cerebral ischemia, bradycardia, and hypotension during manual compression and as long as no cortical venous drainage is present. Manual compression in the presence of cortical venous drainage may increase the risk of intracranial complications. Compression should be performed with the contralateral hand, which would result in immediate cessation of compression should ipsilateral ischemia and contralateral hemiplegia ensue. The patient can start performing compressions for 10 s at a time four to six times an hour and progressively increase their compression time intervals.

However, observation is not recommended when high risk characteristics of CCFs are found on angiographic evaluation. Indications for urgent treatment of indirect CCFs include evidence of cortical venous drainage, presence of a cavernous sinus varix, pseudoaneurysm, epistaxis, and intracranial hemorrhage as these are associated with a worse prognosis [22]. Surgical intervention can also be considered for cosmetically deforming proptosis, obtrusive ophthalmoplegia, intolerable bruit or headache, vision compromise, severe uncontrollable glaucoma, elevated intracranial pressure, and failure to self-resolve after a trial of observation.

Treatment: Surgical Options

Unlike indirect fistulas, direct, high-flow fistulas rarely self-resolve, and surgical intervention is the rule. Historically, surgical treatment of CCFs was achieved by ligating the common or internal carotid artery or by direct surgical exposure and packing of the cavernous sinuses. The advent of endovascular interventional techniques has significantly improved the outcomes and decreased the morbidity of CCF treatment. The goal of treatment is to occlude the communication between the ICA and cavernous sinus while preserving the patency of the ICA. Sacrifice of the ICA is a known risk of surgical embolization. Temporary occlusion of the ICA can be performed to evaluate for the development of neurologic symptoms before permanent occlusion is performed. If collateral flow is insufficient, carotid artery bypass may be required. Fortunately, with the advanced endovascular techniques now available, this is becoming increasingly rare.

The first endovascular embolization involved detachable balloons and was reported by Serbinenko in 1974 [24]. This quickly became the gold standard for treatment, especially for direct fistulas. The high flow rate of direct fistulas provides the ideal conditions for the balloon to traverse the fistula site and enter the cavernous sinus. Unfortunately, the ICA had to be sacrificed in up to 25–37% of reported cases [25, 26]. In 2003, due to problems with balloon valve leaks, detachable balloons were withdrawn from the US market. However, they continue to be used in other countries. Today, embolization can be achieved either transarterially or transvenously with embolic materials such as coils, polyvinyl alcohol, and *n*-butyl cyanoacrylate.

Transarterial access with a microcatheter is achieved through the cervical carotid artery and advanced through the tear in the ICA into the cavernous sinus. From there, embolic material can be deployed into the cavernous sinuses. Transvenous access is achieved through the internal jugular vein to enter the cavernous sinus via the inferior petrosal sinus. If access through the inferior petrosal sinus is unavailable, access through the superior ophthalmic vein via the facial vein can be attempted. Rarely, the services of an orbital surgeon may be elicited to provide direct, transorbital surgical exposure of the superior ophthalmic vein [27].

Transvenous embolization boasts higher clinical and anatomic cure rates than transarterial routes, which often require multiple sessions to achieve complete CCF closure. Angiographic success is achieved in 81–90% of fistulas treated with transvenous embolization [17, 18]. In addition to angiographic success, embolization is associated with high clinical success rates. Kirsch found that vascular complications including glaucoma responded promptly to treatment while neurologic deficits were slower to resolve. Nevertheless, on long-term follow-up, only 5.5% had residual symptoms [17].

Risks of endovascular treatment include aberrant migration of embolic material resulting in transient ischemic attack, permanent neurologic defects from a stroke or intracranial hemorrhage, and rarely death. Ophthalmologically, this could result in blindness if the ophthalmic or central retinal artery or vein was involved. The rate of these complications vary widely based on surgeon and technique, but Keltner's review of multiple studies looking at outcomes of endovascular treatment of CCFs found the average rate of cerebral ischemia was 8%, transient CN palsies 25%, and permanent CN palsies 15% [28]. A more recent series cites lower complication rates with a 2% incidence of ischemia, 14% risk of transient CN palsies, and 7% risk of permanent CN palsies [29].

Many studies have documented the possibility of paradoxical worsening after endovascular treatment. This is thought to reflect thrombosis of the fistula (and thus resolution), and symptoms typically resolve with time. This phenomenon has been documented to occur even in cases without any intervention. The incidence has been reported to be as high as 39.3% [15]; however, a 3–5% incidence is more typical [14, 17].

Recently, stenting has become a popular option for direct fistulas that increases the likelihood of ICA preservation. These stents come in two varieties: porous and nonporous. Porous, non-covered stents are used in conjunction with embolic coils. These stents are deployed across the tear and serve as a barrier to prevent the coils that are placed in the cavernous sinus from refluxing into the ICA. Covered stents are also available and becoming increasingly popular. They are placed to bridge the tear and serve as a conduit for ICA blood flow (Fig. 44.7).

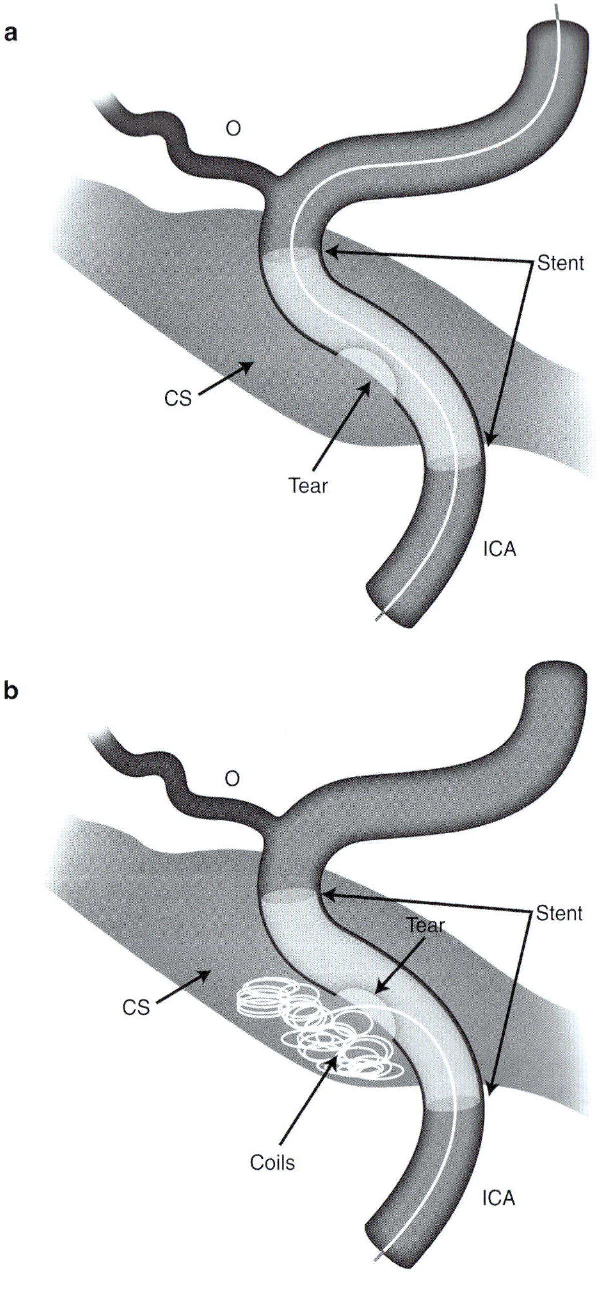

Fig. 44.7 (**a**) Nonporous, covered stents bridge the carotid artery and bypass the fistula. (**b**) Porous stents are used to prevent reflux of coils, which are packed in the cavernous sinus

Stents dedicated to intracranial uses are being produced, but most early experiences have deployed cardiovascular stents. The stiffness of these stents can sometimes pose a challenge in navigating the tortuous ICA, which carries the risk of intimal dissection, thrombus formation, and arterial spasm. In addition, size mismatch especially in cases of long-standing, high flow fistulas may result in endoleak (leakage around the stent) and persistent flow into the fistula. Nevertheless, preliminary studies indicate high success rates (75–100%) with less risk of thromboembolic complications [30–32].

Cavernous ICA Aneurysm

Cavernous ICA aneurysms are a rare, typically benign cause of parasellar syndrome. Aneurysms involving the ICA represent only about 3–5% of all intracranial aneurysms [33]. They can be mycotic, traumatic, or idiopathic. Idiopathic cavernous carotid aneurysms are the most common kind of cavernous carotid aneurysm. Traumatic aneurysms are most commonly associated with basal skull fractures, and mycotic aneurysms are very rare. They most commonly occur in association with infectious endocarditis or meningitis and are accompanied by fever [34].

Clinical Presentation

Like spontaneous CCFs, cavernous carotid aneurysms are commonly found in older women with hypertension. They are often asymptomatic and usually found incidentally on neuroimaging studies performed for other indication. It can also present with painful ophthalmoplegia due to growth of the aneurysm and compressive effect. The abducens nerve is most commonly involved followed by CN 3 and then by CN 4 [33]. Optic nerve involvement can occur if the aneurysm involves the anterior genu of the cavernous ICA and results in decreased vision or visual field defect. Compression of sympathetic fibers can result in Horner's syndrome.

Prognosis

Aneurysm rupture is the most feared complication. The risk of aneurysm rupturecorrelates with its size. The International Study of Unruptured Intracranial Aneurysms [35] found that the 5-year risk of aneurysm rupture was zero if the cavernous ICA aneurysm was <12 mm in diameter. This increased to 3% if the aneurysm was 13–24 mm and 6.4% if >25 mm in diameter. The consequence of aneurysm rupture is determined by whether the aneurysm is intradural or extradural. As previously mentioned, the cavernous carotid artery is anchored at its anterior and posterior extents by dural rings. If it is within the cavernous sinuses, rupture of a cavernous ICA aneurysm usually results in a direct CCF.

Because of this, life-threatening complications such as subarachnoid hemorrhage and cerebral infarction are rare with cavernous ICA aneurysm. There is an estimated risk of 0.19% per patient year of subarachnoid hemorrhage and 0.37% per patient year of cerebral infarction [36]. The risk of life-threatening complications is increased with aneurysms that extend into the subarachnoid space, and catastrophic epistaxis is possible if the ICA aneurysm erodes into the sphenoid sinus.

Treatment

Indications for treatment include progressive ophthalmoplegia, persistent diplopia in primary position, severe pain, concomitant coagulopathy, compression of the optic nerve with progressive vision loss, extension of the aneurysm into the subarachnoid space, and erosion into sphenoid sinus [36, 37]. Treatment is similar to that of CCFs and is achieved by clipping, endovascular embolization, or stenting across the aneurysm. Occasionally, the parent artery cannot be salvaged, and the ICA must be sacrificed. The balloon occlusion test needs to be performed to ensure the patient can tolerate occlusion, and bypass of the involved ICA segment may be required.

While the overall prognosis of ICA aneurysms involving the cavernous segment is benign, it is important to be familiar with high risk characteristics. In addition, close follow-up is recommended to monitor for growth.

Aseptic Cavernous Sinus Thrombosis

Thrombosis of the dural venous sinuses is possible, and when the thrombus involves the cavernous sinuses, the patient can present with signs and symptoms consistent with a parasellar syndrome. Cavernous sinus thrombosis (CST) with or without concurrent superior ophthalmic vein thrombosis is a rare cause of parasellar syndrome. It can be aseptic or septic (reviewed later in this chapter).

Pathogenesis

Aseptic CST can occur because the cerebral dural veins are valveless. Thus, blood flow is determined by pressure gradients and blood flow may stagnate. This creates the setup for Virchow's triad, which is defined by blood flow stasis, vessel wall injury, and hypercoagulability.

Aseptic CST usually occurs in debilitated patients with an underlying hypercoagulable disorder such as anti-thrombin

III deficiency, polycythemia, or use of oral contraceptives. Dehydration and hypotension also predispose to aseptic CST as these conditions allow for cerebral blood flow stagnation. Aseptic CST also can occur secondary to compression and secondary obstruction of blood flow by malignant tumors involving the skull base or nasopharynx.

Clinical Presentation

Patients present with headache, ophthalmoplegia, and signs of venous congestion such as chemosis, proptosis, eyelid edema, and retinal vascular congestion. Unlike cases of septic cavernous sinus thrombosis, there are no signs of infection such as elevated white blood cell count and fever. It may be associated with thrombosis of other dural venous sinuses and can cause elevated intracranial pressure. Aseptic CST often self-resolves and can be clinically confused with Tolosa-Hunt syndrome. However, it does not respond to steroid treatment but rather treatment with anticoagulants.

Though aseptic CST is a rare diagnosis, this is a potential cause of parasellar syndrome. While the diagnosis is benign, evaluation to determine the underlying etiology may reveal other conditions that require more urgent treatment.

Inflammatory Causes

Inflammation can also cause parasellar syndrome and can mimic neoplasia and infection. Like other parasellar syndromes, symptoms include proptosis, eyelid edema and erythema, and ophthalmoplegia. Loss of sensation along CN V1, loss of vision, and sympathetic paralysis are also possible. Pain is a prominent finding. Inflammation can affect the cavernous sinuses, sphenoid sinus, hypophysis, or local pachymeninges surrounding the parasella.

Inflammation can be secondary to an underlying rheumatologic disorder or can be idiopathic. Cases of parasellar syndrome have been reported secondary to systemic inflammation including Wegener's granulomatosis, systemic lupus erythematosus, and sarcoidosis. Thus, if inflammation is suspected, full workup for rheumatologic conditions should be undertaken including CXR, RF, c-ANCA, ANA, anti-dsDNA, ACE, blood sugar, HA1c, RPR, VDRL, and possible lumbar puncture. Since neoplasia and infection are prominent on the differential, neuroimaging is also an important part of the evaluation.

Tolosa-Hunt Syndrome

Idiopathic granulomatous inflammation can occur in the cavernous sinuses and is on a diagnostic continuum with idiopathic orbital inflammation and idiopathic hypertrophic cranial pachymeningitis. Idiopathic cavernous sinus inflammation is more commonly known by its eponym Tolosa-Hunt syndrome (THS).

In 1954, Tolosa described a case of left orbital pain with ipsilateral vision loss, ophthalmoplegia, and reduced sensation over CN V1. Postmortem autopsy demonstrated granulomatous inflammation of carotid and cavernous sinus with narrowing of the ICA [38]. In 1961, Hunt described patients with characteristics similar to that of Tolosa and defined the diagnostic criteria of this syndrome [39]. However, it was not until 1966 that Smith and Taxdal first christened idiopathic cases of granulomatous inflammation involving the cavernous sinuses as Tolosa-Hunt syndrome [40].

Clinical Presentation

The International Headache Society's 2004 revised classifications define THS as a unilateral, painful ophthalmoplegia with motility dysfunction that usually resolves but tends to relapse and remit [41]. Diagnostic criteria include the following:

- One or more episodes of unilateral orbital pain persisting for weeks if untreated.
- Paresis of one or more of the third, fourth, and/or sixth cranial nerves and/or demonstration of granulomas by MRI or biopsy.
- Paresis coincides with the onset of pain or follows it within 2 weeks.
- Pain or paresis resolves within 72 h when treated adequately with corticosteroids.
- Other causes have been excluded by appropriate investigations.

This last criterion is vital to safeguard against missing more sinister causes of parasellar syndrome (specifically lymphoma or other neoplasms as previously discussed).

Tolosa-Hunt syndrome can occur in any age group without any sex predilection. The pain in THS is typically a steady pain behind the eyes that is "pressure-like," "gnawing," or "boring" [4, 42, 43]. While painful ophthalmoplegia is the classic presentation of THS, ophthalmoplegia may sometimes lag in presentation up to 2 weeks after the onset of pain. The oculomotor nerve is the most frequently involved, followed by CN 6 and CN 4 [4, 44]. Proptosis can also occur in a minority of patients and can be bilateral.

Without treatment, symptoms last an average of 8 weeks before resolving. Treatment with steroids should result in resolution of pain and paresis within 72 h according to the International Headache Society (IHS) criteria. However, clinical experience has shown that cranial neuropathy may take an average of 2 weeks to resolve [45, 46]. Despite being characterized by spontaneous remission, residual neurologic deficits may persist. In addition, recurrence can occur in up to 39% of patients after months to years [4, 47]. Recurrence is more likely when inflammation is secondary to an underlying systemic disorder, so repeat rheumatologic evaluation should be considered in recurrent cases especially if patients complain of symptoms on system review.

Neuroimaging

MRI is the preferred mode of neuroimaging for THS as it is more sensitive than CT imaging [44, 46, 48]. Not only is it important for ruling out neoplasia and infection, MRI may demonstrate cavernous sinus fullness causing convexity of the lateral walls. An isointense granulomatous mass on T1-weighted images that enhances homogenously with contrast can also be seen. These neuroimaging changes can be followed and should resolve with steroid therapy.

Despite being the most sensitive imaging modality for THS, MRI may be negative in 21–33% of cases [2, 44, 49]. In these cases, dynamic MRI may prove useful in detecting abnormalities missed on regular MRI. By taking sequential images as contrast is administered, cases of THS have shown progressive enhancement of the granulomatous lesions on dynamic MRI [50]. Other adjunctive studies include venography and angiography. These studies may demonstrate superior ophthalmic vein occlusion with partial or absent filling of the cavernous sinuses and narrowing or displacement of the cavernous ICA [47, 51]. However, these are nonspecific for the diagnosis of THS.

Treatment

The response of THS to corticosteroids is also characteristic of this syndrome. Resolution of symptoms tends to be rapid and is so distinctive that many consider it a diagnostic test. However, caution needs to be taken as other cavernous sinus pathology, most notably lymphoma, can also respond to corticosteroids. The standard treatment for THS is corticosteroids given at high doses (1 mg/kg) daily over 1–3 months. Some advocate starting initially with very high doses of steroids (500–100 mg) for 2–3 days before switching to the standard 1 mg/kg dose as this regimen may reduce the rate of recurrence [45].

If steroids are not tolerated or response to steroids is insufficient, alternative therapies may be employed. These include fractionated radiation of 20–50 Gy divided over ten fractions [52–54]. Other biologic therapies have been explored to treat other causes of ocular inflammation including azathioprine, methotrexate, mycophenolate mofetil, rituximab, and infliximab. These may prove useful in cases of THS as well [55–58].

THS is defined by these strict diagnostic criteria because of the high risk of misdiagnosis. Other more sinister pathologies can mimic THS, so vigilance must be maintained. If a patient with presumed THS fails to respond to corticosteroids within 72 h or has progressive pain and neurologic deficits, further investigation to rule out other pathology is mandatory. In addition, continued follow-up for a minimum of 2 years is recommended by some experts to minimize the shortcomings of incorrect diagnosis [59]. Though THS is benign, knowing the other parasellar syndromes in the differential diagnosis of THS is important to avoid missing another diagnosis.

Hypophysitis

Hypophysitis or inflammation of the pituitary gland is a rare cause of parasellar syndrome. Hypophysitis is part of the differential of sellar masses and causes mass effects such as headache, visual impairment, and hypophyseal dysfunction. Bitemporal visual field defect and symptoms of hypopituitarism are more common, but painful ophthalmoplegia consistent with parasellar syndrome is also possible.

Hypophysitis can be secondary to infectious etiologies or systemic rheumatologic conditions. It can also be a primary diagnosis representing inflammation limited to the pituitary gland without associated systemic disease. Primary hypophysitis is categorized by the type of inflammation. It can be lymphocytic, granulomatous, or xanthomatous. Lymphocytic hypophysitis is more common in pregnant and postpartum women, and it also is the more common histologic subtype in autoimmune hypophysitis.

Hypophysitis most commonly affects women in their 30s and 40s. Surgery is sometimes undertaken when the presentation is misdiagnosed as a neoplasm. However, hypophysitis commonly spontaneously resolves, and conservative treatment with hormonal replacement is often sufficient. However, immunosuppressive therapy such as steroids, azathioprine, methotrexate, and radiation therapy can result in shrinkage of the pituitary mass and improvement of headache and vision.

Hypophysitis is a rare cause of parasellar syndrome but should be suspected in cases of parasellar mass with signs and symptoms of pituitary dysfunction.

Infection

Historically, syphilis was the presumed cause of most cases of parasellar syndrome. Now in the antibiotic era, syphilis and other infections of the parasella are a rare but potentially fatal cause of parasellar syndrome. As with other regions in the body, infections of the parasella can be bacterial (septic cavernous sinus thrombosis), fungal (rhino-orbital-cerebral mucormycosis), or viral (varicella zoster virus (VZV) neuropathy).

Septic Cavernous Sinus Thrombosis

Due to the multiple septations of the cavernous sinuses, bacterial emboli become easily entrapped resulting in septic thrombosis. Septic cavernous sinus thrombosis used to be a uniformly fatal diagnosis [60, 61]. Fortunately, since the discovery of antibiotics, septic CST is now extremely rare with mortality progressively declining over the years to 13–30% today [61, 62]. While mortality rates have significantly improved, morbidity from residual deficits remains an issue due to the number of vital structures in the cavernous sinuses. It is estimated that residual morbidity affects 23–77% of survivors [61, 63].

Infection Sources

The primary sources of infection in septic CST include (1) sphenoid and ethmoid sinusitis, (2) facial infections affecting the middle third of the face, and (3) oral infections affecting dentition or the nasopharynx, such as a paratonsillar abscess. Infections of the middle ear can also cause septic CST if retrograde extension from the sigmoid vein occurs. Because the dural venous system is valveless, septic thrombosis involving any dural veins can result in retrograde or anterograde thrombosis. Thus, concomitant involvement of other dural veins is common with septic CST.

Facial infections, especially nasal furuncles, historically were the most common cause of septic CST. Today, ethmoid and sphenoid sinusitis represents the most common primary source of infection. The sphenoid enjoys a central position within the parasella, and infection can spread directly through communicating veins or indirectly by causing osteomyelitis of the intervening bony wall. Because of its deep location, sphenoid sinusitis has few localizing symptoms and late diagnosis is common. In contrast, infections originating in the ethmoid sinuses spread indirectly through the superior ophthalmic vein after breaching the lamina papyracea. Ethmoid sinusitis can also cause orbital cellulitis. Posterior extension of bacteria through the ophthalmic veins to cause septic CST is also a known complication of orbital cellulitis.

Clinical Presentation

Septic CST can present fulminantly or subacutely. Patients present with fever, chemosis, periorbital edema, proptosis, and painful ophthalmoplegia. Other findings include papilledema, retinal vein dilation, and dysesthesia of the cornea and areas of the face innervated by CN V1 and CN V2. The pupils may be dilated due to CN 3 paralysis or miotic from sympathetic paralysis. Classically, this starts unilaterally and becomes bilateral within 48 h.

When septic CST is unilateral, it can be easily confused with post-septal cellulitis. However, careful evaluation of the motility pattern may demonstrate selective cranial neuropathy rather than the diffuse ophthalmoplegia, which is seen in orbital cellulitis from extraocular muscle edema and infiltration. The abducens nerve is the most susceptible due to its central location in the cavernous sinuses, and abduction deficit is often the first cranial neuropathies to present and the last to resolve. However, severe cases can have total ophthalmoplegia and be difficult to differentiate from orbital infection.

Systemic signs suggestive of sepsis and meningitis may also be present and point to the underlying diagnosis. This includes nuchal rigidity, tachycardia, vomiting, hypotension, confusion, rigors, altered mental status, lethargy, and obtundation. Fevers typically have a "picket fence" pattern characteristic of thrombophlebitis.

Neuroimaging

Neuroimaging helps to clinch the diagnosis and differentiate septic CST from orbital cellulitis. Contrast-enhanced CT with venography is the preferred imaging modality for diagnosis [64]. Expansion of the cavernous sinus results in convex bowing of the lateral wall, which is concave in non-pathologic states. This is best seen on coronal images. Abnormal filling defects within the cavernous sinuses, venous obstruction with dilation of the ipsilateral superior ophthalmic vein, and increased dural enhancement along the lateral wall can also be seen (Fig. 44.8).

Narrowing of the ICA is also frequently documented on neuroimaging and may reflect arteritis, spasm, or compression by the thrombus. This usually resolves with treatment but must be followed closely as ICA occlusion may result in cerebral infarction and hemiparesis. As mentioned previously, although the mortality rate has improved due to the discovery of antibiotics, survivors have a high rate of residual morbidity. Hemiparesis is one of the more devastating potential consequences and can be the result of ICA occlusion, cerebral abscess, or cortical vein thrombosis.

Outcomes and Prognosis

Other intracranial complications include intracranial extension of the infection and progression of the septic thrombophlebitis. Intracranial infection extension can cause meningitis, encephalitis, a subdural empyema, or a brain

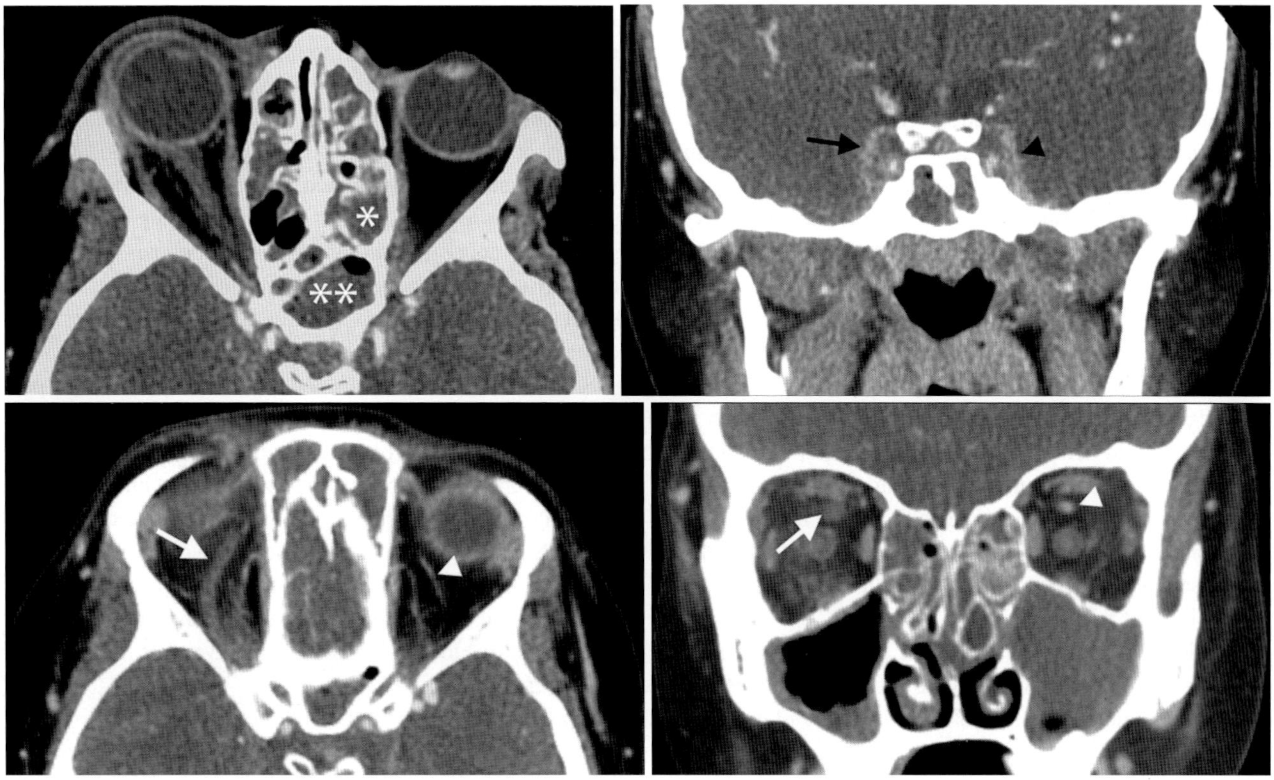

Fig. 44.8 (*Top left*): CT scan of the orbit with contrast, axial view demonstrating proptosis, and retrobulbar fat stranding. Note mucosal thickening and fluid in the ethmoidal (*single asterisk*) and sphenoidal sinuses (*double asterisk*) consistent with acute inflammation. (*bottom left*): CT scan of the orbit with contrast, axial view demonstrating dilated right superior ophthalmic vein (*arrow*) compared with the left (*arrowhead*). (*Bottom right*): CT scan of the orbit with contrast, coronal view demonstrates decreased contrast uptake on the right superior ophthalmic vein (*arrow*) compared with the left (*arrowhead*). (*Top right*): CT scan of the orbit with contrast, coronal view demonstrating subtle rounding and fullness of the cavernous sinus on the right (*arrow*). Compare with the flat, slightly concave appearance of the left (*arrowhead*). (Reproduced from [65]. With permission)

abscess. A brain abscess should be suspected if the patient does not respond to treatment or develops convulsions or systemic neurologic deficits. Progression of the thrombophlebitis to other cortical veins is possible due to the valveless venous connections. This can result in elevated intracranial pressure, especially if the superior sagittal sinus or lateral sinuses are involved, and it increases the risk of hemorrhagic infarction.

Pituitary involvement can cause panhypopituitarism, syndrome of inappropriate ADH (SIADH), diabetes insipidus (DI), and adrenocortical insufficiency that can result in adrenal crisis and systemic collapse. Septic thrombi can also embolize systemically to other organs. This most commonly affects the lungs resulting in pulmonary abscesses, empyemas, pneumonia, pneumothorax, and infarcts [63].

Treatment

If septic CST is diagnosed, prompt hospitalization and treatment is mandatory. High-dose, IV antibiotics are the mainstay of treatment. *Staphylococcus aureus* is most commonly implicated pathogen in septic CST followed by *Streptococcus* species. However, gram-negative and anaerobic organisms have also been documented. Thus, treatment is begun empirically with a third-generation cephalosporin such as ceftriaxone or cefotaxime, metronidazole, and an anti-staphylococcal penicillin such as nafcillin. If there is high risk for methicillin-resistant *S. aureus* or a penicillin allergy, vancomycin is substituted for nafcillin. Antibiotics should be continued for at least 2 weeks after clinical resolution. In addition, close follow-up is required as recurrence has been reported after antibiotics are stopped. Fortunately, this is rare.

Anticoagulation has also been advocated as a treatment adjunct in order to prevent thrombus propagation to other dural venous sinuses, to enhance recanalization, and to improve antibiotic penetration into the thrombus. However, there is a risk for intracranial and systemic bleeding, and central nervous system (CNS) infarction must be ruled out prior to beginning anticoagulation. Anticoagulation is a standard treatment for non-septic dural venous thrombosis, but it has been inadequately studied in septic CST due to the rarity of this diagnosis. Some retrospective reviews have suggested that anticoagulation may reduce mortality [62, 66].

If anticoagulation is instituted, caution is the rule, and hematologic parameters should be closely monitored. In order to minimize the risk of hemorrhagic complications, activated partial thromboplastin time (aPTT) should be maintained between 1.5 and 2.5 and prothrombin time/international normalized ratio (PT/INR) between 2.0 and 3.0. Since anticoagulation only limits additional thrombus formation, it also must be continued for long periods of time until full resolution of the thrombus is achieved.

Steroids are another adjunctive therapy that is more controversial. They certainly have a role should Addisonian crisis develop. However, some advocate more broad use as steroids have been attributed in some case reports with ameliorating cranial nerve dysfunction and orbital inflammation. Naturally, there is concern about using steroids in the setting of this serious infection, and steroids should only be considered once appropriate antibiotics have been started and response has been documented. Even in these cases, steroids have a limited role.

While the treatment of septic CST is largely medical, there is a role for surgery if non-draining sources of infection exist. For example, decompression of infected ethmoid or sphenoid sinuses can accelerate disease resolution. Surgical intervention may also be required if the patient develops an intracranial abscess. By combining these available therapies, the outcomes of patients who develop septic CST have significantly improved. However, despite the rarity nowadays of this diagnosis, it is important to maintain a high clinical suspicion for septic CST since prompt diagnosis and treatment are essential.

Rhino-Cerebral-Orbital Mucormycosis

Fungal infections can extend to involve the parasella and are part of the rhino-cerebral-orbital form of mucormycosis (RCOM). RCOM is an infection of the paranasal sinuses caused by fungi of the Zygomycetes class, Mucorales order, and Mucoraceae family. This includes species in the genera *Rhizopus*, *Rhizomucor*, *Mucor*, and *Absidia*. They are thick walled, nonseptate, branching hyphae that are ubiquitous in nature.

The spore form is frequently aerosolized and inhaled. In normal immunocompetent people, these spores are easily cleared by phagocytosis. In immunocompromised hosts, germination and hypha formation results in infection and vascular invasion. From the sinuses, the fungi can extend locally into the cranial vault and orbit.

Clinical Presentation

RCOM presents with headache, rhinorrhea, facial swelling and pain, fever, and black intranasal or intraoral eschars. Eschar is the classic finding of mucormycotic infection that usually tips the clinician off to the diagnosis. The eschar represents local necrosis due to fungal invasion of the intima and media of the arterial walls causing endothelial damage, fibrin reaction, and thrombosis. This results in local tissue ischemia and infarction, which is clinically manifested as an eschar. Unfortunately, eschar is usually a late finding suggesting advanced disease and a poor prognosis [67]. Thus, maintaining vigilance and keeping fungal etiologies of parasellar syndrome on one's differential is essential for early detection and improved outcomes.

Orbital involvement is found in 75% of RCOM and portends a worse prognosis than cases that do not involve the orbit [68]. Orbital involvement can cause decreased vision, ophthalmoplegia, proptosis, orbital cellulitis, and chemosis. Ophthalmoplegia is usually due to local cranial neuropathy with CN 6 being the most commonly involved followed by CN 3 and CN 4 [69, 70]. CN V1 and CN V2 involvement can cause corneal and perinasal anesthesia, and vision loss can be secondary to either CN 2 involvement or vascular occlusion.

Spread of mucormycotic infection intracranially causes lethargy and meningitis. Mycotic brain abscesses, infectious aneurysms, and carotid artery occlusion are possible sequelae and can cause seizures, massive stroke, and hemiparesis.

In addition to local spread, mucor can embolize systemically to cause other forms of mucormycosis including pulmonary, cutaneous, GI, and disseminated forms. Aspiration can cause pulmonary mucormycosis, which can present with hemoptysis and sudden pleuritic chest pain. Gastrointestinal mucormycosis can be secondary to swallowing mucor hyphae. Clinical symptoms include abdominal pain, diarrhea, constipation, hematemesis, bloody stool, and stigmata of peritonitis. Malnutrition is a major risk factor for GI mucormycosis. Cutaneous mucormycosis occurs secondary to embolization of mucor hyphae to the skin, resulting in necrotic subcutaneous nodules. Disseminated cases of mucormycosis are commonly found in neutropenic patients, especially those with underlying hematologic malignancies.

Risk Factors

Risk factors for developing mucormycosis include immune compromise and metabolic acidosis. This makes diabetics especially susceptible to mucormycotic infection, and diabetes represents the underlying etiology in 60–72% of mucormycosis cases [68, 71, 72]. Other common predisposing conditions include metabolic acidosis secondary to dehydration and diarrhea, renal disease including kidney transplant patients, patients on deferoxamine therapy, and hematologic malignancies. Deferoxamine increases the risk of RCOM because deferoxamine is a natural siderophore from

Streptomyces pilosus and increases iron availability for consumption by fungi.

Acidosis impairs the immune system by decreasing the phagocytic activity of neutrophils, inhibiting mast cell activity, and increasing the proportion of unbound iron, which promotes fungal growth. In addition, *Rhizopus* has its own ketone reductase and thrives in the high glucose environment of diabetic ketoacidosis (DKA). The classic presentation is that of a diabetic patient who presents with unilateral headache, sinusitis, and fever. Another classic presentation is an unresponsive patient in DKA who does not improve, despite reversal of acidosis. Nevertheless, mucormycosis can occur in any immunosuppressed state and even in some immunocompetent patients. Thus, it is important to have a high clinical suspicion for a fungal etiology in atypical cases of sinusitis, especially if the patient does not respond as expected to standard treatment.

Diagnosis

If RCOM is suspected, biopsy is necessary to confirm the diagnosis. Tissue must be sent for fresh, frozen, and permanent sections. Diagnostic yield is improved by taking a biopsy at the junction of well and poorly perfused tissue and including arteries in the sample. Stains with periodic acid-Schiff (PAS), Gomori methenamine, and hematoxylin and eosin (H&E) demonstrate nonseptate branching hyphae as well as tissue necrosis.

Cultures alone are insufficient to make the diagnosis as these fungi are commonly present non-pathogenically. Cultures, however, are helpful in determining speciation and antibiotic sensitivity. Cultures are performed on Sabouraud agar and brain heart infusion broth. Cultures must be maintained for a sufficient period of time to allow growth, and the clinical suspicion for fungal disease must be relayed to the laboratory or they may otherwise disregard positive results as contamination. Neuroimaging is unfortunately nonspecific, demonstrating general signs of sinusitis such as mucosal thickening. Bony destruction and necrosis are suspicious for mucormycosis, but it is also a late finding.

Treatment

The three cornerstones of RCOM treatment are (1) correcting the predisposing condition, (2) administering amphotericin B, and (3) performing surgical debridement of the involved tissues. Despite the relatively high incidence of RCOM in diabetics, it is fortunately also more easily treated due to the reversibility of DKA. Diabetics have three to four times higher survival rates than other underlying condition [67, 68, 71, 72]. Patients with an underlying hematologic malignancy have an especially poor prognosis.

Fortunately, the prognosis of mucormycosis has significantly improved since the discovery of amphotericin B in 1958. From mortality rates of 86–88% [72, 73], mortality has progressively declined to approximately 28.6% [68, 72]. Amphotericin B is produced by the fungus *Streptomyces nodosus*. It binds to steroids in eukaryotic membranes resulting in altered permeability and loss of intracellular cations. It has greater affinity for ergosterol than cholesterol, but its imperfect selectivity results in significant toxicity.

Toxic side effects include renal impairment, hypokalemia, bone marrow suppression, electrolyte abnormalities, local phlebitis, fever, and nausea and vomiting. Amphotericin is first given as a 1-mg test dose followed by a 20-mg therapeutic dose that is increased rapidly by 10–15 mg increments every 12 h until a therapeutic dose of 0.7–1.0 mg/kg/day in two divided doses is reached. Therapy is continued for a cumulative dose of 2–4 g. Amphotericin can be continued as long as creatinine is <3.0 mg/dL and BUN <50 mg/dl. If renal dysfunction exceeds these limits, it is switched to every other day until renal function improves.

More recently, the liposomal form of amphotericin B has been developed as a less toxic alternative. Liposomal encapsulation enhances delivery to fungi in infected organs while also causing less renal toxicity. It is also given as a 1 mg/kg/day dose, but its improved toxicity profile allows greater cumulative doses (>10 g). Regardless of the type of amphotericin B used, prolonged therapy is required because it is fungistatic and not fungicidal. After cessation of amphotericin B therapy, it is important to keep observing for recurrence of infection.

Surgical debridement is carried out to decrease the infectious load of mucormycosis. Debridement usually results in minimal bleeding because of the extensive vaso-occlusion within the tissues. Frozen section-guided surgical debridement similar to Mohs resection has been suggested as a method to limit the extent of resection to only the involved tissues. In mucormycosis, frozen sections have a sensitivity of 85% and a specificity of 100% [74–76]. Post-debridement, close follow-up is recommended as multiple debridements are sometimes necessary.

Traditionally, wide local resection has included exenteration as the standard of care when the orbit is involved. Exenteration improves survival rates [67]. However, cases of patient survival despite refusing exenteration have brought into question whether this cosmetically deforming surgery is required in all cases, especially when there is still some useful vision remaining [68, 77]. While there are as yet no clear guidelines about when exenteration can be safely avoided, preservation of the orbit may be undertaken at the discretion of the surgeon and patient depending on the aggressiveness of presentation, type of underlying disease process, and response to initial therapy. Delivering amphotericin B locally via intraorbital catheter may be a useful adjunct that may increase the likelihood of avoiding exenteration [78].

Hyperbaric oxygen is the primary adjunctive therapy considered for mucormycosis. While still not part of the standard of care, some studies suggest hyperbaric oxygen can improve survival rates [72]. Hundred percent hyperbaric oxygen administered at 1–3 atm has a fungistatic effect. In addition, hyperbaric oxygen can improve the oxygenation of tissues distal to occluded arteries and decrease tissue acidosis [79]. In cases of systemic acidosis, the oxygen-hemoglobin dissociation curve is profoundly shifted to the right limiting the oxygen-binding capacity of hemoglobin (the Bohr effect). Hyperbaric oxygen results in a higher partial pressure of oxygen, which helps increase the oxygen saturation of circulating hemoglobin.

Hyperbaric oxygen increases tissue perfusion both directly and by its effect on acidosis. Hyperbaric oxygen is administered as 100% O_2 at 2–2.5 atm for 90–120 min once or twice daily. However, this requires a special hyperbaric oxygen chamber, and thus, its use is limited. In addition, caution must be used because it is teratogenic and mutagenic. Other toxic side effects include decompression sickness, aeroembolism, spontaneous pneumothorax, seizures from oxygen toxicity, and difficulty equalizing middle ear pressure. Pneumothorax usually self-resolves, but hyperbaric oxygen must be discontinued should this occur.

Other antifungal agents may be used as adjuncts or alternatives to amphotericin B if the patient fails to respond to traditional therapy. Fluconazole and itraconazole are documented to have good CNS penetration and broad-spectrum antifungal activity. However, they lack the track record of amphotericin B and have shown inconsistent in vitro activity. Thus, amphotericin B remains the first-line agent against mucormycosis. Though these treatment modalities have significantly improved the prognosis of RCOM, early diagnosis and prompt treatment are important. High clinical suspicion should be maintained in at risk patients.

Aspergillosis

In addition to the more common RCOM, fungal granulomas can also affect the parasellar region. Fungal granulomas are most commonly due to aspergillosis. These molds belong to the Eurotiomycetes class, Eurotiales order, and Trichocomaceae family. Like the mucor family of fungi, they bear spores and form branching hyphae in tissue. However, unlike mucor, their branches have septations.

Aspergillus is universally present in the air and soil, and their spores are often inhaled. Infection can extend to the orbit and sinuses directly or hematogenously after primary infection of the lungs or intestines. Infection causes granulomatous inflammation and angiitis. Intracranial spread causes chronic granulomatous meningitis and can result in *Aspergillus* abscesses that resemble tumors. The sphenoid sinus is a frequent site for intracranial or orbital invasion and can cause parasellar syndrome.

Clinical Presentation and Treatment

Within humans, there are four major variants of *Aspergillus* infection. The acute fulminant form occurs in immunocompromised and neutropenic patients. An indolent form occurs in immunocompetent patients causing a chronic, noninvasive, circumscribed infection (aspergilloma). This form has a minimal inflammatory response and most commonly exists asymptomatically in the lungs. When it occurs within the paranasal sinuses, it results in sclerotic bony changes rather than bony destruction. *Aspergillus* can also invade locally with aggressive bony destruction and tissue invasion resulting in a purulent mass similar to RCOM. This then causes aggressive destruction of bony structures and can spread to the cavernous sinuses. The final form of aspergillus is the allergic form (allergic bronchopulmonary aspergillosis) where airway inflammation and bronchospasm occur as a hypersensitivity reaction in young, atopic patients.

Thus, *Aspergillus* can cause a more aggressive presentation similar to RCOM or can cause a more indolent, limited form of disease that is more common in immunocompetent patients. Surgical resection of necrotic diseased tissue is usually curative. However, invasive forms may require treatment similar to RCOM including radical surgical resection and amphotericin B.

Zoster Neuropathy

The herpes zoster virus (HZV) is known to cause cranial neuropathies and can sometimes cause a combination of ocular motor neuropathies and proptosis suggestive of parasellar syndrome. HZV is one of the eight herpesviruses that cause disease in humans. Herpesviruses are large double-stranded DNA viruses that have a latent phase within either neural or lymphoid tissue.

Initial infection by HZV causes the childhood exanthem chickenpox. Subsequent to resolution of the initial infection, the virus becomes latent within neural ganglia. Reactivation of the virus occurs in older patients and patients with impaired immunity. It results in a painful vesicular rash with a dermatomal distribution known as shingles. When the trigeminal ganglion is involved, reactivation commonly occurs along the distribution of the ophthalmic division resulting in herpes zoster ophthalmicus (HZO).

In addition to its classic ocular findings of keratitis, uveitis, conjunctivitis, and retinitis, it can also cause neurologic deficits in approximately up to a third of patients [80]. It can cause a meningoencephalitis with altered mental status and focal neurologic defects including optic neuritis and ocular motor palsies. Hemiplegia can occur in severe cases. Neurologic manifestations of HZO are thought to be due to either direct cytopathic effect of the virus on neural tissue or occlusive vasculitis.

Zoster ophthalmoplegia usually occurs 1–2 weeks after the cutaneous manifestations. The oculomotor nerve is the most commonly involved cranial nerve deficit, but multiple cranial nerve involvement with complete ophthalmoplegia, Horner's syndrome, and proptosis are also possible. The prognosis for recovery in 2–3 months is good.

Treatment

The treatment for zoster ophthalmoplegia is anecdotal and lacks strong evidence supporting any specific modality. Acyclovir is the mainstay of treatment in shingles and may be considered in cases of ophthalmoplegia. It is proven to shorten the duration of viral shedding, speed the resolution of presenting signs and symptoms, and reduce the incidence and severity of secondary ocular inflammation [81]. Acyclovir is most effective if started within 72 h of disease onset.

Acyclovir can be given orally at 800 mg five times a day for 7–10 days. Acyclovir is also available for parenteral administration and should be considered especially in immunocompromised patients and patients with disseminated zoster. It is given at 10–15 mg/kg three times daily for 2–3 weeks. Alternatives to acyclovir include valacyclovir 1000 mg TID or famciclovir 500–750 mg TID for 7 days. For cases of zoster ophthalmoplegia, IV acyclovir is usually elected if there is evidence of encephalitis. Acyclovir is most beneficial before significant cytopathic effect and secondary vasculitis can occur.

The use of systemic steroids is controversial for shingles but serves as the mainstay for zoster ophthalmoplegia where it is advocated to counteract the inflammation that results in the neuropathy. Otherwise, systemic steroids should only be considered in immunocompetent patients. They have been shown to decrease the duration of zoster rash and severity of acute pain. However, there is no evidence that steroids affect the incidence or duration of postherpetic neuralgia [82, 83]. Nevertheless, the decision to institute steroids must be weighed against the risks of steroids including the risk of disseminating zoster infection.

Conclusion

The combination of multiple ocular motor neuropathies, headache, and proptosis is suggestive of one of the parasellar syndromes. However, atypical and early presentations may fool the clinician especially if only one cranial nerve is involved. The pathologies that can cause parasellar syndrome are diverse and can be rapidly fatal or benign. Neuroimaging is helpful in differentiating these pathologies. Since early diagnosis can have a significant prognostic impact for many of these pathologies, being familiar with this differential and maintaining a high clinical suspicion are important.

References

1. Tubbs RS, Hill M, May WR, et al. Does the maxillary division of the trigeminal nerve traverse the cavernous sinus? An anatomical study and review of the literature. Surg Radiol Anat. 2008;30:37–40.
2. Fernández S, Godino O, Martínez-Yélamos S, Mesa E, Arruga J, Ramón JM, Acebes JJ, Rubio F. Cavernous sinus syndrome: a series of 126 patients. Medicine (Baltimore). 2007;86:278–81.
3. Lin CC, Tsai JJ. Relationship between the number of involved cranial nerves and the percentage of lesions located in the cavernous sinus. Eur Neurol. 2003;49(2):98–102.
4. Kline LB. The Tolosa-Hunt syndrome. Surv Ophthalmol. 1982;27:79–95.
5. Thomas JE, Yoss RE. The parasellar syndrome: problems in determining etiology. Mayo Clin Proc. 1970;45:617–23.
6. Keane JR. Cavernous sinus syndrome. Analysis of 151 cases. Arch Neurol. 1996;53:967–71.
7. Rush JA, Younge BR. Paralysis of cranial nerves III, IV, and VI. Cause and prognosis in 1,000 cases. Arch Ophthalmol. 1981;99:76–9.
8. Jefferson G. Concerning injuries, aneurysms and tumours involving the cavernous sinus. Trans Ophthalmol Soc U K. 1953;73:117–52.
9. Godtfredsen E, Lederman M. Diagnostic and prognostic roles of ophthalmoneurologic signs and symptoms in malignant nasopharyngeal tumors. Am J Ophthalmol. 1965;59:1063–9.
10. Sibal L, Ball SG, Connolly V, et al. Pituitary apoplexy: a review of clinical presentation, management and outcome in 45 cases. Pituitary. 2004;7:157–63.
11. Kalina P, Black K, Woldenberg R. Burkitt's lymphoma of the skull base presenting as cavernous sinus syndrome in early childhood. Pediatr Radiol. 1996;26:416–7.
12. Rubin MM, Sanfilippo RJ. Lymphoma of the paranasal sinuses presenting as cavernous sinus syndrome. J Oral Maxillofac Surg. 1992;50:749–51.
13. Barrow DL, Spector RH, Braun IF, et al. Classification and treatment of spontaneous carotid-cavernous sinus fistulas. J Neurosurg. 1985;62:248–56.
14. Preechawat P, Narmkerd P, Jiarakongmun P, et al. Dural carotid cavernous sinus fistula: ocular characteristics, endovascular management and clinical outcome. J Med Assoc Thail. 2008;91:852–8.
15. Oishi A, Miyamoto K, Yoshimura N. Etiology of carotid cavernous fistula in Japanese. Jpn J Ophthalmol. 2009;53:40–3.
16. Debrun GM, Viñuela F, Fox AJ, et al. Indications for treatment and classification of 132 carotid-cavernous fistulas. Neurosurgery. 1988;22:285–9.

17. Kirsch M, Henkes H, Liebig T, et al. Endovascular management of dural carotid-cavernous sinus fistulas in 141 patients. Neuroradiology. 2006;48:486–90.
18. Meyers PM, Halbach VV, Dowd CF, et al. Dural carotid cavernous fistula: definitive endovascular management and long-term follow-up. Am J Ophthalmol. 2002;134:85–92.
19. Leonard TJ, Moseley IF, Sanders MD. Ophthalmoplegia in carotid cavernous sinus fistula. Br J Ophthalmol. 1984;68:128–34.
20. Chen CC, Chang PC, Shy CG, et al. CT angiography and MR angiography in the evaluation of carotid cavernous sinus fistula prior to embolization: a comparison of techniques. AJNR Am J Neuroradiol. 2005;26:2349–56.
21. Halbach VV, Hieshima GB, Higashida RT, et al. Carotid cavernous fistulae: indications for urgent treatment. AJR Am J Roentgenol. 1987;149:587–93.
22. Halbach VV, Higashida RT, Hieshima GB, et al. Dural fistulas involving the cavernous sinus: results of treatment in 30 patients. Radiology. 1987;163:437–42.
23. Higashida RT, Hieshima GB, Halbach VV, et al. Closure of carotid cavernous sinus fistulae by external compression of the carotid artery and jugular vein. Acta Radiol Suppl. 1986;369:580–3.
24. Serbinenko FA. Balloon catheterization and occlusion of major cerebral vessels. J Neurosurg. 1974;41:125–45.
25. Lewis AI, Tomsick TA, Tew JM Jr, et al. Long-term results in direct carotid-cavernous fistulas after treatment with detachable balloons. J Neurosurg. 1996;84:400–4.
26. Debrun G, Lacour P, Vinuela F, et al. Treatment of 54 traumatic carotid-cavernous fistulas. J Neurosurg. 1981;55:678–92.
27. Goldberg RA, Goldey SH, Duckwiler G, et al. Management of cavernous sinus-dural fistulas. Indications and techniques for primary embolization via the superior ophthalmic vein. Arch Ophthalmol. 1996;114:707–14.
28. Keltner JL, Satterfield D, Dublin AB, et al. Dural and carotid cavernous sinus fistulas. Diagnosis, management, and complications. Ophthalmology. 1987;94:1585–600.
29. Yoshida K, Melake M, Oishi H, et al. Transvenous embolization of dural carotid cavernous fistulas: a series of 44 consecutive patients. AJNR Am J Neuroradiol. 2010;31:651–5.
30. Morón FE, Klucznik RP, Mawad ME, et al. Endovascular treatment of high-flow carotid cavernous fistulas by stent-assisted coil placement. AJNR Am J Neuroradiol. 2005;26:1399–404.
31. Archondakis E, Pero G, Valvassori L, et al. Angiographic follow-up of traumatic carotid cavernous fistulas treated with endovascular stent graft placement. AJNR Am J Neuroradiol. 2007;28:342–7.
32. Wang C, Xie X, You C, et al. Placement of covered stents for the treatment of direct carotid cavernous fistulas. AJNR Am J Neuroradiol. 2009;30:1342–6.
33. Linskey ME, Sekhar LN, Hirsch W Jr, et al. Aneurysms of the intracavernous carotid artery: clinical presentation, radiographic features, and pathogenesis. Neurosurgery. 1990;26:71–9.
34. Kannoth S, Iyer R, Thomas SV, Furtado SV, Rajesh BJ, Kesavadas C, Radhakrishnan VV, Sarma PS. Intracranial infectious aneurysm: presentation, management and outcome. J Neurol Sci. 2007;256:3–9.
35. Wiebers DO, Whisnant JP, Huston J 3rd, For the International Study of Unruptured Intracranial Aneurysms Investigators, et al. Unruptured intracranial aneurysms: natural history, clinical outcome, and risks of surgical and endovascular treatment. Lancet. 2003;362:103–10.
36. Kupersmith MJ, Stiebel-Kalish H, Huna-Baron R, et al. Cavernous carotid aneurysms rarely cause subarachnoid hemorrhage or major neurologic morbidity. J Stroke Cerebrovasc Dis. 2002;11:9–14.
37. Linskey ME, Sekhar LN, Hirsch WL Jr, et al. Aneurysms of the intracavernous carotid artery: natural history and indications for treatment. Neurosurgery. 1990;26:933–7.
38. Tolosa E. Periarteritic lesions of the carotid siphon with the clinical features of a carotid infraclinoidal aneurysm. J Neurol Neurosurg Psychiatry. 1954;17:300–2.
39. Hunt WE, Meagher JN, Lefever HE, et al. Painful opthalmoplegia. Its relation to indolent inflammation of the carvernous sinus. Neurology. 1961;11:56–62.
40. Smith JL, Taxdal DS. Painful ophthalmoplegia. The Tolosa-Hunt syndrome. Am J Ophthalmol. 1966;61:1466–72.
41. The international classification of headache disorders. ICHD-II. Cephalalgia. 2004;24:131.
42. Hannerz J. Pain characteristics of painful ophthalmoplegia (the Tolosa-Hunt syndrome). Cephalalgia. 1985;5:103–6.
43. Gonzales GR. Pain in Tolosa-Hunt syndrome. J Pain Symptom Manag. 1998;16:199–204.
44. La Mantia L, Curone M, Rapoport AM, Bussone G. Tolosa-Hunt syndrome: critical literature review based on IHS 2004 criteria. Int Headache Soc Cephalalgia. 2006;26(7):772–81.
45. Colnaghi S, Versino M, Marchioni E, et al. ICHD-II diagnostic criteria for Tolosa-Hunt syndrome in idiopathic inflammatory syndromes of the orbit and/or the cavernous sinus. Cephalalgia. 2008;28:577–84.
46. de Arcaya AA, Cerezal L, Canga A, et al. Neuroimaging diagnosis of Tolosa-Hunt syndrome: MRI contribution. Headache. 1999;39:321–5.
47. Muhletaler CA, Gerlock AJ Jr. Orbital venography in painful ophthalmoplegia (Tolosa-Hunt syndrome). AJR Am J Roentgenol. 1979;133:31–4.
48. Goto Y, Goto I, Hosokawa S. Neurological and radiological studies in painful ophthalmoplegia: Tolosa-Hunt syndrome and orbital pseudotumour. J Neurol. 1989;236:448–51.
49. Curone M, Tullo V, Proietti-Cecchini A, et al. Painful ophthalmoplegia: a retrospective study of 23 cases. Neurol Sci. 2009;30:S133–1355.
50. Haque TL, Miki Y, Kashii S, et al. Dynamic MR imaging in Tolosa-Hunt syndrome. Eur J Radiol. 2004;51:209–17.
51. Hannerz J, Ericson K, Bergstrand G. A new etiology for visual impairment and chronic headache. The Tolosa-Hunt syndrome may be only one manifestation of venous vasculitis. Cephalalgia. 1986;6:59–63.
52. Foubert-Samier A, Sibon I, Maire JP, et al. Long-term cure of Tolosa-Hunt syndrome after low-dose focal radiotherapy. Headache. 2005;45:389–91.
53. Mormont E, Laloux P, Vauthier J, et al. Radiotherapy in a case of Tolosa-Hunt syndrome. Cephalalgia. 2000;20:931–3.
54. Furukawa Y, Yamaguchi W, Ito K, et al. The efficacy of radiation monotherapy for Tolosa-Hunt syndrome. J Neurol. 2010;257:288–90.
55. Hatton MP, Rubin PA, Foster CS. Successful treatment of idiopathic orbital inflammation with mycophenolate mofetil. Am J Ophthalmol. 2005;140:916–8.
56. O'Connor G, Hutchinson M. Tolosa-Hunt syndrome responsive to infliximab therapy. J Neurol. 2009;256:660–1.
57. Schafranski MD. Idiopathic orbital inflammatory disease successfully treated with rituximab. Clin Rheumatol. 2009;28:225–6.
58. Smith JR, Rosenbaum JT. A role for methotrexate in the management of non-infectious orbital inflammatory disease. Br J Ophthalmol. 2001;85:1220–4.
59. Förderreuther S, Straube A. The criteria of the International Headache Society for Tolosa-Hunt syndrome need to be revised. J Neurol. 1999;246:371–7.
60. Grove WE. Septic and aseptic types of thrombosis of the cavernous sinus. Arch Otolaryngol. 1936;24:29–50.
61. Yarington CT. The prognosis and treatment of cavernous sinus thrombosis. Review of 878 cases in the literature. Ann Otol Rhinol Laryngol. 1961;70:263–7.

62. Levine SR, Twyman RE, Gilman S. The role of anticoagulation in cavernous sinus thrombosis. Neurology. 1988;38:517–22.
63. Shaw RE. Cavernous sinus thrombophlebitis: a review. Br J Surg. 1952;40:40–8.
64. Schuknecht B, Simmen D, Yüksel C, et al. Tributary venosinus occlusion and septic cavernous sinus thrombosis: CT and MR findings. AJNR Am J Neuroradiol. 1998;19:617–26.
65. Choe CH, Trobe JD. Morning rounds: the potentially fatal red eye. EyeNet. 2009;13(3):69–71.
66. Southwick FS, Richardson EP Jr, Swartz MN. Septic thrombosis of the dural venous sinuses. Medicine (Baltimore). 1986;65:82–106.
67. Hargrove RN, Wesley RE, Klippenstein KA, et al. Indications for orbital exenteration in mucormycosis. Ophthal Plast Reconstr Surg. 2006;22:286–91.
68. Peterson KL, Wang M, Canalis RF. Rhinocerebral mucormycosis: evolution of the disease and treatment options. Laryngoscope. 1997;107:855–62.
69. Fleckner RA, Goldstein JH. Mucormycosis. Br J Ophthalmol. 1969;53:542–8.
70. Schwartz JN, Donnelly EH, Klintworth GK. Ocular and orbital phycomycosis. Surv Ophthalmol. 1977;22:3–28.
71. Blitzer A, Lawson W, Meyers BR, et al. Patient survival factors in paranasal sinus mucormycosis. Laryngoscope. 1980;90:635–48.
72. Yohai RA, Bullock JD, Aziz AA, et al. Survival factors in rhino-orbital-cerebral mucormycosis. Surv Ophthalmol. 1994;39:3–22.
73. Ferry AP. Cerebral mucormycosis (phycomycosis). Ocular findings and review of the literature. Surv Ophthalmol. 1961;6:1–24.
74. Ghadiali MT, Deckard NA, Farooq U, et al. Frozen-section biopsy analysis for acute invasive fungal rhinosinusitis. Otolaryngol Head Neck Surg. 2007;136:714–9.
75. Hofman V, Castillo L, Bétis F, et al. Usefulness of frozen section in rhinocerebral mucormycosis diagnosis and management. Pathology. 2003;35:212–6.
76. Langford JD, McCartney DL, Wang RC. Frozen section–guided surgical debridement for management of rhino-orbital mucormycosis. Am J Ophthalmol. 1997;124:265–7.
77. Songu M, Unlu HH, Gunhan K, et al. Orbital exenteration: a dilemma in mucormycosis presented with orbital apex syndrome. Am J Rhinol. 2008;22:98–103.
78. Kahana A, Lucarelli MJ. Use of radiopaque intraorbital catheter in the treatment of sino-orbito-cranial mucormycosis. Arch Ophthalmol. 2007;125:1714–5.
79. Price JC, Stevens DL. Hyperbaric oxygen in the treatment of rhinocerebral mucormycosis. Laryngoscope. 1980;90:737–47.
80. Marsh RJ, Cooper M. Double-masked trial of topical acyclovir and steroids in the treatment of herpes zoster ocular inflammation. Br J Ophthalmol. 1991;75:542–6.
81. Cobo LM, Foulks GN, Liesegang T, et al. Oral acyclovir in the therapy of acute herpes zoster ophthalmicus. An interim report. Ophthalmology. 1985;92:1574–83.
82. Whitley RJ, Weiss H, Gnann JW Jr, et al. Acyclovir with and without prednisone for the treatment of herpes zoster. A randomized, placebo-controlled trial. The National Institute of Allergy and Infectious Diseases Collaborative Antiviral Study Group. Ann Intern Med. 1996;125:376–83.
83. Wood MJ, Johnson RW, McKendrick MW, et al. A randomized trial of acyclovir for 7 days or 21 days with and without prednisolone for treatment of acute herpes zoster. N Engl J Med. 1994;330:896–900.

Methods for Obtaining and Processing Periocular Tissues for Pathologic Diagnosis

45

Irina V. Koreen and Victor M. Elner

Introduction

Pathologic analysis of ophthalmic specimens relies on the input of oculoplastic specialists who are thoroughly familiar with diseases affecting the periocular tissues, therapeutic modalities, and limitations of treatment. The implications of histopathologic findings can only be ascertained when important clinical information, including age, gender, size, location, predominant signs and symptoms, surgical findings, and extent of surgery, is known to the pathologist. These data are usually transmitted to the pathologist by the pathology request form, which should be completed carefully. When warranted by the complexity and importance of the tissue diagnosis, further direct consultation between the oculoplastic surgeon and the pathologist may be warranted to provide for needed special studies, including frozen section diagnoses during surgery.

The surgical pathologist, on the other hand, must be aware of the clinical implications of pathologic findings. Understanding the surgeon's needs allows the pathologist to respond to issues concerning biopsies and other surgically excised tissues. In considering a specimen, the pathologist must frequently embellish a simple histopathologic diagnosis to inform the surgeon concerning the extent of disease, the adequacy of excision, and the possible therapeutic options and prognostic features that can be gleaned from the pathologic examination of the excised tissue. Such information allows clinicians to correlate the pathologic and clinical findings, thereby contributing to their understanding of reasons for success or failure of therapy and the effects of therapy on normal periocular tissues. For the surgeon, mental preparation for cases, sometimes aided by consultation with the surgical pathologist, yields increased background of knowledge, recognition of specific gross pathologic features at surgery, and clear concepts of the pathogenesis of diseases, all of which will result in good judgment during surgery. With experience, integration of clinical findings with basic knowledge of disease processes allows clinicians to broaden their expertise, recognize those cases in which the pathologist may be of aid, and thereby enhance patient outcomes.

Resection and Handling of Pathologic Specimens

Classification of Pathologic Specimens

Biopsies may be classified in two major categories, incisional biopsy and excisional biopsy. An incisional biopsy consists of a portion of the lesion that is sampled for diagnosis. It is usually performed on large lesions or in regions near small vital structures. Shave biopsy, a type of incisional biopsy, should only be performed on lesions in which diagnostic changes are expected to be present in the epithelium of superficial connective tissue, including lesions such as molluscum contagiosum, seborrheic keratosis, nevus, and actinic keratosis. Curettage is also a type of incisional biopsy that usually yields only scanty material whose architecture is fragmented and distorted. This method, therefore, results in histopathologic material that is the least favorable for diagnosis. If curettage is performed, the best histopathologic material is obtained by a single stroke of the instrument.

Excisional biopsies include the lesion and a small rim of normal tissue. They are usually removed for both diagnostic and therapeutic purposes. They are routinely performed on small lesions when it is logical to resect the entire lesion.

I. V. Koreen (✉)
Eye Physicians of Orange County, P.C., Goshen, NY, USA

V. M. Elner
Eye Plastic and Orbital Surgery Service, Department of Ophthalmology and Visual Sciences, Kellogg Eye Center, University of Michigan, Ann Arbor, MI, USA
e-mail: velner@med.umich.edu

J. J. Servat et al. (eds.), *Smith and Nesi's Ophthalmic Plastic and Reconstructive Surgery*,
https://doi.org/10.1007/978-3-030-41720-8_45

Excisional biopsies are generally not performed on large lesions since the biopsy may disrupt and contaminate large regions of the superficial and deep tissue planes, potentially compromising later, otherwise curative, definitive excision.

In the case of orbital lesions, the decision whether to pursue an excisional or incisional biopsy is guided in part by the differential diagnosis based on the history, examination, and imaging studies. For example, if the preoperative evaluation is consistent with a diagnosis of pleomorphic adenoma XE "Pleomorphic adenoma", every effort should be made to perform an excisional biopsy as partial resection results in increased risk of tumor recurrence. A suspected cavernous hemangioma should also be treated with excisional biopsy. These types of lesions can be thought of as "surgical" orbital disease. However, tumors that are amenable to radiation therapy and/or chemotherapy, such as lymphoma and rhabdomyosarcoma, can be thought of as "medical" orbital disease. Although more complete excision may be beneficial, as in the case of rhabdomyosarcoma, these types of lesions do not require complete excision. The chief purpose of the biopsy is to establish a pathologic diagnosis so that a medical treatment plan can be instituted. Orbital tumors that are very large, that have known lymph node or distant organ metastases, and that appear to be metastatic to the orbit and suspected adenoid cystic carcinoma should also be biopsied using an incisional technique. Complete resection should be delayed until a histologic diagnosis is established, as it may be very disfiguring and without significant survival benefit.

Tissue specimens may also be classified according to the methods used in obtaining them (e.g., needle biopsy or endoscopic biopsy). Each of these techniques renders artifacts in the tissue, and it is important that the pathologist be informed of the type of technique used in obtaining the biopsy. Needle biopsy results in a thin core of tissue that, although small, allows for the preparation of histopathologic material that retains the morphologic architecture of the biopsied tissue. Its principal drawbacks include tumor seeding along the path of the needle, sampling error, and limited material for special pathologic techniques. Endoscopic biopsies are also limited in size, are frequently superficial, and commonly contain crush- and cautery-induced artifacts. Although these methods of tissue sampling in the orbit are not yet routinely used, there is widespread interest in developing less invasive techniques for orbital tissue sampling.

When excising tissue, care must be taken to modify the site, size, and orientation of the biopsy to obtain maximal pathologic material, provide an acceptable functional and cosmetic result, and avoid compromise of a possible subsequent curative surgical excision. In general, biopsy incisions should be as small as possible, have the most direct route to the lesion, and preserve as many tissue planes as possible.

Method of Excision and Handling of Pathologic Specimens

The best biopsy is a cleanly excised, uncrushed piece of tissue that includes the lesion and a small amount of surrounding normal tissue. The biopsy must be of adequate depth so that the normal margin is not included at the expense of representative portions of the lesion. This is especially challenging in the case of deep expanding lesions, particularly those of the orbit and optic nerve, that may form surrounding capsules or elicit hyperplasia of nonneoplastic reactive cells. Failure to obtain an adequately deep biopsy of these types of tumors results in sampling of surrounding normal reactive tissue. Although it may be technically difficult to obtain sufficiently large biopsies for diagnosis, there are instances in which the benefits of more extensive biopsies outweigh the risks of complications to the patient. For example, biopsies of suspected lymphoma should be large enough to provide sufficient tissue for studies such as immunohistochemistry and flow cytometry that would assist in determining the diagnosis. A full-thickness wedge resection of the lid may be required to diagnose sebaceous cell carcinoma in which the only clinical signs are persistent redness and loss of lashes at the lid margin. For suspected pleomorphic adenoma, the entire lesion should be excised en bloc to minimize risk of subsequent recurrence and malignant transformation. Larger biopsies also provide sufficient material for studies such as immunohistochemistry and electron microscopy that may assist in determining the diagnosis.

When excising tissue, the site, size, and orientation of the biopsy must be carefully planned to obtain maximal pathologic material, provide an acceptable functional and cosmetic result, and avoid compromise of a possible curative surgical excision. In general, biopsy incisions should be as small as possible, have the most direct route to the lesion, and preserve as many tissue planes as possible.

Biopsies of orbital lesions are particularly challenging due to the proximity of multiple vital structures that are susceptible to damage during dissection. Often, the best approach is to dissect along a tissue plane between the lesion and adjacent orbital structures and then excise the biopsy by cutting with a curved (e.g., No. 66) blade away from the orbital contents and toward the body orbital wall. This protects the adjacent structures from accidental injury due to poor visualization.

General guidelines in obtaining biopsies (Table 45.1), tailored to individual cases, should provide maximal information from the excised tissue.

Following resection, it is best to submit the fresh specimen immediately to the pathology laboratory in a container with-

Table 45.1 Guidelines for orbital biopsies

1.	Large lesions require several biopsies due to variability at different sites within the lesion
2.	In ulcerated lesions, it is best to biopsy the periphery, including normal and diseased tissue
3.	In partially necrotic lesions, avoid obtaining only the necrotic tissue
4.	The biopsy should extend deep enough into the lesion to obtain representative material, not only peripheral reactive tissue
5.	All tissue fragments should be submitted for microscopic examination since the smallest fragment may be the only one that contains diagnostic material
6.	Crushing or squeezing of tissue during the biopsy or subsequent processing must be avoided to prevent artifacts, rendering the biopsy uninterpretable
7.	The biopsy should be placed promptly into an adequate amount of fixative
8.	To avoid artifacts, the biopsy should not be manipulated or rinsed

Table 45.2 Special techniques in specimen processing

Special histochemical stains
Immunohistochemistry
Cytology
Imprints (touch preparations)
Electron microscopy
Molecular techniques
Enzyme histochemistry
Flow cytometry
Cytogenetics
Culture: bacterial, fungal, viral
Special fixation
Plastic embedding (e.g., bone lesions)
Photography and image processing
Radiography

out adding any fluid. If the specimen must be transported over a distance, desiccation can be avoided by placing the specimen on a Telfa pad moistened with physiologic saline solution. If specimen transport to the pathology laboratory may be delayed, it is best to refrigerate the specimen to reduce the rate of autolysis. Most small biopsies, however, should be placed in fixative immediately to prevent desiccation. The specimen should be handled both at the time of surgery and during pathologic processing with a minimum of trauma to avoid artifacts caused by cautery or by crushing with forceps. The surgeon does not have the prerogative to submit only portions of pathologic specimens but should send all the material so that the pathologist may examine it and select appropriate material for histopathologic assessment.

An advantage of having the specimen received in the pathology laboratory in the fresh state is that, based on the clinical diagnosis and gross pathologic features, special procedures other than routine formalin fixation and paraffin embedding may be initiated (Table 45.2). It should be recognized by both the clinician and the pathologist that routine processing of ophthalmic pathologic specimens may be insufficient to address adequately the probable pathologic diagnoses based on clinical and gross pathologic examination. For example, lymphoproliferative and poorly differentiated orbital lesions may require adjunctive immunohistochemistry for diagnosis. Adequate preoperative consultation with the pathologist and provision of accurate clinical signs, including the probable differential diagnosis, is the best method to allow the pathologist to exercise responsibility in obtaining such special studies when warranted.

Frozen Sections

Frozen sections should be requested when the information so obtained influences the course of the surgical procedure. It is inappropriate to use frozen sections to satisfy curiosity, recognize normal anatomic structures, or be able to render results immediately to the patient or relatives. Appropriate purposes of frozen section diagnosis include the following: (1) to establish the presence and nature of a lesion, (2) to determine the adequacy of surgical excision, and (3) to ascertain that the excised tissue contains diagnostic material. The surgeon must recognize, however, that the frozen sections may not answer any of the foregoing questions. In particular, a diagnosis frequently cannot be established on the frozen section material and must be deferred to interpretation of permanent sections. Given the information gleaned from the frozen sectioned material, the surgeon must decide whether to remove additional material or complete the surgery and wait for a diagnosis based on permanent sections. The surgeon must also recognize that it is wise, if not imperative, that definitive but mutilating surgical therapy be deferred until the final pathologic diagnosis and the possible treatment options are discussed with the patient.

Since frozen sections are used to help determine the extent of surgery, it is appropriate that the surgeon consult with the pathologist concerning the further surgical course. In this role, the pathologist should have knowledge of the clinical history and, in difficult cases, should have had the opportunity to discuss the case with the surgeon prior to surgery. Pathologists should be able to advise which area of the lesion is best to biopsy and to select for histopathologic examination the portion of the excised tissue that is most likely to demonstrate diagnostic microscopic features.

The Mohs technique, which originally involved tissue fixation prior to its excision from the patient, has evolved into a frozen section technique that involves tumor excision with microscopic examination of the surgical margins to ensure complete excision. In this technique, the Mohs surgeon also serves as pathologist and, being human, may not be impartial in microscopic interpretation of the specimens. The sections obtained using this technique may also be difficult to interpret since they are thick and frequently tangentially oriented, resulting in the distinct possibilities of false-positive or false-negative surgical margins. Nevertheless, this technique also has added the important concept of intraoperative histopathologic monitoring of surgical margins using frozen sections, a method that should be employed by all oculoplastic surgeons.

Tissue Fixation

Proper fixation of surgical specimens is an important step that allows preservation of tissue structure and cellular details upon which the histopathologic diagnosis rests. The most common fixative is a 4% phosphate buffer formaldehyde solution (formalin), which is inexpensive, maintains the tissue with minimal artifact, and is compatible with a variety of pathologic techniques. A ratio of approximately 10:1 of formalin to tissue (volume/volume) is necessary to ensure that an adequate concentration of fixative is present in the solution during fixation. This caveat should be observed by both the pathologist and clinician, the latter when submitting specimens placed in fixative immediately following excision.

Other special fixatives are also used in ophthalmic pathology. These include sublimate sodium acetate formalin (B-5) fixative, which contains mercury and is used for optimal preservation of lymphoproliferative lesions, and glutaraldehyde (1–4%) for electron microscopy.

When using any of these fixatives, it is important not only that an adequate volume of fixative be placed in the container harboring the specimen but also that it be placed in a container that allows the fixative to surround the specimen totally and from which the specimen can be removed easily without manipulation. Paper towels or gauze may be used to help wick the fixative around specimens, which have a tendency to either float or sink to the bottom of the container. Once placed in fixative, it is best for fixation to proceed either at room temperature or, in the case of very large specimens, in the refrigerator at 4 °C. Once in fixative, tissue should not be frozen since severe crystal artifacts, which are particularly severe with epithelium, may result. The rate of fixation for 4% buffered formaldehyde (formalin) is approximately 1 mm/h. More rapid fixation may be obtained by heating formalin to 60 °C or, with microwave ovens, by heating the specimen immersed in formalin to 65 °C. Fixation may be hastened in heated formalin solutions when rapid diagnosis is necessary to determine treatment or influence the course of further diagnostic testing.

Labeling of Pathologic Specimens and Completing the Pathology Request Form

The clinician and the pathologist complement each other in obtaining optimal gross pathologic examination of the specimen. It is imperative that all specimens be labeled with the patient's name, date of surgery, and site of excision. It is the responsibility of the surgeon to provide this information, and the surgeon or assistant should be prepared to be called to the laboratory to identify and label the specimen. It is also imperative that the surgical pathology request form contain the patient's name, age, gender, clinical history, type of surgery, and appropriate surgical findings. Again, the surgeon or an assistant must be prepared to provide this information on request prior to specimen processing. If such information is not forthcoming, the pathologist has the option to obtain the clinical record and even examine the patient personally prior to rendering an opinion on the pathologic material. If the pathologist has difficulty with specimen orientation, the surgeon should cooperate in identifying the orientation, surgical landmarks, and surgical margins to enable proper description and submission of material for histopathologic study (Fig. 45.1).

Processing of Pathologic Specimens

Gross Examination of Pathologic Specimens

The processing of a specimen includes gross pathologic examination of the tissue and histopathologic examination of samples derived from the gross specimen. When specimens are small, histopathologic assessment of the entire specimen is commonly performed. Nevertheless, the gross features of a pathologic specimen should not be overlooked since the overall structure of the lesion with respect to the surrounding tissues provides important pathologic clues and places the pathologic diagnosis within the appropriate clinical context. This is particularly true when examining whole eyes, exenteration specimens, and lesions involving bone. In these instances, a gross analysis is important for obtaining specimens for histopathologic examination that will render meaningful information. The gross pathologic examination, if not done adequately prior to further processing for histopathology, cannot be reconstructed, and the information is lost. Complex specimens are best examined and dissected by those with the knowledge and experience to describe and sample the specimen so that the tissue selected for histopathologic analysis provides optimal pathologic information.

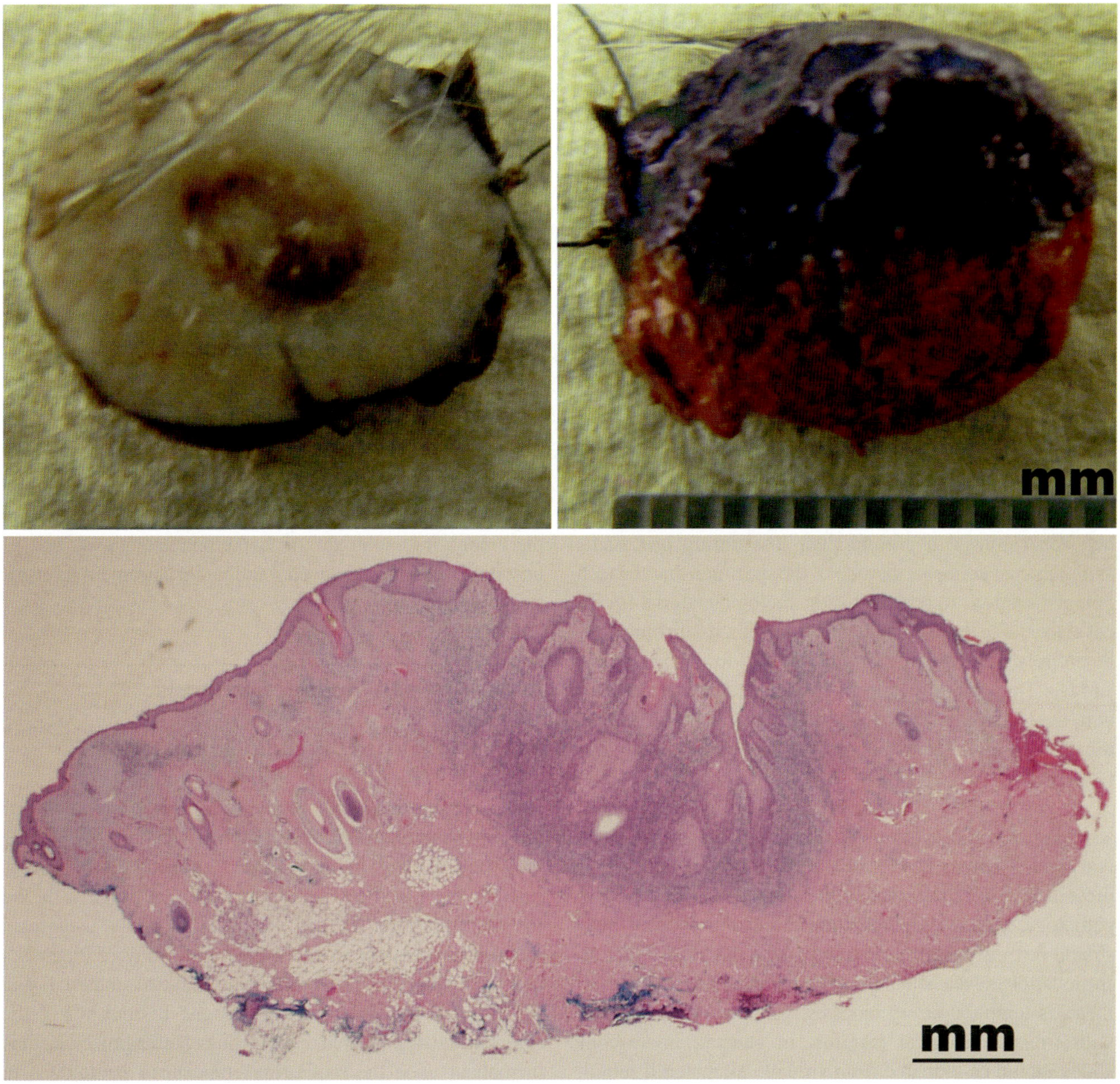

Fig. 45.1 Fixed, excised specimen from brow region oriented by suture placement (*upper left*), with entire cut surface inked superiorly with *blue* and inferiorly with *red* (*upper right*). One of several sequential vertical cross sections demonstrating squamous cell carcinoma with clear margins inked in *blue* and *red* (*bottom*)

Dissection of Pathologic Specimens

The decision of how to dissect the surgical specimen relies on the experience and knowledge of the pathologist. In most cases, large ophthalmic specimens, including whole eyes and exenterations, are best fixed en bloc, making it easier to section the specimen, which is rendered firmer by the fixative. Nonetheless, the specialized techniques that may be necessary for diagnosis may require dissection of the fresh specimen to provide portions for culture, electron microscopy, or immunohistochemistry. Other specimens require dissection with separate processing of portions, such as bone that requires decalcification prior to embedding, sectioning, and staining.

All portions of a specimen are retained until the case is finalized and a surgical pathology report is issued. Even in these cases, it is best to keep any residual wet tissue for at least 3 months, should further questions regarding the pathologic diagnosis arise. For complex specimens, gross photographs of the lesion as a permanent record cannot be overemphasized (Fig. 45.1). Such photographs, together with the gross description, provide permanent documentation and may be used to identify the sites of specimens obtained for histologic processing.

Particularly with respect to ophthalmic specimens, all pathologic material should be examined. Small tissue fragments may be left on sponges, or cotton-tipped applicators, or dried on the underside of the lid of the container. These fragments should all be submitted for histopathologic examination. It is important that the specimen be handled in an area free of tissue debris left from other specimens. The inclusion on histopathologic slides of material from other specimens may result in misdiagnoses that cannot be resolved other than by conjecture.

Sampling for histopathologic examination relies on the pathologist. For ophthalmic specimens, certain caveats are warranted. These specimens frequently are small fragments of tissue that must be wrapped in lens paper or placed between sponges to prevent their loss during processing. With larger specimens, the side of the specimen that the technologist sections to provide histopathologic material is critical since the features borne by one side of a tissue block may be entirely different from those obtained from the opposite surface. Thus, these specimens should be carefully reviewed with the technologist to obtain optimum orientation and histopathologic assessment of grossly observable pathologic features.

To ensure adequate histopathologic assessment, microscopic sections taken at various depths into the tissue embedded in paraffin may be required. If the processed specimen is presumed to contain a lesion that is not seen in the histopathologic slides, deeper sections from the paraffin block should be examined prior to rendering a diagnosis. Sections from various levels should also be examined for such specimens as temporal artery biopsies, whole eyes, and regions with irregular surgical margins. In general, microscopic slides should be prepared from virtually all material submitted for ophthalmic assessment, except for the calottes of routine whole eyes and portions of clinically and pathologically patently benign lesions. When systematic processing of gross ophthalmic pathologic material is not performed, histopathologic slides that are not representative or otherwise not interpretable frequently result.

Identification of Surgical Margins

In addition to describing the specimen as to shape, size, and type, it is also important to identify surgical margins so that the extent of the lesion, the completeness of excision, and the site of possible remaining lesion in the patient may be ascertained. It is therefore important that the surgical margins be accurately located with respect to their site in the living patient. It is also important at this stage to mark the surgical margins with dye (e.g., iodine, India ink) so that histopathologic assessment of the completeness of resection is based on the actual surgical margin of the gross specimen (Fig. 45.1). Prior to dissection of the specimen for processing, it may be helpful to obtain gross photographs. Usually, these consist of the external surface and, most importantly, of the cross section of the lesion.

Mishandling of Pathologic Specimens

Mishandling of specimens may result in tissue that is unsatisfactory for diagnosis or cause difficult-to-recognize artifacts in the cellular detail that may lead to incorrect histologic interpretation, including false-positive or false-negative diagnoses of malignancy. Common types of specimen mishandling include crush artifact, excessive cautery, drying, placement in hypotonic or hypertonic solutions, use of unsuitable fixatives, delayed fixation, or placement in insufficient volume of fixative.

Rendering a Pathologic Diagnosis

Review of Previous Pathologic Material

Prior to interpreting pathologic material, it is important that all previous pathologic material pertinent to the case be reviewed. Review of pathologic specimens from patients referred for treatment is important before surgery or the institution of other therapy that is based on the pathologic diagnosis. Such a practice ensures uniformity of diagnoses and comparison with subsequent surgical material and enables the clinicians and pathologist to understand the extent of the disease. When reviewing challenging cases, it is incumbent upon the requesting clinician or pathologist to have reviewed the clinical history for all pertinent information and intraoperative findings, obtain gross pathologic descriptions and all necessary microscopic slides, and review prior interpretations of the specimens. Furthermore, additional pathologic material in the form of wet or embedded tissue and tissue submitted for special studies (e.g., electron microscopy) should be available. Further clinical findings since the specimen was obtained may also be necessary to place the pathologic findings in the appropriate context.

Histopathologic Diagnosis

The pathologist is required to place the findings in context for the clinician. In situations in which there is a differential diagnosis, caveats concerning the diagnosis, the need for clarification of the diagnosis in the context of clinical findings, or an indication for further clinical testing or definitive treatment, it is important that the pathologist add a comment to the diagnosis lest a false impression be obtained from a brief statement of diagnosis alone. On the other hand, the pathologist should resist coercions of clinicians to extrapolate from inadequate material. The pathologist must also recognize that a diagnosis not be rendered on a disease process that he or she does not recognize, risking morbidity and possible mortality to the patient. Recognition of one's limitations is important so that appropriate expert consultation may be obtained for difficult cases. Prior to such consultation, the complete clinical history and all pathologic material, including the description and interpretation by the initiating pathologist, should be obtained so that patient care, consistency of diagnostic criteria, and self-education are maximized.

Limitations of Histologic Diagnosis

Although histologic examination of lesions is the most valuable technique used to arrive at a diagnosis in ophthalmic pathology, it has important inherent limitations. In many cases, the mere microscopic examination of a portion of tissue cannot, in itself, result in a definitive, well-substantiated diagnosis. Histopathologic findings are frequently only suggestive of a diagnosis or may be nonspecific, particularly in cases such as chronic or subacute inflammation, degenerative conditions, and fibrosing lesions. Conditions that cause difficulty in the diagnosis of neoplasms include lymphoma and reactive lymphoid hyperplasia, squamous cell carcinoma and pseudoepitheliomatous hyperplasia, and malignant melanoma and atypical nevus.

Thus, the pathologist can give the clinician the maximum information only if the specimen is accompanied by all relevant clinical information, including the clinical differential diagnosis. Incomplete clinical information may make an otherwise readily achievable diagnosis difficult, if not impossible. Diagnoses should not be given on small pieces of tissue from ill-defined sources and without clinical information because, even though the pathologist may arrive at the correct diagnosis, in many cases, the diagnosis may be wrong. Prior to biopsy, the clinician may gain valuable information from the pathologist concerning the biological nature of the lesion and the best way to sample it. In difficult diagnostic cases, the pathologist should even be consulted to examine the patient prior to or during surgery. The most meaningful histological material is obtained when the clinical history, physical findings, and exact orientation of the lesion in relation to surrounding anatomy are taken into account.

Issuing Pathology Reports

The surgical pathology report results from an ordered evaluation of the pathologic specimen and contains relevant clinical history, gross and microscopic findings, and the diagnosis. If necessary, a statement of the significance of the pathologic findings relevant to the clinical differential diagnosis, prognosis, or treatment, including recommendations for further clinical testing, may be appended.

The clinical history includes the age, sex, clinical and surgical findings, the type of surgery performed, and prior biopsies or surgeries pertinent to the specimen, including frozen sections at the time of surgery. The gross description is detailed since, except for photographs, it is the only record of the original gross features. Clear descriptions of the size and color of the specimen, including visible lesions, should be recorded in a factual and noninterpretive manner since the actual reasons underlying gross features may not be discernible by gross analysis. The gross description should indicate whether the specimen is fresh or fixed, whether it shows discernible artifact, and how it is submitted for microscopic examination. The microscopic description is optional since it may readily be reconstructed by reexamination of the histopathologic slides and, if necessary, should be brief and to the point.

The diagnosis portion of the report includes (1) the anatomic site, (2) the type of procedure, and (3) the pathologic diagnosis. The last portion of the pathology report is the comment section in which the pathologist may elaborate to the clinician important information such as the differential diagnosis, caveats concerning the pathologic interpretation of the specimen, prognostic and treatment considerations in light of the diagnosis, as well as recommendations for further testing. It is important that the diagnosis and comments be written as clearly as possible in the pathology report and that they be dictated at the time that verbal diagnosis and consultation are rendered to the surgeon since discrepancies may otherwise arise when the clinician interprets and transcribes this information to the chart. This rule pertains not only to permanent sections but also to frozen sections, the diagnosis of which should be recorded immediately. In the case of frozen sections, it is important to corroborate the frozen section diagnoses with the findings on permanent sections to ensure that correct information is conveyed to the clinician.

Medicolegal Considerations of Pathologic Specimens

The basis for medicolegal claims includes the following: (1) misdiagnosis due to misinterpretation of the histologic material, (2) oversight of the pathologic features in the specimen or failure to obtain diagnostic material due to insufficient sampling, and (3) poor wording of the pathologic diagnosis, resulting in misinterpretation by the clinician. Incorrect diagnoses are frequently made on the basis of misinterpretation of inadequate samples. In these cases, it is important for the pathologist to provide a disclaimer indicating that a more or less serious situation may underlie the process seen in the histopathologic material. The pathologist must also guard against inappropriate or inadequate sampling of tissue submitted for pathologic examination. This can be addressed by careful, thoughtful, methodical, and reproducible gross examination of specimens with the submission of adequate material for histopathologic analysis. Misdiagnosis based on histopathologic material is the responsibility of the pathologist, who should exercise the prerogative of consultation with other pathologists in ascertaining the correct diagnosis. To reduce misinterpretation of the diagnosis by clinicians, the pathologist may clarify the pathologic findings to the clinician based on the natural history of the disease and the implications of possible treatment. Although such advice is frequently welcomed by clinicians, the pathologist must keep in mind that the pathologic appearance, both gross and microscopic, is only one of many facts used to determine final clinical therapy. To assist in selecting treatment, the pathologist may also comment upon the difference in behavior of the tumor if left untreated or if treated with different therapies. The pathologist may even indicate a preference on the basis of prior experience and information provided by the clinician, but it is important to realize that the final decision rests with the clinician and the patient.

Special Techniques in Surgical Pathology

Special techniques include special histologic stains, immunohistochemistry, cytology, molecular techniques, and electron microscopy (Table 45.2). These additional methods are used to elucidate etiologic, histogenetic, and pathogenetic features germane to the pathologic diagnosis that cannot be ascertained solely on the basis of routine histopathology. Nevertheless, these studies are useful only when applied in selected cases and when correlated with the histopathologic findings of routinely processed material.

Special Histologic Stains

Special histologic stains are useful in the identification of cellular constituents, including glycogen, intracytoplasmic filaments, hemosiderin, lipid, and mucin (Table 45.3). They are also available in identifying extracellular materials such as elastic fibers, collagen, calcium, and amyloid. Infectious organisms (i.e., bacteria and fungi) may also be identified using special histopathologic stains.

Table 45.3 Special histopathologic stains

Stain	Target substance
Alcian blue	Mucin
Alizarin red	Calcium
Churukian-Schenk	Neurosecretory granules
Congo red	Amyloid
Fontana	Melanin
Giemsa	Bacteria, mast cells
Gomori methenamine silver	Fungi, protozoa
Gram	Bacteria
Oil red O	Neutral lipid
Periodic acid-Schiff (PAS)	Glycogen, basement membrane, mucin, fungi, tumor identification
Perls iron	Hemosiderin
Phosphotungstic acid-hematoxylin (PTAH)	Intracytoplasmic filaments of muscle and glial cells
Trichrome	Collagen, muscle
Verhoeff-van Gieson	Elastic fibers, elastotic degeneration
Warthin-Starry	Spirochetes, melanin
Weigert	Myelin
Ziehl-Neelsen, Fite	Acid-fast bacteria

Immunohistochemistry

Immunohistochemical techniques are an important adjunct in the armamentarium of the surgical pathologist. Immunofluorescence histochemistry provides optimal antigen preservation but is less sensitive than enzymatic techniques, relies on the availability of frozen material, and results in tissue preparations that are not permanent and that lack the morphologic detail present in routinely processed pathologic material. Nevertheless, immunofluorescence of frozen sections is the preferred technique to detect antibody complexes and complement components in the diagnosis of immune-mediated diseases such as cicatricial pemphigoid.

Immunoenzymatic techniques, on the other hand, are extremely sensitive and result in permanent staining that may be correlated and interpreted in the context of the morphologic features normally present in histopathologic material. Immunoenzymatic techniques are compatible with most fixatives, may be performed on routinely processed paraffin-embedded material, even after decalcification, and have been adapted to cytologic preparations. The most commonly utilized of these methods are peroxidase-antiperoxidase (PAP), alkaline phosphatase (AP), alkaline phosphatase-antialkaline phosphatase (APAAP), or avidin-biotin complex (ABC) techniques which are performed on frozen and paraffin sections to detect specific antigens for tumor diagnosis (Tables 45.4 and 45.5). In this role, immunohistochemistry has replaced many traditional histologic stains and has largely supplanted electron microscopy as the procedure of choice when tumors cannot be diagnosed on the basis of routine histopathologic material.

Immunohistochemical staining must be performed using meticulous technique and the proper positive and negative

Table 45.4 Immunohistochemical stains and their corresponding target substances

Antigens stained	Target substance
Chromogranin	Neuroendocrine cells
Cytokeratin	Epithelium Mesothelium Neuroendocrine cells
Desmin	Smooth and striated muscle
Epithelial membrane antigen (EMA)	Epithelium Meningiomas Perineural cells Plasma cells Lymphoma Sarcomas
Estrogen and progesterone receptor	Breast carcinoma
Factor VIII-associated antigen	Vascular endothelium Platelets Megakaryocytes
Glial fibrillary acidic protein (GFAP)	Astrocytes Oligodendrocytes Schwann cells Lacrimal, salivary, and sweat glands
HLA-DR antigens	Mononuclear phagocytes Lymphocytes Langerhans cells
HMB-45	Melanocytes
Immunoglobulin antigens	Plasmacytoma Multiple myeloma Lymphocytes
Leukocyte common antigen (LCA)	Leukocytes
Lymphocyte antigens	Subpopulations of lymphocytes to assist in differentiating lymphoma from reactive lymphoid hyperplasia
Myelin basic protein (MBP)	Schwann cells Granular cell tumors
Myoglobin	Rhabdomyosarcoma Tumors with teratoid elements
Myosin	Rhabdomyosarcoma Tumors with teratoid elements
Neurofilaments	Neuroblastoma Retinoblastoma Neuroendocrine cells
Neuron-specific enolase	Neuroendocrine cells Plasma cells Megakaryocytes Neuroblastoma
S-100 protein	Schwann cells Melanocytes Glial cells Chondrocytes Adipocytes Myoepithelial cells Langerhans cells Sweat glands Breast carcinoma Lung carcinoma
S-antigen	Retinoblastoma Pineal neoplasms

Table 45.4 (continued)

Antigens stained	Target substance
Vimentin	Vascular endothelium Fibroblasts Smooth muscle Chondroblasts Mesothelium Sarcomas Carcinomas (including breast, lung, and squamous)

Table 45.5 Suggested immunohistochemical stains for common and important rare neoplasms

Benign	
Idiopathic inflammatory pseudotumor[a]	n/a
Capillary hemangioma[a]	CD34, factor VIII, *Ulex europaeus* agglutinin, vimentin
Neurilemmoma[a]	Nerve growth factor receptor, S-100, vimentin, HMB-45
Lymphangioma[a]	D2-40 (podoplanin)
Cavernous hemangioma	n/a
Neurofibroma[a]	S-100
Osteoma[a]	n/a
Osteoblastoma	n/a
Lipoma	n/a
Fibroma	n/a
Ossifying fibroma	n/a
Leiomyoma	Smooth muscle actin, muscle-specific actin, desmin, vimentin
Granular cell myoblastoma	S-100, vimentin
Rhabdomyoma	n/a
Chondroma	n/a
Glomus tumor	Smooth muscle actin
Paraganglioma	Chromogranin, neuron-specific enolase, synaptophysin
Juvenile xanthogranuloma	CD68, factor XIIIa, negative S-100
Sinus histiocytosis	CD68, S-100
Teratoma	n/a
Lacrimal gland tumors	
Pleomorphic adenoma (benign mixed tumor)[a]	Cytokeratin, epithelial membrane antigen, smooth muscle actin, ±GFAP
Uncertain behavior	
Reactive lymphoid hyperplasia[a]	n/a
Optic nerve glioma[a]	GFAP, HNK-1, S-100, vimentin
Meningioma[a]	Epithelial membrane antigen, vimentin
Fibrous histiocytoma[a]	CD68, vimentin, α1-antitrypsin, *gene fusion (EWSR1)*
Solitary fibrous tumor	CD34, vimentin
Hemangiopericytoma[a]	CD34, CD99, vimentin, factor XIIIa
Langerhans cell histiocytosis	Leukocyte common antigen, CD1a, S-100
Plasmacytoma	IgG κ and λ chains
Lacrimal gland tumor	

(continued)

Table 45.5 (continued)

Benign lymphoepithelial lesion[a]	n/a
Malignant	
Lymphoma[a]	Leukocyte common antigen, CD3, CD20
Rhabdomyosarcoma[a]	Vimentin, desmin, muscle-specific actin, myoglobin, myosin, CK-M, myogenin, MyoD, *PAX7-FKHR and PAX3-FKHR rearrangements*
Granulocytic sarcoma	Myeloperoxidase, CD43
Multiple myeloma	IgG κ and λ chains
Malignant peripheral nerve sheath tumor	S-100, nerve growth factor receptor
Alveolar soft part sarcoma	TFE3 Ab, *fusion ASPSCR1-TFE3*
Malignant melanoma	S-100, HMB-45, vimentin
Osteosarcoma	Osteocalcin, CD99 (Ewing sarcoma), *translocations (many)*
Fibrosarcoma	Vimentin, *ETV6-NTRK3 translocation*
Leiomyosarcoma	Smooth muscle actin, muscle-specific actin, vimentin, desmin
Chondrosarcoma	S-100, CD99, NSE, CD57, *t(11;22) translocation*
Liposarcoma	S-100, *CHOP-TLS, and CHOP-EWS translocations*
Malignant glioma of optic nerve	GFAP, HNK-1, S-100, vimentin
Endodermal sinus tumor	Alpha fetoprotein
Extension of local tumor	
Paranasal sinus and nasal carcinoma[a]	Pan cytokeratin (AE1/AE3)
Angiosarcoma	CD31, CD34
Esthesioneuroblastoma	NSE, synaptophysin, chromogranin
Uveal melanoma	HMB-45, S-100
Retinoblastoma	NSE, synaptophysin
Eyelid and conjunctival carcinoma	Pan cytokeratin (AE1/AE3)
Retinal anlage tumor	Synaptophysin, NSE, PGP 9.5
Ameloblastoma	Cytokeratins
Metastatic tumor	
Carcinoma	Cytokeratins
Neuroblastoma	NSE, synaptophysin, chromogranin
Nephroblastoma (Wilms tumor)	Cytokeratins, EMA
Malignant melanoma	HMB-45, S-100
Sarcoma	Vimentin
Lacrimal gland tumor	
Adenoid cystic carcinoma[a]	Cytokeratin, EMA
Carcinoma ex pleomorphic adenoma	Cytokeratin, CEA, SMA
Mucoepidermoid carcinoma	Cytokeratin, mucin-type carbohydrate antigens (T, Tn, and syalosyl-Tn)
Poorly differentiated adenocarcinoma	Cytokeratin

[a]Common neoplasms

controls to produce interpretable results. Predigestion of tissue sections with trypsin, pepsin, or other enzymes may improve antibody reactivity with antigens, including those associated with cytoplasmic filaments, immunoglobulin, and factor VIII. The pattern and distribution of reactivity within tissue is an important criterion used to ascertain the specificity of immunohistochemical staining. Staining should correspond to the location of the antigen with which the antibody reacts. Thus, staining for HLA-DR or leukocyte common antigen should be visualized on the cell surface; for S-100 protein and certain lymphoid markers, within the cell nucleus and cytoplasm; and for factor VIII-associated antigen, cytokeratin, or desmin, only in the cell cytoplasm.

Immunohistochemistry is most useful when detecting antigens that are restricted in their cell distribution. For example, leukocyte common antigen and HMB-45 are highly specific for leukocytes and melanocytes, respectively, and may strongly support a histopathologic diagnosis. In contrast, antigens such as vimentin and neuron-specific enolase lack specificity and are not useful by themselves to indicate tumor cell histogenesis. Misinterpretation of positive staining may occur when using antibodies to specific antigens – such as neuron-specific enolase, S-100 protein, vimentin, or epithelial membrane antigen – that originally were thought to be restricted to certain cell types but actually are detectable in many cell types.

Immunohistochemical staining may be performed with either polyclonal or monoclonal antibodies. The main advantage of polyclonal antibodies is that they are composed of a heterogeneous population of antibodies, each reacting with a different antigen epitope, thereby resulting in enhanced immunohistochemical sensitivity. This is particularly helpful when some antigenic sites may have been altered or destroyed by tissue processing. The main disadvantage of polyclonal antibodies is their higher degree of cross-reactivity with epitopes that may be found on unrelated molecules, resulting in false-positive staining. Monoclonal antibodies, on the other hand, consist of a single antigenic epitope, thereby minimizing the possibility of false-positive staining due to binding to unrelated molecules. However, since they bind only to a single antigenic site, loss of antigenicity during tissue processing may produce a false-negative result. Monoclonal antibodies may still cross-react with unrelated antigens, but this is much less common than with polyclonal antibodies.

Regardless of the immunohistochemical technique used, there are a number of pitfalls at each stage of specimen processing and analysis that may result in false-positive or false-negative diagnoses. False-negative diagnoses may result from antigen destruction due to autolysis and inappropriate fixation. For example, formalin fixation destroys many surface markers and some cytoplasmic antigens. False-negative results may also be caused by the use of inappropriate, denatured, or suboptimal antibody concentrations; loss of antigen due to leaching from wet tissue; or seeking antigen that is present at levels below which the immunohistochemical technique is capable of detecting. These reasons for false-negative results indicate that such a result should not be used to eliminate a diagnosis if the other clinical and histopathologic features strongly suggest it. In addition to cross-reactivity of primary antibody with unrelated antigens, false-positive staining may result from nonspecific antibody binding, persistent endogenous peroxidase activity (when using a peroxidase technique), staining of entrapped normal tissue, diffuse staining due to release of soluble antigens that bind nonspecifically to cells and connective tissue, and staining of antigen released by some cells and engulfed by others.

Cytologic Techniques

Fine needle aspiration utilizes a fine needle to aspirate tumor cells that are then spread, fixed, and stained on a microscopic slide for cytologic examination. This technique is an inexpensive, rapid technique that is relatively atraumatic, has a low degree of morbidity, and does not seed tumor cells along the needle track. Its chief drawbacks of sampling error and providing limited pathologic material render it as an unlikely method to use for the definitive diagnosis of primary lesions as false-negative cytologic diagnoses may occur. Nevertheless, it may be useful in demonstrating local recurrence or metastasis of previously diagnosed neoplasms.

Imprints, or touch preparations, are cytologic preparations that are obtained by gently touching to a microscope slide the cross-sectioned surface of tissue suspected of harboring a lymphoproliferative or leukemic tumor. This technique requires very little tissue and allows cytologic examination of the nuclear and cytoplasmic features of the flattened leukocytes to assist in determining the leukocyte subsets and the relative proportions of the leukocyte subsets comprising the lesion. Cytologic material may also be subjected to adjunctive immunohistochemistry and electron microscopy to assist in establishing a diagnosis. Exfoliative cytology is highly reliable but is chiefly a research tool in ophthalmic pathology.

Electron Microscopy

Electron microscopy is most useful when it is used selectively to assist in distinguishing an entity from a limited differential diagnosis. The main applications of electron microscopy, from an orbital pathology standpoint, are for the diagnosis of tumors (Table 45.6). The principal differential diagnoses that may be resolved by ultrastructural examination are distinguishing among (1) carcinoma, melanoma, and sarcoma; (2) undifferentiated rhabdomyosarcoma, lymphoma, neuroendocrine tumors (e.g., neuroblastoma, oat cell carcinoma), and Ewing sarcoma; and (3) spindle cell tumors of soft tissues.

In this technique, representative pieces of tissue less than 1 mm thick should be carefully cut, fixed, and submitted with the expectation of looking for specific characteristics that will assist in formulating a final differential diagnosis. An experienced surgical pathologist reviews light microscopic material prepared from plastic-embedded tissue and selects small areas that are most likely to yield an ultrastructural diagnosis since only small sections may be examined in the electron microscope. These limited areas are then used to prepare thin sections that are mounted on metal grids and placed in the electron microscope for viewing. When diagnostic electron microscopic observations are made, they should be closely correlated with the histopathologic features to assist in formulating a diagnosis.

Table 45.6 Electron microscopic features of neoplasms

Neoplasm	EM feature
Neuroendocrine tumors	Dense-core granules
Neoplasms of cells with granular cytoplasm	Ultrastructural cytoplasmic inclusions (e.g., mitochondria in oncocytomas)
Adenocarcinomas	Glandular differentiation
Squamous cell carcinoma	Intermediate filaments, cytokeratin, desmosomes
Melanocytic neoplasms	Melanosomes
Langerhans cell (histiocytosis X) tumors	Birbeck granules
Vascular endothelial neoplasms	Weibel-Palade bodies
Neoplasms with muscle differentiation	Arrays of cytoplasmic intermediate filaments
Schwann cell tumors (neurilemmomas)	Mesaxons

Electron microscopy has several inherent limitations that restrict its use in routine surgical pathology: (1) it is extremely labor intensive and expensive, (2) it is subject to sampling error since only a small area of lesion can be studied, (3) it often lacks diagnostic specificity since only a few ultrastructural features are limited to certain types of cells, (4) it is limited in distinguishing neoplastic from nonneoplastic and benign from malignant, and (5) it is subject to interpretive error since observations made at such high magnification are difficult to place in the overall context of the lesion and misdiagnosis can occur on the basis of entrapped reactive or normal tissue. Although electron microscopy is still occasionally used, its utility has largely been supplanted by the development of numerous immunohistochemical and molecular techniques.

Although ultrastructural evaluation depends on good fixation of fresh tissue, some diagnostic features, such as the dense-core granules of neuroendocrine tumors, may be identified despite artifacts due to poor fixation or processing in paraffin. When wet formalin-fixed tissue is available, it is best to sample from the periphery of the tissue since this region is likely to be fixed the best. If wet tissue is not available, the paraffin block may be retrieved and the tissue deparaffinized and reprocessed for salvageable ultrastructural characteristics.

Molecular Techniques

Detection of specific genes within the cells relies on the hybridization of enzyme or radiolabeled DNA or RNA probes of specific nucleic acid sequences that are complementary to cellular genetic sequences that may be amplified in vitro. This hybridization may be performed on electrophoretically separated nucleic acids extracted from tissue or directly by in situ hybridization on tissue sections or cells. In situ hybridization allows direct correlation of the detected sequence to the morphologic appearance of the tissue or cell. Hybridization techniques have been employed to detect gene sequences of bacteria and viruses, including herpesvirus and cytomegalovirus in infected cells.

Hybridization techniques are now routinely used to detect gene rearrangements in lymphoproliferative diseases and to demonstrate the histogenesis of endocrine tumors by demonstrating gene expression of specific secretory products.

Cytogenetics

Cytogenetics involves the analysis of structural alterations of chromosomes, including translocations, deletions, or duplications of regions that contain oncogenes that regulate cell growth, development, and differentiation. Qualitative or quantitative alterations in the expression of oncogenes have been shown in a variety of neoplasms and are believed to underlie neoplastic transformation. Examples of ophthalmic tumors with genetic alterations include rhabdomyosarcoma, retinoblastoma, and uveal malignant melanoma. Chromosomal analysis of tumors often requires culture of tumor cells from fresh specimens, followed by fixation and staining (banding) of chromosomes prior to cytogenetic analysis.

Analysis of gene translocations is imperative for the diagnosis and prognostic analysis of lymphomas and sarcomas. Certain tumors are now defined by their gene translocations in addition to histopathologic features. Examples include alveolar subtype of rhabdomyosarcoma, alveolar soft part sarcoma, fibrosarcoma, and Ewing sarcoma. Furthermore, DNA content (i.e., aneuploidy) is a prognostic factor for rhabdomyosarcoma and neuroblastoma.

Flow Cytometry

Flow cytometry is an objective, reproducible, and sensitive technique that provides quantitative assessment of cell populations comprising a tumor. Computer analysis of laser light scattered by cells in suspension allows assessment of such cell features as size, viability, DNA content, surface and cytoplasmic markers, and enzyme content. This technique is particularly useful in analyzing leukemia and lymphoid tumors, the cells of which are easily dispersed, reactive with various fluorescently labeled monoclonal antibodies, and separated by flow cytometry to yield a histogram showing cell sizes and their clonality. In fact, most lymphomas are diagnosed on the basis of flow cytometry.

DNA-binding fluorescent dyes may also be used for flow cytometry of cells isolated from fresh, fixed, or even paraffin-embedded neoplasms to produce histograms that demonstrate the presence of aneuploid cells that correlate with malignancy and tumor aggressiveness. Such flow cytometry studies are useful to support histopathologic diagnoses and assist in determining tumor classification, response to treatment, and relapse.

Other Special Techniques

Enzyme immunohistochemistry may be used diagnostically in the study of myopathies as well as in the identification of different types of leukocytes within tissues and blood smears.

Plastic embedding is used to preserve the architecture of brittle tissues, such as bone, and to provide extremely thin tissue sections that best demonstrate cellular detail in applications such as the histologic examination of bone marrow or poorly differentiated round cell tumors.

Image processing of histopathologic material provides quantitation of lesion thickness, cross-sectional area, and volume. It may also be used in conjunction with other techniques, such as immunohistochemistry, to quantitate the relative proportions of cell types present in lesions. It is an adjunctive tool that may be used to assess prognostic features of lesions.

Radiographic study of ophthalmic tissues is used to identify metallic foreign bodies and calcification that may occur in lesions such as retinoblastoma and phthisis bulbi.

Conclusion

The successful excision, processing, and evaluation of ophthalmic pathologic specimens involve complex, ordered methods involving the coordinated efforts of surgeons, pathologists, and technical staff. At each step in this sequence, there are numerous pitfalls that may compromise the ability to obtain the correct diagnosis and adversely affect patient outcome (Table 45.7). Each person should strive to understand and avoid those pitfalls that fall within his or her realm of responsibility.

Table 45.7 Prevention of pitfalls in ophthalmic pathology

Preoperative assessment
Failure to obtain complete history (e.g., rapidity of onset, unilateral versus bilateral)
Failure to recognize genetic abnormalities or characteristic syndromes (e.g., neurofibromatosis, Goldenhar syndrome)
Failure to recognize extent of disease
Failure to recognize radiologic findings (e.g., bone erosion, margins)
Failure to recognize differential diagnosis
Failure to obtain slides of prior biopsy or resection
Failure to alert pathologist for special pathologic processing techniques
Failure to culture lesion if it may be infectious
Failure to plan to obtain frozen sections for diagnosis or to assess completeness of excision
Failure to consult with the pathologist to view the patient in difficult or unusual cases
Failure to clarify the reason for pathologic consultation (e.g., surgical margins, type of lesion)
Intraoperative and perioperative specimen handling
Failure to recognize features and extent of lesion
Failure to modify biopsy technique to obtain maximal pathologic material and acceptable functional and cosmetic result
Inadequate or nonrepresentative biopsy
Incisional biopsy of lesions requiring excision (e.g., benign mixed tumor of lacrimal gland)
Failure to obtain multiple or map biopsies for diffuse disease (e.g., melanosis, sebaceous carcinoma)
Failure to consult with pathologist intraoperatively
Failure to submit frozen sections
Inappropriate treatment following frozen section diagnosis (e.g., immediate exenteration for adenoid cystic carcinoma before study of permanent sections)
Failure to orient or mark specimens
Traumatic specimen handling resulting in artifacts (e.g., crush, cautery)
Drying artifacts
Inadequate fixation
Failure to complete surgical request form that conveys information to the pathologist
Failure to provide diagrams for complex specimens
Postoperative assessment
Failure to submit representative tissue for histopathologic examination
Failure to obtain needed special studies of pathologic material
Overinterpretation of inadequate material
Misdiagnosis of histopathologic material
Failure to provide differential diagnosis
Failure to obtain pathologic consultation of experts in difficult cases
Failure to issue a clear surgical diagnosis
Lack of clinicopathologic correlation
Failure to correlate pathologic diagnosis with options for treatment or further diagnostic testing
Failure to recognize systemic manifestations associated with the pathologic diagnosis

Suggested Reading

1. Enzinger FM, Weiss SW. Soft tissue tumors. CV Mosby: St. Louis; 1988.
2. Lever WF, Schaumbrug-Lever G. Histopathology of the skin. Philadelphia: JB Lippincott; 1983.
3. Mikel UV. AFIP advance laboratory methods in histology and pathology. Washington, DC: ARP Press; 1994.
4. Prophet EB, Mills B, Arrington JB, Sobin LH. AFIP laboratory methods in histotechnology. Washington, DC: ARP Press; 1992.
5. Rosai J. Ackerman's surgical pathology. CV Mosby: St. Louis; 1989.

Surgical Approaches to the Orbit and Optic Nerve

46

Ayelet Priel, Sang-Rog Oh, Don O. Kikkawa, and Bobby S. Korn

Introduction

In 1888, Kronlein introduced the concept of lateral orbital rim removal to access deep orbital lesions. While this approach is still employed to this day, today's aesthetically oriented orbital surgeon has a myriad of new minimally invasive techniques in their armamentarium. Orbital imaging continues to improve with more sensitive and higher-resolution computed tomography (CT) and magnetic resonance imaging (MRI) scanning technologies. Multidisciplinary collaborations have facilitated newer surgical approaches through the sinuses and transcranial routes. Technological advancements in the instrumentation of today's orbital surgeon have also improved in the 15 years since the last edition of this chapter. Finally, advances in anesthesia techniques have allowed more cases to be performed in an outpatient setting with less sedation.

Preoperative Assessment

Age and Race

Patient age is an important factor in the surgeon's decision-making. An infant's orbital structure is softer than the adult one, allowing the use of different instrumentation if the bone needs to be cut. The infant orbit is also shallow and allows easier access to deep lesions, if necessary, through skin or conjunctival incisions. Particular caution should be exercised to maximize aesthetic outcomes to minimize social factors in a child's development. Surgical wounds should be meticulously reapproximated to reduce scarring of the skin and conjunctival symblepharon formation, which form more exuberantly in younger patients.

Older patients present different considerations. With increasing age, tissues become more lax and fragile. While this increased laxity allows for creation of smaller incisions and greater surgical access, there is a higher tendency for bleeding and postoperative eyelid malpositions. Attention should be paid toward deficiency of the anterior lamella and addressing any eyelid laxity at the time of surgery. Past medical history should be reviewed to understand the immune status of the patient, tendency to bleed, and risks in general anesthesia. Diseases affecting wound healing, such as diabetes, should be taken into consideration when deciding on wound closure and to avoid dehiscence. The shape of the cranium, contour, and bone thickness are influenced by racial characteristics. These differences are well demonstrated in different imaging techniques and may influence decision-making in terms of approach and bone removal.

Patients of Asian descent and those with darker skin are more prone to develop hyperpigmentation, hypertrophic scars, and keloid. If possible, a conjunctival approach should be considered. The use of perioperative antibiotics should be considered in cases with infected sinuses and patients at risk for valvular heart disease.

Use of Anticoagulants

The patient's coagulation status, bleeding history, clotting parameters, and use of any anticoagulants need to be assessed and adjusted to minimize the risk of intraoperative or

A. Priel (✉)
Division of Oculopfacial Plastic and Reconstructive Surgery, Goldschleger Eye Institute, Sheba Medical Center, Ramat Oan, Israel

Sackler School of Medicine, Tel Aviv University, Tel Aviv, Israel

S.-R. Oh
Division of Oculofacial Plastic and Reconstructive Surgery Department of Ophthalmology The Permanente Medical Group, Sacramento, CA, USA

D. O. Kikkawa
Division of Oculofacial Plastic Surgery, Viterbi Family Department of Ophthalmology Shiley Eye Institute University of California San Diego School of Medicine, La Jolla, CA, USA

B. S. Korn
Division of Oculofacial Plastic Surgery, Viterbi Family Department of Ophthalmology Shiley Eye Institute University of California San Diego School of Medicine, La Jolla, CA, USA

J. J. Servat et al. (eds.), *Smith and Nesi's Ophthalmic Plastic and Reconstructive Surgery*,
https://doi.org/10.1007/978-3-030-41720-8_46

postoperative bleeding. Dietary supplements and certain ethnic foods contain endogenous anticoagulants, and these should be ascertained prior to surgery. The more widespread and prolonged use of newer antiplatelet medications, such as clopidogrel, should also be inquired during the preoperative assessment. Up-to-date bleeding profiles should be performed in any patient taking warfarin. Cessation of any anticoagulant must be performed with consent of the primary care physician or cardiologist. The renewal of these medications should likewise be done under supervision of the primary care physician. Consideration of preoperative type and cross-matching of blood should be performed in patients with extreme tendency to bleed.

Imaging

Orbital surgery of any kind requires preoperative planning. Orbital imaging has become a cornerstone in the preoperative assessment. CT and MRI have replaced plain film X-rays as the standard of care. The advantages of CT imaging include visualizing bony structures, including fractures, erosion of bone due to malignant tumors, and calcifications and rapid identification of hemorrhage. CT is contraindicated in pregnant patients. If there is suspicion of ferromagnetic implants or foreign bodies, CT is the modality of choice. At the time of this chapter's composition, the use of CT imaging in children is controversial secondary to the radiation risk.

MRI is the favored modality for assessing apical tumors and identifying soft tissue structures. The surface characteristics and imaging contour of a lesion can determine the surgical approach. Many studies have described the different imaging characteristics between malignant and benign tumors. A malignant process can be suspected when a lesion has an irregular shape or is diffuse in nature, molding around normal orbital structures, has perineural involvement, and shows evidence of bony erosion. Features such as oval shape, hyperostosis, hyperintensity on T2, and hyperdensity or hypodensity on CT are likely to characterize benign tumors.

Ultrasound imaging can be used as an adjunctive modality to CT and MRI. It is especially useful with children since it is easily performed, requires a simple setup, and does not typically require sedation. Ultrasound can add to other imaging modalities in specific cases such as assessing flow in capillary hemangiomas.

Anesthesia and Positioning

Orbital surgery may be performed under local or general anesthesia. Biopsy of anteriorly palpable orbital lesions can generally be performed under local anesthesia. All deep orbital lesions and any bone manipulations should be done under general anesthesia.

Local anesthesia is obtained by infiltration with 2% lidocaine and 1:200,000 epinephrine mixed with an equal part of 0.75% bupivacaine. In cases of local anesthesia with monitored care, the prior instillation of opioid minimizes the sneeze reflex commonly seen after propofol sedation and periocular injection. The local anesthetic is given at least 10 min before preparing for surgery to allow time for maximal vasoconstriction. Additional blocks of the supratrochlear, supraorbital, lacrimal, and infraorbital nerves may be needed for extensive dissection or when the periosteum is involved. IV sedation is used throughout the procedure. The agents employed will depend on the patient's medical status and the preference of the anesthesiologist. Inhalation of a NO/O_2 mixture for 2 min before injection will minimize the sting of local anesthetic agents. If the procedure involves entry into the nasal cavity or sinus, packing of the nose should be done with cocaine or lidocaine and a nasal decongestant. General anesthesia with controlled hypotension is indicated in most patients. Lowering of blood pressure, combined with slight elevation of the head, will decrease operative bleeding and improve operative exposure in the orbital apex.

Instrumentation

Orbital surgery instruments are culled from the ophthalmic, otolaryngologic, and neurosurgical world. The instruments need to be delicate and lengthy to reach deep orbital tissues. The instruments that provide specific needs in orbital surgery are discussed below.

Retractors

Visualization within the tight confines of the orbit is essential for optimal outcomes. A variety of retractors are utilized in orbital surgery. Senn and Desmarres retractors are used for skin and eyelid margin retraction (Fig. 46.1a). The Senn retractor has an extended reach compared to the Desmarres and provides deeper retraction. The curved face of the Desmarres retractor minimizes trauma to the eyelid and is useful for retraction of the lower eyelid for inferior orbitotomy approaches. Silk traction sutures can be placed as needed for further exposure. Malleable retractors of various widths can be bent to shape and used for retraction in the orbit (Fig. 46.1b). Often, prolapse of orbital fat obscures visualization in the orbit. Neurosurgical cottonoids can be placed against the malleable retractor to provide additional retraction of orbital fat (Fig. 46.1c, d).

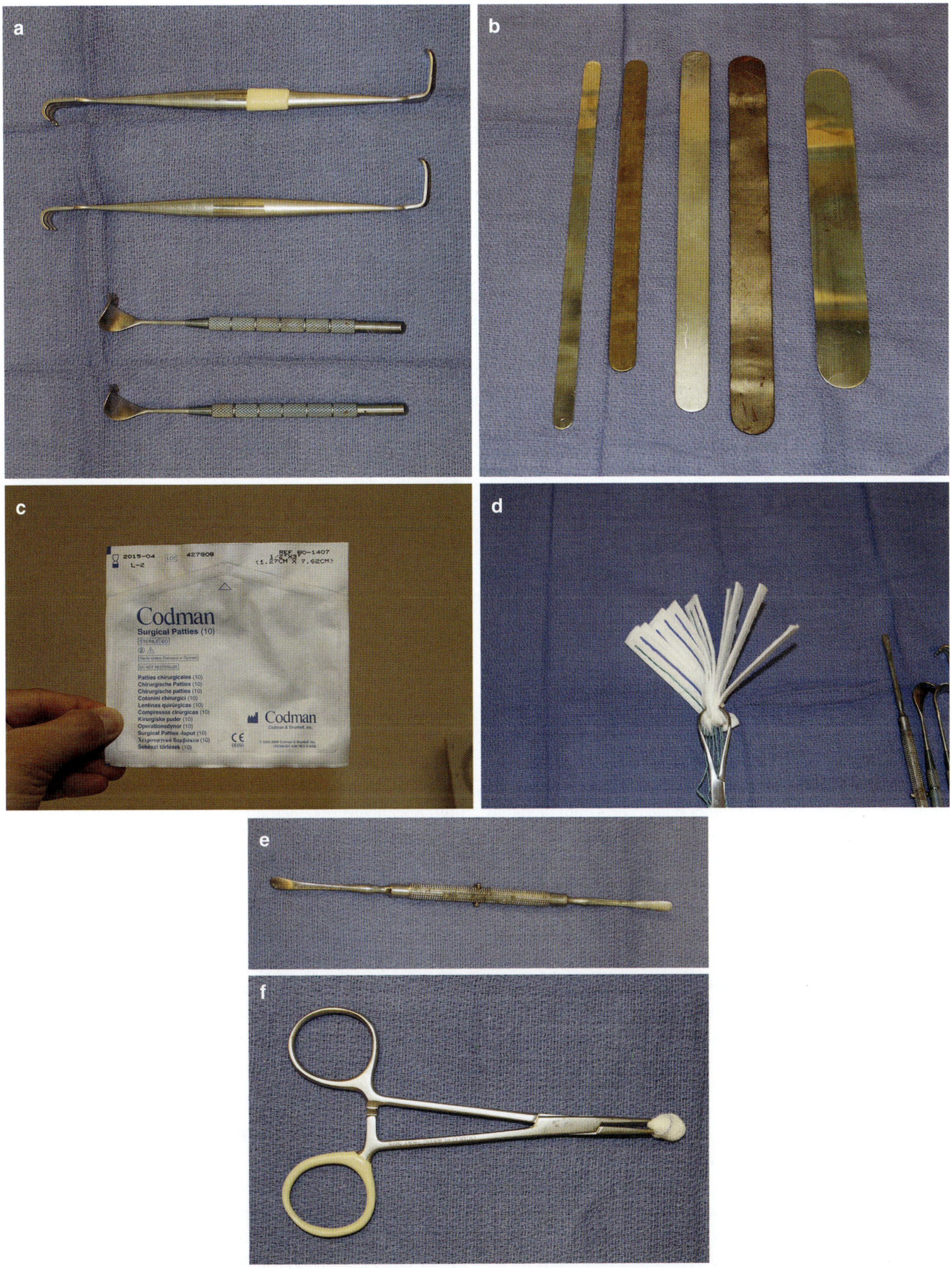

Fig. 46.1 (**a**) Various sizes of Senn (*top*) and Desmarres (*bottom*) retractors useful for orbital exposure. (**b**) Various sizes of malleable retractors used for retraction in the orbit. (**c**, **d**) Neurosurgical cottonoids useful for retraction of orbital fat. (**e**) Freer periosteal elevator with sharp and blunt ends. (**f**) Peanut sponge attached to hemostat clamp (Courtesy of Dr. Arkadi Yakirevitch)

Periosteal Elevator

A variety of sizes of periosteal elevators can be utilized during orbital surgery. Figure 46.1e shows a Freer periosteal elevator which has a blunt and sharp dissecting edge. This instrument provides delicate separation of bone from the periosteum and can also be used to dissect normal orbital structures from pathologic lesions. Two Freer elevators can be simultaneously used to perform dissection through orbital tissues with one elevator providing countertraction, while the other elevator is used for blunt dissection.

Other Dissectors

The dissection in orbital surgery is typically blunt with the goal of keeping a bloodless field. The main goal in keeping a bloodless field is to improve exposure and visualization. A good dissection can help the surgeon identify the anatomical and pathological structures, and that can also shorten the operating time and the length of general anesthesia. The surgeon can use microdissecting instruments, cotton applicators, or peanut sponges for blunt dissection (Fig. 46.1f).

Drills

Bone cutting instruments are used to facilitate bone dissection, reconstruction, and decompression. High-speed bone cutting instruments are used frequently in orbital surgery. Drills are used to sculpt bones or to create tunnels to stabilize the bone with screws, sutures, or implants. The diamond-tipped burr is well suited to sculpt bone. The 4-mm diamond tip is useful during bony decompression as the high speeds (>40,000 rpm) cause thermal coagulation of marrow bleeding, particularly in the deep lateral orbit. When performing any drilling during orbital surgery, caution should be exerted to avoid collateral damage to the surrounding skin, globe, and orbital tissues. Placement of a corneal protector is an absolute requirement in all cases. Malleable retractors should be used to isolate the globe, and frequent saline irrigation is used to dissipate heat generated during drilling.

Endoscope

The use of rigid endoscopes has become an integral part of orbital surgery, especially when approaching through or to the nasal cavity. The endoscope allows a smaller dissection, with better viewing in the deep orbit. The endoscopes are available in different width and several angulations, from 0° to 90°. High-definition video attachment allows good-quality filming for documentation and teaching purposes.

Cryoprobe

The cryoprobe is a useful tool during orbital surgery. It allows stabilization of a mass in the deep orbit, while other dissectors are used to separate the lesion from the surrounding structures. Both the straight- and side-tip probes can be used depending on the location within the orbit. The surgeon freezes the cryoprobe to the mass and dissects it in a "rolling" technique by manipulating it slowly from its surrounding. The use of cryoprobes has been described for benign, encapsulated, or pseudo-encapsulated tumors such as cavernous hemangioma or neuroma.

Image Guidance Procedures

Intraoperative use of image-guided navigation and interactive application of 3D images has been recently acknowledged by orbital surgeons. In orbital fractures, by matching the contours of the mobile segment with the preoperative plan, computer-assisted navigation can be used to guide fracture reduction. In past years, case reports have been published regarding image guidance orbital procedures for removal of deep orbital foreign bodies, mucoceles, and other masses. Future technical developments will likely improve the application of this modality during orbital surgery.

Biopsy Techniques

Orbital biopsy is performed for suspicious lesions, with the goal of obtaining adequate tissue for histologic identification. Specimens obtained during orbital biopsy can be scant and must be treated with exquisite care. Most specimens from excisional and incisional biopsies can be evaluated with conventional stains such as hematoxylin and eosin (H&E) after formalin fixation, but certain specimens should be submitted "fresh" for preservation of cellular epitopes when antibody-based assays are to be used. Hence, these samples should be placed in normal saline instead of fixatives. Communication with the pathologist prior to the biopsy should be performed when there are any concerns about histologic studies.

Fine-Needle Aspiration Biopsy

The use of fine-needle aspiration biopsy in the diagnosis of orbital tumors was introduced in Sweden in 1975. Eligible patients include those with deep orbital lesions not amenable to resection or poor candidates for general anesthesia and wide incision for biopsy. The greatest value of fine-needle aspiration biopsy appears to be in patients with known metastatic disease and a deep orbital lesion suspected of being metastatic. Fine-needle aspiration biopsy can confirm the diagnosis with minimal morbidity and, in some cases, can help the oncologist plan for radiation therapy, chemotherapy, or ablative endocrine therapy. Its use has also been advocated to differentiate meningiomas from low-grade and malignant astrocytomas in patients with optic nerve tumors and blind eyes. In many cases, however, these lesions can be diagnosed by clinical history and CT imaging. Fine-needle aspiration can also be used for muscle biopsies in the orbit. The diagnostic accuracy of fine-needle aspiration biopsy is dependent on the cytopathologist interpreting the material. In skilled hands, there is a diagnostic accuracy of up to 92%.

The technique involves the use of a 22–23-gauge disposable needle on a 20-mL syringe. A needle is introduced into the mass and aspiration is applied. The needle is moved back and forth, producing a cutting action under pressure. Biopsies of intraconal lesions can be performed under simultaneous CT or ultrasonic image guidance. The procedure can be performed under either general or local anesthesia. The needle aspirate is placed on a frosted slide, quickly fixed in 95% alcohol, and stained according to Papanicolaou's technique. The main complications of fine-needle aspiration biopsy are globe perforation, orbital hematoma, and optic nerve injury.

Excisional Biopsy

Excisional biopsy refers to total surgical removal of a mass lesion. This technique typically offers a large tissue sample, with the possibility of defining surgical margins, determining whether the lesion was fully excised, and verifying the presence of a capsule or pseudo-capsule surrounding the lesion. In orbital surgery, excisional biopsies are typically performed for lesions which appear well circumscribed on orbital imaging, such as cavernous hemangioma, hemangiopericytoma, fibrous histiocytoma, or schwannoma.

Incisional Biopsy

An incisional biopsy is partial tissue excision of a mass lesion for histopathologic study without complete removal of the mass. The surgeon should be confident that the amount and quality of the biopsy represent the clinically abnormal tissue. The surgeon must also take care to maintain the gross architecture of the tissue without crushing it or using excess cautery. Fragile tumors such as lymphomas and mesenchymal tumors should be handled delicately, especially when using forceps. Incisional biopsy can be used for muscle biopsies, any diffuse orbital mass, and lesions suspicious for lymphoma. For encapsulated lesions of the lacrimal gland, complete excisional removal with capsular integrity is advocated.

Anterior Orbitotomy

Anterior orbital lesions may be accessed through a transconjunctival or transcutaneous approach. The optimal approach depends on multiple factors including the location of the lesion, history of prior surgery, and status of the anterior lamella and conjunctiva. The incision and approach to the orbit should provide adequate exposure for best visualization and safe manipulation of orbital tissues. The approach should be chosen to minimize collateral damage and to maximize cosmesis.

Superior Orbital Lesions: Transcutaneous Approach

The transcutaneous route is the preferred approach for lesions situated in the anterior and superior orbit (Fig. 46.2a). For lesions located in the subperiosteal space, the dissection plane can be performed along the orbital septum and superiorly to the arcus marginalis while keeping the orbital septum intact. Meticulous care should be taken to avoid damage to the levator, superior oblique muscle, trochlea, lacrimal gland, and sensory nerves and vasculature along the superior orbital rim. Alternatively, the orbital septum can be opened superior

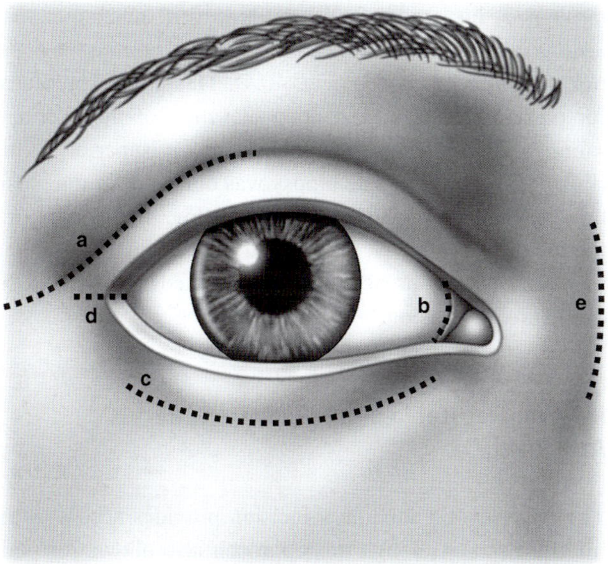

Fig. 46.2 Sites of surgical entry into the orbit. (**a**) Upper eyelid crease. (**b**) Transcaruncular. (**c**) Inferior transconjunctival. (**d**) Lateral canthotomy. (**e**) Frontoethmoidal (Lynch) (remark – not for print) ((**c**) is the *broken line* in the lower lid; (**d**) is the small canthotomy; (**e**) is Lynch drawn vertically between the medial canthus and the bridge of the nose) (Courtesy of Dr. Arkadi Yakirevitch)

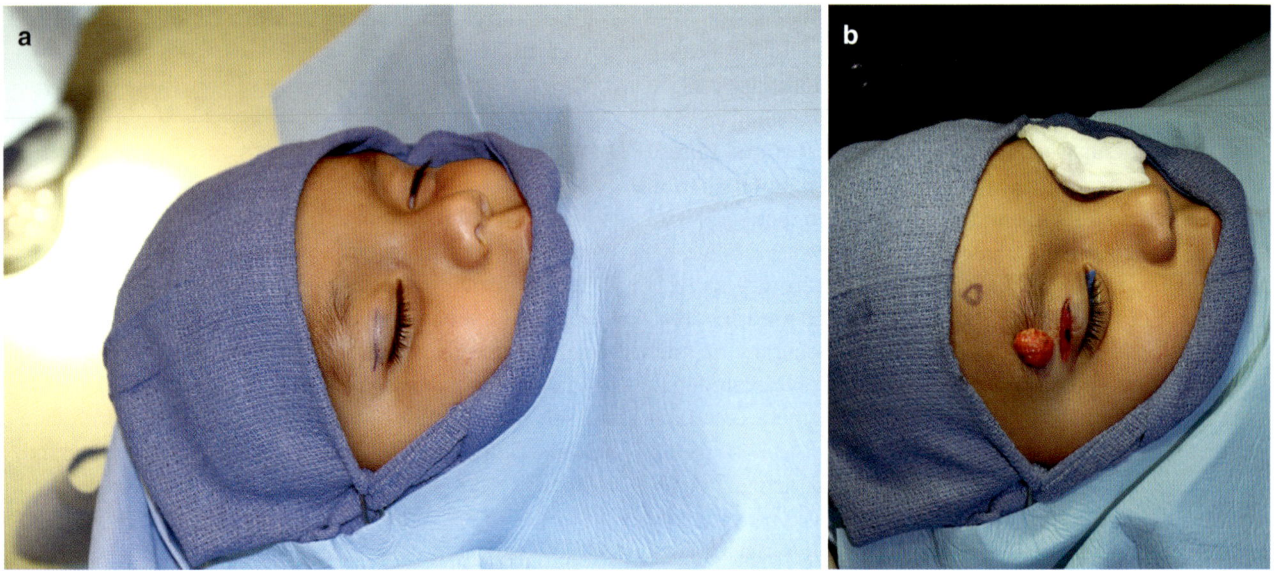

Fig. 46.3 (**a**, **b**) Upper eyelid crease approach for removal of an epibulbar dermoid cyst (Courtesy of Dr. Arkadi Yakirevitch)

to its insertion onto the levator aponeurosis. In this manner, the orbital fat and the lacrimal gland may be exposed. Figure 46.3a, b shows an upper eyelid crease approach for removal of an epibulbar dermoid cyst.

Superior Orbital Lesions: Transconjunctival Approach

The superior transconjunctival approach is less common. Lesions in the superior orbit could be approached usually through a lid crease incision; however, subconjunctival lesions in the superior orbit can be accessed through a superior perilimbal approach (Fig. 46.4). This patient presented for ptosis evaluation, and upon elevation of the eyelid, a salmon-colored lesion was noted in the superior fornix (Fig. 46.5a). An adequate biopsy was obtained for diagnosis through the superior limbal approach (Fig. 46.5b). Of note, the proximity to the lacrimal gland and lacrimal duct openings makes this approach more complicated compared to the eyelid crease incision.

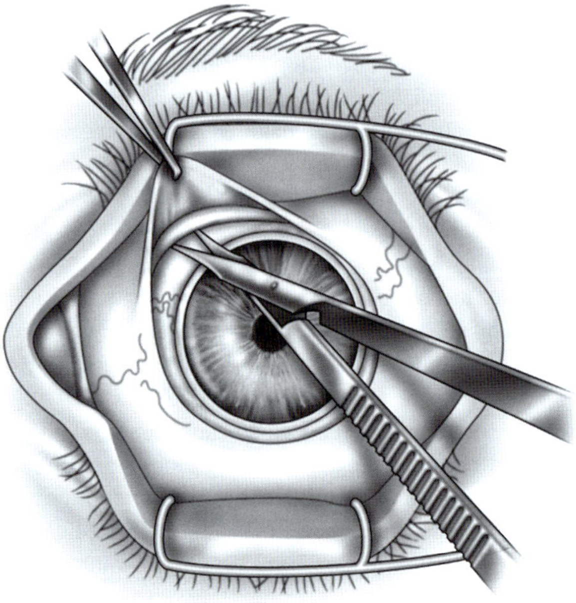

Fig. 46.4 Superior perilimbal approach used to approach subconjunctival lesions in the superior orbit (Courtesy of Dr. Arkadi Yakirevitch)

Inferior Orbital Lesions: Transcutaneous Approach

The lower eyelid subciliary incision provides access to the inferior orbit. Although this approach also allows for wide exposure of the orbital floor, it may be complicated by postoperative eyelid malposition such as ectropion and retraction. In select cases of anophthalmic sockets or cicatrizing conjunctival diseases, the transcutaneous approach is utilized. However, in our experience, the more optimal route for access to the inferior orbit is through the inferior transconjunctival incision.

Inferior Orbital Lesions: Transconjunctival Approach

The conjunctival fornix approach is the preferred approach for inferior orbital lesions (Fig. 46.2c). The transconjunctival incision is typically combined with a lateral

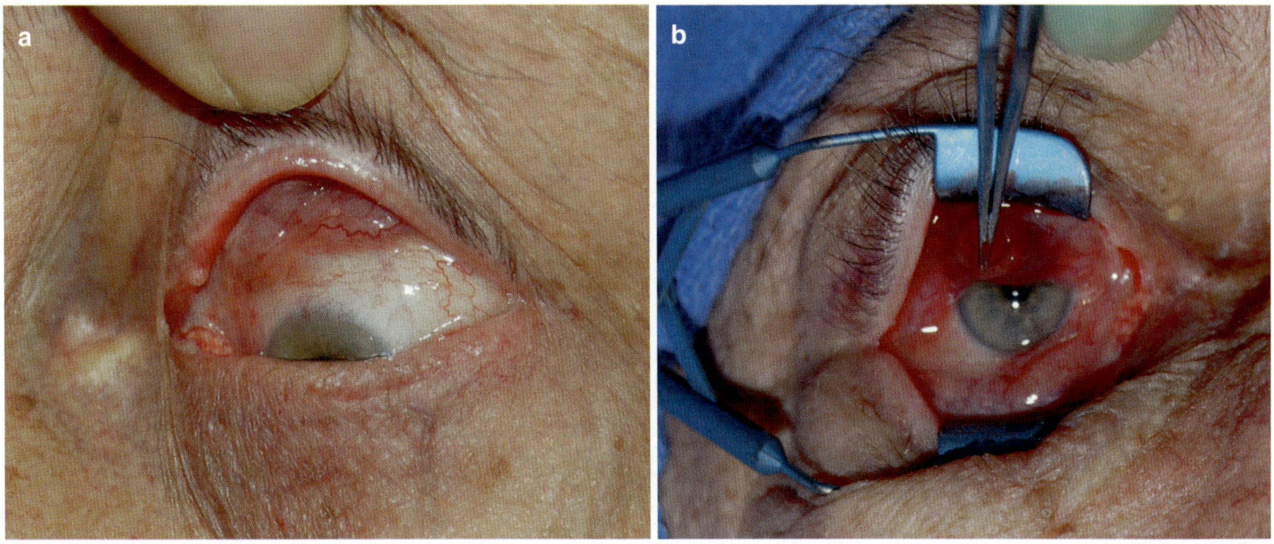

Fig. 46.5 (**a**, **b**) Superior perilimbal approach used during incisional biopsy for a superior salmon patch lesion (Courtesy of Dr. Arkadi Yakirevitch)

canthotomy and cantholysis for added exposure (Fig. 46.6a, b). The subconjunctival tissue is dissected down to the inferior orbital rim by sharp and blunt dissection (Fig. 46.6c). A malleable retractor deep to the orbital rim protects the globe while the dissection is performed. At this point, orbital fat may prolapse anteriorly. An anterior orbital lesion might be visualized at this point. A posterior or extensive orbital lesion will require deeper dissection. For lesions in the inferomedial orbit or when further dissection along the medial wall is desired, the inferior oblique can be imbricated with 6–0 vicryl suture and disinserted (Fig. 46.6d, e). Following the completion of surgery, the muscle is reinserted to its site of origin along the maxillary bone. Figure 46.7a, b shows an orbital MRI of an intraconal, circumscribed lesion in the inferolateral orbit. An inferior transconjunctival approach was used to access the lesion, while a cryoprobe was used to facilitate removal of this cavernous hemangioma. The periosteum is not typically closed to facilitate drainage. The inferior conjunctival incision can be closed with fast-absorbing gut suture. The lateral tarsus should be sutured to the periosteum posterior to the lateral orbital rim or to the superior crus of the lateral canthal ligament. The upper and lower lid margins are reapproximated with 7–0 absorbable sutures at the lateral canthal angle.

Medial Orbital Lesions: Transcutaneous Approach

The Lynch incision can be used to approach lesions near the lacrimal sac, ethmoid sinus, or medial rectus. The incision is made approximately 10 mm medial to the medial canthal angle (Fig. 46.2e). A subperiosteal dissection plane is created while the medial canthal tendon is reflected. The Lynch incision has largely been replaced by the transcaruncular approach or endoscopic approach for drainage of ethmoidal abscesses.

Medial Orbital Lesions: Transconjunctival Approach

Access to the muscle cone can be obtained through a transconjunctival medial orbitotomy. The medial orbitotomy involves a circumlimbal conjunctival incision and disinsertion of the medial rectus muscle (Fig. 46.4). The medial rectus muscle can be tied with a double-armed 6–0 vicryl suture for later reattachment (Fig. 46.8). Sutures (4–0 silk) can be placed at the muscle insertion for traction. Extraconal muscle lesions may not require disinsertion of the rectus muscle. Traction sutures can also be used to retract the eyelids. After exposure of the area to be dissected, blunt-tipped scissors are used to spread the orbital septum and separate vital structures and blood vessels. Retractors should help the dissection by pushing away orbital fat, optimizing visualization creating a bloodless surgical field. Lesions may be removed or biopsy specimens obtained using a cryoprobe or bayonet forceps. The surgeon should avoid crushing the biopsy material since that could cause errors in pathologic diagnosis. The final step in the medial conjunctival approach is to attach all transected muscles back to their insertions. The conjunctiva is closed with 8–0 interrupted absorbable sutures. No pressure dressing should be applied. In cases of large nasal intraconal lesions, it is often mandatory to perform a combined medial and lateral orbitotomy with removal of the lateral orbital wall. That allows displacement of the globe temporally, which improves exposure to the nasal portion of the orbit.

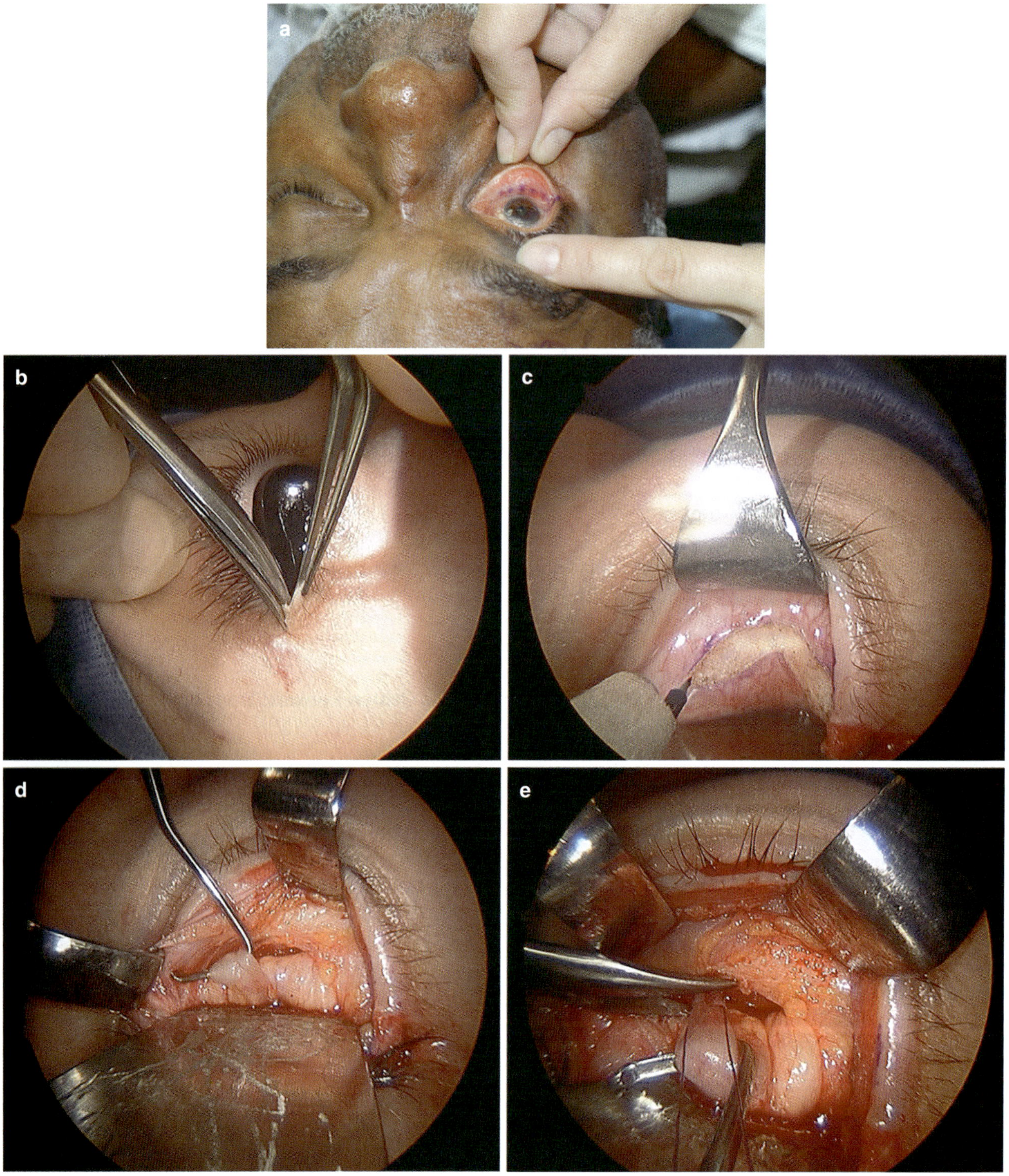

Fig. 46.6 The transconjunctival incision (**a**) is typically combined with a lateral canthotomy and cantholysis (**b**). (**c**) Inferior transconjunctival incision for access to the inferior orbit. (**d**, **e**) Disinsertion of the inferior oblique provides excellent access to the medial and inferomedial orbit (Courtesy of Dr. Arkadi Yakirevitch)

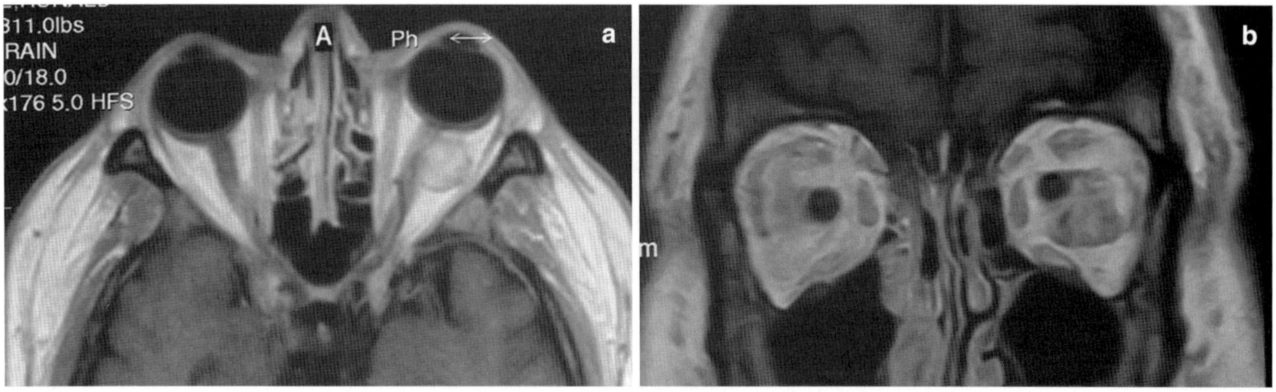

Fig. 46.7 (**a**, **b**) Orbital MRI showing a well-circumscribed intraconal mass in the inferolateral orbit (Courtesy of Dr. Arkadi Yakirevitch)

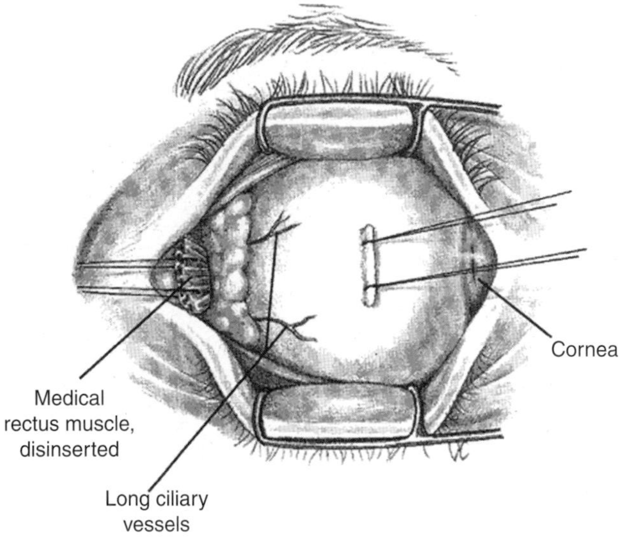

Fig. 46.8 Disinsertion of the medial rectus for access to the medial orbit (Courtesy of Dr. Arkadi Yakirevitch)

Medial Orbital Lesions: Transcaruncular Approach

The transcaruncular approach to the medial orbit begins with a dissection through the caruncle (Fig. 46.2b). Dissection is performed posterior to the lacrimal sac and can be used to gain access to the medial orbital wall for fracture repair, orbital decompression, or abscess drainage (Fig. 46.9a, b). This approach provides excellent cosmesis and surgical exposure. Care should be taken to avoid the lacrimal sac and canalicular system.

Lateral Orbitotomy

Lateral orbitotomy with bone window through a transcutaneous approach provides the best access to the deep orbit (Fig. 46.10). It is ideal for removal of deep masses within the intraconal space, and it aids in reaching small, deep orbital tumors for biopsy. The skin access for a bony orbitotomy can vary depending on the location of the lesion. Berke's modification of the Kronlein operation involves a lateral canthotomy, with dissection of the upper and lower limbs of the lateral canthal tendon from the orbital rim (Fig. 46.2d). The skin is undermined from the temporalis fascia and retracted with silk sutures. The Stallard-Wright incision is curvilinear, extending from the eyebrow cilia to the zygomatic arch through the lateral bony orbital rim. This approach has largely been replaced by the more cosmetically pleasing upper eyelid crease incision (Fig. 46.2a). The superior and inferior skin flaps are undermined to simplify the closure. After the skin incision has been performed, the periosteum is incised with a scalpel or cutting cautery. The periosteal incision should make full use of the exposure gained by the skin incision. The periosteum is then gently dissected from the lateral orbital wall. Stripping the temporalis muscle from its bony fossa requires a blunt dissection. Cutting cautery can be used in the beginning of the dissection with the advantage being minimal hemorrhage in the operative field. Venous bleeding from the temporal bone can be controlled with pressure or bone wax. The periorbita is then elevated from the inner orbital wall using a Freer elevator. This maneuver should be done gently in order to keep the integrity of the periorbita, especially in cases of benign, mixed lacrimal gland tumor. After the lateral orbital rim is fully exposed, malleable retractors are positioned on both sides to protect the surrounding tissues. Drill holes are made on either side of the intended superior and inferior bone cuts. The upper cut is placed above the frontozygomatic suture (Fig. 46.11). The cut is angled 15° caudally to prevent intracranial entry. The lower cut is placed along the upper margin of the zygomatic arch. Slow irrigation prevents heat necrosis of the bone. The lateral rim fragment is gently rocked and removed. Then it is put in sterile saline for later replacement. The bony opening can be enlarged posteriorly by using rongeurs or drilling with a diamond-tipped burr. The intact periorbita is then incised at the intended location. Orbital dissection should proceed gently with blunt dissection using a combination of malleable retractors and

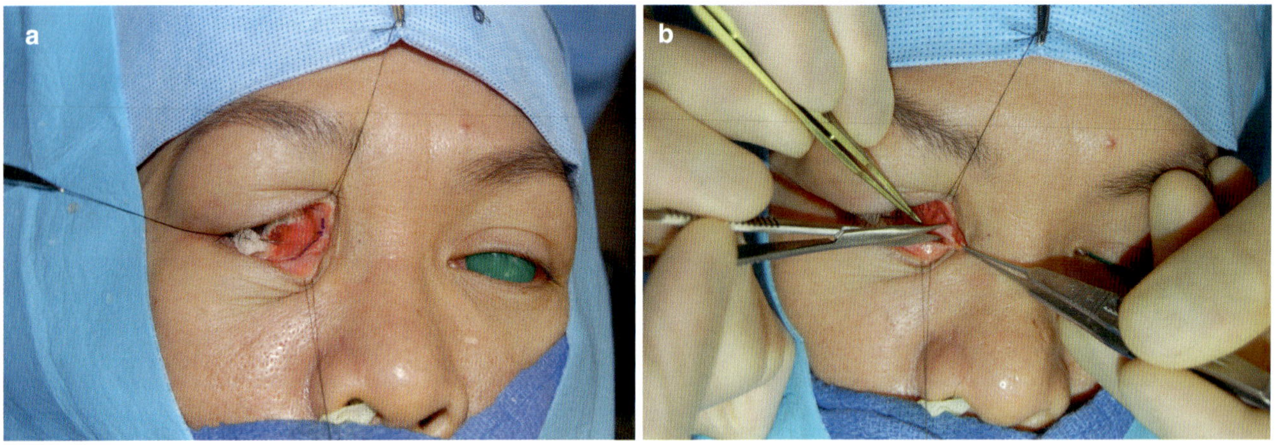

Fig. 46.9 (**a, b**) Transcaruncular approach to the medial orbit (Courtesy of Dr. Arkadi Yakirevitch)

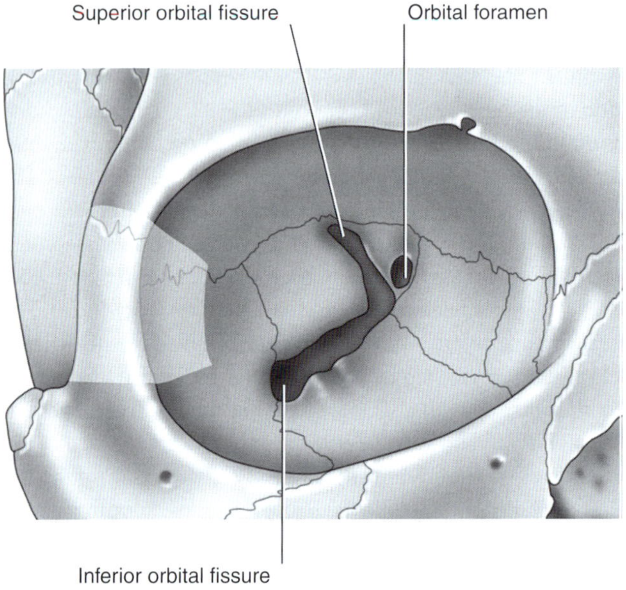

Fig. 46.10 Schematic showing rim removal marked in lateral orbitotomy (Courtesy of Dr. Arkadi Yakirevitch)

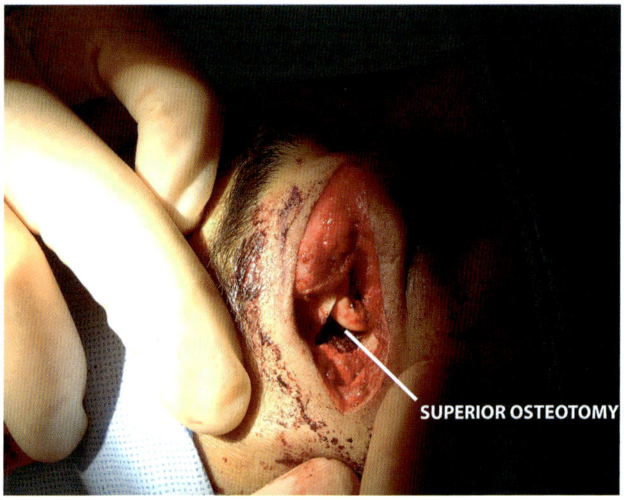

Fig. 46.11 Superior osteotomy is made above the frontozygomatic suture angling inferiorly. (Reproduced with permission from Javier Servat MD)

blunt scissors. The lateral rectus muscle should be identified and retracted for an intraconal mass. Excessive traction should be avoided on the lateral rectus muscle, as it may result in a hematoma or an abduction deficit. Orbital dissection should be performed under direct visualization, and any bleeding should be identified and controlled. It is imperative to maintain a dry surgical field. If an incisional biopsy is performed, only partial exposure may be needed. For an excisional biopsy, complete isolation of the mass from the native structures is needed.

After the tumor has been removed, the surgeon should assess the field and make sure there is no bleeding. The bony fragment of the lateral wall is placed back in position with a stainless steel or silk suture, passed through the previously drilled holes (Fig. 46.12). In specific situations, the surgeon may elect not to place the bone back, and the

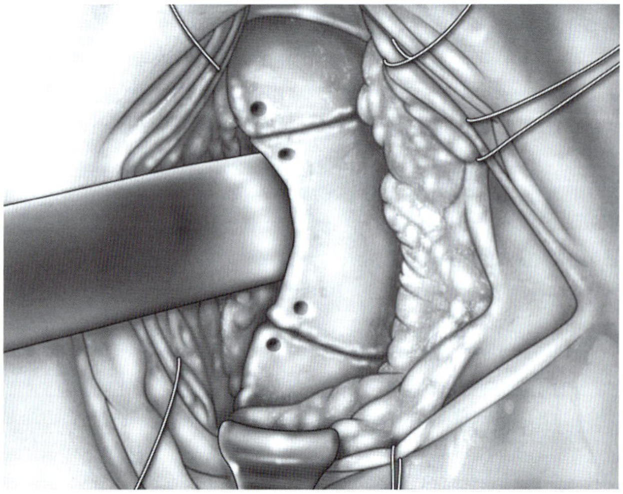

Fig. 46.12 For replacement of the orbital rim, drill holes are placed on both sides of intended bony incision for suture fixation (Courtesy of Dr. Arkadi Yakirevitch)

absent area of the lateral orbital rim will eventually be replaced by fibrous tissue. A suction drainage system can be placed in the fossa of the temporalis muscle in cases of anticipated high wound secretions. The orbicularis is closed with 5–0 vicryl sutures. The skin is closed with a running suture. A light dressing can be applied over the eye and the skin incision, but they can also be left uncovered. Skin sutures should be removed after 7–10 days.

Medial Lid Crease Approach to the Orbit and Optic Nerve

This approach deserves special mention. The superior transcutaneous approach also provides excellent access to the superomedial orbit and optic nerve. The medial one-third of the upper eyelid crease can be incised to gain access through this approach. Following dissection through the orbital septum, the dissection is performed between the nasal and central fat pads in a posterior direction. The medial horn of the levator aponeurosis is pushed laterally, and blunt dissection proceeds under the superior oblique muscle tendon, laterally and inferiorly along the medial sclera, to identify the optic nerve. The vortex veins should be identified and avoided, and the ciliary vessels can be helpful landmarks. Figure 46.13a shows the optic nerve exposed through the superomedial lid crease approach. In this case, the optic nerve sheath is fenestrated in a case of progressive optic neuropathy from idiopathic intracranial hypertension (Fig. 46.13b).

Endoscopic Orbital Surgery

The use of endoscopes in orbital surgery was first described by Norris and Cleasby in 1981. The initial reports described biopsies of orbital tumors and removal of foreign bodies. The advent of endoscopic surgery and intraoperative image guidance has offered a less invasive and more precise approach to the medial and inferior orbit, without crossing the optic nerve. During the past few years, transnasal endoscopic approach have become well established for orbital decompression, orbital medial wall fracture repair, optic canal decompression, and removal of orbital roof lesions. Bleeding from the nasal mucosa, a main concern of the oculoplastic surgeon, is minimal if the nose is prepped with vasoconstrictors. Recent publications show that this approach allows the drainage of a subperiosteal orbital abscess without an external incision. It is also is a preferable one for inferomedial apical lesions due to the lack of neurovascular retraction. Transnasal approach to the orbital apex incudes middle antrostomy followed by a complete ethmoidectomy and optional sphenoidotomy. Lamina papyracea is removed posteriorly to the level of anterior ethmoidal artery and medially to the infraorbital nerve. Next, periorbit is opened. Cautery and trimming of orbital fat is done, and inferior and medial rectus muscles are were dissected and retracted apart. Additional tool can be introduced through the contralateral nostril using temporary cut in the nasal septum. (Fig. 46.14) It allows for bimanual intra orbital manipulation.

The use of a transmaxillary endoscopic approach has also been described for repair of orbital floor fractures.

The primary advantages of the use of the endoscope in the context of orbital surgery are safe visualization in the narrow orbit which may otherwise require bone removal for adequate exposure, excellent depth illumination, magnification, the potential for supervision of trainees, and the ability to engage observers into the operating field.

Complications of endoscopic surgery include uncontrolled bleeding, vision worsening, enophthalmos, hypoglobus and diplopia. Injury to orbital structures and dura with

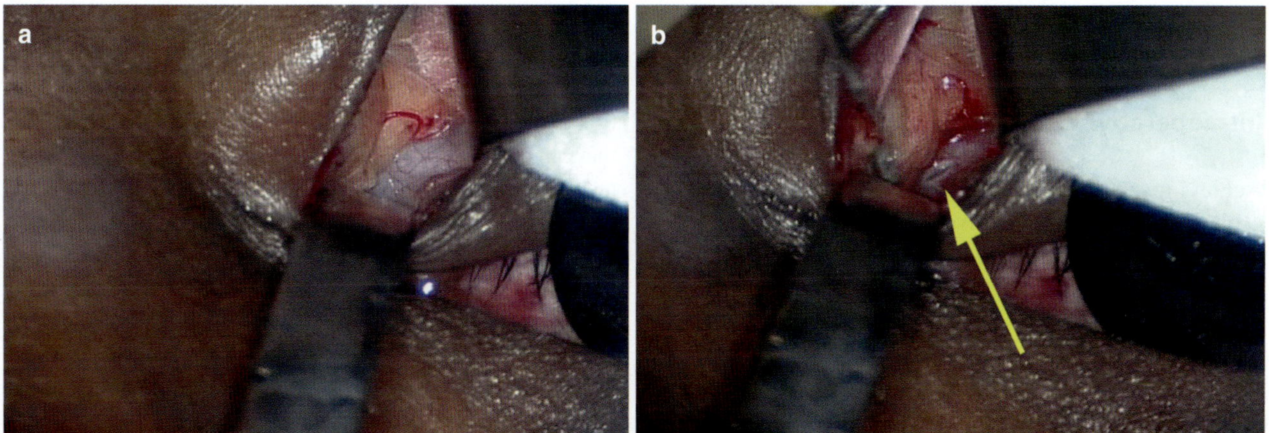

Fig. 46.13 (**a**, **b**) Exposure of the optic nerve through the superomedial lid crease approach. (**b**) *Arrow* pointing to the fenestration created in the optic nerve sheath (Courtesy of Dr. Arkadi Yakirevitch)

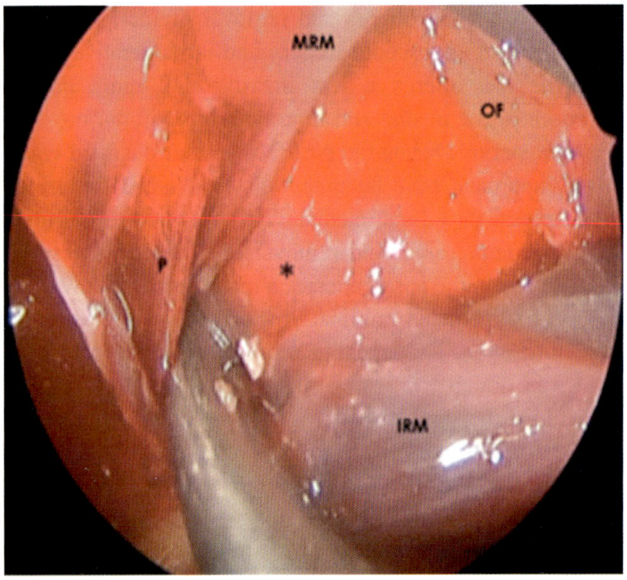

Fig. 46.14 Endoscopic view of transnasal approach for removal of medial orbital apex cavernous hemangioma. P – incised and retracted periorbit; OF – orbital fat; MRM – medial rectus muscle; IRM – inferior rectus muscle; asterix – hemangioma (Courtesy of Dr. Arkadi Yakirevitch)

the instrumentation can be avoided by ensuring good visualization at all times and resting the instrument against a firm surface for stabilization.

Neurosurgical Approach

Neurosurgical approaches to the orbit are utilized during combined surgery with the neurosurgeon and the orbital surgeon. The approach is useful for intracranial lesions that invade into orbit or the optic canal or for deep-infiltrating posterior orbital lesions for which wide exposure is desired. The transcranial neurosurgical approach to the orbit as well as orbital rim reconstruction is discussed in a chapter dedicated to this topic.

Intraoperative Complications

Achieving meticulous hemostasis is vital for successful orbital surgery. Intraoperative bleeding impairs visualization and prolongs operative time. The risk of postoperative hemorrhage with visual loss dictates complete hemostasis before closing the orbital cavity. Pressure packing with gradual removal and hemostasis of oozing vessels can usually be sufficient for soft tissue hemorrhage. Cautery, bone wax, and chemical coagulators are usually sufficient to stop all significant bone bleeding. The anesthesiologist should slowly raise the blood pressure to baseline levels after tumor removal to ensure that no bleeders are missed. Deep extubation should be performed to avoid excessive Valsalva pressure. Nerve laceration or contusion can occur during surgery. It can take as long as 4 weeks for new axons to regenerate across an anastomosis. The patient and the surgeon should wait patiently for recovery of nerve function. Dural penetration with cerebral spinal fluid (CSF) leak should be visualized and managed intraoperatively. Dura mater can be exposed without a tear, and the surgeon needs to carefully observe that it is not lacerated. With good visualization, the surgeon can suture the dura with a silk suture on an atraumatic vascular tapered needle. If overlooked or poorly controlled, a CSF leak can cause postoperative rhinorrhea. Nasolacrimal sac or duct injuries can occur when operating in the area of the medial canthus. The sac is less vulnerable than the canalicular system. If there is any doubt of canalicular laceration, the surgeon should intubate the canaliculi to ensure patency.

Postoperative Complications

Emergent Complications

The most feared complication of orbital surgery is vision loss. Visual loss may result from intraoperative manipulation or postoperative hemorrhage. Perioperative visual loss can occur from direct manipulation of the optic nerve such as seen with surgery on optic nerve sheath meningiomas. Overzealous traction or "blind" dissection of tumors attached to the optic nerve can also produce irreversible posterior optic nerve ischemia. Even moderate traction on an optic nerve for longer than 2 min should be avoided, especially when hypotensive anesthesia is being used. The posterior ciliary arteries also can be damaged when peeling intraconal tumors off the posterior globe. The key to avoiding these complications is meticulous dissection, strict adherence to the knowledge of anatomic landmarks, and good visualization. The use of cautery near the optic nerve should be avoided as much as possible. In the postoperative stage, caution should be made to avoid bleeding or excessive edema that can cause a rise in intraorbital pressure, leading to a posterior ischemic optic neuropathy. This occurs most frequently in elderly patients, who are more susceptible to ischemic optic neuropathy. Since the ischemic event occurs posterior to the cribriform lamina, the optic nerve and retina usually will appear normal despite the visual loss. Retinal artery occlusion and anterior ischemic optic neuropathy can also occur from direct manipulation of the retinal artery or the posterior ciliary arteries.

Tight pressure dressings over the eye are to be avoided due to the threat of causing a "compartment syndrome" of the orbit. A sealed dressing can also delay the finding of acute visual loss in the postoperative state. Infections are not common after orbital surgery. The orbit is well vascularized, and even if the surgery involves the nasal sinuses, infection is rare. During the operation, the anesthesiologist usually infuses a single antibiotic dose, and during the postoperative state, the patient is given a course of oral antibiotics. Infection should be promptly controlled, and signs of possible meningitis should be assessed and addressed urgently.

Non-emergent Complications

Excessive hemorrhage and edema during surgery or in the postoperative state can lead to conjunctival prolapse with conjunctival desiccation. Ophthalmic ointment is applied liberally until the swelling subsides.

Diplopia can be caused by excessive traction on any extraocular muscle (myogenic), damage to a cranial nerve (paresis), or iatrogenic injury to extraocular muscles, leading to scarring (restriction). In most cases, symptomatic diplopia resolves without sequelae.

Ptosis can be seen after orbital surgery, but it generally resolves. Biopsy of superior lesions can cause bleeding into the levator muscle or aponeurosis, resulting in ptosis. Damage to the superior division of the cranial nerve III and hemorrhage in the orbital apex can also cause ptosis. These patients can be observed for up to a year since this condition tends to resolve with time.

Wound dehiscence without any tension can be carefully observed, but resuturing will give the best outcome to any dehisced tissue. Patients with vascular pathology, diabetics, and smokers should be watched carefully to ensure wound closure.

Disturbance of the ciliary ganglion after dissection lateral to the optic nerve, or posterior to the inferior oblique muscle, can result in damage to the pupillary fibers and subsequent irregularity of the pupil.

Total removal of the lacrimal gland for benign, pleomorphic lacrimal gland tumors can cause xerophthalmia in many patients.

Suggested Reading

1. Arya AK, et al. Late periorbital haemorrhage following functional endoscopic sinus surgery: a caution for potential day case surgery. BMC Ear Nose Throat Disord. 2006;6:11.
2. Ben Simon G, et al. Rethinking orbital imaging: establishing guidelines for interpreting orbital imaging studies and evaluating their predictive value in patients with orbital tumors. Ophthalmology. 2005;112(12):2196–207.
3. Berke RN. A modified Kronlein operation. Trans Am Ophthalmol Soc. 1953;51:193.
4. Calcaterra TC. Diagnosis and management of ethmoid cerebrospinal rhinorrhea. Otolaryngol Clin North Am. 1985;18:99–105.
5. Cannon PS, et al. The surgical management and outcomes for spheno-orbital meningiomas: a 7-year review of multi-disciplinary practice. Orbit. 2009;28(6):371–6.
6. Collin R, Rose G. Plastic and orbital surgery. London: BMJ Books; 2001.
7. Hongobo Y, et al. Navigation-guided reduction and orbital floor reconstruction in the treatment of zygomatic-orbital-maxillary complex fractures. J Oral Maxillofac Surg. 2010;68(1):28–34.
8. Jones BR. Surgical approaches to the orbit. Trans Ophthalmol Soc UK. 1970;90:269.
9. Kasperbauer JL, Hinkley L. Endoscopic orbital decompression for Graves' ophthalmopathy. Am J Rhinol. 2005;19:603–6.
10. Kennerdell JS, Dekker A, Johnson BL. Orbital fine needle aspiration biopsy: the results of its use in 50 patients. Neuroophthalomol. 1980;1:117.
11. Kennerdell JS, et al. Fine needle aspiration biopsy: its use in orbital tumors. Arch Ophthalmol. 1979;97:1315.
12. Kennerdell JS, et al. CT-guided fine needle aspiration biopsy of orbital optic nerve tumors. Ophthalmology. 1980;87:491.
13. Krohel GB. Blepharoptosis following traumatic third nerve palsies. Am J Ophthalmol. 1979;88:598.
14. Long JC, Ellis PP. Total unilateral visual loss following orbital surgery. Am J Ophthalmol. 1971;71:218.
15. Norris JL, Cleasby GW. Endoscopic orbital surgery. Am J Ophthalmol. 1981;91:249 52.
16. Norris JL, Stewart WB. Bimanual endoscopic orbital biopsy: an emerging technique. Ophthalmology. 1985;92:34–8.
17. Pelton RW, Patel BCK. Superomedial lid crease approach to the medial intraconal space. Ophthal Plast Reconstr Surg. 2001;17:241–53.
18. Pham AM, Strong EB. Endoscopic management of facial fractures. Curr Opin Otolaryngol Head Neck Surg. 2006;14:234–41.
19. Prabhakaran VC, et al. Orbital endoscopic surgery. Indian J Ophthalmol. 2008;56(1):5–8.
20. Rosen N, Priel A, Ben Simon GJ, Rosner M. Cryo-assisted anterior approach for surgery of retroocular orbital tumours avoids the need for lateral or transcranial orbitotomy in most cases. Acta Ophthalmol. 2010;88:675–80.
21. Reese AB. Tumors of the eye. third ed. New York: Harper & Row; 1976.
22. Reese AB. Expanding lesions of the orbit. Trans Ophthalmol Soc UK. 1971;91:85.
23. Rootman J, Stewart B, Goldberg RA. Orbital surgery – a conceptual approach. Philadelphia: Lippincott Raven; 1995.
24. Schyberg E. Fine needle biopsy of orbital tumors. Acta Ophthalmol Suppl. 1975;125:11.
25. Smith GB. Anesthesia for orbital surgery: observed changes in the visually evoked response at low blood pressures. Mod Probl Ophthalmol. 1975;14:457.
26. Smith JL. Anterolateral approach to the orbit. Trans Am Acad Ophthalmol Otolaryngol. 1971;75:1059.
27. Spoor TC, et al. Orbital fine needle aspiration biopsy with B-scan guidance. Am J Ophthalmol. 1980;89:274.
28. Stallard HB. Surgery of the orbit. Ann R Coll Surg Engl. 1968;43:125.
29. Tanna N, et al. Surgical treatment of subperiosteal orbital abscess. Arch Otolaryngol. 2008;134(7):764–7.
30. Tao J, Nunery W, Kresovsky S, Lister L, Mote T. Efficacy of fentanyl or alfentanil in suppressing reflex sneezing after propofol sedation and periocular injection. Ophthal Plast Reconstr Surg. 2008;24:465–7.
31. Vairavan N, et al. Minimally invasive image-guided removal of retrobulbar intraconal foreign body. Orbit. 2009;28(6):442–3.
32. Westman-Naeser S, Naeser P. Tumors of the orbit diagnosed by fine needle biopsy. Acta Ophthalmol. 1978;56:969.

33. Verity DH, et al. Natural history of periocular capillary haemangiomas: changes in internal blood velocity and lesion volume. Eye. 2006;20(10):1228–37.
34. Write JE. The role of surgery in the management of orbital tumors. Mod Probl Ophthalmol. 1975;14:553.
35. Write JE, Stewart WB, Krohl GB. Clinical presentation and management of lacrimal gland tumors. Br J Ophthalmol. 1979;63:600.
36. Xian J, et al. Value of MR imaging in the differentiation of benign and malignant orbital tumors in adults. Eur Radiol. 2010;20(7):1692–702.
37. Stokken J, Gumber D, Antisdel J, Sindwani R. Endoscopic surgery of the orbital apex: outcomes and emerging techniques. The Laryngoscope 2016;126:20–24.

Transcranial Approach to the Orbit

47

Alon Kahana

Introduction

The transcranial approach to the orbit requires specialized knowledge, skill, and instrumentation. It can be performed by neurosurgeons but is commonly approached collaboratively, with an orbital, skull base, and/or craniofacial plastic surgeon joining the neurosurgical team to provide specialized skills. The role of the ophthalmic plastic surgeon, as an orbital specialist, includes preoperative evaluation and planning, intraoperative anatomic expertise, and postoperative care.

The indication for transcranial orbitotomy includes infiltrative or large posterior orbital tumors and access to tumors that cross the orbitocranial boundary. The goal of treatment is to remove the tumor while preserving normal tissues and reconstruct the orbital walls and rims to restore anatomy and functionality. Occasionally, a transcranial orbitotomy is performed for tumor debulking and orbital decompression, as a palliative approach to non-resectable orbitocranial tumors that are causing severe proptosis and/or optic nerve compression.

The surgical approach is commonly referred to as a frontozygomatic craniotomy. It is commonly approached as a two-step craniotomy – frontal craniotomy that ends 1–2 cm from the superior orbital rim, followed by elevation of a frontozygomatic bar. Because many of these patients may require both an anterior orbital access and a transcranial exposure, a standard craniofacial preoperative prepping and draping is performed, with a full face and scalp prep (Fig. 47.1). This allows alternating between the anterior and posterior approaches to maximize access and assist with reconstruction.

The surgery begins with a standard neurosurgical approach, which is outside the domain of the orbital surgeon and will be recapped only briefly. A bicoronal flap is elevated with preservation of an anteriorly based periosteal flap to utilize as a pericranial flap at the time of closure. The superior and lateral orbital rims are exposed while preserving the supraorbital (and possibly lacrimal) neurovascular bundle. The lateral exposure extends to the zygomatic arch and possibly beyond, depending whether the frontal process of the arch must be removed for access. The temporalis muscle is frequently elevated in order to expose the temporal bone and assist with the lateral osteotomy. Next, a large frontal craniotomy is created. Extending the calvarial osteotomy posteriorly helps to provide more inner table bone for reconstruction of the orbital rims, should that be part of the surgical plans. A medial frontal osteotomy and a lateral rim osteotomy are then performed, the latter below the frontozygomatic suture or lower. Of course, great care is taken to protect the frontal lobe and dura. The medial osteotomy will typically invade the frontal sinus, which will be addressed by the neurosurgeon at the time of closure. Once the frontozygomatic bar is released from the orbital roof, the periorbita is fully exposed (Fig. 47.2).

If a subcranial approach to the skull base is the goal, the skull base surgeon will begin to remove the orbital roof while supporting the frontal lobe. Removal of discreet orbitocranial tumors can proceed via a small frontozygomatic osteotomy, without disturbing the periorbita (Figure 47.3a). Otherwise, the periorbita is carefully incised, and the tumor approached via blunt dissection, with great care to preserve normal orbital tissues. A helpful technique is to preoperatively pass 4–0 silk sutures underneath the insertions of the superior, medial, and/or lateral rectus muscle tendons, which can then be used to safely rotate the globe and aid in orientation. Another technique that helps with orientation is to identify and follow the supraorbital nerve posteriorly to the frontal nerve, which then provides context for surrounding structures (Fig. 47.3b, c).

If transcranial decompression is required, the bone of the greater wing of the sphenoid is carefully removed in a piecemeal approach, using rongeurs, drills, and/or ultrasonic

A. Kahana (✉)
Consultants in Ophthalmic and Facial Plastic Surgery, Southfield, MI, USA
e-mail: akahana@facialworks.com

J. J. Servat et al. (eds.), *Smith and Nesi's Ophthalmic Plastic and Reconstructive Surgery*,
https://doi.org/10.1007/978-3-030-41720-8_47

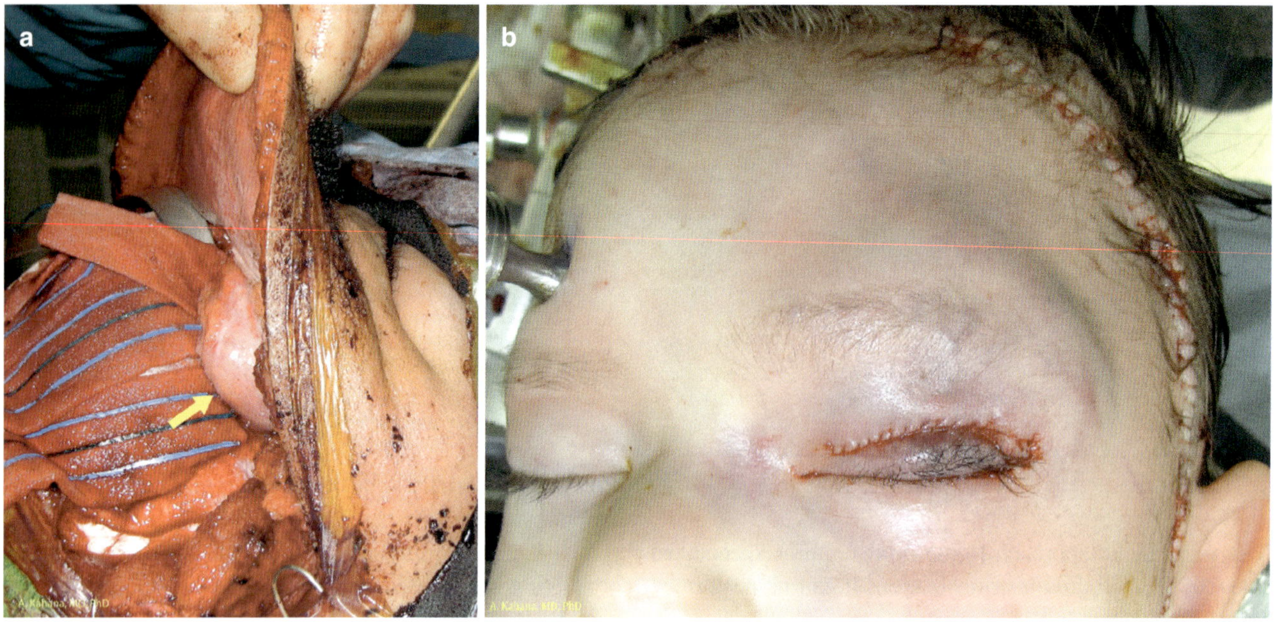

Fig. 47.1 *Craniofacial approach to the orbit*. (**a**) Surgical access to the face and anterior orbit, in addition to the frontal craniotomy, enables a multi-vector approach to the orbital tumor while facilitating reconstruction. The facial flap can be mobilized intraoperatively to accommodate the surgical needs. *Arrow* points to the periorbita as visualized from the cranial side. (**b**) This patient required a transcranial approach to the posterior orbit via a bicoronal incision, as well as an anterior orbitotomy and lid reconstruction. Postoperative picture of the closure of the bicoronal and lid incisions reflects the multi-vector approach

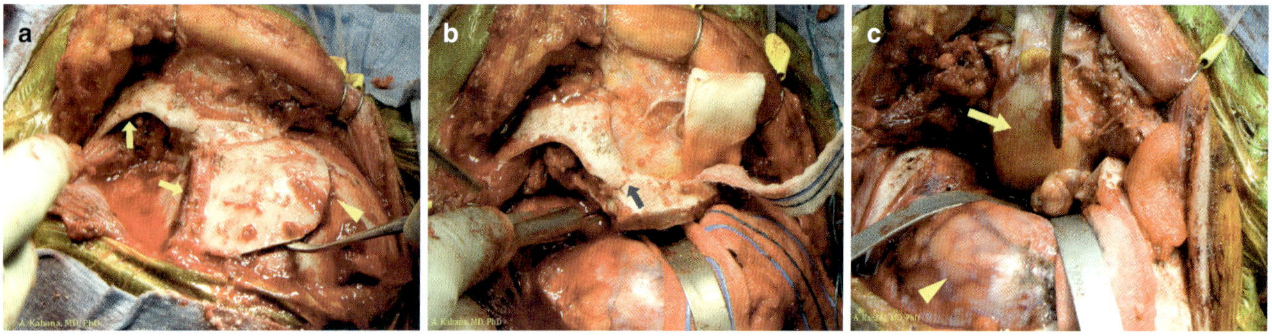

Fig. 47.2 *Transcranial orbitotomy*. (**a**) The calvarial opening can be extended posteriorly to provide additional inner table bone for reconstruction. *Arrows* point to zygomatic arch and *temporal line*. *Arrowhead* points to calvarial osteotomy with elevation of the craniotomy plate. (**b**) Frontozygomatic osteotomy is performed below the frontozygomatic suture (*arrow*). This osteotomy will leave the zygomatic arch intact. (**c**) After elevation of the frontozygomatic orbital bar, the periorbita is fully visualized (*arrow*). *Arrowhead* points to the frontal lobe of the brain

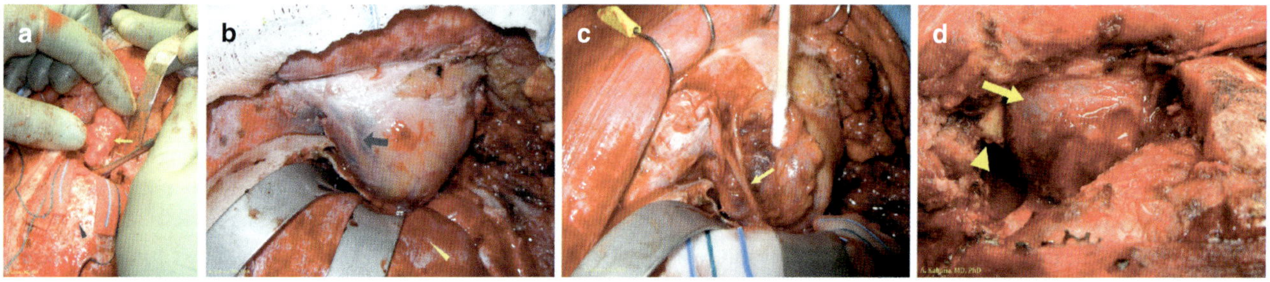

Fig. 47.3 *Orbital exposure and dissection*. (**a**) This orbitocranial osteoma traversed the frontal sinus. It was removed in toto, followed by sinus obliteration and superior orbital bone and roof reconstruction. (**b**) The frontal nerve can be visualized underneath the periorbita (*arrow*) following removal of the frontozygomatic orbital bar. (**c**) After the periorbita is opened, the frontal nerve can be visualized at its bifurcation into the supraorbital and supratrochlear branches (*arrow*). Orienting to the anatomy of the posterior orbit is not trivial, and landmarks such as this can be very helpful. (**d**) This patient underwent transcranial orbitotomy with tumor debulking and orbital decompression. The greater wing of the sphenoid was mostly removed, reducing the proptosis and restoring vision. The *arrow* points to the periorbita wrapped around the ocular contents. *Arrowhead* points at zygomatic edge of osteotomy

instruments (Fig. 47.3d). If optic canal decompression is required, it can also be performed with rongeurs, micro-drill bits, or ultrasonic tools (e.g., Sonopet (Stryker, Kalamazoo, MI) or CUSA (Cavitron Ultrasonic Surgical Aspirator, Integra-Radionics Inc., Burlington, MA). Care must be taken by the orbital surgeon to avoid placing pressure on the brain or inadvertently nick the dura matter.

After removal of the tumor, the frontozygomatic bar is repositioned and secured with titanium plates. The frontal sinus can be cranialized or obliterated if this is required. For obliteration, the sinus mucosa is completely removed, first manually and then with a diamond burr. Failure to completely remove the mucosa can result in a mucocele. Next, the sinus is filled with fat, muscle, bone, fascia, and/or gelfoam. Generally, autogenous fillers are more successful at obliterating the sinus. If orbital rim bone was sacrificed as part of the surgical resection, reconstruction can utilize bone from the calvarial inner table, which can be harvested on a back table using either osteotomes or micro-drill bits (Fig. 47.4). These autografts can then be shaped and combined to reform the proper shape of the orbital rim. Lowering the facial flap to expose the face allows for palpation and assessment of orbital rim contour and position, as well as comparison with the contralateral side. Fixation is achieved via micro-titanium plates (Fig. 47.5).

The craniotomy is then closed using titanium plates. The periosteal flap is commonly placed underneath the calvarial bone flap, to help with protection and reconstruction. Residual small bony defects can be filled with one of several commercially available demineralized bone scaffold agents (Fig. 47.5), which are osteoinductive and osseointegrative. These bone graft substitutes will typically be replaced by newly formed bone within 12 months of surgery. Closure of the bicoronal flap is performed in the usual fashion.

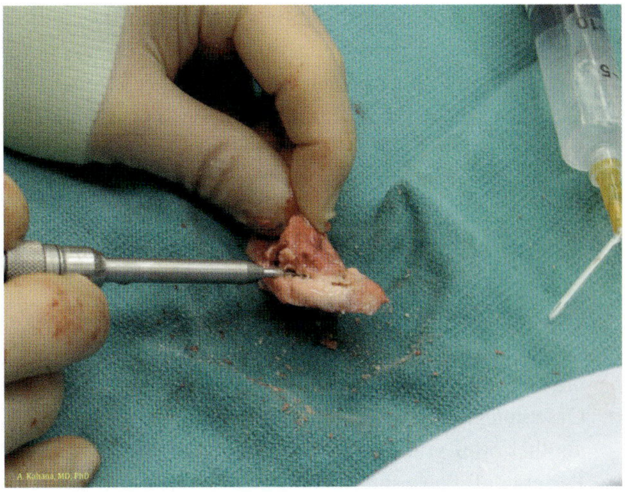

Fig. 47.4 *Inner table calvarial grafts can be harvested and utilized for bony reconstruction.* Osteotomes, drill micro-bits, and harvesting devices can all be used effectively

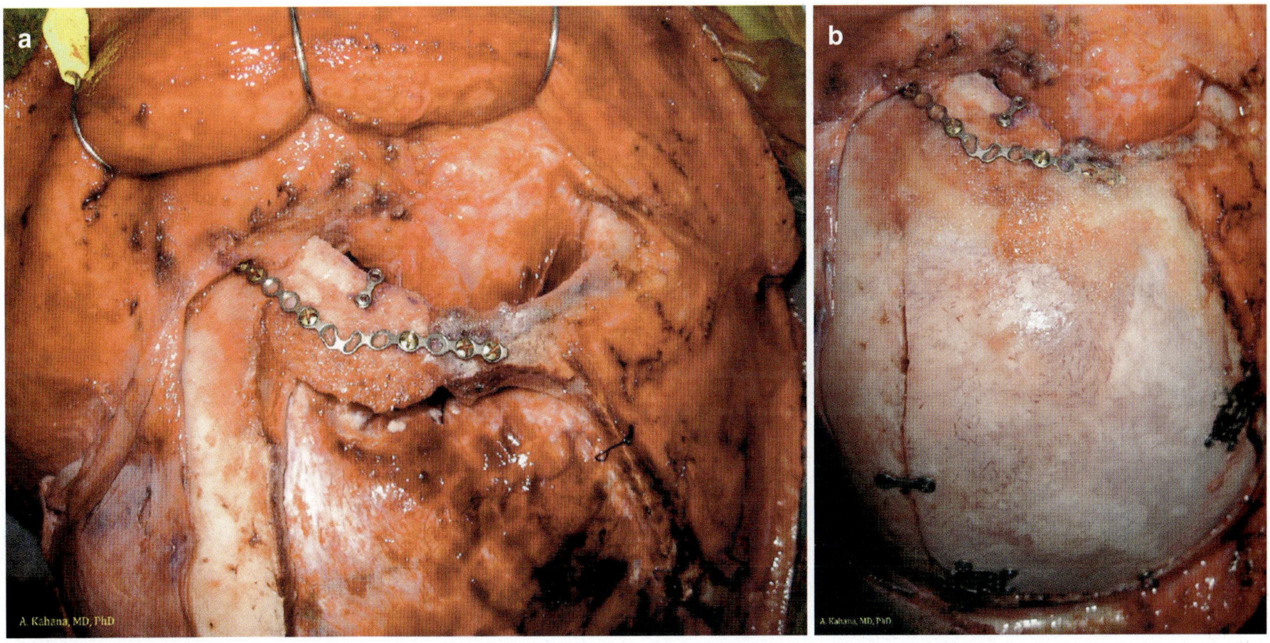

Fig. 47.5 *Reconstruction and closure.* (**a**) Reconstruction of the superior orbital rim and roof using calvarial grafts and titanium microplates. The reconstructed roof (not visualized) is supported by a cantilevered titanium plate. (**b**) After the calvarial bone is repositioned and anchored with titanium microplates, a demineralized bone matrix was used to help fill the residual defects between the grafts and native bone. This bone substitute will serve as a scaffold for new bone growth

Hospital admission to the neurosurgical intensive care unit is required, and the neurosurgical team manages these patients postoperatively. Nevertheless, the ophthalmic plastic surgeon has unique tools to assess visual function and globe position during the postoperative phase. This unique skill set, applied both pre- and postoperatively, is often critical to the overall success of the surgery.

The ophthalmic orbital surgeon is commonly a valuable member of the neurosurgical team that is tackling orbitocranial pathologies. A multidisciplinary approach that utilizes the unique skills and knowledge of different members of the surgical team will maximize outcomes while reducing morbidity. The transcranial orbitotomy approach is an important and useful tool in the treatment of certain orbital lesions.

Definitions

- Osteoconduction = surface bone growth.
- Osteoinduction = recruitment and stimulation of osteoblasts and pre-osteoblasts.
- Osseointegration = stable joining of bone surfaces to one another or of graft to native bone.
- Pericranial flap = anteriorly based scalp periosteal flap that is placed over dura at closure of the craniotomy.
- Sinus cranialization = opening the posterior frontal sinus wall to the cranial cavity, complete removal of all sinus mucosa elements, plugging of the sinus drainage tract with fillers, and allowing the frontal lobe dura matter to rest inside the frontal sinus.
- Sinus obliteration = removal of sinus mucosa and bone and filling the residual cavity with fillers.

Suggested Reading

1. Albrektsson T, Johansson C. Osteoinduction, osteoconduction and osseointegration. Eur Spine J. 2001;10(2):S96–101.
2. Donath A, Sindwani R. Frontal sinus cranialization using the pericranial flap: an added layer of protection. Laryngoscope. 2006;116:1585–8.
3. Lemole GM, Henn JS, Zabramski JM, Spetzler RF. Modifications to the orbitozygomatic approach. Techn Note Neurosurg. 2003;99:924–30.
4. Rootman J, Stewart B, Goldberg RA. Orbital surgery: a conceptual approach. Philadelphia: Lippincott Williams & Wilkins; 1995.
5. Ross DA, Marentette LJ, Moore CE, Switz KL. Craniofacial resection: decreased complication rate with a modified subcranial approach. Skull Base Surg. 1999;9:95–100.
6. Wanibuchi M, Friedman A, Fukushima T. Photo atlas of skull base dissection: techniques and operative approaches. New York: Thieme; 2008.

Evaluation and Management of Lacrimal Gland Diseases

48

David T. Tse

Introduction

The lacrimal gland is the epicenter of a broad spectrum of neoplastic and inflammatory diseases (Table 48.1). Space-occupying lesions of the lacrimal gland and its fossa constitute approximately 5–13% of orbital masses upon biopsy [1–3]. Based primarily on Reese's [4] 1956 clinicopathologic survey of 112 consecutive expanding lesions of the lacrimal gland, most authorities generally report that approximately 50% of the lesions originate from epithelial elements of the lacrimal gland and 50% are of non-epithelial origin [5–7]. Of non-epithelial lesions, 50% are lymphoid tumors and 50% are comprised of various infections and inflammatory pseudotumors. Among the epithelial tumors of the lacrimal gland, approximately 50% are pleomorphic adenomas (benign mixed tumors), 25% adenoid cystic carcinoma, and the remainders are other types of carcinoma. Recent reports, however, suggest that inflammatory lesions and lymphoid tumors are more common and that epithelial malignancies of the lacrimal gland are considerably less frequent than commonly cited, ranging from 22% to 47% [1, 3, 7–10]. Proper differentiation between these two groups is of paramount importance since several of the lesions are life-threatening.

Information from clinical history, physical examination, ultrasonography, and radiographic soft tissue contour analysis forms the foundation in determining which category of disease the lacrimal gland tumor belongs: inflammation, lymphoproliferative disorder, benign epithelial tumor, or malignant epithelial tumor. Acute presentation without contiguous bony changes is suggestive of inflammatory disorders. Insidious, painless onset (less than 1 year) in a senescent age group with radiographic evidence of a lesion molding or conforming to ocular and bony contours, rather than indenting adjacent structures, is a hallmark of lymphoproliferative diseases. Subacute presentation of short duration (usually 4–6 months) and radiographic evidence of

Table 48.1 Diseases of the lacrimal gland

Intrinsic inflammations
Infectious
Viral dacryoadenitis
Bacterial dacryoadenitis
Fungal
Noninfectious
Idiopathic
Systemic inflammation
1. Sjogren's disease
2. Sarcoidosis
3. Wegener's granulomatosis
4. Systemic lupus erythematous
5. Graves' orbitopathy
Lymphoproliferative disorders
Benign lymphoid hyperplasia
Atypical lymphoid hyperplasia
Malignant lymphoma
Benign tumors
Pleomorphic adenoma (benign mixed tumor)
Myoepithelioma
Oncocytoma
Malignant tumors
Adenoid cystic carcinoma
Primary adenocarcinoma (de novo)
Pleomorphic adenocarcinoma (malignant mixed tumor)
Mucoepidermoid carcinoma
Acinic cell carcinoma
Squamous cell carcinoma
Malignant myoepithelial carcinoma
Carcinosarcoma
Miscellaneous
Dacryops
Congenital dermoid cysts
Amyloidosis
Kimura's disease
Warthin's tumor
Solitary fibrous tumor
Hemangiopericytoma
Cavernous hemangioma
Herniated orbital fat

D. T. Tse (✉)
Bascom Palmer Eye Institute, Department of Ophthalmology, Miami, FL, USA
e-mail: dtse@med.miami.edu

J. J. Servat et al. (eds.), *Smith and Nesi's Ophthalmic Plastic and Reconstructive Surgery*,
https://doi.org/10.1007/978-3-030-41720-8_48

infiltration of adjacent structures, calcification, and irregular erosion or destruction of the bone are indicative of malignant epithelial neoplasms. Chronic presentation without pain, associated with radiographic finding of lacrimal fossa remodeling, is suggestive of benign lacrimal gland tumors.

Management protocols based on clinical and radiographic features of lacrimal fossa masses have been well established in the literature [10–14]. Readers are referred to the seminal article by Wright and coworkers, outlining an algorithm for the differentiation and efficacious management of lacrimal gland fossa masses [13]. The intent of this chapter is to review the clinical characteristics, pertinent diagnostic and pathologic features, biological behavior, and conventional management protocols for some of the common lacrimal gland disorders. A new treatment paradigm for adenoid cystic carcinoma will be highlighted.

Intrinsic Inflammations of the Lacrimal Gland

Dacryoadenitis is a general term describing lacrimal gland inflammation without designating an etiology. The lacrimal gland may become inflamed acutely, subacutely, or chronically. The inflammation may have an infectious or noninfectious etiology, either isolated to the lacrimal gland or result from a systemic disorder. Inflammations affecting the lacrimal gland usually have a distinctive, more explosive temporal sequence of presentation that is characterized by pain and discomfort.

Infectious Lesions of the Lacrimal Gland

Acute infectious dacryoadenitis may be secondary to viral, bacterial, or fungal pathogens. The acute infection can affect either the palpebral or orbital lobe of the gland separately or together, presenting with orbital pain and epiphora. The superior sulcus becomes full, and the eyelid is erythematous and edematous and assumes an S-shaped configuration. Edema frequently extends beyond the confines of the lacrimal fossa into the temporalis fossa and cheek. The bulbar conjunctiva is injected, chemotic, and associated with varying amount of mucous discharge. Tenderness of the eyelid often precludes palpation of the lacrimal gland, but swelling of the palpebral lobe lobules has been described as imparting a gritty sensation to touch. Acute orbital dacryoadenitis is much less common than the palpebral form and presents with the same, but accentuated symptoms. Proptosis and limitation of eye movement are frequent findings. The preauricular lymph nodes may be enlarged and tender to palpation. Viral dacryoadenitis is often associated with systemic infections, including infectious mononucleosis, mumps, or herpes zoster. Constitutional symptoms such as fever, chills, sore throat, and malaise offer confirmatory clues for a viral etiology. Tuberculosis, syphilis, histoplasmosis, and trachoma are other infectious diseases known to cause dacryoadenitis.

Bacterial infections of the lacrimal gland are uncommon, presumably related to the constant downward effluence of tears through the ductules and the presence of secretory antibody (IgA) and bacteriostatic lysozymes [15]. However, acute bacterial dacryoadenitis does occur, probably due to an exogenous pathogen ascending the lacrimal ductules through the conjunctiva or as a result of hematogenous spread from a remote site of infection. Bacterial dacryoadenitis may occur as sequelae of trauma. Fever, lymphadenopathy, and leukocytosis will generally be present. A pointing pustule on the palpebral lobe accompanied by purulent conjunctival discharge is a frequent finding with bacterial dacryoadenitis (Fig. 48.1). *Staphylococcus aureus*, *Streptococcus*, and *Neisseria* infections of the lacrimal gland have been reported [16].

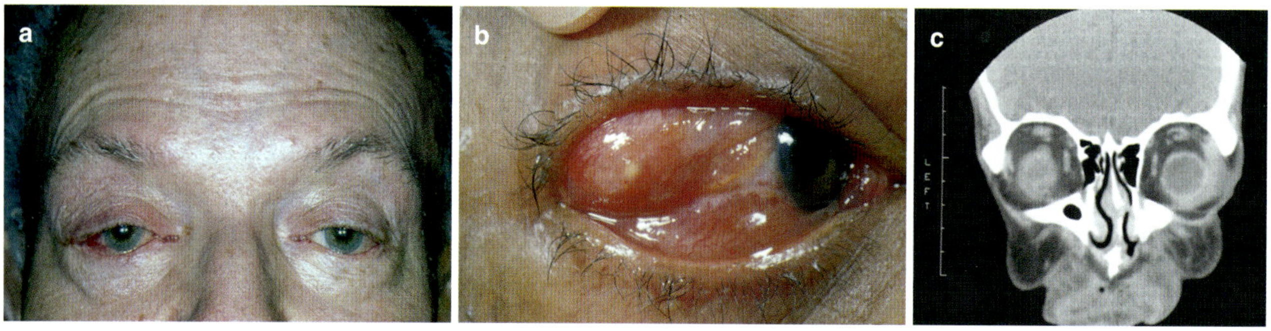

Fig. 48.1 (**a**) A 79-year-old man presented with an acute onset of pain localized to the lacrimal gland fossa region accompanied by lid swelling, erythema, and fullness of the superior sulcus. The lacrimal gland is painful to palpation. (**b**) On eversion of the temporal lid, a yellow pustule is present on the enlarged and erythematous palpebral lobe of the lacrimal gland. Bulbar conjunctival chemosis and injection are present. (**c**) The infection has extended from the palpebral lobe to involve the orbital lobe of the lacrimal gland. Coronal CT scan of the orbit disclosed an enlarged and poorly demarcated orbital lobe molding to the adjacent structures and without destruction of the bone. There is also involvement of the Tenon's capsule, orbital fat, and lateral rectus muscle

The therapy of an infectious dacryoadenitis is determined by the etiology. Dacryoadenitis as a complication of viral disease should be treated symptomatically. Local application of cold compresses offers some relief. Bed rest and salicylates are suggested. If there are no other signs or symptoms of systemic disease and clinical findings are suggestive of a bacterial infection, oral antibiotics are administered. If suppuration occurs, an incision and drainage should be performed. Acute bacterial dacryoadenitis usually will show a clinical response within 48–72 h following appropriate antibiotic therapy and should resolve completely within a few weeks. If the condition persists, a lacrimal gland biopsy must be considered to establish a histopathologic diagnosis. The biopsy should be accomplished through a percutaneous, transseptal approach to avoid injury to the lacrimal gland ductules. If the histopathologic evaluation reveals an inflammatory process, oral corticosteroids are initiated.

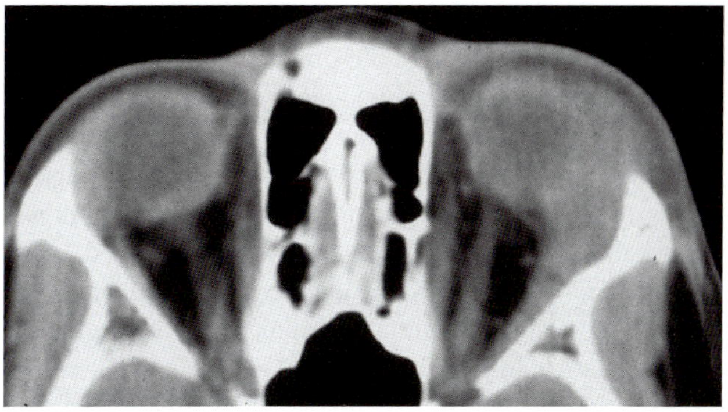

Fig. 48.2 Idiopathic orbital inflammatory disease (*IOID*). The lacrimal gland appears elongated and molded to surrounding structures. Note the absence of bony changes and the rock-hard mass indenting the globe

Noninfectious Lesions of the Lacrimal Gland

Idiopathic Orbital Inflammatory Disease (IOID)

The clinical manifestations of idiopathic orbital inflammatory disease, often referred to as idiopathic inflammatory pseudotumor, are principally determined by the degree of inflammatory response and the particular orbital target tissue under immunologic assault. Orbital inflammation is a tissue response, not a diagnosis. Inflammation may be localized or diffuse and can present acutely, subacutely, or chronically. Idiopathic, noninfectious dacryoadenitis is a specific example of the spectrum of localized forms of orbital pseudotumor, which include anterior or posterior orbit, trochlear [17], and extraocular muscles. Males and females are equally affected, and there is no racial predilection. Lacrimal gland pseudotumors occur most frequently in middle-aged adults, but can affect young children as well as elderly patients.

The disease tends to be unilateral, although it may occur bilaterally, especially in the pediatric population. Typically, patients present with an acute onset of pain localized to the lacrimal fossa region, accompanied by upper eyelid edema and erythema, symptoms similar to other inflammatory conditions. Examination discloses a characteristic S-shape eyelid contour and an exquisitely tender lacrimal gland to palpation. The enlarged palpebral lobe of the lacrimal gland is easily visualized in the supratemporal fornix, and pouting of the lacrimal ductules may be observed. Temporal bulbar conjunctival chemosis and injection are usually present. Adjacent extraocular muscle involvement results in ophthalmoparesis, diplopia, and ptosis. The globe is displaced downward and inward, and proptosis is usually minimal.

Lacrimal gland pseudotumors do not always have an acute, fulminant presentation. Chronic pseudotumors may occur as the sequelae of acute, recurrent orbital inflammations, but more commonly present without a history of acute inflammation. Chronic pseudotumors have signs and symptoms that develop gradually over months to years, and patients present with symptomatic proptosis, diplopia, or decreased vision, with few inflammatory signs. If the sclerosing pseudotumor is localized in the lacrimal gland or anteriorly in the orbit, it may be palpable as a rock-hard mass. This chronic, sclerosing variant is often complicated by permanent motility dysfunction and visual loss and may eventually result in a firm, fixed orbit with an immobile globe.

Computed tomographic imaging usually demonstrates enhancement and enlargement of a poorly demarcated mass in the lacrimal gland fossa region with a surrounding haze (Fig. 48.2). The lacrimal gland appears elongated and molded to surrounding structures. Infiltration of the surrounding tissues is common, manifesting in enlarged extraocular muscles and tendons, thickened Tenon's capsule and sclera, and diffuse irregular opacification of orbital fat. There should be no bony abnormalities on CT imaging. The presence of bony erosion renders the diagnosis of inflammatory pseudotumor unlikely and mandates a reassessment of the situation.

In most cases, an empirical trial of corticosteroids may be initiated without a tissue diagnosis, when the characteristic clinical and radiographic findings for presumed idiopathic inflammatory pseudotumor of the lacrimal gland are present. For isolated lacrimal gland involvement, Rootman and Nugent [18] recommend an initial biopsy due to the high incidence of involvement by systemic and neoplastic processes and the low morbidity of the surgical procedure. Systemic corticosteroid therapy should be given in sufficient strength to achieve rapid suppression of inflammation and in sufficient duration to minimize recrudescence. An initial prednisone dose of 60–100 mg/day is suggested for adults. Normally within 48–72 h of treatment, a dramatic improvement in signs and symptoms associated with inflammatory pseudotumor of the lacrimal gland is observed. The high dose of prednisone is maintained for 2–3 weeks or when echography demonstrates a 50% reduction in the size of the lesion, before commencing a tapering course. The slow tapering process is carried out over the next few weeks, reducing 10 mg/week. If the lesion is refractory to the appropriate steroid treatment regimen, the clinical situation should be reevaluated and a lacrimal gland biopsy performed. Other situations in which biopsy of the lacrimal gland should be considered include recurrence, chronicity of disease, and a discrete mass with bony changes and extraorbital extension.

Radiation therapy is an effective alternative to suppress orbital inflammation. The indications for its use include lesion refractory to corticosteroids therapy, medical contraindications to systemic corticosteroids, and disease relapse during steroid tapering. Low-dose supervoltage radiation in the range of 1000–3000 cGy in fractionated doses delivered over a 10- to 15-day course has been recommended.

For recalcitrant orbital pseudotumor refractory to both corticosteroid therapy and radiotherapy, immunosuppressive agents such as cyclophosphamide and cyclosporine have demonstrated a salutary effect in retarding orbital inflammation. Rootman and coworkers [19] advocate early and aggressive multi-agent immunosuppressive therapy for idiopathic sclerosing orbital pseudotumor. This regimen consists of azathioprine combined with systemic corticosteroids as an initial treatment, with cyclosporine and cyclophosphamide as alternative agents. In a study of 26 patients with lacrimal gland pseudotumor, Mombaerts and coworkers [20] concluded that corticosteroids are not the primary treatment choice for this condition and that surgical excision or debulking is a safe and effective treatment option, including the sclerosing variant.

The histopathologic findings in lacrimal gland pseudotumor are variable, depending on where the biopsy was obtained and when in the course of the disease it was sampled. Classically, there is a mixed inflammatory infiltrate arranged in lymphoid follicles and always associated with varying degree of fibrosis and destruction of acinic and tubular structures. In children, biopsies may exhibit a heavy eosinophilic infiltrate. As the disease progresses, more fibrous tissue is deposited, and inflammatory cells become more widely separated by tracts of collagen. Necrosis of orbital fat may be observed with a resultant granulomatous response. In chronic sclerosing pseudotumor, a paucicellular inflammatory infiltrate with dense fibrous connective tissue is seen.

Systemic Inflammations

Among granulomatous diseases resulting in lacrimal gland inflammation, sarcoidosis and Sjogren's syndrome are the most prominent. A number of inflammatory processes may produce enlargement of the lacrimal gland, simulating a primary tumor. Their detailed clinical and pathologic features are beyond the scope of this chapter. Only few selected systemic conditions will be discussed. In many of these inflammatory processes, there is bilateral lacrimal gland enlargement, whereas primary neoplasms are always unilateral. The lacrimal gland may also experience chronic inflammation and ultimately fibrosis as sequelae to radiation or loss of innervation. The infrequency of reported cases of dacryoadenitis reflects the fact that the lacrimal gland is housed in a bony cavity that is not regularly palpated and can conceal moderate enlargement.

Sjogren's Syndrome

Sjogren's syndrome is an autoimmune disorder of unknown cause characterized by chronic inflammation of the lacrimal and salivary glands with resultant keratoconjunctivitis sicca and xerostomia. The term primary Sjogren's syndrome is used to describe those patients without an underlying connective tissue disorder. Secondary Sjogren's syndrome refers to patients with associated connective tissue disease, such as rheumatoid arthritis, scleroderma, systemic lupus erythematosus, or polymyositis. Sjogren's syndrome most commonly affects middle-aged and elderly women. Infectious agents, such as Epstein-Barr virus and cytomegalovirus, may contribute to the pathogenesis, but the exact role of these agents is not known [21, 22].

Associated systemic manifestations are numerous and include recurrent respiratory infection, salivary gland enlargement, glossitis, peripheral neuropathy, cutaneous vasculitis, and Raynaud's phenomenon. Trigeminal neuropathy increases the risk of sight-threatening corneal complications. Patients are also at increased risk for development of lymphoproliferative disorders such as malignant lymphoma. Positive antinuclear antibodies are found in approximately 70% of patients with Sjogren's syndrome. Positive rheumatoid factor is also frequently found, and SS-A and SS-B antibodies may be present.

Keratoconjunctivitis sicca is the primary ocular manifestation of Sjogren's syndrome due to dysfunction of the lacrimal gland and accessory lacrimal glands. The resultant chronic ocular irritation, characterized by discomfort, burning, gritty sensation, photophobia, and redness, can be very disabling for patients. Physical examination findings include decreased tear meniscus, decreased tear breakup time, conjunctival injection, excess mucus, epithelial keratopathy, and filamentary keratopathy. Occasionally, enlargement of the lacrimal glands is present.

Schirmer testing and tear osmolarity measurements aid in diagnosis, and biopsy of the lacrimal gland or accessory salivary glands of the lip may be performed for confirmation in uncertain cases. The typical histopathologic features include lymphocytic (primarily B-cells and T-helper cells) and plasma cell infiltration, with eventual atrophy of the tubuloacinar elements and fibrosis [21]. Unfortunately, the glandular disease is progressive and refractory to treatment. Current therapy consists mainly of symptomatic treatment for dry eye and xerostomia [23]. Artificial tears or ointment remains the mainstay of therapy in mild cases. Punctal occlusion, bandage contact lens, and even tarsorrhaphy may be considered in severe cases.

Sarcoidosis

Sarcoidosis is an idiopathic, multisystem disease characterized by granulomatous inflammation. The noncaseating granulomas most commonly affect the hilar lymph nodes and lung parenchyma, with radiographic evidence visible in approximately 90% of patients. Women are affected more frequently than men, and African-Americans are affected more frequently than Caucasians. The majority of patients are less than 40 years of age [24]. Ocular manifestations occur in approximately 40% of patients, with anterior uveitis being most common, but any ocular or orbital tissue may be involved [24]. Lacrimal gland enlargement, if present, is usually painless and often bilateral. Chronic inflammation of the lacrimal gland in sarcoidosis can cause keratoconjunctivitis sicca.

While the lacrimal gland is the most frequent site of orbital involvement, only 15.8% of patients with ophthalmic manifestations of sarcoidosis will have clinically detectable enlargement of the gland [24]. However, gallium scanning has identified lacrimal gland involvement in 87% of all patients with systemic sarcoidosis [25]. Of the available serologic tests, serum angiotensin-converting enzyme and serum lysozyme are the most helpful in suggesting a diagnosis of sarcoidosis.

Diagnosis of sarcoidosis is based upon clinical, radiographic, laboratory, and histologic findings. Biopsy of the lacrimal gland via a transconjunctival or lid crease incision may be performed to aid in diagnosis [26]. The characteristic histopathologic finding is noncaseating granulomas containing epithelioid cells surrounded by lymphocytes and macrophages. Multinucleated giant cells are frequently present.

Patients with clinical evidence of active lacrimal gland inflammation may be treated with a short course of oral corticosteroids [27]. Therapy consists of prednisone 0.5–1.0 mg/kg/day, tapered over 8–10 weeks or longer if needed.

Wegener's Granulomatosis

Wegener's granulomatosis (WG) is characterized by granulomatous inflammation and vasculitis classically affecting the upper and lower respiratory tracts and kidneys. This disorder affects men twice as frequently as women, and the incidence peaks in the fifth decade of life. A limited form, more common in females, affects the upper and lower respiratory tract but lacks renal involvement.

Ocular manifestations occur in approximately 40–45% of patients with WG, and orbital involvement accounts for approximately 50% of the cases [28]. Orbital disease, which can be the initial sign of WG, may occur as localized lacrimal gland involvement [29], diffuse orbital inflammation, or midline involvement [30]. Clinical findings that should raise the suspicion of orbital WG include a history of upper or lower respiratory tract ailments, scleritis, keratitis, and bilateral orbital disease [30].

As untreated disseminated WG is generally fatal within 2 years, early diagnosis and treatment is critical. ANCA testing is helpful, with a positive result found in 60–90% of patients with WG. Histopathologic confirmation of the diagnosis is generally recommended, and orbital tissue, the lacrimal gland, or nasal or sinus mucosa may be biopsied. Classic histopathologic changes include vasculitis, granulomatous inflammation, and tissue necrosis. If mixed inflammation with tissue necrosis is seen, the diagnosis of WG should still be considered [30]. Therapy for systemic and local manifestations of the disease usually consists of systemic corticosteroids in combination with cyclophosphamide.

Systemic Lupus Erythematosus

The chronic, multisystem, autoimmune disorder of systemic lupus erythematosus (SLE) may cause a variety of ophthalmic manifestations [31]. SLE occasionally causes orbital inflammation, presenting similar to orbital pseudotumor or myositis [32]. Proptosis secondary to a lacrimal gland mass in the setting of SLE has also been described [33]. Orbital inflammation in the setting of SLE generally responds well to systemic corticosteroids.

Graves' Orbitopathy

Though the pathophysiology of Graves' orbitopathy is yet to be fully elucidated, the classic eye and orbital findings are well-known. As the extraocular muscles appear to be the main target of inflammation and cause of associated findings in Graves' orbitopathy, little attention has been given to the lacrimal gland. Orbital CT scanning of patients with active Graves' orbitopathy reveals enlargement and contrast enhancement of the lacrimal gland [34]. Histopathologic examination reveals infiltration of the lacrimal gland by lymphocytes and plasma cells [34]. Widespread fibrosis and loss of lacrimal gland tissue is not a characteristic finding. Inflammation of the lacrimal gland has been cited as the likely cause of alterations in tear composition found in some Graves' orbitopathy patients [3]. The clinical significance of these findings is not known.

Lymphoproliferative Disorders of the Lacrimal Gland

Lymphoid tumors generally occur in lymph nodes but occasionally may develop in extranodal sites such as the conjunctiva, orbit, lacrimal gland, and eyelids. Anatomic and

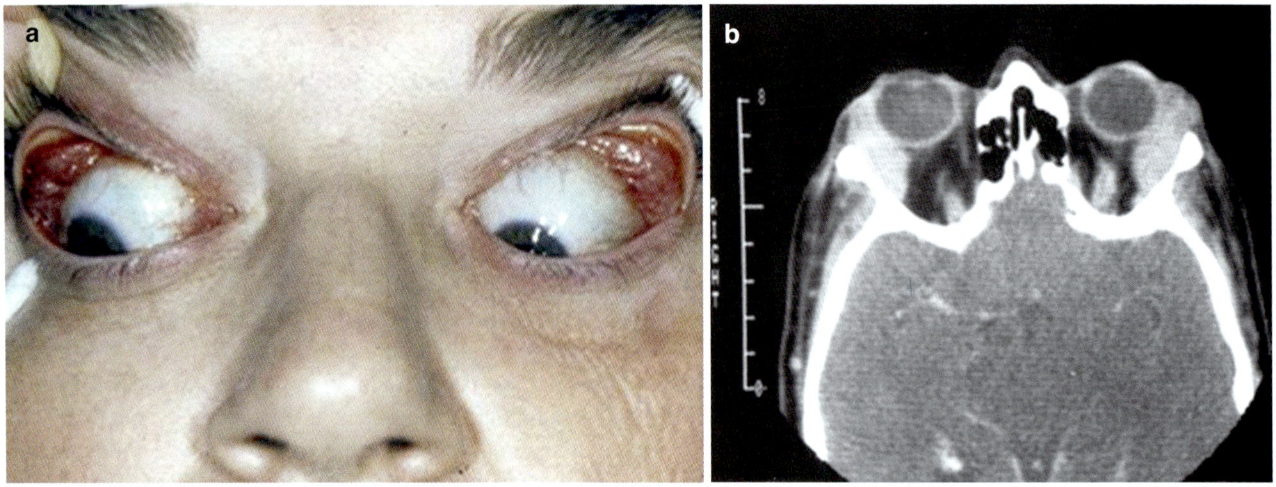

Fig. 48.3 (a) Bilateral painless enlargement of the lacrimal glands referred for evaluation of mechanical ptosis. Eversion of the eyelids disclosed prominent palpebral lobe of the lacrimal gland, with salmon-colored appearance. (b) Axial orbital CT scan shows a homogeneous lacrimal gland mass molding to the surface of the globe and into the contour of the lacrimal fossa. There are no bony destructive changes, and the enlarged lacrimal gland has the characteristic angulated posterior surface. Anterior extension of the mass beyond the orbital rim often indicates concomitant palpebral lobe involvement

immunologic studies disclosed the presence of a native population of lymphocytes within the substantia propria of the conjunctiva and in the interstitium of the lacrimal gland, which are capable of undergoing hyperplasia [35–38]. Lymphoproliferations spawned from these extranodal sites exhibit different biological behavior and prognosis than systemic nodal lymphomas.

Lymphoproliferative lesions of the lacrimal gland encompass a wide spectrum of disorders, ranging from benign reactive lymphoid hyperplasia (RLH) to atypical lymphoid hyperplasia, to malignant lymphoma. Clinically, it is difficult to distinguish between benign and malignant lymphoproliferative disorders. An incisional biopsy is often needed to differentiate benign from malignant infiltrates.

Orbital lymphoid tumors occur almost exclusively in adults and are exceedingly uncommon in children. Any of the orbital tissues may be affected, but there is a predilection for lacrimal gland involvement. Patients are usually in their fifth or seventh decade of life, with a median age in the 1960s [12, 39–41]. They usually present with an insidious onset of painless proptosis, ptosis, motility disturbance, globe displacement, lacrimal gland enlargement, or reduced vision. Most orbital lymphoid tumors are unilateral, with 25% of patients affected bilaterally [42]. Some may be localized to the fossa or diffusely affect the orbit, eyelids, or conjunctiva. Duration of symptoms is usually less than 1 year.

In lymphoproliferative infiltration of the lacrimal gland, a firm, non-tender rubbery mass is palpable in the fossa. Anterior extension of the mass beyond the orbital rim signifies concomitant palpebral lobe involvement, a feature more typical of lymphoid lesions than epithelial tumors of the lacrimal gland.

Computed tomography usually shows a well-defined, homogeneous, oblong orbital mass that molds to the eye and orbital bones without causing bony erosion or excavation and appears isodense to the extraocular muscles (Fig. 48.3). The contours are sharply demarcated, with a posterior perpendicular takeoff from the lateral orbital wall [39, 41]. Orbital lymphoid lesions typically display prominent enhancement with administration of contrast material [41]. Benign and malignant lymphoid lesions appear similar on CT imaging, and magnetic resonance imaging lacks the specificity to differentiate the two. Lymphomas and orbital pseudotumors have similar echographic characteristics. They are regular to slightly irregular in structure, with low to medium reflectivity and low sound attenuation.

Lymphomas of the eye and ocular adnexa are a heterogeneous group of malignancies, comprising approximately 1–2% of non-Hodgkin's lymphomas (NHL) and 8% of extranodal lymphomas. There are two distinct entities of ophthalmic lymphomas. Primary ocular adnexal lymphoma (OAL), arising in the conjunctiva, eyelid, orbit, lacrimal gland, and sac, should be distinguished from primary intraocular lymphomas (PIOL). PIOL, a subtype of primary central nervous system lymphoma, usually affect the retina, uveal tract, vitreous body, or optic nerve head and are almost always diffuse large B-cell lymphomas. Each entity is characterized by fundamentally different clinical features, natural history, therapeutic approaches, and outcome.

The majority of OAL affecting the orbit and ocular adnexa are primary extranodal neoplasms [43–46]. More than 95% is of B-cell origin, and 80% are low-grade lymphomas. The most common subtype, accounting for up to 80% of cases of primary ocular adnexal lymphoma, is extranodal marginal zone lymphoma (EMZL) of mucosal-associated lymphoid tissue (MALT) type.

Novel immunologic and molecular techniques have aided in the distinction between mucosal-associated lymphoid tissue (MALT) lymphoma and other lymphoproliferative disorders. Prior to the advent of immunophenotyping and molecular diagnostic techniques, MALT lymphomas were frequently misdiagnosed as RLH due to their cellular heterogeneity and presence of reactive germinal centers. Histologically, RLH shows a dense infiltration of mature small lymphocytes with scattered histiocytes and plasma cells. In contrast, ocular adnexal MALT lymphoma (OAML) is characterized by a heterogeneous cell population, consisting of monocytoid and plasmacytoid cells, with occasional blasts in the marginal zone surrounding reactive follicles.

Immunophenotypically, OAML have a characteristic profile, which allows for their differentiation from benign lymphoproliferative disorders and other small B-cell lymphomas. They are characterized by the presence of dense CD20+, CD10−, CD23−, and BCL-6 B-cell lymphocytic infiltrates, with few interspersed CD3-positive T lymphocytes. OAML are almost always (95%) negative for CD5, distinguishing them from mantle cell lymphoma and small lymphocytic lymphoma/chronic lymphocytic leukemia.

All patients with lacrimal gland lymphoid lesions, benign or malignant proliferations, must undergo a systemic workup. A complete systemic evaluation should include a general physical examination, hematological evaluation, liver function studies, bone marrow aspiration/biopsy, serum protein electrophoresis, computed tomography scanning of the abdomen, pelvis, and chest, and other appropriate investigations for systemic disease [47].

Management of lacrimal gland lymphoid tumors requires a multidisciplinary team approach involving the ophthalmologist, oncologist, and radiation therapist. Radiation therapy is the mainstay of treatment for orbital lymphoproliferative disorders, including lesions involving the lacrimal gland [48]. Benign lesions usually require 15–20 Gy, whereas malignant lesions require 30–35 Gy [42]. If the tumor is confined to the orbit without evidence of systemic lymphoma, radiation therapy alone is sufficient [47]. If systemic lymphoma is found, chemotherapy is usually initiated. Bilateral orbital disease without systemic disease does not warrant systemic chemotherapy. Close follow-up is essential since systemic disease may develop even years after treatment of the primary orbital lymphoid tumor. If local recurrence develops, a repeat biopsy must be considered to exclude malignancy [41, 49].

Besides radiotherapy and chemotherapy, a variety of new treatment options have emerged in the management of patients with ocular adnexal MALT lymphoma, especially monoclonal antibody therapy and antibiotic therapy against *Chlamydia psittaci*, which has been associated with the pathogenesis of ocular adnexal lymphomas in some parts of the world.

Questions have been raised whether some microbial species may be involved in the pathogenesis of OAML. It was postulated that prolonged antigen stimulation and oxidative damage induced by presence of genotoxic factors, such as infectious agents, could lead to gene mutations that allow for uncontrolled B-cell proliferation. Ferreri et al. [50] demonstrated an association between OAML and infection with *Chlamydia psittaci* (*Cp*) in Italian patients. The presence of *Cp*-DNA was detected in 80% of 40 lymphoma samples, compared with 12% of RLH samples. He treated nine patients with *C. psittaci*-positive marginal-zone B-cell lymphoma of the ocular adnexa at diagnosis or relapse with doxycycline 100 mg, twice daily orally, for 3 weeks. After 1 month of treatment, chlamydial DNA was no longer detectable in peripheral blood mononuclear cells of all four positive patients. Objective response was complete in two patients, partial response (>50%) was observed in two patients, and minimal response (<50%) was observed in three patients.

However, a number of subsequent studies from different countries have failed to show an association between *Cp* infection and OAML [51–58]. A meta-analysis [59] on the association between *Cp* and OAML across geographic regions and between different studies suggested a striking variability in the association between *Cp* and OAML across geographic regions and even between studies from the same geographic regions. Due to variable prevalence of *Cp* infection in OAML, empirical antibiotic treatment without prior testing for chlamydial infection should be discouraged.

Rituximab, a monoclonal chimeric anti-CD20 antibody, has been extensively used in the treatment of B-cell NHL, both as a single agent and in combination with chemotherapy. In patients with follicular and diffuse large B-cell lymphomas, the addition of rituximab to combination chemotherapy has led to significantly improved response rates, progression-free survival, and overall survival. In contrast, there is a limited body of evidence regarding the efficacy of rituximab in patients with MALT lymphoma arising in different organs. Only few case reports using single-agent rituximab in patients with OAML have been published [60–62]. They confirm the high activity of rituximab in both newly diagnosed and relapsed disease, but early recurrence is common [63], particularly in pretreated patients [64].

Benign Tumors of the Lacrimal Gland

Pleomorphic Adenoma (Benign Mixed Tumor)

Pleomorphic adenoma, or benign mixed tumor, is the most common intrinsic lacrimal gland lesion, accounting for approximately 50% of the epithelial tumors. The tumor occurs in virtually every age group, but most commonly in the third through seventh decades of life [13]. The mean age at presentation is about 39 years [65]. There is a slight male to female preponderance. These tumors are derived from lacrimal gland ductules, stroma, and myoepithelial elements. Most arise from the deep orbital lobe; less commonly, the palpebral lobe is the site of origin [66]. Rarely, pleomorphic adenomas arise from accessory [67] or ectopic lacrimal gland tissue [68, 69].

The diagnosis of benign mixed tumor of the orbital lobe can usually be made based on characteristic clinical, echographic, and radiographic information. Typically, the lesion presents as a painless, progressive, slow-growing mass or superotemporal swelling in the upper eyelid, with variable proptosis. Symptoms are usually present for greater than 12 months, but the duration of symptoms may be shorter if the lesion arises from the palpebral lobe and lid swelling becomes more pronounced during early phase of tumor expansion. The direction of globe displacement is dependent on the location of the tumor, with masses situated posterior to the equator inducing proptosis, and more anterior lesions causing downward and inward displacement (Fig. 48.4). Since this tumor is generally well tolerated, patients rarely complain of diplopia or visual decrease. Large tumors indenting the globe, however, may be associated with blurring of vision due to induced astigmatism or myopic shift. Gnawing orbital pain or inflammation is uncharacteristic for this lacrimal fossa mass. Although the lesion is usually painless, pain may occur if there is tumor necrosis or secondary dacryoadenitis.

On examination, mild temporal eyelid ptosis may be present, and palpation of the superotemporal orbital quadrant will reveal a non-tender, firm, well-contoured mass. Less commonly, the palpebral lobe is the site of origin. Due to its anterior location on the eyelid, a benign mixed tumor arising from the palpebral lobe can be misdiagnosed as a hematoma, dermoid, sebaceous cyst, or a dacryops [70].

Axial and coronal CT projections will display a round to oval, well-circumscribed mass in the lacrimal fossa, often with bony expansion and excavation, and an absence of bony destruction (Fig. 48.5). The posterior edge of the lesion typi-

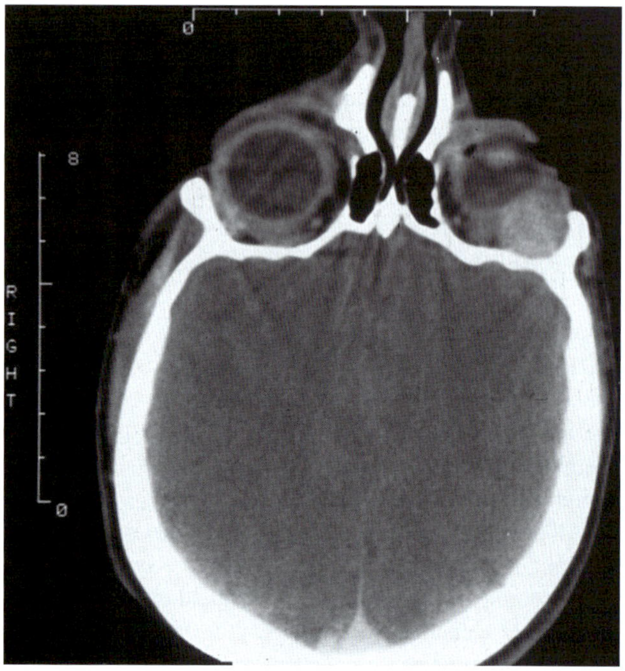

Fig. 48.5 Pleomorphic adenoma possesses a firmer stroma than a lymphoproliferative lesion and is likely to cause well-corticated fossa accentuation of the superolateral roof of the orbit. Axial computed tomographic image reveals an encapsulated, globular-shaped lesion indenting the globe. The posterior surface of the lesion is sharply demarcated and has an arc-like configuration, rather than a perpendicular takeoff contour from the lateral orbital wall of a lymphomatous mass

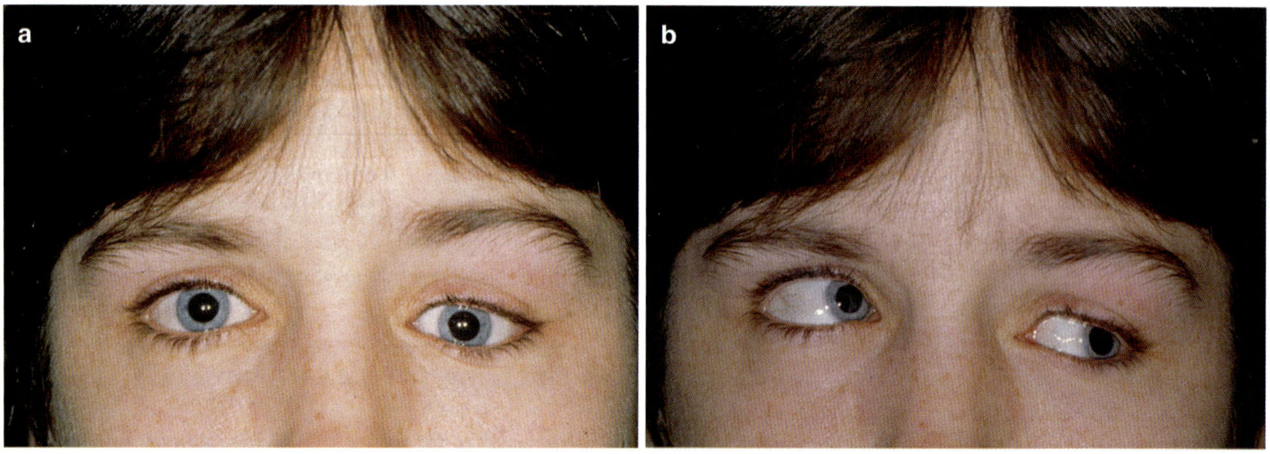

Fig. 48.4 (**a**) A 29-year-old woman presented with a 4-year history of painless, progressive, non-axial proptosis of the left eye. Clinical photograph shows fullness of the temporal superior sulcus and soft S-shape deformity of the upper eyelid. The globe is displaced medially and inferiorly. (**b**) She has difficulty looking up and out

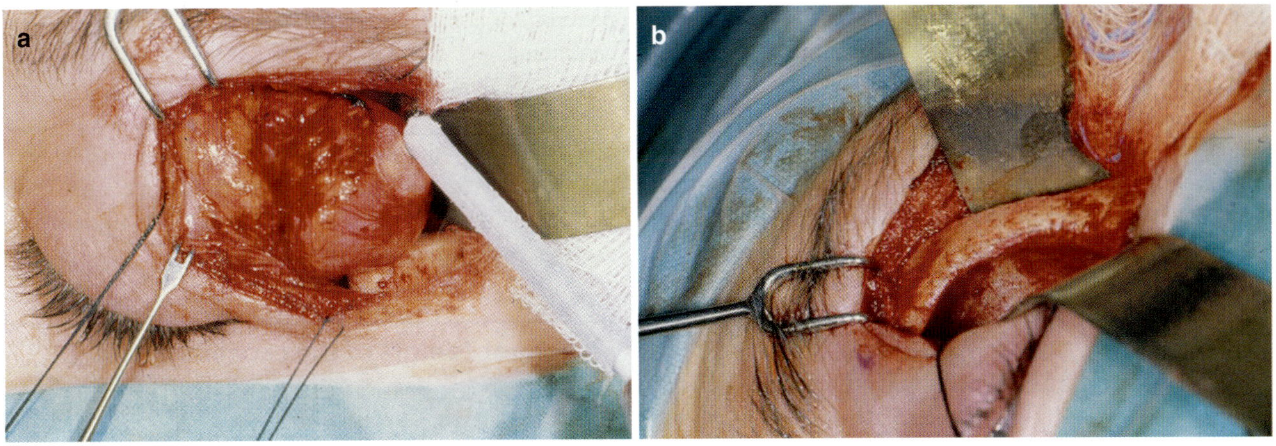

Fig. 48.6 (**a**) Intraoperative view of a benign mixed tumor (pleomorphic adenoma) with its intact capsule being removed through a lateral orbitotomy approach. Multiple projections beyond the surface are referred to as bosselations. (**b**) Intraoperative verification of fossa formation of the orbital bone in the patient depicted in Fig. 48.5. No pitting of the bone within the depression is seen

cally exhibits a curved contact with the adjacent orbital bone. Presence of bone erosion should raise the suspicion of a malignant tumor. Benign mixed tumors do not contour around the globe, like lymphoid or inflammatory lesions. Flattening or indentation of the globe and distortion of the muscle cone may be noted [39]. A-scan ultrasonography exhibits a round to oval mass with medium to high reflectivity and regular internal structure.

Lacrimal gland enlargement may provoke the ophthalmologist to perform a biopsy. The most appropriate management of a pleomorphic adenoma of the lacrimal gland is complete surgical excision of the tumor with an intact pseudocapsule via an anterolateral orbitotomy for orbital lobe lesions, without an antecedent biopsy (Fig. 48.6). Incisional biopsy of the lesion is conducive to seeding of tumor cells into the orbit or lid and clinical recurrence [10, 71]. An anterior orbitotomy approach for an orbital lobe mass is not recommended since it often leads to a subtotal or piecemeal removal of the lesion with possible seeding of the incision site. Small tumor excrescences extending through the pseudocapsule may occasionally be encountered, and removal of a small amount of normal tissue surrounding the neoplasm is advisable. During excision, some surgeons advocate the removal of adjacent periosteum and bone [13]. Rootman recommends a modified lateral orbitotomy and excision using an extraperiosteal approach on the lateral portion, excision of a margin of orbital fat medially, and careful dissection of the palpebral lobe [72]. For anteriorly situated palpebral lobe benign mixed tumor, isolated dacryoadenectomy via a transcutaneous or transconjunctival approach is preferred.

With en bloc removal of the mass within its pseudocapsule, the prognosis is generally excellent. Incomplete or piecemeal removal or rupture of its pseudocapsule results in inevitable recurrence [13, 73]. Recurrence following incomplete excision usually takes a long time to manifest and may be associated with malignant degeneration [74]. Recurrent tumors tend to be widely infiltrative and invariably spread beyond the limits of initial surgical resection, rendering subsequent extirpation difficult.

In most cases of lacrimal gland tumor, management is based on an accurate history supported by characteristic radiographic and A-mode echographic signatures. There are, however, patients with lacrimal gland fossa masses whose clinical and radiologic features do not conform to a particular category of diagnosis. In these atypical cases, an initial incisional biopsy may be necessary because a malignant epithelial tumor and other chronic benign tumors may mimic a painless expanding benign pleomorphic adenoma [75, 76]. In an attempt to avoid tumor spillage in the event an occult benign mixed tumor is incised, Tse and Folberg [77] suggested covering the incision site with several drops of N-butyl-2-cyanoacrylate. The layer of glue acts as an extension of the tumor capsule. The biopsy specimen is then submitted for frozen section examination. If a pleomorphic adenoma is confirmed, the incision can be incorporated into lateral orbitotomy incision for en bloc removal of the tumor. The permanency and bonding strength of the N-butyl-2-cyanoacrylate applied to the biopsy site should permit manipulation of the gland during total excision without disrupting the wound. If the diagnosis of pseudotumor or any other lesion except a pleomorphic adenoma is proven by review of permanent sections, then the presence of N-butyl-2-cyanoacrylate in the incision site should have no adverse effect because the material is biologically inert and has been used in a variety of surgical procedures.

While frozen sections can differentiate inflammatory lesions, lymphoproliferative disorders, and benign and malignant epithelial tumors, three points were emphasized by Tse and Folberg. First, an incisional lacrimal gland biopsy to establish the diagnosis of a benign mixed tumor is contraindicated if the clinical history and radiographic findings clearly support this diagnosis. Second, the routine use of frozen sections to establish the diagnosis of lacrimal gland tumors is not advocated. For example, the definitive surgical management of an adenoid cystic carcinoma should be based only on high-quality permanent sections, not frozen sections. Third, the routine use of tissue adhesive to bond the incision site during lacrimal gland biopsies is not recommended; this method should only be reserved for the scenario in which the possibility of incising into an occult benign mixed tumor exists.

Grossly, pleomorphic adenomas are pseudoencapsulated tumors. They typically exhibit bosselations, which are small projections beyond the surface contour. Histopathologically, the tumor is comprised of two morphologic cell components: benign epithelial cells arranged in a double layer forming ducts and stellate spindle cells contained in a loose stroma. Epithelial cells in the stroma can undergo metaplasia with cartilaginous, osteoid, or myxoid characteristics. The term mixed tumor arose because of the combination of unusual mesenchymal elements (myxoid, chondroid, and osteoid) and double-layered tubular epithelial units. Primary malignant mixed tumors of the lacrimal gland, although much less common, can also occur.

Myoepithelioma

The myoepithelioma differs from the pleomorphic adenoma in that the former is a proliferation of myoepithelial cells, while the latter is comprised of epithelial and myoepithelial cells. Myoepithelial cells are normally found adjacent to the luminal epithelium lining the lacrimal gland ductules. A myoepithelioma may be benign or malignant and consists of myoepithelial cells with up to 10% ductal elements. This tumor is usually considered in discussions of salivary gland tumors, but may rarely affect the lacrimal gland [6, 78, 79].

The biological behavior of lacrimal gland myoepitheliomas is thought to be similar to pleomorphic adenoma. As clinical differentiation is difficult, these lesions should be managed in a similar manner as for pleomorphic adenoma, with the goal of complete surgical removal.

Oncocytoma

Oncocytic lesions are rare tumors consisting of large, eosinophilic cells rich in mitochondria. These tumors arise from the metaplasia of ductular cells of glands such as the salivary, thyroid, parathyroid, pituitary, kidney, and other glands. The term oncocytoma (or oxyphil cell adenoma) is applied when the tumor has oncocytes displaying an adenomatous growth pattern. Lesions may alternatively exhibit patterns of oncocytic hyperplasia or frank oncocytic carcinoma.

These lesions occur predominantly in older adults (greater than 55 years of age) and more commonly affect females. The caruncle is the most common site for ocular adnexal involvement. Occasionally, an oncocytoma may arise from the lacrimal sac, but rarely the lacrimal gland [80]. Surgical excision is the preferred treatment option.

Malignant Tumors of the Lacrimal Gland

Adenoid Cystic Carcinoma

Adenoid cystic carcinoma (ACC) of the lacrimal gland is a rare but devastating disease of the orbit. Its prevalence is estimated to be 1.6% of all orbital tumors, 4.8% of all primary orbital neoplasms, and 25–30% of all epithelial neoplasms of the lacrimal gland [81–84]. Wright [81] has noted a bimodal distribution with peak incidences in the second and fourth decades of life with no apparent sex predilection. This tumor tends to not only affect younger patients but also confers the worst prognosis among the malignant tumors of the lacrimal gland.

Typically, patients with ACC arising from the lacrimal gland complain of periocular pain, mild ptosis, and proptosis, along with downward and inward displacement of the globe. Pain is the predominant symptom due to perineural invasion and bony infiltration by the tumor. Other symptoms include brow numbness and diplopia. These symptoms are typically present for 6 months, and almost always less than 1 year, before the diagnosis is established [13, 39, 81, 82]. Due to the infiltrative growth pattern of this tumor, computed tomography generally reveals a globular lacrimal gland mass with borders that are more irregular than those of an encapsulated pleomorphic adenoma.

Radiographically, an ACC lesion may exhibit features suggestive of a pleomorphic adenoma [85] or simulating a dermoid cyst [86]. Other CT abnormalities include bony erosion, bone destruction, and soft tissue calcification (Fig. 48.7). Contiguous tumor extension toward the medial orbit, apex, and the temporalis fossa is typical of an adenoid cystic carcinoma. Posterior tumor extension toward the superior orbital fissure secondary to retrograde tracking along the lacrimal nerve is another well-recognized aggressive behavior of this malignancy. Ultrasound evaluation often reveals a hard mass, usually within the orbital lobe of the lacrimal gland, which has a slightly irregular structure and medium to high reflectivity.

ACC of the lacrimal gland may also present in an atypical fashion. It is not unusual for a surgeon to have completely removed a well-circumscribed lacrimal gland mass with benign clinical characteristics, only to discover the lesion to

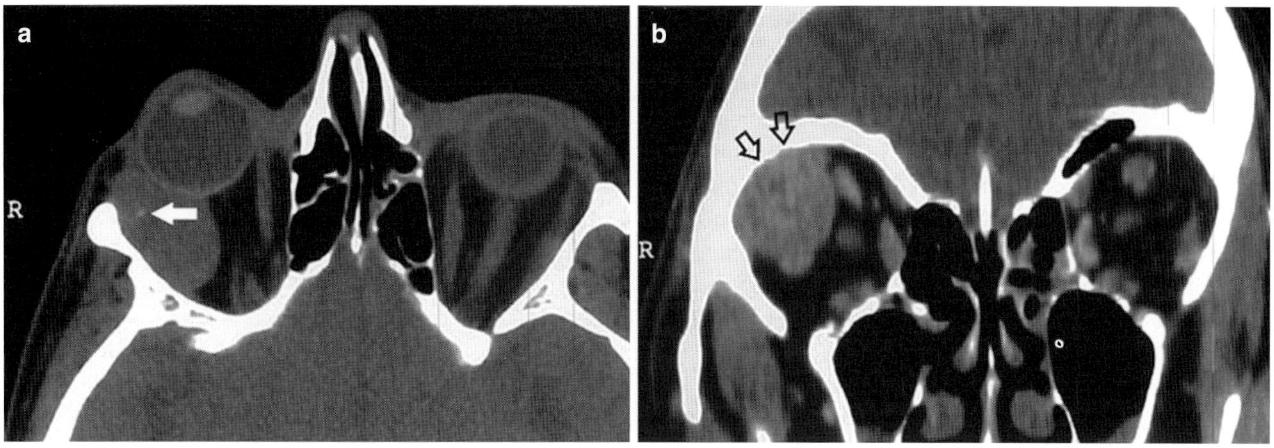

Fig. 48.7 (**a**) CT scan of a patient with adenoid cystic carcinoma of the lacrimal gland, displaying a misleadingly circumscribed lesion that exhibits a more extensive spread medially and posteriorly than is seen with benign mixed tumors. Occasionally, intralesional calcification can be seen (*arrow*). (**b**) Close inspection of the superolateral orbital bone reveals subtle bone erosion (*arrow*)

be an adenoid cystic carcinoma on histopathologic review [86, 87]. Patients presenting with symptoms of an enlarging mass in the lacrimal fossa for more than 3 years prior to the diagnosis of ACC have been reported [88]. Adenoid cystic carcinomas deriving from ectopic lacrimal gland tissue and from the accessory lacrimal gland in the anterosuperonasal orbit have also been reported [85, 89]. Finally, this malignancy may simulate inflammatory pseudotumor of the lacrimal gland, leading to a delay in diagnosis [90–92]. All of these unusual cases shared the common presenting feature of a mass in the lacrimal gland or in the anterior orbit.

Tse and colleagues [93] reported a case of unusual initial presentation of lacrimal gland ACC in the cavernous sinus and orbital apex in the absence of a mass in the lacrimal fossa, a clinical feature that has not been recognized in the past. The first ophthalmic sign may have been an Adie's tonic pupil noted 2 years earlier. The authors believe the ACC cells in this case escaped the lacrimal gland mass in the early phase of tumorigenesis and spread in a retrograde fashion along the lacrimal nerve to reach the ophthalmic nerve (V1) of the trigeminal ganglion in the posterior portion of the cavernous sinus. The proliferative phase of the tumor occurred in the cavernous sinus. The ACC cells then infiltrated the nasociliary division of the ophthalmic nerve and commenced with antegrade extension. After entering the orbit through the annulus of Zinn in the oculomotor foramen, a branch from the nasociliary nerve along the lateral side of the optic nerve enters the ciliary ganglion. The acquired Adie's pupil was most likely due to ACC cells gaining entrance into the ciliary ganglion by the pathway described. Tumor infiltration into the orbital apex and medial orbit may occur either by direct extension through the superior orbital fissure or by tracking along the nasociliary nerve through the annulus of Zinn. In patients presenting with an infiltrative mass in the cavernous sinus or orbital apex, metastatic disease from an occult lacrimal gland ACC should be considered, even with a normal-appearing lacrimal gland.

The histopathologic appearance of adenoid cystic carcinoma is characteristic and consists of sheets of epithelial cells arranged in either solid or cribriform patterns that mimic a glandular structure. Five histopathologic subtypes have been identified: cribriform (Swiss cheese), sclerosing, basaloid, comedocarcinoma, and tubular (ductal). Lower tumor grades are associated with a predominantly cribriform pattern, and patients with this subtype have been reported to have a longer survival [2]. Young patients with adenoid cystic carcinomas have a better prognosis than adult patients. This may be secondary to an increased incidence of tumors with less aggressive histologic features in the younger population [84]. Basaloid pattern connotes a worse prognosis [83].

In patients suspected of having malignant lacrimal gland tumors, an incisional biopsy through a transseptal incision is indicated. An extraperiosteal approach would violate the integrity of the periosteal barrier, potentially increasing the risks of seeding the extraperiosteal space with malignant cells, and should be avoided. Once the diagnosis of ACC is confirmed on permanent histologic sections, a thorough head and neck examination, coupled with a detailed survey of the intracranial compartment, is essential to determine tumor extent at the outset.

Controversy remains regarding the optimal local therapy for ACC of the lacrimal gland confined to the orbit, ranging from local surgical approaches to a radical multidisciplinary intervention. Some practitioners advocate a globe-sparing approach [86, 94–96] with local excision of the orbital mass followed by supplemental external beam radiation therapy, brachytherapy [86, 95, 97], or fast neutron radiotherapy [98, 99]. Other practitioners believe that radical surgery may improve local disease control [81, 100–104]. Most orbital specialists, however, subscribe to the conventional standard local approach of orbital exenteration with or without removal of the contiguous bone, followed by external beam radiation therapy. Rootman [102] advocates a more aggressive surgical tactic for local tumor clearance. In addition to en bloc excision of the orbit and its contents, resection includes the orbital roof, the lateral wall, the lids, and the anterior portion of the temporalis muscle where the zygomaticofrontal and zygomaticotemporal nerves extend. Adjunctive postoperative radiotherapy in a dose of 50–60 Gy may be added for large, advanced lesions.

Despite extensive surgery and radiation therapy, the survival outcome for these patients remains dismal [81, 105–108]. In a clinicopathologic study of 79 patients, Font and Gamel [5] reported an actuarial survival rate of less than 50% at 5 years and 20% at 10 years regardless of treatment regimens, which included local excision alone, exenteration, radiation alone, exenteration combined with radiation, and an unspecified chemotherapeutic protocol. These studies documented a recurrence rate of 55–88%, generally within 5–6 years of diagnosis, and a significant mortality rate with standard local therapies. Local recurrence is common, occurring in nearly half of patients within 2 years, with soft tissues or orbital bone as the most frequent sites. The bone and lung are common foci of distant metastases [82, 109]. The difficulty in achieving a cure in this disease is principally attributable to the complex regional orbital anatomy and the aggressive biological behavior of the tumor with its demonstrated infiltrative growth pattern, distinct propensity for perineural infiltration with retrograde intracranial extension (Fig. 48.8), and tendency for hematogenous [110] and lymphatic invasion (Fig. 48.9). The tumor often infiltrates and spreads through the bone [65, 106, 111] (Fig. 48.10). Frequently, intracranial involvement and metastatic disease are the principal causes of death [65, 82].

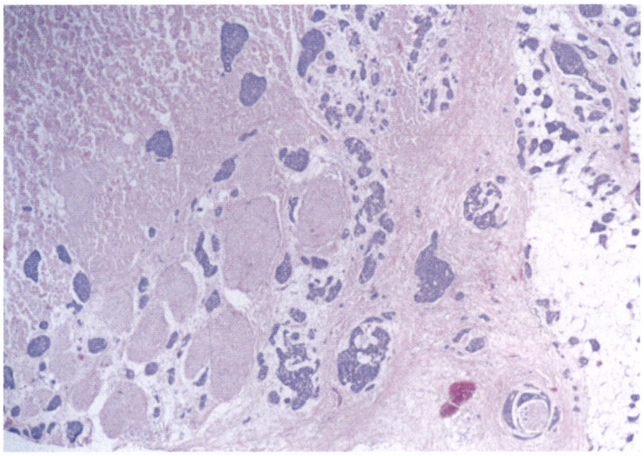

Fig. 48.8 Perineural invasion is a common biological behavior of an adenoid cystic carcinoma of the lacrimal gland, accounting for the frequency of orbital pain that precedes presentation. Note this section of tumor is predominantly basaloid pattern with a cribriform component

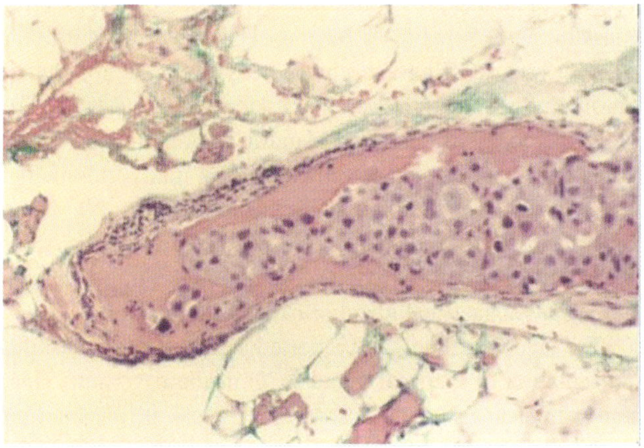

Fig. 48.9 Histopathologic demonstration of adenoid cystic carcinoma cells infiltrating into the lumen of a blood vessel

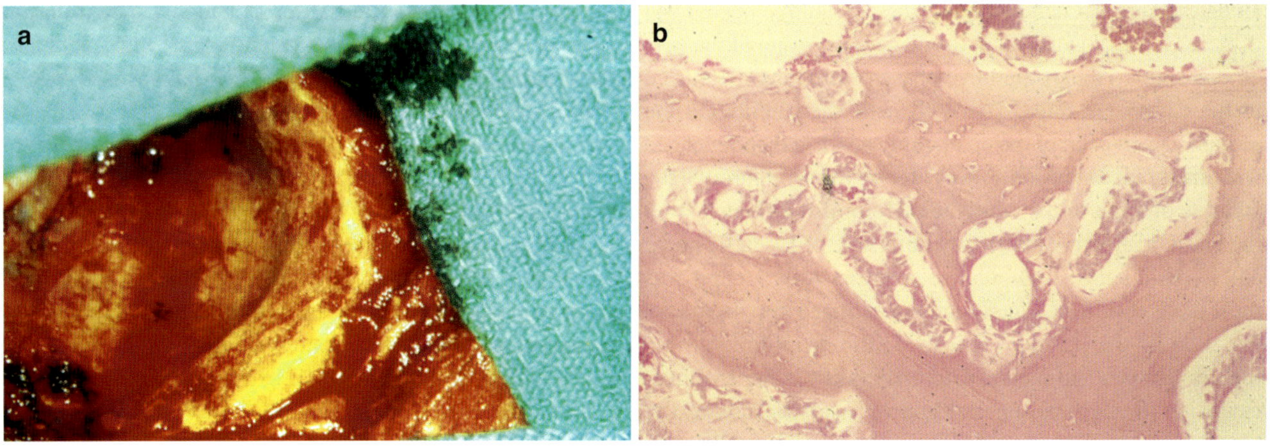

Fig. 48.10 (**a**) Intraoperative view of bone erosion caused by an infiltrative adenoid cystic carcinoma. (**b**) Histopathologic verification of adenoid cystic carcinoma infiltrating into the bone

While surgery and radiation therapy may achieve local disease control in many tumor situations, the early development of occult metastases results in treatment failure. For lacrimal gland ACC, tumor cells may have already escaped the orbit by retrograde extension along the lacrimal nerve or by blood vessel invasion at the time of presentation [106, 111]. The composite series of 94 adult patients from the reports of four major tertiary care centers document a distant metastasis rate of 50% (47/94) at 5 years [14, 76, 82, 109]. Thus, an alteration in outcome may only be possible by addressing the potential for occult metastatic disease early in the disease course.

In an effort to improve patient survival, Meldrum, Tse, and Benedetto [112] introduced the concept of intra-arterial cytoreductive chemotherapy (IACC) as part of a multimodality approach to locally advanced adenoid cystic carcinoma of the lacrimal gland. Since the drug is delivered through the intra-arterial route, the systemic toxicity is limited as a high percentage of the drug is extracted from the capillary bed of the tumor and the remainder is diluted in the systemic venous circulation (Table 48.2).

To optimize drug delivery, the intra-arterial treatment should be performed prior to extirpative surgery or radiation therapy to avoid disruption of blood supply to the lacrimal gland and tumor. The lacrimal gland receives its blood supply from both the internal and external carotid systems. The internal carotid artery gives off the ophthalmic artery, which then branches to form the lacrimal artery. To avoid direct brain perfusion through an internal carotid cannulation, the authors recommend the delivery of chemotherapy via the external carotid artery, relying on the lacrimal artery anastomotic branches to the external carotid system in the orbit and within the eyelids [112].

The choice of chemotherapeutic agents, *cis*-platinum and Adriamycin, was derived from the experience in treating epithelial tumors of the parotid and salivary glands, neoplasms of similar embryogenesis, and biological behavior to adenoid cystic carcinoma of the lacrimal gland. Intravenous *cis*-platinum and Adriamycin have demonstrated efficacy in these tumor types [113, 114].

The treatment protocol consisted of two cycles of preoperative intra-arterial cytoreductive chemotherapy (IACC) and four cycles of postoperative intravenous chemotherapy as an adjunct to conventional orbital exenteration and radiation therapy (Fig. 48.11). The rationale for the six cycles of chemotherapy is based upon the theoretic principle that at diagnosis, a tumor has a population of approximately 10^{12} cells. A highly effective (99%) chemotherapy regimen will kill 10^2 or 2 log-unit cells with each application. Thus, six applications ($10^2 \times 10^2 \times 10^2 \times 10^2 \times 10^2 \times 10^2 = 10^{12}$) would theoretically be required to achieve a "cure." This still leaves 10^0 or 1 cell. It is presumed the host immune defenses will play a role in eradicating small numbers of residual cancer cells, such that a cure is possible. This principle is borne out in the demonstrated efficacy of six cycles of MOPP therapy as curative in Hodgkin's disease, six cycles of CMF (cyclophosphamide, methotrexate, 5-FU) in adjuvant breast cancer, or six cycles of leucovorin and 5-FU in adjuvant colon cancer. The rationale for continued chemotherapy after surgery is to provide adequate therapy to decrease distant disease relapse using a drug protocol known to work in vivo in the same patient.

Aside from the importance of completing all six cycles of chemotherapy, Tse [115] emphasized the importance of surgical clearance of local disease at the time of exenteration – specifically the decision regarding removal of contiguous bone and tumor margin clearance at the apex. In the context of the IACC protocol, apical orbital tissues should be excised for intraoperative frozen section assessment – an orbital form of Mohs microscopically controlled tumor margin surveillance. If biopsy of the apical tissue is positive for residual tumor cells, resection is continued until the superior orbital fissure is reached. A Beaver 66 blade is used to shave off the

Table 48.2 Treatment protocol for adenoid cystic carcinoma of the lacrimal gland

1.	After diagnosis and systemic work-up to exclude distant metastases, the patient is admitted for neoadjuvant chemotherapy
2.	Pretreatment hydration to establish an adequate urine flow of at least 150 cc/h
3.	An intracarotid catheter is inserted into the selected arterial circulation of the lacrimal gland tumor
4.	*Cis*-platinum 100 mg/m^2 diluted in 500 cc normal saline is infused over approximately 60 min in the neuroradiology suite
5.	Maintain hydration for 48 h
6.	Adriamycin 25 mg/m^2/day is administered as intravenous push for 3 days
7.	Neoadjuvant chemotherapy is given for at least two courses separated by 21 days, followed by serial orbital CT scans to assess "radiographic response." Maximal response is defined as complete disappearance of the abnormality or stability between two imaging studies. A third cycle of chemotherapy may be given
8.	Three to four weeks after the last course of chemotherapy and following hematologic recovery (WBC > 2500 cells/mm^3 with adequate polys and a platelet count > 100,000 cells/mm^3), patient undergoes orbital exenteration
9.	Approximately 4–6 weeks after surgery, radiation therapy (5500–6000 cGy) is given in a standard daily fraction protocol
10.	Once each week, and just before receiving the radiation treatment for that day, *cis*-platinum (20 mg/m^2) is infused intravenously over 30 min as a radiation sensitizer. This treatment is preceded and followed by hydration in the outpatient clinic
11.	Two to four weeks after the completion of combined chemotherapy and radiation, intravenous *cis*-platinum (100 mg/m^2) and Adriamycin are given. After radiation, the dose of Adriamycin reduces to 20 mg/m^2/day × 3 days. Chemotherapy administration is in the same manner as the preoperative therapy, but without the intra-arterial approach

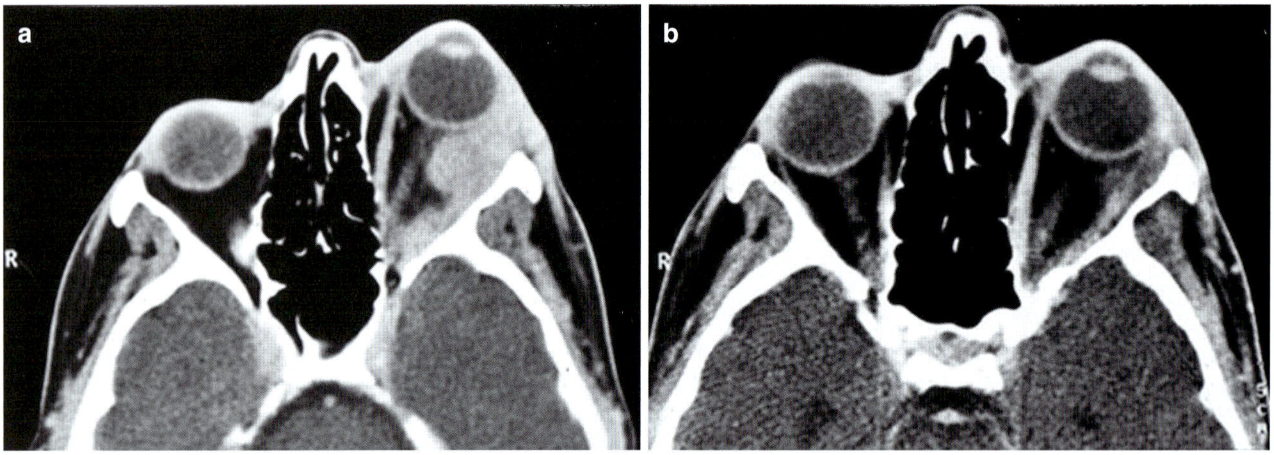

Fig. 48.11 (**a**) Axial orbital CT scan of a 45-year-old woman who complained of crescendo left orbital pain and progressive proptosis of 3 months duration. Biopsy of the lacrimal gland mass confirmed adenoid cystic carcinoma. (**b**) Note the marked shrinkage of the lacrimal gland mass and reduction of axial proptosis of the same patient after completing two cycles of intra-arterial cytoreductive chemotherapy treatment

orbital tissues entering the superior orbital fissure, with the heel of the blade resting flush against the lateral orbital wall so as to avoid the tip of the blade from piercing through the fissure to cause a CSF leak. Given the tumor's proclivity for microscopic retrograde perineural extension, intraoperative frozen section inspection of tissues at the entrance to the superior orbital fissure is an indirect measure of whether the boundary of the proximal-most surgical margin has been breached. Residual chemoresistant tumor cells at the apex will lead to local recurrence and may serve as the source to produce metastasis.

Tse and coworkers [88] reported the outcome of nine consecutive patients with lacrimal gland ACC treated by the above outlined multimodality therapy protocol. This series of nine patients was compared to a series of seven patients treated by conventional local therapies at the same institution. The carcinoma cause-specific death rates between the two treatment groups were significantly different ($p = 0.029$, log-rank test). The cumulative 5-year carcinoma cause-specific death rate in the IACC treated group was 16.7% compared to 57.1% in the conventional treatment group. The cumulative 5-year recurrence rate in the IACC treated group was 23.8% compared to 71.4% in the conventional treatment group. This data suggests that the integration of chemotherapy into the therapy of patients with ACC of the lacrimal gland is associated with a statistically significant reduction in disease relapse and improved overall disease-free survival compared to a historical conventional treatment group.

Tumor suppressor gene loss is a frequent event in many forms of human cancer [116]. Evidence suggests that malignant transformation involves a constellation of gene alterations occurring in a temporal fashion leading to a final pattern of accumulated gene damage characterizing the unique tumor genotype for a given patient [117]. An understanding of genes involved in lacrimal gland adenoid cystic carcinoma tumor development and progression is lacking, and translation of molecular insights from the basic science level into clinical application for this lethal tumor is needed. Tse and colleagues [118] performed gene analysis on microdissected paraffin-embedded fixed-tissue archival samples. Mutational allelotyping targeting 9 genomic loci using 15 polymorphic microsatellite markers situated in proximity to known tumor suppressor genes serve as markers for the presence of gene deletion. Allelic imbalance (loss of heterozygosity [LOH]) for microsatellite markers at 1p36 was the single most common site affected by imbalance in this series, followed by LOH in temporal sequence involving 9p21, 22q12, 10q23, and 9q22. A unique time course for temporal mutation acquisition in lacrimal gland ACC was proposed by the authors, consisting of 1p36 loss first. Allelic loss for microsatellite markers at 1p36 may be a common as well as an early event in ACC formation and progression. Microdissection genotyping holds promise as a clinical tool in integrating molecular analysis into standard histopathology to advance the understanding of lacrimal gland ACC tumorigenesis.

Primary Adenocarcinoma (De Novo)

Primary adenocarcinoma of the lacrimal gland is an uncommon malignancy, comprising only 5–7% of epithelial tumors of the lacrimal gland [73, 96]. These patients have clinical findings similar to those with adenoid cystic carcinoma. They commonly present with a palpable mass in the superotemporal orbit and proptosis, and approximately 40% complain of orbital pain.

Histopathologically, these tumors may represent a poorly or well-differentiated adenocarcinoma. The neoplastic cells are pleomorphic, mitotically active, and arranged in sheets and cords. The tumor may produce mucin or form lumina and undergo sebaceous differentiation, rendering it indistinguishable from carcinoma of the sebaceous glands of the eyelid.

Optimum therapy for this malignancy has not been well-defined due to the small number of reported cases. Exenteration followed by radiation therapy appears to be an effective combination. In a case series of 13 patients in which 7 received exenteration and radiation therapy, 4 were alive without recurrence at 2–16.5 years follow-up. One patient in the treatment group was alive with evidence of local spread of the tumor; two patients died with metastasis.

Adenocarcinomas tend to metastasize early to the lymphatics, in contradistinction to the late dissemination via bloodstream of adenoid cystic carcinomas [15]. Thorough head and neck examination is mandatory. If the regional lymph nodes are involved, radical neck dissection should be considered at the time of orbital surgery [15]. Reported metastatic sites include the liver, lung, bone, and spinal cord.

Pleomorphic Adenocarcinoma (Malignant Mixed Tumor)

Malignant mixed tumor has a reported incidence of 4–15% of primary epithelial neoplasm of the lacrimal gland [90]. The average age at diagnosis is 50 years, but ranges from 15 to 80 years [119]. This tumor may arise de novo, as a consequence of malignant transformation following an incomplete excision of a benign adenoma or as malignant transformation years after diagnosis of a presumed benign adenoma. Shields [120] reported a patient who demonstrated clinical signs and symptoms of a presumed pleomorphic adenoma which had been quiescent for more than 60 years before evolving into malignant growth. Thus, when confronted with a patient with an orbital mass associated with proptosis of several years duration that suddenly develops increased proptosis, the clinician should consider a diagnosis of malignant transformation of a pleomorphic adenoma [121].

Histopathologically, the malignant component may be attached to and arising from the benign mixed aspect of the tumor, yielding a bilobed appearance. The malignancy may be focal and requires extensive sampling to identify or may be readily apparent upon sectioning. Grossly, the tumor is well circumscribed with a pseudocapsule. Microscopically, tumor infiltration into adjacent soft tissues and the bone may be seen [120].

Complete surgical resection is the best treatment approach. Even with complete resection, mortality remains high, with 50% of patients succumbing to the disease by 12 years. Patients with pleomorphic adenocarcinomas transformed from a benign adenoma lived longer (mean 19.2 years) than patients with the de novo type (mean 7.7 years) [119]. Intracranial spread and metastasis to the lung, chest wall, sacrum, and scapula have been reported.

Mucoepidermoid Carcinoma

Mucoepidermoid carcinoma, a common neoplasm in the major salivary glands, rarely affects the lacrimal gland. This tumor originates from the ductal epithelial cells of the lacrimal gland and accounts for only 1–2% of lacrimal gland tumors [122]. A review by Eviatar and Hornblass [123] of the 25 lacrimal gland cases reported to date revealed an average age at presentation of 49 years (ranging 12–79 years), with a male to female ratio of 2:3. The duration or type of presenting symptoms did not appear to correlate with histologic grade of the tumor or prognosis. Bony destruction surrounding the tumor was variably present on CT imaging [124].

Histopathologic examination demonstrates epidermoid and mucus-secreting cells arranged in a pattern of cords and islands. The mucus-secreting cells and cystoid spaces within the specimen stain positively with mucicarmine and alcian blue stains and the periodic acid-Schiff reaction. Well-differentiated (grade 1) neoplasms have prominent mucus-secreting elements. Epidermoid cells predominate in the less differentiated neoplasms (grade 3).

The recommended treatment for grade 1 and 2 lesions includes excision with or without adjuvant radiotherapy. Grade 3 lesions, having a poor prognosis, require exenteration and radiotherapy. Eviatar [123] reported seven of eight patients with low-grade tumors surviving after extirpation, with or without radiation therapy. However, only one of eight patients with high-grade tumors remained tumor-free at 4 years of follow-up. Metastatic work-up for lung and mediastinal involvement is necessary for grade 3 tumors. Intracranial spread has also been reported.

Acinic Cell Carcinoma

Acinic cell carcinoma is an uncommon tumor of major salivary gland origin, with most lesions arising in the parotid gland. It represents 1–3% of salivary gland tumors [125]. The lacrimal gland, considered a minor salivary gland, is an exceedingly rare location to give rise to this type of malignancy. Only three cases of acinic cell carcinoma arising in the lacrimal gland have been described [125, 126].

Histological patterns include solid, microcystic, papillary cystic, or follicular subtypes. Individual cell characteristics include acinar, intercalated duct-like, vacuolated, clear and nonspecific glandular morphologies. As a modified minor salivary gland, the lacrimal gland contains acini that produce zymogen granules. On electron microscopy, characteristic features of acinar cells include cytoplasmic, electron-dense, round to oval, membrane-bound granules analogous to the zymogen granules of serous cells. Radiation therapy is an ineffective method of treatment for lacrimal gland acinic cell carcinoma [125]. Complete surgical resection is the best management approach.

Squamous Cell Carcinoma

Primary squamous cell carcinoma of the lacrimal gland is an extremely rare condition. There have been five cases reported in the literature. Clinically, it often causes bony erosion and pain secondary to perineural invasion. However, it has also been documented to present without pain or bony erosion [127–129].

Squamous cell carcinoma of the lacrimal gland may arise from a pleomorphic adenoma, the ductal epithelium, or an epithelium-lined cyst in the lacrimal gland. It is characterized by a pure proliferation of keratinizing malignant squamous cells that are moderately or well differentiated. No glandular elements are identified. Orbital exenteration is recommended as treatment for this aggressive tumor. Adjuvant radiation therapy may be implemented as well postoperatively [127–130].

Malignant Myoepithelial Carcinoma

Primary epithelial-myoepithelial carcinoma is a very rare, low-grade malignancy with only three cases reported in the literature. Patients usually present with symptoms characteristic of malignancy, including pain and bony erosion. There is one case described, however, in which the patient presented with painless enlargement of the lacrimal gland and a lack of bony erosion on CT scan. Histologic examination reveals variable proportions of ductal and large, clear-staining, myoepithelial differentiated cells. Myoepithelial cells are located between the luminal epithelial cells and the basal lamina of the acini and the intercalated ducts of the lacrimal gland. This characteristic biphasic cellular arrangement of ductal cells and myoepithelial cells helps to differentiate this tumor from other more common conditions such as adenoid cystic carcinoma. Orbital exenteration with adjuvant radiation therapy may be warranted in the treatment of this rare tumor [130, 131].

Carcinosarcoma

Carcinosarcoma may arise from a pleomorphic adenoma. Only two cases have been described. This malignant mixed tumor consists of both carcinomatous and sarcomatous components. This tumor should be considered in the differential diagnosis of a lacrimal gland mass if sarcomatous components are encountered on histologic examination. Management requires complete excision of the lesion [132, 133].

Miscellaneous Conditions

Dacryops

A dacryops is a benign, closed epithelial cyst within the palpebral lobe of the lacrimal gland. It typically presents as a painless, slowly enlarging, and variable-sized mass over the temporal upper eyelid. The cystic lesion may increase in size on exposure to cold or with crying [134]. Eversion of the eyelid will reveal a smooth, bluish cyst situated within the superotemporal conjunctival fornix, corresponding to the openings of the lacrimal gland ductules. On palpation, the mass is non-tender, mobile, and firm but fluctuant. The cystic mass transilluminates well, permitting differentiation from other solid lesions arising from the palpebral lobe. Putative mechanisms of pathogenesis included periductal inflammation with loss of the neuromuscular contractility of the ductules and congenital sequestration or acquired displacement of conjunctival tissue [135, 136]. Small, asymptomatic lesions may be observed, while larger dacryops is usually excised, taking care to avoid damaging the lacrimal ductules [137]. Marsupialization of the cyst is possible. Cysts arising from the ductal epithelium of the accessory lacrimal glands of Wolfring near the superior tarsal border have similar clinical appearance. Wolfring dacryops commonly occurs in patients with a previous history of trachoma [138].

Congenital Dermoid Cysts

Although benign and malignant lacrimal gland tumors in pediatric patients have been reported, primary lacrimal gland neoplasms are rare in the pediatric population. In this age group, space-occupying lesions appearing in the region of the lacrimal gland fossa are most likely congenital dermoid cysts. Dermoid cysts are common benign choristomas that arise from dermal elements pinched off at bony suture lines during embryogenesis. These slow-growing tumors presenting in early childhood occur on the superior temporal orbital rim (the most common site), the superomedial orbit, or the deep orbit. They are usually painless, rubbery in consistency, and often freely movable, as most are located anterior to the orbital septum. Minor trauma with leakage of the cystic contents can incite an acute orbital inflammation resembling orbital cellulitis.

Deep dermoid cysts are more often encountered in older children and adults. The clinical presentation includes slowly progressive, painless proptosis of long duration. CT images of the orbit will reveal a well-defined cystic lesion within the superotemporal orbit with or without pressure remodeling of the orbital bone. Surgical excision of dermoid cysts is the preferred treatment. With complete removal, the prognosis is excellent.

On histopathology, dermoid cysts are lined by stratified squamous epithelium, filled with keratin, and contain adnexal structures such as hair shafts, sebaceous glands, and sweat glands within the cyst wall. Epidermoid cysts are similar in appearance, but do not contain adnexal structures within the cyst wall. There may be signs of granulomatous inflammation within the cyst wall due to previous minor trauma and leakage of the cyst content.

Amyloidosis

Amyloidosis, a form of plasma cell dyscrasia, comprises a group of disorders in which excess amounts of immunoglobulin light chains are deposited in various tissues. These include primary systemic amyloidosis, amyloidosis with myeloma, and localized amyloidosis of the ocular adnexa. Secondary systemic amyloidosis, which affects parenchymal cells, characteristically spares the skin and other mesenchymal tissues. Amyloidosis of the orbit is usually associated with the primary and localized variant of the disorder, less commonly affiliated with the secondary forms of the disease. The localized amyloid of the ocular adnexa involves the infiltration of the extraocular muscles, levator and Muller's muscles, manifesting in ptosis and ophthalmoplegia. Isolated lacrimal gland involvement is rare. Massry and coworkers [139] reported a patient with isolated, primary localized lacrimal gland amyloidosis and reviewed four similar cases from the literature. All affected patients were middle-aged women without any visual morbidity. CT scan soft tissue contour analysis of the lacrimal gland mass demonstrates molding to the adjacent globe and orbital wall without bone destruction. The radiographic characteristics mimic features seen in inflammatory and lymphoproliferative disorders of the lacrimal gland.

Kimura's Disease

Kimura's disease (KD) is a distinct clinicopathologic entity that shares similar clinical and histopathologic features with angiolymphoid hyperplasia with eosinophilia (ALHE). However, based on histologic features, KD and ALHE should best be considered as two separate entities [140]. Kimura's disease is an inflammatory disease characterized by the presentation of violaceous dermal or subcutaneous nodules with a predilection for the preauricular, parotid, and submandibular regions. This is a commonly encountered condition in Asia, affecting predominantly young males. The clinical course is usually indolent, and the subcutaneous lesions may fluctuate in size or regress spontaneously. The etiology of KD is unclear, but thought to be an allergic or autoimmune response due to the associated peripheral-blood eosinophilia, elevated IgE titers, and immune-mediated nephropathy. Histologically, KD is characterized by inflammation with vascular proliferation, lymphoid nodules with germinal centers (T- and B-cells in lymphoid follicles), fibrosis, and aggregates of eosinophils.

Orbital and ocular adnexal involvement by KD is rare, but lesions affecting the eyelid, orbit, and lacrimal gland have been described [140, 141]. Signs and symptoms include eyelid swelling, ptosis, periocular discomfort, pruritis, gradual proptosis, a painless mass in the superior orbit, and motility disturbance. The two cases with orbital involvement reported by Buggage and associates [140] also demonstrated ocular surface damage, elevated intraocular pressure, and optic neuropathy.

Therapeutic options for orbital and adnexal KD include observation, excision, systemic steroids, radiation, and chemotherapy alone or in combination with other modalities [140]. Treatment of a patient with orbital KD with interferon alpha did not effect a permanent response [140]. Severe bleeding on resection and recurrence from incomplete excision has been noted.

Warthin's Tumor

A Warthin's tumor (cystadenolymphoma) is an epithelial neoplasm of the salivary glands, occurring predominantly in the parotid gland. Bonavolonta and coworkers [142] reported a case of Warthin's tumor arising from the lacrimal gland, an unusual extraparotid localization for this tumor. Within the lacrimal gland fossa, this tumor exhibited similar clinical and radiographic characteristics as a pleomorphic adenoma. Microscopically, epithelial columnar cells arranged in solid nests or lining cystic spaces containing an exudative fluid and a lymphoid infiltrate with focal follicular organization characterize the tumor. Management requires complete excision of the globular cystic mass with preservation of the thin capsule, in a similar manner as removing a pleomorphic adenoma.

Solitary Fibrous Tumor

Solitary fibrous tumors are spindle cell neoplasms of mesenchymal origin, which typically arise in the pleura of adults. Orbit, as the extrapleural site of presentation, is exceedingly uncommon. Scott [143] described an elderly man with a solitary fibrous tumor originating from the lacrimal gland fossa. The clinical history, physical examination, and radiographic findings in the reported case shared similar features of a patient with typical pleomorphic adenoma. The recommended treatment is en bloc excision through a lateral orbitotomy approach while employing the same precautions as in managing a benign mixed tumor. The histopathologic appearance of solitary fibrous tumor is varied, and immunohistochemical analysis may help in distinguishing this rare tumor from other lacrimal fossa lesions. The majority of orbital solitary fibrous tumors behave in an indolent manner, but the authors cautioned that lesions displaying hypercellularity, cellular pleomorphism, and high mitotic counts might have a more aggressive clinical behavior.

Hemangiopericytoma

Hemangiopericytoma is a rare soft tissue neoplasm comprised of abnormal proliferating pericytes, cells that are normally in close apposition to the outside of the endothelial cells in capillaries and postcapillary venular channels. This rare vascular tumor is commonly encountered in the lower extremities and retroperitoneum but may also arise from within the muscle cone of the orbit, optic nerve meninges, and lacrimal sacs [144–146]. Redmond and coworkers [147] recently described a highly unusual hemangiopericytoma originating from within the orbital lobe of the lacrimal gland. The patient presented with a short history of painless proptosis, lid swelling, and diplopia. CT scan demonstrated a large well-defined mass in an expanded fossa, but without bony destruction. The lesion was excised in a manner of extirpating a suspected pleomorphic adenoma.

Patients with orbital hemangiopericytoma generally present with progressive proptosis, diplopia, decreased vision, varying degrees of pain, and a palpable mass. There is a predilection for the superior orbit. Computed tomography shows a round to oval, well-circumscribed tumor that enhances with contrast. Within the orbit, the tumor appears pink to violaceous, encapsulated, and with large feeding vessels. The tumor's thin capsule can rupture easily during surgical manipulation. Once the thin capsule is violated and the tumor is incompletely excised, this lesion exhibits a propensity for aggressive local infiltration. These tumors are capable of metastasis, and 15% of patients in the series from the Armed Forces Institute of Pathology died with widespread metastases 6–32 years after initial diagnosis [148].

On microscopic examination, there is a prominent vascular pattern, with sinusoidal spaces forming branching channels, giving a "staghorn" appearance. In addition, there are solid areas of ovoid- to spindle-shaped cells. Tumors are classified as benign, borderline, or malignant, depending on histopathologic features including nuclear atypia and number of mitotic figures. One study demonstrated over 50% of lesions were benign, 15% were borderline, and 33% were malignant on histopathologic examination [148]. Management of orbital hemangiopericytoma includes complete surgical excision with an intact pseudocapsule to prevent recurrence and metastasis. Close follow-up examinations are important due to the unpredictable pattern of behavior and that metastatic disease can occur many years following surgical excision.

Cavernous Hemangioma

Cavernous hemangiomas of the orbit typically present within the intraconal compartment. One case of cavernous hemangioma arising from the lacrimal gland fossa simulating the appearance of a pleomorphic adenoma has been reported [149]. Bony remodeling of the lacrimal fossa was present. En bloc removal of the mass with preservation of the normal lacrimal gland was performed. Cavernous hemangioma emanating from the lacrimal gland parenchyma is rare [150].

Herniated Orbital Fat

An abnormality that may be confused with a lacrimal gland neoplasm is herniated orbital fat, which is visible in the superotemporal conjunctival fornix (Fig. 48.12a). The herniated fat has a similar appearance to a dermolipoma. This abnormality usually appears spontaneously in older patients and is believed to be due to dehiscence in Tenon's capsule, allowing orbital fat to herniate forward. Herniated fat also can present after trauma or surgery. Clinically, the lesion appears as a yellow, soft, indentable mass, with a smooth, convex border, which moves forward and becomes larger on retropulsion of the globe. Dermolipomas, in contrast, are usually pink–white to pink–yellow in color and are flat and diffuse. Additionally, they are not mobile or indentable and have smooth, straight, or slightly concave advancing border (Fig. 48.12b). A dermolipoma will not increase in size with retropulsion of the globe. Vellus hairs are frequently present on the surface of a dermolipoma. Surgical removal of the herniated fat through a fornix-based transconjunctival incision is possible [151].

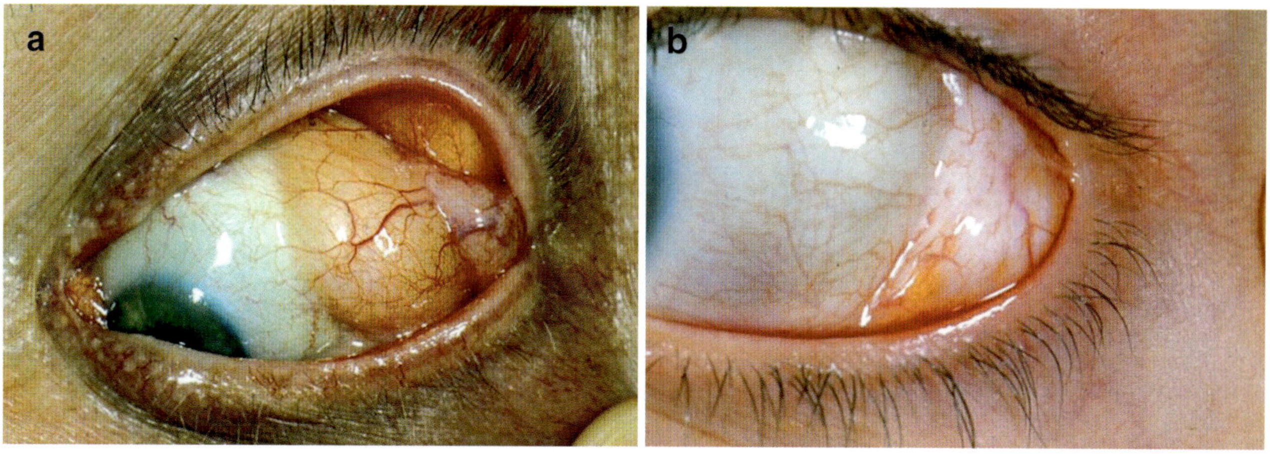

Fig. 48.12 (**a**) Photomicrograph showing herniated orbital fat in a patient referred for evaluation of a presumed lacrimal gland tumor. Subconjunctival herniated orbital fat from the central surgical space typically appears as a yellow, soft, indentable mass, with a smooth, convex leading edge, which moves forward and become larger on retropulsion of the globe. Palpebral lobe of the lacrimal gland is usually firm, lobular, and salmon pink in color. (**b**) A dermolipoma is usually pinkish yellow in color and flat. A distinctive differentiating feature from herniating orbital fat is its concave leading edge

References

1. Shields JA, Bakewell B, Augsburger JJ, Flanagan JC. Classification and incidence of space-occupying lesions of the orbit: a survey of 645 biopsies. Arch Ophthalmol. 1984;102:1606–11.
2. Reese AB. Expanding lesions of the orbit. Bowman lecture. Trans Ophthalmol Soc UK. 1971;91:85–104.
3. Kennedy RE. An evaluation of 820 orbital cases. Trans Am Ophthalmol Soc. 1984;82:134–57.
4. Reese AB. The treatment of expanding lesions of the orbit: with particular regard to those arising in the lacrimal gland. The seventh Arthur J Bedell lecture. Am J Ophthalmol. 1956; 41:3–11.
5. Font RL, Gamel JW. Adenoid cystic carcinoma of the lacrimal gland: a clinicopathologic study of 79 cases. In: Nicholson DH, editor. Ocular pathology update. New York: Mason; 1980. p. 271–5.
6. Goder GJ. Tumours of the lacrimal gland. Orbit. 1982;1:91–6.
7. Rootman J. Diseases of the orbit: a multidisciplinary approach. Philadelphia: Lippincott; 1988. p. 384–405.
8. Shields CL, Shields JA, Eagle RC, Rathwell JP. Clinicopathologic review of 142 cases of lacrimal gland lesions. Ophthalmology. 1989;96:431–5.
9. Jakobiec FA, Font RL. Orbit. In: Spencer WH, editor. Ophthalmic pathology: an atlas and textbook, vol. 3. 3rd ed. Philadelphia: WB Saunders; 1986. p. 2496–525.
10. Stewart WB, Krohel GB, Wright JE. Lacrimal gland and fossa lesions: an approach to diagnosis and management. Ophthalmology. 1979;86:886–95.
11. Wright JE, Ross GE, Garner A. Primary malignant neoplasms of the lacrimal gland. Br J Ophthalmol. 1992;76:401.
12. Hurwitz JJ. A practical approach to the management of lacrimal gland lesions. Ophthalmic Surg. 1982;13:829.
13. Wright JE, Stewart WB, Krohel GB. Clinical presentation and management of lacrimal gland tumours. Br J Ophthalmol. 1979;63:600–6.
14. Font RL, Smith SL, Bryan RG. Malignant epithelial tumors of the lacrimal gland: a clinicopathologic study of 21 cases. Arch Ophthalmol. 1998;116:613.
15. Jakobiec FA. Tumors of the lacrimal gland and lacrimal sac. In: Symposium on diseases and surgery of the lids, lacrimal apparatus, and orbit, Transactions of the New Orleans Academy of Ophthalmology. St. Louis: CV Mosby; 1982. p. 190–202.
16. Milder B. Diseases of the lacrimal gland. In: Milder B, Weil BA, editors. The lacrimal system. Norwalk: Appleton-Century-Croft; 1983. p. 105–10.
17. Tychsen L, Tse DT, Ossoinig K, Anderson RL. Trochleitis with superior oblique myositis. Ophthalmology. 1984;91:1075–9.
18. Rootman J, Nugent R. The classification and management of acute orbital pseudotumors. Ophthalmology. 1982;89:1040–8.
19. Rootman J, McCarthy V, et al. Idiopathic sclerosing inflammation of the orbit: a distinct clinicopathologic entity. Ophthalmology. 1994;101:570–84.
20. Mombaerts I, Schlingemann RO, Goldschmeding R, et al. The surgical management of lacrimal gland pseudotumors. Ophthalmology. 1996;103:1619–27.
21. Pepose JS, Akata RF, Pflugfelder SC, et al. Mononuclear cell phenotypes and immunoglobulin gene rearrangements in lacrimal gland biopsies from patients with Sjögren's syndrome. Ophthalmology. 1990;97:1599–605.
22. Pflugfelder SC, Tseng SCG, Pepose JS, et al. Epstein-Barr virus infection and immunologic dysfunction in patients with aqueous tear deficiency. Ophthalmology. 1990;97:313–23.
23. Bell M, Askari A, Bookman A, et al. Sjögren's syndrome: a critical review of clinical management. J Rheumatol. 1999;26:2051–61.
24. Obenauf CD, Shaw HE, Sydnor CF, et al. Sarcoidosis and its ophthalmic manifestations. Am J Ophthalmol. 1978;86:648–55.
25. Weinreb RN, Yavitz EQ, O'Connor GR. Lacrimal gland uptake of gallium citrate Ga 67. Am J Ophthalmol. 1981;92:16–20.
26. Weinreb RN. Diagnosing sarcoidosis by transconjunctival biopsy of the lacrimal gland. Am J Ophthalmol. 1984;97:573–6.
27. Cook JR, Brubaker RF, Savell J, et al. Lacrimal sarcoidosis treated with corticosteroids. Arch Ophthalmol. 1972;88:513–7.
28. Robin JB, Schanzlin DJ, Meisler DM, et al. Ocular involvement in the respiratory vasculitides. Surv Ophthalmol. 1985;30:127–40.
29. Leavitt JA, Butrus SI. Wegener's granulomatosis presenting as dacryoadenitis. Cornea. 1991;10:542–5.
30. Perry SR, Rootman J, White VA. The clinical and pathologic constellation of Wegener granulomatosis of the orbit. Ophthalmology. 1997;104:683–94.

31. Nguyen QD, Foster CS. Systemic lupus erythematosus and the eye. Int Ophthalmol Clin. 1998;38:33–60.
32. Brenner EH, Shock JP. Proptosis secondary to systemic lupus erythematosus. Arch Ophthalmol. 1974;91:81–2.
33. Burkhalter E. Unique presentation of systemic lupus erythematosus. Arthritis Rheum. 1973;16:428.
34. Trokel SL, Jakobiec FA. Correlation of CT scanning and pathologic features of ophthalmic Graves' disease. Ophthalmology. 1981;88:553–64.
35. Jakobiec FA, Iwamoto T. The ocular adnexa. In: Jakobiec F, editor. Ocular anatomy. Embryology, and teratology. Philadelphia: Harper & Row; 1982. p. 677–732.
36. Wieczorek R, Jakobiec FA, Sacks EH, et al. The immunoarchitecture of the normal lacrimal gland: relevancy for understanding pathologic conditions. Ophthalmology. 1988;95:100–9.
37. Sacks EH, Wieczorek R, Jakobiec FA, et al. Lymphocytic subpopulations in the normal human conjunctiva: a monoclonal antibody study. Ophthalmology. 1986;93:459–71.
38. Rubin PAD, Kent CJ, Jakobiec FA. Orbital and ocular adnexal lymphoid tumors. In: Albert DM, Jakobiec FA, editors. Principles and practice of ophthalmology, vol. 4. Philadelphia: WB Saunders; 1994. p. 3182–97.
39. Jakobiec FA, Yeo JH, Trokel SL, et al. Combined clinical and computed tomographic diagnosis of primary lacrimal fossa lesions. Am J Ophthalmol. 1982;94:785–807.
40. Shields CL, Shields JA, Eagle RC, Rathmell JP. Clinicopathologic review of 142 cases of lacrimal gland lesions. Ophthalmology. 1989;96:431.
41. White V, Rootman J, Quenville N, et al. Orbital lymphoproliferative and inflammatory lesions. Can J Ophthalmol. 1987;22:362.
42. Rootman J, Robertson W, LaPointe JS, White V. Lymphoproliferative and leukemic lesions. In: Rootman J, editor. Diseases of the orbit. A multidisciplinary approach. Philadelphia: JB Lippincott; 1988. p. 205–40.
43. White WL, Ferry JA, Harris NL, et al. Ocular adnexal lymphoma. A clinicopathologic study with identification of lymphomas of mucosa-associated lymphoid tissue type. Ophthalmology. 1995;102:1994–2006.
44. Fung CY, Tarbell NJ, Lucarelli MJ, et al. Ocular adnexal lymphoma: clinical behavior of distinct World Health Organization classification subtypes. Int J Radiat Oncol Biol Phys. 2003;57:1382–91.
45. McKelvie PA, McNab A, Francis IC, et al. Ocular adnexal lymphoproliferative disease: a series of 73 cases. Clin Exp Ophthalmol. 2001;29:387–93.
46. Coupland SE, Hellmich M, Auw-Haedrich C, et al. Plasmacellular differentiation in extranodal marginal zone B cell lymphomas of the ocular adnexa: an analysis of the neoplastic plasma cell phenotype and its prognostic significance in 136 cases. Br J Ophthalmol. 2005;89:352–9.
47. Jakobiec FA, Knowles DM. An overview of ocular adnexal lymphoid tumors. Trans Am Ophthalmol Soc. 1989;LXXXVII:420–44.
48. Jakobiec FA, Font RL. Lymphoid tumors. In: Spencer WH, editor. Ophthalmic pathology: an atlas and textbook. Philadelphia: WB Saunders; 1986. p. 2663–712.
49. Jakobiec FA, McLean I, Font R. Clinicopathologic characteristics of orbital lymphoid hyperplasia. Ophthalmology. 1979;86:948–66.
50. Ferreri AJ, Guidoboni M, Ponzoni M, et al. Evidence for an association between Chlamydia psittaci and ocular adnexal lymphomas. J Natl Cancer Inst. 2004;96:586–94.
51. Ruiz A, Reischl U, Swerdlow SH, et al. Extranodal marginal zone B-cell lymphomas of the ocular adnexa: multiparameter analysis of 34 cases including interphase molecular cytogenetics and PCR for Chlamydia psittaci. Am J Surg Pathol. 2007;31:792–802.
52. Decaudin D, de Cremoux P, Vincent-Salomon A, et al. Ocular adnexal lymphoma: a review of clinicopathologic features and treatment options. Blood. 2006;108:1451–60.
53. Mulder MM, Heddema ER, Pannekoek Y, et al. No evidence for an association of ocular adnexal lymphoma with Chlamydia psittaci in a cohort of patients from the Netherlands. Leuk Res. 2006;30:1305–7.
54. Yakushijin Y, Kodama T, Takaoka I, et al. Absence of chlamydial infection in Japanese patients with ocular adnexal lymphoma of mucosa-associated lymphoid tissue. Int J Hematol. 2007;85:223–30.
55. Gracia E, Froesch P, Mazzucchelli L, et al. Low prevalence of Chlamydia psittaci in ocular adnexal lymphomas from Cuban patients. Leuk Lymphoma. 2007;48:104–8.
56. Vargas RL, Fallone E, Felgar RE, et al. Is there an association between ocular adnexal lymphoma and infection with Chlamydia psittaci? The University of Rochester experience. Leuk Res. 2006;30:547–51.
57. Daibata M, Nemoto Y, Togitani K, et al. Absence of Chlamydia psittaci in ocular adnexal lymphoma from Japanese patients. Br J Haematol. 2006;132:651–2.
58. Liu YC, Ohyashiki JH, Ito Y, et al. Chlamydia psittaci in ocular adnexal lymphoma: Japanese experience. Leuk Res. 2006;30:1587–9.
59. Husain A, Roberts D, Pro B, et al. Meta-analyses of the association between Chlamydia psittaci and ocular adnexal lymphoma and the response of ocular adnexal lymphoma to antibiotics. Cancer. 2007;110:809–15.
60. Morgensztern D, Rosado MF, Serafini AN, et al. Somatostatin receptor scintigraphy in MALT lymphoma of the lacrimal gland treated with rituximab. Leuk Lymphoma. 2004;45:1275–8.
61. Conconi A, Martinelli G, Thieblemont C, et al. Clinical activity of rituximab in extranodal marginal zone B-cell lymphoma of MALT type. Blood. 2003;102:2741–5.
62. Nuckel H, Meller D, Steuhl KP, et al. Anti-CD20 monoclonal antibody therapy in relapsed MALT lymphoma of the conjunctiva. Eur J Haematol. 2004;73:258–62.
63. Yoon JS, Ma KT, Kim SJ, et al. Prognosis for patients in a Korean population with ocular adnexal lymphoproliferative lesions. Ophthal Plast Reconstr Surg. 2007;23:94–9.
64. Ferreri AJ, Ponzoni M, Martinelli G, et al. Rituximab in patients with mucosal-associated lymphoid tissue-type lymphoma of the ocular adnexa. Haematologica. 2005;90:1578–9.
65. Ni C, Cheng SC, Dryja TP, Cheng TY. Lacrimal gland tumors: a clinicopathological analysis of 160 cases. Int Ophthalmol Clin. 1982;22:99–120.
66. Auran J, Jakobiec FA, Krebs W. Benign mixed tumor of the palpebral lobe of the lacrimal gland. Ophthalmology. 1988;95:90–9.
67. Bech K, Jensen OA. Mixed tumor of the lower orbital region. Arch Ophthalmol. 1965;74:226–8.
68. Mueller EC, Borit A. Aberrant lacrimal gland and pleomorphic adenoma within the muscle cone. Ann Ophthalmol. 1979;11:661–3.
69. Mindlin A, Lambert D, Barsky D. Mixed lacrimal gland tumor arising from ectopic lacrimal gland tissue in the orbit. J Pediatr Ophthalmol. 1977;14:44–7.
70. Murphy MB, Rodriques MM. Benign mixed tumor of the (palpebral) lacrimal gland presenting as a nodular eyelid lesion. Am J Ophthalmol. 1974;77:108–11.
71. Jakobiec FA, Font RL. Orbit. In: Spencer WH, Font RL, Green WR, et al., editors. Ophthalmic pathology. an atlas and textbook, vol. 3. 3rd ed. Philadelphia: WB Saunders; 1986. p. 2459–860.
72. Rootman J, Robertson WD. Tumors. In: Rootman J, editor. Diseases of the orbit. Philadelphia: JB Lippincott; 1988.
73. Font RL, Gamel JW. Epithelial tumors of the lacrimal gland: analysis of 265 cases. In: Jakobiec FA, editor. Ocular and adnexal tumors. Birmingham: Aesculapius; 1978. p. 787–805.
74. McPherson SD Jr. Mixed tumor of the lacrimal gland: in a seven-year-old boy. Am J Ophthalmol. 1966;61:561–3.

75. Rose ER, Wright JE. Pleomorphic adenoma of the lacrimal gland. Br J Ophthalmol. 1992;76:395.
76. Wright JE, Rose GE, Garner A. Primary malignant neoplasms of the lacrimal gland. Br J Ophthalmol. 1992;76:401.
77. Tse DT, Folberg R. Technique for incisional biopsy of a lacrimal gland mass when the diagnosis of benign mixed tumor cannot be excluded clinically. Ophthalmic Surg. 1988;19:321–4.
78. Font RL, Garner A. Myoepithelioma of the lacrimal gland: report of a case with spindle cell morphology. Br J Ophthalmol. 1992;76:634–6.
79. Grossniklaus HE, Wojno TH, Wilson MW, et al. Myoepithelioma of the lacrimal gland. Arch Ophthalmol. 1997;115:1588–90.
80. Biggs SL, Font RL. Oncocytic lesions of the caruncle and other ocular adnexa. Arch Ophthalmol. 1977;95:474–8.
81. Wright JE. Factors affecting the survival of patients with lacrimal gland tumours. Can J Ophthalmol. 1982;17:3–9.
82. Lee DA, Campbell RJ, Waller RR, et al. A clinicopathologic study of primary adenoid cystic carcinoma of the lacrimal gland. Ophthalmology. 1985;92:128–34.
83. Gamel JW, Font RL. Adenoid cystic carcinoma of the lacrimal gland: the clinical significance of a basaloid histologic pattern. Hum Pathol. 1982;13:219–25.
84. Tellado MV, McLean JW, Specht CS, Varga J. Adenoid cystic carcinoma s of the lacrimal gland in childhood and adolescence. Ophthalmology. 1997;104:1622–5.
85. Shields JA, Shields CL, Eagle RC Jr, et al. Adenoid cystic carcinoma developing in the nasal orbit. Am J Ophthalmol. 1997;123:398–9.
86. Shields JA, Shields CL, Eagle RC Jr, et al. Adenoid cystic carcinoma of the lacrimal gland simulating a dermoid cyst in a 9-year-old boy. Arch Ophthalmol. 1998;116:1673–6.
87. Wharton JACL, O'Donnell BA. Unusual presentations of pleomorphic adenoma and adenoid cystic carcinoma of the lacrimal gland. Aust N Z J Ophthalmol. 1999;27:145–8.
88. Tse DT, Benedetto P, Dubovy S, Schiffman JC, Feuer WJ. Clinical analysis of the effect of intraarterial cytoreductive chemotherapy in the treatment of lacrimal gland adenoid cystic carcinoma. Am J Ophthalmol. 2006;141:44–53.
89. Duke TG, Fahy GT, Brown LJR. Adenoid cystic carcinoma of the superonasal conjunctival fornix. Orbit. 2000;19:31–5.
90. Henderson JW, Campell RJ, Farrow GM, Garrity JA. Orbital tumors. 3rd ed. New York: Raven; 1994. p. 323–42.
91. Kiratli H, Bilgic S. An unusual clinical course of adenoid cystic carcinoma of the lacrimal gland. Orbit. 1999;18:197–201.
92. Günalp I, Gündüz K. Epithelial tumors of the lacrimal gland. Orbit. 1994;13:147–54.
93. Tse DT, Benedetto P, Morcos JJ, Johnson TE, Weed D, Dubovy S. An atypical presentation of adenoid cystic carcinoma of the lacrimal gland. Am J Ophthalmol. 2006;141:187–9.
94. Saini JS, Mohan K, Khandalavala B. Primary radiotherapy in adenoid cystic carcinoma of the lacrimal gland. Orbit. 1990;9:107–11.
95. Asikin Natanegara IAA, Koornneef L, Veenhof K, et al. An alternative approach for the management of adenocystic carcinoma of the lacrimal gland. Orbit. 1990;9:101–5.
96. Polito E, Leccisotti A. Epithelial malignancies of the lacrimal gland: survival rates after extensive and conservative therapy. Ann Ophthalmol. 1993;25:422–6.
97. Tyl JWM, Blank LECM, Koornneef L. Brachytherapy in orbital tumors. Ophthalmology. 1997;104:1475–9.
98. Buchholz TA, Shimotakahara SG, Weymuller EA Jr, et al. Neutron radiotherapy for adenoid cystic carcinoma of the head and neck. Arch Otolaryngol Head Neck Surg. 1993;119:747–52.
99. Douglas JG, Laramore GE, Austin-Seymour M, et al. Treatment of locally advanced adenoid cystic carcinoma of the head and neck with neutron radiotherapy. Int J Radiat Oncol Biol Phys. 2000;46:551–7.
100. Byers RM, Berkeley RG, Luna M, Jesse RH. Combined therapeutic approach to malignant lacrimal gland tumors. Am J Ophthalmol. 1975;79:53–5.
101. Henderson JW, Neault RW. En bloc removal of intrinsic neoplasms of the lacrimal gland. Am J Ophthalmol. 1976;82:905–9.
102. Rootman J, Lapointe JS. Tumors of the lacrimal gland. In: Rootman J, editor. Diseases of the orbit; a multidisciplinary approach. Philadelphia: JB Lippincott; 1988. p. 384–95.
103. Marsh JL, Wise DM, Smith M, Schwartz H. Lacrimal gland adenoid cystic carcinoma: intracranial and extracranial en bloc resection. Plast Reconstr Surg. 1981;68:577–85.
104. Janecka I, Housepian E, Trokel S, et al. Surgical management of malignant tumors of the lacrimal gland. Am J Surg. 1984;148:539–41.
105. Henderson JW. Adenoid cystic carcinoma of the lacrimal gland, is there a cure? Trans Am Ophthalmol Soc. 1987;85:312–4; discussion 314–9.
106. Henderson JW. Past, present, and future surgical management of malignant epithelial neoplasms of the lacrimal gland. Br J Ophthalmol. 1986;70:727–31.
107. Ashton N. Epithelial tumours of the lacrimal gland. Mod Probl Ophthalmol. 1975;14:306–23.
108. Zimmerman LE, Sanders TE, Ackerman LV. Epithelial tumors of the lacrimal gland: prognostic and therapeutic significance of histologic types. Int Ophthalmol Clin. 1962;2:337–67.
109. Esmaeli B, Ahmadi MA, Youssef A, et al. Outcomes in patients with adenoid cystic carcinoma of the lacrimal gland. Ophthal Plast Reconstr Surg. 2004;20:22–6.
110. Bartley GB, Harris GJ. Adenoid cystic carcinoma of the lacrimal gland: is there a cure…yet? Ophthal Plast Reconstr Surg. 2002;18:315–8.
111. Naugle T Jr, Tepper DJ, Haik BG. Adenoid cystic carcinoma of the lacrimal gland: a case report. Ophthal Plast Reconstr Surg. 1994;10:45–8.
112. Meldrum ML, Tse DT, Benedetto P. Neoadjuvant intracarotid chemotherapy for treatment of advanced adenocystic carcinoma of the lacrimal gland. Arch Ophthalmol. 1998;116:315–21.
113. Sessions RB, Lehane DE, Smith RJ, et al. Intra-arterial cisplatin treatment of adenoid cystic carcinoma. Arch Otolaryngol. 1982;108:221–4.
114. Suen JY, Johns ME. Chemotherapy for salivary gland cancer. Laryngoscope. 1982;92:235–9.
115. Tse DT. Clinical and microdissection genotyping analyses of the effect of intra-arterial cytoreductive chemotherapy in the treatment of lacrimal gland adenoid cystic carcinoma. Trans Am Ophthalmol Soc. 2005;103:337–67.
116. Buendia MA. Genetics of hepatocellular carcinoma. Semin Cancer Biol. 2000;10:185–200.
117. Finkelstein SD, Marsh W, Demetris AJ, et al. Microdissection-based allelotyping discriminates de novo tumor from intrahepatic spread in hepatocellular carcinoma. Hepatology. 2003;37:871–9.
118. Tse DT, Finkelstein SD, Benedetto P, Dubovy S, Schiffman J, Feuer WJ. Microdissection genotyping analysis of the effect of intraarterial cytoreductive chemotherapy in the treatment of lacrimal gland adenoid cystic carcinoma. Am J Ophthalmol. 2006;141:54–61.
119. Henderson JW, Farrow GM. Primary malignant mixed tumors of the lacrimal gland. Ophthalmology. 1980;87:466–75.
120. Shields JA, Shields CL. Malignant transformation of presumed pleomorphic adenoma of lacrimal gland after 60 years. Arch Ophthalmol. 1987;105:1403–5.
121. Font RL, Patipa M, Rosenbaum PS, Smith S, et al. Correlation of computed tomographic and histopathologic features in malignant transformation of benign mixed tumor of lacrimal gland. Surv Ophthalmol. 1990;34:449–52.

122. Reese AB. Tumors of the eye. 2nd ed. New York: Harper & Row; 1963. p. 485–506.
123. Eviatar JA, Hornblass A. Mucoepidermoid carcinoma of the lacrimal gland: 25 cases and a review and update of the literature. OPRS. 1993;9:170–81.
124. Pulitzer DR, Echert ER. Mucoepidermoid carcinoma of the lacrimal gland. Arch Ophthalmol. 1987;105:1406–9.
125. De Rosa G, Zeppa P, Tranfa F, Bonavolonta G. Acinic cell carcinoma arising in a lacrimal gland: first case report. Cancer. 1986;57:1988–91.
126. Rosenbaum PS, Mahadevia PS, Goodman LA, Kress Y. Acinic cell carcinoma of the lacrimal gland. Arch Ophthalmol. 1995;113:781–5.
127. Hotta K, Arisawa T, Mito H, Narita M. Primary squamous cell carcinoma of the lacrimal gland. Clin Exp Ophthalmol. 2005;33:534–5.
128. Su GW, Patipa M, Font RL. Primary squamous cell carcinoma arising from an epithelium-lined cyst of the lacrimal gland. Ophthal Plast Reconstr Surg. 2005;21:383–5.
129. Fenton S, Srinivasan S, Harnett A, Brown I. Squamous cell carcinoma of the lacrimal gland. Eye. 2003;17:424–5.
130. Shields JA, Shields CL, Epstein JA, Scartozzi R. Primary epithelial malignancies of the lacrimal gland: the 2003 Ramon L. Font lecture. Ophthal Plast Reconstr Surg. 2004;20:10–21.
131. Chan WM, Liu DTL, Lam LYM, Choi PCL. Primary epithelial-myoepithelial carcinoma of the lacrimal gland. Arch Ophthalmol. 2004;122:1714–7.
132. Takahira M, Nakamura YM, Shimizu SI, Minato H, et al. Carcinosarcoma of the lacrimal gland arising from a pleomorphic adenoma. Am J Ophthalmol. 2005;140:337–40.
133. Ni C, Kuo KP, Dryja KP. Histopathologic classification of 272 primary epithelial tumors of the lacrimal gland. Chin Med J. 1992;105:481–5.
134. Brownstein S, Belin MW, Krohel GB, Smith RS, et al. Orbital dacryops. Ophthalmology. 1984;91:1424–8.
135. Duke-Elder S, editor. System of Ophthalmology, Vol 13, pt 2: The ocular adnexa: lacrimal, orbital and para-orbital diseases. London: Henry Kimpton; 1974. p. 638–43.
136. Fiander D, Brownstein S, Nicolle D, Jackson WB. Mucosal cyst of lacrimal gland fossa simulating lacrimal gland neoplasm. Can J Ophthalmol. 1980;15:87–90.
137. Bullock JD, Fleishman JA, Rosset JS. Lacrimal ductal cysts. Ophthalmology. 1986;93:1355–60.
138. Weatherhead RG. Wolfring dacryops. Ophthalmology. 1992;99:1575–81.
139. Massry GG, Harrison W, Hornblass A. Clinical and computed tomographic characteristics of amyloid tumor of the lacrimal gland. Ophthalmology. 1996;103:1233–6.
140. Buggage RR, Spraul CW, Wojno TH, Grossniklaus HE. Kimura disease of the orbit and ocular adnexa. Surv Ophthalmol. 1999;44:79–91.
141. Kodama T, Kawamoto K. Kimura's disease of the lacrimal gland. Acta Ophthalmol Scand. 1998;76:374–7.
142. Bonavolonta G, Tranfa F, Staibano S, Di Matteo G, et al. Warthin tumor of the lacrimal gland. Am J Ophthalmol. 1997;124:857–8.
143. Scott IU, Tanenbaum M, Rubin D, Lores E. Solitary fibrous tumors of the lacrimal gland fossa. Ophthalmology. 1996;103:1613–8.
144. Jakobiec F, Howard G, Jones J, et al. Hemangiopericytoma of the orbit. Am J Ophthalmol. 1974;78:816.
145. Boniuk M, Messmer EP, Font RL. Hemangiopericytoma of the meninges of the optic nerve: a clinicopathologic report including electron microscopic observations. Ophthalmology. 1985;92:1780–7.
146. Gurney N, Chalkley T, O'Grady R. Lacrimal sac hemangiopericytoma. Am J Ophthalmol. 1971;71:757–9.
147. Redmond RM, Mannor GE, Garner A, Rose GE. Lacrimal gland hemangiopericytoma. Am J Ophthalmol. 1995;119:99–100.
148. Croxotto JO, Font RL. Hemangiopericytoma of the orbit. A clinicopathologic study of 30 cases. Hum Pathol. 1982;13:210–8.
149. Seiff SR, McFarland JE, Shorr N, Simons KB. Cavernous hemangioma of the lacrimal fossa. Ophthal Plast Reconstr Surg. 1986;2:21.
150. Slem G, Ilcayto R. Hemangioma of the lacrimal glands in an adult. Ann Ophthalmol. 1972;4:77–8.
151. Jordan DR, Tse DT. Herniated orbital fat. Can J Ophthalmol. 1987;22:173–7.

Orbital Inflammation

49

Shivani Gupta, Hakan Demirci, Brian J. Lee, Victor M. Elner, and Alon Kahana

Introduction

Inflammation, from the Latin *inflammare* (to set on fire), represents a complex biological reaction to stimuli of endogenous or exogenous origin. Inflammation of periocular tissues is common and may have local and systemic implications. The varied etiologies of orbital inflammations can make diagnosis and treatment difficult because appropriate treatment is usually dependent on achieving a correct diagnosis.

Orbital inflammation is often a manifestation of systemic disease. Hence, a complete medical evaluation is often necessary in order to narrow the differential diagnosis. Some etiologies, such as bacterial infection, are easier to diagnose and have well-established treatment paradigms. Other etiologies, especially those related to systemic disease, may require systemic evaluation, imaging, and tissue biopsy for pathologic evaluation in order to establish a diagnosis and fashion an appropriate treatment plan. Some inflammatory processes raise the specter of progression to malignancy, and even in the context of a correct diagnosis, the treating physician may need to reevaluate, re-biopsy, and adjust treatment. Most treatments of orbital inflammation divide infectious from noninfectious etiologies, and this chapter will also do so while highlighting shared as well as differentiating features.

Evaluation

Classic teaching of the clinical evaluation of inflammation stresses five cardinal features: *rubor* (redness), *calor* (warmth), *tumor* (swelling), *dolor* (pain), and *functio laesa* (loss of function). The presence of these features only indicates the presence of inflammation but does not illuminate the basic biological processes underpinning the clinical presentations of particular cases that need to be addressed by successful treatment.

The clinical evaluation of the patient involves a history that includes the chief complaint and exploration of the cardinal features of inflammation. For each feature, location, type, severity, and exacerbating/relieving factors should be documented. Timing can be an important clue and should be ascertained with as much accuracy as possible. Pain and tenderness to touch are to be distinguished as the patient can have one without the other.

The evaluation of a patient with orbital inflammatory signs must begin with a complete orbital and ophthalmic examination. This must include assessment of vision, visual field, pupillary responses, extraocular motility, and exophthalmometry and evaluation of ocular adnexa, periocular bony and soft tissue anatomy, cranial nerves, and lacrimal system. Complete intraocular exam is essential, since orbital signs may reflect "spillover" from intraocular inflammation and vice versa. In addition, intraocular manifestations can often help narrow the differential diagnosis and suggest a treatment approach.

The goals of the evaluation are to (1) identify the anatomic compartment that is the primary source of the inflammatory process, i.e., intraocular versus extraocular; (2) differentiate between infectious and noninfectious etiologies; and (3) reveal whether the periocular manifestations are

S. Gupta
Kaiser Permanente, Department of Ophthalmology, Panorama City, CA, USA

H. Demirci (✉)
University of Michigan, Department of Ophthalmology and Visual Sciences, Kellogg Eye Center, Ann Arbor, MI, USA
e-mail: hdemirci@med.umich.edu

B. J. Lee
Maryland Oculoplastic Surgery, Ellicott City, MD, USA

V. M. Elner
Eye Plastic and Orbital Surgery Service, Department of Ophthalmology and Visual Sciences, Kellogg Eye Center, University of Michigan, Ann Arbor, MI, USA

A. Kahana
Consultants in Ophthalmic and Facial Plastic Surgery, Southfield, MI, USA

J. J. Servat et al. (eds.), *Smith and Nesi's Ophthalmic Plastic and Reconstructive Surgery*,
https://doi.org/10.1007/978-3-030-41720-8_49

part of a broader systemic process or are due to a primary process of the ocular region. Evaluation is often not straightforward and commonly requires ancillary tests, including radiological imaging, blood tests, and diagnostic biopsies in order to narrow the differential diagnosis to a manageable short list. In some cases, therapeutic trials may be necessary to establish a presumptive diagnosis. The remainder of this chapter will describe particular entities to arm the clinician with important information useful in addressing these goals.

Orbital Infection

Infection of the ocular adnexal tissues can be preseptal or postseptal (i.e., orbital) and can be caused by a wide variety of bacteria, fungi, parasites, and viruses. Because treatment of each infectious cause is quite different, identifying the cause is critical for proper treatment. In addition, many infections occur in a broader systemic context. Bacterial infections often follow an injury or sinus infection. Fungal infections often signify underlying host immune compromise, and parasitic infections of the orbit suggest a broader colonization that must be treated to achieve therapeutic success. When present, failure to treat the systemic infection will often render the local treatment ineffective.

Bacterial Orbital Cellulitis

Clinical Features

Bacterial orbital cellulitis, the most commonly encountered orbital infection, generally occurs as an extension of adjacent paranasal sinus disease and is most commonly unilateral in presentation. It is distinguished from preseptal cellulitis by involvement posterior to the orbital septum, a fibrous structure that attaches to the periosteum of the orbital rim and separates pre- and postseptal spaces. Orbital cellulitis is more common in the pediatric age group, but all ages may be affected, and studies suggest a bimodal age distribution with slight male predominance [1, 2]. The mean age of pediatric patients with orbital cellulitis has been reported to be greater than those with preseptal cellulitis [3, 4]. In neonates, orbital cellulitis is uncommon with only few case reports in the literature [5].

Extension of paranasal sinusitis accounts for approximately 90% of all cases of orbital cellulitis, with ethmoid sinusitis present in the vast majority of cases [3, 6]. In young children, this is likely to be related to the early development of ethmoid sinuses and absence of frontal and sphenoid sinuses. Additionally, contiguous infection from the maxillary sinus may be less likely due to the thicker orbital floor as compared to the thin lamina papyracea of the medial orbital wall and the dependent location of the inflammatory collection in the maxillary sinus [7]. Factors that are thought to contribute to the spread of infection from the paranasal sinuses to the orbit relate to their intimate anatomic relationship and include the presence of bony foramina conducting blood vessels and nerves that extend between the orbit and adjacent sinuses, valveless veins between the orbit and adjacent structures that allow for bidirectional movement of pathogens, and congenital or acquired bony defects [6, 8]. Orbital cellulitis, however, may also be also associated with contiguous spread from adjacent preseptal infection, antecedent periocular surgery or injection of therapeutic agents, trauma, intraorbital foreign body, conjunctivitis, dacryoadenitis, dacryocystitis, panophthalmic spread of endophthalmitis, odontogenic infection or abscess, and hematologic seeding from underlying bacteremia [6, 9–20].

Diagnosis

A detailed history should be obtained with particular attention paid to the presence of sinusitis or upper respiratory tract infection, preceding preseptal cellulitis or other skin infection, local trauma or retained intraorbital foreign body, ophthalmic surgery, periodontal disease, diabetes, immunocompromised states, and underlying systemic infections. This information, combined with the clinical examination, will lead to a presumptive clinical diagnosis of infectious orbital cellulitis in the majority of patients.

Patients generally present with fever, periocular edema and erythema extending beyond the orbital rim, periocular pain and tenderness, proptosis, pupillary abnormalities, conjunctival injection, chemosis, and ophthalmoplegia. Pain with eye movement is a sensitive, albeit nonspecific sign of orbital inflammation. Hypoesthesia in the distribution of the trigeminal nerve may be noted. Reduced vision and afferent papillary defect may be present due to increased diffuse or localized pressure on the globe, optic nerve, or blood vessels as well as by direct extension of infection to involve these structures or the cavernous sinus. In these cases, optic nerve edema, retinal vascular engorgement, or periphlebitis may be noted on funduscopic examination. Periocular vascular congestion may indicate the presence of superior ophthalmic vein obstruction and impending cavernous sinus thrombosis. In the latter case, patients may also have high fever, headache, nausea, meningismus, severe vision loss, external ophthalmoplegia of the affected side, and progression to involve the contralateral side. Intracranial involvement is suggested by the presence of neurologic signs including altered mental status, focal neurologic deficits, seizures, and radiologic signs of basilar extension or brain abscess [21].

Although orbital cellulitis is often a clinical diagnosis requiring prompt empiric treatment with broad-spectrum antibiotics, imaging of the orbits and surrounding structures should be obtained as soon as possible. High-resolution computed tomography (CT) is the initial imaging study of choice and may help differentiate between preseptal and orbital cellulitis when the clinical picture is unclear. CT also provides useful information regarding the presence, location, and extent of sinus disease, presence of intraorbital foreign bodies, subperiosteal or orbital abscesses, and extraorbital extension that may require surgical intervention. Intraorbital gas or air-fluid levels may suggest the presence of a gas-forming organism or communication with the sinuses [6]. Additionally, clinically silent odontogenic causes, usually of the upper jaw, may be identified on CT by abnormal periapical lucency and widening of the periodontal ligament space [22]. Bony erosion may indicate a neoplastic or fungal process. Because sinus opacification is often an incidental finding in asymptomatic individuals, caution should be used in interpreting sinus findings as the cause of orbital cellulitis in a particular patient [3, 23–25]. MRI provides excellent contrast resolution in the orbit, and it has been suggested as a tool to assess postseptal involvement, cavernous sinus thrombosis, and intracranial extension of orbital cellulitis [26]. Diffusion-weighted imaging is a useful adjunct to contrast-enhanced sequences in identifying orbital abscesses and may provide additional information in patients who have renal failure and in whom gadolinium contrast is contraindicated [26].

Laboratory studies may reveal leukocytosis and elevation of nonspecific inflammatory markers such as C-reactive protein (CRP) and erythrocyte sedimentation rate (ESR). A study by Georgakopoulos et al. [3] reported a statistically significant increase in neutrophils in pediatric patients with orbital cellulitis as compared to preseptal cellulitis and a trend of increased left shift in leukocyte type, elevated serum C-reactive protein, and erythrocyte sedimentation rates. Isolation rates of causative organisms remain fairly low, partly due to the fact that patients often receive antibiotic therapy in the outpatient setting prior to hospital admission. Local cultures including conjunctival, wound (if skin drainage site present), abscess, sinus, and nasopharyngeal swabs should be obtained prior to initiation of treatment when possible and have a much higher rate of positivity as compared to blood cultures [1].

The microbiology of orbital cellulitis is closely linked to the microbiological flora of the associated sinusitis [6]. Harris [27] found that in children less than 9 years of age, single aerobic pathogens were more likely to be the cause of sinusitis and orbital cellulitis compared to older patients from whom multiple pathogens were often isolated. Anatomic changes that occur with facial growth are thought to account for the shift from simple infections due to aerobic organisms that are more commonly seen in young children to complex, polymicrobial infections with mixed aerobic and anaerobic constituents seen in older children and adults [28]. As sinus cavities enlarge with age, their ostia remain the same size. As aerobic bacteria consume the available oxygen, anaerobic bacteria proliferate and colonize low-oxygen regions within the sinuses.

The most commonly isolated organisms in the pediatric population include *S. aureus*, *S. pneumoniae*, *S. epidermidis*, and *H. influenzae* [3]. The relative contributions of these pathogens have changed over time. *H. influenzae*, a virulent pathogen, was most commonly found in culture-positive cases prior to the introduction of *H. influenzae* B (Hib) vaccination and accounted for up to 80% of cases of pediatric preseptal and orbital cellulitis [29, 30]. Orbital infection with *Haemophilus* sp. can lead to devastating complications including meningitis, cavernous sinus thrombosis, severe neurologic impairment, and even death [31]. After the Hib vaccine was introduced, rates of Hib-related periocular and orbital cellulitis have declined significantly and have mirrored the decline in other *H. influenzae*-related diseases [31–33]. More recent studies suggest that, in culture proven cases, *Staphylococcus* and *Streptococcus* species predominate, with increasing prevalence of methicillin-resistant *S. aureus* (MRSA) in up to 73% of *Staphylococcus* isolates in one series [34, 35]. Multiple abscess sites are often seen with MRSA orbital infections. In addition, community-acquired methicillin-resistant *S. aureus* (CAMRSA) has been on the rise as an etiologic agent for community-acquired infections, particularly skin and soft tissue infections among young healthy individuals [36, 37]. Though CAMRSA has a wider susceptibility profile to antibiotics as compared to hospital-acquired MRSA, CAMRSA strains can cause severe infections [37]. Ophthalmic manifestations include conjunctivitis, corneal ulceration, endogenous endophthalmitis, dacryocystitis, blebitis, and orbital cellulitis [37]. One recent series of nine patients with ocular and orbital infections by the USA300 clone of CAMRSA revealed significant morbidity, with seven patients requiring hospitalization, seven requiring surgery or invasive procedures, and one patient with complete blindness in the setting of panophthalmitis despite aggressive treatment [38]. CAMRSA has been reported in several cases of orbital cellulitis [36, 39–41]. Despite appropriate antibiotic treatment, CAMRSA infection has the potential for rapid spread from facial skin or nasal cavity to the orbits, paranasal sinuses, and cavernous sinuses [40]. Consequently, a high index of suspicion should be maintained for this organism, even among otherwise healthy individuals. Necrotizing fasciitis, typically caused by group A β-hemolytic streptococcus, is a rare skin infection that spreads rapidly along subcutaneous tissue planes as bacteria dissect along superficial and deep fasciae [42]. This results in necrosis of skin and subcutaneous tissues. Periocular involvement may result in vision loss from vascular occlusions, and prompt medical and surgical treatment is necessary to prevent vision loss and reduce mortality [42].

Differential Diagnosis

In most cases, patients should be treated with broad-spectrum intravenous antibiotics when orbital cellulitis is suspected, unless clinical presentation and ancillary testing suggest another, specific etiology. Fungi are important microbial pathogens to consider in the differential diagnosis of bacterial cellulitis. Rhino-orbital mucormycosis and invasive *Aspergillus* have the potential for causing aggressive infections with significant morbidity and mortality. Morbidity due to mucormycosis can be secondary to advanced infection and vascular thrombosis within the central nervous system, and mortality rates are high particularly in immunocompromised patients, poorly controlled diabetics with ketoacidosis, and patients with renal disease [30, 43, 44]. See *Fungal Orbital Cellulitis* section for a detailed discussion of fungal diseases affecting the orbit.

An important cause of orbital cellulitis in developing countries is *Mycobacterium tuberculosis*, a highly aerobic acid-fast bacterium. Ocular involvement most commonly affects the choroid, but may affect all ocular and adnexal structures [45–49]. Orbital involvement may be due to hematologic spread or direct spread from the adjacent sinuses [48]. Destruction of orbital bones, osteomyelitic changes, erosion, and rarely sclerotic changes can also be seen. Distinguishing orbital tuberculosis from other etiologies of bacterial cellulitis is important not only to manage the orbital process but to permit systemic treatment. Concurrent orbital and active pulmonary disease is not always seen, and therefore, the diagnosis is often suspected based on clinical suspicion and confirmed by ancillary procedures. Tissue biopsy is generally required for diagnosis, with classic findings of granulomas containing epithelioid histiocytes, Langerhans' giant cells, and caseating necrosis [48]. Acid-fast bacilli present in the tissue sample may be detected by routine stains or immunohistochemistry, culture, or PCR [48]. Tuberculin skin testing or the newer interferon-γ release assays (IGRA) support the diagnosis of tuberculosis infection. Chest radiography and sputum microscopy should also be routinely performed to evaluate for respiratory disease [48].

Table 49.1 Differential diagnosis of orbital cellulitis

Infectious orbital disease
Bacterial
Fungal
Aspergillus
Mucormycosis
Mycobacterial
Tuberculosis
Leprosy
Viral
Herpes zoster
Herpes simplex
Parasitic
Hyatid cyst (echinococcosis)
Cysticercosis
Trichinosis
Insect infestation
Noninfectious inflammatory/autoimmune
Idiopathic orbital inflammation
Scleritis
Thyroid eye disease
Wegener's granulomatosis
Churg-Strauss syndrome
Sarcoidosis
Langerhans' cell histiocytosis
Xanthogranuloma
Erdheim-Chester
Adult-onset xanthogranuloma with or without asthma
Necrobiotic xanthogranuloma
Neoplastic
Rhabdomyosarcoma
Lymphoma
Leukemia
Extension of intraocular tumors
Extension of periocular tumors (e.g., sinus)
Vascular
Carotid cavernous fistula
Cavernous sinus thrombosis
Lymphangioma
Other
Ruptured dermoid or epidermoid cyst
Trauma
Mucocele
Hematic cyst/orbital hemorrhage
Intraorbital foreign body

Other orbital inflammations (Table 49.1) may mimic orbital cellulitis upon initial presentation due to common, nonspecific signs and symptoms. During initial evaluation, distinguishing the inflammatory signs of idiopathic orbital inflammation (IOI) from those of infectious disorders is critical, but often difficult. Features suggesting bacterial orbital cellulitis that may aid in this differentiation include a history of trauma, surgery, or adjacent sinusitis and clinical signs of fever and leukocytosis [50]. Often, the diagnosis of IOI is made after lack of clinical response to a therapeutic trial of antimicrobial treatment for presumed bacterial cellulitis and subsequent rapid response to a trial corticosteroids [50]. Scleritis is a subtype of IOI that typically presents with chemosis, eyelid edema, and pain with eye movement. Scleritis is more likely to have focal tenderness and less likely to cause proptosis. Still, differentiating between IOI/scleritis and infectious cellulitis can be quite challenging at time. Other noninfectious, inflammatory disorders to consider include thyroid eye disease, Tolosa-Hunt syndrome, Wegener's granulomatosis, Churg-Strauss syndrome, sarcoidosis, and Langerhans' cell histiocytosis.

Neoplastic disorders should be considered, and in children, rhabdomyosarcoma is the most common primary orbital malignancy, which may present with significant inflammation, proptosis, eyelid edema, and ptosis and be rapidly progressive. In one review, orbital cellulitis was the initial diagnosis in 15% of rhabdomyosarcoma referrals over a 25-year period [51]. Primary intraocular tumors with orbital invasion, including choroidal melanoma and retinoblastoma, may also be associated with orbital inflammation. Interestingly, necrotic intraocular retinoblastomas and choroidal melanomas without extraocular spread have been reported to have accompanying features of orbital cellulitis [52–55]. In retinoblastoma cases, advanced intraocular tumor growth with extensive necrosis of nonneoplastic ocular tissue was present [55]. Potential theories regarding the mechanism of inflammation are postulated to include leakage of necrotic products as triggers of orbital inflammation [55]. Systemic corticosteroids with or without antibiotics have been shown to improve orbital congestion and edema in these cases and facilitate subsequent enucleation [53, 55].

Metastatic disease to the orbit is uncommon, but, when present, may be confused with orbital cellulitis and represents an important differential diagnosis to consider, particularly in patients with a history of underlying malignancy. In 19% of cases of metastatic disease, however, there is no history of cancer at the time of ophthalmic presentation [56]. Neoplasms most commonly metastatic to the orbit include breast and prostate cancer in adults [56]. In children, neuroblastoma is most commonly implicated [56]. Common presenting signs include ophthalmoplegia, proptosis, ptosis, and a palpable mass [56]. Case reports have described an initial diagnosis of orbital cellulitis in patients with metastatic breast and prostate cancer [57, 58].

Sickle cell disease with bone infarction has, in a few reports, presented with a clinical picture similar to orbital cellulitis with subperiosteal abscess [59, 60]. In patients with sickle cell disease, the absence of sinusitis, negative cultures, presence of hemorrhagic fluid collections, and lack of improvement with antibiotics are helpful in making the diagnosis of orbital compression syndrome secondary to bone infarction [59, 60]. Additionally, radiographic findings on MRI imaging may be helpful in characterizing the hemorrhagic fluid collection and bony changes due to infarction [60].

Trauma with retained intraorbital foreign body may elicit either sterile inflammation that mimics bacterial cellulitis or true infectious orbital cellulitis. Copper-containing foreign bodies often result in suppurative inflammation that may mimic bacterial orbital cellulitis but represent a sterile response. Other inorganic foreign bodies including glass or BB pellets are inert and do not incite inflammatory responses. In contrast, organic matter raises the probability of gas-forming or anaerobic organisms that may result in fulminant infections.

Treatment

Treatment with broad-spectrum antibiotics should be initiated promptly if there is a clinical suspicion for infectious orbital cellulitis, as the potential complications can be sight- and life-threatening. Treatment is generally intravenous, and initial medications should be targeted toward the likely pathogens, if the type of infection has been established. For sinus etiologies, commonly used medications include ampicillin-sulbactam, nafcillin, cefotaxime, and ceftriaxone [3, 6]. Clindamycin should be used in combination with other medications, due to its lack of efficacy against *H. Influenzae* and *M. catarrhalis* [3]. The combination of a third-generation cephalosporin and flucloxacillin or metronidazole can also be considered [35]. If penicillin allergy exists, cefazolin or vancomycin can be used in place of nafcillin [6]. Results of a recent study suggest that the primary use of broad-spectrum oral antibiotics with equivalent bioavailability to intravenous antibiotics may have a role in initial management in select patients [61]. In this study, oral ciprofloxacin and clindamycin were used in combination.

Patients must be monitored closely, and once clinical improvement is clearly demonstrated, treatment can be transitioned to oral antibiotics. Antibiotic treatment should be tailored to culture and drug susceptibility results, when available. Response to treatment is generally assessed by clinical improvement as measured by patient comfort, vision, proptosis, chemosis, extraocular motility, and the cardinal features of inflammation. Caution should be taken in correlating changes in imaging findings over time with clinical status, as these findings may lag clinical improvement [28]. Surgical intervention should be initiated in patients who show progression despite treatment or who have evidence of subperiosteal or soft tissue abscess formation.

Complications

In 1970, Chandler described a modified classification system (Table 49.2) for patients presenting with orbital cellulitis [8]. This provides a framework for evaluating the clinical progression of disease, though time course can be variable and is often rapid. The introduction and evolution of antibiotic therapy have markedly reduced the complications of orbital cellulitis, which prior to this era included death and permanent visual disability in a significant proportion of patients [8].

Complications may occur if the infection is undiagnosed, undergoes delay in treatment, is inadequately treated, or is accompanied by abscess formation.

Table 49.2 Modified orbital cellulitis classification system [8]

Group I	Inflammatory edema
Group II	Orbital cellulitis
Group III	Subperiosteal abscess
Group IV	Orbital abscess
Group V	Cavernous sinus thrombosis

Subperiosteal abscess (SPA) results when purulent material collects between the bone and periosteum (periorbita) [8, 62]. Patients often present with non-axial proptosis, with globe displacement away from the location of the abscess [30]. Rapid expansion may lead to vision loss and intracranial extension [63]. SPA are due to extension of underlying bacterial sinusitis and may present a challenge to medical therapy due to growth arrest of organisms, limited vascular supply, and subsequent poor penetrance of systemically administered antibiotics [27]. The medial orbital wall is the most common location of SPA [6, 7]. Management of SPA is controversial, particularly regarding the choice between immediate surgical drainage or medical management with surgical treatment reserved for nonresponders. Harris, in 1994, proposed a management protocol for patients with CT-diagnosed SPA due to sinusitis based on a review of 37 patients [27]. Using these guidelines, patients younger than 9 years of age with modest-sized SPA localized medially and without expansion to adjacent sinuses or the intracranial cavity and without evidence of optic nerve compromise may be managed with intravenous antibiotics and close observation. The majority of these patients have resolution of their SPA without the need for surgical intervention. Older patients were found significantly more likely to have positive cultures despite antibacterial treatment for 3 days, revealing polymicrobial disease and the presence of anaerobes, suggesting that early evacuation of SPA and drainage of sinuses should be initiated to adequately treat the underlying infection. Other studies have also supported the finding that age is a factor for SPA due to underlying sinusitis, demonstrating that younger patients with isolated medial SPA have better outcomes with medical treatment alone as compared to older patients [64, 65]. Additionally, an increase in the number of cultured organisms with age has been reported [66].

The odds ratio for intracranial involvement secondary to frontal sinusitis has been demonstrated in one review to be as high as 20 compared to cases in which the frontal sinus was not involved [67]. Accordingly, superior SPA associated with frontal sinusitis are more commonly associated with intracranial abscess, and surgical drainage should be expedited. Additionally, any patient with a large SPA causing significant discomfort, mass effect or optic nerve compromise, deteriorating clinical course despite broad-spectrum intravenous antibiotic treatment, or intracranial involvement should undergo prompt surgical drainage. This will not only improve the mass effects of the infection but will aid in identifying causative organisms, reducing bacterial load, improving the oxygen tension, allowing for localized delivery of antibiotics, and improving penetration of systemically administered medications.

The use of corticosteroids in combination with intravenous antibiotics for the treatment of SPA secondary to sinusitis has also been proposed, based on the fact that SPA may be due, in part, to an exuberant inflammatory response to the underlying sinusitis [68]. In one retrospective review, the use of intravenous corticosteroids in combination with broad-spectrum antibiotics was not found to have any adverse effects on clinical outcomes and was associated with a reduced need for intravenous antibiotic therapy following hospital discharge [68]. Results from this study should be interpreted with caution, as corticosteroid administration may result in impaired immune response to infective organisms and, if used in patients with undiagnosed atypical or fungal disease, may result in rapid progression.

SPA unrelated to sinusitis, but with other specific etiology (e.g., odontogenic infection), should be evaluated in a case-specific manner and the underlying etiology addressed, as these SPA often contain polymicrobial or anaerobic infections. All patients should be monitored closely as patients may worsen clinically despite surgical intervention. Caution should be taken in interpreting serial CT scans, which have been shown to worsen in appearance in the first few days of successful medical treatment, even when surgical drainage was not performed and eventual recovery was achieved [28].

True orbital abscesses are less common than SPA [6]. Orbital abscesses develop secondary to extension into the orbital fat and are associated with inflammatory edema, purulence, and fat necrosis [69]. They may develop from preexisting cellulitis, be the precursor for fulminant orbital infection, and occur inside or outside the muscle cone [6, 63]. If intraconal, patients may present with significant proptosis of the globe. Neonatal orbital abscesses, while exceedingly rare, have been documented to result in bacteremia and sepsis [5]. Posterior extension of infection may lead to cavernous sinus thrombosis (CST), a devastating and potentially life-threatening complication of orbital cellulitis. Patients with CST often present with fever, nausea, headache, meningismus, ophthalmoplegia that is often out of proportion to the observed cellulitis, periorbital hypoesthesia, cranial nerve palsies, chemosis, periorbital vascular congestion, and severe vision loss. The contralateral side may become affected as the infection progresses. Pupillary abnormalities may also be noted. In such cases, intravenous antibiotics with good CNS penetration, combined with early surgical drainage of the orbital abscess, is mandatory [63, 70]. Third-generation cephalosporins and vancomycin in high doses are recommended, with the addition of metronidazole in cases of abscess and suspected anaerobic pathogens [70]. The exact role of anticoagulants in the treatment of septic CST remains unclear, with inherent difficulty arising in the extrapolation of information from non-septic venous sinus thrombosis studies to cases of septic CST patients [70]. Subsequently, the potential benefits of arresting further clot formation and facilitating clot lysis must be balanced with risks of intracranial hemorrhage, which may vary depending on severity of disease at presentation.

Intracranial extension of orbital cellulitis is uncommon, but, when present, can result in epidural empyema and/or abscess, meningitis, venous sinus thrombosis, and brain abscess [69]. The mechanism of spread is thought to be by direct extension or via retrograde thrombophlebitis [21, 69]. Intracranial abscess (IA) secondary to orbital cellulitis is a rare but life-threatening complication [21]. It is more commonly associated with superior subperiosteal abscesses, and it may present in the context of pansinusitis [21, 64]. Most patients tend to present late in the course of the disease, and neurological symptoms are not always present initially [21]. When present, they may include fever, altered mental status, and new onset seizures [21]. In patients with IA and sinusitis, concordance between the microbiology of the IA and sinus isolates has been noted, making sinus cultures helpful in refining initial antibiotic regimens [21, 71]. Polymicrobial infection and anaerobic constituents are found in the vast majority of cases. Treatment should include prompt administration of intravenous antibiotics, including β-lactamase-resistant drugs and those with good CNS penetration and anaerobic coverage [71]. Corticosteroid administration may have a role in reducing cerebral edema and the encapsulation process of abscesses, but its use may have adverse effects including rebound effects when discontinued [69]. The combination of medical and surgical intervention is often required in the treatment of IA, and a multidisciplinary approach is recommended.

The most common ocular complications leading to visual loss include optic neuritis and retinal vascular occlusions. A rise in orbital pressure from inflammatory and infectious infiltrates or rapidly expanding subperiosteal abscess may result in orbital compartment syndrome, with subsequent retinal artery ischemia, optic nerve compression, and visual loss [30]. Other ocular morbidities include corneal exposure, neurotrophic keratopathy, glaucoma, septic uveitis or retinitis, and endophthalmitis [6, 72, 73].

Orbital Nocardiosis

Nocardia, a weakly gram-positive filamentous bacteria, has also been reported to cause orbital infections [74, 75]. Chronic, granulomatous infections of the orbit and cerebral involvement concurrent with sino-orbital aspergillosis have been described in the literature [74, 76]. Therapy with Welsh's regimen, consisting of amikacin and cotrimoxazole, or a modification of this regimen has been used in treatment of these infections.

Fungal Orbital Cellulitis

The fungi are ubiquitous saprophytes found in bread, fruit, and vegetable molds and can be cultured from the nose, mouth, throat, and stool of healthy individuals [44]. While in healthy individuals spores are easily cleared by phagocytosis, germination and hyphal proliferation can develop in immunocompromised hosts. Infection of soft tissues leads to vascular invasion, preferentially of arterioles. This results in arteriolar occlusion, which causes tissue ischemia and necrosis that promotes an acidic environment that potentiates spread of the organism. Sinus infection may spread to the orbit, with further extension into the cranium via the superior orbital fissure.

Fungal infections of the orbit, while relatively uncommon, are important to recognize as they are often locally aggressive and have the potential for significant morbidity and mortality, particularly among immunocompromised individuals. The two most common mycoses include aspergillosis and mucormycosis. Other rare causes of fungal orbital infections include *Scedosporium*, *Bipolaris*, *Blastomyces*, *Histoplasma*, and *Sporothrix* species [77]. Therapy should be multipronged: antifungals to fight the infection, surgical debridement to reduce the infectious load, and medical measures to address the causes of any metabolic or immune derangements.

Orbital Aspergillosis

Aspergillus is a ubiquitous fungus found in soil and decaying vegetation, and *Aspergillus* species are common fungal contaminants of the sinuses [78]. They appear as long filamentous fungi with septate hyphae that branch at 45-degree angles and are the most common mycosis caused by filamentous fungi [79, 80]. Most cases of aspergillosis are noninvasive and with good prognosis [81]. Noninvasive colonizations present as either allergic sinusitis or a sinonasal fungal ball with destruction of the sinus mucosa and bony expansion but without invasion of the tissue or bone [82]. Invasive disease is most commonly encountered in immunocompromised patients including those with prolonged neutropenia, advanced HIV infection, inherited immunodeficiency, and patients who have undergone allogeneic hematopoietic stem cell transplantation (HSCT) or lung transplantation [83]. It may also be associated with diabetes, prosthetic devices, and advancing age [78]. Invasive disease may be localized or disseminated and can affect multiple organs [79].

Presentation of orbital aspergillosis is generally nonspecific and may be similar to other orbital inflammatory conditions such as idiopathic orbital inflammation, granulomatous orbital inflammation, Tolosa-Hunt syndrome, bacterial orbital cellulitis, or neoplastic processes [81]. As a result, diagnosis may be delayed due to lack of specific findings. Other systemic signs that may aid in diagnosis include fever, cough, and dyspnea, which may be associated with invasive pulmonary aspergillosis, the most common site of invasive aspergillosis [84]. Orbital imaging of invasive sino-orbital aspergillosis with CT or MRI typically reveals focal soft tissue abnormalities with or without bony erosion [82]. Sphenoid sinus involvement may have only subtle findings and is better evaluated with MRI. Additionally, imaging may be helpful in identifying the extent of disease, presence of intracranial extension, and surgical planning [81]. Biopsy is required for diagnosis and should be repeated if initial biopsy does not reveal any fungal elements when there is a high clinical suspicion for disease, as false-negative biopsies are not uncommon. Diagnosis is critical, particularly in cases where corticosteroid administration would be indicated for other orbital diseases. In cases where corticosteroid treatment is initiated in the setting of undiagnosed orbital aspergillosis, outcomes have generally been poor. Therefore, biopsy is recommended prior to corticosteroid administration when clinical suspicion exists. Serum assays for *Aspergillus* antigen may also aid in the diagnosis of invasive disease.

Treatment of invasive orbital *Aspergillus* consists of debridement combined with systemic antifungal treatment. The most commonly used antifungal in the treatment of orbital aspergillosis has been amphotericin B, a polyene, which is given intravenously. Amphotericin B irrigation may also be performed at the time of debridement to facilitate delivery directly to tissues, and the use of retrobulbar amphotericin B has also been described [85]. Extended use of systemic amphotericin B can result in significant side effects, including renal dysfunction, and consequently newer lipid complex and liposomal formulations that have reduced toxicity may be used. Additionally, itraconazole, an azole antifungal, may have some role in treatment either as monotherapy in select cases or in combination with amphotericin B in patients with orbital aspergillosis [86–88]. Voriconazole has more recently been recommended as the drug of choice in patients with confirmed sinonasal aspergillosis and in patients with CNS disease [83]. Reversal of immunosuppression should also be instituted, and use of adjunctive treatments such as granulocyte and granulocyte-macrophage colony-stimulating factor (G-CSF and GM-CSF) and interferon-gamma should be considered [84].

Orbital Mucormycosis

Mucormycosis is the second most frequent mycosis due to filamentous fungi [79]. Mucormycosis refers to infection by fungi in the class *Zygomycetes* and order *Mucorales*, which display large, broad nonseptate hyphae with right-angle branching [79, 89]. *Mucorales* are ubiquitous saprophytes and can be cultured from the nose, mouth, throat, and stool of healthy individuals [44]. Spores are most commonly inhaled, leading to inoculation of the paranasal sinuses. In healthy individuals, spores are easily cleared. However, germination and hyphae formation can develop in immunocompromised hosts, leading to manifestations of clinical disease [44]. Several clinical forms exist, of which rhino-orbital mucormycosis is the most common [89]. Infection occurs most commonly in immunocompromised patients, poorly controlled diabetics with ketoacidosis, and patients with hematologic malignancies or renal disease [30, 43, 44].

Morbidity and mortality due to rhino-orbital mucormycosis are high and often secondary to advanced infection and vascular thrombosis within the central nervous system. Local invasion is by arteriolar occlusion, leading to necrosis and tissue hypoxia [44]. This creates an acidic environment that may potentiate spread of the organism. The organisms have a predilection for the elastic lamina of arterial vessels, and the internal carotid artery and cavernous sinus are most commonly occluded [89]. Initial signs and symptoms may include fever, nasal mucosal ulceration and necrosis, periorbital and facial swelling, proptosis, reduced vision, ophthalmoplegia, sinusitis, headache, facial pain, and changes in mental status [90]. A black eschar of nasal mucosa, skin, or hard palate may develop as tissue necrosis progresses but is uncommon at initial presentation [90]. Sinus infection may spread to the orbit, with further extension into the cranium via orbital vessels, the superior orbital fissure, or cribriform plate [90]. Cavernous sinus involvement may result in both cavernous sinus thrombosis and progression to carotid artery occlusion and stroke [90]. Orbital imaging is essential to delineate extent of sinus, orbital, and intracranial involvement, if present. Biopsy should be obtained from nasal, sinus, and orbital lesions, when present, to confirm presence of fungal elements.

Patients often have advanced symptoms at the time of presentation, and management consists of aggressive surgical debridement with frozen section monitoring, along with antifungal therapy and treatment of any immune system derangement. Exenteration is only appropriate in very rare cases in which pan-orbital infection is limited to the orbit, and exenteration (i.e., radical excision) would dramatically reduce the infectious load. More commonly, by the time exenteration is seriously contemplated, the infection has already migrated to the cavernous sinus, and orbital exenteration will not alter the intracranial infectious load. Instead, local and systemic antifungal treatment and correction of underlying metabolic or immunologic derangements are essential [44]. Intravenous amphotericin B is the most commonly used systemic antifungal in patients with rhino-orbital mucormycosis. It may also be administered locally into the intraorbital space using infusion catheters and placed into irrigating solutions for enhanced delivery to necrotic and poorly perfused tissues [89, 91, 92]. More recent reports suggest that adjunctive use of systemic posaconazole in addition to systemic amphotericin B in patients who demonstrate progression has promising results [93, 94]. Other adjunctive treatments include interferon-gamma, granulocyte and granulocyte-macrophage colony-stimulating factors (G-CSF and GM-CSF), and hyperbaric oxygen, and in cases of vascular thrombosis, heparin sodium may be used to reduce the risk of stroke [43, 95, 96]. Prompt diagnosis and initiation of treatment are critical, and a multidisciplinary approach is recommended in the treatment of these infections.

Orbital Granulomatous Diseases

The orbit is a common site for granulomatous inflammation, which fall into two broad categories: autoimmune and infectious.

Autoimmune Orbital Granulomatous Disease

Orbital granulomatous inflammations are generally manifestations of systemic autoimmune inflammatory processes. The diagnosis is made on the basis of clinical history and examination, blood tests, and most often, tissue biopsy. These disorders often localize to the lacrimal gland and are discussed in that context elsewhere. The differential diagnosis of autoimmune granulomatous inflammation includes infectious etiologies, typically due to Mycobacteria, Borrelia, fungi, or parasites.

Autoimmune Disorders

Orbital Sarcoidosis

Sarcoidosis is a multisystem, idiopathic granulomatous disease that is characterized by noncaseating granulomata [97]. Although sarcoidosis can affect all races, both sexes, and all ages, it has propensity to adults under the age of 40 years and certain ethnic and racial groups. Age-adjusted annual incidence rate in the United States is estimated to be 10.9 per 100,000 for whites and 35.5 per 100,000 for African-Americans [98]. Similar or higher annual incidence rates have been reported in the studies from Scandinavia and Ireland [98]. Sarcoidosis can affect any organ, but intrathoracic lymph node enlargement is found in more than 90% of patients [99]. Extrathoracic presentations of sarcoidosis, such as erythema nodosum or acute uveitis, may be more common in Puerto Ricans, African-Americans, and Scandinavians. In the ACCESS study, ocular involvement was more frequent in African-American patients than in Caucasians and more common in females than males at 13.9% and 8.2%, respectively [100].

Although granulomatous uveitis is the most common ocular finding, sarcoidosis can involve any part of the eye. In a review of 43 patients with ocular sarcoidosis, Smith and Foster [101] reported that anterior uveitis was the most common manifestation (73%), followed by vitritis (62%), retinal and choroidal lesions (34%), and ocular adnexal and orbital lesions (10%). After reviewing 379 patients with systemic sarcoidosis, Demirci and Christianson reported that 8% of them had orbital and adnexal involvement [102]. Orbital manifestations of sarcoidosis include palpable periocular mass (89%), proptosis (42%), discomfort (31%), ptosis (27%), restricted ocular motility (23%), dry eye (19%), diplopia (15%), and decreased vision (12%) [103]. In the orbit and adnexa, sarcoidosis affects the lacrimal gland (42%), orbit (39%), eyelid (12%), and lacrimal sac (8%) [103]. Orbital and adnexal sarcoidosis can be the initial sign of the systemic disease or develop in patients with known systemic disease. In a review of 30 patients with orbital and adnexal sarcoidosis, Demirci and Christianson [102] found that 37% of patients had known systemic disease, orbital and adnexal involvement was the initial manifestation of systemic disease in 34% of the patients, and 29% of patients had disease limited to the region. Using Kaplan-Meier estimates, systemic sarcoidosis was expected in 8% of the patients who presented with only orbital and adnexal disease by 5 years [102]. No clinical feature was found to be significantly predictive of systemic disease in univariate or multivariate analyses [102].

Imaging of orbital sarcoidosis demonstrates homogenous or lobular enlargement of the lacrimal gland, which molds to the eye or diffuse homogeneous involvement of orbital soft tissue. The diagnosis is usually made based on clinical and radiologic presentation in known cases but requires biopsy for histopathologic diagnosis and exclusion of other possible diseases. Noncaseating granulomatous inflammation is the hallmark pathologic feature. The granulomata may or may not contain giant cells, are usually surrounded by a paucity of lymphoid cells, evoke fibrosis between granulomata, and may exhibit foci of necrosis. A complete medical evaluation should be part of the systemic evaluation; the orbital specialist should have a high level of suspicion and low threshold for referral to an internist in the context of findings suspicious for the disease. Diagnostic evaluation for systemic sarcoidosis is presented in Table 49.3 [97]. Conjunctival biopsy has been reported to be helpful for the diagnosis of systemic sarcoidosis, but biopsy of clinically or radiologically involved tissue has a much higher diagnostic yield for sarcoidosis or diseases in the differential diagnosis [104–106].

Immunosuppression is the mainstay of treatment for orbital sarcoidosis. Corticosteroids have been the traditional standard of care for severe systemic sarcoidosis, and corticosteroid-sparing agents, such as azathioprine and

Table 49.3 Recommended initial evaluation of patients with sarcoidosis [97]

1. History (occupational and environmental exposure, symptoms)
2. Physical examination
3. Posteroanterior chest x-ray
4. Pulmonary function tests: spirometry, diffusing capacity of lung for carbon monoxide (DLCO), rate of carbon monoxide uptake (KCO)
5. Peripheral blood counts: white blood cells, red blood cells, platelets
6. Serum chemistries: calcium, liver enzymes, creatinine, blood urea nitrogen
7. Urine analysis
8. Electrocardiogram
9. Routine ophthalmic examination
10. Tuberculin skin test

methotrexate, have been used successfully in many cases. In orbital cases without active systemic disease, a course of oral prednisone starting at 1 mg/kg of body weight and tapered over 3 months may be considered as initial therapy. In those who fail to respond or are corticosteroid-intolerant, cytotoxic corticosteroid-sparing agents may be used. In localized orbital disease, periocular corticosteroids (1-mL injection of triamcinolone acetonide 40 mg/mL) may be considered. In a multicentric study of 26 patients with orbital and adnexal sarcoidosis, Prabhakaran et al. [103] reported that 73% of patients were treated with systemic corticosteroids and 15% required additional systemic methotrexate therapy. Overall, 85% of these patients showed a good response to therapy. Demirci and Christianson [102] observed that 93% of orbital and adnexal sarcoidosis patients regressed or remained stable following systemic corticosteroid therapy after a mean follow-up of 44 months. The long-term effects of immunosuppression on the natural history of the disease are unclear.

Orbital Wegener's Granulomatosis

Wegener's granulomatosis is a multisystem granulomatous inflammatory disorder of presumed autoimmune origin [107]. It affects Caucasians more commonly, with a peak onset between 40 and 60 years of age [108]. The annual incidence is estimated to be between 4 and 8.5 cases per million [109]. In 1990, the American College of Rheumatology published a set of diagnostic criteria for the purpose of standardizing clinical trials [110]. These were refined at the Chapel Hill Consensus Conference in 1992 and established a diagnostic requirement for (1) granulomatous inflammation of the respiratory system and (2) direct evidence of vasculitis involving small- or medium-sized vessels [110]. Wegener's granulomatosis can affect any organ but has a predilection for the upper respiratory tract, lungs, and kidneys [107]. The upper respiratory tract involvement results in soft tissue, cartilage, and bone destruction with submucosal scarring and stenosis, while lower respiratory involvement causes lower lobe pulmonary masses that may cavitate and cause hemoptysis. Renal involvement is the most serious manifestation and most common cause of death. Its characteristic lesion is of focal, segmental necrotizing glomerulonephritis often with crescents. The term "limited Wegener's granulomatosis" was coined by Carrington and Liebow for disease without renal involvement [111]. Limited Wegener's granulomatosis is also used for disease that appears to spare the classical sites.

In Wegener's granulomatosis, the target of the circulating autoantibodies, termed antineutrophil cytoplasmic antibodies (ANCA), is two leukocyte-associated proteins, proteinase 3 (PR3) and myeloperoxidase (MPO). Antibodies to the former lead to cytoplasmic staining (cANCA), while antibodies to the latter result in perinuclear staining (pANCA) of leukocytes. In systemic Wegener's granulomatosis, high serum titers of cANCA are present in more than 90% of patients with a specificity of almost 100%. In limited disease, as few as 60% of patients show elevated titers of cANCA, making their initial diagnosis more challenging. Pathogenetically, neutrophils bound by ANCA or ANCA-protein complexes attach to or enter the walls of blood vessels and initiate a cascade of severe inflammation that causes endothelial and mural damage and necrosis [112].

Initial signs and symptoms of Wegener's granulomatosis are highly variable, affecting the nose, sinuses, airways, lungs, kidneys, joints, and skin [108]. Nasal symptoms can include rhinitis, epistaxis, and septal perforation (causing "saddle nose deformity"). Respiratory symptoms include shortness of breath secondary to pulmonary nodules and infiltrates, pulmonary cavitary lesions, subglottal stenosis, and oral mucosal ulcerations. Ocular involvement occurs in 50–60% of patients with Wegener's granulomatosis and is the presenting involvement in 15% of Wegener's granulomatosis [108]. It is usually bilateral. Ocular involvement includes keratitis, conjunctivitis, episcleritis, scleritis, choriditis, retinal vasculitis, and optic neuropathy as well as extraocular involvement of muscle, masses involving orbital soft tissue or eyelid structures, dacryocystitis, nasolacrimal duct obstruction, and osteolytic lesions of the orbital walls, in the setting of sinus involvement [108]. The most common presenting feature of orbital involvement is pain, epiphora, and injection. Orbital disease can manifest as a result of primary inflammation or extension of disease from adjacent paranasal sinuses or the nasopharynx. The ocular involvement usually occurs in association with systemic disease, especially sinus disease, but limited Wegener's granulomatosis can involve ocular structures.

The diagnosis of Wegener's granulomatosis is based on histopathological evaluation. It is a part of a spectrum of small- and medium-vessel ANCA vasculitides with Churg-Strauss syndrome and microscopic polyangiitis. All these diseases exhibit acute and chronic granulomatous vasculitis of medium and small arteries and arterioles. They also demonstrate lymphocytic and neutrophilic infiltration of blood vessel walls with fibrinoid necrosis. Soft tissue manifestations include multinucleated giant cells, microabscesses, geographic necrosis, abundant karyorrhectic debris, and fibrosis [113, 114].

Systemic corticosteroids and cyclophosphamide are the mainstay of treatment for Wegener's granulomatosis [111]. Following induction of remission using cyclophosphamide, corticosteroid-sparing immune modulators, such as azathioprine or methotrexate, are used for maintenance [111]. Plasmapheresis may be beneficial in some circumstances, and mycophenolate mofetil, rituximab, and infliximab may also be of benefit in refractory patients. Sulfonamides have been shown to be beneficial, especially in limited disease [111].

It is important to note that while 5-year survival is currently 90%, Wegener's granulomatosis is a deadly disease and should be managed by a rheumatologist with the help of a multidisciplinary medical team [115]. With treatment, 91% of patients with classical system WG are clinically improved, while 75% achieve complete remission. Patients who achieve remission remain in remission 46% of the time on follow-up [115]. The most common long-term complication is chronic renal failure necessitating dialysis [115].

Churg-Strauss Syndrome

Churg-Strauss syndrome (CSS), also known as allergic granulomatosis and angiitis, is a systemic vasculitis characterized by necrotizing granulomatous inflammation, hypereosinophilia, asthma, and allergic rhinitis [116]. Typically, small- to medium-sized vessels are affected. Asthma is a universal feature of CSS and presents at a mean interval of 3 years prior to vasculitis [117]. CSS-associated asthma presents later in life than common asthma, may be more severe, and is more commonly corticosteroid-dependent [117]. Pulmonary infiltrates, nasal polyposis, rhinitis, and sinusitis are also common features of the disease [117]. Constitutional symptoms such as fever, malaise, and weight loss may accompany systemic vasculitis [117, 118]. The systemic vasculitis of CSS is similar to polyarteritis nodosa (PAN); however, renal involvement is generally mild in comparison [117]. Cardiovascular disease accounts for the majority of deaths in patients with CSS, usually secondary to coronary vasculitis and granulomatous infiltration of the myocardium [117]. All organ systems may be affected by vasculitis or by eosinophilic infiltration, however, leading to varied manifestations of disease.

Ophthalmic manifestations of CSS are uncommon but include conjunctival granulomas, subconjunctival swelling, marginal corneal ulceration, amaurosis fugax, periscleritis, anterior ischemic optic neuropathy, branch retinal artery occlusion, central retinal artery occlusion, optic neuritis, cranial nerve palsies, and, rarely, loss of vision [119–126]. Presentation of ophthalmic symptoms may be acute, subacute, or chronic [125]. Several reports of orbital involvement have been described in the literature and include cases of dacryoadenitis, orbital myositis, diffuse bilateral orbital inflammation, eyelid swelling, exophthalmos, and orbital bone destruction [116, 127–133]. Takenashi et al. proposed categorizing the pathologic manifestations as either orbital inflammatory type or ischemic vasculitic type, as these may have implications on visual prognosis [125]. Specifically, the inflammatory types were found to manifest as dacryoadenitis, myositis, periscleritis, perineuritis, conjunctival granuloma, and episcleritis, whereas the ischemic vasculitic types presented as amaurosis fugax, anterior ischemic optic neuropathy, ischemic optic neuropathy, branch retinal artery occlusion, and central retinal artery occlusion [125]. The latter type was found, in a review of published cases, to be more acute in onset, more commonly associated with ANCA positivity, and resulting in worse visual outcomes [125]. These findings indicate that patients with isolated orbital involvement of CSS may have a better prognosis than those with ocular sequelae of ischemic vasculitis.

The pathogenesis of CSS is not clearly defined but likely involves a complex interplay between genetic, immune, and environmental factors. HLA-DRB4 has recently been identified as a potential genetic risk factor for development of disease [134]. Infiltration of eosinophils into tissues is a hallmark of CSS, and it is likely that they play some role in tissue injury [135]. Toxic products of eosinophils can cause tissue damage, resulting in fibrosis and altered function, and exotoxins have been found to be elevated in patients with CSS [135, 136]. T cells, in particular those of the Th2 phenotype, have been generated from CSS patients via in vitro polyclonal stimulation, and lymphocyte targeting immunosuppressive therapies have been found to have some efficacy in CSS patients [135]. Environmental factors that are thought to potentially trigger CSS include inhaled allergens, vaccinations, desensitization, and infections [135, 137, 138]. Asthma therapies, in particular leukotriene modifiers, have also been the focus of much research, yet a definitive link between their use and CSS development has not been elucidated [139].

Diagnosis of CSS is based upon clinical findings in combination with histopathologic features. The combination of asthma, peripheral eosinophilia, and a history of allergies should raise the suspicion of CSS [127]. Peripheral eosinophilia is a crucial feature of CSS and usually exceeds 1.5×10^9/L in peripheral blood [117]. Anemia and elevated erythrocyte sedimentation rates may also be seen, and IgE levels are commonly elevated [117, 118]. Reports of antineutrophil cytoplasm autoantibody positivity in CSS patients range between 40% and 70%, most commonly perinuclear immunofluorescence-labeling pattern (pANCA) and antimyeloperoxidase (anti-MPO) specificity in enzyme-linked immunosorbent assays [117, 140]. The presence of ANCA positivity is not diagnostic for CSS, however, and can be seen in other vasculitides including PAN, Wegener's granulomatosis (WG), and microscopic polyangiitis (MPA). ANCA positivity may have some effect on CSS disease course and progression. ANCA-positive patients have been found to have a higher incidence of purpura, renal involvement, mononeuritis multiplex, and central nervous system (CNS) involvement, whereas ANCA-negative patients had more pulmonary parenchymal and cardiac involvement [140]. Tissue biopsy may aid in diagnosis of CSS. Histopathology, first described by Churg and Strauss, classically reveals (1) necrotizing vasculitis of small- and medium-sized arteries and veins, (2) eosinophil infiltration around involved vessels and in tissues, and (3) extravascular granulomas [141]. It is now recognized that these "classic" features may not always be present simultaneously in patients with CSS, with granulomas being difficult to find in some cases, and in others only eosinophilic perivascular infiltration noted [142]. Imaging studies may reveal pulmonary or sinus abnormalities not elicited by history or evident during examination and should be obtained in patients when CSS is suspected. Additionally, appropriate laboratory testing should be performed to assess systemic involvement.

Among the differential diagnosis of CSS include other vasculitides such as PAN, WG, and MPA. PAN may be differentiated from CSS histopathologically due to the involvement of large caliber vessels in the former [118]. Additionally, neutrophils are more predominantly seen, and extravascular granuloma formation is uncommon in PAN [118]. Of note, histopathologic features of PAN and CSS may overlap in a disorder classified as "polyangiitis overlap syndrome." [118] Orbital involvement in WG is more common than seen with CSS or MPA. A distinguishing feature between WG and CSS is involvement of the nasolacrimal duct. This appears to occur in 7–10% of patients with WG but has not yet been reported with CSS [143]. WG, like CSS, is characterized by granulomatous inflammation but lacks tissue eosinophil infiltration [144]. Additionally, it is more commonly associated with cytoplasmic ANCA with antiproteinase-3 specificity [117]. The orbital signs and symptoms of CSS are nonspecific, and other orbital processes should be considered including idiopathic orbital inflammation (IOI). Presentation and clinical signs of orbital CSS may be identical to those of IOI, and thus, diagnosis is typically made based on pathologic findings and the presence of systemic signs and symptoms in the former. Differentiating the two diseases is critical, since patients with CSS may have multiorgan involvement, thus necessitating systemic workup and, in some cases, more intensive treatments.

Treatment of CSS can potentially reverse disease manifestations, and first-line agents are glucocorticoids at a dose of 1 mg/kg/day [135]. Pulse intravenous corticosteroids may be indicated in patients with acute multiorgan involvement, and cyclophosphamide may be added in combination with corticosteroids in patients with poor prognostic factors [135]. These include proteinuria of greater than 1 g, creatinine elevation above 1.6 mg/dL, cardiomyopathy, gastrointestinal involvement, and CNS involvement [145]. Other adjunctive medications include azathioprine, methotrexate, and intravenous immunoglobulin [135]. Immunomodulatory medications that have been utilized with varying outcomes in ANCA-associated vasculitides include interferon-α, rituximab, and the TNF-α antagonist infliximab [135]. The exact role of these treatments in CSS remains, at present, unclear. Management of orbital disease in CSS has included oral and intravenous pulse corticosteroids and methotrexate, with favorable responses in the overwhelming majority of cases and rapid resolution of disease [116, 125, 127–129, 131, 132].

Sjögren's Syndrome

Sjögren's syndrome is a systemic connective tissue autoimmune disorder and can occur together with rheumatoid arthritis, lupus erythematosus, and scleroderma. Sjögren's syndrome classically manifests with dry eyes (keratoconjunctivitis sicca) as well as dryness of other mucous membranes, including the mouth. Schirmer testing is useful in documenting basal and reflex tear production. Basal tear production of less than 5 mm over 5 min is correlated with Sjögren's syndrome. Diffuse punctate keratopathy and chronic conjunctivitis are also commonly noted on ophthalmic examination. Imaging of the lacrimal glands, using ultrasound, CT scan, or MRI, can be helpful in documenting lacrimal gland enlargement due to diffuse leukocytic infiltration of glandular tissue. Dacryoadenitis is commonly associated with pain and tenderness, although proptosis is usually absent. The patients with Sjögren's syndrome are in a higher risk to develop orbital lymphoma. Thus, biopsy is often performed in cases with atypical findings, including asymmetrical or progressive involvement of lacrimal gland tissue. Histopathologically, diffuse non-granulomatous inflammation with destruction of acini and small ducts together with regenerative ductal epithelial cells are present. Because of background, diffuse, chronic inflammation, the diagnosis of supervening malignant lymphoma may be difficult.

Treatment of Sjögren's syndrome is focused on symptomatic relief, including aggressive lubrication and topical anti-inflammatory medications. Topical cyclosporine is FDA-approved for treatment of dry eyes in the context of Sjögren's syndrome. Punctal plugs or ablation, moisture chambers, warm compresses, and humidifiers, all contribute to the care of patients with Sjögren's syndrome. Blepharotomy may be a surgical option to reduce exposure and improve surface wetting.

Granuloma Annulare

Granuloma annulare is a benign granulomatous disease that usually involves the dermis and is clinically characterized by singularly and annularly grouped papules or nodules that occur in individuals younger than 25 years [146]. The clinical presentation of granuloma annulare may be papular, plaque, annular, perforating, disseminated, or nodular.

Table 49.4 Comparative features in IOI between adult and pediatric patients

	Adults	Children
Bilateral disease	Uncommon	Common
Systemic symptoms (fever, malaise, lymphadenopathy)	Uncommon	Common
Disc edema, uveitis	Uncommon	Common
Tissue eosinophilia	Uncommon	Common
Peripheral eosinophilia	Uncommon	Common
Recurrent disease	Common	Uncommon

Idiopathic Orbital Inflammation

Clinical Features

Idiopathic orbital inflammation (IOI), also known as idiopathic inflammatory pseudotumor, nonspecific orbital inflammation (NSOI), and orbital inflammatory syndrome (OIS), is a noninfectious, inflammatory disorder of the orbit without underlying local or systemic etiology. As diagnosis of exclusion, it remains the third most common orbital disease following thyroid orbitopathy and benign lymphoproliferative lesions [147–150], and reports suggest it represents between 4.7% and 17.6% of all orbital disorders [151–155]. In a review of 1264 orbital tumors and simulating lesions that presented to Wills Eye Hospital over a 30-year period, 11% had inflammatory lesions, of which 74% were diagnosed as orbital pseudotumor with a mean age of presentation at 45 years [152]. Both infectious triggers and autoimmune pathogenesis have been postulated; however, no clear mechanisms have been elucidated [156–159].

IOI is largely a disease of middle-aged adults, with pediatric involvement being uncommon and reports limited to case reports or small case series [149, 150]. No strong racial or gender predilection has been noted, except in cases of myositis and trochleitis where females have been found to be more commonly affected [50, 153, 160, 161]. IOI is most commonly unilateral in adults, with bilaterality suggesting a systemic association. Bilaterality is more common in children than adults and may be associated with systemic disorders, optic neuritis, uveitis, and eosinophilia [156, 162]. Children may present with systemic signs such as fever, malaise, and lymphadenopathy; however, this does not always indicate an identifiable systemic disorder as a cause of the orbital inflammation [149]. Table 49.4 summarizes the differentiating clinical features among adults and children.

Patients often present with orbital pain, conjunctival injection, chemosis, ophthalmoplegia, ptosis, exophthalmos, and impaired vision. With acute lacrimal gland involvement, the upper eyelid may assume a characteristic S-shape configuration with increased edema of the temporal eyelids [163]. This does not typically extend beyond the bony rim, as can be seen with orbital cellulitis. IOI can be subdivided into acute, subacute, or chronic based on symptom onset and duration. Presenting signs are generally related to the underlying orbital structure(s) affected. Inflammation may be diffuse or localized and may involve posterior sclera (posterior scleritis), extraocular muscles (myositis), trochlea (trochleitis), lacrimal gland (dacryoadenitis), optic nerve sheath (perineuritis), and orbital apex (orbital apex syndrome or Tolosa-Hunt syndrome). Contiguous structures and adjacent fibrofatty tissue may be affected, resulting in the varied presentations of this disorder. In chronic or sclerosing variants of IOI, signs of mass effect, including globe displacement and limitation of movement, are more prominent. When affecting the anterior orbit, these variants may be present as a firm, palpable mass [164]. Another framework of evaluation and management of IOI proposed by Rootman [165] divides orbital inflammation into patterns of involvement including myositis, dacryoadenitis, anterior, diffuse, and apical.

Computed tomography (CT) is the initial imaging study of choice and provides inherent contrast between different attenuation values of orbital fat, muscle, bony structures, and air in the paranasal sinuses [164]. Imaging with contrast may reveal thickened and enhanced sclera, extraocular muscles, tendons, and lacrimal gland. Often a homogenous infiltrative orbital mass with mild enhancement and irregular edges is noted. Findings range from subtle infiltrative changes affecting specific orbital structures to almost complete invasion of the orbit [166]. Bony erosion is not characteristic and, when noted, should prompt investigation into an alternate etiology. Magnetic resonance imaging (MRI) and orbital ultrasonography may also be used as adjunct diagnostic imaging tools. MRI shows a reticular pattern of orbital fat that is isointense to muscle in both T1- and T2-weighted images, a feature that may help in distinguishing IOI from orbital cellulitis, which is more commonly hyperintense to muscle in T2 [163]. Ultrasonography may be helpful in assessing extraocular muscle enlargement and tendon involvement with suspected myositis and, in addition, may be used to identify the classic "T sign" associated with scleritis [163]. Extraorbital extension of inflammation is rare but has been reported to occur into the intracranial cavity, paranasal sinuses, and pterygopalatine fossa [167–174] and is best evaluated with MRI.

Biopsy may be undertaken in cases where the diagnosis is uncertain, presentation atypical, or response to medical treatment poor. Histopathology classically reveals an infiltrate of inflammatory cells mainly of mature lymphocytes, admixed with plasma cells, neutrophils, eosinophils, and occasionally macrophages and histiocytes, with tissue eosinophilia seen more commonly in pediatric cases [175, 176]. Extensive variation in the histopathology of IOI specimens exists, and this may be in part reflective of the point in the disease course at which the biopsy was taken. IOI can be pathologically divided into acute, subacute, and chronic forms based on the degree of inflammatory and fibrovascular responses, with increasing amounts of fibrovascular stroma affecting muscles, fat, and glandular elements later in the course of the disease [164, 177]. In acute stages, neutrophils and eosinophils are more numerous and often are present in the orbital septae. With chronic disease, lymphocytes, plasma cells, and macrophages predominate with increasing fibrosis along the septae and honeycombing of orbital fat. Dense fibrosis may result with fixation of orbital structures with recurrent or chronic disease.

Three main histopathological subtypes of IOI have also been proposed including lymphocytic, granulomatous, and sclerosing [167]. This distinction may be useful clinically, especially in sclerosing forms that are generally more aggressive and require prolonged treatment and potential use of steroid-sparing agents or surgical debulking. This subtype, also known as nonspecific orbital inflammation (NSOI), is slowly progressive in its course and may result in worse visual outcomes due to poor response to conventional treatments [50, 178, 179]. NSOI has a predilection for the superior and lateral orbit, with frequent involvement of the lacrimal gland [180]. It is thought to be a distinct clinicopathologic entity from the chronic stage of IOI and is thought to share features with other systemic fibroelastic disorders including retroperitoneal fibrosis and sclerosing mesenteritis [165, 181, 182].

The distinction between lymphoproliferative disorders and IOI may be made clinically and pathologically. Clinically lymphoproliferative disorders tend to be slowly progressive with more insidious onset and more prominent mass effect [156]. Histopathologically, they demonstrate a homogenous monoclonal cell population as compared to the strictly heterogenous nature of the IOI inflammatory cell populations [156]. Metastatic tumors and primary ocular tumors with extrascleral extension such as uveal melanoma or other intraocular neoplasms should also be excluded [50].

In the pediatric population, rhabdomyosarcoma should always be considered in cases of orbital inflammation as this is most common primary orbital malignancy and may be rapidly progressive with significant morbidity. Primary ocular rhabdomyosarcoma also presents with proptosis, eyelid edema, and ptosis, and in one review, IOI was the referring diagnosis to an ocular oncology service for 12% of rhabdomyosarcoma cases over a 25-year period [51]. Retinoblastoma and neuroblastoma may also elicit orbital inflammation and should also be excluded [149]. Other disorders that may be accompanied by a significant inflammatory reaction and can mimic IOI include orbital lymphangioma and ruptured dermoid cysts [50]. A history of trauma and potential intraorbital foreign body causing inflammation should also be investigated. Acute presentation of inflammatory signs, more common in IOI, may assist in differentiating it from other orbital processes such as thyroid-associated orbitopathy or benign lymphoproliferative lesions. However, the clinical diagnosis often remains challenging if the disease is slowly progressive in nature or with the sclerosing variant which may have a more subtle clinical presentation.

Treatment of IOI

Observation or nonsteroidal anti-inflammatory agents may be considered for mild cases that are not vision threatening. Initial treatment, however, typically consists of systemic corticosteroids and usually produces rapid relief of signs and symptoms, which is often used to confirm the initial clinical diagnosis [175]. Caution should be used in making this assumption, however, because thyroid orbitopathy often shows similar improvement and lymphomas and other neoplasms can regress also in response to corticosteroid administration. Systemic steroids can be administered orally or pulsed intravenously. In non-vision-threatening cases and those without optic nerve compression, oral steroids are initiated. The typical starting dose is between 60 and 100 mg of oral prednisone, and a slow taper is recommended over weeks to months to prevent recurrence [183]. Intravenous treatment can be used in atypical cases, those with associated vision loss, or in cases refractory to oral administration [184]. Recurrent disease during or after steroid taper is common in adults, though rarely reported in the pediatric population [150]. Additionally, incomplete resolution of disease and resistance to treatment has been noted [153]. Localized intraorbital injection of steroids can be administered intraoperatively after frozen section confirmation of diagnosis or in the outpatient setting [184]. It has been reported to have efficacy in patients with anterior IOI and in a case of biopsy-proven IOI unresponsive to systemic steroid administration [185, 186]. In addition, it may be used in children or diabetics to reduce the systemic side effects of corticosteroid use.

For patients who are steroid responsive but intolerant, low-dose radiation of 15–20 Gy in divided doses over 10–14 days is often adequate. Orcutt et al. showed a 75% treatment effect at doses of 25 Gy over the course of 15 days, with no significant complications or recurrences during the follow-up period [187]. The use of steroid-sparing agents including antimetabolites, T-cell inhibitors, and alkylating agents has been reported in patients who are not responsive to steroid treatment, have a chronic progressive course, and require long-term immunosuppression, or in combination with steroids as first-line treatment in patients with sclerosing forms of IOI [167, 188–190]. Approximately one third of patients require two or more immunosuppressive medications to adequately control disease [175]. Medications that have been used in IOI patients include methotrexate, azathioprine, mycophenolate mofetil, cyclophosphamide, and cyclosporine [188, 190–194]. No consensus exists regarding the use of these agents, and consultation with a rheumatologist is recommended prior to initiating treatment. Case reports indicate that biologic agents including the monoclonal antibody against TNF-alpha, infliximab, and the anti CD-20 monoclonal antibody rituximab may have some role in the treatment of IOI, but this will require further prospective study and should be used in caution with understanding of their significant side effect profiles [189, 195–199]. Surgical debulking is rarely performed but may have a role in the treatment of sclerosing forms of idiopathic orbital inflammation with significant mass effect, fibrosis, and scarring. Orbital exenteration may be indicated in select cases where diffuse orbital involvement results in vision loss and pain unresponsive to other medical or radiation therapy [153]. In rare cases, IOI may extend intracranially and result in death.

A variant of sclerosing idiopathic orbital inflammation associated with increased levels of IgG4 in serum and affected tissues has been recently reported [200, 201]. Orbital lesions containing immunohistochemically detectable IgG4+ plasma cells have been found in these cases. Patients with IgG4-related disorders can also have involvement of other organs including the pancreas, gallbladder, salivary glands, and retroperitoneum, with histopathologic evidence of chronic inflammation and fibrosis. When present in the orbit, orbital masses or lacrimal gland involvement have been described with uniform clinicopathology consisting of marked lymphoplasmacytic infiltration admixed with dense fibrosis [200]. These patients also have a more guarded prognosis due to the sclerosing nature of the disease.

Orbital Myositis

Myositis affects single or multiple extraocular muscles, is the most common cause of nonthyroid extraocular muscle disease, and is unilateral at presentation in the majority of patients [202]. It has been reported to be more common in women, a feature that distinguishes it from the encompassing group of IOI, which appears to have no gender predilection [161, 202]. Myositis typically presents with painful diplopia exacerbated by extraocular muscle movement, with visual acuity being relatively spared. Symptoms are usually acute or subacute, and accompanying signs of orbital inflammation may be present. Recurrence is common, with multiple muscle involvement and bilateral disease at presentation conferring increased risk of persistent disease or recurrence [202]. Although any muscle may be affected, the horizontal rectus muscles and superior rectus muscle have been found to be most commonly affected [160, 161, 202, 203]. Motility dysfunction can be classified as paretic, restrictive, or a combination of the two [161, 204]. Correlating motility dysfunction with timing of presentation in a large series of patients led Mombaerts et al. to suggest that cases with early presentation may exhibit normal motility [161, 204]. Paresis develops as the muscle belly enlarges with impaired movement in the direction of action of the involved muscle [161]. This may acquire a restrictive component as enlargement continues and inflammation ensues [161]. Additionally, chronic disease may result in restrictive myopathy due to fibrosis of muscles, with restriction of movement in the direction opposite the action of the affected muscle [161].

Diagnosis is made based on history, examination findings, and diagnostic imaging. Biopsy is rarely performed except in atypical cases due to inherent risk of damage to extraocular muscle function. Additionally, biopsy during acute presentation may lead to exacerbation of underlying inflammation [148]. When performed, histopathologic evidence of an inflammatory infiltrate composed of lymphocytes, plasma cells, and eosinophils with varying degrees of fibrosis is present [205]. Echography demonstrates thickened tendons, low reflectivity, and enlarged muscle bellies on standard A-scan, which can provide precise measurements of muscle and tendon sizes [161]. CT and MRI may also demonstrate enlarged muscles with thickened tendons [160]. In one review of enlarged muscles identified on orbital CT scans, myositis was found to be the second most common cause, and enhancement was seen after contrast administration in all cases [206]. The most common cause of enlarged extraocular muscles in this series was Graves' disease, which is the leading consideration in the differential diagnosis of enlarged extraocular muscles. Radiographic findings in Graves' disease include fusiform and prominent enlargement of extraocular muscles, which may be difficult to differentiate from myositis [206]. A few features that may aid in this distinction include the more common presentation of proptosis, lack of tendon thickening, and prolapse of orbital fat in Graves' disease [206]. The borders of extraocular muscles are typically smooth and regular with uniform tapering into tendons, compared to the irregular borders that are often present in patients with myositis [165, 206]. Additionally, in cases of myositis, there may be significant improvement in muscular abnormalities following corticosteroid administration that are demonstrated on CT scan [206, 207]. In patients with bilateral myositis, differentiating the EOM enlargement of myositis and Graves' disease may be difficult, especially when there is no apparent thickening of the muscle tendon, or "tendon sign" [203]. In these cases, clinical features that may aid in the differentiation of these two entities include the acute and subacute onset of myositis symptoms, presence of pain with extraocular movement, absence of eyelid signs such as retraction and lid lag typically associated with Graves' disease, and dramatic improvement that is typically achieved with administration of corticosteroids.

While most commonly idiopathic and "nonspecific," myositis may be associated with underlying systemic disorders and is then termed "specific myositis." Specific myositis has been found to be more commonly bilateral and may be the first presentation of systemic disease [202]. Underlying systemic associations include inflammatory bowel diseases, systemic lupus erythematosus, Wegener's granulomatosis, giant cell arteritis, rheumatoid arthritis, sarcoidosis, psoriatic arthritis, scleroderma, and Kawasaki disease [202, 205, 208–210]. Infectious etiologies have also been implicated, including post-streptococcal, herpes zoster, trichinosis, and Lyme disease [209, 211–214]. Another important differential diagnosis clinically and radiographically is metastatic neoplasms.

Corticosteroids are the mainstay of treatment, with the majority of patients achieving symptomatic relief within 5 days of initiating an initial treatment dose between 60 and 120 mg of prednisone [161]. Corticosteroids should be tapered slowly over several weeks to months. Nonsteroidal anti-inflammatory drugs (NSAIDs) may be initiated for patients with mild disease who have a contraindication to steroid use or in conjunction with steroids. Despite treatment, recurrence rates up to 50% have been described and may affect different muscles in the same orbit or the contralateral orbit [204]. Recurrences are generally treated with a combination of corticosteroids and NSAIDs, the latter allowing for reduced steroid dose. The use of NSAIDs should be accompanied by antacid medications (proton-pump inhibitors or histamine H2-receptor antagonists). For patients with corticosteroid resistance, dependence, or side effects, treatment with 20 Gy of irradiation has been shown to have short-term efficacy. However, long-term recurrences were noted in all irradiated orbits in one series [204]. Cytotoxic immunosuppression, when used to treat atypical, recurrent, or progressive cases, should be done so after biopsy confirmation of disease [205].

Dacryoadenitis

The lacrimal gland is the most frequent orbital structure involved in IOI [147]. It typically affects middle-aged adults, and there appears to be no gender predilection. Dacryoadenitis can present acutely or with chronic signs, be unilateral or bilateral, and may be involved in isolation or in combination with other orbital structures. With acute presentation, the lacrimal gland is tender to palpation, with associated eyelid edema and characteristic S-shape configuration of the upper eyelid. Temporal conjunctival injection may also be present. Chronic presentation is typically due to recurrent inflammation or sclerosing variant of disease and presents with insidious symptoms that may lead to eventual displacement of globe and mass effect with diplopia and reduced visual acuity. Imaging, along with history and examination findings, is typically sufficient to indicate a diagnosis of dacryoadenitis; however, underlying infectious, inflammatory, autoimmune, and neoplastic etiologies of lacrimal gland inflammation should be excluded. Corticosteroids are the mainstay of initial treatment, with radiation therapy and immunosuppressive medications used in cases of corticosteroid failure, dependence, or recalcitrant disease. For a comprehensive review of the evaluation and treatment of dacryoadenitis, refer to Chap. 58.

Trochleitis

Trochleitis is an inflammatory process of the superior oblique tendon trochlea and is an uncommon etiology of periorbital pain [215]. In previously published case reports and series, females appear to be more commonly affected [215, 216]. It is typically idiopathic and infrequently associated with underlying systemic disorders. Trochleitis may occur in isolation or coexistent with inflammation of other orbital structures. In the former case, diagnosis may be facilitated by the lack of redness, chemosis, or proptosis. Findings thought to be consistent with trochleitis include aching pain that may have a sharp or stabbing component, point tenderness posterior to the superonasal orbital rim, pain with supraduction, edema around the superior oblique muscle and trochlea seen on echography, absence of signs of systemic disease, and clinical response to corticosteroids [215, 216]. Patients may also experience ipsilateral headaches [216]. CT imaging may show a soft tissue density in the area of the trochlea, although changes may be subtle when compared to echography [216]. Treatment with peritrochlear injection of dexamethasone and/or triamcinolone is generally effective in cases resistant to oral corticosteroids, with clinical response typically achieved within 48 h [217]. Multiple injections spaced 1–3 months apart may be necessary to achieve remission.

Perineuritis

Optic perineuritis is an inflammatory disorder, distinct from demyelinating optic neuritis, which affects the optic nerve sheath and adjacent structures and may result in orbital pain with associated loss of vision [218]. Patients may also have pain on retrodisplacement of the globe [219]. It occurs commonly in adult females and may recur [50]. The clinical picture may be indistinguishable from retrobulbar optic neuritis, and MRI may be useful in differentiating the two processes radiographically [220]. Contrast enhancement with perineuritis is noted around, not within the substance of, the nerve [218]. On CT and ultrasonography, enhancement of the optic nerve sheath is noted as a diffuse, hazy, inflammatory cuff [219]. Other disorders within the differential diagnosis include infectious optic neuritis, sarcoid optic neuritis, and optic nerve sheath tumors. Response to corticosteroids is typically more dramatic in optic perineuritis as compared to demyelinating optic neuritis, which may also help differentiate these two conditions [218].

Idiopathic Posterior Scleritis

The distinction between posterior scleritis and diffuse anterior IOI is not often clear, with inflammation affecting both the posterior sclera and periocular tissues. Inflammation of the posterior sclera may present with ocular findings in addition to acute orbital inflammatory signs and symptoms. Presenting symptoms include redness, blurred vision, photophobia, and pain with extraocular movement. Ocular findings may include iritis, subretinal fluid, chorioretinal folds, choroidal detachment, and macular and optic disc edema. Narrowing of the anterior chamber angle may be noted with annular ciliochoroidal detachment. On funduscopic examination, choroidal effusion and detachment may resemble a subretinal mass and be confused with benign or malignant neoplastic processes. The diagnosis is typically made by careful history taking and slit lamp and funduscopic examinations in combination with imaging. B-mode ultrasonography is a convenient, low-cost method of assessing scleral thickening with associated sub-Tenon's fascia fluid and the characteristic "ring sign" associated with posterior scleritis. Computed tomography may also be used in this evaluation. Infectious etiologies of scleritis that should be excluded include herpetic, tuberculous, and syphilitic diseases. Systemic evaluation should include laboratory tests for rheumatoid arthritis, Wegener's granulomatosis, systemic lupus erythematosus, and other vasculitides (Table 49.5).

Table 49.5 Autoantibodies detected in patients with connective tissue diseases (Adapted from [221])

Autoantibody	Disease (frequency of autoantibody)	Comments
RF	Rheumatoid arthritis (50–90%), Sjögren's syndrome (75–95%), mixed connective tissue disease (50–60%)	Sensitive but not specific for rheumatoid arthritis; correlates with prognosis of disease severity (not disease activity)
ANA	Systemic lupus erythematosus (99%), drug-induced lupus (100%), other connective tissue diseases	Sensitive but not specific for connective tissue diseases; correlates poorly with disease activity

Table 49.5 (continued)

Autoantibody	Disease (frequency of autoantibody)	Comments
Anti-dsDNA	Systemic lupus erythematosus (60%). Should be tested only in patients with positive ANA	Specific but not sensitive for systemic lupus erythematosus; correlates with lupus nephritis and disease activity
Anti-histone	Drug-induced lupus (90%), systemic lupus erythematosus (50%). Use only in ANA-positive patients with history of exposure to lupus-inducing medications, such as procainamide and isoniazid	Sensitive but not specific for drug-induced lupus
Anti-U1 snRNP	Systemic lupus erythematosus (30–40%), mixed connective tissue disease (100%). Should be tested only in patients with positive ANA	Associated with disease activity in systemic lupus erythematosus
Anti-Ro (anti-SS-A)	Sjögren's syndrome (75%), systemic lupus erythematosus (40%)	Associated with photosensitive skin rash, pulmonary disease, and lymphopenia in systemic lupus erythematosus
Anti-La (anti-SS-B)	Sjögren's syndrome (40%), systemic lupus erythematosus (10–15%)	Associated with late-onset systemic lupus erythematosus, secondary Sjögren's syndrome, and neonatal lupus syndrome
Anti-ribosome	Systemic lupus erythematosus (10–20%)	Highly specific but not sensitive for systemic lupus erythematosus; associated with lupus psychosis
Anti-Jo1	Polymyositis and dermatomyositis (30%)	Associated with pulmonary fibrosis and Raynaud's phenomenon
c-ANCA	Wegener's granulomatosis (>90%). Detects antibodies against proteinase 3	Highly specific and sensitive for Wegener's granulomatosis; correlates with disease activity
p-ANCA	Wegener's granulomatosis (10%), microscopic polyangiitis, glomerulonephritis. Detects antibodies against myeloperoxidase	Sensitivity and specificity quite low in Wegener's granulomatosis

RF rheumatoid factor, *ANA* antinuclear antibody, *anti-dsDNA* anti-double-stranded DNA, *anti-ssDNA* anti-single-stranded DNA, *anti-Sm* anti-Smith, *anti-U1 snRNP* autoantibodies against small nuclear ribonucleoprotein U1, *CREST* calcinosis, Raynaud's phenomenon, esophageal dysmotility, sclerodactyly, and telangiectasias, *c-ANCA* cytoplasmic antineutrophilic cytoplasmic antibodies, *p-ANCA* perinuclear antineutrophilic cytoplasmic antibodies

Neoplastic processes should also be excluded. Treatment of idiopathic posterior scleritis consists of oral corticosteroids. Treatment is multifactorial but usually involves corticosteroids and systemic indomethacin.

Orbital Apex (Tolosa-Hunt) Syndrome

Tolosa-Hunt syndrome is an idiopathic granulomatous disorder that affects the orbital apex, superior orbital fissure, and cavernous sinus and is within the spectrum of orbital inflammatory disease [222, 223]. It shares clinical and pathologic features with IOI, with the main clinical difference pattern of involvement [222]. Patients may also present with painful ophthalmoplegia; however, proptosis, visual loss, and external signs of inflammation are less commonly seen as compared to IOI [147, 222]. Ophthalmoplegia consists of third, fourth, and sixth cranial nerve paresis with hypoesthesia within the distribution of the first division of the trigeminal nerve [147]. Diagnosis is generally made clinically with the aid of CT or MRI imaging which demonstrates a mass lesion within the cavernous sinus and extending into the orbital apex or posterior orbit [224]. Diagnostic biopsy is not frequently performed due to the location of affected structures and close proximity to vital structures. As with IOI, corticosteroids remain the mainstay of treatment, with unresponsive cases requiring radiotherapy or immunosuppressive treatment [223]. Other disorders to consider that may present with acute ophthalmoplegia and orbital apex signs include orbital cellulitis, carotid cavernous fistula, and carotid sinus thrombosis. A high index of suspicion for fungal etiologies such as *Aspergillus* should be maintained, as these may progress rapidly with extracranial extension following corticosteroid administration.

Langerhans' Cell Histiocytosis

Langerhans' cell histiocytosis (LCH) is a group of disorders characterized by a clonal proliferation of Langerhans' cells in single or multiple sites [225]. It is a rare disease of unknown etiology, with an estimated incidence of up to four to five cases per million per year in children [226–228]. The involved age groups vary by clinical presentation. Multisystem LCH usually occurs before 3 years of age, and unifocal disease is more common in later childhood [229]. Males are more frequently affected than females, reaching ratios of 2:1 in some studies [230]. Whether LCH is a reactive proliferation or a neoplastic disorder remains unanswered [231, 232].

Currently, LCH is divided according to the guidelines of the Histiocytosis Society into two major categories: (1) single-system LCH, further subdivided into single site (unifocal bone, skin, or lymph node) or multiple site (multifocal bone or multiple lymph nodes), and (2) multisystem LCH, defined as involvement of two or more organs at diagnosis with or without organ dysfunction. Multisystem LCH is further subdivided into low- and high-risk groups. Involvement of the liver, lungs, spleen, or, diffusely, bone marrow in multisystem LCH is considered high risk because of the high mortality rate associated with this pattern of the disease [233]. In single-system multifocal bone disease, certain sites are considered to be high risk for central nervous system (CNS) disease. One of these sites is the orbit because of the putative risk for delayed-onset diabetes insipidus (DI) [233]. In studies of the Histiocyte Society, patients with orbital lesions had a higher propensity for developing DI, leading the authors to conclude that the orbital involvement is a risk factor for DI [234, 235]. However, all of the cases developing DI had multisystem LCH along with their orbital lesions, and none had unifocal LCH of the orbit. Harris rebutted the conclusion that orbital involvement was risk factor for DI necessitating preventive systemic chemotherapy, stating that he was not aware of any reported case of unifocal LCH of orbit that later developed DI or CNS disease [226]. A recent multivariate meta-analysis by the Histiocytosis Society supports Harris' concept by showing that only auditory system and multisystem diseases are significant risk factors for DI and CNS disease, particularly the pituitary-hypothalamic region [236, 237].

Orbital involvement is by far the most ophthalmic manifestation of LCH, usually occurring during the first two decades of life [238]. Orbital LCH comprises 1% of all orbital tumors and simulating lesions. However, orbital involvement in multisystem LCH may be seen in up to 23% of the patients [152, 238, 239]. Patients usually present with unilateral proptosis, or protuberant frontal bone, often associated with signs of inflammation [238]. Computerized tomography shows marked osteolysis associated with an adjacent soft tissue mass extending into the orbit, anterior cranial fossa, temporal fossa, or forehead [240]. Osteolytic defects of the skull usually display a typical punched-out appearance with scalloped or irregular margins on plain skull radiographs. The differential diagnosis of LCH includes infection, inflammatory diseases, and neoplasia, including neuroblastoma, leukemia, metastatic carcinoma, or fibro-osseous lesions of bone such as aneurismal bone cyst, brown tumor, giant cell tumor, and giant cell reparative granuloma of bone [238].

The diagnosis of LCH requires the presence of Langerhans' cells identified by either positive immunohistochemical staining for CD1a or ultrastructural identification of Birbeck granules. Langerhans' cells are associated with varying proportions of eosinophils, macrophages, multinucleated giant cells, and T lymphocytes [241–243]. Langerhans' cells and these various types of inflammatory cells appear to participate in complex interactions involving secretion of cytokines and binding of cell surface markers that result in a tumor microenvironment characterized by LCH proliferation, osteolysis, and inflammation that cause clinical manifestation of the disease [241, 243].

Management of LCH depends on whether orbital involvement is unifocal bone disease or part of multifocal bone or multisystem disease. Unifocal bone disease runs a benign course and responds favorably to a variety of local interventions, including curettage with or without intralesional corticosteroid or local radiotherapy [238, 244]. Extensive resections are usually unnecessary because most of bone lesions heal spontaneously even if a residual tumor is left after partial surgical debridement [227]. For the patients with extensive unifocal lesions or unifocal lesions that fail to regress after debridement, systemic chemotherapy of vinblastine and prednisone may be used [245]. Patients with multifocal bone disease or multisystem disease are managed with systemic chemotherapy [246].

Adult Xanthogranulomatous Diseases

Adult orbital xanthogranulomatous diseases account for 1% of all orbital tumors and simulating lesions [152]. Included are four types: adult-onset xanthogranuloma, adult-onset asthma and periocular xanthogranuloma, necrobiotic xanthogranuloma, and Erdheim-Chester disease [246, 247].

Adult-onset xanthogranuloma presents with bilateral yellow-orange, elevated, indurated, and non-ulcerated xanthomatous eyelids and/or orbital masses [246, 247]. It is limited to the ocular region, often bilateral, and without systemic involvement. It is a disease of middle-aged to elderly adults without sex predilection. It involves anterior orbit and eyelids, but intraconal involvement can be observed [82, 246]. Histopathological examination shows infiltrating xanthoma cells with scattered Touton giant cells and variable numbers of plasma cells and lymphocytes along with fibrosis. Adult-onset xanthogranuloma is usually self-limited and does not require aggressive treatment. Intralesional corticosteroid injection is successful in controlling adult-onset xanthogranuloma [248].

The presentation of adult-onset asthma and periocular xanthogranuloma is identical to adult-onset xanthogranuloma, occurring in adults of any age with a male predilection of 2:1. Histopathological examination is similar to that of adult-onset xanthogranuloma, often also containing germinal centers and scattered eosinophils [177]. Most patients develop adult-onset asthma within a few months to years after onset of the ocular lesions. Beside asthma, lymphadenopathy, paraproteinemia, and rarely lymphoproliferative disorders may be observed [247, 249]. Surgical debulking is the treatment of choice with 75% of reported cases responding to surgery alone [246, 247]. Systemic corticosteroids are used in unresponsive or recurrent cases.

Necrobiotic xanthogranuloma presents with dermal lesions that have a tendency to ulcerate. It affects adults aged 20–85 years, without sex predilection [246, 247]. Necrobiotic xanthogranuloma is bilateral, involving the eyelids and anterior orbit. Histopathological examination shows necrobiosis of collagen that is surrounded by palisading epithelioid histiocytes. Paraproteinemia, multiple myeloma, or chronic myelogenic leukemia is often associated with necrobiotic xanthogranuloma [246, 247]. Treatment involves surgical excision, systemic or local corticosteroid therapy, systemic immunosuppressive therapy, and radiotherapy [177, 246, 247].

Erdheim-Chester disease is a rare, idiopathic, progressive disorder characterized by infiltrative histiocytic lesions and fibrosis of the orbit, retroperitoneum, bones, and internal organs, including the heart, lungs, brain, and kidneys. It is seen in adults of any age with a male predilection of 2:1 [246, 247]. It often presents with enhancing orbital masses that have a propensity to involve the posterior orbit where they may cause neuropathy [250]. Histopathological examination shows collections of large, markedly xanthomatous histiocytes with dispersed lymphocytes and variable degree of fibrosis which may become extensive. Treatment modalities include systemic corticosteroids, chemotherapy, and radiotherapy [246, 247]. Erdheim-Chester disease is a fatal condition, usually due to cardiomyopathy, severe lung disease, or chronic renal failure.

Kimura Disease and Angiolymphoid Hyperplasia with Eosinophilia

Angiolymphoid hyperplasia with eosinophilia (ALHE) is a rare localized cutaneous condition of the head and neck, which occasionally affects the orbit and ocular adnexa. Young women are more often affected by ocular adnexal ALHE, and symptoms may include painless eyelid swelling and proptosis. Pruritus has been reported in some patients. In decreasing frequency, ALHE can involve the orbit, eyelid, and lacrimal gland [251–257]. The superior orbit is most commonly involved, and bilateral disease has been described. Rare cases of compressive optic neuropathy, spontaneous orbital hemorrhage, or diplopia have been reported [258]. Histopathological evaluation of ALHE lesions shows plump endothelial cells, eosinophilic and lymphocytic infiltrate, and lack of increased mitotic figures or multinucleated cells [259]. Minimal fibrosis and lymphoid follicles help to differentiate ALHE from Kimura disease, a similar condition seen more commonly in Asian patients and associated with systemic eosinophilia, regional lymphadenopathy, and more deeply infiltrating lesions [260]. One case of simultaneous

Kimura disease and ALHE lesions in a patient suggests the possibility of a spectrum of disease [261]. Angiosarcoma can be differentiated from ALHE by increased mitotic figures, areas of necrosis, and absence of eosinophilia [259]. Melkersson-Rosenthal syndrome can be differentiated from ALHE by characteristic granulomatous lymphangitis [262].

Complete surgical excision is recommended for ALHE, and good results without recurrence are typical [259]. Limited lesions of the eyelids or anterior orbit may be treated with excisional biopsy. More extensive or posterior orbital lesions typically require incisional biopsy for diagnosis. If secondary complete excision is not possible without damaging vital orbital structures, debulking is recommended. Reports of lesions not completely excised demonstrate a high frequency of recurrent mild inflammation. For these patients with unresectable lesions, we typically recommend conservative treatment because of the relatively benign natural history of this disease and high side effect profile of systemic steroids.

Intraocular Tumor-Related Orbital Inflammation

Intraocular tumors are usually painless and present with visual complaints or are found during eye examination. Rarely, intraocular tumors, especially uveal melanoma and retinoblastoma, can present with orbital inflammation that may be confused with cellulitis.

Extraocular extension of choroidal melanoma may be accompanied by proptosis, restriction of ocular movements, and orbital inflammation. The poor prognosis in the patients with extraocular extension of uveal melanoma is usually related to cell type, tumor size, and extraocular extension, rather than orbital inflammation. The exact cause of orbital inflammation due to extraocular extension is unknown but may be due to the fact that uveal melanomas often induce inflammation, even when confined within the sclera.

Among uveal melanoma patients, tumor necrosis and extraocular extension may incite scleral/episcleral or orbital inflammation [263–267]. In a histopathological analysis, Moshari et al. reported that 99% of totally necrotic choroidal and ciliary body melanomas and 57% of partially necrotic melanomas developed episcleritis and/or scleritis [268]. Scleritis and necrosis were significant prognostic risk factors for metastasis in univariate statistical analysis but not in multivariate analysis when tumor size was considered. In patients with uveal melanomas, necrosis and scleritis were associated with uveal effusion that is otherwise rare in uveal melanoma. Orbital inflammation in the absence of extraocular extension has been rarely described [264, 266, 269, 270]. It is proposed that necrotic tissue provides a stimulus for orbital inflammation by the release of inflammatory mediators and cytokines, such as tumor necrosis factor and interleukin-1 [267, 268].

Retinoblastoma also can be associated with orbital inflammation. Shields et al. and later Mullaney et al. reported the prevalence of orbital inflammation varied from 1% to 5% in retinoblastoma [54]. Usually, orbital inflammation is seen in cases with advanced (group D) necrotic retinoblastoma with a high incidence of anterior segment involvement [53–55]. The cause of orbital inflammation in retinoblastoma is unknown. It is speculated that large necrotic tumors invading the anterior segment outgrow the blood supply, leading to necrosis and inflammation [55, 271]. Additionally, anterior chamber involvement can cause necrosis of nonneoplastic iris and ciliary body tissue, inducing inflammation of adjacent orbital tissue [271].

The presence of orbital inflammation in retinoblastoma is not indicative of extraocular extension even though the presence of orbital inflammation and thickening of sclera gives the impression of extraocular extension on radiological examination. Thus, Mullaney et al. reported that although 67% of the patients were reported to have possible extrascleral extension on radiological examination, histopathological examination did not confirm the presence of extraocular extension in any of the cases [55]. Systemic corticosteroids, administered for 3–5 days, have been used to decrease the eyelid and orbital inflammation in order to facilitate subsequent enucleation. However, enucleation alone is often preferred in these patients to expedite resolution of the disease process while preventing side effects of systemic corticosteroids.

References

1. Liu IT, Kao SC, Wang AG, Tsai CC, Liang CK, Hsu WM. Preseptal and orbital cellulitis: a 10-year review of hospitalized patients. J Chin Med Assoc. 2006;69(9):415–22.
2. Nageswaran S, Woods CR, Benjamin DK Jr, Givner LB, Shetty AK. Orbital cellulitis in children. Pediatr Infect Dis J. 2006;25(8):695–9.
3. Georgakopoulos CD, Eliopoulou MI, Stasinos S, Exarchou A, Pharmakakis N, Varvarigou A. Periorbital and orbital cellulitis: a 10-year review of hospitalized children. Eur J Ophthalmol. 2010;20(6):1066–72.
4. Israele V, Nelson JD. Periorbital and orbital cellulitis. Pediatr Infect Dis J. 1987;6(4):404–10.
5. Cruz AA, Mussi-Pinhata MM, Akaishi PM, Cattebeke L, Torrano da Silva J, Elia J Jr. Neonatal orbital abscess. Ophthalmology. 2001;108(12):2316–20.
6. Jain A, Rubin PA. Orbital cellulitis in children. Int Ophthalmol Clin. 2001;41(4):71–86.
7. Yang M, Quah BL, Seah LL, Looi A. Orbital cellulitis in children-medical treatment versus surgical management. Orbit. 2009;28(2–3):124–36.
8. Chandler JR, Langenbrunner DJ, Stevens ER. The pathogenesis of orbital complications in acute sinusitis. Laryngoscope. 1970;80(9):1414–28.
9. Youssef OH, Stefanyszyn MA, Bilyk JR. Odontogenic orbital cellulitis. Ophthal Plast Reconstr Surg. 2008;24(1):29–35.
10. Basheikh A, Superstein R. A child with bilateral orbital cellulitis one day after strabismus surgery. J AAPOS. 2009;13(5):488–90.

11. Wilson ME, Paul TO. Orbital cellulitis following strabismus surgery. Ophthalmic Surg. 1987;18(2):92–4.
12. Maheshwari R, Maheshwari S, Shah T. Acute dacryocystitis causing orbital cellulitis and abscess. Orbit. 2009;28(2–3):196–9.
13. Martins MC, Ricardo JR, Akaishi PM, Velasco e Cruz AA. Orbital abscess secondary to acute dacryocystitis: case report. Arq Bras Oftalmol. 2008;71(4):576–8.
14. Kim IK, Kim JR, Jang KS, Moon YS, Park SW. Orbital abscess from an odontogenic infection. Oral Surg Oral Med Oral Pathol Oral Radiol Endod. 2007;103(1):e1–6.
15. Ben Simon GJ, Bush S, Selva D, McNab AA. Orbital cellulitis: a rare complication after orbital blowout fracture. Ophthalmology. 2005;112(11):2030–4.
16. Luemsamran P, Pornpanich K, Vangveeravong S, Mekanandha P. Orbital cellulitis and endophthalmitis in pseudomonas septicemia. Orbit. 2008;27(6):455–7.
17. Decock C, Claerhout I, Kestelyn P, Van Aken EH. Orbital cellulitis as complication of endophthalmitis after cataract surgery. J Cataract Refract Surg. 2010;36(4):673–5.
18. Ang LP, Lee MW, Seah LL, Cheong P, Rootman J. Orbital cellulitis following intralesional corticosteroid injection for periocular capillary haemangioma. Eye. 2007;21(7):999–1001.
19. Hofbauer JD, Gordon LK, Palmer J. Acute orbital cellulitis after peribulbar injection. Am J Ophthalmol. 1994;118(3):391–2.
20. Dahlmann AH, Appaswamy S, Headon MP. Orbital cellulitis following sub-Tenon's anaesthesia. Eye. 2002;16(2):200–1.
21. Hartstein ME, Steinvurzel MD, Cohen CP. Intracranial abscess as a complication of subperiosteal abscess of the orbit. Ophthal Plast Reconstr Surg. 2001;17(6):398–403.
22. Caruso PA, Watkins LM, Suwansaard P, et al. Odontogenic orbital inflammation: clinical and CT findings – initial observations. Radiology. 2006;239(1):187–94.
23. Flinn J, Chapman ME, Wightman AJ, Maran AG. A prospective analysis of incidental paranasal sinus abnormalities on CT head scans. Clin Otolaryngol Allied Sci. 1994;19(4):287–9.
24. Lesserson JA, Kieserman SP, Finn DG. The radiographic incidence of chronic sinus disease in the pediatric population. Laryngoscope. 1994;104(2):159–66.
25. Diament MJ, Senac MO Jr, Gilsanz S, Baker S, Gillespie T, Larsson S. Prevalence of incidental paranasal sinuses opacification in pediatric patients: a CT study. J Comput Assist Tomogr. 1987;11(3):426–31.
26. Sepahdari AR, Aakalu VK, Kapur R, et al. MRI of orbital cellulitis and orbital abscess: the role of diffusion-weighted imaging. AJR Am J Roentgenol. 2009;193(3):W244–50.
27. Harris GJ. Subperiosteal abscess of the orbit. Age as a factor in the bacteriology and response to treatment. Ophthalmology. 1994;101(3):585–95.
28. Harris GJ. Subperiosteal abscess of the orbit: computed tomography and the clinical course. Ophthal Plast Reconstr Surg. 1996;12(1):1–8.
29. Watters EC, Wallar PH, Hiles DA, Michaels RH. Acute orbital cellulitis. Arch Ophthalmol. 1976;94(5):785–8.
30. Kloek CE, Rubin PA. Role of inflammation in orbital cellulitis. Int Ophthalmol Clin. 2006;46(2):57–68.
31. Donahue SP, Schwartz G. Preseptal and orbital cellulitis in childhood. A changing microbiologic spectrum. Ophthalmology. 1998;105(10):1902–5, discussion 1905–06.
32. Ambati BK, Ambati J, Azar N, Stratton L, Schmidt EV. Periorbital and orbital cellulitis before and after the advent of *Haemophilus influenzae* type B vaccination. Ophthalmology. 2000;107(8):1450–3.
33. Barone SR, Aiuto LT. Periorbital and orbital cellulitis in the *Haemophilus influenzae* vaccine era. J Pediatr Ophthalmol Strabismus. 1997;34(5):293–6.
34. McKinley SH, Yen MT, Miller AM, Yen KG. Microbiology of pediatric orbital cellulitis. Am J Ophthalmol. 2007;144(4):497–501.
35. Ferguson MP, McNab AA. Current treatment and outcome in orbital cellulitis. Aust N Z J Ophthalmol. 1999;27(6):375–9.
36. Naimi TS, LeDell KH, Boxrud DJ, et al. Epidemiology and clonality of community-acquired methicillin-resistant *Staphylococcus aureus* in Minnesota, 1996–1998. Clin Infect Dis. 2001;33(7):990–6.
37. Blomquist PH. Methicillin-resistant *Staphylococcus aureus* infections of the eye and orbit (an American Ophthalmological Society thesis). Trans Am Ophthalmol Soc. 2006;104:322–45.
38. Rutar T, Chambers HF, Crawford JB, et al. Ophthalmic manifestations of infections caused by the USA300 clone of community-associated methicillin-resistant *Staphylococcus aureus*. Ophthalmology. 2006;113(8):1455–62.
39. Vazan DF, Kodsi SR. Community-acquired methicillin-resistant *Staphylococcus aureus* orbital cellulitis in a non-immunocompromised child. J AAPOS. 2008;12(2):205–6.
40. Rutar T, Zwick OM, Cockerham KP, Horton JC. Bilateral blindness from orbital cellulitis caused by community-acquired methicillin-resistant *Staphylococcus aureus*. Am J Ophthalmol. 2005;140(4):740–2.
41. Shome D, Jain V, Natarajan S, Agrawal S, Shah K. Community-acquired methicillin-resistant *Staphylococcus aureus* (CAMRSA) – a rare cause of fulminant orbital cellulitis. Orbit. 2008;27(3):179–81.
42. Elner VM, Demirci H, Nerad JA, Hassan AS. Periocular necrotizing fasciitis with visual loss pathogenesis and treatment. Ophthalmology. 2006;113(12):2338–45.
43. Gelston CD, Durairaj VD, Simoes EA. Rhino-orbital mucormycosis causing cavernous sinus and internal carotid thrombosis treated with posaconazole. Arch Ophthalmol. 2007;125(6):848–9.
44. Pelton RW, Peterson EA, Patel BC, Davis K. Successful treatment of rhino-orbital mucormycosis without exenteration: the use of multiple treatment modalities. Ophthal Plast Reconstr Surg. 2001;17(1):62–6.
45. Dewan T, Sangal K, Premsagar IC, Vashishth S. Orbital tuberculoma extending into the cranium. Ophthalmologica. 2006;220(2):137–9.
46. Hughes EH, Petrushkin H, Sibtain NA, Stanford MR, Plant GT, Graham EM. Tuberculous orbital apex syndromes. Br J Ophthalmol. 2008;92(11):1511–7.
47. Sen DK. Tuberculosis of the orbit and lacrimal gland: a clinical study of 14 cases. J Pediatr Ophthalmol Strabismus. 1980;17(4):232–8.
48. Madge SN, Prabhakaran VC, Shome D, Kim U, Honavar S, Selva D. Orbital tuberculosis: a review of the literature. Orbit. 2008;27(4):267–77.
49. Narula MK, Chaudhary V, Baruah D, Kathuria M, Anand R. Pictorial essay: orbital tuberculosis. Indian J Radiol Imaging. 2010;20(1):6–10.
50. Gordon LK. Orbital inflammatory disease: a diagnostic and therapeutic challenge. Eye. 2006;20(10):1196–206.
51. Shields CL, Shields JA, Honavar SG, Demirci H. Clinical spectrum of primary ophthalmic rhabdomyosarcoma. Ophthalmology. 2001;108(12):2284–92.
52. Biswas J, Ahuja VK, Shanmugam MP, Kurian R, Fernandez T. Malignant melanoma of the choroid presenting as orbital cellulitis: report of two cases with a review of the literature. Orbit. 1999;18(2):123–30.
53. Agarwal M, Biswas J. S K, Shanmugam MP. Retinoblastoma presenting as orbital cellulitis: report of four cases with a review of the literature. Orbit. 2004;23(2):93–8.
54. Shields JA, Shields CL, Suvarnamani C, Schroeder RP, DePotter P. Retinoblastoma manifesting as orbital cellulitis. Am J Ophthalmol. 1991;112(4):442–9.
55. Mullaney PB, Karcioglu ZA, Huaman AM, al-Mesfer S. Retinoblastoma associated orbital cellulitis. Br J Ophthalmol. 1998;82(5):517–21.

56. Shields JA, Shields CL, Brotman HK, Carvalho C, Perez N, Eagle RC Jr. Cancer metastatic to the orbit: the 2000 Robert M Curts Lecture. Ophthal Plast Reconstr Surg. 2001;17(5):346–54.
57. Barahimi B, Patel A, Bilyk JR. Orbital metastasis mimicking subperiosteal abscess. Orbit. 2010;29(3):165–7.
58. Fyrmpas G, Televantou D, Papageorgiou V, Nofal F, Constantinidis J. Unsuspected breast carcinoma presenting as orbital complication of rhinosinusitis. Eur Arch Otorhinolaryngol. 2008;265(8):979–82.
59. Douvoyiannis M, Fakioglu E, Litman N. Orbital compression syndrome presenting as orbital cellulitis in a child with sickle cell anemia. Pediatr Emerg Care. 2010;26(4):285–6.
60. Rebsamen SL, Bilaniuk LT, Granet D, et al. Orbital wall infarction in sickle cell disease: MR evaluation. AJNR Am J Neuroradiol. 1993;14(3):777–9.
61. Cannon PS, Mc Keag D, Radford R, Ataullah S, Leatherbarrow B. Our experience using primary oral antibiotics in the management of orbital cellulitis in a tertiary referral centre. Eye. 2009;23(3):612–5.
62. Smith AT, Spencer JT. Orbital complications resulting from lesions of the sinuses. Ann Otol Rhinol Laryngol. 1948;57(1):5–27.
63. Tovilla-Canales JL, Nava A, Tovilla y Pomar JL. Orbital and periorbital infections. Curr Opin Ophthalmol. 2001;12(5):335–41.
64. Greenberg MF, Pollard ZF. Medical treatment of pediatric subperiosteal orbital abscess secondary to sinusitis. J AAPOS. 1998;2(6):351–5.
65. Ryan JT, Preciado DA, Bauman N, et al. Management of pediatric orbital cellulitis in patients with radiographic findings of subperiosteal abscess. Otolaryngol Head Neck Surg. 2009;140(6):907–11.
66. Brown CL, Graham SM, Griffin MC, et al. Pediatric medial subperiosteal orbital abscess: medical management where possible. Am J Rhinol. 2004;18(5):321–7.
67. Hakim HE, Malik AC, Aronyk K, Ledi E, Bhargava R. The prevalence of intracranial complications in pediatric frontal sinusitis. Int J Pediatr Otorhinolaryngol. 2006;70(8):1383–7.
68. Yen MT, Yen KG. Effect of corticosteroids in the acute management of pediatric orbital cellulitis with subperiosteal abscess. Ophthal Plast Reconstr Surg. 2005;21(5):363–6, discussion 366–7.
69. Brook I. Microbiology and antimicrobial treatment of orbital and intracranial complications of sinusitis in children and their management. Int J Pediatr Otorhinolaryngol. 2009;73(9):1183–6.
70. Barahimi B, Murchison AP, Bilyk JR. Forget me not. Surv Ophthalmol. 2010;55(5):467–80.
71. Brook I. Microbiology of intracranial abscesses and their associated sinusitis. Arch Otolaryngol Head Neck Surg. 2005;131(11):1017–9.
72. Okamoto Y, Hiraoka T, Okamoto F, Oshika T. A case of subperiosteal abscess of the orbit with central retinal artery occlusion. Eur J Ophthalmol. 2009;19(2):288–91.
73. Das JK, Choudhury BD, Medhi J. Orbital abscess and hemi-occlusion of the central retinal vein in a child. Orbit. 2007;26(4):295–7.
74. Patil SP, Gautam MM, Sodha AA, Khan KJ. Primary cutaneous nocardiosis with craniocerebral extension: a case report. Dermatol Online J. 2009;15(6):8.
75. Shanbhag NU, Karandikar S, Deshmukkh PA. Disseminated orbital actinomycetoma: a case report. Indian J Ophthalmol. 2010;58(1):60–3.
76. Pieroth L, Winterkorn JM, Schubert H, Millar WS, Kazim M. Concurrent sino-orbital aspergillosis and cerebral nocardiosis. J Neuroophthalmol. 2004;24(2):135–7.
77. Thomas PA. Current perspectives on ophthalmic mycoses. Clin Microbiol Rev. 2003;16(4):730–97.
78. Levin LA, Avery R, Shore JW, Woog JJ, Baker AS. The spectrum of orbital aspergillosis: a clinicopathological review. Surv Ophthalmol. 1996;41(2):142–54.
79. Arndt S, Aschendorff A, Echternach M, Daemmrich TD, Maier W. Rhino-orbital-cerebral mucormycosis and aspergillosis: differential diagnosis and treatment. Eur Arch Otorhinolaryngol. 2009;266(1):71–6.
80. Maiorano E, Favia G, Capodiferro S, Montagna MT, Lo ML. Combined mucormycosis and aspergillosis of the oro-sinonasal region in a patient affected by Castleman disease. Virchows Arch. 2005;446(1):28–33.
81. Choi HS, Choi JY, Yoon JS, Kim SJ, Lee SY. Clinical characteristics and prognosis of orbital invasive aspergillosis. Ophthal Plast Reconstr Surg. 2008;24(6):454–9.
82. Sivak-Callcott JA, Livesley N, Nugent RA, Rasmussen SL, Saeed P, Rootman J. Localised invasive sino-orbital aspergillosis: characteristic features. Br J Ophthalmol. 2004;88(5):681–7.
83. Walsh TJ, Anaissie EJ, Denning DW, et al. Treatment of aspergillosis: clinical practice guidelines of the Infectious Diseases Society of America. Clin Infect Dis. 2008;46(3):327–60.
84. Sherif R, Segal BH. Pulmonary aspergillosis: clinical presentation, diagnostic tests, management and complications. Curr Opin Pulm Med. 2010;16(3):242–50.
85. Wakabayashi T, Oda H, Kinoshita N, Ogasawara A, Fujishiro Y, Kawanabe W. Retrobulbar amphotericin B injections for treatment of invasive sino-orbital aspergillosis. Jpn J Ophthalmol. 2007;51(4):309–11.
86. Massry GG, Hornblass A, Harrison W. Itraconazole in the treatment of orbital aspergillosis. Ophthalmology. 1996;103(9):1467–70.
87. Streppel M, Bachmann G, Arnold G, Damm M, Stennert E. Successful treatment of an invasive aspergillosis of the skull base and paranasal sinuses with liposomal amphotericin B and itraconazole. Ann Otol Rhinol Laryngol. 1999;108(2):205–7.
88. Schaffner A, Bohler A. Amphotericin B refractory aspergillosis after itraconazole: evidence for significant antagonism. Mycoses. 1993;36(11–12):421–4.
89. Warwar RE, Bullock JD. Rhino-orbital-cerebral mucormycosis: a review. Orbit. 1998;17(4):237–45.
90. Yohai RA, Bullock JD, Aziz AA, Markert RJ. Survival factors in rhino-orbital-cerebral mucormycosis. Surv Ophthalmol. 1994;39(1):3–22.
91. Kahana A, Lucarelli MJ. Use of radiopaque intraorbital catheter in the treatment of sino-orbito-cranial mucormycosis. Arch Ophthalmol. 2007;125(12):1714–5.
92. Seiff SR, Choo PH, Carter SR. Role of local amphotericin B therapy for sino-orbital fungal infections. Ophthal Plast Reconstr Surg. 1999;15(1):28–31.
93. Tarani L, Costantino F, Notheis G, et al. Long-term posaconazole treatment and follow-up of rhino-orbital-cerebral mucormycosis in a diabetic girl. Pediatr Diabetes. 2009;10(4):289–93.
94. Yoon YK, Kim MJ, Chung YG, Shin IY. Successful treatment of a case with rhino-orbital-cerebral mucormycosis by the combination of neurosurgical intervention and the sequential use of amphotericin B and posaconazole. J Korean Neurosurg Soc. 2010;47(1):74–7.
95. Abzug MJ, Walsh TJ. Interferon-gamma and colony-stimulating factors as adjuvant therapy for refractory fungal infections in children. Pediatr Infect Dis J. 2004;23(8):769–73.
96. Garcia-Diaz JB, Palau L, Pankey GA. Resolution of rhinocerebral zygomycosis associated with adjuvant administration of granulocyte-macrophage colony-stimulating factor. Clin Infect Dis. 2001;32(12):e145–50.
97. Hunninghake GW, Costabel U, Ando M, et al. ATS/ERS/WASOG statement on sarcoidosis. American Thoracic Society/European Respiratory Society/World Association of Sarcoidosis and other

Granulomatous Disorders. Sarcoidosis Vasc Diffuse Lung Dis. 1999;16(2):149–73.
98. Newman LS, Rose CS, Maier LA. Sarcoidosis. N Engl J Med. 1997;336(17):1224–34.
99. Iannuzzi MC, Rybicki BA, Teirstein AS. Sarcoidosis. N Engl J Med. 2007;357(21):2153–65.
100. Baughman RP, Teirstein AS, Judson MA, et al. Clinical characteristics of patients in a case control study of sarcoidosis. Am J Respir Crit Care Med. 2001;164(10 Pt 1):1885–9.
101. Smith JA, Foster CS. Sarcoidosis and its ocular manifestations. Int Ophthalmol Clin. 1996;36(1):109–25.
102. Demirci H, Christianson M. Orbital and adnexal sarcoidosis: analysis of clinical features and systemic disease in 30 cases. Am J Ophthalmol. 2011;151(6):1074–1080.e1. Epub 2011 Mar 31
103. Prabhakaran VC, Saeed P, Esmaeli B, et al. Orbital and adnexal sarcoidosis. Arch Ophthalmol. 2007;125(12):1657–62.
104. Spaide RF, Ward DL. Conjunctival biopsy in the diagnosis of sarcoidosis. Br J Ophthalmol. 1990;74(8):469–71.
105. Chung YM, Lin YC, Huang DF, Hwang DK, Ho DM. Conjunctival biopsy in sarcoidosis. J Chin Med Assoc. 2006;69(10):472–7.
106. Leavitt JA, Campbell RJ. Cost-effectiveness in the diagnosis of sarcoidosis: the conjunctival biopsy. Eye. 1998;12(Pt 6):959–62.
107. Harman LE, Margo CE. Wegener's granulomatosis. Surv Ophthalmol. 1998;42(5):458–80.
108. Pakrou N, Selva D, Leibovitch I. Wegener's granulomatosis: ophthalmic manifestations and management. Semin Arthritis Rheum. 2006;35(5):284–92.
109. Watts RA, Carruthers DM, Scott DG. Epidemiology of systemic vasculitis: changing incidence or definition? Semin Arthritis Rheum. 1995;25(1):28–34.
110. Bruce IN, Bell AL. A comparison of two nomenclature systems for primary systemic vasculitis. Br J Rheumatol. 1997;36(4):453–8.
111. Carrington CB, Liebow A. Limited forms of angiitis and granulomatosis of Wegener's type. Am J Med. 1966;41(4):497–527.
112. Kallenberg CG. Pathophysiology of ANCA-associated small vessel vasculitis. Curr Rheumatol Rep. 2010;12(6):399–405.
113. Kalina PH, Lie JT, Campbell RJ, Garrity JA. Diagnostic value and limitations of orbital biopsy in Wegener's granulomatosis. Ophthalmology. 1992;99(1):120–4.
114. Fechner FP, Faquin WC, Pilch BZ. Wegener's granulomatosis of the orbit: a clinicopathological study of 15 patients. Laryngoscope. 2002;112(11):1945–50.
115. Danda D, Mathew AJ, Mathew J. Wegener's granulomatosis: a rare presentation. Clin Rheumatol. 2008;27(2):273–5.
116. Pradeep TG, Prabhakaran VC, McNab A, Dodd T, Selva D. Diffuse bilateral orbital inflammation in Churg-Strauss syndrome. Ophthal Plast Reconstr Surg. 2010;26(1):57–9.
117. Cottin V, Cordier JF. Churg-Strauss syndrome. Allergy. 1999;54(6):535–51.
118. Robin JB, Schanzlin DJ, Meisler DM, de Luise VP, Clough JD. Ocular involvement in the respiratory vasculitides. Surv Ophthalmol. 1985;30(2):127–40.
119. Acheson JF, Cockerell OC, Bentley CR, Sanders MD. Churg-Strauss vasculitis presenting with severe visual loss due to bilateral sequential optic neuropathy. Br J Ophthalmol. 1993;77(2):118–9.
120. Alberts AR, Lasonde R, Ackerman KR, Chartash EK, Susin M, Furie RA. Reversible monocular blindness complicating Churg-Strauss syndrome. J Rheumatol. 1994;21(2):363–5.
121. Dagi LR, Currie J. Branch retinal artery occlusion in the Churg-Strauss syndrome. J Clin Neuroophthalmol. 1985;5(4):229–37.
122. Kattah JC, Chrousos GA, Katz PA, McCasland B, Kolsky MP. Anterior ischemic optic neuropathy in Churg-Strauss syndrome. Neurology. 1994;44(11):2200–2.
123. Shields CL, Shields JA, Rozanski TI. Conjunctival involvement in Churg-Strauss syndrome. Am J Ophthalmol. 1986;102(5):601–5.
124. Shintani S, Tsuruoka S, Yamada M. Churg-Strauss syndrome associated with third nerve palsy and mononeuritis multiplex of the legs. Clin Neurol Neurosurg. 1995;97(2):172–4.
125. Takanashi T, Uchida S, Arita M, Okada M, Kashii S. Orbital inflammatory pseudotumor and ischemic vasculitis in Churg-Strauss syndrome: report of two cases and review of the literature. Ophthalmology. 2001;108(6):1129–33.
126. Chumbley LC, Harrison EG Jr, DeRemee RA. Allergic granulomatosis and angiitis (Churg-Strauss syndrome). Report and analysis of 30 cases. Mayo Clin Proc. 1977;52(8):477–84.
127. Billing K, Malhotra R, Selva D, Dodd T. Orbital myositis in Churg-Strauss syndrome. Arch Ophthalmol. 2004;122(3):393–6.
128. Bosch-Gil JA, Falga-Tirado C, Simeon-Aznar CP, Orriols-Martinez R. Churg-Strauss syndrome with inflammatory orbital pseudotumour. Br J Rheumatol. 1995;34(5):485–6.
129. Fujii T, Norizuki M, Kobayashi T, Yamamoto M, Kishimoto M. A case of eosinophilic orbital myositis associated with CSS. Mod Rheumatol. 2010;20(2):196–9.
130. Heine A, Beck R, Stropahl G, Unger K, Guthoff R. Inflammatory pseudotumor of the anterior orbit. A symptom in allergic granulomatous angiitis (Churg-Strauss syndrome). Ophthalmologe. 1995;92(6):870–3.
131. McNab AA. Orbital inflammation in Churg-Strauss syndrome. Orbit. 1998;17(3):203–5.
132. Watanabe R, Ishii T, Harigae H. Churg-strauss syndrome with exophthalmos and orbital bone destruction. Intern Med. 2010;49(14):1463–4.
133. Khan NA, Shenoy PK, McClymont L, Palmer TJ. Exophthalmos and facial swelling: a case of limited Churg-Strauss syndrome. J Laryngol Otol. 1996;110(6):578–82.
134. Vaglio A, Martorana D, Maggiore U, et al. HLA-DRB4 as a genetic risk factor for Churg-Strauss syndrome. Arthritis Rheum. 2007;56(9):3159–66.
135. Grau RG. Churg-Strauss syndrome: 2005–2008 update. Curr Rheumatol Rep. 2008;10(6):453–8.
136. Polzer K, Karonitsch T, Neumann T, et al. Eotaxin-3 is involved in Churg-Strauss syndrome – a serum marker closely correlating with disease activity. Rheumatology (Oxford). 2008;47(6):804–8.
137. Serna-Candel C, Moreno-Perez O, Soriano V, Martinez A. Churg-Strauss syndrome triggered by hyposensitization to *Alternaria* fungus. Clin Rheumatol. 2007;26(12):2195–6.
138. Lane SE, Watts RA, Bentham G, Innes NJ, Scott DG. Are environmental factors important in primary systemic vasculitis? A case-control study. Arthritis Rheum. 2003;48(3):814–23.
139. Harrold LR, Patterson MK, Andrade SE, et al. Asthma drug use and the development of Churg-Strauss syndrome (CSS). Pharmacoepidemiol Drug Saf. 2007;16(6):620–6.
140. Sable-Fourtassou R, Cohen P, Mahr A, et al. Antineutrophil cytoplasmic antibodies and the Churg-Strauss syndrome. Ann Intern Med. 2005;143(9):632–8.
141. Churg J, Strauss L. Allergic granulomatosis, allergic angiitis, and periarteritis nodosa. Am J Pathol. 1951;27(2):277–301.
142. Weller PF, Plaut M, Taggart V, Trontell A. The relationship of asthma therapy and Churg-Strauss syndrome: NIH workshop summary report. J Allergy Clin Immunol. 2001;108(2):175–83.
143. Kubal AA, Perez VL. Ocular manifestations of ANCA-associated vasculitis. Rheum Dis Clin N Am. 2010;36(3):573–86.
144. Pagnoux C, Guillevin L. Churg-Strauss syndrome: evidence for disease subtypes? Curr Opin Rheumatol. 2010;22(1):21–8.
145. Cuchacovich R, Justiniano M, Espinoza LR. Churg-Strauss syndrome associated with leukotriene receptor antagonists (LTRA). Clin Rheumatol. 2007;26(10):1769–71.

146. Wells RS, Smith MA. The natural history of granuloma annulare. Br J Dermatol. 1963;75:199–205.
147. Weber AL, Romo LV, Sabates NR. Pseudotumor of the orbit. Clinical, pathologic, and radiologic evaluation. Radiol Clin N Am. 1999;37(1):151–68, xi
148. Weinstein GS, Dresner SC, Slamovits TL, Kennerdell JS. Acute and subacute orbital myositis. Am J Ophthalmol. 1983;96(2):209–17.
149. Belanger C, Zhang KS, Reddy AK, Yen MT, Yen KG. Inflammatory disorders of the orbit in childhood: a case series. Am J Ophthalmol. 2010;150(4):460–3.
150. Kitei D, DiMario FJ Jr. Childhood orbital pseudotumor: case report and literature review. J Child Neurol. 2008;23(4):425–30.
151. Ho VH, Chevez-Barrios P, Jorgensen JL, Silkiss RZ, Esmaeli B. Receptor expression in orbital inflammatory syndromes and implications for targeted therapy. Tissue Antigens. 2007;70(2):105–9.
152. Shields JA, Shields CL, Scartozzi R. Survey of 1264 patients with orbital tumors and simulating lesions: the 2002 montgomery lecture, part 1. Ophthalmology. 2004;111(5):997–1008.
153. Yuen SJ, Rubin PA. Idiopathic orbital inflammation: distribution, clinical features, and treatment outcome. Arch Ophthalmol. 2003;121(4):491–9.
154. Rubin PA, Foster CS. Etiology and management of idiopathic orbital inflammation. Am J Ophthalmol. 2004;138(6):1041–3.
155. Cruz AAV. Orbital inflammation and infection versus neoplasia. In: Karcioglu ZA, editor. Orbital tumors: diagnosis and treatment. New York: Springer; 2005. p. 441, xv.
156. Mottow LS, Jakobiec FA. Idiopathic inflammatory orbital pseudotumor in childhood. I. Clinical characteristics. Arch Ophthalmol. 1978;96(8):1410–7.
157. Purcell JJ Jr, Taulbee WA. Orbital myositis after upper respiratory tract infection. Arch Ophthalmol. 1981;99(3):437–8.
158. Mombaerts I, Goldschmeding R, Schlingemann RO, Koornneef L. What is orbital pseudotumor? Surv Ophthalmol. 1996;41(1):66–78.
159. Weinstein JM, Koch K, Lane S. Orbital pseudotumor in Crohn's colitis. Ann Ophthalmol. 1984;16(3):275–8.
160. Scott IU, Siatkowski RM. Idiopathic orbital myositis. Curr Opin Rheumatol. 1997;9(6):504–12.
161. Siatkowski RM, Capo H, Byrne SF, et al. Clinical and echographic findings in idiopathic orbital myositis. Am J Ophthalmol. 1994;118(3):343–50.
162. Berger JW, Rubin PA, Jakobiec FA. Pediatric orbital pseudotumor: case report and review of the literature. Int Ophthalmol Clin. 1996;36(1):161–77.
163. Cockerham KP, Hong SH, Browne EE. Orbital inflammation. Curr Neurol Neurosci Rep. 2003;3(5):401–9.
164. Weber AL, Jakobiec FA, Sabates NR. Pseudotumor of the orbit. Neuroimaging Clin N Am. 1996;6(1):73–92.
165. Rootman J. Inflammatory diseases. In: Rootman J, editor. Diseases of the orbit: a multidisciplinary approach. 2nd ed. Philadelphia: Lippincott Williams & Wilkins; 2003. p. 455–506.
166. De Wyngaert R, Casteels I, Demaerel P. Orbital and anterior visual pathway infection and inflammation. Neuroradiology. 2009;51(6):385–96.
167. Zborowska B, Ghabrial R, Selva D, McCluskey P. Idiopathic orbital inflammation with extraorbital extension: case series and review. Eye. 2006;20(1):107–13.
168. Tay E, Gibson A, Chaudhary N, Olver J. Idiopathic orbital inflammation with extensive intra- and extracranial extension presenting as 6th nerve palsy – a case report and literature review. Orbit. 2008;27(6):458–61.
169. de Jesus O, Inserni JA, Gonzalez A, Colon LE. Idiopathic orbital inflammation with intracranial extension. Case report. J Neurosurg. 1996;85(3):510–3.
170. Cruz AA, Akaishi PM, Chahud F, Elias JJ. Sclerosing inflammation in the orbit and in the pterygopalatine and infratemporal fossae. Ophthal Plast Reconstr Surg. 2003;19(3):201–6.
171. Kaye AH, Hahn JF, Craciun A, Hanson M, Berlin AJ, Tubbs RR. Intracranial extension of inflammatory pseudotumor of the orbit. Case report. J Neurosurg. 1984;60(3):625–9.
172. Bencherif B, Zouaoui A, Chedid G, Kujas M, Van Effenterre R, Marsault C. Intracranial extension of an idiopathic orbital inflammatory pseudotumor. AJNR Am J Neuroradiol. 1993;14(1):181–4.
173. Noble SC, Chandler WF, Lloyd RV. Intracranial extension of orbital pseudotumor: a case report. Neurosurgery. 1986;18(6):798–801.
174. Frohman LP, Kupersmith MJ, Lang J, et al. Intracranial extension and bone destruction in orbital pseudotumor. Arch Ophthalmol. 1986;104(3):380–4.
175. Swamy BN, McCluskey P, Nemet A, et al. Idiopathic orbital inflammatory syndrome: clinical features and treatment outcomes. Br J Ophthalmol. 2007;91(12):1667–70.
176. Mottow-Lippa L, Jakobiec FA, Smith M. Idiopathic inflammatory orbital pseudotumor in childhood. II. Results of diagnostic tests and biopsies. Ophthalmology. 1981;88(6):565–74.
177. Jakobiec FA, Mills MD, Hidayat AA, et al. Periocular xanthogranulomas associated with severe adult-onset asthma. Trans Am Ophthalmol Soc. 1993;91:99–125, discussion 125–9.
178. Hsuan JD, Selva D, McNab AA, Sullivan TJ, Saeed P, O'Donnell BA. Idiopathic sclerosing orbital inflammation. Arch Ophthalmol. 2006;124(9):1244–50.
179. Chen YM, Hu FR, Liao SL. Idiopathic sclerosing orbital inflammation – a case series study. Ophthalmologica. 2010;224(1):55–8.
180. Brannan PA. A review of sclerosing idiopathic orbital inflammation. Curr Opin Ophthalmol. 2007;18(5):402–4.
181. Sharma V, Martin P, Marjoniemi VM. Idiopathic orbital inflammation with sclerosing mesenteritis: a new association? Clin Exp Ophthalmol. 2006;34(2):190–2.
182. Levine MR, Kaye L, Mair S, Bates J. Multifocal fibrosclerosis. Report of a case of bilateral idiopathic sclerosing pseudotumor and retroperitoneal fibrosis. Arch Ophthalmol. 1993;111(6):841–3.
183. Jacobs D, Galetta S. Diagnosis and management of orbital pseudotumor. Curr Opin Ophthalmol. 2002;13(6):347–51.
184. Harris GJ. Idiopathic orbital inflammation: a pathogenetic construct and treatment strategy: the 2005 ASOPRS foundation lecture. Ophthal Plast Reconstr Surg. 2006;22(2):79–86.
185. Leibovitch I, Prabhakaran VC, Davis G, Selva D. Intraorbital injection of triamcinolone acetonide in patients with idiopathic orbital inflammation. Arch Ophthalmol. 2007;125(12):1647–51.
186. Skaat A, Rosen N, Rosner M, Schiby G, Simon GJ. Triamcinolone acetonide injection for persistent atypical idiopathic orbital inflammation. Orbit. 2009;28(6):401–3.
187. Orcutt JC, Garner A, Henk JM, Wright JE. Treatment of idiopathic inflammatory orbital pseudotumours by radiotherapy. Br J Ophthalmol. 1983;67(9):570–4.
188. Zacharopoulos IP, Papadaki T, Manor RS, Briscoe D. Treatment of idiopathic orbital inflammatory disease with cyclosporine-A: a case presentation. Semin Ophthalmol. 2009;24(6):260–1.
189. Osborne SF, Sims JL, Rosser PM. Short-term use of Infliximab in a case of recalcitrant idiopathic orbital inflammatory disease. Clin Exp Ophthalmol. 2009;37(9):897–900.
190. Smith JR, Rosenbaum JT. A role for methotrexate in the management of non-infectious orbital inflammatory disease. Br J Ophthalmol. 2001;85(10):1220–4.
191. Hatton MP, Rubin PA, Foster CS. Successful treatment of idiopathic orbital inflammation with mycophenolate mofetil. Am J Ophthalmol. 2005;140(5):916–8.
192. Eagle K, King A, Fisher C, Souhami R. Cyclophosphamide induced remission in relapsed, progressive idiopathic orbital inflammation ('Pseudotumour'). Clin Oncol (R Coll Radiol). 1995;7(6):402–4.

193. Shah SS, Lowder CY, Schmitt MA, Wilke WS, Kosmorsky GS, Meisler DM. Low-dose methotrexate therapy for ocular inflammatory disease. Ophthalmology. 1992;99(9):1419–23.
194. Diaz-Llopis M, Menezo JL. Idiopathic inflammatory orbital pseudotumor and low-dose cyclosporine. Am J Ophthalmol. 1989;107(5):547–8.
195. Sahlin S, Lignell B, Williams M, Dastmalchi M, Orrego A. Treatment of idiopathic sclerosing inflammation of the orbit (myositis) with infliximab. Acta Ophthalmol. 2009;87(8):906–8.
196. Schafranski MD. Idiopathic orbital inflammatory disease successfully treated with rituximab. Clin Rheumatol. 2009;28(2):225–6.
197. Garrity JA, Coleman AW, Matteson EL, Eggenberger ER, Waitzman DM. Treatment of recalcitrant idiopathic orbital inflammation (chronic orbital myositis) with infliximab. Am J Ophthalmol. 2004;138(6):925–30.
198. Wilson MW, Shergy WJ, Haik BG. Infliximab in the treatment of recalcitrant idiopathic orbital inflammation. Ophthal Plast Reconstr Surg. 2004;20(5):381–3.
199. Miquel T, Abad S, Badelon I, et al. Successful treatment of idiopathic orbital inflammation with infliximab: an alternative to conventional steroid-sparing agents. Ophthal Plast Reconstr Surg. 2008;24(5):415–7.
200. Sato Y, Ohshima K, Ichimura K, et al. Ocular adnexal IgG4-related disease has uniform clinicopathology. Pathol Int. 2008;58(8):465–70.
201. Mehta M, Jakobiec F, Fay A. Idiopathic fibroinflammatory disease of the face, eyelids, and periorbital membrane with immunoglobulin G4-positive plasma cells. Arch Pathol Lab Med. 2009;133(8):1251–5.
202. Lacey B, Chang W, Rootman J. Nonthyroid causes of extraocular muscle disease. Surv Ophthalmol. 1999;44(3):187–213.
203. Dresner SC, Rothfus WE, Slamovits TL, Kennerdell JS, Curtin HD. Computed tomography of orbital myositis. AJR Am J Roentgenol. 1984;143(3):671–4.
204. Mombaerts I, Koornneef L. Current status in the treatment of orbital myositis. Ophthalmology. 1997;104(3):402–8.
205. Selva D, Dolman PJ, Rootman J. Orbital granulomatous giant cell myositis: a case report and review. Clin Exp Ophthalmol. 2000;28(1):65–8.
206. Rothfus WE, Curtin HD. Extraocular muscle enlargement: a CT review. Radiology. 1984;151(3):677–81.
207. Slavin ML, Glaser JS. Idiopathic orbital myositis: report of six cases. Arch Ophthalmol. 1982;100(8):1261–5.
208. Cheng S, Vu P. Recurrent orbital myositis with radiological feature mimicking thyroid eye disease in a patient with Crohn's disease. Orbit. 2009;28(6):368–70.
209. Carvounis PE, Mehta AP, Geist CE. Orbital myositis associated with *Borrelia burgdorferi* (Lyme disease) infection. Ophthalmology. 2004;111(5):1023–8.
210. Cornblath WT, Elner V, Rolfe M. Extraocular muscle involvement in sarcoidosis. Ophthalmology. 1993;100(4):501–5.
211. Schoser BG. Ocular myositis: diagnostic assessment, differential diagnoses, and therapy of a rare muscle disease – five new cases and review. Clin Ophthalmol. 2007;1(1):37–42.
212. Nieto JC, Kim N, Lucarelli MJ. Dacryoadenitis and orbital myositis associated with lyme disease. Arch Ophthalmol. 2008;126(8):1165–6.
213. Pendse S, Bilyk JR, Lee MS. The ticking time bomb. Surv Ophthalmol. 2006;51(3):274–9.
214. Holak H, Holak N, Huzarska M, Holak S. Tick inoculation in an eyelid region: report on five cases with one complication of the orbital myositis associated with Lyme borreliosis. Klin Ocz. 2006;108(4–6):220–4.
215. Yanguela J, Sanchez-del-Rio M, Bueno A, et al. Primary trochlear headache: a new cephalgia generated and modulated on the trochlear region. Neurology. 2004;62(7):1134–40.
216. Tychsen L. Trochleitis and migraine headache. Neurology. 2003;61(3):425, author reply 425
217. Zaragoza-Casares P, Gomez-Fernandez T, Gomez de Liano MA, Zaragoza-Garcia P. Bilateral idiopathic trochleitis as a cause of frontal cephalgia. Headache. 2009;49(3):476–7.
218. Purvin V, Kawasaki A, Jacobson DM. Optic perineuritis: clinical and radiographic features. Arch Ophthalmol. 2001;119(9):1299–306.
219. Kennerdell JS, Dresner SC. The nonspecific orbital inflammatory syndromes. Surv Ophthalmol. 1984;29(2):93–103.
220. Fay AM, Kane SA, Kazim M, Millar WS, Odel JG. Magnetic resonance imaging of optic perineuritis. J Neuroophthalmol. 1997;17(4):247–9.
221. Lane SK, Gravel JW Jr. Clinical utility of common serum rheumatologic tests. Am Fam Physician. 2002;65(6):1073–81.
222. Wasmeier C, Pfadenhauer K, Rosler A. Idiopathic inflammatory pseudotumor of the orbit and Tolosa-Hunt syndrome – are they the same disease? J Neurol. 2002;249(9):1237–41.
223. O'Connor G, Hutchinson M. Tolosa-Hunt syndrome responsive to infliximab therapy. J Neurol. 2009;256(4):660–1.
224. Jain R, Sawhney S, Koul RL, Chand P. Tolosa-Hunt syndrome: MRI appearances. J Med Imaging Radiat Oncol. 2008;52(5):447–51.
225. Ladisch S. Langerhans cell histiocytosis. Curr Opin Hematol. 1998;5(1):54–8.
226. Harris GJ. Langerhans cell histiocytosis of the orbit: a need for interdisciplinary dialogue. Am J Ophthalmol. 2006;141(2):374–8.
227. Harris GJ, Woo KI. Is unifocal Langerhans-cell histiocytosis of the orbit a "CNS-Risk" lesion? Pediatr Blood Cancer. 2004;43(3):298–9, author reply 300–1.
228. Stalemark H, Laurencikas E, Karis J, Gavhed D, Fadeel B, Henter JI. Incidence of Langerhans cell histiocytosis in children: a population-based study. Pediatr Blood Cancer. 2008;51(1):76–81.
229. Maccheron LJ, McNab AA, Elder J, et al. Ocular adnexal Langerhans cell histiocytosis clinical features and management. Orbit. 2006;25(3):169–77.
230. Cochrane LA, Prince M, Clarke K. Langerhans' cell histiocytosis in the paediatric population: presentation and treatment of head and neck manifestations. J Otolaryngol. 2003;32(1):33–7.
231. Willman CL. Detection of clonal histiocytes in Langerhans cell histiocytosis: biology and clinical significance. Br J Cancer Suppl. 1994;23:S29–33.
232. da Costa CE, Szuhai K, van Eijk R, et al. No genomic aberrations in Langerhans cell histiocytosis as assessed by diverse molecular technologies. Genes Chromosomes Cancer. 2009;48(3):239–49.
233. Broadbent V, Gadner H. Current therapy for Langerhans cell histiocytosis. Hematol Oncol Clin North Am. 1998;12(2):327–38.
234. Grois N, Flucher-Wolfram B, Heitger A, Mostbeck GH, Hofmann J, Gadner H. Diabetes insipidus in Langerhans cell histiocytosis: results from the DAL-HX 83 study. Med Pediatr Oncol. 1995;24(4):248–56.
235. Haupt R, Nanduri V, Calevo MG, et al. Permanent consequences in Langerhans cell histiocytosis patients: a pilot study from the Histiocyte Society-Late Effects Study Group. Pediatr Blood Cancer. 2004;42(5):438–44.
236. Grois N, Potschger U, Prosch H, et al. Risk factors for diabetes insipidus in langerhans cell histiocytosis. Pediatr Blood Cancer. 2006;46(2):228–33.
237. Grois N, Prayer D, Prosch H, Minkov M, Potschger U, Gadner H. Course and clinical impact of magnetic resonance imaging findings in diabetes insipidus associated with Langerhans cell histiocytosis. Pediatr Blood Cancer. 2004;43(1):59–65.
238. Margo CE, Goldman DR. Langerhans cell histiocytosis. Surv Ophthalmol. 2008;53(4):332–58.
239. Broadbent V, Egeler RM, Nesbit ME Jr. Langerhans cell histiocytosis – clinical and epidemiological aspects. Br J Cancer Suppl. 1994;23:S11–6.

240. Favara BE, Jaffe R. The histopathology of Langerhans cell histiocytosis. Br J Cancer Suppl. 1994;23:S17–23.
241. Laman JD, Leenen PJ, Annels NE, Hogendoorn PC, Egeler RM. Langerhans-cell histiocytosis 'insight into DC biology'. Trends Immunol. 2003;24(4):190–6.
242. Mierau GW, Favara BE. S-100 protein immunohistochemistry and electron microscopy in the diagnosis of Langerhans cell proliferative disorders: a comparative assessment. Ultrastruct Pathol. 1986;10(4):303–9.
243. Jaffe R. The diagnostic histopathology of Langerhans cell histiocytosis. In: Weitzman S, Egeler RM, editors. Histiocytic disorders of children and adults. New York: Cambridge University Press; 2005. p. 14–39.
244. Harris GJ, Woo KI. Eosinophilic granuloma of the orbit: a paradox of aggressive destruction responsive to minimal intervention. Trans Am Ophthalmol Soc. 2003;101:93–103, 1discussion 103–5.
245. Abla O, Egeler RM, Weitzman S. Langerhans cell histiocytosis: current concepts and treatments. Cancer Treat Rev. 2010;36(4):354–9.
246. Guo J, Wang J. Adult orbital xanthogranulomatous disease: review of the literature. Arch Pathol Lab Med. 2009;133(12):1994–7.
247. Sivak-Callcott JA, Rootman J, Rasmussen SL, et al. Adult xanthogranulomatous disease of the orbit and ocular adnexa: new immunohistochemical findings and clinical review. Br J Ophthalmol. 2006;90(5):602–8.
248. Elner VM, Mintz R, Demirci H, Hassan AS. Local corticosteroid treatment of eyelid and orbital xanthogranuloma. Ophthal Plast Reconstr Surg. 2006;22(1):36–40.
249. Hammond MD, Niemi EW, Ward TP, Eiseman AS. Adult orbital xanthogranuloma with associated adult-onset asthma. Ophthal Plast Reconstr Surg. 2004;20(4):329–32.
250. Vick VL, Wilson MW, Fleming JC, Haik BG. Orbital and eyelid manifestations of xanthogranulomatous diseases. Orbit. 2006;25(3):221–5.
251. Lin B, Tan SH, Looi A. Angiolymphoid hyperplasia with eosinophilia of the eyelid with spontaneous regression. Ophthal Plast Reconstr Surg. 2008;24(4):308–10.
252. Thompson MJ, Whitehead J, Gunkel JL, Kulkarni AD. Angiolymphoid hyperplasia with eosinophilia affecting the eyelids. Arch Ophthalmol. 2007;125(7):987.
253. Cook HT, Stafford ND. Angiolymphoid hyperplasia with eosinophilia involving the lacrimal gland: case report. Br J Ophthalmol. 1988;72(9):710–2.
254. Kodama T, Kawamoto K. Kimura's disease of the lacrimal gland. Acta Ophthalmol Scand. 1998;76(3):374–7.
255. Kubo T, Hosokawa K, Kamiji T. Angiolymphoid hyperplasia with eosinophilia of the orbit. Ann Plast Surg. 2000;44(6):683–4.
256. Sanchez-Acosta A, Moreno-Arredondo D, Rubio-Solornio RI, Rodriguez-Martinez HA, Rodriguez-Reyes AA. Angiolymphoid hyperplasia with eosinophilia of the lacrimal gland: a case report. Orbit. 2008;27(3):195–8.
257. Smith DL, Kincaid MC, Nicolitz E. Angiolymphoid hyperplasia with eosinophilia (Kimura's disease) of the orbit. Arch Ophthalmol. 1988;106(6):793–5.
258. Brooks DR, Butnor KJ, Weinberg DA. Spontaneous orbital and periocular hemorrhage in a patient with epithelioid hemangioma. Ophthal Plast Reconstr Surg. 2006;22(6):487–9.
259. Hidayat AA, Cameron JD, Font RL, Zimmerman LE. Angiolymphoid hyperplasia with eosinophilia (Kimura's disease) of the orbit and ocular adnexa. Am J Ophthalmol. 1983;96(2):176–89.
260. Buggage RR, Spraul CW, Wojno TH, Grossniklaus HE. Kimura disease of the orbit and ocular adnexa. Surv Ophthalmol. 1999;44(1):79–91.
261. Esmaili DD, Chang EL, O'Hearn TM, Smith RE, Rao NA. Simultaneous presentation of Kimura disease and angiolymphoid hyperplasia with eosinophilia. Ophthal Plast Reconstr Surg. 2008;24(4):310–1.
262. Cockerham KP, Hidayat AA, Cockerham GC, et al. Melkersson-Rosenthal syndrome: new clinicopathologic findings in 4 cases. Arch Ophthalmol. 2000;118(2):227–32.
263. Fezza J, Chaudhry IA, Kwon YH, Grannum EE, Sinard J, Wolfley DE. Orbital melanoma presenting as orbital cellulitis: a clinicopathologic report. Ophthal Plast Reconstr Surg. 1998;14(4):286–9.
264. Blasi MA, Giammaria D, Balestrazzi E. Necrotic uveal melanoma with orbital inflammation. Eur J Ophthalmol. 2006;16(4):647–50.
265. Goh AS, Francis IC, Kappagoda MB, Filipic M. Orbital inflammation in a patient with extrascleral spread of choroidal malignant melanoma. Clin Exp Ophthalmol. 2001;29(2):97–9.
266. Rose GE, Hoh HB, Harrad RA, Hungerford JL. Intraocular malignant melanomas presenting with orbital inflammation. Eye. 1993;7(Pt 4):539–41.
267. Palamar M, Thangappan A, Shields CL, Ehya H, Shields JA. Necrotic choroidal melanoma with scleritis and choroidal effusion. Cornea. 2009;28(3):354–6.
268. Moshari A, Cheeseman EW, McLean IW. Totally necrotic choroidal and ciliary body melanomas: associations with prognosis, episcleritis, and scleritis. Am J Ophthalmol. 2001;131(2):232–6.
269. Fraser DJ Jr, Font RL. Ocular inflammation and hemorrhage as initial manifestations of uveal malignant melanoma. Incidence and prognosis. Arch Ophthalmol. 1979;97(7):1311–4.
270. Bujara K. Necrotic malignant melanomas of the choroid and ciliary body. A clinicopathological and statistical study. Graefes Arch Clin Exp Ophthalmol. 1982;219(1):40–3.
271. Haik BG, Dunleavy SA, Cooke C, et al. Retinoblastoma with anterior chamber extension. Ophthalmology. 1987;94(4):367–70.

Ocular Adnexal Lymphoproliferative Disease

50

Jurij R. Bilyk and Ann P. Murchison

Introduction

Ocular adnexal lymphoproliferative disease (OALD) represents a variably defined amalgam of pathology that affects the tissues surrounding the eye: the orbit, eyelids, conjunctiva, and lacrimal apparatus. It occurs with such regular frequency in the general population that it is a relatively routine diagnosis for the orbital specialist. Despite this ubiquity, OALD remains a clinical conundrum because of an ever-evolving compendium of classification (immunohistochemical, cytogenetic) and management options. In this chapter, we will concentrate on orbital presentations, which constitute 50–60% of all OALD [1, 2]. Other ocular adnexal sites are covered in detail in Chap. 25.

Recent advances in clinical, histopathologic, and cytogenetic diagnosis have greatly improved the understanding and, hopefully, the management and prognosis of OALD. One of the frustrating features of OALD in the past has been a lack of consensus regarding a consistent classification schema. Prior to the World Health Organization's (WHO) reclassification, OALD was an outlier in a histopathologic order ruled by the Rappaport classification; purely extranodal disease, including OALD, was in essence given a second-class status and forced to align itself, with questionable validity, to existing subtypes of the Rappaport system, which relied exclusively on tumor morphology. The Revised European-American Lymphoma (REAL) classification attempted to define extranodal disease and the mucosa-associated lymphoid tissue (MALT) subtype, and the subsequent introduction of the WHO modifications of REAL brought a welcome and much needed regimentation to extranodal lesions (Table 50.1) [3, 4].

Table 50.1 Classification schema for non-Hodgkin lymphoma

Classification	Year	Basis of diagnosis	Treatment
Rappaport	1970s	Morphology	Uniform across most types
Working Formulation (NIH)	1982	Morphology +/− immunohistochemistry	Uniform across most types
Revised European American Lymphoma (REAL)	1994	Immunohistochemistry +/− cytogenetics	Relatively uniform, classified extranodal sites
World Health Organization (WHO)	2001, 2008, 2016	Cytogenetics	Tailored to type, stage, and known response

Definitions

In general, OALD can be divided into two utilitarian, but oversimplified, categories: a polyclonal, T-cell-rich lymphoid hyperplasia and a monoclonal proliferation (lymphoma), which in the vast majority of cases is of B-cell origin [1, 2]. As an aside, it is possible, especially in this age of PCR amplification techniques, to manifest a clonal population of circulating B cells with no evidence of malignant behavior. In other words, all lymphomas are monoclonal populations, but not all monoclonal populations are lymphomas. Counterintuitively, it is also possible for lymphoma, by definition a malignancy, to be self-limiting and depend on persistent antigenic stimulation for proliferation. These issues are discussed in more detail later in this chapter.

Monoclonal B-cell proliferations can be categorized as either Hodgkin (HL) or non-Hodgkin (NHL) lymphoma. However, it is incorrect to ascribe a sharp delineation

J. R. Bilyk
Attending Surgeon and Professor of Ophthalmology, Oculoplastic and Orbital Surgery Service, Wills Eye Hospital and Thomas Jefferson University Hospital, Philadelphia, PA, USA

A. P. Murchison (✉)
Department of Ophthalmology, Oculoplastic and Orbital Surgery Service and Eye Emergency Room, Wills Eye Hospital and Thomas Jefferson University Hospital, Philadelphia, PA, USA
e-mail: amuchison@willseye.org

J. J. Servat et al. (eds.), *Smith and Nesi's Ophthalmic Plastic and Reconstructive Surgery*,
https://doi.org/10.1007/978-3-030-41720-8_50

between polyclonal lymphoid hyperplasia and monoclonal lymphoma when discussing OALD. A more reasonable approach is to consider these entities as an evolution of disease, ranging from a purely localized and fleeting reactive process in the native lymphocytic population of the conjunctiva through a developing phase of oligoclonality with potential monoclonal transformation into frank lymphoma. Furthermore, relatively indolent subtypes of NHL may transform over time into more aggressive NHL and vice versa [5–7].

It is also important to stress at this juncture that idiopathic orbital inflammatory syndrome (IOIS), previously called inflammatory orbital pseudotumor, is most definitely not part of the spectrum of OALD, and never progresses to monoclonal lesions. This of course assumes that suspected IOIS was correctly diagnosed initially and was not in fact polyclonal OALD that then progressed to lymphoma [8]. Histopathologically, IOIS is described in a somewhat nonspecific fashion as polymorphic, nongranulomatous, and paucicellular but distinctly lacks the dense lymphocytic infiltration typical in OALD and remains a diagnosis of exclusion [8–10].

With regard to lymphoid hyperplasia, one other point of contention needs to be clarified: the use of additional descriptors, which in many cases are misleading, may lull both the clinician and patient into a false sense of security. "Atypical lymphoid hyperplasia," or "pseudolymphoma," is an antiquated term used to describe potentially premalignant or low-grade malignant features seen on light microscopy. The widespread availability and increased diagnostic accuracy of immunohistochemical and cytogenetic markers coupled with specific categorization within the REAL classification and WHO modifications have essentially supplanted this terminology, subsuming most "atypical lymphoid hyperplasia" into the category of extranodal marginal zone lymphoma of mucosa-associated lymphoid tissue (EMZL/MALT) (see below) [11, 12]. As already mentioned, the term "reactive lymphoid hyperplasia" is sometimes used to describe polyclonal OALD with distinct secondary follicle formation. Jakobiec prudently recommends that such terminology, if it is used at all, be limited exclusively to conjunctival lesions, since this adnexal tissue supports a standing population of lymphocytes [11]. However, the term "reactive" should be avoided for other adnexa, including the orbit, which, with the exception of a few scattered lymphocytes in the lacrimal gland [13], does not harbor significant native lymphocytic collections. Similarly, the term "benign lymphoid hyperplasia" is a misnomer, since polyclonal lymphoid transformation into monoclonal lymphoma is not an infrequent occurrence.

Reactive lymphoid hyperplasia also connotes a propensity for spontaneous remission, assuming that the inciting factor is neutralized. On the other hand, ocular adnexal lymphoma (OAL), and presumably an unknown proportion of lymphoid hyperplasia, is in all likelihood autonomous and self-sustaining [11, 14].

In this chapter, we will limit our broad OALD rubrics to two terms: lymphoid hyperplasia and lymphoma. Lymphoma will also be subdivided into two additional categories: primary, defined as lymphoma occurring initially and exclusively in the ocular adnexa, and secondary, defined as spreading to the ocular adnexa from another anatomic site. As we will discuss in more depth later, defining OAL as primary or secondary has its own pitfalls [1, 2, 12].

Finally, OAL is not associated with intraocular, vitreoretinal (large B cell) lymphoma, which is best considered either a harbinger or subset of primary central nervous system lymphoma [11, 15].

Epidemiology

The incidence of NHL is 72,000 cases per year in the United States, resulting in 20,000 disease-specific deaths annually [16]. Overall there has been a 3–4% increase in the incidence of lymphoma, with a doubling noted over the past 20 years [17–22]. The cause for this increased incidence is in all likelihood multifactorial, including changes in classification, earlier diagnosis, more accurate diagnosis, and better reporting. However, a change in risk factors is also contributory, including an increased incidence and survival in AIDS, higher incidence of chronic immunosuppressive medical therapy (e.g., organ transplantation, autoimmune disease, cancer therapy), improved life span, and less proven phenomena such as chronic antigen stimulation and environmental factors [23–27]. Furthermore, there are large, unexplained geographic (and possibly genetic) disparities in the incidence of NHL, ranging from 20–26/100,000 in the United States, Europe, and Australia to only 1.2/100,000 in China [28, 29]. NHL subtypes also vary geographically. As an example, follicular lymphoma (FL) as a percentage of all NHL is more common in the United States and Western Europe than in the rest of the world, while Burkitt lymphoma (BL) is endemic in equatorial Africa [29].

OAL, as a subset of extranodal disease, has been increasing at an even greater rate of 6.3% per year [21, 22, 30] and occurs in approximately 5% of systemic NHL [31]. By contrast, only 0.24% of over 1200 autopsied cases of systemic lymphoma initially presented with OAL, with adnexal involvement increasing to 1.3% by the time of death [32]. The validity of these numbers is less germane at present, since many of the classifications are based on outmoded schema.

OAL accounts for about 10% of all adult orbital neoplasia [11, 33]. The vast majority (98%) of OAL is of B-cell origin [1, 2]. Overall, OAL and orbital lymphoma have a largely equal distribution by sex. By subtype, EMZL/MALT and FL appear to have fairly equal prevalence by sex [34], with some studies showing slight female predominance [1, 2, 12, 35–37], and are most commonly found in older adults [12, 38, 39]. Ocular adnexal mantle cell lymphoma (MCL) has a definite male predonance [1, 2] and also occurs about a decade later than more indolent OAL (e.g., EMZL/MALT, FL). Autoimmune disease is associated with a higher incidence of EMZL/MALT [1, 2, 12, 29, 40], presumably from the evolution of monoclonal B-cell populations from chronic immune stimulation. Similarly, chronic immunosuppression increases the likelihood of OAL, which in some cases can behave aggressively, as typified by the sinoorbital lymphoma seen in HIV/AIDS or after organ transplantation [29]. Of note, with the exception of BL in equatorial Africa, OAL is distinctly rare in the pediatric population, especially when compared to adnexal leukemic infiltrations [11, 35].

Pathogenesis

The pathogenesis of B-cell lymphoma is complex and beyond the scope of this chapter, but several principles are worth reviewing [29]. The innate immune response is managed primarily by T and natural killer (NK) cells, resulting a nonspecific, primitive "first line of defense." Conversely, the adaptive immune response is far more complex, requiring an interaction between T and B cells, resulting in two critical phenomena: specificity and memory [29].

The normal B-cell immune response can be considered as a type of "controlled cancer" – an oligoclonal, self-limiting response to antigen that is occurring constantly. More specifically, the usual background mutation rate in humans is approximately 1 in 10^6 cell divisions. However, during the normal somatic hypermutation that occurs with B-cell clonal expansion in response to antigen, this mutation rate drastically increases to 1:1600 cell divisions. Furthermore, both chronic immune stimulation (e.g., autoimmune disease) and chronic immunosuppression predispose to lymphoma formation. Why then don't all humans develop lymphoma? On a basic level, the answer is that in a normal immune response, clonal proliferation is controlled through a complex system of checks that leads to apoptosis of the vast majority of proliferating clones, allowing for the survival of a handful of clones that produce specific antibody against specific antigen (Fig. 50.1). Specific lymphoma subtypes occur at any phase of B-cell proliferation if a genetic aberration manifests [29], which then allows for uncontrolled clonal proliferation secondary to an oncogene, a suppression of normal apoptosis via a tumor suppressor gene, or both. Specific genetic footprints have been identified for various OAL subtypes, but they are by no means universal [4, 5, 41, 42].

As a general rule, the clinical behavior of lymphoma mirrors that of its B-cell precursor: a naïve B cell will give rise to an aggressive lymphoma (e.g., MCL), whereas more somnolent B cells lead to indolent lymphomas (e.g., EMZL/MALT) (Fig. 50.1). Most subtypes of NHL likely arise from the germinal center [43]. As noted by Coupland, with the exception of MCL and lymphoblastic lymphoma, all NHL either arise from the germinal center or from cells that have arisen from the germinal center (Fig. 50.1) [5]. However, Jaffe et al. stress that "the normal counterpart of the neoplastic cell cannot at this time be the sole basis of the classification" [29].

Normal B-cell maturation can be divided into three simplified stages [15, 44]. In stage I, B cells initially arise from stem cells as progenitor B cells (B-lymphoblasts) and are not affected by foreign antigen. In stage III, fully differentiated plasma cells are the end-product of maturation. In between stages I and III exists a complex, intermediate stage II of foreign antigen exposure and subsequent B-cell development and differentiation which has the potential for lymphoma formation (Fig. 50.1). Naïve B cells (CD5+) occupy the lymph follicle's mantle zone and circulate in peripheral blood. When stimulated, they either transform directly into antibody-secreting short-lived plasma cells or migrate to the germinal center and develop into centroblasts with rapid proliferation. Centroblasts move from the dark zone of the germinal center into the light zone and evolve into centrocytes [5, 29, 43]. Each centrocyte is then re-challenged by antigen. The vast majority of centrocytes that harbor a "low affinity" to the antigen undergo apoptosis. The small minority of centrocytes deemed "high affinity" can revert back into centroblasts or migrate either to the marginal zone as memory B cells or home to the bone marrow as plasma cells. Note that BCL6 is critical in normal functioning of the germinal center – it is first upregulated in the centroblast to facilitate, among other things, somatic hypermutation, and then downregulated to allow centrocyte differentiation into plasma cells, stop proliferation, and restore the DNA-damage response [5].

A critical feature in immune activation is the nuclear factor kappa-light-chain-enhancer of B-cell (NF-κB) pathway (Fig. 50.1). NF-κB is activated by antigenic stimulation through a variety of specific methods and then proceeds to unleash more than 200 genes involved in cellular activation and proliferation [40]. During a normal immune response, NF-κB pathway activation is transient and self-limiting. Transformation into NHL requires additional genetic aberrations. As an example, ocular adnexal EMZL/MALT may harbor translocations that inactivate *A20*, a kind of "molecular brake" of the NF-κB pathway [40]; inactivation of *A20* disinhibits NF-κB, allowing it to function unchecked. *A20* inactivation is also linked to a variety of autoimmune disorders (e.g., rheumatoid arthritis), which are known to have an increased risk of NHL development (see below) [40]. It

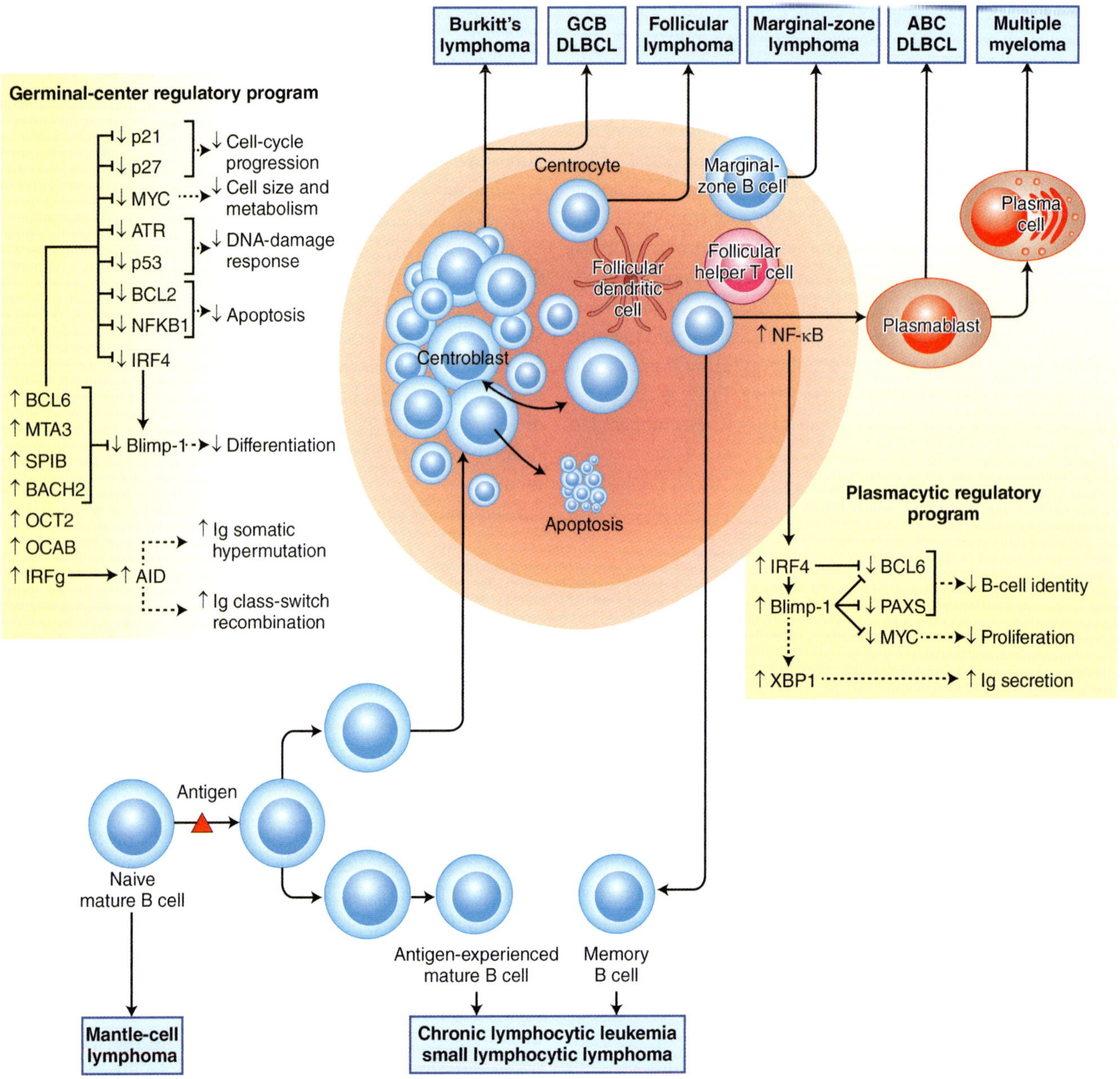

Fig. 50.1 Schematic of the normal B-cell immune response and lymphomagenesis. A naïve B cell is stimulated by a T-cell-dependent antigen, initiating a normal immune response in the germinal center, which is regulated by multiple factors listed in the left box insert (down arrows denote inhibition, whereas up arrows denote upregulation of each specific response). The germinal center response results in heavy chain class switching and somatic hypermutation, resulting in a marked proliferation of centroblasts, most of which undergo apoptosis. The occasional centroblast avoids apoptosis by specific stimulation by antigen on follicular dendritic cells and then reverts back to a centroblast. This allows for the formation of B-cell oligoclones against specific antigen, which can then transform into antibody-secreting plasma cells (regulated by factors in the right box insert) or memory B cells. The specific NHL subtypes arising from B-cell subtypes are also shown. Note that two subtypes of DLBCL arise from different stages of the B-cell immune response. The genetic abnormalities found in NHL combine to promote cell growth and avoid apoptosis. (From Ref. [43])

appears that *A20* inactivation alone will not result in EMZL/MALT formation – additional genetic aberrations and antigenic stimulation are necessary; in other words, EMZL/MALT development may require *both* genetic aberration and surface receptor signaling from chronic immunologic stimulation to flourish (see below).

The activity within the germinal center can be divided into two major fronts: (1) class-switch recombination, in which heavy chain immunoglobulin is converted from IgD and IgM to IgG, IgA or IgE, and (2) somatic hypermutation, wherein mutations occur within the B cell to either increase or decrease the cell's affinity for a particular antigen [5, 43].

This normal, but dramatic, increase in mutation rate in an effort to efficiently deal with a presenting antigen may also give rise to lymphoma.

Once transformation into an autonomous monoclonal population has occurred, the malignant B cells home to specific anatomic sites, mediated by adhesion molecules [45, 46]. The homing mechanism of ocular adnexal EMZL/MALT is as yet not fully understood. As already noted, the conjunctiva contains a well-described native population of lymphocytes secreting immunoglobulin A consistent with mucosa-associated lymphoid tissue (MALT), collectively known as the conjunctiva-associated lymphoid tissue (CALT) [47]. IgA-secreting lymphocytes are also present in the main and accessory lacrimal glands as well as the lacrimal drainage apparatus (lacrimal drainage-associated lymphoid tissue or LDALT) [11, 48]. It is therefore not surprising that ocular adnexal EMZL/MALT occurs with regularity in these structures. However, EMZL/MALT is also found within deeper orbital structures, where no clearly defined lymphocytic population or lymphatic drainage exists. To date, only rudimentary lymphatic channels have been described around the optic nerve and possibly within the intraconal space [49, 50]. The homing mechanisms of non-MALT-related lymphoma to the ocular adnexa remain unclear.

Another fascinating feature of ophthalmic lymphoma is that NHL subtypes tend to prefer certain locations (Fig. 50.2) [6, 42, 51–53]. As example, intravitreal and retinal lesions are typically diffuse large B-cell lymphoma (DLBCL) and behave aggressively, with a significant propensity for simultaneous or subsequent central nervous system involvement [5]. The most common type of ocular adnexal (including the lacrimal gland) is EMZL/MALT; EMZL/MALT is also the most common NHL subtype to affect the choroid (uvea) [5]. However, the lacrimal drainage apparatus seems to harbor NHL that follows the pattern seen in sinonasal lesions – a significant proportion are DLBCLs. This discrepancy has led some authors to distinguish the lacrimal drainage apparatus as a separate entity – the so-called lacrimal drainage-associated lymphoid tissue [48].

The Role of Chronic Immune Stimulation: In Situ Evolution of Lymphoma

Chronic antigenic stimulation from infection or inflammation is postulated to play an important role in the pathogenesis of OAL. The normal lymphocyte environment consists of a fragile détente between T-helper and T-suppressor cells, keeping a potentially volatile B-cell population in check (Fig. 50.3). An antigenic stimulus, especially if chronic, can tilt the balance, causing a preponderance of T-helper cells at the expense of the T-suppressor cells. This leads to the aforementioned somatic hypermutation and frenzied B-cell proliferation, which is maintained by the chronic immune stimulus and in the early stages remains polyclonal (lymphoid hyperplasia). Over time, oligoclones evolve secondary to chromosomal translocations, deletions, and other mutations, which in turn are eventually overwhelmed by a monoclone. This monoclonal proliferation is defined as lymphoma.

The role of infectious agents in chronic antigenic stimulation is discussed below. The role of autoimmune disease in the development of NHL and more specifically lymphoma has been widely reported in the literature. There is an increased risk of developing NHL (especially EMZL) in patients with rheumatoid arthritis, Hashimoto thyroiditis, and systemic lupus erythematosus, among others [54–56]. Autoimmune thyroiditis (Hashimoto disease) appears to predispose for thyroid gland lymphoma, since virtually all such malignancies (especially EMZL) arise in the setting of previous thyroid inflammation [57]. Systemic lupus erythematosus is also associated with higher NHL risk [55, 58]. The association of lymphoma with other rheumatitides (psoriasis, celiac disease, sarcoidosis, etc.) is more controversial [59–61]. There is now a consensus that patients with rheumatoid arthritis have an increased lifetime risk of developing lymphoma when compared to the general population, and this risk is directly related to disease activity [40, 58, 61].

For OAL, the best evidence for this association exists in patients with Sjögren syndrome, who are at 6.5–44 times greater risk for developing NHL when compared to a control population, and a 1000 times greater risk of developing

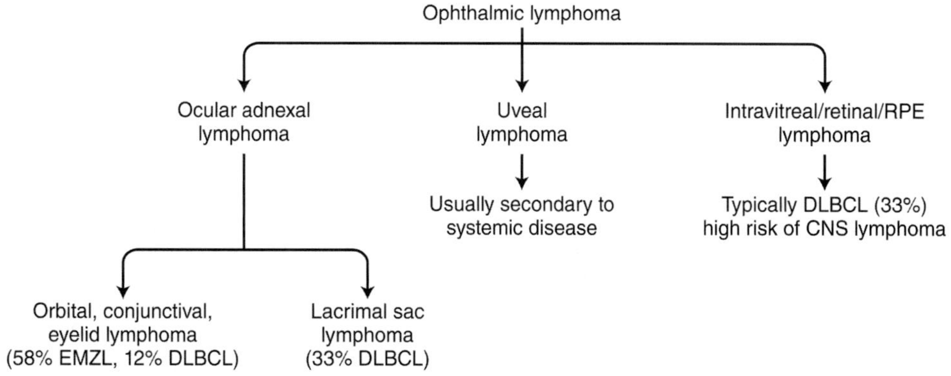

Fig. 50.2 Subtypes of ophthalmic lymphoma. (From Ref. [42])

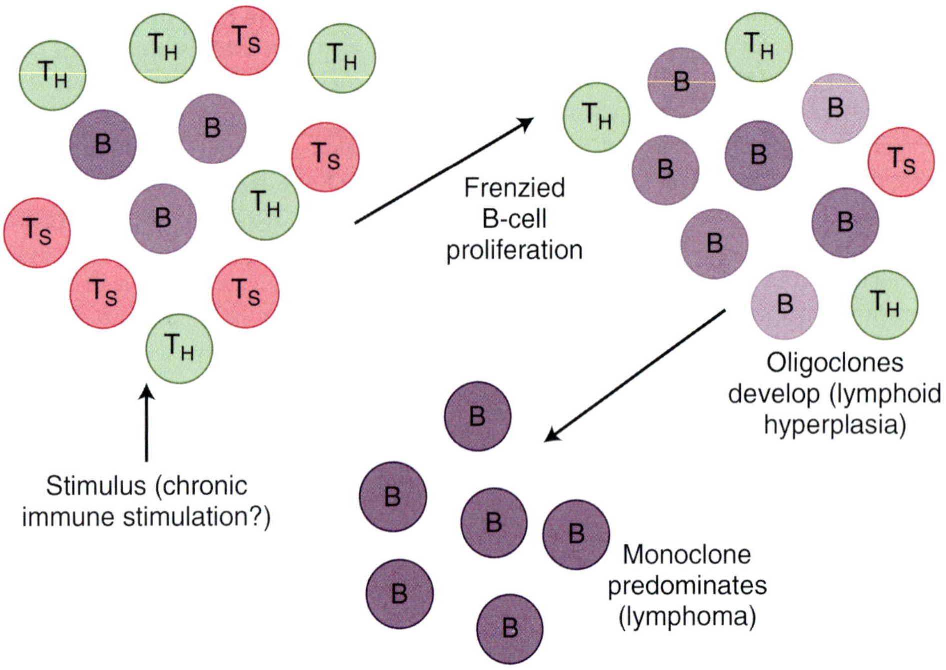

Fig. 50.3 A simplified description of in situ evolution of OAL. A chronic antigenic stimulus shifts the balance of T cells toward a preponderance of helper cells, which in turn cause a polyclonal proliferation of B cells. Over time, B-cell oligoclones form, and, with persistent proliferation, an eventual autonomous and self-sustaining B-cell monoclonality develops

parotid gland EMZL/MALT [25, 59, 62, 63]. Multiple case reports have shown that East Asian patients with IgG4-related orbitopathy may have transformation of their inflammation into EMZL/MALT [64, 65]. One study from the United Kingdom found that patients with OAL had a higher incidence of thyroid eye disease than the overall prevalence of the OAL in the general population [66].

The Role of Immunosuppression

Chronic immunosuppression has long been known to be a risk factor for the development of a variety of malignancies, including lymphoma. This phenomenon was brought to the fore in the 1980s in conjunction with the rise of HIV/AIDS [67]. Chronic immunosuppression results in an increase in NHL (especially DLBCL) for a variety of reasons, including a higher prevalence of EBV which may become activated; decreased immune surveillance of gene mutation and rearrangement due to a breakdown in immune regulation; and effects of other viral pathogens (e.g., HIV, cytomegalovirus, human herpesvirus-8 in conjunctival Kaposi sarcoma) [24, 68, 69]. In addition, when lymphoma manifests in chronic immunosuppression, it tends to behave aggressively, with atypical features both clinically and radiographically.

Chronic immunosuppression can also result in poorly understood lymphoproliferative diseases from iatrogenically induced immunosuppression. Long-term use of methotrexate (MTX) therapy for rheumatoid arthritis appears to result in lymphoproliferative disorders (MTX-LPD), including DLBCL in about 50% of all cases [60]; EBV may play a role in the development of MTX-LPD [58]. Withdrawal of methotrexate may lead to spontaneous resolution of the lymphoproliferative disease [58, 70]. Of note, the role of MTX in MTX-LPD still remains debatable: patients on MTX therapy in all likelihood have a higher disease activity of their rheumatoid arthritis (or other autoimmune disease) and may therefore be at higher risk for developing lymphoproliferative disease; MTX may simply be an epiphenomenon or may indeed play a primary role [58].

Post-transplant lymphoproliferative disorder (*PTLD*), also known as EBV-associated lymphoproliferative disease, is a rare but well-recognized lymphoma associated with the severe immunosuppression seen in transplant recipients [71]. It is especially problematic in allogenic hematopoietic stem cell transplants, with an incidence of 0.45–29%; PTLD occurs in 1–15% of solid organ transplants [72]. Normal immune surveillance typically keeps EBV proliferation in check within a small population of memory B cells. With immunosuppression, EBV proliferation increases, with expression of a variety of latent viral genes, known as the growth program. Activated B cells proliferate into virus-laden memory B cells, which may still be held in check by cytotoxic T cells. If the T cells are also depleted by medications to control graft-versus-host disease, memory B cells proliferate and undergo further genetic transformation, leading to polyclonal, oligoclonal, or monoclonal proliferation.

PTLD may present across a broad spectrum both histopathologically (ranging from plasmocytic hyperplasia to aggressive lymphoma) and clinically (indolent, localized disease to fulminant, disseminated involvement) [72]. Primary EBV infection during transplantation appears to

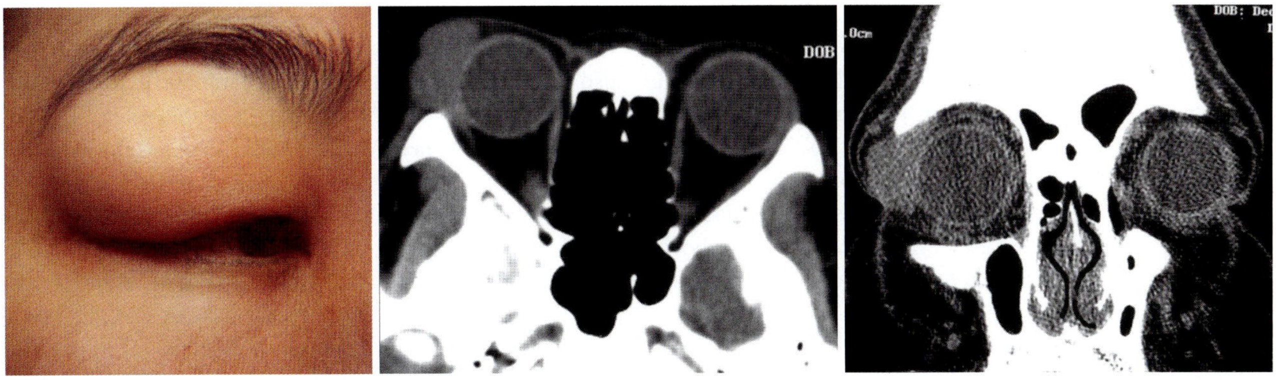

Fig. 50.4 PTLD. Left. A 45-year-old woman presented with progressive painless swelling over a 6-month duration. She had undergone renal transplantation 17 years prior and was on chronic immunosuppressive therapy. Left, external appearance. Center and right, CT soft tissue windows (axial and coronal), of right lacrimal gland infiltration. Excisional biopsy revealed DLBCL with positive EBV in situ hybridization, consistent with PTLD. (Courtesy of Mary A. Stefanyszyn, MD)

predispose to a more aggressive disease [73]. Early diagnosis is critical, as PTLD may in some cases progress rapidly with high mortality (over 80% in some series) [72]. The highest incidence of PTLD occurs during the first 6 months following transplantations but may manifest up to 10 years later. Monitoring of EBV DNA levels for at least 180 days following transplant procedures is now routine in the post-transplant setting, and treatment is either instituted "preemptively" if a critical EBV DNA is reached or "promptly" if a specific EBV DNA level is associated with signs and symptoms of PTLD. Both approaches have markedly reduced PTLD mortality. Treatment has also been improved significantly by chimeric anti-CD20 antibody therapy (rituximab), along with reduction of immunosuppressive regimens, cytotoxic T-cell therapy, chemotherapy, and antiviral agents [72].

Ocular adnexal involvement by PTLD is rare, with fewer than five cases of orbital involvement reported in the literature (Fig. 50.4). In one series of three cases of orbital involvement by Douglas et al. [73], two cases of PTLD presented initially with isolated orbital involvement, while in the third case, orbital and systemic signs occurred simultaneously.

The Role of Infectious Organisms/Chronic Antigenic Stimulation

The issue of chronic antigenic stimulation as well as the role of infectious organisms in systemic malignancies (e.g., human papillomavirus and cervical cancer) has renewed interest in a possible infectious etiology in OAL. The proven role of chronic *Helicobacter pylori* infection in the development of gastric MALToma and the occurrence of EMZL/MALT in the ocular adnexa have initiated an extensive, and sometimes speculative, search of a causative organism in the hopes of a potential antibiotic or antiviral therapy in OALD and OAL. Multiple studies on a variety of possible culprits, including *H. pylori*, *Chlamydia psittaci*, *C. pneumoniae*, *Campylobacter jejuni*, and hepatitis C, have been published [56], sparking heated discussion and much debate.

With the exception of the definitive role of EBV in endemic Burkitt lymphoma (eBL), by far the most impressive and conclusive link between an infectious agent and NHL is certainly the role of *H. pylori* in the development of gastric EMZL/MALT, occurring putatively in about 90% of cases [74–76]. Presumably, chronic antigenic stimulation sustains a reactive lymphoproliferative response that eventually transforms into a monoclonal population. Astoundingly, eradication of the *H. pylori* infection with triple antibiotic therapy will result in complete regression of stage I gastric lymphoma in up to 80% of cases, despite the belief that lymphoma is a self-sustaining and autonomous process [56, 77, 78]. Research has shown that the antigenic stimulation by *H. pylori* infection initially results in a polyclonal response [56]. At some point thereafter, p15 and p16 hypermethylation results in the development of an antigen-specific clone; of note, at this stage, the monoclonal population is still antigen-dependent – if the *H. pylori* infection is cured with antibiotics, the lymphoma resolves. However, with persistent infection additional genetic aberrations (t(11;18), t(1;14), and t(3;14) translocations) occur, resulting in an antigen-independent lymphoma that no longer responds to antibiotic eradication of *H. pylori* [56].

The possible link between *H. pylori* and ocular adnexal (OA) EMZL/MALT was initially inferred because of the shared histopathologic features of EMZL/MALT in the two anatomic sites. It is noteworthy that many antigen-driven (e.g., chronic infection) NHLs occur extranodally and behave indolently [56]. While *H. pylori* is a common infection, occurring in up to 70–90% of the population in developing countries and 25–50% in developed countries [79], there are surprisingly few studies looking at the role of this Gram-negative bacteria in conjunctival EMZL. Only one study reported any evidence of *H. pylori* DNA by polymerase chain reaction (PCR) in conjunctival EMZL/MALT [80]. Two other series, from Denmark [81] and Germany [82], revealed no evidence of *H. pylori*. While these contradictory results may be due to geographic variation of the organism, definitive data to confirm this supposition is lacking. Additionally, while early gastric MALToma has been shown to regress with eradication of *H. pylori* in up to 80% of cases [83], this has not been seen in OAL [84]. Ferreri and co-workers showed no response in treating OAL with anti-*H. pylori* regimens, except for those receiving other concurrent therapies (orbital radiation, doxycycline, or rituximab); conjunctival lesions had no measurable regression [85]. Interestingly, several of the patients with OAL were not only positive for gastric *H. pylori* but also had *C. psittaci*-positive lesions. It is important to remember that despite histopathologic and immunohistochemical similarities of EMZL/MALT from various anatomic locations, the molecular genetic footprint varies significantly depending on the site of origin [5], suggesting that EMZL/MALT may be a manifestation of a single common pathway from varying antigenic stimuli and genetic aberrations that typically regulate NF-κB, a mediator of B-cell activation and immune response regulation [56]. As already noted, in OA EMZL/MALT, the genetic abnormality typically inactivates the *A20* gene, a global inhibitor of NF-κB pathway [5]. The presence of *A20* inactivation is important prognostically for EMZL/MALT [86].

The classic ocular involvement by *Chlamydia* sp. is ocular anterior segment inflammation from *C. trachomatis*; however, all *Chlamydia* sp. tend to cause persistent infections that may be a factor in oncogenesis. *Chlamydia psittaci*, best known to cause the systemic infection psittacosis from exposure to infected birds, has also potentially been associated with OALD. Ferreri and colleagues demonstrated *C. psittaci* DNA in lymphomatous tissue, in peripheral blood, and in reactive lymphadenopathy samples of patients with OA EMZL/MALT, while none of the control groups were positive for the organism. The samples were also negative for *C. pneumoniae* and *C. trachomatis* infections. This data suggested that persistent *C. psittaci* infection in these patients could be related to chronic antigenic stimulation and the oncogenesis of OAL. However, many other studies from a variety of locations have failed to confirm the findings of Ferreri and colleagues [82, 87–92]. This conflicting data suggested, among other factors, a possible geographic variation in *C. psittaci*. Chanudet and colleagues [93] evaluated OA EMZL/MALT from six geographic regions for evidence of *C. psittaci*. The prevalence of *C. psittaci* varied significantly by region but was significantly higher in patients with EMZL than in controls. However, *C. psittaci* was also found in other lymphoma subtypes (non-marginal zone) and non-lymphoproliferative orbital disease. Furthermore, *C. pneumoniae* DNA was also found in 13% of OA EMZL/MALT. The role of infectious agents in periocular EMZL has also been examined in studies using antibiotic treatment with varied results [94–98]. Although the possible role of *C. psittaci* in the pathogenesis of OA EMZL/MALT is intriguing, it is to date inconclusive and may be geographically driven.

Chlamydia pneumoniae, a widespread pathogen, is associated with lung cancer and cutaneous T-cell lymphoma in chronic infections [99–101]. In 2006 the first reported possible association of *C. pneumoniae* and OA EMZL/MALT was published [102]. Other positive associations have since been reported in several countries, both with *C. pneumoniae* in isolation and with *C. psittaci* involvement. However, studies conducted by Ferreri failed to document *C. pneumoniae* evidence, again suggesting a possible geographic variation in the infectious organism [5, 103].

The common pathogenic mechanism of infectious agents providing chronic antigenic stimulation, which in turn promotes clonal B-cell expansion, is also seen with *Campylobacter jejuni*. This infectious agent is known to play a role in small intestine lymphoproliferative disease [104, 105]. While OA EMZL/MALT has not been confirmed with *C. jejuni* infections, ocular inflammation has been reported with this entity [106].

Hepatitis C, an RNA virus, is known as the cause of a benign B-cell proliferative disorder known as mixed cryoglobulinemia. There is a higher prevalence of seropositivity for hepatitis C in patients with B-cell lymphoma [107], as well as an increased risk of developing B-cell NHL in patients with hepatitis C [108]. Chronic infection from hepatitis C as well as interference with signal transduction and apoptosis may contribute to oncogenesis. A small number of patients with OAL have been reported to be positive for hepatitis C [109, 110]. Neither study looked for molecular evidence of infectious RNA in lesions nor the seropositivity differed significantly between studies. Geographic variation may again be a factor in the variation of findings, but further studies are needed to determine the possible role of hepatitis C in OAL.

As it stands, no clear link has been established between OALD/OAL and an infectious agent in a large series. While some of the published series posit intriguing potential associations, at present they must be considered inconclusive and may simply represent an epiphenomenon. When conflicting data arise, the potential for "geographic variability" is immediately proposed, with an arguable degree of validity. Whether a significant local genetic variability occurs in the organism, the host, or both is unknown but is certainly within the realm of possibility. As an example, the link between EBV and eBL in certain environs of Africa is well established [111]. Further study is warranted and in all likelihood will provide better data for interpretation, but based on present evidence, no firm recommendation on the use of antibiotics as first-line therapy for OALD/OAL can be made.

Classification of Lymphoma

Prior to 1994, no global consensus of lymphoma classification existed, and terminology was variably based on morphology: growth pattern, cell type, nuclear characteristics, cell size, and/or degree of differentiation. The initial Rappaport classification spawned several discohesive schema also based exclusively on morphology (Table 50.1). In 1982, the Working Formulation of the National Institutes of Health attempted to not only unify the various approaches but for the first time to also include clinical and early immunohistochemical parameters [78, 112, 113]. The REAL classification, published in 1994 [114], was the first internationally accepted classification and also included extranodal disease (e.g., the ocular adnexa) and MALT. Furthermore, the REAL classification acknowledged the importance of standardized immunophenotyping in lymphoma diagnosis [3].

The WHO then modified the REAL classification system with a variety of deletions and expansions, most recently in 2016 [4]. These alterations are best considered an evolution of the REAL classification; in fact, many of the initial classifications of the REAL system have been preserved within the WHO modifications. Just as the REAL classification emphasized the importance of immunophenotyping, the WHO modifications stressed the inclusion of cytogenetics, further decreasing subjectivity in diagnosis and allowing for a more precise segregation of lymphoma subtypes. The most significant upshots of the WHO modifications for the orbital specialist are the extranodal disease and EMZL/MALT tissue stratifications and modifications. As an example, a retrospective study of OALD using the 2001 WHO modification resulted in over 25% of lesions that had been previously codified as "benign reactive lymphoid hyperplasia" under REAL being reclassified to EMZL or MALT lymphoma (also interchangeably termed "MALToma") [115]. In Ferry et al.'s landmark study, no cases of "reactive" or "atypical" lymphoid hyperplasia were noted, as most if not all such previously characterized lesions were reclassified as EMZL/MALT based on a new understanding of immunohistochemistry and cytogenetics.

The WHO modifications, most recently published in 2017 as a revision 4th edition (Table 50.2), also came to an impor-

Table 50.2 Mature B-cell neoplasms (non-Hodgkin type) from the 2016 WHO revision

Chronic lymphocytic leukemia/small cell lymphoma
Monoclonal B-cell lymphocytosis
B-cell prolymphocytic lymphoma
Splenic marginal zone lymphoma
Hairy cell leukemia
Splenic lymphoma/leukemia, unclassifiable
Splenic diffuse red pulp small B-cell lymphoma
Hairy cell leukemia-variant
Lymphoplasmacytic lymphoma
IgM monoclonal gammopathy of undetermined significance
Heavy chain disease
Alpha heavy chain disease
Gamma heavy chain disease
Mu heavy chain disease
Plasma cell neoplasms
Non-IgM monoclonal gammopathy of undetermined significance
Plasma cell myeloma
Plasma cell myeloma variants (asymptomatic plasma cell myeloma, nonsecretory myeloma, plasma cell leukemia)
Plasmacytoma (solitary plasmycytoma of bone, extraosseous plasmacytoma)
Monoclonal immunoglobulin deposition diseases (primary amyloidosis, light chain and heavy chain deposition diseases)
Plasma cell neoplasms with associated paraneoplastic syndrome (POEMS syndrome, TEMPI syndrome)
Extranodal marginal zone B-cell lymphoma of mucosa-associated lymphoid tissue (MALT lymphoma)
Nodal marginal zone B-cell lymphoma (MZL)
Pediatric type nodal MZL
Follicular lymphoma (grades 1, 2, 3a, 3b)
Testicular follicular lymphoma
In situ follicular neoplasia
Duodenal-type follicular lymphoma
Pediatric-type follicular lymphoma
Large B-cell lymphoma with *IRF4* rearrangement
Primary cutaneous follicle center lymphoma
Mantle cell lymphoma
Leukemic non-nodal mantle cell lymphoma
In situ mantle cell neoplasia
Diffuse large B-cell lymphoma (DLBCL), not otherwise specified (NOS)
T-cell/histiocyte-rich large B-cell lymphoma
Primary DLBCL of the CNS
Primary cutaneous DLBCL, leg type
Epstein-Barr virus (EBV)-positive DLBCL, NOS
EBV-positive mucocutaneous ulcer
DLBLC associated with chronic inflammation
Fibrin-associated DLBCL
Lymphomatoid granulomatosis
Primary mediastinal (thymic) large B-cell lymphoma
Intravascular large B-cell lymphoma
ALK-positive large B-cell lymphoma
Plasmablastic lymphoma
Primary effusion lymphoma
HHV8-associated lymphoproliferative disorders
Multicentric Castleman disease
HHV8-positive DLBCL, NOS
HHV8-positive germinotropic lymphoproliferative disorder
Burkitt lymphoma (BL)
Burkitt-like lymphoma with 11q aberration
High-grade B-cell lymphoma (HGBCL)
HGBCL with *MYC* and *BCL2* and/or *BCL6* rearrangements (double- and triple-hit lymphoma)
HGBCL, NOS
B-cell lymphoma, unclassifiable, with features intermediate between DLBCL and classic Hodgkin lymphoma

Modified from Ref. [4]

Neoplasms in bold type are the most common forms occurring in the ocular adnexa. Italicized neoplasm may present with neuro-ophthalmologic findings and is associated with intraocular (vitreoretinal) lymphoma tant consensus: treatment protocols should be studied within lymphoma subtype and not simply across the entire spectrum of lymphoproliferative disease [3, 4]. Indeed, even the description of lymphoma as a "spectrum" is questionable. Since each subtype of lymphoma represents a clonal proliferation of a specific B-cell (or much less frequently, T cell) stage, each subtype of lymphoma is best thought of as a distinct disease entity, with its own patterns of clinical behavior and response to therapy [3, 116]. This is an important construct to keep in mind, especially when considering the management of OAL: although the WHO modifications emphasize the importance of anatomic site in classification (e.g., central nervous system, skin), the anatomic location (in this case, the ocular adnexa) by no means connotes a uniformity of therapy. For example, under the REAL schema, FL was treated as a single entity both therapeutically and prognostically. The latest WHO modification recognizes that, in fact, grade 1 and 2 FLs behave in a much more indolent fashion than their aggressive grade 3a and 3b counterparts and that, in useful clinical terms, grade 3 follicular lymphoma should be treated as a separate entity [6].

What does this mean practically for the orbital specialist? As just noted, perhaps the most important concept within the WHO modification is that OAL cannot be subsumed as a single, homogenous entity [1, 2, 116]. It would therefore be erroneous to design any therapeutic studies on OAL based on broad and overly inclusive diagnostic brushstrokes, as has been done in the past because of limited immunohistochemical and cytogenetic data. Thus, one should not study OAL based on the flawed assumption that OAL is one entity occupying a single plot of anatomic real estate [117]; while location probably still plays a role, the two most important factors in prognostication and therapy are specific NHL subtype and clinical stage [1, 2].

The 2008 WHO modification of the REAL classification followed by the 2016 revision is now the gold standard in the study of OAL. For the non-pathologist, the breadth of the classification system can be daunting, but when applied critically to OAL, a much narrower list of possibilities emerges: most OAL can be compartmentalized into one of five specific types (Table 50.3) [84, 118–120].

Table 50.3 Distribution of most common systemic and ocular adnexal NHL subtypes

Systemic lymphoma (WHO data)	Ocular adnexal lymphoma ($n = 353$ and 797)
DLBCL (37%)	EMZL (52–57%)
FL (29%)	FL (11–23%)
EMZL (9%)	DLBCL (8–15%)
CLL (12%)	MCL (5–8%)
MCL (7%)	CLL/SCL (1–4%)

Data extracted from Refs. [1, 2, 4, 12, 29]

DLBCL diffuse large B-cell lymphoma, *EMZL* extranodal marginal zone lymphoma, *FL* follicular lymphoma, *CLL/SCL* chronic lymphocytic leukemia/small cell lymphoma, *MCL* mantle cell lymphoma

The vast majority of OAL is B-cell-derived NHL. T-cell lymphoma is uncommon, accounting for fewer than 3% of cases [15]. Burkitt and Hodgkin lymphomas are distinctly rare entities in the ocular adnexa. The most common type of OAL by far is EMZL/MALT. The remaining subtypes occur with differing frequency largely dependent on geographic distribution. In the United States, where follicular lymphoma (FL) is not uncommon, OAL also occurs as follicular lymphoma (FL) (23%), diffuse large B-cell lymphoma (DLBCL) (8%), mantle cell lymphoma (5%), small-cell lymphoma (chronic lymphocytic lymphoma) (4%), and lymphoplasmacytic lymphoma (1%) based on a study by Ferry and colleagues on patients from the United States [12]. In contrast, a recent international, multicenter study concluded that DLBCL occurs more frequently than FL in the ocular adnexa [2]. Interestingly, the distribution of OAL subtypes differs significantly from that of systemic NHL, where DLBCL predominates (Table 50.3).

As mentioned in the previous section, another important concept to stress when considering OAL is that not all lymphomas behave identically because each lymphoma subtype is a distinct disease entity. Therefore, management needs to be individually tailored based on a variety of factors, not least of which is the propensity of aggressive clinical behavior of certain OAL subtypes. In general, it appears that primary OALs tend to behave in a more indolent fashion than secondary OALs [1, 2]. Based on Ferry and co-workers preliminary data analysis as well as publications by Rasmussen, Olsen, and others, one other tenet must be stressed: if a certain subtype (MCL, DLBCL) of OAL is diagnosed histopathologically, in all likelihood it is not primary but has spread from an as yet undetermined anatomic site and represents the first clinical manifestation of a systemic disease [1, 2, 11, 12, 37, 53, 121].

As a somewhat artificial, but clinically useful, sweeping statement, EMZL of the ocular adnexa tend to be a primary lesion, while other low-grade (FL) and most high-grade OALs are generally secondary lesions [12, 84]. Surprisingly, in Ferry et al.'s analysis, only 19% of DLBCL of the ocular adnexa had known systemic involvement, and overall about 50% of DLBCL occurring in the ocular adnexa appeared to be primary lesions, despite aggressive clinical and histopathologic features [12, 14, 91]. However, this analysis was retrospective and based on older technology for systemic evaluation (see below). In addition, some of these patients had prior lower-grade lymphomas, confirming previous findings for a propensity of DLBCL to transform from a more indolent lesion over time [1, 2, 12, 91, 122]. In fact, such "histologic progression" is a well-known feature of lymphoproliferative disorders. In their early phases, many clonal B-cell expansions are difficult to cubbyhole into malignant and benign rubrics and have somewhat unpredictable clinical behaviors; these entities still remain a sticking point in the

Table 50.4 Clinical behavior and management strategies of the most common ocular adnexal NHL subtypes

Aggressive lymphoma	Indolent lymphoma
DLBCL Mantle cell Burkitt	Follicular (grades 1 and 2) EMZL/MALT CLL
Fatal if not cured	Incurable, indolent
Approach to cure	Chronic management

2008 WHO classification and are aptly described as "borderlands of malignancy" by Jaffe [116].

Overall, OA EMZL along with FL and chronic lymphocytic leukemia/small cell lymphoma (CLL/SCL) are less aggressive lesions than DLBCL and mantle cell lymphomas, which in many cases prove fatal (Table 50.4).

Extranodal Marginal Zone B-Cell Lymphoma of Mucosa-Associated Lymphoid Tissue (MALT Lymphoma)

MALT lymphoma, or MALToma, connotes involvement of mucosal tissue arising from indigenous lymphocytic populations (e.g., Peyer's patches, Waldeyer's rings), as first described in the gut and later the respiratory trcc [3, 115, 120, 123–130]. As a gross oversimplification, MALT may be considered as an immunological "early warning system." MALT lines susceptible mucosal surfaces and constitutes about half of all lymphoid tissue of the body. MALT produces IgA (and IgM) as its initial protective response and is intimately connected with the lymph nodal system as a priming mechanism for a more targeted and sustained response against antigen [131]. Memory cells (M cells) are also found along the mucosal surfaces and function as antigen-presenting cells to follicles present at deeper submucosal levels. The B-cell activity within germinal of the follicles results in a more sustained and specific immune response to antigen (see above).

Immunophenotyping of OALD lesions rapidly led to the identification of MALTomas in the ocular adnexa. The term "MALToma" soon became an enthusiastic shibboleth of the orbitologist, used not only to describe NHLs of the conjunctiva but also those exclusively within the orbit with no extension to the conjunctival mucosa or its native lymphocytes. In addition, correctly or not, a rigorous congruity was sought and on occasion forced upon ocular adnexal lesions to bring them "in line" with the clinical behavior of MALTomas elsewhere in the body [11].

It remains unclear whether MALTomas from specific anatomic sites are identical. This is certainly not true from the cytogenetic standpoint: gene translocations found in MALToma vary between anatomic sites [3, 5, 86]. However, there is also evidence that, despite these variations in specific gene translocation, the result is a deregulation of a common molecular pathway of lymphocytes (see above); in other words, the specific gene translocation in MALToma may be a clinically moot point [3]. That said, it is also important to remember that ocular adnexal EMZL/MALT does not necessarily behave in the same manner as MALTomas elsewhere in the body. As an example, there is to date no convincing evidence that ocular adnexal EMZL/MALT responds to the antibiotic regimen that is effective in the treatment of gastric MALToma. As already noted, many gastric MALTomas are not autonomous and self-sustaining processes but instead are at least temporarily dependent on *H. pylori*-activated T cells for survival [3, 54, 56, 116]; no such evidence exists for ocular adnexal EMZL/MALT. Unlike gastric MALToma, which rarely spreads to other anatomic sites, ocular adnexal EMZL/MALT does manifest systemically in a significant minority (16%) of patients [2, 84].

Because of the lack of mucosal involvement in many ocular adnexal MALTomas, the term ocular adnexal EMZL of mucosa-associated lymphoid tissue (OA EMZL/MALT) is more accurate and perhaps preferable (although admittedly more cumbersome), bringing the terminology in line with the 2008 WHO classification. OA EMZL/MALT comprises between 50% and 67% of OAL in the West and up to 90% of OAL in Asia [2, 12, 84, 132].

OA EMZL/MALT is typified by an indolent clinical course (5-month average duration of symptoms), lack of systemic involvement on presentation (78–90% stage IE), and good survival profiles [1, 2, 133]. That said, systemic surveillance is important, since distant relapse rates over 10 years are well-described, occurring in 55% at 10 years, in contradistinction to gastric EMZL [84]. In a recent multicenter study, median duration before relapse or progression for orbital EMZL/MALT was 36 months (range, 2–198 months) [2]. When systemic recurrences manifest, they are typically isolated and are well controlled with local therapy [84]. Disease-specific survival (DSS) for a cohort of 447 patients with orbital EMZL/MALT is listed in Table 50.5 [2]. Overall, DSS for OA EMZL/MALT is good, although relapse or progression portends a worse prognosis [2, 134]. Hindsø et al. found that recurrence or progression rates were related to initial presentation: 28% in stage IE disease and in 48% with disseminated disease [133]. Ten-year DSS was good across multiple studies. Hindsø et al. reported on a large cohort of 679 patients and found that primary OA EMZL/MALT had a 10-year DSS of 93% compared to only 81% for secondary (disseminated or relapsed) disease; stage IE patients has a 20-year DSS of 90% [133]. In a study by Fung and colleagues, patients presenting with stage IE OA EMZL/MALT had a 10-year DSS rate of 100%, compared to only 49% in patients presenting with stage III/IV [84]. However, two more recent studies with larger cohorts (but overlapping data sets) demonstrated that clinical stage at pre-

Table 50.5 Characteristics of the five major subtypes of B-cell *orbital* NHL (data does not include primary conjunctival and eyelid lesions)

OAL subtype	EMZL	FL	DLBCL	MCL	SLL/ CLL
Number of orbital lesions	452	91	118	66	8
Percent of all OAL[a]	57	11	15	8	1
Male sex (%)	50	44	42	73	37
Median age, years (range)	63 (13–100)	62 (39–95)	67 (3–96)	69 (35–90)	NL
Bilateral (%)	12	19	8	45	0
Primary disease (%)	75	58	54	11	75
Initial Ann Arbor stage (%)					
IE	78	55	55	17	88
IIE	6	17	14	3	0
IIIE	2	9	2	4	0
IVE	14	19	29	76	12
AJCC TNM stage (tumor portion)					
T2	97	86	80	100	100
T3	2	10	7	0	0
T4	1	4	13	0	0
Disease-specific survival					
5 years	96	88	54	62	NL
10 years	92	71	41	32	
20 years	84				

Data extracted from Refs. [1, 2]

[a]Includes both B-cell and T-cell lesions. NL = data not listed because of limited data set; see text for additional details. Note that not all subtypes are listed in table

sentation did not influence 10-year DSS [2, 133]. Patient younger than 60 years also fared better than older patients, consistent with findings across other NHL subtypes.

Like FL, EMZL/MALT may transform over time into a more aggressive NHL. In one study of 467 patients with EMZL/MALT, the risk of transformation to DLBCL was 8% but was significantly higher in those patients with systemic versus localized disease (16% vs 4% over 15 years, respectively) [122]. Of note, it appears that the risk of transformation is significantly lower in EMZL/MALT than in FL [122].

Two additional conclusions gleaned from a recent multicenter study are worth noting [133]. First, patients with stage IE disease treated exclusively with external beam radiotherapy (EBRT) at a median total dose of 26 Gy had better outcomes than similarly staged patients treated with systemic chemotherapy. Second, patients with disseminated disease had a better DSS when rituximab was included in the chemotherapeutic regimen.

Follicular Lymphoma

Under the 2008 WHO classification, FL and DLBCL have undergone additional stratification in an effort to further improve diagnostic accuracy and, as a result, presumably improve management options [116]. Early in its conversion to monoclonality, FL is indistinguishable from certain populations of clonal memory B cells (t(14;18)(q32;q21)) that circulate in up to 70% of normal individuals and do not become the autonomous proliferation that would define them as lymphoma [135, 136]. Conversely, so-called "in situ FL" can be identified cytogenetically in otherwise healthy lymph nodes, leading to a subsequent work-up and identification of FL in other anatomic sites about 50% of the time [137]. However, in half of such patients, progression of FL does not occur, once again leaving the question of what actually defines lymphoma a bit up in the air. Certainly, grades 3A and 3B FL are known to behave aggressively and require special attention. Here, then, is yet another example of the strength of the WHO classification schema: grade 3 FL necessitates a different management protocol than the more indolent grades 1 and 2. In previous classifications, all FL would have been lumped together as one entity.

OA FL occurs more frequently in the United States than in either Europe or Asia, but the reasons are unknown [6, 12, 37]. A significant proportion of FLs affecting the ocular adnexa are secondary lesions. In Fung and co-workers' analysis, grades 1 and 2 FL presented as a primary lesion in 75% of cases (usually as stage IE), with the remaining 25% of FL lesions as secondary manifestations. No cases of grade 3 FL were encountered. These findings were buttressed by Olsen et al.'s findings that 28% of orbital FL were stage IIIE/IVE [2]. There was an equal distribution of disease in the conjunctiva, orbit, and lacrimal gland, with only a small minority (6%) occurring exclusively in the eyelid [37]. Of note, conjunctival lesions were associated more frequently with disseminated disease than other ocular adnexal locations in one study, possibly due to lymphocyte recirculation and homing mechanisms [37].

In Rasmussen et al.'s multicenter study, 81% of lesions were categorized as grade 1 or 2, 18% as grade 3A, and 1% as grade 3B [37]. Overall, FL of the ocular adnexa behaves in an indolent fashion, and this is likely due to the lower-grade (1 or 2) histopathology and cytogenetics. As with EMZL/MALT, relapses or progression of adnexal FL may occur (46%) and are more common with grade 3 lesions [37]. In Fung et al.'s series, all stage IE FL lesions were treated with local radiotherapy alone, and 4 (36%) of 11 patients developed relapses at other anatomic sites [84]. No DSS occurred during 10-year follow-up, but, again, no cases of grade 3 FL were noted in this series. DSS data for orbital FL from Olsen et al. are listed in Table 50.5 [2]. Note that both 5- and 10-year DSS were significantly lower than that of orbital EMZL/MALT. The authors also concluded that relapse, progression, or secondary disease at presentation carried a worse prognosis than primary, nonrelapsing, nonprogressive orbital lesions; however, as with orbital EMZL/MALT, there was no difference in 10-year DSS between stage IE/IIE and stage IIIE/IVE cohorts [2]. Of note, it does not appear that any sub-analysis of DSS was made between grade 1/2 and grade 3 lesions [2, 37]. However, a sister study by Rasmussen et al. concluded that grade 3A OA FLs had a shorter maximum survival than grade 1/2 lesions [6]. Survival was also not affected by the presence or absence of the t(14;18) translocation, although patients that were positive for this genetic footprint had more recurrences [6].

One additional point regarding orbital FL should be mentioned. The t(14;18)(q32,q21) gene translocation is found in both FL and in up to 34% of DLBCL. A minority (3% in one study [37]) of FL lesions may transform into DLBCL over time [122, 138].

Diffuse Large B-Cell Lymphoma

DLBCL remains a classification annoyance in the WHO modifications. Although DLBCL is the most common form of adult NHL, cytogenetic outliers have been described (see below) [116]. Some of these intermediate lesions contain the classic MYC translocation of Burkitt lymphoma (see below) but differ from Burkitt lymphoma morphologically. This translocation may also be found in scattered cases of "typical" DLBCL. The WHO classification also includes two specific anatomic distinctions for DLBCL: the central nervous system (CNS) and the skin (Table 50.1).

One additional newly characterized and rare variant of DLBCL, *Epstein-Barr virus (EBV) + DLBCL of the elderly*, has recently been described in the ocular adnexa [139]. This patient presented with stage III disease. It is possible that EBV+ DLBCL of the elderly simply represents an extension of a similar disease process seen in the context of chronic immunosupression (e.g., HIV disease, organ transplantation, and methotrexate therapy for rheumatoid arthritis) and/or is the manifestation of an age-related immunologic deterioration [140].

Despite this first attempt at stratification of DLBCL, a large group of these tumors exists as *not otherwise specified (NOS)*, resulting in difficulties in prognostication and therapeutic recommendation. Early cytogenetic differentiation appears to have prognostic value, but additional insight is certainly needed [116].

Counterintuitively, in a series of 27 ocular adnexal DLBCLs by Ferry and colleagues [12], only 19% had known prior lymphoma, connoting that 81% of ocular adnexal DLBCLs are primary lesions. This seems to argue against the gestalt that histologically and clinically aggressive OALs tend to be secondary lesions but may represent the limitations of a retrospective study spanning 31 years, with the probability of less than ideal systemic work-up (e.g., technological limitations of imaging). Of note, Morley et al. found a similar incidence (21%) of systemic disease at presentation in their cohort of 14 patients presenting more recently over only a 7-year span [141]. A more recent study of OA DLBCL also found stage IE disease in 55–93% of patient with primary OA lesions [2, 53]. Between 27% and 50% of "primary" DLBCLs from these two studies had radiographic evidence of aggressive behavior, including bone destruction and paranasal sinus involvement, begging the question of whether these lesions may have spread from the adjacent sinuses into the orbit secondarily (Fig. 50.5) [12, 141]. Several additional caveats are worth noting. DLBCL is the most common NHL that occurs in association with HIV infection. As noted, bone erosion and involvement of an adjacent anatomic compartment (paranasal sinus, anterior cranial fossa, skull base) may occur [1, 2, 142].

Olsen and co-authors reported on 106 patients with orbital DLBCL in an international, multicenter study [2]. Orbital DLBCL (15%) was the second most frequent orbital NHL encountered after EMZL/MALT (57%); however, Ferry et al.'s study, which included only patients from the United States, found that FL (23%) occurred more frequently in the OA than DLBCL [12]. While 55% of patients presented with stage IE disease, a significant proportion (31%) had stage IIIE/IVE pathology. The duration of symptoms was significantly shorter (2 months) than that described with OA EMZL/MALT, consistent with the aggressive clinical behavior of DLBCL. As expected with this aggressive NHL subtype, most patients with orbital stage IE DLBCL received systemic chemotherapy. Despite this, 44% of patients with primary OA DLBCL suffered either recurrence or progression [53]. DSS is listed in Table 50.5 and reveals a dramatically worse prognosis than that of EMZL/MALT and FL, with 70% dying from a lymphoma-related cause; Kaplan Meier curves for orbital NHLs are shown in Fig. 50.6 [53]. Unlike EMZL/MALT and FL, orbital stage IVE DLBCL had a poorer DSS than lower stage disease; increasing T category also decreased DSS. Male gender portended an earlier disease-related demise, consistent with nodal DLBCL data [53].

One criticism of most publications on OA DLBCL is the same that was leveled at management of OA NHL earlier in this chapter: not all DLBCLs are the same. Furthermore, DLBCL can be difficult to segregate into a clearly distinct subtype (see below), even with the use of immunohistochemistry and molecular genetic analysis.

In general, DLBCL can be divided into three distinct subgroups based on the cell of origin and associated with distinct genetic aberrations: [1, 5, 43]

1. Germinal center B-cell-like (GCB) DLBCL (origin from centroblasts; *BCL2*, *MYC*, *EZH2*, *BCL6*, and *MEF2B* translocations)
2. Activated B-cell-like (ABC) DLBCL (origin from plasmablastic B cells; *BCL2* amplification, NK-κB activation)
3. Primary mediastinal large B-cell lymphoma (origin from thymic B cells)

Each of these subtypes carries its own distinct prognosis [5, 43], but many studies on OA DLBCL do not distinguish between subtypes. In general, GCB-DLBCL carries

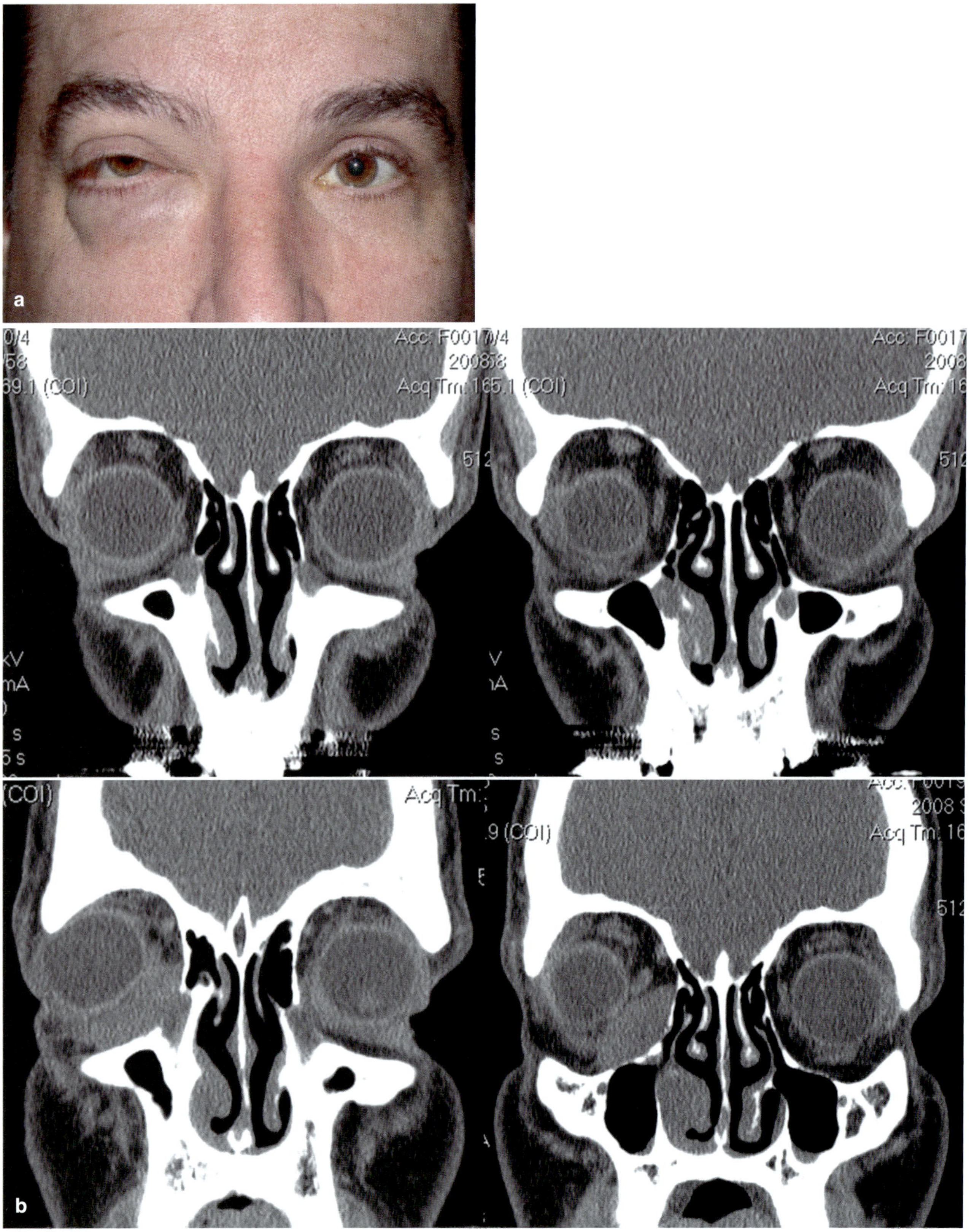

Fig. 50.5 DLBCL of the orbit and lacrimal drainage system. (**a**) Clinical photograph of a 48-year-old male who presented with a 2-month history of right-sided epiphora and medial canthal mass, initially misdiagnosed as dacryocystitis. (**b**) Coronal CT soft tissue views. Top: initial imaging performed elsewhere. Bottom: repeat imaging 2 months later. Note the marked enlargement of the right orbital mass extending along the nasolacrimal duct and involving the inferior turbinate. Biopsy revealed DLBCL. (**c**) PET/CT of the orbital lesion, the SUV is high (red box), measuring 10.81, consistent with the high metabolic activity seen in aggressive lesions. (**d**) Clinical photograph after two cycles of chemotherapy

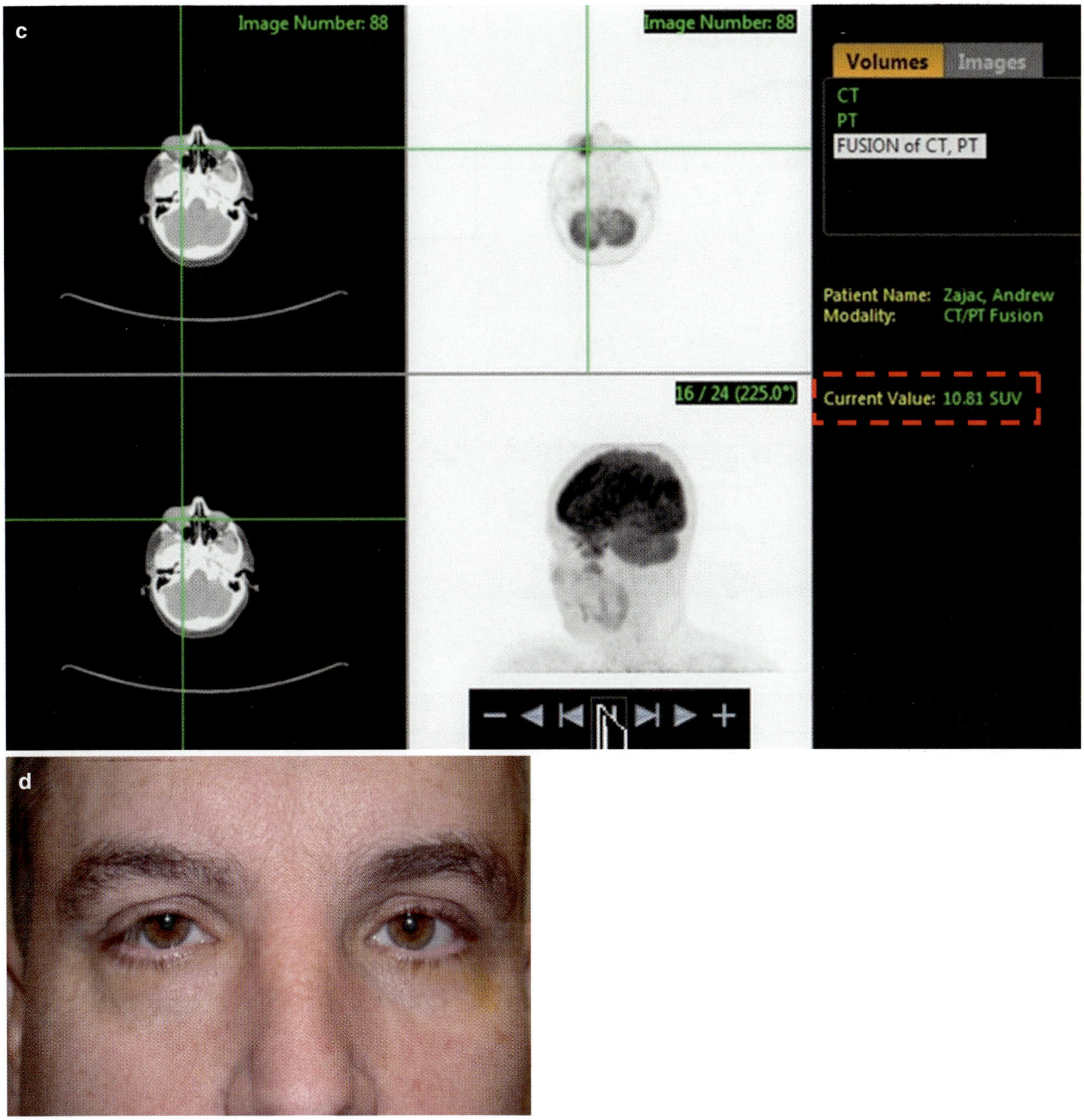

Fig. 50.5 (continued)

a markedly better prognosis than ABC-DLBCL [43]. Two series that studied OA DLBCL subtypes noted that the majority (91%) of OA DLBCL is GBC-DLBCL ("centroblastic"), and, inexplicably when compared to other series on systemic DLBCL, this subtype had similar outcomes as the ABC-DLBCL ("immunoblastic") lesions – this may be due to the small number of ABC-DLBCL in the data set [43, 51, 53].

Despite these shortcomings, an overall picture of ocular adnexal DLBCL is worth summarizing. Prognosis for DLBCL of the ocular adnexa is difficult to predict because of the persistent confusion in DLBCL classification, the relative infrequency of this entity in the ocular adnexa when compared to EMZL, and treatment variability. Even with this limited data, OA DLBCL should be considered an aggressive lesion (3.5-year median overall survival) [53], and the clinician should maintain a high suspicion for systemic involvement, even if initial work-up is unrevealing. OA DLBCL is typically treated with chemotherapy ± radiotherapy, even in stage IE disease limited to the ocular adnexa.

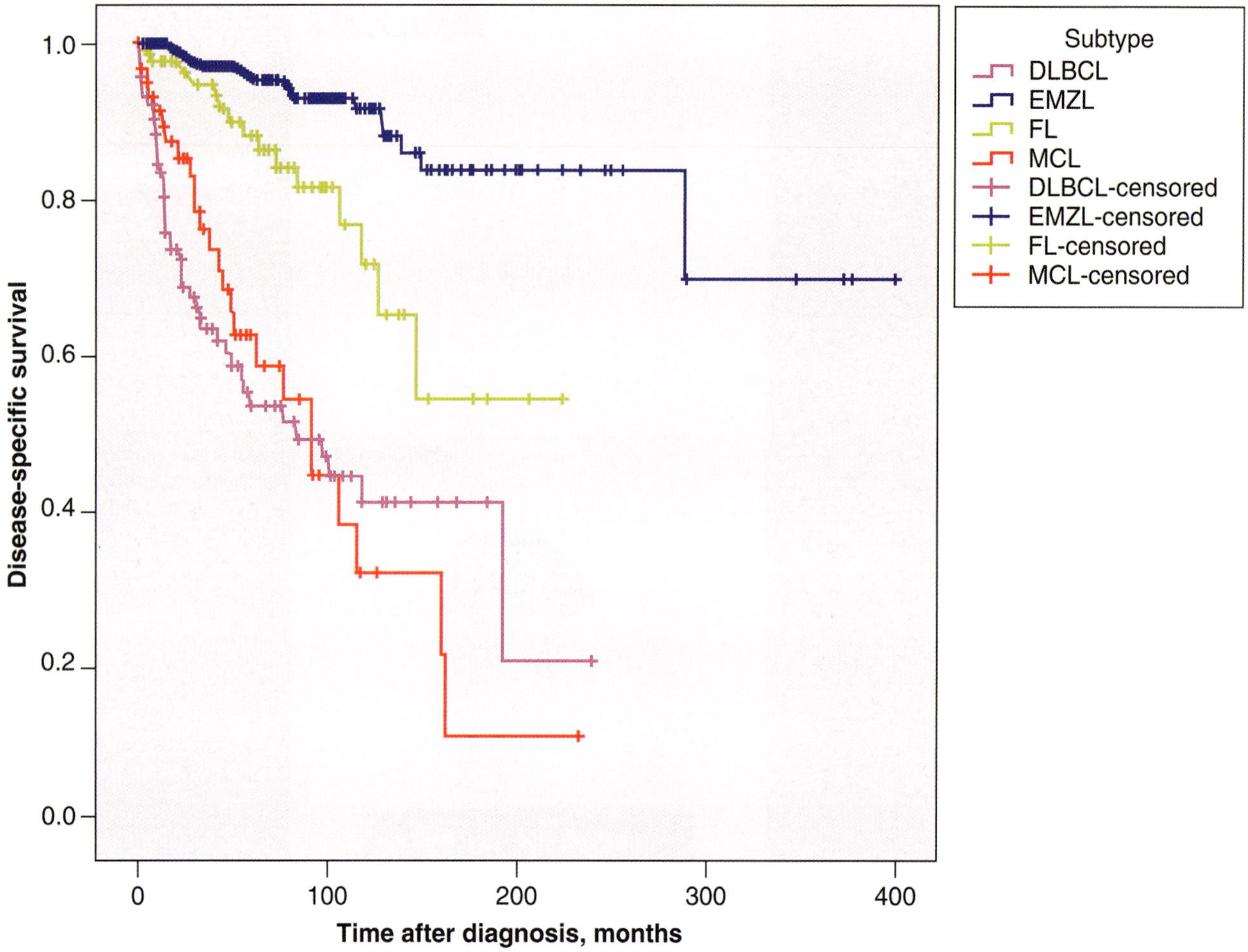

Subtype interval, y	0	5	10	15	20	25	30	35
EMZL (N = 452)								
Patients at risk, No.	444	151	57	21	9	4	3	
Events, No.	10	5	4	0	1	0	0	
FL (N = 91)								
Patients at risk, No.	90	49	13	3	0			
Events, No.	8	5	2	0				
DLBCL (N = 118)								
Patients at risk, No.	115	29	11	3	0			
Events, No.	41	5	0	1				
MCL (N = 66)								
Patients at risk, No.	60	16	4	1				
Events, No.	17	6	2	0				

Fig. 50.6 Disease-specific survival of four subtypes of orbital NHL. EMZL = extranodal marginal zone lymphoma, FL = follicular lymphoma, DLBCL = diffuse large B call lymphoma, MCL = mantle cell lymphoma. (From Ref [2])

Mantle Cell Lymphoma

MCL represents a minority of OAL, subsuming only 2–8% of OAL and 2–7% of all NHL [1, 52, 121, 125]. Despite its infrequency in the ocular adnexa, MCL is a formidable disease with a significant mortality (Table 50.5) [1, 2, 52]. Several studies of MCL in the ocular adnexa have revealed patterns of incidence that can be summarized as the triad of male predominance (76–90%), advanced age (median 64–75 years), and aggressive course (Fig. 50.7) [2, 12, 52, 121, 125]. Duration of symptoms for orbital MCL (3 months) was shorter compared to EMZL [2]. Additional useful data can be gleaned from four studies: [2, 52, 121, 125] the orbit appears to be preferentially affected (58–90%) when compared to other adnexal sites, and bilateral involvement is noted in 45–71% of patients [2]; in a recent multicenter study on ocular adnexal MCL, bilateral involvement correlated with disseminated disease [52]. Although the adnexa may be the initial site of presentation (67–80%), systemic work-up reveals stage III/IV disease in the majority of patients (75–90%), suggesting that ocular adnexal involvement is a secondary, rather than primary, process. Cytogenetic analysis may reveal a composite profile in a minority of cases, once again demonstrating the histopathologic evolution stressed by Jaffe [116]. Aggressive behavior is the hallmark of MCL, and until recently, the prognosis was grim: the median overall survival was 57 months, and the 5-year overall survival was only 39% in a study of 10 patients by Looi and colleagues [125]. Olsen et al. reported a 5- and 10-year DSS of 53% and 22%, respectively, and initial stage of disease did not influence DSS [2]. However, the addition of rituximab to the chemotherapeutic regimen in stage IVE disease appears to markedly improve 5- and 10-year DSS (see below) [2, 52, 121, 143].

Uncommon and Unusual Ocular Adnexal Lymphomas

As noted in the previous sections, the vast majority of OAL are B-cell-derived NHL. The entities described in this section occur with rarity in the ocular adnexa and in many cases exhibit aggressive clinical behavior. They often represent a form of secondary OAL.

Burkitt Lymphoma

Burkitt lymphoma (BL) occurs in three variants in the WHO classification: endemic, sporadic, and immunodeficiency-associated [144–146]. The endemic form (eBL) manifests chiefly in children (boys > girls) in equatorial Africa (where malaria is endemic), is the most common form of NHL in this geographic area, and has an absolute association with Epstein-Barr virus (EBV). An association between eBL and other infectious triggers (e.g., malaria) has never been proved conclusively, but malaria-induced chronic immunosuppression predisposing to more aggressive EBV infection is an interesting hypothesis. eBL usually presents in the mandible and typically affects the orbit secondarily. Conversely, the sporadic form (sBL) found in immunocompetent individuals occurs in non-endemic areas in any age group, without a

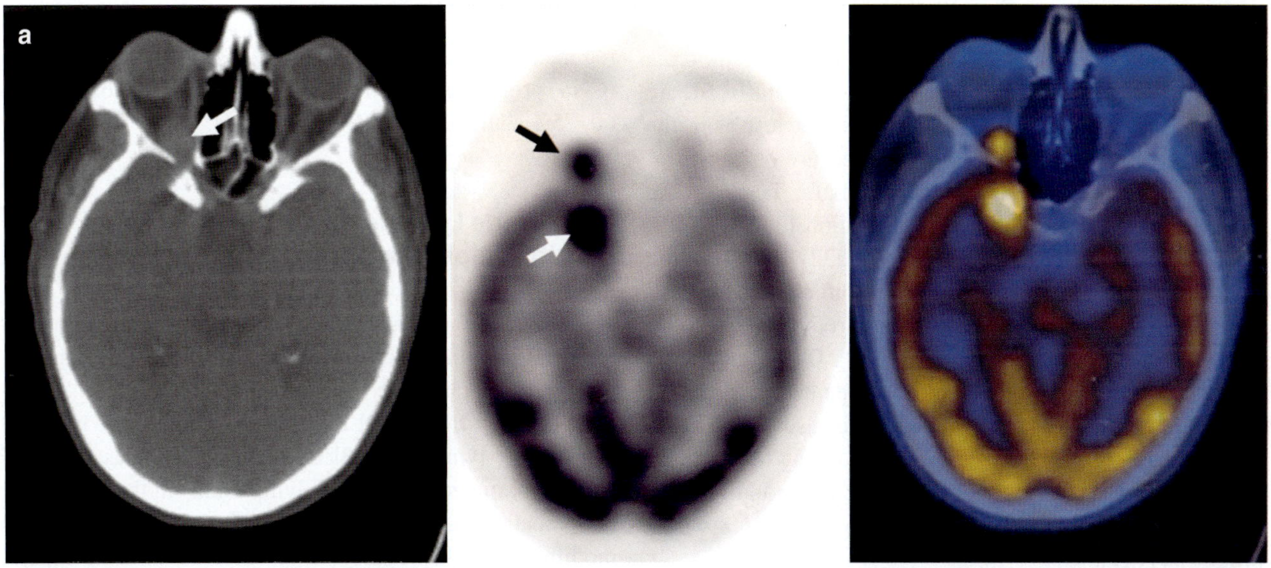

Fig. 50.7 (**a**) Orbital mantle cell lymphoma. An elderly patient presented with slowly progressive diplopia. Initial imaging revealed an orbital apical mass. Left: Low-resolution CT with a right orbital apical mass (arrow). Center, PET demonstrates the orbital mass (black arrow) as well as a metabolically active lesion within the cavernous sinus (white arrow). Right: PET/CT fusion view showing metabolically active lesions. (**b**) Body PET demonstrating widespread metabolic activity in the lymph nodes and spleen with a high SUV. Biopsy diagnosed MCL

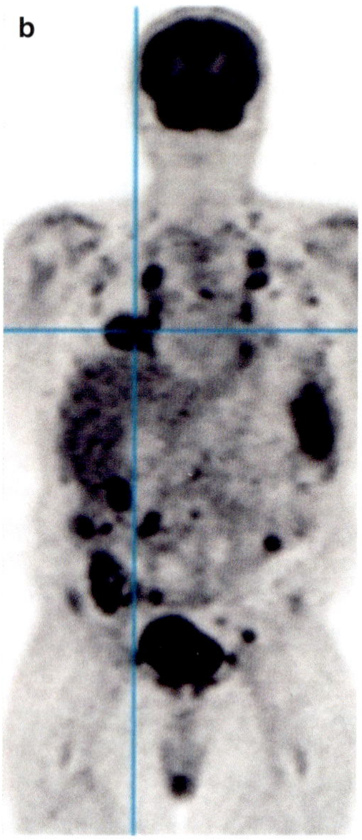

Fig. 50.7 (continued)

proven infectious trigger (only 15–10% EBV+), and typically presents in the abdomen; in the United States and Europe, sBL accounts for 30–50% of all NHL in children [145, 147, 148]. A separate EBV-associated form (immunodeficiency-associated) occurs in conjunction with HIV infection or severe chronic immunosuppressive therapy (e.g., certain allograft regimens) and appears to affect adults more frequently than children [144].

BL is a disease characterized by a high proliferation rate and an aggressive clinical course [145]. All forms of BL are characterized by a genetic translocation that results in the deregulation of the *MYC* oncoprotein because of translocations associated with the immunoglobulin heavy chain (IgH), allowing for fulminant proliferation [3, 145, 149]. Specifically, the classic t(8:14)(q24:q32) translocation transplants the *MYC* proto-oncogene from chromosome 18 and abuts it against the *IgH* gene on chromosome 14; *IgH* then enhances the overexpression of *MYC* [146, 150]. However, the break points for each specific translocation differ among the BL subtypes [145]. It is also important to note that *IgH/MYC* translocation is not unique to BL but is found in other NHL subtypes, including MCL and FL, and the presence of this genetic aberration portends a worse prognosis [145].

The development of BL is variably associated with EBV, but as noted, EBV infection has been implicated in essentially all cases of eBL [144]. As a fascinating historical aside, the suspicion of a viral cause to eBL led to the discovery of EBV. In 1997, based on the available evidence, the carcinogenicity of EBV was deemed a conclusive factor in the development of BL [151].

The association between HIV infection, EBV, and BL is not fully understood. It appears that any EBV effects on B-cell transformation and proliferation are usually kept at bay by normal immune surveillance. Immunosuppression by other factors (HIV infection, pharmacologic/nutritional/environmental factors, etc.) may allow for an unchecked expansion of EBV-infected B-cell populations, increasing the probability of the *MYC* translocation [144]. This hypothesis is tempered by the finding that most patients in Western countries with HIV-associated BL are negative for EBV [144].

BL, regardless of form, has the highest proliferation rate of any known human tumor. In fact, the WHO classification mandates Ki67 (a protein associated with cellular proliferation) staining of >99%, along with *MYC* deregulation, for a diagnosis of BL [144].

In Western countries, orbital BL is typically associated with HIV infection [152]; sBL rarely affects the ocular adnexa [153]. Regardless of the subtype, orbital BL follows an aggressive clinical and radiographic course (Fig. 50.8) [153]. The adjacent paranasal sinuses are frequently involved (50%) and may in fact be the nidus of malignancy. In contradistinction to more indolent forms of OAL, optic neuropathy is a frequent finding in orbital BL (31%). Bone erosion on imaging studies is also common, as is a high incidence of central nervous system (40%) and systemic (80%) involvement [153]. Of note, CNS involvement is distinctly uncommon in BL without orbital involvement. Despite aggressive therapy, the prognosis for orbital BL is guarded, with a significant mortality (54%) within 1 year of presentation. However, the advent of short, intensive chemotherapeutic regimens coupled with intrathecal, central nervous system (CNS) prophylaxis has markedly improved prognosis, with a 60–75% adult cure rate [145, 147, 154].

High-Grade Lymphoma (Including Atypical Burkitt Lymphoma/Burkitt-Like Lymphoma)

A subset of clinical aggressive NHL defies the histopathological, immunohistochemical, and molecular genetic characteristics of classic NHL subtypes and falls into a gray zone between BL and DLBCL; these lesions were known a Burkitt-like lymphoma (BLL) in the REAL classification, "undifferentiated non-Burkitt lymphoma" in the Rappaport classification, and atypical BL/BLL in the 2001 WHO modification [145]. There was disagreement among experts as to whether atypical BL/BLL was a specific entity or simply a biologic continuum between classic BL and DLBCL. In the past, this distinction was likely of little consequence, since treatment was limited and nonspecific. However, with the advent of targeted therapy for each specific NHL subtype, an incorrect shift of a patient with atypical BL/BLL toward either BL or DLBCL treatment may have significant prognostic consequences [145, 155, 156]. In general, atypical BL/BLL has a better prognosis when treated with regimens for BL rather than those used for DLBCL [145].

In 2008, the WHO did away with the "atypical BL/BLL" classification, opting instead for the term "B-cell lymphoma, unclassifiable, with features between BL and DLBCL," and more recently as the self-explanatory and preferred term "high-grade B-cell lymphoma with MYC and BCL2 and/or BCL6 rearrangements" [4]. Note that a second term, "high-grade B-cell lymphoma, not otherwise specified" has also been added by the WHO (Table 50.2) [146]. The upshot of this new schema is that most previous atypical BL/BLL lesions are now shifted to either the classic BL rubric or DLBCL based initially on their morphology and then on their immunohistochemistry and molecular genetic footprint. As an example, an atypical lesion with morphologic features of BL, a Ki-67 proliferation rate of about 100%, and CD10+, BCL6+, BCL2– staining, with only a "single-hit" *IgH/MYC* translocation, would be classified as BL; any additional chromosomal abnormalities should make the diagnosis of BL suspect [4].

Those lesions with a lower Ki67 proliferation and positivity for BCL2 and/or BCL6 now fall under the new terminology and are sometimes called "double-hit" or "two-hit" lymphomas because of the presence of both *IgH/MYC* and *BCL2* or *BLC6* translocations [4]. "Triple-hit" NHL, which carry all three rearrangements, are also possible. Double-hit lymphomas occur most commonly with Ann Arbor stage IV disease in the 6th to 7th decade with no gender preference; CNS involvement may be present [4]. Notably, the dual-hit NHLs carry a grave prognosis (mean survival 4.5–18.5 months), responding poorly to BL regimens and rituximab-based regimens [4, 145].

Currently, any aggressive B-cell lymphoma should first undergo FISH analysis for *MYC* rearrangement, and, if present, *BCL2* and *BCL6* aberrations should then be tested for better characterization into double-hit or triple-hit NHL [146].

a

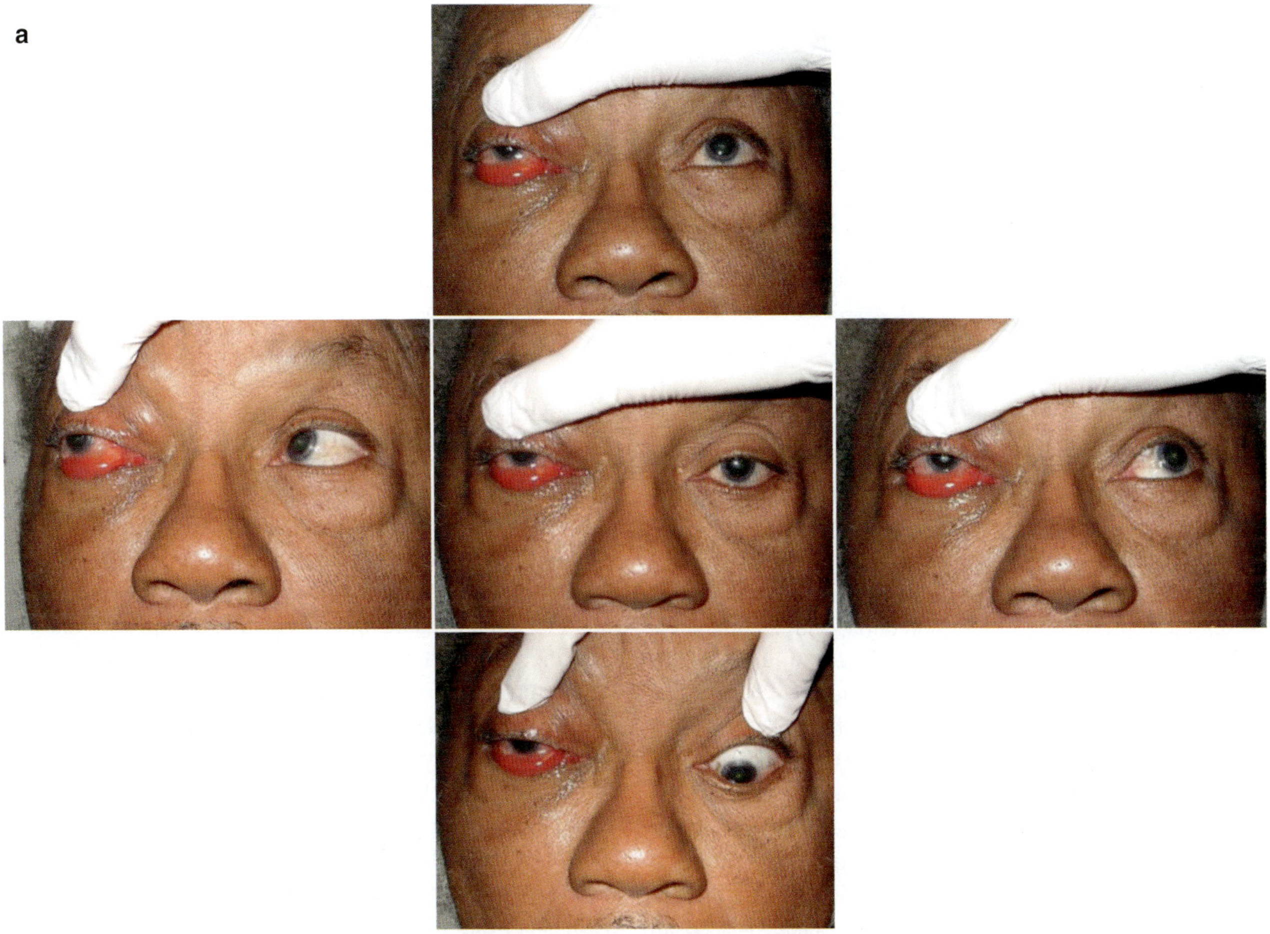

Fig. 50.8 Sporadic Burkitt lymphoma. (**a**) Clinical photographs of a patient presenting with rapidly progressive right proptosis, chemosis, and diplopia. (**b**) CT, axial (left) and coronal (right) soft tissue images. Note that the orbital process is contiguous with the maxillary sinus. Bone remodeling is noted within the sinus (arrows). (**c**) Biopsy specimen demonstrating the "starry sky" appearance of classic BL, confirmed with immunohistochemistry. The patient was HIV negative and responded well to chemoradiotherapy. He remains in remission for over 2 years

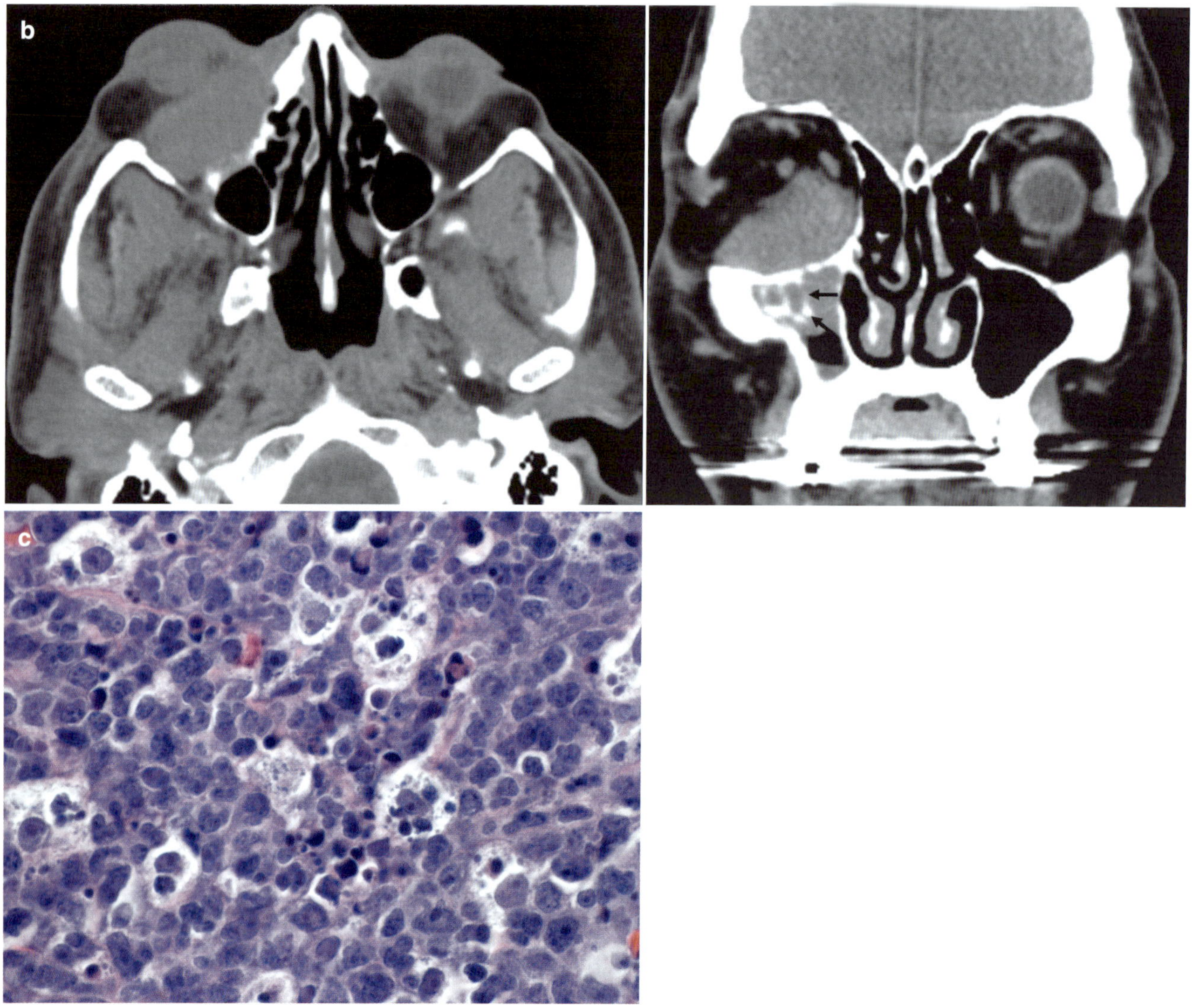

Fig. 50.8 (continued)

AIDS-Related Lymphoma

OAL in the setting of HIV infection deserves specific commentary. HIV-associated NHL is an AIDS-defining diagnosis. The incidence of NHL and CNS lymphoma is markedly increased in the setting of HIV infection, with a cumulative risk of 3–8% [157, 158]. Prior to the advent of highly active antiretroviral therapy (HAART), the incidence of NHL in the HIV-infected population was 40–400 higher than in an age-matched HIV-negative cohort [159, 160]. Although NHL may occur at any stage of HIV/AIDS, three factors have been shown to increase the risk: increasing age, low CD4 count/high viral load, and no prior HAART history [159]. Seventy-two percent of patients with HIV-associated OAL present with a known diagnosis of AIDS [152]. There is also an increased incidence of HL and multiple myeloma (MM) in the HIV-infected population [161].

The cause for this increased incidence is in all likelihood multifactorial [161]. HIV infection represents a chronic state of frantic immune stimulation fighting a losing battle against a retrovirally mediated immune suppression. Chronic antigenic stimulation and immune suppression are known facilitators of lymphomatous transformation, along with chronic cytokine dysregulation and dendritic cell impairment. Furthermore, chronic immune suppression allows for the proliferation of other oncogenic pathogens, including EBV and human herpesvirus 8 (HHV8). A direct oncogenic effect by HIV-1 has also been postulated [160].

AIDS-related lymphoma (ARL) is divided into three categories by the WHO: (1) NHL subtypes also known to occur in HIV-negative individuals (BL, DLBCL); (2) NHL subtypes occurring specifically in HIV-infected individuals (*primary effusion lymphoma, plasmablastic lymphoma*); and (3) NHL that may also occur in other immunodeficiency states (*post-transplant lymphoproliferative disorder*) [161]. The vast majority of ARL are either BL or DLBCL, although double-hit lymphoma may also occur. One unique entity, plasmablastic lymphoma, is a B-cell neoplasm that typically affects the jaw and oral cavity of HIV-infected individuals. Three cases of orbital involvement have been described recently with uniformly rapidly progressive disease and limited survival [141, 162].

CNS lymphoma, more recently renamed *primary cerebral lymphoma* (PCL) or *primary central nervous system lymphoma* (*PCNSL*), typically a rare entity in the immunocompetent population, is also a notable manifestation of HIV/AIDS (Fig 50.9). For therapeutic and prognostic purposes, PCNSL is usually separated out from the compendium of HIV-related NHL. PCNSL is typically an ABC-DLBCL (immunoblastic type) [161]. HIV-related PCNSL is invariably associated with EBV, a very low CD4 count (<50/mm^3), and a poor prognosis [161]. It may present with purely neuro-ophthalmologic signs, including optic neuropathy, optic disk edema, and other cranial neuropathies. Despite recent advances, the prognosis for PCNSL remains guarded, with a median survival of 1.5 years, even with concomitant HAART [161].

Prognosis for HIV-related OAL is also guarded, as aggressive subtypes and advanced stage at presentation are the norm (Fig. 50.10). However, some encouraging recent data has emerged. The incidence of NHL in the HIV-infected population in industrialized countries appears to be declining in large part due to widespread availability of HAART, presumably because immune restoration is protective against lymphoma development, but this finding is debatable [159, 160]. However, there is no difference in clinical presentation of NHL (other than higher CD4) between patients receiving and not receiving HAART therapy; in other words, HAART therapy may be decreasing the incidence of NHL, but not the stage of the lymphoma once it manifests. Paradoxically, while the use of HAART in maintaining some degree of immunocompetence is decreasing the incidence of opportunistic infection and extending survival, the improved life span also allows more time for the emergence of secondary malignancies [161].

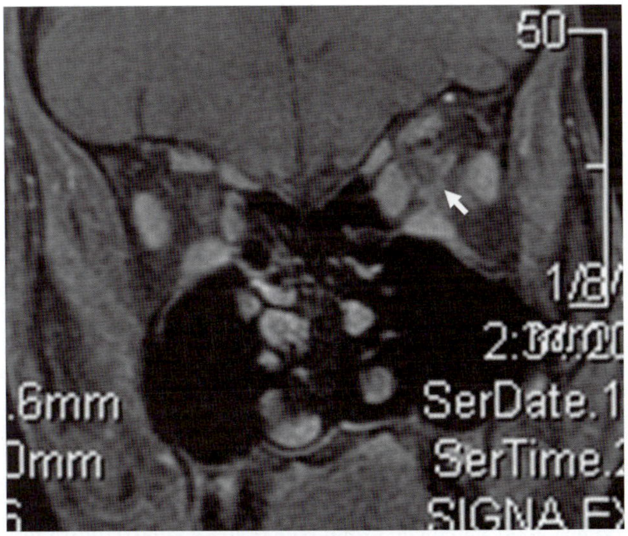

Fig. 50.9 PCNSL of HIV. Coronal MRI of orbital PCNSL infiltration surrounding the optic nerve (arrow) in a patient with AIDS

In general, ARL of the ocular adnexa is clinically aggressive and not infrequently presents with atypical radiographic findings, most notably distortion of native anatomy, bone erosion, and involvement of adjacent paranasal sinuses (Fig. 50.10) [152, 163–165]. For the clinician, these are important characteristics to remember: HIV-related OAL may masquerade as a sinoorbital infectious process, and early confusion with bacterial or fungal (especially sinoorbital aspergillosis) infection is common. Most patients (72%) will present with B symptoms (fever, night sweats, weight loss), and isolated adnexal disease is unlikely [152, 159]. Treatment may be difficult because of toxicity of combined therapies but has shifted from the previous philosophy of palliation alone to attempted cure. Therapy usually consists of a combination of HAART, prophylaxis against opportunistic infections, intrathecal chemotherapeutic prophylaxis, and the usual chemotherapeutic regimen offered to HIV-negative individuals [159]. Impressively, the survival rate of HIV-associated DLBCL is approaching that of the general population [159].

Natural Killer/T-Cell Lymphoma

Non-B-cell lymphomas of the ocular adnexa are rare, estimated to occur in 1–3% of OAL cases [166–168]. Like BL, natural killer/T-cell lymphoma (NKTL) is an EBV-associated malignancy. A natural killer (NK) cell is a unique form of circulating lymphocyte that does not need antigenic priming to mount a cytotoxic reaction to a variety of tumor cells and infectious agents [169, 170].

Orbital involvement by NKTL is most likely secondary to spread from the adjacent sinonasal cavities, which normally harbor a population of NK and cytotoxic T cells (Fig. 50.11) [171]. Of eight cases of ocular adnexal NKTL in a recent study, only three had no evidence of sinonasal disease, with one additional isolated orbital case reported recently [172]. Sinonasal NKTL is characterized by the WHO system as *extranodal NKTL, nasal type*, and does not affect the orbit frequently [173]. Over the years, sinonasal NKTL has had a variety of monikers, including idiopathic midline destructive lesion, angiocentric lymphoma, malignant midline granuloma, and lethal midline granuloma [174]. Ocular adnexal involvement is associated with systemic involvement: of the aforementioned eight patients described by Woog and colleagues, only one had no evidence of systemic disease [169].

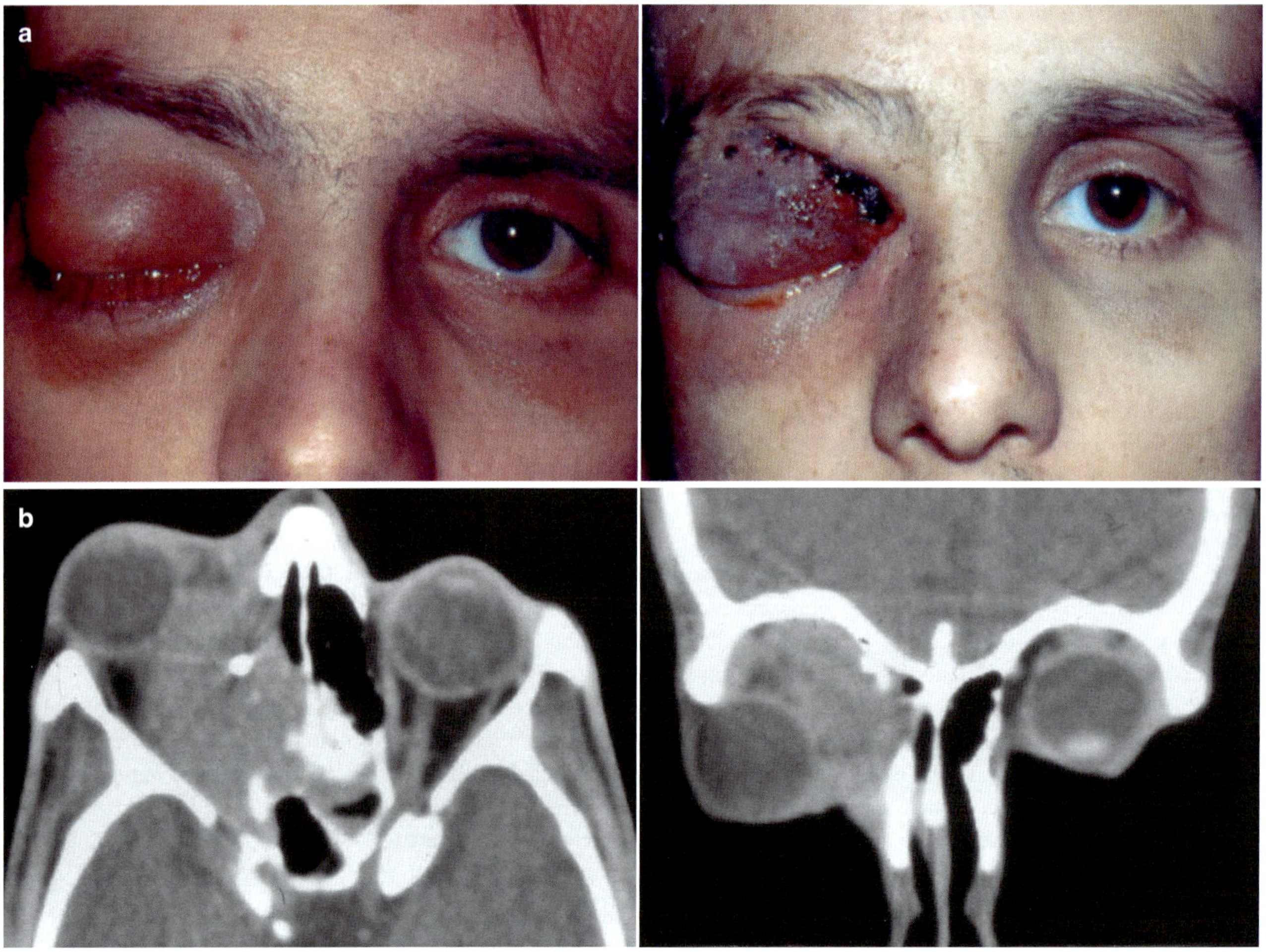

Fig. 50.10 Sinoorbital ARL. (**a**) Clinical photograph of a patient with end-stage AIDS with rapidly progressive proptosis and ptosis over 4 days. Left, on presentation. The patient was also severely anemic and thrombocytopenic. Right, 2 days later, note the marked progression and eyelid necrosis. (**b**) CT, axial (left) and coronal (right) soft tissue views. Note the bone destruction and involvement of the adjacent right ethmoid sinus. Atypical infection was suspected clinically and urgent biopsy was performed, revealing a high-grade B-cell lymphoma. The patient died several weeks later

Of interest, nasal NKTL is rare in Western countries but occurs frequently in Asia and Central America (Fig. 50.11). EBV may play a role in development.

Akin to BL, NKTL involving the ocular adnexa follows an aggressive clinical course, with radiographic features atypical for more indolent forms of OAL: bone erosion was seen on CT in 88% of patients [169]. The disease typically spreads into the orbital cavity with signs of orbitopathy; isolated cranial neuropathies from intracranial spread are distinctly rare [174]. Initial diagnostic biopsy may be difficult and confused with inflammation, since cytokine production by the NK cells may stimulate a significant penumbra of inflammation, camouflaging the true nature of the sinoorbital process; necrotic areas with scant viable tissue are also commonly encountered [174].

As with many other forms of aggressive lymphoma, the prognosis of NKTL is closely related to stage at presentation and is not appreciably affected by a specific treatment regimen [169, 175, 176]. Woog and co-workers reported a mortality of 87.5% spanning between 5 weeks and 17 months after diagnosis; interestingly, their only long-term survivor presented with isolated disease involving the sinonasal cavity and nasolacrimal duct (stage I) [169].

T-Cell Lymphoma

As noted earlier, T-cell lymphoma is uncommon in the periocular regions when compared to its B-cell counterpart, occurring in only 6 of 222 (3%) cases of ocular adnexal NHL in one large series [42]. However, the eyelids appears to harbor a particular propensity for T-cell NHL; this is consistent with the overall propensity of T-cell lymphoma for skin involvement. As a general statement, eyelid lymphoma seems to mirror histopathologic patterns found in skin lymphoma rather than the patterns seen in OAL. In one review of 199 cases of reported

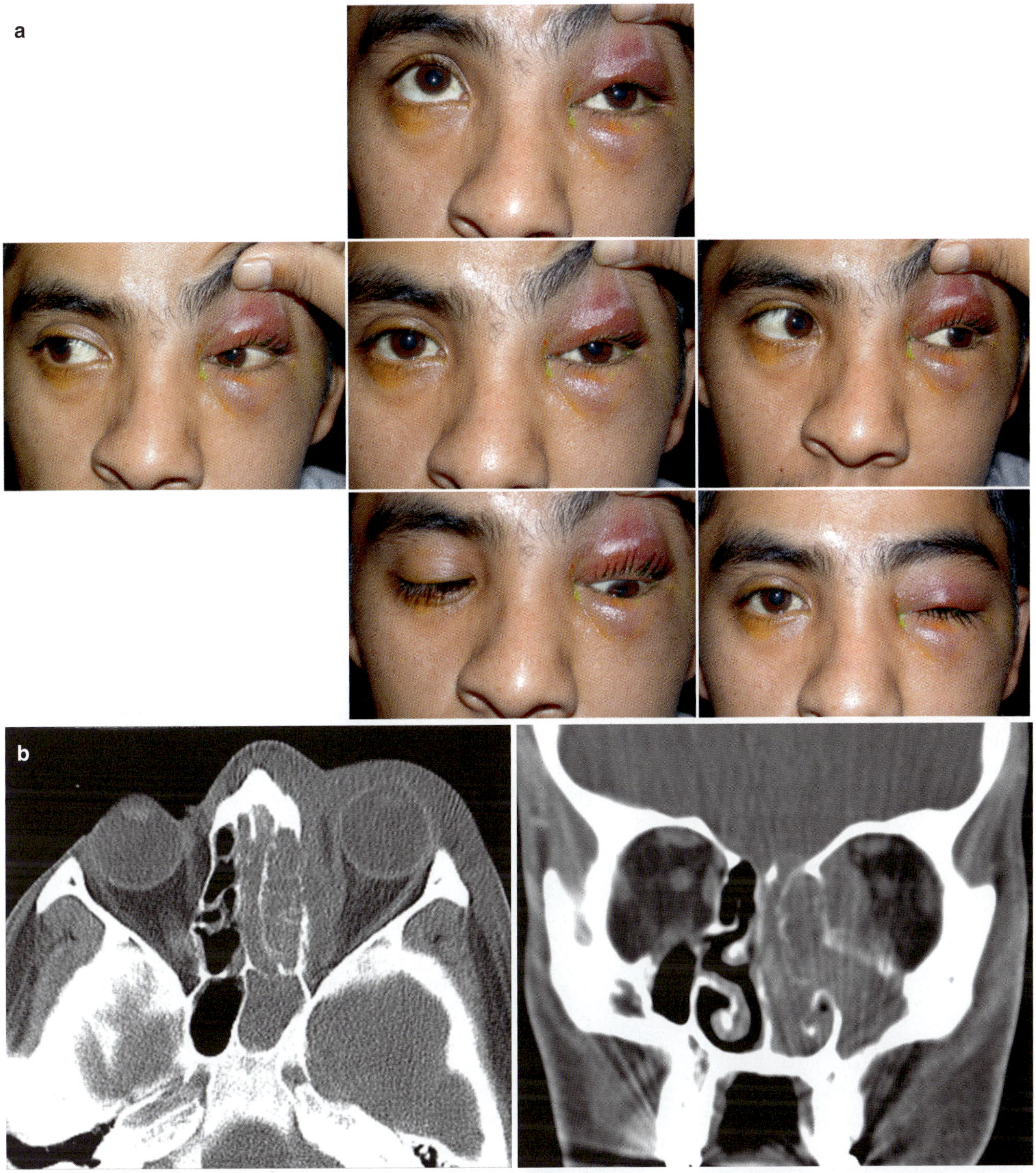

Fig. 50.11 NK/T-cell lymphoma. (**a**) External photographs of a 35-year-old immigrant from Mexico who presented to the emergency room with lid edema of several days duration. (**b**) CT, axial (left) and coronal (right) soft tissue views showing a left paranasal sinus process eroding through the orbital walls and skull base to extend intraorbitally and intracranially

eyelid NHL, 44% were of T-cell origin (12 of 87 cases of T-cell NHL were NK/T-cell lesions) [177]. When compared to B-cell lesion, T-cell lymphoma of the eyelids presents more commonly as ulceration and erythema, with a shorter mean duration of symptoms to presentation, less involvement of orbital anatomy, and unilaterality in 77% of cases [177]. Progression of eyelid T-cell lesions is 36%, with NK-T-cell lesions having the worst prognosis (see previous section) [42].

The most common form of T-cell lymphoma in the eyelids is *mycosis fungoides* (*MF*), occurring in 25% of cases, paralleling its frequency among cutaneous T-cell lymphoma overall [4]. It is typically a disease of adults and the elderly arising from the mature, skin-homing CD4+ T cell [4]. Environmental factors may play a role in MF, as it is found to occur more commonly in certain professions with chronic skin exposure to chemicals (e.g., farming, house painting) [4]. Eyelid MF mirrors the behavior of MF at other skin sites, usually following an indolent course with a good prognosis in cases of limited skin involvement. Eyelid MF has a high rate of recurrence and tends to occur as a secondary lesion to the eyelid from another skin site in most cases (68%) [42].

As with DLBCL, not otherwise specified, *peripheral T-cell lymphoma* (*PTCL*) remains in a classification limbo in the most recent WHO modification [116]. The cytogenetic distinctions of PTCL remain vague, at best. Because of this lack of specificity, therapeutic recommendations are difficult to make, and prognostic predictions may be inaccurate. PTCL may affect the ocular adnexa, occurring typically as an eyelid lesion from either systemic lymphoma or mycosis fungoides [178]. One recent case of isolated orbital PTCL has been reported, but the clinical and cytological descriptions were limited [179]. Svendsen and Heegaard reported PTCL in 3% of all eyelid lymphomas.

Primary cutaneous anaplastic large cell lymphoma (*ALCL*) has been segregated from PTCL, largely due to a distinct clinical profile, with a better prognosis than PTCL [116]. Clinically, ALCL is divided into cutaneous and systemic forms. The cutaneous form is usually a local disease in older patients and responds well to excision and radiotherapy (Fig. 50.12), while systemic ALCL occurs in a younger population and usually requires chemotherapy [178]. Periocular ALCL is the second most common (6%) T-cell NHL in the eyelids after MF and tends to be a low-grade lesion; one unique case of ALCL described both cutaneous (medial canthal) and orbital infiltration [177, 178]. A recent review of eyelid B- and T-cell lymphoma reported that ALCL occurred in 6% of cases [42]. Periocular ALCL has a good prognosis overall (90% 5-year survival) [42].

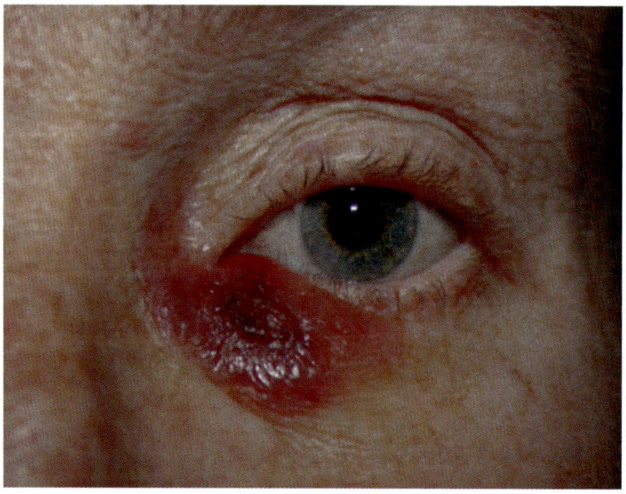

Fig. 50.12 Cutaneous ALCL (T-cell lymphoma). A middle-aged woman presented with a rapidly progressive left lower lid lesion. Biopsy revealed ALCL. Systemic work-up was negative, and the patient was treated with excision and local radiation therapy. A new lesion occurred on the contralateral side several months later and was treated identically. She has had no evidence of recurrence or systemic involvement for over 15 years

Multiple Myeloma

Multiple myeloma (MM) is a plasma cell malignancy manifesting serologically as a monoclonal hypergammaglobulinemia. It is the second most common hematologic cancer following NHL and occurs more frequently in blacks and the elderly [180].

Ocular adnexal involvement is rare and typically presents in one of three ways: (1) *plasmacytoma*, a localized plasma cell proliferation within bone, with a 50% risk of subsequent MM; (2) *primary/solitary extramedullary plasmacytoma*, a localized proliferation affecting soft tissue and, in the case of the orbit, typically spreading from an adjacent paranasal sinus; and (3) *necrobiotic xanthogranuloma*, a histiocytic disease that typically infiltrates cutaneous structures, with a 10% risk of subsequent MM [181–183]. Orbital bone and soft tissue involvement may also occur in patients with a known history of MM.

Median survival with MM is related to clinical stage, spanning from 62 months for stage I disease to only 29 months for stage 3 disease. Overall, isolated orbital lesions (plasmacytoma) have a better prognosis than systemic MM. However, a recent study reviewing plasma cell malignancy affecting the orbit refuted the classic teaching that most orbital lesions are primary and isolated; in fact, of 52 cases found on literature review, 65% of orbital lesions occurred in patients with a known history of MM (Fig. 50.13) [181]. Demographics of patients with orbital lesions mirrored that of systemic MM, and slowly progressive proptosis was the most frequent clinical finding. Radiographically, plasma cell lesions tended to affect the posterior and extraconal orbital spaces, with a distinct predilection for the superolateral orbit and greater sphenoid wing, either abutting adjacent bone with or without osseous erosion or arising from bone (Fig. 50.14) [181]; lesions of the greater sphenoid wing may be initially confused with sphenoid wing meningioma. Although orbital involvement by MM did not change prognosis, for unclear reasons, orbital plasmacytoma carried a worse prognosis than that found in other anatomic locations (28 months vs 8.3 years), but this finding should be considered inconclusive because of the usual potential biases found in retrospective literature reviews.

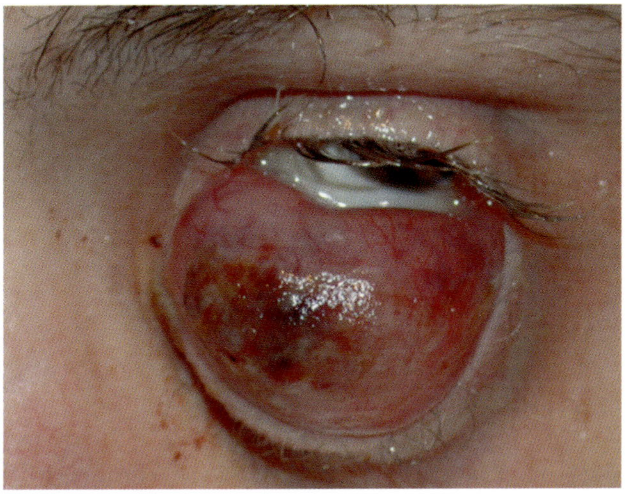

Fig. 50.13 Ocular adnexal multiple myeloma. A patient with a known history of MM presented with an expanding lesion. Biopsy confirmed MM

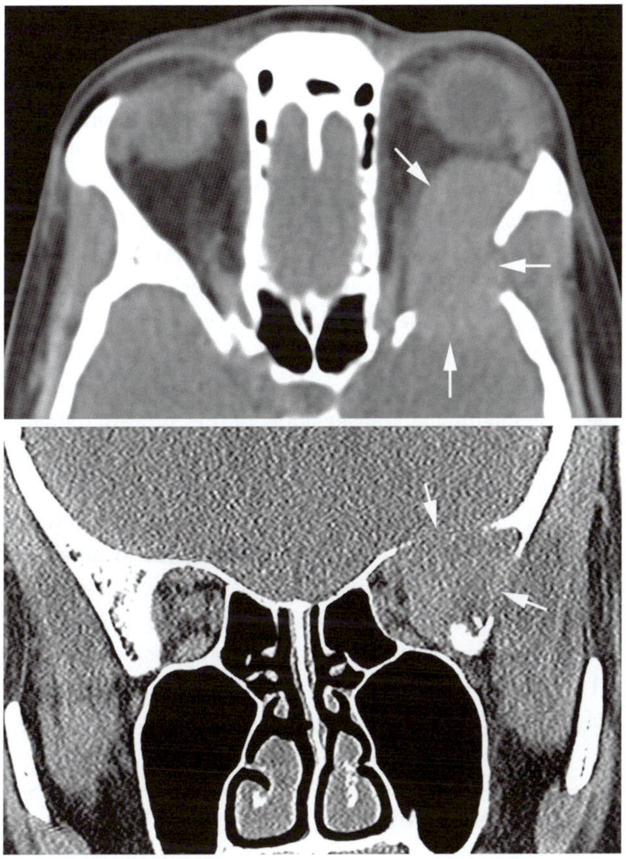

Fig. 50.14 A patient with a known history of multiple myeloma presented with progressive proptosis and an osteolytic lesion centered around the left greater sphenoid wing (arrows). Top: soft tissue axial CT image. Bottom: soft tissue coronal CT image. Hematology/oncology requested biopsy to confirm the diagnosis prior to radiotherapy, and MM was confirmed histopathologically

Pathology, Immunology, and Cytogenetics

The morphologic nuances seen on histopathologic examination of OALD and OAL are beyond the scope of this chapter and are of little practical use to the clinician. Similarly, a listing of immunologic markers found in specific OAL subtypes is an evolving, complex process. The reader is referred to an excellent recent overview by Coupland [5]. However, a broad overview of the subject affords the clinician a basic understanding of the terminology and the recent advances in pathologic diagnosis.

The use of immunohistochemistry is now a standard approach in identifying specific subtypes of OALD. Prior to its availability, diagnosis was based mainly on morphology, which was subject to a high degree of subjectivity among observers. Immunohistochemistry has allowed for the identification of clonality. Flow cytometry provides an even more specific immunophenotyping by allowing for a quantitative analysis of single cells. Immunphenotypic patterns, while certainly not foolproof, contain an inherent objective reproducibility, facilitating a more standardized categorization of OALD. As an example, the immunohistochemical pattern of CD20, CD5, and cyclin D1 positivity is typical and specific for MCL. Table 50.6 summarizes the basic immunohistochemical patterns of B-cell NHL. Note that the data in the table applies to all B-cell NHL and not specifically to OAL.

Cytogenetic aberrations are an important advance in the diagnosis and management of OAL [1, 5]. Analysis of B-cell heavy chain rearrangements can now be identified in small specimens using DNA amplification with polymerase chain reaction (PCR) and fluorescent in situ hybridization (FISH) techniques. Specific nonrandom chromosomal alterations (e.g., translocations) within a polyclonal lesion diagnosed as lymphoid hyperplasia in some cases greatly increase the odds of malignant transformation and may have predictive value as to the subtype of potential lymphoma formation. That said, it remains unclear exactly how predictive the presence of gene rearrangement is with regard to eventual lymphoma formation in a polyclonal lesion: amplification techniques using only small samples of DNA may provide false-positive data [15]. As mentioned earlier, up to 70% of healthy adults may manifest the t(14;18)(q32;q21) clonality in circulating B cells, with no evidence of subsequent malignant proliferation or behavior [3].

As noted previously, certain NHL subtypes harbor characteristic genetic footprints, but they are rarely pathognomonic (Table 50.7). Furthermore, specific genetic mutations vary within an NHL subtype depending on the anatomic location. As an example, the classic gastric and pulmonary EMZL translocations (t(11;18)q24;q21), t(1;14)(p22;q32), t(14;18)(q32;q21), and t(3;14)(p13;q32)), all activators of the NF-κB pathway, occur rarely in the ocular adnexa [40,

Table 50.6 Immunophenotypic analysis of mature B-cell NHL

	CD20 (B-cell marker)	CD3 (T-cell marker)	CD5	CD10	CD23	CD43	BCL2 (germinal center marker)	BCL6 (germinal center marker)	Cyclin D1
EMZL/MALT	+	–	–[a]	–	–	–/+	+/–[b]	–	–
FL	+	–	–[a]	+/–	–/+	–	+/–	+	–
MCL	+	–	+	–	–	+	–/+	–	+
DLBCL	+	–	–[a]	–/+[c]	N/A	–/+	–/+	+/–[c]	–
CLL/SCL	+	–	+	–	+	+	+ [243]	–	–
BL	+	–	–	+	–	–/+	–/+	+	–

Modified from Refs. [4, 241, 242]
+ = >90% of cases; +/– = >50% of cases; –/+ = <50% of cases; – = <10% of cases
[a]Occasional EMZL/MALT, FL, and DLBCL may be CD5+
[b]BCL2 expressed only in low-grade lesions
[c]Germinal center DLBCL are CD10+ and BCL6+

Table 50.7 Molecular genetic footprints for OAL

OAL subtype	Molecular genetic aberration	Percentage of cases
EMZL[a]	Trisomy 3	38
	Trisomy 18	6
	t(11;18)(q21:q21) with API2/MALT1	0–10
	t(14:18)(q32;q21) with IGH/MALT1	0–25
	t(3;14)(p14.1;q32)	14
	t(1:14)(p22;q32) with BCL10/IGH	0
	A20 inactivation (6q23 deletion or mutation)	20
	MYD88 alteration (gain-of-function)	25
FL	t(14:18)(q32;q21) with rearrangement *BCL2* (results in high level of BCL2 protein expression: centrocytes/centroblasts do not undergo usual apoptosis)	50–80
	EZH2 gain-of-function and *ARIDIA* loss of function (chromatin modifiers)	22
DLBCL		
GC-DLBCL	Translocation of *BCL2, BCL6, MYC, MEF2B*	?
	EZH2 gain-of-function and *ARIDIA* loss of	?
	function (chromatin modifying genes)	?
	BCL2 amplification	?
	t(14:18)(q32,q21)	34
	MYC rearrangement	?
ABC-DLBCL	*MYD88* alteration (gain-of-function)	83
MCL	t(11;14)(q13;q32) with upregulation of *BCL1* and cyclin D1 overexpression (enhanced cell proliferation)	79–100

Data modified from Refs. [1, 4, 5, 41, 244, 245]
[a]EMZL translocations appear to be site specific (home to a specific location). *A20* umor necrosis factor, alpha-induced protein 3, *BCL1, 2, 6, 10* B-cell lymphoma 1, 2, 6, 10 gene, respectively, *IGH* immunoglobulin heavy locus, *MYC* proto-oncogene, *MYD88* myeloid differentiation factor 88, *EZH2* enhancer of zeste homolog 2, *ARIDIA* AT-rich interactive domain-containing protein 1A, *MEF2B* myocyte enhancer factor 2B, *?* aberration identified, but inadequate number of cases reported for prevalence analysis

86]. The heterogeneity of genetic variation in EMZL/MALT supports the hypothesis that this disease is a manifestation of a final common pathway from a heterogeneous group of antigenic stimuli.

To put this into an oversimplified context, the majority of OAL genetic aberration target the NF-κB signaling pathway, leading to cellular proliferation (Fig. 50.1). Recent studies have shown that in a subset of OA EMZL/MALT, *A20* inactivation disinhibits the NF-κB pathway, leading to unchecked cellular proliferation. Presence of this aberration portends a worse prognosis and appears to require higher doses of external beam radiation therapy (EBRT) to control [86]. Other aberrations result in decreased apoptosis within the NF-κB pathway – the t(14:18)(q32,q21) of FL causes an overexpression of *BCL2*, an antiapoptotic gene. In the murkiness of DLBCL classification, 15–30% of lesions do not follow easily defined patterns. However, note that the GCL-DLBCL and ABC-DLBCL have distinct footprints based on their specific cell of evolution (Fig. 50.1), leading to a significantly different clinical behavior. Also note that the aforementioned translocation of FL is also found in GCL-DLBCL, explaining why FL has the potential for transformation into GCL-DLBCL.

Finally, some genetic patterns are extremely specific to certain NHL subtypes, regardless of anatomic location. The classic example of an almost pathognomonic aberration is the t(11:14)(q32;q32) translocation, identified in 79–95% of MCL, resulting in cyclin D1 overexpression, whereas the t(14;18) translocation of FL causes an overexpression of bcl-2 (Table 50.7) [184].

Clinical Presentation

The presenting symptoms and signs of patients with OALD are varied. The classic presentation is that of an older individual with few if any symptoms presenting with a well-tolerated, indolent lesion of the ocular adnexa. While this scenario is indeed the norm for OALD, it is by no means the sine qua non. Several series have elucidated other less common but important clinical features of OALD/OAL (Table 50.8); note that these series reported on OAL overall, without a separate analysis for each subtype [1, 2, 185, 186]. In a histopathologic review of 353 cases by Ferry and colleagues using the WHO modification of the REAL classification [12], the mean age was 64 years, mirroring that found in other series [3, 11, 12], but the age range was considerably broader. That said, it is important to once again stress the rarity of OALD/OAL in the pediatric population: only 5 of 353 patients (1.4%) were younger than 21 years. There was no clear gender predilection noted, but this varies by subtype of NHL – as noted, MCL has a distinct male predilection [2, 52]. Overall, the majority (78%) of patients presented with no known history of lymphoma; only one in five patients had a known history of systemic disease. Bilateral lesions were present in 12% of patients. Once again, it must be stressed that much of this "overall" OALD analysis is outdated – when possible, it is best to analyze OALD based on specific subtype (Tables 50.5 and 50.9) [2].

Table 50.8 Clinical characteristics of OAL. Data extracted from Refs. [34, 36, 246]

	Jenkins et al. Moorfields (*n* = 326)	Sullivan et al. Royal Brisbane (*n* = 69)	Demirci et al. Wills Eye (*n* = 106)
Location	Ocular adnexa	Ocular adnexa	Orbit only
Ave. age (range) M:F	66 years (3–90) 1:1	66 years (11–90) 3:4	69 years (2–93) 3:2
Pain Inflammation	7% (soreness in 21%) N/A	20% 30%	8% 6%
Duration before diagnosis	>12 months in 22%	7.4 months	6 months
Incorrect referral diagnosis	N/A	43% (7% as IOIS)	N/A
Systemic disease on presentation	19%	47%	44%

Table 50.9 Distribution of NHL subtypes by ocular adnexal anatomic site

NHL subtype	Orbit (%)	Eyelid (%)	Conjunctiva (%)
EMZL	57	14–37	68
FL	11	5–23	16
DLBCL	15	9–10	5
MCL	8	4–8	7
BL/BLL	1	2	<0.1
NK/T cell	0	6	0
MF	0.3	9–13	0

Data from Refs. [2, 177, 185, 186]
MF mycosis fungoides

With regard to OAL, additional features should be stressed. In all likelihood, these findings can also be extended to OALD in general. It is important to remember that in most patients, it is next to impossible to distinguish polyclonal lymphoid hyperplasia from indolent lymphoma either clinically or radiographically; histopathology (with immunohistochemistry and molecular genetic analysis) remains the gold standard in this regard. First, the duration of symptoms was on average measured in months rather than in days or weeks. This supports the teaching that in most cases, OALD represents an indolent process in the majority of patients. A cautionary finding of pain or soreness was seen in 7–20% of patients, with a trend to more aggressive histopathology; classically, OALD is thought to present in a painless fashion. Also of importance is the finding by Sullivan and colleagues that 43% of patients with an eventual diagnosis of OAL were initially misdiagnosed, with 7% of the total incorrectly diagnosed as IOIS [132].

On examination, OALD may present as a "salmon patch" in the conjunctiva, appearing as a pink lesion that ranges from a flat infiltrate to a nodular mass (Fig. 50.15) [35, 36]. It is extremely important to check the conjunctival cul-de-sacs and tarsal conjunctiva in all patients, as OALD may hide in these areas (Fig. 50.15). Furthermore, subtle involvement of the cul-de-sacs may be missed, especially in elderly patients. Comparison with the contralateral side for asymmetry may be helpful, and palpation of the eyelid and anterior orbit may reveal a rubbery nodularity. Patients may also complain of puffy or swollen eyelids with no other external signs; again, palpation is crucial in such cases. A rubbery mass in the lacrimal gland may be misdiagnosed initially as dacryoadenitis, although significant pain is typically not a feature of lacrimal gland lymphoma (Fig. 50.16); bilateral lacrimal gland enlargement may occur (Fig. 50.17). Axial exophthalmos may also occur, typically without any associated external ophthalmoplegia; nonaxial globe dystopia is much less frequent (Fig. 50.18). Severely restricted extraocular motility is possible, but uncommon in OALD, even with large masses (Fig. 50.19). On occasion, a patient may present with blepharoptosis secondary to OALD involvement of the superior cul-de-sac, the preaponeurotic fat pad, or the levator aponeurosis (Fig. 50.20). Trigeminal dysesthesia and other cranial neuropathies are distinctly uncommon in lymphoma; infiltration along sensory nerves may be seen occasionally and confused with IgG4-related disease (Fig. 50.21). In OALD this would generally occur by direct nerve infiltration when extension to the skull base has occurred [187]. Intraocular vascular occlusion and optic neuropathy are also rare in OALD. However, certain subtypes of OAL (MCL, ARL) can behave in an extremely aggressive fashion, presenting with rapidly progressive orbital and central nervous system signs (Fig. 50.22) [34, 35].

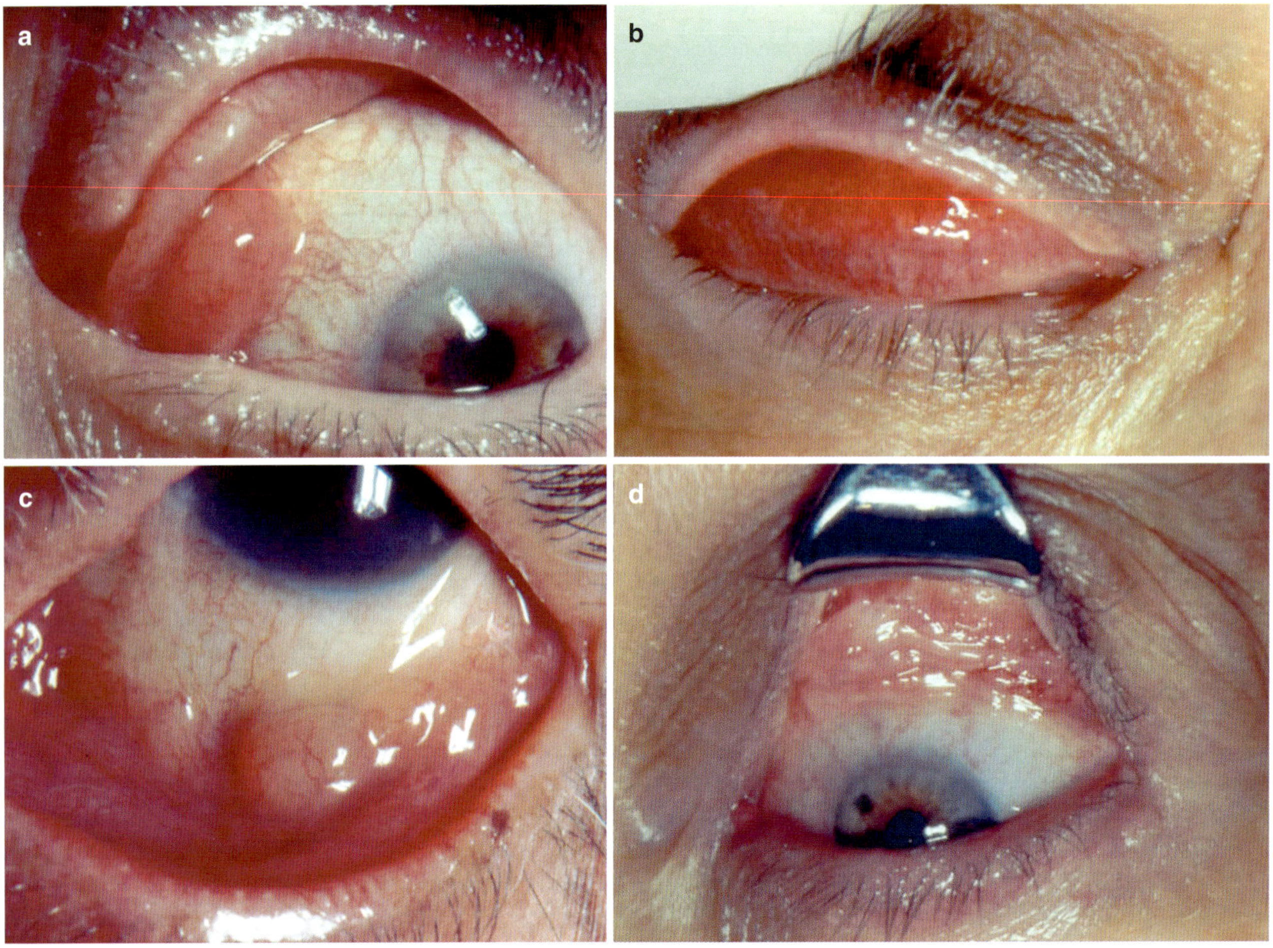

Fig. 50.15 Conjunctival OAL. (**a**) A classic "salmon patch" emanating from the palpebral lobe of the lacrimal gland and extending along the bulbar conjunctiva. (**b**) Infiltration of the tarsal conjunctiva. (**c**) A multifocal, nodular presentation extending from the cul-de-sac onto the globe. (**d**) Infiltration of the superior cul-de-sac

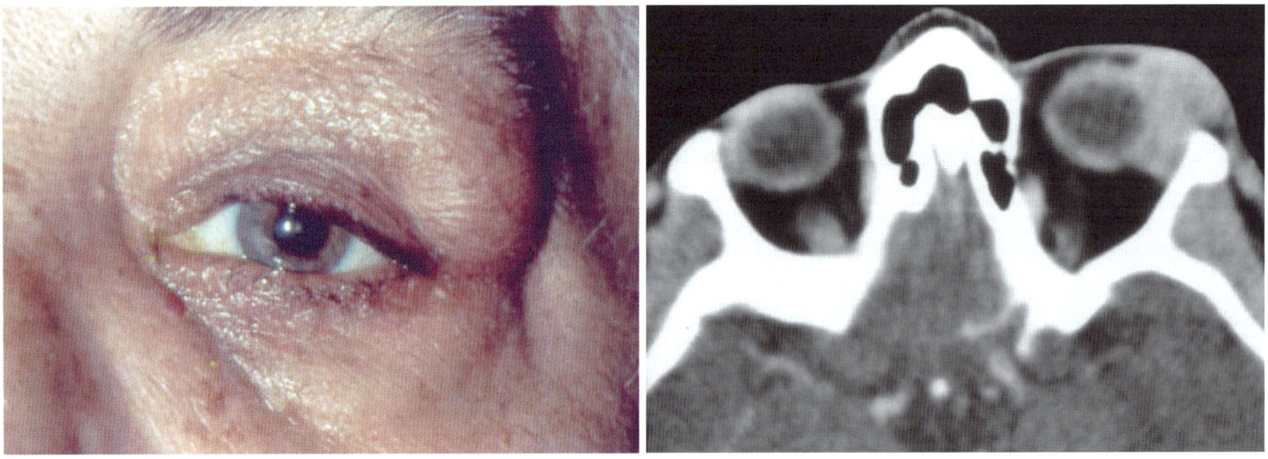

Fig. 50.16 Lacrimal gland enlargement presenting with a rubbery mass and an S-shaped lid (left). Note the lack of overlying skin edema and erythema. Axial CT image, soft tissue window (right) shows a typical pattern for AOL: respect for the native anatomy, no adjacent bone erosion, and involvement of both the orbital and palpebral lobes of the lacrimal gland

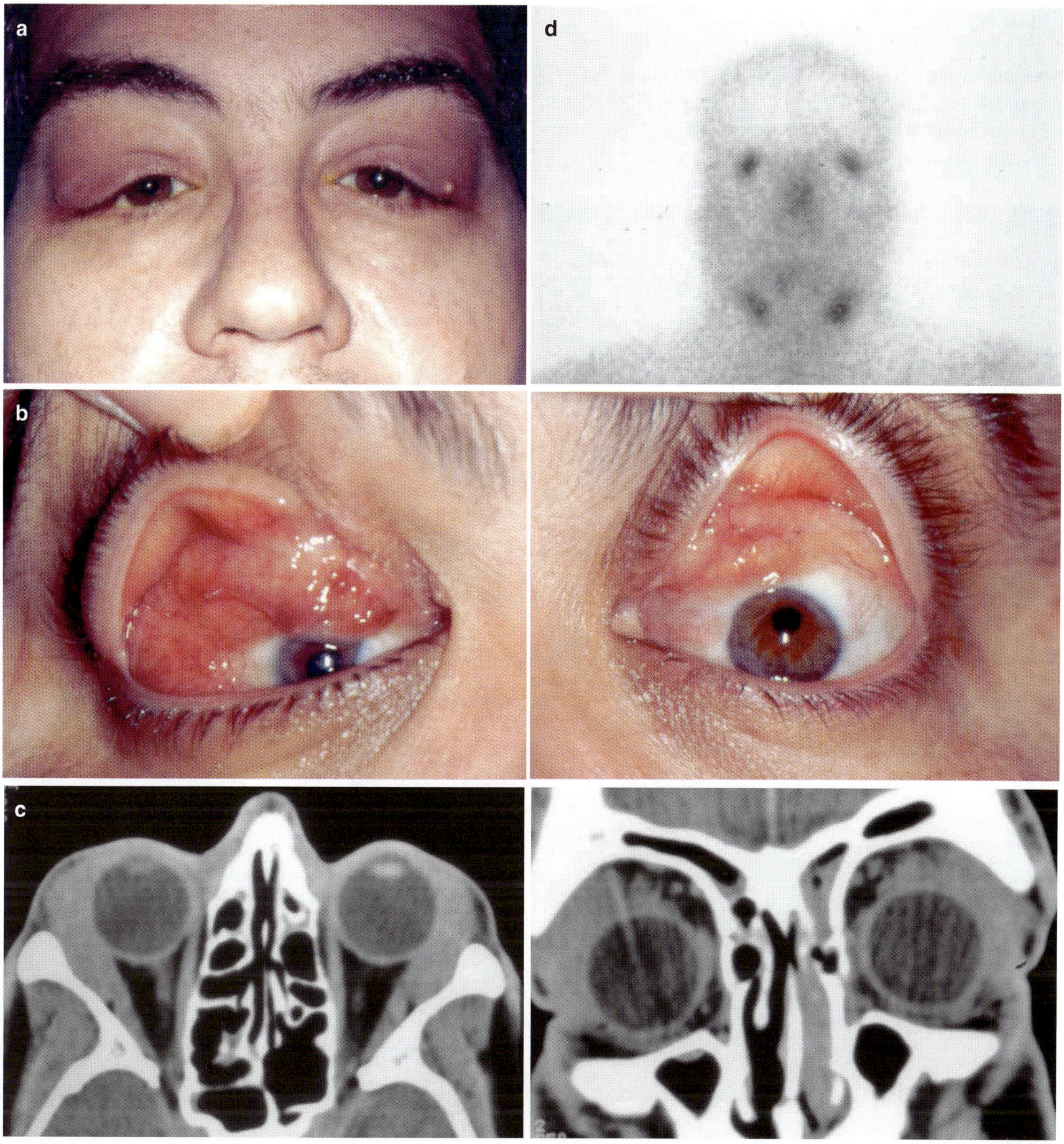

Fig. 50.17 Bilateral lacrimal gland and conjunctival lesions in a patient with a history of ulcerative colitis. (**a**) S-shaped eyelids suggest a lateral anterior orbital process. (**b**) Bilateral conjunctival salmon patches extending from the lacrimal glands. (**c**) CT, axial (left) and coronal (right) soft tissue images show lacrimal gland masses molding to the native anatomy. (**d**) Gallium scan also revealed bilateral cervical adenopathy. Subsequent biopsy showed a polyclonal proliferation consistent with lymphoid hyperplasia

Imaging

Imaging of OALD can be divided into two categories: (1) initial local imaging for diagnosis and surgical planning and (2) subsequent systemic imaging for staging and tumor surveillance.

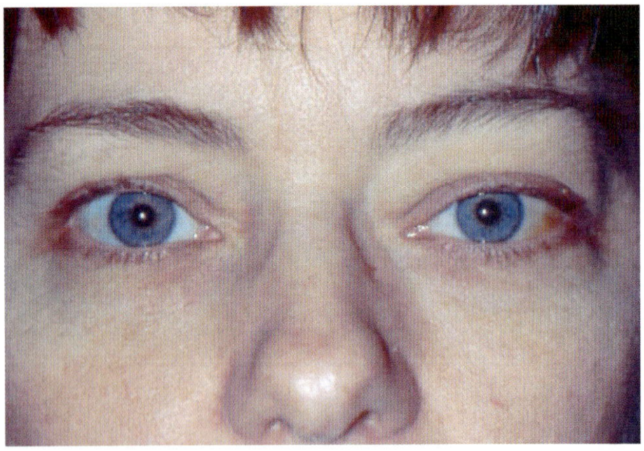

Fig. 50.18 Painless, minimally progressive axial proptosis in a young woman subsequently diagnosed with EMZL/MALT

As a rule, all cases of OALD should undergo orbital imaging. There is a tendency among some clinicians to forego imaging in patients presenting with conjunctival lesions, assuming that this is an isolated finding, when in fact the conjunctival abnormality may only be the proverbial "tip of the iceberg" of a deeper, subclinical orbital process; in one study, orbital involvement was identified with imaging in 50% of patients presenting with conjunctival lesions [188]. Depending on the clinical presentation and to a large degree on personal preference, a clinician may choose either computed tomography (CT) or magnetic resonance imaging (MRI) as the initial modality. The advantages and disadvantages of these technologies are discussed elsewhere [189]. A few brief comments will be made here. CT is preferable when bony anatomy is of importance or when patients are claustrophobic but CT exposes the patient to radiation. MRI is excellent for imaging the orbital apex, cavernous sinus, and skull base but must be performed correctly to optimize the results and lacks the detailed bony anatomy seen on CT; gadolinium and fat suppression (saturation) should be used in all orbital MRI studies. Orbital MRI takes considerably longer to perform than CT (which takes less than 1 min using

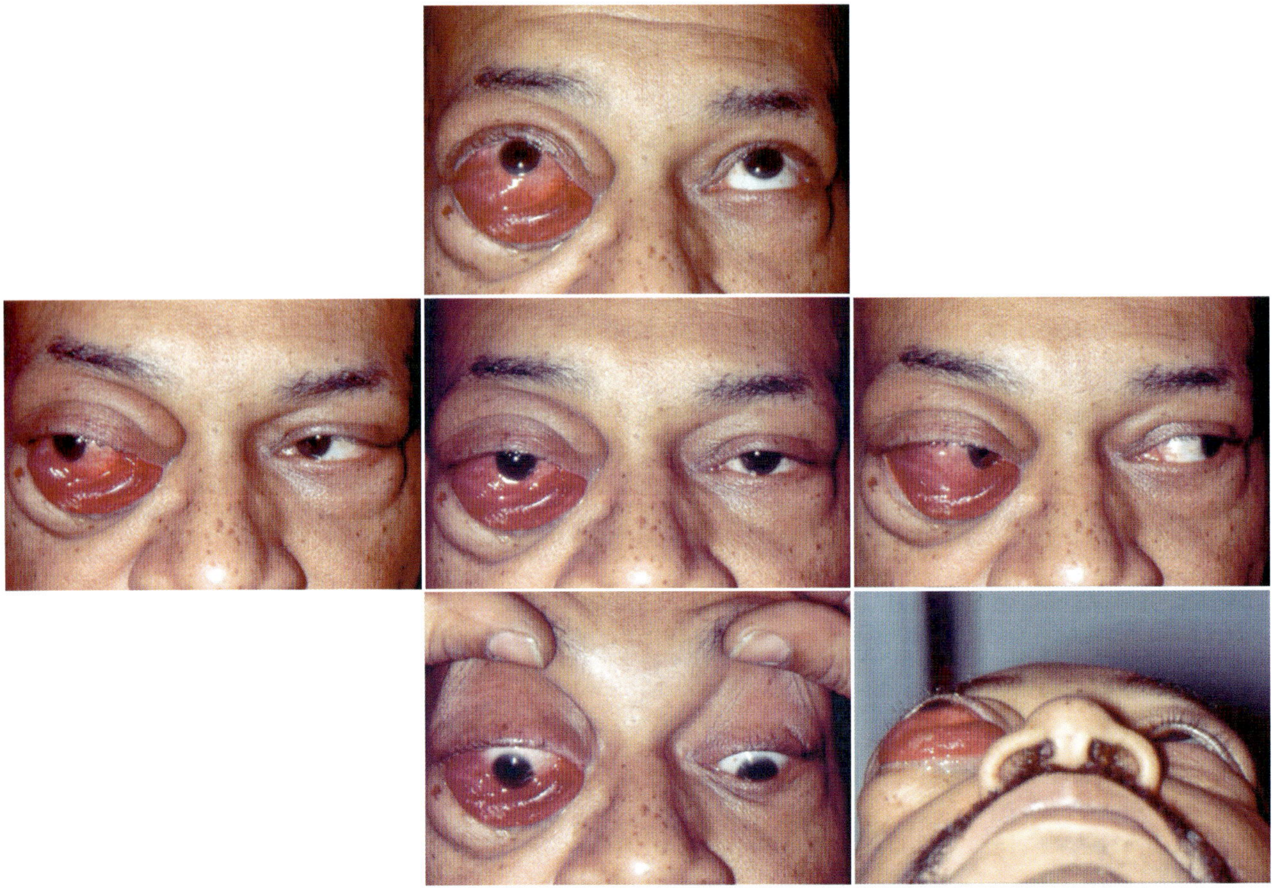

Fig. 50.19 Significant proptosis, orbital congestion, and chemosis in a patient with a neglected orbital process. Biopsy confirmed the clinical suspicion of OAL. Note that despite the impressive orbital signs, no significant external ophthalmoplegia is present, a typical finding in OALD

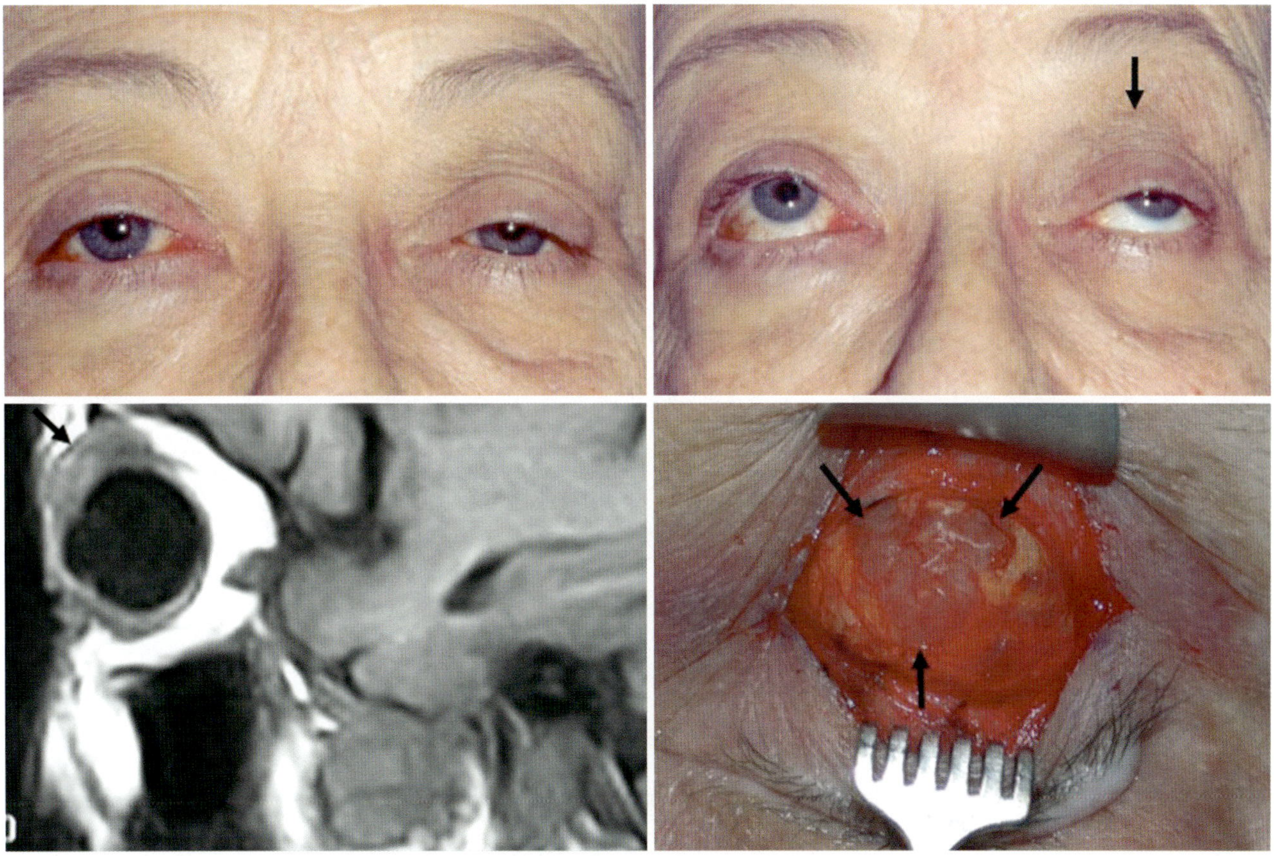

Fig. 50.20 Upper left: an elderly woman was referred for left ptosis repair. Upper right: on upgaze, a nodularity appeared in her superior sulcus (arrow), with a rubbery consistency. Lower left: MRI revealed a mass infiltrating the levator/superior rectus complex (arrow). Lower right: an infiltrating mass (arrows) was noted in the levator aponeurosis and muscle. Histopathology showed EMZL/MALT

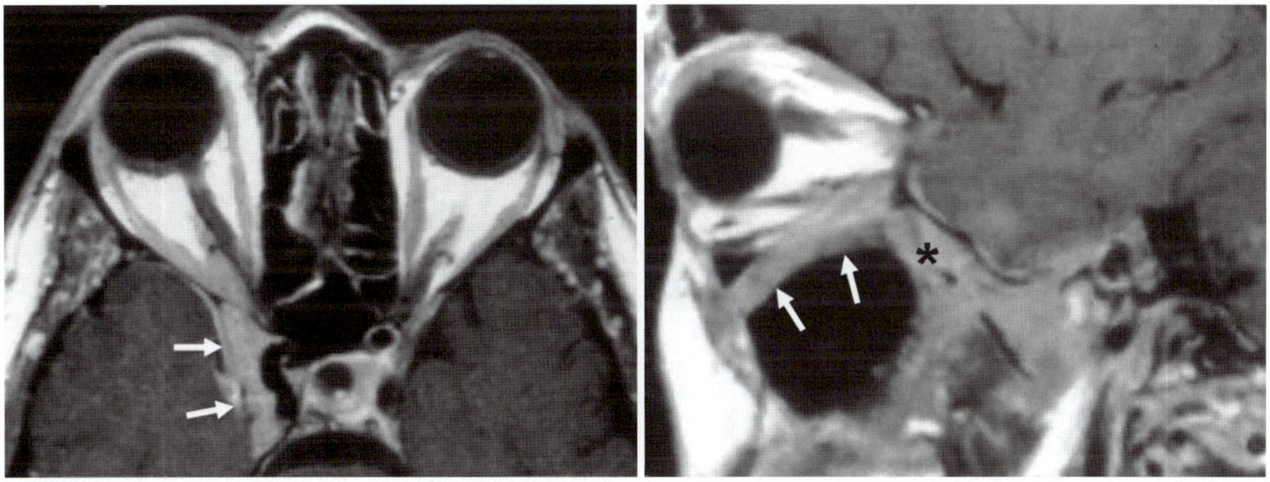

Fig. 50.21 MRI, T1-weighted with fat suppression and contrast. Left, axial, with marked infiltration of the left cavernous sinus (arrows). Right, parasagittal view with OAL infiltration of the infraorbital nerve (arrows), extending into the pterygopalatine fossa (asterisk). Despite this widespread infiltration, the patient had no evidence of cranial neuropathy or sensory abnormalities

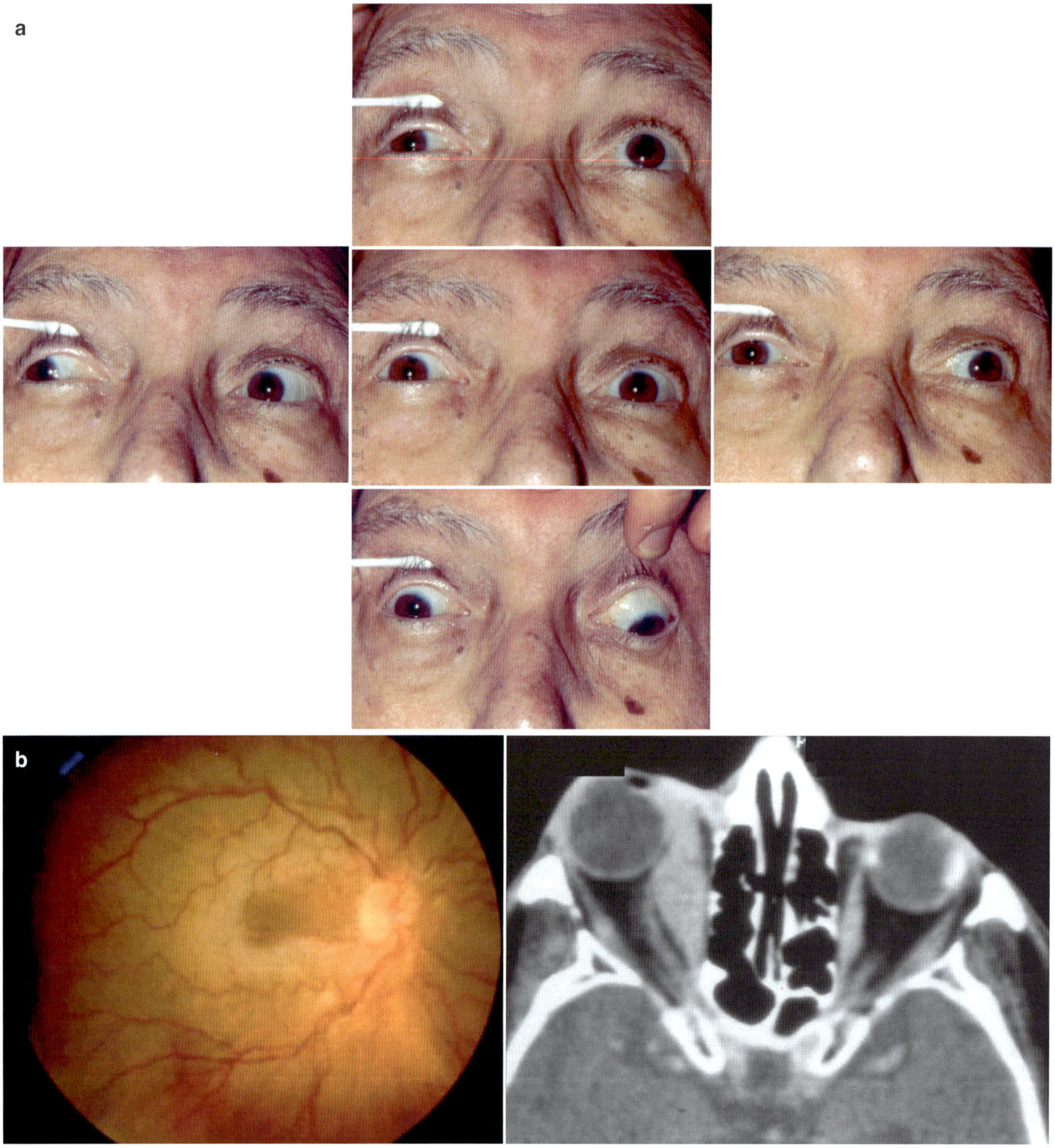

Fig. 50.22 (**a**) An elderly man presented with acute onset right ptosis and visual loss. External photographs demonstrating right CN-III palsy. (**b**) Left, funduscopy revealed a central artery occlusion with cilioretinal artery sparing. Right, enlargement of the medial rectus muscle is seen on this axial CT image, obtained several days later. Biopsy was diagnostic for MCL. (Courtesy of Peter A. D. Rubin, MD)

the newest helical techniques) and is more confining, which may be difficult for patients with claustrophobia. With both CT and MRI, it is important to order an orbital study specifically, since the protocols used for brain imaging may not include adequate orbital views. B-scan ultrasonography is still utilized in some centers for orbital disease and has the advantage of office-based availability, but is useful only for anterior lesions and lacks the anatomic detail available with CT and MRI.

On CT, OALD appears hyperdense to orbital fat and has a homogenous signal distribution. Any orbital structure (lacrimal gland, extraocular muscle, orbital fat, optic nerve) may be involved either in isolation or with adjacent structures (Fig. 50.23). The borders of the lesion may be sharply

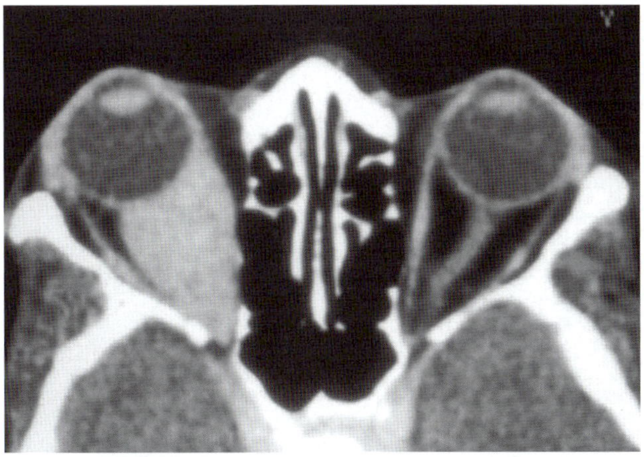

Fig. 50.23 Axial CT image, soft tissue window, of OAL. In this case, infiltration is occurring within the intraconal fat and involving the adjacent medial rectus muscle

delineated or feathery, with infiltration along the fascial planes of the intraconal fat. Less commonly lesions may be inhomogeneous or have calcification and associated bony changes [142]. Bone erosion is distinctly uncommon in OALD; when encountered, it signals the presence of an aggressive OAL (MCL, DLBCL, BL/BLL, ARL) [120, 142, 190].

T1- and T2-weighted MR images are iso- or hypointense to extraocular muscles, with moderate homogenous enhancement with gadolinium (Fig. 50.24). While bony changes are not demonstrated as well with MRI as with CT, extraorbital extension and CNS involvement are more accurately visualized [142, 191]. Diffusion-weighted imaging (DWI), reflecting the macromolecular motion of extracellular water, can be helpful at times in distinguishing lymphoma from other lesions. Lymphoma is highly

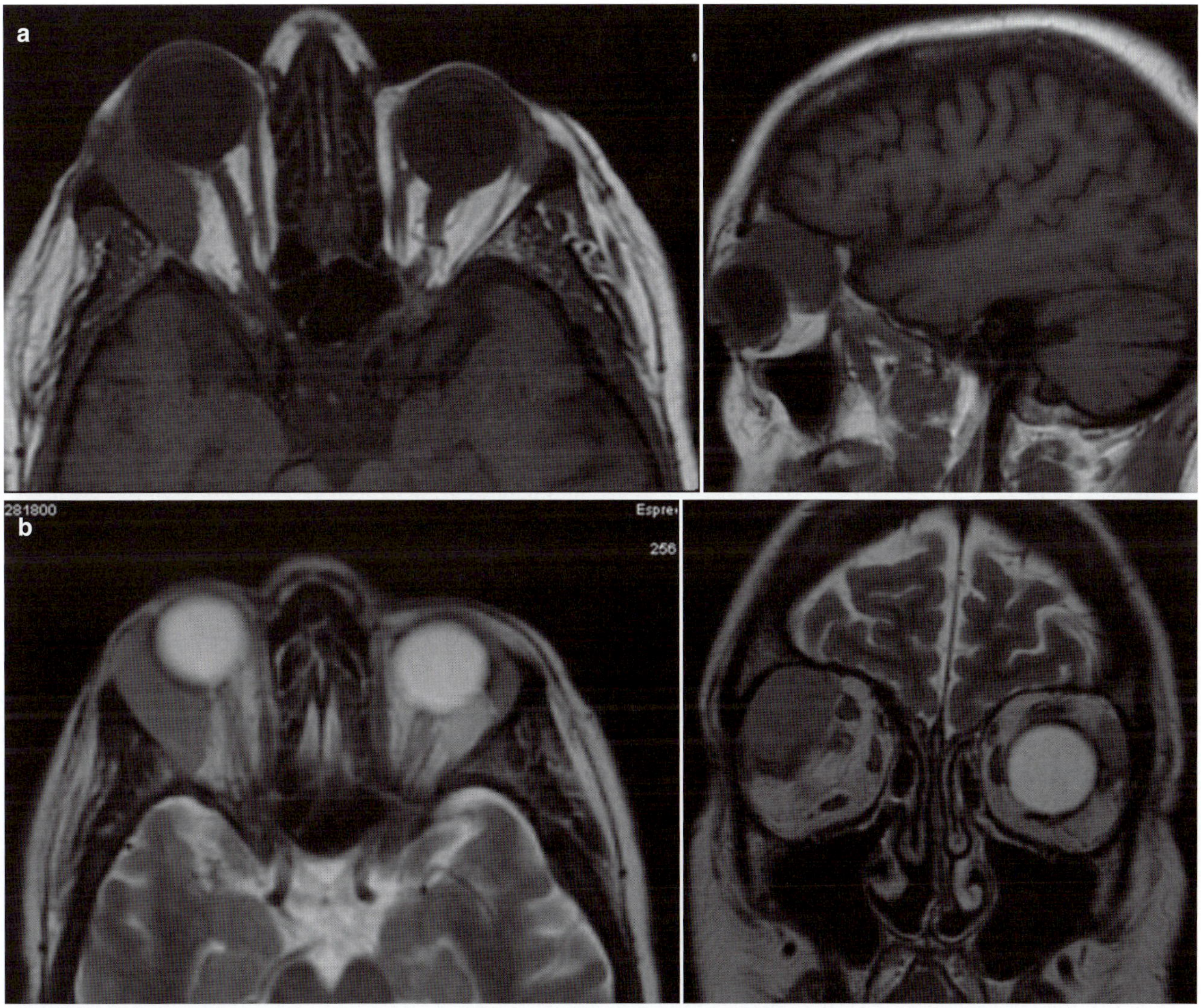

Fig. 50.24 MRI of an orbital lymphoma. (**a**) T1 precontrast axial and parasagittal images demonstrate a lacrimal gland mantle cell lymphoma that is isointense to the extraocular muscles. (**b**) On T2 images (axial and coronal), the lymphoma is slightly hyperintense to the extraocular muscles. In most cases, OALD is hypointense to the muscles, but variations may occur. (**c**) T1 post-contrast axial and coronal images with fat suppression show moderate enhancement of the lesion

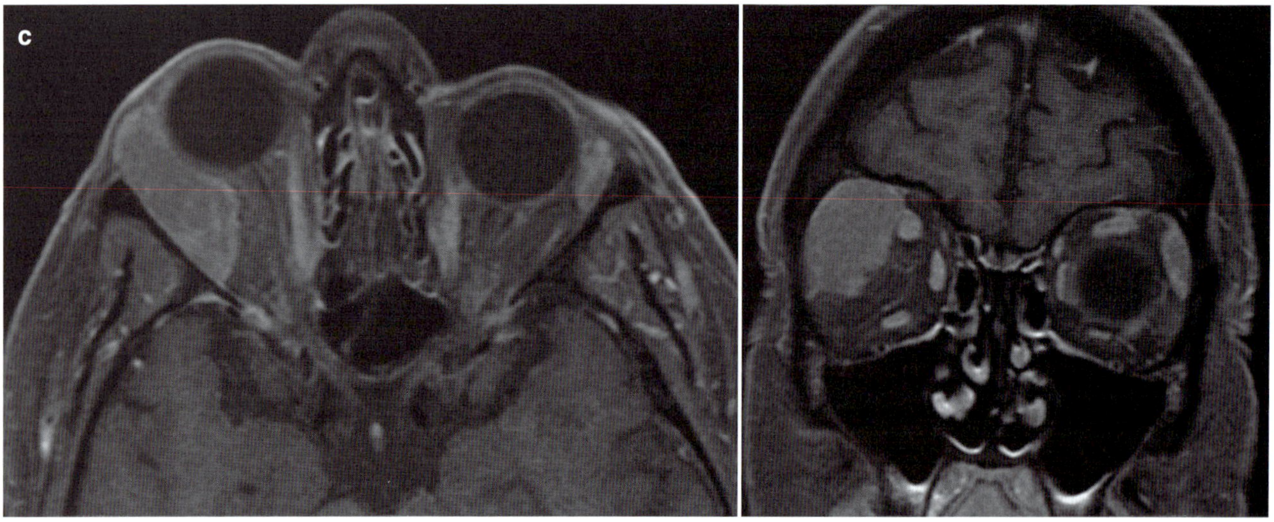

Fig. 50.24 (continued)

cellular, which leads to less Brownian motion of water molecules in the decreased amount of extracellular space. On DWI the tumor would appear hyperintense, and on apparent diffusion coefficient (ADC) maps, hypointensity would be noted (Fig. 50.25). Because DWI measures the cellularity of a lesion and is otherwise nonspecific, OALD often cannot be precisely distinguished from other hypercellular small cell tumors. The minimal ADC values for lymphoma differ from some lesions, but there is overlap with metastases [192]. Perfusion imaging, which can be used to estimate tumoral angiogenesis, may demonstrate the typical increase in intensity-time curve with lymphoma due to contrast leakage [193].

An important finding in two studies on imaging in OAL is worth stressing (Table 50.10) [36, 132]. The classic teaching regarding imaging of OAL is that the lesion invariably molds to the native anatomy, rarely causing significant distortion. In fact, this may occur in only about 50% of cases. OAL may present as a well-circumscribed lesion with distortion of adjacent structures, akin to the long list of other lesions, including cavernous venous malformation, schwannoma, solitary fibrous tumor, and lacrimal gland pleomorphic adenoma (Fig. 50.26).

Positron emission tomography (PET) is rapidly becoming the imaging modality of choice in both the staging and monitoring of systemic lymphoma [194–197]. Unlike conventional imaging with CT and MRI, which provide anatomic data, PET measures metabolic activity. Several basic points about PET are worth mentioning. First, PET is usually used in combination with CT to provide fusion films demonstrating both anatomic and metabolic features (Fig. 50.7). However, the clinician must remember that the CT used in PET/CT is of low resolution and does equal the anatomic detail provided by conventional CT or MRI. Second, metabolic activity in PET is not measured as an all or nothing phenomenon. Rather, the degree of activity is important and is reported as a standard uptake value (SUV). SUVs vary between processes, including inflammation, infection, post-surgical healing, and malignancy. Unfortunately, a significant overlap of SUV occurs among the different diagnoses, and it may be difficult to distinguish, for example, an active inflammation from a low-grade malignancy. On the other hand, the SUV is very helpful in determining the overall metabolic activity of the abnormality being imaged (Fig. 50.27) and is proving to be very useful in not only quantifying the inherent behavior of a lymphoproliferative process but also the response of said process to therapy. As an example, an OAL with systemic involvement, but a very low SUV, may simply be followed conservatively since on PET it is metabolically indolent. Similarly, if an aggressive OAL with systemic involvement fails to improve after 3–4 cycles of systemic therapy, the oncologist may choose to modify the treatment regimen in the hopes of improving response [194–199]. This second feature of PET may be extremely advantageous, allowing for more efficient and individualized therapy. However, to date there is no definitive data that altering therapeutic regimens on the basis of PET improves final patient outcome.

In OALD, and more specifically OAL, the most important advantage of PET/CT is not local imaging [200–202]. In fact, in this regard PET/CT has distinctive disadvantages at present when compared to more conventional anatomic imaging [201, 203]. First, the present limit of resolution for PET is about 5–7 mm. Second, the proximity of the orbit to the brain and its inherently high metabolic activity often limits the ability to distinguish abnormalities, especially at the orbital apex and skull base. PET/CT's greatest strength in the

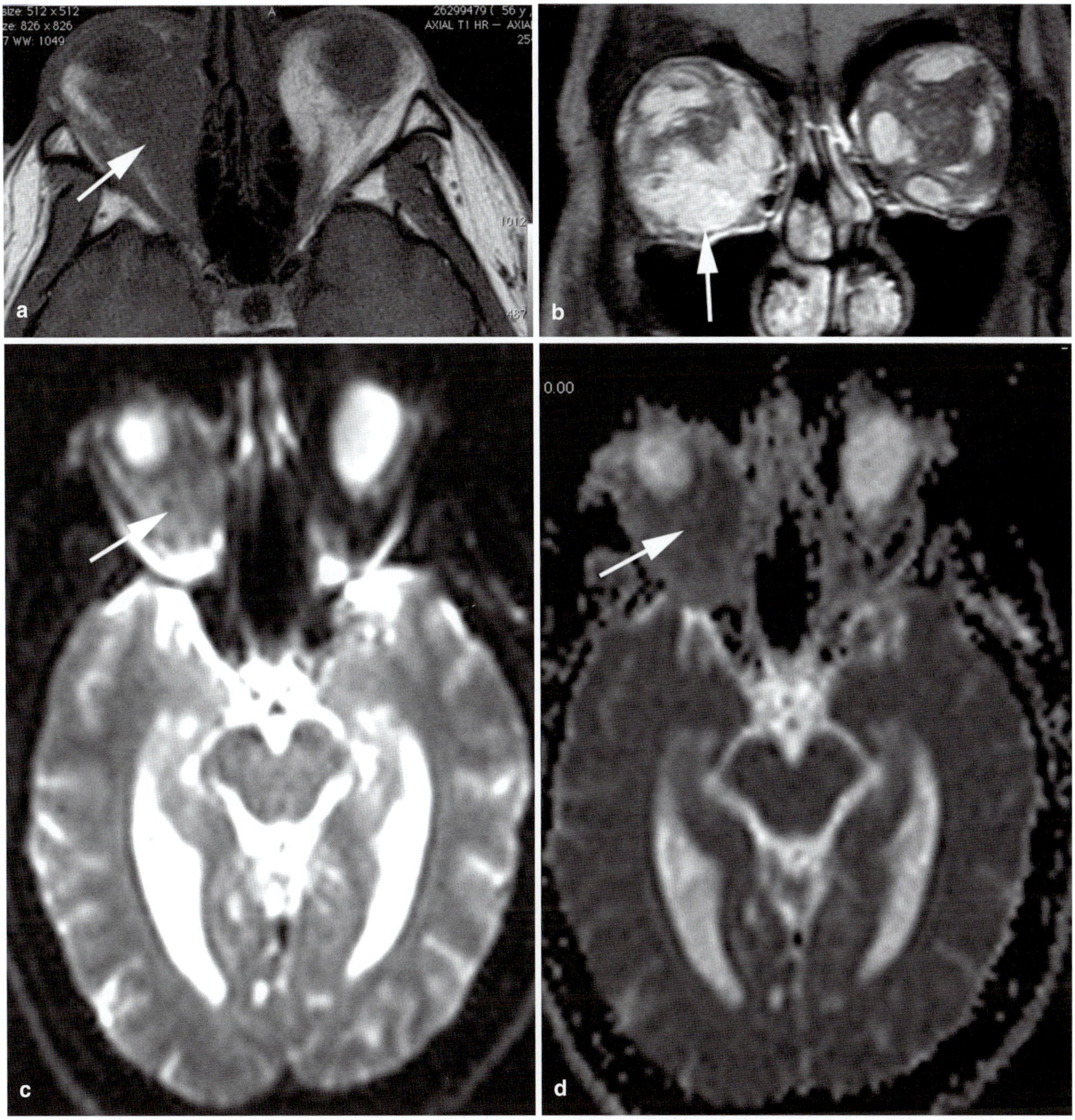

Fig. 50.25 DWI and ADC. (**a**) Precontrast, axial T1-weighted axial MRI of an infiltrating lesion (arrow) in the right inferior orbit. (**b**) Post-contrast, fat-suppressed T1-weighted coronal view of the lesion (arrow). On DWI (**c**) and ADC (**d**) views, the lesion restricts diffusion, consistent with a highly cellular process. Biopsy confirmed EMZL/MALT

Table 50.10 Imaging features of OAL

	Sullivan et al. (*n* = 105)	Demirci et al. (*n* = 106)
Molding	46% (indolent histology)	52%
Well-circumscribed	54%	48%
Bone destruction	9% (aggressive histology)	Diffuse large B cell only
MRI (T1/T2)	Iso/Iso to EOM	Iso/Iso to EOM
PET/CT	Upstaged 71% of cases	N/A

Data extracted from Refs. [36, 142]

management of OALD/OAL is the ability to accurately assess systemic disease [204]. In a small series by Valenzuela and Sullivan, PET/CT upstaged the lymphoma diagnosis more accurately than conventional imaging with CT and MRI [142, 205]. A more recent study from this center not surprisingly also found a higher sensitivity of PET/CT in more aggressive NHL subtypes (DLBCL, MCL) when compared to indolent tumors (EMZL, FL), and this has been confirmed by others [201, 203, 206].

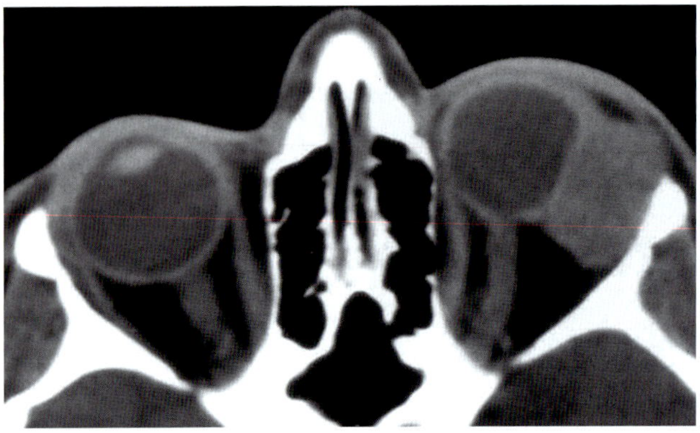

Fig. 50.26 Axial CT, soft tissue window demonstrating a well-circumscribed lacrimal gland mass in the left orbit with distortion of the sclera. The lesion was initially clinically thought to be a pleomorphic adenoma. Excisional biopsy showed OAL

Prognostic Indicators

For decades, the Holy Grail of OALD was the identification of a set of parameters to accurately prognosticate transformation of lymphoid hyperplasia into frank lymphoma, systemic involvement, and disease mortality. To say the least, it has been a bumpy ride. As an example, landmark articles of Knowles and Jakobiec [14, 123, 129] with subsequent confirmation by Jenkins et al. [34] concluded that location of involvement by OALD (Table 50.11), and not histopathology of the lesion, was of paramount importance in predicting eventual systemic lymphoma; these findings directly clashed with studies by Medeiros and Harris, which came to the opposite conclusion [207, 208]. Since that time, significant progress has been made on a number of fronts, including immunohistochemistry, cytogenetics, and accuracy of imaging in staging of disease. Rather than relying on only one parameter, it is best to consider the prognosis of for OALD as being influenced by a combination of clinical, histological, and immunophenotypic findings [209].

With regard to anatomic location, the initial findings by Knowles and Jakobiec still hold true to some degree: eyelid involvement by OALD portends a higher risk for eventual systemic lymphoma than isolated conjunctival involvement, and this is likely due to a higher affinity for more aggressive NHL subtypes in the eyelid, including a variety of T-cell lymphomas; in one study, 24% of eyelid NHL had concomitant systemic disease [177]. Jenkins and colleagues also found that with orbital involvement, lacrimal gland infiltration by OAL worsens the prognosis by increasing the incidence of systemic lymphoma as well as disease-related mortality [34]. Other studies have also concluded that bilateral adnexal and orbital disease significantly increases the risk for systemic lymphoma over time [35, 36]. Yet again, we stress that based on the WHO modification, specific location of OAL is by no means the best prognosticator for systemic disease and disease-related mortality and is likely significantly less important than immunohistochemical and cytogenetic subtype (Table 50.12) [210].

Histopathology of the OAL also has predictive value, although it is difficult to make any definitive statements, because, as stated earlier, many aggressive histopathologies are in all likelihood secondary, and not primary, lesions of the ocular adnexa [209]. Patient age is an extremely important factor in both NHL classification and prognostication, based on the 2008 WHO modification [116]. Put simply, pediatric NHL differs significantly from adult NHL, and the 2008 schema makes specific allowances for this distinction. Although pediatric OAL is notably rare, two variations are worth noting.

First, pediatric FL differs from its adult counterpart both cytogenetically and clinically. Although histologically aggressive, pediatric FL is typically a localized disease with a good prognosis. Interestingly, rare cases of florid reactive lymphoid hyperplasia may contain clonal populations and do not appear to progress to frank lymphoma (Fig. 50.28) [211]. While EMZL is distinctly rare in children, nodal marginal zone lymphoma (MZL) may occur and is afforded a separate category in the 2016 WHO revision (Table 50.2). As just mentioned, pediatric nodal MZL also occurs in the setting of rampant follicular hyperplasia, to the point where a clear distinction from FL is difficult to ascertain [116].

Overall mortality of OAL, whether primary or secondary, is summarized in Table 50.5. Both DLBCL and MCL are considered aggressive lesions with significant mortality (see sections on specific NHL for details).

Additional factors for increased mortality found in clinical series include advanced stage at presentation, MIB-1/Ki-67 staining and proliferation rate, aggressive histology, elevated serum lactate dehydrogenase level (see below), high International Prognostic Index (see below), age over 60 years, cytologic atypia, immunoglobulin heavy chain locus (IGH) gene translocation, bilateral adnexal disease, a local radiotherapy dose of $\leq$20 Gy, pain at presentation, symptoms for less than 1 year, eyelid/lacrimal gland location, and presence of optic neuropathy [34–36, 42, 120, 132, 133, 166, 167, 212–214].

1. *Lactate Dehydrogenase*

Lactate dehydrogenase (LDH, also sometimes abbreviated as LD) is an enzyme involved in anaerobic glycolysis that is found in essentially all body tissues. LDH is released during tissue damage and is therefore a potential marker for a variety of disease states. A variety of nonmalignant conditions (e.g., myocardial infarction, heart failure, hypothyroidism, acute pancreatitis, HIV infection) raise LDH levels

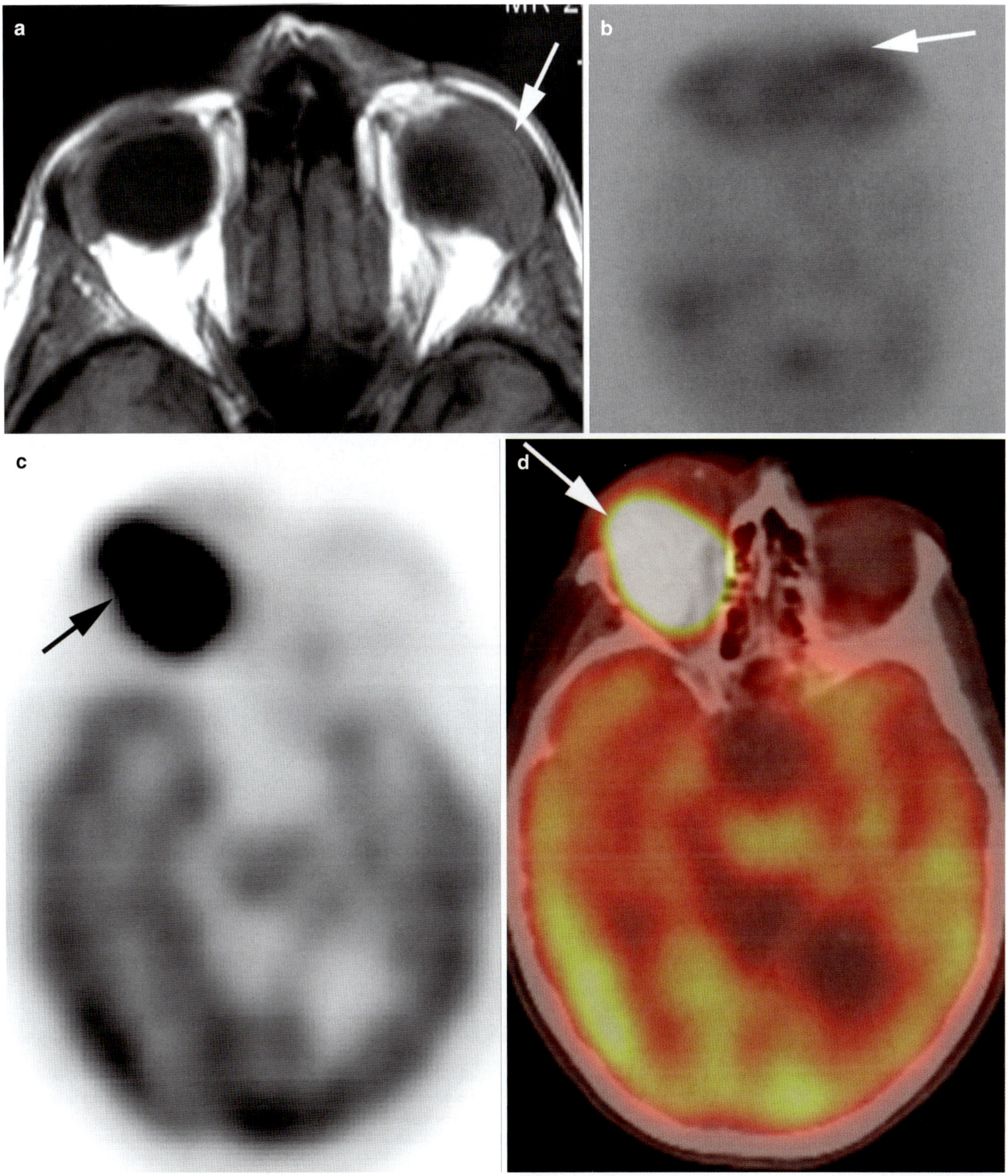

Fig. 50.27 PET for OAL. (**a**) A large lacrimal gland mass (arrow) that proved to be an indolent EMZL/MALT. (**b**) Note the minimal FDG uptake (arrow) on PET (SUV_{max} = 1.83), consistent with low metabolic activity of the tumor. (**c**) PET image with high uptake (arrow) of a neglected FL with rapid recent growth. (**d**) PET/CT fusion image of the same lesion (SUV_{max} = 21.73). The high SUV indicated a highly metabolic lesion. Biopsy confirmed transformation into a DLBCL

Table 50.11 Anatomic location of OALD and risk of systemic lymphoma

	Jakobiec and Knowles Columbia (%)	Jenkins et al. Moorfields (%)
Eyelid	67	50
Deep orbit	35	24
Lacrimal gland		38
Conjunctiva	20	21

Data extracted from Refs. [34, 117]

Table 50.12 Risk of extraorbital involvement at presentation of OAL by subtype

Subtype	Number	Evidence of extraorbital involvement (%)
EMZL/MALT	19	6 (32)
Follicular	9	7 (78)
DLBCL	9	6 (67)
Mantle cell	3	3 (100)
SCL	2	2 (100)
T cell	1	1 (100)
Total	43	25 (58)

Modified from Ref. [210]

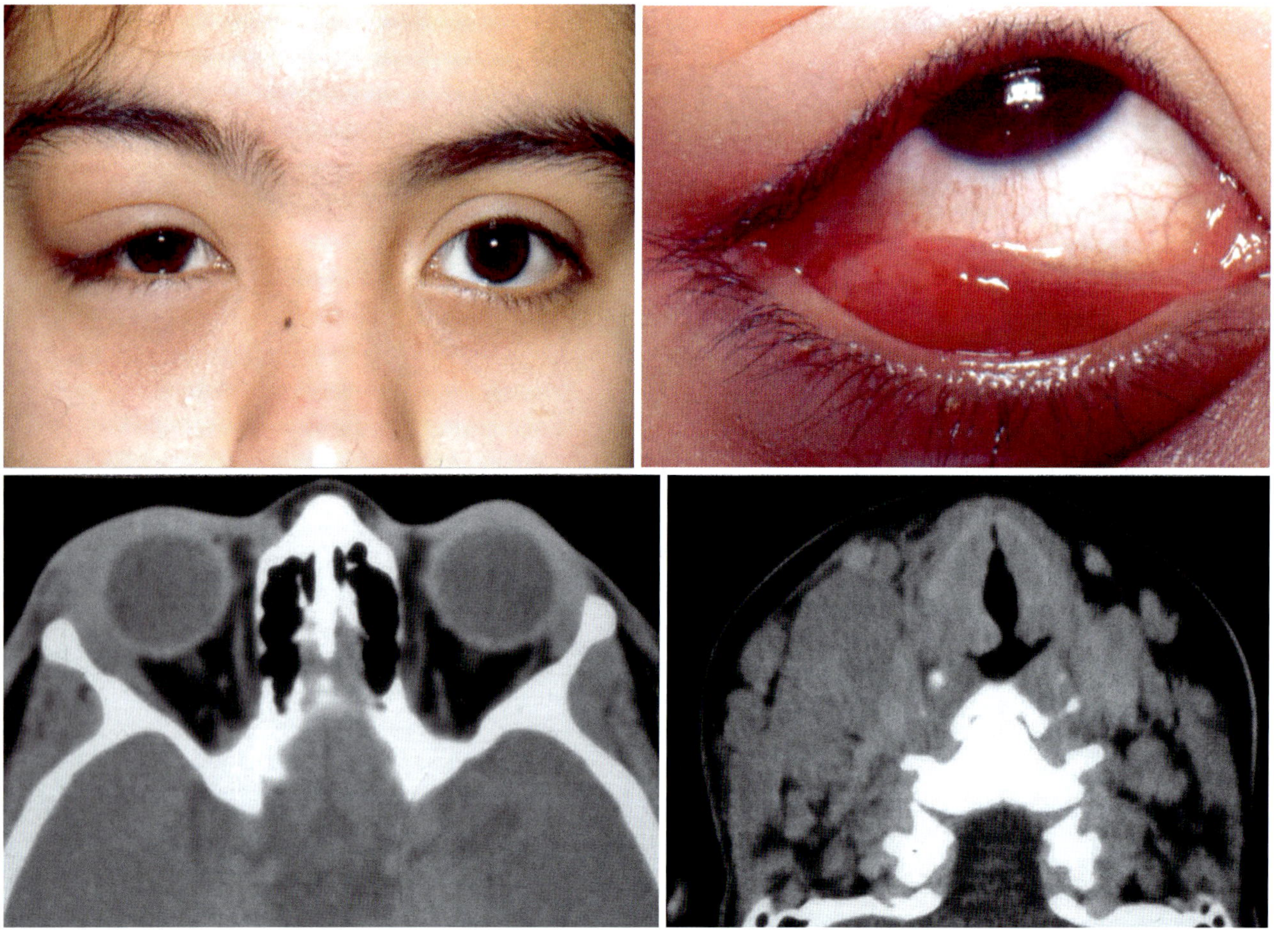

Fig. 50.28 Pediatric follicular hyperplasia. A 7-year-old girl presented with acute lid swelling (top) and marked enlargement of the cervical lymph nodes and parotid gland. Bottom, CT images demonstrate infiltration of the right lacrimal gland, parotid gland, and cervical lymph nodes. Follicular lymphoid hyperplasia was diagnosed on biopsy, and the patient responded to systemic corticosteroid therapy without recurrence or systemic disease

in the blood. However, the primary use of LDH levels is tumor surveillance and response to cancer therapy. Many cancers rely on anaerobic glycolysis preferentially (the Warburg effect) for proliferation, raising LDH levels in the blood [215–217]. Furthermore, cellular damage results in elevated LDH levels. LDH will therefore be elevated in processes with high metabolism, proliferation, and cellular turnover, including many malignancies. Specifically, NHL is often associated with high LDH levels.

In patients presenting with a periocular mass of unknown etiology, a high serum LDH level raises the suspicion for malignancy, including NHL. However, note that LDH is not a reliable marker for a specific cancer type. Furthermore, as already mentioned, LDH can be elevated in a variety of non-malignant processes.

LDH is routinely used as a prognostic marker in NHL, especially in DLBCL. A recent study has concluded that of all of the factors used in the International Prognostic Index

(IPI) for DLBLC, an elevated serum LDH has the highest prognostic impact [218]; patients with an LDH > 311.5 IU/L had a distinctly worse prognosis than those with lower serum LDH. Serum LDH levels are also considered to be a reasonably reliable marker for tumor burden, an important feature in NHL prognostication and response to therapy.

The use of LDH to monitor response to therapy and for tumor surveillance in OAL has not been established. As noted previously, 50–60% of OAL is EMZL/MALT, with another 20–25% comprising other indolent NHL (FL, CLL). Thus, only about 15–20% of OAL comprises aggressive subtypes. It remains unclear whether serum LDH has any role in monitoring progression or recurrence of EMZL/MALT or other indolent OAL subtypes. It may prove helpful in monitoring for transformation of an indolent OAL (e.g., grade 1/2 FL) into a more aggressive DLBCL, but at present this is speculative.

2. *International Prognostic Index*

The IPI was initially developed from clinical data culled from over 2000 patients with aggressive forms of NHL that predated the WHO reclassification to develop a prognostic nomogram [219]. The original IPI assigned one point for each positive finding:

1. Age > 60 years
2. Stage III or IV disease
3. Elevated lactate dehydrogenase (LDH)
4. Eastern Cooperative Oncology Group (ECOG)/WHO/Zubrod performance status of 2, 3, or 4.
5. More than one extranodal site

The sum of these points correlated with prognosis:

1. Low risk (0–1 pt.): 5/10 year survival of 91/71%
2. Intermediate risk (2 pts.): 5/10 year survival of 78/51%
3. High risk (3–5 pts.): 5/10 year survival of 53/36%

Note that these prognostications were made prior to the availability of rituximab, which has markedly changed NHL prognosis. The original IPI has since been modified for age (younger or older than 60 years) and for specific low- and high-grade NHL subtypes, including FL and MCL, and remains an important prognostic tool in the management of NHL.

Management

Tissue Diagnosis

Suspected OALD requires biopsy confirmation in all cases. Unless the surgeon is familiar with the nuances of tissue handling and histologic work-up, a preoperative discussion with the pathologist regarding the amount of tissue and specific tissue handling is of paramount importance. In general, formalin fixation is performed on tissue for conventional (hematoxylin and eosin) staining and immunohistochemistry. *Flow cytometry is performed on fresh (not formalin-fixed) tissue.* The minimum amount of tissue necessary for successful flow cytometry is estimated as the size of a pea. The tissue must be handled carefully and gently.

Staging

OALD, once diagnosed histopathologically, necessitates referral to an oncologist for systemic evaluation and staging, without exception. In a study by Hatef et al., 58% of patients presenting with OAL had evidence of extraorbital involvement, including 32% of EMZL/MALT (Table 50.12) [210]. It is also important to remember and remind the patient that systemic lymphoma can occur even with polyclonal lymphocytic proliferations (lymphoid hyperplasia). In addition to a full physical examination, systemic work-up typically includes blood tests (complete blood count, lactate dehydrogenase and beta-2-microglobulin levels, protein electrophoresis, tests of renal and hepatic function, hepatitis B and C screening, HIV serology), and systemic imaging (see above) [1, 2, 15, 220]. Bone marrow biopsy should be performed in all patients, regardless of NHL subtype; Thuro and colleagues reported that positive bone marrow findings were found at similar rates in indolent (13%) and aggressive (17%) NHL [206]. OAL is generally clinically staged using the Ann Arbor staging system [221]. The first tumor, nodes, metastasis (TNM)-based clinical staging system for OAL was published in 2009 (Table 50.13) [209]. The authors noted that one of the limitations of their staging system remains the difficulty in distinguishing primary from secondary OAL in advanced disease. Regardless, the schema of adnexal tumor classification is based on reasonable conclusions from available data and represents the most detailed and rigid staging currently available; it has been used in multiple recently published multicenter analyses [2, 185, 186].

Repeat staging is performed in all cases of OALD, even in those with isolated, polyclonal proliferations. There are no set guidelines for serial monitoring, and the specifics are usually determined by the oncologist. It is important to remember that the mean time for relapse of OAL is 5 years and long-term monitoring is essential in all patients [15]. Local monitoring of the eye and ocular adnexa is continued by the ophthalmologist on a variable schedule.

As already mentioned, certain indolent OAL subtypes (e.g., EMZL, FL) may transform over time into more aggressive lesions (e.g., DLBCL) [5, 6, 116]. On occasion, additional periocular biopsies may be necessary either at presentation from other anatomic sites of known lymphoma or over time from the initial ocular adnexal location should clinical or radiographic evidence suggest transformation (Fig. 50.27c and d).

Table 50.13 Primary tumor (T) portion of the proposed TNM-based clinical staging system for OAL

TX	Lymphoma extent not specified
T0	No evidence of lymphoma
T1	Lymphoma involving the conjunctiva alone without orbital involvement
T1a	Bulbar conjunctiva only
T1b	Palpebral conjunctiva ± fornix, ± caruncle
T1c	Bulbar and nonbulbar conjunctival involvement
T2	Lymphoma with orbital involvement ± any conjunctival involvement
T2a	Anterior orbital involvement, but no lacrimal gland involvement (± conjunctival disease)
T2b	Anterior orbital involvement with lacrimal gland involvement (± conjunctival disease)
T2c	Posterior orbital involvement (± conjunctival involvement, ± extraocular muscle involvement)
T2d	Nasolacrimal drainage system involvement (± conjunctival involvement but not including nasopharynx)
T3	Lymphoma with preseptal eyelid involvement (± orbital involvement, ± conjunctival involvement)
T4	Orbital adnexal lymphoma extending beyond the orbit to adjacent structures, such as the bone and brain
T4a	Involvement of nasopharynx
T4b	Osseous involvement (including periosteum)
T4c	Involvement of maxillofacial, ethmoidal ± frontal sinuses
T4d	Intracranial spread

Modified from Ref. [209]

Treatment

As with almost all aspects of OALD, specific treatment remains an evolving paradigm and depends of multiple parameters, including morphology and immunohistochemistry of the lesion, systemic involvement, co-morbidities, patient age, local availability of specific therapeutic options, physician experience, and newly published scientific evidence. Specific molecular genetic footprints are increasingly influencing treatment [2, 51, 86]. External beam radiation therapy and chemotherapy in various combinations remain the mainstay of therapy (Fig. 50.29), with the important recent addition of immunomodulating therapy [1, 2, 134]. Older studies have suggested that the combination of chemoradiotherapy is superior to chemotherapy alone in the management of intermediate- or high-grade lymphoma, but this data precedes the availability of monoclonal anti-CD20 antibody (rituximab) therapy and may no longer be valid [222, 223].

The advent of immunotherapy, including interferon and monoclonal antibodies, has led to a shift in lymphoma management. All B cells and most B-cell lymphomas express anti-CD20 antigens. Rituximab, a chimeric (murine/human) monoclonal anti-CD20 antibody, uses the human complement and immune effector cells to activate apoptosis in CD20-positive cells [224–226]. In simple terms, rituximab attaches to all mature B cells (normal and malignant) but not early B cells or plasma cells, causing apoptosis by inducing antibody- and complement-dependent cytotoxicity [227]; stem cells then regenerate the normal B-cell population. Initially, rituximab was approved as a single agent to treat relapsed or refractory FL [228–230] but has since demonstrated benefit for EMZL, DLBCL, CLL/SCL, and lymphoplasmacytic lymphomas [226, 231–234]. This antibody has also been used in combination with chemotherapeutics, both CHOP (cyclophosphamide, doxorubicin, vincristine, and prednisone) and fludarabine, for FL and DLBCL with promising results [226, 235, 236]. Maintenance monotherapy with rituximab is also effective in improving progression-free survival in FL [226]. Early reports of OAL treated with rituximab also show a good response and low side effects [237]. Of note, evidence from clinical series of ocular adnexal MCL found that the addition of monoclonal anti-CD20 antibody (i.e., rituximab) to chemotherapeutic regimens improved the 5-year survival rate [1, 2, 52, 121]. A multicenter study of 689 patients with OA EMZL/MALT also concluded that DSS significantly improved if rituximab was added to older, standard therapy (e.g., CHOP) [133].

One important therapeutic mantra alluded to earlier is that not all NHLs are the same. Certain subtypes behave in an indolent fashion and are incurable, while others behave aggressively with a high mortality rate and therefore require therapy aimed at cure, and not simply tumor control (Table 50.4). In a case of an indolent OA EMZL/MALT with systemic involvement in a frail, elderly patient, the attempted "cure" may be worse than the disease. In such cases, watchful waiting may be in the patient's best interest [238]. On the other hand, aggressive subtypes of OAL are usually secondary lesions. In such cases, aggressive systemic chemotherapy even in the absence of radiographically or clinically documented systemic disease is usually indicated.

In many cases of indolent, isolated OAL, local EBRT is an effective and well-tolerated management option with no systemic toxicity. As noted earlier, one large study of OA EMZL/MALT concluded that patients with stage IE disease had a better DSS when treated with EBRT when compared to systemic chemotherapy [133]. The exact total dose remains controversial [1, 2, 134]. A series by Sullivan and co-workers found that a dose greater than 20 Gy decreased the risk of systemic disease in indolent OAL and to a lesser degree in aggressive OAL [35]. Another study found that local control

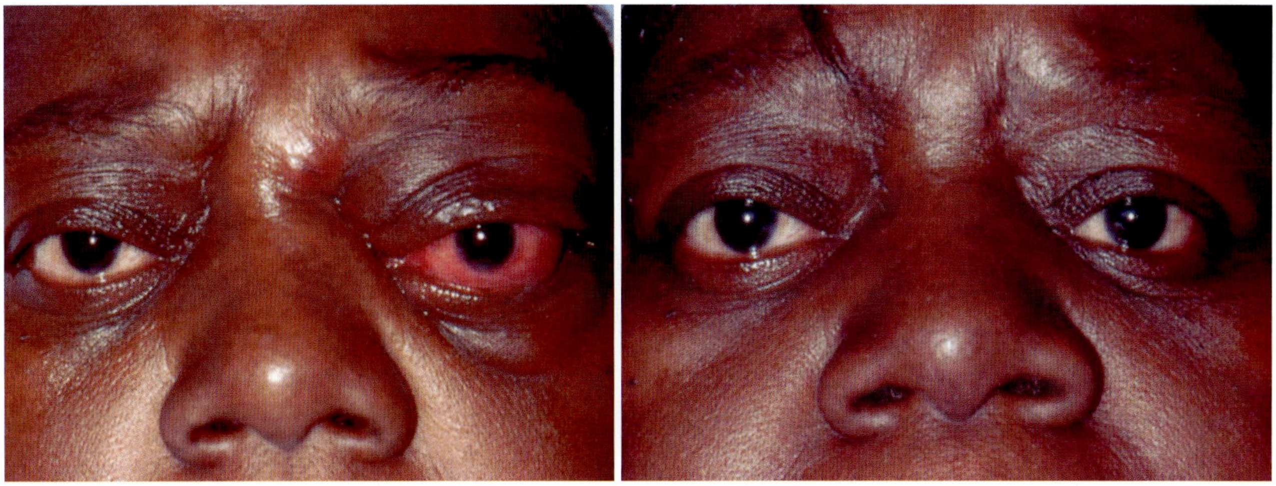

Fig. 50.29 A patient with a slowly progressive orbital process eventually diagnosed as EMZL/MALT. Left, on initial presentation. Right, following left orbital radiation therapy. The patient has had no local or systemic recurrence in over 6 years but is monitored regularly

of OA EMZL/MALT was achieved in 100% of patients treated with a total dose of greater than 30 Gy, compared to 81% with doses of <30 Gy [84]. This was countered in a study by Lowry and colleagues, who concluded that a total dose of 24 GY for low-grade NHL (EMZL/MALT, FL) and 30 Gy for higher-grade lesions (DLBCL) were as effective as a dosages between 40 and 45 Gy, with a trend toward less local toxicity with the lower dose [239]. A recent meta-analysis found that OA EMZL/MALT treated with a mean total EBRT dose of 32.8 Gy resulted in local control of 96% [134]. Two studies have recommended even lower, so-called ultralow-dose EBRT (2 doses of 2 Gy each for total of 4 Gy) for indolent OAL (and in one study, MCL), with complete responses of 85–86% but with relatively short median follow-up. Olsen and colleagues noted a "ratcheting-up" of radiation dose with more aggressive NHL subtypes in their data set [1, 2]. As already discussed, the presence of an *A20* aberration in OA EMZL/MALT may warrant the use of higher EBRT doses [86]. Total EBRT dose must be tempered by the dose-related risks of periocular radiation therapy, including optic neuropathy, retinopathy, xerophthalmia, and cataract formation. Intensity-modulated radiation therapy may enhance treatment effect while reducing local morbidity and clinical trials are ongoing.

The newest advance in lymphoma treatment is radioimmunotherapy. Simply put, a monoclonal antibody is attached to a radioisotope, allowing the radioisotope to bind preferentially to tumor cells expressing the appropriate antigen, while sparing normal tissue (which presumably lacks the specific antigen). This may prove especially useful in OAL, theoretically sparing structures critical for vision (lens, retina, optic nerve). At present, radioimmunotherapy is limited to patients with resistant or relapsing disease, although one series of 12 patients with indolent OAL showed a favorable early outcome utilizing only 1/10th of the standard radiotherapy dose [240].

Conclusions

OALD represents a broad spectrum of pathology with a wide range of therapeutic options and differing prognoses. Lymphoid hyperplasia represents a polyclonal proliferation which, although initially morphologically benign, may progress to systemic lymphoma in a significant percentage of patients; lymphoid hyperplasia should be followed for evidence of systemic lymphoma over the long term. The understanding of NHL, and secondarily OAL, has progressed by leaps and bounds from the purely morphologic classification of the Rappaport system through the immunohistochemical descriptions of the REAL schema to the cytogenetic understanding of the WHO modifications. OAL should never be amalgamated into one unified diagnostic, therapeutic, and prognostic paradigm but rather analyzed within a specific rubric. The role of secondary factors, including chronic immunostimulation and immunosuppression, plays an important role in the evolution of NHL. Although intriguing hypotheses exist, to date there is no convincing evidence that OA EMZL/MALT is caused by a specific, universal infectious agent; however, geographic and genetic factors may play a role in individual susceptibility to specific infectious agents and subsequent OAL.

EMZL/MALT is the most common subtype of OAL, usually presenting as an isolated, primary, and indolent lesion, and the goal of therapy is mostly palliative. However, distant recurrence and more aggressive transformations may occur over years, and the patient must be monitored systemically on a routine basis. While certain subtypes of OAL (e.g., FL) are better characterized in the WHO modification, others are less well-understood, especially DLBCL. Certain aggressive subtypes of lymphoma, including DLBCL and MCL, are either secondary to the ocular adnexa or have a high propensity for systemic involvement and should be treated systemically with complete cure as the goal, rather than simply local disease control.

The prognosis for OAL depends on a variety of factors, including specific location and staging, but is primarily defined by cytogenetic subtype. PET/CT is becoming the norm for both staging and monitoring but at present has limitations of resolution within the ocular adnexa and has yet to prove itself as beneficial for long-term prognosis. Newer therapies, including the introduction of monoclonal anti-CD20 (e.g., rituximab) therapy, have improved the prognosis for certain types of OAL, but therapy still remains tailored to the specific subtype of OAL, the stage, and the co-morbidities of the individual.

References

1. Olsen TG, Heegaard S. Orbital lymphoma. Surv Ophthalmol. 2019;64(1):45–66.
2. Olsen TG, Holm F, Mikkelsen LH, et al. Orbital lymphoma-an international multicenter retrospective study. Am J Ophthalmol. 2019;199:44–57.
3. Jaffe ES, Harris NL, Stein H, Vardiman JW. Pathology and genetics of tumors of the haematopoietic and lymphoid tissues. Lyons: IARC Press; 2001.
4. Swerdlow SH, Campo E, Harris NL, et al. WHO classification of tumors of haematopoietic and lymphoid tissues. Revised 4th ed. Lyon: International Agency for Research on Cancer (IARC); 2017.
5. Coupland SE. Molecular pathology of lymphoma. Eye (Lond). 2013;27(2):180–9.
6. Rasmussen PK, Ralfkiaer E, Prause JU, et al. Follicular lymphoma of the ocular adnexal region: a nation-based study. Acta Ophthalmol. 2015;93(2):184–91.
7. Sagiv O, Thakar SD, Manning JT, et al. Prevalence of a histologic change of ocular adnexal lymphoma in patients with a history of lymphoma. Ophthalmic Plast Reconstr Surg. 2019;35(3):243–6.
8. Mombaerts I, Rose GE, Garrity JA. Orbital inflammation: biopsy first. Surv Ophthalmol. 2016;61(5):664–9.
9. Rose GE. A personal view: probability in medicine, levels of (un)certainty, and the diagnosis of orbital disease (with particular reference to orbital "pseudotumor"). Arch Ophthalmol. 2007;125(12):1711–2.
10. Harris GJ. Idiopathic orbital inflammation: a pathogenetic construct and treatment strategy: the 2005 ASOPRS Foundation Lecture. Ophthal Plast Reconstr Surg. 2006;22(2):79–86.
11. Jakobiec FA. Ocular adnexal lymphoid tumors: progress in need of clarification. Am J Ophthalmol. 2008;145(6):941–50.
12. Ferry JA, Fung CY, Zukerberg L, et al. Lymphoma of the ocular adnexa: a study of 353 cases. Am J Surg Pathol. 2007;31(2):170–84.
13. Wieczorek R, Jakobiec FA, Sacks EH, Knowles DM. The immunoarchitecture of the normal human lacrimal gland. Relevancy for understanding pathologic conditions. Ophthalmology. 1988;95(1):100–9.
14. Jakobiec FA, Knowles DM. An overview of ocular adnexal lymphoid tumors. Trans Am Ophthalmol Soc. 1989;87:420–42; discussion 442–444.
15. Bardenstein DS. Ocular adnexal lymphoma: classification, clinical disease, and molecular biology. Ophthalmol Clin N Am. 2005;18(1):187–97, x.
16. Jemal A, Siegel R, Ward E, et al. Cancer statistics, 2008. CA Cancer J Clin. 2008;58(2):71–96.
17. Clarke CA, Glaser SL. Changing incidence of non-Hodgkin lymphomas in the United States. Cancer. 2002;94(7):2015–23.
18. Fisher SG, Fisher RI. The epidemiology of non-Hodgkin's lymphoma. Oncogene. 2004;23(38):6524–34.
19. Freeman C, Berg JW, Cutler SJ. Occurrence and prognosis of extranodal lymphomas. Cancer. 1972;29(1):252–60.
20. Devesa SS, Fears T. Non-Hodgkin's lymphoma time trends: United States and international data. Cancer Res. 1992;52(19 Suppl):5432s–40s.
21. Margo CE, Mulla ZD. Malignant tumors of the orbit. Analysis of the Florida Cancer Registry. Ophthalmology. 1998;105(1):185–90.
22. Moslehi R, Devesa SS, Schairer C, Fraumeni JF Jr. Rapidly increasing incidence of ocular non-hodgkin lymphoma. J Natl Cancer Inst. 2006;98(13):936–9.
23. Hartage P, Devesa S, Franmeni JF. Hodgkin's and non-Hodgkin's lymphomas. In: Doll R, Fraumeni J, Muir C, editors. Trends in cancer incidence and mortality surveys. Cold Spring Harbor: Cold Spring Harbor Laboratory Press; 1994.
24. Filipovich AH, Mathur A, Kamat D, Shapiro RS. Primary immunodeficiencies: genetic risk factors for lymphoma. Cancer Res. 1992;52(19 Suppl):5465s–7s.
25. Kassan SS, Thomas TL, Moutsopoulos HM, et al. Increased risk of lymphoma in sicca syndrome. Ann Intern Med. 1978;89(6):888–92.
26. Hoover RN. Lymphoma risks in populations with altered immunity – a search for mechanism. Cancer Res. 1992;52(19 Suppl):5477s–8s.
27. Hussell T, Isaacson PG, Crabtree JE, Spencer J. The response of cells from low-grade B-cell gastric lymphomas of mucosa-associated lymphoid tissue to Helicobacter pylori. Lancet. 1993;342(8871):571–4.
28. Harris NL. Mature B-cell neoplasms: Introduction. In: Jaffe ES, Harris N, Stein H, Vardiman JW, editors. Pathology and genetics of tumours of haematopoietic and lymphoid tissue. Lyon: IARC Press; 2001.
29. Jaffe ES, Harris NL, Stein H, Campo E, Pileri SA, Swerdlow SH. Introduction and overview of the classification of the lymphoid neoplasms. In: Swerdlow SH, Campo E, Harris NL, et al., editors. WHO Classification of Tumors of Haematopoietic and Lymphoid Tissues. 4th ed. Lyon: International Agency for Research on Cancer (IARC); 2008. p. 157–66.
30. Sjo LD, Ralfkiaer E, Prause JU, et al. Increasing incidence of ophthalmic lymphoma in Denmark from 1980 to 2005. Invest Ophthalmol Vis Sci. 2008;49(8):3283–8.
31. Bairey O, Kremer I, Rakowsky E, Hadar H, Shaklai M. Orbital and adnexal involvement in systemic non-Hodgkin's lymphoma. Cancer. 1994;73(9):2395–9.
32. Rosenberg SA, Diamond HD, Jaslowitz B, Craver LF. Lymphosarcoma: a review of 1269 cases. Medicine (Baltimore). 1961;40:31–84.
33. Grossniklaus HE, Green WR, Luckenbach M, Chan CC. Conjunctival lesions in adults. A clinical and histopathologic review. Cornea. 1987;6(2):78–116.
34. Jenkins C, Rose GE, Bunce C, et al. Clinical features associated with survival of patients with lymphoma of the ocular adnexa. Eye (Lond). 2003;17(7):809–20.
35. Sullivan TJ, Whitehead K, Williamson R, et al. Lymphoproliferative disease of the ocular adnexa: a clinical and pathologic study with statistical analysis of 69 patients. Ophthal Plast Reconstr Surg. 2005;21(3):177–88.

36. Demirci H, Shields CL, Karatza EC, Shields JA. Orbital lymphoproliferative tumors: analysis of clinical features and systemic involvement in 160 cases. Ophthalmology. 2008;115(9):1626–31, 1631.e1–3.
37. Rasmussen PK, Coupland SE, Finger PT, et al. Ocular adnexal follicular lymphoma: a multicenter international study. JAMA Ophthalmol. 2014;132(7):851–8.
38. Nola M, Lukenda A, Bollmann M, Kalauz M, Petrovecki M, Bollmann R. Outcome and prognostic factors in ocular adnexal lymphoma. Croat Med J. 2004;45(3):328–32.
39. White WL, Ferry JA, Harris NL, Grove AS Jr. Ocular adnexal lymphoma. A clinicopathologic study with identification of lymphomas of mucosa-associated lymphoid tissue type. Ophthalmology. 1995;102(12):1994–2006.
40. Du MQ. MALT lymphoma: many roads lead to nuclear factor-kappa b activation. Histopathology. 2011;58(1):26–38.
41. Streubel B, Simonitsch-Klupp I, Mullauer L, et al. Variable frequencies of MALT lymphoma-associated genetic aberrations in MALT lymphomas of different sites. Leukemia. 2004;18(10):1722–6.
42. Sjo LD. Ophthalmic lymphoma: epidemiology and pathogenesis. Acta Ophthalmol. 2009;87(Thesis 1):1–20.
43. Lenz G, Staudt LM. Aggressive lymphomas. N Engl J Med. 2010;362(15):1417–29.
44. Kuppers R, Klein U, Hansmann ML, Rajewsky K. Cellular origin of human B-cell lymphomas. N Engl J Med. 1999;341(20):1520–9.
45. Pals ST, de Gorter DJ, Spaargaren M. Lymphoma dissemination: the other face of lymphocyte homing. Blood. 2007;110(9):3102–11.
46. Roos E. Adhesion molecules in lymphoma metastasis. Cancer Metastasis Rev. 1991;10(1):33–48.
47. Knop E, Knop N. Lacrimal drainage-associated lymphoid tissue (LDALT): a part of the human mucosal immune system. Invest Ophthalmol Vis Sci. 2001;42(3):566–74.
48. Knop E, Knop N. The role of eye-associated lymphoid tissue in corneal immune protection. J Anat. 2005;206(3):271–85.
49. Gausas RE, Daly T, Fogt F. D2-40 expression demonstrates lymphatic vessel characteristics in the dural portion of the optic nerve sheath. Ophthal Plast Reconstr Surg. 2007;23(1):32–6.
50. Gausas RE, Gonnering RS, Lemke BN, Dortzbach RK, Sherman DD. Identification of human orbital lymphatics. Ophthal Plast Reconstr Surg. 1999;15(4):252–9.
51. Rasmussen PK, Ralfkiaer E, Prause JU, et al. Diffuse large B-cell lymphoma of the ocular adnexal region: a nation-based study. Acta Ophthalmol. 2013;91(2):163–9.
52. Rasmussen P, Sjo LD, Prause JU, Ralfkiaer E, Heegaard S. Mantle cell lymphoma in the orbital and adnexal region. Br J Ophthalmol. 2009;93(8):1047–51.
53. Munch-Petersen HD, Rasmussen PK, Coupland SE, et al. Ocular adnexal diffuse large B-cell lymphoma: a multicenter international study. JAMA Ophthalmol. 2015;133(2):165–73.
54. Teixeira Mendes LS, Wotherspoon A. Marginal zone lymphoma: associated autoimmunity and auto-immune disorders. Best Pract Res Clin Haematol. 2017;30(1–2):65–76.
55. Zintzaras E, Voulgarelis M, Moutsopoulos HM. The risk of lymphoma development in autoimmune diseases: a meta-analysis. Arch Intern Med. 2005;165(20):2337–44.
56. Suarez F, Lortholary O, Hermine O, Lecuit M. Infection-associated lymphomas derived from marginal zone B cells: a model of antigen-driven lymphoproliferation. Blood. 2006;107(8):3034–44.
57. Derringer GA, Thompson LD, Frommelt RA, Bijwaard KE, Heffess CS, Abbondanzo SL. Malignant lymphoma of the thyroid gland: a clinicopathologic study of 108 cases. Am J Surg Pathol. 2000;24(5):623–39.
58. Salliot C, van der Heijde D. Long-term safety of methotrexate monotherapy in patients with rheumatoid arthritis: a systematic literature research. Ann Rheum Dis. 2009;68(7):1100–4.
59. Smedby KE, Askling J, Mariette X, Baecklund E. Autoimmune and inflammatory disorders and risk of malignant lymphomas – an update. J Intern Med. 2008;264(6):514–27.
60. Niitsu N, Okamoto M, Nakamine H, Hirano M. Clinicopathologic correlations of diffuse large B-cell lymphoma in rheumatoid arthritis patients treated with methotrexate. Cancer Sci. 2010;101(5):1309–13.
61. Cuttner J, Spiera H, Troy K, Wallenstein S. Autoimmune disease is a risk factor for the development of non-Hodgkin's lymphoma. J Rheumatol. 2005;32(10):1884–7.
62. Schmid U, Helbron D, Lennert K. Development of malignant lymphoma in myoepithelial sialadenitis (Sjogren's syndrome). Virchows Arch A Pathol Anat Histol. 1982;395(1):11–43.
63. Hyjek E, Smith WJ, Isaacson PG. Primary B-cell lymphoma of salivary glands and its relationship to myoepithelial sialadenitis. Hum Pathol. 1988;19(7):766–76.
64. McNab AA, McKelvie P. IgG4-related ophthalmic disease. Part II: clinical aspects. Ophthalmic Plast Reconstr Surg. 2015;31(3):167–78.
65. McNab AA, McKelvie P. IgG4-related ophthalmic disease. Part I: background and pathology. Ophthalmic Plast Reconstr Surg. 2015;31(2):83–8.
66. Nutting CM, Shah-Desai S, Rose GE, Norton AP, Plowman PN. Thyroid orbitopathy possibly predisposes to late-onset of periocular lymphoma. Eye (Lond). 2006;20(6):645–8.
67. Goedert JJ. The epidemiology of acquired immunodeficiency syndrome malignancies. Semin Oncol. 2000;27(4):390–401.
68. Kinlen L. Immunosuppressive therapy and acquired immunological disorders. Cancer Res. 1992;52(19 Suppl):5474s–6s.
69. Verma V, Shen D, Sieving PC, Chan CC. The role of infectious agents in the etiology of ocular adnexal neoplasia. Surv Ophthalmol. 2008;53(4):312–31.
70. Hoshida Y, Xu JX, Fujita S, et al. Lymphoproliferative disorders in rheumatoid arthritis: clinicopathological analysis of 76 cases in relation to methotrexate medication. J Rheumatol. 2007;34(2):322–31.
71. Meijer E, Cornelissen JJ. Epstein-Barr virus-associated lymphoproliferative disease after allogeneic haematopoietic stem cell transplantation: molecular monitoring and early treatment of high-risk patients. Curr Opin Hematol. 2008;15(6):576–85.
72. Styczynski J, Einsele H, Gil L, Ljungman P. Outcome of treatment of Epstein-Barr virus-related post-transplant lymphoproliferative disorder in hematopoietic stem cell recipients: a comprehensive review of reported cases. Transpl Infect Dis. 2009;11(5):383–92.
73. Douglas RS, Goldstein SM, Katowitz JA, et al. Orbital presentation of posttransplantation lymphoproliferative disorder: a small case series. Ophthalmology. 2002;109(12):2351–5.
74. Wotherspoon AC, Ortiz-Hidalgo C, Falzon MR, Isaacson PG. Helicobacter pylori-associated gastritis and primary B-cell gastric lymphoma. Lancet. 1991;338(8776):1175–6.
75. Parsonnet J, Hansen S, Rodriguez L, et al. Helicobacter pylori infection and gastric lymphoma. N Engl J Med. 1994;330(18):1267–71.
76. Kuo SH, Wu MS, Yeh KH, et al. Novel insights of lymphomagenesis of Helicobacter pylori-dependent gastric mucosa-associated lymphoid tissue lymphoma. Cancers (Basel). 2019;11(4):547.
77. Isaacson PG. Mucosa-associated lymphoid tissue lymphoma. Semin Hematol. 1999;36(2):139–47.
78. Lukes RF, Collins R. New observations on follicular lymphoma. In: Akazaki K, editor. Malignant diseases of the hematopoietic system; No. GANN Monograph on Cancer Research No. 15. Tokyo: University Park Press; 1973.
79. Dunn BE, Cohen H, Blaser MJ. Helicobacter pylori. Clin Microbiol Rev. 1997;10(4):720–41.
80. Chan CC, Shen D, Mochizuki M, et al. Detection of Helicobacter pylori and Chlamydia pneumoniae genes in primary orbital lymphoma. Trans Am Ophthalmol Soc. 2006;104:62–70.

81. Sjo NC, Foegh P, Juhl BR, et al. Role of Helicobacter pylori in conjunctival mucosa-associated lymphoid tissue lymphoma. Ophthalmology. 2007;114(1):182–6.
82. Goebel N, Serr A, Mittelviefhaus H, Reinhard T, Bogdan C, Auw-Haedrich C. Chlamydia psittaci, Helicobacter pylori and ocular adnexal lymphoma-is there an association? The German experience. Leuk Res. 2007;31(10):1450–2.
83. Wotherspoon AC. Gastric lymphoma of mucosa-associated lymphoid tissue and Helicobacter pylori. Annu Rev Med. 1998;49:289–99.
84. Fung CY, Tarbell NJ, Lucarelli MJ, et al. Ocular adnexal lymphoma: clinical behavior of distinct World Health Organization classification subtypes. Int J Radiat Oncol Biol Phys. 2003;57(5):1382–91.
85. Ferreri AJ, Ponzoni M, Viale E, et al. Association between Helicobacter pylori infection and MALT-type lymphoma of the ocular adnexa: clinical and therapeutic implications. Hematol Oncol. 2006;24(1):33–7.
86. Bi Y, Zeng N, Chanudet E, et al. A20 inactivation in ocular adnexal MALT lymphoma. Haematologica. 2012;97(6):926–30.
87. de Cremoux P, Subtil A, Ferreri AJ, et al. Re: Evidence for an association between Chlamydia psittaci and ocular adnexal lymphomas. J Natl Cancer Inst. 2006;98(5):365–6.
88. Daibata M, Nemoto Y, Togitani K, et al. Absence of Chlamydia psittaci in ocular adnexal lymphoma from Japanese patients. Br J Haematol. 2006;132(5):651–2.
89. Gracia E, Froesch P, Mazzucchelli L, et al. Low prevalence of Chlamydia psittaci in ocular adnexal lymphomas from Cuban patients. Leuk Lymphoma. 2007;48(1):104–8.
90. Mulder MM, Heddema ER, Pannekoek Y, et al. No evidence for an association of ocular adnexal lymphoma with Chlamydia psittaci in a cohort of patients from the Netherlands. Leuk Res. 2006;30(10):1305–7.
91. Rosado MF, Byrne GE Jr, Ding F, et al. Ocular adnexal lymphoma: a clinicopathologic study of a large cohort of patients with no evidence for an association with Chlamydia psittaci. Blood. 2006;107(2):467–72.
92. Vargas RL, Fallone E, Felgar RE, et al. Is there an association between ocular adnexal lymphoma and infection with Chlamydia psittaci? The University of Rochester experience. Leuk Res. 2006;30(5):547–51.
93. Chanudet E, Zhou Y, Bacon CM, et al. Chlamydia psittaci is variably associated with ocular adnexal MALT lymphoma in different geographical regions. J Pathol. 2006;209(3):344–51.
94. Abramson DH, Rollins I, Coleman M. Periocular mucosa-associated lymphoid/low grade lymphomas: treatment with antibiotics. Am J Ophthalmol. 2005;140(4):729–30.
95. Ferreri AJ, Ponzoni M, Guidoboni M, et al. Regression of ocular adnexal lymphoma after Chlamydia psittaci-eradicating antibiotic therapy. J Clin Oncol. 2005;23(22):5067–73.
96. Ferreri AJ, Ponzoni M, Guidoboni M, et al. Bacteria-eradicating therapy with doxycycline in ocular adnexal MALT lymphoma: a multicenter prospective trial. J Natl Cancer Inst. 2006;98(19):1375–82.
97. Grunberger B, Hauff W, Lukas J, et al. "Blind" antibiotic treatment targeting Chlamydia is not effective in patients with MALT lymphoma of the ocular adnexa. Ann Oncol. 2006;17(3):484–7.
98. Ferreri AJ, Dolcetti R, Magnino S, Doglioni C, Ponzoni M. Chlamydial infection: the link with ocular adnexal lymphomas. Nat Rev Clin Oncol. 2009;6(11):658–69.
99. Abrams JT, Balin BJ, Vonderheid EC. Association between Sezary T cell-activating factor, Chlamydia pneumoniae, and cutaneous T cell lymphoma. Ann N Y Acad Sci. 2001;941:69–85.
100. Kocazeybek B. Chronic Chlamydophila pneumoniae infection in lung cancer, a risk factor: a case-control study. J Med Microbiol. 2003;52(Pt 8):721–6.
101. Littman AJ, Jackson LA, Vaughan TL. Chlamydia pneumoniae and lung cancer: epidemiologic evidence. Cancer Epidemiol Biomark Prev. 2005;14(4):773–8.
102. Shen D, Yuen HK, Galita DA, Chan NR, Chan CC. Detection of Chlamydia pneumoniae in a bilateral orbital mucosa-associated lymphoid tissue lymphoma. Am J Ophthalmol. 2006;141(6):1162–3.
103. Ferreri AJ, Guidoboni M, Ponzoni M, et al. Evidence for an association between Chlamydia psittaci and ocular adnexal lymphomas. J Natl Cancer Inst. 2004;96(8):586–94.
104. Du MQ. MALT lymphoma: recent advances in aetiology and molecular genetics. J Clin Exp Hematop. 2007;47(2):31–42.
105. Shaye OS, Levine AM. Marginal zone lymphoma. J Natl Compr Cancer Netw. 2006;4(3):311–8.
106. Saari KM, Kauranen O. Ocular inflammation in Reiter's syndrome associated with Campylobacter jejuni enteritis. Am J Ophthalmol. 1980;90(4):572–3.
107. Gisbert JP, Garcia-Buey L, Pajares JM, Moreno-Otero R. Prevalence of hepatitis C virus infection in B-cell non-Hodgkin's lymphoma: systematic review and meta-analysis. Gastroenterology. 2003;125(6):1723–32.
108. De Vita S, Sacco C, Sansonno D, et al. Characterization of overt B-cell lymphomas in patients with hepatitis C virus infection. Blood. 1997;90(2):776–82.
109. Ferreri AJ, Viale E, Guidoboni M, et al. Clinical implications of hepatitis C virus infection in MALT-type lymphoma of the ocular adnexa. Ann Oncol. 2006;17(5):769–72.
110. Arnaud P, Escande MC, Lecuit M, et al. Hepatitis C virus infection and MALT-type ocular adnexal lymphoma. Ann Oncol. 2007;18(2):400–1; author reply 401–403.
111. Allday MJ. How does Epstein-Barr virus (EBV) complement the activation of Myc in the pathogenesis of Burkitt's lymphoma? Semin Cancer Biol. 2009;19(6):366–76.
112. Rappaport H, editor. Tumors of hematopoietic system, Atlas of tumor pathology, 1st series. Washington, DC: Armed Forces Institute of Pathology; 1966.
113. Lennert K, Mohri N, Kaiserling E, et al., editors. Malignant lymphomas other than Hodgkin's disease. Berlin: Springer-Verlag; 1978.
114. Harris NL, Jaffe ES, Stein H, et al. A revised European-American classification of lymphoid neoplasms: a proposal from the International Lymphoma Study Group. Blood. 1994;84(5):1361–92.
115. Auw-Haedrich C, Coupland SE, Kapp A, Schmitt-Graff A, Buchen R, Witschel H. Long term outcome of ocular adnexal lymphoma subtyped according to the REAL classification. Revised European and American Lymphoma. Br J Ophthalmol. 2001;85(1):63–9.
116. Jaffe ES. The 2008 WHO classification of lymphomas: implications for clinical practice and translational research. Hematology Am Soc Hematol Educ Program. 2009;2009:523–31.
117. Knowles DM, Jakobiec FA, McNally L, Burke JS. Lymphoid hyperplasia and malignant lymphoma occurring in the ocular adnexa (orbit, conjunctiva, and eyelids): a prospective multiparametric analysis of 108 cases during 1977 to 1987. Hum Pathol. 1990;21(9):959–73.
118. Isaacson PG. Lymphomas of mucosa-associated lymphoid tissue (MALT). Histopathology. 1990;16(6):617–9.
119. Bhatia S, Paulino AC, Buatti JM, Mayr NA, Wen BC. Curative radiotherapy for primary orbital lymphoma. Int J Radiat Oncol Biol Phys. 2002;54(3):818–23.
120. Jenkins C, Rose GE, Bunce C, et al. Histological features of ocular adnexal lymphoma (REAL classification) and their association with patient morbidity and survival. Br J Ophthalmol. 2000;84(8):907–13.
121. Knudsen MKH, Rasmussen PK, Coupland SE, et al. Clinicopathological features of ocular adnexal mantle-cell lymphoma in an international multicenter cohort. JAMA Ophthalmol. 2017;135(12):1367–74.
122. Maeshima AM, Taniguchi H, Toyoda K, et al. Clinicopathological features of histological transformation from extranodal marginal

zone B-cell lymphoma of mucosa-associated lymphoid tissue to diffuse large B-cell lymphoma: an analysis of 467 patients. Br J Haematol. 2016;174(6):923–31.
123. Jakobiec FA, Iwamoto T, Patell M, Knowles DM 2nd. Ocular adnexal monoclonal lymphoid tumors with a favorable prognosis. Ophthalmology. 1986;93(12):1547–57.
124. Sharara N, Holden JT, Wojno TH, Feinberg AS, Grossniklaus HE. Ocular adnexal lymphoid proliferations: clinical, histologic, flow cytometric, and molecular analysis of forty-three cases. Ophthalmology. 2003;110(6):1245–54.
125. Looi A, Gascoyne RD, Chhanabhai M, Connors JM, Rootman J, White VA. Mantle cell lymphoma in the ocular adnexal region. Ophthalmology. 2005;112(1):114–9.
126. Decaudin D, de Cremoux P, Vincent-Salomon A, Dendale R, Rouic LL. Ocular adnexal lymphoma: a review of clinicopathologic features and treatment options. Blood. 2006;108(5):1451–60.
127. Kubota T, Moritani S. High incidence of autoimmune disease in Japanese patients with ocular adnexal reactive lymphoid hyperplasia. Am J Ophthalmol. 2007;144(1):148–9.
128. Isaacson P, Wright DH. Malignant lymphoma of mucosa-associated lymphoid tissue. A distinctive type of B-cell lymphoma. Cancer. 1983;52(8):1410–6.
129. Knowles DM 2nd, Jakobiec FA. Cell marker analysis of extranodal lymphoid infiltrates: to what extent does the determination of mono- or polyclonality resolve the diagnostic dilemma of malignant lymphoma v pseudolymphoma in an extranodal site? Semin Diagn Pathol. 1985;2(3):163–8.
130. Isaacson PG, Du MQ. Gastrointestinal lymphoma: where morphology meets molecular biology. J Pathol. 2005;205(2):255–74.
131. Borie R, Wislez M, Antoine M, Copie-Bergman C, Thieblemont C, Cadranel J. Pulmonary mucosa-associated lymphoid tissue lymphoma revisited. Eur Respir J. 2016;47(4):1244–60.
132. Sullivan T. Ocular adnexal lymphoproliferative disease. In: Guthoff RF, Katowitz JA, editors. Oculoplastics and orbit. 3rd ed. Berlin: Springer-Verlag; 2010.
133. Hindso TG, Esmaeli B, Holm F, et al. International multicentre retrospective cohort study of ocular adnexal marginal zone B-cell lymphoma. Br J Ophthalmol. 2020;104(3):357–62.
134. Yen MT, Bilyk JR, Wladis EJ, Bradley EA, Mawn LA. Treatments for ocular adnexal lymphoma: a report by the American Academy of Ophthalmology. Ophthalmology. 2018;125(1):127–36.
135. Limpens J, de Jong D, van Krieken JH, et al. Bcl-2/JH rearrangements in benign lymphoid tissues with follicular hyperplasia. Oncogene. 1991;6(12):2271–6.
136. Roulland S, Navarro JM, Grenot P, et al. Follicular lymphoma-like B cells in healthy individuals: a novel intermediate step in early lymphomagenesis. J Exp Med. 2006;203(11):2425–31.
137. Cong P, Raffeld M, Teruya-Feldstein J, Sorbara L, Pittaluga S, Jaffe ES. In situ localization of follicular lymphoma: description and analysis by laser capture microdissection. Blood. 2002;99(9):3376–82.
138. Montgomery ND, Mathews SP. Transformation in low-grade B-cell neoplasms. Surg Pathol Clin. 2016;9(1):79–92.
139. Tsuji H, Tamura M, Yokoyama M, Takeuchi K, Mimura T. Ocular involvement by Epstein-Barr virus-positive diffuse large B-cell lymphoma of the elderly: a new disease entity in the world health organization classification. Arch Ophthalmol. 2010;128(2):258–9.
140. Purtilo DT, Tatsumi E, Monolov G, Monolova Y, Harada S, Lipscom H. Epstein-Barr virus as an etiological agent in the pathogenesis of lymphoproliferative and aproliferative diseases in immune deficient patients. In: Richter GW, Epstein M, editors. International review of experimental pathology. Orlando: Academic Press; 1985.
141. Morley AM, Verity DH, Meligonis G, Rose GE. Orbital plasmablastic lymphoma – comparison of a newly reported entity with diffuse large B-cell lymphoma of the orbit. Orbit. 2009;28(6):425–9.
142. Sullivan TJ, Valenzuela AA. Imaging features of ocular adnexal lymphoproliferative disease. Eye (Lond). 2006;20(10):1189–95.
143. Witzig TE. Current treatment approaches for mantle-cell lymphoma. J Clin Oncol. 2005;23(26):6409–14.
144. Orem J, Mbidde EK, Lambert B, de Sanjose S, Weiderpass E. Burkitt's lymphoma in Africa, a review of the epidemiology and etiology. Afr Health Sci. 2007;7(3):166–75.
145. Thomas DA, O'Brien S, Faderl S, et al. Burkitt lymphoma and atypical Burkitt or Burkitt-like lymphoma: should these be treated as different diseases? Curr Hematol Malig Rep. 2011;6(1):58–66.
146. Rimsza L, Pittaluga S, Dirnhofer S, et al. The clinicopathologic spectrum of mature aggressive B cell lymphomas. Virchows Arch. 2017;471(4):453–66.
147. Blum KA, Lozanski G, Byrd JC. Adult Burkitt leukemia and lymphoma. Blood. 2004;104(10):3009–20.
148. Kutok JL, Wang F. Spectrum of Epstein-Barr virus-associated diseases. Annu Rev Pathol. 2006;1:375–404.
149. Pelengaris S, Khan M, Evan G. c-MYC: more than just a matter of life and death. Nat Rev Cancer. 2002;2(10):764–76.
150. Hecht JL, Aster JC. Molecular biology of Burkitt's lymphoma. J Clin Oncol. 2000;18(21):3707–21.
151. IARC. Epstein-Barr virus and Kaposi's sarcoma herpesvirus/human herpesvirus 8, vol. 70. Lyon: IARC Monographs on the Evaluation of Carcinogenic Risk to Humans; 1997. p. 524.
152. Reifler DM, Warzynski MJ, Blount WR, Graham DM, Mills KA. Orbital lymphoma associated with acquired immune deficiency syndrome (AIDS). Surv Ophthalmol. 1994;38(4):371–80.
153. Baker PS, Gold KG, Lane KA, Bilyk JR, Katowitz JA. Orbital Burkitt lymphoma in immunocompetent patients: a report of 3 cases and a review of the literature. Ophthal Plast Reconstr Surg. 2009;25(6):464–8.
154. Kenkre VP, Stock W. Burkitt lymphoma/leukemia: improving prognosis. Clin Lymphoma Myeloma. 2009;9(Suppl 3):S231–8.
155. Dave SS, Fu K, Wright GW, et al. Molecular diagnosis of Burkitt's lymphoma. N Engl J Med. 2006;354(23):2431–42.
156. Hummel M, Bentink S, Berger H, et al. A biologic definition of Burkitt's lymphoma from transcriptional and genomic profiling. N Engl J Med. 2006;354(23):2419–30.
157. Fauci AS, Macher AM, Longo DL, et al. NIH conference. Acquired immunodeficiency syndrome: epidemiologic, clinical, immunologic, and therapeutic considerations. Ann Intern Med. 1984;100(1):92–106.
158. Hamilton-Dutoit SJ, Pallesen G, Franzmann MB, et al. AIDS-related lymphoma. Histopathology, immunophenotype, and association with Epstein-Barr virus as demonstrated by in situ nucleic acid hybridization. Am J Pathol. 1991;138(1):149–63.
159. Bower M, Palmieri C, Dhillon T. AIDS-related malignancies: changing epidemiology and the impact of highly active antiretroviral therapy. Curr Opin Infect Dis. 2006;19(1):14–9.
160. Barbaro G, Barbarini G. HIV infection and cancer in the era of highly active antiretroviral therapy (review). Oncol Rep. 2007;17(5):1121–6.
161. Cheung MC, Pantanowitz L, Dezube BJ. AIDS-related malignancies: emerging challenges in the era of highly active antiretroviral therapy. Oncologist. 2005;10(6):412–26.
162. Valenzuela AA, Walker NJ, Sullivan TJ. Plasmablastic lymphoma in the orbit: case report. Orbit. 2008;27(3):227–9.
163. Desai UR, Peyman GA, Blinder KJ, Alturki WA, Paris CL, Nelson NC Jr. Orbital extension of sinus lymphoma in AIDS patient. Jpn J Ophthalmol. 1992;36(2):205–14.
164. Font RL, Laucirica R, Patrinely JR. Immunoblastic B-cell malignant lymphoma involving the orbit and maxillary sinus in a patient with acquired immune deficiency syndrome. Ophthalmology. 1993;100(6):966–70.

165. Turok DI, Meyer DR. Orbital lymphoma associated with acquired immunodeficiency syndrome. Arch Ophthalmol. 1992;110(5):610–1.
166. Coupland SE, Foss HD, Assaf C, et al. T-cell and T/natural killer-cell lymphomas involving ocular and ocular adnexal tissues: a clinicopathologic, immunohistochemical, and molecular study of seven cases. Ophthalmology. 1999;106(11):2109–20.
167. Coupland SE, Krause L, Delecluse HJ, et al. Lymphoproliferative lesions of the ocular adnexa. Analysis of 112 cases. Ophthalmology. 1998;105(8):1430–41.
168. Henderson JW, Banks PM, Yeatts RP. T-cell lymphoma of the orbit. Mayo Clin Proc. 1989;64(8):940–4.
169. Woog JJ, Kim YD, Yeatts RP, et al. Natural killer/T-cell lymphoma with ocular and adnexal involvement. Ophthalmology. 2006;113(1):140–7.
170. Raulet DH. Natural killer cells. In: Paul WE, editor. Fundamental immunology. 5th ed. Philadelphia: Lippincott Williams & Wilkins; 2003.
171. Chan JKC, Jaffe ES, Ralfkiaer E. Extranodal NK/T-cell lymphoma, nasal type. In: Jaffe ES, Harris N, Stein H, Vardiman JW, editors. World Health Organization classification of tumors: tumours of haematopoietic and lymphoid tissues. Lyons: IARC; 2001.
172. Ely A, Evans J, Sundstrom JM, Malysz J, Specht CS, Wilkinson M. Orbital involvement in extranodal natural killer T cell lymphoma: an atypical case presentation and review of the literature. Orbit. 2012;31(4):267–9.
173. Davison SP, Habermann TM, Strickler JG, DeRemee RA, Earle JD, McDonald TJ. Nasal and nasopharyngeal angiocentric T-cell lymphomas. Laryngoscope. 1996;106(2 Pt 1):139–43.
174. Chen CS, Miller NR, Lane A, Eberhart C. Third cranial nerve palsy caused by intracranial extension of a sino-orbital natural killer T-cell lymphoma. J Neuroophthalmol. 2008;28(1):31–5.
175. Cheung MM, Chan JK, Lau WH, et al. Primary non-Hodgkin's lymphoma of the nose and nasopharynx: clinical features, tumor immunophenotype, and treatment outcome in 113 patients. J Clin Oncol. 1998;16(1):70–7.
176. Kuwabara H, Tsuji M, Yoshii Y, et al. Nasal-type NK/T cell lymphoma of the orbit with distant metastases. Hum Pathol. 2003;34(3):290–2.
177. Svendsen FH, Heegaard S. Lymphoma of the eyelid. Surv Ophthalmol. 2017;62(3):312–31.
178. Koreen IV, Cho RI, Frueh BR, Elner VM. Primary cutaneous anaplastic large cell lymphoma of the medial canthus and orbit. Ophthal Plast Reconstr Surg. 2009;25(1):63–5.
179. Chen YJ, Chen JT, Lu DW, Gao HW, Tai MC. Primary peripheral T-cell lymphoma of the orbit. Arch Ophthalmol. 2009;127(8):1070–2.
180. Landgren O, Weiss BM. Patterns of monoclonal gammopathy of undetermined significance and multiple myeloma in various ethnic/racial groups: support for genetic factors in pathogenesis. Leukemia. 2009;23(10):1691–7.
181. Burkat CN, Van Buren JJ, Lucarelli MJ. Characteristics of orbital multiple myeloma: a case report and literature review. Surv Ophthalmol. 2009;54(6):697–704.
182. Maheshwari R, Maheshwari S. Extramedullary pasmacytoma masquerading as chalazion. Orbit. 2009;28(2–3):191–3.
183. Knecht P, Schuler R, Chaloupka K. Rapid progressive extramedullary plasmacytoma in the orbit. Klin Monatsbl Augenheilkd. 2008;225(5):514–6.
184. Raffeld M, Jaffe ES. bcl-1, t(11;14), and mantle cell-derived lymphomas. Blood. 1991;78(2):259–63.
185. Svendsen FH, Rasmussen PK, Coupland SE, et al. Lymphoma of the eyelid – an international multicenter retrospective study. Am J Ophthalmol. 2017;177:58–68.
186. Kirkegaard MM, Rasmussen PK, Coupland SE, et al. Conjunctival lymphoma – an international multicenter retrospective study. JAMA Ophthalmol. 2016;134(4):406–14.
187. Kelly JJ, Karcher DS. Lymphoma and peripheral neuropathy: a clinical review. Muscle Nerve. 2005;31(3):301–13.
188. Stafford SL, Kozelsky TF, Garrity JA, et al. Orbital lymphoma: radiotherapy outcome and complications. Radiother Oncol. 2001;59(2):139–44.
189. Lee AG, Johnson MC, Policeni BA, Smoker WR. Imaging for neuro-ophthalmic and orbital disease – a review. Clin Exp Ophthalmol. 2009;37(1):30–53.
190. Yeo JH, Jakobiec FA, Abbott GF, Trokel SL. Combined clinical and computed tomographic diagnosis of orbital lymphoid tumors. Am J Ophthalmol. 1982;94(2):235–45.
191. Haque S, Law M, Abrey LE, Young RJ. Imaging of lymphoma of the central nervous system, spine, and orbit. Radiol Clin N Am. 2008;46(2):339–61, ix.
192. Calli C, Kitis O, Yunten N, Yurtseven T, Islekel S, Akalin T. Perfusion and diffusion MR imaging in enhancing malignant cerebral tumors. Eur J Radiol. 2006;58(3):394–403.
193. Hartmann M, Heiland S, Harting I, et al. Distinguishing of primary cerebral lymphoma from high-grade glioma with perfusion-weighted magnetic resonance imaging. Neurosci Lett. 2003;338(2):119–22.
194. Surbone A, Longo DL, DeVita VT Jr, et al. Residual abdominal masses in aggressive non-Hodgkin's lymphoma after combination chemotherapy: significance and management. J Clin Oncol. 1988;6(12):1832–7.
195. Jerusalem G, Beguin Y, Fassotte MF, et al. Whole-body positron emission tomography using 18F-fluorodeoxyglucose for posttreatment evaluation in Hodgkin's disease and non-Hodgkin's lymphoma has higher diagnostic and prognostic value than classical computed tomography scan imaging. Blood. 1999;94(2):429–33.
196. Romer W, Hanauske AR, Ziegler S, et al. Positron emission tomography in non-Hodgkin's lymphoma: assessment of chemotherapy with fluorodeoxyglucose. Blood. 1998;91(12):4464–71.
197. Spaepen K, Stroobants S, Dupont P, et al. Prognostic value of positron emission tomography (PET) with fluorine-18 fluorodeoxyglucose ([18F]FDG) after first-line chemotherapy in non-Hodgkin's lymphoma: is [18F]FDG-PET a valid alternative to conventional diagnostic methods? J Clin Oncol. 2001;19(2):414–9.
198. Gallamini A, Rigacci L, Merli F, et al. The predictive value of positron emission tomography scanning performed after two courses of standard therapy on treatment outcome in advanced stage Hodgkin's disease. Haematologica. 2006;91(4):475–81.
199. Hutchings M, Loft A, Hansen M, Ralfkiaer E, Specht L. Different histopathological subtypes of Hodgkin lymphoma show significantly different levels of FDG uptake. Hematol Oncol. 2006;24(3):146–50.
200. Lane KA, Bilyk JR. Preliminary study of positron emission tomography in the detection and management of orbital malignancy. Ophthal Plast Reconstr Surg. 2006;22(5):361–5.
201. Zanni M, Moulin-Romsee G, Servois V, et al. Value of 18FDG PET scan in staging of ocular adnexal lymphomas: a large single-center experience. Hematology. 2012;17(2):76–84.
202. Hui KH, Pfeiffer ML, Esmaeli B. Value of positron emission tomography/computed tomography in diagnosis and staging of primary ocular and orbital tumors. Saudi J Ophthalmol. 2012;26(4):365–71.
203. English JF, Sullivan TJ. The role of FDG-PET in the diagnosis and staging of ocular adnexal lymphoproliferative disease. Orbit. 2015;34(5):284–91.
204. Juweid ME, Wiseman GA, Vose JM, et al. Response assessment of aggressive non-Hodgkin's lymphoma by integrated International

Workshop Criteria and fluorine-18-fluorodeoxyglucose positron emission tomography. J Clin Oncol. 2005;23(21):4652–61.
205. Valenzuela AA, Allen C, Grimes D, Wong D, Sullivan TJ. Positron emission tomography in the detection and staging of ocular adnexal lymphoproliferative disease. Ophthalmology. 2006;113(12):2331–7.
206. Thuro BA, Ning J, Peng SA, et al. Rates of positive findings on positron emission tomography and bone marrow biopsy in patients with ocular adnexal lymphoma. Ophthalmic Plast Reconstr Surg. 2017;33(5):355–60.
207. Medeiros LJ, Harris NL. Lymphoid infiltrates of the orbit and conjunctiva. A morphologic and immunophenotypic study of 99 cases. Am J Surg Pathol. 1989;13(6):459–71.
208. Medeiros LJ, Harmon DC, Linggood RM, Harris NL. Immunohistologic features predict clinical behavior of orbital and conjunctival lymphoid infiltrates. Blood. 1989;74(6):2121–9.
209. Coupland SE, White VA, Rootman J, Damato B, Finger PT. A TNM-based clinical staging system of ocular adnexal lymphomas. Arch Pathol Lab Med. 2009;133(8):1262–7.
210. Hatef E, Roberts D, McLaughlin P, Pro B, Esmaeli B. Prevalence and nature of systemic involvement and stage at initial examination in patients with orbital and ocular adnexal lymphoma. Arch Ophthalmol. 2007;125(12):1663–7.
211. Kussick SJ, Kalnoski M, Braziel RM, Wood BL. Prominent clonal B-cell populations identified by flow cytometry in histologically reactive lymphoid proliferations. Am J Clin Pathol. 2004;121(4):464–72.
212. Coupland SE, Hellmich M, Auw-Haedrich C, Lee WR, Stein H. Prognostic value of cell-cycle markers in ocular adnexal lymphoma: an assessment of 230 cases. Graefes Arch Clin Exp Ophthalmol. 2004;242(2):130–45.
213. Tanimoto K, Kaneko A, Suzuki S, et al. Primary ocular adnexal MALT lymphoma: a long-term follow-up study of 114 patients. Jpn J Clin Oncol. 2007;37(5):337–44.
214. Armitage JO. Staging non-Hodgkin lymphoma. CA Cancer J Clin. 2005;55(6):368–76.
215. Bertram JS. The molecular biology of cancer. Mol Asp Med. 2000;21(6):167–223.
216. Grander D. How do mutated oncogenes and tumor suppressor genes cause cancer? Med Oncol. 1998;15(1):20–6.
217. Warburg O. On the origin of cancer cells. Science. 1956;123(3191):309–14.
218. Park J, Yoon D, Kim D, et al. The highest prognostic impact of LDH among International Prognostic Indices (IPIs): an explorative study of five IPI factors among patients with DLBCL in the era of rituximab. Ann Hematol. 2014;93(10):1755–64.
219. International Non-Hodgkin's Lymphoma Prognostic Factors Project. A predictive model for aggressive non-Hodgkin's lymphoma. N Engl J Med. 1993;329(14):987–94.
220. Tsang RW, Gospodarowicz MK, O'Sullivan B. Staging and management of localized non-Hodgkin's lymphomas: variations among experts in radiation oncology. Int J Radiat Oncol Biol Phys. 2002;52(3):643–51.
221. Carbone PP, Kaplan HS, Musshoff K, Smithers DW, Tubiana M. Report of the committee on Hodgkin's disease staging classification. Cancer Res. 1971;31(11):1860–1.
222. Miller TP, Dahlberg S, Cassady JR, et al. Chemotherapy alone compared with chemotherapy plus radiotherapy for localized intermediate- and high-grade non-Hodgkin's lymphoma. N Engl J Med. 1998;339(1):21–6.
223. Cosset JM. Chemoradiotherapy for localized non-Hodgkin's lymphoma. N Engl J Med. 1998;339(1):44–5.
224. Coiffier B, Haioun C, Ketterer N, et al. Rituximab (anti-CD20 monoclonal antibody) for the treatment of patients with relapsing or refractory aggressive lymphoma: a multicenter phase II study. Blood. 1998;92(6):1927–32.
225. Cartron G, Watier H, Golay J, Solal-Celigny P. From the bench to the bedside: ways to improve rituximab efficacy. Blood. 2004;104(9):2635–42.
226. Keating GM. Rituximab: a review of its use in chronic lymphocytic leukaemia, low-grade or follicular lymphoma and diffuse large B-cell lymphoma. Drugs. 2010;70(11):1445–76.
227. Schioppo T, Ingegnoli F. Current perspective on rituximab in rheumatic diseases. Drug Des Devel Ther. 2017;11:2891–904.
228. Hiddemann W, Kneba M, Dreyling M, et al. Frontline therapy with rituximab added to the combination of cyclophosphamide, doxorubicin, vincristine, and prednisone (CHOP) significantly improves the outcome for patients with advanced-stage follicular lymphoma compared with therapy with CHOP alone: results of a prospective randomized study of the German Low-Grade Lymphoma Study Group. Blood. 2005;106(12):3725–32.
229. McLaughlin P, Grillo-Lopez AJ, Link BK, et al. Rituximab chimeric anti-CD20 monoclonal antibody therapy for relapsed indolent lymphoma: half of patients respond to a four-dose treatment program. J Clin Oncol. 1998;16(8):2825–33.
230. Marcus R, Imrie K, Solal-Celigny P, et al. Phase III study of R-CVP compared with cyclophosphamide, vincristine, and prednisone alone in patients with previously untreated advanced follicular lymphoma. J Clin Oncol. 2008;26(28):4579–86.
231. Cheson BD, Leonard JP. Monoclonal antibody therapy for B-cell non-Hodgkin's lymphoma. N Engl J Med. 2008;359(6):613–26.
232. Foran JM, Rohatiner AZ, Cunningham D, et al. European phase II study of rituximab (chimeric anti-CD20 monoclonal antibody) for patients with newly diagnosed mantle-cell lymphoma and previously treated mantle-cell lymphoma, immunocytoma, and small B-cell lymphocytic lymphoma. J Clin Oncol. 2000;18(2):317–24.
233. Nguyen DT, Amess JA, Doughty H, Hendry L, Diamond LW. IDEC-C2B8 anti-CD20 (rituximab) immunotherapy in patients with low-grade non-Hodgkin's lymphoma and lymphoproliferative disorders: evaluation of response on 48 patients. Eur J Haematol. 1999;62(2):76–82.
234. Treon SP, Agus DB, Link B, et al. CD20-directed antibody-mediated immunotherapy induces responses and facilitates hematologic recovery in patients with Waldenstrom's macroglobulinemia. J Immunother. 2001;24(3):272–9.
235. Czuczman MS, Weaver R, Alkuzweny B, Berlfein J, Grillo-Lopez AJ. Prolonged clinical and molecular remission in patients with low-grade or follicular non-Hodgkin's lymphoma treated with rituximab plus CHOP chemotherapy: 9-year follow-up. J Clin Oncol. 2004;22(23):4711–6.
236. Czuczman MS, Koryzna A, Mohr A, et al. Rituximab in combination with fludarabine chemotherapy in low-grade or follicular lymphoma. J Clin Oncol. 2005;23(4):694–704.
237. Sokol JA, Landau L, Lauer SA. Rituximab immunotherapy for ocular adnexal lymphoma: clinicopathologic correlation with 5-year follow-up. Ophthal Plast Reconstr Surg. 2009;25(4):322–4.
238. Decaudin D, Dendale R, Lumbroso-Le RL. Treatment of mucosa-associated lymphoid tissue-type ocular adnexal lymphoma. Anti-Cancer Drugs. 2008;19(7):673–80.
239. Lowry L, Smith P, Qian W, et al. Reduced dose radiotherapy for local control in non-Hodgkin lymphoma: a randomised phase III trial. Radiother Oncol. 2011;100(1):86–92.
240. Esmaeli B, McLaughlin P, Pro B, et al. Prospective trial of targeted radioimmunotherapy with Y-90 ibritumomab tiuxetan (Zevalin) for front-line treatment of early-stage extranodal indolent ocular adnexal lymphoma. Ann Oncol. 2009;20(4):709–14.
241. Mahmoud HM, El-Sakhawy YN. Significance of Bcl-2 and Bcl-6 immunostaining in B-non Hodgkin's lymphoma. Hematol Rep. 2011;3(3):e26.

242. Navratil E, Gaulard P, Kanavaros P, et al. Expression of the bcl-2 protein in B cell lymphomas arising from mucosa associated lymphoid tissue. J Clin Pathol. 1995;48(1):18–21.
243. Zaja F, Di Loreto C, Amoroso V, et al. BCL-2 immunohistochemical evaluation in B-cell chronic lymphocytic leukemia and hairy cell leukemia before treatment with fludarabine and 2-chloro-deoxy-adenosine. Leuk Lymphoma. 1998;28(5–6):567–72.
244. Sjo LD, Heegaard S, Prause JU, Petersen BL, Pedersen S, Ralfkiaer E. Extranodal marginal zone lymphoma in the ocular region: clinical, immunophenotypical, and cytogenetical characteristics. Invest Ophthalmol Vis Sci. 2009;50(2):516–22.
245. Cani AK, Soliman M, Hovelson DH, et al. Comprehensive genomic profiling of orbital and ocular adnexal lymphomas identifies frequent alterations in MYD88 and chromatin modifiers: new routes to targeted therapies. Mod Pathol. 2016;29(7):685–97.
246. Sullivan TJ, Whitehead K, Williamson R, et al. Lymphoproliferative disease of the ocular adnexa: a clinical and pathologic study with statistical analysis of 69 patients. Ophthalmic Plast Reconstr Surg. 2005;21(3):177–88.

Orbital Vascular Anomalies

51

Anaïs L. Carniciu and Alon Kahana

Introduction

Vascular anomalies are classified into vascular tumors and vascular malformations based on the classification system of the International Society for the Study of Vascular Anomalies (ISSVA) [1–3]. Vascular *tumors* are characterized by proliferation and tumor enlargement, and the most common vascular tumor is infantile hemangioma, while a less common vascular tumor is hemangiopericytoma. Vascular *malformations* consist of nonproliferating vascular lesions in which blood flow is misdirected through anomalous channels. Malformations exist on a spectrum, ranging from high-flow arteriovenous malformation (AVM), low-flow venous (varix) and lympho-venous malformations, and capillary-venous malformations. Flow characteristics influence the natural history of vascular anomalies and are helpful in making the correct diagnosis.

In the orbit, vascular anomalies represent a special challenge because of the risk of compartment syndrome from a distensible mass or a hemorrhage and because the tumor mass can deform the eye and surrounding structures, leading to irregular astigmatism, eyelid ptosis, or even optic nerve compression. Treatment of symptomatic orbital vascular anomalies requires an accurate understanding of the anatomy, including the extent of the anomaly and its relationship to surrounding structures. The orbit offers little room for error, and careful preoperative planning, adequate exposure, and outstanding hemostasis are required to achieve an optimal result [4–8]. Recent advances in medical therapy, including beta-blocker treatment and anti-VEGF therapy for certain vascular anomalies, have improved the safety profile of managing vascular anomalies [9–11].

Digital subtraction angiography has been the "gold standard" for the evaluation of vascular malformations. However, vascular access in the orbit is limited, and endovascular catheters can compromise blood flow to the eye. In addition, digital subtraction angiography cannot visualize the surrounding soft tissues, and visualization of all the relevant vascular channels of complex malformations may not be possible without increasing the risks of vascular compromise and radiation exposure.

Dynamic noninvasive imaging using magnetic resonance imaging (MRI) or computed tomography (CT) technology are excellent alternatives for imaging vascular malformations of the orbit. Both modalities provide a comprehensive assessment of blood flow channels as well as surrounding soft tissue anatomy. MRI is better for assessing soft tissue abnormalities and has reduced radiation and contrast-related risks. However, MRIs are more expensive, require specialized equipment and software, and require a much-longer acquisition time. Dynamic CT scans provide excellent visualization of blood flow and soft tissue, and are quicker to perform, but require extended radiation times as well as radiopaque contrast, to which many patients are allergic.

All three major MRI technology companies market dynamic contrast-enhanced magnetic resonance angiography (MRA) systems: "TRICKS" (General Electric Healthcare, Milwaukee, Wisconsin), "4D-TRAK" (Philips Medical Systems, Best, Netherlands), and "syngo-TWIST" (Siemens Medical Solutions, Iselin, New Jersey). Orbital surgeons should become familiar with the image modalities available to them.

Arteriovenous Malformation (AVM)

Blood circulation depends on three elements that together constitute the vascular channel: arteries to carry high-pressure flow, veins to carry low-pressure flow, and capillaries in between to promote nutrient and oxygen exchange. AVMs are

A. L. Carniciu · A. Kahana (✉)
Consultants in Ophthalmic and Facial Plastic Surgery, Southfield, MI, USA
e-mail: akahana@facialworks.com

J. J. Servat et al. (eds.), *Smith and Nesi's Ophthalmic Plastic and Reconstructive Surgery*, https://doi.org/10.1007/978-3-030-41720-8_51

high-flow congenital vascular malformations in which arterial blood flows directly into a venous channel, without a capillary network in between. These anomalies center on a "nidus," site of the vascular "short circuit." Treatment of AVMs must address the nidus in order to prevent a recurrence. Direct high-pressure blood flow from an arterial feeder into a draining vein results in arterialization of the vein, consisting of myointimal thickening with matrix deposition, adventitial remodeling, and vascular dilatation. Scientific studies of AVMs utilize AV fistulization, focusing on venous grafts for vascular reconstruction as well as dialysis ports. Indirectly, these studies reveal that while veins lose some of their venous characteristics, they do not become true arteries, resulting in an acquired bioactive vascular anomaly that changes over time [12]. In congenital AVMs, the signals that control vessel identity (artery or vein) become misregulated, so congenital and acquired fistulas are not equivalent: acquired fistulas contain normal veins that become arterialized, whereas congenital malformations contain embryologically abnormal arterial and venous channels. Aberrant Notch signaling has been implicated in this process [12]. AVMs present to the orbital surgeon with complaints of proptosis or periocular deformity, occasionally with a history of bleeding, and possibly with secondary symptoms such as decreased vision, diplopia, and eyelid malposition.

Diagnosis of AVMs requires identification of both a feeding vessel (artery) and a draining vessel (vein). Multiple draining channels are commonly encountered, and mixed anomalies are the rule, rather than the exception (Fig. 51.1).

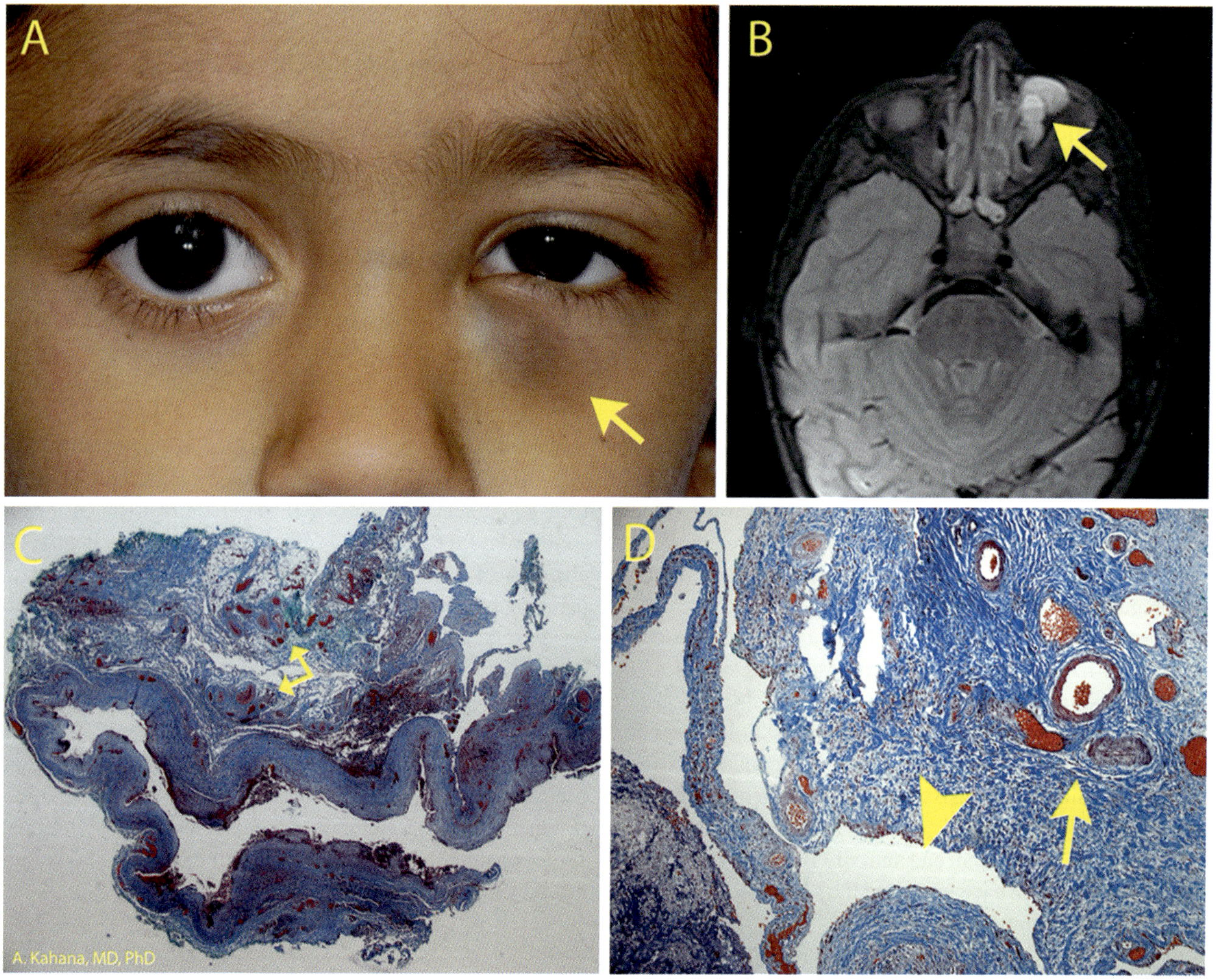

Fig. 51.1 Mixed vascular malformation. Patient is a 3 year-old who presented with recurrent orbital hemorrhage and decreased vision in the left eye from induced astigmatism (**a**). MR imaging revealed large cystic spaces and a fluid level, consistent with a lymphangioma (**b**). Dynamic MRA revealed trace mid-phase flow, more consistent with a venous or arteriovenous malformation (not shown). Histopathologic evaluation (Masson trichrome) revealed clusters of arterioles and venules (**c** and **d** – arrows), and large dilated cyst-like veins (**d** – arrowhead). The cystic spaces had ample smooth muscle actin on immunohistochemistry (not shown), and there was patchy D2–40 staining (not shown). There were a few clusters of lymphocytes but no germinal centers, and different portions of the excised tissue displayed somewhat different characteristics or combinations thereof. This malformation contains elements of both AVM and lymphovenous malformation (LVM), but is predominantly venous in nature. It is a good example of the shared origins and mixed features of vascular malformations

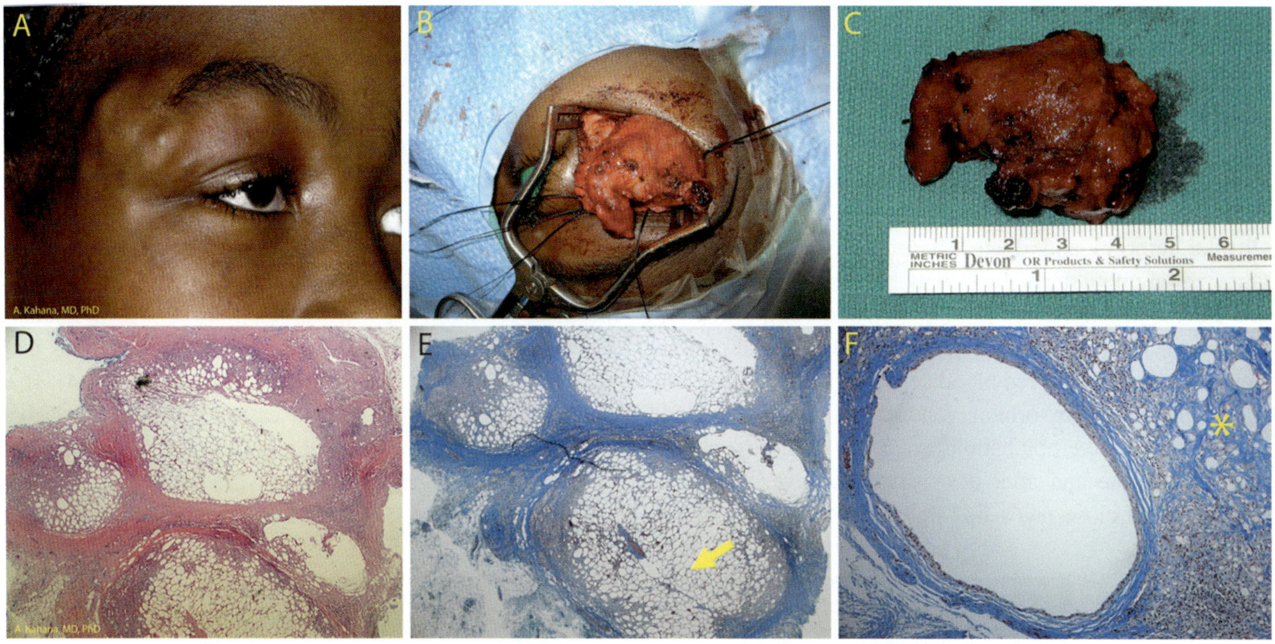

Fig. 51.2 Arteriovenous malformation (AVM). Patient was a child who presented with a pulsatile mass, a history of growth, and multiple restrictions on activity at school (**a**). Following percutaneous and endovascular embolization with glue and Onyx, the nidus was surgically excised (**b**, **c**). Residual feeder vessels were identified preoperatively on dynamic MRA and ligated intraoperatively (silk sutures in **b**). Histopathologic examination revealed arteries and arterialized veins, embolized spaces with glue remnants (**d**: H&E; **e**: Masson trichrome), and clusters of arterioles and venules (**f**, asterisk). Arrow in (**e**) points to glue within the lumen of an embolized vessel

The "gold standard" of diagnostic tests is the invasive angiogram, with direct catheterization (endovascular or percutaneous), and injection of contrast dye under fluoroscopy. This allows identification of the flow channels that center on the catheter tip. However, because AVMs contain anomalous channels, the angiogram operator must be extremely careful about movement of the catheter tip within the nidus. Needless to say, catheterization of the ophthalmic artery is both difficult and dangerous. Hence, dynamic contrast-enhanced imaging is particularly helpful with orbital AVMs, revealing the vascular channels and the soft tissue context noninvasively. With dynamic CT angiography and dynamic contrast-enhanced MR angiography, adjunctive virtual dynamic angiogram is very useful for both diagnosis and pre-treatment planning [13]. The virtual angiogram provides a view of feeding and draining channels that is independent of cannula tip positioning and adds soft tissue visualization. In addition, when planning a staged treatment approach (embolization followed days later by surgical excision of the nidus), dynamic virtual imaging can reveal the extent of embolization, suggest the appropriate surgical approach, and identify any residual high-flow channels requiring surgical clipping or tie-off.

Treatment of orbital AVMs is complex because of the tight space of the orbit, the proximity of critical tissues, and the small-gauge vasculature that supplies the retina with minimal collateral circulation. The goal of treatment remains excision of the nidus. This is often preceded by endovascular or percutaneous embolization, either preoperatively or intraoperatively, in order to reduce the risk of a significant hemorrhage (Fig. 51.2). Using a combination of dilute and viscous Onyx (Onyx 18 and Onyx 36, respectively; ev3, Inc., Plymouth, MN), as well as liquid glue, the endovascular surgeon can penetrate and embolize even small-diameter vessels, as small as 5 um [14]. Optimizing surgical exposure and maintaining meticulous hemostasis are essential for successful surgical outcomes. If a lesion is limited to the anterior orbit, then surgical access is straightforward. However, if the lesion is located in the posterior orbit, or extends and infiltrates throughout the orbit, then a lateral orbitotomy with removal of the lateral orbital rim, or a trans-cranial orbitotomy with assistance from a neurosurgeon, may be necessary for optimizing exposure. If a lesion has intracranial involvement, then a neurosurgical approach would be required, and the ophthalmic orbital surgeon will generally be helpful with the intra-orbital elements of the surgery, pre- and postoperative ophthalmic evaluations, and any necessary eyelid, fornix, and canthal reconstructive procedures.

Venous Malformation

Pure venous malformations (often referred to as "varices") are formed by dilated anomalous venous channels, with low-pressure blood flow. They may be divided into two broad categories: distensible and non-distensible. Maybe counter-intuitively, non-distensible venous malformations may be more likely to hemorrhage and become symptomatic because they cannot accommodate alterations in local venous pressure. Venous malformations can be local or extensive and may be part of a more complex mixed vascular anomaly (see below).

Histopathologically, venous malformations have irregular attenuated smooth muscle cells within their walls, with both slit-like (empty) and dilated lumina containing thrombi. Older intraluminal thrombosis may be organized with collagen fibers, which are prone to calcification and phlebolith formation. Hemosiderin deposition and cholesterol clefting (residuals of necrosed red blood cells) are common.

Evaluation of an orbital venous malformation should include a complete ophthalmic exam, including exophthalmometry before and after a valsalva maneuver. A simple instruction to close one's lips tightly around a thumb and blow through the mouth should elicit a robust Valsalva effect. Multiple imaging modalities can be successfully utilized, although magnetic resonance imaging is the best tool for delineating the anatomy of the venous malformation and its relationship to surrounding structures. Dynamic magnetic resonance angiography (MRA) with contrast enhancement will reveal the location and flow characteristics of the lesion (Fig. 51.3). Contrast-enhanced CT scanning can also provide rapid visualization of blood flow, although it requires increased radiation exposure. Combining a valsalva maneuver with contrast-enhanced imaging can reveal venous distention and effects on surrounding tissues (Fig. 51.4). If a patient requires anesthesia and cannot produce a valsalva maneuver, the anesthesiologist can be asked to produce the valsalva effect. Hence, this maneuver can be performed in young children undergoing MRI under general anesthesia.

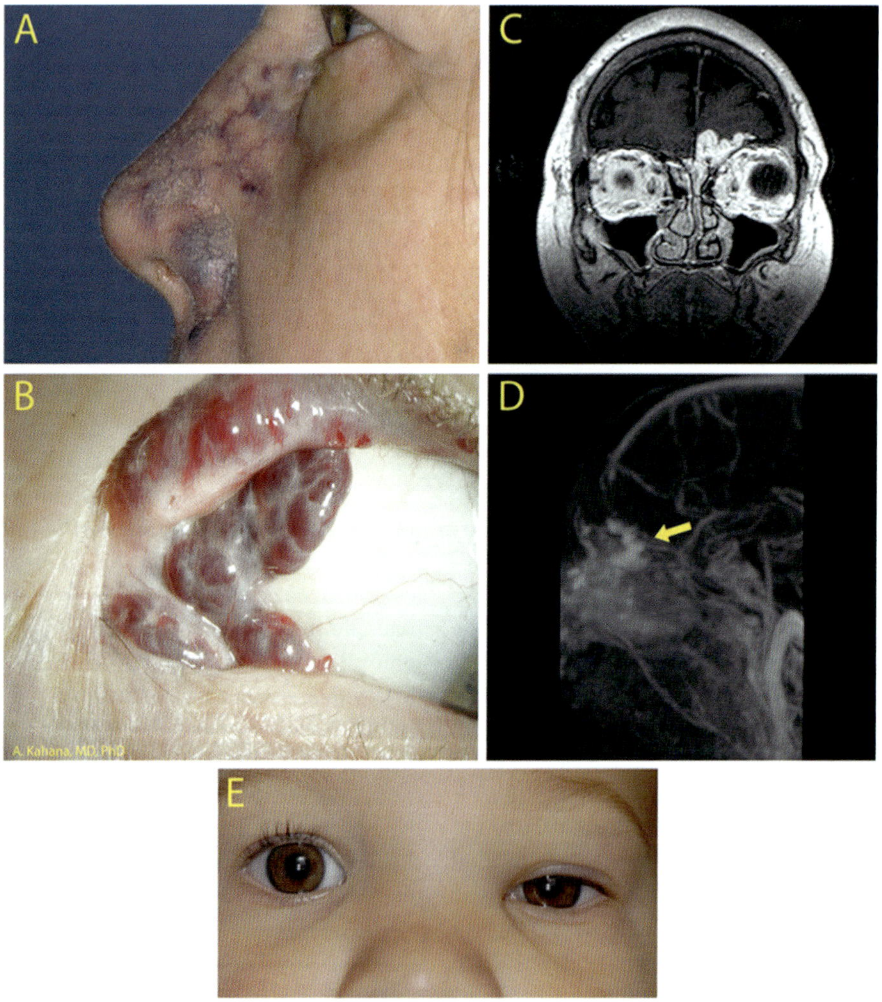

Fig. 51.3 Mixed venous malformation. Patient in top panels (**a**–**d**) has a venous malformation that respects the midline and is associated with a forme fruste port-wine stain that was laser-treated by a dermatologist (**a** and **b**). CT scan revealed a phlebolith (not shown), and the lesion had remained stable for many years. MRI (**c**) reveals both orbital and intracranial components. Dynamic MRA (**d**) reveals a slow-filling vascular malformation (arrow). In the course of evaluation, this patient was also found to have a cerebral aneurysm and was referred to the neurosurgery service for further work-up. Patient in bottom panels (**e**–**k**) is a girl who presented with ptosis (**e**). Dynamic MRA (axial **f**–**h** and sagittal **i**–**k**) reveals early venous phase enhancement that increases slowly with late-phase imaging, consistent with a predominantly venous malformation. The lesion has never bled and is distensible

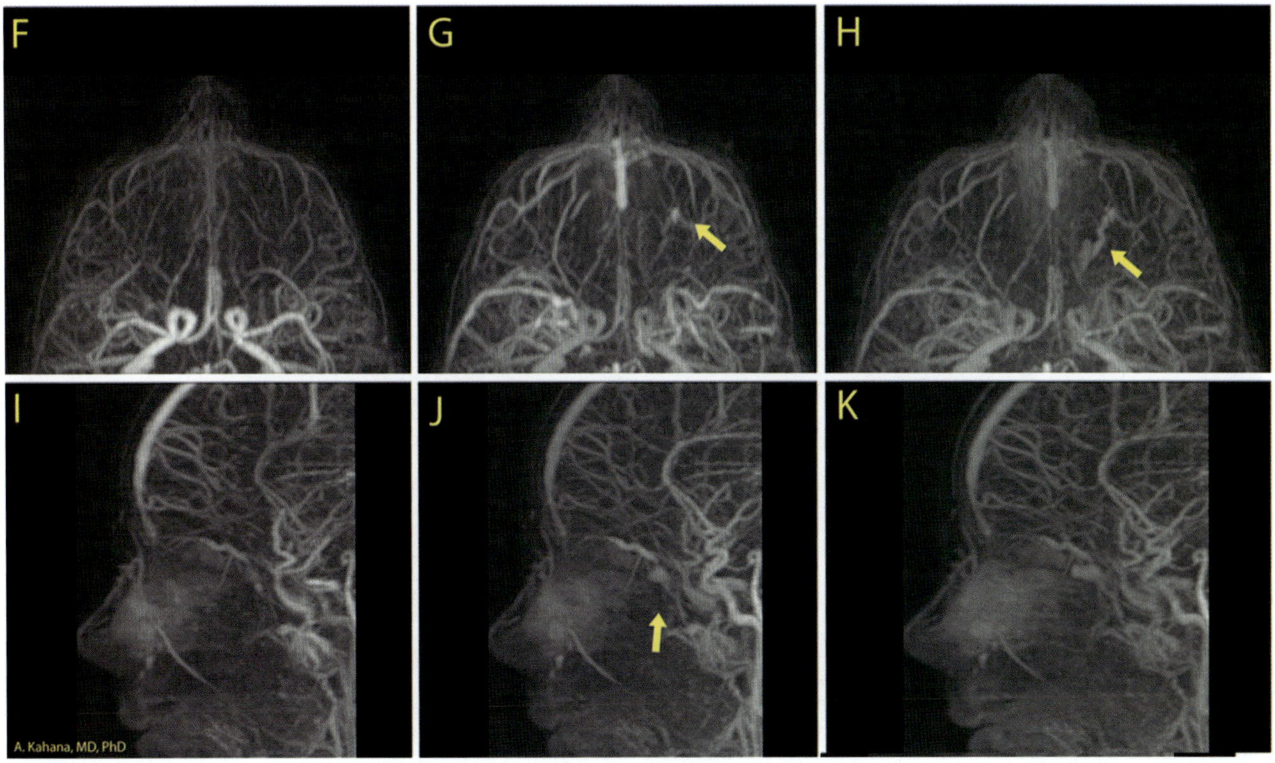

Fig. 51.3 (continued)

Management of most symptomatic slow-flow lesions, including venous malformations, involves percutaneous sclerotherapy [15–17]; surgery is now rarely necessary. The decision to excise an orbital venous malformation refractive to sclerotherapy depends on the extent of the symptoms and the weighted risks between progression of the lesion and surgical excision. Many distensible varices are discovered incidentally, are fairly asymptomatic low-flow lesions, and may only require some mild lifestyle modifications, such as alterations in exercise habits to avoid unnecessary valsalva maneuvers or dependent head positions. However, patients with varices that bleed repeatedly or cause significant proptosis, diplopia, or vision changes would typically benefit from treatment. Surgical approaches are quite similar to those used for AVMs, and pre- or intraoperative percutaneous embolization of the malformation can be beneficial. Exact delineation of the main channels into and out of the varix is very helpful, as these channels should be surgically exposed and ligated with silk sutures or clips prior to excision. The use of fibrin sealants and hemostatic surgical devices can be helpful with venous lesions in a way in which they cannot with arterial lesions: venous blood flow is slow enough that clot promotion can help reduce both intra- and postoperative bleeding. Devices that combine tissue matrix with thrombin with or without fibrinogen are particularly helpful. Examples include recombinant thrombin, gelatin sponge, thrombin/fibrinogen tissue sealants, and gelatin granules coated with thrombin.

Lympho-venous Malformation (Lymphangioma)

Mixed venous malformations are common, and among the most common manifestations is the lympho-venous malformation (LVM, a.k.a. lymphangioma). Despite the common proliferation of lymphocytes within these lesions, and the growth that can occur over time, these lesions are considered anomalies rather than tumors. These lesions can be challenging to classify, because both clinically and histopathologically they can manifest multiple features (Figs. 51.1, 51.5, and 51.6). The use of immunohistochemistry can be helpful, but should only be used to support and validate the clinical and histologic diagnosis. For example, while D2–40 antibodies bind to endothelial cells of lymphatic channels, they can also interact with cells within venous malformations, underscoring the relationship of venous and lymphatic anomalies.

LVMs, and especially lymphatic-predominant LVMs, have little to no blood flow through the anomalous channels. They can transiently expand and contract based on immune-

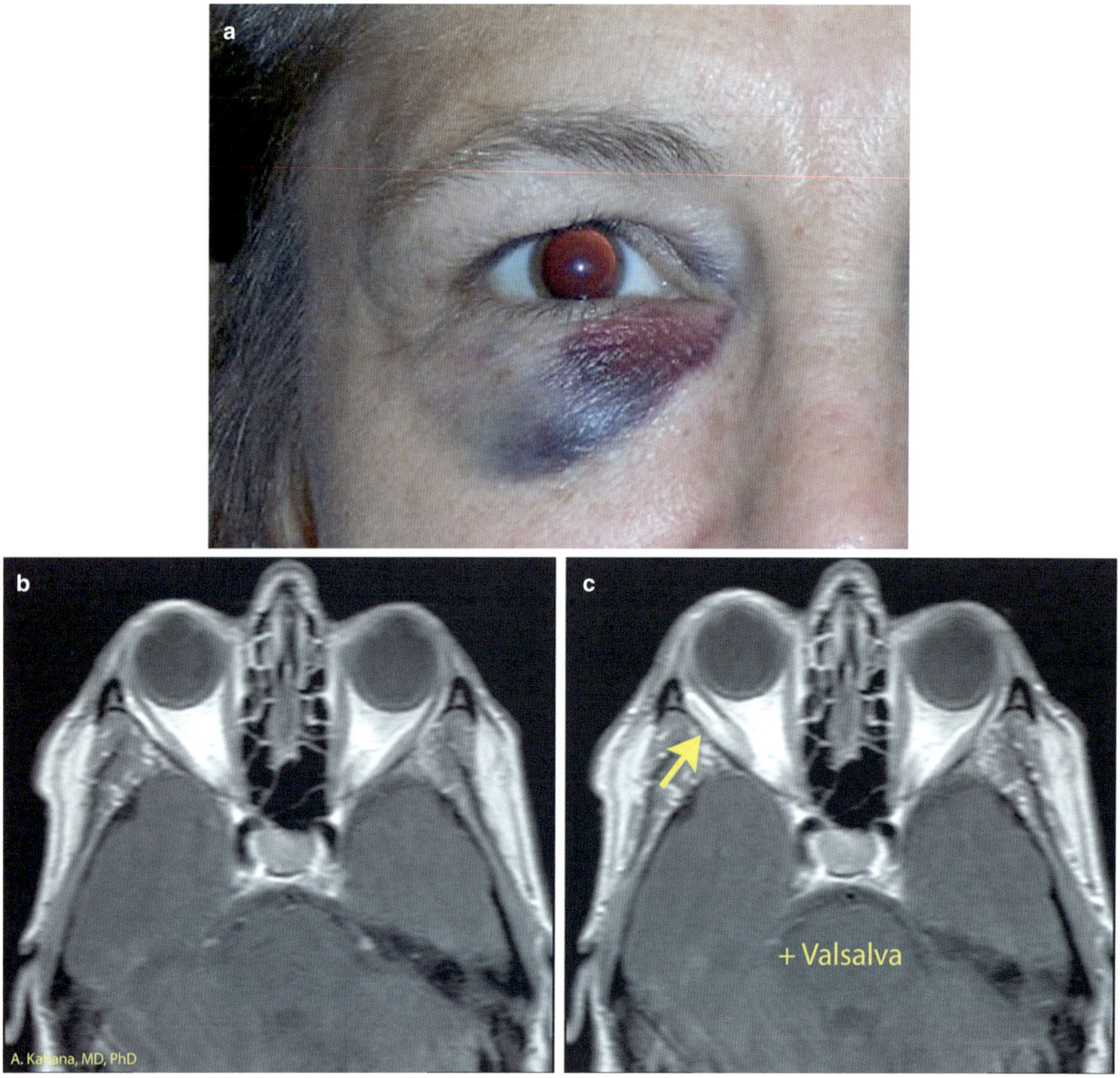

Fig. 51.4 Venous malformation. This patient presented with spontaneous orbital hemorrhage (**a**) and a history of orbital pressure with exercise. MRI without (**b**) and with (**c**) valsalva maneuver revealed distensibility of a mass located between the lateral rectus muscle and the lateral orbital wall (**c**, arrow). Dynamic MRA revealed uniform slow-filling lesion, consistent with a pure venous malformation (commonly referred to as a "varix")

mediated signals that interact with lymphocytes within the lesions (note abundance of germinal centers in Fig. 51.6). Sudden local expansion can lead to capillary breaks and accumulation of blood within the dead-end channels of the anomaly, leading to hemorrhagic (chocolate) cysts and fluid interfaces that are commonly noted on imaging (Figs. 51.1 and 51.5). A common presentation is of a child or young adult with a viral upper respiratory infection who suddenly notes a small mass under the lid, with bluish discoloration, and eventually a frank bruise (Fig. 51.1). LVMs may respond to glucocorticoid administration, but any response is only transient, providing temporary improvement, while the blood is allowed to resorb or surgical debulking is performed.

Treatment of LVMs can be quite challenging. There are no vascular channels to embolize, yet they can bleed profusely intraoperatively from the broad vascular network. The malformations are commonly found to be intimately associated with vital orbital structures, and complete excision is typically impossible to achieve without significant collateral damage. Following debulking surgery, residual LVM ele-

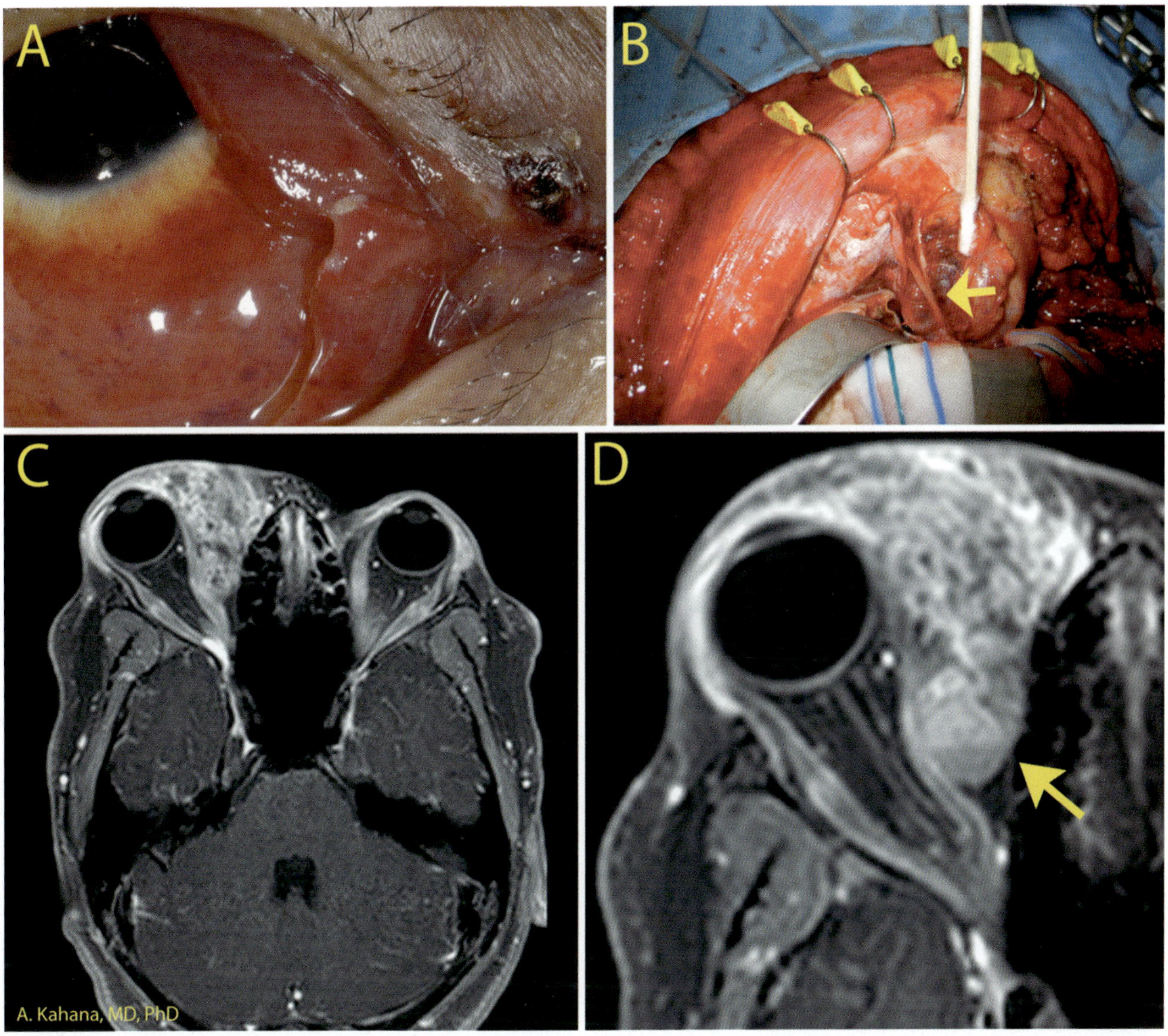

Fig. 51.5 Lymphangioma (lymphatic-predominant LVM). This patient presented with recurrent periocular hemorrhages (**a**), severe proptosis, diplopia, and decreased vision. Symptoms were worst in the context of viral respiratory infections, and there was transient response to oral corticosteroid treatment. With worsening symptoms, a transcranial orbitotomy was performed (**b**), with successful debulking of the lesion and sclerosis of residual anomalous tissue. (**b**) arrow points at frontal nerve. (**c**, **d**) MRI of right orbital mass, revealing cystic spaces, fluid levels (arrow), and gross deformity of the orbital contents

ments can grow and repopulate, in line with a more tumor-like behavior.

Sclerosing agents have been shown to successfully cause involution of LVMs [16–18]. Anterior orbital LVMs can be successfully treated with sclerosing agents alone, e.g., 5% sodium morrhuate [19]. However, non-surgical treatment of deep orbital LVMs through injection of sclerosing agents can lead to significant inflammation, deep orbital scarring, and visual compromise. In our experience, combining intraoperative sclerosis with surgical debulking can achieve excellent results even with particularly complex lesions [20]. Because LVMs can contain venous channels with low blood flow, it is important to characterize the venous channels prior to injection of sclerosing agents, which can be carried away by venous blood and cause damage beyond the confines of the lesion.

Cavernous Malformation (Cavernous Hemangioma)

Adult cavernous hemangioma, also known as a cavernous vascular malformation, is the most common primary orbital tumors that cause exophthalmos. It is a very low-flow, slow-

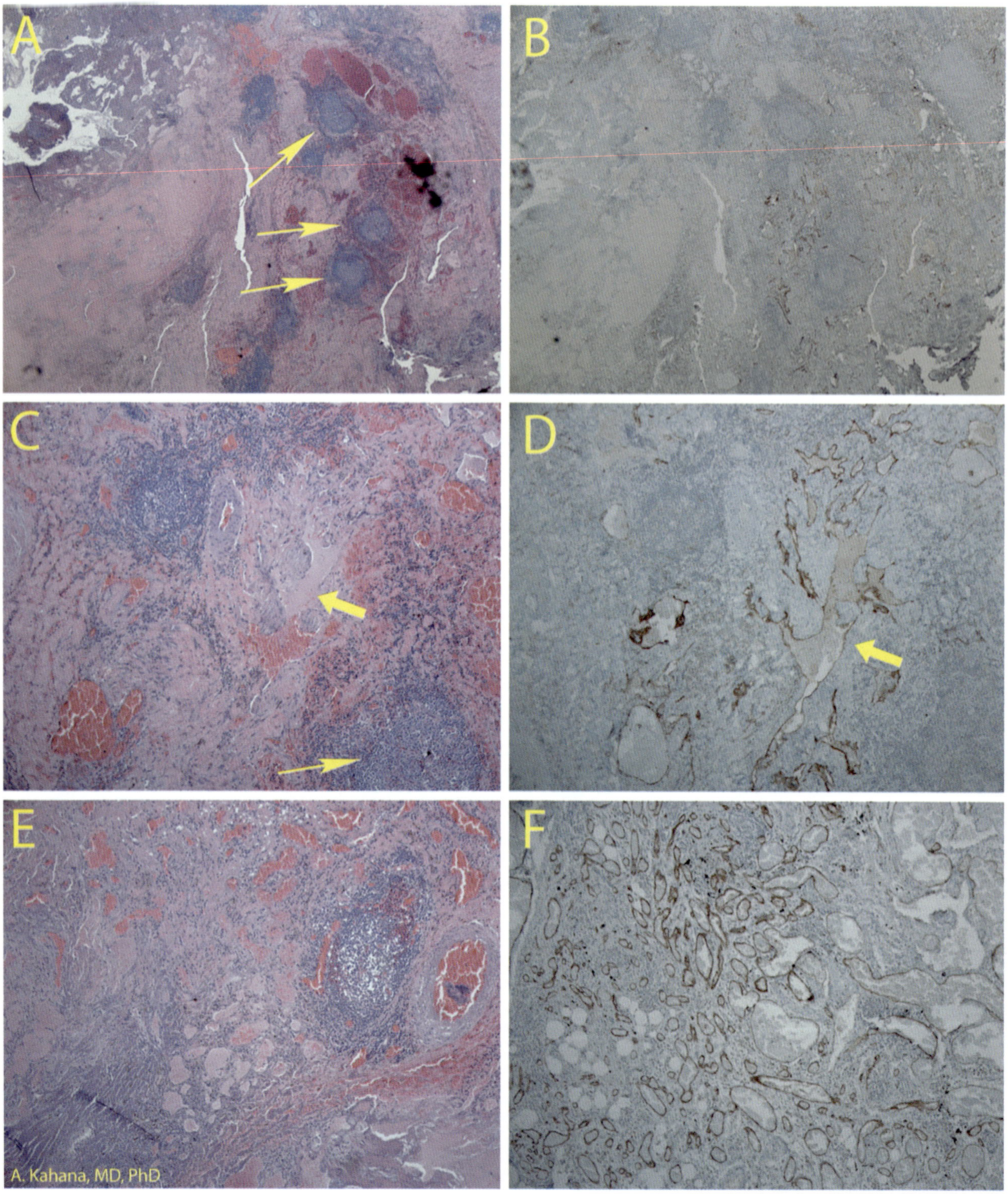

Fig. 51.6 Histopathology of lymphangioma from previous figure. (**a**, **c**, **e**) Masson trichrome staining reveals germinal centers (thin arrows) and fluid-filled (presumably lymph) cystic spaces (arrow). (**b**, **d**, **f**) Corresponding IHC with D2–40 reveals endothelial staining of the fluid-filled and blood-filled spaces

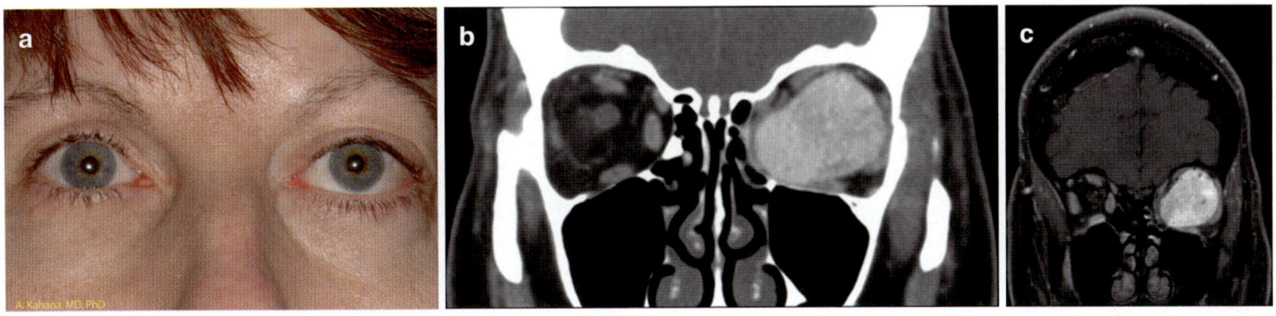

Fig. 51.7 Hemangiopericytoma. This patient presented with rapid proptosis on the left (**a**), with hyperopic shift. CT (**b**) and MR (**c**) imaging revealed a large enhancing mass in the muscle cone, causing axial proptosis. Initial diagnosis was a cavernous hemangioma. However, flow voids on the MRI suggested high-flow and large blood vessels, inconsistent with a cavernous hemangioma. Dynamic MRA revealed arterial-phase blood flow (not shown), and the diagnosis was changed to hemangiopericytoma. This was confirmed on histopathologic examination following excision

growing, well-encapsulated vascular anomaly that occurs commonly in the orbit. Their exact nature is not fully understood. Some consider them cavernous venous malformations, whereas others consider them low-flow AVMs. They appear to grow by slow proliferation, which is more suggestive of tumorlike behavior.

Cavernous malformations bleed rarely, in which case they can give rise to a hematic cyst. When in contact with the globe, they can cause retinal striae. Histopathologically, cavernous malformations are characterized by single-layer endothelial walls that form large cavities filled with stagnant blood. Most cavernous hemangiomas are asymptomatic and discovered incidentally following orbital imaging. Clinical symptoms of orbital cavernous hemangiomas include proptosis, induced hypermetropia, diplopia, blurred vision, orbital pain, and rarely orbital bleeding.

On imaging, cavernous hemangioma will enhance robustly, albeit slowly if dynamic imaging is used. It enhances as a distinct, well-circumscribed entity with no feeding or draining vessels, and any deviation from this description, or a history of rapid growth, should alert the clinician to other possibilities such as hemangiopericytoma (which enhance quickly and contain large vascular channels with flow voids; Fig. 51.7).

Symptomatic or deforming cavernous hemangiomas can be surgically removed, and the challenge is to obtain access and sufficient surgical exposure. The use of cryoextraction with an ophthalmic cryoprobe can be extremely helpful with these lesions [21]. They are modestly compressible, which allows retrieval through small surgical openings, and typically do not bleed. The exception includes intraosseous orbital hemangiomas, which can bleed from perforating bone vessels, and embolization with glue or sclerosing agent can be very helpful.

Infantile Hemangioma

Infantile hemangiomas (IH) are known by a variety of names, including "capillary hemangioma." This is a common benign vascular tumor that grows rapidly in early infancy (through cellular proliferation), followed by a period of involution over several years (commonly 5–10 years) [2]. Hemangioma is by definition a congenital/infantile tumor and cannot arise spontaneously in an adult. However, two overlapping entities should be distinguished: *infantile* hemangioma, which is barely observable at birth but grows rapidly over the ensuing post-natal days and weeks and involutes slowly over years (GLUT1 positive on immunohistochemistry), and *congenital nonprogressive* hemangioma, which is fully grown at birth and usually involutes rapidly (GLUT1 negative) [22]. The biological cause of hemangiomas is not known, but they have a placenta-like microvascular architecture [23], which suggests the intriguing possibility that these tumors represent in utero migration of placental cells. Commonly, patients with one infantile hemangioma will also have at least another somewhere else on (or within) the body, which can include the liver, intestines, and brain. There is a significant predilection for girls over boys.

Infantile hemangiomas can also occur in a syndromic context, the most common of which is PHACE(S) syndrome, reflecting: *p*osterior fossa anomalies, *h*emangiomas, cranial *a*rterial anomalies, *c*oarctation of the aorta, *e*ye abnormalities, and *s*ternal or *s*upraumbilical malformations. The most serious complications from PHACES involve cerebral infarctions and cardiac dysfunction, which can occur at any time from infancy to adulthood.

Diagnosis of IH is typically based on the clinical evaluation, especially in an infant. MRI scans can be helpful if there is suspicion of a complex mixed lesion or intracranial

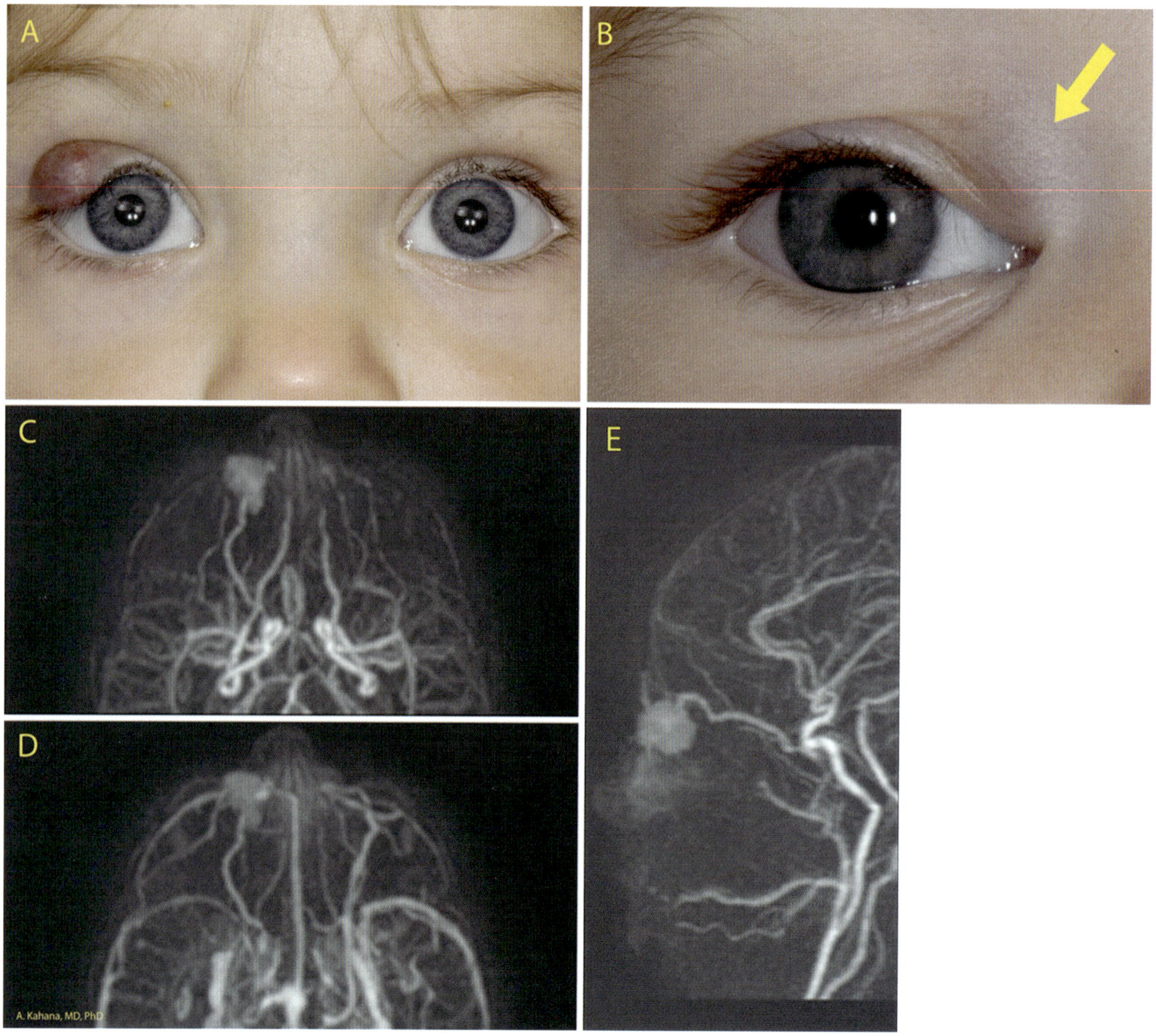

Fig. 51.8 Infantile hemangioma. Patient in (**a**) presented with a classic superficial hemangioma, without affecting the visual axis. The patient was followed carefully and is doing well with observation alone. Patient in (**b**) presented with ptosis a few weeks after birth, with a deformity of the medial right upper lid (**b**, arrow). Worsening of the ptosis led to dynamic MRA, revealing a vascular lesion that extends into the orbit, with arterial-phase filling and venous drainage (**c** axial early phase, **d** axial mid-phase, **e** sagittal early phase). These features are generally consistent with AVM. However, in the context of rapid growth following birth, reaching a peak at approximately 6 months of age, followed by stabilization and involution, this represents an infantile hemangioma

extension. Dynamic MRA will reveal rapid flow, with clear feeders, but typically without a clear draining vessel. The presence of a draining vessel would be more consistent with an AVM, although complex mixed lesions can occur (Fig. 51.8). Ultrasound Doppler evaluation can be very helpful, although it cannot differentiate between IH and AVM because both have rapid blood flow.

Treatment of IH is typically supportive. These lesions are usually minimally or non-symptomatic and will involute without intervention. However, periocular lesions that are amblyogenic because they cover the visual axis or cause ocular misalignment should be treated. Treatment can be divided into medical and surgical approaches.

In the medical treatment of IH, beta-blockers are the first-line therapy and have shown an acceptable side effect profile [10, 24]. Topical timolol is often effective for superficial capillary hemangiomas, while oral propranolol may be used to target deeper lesions. It has been suggested that propranolol works by downregulating vascular endothelial growth factor (VEGF) [11] and other pro-angiogenic signals by inhibiting the RAF-MAP kinase pathway [10], renin/angiotensin signaling [25], or directly inducing apoptosis of capillary endothelial cells [26]. Complications from propranolol treatment can be significant, including hypoglycemia, cardiac and renal dysfunction, and breathing irregularities. Treatment should be initiated under observation of an experienced pediatric medical team, with support from the orbital specialist and ophthalmologist. Oral glucocorticoids may be used to treat refractory lesions. Periocular IH can also be injected with triamcinolone suspension, as described by Burton Kushner [27, 28], although rare instances of ophthalmic artery particulate embolization leading to vision loss have been reported.

Surgical treatment has traditionally involved direct excision, cryotherapy, pulsed dye lasers, and rarely adjunctive embolization. Surgical treatment carries significant risks, similar to those with AVMs, but with more friable tissue and in younger patients. Hence, surgery should be considered with extreme caution and only under unique circumstances, such as amblyopic lesions not responsive to medical therapy.

In summary, while IH is quite common, it is usually self-limiting and minimally symptomatic and, when necessary, can be successfully treated medically in most cases.

Hemangiopericytoma/Solitary Fibrous Tumor

Hemangiopericytomas (HPC) are mesenchymal tumors containing extensive vascular networks and aberrant pericyte differentiation. They are uncommonly found in the orbit and can resemble cavernous hemangiomas on imaging. Pathologically, they are thought to be part of a spectrum of mesenchymal tumors that includes solitary fibrous tumor (SFT), and histopathologic differentiation may be somewhat arbitrary [29]. Importantly, hemangiopericytoma can undergo malignant degeneration, and local control may require both complete surgical excision with clear margins and adjuvant radiation and chemotherapy.

Most patients present with proptosis and found to have an orbital mass on imaging (Fig. 51.7). The mass is usually well defined within a pseudocapsule and strongly resembles cavernous hemangiomas. However, there are key signs that should point the orbital specialist away from hemangioma and toward the diagnosis of hemangiopericytoma/solitary fibrous tumor: [1] rapid growth is characteristic of HPC, while cavernous hemangiomas grow very slowly; [2] while both lesions strongly enhance with contrast on imaging, dynamic imaging will reveal that HPCs display very rapid (arterial) flow, while hemangiomas have very low blood flow; and [3] HPC contain flow voids that correspond to the classic "stag-horn" vessels that are notable on histopathology [13]. When confronted with a patient reporting rapid progression of proptosis, and in which orbital imaging reveals large intra-lesional blood vessels, the orbital specialist should have a low threshold for suspecting the diagnosis of HPC/SFT.

Treatment consists of complete excision. Like cavernous hemangiomas, HPCs can be removed using cryoprobe extraction. However, any technique may leave residual tumor behind, which can result in recurrence and malignant transformation. Adjuvant radiation therapy is usually reserved for patients with a recurrence or in whom complete excision is impossible or unacceptable. Further studies are required to assess long-term outcomes following orbital radiation therapy for HPC/SFT. Overall prognosis is good, so conservative management is typically appropriate.

Carotid-Cavernous Fistulas

Carotid-cavernous fistula (CCF) describes an abnormal communication between the cavernous sinus and the carotid artery. CCFs are classified based on blood flow velocity (high vs. low flow), etiology (traumatic vs. spontaneous), and anatomy (internal vs. external carotid, and direct vs. dural). CCFs occur when the wall of the artery is damaged, causing a short circuit between arterial and venous blood. The most common presentation is proptosis, with or without pulsation, with subconjunctival vascular dilatation, changes in vision, diplopia, and occasionally a bruit noted by the patient. On imaging, orbital venous congestion/dilatation is noted, suggestive of the underlying diagnosis. Findings on imaging may be similar to those with thyroid-related orbitopathy, namely, proptosis, congestion, and extraocular muscle thickening. It is important to assess the superior ophthalmic vein and to maintain a high level of clinical suspicion.

Most CCFs that come to the attention of the ophthalmologist are traumatic high-flow direct communications between the internal carotid artery and the cavernous sinus. Indirect (dural vein) CCFs are less common, typically low-flow, and reflect a communication between a dural vein and a meningeal branch of either the internal or external carotid artery. The indirect CCFs are typically caused by systemic or local vascular abnormalities, such as atherosclerosis and hypertension, collagen vascular disease (such as Ehlers-Danlos syndrome), or congenital arteriovenous malformations (AVM). The main risks of CCFs are intracranial hemorrhage, vascular steal causing cerebral infarction, and vision loss. Upstream of the CCF, one can find edema and tissue engorgement, while downstream of the CCF, one finds venous dilation and thrombosis (including retinal vein thrombosis causing vision loss).

Work-up begins with a complete ophthalmic examination. Special attention should be paid to the retinal exam, looking for signs of hemorrhage or vascular occlusion. A bruit may be heard using the bell of a stethoscope placed over a closed lid. Imaging with contrast, whether CT or MRI, will reveal dilation of the superior ophthalmic vein(s), orbital congestion with extraocular muscle enlargement, and potentially enlarged cavernous sinus. The "gold-standard" for diagnosis is the invasive subtraction angiogram (Fig. 51.9), although

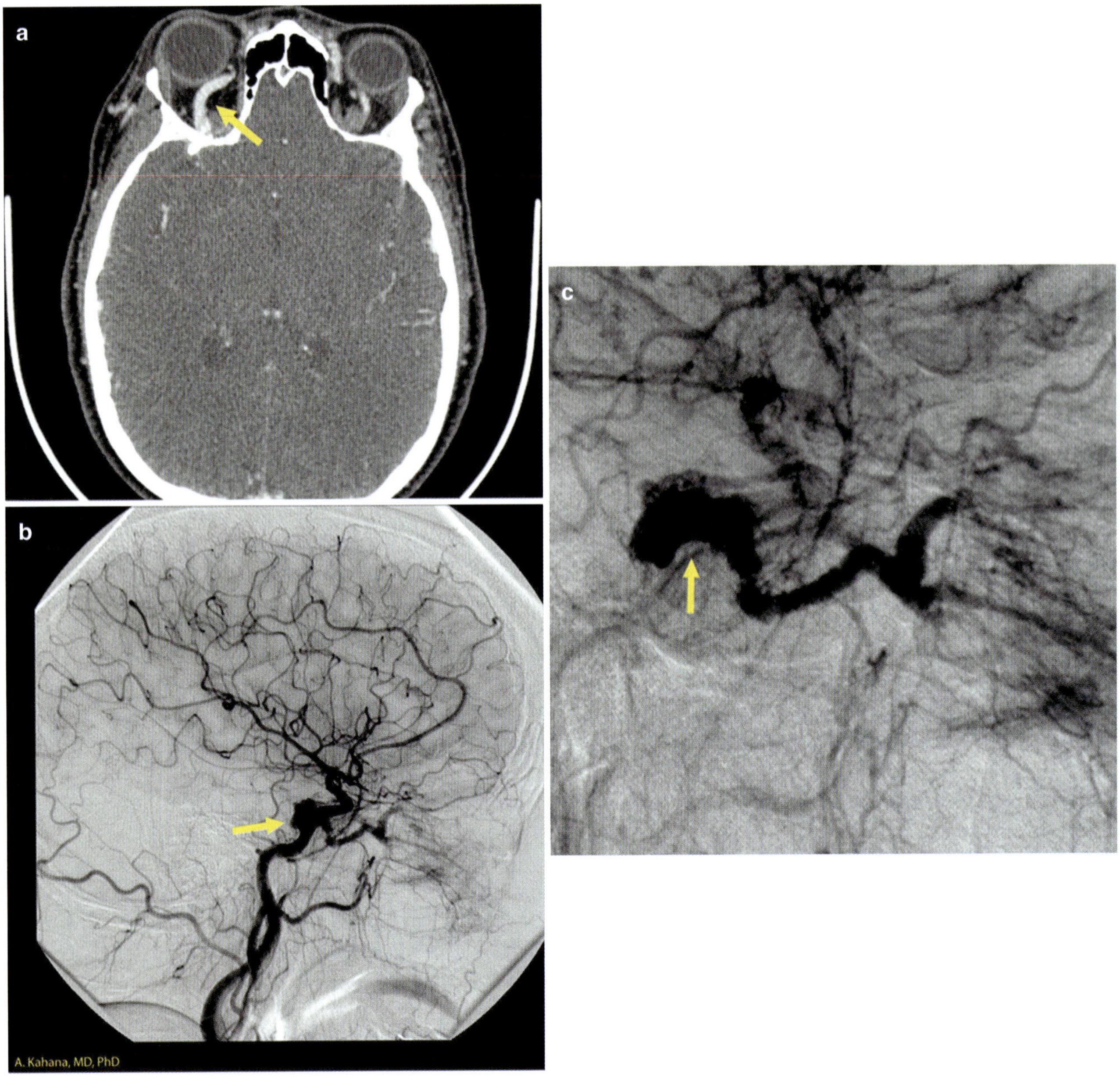

Fig. 51.9 High-flow direct carotid-cavernous fistula. This patient presented with right proptosis and vision loss. CT imaging revealed a dilated superior ophthalmic vein (**a**, arrow). Angiogram revealed early enhancement of the right cavernous sinus (**b**, arrow), coincident with early filling of the cerebral arterial tree. Blood and contrast flow out of the carotid artery uncovers the full extent of the dilated cavernous sinus (**c**, arrow) and superior ophthalmic vein, which is filling by retrograde flow. The CCF thrombosed spontaneously, and the patient fully recovered vision

noninvasive dynamic imaging may provide most of the needed information.

Treatment requires closure of the fistula. CCFs may close spontaneously, especially the low-flow type. If intervention is required, endovascular occlusion and embolization are the preferred approaches. The orbital surgeon may occasionally be asked by the endovascular surgeon to obtain access to the vascular channels through the orbit. A dilated superior ophthalmic vein is typically exposed and cannulated just below and next to the superior rectus muscle, via an anterior orbitotomy through a lid-crease incision. After securing the cannula and closing the incision, the patient is transferred to the fluoroscopy suite, where the endovascular procedure can proceed. There is a risk for intraoperative hemorrhage, and the orbital surgeon must remain available for emergent surgical intervention should it be needed.

Conclusion

Treatment of orbital vascular anomalies is complex and depends on making an accurate diagnosis based on history, clinical exam, and imaging studies. The key points to consider are location within the orbit, blood flow characteristics, age of patient, and symptoms. Once the diagnosis is made, the natural history of the lesion should be considered when contemplating intervention. Careful observation is commonly the most appropriate recommendation, in keeping with the old adage, "primum non nocere."

References

1. Al-Adnani M, Williams S, Rampling D, Ashworth M, Malone M, Sebire NJ. Histopathological reporting of paediatric cutaneous vascular anomalies in relation to proposed multidisciplinary classification system. J Clin Pathol. 2006;59(12):1278–82.
2. Enjolras O, Wassef M, Chapot R. Color atlas of vascular tumors and vascular malformations. Cambridge/New York: Cambridge University Press; 2007.
3. Rootman J, Heran MK, Graeb DA. Vascular malformations of the orbit: classification and the role of imaging in diagnosis and treatment strategies*. Ophthalmic Plast Reconstr Surg. 2014;30(2):91–104.
4. Harris GJ. Orbital vascular malformations: a consensus statement on terminology and its clinical implications. Orbital Society. Am J Ophthalmol. 1999;127(4):453–5.
5. Rootman J. Diseases of the orbit: a multidisciplinary approach. Philadelphia: Lippincott; 1988.
6. Rootman J. Vascular malformations of the orbit: hemodynamic concepts. Orbit. 2003;22(2):103–20.
7. Smoker WR, Gentry LR, Yee NK, Reede DL, Nerad JA. Vascular lesions of the orbit: more than meets the eye. Radiographics. 2008;28(1):185–204; quiz 325.
8. Stacey AW, Gemmete JJ, Kahana A. Management of orbital and periocular vascular anomalies. Ophthalmic Plast Reconstr Surg. 2015;31(6):427–36.
9. Kahana A, Lee BJ, Flint A, Elner VM. Periocular epithelioid hemangioma: response to bevacizumab and vascular pathogenesis. Arch Ophthalmol. 2012;130(9):1209–12.
10. Leaute-Labreze C, Dumas de la Roque E, Hubiche T, Boralevi F, Thambo JB, Taieb A. Propranolol for severe hemangiomas of infancy. N Engl J Med. 2008;358(24):2649–51.
11. Atchison EA, Garrity JA, Castillo F, Engman SJ, Couch SM, Salomao DR. Expression of vascular endothelial growth factor receptors in benign vascular lesions of the orbit: a case series. Ophthalmology. 2016;123(1):209–13.
12. Aitsebaomo J, Portbury AL, Schisler JC, Patterson C. Brothers and sisters: molecular insights into arterial-venous heterogeneity. Circ Res. 2008;103(9):929–39.
13. Kahana A, Lucarelli MJ, Grayev AM, Van Buren JJ, Burkat CN, Gentry LR. Noninvasive dynamic magnetic resonance angiography with Time-Resolved Imaging of Contrast KineticS (TRICKS) in the evaluation of orbital vascular lesions. Arch Ophthalmol. 2007;125(12):1635–42.
14. Natarajan SK, Born D, Ghodke B, Britz GW, Sekhar LN. Histopathological changes in brain arteriovenous malformations after embolization using Onyx or N-butyl cyanoacrylate. Laboratory investigation. J Neurosurg. 2009;111(1):105–13.
15. Chiramel GK, Keshava SN, Moses V, Mammen S, David S, Sen S. Percutaneous sclerotherapy of congenital slow-flow vascular malformations of the orbit. Cardiovasc Intervent Radiol. 2015;38(2):270–9.
16. Colletti G, Biglioli F, Poli T, et al. Vascular malformations of the orbit (lymphatic, venous, arteriovenous): diagnosis, management and results. J Craniomaxillofac Surg. 2019;47(5):726–40.
17. Sundar G. Vascular lesions of the orbit: conceptual approach and recent advances. Indian J Ophthalmol. 2018;66(1):3–6.
18. Hill RH 3rd, Shiels WE 2nd, Foster JA, et al. Percutaneous drainage and ablation as first line therapy for macrocystic and microcystic orbital lymphatic malformations. Ophthalmic Plast Reconstr Surg. 2012;28(2):119–25.
19. Schwarcz RM, Ben Simon GJ, Cook T, Goldberg RA. Sclerosing therapy as first line treatment for low flow vascular lesions of the orbit. Am J Ophthalmol. 2006;141(2):333–9.
20. Kahana A, Bohnsack BL, Cho RI, Maher CO. Subtotal excision with adjunctive sclerosing therapy for the treatment of severe symptomatic orbital lymphangiomas. Arch Ophthalmol. 2011;129(8):1073–6.
21. Rosen N, Priel A, Simon GJ, Rosner M. Cryo-assisted anterior approach for surgery of retroocular orbital tumours avoids the need for lateral or transcranial orbitotomy in most cases. Acta Ophthalmol. 2010;88(6):675–80.
22. North PE, Waner M, James CA, Mizeracki A, Frieden IJ, Mihm MC Jr. Congenital nonprogressive hemangioma: a distinct clinicopathologic entity unlike infantile hemangioma. Arch Dermatol. 2001;137(12):1607–20.
23. North PE, Waner M, Mizeracki A, et al. A unique microvascular phenotype shared by juvenile hemangiomas and human placenta. Arch Dermatol. 2001;137(5):559–70.
24. Sullivan TJ. Vascular anomalies of the orbit – a reappraisal. Asia Pac J Ophthalmol (Phila). 2018;7(5):356–63.
25. Itinteang T, Brasch HD, Tan ST, Day DJ. Expression of components of the renin-angiotensin system in proliferating infantile haemangioma may account for the propranolol-induced accelerated involution. J Plast Reconstr Aesthet Surg. 2011;64(6):759–65.
26. Sommers Smith SK, Smith DM. Beta blockade induces apoptosis in cultured capillary endothelial cells. In Vitro Cell Dev Biol Anim. 2002;38(5):298–304.
27. Kushner BJ. The treatment of periorbital infantile hemangioma with intralesional corticosteroid. Plast Reconstr Surg. 1985;76(4):517–26.
28. Kushner BJ, Lemke BN. Bilateral retinal embolization associated with intralesional corticosteroid injection for capillary hemangioma of infancy. J Pediatr Ophthalmol Strabismus. 1993;30(6):397–9.
29. Furusato E, Valenzuela IA, Fanburg-Smith JC, et al. Orbital solitary fibrous tumor: encompassing terminology for hemangiopericytoma, giant cell angiofibroma, and fibrous histiocytoma of the orbit: reappraisal of 41 cases. Hum Pathol. 2011;42(1):120–8.

Pediatric Orbital Disease

52

Mithra O. Gonzalez, Natalie A. Homer, and Vikram D. Durairaj

Introduction

The pediatric orbit is an enlarging bony cave wherein the globe and its accompanying soft tissue are found. Treatment of pediatric orbital disease requires sensitivity to the unique properties of the developing pediatric face, as well as detailed knowledge orbital diseases inherent to the pediatric population.

Pediatric Orbital Development and Anatomy

The pediatric orbit is an enlarging bony cave wherein the globe and its accompanying soft tissue are found. Not only does the pediatric orbit differ in size from the adult version, but the bones are more pliable, the adjacent sinuses are only just beginning to pneumatize, and there is an increased craniofacial ratio.

The infantile bony orbit is 17.3% to that of an adult [1]. With regard to the skeletal properties of the pediatric face, there is a high ratio of cancellous to cortical bone, as well as active growth centers of both bone and dentition [2]. Given the relative paucity of skeletal mineralization, the pediatric facial skeleton is remarkably malleable. Thus pediatric facial fractures should alert practitioners to the possibility of high-energy trauma, and patients should be assessed for signs of soft tissue entrapment within elastic fracture sites [2].

M. O. Gonzalez
University of Rochester Department of Ophthalmology, Oral and Maxillofacial Surgery, Otolaryngology, Plastic and Reconstructive Surgery, Rochester, NY, USA

N. A. Homer
Ophthalmic Plastic and Reconstructive Surgery, TOC Eye and Face, Austin, TX, USA

V. D. Durairaj (✉)
Dell Medical School – University of Texas at Austin, TOC Eye and Face, Austin, TX, USA

Ophthalmic Plastic and Reconstructive Surgery, TOC Eye and Face, Austin, TX, USA
e-mail: vdurairaj@tocaustin.com

The paranasal sinuses of the pediatric face enlarge and pneumatize throughout childhood [3, 4]. The ethmoid and maxillary sinuses are present at birth in an immature form [3, 4]. The ethmoid sinuses continue to mature and pneumatize from birth to 8 years of life [3, 4]. The maxillary sinuses, present at birth, enlarge from age 7 to 18 [3, 4]. The sphenoid sinuses are next to appear yet do not fully pneumatize until the age of 12. The frontal sinuses cannot be seen radiographically until 1–6 years of age [3, 4]. The delayed pneumatization of the frontal sinus leads to higher rates of orbital roof fractures in the pediatric population.

The pediatric orbit has an increased craniofacial ratio, compared to that of an adult. The infant cranium to facial skeleton ratio is 8:1, while the adolescence ratio is 2:1 [2]. Between the ages of 5 and 7 years of life, the cranio–orbito–zygomatic skeleton reaches approximately 85% of its adult size [2, 5]. The increased craniofacial ratio influences location and frequency of pediatric facial fractures.

Variations in orbital soft tissue in the pediatric population also contribute to commonly seen pathology in this age group. Certain soft tissue lesions are found nearly exclusively in this patient population (e.g., rhabdomyosarcoma), while other disorders occur less commonly (e.g., thyroid orbitopathy) than in their adult counterparts. Anatomical differences also may have surgical implications. For instance, at birth, the distance from the rectus muscle insertions to the corneal limbus is roughly 2 mm less than in adults, and does not reach the ultimate distance until 20 months of age [1].

The evaluation of the pediatric patient, especially the extremely young, can be challenging and unreliable and therefore requires a heightened index of suspicion and a broad differential diagnosis. Management of these disease processes requires an understanding of the growing face and sensitivity to the long-term impact of intervention. Fortunately, the pediatric orbit is highly resilient. The aim of this chapter is to provide information about pediatric orbital disease processes with emphasis placed on features that distinguish them from their adult counterparts.

J. J. Servat et al. (eds.), *Smith and Nesi's Ophthalmic Plastic and Reconstructive Surgery*,
https://doi.org/10.1007/978-3-030-41720-8_52

Infectious Orbital Disease

Periorbital inflammation and infection may be classified as preseptal or postseptal, based on anatomical extent of disease. The orbital septum is a thin areolar tissue that originates at the arcus marginalis of the orbital rim and extends to attach at upper and lower eyelid tarsus. The arcus marginalis is continuous with the periorbita posteriorly. The distinction of pre- or postseptal cellulitis has significant management and prognostic implications. In the majority of cases, infectious preseptal or orbital cellulitis is caused by bacteria, although can rarely arise from mycotic or viral infections.

Bacterial Preseptal Cellulitis

Bacterial preseptal cellulitis is more common than postseptal cellulitis, accounting for 65–84% of pediatric periorbital infections [6–9]. It is commonly associated with skin trauma but may be result from upper respiratory tract infections and dacryocystitis [7, 10]. Typical signs and symptoms include erythema, pain, warmth, and swelling of the eyelid with possible extension to the brow or cheek. *Haemophilus influenzae* (H. flu) was historically the most common pathogen of preseptal cellulitis and was associated with a high level of bacteremia (80%), because of its ability to cause central nervous system (CNS) sequelae including meningitis and death [6, 11–13]. Since the advent of the H. flu type B vaccine in 1985, the incidence of H. flu-derived preseptal cellulitis has decreased [6, 13, 14]. *Staph.* and *Strep.* species have now become the most common pathologic isolates [6, 7, 13].

Mild afebrile cases of preseptal cellulitis may be managed as an outpatient with oral antibiotics that cover empiric pathogens (e.g., amoxicillin/clavulanate or trimethoprim/sulfamethoxazole) [15]. The patient should be followed daily until symptomatic resolution is observed. Admission should be considered in children less than 5 years of age, those with confirmed H. flu, and in patients with moderate-to-severe edema, constitutional symptoms, unreliable follow-up, or failure to improve within 24–48 hours of oral antibiotic initiation [15].

Bacterial Orbital Cellulitis

Bacterial orbital cellulitis has significant associated morbidity and thus needs to be distinguished from its more common preseptal counterpart. A thorough ophthalmic evaluation with particular attention to orbital signs will allow for differentiation between preseptal cellulitis and orbital cellulitis. The differential diagnosis includes mycotic orbital infection, thyroid eye disease, noninfectious inflammation, trauma-related edema, as well as vascular, congenital, and neoplastic pathologies.

Signs such as exophthalmos/proptosis, diplopia, chemosis, and a relative afferent papillary defect suggest an orbital process and have been associated with orbital cellulites [7, 16]. Many of these signs result from soft tissue volume increase (i.e., edema or abscess) within the bony orbital confines, resulting anterior subluxation of the globe and optic nerve. Globe proptosis is seen in 61–99% of orbital cellulitis cases [7]. A collection of purulent material often collects between the periosteum and bony orbit (i.e., subperiosteal abscess), typically adjacent to the superomedial ethmoid sinuses, and may induce globe displacement and motility limitations in the direction of the abscess [17].

A myriad of morbid sequelae may result from orbital cellulitis. Vision loss from optic nerve or retina compromise may occur from a variety of mechanisms, including orbital compartment syndrome, direct mass effect, vascular occlusion, or collateral inflammation (sphenoethmoid sinusitis) [18–20]. Additional sequelae may include gaze paresis, exposure keratopathy, retinitis, uveitis, exudative retinal detachment, and endophthalmitis [21]. The orbit's propinquity to the central nervous system also places patients at risk for developing cavernous sinus thrombosis, meningitis, subdural empyema, and epidural abscess [22].

Diagnostic testing often includes a complete blood count (CBC), blood cultures, and an imaging study. Computerized tomography (CT) is generally safe and the most commonly employed imaging modality of orbital cellulites, although enthusiasm for its uses has been tempered by safety concerns in the pediatric population [23, 24]. Contrast-enhanced imaging enables detection of subperiosteal and orbital abscesses. Imaging typically reveals paranasal sinusitis (84–100%), usually involving the ethmoid air cells [7, 8, 16] (Fig. 52.1).

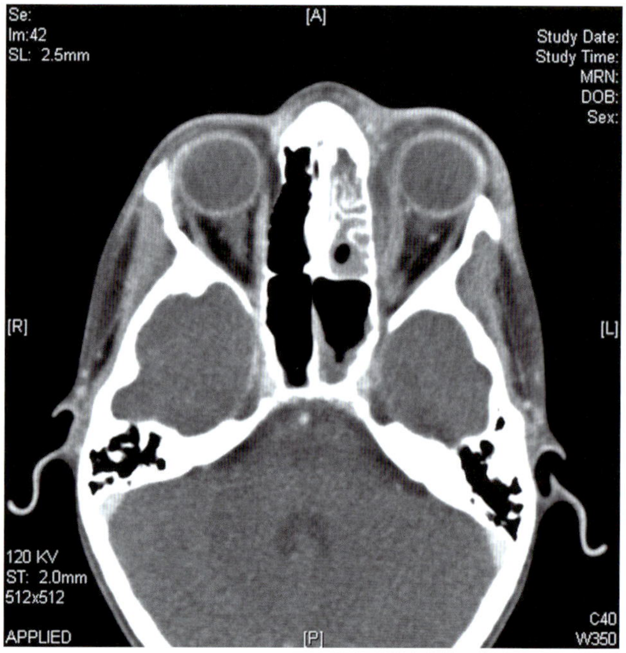

Fig. 52.1 Axial CT scan showing extensive left ethmoid sinusitis and subperiosteal abscess with lateral displacement of medial rectus

Organisms of preseptal cellulitis are also the common pathogens of orbital cellulitis, namely, *Staph.* and *Strep.* species [6, 7, 13, 17, 25]. Methicillin-resistant *Staphylococcus aureus* (MRSA), either community or hospital acquired, is of increasing concern in all periocular cellulites [26–28]. MRSA was the most common pathogen isolated from rare neonatal orbital abscesses [27, 29].

Management may consist of both medical and surgical interventions. Broad spectrum intravenous (IV) antibiotics, such as combinations of vancomycin and ampicillin–sulbactam or piperacillin–tazobactam, are used. In children less than 9 years of age, ceftriaxone is often used singularly [15, 21]. Current recommendations are for IV antibiotics, for a minimum of 3 days or until a clinical improvement is observed, followed by 7–10 days of oral antibiotics [15, 21]. Microbial sensitivity is dynamic, and an infectious disease consultation may provide considerable benefit. Initiation of systemic steroids at dose of 1 mg/kg/day, once the patient demonstrates clinical improvement or has C-reactive protein less than 4 mg/dl on antibiotics, has been shown to decrease length of hospital stay [30, 31]. Nasal decongestants may also be beneficial.

The timing of surgical interventions is a contentious subject and, consequently, the subject of extensive research. Some groups have advocated for immediate drainage of all subperiosteal abscesses and adjacent sinuses reasoning to decrease chance of extraorbital spread [32, 33]. Others have found that subperiosteal abscesses can resolve with IV antibiotics alone and that surgical intervention risks seeding of infection to the CNS [17, 34]. Harris found that subperiosteal abscesses become increasingly aggressive with age and that children greater than 15 years of age were more likely to be unresponsive to IV antibiotics, require surgical intervention, and have polymicrobial disease [17].

Jain and Rubin proposed a series of recommendations to guide management in setting of abscess [21]. Emergent drainage should be performed on patients with optic nerve or retina compromise. This should be preceded by an immediate canthotomy and cantholysis in setting of elevated intraocular pressure and taught swollen eyelids, suggestive of orbital compartment syndrome [21]. Urgent drainage is performed on patients with large subperiosteal abscesses associated with significant pain, intracranial complications, or frontal sinusitis. Expectant observation may be offered to patients with subperiosteal abscesses less than 9 years of age who are admitted and treated with IV antibiotics. These patients should be closely monitored at 6-hour intervals with special attention to the pupillary reflex [14].

Mycotic Orbital Cellulitis

Although a rare cause of orbital infections, mycotic orbital cellulitis is associated with high morbidity and a mortality rate of at least 66% [35]. Fungus of the *Mucoraceae* family such as *Mucor*, *Rhizopus*, and *Absidia* and mold *Aspergillus* and *Candida* are organisms isolated from these mycotic infections. *Mucor* and *Aspergillus* invade blood vessels which leads to local and disseminated thromboembolic events [36].

In the United States, mycotic orbital cellulitis is primarily seen in immunocompromised patients, while other countries have reported more extensively of infections occurring in immunocompetent individuals [36–39]. Risk factors for *Aspergillus* infections include total neutrophil count ≤1000/mm^3, AIDS, defective phagocytosis, hematologic malignancy, steroid or other immunosuppressive medication use, diabetes mellitus, prosthetic devices, trauma, and environmental exposure to building demolition, compost heaps, or endemic areas (e.g., Sudan) [39]. Although *Aspergillus* infections may be more common than *Mucor* in the immunocompromised population, both can produce opportunistic infections [36]. Beyond immunosuppression, specific risk factors for *Mucor* infections include diabetes mellitus, hematologic malignancy, renal disease, steroids, antimetabolites, and burns [36].

As many of the infected patients are immunocompromised, signs and symptoms may be minimal to nonspecific and include periorbital edema, facial pain, and headache until late in the disease course [38]. Others signs and symptoms may include nasal obstruction, exophthalmos, ptosis, decreased visual acuity, cranial nerve palsy, fever, altered/loss of consciousness, facial induration, and skin necrosis [36, 40–42].

A high index of suspicion in setting of the aforementioned signs, symptoms, and risk factors is required to accurately diagnose mycotic orbital cellulitis. Both CT and magnetic resonance (MR) imaging have been successfully employed. As with most orbital cellulitis, mycotic orbital cellulitis most commonly spreads from paranasal ethmoid or maxillary sinusitis [36, 42]. CT findings may include soft tissue contrast enhancement, bony erosion, thickening of the sinus linings, absence of fluid levels, small foci of gas or calcification, and areas of hypodensity [36, 42]. MRI may provide superior delineation of involved soft tissue including brain and cavernous sinus [37, 40]. Chest imaging should additionally be considered due to a high incidence of pulmonary involvement [40].

Management of mycotic orbital cellulitis is complex and requires a multidisciplinary team to treat often medically complicated patients with concurrent mycotic sinus and brain disease [36, 37, 42, 43]. Despite rapid diagnosis and treatment and a combination of aggressive medical and surgical interventions, mortality remains high [37]. IV antifungal therapy includes amphotericin B, liposomal amphotericin B, itraconazole, voriconazole, echinocandins, caspsofungin, and micafungin. Immune reconstitution is occasionally attempted [40]. When possible, a biopsy should be obtained via a direct or endoscopic approach. Focal areas of hypodensity within apical infiltrates on CT with contrast may correlate with abscesses and be targeted for biopsy [38]. Surgical debridement of involved orbital and sinus tissues, and sometimes complete orbital exenteration, is indicated [39, 43]. More recently intraorbital injections of liposomal amphotericin have been utilized with some success [44]. Repeat biopsy and debridement are not uncommon [37].

Pediatric Orbital Inflammatory Disease

Pediatric orbital inflammatory diseases may be seen in the pediatric population and are often diagnoses of exclusion, once infection and neoplasm have been ruled out. These etiologies often follow a similar presentation and course of to their adult counterparts, with some exceptions.

Idiopathic Orbital Inflammation

Also known as orbital pseudotumor, idiopathic orbital inflammation is a noninfectious, nonneoplastic inflammatory disease of unknown etiology. In the adult population, it follows thyroid eye disease (TED) and lymphoproliferative disease as the third most common orbital disease, accounting for 4.7–16% of cases [45, 46]. Orbital pseudotumor in children is rare, with only 68 reported cases in the literature [46]. Biopsy-proven orbital inflammation has been reported in children as young as 10 months of age [47].

On presentation, the most common signs and symptoms include edema, pain, redness, palpable mass, and diplopia/motility restriction that has developed over hours to days and, occasionally, weeks [46, 48, 49]. Unlike their adult counterparts, the pediatric population may display constitutional symptoms such as headache, emesis, sore throat, lethargy, and weight loss [49]. The pediatric population is more likely to have bilateral disease, uveitis, disc edema, and preceding trauma [49, 50]. Clinical presentations include dacryoadenitis (21%), myositis (19%), dacryoadenitis and myositis (5%), orbital apex (6%), and more generalized inflammation of the orbital soft tissues and/or optic nerve (14%) [45].

The differential diagnosis of idiopathic orbital inflammation differs slightly from that of adults and includes infectious orbital cellulitis, congenital abnormalities (e.g., dermoid cyst, sinus mucocoele), and other inflammatory diseases such as sarcoidosis, Wegener's granulomatosis, TED, traumatic diseases, and neoplastic diseases (e.g., rhabdomyosarcoma, leukemia, lymphoma, retinoblastoma, optic nerve glioma) [46, 47].

Diagnostic testing includes a CBC, erythrocyte sedimentation rate (ESR), thyroid function studies, and CT imaging [47]. In the setting of idiopathic orbital inflammation, serum studies are normal with the exception of an occasionally elevated leukocyte count, eosinophil count, and ESR [49]. Typical neuroimaging features of idiopathic orbital inflammation include exophthalmos, contrast enhancement, and infiltration of the orbital tissue, extraocular muscle enlargement (classically with tendon involvement), and the notable absence of contiguous paranasal sinus disease, bony erosion, or distortion of orbital contents [45, 47]. MRI imaging can be employed to further define tissue involvement and should be utilized if evidence of extraorbital extension [51].

Treatment often consists of corticosteroids, 1.0–1.5 mg/kg/day with a clinical response expected within 24–48 h [47]. Orbital biopsy is usually unnecessary, except for in atypical or refractory cases and when orbital malignancy is suspected [45–47]. Severe inflammation should raise suspicion for idiopathic sclerosing orbital inflammation, may be confirmed with biopsy, and often requires additional therapies [53]. Recurrences are seen in up to 37% of pediatric cases [50]. Additional therapies for refractory cases or those intolerant to steroids include radiotherapy and immunomodulation [48, 49, 52].

Pediatric Thyroid Eye Disease

Graves' disease is rare in children and, excluding neonatal Graves' disease, is estimated to have an incidence between 6.5 per 100,000 children, with 1 per million in children under 4 years of age and 38 per million in older children [54, 55]. Findings such as goiters, tachycardia, nervousness, hypertension, polyphagia, tremor, weight loss, heat intolerance, insomnia, behavioral issues, and nocturnal enuresis may be seen in those affected [55]. Pediatric thyroid eye disease (TED) is found in a subset (between 52% and 54%) of those with Graves' disease [56]. In the cohort of pediatric TED, there is a notable female predominance of 7:1 in some studies [55–57]. Nonneonatal disease has been reported in children as young as 4 months of age, with median age of diagnosis between 11 and 13.9 years [54, 55, 57]. Of those with TED, thyroid status varies with some reports having found hyperthyroid in 88.6%, euthyroid in 8.6%, and hypothyroid in 2.9%, while other studies report that pediatric patients with TED are predominately euthyroid (89%) [56, 57].

Pediatric patients with TED typically are more mildly affected in comparison to adults. Signs and symptoms often include eyelid retraction (38–82%), exophthalmos (23–80%), lid lag (74–86%), conjunctival injection (48%), lagophthalmos (37%), foreign body sensation (37%), photophobia (28%) and pain (25%), diplopia (17%), superior limbic keratitis (17%), and extraocular motility defects (11–24%) [55–57] (Fig. 52.2). Postpubescent patients tend to have similar signs and symptoms to their adult counterparts, where prepubescent children display more mild disease, suggesting a hormonal correlation [56]. Specifically, postpubescent TED patients more commonly have proptosis (80% vs. 50%), strabismus (24% vs. 0%), and periorbital

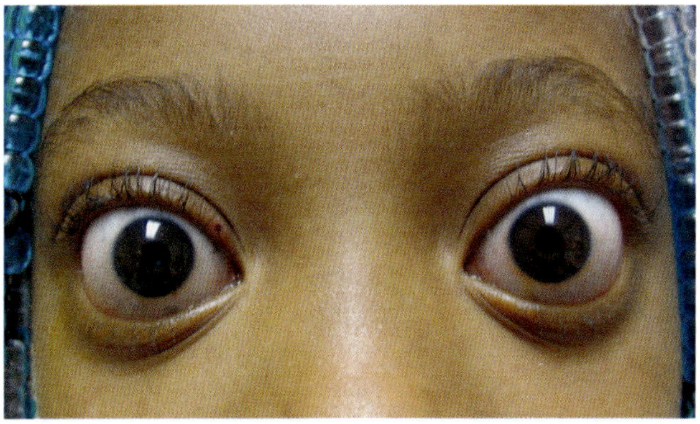

Fig. 52.2 An 8-year-old girl with pediatric thyroid eye disease manifested by exophthalmos and eyelid retraction

fullness (7% vs. 0%), when compared to the prepubescent age group [56]. Orbital radiologic imaging may demonstrate increased orbital fat volume and/or tendon-sparing enlargement of the rectus muscles, most commonly the medial and inferior rectus [56].

The differential diagnosis of pediatric TED may include infectious, neoplastic, traumatic, congenital, and other inflammatory disorders. Pediatric lid retraction may also result from disease of the dorsal midbrain (e.g., pinealoma, hydrocephalus, meningitis, cyclic oculomotor spasm, Duane syndrome), peripheral nervous system (e.g., aberrant cranial nerve III regeneration, overactive sympathetic system, Marcus Gunn jaw-winking), neuromuscular junction (e.g., drugs, myasthenia gravis), muscle (e.g., thyroid, hyperkalemic periodic paralysis, chronic systemic corticosteroid use, congenital levator fibrosis), or other nonspecific etiologies [58].

Initial diagnostic testing includes serum thyroid function studies. CT and MR imaging may be performed, although are often not needed. Children with TED tend to have a pattern of orbital fat enlargement without significant muscle enlargement [59].

Treatment in the vast majority of pediatric TED patients is supportive [55–57]. Ocular lubricants and sunglasses may relieve ocular surface discomfort [57]. Stabilization of the patient's thyroid function is of great importance to the child's systemic health and has correlated with a reduction in eyelid retraction [55]. In rare cases, surgical correction of the orbit, extraocular muscles, or eyelids may be necessary to address disfiguring proptosis, exposure keratopathy, or diplopia [55–57]. TED-induced optic neuropathy is exceedingly rare [55–57]. Steroids, immunomodulators, and radiation are not often utilized in the pediatric population [57].

Pediatric Granulomatosis with Polyangiitis

Pediatric orbital granulomatosis with polyangiitis (GPA; formerly Wegener's granulomatosis) is rare, with 13 total cases reported in the literature [60]. Ocular involvement is noted in approximately 50% of adults with GPA [61]. Signs and symptoms may include proptosis, optic neuritis, nasolacrimal duct obstruction, altered motility, orbital inflammation, conjunctivitis, episcleritis, scleritis, uveitis, and vasculitis of the retina, choroid, and optic nerve [64]. The differential diagnosis is similar to that of other pediatric orbital processes. Antineutrophil cytoplasmic antibody testing (ANCA) or biopsy may be used to diagnosis GPA [60, 62]. In the largest retrospective review reported, six children were diagnosed with ocular GPA, five of whom were found to have systemic disease (e.g., respiratory, renal, or both). This is of significance because if untreated, GPA can have life-threatening consequences [60]. The ocular signs and symptoms of GPA respond well to prompt steroid initiation, although other immunomodulators such as methotrexate, cyclophosphamide, and infliximab may be required [60].

Systemic Lupus Erythematosus

Systemic lupus erythematosus (SLE) is a disease thought to result from immune complex deposition throughout the body [63]. The common and severe ocular and periocular findings of SLE include keratoconjunctivitis sicca, periorbital edema, retinal microangiopathy, optic neuropathy, extraocular dysmotility, chronic blepharitis/eczema, and orbital changes [63]. There are few reports of SLE orbital disease in the pediatrics literature [64, 65]. When it does occur, SLE-associated orbital inflammation may mimic idiopathic orbital inflammation or myositis [66]. Lupus profundus is a panniculitis (adipose inflammation) that pathologically appears as lymphocytic infiltrate of the subcutaneous connective tissue and orbital fat with vasculitis [63, 66–68]. Lupus profundus often presents with globe proptosis and be the initial finding of SLE [67]. Although exceedingly rare, SLE-associated panniculitis may progress into orbital infarction syndrome that results in limited extraocular movements, chronic fistula formation, complete loss of vision, and orbital soft tissue necrosis [69]. Biopsy is necessary to confirm the diagnosis. Medical treatment options include steroids, nonsteroidal anti-inflammatory drugs, antimalarial and other immunomodulators, and plasmapheresis [63].

Periarteritis Nodosa/Polyarteritis Nodosa

Periarteritis nodosa or polyarteritis nodosa (PAN) is a systemic necrotizing vasculitis that affects small- to medium-sized vessels, originally described in 1866 by Kussmaul and Maier [70]. It is uncommon in all age groups but, when described, typically affects males between the ages of 40 and 60 [71]. Ten to 20 percent of patients with PAN have ocular disease such as retinal artery occlusions, ischemic optic neuropathy, scleritis, extraocular nerve pareses, and orbital inflammation [71]. Although orbital inflammation with proptosis is a known phenomenon in PAN, it is an uncommon presentation [70–72]. Rarely, muscle involvement may lead to clinical and radiographic findings similar to TED [70]. Diagnostic testing includes perinuclear antinuclear cytoplasmic antibody assay, arteriography, and biopsy [71]. Treatment is with steroids and other immunosuppressive agents [71].

Sarcoidosis

Sarcoidosis has three primary clinical variations in the pediatric population. Children younger than 5 years of age and (typically during the first year of life) may develop "early-onset sarcoidosis" (EOS), which consists of the clinical trial of exanthema, arthritis, and uveitis and rarely has accompanying pulmonary disease [73]. Blau syndrome, an autosomal dominant granulomatous disease consisting of dermatitis, arthritis, and uveitis, is a second variant of pediatric sarcoidosis [74]. Mutations in the gene NOD2 (nucleotide-binding oligomerization domain 2) have been reported in both EOS and Blau syndrome, suggesting a shared disease process [75]. Some have placed the two disease processes under the unifying rubric of "pediatric granulomatous arthritis" [76]. The third variant, termed pediatric sarcoidosis, typically affects children older than 5 years of age and presents similarly to that of the adult disease [73, 78, 79]. Correspondingly, findings of bilateral hilar lymphadenopathy and pulmonary infiltration are commonly seen [78, 79].

The prevalence of adult sarcoidosis is between 10 and 40 cases per 100,000, while pediatric sarcoidosis occurs much more rarely in 0.22 to 0.27 per 100,000 children [78]. The age of pediatric sarcoidosis onset ranges between 13 and 15 years of age and, unlike the adult variant, does not have a sexual predilection [78]. Within the southeastern United States, African Americans have a higher incidence of disease [78]. The etiology of sarcoidosis is unknown, although experts often invoke a combined mechanism hypothesis of genetic susceptibility and environmental exposure [78, 80].

The clinical presentation of pediatric sarcoidosis varies by disease variant. EOS and Blau syndrome lack pulmonary involvement and instead present with dermatitis, arthritis, and/or uveitis [73, 77, 78, 80]. Pediatric sarcoidosis in the older population most commonly presents with pulmonary symptoms, including chest pain, dyspnea, and cough, along with lymphadenopathy, arthritis, rash, and parotid gland enlargement [78, 80]. Between 24% and 58% of those with pediatric sarcoidosis have ocular disease such as uveitis (30–70%), conjunctival or eyelid granuloma (40%), dacryoadenitis, and optic neuropathy [78, 80]. Of those with isolated orbital sarcoidosis, the most common signs and symptoms were palpable mass/swelling (65–88.5%), ptosis (27–45%), and proptosis/globe displacement (25–42%) [81, 82]. Although not common to pediatric literature, other orbital manifestations of sarcoidosis have been reported in the adult literature [81, 82]. Radiographic orbital sarcoid disease may include lacrimal gland infiltration (42–55%), orbital mass (20–39%), optic nerve sheath and dural inflammation (20%), and extraocular muscle enlargement (3–5%) [81, 82].

As no single diagnostic test to confirm sarcoid disease, sarcoidosis remains a diagnosis of exclusion [78, 80]. Clinical findings and radiographic or serologic evidence, coupled with a biopsy demonstrating noncaseating epithelioid granulomatous inflammation, are usually diagnostically sufficient [80]. Similar biopsy findings may also be seen in tuberculosis, leprosy, Sjogren's syndrome, Behcet's disease, and berylliosis [80, 82]. Chest radiographs have been reported as abnormal in up to 80–90% of those with sarcoidosis [78, 80]. Chest CT imaging has also been used to determine pulmonary involvement. Angiotensin-converting enzymes (ACE) levels, which are thought to correlate with an individual's total granuloma burden, are elevated in up to 50% of children with pediatric sarcoidosis [78]. In addition to elevated ACE levels, blood work may show serum elevations in lysozyme and calcium [82]. When sarcoidosis affects orbital tissue, CT or MR imaging of the orbit and, possibly, a gallium scan may be of use [82]. Conceivably, genetic testing could be of use in those individuals with Blau syndrome or EOS.

Immunosuppression with corticosteroids is the first-line agent in the treatment of pediatric sarcoidosis [78, 80]. Other immunosuppressive agents, such as methotrexate, mycophenolate, and infliximab, have been used in refractory cases and those intolerant to steroids [78]. In addition to immunosuppression, orbital cases specifically have been treated with systemic, cyclosporine, hydroxychloroquine and azathioprine, intraorbital and intralesional steroid injection, surgical debulking, and observation [81, 82].

Pediatric Crohn's Disease

Inflammatory bowel disease (IBD) consists of ulcerative colitis (UC), Crohn's disease (CD), and inflammatory disorders of unknown cause. UC and CD are affecting both males and females in early and late adulthood, with incidence of approximately 5.6–10.4 per 100,000 [83]. Although the etiology remains unclear, environmental factors, combined with a genetic predisposition, seem to play a role [83, 84]. Ocular involvement of Crohn's disease is seen in approximately 10% of cases. Dry eye is the most common reported manifestation (50%), although steroid-induced cataract (30%), uveitis (11.5%), scleritis, episcleritis (8%), and conjunctivitis are also seen [83–85]. Optic neuritis, papillitis, and neuroretinitis have been associated with Crohn's disease [83, 84]. Orbital findings of inflammation, myositis, acute dacryoadenitis, blepharitis, and lid swelling may also be seen [83, 84, 86–89]. Treatment of Crohn's disease includes immunosuppression with steroids, antimetabolites, T-cell inhibitors, alkylating agent, and antitumor necrosis factor [83]. Orbital inflammation typically responds well to steroids, although recurrence is not uncommon [83].

Sjogren's Syndrome

Sjogren's syndrome is a chronic disease of the exocrine glands. It may occur in isolation (i.e., primary Sjogren's syndrome) or may develop in the setting of other autoimmune conditions, such as rheumatoid arthritis, SLE, and progressive systemic sclerosis. The latter is known as secondary Sjogren's syndrome. Sjogren's syndrome affects females nine times more frequently than males, often presenting in the third and fourth decade of life [90]. Patients may complain of ocular or oral symptoms. Most commonly, patients present with symptoms of ocular surface dryness and are found clinically to have positive corneal staining or a decreased Schirmer's I test [90]. In rare cases the lacrimal glands may enlarge and be found as palpable masses [91, 92]. Biopsy reveals nonspecific lymphocytic infiltration [92]. In 5% of cases, a malignant lymphoma may develop [92]. Sjogren's syndrome rarely affects the pediatric age group, with very few reports in the pediatric literature [93].

Orbital Tumors

Congenital Orbital Tumors and Cysts

Hamartomas and Choristomas

A hamartoma is a nonneoplastic, disorganized collection of tissue that is native to the site where it is located. A choristoma is a collection of normal tissue located in abnormal site (i.e., ectopic). Like hamartoma, choristoma is nonneoplastic. Hamartoma types include neural-glial, vascular, soft tissue, and bone [94–99]. Vascular hamartomas including hemangiomas and lymphangiomas will be discussed in a later section [99]. Soft tissue hamartomas may include smooth muscle, adipose, and mesenchyme [97, 98]. Choristomas of both nervous and soft tissue types have been reported. Choristomatous neural tissue has included brain, cerebellar, glial, and meningeal tissue [100–103]. Soft tissue choristomas have included lacrimal gland, respiratory epithelium, and conjunctiva [104–106].

Clinical presentation of these lesions depends on the location and the tissue involved. Stationary and dynamic proptosis, anisocoria, pain, diplopia/strabismus, vision loss, epiphora, and palpable mass have been reported [94, 96, 97, 107–109]. Most congenital orbital hamartomas present during childhood. Imaging studies help to narrow the differential diagnosis. Tissue biopsy is necessary for definitive diagnosis. If treatment is indicated, surgical resection is the mainstay option.

Orbital cysts, which are often choristomas, are common to the pediatric population. Epidermal dermoid cysts accounted for up to 46% of all pediatric orbital lesions and 89% of all pediatric cystic lesions in a large review [110]. They may occur primarily (most common) or secondarily following surgery or trauma [110–112]. Shields and Shields devised a useful classification schema of orbital cystic lesions, which includes surface epithelium cysts, teratomatous cysts, neural cysts, secondary cysts, and inflammatory cysts [110].

Histopathologically, simple orbital epithelial cysts are comprised of epithelial tissue with characteristics of the skin, lung, or conjunctiva and, by definition, lack adnexal structures like hair shafts, sebaceous, and sweat glands. Epidermal dermoid cysts, alternatively, contain adnexal structures [110]. Teratomas classically contain histologic features of all embryonic germ layers including ectoderm, mesoderm, and endoderm [110]. Neural colobomatous cysts are commonly seen in the setting of microphthalmos, resulting from a failure of primary embryonic fissure [110]. Orbital neural cysts, associated with brain or meningeal tissue, may result from bony defects that lead to cephalocele or in the absence of a bony defect, ectopic brain [110]. Although rare, meningocele of the optic nerve has also been reported. Orbital cysts may result from activity in adjacent structures such as the sinuses (mucoceles) or teeth (dentigerous cyst). Rarely, orbital cysts can be seen in the setting of parasitic infection or neoplastic process [110].

Orbital dermoid cysts, also known as "dermoids," are the most common type of orbital cyst (89%) in the pediatric population [110]. Dermoid cysts are congenital nests of epithelial and subepithelial tissue with an epithelial lining containing dermal appendages, believed to have become trapped during embryonic development [110]. These cysts present over the first decade of life. In the orbit, dermoids are typically located in the superior lateral or superior medial spaces near the frontozygomatic or frontoethmoidal suture, respectively [110, 111] (Fig. 52.3). They are also commonly found at the lateral canthus [112]. Orbital dermoid cysts may be classified as simple versus complicated, or superficial versus deep [111]. Occasionally, a single dermoid cyst presents with both intraorbital and extraorbital components across a given suture, forming a "dumbbell dermoid" [110]. Most asymptomatic simple superficial lesions are found in younger children, while symptomatic complicated deep dermoids with bony erosion and tissue invasion are more often seen in adolescents and adults [111, 113]. Signs and symptoms of dermoids may include palpable mass, ptosis, diplopia, orbital inflammation (if cyst ruptures), fistulae, nasolacrimal duct

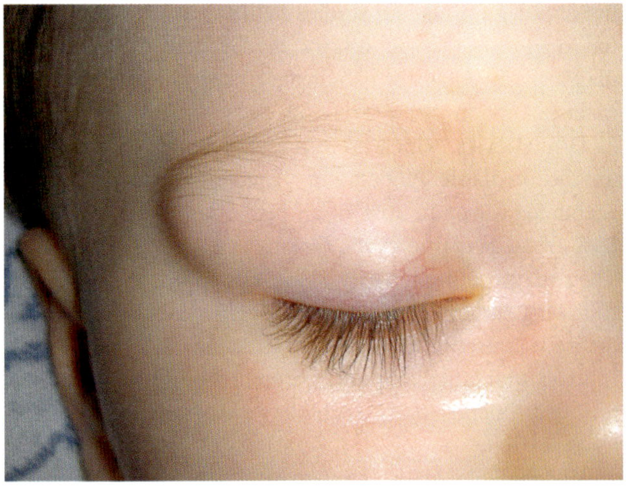

Fig. 52.3 Right dermoid cyst at the level of the frontozygomatic suture

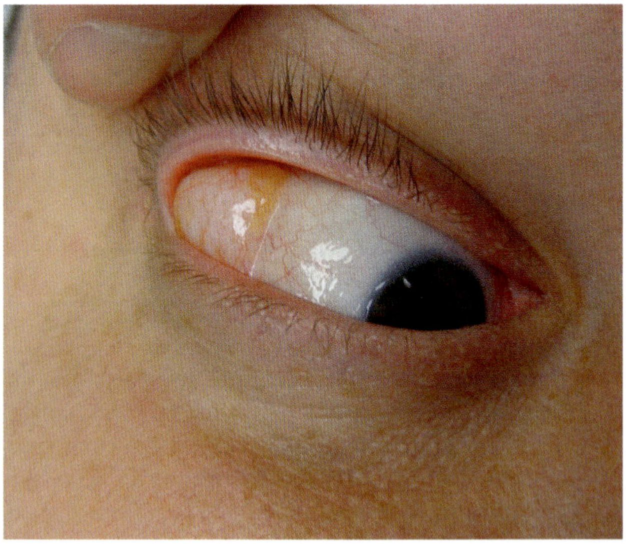

Fig. 52.4 Dermolipoma in superior lateral fornix

obstruction, extraocular rectus enlargement, choroidal folds, and proptosis [110, 111, 114, 115]. CT and MR imaging studies may be of use, especially when deep complicated dermoid cysts are suspected. In such imaging studies, bony changes are reported in up to 85% of patients, while 61% where noted to have a visible cystic wall [112, 116]. Calcification, fluid level, and orbital fat congestion are uncommonly seen [112]. Treatment depends on signs and symptoms. Asymptomatic dermoids may be observed, although parents should be warned about risk of cyst rupture. Most commonly surgical resection via en bloc cyst excision without wall disruption is recommended [110, 111]. In cases where surgical resection is not possible, percutaneous fluoroscopy-guided drainage and chemical ablation have been used [115].

Dermolipomas are another type of choristoma that are composed of adipose tissue and dense connective tissue [117]. They are often found in the superior lateral fornix and appear as yellow-colored mass with cilia or pilosebaceous structures [117] (Fig. 52.4). Dermolipomas adhere firmly to the overlying conjunctiva and may be contiguous with orbital fat. The masses can be irritating and deform the lateral canthus, prompting surgical excision. The differential diagnosis includes prolapsed orbital fat, lacrimal gland cyst, lymphangioma, and lymphoma [117]. Imaging studies are rarely necessary. Surgical resection is often the treatment of choice, although conservative resection is advised as complications including blepharoptosis, keratoconjunctivitis sicca, diplopia, symblepharon, and restrictive strabismus have been reported [117].

Teratomas or teratomatous cyst are rare congenital orbital tumors derived from the three germinal layers (endoderm, mesoderm, and ectoderm) [110]. Children typically present with massive unilateral proptosis progressing over days to weeks and may result in vision loss and severe facial deformation [110, 119, 120]. Malignant transformation has been reported in rare cases [110]. MR or CT imaging is helpful in the management and may reveal cystic changes [119]. Surgical excision is the definitive therapy and is often required, while aspiration has been used as a temporizing measure [110, 118–120].

Pediatric Orbital Neural Tumors

Optic Pathway Glioma

Optic pathway gliomas (OPGs) are the most frequent primary neoplasm of the optic pathway, often presenting in children (mean age of 8.8 years) and accounting for approximately 4–8% of all pediatric brain tumors [121–124]. Of OPGs, 24% are found along the optic nerve, termed optic nerve gliomas (ONG), while the remainder are chiasmal or retrochiasmal [124]. Between 30% and 50% of all OPGs are associated with neurofibromatosis type 1 (NF1); the remainder are sporadic [124].

Due to the increased incidence of OPGs among those with NF1 (15–20%), the majority of the research has focused on OPG in this setting [123]. Some studies have found that ONGs are more common in those with NF1, while postchiasmal involvement was more common to the sporadic variety [122]. According to some reports, OPG associated with NF1 have a more favorable prognosis compared to their sporadic counterpart. This may reflect an ascertainment bias as those with NF1 are screened for OPG, while those who develop sporadic OPG may have delayed presentation.

Signs and symptoms of OPG depend on the location of the lesion and include vision loss (87.5%), bitemporal hemianopsia, homonymous hemianopsia, diplopia, proptosis, relative afferent pupillary defect (RAPD), optic disc edema (35%) or atrophy (59%), choroidal folds, ophthalmoplegia,

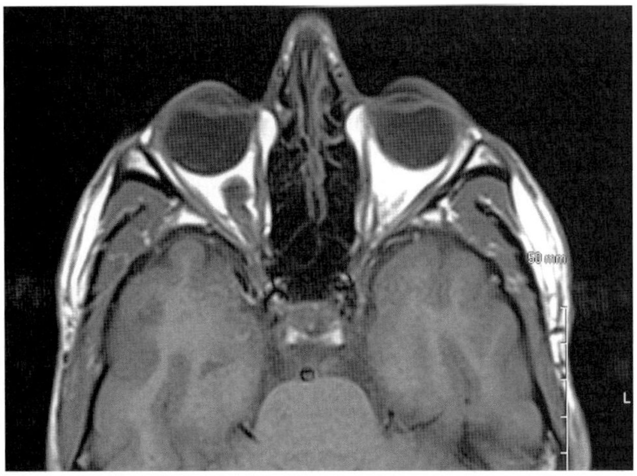

Fig. 52.5 MRI of right optic nerve glioma with multilobulated enlargement of optic nerve

nystagmus (23%), and hypothalamic signs (26%) [123, 124]. Accelerated linear growth, precocious puberty, headache, nausea, emesis, and hydrocephalus may be signs of hypothalamic involvement [124]. The growth rate of OPG is variable and can be rapid.

Diagnosis can often be made with imaging studies such as CT or MR imaging and without a biopsy [124] (Fig. 52.5). According to the World Health Organization, OPGs are, by histologic classification, most commonly grade I astrocytomas, although grade II fibrillary astrocytomas have been reported [122]. Classically, a well-demarcated fusiform enlargement or kinking of the optic nerve, as well as enlargement or enhancement of the optic chiasm or retrochiasmal visual pathway, may be observed [124]. Occasionally, lesions may have cystic components [123]. Once an OPG is suspected, a patient's neurofibromatosis status should be determined.

Management of OPGs is controversial, though with some consistent recommendation patterns. Prognosis is based primarily on location, with the highest morbidity rates associated with hypothalamic gliomas, followed by optic chiasmal gliomas (OCG). Optic nerve gliomas portend the best prognosis. Mortality of all patients with OPG is reported to be 30–33%, while those with ONG have a 6% mortality rate [124]. In the setting of ONG, the primary objective is vision preservation, and thus, surgical intervention is often limited to those cases that show either radiologic or ophthalmologic progression [122–124]. Other indications for treatment of OPG include obstructive hydrocephalus, exposure keratopathy, and cosmetically unacceptable proptosis [123]. The desire to perform surgery is tempered by its associated morbidity – vision loss [124]. Fortunately, stable vision and visual fields may be seen with observation in as many as 78% over a decade, although clinical and radiographic progression many be seen in as high as 40%. Treatment for unacceptable proptosis or exposure issues may involve surgical debulking [122]. Optic chiasmal gliomas and retrochiasmal gliomas are typically not amenable to complete surgical resection, and therefore radiation and chemotherapy may be employed [124]. Special consideration of treatment-related side effects should be taken in the pediatric population [123, 124]. Radiation therapy, for example, has been associated with numerous pediatric complications including intelligence impairment, endocrine dysfunction, and cerebral vasculopathy [123]. Chemotherapy, including carboplatin and vincristine, is often the first-line therapy for progressive lesions. Side effects include neutropenia, thrombocytopenia, and allergic reactions [124].

Orbital Neurofibroma

Orbital neurofibromas are the most common facial hamartomas, particularly frequent in 40–94% of patients with NF1 [125, 126]. The classification of neurofibromas is not formalized, although a commonly used system includes five subtypes: localized cutaneous, diffuse cutaneous, localized intraneural, plexiform, and massive soft tissue neurofibromas [127]. Localized cutaneous neurofibromas are extraneural tumors of less than 2 cm diameter and exhibit painless slow growth [127]. Localized intraneural neurofibromas affect peripheral nerves, particularly the spinal and cranial nerves and may be "dumbbell-shaped" [127]. They are the second most common type of neurofibroma. Diffuse cutaneous neurofibromas slowly spread along the planes of connective and adipose tissue in a plaque-like manner and are typically found on the head and neck [127]. They are found in 10% of those with NF1 [127]. Plexiform neurofibromas are more sensitive for NF1 and only rarely occur in a sporadic fashion [127]. Often located along large nerves, these proliferations of nerve sheath cells are capable of local destruction and compression [127]. Of the five types of neurofibromas, plexiform neurofibromas have shown to carry a risk of malignant transformation, further increased by the presence of NF1 and irradiation [127, 128]. Some believe that malignant transformation may occur with any neurofibroma [129]. The resulting highly aggressive malignant neoplasm is called a malignant peripheral nerve sheath tumor (MPNST) and may occur in between 1% and 5% of those with NF1 [127]. The rare fifth type of neurofibroma, a massive soft tissue neurofibroma, invades soft tissue and muscle, producing disfigurement [127].

Orbitotemporal neurofibromatosis was classified by Jackson into three groups: group I, soft tissue involvement with seeing eye; group II, soft tissue and significant bony involvement with seeing eye; and group III, soft tissue and bony involvement with blind or absent eye [130].

Ocular and orbital signs of neurofibromas depend on the location of the lesion and include ptosis (S-shaped deformity), brow ptosis, lateral canthus disinsertion, conjunctival/lacrimal gland infiltration, myopia, ocular pain/irritation, epiphora, exophthalmos, vision loss, and diplopia/strabismus [125, 126, 131, 132]. MPNST may be difficult to detect clinically because signs and symptoms can overlap with their nonmalignant counterpart, specifically pain, increasing size, and focal neurological deficit [129]. In the setting of NF1, a hypoplastic or absent sphenoid wing may result in pulsatile exophthalmos or enophthalmos [133].

CT and MR imaging studies may provide information about the extent and type of neurofibroma and thus inform the surgical risks and objectives. Neurofibromatous lesions may be encapsulated, infiltrative, solid, cystic, or heterogeneous [134]. MPNST appear similar to other sarcomas and are characteristically large, unencapsulated, and fusiform [128]. The sphenoid wing should be closely observed because of the dysplastic association with NF1. Biopsy is usually not necessary [126].

Treatment of orbitotemporal neurofibromas, which includes both pre- and postseptal neurofibromas, is challenging because infiltration is common, complete resection is rare, and, therefore, recurrence is frequent [126, 133]. If a neurofibroma is stable and does not cause significant psychosocial distress, it may be safely observed [133]. Indications for surgery include disfigurement, pain, dysfunction (i.e., amblyopia), suspicion for malignant transformation, and biopsy in the setting of diagnostic uncertainty [126]. Many surgeons recommend early intervention to prevent deformation and dysfunction [133]. When compelled, surgery is the treatment of choice, although radiotherapy has been used in some cases of subtotal resection [126, 127]. Although often impossible, complete resection is recommended to decrease the risk of malignant transformation and recurrence [133]. Among a cohort of children with NF1, those most likely to experience progression had surgery before age 10 (presumably because of inherently more aggressive lesions) and underwent subtotal resections [126]. In the setting of a seeing eye and a sphenoid wing defect, a combined transcranial orbitotomy in combination with neurosurgery may be preferred [133]. In patients with severe disfigurement and a non-seeing eye, orbital exenteration may reduce the risk of progression and malignant transformation and provide dramatically improved cosmesis [133]. Caution should be exhibited prior to embarking on these surgeries as a great number of complications have been reported, including intraoperative hemorrhage, poor healing, facial nerve palsy, blindness, and cerebral edema [133].

Orbital Meningioma

Orbital meningiomas may be primary or secondary and are comprised of meningothelial cap cells of the arachnoid villi [135, 136]. Primary orbital meningiomas originate from the optic nerve sheath, while secondary orbital meningiomas arise from the inner or outer aspect of the sphenoid wing or from within the cranium [135, 136]. Two to nine percent of all orbital tumors are meningiomas, with the secondary type predominating (90%) [135, 137]. Meningiomas may be unilateral, bilateral, or multifocal and associated with neurofibromatosis type 2 (NF2) [136]. Overall, there is a female proclivity, but there are conflicting reports as to whether this is true in children [135, 137]. Moreover, the exact prevalence within the pediatric age group is unclear, although pediatric optic nerve sheath meningiomas (ONSM) are estimated to occur between 1 in 95,000–525,000 [137]. Recent literature has suggested that pediatric meningiomas are more aggressive and display rapid growth, as compared to adult meningiomas [138].

Signs and symptoms of orbital meningiomas may include acute or gradual visual loss (65–100%), transient visual obscurations, RAPD, visual field defect (48%), exophthalmos (68%), optic disc changes (edema/atrophy or pallor) (63%), contiguous macular edema, optociliary shunt vessels (28%), choroidal folds, diplopia/strabismus (9–100%), and pain, along with increased intracranial pressure and its sequelae [135, 137]. The Hoyt–Spencer triad of disk swelling, optic atrophy, and optociliary shunt vessels does not appear to be sensitive or specific for pediatric primary ONSM [135].

Both CT and MR imaging are useful, although fat-suppressed MRI sequence with gadolinium is considered the gold standard for diagnosis [136, 139]. Meningiomas are homogeneous contrast-enhancing masses, often with calcific changes [135]. ONSM often have the "tram-tracking" sign [136]. When bone is involved, hyperostosis or erosion can be seen [135]. Several radiographic patterns have been described with different frequencies within the adult population including a tubular configuration (63%), globular (23%), fusiform (11%), and focal enlargement (4%); it is unclear if these frequencies hold true in the pediatric population [137].

Management of orbital meningiomas is a function of the patient's clinical status and the lesion location [136]. Pediatric orbital meningiomas are noted to be more aggressive than their adult counterparts [135, 136, 139]. Mortality from orbital meningiomas is extremely rare. Thus, in most cases, visual preservation is the primary objective [136]. In the setting of a well-seeing eye, observation with imaging evaluations performed at least every 6 months for 1–2 years is recommended [139]. Clinical metrics such as visual acuity, color vision, and visual fields are followed. When indicated,

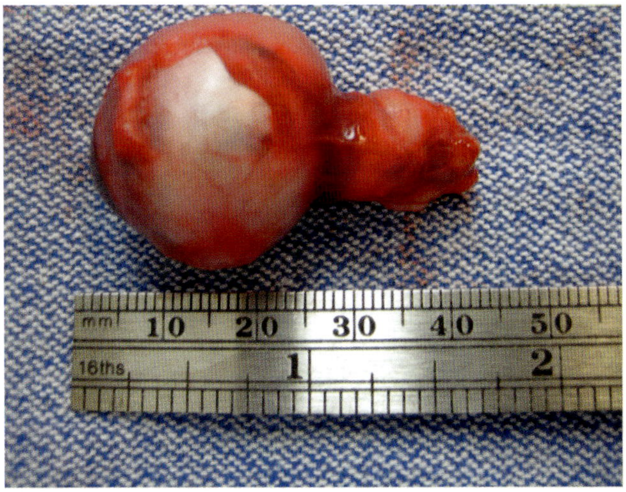

Fig. 52.6 Gross photo of optic nerve sheath meningioma in a 7-year-old boy with a blind painful eye and posterior extension of optic nerve meningioma

surgical resection is the treatment of choice within the pediatric age group. This often requires a multispecialty approach and results in high morbidity, including loss of visual function [135, 137]. Indications for surgery may include loss of functional vision with simultaneous cosmetic concerns or intracranial extension with growth toward the contralateral optic nerve [139] (Fig. 52.6). Surgery of ONSM is especially challenging because of intimate involvement of the lesions to the nerve and its vascular networks [139]. Therefore, preoperative embolization has been used prior to resection [135]. For the goal of preserving vision, fractionated radiation therapy is currently recommended in nondiabetic adults [136]. There is heightened concern for radiation-related side effects in the pediatric population, and thus the role of radiation in pediatric orbital meningioma management has not been completely elucidated [137].

Orbital Schwannoma

Orbital schwannomas are relatively rare, accounting for approximately 1–2% of all orbital tumors [140]. They typically occur in adults between 20 and 50 years of age and may be associated with neurofibromatosis type 2 (NF2) [140]. Patients typically present with slowly progressive proptosis and diplopia, with preserved vision [141, 142]. Schwannomas arise [142] from peripheral sensory nerves, most commonly the supratrochlear or supraorbital branches of CN V [140, 141]. In a large case series, the majority of schwannomas were found in the superior (27%) and superomedial (19%) orbit [140]. Histologically, Antoni A and Antoni B cellular patterns are characteristic of schwannomas. These patterns that may account for the variability observed in MR imaging [140]. MRI with gadolinium is the imaging modality of choice and most commonly reveals a well-encapsulated mass that can be cone-shaped (26%), dumbbell-shaped (16%), oval (15%), or round (13%) [140]. Enhancement patterns vary considerably and may lead to diagnostic confusion with hemangiomas [140]. Malignant schwannomas have been reported but are unusual in the orbit [141]. When treatment is required for either cosmetic or functional reasons, en bloc excision can provide a definitive diagnosis. Recurrence is rare [143].

Pediatric Orbital Vascular Tumors

Infantile Hemangioma

Periocular infantile hemangiomas, also known as capillary hemangiomas, are hamartomas composed of capillary endothelium with basement membranes, fibroblasts, mast cells, and macrophages. These lesions lack a formal capsule and are typically located in the eyelid although are occasionally found in the orbit [144]. They are the most common vascular lesion of childhood occurring in 1–2.6% of the general newborn population, most commonly in females and those born prematurely [144–146]. Clinically, infantile hemangiomas tend to present during infancy and enlarge over the course of 3–6 months in what is called the "proliferative phase" [146]. If observed, spontaneous involution typically occurs with approximately 50%, completely resolving by 5 years and 70–90% by 7 years [146, 147]. Histologically, the involutional phase is associated with the development of fibrofatty tissue around lobules which incites fibrosis and collapse of the hemangioma [146]. The tendency toward spontaneous involution helps distinguish infantile hemangiomas from other vascular lesions of childhood, such as lymphangiomas and arteriovenous malformations which persist into adulthood [147]. While several classification systems have been proposed, their ability to guide treatment decisions was limited. A more recent schema developed by Schwartz et al. does provide such utility [146].

- Group 1: Hemangiomas less than 1 cm.
- Group 2: Hemangiomas greater than 1 cm and measurable.
- Group 3: Diffuse hemangiomas involving the eyelid and orbit.
- Group 4: Diffuse hemangiomas involving the eyelid and orbit and associated with PHACES (Posterior fossa malformations, Hemangiomas, Arterial anomalies, Cardiac defects and coarctation of the aorta, Eye abnormalities, and Sternal abnormalities or midline developmental defects).

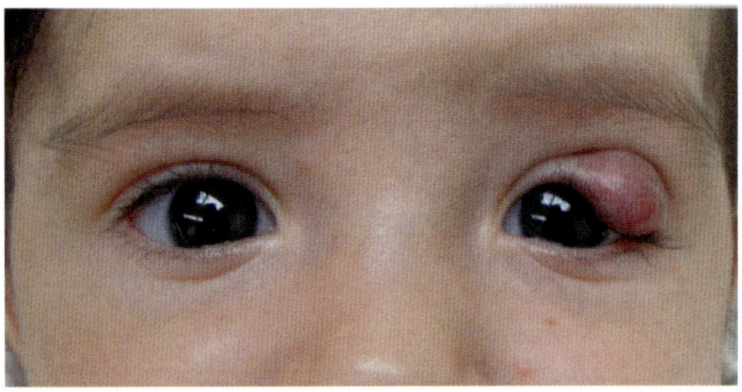

Fig. 52.7 Left upper eyelid infantile hemangioma in a 6-month-old girl resulting in anisometropic amblyopia and mechanical ptosis

Infantile hemangiomas often produce a discolored mass that is typically reddish to dark blue, though, when deep, may present without discoloration [146] (Fig. 52.7). Other mechanical mass effects may include blepharoptosis (13–72%), eyelid margin deformation (16–100%), globe displacement (0–17%), proptosis (0–29%), strabismus (9–71%), amblyopia (0–78%), astigmatism (0–67%), and pupil occlusion (0–43%); larger lesions are more commonly associated with the mechanical effects and their sequelae [144, 146, 148]. Although temporary cosmetic concerns are most common, the risk of both depravation and astigmatic amblyopia is significant (46–80%), and thus, careful observation is necessitated [146]. Orbital infantile hemangiomas are usually located in the superior orbit and may produce blepharoptosis, proptosis, exposure keratopathy, anisometropia (in up to 100%), and optic neuropathy [144, 146].

MR imaging provides the greatest detail, although CT imaging and ultrasonography have been utilized [149]. Regarding ultrasonography, the proliferative phase of an infantile hemangioma is characterized by its smooth contour and variable echogenicity, while Doppler imaging studies demonstrate a high arterial flow lesion [149]. In the proliferative phase, most lesions are well demarcated, isointense to muscle, homogenous, and extraconal [149]. Lesions may cause bony expansion or scalloping but rarely invade bone or display calcification. Contrast may reveal lobulated enhancement that occurs early and persists, while involuting lesions may become increasingly heterogeneous with less-prominent enhancement [149].

First-line treatment of periocular hemangiomas usually entails intralesional steroid (20 mg methylprednisolone and 4 mg dexamethasone injected into three to five areas) or oral steroid (prednisone 1–2 mg/kg/day) [145]. Repeat treatments are not uncommon (50%). Patients often require refractive correction (50%) and occlusion therapy (37.5%) for amblyopia prevention [145]. Other therapies for refractory cases have included surgical debulking or laser therapy [146]. Oral propranolol has been recently used with remarkable success [148, 150, 151]. The regimen of choice has yet to be determined, but gradual escalation and de-escalation are commonly employed. For example, Harper et al. described starting with 1 mg/kg divided into three doses for 1 week and increasing to 2 mg/kg thereafter [150]. Responses could be seen as early as 24–48 hours after initiation of therapy. Regardless of the exact regimen, it is important to coordinate with a pediatric cardiologist as several protocols have recommended in-house monitoring over the first few hours of administration [150, 152]. Adverse side effects of beta-blockers can include bradycardia, bronchospasm, vasospasm, heart block, congestive heart failure, and hypoglycemia [153]. Consequently, there has been recent interest in the use of a topical beta-blocker in the treatment of infantile capillary hemangioma [153]. Two drops of topical timolol maleate 0.5% ophthalmic solution was applied, twice per day to the surface of the hemangioma and spread over the lesion's surface [153]. The topical regimen was continued for seven weeks and resulted in marked improvement in the size of the lesion, as well as the resulting cycloplegic refraction [153]. Oral cyclophosphamide and subcutaneous interferon alfa-2a have both shown success in treating orbital capillary hemangiomas [144, 148].

Orbital Lymphangiomas

Like capillary hemangiomas, orbital lymphangiomas are hamartomatous lesions that often present during childhood [154]. Accounting for approximately 20% of periocular masses and less than 2% of orbital biopsies, orbital lymphangiomas histologically lack a capsule and are composed of lymphocytes and lymphoid aggregates and endothelium-lined cysts containing proteinaceous or hemorrhagic material. Intraoperatively they appear as dark-fluid filled "chocolate cysts" [154].

Orbital lymphangiomas are clinically characterized by an orbital process presenting in a female (77%) patient between the ages of 0 and 20 years (92%) [154]. There may be precipitating upper respiratory tract infection (URI) or mild trauma. Some have theorized that the URI may incite a lymphocytic reaction within the lymphangioma, leading to symptomatic lesion enlargement. Trauma may induce intralesional hemorrhage with formation of "chocolate cysts," [155]. Signs and symptoms include proptosis (85%), blepharoptosis (73%), strabismus (46%), ocular pain, amblyopia, retinal folds, and optic neuropathy [154, 156, 157] (Fig. 52.8). Lesions may enlarge with Valsalva maneuver [158].

Most lymphangiomas may be diagnosed purely from clinical and radiographic findings [159]. Although both CT and MR imaging have both been successfully used to evaluate orbital lymphangiomas, contrast-enhanced MR imaging better delineates these lesions [160]. At least one study has found an increased frequency of intracranial vascular anomalies in those with periocular lymphatic and lymphaticovenous malformations, and therefore, the authors recommend

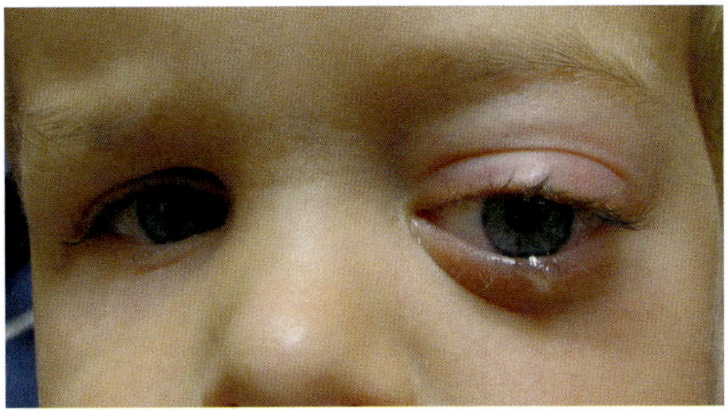

Fig. 52.8 Acute left proptosis associated with orbital lymphangioma with intralesional hemorrhage in a 3-year-old boy

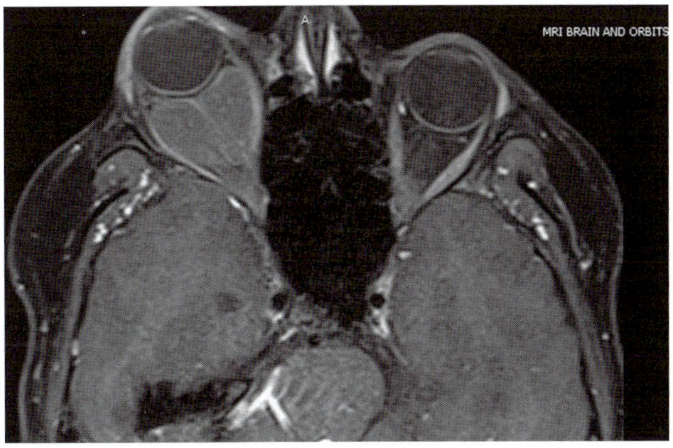

Fig. 52.9 MRI brain and orbits axial T1 fat suppression showing intraconal lymphangioma with intralesional hemorrhage

MR imaging of the brain as well as the orbit [160]. Lesions may be intra- or extraconal or encompassing both spaces and termed a "diffuse lymphangioma." Diffuse lymphangiomas predominate and account for 86% of orbital lymphangiomas [154]. As lymphangiomas are cystic lesions, other orbital lesions with cystic components, including adenoid cystic carcinoma of the lacrimal gland, rhabdomyosarcoma, varix, and optic nerve glioma, should be excluded [158]. The characteristic imaging finding of lymphangioma is a fluid–fluid levels on contrast-enhanced MR imaging, which develops as a consequence of variously aged blood products, aka "chocolate cyst." This feature helps to distinguish lymphangiomas from other cyst-containing lesions [158]. Of note, there may be an increased risk of recurrence in those with definite "chocolate cyst" on MRI [154]. Most lesions enhance with contrast to some degree [158] (Fig. 52.9).

Management goals of orbital lymphangiomas include preservation of visual function and cosmesis [154]. Surgical resection, although challenging and with frequent recurrence, has emerged as the primary treatment modality. The surgical challenges stem from the diffuse nature of lymphangiomas, as well as their friable and unencapsulated composition. Complete resection is therefore not always possible, and debulking may become the resultant objective. In a series of 26 cases reported by Char et al., symptomatic recurrence occurred in 54% of individuals at approximately 3.4 years [154]. Of the original 26 patients, 23% recurred a second surgery, of whom 20% required a third surgery. Various enhancing techniques have been employed to improve surgical success rates such as the use of intralesional injection of Tisseel fibrin glue before resection or carbon dioxide laser [154, 155]. Percutaneous sclerosing therapy with OK-432 and sodium morrhuate 5% has been effectively used to treat lymphangiomas [159, 161]. Long-term follow-up of these agents has not been determined. During episodes with acute symptomatic exacerbation, often following minor trauma or URI, systemic steroids have been used with inconsistent success [156, 162]. In the management of the pediatric patient with orbital lymphangioma, one should note that early presentation may be associated with an increased risk of amblyopia, strabismus, and compressive optic neuropathy [154].

Pediatric Orbital Mesenchymal Tumors

Rhabdomyosarcoma

Rhabdomyosarcoma (RMS) is the most common orbital sarcoma of childhood. Orbital RMS represents about 10% of all rhabdomyosarcoma [163]. These tumors, historically incorrectly believed to of muscle origin, are derived from undifferentiated mesenchymal cells capable of producing striated muscle. The four major subtypes of RMS include embryonal (ERMS; 57–90%), alveolar (ARMS; 9–19%), botryoid (BRMS; 1–6%), pleomorphic (PRMS; 1%), and those too undifferentiated (UDS) or heterogeneous to be further classified (1–7%) [164].

In 1972, a collaborative effort known as the Intergroup Rhabdomyosarcoma Study Group (IRSG) was formed and has since concluded four major trials that have advanced survival rates of orbital RMS from 30% to 94% at 3 years [164]. Moreover, exenteration, which played a primary role in the treatment of orbital RMS prior to 1972, has been supplanted by therapies with far less morbidity.

The original IRSG classification included four *groups* based on surgical outcomes and systemic evaluation. Group I consisted of patients who had complete excision of localized disease, accounting for 3% of those with orbital RMS, with a 90% survival rate. Group II consisted of patients who had gross resection of localized disease, with or without regional lymph node involvement and/or microscopic residual disease, accounting for 20% of orbital RMS, with an 85% survival rate. Group III consisted of patients with residual gross disease, accounting for 74% with orbital RMS, with a 70% survival rate. Group IV consisted of patients with distant metastatic disease, accounting for 3% of orbital RMS, with a 40% survival rate. The data of Intergroup Rhabdomyosarcoma Study (IRS)-II afforded the development of a new staging system that took into account the primary tumor, regional lymph nodes, and distant metastasis, known as the TNM system [165]. In the IRS-IV protocol, the group classification assigned radiation therapy, while the study stage was used to assign chemotherapeutic regiments [165].

The current IRS iteration (IRS-V) creates patient cohorts of similar risk of relapse and treatment requirements and categorizes by tumor histology, group, and stage [165]. Patients at low risk have a defined 3-year failure-free survival (FFS) rate of 88%, include those with localized ERMS and botryoid or spindle-cell ERMS, and are divided into two subgroups. Subgroup A consists of patients with localized stage 1 tumors that have been grossly resected or arisen in the orbit and those with stage 2 tumors that have been completely resected. Subgroup B includes patients with stage 1, 2, or 3 tumors that have been grossly resected and with microscopic residual disease with or without regional disease-positive lymph nodes. Intermediate risk patients are those who have a 55–76% 3-year FFS rate [165]. These intermediate risk patients have stage 1 through 3 localized ARMS or UDS, stage 2 and 3 ERMS with gross residual disease, or stage 4 ERMS in children less than 10 years of age [165]. High-risk patients have a less than 30% 3-year FFS rate which are characterized by stage 4 ARMS/UDS or ERMS in those older than 10 years of age [165].

Orbital embryonal RMS (ERMS), although most common, has the best 5-year survival rate at 94%, while the 5-year survival rate of orbital alveolar RMS (ARMS) is reportedly around 74% [163]. The orbital caveat should be emphasized as it is considered a more favorable site with a better prognosis, i.e., unfavorably located ARMD or undifferentiated sarcoma group I or II has a 66% 5-year FFS rate, while group III has a 45% 5-year FFS rate [166]. Age is also a prognostic indicator in some groups, i.e., stage 1 or 2, group III ARMS/UDS and ERMS subgroup A with children 10 years of age or greater having a worse prognosis [166].

Orbital RMS tends to affect males more than females with the mean age of presentation between 8 and 10 years [163, 164]. These masses are often found in the superior nasal quadrant of the orbit if of the embryonal subtype, while alveolar masses tend to occur in the inferior orbit. A story of mild trauma may accompany the initial presentation and distract from the diagnosis of orbital RMS, and thus, one must have a high index of suspicion for orbital RMS in a child with rapidly progressive unilateral exophthalmos [163]. Signs and symptoms include proptosis (79%), eyelid edema (64%), blepharoptosis (18%), conjunctival congestion (9%), visible mass (6%), disc edema, choroidal folds, and strabismus [163, 164] (Fig. 52.10). CT imaging with

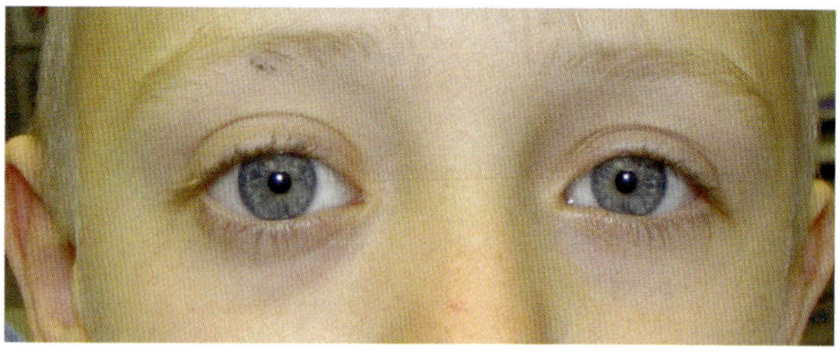

Fig. 52.10 Sub-acute right proptosis in an 8-year-old. Anterior orbitotomy with incisional biopsy showed rhabdomyosarcoma

contrast often demonstrates a soft tissue noncalcified contrast-enhancing mass. Rarely, masses have cystic regions. MR imaging similarly reveals a soft tissue contrasting enhancing mass.

Treatment for orbital RMS is ever evolving and depends on the location and extent of disease, although most primary protocols use a combination of chemotherapy and radiotherapy after an excisional biopsy has been performed [164]. Some centers perform extensive surgical debulking, reasoning that group I disease has a significantly improved survival rate, while others perform tumor excision that spares vital structures of the orbit and employ tumor control by external beam radiation and chemotherapy, thus reducing morbidity [163]. Orbital exenteration is often applied to recurrent tumors [164]. Considerable discussion has been given to the long-term side effects of radiotherapy, with late effects such as cataract (55–82%), decreased visual acuity (70%), orbital hypoplasia (59%), dry eye (30–36%), and chronic keratoconjunctivitis (27%) [164].

Fibrous Dysplasia

Originally described by von Recklinghausen as *osteitis fibrosa generalisata* in 1891, fibrous dysplasia (FD) is a benign neoplastic disorder of bone that accounts for approximately 2.5% of all bone neoplasia [167, 168]. The disease may be localized to one bone (monostotic) or affect several bones (polyostotic). The labeling, however, can be confusing as some authors may term a craniofacial process which involves a single craniofacial region, though multiple bones as monostotic when it has only one locus of disease, thus reserving the term polyostotic for disease that affects multiple bones of the appendicular skeleton [168].

FD is caused by a somatic mutation in *GNAS1* and results in small irregular spicules of immature bone that has been described as "woven bone" [167]. The malignant potential is low at 0.5%, but may increase to 44% in those treated with radiotherapy [167, 169]. Sarcomas, such as osteosarcoma, fibrosarcoma, chondrosarcoma, and malignant fibrohistiocytoma, have all been reported as the consequence of such malignant transformation [167].

Signs and symptoms of FD include exophthalmos, dystopia, periocular facial asymmetry, strabismus, pain, epiphora, visual impairment, and optic neuropathy/vision loss [167–170]. The disease typically presents before the third decade of life and has a tendency to affect the craniofacial region in 50–100% of those with the polyostotic form and 10–30% of those with the monostotic form [167, 170]. Vision loss from FD has been attributed to optic nerve traction, mucocele formation, orbital compartment syndrome, spontaneous hemorrhage, stenosis of the optic canal, and bone cyst formation [167]. In some reports, cystic degeneration was the most common cause of visual impairment [167, 168]. When polyostotic disease is associated both with café au lait spots and precocious puberty, the disease process is termed McCune–Albright syndrome [167, 168]. FD is thought to be most active during puberty and pregnancy, although progression has been reported in a wide range of age groups [169].

Radiographically, FD is described in three categories: cystic (25%), sclerotic (35%), or mixed (40%) [167]. CT imaging well characterizes the bony involvement, while MR imaging aides in revealing the degree to which soft tissue is affected [167] (Fig. 52.11). The cystic and mixed variant have a relatively heterogeneous textured appearance within expanding bone, while the sclerotic form is said to resemble "ground glass," in appearance [167]. Lytic lesions may suggest malignant degeneration [167]. The differential diagnosis of these bony lesions may include osteomas and osteoblastomas which may resemble FD on CT imaging studies.

Management of FD continues to evolve, and no single approach is universally embraced. As a result of the increased rate of malignant transformation in those treated with radiotherapy, this treatment modality is not advised [167]. Although several medications have been used, none are proven in the treatment of FD. Systemic steroids have

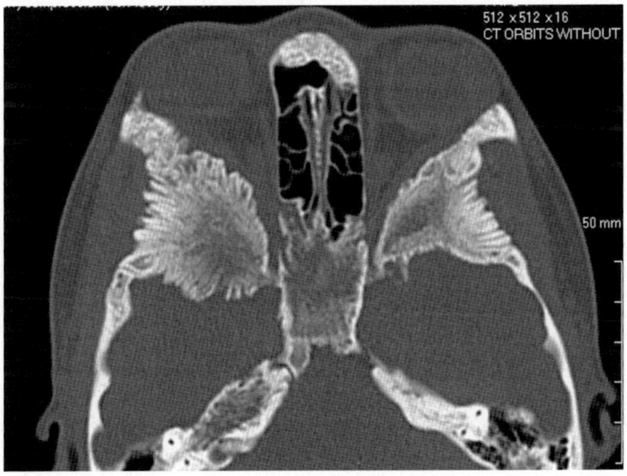

Fig. 52.11 A 15-year-old girl with fibrous dysplasia and evidence of bilateral optic canal narrowing on axial CT scan

been used as a temporizing measure to treat acute vision loss [167]. Indications for surgery include unacceptable cosmetic deformity and vision loss [167, 168]. Controversies arise in the setting of radiographically apparent optic canal stenosis in a child with normal vision and FD. Some authors recommend prophylactic decompression, which carries a high risk of vision loss [168]. Other authors recommend that intralesional cysts merit surgery because of their relatively high risk of vision compromise [168]. Other experts recommend aggressive management of eye dystopia or exophthalmos and conservative management of FD with apex involvement [168]. Recurrence after surgery is not uncommon and may occur more frequently with conservative surgical approaches, thus requiring some patients to undergo multiple surgeries [169].

Orbital Soft Tissue Sarcomas

Orbital soft tissues sarcomas are neoplasias derived from mesenchymal cells [171]. Within specific tissue types, there are several distinct sarcoma types. Of the more than 14 different subtypes, malignant fibrous histiocytoma, dermatofibrosarcoma protuberans, angiosarcoma, and rhabdomyosarcoma were the most common sarcomas of the craniofacial region in one series of 802 head and neck sarcomas [172]. Orbital sarcomas may also include osteogenic sarcomas, leiomyosarcoma, fibrosarcoma, primary synovial sarcoma, and alveolar soft part sarcoma [171]. The optimal treatment of most of these orbital lesions is unclear because of their rarity. In most cases, surgical resection with wide margins is recommended, often with adjuvant chemo- or radiotherapy [172].

Ewing Sarcoma

James Ewing originally described what is now known as Ewing's sarcoma (ES) in 1921 [173]. Often considered a neoplasm of childhood (75% in patients $\leq$20 years of age), ES results account for about 20% of all malignant bone neoplasia [174]. White males between the ages of 5 and 13 are most commonly affected [173]. ES primarily affects long bones (47%) and rarely craniofacial bones (1–6%) [173, 174]. Orbital bone involvement suggests metastatic disease, as primary orbital ES is exceedingly rare [173, 174]. Clinical features of primary ES of the orbit include exophthalmos, headache, cranial exostosis, vision loss, papillary abnormalities, somnolence, disc edema, strabismus, pain, and a medial canthus mass [173]. Histologically, ES is part of the small round cell tumors (SRCT) of childhood and adolescents [175]. The biopsy specimen must often undergo electron microscopy and immunohistochemistry analysis to distinguish it from other neoplasia within the (SRCT) category, e.g., neuroblastomas, embryonal and alveolar rhabdomyosarcoma, and various hematolymphoid malignancies [175]. Imaging studies typically reveal a diffuse unevenly enhancing mass with bony destruction and areas of hypodensity that may correlate with hemorrhage and necrosis [173]. MR imaging may reveal the heterogeneous lesion with enhancement, bony destruction, and occasional fluid–fluid levels [174]. Treatment typically includes radical excision with subsequent radio- and chemotherapy [173, 174].

Histiocytic Tumors

Histiocytosis of childhood has included such diseases as histiocytosis X, juvenile xanthogranuloma (JXG), and histiocytic lymphoma [176, 177]. The Histiocyte Society has created a classification system based on the number of sites and organ systems involved and has improved diagnostic and therapeutic implications [176]. Class I consists of Langerhans cell histiocytosis (LCH), which was originally termed histiocytosis X by Lichtenstein in 1953 [176]. Lichtenstein's original description included three entities, namely, eosinophilic granuloma, Hand–Schuller–Christian disease, and Letterer–Siwe disease, which were thought to share the same pathogenesis [176]. Class II includes JXG, histiocytosis of mononuclear phagocytes other than LCH, hemophagocytic lymphohistiocytosis (familial and reactive), sinus histiocytosis with massive lymphadenopathy (Rosai–Dorfman disease), and reticulohistiocytoma. Class III consists of the malignant histiocytic processes and includes acute monocytic leukemia, malignant histiocytosis, and true histiocytic lymphoma.

LCH, although rare, is the most common histiocytosis of childhood and occurs in approximately 3–7 per one million children each year, therefore accounting for fewer than 1% of orbital tumors in the general population [178]. As the name implies, Langerhans cells (LC) pathologically characterize the LCH, although their appearance differs from normal LC [178]. Specifically, the LC of LCH lack dendritic processes and tend to have an ovoid epithelioid morphology [178]. LC derive from pluripotent stem cells and develop into either antigen-processing macrophages or dendritic cells as a consequence of cytokine exposure [178]. They express CD1a and S-100 surface protein, which aids in the diagnosis [176, 178]. According the Histiocyte Society, definitive diagnosis requires light microscopy findings plus positive surface staining and Birbeck granules when examined with electron microscopy [176].

The clinical presentation varies with the type of LCH encountered but usually occurs during the first or second decade [179]. Eosinophilic granuloma (EG) is described as a unifocal variant, whereas Hand–Schuller–Christian syndrome (HSCS) involves multiple systems with chronic intermediate severity, while Letterer–Siwe disease (LSD) is acute, disseminated, and often lethal [180]. Ophthalmic manifestations of LCH are thought to be present in 10–23% of those with LCH and are more common in those with EG and HSCS [178]. Isolated orbital unifocal LCH, aka EG, accounts for 4% of all LCH patients [178]. Signs and symptoms may include upper lateral palpebral swelling with associated erythema and tenderness that develops over weeks to months, although acute presentations are possible. The propensity for the anterolateral frontal bone is thought to result from continued hematopoietic activity of the frontal bone marrow in the pediatric population [176, 177, 179]. Neuro-ophthalmic disease such as papilledema, optic atrophy, ptosis, cranial nerve VII palsy, and cavernous sinus disease has been rarely reported [176]. Interestingly, exophthalmos occurs in only 50% of cases, the paucity of which is hypothesized to result from the relative orbital decompression that results from the osteolytic lesions [178].

CT imaging is highly valuable in the diagnosis of LCH and typically demonstrates an enhancing osteolytic lesion with well-defined borders and an associated soft tissue mass [178]. Neuroblastoma, Ewing sarcoma and Wilms' tumor, among others, may have a similar imaging appearance [178, 179]. If LCH is suspected, many authors recommend open biopsy over fine-needle aspiration [178, 179] (Fig. 52.12).

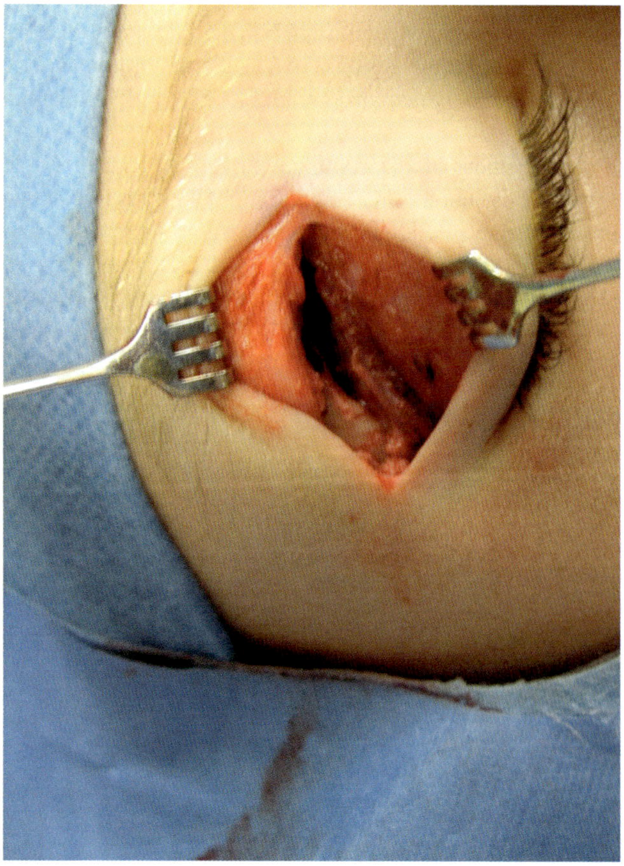

Fig. 52.12 Lateral orbitotomy with incisional biopsy in a 6-year-old boy. Histopathological analysis showed Langerhans cell histiocytosis

Intraoperatively, frozen section may be suggestive of LCH and allow the surgeon to confidently perform a limited curettage with subsequent intralesional steroid injection [179]. The patient must be evaluated by a pediatric oncologist as multifocal/multisystem disease may initially present within the orbit, although EG is more likely [176, 178, 179]. Typical systemic evaluation includes skeletal radiographic survey, radionuclide bone scan, brain MR imaging, blood work, and urine osmolality (given the possibility of diabetes insipidus) [178, 179]. Beyond curettage and steroid injection, pediatric oncologists have recommended chemotherapy. Although successfully used in the past, radiotherapy has become increasingly uncommon in the treatment of LCH [178–180]. Recurrence has been reported in up to 18% of patients, often in the initial 3 weeks to 25 months following treatment. Thus, long-term follow-up by the patient's ophthalmologist, pediatrician, and oncologist is recommended with possible serial CT imaging [179].

Lymphoproliferative Tumors

Orbital lymphomas are most commonly non-Hodgkin's B-cell lymphomas affecting older individuals, although younger patients may be affected in the setting of a compromised immune system or in the case of Burkitt lymphoma [181]. Signs and symptoms of orbital lymphoma may include painless exophthalmos with increased resistance to retropulsion with or without a palpable rubbery mass, diplopia, vision loss, and visual field abnormality [181, 184]. Additional ocular and periocular disease may be observed in the conjunctiva (i.e., salmon patch) (28%) and eyelids (8%), although the superior retrobulbar orbit is the most common (64%) [182]. Bilateral disease may be seen and when present is often simultaneous [182]. Ocular and periocular disease may be associated with systemic disease in up to 35% of patients, and thus evaluation by a pediatric oncologist is recommended. CT or MR imaging demonstrates an ovoid mass that tends to mold to adjacent orbital structures [181]. Biopsy is essential to confirm the diagnosis, and subsequent systemic staging should be performed. In the absence of systemic disease, radiotherapy has been used, although its use in the pediatric population is somewhat controversial. Chemotherapy remains a viable treatment option. The use of systemic steroids can be useful, although rebound or recurrence has been reported [181, 182]. Follow-up by the pediatrician or pediatric oncologist is recommended to monitor for systemic lymphoma.

Burkitt Lymphoma

Burkitt lymphoma (BL) is a non-Hodgkin's lymphoma that presents in three major forms: endemic (African) form, sporadic form, and the form associated with immunodeficiency [181, 183]. The endemic form occurs in 50–100 cases per million, has been associated with Epstein–Barr virus infections (up to 95% of affected individuals), and tends to affect the facial bones including those of the orbit, mandible, and maxilla [183]. Orbital soft tissue as well as the eye can be affected [181, 183]. The sporadic form affects two to three patients per million and rarely involves the orbit or eye. The third form is often associated with HIV infections and AIDS [183]. BL typically presents as an abdominal mass with bone marrow involvement [183]. Common signs and symptoms of orbital disease may include exophthalmos, eyelid edema, blepharoptosis, visible eyelid mass, and less commonly, optic neuropathy, cavernous sinus disease, and concomitant paranasal sinus disease [181, 182, 184]. In a literature review of sporadic BL, Baker et al. found that children are most commonly affected and that when orbital and ocular disease occurs, systemic disease is found in more than 80% of individuals of whom 40% have CNS involvement [183]. CT imaging may reveal a mass with bony erosion. Biopsy is required and characteristically demonstrates a lymphoid lesion with a "starry sky pattern," as well as compatible immunohistochemical staining, is needed [57, 183]. Patients require a systemic evaluation by pediatric oncology and treatment consists of systemic chemotherapy.

Lacrimal Gland Tumors

Adenoid Cystic Carcinoma

Adenoid cystic carcinoma (ACC) is the most common malignant epithelial tumor of the lacrimal gland [185]. Typically occurring about the fourth decade of life, this lesion is rarely observed in the pediatric population [185, 186]. Signs and symptoms of the few reported cases in the pediatric literature include downward globe displacement, pain, edema, or a palpable mass around the superolateral orbital rim [185, 186]. In one case report, the child was mistakenly believed to have a dermoid cyst, and in the other, symptoms were incorrectly attributed to sinus disease [185, 186]. CT imaging of ACC may reveal a cystic mass that enhances circumferentially, with an associated smooth bony fossa formation [185, 186]. Pathologic evaluation reveals an encapsulated mass with small densely packed cells and numerous cyst-like spaces that produced a cribriform or "swiss cheese" pattern [185, 186]. ACC is considered highly malignant because of their invasive, recurrent, and metastatic tendencies [186]. Accordingly, radical orbital exenteration following confirmed diagnosis has been advocated, with possible adjuvant radio- or chemotherapy [186]. Neoadjuvant intra-arterial chemotherapy has also shown to optimize outcomes [187]. However, more recently, globe-sparing therapy has been advocated. Lesion excision with postoperative chemoradiation therapy and orbital plaque brachytherapy has been successfully utilized [185, 188] Due to its rarity, long-term treatment outcomes of ACC in the pediatric population are not fully known.

Metastatic Tumors

Neuroblastoma

Neuroblastomas are the most common extracranial solid tumor of childhood and may account for 7.5–10% of all childhood neoplasms [189]. Derived from sympathetic nervous tissue of the adrenal medulla or the paraspinal ganglion, 90% present before the age of 10 years of age with a mean presentation of 2 years [189]. Of these, 10–20% will have orbital metastasis that often presents with exophthalmos and/or periorbital ecchymosis ("raccoon or panda eyes") with subsequent unilateral Horner's syndrome and opsoclonus [190]. Restrictive strabismus, globe displacement or blindness, and systemic symptoms such as cerebellar ataxia and myoclonus have been reported with less frequency [189]. Bilateral symptoms have been reported in 20–50% of cases, with the abdomen being the most common primary site of these neoplasms [189]. Palpation of the abdomen should therefore be performed to assess for tumor. A high index of suspicion should be exercised, as early detection profoundly impacts prognosis. Those patients diagnosed before the age of 1 year having a 75% 2-year relapse-free survival rate, while those diagnosed after 2 years age having a 12% 2-year relapse-free survival rate [189]. Up to 20% of patients with neuroblastoma present initially with ophthalmic involvement [189].

The ophthalmologist plays a vital role in diagnosing, staging (via biopsy), monitoring visual involvement, and assessing treatment response [190]. CT imaging may be useful in revealing a heterogeneously enhancing lesion with associated lytic bony erosions, while MR imaging may demonstrate an isointense enhancing mass with some variance depending on the state of intralesional hemoglobin decay [189] (Fig. 52.13). Immunohistochemistry facilitates in distinguishing neuroblastoma from other small cell tumors [189].

Current treatment is based on the Children's Oncology Group Neuroblastoma Risk Group Assignment Schema of low, intermediate, or high [190]. Orbital involvement qualifies for the high-risk category and multiagent high-dose chemotherapy is indicated. After induction and consolidation of the tumor, resection is often attempted, followed by myeloablative chemotherapy [190]. Radiotherapy is sometimes used at the primary site. Treatment is additionally supplemented by oral 13-*cis*-retinoic acid treatment. Ophthalmic side effects are common with these therapies, and careful monitoring is advised. Unfortunately, the 3-year survival rate is only 11% with current management [189].

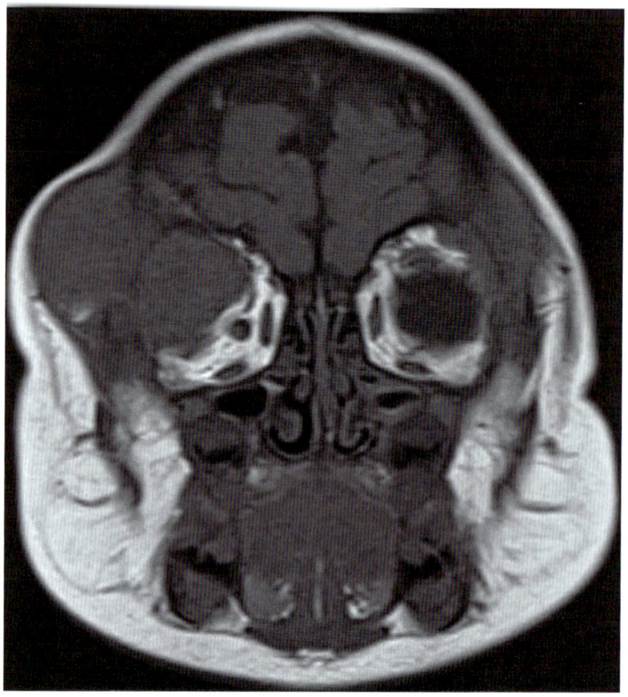

Fig. 52.13 A 9-month-old girl with bilateral orbital involvement from metastatic neuroblastoma

Leukemic Neoplasia

Leukemia is known to cause mass lesions throughout the body that sometimes occur in and/or affect the orbit. Originally described by Allen Burns in 1811 or Dock in 1893 as "green tumors" or chloromas, these lesions are now referred to as granulocytic sarcoma, myeloblastoma, megakaryoblastoma, or, as the World Health Organizations favors, myeloid sarcoma [181, 191, 192]. A green appearance, seen in 70% of lesions, results from a reaction between myeloperoxidase and ultraviolet light [191]. Although all forms of leukemia can manifest as orbital lesions through extramedullary activity, acute myelogenous leukemia (AML) does so most commonly [186, 192]. In a retrospective study of 27 patients with orbital leukemic tumors over 22 years, Haik et al. found that 77.8% were AML, 18.5% were acute lymphocytic leukemia, and 3.7% were chronic myelogenous leukemia [192]. These neoplastic masses are thought to occur more frequently in male children of African, Middle Eastern, East Asian, or Latin American descent between 7 and 8 years of age [192]. The orbital process may occur prior to diagnosed systemic leukemia (85.2%) or secondary to known leukemia. Patients commonly present with exophthalmos which may be acute, periocular cellulitis, as well as mass lesions of the lacrimal gland, eyelid, iris, conjunctiva, or sclera [191].

Workup is largely directed by the patient's leukemic status. Specifically, if the patient is known to have leukemia, CT and/or MR imaging studies are often sufficient to diagnosis myeloid sarcoma [192]. Imaging studies often demonstrate a mildly enhancing homogenous mass commonly in the lateral orbital wall without bony destruction [192]. However, in the absence of known leukemia, imaging studies are incapable of adequately distinguishing myeloid sarcoma from other orbital tumors such as rhabdomyosarcoma, neuroblastoma, and other poorly differentiated neoplastic masses of childhood [191]. Thus, a biopsy is performed and submitted in fresh solution to undergo light microscopy and immunohistochemical analysis, with particular emphasis placed on the Leder stain [191]. Treatment involves multiagent chemotherapy, with or without radiation, resulting in a survival between 8.7 months and 6.5 years [192].

Pediatric Facial Trauma

Facial fractures are less common in children than adults but warrant special consideration [193]. Facial fractures include craniofacial, orbital fractures, and midface (maxillofacial and mandibular) fractures. Several studies have found an increased frequency of skull fractures compared to other facial fractures within the pediatric population when compared to their adult counterparts. This observation has been explained by the relatively large skull to face ratio [193]. The pneumatization of the paranasal sinuses may also impact facial fractures. The pediatric population is more likely to sustain orbital roof fracture due to the delayed pneumatization of the frontal sinus. In a large review of traumatic pediatric fractures, orbital roof fractures were most common in patients younger than 8 years of age, whereas orbital floor fractures predominated in patients older than 8 years [194]. Dentition must always be considered when treating maxillary and mandibular fractures, as the tooth buds grow within these bones and may limit surgical treatment options [193]. Lastly, the structure of the pediatric bone differs from adult bone by virtue of its low mineralization, abundance of cartilage, and cancellous bone and flexible suture lines, all of which afford greater elasticity and make "trapdoor" or "greenstick" fractures with soft tissue herniation more likely [193].

Clinical and radiographic examination of the pediatric population presents unique challenges. Radiation exposure must always be considered. Careful radiographic evaluation for small "trapdoor" fractures should be performed, which require emergent surgical soft tissue reduction and fracture repair. Orbital roof fractures typically do not require surgical repair [194]. Conservative management is preferred when possible [193, 195]. When necessary, however, both open and closed reduction surgery can be done with low risk and good results.

Midfacial Fractures

Midfacial or maxillofacial fractures are relatively uncommon in the pediatric population. For example, children under the age of 10 contribute only 2.8–14% of all patients with maxillofacial fractures [196]. Depending on the study, midfacial fractures include fractures of the alveolar, mandible (condyle, ramus, angle, body, symphysis/parasymphysis), Le Fort, nasal, hard palate, and isolated zygomatic fracture [197, 198]. In many series, orbital fractures are included under the rubric of midfacial fractures, but in this chapter, they will be addressed separately [196–198]. Most fractures affect males (74–77%) with a positive correlation between frequency of fracture and age [193, 196–198]. In two large studies of 521 and 492 pediatric patients with midfacial fractures, the average age was 13 with an increased incidence between the ages of 11 and 16, respectively [197, 198]. Midfacial fractures often result from motor vehicle accidents, bicycle accidents, fall, and sports [193, 196–198]. Associated injury such as brain contusion, intracranial hemorrhage, ocular injury, lacerations, and other nonfacial injuries are not uncommon and must be considered [193, 197, 198]. The evaluation and treatment of midfacial fractures will be discussed in the trauma section of this book.

Orbital Fractures

Orbital Floor Fractures

Orbital floor fractures are commonly seen in the pediatric population [199]. In a review of 96 pediatric patients with orbital fractures, Hatton found that orbital floor fractures accounted for the majority of orbital fractures (66.7%) and that they predominately affected males (81%) and were most commonly associated with sports (44%), assault (24%), motor vehicle trauma (27.7%), and accidents during play (11–14%) [199]. Other large studies of facial fractures have found that motor vehicle trauma and fall are the commonest mechanisms [193, 197, 198]. Orbital floor fractures may be direct or indirect. Those that involve the orbital rim are called direct orbital floor fractures. If the orbital floor fracture does not involve the inferior orbital rim, it may be called indirect, blowout, or pure internal floor fracture.

Signs and symptoms of orbital floor include periorbital ecchymosis, infraorbital nerve anesthesia, facial deformity, enophthalmos, difficulty with mastication, epiphora, and ocular injuries like hyphema, vitreous hemorrhage, globe rupture, diplopia, strabismus with extraocular muscle restriction, and pupillary abnormalities [200].

Children are somewhat unique because, in addition to the aforementioned signs and symptoms, pediatric patients

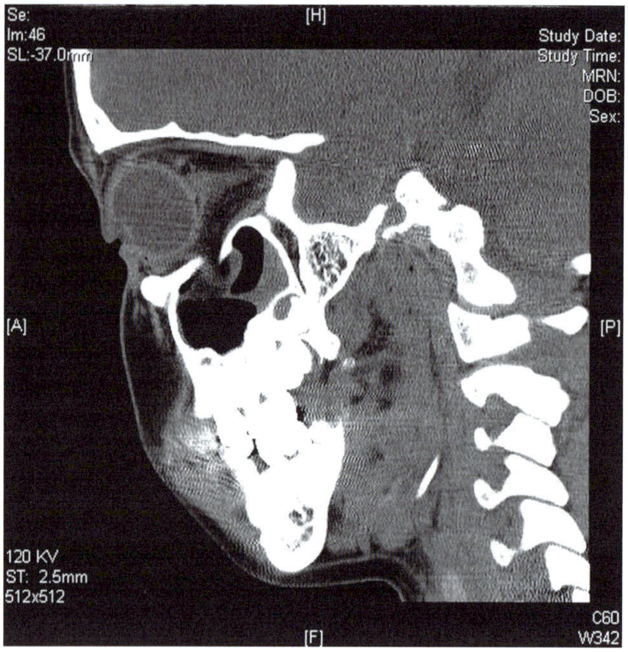

Fig. 52.14 Sagittal CT scan demonstrating entrapped inferior rectus

are also subject to systemic findings such as nausea, emesis, and bradycardia from the oculocardiac reflex which are suggestive of the so-called white-eyed blowout fractures [201]. "White-eyed blowout fractures" were so named because their original description was of pediatric patients with a history of trauma, but minimal clinically apparent ecchymosis, yet profound vertical motility restriction. The fracture pattern of the clinically described "white-eyed blowout fracture" was commonly that of a trapdoor fracture. If apparent at all, the fracture appeared small with associated mild inferior rectus muscle deformation or the report of a maxillary sinus cyst. Intraoperatively, an incomplete orbital floor fracture could be seen as a hinge, with the inferior rectus muscle trapped within the hinged fracture site. CT imaging revealed minimal if any fracture (Fig. 52.14). The report of a maxillary sinus cyst corresponded to entrapped muscle or perimuscular soft tissue. "White-eyed blowout fractures" are rarely seen in adults, a fact attributed to the elastic immature bones of the pediatric skeleton, as compared to their more brittle adult counterparts.

Management of orbital floor fractures varies according to the service managing them. Evaluation with CT imaging helps further characterize the fracture and assist in surgical planning when indicated. When possible, conservative management includes antibiotics, tetanus prophylaxis, nasal decongestant, ice packs, and avoidance of nose blowing. Conservative management may be recommended in those with minimal diplopia (not in primary or downgaze), good ocular motility, and no significant deformity, i.e., hypoophthalmos or enophthalmos [200].

Surgical indications have been well characterized by Burnstein [200], in which he describes those orbital floor fractures that require immediate repair (within 24–48 h) and those that require early repair. Immediate repair is recommended for those with diplopia, CT evidence of entrapment, and a nonresolving oculocardiac reflex. "White-eyed blowout fractures" that tend to occur in patients less than 18 years of age with extraocular motility restriction and a history of trauma, minimal ecchymosis, marked vertical motility restriction, and CT findings consistent with muscle or perimuscular soft tissue entrapment should also receive immediate repair. Early repair (within 2 weeks) is recommended for those with (1) symptomatic diplopia and positive forced duction testing and CT evidence of inferior rectus muscle or perimuscular soft tissue entrapment and minimal improvement over 2 weeks, (2) significant hypoglobus, and (3) large floor fractures (≥50%). Recently, two studies have suggested that the same results can be obtained if the surgical repair is done within 14 days or 29 days [202, 203].

Orbital Medial Wall Fractures

Isolated orbital medial wall fractures are rare where as they have been found to accompany 7–53% of orbital floor fractures [204]. As a result, they are less well represented in the literature. Fracture of the medial wall could include the lacrimal or ethmoid bone. In a study of 304 medial wall fractures, the mechanisms of injury included assault (78%), motor vehicle trauma (14%), fall (6%), and other causes (2%). Signs and symptoms of orbital medial wall fractures include periorbital edema, ecchymosis, subcutaneous emphysema, epistaxis, enophthalmos, restriction of adduction or abduction, and "pseudo-Duane syndrome" [204–206]. A complete ophthalmic examination is necessary as there is a high incidence of associated ocular injury (27–76%) [206]. Medial rectus muscle incarceration within the rare isolated medial orbital wall fracture is extremely rare but may occur in "blowout" mechanisms that develop trapdoor fractures [204, 205]. These types of fractures tend to affect younger patients and have been described as orbital medial wall white-eyed blowout fractures [205]. When an orbital fracture is suspected, CT imaging is preferable, rapid, and accurate. The complete evaluation and management of medial wall orbital fractures will be discussed in the trauma chapter of this text.

Orbital Roof Fractures

Compared to other facial fractures, orbital roof fractures are rare regardless of age or population [207]. There is an increased frequency of these fractures among children which has been attributed to the lack of pneumatized frontal sinuses and an increased craniofacial proportion [193]. Most epidemiologic studies have found frequencies of 1–9% of all facial fractures and between 3.2% and up to 36% of all pediatric facial fractures [196, 207, 208]. Adult orbital roof fractures are often associated with high-energy trauma, while pediatric orbital roof fractures may result from seemingly mild trauma [207]. Within the pediatric population, orbital roof fractures typically occur around the age of 8 in both males and females [207, 209]. Motor vehicle trauma, falls, and assault are recurrent mechanisms of injury reported in the literature [207, 209]. Orbital roof fractures may be associated with multisystem potentially life-threatening injury (61–86%), the evaluation of which is critical [207].

Signs and symptoms of orbital roof fractures include exophthalmos, enophthalmos, strabismus, vertical diplopia, periorbital edema, epiphora, supraorbital paresthesia, vision loss, rhinorrhea, meningitis, and altered mental status [207, 209, 210]. In those with suspected orbital roof fractures, CT imaging is preferable to evaluate the orbital and cranial bones, and one should at least consider a CT imaging study of the brain given the high incidences of intracranial complications (Fig. 52.15). In addition to an obvious fracture seen on imaging studies, pneumocephalus indicates a dural tear and thus an increased risk of meningitis and should alert the clinician to the possibility of an orbital roof fracture [210]. However, when there is pulsatile exophthalmos, an MR imaging study should be considered for the evaluation of a traumatic encephalocele [210]. Various cadres describing orbital roof fractures have been presented through Haug classification and are especially useful in guiding treatment [207, 210].

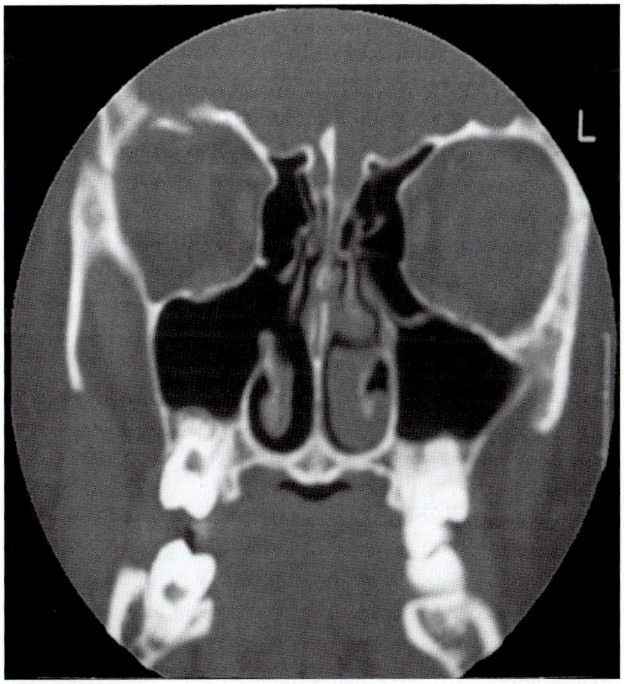

Fig. 52.15 Right orbital roof fracture with impingement of levator/superior rectus complex by fractured bone

Haug CT Classification of Orbital Roof Fractures

- Nondisplaced
- Isolated blow-in (roof displaced inferiorly)
- Isolated blow-up (roof displaced superiorly)
- Supraorbital rim involvement (without the frontal sinus)
- Frontal sinus involvement
- Combinations

Management of these injuries often requires a multidisciplinary approach [207]. Like other facial fractures, conservative management is preferred when possible and most orbital roof fractures may be managed in this fashion [209]. Even those with CSF leaks can be managed with intravenous antibiotics, as 80% of leaks close spontaneously [209]. According to Haug et al., beyond repair of soft tissue injury, nondisplaced orbital roof fractures can be managed with observation and close monitoring of neurologic status because of the risk of associated intracranial injury. Isolated blow-in fractures with exophthalmos or restrictive strabismus are candidates for open reduction and fixation. Haug et al. recommended the use of titanium plates and microscrews, with layered closure and intraoperative IV antibiotics such as nafcillin, gentamicin, or cefazolin [207]. Isolated blow-up fractures without ocular symptoms may be observed similarly to nondisplaced fractures, while those with symptoms without intracranial involvement may be managed as blow-in fractures. Those with suspected intracranial involvement benefit from an intracranial approach followed by the same plating, closure, and antibiotics. Supraorbital rim involved orbital roof fractures may be managed as isolated blow-in fractures excepting the initial stabilization of the orbital rim and subsequent reconstruction of the roof. When the frontal sinus is involved in a roof fracture, both sites are commonly treated in the same operative session. Reconstruction of the orbital rim usually precedes management of the frontal sinus fracture which often involves its obliteration or cranialization in the same operative session.

Lateral Orbital Wall Fractures

Lateral wall fractures in isolation may involve the zygoma and/or the greater wing of sphenoid bones forming the anterior and posterior aspects of the lateral wall, respectively. Compared to other types of orbital fractures, there is a relative paucity of data about isolated lateral orbital wall fractures. In many cases, additional fractures may be seen and may form what is called a zygomaticomaxillary complex (ZMC) fracture. ZMC fractures will be discussed in a separate section. Signs and symptoms may include decreased or loss of vision, strabismus, periocular ecchymosis, lacerations, proptosis, and, mostly, any variety of ocular trauma [211]. Some displaced fractures may impinge upon either the rectus muscles or the optic nerve [211, 212]. In some cases, the middle cranial fossa may be involved. CT imaging is useful in the initial fracture evaluation, although an MRI may be useful if nervous tissue (e.g., brain or optic nerve) injury is suspected. The evaluation and treatment of lateral wall orbital fractures will be discussed in the trauma chapter.

Zygomaticomaxillary Complex Fractures

Zygomaticomaxillary complex (ZMC) fractures are common and account for between 6% and 20% of all pediatric facial fracture and about 36% of midfacial fractures [196, 208, 213] (Fig. 52.16). As with most facial fracture, males are overrepresented (77%) [213]. The evaluation and management will be discussed in the trauma chapter.

Intraorbital Foreign Body

Intraorbital foreign bodies (IOFB) disproportionately affect younger patients (mean of 24.6 years of age) [214, 215]. They may result from seemingly minor to overt multisystem trauma [214, 215]. Mechanisms of injury include shootings, children's play/fall, industrial accidents, assault, gardening, and motor vehicle accidents [214–217]. Evaluation for a metallic IOFB should be performed with CT imaging. Further evaluation and management will be discussed in the trauma chapter.

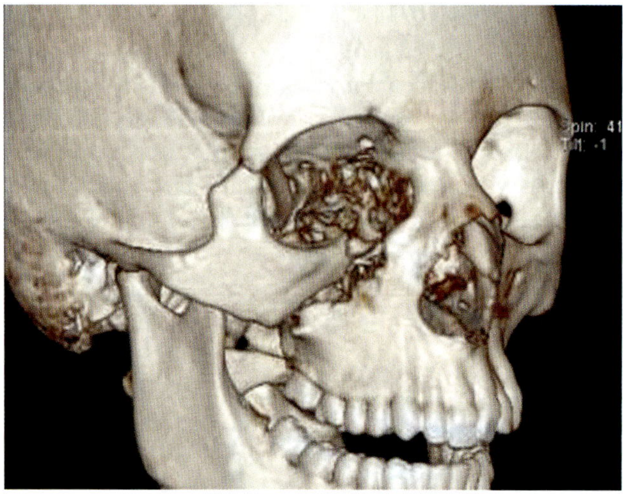

Fig. 52.16 Three-dimensional reconstruction of depressed right zygomaticomaxillary complex fracture

Orbital Hemorrhage

Orbital hemorrhage may be either intraorbital or subperiosteal [218]. Commonly, there is a history of recent surgery, trauma, chronic sinusitis, or blood dyscrasia [219]. Prescription and nonprescription drugs that may predispose an individual to orbital hemorrhages include antiplatelets, blood thinners, thrombolytics, chronic corticosteroids, cold/flu preparations, ginkgo biloba, ginseng, and garlic [219]. Signs and symptoms may develop over minutes to hours and include decreased vision, pain, exophthalmos, RAPD, elevated IOP, strabismus, "tense lids," "a tight orbit," subconjunctival hemorrhage, optic nerve edema, retinal venous congestion, central retinal artery pulsations or occlusion, and retinal edema. The diagnosis is primarily clinical, and therapeutic intervention is not predicated on imaging studies as this may result in devastating and irreversible vision loss [219].

The vision loss associated with orbital hemorrhages results from orbital compartment syndrome (OCS). OCS results from an increased volume within the bony confines of the orbit. The resulting increase in orbital pressure may cause injury to ocular or orbital tissues. The described mechanisms of injury fall largely into vascular occlusion to various tissues and compressive optic neuropathy [219]. Other causes of OCS include orbital emphysema, orbital cellulitis, orbital edema, and foreign materials [219].

Although facial trauma is a common cause of orbital hemorrhage, surgery (e.g., eyelid, orbital, lacrimal, endoscopic sinus, orthognathic, and neurosurgery), blood dyscrasias, drugs, retrobulbar injections, and lesions with hemorrhagic predispositions may also be causative [219]. Children, particularly, may present with orbital hemorrhages and OCS as a result of vascular lesions, such as venous and lymphatic anomalies. In some cases, the orbital hemorrhage may develop in a perinatal fashion with or without an associated complicated birth history or known clotting disorder; these orbital perinatal orbital hemorrhages tend to be subperiosteal [218, 220]. Although rare, orbital hemorrhage may be a complication of strabismus surgery [221]. Orbital hemorrhage has been reported in a child with scurvy as well [222].

CT or MR imaging studies may demonstrate a biconvex, well-defined, non-enhancing homogeneous mass with density slightly higher than the brain located in the superior aspect of the orbit in the setting of a subperiosteal hemorrhage or more diffuse or localized areas of high intensity located either intra- or extraconal depending on the etiology [218]. Tenting of the globe is associated with poorer prognosis [219]. Imaging studies may be especially useful in the pediatric population where subjective examination is limited or unreliable. MR imaging sequences can characterize the age of a given hematoma by virtue of its decaying blood products [220]. Magnetic resonance angiography (MRA) and magnetic resonance venography (MRV) are useful when a lesion with hemorrhagic predisposition is suspected. In the setting of spontaneous orbital hemorrhages, coagulation studies are recommended.

In the setting of an orbital hemorrhage and OCS, a bedside lateral canthotomy and inferior cantholysis are recommended [219]. If elevated orbital pressure does not improve within minutes, then a superior cantholysis is recommended, followed by, if further failing to improve, disinsertion of the orbital septum from the orbital rim via a transconjunctival or transcutaneous/anterior approach [219]. Were these techniques to fail, urgent consultation with an orbital surgeon is recommended for possible bony decompression. Most subperiosteal orbital hemorrhages without OCS may be managed with close observation, although some may require surgical drainage [218, 220]. If no OCS is present, exact follow-up depends on the extent, location and mechanism of the orbital hemorrhage. With regard to prognosis, younger patients tend to recover more completely [219].

Pediatric Traumatic Optic Neuropathy

Traumatic optic neuropathy (TON) is the consequence of direct or indirect trauma to the optic nerve. This trauma may be accidental or iatrogenic, endoscopic sinus surgery, orbital apex surgery, retrobulbar injection-induced orbital hemorrhage, or repair of midface fractures [223]. It occurs in 0.5–5% of patients following head trauma and may result instant or delayed visual loss [224]. Most TON articles focus on adults, although some have been published specifically pertaining to the pediatric population. Repka looked at 40 children with TON [224]. In their study of pediatric TON, they found that the mean age was 11.6 years, predominately male, and that the most common mechanisms were motor vehicle accidents (62%) and sports injuries (22%). Visual acuity ranged from no light perception (NLP) to 20/80. An otolaryngology group of Malhotra et al. also studied TON in the pediatric population [227]. The characteristics of their groups were predominately males, with a mean age of 9.67 years and common mechanisms of injury including fall (83.87%), sports injuries (12.9), and intranasal injury by a blunt object (3.23%). Generally speaking, the work of Repka et al. demonstrated that the pediatric TON behaves similarly to its adult counterpart and that steroids do not improve visual outcomes [226]. Spontaneous recovery is more commonly seen in the pediatric population, with studies reporting recovery rates of 29–44%. The evaluation and treatment of pediatric TON will be discussed in another chapter.

Conclusion

The evaluation and treatment of pediatric orbital disease is both challenging and rewarding. Nonverbal patients depend on the clinical and diagnostic acumen of the clinician. The pediatric facial skeleton is not merely a smaller version of the adults but rather a maturing unit that requires a specialized therapeutic paradigm. Treatment of pediatric orbital disease requires sensitivity to the growing pediatric face as well as the special differential diagnoses inherent to the pediatric population. Some pediatric orbital diseases are almost exclusively found in the pediatric population while others affect both child and adults. Other diseases present during childhood and remain problematic throughout life. Pediatric orbital disease is challenging but many cases can be treated successfully. It is this property of such a special population that makes their care so rewarding.

References

1. Eustis HS, Guthrie MA, Wright KW, Spiegel PH. Postnatal development. In: Pediatric ophthalmology and strabismus. New York, NY: Springer; 2013. p. 39–53.
2. Costello BJ, Papadopoulos H, Ruiz R. Pediatric craniomaxillofacial trauma. Clin Ped Emerg Med. 2005;6:32–40.
3. Shah RK, et al. Paranasal sinus development: a radiographic study. Laryngoscope. 2003;113(2):205–9.
4. Van Cauwenberge P, et al. Anatomy and physiology of the nose and the paranasal sinuses. Immunol Allergy Clin N Am. 2004;24(1):1–17.
5. Waitzman AA, et al. Craniofacial skeletal measurements based on computed tomography: part II. Normal values and growth trends. Cleft Palate Craniofac J. 1992;29(2):118–28.
6. Donahue SP, Schwartz G. Preseptal and orbital cellulitis in childhood. A changing microbiologic spectrum. Ophthalmology. 1998;105(10):1902–5; discussion 1905–6.
7. Botting AM, McIntosh D, Mahadevan M. Paediatric pre- and post-septal peri-orbital infections are different diseases. A retrospective review of 262 cases. Int J Pediatr Otorhinolaryngol. 2008;72(3):377–83.
8. Uzcategui N, et al. Clinical practice guidelines for the management of orbital cellulitis. J Pediatr Ophthalmol Strabismus. 1998;35(2):73–9, quiz 110–1.
9. Jackson K, Baker SR. Periorbital cellulitis. Head Neck Surg. 1987;9(4):227–34.
10. Chaudhry IA, et al. Inpatient preseptal cellulitis: experience from a tertiary eye care Centre. Br J Ophthalmol. 2008;92(10):1337–41.
11. Patt BS, Manning SC. Blindness resulting from orbital complications of sinusitis. Otolaryngol Head Neck Surg. 1991;104(6):789–95.
12. Smith TF, O'Day D, Wright PF. Clinical implications of preseptal (periorbital) cellulitis in childhood. Pediatrics. 1978;62(6):1006–9.
13. Schwartz GR, Wright SW. Changing bacteriology of periorbital cellulitis. Ann Emerg Med. 1996;28(6):617–20.
14. Ambati BK, et al. Periorbital and orbital cellulitis before and after the advent of Haemophilus influenzae type B vaccination. Ophthalmology. 2000;107(8):1450–3.

15. Ehlers JP, Shah CP, et al., editors. The wills eye manual: office and emergency room diagnosis and treatment of eye disease. 5th ed. Philadelphia: Lippincott Williams & Wilkins; 2008.
16. Nageswaran S, et al. Orbital cellulitis in children. Pediatr Infect Dis J. 2006;25(8):695–9.
17. Harris GJ. Age as a factor in the bacteriology and response to treatment of subperiosteal abscess of the orbit. Trans Am Ophthalmol Soc. 1993;91:441–516.
18. Kloek CE, Rubin PA. Role of inflammation in orbital cellulitis. Int Ophthalmol Clin. 2006;46(2):57–68.
19. Rothstein J, et al. Relationship of optic neuritis to disease of the paranasal sinuses. Laryngoscope. 1984;94(11 Pt 1):1501–8.
20. Youssef OH, Stefanyszyn MA, Bilyk JR. Odontogenic orbital cellulitis. Ophthal Plast Reconstr Surg. 2008;24(1):29–35.
21. Jain AAR, Rubin PAD. Orbital cellulitis in children. Int Ophthalmol Clin. 2006;47:71–86.
22. Reynolds DJ, et al. Intracranial infection associated with preseptal and orbital cellulitis in the pediatric patient. J AAPOS. 2003;7(6):413–7.
23. Brenner D, et al. Estimated risks of radiation-induced fatal cancer from pediatric CT. AJR Am J Roentgenol. 2001;176(2):289–96.
24. Jaffurs D, Denny A. Diagnostic pediatric computed tomographic scans of the head: actual dosage versus estimated risk. Plast Reconstr Surg. 2009;124(4):1254–60.
25. McKinley SH, et al. Microbiology of pediatric orbital cellulitis. Am J Ophthalmol. 2007;144(4):497–501.
26. Blomquist PH. Methicillin-resistant Staphylococcus aureus infections of the eye and orbit (an American ophthalmological society thesis). Trans Am Ophthalmol Soc. 2006;104:322–45.
27. Cruz AA, et al. Neonatal orbital abscess. Ophthalmology. 2001;108(12):2316–20.
28. Yen MT, Yen KG. Effect of corticosteroids in the acute management of pediatric orbital cellulitis with subperiosteal abscess. Ophthal Plast Reconstr Surg. 2005;21(5):363–6; discussion 366–7.
29. Miller A, et al. Infantile orbital cellulitis. Ophthalmology. 2008;115(3):594.
30. Pushker N, Tejwani LK, Bajaj MS, Khurana S, Velpandian T, Chandra M. Role of Oral corticosteroids in orbital cellulitis. Am J Ophthalmol. 2013;156(1):178–83.
31. Davies BW, Smith JM, Hink EM, Duriaraj VD. C-reactive protein as a marker for initiating steroid treatment in children with orbital cellulitis. Ophthalmic Plast Reconstr Surg. 2015;31(5):364–8.
32. Hornblass A, et al. Orbital abscess. Surv Ophthalmol. 1984;29(3):169–78.
33. Eustis HS, et al. Staging of orbital cellulitis in children: computerized tomography characteristics and treatment guidelines. J Pediatr Ophthalmol Strabismus. 1986;23(5):246–51.
34. Souliere CR Jr, et al. Selective non-surgical management of subperiosteal abscess of the orbit: computerized tomography and clinical course as indication for surgical drainage. Int J Pediatr Otorhinolaryngol. 1990;19(2):109–19.
35. Denning DW. Therapeutic outcome in invasive aspergillosis. Clin Infect Dis. 1996;23(3):608–15.
36. Centeno RS, Bentson JR, Mancuso AA. CT scanning in rhinocerebral mucormycosis and aspergillosis. Radiology. 1981;140(2):383–9.
37. McCarty ML, et al. Manifestations of fungal cellulitis of the orbit in children with neutropenia and fever. Ophthal Plast Reconstr Surg. 2004;20(3):217–23.
38. Sivak-Callcott JA, et al. Localised invasive sino-orbital aspergillosis: characteristic features. Br J Ophthalmol. 2004;88(5):681–7.
39. Levin LA, et al. The spectrum of orbital aspergillosis: a clinicopathological review. Surv Ophthalmol. 1996;41(2):142–54.
40. Robinson MR, et al. Sino-orbital-cerebral aspergillosis in immunocompromised pediatric patients. Pediatr Infect Dis J. 2000;19(12):1197–203.
41. Sohail MA, et al. Acute fulminant fungal sinusitis: clinical presentation, radiological findings and treatment. Acta Trop. 2001;80(2):177–85.
42. Hussain S, et al. Rhinocerebral invasive mycosis: occurrence in immunocompetent individuals. Eur J Radiol. 1995;20(2):151–5.
43. Dhiwakar M, Thakar A, Bahadur S. Invasive sino-orbital aspergillosis: surgical decisions and dilemmas. J Laryngol Otol. 2003;117(4):280–5.
44. Seiff SR, Choo PH, Carter SR. Role of local amphotericin B therapy for sino-orbital fungal infections. Ophthalmic Plast Reconstr Surg. 1999;15(1):28–31.
45. Yuen SJ, Rubin PA. Idiopathic orbital inflammation: distribution, clinical features, and treatment outcome. Arch Ophthalmol. 2003;121(4):491–9.
46. Kitei D, DiMario FJ Jr. Childhood orbital pseudotumor: case report and literature review. J Child Neurol. 2008;23(4):425–30.
47. Stevens JL, et al. Pseudotumor of the orbit in early childhood. J AAPOS. 1998;2(2):120–3.
48. Mottow LS, Jakobiec FA. Idiopathic inflammatory orbital pseudotumor in childhood. I Clinical characteristics Arch Ophthalmol. 1978;96(8):1410–7.
49. Mottow-Lippa L, Jakobiec FA, Smith M. Idiopathic inflammatory orbital pseudotumor in childhood. II. Results of diagnostic tests and biopsies. Ophthalmology. 1981;88(6):565–74.
50. Spindle J, Tang SX, Davies B, Wladis EJ, Piozzi E, Pellegrini M, Lally SE, Shields C, Shinder R. Pediatric idiopathic orbital inflammation: clinical features of 30 cases. Ophthalmic Plast Reconstr Surg. 2016;32(4):270–4.
51. Weber AL, Romo LV, Sabates NR. Pseudotumor of the orbit. Clinical, pathologic, and radiologic evaluation. Radiol Clin N Am. 1999;37(1):151–68, xi.
52. Wilson MW, Shergy WJ, Haik BG. Infliximab in the treatment of recalcitrant idiopathic orbital inflammation. Ophthal Plast Reconstr Surg. 2004;20(5):381–3.
53. Hsuan JD, et al. Idiopathic sclerosing orbital inflammation. Arch Ophthalmol. 2006;124(9):1244–50.
54. Chan W, et al. Ophthalmopathy in childhood graves' disease. Br J Ophthalmol. 2002;86(7):740–2.
55. Goldstein SM, et al. Pediatric thyroid-associated orbitopathy: the children's hospital of Philadelphia experience and literature review. Thyroid. 2008;18(9):997–9.
56. Holt H, et al. Pediatric graves' ophthalmopathy: the pre- and post-pubertal experience. J AAPOS. 2008;12(4):357–60.
57. Durairaj VD, Bartley GB, Garrity JA. Clinical features and treatment of graves ophthalmopathy in pediatric patients. Ophthal Plast Reconstr Surg. 2006;22(1):7–12.
58. Shields CL, et al. Neonatal graves' disease. Br J Ophthalmol. 1988;72(6):424–7.
59. Antoniazzi F, et al. Graves' ophthalmopathy evolution studied by MRI during childhood and adolescence. J Pediatr. 2004;144(4):527–31.
60. Levi M, et al. Ocular involvement as the initial manifestation of Wegener's granulomatosis in children. J AAPOS. 2008;12(1):94–6.
61. Parelhoff ES, Chavis RM, Friendly DS. Wegener's granulomatosis presenting as orbital pseudotumor in children. J Pediatr Ophthalmol Strabismus. 1985;22(3):100–4.
62. Spalton DJ, et al. Ocular changes in limited forms of Wegener's granulomatosis. Br J Ophthalmol. 1981;65(8):553–63.
63. Davies JB, Rao PK. Ocular manifestations of systemic lupus erythematosus. Curr Opin Ophthalmol. 2008;19(6):512–8.
64. Amirlak I, Narchi H. Isolated orbital pseudotumor as the presenting sign of systemic lupus erythematosus. J Pediatr Ophthalmol Strabismus. 2008;45(1):51–4.
65. Koch M, Langmann A. Diplopia as the presenting sign of systemic lupus erythematosus: the chameleon diagnosis. J AAPOS. 2006;10(2):184–5.

66. Grimson BS, Simons KB. Orbital inflammation, myositis, and systemic lupus erythematosus. Arch Ophthalmol. 1983;101(5):736–8.
67. Jordan DR, et al. Orbital panniculitis as the initial manifestation of systemic lupus erythematosus. Ophthal Plast Reconstr Surg. 1993;9(1):71–5.
68. Siebert S, Srinivasan U. Proptosis can be the presenting feature of systemic lupus erythematosus. Ann Rheum Dis. 2004;63(8):908–9.
69. Arthurs BP, et al. Orbital infarction and melting in a patient with systemic lupus erythematosus. Ophthalmology. 1999;106(12):2387–90.
70. Koike R, et al. Polyarteritis nodosa (PN) complicated with unilateral exophthalmos. Intern Med. 1993;32(3):232–6.
71. Hsu CT, et al. Choroidal infarction, anterior ischemic optic neuropathy, and central retinal artery occlusion from polyarteritis nodosa. Retina. 2001;21(4):348–51.
72. Garner A. Pathology of 'pseudotumours' of the orbit: a review. J Clin Pathol. 1973;26(9):639–48.
73. Ohga S, et al. Early-onset sarcoidosis mimicking refractory cutaneous histiocytosis. Pediatr Blood Cancer. 2008;50(3):723–6.
74. Blau EB. Familial granulomatous arthritis, iritis, and rash. J Pediatr. 1985;107(5):689–93.
75. Rose CD, et al. Blau syndrome mutation of CARD15/NOD2 in sporadic early onset granulomatous arthritis. J Rheumatol. 2005;32(2):373–5.
76. Rose CD, et al. Pediatric granulomatous arthritis: an international registry. Arthritis Rheum. 2006;54(10):3337–44.
77. Rybicki BA, et al. The Blau syndrome gene is not a major risk factor for sarcoidosis. Sarcoidosis Vasc Diffuse Lung Dis. 1999;16(2):203–8.
78. Shetty AK, Gedalia A. Childhood sarcoidosis: a rare but fascinating disorder. Pediatr Rheumatol Online J. 2008;6:16.
79. Shetty AK, Gedalia A. Sarcoidosis: a pediatric perspective. Clin Pediatr (Phila). 1998;37(12):707–17.
80. Rothova A. Ocular involvement in sarcoidosis. Br J Ophthalmol. 2000;84(1):110–6.
81. Mavrikakis I, Rootman J. Diverse clinical presentations of orbital sarcoid. Am J Ophthalmol. 2007;144(5):769–75.
82. Prabhakaran VC, et al. Orbital and adnexal sarcoidosis. Arch Ophthalmol. 2007;125(12):1657–62.
83. Taylor SR, McCluskey P, Lightman S. The ocular manifestations of inflammatory bowel disease. Curr Opin Ophthalmol. 2006;17(6):538–44.
84. Mintz R, et al. Ocular manifestations of inflammatory bowel disease. Inflamm Bowel Dis. 2004;10(2):135–9.
85. Felekis T, et al. Spectrum and frequency of ophthalmologic manifestations in patients with inflammatory bowel disease: a prospective single-center study. Inflamm Bowel Dis. 2009;15(1):29–34.
86. Leibovitch I, Galanopoulos A, Selva D. Suppurative granulomatous myositis of an extra-ocular muscle in Crohn's disease. Am J Gastroenterol. 2005;100(9):2136–7.
87. Ramalho J, Castillo M. Imaging of orbital myositis in Crohn's disease. Clin Imaging. 2008;32(3):227–9.
88. Weinstein JM, Koch K, Lane S. Orbital pseudotumor in Crohn's colitis. Ann Ophthalmol. 1984;16(3):275–8.
89. Dutt S, Cartwright MJ, Nelson CC. Acute dacryoadenitis and Crohn's disease: findings and management. Ophthal Plast Reconstr Surg. 1992;8(4):295–9.
90. Fox RI. Sjogren's syndrome. Lancet. 2005;366(9482):321–31.
91. Parkin B, et al. Lymphocytic infiltration and enlargement of the lacrimal glands: a new subtype of primary Sjogren's syndrome? Ophthalmology. 2005;112(11):2040–7.
92. Wilson C, Nigar E, Lee V. An atypical case of Sjogren's syndrome causing unilateral severe lacrimal gland enlargement and hypoglobus. Orbit. 2007;26(1):49–51.
93. Deprettere AJ, et al. Diagnosis of Sjogren's syndrome in children. Am J Dis Child. 1988;142(11):1185–7.
94. Goldstein SM, et al. Orbital neural-glial hamartoma associated with a congenital tonic pupil. J AAPOS. 2002;6(1):54–5.
95. Gunduz K, et al. Primary chondromesenchymal hamartoma of the orbit. Ophthal Plast Reconstr Surg. 2009;25(4):324–7.
96. Abel A, et al. Bony hamartoma of the inferior orbital rim in a patient with tuberous sclerosis. Arch Ophthalmol. 2004;122(5):780–2.
97. Roper GJ, Smith MS, Lueder GT. Congenital smooth muscle hamartoma of the conjunctival fornix. Am J Ophthalmol. 1999;128(5):643–4.
98. Brown HH, Kersten RC, Kulwin DR. Lipomatous hamartoma of the orbit. Arch Ophthalmol. 1991;109(2):240–3.
99. Nath K, et al. Vascular hamartoma and vascular tumours of orbit. Indian J Ophthalmol. 1977;25(1):18–23.
100. Mihora LD, et al. Ectopic orbital brain diagnosed 20 years after symptomatic presentation. Orbit. 2009;28(2–3):185–7.
101. Kiratli H, Sekeroglu MA, Tezel GG. Orbital heterotopic glial tissue presenting as exotropia. Orbit. 2008;27(3):165–8.
102. Farah SE, et al. Ectopic orbital meningioma: a case report and review. Ophthal Plast Reconstr Surg. 1999;15(6):463–6.
103. Call NB, Baylis HI. Cerebellar heterotopia in the orbit. Arch Ophthalmol. 1980;98(4):717–9.
104. Newton C, Dutton JJ, Klintworth GK. A respiratory epithelial choristomatous cyst of the orbit. Ophthalmology. 1985;92(12):1754–7.
105. Guy JR, Quisling RG. Ectopic lacrimal gland presenting as an orbital mass in childhood. AJNR Am J Neuroradiol. 1989;10(5 Suppl):S92.
106. West JA, Drewe RH, McNab AA. Atypical choristomatous cysts of the orbit. Aust N Z J Ophthalmol. 1997;25(2):117–23.
107. Mavrikakis I, et al. Orbital mesenchymal hamartoma with rhabdomyomatous features. Br J Ophthalmol. 2007;91(5):692–3.
108. Islam N, Mireskandari K, Rose GE. Orbital varices and orbital wall defects. Br J Ophthalmol. 2004;88(8):1092–3.
109. Verb SP, et al. Phakomatous choristoma: a rare orbital tumor presenting as an eyelid mass with obstruction of the nasolacrimal duct. J AAPOS. 2009;13(1):85–7.
110. Shields JA, Shields CL. Orbital cysts of childhood–classification, clinical features, and management. Surv Ophthalmol. 2004;49(3):281–99.
111. Sherman RP, Rootman J, Lapointe JS. Orbital dermoids: clinical presentation and management. Br J Ophthalmol. 1984;68(9):642–52.
112. Chawda SJ, Moseley IF. Computed tomography of orbital dermoids: a 20-year review. Clin Radiol. 1999;54(12):821–5.
113. Giulio B, Tranfa F, de Concilis C, Strianese D. Dermoid cysts: 16-year survey. Ophthalmic Plast Reconstr Surgery. 1995;11(3):187–92.
114. Meyer DR, et al. Primary temporal fossa dermoid cysts. Characterization and surgical management. Ophthalmology. 1999;106(2):342–9.
115. Golden RP, et al. Percutaneous drainage and ablation of orbital dermoid cysts. J AAPOS. 2007;11(5):438–42.
116. Sathananthan N, et al. The frequency and clinical significance of bone involvement in outer canthus dermoid cysts. Br J Ophthalmol. 1993;77(12):789–94.
117. Fry CL, Leone CR Jr. Safe management of dermolipomas. Arch Ophthalmol. 1994;112(8):1114–6.
118. Barber JC, et al. Congenital orbital teratoma. Arch Ophthalmol. 1974;91(1):45–8.
119. Gnanaraj L, et al. Massive congenital orbital teratoma. Ophthal Plast Reconstr Surg. 2005;21(6):445–7.
120. Ide CH, Davis WE, Black SP. Orbital teratoma. Arch Ophthalmol. 1978;96(11):2093–6.
121. Kaufman LM, Doroftei O. Optic glioma warranting treatment in children. Eye (Lond). 2006;20(10):1149–64.
122. Listernick R, et al. Optic pathway gliomas in neurofibromatosis-1: controversies and recommendations. Ann Neurol. 2007;61(3):189–98.

123. Shamji MF, Benoit BG. Syndromic and sporadic pediatric optic pathway gliomas: review of clinical and histopathological differences and treatment implications. Neurosurg Focus. 2007;23(5):E3.
124. Lee AG. Neuroophthalmological management of optic pathway gliomas. Neurosurg Focus. 2007;23(5):E1.
125. Lee V, Ragge NK, Collin JR. Orbitotemporal neurofibromatosis. Clinical features and surgical management. Ophthalmology. 2004;111(2):382–8.
126. Needle MN, et al. Prognostic signs in the surgical management of plexiform neurofibroma: the children's hospital of Philadelphia experience, 1974–1994. J Pediatr. 1997;131(5):678–82.
127. Chopra R, et al. Radiotherapy and radiosurgery for benign neurofibromas. Am J Clin Oncol. 2005;28(3):317–20.
128. Dutton JJ, et al. Multiple recurrences in malignant peripheral nerve sheath tumor of the orbit: a case report and a review of the literature. Ophthal Plast Reconstr Surg. 2001;17(4):293–9.
129. Ragge NK. Clinical and genetic patterns of neurofibromatosis 1 and 2. Br J Ophthalmol. 1993;77(10):662–72.
130. Jackson IT, et al. Orbitotemporal neurofibromatosis: classification and treatment. Plast Reconstr Surg. 1993;92(1):1–11.
131. Earley MJ, Moriarty P, Yap LH. Isolated bilateral orbital neurofibromatosis in a twelve-year-old. Br J Plast Surg. 2001;54(2):162–4.
132. Chen JY, Muecke JS, Brown SD. Orbital plexiform neurofibroma and high axial myopia. Ophthal Plast Reconstr Surg. 2008;24(4):284–6.
133. Erb MH, et al. Orbitotemporal neurofibromatosis: classification and treatment. Orbit. 2007;26(4):223–8.
134. Park WC, et al. The role of high-resolution computed tomography and magnetic resonance imaging in the evaluation of isolated orbital neurofibromas. Am J Ophthalmol. 2006;142(3):456–63.
135. Boulos PT, et al. Meningiomas of the orbit: contemporary considerations. Neurosurg Focus. 2001;10(5):E5.
136. Turbin RE, Pokorny K. Diagnosis and treatment of orbital optic nerve sheath meningioma. Cancer Control. 2004;11(5):334–41.
137. Harold Lee HB, et al. Primary optic nerve sheath meningioma in children. Surv Ophthalmol. 2008;53(6):543–58.
138. Grob SR, Jakobiec FA, Rashid A, MacIntosh P, Kelly H, Fay A. Pediatric optic nerve meningioma: diagnostic and therapeutic challenges. Ophthalmic Plast and Reconst Surgery. 2016;32(6):e160–4.
139. Eddleman CS, Liu JK. Optic nerve sheath meningioma: current diagnosis and treatment. Neurosurg Focus. 2007;23(5):E4.
140. Wang Y, Xiao LH. Orbital schwannomas: findings from magnetic resonance imaging in 62 cases. Eye (Lond). 2008;22(8):1034–9.
141. Cantore WA. Neural orbital tumors. Curr Opin Ophthalmol. 2000;11(5):367–71.
142. Tanaka A, et al. Differentiation of cavernous hemangioma from schwannoma of the orbit: a dynamic MRI study. AJR Am J Roentgenol. 2004;183(6):1799–804.
143. Kapur R, et al. Orbital schwannoma and neurofibroma: role of imaging. Neuroimaging Clin N Am. 2005;15(1):159–74.
144. Wilson MW, et al. Low-dose cyclophosphamide and interferon alfa 2a for the treatment of capillary hemangioma of the orbit. Ophthalmology. 2007;114(5):1007–11.
145. O'Keefe M, Lanigan B, Byrne SA. Capillary haemangioma of the eyelids and orbit: a clinical review of the safety and efficacy of intralesional steroid. Acta Ophthalmol Scand. 2003;81(3):294–8.
146. Schwartz SR, et al. Risk factors for amblyopia in children with capillary hemangiomas of the eyelids and orbit. J AAPOS. 2006;10(3):262–8.
147. Rosca TI, et al. Vascular tumors in the orbit–capillary and cavernous hemangiomas. Ann Diagn Pathol. 2006;10(1):13–9.
148. Taban M, Goldberg RA. Propranolol for orbital hemangioma. Ophthalmology. 2010;117(1):195 e4.
149. Chung EM, et al. From the archives of the AFIP: pediatric orbit tumors and tumorlike lesions: nonosseous lesions of the extraocular orbit. Radiographics. 2007;27(6):1777–99.
150. Manunza F, et al. Propranolol for complicated infantile haemangiomas: a case series of 30 infants. Br J Dermatol. 2010;162(2):466–8.
151. Leaute-Labreze C, et al. Propranolol for severe hemangiomas of infancy. N Engl J Med. 2008;358(24):2649–51.
152. Siegfried EC, Keenan WJ, Al-Jureidini S. More on propranolol for hemangiomas of infancy. N Engl J Med. 2008;359(26):2846, author reply 2846–7.
153. Guo S, Ni N. Topical treatment for capillary hemangioma of the eyelid using beta-blocker solution. Arch Ophthalmol. 2010;128(2):255–6.
154. Tunc M, Sadri E, Char DH. Orbital lymphangioma: an analysis of 26 patients. Br J Ophthalmol. 1999;83(1):76–80.
155. Boulos PR, et al. Intralesional injection of Tisseel fibrin glue for resection of lymphangiomas and other thin-walled orbital cysts. Ophthal Plast Reconstr Surg. 2005;21(3):171–6.
156. Sires BS, et al. Systemic corticosteroid use in orbital lymphangioma. Ophthal Plast Reconstr Surg. 2001;17(2):85–90.
157. Reeves SW, et al. Retinal folds as initial manifestation of orbital lymphangioma. Arch Ophthalmol. 2005;123(12):1756–8.
158. Gunduz K, et al. Correlation of surgical outcome with neuroimaging findings in periocular lymphangiomas. Ophthalmology. 2006;113(7):1231 e1–8.
159. Schwarcz RM, et al. Sclerosing therapy as first line treatment for low flow vascular lesions of the orbit. Am J Ophthalmol. 2006;141(2):333–9.
160. Bisdorff A, et al. Intracranial vascular anomalies in patients with periorbital lymphatic and lymphaticovenous malformations. AJNR Am J Neuroradiol. 2007;28(2):335–41.
161. Suzuki Y, et al. Management of orbital lymphangioma using intralesional injection of OK-432. Br J Ophthalmol. 2000;84(6):614–7.
162. Tawfik HA, Budin H, Dutton JJ. Lack of response to systemic corticosteroids in patients with lymphangioma. Ophthal Plast Reconstr Surg. 2005;21(4):302–5.
163. Karcioglu ZA, et al. Orbital rhabdomyosarcoma. Cancer Control. 2004;11(5):328–33.
164. Shields CL, et al. Clinical spectrum of primary ophthalmic rhabdomyosarcoma. Ophthalmology. 2001;108(12):2284–92.
165. Raney RB, et al. Rhabdomyosarcoma and undifferentiated sarcoma in the first two decades of life: a selective review of intergroup rhabdomyosarcoma study group experience and rationale for intergroup rhabdomyosarcoma study V. J Pediatr Hematol Oncol. 2001;23(4):215–20.
166. Meza JL, et al. Analysis of prognostic factors in patients with nonmetastatic rhabdomyosarcoma treated on intergroup rhabdomyosarcoma studies III and IV: the children's oncology group. J Clin Oncol. 2006;24(24):3844–51.
167. Dumont AS, et al. Cranioorbital fibrous dysplasia: with emphasis on visual impairment and current surgical management. Neurosurg Focus. 2001;10(5):E6.
168. Cruz AA, et al. Apical involvement with fibrous dysplasia: implications for vision. Ophthal Plast Reconstr Surg. 2007;23(6):450–4.
169. Bibby K, McFadzean R. Fibrous dysplasia of the orbit. Br J Ophthalmol. 1994;78(4):266–70.
170. Goisis M, et al. Fibrous dysplasia of the orbital region: current clinical perspectives in ophthalmology and cranio-maxillofacial surgery. Ophthal Plast Reconstr Surg. 2006;22(5):383–7.
171. Castillo BV Jr, Kaufman L. Pediatric tumors of the eye and orbit. Pediatr Clin N Am. 2003;50(1):149–72.
172. Sturgis EM, Potter BO. Sarcomas of the head and neck region. Curr Opin Oncol. 2003;15(3):239–52.
173. Dutton JJ, et al. Orbital Ewing's sarcoma of the orbit. Ophthal Plast Reconstr Surg. 2000;16(4):292–300.
174. Sharma A, et al. Primary Ewing's sarcoma of the sphenoid bone with unusual imaging features: a case report. Clin Neurol Neurosurg. 2005;107(6):528–31.

175. Wilson DJ, et al. Primary Ewing sarcoma of the orbit. Ophthal Plast Reconstr Surg. 2001;17(4):300–3.
176. Levy J, et al. Ophthalmic manifestations in Langerhans cell histiocytosis. Isr Med Assoc J. 2004;6(9):553–5.
177. Freyer DR, et al. Juvenile xanthogranuloma: forms of systemic disease and their clinical implications. J Pediatr. 1996;129(2):227–37.
178. Lee Y, Fay A. Orbital Langerhans cell histiocytosis. Int Ophthalmol Clin. 2009;49(1):123–31.
179. Woo KI, Harris GJ. Eosinophilic granuloma of the orbit: understanding the paradox of aggressive destruction responsive to minimal intervention. Ophthal Plast Reconstr Surg. 2003;19(6):429–39.
180. Harris GJ. Langerhans cell histiocytosis of the orbit: a need for interdisciplinary dialogue. Am J Ophthalmol. 2006;141(2):374–8.
181. Shields JA, Shields CL. Atlas of orbital tumors. Philadelphia: Lippincott Williams & Wilkins; 1999. p. xvi. 240 p
182. Jakobiec FA, Knowles DM. An overview of ocular adnexal lymphoid tumors. Trans Am Ophthalmol Soc. 1989;87:420–42, discussion 442–4.
183. Baker PS, et al. Orbital Burkitt lymphoma in immunocompetent patients: a report of 3 cases and a review of the literature. Ophthal Plast Reconstr Surg. 2009;25(6):464–8.
184. Prall FR, et al. Rapid onset proptosis and vision loss as the initial presentation of Burkitt lymphoma. Ophthalmic Surg Lasers Imaging. 2008;39(4):331–4.
185. Shields JA, et al. Adenoid cystic carcinoma of the lacrimal gland simulating a dermoid cyst in a 9-year-old boy. Arch Ophthalmol. 1998;116(12):1673–6.
186. Dagher G, et al. Adenoid cystic carcinoma of the lacrimal gland in a child. Arch Ophthalmol. 1980;98(6):1098–100.
187. Tse DT, Kossler AL, Feuer WJ, Benedetto PW. Long-term outcomes of Neoadjuvant intra-arterial Cytoreductive chemotherapy for lacrimal gland adenoid cystic carcinoma. Ophthalmology. 2013;120(7):1313–23.
188. Esmaeli B, Yin VT, Hanna EY, Kies MS, William WN, Bell D, Frank SJ. Eye-sparing multidisciplinary approach for the management of lacrimal gland carcinoma. Head Neck. 2016;38(8):1258–62.
189. Karcioglu ZA, editor. Orbital tumors: diagnosis and treatment. New York: Springer; 2005.
190. Ahmed S, et al. Neuroblastoma with orbital metastasis: ophthalmic presentation and role of ophthalmologists. Eye (Lond). 2006;20(4):466–70.
191. Stockl FA, et al. Orbital granulocytic sarcoma. Br J Ophthalmol. 1997;81(12):1084–8.
192. Bidar M, et al. Clinical and imaging characteristics of orbital leukemic tumors. Ophthal Plast Reconstr Surg. 2007;23(2):87–93.
193. Alcala-Galiano A, et al. Pediatric facial fractures: children are not just small adults. Radiographics. 2008;28(2):441–61, quiz 618.
194. Hink EM, Wei LA, Durairaj VD. Clinical features and treatment of pediatric orbit fractures. Ophthal Plast Reconstr Surg. 2014;30(2):124–31.
195. Eggensperger Wymann NM, et al. Pediatric craniofacial trauma. J Oral Maxillofac Surg. 2008;66(1):58–64.
196. Thoren H, et al. Changing trends in causes and patterns of facial fractures in children. Oral Surg Oral Med Oral Pathol Oral Radiol Endod. 2009;107(3):318–24.
197. Ferreira P, et al. Midfacial fractures in children and adolescents: a review of 492 cases. Br J Oral Maxillofac Surg. 2004;42(6):501–5.
198. Rahman RA, et al. Maxillofacial trauma of pediatric patients in Malaysia: a retrospective study from 1999 to 2001 in three hospitals. Int J Pediatr Otorhinolaryngol. 2007;71(6):929–36.
199. Hatton MP, Watkins LM, Rubin PA. Orbital fractures in children. Ophthal Plast Reconstr Surg. 2001;17(3):174–9.
200. Burnstine MA. Clinical recommendations for repair of orbital facial fractures. Curr Opin Ophthalmol. 2003;14(5):236–40.
201. Bansagi ZC, Meyer DR. Internal orbital fractures in the pediatric age group: characterization and management. Ophthalmology. 2000;107(5):829–36.
202. Dal Canto AJ, Linberg JV. Comparison of orbital fracture repair performed within 14 days versus 15 to 29 days after trauma. Ophthal Plast Reconstr Surg. 2008;24(6):437–43.
203. Simon GJ, et al. Early versus late repair of orbital blowout fractures. Ophthalmic Surg Lasers Imaging. 2009;40(2):141–8.
204. Brannan PA, Kersten RC, Kulwin DR. Isolated medial orbital wall fractures with medial rectus muscle incarceration. Ophthal Plast Reconstr Surg. 2006;22(3):178–83.
205. Tse R, Allen L, Matic D. The white-eyed medial blowout fracture. Plast Reconstr Surg. 2007;119(1):277–86.
206. Nolasco FP, Mathog RH. Medial orbital wall fractures: classification and clinical profile. Otolaryngol Head Neck Surg. 1995;112(4):549–56.
207. Haug RH, Van Sickels JE, Jenkins WS. Demographics and treatment options for orbital roof fractures. Oral Surg Oral Med Oral Pathol Oral Radiol Endod. 2002;93(3):238–46.
208. Chapman VM, et al. Facial fractures in children: unique patterns of injury observed by computed tomography. J Comput Assist Tomogr. 2009;33(1):70–2.
209. Fulcher TP, Sullivan TJ. Orbital roof fractures: management of ophthalmic complications. Ophthal Plast Reconstr Surg. 2003;19(5):359–63.
210. Antonelli V, et al. Traumatic encephalocele related to orbital roof fractures: report of six cases and literature review. Surg Neurol. 2002;57(2):117–25.
211. Stanley RB Jr. The temporal approach to impacted lateral orbital wall fractures. Arch Otolaryngol Head Neck Surg. 1988;114(5):550–3.
212. Koo L, Hatton MP, Rubin PA. Traumatic blindness after a displaced lateral orbital wall fracture. J Trauma. 2007;62(5):1288–9.
213. Ellis E 3rd, Kittidumkerng W. Analysis of treatment for isolated zygomaticomaxillary complex fractures. J Oral Maxillofac Surg. 1996;54(4):386–400; discussion 400–1.
214. Fulcher TP, McNab AA, Sullivan TJ. Clinical features and management of intraorbital foreign bodies. Ophthalmology. 2002;109(3):494–500.
215. Ho VH, et al. Retained intraorbital metallic foreign bodies. Ophthal Plast Reconstr Surg. 2004;20(3):232–6.
216. Ho VT, McGuckin JF Jr, Smergel EM. Intraorbital wooden foreign body: CT and MR appearance. AJNR Am J Neuroradiol. 1996;17(1):134–6.
217. Yoshii M, et al. Intraorbital wooden foreign body. Acta Ophthalmol Scand. 2004;82(4):492–3.
218. Atalla ML, et al. Nontraumatic subperiosteal orbital hemorrhage. Ophthalmology. 2001;108(1):183–9.
219. Lima V, et al. Orbital compartment syndrome: the ophthalmic surgical emergency. Surv Ophthalmol. 2009;54(4):441–9.
220. Ezzadin EM, et al. Bilateral orbital hemorrhage in a newborn. Am J Ophthalmol. 2000;129(4):531–3.
221. Ares C, Superstein R. Retrobulbar hemorrhage following strabismus surgery. J AAPOS. 2006;10(6):594–5.
222. Sloan B, Kulwin DR, Kersten RC. Scurvy causing bilateral orbital hemorrhage. Arch Ophthalmol. 1999;117(6):842–3.
223. Steinsapir KD. Traumatic optic neuropathy. Curr Opin Ophthalmol. 1999;10(5):340–2.
224. Goldenberg-Cohen N, Miller NR, Repka MX. Traumatic optic neuropathy in children and adolescents. J AAPOS. 2004;8(1):20–7.
225. Gupta AK, Gupta A, Malhotra SK. Traumatic optic neuropathy in pediatric population: early intervention or delayed intervention? Int J Pediatr Otorhinolaryngol. 2007;71(4):559–62.

Orbital Exenteration

53

Raymond I. Cho and Alon Kahana

Introduction

Orbital exenteration is defined as the surgical excision of the ocular globe, orbital soft tissues, and ocular adnexa. Total exenteration entails removing the orbital contents in their entirety, whereas a subtotal exenteration spares some portion of the posterior orbital soft tissues. In extended exenteration, removal of bone and/or adjacent structures is also performed. Because the operation results in permanent vision loss and significant facial deformity, it is usually reserved for the treatment of life-threatening or progressively destructive disease processes, such as high-grade or advanced malignancies or invasive infections. In cases where exenteration is contemplated, consideration should be given to management alternatives, including medical therapy and chemotherapy, radiation therapy, or observation.

Georg Bartisch, the father of German ophthalmology, is credited with performing the first exenteration procedure and described it in his 1583 textbook. In that operation, much of the contents of the orbit were removed, and the eyelids were preserved. The lack of anesthesia, blood replacement, antibiotics, and sterile surgical techniques made the operation and follow-up, at best, a significant risk and challenge for patient and surgeon. Present-day surgical techniques and preoperative and postoperative management make the operation one with a more acceptable rate of morbidity and mortality.

As a result of modern advances in the diagnosis and treatment of orbital disease, the need for exenteration has become less frequent. Computed tomography (CT) and magnetic resonance imaging (MRI) have become invaluable tools in the diagnosis and surveillance of orbital tumors and disease processes, and positron emission tomography (PET) [1] is also becoming more widely utilized. Alternative treatment strategies have also emerged for many tumors and disease processes which historically would have led to exenteration [2]. For example, exenteration was once considered standard treatment for orbital rhabdomyosarcoma, but tremendous advances in chemotherapy and radiation therapy over the past several decades have greatly reduced the need to resect this malignancy in such an aggressive manner [3]. Uveal melanoma with extrascleral extension was, at one time, a frequent cause for exenteration, but alternative treatments such as brachytherapy and modified enucleation have become more commonly favored [4]. Orbital mucormycosis and aspergillosis have also, in the past, been thought to necessitate exenteration but are now often treated with globe-sparing approaches such as surgical debridement with frozen section control, systemic and intraorbital antifungal therapy, hyperbaric oxygen therapy, and treatments aimed at boosting the patient's immune system [5–9]. Nonetheless, despite these advances, the occasion still arises for which exenteration is the most effective means of controlling orbital disease, extending patient survival, or improving quality of life.

Indications for Orbital Exenteration

The indications for orbital exenteration include the following:

1. Malignant primary orbital tumors
2. Malignant eyelid or ocular adnexal tumors with orbital invasion
3. Malignant secondary orbital tumors invading from the paranasal sinuses or cranium
4. Malignant intraocular tumors with extrascleral extension
5. Life-threatening invasive orbital infections
6. Severe trauma or orbital contracture

R. I. Cho
Ophthalmic Plastic and Reconstructive Surgery, The Ohio State University Wexner Medical Center, Department of Ophthalmology and Visual Science, Columbus, OH, USA

A. Kahana (✉)
Consultants in Ophthalmic and Facial Plastic Surgery, Southfield, MI, USA
e-mail: akahana@facialworks.com

J. J. Servat et al. (eds.), *Smith and Nesi's Ophthalmic Plastic and Reconstructive Surgery*,
https://doi.org/10.1007/978-3-030-41720-8_53

7. Massive or debilitating benign tumors of the orbit
8. Congenital deformities of the eye and orbit

This list, while not all-inclusive, accounts for the vast majority of conditions for which exenteration is performed.

Malignant tumors are the most common indication for orbital exenteration [10–16]. Examples include basal cell carcinoma, squamous cell carcinoma, melanoma (eyelid, conjunctival, and uveal), sebaceous cell carcinoma, adenoid cystic carcinoma, sarcoma, and retinoblastoma. In general, indolent tumors such as basal cell carcinoma only require exenteration if they have grown to such a size or invaded orbital tissues to such an extent that complete resection with clear margins cannot be accomplished without sacrificing the globe or its supporting structures [17]. However, the long-term prognosis after exenteration with clear margins is generally good. By contrast, high-grade malignancies such as adenoid cystic carcinoma often prompt exenteration even when the tumor size is relatively small, in an effort to decrease the risk of metastasis and improve patient survival [18]. Unfortunately, tumor recurrence or metastasis can still occur after exenteration in far too many cases, even with the use of adjunctive radiation and chemotherapy [19]. Consequently, the decision to treat any orbital malignancy must take into account its histologic type and natural history, tumor size and stage, the current status of the globe and visual function, overall patient health along with any comorbidities, and the expectations of the patient and family. Exenteration will not improve survival for orbital malignancies with known metastasis but, in selected cases, may provide palliation and improved quality of life. The importance of definitive histopathologic diagnosis from permanent sections before committing to exenteration cannot be overemphasized. This operation should never be performed on the basis of clinical impression or pathologic frozen sections.

Benign orbital tumors are rarely the cause for exenteration. Even in the case of massive congenital teratomas, it is sometimes possible to perform a globe-sparing resection and achieve a satisfactory aesthetic outcome [20]. However, the operative risks incurred by such a strategy must be taken into account, particularly when a neurosurgical approach is considered. Disfigurement, intractable pain, or intracranial extension are other potential factors which might lead one to consider exenteration for a benign tumor or inflammatory process [21–23].

Significant controversy and practice variation exist regarding exenteration for invasive orbital fungal infections. Because of the potential mortality from intracranial spread of organisms such as *Mucorales* and *Aspergillus*, aggressive surgical debridement of all infected tissue is widely accepted as an important component of treatment [24]. However, subtotal or total exenteration has not been definitively shown to improve the chance of survival in these patients, and no practical guidelines or predictive features have been identified to indicate which patients might benefit from exenteration [25]. Extensive counseling of the patient and family members is required, taking into account all clinical, emotional, and psychosocial factors during the decision-making process.

Periocular necrotizing fasciitis is a rare but potentially fatal infection which is usually caused by group A β-hemolytic *Streptococcus*. Systemic antibiotic therapy and subcutaneous debridement of involved tissue can sometimes spare the patient's globe and life, but exenteration may be necessary if orbital invasion is present [26].

Severe trauma resulting in loss of a significant portion of the orbital bone and/or soft tissues may necessitate some form of exenteration when orbital reconstruction is impossible. However, trauma of such severity is uncommon and often nonsurvivable, and every attempt should be made to salvage any remaining periocular and orbital tissues, however severely traumatized, before resorting to exenteration. If severe orbital contracture results from trauma or prior surgery, exenteration may be indicated to rehabilitate the orbit [27]. The suboptimal aesthetic results of this procedure must be kept in mind when considering treatment options for these patients. The effectiveness of exenteration for the treatment of chronic pain in anophthalmic sockets has not been clearly demonstrated.

Preoperative Evaluation and Planning

It goes without saying that a complete ocular examination is essential in the preoperative evaluation of the exenteration patient. The effects of the orbital process on the patient's vision, ocular motility, globe position, and eyelids and ocular adnexa should be clearly documented. Other possible pertinent findings include facial abnormalities, lymphadenopathy, signs of lacrimal outflow obstruction, or sensory deficit in the distributions of the ophthalmic (V1) or maxillary (V2) divisions of the trigeminal nerve. Malignancies with the potential for metastatic spread must undergo a complete metastatic workup. In certain cases, such as with periocular melanoma or sebaceous cell carcinoma, sentinel lymph node biopsy may provide useful information in guiding the patient's management [28, 29]. In most cases, CT or MRI images of the orbit have already been obtained during the initial evaluation of the orbital process in question, and these studies can provide information which is invaluable both preoperatively and intraoperatively. In particular, evidence of extraorbital extension of tumor or disease should be noted, as this may necessitate additional resection of bone and adjacent structures. In cases where resection of tissue adjacent to or invading the sinuses or cranial vault is anticipated, collaboration with other specialists such as otolaryngologists or neurosurgeons is useful, and even essential. This is especially important when considering an extraorbital surgical route, such as transnasal or transcranial. An example of a tumor commonly requiring transcranial exenteration is adenoid cystic carcinoma of the lacrimal gland with involvement of the orbital roof [18]. In order to safely remove the involved portion of frontal bone, a frontal craniotomy performed by neurosurgery will provide optimal surgical exposure and protect the dura and brain during resection.

Reconstruction of the exenterated orbit must also be considered during preoperative planning. As will be discussed later in this chapter, skin grafts, bone grafts, transfer flaps, or microvascular free flaps can all be utilized to reconstruct various orbital defects, and consultation with a facial plastic surgery specialist may be very useful in some of these cases.

Finally, the importance of postoperative follow-up, the options for rehabilitation, and, in many cases, the need for adjunctive therapy should be discussed carefully with patients and their families. Preoperative consultation with an orbital prosthetic specialist (anaplastologist) can often be quite reassuring and may go a long way toward preparing the patient emotionally for the operation and its aftermath. In cases of malignant orbital tumors in which adjunctive chemotherapy or radiation is indicated, a team-oriented approach is necessary, and good communication with hematology/oncology and radiation oncology is essential.

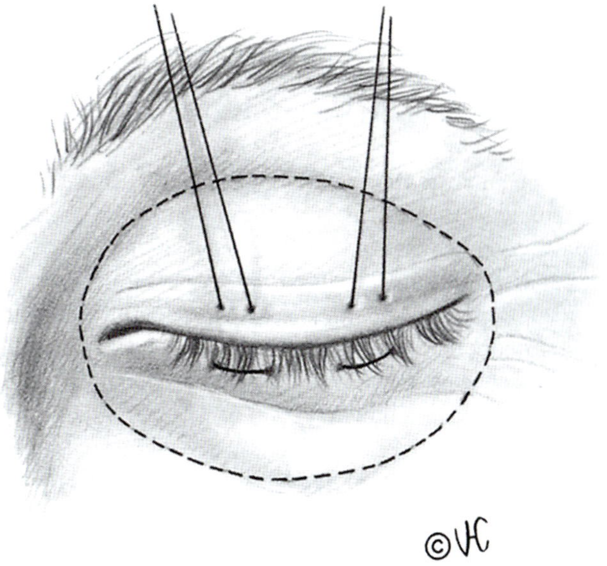

Fig. 53.1 Initial incision for total orbital exenteration

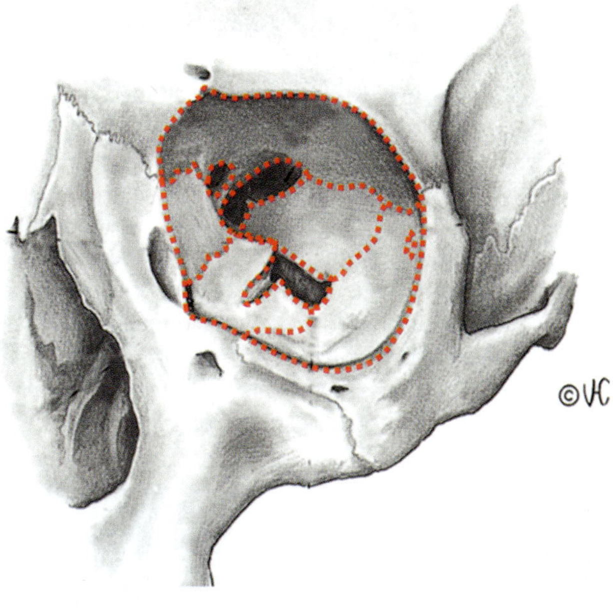

Fig. 53.2 Bony anatomy of the orbit showing points of increased periosteal adherence

Exenteration Techniques

From a technical standpoint, orbital exenteration can be thought of as several different techniques or as one basic technique with several variations. The latter approach will be presented here, describing first the total exenteration and then proceeding to the various modifications with their potential indications.

Total Exenteration

Exenterations should be performed under general anesthesia whenever possible. Local infiltration anesthesia is helpful for hemostasis in the eyelid, but intraorbital or retrobulbar injections are not generally useful and should be particularly avoided in the presence of an orbital malignancy. At the beginning of the case, sutures (e.g., 3-0 silk) can be placed around the rectus muscles or through the upper and lower tarsi to provide traction on the orbital contents. An elliptical incision is made with a scalpel blade or electrocautery through the skin overlying the orbital rim (Fig. 53.1). Dissection is then carried to the orbital rim, and the periosteum just outside the arcus marginalis is incised. Periosteal elevators are used to dissect the periorbita from the bony orbit, beginning at the orbital rim and continuing all the way back to the orbital apex. Most of the periorbita is loosely adherent to the bone, but it is more tightly adherent at several anatomic locations, including the anterior and posterior lacrimal crests, lateral orbital tubercle, trochlea, inferior oblique origin, and superior and inferior orbital fissures (Fig. 53.2). If disease involvement of the lacrimal sac is not suspected, the sac can be spared by dissecting lateral to it and dividing the common canaliculus and orbicularis attachments. Subperiosteal dissection can then proceed from the posterior lacrimal crest and beyond. If the lacrimal sac is to be removed, it is dissected from the lacrimal sac fossa and divided from the nasolacrimal duct with electrocautery. The exposed nasolacrimal duct can be obliterated with fat, muscle, or soft tissue to decrease the risk of postoperative fistula formation.

Throughout the course of the subperiosteal dissection, the supraorbital, supratrochlear, anterior and posterior ethmoidal, zygomaticofacial, and zygomaticotemporal neurovascular bundles are identified, cauterized or ligated, and divided. Dissection should be performed carefully along the orbital floor and medial wall, so as to not fracture the thin bone and create a communication with the ethmoid or maxillary sinuses. In the inferotemporal orbit, the inferior orbital fissure is encountered and penetrating vessels divided with electrocautery. The infraorbital nerve should be preserved unless it must be sacrificed to achieve the intended result. Once the periorbita has been dissected to the apex, gently curved scissors are introduced into the posterior orbit and the optic nerve, and superior orbital fissure contents and posterior orbital tissues are cut (Fig. 53.3). If desired, a clamp may be placed across the apical tissues prior to cutting in order to aid in hemostasis. If the ophthalmic artery is identified, it can be cauterized, suture-ligated, or clipped. Additional hemostasis may be obtained with ice-cold wet gauze, pressure, and cautery. As discussed in detail later in this chapter, the orbit may be left to granulate or covered with a skin graft or tissue flap. The orbit is then packed with petrolatum gauze and a pressure patch placed.

In cases of tumor resection, clearance of surgical margins using either frozen or permanent sections is often advisable. The location of these specimens is, of course, dependent on the location and characteristics of the original tumor, and intraoperative findings such as bony erosion or apparent periocular soft tissue invasion may prompt the biopsy of additional anatomic locations as deemed appropriate.

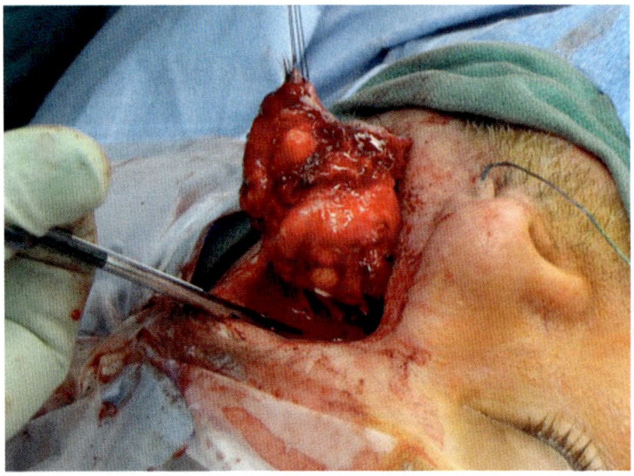

Fig. 53.3 Intraoperative photograph during total exenteration. Following complete subperiosteal dissection to the orbital apex, curved scissors are used to cut the posterior orbital tissues

Eyelid-Sparing Exenteration

In cases where the orbital disease process does not involve the eyelids, a lid-sparing technique, as popularized by Coston and Small [30], can be utilized. The total exenteration technique described above is modified by placing the initial skin incisions just outside the upper and lower lid lash lines and joining them at the medial and lateral commissures (Fig. 53.4). Dissection is then carried in the preorbicularis or preseptal plane to the orbital rim (Fig. 53.5), after which point the exenteration technique remains unchanged. Dissecting in the preorbicularis plane decreases

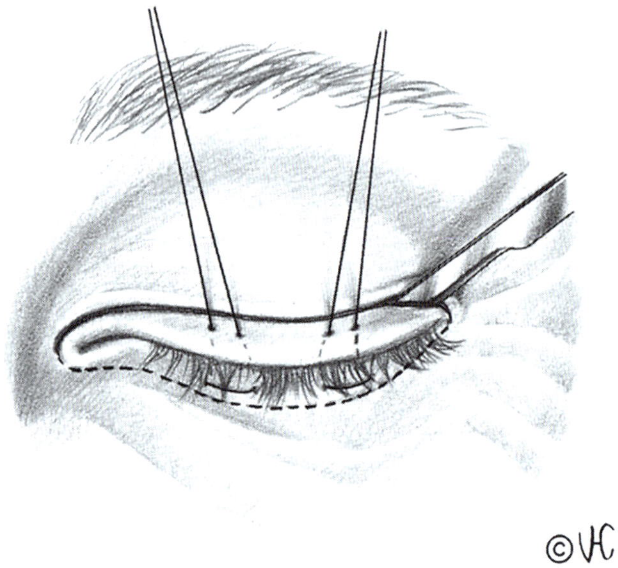

Fig. 53.4 Initial incision for eyelid-sparing exenteration

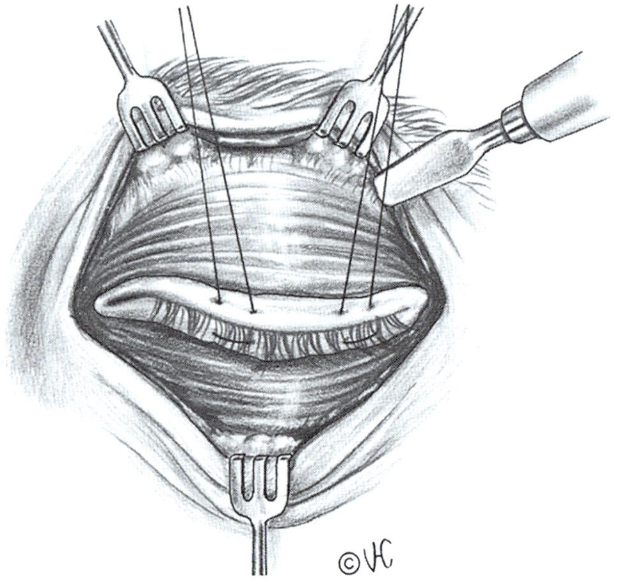

Fig. 53.5 The lid skin is dissected in the preorbicularis plane to the orbital rim

the likelihood of violating the orbital septum, which is undesirable if tumor is present in the anterior orbit. Alternatively, dissecting in the preseptal plane spares the orbicularis muscle, which provides an excellent vascular supply to the skin flap. It should be noted that the term "lid-sparing" is somewhat of a misnomer since only the anterior lamella is spared, while the lashes, tarsus, septum, levator, and conjunctiva are all resected.

The advantage of sparing the lid skin is that it provides some coverage for the bone of the anterior orbit [31]. For total exenterations, this amount of skin will typically provide only partial coverage, and the remainder of the socket will need to be grafted or left to granulate. However, in cases of subtotal exenteration (as discussed below), the eyelid skin may be enough to provide complete coverage of the socket.

Subtotal Exenteration

For diseases that involve only the anterior orbit or conjunctiva, subtotal exenteration may be considered [32]. Conjunctival melanoma or sebaceous cell carcinoma without evidence of deep orbital invasion can potentially be treated in this manner. The advantage of subtotal exenteration is that soft tissue is left in the posterior orbit which can be covered with eyelid skin (if spared) or a skin graft. However, secure fixation of an orbital prosthesis may be more difficult postoperatively since the socket is left shallow (Fig. 53.6). There is also a theoretically increased risk of recurrence if residual tumor or disease is inadvertently left in the posterior orbital tissues.

The technique for subtotal exenteration proceeds as with total exenteration, except that subperiosteal dissection is only carried as far posteriorly as deemed necessary. The orbital tissues are clamped and cut at the level chosen by the surgeon, ensuring that the optic nerve is cut posterior to the globe. The orbit can then be lined with a skin flap or split-thickness skin graft if desired.

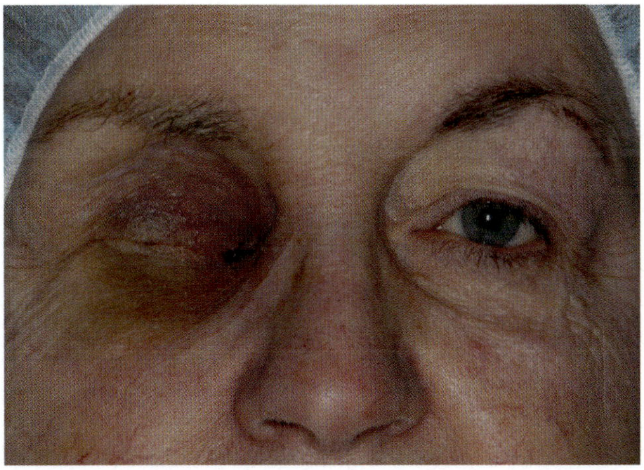

Fig. 53.6 Early postoperative photograph following eyelid-sparing subtotal exenteration. Because the posterior orbital tissues were preserved, the lid skin was sufficient to completely cover the orbital defect

Extended Exenteration with Bone Removal and/or Additional Resection

For particularly high-grade malignancies or destructive osteolytic processes, total exenteration with removal of a portion of the bony orbit may be indicated. The location and extent of bony resection is dictated by the primary tumor location, gross or microscopic evidence of bony invasion, perineural tumor spread, and/or involvement of the orbital fissures and foramina. When resection involves the orbital roof or other portions of the skull base, a transcranial approach in collaboration with neurosurgery should be utilized [33–35]. For tumors arising from or involving the paranasal sinuses, an otolaryngologist can provide invaluable assistance in navigating the complex anatomy of this region and resecting tumor-involved portions of the midface using open or endoscopic surgical techniques [36].

Primary Reconstruction of the Exenterated Orbit

A plethora of surgical options are available for reconstructing the exenterated socket [37–39]. The decision on which method is used primarily depends upon whether an "open" or "closed" cavity is planned [40]. Open cavities are generally preferred in patients who desire rehabilitation with an orbital prosthesis, and spontaneous epithelialization, skin grafts, or thin local flaps can all achieve this goal (Fig. 53.7a, b). Closed cavities in which the orbit is filled with soft tissue (microvascular free flap or muscle flap) up to the level of the orbital rim may be preferred when prosthesis use is not planned or may be helpful after extended exenteration resulting in communication with the cranial fossa or paranasal sinuses (Fig. 53.8). Modern imaging technologies allow for detection of tumor recurrence even posterior to a vascular flap, and this subject should be discussed with the patient and among the medical team members.

Spontaneous Granulation

An open socket with exposed bone may be allowed to spontaneously granulate and epithelialize postoperatively [41]. Although this approach entails the least operative time and no additional surgical sites, it does require intensive cooperation and perseverance on the part of the patient. Regular dressing changes with petrolatum gauze, typically three

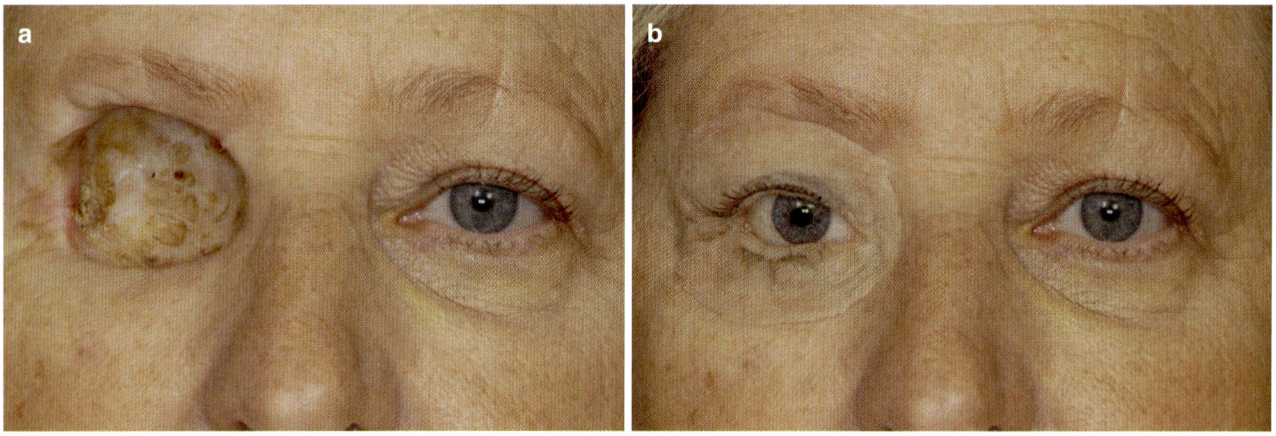

Fig. 53.7 (a) Open cavity following total orbital exenteration with split-thickness skin graft. (b) Same patient with an orbital prosthesis

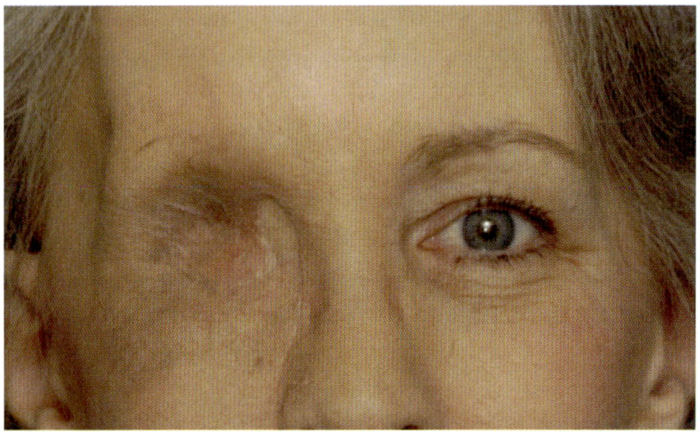

Fig. 53.8 Closed cavity following extended transcranial exenteration with maxillectomy and primary reconstruction with scapular free flap

times a week, should be performed by a home health nurse or other trained caregiver. Granulation tissue begins to appear within a week postoperatively, and epithelialization progresses over a period of 3–6 months. Orbital radiation can significantly delay the healing process. The opposite is also true – a slowly healing, granulating socket may delay initiation of needed radiation. If desired, the patient may be fit with an orbital prosthesis once complete epithelialization has occurred.

Skin Grafting

Although the harvesting of a skin graft necessitates an additional operative site, the placement of such facilitates much more rapid healing of the socket and earlier rehabilitation compared to spontaneous granulation. While full-thickness skin grafts are acceptable, split-thickness grafts are more commonly used in this setting due to the need for relatively large grafts to cover the surface area inside the orbit [42]. Split-thickness grafts are also more likely than full-thickness grafts to successfully take onto the bare bone surface of the orbit.

Split-thickness skin grafts can be harvested from the thigh or other suitable location with an automated dermatome (Fig. 53.9). The graft may be meshed if desired, or alternatively, several slits can be made with a scalpel or scissors to allow for fluid drainage and increased stretching of the graft. For optimal cosmesis, any meshed graft should be limited to the confines of the socket and avoid any areas that will not eventually be covered by a prosthesis or patch. After the graft is trimmed to an appropriate size and shape, it is placed in the socket and the edges secured with absorbable sutures (Fig. 53.10). The socket is packed with petrolatum gauze and a pressure dressing placed. The first dressing change is performed approximately 1 week postoperatively, followed by dressing changes every other day for up to another week. If desired, a cotton-tipped applicator soaked in hydrogen peroxide may be used to carefully clean the socket during this period. Once good graft take is observed, the orbit can simply be covered with an eye patch until a prosthesis is made, and the patient should be instructed to clean the socket periodically with soap and water. The skin graft donor site can be covered with a single layer of fine mesh gauze and allowed to dry. The dressing will spontaneously separate once the wound has healed in about 3 weeks.

The dermis-fat graft has also been described as an alternative method of covering the exenterated socket, both with and without a temporalis muscle transfer flap [16, 43]. This provides a substrate for epithelialization and partially replaces the lost orbital soft tissue while still potentially leaving room for a prosthesis.

Soft Tissue Reconstruction

In lieu of rehabilitation with an orbital prosthesis, some surgeons advocate primary reconstruction of exenterated sockets by replacing the lost orbital soft tissue volume and periocular skin with pedicled or microvascular free flaps.

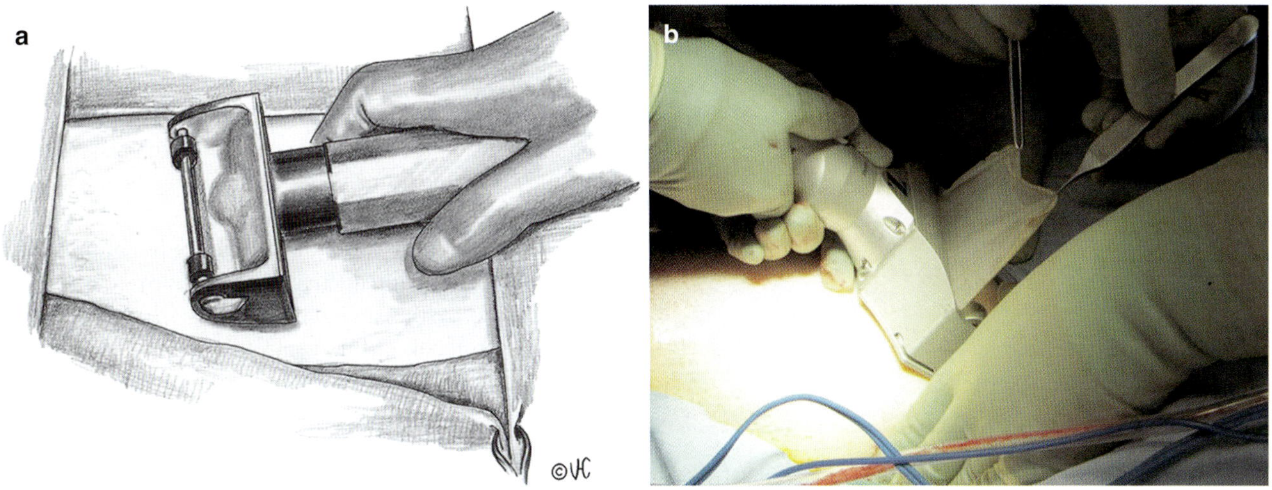

Fig. 53.9 Split-thickness skin graft is harvested from the thigh with an automated dermatome. (**a**) Line drawing. (**b**) Intraoperative photograph showing a split-thickness graft harvested from the thigh

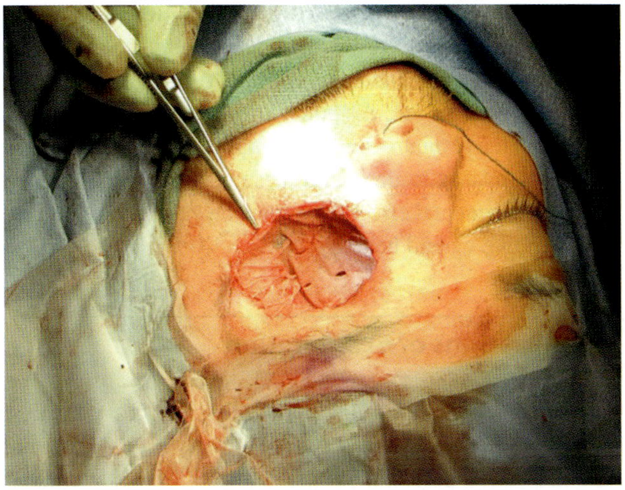

Fig. 53.10 Intraoperative photograph showing exenterated orbit lined with split-thickness skin graft. The graft was meshed with a #15 scalpel blade prior to being placed, and the edges are secured with 6-0 chromic sutures

Because these techniques do not attempt to recreate the appearance of the eyelids and globe, their aesthetic outcome is admittedly unnatural. Potential donor site morbidity is another disadvantage. However, postoperative orbital healing takes place quite rapidly, and the problems associated with orbital prostheses are eliminated. Vascularized flaps are also advantageous for covering any grafts or alloplastic implants that may be utilized for bony reconstruction, as discussed below.

Many local flaps have been described for orbital reconstruction, such as temporoparietal fascia, temporalis muscle, frontalis muscle, and myocutaneous flaps from the forehead, scalp, and cervicofacial region [38, 39, 43–46]. In some cases of lid-sparing exenteration, mucous membrane grafts have been placed over vascularized flaps to create a cavity suitable for wear of an ocular prosthesis [38].

Microvascular free flaps which have been utilized for reconstruction of the exenterated socket include radial forearm, latissimus dorsi, rectus abdominus, lateral arm, and anterolateral thigh flaps [47–50]. An additional advantage of free flaps is the potential for bony reconstruction with vascularized osseocutaneous flaps such as radial forearm, scapular, or fibular free flaps [49, 51, 52]. Free flap reconstructions are typically performed by facial or general plastic surgeons trained in microvascular surgery, and postoperative hospitalization is required.

It should be noted that these methods of soft tissue reconstruction can potentially affect postoperative tumor surveillance [37]. Their size and bulk will mask the direct clinical observation of recurrent tumor, necessitating the use of periodic imaging studies in these patients, in contrast with orbits covered with skin alone, where tumor recurrence can more readily be detected on clinical exam. MRI would typically be the imaging modality of choice for surveillance of soft tissues.

Bony Reconstruction

When orbital bone is either destroyed by the primary disease process or resected during exenteration, reconstruction of the bony orbit may be necessary to achieve an optimal outcome. Whenever possible, defects of the orbital rim should be reconstructed to maintain the continuity and bony contour of the upper and midface (Fig. 53.11). Defects of the orbital roof may not require reconstruction unless more than half of the roof is involved. Likewise, lateral orbital wall defects do not typically require reconstruction, with the possible excep-

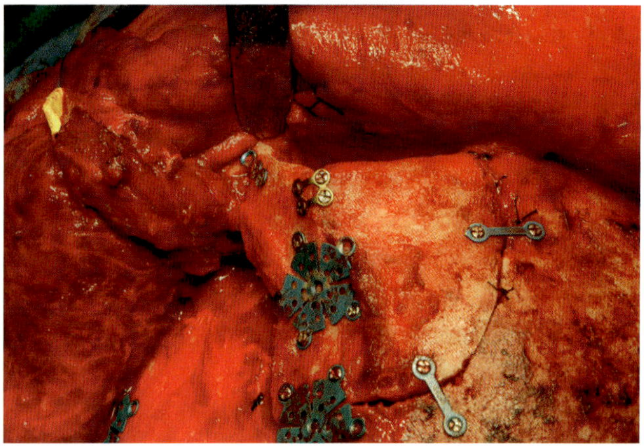

Fig. 53.11 Bony reconstruction of the superotemporal orbital rim with autogenous calvarial bone graft, following extended transcranial exenteration with removal of the orbital roof and lateral wall

tion of cases in which the entire greater sphenoid wing is removed. Reconstruction of the orbital floor and medial wall can be problematic due to the paucity of bony support and vascularized tissue within the ethmoid and maxillary sinuses. The necessity and type of such reconstruction largely depend on the chosen method of soft tissue coverage. Spontaneous epithelialization will not take place within an exposed sinus, and skin grafts are likely to fail if placed either over the defect, within the sinus, or over a reconstructed orbital wall. In these cases, microvascular free flaps are typically used to reconstruct or obliterate the open sinus.

A variety of materials can be utilized for reconstruction of the bony orbit. Autogenous bone grafts, such as split calvarium or iliac crest, are ideal for this purpose due to their biocompatibility and longevity. A microvascular free flap with a bony component is also an excellent choice. Irradiated cadaver bone is suitable but less optimal due to its propensity for absorption. Alloplastic implants, while readily available, are more prone to exposure and infection and require adequate coverage with well-vascularized tissue. Standard titanium plates and screws can be used to fixate grafts or implants during bony reconstruction.

Special Clinical Considerations

The orbital diseases which require treatment by exenteration are typically severe and complex. Many of the malignant tumors, by virtue of their size, invasiveness, or propensity for metastasis, will require adjunctive treatment with chemotherapy or radiation. In an orbit that has undergone radiation prior to exenteration, the surgeon must keep in mind the fibrosing and devascularizing effects of radiation on orbital tissues and their potentially detrimental effects on postoperative healing. By the same token, when the administration of postoperative radiation is anticipated, consideration may be given to the use of thicker or more vascularized reconstructive soft tissue flaps, as radiation-induced necrosis is more likely with skin grafts or thinner flaps [53]. Coordination should also take place with the radiation oncologist to determine the ideal time frame to initiate radiation treatment once adequate healing has occurred.

Recent research by Tse et al. [54]. in the use of preoperative intra-arterial cytoreductive chemotherapy for lacrimal gland adenoid cystic carcinoma deserves specific mention. Under this protocol, chemotherapeutic agents are administered via the external carotid artery directly to the orbital tissues. Following completion of this therapy, the orbit is exenterated with or without bone removal, and postoperative radiation is administered as indicated. Early data suggests that this treatment strategy may increase survival for patients with this highly malignant tumor. (Please see "Lacrimal Gland" chapter in this book for additional reading.)

Exenteration of the post-traumatic orbit can be particularly challenging. Extensive scarring, distortion of anatomic landmarks, and bony loss with paranasal sinus communication are commonly encountered. In addition, if the orbital roof has been violated, the potential exists for intraoperative or postoperative neurosurgical complications. The surgeon must be prepared to deal with these potential issues, along with the detrimental effects of trauma on vascular supply and postoperative wound healing.

Complications of Exenteration

As with all surgical procedures, bleeding, infection, damage to surrounding structures, and an unsatisfactory aesthetic outcome are potential complications of exenteration. Hemostasis can be particularly difficult following division of the major vessels of the orbit, the ophthalmic artery in particular. Violation of the ethmoid or maxillary sinuses can also increase the risk of microbial contamination and infection. The usefulness of prophylactic antibiotics for exenteration has not been demonstrated, but they may be prescribed at the surgeon's discretion.

An unavoidable side effect of exenteration is postoperative numbness in the distribution of the ophthalmic division of the trigeminal nerve (V1) due to resection of the supraorbital, supratrochlear, infratrochlear, and ethmoidal nerves. Preoperative counseling is important to ensure that this unpleasant effect is fully expected by the patient. Return of sensation is unpredictable but may take place over many months. Numbness in the V2 distribution is also common due to division of the zygomatic nerves but is usually much less noticeable and shorter-lived. Infraorbital nerve injury is unusual unless the orbital floor is inadvertently violated along the course of the infraorbital canal.

Fistular communication with the paranasal sinuses can result from violation of the orbital floor or medial wall, either as a result of the orbital disease or from intraoperative trauma [55]. The nasolacrimal duct is also a potential cause of fistulas, and intraoperative obliteration of the proximal nasolacrimal duct with fat or muscle may decrease the risk of this complication. While smaller bony defects may spontaneously epithelialize with proper socket care, larger defects more commonly result in fistulas causing discharge, crusting, and possible difficulty maintaining an orbital prosthesis. Orbital radiation also increases the risk of sino-orbital fistulas. Skin grafts or vascularized flaps can be used primarily to prevent fistulas or secondarily to treat persistent, symptomatic fistulas [56]. The use of an extraocular muscle and orbital fat graft has also been described to primarily fill orbital wall defects during exenteration [57].

Cerebrospinal fluid (CSF) leaks can potentially complicate exenteration due to violation of the orbital roof, cribriform plate, or greater sphenoid wing [58, 59]. In many cases, CSF leaks that are recognized intraoperatively can be controlled with bone wax if the bony defect is small. However, consultation with a neurosurgeon is advisable if the leak persists despite attempted repair by the orbital surgeon. Intracranial infection can also complicate orbital exenteration with bone removal, with or without a CSF leak. This risk can be decreased by primary obliteration of the socket with soft tissue grafts or flaps [60].

Tumor recurrence can follow exenteration for malignant or benign lesions. This risk increases when residual gross or microscopic tumor is left and can be minimized through careful operative planning and surgical margin control. However, clear surgical margins do not preclude the possibility of tumor recurrence or metastasis, and the occurrence of such does not necessarily imply any failure on the part of the surgeon, particularly with high-grade malignancies such as adenoid cystic carcinoma or melanoma. As mentioned above, periodic postoperative imaging is essential for tumor surveillance after reconstruction with thick vascularized tissue flaps.

Rehabilitation of the Exenterated Socket

There is no escaping the significant facial deformity that follows orbital exenteration [61]. There are many ways to mitigate the undesirable aesthetic outcome of this procedure, but none of them are ideal. The simplest way to mask the post-exenteration orbit is by patching, which some patients may, for various reasons, find preferable to the other available options [39]. Custom orbital prostheses may arguably produce the most anatomically natural appearance, but the silicone material can never perfectly reproduce the color and texture of the lid and periocular skin, and there is no dynamic movement of the prosthetic eyelids and globe. The social ramifications of an inadvertently dislocated orbital prosthesis in a public setting can also be very disturbing, particularly for schoolchildren. As discussed above, coverage of the socket with vascularized tissue flaps provides natural skin in the periocular region but complete absence of the appearance of ocular structures.

Orbital Prosthetics

The creation of orbital prostheses [62, 63] is a highly specialized field and, in many cases, is performed by an anaplastologist who works with an ocularist, as completely different materials and techniques are utilized by each. Because of the relatively small number of these specialists, it is often necessary for the patient to travel long distances to enlist their services. However, the significant cost and effort involved is far outweighed in many people's minds by the dramatic aesthetic improvement and psychosocial benefits of an orbital prosthesis.

An impression of the orbit is typically made with hydrocolloid, which is then used to create a plaster cast (Fig. 53.12). A custom ocular prosthesis is positioned in the cast, and clay is molded into the "orbit" and around the prosthesis. The clay is then placed into the patient's orbit and sculpted to match the contour and appearance of the contralateral eyelids and periocular region (Fig. 53.13). A plaster mold is made from the sculpted clay and used to create the silicone prosthesis within which the ocular prosthesis is placed (Fig. 53.14). Dental thermal molding material can also be used to line the posterior prosthesis surface to prevent microbial infiltration of the silicone. The prosthesis is trimmed to fit the patient's socket, and eyelashes are added. If desired, the patient may wear spectacles to camouflage the silicone-to-skin interface.

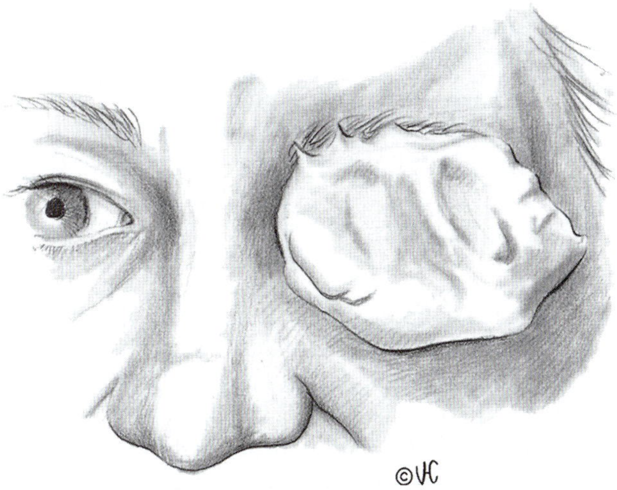

Fig. 53.12 A hydrocolloid impression is made from the orbit for creation of an orbital prosthesis

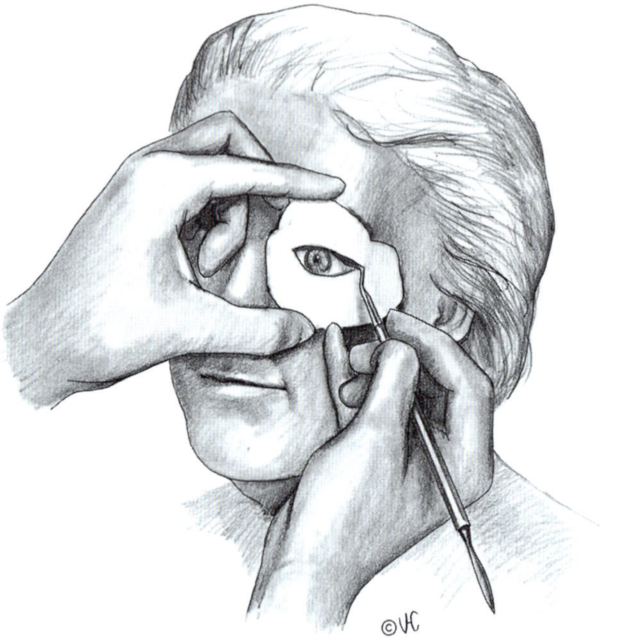

Fig. 53.13 The ocular prosthesis is placed within the clay mold, which is then sculpted to match the fellow eye

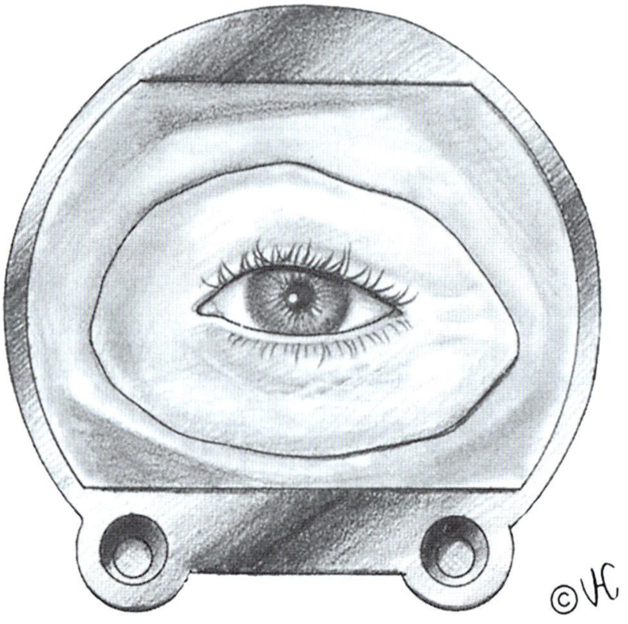

Fig. 53.14 Completed orbital prosthesis within the opened molding flask

Some orbital prostheses may be prone to dislodgement, particularly in shallower orbits. Adhesives or solvents may aid in retention but can also have detrimental effects on the prosthesis or the patient's skin. Support of the prosthesis with spectacles is another option. Magnetic coupling to osseointegrated screws can be very effective but requires additional surgery, typically performed several months postoperatively after epithelialization is complete [64].

As with any other type of prosthesis, care is required by the patient to maintain the prosthesis and keep the orbit clean. Regular follow-up with the prosthetist is important to optimize the comfort, appearance, and longevity of the prosthesis.

Conclusion

Orbital exenteration is an uncommon operation that is thankfully becoming even more rare, thanks to advances in the medical and surgical care of complex orbital disorders. Nevertheless, it has importance in the management of certain conditions and may literally be lifesaving. Modern prosthetic and reconstructive techniques are very helpful in rehabilitation efforts, and a team-oriented approach is recommended for these patients.

References

1. Lane KA, Bilyk JR. Preliminary study of positron emission tomography in the detection of orbital malignancy. Ophthal Plast Reconstr Surg. 2006;22:361–5.
2. Hsu A, Frank SJ, Esmaeli B, et al. Postoperative adjuvant external-beam radiation for cancers of the eyelid and conjunctiva. Ophthal Plast Reconstr Surg. 2008;24:444–9.
3. Shields JA, Shields CL. Rhabdomyosarcoma: review for the ophthalmologist. Surv Ophthalmol. 2003;48:39–57.
4. Shields JA, Shields CL, DePotter P, Singh AD. Diagnosis and treatment of uveal melanoma. Semin Oncol. 1996;23:763–7.
5. Ochi JW, Harris JP, Feldman JI, Press GA. Rhinocerebral mucormycosis: results of aggressive surgical debridement and amphotericin B. Laryngoscope. 1988;98:1339–42.
6. Yohai RA, Bullock JD, Aziz AA, Markert RJ. Survival factors in rhino-orbital-cerebral mucormycosis. Surv Ophthalmol. 1994;39:3–22.
7. Levin LA, Avery R, Shore JW, et al. The spectrum of orbital aspergillosis: a clinicopathological review. Surv Ophthalmol. 1996;41:142–54.
8. Kahana A, Lucarelli MJ. Use of radiopaque intraorbital catheter in the treatment of sino-orbito-cranial mucormycosis. Arch Ophthalmol. 2007;125:1714–5.
9. Taxy JB, El-Zayaty S, Langerman A. Acute fungal sinusitis. Am J Clin Pathol. 2009;132:86–93.
10. Bartley GB, Garrity JA, Waller RR, et al. Orbital exenteration at the Mayo Clinic: 1967–1986. Ophthalmology. 1989;96:468–73.
11. Levin PS, Dutton JJ. A 20-year series of orbital exenteration. Am J Ophthalmol. 1991;112:496.
12. Kennedy RE. Indications and surgical techniques for orbital exenteration. Adv Ophthalmic Plast Reconstr Surg. 1992;9:163–73.
13. Günalp I, Gündüz K, Dürük K. Orbital exenteration: review of 429 cases. Int Ophthalmol. 1995/1996;19:177–84.
14. Ben Simon GJ, Schwarcz RM, Douglas R, et al. Orbital exenteration: one size does not fit all. Am J Ophthalmol. 2005;139:11–7.
15. Rahman I, Cook AE, Leatherbarrow B. Orbital exenteration: a 13 year Manchester experience. Br J Ophthalmol. 2005;89:1335–40.
16. Nemet AY, Martin P, Benger R, et al. Orbital exenteration: a 15-year study of 38 cases. Ophthal Plast Reconstr Surg. 2007;23:468–72.
17. Nassab RS, Thomas SS, Murray D. Orbital exenteration for advanced periorbital skin cancers: 20 years experience. J Plast Reconstr Aesthet Surg. 2007;60:1103–9.

18. Esmaeli B, Golio D, Kies M, DeMonte F. Surgical management of locally advanced adenoid cystic carcinoma of the lacrimal gland. Ophthal Plast Reconstr Surg. 2006;22:366–70.
19. Rahman I, Maino A, Cook AE, Leatherbarrow B. Mortality following exenteration for malignant tumours of the orbit. Br J Ophthalmol. 2005;89:1445–8.
20. Gnanaraj L, Skibell BC, Coret-Simon J, et al. Massive congenital orbital teratoma. Ophthal Plast Reconstr Surg. 2005;21:445–7.
21. Smith B, Guberina C, Rees T. Radical approach in the treatment of neurofibroma. Orbit. 1982;1:267.
22. Rose GE, Wright JE. Exenteration for benign orbital disease. Br J Ophthalmol. 1994;78:14–8.
23. Pribila JT, Cornblath WT, Elner VM, et al. Glomus cell tumor of the orbit. Arch Ophthalmol. 2010;128:144–6.
24. Schwarz JN, Donnelly EH, Klintworth GK. Ocular and orbital phycomycosis. Surv Ophthalmol. 1977;22:3–28.
25. Hargrove RN, Wesley RE, Klippenstein KA, et al. Indications for orbital exenteration in mucormycosis. Ophthal Plast Reconstr Surg. 2006;22:286–91.
26. Elner VM, Demirci H, Nerad JA, Hassan AS. Periocular necrotizing fasciitis with visual loss: pathogenesis and treatment. Ophthalmology. 2006;113:2338–45.
27. Small RG, LaFuente H. Exenteration of the orbit in selected cases of severe orbital contracture. Ophthalmology. 1983;90:236.
28. Ho VH, Ross MI, Esmaeli B, et al. Sentinel lymph node biopsy for sebaceous cell carcinoma and melanoma of the ocular adnexa. Arch Otolaryngol Head Neck Surg. 2007;133:820–6.
29. Savar A, Ross MI, Esmaeli B, et al. Sentinel lymph node biopsy for ocular adnexal melanoma: experience in 30 patients. Ophthalmology. 2009;116:2217–23.
30. Coston TO, Small RG. Orbital exenteration simplified. Trans Am Ophthalmol Soc. 1981;79:136.
31. Shields JA, Shields CL, Demirci H, et al. Experience with eyelid-sparing orbital exenteration: the 2000 Tullos O. Coston Lecture. Ophthal Plast Reconstr Surg. 2001;17:355–61.
32. Yeatts RP, et al. Removal of the eye with socket ablation: a limited subtotal exenteration. Arch Ophthalmol. 1991;109:1306.
33. Sypert SW, Habal MB. Combined cranio-orbital surgery for extensive malignant neoplasms of the orbit. J Neurosurg. 1978;2:8.
34. Schramm VL, Myers EN, Maroon JC. Anterior skull base surgery for benign and malignant disease. Laryngoscope. 1979;89:1077.
35. Shah JP, et al. Craniofacial resection of tumors involving the anterior skull base. Otolaryngol Head Neck Surg. 1992;106:387.
36. Conley J, Baker DC. Management of the eye socket in cancer of the paranasal sinuses. Arch Otolaryngol. 1979;105:702.
37. Levin PS, Ellis DS, Stewart WB, Toth BA. Orbital exenteration: the reconstructive ladder. Ophthal Plast Reconstr Surg. 1991;7:84–92.
38. Mohr C, Esser J. Orbital exenteration: surgical and reconstructive strategies. Graefes Arch Clin Exp Ophthalmol. 1997;235:288–95.
39. Goldberg RA, Kim JW, Shorr N. Orbital exenteration: results of an individualized approach. Ophthal Plast Reconstr Surg. 2003;19:229–36.
40. Hanasono MM, Lee JC, Yang JS, et al. An algorithmic approach to reconstructive surgery and prosthetic rehabilitation after orbital exenteration. Plast Reconstr Surg. 2009;123:98–105.
41. Putterman AM. Orbital exenteration with spontaneous granulation. Arch Ophthalmol. 1986;104:139.
42. Mauriello JA, Han KH, Wolfe R. The use of autogenous split-thickness dermal graft for reconstruction of the lining of the exenterated orbit. Am J Ophthalmol. 1985;100:465.
43. Looi A, Kazim M, Cortes M, Rootman J. Orbital reconstruction after eyelid- and conjunctiva-sparing orbital exenteration. Ophthal Plast Reconstr Surg. 2006;22:1–6.
44. Dortzbach DK, Hawes MJ. Midline forehead flap in reconstructive procedures of the eyelids and exenterated socket. Ophthalmic Surg. 1981;12:257.
45. Bonavolontà G. Frontalis muscle transfer in the reconstruction of the exenterated orbit. Adv Ophthalmic Plast Reconstr Surg. 1992;9:239–42.
46. Lai A, Cheney ML. Temporoparietal fascial flap in orbital reconstruction. Arch Facial Plast Surg. 2000;2:196–201.
47. Ariyan S, Cuono CB. Use of the pectoralis major myocutaneous flap for reconstruction of large cervical, facial or cranial defects. Am J Surg. 1980;140:503.
48. Donahue PJ, et al. Reconstruction of orbital cavities: the use of the latissimus dorsi myocutaneous free flap. Arch Ophthalmol. 1989;107:1681.
49. Chepeha DB, Wang SJ, Marentette LJ, et al. Restoration of the orbital aesthetic subunit in complex midface defects. Laryngoscope. 2004;114:1706–13.
50. Pryor SG, Moore EJ, Kasperbauer JL. Orbital exenteration reconstruction with rectus abdominus microvascular free flap. Laryngoscope. 2005;155:1912–6.
51. Chang DW, Langstein HN. Use of the free fibula flap for restoration of orbital support and midfacial projection following maxillectomy. J Reconstr Microsurg. 2003;19:147–52.
52. Kosutic D, Uglesic V, Knezevic P, et al. Latissimus dorsi-scapula free flap for reconstruction of defects following radical maxillectomy with orbital exenteration. J Plast Reconstr Aesthet Surg. 2008;61:620–7.
53. Savar DE. High-dose radiation to the orbit: a cause of skin graft failure after exenteration. Arch Ophthalmol. 1982;100:1755.
54. Tse DT, Benedetto P, Dubovy S, et al. Clinical analysis of the effect of intraarterial cytoreductive chemotherapy in the treatment of lacrimal gland adenoid cystic carcinoma. Am J Ophthalmol. 2006;141:44–53.
55. Limawararut V, Leibovitch I, Davis G, et al. Sino-orbital fistula: a complication of exenteration. Ophthalmology. 2007;114:355–61.
56. Tse DT, Bumsted RM. A two-layer closure of sino-orbital fistula. Ophthalmology. 1989;96:1673–8.
57. Bartley GB, Kasperbauer JL. Use of a flap of extraocular muscle and fat during subtotal exenteration to repair bony orbital defects. Am J Ophthalmol. 2002;134:787–8.
58. Wulc AE, Adams JL, Dryden RM. Cerebrospinal fluid leakage complicating orbital exenteration. Arch Ophthalmol. 1989;107:827.
59. Limawararut V, Valenzuela AA, Sullivan TJ, et al. Cerebrospinal fluid leaks in orbital and lacrimal surgery. Surv Ophthalmol. 2008;53:274–84.
60. Spiegel JH, Varvares MA. Prevention of postexenteration complications by obliteration of the orbital cavity. Skull Base. 2007;17:197–203.
61. Bonanno A, Esmaeli B, Fingeret MC, et al. Social challenges of cancer patients with orbitofacial disfigurement. Ophthal Plast Reconstr Surg. 2010;26:18–22.
62. Joneja OP, et al. Orbital prostheses. J Prosthet Dent. 1976;36:306.
63. Shifman A, et al. Prosthetic restoration of orbital defects. J Prosthet Dent. 1979;42:543.
64. Larson JSM, Nerad JA. The use of osseointegration and rare earth magnetic coupling for oculofacial prosthesis retention in the exenterated orbit. Curr Opin Ophthalmol. 2009;20:412–6.

Image-Guided Orbital Surgery

54

Anaïs L. Carniciu and Alon Kahana

Introduction

Stereotaxy involves the use of computerized technology to identify a point in three dimensions using a Cartesian coordinate system, which can be used for preoperative surgical planning and intraoperative computer-assisted surgical navigation. Stereotactic technology allows for the visualization of surgical anatomy and instrument placement intraoperatively in real-time on preoperatively acquired images, typically computed tomography (CT), magnetic resonance imaging (MRI), or CT-MRI fusion studies [1, 2]. Image-guided surgery has modernized a variety of surgical interventions, including radiosurgery, biopsy, implantation, resection, stimulation, and reconstruction [3–10]. Although neurosurgery is the field that most frequently utilizes stereotaxy, skull base surgery, otolaryngology, oral and maxillofacial surgery (OMFS), orthopedic surgery, and other medical specialties have also appropriated image-guided surgery into their armamentarium, with notable improvements in patient outcomes [5, 11–21]. Importantly, the use of stereotactic navigation has been extended to orbital surgery by neurosurgeons, skull base surgeons, and OMF surgeons – a natural extension of this useful surgical tool.

In the past decade, navigated surgery has become increasingly used in orbital surgery by oculoplastic surgeons [22–25]. Since the orbit has relatively fixed intraorbital and bony surgical targets, the orbital anatomy lends itself quite nicely to registration and computer-assisted navigation. Stereotactic surgery has a variety of applications in orbital surgery, including orbital decompression for thyroid eye disease (TED) [24, 26, 27], orbital fracture repair [28, 29], and excision/debulking of intraorbital tumors [2, 30]. The increasing adoption of stereotaxy in modern orbital surgery has resulted in greater surgical safety and efficiency in orbital cases through improved anatomical localization, fewer complications, and shorter surgical times for experienced surgeons [23, 24, 31]. Importantly, a retrospective analysis of a high-volume orbital decompression practice revealed improved surgical outcomes related to use of intraoperative navigation, in the form of reduced post-operative strabismus, reduced need for post-operative strabismus surgery, and improved proptosis reduction [32].

Different modalities of stereotaxy systems are currently available, including electromagnetic (EM) and optical options. Similarities and differences exist among the navigation platforms developed by the main manufacturers, including Brainlab (Westchester, IL), Medtronic (Minneapolis, MN), and Stryker (Kalamazoo, MI). Given the cost of acquisition, a good understanding of the various options available and their key features is important when selecting a navigation system.

Science of Stereotaxy

The original stereotactic systems developed were frame-based, which involves a stereotactic device that maintains the patient's head in fixed position in reference to a three-coordinate system. The head is then imaged by CT or MRI, and the lesion of interest is plotted relative to the external frame. The distance of the target from the reference point on the frame is then measured in each dimension on the radiographic image. Surgical instruments are tracked to the three-dimensional Cartesian coordinates of the lesion, which can then be approached with greater precision utilizing computer software. This early frame-based approach to image-guided surgery became popular in neurosurgery in the 1980s [33–35].

Frame-based stereotaxy is used less commonly now that modern, frameless systems are available. With frameless platforms, imaging markers are attached to the scalp or forehead, thereby eliminating the need for a mounted frame [24, 36–39]. Optical frameless navigation platforms were developed first. In these systems, reflecting spheres or light-emitting diodes are fixed to the patient and to probes on

A. L. Carniciu · A. Kahana (✉)
Consultants in Ophthalmic and Facial Plastic Surgery, Southfield, MI, USA
e-mail: akahana@facialworks.com

J. J. Servat et al. (eds.), *Smith and Nesi's Ophthalmic Plastic and Reconstructive Surgery*,
https://doi.org/10.1007/978-3-030-41720-8_54

surgical instruments and then tracked in space via triangulation with an infrared camera system [40]. One notable disadvantage to optical navigation is the need for a constant line-of-sight between the operating field and camera system to track the reference frame and the navigated instruments; this can be challenging when surgical fields are cluttered with equipment. However, optical navigation also has an important advantage, namely, that interference with the signal occurs only if the line-of-sight is broken. EM navigation was subsequently developed as an alternative to optical-based tracking; it is particularly useful when the line-of-sight limitation of optical tracking is too restrictive. An emitter generates an EM field, and the position is detected either actively by coils in the instrument or passively through a wireless instrument that induces distortions that are measured by the emitter. The main disadvantage of EM-based stereotaxy is the potential for degradation of accuracy and reliability by the presence of metallic objects in the operating field [40].

Today, EM-based navigation systems are primarily used when the surgical exposure is wide and the use of metallic instruments can be avoided during stereotaxy. Alternatively, optical navigation systems have become particularly useful for small-incision surgical approaches that require retractors, suction, and other surgical tools to expose the surgical field during stereotaxy. A prime example of the latter is orbital surgery.

History of Stereotactic Surgery

The first reported surgical use of stereotaxy in humans was by neurosurgeons Spiegel and Wycis in 1947, using X-ray images and a Cartesian coordinate system [41]. In 1949, Leksell developed a semicircular stereotactic system based on the principle of "center-of-arc" which allowed for greater flexibility in probe positioning utilizing three polar coordinates: angle, depth, and anterior-posterior location [42]. Stereotactic navigation did not gain widespread clinical use until later in the twentieth century when Brown, a third year medical student, developed the N-localizer stereotactic frame [43, 44]. This technology enabled the development of frame-based image-guided surgery via CT, MRI, and PET scan [45–50].

Frame-based systems can be cumbersome to use due to the bulkiness of the frame itself, which may interfere with the surgical approach. As such, frame-based systems are less practical in orbital surgery. The development of frameless systems in the 1990s revolutionized neurological surgery [51–54]. Frameless stereotactic technology has been shown to be comparable or superior to frame stereotaxy [55] and has enabled the growth of image-guided surgery in the field of ophthalmic plastic and reconstructive surgery in the twenty-first century.

Stereotaxy in Orbital Surgery

The orbit is a site of challenging regional anatomy in which the ocular globe is surrounded by tightly organized muscles, cranial nerves, the lacrimal apparatus, and vascular structures. Importantly, because the globe occupies much of the volume within the anterior orbit, exposure of the posterior orbit necessitates a surgical approach around the globe with limited exposure and visualization – something that orbital surgeons spend years learning to perform. This unique anatomy makes orbital surgery an ideal discipline for utilizing image-guided perioperative planning and intraoperative navigation [56].

As early as the 1990s, the benefit of a stereotactic approach to the orbit was described for reconstruction of complex craniofacial and orbital defects [57, 58]. Around the same time, stereotactic-assisted orbital biopsy was also reported [59]. A case series by Camara and colleagues described the successful use of computer-assisted image guidance in a variety of orbital procedures, including orbital fracture repair, tumor excision, and orbital decompression. Although the frame-based navigation system utilized in these cases was designed for rhinology and more cumbersome to utilize than modern platforms, it demonstrated a clear utility of stereotaxy in orbital surgery [60]. The benefit of intraoperative stereotactic assistance was further described in the sino-orbital approach to an extensive orbital osteoma [61], fronto-orbital approach to a cavernous hemangioma in the orbital apex [62], and removal of other orbital tumors [63]. More recently, image guidance has been used in orbital reconstruction cases to confirm safe and successful positioning of orbital implants [10, 64], even when the defect is in proximity to the optic nerve [28].

Image guidance is highly beneficial in orbital decompression for TED, where knowledge of real-time location within the orbit is of paramount importance. A case-controlled study of seven patients by Millar and Maloof reported an approximate 9 mm reduction in proptosis without complications using a balanced orbital decompression with maximal lateral wall debulking under image guidance. In these cases, stereotactic guidance allowed surgeons to more confidently determine the maximal decompression possible with planned exposure of dura [25]. When posterior medial wall decompression is performed, stereotactic guidance can help the surgeon avoid optic nerve injury [56]. Furthermore, stereotactic assistance is particularly helpful when a deep and effective lateral wall decompression is desired [24, 65]. Servat and colleagues advocated for the use of stereotaxy in orbital surgery to reduce the risk associated with cases in which aggressive decompression is planned [26]. A large 7-year retrospective series of deep lateral orbital wall decompression surgeries for TED demonstrated the efficiency of using a microdebrider with built-in stereotaxy. This surgical instrument functioned as an "all-in-one" handpiece, microdebrider, irrigator, retractor, and suction device with an integrated tissue guard, which enhanced anatomical localization and safety during orbital decompression [27]. Beyond efficiency and surgeon confidence, the ability to precisely target bone removal using image guidance also enables more predictable and consistent decompressions. Mahoney et al. utilized three-dimensional CT for surgical planning and intraoperative navigation during orbital decompression for asymmetric exophthalmos. Image guidance allowed for assessment of pre-existing variation in orbital anatomy to better determine the surgical plan. Additionally, navigation software allows for an objective measure of orbital decompression outcome using preoperative and postoperative CT image analysis to quantify the magnitude of decompression and better assess surgical results [56].

Overall, the enhanced surgical precision and safety afforded during orbital surgery [23] as well as deceased rates of postoperative complications and need for repeat surgery make stereotactic guidance an appealing enhancement to orbital surgery [31].

Stereotactic Platforms

Several types of frameless stereotactic systems are currently available for use in orbital surgery. The main difference among the various platforms is the mode by which localization of a target is achieved. Optical, EM, and combination systems that can alternate between optical and EM modes are available.

Optical image guidance utilizes light-emitting diodes (LEDs) that are visible to the infrared camera of the navigation system workstation. The combination of the LEDs and unique anatomical landmarks of the face allows for automatic surface registration without the need for fiducial markers [66, 67]. Intraoperatively, a guidance probe is used to identify anatomical landmarks to assess registration accuracy. Optical systems have the advantage of relative ease of setup and implementation, but require a clear path between operating field and camera system to function. Hence, their use can be challenging in the setting of a crowded operating room [66, 67]. Optical navigation is used by the Stryker Navigation System III (Stryker, Kalamazoo, Michigan) and Brainlab's Kick and Curve (Brainlab, Westchester, IL) platforms, which transmit intraoperative location of instruments onto preoperative CT or MR imaging studies [24].

Like optical navigation platforms, EM-based stereotaxy enables preoperative imaging studies to be loaded into a planning software that aligns images and identifies anatomical targets to help virtually plan customized surgery. These images as well as real-time navigation are available intraoperatively to execute surgical goals. EM platforms are based on the principle of EM field generation, which is achieved by special equipment in the navigation system: an emitter that generates an EM field around the patient's head and instruments containing coils that are detected by the system. The Kick EM navigation system manufactured by Brainlab (Westchester, IL) uses these principles to provide real-time intraoperative image guidance. EM systems avoid the line-of-sight issues that may be problematic with optical systems; however, the presence of metallic objects within the operating field will degrade the signal, reducing the utility of this tool for small-incision orbital surgery in which retractors and suction are critical to deep exposure.

Both optical modes and EM capabilities can be available in a single navigation system, such as the Medtronic StealthStation™ (Medtronic, Minneapolis, MN) and TargetGuided Surgery™ (TGS) Navigation System (Stryker, Kalamazoo, MI). A study by Ali et al. found no difference in the accuracy of anatomic localization within the orbit between optical and EM navigation modes [68].

Approach to Stereotactic Orbital Surgery

Getting Started

An orbital surgeon has several considerations when deciding to transition to image-guided orbital surgery. Prior to getting started with stereotaxy, it is important to research the available navigation systems and select a system that is best for one's needs. If the goal is to use stereotactic navigation to assist with small-incision deep orbital surgeries, such as medial orbital decompression or floor fracture repair, then an optical system would have significant advantages over an EM system for which all metallic instruments, including retractors and suction, must be removed from the surgical field every time that navigation is utilized. In academic centers, stereotactic navigation is likely already in use by other specialties, such as otolaryngology and neurosurgery. Academic orbital surgeons would therefore benefit from talking to colleagues in other fields and observing their navigated surgeries to learn from their experience with stereotaxy. Similarly, it is worth conferring with oculoplastic surgery colleagues who utilize image guidance at other institutions to gain a better understanding of the technology. If working in a setting where stereotaxy is not already in use by other services, it is beneficial to touch base with the local stereotactic device representative to assist with setup and general approach to initial cases. A surgeon who is just beginning to perform navigated surgery should be prepared to face the learning curve and anticipate longer cases initially as one adjusts to using the equipment. Ophthalmology operating room staff, who may not have any prior experience with stereotactic equipment, should be educated about setup and troubleshooting. Device representatives are usually available to provide in-service sessions as needed. In addition, all device manufacturers sponsor hands-on training courses taught by surgeons experienced with navigation. Such courses can be invaluable when starting to use navigation in orbital surgery.

Basic Technique

Appropriate imaging (i.e., non-contrast facial bone CT scan) is obtained preoperatively with a device-specific navigation protocol and uploaded into the navigation program. The protocol usually specifies the slice thickness and requires that the nose, ears, and cranial vertex to be included. Preoperative surgical planning is accomplished using navigation device compatible software that can segregate anatomical areas of interest and color code different targets. Orbital surgery is performed under general anesthesia. After patient induction by the anesthesia team, the surgical team prepares the patient for image-guided surgery. Prepping the patient's face requires extending the prep area into the hairline and to the upper lip and ears. A reference frame is placed on the patient's head; in the absence of any surgical field restrictions, the forehead is usually a good location. A study by Ali et al. determined that the location of reference frame placement does not affect the accuracy of anatomic localization. Therefore, the reference frame can be placed out of the way from the surgical field [68]. The registration process correlates the image space on the navigation device obtained from the preoperative CT or MR images and the patient's location. The accuracy of registration can be confirmed by the surgeon with a stereotactic probe. After ensuring the navigation equipment is functioning properly, the surgeon may proceed with surgery using the stereotactic system (Fig. 54.1).

Benefits of Stereotaxy

In the authors' opinion, the benefits of navigated surgery far outweigh any potential drawbacks. Stereotactic surgery affords better anatomical localization and lesion targeting, enhanced safety through potentially smaller incisions, reduced surgical stress, and decreased need for secondary revision procedures [24]. Additionally, image guidance can

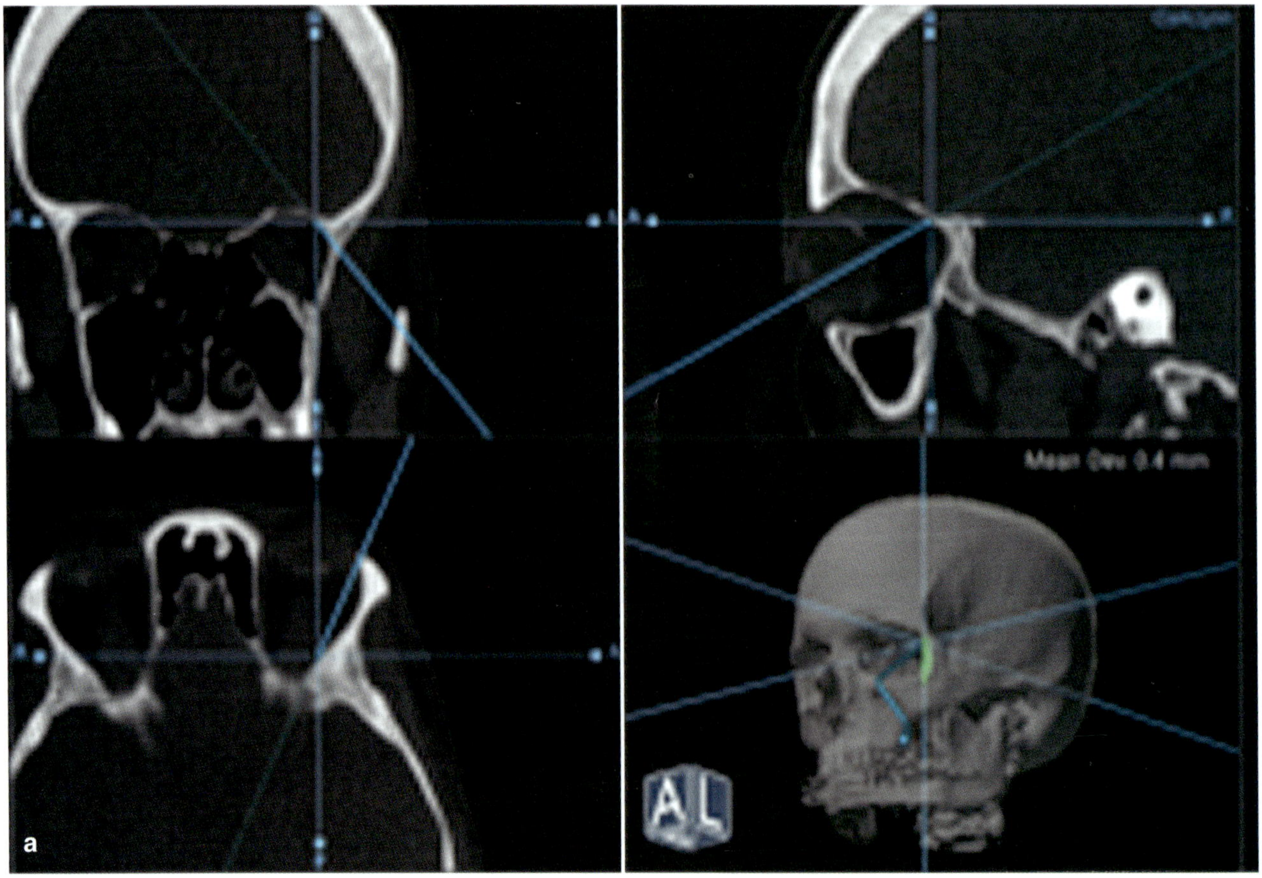

Fig. 54.1 Stereotactic navigation during orbital decompression for thyroid eye disease (**a**) Localization of superomedial aspect of sphenoid trigone prior to decompression. (**b**) Inferolateral boundary of sphenoid trigone prior to decompression. (**c**) Deep lateral wall decompression prior to removal of sphenoid trigone. (**d**) Posterior boundary of sphenoid trigone after maximal decompression

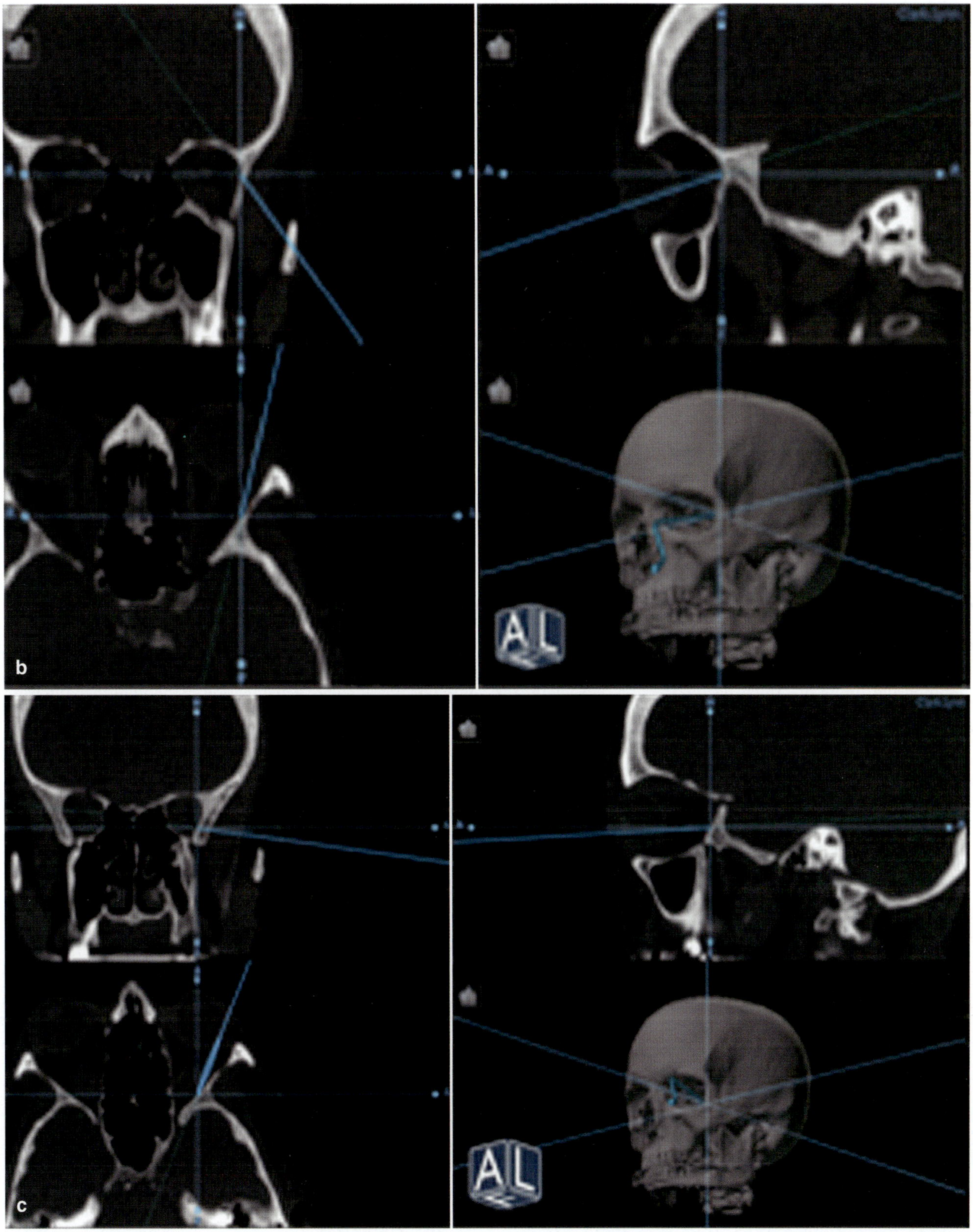

Fig. 54.1 (continued)

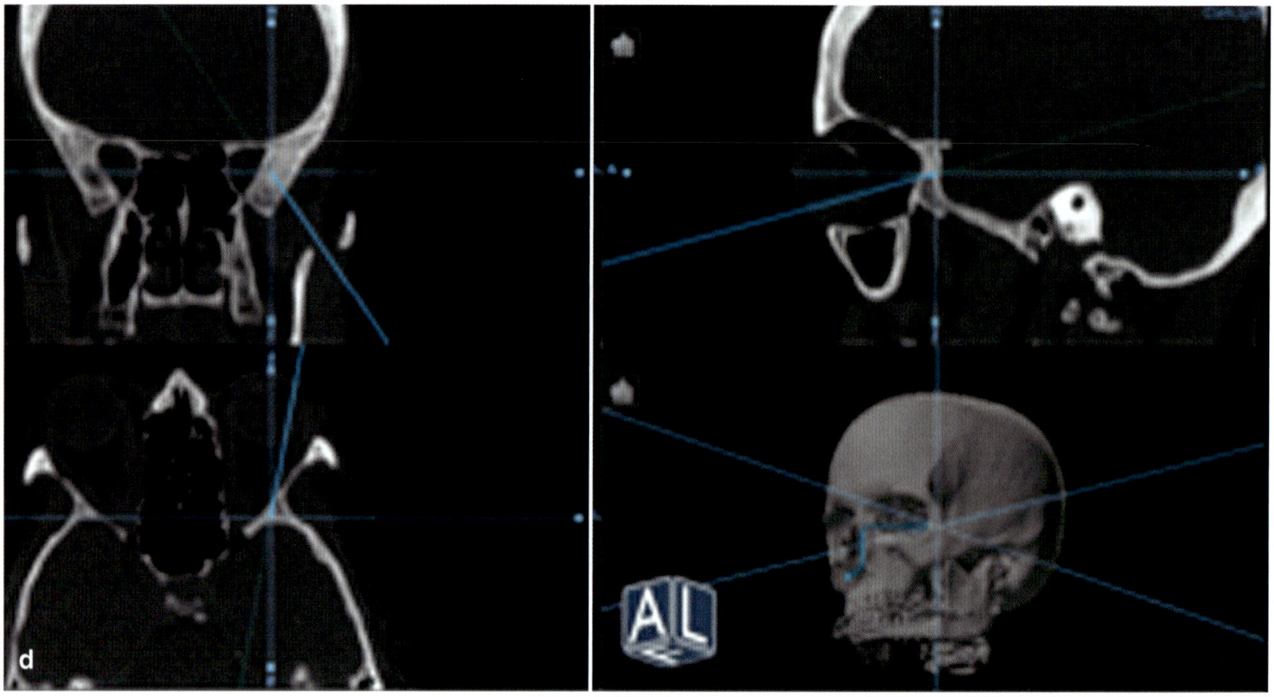

Fig. 54.1 (continued)

provide valuable assistance in orbital surgery training [24, 68]. Preoperative surgical planning software can assist in defining the limits of orbital decompression, especially for deep lateral decompressions, leading to increased surgical efficiency [24, 27]. Although operating times may extend initially, during the learning curve, the duration of surgery and total operating room time become rapidly shorter with surgeon experience. Up to 24 minutes of time can be saved per case [24]. Most importantly, for orbital decompression surgery there is now good evidence that intraoperative stereotactic navigation may improve surgical outcomes; facilitating more precise bone removal appears to reduce the rate and severity of postoperative strabismus while enhancing proptosis reduction [32]. Disadvantages include the expense, equipment availability, learning curve, and longer setup times [22, 24, 25]. Still, stereotactic navigation is considered the standard of care for all skull base surgeries. Ophthalmic orbital surgeons have been somewhat late in adopting this technology, but there should be no artificial impediments to its use given a long track record of efficacy and safety.

Summary

Navigated surgery is an important tool in the orbital surgeon's armamentarium, with growing availability and utilization. Image guidance can assist with optimizing orbital decompressions, complex orbital reconstructions, and tumor resections. It is also an outstanding teaching tool – for self-improvement as well as for the benefit of trainees. Surgeons utilizing intraoperative navigation technology benefit from improved safety, efficiency, and confidence.

References

1. Geevarghese R, O'Gorman Tuura R, Lumsden DE, Samuel M, Ashkan K. Registration accuracy of CT/MRI fusion for localisation of deep brain stimulation electrode position: an imaging study and systematic review. Stereotact Funct Neurosurg. 2016;94(3):159–63.
2. Nemec SF, Peloschek P, Schmook MT, et al. CT-MR image data fusion for computer-assisted navigated surgery of orbital tumors. Eur J Radiol. 2010;73(2):224–9.
3. Yang I, Udawatta M, Prashant GN, et al. Stereotactic radiosurgery for neurosurgical patients: a historical review and current perspectives. World Neurosurg. 2019;122:522–31.
4. Mok ST, Kam MK, Tsang WK, et al. Frameless stereotactic radiosurgery for brain metastases: a review of outcomes and prognostic scores evaluation. Hong Kong Med J. 2017;23(6):599–608.
5. Bahl M, Maunglay M, D'Alessandro HA, Lehman CD. Comparison of upright digital breast tomosynthesis-guided versus prone stereotactic vacuum-assisted breast biopsy. Radiology. 2019;290(2):298–304.
6. Mohyeldin A, Elder JB. Stereotactic biopsy platforms with intraoperative imaging guidance. Neurosurg Clin N Am. 2017;28(4):465–75.
7. Toossi A, Everaert DG, Seres P, et al. Ultrasound-guided spinal stereotactic system for intraspinal implants. J Neurosurg Spine. 2018;29(3):292–305.
8. Sayyahmelli S, Aydin I, Wheeler B, Baskaya MK. Mapping of the internal capsule with subcortical stimulation for gross-

total resection of a thalamic metastatic tumor. Neurosurg Focus. 2018;45(VideoSuppl2):V7.
9. Jakobs M, Krasniqi E, Kloß M, et al. Intraoperative stereotactic magnetic resonance imaging for deep brain stimulation electrode planning in patients with movement disorders. World Neurosurg. 2018;119:e801–8.
10. Choi KJ, Sajisevi MB, McClennen J, Kaylie DM. Image-guided placement of osseointegrated implants for challenging auricular, orbital, and rhinectomy defects. Ann Otol Rhinol Laryngol. 2016;125(10):801–7.
11. Kelly PJ. Stereotactic technology in tumor surgery. Clin Neurosurg. 1989;35:215–53.
12. Gunkel AR, Freysinger W, Martin A, et al. Three-dimensional image-guided endonasal surgery with a microdebrider. Laryngoscope. 1997;107(6):834–8.
13. Kacker A, Komisar A, Huo J, Mangiardi J. Transsphenoidal surgery utilizing computer-assisted stereotactic guidance. Rhinology. 2001;39(4):207–10.
14. Marcus HJ, Vakharia VN, Ourselin S, Duncan J, Tisdall M, Aquilina K. Robot-assisted stereotactic brain biopsy: systematic review and bibliometric analysis. Childs Nerv Syst. 2018;34:1299.
15. Jagannathan J, Prevedello DM, Ayer VS, Dumont AS, Jane JA, Laws ER. Computer-assisted frameless stereotaxy in transsphenoidal surgery at a single institution: review of 176 cases. Neurosurg Focus. 2006;20(2):E9.
16. Caversaccio F. Computer assistance for intraoperative navigation in ENT surgery. Minim Invasive Ther Allied Technol. 2003;12(1):36–51.
17. Klimek L, Mösges R, Schlöndorff G, Mann W. Development of computer-aided surgery for otorhinolaryngology. Comput Aided Surg. 1998;3(4):194–201.
18. Bobek SL. Applications of navigation for orthognathic surgery. Oral Maxillofac Surg Clin North Am. 2014;26(4):587–98.
19. Collyer J. Stereotactic navigation in oral and maxillofacial surgery. Br J Oral Maxillofac Surg. 2010;48(2):79–83.
20. Correia MM, Jesus JP, Feitosa R, Oliveira DA. The introduction of navigation in liver surgery in Brazil. Rev Col Bras Cir. 2014;41(6):451–4.
21. Atallah S, Nassif G, Larach S. Stereotactic navigation for TAMIS-TME: opening the gateway to frameless, image-guided abdominal and pelvic surgery. Surg Endosc. 2015;29(1):207–11.
22. Lee KY, Ang BT, Ng I, Looi A. Stereotaxy for surgical navigation in orbital surgery. Ophthalmic Plast Reconstr Surg. 2009;25(4):300–2.
23. Ali MJ, Naik MN, Kaliki S, Dave TV, Dendukuri G. Interactive navigation-guided ophthalmic plastic surgery: the techniques and utility of 3-dimensional navigation. Can J Ophthalmol. 2017;52(3):250–7.
24. Wu CY, Kahana A. Stereotactic navigation with a registration mask in orbital decompression surgery: preliminary results. Ophthalmic Plast Reconstr Surg. 2015;31(6):440–4.
25. Millar MJ, Maloof AJ. The application of stereotactic navigation surgery to orbital decompression for thyroid-associated orbitopathy. Eye (Lond). 2009;23(7):1565–71.
26. Servat JJ, Elia MD, Gong D, Manes RP, Black EH, Levin F. Electromagnetic image-guided orbital decompression: technique, principles, and preliminary experience with 6 consecutive cases. Orbit. 2014;33(6):433–6.
27. Nguyen J, Fay A, Yadav P, MacIntosh PW, Metson R. Stereotactic microdebrider in deep lateral orbital decompression for patients with thyroid eye disease. Ophthalmic Plast Reconstr Surg. 2014;30(3):262–6.
28. Kim YH, Jung DW, Kim TG, Lee JH, Kim IK. Correction of orbital wall fracture close to the optic canal using computer-assisted navigation surgery. J Craniofac Surg. 2013;24(4):1118–22.
29. Andrews BT, Surek CC, Tanna N, Bradley JP. Utilization of computed tomography image-guided navigation in orbit fracture repair. Laryngoscope. 2013;123(6):1389–93.
30. Miller NR, Agrawal N, Sciubba JJ, Lane AP. Image-guided transnasal endoscopic resection of an orbital solitary fibrous tumor. Ophthalmic Plast Reconstr Surg. 2008;24(1):65–7.
31. Cai EZ, Koh YP, Hing EC, et al. Computer-assisted navigational surgery improves outcomes in orbital reconstructive surgery. J Craniofac Surg. 2012;23(5):1567–73.
32. Heisel CJ, Tuohy MM, Riddering AL, Sha C, Kahana A. Stereotactic Navigation Improves Outcomes of Orbital Decompression Surgery for Thyroid Associated Orbitopathy. Ophthalmic Plastic and Reconstructive Surgery, 2020. [Epub ahead of print.] PubMed PMID: 32134770.
33. Perry JH, Rosenbaum AE, Lunsford LD, Swink CA, Zorub DS. Computed tomography/guided stereotactic surgery: conception and development of a new stereotactic methodology. Neurosurgery. 1980;7(4):376–81.
34. Kelly PJ, Alker GJ, Kall BA, Goerss S. Method of computed tomography-based stereotactic biopsy with arteriographic control. Neurosurgery. 1984;14(2):172–7.
35. Peters TM, Clark J, Pike B, Drangova M, Olivier A. Stereotactic surgical planning with magnetic resonance imaging, digital subtraction angiography and computed tomography. Appl Neurophysiol. 1987;50(1–6):33–8.
36. Ryan MJ, Erickson RK, Levin DN, Pelizzari CA, Macdonald RL, Dohrmann GJ. Frameless stereotaxy with real-time tracking of patient head movement and retrospective patient-image registration. J Neurosurg. 1996;85(2):287–92.
37. Germano IM, Queenan JV. Clinical experience with intracranial brain needle biopsy using frameless surgical navigation. Comput Aided Surg. 1998;3(1):33–9.
38. Roessler K, Ungersboeck K, Aichholzer M, et al. Frameless stereotactic lesion contour-guided surgery using a computer-navigated microscope. Surg Neurol. 1998;49(3):282–8. discussion 288-289
39. Barnett GH, Miller DW, Weisenberger J. Frameless stereotaxy with scalp-applied fiducial markers for brain biopsy procedures: experience in 218 cases. J Neurosurg. 1999;91(4):569–76.
40. Kral F, Puschban EJ, Riechelmann H, Freysinger W. Comparison of optical and electromagnetic tracking for navigated lateral skull base surgery. Int J Med Robot. 2013;9(2):247–52.
41. Spiegel EA, Wycis HT, Marks M, Lee AJ. Stereotaxic apparatus for operations on the human brain. Science. 1947;106(2754):349–50.
42. Leksell L. A surgical procedure for atresia of the aqueduct of Sylvius. Acta Psychiatr Neurol. 1949;24(3–4):559–68.
43. Brown RA. A stereotactic head frame for use with CT body scanners. Investig Radiol. 1979;14(4):300–4.
44. Brown RA, Nelson JA. The origin and history of the N-localizer for stereotactic neurosurgery. Cureus. 2015;7(9):e323.
45. Thomas DG, Anderson RE, du Boulay GH. CT-guided stereotactic neurosurgery: experience in 24 cases with a new stereotactic system. J Neurol Neurosurg Psychiatry. 1984;47(1):9–16.
46. Coffey RJ, Lunsford LD. Diagnosis and treatment of brainstem mass lesions by CT-guided stereotactic surgery. Appl Neurophysiol. 1985;48(1–6):467–71.
47. Debaene A, Gomez A, Lavieille J, Alessandri C, Legre J. Stereotactic CT localization and biopsy of brain tumours using the Leksell frame. A study of 45 cases. J Neuroradiol. 1988;15(3):266–75.
48. Kelly PJ, Sharbrough FW, Kall BA, Goerss SJ. Magnetic resonance imaging-based computer-assisted stereotactic resection of the hippocampus and amygdala in patients with temporal lobe epilepsy. Mayo Clin Proc. 1987;62(2):103–8.
49. Heilbrun MP, Sunderland PM, McDonald PR, Wells TH, Cosman E, Ganz E. Brown-Roberts-Wells stereotactic frame modifications to accomplish magnetic resonance imaging guidance in three planes. Appl Neurophysiol. 1987;50(1–6):143–52.
50. Maciunas RJ, Kessler RM, Maurer C, Mandava V, Watt G, Smith G. Positron emission tomography imaging-directed stereotactic neurosurgery. Stereotact Funct Neurosurg. 1992;58(1–4):134–40.

51. Barnett GH, Kormos DW, Steiner CP, Morris H. Registration of EEG electrodes with three-dimensional neuroimaging using a frameless, armless stereotactic wand. Stereotact Funct Neurosurg. 1993;61(1):32–8.
52. Laborde G, Klimek L, Harders A, Gilsbach J. Frameless stereotactic drainage of intracranial abscesses. Surg Neurol. 1993;40(1):16–21.
53. Ungersböck K, Aichholzer M, Günthner M, Rössler K, Görzer H, Koos WT. Cavernous malformations: from frame-based to frameless stereotactic localization. Minim Invasive Neurosurg. 1997;40(4):134–8.
54. Moriarty TM, Quinones-Hinojosa A, Larson PS, et al. Frameless stereotactic neurosurgery using intraoperative magnetic resonance imaging: stereotactic brain biopsy. Neurosurgery. 2000;47(5):1138–45; discussion 1145-1136.
55. Dorward NL, Paleologos TS, Alberti O, Thomas DG. The advantages of frameless stereotactic biopsy over frame-based biopsy. Br J Neurosurg. 2002;16(2):110–8.
56. Mahoney N, Grant MP, Susarla SM, Merbs S. Computer-assisted three-dimensional planning for orbital decompression. Craniomaxillofac Trauma Reconstr. 2015;8(3):211–7.
57. Fialkov JA, Phillips JH, Gruss JS, Kassel EE, Zuker RM. A stereotactic system for guiding complex craniofacial reconstruction. Plast Reconstr Surg. 1992;89(2):340–5. discussion 346-348
58. Frodel JL, Pacheco E. The use of intraoperative image-guided surgical techniques for reconstruction of orbital and zygomatic deformities. Facial Plast Surg. 1999;15(1):83–9.
59. Novák Z, Nádvorník LP, Chrastina J. [Stereotaxic biopsy of orbital tumors]. Cesk Slov Oftalmol. 1997;53(4):220–222.
60. Camara JG, Nguyen LT, Fernandez-Suntay JP, Nardin GF, Sua AS. The use of a computer-assisted image-guided system (InstaTrak) in orbital surgery. Ophthalmic Plast Reconstr Surg. 2001;17(6):447–51.
61. Selva D, Chen C, Wormald PJ. Frontoethmoidal osteoma: a stereotactic-assisted sino-orbital approach. Ophthalmic Plast Reconstr Surg. 2003;19(3):237–8.
62. Papalkar D, Francis IC, Stoodley M, et al. Cavernous haemangioma in the orbital apex: stereotactic-guided transcranial cryoextraction. Clin Exp Ophthalmol. 2005;33(4):421–3.
63. Karcioglu ZA, Mascott CR. Computer-assisted image-guided orbit surgery. Eur J Ophthalmol. 2006;16(3):446–52.
64. Varley I, White L, Salvi SM, Lee N. Digital import of orbital implants to enhance navigation in reconstruction of the deep orbit. Orbit. 2016;35(1):20–3.
65. Patel BC. Stereotactic navigation for lateral orbital wall decompression. Eye (Lond). 2009;23(7):1493–5.
66. Makiese O, Pillai P, Salma A, Sammet S, Ammirati M. Accuracy validation in a cadaver model of cranial neuronavigation using a surface autoregistration mask. Neurosurgery. 2010;67(3 Suppl Operative):ons85–90; discussion ons90.
67. Amin DV, Lozanne K, Parry PV, Engh JA, Seelman K, Mintz A. Image-guided frameless stereotactic needle biopsy in awake patients without the use of rigid head fixation. J Neurosurg. 2011;114(5):1414–20.
68. Ali MJ, Naik MN, Girish CM, et al. Interactive navigation-guided ophthalmic plastic surgery: assessment of optical versus electromagnetic modes and role of dynamic reference frame location using navigation-enabled human skulls. Clin Ophthalmol. 2016;10:2383–90.

Silent Sinus Syndrome

55

Steven E. Katz, Bryan R. Costin, and Mark R. Levine

Introduction

A rare condition of painless acquired unilateral enophthalmos and hypoglobus was first described by Montgomery et al. in 1964 [1]. The term "silent sinus syndrome" (SSS) was coined by Soparker et al. in 1994 [2]. Other names for SSS include "the imploding antrum" and "chronic maxillary sinus atelectasis." The exact etiology remains unclear, but it is thought to revolve around the creation of a vacuum within the maxillary sinus by occlusion of the sinus outflow tract. Negative pressure within the sinus may cause bone resorption of the sinus walls leading to their retraction and subsequent downward displacement of orbital contents [2–8].

SSS is diagnosed clinically by the characteristic history, physical examination, and radiographic evidence to confirm the diagnosis and to rule out life-threatening causes of enophthalmos and hypoglobus such as malignancy. Treatment typically involves surgical intervention with two goals: restoration of normal sinus drainage and correction of enophthalmos and hypoglobus. The silent sinus syndrome is a rare disorder, but possibly underdiagnosed because of a lack of recognition on the part of clinicians and also due to patients' "silent" symptoms which may not incite them to seek medical consultation [5].

S. E. Katz
Ocular & Orbital Traume Service, Riverside Methodist Hospital, Department of Opthalmology, Columbus, OH, USA

B. R. Costin
Department of Oculoplastics, Cleveland Eye Clinic, Brecksville, OH, USA

M. R. Levine (✉)
University Hospitals of Cleveland, Department of Ophthalmology, Cleveland, OH, USA
e-mail: mlevine@eye-lids.com

Epidemiology

SSS is relatively uncommon with the largest study containing only 22 cases [7]. Incidence is unknown, but the age at presentation is around the fourth decade of life, and there does not appear to be a predilection with respect to race or gender [2–8]. Soparkar et al. suggested that a history of previous facial or orbital trauma and/or surgery precludes the diagnosis of the silent sinus syndrome [2]. Other authors suggest a history of congenital abnormalities of the face or sinuses or a history of sinusitis must not be present in order to make this diagnosis [6]. However, some authors have suggested that trauma, surgery, and sinus disease may be risk factors for the development of this condition [5].

The condition seems to be exclusively unilateral, without reports of bilateral cases in review of the literature. It is unclear whether the silent sinus syndrome is a purely acquired condition or whether there is a congenital component. There appears to be a mild maxillary sinus hypoplasia found in many patients with the silent sinus syndrome, which might suggest an abnormality in sinus development, but whether the sinus hypoplasia occurred first and predisposed to sinus disease or the sinus disease and hypoplasia are unrelated is unclear [2]. Other possible predisposing anatomic features may include a congenitally narrow or slit-shaped ostium, nasal septal deviation, nasal polyps, antral polyps, chronic inflammation, and a retention cyst or a pseudocyst at the edge of the ostium [2].

Pathophysiology

The exact pathophysiology of the silent sinus syndrome is not known, but several theories have been proposed to explain the collapse of the maxillary sinus roof and the resulting enophthalmos and hypoglobus. The leading theory of pathogenesis revolves around a chronic obstruction of the maxillary sinus by occlusion of the sinus ostium or

J. J. Servat et al. (eds.), *Smith and Nesi's Ophthalmic Plastic and Reconstructive Surgery*, https://doi.org/10.1007/978-3-030-41720-8_55

infundibulum [4]. Occlusion is usually caused by retraction of the uncinate process against the sinus wall, but there are examples of other entities, such as mucus plugging of the maxillary sinus ostium. Regardless of the cause, this obstruction takes the maxillary sinus out of communication with the nasal cavity and leads to a chronic hypoventilation of the cavity and accumulation of mucus.

Eventually, mucus fills the sinus, but air is still present, and this gas is thought to resorb across the walls of the sinus, leading to a negative pressure gradient [8]. The resulting vacuum is thought to induce the osteolysis, osteopenia, and bone remodeling seen in sinus wall specimens, but a low-grade chronic inflammation, which is found in mucosal specimens, could also be responsible for the thinning of the sinus walls [2]. Kass et al. demonstrated negative intrasinus pressures in patients with the silent sinus syndrome [8]. The sinus walls, thinned by inflammation or gas resorption or both, are pulled into the sinus by negative sinus pressure, and the orbital contents settle down into the maxillary sinus [2].

A pathophysiological comparison is often made between the silent sinus syndrome and middle ear atelectasis. In this condition, the tympanic membrane retracts due to chronic Eustachian tube obstruction which results in occlusion of a mucus-membrane-lined cavity, gas resorption, and negative pressure formation [4]. Indeed, the silent sinus syndrome is also called "chronic maxillary sinus atelectasis" and referred to as a process of sinus atelectasis. Atelectasis is defined as decreased or absent air in a part of the lung, with resulting loss of lung volume. Resorption atelectasis is a specific form of atelectasis and is perhaps a better analogy to the collapse of the maxillary sinus that occurs when communication to the nasal cavity via the sinus ostium is obstructed. In resorption atelectasis, a slow, partial collapse of a lobe occurs when communication between alveoli and the trachea is obstructed.

Although this model seems to be a good explanation for the development of the silent sinus syndrome, several questions remain unanswered. Most obvious is the disparity between maxillary sinus obstruction, a very common condition, and the silent sinus syndrome, a very rare condition [5]. The theory also fails to offer an explanation for the exclusive involvement of the maxillary sinus, although concomitant ethmoidal involvement has been reported as well [9].

Routine fungal and bacterial cultures, as well as cytology studies performed on the mucoid material recovered from the maxillary sinus in patients with silent sinus syndrome, are negative [2]. This finding is not surprising given the negative pressure and hypoventilation within the maxillary sinus and the inhibitory effects that a vacuum and low oxygen content exert on most microorganisms. Histopathology of the sinus mucosa in patients with silent sinus syndrome show mild, non-specific, chronic, and inflammatory cell infiltrates. Bone specimens from the sinus walls demonstrate reparative bone changes with increased osteoblastic activity and no evidence of inflammation or other alterations [2].

Presentation

The typical patient with the silent sinus syndrome is an adult in the third to fifth decades of life who presents to the ophthalmologist or otolaryngologist with complaints of a spontaneous, progressive, and painless eye or facial asymmetry [4]. Vertical diplopia secondary to hypoglobus and mechanical strabismus can also lead the patient to seek medical attention [6]. A painlessness presentation is the sine qua non of the silent sinus syndrome.

Diagnosis

There are no established criteria for making the diagnosis of the silent sinus syndrome. The diagnosis of this condition involves clinical and radiographic evidence, but certain prerequisites must be met before a diagnosis of silent sinus syndrome can be made. The patient must have no prior history of trauma, chronic rhinosinusitis, or sinus surgery; no episodes of acute rhinosinusitis in the last 6 months; no prior history of enophthalmos; and no documented congenital deformity or anatomic anomalies of the sinus or orbital cavity [2, 8].

The patient's history reveals a chronic, progressive, and painless facial asymmetry. Aside from enophthalmos and hypoglobus, physical examination may reveal upper lid retraction, deepened upper lid sulcus, malar depression, facial asymmetry, orbital asymmetry, disappearance of the palpebral fold line, and palpebral retraction [6] (Fig. 55.1). Enophthalmos is typically between 2 and 4 mm by Hertel exophthalmometer in comparison with the contralateral eye. Vertical diplopia may occur to varying degrees, but typically, the visual acuity, intraocular pressure, and ocular movements are preserved [6]. To confirm the diagnosis, radiologic studies are next obtained to visualize the paraorbital sinuses and orbits and to exclude orbital tumor or evidence of trauma [4].

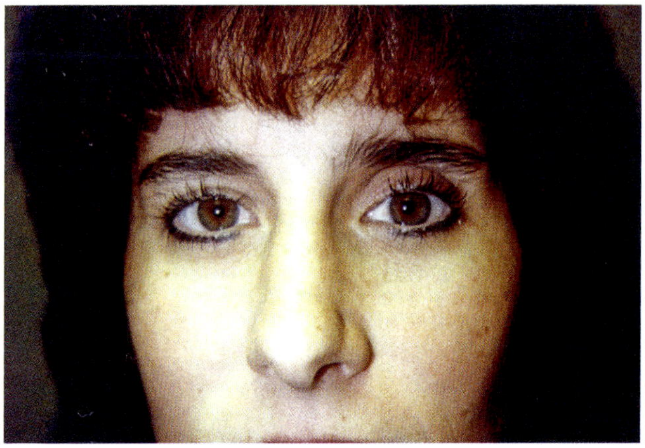

Fig. 55.1 A patient with left upper sulcus deformity and hypoglobus

Differential Diagnosis

Spontaneous enophthalmos and hypoglobus can be ominous signs. These findings may be associated with life-threatening conditions such as primary or metastatic malignancy (i.e., breast), osteomyelitis, and severe collagen vascular disease [2]. It is imperative that these entities be ruled out before the patient can be diagnosed with the silent sinus syndrome. Once these more serious conditions have been ruled out, other causes of enophthalmos and hypoglobus should be considered. These include hypoplastic maxillary sinus, trauma, iatrogenic (i.e., previous surgery), systemic inflammatory disease (i.e., Wegener granulomatosis), neurofibromatosis, chronic sinusitis, maxillary mucocele, orbital varices, and benign tumors. Burroughs et al. reported 19 cases of spontaneous enophthalmos erroneously diagnosed as silent sinus syndrome in a retrospective case series; they called particular attention to Parry-Romberg syndrome and linear scleroderma as entities of inflammatory-mediated spontaneous enophthalmos that must be differentiated from SSS [10].

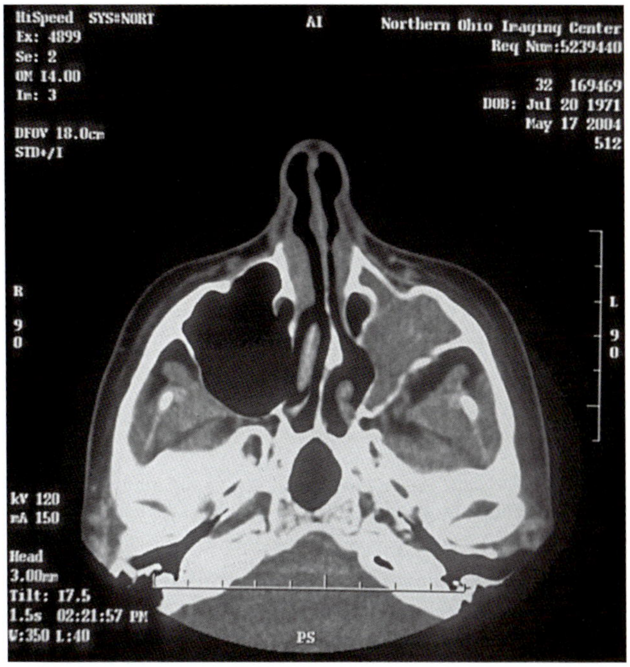

Fig. 55.2 An axial CT scan showing clouding of the maxillary sinus with bowing inward of the maxillary sinus walls

Imaging

Once a clinical history and physical examination have suggested a diagnosis of silent sinus syndrome, radiographic evidence, specifically a contrasted CT of the face and orbits, is obtained to confirm the diagnosis by ruling out more sinister entities. Imaging findings in the silent sinus syndrome are characteristic. The primary finding is retraction of the maxillary roof or orbital floor, causing enophthalmos and hypoglobus. Typically, all four walls of the maxillary sinus are retracted, though one of the medial, anterior, or posterolateral walls may be spared [4]. In addition to being retracted, the sinus walls are usually dramatically thinned or sometimes completely resorbed in the case of the maxillary roof, but the thickness of the other walls may be normal or even slightly thickened [5]. A second finding on imaging is that the sinus is partially or completely opacified and may have air/fluid levels (Figs. 55.2 and 55.3).

Finer radiographic features that may be appreciated include occlusion of the maxillary sinus infundibulum, which is always present in the silent sinus syndrome. Occlusion of the infundibulum is usually caused by lateral retraction of the uncinate process with apposition of the uncinate process against the inferomedial aspect of the orbital wall [4]. The adjacent middle meatus is correspondingly enlarged with varying degrees of lateral retraction of the middle turbinate [4].

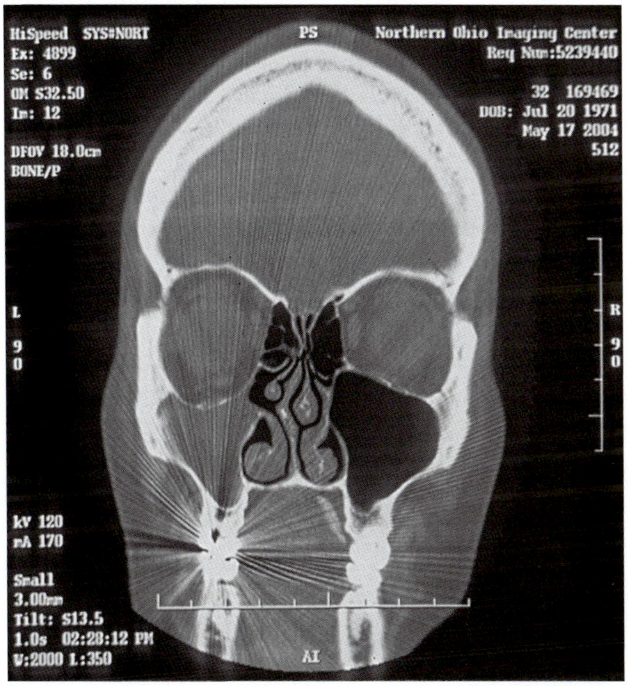

Fig. 55.3 A coronal view showing the same

Treatment

The treatment of the silent sinus syndrome is surgical, with the goals for surgery being (1) to restore communication between the maxillary sinus and nasal cavity and (2) to correct enophthalmos by repairing the orbital floor. For correction of sinus obstruction, endoscopy with sinus drainage, uncinectomy, and intranasal antrostomy are the gold standards for restoring sinus outflow, which arrests disease progression [6]. No agreement exists on whether the orbital floor repair should occur simultaneously or sequentially in a staged fashion (Fig. 55.4).

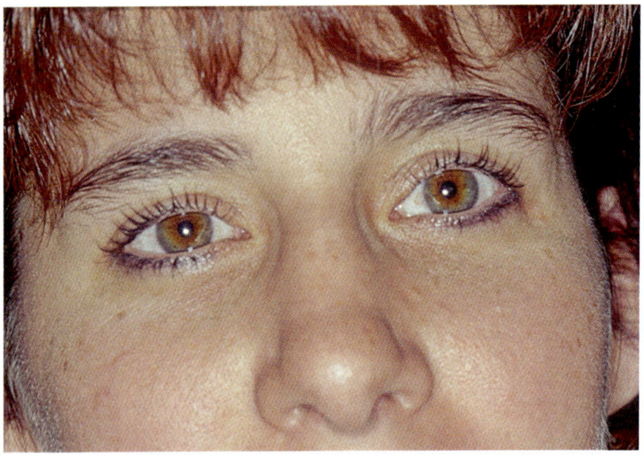

Fig. 55.4 The same patient post-op endoscopic sinus drainage and restoration, followed by an orbital floor implant at a later date

Most reports suggest a 2-month waiting period between the sinus surgery and orbital floor repair based on the idea that restoring sinus drainage and aeration may correct, at least in part, enophthalmos, and immediate floor repair could lead to overcorrection. A single-stage operation is indicated when severe enophthalmos, diplopia, and cosmetic disfigurement are present, as reconstruction of the orbital floor is mandatory and performing floor reconstruction with sinus surgery reduces morbidity, costs, and hospitalizations [6].

Postoperatively, maxillary sinus configuration may remain unchanged, improve slightly, or return to a normal shape over time [4]. There are no reports of medical management of the sinus silent syndrome, although there are reports of patients who deferred surgical treatment. In these cases, it was not reported if enophthalmos and hypoglobus worsened or if symptoms and signs reached a plateau.

Summary

In summary, the silent sinus syndrome is a rare condition characterized by painless, progressive enophthalmos and hypoglobus due to thinning and retraction of the orbital floor into the maxillary sinus and enlargement of the orbit with downward displacement of its contents. The retraction of the floor and possibly other maxillary walls is due to a negative pressure gradient and possibly a low-grade, chronic inflammatory reaction which are both results of obstruction of the maxillary ostium and separation from the nasal cavity. The diagnosis is made clinically by history and physical examination, with radiographic findings involving the maxillary sinus and orbit, confirming the diagnosis of the silent sinus syndrome. Although rare, it is likely underdiagnosed because of its subtle features and hallmark painlessness. Restoration of maxillary sinus ventilation and reconstruction of the orbital floor are key features in the surgical treatment of the silent sinus syndrome.

References

1. Montgomery WW. Mucocele of the maxillary sinus causing enophthalmos. Eye Ear Nose Throat Mon. 1964;43:41–4.
2. Soparkar CN, Patrinely JR, Cuaycong MJ, Dailey RA, Kersten RC, Rubin PA, et al. The silent sinus syndrome: a cause of spontaneous enophthalmos. Ophthalmology. 1994;101:772–8.
3. Soparkar CN, Patrinely JR, Davidson JK. Silent sinus syndrome: new perspectives? Ophthalmology. 2004;111:414–5, author reply 415–416.
4. Illner A, Davidson HC, Harnsberger HR, Hoffman J. The silent sinus syndrome: clinical and radiographic findings. Am J Roentgenol. 2002;178:503–6.
5. Hourany R, Aygun N, Della Santina CC, Zinreich SJ. Silent sinus syndrome: an acquired condition. Am J Neuroradiol. 2005;26:2390–3.
6. Sesenna E, Oretti G, Anghinoni ML, Ferri A. Simultaneous management of enophthalmos and sinus pathology in silent sinus syndrome: a report of three cases. J Craniomaxillofac Surg. 2010;38:1–4.
7. Kass ES, Salman S, Rubin PAD, Weber AL, Montgomery WW. Chronic maxillary atelectasis. Ann Otol Rhinol Laryngol. 1997;106:109–16.
8. Kass ES, Salman S, Montgomery WW. Manometric study of complete ostial occlusion in chronic maxillary atelectasis. Laryngoscope. 1996;106:1255–8.
9. Braganza A, Khooshabeh R. Ethmoidal involvement in "imploding" (silent) sinus syndrome. Ophthalmic Plast Reconstr Surg. 2005;21:305–6.
10. Burroughs JR, Hernandez Cospin JR, Soparker CN, Patrinely JR. Misdiagnosis of silent sinus syndrome. Ophthalmic Plast Reconstr Surg. 2003;19:449–54.

Orbital Tumors

56

Jonathan J. Dutton, Daniel T. Sines, and Victor M. Elner

Introduction

The orbit and ocular adnexa are important sites for primary and secondary orbital diseases [16, 52, 55, 61]. All tissue types including bone, vascular, neural, muscular, and glandular tissues may be involved with specific pathologies. Tumors or inflammations can secondarily invade the orbit from periorbital regions such as the paranasal sinuses, eyelids, and intracranial compartment. The volume of the orbit is small and confined by bony walls on all sides except anteriorly, and within this space, numerous structures subserve visual functions. It is not surprising, therefore, that ophthalmic symptoms are common presenting findings with most orbital diseases. In this chapter, we will restrict our discussion to benign and malignant tumors and to some of the more common nonneoplastic lesions.

Clinical Evaluation

The initial examination of any patient with a suspected orbital lesion is critical and serves to create a narrow differential diagnosis. The latter will direct the clinician to perform specific laboratory and diagnostic tests that will further narrow the list or, in some cases, make a firm diagnosis. They will also help guide the treating physician in establishing the most appropriate medical or surgical treatment plan.

Ophthalmic and Medical History

A careful and complete ophthalmic and systemic history should include the patient's chief complaint, major ophthalmic symptoms, nature of onset, and duration of symptoms [16]. Past ocular history may uncover a history of trauma, prior periorbital surgery, or periocular tumors that could relate to the present illness. A history of intraocular malignancy such as malignant melanoma might point to the possibility of orbital extension or metastasis. The past general medical history may elicit important diagnostic information. For example, a history of cancer might suggest an etiology for new-onset proptosis. A history of systemic inflammatory disease such as sarcoidosis or hyperthyroidism should raise concern for a related orbital inflammatory process.

Ophthalmic Examination

A thorough ophthalmic examination is essential in the evaluation of any patient with suspected orbital disease. Radiologic imaging and diagnostic ultrasound are valuable adjunctive tests, but they should never be used as a substitute for a comprehensive physical examination. The clinician should be familiar with the typical presenting characteristics of different lesions and their time course, as well as such features as the usual age at presentation, any sexual preferences, and characteristic anatomic locations of occurrence.

A differential diagnosis is established based on the initial physical findings and history and will form the basis of deciding on specific ancillary studies that will provide useful additional information. For example, if the examination suggests the involvement of orbital bone, computerized tomography with bone window settings is likely to provide information that is of greater diagnostic value than an MRI. Likewise, for suspected extraocular extension of choroidal lesions, ultrasound would be an appropriate initial study.

J. J. Dutton
University of North Carolina, Department of Ophthalmology, Chapel Hill, NC, USA

D. T. Sines (✉)
Boozman Hof Regional Eye Clinic, Rogers, AR, USA

V. M. Elner
Eye Plastic and Orbital Surgery Service, Department of Ophthalmology and Visual Sciences, Kellogg Eye Center, University of Michigan, Ann Arbor, MI, USA

J. J. Servat et al. (eds.), *Smith and Nesi's Ophthalmic Plastic and Reconstructive Surgery*,
https://doi.org/10.1007/978-3-030-41720-8_56

A complete ophthalmic physical examination should include evaluation of the eyelids, eye, anterior orbit, and periorbital tissues. At a minimum, the examination should include best-corrected visual acuity, pupillary reactions, visual fields, slit lamp examination of the anterior ocular segment, corneal and periorbital sensory function, ocular motility, periorbital palpation, exophthalmometry, and a dilated fundus examination. Each of these may uncover findings suggestive of orbital disease and provide useful clues as to etiology.

Signs and Symptoms of Orbital Disease

Proptosis

Proptosis refers to displacement of the globe relative to the orbital rims. It is usually measured with an exophthalmometer as the distance in millimeters from the lateral orbital rim to the anterior corneal surface. The normal values are 14–21 mm. However, the degree of proptosis in any given individual patient largely depends upon what was normal for that patient. Thus, a measurement of 19 mm, while well within the normal range, could represent significant proptosis for a patient whose normal baseline measurement was 15 mm. Examination of old photographs is often helpful in evaluating proptosis.

Because the bony orbit is a closed space open only at the front, proptosis is the most common clinical finding associated with a retrobulbar mass lesion. The pattern of proptosis depends largely on the location of the lesion, and this can be of great value in developing a differential diagnosis. The clinician should envision the anatomic structures situated in various parts of the orbit or paraorbital regions when evaluating proptosis. Axial proptosis refers to the condition where the eye is displaced straight outward along the anteroposterior orbital axis. It is typically seen with intraconal masses such as optic nerve tumors or an intraconal hemangioma.

When the eye is pushed outward and also displaced off the central axis, this is called abaxial proptosis. This situation occurs when the mass lesion lies largely outside the muscle cone. The direction of globe displacement typically suggests one or several possible anatomical sites of origin. Since most orbital mass lesions occur in the superior orbit, the eye is often displaced downward. Causative lesions include schwannomas, neurofibromas, and lymphomas. Lacrimal gland tumors will usually displace the globe downward and medially. Lesions situated in the medial orbit, such as an ethmoid mucocele or subperiosteal abscess, will displace the globe laterally. Metastatic tumors to the inferior rectus muscle, maxillary sinus tumors invading the orbit, or orbital floor hematomas associated previously placed implants for blow out fracture repair will displace the eye upward.

Ocular Motility

The extraocular rectus muscles extend from their origin within the annulus of Zinn at the orbital apex to their insertions just anterior to the ocular equator. Along their course, they are invested with a thin connective tissue sheath that is part of the vast orbital fascial connective tissue and pulley systems. The latter are a network of suspensory membranes that interconnect the muscles to each other, to the adjacent orbital walls, and to the optic nerve and posterior Tenon's capsule. Mass lesions or inflammatory processes in the orbit that expand or restrict these fascial layers may exert traction on the muscles resulting in motility disturbance and subjective diplopia.

Less commonly neuropathic ophthalmoplegia may result from malignant tumor infiltrating or compressing cranial nerves that supply the extraocular muscles, either in the orbital apex or in the cavernous sinus. Occasionally, diplopia may be the initial symptom of orbital disease before any other findings such as proptosis become obvious.

Loss of Vision

Visual loss is an uncommon finding with most orbital diseases. When present, it is often associated with compression of the optic nerve by intrinsic lesions such as meningiomas or optic nerve gliomas. In these cases, visual loss is often severe, associated with decreased color vision and a relative afferent papillary defect. Similarly, vision loss may be profound with small nonneural tumors located in the orbital apex, such as a hemangioma. Benign tumors in the midorbital muscle cone rarely cause visual problems unless they become very large. Symmetrical enlargement of multiple extraocular muscles, as with Graves' disease, may be associated with compressive optic neuropathy especially with increased muscle mass in the orbital apex.

Orbital Pain

Pain is not a typical feature of most orbital diseases. Even when very large, most slow-growing benign tumors such as cavernous hemangiomas and schwannomas do not cause significant pain. However, pain can be a significant symptom of acute inflammations and infections. Pain is also a feature of some malignant tumors that show perineural spread, such as adenoid cystic carcinoma of the lacrimal gland.

Periorbital Inflammation

Inflammatory signs of the eyelids and conjunctiva are associated with infections and acute inflammatory diseases. Inflammation can also be seen with debris as from a ruptured dermoid cyst. Inflammatory signs include erythema, edema, chemosis, dilated vessels, and tenderness. However, most orbital tumors are not associated with an inflammatory process.

Laterality

Orbital disease can be unilateral or bilateral. Most benign and malignant tumors, cysts, and structural vascular anomalies occur in only one orbit. Some orbital inflammations may be bilateral either simultaneously or sequentially. Graves' orbitopathy is always a bilateral disease, but can be very asymmetric with one side appearing nearly normal.

Other Key Features

In addition to presenting symptoms and clinical signs, other features uncovered in the history can offer important clues as to the nature of the disease process.

Nature of Onset

The onset of orbital disease may vary from sudden to insidious. This can often provide useful information on the likely nature of the pathology. Catastrophic onset over hours to days is typically associated with trauma, hemorrhage, and sometimes infections (Table 56.1). Chronic onset, over months to years, is more likely associated with slow-growing lesions such as neurogenic tumors, vascular tumors, and lymphoproliferative disorders.

Age at Onset

The age at the onset of orbital symptoms can vary with the specific orbital disease. Although there is considerable overlap in the age at presentation, some diseases occur more commonly in specific age groups (Table 56.2). Dermoid cysts, for example, can be seen into middle age, but the vast majority present within the first decade of life. Other lesions such as lacrimal gland tumors, metastatic carcinomas, and cavernous hemangiomas more commonly present in adulthood. Orbital lymphoma is a disease seen almost exclusively in patients beyond the fourth to fifth decades. While age alone cannot absolutely rule out any specific disease, nevertheless, the patient's age at presentation should direct the physician to a narrower differential.

Unusual Features

Some uncommon features can point to a specific diagnosis. Dilated tortuous episcleral vessels associated with increased intraocular pressure and signs of orbital congestion are highly suggestive of vascular anomalies such as a carotid-cavernous fistula. In patients with orbital neurofibromatosis, bony defects in the orbital roof can cause pulsating proptosis. Intermittent proptosis, especially when associated with bending forward or with Valsalva, is a common finding with orbital varices. Similarly, Valsalva associated with crying can cause enlargement of a mass with increased proptosis from a capillary hemangiomas in

Table 56.1 Temporal onset of common orbital diseases

Hours	Days	Weeks	Months	Years
Traumatic	Inflammatory	Inflammatory	Neoplastic	Neoplastic
Hemorrhagic	Infectious	Neoplastic	Lymphoid	Degenerative
Infectious	Traumatic	Traumatic	Vascular	Lymphoid
	Hemorrhagic	Lymphoid	Inflammatory	Vascular
	Vascular	Vascular	Degenerative	Inflammatory

Table 56.2 Age distribution of common orbital diseases

	Childhood and adolescence (0–20 years) (%)	Middle age (21–60 years) (%)	Later adult life (61–90+ years) (%)
Thyroid orbitopathy	4	81	15
Infectious processes	35	50	15
Inflammatory lesions	12	67	21
Cystic lesions	77	18	5
Vascular neoplastic lesions	54	38	8
Secondary and metastatic tumors	6	35	59
Mesenchymal lesions	25	50	25
Lymphoproliferative diseases	5	45	50
Neurogenic tumors	33	55	12
Lacrimal gland fossa lesions	9	82	9

young children. In the presence of upper respiratory infections, orbital lymphangiomas often produce intermittent exacerbation of proptosis.

Ancillary Imaging Techniques

Radiographic examination is a crucial step in the evaluation of any patient with suspected orbital disease. Such studies may contribute to a specific diagnosis and often will provide guidance in planning the most appropriate medical therapy or surgical approach.

Computed Tomography

Computerized tomography (CT) utilizes an array of thin collimated X-ray beams that pass through tissue along the rows and columns of a complex intersecting matrix. As the X-ray beams traverse tissue, they are attenuated or weakened according to the density of the tissues through which they pass, and this attenuation is proportional to the relative density of the tissue with respect to the passage of X-rays. Less dense tissues, such as water, allow more X-rays to pass through producing a darker region on the final image. More dense tissues, such as bone, attenuate the X-rays to a greater extent resulting in a lighter or white area on the final image [13, 15]. Iodinated intravenous contrast agents are frequently used to improve contrast by increasing the attenuation of blood vessels or highly vascularized tissues. Such agents may help outline normal anatomy and can more accurately define pathologic processes.

Orbital CT should routinely include scans in both the axial and coronal planes. Unless contraindicated because of iodine allergy, a contrast series should be included in all orbital scans. For any suspected bony involvement, bone windows should also be included. Orbital mass lesions generally appear as an abnormal density within the typically low-density orbital fat [1, 11]. The lesion may be well defined with sharp borders as with a cavernous hemangioma or infiltrative with diffuse borders that merge with or surround normal anatomic structures as with inflammatory pseudotumor.

Magnetic Resonance Imaging

Magnetic resonance imaging (MRI) is a valuable technique for orbital evaluation that does not rely on the passage of X-rays through tissue. The magnetic resonance signal is generated by spinning proton nuclei within biological tissues whose rotational axes are deformed in an externally applied magnetic field. Under the influence of an RF pulse, reorientation of spinning axes occurs perpendicular to the external magnetic field. The spinning proton axes return to baseline when the RF pulse is removed and, in the process, produce the T1 and T2 resonance signals that are used to create an image [15]. Tissue contrast can be adjusted by modification of the RF pulse sequence allowing a high degree of tissue differentiation based on biochemical differences. Gadolinium is a paramagnetic element that can increase the relative contrast of vascular tissues when injected intravenously. In addition, various fat suppression techniques permit the visualization of gadolinium-enhanced lesions that otherwise would be difficult to see within orbital fat.

Magnetic resonance imaging offers several advantages over CT. Soft tissue visualization in the region of the orbital apex, optic canal, and cavernous sinus is not degraded by dense surrounding bone, as it is in CT scans, because of the low-resonance signal generated from bone [9, 10, 43]. Also, with manipulation of resonance signals from various tissues, contrast variability and tissue differentiation can be achieved that are unobtainable with any X-ray technique.

Incidence of Orbital Disease

The incidence of various orbital diseases varies considerably in the literature depending upon the source of the patient population [7, 16, 24, 30–32, 36, 42, 46–48, 52, 55, 57, 58, 61]. Studies based primarily on pediatric patients will show different lesions and different frequencies of occurrence than those based on adults. Likewise, series based on histopathologic material may yield different results from those determined from clinical material, some of which may not have histopathologic confirmation.

The frequency of orbital lesions noted in this chapter is from Dutton et al. and is based on 3 large series of orbital lesions totaling 1635 patients [16]. While these series undoubtedly have some inherent referral biases, nevertheless, our numbers are similar to those published in other ophthalmic reports.

Table 56.3 shows the frequency of the major categories of orbital diseases. Graves' orbital disease accounts for

Table 56.3 Frequency of orbital lesions by major diagnostic group

Inflammatory lesions	22%
Cystic lesions	20%
Lymphoproliferative diseases	11%
Secondary tumors	9%
Vascular lesions	8%
Mesenchymal lesions	7%
Neurogenic tumors	6%
Metastatic tumors	4%
Lacrimal gland tumors	3%
Other and unclassified	10%

nearly half of these (47%). Mass lesions make up 53% of the total. Among the non-Graves' space-occupying mass lesions in the orbit, inflammatory lesions account for the majority (22%). These are followed by cystic lesions (20%), lymphoproliferative tumors and infiltrates (11%), vascular lesions (8%), secondary tumors (9%), mesenchymal and adipose lesions (7%), neurogenic tumors (6%), metastatic tumors (4%), and lacrimal gland tumors and infiltrates (3%). Specific lesions within each of these groups will be discussed later in this chapter or in other chapters in this book.

Cystic Lesions

The most common cystic lesions in the orbit are cutaneous and conjunctival dermoid cysts, which represent 62% of the total (Table 56.4) [2, 53, 55, 374]. Mucoceles, primarily ethmoid and frontal, represent 20%. Other less common cysts include simple epithelial cysts, lacrimal cysts, hematic cysts, parasitic cysts, rare colobomatous cysts associated with microphthalmos, and cystic teratomas.

Inflammatory Lesions

Orbital inflammatory lesions account for 22% of all non-Graves' orbital mass lesions. By far, the most common forms are the various idiopathic inflammations [26] (53%), including orbital pseudotumor and myositis. Dacryoadenitis accounts for 20% of orbital inflammations. Infectious etiologies from adjacent sinusitis or hematogenous sources constitute 21% of orbital inflammatory processes. Other lesions include sarcoidosis and Wegener's granulomatosis. Inflammatory lesions will be discussed in a separate chapter.

Vascular Lesions

Lesions of vascular origin can be divided into structural malformations and neoplastic lesions [3, 4, 23, 28, 33, 50, 51, 62]. Among the structural malformations, we include varices and arteriovenous shunts, which account for 26% of all vascular lesions (Table 56.5). The remaining 74% are neoplastic vascular tumors, of which the most common are the cavernous hemangioma in adults (26%) and the capillary hemangiomas primarily in children (24%). Lymphangiomas represent 17% of this group. Hemangiopericytomas (solitary fibrous tumors) are rare vascular tumors seen principally in adults (1%).

Table 56.4 Common cystic lesions of the orbit

Dermoid cyst	62%
Mucocele	20%
Epithelial cyst	8%
Lacrimal gland cysts	5%
Microphthalmos with cyst	2%
Colobomatous cyst	<1%
Parasitic cyst	<1%
Hematic cyst	<1%

Neural Tumors

Tumors arising from nerve can be considered in two categories: those originating from the optic nerve [5, 8, 12, 13, 17, 27, 39–41, 49] and those from other neural tissues including cranial nerves, meninges, and other neural tissues. Cranial nerve and meningeal tumors account for 69% of all neural mass lesions and include sphenoid wing meningiomas (30%), neurofibromas (19%), and schwannomas (9%) (Table 56.6). Rare lesions include malignant peripheral nerve sheath tumor, amputation neuroma, and alveolar soft part sarcoma.

Optic nerve tumors account for 33% of all orbital neural lesions. Optic nerve gliomas make up 66% of these and occur primarily in children, whereas optic sheath meningiomas account for 33% and are seen predominantly in adults.

Mesenchymal Lesions

Mesenchymal tumors constitute an important group in both children and adults and include several malignant neoplasms [22, 33, 35, 44, 45, 54]. Together, mesenchymal

Table 56.5 Frequency of the commonest vascular orbital lesions

Cavernous hemangioma	26%
Capillary hemangioma	24%
Lymphangioma	17%
Orbital varices	13%
AV shunt	13%
Hemangiopericytoma	1%
Other	5%

Table 56.6 Frequency of the commonest neurogenic orbital tumors

Sphenoid wing meningioma	30%
Optic nerve glioma	22%
Neurofibroma	19%
Optic sheath meningioma	11%
Schwannoma	9%
Other	4%
Carcinoid tumor	<1%
Malignant peripheral nerve tumor	<1%
Neuroblastoma	<1%

tumors account for 7% of all orbital mass lesions. Dermolipomas are the most common lesions (44%), seen mostly in childhood, and although most are superficial, some can extend posteriorly into the orbit (Table 56.7). Other important lesions include fibrous histiocytomas (22%), fibrous dysplasia (10%), osteomas (9%), and fibromas (4%). Rare tumors in the orbit include liposarcomas, myxomas, leiomyomas, and leiomyosarcomas. Rhabdomyosarcoma is the most common malignant mesenchymal tumor of childhood and accounts for 22% of all orbital mesenchymal lesions.

Tumors of Bone

Tumors arising from bone are not very common, making up about 1.5–2% of orbital mass lesions [16]. Along with other nonneoplastic processes, bone lesions account for about 10% of all orbital lesions. Bone tumors are difficult to classify appropriately, and many might be placed among mesenchymal, vascular, or other categories. Many are slow-growing expansile dysplasia noninfiltrating lesions such as fibrous dysplasia, osteoma, and ossifying fibroma. Reactive lesions tend to show bone erosion and a more rapid growth pattern. These include reparative granuloma, aneurysmal bone cyst, and brown tumor. Neoplasms, such as osteogenic sarcoma, chondrosarcoma, and Ewing sarcoma, show tissue infiltration with relentless progression and a metastatic potential. The most common tumor of bone is the osteoma, accounting for 39% of the total, followed by Ewing sarcoma (14%), aneurysmal bone cyst (11%), and ossifying fibroma (11%) (Table 56.8).

Table 56.7 Frequency of the commonest mesenchymal orbital tumors

Dermolipoma	44%
Rhabdomyosarcoma	22%
Fibrous histiocytoma	20%
Liposarcoma	4%
Fibrosarcoma	3%
Leiomyosarcoma	<1%
Juvenile xanthogranuloma	<1%
Lipoblastomatosis	<1%
Lipoma	<1%

Table 56.8 Frequency of the commonest orbital tumors of bone

Osteoma	39%
Ewing sarcoma	14%
Aneurysmal bone cyst	11%
Ossifying fibroma	11%
Fibrous dysplasia	7%
Osteosarcoma	7%
Brown tumor	7%
Chondrosarcoma	4%

Lacrimal Gland Lesions

A variety of primary and secondary lesions can involve the lacrimal gland [20, 21, 25, 59, 63]. Together, lacrimal lesions represent 3% of all orbital mass lesions. These are often divided into those arising from the lacrimal epithelium (30%) and nonepithelial infiltrative lesions (70%) (Table 56.9). Among epithelial tumors, the pleomorphic adenoma (benign mixed tumor) represents 58%, and adenoid cystic carcinoma accounts for 36%. Other rare epithelial lesions include pleomorphic adenocarcinoma and mucoepidermoid carcinoma. Of the nonepithelial infiltrations affecting the lacrimal gland, dacryoadenitis is the most common accounting for 70% of the total. This is followed by benign lymphoid hyperplasia (15%), lymphoma (6%), and occasionally sarcoidosis.

Metastatic Tumors

Metastatic tumors to the orbit account for 4% of all orbital lesions [19, 29, 60]. The most common primary site is the breast which represents 49% of the total (Table 56.10). Other sources include prostate (11%), gastrointestinal tumors (9%), malignant melanoma (6%), thyroid carcinoma (5%), and lung carcinoma (5%), as well as a variety of sarcomas.

Lymphoproliferative Lesions

Lymphoid tumors are reasonably common in the orbit, representing 6% of all orbital lesions [6, 18, 34, 37]. Lymphoma

Table 56.9 Frequency of lacrimal fossa lesions

Dacryoadenitis	49%
Pleomorphic adenoma	18%
Reactive lymphoid hyperplasia	11%
Adenoid cystic carcinoma	11%
Dacryops (epithelial cyst)	5%
Lymphoma	4%
Mucoepidermoid carcinoma	<%
Pleomorphic adenocarcinoma	<1%
Plasmacytoid lesions	<1%

Table 56.10 Primary origins of metastatic tumors to the orbit

Breast	49%
Prostate	11%
Gastrointestinal	9%
Melanoma	6%
Lung	5%
Thyroid	5%
Sarcomas and other	15%

Table 56.11 Frequency of lymphoproliferative diseases of the orbit

Lymphoma	51%
Reactive and atypical lymphoid hyperplasia	35%
Leukemia	5%
Plasma cell dyscrasias	5%
Histiocytoses	3%
Leukemia	<1%

is the most common tumor (51%), followed by benign reactive lymphoid hyperplasia (35%) (Table 56.11). Other less common diagnoses include plasma cell tumors, eosinophilic granuloma, and leukemia. Lymphoproliferative diseases will be discussed in a separate chapter.

Secondary Tumors

Secondary tumors are those that extend into the orbit from adjacent sites such as the eyelids or paranasal sinuses. They account for 4% of all orbital lesions. The majority are from cutaneous eyelid and conjunctival tumors such as basal cell and squamous cell carcinomas. Sebaceous cell tumors and epithelial melanomas are less common but important because of their relatively poor prognosis. Extrascleral extension of intraocular tumors, most frequently uveal melanoma, represents 25% of secondary lesions.

Cystic Lesions

Dermoid Cyst

Clinical Pearls

- Dermoid cysts are the most common cystic lesion of the orbit.
- The dermoid cyst is lined by skin and skin appendages and may contain keratin, hair, or sebum.
- Orbital dermoid cysts most commonly present in childhood as a slow-growing, painless, subcutaneous mass along the frontozygomatic suture.
- If the cyst capsule spontaneously ruptures, an intense inflammatory reaction may result.
- Surgical excision typically results in complete resolution.

The most common cystic lesion of the orbit is the dermoid. The pathogenesis of this choristoma results from embryonic ectoderm becoming trapped within bony sutures or from the failed separation of surface ectoderm from the neural tube. The dermoid cyst is lined by skin and skin appendages and may contain keratin, hair, or

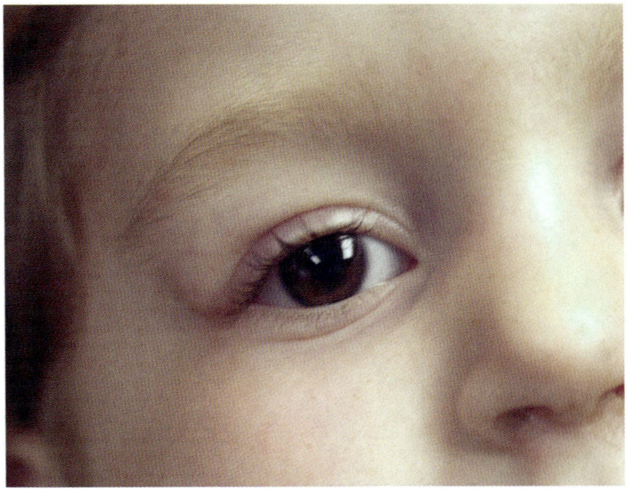

Fig. 56.1 Dermoid cyst on the lateral orbital rim at the frontozygomatic suture of the right orbit

sebum. When the lesion is exophytic, it tends to present in childhood. Endophytic lesions may invade the adjacent bone or orbital tissues and are more likely to be discovered later in life.

Clinical Presentation

Orbital dermoid cysts most commonly present in childhood, but can present at any age. Ninety percent of cases present as a slow-growing, painless, subcutaneous mass. Seventy-five percent of dermoids occur adjacent to the frontozygomatic suture within the superotemporal orbit (Fig. 56.1), but may also occur adjacent to the frontoethmoid, frontolacrimal, or sphenozygomatic sutures. Given their superotemporal location, they may mimic a lacrimal gland tumor. The lesions may range from firm to fluctuant. When rupture of the cyst wall occurs, an intense inflammatory reaction may follow. Rarely do dermoids cause globe displacement or decreased vision. However, proptosis and ocular motility disturbance may occur with deep orbital or intraconal dermoids. Rarely these lesions may lie within extraocular muscles or lacrimal gland, extend within the temporal fossa, or extend intracranially.

Computed Tomography

Dermoids appear as round to oval, well-defined, cystic lesions, typically in the anterior superotemporal orbit. They are usually extraconal. The lesion typically has a low-density cystic center, which may be very low with high fat content (Fig. 56.2). Denser foci within the cyst represent flecks of keratin and sebum. The cyst is surrounded by a thin rim of tissue that may be partially calcified. Changes of adjacent bone, such as orbital contour

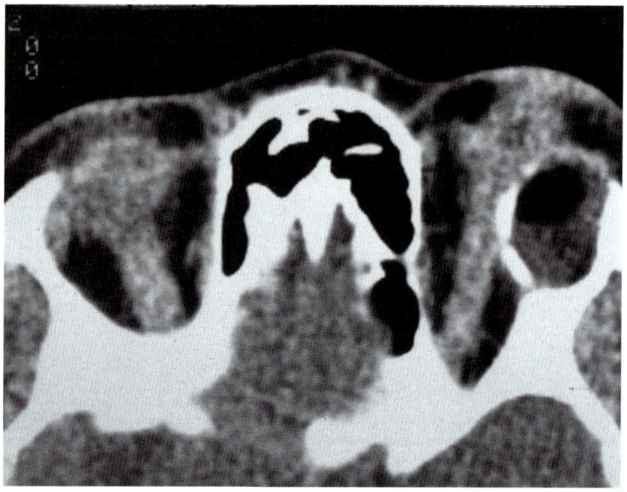

Fig. 56.2 Tissue window CT scan with an intraosseous dermoid cyst along the left orbital wall

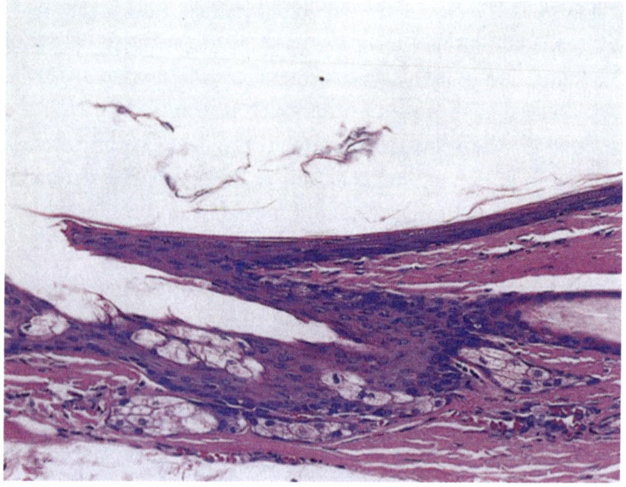

Fig. 56.3 Dermoid cyst with keratin in lumen, squamous epithelial lining, and pilosebaceous unit in wall

abnormalities and bone remolding, may occur in up to 85% of patients. Occasionally, the cystic cavity will extend across bones into the temporal or intracranial fossa. Contrast administration produces enhancement of the cyst rim, but not of the lumen.

Magnetic Resonance Imaging

On T1-weighted images, the cyst cavity produces a relatively low signal because of its water content. It is isointense or slightly hyperintense to vitreous and orbital muscle and hypointense to fat. On T2-weighted sequences, the signal is isointense or hypointense with respect to vitreous and hyperintense to fat. Images may be homogeneous to heterogeneous depending upon the cyst contents. A fat-fluid level is seen in some cases, with the upper lipid layer giving a brighter signal on T1 and a lower signal on T2 relative to the lower water-keratin layer. Calcifications appear as signal voids. With gadolinium, the cyst rim shows moderate enhancement, but the lumen does not enhance. Rupture of CNS dermoids results in a chemical meningitis with multiple fat globules in the subarachnoid space.

Histopathology

Dermoid cysts are lined by keratinized, stratified squamous epithelium, identical to that of the epidermis, with adnexal structures including sebaceous glands, eccrine glands, and hair follicles (Fig. 56.3). Most dermoids arise from keratinized squamous epithelium, but occasionally can originate from conjunctival epithelium. The cysts most commonly contain keratin, hair shafts, and sebaceous secretions, but may also include cholesterol, lipid, calcium, hemosiderin, macrophages, and other inflammatory cells. More than half of cases show histologic evidence of leakage and associated inflammation. If the cyst ruptures, it typically incites an intense granulomatous inflammatory response.

Treatment

Appropriate management is complete surgical excision. Surgical approach will vary depending upon location of lesion. Since microscopic examination frequently shows leakage and associated inflammation, early removal is indicated to prevent tissue fibrosis. A cryoprobe may be used to assist manipulation of the cyst. With very large cysts, the contents can be aspirated before the lesion is resected. Following loss of cyst contents, the orbital site should be copiously irrigated to remove particles of lipid and keratin debris. The underlying bone should be inspected for the remaining epithelium.

Prognosis

The prognosis is usually excellent. Surgical excision typically results in complete resolution. If the cyst capsule spontaneously ruptures, an intense inflammatory reaction may result. This can be treated effectively with systemic corticosteroids. In rare cases, spontaneous rupture can result in orbital fibrosis and permanent dysfunction.

Dermoid Cyst of Conjunctival Origin

Clinical Pearls

- Dermoid cysts of conjunctival origin occur most commonly in the nasal or superonasal orbit of young adults.
- These tumors present as a firm or fluctuant mass.
- The tumor is lined with non-keratinized squamous or low cuboidal epithelium associated with goblet cells.
- Surgical excision is generally curative.

These uncommon variants of the dermoid cyst typically present in the nasal or superonasal orbit of young adults.

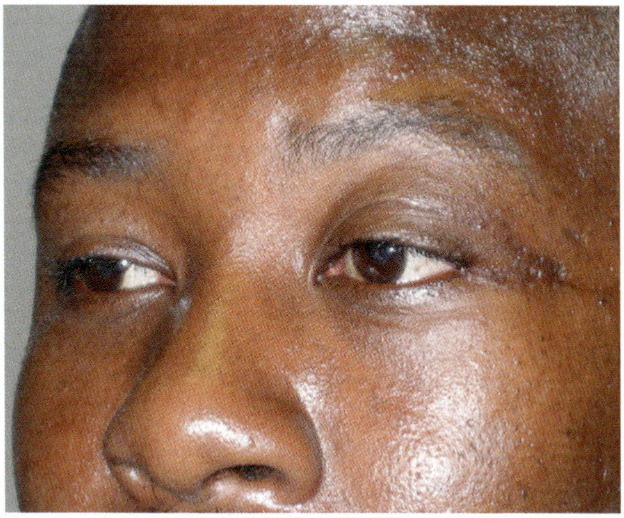

Fig. 56.4 Dermoid cyst of conjunctival origin in the left orbit, causing proptosis

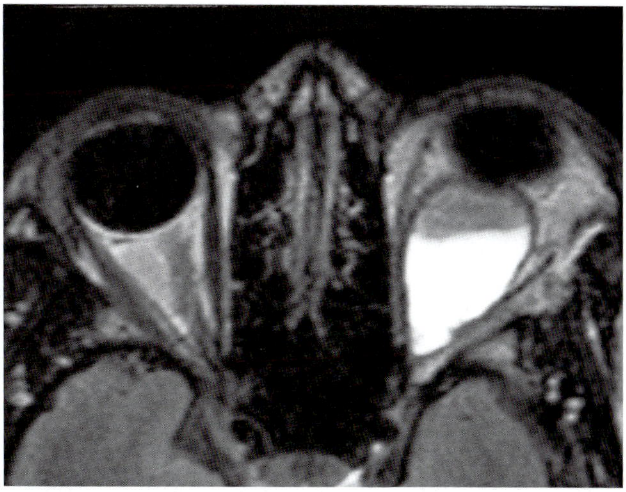

Fig. 56.5 T1-weighted fat suppressed MRI of a dermoid cyst of conjunctival origin, showing a fluid-fat interface

Unlike dermoid cysts of cutaneous origin, this tumor is lined with non-keratinized squamous or low cuboidal epithelium typically associated with goblet cells. This accounts for 5% of dermoid cysts. Unlike simple conjunctival cysts, these contain adnexal structures. The lack of cilia suggests that these do not originate from sinus mucosa. The etiology is felt to be developmental sequestration of primitive epithelium that is destined to become conjunctiva or, more likely, the caruncle.

Clinical Presentation

Dermoid cysts of conjunctival origin typically present as a firm or fluctuant mass within the nasal or superonasal orbit of young adults (Fig. 56.4). These tumors tend to be localized to soft tissues, although, when very large, they can cause adjacent bone erosion. Cases have been reported in which the tumor is attached to the superior oblique tendon, levator palpebralis sheath, superior rectus sheath, and even the optic nerve.

Computed Tomography

The conjunctival dermoid appears as a well-defined hypodense to isodense cystic mass in the medial extraconal or intraconal space. The lamina papyracea may be remolded, and proptosis may occur in larger lesions. Optic nerve displacement may occur with intraconal lesions.

Magnetic Resonance Imaging

The MRI demonstrates a sharply circumscribed cystic orbital mass (Fig. 56.5). Displacement of the optic nerve, extraocular muscles, and globe may be seen. The lesion has low signal intensity on T1 sequences and high intensity on T2 images. A fat-fluid level may be present which appears as a hyperintense fat signal above a less intense water signal on T1-weighted images. On fat suppressed (fat saturation) images, the fat signal is reduced.

Histopathology

Dermoid cysts of conjunctival origin are lined with non-keratinized squamous or low cuboidal epithelium typically associated with goblet cells. Goblet cells may not be present in every section, making careful evaluation necessary for definitive diagnosis. Unlike simple conjunctival cysts, these have been reported to contain adnexal elements. They have been reported to contain hair shafts, sebaceous glands, apocrine glands, lacrimal gland, smooth muscle, and cartilage. Oncocytic changes in some dermoids have been reported.

Treatment

Appropriate management is complete surgical excision. Surgical approach will vary depending upon location of lesion. Because the tumor is most commonly located anteriorly within the nasal or superonasal orbit, a conjunctival or skin incision may be used. Recurrence may occur with incomplete resection. With very large cysts, the contents can be aspirated prior to resection. Following loss of cyst contents, the orbital site should be copiously irrigated.

Prognosis

The prognosis is usually excellent. Surgical excision typically results in complete resolution. When dermoids are adjacent to structures such as the optic nerve or extraocular muscles, careful and sometimes incomplete resection may be required to prevent damage resulting in vision loss or diplopia.

Epithelial Cyst

Clinical Pearls

- Epithelial cysts are thought to occur as a congenital sequestration of epithelial tissue or from trauma or surgery.
- Histologically, epithelial cysts contain keratin and do not contain dermal appendages.
- These most often present in adolescents or young adults as a fluctuant nontender palpable mass in the superonasal or superotemporal orbit.
- Surgical excision is generally curative.

The congenital sequestration of epithelial tissue may result in the formation of this congenital choristoma. Epithelial cysts may also occur following the implantation of epidermal tissue following trauma, surgery, or the obstruction of lacrimal epithelial ducts or accessory glands. Histologically, epidermoid cysts contain keratin and do not contain dermal appendages, helping to differentiate them from dermoid cysts. Most epidermoid cysts occur in the eyelids, but they may present in the orbit via posterior extension or as a primary lesion.

Clinical Presentation

Simple epithelial cysts are most commonly seen in adolescents and young adults, but may occur at any age. This may present as a fluctuant nontender palpable mass in the superonasal or superotemporal orbit (Fig. 56.6). Symptoms usually include slowly progressive upper eyelid swelling, globe displacement, and occasional diplopia. With large cysts, proptosis is usually mild and may result in the formation of choroidal folds. In enucleated sockets, inability to retain a prosthesis may be the initial symptom. CNS epithelial cysts arise from inclusion of ectodermal squamous epithelial rests during closure of the embryonic neural tube. They present in the fourth and fifth decades as they enlarge from accumulation of keratin debris. Epithelial cysts can be intra- or extradural and tend to occur more commonly in the cerebellopontine angle and in a parasellar location. They have a tendency to insinuate and surround normal neural structures.

Computed Tomography

Epithelial cysts appear as a well-defined, multiloculated cyst within the orbital soft tissues (Fig. 56.7). Bone destruction has been reported, although most bony changes are the results of well-corticated remolding in larger long-standing lesions. The cyst shows low attenuation and may be difficult to distinguish from a dermoid cyst unless the latter has a significant fat content or areas of calcification. While it is usually homogeneous in texture, some large conjunctival cysts can show a fluid level. There is no enhancement of cyst contents. Intracranial epithelial cysts are lobulated masses with irregular borders. They are hypodense and may contain some calcifications along the margin. They do not enhance with contrast agents.

Magnetic Resonance Imaging

The MRI demonstrates a well-circumscribed multicystic scalloped mass. On the T1-weighted imaging, the signal is isointense to vitreous, slightly hypointense to muscle, and markedly hypointense to fat. The T2-weighted image produces a high signal that is isointense to vitreous and hyperintense to muscle and fat, similar to CSF. This is because of the high water content of the cyst. With some larger conjunctival cysts, a layered fat-water interface can be seen similar to that of a dermoid cyst. With gadolinium there is no enhancement of the cyst contents, but there may be some increased signal from the cyst wall.

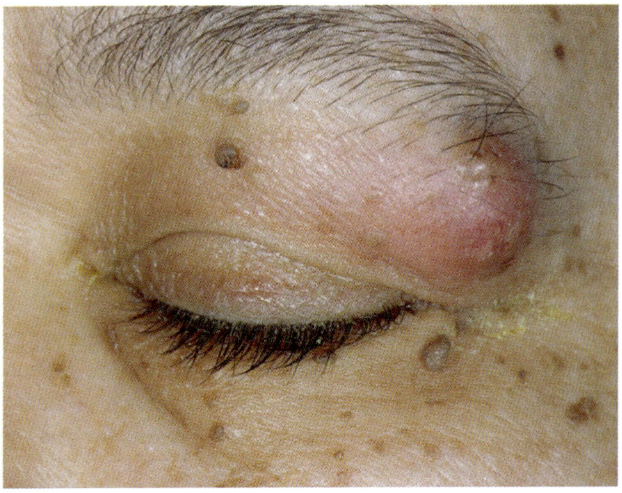

Fig. 56.6 Epithelial cyst at the left brow and anterior orbit

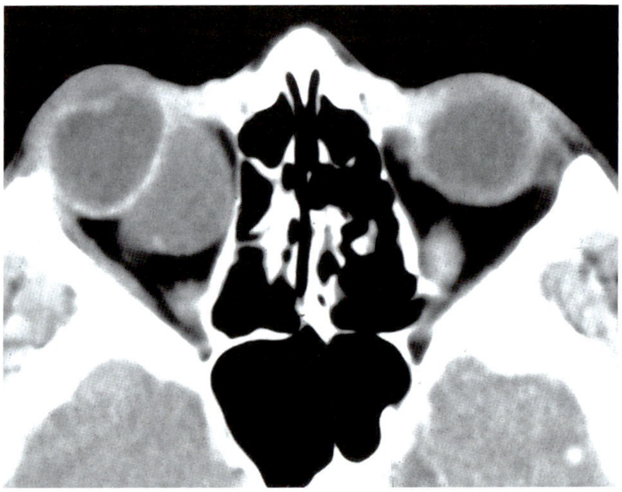

Fig. 56.7 CT scan with an epithelial cyst in the right medial orbit

Histopathology

Epithelial cysts of the orbit may have diverse histologic characteristics because they may arise from cutaneous, conjunctival, respiratory, or lacrimal gland epithelium. Epithelial cysts are lined by keratinized, stratified squamous epithelium nearly identical to epidermis. Adnexal structures are absent from the cyst lining. The lumen is filled with laminated keratin. The respiratory cyst is lined with pseudostratified ciliated columnar epithelium containing goblet cells. The lumen is filled with thick mucoid acellular debris. Conjunctival cysts have walls of cuboidal epithelium with goblet cells. Epithelial cysts of the lacrimal gland represent ectatic excretory ductules. The cyst lining is a double layer of cells, similar to normal major ducts of this gland. The inner cell layer tends to be cuboidal or low columnar, while the outer layer is more flattened. Occasional mucus-secreting goblet cells are evident in the inner layer.

Treatment

Epithelial cysts may be observed. When symptoms become bothersome, surgical excision is generally curative. Aspiration and collapse of large cysts can facilitate removal through small anterior transconjunctival incisions. In the anophthalmic socket, large cysts can be marsupialized to the surface with surgery or argon laser, or they can be injected with absolute alcohol without further excision.

Prognosis

The prognosis for vision is excellent, and there is rarely any functional disturbance.

Respiratory Epithelial Cyst

Clinical Pearls

- Respiratory cysts are rare congenital choristomas arising from the respiratory epithelium that is sequestered within the temporal orbit.
- Secondary respiratory cysts may occur following sinusitis, trauma, or surgery.
- Young adult patients most commonly present with upper eyelid swelling, proptosis, and globe displacement.
- Intermittent episodes of orbital pain and increased proptosis may be associated with respiratory infections.
- Treatment is by complete surgical excision.
- There is a thin cyst wall lined with pseudostratified ciliated columnar epithelium containing goblet cells.

Respiratory cysts are rare congenital choristomas that arise from respiratory epithelium that is sequestered within the temporal orbit. Secondary respiratory cysts, which are far less common, typically occur following sinusitis, trauma, or surgery. Unlike mucoceles, which they resemble histologically, primary respiratory cysts do not communicate with the nasal cavity or paranasal sinuses.

Clinical Presentation

Respiratory cysts can occur at any age, but tend to present in younger adults. Symptoms include slowly progressive upper eyelid swelling, proptosis, globe displacement, and occasional diplopia. Proptosis is typically mild, even with large cysts (Fig. 56.8). A fluctuant nontender palpable mass may be present beneath the orbit rim. Indentation of the eye can be seen, but visual acuity is usually normal. Intermittent episodes of orbital pain and increased proptosis may be associated with respiratory infections.

Computed Tomography

There is typically a well-defined cyst cavity in the orbital soft tissues (Fig. 56.9). There is no destruction of bone, but

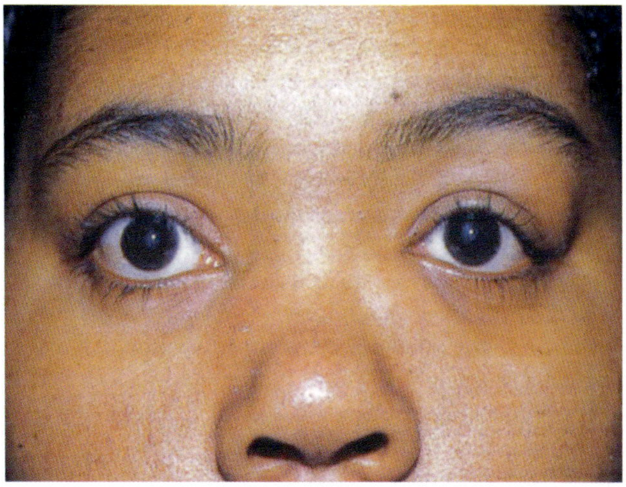

Fig. 56.8 Respiratory epithelial cyst in the right orbit with minimal proptosis

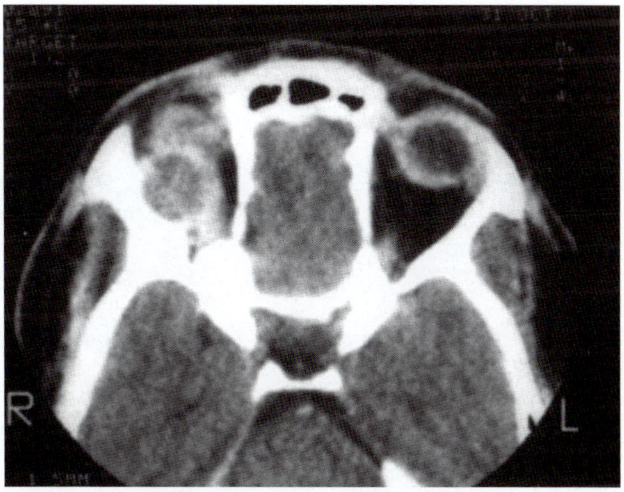

Fig. 56.9 CT scan showing a respiratory epithelial cyst in the retrobulbar space of the right orbit

remolding can be seen with long-standing lesions. The lesion is not related anatomically to the paranasal sinuses. A dense surface rim represents the fibrous capsule, but the cyst cavity shows low internal attenuation that may be difficult to distinguish from a dermoid cyst. With contrast administration, there is no enhancement of cyst contents.

Magnetic Resonance Imaging

Orbital respiratory cysts have not been described on MRI. It would likely appear similar to a mucocele without connection to the sinuses. On the T1-weighted image, the signal should be isointense to vitreous, slightly hypointense to muscle, and markedly hypointense to fat. The T2-weighted image should produce a high signal that is isointense to vitreous and isointense to muscle and fat. This is because of the high water content of the cyst. With gadolinium there should be no enhancement.

Histopathology

The lesion demonstrates a thin cyst wall lined with pseudostratified ciliated columnar epithelium containing goblet cells (Fig. 56.10). Some of the lining may consist of flattened, non-ciliated, non-keratinized low cuboidal epithelium. The basal cells of the epithelial lining stain positively for keratin. The fibrous capsule is variably thickened and may contain tiny foci of granulomatous inflammation. The cyst cavity contains acellular material that stains positively with the periodic acid-Schiff stain and Hale's colloidal iron techniques, but does not demonstrate keratin staining on immunohistochemistry. Rare polymorphonuclear leukocytes, lymphocytes, plasma cells, and macrophages are seen.

Treatment

Treatment is by complete surgical excision, which is curative. Aspiration of cyst contents can facilitate the surgical removal of large cysts through a small anterior transconjunctival incision. Aspiration as a primary treatment is likely to leave retained epithelium, which generally results in recurrence.

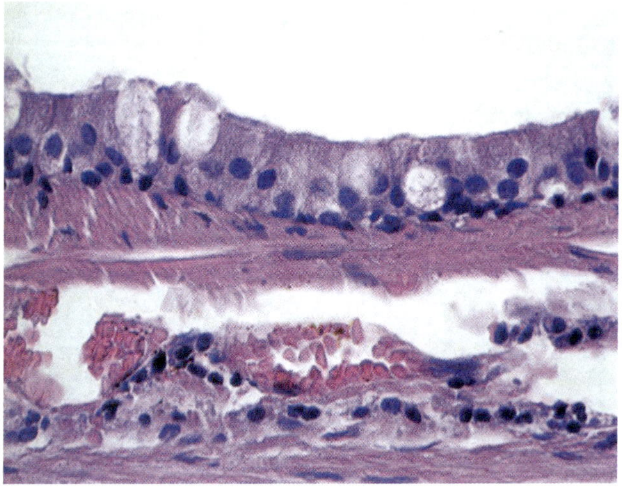

Fig. 56.10 Respiratory epithelial cyst wall lined by pseudostratified ciliated epithelium containing goblet cells

Prognosis

The prognosis for vision and life is excellent. Removal is easily accomplished with only rare functional disturbance.

Mucocele and Mucopyocele

Clinical Pearls

- Mucoceles most commonly arise in the frontal, frontoethmoid, and ethmoid sinuses.
- These lesions are associated with chronic inflammation, previous trauma, or mechanical obstruction to drainage.
- Abaxial proptosis is common, with downward and lateral displacement of the globe.
- Mucopyoceles commonly present with symptoms related to the presence of orbital cellulitis.
- Treatment is usually with surgical drainage and exenteration of the involved sinus.

Mucoceles are cysts originating in the paranasal sinuses. They most commonly arise in the frontal, frontoethmoid, and ethmoid sinuses, but also have been reported to arise in the maxillary and sphenoid sinuses. These lesions are associated with chronic inflammation, previous trauma, or mechanical obstruction to drainage. As mucous and inflammatory debris accumulate, the cyst slowly enlarges. Thinning of the overlying orbital bones allows for expansion of the mucocele into the orbit. Mucoceles represent 4% of all orbital mass lesions. Occasionally, the mucocele becomes infected to form a mucopyocele filled with purulent material. Most cases involve adults, but young children with cystic fibrosis are prone to develop mucoceles.

Clinical Presentation

Patients frequently have a history of chronic sinusitis, often with headache and visual complaints. Abaxial proptosis is common, with downward and lateral displacement of the globe. A nontender, fluctuant mass may be palpable at the superomedial orbital rim. Occasionally, a frontoethmoid mucocele can erode through an ethmoidal artery to present as a subperiosteal hemorrhage. Other findings may include blepharoptosis, eyelid swelling, and orbital pain (Fig. 56.11). Mucoceles arising in the sphenoid sinus are rare. These may cause early vision loss without obvious proptosis or diplopia due to isolated oculomotor nerve palsy. Patients with mucopyoceles commonly present with symptoms of orbital cellulitis.

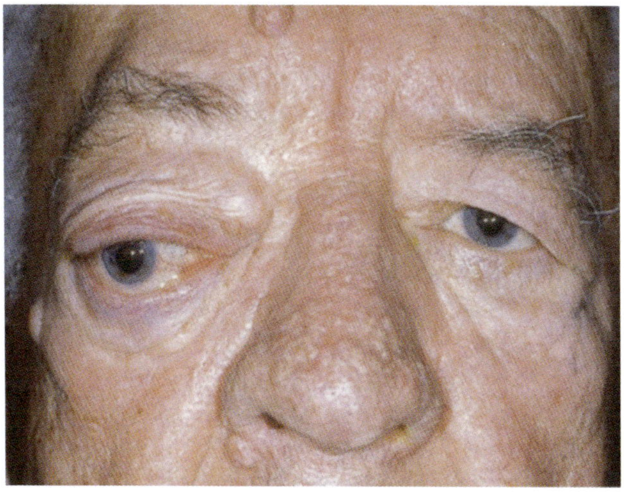

Fig. 56.11 Right frontoethmoid mucocele displacing the globe inferolaterally

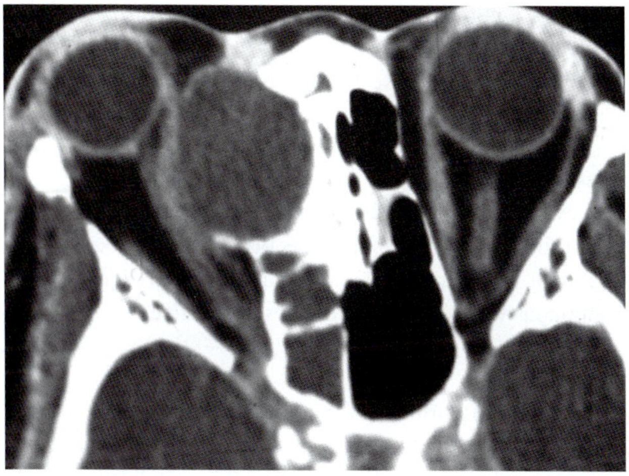

Fig. 56.12 CT scan showing a right frontoethmoid mucocele extending into the right orbit

Computed Tomography

One or more sinuses are opacified with extension of a well-defined, rounded cystic mass into the orbit. The intervening bone may be destroyed or remolded as a thin shell around the perimeter of the cystic exostosis (Fig. 56.12). Orbital structures are displaced, depending upon the location of the lesion. The cyst is filled with a homogeneous low-density mucoid material, but when the contents are viscid, the cyst may image as dense as muscle. There is no enhancement with contrast administration.

Magnetic Resonance Imaging

On MRI, mucoceles have a variable appearance, depending upon the state of hydration of its contents. In early stages, when the water content of mucoid secretions is high, the T1-weighted image shows a well-defined cyst of low signal intensity relative to muscle. On T2-weighted sequences, the cyst contents produce a hyperintense signal relative to muscle and fat. As water is absorbed and protein is concentrated, the signal becomes hyperintense on both the T1- and T2-weighted images. With continued desiccation and increasing protein concentration, the signal becomes lower again, becoming hypointense to muscle on both the T1- and T2-weighted sequences. Bone destruction or remodeling is difficult to assess due to the signal void of bone. There is no enhancement with gadolinium.

Histopathology

The mucocele is classically lined by ciliated pseudostratified respiratory epithelium. Goblet cells and basal cells are also incorporated within the epithelium. Mucous secreted by the epithelium causes increase in the size of the lesion. Epithelial characteristics change with expansion of the mucocele. Squamous metaplasia of the epithelium commonly results from the chronic sinusitis that caused the mucocele. Goblet cells are often absent in expansive mucoceles that may have only scattered flattened epithelial cells. Macrophages with ingested mucus are often adherent to the epithelial surface. The subepithelial connective tissue is usually chronically inflamed or fibrotic, and eosinophils may be prominent.

Treatment

Treatment is usually with surgical drainage, exenteration, and fat obliteration of the involved sinus. Any displaced orbital bone is removed. Appropriate drainage is reestablished between the sinus and the nose. Endoscopic drainage using image guidance has been reported for repair of paranasal sinus mucoceles with orbital bony erosion. In patients with frontoethmoid mucoceles with orbital extension, sinus surgery alone may result in resolution of the orbital symptoms without the need for orbital reconstruction. Mucopyoceles should be treated with broad-spectrum antibiotics prior to treatment. Cultures should be used to guide specific antibiotic therapies.

Prognosis

The prognosis for both life and vision is typically excellent with appropriate therapy. Surgical excision is usually curative, although recurrences have been reported in up to 26% of patients. With long-standing mucoceles, especially those arising in the sphenoid sinus, optic nerve atrophy with permanent visual loss may result.

Colobomatous Cyst

Clinical Pearls

- Colobomatous cysts develop from failure of closure of the embryonic fissure.
- They are often associated with a microphthalmic deformed eye with little visual potential.

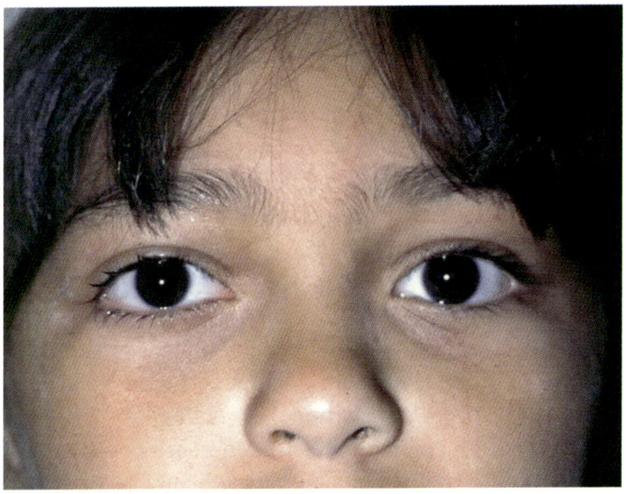

Fig. 56.13 Mild microphthalmos of the right eye with minimal proptosis

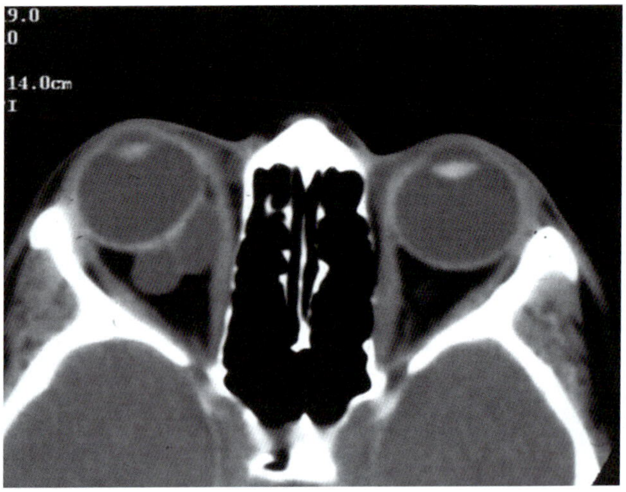

Fig. 56.14 CT scan of the same patient as in Fig. 56.10 showing a colobomatous cyst associated with a microphthalmic eye

- In some cases, the eye is near normal with good vision.
- Treatment is with aspiration of cyst contents or surgical excision with ligation of the pedicle connecting it to the globe or optic nerve.

Colobomatous cyst is a developmental malformation of the globe associated with cyst formation. It results from failure of closure of the embryonic fissure during invagination of the optic vesicle and stalk. It can be seen as an isolated phenomenon or as part of a genetic syndrome. The globe is usually microphthalmic to varying degrees, but is at least 3 mm smaller than the normal eye. The condition may be bilateral in up to 20% of cases. The cyst is inferior in the region of the embryonic fissure.

Clinical Presentation

The patient presents at birth or early thereafter because of the microphthalmic eye. However, the eye can be near normal in size, presenting with proptosis or globe displacement caused by the orbital cyst (Fig. 56.13). The cyst may be palpable through the lower eyelid where it is fluctuant and easily transilluminates. Strabismus may be an associated finding.

Computed Tomography

On CT scan, the globe may be seen to be smaller than normal and may be deformed in shape. A cyst of low attenuation is seen in the inferior orbit in contact with the posterior sclera or distal optic nerve (Fig. 56.14). The bony orbit may be enlarged from mass effect. There is no enhancement of the cyst contents or its enclosing wall.

Magnetic Resonance Imaging

The MRI shows a multilobulated cystic mass in the inferior orbit. The globe may be smaller than normal and may show a deformed contour. On the T1-weighted image, the cyst produces a homogeneous low signal that varies from isointense to hypointense to brain. On the T2-weighted image, the cyst is hyperintense to both brain and fat. There is no enhancement with gadolinium.

Histopathology

The cyst wall is composed of two layers. An inner layer contains primitive neuroretinal tissues that may show some degree of retinal or ciliary epithelial architecture. An outer layer is continuous with sclera and contains connective tissue.

Treatment

Conservative treatment is recommended if the eye is near normal in size and has good visual function. When the cyst is large, aspiration of its contents will result in collapse. While permanent cure has been reported with simple aspiration alone, recurrence is typical. When vision is good, the cyst can sometimes be excised with ligation of the pedicle. However, in the face of a microphthalmic severely deformed eye, enucleation of the eye and cyst may be indicated.

Prognosis

The prognosis depends on the degree of deformity of the eye. If the eye is near normal and vision is good, the prognosis for vision is excellent.

Vascular Lesions

Capillary Hemangioma

Clinical Pearls

- Capillary hemangiomas are congenital hamartomas of small vascular channels.
- They are usually characterized by an initial proliferative phase of rapid growth, followed by gradual involution.

- Clinically capillary hemangiomas tend to enlarge with crying or Valsalva.
- Histologically, they are formed by capillaries lined by plump endothelial cells and separated by fibrous septae.
- Treatment is usually conservative, since most will involute with minimal sequellae.
- When amblyopia is present, intralesional corticosteroids or systemic propranolol may result in reduction in tumor volume.

Capillary hemangiomas are congenital hamartomas of vascular channels. In the orbit, they represent the most common vascular tumors of childhood. They may involve the eyelid skin or deep orbit, but nearly always include an anterior component. Typically, there is a proliferative phase characterized by a period of rapid growth during the first 6–12 months of life. There then usually follows an involutional phase of slow regression seen in 75% of cases by age 7 years.

Clinical Presentation

This lesion presents within 6 weeks of birth in 88% of cases. The remaining cases occur within the first year of life. The most common location is in the upper eyelid and superior orbit, and females are affected more than males. Lesions vary from small, isolated, and clinically insignificant to large and disfiguring masses with visual impairment. When anterior in location, the mass is fluctuant to palpation and reddish in color (Fig. 56.15). About half of cases show enlargement in tumor size on crying or Valsalva. In more than half of cases, ptosis, strabismus, and anisometropia may result in amblyopia.

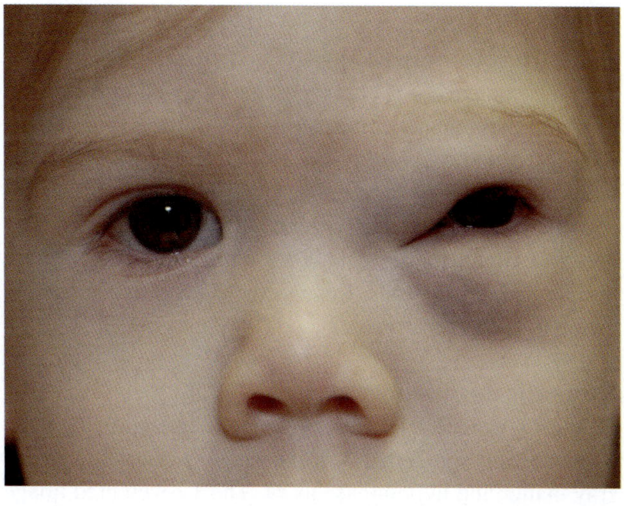

Fig. 56.15 Child with a capillary hemangioma in the anterior inferior orbit

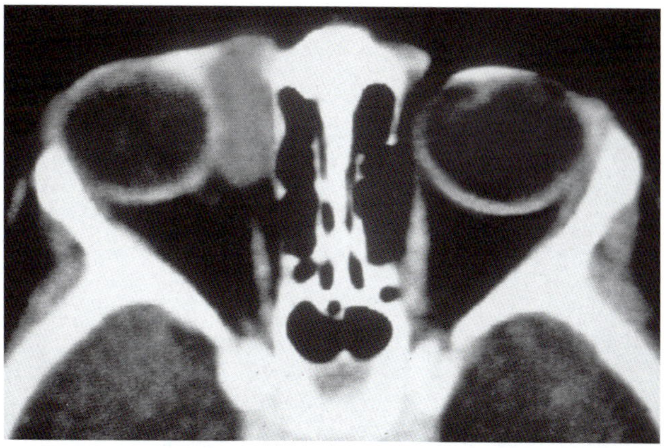

Fig. 56.16 CT scan showing a medium-density capillary hemangioma in the medial anterior orbit

Computed Tomography

On CT scan, orbital capillary hemangioma appears as a well-defined to infiltrating mass. It may be intraconal or extraconal in location and can extend forward into the eyelids (Fig. 56.16). Rarely, these lesions may occur as an intraosseous lesion forming an expansile mass with intact inner and outer tables. With contrast administration, enhancement is moderate to marked.

Magnetic Resonance Imaging

On the T1-weighted image, capillary hemangioma gives a heterogeneous signal, hyperintense to muscle, and hypointense to fat. On T2-weighted sequences, the signal remains heterogeneous with areas of both high and low intensity. Stagnant blood images as hyperintense to fat, whereas blood with a high flow rate produces a signal void that is hypointense to other orbital tissues. With gadolinium, there is diffuse heterogeneous enhancement, best demonstrated with fat suppression algorithms.

Histopathology

Closely packed capillaries lined by plump endothelial cells form lobules that are separated by thin fibrous septa (Fig. 56.17). With involution, the capillaries may be lined by flattened endothelium and assume a cavernous appearance. Tumors with cavernous vessels are often well circumscribed by fibrous connective tissue, making them amenable to resection.

Treatment

In most cases, the appropriate treatment is observation. When lesions are large and causing amblyopia, radiotherapy or intralesional corticosteroids are indicated and generally result in dramatic regression. Corticosteroids appear to reduce vascular flow with transient reduction in tumor volume. For small, localized, and noninfiltrative lesions, surgical excision can be effective. Recombinant interferon

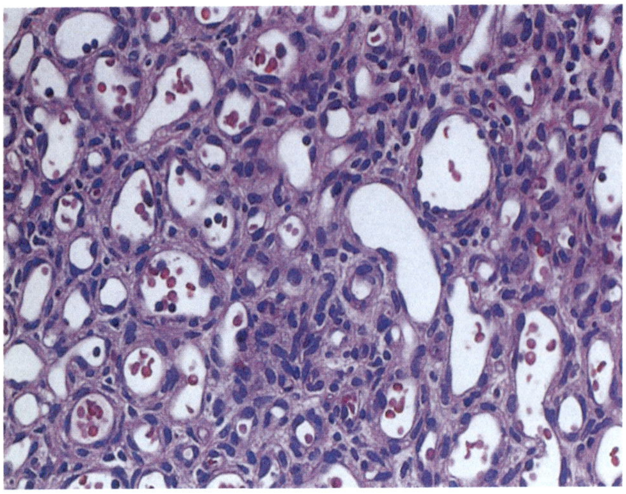

Fig. 56.17 Capillary hemangioma consisting of variably small blood vessels, the smallest lined by plump endothelium

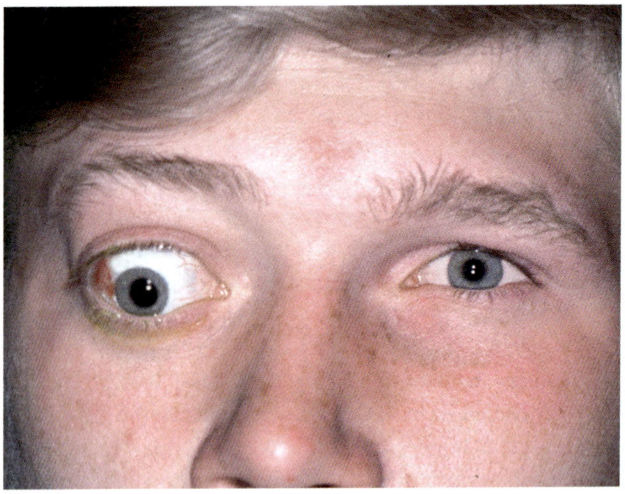

Fig. 56.18 Teenage boy with proptosis and downward displacement of the right

alpha-2 has also been used as an alternative treatment with good results. Interstitial Nd:YAG laser photocoagulation has also been reported to achieve 20–98% reduction in size. More recently, systemic propranolol has been shown to be useful in reducing the size of capillary hemangiomas in the proliferative phase, although its exact mechanism of action is not yet clear. Bradycardia and hypotension are potential complications, and propranolol can mask clinical signs of early cardiac failure from high-output cardiac compromise in infants with large tumors.

Prognosis

Most capillary hemangiomas resolve spontaneously by the age of 7 years. Intralesional corticosteroid injection is effective but can be associated with serious complications from intravascular injection and hemodynamic continuity between the hemangioma and systemic circulation. Local corticosteroids can also cause skin depigmentation. Surgery can result in significant bleeding and cosmetic deformity.

Cavernous Hemangioma

Clinical Pearls

- Cavernous hemangiomas are vascular proliferations composed of large vascular channels.
- They usually present as a slowly progressive orbital mass in young to middle-aged adults.
- Histologically, they are well circumscribed and noninfiltrative.
- When symptomatic, treatment is with complete surgical excision.

The cavernous hemangioma is a benign noninfiltrative, slowly progressive vascular tumor of large endothelial-lined channels. It presents most commonly in early middle-aged adults from 20 to 60 years of age. Females are affected more commonly than males. The most frequent orbital location is intraconal, often lateral to optic nerve. Larger lesions extend into the extraconal space. Rarely, cavernous hemangioma may be intraosseous. Growth occurs by budding of capillary channels into the surrounding interstitium.

Clinical Presentation

The most common symptom is slowly progressive painless proptosis (Fig. 56.18). The usual duration of symptoms prior to presentation is 6 months to 2 years. With large lesions, extraocular muscle restriction and diplopia may be prominent features. Decreased vision can result from induced hyperopia or from optic nerve compression. Gaze-evoked amaurosis has been reported. Lesions are occasionally multiple within one orbit or can be bilateral. Rarely, many tumors can be widely distributed in the head and neck.

Computed Tomography

On CT scan, cavernous hemangioma is a well-defined oval to round, homogeneous mass that has a density somewhat greater than muscle (Fig. 56.19). It is typically located within the intraconal space, but larger lesions extend extraconally. Bone remodeling is seen with large lesions of long duration. Small foci of calcification are sometimes present in long-standing lesions. Enhancement is mild to moderate owing to the generally low blood flow.

Magnetic Resonance Imaging

On the T1-weighted images, cavernous hemangioma gives a homogeneous signal that is isointense to muscle and cortical gray matter and hypointense to fat. The T2-weighted image produces a high signal that is hyperintense to fat and brain. With gadolinium, there is an initial central patchy area of enhancement, with later total homogeneous enhancement.

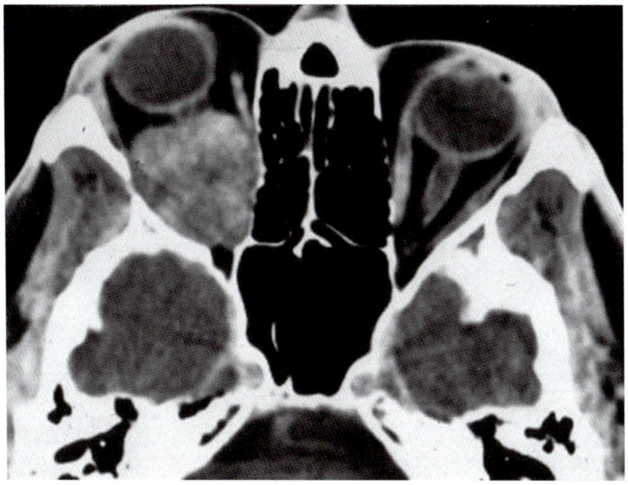

Fig. 56.19 CT scan of the same patient as in Fig. 56.15 showing a large intraconal cavernous hemangioma

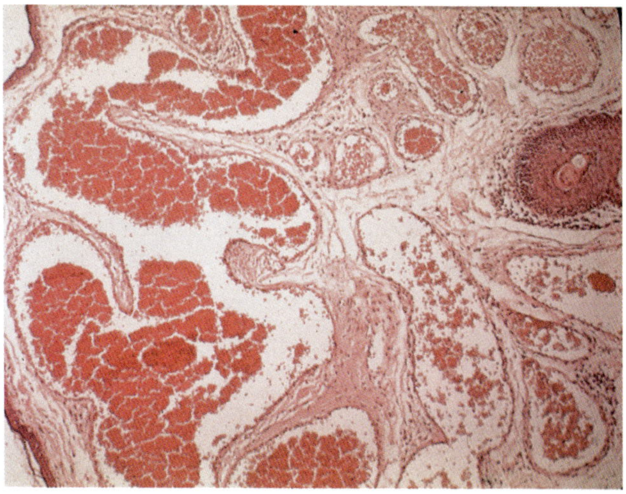

Fig. 56.20 Cavernous hemangioma containing ectatic vascular spaces lined by flattened endothelium and separated by septae containing smooth muscle

Dynamic MRI with rapid infusion of gadolinium shows a point of enhancement initially, followed by diffuse homogeneous enhancement of the entire lesion. The initial point of enhancement represents the connecting point of feeder vessels.

Histopathology

Cavernous hemangiomas are well-circumscribed lesions formed of large, cavernous vascular spaces separated by distinct fibrous connective tissue septae. The vascular spaces are lined by flattened endothelial cells and are surrounded by one to five layers of smooth muscle cells that stain red with Masson's trichrome (Fig. 56.20). The vascular spaces are partly or completely filled with blood. Intravascular thrombosis is common due to stagnant circulation within the tumor. The tumor is circumscribed by a fibrous pseudocapsule through which feeder vessels pass.

Treatment

For symptomatic lesions causing diplopia or visual disturbance, surgical excision is appropriate. Hemangiomas in the anterior two-thirds of the orbit can be removed through an anterior eyelid, transconjunctival, or transcaruncular approach. For deep lesions, a lateral orbitotomy may be required. Apical tumors usually require a craniotomy route. Tumors typically shell out easily, even when large. A cryoprobe facilitates removal with little bleeding. Recent studies have demonstrated the value of stereotactic radiosurgery for symptomatic extraconal cavernous hemangiomas.

Prognosis

The prognosis for vision typically is excellent following surgical removal. Occasionally, visual loss can be a complication of surgery from injury to cilioretinal or central retinal arteries. Recurrence may occur with incomplete excision. Occasionally, recurrences may be multiple and relentless. Relative hyperopia can sometimes persist despite complete excision.

Lymphangioma

Clinical Pearls

- These are congenital lesions of low flow hemodynamically isolated lymphatic channels.
- They typically present with painless proptosis in children.
- Hemorrhagic events often cause an abrupt painful increase in proptosis, with motility disturbance and sometimes decreased vision.
- Treatment is usually conservative, but for loss of vision, hemorrhagic cysts can be drained and bleeding vessels ligated.

Lymphangiomas are lesions of abortive vascular elements that arborize among normal structures. They represent hamartomas of venous-lymphatic channels. Although this lesion is hemodynamically isolated from large-flow vessels of the arteriovenous system, they are prone to intrinsic hemorrhage from small vessels. Such events expand portions of the vascular network into large "chocolate" cysts, leading to clinical urgency. Orbital lesions may be deep or combined with a superficial component. Lymphangiomas present most commonly in children and teens.

Clinical Presentation

Affected children typically present with progressive painless proptosis. Deep lesions may not be clinically apparent until there is a sudden hemorrhage (Fig. 56.21). Such events

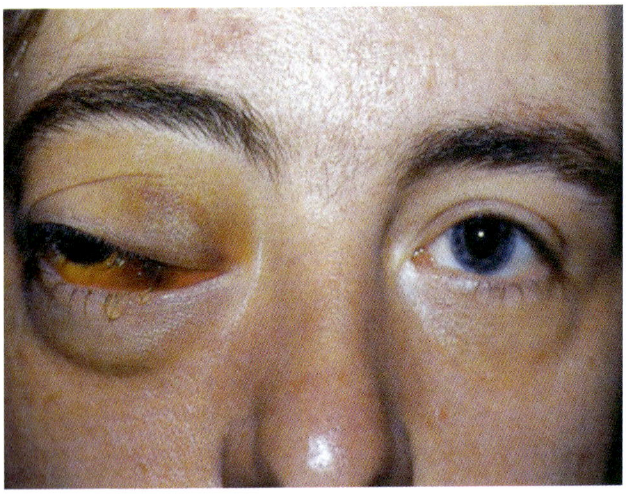

Fig. 56.21 Proptosis and globe displacement of the right eye from an extensive lymphangioma

can be associated with motility impairment or compressive optic neuropathy. Increased intraocular pressure can cause nausea and vomiting, and excessive vagal stimulation can result in bradycardia and somnolence through the oculocardiac reflex. More superficial components of the lymphangioma in the conjunctiva may appear as clear fluid-filled channels and cysts. Periorbital and facial swelling are sometimes associated with upper respiratory infections. Recurrent hemorrhages are seen in about half of cases, and the interval between events may be weeks to decades. Hemorrhagic cysts usually resolve spontaneously, but in some cases will require surgical drainage. Large lesions can extend intracranially resulting in hydrocephalus.

Computed Tomography

The CT scan shows an irregular heterogeneous and poorly defined density that infiltrates among normal orbital structures. Lymphangiomas cross anatomical boundaries such as the orbital septum and fascial layers. Low-density cystic areas are present, and, occasionally, phleboliths may be seen (Fig. 56.22). With contrast administration, enhancement is variable from patchy to diffuse. Larger lesions may extend into adjacent sinuses, into the middle cranial fossa, or through the inferior orbital fissure into the infratemporal fossa.

Magnetic Resonance Imaging

A diffuse infiltrative mass is often seen on MRI and may contain one or more distinct cystic cavities. The T1-weighted image produces a heterogeneous signal that is mildly hyperintense to muscle and hypointense to fat. The T2-weighted image is highly variable with blood cysts generally showing a high signal intensity that is hyperintense to fat. Serpentine zones of signal voids in the orbit represent vessels containing rapidly flowing blood. Within cysts,

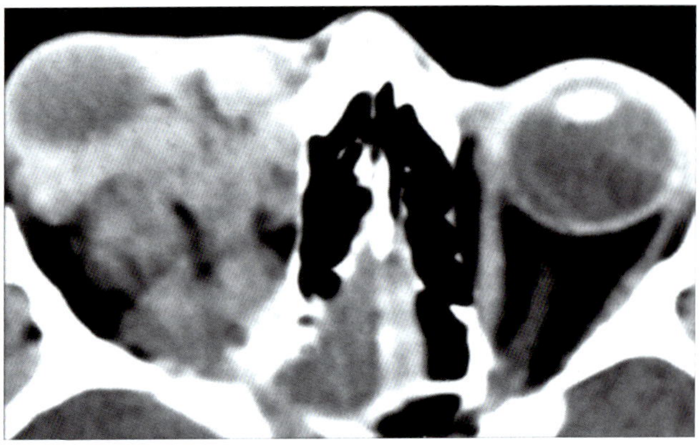

Fig. 56.22 CT scan showing a large medium-density lymphangioma in the right orbit

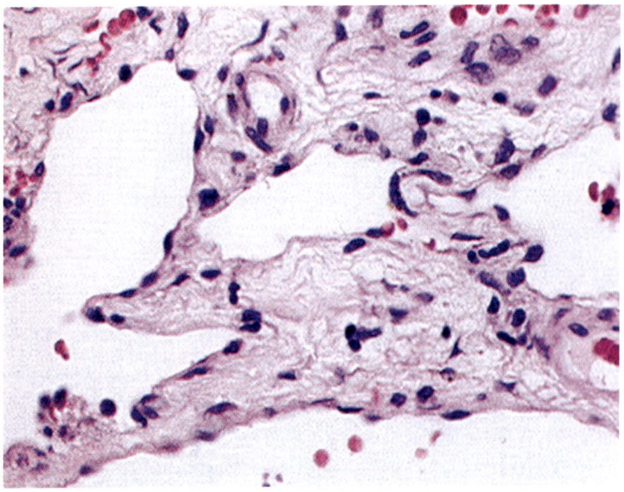

Fig. 56.23 Lymphangioma containing delicate vascular spaces lined by attenuated endothelium and containing proteinaceous material and scant erythrocytes

acute hemorrhage is hypointense to muscle on T1-weighted images; older blood is hyperintense on both T1- and T2-weighted sequences because of the presence of paramagnetic methemoglobin. With further degradation of the blood to ferritin and hemosiderin, low signal intensity is seen on the T1- and T2-weighted images.

Histopathology

Orbital lymphangiomas are infiltrative lesions having wide variation in the size of the lymphatic channels. The channels in a given lesion vary from the size of capillaries to cavernous spaces. Attenuated endothelium resembling that of normal lymphatic vessels lines the channels. The adventitial coat of the lymphatic spaces is inconspicuous in most orbital lymphangiomas (Fig. 56.23). The lymphatic spaces contain proteinaceous (eosinophilic) fluid, but erythrocytes may be present and reflect spontaneous hemorrhage into the tumor. The stroma between lymphatic channels is loose fibrous connective tissue that may contain lymphoid aggregates. Older or reoperated lesions have a fibrotic stroma, often with hemosiderin deposits from prior bleeding. There is a histopathologic continuum between lymphangiomas, varices, and arteriovenous malformations. Immunohistochemistry may assist in identifying lymphatic endothelium.

Treatment

For most cases, conservative observation is the best course of action. Because of the highly infiltrative nature of these lesions, attempted complete surgical excision is hazardous and may lead to significant damage to normal orbital structures. Acute hemorrhagic cysts may require surgical evacuate because of visual dysfunction. Drainage with partial resection of the cyst or ligation of feeding vessels should be the goal rather than any attempt at complete resection. For large visually symptomatic lesions, subtotal resection has been shown to be a feasible modality with good functional and aesthetic results. Intralesional sclerosing therapy has also been shown to be effective in some cases with few orbital complications.

Prognosis

Except for rare cases, complete resection is usually not possible. Recurrent hemorrhages occur in half of cases over many years. Severe amblyopia unresponsive to therapy and disfiguring cosmesis are common sequellae. Relentless orbital bleeding with severe pain may require orbital exenteration for palliation. Poor visual outcome is associated with multiple surgeries.

Varices

Clinical Pearls

- Varices are developmental anomalies of the venous system.
- They present with slowly progressive proptosis, sometimes associated with ophthalmoplegia.
- Acute hemorrhage can be mistaken for a rapidly growing tumor.
- Surgical excision can be difficult, but hemorrhagic cysts can be ligated, or the vascular channels can be embolized.
- Treatment is usually conservative, since most will involute with minimal sequellae.

Orbital varices are dilated venous channels, most commonly involving the superior ophthalmic vein or its tributaries. They are considered to represent one end of the spectrum of developmental venous anomalies that also includes lymphangiomas. Varices are prone to spontaneous hemorrhage and thrombosis formation.

Clinical Presentation

Varices typically present with slowly progressive intermittent proptosis. Ophthalmoplegia and pain are variable findings depending upon the size and location of the varix and on the presence or absence of thrombosis. Lesions often will enlarge with bending forward or with Valsalva (Fig. 56.24). Acute hemorrhage can be mistaken for a rapidly growing tumor. Symptoms frequently are exacerbated by changes in head position, bending forward, or Valsalva maneuver. Optic nerve compression and visual compromise may be associated with larger lesions. Anterior varices are sometimes visible as a vermiform subconjunctival mass. When located at the medial canthus, the cystic varix can mimic dacryocystitis.

Computed Tomography

On CT, dilated varices appear as serpiginous areas of increased density (Fig. 56.25). The vascular channels can be seen to

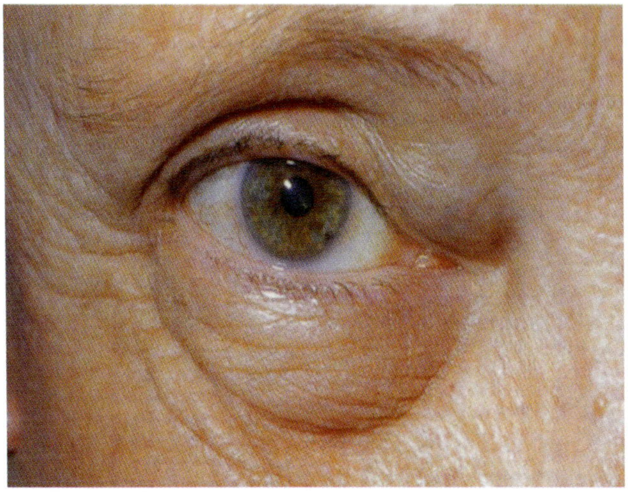

Fig. 56.24 Superomedial orbital varix enlarging with Valsalva

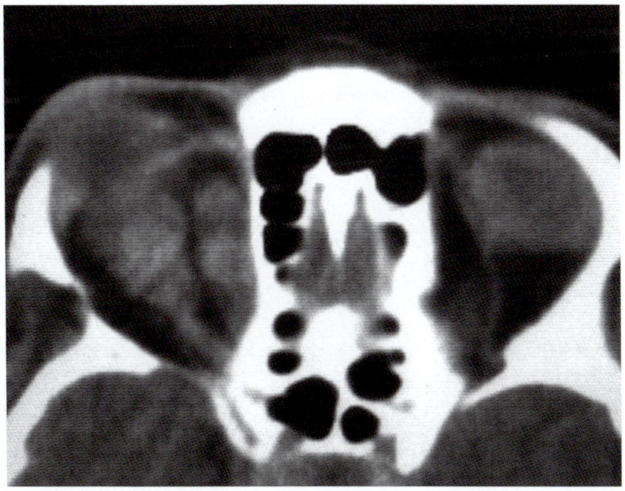

Fig. 56.25 CT scan showing several dilated tubular varices in the right orbit

enlarge with Valsalva maneuver, even in patients without orbital symptoms. With contrast, there is marked patchy enhancement where the vascular channels are patent to blood flow. Regions of thrombus formation and phleboliths do not show enhancement resulting in marked heterogeneity. Expansion of the bony walls can be seen, especially in children.

Magnetic Resonance Imaging

On T1-weighted images, the varix produces a low signal that is isointense to muscle. With Valsalva maneuver, the mass typically shows marked enlargement in size. The signal may be heterogeneous because of the presence of flowing blood, various degradation products of hemoglobin, and thrombus formation. On T2-weighted images, flowing blood produces a dark signal void. Fresh but stagnant blood gives a high signal intensity that is hyperintense to fat. Areas of thrombus formation are variably hypointense to muscle depending upon the presence of hemoglobin degradation products. With gadolinium, enhancement is marked except in areas of thrombus formation where there is little or no enhancement.

Histopathology

A single large vessel may dominate an orbital varix, or there may be multiple ectatic veins. The vessel walls, lined by endothelium, may be thickened and fibrotic, and the lumina may be thrombosed or contain phleboliths resulting from calcification of old thrombus (Fig. 56.26). Thrombi may be recanalized.

Treatment

No treatment is required if symptoms are mild. For more severe orbital symptoms, surgical evacuation of clots and partial excision of ectatic venous channels may be necessary. Dissection can be difficult, and injury to normal orbital structures is a potential risk. Embolization with glue or coils may limit traumatic dissection.

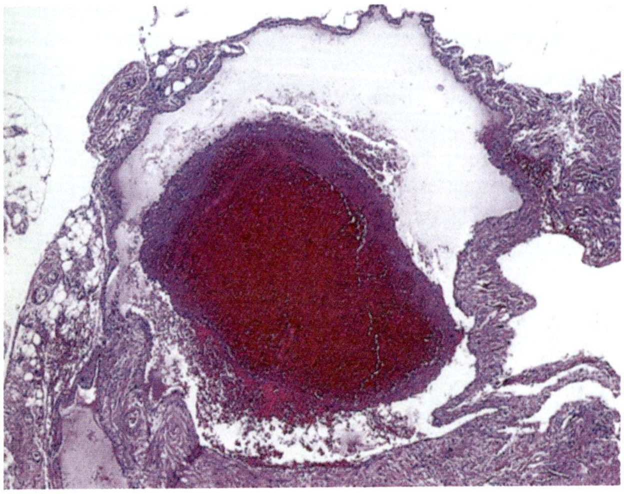

Fig. 56.26 Varix containing ectatic venous channels lined by endothelium and containing thrombus

Prognosis

The prognosis for vision is generally good. With very large lesions, visual loss can result from prolonged optic nerve compression.

Angiosarcoma

Clinical Pearls

- Angiosarcomas are highly malignant vascular tumors arising from endothelial cells.
- Presentation is nonspecific, similar to other orbital tumors with proptosis and ophthalmoplegia.
- Treatment is best with wide surgical excision, with adjunctive radiotherapy and or chemotherapy.
- Prognosis is poor with a high mortality rate.

Angiosarcomas are malignant vascular neoplasms that may originate from endothelial cells of blood vessels. It accounts for 1% of all soft tissue sarcomas, and 50% occur in the head and neck. Orbital tumors have a predilection for males. Presentation is insidious, and symptoms may be delayed until the disease is quite advanced. Eventually, a growing mass is seen with compression of adjacent structures. Proptosis, globe displacement, ptosis, and ophthalmoplegia are common findings. More anterior lesions present as a growing subcutaneous mass with local edema. Even with radical surgery, tumor control is difficult, and the 5-year mortality is about 80%. These tumors have a high rate of local recurrence rate and metastasis because of their intrinsic biologic properties and because they are often misdiagnosed.

Clinical Presentation

These tumors may be localized or diffuse within the orbit. Patients present with progressive proptosis and abaxial displacement of the globe (Fig. 56.27). Upper eyelid ptosis is typical as is reduced ocular motility and diplopia. The rate of lymphatic metastasis is as high as 45% so that regional lymph nodes are frequently enlarged.

Computed Tomography

On CT, angiosarcoma appears as a nonspecific infiltrating soft tissue mass. It is hyperdense with attenuation values similar to that of muscle (Fig. 56.28). With bone involvement, on bone window images, there may be lytic bone lesions. Heterogeneous enhancement varied from minimal to moderate.

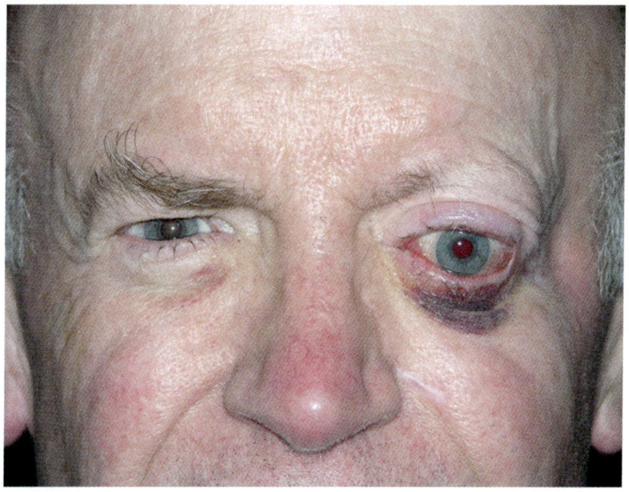

Fig. 56.27 Angiosarcoma of the left orbit with proptosis and eyelid ecchymosis

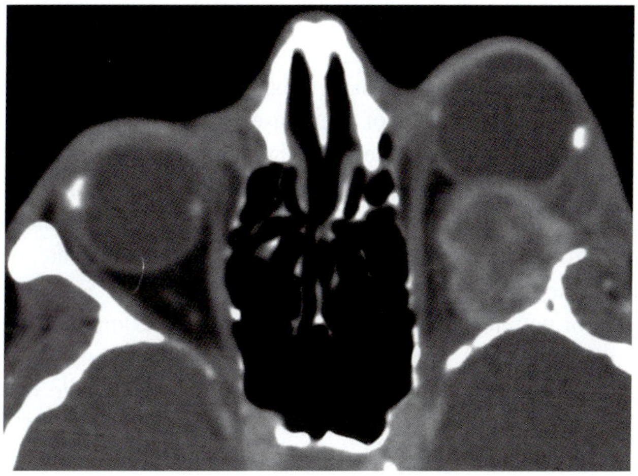

Fig. 56.28 CT scan with a large heterogeneous angiosarcoma in the lateral left orbit

Magnetic Resonance Imaging

The MRI shows an isointense to hypointense signal to muscle and gray brain matter on T1WI. On T2WI, the tumor mass is heterogeneous and hyperintense, with a very bright surrounding signal if vasogenic edema is associated. With gadolinium there is moderate diffuse enhancement. Areas of low signal intensity on both T1 and T2 images suggest organized hemorrhage.

Histopathology

Tumors are composed of atypical endothelial cells lining narrow and ectatic vascular spaces that are separated by fibrous connective tissue. Fronds of endothelial cells may grow into the vessel lumina. Higher-grade lesions are more cellular, with enlarged pleomorphic cells and atypical mitoses. Angiosarcoma may be confused with other vascular tumors of intermediate malignancy, and in its more benign form, it may be confused with hemangiomas. Immunohistochemistry is useful in determining the malignant endothelial component of the tumor.

Treatment

Angiosarcoma is treated with wide surgical resection, often requiring orbital exenteration. Adjunctive radiotherapy of 50–60 Gy has been advocated, but data supporting its efficacy are lacking. Ancillary chemotherapy with doxorubicin or multiple agents prior to surgery may help reduce the size of the tumor.

Prognosis

Angiosarcoma is a high-grade sarcoma that tends to recur locally and spread widely, with a high rate of death and short survival time. Despite aggressive treatment, the prognosis is poor with a 5-year survival rate of less than 20%.

Neural Tumors

Carcinoid

Clinical Pearls

- Carcinoids are slow-growing malignant tumors originating from neuroendocrine cells, most commonly within the gastrointestinal and bronchopulmonary tracts.
- The most common signs of orbital carcinoid include painless proptosis and extraocular motility restriction.
- Associated carcinoid syndrome may include the following symptoms: cutaneous flushing, diarrhea, abdominal cramps, bronchoconstriction, systemic blood pressure fluctuations, light headedness, palpitations, and valvular fibrosis.
- Scintigraphic testing with ^{111}In-DTPA-octreotide has 96% sensitivity in identifying carcinoid tumors and metastasis.
- Surgical treatment depends upon the presence and extent of metastasis.

Carcinoids are slow-growing malignant tumors originating from neuroendocrine cells. The majority of tumors occur within the gastrointestinal and bronchopulmonary tracts, where they are most common in the small intestine (45%), appendix (17%), colon (11%), and bronchus (11%). Other sites include the stomach, lung, trachea, mediastinum, thymus, thyroid, ovaries, testes, liver, and pancreas. Several cases of supposed primary orbital carcinoid have been reported, but these cases are likely to represent metastasis from silent primary carcinoids. Although rare, aggressive and metastatic disease does occur. For tumors larger than 2 cm in size, there is an 80% likelihood of metastasis, while tumors smaller than 1 cm have less than a 2% chance of metastasis. The most frequent sites of metastasis include the lymph nodes, liver, and bone marrow. Orbital metastases have rarely been described, and the majority of them involve the choroid rather than orbital structures. Orbital metastases most often arise from primary ileal carcinoid, while choroidal metastases most often arise from primary bronchial carcinoid. Depending upon the size and location of tumors, patients may present with paraneoplastic carcinoid syndrome. Carcinoid syndrome results from the overproduction of serotonin and vasogenic amines released into the systemic circulation. 5-Hydroxyindoleacetic acid is typically elevated in the urine. This syndrome may include the following symptoms: cutaneous flushing, diarrhea, abdominal cramps, bronchoconstriction, systemic blood pressure fluctuations, light headedness, palpitations, and valvular fibrosis. Symptomatic patients have a 93% rate of metastasis, while incidentally found tumors have only a 9% rate of metastasis. Scintigraphic testing with ^{111}In-DTPA-octreotide has 96% sensitivity in identifying carcinoid tumors and metastasis. Metaiodobenzylguanidine (mIBG) scintigraphy may also be utilized, but has a sensitivity of only 60–70%.

Presentation

The most common signs of orbital carcinoid include painless proptosis and extraocular motility restriction. Metastases often infiltrate extraocular muscles. Decreased vision may result from compressive optic neuropathy. Recurrent and relapsing unilateral orbital and ocular adnexal inflammation may occur. Associated eyelid swelling and ptosis also occurs. Retinal and choroidal vasospasm results from release of vasogenic peptides. Tumors may invade bone and extend in the anterior cranial fossa. Symptoms of headache, seizures, and neurologic deficits may be caused by mass effect from brain metastases.

Computed Tomography

Carcinoid tumors may appear as either well-circumscribed or ill-defined infiltrative masses. Approximately 50% of cases involve an extraocular muscle, and 33% form a discreet mass. The mass is heterogeneous and hypodense to muscle, with peripheral enhancement. Low-density foci of necrosis and high-density calcification may be seen. Bone erosion can result in extension into the intracranial or temporalis fossa.

Magnetic Resonance Imaging

The MRI shows a heterogeneous mass lesion that is usually isointense to hypointense on both T1- and T2-weighted images. With gadolinium, circumferential enhancement is seen. Focal areas of increased T2 signal represent zones of necrosis.

Histopathology

The tumors are composed of nests and trabeculae of small monomorphous, polygonal cells with large, round, hyperchromatic nuclei and scant cytoplasm. The nuclei have a characteristic stippled chromatin pattern. Well-defined connective tissue divides these nests. Malignant changes such as anaplasia, necrosis, and mitoses are rare. Evidence of local invasion and infiltration is evidence of malignancy. Ki-67 labeling can be used to determine the degree of proliferation and possibly tumor behavior. Areas of mucinous differentiation may be present. Midgut carcinoids are more likely to be arranged in nests and are argentaffinic. Foregut carcinoids are more likely to be arranged in nests and are argyrophilic. Electron microscopy demonstrates dense core granules and membrane-bound secretory granules within the cytoplasm. Immunohistochemical staining is generally positive for cytokeratins, CK-7 or CK-20, chromogranin, neuron specific enolase, and serotonin.

Treatment

Treatment of orbital carcinoid tumors is often dictated by the presence and number of metastases. Careful examination and imaging should be performed to assess for presence of a primary or additional metastatic tumors prior to planning a treatment regimen. Symptomatic treatment for carcinoid syndrome may include octreotide, methysergide maleate, or cyproheptadine.

For patients with isolated orbital tumors, complete surgical resection is the only way to achieve a cure. For patients with widely metastatic disease, cytoreductive surgery may result in an improved 5-year survival rate (>70%) and carcinoid symptoms (86%). Patients with isolated orbital or lymph node metastasis and small primary tumors may benefit from complete surgical resection, although cure is unlikely. Mechanical manipulation of carcinoid tumors intraoperatively may result in the release of vasoactive compounds and subsequent systemic hypertension. Adjunctive chemotherapy with interferon alpha or combination cytotoxic regimens has been reported, although efficacy is limited. Adjunctive radiotherapy has been reported but remains controversial. Radiotherapy and chemotherapy modalities are most frequently used for palliative purposes.

Prognosis

The 5-year survival rate for isolated primary tumors may be as high as 95%. The 5-year survival rate for metastatic carcinoid tumors may be as low as 20–41%. Studies suggest that tumor cytoreduction improves the 5-year survival rate significantly.

Malignant Peripheral Nerve Sheath Tumor

Clinical Pearls

- It is seen in patients between 20 and 50 years of age, but occurs earlier in patients with neurofibromatosis.
- It may develop de novo, following radiotherapy, or from a preexisting plexiform neurofibroma.
- Neurofibromatosis is an associated finding in about half of patients with MPNST.
- Progressive gradual proptosis and globe displacement are often followed by rapidly progressing symptoms when a MPNST develops in a preexisting neurofibroma.
- Wide surgical resection is necessary for any attempted cure.
- Progression is typically relentless despite all forms of therapy.

Malignant peripheral nerve sheath tumor (MPNST) is a rare neoplasm of the peripheral nerve sheath. MPNST refers to any malignant tumor that arises from cells of the peripheral or cranial nerve sheath. Malignant neurilemmoma, neurofibrosarcoma, malignant schwannoma, and neurogenic sarcoma are names that have been associated with these tumors in the past. It may develop de novo, following radiotherapy, or from preexisting plexiform neurofibromas. Patients without NF-1 developing MPNST following radiotherapy have an average latent period of 17 years. Neurofibromatosis is an associated finding in about half of patients with MPNST, with an overall incidence of MPNST in 4% of patients with NF-1. This tumor is more common in individuals between 20 and 50 years of age, but in patients with neurofibromatosis, the mean age at presentation is in the second decade. In the orbit, there is a tendency for these tumors to involve the supraorbital nerve, but they may also occur along the oculomotor, abducens, branches of the trigeminal nerves, or autonomic nerve fibers. Progression tends to occur relentlessly, with invasion of the brain and metastasis to cervical lymph nodes and the lungs.

Clinical Presentation

The onset of symptoms is typically slow. Since many patients also have neurofibromatosis, the diagnosis is frequently initially assumed to be neurofibroma or optic nerve glioma. After some years of gradual proptosis and displacement of the globe, symptoms may evolve much more rapidly, heralding malignant transformation. Periorbital pain, regional hypesthesia, ptosis, and vision loss are more common findings (Fig. 56.29). Diplopia, extraocular muscle restriction, keratopathy, papilledema, optic atrophy, and headaches are less common findings. The tumor may extend through the superior orbital fissure to involve the Gasserian ganglion.

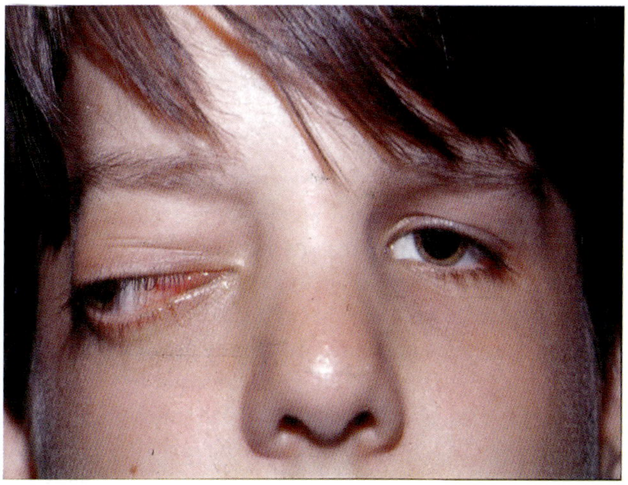

Fig. 56.29 Large malignant peripheral nerve sheath tumor displacing the right globe laterally

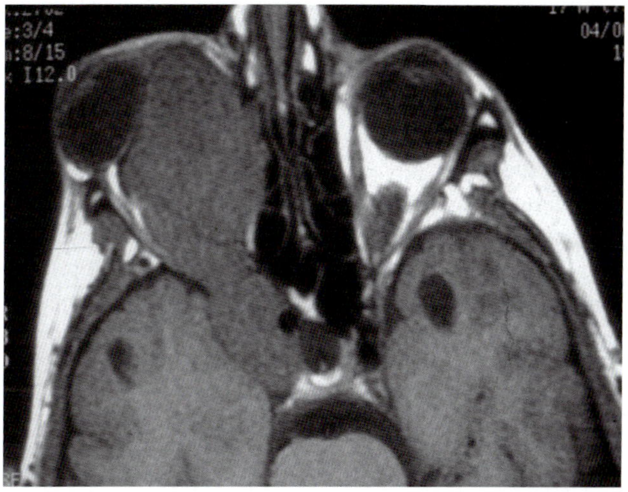

Fig. 56.30 T1-weighted MRI of the same patient as in Fig. 56.29; the MPNST extends into the right cavernous sinus

Computed Tomography

This tumor appears as an irregular nodular or bulbous mass that is usually poorly defined, but may be well demarcated in about 20% of cases. Density is generally low on unenhanced studies. It can be associated with bone destruction or enlargement of the superior orbital fissure. There is a distinct tendency for these tumors to grow along the supraorbital nerve, through the superior orbital fissure to the Gasserian ganglion, and even to the trigeminal rootlets at the pons. Following contrast administration, enhancement is moderate and usually heterogeneous.

Magnetic Resonance Imaging

On T1-weighted images, the tumor produces a heterogeneous signal that is isointense or slightly hyperintense to muscle and hypointense to fat (Fig. 56.30). The T2-weighted sequence yields a variable signal that is hyperintense to both muscle and fat. Atrophy of muscles is seen with large tumors, and orbital fat may be completely replaced. With gadolinium, there is variable heterogeneous enhancement.

Histopathology

Malignant peripheral nerve sheath tumors are often large unencapsulated, fusiform masses that resemble other soft tissue sarcomas. Spindle-shaped cells with hyperchromatic tapered to oval nuclei, prominent nucleoli, and amphophilic cytoplasm are often arranged into densely packed cellular fascicles, loosely packed myxoid zones, nodular aggregates, or whorls (Fig. 56.31). Frequent atypical mitoses, scattered giant tumor cells, and focal necrosis are commonly seen. In contrast to fibrosarcoma, a herringbone pattern is usually not prominent in malignant peripheral nerve sheath tumors. Moreover, the nuclei of malignant peripheral nerve sheath tumors are less elongated, oval, and symmetric than those of fibrosarcomas and are often twisted, wavy, or buckled. Nerve sheath differentiation may be confirmed in paraffin sections using immunostains for S-100 protein, Leu-7, and myelin basic protein. Because MPNST may arise from various cell types composing the peripheral nerve sheath, none of these is entirely specific or present in all tumors. S-100 is positive in 50% of tumors, so the use of a panel of antibodies is recommended. Evaluation by electron microscopy demonstrating long cytoplasmic processes with cells surrounded by basement membrane suggests a Schwann cell or perineural cell origin.

Treatment

Wide surgical margins are necessary for any attempted cure. Because MPNST has a tendency to eventually invade intracranial structures, orbital exenteration is often considered the best treatment option. Multidisciplinary surgical approaches are required for many patients. The tumors tend to be radioresistant, and therefore, radiotherapy is typically utilized only for palliation. Successful use of adjuvant chemotherapy has not been reported. Recurrences are typical, and surgery can stimulate alarmingly rapid regrowth over months or even weeks. In rare cases, recurrence may be seen after years without any symptoms.

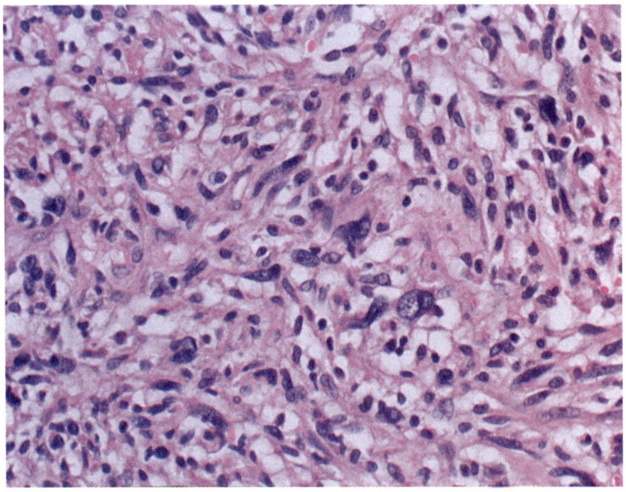

Fig. 56.31 Malignant peripheral nerve sheath tumor containing nerve fibers replete with nodes of Ranvier (*left center bottom*), indicating Schwann cell component and containing pleomorphic cells with enlarged hyperchromatic nuclei

Prognosis

Progression is typically relentless despite all forms of therapy. The prognosis for life is poor, with the 5-year mortality rate exceeding 70%. Recurrence rates for nonorbital tumors are greater than 50%. Metastasis may occur via hematogenous or lymphatic spread. Most patients die from intracranial extension or pulmonary metastases, although metastases have been reported to soft tissues, bones, liver, abdomen, adrenal gland, diaphragm, mediastinum, ovary, and kidney. Survival is better following total resection, but incomplete surgery may accelerate recurrence. Adjuvant chemotherapy and radiotherapy does not appear to improve survival.

Meningocele (Meningoencephalocele)

Clinical Pearls

- A meningocele results from failure in closure of the neural tube or defective basilar ossification.
- The defect usually occurs in the skull midline.
- This typically presents in infancy or childhood as a smooth medial canthal mass.
- CT scan best demonstrates the bony defect that is present.
- Pulsation may be present with lesions of adequate size.
- Reconstruction of the orbital bones varies depending upon the location and size of the defect.

A meningocele results from failure in closure of the neural tube or from defective basilar ossification leading to a bony defect in the skull through which brain and/or meninges herniate. The defect usually occurs in the skull midline and can be seen anywhere from the nose to the occipital bone. If the displaced cerebral tissues lack meninges, it is an encephalocele, and if only meninges herniate through the bony defect, the lesion is a meningocele. Ectopic brain tissue may have the same general appearance as a meningoencephalocele without a direct connection to the brain.

Clinical Presentation

Abnormalities of the anterior cranium, such as the cribriform plate or planum sphenoidale, may result in displacement of cerebral tissue into the orbit, ethmoid sinus, and sphenoid sinus, externally at the bridge of the nose, or between the frontal bones. Anterior meningoceles occur via a defect between the lacrimal and frontal bones. These typically present in infancy or childhood as a smooth medial canthal mass. Posterior meningoceles typically enter the orbit via abnormalities in the optic foramen, superior orbital fissure, or greater wing of sphenoid. Posterior lesions tend to present later than anterior lesions. Patients can present with abaxial proptosis, which varies depending upon the size of the lesion. Pulsation may be present with larger lesions. Dysplasia of the greater wing of sphenoid has been associated with neurofibromatosis. Other rare associations have been made including morning glory syndrome, cryptophthalmia, colobomas, anophthalmia, and microphthalmia.

Computed Tomography

CT scan best demonstrates the bony defect that is present. Three-dimensional reconstruction can be helpful to better assess the nature of the defect. Associated soft tissue elements are not well imaged although a tissue density mass is generally observed projecting through the bony defect. With a meningocele, the mass is of CSF density.

Magnetic Resonance Imaging

MRI is the preferred imaging modality because of its superior soft tissue differentiation. It can demonstrate soft tissue herniation and can distinguish CSF fluid from brain tissue. On T1 and T2 scans, tissue images similar to that of normal brain, but sometimes the herniating tissue is disorganized and images with a more heterogeneous signal. MRI is also useful in the evaluation of associated CNS anomalies such as Chiari malformations in the posterior fossa.

Histopathology

Parenchymal brain tissue, meningeal tissue, or both may be included in these lesions that often contain tortuous ectatic and thick-walled vessels. Chronic changes of meninges may include fibrosis. The ectopic brain tissue, containing visible neurons and glial cells, is often disorganized, and parts of it may be infarcted. Chronic changes to the parenchymal brain tissue may include edema, psammomatous calcifications, or degeneration.

Treatment

A multidisciplinary approach is recommended for surgical management of these lesions. Successful reconstruction of the orbital bones varies depending upon the location and size of the defect. Observation is reasonable for small lesions in patients without significant symptoms.

Prognosis

The prognosis for these lesions depends upon the size and character of the lesion. Smaller lesions generally have a better prognosis.

Neuroblastoma

Clinical Pearls

- Neuroblastoma is the most frequent extracranial solid tumor and the most common tumor metastatic to the orbit in children.
- These tumors represent a malignant neoplasm of neuroblasts derived from primitive neural crest cells.
- Most cases with orbital involvement are metastatic, with 90% originating in the abdomen.
- The child typically presents with rapidly progressive proptosis and periorbital ecchymosis over several weeks.
- The principle treatment is chemotherapy. Radiotherapy may be warranted in some patients.

In children, neuroblastoma is the most frequent extracranial solid tumor and the most common tumor metastatic to the orbit. It represents a malignant neoplasm of neuroblasts derived from primitive neural crest cells, which normally differentiate into sympathetic nerves and ganglia. The tumor usually arises during the first 2 years of life, with the primary tumor located in the adrenal medulla (55%) and the sympathetic or parasympathetic tissues of the abdomen or chest. Most tumors develop before the age of 8, but rare cases in adults have been reported. Most cases with orbital involvement are metastatic, with 90% originating in the abdomen. In 92–97% of cases, the presence of a primary tumor in the chest or abdomen is already known prior to onset of orbital symptoms. In 90% of patients, an increase of catecholamine metabolites can be found in their urine. A variety of scintigraphic studies are often used to determine the presence or extent of metastasis. In very rare instances, neuroblastoma can occur as a primary tumor in the orbit of adults.

Clinical Presentation

Ophthalmic involvement develops in 10–20% of children with neuroblastoma. Symptoms are bilateral in 20–50% of cases. Neuroblastoma metastases typically arise in the marrow of the orbital roof or orbital walls. These tumors are usually extraconal and may be contained by overlying periosteum. Children present with rapidly progressive proptosis and periorbital ecchymosis over several weeks (Fig. 56.32). Eyelid edema, Horner's syndrome, ptosis, and displacement of the globe are also common findings. Horner's syndrome occurs as a result of tumor in the cervical sympathetic chain. Less common findings may include subconjunctival hemorrhage, motility disturbance, and opsoclonus myoclonus. Visual loss may be seen either as an early finding or because of treatment. On funduscopic examination, papilledema, optic atrophy, or dilated retinal vessels may be seen. Increased intracranial pressure and separation of bony sutures are associated with intracranial metastases.

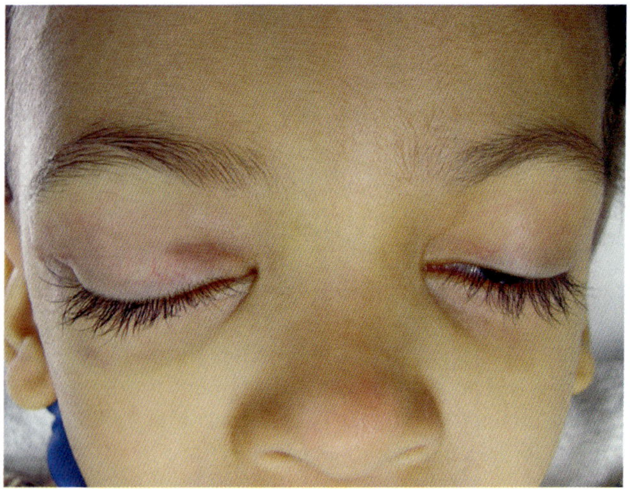

Fig. 56.32 Neuroblastoma of the right orbit associated with eyelid ecchymosis

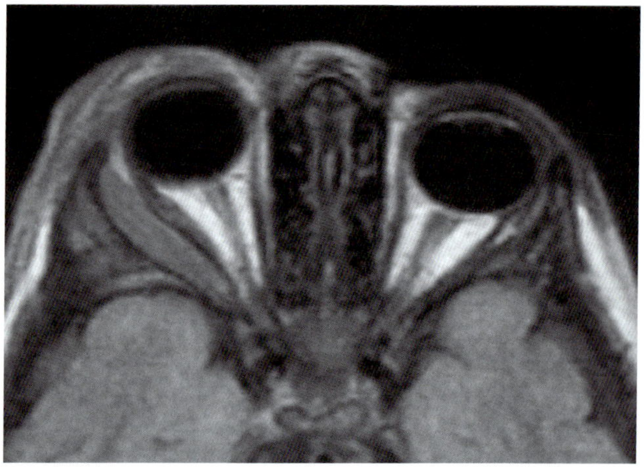

Fig. 56.33 T1-weighted MRI of the same patient as in Fig. 56.32; the neuroblastoma extends along the medial orbital wall

Computed Tomography

On CT scan, neuroblastomas appear as large, irregular, lobulated, and poorly defined orbital masses. They can be unilateral or bilateral. The tumor is hyperdense, but lower attenuating, more lucent areas within the lesion represent sites of tumor necrosis and hemorrhage. Eighty percent of lesions demonstrate stippled calcifications. Spiculated thickening or destruction of adjacent bone is seen on bone window settings.

Magnetic Resonance Imaging

The MRI appearance is of a mass with ill-defined margins from infiltration into adjacent orbital structures such as the extraocular muscles (Fig. 56.33). On the T1-weighted image, the resonance signal is heterogeneous or homogeneous and hypointense to cortical gray matter and muscle. Areas of hemorrhage are hyperintense. The T2-weighted image is isointense or slightly hyperintense to gray matter and muscle. Calcifications appear as signal voids. With gadolinium, heterogeneous enhancement is typically seen.

Histopathology

Most tumors contain small round primitive neuroblasts with hyperchromatic speckled nuclei and scant cytoplasm (Fig. 56.34). Neuroblasts with greater differentiation are often arranged into characteristic Homer-Wright rosettes. Schwann cells are sometimes present within a network of fibrovascular tissue. Well-differentiated tumors may be comprised of ganglion and Schwann cells. Neuron-specific enolase is positive in many of these tumors. Immunohistochemistry studies may be positive for S-100, chromogranin, vasoactive intestinal peptide, gene product 9.5, or synaptophysin.

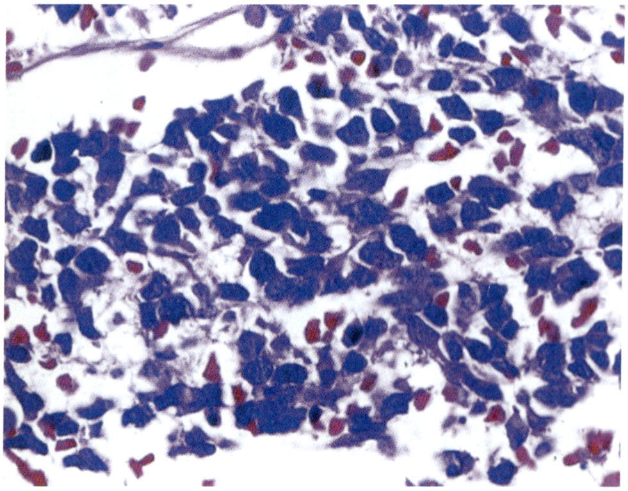

Fig. 56.34 Neuroblastoma consisting of cells with large hyperchromatic nuclei with stippled chromatin and scant cytoplasm

Treatment

The principal treatment is chemotherapy. Combinations of cyclophosphamide, vincristine, doxorubicin, cisplatin, dacarbazine, and teniposide have been employed with a rapid response reported over 4–6 months. Supplemental radiotherapy is recommended at doses ranging from 1000 to 1500 cGy for children less than 1 year old. For children over 4 years of age, up to 4000 cGy is used. Total body radiotherapy with bone marrow transplantation has been advocated.

Prognosis

Most cases have widespread metastasis at presentation. Management of treatment is conducted in coordination with pediatric oncologists. Fifteen to twenty percent of children with orbital neuroblastoma develop visual loss either as a direct consequence of tumor or secondary to treatment. Once orbital metastases develop, the overall prognosis is generally poor. Even with maximal therapy, 90% of patients suffer recurrence over 1–2 years. Despite aggressive treatment with chemotherapy and radiotherapy, the 3-year survival rate is 11%. Prognosis for patients under 1 year of age with disseminated disease is significantly better and may be associated with tumor differentiation.

Optic Pathway Glioma

Clinical Pearls

- Optic pathway gliomas are neoplasms of astrocytic glia called pilocytic astrocytomas.
- About 29% of children with optic pathway gliomas will have neurofibromatosis type 1.
- Clinically, most children show visual loss that tends to stabilize.
- Seventy-six percent of cases involve the optic chiasm, and 24% are confined to the optic nerve.
- Treatment may be conservative if only the optic nerve is involved.
- With progressive posterior extension or invasion of the optic chiasm or hypothalamus, the prognosis diminishes, and treatment is initiated with chemotherapy for younger children and/or radiotherapy for children over 10 years of age.

Optic gliomas are uncommon neoplasms of astrocytic glia located along the visual pathways. They represent 1.5–3.5% of all orbital tumors and 66% of primary optic nerve tumors. Gliomas are seen most commonly in children, with a mean age of 9 years at presentation. Males and females are equally affected. The optic nerve alone is involved in 24% of cases and the chiasm in 76% of cases, and in 46% of patients, invasion of the midbrain or third ventricle is present. About 29% of optic gliomas are seen in the setting of neurofibromatosis. Among children with NF1, optic nerve gliomas may be discovered in 15% (range 2–25%) of cases, most of which may be asymptomatic. Gliomas in children with NF1 tend to have a lower incidence of chiasmal involvement and run a more indolent course. Spontaneous regression has been reported, but is uncommon.

Clinical Presentation

Most children present with slowly progressive decreased vision. More than 55% have visual acuity of 20/300 or worse in the affected eye. Proptosis is frequent with gliomas involving the optic nerve (Fig. 56.35), but is uncommon when the lesion is primarily in the chiasm. Motility disturbance or nystagmus may occur in 25% of cases. Optic atrophy is a typical finding, but one-third of cases present with disc edema. Chiasmal tumors can be associated with increased intracranial pressure and with hypothalamic signs including precocious puberty, diabetes insipidus, and panhypopituitarism. Sudden enlargement of the tumor and resultant rapidly increasing proptosis may result from the hydrophilia of mucoid degenerated stroma within the tumor rather than from cellular proliferation.

Computed Tomography

A normal CT scan in children with neurofibromatosis does not preclude future development of an optic nerve glioma. On CT, the orbital glioma appears as a well-outlined enlargement of the optic nerve that is usually fusiform, but may be more rounded or even multilobulated (Fig. 56.36). Increased tortuosity or kinking of the nerve is a common finding. The tumor is isodense to brain, but typically shows a heterogeneous structure. Less dense cystic spaces correspond to areas of mucinous accumulation. Small high-attenuation

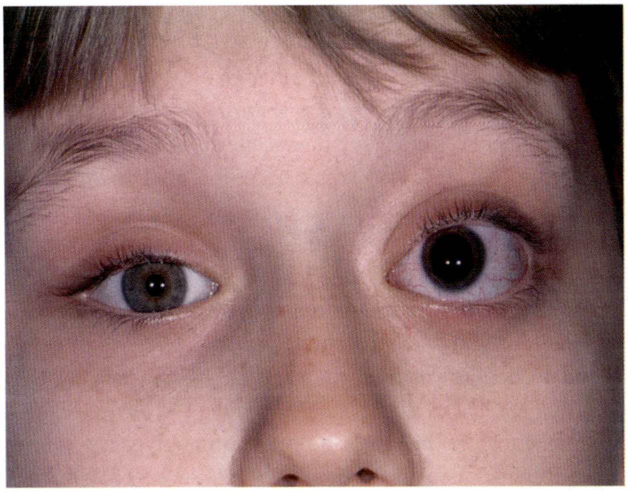

Fig. 56.35 Left optic nerve glioma in a child with proptosis and eyelid retraction

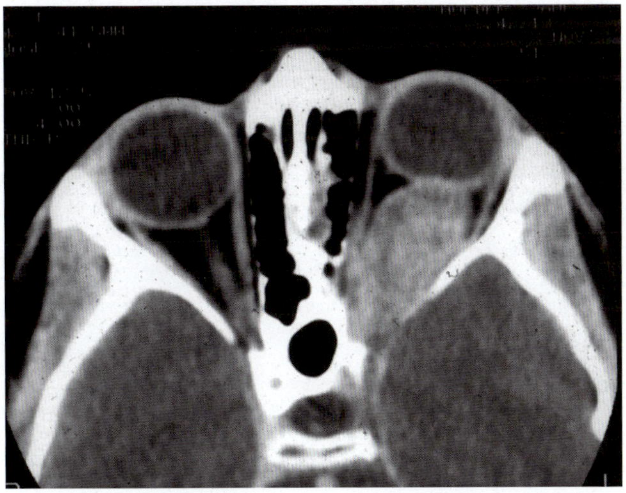

Fig. 56.36 CT scan showing a glioma of the left optic nerve

foci of calcification are rare. Following contrast administration, enhancement is heterogeneous and variable from imperceptible to moderate.

Magnetic Resonance Imaging

On the T1-weighted image, gliomas are isointense or slightly hypointense with respect to cortical gray matter. A dilated subarachnoid space filled with CSF may image as a hypointense zone surrounding the tumor. Low signal hypointense regions within the lesion may represent cystic areas of mucinous degeneration. On T2-weighted images, the signal may be more variable. Small fusiform tumors can be homogeneously hyperintense due to the proton-rich water component and prolonged relaxation time. Larger lesions are usually heterogeneous with a peripheral zone of hyperintense arachnoidal hyperplasia and CSF and a hypointense inner zone of optic nerve and glial cells. There is mild to moderate enhancement with gadolinium, but less than seen with meningiomas.

Histopathology

The histologic picture is that of a benign pilocytic ("hairlike") astrocytoma. Elongated spindle-shaped astrocytes with uniform oval nuclei form wavy intersecting bundles that distend the fibrous pial septa of the optic nerve that contain proliferating meningothelial cells. The astrocytes are cytologically benign, and mitotic figures are absent. In most tumors, there are some astrocytes with spherical (when cut transversely) or cylindrical (when cut longitudinally), swollen cell processes that stain brightly eosinophilic (Rosenthal fibers) that correspond to bundles of glial filaments (Fig. 56.37). There are usually pale cystic areas scattered among the astrocytes that contain hematoxiphilic mucin (glycosaminoglycans) that can be highlighted using histochemical stains such as alcian blue. Mucin may be particularly prominent in long-standing tumors. If the tumor is infiltrated by surrounding proliferating meningothelial cells, then the astrocytes may be interspersed with fibroblasts and meningothelial cells. Though not usually necessary for diagnosis, the astrocytic nature of the neoplasm can be immunohistochemically confirmed in paraffin sections using antibodies against glial fibrillary acidic protein (GFAP). Superficial biopsies of the optic nerve may only contain the reactive meningothelial cells and may lead to an incorrect diagnosis of meningioma.

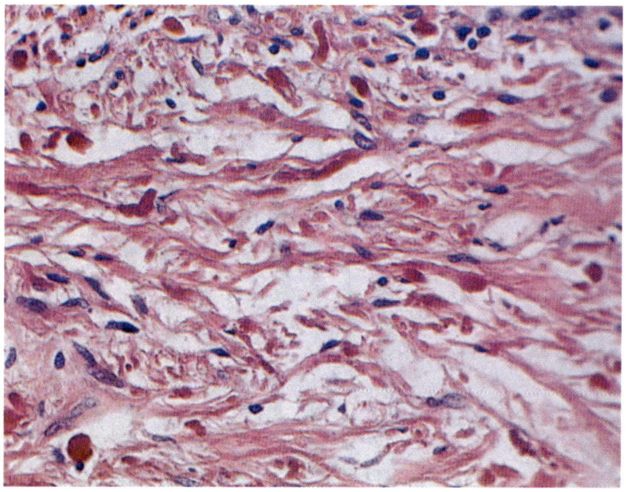

Fig. 56.37 Optic nerve glioma composed of wavy pilocytic astrocytes with small oval to wavy nuclei and cytoplasm containing bundles of intensely eosinophilic glial filaments (Rosenthal fibers)

Treatment

For children with NF1, a baseline exam with neuroimaging is appropriate with annual exams until the age of 8 years. Thereafter, the risk of developing an optic glioma diminishes. For all patients with a documented glioma and lesions confined to the orbit with good vision and minimal proptosis, observation with serial MR imaging is appropriate. With posterior extension, surgical excision should be considered and may be curative. For large chiasmal tumors, surgical debulking followed by adjunctive therapy may delay other CNS complications. Radiotherapy may be effective in advanced cases or where progression is documented, but may cause significant morbidity in young children. This includes endocrine disorders such as growth hormone deficiency, CNS atrophy, and Moyamoya syndrome. Secondary malignancies have been reported in up to 50% of NF1 patients treated with CNS radiotherapy. This is especially significant in children younger than 5–10 years of age. While the optimal role of chemotherapy for optic pathway gliomas has not been determined, multiple agent therapy, such as with vincristine and carboplatin, for chiasmatic or recurrent tumors may shrink the tumor and delay progression, with only mild toxicity. Chemotherapy is now preferable in children younger than 10 years of age in order to delay radiotherapy.

Prognosis

After initial visual deterioration seen in 80% of patients, vision tends to stabilize. In 26% of cases, vision remains better than 20/40, and in 45%, better than 20/200. Radiotherapy for chiasmal tumors is associated with multiple endocrinologic deficiencies in younger children. For orbital lesions, prognosis for life is excellent with mortality less than 5%. With chiasmal involvement, mortality is 20%. Midbrain invasion carries a 55% mortality rate over 10 years.

Optic Nerve Sheath Meningioma

Clinical Pearls

- Optic nerve sheath meningiomas are neoplasms arising from meningothelial cap cells of arachnoid tissue surrounding the optic nerve.

- Meningiomas are seen most commonly in middle-aged individuals between 30 and 50 years old.
- Patients most commonly present with painless, progressive gradual visual loss and visual field disturbance over years.
- The classic triad of optic atrophy, visual loss, and optociliary shunt vessels is present in only a minority of patients.
- "Tram-tracking" is often evident on axial views, while the "doughnut" or "ring" sign is evident on coronal views.
- Close observation is appropriate if the patient has no significant visual dysfunction, progressive visual loss, or intracranial tumor spread.
- Surgical resection of ONSM is warranted in patients with aggressive intracranial extension, extension near the contralateral optic nerve, or blindness with disfiguring proptosis.
- Both conventional and stereotactic radiotherapy have been demonstrated to result in tumor control or stabilization.

Optic nerve sheath meningiomas (ONSM) are neoplasms arising from meningothelial cap cells of arachnoid tissue surrounding the optic nerve. True ONSM extend between the arachnoid and dural sheaths, ultimately compromising optic nerve blood supply and axonal transport. Secondary ONSM arise intracranially near the planum sphenoidale and spread into this space. Rare extension and infiltration of orbital fat, extraocular muscles, and bone may occur. ONSM represent between 1% and 2% of orbital tumors and 33% of optic nerve tumors. Optic nerve sheath meningiomas occur anywhere along the orbital optic nerve. For primary ONSM, 92% arise from the intraorbital nerve sheath, 8% are intracanalicular, and 15% may extend intracranially. Of the 5% of patients with bilateral tumors, 65% are intracanalicular. Meningiomas are seen most commonly in middle-aged individuals between 30 and 50 years old, with a mean of 41 years. Four to seven percent of ONSM occur within the pediatric population, where they are more aggressive, more likely to recur, and more likely to be bilateral and to extend intracranially. Females are affected more frequently than males in a ratio of 3:2. In 9% of tumors, an association with neurofibromatosis is found.

Clinical Presentation

The classic triad of optic atrophy, visual loss, and optociliary shunt vessels is present in only a minority of patients. Patients most commonly present with painless, progressive visual loss and visual field disturbance over years (Fig. 56.38). Initially visual impairment is usually mild, with half of patients presenting with 20/60 acuity or better. Decreased visual acuity, dyschromatopsia, scotomas, and

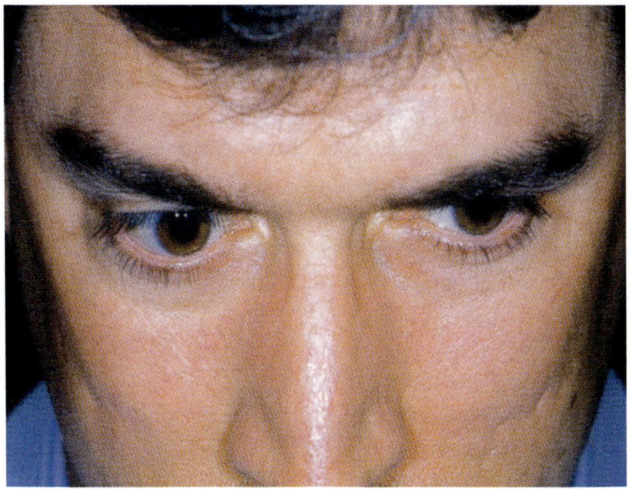

Fig. 56.38 Right optic nerve sheath meningioma with mild proptosis of the right eye

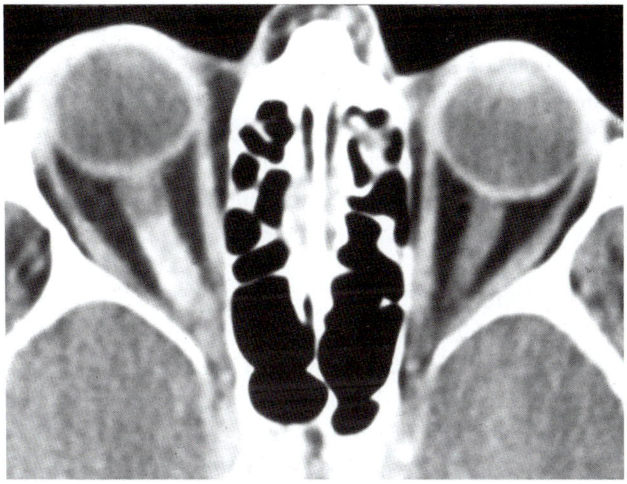

Fig. 56.39 CT scan showing thickening and enhancement of the right optic nerve sheath from a meningioma

visual field defects usually develop over time. Transient visual obscurations are common and often gaze-evoked. Mild to moderate painless axial proptosis usually follows early visual loss and progresses slowly. Compressive optic neuropathy as evidenced by optic atrophy, papilledema, or relative afferent pupillary defects can be demonstrated in almost all patients. Optociliary shunt vessels are reported in 30% of cases. Patients may also present with ocular motility restriction, headaches, or orbital pain. In bilateral cases, involvement of the two eyes is generally separated by several years.

Computed Tomography

The optic nerve typically shows a smooth tubular enlargement (Fig. 56.39). Less commonly, the meningioma may be fusiform in shape or globular when it breaks through the dura. The lesion is isodense to cortical gray matter and may show high-attenuation foci of calcification in 20–50% of cases. Contrast administration produces marked homogeneous enhancement of the tumor, often with a linear central zone of lower density representing the optic nerve (tram-tracking sign). Expansion of the bony orbital walls is seen with very large, long-standing tumors. Somatostatin receptor scintigraphy, with 100% sensitivity and 97% specificity at a threshold uptake ratio of 5.9, can be helpful in further classifying these tumors.

Magnetic Resonance Imaging

On the T1-weighted image, meningiomas generally produce an isointense signal with respect to normal optic nerve and cortical gray matter. "Tram-tracking" is often evident on axial views, while the "doughnut" or "ring" sign is evident on coronal views. The T2-weighted image is heterogeneous and variable from slightly hypointense to slightly hyperintense to gray matter. The hypointense areas reflect foci of calcium, and the hyperintense regions may correspond to collections of CSF that sometimes form perineural cysts. The postgadolinium T1-weighted image shows marked enhancement of the tumor surrounding an optic nerve of lower signal intensity. This is best distinguished on fat suppression sequences. Subtle intracranial extension may only be visible on the contrasted image.

Histopathology

Biopsies should include adequate dural sheath and subdural tissue without violating the nerve. Care should be taken to avoid mischaracterization of tumors as meningiomas due to the presence of meningeal hyperplasia, which is often present within optic nerve gliomas. Meningiomas of the optic nerve are usually of the meningothelial type, with distinctive small nests of tumor cells having a whorled pattern (Fig. 56.40). The tumor cells have round to oval nuclei, with inconspicuous or unapparent nucleoli, moderate amounts of lightly eosinophilic cytoplasm, and indistinct cell borders. Intranuclear vacuoles, resulting from cytoplasmic invagination, are a characteristic feature of the meningothelial cells. Mitoses are rare. Psammomatoid meningiomas contain psammoma bodies (laminated calcified concretions that are deeply basophilic) of variable frequencies that develop from hyalinization and deposition of calcium within tumor cells forming whorls. On rare occasions, meningiomas of the optic nerve may appear fibroblastic ("fibroblastic meningioma") or may be a combination of fibroblastic and meningothelial types ("transitional meningioma").

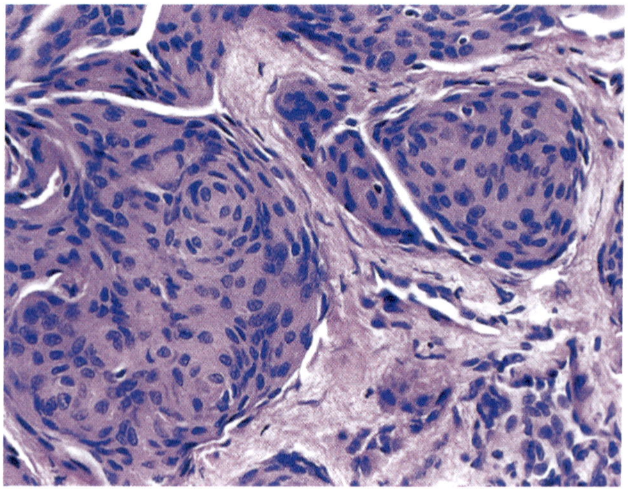

Fig. 56.40 Optic nerve sheath meningioma containing tumor nests composed of whorls of cells with bland nuclei

Treatment

Close observation of ONSM with serial examination and MR imaging is appropriate if the patient has no significant visual dysfunction, progressive visual loss, or intracranial tumor spread. Surgical resection of ONSM is warranted in patients with aggressive intracranial extension, extension near the contralateral optic nerve, or blindness with disfiguring proptosis. In patients with significant proptosis and intraocular invasion, exenteration may be considered. Even with some vision, surgical excision should be considered for lesions that approach the optic canal because of the small chance of spread to the opposite optic nerve. Surgical excision of ONSM usually results in postoperative blindness (78%), ophthalmoparesis, and ptosis. Only 5% of patients show an improvement of visual acuity following surgical resection, with most being small anterior tumors. Although patients often have improved visual acuity following optic nerve sheath fenestration, the improvement tends to be temporary due to the continued tumor growth. Because of this, the use of optic nerve sheath fenestration has only been advocated when followed by radiotherapy. Both conventional and stereotactic radiotherapy have been demonstrated to result in tumor control or stabilization in most patients and improvement of visual acuity (54–86%), diplopia, and proptosis. Patients treated with conventional radiotherapy have been reported to develop radiation retinopathy, retinal vascular occlusion, persistent iritis, and temporal lobe atrophy. Stereotactic fractionated radiotherapy delivers radiation in a more focused manner than conventional fractionated radiation therapy, although radiation-related optic neuropathy, dry eye, iritis, cataracts, pituitary dysfunction, and small vessel ischemic disease can still develop following this treatment. Radiotherapy may be the most appropriate option for patients with progressive or advanced disease.

Prognosis

The prognosis for life is excellent, as no patient has been reported to die directly from an optic nerve sheath meningioma. The outlook for vision is poor, with relentless progression to blindness over many years. Timely surgical intervention of selected meningiomas can achieve stability or even improve vision. The WHO classifies tumors as benign, atypical, and malignant, with recurrence rates of 7%, 35%, and 73%, respectively.

Plexiform Neurofibroma

Clinical Pearls

- Plexiform neurofibromas are the most common benign peripheral nerve tumors occurring in the eyelid and orbit.
- Plexiform neurofibromas have been considered pathognomonic for neurofibromatosis.
- These tumors typically present in children during the first decade of life.
- Most often involves sensory nerves in the superior orbit and eyelid.
- Thickened nerve bundles have been described as a "bag of worms."
- On CT, hypodense tubular masses are seen branching and extending through orbital tissues.
- The tumors are infiltrative, making complete excision difficult.
- Recurrences are frequent.

The plexiform neurofibroma represents 1–2% of all orbital tumors. It is the most common benign peripheral nerve tumor occurring in the eyelid and orbit. Historically, plexiform neurofibromas have been considered pathognomonic for neurofibromatosis, although several cases without associated neurofibromatosis have been reported. The lesion arises from and grows as an expansion of any peripheral nerve, but in the orbit, it most often involves sensory cranial nerves in the superior orbit and eyelid. Plexiform neurofibromas typically present in children during the first decade of life, with one-third involving the eyelids. It may be associated with widening of the superior orbital fissure or defects in the greater sphenoid wing.

Clinical Presentation

When the eyelid is involved, it has a characteristic S-shape due to thickening and horizontal redundancy and to proliferation of connective tissue in response to the tumor (Fig. 56.41). On palpation the tortuous, interwoven, and thickened nerve bundles have been described as a "bag of worms." Mechanical ptosis can be profound and, in younger children, may result in deprivation amblyopia. Tumors involving branches of the trigeminal nerves may result in sensory deficits, neuralgias, paresthesias, and decreased corneal sensation. Increased levels of ankyrin G may result in hyperexcitable axonal membranes and increased pain. With orbital tumors, the globe can be proptotic or enophthalmic depending upon the presence of the greater sphenoid wing and the degree of bony expansion of the orbit. With large defects in the sphenoid bone, pulsatile exophthalmos may be present. Orbital lesions have been associated with uveal neurofibromas (50%), iris (Lisch) nodules (77%), prominent corneal nerves (25%), or optic nerve gliomas (10–15%).

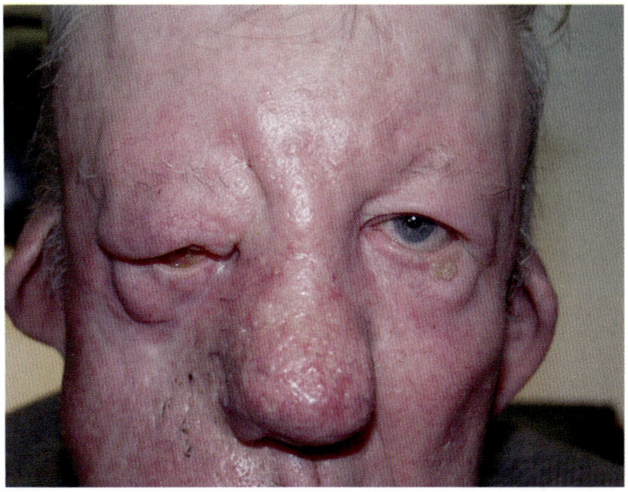

Fig. 56.41 Plexiform neurofibromatosis involving the right eyelids and face

Computed Tomography

On CT, the plexiform neurofibroma appears as a moderately dense, irregular, diffuse mass that crosses multiple tissue planes. Hypodense tubular masses are seen branching and extending through the tissues. There is thickening of eyelids and periorbital soft tissues, increased density of intraconal fat which may be due to tumor involvement of small intraconal nerves, irregular nodular thickening of optic nerve sheath from tumor involving the posterior ciliary nerves, and thickening of sclera or choroid from tumor within these structures. The tumor infiltrates normal orbital structures and may be inseparable from extraocular muscles. Involvement of cranial nerves III, IV, V, and VI has been reported. The orbital contour and superior orbital fissure are frequently enlarged. Tumors may extend into the cavernous sinus, nasopharynx, or pterygomaxillary fissure. When large regions of the sphenoid bone are absent, a meningoencephalocele may prolapse into the obit. With contrast administration, the tumor shows moderate enhancement.

Magnetic Resonance Imaging

On MRI, plexiform neurofibromas appear as an ill-defined irregular mass resulting from multiple thickened nerves within the orbit or eyelid. On T1-weighted images, the tumor produces a heterogeneous, hypointense to isointense

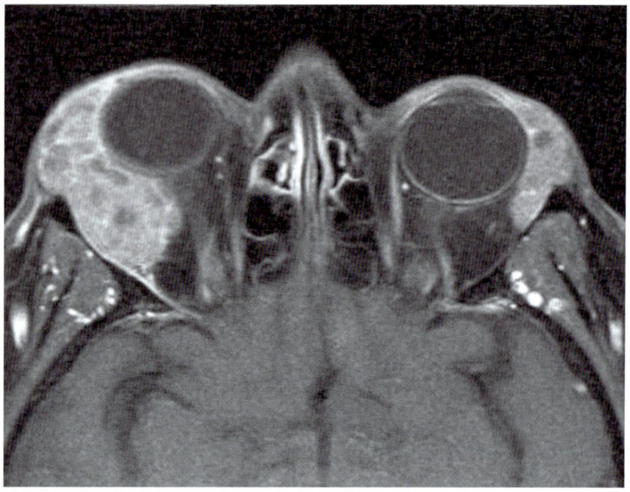

Fig. 56.42 T1-weighted MRI showing a heterogeneously hyperintense mass in the right and left eyelids

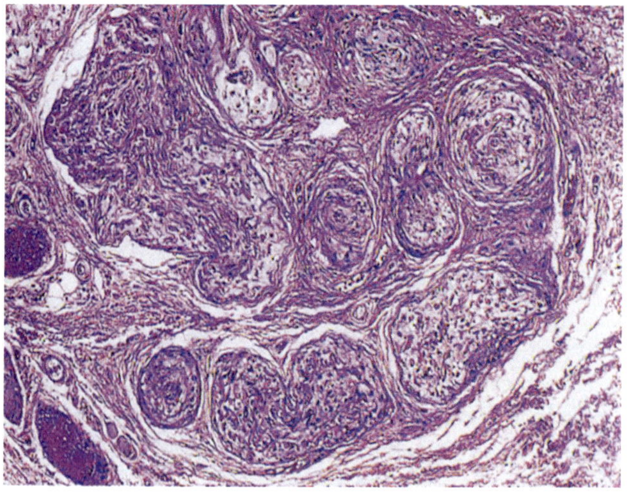

Fig. 56.43 Plexiform neurofibroma containing expanded nerve fascicles composed of variable numbers of neurites, Schwann cells, and fibroblasts in a myxoid matrix richly supplied with blood vessels

signal with respect to muscle (Fig. 56.42). Signal intensity is increased on T2-weighted sequences where the tumor is hyperintense to muscle and isointense or slightly hyperintense to fat. It is best demonstrated using STIR T2 fat suppression techniques. A target-like appearance has been seen in some deep plexiform neurofibromas caused by darker central nerve fibers surrounded peripherally by brighter myxoid matrix. With gadolinium, enhancement is variable from mild to moderate.

Histopathology

In plexiform neurofibromas, large fascicles of peripheral nerve become convoluted and appear like a "bag of worms" macroscopically. Microscopically, there is a tortuous mass of expanded nerve branches, containing all of the cell types normally found in peripheral nerve – nerve cells, perineural cells, Schwann cells, and fibroblasts (Fig. 56.43). Proliferated nerve bundles may be enlarged by endoneural accumulation of myxoid (glycosaminoglycan-rich) matrix. As the lesions age, Schwann cells proliferate, and fibroblast-derived collagen accumulates within the nerves. There is usually a rich plexus of thin-walled blood vessels intermixed with the neural proliferation. Immunohistochemical analysis, including S-100 positivity, can be utilized to identify these tumors.

Treatment

Management is usually frustrating and disappointing because of the infiltrative nature and vascularity of this tumor. Neurofibromas often arise along nerve trunks, resulting in entrapment of nerve fibers within the tumor, making it impossible to separate the tumor from the nerve. Multidisciplinary approaches are often required for adequate tumor resection and preservation of important neural structures. Recurrences are typical, resulting from subtotally resected tumors. Repeated surgical debulking may be necessary to maintain visual function and for some cosmetic improvement. In cases of severe proptosis and orbital pain, exenteration may be considered. Plans for reconstruction should be considered during surgical planning. The role of radiotherapy and radiosurgery is limited.

Prognosis

The overall prognosis for life is good. Rarely, the tumor can erode into the cranial cavity with fatal results, and patients with neurofibromatosis carry a significant risk of secondary malignant tumors including malignant peripheral nerve sheath tumors. The prognosis for vision depends upon the extent of tumor invasion as well as the potential complications of surgical intervention.

Schwannoma (Neurilemoma)

Clinical Pearls

- Schwannomas are benign tumors arising for peripheral nerve sheaths.
- They are most common in young to middle-aged adults.
- They are slow growing, presenting with proptosis and abaxial displacement of the globe.
- Treatment is with surgical excision.
- Prognosis is excellent and recurrences are uncommon.

The schwannoma is a benign tumor of nerve sheaths, arising from Schwann cells of neural crest origin. These benign tumors are well encapsulated, occurring most frequently within the superior orbit along the supraorbital and supratrochlear nerves. These tumors may occur both intra- and extraconally within the orbit and have been reported to occur within the conjunctiva, extraocular muscles, paranasal sinuses, lacrimal gland fossa, and the eyelids. Schwannomas account for 1–6.5% of all orbital tumors and 35–61% of

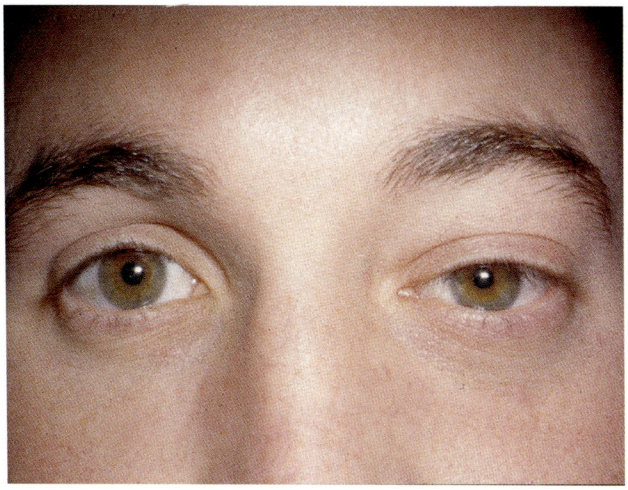

Fig. 56.44 Right orbital schwannoma with proptosis

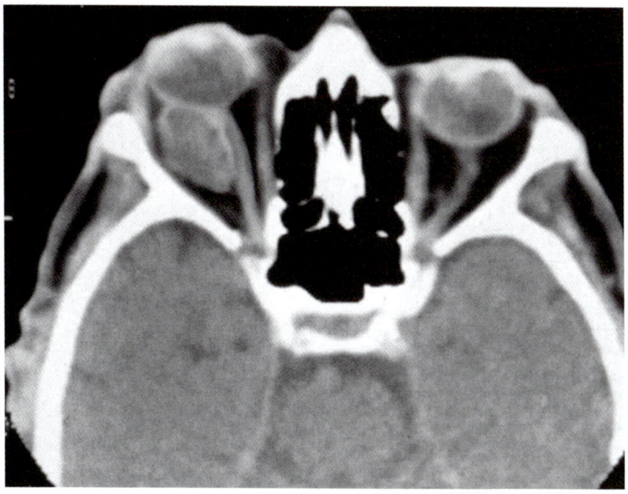

Fig. 56.45 CT scan showing a fusiform schwannoma in the right lateral orbit

peripheral nerve lesions within the orbit in large tumor series. They occur most frequently in patients between 20 and 60 years of age. Ten to eighteen percent of cases are associated with neurofibromatosis. Schwannomas rarely undergo malignant transformation.

Clinical Presentation

Schwannomas typically present as insidious, slow-growing lesions. They most commonly present with painless proptosis, eyelid edema, and globe displacement. The majority of lesions occur in the superior orbit or within the muscle cone so that the globe is usually displaced forward or downward (Fig. 56.44). Isolated motility disturbance can be seen with involvement of the third, fourth, or sixth cranial nerves and from tumors involving the cavernous sinus. Tumors adjacent to or arising within extraocular muscles also cause motility restriction. Larger tumors may cause globe indentation, choroidal folds, and optic nerve edema and atrophy, which are frequently associated with visual acuity and visual field loss. Very rarely, large tumors may extend from the orbit to the paranasal sinus and anterior cranial fossa.

Computed Tomography

On CT scan, orbital lesions appear as a smoothly contoured, sharply defined dense mass, usually in the superior orbit. Schwannomas are ovoid, elongated, or fusiform in shape, aligned anteroposteriorly along the involved nerve (Fig. 56.45). Areas of mucinous cystic degeneration are seen as darker, low attenuating regions that can coalesce causing the tumor to mimic the appearance of an inclusion cyst. The cystic areas are thought to form as the result of cellular necrosis, hemorrhagic debris, and hyaline degeneration of blood vessels within the tumor causing vascular thromobosis and hemorrhage. Foci of calcification are occasionally seen in larger tumors. Adjacent bone can be thinned and remodeled. The epicenter can arise in a paranasal sinus with secondary extension into the orbit. Pleomorphic adenoma should be considered in the differential diagnosis of tumors occurring within the lacrimal gland fossa. Lesions arising from the intracranial trigeminal nerve or ganglion may be contiguous with the orbit through the superior orbital fissure. Cranial foramina can be enlarged from intracranial schwannomas extending anteriorly. Contrast administration typically shows moderate enhancement but can be marked in some cases.

Magnetic Resonance Imaging

MRI shows a well-circumscribed, elongated, fusiform, or oval mass with heterogeneous signal intensity. On T1-weighted images, the more cellular portions of the tumor produce an isointense or slightly hyperintense signal compared to muscle. Mucinous regions are hyperintense to muscle and hypointense to fat. Areas of cystic degeneration give low signals, isointense or hypointense to muscle, and do not enhance with contrast. On T2-weighted sequences, the cellular zones appear slightly hyperintense to muscle and fat, while the more mucinous regions are markedly hyperintense to fat. Antoni A portions of the tumor consist of densely packed Schwann cells that appear darker on T2-weighted images. Antoni B regions are more loosely packed with mucinous degeneration that images with higher signal intensity. Loss of the usual signal void around the orbit suggests thinning or erosion of bone. Calcification and intralesional hemorrhage is not common but can be seen in some cases. With gadolinium, enhancement is moderate to marked, more so in mucinous areas.

Histopathology

Schwannomas are encapsulated masses with distinctive patterns of Antoni A and B areas. Antoni A areas are solid cellular regions with fascicles of fusiform cells having twisted nuclei and indistinct cell borders (Fig. 56.46). Highly differentiated Antoni A areas may exhibit cellular palisad-

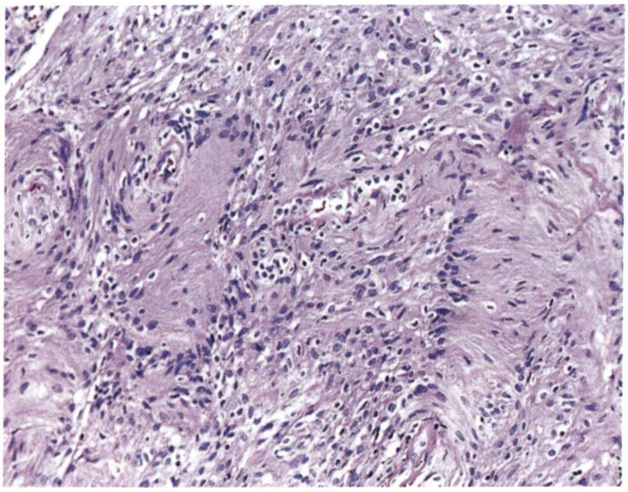

Fig. 56.46 Schwannoma (neurilemmoma) containing palisades of Schwann cells forming Verocay bodies and areas of mucinous degeneration

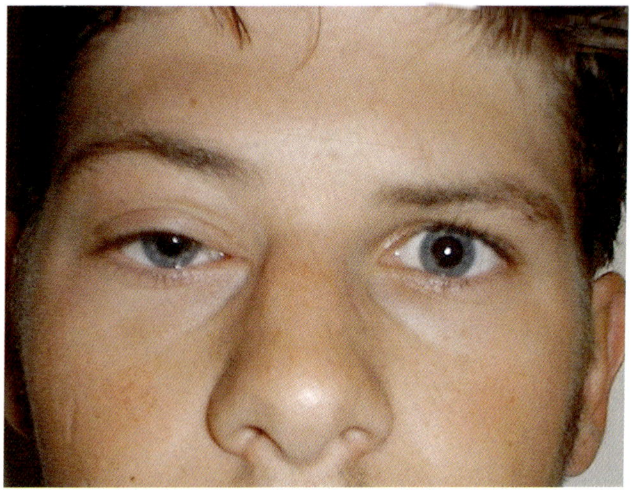

Fig. 56.47 Solitary neurofibroma in the right superior orbit, displacing the globe downward

ing known as Verocay bodies, formed by rows of aligned nuclei separated by fibrillar cytoplasmic processes. Antoni B areas are loose mucinous regions that are less cellular and less orderly than the Antoni A areas. Microcysts are frequently encountered in the Antoni B domains. Macrophages, hemorrhage, and calcifications are occasionally present. On immunohistochemical analysis, the tumors are strongly positive for S-100. Malignant schwannomas fall in the spectrum of malignant peripheral nerve sheath tumors.

Treatment

These tumors progressively grow, and surgical excision is indicated for symptomatic lesions. The tumor can sometimes be stripped off its nerve of origin with preservation of function. Multidisciplinary approaches are often required for complete surgical resection. Schwannomas are relatively radioresistant, offering little benefit from this treatment. Recurrences are rare for benign tumors, but occur frequently following resection of malignant schwannomas.

Prognosis

The prognosis for life is excellent, and recurrences are rare, even after partial excision. With larger, long-standing tumors, permanent visual loss may result from optic nerve compression.

Solitary Neurofibroma

Clinical Pearls

- Solitary neurofibromas result from a nonhereditary proliferation of Schwann cells derived from the neural crest.
- Only 10–28% of patients have clinical signs or a family history of neurofibromatosis.
- Tumors are more commonly seen in middle-aged adults, between 20 and 60 years old within the superior orbit.
- The major clinical symptom is mild, slowly progressive, painless proptosis.
- Tumors have an elongated axis oriented in the anteroposterior direction along the nerve of origin.
- Isolated neurofibromas can be followed conservatively in many cases. For tumors with significant growth or bothersome symptoms, surgical excision is appropriate.

The isolated or solitary neurofibroma is a nonhereditary proliferation of neurons, Schwann cells, fibroblasts, and perineural cells derived from peripheral nerves. The solitary neurofibromas represent less than 1% of orbital tumors. Unlike the plexiform variety, only 10–28% of patients have clinical signs or a family history of neurofibromatosis. Isolated neurofibromas may be multiple in the same orbit.

Multilobulated or multiple tumors are thought to represent a localized, forme fruste neurofibromatosis. Solitary neurofibromas are more commonly seen in middle-aged adults, between 20 and 60 years old. The tumor has a propensity for the superior orbit. It arises primarily along cranial or peripheral sensory nerves, typically branches of the frontal, supraorbital, or supratrochlear nerves.

Clinical Presentation

The major clinical symptom is mild, slowly progressive, painless proptosis. The globe may be displaced downward because of the predilection of this lesion to occur in the superior orbit (Fig. 56.47). Paresthesias or even anesthesia can

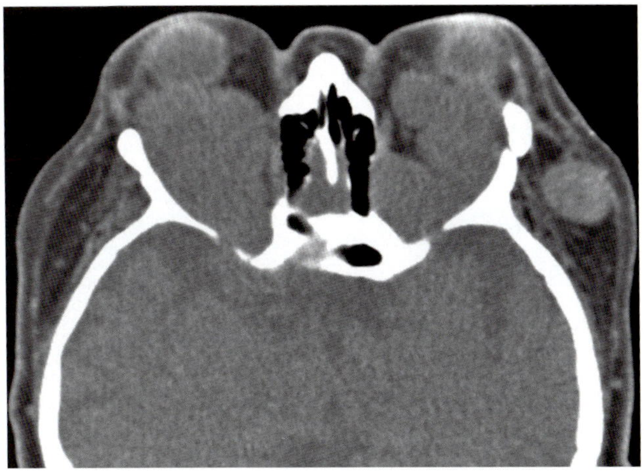

Fig. 56.48 CT scan showing multiple neurofibromas in both orbits

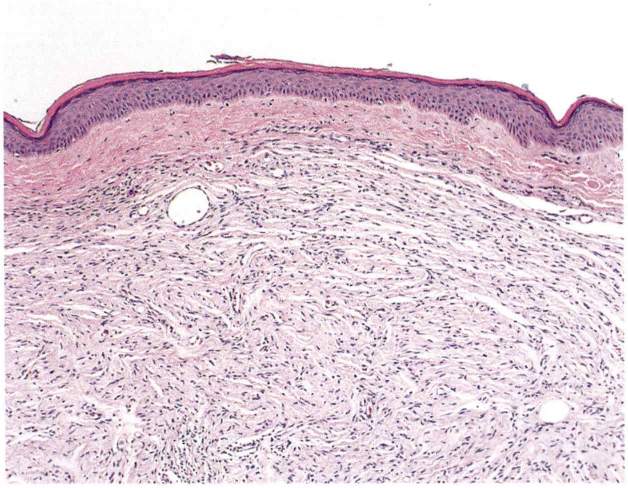

Fig. 56.49 Solitary neurofibroma containing neurites, fibroblasts, and Schwann cells with interspersed mast cells

often be demonstrated in the distribution of the affected nerve. Lesions in the lacrimal gland fossa may be indistinguishable clinically from a benign lacrimal gland tumor. Limitation of ocular motility and diplopia can occur in larger tumors. Decreased visual acuity typically does not occur unless the tumors are quite large or compressing the optic nerve.

Computed Tomography

The CT image shows a round to ovoid well-defined, homogeneously isodense, or slightly hyperdense mass with respect to muscle (Fig. 56.48). It is typically located in the superior or medial orbit with the elongated axis oriented in the anteroposterior direction along the nerve of origin. Low attenuating areas of cystic degeneration appear darker, and bright foci of calcification can be seen. Following contrast administration, enhancement is mild and uniform. Adjacent orbital bone remodeling may be seen. Multilobulation (46%) or multiple tumors may be present within the same orbit. High-resolution CT and MRI provide information that is helpful with diagnosis and surgical planning.

Magnetic Resonance Imaging

On T1-weighted imaging, the isolated neurofibroma yields a smooth, well-defined homogeneous to heterogeneous signal that is isointense or slightly hyperintense to muscle and hypointense to fat. The T2-weighted image produces a higher signal that is hyperintense to both muscle and fat. Moderate to marked heterogeneous enhancement is seen with intravenous gadolinium. Cysts with myxomatous degeneration appear more hypointense on T1WI and more hyperintense on T2WI and do not enhance with gadolinium. Imaging features such as a ring configuration, multilobulation, or multiple tumors are often noted.

Histopathology

The tumors are often surrounded by a pseudocapsule. Interlacing bundles of spindle-shaped cells with uniform dark-staining comma-shaped and tapered nuclei epitomize the solitary neurofibroma, which may be intraneural or diffusely infiltrative (Fig. 56.49). Cellular atypia and mitotic figures are absent. Thin wire-like strands of collagen are associated with the tumor cells, and a small to moderate amount of myxoid stroma with scattered mast cells and lymphocytes accompanies the cells and their associated collagenous strands. Blood vessels are usually located at the tumor periphery. Some tumors have a predominantly collagenous stroma and are more cellular, giving an atypical appearance. Diagnosis can be verified with silver staining of nerve axons or immunohistochemical staining typically for S-100 antigen. Electron microscopy reveals nerve axons, Schwann-like cells, perineural cells, fibroblast-like cells, and intermediate cells.

Treatment

Isolated neurofibromas can be followed conservatively in many cases. For tumors with significant growth or bothersome symptoms, surgical excision is appropriate. Identification of the involved nerve should be verified prior to excision. Complete surgical excision is generally obtainable due to the solid nature of most tumors. The capsule may be adherent to adjacent structures, or the tumor may represent an expansion of a nerve in which case the involved nerve must be sacrificed. Following complete resection, recurrence is rare.

Prognosis

The prognosis for life and vision is excellent. Rare recurrences have been reported, most often resulting from additional unrecognized tumors.

Sphenoid Wing Meningioma

Clinical Pearls

- Meningiomas represent nearly 95% of all benign brain tumors, with 14–18% located within the sphenoid wing.
- They arise from meningothelial cells of the arachnoid.
- Sphenoid wing meningiomas most commonly present with proptosis in middle-aged women.
- Some compromise of vision is seen in 50% of cases.
- Surgical excision typically occurs in a piecemeal fashion.
- There are high rates of local recurrence, risk of compression of orbital structures, and need for repeated surgeries.

The majority of meningiomas that involve the orbit are secondary tumors of intracranial origin. Meningiomas represent nearly 95% of all benign brain tumors, with 14–18% located within the sphenoid wing. Meningiomas are atypical in 5–7% and malignant in 1–3% of cases. They arise from meningothelial cells of the arachnoid. Tumors of the olfactory groove, the suprasellar area, and particularly the greater sphenoid wing are most likely to result in ophthalmic symptoms. Meningiomas tend to occur in adults during the fourth or fifth decade of life, generally an older group than for optic nerve sheath meningiomas. Females are affected more commonly than males in a ratio of 3:1.

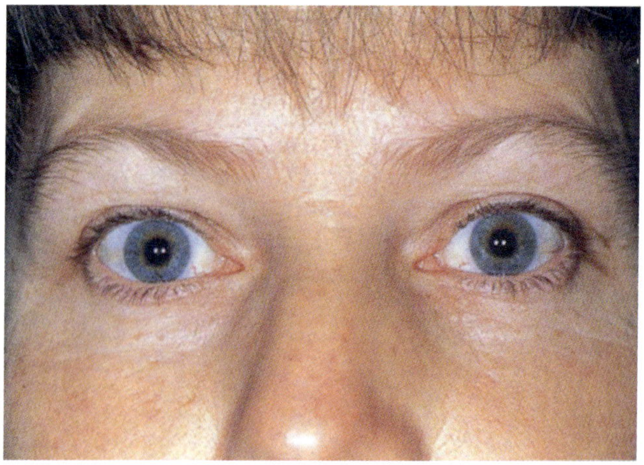

Fig. 56.50 Sphenoid wing meningioma of the left orbit with minimal proptosis

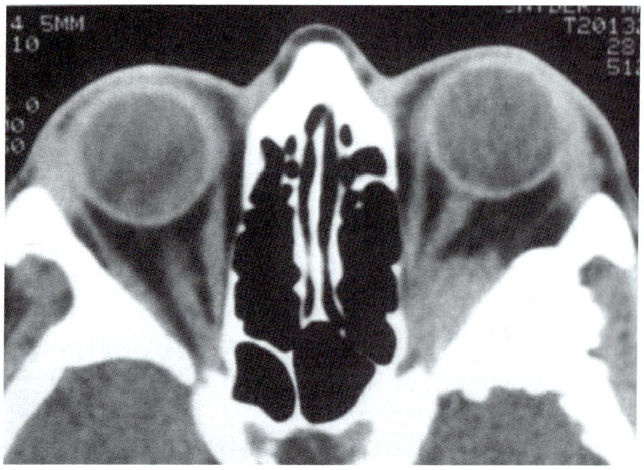

Fig. 56.51 CT scan of a left wing meningioma with thickening of the greater sphenoid wing and an apical soft tissue mass

Clinical Presentation

Sphenoid wing meningiomas most commonly present with proptosis in middle-aged women. Symptoms result from tumor expansion into the posterior orbit or from a mass effect on the intracranial portions of the optic nerve, chiasm, or hypothalamus. Lesions centered in the lateral part of the greater sphenoid wing extend along the lateral orbital wall resulting in early proptosis and a temporal fossa mass (Fig. 56.50). Tumors arising from the medial portion of the sphenoid wing produce early optic neuropathy with vision loss, relative afferent pupillary defects, color vision defects, and visual field deficits. Associated cranial nerve palsies and venous obstruction occur from involvement of the superior orbital fissure. Overall, some compromise of vision is seen in 50% of cases and tends to be progressive. With olfactory groove or suprasellar meningiomas, bilateral visual disturbance is common.

Computed Tomography

On unenhanced CT scans, meningiomas are well defined and are usually isodense or slightly hyperdense to normal brain. In 20–25% of cases, small dense areas of calcification may be seen. Occasionally, fatty degeneration is seen as a low-density area within the tumor. The density of the tumor may not differ significantly from adjacent muscle or optic nerve so that it may not be possible to distinguish meningioma from a primary tumor of the orbit. Hyperostosis of adjacent bone is seen as bone thickening with hyperdensity adjacent to the soft tissue mass (Fig. 56.51). There may be narrowing of the optic canal or superior orbital fissure. Contrast administration results in intense homogeneous enhancement.

Magnetic Resonance Imaging

MRI is the preferred imaging modality because of its ability to distinguish edema and vascularity. On T1-weighted images, the tumor is isointense to slightly hypointense to muscle and cortical gray matter. With more extensive intraosseous tumor invasion, the bone signal can be somewhat brighter and more homogeneous. On T2-weighted images, the signal is more heterogeneous. The extraosseous component produces signals that are isointense or hypointense to muscle, but the intraosseous portion remains significantly hypointense. Following gadolinium administration, the soft tissue components show marked enhancement. Mottled enhancement of medullary bone demonstrates tumor invasion, and enhancement only in the periphery occurs in the presence of extensive calcification.

Histopathology

Intracranial meningiomas exhibit a variety of histological patterns, with 11 subtypes of meningiomas recognized by the World Health Organization. Multiple tumor subtypes may be present within a single tumor. Atypical (5–7%) and malignant tumors (1–3%) may be seen. Most commonly, sphenoid wing meningiomas exhibit the meningothelial, fibroblastic, transitional, and psammomatoid variants. Fibroblastic, or fibrous, meningiomas are composed of parallel and interlacing bundles of elongated cells resembling fibroblasts. Intranuclear vacuoles resulting from invaginated cytoplasm are present in some cells of the meningothelial and psammomatoid variants. Transitional meningiomas are a composite of meningothelial and fibrous types with islands of whorled meningothelial cells alternating with interlacing bundles of spindle-shaped cells. Psammomatous meningiomas, as the name implies, feature numerous psammoma bodies (laminated calcific concretions). These tumors may be sparsely cellular. Immunostaining for the epithelial membrane antigen (EMA) may be helpful in arriving at a diagnosis.

Treatment

A multidisciplinary surgical approach is typically required for complete surgical resection, which typically occurs in a piecemeal fashion. The traditional surgical approach remains the frontopterional craniotomy, which allows for extensive resections of the lateral orbital wall and orbital roof. These lesions have a propensity to crowd structures in the orbital apex, cavernous sinus, and carotid artery, making complete surgical excision difficult. Complete surgical resection is possible in only as few as 63% cases. Stereotactic image guidance can be helpful during these complicated surgeries. Additional surgical goals should include restoring ophthalmic function and improving overall cosmesis. Spheno-orbital reconstruction may include a variety of materials, including split calvarial grafts, rib grafts, iliac crest, titanium mesh, and synthetic materials, some of which are computer engineered. The 5-year recurrence rates following gross total resection (4–33%) and subtotal resection (19–63%) emphasize the importance of complete surgical resection. Recurrence rates are higher with atypical or undifferentiated tumors at any site. Adjuvant radiation has been shown to decrease significantly the 5-year recurrence rates in patients with subtotal resection. Chemotherapy is generally ineffective. Tumor growth is often slow, and recurrences may not be seen for many years. Close clinical follow-up should occur for 10–20 years and typically includes radiographic testing, Hertel exophthalmometry, color vision testing, visual field testing, and extraocular motility examination.

Prognosis

The prognosis for vision is guarded because of the high rates of local recurrence, risk of compression of orbital structures, and need for repeated surgeries. Overly aggressive attempts at surgical extirpation can result in further vision loss as well as endocrine dysfunction. The 5-year survival rates for benign (85%) and malignant (58%) intracranial meningiomas may not apply to sphenoid wing meningiomas. Long-term survival is related to the presence of intracranial complications.

Mesenchymal Tumors

Fibrosarcoma

Clinical Pearls

- Infantile, juvenile, and adult forms of primary orbital fibrosarcoma have been described and may involve any orbital wall.
- Fibrosarcoma of the orbit is the second most common sarcoma to occur following radiotherapy treatment for hereditary retinoblastoma.
- Patients often present with moderately progressive proptosis.
- Fibrosarcomas are highly cellular tumors with closely packed malignant fibroblastic cells that are arranged in into fascicles and bundles (herringbone pattern).
- On CT scan, fibrosarcomas appear as lytic lesions within bone with nonspecific attenuation of unmineralized soft tissue.
- Wide surgical excision is recommended for confirmed fibrosarcomas.

Fibrosarcomas are mesenchymal tumors that may involve soft tissue or bone. In bone, they represent about 10% of musculoskeletal sarcomas and 5% of all primary bone tumors. Primary orbital or craniofacial tumors are rare. Most fibrosarcomas occur in the limbs or hip. Fibrosarcomas originating from the paranasal sinuses or nasal cavity may invade the orbit. Primary development within the scleral stroma has been reported. Orbital spread of ameloblastic forms originating in the jaw has been described. Fibrosarcoma of the orbit is the second most common sarcoma to occur following radiotherapy treatment of hereditary retinoblastoma.

Clinical Presentation

Fibrosarcomas of the orbit often present with moderately progressive proptosis. Infantile, juvenile, and adult forms of primary orbital fibrosarcoma have been described. Tumors have involved all orbital walls. The sinonasal type most often presents within the superonasal orbit. Sinonasal fibrosarcomas with orbital spread occur most commonly in males between 30 and 40 years of age. Common symptoms include globe displacement, ophthalmoplegia, blepharoptosis, retroorbital pain, sinonasal obstruction, and decreased visual acuity. Extension to the orbital apex occurs frequently. Extension to the skull base, cavernous sinus, and paranasal sinuses has been reported.

Computed Tomography

Fibrosarcomas appear as lytic lesions within bone with nonspecific attenuation of unmineralized soft tissue. Bony erosion through paranasal sinuses and orbital walls is frequently seen and is best evaluated with bone window settings. The tumor is isodense to normal muscle.

Magnetic Resonance Imaging

MRI is better for defining the intraosseous and extraosseous components of the tumor. Fibrosarcoma images on MRI like other lytic lesions of bone. Fibrosarcomas are well demarcated. On T1WI, the signal is of low intensity. The T2WI shows a heterogeneous signal of high intensity that varies with the degree of tissue cellularity, necrosis, and intralesional hemorrhage. Infantile and juvenile fibrosarcomas may be more benign appearing than adult fibrosarcomas.

Histopathology

Fibrosarcomas are highly cellular tumors with closely packed malignant fibroblasts that are arranged in interlacing fascicles and bundles classically forming a herringbone pattern. The cells have elongated or ovoid hyperchromatic nuclei that demonstrate coarse chromatin and atypia. Mitotic activity may be brisk. Extracellular collagen is present. On immunohistochemistry, fibrosarcomas are usually positive for vimentin and variably positive for CD34.

Treatment

Wide surgical excision is recommended for confirmed fibrosarcomas. Many surgeons would recommend total orbital exenteration at the time of diagnosis. Frozen section evaluation should be utilized to confirm tumor margins, as there is a high rate of recurrence with incomplete excision. Multidisciplinary surgical approaches are often required for complete excision. Fractionated radiotherapy may be utilized following surgical excision, especially for incompletely resected tumors. Chemotherapy may be useful for patients with recurrent or widespread disease.

Prognosis

Fibrosarcomas have up to a 50% chance of local recurrence with less than 8% chance of metastasis. Infantile and juvenile fibrosarcomas have a more favorable prognosis than adult forms. Adult fibrosarcoma tends be more infiltrative. Death may result from the intracranial extension of a persistent or recurrent tumor. Orbital tumor survival rates have not been reported. Nonorbital fibrosarcomas have a 60% 5-year survival rate.

Fibrous Histiocytoma

Clinical Pearls

- Fibrous histiocytoma has classically been considered the most common mesenchymal orbital tumor.
- The tumors arise from pleuripotential mesenchymal cells within fascia, muscle, or other soft tissues.
- It is seen most commonly in middle-aged adults between 30 and 60 years of age.
- Tumors most commonly occur within the superonasal orbit.
- Patients most commonly present with progressive proptosis with associated inferolateral globe displacement.
- The type of surgical approach should be directed by individual tumor characteristics.
- Many of these tumors have been reclassified as solitary fibrous tumors.

Pleuripotential mesenchymal cells are thought to result in the formation of fibrous histiocytomas within fascia, muscle, or other soft tissues. It may be seen as a primary tumor of the eyelid, conjunctiva, or orbit or, rarely, as a metastatic lesion from a distant site. Fibrous histiocytoma is the most common mesenchymal orbital tumor in adults representing about 1% of all such neoplasms. It is seen most commonly in middle-aged adults between 30 and 60 years of age, but can occur at any age, including infancy. Reports indicate that 3–10% of tumors occur in children. Tumors in the pediatric population may follow orbital radiotherapy for retinoblastoma. There is no sex predilection. Fibrous histiocytomas range clinically and histologically from benign (63%), to locally aggressive (26%), to malignant (11%).

Clinical Presentation

The superonasal orbital quadrant is the most frequent site of occurrence. Progressive proptosis is the most common clinical feature (Fig. 56.52). Associated globe displacement and pain may be present. Ptosis, eyelid edema, chemosis, and extraocular muscle palsy are seen with larger tumors. Retrobulbar lesions can be associated with retinal striae, optic neuropathy, and visual loss. When located in the superolateral orbit, fibrous histiocytoma may mimic a

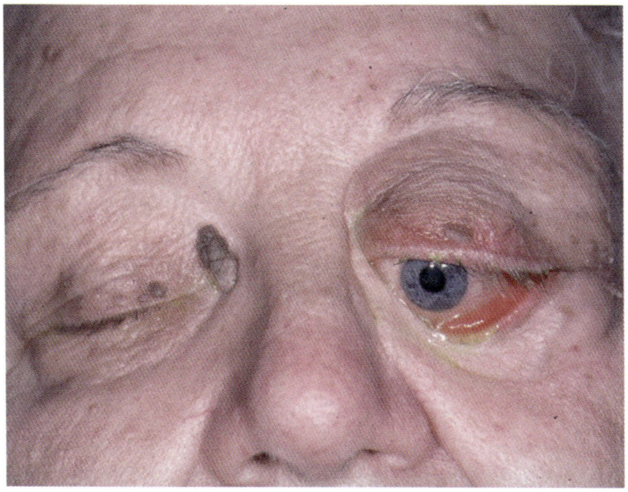

Fig. 56.52 Massive left proptosis from a long-standing fibrous histiocytoma

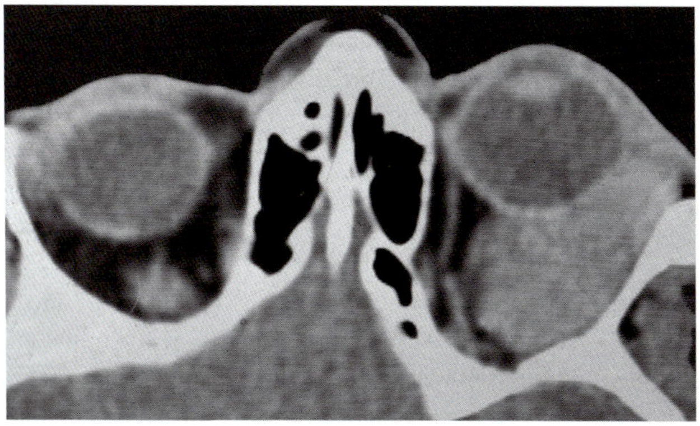

Fig. 56.53 CT scan of the same patient as in Fig. 56.39, showing a large irregular mass in the left lateral orbit

lacrimal gland tumor. The lacrimal sac may be involved, resulting in epiphora or dacryocystitis. Occasional involvement of paranasal sinuses has been reported. Symptoms may progress slowly in the more benign variants, but more malignant tumors can advance rapidly and be locally aggressive.

Computed Tomography

These are well-defined, rounded to irregular masses of uniform density (Fig. 56.53). In this regard, it appears similar to other benign lesions such as schwannomas or cavernous hemangiomas. Bone erosion and enlargement of the orbit are rare, but may be seen with recurrent or malignant tumors using extended window settings. Globe indentation and displacement may be seen with large tumors.

Magnetic Resonance Imaging

Fibrous histiocytomas are rounded to oval, well-circumscribed masses on MRI. The T1-weighted image

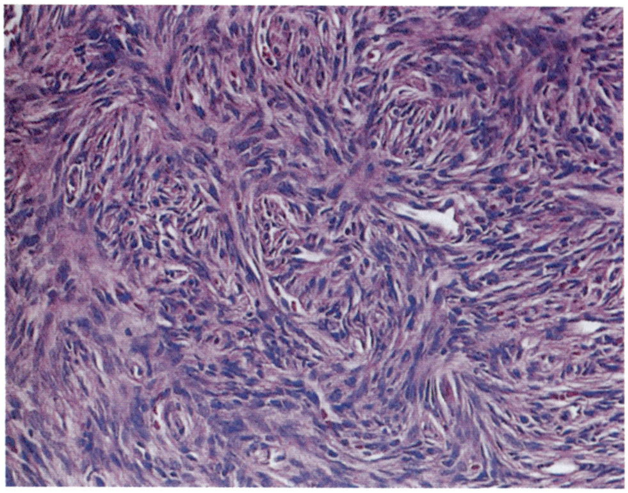

Fig. 56.54 Benign fibrous histiocytoma demonstrating storiform arrangement of interlacing fibroblasts and containing blood vessels with plump endothelium

shows a lesion that is heterogeneous in density. It is isointense to slightly hyperintense relative to muscle and hypointense to fat. A capsule may image as a low-intensity rim. On T2-weighted sequences, collagenous regions remain hypointense, but more cellular areas show a higher hyperintense signal. Marked heterogeneous enhancement is seen following gadolinium administration.

Histopathology

Benign fibrous histiocytomas of the orbit have poorly defined margins. They contain a mixture of cells resembling fibroblasts and histiocytes. The spindle-shaped fibroblasts form an irregular whorled (storiform) pattern (Fig. 56.54). Variable capillary networks may be seen. Approximately one-third of orbital fibrous histiocytomas have vascular areas replete with sinusoidal or staghorn-shaped vessels indistinguishable from those of benign hemangiopericytomas. Benign fibrous histiocytomas must be differentiated from those that are locally aggressive or malignant. Locally aggressive forms have more infiltrative margins, nuclear hyperchromasia, areas of hypercellularity, and mitotic figures of more than 5 per 40 high-power fields. Atypical mitoses without associated necrosis may be present. Malignant forms have infiltrating edges, nuclear pleomorphism and atypia, areas of necrosis, bizarre multinucleated giant cells, and increased number of mitoses. Myxoid fibrous histiocytomas are a variant of these tumors, but they are rare in the orbit. The content of histiocytes is highly variable, and they are often inapparent without the use of immunohistochemical staining. Immunohistochemical testing often reacts positively for vimentin, α-antitrypsin, factor XIIIA, smooth muscle actin, and CD68.

Treatment

Local excision is advocated for well-circumscribed benign lesions, but there is a tendency for local recurrence. For lesions showing infiltration or more aggressive histologies, wide surgical excision is preferred since the ultimate behavior of these tumors cannot be predicted on histopathology. Recurrent benign lesions often require repeated resections. For those that appear frankly malignant on biopsy, radical surgery is appropriate, including orbital exenteration. Radiotherapy has been reported as ineffective. Use of adjunctive chemotherapy regimens has been reported. Positron emission tomography can help to identify malignant and metastatic lesions.

Prognosis

Approximately 63% of lesions are benign, 26% are locally aggressive, and 11% are considered malignant. Following surgical resection, tumor occurrence has been reported to be 31% for benign tumors and 64% for malignant tumors. For benign tumors, the prognosis for life is excellent, with a 10-year survival rate of 100% following complete resection. Locally aggressive tumors and malignant tumors carry 10-year mortality rates of 8% and 78%, respectively.

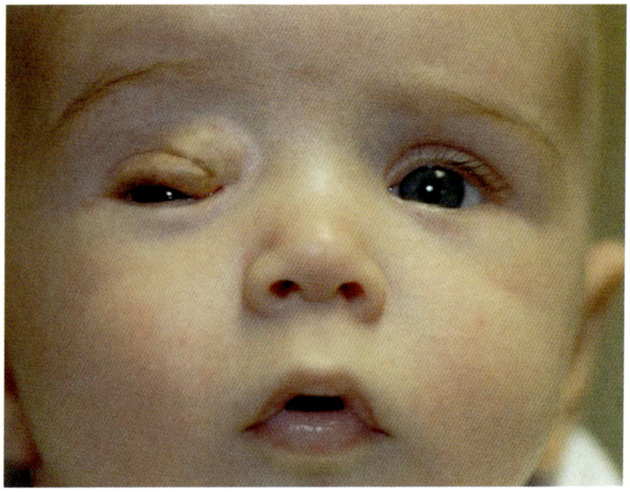

Fig. 56.55 A child with right upper eyelid and anterior orbital juvenile xanthogranuloma

Juvenile Xanthogranuloma

Clinical Pearls

- Juvenile xanthogranuloma is a disease of non-Langerhans cell histiocytes that occurs in children.
- This tumor is characterized by one or more yellow to orange, well-demarcated cutaneous nodules appearing within the first several months to years of life.
- Systemic involvement is possible and often results in fever and malaise.
- Most lesions will resolve within 1–2 years under close clinical observation.
- Treatment, most often with corticosteroids or low-dose radiotherapy, is warranted for patients with vision loss or development of amblyopia.

Juvenile xanthogranuloma (JXG) is a systemic childhood disease of non-Langerhans cell histiocytes. It is generally characterized by one or more yellow to orange, well-demarcated cutaneous nodules appearing within the first several months to years of life. Though usually a benign process, systemic or visceral involvement by JXG has been reported to be associated with chronic myelogenous leukemia, urticaria pigmentosa, type I diabetes mellitus, neurofibromatosis type I, and possibly cytomegalovirus infection. Extracutaneous involvement may involve any site, including the liver, spleen, central nervous system, and lung, but there is a predilection for subcutaneous soft tissue and ocular tissues. While iris lesions are the most common, ocular involvement can also include the orbit, conjunctiva, cornea, episclera, ciliary body, or optic nerve, with 85% presenting before 1 year of age. Solitary JXG lesions usually involute over months to years.

Clinical Presentation

Orbital JXG most commonly presents with unilateral lesions, although bilateral involvement has been reported. The cutaneous lesions are isolated yellow-orange firm nodules, generally less than 2 cm in size (Fig. 56.55). Patients with orbital involvement often present with eyelid swelling, ptosis, mild proptosis, and rarely globe displacement. The lesions are usually located within the anterior orbit where they are palpable along the orbital rim. Even without systemic disease, patients can present with fever and malaise. While ocular and orbital disease is much more likely to occur in isolation, systemic involvement may be present in up to 5% of patients. When systemic JXG is present, it often involves two or more organ systems with an unpredictable number of lesions and sites.

Computed Tomography

On CT, the mass appears as a homogeneous to heterogeneous isodense infiltrative mass in the eyelid or anterior orbit. There may be molding around the globe and other structures. With contrast administration enhancement is moderate. Rarely, bony destruction or intracranial extension may be noted.

Magnetic Resonance Imaging

MRI reveals thickening of the eyelid or a soft tissue mass extending into the anterior orbit (Fig. 56.56). On T1 images,

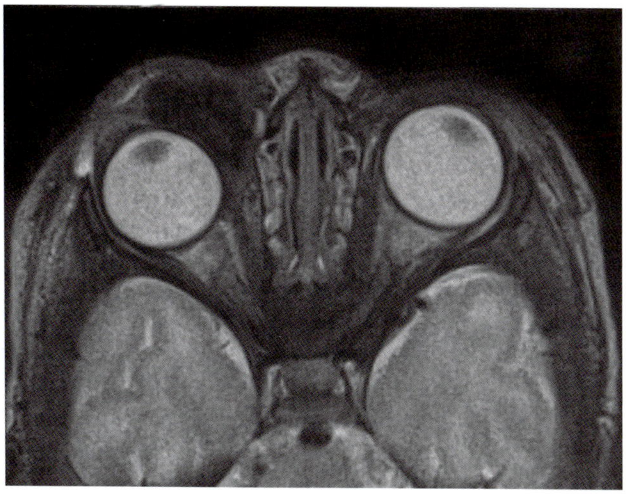

Fig. 56.56 T2-weighted MRI showing a hypointense mass in the right medial orbit

the mass is isointense to muscle with moderate to marked enhancement. The T2 image is homogeneous and of low signal intensity.

Histopathology

JXG is identified by the presence of lipid-laden histiocytes, variable lymphocytic/eosinophilic infiltration, and Touton giant cells. Touton giant cells have a central wreath of nuclei and a peripheral rim of eosinophilic cytoplasm. Rare mitoses are occasionally noted. Vessels may have a perivascular cuffing of lymphocytes. Birbeck granules are not found on electron microscopy. Due to the variable histology, immunohistochemical stains are often used to classify this lesion. The lesions are usually positive for vimentin, HAM-56, HHF-35, CD68, CD14, fascin, and factor XIIIa.

Treatment

Patients with JXG should undergo a multidisciplinary evaluation for other lesions. If the patient has clinical findings suggestive of systemic disease, a directed workup may include diagnostic testing, CT/MRI of the brain and orbits, chest X-ray, CT or ultrasound of the abdomen, skeletal survey, or radionuclide bone scan. Most lesions will resolve within 1–2 years under close clinical observation. Treatment is warranted for patients with orbital or periorbital disease that may result in vision loss or development of amblyopia. Injection with triamcinolone/dexamethasone has been reported to have good success. Treatment with systemic corticosteroids or immunosuppressive agents should be limited to patients with severe systemic disease. Rarely, surgical debulking may be necessary. Treatment with radiotherapy has been reported, but the long-term risks may outweigh any potential benefit.

Prognosis

Most lesions resolve spontaneously over a period of 1–2 years. For vision-threatening lesions, periocular corticosteroid injection, systemic corticosteroids, and surgical debulking are highly effective treatments. Surgically excised lesions have a low rate of recurrence. The prognosis for vision and life is very good.

Leiomyosarcoma

Clinical Pearls

- Leiomyosarcomas arise from smooth muscle in blood vessels; from Muller's muscle, along orbital fascial septa; or de novo from smooth muscle precursor cells.
- These tumors occur primarily in patients 30–90 years of age.
- Patients typically present with progressive painless proptosis of variable duration.
- Aggressive surgical resection with wide margins, including adjacent bone or complete orbital exenteration, is warranted for most tumors.
- Adjuvant chemotherapy and radiotherapy is often used.

Leiomyosarcomas are rare malignant tumors. Ten primary orbital tumors have been reported, although additional cases of tumors metastatic to the orbit have been reported. The incidence of primary orbital lesions is greater in women, and these are generally located within the extraconal space. Radiation-induced lesions have been reported to occur in younger adults and children, but can develop years or decades following exposure. HIV and Epstein-Barr virus infections have been associated with tumor development. Tumors arise from smooth muscle in blood vessels; from Muller's muscle, along orbital fascial septa; or de novo from smooth muscle precursor cells. Most reports have involved patients between 30 and 90 years of age. Few pediatric cases have been reported.

Clinical Presentation

Duration of symptoms may be as short as 6 weeks or more protracted over 12–18 months. Patients most often present with progressive painless proptosis. Abaxial displacement of the globe is seen with anterior lesions, which may be palpable beneath the orbital rim (Fig. 56.57). Axial proptosis may be seen with apical tumors. Motility disturbance and visual loss are seen with larger tumors. Blepharoptosis, conjunctival hyperemia, choroidal folds, papilledema, retinal venous stasis, and peripapillary hemorrhages have been reported.

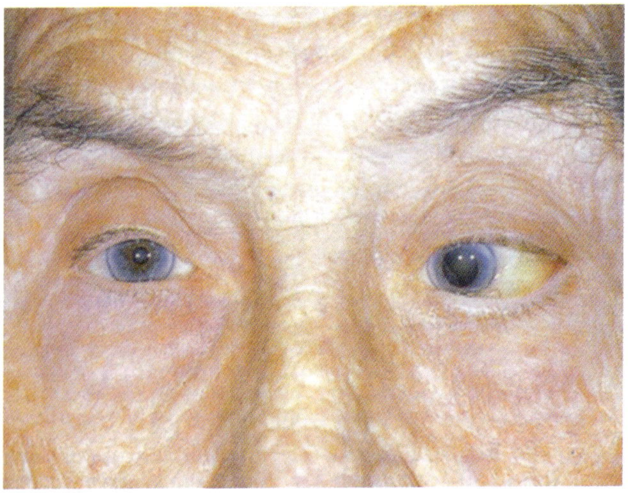

Fig. 56.57 Displacement of the globe from a malignant leiomyosarcoma

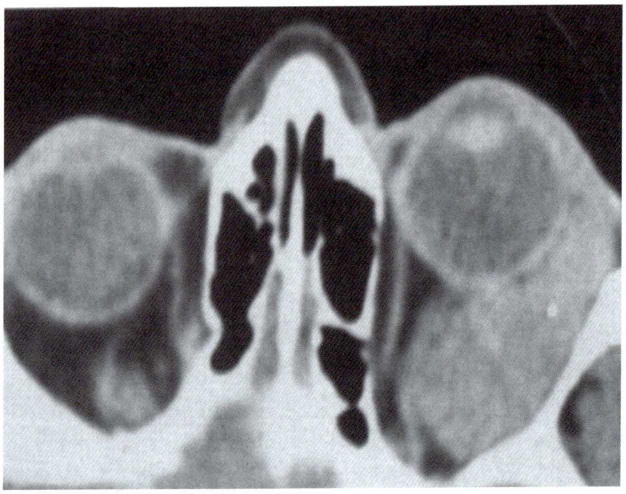

Fig. 56.58 CT scan with a large leiomyosarcoma filling the lateral orbit and apex

Computed Tomography

Leiomyosarcomas appear as a heterogeneously dense, moderately well-defined, multilobulated mass within the orbital soft tissue on CT (Fig. 56.58). When the tumor is infiltrative, the lesion borders are more diffuse and may mold around the globe. Destruction of adjacent bone or extension into adjacent sinuses is sometimes seen. The lesion demonstrates moderate contrast enhancement.

Magnetic Resonance Imaging

On T1-weighted images, the signal is intermediate, being isointense to muscle and cerebral cortex and hypointense to fat. The tumor is mostly homogeneous, but heterogeneity can be seen depending upon the degree of vascularizations, hemorrhage, or necrosis. The T2-weighted image produces a heterogeneous signal that is isointense to muscle and hypointense to cerebral cortex, with areas of more

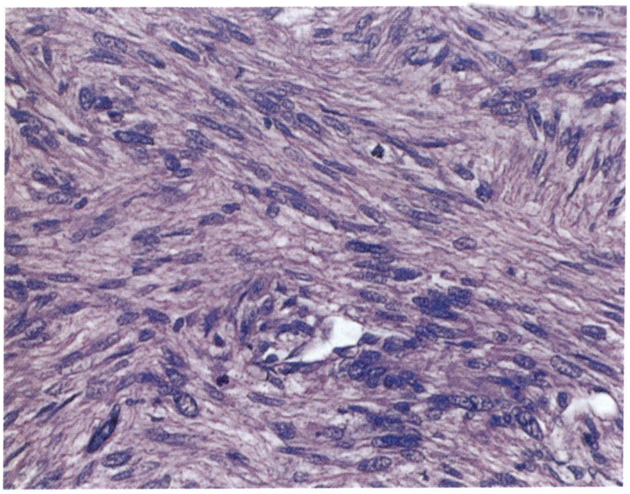

Fig. 56.59 Leiomyosarcoma consisting of interlacing fascicles of cells with eosinophilic fibrillar cytoplasm, pleomorphic nuclei, and mitotic figures. Tumors immunostain for smooth muscle-specific antigen

hyperintense signal. Following gadolinium, the tumor demonstrates moderate heterogeneous enhancement with occasional rim enhancement.

Histopathology

Leiomyosarcomas are nonencapsulated. Their appearance is variable, depending upon their degree of differentiation. Well-differentiated tumors have intersecting fascicles of tumor cells similar to leiomyomas. The cells are fusiform with regular, central cigar-shaped nuclei and eosinophilic fibrillar cytoplasm (Fig. 56.59). Nuclear irregularity is present, and staining intensity increases as the tumors become more poorly differentiated. Multinucleated tumor giant cells are frequent in poorly differentiated leiomyosarcomas. Masson trichrome stain reveals parallel myofibrils in well-differentiated tumor cells, but the striations may be difficult or impossible to identify in poorly differentiated tumors. Fibrous or myxoid change is seen occasionally, and necrosis occurs in larger tumors. Immunohistochemical staining for actin allows for identification of these tumors without the need for transmission electron microscopy. These tumors express smooth muscle-specific antigen (SMA), but do not demonstrate S-100, CD34, CD68, or HMB positivity, and may rarely express desmin or vimentin. Distinguishing a soft tissue leiomyoma from a well-differentiated leiomyosarcoma relies on counting mitotic figures: 1–4 mitoses/10 high-power fields (HPF) indicate potential malignancy, and 5 or more mitoses/10 HPF should be considered malignant.

Treatment

Standard orbital or multidisciplinary approaches may allow for complete surgical excision. Leiomyosarcomas are frequently infiltrative into adjacent orbital tissues, resulting in frequent local recurrence. Aggressive surgical resection with wide margins, including adjacent bone or complete orbital exenteration, is warranted for most tumors. Local resection with adjunctive radiotherapy has been advocated for small or well-circumscribed lesions. Adjuvant chemotherapy has been reported. Chemotherapy is indicated for treatment of systemic metastases.

Prognosis

Following local resection alone, orbital recurrence may be seen in 60% of cases within 5–36 months. Further management after recurrence, including orbital exenteration, does not appear to influence the development of metastases to the lungs, liver, kidney, and brain. Overall prognosis for life remains poor, with a reported mortality rate of 50–75%.

Lipoblastoma

Clinical Pearls

- Lipoblastomas are rare, benign, soft tissue tumors of embryonal white fat.
- Seventy to ninety percent of tumors occur in children less than 3 years of age.
- Patients most commonly present with eyelid fullness, which may be associated with swelling and erythema.
- Complete surgical excision is generally curative.
- Recurrence is likely with incomplete resection.

Lipoblastomatosis and lipoblastomas are rare, benign, soft tissue tumors of embryonal white fat. Approximately, 70–90% of tumors occur in children less than 3 years of age with nearly all occurring in children under 10 years of age. While these two entities are histologically identical, lipoblastoma is a well-circumscribed encapsulated lesion, whereas lipoblastomatosis is more diffuse and infiltrative. These tumors occur rarely within the orbit and eyelids, with most tumors arising in the extremities, trunk, abdomen, head, and neck. The tumors have a propensity to spread locally and do not metastasize. The cellular characteristics of lipoblastomas mimic the mesenchymatous fat lobule of embryos. Orbital lipoblastomas have rarely been associated with other syndromes. Systemic lipoblastomas have been associated with diffuse lipomatosis, Michelin tire baby syndrome, encephalocraniocutaneous lipomatosis, epiploic lipomatosis, mediastinal lipomatosis, Bannayan-Zonana syndrome, nevus lipomatosus cutaneous superficialis, Proteus syndrome, and facial lipomatosis.

Clinical Presentation

Patients most commonly present with eyelid fullness, which may be associated with swelling and erythema (Fig. 56.60). The lesions are usually located anteriorly and are often palpable. Proptosis, globe displacement, extraocular motility disturbance, and diplopia are associated symptoms. Cases of patients with intranasal extension or absent canaliculi and puncta have been reported.

Computed Tomography

CT scan of the orbits shows thickening of the eyelid. The surrounding eyelid appears hyperdense with an associated low-density mass.

Magnetic Resonance Imaging

T1-weighted images reveal a heterogeneous density with areas of low signal intensity (Fig. 56.61). Areas of increased intensity are seen on fat saturation sequence images. The T2 images show areas of high signal intensity comparable to fat. The fibrous architecture within the tumor does not enhance, making the tumor heterogeneous.

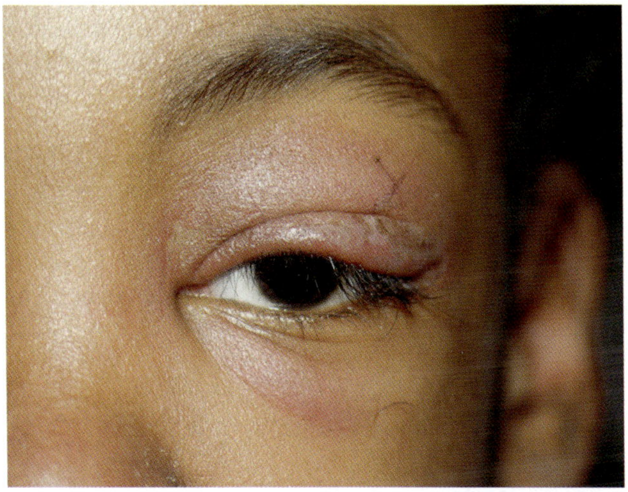

Fig. 56.60 Left upper eyelid swelling from a lipoblastoma

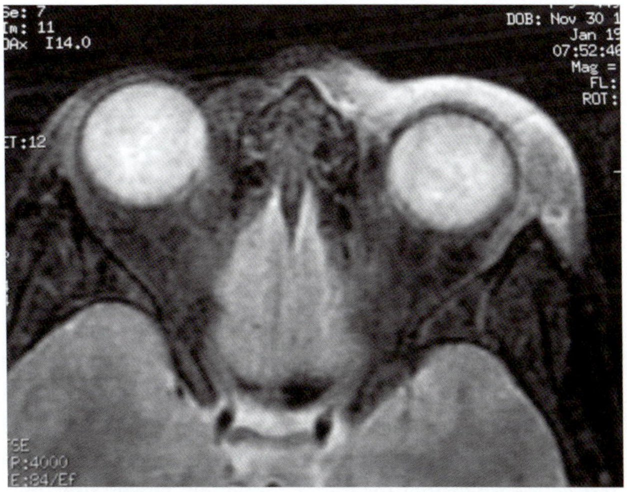

Fig. 56.61 T2-weighted MRI showing a hyperintense thickening of the left upper eyelid

Histopathology

Grossly the lesions present as yellow to red lobulated masses, occasionally having a thin fibrous pseudocapsule. Lipoblastomatosis and lipoblastomas contain an admixture of mature adipocytes and multivacuolated lipoblasts, an abundant myxoid stroma, and a sparse plexiform vascular network. The embryonic lipoblasts have varying degrees of maturation throughout the tumor. The cells are vacuolated with centrally located nuclei, without evidence of anaplasia or atypia. The myxoid stroma may contain undifferentiated spindle cells. The adipose tissue is arranged into lobules by collagenous fibrous septa in lipoblastomas, helping to differentiate this tumor from lipomas. Studies have found chromosomal abnormalities in most tumors, commonly involving chromosome 8.

Treatment

Complete surgical excision is generally curative. Meticulous surgical technique is required for resection of more infiltrative tumors to ensure complete excision with preservation of normal tissues. Recurrence is likely with incomplete resection.

Prognosis

The prognosis for vision and life is excellent. Complete surgical excision is generally curative. Recurrence for orbital tumors has not been reported, but systemic tumor recurrence has been found to range from 14% to 25%.

Benign Cartilaginous Tumors

Clinical Pearls

- These tumors occur most frequently in children and young adults.
- Patients most commonly present with a slow-growing palpable superomedial mass resulting in mild proptosis.
- Lesions are often associated with the trochlea, resulting in ocular motility disturbances such as Brown's syndrome.
- Surgical excision is generally curative.

Cases of benign cartilaginous tumors within the orbit have rarely been reported. These have been classified as fibrochondromas, chondromas, enchondromas, osteochondromas, and cartilaginous hamartomas. Most lesions occur within the superomedial orbit near the orbital rim or the trochlea. These tumors occur most frequently in children and young adults. The only cartilaginous structure within the orbit is the trochlea, and it is the presumed site for cartilage rest cells responsible for tumor formation. Other cases outside the superomedial orbit are thought to arise from primitive mesenchymal cells with the potential for cartilaginous differentiation. Rare cavernous sinus lesions have been reported. These tumors may be a part of Ollier or Maffucci syndromes.

Clinical Presentation

Patients most commonly present with a slow-growing palpable superomedial mass resulting in mild proptosis. Given the association with the trochlea, ocular motility disturbances such as Brown's syndrome are frequent. Other clinical findings may include ptosis, globe displacement, diplopia, headache, and sinus obstruction. Optic nerve changes resulting in vision loss are exceedingly rare. Involvement of the skull base or cavernous sinus is often associated with cranial nerve palsies.

Computed Tomography

The benign cartilaginous tumors often appear as well-circumscribed lesions on CT scan. The lesion is usually homogenous and isodense to soft tissue with the presence of occasional calcifications. Occasional lobulations or cysts may be seen. Bone remodeling is commonly seen, but bony destruction is rarely noted. The lesions have little or no contrast enhancement.

Magnetic Resonance Imaging

These appear as well-circumscribed, heterogeneous, multicystic masses. On T1-weighted images, the lesions have moderate signal intensity. The solid components of the tumor are isointense to brain. The cystic components are isointense to CSF. Calcified or ossified portions of the tumor may be seen. On T2-weighted images, these lesions have increased signal intensity.

Histopathology

Chondromas are well-differentiated cartilaginous tumors that are often well demarcated. Lobules of hyaline and cartilaginous matrix coalesce in scattered lacunae with round or polygonal mononuclear chondrocytes that are increased in number and are more irregularly arranged than in normal cartilage. The nuclei are round without mitotic figures or signs of anaplasia, but mild nuclear atypia may be present. These lesions are typically hypovascular. Enchondromas have hypocellular lobules of cartilage enclosed by lamellar bone without evidence of infiltration. Osteochondromas have a mixture of immature osteoid and cartilaginous tissue. Chondromesenchymal hamartomas have immature and mature cartilage present within a fibrous stroma. Partial calcification may be seen. The stroma may contain fibroblasts and myofibroblasts.

Treatment

Complete surgical resection is the primary mode of treatment for these benign cartilaginous tumors. Given the anterior location of most tumors, complete resection is feasible through an anterior orbitotomy. Careful dissection should be performed to prevent inadvertent injury to the superior oblique muscle or trochlea. The risk of recurrence is low.

Prognosis

The prognosis for life and vision is excellent. Surgical excision is generally curative, and recurrences are rare.

Lipodermoid (Dermolipoma)

Clinical Pearls

- Lipodermoids are a common congenital tumor that arises as a dysgenetic choristoma associated with the second branchial arch.
- These tumors present within the superotemporal fornix or lateral canthus as a pink to yellow, soft, rounded mass.
- CT can be useful in delineating the posterior extent of the tumor and in planning treatment.
- The tumors are generally managed by observation. Symptomatic or cosmetically unacceptable tumors may be resected transconjunctivally.
- Tumor proximity to the lacrimal excretory ductules and lateral rectus muscle can result in injury during resection.

Lipodermoids are a common congenital tumor that arise as a dysgenetic choristoma associated with the second branchial arch. These tumors have been reported to represent 3% of all orbital lesions in adults and 5% in children. These most often present within the superotemporal fornix or lateral canthus as a pink to yellow, soft, rounded mass. Lipodermoids may slowly enlarge, but generally retain a stable clinical appearance.

These tumors may be associated with developmental anomalies of the second arch such as Goldenhar's syndrome.

Clinical Presentation

Tumors usually present within the superotemporal fornix. They present as a pink to yellow, soft, rounded mass and can be confused with a dermoid cyst (Fig. 56.62). Dermolipomas are typically unilateral, but bilateral lesions have been reported. These tumors are located beneath the conjunctiva with extension into the anterior orbit, where they may be associated with the lateral rectus, lacrimal gland, levator, and other orbital structures. Extension to the corneal limbus can occur. Unlike orbital fat herniation, which has a convex shape, lipodermoids tend to have a concave shape. Small hairs, keratinization, and lipid globules may be visible. Dermolipomas generally remain stable in size, although rarely they can enlarge slowly.

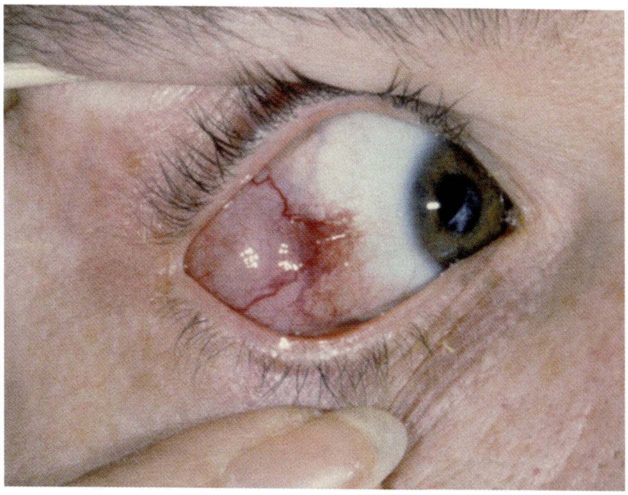

Fig. 56.62 Dermolipoma of the right anterior orbit with dilated anterior ciliary arteries

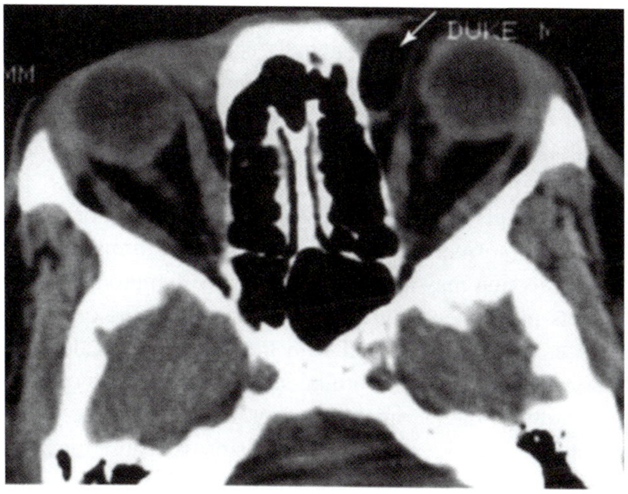

Fig. 56.63 CT scan showing a low-density dermolipoma in the left medial orbit

Computed Tomography

CT is useful in delineating the posterior extent of the tumor and in planning treatment. Lesions appear as a well-defined oval low-density mass in the superomedial or superotemporal orbit. Some tumors extend back to the equator. Attenuation is very low, similar to orbital fat (Fig. 56.63).

Magnetic Resonance Imaging

On MRI, the dermolipoma is an oval mass in the anterior orbit adjacent to the globe. The T1-weighted signal is isointense to fat. On T2-weighted sequences, the signal remains isointense to fat. There is no enhancement with gadolinium.

Histopathology

Dermolipomas are lined by stratified squamous epithelium. They are composed of mature adipose and thick bundles of

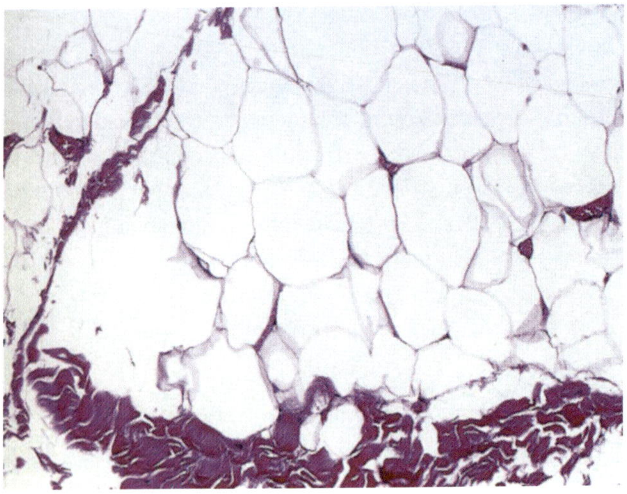

Fig. 56.64 Dermolipoma consisting of fat and lipoblast-like cells, which are multinucleated

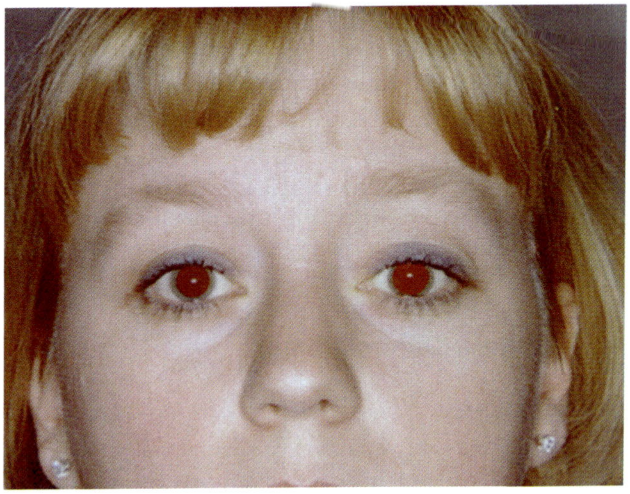

Fig. 56.65 Left orbital lipoma

dense collagenous tissue (Fig. 56.64). Pilosebaceous units are commonly seen. Occasionally cartilage, bone, or glandular acini may be identified. The conjunctival epithelium may be irregularly thickened, or it may be thin and smooth.

Treatment

Lipodermoids are best managed by observation. For symptomatic or cosmetically unacceptable tumors, transconjunctival resection may significantly improve symptoms. These lesions may extend significantly deep within the orbit and may be closely associated with the lateral rectus, levator, lacrimal gland, or other orbital structures. Because of their proximity to the lacrimal excretory ductules and the insertion of the lateral rectus muscle, excision can cause injury to these structures. Given the potential risk of keratoconjunctivitis sicca, diplopia, or ptosis, resection should be limited to the subconjunctival portion of the tumor.

Prognosis

The prognosis for vision is usually excellent, and there is no malignant potential. Subconjunctival resection typically provides improvement of symptoms and cosmesis for these patients, but the subconjunctival component may recur following resection. Deeper orbital resections should be avoided as the complications of surgery can include restrictive symblepharon, diplopia, ptosis, and keratoconjunctivitis sicca from damage to the lacrimal gland or its ductules.

Lipoma

Clinical Pearls

- Lipomas are a frequently occurring mesenchymal neoplasm that occurs rarely in the orbit.
- Patients most commonly present with painless proptosis and eyelid fullness.
- B-scan characteristics reveal a regular hypoechoic mass.
- Most lesions do not result in significant visual symptoms and may be observed clinically.

Lipomas are frequently occurring mesenchymal neoplasms, typically occurring in the subcutaneous tissues of the extremities or trunk. Only 20–25% of all lipomas occur within the head. While fat contributes significantly to orbital volume, true intraorbital lipomas are very rare. The incidence of lipomas within orbital tumor series has ranged from 0% to 11% of orbital tumors, with a mean of 0.6% for all series.

Clinical Presentation

Patients most commonly present with slowly progressive enlargement of the mass resulting in mild painless proptosis and eyelid fullness (Fig. 56.65). Many lesions are anterior and can be palpable. If the lesions are quite large, the patients may develop globe displacement, extraocular motility disturbance, and optic atrophy. Lipomas should be distinguished from prolapsed orbital fat, which is occasionally seen subconjunctivally adjacent to the lacrimal gland.

Computed Tomography

Lipomas appear as a well-circumscribed orbital mass with low attenuation. These tumors often mold to orbital structures. Lipomas do not enhance with contrast administration. Bony destruction is not seen. Cystic areas will appear radiolucent.

Magnetic Resonance Imaging

On T1-weighted imaging, lipomas appear hypointense to muscle and isointense to fat (Fig. 56.66). On T2-weighted imaging, lipomas are hyperintense to muscle and isointense

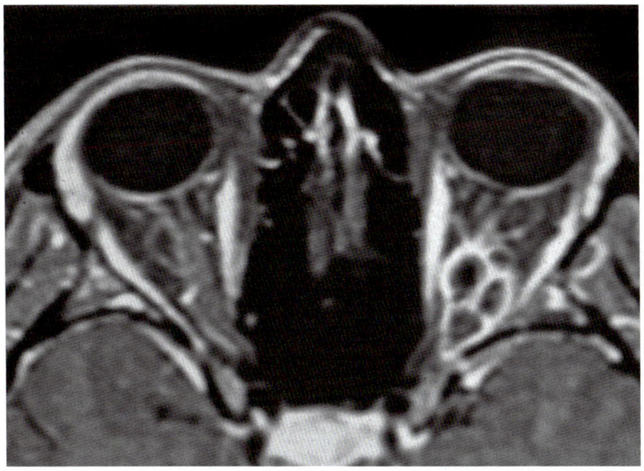

Fig. 56.66 T1-weighted fat-saturated MRI with a multilobulated low-density lipoma in the left orbit

to fat. Molding around orbital structures may be seen. Rarely, the capsule may be visible. The tumor does not enhance with administration of contrast.

Histopathology

Lipomas are noted to be soft, smooth, lobulated masses following resection. A fibrous capsule may be present. Lipomas are characterized by the presence of mature adipocytes, which may be slightly larger than those of normal orbital fat. Vessels are seen within the fine collagenous septae. Multinucleated giant cells with overlapping nuclei (floret) can be found in some tumors. Peripherally placed nuclei have no evidence of mitotic activity or anaplasia. Spindle cell, angiolipoma, and pleomorphic variants have been reported. Immunohistochemical testing may be positive for CD34, vimentin, and S-100. Many lipomas demonstrate chromosomal translocations.

Treatment

Most lesions do not result in significant visual symptoms and should be observed clinically. Complete surgical excision is curative, although recurrence frequently occurs with incomplete excision. Brisk bleeding has been reported during resection of some lipomas.

Prognosis

The prognosis for life and vision is excellent. Surgical excision is generally curative.

Liposarcoma

Clinical Pearls

- Liposarcomas arise from primitive mesenchymal lipoblasts.
- Primary tumors are most likely to occur in middle-aged individuals (age range 5–77).

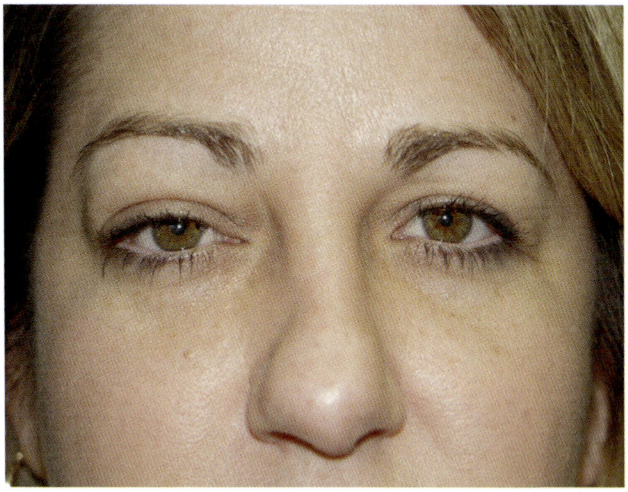

Fig. 56.67 Right-sided ptosis and minimal proptosis from a liposarcoma of the superior oblique muscle

- Patients present with slowly progressive painless proptosis and globe displacement.
- Clinical behavior is dependent upon the tumor subtype.
- Radical surgery with wide surgical margins, usually including complete orbital exenteration, is required.
- Recurrence occurs in 20–50% of cases.

Liposarcomas are the most common soft tissue sarcoma, representing approximately 20% of all sarcomas. These malignant tumors arise from primitive mesenchymal lipoblasts. Liposarcomas occur most commonly in the thigh and retroperitoneum. Rare metastasis to the orbit has been reported. More than 30 primary orbital liposarcomas have been reported in the literature. They have represented up to 0.3% of orbital tumors in some series. Primary orbital tumors have occurred in individuals ranging from 5 to 77 years of age, with most occurring in middle-aged individuals.

Clinical Presentation

Patients with liposarcomas most frequently present with slowly progressive painless proptosis and globe displacement (Fig. 56.67). Decreased visual acuity, signs of optic nerve compromise, and pain may occur if located near the orbital apex. The lesions can grow quite large, resulting in extraocular motility disturbance and diplopia. When located anteriorly, a rubbery mass may be palpable.

Computed Tomography

On CT, a liposarcoma is a well-defined, often lobulated mass. Imaging features often vary depending upon the individual tumor characteristics. Hypodense fat attenuation with denser septae is noted within the lesion. With contrast administration, moderate to marked enhancement that is heterogeneous in nature is noted.

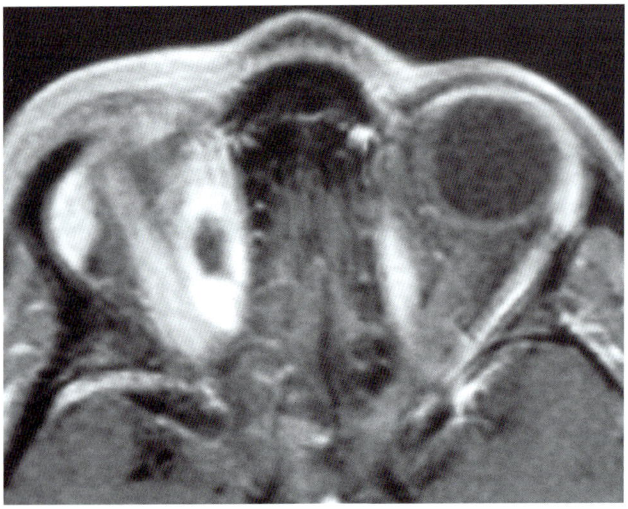

Fig. 56.68 T1-weighted MRI showing a hyperintense superior oblique muscle with a hypointense center

Magnetic Resonance Imaging

On T1-weighted images, the lesion is isointense to hyperintense to muscle. The T2-weighted imaging shows a well-differentiated homogeneous to heterogeneous mass that is hyperintense to muscle. Septae appear as low-intensity lines. Enhancement is diffuse and variable, mild in myxoid liposarcomas, and marked in more aggressive pleomorphic liposarcomas. Enhancement is greater at the periphery, with nodular enhancement in the center. The tumor may be adjacent to or invade extraocular muscles (Fig. 56.68).

Histopathology

Grossly, the tumors are yellow white to gray in color. The degree of tumor differentiation correlates well with clinical behavior. Several subtypes have been identified and include myxoid, round cell, pleomorphic, dedifferentiated, and well-differentiated tumors. The well-differentiated and myxoid tumors are the most common subtypes. Well-differentiated liposarcomas contain immature adipocytes with nuclear pleomorphism, varying numbers of vacuolated lipoblasts, and hyperchromatic multinucleated cells. Myxoid and round cell tumors consist of uniform round to oval-shaped primitive mesenchymal cells and small lipoblasts with lipid droplets displacing nuclei, resulting in a signet-ring appearance. There is a myxomucinous stroma with a variable fibrillar network containing an arborizing plexiform capillary network. Myxoid and round subtypes tend to have a balanced chromosome translocation t(12;16), with the round subtype likely representing a more poorly differentiated myxoid tumor. The dedifferentiated type contains areas of well-differentiated liposarcoma and cellular nonlipogenic spindle cell or pleomorphic sarcoma. Pleomorphic subtypes are characterized by a disorderly growth pattern or grow in fascicles, with increased cellularity, nuclear pleomorphism, and pleomorphic multinucleated lipoblasts. More malignant types are often noted to have increased mitoses, necrosis, and hemorrhage. All subtypes have a lobulated appearance and may have osseous or cartilaginous metaplasia present. Immunohistochemistry studies vary depending upon the tumor subtype with S-100 positivity of lipoblasts. The well-differentiated and myxoid subtypes have a more indolent course. Well-differentiated tumors typically do not metastasize. The pleomorphic and round cell subtypes behave more aggressively, tend to recur, and have a worse prognosis.

Treatment

Multidisciplinary approach should be utilized for management of this malignancy. Radical surgery with wide surgical margins, usually including complete orbital exenteration, provides the greatest opportunity for local control of primary liposarcomas. The posterior margin of resection should be carefully evaluated to ensure that no residual tumor remains in the specimen. There is an 85% chance of recurrence with subtotal excision. With wide surgical margins, the recurrence rate may be between 20% and 50%. Five percent of recurrent tumors dedifferentiate into more malignant subtypes. Radiotherapy use remains controversial and is most commonly used for tumor recurrences. Most tumors are resistant to treatment with chemotherapeutic agents. Cytostatic drugs have been utilized in the treatment of metastatic disease, resulting in a 40% remission rate.

Prognosis

The prognosis for life and vision is guarded. The overall survival rate for systemic liposarcomas has ranged from 50% to 85%. Primary orbital tumors appear to have a more favorable prognosis. Regional or distant metastases occur rarely. Recurrence with local spread can be difficult to manage.

Rhabdomyosarcoma

Clinical Pearls

- Rhabdomyosarcoma is the most common soft tissue mesenchymal tumor and malignancy of the orbit in children.
- This tumor frequently presents with acute to subacute rapidly progressive proptosis over days to weeks.
- The eyelids often have a blue or reddish color that may mimic an acute infection.
- Immediate biopsy followed by definitive therapy is mandatory.
- Complete surgical excision, if possible, generally improves prognosis.
- Chemotherapy and radiotherapy are recommended as primary treatments in most patients.

Rhabdomyosarcoma (RMS) is the most common soft tissue mesenchymal tumor and malignancy of the orbit in children. It represents about 4% of all childhood orbital mass lesions and 1% of all orbital tumors. RMS arises from pleuripotential mesenchymal precursors that normally dif-

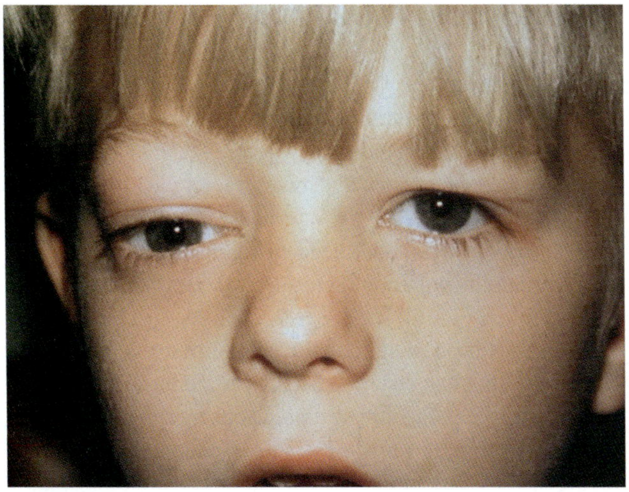

Fig. 56.69 Rhabdomyosarcoma of the right orbit, displacing the globe downward

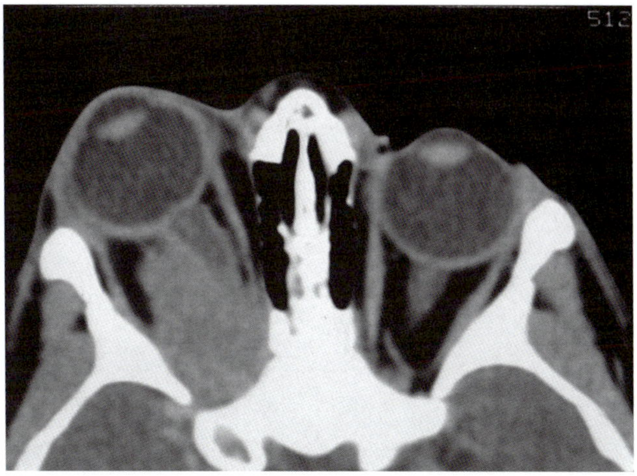

Fig. 56.70 CT scan with a retrobulbar rhabdomyosarcoma around the optic nerve

ferentiate into striated muscle. Cases have been reported in young children and older adults, but the median age of presentation is age 8–9. Males are more commonly affected than females in a ratio of 5:3. Occasionally, RMS can metastasize to the orbit from a systemic location.

Clinical Presentation

This tumor frequently presents with acute to subacute rapidly progressive proptosis over days to weeks. The eyelids often have a blue or reddish color that may mimic an acute infection. It is frequently associated with ptosis, eyelid edema, and ocular motility disturbance (Fig. 56.69). The lesion is most commonly located within the superomedial orbit, resulting in abaxial proptosis and inferolateral displacement of the globe. A firm mass is palpable in only 25% of cases. Larger tumors may be associated with choroidal folds and papilledema. RMS arising in the paranasal sinuses can simultaneously involve both orbits.

Computed Tomography

CT scans show an irregular, but moderately well-defined soft tissue mass. Most tumors occupy the extraconal space, with about half extending into the intraconal compartment. Two-thirds of tumors are in the superonasal quadrant. The density is similar to muscle, but may be heterogeneous due to areas of focal hemorrhage. The tumor may conform to adjacent bony walls and orbital structures such as the globe or optic nerve (Fig. 56.70). Bony erosion or destruction is unusual, but is more common with large tumors where it can be seen in up to 40% of cases. If bony destruction of the skull base occurs, MRI is indicated to determine the extent of intracranial spread, which worsens the prognosis. With contrast administration, there is mild to moderate uniform enhancement.

Magnetic Resonance Imaging

Relaxation times in RMS are generally long. The MRI shows a heterogeneous or homogeneous irregular mass that is isointense to slightly hypointense with respect to muscle and hypointense to fat on T1-weighted images. Chronic hemorrhage produces areas of low intensity. Postcontrast fat-suppressed images show a higher signal intensity of the tumor. On T2-weighted sequences, the tumor signal is higher, being hyperintense to both muscle and fat. Areas of subacute hemorrhage produce focal areas of increased signal intensity on both T1-weighted and T2-weighted images. Moderate to marked enhancement is seen following gadolinium administration.

Histopathology

Rhabdomyosarcomas are divided histologically into embryonal, alveolar, and pleomorphic variants. Embryonal tumors are the most common variant. Embryonal tumors usually have highly cellular areas alternating with less cellular myxoid areas. They have an admixture of undifferentiated round cells, spindle-shaped cells, and rhabdomyoblasts, which are differentiated cells with eosinophilic, granular to fibrillar cytoplasm. Rhabdomyoblasts may be larger eosinophilic cells with a strap, ribbon, tadpole, or racquet shapes that rarely have cross striations that may be visualized with the Masson trichrome stain (Fig. 56.71). Alveolar rhabdomyosarcomas have a network of fibrous septa dividing poorly differentiated, round, or oval tumor cells into aggregates. The tumor cells lack cellular cohesion, and degeneration of the cells in the center of the aggregates creates the alveolar pattern. Tumor giant cells with multiple peripheral nuclei are often seen. Pleomorphic rhabdomyosarcoma, the least common variant of these tumors, has numerous large, often multinucleate, round, or pleomorphic cells with intensely eosinophilic cytoplasm. The diagnosis of all variants of rhabdomyosarcoma may be confirmed by immunohistochemistry of paraffin sections using antibodies to muscle-specific actin, desmin, myogenin, or MyoD. Alveolar rhabdomyosarcomas demonstrate unique chromosomal translocations in 80% of cases as well as increased immunopositivity for MyoD and myogenin.

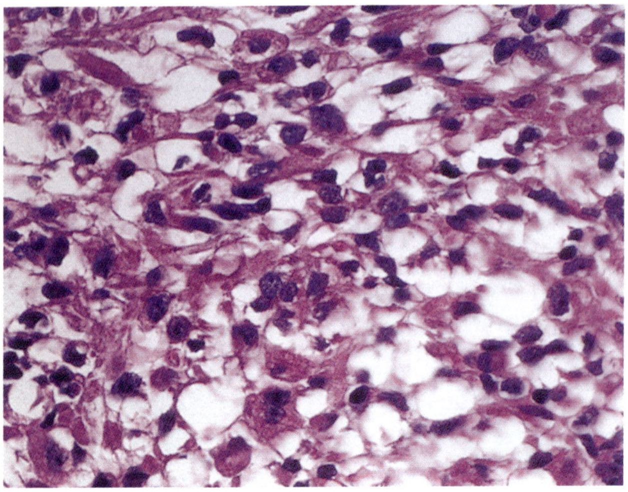

Fig. 56.71 Embryonal rhabdomyosarcoma containing rhabdomyoblasts with intensely staining eosinophilic cytoplasm and enlarged pleomorphic nuclei with prominent nucleoli

Treatment

Immediate biopsy followed by definitive therapy is mandatory. The Intergroup Rhabdomyosarcoma Study (IGRS) has classified patients as follows: Group I as localized disease, completely resected; Group II as total gross resection with evidence of regional spread; Group III as incomplete resection with gross residual disease; and Group IV distant metastatic disease or intracranial spread present at onset. Complete surgical excision generally provides the best chance for cure. Combination chemotherapy (vincristine, actinomycin D, and cyclophosphamide) has been recommended by the International Rhabdomyosarcoma Study Group. In patients with Group I embryonal rhabdomyosarcoma, there is no proven benefit from XRT. All other patients should receive graded dosing of radiotherapy depending upon the grade, type, and location of the tumor. In patients with unresectable tumors, primary chemotherapy followed by XRT was the recommended approach for orbital treatment by the IGRS. Following treatment, shrinkage of the tumor occurs, possibly allowing for complete excision of an initially unresectable tumor. Radiotherapy alone has been successful, but carries the risk for radiation-induced orbital malignancies in young children. For local treatment failures, exenteration may be necessary.

Prognosis

With appropriate treatment, the 5-year survival for embryonal rhabdomyosarcomas of the orbit is about 90%. Group I patients have the best overall survival, while Group IV have the worst prognosis. IGRS Group III local failure rates were 2%, but other reports have been as high as 5–10%. Hematogenous metastases to the lung and bones carry a 3-year survival rate of 70%. Alveolar variant carries a worse prognosis, particularly in Groups III and IV. The prognosis for vision is guarded following radiotherapy.

Solitary Fibrous Tumor

Clinical Pearls

- Solitary fibrous tumor is an uncommon benign spindle cell tumor or mesenchymal origin.
- They present at any age but typically in middle-aged individuals.
- They are vascular and bleed easily during surgery.
- Treatment is with complete surgical excision.

Solitary fibrous tumor is an uncommon benign spindle cell tumor that has been reported with increasing frequency in the orbit. It is thought to arise from mesenchymal cells, some differentiation toward vascular endothelial cells and giving rise to the closely related giant cell angiofibroma. In the past it has been confused with other spindle cell tumors and in particular with hemangiopericytoma in the orbit. Here, we elect to classify this lesion with the mesenchymal tumors.

Clinical Presentation

Solitary fibrous tumor occurs in children and adults, but most commonly between the ages of 30 and 50 years. Patients present with slowly progressive painless proptosis and globe displacement (Fig. 56.72). Vision may be normal or decreased. The tumor has a predilection for the superior orbit, although it can occur in any quadrant of the orbit. Eyelid swelling and motility disturbance are common, but visual loss is infrequent. Malignant transformation has been reported in the orbit.

Computed Tomography

On CT scan, the tumor appears as a well-defined heterogeneous round to elongated mass of moderate density (Fig. 56.73). Up to 25% may have focal areas of calcification. Bone erosion is uncommon but may be seen with long-

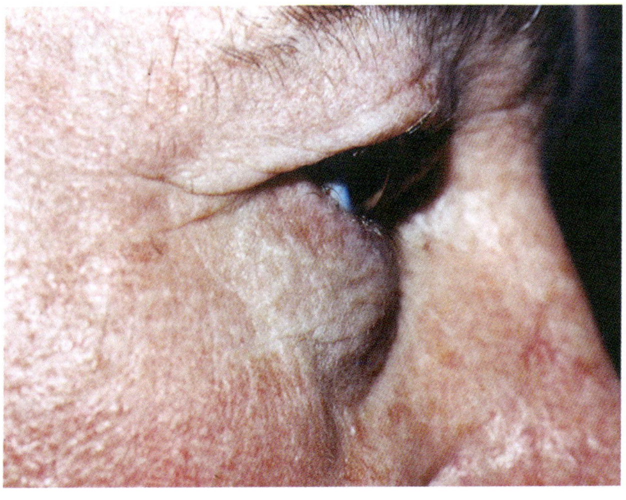

Fig. 56.72 Solitary fibrous tumor of the right inferior orbit

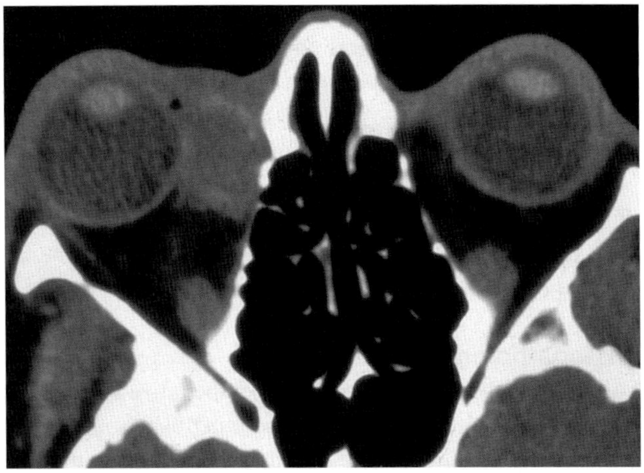

Fig. 56.73 CT scan showing a medium-density solitary fibrous tumor in the right medial orbit

standing lesions. Enhancement is moderate to marked and dynamic CT may show prominent feeder vessels.

Magnetic Resonance Imaging

The MRI shows a round to oval well-defined mass. On the T1-weighted image, the signal is isointense to gray matter and muscle and hypointense to fat. On the T2-weighted image, the tumor is hypointense to gray matter and hyperintense to fat. Low-intensity signal voids represent large blood vessels with rapidly flowing blood or cystic spaces. With gadolinium, there is moderate to marked homogeneous enhancement.

Histopathology

This tumor has been confused with other spindle cell tumors. In the orbit, many tumors previously referred to as fibrous histiocytoma or hemangiopericytoma have been reclassified by some authors and pathologists as solitary fibrous tumor. Histologically, SFT is well circumscribed with a pseudocapsule and shows a "patternless pattern" with thick bands of collagen alternating with hypercellular and hypocellular areas. They are characterized by fibrocollagenous tissue and spindle-shaped cells arranged in a fascicular pattern with occasional myxoid stroma. Numerous vascular channels with a pericytoma-like arrangement may be seen in some tumors. On immunohistochemistry, the cytoplasm stains positive for CD34 and vimentin. Giant cell angiofibromas appear to be a variant of solitary fibrous tumor with myxoid areas and giant cells.

Treatment

Complete surgical excision is the treatment of choice. These tumors tend to be less cohesive than other tumor so that en bloc excision can be difficult. Bleeding is common since these are rather vascular lesions.

Prognosis

Solitary fibrous tumors usually behave in a benign manner and generally do not metastasize. However, malignant transformation has been reported. Even after adequate resection, recurrence rates of up to 20–30% have been seen. With recurrence, these tumors tend to become more invasive into surrounding tissues.

Tumors of Bone

Aneurysmal Bone Cyst

Clinical Pearls

- Aneurysmal bone cyst is an expansile, multicystic, non-neoplastic reactive lesion of bone that may follow trauma or vascular disturbance.
- Lesions most often occur in adolescents along the orbital roof.
- Clinical manifestations include proptosis, globe displacement, and diplopia from cranial nerve palsy.
- Progressive pain is due to stretching of periosteum.
- CT scans show an expansile, irregular lytic lesion of bone with cortical destruction.
- Complete removal with surgical curettage results in an excellent prognosis.

Aneurysmal bone cyst is an expansile, multicystic, non-neoplastic reactive lesion of bone. This lesion may occur in nearly all bones, but occurs uncommonly in the orbit. It may arise secondary to trauma or perhaps a local vascular disturbance. In approximately 30% of cases, the cyst may be associated with underlying bone lesions such as fibrous dysplasia, non-ossifying fibroma, giant cell tumor, osteoblastoma, osteoclastoma, osteosarcoma, chondroblastoma, fibrous histiocytoma, and other lesions. Clinical onset is typically in adolescence, but may sometimes be seen in young children and middle-aged adults. Most commonly, the orbital roof is involved and may be associated with intracranial involvement.

Clinical Presentation

Common clinical manifestations include proptosis and variable globe displacement (Fig. 56.74). Larger lesions can result in cranial nerve palsies with resultant diplopia. Progressive pain is due to stretching of the overlying periosteum. Refractive changes resulting in visual disturbance have been reported to occur prior to onset of proptosis. Onset of symptoms may be sudden or gradual over months. Orbital pain, headache, and local swelling are often prominent features. Compressive optic neuropathy, papilledema, and visual loss are rare complications.

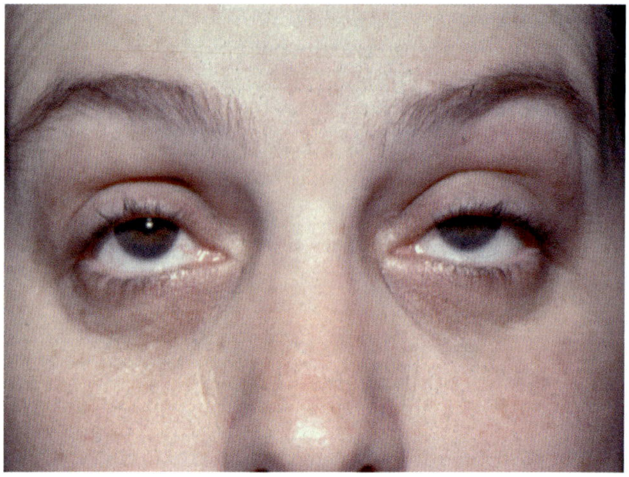

Fig. 56.74 Aneurysmal bone cyst of the left orbit, causing mild ptosis

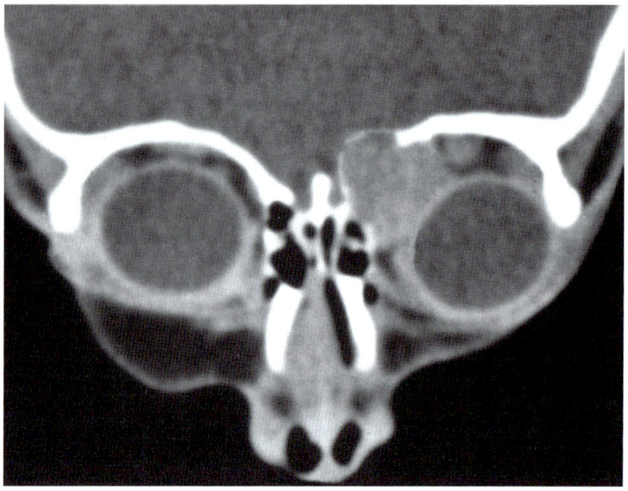

Fig. 56.75 Coronal CT scan showing a cystic mass in the left superomedial orbit extending into the anterior cranial fossa

Computed Tomography

CT scans show an expansile, irregular lytic lesion of bone with cortical destruction (Fig. 56.75). The lesion appears cystic and loculated. There is mild patchy enhancement of the soft tissue component following contrast administration. A fluid-fluid level may be seen within the cyst cavities representing hemorrhage with settled blood products. Subtle periosteal calcification can sometimes be appreciated at the margins of the lesion.

Magnetic Resonance Imaging

On MRI, the aneurysmal bone cyst appears as a multicystic mass associated with bone destruction. A fluid-fluid level may be demonstrated with heterogeneous signal intensity depending upon the state of the included blood. Fresh oxygenated blood appears hypointense or isointense to brain on T1-weighted images and is hyperintense on T2-weighted acquisitions. Deoxygenated blood shortens the relaxation times resulting in a more hyperintense signal on the T1-weighted image and a more hypointense signal on the T2-weighted sequence. As cell lysis occurs and iron is broken down, the T1-weighted image becomes hyperintense, whereas the T2-weighted signal intensity decreases even further. In general, the upper level shows a brighter image than the lower level. Fluid level characteristics and intensities may vary from one cavity to another.

Histopathology

Aneurysmal bone cysts have nonendothelialized cavernous spaces filled with blood and/or more cellular, solid, areas. The cavernous spaces have fibrous septa of variable thickness containing fibroblasts, histiocytes, osteoclast-like giant cells, and irregular bone trabeculae with a prominent osteoblastic rimming and osteoclastic-type giant cells. Mitotically, active granulation tissue may be present. The fibrous wall and solid portions of the tumor appear similar to the septa, with the addition of dilated, engorged blood vessels. Mitotic figures, without atypia, may be numerous in the fibrous wall and solid areas. Calcified matrix is present in the walls or solid areas in approximately one-third of aneurysmal bone cysts. Hemosiderin-laden macrophages may be present.

Treatment

The surgical approach of the tumor will depend upon tumor location. Once identified, complete removal with surgical curettage is the treatment of choice. Recurrence is likely following incomplete resection. Supplemental radiotherapy may be useful; however, this carries a risk of radiation-induced secondary sarcomas in young patients. Selective embolization of inaccessible lesions has been reported to result in progressive ossification.

Prognosis

For aneurysmal bone cysts involving the orbit, the prognosis is generally excellent. Complete surgical excision is generally curative. Permanent visual compromise is unusual.

Cholesterol Granuloma

Clinical Pearls

- Young adult males typically present with an insidious history of painless proptosis.
- Remote trauma is the most likely origin of these lesions.
- The lesion characteristically occurs within or just behind the superotemporal orbital rim.
- CT scan demonstrates a well-circumscribed, noncalcified extraconal soft tissue mass associated with an expansile, lytic bone defect.

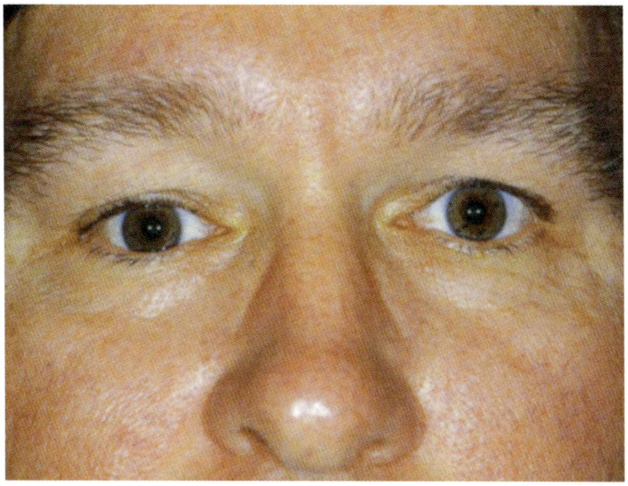

Fig. 56.76 Right cholesterol granuloma with minimal ptosis

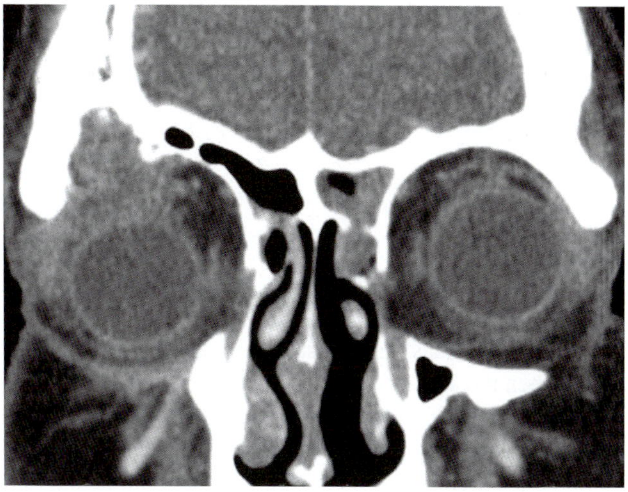

Fig. 56.77 Coronal CT scan with a lytic lesion in the right lateral superior orbit, representing a cholesterol granuloma

- The most appropriate treatment is surgical drainage followed by careful curettage or burring of abnormal tissue and bone.

Cholesterol granulomas are rare lesions arising in bone. Their precise etiology remains a matter of debate. In the nonpneumatized orbital bones, remote trauma is the most likely origin of these lesions. Others have speculated that a bony abnormality that is dysplastic, pagetoid, or vascular in nature may result in formation of these lesions. Hemorrhage and tissue edema occurs within the bone, and sluggish blood flow allows time for cholesterol crystals to precipitate. These act as a foreign body, inciting a granulomatous reaction. Enlargement erodes through the bone into the orbit. The lesion characteristically occurs behind the superotemporal orbital rim.

Clinical Presentation

Presentation typically is in young adults, a majority of which are males, with an insidious history of painless proptosis. These tumors are most frequently located within the superotemporal orbit within the lacrimal gland fossa, often resulting in inferonasal displacement of the globe (Fig. 56.76). Other symptoms may include ptosis, dystopia, extraocular motility restriction, diplopia, decreased vision, or choroidal folds. Symptoms develop over years, and, frequently, a history of trauma cannot be elicited. A soft mass may be palpable along or behind the superotemporal orbital rim, sometimes associated with a jagged bony defect.

Computed Tomography

The CT generally demonstrates a well-circumscribed, noncalcified extraconal soft tissue mass that is associated with an expansile, lytic bone defect (Fig. 56.77). Thinning of both the inner and outer tables is seen, and the lesion may extend intracranially or into the orbit. On bone windows, there is no sclerosis of the bony margins. The lesion has homogeneous attenuation with a density equal to brain and muscle. Enhancement is not seen with contrast administration.

Magnetic Resonance Imaging

Because the lesion contains blood breakdown products, the MR resonance is characteristically high. On T1-weighted images, the signal is heterogeneous due to the presence of secondary inflammation and granulation tissue. The signal is bright and isointense to orbital fat. On the T2-weighted sequence, the image remains isointense to fat. With gadolinium, there is no enhancement.

Histopathology

The cystic cavity in a cholesterol granuloma contains numerous cholesterol clefts, resulting from cholesterol dissolved during processing. The key feature differentiating the cholesterol granuloma from the cholesteatoma is the absence of an epithelial lining in the cholesterol granuloma. Granulomatous inflammation with epithelioid histiocytes and multinucleated giant cells containing cholesterol clefts surrounds the cavity. Hemosiderin-laden macrophages are also common. As the lesion ages, the cyst wall becomes progressively fibrotic.

Treatment

The most appropriate treatment is surgical drainage followed by careful curettage of abnormal cyst contents. Burring of abnormal bone may be performed, but the underlying bone is frequently thinned, so care should be taken during surgery to avoid inadvertently damaging underlying dura. Endoscopic approaches to this tumor have been reported. Recurrences have rarely been reported, but can occur with incomplete resection. Displaced bony fragments and spurs should be removed. If the defect is very large, a fat graft can be placed to fill the void.

Prognosis

Surgical removal is generally curative. The prognosis for both vision and life is excellent, and recurrences are rare.

Ewing Sarcoma

Clinical Pearls

- Ewing sarcoma may represent undifferentiated cells of neuroectodermal origin.
- Ewing sarcomas are most likely to occur in males between the ages of 5 and 13.
- Patients present with slowly worsening ophthalmoplegia, diplopia, ptosis, proptosis, or globe displacement.
- Systemic symptoms of fever, fatigue, anorexia, and weight loss are associated with disseminated metastases.
- The combination of multiagent chemotherapy, surgical resection, and radiotherapy results in improved survival.

Ewing sarcoma is a distinctive neoplasm consisting of undifferentiated small round cells arising in bone, but extraskeletal primary tumors occur. The cell of origin remains controversial, but some evidence suggests that Ewing sarcoma may develop from undifferentiated cells of neuroectodermal origin. The tumor classically involves the limbs, ribs, and pelvis. Ewing sarcoma is responsible for 10% of primary malignant bone tumors, with greater than 75% of cases having metastasis within 2 years of diagnosis. Peak incidence of Ewing sarcoma occurs between the ages of 5 and 13. Ninety percent of patients are less than 30 years old, and 75% are less than 20 years old. This is a disease primarily of Caucasians, and males are more frequently affected than females in a ratio of 1.6:1. Orbital involvement is typically the result of metastasis from a distant site or extension from an adjacent tumor, although primary orbital tumors have been reported.

Clinical Presentation

Tumor growth is usually insidious, with ophthalmic symptoms that develop over several months. Common findings include ophthalmoplegia, diplopia, ptosis, proptosis, and globe displacement (Fig. 56.78). Less common findings include decreased vision, optic nerve edema, choroidal folds, and headache. A soft nontender mass may be palpable beneath the orbital rim. Hemorrhagic necrosis may cause erythema and local warmth simulating osteomyelitis. Systemic symptoms of fever, fatigue, anorexia, and weight loss are associated with disseminated metastases, seen in 10–30% of patients at initial diagnosis.

Computed Tomography

The CT scan reveals an irregular heterogeneous cystic mass. Adjacent bone shows mottled destruction (Fig. 56.79). The mass frequently extends from the maxillary sinus or mandible. Patchy hypodense areas correlate with old hemorrhage and necrosis. Enhancement with contrast administration is variable.

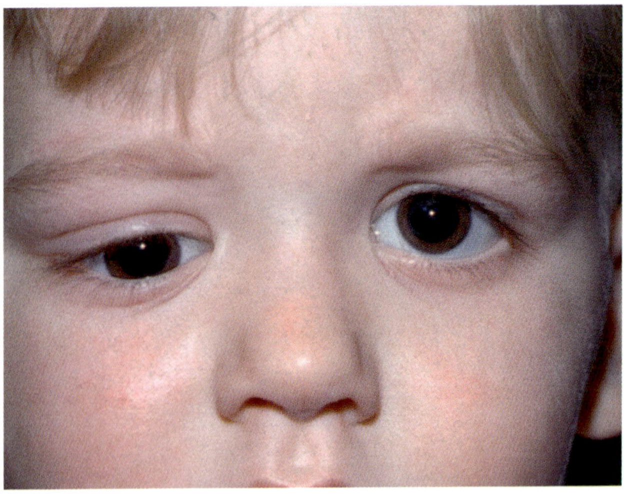

Fig. 56.78 Child with proptosis and downward displacement of the right globe from a Ewing sarcoma

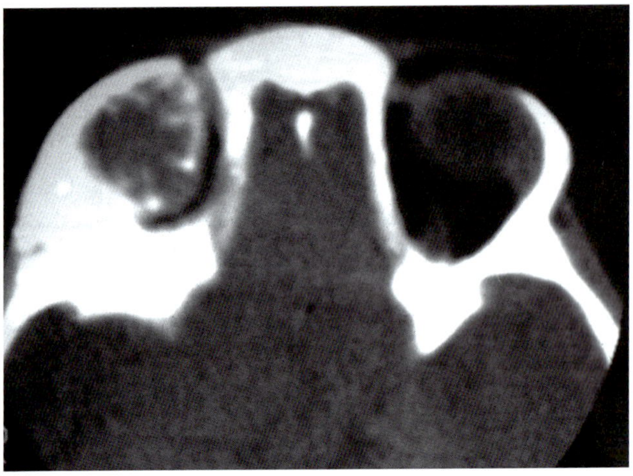

Fig. 56.79 Axial CT scan of the patient in Fig. 56.78 with a lytic expansile mass lesion in the right superolateral orbital rim

Magnetic Resonance Imaging

On MRI, an extraosseous mass is seen contiguous with bone destruction. The T1-weighted signal is low, being hypointense to both fat and muscle. On the T2-weighted sequence, the signal is high, imaging isointense to fat and hyperintense to muscle. Heterogeneity is due to areas of necrosis that produce lower signal intensity. There is generally no significant periosteal reaction. With gadolinium, only the cellular areas enhance.

Histopathology

The most common pattern is seen as sheets and nests of monomorphic, small, round cells with scant cytoplasm (Fig. 56.80). Round tumor cells are slightly larger than lym-

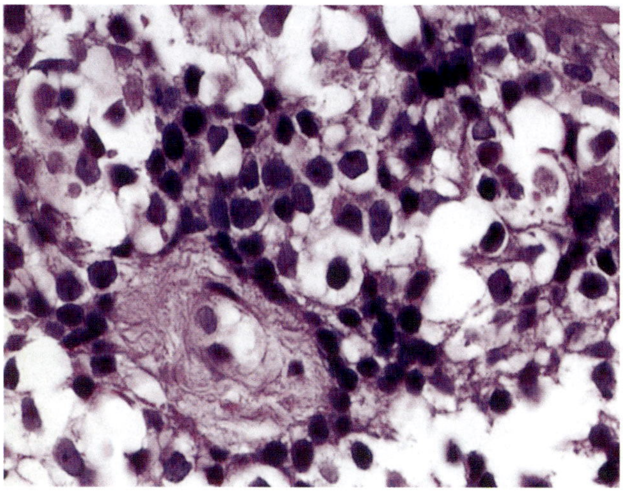

Fig. 56.80 Ewing sarcoma consisting of cells with enlarged hyperchromatic nuclei and scant cytoplasm. These tumors are CD99 immunopositive

phocytes and have a round nucleus (often with indentations) containing open, finely dispersed chromatin and one or two small nucleoli. The cytoplasm is pale or vacuolated due to the presence of glycogen that stains with the periodic acid-Schiff stain. Numerous mitoses may be present. These cells may be surrounded by fine fibrous tissue. The dark cells have denser and more elongated nuclei and tend to form aggregates. Immunohistochemical stains help to differentiate Ewing sarcoma from other round cell tumors such as rhabdomyosarcoma, lymphoma, and neuroblastoma. Positive staining using antibodies that detect the MIC2 gene product in paraffin sections supports a diagnosis of Ewing sarcoma, though the antibody is not specific for this entity. Strong membranous staining with CD99 supports the diagnosis.

Treatment

Since orbital disease is usually metastatic or secondary, treatment must include aggressive multiagent chemotherapy. Chemotherapy regimens may include variable combinations of vincristine, adriamycin, cyclophosphamide, doxorubicin, etoposide, or ifosfamide. Several cycles of the selected chemotherapy regimen are typically given prior to planned surgical excision, enabling one to obtain improved surgical margins. Adjunctive radiotherapy at 4500–5200 cGy may also be used.

Prognosis

Until recently, treatment with surgery and radiotherapy alone gave a 5-year survival rate of only 10%. The combination of multiagent chemotherapy, surgical resection, and radiotherapy has increased the 5-year survival rate to 45–75% and decreased local recurrence to approximately 5%. Poor prognosis has been associated with metastasis at diagnosis, systemic symptoms, symptoms greater than 6 months, and central tumor location.

Fibrous Dysplasia

Clinical Pearls

- Fibrous dysplasia is a hamartomatous malformation resulting from the arrest of maturation at the woven bone stage.
- Fibrous dysplasia most frequently affects children, adolescents, and young adults.
- Progressive orbital dystopia and facial asymmetry occur from thickening of orbital bones.
- Slowly progressive visual loss from optic nerve compression is seen in up to 50% of cases.
- CT scans show a narrowed orbital contour and replacement of adjacent sinuses with dense bone. The thickened bone is sclerotic, with a "ground-glass" appearance.
- Surgery is indicated to debulk the bone and open foramina in cases of progressive nerve compression and for cosmetic improvement of facial asymmetry.

Fibrous dysplasia is a benign developmental fibro-osseous lesion. This is a hamartomatous malformation resulting from the arrest in maturation at the woven bone stage. Bone is replaced with abnormal fibrous tissue containing dysplastic bony trabeculae. Fibrous dysplasia most frequently affects children, adolescents, and young adults. The orbit is affected in 20–39% of patients with craniofacial disease. The lesion is usually mono-ostotic (70–80%) around the orbit, but may involve multiple adjacent bones, especially when associated with McCune-Albright's syndrome. The latter occurs mostly in women and often presents with polyostotic fibrous dysplasia, sexual precocity, endocrine dysfunction, and cutaneous pigmentation. Occurrence is more common in children and young adults and is progressive into the second or third decade of life. Malignant degeneration may occur in 0.5–1% of cases.

Clinical Presentation

Progressive orbital dystopia and facial asymmetry occur from thickening of orbital bones. The frontal bone is most commonly involved, resulting in unilateral proptosis, ptosis, and a downward displacement of the orbit and globe (Fig. 56.81). The sphenoid is the second most commonly involved bone and can result in compression of structures within the orbital apex. Proptosis may be severe enough to cause corneal exposure and ulceration. Epiphora can result from involvement of the nasolacrimal duct. Sensory loss due to narrowing of the infraorbital and supraorbital foramina can occur. Progressive constriction of orbital foramina and canals of the cranial base may cause cranial nerve palsies and trigeminal neuralgia. Slowly progressive visual loss from optic nerve compression is seen in up to 50% of cases. Acute vision loss occurs secondary to intralesional hemorrhage, sphenoidal mucocele, or aneurysmal bone

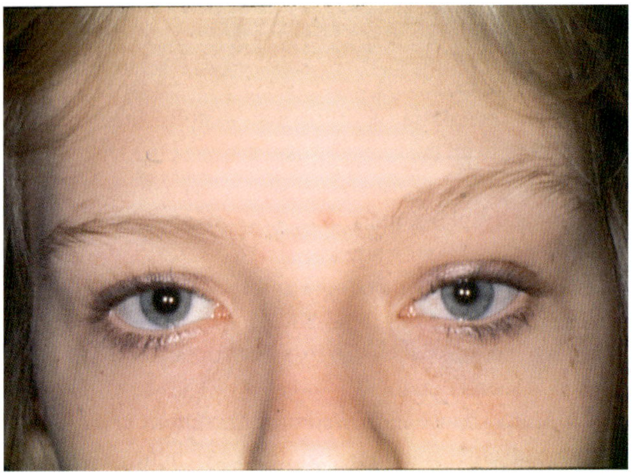

Fig. 56.81 A young female with ptosis and mild proptosis of the left eye from fibrous dysplasia

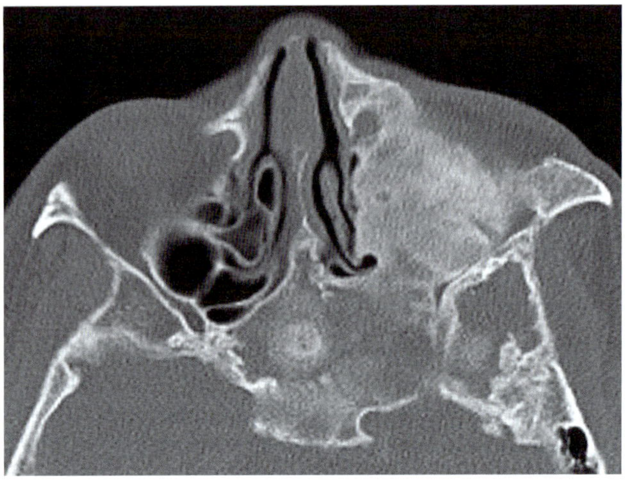

Fig. 56.82 Bone window axial CT scan showing thickened ground-glass appearance of the left sphenoid, ethmoid, and zygomatic bones

cyst. The lesion has been associated with sensorineural hearing loss, vertigo, temporomandibular joint dysfunction, mucocele, and dental malocclusion.

Computed Tomography

On CT scans, orbital fibrous dysplasia shows a narrowing of the orbital contour and replacement of adjacent sinuses with dense bone. The involved bone is thickened and sclerotic, with a "ground-glass" appearance of increased density (Fig. 56.82). Heterogeneous density represents mixed areas of ossified and unossified fibrous tissue. There may be regions of cystic lucency or increased density. The distorted internal bony architecture can be seen with extended window settings. The lesion can cross suture lines and extend across the midline. Small areas of high attenuation reflect the presence of microscopic calcification within the abnormal fibrous tissue. Other areas of low attenuation may reflect zones of poorly calcified trabeculae.

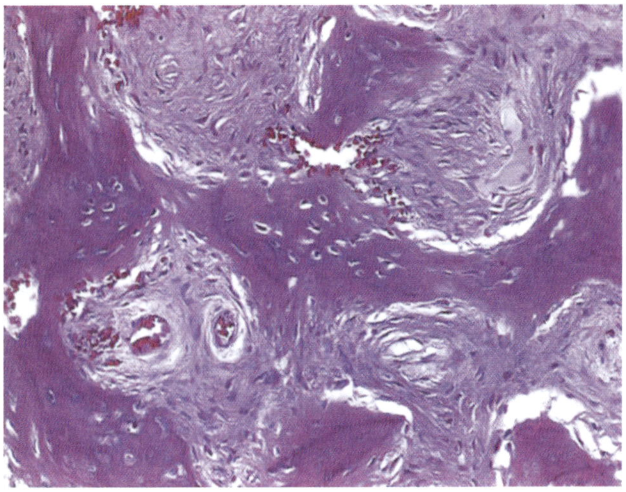

Fig. 56.83 Fibrous dysplasia showing interlacing trabeculae of woven bone with interspersed fibrous matrix

Magnetic Resonance Imaging

Normal bone appears as a very dark signal void. Involved orbital bones are thickened with a homogenous low signal that is hypointense to isointense with respect to muscle on T1-weighted images. On T2-weighted sequences, the signal is mildly heterogeneous and generally hyperintense to muscle with lower signal linear septae. Less calcified areas of vascularized fibrous stroma may show foci of more hyperintense signals. Areas of cystic degeneration demonstrate brighter fluid signal intensity or a fluid-fluid level. With gadolinium, there is most often mild central enhancement (73%), although peripheral rim enhancement may be seen in 27%. Hyperostotic meningioma may be distinguished from fibrous dysplasia by enhancing soft tissue component seen on T1 and T2 images that are isointense to gray matter.

Histopathology

The bony trabeculae appear as round islands and interconnected irregular networks, curves, or serpiginous forms referred to as "Chinese characters." Osteoblastic rimming of the bony trabeculae is typically absent, but occasionally may be seen. Within a fibrous stroma composed of small spindle cells are irregularly distributed trabeculae of immature bone (Fig. 56.83). The stromal spindle cells have oval nuclei and indistinct cytoplasmic borders. Anaplasia and mitotic figures are absent. The fibrous tissue may appear whorl-like, but typically lacks a characteristic pattern of organization. The fibrous stroma may demonstrate areas with cartilaginous nodules, myxomatous changes, lamellar bone, and aneurismal bone cysts. Foam cells (lipid-laden histiocytes) and giant cells may be associated with foci of hemorrhage in the stroma.

Treatment

Surgery is indicated to debulk and open foramina in cases of progressive nerve compression and for cosmetic improvement of facial asymmetry. Bleeding can be a significant problem during surgery. Multidisciplinary approaches may allow for maximal resection of abnormal bone, followed by reconstruction. Concurrent cranial reconstruction with bone grafts offers the best chances for a successful cosmetic result. Complete excision is usually not possible, and repeat surgery is typical. Intravenous pamidronate has been reported to increase bone density and decrease bone remodeling, offering some help to those with severe forms of the diseases. Radiotherapy may be useful, but carries the risk of malignant degeneration.

Prognosis

With sphenoid bone involvement, early aggressive intervention is required to prevent permanent visual loss. Visual recovery has been reported with timely decompression of the optic canal. Malignant transformation to osteosarcoma, fibrosarcoma, chondrosarcoma, and giant cell sarcoma is often heralded by rapid progression and worsening pain. This transformation occurs in less than 0.5% of patients, but increases up to 15% following radiotherapy.

Giant Cell Reparative Granuloma

Clinical Pearls

- Giant cell reparative granulomas are benign proliferative lesions which likely result from intraosseous hemorrhage associated with local trauma or sinusitis.
- These lesions tend to occur more commonly during the first and second decades of life.
- Proptosis and abaxial displacement of the globe can occur rapidly, but usually progresses gradually.
- On CT scan, the giant cell granuloma appears as an osteolytic, expansile lesion of bone with cortical erosion and focal destruction.
- The lesion contains multinucleated giant cells and mononuclear spindle-shaped cells without evidence of nuclear atypia.
- Therapy consists of aggressive surgical curettage and resection of the adjacent bony margin.

The giant cell reparative granulomas are benign proliferative lesions representing an exuberant reparative response to intraosseous hemorrhage associated with local trauma or sinusitis. Expansion of this granulomatous mass occurs by proliferation of its stromal component. Lesions tend to occur more commonly during the first and second decades of life, although cases have been reported in older patients. The granuloma most commonly affects the mandible and maxilla. Orbital involvement occurs via extension from the sphenoid, ethmoid, or frontal bones. Associated bony destruction and intracranial extension may be found. Differentiating this tumor from osteoclastoma, eosinophilic granuloma, and aneurysmal bone cyst may be difficult, but differences in patient demographics and radiologic features are often helpful with classification. Serum calcium and phosphate levels should be performed to rule out brown tumor of hyperparathyroidism.

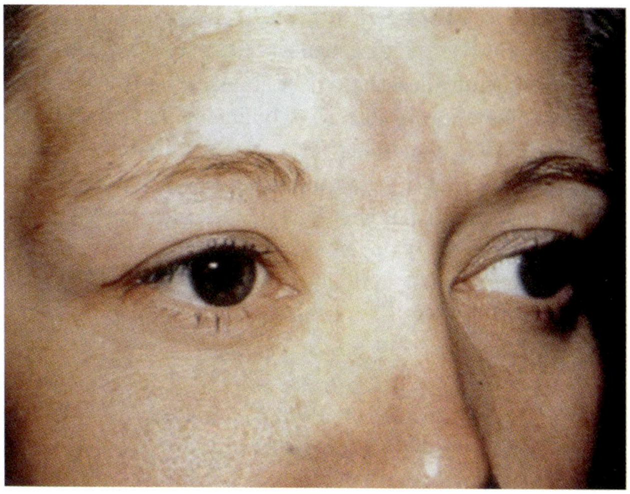

Fig. 56.84 Swelling of the right lateral orbital rim from a giant cell reparative granuloma

Clinical Presentation

Intraosseous hemorrhage results in cortical lysis and formation of a soft tissue mass (Fig. 56.84). Proptosis and abaxial displacement of the globe can occur as a catastrophic event, but usually progresses gradually. Symptoms of retrobulbar pain are associated with stretching of periorbita. Anterior lesions are palpable as a firm mass. Lesions involving the orbital apex can present with optic nerve compression, papilledema, and visual field defects. Invasion of adjacent orbital soft tissues rarely occurs, resulting in motility restriction and diplopia.

Computed Tomography

Giant cell granulomas appear as an osteolytic, expansile lesion of bone with cortical erosion and focal destruction. Density is heterogeneous, with lower attenuating darker regions representing areas of hemorrhage. Patchy areas of moderate contrast enhancement may be seen within the large nonenhancing cystic mass. The cortical bone is thinned, but there is no periosteal reaction of reactive sclerosis.

Magnetic Resonance Imaging

The reparative granuloma appears as a well-defined mass associated with destruction of bone. On T1-weighted images, the mass is isointense to brain and may show linear streaks of lower signal intensity representing fibrous septa. Trapped secretions in adjacent sinuses produce more hyperintense signals. On T2-weighted images, the mass remains hypointense to the brain. Moderate homogeneous enhancement is seen on postgadolinium T1 scans.

Histopathology

The moderately cellular stroma of reparative granulomas has significant collagen deposition and hemorrhage. The lesion contains multinucleated osteoclast-type giant cells (10–15 nuclei) and reactive mononuclear spindle-shaped cells resembling myofibroblasts. They show no evidence of nuclear atypia. Vascularization of these lesions is often noted. The number of osteoclast-like giant cells in the stroma is highly variable, with a tendency for the giant cells to congregate in areas of hemorrhage. Hemosiderin and hemosiderin-laden macrophages are associated with stromal hemorrhages. Focal areas of bony erosion, osteoid, and reactive bone formation may also be found. Irregular trabeculae of woven bone lined by osteoblasts may be present.

Treatment

Therapy consists of surgical curettage and resection of the adjacent bony margin. Multidisciplinary approaches may be required for complete resection of the lesion. The rate of local recurrence following surgical resection is 10–15%. These recurrences are thought to be the result of incomplete removal, although partial resection has been reported to result in spontaneous resolution. Adjunctive radiotherapy has been advocated, but has been associated with sarcomatous tumors in young patients.

Prognosis

The prognosis for life and vision is excellent. Where optic nerve compression has resulted in optic atrophy, some visual loss may be permanent.

Ossifying Fibroma

Clinical Pearls

- Ossifying fibromas may arise in any of the orbital bones, but most tumors invade the orbit secondarily.
- Orbital ossifying fibromas most commonly occur in the ethmoid region, tend to be mono-ostotic, and do not cross suture lines.
- The tumor occurs most commonly presents with slowly progressive proptosis during the first to third decades of life.
- The CT scan shows enlargement of the involved bone, with well-defined rounded borders.
- Because of the aggressive nature and risk of recurrence, tumors should be completely resected surgically.

Ossifying fibroma is a benign acquired fibro-osseous tumor that most commonly arises within the paranasal sinuses. This tumor may arise in any of the orbital bones, but usually invades the orbit secondarily. Ossifying fibromas involving the orbit most commonly arise from the ethmoid region or superior orbital plate of the frontal bone. It is mono-ostotic and does not cross suture lines. Young individuals in the first to third decades of life are primarily affected, without any sex predilection.

Clinical Presentation

Slowly progressive proptosis is the most common symptom, with associated globe displacement. Other associated symptoms include decreased visual acuity, extraocular motility disturbance, headache, sinusitis, nasal obstruction, facial swelling, and even inflammation mimicking orbital cellulitis (Fig. 56.85). Anterior lesions may be palpable as a smooth, nontender, firm mass. Apical tumors are often associated with optic nerve compression, decreased vision, and visual field defects. Lesion arising from the ethmoid bone may present with epiphora from nasolacrimal duct obstruction. Intracranial extension does occur, but typically does not result in neurologic symptoms due to its slow growth.

Computed Tomography

The CT scan shows enlargement of the involved bone, with well-defined smooth borders. On tissue window settings, the mass demonstrates heterogeneous bone density due to the presence of osteoblastic and osteoclastic regions within a

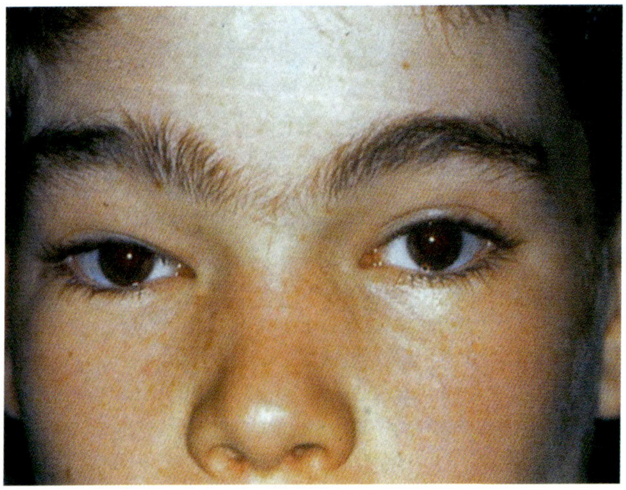

Fig. 56.85 Child with ptosis and downward displacement of the right eye from an ossifying fibroma

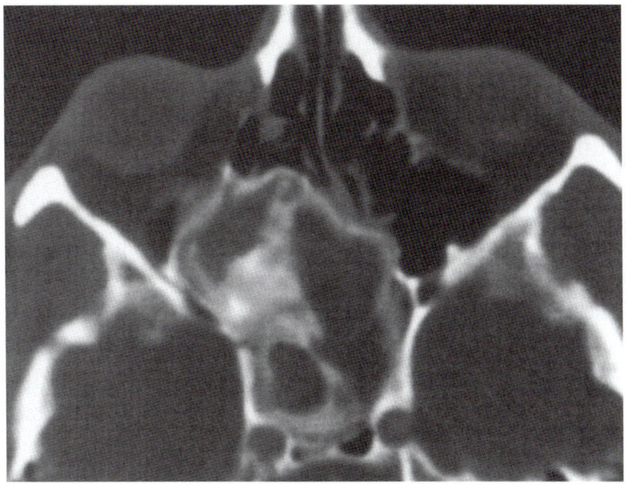

Fig. 56.86 Bone window axial CT showing an ossifying fibroma of the sphenoid bone

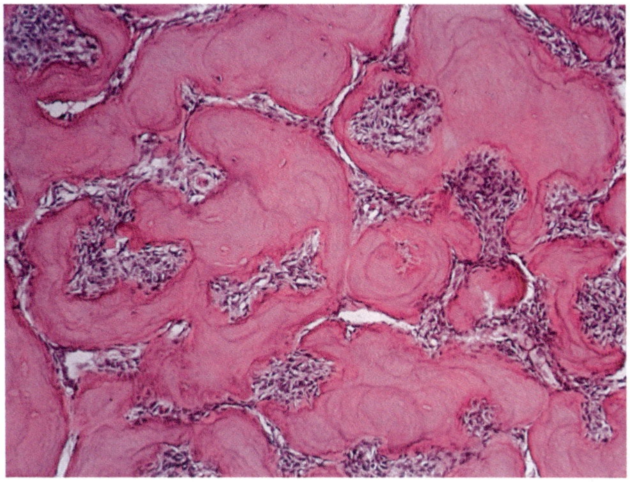

Fig. 56.87 Ossifying fibroma demonstrating bony trabeculae composed of lamellar bone, some lined by plump osteoblasts, interspersed with cellular fibrous stroma

hyperdense thin sclerotic rim (Fig. 56.86). Focal areas of mineralization or calcification are often noted. There may be focal radiodense areas representing bone spicules and radiolucent regions of nonossified matrix or cysts. With lesions that arise in a paranasal sinus, there can be an associated mucocele.

Magnetic Resonance Imaging

Because of the overall low proton density of bone, ossifying fibroma produces a heterogeneous low to intermediate signal intensity on T1-weighted images that is generally isointense to muscle. On T2-weighted sequences, ossified regions give a low, hypointense signal intensity compared to adjacent bone and muscle. Areas of nonossified matrix or cysts may appear more hyperintense. With gadolinium, minimal to moderate enhancement is seen within areas of fibrous matrix. Inspisated secretions associated with mucoceles produce a hyperintense signal on T2-weighted images and only an enhancing rim of tissue on postcontrast T1-weighted scans.

Histopathology

The aggressive psammomatoid variant of ossifying fibroma is the most common form. This variant is characterized by the presence of ovoid and cementum-like spherules or osteoid spicules that are hypocellular or acellular and lie within a highly vascularized stroma or within bony trabeculae (Fig. 56.87). In contrast to fibrous dysplasia, bony trabeculae are composed of lamellar bone lined by osteoblasts. This myxomatous stroma contains round and spindle-shaped cells with prominent nuclei that have rare mitoses. The spherules are reminiscent of the psammoma bodies in meningiomas, leading to the term "psammomatoid ossifying fibroma." The trabecular variant is characterized by bands of cellular osteoid and trabeculae of immature bone lined with osteoblasts.

Treatment

Because these tumors can be locally aggressive, they should be surgically resected. Complete excision is recommended because of the tendency of this tumor to recur following incomplete resections. The exact approach will depend upon the individual bone involved and generally includes a multidisciplinary team of specialists.

Prognosis

The prognosis for life is excellent. No metastases have been reported. With timely therapy, the prognosis for vision should be very good.

Osteoblastoma

Clinical Pearls

- Approximately 20% of osteoblastomas occur within craniofacial bones.
- Osteoblastomas of the orbit have a peak incidence in the second and third decades of life.
- Osteoblastomas of the orbit usually also involve the ethmoid or frontal sinus or the orbital roof.
- Symptoms include headache, epistaxis, proptosis, globe displacement, and eyelid swelling.
- Management is complete excision and reconstruction.
- The prognosis is excellent.

Osteoblastoma is an uncommon primary benign neoplasm of bone. The etiology is unknown, but histologically, osteoblastomas are similar to osteoid osteomas, producing both osteoid and primitive woven bone within a fibrovascular connective tissue matrix. Although usually considered benign, a controversial aggressive variant has been described with histologic features similar to those of malignant tumors such as an osteosarcoma and has been associated with metastasis and death. Osteoblastoma affects males more than females in a ratio of 2–3:1. Osteoblastoma can occur at any age, but about 80% occur in patients under the age of 30 years.

Clinical Presentation

The tumor generally results in slowly progressive abaxial proptosis with the globe displaced inferiorly. Focal tenderness to touch and periorbital and eyelid swelling may be present. Epistaxis can be seen with sinus involvement. Visual loss is not common, but has been reported.

Computed Tomography

CT usually demonstrates typical radiographic features of a central nidus and surrounding reactive bone. An expansile lobulated mass is seen extending into adjacent tissues with significant bone destruction. Portions of the tumor may be less dense with a ground-glass appearance.

Magnetic Resonance Imaging

Unenhanced T1-weighted images show a ground-glass appearance with low signal intensity. Dense osseous lesions reveal darker signal voids on both T1- and T2-weighted images. With gadolinium, there is only minimal enhancement.

Histopathology

The tumor consists of interlacing trabeculae of woven bone lined by plump osteoblasts and a few osteoclasts. The trabeculae are distributed in a loose richly vascular stroma containing bland fibroblastic spindle cells. The osteoblast nuclei show occasional mitoses.

Treatment

Treatment is with en bloc excision that often requires a multidisciplinary surgical team, including a skull base surgeon. Incomplete resections result in recurrences of more than 25% of cases. Following resection reconstruction with split-thickness bone grafts is often necessary. The role of radiotherapy has not been established but has been used in cases of incomplete resection.

Prognosis

Complete resection yields an excellent prognosis with overall recurrence rates of less than 15%. Malignant transformation is rare.

Osteoma

Clinical Pearls

- Osteomas are the most common bony tumor of the orbit.
- Tumors occur more commonly in men during the second to fifth decades.
- Slowly progressive proptosis is the most common finding.
- CT shows a sharply defined, very dense, rounded, lobulated, or pedunculated heterogeneous mass arising from bone.
- The management of a symptomatic osteoma involving the orbit is surgical excision.

Osteomas are well-differentiated, slow-growing, benign tumors of bone. They are the most common bony tumor of the orbit, representing 1–2% of all orbital tumors. Most arise in the paranasal sinuses, with about 15% resulting in orbital symptoms. Males are affected more than females, with symptoms most often presenting in the second to fifth decades of life. Although controversial, osteomas are likely related to developmental, traumatic, or infectious etiologies. Multiple osteomas may be seen in association with Gardner's syndrome (familial polyposis coli).

Clinical Presentation

Slowly progressive proptosis is the most common sign of orbital involvement. Patients often present with a history of sinusitis and facial pain. Other common symptoms include headache, facial deformity, dizziness, and diplopia. Anteriorly placed tumors are often palpable as a rock hard mass (Fig. 56.88). The globe is typically displaced downward and laterally, since most orbital osteomas arise in the frontal or ethmoid sinuses. Osteomas occur less commonly within the maxillary and sphenoid sinuses. Nasolacrimal duct obstruction or rhinorrhea may occur with maxillary sinus lesions. Pain on ocular movement, amaurosis fugax, papilledema, optic atrophy, and visual loss can be associated with sphenoid bone involvement. Rarely, erosion through periorbita can result in orbital emphysema and cellulitis.

Computed Tomography

Osteomas are sharply defined, very dense, rounded, lobulated, or pedunculated heterogeneous masses arising from bone (Fig. 56.89). In the fibrous type of osteoma, a low-

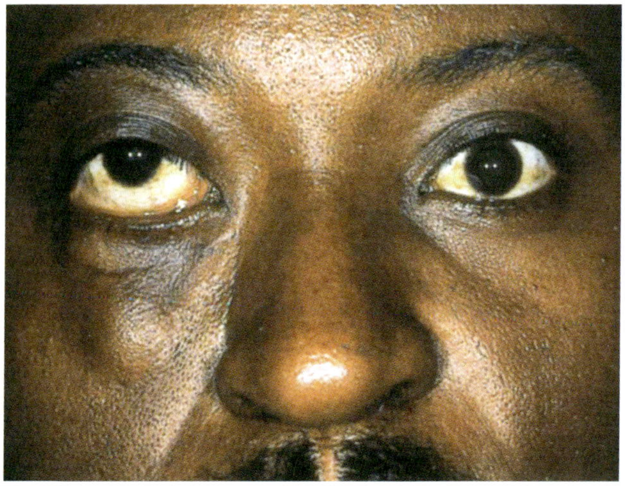

Fig. 56.88 Bony osteoma of the right maxillary bone

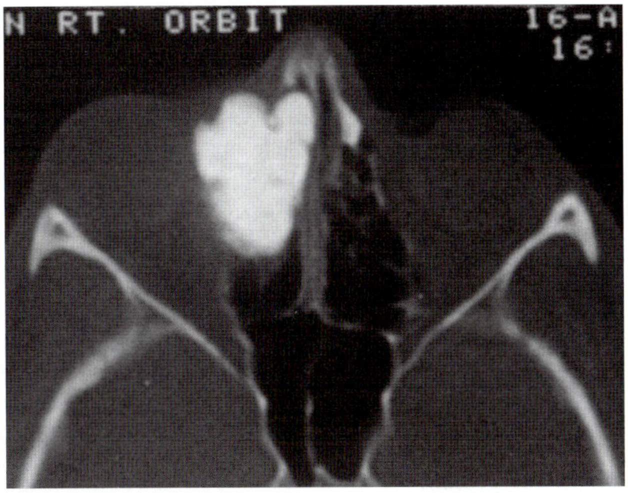

Fig. 56.89 Bone window CT with a dense osteoma of the right ethmoid bone

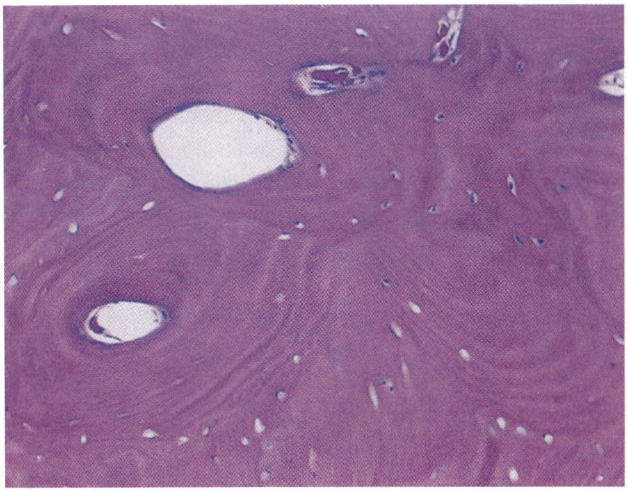

Fig. 56.90 Ivory osteoma consisting of compact bone with osteocytes, Haversian canals, and scanty fibrous stroma

density, ground-glass appearance may be more similar to fibrous dysplasia. Scattered or confluent islands of dense bone formation are seen within the mass. The involved paranasal sinus is frequently opacified from secondary drainage obstruction, sometimes with mucocele formation. On bone window settings, the lesion appears as dense sclerotic compact bone. The central area may sometimes show a radiolucent, low-density fibrous trabecular nidus.

Magnetic Resonance Imaging

On the MRI, regions of cortical bone are relatively devoid of resonance signal. They appear as a signal void on both T1-weighted and T2-weighted sequences. The central nidus of osteoid-rich fibrovascular tissue produces brighter regions within the signal void that are hypointense to hyperintense with respect to muscle. Following gadolinium administration, the nidus may show moderate to marked enhancement.

Histopathology

Osteomas represent an overgrowth of bone. These tumors may be classified as compact, cancellous, or fibrous. Compact (ivory) osteomas are composed of dense, lamellar, or woven cortical bone with small Haversian canals. Mature osteomas contain thinner, cancellous, trabecular bone lined by osteoblasts and osteoclasts with a loose fibrovascular matrix (Fig. 56.90). A cartilaginous component is absent, and a thin layer of spindle cells covers the lesion. Mature osteomas need to be distinguished from ossifying fibroma and fibrous dysplasia.

Treatment

The management of a symptomatic osteoma involving the orbit is surgical excision. When sinus obstruction or mucocele is present, sinus drainage is necessary. Endoscopic resection and reconstruction has been reported. More extensive lesions may require a multidisciplinary approach involving neurosurgery, otolaryngology, and ophthalmology.

Prognosis

The prognosis is generally very good except in cases of long-standing optic nerve compression associated with sphenoid bone lesions. Rare complications such as pneumatocele, pneumocephalus with meningitis, and CSF leaks have been reported.

Osteosarcoma

Clinical Pearls

- Osteosarcoma is the most common malignant bone tumor.
- The tumor arises from primitive mesenchymal bone-forming cells and classically produces malignant osteoid.
- Orbital involvement most often occurs as the result of invasion from paranasal sinuses and the nasal cavity.
- Children, adolescents, or young adults typically present with rapidly progressive proptosis with globe displacement.
- Aggressive surgical resection followed by adjuvant chemotherapy and/or radiotherapy may improve outcome.

Osteosarcomas are the most common malignant bone tumor and represent 0.5–1.0% of orbital tumors. Osteosarcomas can occur in any bone, usually in the extremities of long bones near metaphyseal growth plates. Orbital involvement most often occurs as the result of invasion from paranasal sinuses or the nasal cavity. Distant metastases to the orbit and primary orbital tumors have been reported. Osteosarcomas may arise in a solitary fashion or more rarely in multiple sites over a period of 6 months or more. Metastasis occurs via hematogenous spread, most commonly to the lungs and bones. Osteosarcoma is thought to arise from primitive mesenchymal bone-forming cells, and its histologic hallmark is the production of malignant osteoid. Approximately 10% of patients have a history of radiotherapy to the area where osteosarcoma develops. Tumor development has been associated with Paget's disease, fibrous dysplasia, giant cell tumors, and osteochondromas. Patients with familial retinoblastoma have a 10% risk of developing ostosarcoma by age 25. Most osteosarcomas are reported to occur in children, adolescents, and young adults. Craniofacial osteosarcomas tend to affect individuals between 26 and 40 years of age, on average 10 years older than patients with tumors of long bones.

Clinical Presentation

Patients with orbital involvement typically present with rapidly progressive proptosis with globe displacement. Other common symptoms include pain, chemosis, sensory nerve paresthesias, and soft tissue swelling. The mass may be palpable if located anteriorly. Patient may complain of epiphora, epistaxis, nasal obstruction, headache, and diplopia. Globe indentation, extraocular motility disturbance, and facial and eyelid swelling may be noted on examination.

Computed Tomography

The appearance on CT scan may vary in density from case to case depending upon the amount of osseous, cartilaginous, and fibrous tissue components. The tumor is an irregular invasive and often destructive sclerotic mass. Density is high when osteoid predominates but areas of increased fibrovascular tissue image as lower density than bone. There may be focal areas of increased density representing calcification. Fine linear shadows of new bone formation may be seen radiating from the nidus. The tumor often breaches the cortex, incites a periosteal reaction, and invades soft tissue. With contrast administration, there is marked enhancement.

Magnetic Resonance Imaging

MRI is the preferred modality for delineating any associated soft tissue component. An intramedullary expansile lesion is seen that is heterogeneous and hyperintense to muscle on T1-weighted imaging and hypointense or mixed in signal intensity on T2-weighted imaging. STIR sequences can overestimate the disease because the high signal intensity of surrounding edema can simulate tumor. Cystic blood spaces appear as focal areas of increased signal intensity on T2-weighted imaging. With gadolinium, there is heterogeneous enhancement.

Histopathology

Osteoblastic, chondroblastic, and fibroblastic variants are the most common. Most tumors contain areas of osteogenic, chondroblastic, and fibroblastic differentiation. To identify malignant osteoid, adequate sampling of the tumor is mandatory. Sheets of atypical or pleomorphic osteoblasts invariably surround islands of osteoid. The cells tend to be spindle or polygonal in shape with variable anaplasia, increased mitoses, and hyperchromatic nuclei. The surrounding matrix is usually fibromatous or cartilaginous. Foci of calcifications, areas of necrosis, and vascular invasion may be seen. Less common histologic variants include small-cell osteosarcoma containing hyperchromatic cells with scant cytoplasm and telangiectasis with ectatic vascular spaces, the walls of which contain the pleomorphic cells and associated osteoid.

Treatment

Careful examination and imaging should be performed prior to the initiation of treatment in order to rule out metastasis or advanced disease, with the involvement of an oncologist. Multiagent chemotherapy is often utilized prior to surgery and may include the following: doxorubicin, cyclophosphamide, dacarbazine, cisplatin, or methotrexate. Patients treated only with chemotherapy for metastatic disease or advanced disease typically have poor outcomes. Chemotherapy following aggressive surgical excision has been reported to improve survival. Osteosarcomas are also frequently treated with surgical excision followed by radiotherapy. External beam radiotherapy may be helpful for patients who refuse surgery, have incomplete surgical resection, or have unresectable tumors. There have been no prospective trials comparing the most beneficial forms of treatment for orbital or craniofacial osteosarcomas.

Prognosis

Historically, 80–90% of patients with osteosarcomas have died as a result of pulmonary metastasis. Multiagent chemotherapy combinations have dramatically increased the disease-free survival from 20% to 70% for long bone osteosarcomas. Patients with craniofacial tumors have been reported to have a 2-year survival rate of 66% and a 5-year survival rate of 55%. However, the presence of craniofacial tumors outside the maxilla or mandible portends a worse prognosis, with a survival rate approaching 10%. In craniofacial disease, local invasion and spread is the most common cause of death. Those with high-grade tumors or necrosis have a worse survival rate.

Lacrimal Gland Tumors

Adenocarcinoma

Clinical Pearls

- Primary adenocarcinoma is a very rare epithelial tumor of the lacrimal gland, with prognosis and treatment often compared to salivary tumors.
- Patients commonly present with a firm, nontender palpable mass or nodule within the superotemporal orbit or eyelid.

- Adenocarcinomas behave aggressively, with early metastasis and high local recurrence rates.
- Patients should be evaluated for systemic metastasis prior to undergoing aggressive surgical resection.
- Prognosis is poor, with tumor-related mortality approaching 70%.

Primary adenocarcinoma is a very rare epithelial tumor of the lacrimal gland that has glandular or ductal differentiation. Histologically and immunohistochemically, these tumors are similar to salivary duct adenocarcinomas. These lacrimal tumors tend to behave aggressively, with early metastasis and high local recurrence rates, similar to salivary ductal carcinomas. Primary adenocarcinomas of salivary glands have been classified into subtypes that have different clinical appearance and prognosis. The salivary gland tumors present most commonly in men (3:1) within the sixth decade.

Clinical Presentation

Patients commonly present with a firm, nontender palpable mass or nodule within the superotemporal orbit or eyelid, often resulting blepharoptosis. Slowly progressive proptosis and inferonasal globe displacement are frequently found. In more advanced tumors, optic neuropathy, vision changes, sensory hypesthesia, and extraocular motility disturbances may be noted. Excessive lacrimation is occasionally reported.

Computed Tomography

Primary ductal adenocarcinomas have been reported to be an isodense homogenously enhancing lesion with ill-defined margins located in the superotemporal orbit. The mass often displaces the globe inferonasally and may extend intraconally. Remodeling of orbital walls is often noted, but bony destruction is rare. Calcifications may be seen adjacent to the tumor.

Magnetic Resonance Imaging

This tumor has been reported as a superotemporal orbital mass that has ill-defined borders on MRI. There is diffuse homogenous enhancement in the region of the lacrimal gland following contrast administration.

Histopathology

Primary ductal adenocarcinomas are composed of dilated glandular or duct-like structures with papillary, comedonecrosis, cribriform, or solid patterns. The infiltrative component may be composed of trabeculae, ductules, nests, or sheets of neoplastic cells surrounded by desmoplastic stroma. Tumor cells are large and polygonal with amphophilic cytoplasm. They contain round vesicular nuclei with prominent nucleoli. Frequent mitoses (10–15 per HPF) are often noted. Mucicarmine or alcian blue histochemical staining helps to identify the presence of mucin production. Perineural and vascular invasion are frequently noted. Immunohistochemical staining is often positive for cytokeratin (7, 10, 18, or 19), epithelial membrane antigen, and carcinoembryonic antigen. Electron microscopy reveals tumor cells with well-developed lumina and microvilli.

Treatment

Because of the aggressive nature of these tumors, aggressive surgical excision is often required. Some cases may require a multidisciplinary approach for complete resection. Some surgeons have advocated primary exenteration followed by radiotherapy as primary treatment. There is a high rate of recurrence. Chemotherapy for systemic metastasis has been reported to be largely ineffective. Because of the likelihood of early metastasis, every patient should be carefully evaluated prior to considering aggressive surgical intervention. Patients should be closely followed postoperatively for signs of recurrence.

Prognosis

The prognosis for life is poor. Based on case reports of lacrimal primary ductal adenocarcinomas, tumor recurrences are frequent and may occur up to 10 years following initial treatment. Frequent metastases have been reported to distant sites such as the brain, lungs, liver, pancreas, bones, and common bile duct. Because primary ductal adenocarcinoma of the lacrimal gland is so rare, its clinical behavior should be compared to salivary duct carcinoma. The tumor-related mortality of salivary duct carcinoma is 70%, usually occurring within 2–3 years following diagnosis.

Adenoid Cystic Carcinoma

Clinical Pearls

- Adenoid cystic carcinoma is the most common primary malignancy of the lacrimal gland.
- The tumor occurs most commonly in the fourth decade of life.
- Patients typically present with abaxial proptosis with inferomedial displacement of the globe.
- Orbital pain from perineural invasion is common.
- The cribriform pattern is the most common and has a Swiss cheese-like appearance.
- Management typically requires en bloc orbital exenteration with wide margins, including adjacent bone.
- The mean survival is 5 years, with a mortality rate of 60%.

Adenoid cystic carcinoma is the most common primary malignancy of the lacrimal gland. It constitutes about 30% of all epithelial lacrimal gland tumors. This tumor may occur at any age, but is seen most commonly in the fourth decade of life. Males and females are equally affected. Metastasis or invasion of the orbit from other primary sites such as the maxillary sinuses, ethmoid sinuses, oral cavity, nasal cavity, lacrimal sac, and parotid gland have been reported. Secondary orbital involvement has been reported to be at least as frequent as the primary tumors of the orbit.

Clinical Presentation

Patients typically present with abaxial proptosis with downward and medial displacement of the globe. Secondary tumors may present differently depending upon location of the tumor. Ptosis, diplopia, visual loss, and periorbital paresthesias may be associated findings (Fig. 56.91). Orbital pain is common from perineural invasion and may be reported in 10–40% of patients. The duration of symptoms is usually short, frequently less than 6 months and usually less than 1 year.

Computed Tomography

CT demonstrates a mass with heterogeneous density in the lacrimal gland fossa. It can be irregular and poorly demarcated, round to oval, and well outlined (Fig. 56.92). Larger tumors can extend along the lateral orbital wall to the orbital apex. Foci of calcification are frequently present within the lesion. Destruction or sclerosis of adjacent bone is common, especially with larger tumors. With contrast administration, there are often areas of marked focal enhancement.

Magnetic Resonance Imaging

On MRI, adenoid cystic carcinoma appears as a well-defined, irregular mass that may infiltrate along the lateral rectus muscle. The lesion gives a heterogeneous signal on T1-weighted images, hyperintense to muscle and hypointense to fat. The signal becomes hyperintense to orbital fat on the T2-weighted images. Central necrosis may be seen as an area of increased signal intensity on T2-weighted imaging. Hypointense areas within the tumor represent foci of calcification. Subtle bone destruction may be difficult to detect on MRI because of its signal void. Moderate enhancement is seen with gadolinium, but there may be focal areas of more intense enhancement.

Histopathology

Adenoid cystic carcinomas are composed of deceptively bland small cells that have dark, round-oval nuclei and scant cytoplasm (Fig. 56.93). There are five histological patterns: cribriform, sclerosing, basaloid (solid), comedocarcinoma (basaloid pattern with central areas of necrosis), and tubular. An individual tumor may have a combination of patterns. The cribriform pattern is the most common,

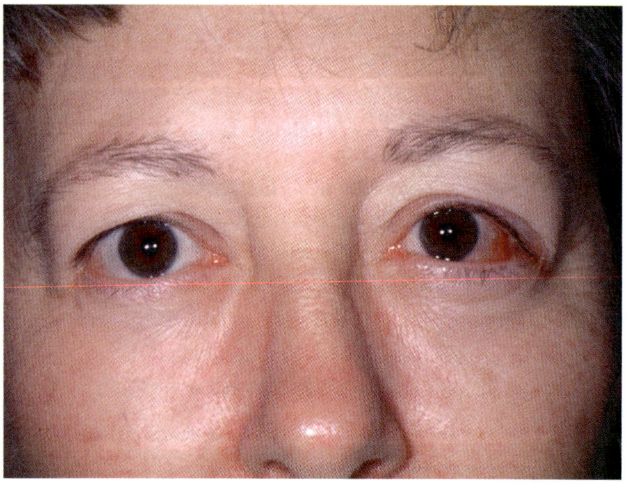

Fig. 56.91 Adenoid cystic carcinoma of the left orbit

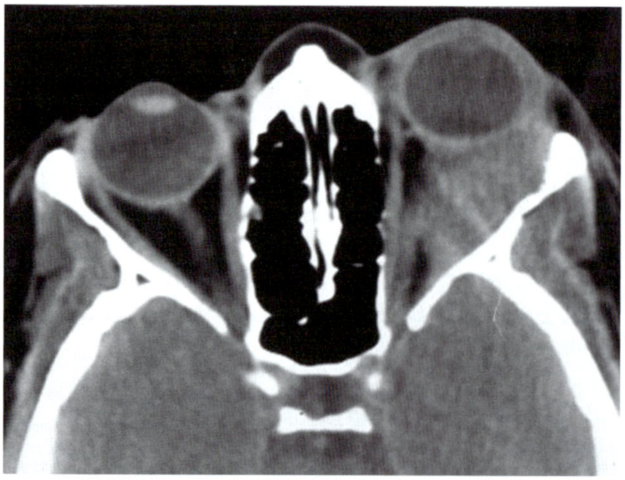

Fig. 56.92 CT scan with a large medium-density mass along the left lateral orbit

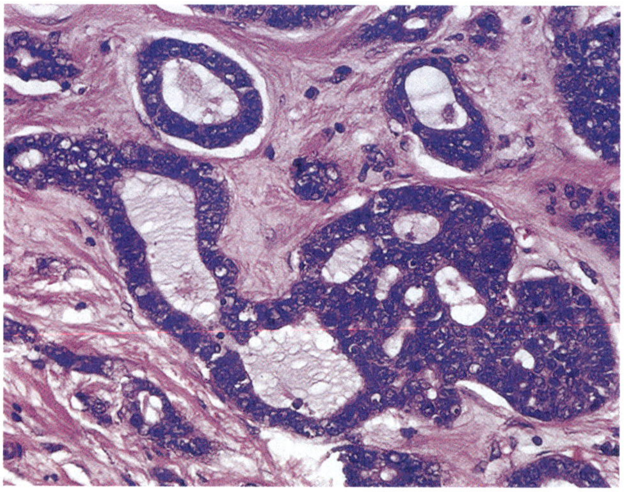

Fig. 56.93 Adenoid cystic carcinoma of the lacrimal gland demonstrating tubular and comedo patterns of growth. The hyperchromatic cells also demonstrate single cell invasion of the stroma

with cystic spaces containing myxoid material that gives the tumor a Swiss cheese-like appearance. The sclerosing pattern has epithelial cords surrounded by a hyalinized stroma. The basaloid pattern has lobules containing large basophilic nuclei with little cytoplasm. The comedocarcinoma pattern has lobules with large central areas of necrosis. The tubular pattern has elongated epithelial tubules. The presence of basaloid histologic pattern correlates with a worse prognosis. In any of these histologic patterns, single cell invasion of the stroma and bone surrounding the tumor cells may be seen. The tumor has a propensity for perineural and intraneural extension, accounting for the pain that commonly accompanies the tumor. The propensity for single cell tumor invasion and perineural spread often results in skip lesions some distance from the primary tumor.

Treatment

Suspicious lesions should be biopsied through an eyelid crease incision. Management typically requires en bloc resection or orbital exenteration with wide margins, including adjacent bone. Although a conservative resection has been advocated for some cases, clinical support for this approach is limited. While irradiation does not appear to be useful as a primary modality, adjunctive radiotherapy for advanced tumors may offer some benefit. Descriptions of external beam, gamma knife, and brachytherapy for treatment have all been reported. Intracarotid chemotherapy (doxorubicin and cisplatin) prior to surgical resection has been reported with encouraging results.

Prognosis

Even with radical surgery, the local recurrence rate is high, and intracranial extension is common. The mean survival is 5 years, with a mortality rate of 60%. The 10-year survival rate has been reported to be 20% despite extensive surgery and postoperative radiation. Regardless of treatment, the prognosis for life remains dismal. Young patients may have a better prognosis, possibly due to their tumors having less aggressive histologic features. Patients with basaloid variants have a worse prognosis.

Mucoepidermoid Carcinoma

Clinical Pearls

- Mucoepidermoid carcinomas are believed to arise from ductal epithelium within the lacrimal gland and accessory conjunctival glands.
- Conjunctival tumors are more common than lacrimal tumors.
- The tumors occur most commonly in older males with a mean age at onset of 63 years.
- Lacrimal tumors often present with painless proptosis and inferonasal displacement of the globe.
- The tumor has a propensity for local infiltration, but tends to be less aggressive than adenoid cystic carcinoma or undifferentiated adenocarcinoma.
- Wide surgical excision is necessary, often requiring enucleation or exenteration.

Mucoepidermoid carcinoma is the most common salivary gland tumor, but does rarely occur within the lacrimal gland (accounting for 4% of tumors), conjunctiva, and lacrimal sac. These tumors are believed to arise from ductal epithelium within the lacrimal gland and accessory glands, where they contain an admixture of mucoid, epidermoid, intermediate, columnar, and clear cells. Clinically and histologically, they resemble squamous cell carcinoma. The tumor has a propensity for local infiltration, but tends to be less aggressive than adenoid cystic carcinoma or undifferentiated adenocarcinoma. Conjunctival lesions occur most commonly in older men (mean 63 years of age) or in immunosuppressed individuals, including in those with HIV; they are most frequent in the limbal or perilimbal regions. Lacrimal gland tumors have occasionally been reported in young adults and children.

Clinical Presentation

Mucoepidermoid carcinoma is a rare tumor that usually presents as a conjunctival lesion. The clinical presentation of conjunctival tumors has been described as nodular, leukoplakic, infiltrative, ulcerative, and papillomatous. When the primary tumor is located within the lacrimal gland, patients often present with painless proptosis and inferonasal displacement of the globe (Fig. 56.94). A palpable nodule is often present along the superior orbital rim, which may be

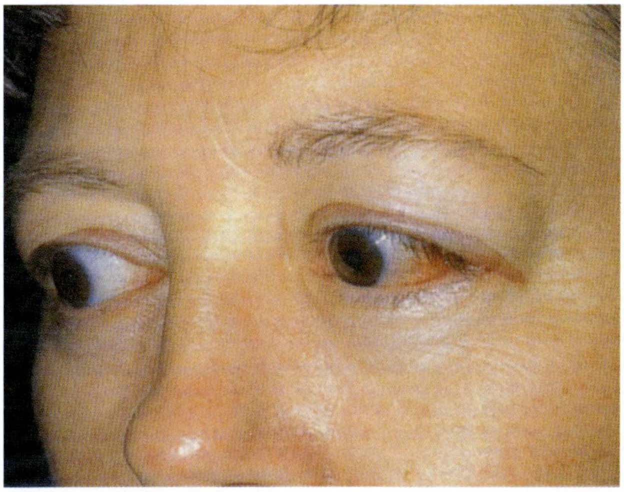

Fig. 56.94 Left orbital mass in the upper lateral orbit from a mucoepidermoid carcinoma

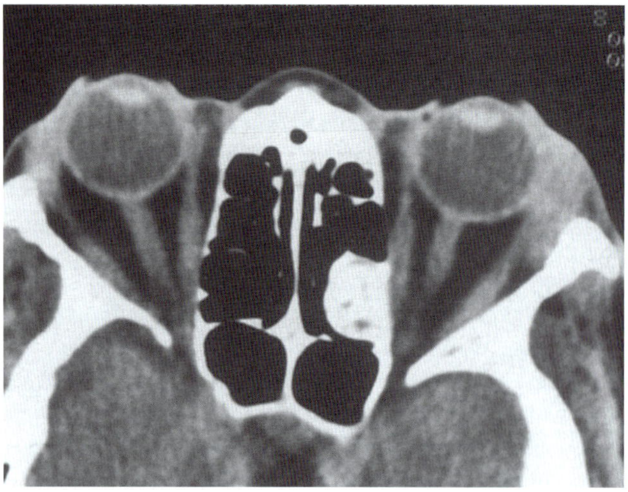

Fig. 56.95 CT scan showing an enlarged left lacrimal gland

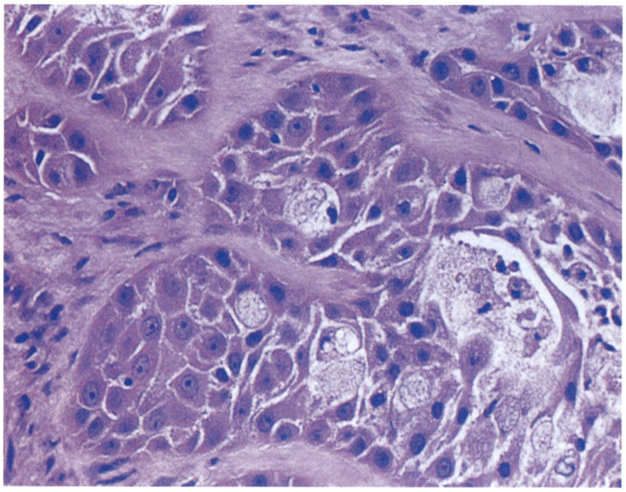

Fig. 56.96 Mucoepidermoid carcinoma of the lacrimal gland demonstrating biphasic appearance of squamous cells with intensely eosinophilic cytoplasm and intercellular bridges, and cells containing large mucin droplets, all in nests invading reactive stroma

indurated. These tumors are frequently aggressive locally, with massive infiltration of the eyelids, orbit, paranasal sinuses, or eye.

Computed Tomography

With orbital involvement, CT demonstrates a heterogeneous mass that may be centered in the lacrimal gland fossa or diffusely invasive from the conjunctiva (Fig. 56.95). It can be irregular and poorly demarcated, or round to oval, and well outlined where it can resemble a pleomorphic adenoma of the lacrimal gland. With contrast administration, there are often areas of focal enhancement.

Magnetic Resonance Imaging

On MRI, mucoepidermoid carcinoma appears as a diffuse to well-defined, irregular mass that may be deeply infiltrative. The lesion gives a heterogeneous signal on T1-weighted images, hyperintense to muscle but hypointense to fat. The signal becomes hyperintense to orbital fat on T2-weighted images. Subtle bone destruction may be present. Moderate enhancement is seen with gadolinium, but there may be focal areas of more intense enhancement.

Histopathology

Mucoepidermoid carcinoma appears similar whether it arises in the lacrimal gland or extends into the orbit from the conjunctiva or paranasal sinuses. A mixture of squamous epithelial cells and mucus-producing goblet cells form lobules (Fig. 56.96). The cytoplasm has a vacuolated appearance. Because cells contain mucin, they often demonstrate positive staining with PAS (following diastase treatment) and mucicarmine. The cells contain vesicular oval nuclei with a high mitotic rate and prominent nucleoli. Goblet cells predominate in well-differentiated tumors, and squamous epithelium is more prominent in poorly differentiated neoplasms. Areas of perineural spread are often identified. Mucoepidermoid carcinomas spreading along the cornea or sclera demonstrate a propensity to invade the eye, especially when recurrent. Immunohistochemical analysis with CEA, CK7, and CK20 can help to differentiate these tumors from squamous cell carcinoma.

Treatment

Mucoepidermoid carcinomas tend to invade local tissues aggressively and show a propensity for local recurrence. Wide surgical excision is necessary, often requiring enucleation or exenteration. Frozen section-guided surgical excision can help to improve results. Radiotherapy, including episcleral plaque application for conjunctival lesions, may offer good local control in some cases. Frequent follow-up is required postoperatively due to the high recurrence rates.

Prognosis

Rapid and relentless recurrence is the rule regardless of treatment. In conjunctival tumors, up to 79% of tumors may recur within 6 months. The ultimate prognosis is guarded, with at least 25% 5-year mortality.

Pleomorphic Adenoma

Clinical Pearls

- Pleomorphic adenomas are the most common epithelial tumors of the lacrimal gland.
- Tumors usually occur between the second and fifth decades of life.
- Symptoms of progressive painless abaxial proptosis and inferomedial globe displacement are often present for more than 1 year.
- Associated inflammation or pain may be indicative of malignant transformation.

- Complete removal with an intact pseudocapsule results in complete cure in almost all cases.
- Following biopsy or pseudocapsule rupture, the recurrence rates increase significantly.

Pleomorphic adenoma or benign mixed cell tumor accounts for 3–5% of all orbital tumors. It represents 12–40% of all lacrimal gland mass lesions and more than 50% of tumors arising from the lacrimal epithelium. Pleomorphic adenomas occur primarily in the orbital lobe, but can involve the palpebral lobe. These tumors usually occur between the second and fifth decades of life, with a mean age at presentation of 40 years. Males are affected slightly more frequently than females. Tumors rarely arise from accessory glands of Wolfring or Krause.

Clinical Presentation

Patients typically have symptoms for 1 year or more before presenting for medical attention. The most common clinical features include slowly progressive painless abaxial proptosis and inferomedial globe displacement (Fig. 56.97). Ptosis, choroidal folds, decreased vision, diplopia, and extraocular motility restriction may be seen. A firm mobile palpable mass is usually present beneath the superolateral orbital rim. Associated inflammation or pain is most often indicative of malignant transformation.

Computed Tomography

On CT scan, this tumor appears as a well-circumscribed, dense, and round to oval nodular mass. It is characteristically located in the anterior superotemporal extraconal orbit (Fig. 56.98). When very large, the globe and extraocular muscles are displaced medially and downward. Nonhomogenous areas are due to the presence of cystic degeneration, mesenchymal stroma, necrosis, or mucinous degeneration. Occasionally, small calcific or cartilaginous foci are present. Remodeling of adjacent bone without destruction is common.

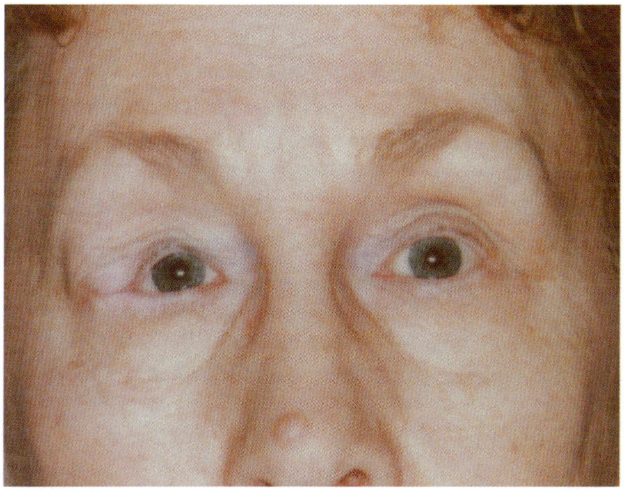

Fig. 56.97 Pleomorphic adenoma with fullness of the superolateral right orbit

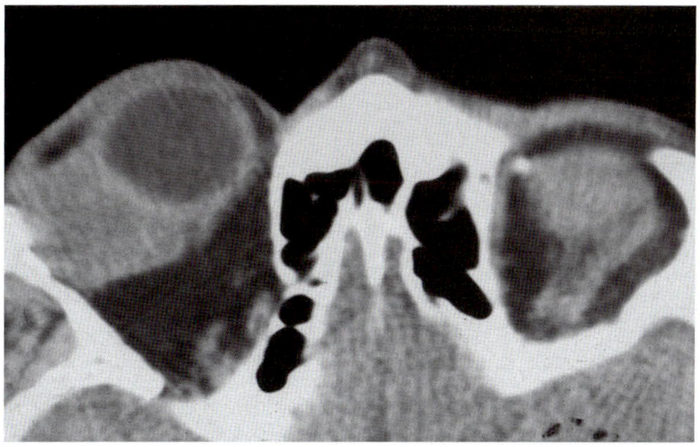

Fig. 56.98 CT scan with a well-defined enlargement of the right lacrimal gland

Magnetic Resonance Imaging

Pleomorphic adenomas are well-circumscribed masses in the superotemporal anterior orbit, most commonly occurring within the orbital lobe of the lacrimal gland. On T1-weighted sequences, the signal may be heterogeneous or homogeneous and is hypointense to extraocular muscles and gray matter. The signal appears hyperintense to extraocular muscle and gray matter on T2-weighted images. Moderate enhancement is demonstrated with gadolinium.

Histopathology

Heterogeneity is the dominant histological feature of this tumor, with both epithelial and mesenchymal features being prominent. The pseudocapsule varies significantly in overall thickness. Cellular atypia, nuclear pleomorphism, and mitotic figures are not present. Epithelial cells form ducts, irregular tubules, and sheets of cells (Fig. 56.99). The neoplastic ducts have an inner layer of cuboidal to columnar cells surrounded by flattened to spindle-shaped myoepithelial cells. Squamous metaplasia of the epithelial cells is common. Strands of myoepithelial cells often extend outward into the adjacent myxomatous mesenchyme, which they participate in forming. Myxoid fibrous stroma is the most common in pleomorphic adenomas, but cartilaginous or even osseous differentiation may be seen focally. Recurrent tumors are often characterized by multifocal and multinodular growth. The risk of malignant transformation appears to be related to tumor age and degree of hyalinization. Malignant pleomorphic adenomas of the lacrimal gland are rare, and the malignancy is usually limited to the epithelial component in a portion of the tumor, resulting in malignant mixed tumors termed carcinoma ex pleomorphic adenoma.

Treatment

Pleomorphic adenomas should be excised completely with the pseudocapsule intact. Total removal with intact

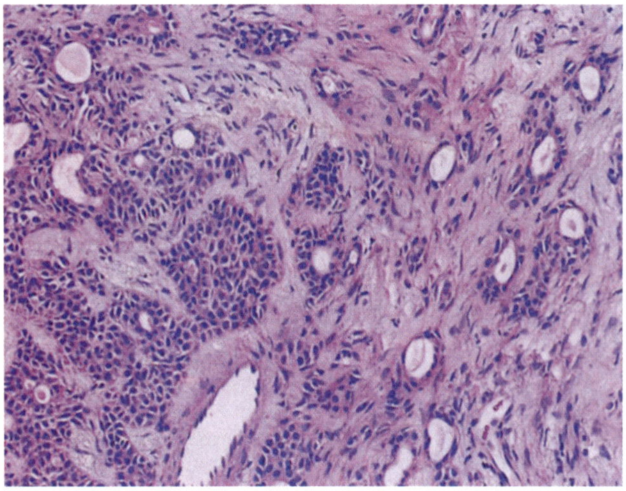

Fig. 56.99 Pleomorphic adenoma (benign mixed tumor) of the lacrimal gland consisting of bland epithelial cells and myofibroblastic cells that interdigitate with fibrous stroma

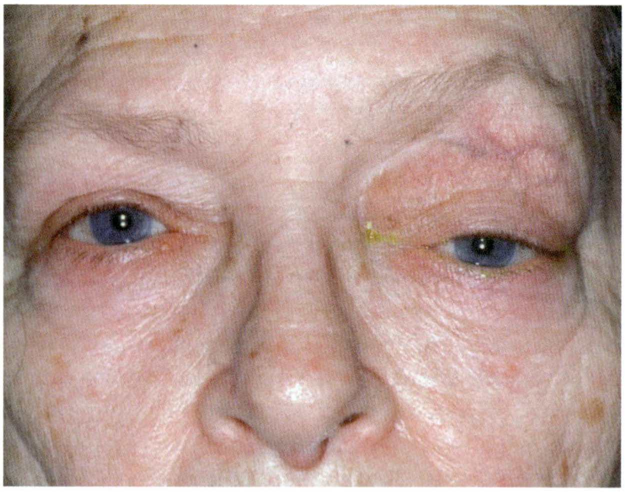

Fig. 56.100 Metastatic breast carcinoma to the superior left orbit

pseudocapsule results in complete cure in almost all cases. Following biopsy or pseudocapsule rupture, recurrence rates range from 21% to 32%. This increased rate of recurrence is likely due to spillage of tumor cells. Recent studies have reported a low rate of recurrence following fine needle aspiration biopsy. However, the follow-up intervals were short, and recurrence for this tumor can be seen after 10–15 years. Patients who inadvertently undergo incisional biopsy should have additional excision along the biopsy tract. Recurrent growth may be infiltrative and carries a risk of malignant degeneration of about 10% per decade. Postoperative radiotherapy may further add to this risk.

Prognosis

With complete excision, the prognosis is excellent, and cure rates approaching 99% are typical. Rupture of the pseudocapsule or prior biopsy carries a risk of multiple recurrences. Tumor recurrence and radiotherapy use have been associated with malignant degeneration. Vision remains normal in most cases. Repeated surgeries can result in significant orbital scarring and extraocular motility disturbance.

Metastatic Tumors

Breast Carcinoma

Clinical Pearls

- Breast carcinoma is the most common tumor to metastasize to the orbit.
- Orbital metastases from the breast are usually seen in women most commonly between 40 and 60 years of age.
- Typically, there is a rapid onset of proptosis, diplopia, chemosis, and visual loss.
- Scirrhous adenocarcinoma results in fibrosis of extraocular muscles and other orbital structures, often resulting in enophthalmos and decreased extraocular motility.
- The management of metastatic breast carcinoma most commonly involves the use of chemotherapeutic agents.
- Radiotherapy is often palliative.

Breast carcinoma is the most common tumor to metastasize to the orbit, accounting for approximately 50% of all orbital metastases. These metastases occur via hematogenous spread and commonly present years after the diagnosis of the primary tumor. In about 20% of cases, the orbital lesions may be bilateral.

Clinical Presentation

Orbital metastases from the breast are usually seen in women between 40 and 60 years of age. Rarely, cases have been reported in males. Most patients have a prior history of treatment for breast cancer, generally 2–5 years earlier, but orbital involvement may occur decades following initial treatment. The orbital symptoms can be the initial presentation of the disease. Typically, there is a rapid onset of proptosis, diplopia, chemosis, and visual loss (Fig. 56.100). Infiltration of the eyelids can result in ptosis, lagophthalmos, or edema. In scirrhous adenocarcinoma of the breast, fibrosis of extraocular muscles and other structures within the orbit may cause enophthalmos and decreased extraocular motility. Pain is often a prominent feature. The association of rapid progression and pain may mimic orbital inflammatory disease, causing a delay in diagnosis. When located in the anterior orbit, a firm mass may be palpable beneath the orbital rim.

Computed Tomography

On CT scan, an ill-defined, infiltrative mass is seen that may result in enlargement of extraocular muscles, the lacrimal gland, or optic nerve (Fig. 56.101). The lesion shows

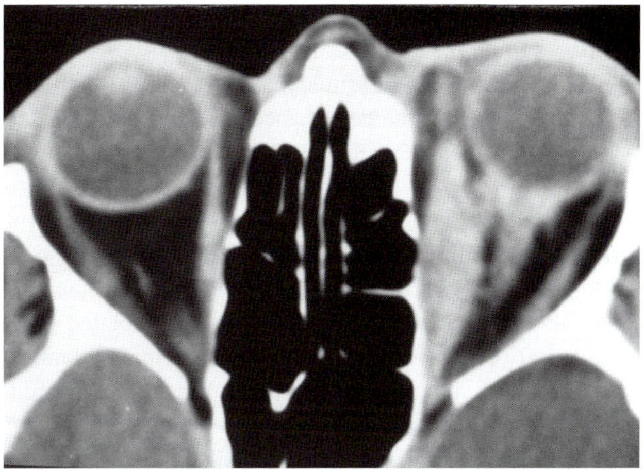

Fig. 56.101 Axial CT scan showing a metastatic breast carcinoma to the left medial rectus muscle

moderate density similar to muscle. Bone destruction may be present, especially when the metastasis is localized to bone. There is usually some degree of enhancement with contrast administration.

Magnetic Resonance Imaging

Metastatic breast carcinoma is a diffusely infiltrating mass that is moderately well defined. It may involve any structure in the orbit including the bony walls. The T1-weighted signal is isointense to muscle and hypointense to fat. On the T2-weighted image, the signal is increased and is hyperintense to both muscle and fat. In the presence of intralesional hemorrhage, the signal becomes more heterogeneous with specific MR characteristics depending upon the degree of blood degradation. There is moderate to marked enhancement following gadolinium administration, best seen on fat suppression sequences.

Histopathology

Metastatic breast carcinomas have a variety of histologic patterns that are often similar to the characteristics of the primary tumor. Invasive (infiltrating) ductal carcinoma has cords, solid nests, tubules, and anastomosing islands of tumor cells in a dense fibrous stroma. The tumor cells vary from small cells with regular nuclei to large cells with irregular, hyperchromatic nuclei. Invasive lobular carcinoma has strands of tumor cells, often one cell thick. The cells tend to be small with little nuclear pleomorphism. Signet-ring cells are common.

Treatment

Specific tumor markers, especially the presence or absence of progesterone and HER2/neu (ErbB-25) receptors, are used to guide treatment. The management of metastatic breast carcinoma most commonly involves the use of chemotherapeutic agents such as doxorubicin, cisplatin, and cyclophosphamide. Therapeutic drug combinations including paclitaxel, docetaxel, methotrexate, fluorouracil, and epirubicin have been reported. Nonsteroidal, antiestrogen tamoxifen, either alone or in combination with other agents, may improve survival in receptor positive patients. For isolated orbital or choroidal metastases, local radiotherapy at 30–40 Gy is a useful palliative modality.

Prognosis

The prognosis for vision is poor, and most patients maintain some degree of visual loss following treatment. In addition to the orbit metastasis, there is often widespread systemic metastasis, resulting in a dismal prognosis for life. Median survival is only 1–2 years after the diagnosis of orbital metastasis.

Bronchogenic Carcinoma

Clinical Pearls

- Lung cancer is the second most common carcinoma to metastasize to the orbit.
- It occurs most commonly in persons 40–60 years of age.
- Orbital metastases from bronchogenic carcinoma may present before or concurrent with the pulmonary disease in more than half of cases.
- Proptosis tends to occur rapidly.
- Treatment is with systemic chemotherapy. Radiotherapy is used for palliation.

Bronchogenic carcinoma is a common form of lung cancer and the leading cause of death from cancer in males. Lung cancer is the second most common carcinoma to metastasize to the orbit, causing 8–12% of all orbital metastases, second only to breast carcinoma. It occurs most commonly in persons 40–60 years of age, typically with a history of heavy smoking. Bronchogenic carcinoma tends to metastasize early and rapidly.

Clinical Presentation

Unlike breast cancer, orbital metastases from bronchogenic carcinoma may present before or concurrent with the pulmonary disease in more than half of cases. The most common clinical symptom is proptosis, seen in about 80% of patients. Proptosis tends to occur rapidly and may be axial or abaxial depending upon tumor location. Ptosis, eyelid swelling, ophthalmoplegia, orbital pain, and facial pain or paresthesias are less frequent findings. An anterior mass is palpable in 20% of cases. The orbital lesion can occur concurrently with choroidal metastases manifesting with visual loss, retinal detachment, or glaucoma.

Computed Tomography

The CT scan shows an ill-defined infiltrating mass of moderate density. Metastases can be isolated to individual orbital structures. In such cases, they may appear only as an enlargement of the lacrimal gland, optic nerve, or extraocular muscle. However, the borders of these structures are typically irregular. Bone destruction is seen with metastases to the bones themselves or with those involving periorbita. With contrast administration, enhancement is usually mild to moderate.

Magnetic Resonance Imaging

The T1-weighted image usually shows an irregular enlargement of extraocular muscle or other structures. The resonance signal from the tumor is high, being isointense or slightly hyperintense to normal optic nerve and muscle, but hypointense to fat. On the T2-weighted sequence, the tumor is hyperintense to nerve, muscle, and fat. Moderate to marked enhancement is seen with gadolinium, best seen on fat suppression sequences.

Histopathology

Small-cell carcinoma is the most frequent type of bronchogenic carcinoma to metastasize to the orbit. In small-cell carcinoma, the tumor cells are small, are deeply basophilic, have scant cytoplasm, and are round to oval in shape. The cells grow in sheets or trabeculae, and areas of necrosis are common. Undifferentiated large-cell carcinoma is the second most common type to metastasize to the orbit. Squamous cell carcinoma and adenocarcinoma may also metastasize to the orbit, but with much less frequency. The tumors are cytokeratin and TTF positive on immunohistochemical staining.

Treatment

With bronchogenic carcinoma, widely disseminated metastases are often present by the time orbital symptoms occur. Treatment is with systemic chemotherapy, which varies depending upon the type of carcinoma present. Local radiotherapy can be useful for palliation of orbital symptoms.

Prognosis

With bronchogenic carcinoma, the presence of metastases heralds a very poor prognosis for life. The presence of p53 mutation or inactivation is present in most types of lung cancer and is associated with a poorer prognosis in non-small-cell lung cancers. Most patients die from visceral disease within 1 year.

Malignant Melanoma

Clinical Pearls

- Extension of primary uveal or conjunctival melanomas is the most common causes of orbital malignant melanoma.
- Orbital symptoms in patients with ocular melanocytosis should be evaluated for an orbital melanoma.
- Biopsy should be avoided in patients with suspected primary orbital melanomas.
- Complete excision of primary and secondary orbital melanomas provides the best chance of cure.
- Cutaneous metastatic melanomas have a poor prognosis.

Malignant melanoma of the orbit can be classified as primary, secondary, or metastatic. Melanomas are responsible for 5–7% of orbital tumors. Primary orbital melanomas (POM) are very rare and are associated with congenital ocular melanocytosis, oculodermal melanocytosis, orbital melanocytosis, and hypercellular blue nevus. In rare instances, POM may arise de novo. A predisposing pigmentary condition is found in 90% of patients with POM. Patients with POM have a mean age of 42 years. Secondary orbital melanomas result from the extension of conjunctival, eyelid, or uveal melanomas and are responsible for most orbital melanomas. They may spread through emissary canals in the sclera or less commonly through the lamina cribrosa around the optic nerve. Extrascleral extension of uveal melanomas may be seen in 8–10% of enucleated eyes. Patients with choroidal melanoma are typically older, between 50 and 70 years of age. Melanoma arising in primary acquired melanosis (PAM) is the most common cause of orbital melanoma originating in the conjunctiva. It is most common in middle-aged adults. Occasionally, malignant melanoma may metastasize to orbital structures, including bone, from distant sites. Spread to the orbit occurs via hematogenous spread. Patients with orbital metastases have a mean age of 54 years. Primary lesions are most commonly found on the trunk (39%), upper extremities (24%), and lower extremities (21%). Nearly all patients have a history of primary cutaneous melanoma prior to the development of orbital disease. There is often advanced metastatic disease at the time of diagnosis.

Clinical Presentation

Patients with POM often have evidence of ocular and periocular abnormal pigmentary changes. The onset of orbital symptoms should initiate a regional and systemic workup for orbital melanoma. Congenital nevi evolving into malignant melanomas exhibit increased nodularity, variegated pigmentation, bleeding, or inflammation. Orbital extension of choroidal melanomas may be microscopic without any orbital symptoms. The development of orbital symptoms months or years following treatment is often the first indication of extrascleral spread (Fig. 56.102). Patients with PAM may have diffuse perilimbal or forniceal pigmentation that evolves over years into darker, nodular melanomas that spread to lymphatics and extends posterior to the orbital septum. Metastatic cutaneous melanomas are usually more aggressive and grow more rapidly than uveal melanomas. Metastatic tumors are more likely to have

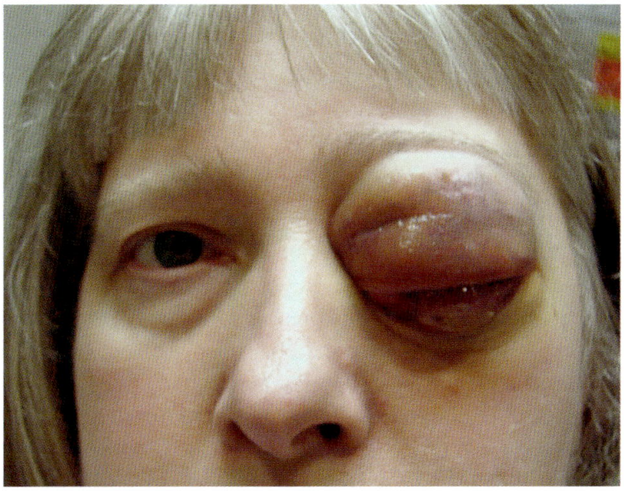

Fig. 56.102 Massive malignant melanoma of the left orbit from extrascleral extension of a uveal tumor

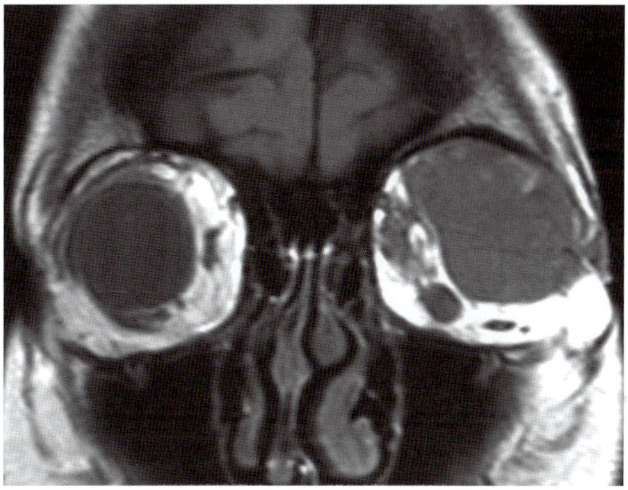

Fig. 56.103 Coronal T1-weighted MRI with a hypointense melanoma in the left orbit

proptosis with involvement of extraocular muscles, resulting in diplopia. Patients with metastatic orbital tumors often have multiple systemic metastasis at the time of presentation, which most commonly include cutaneous or subcutaneous (45%), lymph node (38%), CNS (34%), lung (27%), and liver (25%) lesions. Advanced orbital melanomas may present with proptosis, globe displacement, optic nerve compression, and associated changes, ptosis, chemosis, retinal striae, and pain.

Computed Tomography

The CT demonstrates a homogeneous orbital mass of moderate density. When extension is from the choroid, the mass is typically intraconal and may be infiltrative around orbital structures. A similar and contiguous mass may be seen as a dome or collar-button density within the globe. However, in the presence of diffuse choroidal melanoma, an intraocular component may not be obvious. In cases of prior enucleation for intraocular melanoma, the orbital implant may be displaced forward by the tumor. With conjunctival primaries, an irregular density is seen in the anterior orbit continuous with the conjunctival mass. The lesion may be seen to extend along extraocular muscles or around the globe.

Magnetic Resonance Imaging

On MRI, uveal melanomas appear with domed or collar-button configuration. Rarely, a nodule or extrascleral extension can be appreciated. Orbital melanomas image as a moderately defined to infiltrative mass that may be intraconal or anterior just behind the orbital septum, depending upon the primary site or origin. The tumor may appear heterogeneous in the presence of necrosis or intralesional hemorrhage (Fig. 56.103). The signal characteristics are believed to relate to the paramagnetic properties of melanin, which shortens both the T1 and T2 relaxation times. This will produce a high signal on T1-weighted images that is hyperintense to vitreous and hypointense to fat. When associated with a serous retinal detachment, the melanoma is hyperintense to vitreous but hypointense to the brighter subretinal fluid. Melanomas show moderate enhancement with gadolinium and may appear brighter than subretinal fluid on T1-weighted images since the serous fluid does not enhance. The signal is increased on fat saturation sequences. On the T2-weighted imaging, melanomas give a high heterogeneous signal that is hyperintense to both fat and muscle, but hypointense to vitreous.

Histopathology

POM is most commonly of a mixed cell type. Choroidal melanoma extending into the orbit through a scleral canal will have the appearance of the primary uveal tumor. In contrast, melanoma recurrent in the orbit may be composed solely of amelanotic, polygonal, or spindle-shaped tumor cells. The presence of a large nucleolus within a round to oval nucleus is a clue to the diagnosis of recurrent melanoma (Fig. 56.104). Metastatic cutaneous melanomas most often contain epithelioid cells. Spindle cell type and low mitotic rate are better prognostic factors. Paraffin sections can be immunostained for S-100 protein and/or HMB-45, melan A, or other melanoma-associated antigens to confirm the diagnosis.

Treatment

The best treatments have not been firmly established. Although local resection has been advocated for some well-defined low-grade tumors arising from blue nevi, in most cases a more radical procedure will be needed for cure. Biopsy of tumors associated with ocular melanocytosis should be avoided to prevent liberation of any malignant cells and opening of routes for tumor spread. Treatment modalities for POM include complete surgical

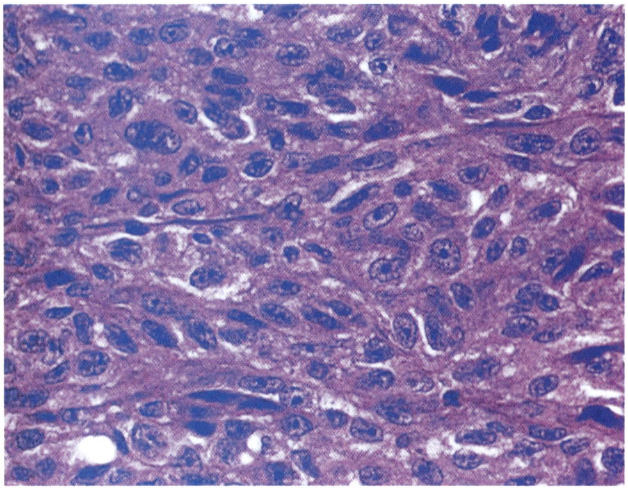

Fig. 56.104 Amelanotic malignant melanoma consisting of pleomorphic cells with eosinophilic cytoplasm and enlarged hyperchromatic nuclei with prominent nucleoli. Immunostain for melanin-associated antigen is usually essential in establishing the diagnosis

resection with an intact capsule that may require orbital exenteration, surgical debulking for tumors not amenable to complete resection, adjuvant radiation, and chemotherapy. Following surgical excision, map biopsies of melanocytic areas should be performed. Extension of uveal melanomas can be treated with a modified enucleation, where the extraocular nodule is resected with associated involved orbital tissue. Globe sparing treatment with episcleral plaque brachytherapy has been reported for small localized tumors. More advanced extension should be treated primarily with an eyelid sparing orbital exenteration. Extension of eyelid and conjunctival melanomas are generally treated by orbital exenteration. Small tumors may be treated by local resection with wide surgical margins followed by radiotherapy. Patients with metastatic cutaneous melanomas generally have a poor prognosis. The most common treatment is with surgical excision or resection (58%), radiotherapy (47%), or chemotherapy (93%). Palliative measures such as surgical debulking or irradiation can be utilized for patients with diffuse metastatic disease and extraorbital extension.

Prognosis

Localized orbital melanomas can sometimes be resected with a permanent cure, especially those arising from congenital blue nevi. In patients with orbital melanoma arising from an intraocular site or associated with oculodermal melanocytosis, the prognosis is not as good. The 5-year incidence of metastasis from POM is 38%. Stage IV disease of cutaneous melanoma has a 5-year survival rate of 22%. Patients with orbital metastasis have an average survival of 9–20 months.

Secondary Tumors

Basal Cell Adenocarcinoma

Clinical Pearls

- Basal cell adenocarcinomas are a very rare within the lacrimal gland. Treatment and prognosis are based on similar tumors of the major and minor salivary gland tumors.
- Patients most commonly present with slowly progressive proptosis and inferomedial globe displacement.
- Basal cell adenocarcinomas are characterized by two types of basaloid cells, which can be confused with basaloid adenoid cystic carcinomas.
- The clinical course and prognosis are much better for basal cell adenocarcinomas than for adenoid cystic carcinomas and can therefore be managed with less radical surgery.
- The primary treatment recommendation for these tumors is wide surgical excision. Additional postoperative radiotherapy may be considered in certain cases.

Basal cell adenocarcinomas are a very rare and likely under-recognized epithelial tumor of the lacrimal gland. The treatment and prognosis for this tumor are based on the characteristics of major and minor salivary gland tumors. Basal cell adenocarcinomas appear histopathologically similar to basaloid monomorphic adenomas, except for the presence of tissue infiltration, local destruction, and slight potential for metastasis. The majority of basal cell adenocarcinomas likely arise de novo, with the remainder developing within basal cell adenomas. Basal cell adenocarcinomas are responsible for approximately 3% of malignant epithelial salivary gland tumors and less than 1% of minor salivary gland tumors. The distribution of these tumors is as follows: 80% in the parotid gland, 9% in the submandibular gland, and 11% occur in the minor salivary glands. The WHO has classified these salivary gland tumors as low-grade tumor with a favorable prognosis. Basal cell adenocarcinomas of the salivary glands typically present between the fourth and ninth decades, with a mean age of 58 and peak incidence during the eighth decade.

Clinical Presentation

Patients typically present with progressive proptosis due to a mass within the superotemporal orbit. This may be associated with left upper eyelid fullness, swelling, or discomfort. The globe may be displaced inferomedially. An irregular, firm mass is often palpable anteriorly, which is often irregular and rubbery. Significant visual or optic nerve compromise has not been reported.

Computed Tomography

These tumors appear as a homogenous enhancing mass within the superotemporal orbit, which is continuous with the lacrimal gland. Cystic spaces may be noted within the tumor. No bony erosion has been reported, although remodeling has been noted. The lesion has not been reported to infiltrate the globe or extraocular muscles.

Magnetic Resonance Imaging

The only MR reported of basal cell adenocarcinoma involving the lacrimal gland contained cystic spaces. The tumor was found to be heterogeneously enhancing within the superotemporal orbit. Tumor mass effect resulted in depression of the globe.

Histopathology

Basal cell adenocarcinomas are characterized by two types of basaloid cells. The majority are large uniform cells with abundant eosinophilic cytoplasm, indistinct cell borders, and pale, round or oval, basophilic nuclei. Fewer small cells with less cytoplasm and intense basophilic nuclei are oriented along the periphery of epithelial nests or islands. Surrounding the nests or islands is a basal membrane-like structure that separates these cells from the surrounding connective tissue. There is a slight increase of cytologic atypia compared to basal cell adenomas. Some peripheral palisading of nuclei along the stromal interface is present, but is less prominent in basal cell adenocarcinomas than in basal cell adenomas Necrosis is occasionally present and suggests a malignant process. Squamous differentiation with or without keratin production is present in many tumors. Ductal and myoepithelial differentiation is evident on electron microscopy (AFIP). Immunohistochemical evaluation reveals the following: all tumors are reactive to cytokeratins; vimentin stains diffusely, while actin stains peripherally; most tumors are reactive to CK14; and many tumors will be positive for EMA and CEA.

Basal cell adenocarcinoma can be easily confused histologically with the basaloid variant of adenoid cystic carcinoma, which represents approximately 20% of adenoid cystic carcinomas. The clinical course and prognosis are much better for basal cell adenocarcinomas than for adenoid cystic carcinomas and can therefore be managed with less radical surgery. Basaloid adenoid cystic carcinomas are characterized by myoepithelial cells with irregular or angular nuclei. Unlike basal cell adenocarcinomas, there is variable staining for cytokeratins and positive staining for smooth muscle actin. The cystic spaces within basaloid adenoid cystic carcinomas stain positive with alcian blue, whereas basal cell carcinomas do not. Squamous differentiation is not seen, while cribriform or tubular foci are seen in most basaloid adenoid cystic carcinomas. Perineural invasion is a constant feature of basaloid adenoid cystic carcinomas, but is present in only 25% of basal cell adenocarcinomas. Any lacrimal tumor identified as basaloid adenoid cystic carcinoma should be studied more extensively to rule out basal cell adenocarcinoma.

Treatment

Given the rarity of basal cell adenocarcinomas within the lacrimal gland, the treatment and prognosis are largely based on results from major and minor salivary gland tumor studies. The primary treatment recommendation for these tumors is wide surgical excision. Postoperative radiation should be considered for tumors that are large, have close surgical margins, are recurrent, or have intracranial spread.

Prognosis

The prognosis for vision and life is good. For patients with salivary tumors, the rate of local recurrence ranges from 28% to 50%. Metastasis to regional lymph nodes has occurred in 8–12%. Distant metastasis has been reported in 4–8%. The 10–15-year mortality rate likely ranges between 3% and 10%. Of the three patients reported with lacrimal tumors, none have died as a result of their tumors.

Basal Cell Carcinoma

Clinical Pearls

- Basal cell carcinoma is the most common malignancy of the eyelids and the most frequent secondary tumor involving the orbit.
- Most patients are older than 50 years of age and have a history of a previous skin cancer.
- Lesions originating in the medial canthus are more likely to invade the orbit.
- The rate of recurrence increases once orbital invasion occurs.
- Complete surgical excision is the goal. Less aggressive excision can result in orbital recurrences with possible intracranial or sinus invasion.
- Radiotherapy may be used for nonsurgical tumors and can result in remissions.

Basal cell carcinoma is the most common malignancy of the eyelids, accounting for 87% of cutaneous eyelid tumors. Although it is a true malignancy, basal cell carcinoma only rarely metastasizes to distant sites. When neglected, this lesion can be very destructive locally, resulting in orbital, sinus, or even intracranial invasion. Basal cell carcinoma is the most frequent secondary tumor involving the orbit. Orbital involvement has been reported during initial

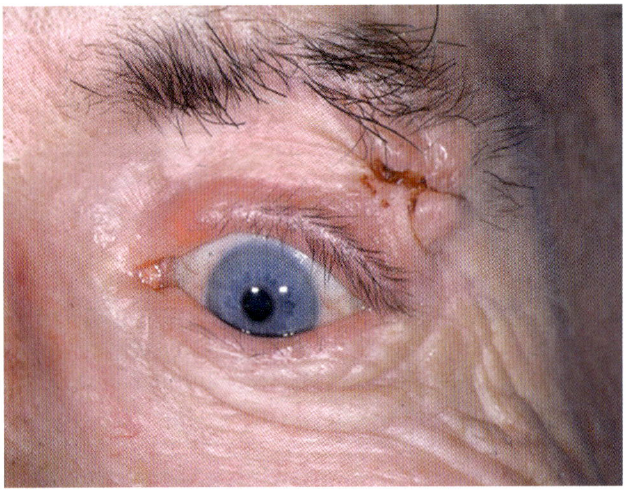

Fig. 56.105 Basal cell carcinoma of the left upper eyelid and brow, extending into the left orbit

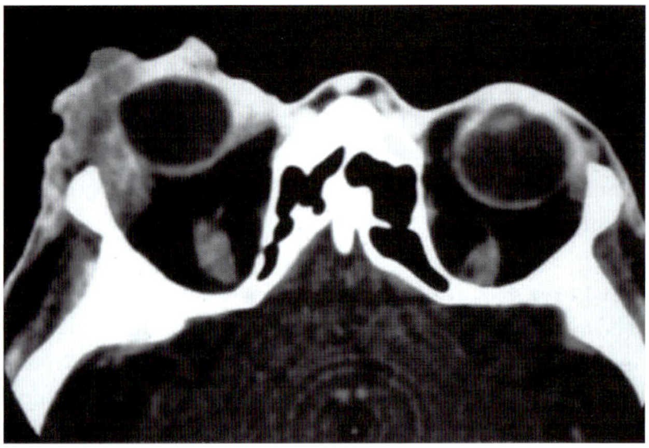

Fig. 56.106 CT scan showing a right lobulated basal cell carcinoma extending into the lateral orbit

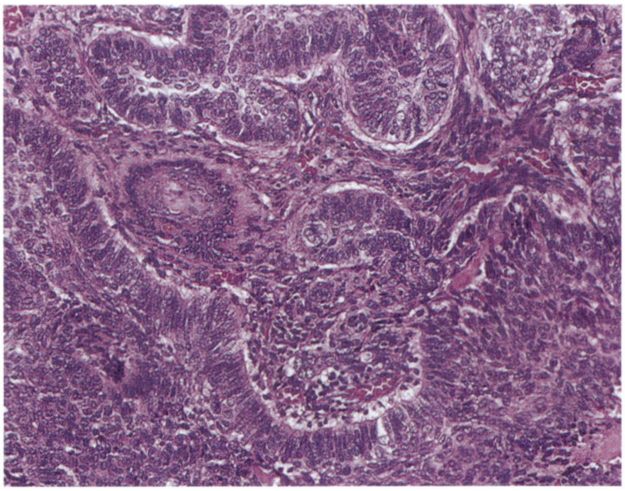

Fig. 56.107 Basal cell carcinoma demonstrating intensely hematoxiphilic cells with hyperchromatic nuclei, peripheral palisading of cells, and retraction artifact in paraffin sections

presentation, but is most commonly associated with cutaneous recurrence. Lesions originating along the medial canthus are more likely to invade the orbit because of anatomic discontinuities in the orbital septal complex.

Clinical Presentation

Most patients are older than 50 years of age and have a history of a previous skin cancer on the eyelids or forehead. This tumor occurs most commonly along the lower eyelid and medial canthal areas, but can involve the brow also (Fig. 56.105). Eyelid malpositions such as ectropion, entropion, and dystopias are commonly seen. In many cases, an irregular, ulcerated, often friable cutaneous mass is present that is fixed to periosteum. In advanced cases, there may be ocular motility restriction or globe displacement. With some tumors, orbital symptoms can be seen without obvious cutaneous recurrence, presenting with complaints of diplopia, ptosis, and orbital pain. Typically, basal cell carcinoma progresses very slowly over years.

Computed Tomography

Orbital basal cell carcinoma appears as irregular, often lobulated, but well-defined densities involving tissues anterior to the orbital septum and extending into the retroseptal space (Fig. 56.106). Tumor may extend down the nasolacrimal duct, along extraocular muscles, or conform to the globe. Less dense cystic spaces can be present that mimic a mucocele, inclusion cyst, or necrotic metastasis. Enhancement is moderate.

Magnetic Resonance Imaging

The T1-weighted image shows a lesion of homogeneous low signal intensity that is isointense to slightly hyperintense with reference to muscle and hypointense to fat. On the T2-weighted image, the tumor produces a somewhat brighter image that remains isointense to muscle and becomes hyperintense to fat. There is marked enhancement with gadolinium that is best visualized with fat suppression algorithms.

Histopathology

The tumor cells are basophilic with hyperchromatic nuclei and form irregular lobules. Along the lobules, cells are arranged radially, with their long axes parallel to each other, creating so-called peripheral palisading (Fig. 56.107). The stroma surrounding the tumor is often mucinous and artifactually shrinks away from the tumor islands during histological processing, creating thin clefts. The clefts and mucinous matrix help to distinguish poorly differentiated basal cell carcinoma from poorly differentiated squamous cell carcinoma invading the orbit. Sometimes, the tumor lobules have central necrosis or a prominent adenoid pattern. Basal cell carcinoma infiltrating the orbit may also have strands of basaloid cells in a dense fibrous stroma, recapitulating the morphea (sclerosing) pattern in the skin.

Treatment

Complete surgical excision of cutaneous lesions with clear margins is generally curative. Medial canthal lesions are the most likely to extend posteriorly within the orbit because of the discontinuous nature of the orbital septum in that location. Localized lesions in the anterior orbit should be excised when possible. Less aggressive excision can result in orbital recurrences with possible intracranial or sinus invasion. Heroic attempts to retain visual function frequently result in scarring and globe fixation. Deep orbital tumors that invest the globe require limited or radical orbital exenteration. Radiotherapy is not generally considered a primary therapeutic option. For widespread nonsurgical tumors, radiotherapy at 3000–4000 cGy can result in local tumor remission.

Prognosis

Prognosis for life is good. Recent reports suggest that surgically excised cutaneous tumors with histologically clear margins have less than a 1% chance of recurrence. Following orbital invasion, the likelihood of recurrence increases. Invasion of the brain or sinuses is associated with a poor prognosis, and these lesions are almost impossible to cure. However, the course is indolent so that tumor-related mortality is relatively low. Recurrences may be seen after many years. Relentless orbital and mid-facial destruction is not an uncommon outcome.

Inverted Papilloma

Clinical Pearls

- Inverted papillomas are caused by polypoid proliferation of schneiderian respiratory epithelium along the nasal and paranasal sinus mucosa.
- Inverted papillomas are benign histologically but often behave aggressively with invasion, destruction, and frequent recurrence.
- Tumors most commonly occur along the lateral nasal wall.
- These tumors occur most commonly in men (3:1) with a median age of 66 years.
- Patients commonly present with nasal obstruction, epistaxis, rhinorrhea, and pressure sensation.
- Complete resection with complete pathologic margins is the standard of care.

These rare tumors result from polypoid proliferation of schneiderian respiratory epithelium along the nasal and paranasal sinus mucosa. Inverted papillomas are benign histologically but often behave aggressively with invasion, destruction, and frequent recurrence (27–71%). The tumor's name comes from its downward extension into mucosa, unlike other tumors that exhibit exophytic growth patterns. The tumor etiology is unknown, but has been associated with HPV or EBV infection, sinusitis, allergy, chronic inflammation, environmental carcinogens, and proliferation of nasal polyps. Tumors most commonly occur along the lateral nasal wall, followed by the maxillary and ethmoid sinuses. Papillomas occur less commonly along the vestibule, septum, floor of the nasopharynx, sphenoid and frontal sinus, and the lacrimal sac. Inverted papillomas account for 0.5–4% of nasal tumors, with only 2.7% resulting in orbital invasion. Inverted papillomas invading the orbit are more likely to undergo malignant degeneration, most commonly to squamous cell or transitional cell carcinomas.

Clinical Presentation

Inverted papillomas occur more commonly in men (3:1) with a median age of 66 years. Patients commonly present with nasal obstruction, epistaxis, rhinorrhea, and pressure sensation. With orbital invasion, patients often complain of proptosis, epiphora, diplopia, decreased vision, and periorbital pain. Less common symptoms include hypoesthesia, hyponasal speech, anosmia, headache, and facial pruritus. Clinical examination may reveal nasolacrimal duct obstruction, globe displacement, extraocular motility disturbance, visual field defects, and palpable medial canthal mass.

Computed Tomography

The most common CT findings include a unilateral mass with a lobulated surface occupying the middle nasal meatus and extending into one or more of the adjacent sinuses (Fig. 56.108). Opacification of the sinuses and mucosal

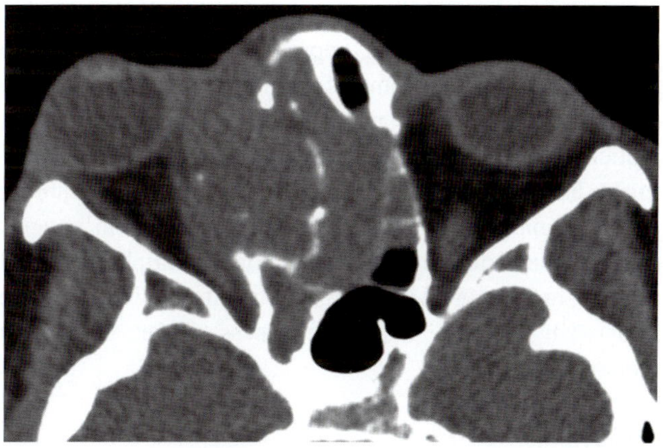

Fig. 56.108 Axial CT scan showing an inverted papilloma in the right ethmoid sinus, extending into the right orbit

thickening may be seen, as well as bony thinning, remodeling, or erosion.

Magnetic Resonance Imaging
MRI is superior to CT for distinguishing papillomas from inflammatory lesions, and it provides better delineation of lesions in contrast to surrounding soft tissue. On T1-weighted images, inverted papillomas are isointense to slightly hyperintense to muscle and homogenous. On T2-weighted images, inverted papilloma has intermediate signal intensity, whereas inflammatory polyps and inspissated material in the sinuses secondary to obstruction by papilloma are hyperintense.

Histopathology
Inverted papillomas are the most common type of Schneiderian papilloma, characterized by an endophytic pattern of downward growth into the underlying stroma. There is a non-keratinized multilayered squamous epithelium or respiratory epithelium containing goblet cells associated with serous and/or mucous glands and ducts. A keratinized surface is noted in 10% of lesions. The cells demonstrate oval nuclei with a low mitotic rate, dense chromatin, and small nucleoli. Smaller numbers of transitional cells and clear cells containing glycogen may be seen. Inflammatory cells, edema, or fibrosis is often seen within the stroma. Atypia is seen preceding malignancy, while malignant transformation may be seen in 10% of sinonasal cases. Malignant foci are seen in almost all cases with orbital extension, most commonly squamous cell carcinoma. Immunohistochemical expression of various cytokeratins, including high molecular weight keratin, is often found. Attenuated expression of CK14 is related to increased risk of recurrence.

Treatment
Because of this tumor's aggressive nature, recurrence rate, and risk of malignant transformation, complete resection with clear surgical margins is the standard of care. Multidisciplinary surgical approaches are most likely to result in optimal outcomes for patients. In certain cases, endoscopic approaches may allow for complete excision. Patients with incomplete tumor resection and orbital involvement have higher recurrence rates, with some requiring exenteration. Radiotherapy may be considered in patients with incompletely resectable tumors, multiple recurrent tumors, and tumors with malignant transformation, although long-term studies of effectiveness have not been demonstrated.

Prognosis
The risk for recurrence has been reported to range from 28% to 80%. Recurrent tumors and those with orbital invasion are more likely to have malignant changes. Mortality has been reported to be as high as 30% in patients with orbital involvement, although malignant transformation and intracranial extension significantly increase the usual risks. The best chance for cure is complete excision during the initial resection.

Sinonasal Carcinoma

Clinical Pearls
- Sinonasal carcinoma is a rare infiltrative tumor of the nasopharyngeal epithelium.
- The prevalence is greater in China and Southeast Asia.
- Patients in the United States are older and often present with proptosis, associated globe displacement, and other nasopharyngeal symptoms.
- MRI often shows focal or diffuse thickening of the nasal and sinus mucosa and cervical lymphadenopathy.
- Radiotherapy has been the primary treatment for sinonasal carcinoma with orbital extension and regional lymph nodal metastasis.
- The 5-year survival has been reported to be 28% with orbital extension.

Nasopharyngeal and sinonasal carcinoma is a rare infiltrative tumor arising from the epithelium of the nasopharynx. The prevalence of sinonasal carcinoma in areas of China and Southeast Asia is significantly higher, accounting for up to 25% of all tumors and 3% of orbital tumors. Three subtypes of NPC are recognized in the World Health Organization (WHO) classification: (1) squamous cell carcinoma, (2) nonkeratinizing carcinoma, and (3) undifferentiated carcinoma, which is the most frequent type worldwide. Possible etiologies include environmental factors, infection with Epstein-Barr virus (EBV), and genetic susceptibility. Rare orbital invasion occurs most commonly as the result of recurrent tumors entering through orbital fissures or through bones. Tumors within the pterygopalatine fossa extend to the infratemporal fossa, entering the orbit through orbital fissures or through bones. Tumors extending into the ethmoid or sphenoid sinuses can erode the lamina papyracea, resulting in medial orbital extension. Invasion of the skull base occurs in 12–31% of cases. These tumors rarely come to medical attention before they have spread to regional lymph nodes.

Clinical Presentation
In the United States, sinonasal carcinoma typically presents in older patients. Patients present with orbital invasion usually into the inferior orbit most commonly associated with proptosis and associated globe displacement (Fig. 56.109). Patients may complain of diplopia, blurred

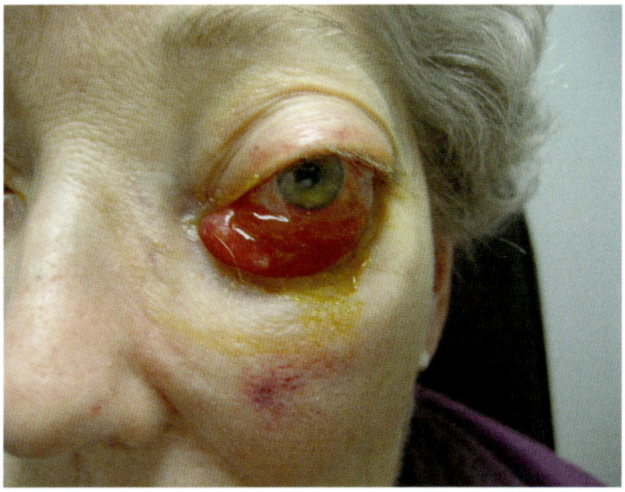

Fig. 56.109 Naso-sinus tumor extending into the inferior left orbit

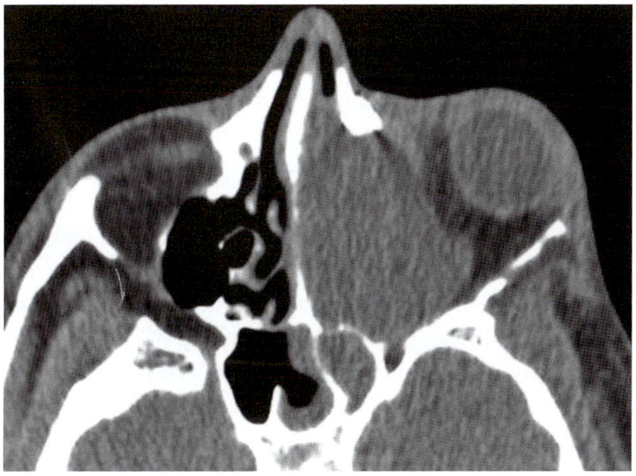

Fig. 56.110 Axial CT scan with a large passion tumor extending into the left orbit

vision, and orbital pain. Clinical findings often include visual field changes, motility restriction, palpable lid mass, papilledema, and optic atrophy. Symptoms related to the location of the primary tumor include trismus, pain, otitis media, and nasal regurgitation due to paresis of the soft palate, hearing loss, and cranial nerve palsies from extension of tumor into the skull base. Larger growths may produce nasal obstruction or bleeding and a "nasal twang" to speech.

Computed Tomography

CT scan shows an ill-defined isodense to slightly hyperdense irregular soft tissue mass with destruction of bone and invasion into the orbit (Fig. 56.110). Masses with orbital extension often involve the infratemporal fossa or paranasal sinuses. Sinus mucosal thickening and enlargement of local lymph nodes are common findings. With contrast administration there is usually heterogeneous enhancement.

Magnetic Resonance Imaging

The MR image shows focal or diffuse thickening of the nasopharyngeal mucosa and cervical lymphadenopathy. The tumor mostly shows a poorly defined hypointense to isointense signal intensity relative to muscle on T1-weighted images. Osseous destruction may be seen, and the normal high marrow signal on T1 is replaced with an intermediate signal. Heterogeneous enhancement is seen with gadolinium. On T2-weighted images, this lesion remains hypointense to isointense and shows moderate to intense homogeneous enhancement on contrast-enhanced sequences. MRI has been shown to be more accurate in identifying the extent of tumor involvement in the nasopharynx, skull base, and orbit than PET/CT.

Histopathology

Nasopharyngeal carcinoma has three WHO classified subtypes: squamous cell carcinoma (SCC), nonkeratinizing carcinoma (NKC), and undifferentiated carcinoma (UC). These subtypes may be further classified as well, moderately, or poorly differentiated. The SCC subtype demonstrates squamous differentiation, as evidenced by the presence of intercellular bridges and keratin production. The cells are often spindle-shaped and may be arranged into islands. Prominent nuclei with moderate amounts of eosinophilic cytoplasm are seen. Lymphocytes and keratin whorls are often present in the surrounding stroma. The NKC and UKC subtypes have no squamous differentiation, with most tumors having lymphohistiocytic infiltrates. The UC subtype has indistinct cell margins that form sheet-like masses. Prominent nucleoli and vesicles are noted within nuclei. The NKC subtype may have a stratified, sheet-like, or cord-like configuration with distinct cell margins. The NKC and UC subtypes are most commonly associated with the presence of the Epstein-Bar virus. These tumors exhibit positive immunostaining for cytokeratin.

Treatment

Radiotherapy has been the primary treatment for sinonasal carcinoma with orbital extension and regional lymph node metastasis. Combined radiotherapy and chemotherapeutic regimens have been used for advanced lymph node and visceral metastasis. Even with well-planned multidisciplinary approaches, complete surgical resection of these tumors is often impossible. Orbital decompression may provide relief of symptoms and improve visual acuity. Radioresistant lymph nodes may need to be removed by radical neck dissection; otherwise, the surgical role for treatment of this tumor is limited.

Prognosis

The patient's risk can be stratified based on the size, type, and staging of the tumor. The 5-year survival has been reported to be 30–35% with intracranial extension and 28% with orbital extension. Orbital involvement is also a risk factor for development of distant metastasis.

Squamous Cell Carcinoma

Clinical Pearls

- Squamous cell carcinomas are the second most common eyelid malignancy.
- Periocular squamous cell carcinomas most often present as a painless nodule or plaque with irregular pearly margins.
- Extension may proceed along extraocular muscles, via perineural extension, and via invasion of other orbital structures.
- Squamous cell tumors tend to be locally invasive, with skip lesions occurring as the result of perineural spread.
- Radical surgery with wide margins is generally recommended, including exenteration with adjacent bone removal.
- Postoperative radiotherapy is indicated for patients with significant sinus involvement, incomplete resections, or evidence of perineural spread.

Squamous cell carcinoma of the orbit occurs by extension of periocular skin tumors, by extension of conjunctival tumors, or by invasion of paranasal sinus tumors. Rare metastases to the orbit from a distant primary tumor have been reported. Periorbital skin tumors are a relatively rare malignant epithelial tumor that typically affects elderly fair-skinned individuals. Squamous cell carcinomas are the second most common eyelid malignancy, accounting for approximately 5% of all eyelid neoplasms. These tumors occur most commonly in sun-exposed areas, frequently along the lower eyelid, medial canthus, and upper eyelid. Extension from lesions of the brow or lacrimal sac has been reported. Risk factors for development include actinic keratosis, xeroderma pigmentosa, previous radiotherapy, HPV infection, HIV infection, or immunosuppression. Orbital invasion of periocular squamous cell carcinoma reportedly occurs in 6% of tumors.

Squamous cell carcinoma is the most common neoplasm of the conjunctival epithelium. They most frequently present as a slow-growing lesion in elderly patients. Risk factors for conjunctival tumors include HPV infection, HIV infection, sun exposure, and immunosuppression. There have been several reports of tumors occurring in patients with anophthalmic sockets, thought to be the result of chronic inflammation from prosthetic wear.

Orbital invasion by squamous cell carcinomas from the adjacent maxillary sinuses, ethmoid sinuses, and nasal cavity does occur. Reported risk factors include previous radiotherapy, chronic sinusitis, and inhalation of certain dusts, nickel, chromium, radium, mustard gas, or cigarette smoke. When the ethmoid sinuses are involved, extension into the orbit has been reported in 35–72% of cases. Rarely, tumors may spread from other sites on the head via anterograde extension along the skull base. Metastasis may occur by lymphatic or hematogenous spread.

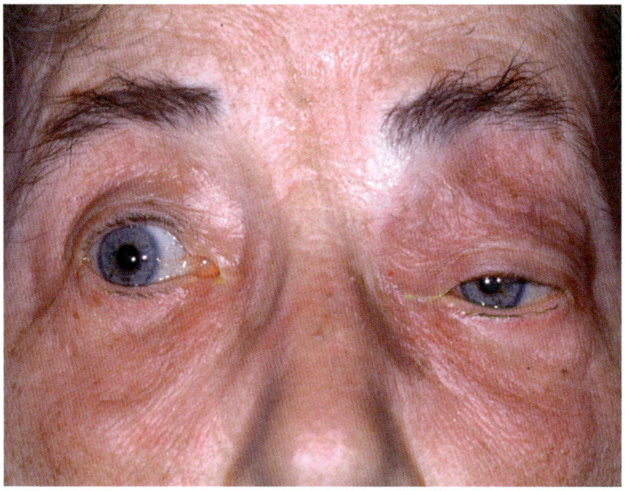

Fig. 56.111 Recurrent squamous cell carcinoma of the medial upper eyelid with orbital extension

Clinical Presentation

Periocular squamous cell carcinomas most often present as a painless nodule or plaque with irregular pearly margins, scaling and crusting, fissuring or central ulceration, and telangiectasias (Fig. 56.111). Conjunctival tumors are slow growing and most frequently located along the limbus. Patients often complain of conjunctival irritation and redness. The lesions have variable appearances that are described as gelatinous, velvety, papilliform, leukoplakic, nodular, or diffuse. A palpable mass along the preauricular nodes may provide evidence of early lymphatic spread. Extension may proceed along extraocular muscles by perineural extension (sensory, motor, and optic) or by invasion of other orbital structures. Anterior masses are often palpable. Vision loss, epiphora, headache, periorbital paresthesias or pain, and eyelid swelling are sometimes found. Extraocular muscle disturbance and diplopia may be noted. Patients with orbital tumors originating in the sinuses or nasal cavity are more likely to present with proptosis, globe displacement, and pain. Additional symptoms indicating sinus involvement include rhinorrhea, nasal obstruction, paresthesias, nasal obstruction, orbital apex syndrome, epistaxis, and hyposmia.

Computed Tomography

On CT scan, squamous cell carcinoma appears as an irregular, solid, but well-circumscribed density in the eyelid and orbit and may extend into the retrobulbar space (Fig. 56.112). Tumors may extend down the nasolacrimal duct, along orbital nerves to the orbital apex, or may mold to the globe or extraocular muscles. Bony destruction is commonly seen. Enhancement is moderate.

Magnetic Resonance Imaging

On MRI, the T1-weighted image shows a homogeneous mass of low signal intensity that is isointense to slightly

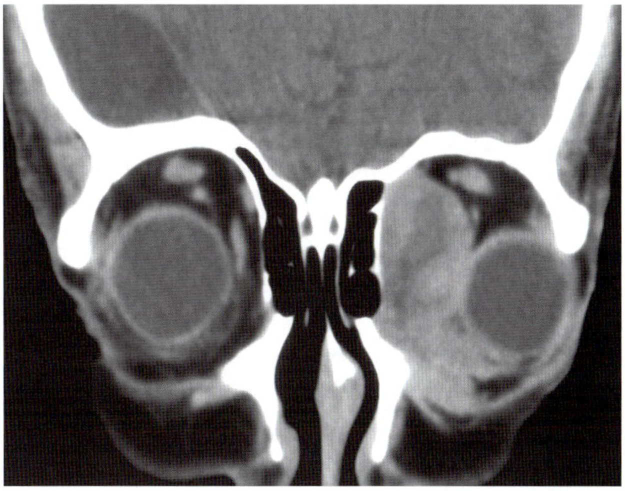

Fig. 56.112 Coronal CT scan showing a large squamous cell carcinoma invading the left medial orbit

hyperintense to muscle and hypointense to fat. On the T2-weighted image, the tumor produces a more intense image that remains isointense to muscle and becomes hyperintense to fat. There is marked enhancement with gadolinium that is best seen on fat suppression sequences. MRI is able to detect the presence of perineural spread (95% sensitivity), but not necessarily the extent (63% sensitivity).

Histopathology

Squamous cell carcinomas are characterized by cells with large atypical nuclei with prominent nucleoli. Tumors may be characterized as well differentiated (59%), moderately differentiated (29%), or poorly differentiated (11.8%). Well-differentiated tumors have polygonal shaped cells arranged into distinct nests or lobules with cells showing keratinization, intercellular bridges, or pearl formation. Poorly differentiated tumors have highly anaplastic rounded cells with foci of necrosis and rare keratinization. Cutaneous tumors tend to be well differentiated, while nasal or sinus tumors are more likely to be poorly differentiated. Perineural spread is frequently seen along the facial, trigeminal, extraocular, and optic nerves. Immunohistochemical studies are usually positive for cytokeratin and epithelial membrane antigen.

Treatment

Squamous cell tumors tend to be locally invasive, with skip lesions occurring as the result of perineural spread. Management will vary depending upon tumor size, location, grade, histological subtype, and the presence of recurrence or perineural invasion. Radical surgery with wide margins is generally recommended, including exenteration with adjacent bone removal. Multidisciplinary approaches are often utilized for patients requiring orbitectomy, maxillectomy, or craniofacial resections. Postoperative radiotherapy is indicated for patients with significant sinus involvement, incomplete resections, or evidence of perineural spread. Adjuvant chemotherapy is used with less frequency. Patients with multiple lesions may require combination therapy with cisplatin, doxorubicin, bleomycin, peplomycin, methotrexate, or 5-fluorouracil. Combined radiotherapy and chemotherapy may be used for palliative care and may actually improve survival. The potential for distant metastatic spread has ranged from 6% to 43% in various studies of periocular and orbital tumors. Complete physical examination, laboratory evaluation (CBC, chemistry panel, and liver enzymes), and imaging (chest, abdomen, and pelvis) should be performed in all patients to rule out systemic metastasis.

Prognosis

The prognosis is often dependent upon the completeness of the surgical resection. The prognosis for vision and life is poor for patients with orbital spread. Patients with primary skin tumors live nearly twice as long compared to patients with primary sinus tumors. The mortality rate for patients having orbital extension of sinus tumors is 60% at 5 years. Patients with metastases to lymph nodes have a 55–80% mortality rate at 5 years. With orbital involvement, the rate of recurrence or presence of residual tumor ranges from 35% to 49%. In cases of locally recurrent tumors, the risk of recurrence and metastasis increases significantly. In cases with intracranial spread, the 5-year mortality rates exceed 50%. Patients with a delay in care or tumor recurrence have a much worse prognosis. Other poor prognostic indicators include lesion greater than 2 cm or greater than 4 mm depth, poorly differentiated tumors, perineural invasion, and immunosuppression. The presence of a peritumorous lymphocytic infiltrate portends an improved prognosis.

Suggested Reading

Introduction

1. Armington WG, Bilaniuk LT. The radiologic evaluation of the orbit: conal and intraconal lesions. Semin Ultrasound CT MRI. 1988;9:455–73.
2. Avery G, Tang RA, Close LG. Ophthalmic manifestations of mucoceles. Ann Ophthalmol. 1983;15:734–7.
3. Bilaniuk LT. Vascular lesions of the orbit in children. Neuroimaging Clin N Am. 2005;15:107–20.
4. Buckmiller LM. Update on hemangiomas and vascular malformations. Curr Opin Otolaryngol Head Neck Surg. 2004;12:476–87.
5. Cantore WA. Neural orbital tumors. Curr Opin Ophthalmol. 2000;11:367–71.
6. Coupland SE. Lymphoproliferative lesions of the ocular adnexa. Differential diagnostic guidelines. Ophthalmologe. 2004;101:197–215.
7. Crawford JS. Diseases of the orbit. In: Toronto Hospital for Sick Children, Department of Ophthalmology, editor. The eye in childhood. Chicago: Year Book; 1967.
8. Della Rocca RC, Roen J, Labay JR, et al. Isolated neurofibroma of the orbit. Ophthalmic Surg. 1985;16:634–8.
9. DePotter P, Shields JA, Shields CL. MRI of the eye and orbit. Philadelphia: J.B. Lippincott; 1995. p. 3–17.

10. Dortzbach RK, Kronish JW, Gentry LR. Magnetic resonance imaging of the orbit. Part II. Clinical applications. Ophthal Plast Reconstr Surg. 1989;5:160–70.
11. Dutton JJ. Radiographic evaluation of the orbit. In: Doxanas MT, Anderson RL, editors. Clinical orbital anatomy. Baltimore: Williams & Wilkins; 1984. p. 35–56.
12. Dutton JJ. Gliomas of the anterior visual pathways. Surv Ophthalmol. 1993;38:427–52.
13. Dutton JJ. Atlas of clinical and surgical orbital anatomy. Philadelphia: W.B. Saunders; 1994. p. 201–32.
14. Dutton JJ. Optic nerve sheath meningiomas. Surv Ophthalmol. 1994;37:167–83.
15. Dutton JJ. Radiology of the orbit and visual pathways. London: Saunders, Elsevier; 2010. 408 pp.
16. Dutton JJ, Byrne SF, Proia AD. Diagnostic atlas of orbital diseases. Philadelphia: W.B. Saunders; 2000.
17. Dutton JJ, Tawfik HA, DeBacker CM, Lipham WJ, et al. Multiple recurrences in malignant peripheral nerve sheath tumor of the orbit: a case report and a review of the literature. Ophthal Plast Reconstr Surg. 2001;17:293–9.
18. Ellis JH, Banks PM, Campbell RJ, et al. Lymphoid tumors of the ocular adnexa. Clinical correlation with the working formulation, classification and immunoperoxidase staining of paraffin sections. Ophthalmology. 1985;92:1311–24.
19. Ferry AP, Font RL. Carcinoma metastatic to the eye and orbit. I. A clinicopathologic study of 227 cases. Arch Ophthalmol. 1974;92:276–86.
20. Font RL, Gamel JW. Epithelial tumors of the lacrimal gland: an analysis of 265 cases. In: Jakobiec FA, editor. Ocular and adnexal tumors. Birmingham: Aesculapius; 1978.
21. Font RL, Gamel JW. Adenoid cystic carcinoma of the lacrimal gland. A clinicopathologic study of 79 cases. In: Nicholson DH, editor. Ocular pathology update. New York: Masson; 1980. p. 277–83.
22. Font RL, Hidayat AA. Fibrous histiocytoma of the orbit. A clinicopathologic study of 150 cases. Hum Pathol. 1982;13:199–209.
23. Forbes G. Vascular lesions of the orbit. Neuroimaging Clin N Am. 1996;6:113–22.
24. Forrest AW. Intraorbital tumors. Arch Ophthalmol. 1942;41:198–232.
25. Forrest AW. Lacrimal gland tumors. In: Jones IS, Jakobiec FA, editors. Diseases of the orbit. Hagerstown: Harper and Row; 1979. p. 355.
26. Gordon LK. Diagnostic dilemmas in orbital inflammatory disease. Ocul Immunol Inflamm. 2003;11:2–15.
27. Harold Lee HB, Garrity JA, Cameron JD, Strianese D, Bonavolonta G, Patrinely JR. Primary optic nerve sheath meningioma in children. Surv Ophthalmol. 2008;53:543–58.
28. Harris GJ. Orbital vascular malformations: a consensus statement on terminology and its clinical implications. Orbital Society. Am J Ophthalmol. 1999;127:453–5.
29. Hart WM. Metastatic carcinoma to the eye and orbit. In: Zimmerman LE, editor. Tumors of the eye and adnexa, Int Ophthalmol Clin, vol. 2; 1962. p. 465–82.
30. Henderson JW, Farrow GM. Orbital tumors. 2nd ed. New York: Brian C. Decker (Thieme-Stratton); 1980. p. 67–74.
31. Iliff CE, Ossofsky HJ. Tumors of the orbit. Trans Am Ophthalmol Soc. 1957;55:505–41.
32. Ingalis RG. Tumors of the orbit and allied pseudo tumors. Charles C. Thomas: Springfield; 1953.
33. Jakobiec FA, Jones IS. Vascular tumors, malformations and degenerations. In: Jones IS, Jakobiec FA, editors. Diseases of the orbit. Hagerstown: Harper & Row; 1979. p. 269–308.
34. Jakobiec FA, Iwamoto T, Knowles DM II. Ocular adnexal lymphoid tumors. Correlative ultrastructural and immunologic marker studies. Arch Ophthalmol. 1982;100:84–98.
35. Karcioglu ZA, Hadjistilianou D, Rozans M, DeFrancesco S. Orbital rhabdomyosarcoma. Cancer Control. 2004;11:328–33.
36. Kennedy RE. An evaluation of 820 orbital cases. Trans Am Ophthalmol Soc. 1984;82:134–57.
37. Kincaid MC, Green WR. Ocular and orbital involvement in leukemia. Surv Ophthalmol. 1983;27:211–32.
38. Knowles DM II, Jakobiec FA. Ocular adnexal lymphoid neoplasms: clinical, histopathologic, electron microscopic, and immunologic characteristics. Hum Pathol. 1982;13:148–62.
39. Konrad GB, Thiel HJ. Schwannoma of the orbit. Ophthalmologica. 1984;188:118–27.
40. Korbin EA, Blodi FC, Weingeist TA. Ocular and orbital manifestations of neurofibromatosis. Surv Ophthalmol. 1984;188:118–27.
41. Lee AG. Neuroophthalmological management of optic pathway gliomas. Neurosurg Focus. 2007;23:E1.
42. MacCarty CS, Brown DN. Orbital tumors in children. Clin Neurosurg. 1964;11:76–93.
43. Mafee MF, Putterman A, Valvassori GE, Campos M, Capek V. Orbital space-occupying lesions: role of computed tomography and magnetic resonance imaging. Radiol Clin N Am. 1987;25:529–59.
44. Meekins B, Dutton JJ, Proia AD. Primary orbital leiomyosarcoma: a case report and review of the literature. Arch Ophthalmol. 1988;106:82–6.
45. Mortada A. Fibroma of the orbit. Br J Ophthalmol. 1971;55:350–2.
46. Moss MH. Expanding lesions of the orbit: a clinical study of 230 consecutive cases. Am J Ophthalmol. 1962;54:761–70.
47. Porterfleld JF. Orbital tumors in children: a report on 214 cases. Int Ophthalmol Clin. 1962;2:319–35.
48. Reese AB. Expanding lesions of the orbit. Trans Ophthalmol Soc UK. 1971;91:85–104.
49. Rootman J, Goldberg C, Robertson W. Primary orbital schwannomas. Br J Ophthalmol. 1982;66:194–204.
50. Rootman J, Hay E, Graebo D, et al. Orbital-adnexal lymphangiomas: a spectrum of hemodynamically isolated vascular hamartomas. Ophthalmology. 1986;93:1558–70.
51. Rootman J. Vascular malformations of the orbit: hemodynamic concepts. Orbit. 2003;22:103–20.
52. Rootman J. Diseases of the orbit. A multidisciplinary approach. Philadelphia: J.B. Lippincott; 1988.
53. Sherman RP, Rootman J, LaPointe JS. Orbital dermoids: clinical presentation and management. Br J Ophthalmol. 1986;101:726–9.
54. Shields JA. Rhabdomyosarcoma of the orbit. In: Hornblass A, editor. Ophthalmic plastic and reconstructive surgery. Baltimore: Wiliams & Wilkins; 1987.
55. Shields JA. Diagnosis and management of orbital tumors. Philadelphia: W.B. Saunders; 1989. p. 89–122.
56. Shields JA, Shields CL. Orbital cysts of childhood – classification, clinical features, and management. Surv Ophthalmol. 2004;49:281–99.
57. Shields JA, Bakewell B, Augsburger JJ, et al. Classification and incidence of space-occupying lesions of the orbit. A survey of 645 biopsies. Arch Ophthalmol. 1984;102:1606–11.
58. Shields JA, Bakewell B, Augsburger JJ, et al. Space-occupying orbital masses in children: a review of 250 consecutive biopsies. Ophthalmology. 1986;93:379–84.
59. Shields JA, Shields CL, Eagle RC, et al. Pleomorphic adenoma ("benign mixed tumor") of the lacrimal gland. Arch Ophthalmol. 1987;105:560–1.
60. Shields CL, Shields JA, Peggs M. Metastatic tumors to the orbit. Ophthalmic Reconstr Plast Surg. 1988;4:73–80.
61. Shields JA, Shields CL, Scartozzi R. Survey of 1264 patients with orbital tumors and simulating lesions: the 2002 Montgomery Lecture, part I. Ophthalmology. 2004;111:997–1008.
62. Smoker WR, Gentry LR, Yee NK, Reede DL, Nerad JA. Vascular lesions of the orbit: more than meets the eye. Radiographics. 2008;28:185–204.
63. Zimmerman LA, Sanders TE, Ackerman LV. Epithelial tumors of the lacrimal gland: prognostic and therapeutic significance of histologic types. Int Ophthalmol Clin. 1962;2:337–67.

Cystic Lesions: Dermoid Cyst

64. Bartlett SP, Lin KY, Kilowatts J. The surgical management of orbit facial dermoids in the pediatric patient. Plast Reconstr Surg. 1993;91:1208–15.
65. Blei L, Chambers JT, Liotta LA, Di Chiro G. Orbital dermoid diagnosed by computed tomographic scanning. Am J Ophthalmol. 1978;85:58–61.
66. Bonavolonta G, Tranfa F, de Conciliis C, Strainers D. Dermoid cysts: 16-year survey. Ophthal Plast Reconstr Surg. 1995;11:187–92.
67. Chawda SJ, Moseley IF. Computed tomography of orbital dermoids. A 20 year review. Clin Radiol. 1999;54:821–5.
68. Colombo F, Holback LM, Naumann GO. Chronic inflammation in dermoid cysts: a clinicopathologic study of 115 patients. Orbit. 2000;19(2):97–107.
69. De Potter P, Flanders AE, Shields CL, Shields JA. Magnetic resonance imaging of orbital tumors. Int Ophthalmol Clin. 1993;33:163–73.
70. Emerick GT, Shields CL, Shields JA, et al. Chewing-induced visual impairment from a dumbbell dermoid cyst. Ophthal Plast Reconstr Surg. 1997;13:57–61.
71. Grove AS Jr. Giant dermoid cysts of the orbit. Ophthalmology. 1979;86:1513–20.
72. Howard GR, Nerad JA, Bonavolonta G, Tranfa F. Orbital dermoid cysts located within the lateral rectus muscle. Ophthalmology. 1994;101:767–71.
73. Kersten RC. The eyelid crease approach to superficial lateral dermoid cysts. J Pediatr Ophthalmol Strabismus. 1988;25:48–51.
74. Kiratli H, Bilgic S, Tezel GG. Dermoid cyst of the lacrimal gland. Orbit. 2005;24(2):145–8.
75. Lane CM, Erhich WW, Wright JE. Orbital dermoid cyst. Eye. 1987;1:504–11.
76. Leonardo D, Shields CL, Shields JA, Nelson LB. Recurrent giant orbital dermoid of infancy. J Pediatr Ophthalmol Strabismus. 1994;31:50–2.
77. McCollough ML, Glover AT, Grabski WJ, Berger TG. Orbital dermoid cysts showing conjunctival epithelium. Am J Dermatopathol. 1991;13:611–5.
78. Meyer DR, Lessner AM, Yeatts RP, et al. Primary temporal fossa dermoid cysts. Characterization and surgical management. Ophthalmology. 1999;106:342–9.
79. Nevrekar D, Abdu E, Selden NR. Craniectomy for a bilobed dermoid cyst in the temporal fossa and greater wing of sphenoid bone. Pediatr Neurosurg. 2009;45:46–8.
80. Nugent RA, Lapointe JS, Rootman J, Robertson WD, Graeb DA. Orbital dermoids: features on CT. Radiology. 1987;165:475–8.
81. Pollard ZF, Harley RD, Calhoun J. Dermoid cysts in children. Pediatrics. 1976;57:379–82.
82. Sagoo MS, Shields CL, Marr BP, Eagle RC Jr, Shields JA. Orbital conjunctival dermoid cyst with oncocytic differentiation. Ophthal Plast Reconstr Surg. 2008;24(1):69–71.
83. Samuleson TW, Margo CE, Levy MH, Pusateri TJ. Zygomaticofrontal suture defect associated with orbital dermoid cyst. Surv Ophthalmol. 1988;33:127–30.
84. Sathananthan N, Moseley IF, Rose GE, Wright JE. The frequency and clinical significance of bone involvement in outer canthus dermoid cysts. Br J Ophthalmol. 1993;77:789–94.
85. Sherman RP, Rootman J, LaPointe JS. Orbital dermoids: clinical presentation and management. Br J Ophthalmol. 1984;68:642–52.
86. Shields JA, Augsburger JJ, Donoso LA. Orbital dermoid cyst of conjunctival origin. Am J Ophthalmol. 1986;101:726–9.
87. Shields JA, Kaden IH, Eagle RC Jr, Shields CL. Orbital dermoid cysts: clinicopathologic correlations, classification, and management. The 1997 Josephine E. Schuleler Lecture. Ophthalmic Plast Reconstr Surg. 1997;13:265–76.
88. Traboulsi EI, Azar DT, Khattar J, Salamoun SG. A-scan ultrasonography in the diagnosis of orbital dermoid cysts. Ann Ophthalmol. 1988;20:229–32.
89. Wilkins RB, Byrd WA. Intraconal dermoid cyst. A case report. Ophthal Plast Reconstr Surg. 1986;2:83–7.

Cystic Lesions: Dermoid Cyst of Conjunctival Origin

90. Bartlett SP, Lin KY, Katowitz J. The surgical management of orbitofacial dermoids in the pediatric patient. Plast Reconstr Surg. 1993;91:1208–15.
91. Dutton JJ, Byrne SF, Proia AD. Diagnostic atlas of orbital diseases. Philadelphia: WB Saunders; 2004. p. 4–7.
92. Jakobiec FA, Bonanno PA, Sigelman J. Conjunctival adnexal cysts and dermoids. Arch Ophthalmol. 1978;96:1404–9.
93. Lane CM, Ehrlich WW, Wright JE. Orbital dermoid cyst. Eye. 1987;1:504–11.
94. Shields JA, Shields CL. Orbital cysts of childhood: classification, clinical features and management. Surv Ophthalmol. 2004;49:281–99.
95. Shields JA, Kaden IH, Eagle RC, Shields CL. Orbital dermoid cysts: clinicopathologic correlations, classification and management: the 1997 Josephine E. Schuler Lecture. Ophthalmic Plast Reconstr Surg. 1997;13:256–76.

Cystic Lesions: Epidermoid Cyst

96. Blanco G, Esteban R, Falarreta D, Saornil A. Orbital intradiploic giant epidermoid cyst. Arch Ophthalmol. 2001;119:771–3.
97. Bradey N, Hayward JM. Case report: bilateral lacrimal gland enlargement: an unusual manifestation of dacryops. Clin Radiol. 1991;43:280–1.
98. Brownstein S, Belin MW, Krohel GB, et al. Orbital dacryops. Ophthalmology. 1984;91:1424–8.
99. Bullock JD, Fleishman JA, Rosset JS. Lacrimal ductal cysts. Ophthalmology. 1986;93:1355–60.
100. Eggert JE, Harris GJ, Caya JG. Respiratory epithelial cyst of the orbit. Ophthal Plast Reconstr Surg. 1988;4:101–4.
101. Eijpe AA, Koornneef L, Verbeeten B, et al. Intradiploic epidermoid cysts of the bony orbit. Ophthalmology. 1991;98:1737–43.
102. Haik BG, St Louis L. Radiologic recognition of orbital dacryops. Am J Neuroradiol. 1989;10:S89–90.
103. Hanig CJ, Hornblass A. Treatment of postenucleation orbital cysts. Ann Ophthalmol. 1986;18:191–3.
104. Ho VT, Rao VM, Flanders AE. Postsurgical conjunctival epithelial cysts. Am J Neuroradiol. 1994;15:1181–3.
105. Johnson DW, Bartley GB, Garrity JA, Robertson DM. Massive epithelium-lined cysts after scleral buckling. Am J Ophthalmol. 1992;113:439–42.
106. Monica M, Long DA, Karciougl u ZA. Bilateral dacryops. Ann Ophthalmol. 1988;20:259–63.
107. Morax S, Herdan ML, Chouard B. Kystes orbitaires par inclusion conjunctivale après chirurgie orbito-oculopalpebrale. J Fr Ophtalmol. 1987;10:41–9.
108. Nerad JA, Carter K, Folberg R. Simple dacryops. Arch Ophthalmol. 1988;106:1129.
109. Newton C, Dutton JJ, Klintworth GK. A respiratory epithelial choristomatous cyst of the orbit. Ophthalmology. 1985;12:1754–7.
110. Pantaleoni FB, Spagnolo S, Martini A, et al. Argon laser photocoagulation in the treatment of the palpebral lobe cysts of the lacrimal gland (dacryops). Ophthalmic Surg Lasers. 1997;28:690–2.
111. Rumelt S, Harsh GR IV, Rubin PAD. Giant epidermoid involving 3 cranial bones. Arch Ophthalmol. 1997;115:922–4.

112. Scholte T, Nagel G, Vecsei PV, Herzau V, Rohrbach JM. Conjunctival cysts of the orbits: clinical aspects and histology in 4 patients. Klin Monatsbl Augenheilkd. 1998;213:117–20.

Cystic Lesions: Mucocele

113. Aoki H, Tanaka Y, Niki Y, Kamada K, Fujita T. Intraorbital subperiosteal hematoma due to paranasal mucocele – case report. Neurol Med Chir (Tokyo). 1997;37:627–9.
114. Barat JL, Marchal JC, Bracard S, Auque J, Lepoire J. Mucoceles of the sphenoidal sinus. Report of six cases and review of the literature. J Neuroradiol. 1990;17:135–51.
115. Hejazi N, Witzmann A, Hassler W. Ocular manifestations of sphenoid mucoceles: clinical features and neurosurgical management of three cases and review of the literature. Surg Neurol. 2001;56:338–43.
116. Iliff CE. Mucoceles in the orbit. Arch Ophthalmol. 1973;89:392–5.
117. Knipe TA, Gandhi PD, Fleming JC, Chandra RK. Transblepharoplasty approach to sequestered disease of the lateral frontal sinus with ophthalmologic manifestations. Am J Rhinol. 2007;21(1):100–4.
118. Moriyama H, Nakajima T, Honda Y. Studies on mucoceles of the ethmoid and sphenoid sinuses analysis of 47 cases. J Laryngol Otol. 1992;106:23–7.
119. Ormerod LD, Weber AL, Rauch SD, Feldon SE. Ophthalmic manifestations of maxillary sinus mucoceles. Ophthalmology. 1987;94:1013–9.
120. Palmer-Hall AM, Anderson SF. Paraocular sinus mucoceles. J Am Optom Assoc. 1997;68:725–33.
121. Sautter NB, Citardi MJ, Perry J, Batra PS. Paranasal sinus mucoceles with skull-base and/or orbital erosion: is the endoscopic approach sufficient? Otolaryngol Head Neck Surg. 2008;139(4):570–4.
122. Sethi DS, Lau DP, Chan C. Sphenoid sinus mucocele presenting with isolated oculomotor nerve palsy. J Laryngol Otol. 1997;111:471–3.
123. Shah A, Meyer DR, Parnes S. Management of frontoethmoidal mucoceles with orbital extension: is primary orbital reconstruction necessary? Ophthal Plast Reconstr Surg. 2007;23(4):267–71.
124. Stanton MB. Sphenoid sinus mucocele. Am J Ophthalmol. 1970;70:991–4.
125. Van Tassel P, Lee YY, Jing BS, De Pena CA. Mucoceles of the paranasal sinuses: MR imaging with CT correlation. Am J Neuroradiol. 1989;10:607–12.

Cystic Lesions: Respiratory Cyst

126. Eggert JE, Harris GJ, Caya JG. Respiratory epithelial cyst of the orbit. Ophthal Plast Reconstr Surg. 1988;4:101–4.
127. Hanke V, Gotzfried H. Rhinoepithelial, cystic choristoma of the orbit. Klin Monatsbl Augenheilkd. 1987;190:192–5.
128. James CR, Lyness R, Wright JE. Respiratory epithelium lines cysts presenting in the orbit without associated mucocele formation. Br J Ophthalmol. 1986;70:387–90.
129. Mee JJ, McNab AA, McKelvie P. Respiratory epithelial orbital cysts. Clin Exp Ophthalmol. 2004;30:356–60.
130. Morris WR, Fleming JC. Respiratory choristomatous cysts in the temporal orbit. Ophthal Plast Reconstr Surg. 2001;17:462–4.
131. Neves RB, Yeatts RP, Martin TJ. Pneumonia-orbital cysts after orbital fracture repair. Am J Ophthalmol. 1998;125:879–80.
132. Newton C, Dutton JJ, Klintworth GK. A respiratory epithelial choristomatous cyst of the orbit. Ophthalmology. 1985;12:1754–7.
133. Schelper RL, Kagan-Hallet KS, Huntington HW. Brainstem subarachnoid respiratory epithelial cysts: report of two cases and review of the literature. Hum Pathol. 1986;17:417–22.

Vascular Lesions: Capillary Hemangioma

134. Balchunas ER, Quencer RM, Byrne SF, et al. Correlative of the computed tomographic, ultrasonographic, and pathological characteristics of cavernous versus capillary hemangiomas of the orbit. J Clin Neuroophthalmol. 1983;6:14.
135. Clymer MA, Fortune DS, Reinisch L, et al. Interstitial Nd:YAG photocoagulation for vascular malformations and hemangiomas in childhood. Arch Otolaryngol Head Neck Surg. 1998;124:431–6.
136. Cogen MS, Elsas FJ. Eyelid depigmentation following corticosteroid injection for infantile ocular adnexal hemangioma. J Pediatr Ophthalmol Strabismus. 1989;26:35–8.
137. Deans RM, Harris GJ, Kivlin JD. Surgical dissection of capillary hemangiomas. An alternative to intralesional corticosteroids. Arch Ophthalmol. 1992;110:1743–7.
138. Gdal-On M, Gelfand YE. Cryoextraction of orbital capillary hemangioma diagnosed by technetium-99 labeled red blood cell scintigraphy. Ophthalmic Surg Lasers. 1997;28:954–6.
139. Gundalp I, Gunduz K. Vascular tumors of the orbit. Doc Ophthalmol. 1995;89:337–45.
140. Haik BG, Jakobiec FA, Ellsworth RM, Jones IS. Capillary hemangioma of the lids and orbit: an analysis of the clinical features and therapeutic results in 101 cases. Ophthalmology. 1979;86:760–92.
141. Haik BG, Karcioglu ZA, Goson RA, Pechous BP. Capillary hemangioma (infantile periocular hemangioma). Surv Ophthalmol. 1994;38:399–426.
142. Harris GJ, Jakobiec FA. Cavernous hemangioma of the orbit. J Neurosurg. 1979;51:219–28.
143. Léauté-Labrèze C, Dumas de la Roque E, Hubiche T, et al. Propranolol for severe hemangiomas of infancy. N Engl J Med. 2008;358:2649–51.
144. Milot J, Saurel P. Peri-ocular hemangioma in children. Apropos of 25 cases. Chir Pediatr. 1989;30:43–6.
145. O'Keefe M, Lanigan B, Byrne SA. Capillary haemangioma of the eyelids and orbit: a clinical review of the safety and efficacy of intralesional steroid. Acta Ophthalmol Scand. 2003;81:294–8.
146. Orawiec B, Stefanczyk L, Czajkowski J, Bogorodzki B, Gralek M. Periorbital capillary hemangiomas in children – treatment and monitoring of treatment. Klin Ocz. 1996;98:217–20.
147. Siegfried EC, Keenan WJ, Al-Jureidini S, et al. More on propranolol for hemangiomas in infancy. N Engl J Med. 2008;359:2846–7.
148. Sklar EL, Quencer RM, Byrne SF, Sklar VE. Correlative study of the computed tomographic, ultrasonographic, and pathological characteristics of cavernous versus capillary hemangiomas of the orbit. J Clin Neuroophthalmol. 1986;6:14–21.
149. Sweet C, Silbergleit R, Mehta B. Primary intraosseous hemangioma of the orbit: CT and MRI appearance. Am J Neuroradiol. 1997;18:379–81.
150. Taban M, Goldberg RA. Propranolol for orbital hemangioma. Ophthalmology. 2010;117:195–195.e4.
151. Teske S, Ohlrich SJ, Gole G, et al. Treatment of orbital capillary haemangioma with interferon. Aust N Z J Ophthalmol. 1994;22:13–7.
152. Verity DH, Restori M, Rose GE. Natural history of periocular capillary haemangiomas: changes in internal blood velocity and lesion volume. Eye. 2006;20:1228–37.
153. Verity DH, Rose GE, Restori M. The effect of intralesional steroid injections on the volume and blood flow in periocular capillary haemangiomas. Orbit. 2008;27:41–7.

154. Walker RS, Custer PL, Nerad JA. Surgical excision of periorbital capillary hemangiomas. Ophthalmology. 1994;101:1333–40.

Vascular Lesions: Cavernous Hemangioma

155. Acciarri N, Padovani R, Giulioni M, Gaist G, Acciarri R. Intracranial and orbital cavernous angiomas: a review of 74 surgical cases. Br J Neurosurg. 1993;7:529–39.
156. Acciarri N, Giulioni M, Padovani R, et al. Orbital cavernous angiomas: surgical experience on a series of 13 cases. J Neurosurg Sci. 1995;39:203–9.
157. Alfred PR, Char DH. Cavernous hemangiomas of the orbit. Orbit. 1996;15:59–66.
158. Ansari SA, Mafee MF. Orbital cavernous hemangioma: role of imaging. Neuroimaging Clin N Am. 2005;15:137–58.
159. Balchunas ER, Quencer RM, Byrne SF, et al. Correlative of the computed tomographic, ultrasonographic, and pathological characteristics of cavernous versus capillary hemangiomas of the orbit. J Clin Neuroophthalmol. 1983;6:14.
160. Davis KR, Hesselink JR, Dallow RL, Grove AS Jr. CT and ultrasound in the diagnosis of cavernous hemangioma and lymphangioma of the orbit. CT. 1980;4:98–104.
161. Fries PD, Char DH, Norman D. MR imaging of orbital cavernous hemangioma. J Comput Assist Tomogr. 1987;11:418–21.
162. Fries PD, Char DH. Bilateral orbital cavernous haemangiomas. Br J Ophthalmol. 1988;72:871–3.
163. Gdal-On M, Gelfand YA. Surgical outcome of transconjunctival cryosurgical extraction of orbital cavernous hemangioma. Ophthalmic Surg Lasers. 1998;29:969–73.
164. Goldberg RA, Shorr N, Arnold AC, Garcia GH. Deep transorbital approach to the apex and cavernous sinus. Ophthal Plast Reconstr Surg. 1998;14:336–41.
165. Harris GJ, Jakobiec FA. Cavernous hemangioma of the orbit: a clinicopathologic analysis of sixty-six cases. In: Jakobiec FA, editor. Ocular and adnexal tumors. Birmingham: Aesculapius; 1977. p. 741–81.
166. Harris GJ, Jakobiec FA. Cavernous hemangioma of the orbit. J Neurosurg. 1979;51:219–28.
167. Hashimoto M, Ohtsuka K, Nakamura Y, Nakagawa T. Diagnostic imaging of orbital cavernous hemangioma. Jpn J Clin Ophthalmol. 1997;51:1613–7.
168. Khan AA, Niranjan A, Kano H, et al. Stereotactic radiosurgery for cavernous sinus or orbital hemangiomas. Neurosurgery. 2009;65:914–8.
169. Kopelow SM, Foos RY, Straatsma BR, Helper RS, Pearlman JT. Cavernous hemangioma of the orbit. Int Ophthalmol Clin. 1971;11:113–24.
170. Leatherbarrow B, Noble JL, Lloyd IC. Cavernous haemangioma of the orbit. Eye. 1989;3:90–9.
171. Mawn LA, Jordan DR, Gilberg SM. Cavernous hemangiomas of the orbital apex with intracranial extension. Ophthalmic Surg Lasers. 1998;29:680–4.
172. McNab AA, Wright JE. Cavernous haemangiomas of the orbit. Aust N Z J Ophthalmol. 1989;17:337–45.
173. Ohtsuka K, Hashimoto M, Akiba H. Serial dynamic magnetic resonance imaging of orbital cavernous hemangioma. Am J Ophthalmol. 1997;123:396–8.
174. Orcutt JC, Wulc AE, Mills RP, Smith CF. Asymptomatic orbital cavernous hemangiomas. Ophthalmology. 1991;98:1257–60.
175. Ossoinig KC. Echographic differentiation of vascular tumors in the orbit. In: Thijssen JM, Verbeek A, editors. Ultrasonography in ophthalmology. Dordrecht: Dr W Junk; 1981. p. 283.
176. Ruchman MC, Flannagan J. Cavernous hemangiomas of the orbit. Ophthalmology. 1983;90:1328–36.
177. Shields JA, Shields CL, Eagle RC. Cavernous hemangioma of the orbit. Arch Ophthalmol. 1987;105:853.
178. Sklar EL, Quencer RM, Byrne SF, Sklar VE. Correlative study of the computed tomographic, ultrasonographic, and pathological characteristics of cavernous versus capillary hemangiomas of the orbit. J Clin Neuroophthalmol. 1986;6:14–21.
179. Sullivan TJ, Aylward GW, Wright JE, Moseley IF, Garner A. Bilateral multiple cavernous haemangiomas of the orbit. Br J Ophthalmol. 1992;76:627–9.
180. Wilms G, Raat H, Dom R, et al. Orbital cavernous hemangioma: findings on sequential Gd-enhanced MRI. J Comput Assist Tomogr. 1995;19:548–51.
181. Yan J, Wu Z. Cavernous hemangioma of the orbit: analysis of 214 cases. Orbit. 2004;23:33–40.

Vascular Lesions: Lymphangioma

182. Berthout A, Jacomet PV, Putterman M, et al. Surgical treatment of diffuse adult orbital lymphangioma: two case studies. J Fr Ophtalmol. 2008;31:1006–17.
183. Bond JB, Haik BG, Taveras JL, et al. Magnetic resonance imaging of orbital lymphangioma with and without gadolinium contrast enhancement. Ophthalmology. 1992;99:1318–24.
184. Gelbert F, Riche MC, Reizine D, et al. MR imaging of head and neck vascular malformations. J Magn Reson Imaging. 1991;1:579–84.
185. Graeb DA, Rootman J, Robertson WD, et al. Orbital lymphangiomas: clinical, radiologic, and pathologic characteristics. Radiology. 1990;175:417–21.
186. Gunduz K, Demirel S, Yagmurlu B, Erden E. Correlation of surgical outcome with neuroimaging findings in periocular lymphangiomas. Ophthalmology. 2006;113:1231.e1–8.
187. Harris GJ, Sakol PJ, Bonavolonta GT, De Conciliis C. An analysis of thirty cases of orbital lymphangioma. Pathophysiologic considerations and management recommendations. Ophthalmology. 1990;97:1583–92.
188. Hemmer KM, Marsh JL, Milder B. Orbital lymphangioma. Plast Reconstr Surg. 1988;82:340–3.
189. Huckabee RE, Raila FA. MRI and CT comparison of an orbital cavernous lymphangioma. J Miss State Med Assoc. 1991;32:371–3.
190. Iliff EJ, Green WR. Orbital lymphangiomas. Ophthalmology. 1979;86:914–29.
191. Katz SE, Rootman J, Vangveeravong S, Graeb D. Combined venous lymphatic malformations of the orbit (so-called lymphangiomas). Associated with noncontiguous intracranial vascular anomalies. Ophthalmology. 1998;105:176–84.
192. Kazim M, Kennerdell JS, Rothfus W, Marquardt M. Orbital lymphangioma. Correlation of magnetic resonance images and intraoperative findings. Ophthalmology. 1992;99:1588–94.
193. Morax S, Cochetel C. Orbital lymphangioma. Apropos of 2 uncommon cases. Ann Chir Plast Esthet. 1991;36:306–12.
194. Schwarcz RM, Ben Simon GJ, Cook T, Goldberg RA. Sclerosing therapy as first line treatment for low flow vascular lesions of the orbit. Am J Ophthalmol. 2006;141:333–9.
195. Westerling D, Blohma J, Stigmar G. Orbital mass in a child causing somnolence, nausea and bradycardia. Can J Anaesth. 1998;45:777–80.
196. Wilson ME, Parker PL, Chavis RM. Conservative management of childhood orbital lymphangioma. Ophthalmology. 1989;96:484–9.
197. Wright JE, Sullivan TJ, Garner A, Wulc AE, Moseley IF. Orbital venous anomalies. Ophthalmology. 1997;104:905–13.
198. Zucker JL, Assaad M, Levine MR. Orbital lymphangioma with intracranial extension. Ophthal Plast Reconstr Surg. 1995;11:22–6.

Vascular Lesions: Varices

199. Beyer R, Levine MR, Sternberg I. Orbital varices: a surgical approach. Ophthal Plast Reconstr Surg. 1985;1:205–10.
200. Bullock JD, Goldberg SH, Connelly PJ. Orbital varix thrombosis. Ophthalmology. 1990;97:251–6.
201. Garrity JA. Orbital venous anomalies. A long-standing dilemma. Ophthalmology. 1997;104:903–4.
202. Islam N, Mireskandari K, Rose GE. Orbital varices and orbital wall defects. Br J Ophthalmol. 2004;88:833–4.
203. Kim YJ, Kim YD. Orbital venous anomaly presenting with orbital hemorrhage. Jpn J Ophthalmol. 2009;53:408–13.
204. Lieb WE, Merton DA, Shields JA, et al. Colour Doppler imaging in the demonstration of an orbital varix. Br J Ophthalmol. 1990;74:305–8.
205. Lloyd GA. Phleboliths in the orbit. Clin Radiol. 1965;16:339–46.
206. Lloyd GA. Vascular anomalies in the orbit: CT and angiographic diagnosis. Orbit. 1982;1:45–54.
207. Nasr AM, Huaman AM. Anterior orbital varix presenting as a lacrimal sac mucocele. Ophthal Plast Reconstr Surg. 1998;14:193–7.
208. Phan IT, Hoyt WF, McCulley TJ, Hwang TN. Blindness from orbital varices: case report. Orbit. 2009;28:303–5.
209. Rubin PA, Remulla HD. Orbital venous anomalies demonstrated by spiral computed tomography. Ophthalmology. 1997;104:1463–70.
210. Shields JA, Eagle RC Jr, Shields CL, De Potter P, Shapiro RS. Orbital varix presenting as a subconjunctival mass. Ophthal Plast Reconstr Surg. 1995;11:37–8.
211. Tsai AS, Fong KS, Lim W, et al. Bilateral orbital varices: an approach to management. Ophthal Plast Reconstr Surg. 2008;24:486–8.
212. Weill A, Cognard C, Castaings L, Robert G, Moret J. Embolization of an orbital varix after surgical exposure. Am J Neuroradiol. 1998;19:921–3.
213. Wildenhain PM, Leher SC, Dastur KJ. Dodd 3rd GD. Orbital varix: color flow imaging correlated with CT and MRI studies. J Comput Assist Tomogr. 1991;15:171–3.
214. Wright JE, Sullivan TJ, Garner A, Wulc AE, Moseley IF. Orbital venous anomalies. Ophthalmology. 1997;104:905–13.
215. Yeatts RP, Driver PJ. Orbital varix. Arch Ophthalmol. 1993;111:702–3.

Vascular Lesions: Angiosarcoma

216. Brush M, Zhang J, Schuetze S, Sires B. Angiosarcoma metastatic to the orbit. Ophthal Plast Reconstr Surg. 2006;22:62–4.
217. Burnstein MA, Frueh BR, Elner VM. Angiosarcoma metastatic to the orbit. Arch Ophthalmol. 1996;114:93–6.
218. De Keizer RJ, de Wolff-Rouendaal D, Nooy MA. Angiosarcoma of the eyelid and periorbital region. Experience in Leiden with iridium192 brachytherapy and low-dose doxorubicin chemotherapy. Orbit. 2008;27:5–12.
219. Günalp I, Günalp K. Vascular tumors of the orbit. Doc Ophthalmol. 1995;89:337–45.
220. Hufnagel T, Ma L, Kuo TT. Orbital angiosarcoma with subconjunctival presentation. Report of a case and literature review. Ophthalmology. 1987;94:72–7.
221. Lopes M, Duffau H, Fleuridas G. Primary spheno-orbital angiosarcoma: case report and review of the literature. Neurosurgery. 1999;44:405–7.
222. Mehrens C, Anvari L, Grezebach UH, Metze D. Unilateral eyelid swelling as an initial manifestation of angiosarcoma. Hautarzt. 2000;51:419–22.
223. Messmer EP, Font RL, McCrary JA 3rd, Murphy D. Epithelioid angiosarcoma of the orbit presenting as Tolosa-Hunt syndrome. A clinicopathologic case report with review of the literature. Ophthalmology. 1983;90:1414–21.
224. Sasaki R, Soejima T, Kishi K, et al. Angiosarcoma treated with radiotherapy: impact of tumor type and size on outcome. Int J Radiat Ocol Boil Phys. 2002;15:1032–40.
225. Siddens JD, Fishman JR, Jackson IT, et al. Primary orbital angiosarcoma: a case report. Ophthal Plast Reconstr Surg. 1999;15:454–9.

Neural Tumors: Carcinoid

226. Aburn NS, Whitehead K, Sullivan TJ. Bronchopulmonary atypical carcinoid tumour metastatic to the orbit. Aust N Z J Ophtalmol. 1995;23:241–4.
227. Borota OC, Kloster R, Lindal S. Carcinoid tumour metastatic to the orbit with infiltration to the extraocular orbital muscle. APMIS. 2005;113:165–7.
228. Braffman BH, Bilaniuk LR, Eagle RC, et al. MR imaging of a carcinoid tumor metastatic to the orbit. J Comput Assist Tomogr. 1987;11:891–4.
229. Couch DA, O'Halloran HS, Hainsworth KM, et al. Carcinoid metastasis to extraocular muscles: case reports and review of the literature. Orbit. 2000;19:263–9.
230. Divine RD, Anderson RL, Ossoinig KC. Metastatic carcinoid unresponsive to radiation therapy presenting as a lacrimal fossa mass. Ophthalmology. 1982;89:516–20.
231. El-Toukhy E, Levine MR, Abdul-Karim FW, et al. Carcinoid tumors of the orbit: a dilemma of diagnosis and treatment. Ophthal Plast Reconstr Surg. 1996;12:279–83.
232. Fan JT, Buettner H, Bartley GB, Bolling JP. Clinical features and treatment of seven patients with carcinoid tumor metastatic to the eye and orbit. Am J Ophtalmol. 1995;119:211–8.
233. Ferry AP, Font RL. Carcinoma metastatic to the eye and orbit, I: a clinicopathologic study of 227 cases. Arch Ophthalmol. 1974;92:276–86.
234. Harris AL, Montgomery A. Orbital carcinoid tumor. Am J Ophtalmol. 1980;90:875–6.
235. Isidori AM, Kaltsas G, Frajese V, Kola B, Whitelocke RA, Plowman PN, et al. Ocular metastases secondary to carcinoid tumors: the utility of imaging with [(123)I]meta-iodobenzylguanidine and [(111)In]DTPA pentetreotide. J Clin Endocrinol Metab. 2002;87:1627–33.
236. Kiratli H, Yilmaz PT, Yildiz ZI. Metastatic atypical carcinoid tumor of the inferior rectus muscle. Ophthal Plast Reconstr Surg. 2008;24:482–4.
237. Knox RJ, Gigantelli JW, Arthurs BP. Recurrent orbital inflammation from metastatic orbital carcinoid tumor. Ophthal Plast Reconstr Surg. 2001;17:137–9.
238. Pinchot SN, Holen K, Sippel RS, Chen H. Carcinoid tumors. Oncologist. 2008;13:1255–69.
239. Riddle PJ, Font RL, Zimmerman LE. Carcinoid tumours of the eye and orbit: a clinicopathologic study of 15 cases, with histochemical and electron microscopic observations. Hum Pathol. 1982;13:459–69.
240. Rush JA, Waller RR, Campbell RJ. Orbital carcinoid tumor metastatic from the colon. Am J Ophtalmol. 1980;189:636–40.
241. Shetlar DJ, Font RI, Ordonez N, et al. A clinicopathologic study of three carcinoid tumors metastatic to the orbit. Immunohistochemical, ultrastructural, and DNA flow cytometric studies. Ophthalmology. 1990;97:257.64.
242. Takemoto Y, Nishida N, Kjiro S, et al. Metastatic carcinoid tumor in the orbit. Kurume Med J. 2003;50:165–7.
243. Zimmerman LE, Stangl R, Riddle PJ. Primary carcinoid tumor of the orbit. A clinicopathologic study with histochemical and electron microscopic observations. Arch Ophthalmol. 1983;101:1395–8.

Neural Tumors: Malignant Peripheral Nerve Sheath Tumor

244. Aydin MD, Yildrim U, Gundogdu C, et al. Malignant peripheral nerve sheath tumor of the orbit: case report and literature review. Skull Base. 2004;14:109–13.
245. Beegun I, Bottrill ID, Hollowood K. Malignant peripheral nerve sheath tumours of the infraorbital nerve: case report and literature review. J Laryngol Otol. 2009;123:466–70.
246. Bhargava R, Parham DM, Lasater OE, et al. MR imaging differentiation of benign and malignant peripheral nerve sheath tumors: use of the target sign. Pediatr Radiol. 1997;27:124–9.
247. Cheng SF, Chen YI, Chang CY, et al. Malignant peripheral nerve sheath tumor of the orbit: malignant transformation from neurofibroma without neurofibromatosis. Ophthal Plast Reconstr Surg. 2008;24:413–5.
248. Chibbaro S, Herman P, Povlika M, George B. Malignant trigeminal schwannoma extending into the anterior skull base. Acta Neurochir. 2008;150:599–604.
249. Erzurum SA, Melen O, Lissner G, et al. Orbital malignant peripheral nerve sheath tumors. Treatment with surgical resection and radiation therapy. J Clin Neuroophthalmol. 1993;13:1–7.
250. Eviatar JA, Hornblass A, Herschorn B, Jakobiec FA. Malignant peripheral nerve sheath tumor of the orbit in a 15-year-old child. Nine-year survival after local excision. Ophthalmology. 1992;99:1595–9.
251. Fezza JP, Wolfley DE, Flynn SD. Malignant peripheral nerve sheath tumor of the orbit in a newborn: a case report and review. J Pediatr Ophthalmol Strabismus. 1997;34:128–31.
252. Grinberg MA, Levy NS. Malignant neurilemoma of the supraorbital nerve. Am J Ophthalmol. 1974;78:489–92.
253. Jakobiec FA, Font RL, Zimmerman LE. Malignant peripheral nerve sheath tumors of the orbit: a clinicopathologic study of eight cases. Trans Am Ophthalmol Soc. 1985;83:332–66.
254. Lyons CJ, McNab AA, Garner A, Wright JE. Orbital malignant peripheral nerve sheath tumours. Br J Ophthalmol. 1989;73:731–8.
255. Miliaras G, Tsitsopoulos PP, Asproudis I, et al. Malignant orbital schwannoma with massive intracranial recurrence. Acta Neurochir. 2008;150:1291–4.
256. Mortada A. Solitary orbital malignant neurilemmoma. Br J Ophthalmol. 1968;52:188–90.
257. Morton AD, Elner VM, Frueh B. Recurrent orbital malignant peripheral nerve sheath tumor 18 years after initial resection. Ophthal Plast Reconstr Surg. 1997;13:239–43.
258. Prescott DK, Racz MM, Ng JD. Epithelioid malignant peripheral nerve sheath tumor in the infraorbital nerve. Ophthal Plast Reconstr Surg. 2006;22:150–1.
259. Stull MA, Moser RP Jr, Kransdorf MJ, Bogumill GP, Nelson MC. Magnetic resonance imaging appearance of peripheral nerve sheath tumors. Skelet Radiol. 1991;20:9–14.

Neural Tumors: Meningocele

260. Clauser L, Carinci F, Galie M. Neurofibromatosis of the orbit and skull base. J Craniofac Surg. 1998;9:280–4.
261. Holmes AD, Meara JG, Kolker AR, et al. Frontoethmoidal encephaloceles: reconstruction and refinements. J Craniofac Surg. 2001;12:6–18.
262. Hershewe GL, Corbett JJ, Ossoinig KC, et al. Optic nerve compression from a basal encephalocele. J Neuroophthalmol. 1995;15:161–5.
263. Islam N, Mireskandari K, Burton BJ, Rose GE. Orbital varices, cranial defects, and encephaloceles: an unrecognized association. Ophthalmology. 2004;111(6):1244–7.
264. Lieb W, Rochels R, Kretzschmar K. Sonography and computed tomography in the diagnosis of orbitocranial malformations and tumors. Neurosurg Rev. 1987;10(2):93–101.
265. Macfarlane R, Rutka JT, Armstrong D, et al. Encephaloceles of the anterior cranial fossa. Pediatr Neurosurg. 1989;23:148–58.
266. Nasu W, Kobayashi S, Kashiwa K, Honda T. Secondary craniofacial reconstruction of huge frontoethmoidal encephalomeningocele after primary neurosurgical repair. J Craniofac Surg. 2008;19(1):171–4.
267. Newman NJ, Miller NR, Green WR. Ectopic brain in the orbit. Ophthalmology. 1986;93:268–72.
268. Shields JA, Shields CL. Orbital cysts of childhood–classification, clinical features, and management. Surv Ophthalmol. 2004;49(3):281–99.
269. Songur E, Mutluer S, Gurler T, et al. Management of frontoethmoidal encephalocele. J Craniofac Surg. 1999;10:135–9.
270. Spooler JC, Cho D, Ray A, Zouros A. Patient with congenital optic nerve meningocele presenting with left orbital cyst. Childs Nerv Syst. 2009;25(2):267–9.
271. Sugawara Y, Harii K, Hirabayashi S, et al. A spheno-orbital encephalocele with unilateral exophthalmos. Ann Plast Surg. 1996;36:410–2.

Neural Tumors: Neuroblastoma

272. Alfano JE. Ophthalmological aspects of neuroblastomatosis: a study of 53 verified cases. Trans Am Acad Ophthalmol Otolaryngol. 1968;72:830–48.
273. Apple DJ. Metastatic orbital neuroblastoma originating in the cervical sympathetic ganglion chain. Am J Ophthalmol. 1969;68:1093–5.
274. Belgaumi AF, Kauffman WM, Jenkins JJ, et al. Blindness in children with neuroblastoma. Cancer. 1997;80:1997–2004.
275. Boubaker A, Bischof-Delaloye A. Nuclear medicine procedures and neuroblastoma in childhood: their value in the diagnosis, staging and assessment of response to therapy. Q J Nucl Med. 2003;47:31–40.
276. Bullock JD, Goldberg SH, Rakes SM, Felder DS, Connelly PJ. Primary orbital neuroblastoma. Arch Ophthalmol. 1989;107:1031–3.
277. Chung EM, Murphey MD, Specht CS, et al. From the archives of the AFIP pediatric obit tumors and tumor like lesions: osseous lesions of the orbit. Radiographics. 2008;28:1193–214.
278. Gallet BL, Egelhoff JC. Unusual CNS and orbital metastases of neuroblastoma. Pediatr Radiol. 1989;19:287–9.
279. Jakobiec FA, Klepach GL, Crissman JD, Spoor TC. Primary differentiated neuroblastoma of the orbit. Ophthalmology. 1987;94:255–66.
280. Kai T, Ishii E, Matsuzaki A, et al. High-dose chemotherapy and autologous blood stem transplantation in children with metastatic neuroblastoma. Acta Paediatr Jpn. 1997;39:54–60.
281. Laforest C, Selva D, Cromptom J, Leibovitch I. Orbital invasion by esthesioneuroblastoma. Ophthal Plast Reconstr Surg. 2005;21:435–40.
282. Latchaw RE, L'Heureux PR, Young G, Priest JR. Neuroblastoma presenting as central nervous system disease. Am J Neuroradiol. 1982;3:623–30.
283. Lau JJ, Trobe JD, Ruiz RE, et al. Metastatic neuroblastoma presenting with binocular blindness from intracranial compression of the optic nerves. J Neuroophthalmol. 2004;24:119–24.
284. Lonergan GJ, Schwab CM, Suarez ES, Carlson CL. Neuroblastoma, ganglioneuroblastoma, and ganglio-

neuroma: radiologic-pathologic correlation. Radiographics. 2002;22:911–34.
285. Mehta A, Chandra M. Rare orbitocranial tumour in an adult. Orbit. 2009;28:285–9.
286. Mortada A. Clinical characteristics of early orbital neuroblastoma. Am J Ophthalmol. 1967;63:1787–93.
287. Musarella M, Chan HSL, DeBoer G, et al. Ocular involvement in neuroblastoma: prognostic implications. Ophthalmology. 1984;91:936–40.
288. Reim M, Muther HC, Karstens JH, Sieverts H. Pediatric neuroblastoma with early bilateral blindness. Klin Monatsbl Augenheilkd. 1988;192:33–6.
289. Schubert EE, Oliver GL, Jaco NT. Metastatic neuroblastoma causing bilateral blindness. Can J Ophthalmol. 1969;4:100–3.
290. Slamovits TL, Rosen CE, Suhrland MJ. Neuroblastoma presenting as acute lymphoblastic leukemia but correctly diagnosed after orbital fine-needle aspiration biopsy. J Clin Neuroophthalmol. 1991;11:158–61.

Neural Tumors: Optic Pathway Glioma

291. Alshail E, Rutka JT, Becker LE, Hoffman HJ. Optic chiasmatic-hypothalamic glioma. Brain Pathol. 1997;7:799–806.
292. Aoki S, Barkovich AJ, Nishimura K, et al. Neurofibromatosis type 1 and 2: cranial MR findings. Radiology. 1989;172:527–34.
293. Azar-Kia B, Naheedy MH, Elias DA, Mafee MF, Fine M. Optic nerve tumors: role of magnetic resonance imaging and computed tomography. Radiol Clin N Am. 1987;25:561–81.
294. Barnes PD, Robson CD, Robertson RL, Poussaint TY. Pediatric orbital and visual pathway lesions. Neuroimaging Clin N Am. 1996;6:179–98.
295. Collet-Solberg PF, Sernyak H, Satin-Smith M, et al. Endocrine outcome in long-term survivors of low-grade hypothalamic/chiasmatic glioma. Clin Endocrinol. 1997;47:79–85.
296. Dutton JJ. Gliomas of the anterior visual pathway. Surv Ophthalmol. 1994;38:427–52.
297. Es SV, North KN, McHugh K, Silva MD. MRI findings in children with neurofibromatosis type 1: a prospective study. Pediatr Radiol. 1996;26:478–87.
298. Garvey M, Packer RJ. An integrated approach to the treatment of chiasmatic hypothalamic gliomas. J Neuro-Oncol. 1996;28:167–83.
299. Grill J, Bhangoo NR. Recent developments in chemotherapy of paediatric brain tumors. Curr Opin Oncol. 2007;19:612–5.
300. Haik BG, Saint-Louis L, Bierly J, et al. Magnetic resonance imaging in the evaluation of optic nerve glioma. Ophthalmology. 1987;94:709–17.
301. Holman RE, Grimson BS, Drayer BP, Buckley EG, Brennan MW. Magnetic resonance imaging of optic nerve gliomas. Am J Ophthalmol. 1985;100:596–601.
302. Imes RK, Hoyt WF. Magnetic resonance imaging signs of optic nerve gliomas in neurofibromatosis. Am J Ophthalmol. 1991;111:729–34.
303. Jakobiec FA, Depot MJ, Kennerdell JS, et al. Combined clinical and computed tomographic diagnosis of orbital glioma and meningioma. Ophthalmology. 1984;91:137–55.
304. Janss AJ, Grundy R, Cnaan A, et al. Optic pathway and hypothalamic/chiasmatic gliomas in children younger than 5 years with a 6-year follow-up. Cancer. 1995;75:1051–9.
305. Lama G, Espisito Salsano M, Grassia C, et al. Neurofibromatosis type I and optic pathway glioma, a long-term follow-up. Minerva Pediatr. 2007;59:13–21.
306. Listernick R, Louis DN, Packer RJ, Gutmann DH. Optic pathway gliomas in children with neurofibromatosis 1: consensus statement from the NF1 Optic Pathway Glioma Task Force. Ann Neurol. 1997;41:143–9.
307. Listernick R, Ferner RE, Liu GT, Gutmann DH. Optic pathway gliomas in neurofibromatosis-1: controversies and recommendations. Ann Neurol. 2007;61:189–98.
308. Lloyd LA. Gliomas of the optic nerve and chiasm in childhood. Trans Am Ophthalmol Soc. 1973;71:488–535.
309. Mahoney DHJ, Cohen ME, Friedman HS, et al. Carboplatin is effective therapy for young children with progressive optic pathway tumors: a Pediatric Oncology Group phase II study. Neuro-Oncology. 2000;2:213–20.
310. Marquardt MD, Zimmerman LE. Histology of meningiomas and gliomas of the optic nerve. Hum Pathol. 1982;13:226–34.
311. Massry GG, Morgan CF, Chung SM. Evidence of optic pathway gliomas after previously negative neuroimaging. Ophthalmology. 1997;104:930–5.
312. Miller NR. Primary tumours of the optic nerve and its sheaths. Eye. 2004;18:1026–37.
313. Packer RJ, Ater J, Allen J, et al. Carboplatin and vincristine for children with newly diagnosed progressive low-grade gliomas. J Neurosurg. 1997;86:747–54.
314. Parsa CF, Hoyt CS, Lesser RL, et al. Spontaneous regression of optic gliomas: thirteen cases documented by serial imaging. Arch Ophthalmol. 2001;119:516–29.
315. Piccirilli M, Lenzi J, Delfinis C, et al. Spontaneous regression of optic pathway gliomas in three patients with neurofibromatosis type 1 and critical review of the literature. Childs Nerv Syst. 2006;22:1332–7.
316. Seiff SR, Brodsky MC, MacDonald G, et al. Orbital optic glioma in neurofibromatosis. Magnetic resonance diagnosis of perineural arachnoidal gliomatosis. Arch Ophthalmol. 1987;105:1689–92.
317. Sharif S, Ferner R, Birch JM, et al. Second primary tumors in neurofibromatosis 1 patients treated for optic nerve glioma: substantial risks after radiotherapy. J Clin Oncol. 2006;24:2570–5.
318. Spencer WH. Diagnostic modalities and natural behavior of optic nerve gliomas. Ophthalmology. 1979;86:881–5.
319. Stern J, Jakobiec FA, Housepian EM. The architecture of optic nerve gliomas with and without neurofibromatosis. Arch Ophthalmol. 1980;98:505–11.
320. Stieber VW. Radiation therapy for visual pathway gliomas. J Neuroophthalmol. 2008;28:222–30.
321. Sylvester CL, Drohan LA, Sergott RC. Optic-nerve gliomas, chiasmal gliomas and neurofibromatosis type 1. Curr Opin Ophthalmol. 2006;17:7–11.
322. Tao ML, Barnes PD, Billett AL, et al. Childhood optic chiasm gliomas: radiographic response following radiotherapy and long-term clinical outcome. Int J Radiat Oncol Biol Phys. 1997;39:579–87.
323. Thompson CR, Lessell S. Anterior visual pathway gliomas. Int Ophthalmol Clin. 1997;37:261–79.

Neural Tumors: Optic Nerve Sheath Meningioma

324. Andrews DW, Faroozan R, Yang BP, et al. Fractionated stereotactic radiotherapy for the treatment of optic nerve sheath meningiomas: preliminary observations of 33 optic nerves in 30 patients with historical comparison to observation with or without prior surgery. Neurosurgery. 2002;51:890–904.
325. Arvold ND, Lessell S, Bussiere M, et al. Visual outcome and tumor control after conformal radiotherapy for patients with optic nerve sheath meningioma. Int J Radiat Oncol Biol Phys. 2009;75:1166–72.
326. Baumert BG, Villa S, Studer G, et al. Early improvements in vision after fractionated stereotactic radiotherapy for primary optic nerve sheath meningioma. Radiother Oncol. 2004;72:169–74.
327. Bleeker GM. Orbital meningioma. Orbit. 1984;3:3–17.

328. Carrasco JR, Penne RB. Optic nerve sheath meningiomas and advanced treatment options. Curr Opin Ophthalmol. 2004;15:406–10.
329. Clark WC, Theofilos CS, Fleming JC. Primary optic nerve sheath meningiomas. Report of nine cases. J Neurosurg. 1989;70:37–40.
330. Cohn EM. Optic sheath meningioma. Neuroradiologic findings. J Clin Neuroophthalmol. 1983;3:85–9.
331. Cristine L. Surgical treatment of meningiomas of the optic canal: a retrospective study with particular attention to the visual outcome. Acta Neurochir. 1994;126:27–32.
332. Dutton JJ. Optic nerve sheath meningiomas. Surv Ophthalmol. 1992;37:167–83.
333. Eddelman CS, Liu JK. Optic nerve sheath meningioma: current diagnosis and treatment. Neurosurg Focus. 2007;23:E4.
334. Elster AD, Challa VR, Gilbert TH, Richardson DN, Contento JC. Meningiomas: MR and histopathologic features. Radiology. 1989;170:857–62.
335. Imes RK, Schatz H, Hoyt WF, et al. Evolution of optociliary veins in optic nerve sheath meningioma. Arch Ophthalmol. 1985;103:59–60.
336. Jakobiec FA, Depot MJ, Kennerdell JS, et al. Combined clinical and computed tomographic diagnosis of orbital glioma and meningioma. Ophthalmology. 1984;91:137–55.
337. Jew SY, Bartley GB, Garrity JA, et al. Radiation-induced meningiomas involving the orbit. Ophthal Plast Reconstr Surg. 2001;17:362–8.
338. Kennerdell JS, Maroon JC, Malton M, Warren FA. The management of optic sheath meningiomas. Am J Ophthalmol. 1988;106:450–7.
339. Kim JW, Rizzo JF, Lessell S. Controversies in the management of optic nerve sheath meningiomas. Int Ophthalmol Clin. 2005;45:15–23.
340. Lee AG, Woo SY, Miller NR, et al. Improvement in visual function in an eye with a presumed optic nerve sheath meningioma after treatment with three-dimensional conformal radiation therapy. J Neuroophthalmol. 1996;16:247–51.
341. Lieb WE, Rochels R, Wallenfang T, Ahl G. Ophthalmologic symptoms in meningioma of the orbits and in the anterior and medial cranial fossa. Fortschr Ophthalmol. 1994;91:341–5.
342. Lindblom B, Norman D, Hoyt WF. Perioptic cyst distal to optic nerve meningioma: MR demonstration. Am J Neuroradiol. 1992;13:1622–4.
343. Lindblom B, Truwit CL, Hoyt WF. Optic nerve sheath meningioma. Definition of intraorbital, intracanalicular, and intracranial components with magnetic resonance imaging. Ophthalmology. 1992;99:560–6.
344. Louis DN, Scheithauer BW, Budka H, et al. Meningiomas. In: Kleihues P, Cavenee WK, editors. World health organization classification of tumours. Pathology and genetics. Tumours of the nervous system. Lyon: IARC Press; 2000. p. 176–84.
345. McNab AA, Wright JE. Cysts of the optic nerve three cases associated with meningioma. Eye. 1989;3:355–9.
346. Milker-Zabel S, Huber P, Schlegel W, et al. Fractionated stereotactic radiation therapy in the management of primary optic nerve sheath meningiomas. J Neuro-Oncol. 2009;94:419–24.
347. Miller NR. New concepts in the diagnosis and management of optic nerve sheath meningioma. J Neuro-Oncol. 2006;26:200–8.
348. Moyer PD, Golnik KC, Breneman J. Treatment of optic nerve sheath meningioma with three-dimensional conformal radiation. Am J Ophthalmol. 2000;129:694–6.
349. Oritz O, Schochet SS, Kotzan JM, Kostick D. Radiologic-pathologic correlation. Meningioma of the optic nerve sheath. Am J Neuroradiol. 1996;17:901–6.
350. Saeed P, Rootman J, Nugent RA, et al. Optic nerve sheath meningiomas. Ophthalmology. 2003;110:2019–30.
351. Saeed P, Tanck MW, Freling N, et al. Somatostatin receptor scintigraphy for optic nerve sheath meningiomas. Ophthalmology. 2009;116:1581–6.
352. Sarkies NJ. Optic nerve sheath meningioma: diagnostic features and therapeutic alternatives. Eye. 1987;1:597–602.
353. Schick U, Dott U, Hassler W. Surgical management of meningiomas involving the optic nerve sheath. J Neurosurg. 2004;101:951–9.
354. Sibony PA, Krauss HR, Kennerdell JS, Maroon JC, Slamovits TL. Optic nerve sheath meningioma. Clinical manifestations. Ophthalmology. 1984;91:1313–26.
355. Smee RI, Schneider M, Williams JR. Optic nerve sheath meningiomas – non-surgical treatment. Clin Oncol. 2009;21:8–13.
356. Smith JL, McCrary JA III, Ray BS, et al. Managing menacing meningiomas. J Clin Neuroophthalmol. 1983;3:169–79.
357. Spagnoli MV, Goldberg HI, Grossman RI, et al. Intracranial meningiomas: high-field MR imaging. Radiology. 1986;161:369–75.
358. Turbin RE, Pokorny K. Diagnosis and treatment of orbital optic nerve sheath meningioma. Cancer Control. 2004;11:334–41.
359. Turbin RE, Thompson CR, Kennerdell JS, et al. A long-term visual outcome comparison in patients with optic nerve sheath meningioma managed with observation, surgery, radiotherapy, or surgery and radiotherapy. Ophthalmology. 2002;109:890–900.
360. Wilson WB. Meningiomas of the anterior visual system. Surv Ophthalmol. 1981;26:109–27.
361. Wright JE. Primary optic nerve meningiomas: clinical presentation and management. Ophthalmology. 1977;83:617–25.
362. Wright JE, Call NB, Liaricos S. Primary optic nerve meningioma. Br J Ophthalmol. 1980;64:553–8.
363. Wright JE, McNab AA, McDonald WI. Primary optic nerve sheath meningioma. Br J Ophthalmol. 1989;73:960–6.
364. Zimmerman CF, Schatz NJ, Glaser JS. Magnetic resonance imaging of optic nerve meningiomas. Enhancement with gadolinium-DTPA. Ophthalmology. 1990;97:585–91.

Neural Tumors: Plexiform Neurofibroma

365. Chopra R, Morris CG, Friedman WA, et al. Radiotherapy and radiosurgery for benign neurofibromas. Am J Clin Oncol. 2005;28:317–20.
366. Farris SR, Grove AS Jr. Orbital and eyelid manifestations of neurofibromatosis: a clinical study and literature review. Ophthal Plast Reconstr Surg. 1996;12:245–59.
367. Garrity JA, Henderson JW. Henderson's orbital tumors edition. 4th ed. Philadelphia: Lippincott Williams and Wilkins; 2007.
368. Gurland JE, Tenner M, Hornblass A, et al. Orbital neurofibromatosis. Arch Ophthalmol. 1976;94:1723–5.
369. Kobrin JL, Blodi FC, Weingeist TA. Ocular and orbital manifestations of neurofibromatosis. Surv Ophthalmol. 1979;24:45.
370. Kretschmer T, Nguyen DH, Beuerman RW, et al. Elevated ankyrin G in a plexiform neurofibroma and neuromas associated with pain. J Clin Neurosci. 2004;11:6–9.
371. McCarron KF, Goldblum JR. Plexiform neurofibroma with and without associated malignant peripheral nerve sheath tumor: a clinicopathologic and immunohistochemical analysis of 54 cases. Mod Pathol. 1998;11:612–7.
372. Reed D, Robertson WD, Rootman J, Douglas G. Plexiform neurofibromatosis of the orbit: CT evaluation. Am J Neuroradiol. 1986;7:259–63.
373. Santaolalla F, Sanchez JM, Ereno C, et al. Severe exophthalmos in trigeminal plexiform neurofibroma involving the orbit and infratemporal fossa. J Clin Neurosci. 2009;16:970–2.
374. Shields JA, Shields CL, Scartozzi R. Survey of 1264 patients with orbital tumors and simulating lesions: the 2002 Montgomery Lecture, part 1. Ophthalmology. 2004;11:997–1008.

375. Tada M, Sawamura Y, Ishii N, Chin S, Abe H. Massive plexiform neurofibroma in the orbit in a child with von Recklinghausen's disease. Childs Nerv Syst. 1998;14:210–2.
376. Woog JJ, Albert DM, Solt LC, et al. Neurofibromatosis of the eyelid and orbit. Int Ophthalmol Clin. 1982;22:157.
377. Wood JJ, Albert DM, Solt LC, Hu DN, Wang WJ. Neurofibromatosis of the eyeball and orbit. Int Ophthalmol Clin. 1982;22:157–87.
378. Zimmerman RA, Bilaniuk LT, Metzger RA, et al. Computed tomography of orbital facial neurofibromatosis. Radiology. 1983;146:113–6.

Neural Tumors: Schwannoma

379. Allman M, Frayer W, Hedges T. Orbital neurilemoma. Ann Ophthalmol. 1977;9:1409–13.
380. Bavetta S, McFall MR, Afshar F, Hutchinson I. Schwannoma of the anterior cranial fossa and paranasal sinuses. Br J Neurosurg. 1993;7:697–700.
381. Bergin DJ, Parmley V. Blepharochalasis. Arch Ophthalmol. 1988;106:414–5.
382. Butt ZA, McNab AA. Orbital neurilemmoma: report of seven cases. J Clin Neurosci. 1998;5:390–3.
383. Cantore G, Ciappetta P, Raco A, Lunardi P. Orbital schwannomas: report of nine cases and review of the literature. Neurosurgery. 1986;19:583–8.
384. Capps DH, Brodsky MC, Rice CD, et al. Orbital intramuscular schwannoma. Am J Ophthalmol. 1990;110:535–9.
385. Celli P, Ferrante L, Acqui M, et al. Neurinoma of the third, fourth, and sixth cranial nerves: a survey and report of a new fourth nerve case. Surg Neurol. 1992;38:216–24.
386. Chisholm IA, Polyzoidis K. Recurrence of benign orbital neurilemmoma (schwannoma) after 22 years. Can J Ophthalmol. 1982;17:271–3.
387. De Silva DJ, Tay E, Rose GE. Schwannomas of the lacrimal gland fossa. Orbit. 2009;28:433–5.
388. Faucett DC, Dutton JJ, Bullard DE. Gasserian ganglion schwannoma with orbital extension. Ophthal Plast Reconstr Surg. 1989;5:235–8.
389. Jakobiec FA, Font RL, et al. Peripheral nerve sheath tumors. In: Spencer WH, Font RL, Green WR, editors. Ophthalmic pathology. An atlas and textbook. Philadelphia: WB Saunders; 1986. p. 2603–32.
390. Kansu T, Ozcan OE, Ozdirim E, et al. Neurinoma of the oculomotor nerve. J Clin Neuroophthalmol. 1982;2:271–2.
391. Kashyap S, Pushker N, Meel R, et al. Orbital schwannoma with cystic degeneration. Clin Exp Ophthalmol. 2009;37:293–8.
392. Kiratli H, Yildiz S, Soylemezoglu F. Neurofibromatosis type 2: optic nerve sheath meningioma in one orbit, intramuscular schwannoma in the other. Orbit. 2008;27:451–4.
393. Lam DS, Ng JS, To KF, et al. Cystic schwannoma of the orbit. Eye. 1997;11:798–800.
394. Shen WC, Yang DY, Ho WL, Ho YJ, Lee SK. Neurilemmoma of the oculomotor nerve presenting as an orbital mass: MR findings. Am J Neuroradiol. 1993;14:1253–4.
395. Shields JA, Kapustiak J, Arbizo V, Augsburger JJ, Schnitzer RE. Orbital neurilemoma with extension through the superior orbital fissure. Arch Ophthalmol. 1986;104:871–3.
396. Simpson RK, Harper RL, Kirkpatrick JB, et al. Schwannomas of the optic nerve sheath. J Clin Neuroophthalmol. 1987;7:219–22.

Neural Tumors: Solitary Neurofibroma

397. De Potter P, Shields CL, Shields JA, et al. The CT and MRI features of an unusual case of isolated neurofibroma. Ophthal Plast Reconstr Surg. 1992;8:221–7.
398. DePotter P, Shields CL, Shields JA. The CT features of an unusual case of isolated orbital neurofibroma. Ophthal Plast Reconstr Surg. 1992;8:221–7.
399. Garrity JA, Henderson JW. Henderson's orbital tumors edition: 4th ed. Philadelphia: Lippincott Williams and Wilkins; 2007.
400. Kottler UB, Conway RM, Schlotzer-Schrehardt U, Holbach LM. Isolated neurofibroma of the orbit with extensive myxoid changes: a clinicopathologic study including MRI and electron microscopic findings. Orbit. 2004;23:59–64.
401. Krohl GB, Rosenberg PN, Wright JE, Smith RS. Localized orbital neurofibromas. Am J Ophthalmol. 1985;100:458–64.
402. Lee LR, Gigantelli JW, Kincaid MC. Localized neurofibroma of the orbit: a radiographic and histopathologic study. Ophthal Plast Reconstr Surg. 2000;16:241–6.
403. Linder B, Campos M, Schafer M. CT and MRI of orbital abnormalities in neurofibromatosis and selected craniofacial anomalies. Radiol Clin N Am. 1987;25:787–802.
404. Meyer DR, Wobig JL. Bilateral localized orbital neurofibromas. Ophthalmology. 1992;99:1313–7.
405. Park WC, White WA, Woog JJ, et al. The role of high-resolution computed tomography and magnetic resonance imaging in the evaluation of isolated orbital neurofibromas. Am J Ophthalmol. 2006;142:456–63.
406. Shields JA, Shields CL, Lieb WE, Eagle RC. Multiple orbital neurofibromas unassociated with von Recklinghausen's disease. Arch Ophthalmol. 1990;108:80–3.

Neural Tumors: Sphenoid Wing Meningioma

407. Anderson D, Khalil M. Meningiomas and the ophthalmologist. A review of 80 cases. Ophthalmology. 1981;88:1004–9.
408. Anderson D, Khalil MK. Meningioma and the ophthalmologist: diagnostic pitfalls. Can J Ophthalmol. 1981;16:10–5.
409. Basso A, Carrizo AG, Duma C. Sphenoid wing meningiomas. In: Sweet WH, editor. Operative neurosurgical techniques, vol. 1. Philadelphia: Saunders; 2000. p. 316–24.
410. Black PM. Meningiomas. Neurosurgery. 1993;32:643–57.
411. Bleeker GM. Orbital meningioma. Orbit. 1984;3:3–17.
412. Bydder GM, Kingsley DPE, Brown J, Niendorf HP, Young IR. MR imaging of meningiomas including studies with and without gadolinium-DTPA. J Comput Assist Tomogr. 1985;9:690–7.
413. Elster AD, Challa VR, Gilbert TH, Richardson DN, Contento JC. Meningiomas: MR and histopathologic features. Radiology. 1989;170:857–62.
414. Goldsmith BJ, Wara WM, Wilson CB, Larson DA. Postoperative irradiation for subtotally resected meningiomas. A retrospective analysis of 140 patients treated from 1967 to 1990. J Neurosurg. 1994;80:195–201.
415. Heufelder MJ, Sterker I, Trantakis C, et al. Reconstructive and ophthalmologic outcomes following resection of spheno-orbital meningiomas. Ophthal Plast Reconstr Surg. 2009;25:223–6.
416. Jakobiec FA, Depot MJ, Kennerdell JS, et al. Combined clinical and computed tomographic diagnosis of orbital glioma and meningioma. Ophthalmology. 1984;91:137–55.
417. Lee S, Maronian N, Most SP, et al. Porous high-density polyethylene for orbital reconstruction. Arch Otolaryngol Head Neck Surg. 2005;131:446–50.
418. Lieb WE, Rochels R, Wallenfang T, Ahl G. Ophthalmologic symptoms in meningioma of the orbits and in the anterior and medial cranial fossa. Fortschr Ophthalmol. 1994;91:41–5.
419. Mathiesen T, Lindquist C, Kihlstrom L, Karlsson B. Recurrence of cranial base meningiomas. Neurosurgery. 1996;39:2–7.
420. McGovern SL, Aldape KD, Munsell MF, et al. A comparison of World Health Organization tumor grades at recurrence in patients with non-skull base and skull base meningiomas. J Neurosurg. 2010;112:925–33.

421. Newall FW, Beaman TC. Ocular signs of meningioma. Trans Am Ophthalmol Soc. 1957;55:297–312.
422. Peele KA, Kennerdell JS, Maroon JC, Kalnicki S, et al. Role of postoperative irradiation in the management of sphenoid wing meningiomas. A preliminary report. Ophthalmology. 1996;103:1766–7.
423. Pritz MB, Burgett RA. Spheno-orbital reconstruction after meningioma resection. Skull Base. 2009;19:163–7.
424. Rodrigues MM, Savino PJ, Schatz NJ. Spheno-orbital meningioma with optociliary veins. Am J Ophthalmol. 1976;81:666–70.
425. Sandalcioglu IE, Gasser T, Mohr C, et al. Spheno-orbital meningiomas: interdisciplinary approach, resectability and long-term results. J Craniomaxillofac Surg. 2005;33:260–6.
426. Schick U, Bleyen J, Bani A, Hassler W. Management of meningiomas en plaque of the sphenoid wing. J Neurosurg. 2006;104:208–14.
427. Spagnoli MV, Goldberg HI, Grossman RI, et al. Intracranial meningiomas: high-field MR imaging. Radiology. 1986;161:369–75.
428. Stafford SL, Pollock BE, Foote RL, et al. Meningioma radiosurgery: tumor control, outcomes, and complications among 190 consecutive patients. Neurosurgery. 2001;49:1029–37.
429. Terstegge K, Schorner W, Henkes H, et al. Hyperostosis in meningiomas: MR findings in patients with recurrent meningioma of the sphenoid wings. Am J Neuroradiol. 1994;15:55–560.
430. Wilson WB. Meningiomas of the anterior visual system. Surv Ophthalmol. 1981;26:109–27.
431. Wilson WB, Gordon M, Lehman RAW. Meningiomas confined to the optic canal and foramina. Surg Neurol. 1979;12:21–8.
432. Yao YT. Clinicopathologic analysis of 615 cases of meningioma with special reference to recurrence. J Formos Med Assoc. 1994;93:145–52.

Mesenchymal Tumors: Fibrosarcoma

433. Dallet RW. Fibrous histiocytoma and fibrous tissue tumors of the orbit. Radiol Clin N Am. 1999;37:185–94.
434. Eifrig DE, Foos RY. Fibrosarcoma of the orbit. Am J Ophthalmol. 1969;67:244–8.
435. Guthikonda B, Hanna EY, Skoracki RJ, et al. Ameloblastic fibrosarcoma involving the anterior and middle skull base with intradural extension. J Craniofac Surg. 2009;20:2087–90.
436. Lee MJ, Cairns RA, Munk PL, Poon PY. Congenital-infantile fibrosarcoma: magnetic resonance imaging findings. Can Assoc Radiol J. 1996;47:121.
437. Ohtsuka K, Saito K. Primary orbital fibrosarcoma developing in the scleral stroma. Br J Ophthalmol. 1996;80:932–3.
438. Plaza G, Ferrando J, Pinedo F. Sinonasal fibrosarcoma: a case report. Eur Arch Otorhinolaryngol. 2006;263:641–3.
439. Scott SM, Reiman HM, Ppritchard DJ, et al. Soft tissue fibrosarcoma: a clinicopathologic study of 132 cases. Cancer. 1989;64:225–31.
440. Weiner JM, Hidayat AA. Juvenile fibrosarcoma of the orbit and eyelid: a study of five cases. Arch Ophthalmol. 1983;101:253–9.
441. Yanoff M, Scheie HG. Fibrosarcoma of the orbit: report of two patients. Cancer. 1966;19:1711–6.

Mesenchymal Tumors: Fibrous Histiocytoma

442. Al-Hazzaa SA, Specht CS, McLean IW, Holds JB, Anderson RL. Benign orbital fibrous histiocytoma simulating a lacrimal gland tumor. Ophthalmic Surg Lasers. 1996;27:140–2.
443. Arora R, Monga S, Mehta DK, et al. Malignant fibrous histiocytoma of the conjunctiva. Clin Exp Ophthalmol. 2006;34:275–8.
444. Bajaj MS, Pushker N, Kashyap S, et al. Fibrous histiocytoma of the lacrimal gland. Ophthal Plast Reconstr Surg. 2007;23:145–7.
445. Balestrazzi E, Ventura T, Delle Noci N, et al. Malignant conjunctival epibulbar fibrous histiocytoma with orbital invasion. Eur J Ophthalmol. 1991;1:23–7.
446. Biedner B, Rothkoff L. Orbital fibrous histiocytoma in an infant. Am J Ophthalmol. 1978;85:548–50.
447. Boehilke CS, Frueh BR, Flint A, Elner VM. Malignant fibrous histiocytoma of the lateral conjunctiva and anterior orbit. Ophthal Plast Reconstr Surg. 2007;23:338–40.
448. Boynton JR, Markowitch W Jr, Searl SS, Presser SE, Quatela VC. Periocular malignant fibrous histiocytoma. Ophthal Plast Reconstr Surg. 1989;5:239–46.
449. Caballero LR, Rodriguez AC, Sopelana AB. Angiomatoid fibrous histiocytoma of the orbit. Am J Ophthalmol. 1981;92:13–5.
450. Char D, Caputo G, Miller T. Orbital fibrous histiocytomas. Orbit. 2000;19:155–9.
451. Cole SH, Ferry AP. Fibrous histiocytoma (fibrous xanthoma) of the lacrimal sac. Arch Ophthalmol. 1978;96:1647–9.
452. Font RL, Hidayat AA. Fibrous histiocytoma of the orbit. A clinicopathologic study of 150 cases. Hum Pathol. 1982;13:199–209.
453. Gupta VP, Saxena T, Dev G. Fibrous histiocytoma in primary pterygium. Orbit. 2002;21:217–21.
454. Hirano N, Sasaki A, Watanabe T, et al. Malignant fibrous histiocytoma of the lateral wall of the orbit. Neurol Med Chir (Tokyo). 1996;36:246–50.
455. Jacomb-Hood J, Moseley IF. Orbital fibrous histiocytoma: computed tomography in 10 cases and a review of radiologic findings. Clin Radiol. 1991;43:117–20.
456. Jakobiec FA, Howard GM, Jones IS, et al. Fibrous histiocytoma of the orbit. Am J Ophthalmol. 1974;77:333–45.
457. Jakobiec FA, Klapper D, Maher E, Krebs W. Infantile subconjunctival and anterior orbital fibrous histiocytoma. Ultrastructural and immunohistochemical studies. Ophthalmology. 1988;95:516–25.
458. John T, Yanoff M, Scheie HG. Eyelid fibrous histiocytoma. Ophthalmology. 1981;88:1193–5.
459. Krohel GB, Gregor D. Fibrous histiocytoma. J Pediatr Ophthalmol. 1980;17:37–9.
460. Larkin DF, O'Donoghue HN, Mullaney J, Breatnach F. Orbital fibrous histiocytoma in an infant. Acta Ophthalmol. 1988;66:585–8.
461. Lui D, McCann P, Kini RK, Joliat TL. Malignant fibrous histiocytoma of the orbit in a 3-year-old girl. Arch Ophthalmol. 1987;105:895–6.
462. Marback RL, Kincaid MC, Green WR, et al. Fibrous histiocytoma of the lacrimal sac. Am J Ophthalmol. 1982;93:511–7.
463. Milman T, Finger PT, Iacob C, et al. Fibrous histiocytoma. Ophthalmology. 2007;114:2369–70.
464. Milman T, Finger PT, Iacob C, et al. Fibrous histiocytoma. Ophthalmologica. 2007;114:2369.
465. Paglen PG, Kracher DS, McMahon RT. Fibrous histiocytoma of the conjunctiva. Ann Ophthalmol. 1980;12:522–5.
466. Rodriguez MM, Furgiuele FP, Weinreb S. Malignant fibrous histiocytoma of the orbit. Arch Ophthalmol. 1977;95:2025–8.
467. Ros PR, Kursunoglu S, Battle JF, Sheldon JJ, Glaser J. Malignant fibrous histiocytoma of the orbit. J Clin Neuroophthalmol. 1985;5:116–9.
468. Shields JA, Husson M, Chields CL, et al. Orbital malignant fibrous histiocytoma following irradiation for retinoblastoma. Ophthal Plast Reconstr Surg. 2001;17:58–61.
469. Stewart WB, Newman NM, Cavender JC, Spencer WH. Fibrous histiocytoma metastatic to the orbit. Arch Ophthalmol. 1978;96:871–3.
470. Verity MA, Ebert JT, Helper RS. Atypical fibrous histiocytoma of the orbit: an electron-microscopic study. Ophthalmologica. 1977;175:73–9.

Mesenchymal Tumors: Juvenile Xanthogranuloma

471. Borrego O, Hidayat AA. Solitary juvenile xanthogranuloma of the orbit. Orbit. 1996;15:41–5.
472. Freyer DR, Kennedy R, Bostrom BC, et al. Juvenile xanthogranuloma: forms of systemic disease and their clinical implications. J Pediatr. 1996;129:227–37.
473. Kaur H, Cameron JD, Mohney BG. Severe astigmatic amblyopia secondary to subcutaneous juvenile xanthogranuloma of the eyelid. J AAPOS. 2006;10:277–8.
474. Kuruvilla R, Escaravage GK, Finn AJ, Dutton JJ. Infiltrative subcutaneous juvenile xanthogranuloma of the eyelid in a neonate. Ophthal Plast Reconstr Surg. 2009;25:330–2.
475. Miszkiel KA, Sohaib SA, Rose GE, et al. Radiological and clinicopathological features of orbital xanthogranuloma. Br J Ophthalmol. 2000;84:251–8.
476. Schwartz TL, Carter KD, Judisch F, et al. Congenital macronodular juvenile xanthogranuloma of the eyelid. Ophthalmology. 1991;98:1230–3.
477. Shields CL, Shields JA, Buchanon HW. Solitary orbital involvement with juvenile xanthogranuloma. Arch Ophthalmol. 1990;108:1587–9.
478. Shin HT, Harris MB, Orlow SJ. Juvenile myelomonocytic leukemia presenting with features of hemophagocytic lymphohistiocytosis in association with neurofibromatosis and juvenile xanthogranulomas. J Pediatr Hematol Oncol. 2004;26:591–5.
479. Sonoda T, Hashimoto H, Enjoji M. Juvenile xanthogranuloma. Clinicopathologic analysis and immunohistochemical study of 57 patients. Cancer. 1985;56:2280–6.
480. Weitzman S, Jaffe R. Uncommon histiocytic disorders: the non-Langerhans cell histiocytosis. Pediatr Blood Cancer. 2005;45:256–64.
481. Zimmerman LE. Ocular lesions of juvenile xanthogranuloma. Nevoxanthoendotheiloma. Am J Ophthalmol. 1965;60:1011–35.

Mesenchymal Tumors: Leiomyosarcoma

482. Arora R, Betharia SM. Aspiration cytology of smooth-muscle tumours of the orbit. Orbit. 1990;9:35–41.
483. Bakri SJ, Krohel GB, Peters GB, Farber MG. Spermatic cord leiomyosarcoma metastatic to the orbit. Am J Ophthalmol. 2003;136:213–5.
484. Conlon MR, Rubin PA, Samy CN, Albert DM. Metastatic orbital leiomyosarcoma. Can J Ophthalmol. 1994;29:85–9.
485. Das DK, Das J, Kumar D, et al. Leiomyosarcoma of the orbit: diagnosis of its recurrence by fine-needle aspiration cytology. Diagn Cytopathol. 1992;8:609–13.
486. Folberg R, Cleaseby G, Flanagan JA, Spencer WH, Zimmerman LE. Orbital leiomyosarcoma after radiation therapy for bilateral retinoblastoma. Arch Ophthalmol. 1983;101:1562–5.
487. Font RL, Jurco S III, Brechner RJ. Postradiation leiomyosarcoma of the orbit complicating bilateral retinoblastoma. Arch Ophthalmol. 1983;101:1557–61.
488. Hou LC, Murphy MA, Tung GA. Primary orbital leiomyosarcoma: a case report with MRI findings. Am J Ophthalmol. 2003;135(3):408–10.
489. Jakobiec FA, Howard G, Rosen M, et al. Leiomyoma and leiomyosarcoma of the orbit. Am J Ophthalmol. 1975;80:1028–42.
490. Jakobiec FA, Mitchell JP, Chauhan PM, Iwamoto T. Mesectodermal leiomyosarcoma of the antrum and orbit. Am J Ophthalmol. 1978;85:51–7.
491. Kaltreider SA, Destro M, Lemke BN. Leiomyosarcoma of the orbit. A case report and review of the literature. Ophthal Plast Reconstr Surg. 1987;3:35–41.
492. Logrono R, Inhorn SL, Dortzbach RK, Kurtycz DF. Leiomyosarcoma metastatic to the orbit: diagnosis of fine-needle aspiration. Diagn Cytopathol. 1997;17:369–73.
493. Meekins BB, Dutton JJ, Proia AD. Primary orbital leiomyosarcoma. Arch Ophthalmol. 1988;106:82–6.
494. Mihara F, Gupta KL, Kartchner ZA, Kogutt MS, Robinson AE. Leiomyosarcoma after retinoblastoma radiotherapy. Radiat Med. 1991;9:183–4.
495. Minkovitz JB, Dickersin GR, Dallow RL, Albert DM. Leiomyosarcoma metastatic to the orbit. Arch Ophthalmol. 1990;108:1525–6.
496. Suankratay C, Shuangshoti S, Mutirangura A, et al. Epstein-Barr virus infection-associated smooth muscle tumors in patients with AIDS. Clin Infect Dis. 2005;40:1521–8.
497. Tanaka H, Westesson PL, Wilbur DC. Leiomyosarcoma of the maxillary sinus: CT and MRI findings. Br J Radiol. 1998;71:221–4.
498. Voros GM, Birchall D, Ressiniotis T, Neoh C, Owen RI, Strong NP. Imaging of metastatic orbital leiomyosarcoma. Ophthal Plast Reconstr Surg. 2005;21(6):453–5.
499. Wiechens B, Werner JA, Luttges J, et al. Primary orbital leiomyoma and leiomyosarcoma. Ophthalmologica. 1999;213:159–64.
500. Wojno T, Tenzel RR, Nadji M. Orbital leiomyosarcoma. Arch Ophthalmol. 1983;101:1566–8.

Mesenchymal Tumors: Lipoblastomatosis

501. Adams RJ, Drwiega PJ, Rivera CA. Congenital orbital lipoblastoma: a pathologic and radiologic study. J Pediatr Ophthalmol Strabismus. 1997;34:194–6.
502. Chung EB, Enzinger FM. Benign lipoblastomatosis: an analysis of 35 cases. Cancer. 1973;32:482–92.
503. Dilley AV, Patel DL, Hicks MJ, Brandt ML. Lipoblastoma: path physiology and surgical management. J Pediatr Surg. 2001;36(1):229–31.
504. Enghardt MH, Warren RC. Congenital palpebral lipoblastoma. First report of a case. Am J Dermatopathol. 1990;12:408–11.
505. Greco MA, Garcia RL, Vuletin JC. Benign lipoblastomatosis: ultrastructure and histogenesis. Cancer. 1980;45:511–5.
506. Hicks J, Dilley A, Patel D, et al. Lipoblastoma and lipoblastomatosis in infancy and childhood: histopathologic, ultrastructural, and cytogenetic features. Ultrastruct Pathol. 2001;25(4):321–33.
507. Jung SM, Chang PY, Luo CC, et al. Lipoblastoma/lipoblastomatosis: a clinicopathologic study of 16 cases in Taiwan. Pediatr Surg Int. 2005;21:809–12.
508. Seider N, Gilboa M, Barishak YR, Miller B. Congenital combined orbito-nasal lipoblastoma: clinico-pathologic study. Orbit. 2007;26:125–7.

Mesenchymal Tumors: Benign Cartilaginous Tumors

509. Albert DM, Ni C, Sebag J, Renna T. Rare orbital tumors. Int Ophthalmol Clin. 1981;22:183–204.
510. Blodi FC. Pathology of orbital bones. The XXXII Edward Jackson Memorial Lecture. Am J Ophthalmol. 1976;81:1–26.
511. Bowen JH, Christensen FH, Klintworth GK, Sydnor CF. A clinicopathologic study of a cartilaginous hamartoma of the orbit: a rare cause of proptosis. Ophthalmology. 1981;88:135–60.
512. Harrison A, Loftus S, Pambuccian S. Orbital chondroma. Ophthal Plast Reconstr Surg. 2006;22:484–5.
513. Jepson CN, Wetzig PC. Pure chondroma of the trochlea; a case report. Surv Ophthalmol. 1966;11:656–9.
514. Pasternak S, O'Connell JX, Verchere C, Rootman J. Enchondroma of the orbit. Am J Ophthalmol. 1996;122:444–5.

515. Selva D, White VA, O'Connell JX, Rootman J. Primary bone tumors of the orbit. Surv Ophthalmol. 2004;49:328–42.
516. Tashiro T, Inoue Y, Nemoto Y, Shakudo M, et al. Magnetic resonance imaging of chordoma and chondroma in the skull base. Differential diagnosis by IR sequence. Nippon Acta Radiologica. 1992;52:589–93.
517. Terasaka S, Sawamura Y, Abe H. Surgical removal of a cavernous sinus chondroma. Surg Neurol. 1997;48:153–9.

Mesenchymal Tumors: Lipodermoid

518. Beard C. Dermolipoma surgery, or, "an ounce of prevention is worth a pound of cure". Ophthal Plast Reconstr Surg. 1990;6:153–7.
519. Craitoiu S. Goldenhar's oculoauricular dysplasia, limbic dermoid and conjunctival dermolipoma. Oftalmologia. 1992;36:357–61.
520. Economidis I, Tragakis M, Mangouritsas N, Papademetriou D. Keratoconjuntivitis sicca following excision of a dermolipoma of the lacrimal gland. Ann Ophthalmol. 1978;10:1273–8.
521. Eijpe AA, Koornneef L, Bras J, et al. Dermolipoma: characteristic CT appearance. Doc Ophthalmol. 1990;74:321–8.
522. Francois P, Lekieffre M, Woillez M, Ryckewaert M. Complications of dermolipoma ablation. Bull Soc Ophtalmol Fr. 1989;89:289–90.
523. Fry CL, Leone CR Jr. Safe management of dermolipomas. Arch Ophthalmol. 1994;112:1114–6.
524. Kim YD, Goldberg RA. Orbital fat prolapse and dermolipoma: two distinct entities. Korean J Ophthalmol. 1994;8:42–3.
525. McNab AA, Wright JE, Caswell AG. Clinical features and surgical management of dermolipomas. Aust N Z J Ophthalmol. 1990;18:159–62.
526. Paris GL, Beard C. Blepharoptosis following dermolipoma surgery. Ann Ophthalmol. 1973;5:697–9.
527. Rootman J. Structural lesions. Dermolipoma. Diseases of the orbit. 2nd ed. Philadelphia: Lippincott, Williams and Wilkins; 2003. p. 298–301.
528. Shields CL, Shields JA. Tumors of the conjunctiva and cornea. Surv Ophthalmol. 2004;49:3–24.
529. Shields CL, Shields JA. Conjunctival tumors in children. Curr Opin Ophthalmol. 2007;18(5):351–60.
530. Shields CL, Dermirci H, Karatza E, et al. Clinical survey of 1643 melanocytic and nonmelanocytic tumors of the conjunctiva. Ophthalmology. 2004;111:1747–54.

Mesenchymal Tumors: Lipoma

531. Bartley GB, Yeatts RP, Garrity JA, et al. Spindle cell lipoma of the orbit. Am J Ophthalmol. 1985;100:605–9.
532. Behrendt S, Werner JA, Janig U. Lipoma of the orbit. Orbit. 1996;15:101–4.
533. Brown HH, Kersten RC, Kulwin DR. Lipomatous hamartoma of the orbit. Arch Ophthalmol. 1991;109:240–3.
534. Daniel CS, Beaconsfield M, Rose GE, et al. Pleomorphic lipoma of orbit: a case series and review of literature. Ophthalmology. 2003;110:101–5.
535. Dutton JJ, Wright JJ. Intramuscular lipoma of the superior oblique muscle. Orbit. 2006;25:227–33.
536. Feinfield RE, Hesse RJ, Scharfenberg JC. Orbital angiolipoma. Arch Ophthalmol. 1988;106:1093–5.
537. Iliff WJ, Green WR. Orbital tumors in children. In: Jakobiec FA, editor. Ocular and adnexal tumors. Birmingham: Aesculapius; 1978. p. 669–84.
538. Johansen S, Heegaard S, Bogeskov L, Prause JU. Orbital space-occupying lesions in Denmark 1974–1997. Acta Ophthalmol Scand. 2000;78:547–52.
539. Mawn LA, Jordan DR, Olberg B. Spindle-cell lipoma of the preseptal eyelid. Ophthal Plast Reconstr Surg. 1998;14:174–7.
540. Shah NB, Chang WY, White VA, et al. Orbital Lipoma: 2 cases and review of literature. Ophthal Plast Reconstr Surg. 2007;23:202–5.
541. Shields JA, Shields CL, Scartozzi R, et al. Survey of 1264 patients with orbital tumors and simulating lesions: the 2002 Montgomery Lecture, part 1. Ophthalmology. 2004;111:997–1008.
542. Silva D. Orbital tumors. Am J Ophthalmol. 1968;65:318–39.

Mesenchymal Tumors: Liposarcoma

543. Abdalla MI, Ghaly AF, Hosni F. Liposarcoma with orbital metastases: case report. Br J Ophthalmol. 1966;50:426–8.
544. Cai YC, McMenamin ME, Rose G, et al. Primary liposarcoma of the orbit: a clinicopathologic study of seven cases. Ann Diagn Pathol. 2001;5:255–6.
545. Cockerman KP, Kennerdell JS, Celin SE, FEchter HP. Liposarcoma of the orbit: a management challenge. Ophthal Plast Reconstr Surg. 1998;14:370–4.
546. Enterline HT, Culberson JD, Rochlin DB, et al. Liposarcoma: a clinical and pathological study of 53 cases. Cancer. 1960;13:932–50.
547. Fabi A, Salesi N, Vidiri A, Mirri A, et al. Retroperitoneal liposarcoma with metastasis to both orbits: an unusual metastatic site. Anticancer Res. 2005;25:4769–71.
548. Favrot SR, Ridley MB, Older JJ, et al. Orbital liposarcoma. Otolaryngol Head Neck Surg. 1994;111:111–5.
549. Fezza J, Sinard J. Metastatic liposarcoma to the orbit. Am J Ophthalmol. 1997;123:271–2.
550. Jakobiec FA, Rini F, Char D, et al. Primary liposarcoma of the orbit: problems in the diagnosis and management of five cases. Ophthalmology. 1989;86:180–91.
551. McNab AA, Moseley I. Primary orbital liposarcoma: clinical and computed tomographic features. Br J Ophthalmol. 1990;74:437–9.
552. Montiero MLR. Liposarcoma of the orbit presenting as an enlarged medial rectus muscle on CT scan. Br J Ophthalmol. 2002;86:1450.
553. Mridha AR, Sharma MC, Sarkar C, et al. Primary liposarcoma of the orbit: a report of two cases. Can J Ophthalmol. 2007;42:481–3.
554. Nasr AM, Ossoinig KC, Kersten RF, Blodi FC. Standardized echographic-histopathologic correlations in liposarcoma. Am J Ophthalmol. 1985;99:193–200.
555. Saeed MU, Chang BY, Atherley C, et al. A rare diagnosis of dedifferentiated liposarcoma of the orbit. Orbit. 2007;26:43–5.
556. Wagle MA, Biswas J, Subramaniam N, et al. Primary liposarcoma of the orbit: a clinicopathologic study. Orbit. 1999;18:1213–23.

Mesenchymal Tumors: Rhabdomyosarcoma

557. Abramson DH, Notis CM. Visual acuity after radiation for orbital rhabdomyosarcoma. Am J Ophthalmol. 1994;118:808–9.
558. Boparai MS, Dash RG. Clinical, ultrasonographic and CT evaluation of orbital rhabdomyosarcoma with management. Indian J Ophthalmol. 1991;39:129–31.
559. Breen LA, Kline LB, Hart WM Jr, Burde RM. Rhabdomyosarcoma causing rapid bilateral visual loss in children. J Clin Neuroophthalmol. 1984;4:185–8.
560. Fekrat S, Miller NR, Loury MC. Alveolar rhabdomyosarcoma that metastasized to the orbit. Arch Ophthalmol. 1993;111:1662–4.
561. Frilling R, Marcus M, Monos T, Moses M, Yassur Y. Rhabdomyosarcoma invading the orbit in an adult. Ophthal Plast Reconstr Surg. 1994;10:283–6.
562. Ghafoor SY, Dudgeon J. Orbital rhabdomyosarcoma: improved survival with combined pulsed chemotherapy and irradiation. Br J Ophthalmol. 1985;69:557–61.

563. Hatton MP, Green L, Boulos PR, Rubin PA. Rhabdomyosarcoma metastases to all extraocular muscles. Ophthal Plast Reconstr Surg. 2008;24(4):336–8.
564. Huh WW, Beverly RR. Orbital metastasis in patients with rhabdomyosarcoma: case series and review of the literature. J Pediatr Hematol Oncol. 2006;28(10):684–7.
565. Humpl T, Bruhl K, Pitz S, et al. Rhabdomyosarcoma of the orbits in childhood. Ophtalmologie. 1997;94:914–9.
566. Jones IS, Reese AB, Kraut J. Orbital rhabdomyosarcoma: an analysis of sixty-two cases. Trans Am Ophthalmol Soc. 1965;63:223–55.
567. Judmaier W, Birbamer G, Buchberger W, et al. MR imaging of late onset orbital rhabdomyosarcoma with intracranial extension. Magn Reson Imaging. 1993;11:285–8.
568. Knowles DM, Jakobiec FA, Potter GD, Jones IS. Ophthalmic striated muscle neoplasms. Surv Ophthalmol. 1976;21:219–61.
569. Kodet R, Newton WA, Hamoudi AB, et al. Orbital rhabdomyosarcoma and related tumors in childhood: relationship of morphology to prognosis – an Intergroup Rhabdomyosarcoma study. Med Pediatr Oncol. 1997;29:51–60.
570. Mamalis N, Grey AM, Good JS, McLeish WM, Anderson RL. Embryonal rhabdomyosarcoma of the orbit in a 35-year-old man. Ophthalmic Surg. 1994;25:332–5.
571. Mannor GE, Rose GE, Plowman PN, et al. Multidisciplinary management of refractory orbital rhabdomyosarcoma. Ophthalmology. 1997;104:1198–202.
572. McDonald MW, Esiashvili N, George BA, Katzenstein HM, Olson TA, Rapkin LB, et al. Intensity-modulated radiotherapy with use of cone-down boost for pediatric head-and-neck rhabdomyosarcoma. Int J Radiat Oncol Biol Phys. 2008;72(3):884–91.
573. Meza JL, Anderson J, Pappo AS, Meyer WH, Children's Oncology Group. Analysis of prognostic factors in patients with nonmetastatic rhabdomyosarcoma treated on intergroup rhabdomyosarcoma studies III and IV: the Children's Oncology Group. J Clin Oncol. 2006;24(24):3844–51.
574. Notis CM, Abramson DH, Sagerman RH, Ellsworth RM. Orbital rhabdomyosarcoma: treatment or overtreatment. Ophthalmic Genet. 1995;16:159–62.
575. Porterfield JF, Zimmerman LE. Rhabdomyosarcoma of the orbit. Virchows Arch [A]. 1962;335:329–44.
576. Raney RB, Maurer HM, Anderson JR, et al. The Intergroup Rhabdomyosarcoma Study Group (IRSG): major lessons from the IRS-I through IRS-IV studies as background for the current IRS-V treatment protocols. Sarcoma. 2001;5:9–15.
577. Shields JA, Shields CL. Rhabdomyosarcoma of the orbit. Int Ophthalmol Clin. 1993;33:203–10.
578. Shields JA, Shields CL, Eagle RC Jr, Nowinski T. Orbital rhabdomyosarcoma. Arch Ophthalmol. 1987;105:700–1.
579. Sohaib SA, Moseley I, Wright JE. Orbital rhabdomyosarcoma – the radiologic characteristics. Clin Radiol. 1998;53:357–62.
580. Vade A, Armstrong D. Orbital rhabdomyosarcoma in childhood. Radiol Clin N Am. 1987;25:701–14.
581. Walton RC, Ellis GS Jr, Haik BG. Rhabdomyosarcoma presumed metastatic to the orbit. Ophthalmology. 1996;103:1512–6.
582. Wharam M, Beltangady M, Hays D, et al. Localized orbital rhabdomyosarcoma. An interim report of the Intergroup Rhabdomyosarcoma Study Committee. Ophthalmology. 1987;94:251–4.

Mesenchymal Tumors: Solitary Fibrous Tumor

583. Alexandrakis G, Johnson TE. Recurrent orbital solitary fibrous tumor in a 14-year-old girl. Am J Ophthalmol. 2000;130:373–6.
584. Bernardini FP, de Conciliis C, Schneider S, et al. Solitary fibrous tumor of the orbit: is it rare? Report of a case series and review of the literature. Ophthalmology. 2003;110:1442–8.
585. Carrera M, Prat J, Quintana M. Malignant solitary fibrous tumor of the orbit. Report of a case with 8 years of follow-up. Eye. 2001;15:102–4.
586. Dailey RW. Fibrous histiocytoma and fibrous tissue tumors of the orbit. Radiol Clin N Am. 1999;37:185–94.
587. DeBacker CM, Bodker F, Putterman AM, Beckmann E. Solitary fibrous tumor of the orbit. Am J Ophthalmol. 1996;121:447–9.
588. Dorfman DM, To K, Dickersin GR, et al. Solitary fibrous tumor of the orbit. Am J Surg Pathol. 1994;18:281–7.
589. Giuffre I, Faiola A, Bonanno E, Liccardo G. Solitary fibrous tumor of the orbit. Case report and review of the literature. Surg Neurol. 2001;56:242–6.
590. Ing EB, Kennerdell JS, Olson PR, Ogino S, Rothfus WE. Solitary fibrous tumor of the orbit. Ophthal Plast Reconstr Surg. 1998;14:57–61.
591. Kim HJ, Kim H-J, Kim Y-D, et al. Solitary fibrous tumor of the orbit: CT and MRI imaging findings. Am J Neuroradiol. 2008;29:857–62.
592. Krishnakumar S, Ubramanian N, Mohan ER, et al. Solitary fibrous tumor of the orbit: a clinicopathologic study of six cases with review of the literature. Surv Ophthalmol. 2003;48:544–54.
593. Leoncini G, Maio V, Puccioni M, et al. Orbital solitary fibrous tumor: a case report and review of the literature. Pathol Oncol Res. 2008;14:213–7.
594. Mascarenhas L, Lopes M, Duarte AM, et al. Histologically malignant solitary fibrous tumor of the orbit. Neurochirurgie. 2006;52:415–8.
595. Meyer D, Riley F. Solitary fibrous tumor of the orbit: a clinicopathologic entity that warrants both a heightened awareness and a traumatic surgical removal technique. Orbit. 2006;25:45–50.
596. Romer M, Bode B, Schuknecht B, Schmid S. Solitary fibrous tumor of the orbit; two cases and a review of the literature. Eur Arch Otorhinolaryngol. 2005;262:81–8.
597. Suzuki S. A case of malignant solitary fibrous tumor presenting with exophthalmos. Jpn J Clin Oncol. 2007;37:401.
598. Tam ES, Chen EC, Nijhawan N, et al. Solitary fibrous tumor of the orbit: a case series. Orbit. 2008;27:426–31.

Tumors of Bone: Aneurysmal Bone Cyst

599. Bealer LA, Cibis GW, Barker BF, et al. Aneurysmal bone cyst: report of a case mimicking orbital tumor. J Pediatr Ophthalmol Strabismus. 1993;30:199–200.
600. Borkar SA, Kasliwal MK, Sinha S, Sharma BS. MR imaging in aneurismal bone cyst of the orbit. Turk Neurosurg. 2008;18:183–6.
601. Citardi MJ, Janjua T, Abrahams JJ, Sasaki CT. Orbitoethmoid aneurysmal bone cyst. Otolaryngol Head Neck Surg. 1996;114:466–70.
602. Cory DA, Fritsch SA, Cohen MD, et al. Aneurysmal bone cysts: imaging findings and embolotherapy. Am J Roentgenol. 1989;153:369–73.
603. Fite JD, Schwarts JF, Calhoun FP. Aneurysmal bone cyst of the orbit. A clinicopathologic case report. Trans Am Acad Ophthalmol Otolaryngol. 1968;72:614–8.
604. Hino N, Ohtsuka K, Hashimoto M, Sakata M. Radiographic features of an aneurysmal bone cyst of the orbit. Ophthalmologica. 1998;212:198–201.
605. Hunter JV, Yokoyama C, Moseley IF, Wright JE. Aneurysmal bone cyst of the sphenoid with orbital involvement. Br J Ophthalmol. 1990;74:505–8.
606. Iraci G, Giordano R, Fiore D, et al. Exophthalmos from aneurysmal bone cyst of the orbital roof. Childs Brain. 1980;6:206–17.
607. Johnson TE, Bergin DJ, McCord CD. Aneurysmal bone cyst of the orbit. Ophthalmology. 1988;95:86–9.
608. Klepach GL, Ho RE, Kelly JK. Aneurysmal bone cyst of the orbit. A case report. J Clin Neuroophthalmol. 1984;4:49–52.

609. Marcol W, Mander M, Milnoska I, et al. Aneurysmal bone cyst of the orbit. Pediatr Neurosurg. 2006;42:325–7.
610. O'Gorman AM, Kirkham TH. Aneurysmal bone cyst of the orbit with unusual roentgenographic features. Am J Roentgenol. 1976;126:896–9.
611. Patel BC, Sabir DI, Flaharty PM, Anderson RL. Aneurysmal bone cyst of the orbit and ethmoid sinus. Arch Ophthalmol. 1993;111:586–7.
612. Powell JO, Glaser JS. Aneurysmal bone cyst of the orbit. Arch Ophthalmol. 1975;93:340–2.
613. Ronner HJ, Jones IS. Aneurysmal bone cyst of the orbit: a review. Ann Ophthalmol. 1983;15:626–9.
614. Senol U, Karaali K, Akyuz M, et al. Aneurysmal bone cyst of the orbit. Am J Neuroradiol. 2002;23:319–21.
615. Yuen VH, Jordan DR, Jabi M, Agbi C. Aneurysmal bone cyst associated with fibrous dysplasia. Ophthal Plast Reconstr Surg. 2002;18:471–4.

Tumors of Bone: Cholesterol Granuloma

616. Aferzon M, Millman B, O'Donnell TR. Cholesterol granuloma of the frontal bone. Otolaryngol Head Neck Surg. 2002;127:578–81.
617. Arat YO, Chaudhry IA, Boniuk M. Orbitofrontal cholesterol granuloma: distinct diagnostic features and management. Ophthal Plast Reconstr Surg. 2003;19:382–7.
618. Chow LP, McNab AA. Orbitofrontal cholesterol granuloma. J Clin Neurosci. 2005;12:206–9.
619. Daus W, Vogcs J, Schwechheimer K, et al. Cholesterol granuloma of the orbit. Klin Monatsbl Augenheilkd. 1988;193:195–9.
620. Dickey JB, Mullenix CD, O'Grady RB. Atypical magnetic resonance findings in an orbitofrontal cholesterol granuloma. Ophthal Plast Reconstr Surg. 1992;8:215–20.
621. Dobben GD, Philip B, Mafee MF, et al. Orbital subperiosteal hematoma, cholesterol granuloma, and infection. Radiol Clin N Am. 1998;36:1185–200.
622. Eijpe AA, Koornneef L, Verbeeten B Jr, et al. Cholesterol granuloma of the frontal bone: CT diagnosis. J Comput Assist Tomogr. 1990;14:914–7.
623. Elmaleh C, D'Hermies F, Barraco P, Pouliquen Y. Cholesteatoma of the orbit: a rare etiology of orbital tumor. J Fr Ophtalmol. 1989;12:139–42.
624. Fukata K, Jackson IT. Epidermal cyst and cholesterol granuloma of the orbit. Br J Surg. 1990;43:521–7.
625. Hill CA, Moseley IF. Imaging of orbitofrontal cholesterol granuloma. Clin Radiol. 1992;46:237–42.
626. Jordan DR, Spitellie P, Brownstein S. Orbital cholesterol granuloma and cholesteatoma: significance of differentiating the two. Ophthal Plast Reconstr Surg. 2007;23:415–7.
627. Kersten RC, Kersten JL, Bloom BR, Kulwin DR. Chronic hematic cyst of the orbit. Role of magnetic resonance imaging in diagnosis. Ophthalmology. 1988;95:1549–53.
628. McNab AA, Wright GE. Orbitofrontal cholesterol granuloma. Ophthalmology. 1990;97:28–32.
629. Ong LY, McNab AA. Recurrent orbital cholesterol granuloma. Orbit. 2008;27:119–21.
630. Parke DW 2nd, Font RL, Boniuk M, McCrary JA 3rd. Cholesterol granuloma of the orbit. Arch Ophthalmol. 1992;100:612–6.
631. Prabhakaran VC, Hsuan J, Selva D. Endoscopic-assisted removal of orbital roof lesions via a skin crease approach. Skull Base. 2007;17:341–5.
632. Selva D, Chen C. Endoscopic approach to orbitofrontal cholesterol granuloma. Orbit. 2004;23:49–52.
633. Selva D, Phipps SE, O'Connell JX. Pathogenesis of orbital cholesterol granuloma. Clin Exp Ophthalmol. 2003;31:78–82.
634. Wiot JG, Pleatman CW. Chronic hematic cysts of the orbit. Am J Neuroradiol. 1989;10:37–9.

Tumors of Bone: Ewing's Sarcoma

635. Bajaj MS, Pushker N, Sen S, et al. Primary Ewing's sarcoma of the orbit: a rare presentation. J Pediatr Ophthalmol Strabismus. 2003;40:101–4.
636. Dutton JJ, Rose JG Jr, DeBacker CM, Gayre G. Orbital Ewing's sarcoma of the orbit. Ophthal Plast Reconstr Surg. 2000;16:292–300.
637. Eggli KD, Quiogue TM, Moser RP. Ewing's sarcoma. Radiol Clin N Am. 1993;31:325–37.
638. Frandsen E. Ewing's sarcom I orbiti. Nord Med. 1952;48:1673.
639. Green DM, Marinello MJ, Fisher J, et al. Ewing's sarcoma of the scapula with metastases to the lung and eye. Am J Pediatr Hematol Oncol. 1986;8:134–43.
640. Guzowski M, Tumuluri K, Walker DM, Maloof A. Primary orbital Ewing sarcoma in a middle-aged man. Ophthal Plast Reconstr Surg. 2005;21:449–51.
641. Harbert F, Tabor GL Jr. Ewing's tumor of the orbit. Am J Ophthalmol. 1950;33:1219–55.
642. Henk CB, Grampp S, Wiesbauer P, et al. Ewing sarcoma. Diagnostic imaging. Radiologe. 1998;38:509–22.
643. Jereb B, Ong RL, Mohan M, Caparros B, Exelby P. Redefined role of radiation in combined treatment of Ewing's sarcoma. Pediatr Hematol Oncol. 1986;3:11–118.
644. Kissane JM, Askin FB, Foulkes M, Stratton LB, Shirley SF. Ewing's sarcoma of bone: clinicopathologic aspects of 303 cases from the intergroup Ewing's sarcoma study. Hum Pathol. 1983;14:773–9.
645. Li T, Goldberg RA, Becker B, McCann J. Primary orbital extraskeletal Ewing sarcoma. Arch Ophthalmol. 2003;121:1049–51.
646. Mansfield JB. Primary Ewing's sarcoma of the skull. Surg Neurol. 1982;18:286–8.
647. Pang NK, Bartley GB, Giannini C. Primary Ewing sarcoma of the orbit in an adult. Ophthal Plast Reconstr Surg. 2007;23:153–4.
648. Rootman J. Diseases of the orbit: a multidisciplinary approach. 2nd ed. Philadelphia: Lippincott Williams & Wilkins; 2003. p. 299–301.
649. Sharma A, Garg A, Mishra NK, Gaikwad SB, et al. Primary Ewing's sarcoma of the sphenoid bone with unusual imaging features: a case report. Neurol Neurosurg. 2005;107:528–31.
650. Wilson DJ, Dailey RA, Griffeth MT, Newton CJ. Primary Ewing sarcoma of the orbit. Ophthal Plast Reconstr Surg. 2001;17:300–3.
651. Woodruff G, Thorner P, Skarf B. Primary Ewing's sarcoma of the orbit presenting with visual loss. Br J Ophthalmol. 1988;72:786–92.

Tumors of Bone: Fibrous Dysplasia

652. Bibby K, McFadzean R. Fibrous dysplasia of the orbit. Br J Ophthalmol. 1994;78:266–70.
653. Casselman JW, De Jonge I, Neyt L, De Clercq C, D'Hont G. MRI in craniofacial fibrous dysplasia. Neuroradiology. 1993;35:234–7.
654. Chung EM, Murphey MD, Specht CS, et al. From the archives of the AFIP. Pediatric orbit tumors and tumorlike lesions: osseous lesions of the orbit. Radiographics. 2008;28:1193.
655. Cruz AA, Constanzi M, de Castro FA, dos Santos AC. Apical involvement with fibrous dysplasia: implications for vision. Ophthal Plast Reconstr Surg. 2007;23:450–4.
656. Daffner RH, Kirks DR, Gehweiler JA, Heaston DK. Computed tomography of fibrous dysplasia. Am J Roentgenol. 1982;139:943–8.
657. Donoso LA, Margargal LE, Eiferman RA. Fibrous dysplasia of the orbit with optic nerve decompression. Ann Ophthalmol. 1982;14:80–3.
658. Gass JDM. Orbital and ocular involvement in fibrous dysplasia. Case report. South Med J. 1965;58:324–9.

659. Giordano F, Serio P, Savasta S, et al. Craniofacial surgery in fibrous dysplasia. J Pediatr Endocrinol Metab. 2006;19:595–604.
660. Goisis M, Biglioli F, Guareschi M, et al. Fibrous dysplasia of the orbital region: current clinical perspectives in ophthalmology and cranio-maxillofacial surgery. Ophthal Plast Reconstr Surg. 2006;22:383–7.
661. Katz BJ, Nerad JA. Ophthalmic manifestations of fibrous dysplasia: a disease of children and adults. Ophthalmology. 1998;105:2207–15.
662. Liakos GM, Walker CB, Carruth JAS. Ocular complications in craniofacial fibrous dysplasia. Br J Ophthalmol. 1979;63:611–6.
663. McCluskey P, Wingate R, Benger R, McCarthy S. Monostotic fibrous dysplasia of the orbit: an unusual lacrimal fossa mass. Br J Ophthalmol. 1993;77:54–6.
664. Melen O, Weinberg PE, Kim KS, et al. Fibrous dysplasia of bone with active visual loss. Ann Ophthalmol. 1980;12:734–9.
665. Moore RT. Fibrous dysplasia of the orbit. Review. Surv Ophthalmol. 1969;13:321–34.
666. Moore AT, Buncic JR, Munro IR. Fibrous dysplasia of the orbit in childhood. Clinical features and management. Ophthalmology. 1985;92:12–20.
667. Papay FA, Morlaes L Jr, Flaharty P, Smith SJ, et al. Optic nerve decompression in cranial base fibrous dysplasia. J Craniofac Surg. 1995;6:5–10. Discussion 11–14.
668. Ronner HJ, Trokel SL, Hilal SK. Acute blindness in a patient with fibrous dysplasia. Orbit. 1982;1:231–4.
669. Seiff SR. Optic nerve decompression in fibrous dysplasia: indications, efficacy, and safety. Plast Reconstr Surg. 1997;100:1611–2.
670. Selva D, White VA, O'Connell JX, Rootman J. Primary bone tumors of the orbit. Surv Ophthalmol. 2004;49:328–42.
671. Weisman JS, Hepler RS, Vinters HV. Reversible visual loss caused by fibrous dysplasia. Am J Ophthalmol. 1990;110:244–9.
672. Yuen VH, Jordan DR, Jabi M, Agbi C. Aneurysmal bone cyst associated with fibrous dysplasia. Ophthal Plast Reconstr Surg. 2002;18:471–4.

Tumors of Bone: Giant Cell Reparative Granuloma

673. D'Ambrosio AL, Williams SC, Lignelli A, et al. Clinicopathological review: giant cell reparative granuloma of the orbit. Neurosurgery. 2005;57:773–8.
674. Font RL, Blanco G, Soparkar CN, et al. Giant cell reparative granuloma of the orbit associated with cherubism. Ophthalmology. 2003;110:1846–9.
675. Hirschl S, Katz A. Giant cell reparative granuloma outside the jawbone. Diagnostic criteria and review of the literature with the first case description in the temporal bone. Hum Pathol. 1974;5:171–81.
676. Hoopes PC, Anderson RL, Blodi FC. Giant cell (reparative) granuloma of the orbit. Ophthalmology. 1981;88:1361–6.
677. Hyver SW, Ellis DS, Stewart WB, Spencer WH, Bartlett PC. Sino-orbital giant cell reparative granuloma. Ophthal Plast Reconstr Surg. 1998;14:178–81.
678. Mercado GV, Shields CL, Gunduz K, et al. Giant cell reparative granuloma of the orbit. Am J Ophthalmol. 1999;127:485–7.
679. Pherwani AA, Brooker D, Lacey B. Giant cell reparative granuloma of the orbit. Ophthal Plast Reconstr Surg. 2005;21:463–5.
680. Sebag J, Chapman P, Truman J, Riemersma RR. Giant cell granuloma of the orbit with intracranial extension. Neurosurgery. 1985;16:75–8.
681. Spraul CW, Wojno TH, Grossniklaus HE, Lang GK. Reparative giant cell granuloma with orbital involvement. Klin Monatsbl Augenheilkd. 1997;21:133–4.

Tumors of Bone: Ossifying Fibroma

682. Baumann I, Zimmerman R, Dammann F, et al. Ossifying fibroma of the ethmoid involving the orbit and the skull base. Otolaryngol Head Neck Surg. 2005;133:158–9.
683. Chung EM, Murphey MD, Specht CS, et al. From the archives of the AFIP pediatric obit tumors and tumorlike lesions: osseous lesions of the orbit. Radiographics. 2008;28:1193–214.
684. Cruz AA, Alencar VM, Figueiredo AR, et al. Ossifying fibroma: a rare cause of orbital inflammation. Ophthal Plast Reconstr Surg. 2008;24:107–12.
685. Fakadej A, Boynton JR. Juvenile ossifying fibroma of the orbit. Ophthal Plast Reconstr Surg. 1996;12:174–7.
686. Hartstein ME, Grove AS Jr, Woog JJ, Shore JW, Joseph MP. The multidisciplinary management of psammomatoid ossifying fibroma of the orbit. Ophthalmology. 1998;105:591–5.
687. Jordan DR, Farmer J, DaSilva V. Psammomatoid ossifying fibroma of the orbit. Can J Ophthalmol. 1992;27:194–6.
688. Khalil MK, Leib ML. Cemento-ossifying fibroma of the orbit. Can J Ophthalmol. 1979;14:195–200.
689. Margo CE, Ragsdale BD, Perman KI, Zimmerman LE, Sweet DE. Psammomatoid (juvenile) ossifying fibroma of the orbit. Ophthalmology. 1985;92:150–9.
690. Margo CE, Weiss A, Habal MB. Psammomatoid ossifying fibroma. Arch Ophthalmol. 1986;104:1347.
691. Shields JA, Nelson LB, Brown JF, Dolinskas C. Clinical, computed tomographic, and histopathologic characteristics of juvenile ossifying fibroma with orbital involvement. Am J Ophthalmol. 1983;96:650–3.
692. Shields JA, Peyster RG, Handler SD, Augsburger JJ, Kapustiak J. Massive juvenile ossifying fibroma of maxillary sinus with orbital involvement. Br J Ophthalmol. 1985;69:392–5.
693. Tunc M, Char DH. Ossifying fibroma of the later orbital wall in an adult. Orbit. 1999;18:291–3.

Tumors of Bone: Osteoma

694. Alper M, Gurler T, Bilkay U, Songur E, Mutluer S. Intraorbital osteoma and surgical strategy. J Craniofac Surg. 1998;9:464–7.
695. Grove AS Jr. Osteomas of the orbit. Ophthalmic Surg. 1978;9:23–39.
696. Jack LS, Smith TL, Ng JD. Frontal sinus osteoma presenting with orbital emphysema. Ophthal Plast Reconstr Surg. 2009;25:155–7.
697. Lachanas VA, Koutsopoulos AV, Hajiioannou JK, et al. Osteoid osteoma of the ethmoid bone associated with dacryocystitis. Head Face Med. 2006;2:23.
698. Livaoglu M, Cakir E, Karacal N. Large orbital osteoma arising from orbital roof: excision through an upper blepharoplasty incision. Orbit. 2009;28:200–2.
699. Maiuri F, Iaconetta G, Giamundo A, Stella L, Lamaida E. Fronto-ethmoid and orbital osteomas with intracranial extension. Report of two cases. J Neurosurg Sci. 1996;40:65–70.
700. McNab AA. Orbital osteoma in Gardner's syndrome. Aust N Z J Ophthalmol. 1998;26:169–70.
701. Miller NR, Gray J, Snip R. Giant mushroom-shaped osteoma of the orbit originating from the maxillary sinus. Am J Ophthalmol. 1977;83:587–91.
702. Milman MC, Bayindir T, Akarcay M, et al. Endoscopic removal technique of a huge ethmoido-orbital osteoma. J Craniofac Surg. 2009;20:1403–6.
703. Mortada A. Orbital osteoma within the domain of ophthalmic surgery. Can J Ophthalmol. 1969;68:258–65.
704. Rawe SE, VanGilder JC. Surgical removal of orbital osteoma; case report. J Neurosurg. 1976;44:233–6.

705. Saetti R, Silvestrini M, Narne S. Ethmoid osteoma with frontal and orbital extension: endoscopic removal and reconstruction. Acta Otolaryngol. 2005;125:1122–5.
706. Selva D, Chen C, Wormald PJ. Frontoethmoidal osteoma: a stereotactic-assisted sino-orbital approach. Ophthal Plast Reconstr Surg. 2003;19:237–8.
707. Selva D, Shite VA, O'Connell JX, Rootman J. Primary bone tumor of the orbit. Surv Ophthalmol. 2004;49:328–42.
708. Whitson WE, Orcutt JC, Walkinshaw MD. Orbital osteoma in Gardner's syndrome. Am J Ophthalmol. 1986;101:236–41.
709. Wilkes SR, Trautmann JC, DeSantos LW, Campbell RJ. Osteoma: an unusual cause of amaurosis fugax. Mayo Clin Proc. 1979;54:258–60.

Tumors of Bone: Osteosarcoma

710. Anderson PM. Effectiveness of radiotherapy for osteosarcoma that responds to chemotherapy. Mayo Clin Proc. 2003;78:145–6.
711. Attili SV, Jain A, Saini KV, et al. Orbital metastasis: a rare presentation of osteosarcoma. Int Ophthalmol. 2008;28:433–6.
712. Chalvatzis NT, Kalantzis G, Manthou ME, et al. Parosteal osteosarcoma of the orbit. Ophthal Plast Reconstr Surg. 2008;24:229–31.
713. Dhir SP, Munjal VP, Jain IS, et al. Osteosarcoma of the orbit. J Pediatr Ophthalmol Strabismus. 1980;17:312–4.
714. Draper GJ, Sanders BM, Kingston JE. Second primary neoplasms in patients with retinoblastoma. Br J Cancer. 1986;53:661–71.
715. Epley KD, Lasky JB, Karesh JW. Osteosarcoma of the orbit associated with Paget disease. Ophthal Plast Reconstr Surg. 1998;14:62–6.
716. Goldberg S, Slamovits TL, Dorfman HD, et al. Sarcomatous transformation of the orbit in a patient with Paget's disease. Ophthalmology. 2000;107:1464–7.
717. Ha PK, Eisele DW, Frassica FJ, et al. Osteosarcoma of the head and neck: a review of the Johns Hopkins experience. Laryngoscope. 1999;109:964–9.
718. Hayashi T, Kuroshima Y, Yoshida K, et al. Primary osteosarcoma of the sphenoid bone with extensive periosteal extension-case report. Neurol Med Chir. 2000;40:419–22.
719. Jacob R, Abraham E, Jyothirmayi R, Nair MK. Extraskeletal osteosarcoma of the orbit. Sarcoma. 1998;2:121–4.
720. Lin PY, Chen WM, Hsieh YL, et al. Orbital metastatic osteosarcoma. J Chin Med Assoc. 2005;68:286–9.
721. Malawer MM, Helman LJ, O'Sullivan B. Sarcomas of bone. In: DeVita Jr VT, Hellman S, Rosenberg SA, editors. Cancer principles and practice of oncology. 7th ed. New York: Lippincott Williams & Wilkins; 2006. p. 1638–87.
722. Misra A, Misra S, Chaturvedi A, et al. Osteosarcoma with metastasis to the orbit. Br J Ophthalmol. 2001;85:1387–8.
723. Mohadjer Y, Wilson MW, Fuller CE, Haik BG. Primary pelvic telangiectatic osteosarcoma metastatic to both orbits. Ophthal Plast Reconstr Surg. 2004;20:77–9.
724. Parmar DN, Luthert PJ, Cree IA, et al. Two unusual osteogenic orbital tumors: presumed parosteal osteosarcomas of the orbit. Ophthalmology. 2001;108:1452–6.
725. Trevisani MG, Fry GL, Hesse RJ, et al. A rare case of orbital osteogenic sarcoma. Arch Ophthalmol. 1996;114:494–5.
726. Wenig BM, Mafee MF, Ghosh L. Fibro-osseous, osseous, and cartilaginous lesions of the orbit and paraorbital region: correlative, clinicopathologic and radiographic features, including the diagnostic role of CT and MR imaging. Radiol Clin N Am. 1998;36:1241–59.

Lacrimal Gland Tumors: Adenocarcinoma

727. Gong H, Hayashida H, Kitaoka T, Amemiya T. Ultrastructural study of primary lacrimal adenocarcinoma. Eur J Ophthalmol. 2001;11:301–5.
728. Heaps RS, Miller NR, Albert DM, et al. Primary adenocarcinoma of the lacrimal gland. Ophthalmology. 1993;100:1856–60.
729. Ishida M, Hotta M, Kushima R, et al. Case of ductal adenocarcinoma ex pleomorphic adenoma of the lacrimal gland. Rinsho Byori. 2009;57:746–51.
730. Katz SE, Rootman J, Dolman PJ, et al. Primary ductal adenocarcinoma of the lacrimal gland. Ophthalmology. 1996;103:157–62.
731. Kurisu Y, Shibayama Y, Tsuji M, et al. A case of primary ductal adenocarcinoma of the lacrimal gland: histopathological and immunohistochemical study. Pathol Res Pract. 2005;201:49–53.
732. Kim MJ, Hanmantgad S, Holdny AI. Novel management and unique pattern of primary ductal adenocarcinoma of the lacrimal gland. Clin Exp Ophthalmol. 2008;36:194–6.
733. Krishnakumar S, Subramanian N, Mahesh L, et al. Primary ductal adenocarcinoma of the lacrimal gland in a patient with neurofibromatosis. Eye. 2003;17:843–5.
734. Lee YJ, Oh YH. Primary ductal adenocarcinoma of the lacrimal gland. Jpn J Ophthalmol. 2009;53:268–70.
735. Milman T, Shields JA, Husson M, et al. Primary ductal adenocarcinoma of the lacrimal gland. Ophthalmology. 2005;112:2048–51.
736. Nasu M, Haisa T, Kondo T, Matsubara O. Primary ductal adenocarcinoma of the lacrimal gland. Pathol Int. 1998;48:981–4.
737. Shields JA, Shields CL, Epstein JA, et al. Primary epithelial malignancies of the lacrimal gland: the 2003 Ramon L. Font lecture. Ophthalmic Plast Reconstr Surg. 2004;20:10–21.

Lacrimal Gland Tumors: Adenoid Cystic Carcinoma

738. Ashton N. Epithelial tumours of the lacrimal gland. Mod Probl Ophthalmol. 1975;14:306–23.
739. Bartley GB, Harris GJ. Adenoid cystic carcinoma of the lacrimal gland: is there a cure, yet? Ophthal Plast Reconstr Surg. 2002;18:315–8.
740. Font RL, Smith SL, Bryan RG. Malignant epithelial tumors of the lacrimal gland: a clinicopathologic study of 21 cases. Arch Ophthalmol. 1998;116:613–6.
741. Galliani CA, Faught PR, Ellis FD. Adenoid cystic carcinoma of the lacrimal gland in a six-year old girl. Pediatr Pathol. 1993;13:559–65.
742. Gamel JW, Font RL. Adenoid cystic carcinoma of the lacrimal gland: the clinical significance of a basaloid histologic pattern. Hum Pathol. 1982;13:219–25.
743. Garrity JA, Henderson JW. Orbital tumors. 4th ed. Philadelphia: Lippincott Williams & Wilkins; 2007. p. 23–32.
744. Henderson JW. Adenoid cystic carcinoma of the lacrimal gland, is there a cure? Trans Am Ophthalmol Soc. 1987;85:312–9.
745. Hendrix LE, Massaro BM, Daniels DL, Smith DF, Haughton VM. Surface coil MR evaluation of a lacrimal gland carcinoma. J Comput Assist Tomogr. 1988;12:866–8.
746. Jung WS, Ahn KJ, Park MR, Kim JY, Choi JJ, Kim BS, et al. The radiological spectrum of orbital pathologies that involve the lacrimal gland and the lacrimal fossa. Korean J Radiol. 2007;8:336–42.
747. Lee AG, Phillips PH, Newman NJ, et al. Neuro-ophthalmic manifestations of adenoid cystic carcinoma. J Neuroophthalmol. 1997;17:183–8.

748. Levartovsky S, Milstein A, Nissim F, Loven D, Shani A. An unusual presentation of adenoid cystic carcinoma of the lacrimal gland. Ophthal Plast Reconstr Surg. 1993;9:47–50.
749. Mafee MF, Haik BG. Lacrimal gland and fossa lesions: role of computed tomography. Radiol Clin N Am. 1987;25:767–80.
750. Marsh JL, Wise DM, Smith M, Schwartz H. Lacrimal gland adenoid cystic carcinoma: intracranial and extracranial en bloc resection. Plast Reconstr Surg. 1981;68:577–85.
751. Meldrum ML, Tse DT, Benedetto P. Neoadjuvant intracarotid chemotherapy for treatment of advanced adenoid cystic carcinoma of the lacrimal gland. Arch Ophthalmol. 1998;116:315–21.
752. Mizokami H, Inokuchi A, Sawatsu M, et al. Adenoid cystic carcinoma of the lacrimal gland with wide and severe myoepithelial differentiation. Auris Nasus Larynx. 2002;29:77–82.
753. Naugle T Jr, Tepper DJ, Haik BG. Adenoid cystic carcinoma of the lacrimal gland: a case report. Ophthal Plast Reconstr Surg. 1994;10:45–8.
754. Portis JM, Krohl GB, Steward WB. Calcifications in lesions of the fossa of the lacrimal gland. Ophthal Plast Reconstr Surg. 1985;1:137–44.
755. Shields CL, Shields JA. Lacrimal gland tumors. Int Ophthalmol Clin. 1993;33:181–8.
756. Shields JA, Shields CL, Eagle RC Jr, Adkins J, De Potter P. Adenoid cystic carcinoma developing in the nasal orbit. Am J Ophthalmol. 1997;123:398–9.
757. Shields JA, Shields CL, Eagle RC Jr, et al. Adenoid cystic carcinoma of the lacrimal gland simulating a dermoid cyst in a 9-year-old boy. Arch Ophthalmol. 1998;116:1673–6.
758. Shields JA, Shields CL, Epstein JA, et al. Primary epithelial malignancies of the lacrimal gland: the 2003 Ramon L. Font Lecture. Ophthalmic Plast Reconstr Surg. 2004;20(1):10–21.
759. Tellado MV, McLean IW, Specht CS, Varga J. Adenoid cystic carcinomas of the lacrimal gland in childhood and adolescence. Ophthalmology. 1997;104:1622–5.
760. Tse DT, Neff AG. Recent developments in the evaluation and treatment of lacrimal gland tumors. Ophthalmol Clin N Am. 2000;13:663–81.
761. Vaidhyanath R, Kirke R, Brown L, Sampath R. Lacrimal fossa lesions: pictorial review of CT and MRI features. Orbit. 2008;27(6):410–8.
762. Wright JE, Rose GE, Garner A. Primary malignant neoplasms of the lacrimal gland. Br J Ophthalmol. 1992;76:401–7.

Lacrimal Gland Tumors: Mucoepidermoid Carcinoma

763. Carrau RL, Stillman E, Canaan RE. Mucoepidermoid carcinoma of the conjunctiva. Ophthal Plast Reconstr Surg. 1994;10:163–8.
764. Dhermy P, Pouliquen Y, Haye C, Parent A. Mucoepidermoid carcinoma of the conjunctiva. Clinical, histologic and ultrastructural study. J Fr Ophtalmol. 1983;6:553–63.
765. Dithmar S, Wojno TH, Washington C, Grossniklaus HE. Mucoepidermoid carcinoma of an accessory lacrimal gland with orbital invasion. Ophthal Plast Reconstr Surg. 2000;16:162–6.
766. Gamel JW, Eiferman RA, Guibor P. Mucoepidermoid carcinoma of the conjunctiva. Arch Ophthalmol. 1984;102:730–1.
767. Gunduz K, Shields CL, Shields JA, Mercado G, Eagle RC Jr. Intraocular neoplastic cyst from a mucoepidermoid carcinoma of the conjunctiva. Arch Ophthalmol. 1998;116:1521–3.
768. Hwang IP, Jordan DR, Brownstein S, et al. Mucoepidermoid carcinoma of the conjunctiva: a series of three cases. Ophthalmology. 2000;107:801–5.
769. Lawton AW, Karesh JW. Mucoepidermoid carcinoma of the lacrimal gland fossa: confirmation by ultrastructural study. South Med J. 1989;82:643–6.
770. Levin LA, Popham J, To K, et al. Mucoepidermoid carcinoma of the lacrimal gland. Report of a case with oncocytic features arising in a patient with chronic dacryops. Ophthalmology. 1991;98:1551–5.
771. Margo CE, Weitzenkorn DE. Mucoepidermoid carcinoma of the conjunctiva: report of a case in a 36-year-old with paranasal sinus invasion. Ophthalmic Surg. 1986;17:151–4.
772. Panda A, Sharma N, Sen S, et al. Mucoepidermoid carcinoma of the conjunctiva managed by frozen section-guided excision and lamellar keratoplasty. Clin Exp Ophthalmol. 2003;31:275–7.
773. Pulitzer DR, Eckert ER. Mucoepidermoid carcinoma of the lacrimal gland. An oxyphilic variant. Arch Ophthalmol. 1987;105:1406–9.
774. Rao NA, Font RL. Mucoepidermoid carcinoma of the conjunctiva: a clinicopathologic study of five cases. Cancer. 1976;38:1699–709.
775. Robinson JW, Brownstein S, Jordan DR, Hodge WG. Conjunctival mucoepidermoid carcinoma in a patient with ocular cicatricial pemphigoid and a review of the literature. Surv Ophthalmol. 2006;51:513–9.
776. Sofinski SJ, Brown BZ, Rao N, Wan WL. Mucoepidermoid carcinoma of the lacrimal gland. Case report and review of the literature. Ophthal Plast Reconstr Surg. 1986;2:147–51.
777. Stefanyszyn MA, Hidayat AA, Pe'er JJ, Flanagan JC. Lacrimal sac tumors. Ophthal Plast Reconstr Surg. 1994;10:169–84.
778. Ullman S, Augsburger JJ, Brady LW. Fractionated epibulbar I-125 plaque radiotherapy for recurrent mucoepidermoid carcinoma of the bulbar conjunctiva. Am J Ophthalmol. 1995;119:102–3.
779. Wagoner MD, Chuo N, Gonder JR, et al. Mucoepidermoid carcinoma of the lacrimal gland. Ann Ophthalmol. 1982;14:383–5.

Lacrimal Gland Tumors: Pleomorphic Adenoma

780. Alyahya GA, Stenman G, Persson F, et al. Pleomorphic adenoma arising in an accessory lacrimal gland of Wolfring. Ophthalmology. 2006;113:879–82.
781. Auran J, Jakobiec FA, Krebs W. Benign mixed tumor of the palpebral lobe of the lacrimal gland. Clinical diagnosis and appropriate surgical management. Ophthalmology. 1988;95:90–9.
782. Balchunas WR, Quencer RM, Byrne SF. Lacrimal gland and fossa masses: evaluation by computed tomography and A-mode echography. Radiology. 1983;149:751–8.
783. Bernardini FP, Devoto MH, Croxatto JO. Epithelial tumors of the lacrimal gland: an update. Curr Opin Ophthalmol. 2008;19:409–13.
784. Currie ZI, Rose GE. Long term risk of recurrence after intact excision of pleomorphic adenomas of the lacrimal gland. Arch Ophthalmol. 2007;1125:1643–6.
785. D'Hermies F, Mourier L, Wastl JP, et al. Palpebral form of mixed tumor of the lacrimal gland. Apropos of a case. J Fr Ophtalmol. 1992;15:220–3.
786. Faktorovitch EG, Crawford JB, Char DH, Kong C. Benign mixed tumor (pleomorphic adenoma) of the lacrimal gland in a 6-year old boy. Am J Ophthalmol. 1996;122:446–7.
787. Font RL, Gamel JW. Epithelial tumors of the lacrimal gland: an analysis of 265 cases. In: Jakobiec FA, editor. Ocular and adnexal tumors. Birmingham: Aesculapius; 1978. p. 787.
788. Gunduz K, Shields CL, Gunalp I, Shields JA. Magnetic resonance imaging of unilateral lacrimal gland lesions. Graefes Arch Clin Exp Ophthalmol. 2003;241:907–13.
789. Jakobiec FA, Trokel SL, Abbott GF, et al. Combined clinical and computed tomographic diagnosis of primary lacrimal fossa lesions. Am J Ophthalmol. 1982;94:785–807.
790. Jakobiec FA, Font RL. Lacrimal gland tumors. In: Spencer WH, Font RL, Green WR, et al., editors. Ophthalmic pathol-

ogy. An atlas and textbook. Philadelphia: WB Saunders; 1986. p. 2496–2525.
791. Lacrimal Gland Tumor Study Group. An epidemiological survey of lacrimal fossa lesions in Japan: number of patients and their sex ratio by pathological diagnosis. Jpn J Ophthalmol. 2005;49:343–8.
792. Lai T, Prabhakaran VC, Malhortra R, Selva D. Pleomorphic adenoma of the lacrimal gland: is there a role for biopsy. Eye. 2009;23:2–6.
793. Lemke AJ, Hosten N, Neumann K, Grote A, Felix R. Space-occupying lesions of the lacrimal gland in CT and MRI exemplified by 4 cases. Aktuelle Radiol. 1995;5:363–6.
794. Mercado GJ, Gunduz K, Shields CL, Shields JA, Eagle RC Jr. Pleomorphic adenoma of the lacrimal gland in a teenager. Arch Ophthalmol. 1998;116:962–3.
795. Mindlin A, Lamberts D, Barsky D. Mixed lacrimal gland tumor arising in ectopic lacrimal gland tissue. J Pediatr Ophthalmol. 1977;14:44–7.
796. Rose GE, Wright JE. Pleomorphic adenoma of the lacrimal gland. Br J Ophthalmol. 1992;76:395–400.
797. Shields CL, Shields JA. Review of lacrimal gland lesions. Trans Pa Acad Ophthalmol Otolaryngol. 1990;42:925–30.
798. Tong JT, Flanagan JC, Eagle RC Jr, Mazzoli RA. Benign mixed tumor arising from an accessory lacrimal gland of Wolfring. Ophthal Plast Reconstr Surg. 1995;11:136–8.
799. Verma K, Kapila K. Role of the aspiration cytology in diagnosis of pleomorphic adenomas. Cytopathology. 2002;13:121–7.
800. Weis E, Rootman J, Joly TJ, et al. Epithelial lacrimal gland tumors: pathologic classification and current understanding. Arch Ophthalmol. 2009;127:1016–28.

Metastatic Tumors: Breast Carcinoma

801. Bullock JD, Yanes B. Ophthalmic manifestations of metastatic breast cancer. Ophthalmology. 1980;87:961–73.
802. Burmeister BH, Benjamin CS, Childs WJ. The management of metastases to the eye and orbit from carcinoma of the breast. Aust N Z J Ophthalmol. 1990;18:187–90.
803. Char DH, Miller T, Kroll S. Orbital metastases: diagnosis and course. Br J Ophthalmol. 1997;81:386–90.
804. Crown J. Evolution in the treatment of advanced breast cancer. Semin Oncol. 1998;25:12–7.
805. Font RL, Ferry AP. Carcinoma metastatic to the eye and orbit III. A clinicopathologic study of 28 cases metastatic to the orbit. Cancer. 1976;38:1326–35.
806. Freedman MI, Folk JC. Metastatic tumors to the eye and orbit. Patient survival and clinical characteristics. Arch Ophthalmol. 1987;105:1215–9.
807. Garcia GH, Weinberg DA, Glasgow BJ, et al. Carcinoma of the male breast to both orbits. Ophthal Plast Reconstr Surg. 1998;14:130–3.
808. Hesselionk JR, Davis KR, Weber AL, et al. Radiological evaluation of orbital metastases, with emphasis on computed tomography. Radiology. 1980;137:363–6.
809. Kuo SC, Hsiao SC, Chiou CC, et al. Metastatic carcinoma of the breast: a case with the unusual presentation of unilateral periorbital edema. Jpn J Ophthalmol. 2008;52:305–7.
810. Manor RS. Enophthalmos caused by orbital metastatic breast carcinoma. Acta Ophthalmol. 1974;52:881–4.
811. Milman T, Pliner L, Lnager PD. Breast carcinoma metastatic to the orbit: an unusually late presentation. Ophthal Plast Reconstr Surg. 2008;24:480–2.
812. Peyster RG, Shapiro MD, Haik BG. Orbital metastasis: role of magnetic resonance imaging and computed tomography. Radiol Clin N Am. 1987;25:647–62.
813. Po SM, Custer PL, Smith ME. Bilateral lagophthalmos. An unusual presentation of metastatic breast carcinoma. Arch Ophthalmol. 1996;114:1139–41.
814. Ratanatharathorn V, Powers WE, Grimm J, et al. Eye metastasis from carcinoma of the breast: diagnosis, radiation treatment and results. Cancer Treat Rev. 1991;18:261–76.
815. Reeves D, Levine MR, Lash R. Nonpalpable breast carcinoma presenting as orbital infiltration: case presentation and literature review. Ophthal Plast Reconstr Surg. 2002;18:84–8.
816. Reifler DM, Davison P. Histochemical analysis of metastatic breast carcinoma to the orbit. Ophthalmology. 1986;93:254–9.
817. Shields CL, Shields JA. Metastatic tumors of the orbit. Int Ophthalmol Clin. 1993;33:189–202.
818. Shields CL, Shields JA, Peggs M. Tumors metastatic to the orbit. Ophthalmic Reconstr Plast Surg. 1988;4:73–80.
819. Shields CL, Stopyra GA, Marr BP, Moster ML, Shields JA. Enophthalmos as initial manifestation of occult, mammogram-negative carcinoma of the breast. Ophthalmic Surg Lasers Imaging. 2004;35:56–7.
820. Stephanyszyn MA, DeVita EG, Flanagan JC. Breast carcinoma metastatic to the orbit. Ophthal Plast Reconstr Surg. 1987;3:43–7.
821. Valenzuela AA, Archibald CW, Fleming B, et al. Orbital metastasis: clinical features, management and outcome. Orbit. 2009;28:153–9.
822. Watkins LM, Rubin PA. Metastatic tumors of the eye and orbit. Int Ophthalmol Clin. 1998;38:117–28.

Metastatic Tumors: Bronchogenic Carcinoma

823. Ahmad SM, Esmaeli B. Metastatic tumors of the orbit and ocular adnexa. Curr Opin Ophthalmol. 2007;18:405–13.
824. Buys R, Abramson DH, Kitchin FD, Gottielb F, Epstein M. Simultaneous ocular and orbital involvement from metastatic bronchogenic carcinoma. Ann Ophthalmol. 1982;14:1165–7, 1170–1.
825. Campling BE, El-Deiny WS. Clinical implication of p53 mutations. In: Driscoll B, editor. Lung cancer: methods in molecular medicine. 2nd ed. Totowa: Humana Press; 2003. p. 57–77.
826. Dunaway RL. Ptosis as the presenting sign of orbital involvement from metastatic bronchogenic carcinoma. Am J Optom Physiol Optic. 1985;62:908–12.
827. Ferry AP, Font RL. Carcinoma metastatic to the orbit. Mod Probl Ophthalmol. 1975;14:377–81.
828. Ferry AP, Naghdi MR. Bronchogenic carcinoma metastatic to the orbit. Arch Ophthalmol. 1967;77:214–6.
829. Jordan DR, Lee-Wing MW. Metastatic large-cell lung carcinoma to the orbit in a 25-year-old nonsmoker. Ophthalmic Surg Lasers. 2002;33:488–90.
830. Macedo JE, Machado M, Araujo A, et al. Orbital metastasis as a rare form of clinical presentation of nonsmall cell lung cancer. J Thorac Oncol. 2007;2:166–7.
831. Shields JA, Shields CL, Eagle RC Jr, Lin B. Diffuse ocular metastases as an initial sign of metastatic lung cancer. Ophthalmic Surg Lasers. 1998;29:598–601.
832. Spaide RF, Granger E, Hammer BD, Negron FJ, Paglen PG. Rapidly expanding exophthalmos: as unusual presentation of small cell lung cancer. Br J Ophthalmol. 1989;73:461–2.
833. Tibolt RE, Meyer DR, Wobig JL. Small-cell carcinoma metastatic to the lacrimal gland. Arch Ophthalmol. 1991;109:921–2.
834. Whyte AM. Bronchogenic carcinoma metastasizing to the orbit. A case report. J Maxillofac Surg. 1978;6:277–80.

Metastatic Tumors: Malignant Melanoma

835. Conill C, Morilla I, Malvehy J, et al. Secondary orbital metastases from cutaneous melanoma. Melanoma Res. 2004;14:437–8.
836. Coppeto JR, Jaffe R, Gillies CG. Primary orbital melanoma. Arch Ophthalmol. 1978;96:2255–8.
837. Di Bernardo C, Pacheco EM, Hughes JR, Iliff WJ, Byrne SF. Echographic evaluation and findings in metastatic melanoma to extraocular muscles. Ophthalmology. 1996;103:1794–7.
838. Drummond SR, Fenton S, Pantilidis EP, et al. A case of cutaneous melanoma metastatic to the right eye and left orbit. Eye. 2003;17:420–2.
839. Dutton JJ, Anderson RL, Schelper RL, et al. Orbital malignant melanoma and oculodermal melanocytosis. Report of two cases and review of the literature. Ophthalmology. 1984;91:497–505.
840. Folberg R, McLean IW, Zimmerman LE. Malignant melanoma of the conjunctiva. Hum Pathol. 1985;16:136–43.
841. Gonder JR, Shields JA, Albert DM, et al. Uveal malignant melanoma associated with ocular and oculodermal melanocytosis. Ophthalmology. 1982;89:953–60.
842. Gunduz K, Shields JA, Shields CL, Eagle RC Jr. Periorbital cellular blue nevus leading to orbitopalpebral and intracranial melanoma. Ophthalmology. 1998;105:2046–50.
843. Henderson JW, Farrow GM. Malignant melanoma primary in the orbit. Report of a case. Trans Am Acad Ophthalmol Otolaryngol. 1972;76:1487–90.
844. Jakobiec FA, Ellsworth RM, Tannenbaum M. Primary orbital melanoma. Am J Ophthalmol. 1974;78:24–39.
845. Mahoney NR, Engleman T, Morgenstern KE. Primary malignant melanoma of the orbit in an African-American man. Ophthal Plast Reconstr Surg. 2008;24:475–7.
846. Odashiro AN, Arthurs B, Pereira PR, et al. Primary orbital melanoma associated with a blue nevus. Ophthal Plast Reconstr Surg. 2005;21:247–8.
847. Orcutt JC, Char DH. Melanoma metastatic to the orbit. Ophthalmology. 1988;95:1033–7.
848. Paridaens AD, McCartney AC, Minassian DC, Hungerford JL. Orbital exenteration in 95 cases of primary conjunctival malignant melanoma. Br J Ophthalmol. 1994;78:520–8.
849. Rini FJ, Jakobiec FA, Hornblass A, Beckman BL, Anderson RL. The treatment of advanced choroidal melanoma with massive orbital extension. Am J Ophthalmol. 1987;104:634–40.
850. Rosenberg C, Finger PT. Cutaneous malignant melanoma metastatic to the eye, lids, and orbit. Surv Ophthalmol. 2008;53:187–202.
851. Scott IU, Murray TG, Hughes JR. Evaluation of imaging techniques for detection of extraocular extension of choroidal melanoma. Arch Ophthalmol. 1998;116:897–9.
852. Shields JA, Sheilds CL. Massive orbital extension of posterior uveal melanomas. Ophthal Plast Reconstr Surg. 1991;7:238–51.
853. Shields JA, Shields CL. Current management of posterior uveal melanoma. Mayo Clin Proc. 1993;68:1196–200.
854. Shields JA, Shields CL. Orbital malignant melanoma. The 2002 Sean B. Murphy Lecture. Ophthal Plast Reconstr Surg. 2003;19:62–9.
855. Shields JA, Perez N, Shields CL, et al. Orbital melanoma metastatic from contralateral choroid: management by complete surgical resection. Ophthalmic Surg Lasers. 2002;33:416–20.
856. Spencer WH. Optic nerve extension of intraocular neoplasms. Am J Ophthalmol. 1975;80:465–71.
857. Tellada M, Specht CS, McLean IW, Grossniklaus HE, Zimmerman LE. Primary orbital melanomas. Ophthalmology. 1996;103:929–32.
858. Zografos L, Ducrey N, Beati D, et al. Metastatic melanoma in the eye and orbit. Ophthalmology. 2003;110:2245–56.

Secondary Tumors: Basal Cell Adenocarcinoma

859. Barnes L, Eveson JW, Reichart P, Sidransky D. Pathology and genetics of tumours of the head and neck. In: World Health Organization classification of tumours, vol. 9. Lyon: IARC Press; 2005.
860. Buchholz TA, Laramore GE, Griffin BR, Koh W-J, Griffin TW. The role of fast neutron radiation therapy in the management of advanced salivary gland malignant neoplasms. Cancer. 1992;69:2779–88.
861. Buchner A, Merrell PW, Carpenter WM. Relative frequency of intra-oral minor salivary gland tumors: a study of 380 cases from northern California and comparison to reports from other parts of the world. J Oral Pathol Med. 2007;36:207–14.
862. Ellis GL, Auclair PL. Tumor of the salivary glands. In: AFIP Atlas of tumor pathology. Fourth series. Fasc 9. Washington: Armed Forces Institute of Pathology; 2008. p. 269–81.
863. Ellis GL, Wiscovitch JG. Basal cell adenocarcinomas of the major salivary glands. Oral Surg Oral Med Oral Pathol. 1990;69:461–9.
864. Font RL, Gamel JW. Epithelial tumors of the lacrimal gland. In: Jakobiec FA, editor. Ocular and adnexal tumors. Birmingham: Aesculapius; 1978. p. 787–805.
865. Forrest AW. Epithelial lacrimal gland tumors: pathology as a guide to prognosis. Trans Am Acad Ophthalmol Otolaryngol. 1954;58:848–65.
866. Garrity JA, Henderson JW. Primary epithelial neoplasms. In: Garrity JA, Henderson JW, Cameron JD, editors. Henderson's orbital tumors. 4th ed. Philadelphia: Lippincott Williams and Wilkins; 2007. p. 279–96.
867. Hirai H, Harada H, Okada N, et al. A case of basal cell adenocarcinoma of the upper gingival. Oral Surg Oral Med Oral Pathol Oral Radiol Endod. 2009;107:542–6.
868. Jakobiec FA, Font RL. Orbit. In: Spencer WH, editor. Ophthalmic pathology. An atlas and textbook, vol. 3. 3rd ed. Philadelphia: WB Saunders; 1986. p. 2459–860.
869. Khalil M, Arthurs B. Basal cell adenocarcinoma of the lacrimal gland. Ophthalmology. 2000;107:164–8.
870. Muller S, Barner L. Basal cell adenocarcinoma of the salivary glands: report of seven cases and review of the literature. Cancer. 1996;78:2471–7.
871. Parashar P, Baron E, Papadimitriou JC, et al. Basal cell adenocarcinoma of the oral minor salivary glands: review of the literature and presentation of two cases. Oral Surg Oral Med Oral Pathol Oral Radiol Endod. 2007;103:77–84.
872. Raslan WF, Leonetti JP, Sawyer DR. Basal cell adenocarcinoma of the parotid gland: a case report with immunohistochemical, ultrastructural findings and review of the literature. Oral Maxillofac Surg. 1995;53:1456–62.
873. Sanders TE, Ackerman LV, Zimmerman LE. Epithelial tumors of the lacrimal gland. A comparison of the pathologic and clinical behavior with those of the salivary glands. Am J Surg. 1962;104:657–65.
874. Shields CL, Shields JA, Eagle RC, Rathmell JP. Clinicopathologic review of 142 cases of lacrimal gland lesions. Ophthalmologica. 1989;96:431–5.
875. Speight PM, Barrett AW. Salivary gland tumours. Oral Dis. 2002;8:229–40.
876. Tilakaratne WM, Jaysooriya PR, Tennakoon TMPB, Saku T. Epithelial salivary tumors in Sri Lanka: a retrospective study of 713 cases. Oral Maxillofac Pathol. 2009;108:90–8.
877. Ward BK, Seethala RR, Barnes EL, Lai SY. Basal cell adenocarcinoma of a hard palate minor salivary gland: case report and review of the literature. Head Neck Oncol. 2009;1(1):31. [Epub ahead of print].
878. Wright JE, Rose GE. Primary malignant neoplasms of the lacrimal gland. Br J Ophthalmol. 1992;76:401–7.

Secondary Tumors: Basal Cell Carcinoma

879. Aurora AL, Blodi FC. Lesions of the eyelids. A clinicopathologic study. Surv Ophthalmol. 1970;15:94–104.
880. Baker HE, Berry-Brincat A, Zaki I, Cheung D. Three different consecutive manifestations of BCC in the same patient: presenting first as ectropion, then entropion, and finally medial canthal dystopia with epicanthus inversus. Orbit. 2008;19:1154–8.
881. Doxanas MT, Green WR, Iliff CE. Factors in the successful management of basal cell carcinoma of the eyelids. Am J Ophthalmol. 1981;91:726–36.
882. Gunalp I, Gunduz K. Secondary orbital tumors. Ophthal Plast Reconstr Surg. 1997;13:31–5.
883. Hornblass A, Rosen JL. A combined facial, orbital, and intracranial resection of extensive basal cell carcinoma arising in the eyelid. Ophthalmic Surg. 1985;16:769–73.
884. Karcioglu ZA. al-Hussain H, Svedberg AH. Cystic basal cell carcinoma of the orbit and eyelids. Ophthal Plast Reconstr Surg. 1998;14:134–40.
885. Katirciuglu YA, Yildiz EH, Kocaoglu FA, et al. Basal cell carcinoma in the lacrimal sac. Orbit. 2007;26:303–7.
886. Kleydman Y, Manolidis S, Ratner D. Basal cell carcinoma with intracranial invasion. J Am Acad Dermatol. 2009;60:1045–9.
887. Leshin B, Yeatts P, Anscher M, Montano G, Dutton JJ. Management of periocular basal cell carcinoma: Moths' micrographic surgery versus radiotherapy. Surv Ophthalmol. 1993;38:193–212.
888. Lindgren G, Lark O. Long-term follow-up of cryosurgery of basal cell carcinoma of the eyelids. J Am Acad Dermatol. 1997;36:742–6.
889. Margo CE, Waltz K. Basal cell carcinoma of the eyelids and periorbital skin. Surv Ophthalmol. 1993;38:169–92.
890. McDougall AL, Chaplin AJ, Jones RL. Infiltration of the supraorbital nerve by basal cell carcinoma. Am J Dermatol Pathol. 1983;5:381–4.
891. Ly O, Lane CM. Eyelid contracture may indicate recurrent basal cell carcinoma, even after Mohs' micrographic surgery. Orbit. 2009;28:29–33.
892. Payne J, Duke J, Butner R, et al. Basal cell carcinoma of the eyelids. A long-term follow-up study. Arch Ophthalmol. 1969;81:553–8.
893. Selva D, Hale L, Bouskill K, et al. Recurrent morphoeic basal cell carcinoma at the lateral canthus with orbitocranial invasion. Aust J Dermatol. 2003;44:126–8.
894. Shah HA, Lee HB, Nunery WR. Neglected basal cell carcinoma in a schizophrenic patient. Ophthal Plast Reconstr Surg. 2008;24:495–7.
895. Sigurdsson H, Agnarsson BA. Basal cell carcinoma of the eyelid. Risk of recurrence according to adequacy of surgical margins. Acta Ophthalmol Scand. 1998;76:477–80.
896. Steinkogler FJ, Schoda CD. The necessity of long-term follow up after surgery for basal cell carcinomas of the eyelid. Ophthalmic Surg. 1993;24:755–8.
897. Stefanous S. Five-year cycle of basal cell carcinoma management re-audit. Orbit. 2009;28:264–9.
898. Weimar VM, Ceilley RI. Basal cell carcinoma of the medial canthus with invasion of supraorbital and supratrochlear nerves: report of a case treated by Mohs' technique. J Dermatol Surg Oncol. 1979;5:279–82.

Secondary Tumors: Inverted Papilloma

899. Anderson KK, Lessner AM, Hood I, et al. Invasive transitional cell carcinoma of the lacrimal sac arising in an inverted papilloma. Arch Ophthalmol. 1994;112:306–7.
900. Bajaj MS, Pushker N. Inverted papilloma invading the orbit. Orbit. 2002;21:155–9.
901. Elner VM, Burnstine MA, Goodman ML, Dortzbach RK. Inverted papillomas that invade the orbit. Arch Ophthalmol. 1995;113:1178–83.
902. Golub JS, Parikh SL, Budnick SD, et al. Inverted papilloma of the nasolacrimal system invading the orbit. Ophthal Plast Reconstr Surg. 2007;23:151–3.
903. Gomez JA, Mendenhall WM, Tannehill SP, et al. Radiation therapy in inverted papillomas of the nasal cavity and paranasal sinuses. Am J Otolaryngol. 2000;21:174–8.
904. Karcioglu ZA, Wesley RE, Greenidge KC, McCord CD. Proptosis and pseudocyst formation from inverted papilloma. Ann Ophthalmol. 1982;14:443–8.
905. Klimek T, Atai E, Schubert M, Glanz H. Inverted papilloma of the nasal cavity and paranasal sinuses: clinical data, surgical strategy and recurrence rates. Acta Otolaryngol. 2000;120:267–72.
906. Krouse JH. Endoscopic treatment of inverted papilloma: safety and efficacy. Am J Otolaryngol. 2001;22:87–99.
907. Lawson W, Kaufman MR, Biller HF. Treatment outcomes in the management of inverted papilloma: an analysis of 160 cases. Laryngoscope. 2003;113:1548–56.
908. Macdonald MR, Le KT, Freeman J, et al. A majority of inverted sinonasal papillomas carries Epstein-Barr virus genomes. Cancer. 1995;75:2307–12.
909. Moss AL. Inverted papilloma of the nose: an unusual cause of a medial canthal mass. Br J Plast Surg. 1983;36:254–7.
910. Perez-Ordonez B. Hamartomas, papillomas, and adenocarcinomas of the sinonasal tract and nasopharynx. J Clin Pathol. 2009;62:1085–95.
911. Raemdonck TY, Van den Broecke CM, Claerhout I, Decock CE. Inverted papilloma arising primarily from the lacrimal sac. Orbit. 2009;28:181–4.

Secondary Tumors: Nasopharyngeal Carcinoma

912. Au JS, Law CK, Foo W, Lau WH. In-depth evaluation of the AJCC/UICC 1997 staging system of nasopharyngeal carcinoma: prognostic homogeneity and proposed refinements. Int J Radiat Oncol Biol Phys. 2003;56:413–26.
913. Bass IS, Haller JO, Berdon WE, et al. Nasopharyngeal carcinoma: clinical and radiographic findings in children. Radiology. 1985;156:651–4.
914. Bernardini FP, Croxatto JO, Orcioni GF, Bianchi S. Visual loss secondary to orbital apex invasion as the first manifestation of recurrent nasopharyngeal carcinoma. Ophthal Plast Reconstr Surg. 2009;25:248–50.
915. Hsu MM, Tsu SM. Nasopharyngeal carcinoma in Taiwan. Clinical manifestations and results of therapy. Cancer. 1983;52:362–8.
916. Hsu WM, Wang AG. Nasopharyngeal carcinoma with orbital invasion. Eye. 2004;18:833–8.
917. King AD, Ma BB, Yau YY, et al. The impact of 18 F-FDG PET/CT on assessment of nasopharyngeal carcinoma at diagnosis. Br J Radiol. 2008;81:291–8.
918. Lee KYC, Seah LL, Tow S, et al. Nasopharyngeal carcinoma with orbital involvement. Ophthal Plast Reconstr Surg. 2008;24:185–9.
919. Pathmanathan R, Prasad U, Chandrika G, et al. Undifferentiated, nonkeratinizing, and squamous cell carcinoma of the nasopharynx. Variants of Epstein-Barr virus-infected neoplasia. Am J Pathol. 1995;146:1355–67.
920. Sham JS, Choy D. Prognostic factors of nasopharyngeal carcinoma: a review of 759 patients. Br J Radiol. 1990;63:51–8.
921. Zhang H, Yan JH, Wu ZY, Li YP. Clinical analysis of orbital metastasis from nasopharyngeal carcinoma. Zhonghua Yan Ke Za Zhi. 2006;42:318–22.

Secondary Tumors: Squamous Cell Carcinoma

922. Carrillo JF, Guemes A, Ramirez-Ortega MC, Onate-Ocana LF. Prognostic factors in maxillary sinus and nasal cavity carcinoma. Eur J Surg Oncol. 2005;31:1206–12.
923. Cook BE Jr, Bartley GB. Treatment options and future prospects for the management of eyelid malignancies: an evidence based update. Ophthalmology. 2001;108:2088–100.
924. De Keizer RJ, Padberg GW, de Wolff-Rouendaal D. Superior orbital fissure syndrome caused by intraorbital spread of cutaneous squamous cell carcinoma and not detected on computed tomography and magnetic resonance imaging. Jpn J Ophthalmol. 1997;41:104–10.
925. Dulguerov P, Jacobsen MS, Allal AS, et al. Nasal and paranasal sinus carcinoma: are we making progress? A series of 220 patients and a systematic review. Cancer. 2001;92:3012–29.
926. Finger PT, Tran HV, Turbin RE, et al. High-frequency ultrasonographic evaluation of conjunctival intraepithelial neoplasia and squamous cell carcinoma. Arch Ophthalmol. 2003;121:168–72.
927. Gokmen SH, Ardic F. Malignant conjunctival tumors invading the orbit. Ophthalmologica. 2008;222:338–43.
928. Howard GR, Nerad JA, Carter KD, et al. Clinical characteristics associated with orbital invasion of cutaneous basal cell and squamous cell tumors of the eyelid. Am J Ophthalmol. 1992;113:123–33.
929. Johnson TE, Tabbara KF, Weatherhead RG, et al. Secondary squamous cell carcinoma of the orbit. Arch Ophthalmol. 1997;115:75–8.
930. Johnson LN, Krohel GB, Yeon EB, Parnes SM. Sinus tumors invading the orbit. Ophthalmology. 1984;91(3):209–17.
931. Limawararut V, Hoyama E, Selva D, Davis G. Squamous cell carcinoma presenting as an orbital cyst with radiologic evidence of perineural invasion. Eur J Ophthalmol. 2007;17:970–2.
932. Limawararut V, Leibovitch I, Sullivan T, Selva D. Periocular squamous cell carcinoma. Clin Exp Ophthalmol. 2007;35:174–85.
933. Malhatra R, Huilgol SC, Huynh NT, et al. The Australian Mohs database. Periocular squamous cell carcinoma. Ophthalmology. 2004;111:617–23.
934. McCord CD Jr, Cavanagh HD. Microscopic features and biologic behavior of eyelid tumors. Ophthalmic Surg. 1980;11:671–81.
935. McNab AA, Francis JC, Benger R, et al. Perineural spread of cutaneous squamous cell carcinoma via the orbit. Clinical features and outcome in 21 cases. Ophthalmology. 1997;104:1457–62.
936. Nemzek WR, Hecht S, Gandour-Edwards R, et al. Perineural spread of head and neck tumors: how accurate is MR imaging? Am J Neuroradiol. 1998;19:701–6.
937. Nguyen J, Ivan D, Esmaeli B. Conjunctival squamous cell carcinoma in the anophthalmic socket. Ophthal Plast Reconstr Surg. 2008;24:98–101.
938. Nieto EJ, Medel JR, Huguet RP. Undiagnosed squamous cell carcinoma of the forehead presenting as a Tolosa-Hunt syndrome. Orbit. 2009;28:290–2.
939. Soysal HG, Markoc F. Invasive squamous cell carcinoma of the eyelids and periorbital region. Br J Ophthalmol. 2007;91:325–9.
940. Veness MJ, Biankin S. Perineural spread leading to orbital invasion from skin cancer. Australas Radiol. 2000;44:296–302.

Pathogenesis and Medical Management of Thyroid Eye Disease

57

Anaïs L. Carniciu and Alon Kahana

Introduction

Thyroid eye disease (TED) is caused by an inflammatory process involving the orbit and periorbital tissues in the setting of autoimmune thyroiditis. TED has been shown not only to impact visual and social functioning but also to reduce patients' quality of life [1, 2]. Thyroid dysfunction in TED most frequently involves hyperthyroidism secondary to Graves' disease (GD); hypothyroidism secondary to Hashimoto's thyroiditis, or subclinical inflammation, are involved less commonly [3]. Approximately 25–50% of patients with GD will develop clinically apparent TED some time during their lifetime. Sight-threatening disease is infrequent and occurs in approximately 3–5% of patients [4, 5]. In contrast, subclinical manifestations, including radiographic evidence of enlargement of extraocular muscles, may be present in a larger subset of patients [5, 6]. Regardless of whether thyroid gland dysfunction or TED presents first, the other manifestation usually becomes apparent within 18 months [7]. Additionally, it has been shown that the phenotype of TED is similar regardless of the underlying thyroid disease [8]. Since the disease can coexist with hyper-, hypo-, and euthyroid endocrine states, the direct role of endocrine dysfunction in the pathogenesis of TED is controversial. It is generally accepted, however, that normalization of the endocrine disease is a prerequisite to proper control and management of the ophthalmopathy [9].

Although the term "TED" is used in this chapter to discuss this inflammatory process, there is currently no universally accepted nomenclature for this disorder. Various descriptors, including "Graves'," "thyroid," or "thyroid-associated," are typically combined with the terms "orbitopathy," "ophthalmopathy," or "eye disease." We have selected to use the term TED throughout this chapter for clarity and consistency, although the term "thyroid-associated orbitopathy" may be the more accurate term.

The clinical features of TED are well-documented and include eyelid retraction, periorbital edema and erythema, exophthalmos, chemosis, expansion of orbital fat, orbital congestion, and infiltration and enlargement/fibrosis of extraocular muscles. The combination of these features often causes facial disfigurement. Additionally, these changes may lead to secondary ophthalmic manifestations, including increased intraocular pressure, exposure keratopathy and dry eye, chronic conjunctivitis, restrictive strabismus/diplopia, orbital pressure pain, and compressive optic neuropathy. While reconstructive surgery can achieve at least partial restoration of form and function, the ultimate goal of treatment is to halt the disease process in its early stages and possibly avoid the onset of TED altogether.

Variability in clinical presentation is a hallmark of TED. Some patients experience only mild ocular discomfort, while others experience significant vision loss. Despite this considerable heterogeneity, the clinical course of TED is biphasic and can be divided into active versus inactive, or stable, disease. Active disease exhibits time-dependent changes in the clinical features and prominent immune infiltration of the orbit. Rarely, loss of sight from optic nerve compression complicates active disease. Active disease can be targeted by medical therapy and typically lasts from 6 months to 2 years, though it may persist longer in smokers. The stable phase follows, during which proptosis, eyelid retraction, and restrictive strabismus remain unchanged or, rarely, improve. In stable disease, inflammation and its associated symptoms resolve, although ocular exposure and some measure of orbital congestion with pressure pain may remain. Although active TED is self-limiting, there is a 5–10% risk of recurrence in patients who were previously

A. L. Carniciu · A. Kahana (✉)
Consultants in Ophthalmic and Facial Plastic Surgery, Southfield, MI, USA
e-mail: akahana@facialworks.com

J. J. Servat et al. (eds.), *Smith and Nesi's Ophthalmic Plastic and Reconstructive Surgery*,
https://doi.org/10.1007/978-3-030-41720-8_57

quiescent, particularly in smokers or in patients with unstable endocrine disease [9–12].

The choice and timing of medical treatment in patients with autoimmune thyroiditis are well-known to affect the clinical course of TED. Various treatment options for TED have been utilized, ranging from medical to surgical depending on the severity of the disease. Overall, the high prevalence of TED and its significant impact on visual function and quality of life make it a high priority for research and improved approaches to treatment [13].

Pathogenesis

The pathogenesis of TED has yet to be fully elucidated. Susceptibility genes and environmental factors alike predispose individuals to both thyroid gland dysfunction and TED. Cigarette smoking, a modifiable environmental risk factor, has the strongest association between an acquired factor and the development and progression of TED. Smokers exhibit more severe TED with a more aggressive disease process following radioactive iodine thyroid ablation and may be less responsive to treatment [14–16]. The detrimental effect of smoking on TED is dose-dependent [17] and has been demonstrated to also worsen the course of other autoimmune diseases as well [18–21]. Potential mechanisms for the impact of smoking on TED include generation of free radicals and hypoxia within orbital tissues in close proximity to the sinuses, as well as increasing glycosaminoglycan production, adipogenesis, and expression of adhesion molecules and cytokines such as IL-1 and HLA–DR in orbital fibroblasts [15, 22, 23]. Genetic factors contribute to susceptibility to both GD and TED, as evidenced by increased concordance among monozygotic twins [24–26]. Identification of specific genetic modifications in GD and TED is an ongoing process. Major histocompatibility complex (MHC) class II, protein tyrosine phosphatase-22, CD40, cytotoxic T-lymphocyte antigen 4 (CTLA4), FOXP3, MCP/CCL12, and IL-12 are each thought to have a role in disease development [26–31]. Research is ongoing to determine the underlying genetic factors that could distinguish the patients that develop TED from those who manifest GD without orbital pathology. Though no specific factors have yet received consistent support, there is a potential for certain genetic haplotypes to play a role in modulating the clinical phenotype of orbitopathy in GD [32].

GD, both with and without TED, is more common in women, with female to male incidence rates of approximately 10:1 [33, 34]. However, men with GD may develop a more severe version of TED. Radioiodine ablation of the thyroid gland is associated with worsening of TED in at least 10–15% of patients [35, 36]. Untreated hypothyroidism resulting from radioiodine ablation may increase the risk of developing TED or enhance its progression. Therefore, maintenance of a euthyroid state is important [35, 37, 38].

Immunology

Adults normally exhibit immunologic tolerance to antigens that are recognized as "self." Autoimmune thyroid disease is marked by the development of antibodies against thyroid-related antigens and exists on an immunologic spectrum marked by a collection of antibodies that can either activate (GD) or inhibit (Hashimoto's) thyroid gland function [39]. In GD, loss of immunologic tolerance leads to the development of autoantibodies stereotypically targeting the thyrotropin receptor (TSHR) [40]. Thyroid-stimulating antibodies (e.g., TSI) bind to and activate TSHR, leading to stimulation of thyroid hormone synthesis that is uncoupled from the hypothalamic-pituitary axis [41]. Detecting these antibodies can be useful in cases of the euthyroid ophthalmopathy or when the diagnosis of GD is uncertain [42]. In addition to TSI, blocking antibodies can also bind TSHR. Laboratory testing currently in use to identify the presence of these antibodies includes the thyroid-stimulating hormone-binding inhibiting immunoglobulin assay, which identifies TSHR autoantibodies in a competitive manner, and the thyroid-stimulating immunoglobulin assay, which measures the biologic activity of the stimulating TSHR antibodies [42]. Other autoantibodies frequently encountered in GD include antibodies against thyroglobulin (TG) and thyroid peroxidase (TPO), though these are nonspecific and are commonly found in patients with Hashimoto's thyroiditis [43]. Interestingly, although they are not predictive of TED, anti-TPO and anti-TG antibodies are positive in the presence of ophthalmopathy in 90% and 50% of patients, respectively [44, 45]. Recent discovery that patients with GD have antibodies against the insulin-like growth factor-1 (IGF-1) receptor has led to the testing of drugs that target this pathway as potential modulators of disease activity [46].

The active phase of TED is characterized by inflamed orbital and periorbital fatty connective tissue with a shared embryologic origin in the neural crest [47]. The inflammatory process appears to be driven by orbital infiltration of lymphocytes and other bone marrow-derived cells [48, 49]. Examination under electron and light microscopy demonstrates integrity of extraocular muscle cells early in the disease. Microscopy reveals infiltration of T lymphocytes, mast cells, and occasional B lymphocytes in between cells [50–54]. These findings suggest that connective tissues and not extraocular muscles represent the primary immune targets in active TED [40, 55, 56]. Affected orbital tissues demonstrate cytokine activity involving interferon-γ (IFN-γ), tumor necrosis factor-α (TNF-α), interleukin-1α (IL-1α), interleukin-1β (IL-1 β), and monocyte chemoattractant protein-1 (MCP1/CCL2), which are produced by infiltrating mononuclear cells and fibroblasts [40, 57]. These cytokines subsequently mediate T lymphocyte and fibroblast interactions which promote the synthesis of extracellular matrix proteins and fibroblast differentiation and proliferation [58–60].

In addition to inflammation and fibrosis, expansion of orbital tissues has also been ascribed to deposition of hyaluronan and to increased adipogenesis [52, 61–65]. These processes occur through the stimulation of the TSHR and a second receptor, insulin-like growth factor-1 receptor (IGF-1R), which is present at higher levels in orbital fibroblasts than in fibroblasts in other parts of the body. IGF-1R stimulation may lead to adipogenesis, hyaluronan synthesis, and production of the chemokines which may facilitate lymphocyte trafficking into the orbit [66]. The association between the insulin growth factor-1 (IGF-1) pathway, inflammation, and thyroid eye disease has recently been proposed [67–71]. It is thought that IGF-1R may be involved in TED via its interactions with anti-IGF-1R antibodies generated in GD, complex formation with TSHR, and regulation of downstream signaling [71–73].

Following the active phase inflammation, TED enters the fibrotic phase [74–76]. The mechanism involved in dampening inflammation in the orbit remains uncertain but could reflect a shift in cytokine profiles. Specifically, Th1 cytokines (IFN-γ, IL-2, TNF-α) may dominate the cytokine milieu during active disease, while Th2 cytokines (IL-4, IL-5, and IL-13) may become more abundant as the orbitopathy becomes less inflamed and more fibrotic [77, 78]. Shifts in the cytokine environment may alter immune cell trafficking, promoting tissue fibrosis [40, 79]. Other factors that may affect the transition from active to stable disease include reduced autoantigen abundance or presentation [80, 81]. The absence of lymphoid structures and lack of lymphoid neogenesis in the orbit may also contribute to this transition, unlike autoimmune processes where sustained immune reactivity might derive from more complete lymphoid structures and function [40]. Although the clinical picture of TED overwhelmingly presents with fibrotic disease that follows a period of active inflammation, there have been reports of progressive fibrosis without prior inflammation [82].

Role of Orbital Fibroblasts

Fibroblasts respond to immune stimulation and actively participate in inflammatory pathways through their synthesis of chemokines, cytokines, and lipid mediators [48]. Orbital fibroblasts exhibit unique responses to several proinflammatory cytokines, particularly in those derived from patients with GD [83–85]. Additionally, the unique orbital fibroblast phenotype may contribute to the anatomic site-selective manifestations of GD [71, 83, 86, 87]. Importantly, orbital fibroblasts are embryologically distinct from dermal fibroblasts in that the former are derived from neural crest stem cells – a transient migratory collection of neuroepithelial cells that is responsible for much of the connective tissues of the eye and periocular structures [88–90]. Unlike dermal fibroblasts, orbital fibroblasts do not generate adequate levels of soluble IL-1 receptor antagonist, which results in unopposed signaling by IL-1β [40, 91]. In addition, GD orbital fibroblasts overproduce prostaglandin E_2 (PGE_2) in response to IL-1β, CD154, and leukoregulin due to the induction of prostaglandin-endoperoxide H synthase-2 (PGHS-2) and microsomal PGE_2 synthase genes [40, 91–93]. These cytokines signal the increased production of the extracellular matrix component hyaluronic acid and other glycosaminoglycans (GAGs) by fibroblasts, resulting in orbital tissue expansion and remodeling. The characteristic TED phenotypic appearance is promoted by the hydrophilic nature of GAGs, which contributes to periorbital edema and proptosis [94]. Consequently, orbital fibroblasts are central both as proinflammatory molecules and as macromolecules that participate in the tissue-remodeling characteristic of TED [62, 95].

Orbital fibroblasts are activated in part through interactions between the antigen CD40 and the CD40 ligand (CD40L, aka CD154). CD40 expressed by orbital fibroblasts binds to CD40L on T lymphocytes, which results in upregulation of glycosaminoglycan and prostaglandin synthesis [48, 96]. The CD40–CD40L interaction provides T-lymphocyte co-stimulation and can result in clonal expansion of naïve T lymphocytes and the production of proinflammatory cytokines, including IL-1, IL-6, and IL-8 [97]. These actions can in turn activate the expression of the prostaglandin PGHS-2, hyaluronan synthase (HAS), and UDP-glucose dehydrogenase (UGDH) genes in fibroblasts. These enzymes stimulate the production of hyaluronan. Therefore, the CD40–CD40L might be successfully exploited as a potential therapeutic target in TED, as it has been in other diseases [98–100]. More broadly, the key role of T cells in the pathogenesis of TED has now been more fully appreciated (see below) [100].

Inflammasomes also participate in the underlying proinflammatory environment. Nucleotide-binding oligomerization domain-like receptor pyrin domain-containing-3 (NLRP3) inflammasome activity contributes to the inflammatory process by promoting the release IL-1β and IL-18 via caspase-1 activation [101, 102]. Inflammasomes can contribute to the pathology of autoimmune and inflammatory diseases [102] and may also play a role in the development of major retinal degenerative diseases, including age-related macular degeneration and diabetic retinopathy [103–105].

Additionally, retinoids can modulate orbital inflammation. Retinoid acid receptor-alpha (RARα) appears to be associated with inflammation and adipocyte differentiation. Orbital fibroblasts in TED have been shown to express the RARα gene [106, 107]. All-trans retinoic acid may induce morphologic changes, apoptosis, and inhibition of cell growth in orbital fibroblasts from TED patients through its effect on the retinoic acid receptor [107]. Additionally, retinol has been shown to reduce IL-1β, glutathione disulfide (a parameter of oxidative stress), and IFN-γ in fibroblasts from TED and control subjects [108]. These findings suggest an antioxidant role for retinol in the setting of TED.

Within orbital connective tissue, fibroblast subsets with specific phenotypic attributes may account for the varied clinical presentation of TED. Expression of the glycoprotein Thy-1 has been utilized to characterize this diversity. Perimysial fibroblasts uniformly express Thy-1 and have the capacity to differentiate into myofibroblasts [83, 109, 110]. Orbital connective tissue contains both Thy-1^+ and Thy-1– fibroblasts [111]. Orbital fat expansion in TED results from the differentiation of Thy-1– fibroblasts into adipocytes [111], which is triggered by the activation of peroxisome proliferator-activated receptor γ (PPARγ) [112, 113]. This differentiation leads to the proliferation of orbital adipose tissue, which has been associated with compressive optic neuropathy in TED [111]. Conversely, orbital Thy-1^+ fibroblasts can evolve into a different mature cell type, myofibroblasts, in the presence of TGF-β. Expansion of fibroblasts with a mature myofibroblast phenotype enhances fibrosis, which can lead to restrictive myopathy [109, 111]. The balance between Thy-1– and Thy-1^+ fibroblasts in the orbit may be important to maintain normal connective tissue functions in the healthy orbit [48].

The role of hypoxia on orbital fibroblasts offers a potential molecular explanation for the harmful effects of smoking on the course of TED. Hypoxia induces adipogenesis and angiogenesis in orbital fibroblasts [114]. These changes occur as hypoxia drives tissue remodeling through activation of hypoxia-inducible factor-1 (HIF-1)-dependent pathways in orbital fibroblasts [115]. Recently, a study has shown a role for the hypoxia-inducible factor-2α (HIF-2α)-lysyl oxidase (LOX) pathway in orbital fibrotic tissue remodeling. HIF2α appears to accelerate extracellular matrix deposition by inducing LOX, a collagen-crosslinking enzyme, thereby promoting fibrosis [116]. This pathway may serve as a potential therapeutic target for TED.

Role of Lymphocytes

The active stage of TED is characterized by infiltration of orbital tissues with macrophages, mast cells, and T lymphocytes. Activated CD4+ T lymphocytes produce cytokines and chemoattractants that further amplify the inflammatory response [117, 118]. Endogenous ligation of the T-cell receptor (TCR) alone in the absence of co-stimulation is insufficient for cell activation and can lead to T-cell depletion, anergy, or tolerance [119, 120]. Thus, T cells require dual signals, including those provided by interactions between CD28 and costimulatory molecules on antigen-presenting cells [48]. This interplay may be modulated by the CD40–CD40L pathway [48]. CD40 and CD40L form a molecular bridge allowing T-/B-cell interactions and immunoglobulin class switching [48, 118]. This bridge has been implicated in the cross talk between T lymphocytes and several other cell types, including orbital fibroblasts [118]. A subset of T lymphocytes that serve a regulatory function, known as regulatory T cells (Treg), may be involved in attenuating the inflammatory response in TED [121, 122]. Given the diverse roles attributed to T cells, they offer a potential therapeutic target for controlling the inflammatory response [123, 124]. In particular, therapies that specifically target T-cell function or the molecules through which they interact may prove effective in treating TED [60].

B lymphocytes also serve a critical role in the inflammatory pathway and therefore are an important mediator in TED. B cells are precursors to antibody-producing plasma cells and further stimulate the immune response by presenting antigens and expressing cytokines. Autoantibody generation is dependent on the complex interplay between B and T cells. B cells are central to the pathogenesis of GD by providing support for the function of both T lymphocytes and fibroblasts [125]. B lymphocytes are a key player in the initiation of autoimmunity in TED, as demonstrated by the inability of B-cell-deficient mice to elicit T-cell responses following immunization with TSHR [126, 127]. Survival of plasma cell precursors is mediated through B-cell-activating factor receptors, which are fundamental to autoantibody production [127, 128]. Regulatory B lymphocytes may play a role in restraining inflammation in TED via the production of IL-10 and inhibitory interactions with T cells [129, 130]. Thus, the B cell has emerged as a valuable potential therapeutic target in TED and other autoimmune diseases.

Diagnosis and Role of Autoantigens in TED

The lack of direct correlation between thyroid dysfunction and the presence of TED creates somewhat of a diagnostic conundrum. While TED most frequently occurs in the context of autoimmune hyperthyroidism (i.e., Graves' disease), it can also occur in the context of hypothyroidism (i.e., Hashimoto's thyroiditis) and in the euthyroid state [74]. Irrespective of the thyroid function status in most of these cases, serum autoantibodies can be detected. One of these antibodies, TSI, mimics the activity of thyroid-stimulating hormone (TSH) when binding to TSHR. TSI is the most diagnostic of the activity and severity of GD among the autoantibodies [131–135]. A positive TSI with appropriate ophthalmologic findings indicates a diagnosis of Graves' orbitopathy even if thyroid function tests (TFTs) are otherwise normal. While elevation of TSI titers is diagnostic for Graves' disease, the majority of patients with elevated TSI levels will not develop clinically significant TED. However, among those who do develop orbitopathy, moderate-to-high TSI titers (e.g., >4.5 on the Mayo scale, reference value ≤1.3 TSI index) tend to predict a more aggressive, symptomatic course of TED [131]. A moderate-to-high TSI titer should raise concern for the risk of TED and prompt an explicit conversation with patients about TED, including the rationale for smoking cessation and controlling the thyroid hormone level, and may be used to assess the risks of ablative therapy.

Autoantibodies against another key player, IGF-1R, have also been shown to partake in TED pathogenesis [73, 87]. Higher levels of IGF-1R have been found on cultured orbital fibroblasts from patients with GD [68, 69, 136]. Treatment of these fibroblasts with IGF-1 results in the generation of hyaluronan and the synthesis of the T-cell chemoattractants IL-16 and RANTES [68, 87, 137]. IGF-1R has been shown to form a physical and functional complex with TSHR in thyroid tissue and orbital fibroblasts. Additionally, TSHR signaling can be attenuated by an IGF-1R-blocking antibody via an intermediate kinase (Erk) [138–140]. The synergistic effect of IGF-1 and TSH has specifically been demonstrated in TED, where TSHR/IGF-1 cross talk is an important regulator of fibroblast proliferation and transdifferentiation [141–143]. Although research involving this pathway in TED is promising, diagnostic testing and medical therapy targeting IGF-1 are not yet commercially available [46, 73, 144].

Positive serum titers of other thyroid antibodies, including TPO and TG, do not appear to positively correlate with disease progression or severity of TED. Some reports have actually found that these antibodies may be inversely related to TED [145, 146], while others have found that they are often positive in the presence of ophthalmopathy [44, 45]. Other potential autoantigens expressed by extraocular muscles include the G2s terminal portion of transcription factor FOXP1, tropomodulin, and the calcium-binding protein calsequestrin [147]. Though antibodies targeting these antigens have been detected in patients with GD, they are most likely nonpathogenic. Additionally, antibodies to acetylcholinesterase, which share physical attributes with TG, were detected in 8% of patients with TED. None of these other autoantigens appear proximately related to TED since the levels of antibodies directed against them do not correlate with disease activity [147, 148].

Clinical Monitoring and Classification Systems

Several classification systems have been used to categorize patients with TED. While their utility in patient management is not clear, they are important tools in clinical research of TED and hence are important to understand. The "no signs and symptoms, only signs, soft tissue involvement, proptosis, extraocular muscle involvement, corneal involvement, and sight loss" (NOSPECS) system, developed by Werner et al., grades TED by the clinical characteristics at disease presentation [149, 150]. The NOSPECS classification system is helpful as a broad descriptor to characterize TED signs and symptoms, though it has limited clinical value for assessing disease severity and guiding management.

The European Group on Graves' Orbitopathy (EUGOGO) classification determines the severity of TED based on the following parameters: presence of an afferent pupillary defect (APD), eyelid retraction, Hertel exophthalmometry, and risk of corneal ulceration (increased in the presence of lagophthalmos and absent Bell's phenomenon). Important considerations when using this system include the variation of normal exophthalmometry measurements based on ethnicity and gender [151] and the potential absence of relative afferent pupillary defect in bilateral disease. Additionally, EUGOGO has classified TED as mild, moderate-to-severe, and sight-threatening based on specific disease features [152, 153] (Table 57.1).

The clinical activity score (CAS), developed by Mourits et al., is based on TED activity and used to identify patients who are more likely to respond to corticosteroids or orbital radiation [154]. This scale formulates an overall score based

Table 57.1 European Group on Graves' Orbitopathy (EUGOGO) grading of TED severity

Category	Features	Recommended management
Sight-threatening TED	Dysthyroid optic neuropathy Corneal breakdown	Immediate intervention
Moderate-to-severe TED	Lid retraction ≥2 mm Moderate or severe soft tissue involvement Exophthalmos ≥3 mm above normal for race and gender Inconstant or constant diplopia	Immunosuppression (if active) or surgical intervention (if inactive)
Mild TED	Mild lid retraction (<2 mm) Mild soft tissue involvement Exophthalmos <3 mm above normal for race and gender Transient or no diplopia Corneal exposure responsive to lubricants	Conservative

on symptoms and signs, including retrobulbar or peribulbar pain/pressure, eyelid erythema, conjunctival injection, chemosis, caruncle swelling, and eyelid edema. One point is assigned for each clinical feature that is present, and the total is summed to determine the score. A score of ≥3 was found to correlate with active TED, and a score of ≥4 carries high predictive value for response to immunosuppressive treatment [155, 156]. Some have criticized this system because "activity" can be easily confused with "congestion," and CAS levels did not appear to correlate with sight-threatening disease in a recent report [157].

The "vision, inflammation, strabismus, and appearance/exposure" (VISA) system by Dolman et al. uses four disease end points to classify disease activity and severity [158]. Each end point is assigned a severity score, which can then be assessed longitudinally and used to identify time-dependent changes.

Both CAS and VISA classifications are useful in tracking changes – a very important element of active orbitopathy. However, while the CAS and VISA classification systems are useful in research, their utility in routine clinical care of TED patients is unknown [157], particularly in their ability to detect vision-threatening disease or differentiate between inflammation and orbital congestion/compartment syndrome. A less systematic but still reliable method of monitoring disease activity involves noting changes in the clinical findings on ophthalmic exam (e.g., worsening proptosis, extraocular muscle (EOM) restriction, visual fields, etc.) at baseline and routine follow-up visits.

Endocrine Management of Systemic Graves' Disease

Thioamide Drugs

Upon diagnosis of systemic GD, patients are typically prescribed a thioamide drug for hyperthyroidism and a beta-blocker for symptomatic tachycardia. Methimazole and propylthiouracil (PTU) are members of the thioamide drug class and exert their function by inhibiting thyroid peroxidase to prevent iodinization of thyroglobulin. Thioamides do not block the action of sodium-dependent iodide transporters and have minimal, if any, effect on the underlying autoimmune process, which continues unabated. Importantly, even when thioamide treatment successfully restores the euthyroid state, the thyroid gland can continue to enlarge in response to autoantibody stimulation and immune cell infiltration; this may lead to a worsening goiter and further inflammatory activity. Patients can remain on thioamide therapy with a goal of achieving remission, defined as normalized thyroid function while off thioamide therapy, or converting to the hypothyroid state. The rate of sustained remission, lasting over 2 years, can be quite low. Relapse rates are high even while on antithyroid medication, with a meta-analysis revealing relapse rates of 53% with antithyroid drugs, 15% following RAI, and 10% following thyroidectomy surgery [159, 160]. While methimazole can be used indefinitely with reasonable systemic endocrine results, its side effect profile is not benign: hepatitis, thrombocytopenia, gastrointestinal irritation, skin rash, joint and muscle pain, birth defects, and adverse interactions with other prescription drugs, including anticoagulants, diabetes medications, and cardiac medications, have all been reported [161–164].

Prolonged hypothyroidism is also associated with TED, albeit usually a milder form. Nevertheless, a prolonged hypothyroid state should be avoided at least as much as a prolonged hyperthyroid state [165–167]. In the hypothyroid state, the elevation in circulating TSH levels leads to increased activation of TSH receptors, thereby driving intra- and intercellular signaling pathways that promote cytokine release and inflammation [168–171]. Patients may present with inflammatory orbitopathy in the context of Hashimoto's disease and elevated TSH levels without elevation of TSI titer. Hence, thyroid hormone replacement with levothyroxine in the prolonged hypothyroid state is critical [172]. Additionally, significant fluctuation in thyroid hormone levels may itself be a risk factor for TED. Therefore, efforts should be made to stabilize TFTs as soon as possible after diagnosis.

Radioactive Iodine (RAI)

In lieu of indefinite thioamide therapy, ablative therapy with radiation is often utilized for long-term systemic control of GD. The relative accumulation of iodine in thyroid tissue has led to the use of iodine-131 to deliver a necrosis-inducing dose of targeted radioactivity to the diseased gland. In smaller- and medium-sized thyroid glands, a radioactive uptake test can be used to calculate the dose needed for complete versus partial thyroid ablation. Partial thyroid ablation reduces the need for posttreatment levothyroxine supplement. However, the residual thyroid gland may continue to stimulate production of autoantibodies and subsequent inflammation in GD. Moreover, there is an increased likelihood of difficult-to-control fluctuations in serum thyroid hormone levels in such patients. Consequently, planned partial thyroid ablation with lower doses of I-131 is discouraged for most patients with access to levothyroxine replacement therapy.

Since RAI can negatively impact the status of TED, it is critical that dosing is determined precisely. Empiric doses are much more likely to result in partial thyroid ablation, persistent hyperthyroidism, and perpetuation of autoimmune orbitopathy. Therefore, the practice of using empiric fixed dose of 131-I activity (i.e., 15–20 mCi) that is not adjusted based on gland size or radioiodine uptake testing (RAIU) should be discouraged. These risks increase with larger thyroid gland sizes (>60–80 grams, or 3–4 times the normal gland size) and with low RAIU values, which is commonly seen with high dietary iodine content. Additionally, repeat treatments are more often necessary, as high as nearly 50%, with empiric- or low-dose RAI [173]. While some centers still prescribe 80–100 microCi/gram of thyroid tissue (low dose), other centers now recommend 200 microCi/gram of thyroid tissue based on RAIU in order to ensure complete ablation.

RAI treatment leads to tissue necrosis, cytokine release [174], and increase of both thyroid hormone and thyroid tissue antigens into the bloodstream. Pre-treatment with lithium can deplete intrathyroidal thyroid store and decrease the latter [175], although lithium has its own set of side effects and is not routinely used for this purpose. Usually, within 4–8 weeks after RAI, circulating levels of T4 and T3 decline, and hormone replacement therapy may be considered. Since the timing for replacement therapy is variable among patients, and post-ablative hypothyroidism is a major risk for progressive orbitopathy [165–167], it is critical to carefully monitor post-RAI patients to properly time initiation of hormone replacement therapy. Usually, the recommended approach is to obtain blood tests at 4 weeks post-RAI and then every 1–2 weeks until hypothyroidism is detected, at which time levothyroxine is initiated.

RAI treatment has been associated with significant worsening of orbitopathy, with up to 15% of patients developing new or worsening orbitopathy following treatment [9, 176]. Along with smoking and prolonged hypothyroidism, RAI is a key risk factor for progression to moderate-to-severe orbitopathy [16, 35, 167, 177–179]. Although the mechanism for this association has yet to be fully elucidated, one theory is that thyroid tissue necrosis and antigen release in the setting of sudden thyroid hormone fluctuation lead to progressive orbitopathy. This increased risk is lowered with the use of post-ablative corticosteroids [180–182]. Many orbital specialists recommend daily oral or weekly intravenous corticosteroid administration for most patients undergoing RAI, regardless of the current orbitopathy status. Corticosteroid treatment duration usually ranges from 2 to 6 weeks post ablation but can be administered as long as 12 weeks, with starting doses of 0.2–0.5 mg/kg/day [180–183]. In cases of RAI without post-ablative corticosteroid administration, poor orbital outcomes can be seen [184]. In contrast, low-dose and pulsed IV steroids appear to be efficacious with fewer side effects [180–182]. Thus, for the majority of patients undergoing RAI, the low risks associated with a 1- to 3-month treatment with corticosteroids are outweighed by the potential benefits of orbitopathy risk reduction [183].

However, RAI is a less desirable option for smokers with GD due to the additive and potentially synergistic risks of smoking and RAI on orbitopathy. These patients are at higher risk of developing moderate-to-severe orbitopathy and are also at higher risk for reactivation after the quiescent phase of the disease is achieved. Furthermore, smoking is also associated with poorer response to treatment for TED [16, 185–187].

Surgical Thyroidectomy

Another option for thyroid ablation, surgical thyroidectomy, involves partial or complete removal of the thyroid gland. Historically, partial thyroidectomy was more commonly performed, despite this more conservative approach often resulting in treatment failures. From the endocrinologist's perspective, surgical ablation has therefore been considered a final treatment option of last resort when other therapies have failed. However, advances in surgical science and the realization that total thyroidectomy is superior to partial thyroidectomy [188], along with the increased experience with total thyroidectomies in the context of early detection of thyroid cancer, have made this procedure a much safer option. Patients who have undergone total surgical thyroidectomy have the benefit of starting hormone replacement therapy upon hospital discharge, thereby avoiding hypothyroidism and the associated risk of worsening orbitopathy [166, 167, 178]. Additionally, these patients experience faster resolution of thyroid hormone imbalance and associated symptoms of dysthyroidism [178, 189–193]. From the ophthalmic perspective, complete surgical thyroidectomy can be considered the preferred first-line therapeutic option for hyperthyroidism in GD due to the orbital risks of RAI, particularly in patients at risk for significant TED (i.e., older age, positive smoking status, and high TSI titer). Indeed, better outcomes have resulted in patients who underwent early thyroidectomy when compared with those who underwent RAI [184].

Surgical treatment is not without risks, however. Complex regional anatomy and potential damage to critical nearby structures, including the trachea, recurrent laryngeal nerves, external branch of the superior laryngeal nerve, and parathyroid glands, along with the highly vascular nature of inflamed thyroid tissue, can make complete surgical thyroidectomy challenging. These risks are partially mitigated by training and experience [194], and modern knowledge and technology have further improved the safety profile. Patients are typically prescribed inorganic iodine solution (i.e., Lugol's solution [195]) based on results of duplex ultrasound for blood flow analysis, which has been shown to reduce blood flow and bleeding risk and thus lowers the risk of damage to nearby critical structures. Real-time intraoperative nerve monitoring can additionally reduce the risk of injury to the recurrent laryngeal nerve [196]. Furthermore, the development of modern techniques in parathyroid gland autotransplantation has reduced the risks of post-thyroidectomy hypoparathyroidism [197]. All of these factors combined have made complete surgical thyroidectomy a much safer and feasible option for systemic GD management.

Total thyroidectomy may also be followed by RAI, a therapeutic option known as total thyroid ablation. The goal of this treatment is to completely remove thyroid antigens and thyroid-infiltrating lymphocytes, which is thought to reduce the autoimmune reaction in the orbit and thereby reduce the severity of TED. Total thyroid ablation may improve the time to resolution of TED symptoms, although the end result of therapy may be equal to that of total thyroidectomy alone [190, 191, 198].

Medical Management of TED

Conservative Measures

Management of TED is guided by its severity and level of activity. Many patients have self-limited disease and will undergo spontaneous improvement [199]. Patients should be educated on maintaining a euthyroid state and eliminating modifiable risk factors. In any patients with active TED or those with GD at risk for developing TED, smoking cessation is a modifiable risk factor of paramount importance. Mild disease can be treated with supportive care that addresses ocular surface compromise and diplopia. The conservative measures include ocular lubrication (artificial tears or lubricating ointments), punctal occlusion, moisture chambers, and prismatic correction. In patients with nocturnal lagophthalmos, eyelid taping may reduce desiccation of the ocular surface. For patients with more severe TED, including optic neuropathy, disfiguring proptosis, or intractable exposure keratopathy, conservative measures will not suffice, and medical and/or surgical intervention is warranted.

Supplementation with the antioxidant selenium may be a low risk, helpful intervention for reducing the symptoms associated with TED. Oral sodium selenite at a dose of 100 micrograms administered twice daily appeared to decreased the risk of worsening TED when initiated within 6 months of Graves' disease diagnosis in patients with mild orbitopathy and selenium deficiency [200]. Studies have shown that a 6-month treatment course can improve the symptoms of mild TED and prevent deterioration when compared with placebo [201]. Due to the low-risk profile of selenium, many endocrinologists and ophthalmologists have begun routinely incorporating this supplement into their management of TED patients. Selenium deficiency may be a modifiable risk factor for the disease, as low selenium levels have been associated with a higher community prevalence of TED [202]. However, additional research is needed to confirm the value of supplementation in selenium replete regions and to identify selenium deficiency as predictor of progressive TED.

Corticosteroids

Systemic steroids, with or without radiation, are the mainstay of treatment for moderate-to-severe, sight-threatening TED in the active stage. Based on the European Group on Graves' Orbitopathy (EUGOGO) classification, patients with moderate-to-severe TED present with one or more of the following: lid retraction ≥2 mm, moderate or severe soft tissue involvement, exophthalmos ≥3 mm above normal for race and gender, and diplopia [156]. Steroids reduce the inflammatory orbitopathy seen in TED through modulation of cytokine production by targeting resident macrophages and fibroblasts [203]. Oral (PO) and intravenous (IV) systemic steroid preparations are available [204], though the decreased side effect profile of IV formulations makes IV treatment preferable. PO steroids typically require high doses, 1 mg/kg, over prolonged treatment periods and carry a large side effect profile. In contrast, studies have shown pulsed IV methylprednisolone protocols have demonstrated superior efficacy, even at lower cumulative doses, with reduced risks compared to PO steroids [205–207]. However, a meta-analysis of several studies failed to identify any difference in long-term outcome with the two routes of administration [208]. When considering the IV route, cumulative doses must remain below 8 gm per course of therapy to avoid acute liver damage [209].

Apart from their use in active TED, IV steroids can also be used to prevent the development or worsening of TED following RAI therapy [206]. This is especially true in patients with active TED and those with risk factors for TED, including smoking, high TSH, and elevated serum FT3 levels [182]. Lower doses of prophylactic steroids (<0.3 mg/kg) following RAI have been shown to be just as effective as traditional, larger doses (>0.3 mg/kg) even with a relatively short treatment course of 6 weeks post-RAI [181]. While there is strong evidence for the use of prophylactic steroids in patients with active TED and in patients with risk factors for developing TED, the question remains whether to treat patients without TED and no risk factors with steroids following RAI. Some assert that given the low risk, these patients do not require steroid prophylaxis [181]. However, the argument can also be made to discuss the advantages and disadvantages of steroid prophylaxis following RAI on an individual basis with low-risk patients due to the invalidating and disfiguring nature of TED if it does indeed occur [210].

Negative systemic effects of corticosteroid use are well-documented and include hyperglycemia, mood lability, hypertension, weight gain, reduced bone mineral density, increased susceptibility to infections, and Cushing's syndrome. For patients who wish to avoid systemic steroid effects, localized steroid administration is an option. Intraorbital steroid injections can also be considered for symptomatic patients with TED, but this option is less effective than PO or IV steroid treatments [211].

Targeted Immunotherapies

Studies have also examined the efficacy of alternate immunosuppressive therapy in TED. The existing research has focused on patients who had previously failed the mainstay treatment of corticosteroids and/or radiotherapy.

Cyclosporine, a drug frequently used to prevent organ transplant rejection, reduces T-cell activity via cytokine interference. Cyclosporine monotherapy was found to be less efficacious at curbing TED than steroids alone; however, cyclosporine in combination with steroids may provide a beneficial therapeutic adjunct [212–214]. Despite the potential role of combination therapy with cyclosporine, it is not frequently used in TED management due to its unwanted side effects of irreversible plasma creatinine elevation and systemic hypertension [215].

Few published studies involving the cytostatic agents' methotrexate (MTX) and azathioprine have been conducted. MTX monotherapy has been shown to be a successful steroid-sparing option in certain patients who are steroid resistant, tolerant, or dependent [216–218]; however, MTX has not achieved wide use for TED. Trials of the purine antagonist azathioprine for moderate-to-severe TED have not shown promise as a single agent [208, 219], though it may be efficacious in combination with radiation or steroids [220, 221]. However, potential bone marrow suppression limits the safety profile of azathioprine use.

Mycophenolate mofetil (MMF) blocks the proliferation of lymphocytes via guanosine monophosphate synthesis inhibition. This drug has a safer safety profile compared to azathioprine, but its use in TED has been limited. One study of patients with moderate-to-severe TED showed promising results for those treated with MMF monotherapy compared to steroids and absence of disease reactivation [222]. Further studies are warranted to further elucidate its role in TED.

Antibody Therapy

For patients who have failed conventional treatment for TED, various biologic therapies have been trialed.

Rituximab, an anti-CD20 monoclonal antibody, targets B cells maturation and proliferation [223]. Although rituximab is used routinely with success in other autoimmune conditions, notably systemic lupus erythematosus (SLE) and rheumatoid arthritis (RA), its use in TED has produced inconsistent results [215]. Early retrospective studies found improvement in orbital inflammation with use of rituximab in patients who previously failed steroids [224–226]. However, a 2013 Cochrane review found insufficient evidence to support the use of rituximab in patients with TED, citing the need for larger randomized control studies investigating its use compared to placebo or steroids [227]. In the ensuing years, RTX has been more widely studied. One randomized controlled study found evidence for better therapeutic outcomes (ocular motility, visual functioning, and fewer surgical procedures) with RTX in active moderate-to-severe TED compared to IV steroids, even at lower RTX doses [228]. In contrast, another controlled trial comparing RTX to placebo showed no statistically significant difference in outcomes in patients with moderate-to-severe TED and in fact demonstrated a higher incidence of adverse events in the RTX group [229]. Two recent meta-analyses found promising preliminary effects of RTX treatment on TED, particularly in moderate-to-severe patients who have failed steroids [230, 231]. However, both studies recommended larger sampled studies to further assess the use of rituximab in TED. Adverse effects associated with RTX include transient hypotension, cough, pruritis, transient fevers, and increased infection risk [232]. Additionally, RTC carries a "black box" warning in the United States for progressive multifocal leukoencephalopathy with chronic therapy for other diseases. The risks of treatment and high cost may limit its use [233].

Active TED may be associated with increased serum levels of tumor necrosis factor alpha (TNF-α) [234, 235]. Therefore, agents that inhibit TNF-α (infliximab, adalimumab, and etanercept) may also play in a role in treating TED. Infliximab and adalimumab are monoclonal antibodies, and etanercept is a recombinant human soluble TNF-α receptor fusion protein. These anti-cytokine drugs have shown potential benefit in case reports and small studies. Infliximab has demonstrated potential to improve signs and symptoms of TED in two reports, though it has not achieved widespread clinical use [236, 237]. In one patient, infliximab was shown to resolve orbital inflammation within 3 days with subsequent improvement in visual acuity and color vision over the following week [236]. In another, a single dose of infliximab improved inflammatory signs [237]. Etanercept has been trialed in a small pilot study of ten patients with active mild-to-moderate TED and shown potential to improve inflammatory symptoms without serious side effects at 18 months, though recurrence occurred in 30% following treatment cessation [238]. A small pilot study of ten patients showed adalimumab may potentially improve symptoms of TED, particularly in patients with a strong inflammatory component, though there was no statistically significant change in inflammatory index after 3 months of treatment [239]. These preliminary reports and pilot studies should be followed with larger randomized control studies to further determine the efficacy and safety of anti-cytokine monotherapy in TED.

Tocilizumab, an antibody against IL-6, is used for RA and juvenile idiopathic arthritis (JIA), particularly in cases where traditional disease-modifying antirheumatic drugs and TNF-α blockers have failed or are not tolerated. In preliminary studies, tocilizumab was reported to be an effective therapy for moderate-to-severe thyroid eye disease in patients resistant to IV steroids [240, 241]. In a nonrandomized prospective study of 18 patients, extraocular motility improved in 83%, proptosis was reduced in 72%, and diplopia resolved in 54% of patients; no severe side effects or relapse of active TED occurred [240]. A larger double-blinded, randomized control study of 32 adults demonstrated reduction in TED signs and symptoms at 16 weeks in 93% of patients treated with tocilizumab [241]. Another report of two cases of severe TED refractory even to orbital decompression showed clinical improvement in both patients with minimal side effects after tocilizumab therapy [242].

Teprotumumab, a human monoclonal antibody that targets IGF-1R, is another experimental drug with promising results. In a large double-blinded randomized controlled study of 88 patients, a 24-week course of teprotumumab was shown to be superior to placebo in patients with active, moderate-to-severe TED [46]. Teprotumumab was shown to improve clinical signs and symptoms of TED, reduce proptosis, and improve quality of life in TED patients. Though hyperglycemia was noted in diabetic patients receiving the experimental drug, no major adverse effects were reported [46]. A phase III trial of teprotumumab is underway; if successful, the inhibition of IGF-IR may be a novel therapeutic option for patients with active TED [144].

Orbital Radiotherapy

For patients with active TED, orbital radiotherapy can target the inflammatory milieu through its actions on orbital fibroblasts and lymphocytes, though the exact anti-inflammatory mechanism is unclear [243, 244]. Radiation can reduce the duration and severity of active disease, particularly when administered in combination with steroid therapy [243, 245]. Additionally, radiotherapy can minimize the dose and duration of corticosteroid therapy for TED while improving ocular symptoms of proptosis and diplopia [246]. Reduced soft tissue signs and improved ocular motility usually occur within 2–3 weeks of treatment, but improvement can continue for several months [203].

A response rate to orbital radiation of approximately 60% was reported in one uncontrolled study [247]. In another randomized, prospective trial, patients with moderate-to-severe TED had improved ocular motility and a reduced need for strabismus surgery following the administration of radiotherapy (20 Gy in 10 fractions over 12 days) compared to sham controls [203]. A single prospective randomized controlled study found no significant benefit with orbital radiation, though several patients were previously nonresponsive to steroids and others had inactive TED [248]. The CIRTED study, a large multicenter double-blind study of 126 patients, investigated the use of combined immunosuppression and radiation. This study found that radiotherapy had no added benefit in patients receiving oral prednisolone for 24 weeks; however, these results were limited by the high number of patients who withdrew from treatment [249].

Despite some inconsistent results, radiotherapy has generally shown to be an effective treatment and has achieved widespread acceptance for moderate-to-severe TED. A meta-analysis of 18 studies determined that orbital radiotherapy is be efficacious in the treatment of TED, especially when combined with intravenous corticosteroids [250]. A large retrospective review found strong evidence for the use of orbital radiotherapy in patients with TED-compressive optic neuropathy responsive to steroids, with radiation preventing recurrent compressive optic neuropathy after corticosteroid withdrawal. In this study, radiotherapy was found to eliminate the need for urgent orbital decompression in 98% of patients in the active phase, and only 37% of patients elected to pursue any surgical intervention during the inactive phase [251].

Orbital radiation therapy is generally safe and well tolerated [252]. Treatment doses should typically approach 20 Gy, but lower doses may be considered in younger patients without significant dysmotility [253]. Side effects of radiation are often minimal but can include dry eye, cataract formation, retinopathy, and optic neuropathy. Consequently, irradiation is relatively contraindicated in patients with diabetes or hypertensive retinopathy [243]. Side effects of secondary malignancies are rare but have been reported [254].

Conclusions

TED is a common manifestation of thyroid autoimmune disease. Primary treatment of the systemic endocrine disease provides resolution of the thyroid hormone imbalance. However, the orbitopathy associated with autoimmune thyroid diseases is progressive and often irreversible, leading to disfigurement, loss of visual function, and chronic pain. The mainstay of nonsurgical treatment for active TED is corticosteroid treatment with or without orbital radiotherapy. As the understanding of the underlying pathophysiology of TED continues to expand, so does the development of new therapeutic options to potentially revolutionize the management of this complex disease.

References

1. Terwee C, Wakelkamp I, Tan S, Dekker F, Prummel MF, Wiersinga W. Long-term effects of Graves' ophthalmopathy on health-related quality of life. Eur J Endocrinol. 2002;146(6):751–7.
2. Yeatts RP. Quality of life in patients with Graves ophthalmopathy. Trans Am Ophthalmol Soc. 2005;103:368–411.
3. Smith TJ, Hegedüs L. Graves' disease. N Engl J Med. 2016;375(16):1552–65.
4. Heufelder AE, Dutton CM, Sarkar G, Donovan KA, Bahn RS. Detection of TSH receptor RNA in cultured fibroblasts from patients with Graves' ophthalmopathy and pretibial dermopathy. Thyroid. 1993;3(4):297–300.
5. Wiersinga WM, Bartalena L. Epidemiology and prevention of Graves' ophthalmopathy. Thyroid. 2002;12(10):855–60.
6. Bahn RS. Graves' ophthalmopathy. N Engl J Med. 2010;362(8):726–38.
7. Marcocci C, Bartalena L, Bogazzi F, Panicucci M, Pinchera A. Studies on the occurrence of ophthalmopathy in Graves' disease. Acta Endocrinol. 1989;120(4):473–8.
8. Leo M, Menconi F, Rocchi R, et al. Role of the underlying thyroid disease on the phenotype of Graves' orbitopathy in a tertiary referral center. Thyroid. 2015;25(3):347–51.
9. Bartalena L, Marcocci C, Bogazzi F, et al. Relation between therapy for hyperthyroidism and the course of Graves' ophthalmopathy. N Engl J Med. 1998;338(2):73–8.
10. Patel P, Khandji J, Kazim M. Recurrent thyroid eye disease. Ophthalmic Plast Reconstr Surg. 2015;31(6):445–8.
11. Wiersinga WM. Smoking and thyroid. Clin Endocrinol. 2013;79(2):145–51.
12. Anagnostis P, Adamidou F, Polyzos SA, et al. Predictors of long-term remission in patients with Graves' disease: a single center experience. Endocrine. 2013;44(2):448–53.
13. Ponto KA, Merkesdal S, Hommel G, Pitz S, Pfeiffer N, Kahaly GJ. Public health relevance of Graves' orbitopathy. J Clin Endocrinol Metab. 2013;98(1):145–52.
14. Prummel MF, Wiersinga WM. Smoking and risk of Graves' disease. JAMA. 1993;269(4):479–82.
15. Mack WP, Stasior GO, Cao HJ, Stasior OG, Smith TJ. The effect of cigarette smoke constituents on the expression of HLA-DR in orbital fibroblasts derived from patients with Graves ophthalmopathy. Ophthalmic Plast Reconstr Surg. 1999;15(4):260–71.
16. Bartalena L, Marcocci C, Tanda ML, et al. Cigarette smoking and treatment outcomes in Graves ophthalmopathy. Ann Intern Med. 1998;129(8):632–5.
17. Cawood TJ, Moriarty P, O'Farrelly C, O'Shea D. Smoking and thyroid-associated ophthalmopathy: a novel explanation of the biological link. J Clin Endocrinol Metab. 2007;92(1):59–64.
18. Seksik P, Nion-Larmurier I, Sokol H, Beaugerie L, Cosnes J. Effects of light smoking consumption on the clinical course of Crohn's disease. Inflamm Bowel Dis. 2009;15(5):734–41.
19. Harrison BJ, Silman AJ. Does smoking influence disease outcome in patients with rheumatoid arthritis? J Rheumatol. 2000;27(3):569–70.
20. Harrison BJ, Silman AJ, Wiles NJ, Scott DG, Symmons DP. The association of cigarette smoking with disease outcome in patients with early inflammatory polyarthritis. Arthritis Rheum. 2001;44(2):323–30.
21. Silman AJ, Newman J, MacGregor AJ. Cigarette smoking increases the risk of rheumatoid arthritis. Results from a nationwide study of disease-discordant twins. Arthritis Rheum. 1996;39(5):732–5.
22. Metcalfe RA, Weetman AP. Stimulation of extraocular muscle fibroblasts by cytokines and hypoxia: possible role in thyroid-associated ophthalmopathy. Clin Endocrinol. 1994;40(1):67–72.
23. Wakelkamp IM, Gerding MN, van der Meer JW, Prummel MF, Wiersinga WM. Smoking and disease severity are independent determinants of serum adhesion molecule levels in Graves' ophthalmopathy. Clin Exp Immunol. 2002;127(2):316–20.
24. Ringold DA, Nicoloff JT, Kesler M, Davis H, Hamilton A, Mack T. Further evidence for a strong genetic influence on the development of autoimmune thyroid disease: the California twin study. Thyroid. 2002;12(8):647–53.
25. Brix TH, Petersen HC, Iachine I, Hegedüs L. Preliminary evidence of genetic anticipation in Graves' disease. Thyroid. 2003;13(5):447–51.
26. Prabhakar BS, Bahn RS, Smith TJ. Current perspective on the pathogenesis of Graves' disease and ophthalmopathy. Endocr Rev. 2003;24(6):802–35.
27. Han S, Zhang S, Zhang W, et al. CTLA4 polymorphisms and ophthalmopathy in Graves' disease patients: association study and meta-analysis. Hum Immunol. 2006;67(8):618–26.
28. Gianoukakis AG, Smith TJ. Recent insights into the pathogenesis and management of thyroid-associated ophthalmopathy. Curr Opin Endocrinol Diabetes Obes. 2008;15(5):446–52.
29. Tomer Y. Genetic susceptibility to autoimmune thyroid disease: past, present, and future. Thyroid. 2010;20(7):715–25.
30. Pawlowski P, Wawrusiewicz-Kurylonek N, Eckstein A, et al. Disturbances of modulating molecules (FOXP3, CTLA-4/CD28/B7, and CD40/CD40L) mRNA expressions in the orbital tissue from patients with severe Graves' ophthalmopathy. Mediat Inflamm. 2015;2015:340934.
31. Wu T, Mester T, Gupta S, Sun F, Smith TJ, Douglas RS. Thyrotropin and CD40L stimulate interleukin-12 expression in fibrocytes: implications for pathogenesis of thyroid-associated ophthalmopathy. Thyroid. 2016;26(12):1768–77.
32. Pawlak-Adamska E, Frydecka I, Bolanowski M, et al. CD28/CTLA-4/ICOS haplotypes confers susceptibility to Graves' disease and modulates clinical phenotype of disease. Endocrine. 2017;55(1):186–99.
33. Burch HB, Wartofsky L. Graves' ophthalmopathy: current concepts regarding pathogenesis and management. Endocr Rev. 1993;14(6):747–93.
34. Melmed S, Polonsky KS, Larsen PR, Kronenberg H. Williams textbook of endocrinology. 13th ed. Philadelphia: Elsevier; 2016.
35. Kung AW, Yau CC, Cheng A. The incidence of ophthalmopathy after radioiodine therapy for Graves' disease: prognostic factors and the role of methimazole. J Clin Endocrinol Metab. 1994;79(2):542–6.
36. Acharya SH, Avenell A, Philip S, Burr J, Bevan JS, Abraham P. Radioiodine therapy (RAI) for Graves' disease (GD) and the effect on ophthalmopathy: a systematic review. Clin Endocrinol. 2008;69(6):943–50.
37. Bartalena L, Marcocci C, Pinchera A. Graves' ophthalmopathy: a preventable disease? Eur J Endocrinol. 2002;146(4):457–61.
38. Prummel MF, Wiersinga WM, Mourits MP, Koornneef L, Berghout A, van der Gaag R. Effect of abnormal thyroid function on the severity of Graves' ophthalmopathy. Arch Intern Med. 1990;150(5):1098–101.
39. Ludgate M, Baker G. Unlocking the immunological mechanisms of orbital inflammation in thyroid eye disease. Clin Exp Immunol. 2002;127(2):193–8.
40. Naik VM, Naik MN, Goldberg RA, Smith TJ, Douglas RS. Immunopathogenesis of thyroid eye disease: emerging paradigms. Surv Ophthalmol. 2010;55(3):215–26.
41. McKenzie JM, Zakarija M, Sato A. Humoral immunity in Graves' disease. Clin Endocrinol Metab. 1978;7(1):31–45.
42. Kotwal A, Stan M. Thyrotropin receptor antibodies-an overview. Ophthalmic Plast Reconstr Surg. 2018;34(4S Suppl 1):S20–7.

43. Soh SB, Aw TC. Laboratory testing in thyroid conditions – pitfalls and clinical utility. Ann Lab Med. 2019;39(1):3–14.
44. Kumar S, Schiefer R, Coenen MJ, Bahn RS. A stimulatory thyrotropin receptor antibody (M22) and thyrotropin increase interleukin-6 expression and secretion in Graves' orbital preadipocyte fibroblasts. Thyroid. 2010;20(1):59–65.
45. Eckstein AK, Plicht M, Lax H, et al. Thyrotropin receptor autoantibodies are independent risk factors for Graves' ophthalmopathy and help to predict severity and outcome of the disease. J Clin Endocrinol Metab. 2006;91(9):3464–70.
46. Smith TJ, Kahaly GJ, Ezra DG, et al. Teprotumumab for thyroid-associated ophthalmopathy. N Engl J Med. 2017;376(18):1748–61.
47. Tao W, Ayala-Haedo JA, Field MG, Pelaez D, Wester ST. RNA-sequencing gene expression profiling of orbital adipose-derived stem cell population implicate HOX genes and WNT signaling dysregulation in the pathogenesis of thyroid-associated orbitopathy. Invest Ophthalmol Vis Sci. 2017;58(14):6146–58.
48. Lehmann GM, Feldon SE, Smith TJ, Phipps RP. Immune mechanisms in thyroid eye disease. Thyroid. 2008;18(9):959–65.
49. Lehmann GM, Garcia-Bates TM, Smith TJ, Feldon SE, Phipps RP. Regulation of lymphocyte function by PPARgamma: relevance to thyroid eye disease-related inflammation. PPAR Res. 2008;2008:895901.
50. Prummel MF. Pathogenetic and clinical aspects of endocrine ophthalmopathy. Exp Clin Endocrinol Diabetes. 1999;107(Suppl 3):S75–8.
51. Hufnagel TJ, Hickey WF, Cobbs WH, Jakobiec FA, Iwamoto T, Eagle RC. Immunohistochemical and ultrastructural studies on the exenterated orbital tissues of a patient with Graves' disease. Ophthalmology. 1984;91(11):1411–9.
52. Tallstedt L, Norberg R. Immunohistochemical staining of normal and Graves' extraocular muscle. Invest Ophthalmol Vis Sci. 1988;29(2):175–84.
53. Prummel MF, Bakker A, Wiersinga WM, et al. Multi-center study on the characteristics and treatment strategies of patients with Graves' orbitopathy: the first European Group on Graves' Orbitopathy experience. Eur J Endocrinol. 2003;148(5):491–5.
54. Rotondo Dottore G, Torregrossa L, Caturegli P, et al. Association of T and B cells infiltrating orbital tissues with clinical features of Graves orbitopathy. JAMA Ophthalmol. 2018;136(6):613–9.
55. Weetman AP, Cohen S, Gatter KC, Fells P, Shine B. Immunohistochemical analysis of the retrobulbar tissues in Graves' ophthalmopathy. Clin Exp Immunol. 1989;75(2):222–7.
56. Wegelius O, Asboe-Hansen G, Lamberg BA. Retrobulbar connective tissue changes in malignant exophthalmos. Acta Endocrinol. 1957;25(4):452–6.
57. Heufelder AE, Bahn RS. Detection and localization of cytokine immunoreactivity in retro-ocular connective tissue in Graves' ophthalmopathy. Eur J Clin Investig. 1993;23(1):10–7.
58. Han R, Smith TJ. Induction by IL-1 beta of tissue inhibitor of metalloproteinase-1 in human orbital fibroblasts: modulation of gene promoter activity by IL-4 and IFN-gamma. J Immunol. 2005;174(5):3072–9.
59. Li B, Smith TJ. Regulation of IL-1 receptor antagonist by TSH in fibrocytes and orbital fibroblasts. J Clin Endocrinol Metab. 2014;99(4):E625–33.
60. Feldon SE, Park DJ, O'Loughlin CW, et al. Autologous T-lymphocytes stimulate proliferation of orbital fibroblasts derived from patients with Graves' ophthalmopathy. Invest Ophthalmol Vis Sci. 2005;46(11):3913–21.
61. Kahaly G, Förster G, Hansen C. Glycosaminoglycans in thyroid eye disease. Thyroid. 1998;8(5):429–32.
62. Kaback LA, Smith TJ. Expression of hyaluronan synthase messenger ribonucleic acids and their induction by interleukin-1beta in human orbital fibroblasts: potential insight into the molecular pathogenesis of thyroid-associated ophthalmopathy. J Clin Endocrinol Metab. 1999;84(11):4079–84.
63. Martins JR, Furlanetto RP, Oliveira LM, et al. Comparison of practical methods for urinary glycosaminoglycans and serum hyaluronan with clinical activity scores in patients with Graves' ophthalmopathy. Clin Endocrinol. 2004;60(6):726–33.
64. Pappa A, Jackson P, Stone J, et al. An ultrastructural and systemic analysis of glycosaminoglycans in thyroid-associated ophthalmopathy. Eye (Lond). 1998;12(Pt 2):237–44.
65. Shishido M, Kuroda K, Tsukifuji R, Fujita M, Shinkai H. A case of pretibial myxedema associated with Graves' disease: an immunohistochemical study of serum-derived hyaluronan-associated protein. J Dermatol. 1995;22(12):948–52.
66. Khong JJ, McNab AA, Ebeling PR, Craig JE, Selva D. Pathogenesis of thyroid eye disease: review and update on molecular mechanisms. Br J Ophthalmol. 2016;100(1):142–50.
67. Weightman DR, Perros P, Sherif IH, Kendall-Taylor P. Autoantibodies to IGF-1 binding sites in thyroid associated ophthalmopathy. Autoimmunity. 1993;16(4):251–7.
68. Pritchard J, Han R, Horst N, Cruikshank WW, Smith TJ. Immunoglobulin activation of T cell chemoattractant expression in fibroblasts from patients with Graves' disease is mediated through the insulin-like growth factor I receptor pathway. J Immunol. 2003;170(12):6348–54.
69. Pritchard J, Horst N, Cruikshank W, Smith TJ. Igs from patients with Graves' disease induce the expression of T cell chemoattractants in their fibroblasts. J Immunol. 2002;168(2):942–50.
70. Smith TJ. Is IGF-I receptor a target for autoantibody generation in Graves' disease? J Clin Endocrinol Metab. 2013;98(2):515–8.
71. Smith TJ, Janssen JAMJ. Insulin-like growth factor-I receptor and thyroid-associated ophthalmopathy. Endocr Rev. 2019;40(1):236–67.
72. Mohyi M, Smith TJ. IGF1 receptor and thyroid-associated ophthalmopathy. J Mol Endocrinol. 2018;61(1):T29–43.
73. Smith TJ, Janssen JA. Building the case for insulin-like growth factor receptor-I involvement in thyroid-associated ophthalmopathy. Front Endocrinol (Lausanne). 2016;7:167.
74. Bartley GB. The epidemiologic characteristics and clinical course of ophthalmopathy associated with autoimmune thyroid disease in Olmsted County, Minnesota. Trans Am Ophthalmol Soc. 1994;92:477–588.
75. Bartley GB, Fatourechi V, Kadrmas EF, et al. Clinical features of Graves' ophthalmopathy in an incidence cohort. Am J Ophthalmol. 1996;121(3):284–90.
76. Bartley GB, Fatourechi V, Kadrmas EF, et al. Chronology of Graves' ophthalmopathy in an incidence cohort. Am J Ophthalmol. 1996;121(4):426–34.
77. Han R, Smith TJ. T helper type 1 and type 2 cytokines exert divergent influence on the induction of prostaglandin E2 and hyaluronan synthesis by interleukin-1beta in orbital fibroblasts: implications for the pathogenesis of thyroid-associated ophthalmopathy. Endocrinology. 2006;147(1):13–9.
78. Aniszewski JP, Valyasevi RW, Bahn RS. Relationship between disease duration and predominant orbital T cell subset in Graves' ophthalmopathy. J Clin Endocrinol Metab. 2000;85(2):776–80.
79. Hiromatsu Y, Kaku H, Miyake I, Murayama S, Soejima E. Role of cytokines in the pathogenesis of thyroid-associated ophthalmopathy. Thyroid. 2002;12(3):217–21.
80. Drayton DL, Liao S, Mounzer RH, Ruddle NH. Lymphoid organ development: from ontogeny to neogenesis. Nat Immunol. 2006;7(4):344–53.
81. Aloisi F, Pujol-Borrell R. Lymphoid neogenesis in chronic inflammatory diseases. Nat Rev Immunol. 2006;6(3):205–17.
82. Ugradar S, Rootman DB. Case series: noninflammatory thyroid eye disease. Ophthalmic Plast Reconstr Surg. 2019;35(5):461–4.

83. Smith TJ. Orbital fibroblasts exhibit a novel pattern of responses to proinflammatory cytokines: potential basis for the pathogenesis of thyroid-associated ophthalmopathy. Thyroid. 2002;12(3):197–203.
84. Chen B, Tsui S, Boeglin WE, Douglas RS, Brash AR, Smith TJ. Interleukin-4 induces 15-lipoxygenase-1 expression in human orbital fibroblasts from patients with Graves disease. Evidence for anatomic site-selective actions of Th2 cytokines. J Biol Chem. 2006;281(27):18296–306.
85. Young DA, Evans CH, Smith TJ. Leukoregulin induction of protein expression in human orbital fibroblasts: evidence for anatomical site-restricted cytokine-target cell interactions. Proc Natl Acad Sci U S A. 1998;95(15):8904–9.
86. Smith RS, Smith TJ, Blieden TM, Phipps RP. Fibroblasts as sentinel cells. Synthesis of chemokines and regulation of inflammation. Am J Pathol. 1997;151(2):317–22.
87. Smith TJ. The putative role of fibroblasts in the pathogenesis of Graves' disease: evidence for the involvement of the insulin-like growth factor-1 receptor in fibroblast activation. Autoimmunity. 2003;36(6–7):409–15.
88. Sasaki T, Ito Y, Bringas P, et al. TGFbeta-mediated FGF signaling is crucial for regulating cranial neural crest cell proliferation during frontal bone development. Development. 2006;133(2):371–81.
89. Tawfik HA, Dutton JJ. Embryologic and fetal development of the human orbit. Ophthalmic Plast Reconstr Surg. 2018;34(5):405–21.
90. Bohnsack BL, Gallina D, Thompson H, et al. Development of extraocular muscles requires early signals from periocular neural crest and the developing eye. Arch Ophthalmol. 2011;129(8):1030–41.
91. Cao HJ, Smith TJ. Leukoregulin upregulation of prostaglandin endoperoxide H synthase-2 expression in human orbital fibroblasts. Am J Phys. 1999;277(6):C1075–85.
92. Han R, Tsui S, Smith TJ. Up-regulation of prostaglandin E2 synthesis by interleukin-1beta in human orbital fibroblasts involves coordinate induction of prostaglandin-endoperoxide H synthase-2 and glutathione-dependent prostaglandin E2 synthase expression. J Biol Chem. 2002;277(19):16355–64.
93. Paik JS, Cho WK, Oh EH, Lee SB, Yang SW. Palmitate induced secretion of IL-6 and MCP-1 in orbital fibroblasts derived from patients with thyroid-associated ophthalmopathy. Mol Vis. 2012;18:1467–77.
94. Korducki JM, Loftus SJ, Bahn RS. Stimulation of glycosaminoglycan production in cultured human retroocular fibroblasts. Invest Ophthalmol Vis Sci. 1992;33(6):2037–42.
95. Smith TJ, Wang HS, Evans CH. Leukoregulin is a potent inducer of hyaluronan synthesis in cultured human orbital fibroblasts. Am J Phys. 1995;268(2 Pt 1):C382–8.
96. Sempowski GD, Rozenblit J, Smith TJ, Phipps RP. Human orbital fibroblasts are activated through CD40 to induce proinflammatory cytokine production. Am J Phys. 1998;274(3 Pt 1):C707–14.
97. Ramsdell F, Seaman MS, Clifford KN, Fanslow WC. CD40 ligand acts as a costimulatory signal for neonatal thymic gamma delta T cells. J Immunol. 1994;152(5):2190–7.
98. Durie FH, Foy TM, Noelle RJ. The role of CD40 and its ligand (gp39) in peripheral and central tolerance and its contribution to autoimmune disease. Res Immunol. 1994;145(3):200–5; discussion 244–209.
99. Mohan C, Shi Y, Laman JD, Datta SK. Interaction between CD40 and its ligand gp39 in the development of murine lupus nephritis. J Immunol. 1995;154(3):1470–80.
100. Bour-Jordan H, Salomon BL, Thompson HL, Szot GL, Bernhard MR, Bluestone JA. Costimulation controls diabetes by altering the balance of pathogenic and regulatory T cells. J Clin Invest. 2004;114(7):979–87.
101. Gu ZX, Zhang Y, Dou ZX, Zhao SZ. Research progress on the role of NLRP3 inflammasome in ocular diseases. Zhonghua Yan Ke Za Zhi. 2018;54(5):396–400.
102. Yerramothu P, Vijay AK, Willcox MDP. Inflammasomes, the eye and anti-inflammasome therapy. Eye (Lond). 2018;32(3):491–505.
103. Akhtar-Schäfer I, Wang L, Krohne TU, Xu H, Langmann T. Modulation of three key innate immune pathways for the most common retinal degenerative diseases. EMBO Mol Med. 2018;10(10):e8259.
104. Chaurasia SS, Lim RR, Parikh BH, et al. The NLRP3 inflammasome may contribute to pathologic neovascularization in the advanced stages of diabetic retinopathy. Sci Rep. 2018;8(1):2847.
105. Kerur N, Fukuda S, Banerjee D, et al. cGAS drives noncanonical-inflammasome activation in age-related macular degeneration. Nat Med. 2018;24(1):50–61.
106. Cury SS, Oliveira M, Síbio MT, et al. Graves' ophthalmopathy: low-dose dexamethasone reduces retinoic acid receptor-alpha gene expression in orbital fibroblasts. Arch Endocrinol Metab. 2018;62(3):366–9.
107. Pasquali D, Bellastella A, Colantuoni V, et al. All-trans retinoic acid- and N-(4-hydroxyphenil)-retinamide-induced growth arrest and apoptosis in orbital fibroblasts in Graves' disease. Metabolism. 2003;52(11):1387–92.
108. Rotondo Dottore G, Ionni I, Menconi F, et al. Antioxidant effects of β-carotene, but not of retinol and vitamin E, in orbital fibroblasts from patients with Graves' orbitopathy (GO). J Endocrinol Investig. 2018;41(7):815–20.
109. Koumas L, Smith TJ, Feldon S, Blumberg N, Phipps RP. Thy-1 expression in human fibroblast subsets defines myofibroblastic or lipofibroblastic phenotypes. Am J Pathol. 2003;163(4):1291–300.
110. Sorisky A, Pardasani D, Gagnon A, Smith TJ. Evidence of adipocyte differentiation in human orbital fibroblasts in primary culture. J Clin Endocrinol Metab. 1996;81(9):3428–31.
111. Smith TJ, Koumas L, Gagnon A, et al. Orbital fibroblast heterogeneity may determine the clinical presentation of thyroid-associated ophthalmopathy. J Clin Endocrinol Metab. 2002;87(1):385–92.
112. Adams M, Montague CT, Prins JB, et al. Activators of peroxisome proliferator-activated receptor gamma have depot-specific effects on human preadipocyte differentiation. J Clin Invest. 1997;100(12):3149–53.
113. Valyasevi RW, Harteneck DA, Dutton CM, Bahn RS. Stimulation of adipogenesis, peroxisome proliferator-activated receptor-gamma (PPARgamma), and thyrotropin receptor by PPARgamma agonist in human orbital preadipocyte fibroblasts. J Clin Endocrinol Metab. 2002;87(5):2352–8.
114. Chng CL, Lai OF, Chew CS, et al. Hypoxia increases adipogenesis and affects adipocytokine production in orbital fibroblasts-a possible explanation of the link between smoking and Graves' ophthalmopathy. Int J Ophthalmol. 2014;7(3):403–7.
115. Görtz GE, Horstmann M, Aniol B, et al. Hypoxia-dependent HIF-1 activation impacts on tissue remodeling in Graves' ophthalmopathy-implications for smoking. J Clin Endocrinol Metab. 2016;101(12):4834–42.
116. Hikage F, Atkins S, Kahana A, Smith TJ, Chun TH. HIF2A-LOX pathway promotes fibrotic tissue remodeling in thyroid-associated orbitopathy. Endocrinology. 2019;160(1):20–35.
117. Fang S, Huang Y, Wang S, et al. IL-17A exacerbates fibrosis by promoting the proinflammatory and profibrotic function of orbital fibroblasts in TAO. J Clin Endocrinol Metab. 2016;101(8):2955–65.
118. Bacchetta R, Gregori S, Roncarolo MG. CD4+ regulatory T cells: mechanisms of induction and effector function. Autoimmun Rev. 2005;4(8):491–6.
119. Bluestone JA. Regulatory T-cell therapy: is it ready for the clinic? Nat Rev Immunol. 2005;5(4):343–9.
120. Hwang CJ, Afifiyan N, Sand D, et al. Orbital fibroblasts from patients with thyroid-associated ophthalmopathy overexpress

CD40: CD154 hyperinduces IL-6, IL-8, and MCP-1. Invest Ophthalmol Vis Sci. 2009;50(5):2262–8.
121. Li C, Yuan J, Zhu YF, et al. Imbalance of Th17/Treg in different subtypes of autoimmune thyroid diseases. Cell Physiol Biochem. 2016;40(1–2):245–52.
122. Lv M, Shen J, Li Z, et al. Role of Treg/Th17 cells and related cytokines in Graves' ophthalmopathy. Nan Fang Yi Ke Da Xue Xue Bao. 2014;34(12):1809–13.
123. Kohm AP, Williams JS, Bickford AL, et al. Treatment with nonmitogenic anti-CD3 monoclonal antibody induces CD4+ T cell unresponsiveness and functional reversal of established experimental autoimmune encephalomyelitis. J Immunol. 2005;174(8):4525–34.
124. Herold KC, Hagopian W, Auger JA, et al. Anti-CD3 monoclonal antibody in new-onset type 1 diabetes mellitus. N Engl J Med. 2002;346(22):1692–8.
125. Naik V, Khadavi N, Naik MN, et al. Biologic therapeutics in thyroid-associated ophthalmopathy: translating disease mechanism into therapy. Thyroid. 2008;18(9):967–71.
126. Avery DT, Kalled SL, Ellyard JI, et al. BAFF selectively enhances the survival of plasmablasts generated from human memory B cells. J Clin Invest. 2003;112(2):286–97.
127. Tuscano JM, Harris GS, Tedder TF. B lymphocytes contribute to autoimmune disease pathogenesis: current trends and clinical implications. Autoimmun Rev. 2003;2(2):101–8.
128. Macht LM, Corrall RJ, Banga JP, Elson CJ. Control of human thyroid autoantibody production in SCID mice. Clin Exp Immunol. 1993;91(3):390–6.
129. Yoshizaki A, Miyagaki T, DiLillo DJ, et al. Regulatory B cells control T-cell autoimmunity through IL-21-dependent cognate interactions. Nature. 2012;491(7423):264–8.
130. Ding YG, Chen G, Li Q, Wen XF, Wei L, Yang HS. Frequency of IL-10-producing regulatory B cells associated with disease activity in thyroid-associated orbitopathy. Int J Ophthalmol. 2018;11(9):1458–62.
131. Jang SY, Shin DY, Lee EJ, Lee SY, Yoon JS. Relevance of TSH-receptor antibody levels in predicting disease course in Graves' orbitopathy: comparison of the third-generation TBII assay and Mc4-TSI bioassay. Eye (Lond). 2013;27(8):964–71.
132. Woo YJ, Jang SY, Lim TH, Yoon JS. Clinical association of thyroid stimulating hormone receptor antibody levels with disease severity in the chronic inactive stage of Graves' orbitopathy. Korean J Ophthalmol. 2015;29(4):213–9.
133. Takakura A, Kirkeby K, Earle K, Silkiss RZ. Predicting the development of orbitopathy in Graves thyroidopathy patients: the potential role of TSI testing. Ophthal Plast Reconstr Surg. 2015;31(5):369–72.
134. Yin X, Latif R, Bahn R, Tomer Y, Davies TF. Influence of the TSH receptor gene on susceptibility to Graves' disease and Graves' ophthalmopathy. Thyroid. 2008;18(11):1201–6.
135. Diana T, Kahaly GJ. Thyroid stimulating hormone receptor antibodies in thyroid eye disease-methodology and clinical applications. Ophthalmic Plast Reconstr Surg. 2018;34(4S Suppl 1):S13–9.
136. Pritchard J, Tsui S, Horst N, Cruikshank WW, Smith TJ. Synovial fibroblasts from patients with rheumatoid arthritis, like fibroblasts from Graves' disease, express high levels of IL-16 when treated with Igs against insulin-like growth factor-1 receptor. J Immunol. 2004;173(5):3564–9.
137. Smith TJ, Hoa N. Immunoglobulins from patients with Graves' disease induce hyaluronan synthesis in their orbital fibroblasts through the self-antigen, insulin-like growth factor-I receptor. J Clin Endocrinol Metab. 2004;89(10):5076–80.
138. Sachdev D, Yee D. Inhibitors of insulin-like growth factor signaling: a therapeutic approach for breast cancer. J Mammary Gland Biol Neoplasia. 2006;11(1):27–39.
139. Hartog H, Wesseling J, Boezen HM, van der Graaf WT. The insulin-like growth factor 1 receptor in cancer: old focus, new future. Eur J Cancer. 2007;43(13):1895–904.
140. Paz K, Hadari YR. Targeted therapy of the insulin-like growth factor-1 receptor in cancer. Comb Chem High Throughput Screen. 2008;11(1):62–9.
141. Krieger CC, Place RF, Bevilacqua C, et al. TSH/IGF-1 receptor cross talk in Graves' ophthalmopathy pathogenesis. J Clin Endocrinol Metab. 2016;101(6):2340–7.
142. Krieger CC, Perry JD, Morgan SJ, Kahaly GJ, Gershengorn MC. TSH/IGF-1 receptor cross-talk rapidly activates extracellular signal-regulated kinases in multiple cell types. Endocrinology. 2017;158(10):3676–83.
143. Smith TJ, Hegedüs L, Douglas RS. Role of insulin-like growth factor-1 (IGF-1) pathway in the pathogenesis of Graves' orbitopathy. Best Pract Res Clin Endocrinol Metab. 2012;26(3):291–302.
144. Smith TJ. New advances in understanding thyroid-associated ophthalmopathy and the potential role for insulin-like growth factor-I receptor. F1000Res. 2018;7:134.
145. Lantz M, Planck T, Asman P, Hallengren B. Increased TRAb and/or low anti-TPO titers at diagnosis of graves' disease are associated with an increased risk of developing ophthalmopathy after onset. Exp Clin Endocrinol Diabetes. 2014;122(2):113–7.
146. Srinivasan A, Kleinberg TT, Murchison AP, Bilyk JR. Laboratory investigations for diagnosis of autoimmune and inflammatory periocular disease: part I. Ophthal Plast Reconstr Surg. 2016;32(5):321–8.
147. Eckstein AK, Plicht M, Lax H, et al. Clinical results of anti-inflammatory therapy in Graves' ophthalmopathy and association with thyroidal autoantibodies. Clin Endocrinol. 2004;61(5):612–8.
148. Gerding MN, van der Meer JW, Broenink M, Bakker O, Wiersinga WM, Prummel MF. Association of thyrotrophin receptor antibodies with the clinical features of Graves' ophthalmopathy. Clin Endocrinol. 2000;52(3):267–71.
149. Wiersinga WM, Prummel MF, Mourits MP, Koornneef L, Buller HR. Classification of the eye changes of Graves' disease. Thyroid. 1991;1(4):357–60.
150. Werner SC. Classification of the eye changes of Grave's disease. J Clin Endocrinol Metab. 1969;29(7):982–4.
151. Dunsky IL. Normative data for hertel exophthalmometry in a normal adult black population. Optom Vis Sci. 1992;69(7):562–4.
152. Stan MN, Garrity JA, Bahn RS. The evaluation and treatment of graves ophthalmopathy. Med Clin North Am. 2012;96(2):311–28.
153. Bartalena L, Baldeschi L, Dickinson AJ, et al. Consensus statement of the European group on Graves' orbitopathy (EUGOGO) on management of Graves' orbitopathy. Thyroid. 2008;18(3):333–46.
154. Mourits MP, Koornneef L, Wiersinga WM, Prummel MF, Berghout A, van der Gaag R. Clinical criteria for the assessment of disease activity in Graves' ophthalmopathy: a novel approach. Br J Ophthalmol. 1989;73(8):639–44.
155. Mourits MP, Prummel MF, Wiersinga WM, Koornneef L. Clinical activity score as a guide in the management of patients with Graves' ophthalmopathy. Clin Endocrinol. 1997;47(1):9–14.
156. Bartalena L, Baldeschi L, Dickinson A, et al. Consensus statement of the European Group on Graves' orbitopathy (EUGOGO) on management of GO. Eur J Endocrinol. 2008;158(3):273–85.
157. Kauh CY, Gupta S, Douglas RS, et al. Compressive optic neuropathy and repeat orbital decompression: a case series. Ophthalmic Plast Reconstr Surg. 2015;31(5):385–90.
158. Dolman PJ, Rootman J. VISA classification for graves orbitopathy. Ophthalmic Plast Reconstr Surg. 2006;22(5):319–24.
159. Sundaresh V, Brito JP, Thapa P, Bahn RS, Stan MN. Comparative effectiveness of treatment choices for Graves' hyperthyroidism: a historical cohort study. Thyroid. 2017;27(4):497–505.
160. Sundaresh V, Brito JP, Wang Z, et al. Comparative effectiveness of therapies for Graves' hyperthyroidism: a systematic

review and network meta-analysis. J Clin Endocrinol Metab. 2013;98(9):3671–7.
161. Akmal A, Kung J. Propylthiouracil, and methimazole, and carbimazole-related hepatotoxicity. Expert Opin Drug Saf. 2014;13(10):1397–406.
162. Andersen SL, Laurberg P. Antithyroid drugs and congenital heart defects: ventricular septal defect is part of the methimazole/carbimazole embryopathy. Eur J Endocrinol. 2014;171(5):C1–3.
163. Laurberg P, Andersen SL. Therapy of endocrine disease: antithyroid drug use in early pregnancy and birth defects: time windows of relative safety and high risk? Eur J Endocrinol. 2014;171(1):R13–20.
164. Heidari R, Niknahad H, Jamshidzadeh A, Abdoli N. Factors affecting drug-induced liver injury: antithyroid drugs as instances. Clin Mol Hepatol. 2014;20(3):237–48.
165. Meyer Zu Horste M, Pateronis K, Walz MK, et al. The effect of early thyroidectomy on the course of active Graves' orbitopathy (GO): a retrospective case study. Horm Metab Res. 2016;48(7):433–9.
166. Tallstedt L, Lundell G, Blomgren H, Bring J. Does early administration of thyroxine reduce the development of Graves' ophthalmopathy after radioiodine treatment? Eur J Endocrinol. 1994;130(5):494–7.
167. Stan MN, Durski JM, Brito JP, Bhagra S, Thapa P, Bahn RS. Cohort study on radioactive iodine-induced hypothyroidism: implications for Graves' ophthalmopathy and optimal timing for thyroid hormone assessment. Thyroid. 2013;23(5):620–5.
168. Heufelder AE. Involvement of the orbital fibroblast and TSH receptor in the pathogenesis of Graves' ophthalmopathy. Thyroid. 1995;5(4):331–40.
169. Kloprogge SJ, Busuttil BE, Frauman AG. TSH receptor protein is selectively expressed in normal human extraocular muscle. Muscle Nerve. 2005;32(1):95–8.
170. Otto E, Forster G, Kuhlemann K, Hansen C, Kahaly GJ. TSH receptor in endocrine autoimmunity. Clin Exp Rheumatol. 1996;14(Suppl 15):S77–84.
171. Wakelkamp IM, Bakker O, Baldeschi L, Wiersinga WM, Prummel MF. TSH-R expression and cytokine profile in orbital tissue of active vs. inactive Graves' ophthalmopathy patients. Clin Endocrinol. 2003;58:280–7.
172. Jonklaas J, Bianco AC, Bauer AJ, et al. Guidelines for the treatment of hypothyroidism: prepared by the american thyroid association task force on thyroid hormone replacement. Thyroid. 2014;24(12):1670–751.
173. Tallstedt L, Lundell G, Torring O, et al. Occurrence of ophthalmopathy after treatment for Graves' hyperthyroidism. The Thyroid Study Group. N Engl J Med. 1992;326(26):1733–8.
174. Jones BM, Kwok CC, Kung AW. Effect of radioactive iodine therapy on cytokine production in Graves' disease: transient increases in interleukin-4 (IL-4), IL-6, IL-10, and tumor necrosis factor-alpha, with longer term increases in interferon-gamma production. J Clin Endocrinol Metab. 1999;84(11):4106–10.
175. Bogazzi F, Bartalena L, Campomori A, et al. Treatment with lithium prevents serum thyroid hormone increase after thionamide withdrawal and radioiodine therapy in patients with Graves' disease. J Clin Endocrinol Metab. 2002;87(10):4490–5.
176. Bartalena L, Marcocci C, Bogazzi F, Panicucci M, Lepri A, Pinchera A. Use of corticosteroids to prevent progression of Graves' ophthalmopathy after radioiodine therapy for hyperthyroidism. N Engl J Med. 1989;321(20):1349–52.
177. Thornton J, Kelly SP, Harrison RA, Edwards R. Cigarette smoking and thyroid eye disease: a systematic review. Eye. 2007;21(9):1135–45.
178. Wu VT, Lorenzen AW, Beck AC, et al. Comparative analysis of radioactive iodine versus thyroidectomy for definitive treatment of Graves' disease. Surgery. 2017;161(1):147–55.
179. Rasmussen AK, Nygaard B, Feldt-Rasmussen U. (131) I and thyroid-associated ophthalmopathy. Eur J Endocrinol. 2000;143(2):155–60.
180. Bartalena L, Baldeschi L, Boboridis K, et al. The 2016 European Thyroid Association/European Group on Graves' Orbitopathy guidelines for the management of Graves' orbitopathy. Eur Thyroid J. 2016;5(1):9–26.
181. Lai A, Sassi L, Compri E, et al. Lower dose prednisone prevents radioiodine-associated exacerbation of initially mild or absent Graves' orbitopathy: a retrospective cohort study. J Clin Endocrinol Metab. 2010;95(3):1333–7.
182. Vannucchi G, Campi I, Covelli D, et al. Graves' orbitopathy activation after radioactive iodine therapy with and without steroid prophylaxis. J Clin Endocrinol Metab. 2009;94(9):3381–6.
183. Shiber S, Stiebel-Kalish H, Shimon I, Grossman A, Robenshtok E. Glucocorticoid regimens for prevention of Graves' ophthalmopathy progression following radioiodine treatment: systematic review and meta-analysis. Thyroid. 2014;24(10):1515–23.
184. Stein JD, Childers D, Gupta S, et al. Risk factors for developing thyroid-associated ophthalmopathy among individuals with Graves' disease. JAMA Ophthalmol. 2015;133(3):290–6.
185. Tallstedt L, Lundell G, Taube A. Graves' ophthalmopathy and tobacco smoking. Acta Endocrinol. 1993;129(2):147–50.
186. Tellez M, Cooper J, Edmonds C. Graves' ophthalmopathy in relation to cigarette smoking and ethnic origin. Clin Endocrinol. 1992;36(3):291–4.
187. Winsa B, Mandahl A, Karlsson FA. Graves' disease, endocrine ophthalmopathy and smoking. Acta Endocrinol. 1993;128(2):156–60.
188. Sung TY, Lee YM, Yoon JH, Chung KW, Hong SJ. Long-term effect of surgery in Graves' disease: 20 years experience in a single institution. Int J Endocrinol. 2015;2015:542641.
189. Marcocci C, Bartalena L, Pinchera A. Ablative or non-ablative therapy for Graves' hyperthyroidism in patients with ophthalmopathy? J Endocrinol Investig. 1998;21(7):468–71.
190. Menconi F, Leo M, Vitti P, Marcocci C, Marino M. Total thyroid ablation in Graves' orbitopathy. J Endocrinol Investig. 2015;38(8):809–15.
191. Menconi F, Marino M, Pinchera A, et al. Effects of total thyroid ablation versus near-total thyroidectomy alone on mild to moderate Graves' orbitopathy treated with intravenous glucocorticoids. J Clin Endocrinol Metab. 2007;92(5):1653–8.
192. Gauthier JM, Mohamed HE, Noureldine SI, Nazari-Shafti TZ, Thethi TK, Kandil E. Impact of thyroidectomy on cardiac manifestations of Graves' disease. Laryngoscope. 2016;126(5):1256–9.
193. Vital D, Morand GB, Meerwein C, et al. Early timing of thyroidectomy for hyperthyroidism in Graves' disease improves biochemical recovery. World J Surg. 2017;41(10):2545–50.
194. Sosa JA, Bowman HM, Tielsch JM, Powe NR, Gordon TA, Udelsman R. The importance of surgeon experience for clinical and economic outcomes from thyroidectomy. Ann Surg. 1998;228(3):320–30.
195. Erbil Y, Ozluk Y, Giris M, et al. Effect of Lugol's solution on thyroid gland blood flow and microvessel density in the patients with Graves' disease. J Clin Endocrinol Metab. 2007;92(6):2182–9.
196. Sun W, Liu J, Zhang H, et al. A meta-analysis of intraoperative neuromonitoring of recurrent laryngeal nerve palsy during thyroid reoperations. Clin Endocrinol. 2017;87(5):572–80.
197. Karakas E, Osei-Agyemang T, Schlosser K, et al. The impact of parathyroid gland autotransplantation during bilateral thyroid surgery for Graves' disease on postoperative hypocalcaemia. Endocr Regul. 2008;42(2–3):39–44.
198. Leo M, Marcocci C, Pinchera A, et al. Outcome of Graves' orbitopathy after total thyroid ablation and glucocorticoid treatment: follow-up of a randomized clinical trial. J Clin Endocrinol Metab. 2012;97(1):E44–8.

199. El-Kaissi S, Frauman AG, Wall JR. Thyroid-associated ophthalmopathy: a practical guide to classification, natural history and management. Intern Med J. 2004;34(8):482–91.
200. Marcocci C, Kahaly GJ, Krassas GE, et al. Selenium and the course of mild Graves' orbitopathy. N Engl J Med. 2011;364(20):1920–31.
201. Marinò M, Menconi F, Rotondo Dottore G, Leo M, Marcocci C. Selenium in Graves hyperthyroidism and orbitopathy. Ophthalmic Plast Reconstr Surg. 2018;34(4S Suppl 1):S105–10.
202. Wu Q, Rayman MP, Lv H, et al. Low population selenium status is associated with increased prevalence of thyroid disease. J Clin Endocrinol Metab. 2015;100(11):4037–47.
203. Modjtahedi SP, Modjtahedi BS, Mansury AM, et al. Pharmacological treatments for thyroid eye disease. Drugs. 2006;66(13):1685–700.
204. Zoumalan CI, Cockerham KP, Turbin RE, et al. Efficacy of corticosteroids and external beam radiation in the management of moderate to severe thyroid eye disease. J Neuroophthalmol. 2007;27(3):205–14.
205. Kahaly GJ, Pitz S, Hommel G, Dittmar M. Randomized, single blind trial of intravenous versus oral steroid monotherapy in Graves' orbitopathy. J Clin Endocrinol Metab. 2005;90(9):5234–40.
206. Macchia PE, Bagattini M, Lupoli G, Vitale M, Vitale G, Fenzi G. High-dose intravenous corticosteroid therapy for Graves' ophthalmopathy. J Endocrinol Investig. 2001;24(3):152–8.
207. Aktaran S, Akarsu E, Erbağci I, Araz M, Okumuş S, Kartal M. Comparison of intravenous methylprednisolone therapy vs. oral methylprednisolone therapy in patients with Graves' ophthalmopathy. Int J Clin Pract. 2007;61(1):45–51.
208. Stiebel-Kalish H, Robenshtok E, Hasanreisoglu M, Ezrachi D, Shimon I, Leibovici L. Treatment modalities for Graves' ophthalmopathy: systematic review and metaanalysis. J Clin Endocrinol Metab. 2009;94(8):2708–16.
209. Weissel M, Hauff W. Fatal liver failure after high-dose glucocorticoid pulse therapy in a patient with severe thyroid eye disease. Thyroid. 2000;10(6):521.
210. Bartalena L. Steroid prophylaxis after radioiodine treatment for Graves' hyperthyroidism: selective or universal? Thyroid. 2014;24(10):1441–2.
211. Ebner R, Devoto MH, Weil D, et al. Treatment of thyroid associated ophthalmopathy with periocular injections of triamcinolone. Br J Ophthalmol. 2004;88(11):1380–6.
212. Kahaly G, Schrezenmeir J, Krause U, et al. Ciclosporin and prednisone v. prednisone in treatment of Graves' ophthalmopathy: a controlled, randomized and prospective study. Eur J Clin Investig. 1986;16(5):415–22.
213. Leövey A, Bakó G, Szabó J, Kálmán K, Fórizs E. Combined cyclosporin-A and methylprednisolone treatment of Graves' ophthalmopathy. Acta Med Hung. 1992;49(3–4):179–85.
214. Prummel MF, Mourits MP, Berghout A, et al. Prednisone and cyclosporine in the treatment of severe Graves' ophthalmopathy. N Engl J Med. 1989;321(20):1353–9.
215. Strianese D. Efficacy and safety of immunosuppressive agents for thyroid eye disease. Ophthalmic Plast Reconstr Surg. 2018;34(4S Suppl 1):S56–9.
216. Smith JR, Rosenbaum JT. A role for methotrexate in the management of non-infectious orbital inflammatory disease. Br J Ophthalmol. 2001;85(10):1220–4.
217. Strianese D, Iuliano A, Ferrara M, et al. Methotrexate for the treatment of thyroid eye disease. J Ophthalmol. 2014;2014:128903.
218. Rivera-Grana E, Lin P, Suhler EB, Rosenbaum JT. Methotrexate as a corticosteroid-sparing agent for thyroid eye disease. J Clin Exp Ophthalmol. 2015;6(2)422. https://www.longdom.org/open-access/methotrexate-as-a-corticosteroidsparing-agent-for-thyroid-eye-disease-2155-9570-1000422.pdf.
219. Perros P, Weightman DR, Crombie AL, Kendall-Taylor P. Azathioprine in the treatment of thyroid-associated ophthalmopathy. Acta Endocrinol. 1990;122(1):8–12.
220. Rajendram R, Lee RW, Potts MJ, et al. Protocol for the combined immunosuppression & radiotherapy in thyroid eye disease (CIRTED) trial: a multi-centre, double-masked, factorial randomised controlled trial. Trials. 2008;9:6.
221. Chalvatzis NT, Tzamalis AK, Kalantzis GK, El-Hindy N, Dimitrakos SA, Potts MJ. Safety and efficacy of combined immunosuppression and orbital radiotherapy in thyroid-related restrictive myopathy: two-center experience. Eur J Ophthalmol. 2014;24(6):953–9.
222. Ye X, Bo X, Hu X, et al. Efficacy and safety of mycophenolate mofetil in patients with active moderate-to-severe Graves' orbitopathy. Clin Endocrinol. 2017;86(2):247–55.
223. Stan MN, Salvi M. Management of Endocrine Disease: rituximab therapy for Graves' orbitopathy – lessons from randomized control trials. Eur J Endocrinol. 2017;176(2):R101–9.
224. Salvi M, Vannucchi G, Campi I, et al. Efficacy of rituximab treatment for thyroid-associated ophthalmopathy as a result of intraorbital B-cell depletion in one patient unresponsive to steroid immunosuppression. Eur J Endocrinol. 2006;154(4):511–7.
225. Khanna D, Chong KK, Afifiyan NF, et al. Rituximab treatment of patients with severe, corticosteroid-resistant thyroid-associated ophthalmopathy. Ophthalmology. 2010;117(1):133–139.e132.
226. El Fassi D, Nielsen CH, Hasselbalch HC, Hegedüs L. Treatment-resistant severe, active Graves' ophthalmopathy successfully treated with B lymphocyte depletion. Thyroid. 2006;16(7):709–10.
227. Minakaran N, Ezra DG. Rituximab for thyroid-associated ophthalmopathy. Cochrane Database Syst Rev. 2013;(5):CD009226.
228. Salvi M, Vannucchi G, Currò N, et al. Efficacy of B-cell targeted therapy with rituximab in patients with active moderate to severe Graves' orbitopathy: a randomized controlled study. J Clin Endocrinol Metab. 2015;100(2):422–31.
229. Stan MN, Garrity JA, Carranza Leon BG, Prabin T, Bradley EA, Bahn RS. Randomized controlled trial of rituximab in patients with Graves' orbitopathy. J Clin Endocrinol Metab. 2015;100(2):432–41.
230. Shen WC, Lee CH, Loh EW, Hsieh AT, Chen L, Tam KW. Efficacy and safety of rituximab for the treatment of Graves' orbitopathy: a meta-analysis of randomized controlled trials. Pharmacotherapy. 2018;38(5):503–10.
231. Wang C, Ning Q, Jin K, Xie J, Ye J. Does rituximab improve clinical outcomes of patients with thyroid-associated ophthalmopathy? A systematic review and meta-analysis. BMC Ophthalmol. 2018;18(1):46.
232. Cooper N, Stasi R, Cunningham-Rundles S, et al. The efficacy and safety of B-cell depletion with anti-CD20 monoclonal antibody in adults with chronic immune thrombocytopenic purpura. Br J Haematol. 2004;125(2):232–9.
233. Ahn ES, Subramanian PS. Treatment modalities of thyroid related orbitopathy. Indian J Ophthalmol. 2014;62(10):999–1002.
234. Rothe A, Power BE, Hudson PJ. Therapeutic advances in rheumatology with the use of recombinant proteins. Nat Clin Pract Rheumatol. 2008;4(11):605–14.
235. Peyrin-Biroulet L, Deltenre P, de Suray N, Branche J, Sandborn WJ, Colombel JF. Efficacy and safety of tumor necrosis factor antagonists in Crohn's disease: meta-analysis of placebo-controlled trials. Clin Gastroenterol Hepatol. 2008;6(6):644–53.
236. Durrani OM, Reuser TQ, Murray PI. Infliximab: a novel treatment for sight-threatening thyroid associated ophthalmopathy. Orbit. 2005;24(2):117–9.
237. Komorowski J, Jankiewicz-Wika J, Siejka A, et al. Monoclonal anti-TNFalpha antibody (infliximab) in the treatment of patient with thyroid associated ophthalmopathy. Klin Ocz. 2007;109(10–12):457–60.

238. Paridaens D, van den Bosch WA, van der Loos TL, Krenning EP, van Hagen PM. The effect of etanercept on Graves' ophthalmopathy: a pilot study. Eye (Lond). 2005;19(12):1286–9.
239. Ayabe R, Rootman DB, Hwang CJ, Ben-Artzi A, Goldberg R. Adalimumab as steroid-sparing treatment of inflammatory-stage thyroid eye disease. Ophthalmic Plast Reconstr Surg. 2014;30(5):415–9.
240. Pérez-Moreiras JV, Alvarez-López A, Gómez EC. Treatment of active corticosteroid-resistant Graves' orbitopathy. Ophthalmic Plast Reconstr Surg. 2014;30(2):162–7.
241. Perez-Moreiras JV, Gomez-Reino JJ, Maneiro JR, et al. Efficacy of tocilizumab in patients with moderate to severe corticosteroid resistant Graves' orbitopathy: a randomized clinical trial. Am J Ophthalmol. 2018;195:181–90.
242. Sy A, Eliasieh K, Silkiss RZ. Clinical response to tocilizumab in severe thyroid eye disease. Ophthalmic Plast Reconstr Surg. 2017;33(3):e55–7.
243. Bartalena L, Marcocci C, Tanda ML, et al. Orbital radiotherapy for Graves' ophthalmopathy. Thyroid. 2002;12(3):245–50.
244. Mourits MP, van Kempen-Harteveld ML, García MB, Koppeschaar HP, Tick L, Terwee CB. Radiotherapy for Graves' orbitopathy: randomised placebo-controlled study. Lancet. 2000;355(9214):1505–9.
245. Sisti E, Menconi F, Leo M, et al. Long-term outcome of Graves' orbitopathy following high-dose intravenous glucocorticoids and orbital radiotherapy. J Endocrinol Investig. 2015;38(6):661–8.
246. Hahn E, Laperriere N, Millar BA, et al. Orbital radiation therapy for Graves' ophthalmopathy: measuring clinical efficacy and impact. Pract Radiat Oncol. 2014;4(4):233–9.
247. Behbehani R, Sergott RC, Savino PJ. Orbital radiotherapy for thyroid-related orbitopathy. Curr Opin Ophthalmol. 2004;15(6):479–82.
248. Gorman CA, Garrity JA, Fatourechi V, et al. A prospective, randomized, double-blind, placebo-controlled study of orbital radiotherapy for Graves' ophthalmopathy. Ophthalmology. 2001;108(9):1523–34.
249. Rajendram R, Taylor PN, Wilson VJ, et al. Combined immunosuppression and radiotherapy in thyroid eye disease (CIRTED): a multicentre, 2 × 2 factorial, double-blind, randomised controlled trial. Lancet Diabetes Endocrinol. 2018;6(4):299–309.
250. Wei RL, Cheng JW, Cai JP. The use of orbital radiotherapy for Graves' ophthalmopathy: quantitative review of the evidence. Ophthalmologica. 2008;222(1):27–31.
251. Gold KG, Scofield S, Isaacson SR, Stewart MW, Kazim M. Orbital radiotherapy combined with corticosteroid treatment for thyroid eye disease-compressive optic neuropathy. Ophthalmic Plast Reconstr Surg. 2018;34(2):172–7.
252. Chundury RV, Weber AC, Perry JD. Orbital radiation therapy in thyroid eye disease. Ophthalmic Plast Reconstr Surg. 2016;32(2):83–9.
253. Godfrey KJ, Kazim M. Radiotherapy for active thyroid eye disease. Ophthalmic Plast Reconstr Surg. 2018;34(4S Suppl 1):S98–S104.
254. Gillis CC, Chang EH, Al-Kharazi K, Pickles T. Secondary malignancy following radiotherapy for thyroid eye disease. Rep Pract Oncol Radiother. 2016;21(3):156–61.

Surgical Management of Thyroid Eye Disease

58

Anaïs L. Carniciu, Raymond I. Cho, and Alon Kahana

Introduction

Surgical management of thyroid eye disease (TED) has two general aims: (1) relieve symptoms of orbital congestion and fibrosis, including possibly compressive optic neuropathy, and (2) reconstruct the periocular region to reduce deformity and renormalize appearance. Surgical management follows a sequence that is tailored to individual patient needs. The signs and symptoms of TED that can be addressed surgically include proptosis, orbital pressure/pain, orbital inflammatory signs, diplopia secondary to restrictive strabismus, ocular surface exposure secondary to lagophthalmos, and eyelid retraction. Because orbital decompression surgery can improve lagophthalmos and eyelid retraction, and can affect strabismus (positively or negatively), these issues are traditionally addressed sequentially by orbital decompression first, followed by strabismus surgery, and finally eyelid retraction repair, as needed. In this chapter, we focus primarily on orbital decompression surgery and eyelid surgery, although key aspects of strabismus surgery are also discussed.

Thyroid eye disease follows a sequence that is tailored to patient needs. The key issues addressed by surgery include proptosis, orbital pressure/pain, orbital inflammatory signs, diplopia secondary to restrictive strabismus, ocular surface exposure secondary to lagophthalmos, and eyelid retraction. These are traditionally addressed sequentially by orbital decompression, strabismus surgery, and eyelid retraction repair surgery. The extent of surgical rehabilitation is patient specific and customized to the needs of each patient. Coordination and proper sequencing of surgical intervention is key to promoting good outcomes. In this chapter, we focus primarily on orbital decompression and eyelid surgery – the two main reconstructive surgeries performed by oculoplastic surgeons for patients with TED.

Orbital decompression surgery is performed to address the tight compartment caused by expansion of orbital soft tissues. The surgery essentially rebalances the contents to the size of the bony orbit, thereby reducing orbital pressure, proptosis, and, when present, compressive optic neuropathy. Surgical techniques include different approaches to removing orbital bone in order to enlarge the space within the orbital compartment, as well as removal of scarred fat and connective tissue to reduce the volume of orbital soft tissue.

Strabismus surgery is performed following orbital decompression surgery, but prior to eyelid retraction surgery. This is done for three reasons: (1) orbital decompression must be performed first because it can alter mechanical vectors of extraocular muscle function, leading to changes in eye alignment; (2) restrictive strabismus can lead to secondary eyelid retraction – essentially a pseudoretraction that can be reduced by releasing the extraocular muscle restriction; and (3) strabismus surgery can itself cause eyelid retraction, particularly of the lower eyelids, secondary to the relationship of the lower eyelid retractors to the inferior rectus and oblique muscles.

It is important to note that recession of fibrotic inelastic muscles frequently causes worsening proptosis [1]. Therefore, it is important to provide sufficient decompression to account for the expected increase in proptosis following strabismus surgery and to properly counsel patients.

Eyelid retraction repair is performed last – once proptosis is reduced to an acceptable level, any compressive issues are addressed, and strabismus is resolved. Upper eyelid retraction repair typically requires release of eyelid retractors,

A. L. Carniciu · A. Kahana (✉)
Consultants in Ophthalmic and Facial Plastic Surgery, Southfield, MI, USA
e-mail: akahana@facialworks.com

R. I. Cho
Ophthalmic Plastic and Reconstructive Surgery, The Ohio State University Wexner Medical Center, Department of Ophthalmology and Visual Science, Columbus, OH, USA

J. J. Servat et al. (eds.), *Smith and Nesi's Ophthalmic Plastic and Reconstructive Surgery*,
https://doi.org/10.1007/978-3-030-41720-8_58

which undergo fibrosis as part of the orbitopathy process. This can be done via anterior or posterior surgical approaches and may involve levator muscle, Müller's muscle, and/or conjunctiva. Lower eyelid retraction repair frequently requires a spacer graft, which can be autologous (e.g., hard palate, ear cartilage, dermis), allograft or xenograft (e.g., decellularized dermis), or alloplastic material.

In this chapter, we will describe the diagnostic process for customizing a surgical plan, perioperative planning, surgical techniques and postoperative considerations.

Orbital Decompression

History

Orbital decompression has evolved since its inception in the early twentieth century. Dollinger first described orbital bone decompression for TED in 1911 by removing the lateral wall [2, 3]. Orbital roof decompression was advocated by Naffziger, a neurosurgeon, in 1931. The procedure allowed access to both orbital apices in cases of bilateral optic neuropathy, though it provided minimal volumetric decompression [2]. Direct external ethmoidectomy for decompression of the medial wall was described by Sewall, an otolaryngologist, in 1936 [2, 4]. The combined approach to the medial wall and floor of the orbit was described by Walsh and Ogura, otolaryngologists, in 1957, and performed via a transantral approach [2, 4]. This was the procedure of choice until the early 1980s, when more direct orbital approaches, including the swinging eyelid, transconjunctival, transcaruncular, and endoscopic approaches to the lateral wall, floor, and medial wall were described [5–9]. Decompression of the orbital roof has generally been avoided due to its potential complications, including cerebrospinal fluid leak and pulsating proptosis from transmission of intracranial pressure changes [10].

Currently, the most common surgical approaches to orbital decompression surgery include (1) lateral decompression through an extended lateral upper eyelid crease or a lateral canthotomy approach to the lateral orbit, lateral roof, and lateral floor (avoiding injury to the lateral commissure); (2) medial transconjunctival approach to the orbit (allows access to the medial orbit and posterior floor); and (3) inferior fornix approach to the anterior floor and orbital fat [11–14]. Endonasal surgery is a reasonable option to access the medial wall and floor [15, 16], although this approach has several important limitations, including extended length of surgery [17], removal of tissue while moving toward the globe instead of away from the globe (increasing risk of inadvertent injury), and a more limited access to the orbital process of the palatine bone at the orbital apex [18].

With improved techniques and better fellowship training, the trend in surgical decompression has been toward more nuanced customizable techniques that enhance outcomes and decrease morbidity [19–37]. Each surgery for TED is individually tailored based on patient characteristics and surgeon experience. Given the lack of randomized controlled trials comparing surgical techniques for orbital decompression, no particular method has been deemed scientifically superior [35, 38]. However, with improved understanding of the goals of surgery, some techniques have been abandoned by most orbital surgeons. This includes the misguided technique of discarding the lateral orbital rim in the hope of providing additional decompression; this technique not only damages the lateral canthal tendon attachments, leading to disfigurement and eyelid instability, but also provides no decompression where it is most needed – at the orbital apex. Instead, improved understanding of how to deeply contour the diploic spaces within the sphenoid, frontal, and zygomatic bones has led to excellent results with dramatic improvements in proptosis reduction through smaller incisions and without damaging the lateral orbital rim. Indeed, many orbital surgeons no longer remove the orbital rim at all during a lateral decompression surgery, choosing instead to create the window to the temporalis fossa from within the orbit, prior to initiating removal of diploe for apical decompression.

Customization of orbital decompression can be accomplished through the number and choice of orbital walls removed, augmenting the decompression with excision of hypertrophied and fibrotic orbital fat, varying the extent of ethmoidectomy (medial decompression) or deep bone removal (lateral decompression), targeting the posterior inferomedial strut and orbital process of the palatine bone, and timing of surgery. The development of modern techniques has been made possible by advancements in noninvasive imaging [39, 40], preoperative analysis of the orbital anatomy [41, 42], stereotactic image-guided surgical navigation devices [43–47], piezoelectric technology that minimizes tissue damage [48], and an improved understanding of the spectrum of orbital pathology represented by thyroid eye disease (TED) [49–51]. Additionally, the expansion of accepted indications for decompression, the growing referral pattern of most advanced TED patients to academic medical centers, and the significant increase in the number of orbital surgery fellowships over the past decade have resulted in more orbital surgeons who have better surgical training and experience with decompression. Hence, the clinical threshold for performing orbital decompression surgery has decreased, leading to earlier and more robust interventions with good outcomes.

Surgical Timing

The acute phase of TED is marked by congestive and inflammatory signs, such as chemosis, caruncular edema, eyelid edema, orbital pain, and progressive strabismus. For many years, conventional wisdom ruled that orbital decompression should be avoided in patients in the acute phase of TED, limiting treatment to medical measures, including topical lubrication, salt restriction, head elevation, prism glasses, corticosteroids (oral, intravenous, or intraorbital), and low-dose external beam radiotherapy [52]. Details of medical therapy, including new potential therapeutic modalities, are described in the previous chapter. However, with the understanding that congestion and inflammation cannot be differentiated based on clinical exam, and the further understanding that orbital congestion leads to venous stasis and accumulation of cytokines within the orbit, some surgeons began to perform orbital decompression surgery for orbits with acute-phase signs and symptoms – with excellent results [53, 54]. These outcomes may be related to improved techniques that allow for excellent decompression of the orbital apex, where the ophthalmic venous system drains, through smaller incisions and less invasive surgical approaches. Since there are no good randomized clinical trials of orbital decompression techniques, surgeons are mostly left to their own device regarding the best approach to the timing and technique of orbital decompression surgery. However, operating on the acutely involved orbit with signs of congestion and inflammation is progressively gaining wider acceptance, and the decision rests with the surgeon and patient based on a personalized, customized approach to the rehabilitation process.

TED with imminent visual threat due to dysthyroid compressive optic neuropathy (CON) occurs in approximately 6% of patients [55] and represents a unique, more urgent situation. These orbits will typically require decompression surgery. However, the urgency of surgery is not clear. Many surgeons may choose to "buy time" using pulsed intravenous corticosteroids [56] and/or low-dose orbital radiation. These options are particularly important when patients are medically unstable or not fully optimized for surgical anesthesia. Importantly, unlike other causes of optic neuropathy, such as microvascular disease, visual field loss from CON is often reversible [57], revealing a unique resilience in retinal ganglion cells and axons that may have to do with axonal stasis. Still, that resilience should not be tested without important medical reasons, and orbital decompression is often required at the earliest opportunity for optimal outcomes.

In patients whose vision is not acutely threatened, the decision regarding when to perform orbital decompression is more nuanced. A single pulse of intravenous corticosteroids may serve as a therapeutic trial that can differentiate the inflammatory and congestive processes in the acute phase: inflammatory orbitopathy improves following corticosteroid administration, while congestive orbitopathy is usually unresponsive [58]. Early orbital decompression may have beneficial effects on the overall course of the orbitopathy by relieving the orbital congestion and improving blood flow to orbital tissues in patients with symptomatic orbital congestion [53, 54]. Hence, orbital decompression surgery is no longer relegated to a rehabilitative stage once the disease has become quiescent, but is rather considered a key stage of a multistep approach to control TED and avoid its more significant consequences.

Although early decompression may be beneficial, orbital decompression surgery should not be undertaken prior to the stabilization of endocrine disease. Conventional wisdom is that the thyroid status is not directly related to the orbit. Our clinical experience and an extensive nuanced reading of the literature [59–61] have revealed that this is not necessarily true. In particular, we have found that in patients who have successfully ceased smoking and whose thyroid function tests are stable prior to (and following) decompression, a primary decompression is frequently successful, with rare need for additional decompressions at a later date. Thus, to obtain the best surgical result, the patient's endocrine status needs to be normal and stable. Furthermore, the presence of TED is a contraindication for RAI therapy, which may provoke a recurrence or worsening of the orbitopathy.

Preoperative Planning

Selection of the surgical procedure is customized through an analysis of the clinical examination, orbital imaging studies, and premorbid facial photographs. The clinical examination focuses on the exophthalmometry measurements, lid retraction, ocular motility, the amount of lagophthalmos, and degree of corneal exposure. By reviewing the premorbid photos in conjunction with clinical measurements, an assessment of the amount of proptosis reduction that would be required to return to the normal state can be made.

CT or MR imaging in the axial and coronal planes is analyzed to determine the relative contribution of the enlargement of the extraocular muscles to the observed proptosis [19, 39]. TED can be divided into three categories based on the radiographic appearance: fat-predominant disease, muscle-predominant disease, and disease with mixed fat and muscle expansion (Figs. 58.1 and 58.2).

Image analysis should also consider the size of the paraorbital sinuses and thickness of the diploic spaces of the sphenoid, lateral frontal, and zygomatic bones, which can vary considerably and impact the success of orbital decompression. Additionally, the surgeon should review the radiographic images for potential coexisting orbital or sinus pathology.

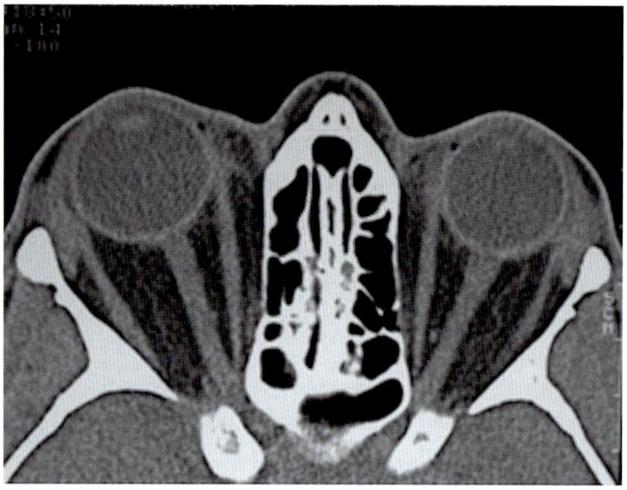

Fig. 58.1 Normal extraocular muscles, proptosis due to expansion of the fat compartment

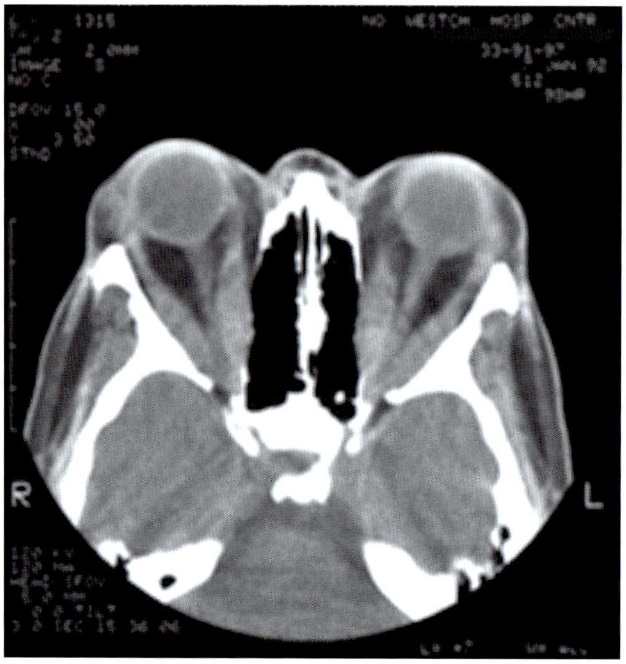

Fig. 58.2 Predominantly enlarged extraocular muscles

In fat-predominant TED, fat decompression alone may be beneficial. In these patients, an average reduction of proptosis of as much as 3–4 mm can be expected. The greatest mean proptosis reduction, 4.7 mm, is expected in patients with preoperative Hertel measurements over 25 mm, whereas the smallest mean proptosis reduction, 1.5 mm, is achieved in patients whose preoperative Hertel measurements are less than 20 mm [62]. Fat decompression in these patients is most effective when the fat is thick and fibrotic, as opposed to soft, supple fat lobules that characterize the normal orbit [63].

In contrast, patients with predominately enlarged EOMs typically benefit most from bone decompression. The amount of proptosis reduction achieved by a given decompression is highly variable and depends on both individual patient anatomy and the surgeon's technique. Based on published data, one can expect an average of 3.5–6.3 mm of proptosis reduction from a lateral wall decompression [33, 64–66], 2.5–4.5 mm from an extended medial wall decompression with removal of the posterior floor [29, 64, 67–69], and a somewhat smaller effect from an anterior floor decompression [70]. Importantly, significant decompression can be achieved with minimal reduction in proptosis secondary to the stiff EOMs resisting the posterior repositioning of the globe within a decompressed orbit. Hence, proptosis reduction is only one variable when assessing outcomes of orbital decompression surgery, with other variables that include conjunctival chemosis and orbital pressure pain, both of which assess improvement in orbital congestion. Both lateral and medial decompression can achieve a good decompression of the orbital apex. Because the optic foramen is located within the lesser wing of the sphenoid at the posterior edge of the medial wall, a posterior medial decompression has historically been thought to be the most effective approach to treating CON [71]. However, it has been demonstrated that a full lateral decompression with deep bone removal can be just as effective in treating CON as a medial decompression [64] (Tables 58.1 and 58.2).

Table 58.1 Indications for decompression

Indication	Surgical approach
Mild proptosis (no greater than 2 mm) with lower eyelid fat herniation	Fat-only decompression
Asymmetric proptosis, moderate EOM enlargement, moderate proptosis without strabismus	Lateral approach with fat decompression
Asymmetric proptosis, moderate EOM enlargement, moderate proptosis with strabismus	Lateral +/− medial approach with fat decompression
Optic neuropathy, severe EOM enlargement, severe proptosis	Combined medial and deep lateral approach with fat decompression +/− orbital floor

Modified from Kacker et al. [44]

Table 58.2 Proptosis reduction using various surgical procedures

Fat (no significant EOM enlargement or CON)	2–4 mm
Medial	2–3 mm
Medial + floor	3–5 mm
Lateral (including deep bone removal)	4–6 mm
Lateral + fat	5–8 mm
Lateral + medial	6–9 mm
Lateral + fat + medial	7–11 mm
Lateral + fat + medial + floor	8–13 mm

Modified from published data [20, 21, 35, 43, 44]

Surgical Techniques

In all orbital decompression, we recommend preoperative administration of intravenous steroids, e.g., 8–10 mg of dexamethasone. Consideration should also be given to preoperative antibiotics. To reduce bleeding during decompression into the sinus cavities, patients can be given preoperative oxymetazoline spray (1–2 puff into the nostrils 3 times over 15 minutes), and their nasal passages are packed with neurosurgical patties soaked in a vasoconstrictor such as oxymetazoline, epinephrine, or cocaine.

Orbital Fat Decompression

The main surgical approach for orbital fat decompression is through the inferior fornix and usually does not require a canthotomy/cantholysis [6, 7, 38, 72, 73]. This approach allows good access to both intra- and extraconal fat, particularly inferolaterally, with reduced risk of collateral injury to important periocular structures. It is important to point out that removal of the preaponeurotic fat through an upper lid blepharoplasty approach does not qualify as an orbital fat decompression. While it can provide cosmetic rehabilitation (important as that might be), it does not reduce proptosis or orbital congestion. In general, extended dissection through the soft tissues of the superior orbit carries significant risk for collateral damage, including to the lacrimal gland and levator muscle. Fat decompression can usually be performed under conscious sedation and local anesthesia, with rapid recovery, and has relatively low risk of inducing new-onset strabismus.

The surgical approach to the inferolateral orbital fat compartments involves a conjunctival incision at least 4 mm inferior to the inferior edge of the tarsal plate, in a manner similar to the surgical approach to the orbital floor for fracture repair, or to the anterior fat pads for lower eyelid blepharoplasty. The anatomic boundaries for fat removal are the lateral orbital wall (consisting of the zygoma and greater wing of the sphenoid), lateral orbital floor (zygoma and maxillary bones), the lateral rectus muscle superiorly, the inferior rectus muscle medially, and the globe superonasally. Blunt dissection is used the release fibrotic clumps of fat from surrounding tissue followed by piecemeal excision while directly observing the rectus muscles to avoid injury. Some surgeons use a hemostat to clamp fat prior to excision, but care must be taken because muscle tissue can inadvertently get caught within the clamp. Usually, 2–3 mL of fibrotic fat can be excised, and we routinely measure this volume using a 3 or 5 mL syringe. Hemostasis is critical and can be obtained with bipolar cautery or other hemostatic agents such as thrombin-soaked surgical foam or fibrin sealant. Once hemostasis is obtained, the surgical incision is closed with suture.

Lateral Wall Decompression

Decompression of the lateral wall may be approached through a lateral upper eyelid crease incision or through a canthotomy/cantholysis. The authors have utilized both approaches and find the laterally extended upper eyelid crease approach to be superior regarding with the postoperative healing and avoiding unnecessary injury to key structures of the lateral commissure and canthal tendon.

Following infiltration with local anesthetic mix of the surgeon's choice, dissection is carried down to the lateral orbital rim. Once the lateral orbital rim periosteum is exposed, it is incised with monopolar cautery and elevated off of the bony rim. A periosteal elevator is used to elevate the lateral periorbita to expose the perforating zygomaticotemporal and zygomaticofacial neurovascular bundles. These can be cauterized and divided with bipolar and monopolar cautery. With a malleable ribbon retractor in place, the lateral wall periorbita is elevated to expose the zygoma, sphenoid, and lateral frontal bones.

If desired, additional exposure can be obtained to the external lateral wall through the temporalis fossa. This is achieved by dissecting the periosteum from the lateral orbital rim to the insertion of the superficial and deep layers of the temporalis fascia and then sharply separating the fascia from the bone with monopolar cautery to expose the temporalis muscle. The fascia is then opened horizontally in a T-fashion with monopolar cautery at the level of the lateral commissure, taking care to stay less than 25 mm from the lateral rim to avoid the temporal branch of the facial nerve. The muscle is then carefully dissected from the lateral surface of the zygomatic bone with a sharp periosteal elevator, taking care to avoid excessive damage to the muscle fibers. This temporalis fossa dissection can greatly aid in maximizing exposure to the deep lateral orbit and provides another angle of approach for deep bone removal. It is particularly helpful in cases where the lateral orbital rim is kept in place intraoperatively.

The lateral orbital rim can be removed to enhance exposure, although we do not find this maneuver to be necessary in most cases. If removed, the lateral orbital rim itself should always be preserved and repositioned at the end of the surgery, as it serves an important protective and structural role for the globe and periocular tissues. Discarding the lateral rim does not provide any significant decompressive effect but only contributes to facial disfigurement and can aggravate eyelid malpositioning. Rim-sparing orbital decompression has been shown to provide efficacious outcomes while preserving the integrity of the lateral vertical buttress, and greater improvements in patient quality of life are reported compared to the rim-removal technique [74].

Removal of bone can be achieved with a combination of osteotomes and bone rongeurs for the thinner anterior portion of the lateral wall, and a high-speed drill or ultrasonic bone aspirator (e.g., Sonopet, Stryker Corp.) for deep bone removal [75] (Fig. 58.3). Several tips are available for both the drill and the ultrasonic aspirator, and surgeons should be sure to develop a good understanding of different tips prior to surgical use. In general terms, more aggressive tips such as the cutting burr or the ultrasonic Payner 360° tip remove bone faster but are more likely to damage soft tissue, whereas the reverse is true for less aggressive tips such as the diamond burr or ultrasonic Spetzler claw. The order of bone removal is dictated by surgeon preference, but most surgeons well start with the posterior zygoma, which is the thinnest portion of the lateral wall and is amenable to removal with osteotomes and Kerrison rongeurs. When using the osteotome, care must be taken to create the osteotomies anterior and inferior enough to avoid direct or indirect damage to the temporal and frontal lobes of the brain (Fig. 58.4). Complete removal of the posterior zygomatic bone provides excellent access to the sphenoid and frontal trigones. An alternative strategy, as described by Chang et al. [76], is to start the bone removal with the drill or ultrasound through the temporalis

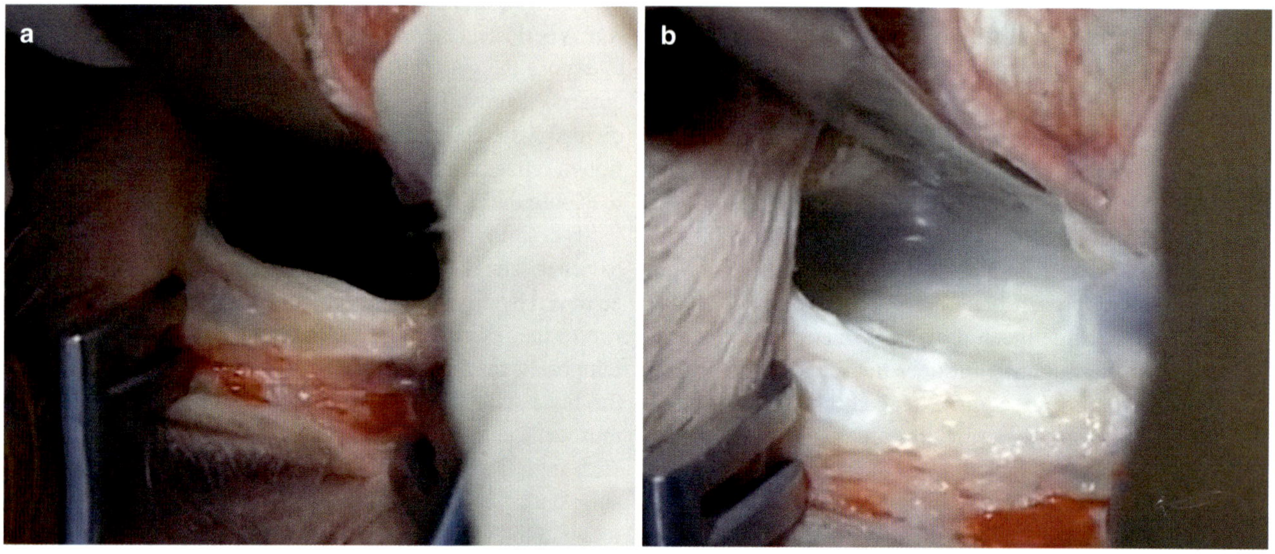

Fig. 58.3 Intraoperative view of lateral orbital decompression. (**a**) The lateral rim periosteum is exposed and elevated. (**b**) The Sonopet ultrasonic aspirator (Stryker, Kalamazoo, MI) is used to contour the lateral orbital wall

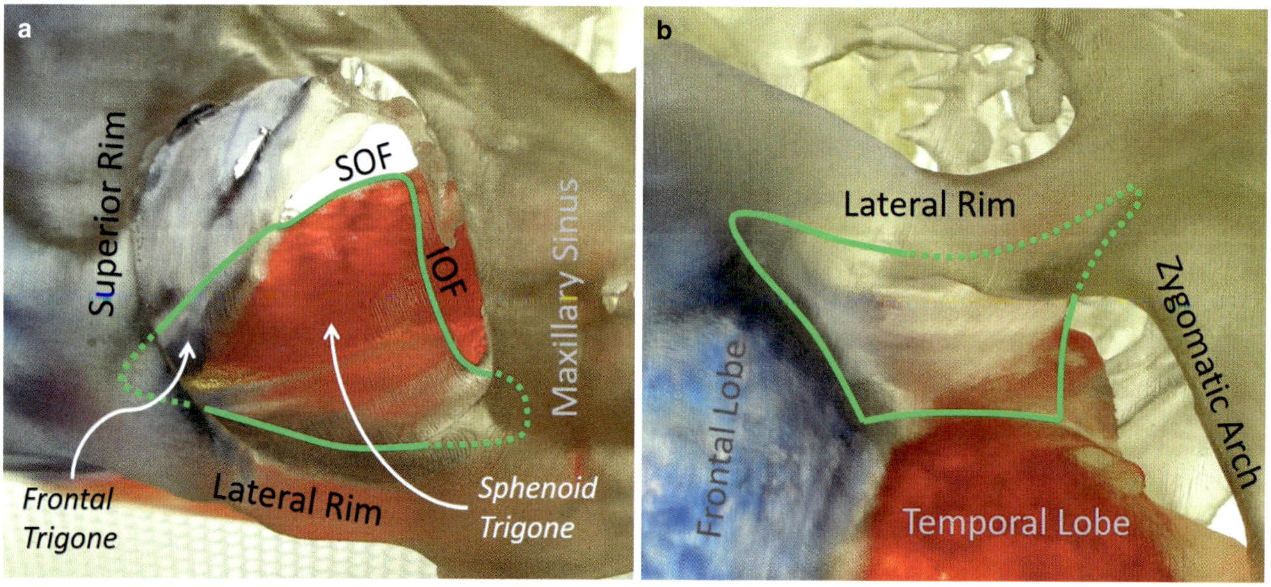

Fig. 58.4 Stereolithographic model of the right orbit, frontal view (**a**) and lateral view (**b**). The area of potential bone removal for lateral decompression is outlined in green. The intracranial surface of the anterior cranial fossa has been colored blue, and the middle cranial fossa has been colored red

fossa approach posteriorly at the base of the sphenoid trigone and immediately expose the dura over the temporal lobe. This gives the surgeon a definitive posterior limit very early in the case, and bone removal proceeds only anteriorly from that point. However, exposure of dura can be unnecessarily risky, and there are other safer methods for assessing the extent of needed bone removal.

One may argue that dura should never be in contact with orbital muscle and connective tissues since dura is highly vascular and bioactive, releasing multiple neuropeptides that can lead to postoperative muscle enlargement, orbital inflammation, and swelling [77–80]. Indeed, the dura mater is highly biologically active tissue that in nature is never in contact with muscle or orbital connective tissue. Not only is the external dura highly vascular compared to internal dura – the reason why dural switch works for treating Moyamoya disease [81] – but the external dura also interacts robustly with the cranial bones and cranial sutures during development, to drive bone growth and suture closure timing [82, 83]. It does that by releasing TGF-beta, collagen I and III, osteocalcin, FGF, and other osteogenic cytokines. Furthermore, the dura is highly sensitive to mechanical tension changes [77], such as what would happen when you suddenly remove bone and leave a large surface area abutting orbital fat and muscle. Such tension changes can cause release of bioactive cytokines [78, 79]. Lastly, the dura is highly innervated [79, 84, 85], particularly with C fibers expressing CGRP intertwined with noradrenergic sympathetic fibers and non-peptidergic unmyelinated "C-like" A-delta fibers expressing NF200. These dural nerves respond to CGRP as well as substance P, neuropeptide Y, and serotonin, which regulate blood flow – an important potential regulator of tissue swelling. Substance P in particular is known to cause tissue swelling through a histamine-independent mechanism [86].

Once the trigone is exposed, bone removal is performed through the anterior cortical bone to expose the diploic space, which is filled with cancellous bone (Figs. 58.5 and 58.6). Bone removal continues through the diploe, during which time brisk bleeding is typically encountered and can be controlled intermittently with bone wax. An effective technique for application of bone wax is to place a small pea-sized sphere of wax on the wooden end of a cotton-tipped applicator (CTA) and use the CTA to loosely apply the wax to the bone surface. The CTA is then turned over and the cotton end used to press the wax firmly into the bleeding crevices of bone. Once the cancellous bone is removed and the cortical bone covering the temporal and frontal lobes is reached, the bleeding typically abates. The diploic space of the sphenoid is continuous with the diploe of the lateral frontal bone. To achieve a maximal decompression, the diploic space should be removed entirely to expose the inner cortical table of bone covering the temporal lobe posteriorly and the frontal lobe superiorly. Depending on the surgeon's comfort level, the inner cortical table can be focally thinned to expose dura of the frontal and temporal lobes, thus ensuring that the limits of bone removal have been reached. However, exposure of large areas of dura is unnecessary and increases the risk of CSF leakage as well as the potential for altering orbital tissue biology through non-physiologic contact with dura mater, as described earlier [77–79]. Alternatively, intraoperative navigation can be used to confirm that maximal bone removal has been achieved without the need to expose dura. In addition to the sphenoid and frontal trigones, significant bone removal can be accomplished along the inferior orbital fissure and extend to the inferolateral orbital floor. Occasionally, the roof

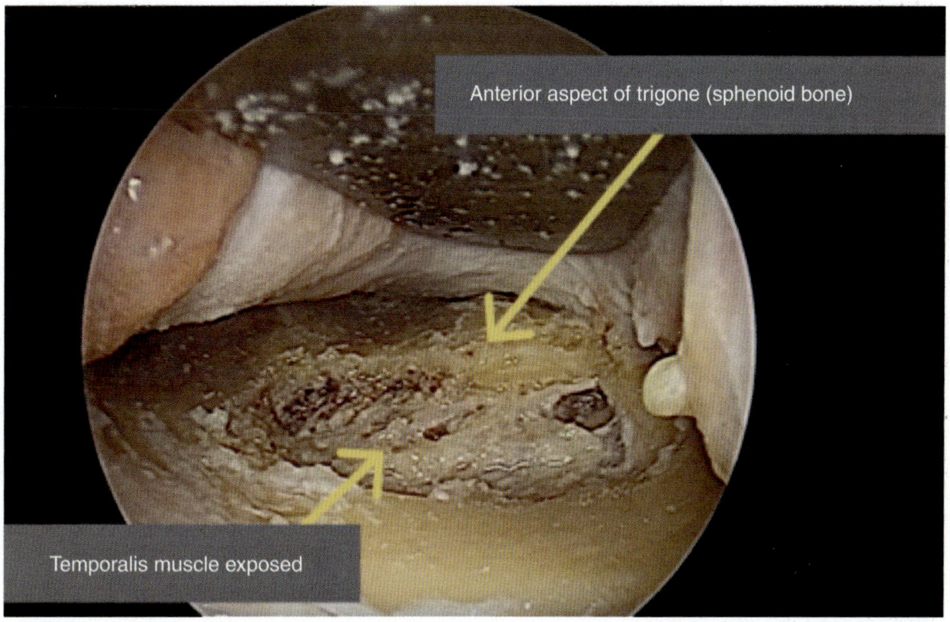

Fig. 58.5 Intraoperative view of temporalis muscle exposure during lateral orbital decompression. Once the anterior aspect of the sphenoid trigone is adequately debulked internally, the external muscle fibers are visible

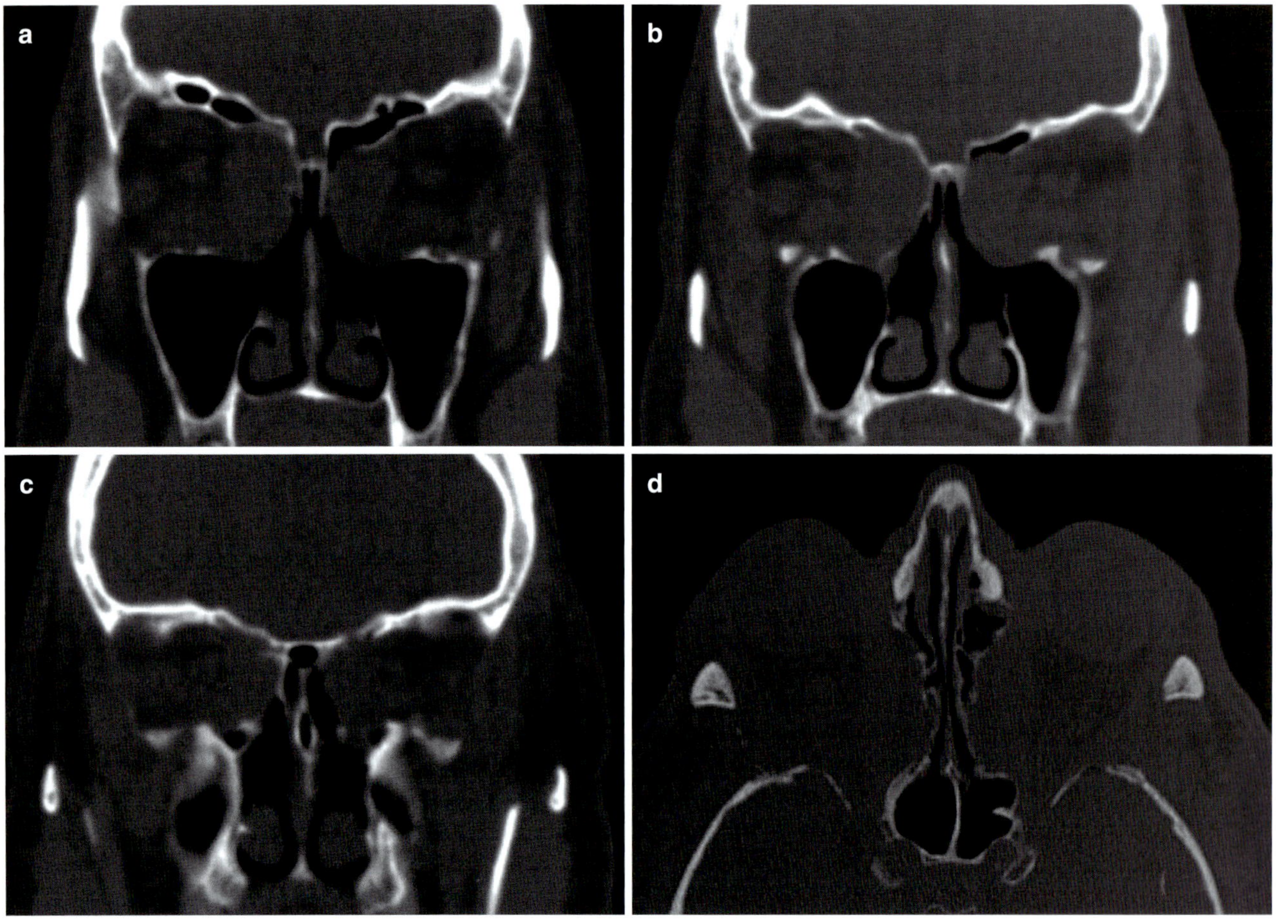

Fig. 58.6 Coronal (**a–c**) and axial (**d**) CT orbits following medial and lateral orbital decompressions in a single patient

of the maxillary sinus may be exposed. Superolaterally, the bone above the lacrimal gland fossa can also be removed.

Decompression of the orbital floor, whether directly or through inferior extension of a lateral decompression, can lead to inferior globe displacement. The combination of posterior and inferior displacement of the globe has the secondary effect of reducing lower eyelid retraction while increasing upper eyelid retraction and can be customized to patients' needs and overall surgical plan.

At this point, the periorbita is opened sharply to allow for herniation of soft tissue into the newly created space (Figs. 58.7 and 58.8). Adjunctive fat excision can now be performed, with excellent access to both inferolateral and superolateral fat compartments. Because of the increased risk of bleeding and injury to the lacrimal gland, superolateral fat debulking is usually reserved for the most severe cases of orbitopathy. However, the authors routinely debulk inferolateral orbital fat, with good effect on both proptosis and lower eyelid contour/fullness.

If the rim was removed, it can now be repositioned with either titanium plates or screws or sutured through pre-drilled holes. The periosteum is closed over the rim with absorbable sutures, and the surgical incision is closed using sutures of the surgeon's choice.

Medial Transconjunctival Approach to the Orbit

The medial transconjunctival approach to orbital decompression was developed by Shorr et al. in the 1990s [27]. While the incision was originally described as being made through the lateral third of the caruncle ("transcaruncular"), most surgeons now place the incision immediately lateral to the caruncle, for which some use the term "retrocaruncular." While the terms "transcaruncular" and "retrocaruncular" refer to slightly different locations of incision placement, they are often used interchangeably. In this chapter, we will refer to both of these approaches jointly as the medial transconjunctival approach to the orbit. Prior to the introduction of the medial transconjunctival approach, the transcutaneous Lynch incision was the most common approach to the medial orbit, but its use has largely been abandoned by orbital surgeons.

Following infiltration of local anesthetic of the surgeon's choice, the caruncle and plica semilunaris are grasped and retracted away from one another. Westcott scissors are used

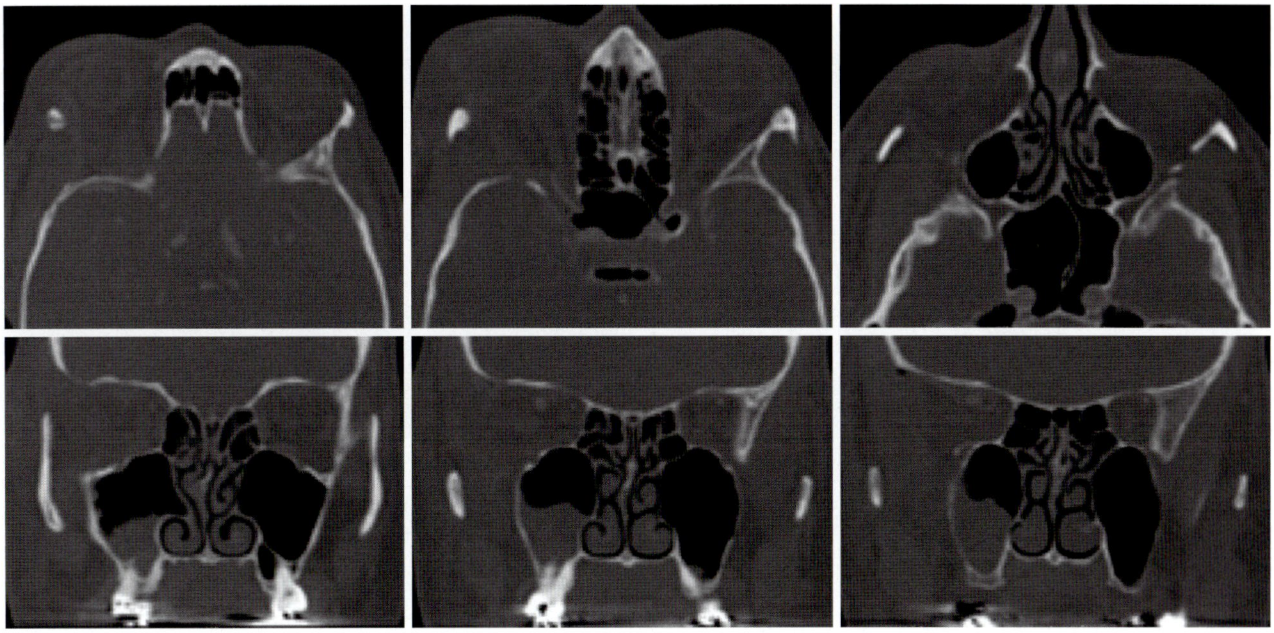

Fig. 58.7 Postoperative axial (upper row) and coronal (lower row) CT scans following lateral orbital decompression demonstrating increased orbital volume for soft tissue herniation

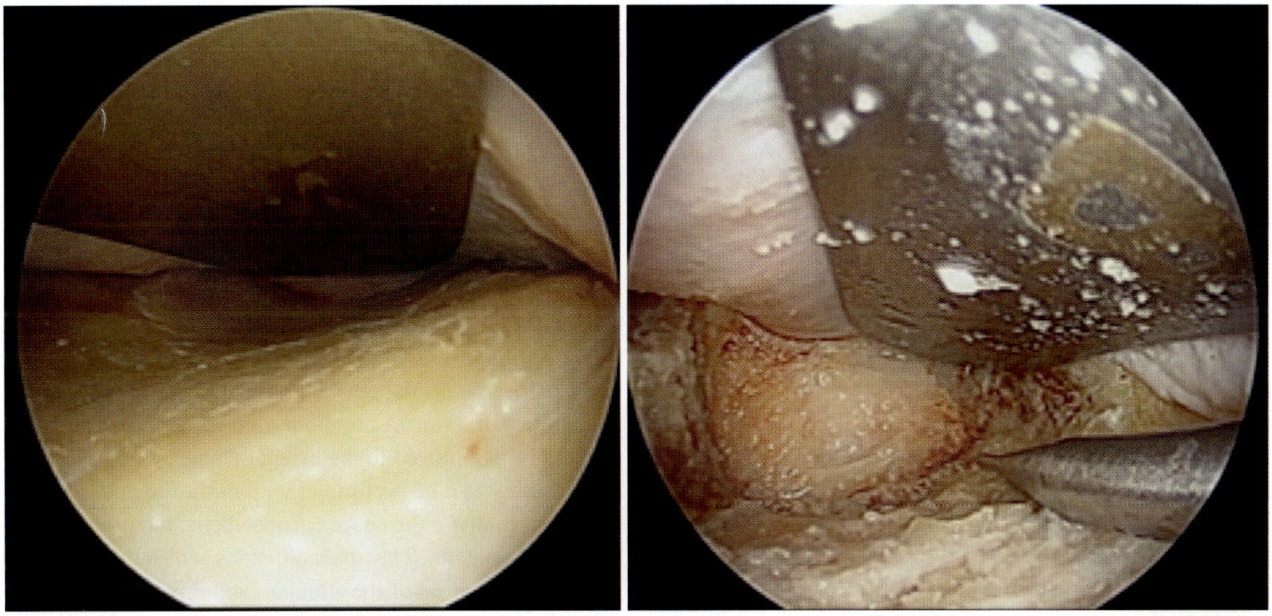

Fig. 58.8 Intraoperative view before (left image) and after (right image) decompression of the lateral orbital wall. In the right image, the lateral wall has been contoured to allow for increased orbital volume into which the orbital contents can expand

to make the conjunctival incision between these structures (i.e., retrocaruncular), curving the incision supero- and inferolaterally to follow the contour of the plica. Curved Stevens scissors are placed through the incision in a posteromedial direction at a 45° angle in the axial plane and used to bluntly dissect tissue down to the posterior lacrimal crest, while the globe is retracted with a small malleable ribbon retractor and the caruncle with a small retractor or skin hook. This dissection should be tangential to the globe to prevent damage of the (frequently enlarged) medial rectus muscle (Fig. 58.9). Once exposed, the periosteum over the posterior lacrimal crest is incised vertically and carefully elevated to expose the medial orbital wall (Fig. 58.10). Subperiosteal dissection is then carried along the lamina papyracea with periosteal elevators and malleable ribbon retractors. Every effort should be made to keep the periorbita intact during this dissection,

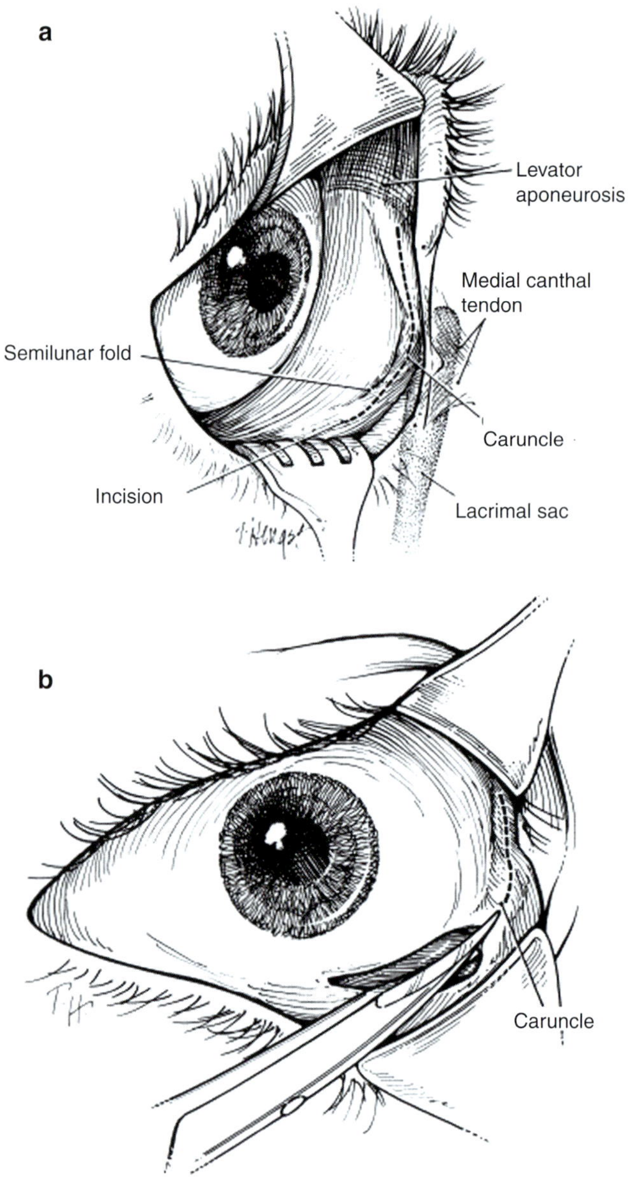

Fig. 58.9 Medial transconjunctival wall decompression. (Reproduced with permission from [27])

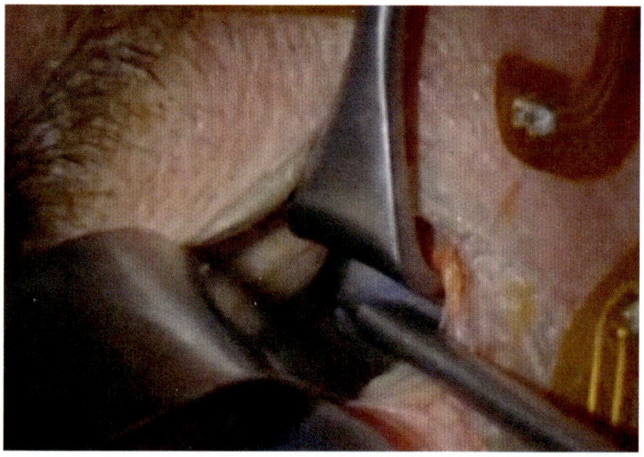

Fig. 58.10 Retrocaruncular approach to medial orbital decompression. An incision is made just lateral to the caruncle, and dissection is carried down to expose the medial orbital wall

as this can improve visualization and decrease the risk of damage to intraorbital structures. A critical aspect of this surgical approach is the identification of the anterior and posterior ethmoidal foramina, which typically demarcate the frontoethmoidal suture and with it the superior boundary of decompression (Fig. 58.11). Any bone removal above this suture line may result in entry into the anterior cranial fossa. The anterior ethmoidal neurovascular bundle is cauterized and may be divided with bipolar and monopolar cautery. The posterior ethmoidal neurovascular bundle is located only 4–7 mm away from the optic foramen, and may or may not be divided, depending on surgeon preference. This important landmark usually demarcates the posterior superior edge of the bone removal. It should be noted that variations exist in the anatomic position of the ethmoidal vessels, so the frequently quoted 24-12-6 rule, as well as their location at the frontoethmoidal suture, cannot be considered absolute [87]. Careful study of a preoperative CT scan, and possibly use of stereotactic navigation, can greatly assist with identifying and utilizing appropriate landmarks.

Decompression begins by fracturing the lamina papyracea with an elevator or suction tip and removing the thin medial wall with nasal forceps (e.g., Takahashi or Blakesley). As the bone becomes thicker near the frontoethmoidal suture or inferomedial strut, rongeurs or an ultrasonic bone aspirator can be used if necessary. A useful surgical approach is to remove the posterior part of the medial orbital wall first, since the sinus mucosa on the other side can bleed and anterior bleeding will accumulate posteriorly, obscuring good visualization of the orbital apex. By extension, the best time to visualize the orbital apex and to plan out the deep part of the surgery is prior to any bone removal. Once the lamina papyracea is removed to the extent planned, a complete ethmoidectomy can be performed with nasal forceps to reduce bleeding, improve the space enhancement, and prevent postoperative sinusitis. The sphenoid sinus will be encountered at the posterior end of the ethmoid, and this defines the posterior limit of bone removal. Venturing further into the sphenoid sinus does not add appreciably to the decompressive effect and carries a high risk of damage to the optic nerve and internal carotid artery. Once the ethmoidectomy is complete, the orbital process of the palatine bone and the inferomedial strut can be visualized and removed with an osteotome or ultrasonic aspirator. If using an osteotome, care must be taken to direct energy away from the optic foramen and fovea ethmoidalis. If floor decompression is planned in conjunction with the medial wall, the posterior half to two-thirds of the floor can be removed with nasal forceps up to the infraorbital canal. Leaving the anterior third of the floor

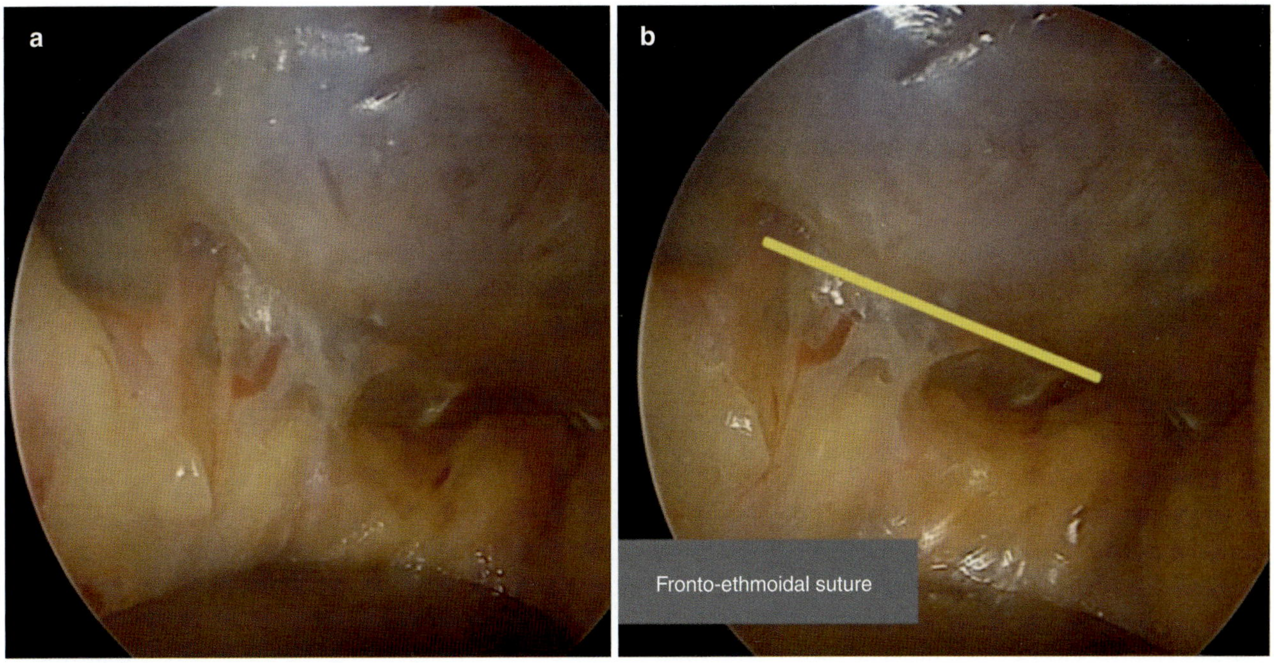

Fig. 58.11 Intraoperative view of medial orbital decompression. (**a**) The medial orbital wall is exposed. (**b**) The frontoethmoidal suture, demarcated by the anterior and posterior ethmoidal foramina, identifies the superior boundary of planned decompression

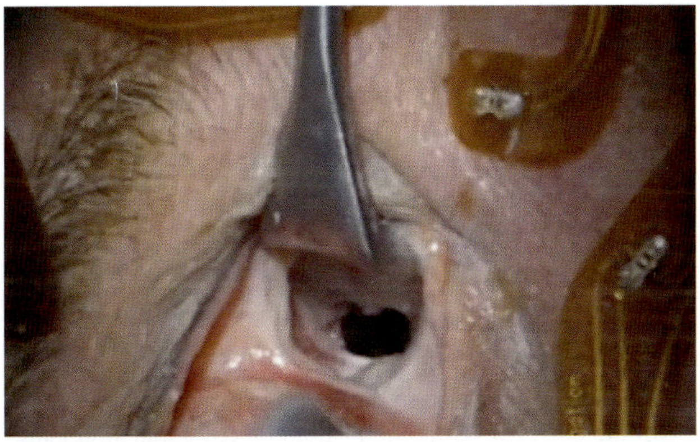

Fig. 58.12 Medial orbital decompression. The medial orbital wall is exposed and debulked, taking care to not surpass the anterior boundary of decompression at the level of the anterior ethmoid foramen

intact is thought to decrease the risk of postoperative diplopia and globe dystopia.

An important consideration of medial orbital decompression is strabismus, as this technique is known to be associated with greater degree of induced strabismus [88, 89]. The authors have noted that leaving 10–12 mm of anterior medial wall posterior to the posterior lacrimal crest reduces significantly the risk of induced severe strabismus. Our current approach in most patients is to set the anterior boundary of the medial decompression at the level of the anterior ethmoid foramen (Fig. 58.12).

Once the bony decompression is completed, the periorbita is opened sharply with scissors or a sickle blade to allow for soft tissue herniation into the newly created space. The medial transconjunctival incision may be left to heal by secondary intention or closed with a buried absorbable suture [90].

Orbital Floor Decompression

The orbital floor can be accessed via an inferior fornix approach, similar to repair of an orbital blowout fracture repair. Because this is a very familiar approach to most orbital surgeons, it is a commonly used technique for decompression. And because the bone is thin, bone removal can be easily achieved with minimal instrumentation while avoiding injury to the infraorbital nerve. However, it is more likely to cause worsening strabismus and globe dystopia, carries a high risk of infraorbital hypoesthesia, and does not provide good access to the orbital apex. As a result, most specialists in thyroid eye disease prefer to decompress the lateral and medial walls, in what has been referred to as a "balanced" decompression [20, 44, 91–93]. The floor decompression has now become more of an adjunctive procedure for patients in whom a balanced decompression provides insufficient proptosis reduction or in whom the compartment syndrome is so severe that maximal decompression is required.

Endonasal Endoscopic Orbital Decompression (Medial Wall and Floor)

The endonasal approach to orbital decompression is frequently performed by otolaryngologists, often with some involvement by an ophthalmologist. It is a good approach that offers good visualization and access to the medial orbital wall, orbital floor, and the orbital apex [10, 32]. When an orbital surgeon is not easily available, this approach provides a good alternative for many patients. Once the nasal passages are vasoconstricted, the endoscope is introduced into the nose, the middle turbinate is endoscopically medialized, and an uncinectomy performed. A complete endoscopic ethmoidectomy is then performed with sinus forceps and/or a microdebrider. The anatomic limits of the dissection are the frontal sinus ostium anteriorly, sphenoid sinus posteriorly, fovea ethmoidalis superiorly, lamina papyracea laterally, and middle turbinate medially. A frontal sinusotomy can be done to ensure patency of the ostium. The sphenoid sinus may be entered using a sphenoid punch to create a 4 × 4 mm opening, although entering the sphenoid sinus is usually not necessary for an orbital decompression. Nasal antral windows are fashioned by cannulating and expanding the natural ostium of the maxillary sinus. Endonasal access is now complete, allowing for removal of bone from the medial orbital wall and floor. The periorbita is then opened to allow herniation of soft tissue into the newly created space. Extreme care must be taken to avoid injury to the extraocular muscles. Additional care must be taken to avoid removal of the anterior aspect of the inferomedial strut, in order to reduce the risk of worsening strabismus and globe dystopia [94, 95].

Although endoscopic decompression with inferomedial strut preservation was once considered technically difficult due to concerns of potential limited orbital floor access [96], advances in endoscopic surgery have demonstrated the feasibility of accessing the orbital floor with this technique [97]. A modification of this method, with selective endoscopic removal of the posterior inferomedial strut and preservation of the anterior aspect of the strut, can provide deeper decompression and reduce diplopia [98]. However, the level of expertise required is higher. In general, a direct orbital approach to decompression is usually favored unless not available to the patient.

Postoperative Considerations

Following orbital decompression surgery, patients are prescribed oral analgesic medication and cold compresses for 3–5 days, along with the usual regimen of incisional care including an antibiotic ointment. They should be instructed to avoid exertion, bending, or lifting for at least 2–3 days postoperatively – the key time period for postoperative bleeding. Following surgery in the sinuses, nasal saline spray can be prescribed to facilitate healing and reduce postoperative congestive symptoms.

Overall, the list of potential complications of orbital decompression is quite long [65, 99, 100] and may vary based on surgical technique [101]. The most important and common risks include infection, worsened strabismus/diplopia, and postoperative hemorrhage causing an acute compartment syndrome. Temporary postoperative hypoesthesia has been reported in up to 29% of lateral decompressions and 17% of other bony decompressions [65]. CSF leak is a rare, potentially morbid, complication; it may be more common in lateral than medial approaches [102, 103], but because the lateral exposure is greater and orbital tissues can tamponade a leak, the medial CSF leak is usually considered more consequential. Additionally, temporal wasting may occur, particularly in patients undergoing a coronal approach [102]. While the risk of postoperative new-onset strabismus is present for any decompression surgery, this risk appears to be highest with medial and floor decompression and lowest with lateral and fat decompression surgery [88, 104, 105]. Diligent follow-up of patients in the postoperative period is critical in order to detect potential complications and monitor healing.

Strabismus Surgery

Extraocular muscle surgery for TED is routinely performed by a pediatric ophthalmologist or neuro-ophthalmologist to address ocular misalignment and any associated diplopia. Ocular misalignment may be affected by orbital decompression surgery – positively or, more commonly, negatively [35, 80, 88, 104, 105]. Hence, patients who need orbital decompression should undergo that procedure prior to any strabismus surgery. Ideally, the orbital and strabismus surgery teams work closely together to optimize outcomes through proper sequencing and timing of surgeries. When available, orthoptic examinations before and after decompression surgery can provide useful information for planning eventual strabismus surgery.

In the past, conventional wisdom dictated that strabismus surgery should be delayed at least 6 months after decompression surgery. However, with improved coordination between orbital and strabismus surgeons, availability of more frequent orthoptic measurements, and the more modern surgical techniques for orbital decompression (as outlined above), strabismus surgery may be performed as early as 6–8 weeks after decompression surgery, with good results as long as measurements were stable postoperatively.

Once a patient is ready for strabismus surgery, muscle recession is usually performed in TED to weaken the action of fibrotic muscles. The most commonly affected muscles are the inferior and medial rectus muscles, and these are often the targets of muscle recession surgery. Restrictive EOM disease can be challenging to treat since the altered muscles may not respond to surgery in a predictable fashion [106]. Additionally, recessing fibrotic muscles may worsen proptosis [1] and potentially even induce optic nerve stretching, which is a risk for vision loss. More frequently, it may worsen lower eyelid retraction [107, 108].

Optimal outcomes for strabismus surgery necessitate stability in ocular alignment measurements as documented over time. Since patients who smoke often have a less stable disease course, achieving optimal alignment in smokers with TED may be impossible. Patients should therefore be strongly encouraged to cease smoking prior to initiation of surgical rehabilitation.

A full discussion of the techniques involved in strabismus surgery for TED is beyond the scope of this chapter. There are many variations in use of absorbable versus nonabsorbable and adjustable versus nonadjustable sutures, but overall the success rate of allowing patients to fuse without prisms or with less than 4 prism diopter correction is quite high in experienced hands.

An important consideration is the effect of strabismus surgery on eyelid position. In patients with a restricted inferior rectus muscle, attempting to bring the eye to primary position results in secondary upper eyelid retraction. Such retraction is improved following inferior rectus recession. However, recessing the inferior rectus can worsen lower eyelid retraction, which can be partially mitigated by carefully separating the inferior rectus muscle from the lower eyelid retractors during the recession surgery.

Eyelid Surgery

Etiology of Eyelid Changes in TED

Eyelid retraction is the most common feature of TED. The etiology of upper eyelid retraction is multifactorial, including fibrosis of the upper eyelid retractors (similar to EOMs), increased sympathetic tone, and extreme effort to supraduct the globe against a restricted inferior rectus muscle (i.e., pseudoretraction) [109–111]. Lower eyelid retraction is also multifactorial, including fibrosis of the lower eyelid retractors, increased sympathetic tone, or globe malposition/proptosis. It may be exacerbated by malar hypoplasia, and assessment of photos from prior to disease onset can be very helpful in assessing the patient's natural lower eyelid position.

Whenever ptosis is noted in a patient with TED, the diagnosis of myasthenia gravis must be considered, since it occurs in approximately 5% of patients with TED [112]. Other eyelid findings that may be encountered in TED include dermatochalasis, anterior herniation of the orbital fat pads, and periorbital soft tissue expansion (i.e., thyroid periorbitopathy [113]) (Fig. 58.13).

While many surgical techniques for eyelid reconstruction can be employed, the role of a good decompression in improving eyelid position is important [114]. An effective decompression can reduce axial proptosis and sometimes reduce or even eliminate lower lid retraction without any additional lower lid surgery [115, 116].

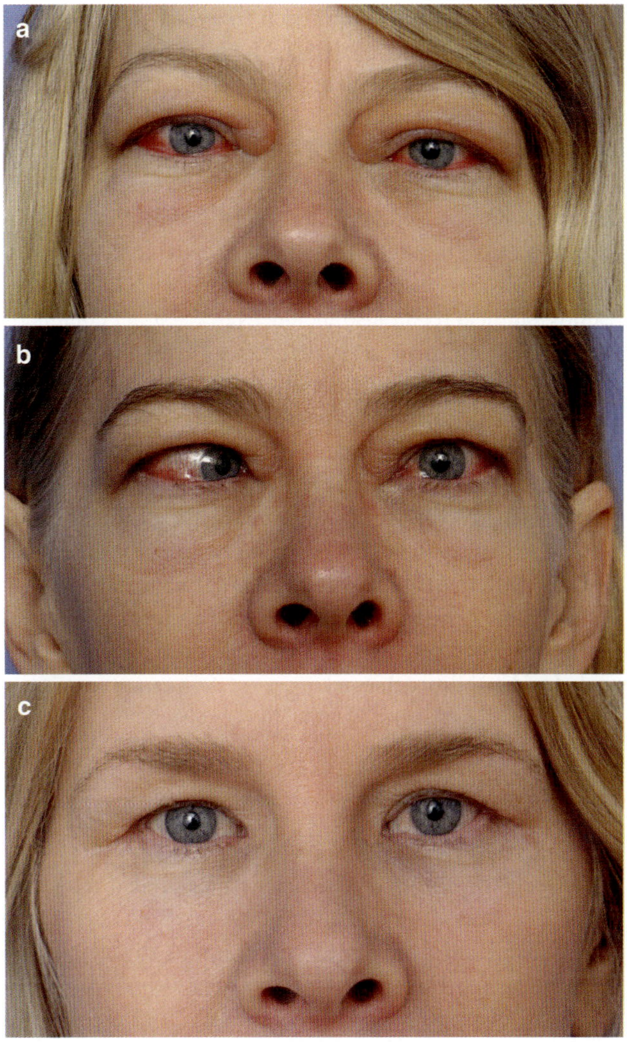

Fig. 58.13 Patient with active thyroid eye disease at presentation (**a**), following thyroidectomy (**b**), and following orbital decompression and strabismus surgery performed during the active stage (**c**). The patient did not require eyelid retraction repair

Alternatives to surgery, such as the historic use of the topical sympatholytic guanethidine [117, 118] and local injection of botulinum toxin or hyaluronic acid filler [119–121], are limited by additional corneal surface toxicity and temporary effect, respectively. Additionally, botulinum toxin has the known side effects of ptosis and diplopia from iatrogenic extraocular muscle palsy.

Eyelid retraction surgery is required when medical therapy, including topical lubricant drops and ointments, patching, and moisture chambers, is unsuccessful in addressing corneal compromise in TED [122]. In addition, the psychosocial effects of disfigurement secondary to eyelid retraction should not be underestimated [123].

The simplest surgical approach to eyelid retraction is a tarsorrhaphy – lateral, medial, or both. However, this is a disfiguring surgery that should only be used when patients are not good candidates for more definitive and physiological surgery.

The standard approach to eyelid retraction surgery is a lid-lengthening procedure. In the upper eyelids, this involves recession of the upper lid retractors. There is rarely (if ever) a need to place a spacer graft in the upper eyelid. In the lower eyelids, surgical repair also includes retractor and conjunctival recession. However, a spacer graft is sometimes required.

Blepharoplasty, brow lift, and sub-brow fat debulking are all excellent adjunctive procedures that can be performed as part of the surgical rehabilitation of patients with TED. These techniques are not TED-specific and have been described well elsewhere [124–128]. Importantly, they should not be combined with eyelid retraction surgery since the additional scarring may undermine the surgical effort to release scar tissue. Eyelid retraction repair should be performed first, and adjunctive procedures can be performed once the patient has healed and stability achieved.

Surgical Techniques

Upper Eyelid Recession

There are two general approaches to upper eyelid retraction repair: percutaneous and transconjunctival. Both approaches can be successful, and each technique has its advantages and disadvantages. The percutaneous approach (e.g., full-thickness blepharotomy) is more likely to raise the lid crease – an acceptable result in many women but potentially unacceptable in men. It also injures the orbicularis muscle, which functions to close the eyelid, and hence its preservation can be important. The septum may be opened in the percutaneous technique, which can cause additional scarring as the eyelid heals. Nevertheless, this approach offers excellent exposure, ease of hemostasis, and full control of eyelid contour. The posterior approach is technically more demanding, with reduced exposure and more challenging hemostasis. However, it avoids a cutaneous scar and injury to the orbicularis or septum. For both techniques, the ability to sit the patient intraoperatively and make final adjustments with the patient awake and alert can be extremely helpful.

Anterior Approach (Full-Thickness Blepharotomy)

The incision is made at the desired position of the eyelid crease, although final length of the incision can vary significantly. In the standard approach, each tissue layer is incised in turn until the conjunctiva is encountered, with retention of a bridge of tissue that would form the peak of the eyelid and with careful consideration of eyelid margin contour. In the variant introduced by Leo Koornneef and popularized by Elner et al. [129], a protective plate is introduced under the eyelid, and a #15 blade is used to make a full-thickness incision medial to lateral through the skin, muscle, septum, levator, Müller, and conjunctiva while still leaving a small bridge at the desired point of an eyelid peak. Both approaches offer excellent control. Overcorrection can be repaired by suturing conjunctiva and/or retractors with 6-0 Vicryl suture. Adjustments should be made with the patient in a sitting position. Wound closure can be layered (orbicularis and skin) or just skin.

Posterior Approach

The posterior approach involves a palpebral conjunctival incision. The fornix is infiltrated with a small amount of local anesthetic, and the presence or absence of epinephrine depends on surgeon preference. Presence of epinephrine can alter eyelid height, which needs to be compensated for based on experience. Additional anesthesia can be injected along the frontal nerve, as a nerve block that will only minimally affect eyelid position.

A traction suture is placed through the central upper eyelid, and the lid everted over a baby Desmarres retractor (in a manner similar to performing a Mullerectomy surgery for ptosis repair). Westcott scissors are used to incise conjunctiva 4–5 mm superior to the superior tarsal border on either side of the centrally placed traction suture. Westcott scissors are then used to carefully incise eyelid retractors in a graded fashion, with frequent assessment of eyelid height and contour with patient cooperation. Bipolar cautery is used for hemostasis. Once eyelid height and contour are close to ideal, the patient is brought to a sitting position and final adjustments made. Overcorrection can be repaired with 6-0 Vicryl suture to the conjunctiva and/or retractors. Once ideal eyelid height, contour, and symmetry are achieved, the traction suture is cut, and the operation is over – there is no need to close the surgical incision.

Lower Eyelid Retraction Repair

As in upper eyelid retraction repair, the lower eyelid can be lengthened either through an anterior or posterior approach. It is technically easier to perform the posterior, transconjunctival approach for the lower eyelid. Spacer graft materials are more frequently needed in the lower lid and can provide 3–4+ mm of elevation. Examples of lower eyelid donor materials include autologous cartilage (ear or nasal septum), autologous hard palate, donor sclera, acellular dermis (human, bovine or porcine), or an alloplastic material such as porous polyethylene [130–137].

Regardless of the spacer material used, a similar surgical approach is employed. First, the lower eyelid is injected with lidocaine +/– epinephrine. An incision is then made in the conjunctiva 2–4 mm inferior to the inferior border of the tarsus (Fig. 58.14). This may be combined with a lateral canthotomy and inferior cantholysis if lateral eyelid tightening is required. The lower eyelid retractors are then identified and disinserted from the tarsus. A spacer graft is placed into the newly created pocket between the retractors and tarsal border and sutured into position with an absorbable suture such as 6-0 Vicryl, keeping the knots away from the ocular surface. A double-armed bolster suture is placed through the spacer graft, exiting on skin and tied over a bolster of the surgeon's choosing. If a lateral tarsal suspension is required, a sufficiently long lateral tarsal strip is then created to allow for appropriate tightening of the lower lid margin. The lateral tarsal strip is fixed to the periosteum of the lateral orbital rim in the usual fashion.

Spacer Graft Materials

A variety of spacer graft materials are available for use in eyelid retraction repair. The choice of graft material varies by surgeon, though the most frequently utilized grafts in modern practice are autologous cartilage, hard palate, and acellular dermis. Dermis fat graft (DFG) is a reasonable option for some patients, but because the fat compartment of TED patients is already expanded, DFG is usually not the first option in most patients with lower eyelid retraction.

Autologous Auricular Cartilage

Autologous auricular cartilage has the benefit of producing predictable postoperative results due to minimal graft shrinkage and postoperative inflammation. Auricular cartilage is harvested from the superior aspect of the ear, using the flattest area between the helix and antihelix (Fig. 58.15). Either anterior or posterior approaches can be used for the harvest. After administration of local anesthesia, a curved 15–20 mm skin incision is made just behind the helix, and the cartilage is exposed with blunt dissection. The graft is then harvested with a no. 15 Bard-Parker blade or razor blade knife. For graft sizing, a 1:1 vertical graft height to lower eyelid elevation ratio is typically used. Minimal cautery is used for hemostasis, with care to avoid cautery to the cartilage, which can lead to significant postoperative pain. Primary closure of the ear skin incision is then performed.

Because ear cartilage has a curve to it, the cartilage needs to be treated to reduce its rigidity and curvature. This can be

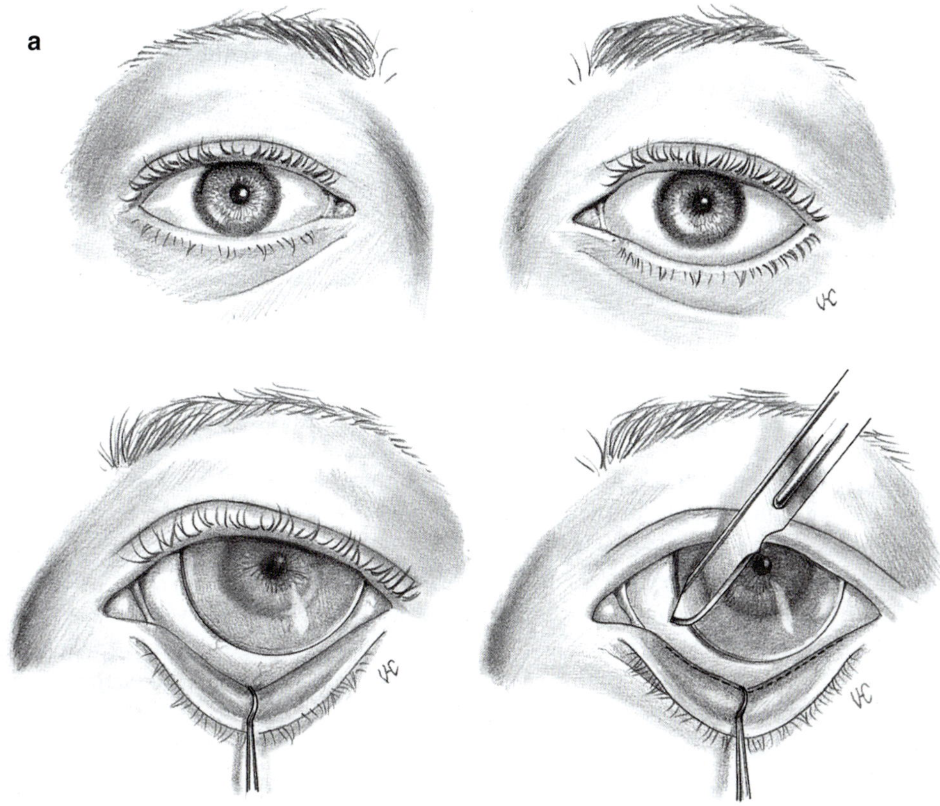

Fig. 58.14 (**a**) Lower eyelid retraction secondary to adhesions in and around the capsulopalpebral fascia. Lower eyelid retraction (**b**) is approached internally. A skin hook is placed beneath the inferior tarsal border, and the lower eyelid is everted. A conjunctival incision is made beneath the inferior tarsal border (dotted line) (**c**). A sagittal view demonstrates the severance of the capsulopalpebral fascia from the inferior tarsal border (**d**). A spacer graft is inserted beneath the inferior border of the tarsus and the advancing recessed edge of the retractors. The graft does not need to be sutured in its entirety but stabilized with a percutaneous through-and-through mattress suture (**e**). Two mattress sutures are used to stabilize the graft nasally and temporally and tied over bolsters (**f**)

b

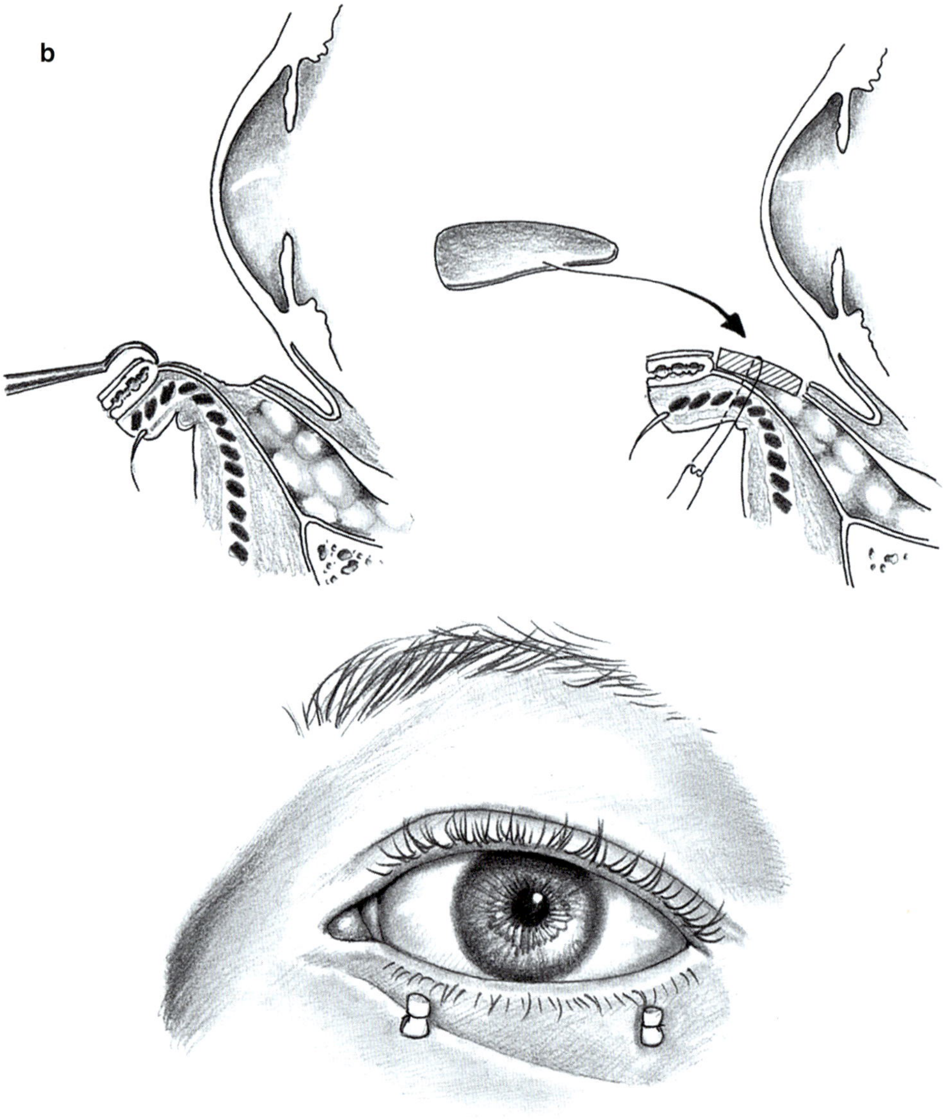

Fig. 58.14 (continued)

done with a Septal Morselizer (available from numerous manufacturers) or by scoring with a #15 blade. The cartilage is then placed into the posterior lamellar pocket of the treated eyelid and sutured into position using buried interrupted 6-0 Vicryl sutures. One edge of the graft should be sutured to retractors and the other to the edge of tarsus. Since auricular cartilage is not epithelialized, the graft should be covered posteriorly with conjunctiva. If two eyelids need to be treated simultaneously, the graft can be divided to provide two right triangles. A key maneuver in the grafting of ear cartilage to the eyelid is the placement of a bolster suture in a horizontal mattress fashion through the center of the graft, exiting on skin where it is tied over a bolster. A 5-0 Prolene is usually used for this purpose, to make sure that the surface of the cartilage graft is tightly adherent to the septum and will not be displaced toward the eye during the acute healing process.

Hard Palate Mucosa

When used as a lower eyelid spacer, hard palate mucosa offers the advantages of an epithelial lining, minimal postoperative graft shrinkage, and ready availability [131]. Hard palate mucosa is similar in structure to native tarsus. The graft is taken from the hard palate between the gingival processes and the midline raphe (Fig. 58.16). The prospective site is marked and submucosally injected with local anesthetic. During dissection, care is taken to avoid the incisive and greater palatine foramina, which transmit the nasopalatine and greater palatine neurovascular bundles, respectively.

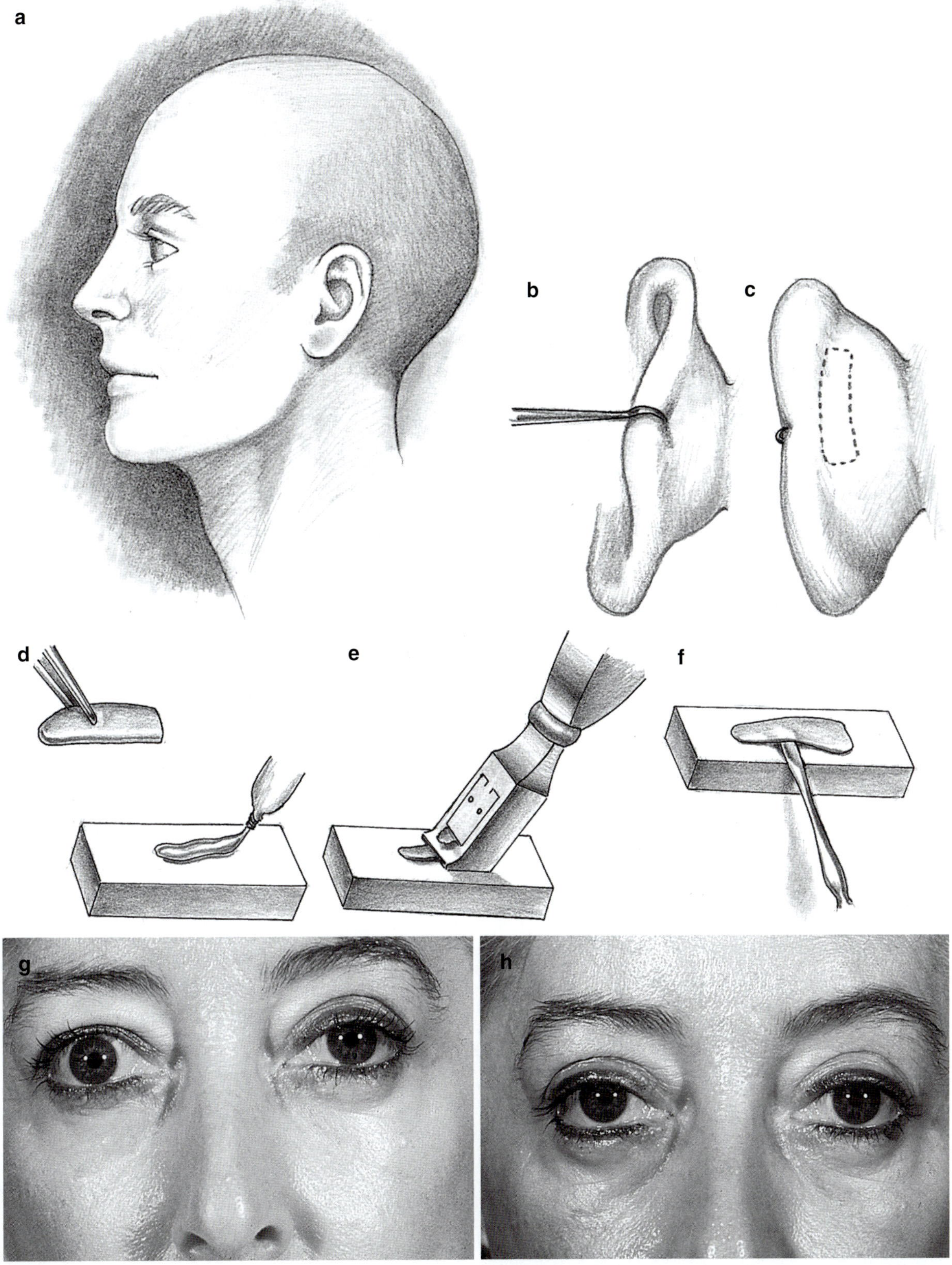

Fig. 58.15 Auricular cartilage is much thicker than other spacers and certainly much thicker than an eyelid that has undergone only levator recession. The flattened portion of the posterior ear at the junction between the ear and skull is used (**a**–**c**). The graft is difficult to thin, because it is brittle and friable. It is possible to thin the graft by stabilizing it to a cutting block with sterile cyanoacrylate glue or even Mastisol (**d**). The graft is then shaved with mucotome or dermatome to thin it without breakage (**e**). The graft is elevated off the cutting block with a Freer elevator (**f**) to break the temporary adhesive connection. (**g**) Preoperative retraction. (**h**) Postoperative view at 2 months after auricular cartilage spacer utilization

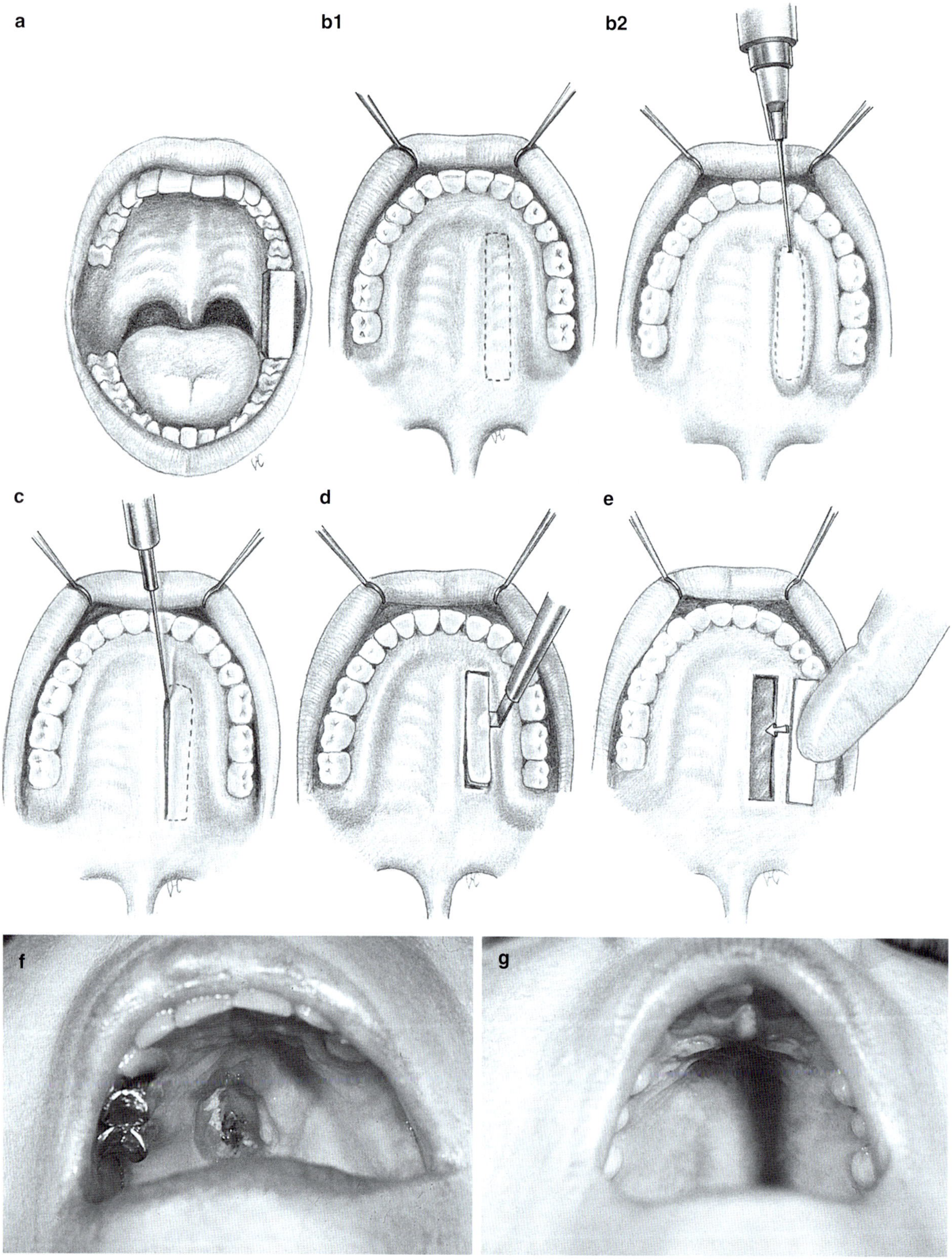

Fig. 58.16 Hard palate mucosal grafting. (**a**) A bite plate or silicone block is used to stabilize the mouth. (**b1**) The prospective donor site is marked and injected with local anesthetic with epinephrine. The naso-palatine neurovascular bundle is avoided, and the greater palatine vascular bundle is also avoided. (**b2**) Demonstrates the ballooning of the hard palate mucosal graft with local anesthesia with adrenaline. It is preferred to allow 2–5 min for vasoconstrictive effect. (**c**) The graft is harvested by outlining the mucosal site with a cutting Bovie on a sharp-pointed tip such as a Colorado needle. (**d**) The graft is harvested using a right-angle sharp blade such as a super blade or crescent knife or #57 Beaver blade. The graft is undermined, but an attempt is made to keep it thin. (**e**) Hemostasis is obtained with cautery or a bone wax pledget. (**f**) Immediate appearance of the hard palate mucosal grafting site. (**g**), Appearance at 1 month after surgery

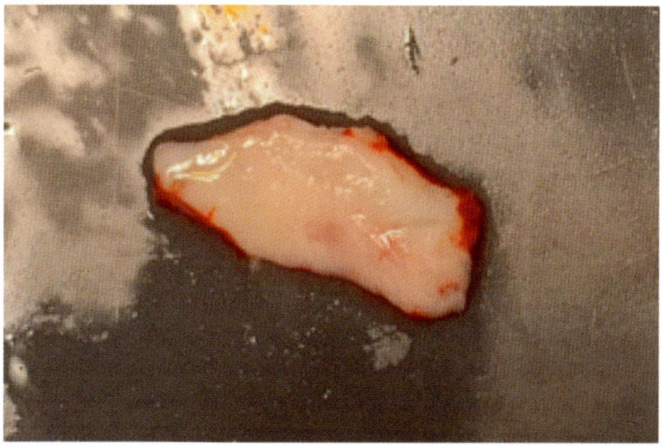

Fig. 58.17 Hard palate graft. This graft has been harvested from the patient intraoperatively and will be sized to provide lower eyelid support for the treatment of retraction

The desired graft size is harvested with a #57 Beaver blade and dissected from the underlying submucosa with a crescent-shaped blade (Fig. 58.17). Electrocautery should be avoided as much as possible, and gel foam may be placed in the donor bed to control bleeding. The graft is then thinned with a pair of curved Stevens scissors and sewn into position in the recipient bed with 6-0 chromic or Vicryl sutures (Fig. 58.18). The lower eyelid is then placed on upward stretch with a Frost suture for 1 week. The donor site heals in the postoperative state by reepithelialization (Fig. 58.19). A pre-made dental splint can be used postoperatively to reduce discomfort while eating.

Acellular Dermis

Acellular human, porcine, and bovine dermal matrices are available as viable alternatives for autogenous upper

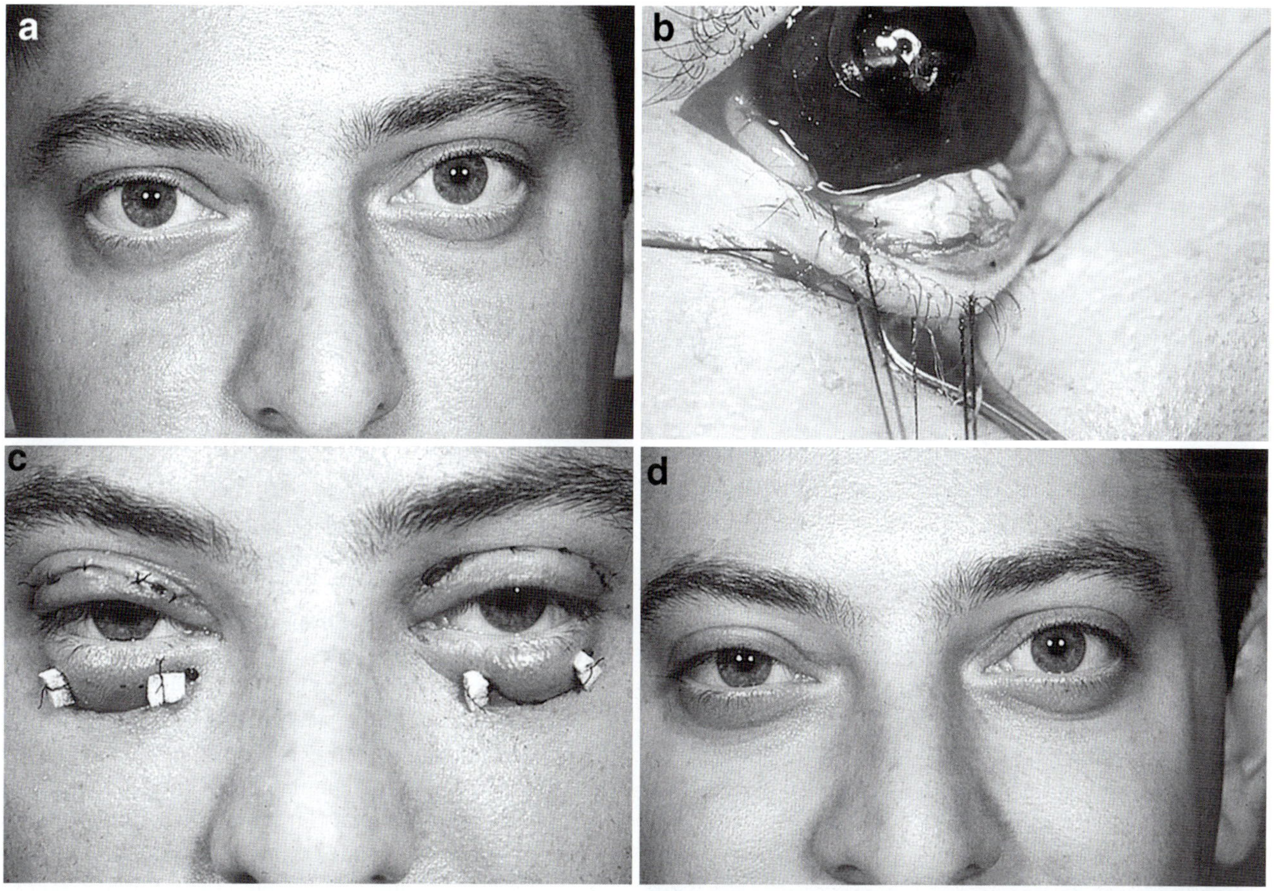

Fig. 58.18 (**a**) The graft must be debulked by thinning with a curved Stevens scissors and removing all subcutaneous tissue. (**b**) This spacer can be used in either upper or lower eyelids, but sutures are avoided on the posterior surface. The graft is located in its interpositional space, and a double-armed 6-0 suture is led through the graft to be tied externally over bolsters or up through the upper eyelid to keep the grafted lid on the stretch and then secured over a bolster (**c**). Preoperative appearance of a patient with thyroid eye disease and slight lower eyelid retraction. This was objectionable to the patient aesthetically, and he underwent a hard palate mucosal graft (**d**) tied over bolsters (**e**). His appearance at 1 month after surgery demonstrates an elevation of both lower eyelids of approximately 2 mm (**f**). His lids are now above the inferior limbus compared with 1–2 mm of lower eyelid retraction preoperatively (**g**)

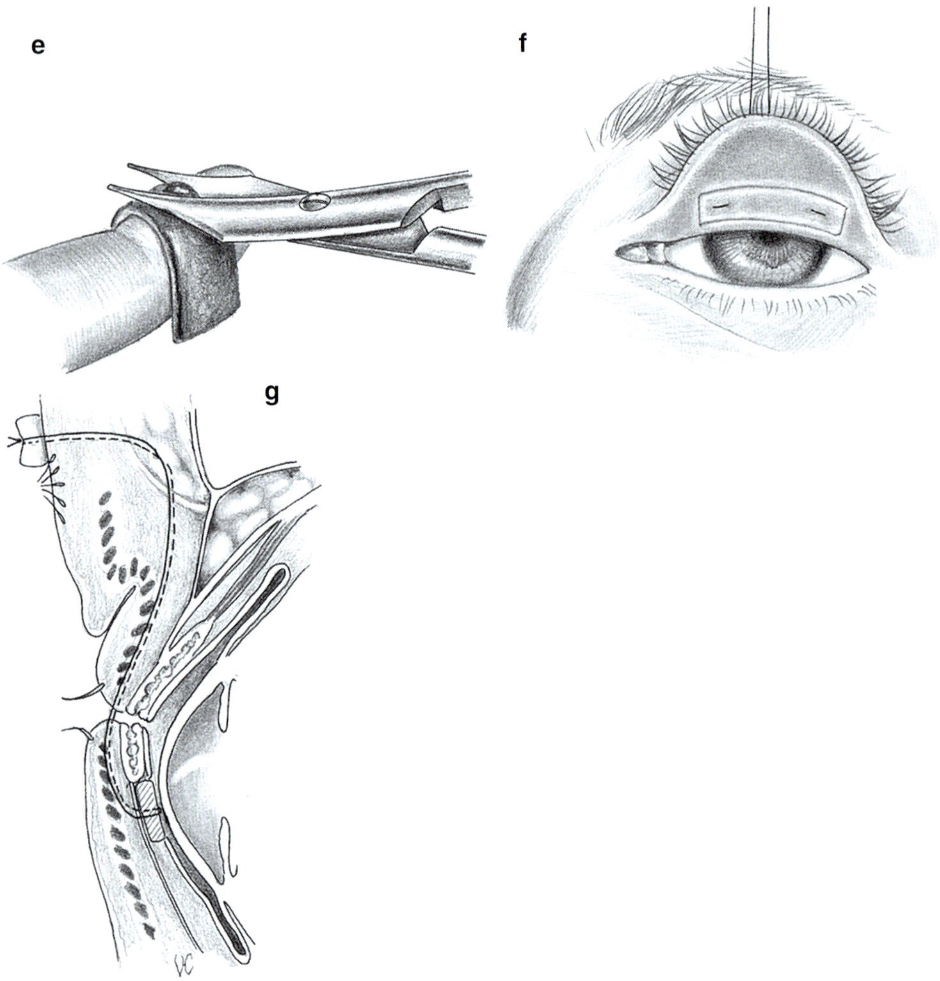

Fig. 58.18 (continued)

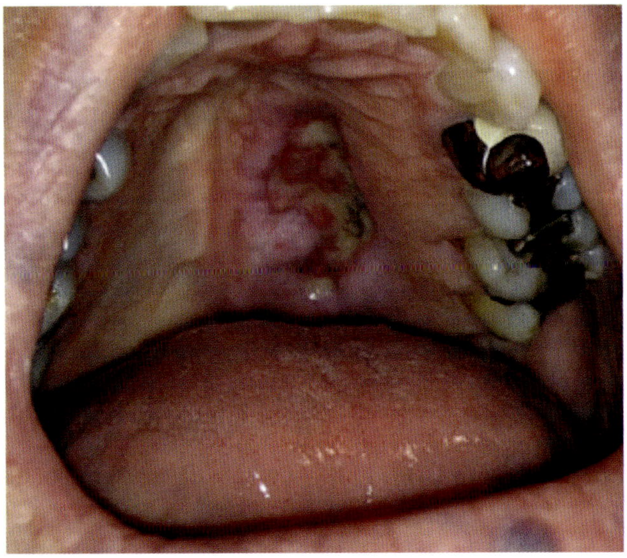

Fig. 58.19 Hard palate donor site healing at 10 days postoperatively

[136, 138] and lower eyelid [137, 139] spacer grafts. These materials are derived from cadaveric human, porcine, or bovine dermis and are immunologically inert. They offer enough structural rigidity to replace tarsus while allowing for conjunctival epithelial migration and graft surface repopulation [133, 137, 140, 141]. Unlike autogenous human tissue, acellular human dermis avoids the need for tissue harvesting at time of surgery. Although this material has excellent handling properties and is associated with minimal inflammation, its long-term effects may not be as long lasting as seen with hard-palate grafting due to graft shrinkage [141]. Porcine acellular dermis is available ready for use as a prehydrated dermal matrix. Bovine acellular dermal matrix is also available, though this material needs to be hydrated prior to use. These materials are both relatively straightforward to use surgically since neither has a particular orientation [137].

Free Tarsal Grafts

In TED, use of free tarsal grafts for lower lid retraction requires that the upper eyelid from which the graft is taken is not retracted, as this would worsen the retraction by shortening the posterior lamella. Therefore, this approach is typically avoided in TED due to the potential for contralateral eye involvement.

A free tarsal graft is prepared by everting the donor upper eyelid on a Desmarres retractor. Then, a straight incision is made parallel to the lid margin 3 mm superior to the margin at the same horizontal length as the corresponding lower eyelid conjunctival incision. At least 3 mm of vertical tarsal height must remain to maintain the structural integrity of the upper lid. A second incision is made 4–5 mm superior to the first to form an ellipse of tarsus, which is dissected from the upper lid. The tarsal graft is then sutured into the recipient bed in the lower eyelid with interrupted or running 6-0 suture (usually gut or Vicryl) (Fig. 58.20).

Alloplastic Material

Alloplastic material, such as porous polyethylene, can effectively raise the lower lid height and has been shown to biointegrate on a histopathologic level [142, 143]. However, there is a high incidence of complications with this material, including revision and exposure. Therefore, porous polyethylene spacers are best used in refractory cases not responding to other techniques [142, 143].

a

b

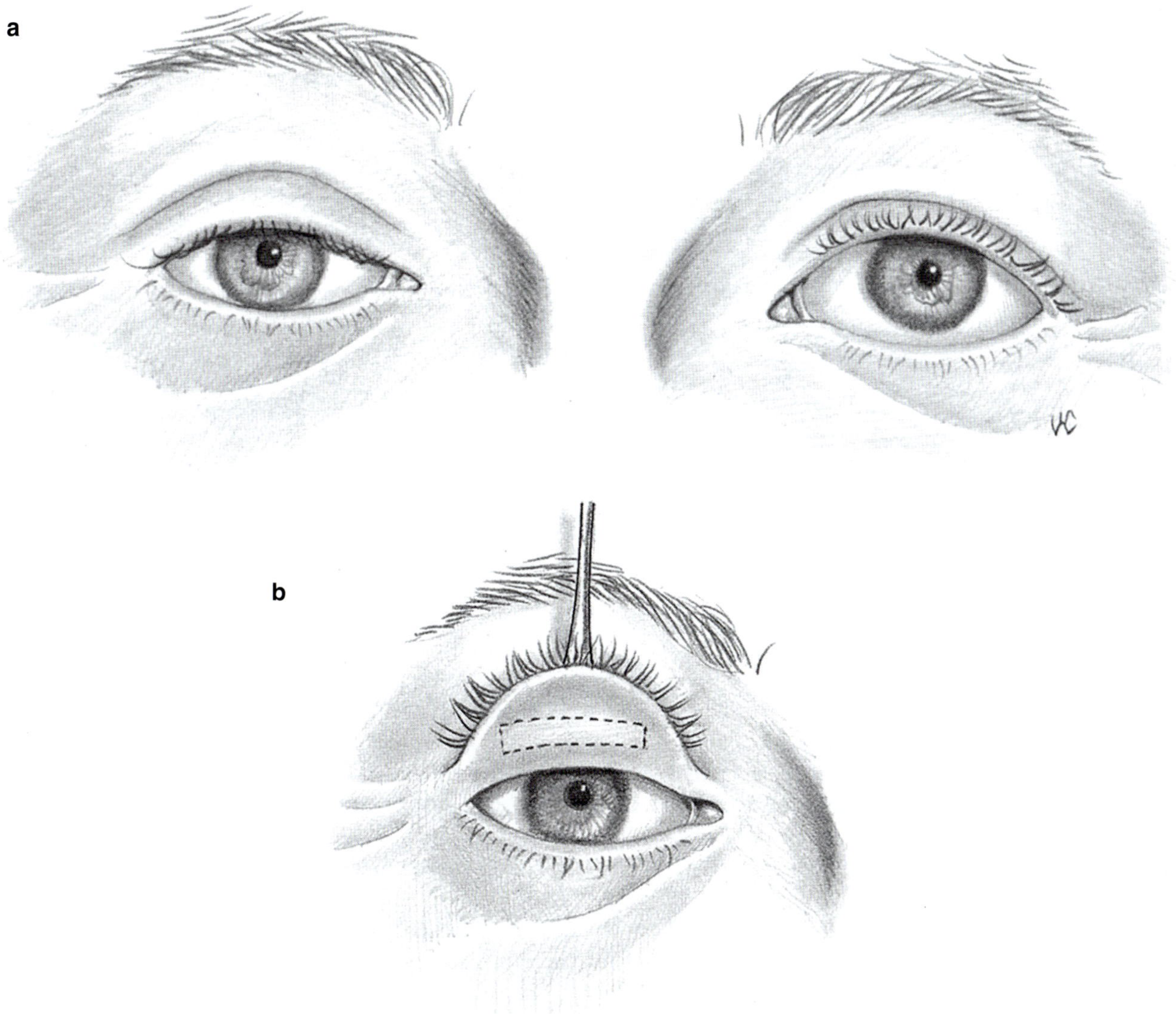

Fig. 58.20 Free tarsal grafts can be used to elevate a retracted lower eyelid if the patient happens to have unilateral ptosis (**a**). A free tarsal graft can be harvested, similar to a Fasanella-Servat specimen (**b**). This is transferred to a similar incision as produced in Fig. 58.14, to recess the retractors and space the gap (**c**). The conjunctival incision does not need to be closed because this is a composite graft with conjunctiva intact. (**d**) This graft also is stabilized nasally and temporally and tied over external bolsters with a mattress suture of 6-0 silk. The conjunctiva is not sutured closed but is left well opposed to the surrounding conjunctival edges

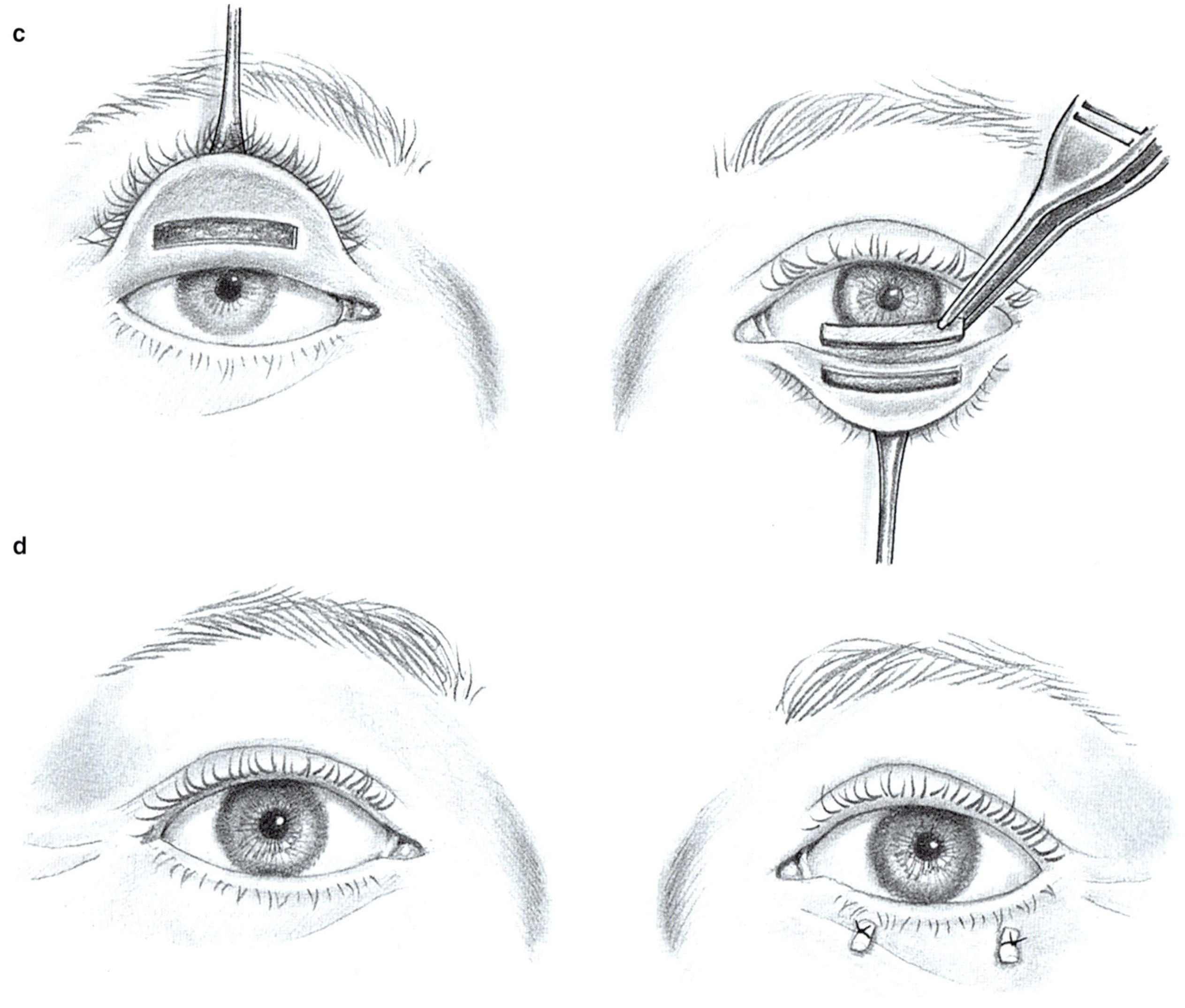

Fig. 58.20 (continued)

Banked Sclera

Sclera was historically used for spacer grafts, though it has fallen out of favor in modern practice as the more desirable aforementioned options have become available.

Results

Limited studies are currently available that analyze the surgical results of these various spacer graft materials. With regard to surgical outcomes comparing autogenous auricular cartilage, bovine acellular matrix, and porcine acellular matrices for lower lid retraction repair, a recent prospective, randomized study by Barmettler and Heo found no significant difference among the three groups [137].

Postoperative Considerations

Following lid retraction surgery, patients are discharged the same day and instructed to follow up in a clinic for re-evaluation within 1 week. An antibiotic or a combination of antibiotic-steroid ointment is prescribed topically for the surgical wounds. If an underlying corneal epithelial disease is present, the patient should continue ocular surface treatment as per the managing ophthalmologist.

In the event that initial eyelid retraction surgery results in postoperative ptosis or residual retraction, additional surgery may be needed depending on the level of patient satisfaction and functional outcome. Among the surgical options available, repeat posterior lamellar grafting [144] for persistent retraction and "hang-back" suture repair of secondary ptosis [145] may be considered. In general, it is always easier to address an undercorrected upper eyelid than an eyelid that becomes ptotic following retraction surgery. The fibrosis of the retractors makes ptosis surgery more challenging. Hence, we recommend that surgeons err on the side of undercorrecting vs. overcorrecting upper eyelid retraction. With spacer grafts, lower eyelids typically remain where the surgeons placed them, with good consistency of outcomes.

Summary

Surgical management of the TED begins with careful assessment of the patient and thoughtful planning regarding the timing and approach to surgical rehabilitation. A variety of surgical techniques have been developed to address the functional and cosmetic complications of TED, and these approaches can be tailored to the needs of the individual patient. Traditionally, surgery is performed in a stepwise fashion, first with orbital decompression, followed by strabismus surgery, then lastly, eyelid repositioning. Careful selection of patients for surgery and clear explanation of the limitations and possible complications of surgery will maintain patient satisfaction and maximize successful surgical results.

References

1. Gomi CF, Yang SW, Granet DB, et al. Change in proptosis following extraocular muscle surgery: effects of muscle recession in thyroid-associated orbitopathy. J AAPOS. 2007;11(4):377–80.
2. Lund VJ, Larkin G, Fells P, Adams G. Orbital decompression for thyroid eye disease: a comparison of external and endoscopic techniques. J Laryngol Otol. 1997;111(11):1051–5.
3. van der Wal KG, de Visscher JG, Boukes RJ, Smeding B. Surgical treatment of Graves orbitopathy: a modified balanced technique. Int J Oral Maxillofac Surg. 2001;30(4):254–8.
4. Rizk SS, Papageorge A, Liberatore LA, Sacks EH. Bilateral simultaneous orbital decompression for Graves' orbitopathy with a combined endoscopic and Caldwell-Luc approach. Otolaryngol Head Neck Surg. 2000;122(2):216–21.
5. Weisman RA, Osguthorpe JD. Orbital decompression in Graves' disease. Arch Otolaryngol Head Neck Surg. 1994;120(8):831–4.
6. Lyons CJ, Rootman J. Orbital decompression for disfiguring exophthalmos in thyroid orbitopathy. Ophthalmology. 1994;101(2):223–30.
7. McCord CD. Current trends in orbital decompression. Ophthalmology. 1985;92(1):21–33.
8. Kennerdell JS, Maroon JC. An orbital decompression for severe dysthyroid exophthalmos. Ophthalmology. 1982;89(5):467–72.
9. Paridaens DA, Verhoeff K, Bouwens D, van Den Bosch WA. Transconjunctival orbital decompression in Graves' ophthalmopathy: lateral wall approach ab interno. Br J Ophthalmol. 2000;84(7):775–81.
10. Tyler MA, Zhang CC, Saini AT, Yao WC. Cutting-edge endonasal surgical approaches to thyroid ophthalmopathy. Laryngoscope Investig Otolaryngol. 2018;3(2):100–4.
11. Zhang-Nunes SX, Dang S, Garneau HC, et al. Characterization and outcomes of repeat orbital decompression for thyroid-associated orbitopathy. Orbit. 2015;34(2):57–65.
12. Korkmaz S, Konuk O. Surgical treatment of dysthyroid optic neuropathy: long-term visual outcomes with comparison of 2-wall versus 3-wall orbital decompression. Curr Eye Res. 2016;41(2):159–64.
13. Bernardini FP, Nerad J, Fay A, Zambelli A, Cruz AA. The revised direct transconjunctival approach to the orbital floor. Ophthalmic Plast Reconstr Surg. 2017;33(2):93–100.
14. Cruz AA, Leme VR. Orbital decompression: a comparison between trans-fornix/transcaruncular inferomedial and coronal inferomedial plus lateral approaches. Ophthalmic Plast Reconstr Surg. 2003;19(6):440–5; discussion 445
15. Abuzayed B, Tanriover N, Gazioglu N, Eraslan BS, Akar Z. Endoscopic endonasal approach to the orbital apex and medial orbital wall: anatomic study and clinical applications. J Craniofac Surg. 2009;20(5):1594–600.
16. White WA, White WL, Shapiro PE. Combined endoscopic medial and inferior orbital decompression with transcutaneous lateral orbital decompression in Graves' orbitopathy. Ophthalmology. 2003;110(9):1827–32.
17. Ference EH, Sindwani R, Tan BK, et al. Open versus endoscopic medial orbital decompression: utilization, cost, and operating room time. Am J Rhinol Allergy. 2016;30(5):360–6.
18. Mueller SK, Freitag SK, Bleier BS. Morphometric analysis of the orbital process of the palatine bone and its relationship to endoscopic orbital apex surgery. Ophthalmic Plast Reconstr Surg. 2018;34(3):254–7.
19. Leone CR, Piest KL, Newman RJ. Medial and lateral wall decompression for thyroid ophthalmopathy. Am J Ophthalmol. 1989;108(2):160–6.
20. Shepard KG, Levin PS, Terris DJ. Balanced orbital decompression for Graves' ophthalmopathy. Laryngoscope. 1998;108(11 Pt 1):1648–53.
21. Kikkawa DO, Pornpanich K, Cruz RC Jr, Levi L, Granet DB. Graded orbital decompression based on severity of proptosis. Ophthalmology. 2002;109(7):1219–24.
22. Richter DF, Stoff A, Olivari N. Transpalpebral decompression of endocrine ophthalmopathy by intraorbital fat removal (Olivari technique): experience and progression after more than 3000 operations over 20 years. Plast Reconstr Surg. 2007;120(1):109–23.
23. Kazim M, Trokel SL, Acaroglu G, Elliott A. Reversal of dysthyroid optic neuropathy following orbital fat decompression. Br J Ophthalmol. 2000;84(6):600–5.
24. Goldberg RA. Advances in surgical rehabilitation in thyroid eye disease. Thyroid. 2008;18(9):989–95.
25. Graham SM, Thomas RD, Carter KD, Nerad JA. The transcaruncular approach to the medial orbital wall. Laryngoscope. 2002;112(6):986–9.
26. Gockeln R, Winter R, Sistani F, Kretschmann U, Hussein S. Minimal invasive decompression of the orbit in Graves' orbitopathy. Strabismus. 2000;8(4):251–9.
27. Shorr N, Baylis HI, Goldberg RA, Perry JD. Transcaruncular approach to the medial orbit and orbital apex. Ophthalmology. 2000;107(8):1459–63.
28. Schaefer SD, Soliemanzadeh P, Della Rocca DA, et al. Endoscopic and transconjunctival orbital decompression for thyroid-related orbital apex compression. Laryngoscope. 2003;113(3):508–13.
29. Wee DT, Carney AS, Thorpe M, Wormald PJ. Endoscopic orbital decompression for Graves' ophthalmopathy. J Laryngol Otol. 2002;116(1):6–9.

30. Tooley AA, Godfrey KJ, Kazim M. Evolution of thyroid eye disease decompression-dysthyroid optic neuropathy. Eye (Lond). 2019;33(2):206–11.
31. Cubuk MO, Konuk O, Unal M. Orbital decompression surgery for the treatment of Graves' ophthalmopathy: comparison of different techniques and long-term results. Int J Ophthalmol. 2018;11(8):1363–70.
32. Kingdom TT, Davies BW, Durairaj VD. Orbital decompression for the management of thyroid eye disease: an analysis of outcomes and complications. Laryngoscope. 2015;125(9):2034–40.
33. Mehta P, Durrani OM. Outcome of deep lateral wall rim-sparing orbital decompression in thyroid-associated orbitopathy: a new technique and results of a case series. Orbit. 2011;30(6):265–8.
34. Boboridis KG, Uddin J, Mikropoulos DG, et al. Critical appraisal on orbital decompression for thyroid eye disease: a systematic review and literature search. Adv Ther. 2015;32(7):595–611.
35. Wu CY, Niziol LM, Musch DC, Kahana A. Thyroid-related orbital decompression surgery: a multivariate analysis of risk factors and outcomes. Ophthal Plast Reconstr Surg. 2017;33(3):189–95.
36. Wu CY, Stacey AW, Kahana A. Simultaneous versus staged balanced decompression for thyroid-related compressive optic neuropathy. Ophthal Plast Reconstr Surg. 2016;32(6):462–7.
37. Prat MC, Braunstein AL, Dagi Glass LR, Kazim M. Orbital fat decompression for thyroid eye disease: retrospective case review and criteria for optimal case selection. Ophthal Plast Reconstr Surg. 2015;31(3):215–8.
38. Braun TL, Bhadkamkar MA, Jubbal KT, Weber AC, Marx DP. Orbital decompression for thyroid eye disease. Semin Plast Surg. 2017;31(1):40–5.
39. Trokel SL, Jakobiec FA. Correlation of CT scanning and pathologic features of ophthalmic Graves' disease. Ophthalmology. 1981;88(6):553–64.
40. Peyster RG, Ginsberg F, Silber JH, Adler LP. Exophthalmos caused by excessive fat: CT volumetric analysis and differential diagnosis. AJR Am J Roentgenol. 1986;146(3):459–64.
41. Goldberg RA, Kim AJ, Kerivan KM. The lacrimal keyhole, orbital door jamb, and basin of the inferior orbital fissure. Three areas of deep bone in the lateral orbit. Arch Ophthalmol. 1998;116(12):1618–24.
42. Spalthoff S, Jehn P, Zimmerer R, Rana M, Gellrich NC, Dittmann J. Modified lateral orbital wall decompression in Graves' orbitopathy using computer-assisted planning. Int J Oral Maxillofac Surg. 2018;47(2):167–74.
43. Dubin MR, Tabaee A, Scruggs JT, Kazim M, Close LG. Image-guided endoscopic orbital decompression for Graves' orbitopathy. Ann Otol Rhinol Laryngol. 2008;117(3):177–85.
44. Kacker A, Kazim M, Murphy M, Trokel S, Close LG. "Balanced" orbital decompression for severe Graves' orbitopathy: technique with treatment algorithm. Otolaryngol Head Neck Surg. 2003;128(2):228–35.
45. Wu CY, Kahana A. Stereotactic navigation with a registration mask in orbital decompression surgery: preliminary results. Ophthalmic Plast Reconstr Surg. 2015;31(6):440–4.
46. Servat JJ, Elia MD, Gong D, Manes RP, Black EH, Levin F. Electromagnetic image-guided orbital decompression: technique, principles, and preliminary experience with 6 consecutive cases. Orbit. 2014;33(6):433–6.
47. Lee KY, Ang BT, Ng I, Looi A. Stereotaxy for surgical navigation in orbital surgery. Ophthalmic Plast Reconstr Surg. 2009;25(4):300–2.
48. Naik MN, Nema A, Ali MH, Ali MJ. Piezoelectric surgery versus mechanical drilling for orbital floor decompression: effect on infraorbital hypoaesthesia. Orbit. 2019;38(3):184–6.
49. Siracuse-Lee DE, Kazim M. Orbital decompression: current concepts. Curr Opin Ophthalmol. 2002;13(5):310–6.
50. Sisler H, Jakobiec F, Trokel S. Ocular abnormalities and orbital changes of Graves' disease. In: Tasman W, Jaeger E, editors. Duane's clinical ophthalmology, rev. ed, vol. 2. Philadelphia: JB Lippincott; 1992.
51. Prat MC, Braunstein AL, Dagi Glass LR, Kazim M. Orbital fat decompression for thyroid eye disease: retrospective case review and criteria for optimal case selection. Ophthalmic Plast Reconstr Surg. 2015;31(3):215–8.
52. Bhatti MT, Dutton JJ. Thyroid eye disease: therapy in the active phase. J Neuroophthalmol. 2014;34(2):186–97.
53. Onaran Z, Konuk O, Oktar SO, Yucel C, Unal M. Intraocular pressure lowering effect of orbital decompression is related to increased venous outflow in Graves orbitopathy. Curr Eye Res. 2014;39(7):666–72.
54. Perez-Lopez M, Sales-Sanz M, Rebolleda G, et al. Retrobulbar ocular blood flow changes after orbital decompression in Graves' ophthalmopathy measured by color Doppler imaging. Invest Ophthalmol Vis Sci. 2011;52(8):5612–7.
55. Neigel JM, Rootman J, Belkin RI, et al. Dysthyroid optic neuropathy. The crowded orbital apex syndrome. Ophthalmology. 1988;95(11):1515–21.
56. Kahaly GJ, Pitz S, Hommel G, Dittmar M. Randomized, single blind trial of intravenous versus oral steroid monotherapy in Graves' orbitopathy. J Clin Endocrinol Metab. 2005;90(9):5234–40.
57. Kauh CY, Gupta S, Douglas RS, et al. Compressive optic neuropathy and repeat orbital decompression: a case series. Ophthalmic Plast Reconstr Surg. 2015;31(5):385–90.
58. MacAndie K, Harnett AN, Kyle P. Restoration of vision by radiotherapy for severe, acute, steroid-refractory, congestive thyroid orbitopathy. Clin Oncol (R Coll Radiol). 2000;12(3):188–91.
59. Kotwal A, Stan M. Current and future treatments for Graves' disease and Graves' ophthalmopathy. Horm Metab Res. 2018;50(12):871–86.
60. Genere N, Stan MN. Current and emerging treatment strategies for Graves' orbitopathy. Drugs. 2019;79(2):109–24.
61. Soeters MR, van Zeijl CJ, Boelen A, et al. Optimal management of Graves orbitopathy: a multidisciplinary approach. Neth J Med. 2011;69(7):302–8.
62. Trokel S, Kazim M, Moore S. Orbital fat removal. Decompression for Graves orbitopathy. Ophthalmology. 1993;100(5):674–82.
63. Rajabi MT, Papageorgiou K, Taban M, et al. Ultrasonographic motion analysis of lower eyelid compartments in patients with chronic thyroid associated ophthalmopathy. J Curr Ophthalmol. 2017;29(4):310–7.
64. Choe CH, Cho RI, Elner VM. Comparison of lateral and medial orbital decompression for the treatment of compressive optic neuropathy in thyroid eye disease. Ophthalmic Plast Reconstr Surg. 2011;27(1):4–11.
65. Jefferis JM, Jones RK, Currie ZI, Tan JH, Salvi SM. Orbital decompression for thyroid eye disease: methods, outcomes, and complications. Eye (Lond). 2018;32(3):626–36.
66. Choi SU, Kim KW, Lee JK. Surgical outcomes of balanced deep lateral and medial orbital wall decompression in Korean population: clinical and computed tomography-based analysis. Korean J Ophthalmol. 2016;30(2):85–91.
67. Liao SL, Chang TC, Lin LL. Transcaruncular orbital decompression: an alternate procedure for Graves ophthalmopathy with compressive optic neuropathy. Am J Ophthalmol. 2006;141(5):810–8.
68. Woo KI, Kim YD. Isolated caruncular approach for orbital decompression. Jpn J Ophthalmol. 2004;48(4):397–403.
69. Borumandi F, Hammer B, Kamer L, von Arx G. How predictable is exophthalmos reduction in Graves' orbitopathy? A review of the literature. Br J Ophthalmol. 2011;95(12):1625–30.
70. Ben Simon GJ, Schwarcz RM, Mansury AM, Wang L, McCann JD, Goldberg RA. Minimally invasive orbital decompres-

sion: local anesthesia and hand-carved bone. Arch Ophthalmol. 2005;123(12):1671–5.
71. Blandford AD, Zhang D, Chundury RV, Perry JD. Dysthyroid optic neuropathy: update on pathogenesis, diagnosis, and management. Expert Rev Ophthalmol. 2017;12(2):111–21.
72. Olivari N. Transpalpebral decompression of endocrine ophthalmopathy (Graves' disease) by removal of intraorbital fat: experience with 147 operations over 5 years. Plast Reconstr Surg. 1991;87(4):627–41; discussion 642–623
73. Wu CH, Chang TC, Liao SL. Results and predictability of fat-removal orbital decompression for disfiguring graves exophthalmos in an Asian patient population. Am J Ophthalmol. 2008;145(4):755–9.
74. Zhang S, Li Y, Wang Y, et al. Comparison of rim-sparing versus rim-removal techniques in deep lateral wall orbital decompression for Graves' orbitopathy. Int J Oral Maxillofac Surg. 2019;48(4):461–7.
75. Cho RI, Choe CH, Elner VM. Ultrasonic bone removal versus high-speed burring for lateral orbital decompression: comparison of surgical outcomes for the treatment of thyroid eye disease. Ophthalmic Plast Reconstr Surg. 2010;26(2):83–7.
76. Chang EL, Piva AP. Temporal fossa orbital decompression for treatment of disfiguring thyroid-related orbitopathy. Ophthalmology. 2008;115(9):1613–9.
77. Fong KD, Warren SM, Loboa EG, et al. Mechanical strain affects dura mater biological processes: implications for immature calvarial healing. Plast Reconstr Surg. 2003;112(5):1312–27.
78. Valdivia-Gandur I, Engelke W, Beltrán V, Borie E, Fuentes R, Manzanares-Céspedes MC. Novel use of cranial epidural space in rabbits as an animal model to investigate bone volume augmentation potential of different bone graft substitutes. Head Face Med. 2016;12(1):35.
79. Keller JT, Marfurt CF. Peptidergic and serotoninergic innervation of the rat dura mater. J Comp Neurol. 1991;309(4):515–34.
80. Gupta A, Nobori A, Wang Y, Rootman D, Goldberg R. Lateral rectus muscle expands more than medial rectus following maximal deep balanced orbital decompression. Ophthal Plast Reconstr Surg. 2017;34(2):140–2.
81. Dauser RC, Tuite GF, McCluggage CW. Dural inversion procedure for moyamoya disease. Technical note. J Neurosurg. 1997;86(4):719–23.
82. Greenwald JA, Mehrara BJ, Spector JA, et al. Regional differentiation of cranial suture-associated dura mater in vivo and in vitro: implications for suture fusion and patency. J Bone Miner Res. 2000;15(12):2413–30.
83. Greenwald JA, Mehrara BJ, Spector JA, et al. Immature versus mature dura mater: II. Differential expression of genes important to calvarial reossification. Plast Reconstr Surg. 2000;106(3):630–8; discussion 639
84. Rice FL, Xie JY, Albrecht PJ, et al. Anatomy and immunochemical characterization of the non-arterial peptidergic diffuse dural innervation of the rat and Rhesus monkey: Implications for functional regulation and treatment in migraine. Cephalalgia. 2017;37(14):1350–72.
85. Baillie LD, Ahn AH, Mulligan SJ. Sumatriptan inhibition of N-type calcium channel mediated signaling in dural CGRP terminal fibres. Neuropharmacology. 2012;63(3):362–7.
86. Cappugi P, Tsampau D, Lotti T. Substance P provokes cutaneous erythema and edema through a histamine-independent pathway. Int J Dermatol. 1992;31(3):206–9.
87. Abed SF, Shams P, Shen S, Adds PJ, Uddin JM. A cadaveric study of ethmoidal foramina variation and its surgical significance in Caucasians. Br J Ophthalmol. 2012;96(1):118–21.
88. Fabian ID, Rosen N, Ben Simon GJ. Strabismus after inferior-medial wall orbital decompression in thyroid-related orbitopathy. Curr Eye Res. 2013;38(1):204–9.
89. Zloto O, Ben Simon G, Didi Fabian I, et al. Association of orbital decompression and the characteristics of subsequent strabismus surgery in thyroid eye disease. Can J Ophthalmol. 2017;52(3):264–8.
90. Verity DH, Rose GE. Acute thyroid eye disease (TED): principles of medical and surgical management. Eye (Lond). 2013;27(3):308–19.
91. Alsuhaibani AH, Carter KD, Policeni B, Nerad JA. Orbital volume and eye position changes after balanced orbital decompression. Ophthalmic Plast Reconstr Surg. 2011;27(3):158–63.
92. Unal M, Leri F, Konuk O, Hasanreisoğlu B. Balanced orbital decompression combined with fat removal in Graves ophthalmopathy: do we really need to remove the third wall? Ophthalmic Plast Reconstr Surg. 2003;19(2):112–8.
93. Unal M, Ileri F, Konuk O, Hasanreisoğglu B. Balanced orbital decompression in Graves' orbitopathy: Upper eyelid crease incision for extended lateral wall decompression. Orbit. 2000;19(2):109–17.
94. Wright ED, Davidson J, Codere F, Desrosiers M. Endoscopic orbital decompression with preservation of an inferomedial bony strut: minimization of postoperative diplopia. J Otolaryngol. 1999;28(5):252–6.
95. Finn AP, Bleier B, Cestari DM, et al. A retrospective review of orbital decompression for thyroid orbitopathy with endoscopic preservation of the inferomedial orbital bone strut. Ophthalmic Plast Reconstr Surg. 2017;33(5):334–9.
96. Metson R, Samaha M. Reduction of diplopia following endoscopic orbital decompression: the orbital sling technique. Laryngoscope. 2002;112(10):1753–7.
97. Bleier BS, Lefebvre DR, Freitag SK. Endoscopic orbital floor decompression with preservation of the inferomedial strut. Int Forum Allergy Rhinol. 2014;4(1):82–4.
98. Yao WC, Sedaghat AR, Yadav P, Fay A, Metson R. Orbital decompression in the endoscopic age: the modified inferomedial orbital strut. Otolaryngol Head Neck Surg. 2016;154(5):963–9.
99. Goldberg RA, Perry JD, Hortaleza V, Tong JT. Strabismus after balanced medial plus lateral wall versus lateral wall only orbital decompression for dysthyroid orbitopathy. Ophthalmic Plast Reconstr Surg. 2000;16(4):271–7.
100. Ben Simon GJ, Wang L, McCann JD, Goldberg RA. Primary-gaze diplopia in patients with thyroid-related orbitopathy undergoing deep lateral orbital decompression with intraconal fat debulking: a retrospective analysis of treatment outcome. Thyroid. 2004;14(5):379–83.
101. Boboridis KG, Bunce C. Surgical orbital decompression for thyroid eye disease. Cochrane Database Syst Rev. 2011(12):CD007630.
102. Sellari-Franceschini S, Dallan I, Bajraktari A, et al. Surgical complications in orbital decompression for Graves' orbitopathy. Acta Otorhinolaryngol Ital. 2016;36(4):265–74.
103. Massoud VA, Fay A, Yoon MK. Cerebrospinal fluid leak as a complication of oculoplastic surgery. Semin Ophthalmol. 2014;29(5–6):440–9.
104. Rootman DB, Golan S, Pavlovich P, Rootman J. Postoperative changes in strabismus, ductions, exophthalmometry, and eyelid retraction after orbital decompression for thyroid orbitopathy. Ophthal Plast Reconstr Surg. 2017;33(4):289–93.
105. Wu CY, Kahana A. Geriatric patients are predisposed to strabismus following thyroid-related orbital decompression surgery: a multivariate analysis. Orbit. 2017;36(2):95–101.
106. Thomas SM, Cruz OA. Comparison of two different surgical techniques for the treatment of strabismus in dysthyroid ophthalmopathy. J AAPOS. 2007;11(3):258–61.
107. Pacheco EM, Guyton DL, Repka MX. Changes in eyelid position accompanying vertical rectus muscle surgery and prevention of lower lid retraction with adjustable surgery. J Pediatr Ophthalmol Strabismus. 1992;29(5):265–72.

108. Flanders M, Hastings M. Diagnosis and surgical management of strabismus associated with thyroid-related orbitopathy. J Pediatr Ophthalmol Strabismus. 1997;34(6):333–40.
109. Bartley GB, Fatourechi V, Kadrmas EF, et al. Clinical features of Graves' ophthalmopathy in an incidence cohort. Am J Ophthalmol. 1996;121(3):284–90.
110. Bartley GB. The differential diagnosis and classification of eyelid retraction. Ophthalmology. 1996;103(1):168–76.
111. Byun JS, Lee JK. Relationships between eyelid position and levator-superior rectus complex and inferior rectus muscle in patients with Graves' orbitopathy with unilateral upper eyelid retraction. Graefes Arch Clin Exp Ophthalmol. 2018;256(10):2001–8.
112. Marinó M, Ricciardi R, Pinchera A, et al. Mild clinical expression of myasthenia gravis associated with autoimmune thyroid diseases. J Clin Endocrinol Metab. 1997;82(2):438–43.
113. Papageorgiou KI, Hwang CJ, Chang SH, et al. Thyroid-associated periorbitopathy: eyebrow fat and soft tissue expansion in patients with thyroid-associated orbitopathy. Arch Ophthalmol. 2012;130(3):319–28.
114. Rajabi MT, Jafari H, Mazloumi M, et al. Lower lid retraction in thyroid orbitopathy: lamellar shortening or proptosis? Int Ophthalmol. 2014;34(4):801–4.
115. Pieroni Goncalves AC, Gupta S, Monteiro MLR, Douglas RS. Customized minimally invasive orbital decompression surgery improves lower eyelid retraction and contour in thyroid eye disease. Ophthalmic Plast Reconstr Surg. 2017;33(6):446–51.
116. Cho RI, Elner VM, Nelson CC, Frueh BR. The effect of orbital decompression surgery on lid retraction in thyroid eye disease. Ophthalmic Plast Reconstr Surg. 2011;27(6):436–8.
117. Gay AJ, Wolkstein MA. Topical guanethidine therapy for endocrine lid retraction. Arch Ophthalmol. 1966;76(3):364–7.
118. Cant JS, Lewis DR. Unwanted pharmacological effects of local guanethidine in the treatment of dysthyroid upper lid retraction. Br J Ophthalmol. 1969;53(4):239–45.
119. Morgenstern KE, Evanchan J, Foster JA, et al. Botulinum toxin type a for dysthyroid upper eyelid retraction. Ophthalmic Plast Reconstr Surg. 2004;20(3):181–5.
120. Salour H, Bagheri B, Aletaha M, et al. Transcutaneous dysport injection for treatment of upper eyelid retraction associated with thyroid eye disease. Orbit. 2010;29(2):114–8.
121. Uddin JM, Davies PD. Treatment of upper eyelid retraction associated with thyroid eye disease with subconjunctival botulinum toxin injection. Ophthalmology. 2002;109(6):1183–7.
122. MacCarthy CF, Hollenhorst RW. Protective moist-chamber eye dressing. Am J Ophthalmol. 1971;71(6):1333–4.
123. Terwee CB, Gerding MN, Dekker FW, Prummel MF, Wiersinga WM. Development of a disease specific quality of life questionnaire for patients with Graves' ophthalmopathy: the GO-QOL. Br J Ophthalmol. 1998;82(7):773–9.
124. Yang P, Ko AC, Kikkawa DO, Korn BS. Upper eyelid blepharoplasty: evaluation, treatment, and complication minimization. Semin Plast Surg. 2017;31(1):51–7.
125. Codner MA, Kikkawa DO, Korn BS, Pacella SJ. Blepharoplasty and brow lift. Plast Reconstr Surg. 2010;126(1):1e–17e.
126. Georgescu D, Anderson RL, McCann JD. Brow ptosis correction: a comparison of five techniques. Facial Plast Surg. 2010;26(3):186–92.
127. Arneja JS, Larson DL, Gosain AK. Aesthetic and reconstructive brow lift: current techniques, indications, and applications. Ophthalmic Plast Reconstr Surg. 2005;21(6):405–11.
128. McCord CD, Doxanas MT. Browplasty and browpexy: an adjunct to blepharoplasty. Plast Reconstr Surg. 1990;86(2):248–54.
129. Elner VM, Hassan AS, Frueh BR. Graded full-thickness anterior blepharotomy for upper eyelid retraction. Arch Ophthalmol. 2004;122(1):55–60.
130. Doxanas MT, Dryden RM. The use of sclera in the treatment of dysthyroid eyelid retraction. Ophthalmology. 1981;88(9):887–94.
131. Oestreicher JH, Pang NK, Liao W. Treatment of lower eyelid retraction by retractor release and posterior lamellar grafting: an analysis of 659 eyelids in 400 patients. Ophthalmic Plast Reconstr Surg. 2008;24(3):207–12.
132. Cohen MS, Shorr N. Eyelid reconstruction with hard palate mucosa grafts. Ophthalmic Plast Reconstr Surg. 1992;8(3):183–95.
133. Chang EL, Rubin PA. Upper and lower eyelid retraction. Int Ophthalmol Clin. 2002;42(2):45–59.
134. Rubin PA, Fay AM, Remulla HD, Maus M. Ophthalmic plastic applications of acellular dermal allografts. Ophthalmology. 1999;106(11):2091–7.
135. Baylis HI, Perman KI, Fett DR, Sutcliffe RT. Autogenous auricular cartilage grafting for lower eyelid retraction. Ophthalmic Plast Reconstr Surg. 1985;1(1):23–7.
136. McCord C, Nahai FR, Codner MA, Nahai F, Hester TR. Use of porcine acellular dermal matrix (Enduragen) grafts in eyelids: a review of 69 patients and 129 eyelids. Plast Reconstr Surg. 2008;122(4):1206–13.
137. Barmettler A, Heo M. A prospective, randomized comparison of lower eyelid retraction repair with autologous auricular cartilage, bovine acellular dermal matrix (surgimend), and porcine acellular dermal matrix (enduragen) spacer grafts. Ophthalmic Plast Reconstr Surg. 2018;34(3):266–73.
138. Sun J, Liu X, Zhang Y, et al. Bovine acellular dermal matrix for levator lengthening in thyroid-related upper-eyelid retraction. Med Sci Monit. 2018;24:2728–34.
139. Lee EW, Berbos Z, Zaldivar RA, Lee MS, Harrison AR. Use of DermaMatrix graft in oculoplastic surgery. Ophthalmic Plast Reconstr Surg. 2010;26(3):153–4.
140. Li TG, Shorr N, Goldberg RA. Comparison of the efficacy of hard palate grafts with acellular human dermis grafts in lower eyelid surgery. Plast Reconstr Surg. 2005;116(3):873–8; discussion 879–880
141. Sullivan SA, Dailey RA. Graft contraction: a comparison of acellular dermis versus hard palate mucosa in lower eyelid surgery. Ophthalmic Plast Reconstr Surg. 2003;19(1):14–24.
142. Tan J, Olver J, Wright M, Maini R, Neoh C, Dickinson AJ. The use of porous polyethylene (Medpor) lower eyelid spacers in lid heightening and stabilisation. Br J Ophthalmol. 2004;88(9):1197–200.
143. Mavrikakis I, Francis N, Poitelea C, Parkin B, Brittain P, Olver J. Medpor lower eyelid spacer: does it biointegrate? Orbit. 2009;28(1):58–62.
144. McAlister CN, Oestreicher JH. Repeat posterior lamellar grafting for recalcitrant lower eyelid retraction is effective. Orbit. 2012;31(5):307–12.
145. Shah-Desai S, Azarbod P, Szamocki S, Rose GE. Nylon Hang back sutures in the repair of secondary ptosis following overcorrected dysthyroid upper eyelid retraction. Ophthalmic Plast Reconstr Surg. 2016;32(1):61–4.

Part IX

Socket Surgery

David R. Jordan

Enucleation, Evisceration, and Secondary Orbital Implantation

59

David R. Jordan and Stephen R. Klapper

Introduction

Enucleation or evisceration of an eye may be indicated for management of a malignant ocular tumor, removal of a disfigured globe following severe penetrating trauma, or because of degenerative changes resulting from end-stage ocular disease. Loss of binocular visual function with reduced peripheral field and loss of some depth perception may result in difficulties with activities of daily living and impose various vocational restrictions [1–6]. Affected individuals may experience a sense of facial disfigurement and diminished self-esteem as a result of the lost body part [3, 4, 6]. Because eye contact and facial appearance are an essential part of human interaction, it is important for the anophthalmic patient to maintain a natural, normal-appearing prosthetic eye.

Characteristics of the ideal anophthalmic socket include [7]:

1. A centrally placed, well-covered, buried implant of adequate volume, fabricated from a bioinert material that transmits motility from the implant to the overlying prosthesis.
2. A socket lined with healthy conjunctiva and fornices deep enough to retain the prosthesis and permit horizontal and vertical excursions of the artificial eye.
3. Normal eyelid and eyelash position, appearance, and tone.
4. A supratarsal eyelid fold that is symmetric with that of the contralateral eyelid.
5. A comfortable ocular prosthesis that looks similar to the sighted, contralateral globe and in the same horizontal and anterior-posterior plane.

Currently, no surgical procedure satisfies all of the above criteria. Over the past three decades, there have been numerous developments and refinements in anophthalmic socket surgery with respect to implant material and design, implant wrapping, implant-prosthesis coupling, and socket volume considerations. Success in anophthalmic surgery is characterized by a painless, noninflamed eye socket with adequate volume restoration and an artificial eye that looks and moves almost as naturally as a normal eye (Fig. 59.1a, b).

Historical Perspective

The ancient Egyptians, in the process of mummification, would remove the eyes, fill the orbit with wax, and use precious stones to simulate the iris color [8]. Around 500 BCE Egyptians and Romans wore external ocular prostheses (made of clay) designed by pagan priests, who also practiced as physicians. These ocular prostheses were placed outside the socket over phthisical or disfigured globes as an external cosmetic covering and held in place by an adhesive substance or a thong [9, 10]. There were no recorded techniques of enucleation or evisceration in the living human until the late sixteenth century in Europe. George Bartisch, a Saxon, in 1583 is credited with the first recorded description of removal of an eye for treatment of severe ocular disease [8, 11–14]. The extirpation procedure was performed without anesthesia and required the patient to be bound and held in position (Fig. 59.2a). An instrument (Fig. 59.2b) sharpened like a razor and with the best fit in one's hand was quickly pressed up under the upper eyelid very fast toward the bone as far posteriorly as possible [14]. The goal was to expeditiously encompass the entire eye so that the eye is freed from all of its attachments with the greatest speed [14].

The authors of this study do not have a commercial or proprietary interest in any of the products reviewed in this manuscript.

D. R. Jordan (✉)
Ottawa Hospital – General Campus, Eye Institute,
Ottawa, ON, Canada

S. R. Klapper
Ophthalmology/Oculoplastic Surgery, Klapper Eyelid and Facial Plastic Surgery, Carmel, IN, USA

J. J. Servat et al. (eds.), *Smith and Nesi's Ophthalmic Plastic and Reconstructive Surgery*,
https://doi.org/10.1007/978-3-030-41720-8_59

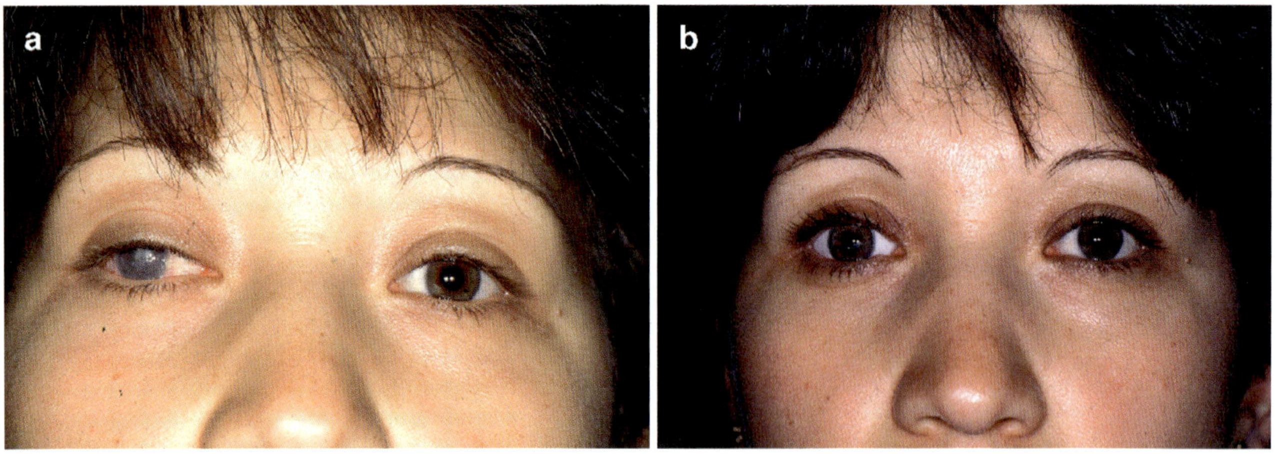

Fig. 59.1 A 28-year-old female pre-evisceration surgery with blind painful unsightly eye. Post evisceration with a porous orbital implant

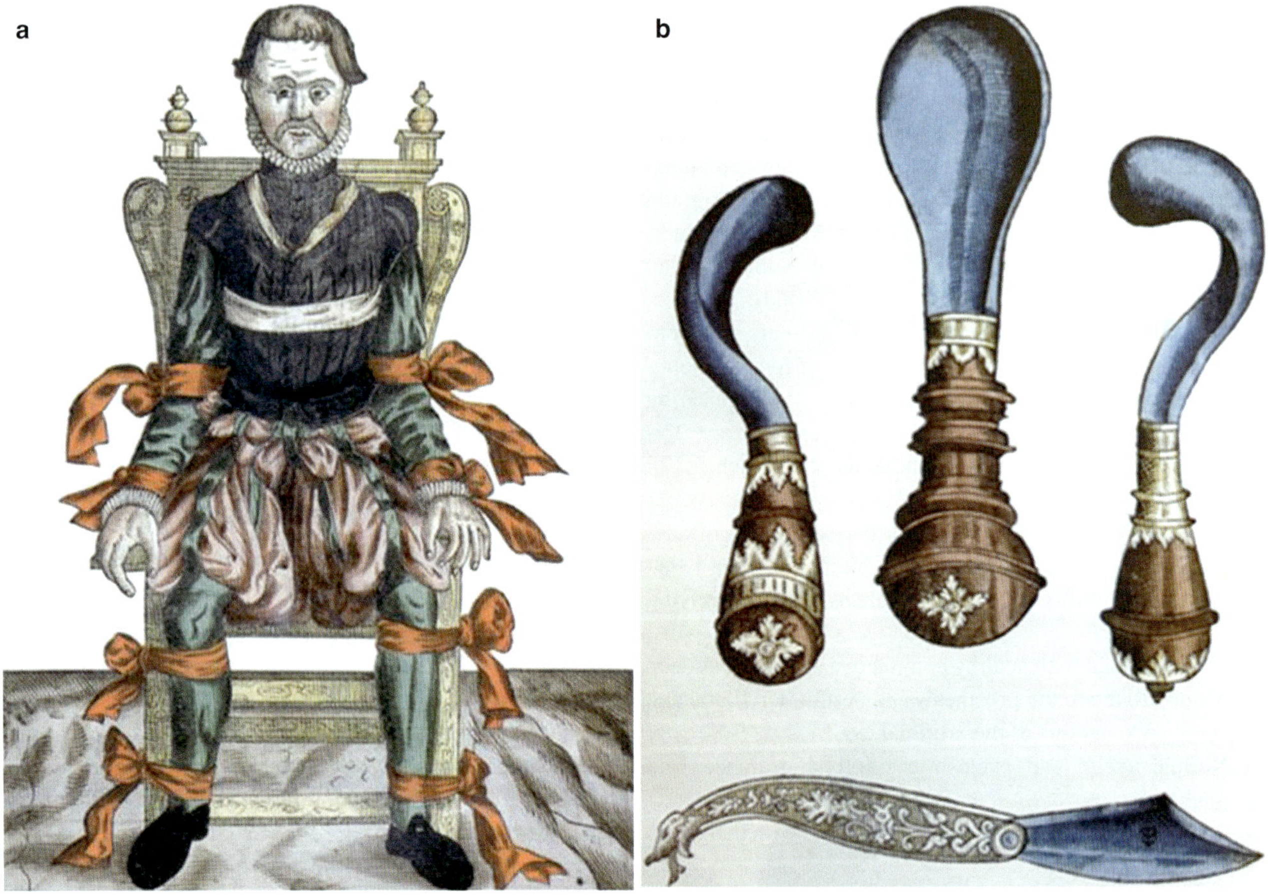

Fig. 59.2 Artist's conception. (**a**) Presurgical positioning of patient with arms and legs bound. (**b**) Instruments used for removal of the eye. (From Blanchard [14])

The extirpation procedure has been described as one of the most severe and repulsive operations in surgery [10–12]. The remaining eye socket deformity often made it impossible to successfully wear a prosthesis. Extirpation of the eye went on with little change for the next 265 years [8]. In 1826, Cleobury described a simple enucleation procedure that fell into disuse only to be described again independently by O'Ferrall (Dublin) and Bonnet (Paris) only weeks apart in 1841 [8]. The introduction of controlled general anesthesia (1874) dramatically changed the field of surgery and certainly had an impact on further advance in ophthalmic surgery [9, 10].

The first recorded evisceration is credited to James Bear in 1817 [15]. While performing an iridectomy for acute glaucoma, the procedure was complicated by an expulsive hemorrhage making it necessary for him to remove the entire contents of the globe [15]. Noyes (1874) was the first to perform a planned evisceration and published a review of his procedures in cases of severe ocular infection [8, 16]. In 1884, P.H. Mules inserted a hollow glass sphere into the scleral cavity following removal of the intraocular contents [16]. A year later W.A. Frost introduced a similar implant into Tenon's capsule following an enucleation procedure [8, 9]. The Mules sphere revolutionized anophthalmic socket surgery by replacing lost orbital volume with a buried orbital implant. Complications including migration, extrusion, and implant shattering became evident as use of these novel implants increased [9, 10]. Sponge, rubber, paraffin, ivory, wool, cork, bone, cartilage, silver, gold, and many other buried orbital implant materials were utilized with little success over the next several decades [8]. The idea of coupling an orbital implant to the overlying prosthetic eye to improve motility was first reported in 1945 (Rudemann) and was followed by several other unique designs that allowed direct attachment of the orbital implant (via a peg) to an overlying prosthetic eye [9, 17]. Unfortunately, with time and increased use, their complications became more evident, and most coupled implants eventually extruded due to chronic infection [9, 17, 18]. By the 1950s completely buried implants gained wide acceptance [8–10]. A variety of implant designs attempting to indirectly couple the buried implant to an overlying prosthetic eye by modifying the anterior implant surface, a type of quasi-integration became available (e.g., Iowa implant, Allen implant), as did paired magnets in the implant and prosthetic eye (Fig. 59.3a–g) [10, 19–22]. Despite initial acceptance prosthetic fitting and implant exposure problems plagued these designs [4, 19–23]. Many surgeons returned to simpler spherical buried implants associated with a lower risk of socket complications [8–10]. By 1989 spherical implants made of silicone, polymethylmethacrylate (PMMA), or glass were the implants most widely used by ophthalmic plastic surgeons (Fig. 59.3h, i) [23].

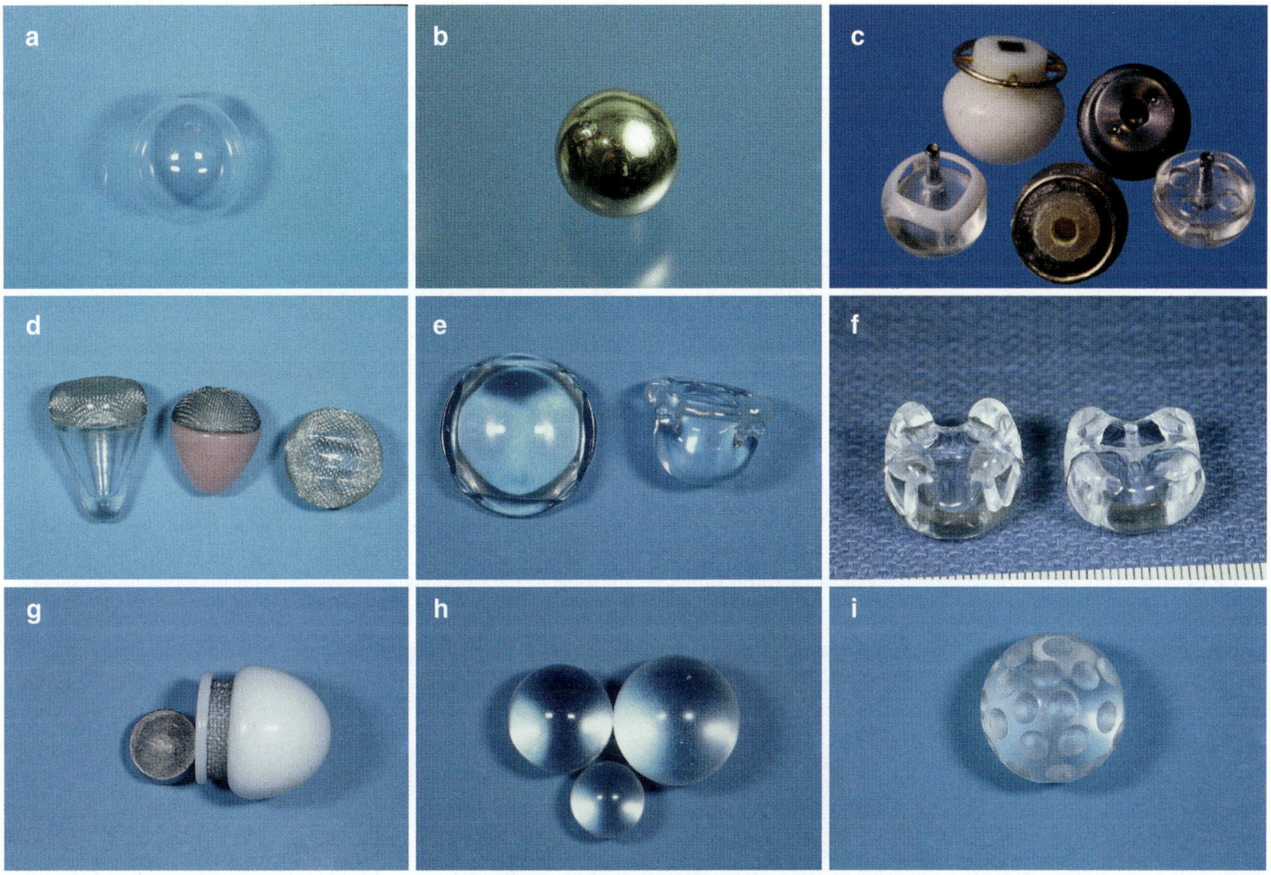

Fig. 59.3 Sampling of orbital implants from the past. (**a**) This hollow plastic sphere is similar in appearance to the original Mules glass sphere. (**b**) Hollow gold sphere. (**c**) Example of an integrated implant from the 1940s. Each implant had a male or female end protruding through the conjunctiva to attach to the overlying prosthesis, (**d**) Tantalum mesh-covered implants. (**e**) The Allen implant. (**f**) The Iowa implant, with steep mounds (left), and the Universal implant, with shallower mounds (right). (**g**) Example of a buried magnetic implant. Both the orbital implant and prosthesis had magnets within their surface. (**h**) Smooth spherical polymethylmethacrylate implants. (**i**) Spherical polymethylmethacrylate implant with multiple indentations designed to try and increase tissue fixation and decrease implant migration

Just as surgeons have sought to advance anophthalmic socket surgery, ocularists have strived to improve the lifelike qualities of prostheses. The French military surgeon Ambroise Pare (1579) described the first in-socket prosthetic eye which was made of metal and coated with paint and enamel [8]. Venetian glass artisans produced the first glass eyes around the same time period after they discovered a formula that could be tolerated within the eye socket [8, 24]. Although these early glass eyes were crude, uncomfortable, and very fragile, the "Venetian method" was considered the finest in the world. Their methods and materials were kept a secret until the eighteenth century. German doll maker Ludwig Muller-Uri's invention of cryolite glass (a superior glass formula) in 1835 allowed for well-tolerated lifelike hollow glass eyes [24]. After Muller-Uri refined the design of the artificial glass eye, Dutch ophthalmologist Snellen popularized its use throughout the Western Hemisphere in the late 1890s. During World War II, the imported cryolite glass for making prosthetic eyes became unavailable from Germany. With so many injured Allied soldiers needing artificial eyes, the US government searched for a replacement material. Medical plastics were already being used in the dental field, and synthetic dental methylmethacrylate became a substitute for the cryolite glass in the Americas [24]. The standard technique for making a prosthesis from medical grade acrylic plastic was developed in 1944 and is still used today throughout most of the developed world.

Current Perspective: Porous Orbital Implants

Hydroxyapatite Implants

In an effort to design a biocompatible, integrated orbital implant, Perry (1985) introduced coralline (sea coral) hydroxyapatite (HA) spheres (Bio-Eye, Integrated Orbital Implants, San Diego, CA) [25]. The HA implants (FDA approved in 1989) represented a new generation of buried, biointegrated spheres with a regular system of interconnecting pores that allowed host fibrovascular ingrowth (Figs. 59.4 and 59.5a–c) [25, 26]. Implant fibrovascularization theoretically was thought to reduce the risk of migration, extrusion, and infection [26]. The HA implant also allowed secure attachment of the extraocular muscles, which was suggested to potentially improve implant motility [25, 26]. By drilling into the HA implant, inserting a peg, and coupling the peg to the prosthetic eye, an improved range of movement as well as fine darting eye movements (seen during conversation) were possible, permitting a more naturally appearing artificial eye.

Although HA implants represented a significant advance in anophthalmic surgery, experience with HA over the last few decades has expanded our understanding of its limitations. Reported complications are not uncommon and include implant exposure, conjunctival thinning, socket discharge, pyogenic granuloma formation, implant infection, and persistent pain or discomfort [27–33].

The introduction of HA as an orbital implant significantly raised the costs associated with enucleation, evisceration, and secondary orbital implant procedures. The Bio-Eye™ HA

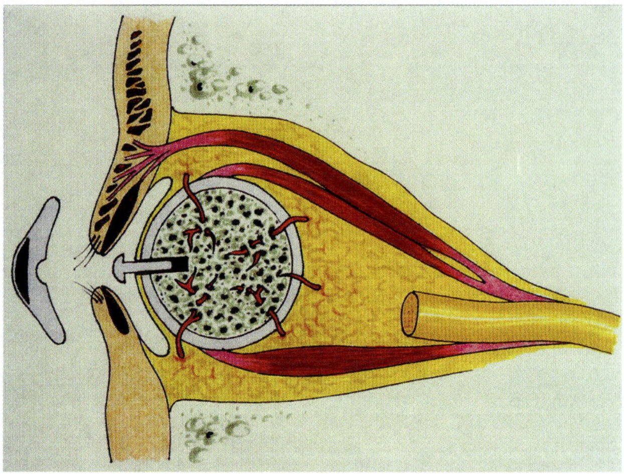

Fig. 59.4 Artist's conception of a porous orbital implant showing fibrovascular ingrowth. A round-headed peg has been inserted into the implant to show the coupling effect with the overlying prosthetic eye

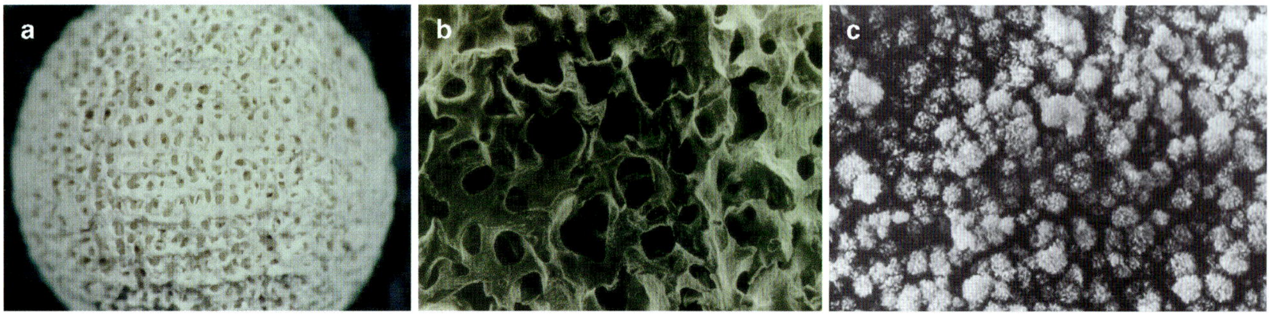

Fig. 59.5 (**a**) The porous architecture of the Bio-Eye™ hydroxyapatite implant is well visualized. (**b**) Scanning electron microscopy illustrating the porous architecture (222×10^1). (**c**) High-power scanning electron microscopy (230×10^3) illustrating the rough surfaced microcrystals making up the Bio-Eye™

implant cost is much higher than traditional silicone or polymethylmethacrylate (PMMA) spherical implants ($30–$60 US). Additional expenses associated with HA placement include an implant wrap material, assessment of implant vascularization with a confirmatory magnetic resonance (MR) imaging study, a secondary drilling procedure with peg placement, and prosthetic modifications. In the search for porous orbital implants with a reduced complication profile and diminished surgical and postoperative costs, numerous alternative implant materials have been introduced worldwide.

Porous Polyethylene Implants

Synthetic porous polyethylene (MEDPOR®, Stryker Craniomaxillofacial, Kalamazoo, Michigan, 49002, USA) implants were introduced over two decades ago (MEDPOR®, Porex Surgical Inc., Newnan, GA, USA) for use in the orbit and have been widely accepted as an alternative to the Bio-Eye™ HA [34–38]. Porous polyethylene implants although less biocompatible than HA are typically well tolerated by orbital soft tissue [39]. They have a smoother surface than HA implants which permits easier implantation and potentially less irritation of the overlying conjunctiva following placement (Fig. 59.6a–c). These implants have a high tensile strength yet are malleable which allows sculpting of the anterior surface of the implant. Although the rectus muscles may be sutured directly to the implant, many surgeons may find this challenging without predrilled holes and prefer to use wrapping material to facilitate extraocular muscle attachment. Porous polyethylene implants are available in spherical, egg, conical, and mounded shapes (Quad implant) [35–37]. The anterior surface can also be manufactured with a smooth, nonporous surface to potentially minimize irritation of the overlying tissue (e.g., MEDPOR® smooth surface tunnel implant, SST™) while retaining a larger pore size posteriorly to facilitate fibrovascular ingrowth. The addition of Bioglass (US biomaterials Corp, Alachua, FL, USA) to the MEDPOR® implant may help stimulate early vascular ingrowth [33]. The MEDPOR® implant costs vary depending upon what model is used and the quantity purchased but are priced slightly less than the Bio-Eye™.

Synthetic Hydroxyapatite Implants

Synthetic HA implants developed by FCI (Issy-les-Moulineaux,Cedex, France) have an identical chemical composition to that of the Bio-Eye™, although scanning electron microscopy (SEM) has revealed decreased pore uniformity and interconnectivity and the presence of blind pouches (Fig. 59.7a–c) [40]. Central implant fibrovascularization in a

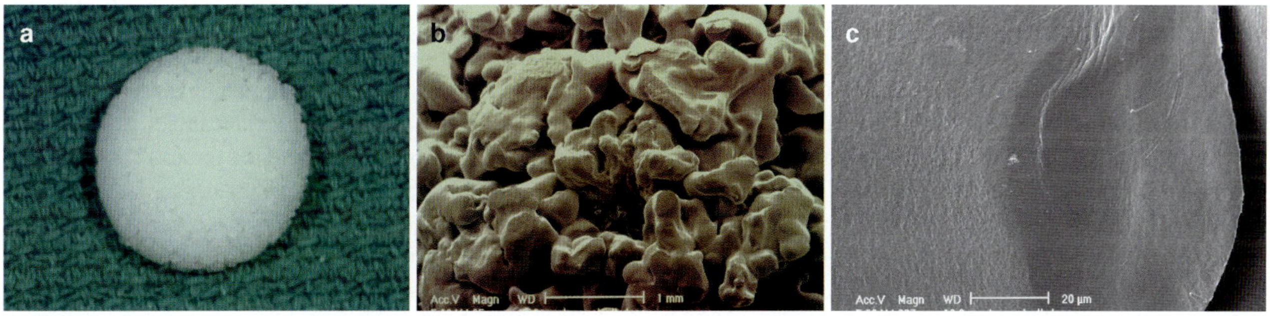

Fig. 59.6 (**a**) The porous architecture of the synthetic porous polyethylene (MEDPOR®) implant is slightly different than the other porous implants. (**b**) Scanning electron microscopy illustrating numerous large channels rather than pores (222×10^1). (**c**) High-power scanning electron microscopy (230×10^3) illustrating the smooth-surfaced porous polyethylene rather than a microcrystalline structure (230×10^3)

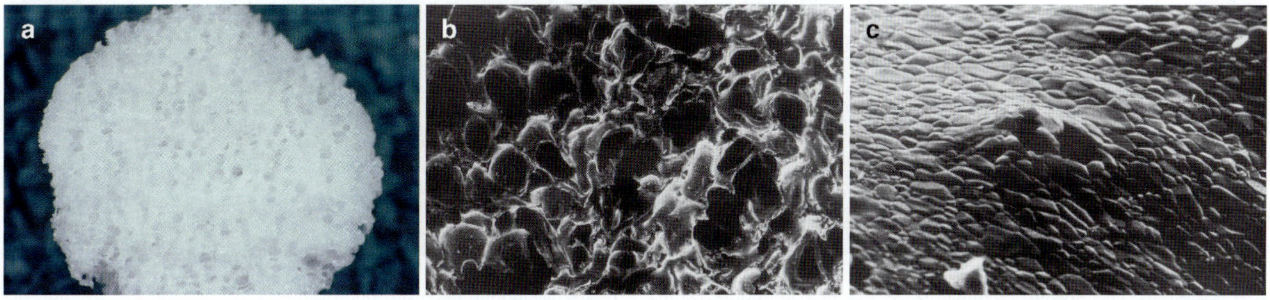

Fig. 59.7 (**a**) The porous architecture of the FCI synthetic hydroxyapatite implant is well visualized. (**b**) Scanning electron microscopy illustrating the porous architecture (222×10^1) with multiple blind-ended pores. (**c**) High-power scanning electron microscopy (230×10^3) illustrating the smooth-surfaced microcrystals making up the FCI synthetic hydroxyapatite implant (230×10^3)

rabbit model still appears to occur in a similar manner in both the Bio-Eye™ and FCI_3 implants [41]. The synthetic FCI_3 implant has gained in popularity in many parts of the world over the past 20 years; however, it is not yet available in the United States. The problems and complications associated with the synthetic FCI_3 implant are similar to that of the Bio-Eye™ [42]. It is typically less expensive than the Bio-Eye™.

Other forms of HA implants in use around the world include the Chinese HA and the Brazilian HA implants [43, 44]. Although less expensive than the Bio-Eye™, these implants have impurities or poor porous structure that make them inferior products [43, 44]. Other implant designs continue to be developed, some of which offer little added value while others have only been in use for a short time and their advantages/disadvantages have not been elucidated [45, 46].

Bioceramic Implants

Aluminum oxide (Al_2O_3) is a ceramic implant biomaterial that has been used in orthopedic surgery and dentistry for more than 30 years. Spherical and egg-shaped Bioceramic Orbital Implants (FCI, Issy-Les-Moulineaux, Cedex, France) have been available in North America for over 15 years [47, 48]. Aluminum oxide is a porous, inert substance and has been suggested as a standard reference material in studies of implant biocompatibility [49]. These implants permit host fibrovascular ingrowth similar to the Bio-Eye™ [47, 48]. Human fibroblasts and osteoblasts proliferate more rapidly on aluminum oxide than HA suggesting it is a more biocompatible substance than HA [39, 49]. The Bioceramic implant is lightweight and has a uniform pore structure and excellent pore interconnectivity (Fig. 59.8a, b) [40]. The microcrystalline structure is smoother than the rough surfaced Bio-Eye™ (Fig. 59.8c). Although sockets with the aluminum oxide implants may initially be quieter than those with HA, the same complications as other porous implants (e.g., primarily exposure) may be seen [50]. Long-term follow-up is important with any porous implant as late complications (years after implantation) are known to occur [50–53]. As with most of the other available porous orbital implants, aluminum oxide implants are less expensive than the Bio-Eye™.

Porous Versus Nonporous Implants: Which to Use?

A new era in anophthalmic socket surgery began with the introduction of coralline hydroxyapatite (HA) by Dr. A. Perry previously discussed [25]. In 1989, HA accounted for only 1.5% of implants used, but by 1992 it had become the anophthalmic orbital implant of choice [23]. Over the next several years, additional porous implants (e.g., synthetic hydroxyapatite, porous polyethylene, aluminum oxide) entered the market place and were widely promoted [48]. Implant companies often portrayed their porous implant as better than competitors, frequently without little scientific support. Marketing slogans such as "the original, the leader, the total solution," "take a closer look at a better material," and "the best choice for implantation candidates" became common at oculoplastic surgery meetings and in ophthalmic plastic surgery journals [55]. During this same time period, we and many others reported our experience with a variety of porous orbital implants including their problems and complications [27–34, 42, 50, 52, 53, 56–58]. It remained difficult to determine whether one porous implant was truly superior than another [29, 34, 42, 50, 52, 53, 56, 57]. However, it became clear that all porous implants had potential complications including conjunctival thinning, implant exposure, pyogenic granulomas, socket discharge, implant infection, persistent pain and discharge, as well as pegging issues [27–29, 34, 50, 52, 56, 57]. With time, some surgeons began to question the use of porous implants and advocated a return to nonporous spheres because of their overall low complication rate [58–61]. Spirited debate centered on multiple questions including which porous implant is the best, should they be wrapped, which wrap is the best, should they be pegged, which peg

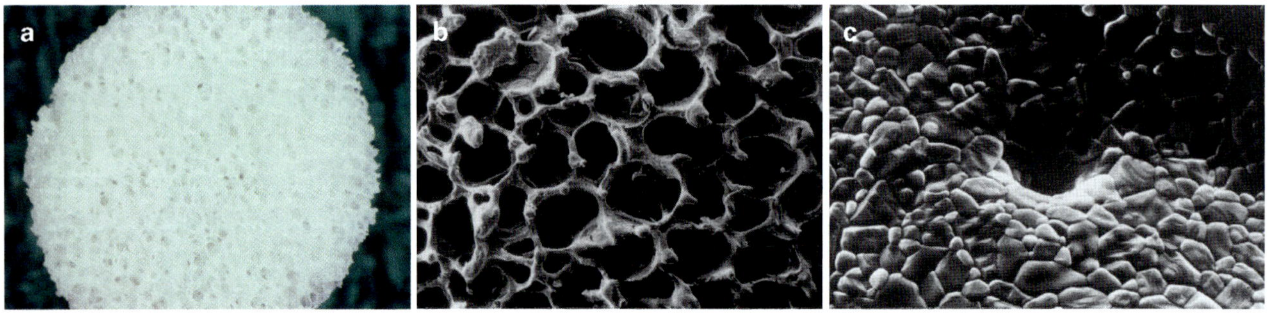

Fig. 59.8 (**a**) The porous architecture of the FCI aluminum oxide (Bioceramic) implant is well visualized. (**b**) Scanning electron microscopy illustrating the uniform porous architecture (222×10^1). (**c**) High-power scanning electron microscopy (230×10^3) illustrating the smooth-surfaced microcrystals making up the Bioceramic implant (230×10^3)

system is the best, who should be pegged, when should pegging be done, are porous implants truly advantageous, do they have a lower migration rate, do they have a lower extrusion rate, is there resistance to infection, and is there any motility advantage? [62]

With respect to implant migration, an early enucleation technique by Frost Lange involved imbricating the extraocular muscles over unwrapped polymethylmethacrylate (PMMA) or silicone spheres [63]. It is now well established that this technique leads to *superotemporal* implant migration in 16% or more of patients over 8–10 years, so it has largely been abandoned [56, 64–66]. Nunnery, Wells, and others have shown that attaching the rectus muscles in their normal anatomic position to nonporous spheres (e.g., PMMA, silicone) results in a very low *superotemporal* migration rate (0–1.3%) and is stable over many years [65–67]. Reports of *superotemporal* migration with porous orbital implants are not significantly different (0.5–1.7%) [23, 59]. However, if one considers *anterior migration* of porous implants, the overall rate of implant migration may be higher with porous implants as this type of implant migration is seldom discussed. A*nterior migration* manifests as implant exposure. These cases are often grouped with other cases of implant exposure that may be due to a variety of other factors (e.g., inadequate or poor surgical wound closure, infection, mechanical or inflammatory irritation from the rough anterior surface of the porous implant, delayed ingrowth of fibrovascular tissue with subsequent tissue breakdown, and pressure points from a poorly fit prosthesis) [42]. *Anterior migration* is most often secondary to improper seating of the porous implant. Porous implants have a rough surface and drag tissue inward as they are placed into the orbit; this "Velcro®" effect makes implantation technically more demanding [60]. An inserter, tissue glide, and/or implant wrap may help avoid the posterior drag of anterior tissue [68]. The overlying tissue may be closed successfully over the implant, but with time the tissues dragged inward may try to return to their original relaxed position – a natural restitution of tissue (cactus syndrome) [68]. As this occurs, a gradual migration of the implant anteriorly with progressive conjunctival thinning and eventual tissue breakdown over the anterior implant surface (exposure) occurs [68]. Fibrovascular ingrowth has not been shown to diminish implant exposure risk [67]. Thus, there is little evidence that implant migration is less with porous orbital implants; it may actually be more common if one also considers anterior implant migration.

With respect to implant extrusion, when nonporous implants become exposed, they typically extrude from the socket [57, 58]. When porous orbital implants become exposed, the fibrovascular ingrowth helps retain them within the orbit, often preventing complete extrusion. Although porous implant exposures can be surgically repaired by a variety of techniques, large, recurrent, or persistent exposures may require implant removal which essentially is a delayed extrusion (iatrogenic). Rather than ask whether porous orbital implants have a decreased extrusion rate, it is more prudent to ask whether they have a "decreased exposure rate" [65]. Implant exposure is the most frequent and challenging problem associated with porous orbital implants [58]. Reported exposure rates for nonporous spherical implants (e.g., PMMA/silicone) are typically low (0–3%) [23, 29, 58, 65–67]. Exposure rates for porous orbital implants are also generally low but can vary from 0% to 50% [23, 50, 52, 59, 67]. Custer et al. reviewed pooled data and found a 6.6% exposure rate in 3012 porous orbital implants compared to 2.9% in 615 nonporous implants [58]. More recently, Wladis et al. reported that rates of exposure (and extrusion) are generally comparable between porous and nonporous implants, suggesting the choice of implant may not result in a dramatic difference in this complication [67]. Thus, there is little evidence that porous implants have a reduced extrusion or exposure rate, and in fact, it may be higher [58, 59]. Porous implant exposures can occur anytime, and with the longer the follow-up, the greater the number of exposures [52, 57, 58].

With respect to infection, nonporous implants (e.g., PMMA/silicone) have been shown to have a low infection rate (0–1%) [23, 66, 67]. Unpegged porous orbital implants also have a low infection rate (0–2%) [42, 50, 52, 53, 59, 67]. Pegging porous implants is associated with an increased number of complications including infections, reported in up to 20% of pegged orbital implants in one study [52, 57]. Fibrovascular ingrowth has not been shown to afford protection against infection [67]. Thus, there is little evidence to support the suggestion that porous orbital implants have a reduced infection rate; it appears to be similar to nonporous implants and potentially higher with a peg [52, 57].

With respect to enhanced motility, peg placement has been shown to improve horizontal gaze movements in the artificial eye [26, 69–71]. There is also a more natural movement to the prosthesis because of the fine darting eye movements retained with direct prosthesis coupling to an implant peg [26, 60]. However, without a peg in place, there is no proven motility advantage of porous over nonporous implants [58, 67, 69–71].

As with innovative implant designs from the past (e.g., Mules, Rudemann, Cutler), the initial wave of enthusiasm with porous implants has been tempered as an increasing number of surgeons recognize that the touted advantages have little scientific data to support them and that these implants are associated with numerous risks and complications that may be challenging to manage [23, 27, 29, 42, 52–58]. Porous implants may not be the presumptive "gold standard" as often marketed [55], and continued research is essential to develop improved materials and techniques to further minimize the complications associated with anophthalmic surgery.

Current Classification of Implants and Terminology (Table 59.1)

Orbital implants can be classified as porous or nonporous, and in either category, the implants are non-integrated, integrated, or quasi-integrated depending on how the implant is connected to the overlying prosthetic eye. Porous implants (hydroxyapatite, porous polyethylene, aluminum oxide) allow fibrovascular ingrowth, while nonporous implants (silicone, polymethylmethacrylate) do not. Non-integrated implants have no connection with the prosthetic eye, whereas integrated implants can be directly coupled to the prosthetic eye through a peg system. Quasi-integrated (or indirectly integrated) implants may be porous or nonporous and because of their irregular anterior surface are partially coupled to the overlying prosthetic eye (e.g., Allen, Iowa, Universal, MEDPOR® Quad implant). These quasi-integrated implants remain buried. Extraocular muscles are attached to their surface by passing the muscles through tunnels in the implant (Allen implant) or through grooves in the implant created by mounds on the anterior aspect (Iowa and Universal implants, MEDPOR® Quad). The broad flat surface of the Allen implant or the protruding mounds of the Iowa/Universal/MEDPOR® Quad which have corresponding indentations on the posterior surface of the prosthetic eye move the prosthesis because of this "quasi-integration." The movement is often better than a standard spherical implant, but may not be as good as a porous integrated implant coupled to the overlying prosthesis through a peg system.

Implant Selection in Adults and Children

There continues to be little consensus regarding orbital implant material and design preference [66]. Surgeons have their own preferences regarding porous versus nonporous, spherical versus shaped implants, wrapped versus unwrapped implants, and pegged versus unpegged implants. Implant cost, surgery center and hospital budgets, and marketing pressures also play a role in implant selection.

When deciding upon an implant to use, we divide the various implants into three useful categories:

(a) Porous spheres that may potentially be pegged (HA – coralline or synthetic, porous polyethylene (MEDPOR®), aluminum oxide (Bioceramic))
(b) Quasi-integrated implants (Universal implant, Durette® implant, Quad MEDPOR®)
(c) Standard nonporous sphere (polymethylmethacrylate, silicone)

Table 59.1 Terminology in anophthalmic socket surgery

Anophthalmic implant: Material or substance used to replace an enucleated or eviscerated globe (e.g., polymethylmethacrylate, silicone, hydroxyapatite, aluminum oxide, porous polyethylene, etc.)
Porous implant: An implant with numerous interconnected pores or channels throughout its structure that permit fibrovascular ingrowth (e.g., hydroxyapatite, aluminum oxide, porous polyethylene)
Nonporous implant: An implant that is solid and does not allow fibrovascular ingrowth (e.g., polymethylmethacrylate, silicone)
Conformer: A clear shell (typically acrylic) with or without holes placed over the closed bulbar conjunctival wound that extends into the conjunctival fornices behind the eyelids following implant placement in enucleation, evisceration, or secondary implant surgery
Scleral shell: A thin ocular prosthesis that fits over a non-painful, blind, atrophic eye (with or without shrinkage, i.e., phthisis)
Prosthesis, prosthetic eye, artificial eye: A ceramic shell placed in the anophthalmic socket conjunctival fornices that is typically fabricated to look like the patient's contralateral healthy eye to provide a symmetric ocular appearance
Buried implant: An implant that has been placed within the anophthalmic socket with an overlying closed, smooth, uninterrupted conjunctival surface completely covering the implant
Exposed implant: An implant that does not have an overlying closed, smooth uninterrupted surface completely covering it. An exposed implant is an unwanted complication postoperatively with any implant
Non-integrated implant: An implant that has been placed within the anophthalmic socket that has no connection with the overlying prosthetic eye. There is a closed, smooth, uninterrupted conjunctival surface completely covering the anophthalmic implant. Also known as a "buried non-integrated implant"
Integrated implant: An implant that can be directly coupled to the overlying prosthetic eye with a peg system. As there is a small break in the overlying conjunctiva through which the peg protrudes, there is some debate whether this type of implant should also be known as a partially "exposed integrated implant"
Quasi-integrated implant: An implant that has been placed within the anophthalmic socket with a closed, uninterrupted conjunctival surface completely covering an anophthalmic implant and has an irregular anterior surface allowing indirect coupling ("quasi-integration") of the implant to the overlying, modified prosthesis (e.g., Allen, Iowa, Universal, MEDPOR Quad implants). Also known as a "buried integrated implant" or an "indirectly integrated implant"
Peg: A motility coupling post, currently made of titanium, which permits direct coupling of the implant movement to an overlying prosthesis. Pegs may be inserted within sleeves that are drilled into the anterior aspect of the implant. Some implant-peg systems are designed for placement at the time of enucleation/evisceration, whereas others are inserted once implant fibrovascularization occurs, typically around 6 months postoperatively
Secondary orbital implant: An orbital implant (of any type) that is placed into the anophthalmic socket at a time other than the initial enucleation or evisceration procedure

Ophthalmic surgeons currently favor the use of porous implants even though unpegged porous implants have no apparent advantage over nonporous spheres [59, 67, 69, 71–73]. The decision to use a porous or nonporous implant is up to the surgeon and his/her patient. Porous implants are not for every patient [60, 61]. If the patient is healthy and roughly between the ages of 15 and 70 years, a porous implant (e.g., hydroxyapatite, aluminum oxide implant) that can potentially be pegged is initially considered [48, 50]. Those with chronic systemic disease (e.g., collagen vascular disease, autoimmune disorders, diabetes mellitus, peripheral vascular disease) or who use immunosuppressive medication (e.g., prednisone, methotrexate, etc.) or have undergone prior socket radiation are generally poor candidates [56, 57]. Porous orbital implants are also not for every ophthalmic surgeon [60, 61]. Implantation requires experience and skill to appreciate technical nuances critical for a successful outcome. We *only* consider porous implant use in healthy, adult patients wanting maximal prosthetic motility (pegging) and willing to accept the potential increased risk of complications. Ideally, the patient *should* live within a reasonable travel distance to maintain regular follow-up visits so that any minor implant problems can be promptly addressed. Continued follow-up (typically every 1–2 years) is essential for porous implants (pegged or unpegged) as small problems (e.g., implant exposure) can often be handled within the office/minor room setting before they develop into a more extensive problem (e.g., implant infection), requiring additional surgery and potentially implant removal [50, 52]. If peg placement is not a consideration, a nonporous implant (sphere or mounded) may be preferred. Nonporous spherical implants can be used effectively during a primary enucleation or evisceration, and the surgical techniques required for a successful outcome are more easily accomplished by most ophthalmic surgeons. Direct anatomic fixation of the rectus muscles to a solid silicone sphere or a wrapped PMMA sphere provides implant stability and good prosthesis movement [66]. Motility results are similar to that of non-pegged porous implants [66, 67, 69–72]. Nonporous implants are inexpensive, and in a healthcare era in which the global expense of a patient's anophthalmic socket rehabilitation should be considered, a cost-conscious primary procedure with a low incidence of complications may be desirable [66].

A quasi-integrated implant such as the Universal or Durette® (PMMA) or the MEDPOR® Quad mounded implant are alternative considerations to the porous or nonporous spherical implants as the mounded surface of the implant potentially offers improved motility over a standard sphere as a result of the partial coupling that occurs between the mounds on the implant and the posterior surface of the prosthesis [37]. Correct implant placement is technique sensitive and may require considerable surgeon experience with enucleation and secondary implant placement.

In a young child (less than 5 years old), a wrapped nonporous sphere (PMMA, silicone) centered within the muscle cone and connected to the four-rectus muscles and the inferior oblique muscle or a PMMA mounded implant (Universal or Durette®) is preferred. Implant exchange with a porous orbital implant that can potentially be pegged is considered at a later age (typically >15 years old). An additional factor to consider in children undergoing eye removal is the need for further growth of the orbit. Eighty percent of adult orbital volume is reached around 5 years of age, with adult volume achieved by 12–14 years [74, 75]. Orbital soft tissue volume is a critical factor in continued orbital and facial bone growth, and thus adequate socket volume replacement following enucleation or evisceration surgery is important. The ocular prosthesis is also believed to be an important factor that helps minimize orbital growth retardation and prevent significant periorbital asymmetries following enucleation or evisceration. Autogenous dermis-fat grafts are an alternative to the above described orbital implants in children under 5 years of age for volume replacement. These grafts may undergo hypertrophy and help stimulate orbital bone growth (see dermis fat graft discussion) [76–83].

Socket Volume Considerations

Removal of an eye following enucleation or evisceration creates an orbital soft tissue volume deficiency. Insufficient volume replacement often results in an abnormally deep superior sulcus, upper eyelid ptosis, and enophthalmos and may require a larger than desirable prosthesis (the "anophthalmic socket syndrome") [84–90].

The ideal implant volume may be estimated either preoperatively from the axial length of the eye or intraoperatively by determining the volume of fluid the enucleated eye displaces in a graduated cylinder [86–90]. Several investigators have reported that the variability of axial length and globe volume may vary between 6.9 and 9.0 mL [87, 88]. Calculated implant volumes can be greater than 22 mm in some cases; however, implants larger than 22 mm may be unavailable, are difficult to insert in the socket, frequently limit socket excursion, have a higher exposure rate, and hinder fitting of an acceptable custom prosthesis [84–88].

Ideally, 70–80% of the volume of an individual's normal globe should be replaced with the orbital implant [85, 87]. This generally allows for a prosthetic volume that is approximately 2 ml [84]. Larger prostheses often result in progressive lower eyelid laxity and malposition due to the weight of the prostheses on the eyelid. Larger prostheses may also have limited socket excursion [84].

In most adults, 20–22 mm spherical implants are typically used following enucleation and 18–20 mm implants following evisceration. In pediatric patients slightly smaller implants (16–18 mm) may be sufficient, depending on the patient's age and orbital bone development. Individualization of the implant size is important in optimizing orbital volume replacement and in achieving the best possible functional and aesthetic result [84–88].

Orbital Implant Wrapping

Placement of an HA implant or Bioceramic implant within the soft tissue of the eye socket is facilitated by a smooth wrapping material which diminishes tissue drag and facilitates precise anatomic fixation of the rectus muscles to the implant surface [25, 68]. Implant wraps may also provide a barrier function over the spiculated porous implant surface [25, 51], although there is some debate as to whether exposure is truly minimized by an avascular implant covering [91–94]. Suggested advantages of placing an unwrapped implant include simplification of the procedure, decreased operating room time, reduced cost, elimination of a second surgical site for harvesting autogenous wrap, avoidance of a possible barrier to fibrovascular ingrowth, and decreased risk of disease transmission [92–94].

Human donor sclera was historically the first choice of implant wrapping material for most orbital surgeons [25, 26]. The use of human donor material, however, carries the risk of transmission of viruses (e.g., human immunodeficiency virus (HIV), hepatitis B or C) and other pathogens (prions) that may be responsible for a variety of infectious and neurodegenerative disorders [95]. Although we are not aware of any reports of disease transmission from donor sclera, segments of the HIV-1 genome have been identified in preserved human sclera [96]. Creutzfeldt-Jakob disease (prion) transmission from dural and corneal transplants has been reported [97–99]. In addition, seronegative organ and tissue donors may transmit HIV [100]. Many eye banks charge a substantial fee to provide donor sclera.

Specially processed human donor pericardium, fascia lata, and sclera are marketed (Biodynamics International (USA), Inc., Tampa, FL) as safe alternative implant wraps to preserved human donor tissues. These wraps have the convenience of a long (up to 5 years) shelf life; however, their cost may exceed that of the implant.

Processed bovine pericardium (Peri-Guard® or Ocu-Guard™ Supple, Bio Vascular Inc., Saint Paul, MN, USA) is FDA approved and also available as an implant wrap material [101, 102]. Although there have been only a few cases of bovine spongiform encephalopathy (BSE) in American cattle to date, reports of infected cattle in Alberta, Canada, have surfaced in the past few decades, and the potential for the disease to occur with possible prion transmission still exists [93].

Autologous temporalis fascia [103], fascia lata [104], rectus abdominis sheath [105, 106], and posterior auricular muscle complex graft [100] have been tried as orbital implant wrapping materials. Use of these tissues requires a second operative site, prolonged operative time, and a potentially increased risk of morbidity.

Microporous expanded polytetrafluoroethylene (e-PTFE) (Gore-Tex, W.L. Gore & Associates, Flagstaff, AZ) has also been advocated as an implant wrapping material (Oculo-Plastik, Montreal, Quebec, Canada); however, complications with its use have made it undesirable [107–109].

Undyed polyglactin 910 mesh (Vicryl mesh, Ethicon, Somerville, NJ, USA) is a bioabsorbable synthetic material and is our preference as a wrapping material for porous orbital implants (Fig. 59.9a–c) [110–112]. Vicryl mesh eliminates the risk of infectious disease transmission, does not require a second surgical site, and is readily available and simple to use. Bioceramic implants prewrapped with Vicryl mesh are convenient and cost-efficient. Vicryl mesh-wrapped HA implants have been shown to permit rapid implant fibrovascularization in an animal model and may provide a potential advantage of permitting fibrovascular ingrowth over the entire implant surface unlike implants completely wrapped in sclera [113, 150]. We have reported a 2.1% incidence of implant exposure in 187 consecutive patients receiving Vicryl mesh-wrapped HA orbital implants [114]. Oestreicher

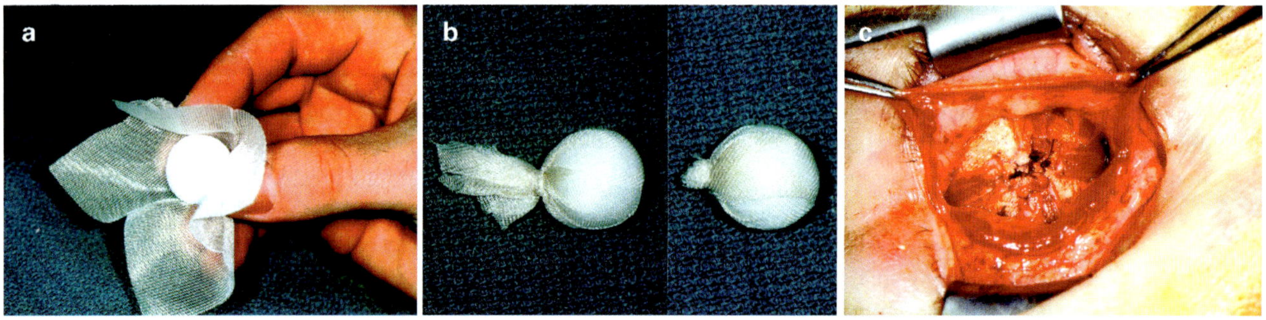

Fig. 59.9 (**a**) Bioceramic implant resting and a Vicryl mesh ready to wrap around it. (**b**) Bioceramic implant wrapped in Vicryl mesh (left, Vicryl mesh has been tied; right, excess Vicryl has been trimmed. (**c**) Vicryl mesh-wrapped Bioceramic implant in position within the right eye socket showing extraocular muscles at least 5 mm anterior to their normal anatomic insertion sites

et al. [32] also reported a low exposure incidence using a similar bioabsorbable wrapping material composed of polyglycolic acid (Dexon mesh style No. 8, non-stretch, medium-weight closed tricot, Davis & Geck, Manati, Puerto Rico). Despite our success with polyglactin 910 mesh as an implant wrap material, some surgeons continue to believe that it is associated with a higher rate of implant exposure [115, 116]. It remains our view that high exposure rates with Vicryl mesh-wrapped implants are a technique-related problem that can be significantly mitigated with correct implant insertion and meticulous tension-free wound closure. We also now routinely use a 13–15 mm diameter cap of donor sclera over the anterior surface of the mesh-wrapped implant to potentially further minimize the risk of implant exposure [51].

Pegging Porous Orbital Implants

Motility peg placement improves horizontal gaze movements in the artificial eye (Fig. 59.10a–f) [72]. Despite the improved motility, many surgeons and patients elect to avoid peg placement due to the satisfactory results without pegging and the possibility of peg-related complications [117–124]. Complications with implant pegging may include discharge,

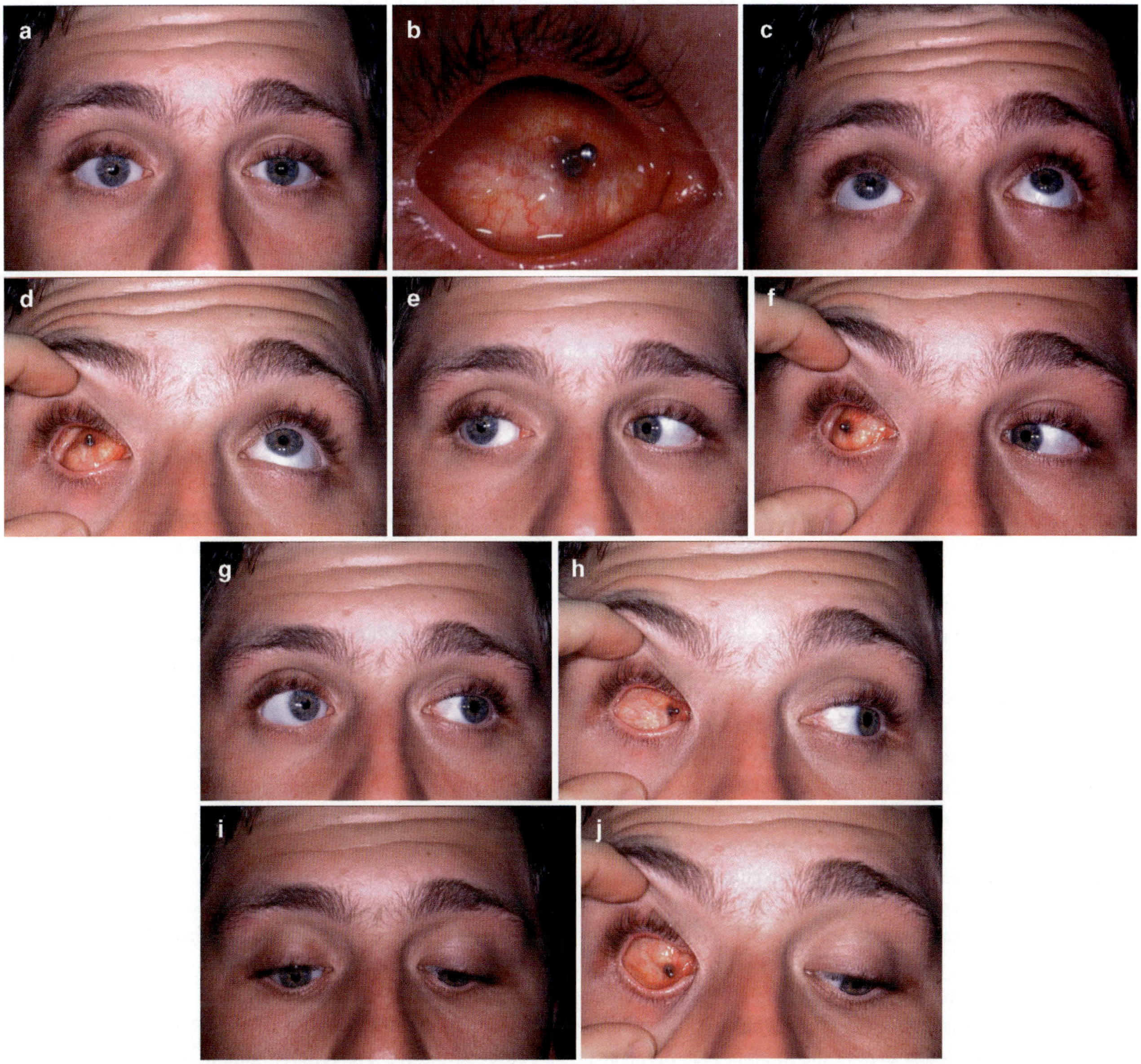

Fig. 59.10 (**a**, **b**) A 26-year-old male following evisceration with placement of a Bioceramic orbital implant and titanium peg and sleeve (**c**, **d**), up-gaze; (**e**, **f**), gaze right; (**g**, **h**), gaze left; (**i**, **j**), down-gaze

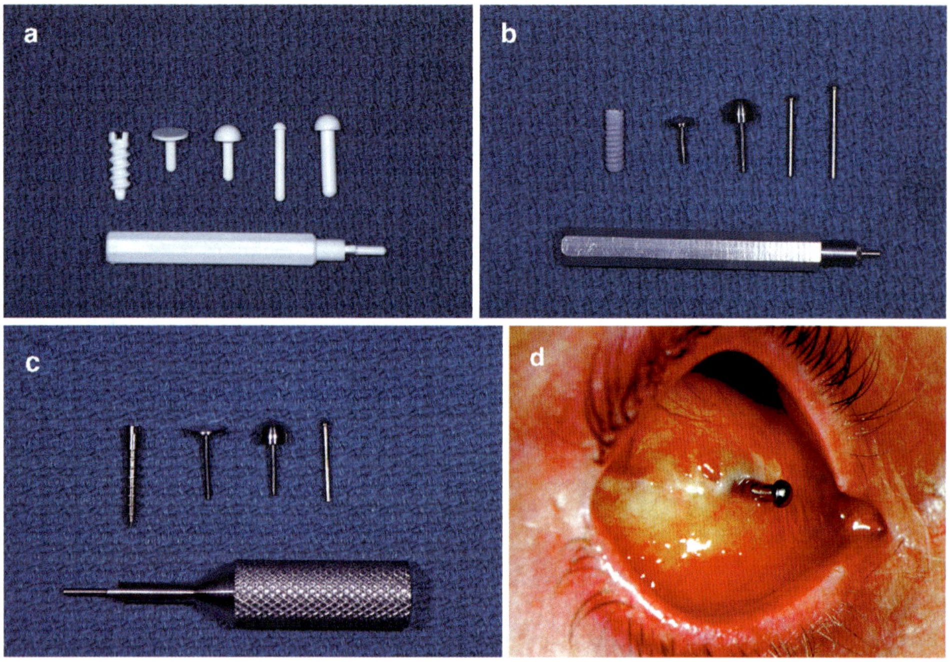

Fig. 59.11 (**a**) Original polycarbonate peg (large peg on far right)) with polycarbonate peg and sleeve system to the left and screwdriver for sleeve below. (**b**) FCI hydroxyapatite-coated titanium sleeve with titanium pegs and screwdriver below. (**c**) Dr. A Perry's PK titanium peg system produced for the Bio-Eye ™. (**d**) A well-positioned titanium peg (FCI type) with a quiet conjunctival interface

recurrent pyogenic granulomas, implant exposure around the peg, implant infection, tissue overgrowth, peg dislocation, audible clicking, and various fitting problems [117]. Refitting the prosthesis, scleral patch grafting, peg removal, and occasionally implant removal may be required [117].

Although the use of pegging has declined dramatically over the past few years, a precise and meticulous technique [123] in the appropriately selected individual can yield a successful outcome. Johnson [124] and others [32, 52, 117, 123] have also shown largely positive results, validating the efficacy of pegging porous orbital implants (e.g., hydroxyapatite, Bioceramic) with minimal risk of significant complications.

Proper care of the artificial eye and regular follow-up visits with the ocularist and ophthalmic plastic surgeon are important. Watching for small problems (e.g., exposure around the peg) and management of these minor issues at an early stage can often avoid more serious problems with the peg and implant later. If the patient is unlikely or unable to adhere to timely follow-up visits, pegging should be avoided. Children (less than 15 years old), older adults (over 70 years old), or individuals of any age with a chronic illness (diabetes mellitus, collagen vascular disease, autoimmune disorder, peripheral vascular disease, or immunosuppression) in our view should not be considered for pegging.

Peg systems were generally designed for peg placement once fibrovascularization of the implant has been completed. Drilling into an avascular area of the implant may predispose the implant to infection [125]. Gadolinium-enhanced MR imaging is currently the recommended method of assessing the extent of implant vascularization [126]. Fibrovascular ingrowth may occur at varying rates in different patients. Implant drilling and peg insertion are generally deferred until 10–12 months following HA implant placement.

Several titanium peg systems were previously available for the various porous orbital implants (Fig. 59.11a–d) [123]. The only system available at this time is the PK titanium peg for the Bio-Eye™ and supplied by Integrated Orbital Implants (11230 Sorrento Valley Road, suite 135, San Diego, CA, 92121). Titanium is more biocompatible and better tolerated by human soft tissue than the original peg systems made of polycarbonate [127]. The once available FCI peg system utilized a hydroxyapatite-coated titanium sleeve [123]. The HA coating potentially allowed for stronger interface bonding with the orbital fibroblasts than the uncoated PK system supplied for use with the Bio-Eye™. The MEDPOR® motility coupling post (MCP) which is also no longer available was a titanium screw that could be screwed directly into porous polyethylene implants [128, 129]. Some authors use to advocate primary placement of the MCP at the time of implant insertion; however, this practice was controversial, and most surgeons deferred implant pegging for more than 6 months after implant placement [130, 131].

Preoperative Preparation for Enucleation and Evisceration Surgery

1. A careful ophthalmic history and examination to identify indications for eye removal and whether evisceration is appropriate or enucleation is more prudent.
2. Assess medical history and perioperative surgical risks; e.g., cardiac or pulmonary disease, vasculopathies, and coagulopathies (including anticoagulation medications).

3. Review the goals of surgery with the patient (and family): removal of the diseased eye, restoration of orbital volume, providing of movement to the ocular prosthesis, and fabrication of an ocular prosthesis.
4. Review the surgical procedure with the patient (and family) including the temporary closure of the eyelids and use of a conformer until custom prosthesis fitting, typically 6 weeks following surgery. Review monitored anesthesia care (MAC) versus general anesthesia, expected postoperative pain and nausea, potential time away from work, and follow-up visits required. The potential complications of implant infection, exposure, extrusion, and migration should be discussed.
5. Discuss the relative advantages and disadvantages of enucleation versus evisceration surgery, and select a technique that is most suitable for the clinical situation.
6. Decide on the orbital implant to use (porous versus nonporous). Proper selection of implant volume helps minimize the potential for a superior sulcus deformity and enophthalmos of the prosthesis. In general, a 20–22-mm-diameter sphere allows reasonable volume to return following enucleation surgery in the adult, whereas an 18–20-mm-diameter sphere is typically sufficient for evisceration procedures. Anterior and posterior sclerotomies are routinely performed with evisceration surgery permitting placement of a larger implant and minimizing tension on wound closure.
7. For enucleation cases, select the type of implant wrapping material. A wrap facilitates placement of a porous implant in the eye socket and allows precise fixation of the extraocular muscles to the implant surface. It may also act as a barrier to the rough porous implant surface. A porous polyethylene implant modified on the anterior surface for placement without a wrap is available. Wraps are also useful with nonporous spheres to allow reattachment of the extraocular muscles. Prewrapped implants are often more efficient and less expensive than wrapping materials provided separately.

Indications for Enucleation

Enucleation involves removal of the entire globe while preserving the remaining adnexal and orbital tissues. The primary indications for enucleation include:

1. Primary intraocular malignancies (e.g., uveal melanoma, retinoblastoma) not amenable to alternative modes of therapy such as external or proton beam irradiation or episcleral plaque brachytherapy.
2. Blind, painful, ± disfigured, or deformed eyes where the past ophthalmic history is not entirely clear and an intraocular tumor cannot be ruled out.
3. Historically, enucleation was considered within the first 10–14 days for the severely traumatized eye with extensive prolapse of uveal tissue. Because the concern for sympathetic ophthalmia and harm to the remaining eye was thought to be greater than the likelihood of recovering useful vision in the traumatized eye, enucleation was recommended [132]. As sympathetic ophthalmia affecting the non-traumatized eye is exceedingly rare and successful uveitis treatment options are available, prophylactic enucleation is now a debateable practice [133, 134]. Retention of the patients eye, even if nonfunctional and phthisical, is important as it allows the patient to keep their body part (the eye) [1–6]. Removal may have unwanted psychological effects on the patient as a result of losing a body part (sense of facial disfigurement, loss of self-esteem, depression) [3, 4, 6]. It is our approach to preserve the eye whenever possible, even though there may be no visual potential. Retention of the traumatized eye allows the patient to recover from their trauma and emotionally prepare for removal, if needed, of a blind eye. If removal is not indicated, a non-painful, phthisical eye may be a good platform for an overlying prosthetic eye (scleral shell). If the eye becomes painful at any time in the future, removal remains a management option.

Indications for Evisceration

Evisceration involves removal of the entire intraocular contents of the eye, leaving the scleral shell intact. It is typically preformed with complete keratectomy, but the cornea may be retained. Evisceration is contraindicated if an intraocular tumor is present or suspected or a complete histopathologic examination of the globe and its contents is required [135]. It is also contraindicated in severe cases of phthisis (atrophic bulbi – see below).

The primary indications for evisceration surgery include:

1. A blind, painful eye with a well documented past ocular history that excludes an intraocular tumor. A thorough examination of the iris and fundus should be performed, or, in cases of opacified media, imaging (B-scan ultrasound, CT/MR) should be arranged to help confirm the absence of an intraocular mass.
2. In cases with minimal globe shrinkage (mild phthisis), a standard evisceration can be performed. Ultrasonography, with or without neuroimaging (CT/MR), is indicated prior to consideration of evisceration. If there is severe phthisis with significant shrinkage present (atrophic bulbi), then large anterior and posterior sclerotomies may be required or a complete sclerotomy where the scleral shell is bisected into two complete halves (from superotemporal quadrant to inferonasal quadrant). In others, one

may be able to place the implant immediately behind the sclera (i.e., posterior to posterior Tenon's capsule in order to put in a large diameter implant). A variety of modifications of the traditional evisceration technique using various types of sclerotomies to increase the scleral volume have been previously described in normal sized and phthisical eyes [136–142].

Enucleation Versus Evisceration

The decision to perform evisceration or enucleation has stimulated controversy over the years [143]. Dramatic relief from discomfort can be achieved with either technique. Since evisceration minimizes the disruption of the sclera, Tenon's capsule, extraocular muscle attachments, orbital connective tissue framework, and suspensory ligaments, evisceration is thought to be associated with better postoperative appearance and motility than with enucleation surgery (regardless of implant type) [139, 144]. Evisceration is also simpler and quicker to perform than enucleation. During evisceration surgery it may be difficult to confirm that all the uveal tissue has been removed from the scleral shell. As a result, the potential for sympathetic ophthalmia theoretically remains [134, 145, 146]. Jonathan Dutton, MD, PhD, has reviewed the relative risk of sympathetic ophthalmia following evisceration and contrasted this risk with other ophthalmic surgeries as well as other possible catastrophic life events (Dutton JJ, Sympathetic Ophthalmia: relevance to oculoplastic surgery, Presented at the 45th Sally Letson Symposium; Ottawa, Canada, Sept 19-21,2013). The relative risk of sympathetic ophthalmia following evisceration surgery is estimated to be 1:62,000 versus 1:1600 after vitrectomy surgery, a 40-fold increase in risk with this more common ophthalmic procedure. The lifetime risk of dying in a car accident (1:237), perishing in a plane crash (1:5051), drowning (1:9097), electrocuted from an electric transmission line (1:39,042), or being eaten by a wild animal (1:48,052) are all more common than the risk of sympathetic ophthalmia post evisceration. Thus, although the risk of sympathetic ophthalmia following evisceration exists, it is exceedingly rare, and most ophthalmologists will never see a case in their professional careers [134]. Furthermore, should this inflammatory condition develop, it may be treated with corticosteroids, or other immunosuppressive or biologic agents that offer effective treatment options unavailable years ago when concern about sympathetic ophthalmia kept many surgeons from offering evisceration to their patients.

Nonsurgical Management of the Blind, Painful Eye

For those debilitated patients with blind, painful eyes unable to undergo surgery and rehabilitation or psychologically not ready to have their eye removed, a retrobulbar injection of ethanol or chlorpromazine may, in some cases, provide adequate pain relief [147–153]. Several reports have suggested that chlorpromazine produces superior pain control with fewer complications [152, 153]. However, severe periorbital inflammation can result from retrobulbar chlorpromazine and may manifest as chemosis, proptosis, limited ocular motility, and facial swelling that may extend beyond the eyelids [152, 153]. Retrobulbar injections should be avoided in patients that may be considering enucleation or evisceration surgery as socket motility may be impaired by these toxic medications.

Alternatively, the patient with a phthisical eye without significant discomfort and with no suspicion of an intraocular tumor may be a candidate for a scleral shell (a thin ocular prosthesis that fits over the blind eye). The shell provides a natural appearance and allows the patient to retain their own eye. If some globe shrinkage is not present, a scleral shell will frequently make the prosthetic eye appear proptotic and may not be a good aesthetic option. A cosmetic painted contact lens may occasionally be an alternative in these patients.

Enucleation Surgical Technique

1. Develop a presurgery routine to ensure the correct eye is removed. The patient should identify the eye to be removed by pointing to it or touching the eye to be removed. Confirm that this eye corresponds to the informed consent and to office chart notes. Large arrows using a surgical marking pen should be placed within the visible surgical field around the eye to be removed. If there is a tumor in the eye, dilate the eye in the preoperative holding area so you can carry out direct visualization of the mass when the patient arrives in the operating room. A standard "timeout session" or "preoperative pause" should be performed with all staff in the operating room to reverify that the marked side of surgery corresponds to the informed consent.
2. Local anesthesia with intravenous sedation (MAC) or general anesthesia can be used. If MAC is used, then the upper and lower eyelids are blocked with 2% lidocaine in combination with 1:100,000 epinephrine mixed 50:50 with bacteriostatic saline (approximately 1.5–2.0 ml in

each eyelid and lateral canthal area). In all cases a retrobulbar, intraconal injection of 2% lidocaine in combination with 1:100,000 epinephrine, half-and-half with 0.75% bupivacaine, is administered (5–7 ml), followed by pressure application to the orbit for 5 min.

3. Instill Neo-Synephrine 2.5% eye drops onto the operative eye.
4. Prep and drape the patient in standard sterile fashion taking particular care to adequately sterilize the lid margin and eyelashes. We prefer not to cover the unoperated eye; others may tape and apply a shield.
5. Place an eyelid speculum.
6. Perform a 360° conjunctival limbal peritomy using Wescott scissors.
7. Dissect Tenon's tissue away from the globe in each oblique quadrant using Stevens' tenotomy scissors (Fig. 59.12a).
8. Localize each rectus muscle on a large muscle hook to ensure that the entire muscle insertion is isolated. Gently apply cautery to the arteries at the muscle insertion.
9. Pass a double-armed 5-0 polyglactin (Vicryl) suture in whiplock fashion on either side of the muscle near its insertion (Fig. 59.12b).
10. Sever each rectus muscle from the globe. A 1–2 mm stump of muscle tendon is left attached to the globe over the medial and lateral rectus insertions so that traction sutures or forceps can be applied to grasp the eye during removal. Clamp sutures away from the field (e.g., bulldog-type clamp). As an alternative technique, each rectus muscle can be localized with the muscle hook as described in step 8. Rather than passing a suture into the muscles (step 9), they are simply cut away from the globe leaving a 1–2 mm stump of muscle tendon attached to the globe over the medial and lateral rectus as described in step 10. Contrary to common belief, the recti muscles do not retract into the orbit but remain in their anatomic position [154]. Once the globe has been removed (step 14) and the implant inserted (step 17), the rectus muscles are ready to be attached to the wrapped implant (step 18). With conjunctiva and Tenon's tissue held on gentle traction anteriorly in the area of each rectus muscle, the muscle tendon stumps are readily visualized sitting exactly where they were detached [154]. A double-armed 5-0 Vicryl suture can be used to engage them in a locking-type stitch or even a simple stitch and reconnect them to the wrapped implant surface. This "hook and release" technique avoids any risk of globe penetration in step 9 when the stitch is placed while the rectus muscle is still attached to globe. It may be a little faster and is most helpful when teaching enucleation surgery to resident staff as it eliminates a challenging part of the procedure for the novice surgeon [154].
11. Hook the inferior oblique muscle in the inferotemporal quadrant with the tip of the muscle hook sweeping from posterior to anterior (staying adjacent to the globe) toward the inferior rectus muscle. The muscle is then held between two muscle hooks, clamped with a straight hemostat, cauterized in the clamped section, and cut and cauterized again if the muscle stumps are still bleeding (Fig. 59.12c). Secure the inferior oblique with a double-armed 5-0 polyglactin suture in a similar manner as described for the rectus muscles for later reattachment to the implant.
12. The superior oblique tendon is located in the superonasal quadrant by sweeping the muscle hook from anterior to posterior (staying adjacent to the globe) toward the superior rectus muscle (Fig. 59.12d). The superior oblique tendon is cut and left untagged.
13. Attach a 4-0 silk suture to the lateral and/or medial rectus insertion sites or grasp with a forceps to allow traction of the globe anteriorly during removal.
14. Place the closed enucleation scissors behind the globe and localize the optic nerve by strumming the nerve with the closed scissors. Gentle blunt dissection is carried out on either side of the optic nerve, and the open scissor tips are placed on either side of the optic nerve (Fig. 59.12e). To include as much optic nerve stump as possible, direct the scissor tips posteriorly for several millimeters. As the optic nerve is cut posteriorly, directed pressure prevents the scissor tips from sliding off the optic nerve. Once the nerve is transected, the entire globe moves forward. Cut the remaining Tenon's tissue away from the globe staying as close as possible to the globe to avoid inadvertent soft tissue or muscle injury and to avoid cutting the preplaced polyglactin sutures (Fig. 59.12f). Clamping of sutures and the aid of a surgical assistant are helpful to retract the preplaced muscle sutures away from the field during optic nerve transaction and globe delivery. Some surgeons prefer cutting the optic nerve from the medial side of the globe.
15. Once the globe has been removed, apply pressure to the socket with cotton sponges soaked in thrombin, 4% cocaine, or simply saline for 5 min to assist in hemostasis.
16. Following socket tamponade, gently remove some but not all of the gauze packing used in step 15. Insert malleable ribbon retractors into the orbit between the medial rectus and remaining gauze. Apply gentle traction on the retractors while looking for the optic nerve stump and active bleeders within the orbit. For any prolapsing fat, use 1 in. by ½ inch moistened neurosurgical gauze paddies to gently retract it away from the optic nerve stump. Cauterize active bleeders in this area under direct visualization with neurosurgical type Bayonet bipolar cautery forceps.

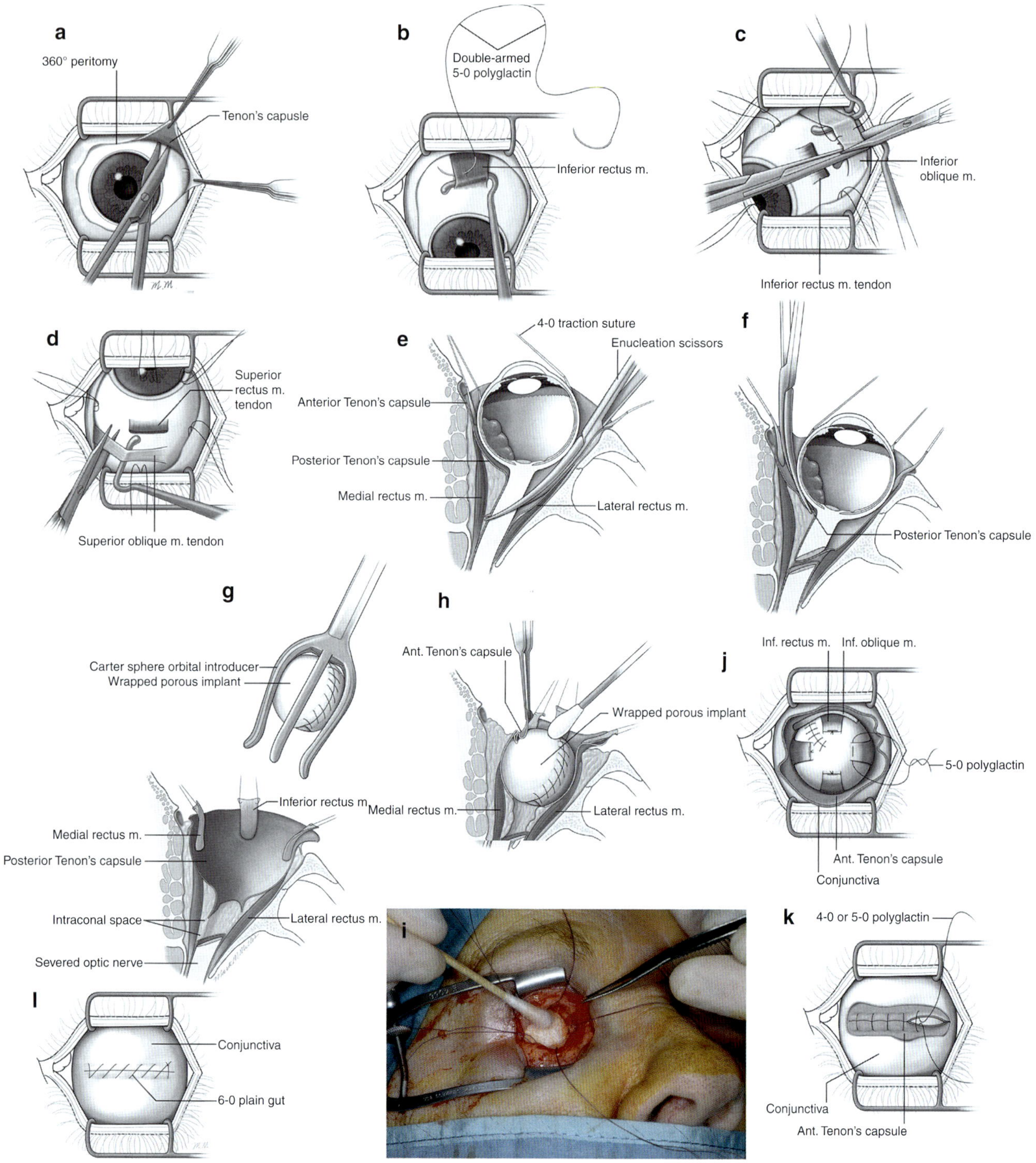

Fig. 59.12 (**a**) Tenon's tissue is dissected away from globe. (Figs. 59.12 and 59.13 – Reproduced, with permission, from Dunn, Langer PD (eds), Basic Techniques of Ophthalmic Surgery, American Academy of ophthalmology, 2009. Illustrations courtesy of Mark Miller). (**b**) A double-armed 5-0 polyglactin suture is passed, locked on either side of the muscle. (**c**) The inferior oblique tendon is cut. (**d**) The superior oblique tendon is cut. (**e**) The tips of the enucleation scissors are positioned on either side of the optic nerve. (**f**) Once the optic nerve has been transected, the entire globe moves forward. (**g**) Placing the implant in the socket with the Carter sphere orbital introducer. (**h**) Applying posterior pressure to the implant to "seat" the implant within Tenon's tissue space. (**i**) Tenon's tissue retracted with a toothed forceps while pressure is being applied posterior to seat the implant (as illustrated in Fig. 59.12h). (**j**) The rectus muscle sutures are secured to the anterior portion of the wrapped implant. (**k**) Anterior Tenon's is closed under no tension. (**l**) The conjunctiva is closed with a running plain gut suture

17. If a porous implant such as hydroxyapatite or aluminum oxide is being used, a 25 gauge needle is used to place several drill holes to the core of a porous implant around the equator of the implant. A drill hole is also placed posteriorly. These holes facilitate implant fibrovascular ingrowth.
18. Prior to insertion of a porous implant, the implant is immersed in an antibiotic solution (e.g., 500 mg of cefazolin or bacitracin in 500 ml of normal saline) within a 60 ml syringe, and an air-fluid exchange is performed.
19. Vicryl mesh (or other wrap per surgeon's preference) is placed around the implant, twisting the excess mesh around the posterior aspect of the implant and securing the mesh to the implant with a 4-0 polyglactin suture tied around the twisted mesh. The excess mesh is then cut (Fig. 59.9a, b). Prewrapped implants eliminate this step.
20. The wrapped implant is placed within a Carter sphere introducer (Fig. 59.12g), glide or sleeve with the anterior aspect of the implant appropriately oriented. The orbital implant is inserted partly within Tenon's capsule and the intraconal space. Other surgeons prefer placing the implant entirely within the intraconal space (behind posterior Tenon's). Anterior Tenon's capsule should be retracted by a surgical assistant to avoid dragging anterior Tenon's tissue posteriorly with implant insertion (a common problem with porous orbital implants). A tissue glide may also be useful to prevent posterior drag of anterior tissue. Once the implant is placed into the orbit, it is important to position or "seat" the implant. To perform this maneuver, apply gentle posterior pressure to the anterior implant surface using a cotton-tipped applicator while an Adson toothed forceps is used to unravel any rolled Tenon's edges for 360°. Additional posterior pressure is applied to the implant with a cotton-tipped applicator while pulling anteriorly on Tenon's if the surgeon would like to place the implant deeper within the orbital cavity (Fig. 59.12h, i).
21. Secure the rectus muscle sutures to the wrapped implant, just anterior to their normal anatomic insertion sites approximately 5–10 mm away from the antagonist rectus muscle. Rarely, these muscles may be in close proximity, but imbrication (or overlapping) of the rectus muscles is avoided (Figs. 59.12j, 59.9c). The inferior oblique muscle is secured to the implant just inferior to the lateral rectus muscle attachment site.
22. Meticulously close anterior Tenon's tissue with a buried 4-0 or 5-0 polyglactin suture in an interrupted fashion. It is extremely important that Tenon's tissue not be closed under tension (Fig. 59.12k).
23. Tension-free closure of the conjunctiva is performed with a running suture (6-0 plain gut) in a locking or non-locking fashion. Rapid absorbing 6-0 plain gut suture is avoided due to the risk of early wound dehiscence (Fig. 59.12l).
24. Apply antibiotic ointment to the eye socket, and insert a small, medium, or large acrylic conformer with holes depending upon the forniceal volume. A temporary suture tarsorrhaphy is often helpful to maintain the conformer during the first 1–2 weeks following surgery. A single, simple suture using the remaining 6-0 plain can be placed through the upper and lower lid margin and left in place until it dissolves over 7–10 days. Alternatively, a double-armed suture (e.g., 4-0 silk) can be passed over a cotton or red rubber bolster to secure the eyelids.
25. Firmly apply two eye patches which are generally left in place for 3–5 days.

Evisceration Surgical Technique (with Keratectomy)

1–6. See enucleation surgical technique.

7. Undermine the conjunctiva by approximately 5 mm for 360° (Fig. 59.12a).
8. Enter the anterior chamber with a No. 11 scalpel blade passed horizontally through the limbus. A 360° keratectomy with the scalpel blade and curved Westcott scissors is performed (Fig. 59.13a).
9. Place an evisceration spoon into the potential space between the choroid and sclera, and attempt to remove the intraocular contents en bloc (although it often comes out piecemeal). Once the intraocular contents have been completely removed, maintain hemostasis with suction and bipolar cautery (Fig. 59.13b).
10. Wipe the entire internal scleral surface with cotton-tipped applicators soaked with absolute alcohol (Fig. 59.13c). This technique is thought to denature any residual uveal pigment remaining that may potentially contribute to the development of sympathetic ophthalmia (see prior discussion). This technique is likely ineffective in eliminating uveal pigment deeper within the scleral wall along tracts of various nerves and blood vessels. There is no scientific evidence to support the use of alcohol, and as a result, many surgeons have eliminated this step.
11. With a straight Stevens tenotomy scissors, remove a V-shaped piece of sclera 3–6 mm in length at the 3 o'clock and 9 o'clock positions; these anterior sclerectomies can be increased in length as required up to the insertions of the medial and lateral rectus muscles to accommodate a large implant (Fig. 59.13d).

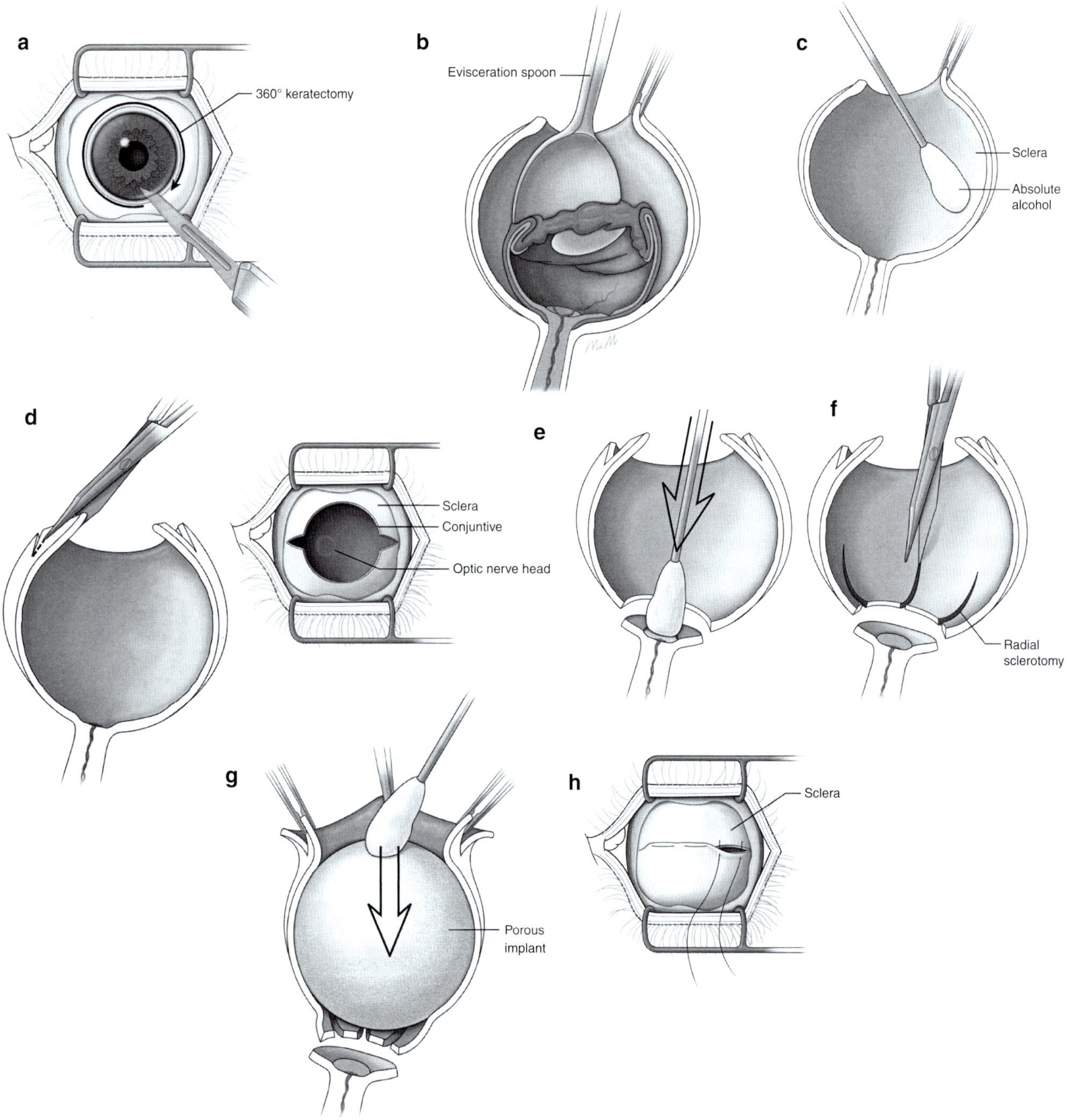

Fig. 59.13 (**a**) Evisceration with keratectomy. The conjunctiva is undermined. (**b**) An evisceration spoon is placed prior to the removal of the intraocular contents. (**c**) The entire internal scleral surface is cleaned with cotton-tipped applicators soaked with absolute alcohol. (**d**) A V-shaped piece of sclera is removed 3–6 mm in length at the 3 and 9 o'clock positions. (**e**) Posterior sclerotomy. A small scleral incision is made posteriorly, about 5–10 mm away from the optic nerve head with a number 11 scalpel blade. The posterior sclera (with attached optic nerve) is pushed into the retrobulbar space with a cotton-tipped applicator. (**f**) Radial sclerotomies are created to allow placement of the implant and facilitate vascularization into the posterior surface of the implant. (**g**) The implant is pushed posteriorly until the anterior scleral edges can be closed without tension. (**h**) The anterior scleral wound is closed with three equally spaced double-armed 5-0 polyglactin sutures passed in horizontal mattress fashion so that the scleral edges are overlapped by 5 mm and are under no tension

12. Perform a posterior sclerotomy as a volume enhancing step. Several techniques are available [135–142]. As an example, a No. 11 scalpel blade is used to create a posterior sclerotomy about 5–10 mm away from the optic nerve head [136]. Incise the posterior sclera for 360° around the nerve head with the No. 11 blade and/or Stevens scissors. Prolapse the posterior sclera (with attached optic nerve) into the retrobulbar space with a

cotton-tipped applicator (Fig. 59.13e). Bleeding may occur once the 360° incision and radial sclerotomies are made. A headlight, cotton-tipped applicators and neurosurgical bipolar forceps are very helpful in obtaining hemostasis.

13. Make several 10–15 mm radial scleral incisions with Stevens scissors in the 4–6 positions around the posterior sclerotomy site (Fig. 59.13f) [136]. The radial sclerotomies open the posterior scleral shell widely, to allow placement of a larger implant (e.g., a 20 mm sphere) and facilitate fibrovascularization of the posterior surface of the implant. Alternatively, a complete posterior sclerotomy can be performed [141]. The sclera is transected from the superior nasal scleral edge posteriorly toward the optic nerve and from the inferior temporal scleral edge posteriorly toward the optic nerve. Sclera is then trimmed away from the optic nerve, and the optic nerve is gently moved posteriorly with a cotton-tipped applicator. This technique will allow placement of even larger orbital implants (e.g., 21, 22 mm spheres). Another posterior sclerotomy technique (the four-petal sclerotomy) involves sectioning sclera into four petals by transecting sclera between each rectus muscle and incising the sclera to the level of the optic nerve [142]. Once the four petals have been created, they are cut away from the optic nerve which is then gently pushed posteriorly with a cotton-tipped applicator [142].
14. Place an implant into a Carter sphere introducer (or similar plunger device) and insert the implant into the scleral cavity while a surgical assistant retracts the sclera (Fig. 59.12g). If the anterior scleral opening is too small to allow entry of the implant, the V-shaped sclerotomies are opened further using a scissors or a No. 11 scalpel blade to incise sclera immediately beneath the medial and lateral rectus insertion sites. An unwrapped porous implant often sticks to the scleral walls as it is being injected into the scleral shell and may not completely enter the shell. To position or "seat" the implant within the scleral shell so that the anterior scleral edges can be apposed without tension, an Adson toothed forceps are used to retract the anterior scleral lip while pressure is applied to the implant with a cotton-tipped applicator (Fig. 59.13g). The implant is not pushed posterior to the posterior sclerotomy at this stage although this is another technique available [138]. Any bits of cotton fluff are removed from the surface of the implant, and the surface is irrigated with an antibiotic solution.
15. Close the anterior scleral edges with three equally spaced double-armed 5-0 polyglactin sutures passed in horizontal mattress fashion so that the scleral edges are overlapped by approximately 5 mm and are under no tension. Between each 5-0 polyglactin suture, 4-0 polyglactin sutures are placed in interrupted fashion through the apposing edges of sclera to reinforce the closure (Fig. 59.13h). If a four-petal posterior sclerotomy has been performed, the medial and lateral petals are closed with an overlap of approximately 5 mm of the scleral edges followed by closure of the superior and inferior petals with the same overlap of the scleral edges [142]. If a complete sclerotomy has been performed, the scleral edges are also overlapped during closure by approximately 5 mm [141].
16. Approximate the conjunctiva and Tenons' tissue and close them together without tension using a running 6-0 plain gut suture (locking or non-locking suture technique). Some physicians prefer closing Tenons' and conjunctiva as separate layers. Rapid absorbing 6-0 plain gut suture is avoided due to the risk of early wound dehiscence (Fig. 59.12k, l).
17. Apply antibiotic ointment to the eye socket, and insert a small, medium, or large conformer. A temporary suture tarsorrhaphy is helpful to maintain the conformer in place during the first 1 to 2 weeks following surgery. A single suture using the remaining 6-0 plain can be placed through the upper and lower lid margin and left in place until it dissolves over 7–10 days. Alternatively, a double-armed suture (e.g., 4-0 silk) can be passed over a cotton or red rubber bolster to secure the eyelids.
18. Firmly apply two eye patches and leave in place for 3–5 days.

Secondary Orbital Implants

In North America and most developed countries, an orbital implant is placed into the socket after enucleation or evisceration in almost all cases. In rare patients with severe endophthalmitis, implant placement may be delayed until the tissue swelling settles or a gross infection resolves. In those individuals without an orbital implant, the term "secondary implant" is used when the implant is placed into the socket at a time other than the initial enucleation/evisceration procedure. An orbital implant exchange is required in some sockets that already have an implant in position, and this too is considered a "secondary implant." Five clinical scenarios exist where an implant exchange might be considered:

1. To improve motility
2. To reposition a migrated implant
3. To replace an exposed implant
4. To increase orbital volume
5. To replace an infected porous implant

Prior to the widespread use of porous orbital implants, orbital implants were often placed into the socket without a wrapping material or attachment to the extraocular muscles. Improvement in prosthetic motility may be possible by removing the previously placed implant, localizing the extraocular muscles, and reattaching them to a porous orbital implant (aluminum oxide, hydroxyapatite, porous polyethylene) [155]. Similarly, if an implant migrates or rotates into a position that does not allow custom fitting of a prosthesis, the original implant can be removed and a new one placed. For large exposures that have failed previous free graft patch repair (i.e., scleral or temporalis fascia) or local tarsoconjunctival flap repair, an implant exchange may be required.

An attempt should be made to localize the extraocular muscles so that the secondary implant can be placed within the muscle cone (the ideal anatomical position) to allow some implant motility. A common misconception is that the extraocular muscles once transected (in an earlier enucleation procedure) from the globe retract deep into the posterior orbit, precluding their later localization. Fortunately, the fibrous connective tissue framework remains intact and often prevents the extraocular muscles from retracting into the posterior eye socket. The extraocular muscles are usually straightforward to localize in the majority of anophthalmic sockets without an implant [154].

Secondary Orbital Implant Placement Surgical Technique (Fig. 59.14)

1. Prior to administering local or systemic anesthesia, a topical anesthetic and vasoconstrictor (topical 2.5% neosynephrine) is applied to the conjunctiva. General anesthesia is preferred, but surgery may be done under local injection with intravenous sedation.
2. The patient is asked to look in the direction of each rectus muscle. A gentian violet mark is placed on the conjunctiva over the area of strongest conjunctival retraction (Fig. 59.14c).
3. After injecting 3 ml of lidocaine 2% with epinephrine into the muscle cone and waiting for 5 min to allow for vasoconstriction, a horizontal incision is made in the conjunctiva, and Tenon's capsule and the implant (if present) are removed, leaving the implant pseudocapsule (Fig. 59.14d). The conjunctival edges are placed on traction, and the surgeon uses cotton-tipped applicators to gently dissect into the area previously marked with gentian violet (Fig. 59.14e, f).
4. Once the rectus muscle is identified (Fig. 59.14g, h), it is dissected from the surrounding tissue and tagged with a 5-0 polyglactin suture passed in whiplock fashion (Fig. 59.14i). Once all four rectus muscles have been tagged, a central pocket is created, and a secondary implant is placed into the muscle cone using a Carter sphere introducer as previously described for enucleation and evisceration.
5. For those patients having had an evisceration without an implant, there are two options: (1) the shrunken eviscerated scleral remnant can be enucleated after identifying and tagging the extraocular muscles. A secondary implant is then put in place and attached to the extraocular muscles, or (2) the scleral remnant can be opened by incising it from the superonasal quadrant to the inferotemporal quadrant and from the superotemporal quadrant to the inferonasal quadrant [137]. A 5-0 polyglactin suture is attached to each of these scleral remnants (as if they represented extended rectus muscle tendons). Transecting the sclera like this allows exposure to the muscle cone. A wrapped nonporous or porous implant can be placed into the muscle cone posterior to the four scleral remnants that have been created. The scleral remnants pieces can then be reattached to the wrapped implant 4–5 mm anterior to the normal extraocular muscle attachment sites, or in some cases, they may be reconnected to the opposing remnant, creating a barrier of sclera over the implant.
6. Tenon's capsule and conjunctiva are closed in layered fashion without tension as described previously for enucleation and evisceration.

Postoperative Care Following Enucleation, Evisceration, and Secondary Orbital Implant Surgery

1. Pain is typically managed with moderate analgesics (acetaminophen with or without codeine, hydrocodone, morphine, etc.). Severe pain not adequately managed by moderate analgesia is unusual and may require more intensive oral or intramuscular pain medication administration.
2. Nausea is not uncommon due to general anesthesia and discomfort associated with the socket surgery and as a vasovagal response as often seen with strabismus surgery. If intraoperative and recovery area antiemetic therapies do not adequately relieve postoperative nausea, then sublingual, oral, or suppository antiemetic medications should be prescribed prior to discharge. Placement of a scopolamine patch prior to surgery may be helpful in patients with a known perioperative nausea.
3. Once the eye patches are removed in 3–5 days, there is no special cleaning required. Showering and gentle face washing are acceptable.
4. Topical antibiotic-steroid eye drops or ointment (e.g., tobramycin-dexamethasone) is started 3–4 times daily for 1–3 weeks following patch removal. A broad-spectrum oral

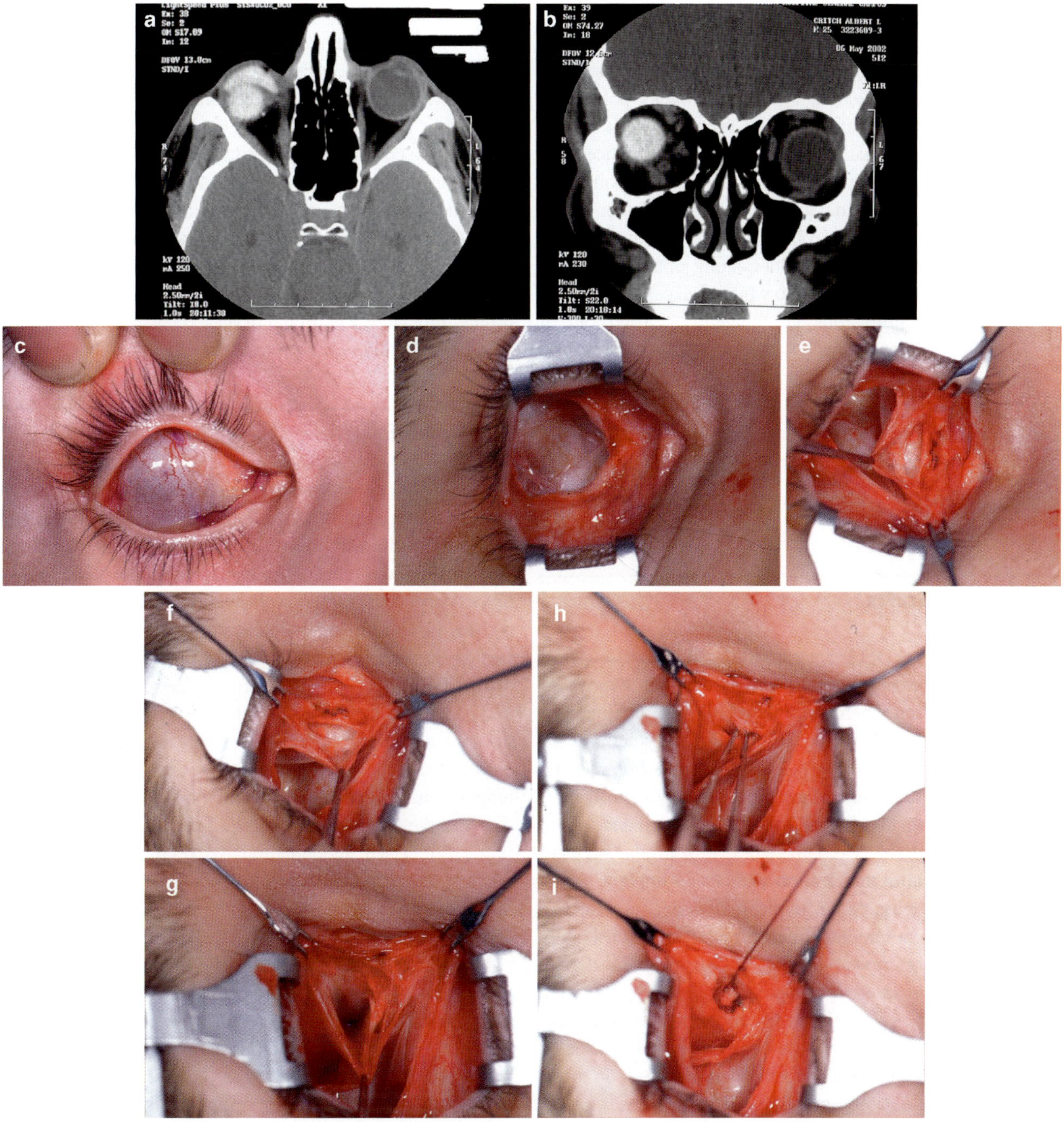

Fig. 59.14 (**a**, **b**) A migrated polymethylmethacrylate orbital implant is seen in the axial and coronal view. (**c**) A gentian violet mark has been placed in the area of the strongest conjunctival retraction when looking up, down, left, and right – indicating the location of the rectus muscles. (**d**) The migrated implant has been removed, and the implant pseudocapsule is well seen. (**e**) The conjunctival edges have been placed on traction with double-pronged retractors, and a cotton-tipped applicator has been used to tease the tissues away. The connective tissue "tunnels" of the fibrous connective tissue framework are seen end on [155]. A small amount of gentian violet maker has been placed where the medial rectus is likely to be found. (**f**) Surgeons view of Fig. 59.14e. (**g**) Further gentle dissection down one of the "connective tissue tunnels" with the cotton-tipped applicator is shown, and the belly of the medial rectus has been identified in one of the tunnels. (**h**) The medial rectus is grasped with a forcep. (**i**) A 5-0 polyglactin suture has been placed through the end of the medial rectus

antibiotic is used by some surgeons, but there is no scientific evidence that it is beneficial, and the trend is away from using prolonged use of prophylactic antibiotics.

5. Cool compresses may be applied for 10–15 min four times daily for a few days following patch removal to help with swelling and also socket discomfort.

6. The temporary acrylic conformer is left in the socket until the patient is evaluated by the ocularist for an "impression-fitted" custom prosthesis once the conjunctival chemosis has adequately resolved, typically 6 weeks postoperatively. If the conformer falls out prematurely, it can be reinserted by the patient or in the surgeon's office after the application of a lubricating or antibiotic eye ointment to the edges and inside surface of the conformer. If the conjunctival chemosis prolapses out of the lid fissure, it must be kept moist with a lubricating ophthalmic ointment applied every 1–2 h two while awake.
7. Follow-up examinations are generally carried out at 1 week postoperatively, 3–4 weeks postoperatively, and again a few weeks following fitting of the artificial eye. Patients are reevaluated at 6–12 months and annually thereafter. More frequent assessments may be indicated if any socket or eyelid malposition issues require more urgent management.

Dermis Fat Grafts

Dermis fat grafts (DFG) have traditionally been used most frequently after extrusion of an orbital implant or removal of a migrated implant where there is some loss of conjunctival tissues and shortened fornices. Conjunctival epithelium will migrate over the anterior surface of the dermis fat graft and expand the conjunctival surface area. Dermis fat grafts have also been used for the following indications: expand orbital volume, treat partially contracted eye sockets, augment socket volume after enucleation without an implant, repair extrusion of an evisceration implant, augment superior sulcus deformities in anophthalmic patients, and occasionally used as a primary implant [76–79]. Disadvantages of dermis fat grafts include an unpredictable rate of absorption with a resulting superior sulcus deformity and orbital volume deficiency. In addition, there is little or no transfer of eye socket movement to the overlying prosthesis resulting in an artificial eye with little natural motility.

Autogenous dermis fat grafts have been very useful in children with anophthalmia and microphthalmia [80]. Approximately 80% of orbital growth occurs by 5 years of age, so it is critical to initiate effective treatment as young as possible [81, 82]. The goal of treatment is to enlarge the bony orbit, forniceal depth, and palpebral fissure length and thus promote facial symmetry and prosthesis fitting. Initially, serial enlarged conformers can be used to stimulate orbital volume and conjunctival development. This requires good parental and child cooperation with the ocularist. At approximately 2–3 years of age, the limit of expanding conformers is reached, and a surgical procedure to expand the conjunctiva and socket is usually required as a next step. Volume expansion of the orbit may be achieved by several methods. A silicone or polymethylmethacrylate implant may be placed in the socket. By 2–3 years of age, a 16- or 18-mm diameter implant can usually be placed. Another good implant option is a dermis fat graft. A DFG has the advantage of providing both volume and surface area to the socket. When placed in a child under the age of 4 years, the implant often grows with the patient, providing excellent volume expansion [76, 77, 80]. Other options to expand the socket include placement of a soft tissue expander within the orbit that has a subcutaneous injection port in the temporalis fossa to expand the orbital implant or a hydrogel tissue expander (hemispherical or spherical) [83].

The Ocularist

Close collaboration between the orbital surgeon and the ocularist is essential in order to obtain the best functional and cosmetic results with an ocular prosthesis in an anophthalmic socket and a reduced frequency of reoperations or secondary procedures. The well-qualified ocularist will also provide invaluable anophthalmic patient support and education. A prosthesis is generally not fit until approximately 6 weeks after anophthalmic surgery. The delay is necessary to allow tissue healing and suture absorption and to permit the conjunctival chemosis to subside so that the ocularist can correctly size the prosthetic eye. Stock prosthesis should no longer be used in developed countries. The modified impression technique is currently the best means of prosthetic fitting [156]. Each anophthalmic socket has an impression made of its size and dimension. A custom-made ocular prosthesis is then designed. In an uncooperative child, the conformer put in place immediately after the surgery can be used as a template for the prosthesis with good results. Artificial eye patients often require some adjustment to the prosthesis after the initial fitting and are typically seen again in about 1 month. Following the initial fitting process, periodic visits to the ocularist once or twice per year are recommended to polish the prosthesis to keep it smooth, to limit biofilm development, and to check the appropriate fit. A poorly maintained or ill-fitting prosthesis may cause socket irritation and discomfort, which may lead to mucous production, pyogenic granuloma formation, or implant exposure. Chronic socket discharge may be caused by a poorly fitted prosthesis that allows pooling of secretions behind it. Modifying the prosthesis at an annual checkup or refitting the socket with a new prosthesis (generally every 5 years) may help prevent these problems. The upper and lower eyelid as well as the superior sulcus may change with time (ptosis, lower lid laxity with retraction or ectropion, deep superior sulcus) as a result of the weight of the prosthetic eye, anatomic changes within the socket, and periodic removal of the artificial eye [86, 87, 89,

90]. These abnormalities may require surgical intervention, but the ocularist may also be able to reduce them with prosthetic modification.

Summary

Loss of an eye to malignancy, trauma, or end-stage ocular disease is a devastating circumstance. There is a loss of binocular vision, reduced depth perception, reduced visual field, as well as various job restrictions. The psychological trauma (e.g., sense of facial disfigurement, loss of self-esteem, depression, etc.) may be worse than the physical disability in some patients. Few operations in ophthalmic surgery require as much compassion on the part of the ophthalmologist as that needed to counsel a patient preparing to undergo removal of an eye. The surgeon must outline the expected postoperative care and appearance, review potential problems, and provide emotional assistance in returning the patient to a productive life. Anophthalmic surgery is not simply about replacing a diseased eye with an orbital implant. Ophthalmic surgeons and ocularists are increasingly focused on restoring a patient's appearance and prosthetic motility to as near normal as possible. Evisceration surgery is favored by many surgeons because of the simplicity of the technique, minimal disruption to the socket anatomy, and excellent cosmetic results. Enucleation is still required in patients with known or potentially occult ocular malignancies as well as blind, painful, and/or unsightly eyes with opaque media and unknown or poorly documented past ocular histories [139].

While there have been many advances in anophthalmic surgical techniques and implant materials over the past three decades, it will require continued research and collaboration to identify more advantageous implants and procedures to optimally rehabilitate the anophthalmic socket.

References

1. Coday MP, Warner MA, Jarling KU, Rubin PA. Acquired monocular vision, functional consequences form the patients perspective. Ophthal Plast Reconstr Surg. 2002;18:55–63.
2. Bohman E, Roed Rassmussen ML, Dafgard KE. Pain and discomfort in the anophthalmic socket. Curr Opin Ophthalmol. 2014;25:455–60.
3. Rasmussen ML, Ekholm O, Prause JU, Toft PB. Quality of life of eye amputated patients. Acta Ophthalmol. 2012;90:435–40.
4. Ahn JM, Lee SY, Yoon JS. Health related quality of life and emotional status of anophthalmic patients in Korea. Am J Ophthalmol. 2010;149:1005–11.
5. Dolman P, Masdottir S, Sahlin S. Patient satisfaction and results after evisceration with a split-sclera technique. Orbit. 2007;26:241–7.
6. McBain HB, Ezra DG, Rose GE, Newman SP. The psychological impact of living with an ocular prosthesis. Orbit. 2014;33:33–9.
7. Jordan DR, Klapper SR, Mawn LA. Chaptter 36: the anophthalmic socket and complications. In: Fay A, Dolman P, editors. Diseases and disorders of the orbit and ocular adnexa. Edinburgh: Elsevier; 2017. p. 657–75.
8. Kelley JJ. History of ocular prosthesis. Int Ophthalmol Clin. 1970;10(4):713–9.
9. Gougelmann HP. The evolution of the ocular motility implant. Int Ophthalmol Clin. 1970;10(4):689–711.
10. Luce CM. A short history of enucleation. Int clinics North America. Int Ophthalmol Clin. 1970;10:681–7.
11. Snyder C. An operation designated the extirpation of an eye. Arch Ophthalmol. 1965;74:429–34.
12. Grinsdale H. Notes on early cases of Mules' operation. Br J Ophthalmol. 1919;8:452–6.
13. Sami D, Young S, Petersen R. Perspective on orbital enucleation implants. Surv Ophthalmol. 2007;52(3):244–65.
14. Blanchard DL, editor. Ophtalmodouleia. Ostend: J.F. Wayenborgh; 1996.
15. Rudemann AD. Modified Burch type evisceration with scleral implant. Am J Ophthalmol. 1960;49:41–4.
16. Mules PH. Evisceration of the globe, with artificial vitreous. Adv Ophthalmic Plast Reconstr Surg. 1885;5:200–6.
17. Cutler NL. A positive contact ball and ring implant for use after enucleation. Arch Ophthalmol. 1947;37:73–8.
18. Beard C. Remarks on historical and newer approaches to orbital implants. Ophthal Plast Reconstr Surg. 1995;11(2):89–90.
19. Allen JH, Allen L. A buried muscle cone implant: development of a tunneled hemispherical type. Arch Ophthalmol. 1950;43:879–90.
20. Allen LH, Ferguson EC III, Braley AE. A quasi integrated buried muscle cone implant with good motility and advantages foe prosthetic fitting. Trans Am Acad Ophthalmol Otolaryngol. 1960;64:272–8.
21. Spivey BE, Allen LH, Burns CA. The Iowa enucleation implant: a ten year evaluation of techniques and results. Am J Ophthalmol. 1969;67:171–81.
22. Jordan DR, Anderson RL, Nerad JA, Allen L. A preliminary report on the universal implant. Arch Ophthalmol. 1987;105:1726–31.
23. Hornblass A, Biesman BS, Eviator JA. Current techniques of enucleation: a survey of 5,439 intraorbital implants and a review of the literature. Ophthal Plast Reconstr Surg. 1995;11:77–88.
24. Martin O, Clodius L. The history of the artificial eye. Ann Plast Surg. 1979;3(2):168–71.
25. Perry AC. Advances in enucleation. Ophthal Clin NA. 1991;4:173–82.
26. Dutton JJ. Coralline hydroxyapatite as an ocular implant. Ophthalmology. 1991;98:370–7.
27. Nunery WR, Heinz GW, Bonnin JM, Martin RT, Cepela MA. Exposure rate of hydroxyapatite spheres in the anophthalmic socket: histopathologic correlation and comparison with silicone sphere implants. Ophthalmic Plast Reconstr Surg. 1993;9:96–104.
28. Goldberg RA, Holds JB, Ebrahimpour J. Exposed hydroxyapatite orbital implants: report of six cases. Ophthalmology. 1992;99:831–6.
29. Buettner H, Bartley GB. Tissue breakdown and exposure associated with orbital hydroxyapatite implants. Am J Ophthalmol. 1992;113:669–73.
30. Kim YD, Goldberg RA, Shorr N, Steinsapir KD. Management of exposed hydroxyapatite orbital implants. Ophthalmology. 1994;101:1709–15.
31. Remulla HD, Rubin PAD, Shore JW, Sutula FC, Townsend DJ, Woog JJ, Jahrling KV. Complications of porous spherical orbital implants. Ophthalmology. 1995;102:586–93.
32. Oestreicher JH, Liu E, Berkowitz M. Complications of hydroxyapatite orbital implants: a review of 100 consecutive cases and a comparison of Dexon mesh (polyglycolic acid) with scleral wrapping. Ophthalmology. 1997;104:324–9.

33. Jordan DR, Brownstein S, Jolly SS. Abscessed hydroxyapatite orbital implants: a report of two cases. Ophthalmology. 1996;103:1784–7.
34. Blaydon SM, Shepler TR, Neuhaus RW, White WL, Shore JW. The porous polyethylene (Medpor) spherical orbital implant: a retrospective study of 136 cases. Ophthal Plast Reconstr Surg. 2003;19:364–74.
35. Karesh JW, Dresner SC. High density porous polyethylene (Medpor) as a successful anophthalmic implant. Ophthalmology. 1994;101:1688–96.
36. Rubin PAD, Popham J, Rumeldts S, et al. Enhancement of the cosmetic and functional outcomes of enucleation with the conical orbital implant. Ophthalmology. 1998;105:919–25.
37. Anderson RL, Yen MT, Lucci LM, et al. The quasi-integrated porous polyethylene orbital implant. Ophthal Plast Reconstr Surg. 2002;18:50–5529.
38. Ma Y, Schou KR, Maloney-Schou M, Harwin FM, NG J. The porous polyethylene/Bioglass spherical orbital implant: a retrospective study of 170 cases. Ophthal Plast Reconstr Surg. 2011;27:21–7.
39. Mawn LA, Jordan DR, Gilberg S. Proliferation of human fibroblasts in vitro after exposure to orbital implants. Can J Ophthalmol. 2001;36:245–51.
40. Mawn L, Jordan DR, Gilberg S. Scanning electron microscopic examination of porous orbital implants. Can J Ophthalmol. 1998;33:203–9.
41. Jordan DR, Munro SM, Brownstein S, Gilberg SM, Grahovac SZ. A synthetic hydroxyapatite implant: the so-called counterfeit implant. Ophthalmic Plast Reconstr Surg. 1998;14(4):244–9.
42. Jordan DR, Bawazeer A. Experience with 120 synthetic hydroxyapatite implants (FCI_3). Ophthalmic Plast Reconstr Surg. 2001;17:184–90.
43. Jordan DR, Pelletier C, Gilberg SM, Brownstein S, Grahovac SZ. A new variety of hydroxyapatite: the Chinese Implant. Ophthal Plast Reconstr Surg. 1999;15(6):420–4.
44. Jordan DR, Hwang I, McEachren TM, Brownstein S, Gilberg SM, Grahovac SZ, Mawn L. Brazilian hydroxyapatite implant. Ophthalmic Plast Reconstr Surg. 2000;16:363–9.
45. Jordan DR, Brownstein S, Gilberg S, Matthew B, Mawn L, Khouri L. Investigation of a bioresorbable orbital implant. Ophthalmic Plast Reconstr Surg. 2002;18:342–8.
46. Klett A, Guthoff R. Deckung von Orbitaimplantaten mit muskelgestielter autologer sklera. Ophthalmologe. 2003;100:449–52.
47. Jordan DR, Mawn L, Brownstein S, McEachren TM, Gilberg SM, Hill V, Grahovac SZ, Adenis JP. The bioceramic orbital implant: a new generation of porous implants. Ophthalmic Plast Reconstr Surg. 2000;16:347–55.
48. Jordan DR, Gilberg S, Mawn LA. The bioceramic orbital implant: experience with 107 implants. Ophthalmic Plast Reconstr Surg. 2003;19:128–35.
49. Christel P. Biocompatibility of alumina. Clin Orthop. 1992;282:10–8.
50. Jordan DR, Klapper SK, Gilberg SM, Dutton JJ, Wong A, Mawn L. The bioceramic implant: evaluation of implant exposures in 419 implants Ophthalmic. Plast Reconstr Surg. 2010;26:80–2.
51. Wang JK, Lai PC, Liao SL. Late exposure of the bioceramic orbital implant. Am J Ophthalmol. 2009;147:162–70.
52. Karslioglu SK, Buttanri IB, Fazil K, Serin D, Akbaba M. Long-term outcomes of pegged and unpegged bioceramic orbital implants. Ophthalmic Plast Reconstr Surg. 2012;28:264–7.
53. Jordan DR, Gilberg SM, Bawazeer A. The coralline hydroxyapatite orbital implant (Bio-Eye™): experience with 170 Patients. Ophthal Plast Reconstr Surg. 2004;20(1):69–71.
54. Jordan DR. Anophthalmic orbital implants. Ophthal Clinics NA. 2000;13(4):587–608.
55. Integrated Orbital Implants, Inc. Advertisement. Ophthal Plast Reconstr Surg. 2017;33:2.
56. Jordan DR, Brownstein S, Faraji H. Clinicopathologic analysis of 15 explanted hydroxyapatite implants. Ophthal Plast Reconstr Surg. 2004;20(4):285–90.
57. Jordan DR, Chan S, Mawn L, et al. Complications associated with pegging hydroxyapatite orbital implants. Ophthalmology. 1999;106:505–12.
58. Custer PL, Trinkhaus KM. Porous implant exposure: incidence, management and morbidity. Ophthal Plast Reconstr Surg. 2007;23(1):1–7.
59. Su GW, Yen MT. Current trends in managing the anophthalmic socket after primary enucleation and evisceration. Ophthal Plast Reconstr Surg. 2004;20(4):274–80.
60. Goldberg RA. Who should have hydroxyapatite orbital implants? Arch Ophthalmol. 1995;113:566–7.
61. Codere F. Hydroxyapatite implants: a rational approach. Can J Ophthalmol. 1995;30:235–7.
62. Jordan DR. Porous orbital implants; are they advantageous and anyone still pegging? American Society of Ophthalmic Plastic and Reconstructive Surgery Meeting, Fairmont, Waterfront Hotel, Vancouver, British Columbia, June 23–25, 2017.
63. Allen L. The argument against imbricating the rectus muscles over spherical orbital implants after enucleation. Ophthalmology. 1983;90:1116–20.
64. Trichopoulos N, Augsberger JJ. Enucleation with unwrapped porous and nonporous orbital implants: a 15-year experience. Ophthal Plast Reconst Surg. 2005;21(5):331–6.
65. Nunery WR, Cepela MA, Heinz GW, et al. Extrusion rate of silicone spherical anophthalmic socket implants. Ophthal Plast Reconstr Surg. 1993;9:290–4.
66. Wells ST, Harris GJ. Direct fixation of extraocular muscles to a silicone sphere: a cost-sensitive, low risk enucleation procedure. Ophthal Plast Reconstr Surg. 2011;27:364–7.
67. Wladis EI, Aakalu VK, Sobel RK, et al. Orbital implants in enucleation surgery; a report by the American academy of ophthalmology. Ophthalmology. 2018;125(2):311–7. https://doi.org/10.1016/j.ophtha.2017.08.006. [Epub ahead of print].
68. Sagoo MS, Rose GE. Mechanisms and treatment of extruding intraconal implants. Arch Ophthalmol. 2007;125(12):1116–620.
69. Custer PL, Trinkaus KM, Fornoff J. Comparative motility of hydroxyapatite and alloplastic enucleation implants. Ophthalmology. 1999;106:513–6.
70. Guillinta P, Vasani SN, GRanet DB, et al. Prosthetic motility in pegged and unpegged integrated porous orbital implants. Ophthal Plast Reconstr Surg. 2000;19:119–22.
71. Colen TP, Paridaens DA, Lemij HG, et al. Comparison of artificial eye amplitudes with acrylic and hydroxyapatite spherical enucleation implants. Ophthalmology. 2000;107:1889–94.
72. Guillinta P, Vasani SN, Granet DB, Kikkawa DO. Prosthetic motility in pegged versus unpegged integrated porous orbital implants. Ophthal Plast Reconstr Surg. 2000;19:119–22.
73. Custer PL, Kennedy RH, Woog JJ, Kaltreider SA, Meyer DA. Orbital implants in enucleation surgery, a report by the American Academy of Ophthalmology. Ophthalmology. 2003;110:2054–61.
74. Bentley RP, Sgouros S, Natarajan K, et al. Normal changes in orbital volume during childhood. J Neurosurg. 2002;96:742–6.
75. Yago K, Furuta M. Orbital growth after unilateral enucleation in infancy without an orbital implant. Jpn J Ophthalmol. 2001;45:648–52.
76. Heber KL, Katowitz JA, Low JE. Unilateral dermis-fat graft implantation in the pediatric orbit. Ophthal Plast Reconstr Surg. 1998;14:81–8.
77. Mitchell KT, Holster DA, White WL. The autogenous dermis-fat orbital implant in children. JAAPOS. 2001;5:367–9.

78. Nunery WR, Hetzler KJ. Dermal-fat graft as a primary enucleation technique. Ophthalmology. 1985;92:1256–61.
79. Migliori ME, Putterman AM. The domed dermis-fat graft orbital implant. Ophthal Plast Reconstr Surg. 1991;7:23–30.
80. Katowitz JA. Pediatric oculoplastic surgery. New York: Springer Verlag; 2002. p. 180–3.
81. Fargas LG, et al. Growth patterns in the orbital region. Cleft Palate Craniofac J. 1992;29:315–8.
82. Osaki TH, Fay A, Mehta M, et al. Orbital development as a function of age in indigenous North American skeletons. Ophthal Plast Reconstr Surg. 2013;29(2):131–6.
83. Gundlach KK, et al. Expansion of the socket and orbit for congenital clinical anophthalmia. Plast Reconstr Surg. 2005;116:1214–22.
84. Kaltreider SA. The ideal ocular prosthesis: analysis of prosthetic volume. Ophthalmic Plast Reconstr Surg. 2000;16:388–92.
85. Kaltreider SA, Lucarelli MJ. A simple algorithm for selection of implant size for enucleation and evisceration. Ophthalmic Plast Reconstr Surg. 2002;18:336–41.
86. Custer PL, Trinkaus KM. Volumetric determination of enucleation implant size. Am J Ophthalmol. 1999;128:489–94.
87. Thaller VT. Enucleation volume measurement. Ophthal Plast Reconstr Surg. 1997;13:18–20.
88. Kaltreider SA, Jacobs JL, Hughes MO. Predicting the ideal implant size before enucleation. Ophthal Plast Reconstr Surg. 1999;15(3):37–43.
89. Shah CT, Hughes MO. Kirzhmer. Anophthalmic socket syndrome, a review of the management. Ophthal Plast Reconstr Surg. 2014;30(30):361–5.
90. Choi BH, Lee SH, Chung WS. Correction of superior sulcus deformity and enophthalmos with porous high-density polyethylene sheet in anophthalmic patients. Koreon J OPhthalmol. 2005;19:168–73.
91. Trichopoulas N, Augsburger JJ. Enucleation with unwrapped porous and non-porous implants: a 15 year experience. Ophthalmic Plast Reconstr Surg. 2005;21:331–6.
92. Perry JD. Hydroxyapatite implants (letter). Ophthalmology. 2003;110:1281.
93. Long JA, Tann TM, Bearden WH, Callahan MA. Enucleation: is wrapping the implant necessary for optimal motility. Ophthalmic Plast Reconstr Surg. 2003;19(3):194–7.
94. Perry JD, Tam RC. Safety of unwrapped spherical orbital implants. Ophthal Plast Reconstr Surg. 2004;20:281–4.
95. Nunery WR. Risk of prion transmission with the use of xenografts and allografts in surgery. Ophthalmic Plast Reconstr Surg. 2003;17:389–94.
96. Seiff SR, Chang JS Jr, Hurt MH, Khayam-Bashi H. Polymerase chain reaction identification of human immunodeficiency virus-1 in preserved human sclera. Am J Ophthalmol. 1994;118:528–9.
97. Long CJ, Heckman JG, Neunderfer B. Creutzfeldt-Jakob disease via dural and corneal transplants. J Neurol Sci. 1998;160:128–39.
98. Hogan RN, Brown P, Heck E, Cavanagh H. Risk of prion disease transmission from ocular donor tissue transplantation. Cornea. 1999;18:2–11.
99. Heckman JG, Lang CJ, Petruch F, et al. Transmission of Creutzfeldt-Jakob disease via a corneal transplant. J Neurol Neurosurg Psychiatry. 1997;63:388–90.
100. Simonds RJ, Holmberg SD, Hurwitz RL, Coleman TR, Bottenfield S, Conley LJ, Kohlenberg SH, Castro KG, Dahan BA, Schable CA, Rayfield MA, Rogers MF. Transmission of human immunodeficiency virus type 1 from a seronegative organ and tissue donor. N Engl J Med. 1992;326:726–32.
101. Arat YO, Shetlar DJ, Boniuk M. Bovine pericardium versus homologous sclera as a wrapping for hydroxyapatite orbital implants. Ophthalmic Plast Reconstr Surg. 2003;19:189–93.
102. Gayre GS, DeBacker CM, Lipham W, Tawfik HA, Holck DEE, Dutton JJ. Bovine pericardium as a wrapping for orbital implants. Ophthalmic Plast Reconstr Surg. 2001;17:381–7.
103. Pelletier C, Gilberg S, Jordan DR. Use of Temporalis fascia for management of exposed hydroxyapatite implants. Ophthal Plast Reconstr Surg. 1998;14:198–203.
104. Naugle TC Jr, Fry CL, Sabatier RE, Elliot LF. High leg incision fascia lata harvesting. Ophthalmology. 1997;104:1480–8.
105. Kao SCS, Chen S. The use of rectus abdominis sheath for wrapping of the hydroxyapatite orbital implants. Ophthalmic Surg Lasers. 1999;30:69–71.
106. Naugle TC Jr, Lee AM, Haik BG, Callahan MA. Wrapping hydroxyapatite orbital implants with posterior auricular muscle complex grafts. Am J Ophthalmol. 1999;128:495–501.
107. Karesh JW. Polytetrafluoroethylene as a graft material in ophthalmic plastic and reconstructive surgery: an experimental and clinical study. Ophthalmic Plast Reconstr Surg. 1987;3:179–85.
108. Choo PH, Carter SR, Crawford JB, Seiff SR. Exposure of expanded polytetrafluoroethylene-wrapped hydroxyapatite orbital implant: a report of two patients. Ophthalmic Plast Reconstr Surg. 1999;15:77–8.
109. Kao L. Polytetrafluoroethylene as a wrapping material for a hydroxyapatite orbital implant. Ophthalmic Plast Reconstr Surg. 2000;16:286–8.
110. Jordan DR, Allen LH, Ells A, Gilberg S, Brownstein S, Munro S, Grahovac S, Raymond F. The use of vicryl mesh (polyglactin 910) for implantation of hydroxyapatite orbital implants. Ophthalmic Plast Reconstr Surg. 1995;11:95–9.
111. Jordan DR, Ells A, Brownstein S, Munro S, Grahovac S, Raymond F, Allen LH. Vicryl-mesh wrap for the implantation of hydroxyapatite orbital implants:an animal model. Can J Ophthalmol. 1995;30:241–6.
112. Klapper SR, Jordan DR, Punja K, Brownstein S, Gilberg SM, Mawn L, Grahovac SZ. Hydroxyapatite implant wrapping materials: analysis of fibrovascular ingrowth in an animal model. Ophthalmic Plast Reconstr Surg. 2000;16:278–85.
113. Gayre GS, Lipham W, Dutton JJ. A comparison of rates of fibrovascular ingrowth in wrapped versus unwrapped hydroxyapatite spheres in a rabbit model. Ophthalmic Plast Reconstr Surg. 2002;18:275–28.
114. Jordan DR, Klapper SR, Gilberg SM. The use of vicryl mesh in 200 porous orbital implants. Ophthalmic Plast Reconstr Surg. 2003;19:53–61.
115. Custer PL. Enucleation: past, present, and future. Ophthalmic Plast Reconstr Surg. 2000;16:316–21.
116. Custer PL. Reply to Dr. D.R. Jordan's letter on polyglactin mesh wrapping of hydroxyapatite implants. Ophthalmic Plast Reconstr Surg. 2001;17:222–3.
117. Jordan DR, Chan S, Mawn L, Gilberg SM, Brownstein S, Hill V. Complications associated with pegging hydroxyapatite orbital implants. Ophthalmology. 1999;106:505–12.
118. Edelstein C, Shields CL, DePotter P, Shields JA. Complications of motility peg placement for the hydroxyapatite orbital implant. Ophthalmology. 1997;104:1616–21.
119. Lin CJ, Lio SL, Jou JR, Kao SC, Hou PK, Chen MS. Complications of motility peg placement for porous hydroxyapatite orbital implants. Br J Ophthalmol. 2002;86:394–6.
120. Jordan DR. Spontaneous loosening of hydroxyapatite peg sleeves. Ophthalmology. 2001;108:2041–4.
121. Cheng MS, Lio SL, Lin L. Late porous polyethylene implant exposure after motility coupling post placement. Am J Ophthalmol. 2004;138:420–4.
122. Lee SY, Jang JW, Lew H, Kim SJ, Kim HY. Complications in motility peg placement for hydroxyapatite orbital implants in anophthalmic socket. Jpn J Ophthalmol. 2002;46:103–7.

123. Jordan DR, Klapper SR. A new titanium peg system for hydroxyapatite orbital implants. Ophthalmic Plast Reconstr Surg. 2000;16:380–7.
124. Johnson RLC, Ramstead CL, Nathoo N. Pegging the porous implant. Ophthalmic Plast Reconstr Surg. 2011;27:74–5.
125. Ainbinder DJ, Haik BG, Tellado M. Hydroxyapatite orbital implant abscess: histopathologic correlation of an infected implant following evisceration. Ophthalmic Plast Reconstr Surg. 1994;10:267–70.
126. Klapper SR, Jordan DR, Ells A, Grahovac SZ. Hydroxyapatite orbital implant vascularization assessed by magnetic resonance imaging. Ophthalmic Plast Reconstr Surg. 2003;19:46–5.
127. Cook S, Dalton J. Biocompatibility and biofunctionality of implanted materials. Alpha Omegan. 1992;85:41–7.
128. Choi JC, Iwamoto MA, Bstandig S, Rubin PA, Shore J. Medpor motility coupling post: a rabbit model. Ophthalmic Plast Reconstr Surg. 1999;15:190–201.
129. Rubin PAD, Fay AM, Remulla HD. Primary placement of motility coupling post in porous polyethylene orbit implants. Arch Ophthalmol. 2000;118:826–32.
130. Hsu WC, Green JP, Spilker MH, Rubin PAD. Primary placement of a titanium motility post in a porous polyethylene orbital implant. Ophthalmic Plast Reconstr Surg. 2003;16:370–9.
131. Tawfik HA, Dutton JJ. Primary peg placement in evisceration with the spherical porous polyethylene orbital implant. Ophthalmology. 2004;111:1401–6.
132. Chen WP-D. Chapter 119: Enucleation, evisceration, and exenteration. In: McCord Jr CD, Tanenbaum M, Nunery WR, editors. Oculoplastic surgery. New York: Raven Press; 1995. p. 581.
133. Jordan DR, Mawn L. Chapter 53: enucleation, evisceration, and exenteration. In: Dunn JP, Langer PD, editors. Basic techniques of ophthalmic surgery. San Francisco: American Academy of Ophthalmology Manual; 2015. p. 305–28.
134. Levine MR, Pou CR, Lesh RH. The 1998 Wendell Hughes lecture. Evisceration: is sympathetic ophthalmia a concern in the new millennium? Ophthal Plast Reconstr Surg. 1999;15:4–8.
135. Jordan DR, Mawn L. Enucleation, evisceration, and Exenteration. In basic techniques of ophthalmic surgery, American Academy of ophthalmology manual, eds. JP Dunn, PD Langer. Chpt. 2015;53:305–28.
136. Jordan DR, Khouri LM. Evisceration with posterior sclerotomies. Can J Ophthalmol. 2001;3(7):404–7.
137. Jordan DR, Parisi J. The scleral fillet technique for secondary orbital implantation. Can J Ophthalmol. 1996;3(7):356–60.
138. Jordan DR, Stoica B. Evisceration with implant placement posterior to posterior sclera. Ophthal Plast Reconstr Surg. 2016;32(3):178–82.
139. Timothy NH, Feilich DE, Linberg JV. Perspective: evisceration versus enucleation, the ocularists standpoint. Ophthal Plast Reconstr Surg. 2003;19(6):417–20.
140. Long JA, Tann TM III, Girgin CA. Evisceration: a new technique of trans scleral implant placement. Ophthal Plast Reconstr Surg. 2000;5(3):322–5.
141. Massry GG, Holds JB. Evisceration with scleral modification. Ophthal Plast Reconstr Surg. 2001;17:42–7.
142. Sales-Sanz M, Sanz-Lopez A. Four-petal evisceration: anew technique. Ophthal Plast Reconstr Surg. 2007;23:389–92.
143. Stephenson CM. Evisceration of the eye with expansion sclerotomies. Ophthal Plast Reconstr Surg. 1987;3:249–51.
144. Ben NT, Simon GY, Douglas RS. Comparing outcomes of enucleation and evisceration. Ophthalmology. 2006;113:2270–5.
145. Green WR, Maumenee AE, Sanders TE, Smith ME. Sympathetic uveitis following evisceration. Trans Am Acad Ophthalmol Otolaryngol. 1972;76:625–44.
146. Rudemann AD Jr. Sympathetic ophthalmia after evisceration. Trans Am Ophthalmol Soc. 1963;16:274–314.
147. Maumanee AE. Retrobulbar alcohol injection:relief of ocular pain in eyes with and without vision. Am J Ophthalmol. 1949;32:1502–8.
148. Al-Faran MF, Al-Omar O. Retrobulbar alcohol injection in blind painful eyes. Ann Ophthalmol. 1990;22:460–2.
149. Olurin O, Osuntokun O. Complications of retrobulbar alcohol injections. Ann Ophthalmol. 1978;10:474–6.
150. Chen TC, Ahn Yuen SJ, Sangaalang MA, Fernando RE, Luenberger EU. Retrobulbar chlorpromazine injections for management of blind and seeing eyes. J Glaucoma. 2002;11:209–13.
151. Estafanous MFG, Kaiser PK, Baerveldt G. Retrobulbar chlorpromazine in blind and seeing eyes. Retina. 2000;20:555–8.
152. McCulley TJ, Kersten RC. Periocular inflammation after retrobulbar chlorpromazine (Throzine) injection. Ophthal Plast Reconstr Surg. 2006;4:283–5.
153. Cotliar JM, Shields CL, Meyer DR. Chronic orbital inflammation and fibrosis after retrobulbar alcohol and chlorpromazine injections in a patient with choroidal melanoma. Ophthal Plast Reconstr Surg. 2008;24:410–1.
154. Jordan DR, Stoica B, Dutton J. The hook and release technique for enucleation surgery. Ophthal Plast Reconstr Surg. 2018;34:31–6.
155. Jordan DR. Localization of extraocular muscles during secondary orbital implantation surgery: the tunnel technique. Experience in 100 patients. Ophthalmology. 2004;111:1048–54.
156. Spivey BE, et al. The Iowa enucleation implant: a 10 year evolution of technique and results. Am J Ophthalmol. 1969;67:171–7.

Evaluation and Management of the Anophthalmic Socket and Socket Reconstruction

60

David R. Jordan and Stephen R. Klapper

Introduction

The absence or loss of an eye due to a congenital malformation, tumor, trauma, or end-stage ocular disease can be an exceptionally difficult situation for patients, and the management of the anopthalmic socket has long been a challenge for the ophthalmologist and ocularist. Loss of binocular visual function with reduced peripheral visual field and loss of depth perception may result in difficulties with activities of daily living and have various vocational restrictions [1–6]. Individuals may experience a sense of facial disfigurement and poor self-esteem as a result of the "lost body part." [3–7]. In the past three decades, there have been numerous developments and refinements in anophthalmic socket surgery with respect to implant material and design, implant wrapping, implant-prosthesis coupling, and socket volume considerations. Anophthalmic surgery is no longer simply about replacing a diseased eye with an orbital implant and delegating the procedure to junior resident staff. As with other microsurgical ophthalmic procedures, enucleation and eviscerations should be performed meticulously to attain the best functional and cosmetic result and to avoid deformities that may compound the patients' already challenging situation. Because eye contact is such an essential part of human interaction, it is extremely important for the patient with an artificial eye to maintain a natural, normal-appearing prosthetic eye.

Characteristics of the ideal anophthalmic socket include [8, 9].

1. A centrally placed, well-covered, buried implant of adequate volume, fabricated from a bioinert material that transmits motility from the implant to the overlying prosthesis.
2. A socket lined with healthy conjunctiva and fornices deep enough to retain a prosthesis and to permit horizontal and vertical excursion of an artificial eye.
3. Normal eyelid and eyelash position, appearance, and eyelid tone.
4. A supratarsal eyelid fold that is symmetric with that of the contralateral eyelid.
5. A comfortable ocular prosthesis that looks similar to the sighted, contralateral globe and in the same horizontal and anterior-posterior plane.

Close collaboration between the ophthalmologist and the ocularist is essential in order to obtain the best functional and cosmetic results with an ocular prosthesis in an anophthalmic socket and to reduce the frequency of secondary periorbital procedures. Excellent cosmetic results and long-term control of socket problems are the ideal but may be difficult to achieve in some cases. Secondary procedures are often helpful but can be challenging and unsatisfactory for both the patient and surgeon. Successful anophthalmic socket surgery is achieved when the anophthalmic patient obtains a painless, non-inflamed eye socket with adequate volume restoration and an artificial eye that looks and moves almost as naturally as a normal eye. When the patient reports that their friends and colleagues "don't know which is the prosthetic eye," a primary goal of surgery has been achieved. Yearly follow-up examinations with the ocularist for prosthesis polishing and implant fit evaluation, as well as with the ophthalmologist to examine any socket issues that are more easily addressed when identified at an early stage (e.g., implant exposure) are important. This chapter focuses on the clinical assessment of the anophthalmic socket and some of the common problems and complications encountered following enucleation and evisceration surgery.

The authors of this study do not have a commercial or proprietary interest in any of the products reviewed in this manuscript.

D. R. Jordan (✉)
Ottawa Hospital – General Campus, Eye Institute, Ottawa, ON, Canada

S. R. Klapper
Ophthalmology/Oculoplastic Surgery, Klapper Eyelid and Facial Plastic Surgery, Carmel, IN, USA

J. J. Servat et al. (eds.), *Smith and Nesi's Ophthalmic Plastic and Reconstructive Surgery*,
https://doi.org/10.1007/978-3-030-41720-8_60

Changes Associated with Anophthalmic Socket

In addition to the absence of the globe, the anophthalmic socket has other anatomic differences from a normal orbit. Postoperative socket changes begin a complex sequence of interrelationships that affects both the appearance of the socket and the function of the socket with a prosthesis. Progressive intraorbital volume loss following an enucleation or evisceration procedure results in rotary displacement of the orbital contents from superior to posterior and from the posterior to the inferior orbit [10, 11]. There is retraction of the superior rectus/levator muscle complex, a downward and forward redistribution of the orbital fat, and an upward movement of the distal end of the inferior rectus muscle resulting in a shallow inferior fornix and potential tilting of the prosthesis. The superior sulcus may deepen, and upper eyelid ptosis may develop (Fig. 60.1a–d).

Progressive lower eyelid laxity of senescence may be aggravated by the weight of an artificial eye. Loss of lower eyelid support and inferior fornix volume may make fitting and wearing of the custom prosthesis more difficult. Insufficient volume replacement, rotational socket changes, and tissue laxity associated with aging result in the "post-enucleation socket syndrome" or "anophthalmic socket syndrome" (deep superior sulcus, upper eyelid ptosis, an enophthalmic appearance, lower eyelid malposition) and may require a larger than desirable prosthesis [12–16].

Proper implant volume at the time of enucleation or evisceration may be determined either preoperatively or intraoperatively (enucleation cases) from the axial length of the eye or by determining the volume of fluid the enucleated eye displaces in a graduated cylinder [14–16]. Approximately 70–80% of the volume of an individual's normal globe ideally should be replaced with an orbital implant [14, 16]. This generally allows for a prosthetic volume that is 2.0–2.5 ml [13]. While the upper limit of prosthetic volume is approximately 4.0 ml, larger prostheses often result in progressive lower lid laxity and malposition due to the weight of the prostheses on the eyelid and the projection of the anterior surface of the artificial eye. Larger prostheses may also have limited socket excursion [14]. The preoperative or intraoperative calculated implant size is often greater than 22 mm [14–16]. Unfortunately, implants larger than 22 mm may have a higher exposure rate and if too large will hinder fitting of an acceptable custom prosthesis [14, 16]. In most adults, we typically use 20–22 mm spherical implants following enucleation and 18–20 mm implants in evisceration procedures. Individualization of the implant size is important in optimizing orbital volume replacement and in achieving the best possible functional and aesthetic results [13–16].

Fabrication, Care, and Maintenance of the Artificial Eye

Following enucleation, evisceration, or secondary orbital implant surgery, an acrylic (polymethyl methacrylate) conformer is placed in the conjunctival fornices to maintain the conjunctival space during the early postoperative healing phase. An anophthalmic socket without a conformer may be at risk for contraction, potentially compromising placement of an adequately sized prosthesis. The conformer is replaced with a custom-made ocular prosthesis typically fashioned in 6–8 weeks following socket surgery. Prefabricated or "stock eyes" (still used in underdeveloped countries) are unsatisfactory as they are generally not cosmetically optimal, limit motility, may trap secretions between the socket and prosthesis, and may not position well in the socket resulting in rotation and extrusion (Fig. 60.1d). The ideal prosthetic eye is custom fit to the dimensions of the conjunctival fornices of each individual patient using the "modified impression technique" [17]. An impression of the socket is taken in a similar fashion to that used in fitting dentures. The initial impression is made of a paste-like material composed of highly refined alginate mixed with water [17]. Once the impression material sets to a firm consistency, the shape is copied into a wax mold. A prepared iris-cornea piece is polished on the front surface of the wax pattern. The wax mold is placed into the socket and reshaped for comfort and to improve cosmesis. The wax shape is then changed (using additional molds) into fine-quality acrylic (from methyl methacrylate resin) painted, cured, and polished. The patient's remaining eye is used as a template to match the size and shape of the pupil, iris color, as well as superficial vascular network on the sclera, episcleral, and conjunctiva [17].

The time required for an individual patient to get used to the prosthetic eye is variable [18]. Some will be accustomed to it in a matter of hours; others may require days to weeks, and a few never adjust comfortably. Ideally the prosthetic eye should not be removed from the socket unless a foreign body (e.g., eyelash) is being removed or the prosthesis is being professionally cleaned or adjusted. If the artificial eye is left out while sleeping or for other reasons, it should be stored in soft contact lens saline solution. If the prosthesis is allowed to remain dry, the painted layers may separate and degrade.

Pine et al. have recently proposed a three-phase model that describes the response of the socket microenvironment to prosthetic eye wear [19–23]. The three phases include an "initial phase" of wear of a new (or recently polished) prosthesis when homeostasis is being established (or reestablished) within the socket (conjunctival mucous coating of the prosthesis and tear balance); a second homeostatic phase, the "equilibrium phase" when beneficial surface deposits that

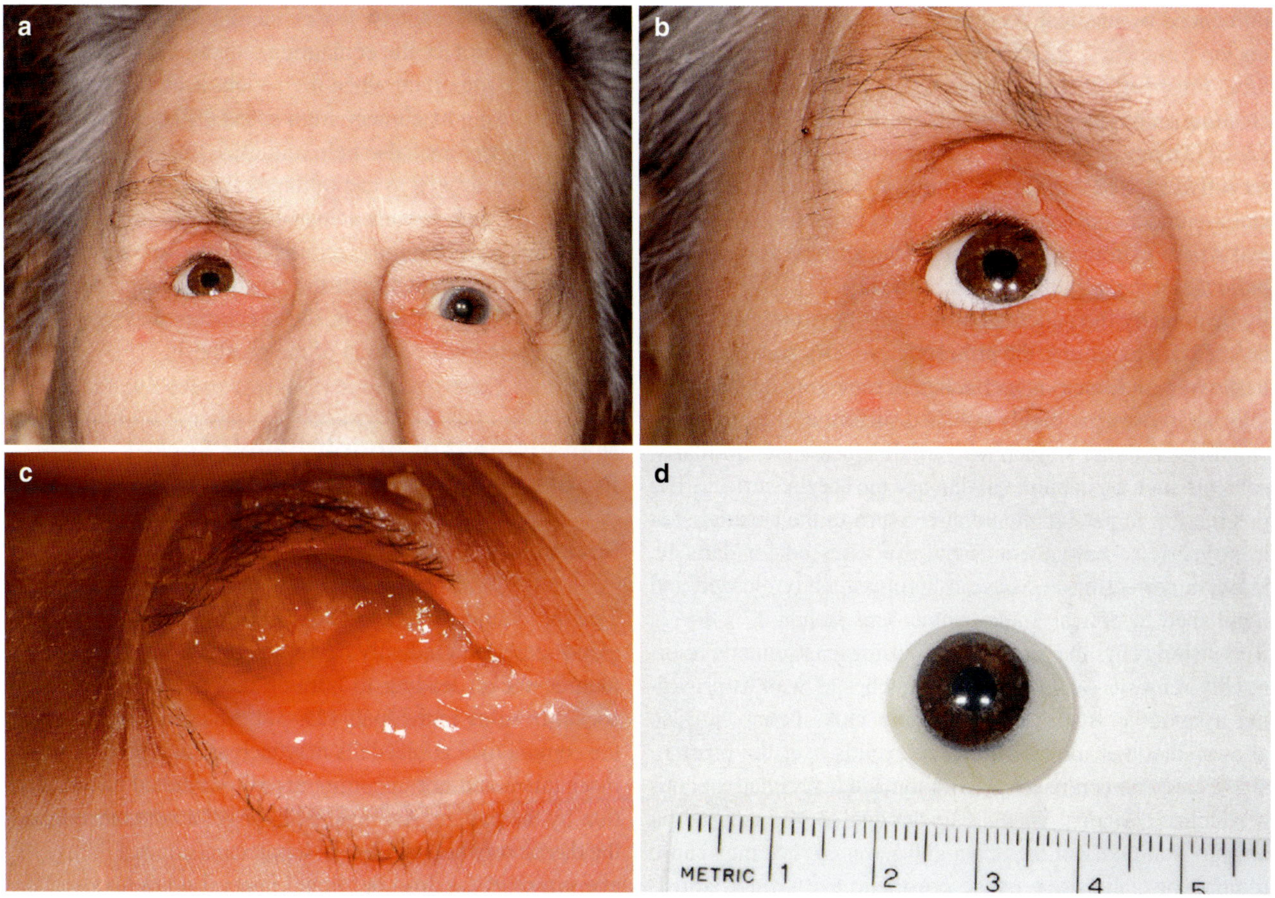

Fig. 60.1 An 80-year-old female presented with difficulty wearing her prosthesis. The eye had been lost 50 years earlier. Following enucleation without a socket implant, she was fit with a stock eye that had a fairly good color match to the normal eye and felt comfortable. It fit well until the last few years when it would spontaneously fall out. (**a**) The right socket is enophthalmic with a very deep superior sulcus as a result of volume loss. (**b**) The superior edge of the prosthesis is tilted posteriorly, and the inferior edge is pushed up against the lower lid as a result of the rotary migration of the orbital tissue. (**c**) The superior and inferior fornices are shortened, and the inferior fornix shows a bulge as a result of the inferior rectus/oblique muscles migrating forward. (**d**) The stock eye does not have a custom fit and is small and lost its luster. It has not been changed or polished in over 50 years

facilitate wettability of the prosthesis buildup on the prosthesis and wear is comfortable; and a third phase or "breakdown phase" where there is an increasing likelihood of irritation from continued wear. The proposed model also provides a rationale for prosthesis cleaning to help manage non-specific mucoid discharge [19].

The initial phase of wear when physiological homeostasis is being established within the socket is approximately a month [19]. The prosthetic eye then enters an equilibrium phase when a homeostatic period exists, and the artificial eye is comfortable to wear and discharge is minimal - mild. The length of time beyond this homeostatic phase (or equilibrium phase) when the microenvironment starts to break down varies between individuals but is several months (generally 6–12 months) in duration. Artificial eye patients usually know when their equilibrium phase is ending as the artificial eye starts to have increased discharge and some irritation [18]. Frequent removal and manipulation of the artificial eye (e.g., daily or weekly) never allow the artificial eye and socket microenvironment to enter the homeostatic or equilibrium phase when it's comfortable to wear the prosthetic eye. As a result, discharge is often more of a problem [19]. Frequent removal of the artificial eye also roughens the fine polished surface of the prosthesis and may lead to microtrauma of the conjunctiva with resultant socket irritation and discharge.

If the prosthetic eye has to be removed by the patient (e.g., to remove lashes trapped behind it or other foreign bodies), proper cleaning and handling of the prosthetic eye are important. Cleaning (by the patient) approximately every 6 months is also suggested as prosthetic deposits accumulate continuously and after 6 months of wear may be thick enough to irritate the conjunctiva and cause discharge [19–21]. The ideal cleaning regimen for most individuals will also be influenced by medical conditions (e.g., allergies), the wearing environment (e.g., dust, dirt, wind), and the standard surface finish of the prosthesis [19]. Although numerous cleaning techniques have been suggested over the years [18, 24–28] (many of which are contradictory), Pine et al. have recently reported that simply wiping all surfaces of the artificial eye under cool tap water with a wet paper towel is simple and works extremely well to clean the surface deposits that build up on the artificial eye over time [19–21]. This can easily be done by the patient in almost any environment should he/she have to remove the prosthetic eye. Dry paper towel or tissue (e.g., Kleenex) is ineffective in removing deposits and may wear away the highly polished surface of the prosthesis creating a rougher surface with a dull appearance. Similarly, solvents such as alcohol will damage the acrylic surface. The prosthetic eye patient should also return to their ocularist at least yearly to have the artificial eye assessed for damage, reassess correct fit, and have it "professionally cleaned and repolished to optical grade contact lens standard." [19–21] Repolishing by the ocularist's buffing instruments thoroughly removes deposits, microscratches as well as providing a smoother surface that not only looks better but also allows smoother movement of the eyelids over the prosthesis, decreasing conjunctival irritation and associated mucous production. Gradual changes to the eye socket such as fat atrophy and laxity of the upper and lower eyelids may cause rotation or malposition of the prosthetic eye. Minor adjustments in the shape or thickness of the artificial eye may provide the patient with a more comfortable fit and improve cosmesis [19]. Yearly checkups with an ophthalmologist allows assessment for post-enucleation socket syndrome or other complications (e.g., implant exposure) that are easier to repair if identified early.

Living with a Prosthetic Eye

It is important for prosthetic eye patients to avoid focusing on the presence of their prosthesis. An unhealthy level of self-consciousness can lead to chronic anxiety [3–7]. The ocularist and ophthalmologist have a critical role in helping the patient to cope with their disability by keeping a natural-appearing prosthetic eye and comfortable socket. The patient's primary care physician and or psychologist/psychiatrist may also play a role in helping the monocular patient adjust to life with an artificial eye [6, 7].

All ocular prostheses inherently have some limited motility. It is beneficial for patients to learn to turn their head and shoulders in the direction of gaze to maintain primary ocular gaze and minimize ocular asymmetries present with horizontal and/or vertical gaze. Facial expressions, such as smiling, animate the periorbital muscles and distract attention from the artificial eye [7].

Polycarbonate safety lenses should be worn whenever possible to protect the remaining, functioning eye. This is particularly important when the patient is involved in sports activities, using machinery, high-speed drills, etc. Spectacles with a light tint may also help minimize imperfections in the artificial eye, as well as camouflage asymmetries of the superior sulcus and eyelids. Cosmetic optics, involving plus (magnification) or minus (minification) lenses, are useful in altering the apparent size of the prosthesis and palpebral fissure. In addition, prisms in the spectacles may be used to alter the perceived position of the prosthesis.

Management of Anophthalmic Socket Problems

Socket Dryness

Tear production (basic and reflex) as well as meibomian gland secretion gradually decreases over time in the anophthalmic socket leading to burning and irritation within the socket in some individuals [29–31]. Mucous secretion from the conjunctival goblet cells may increase as a compensatory mechanism and not uncommonly is interpreted as an infection by the patient. Artificial tears or gel applied throughout the day is very helpful. If tear supplements do not relieve dry eye symptoms, a drop of "light" mineral oil (a laxative purchased at any pharmacy) can be used on the artificial eye surface to allow the eyelids to glide smoothly over the prosthesis. Topical silicone oil (e.g., Sil-Ophtho – Stony Brook, Inc., Davenport, Iowa) may also be used and is often available through ocularists' offices.

Discharge and Irritation

Mucoid discharge with prosthetic eye wear often develops to some degree with time and can be a distressing condition that affects the quality of life of people who have lost an eye [19–22, 27, 28]. Alterations in tear production following enucleation or evisceration and the presence of a foreign body (the artificial eye) stimulate mucous secretion from the conjunctival goblet cells (see earlier) simulating infection. Frequent handling of the prosthesis may retard the normal prosthesis socket microenvironment development and also result in damage to the highly polished prosthetic surface [19, 20]. Similarly, a prosthesis older than 5 years may develop an irregular surface leading to further mucous production. A poorly fit prosthetic eye may also have a sizeable dead space between the posterior surface of the prosthesis and the conjunctiva where mucoid debris (i.e., stagnant tears, dust particles, eyelashes) often accumulates giving the patient the impression they have a socket infection [32–34].

When assessing the prosthetic eye patient with discharge, it is important for the physician to determine the age of the prosthesis and the patient's routine of prosthetic hygiene. Minimizing handling of the prosthesis should be encouraged. Prosthesis irregularities (e.g., nicks, scratches) and poor surface quality (loss of luster) are usually obvious at the slit lamp or when the prosthesis is taken out to assess the eye socket (Fig. 60.1d). Lubrication of the prosthesis should be evaluated as socket dryness with burning is not uncommon and artificial tear gels or other lubricants can be suggested. Frequency of ocularist's visits should be determined, and appropriate intervals of ocularist care encouraged. The ocularist will evaluate the surface of the prosthesis for nicks and scratches as well as assess the fit of the artificial eye, being sure it is the appropriate size and that there is no dead space between the prosthesis and orbital implant where mucous and other debris can accumulate. Most patients require annual polishing of the prosthesis, but some sockets require semiannual polishing of the artificial eye to smooth the surface and remove the protein deposits. The average life of an artificial eye is typically 5–7 years but varies from socket to socket and is impacted by the frequency and method of a patient's socket hygiene routine. If discharge is still a problem after assessment by the ophthalmologist and ocularist, then treatment with a mild corticosteroid drop (i.e, fluorometholone (FML)) or a combined antibiotic/steroid drop (e.g., tobramycin- dexamethasone) once or twice daily often diminishes the discharge.

When more excessive discharge is present, a conjunctival infection (viral or bacterial) should be considered. Usually there are accompanying signs of acute or chronic conjunctivitis including edematous eyelids, conjunctival chemosis, hyperemia, and mucopurulent discharge in the conjunctival fornices. Conjunctival cultures are helpful in guiding appropriate antibiotic treatment of bacterial infections.

There is also a subset of anophthalmic patients that have an exceptionally deep superior fornix, chronic conjunctival discharge, and ptosis [34]. The deep fornix and low-grade conjunctival inflammation lead to buildup of a protein exudate that becomes colonized by bacteria leading to recurrent discharge [33, 34]. Rose described this "giant fornix syndrome" and suggested a cycle of progressively worsening symptoms that may not be responsive to frequent topical and or systemic antibiotics [33, 34]. Jones et al. proposed eliminating the potential space harboring the chronic mucopurulent coagulum by shortening the fornix and concomitantly repairing the ptosis through a posterior surgical approach [34]. The superior conjunctivoplasty-Mullerectomy procedure resulted in significant improvement in their patients' chronic socket discharge [34].

A pyogenic granuloma may also be the cause of recurrent or chronic socket discharge. Intermittent bleeding is often reported, and these vascular lesions are typically present along the conjunctival closure site or around an implant peg (Fig. 60.17b). Pyogenic granulomas are a sign of local irritation or microtrauma and may also indicate an underlying implant exposure and/or infection [34, 35].

Recurrent and chronic socket discharge is also a distinguishing feature of giant papillary conjunctivitis or "GPC" [36, 37]. The etiology of GPC is not fully understood but is believed to be an immunologic reaction to an antigen present on the surface of the prosthesis. Giant papillae (>1 mm) on the tarsal conjunctiva of the upper eyelid is the hallmark of GPC (Fig. 60.2a, b). In severe cases, GPC may significantly limit the amount of time the patient can wear the prosthesis. Treatment can be difficult and may involve corticosteroid eye drops in conjunction with allergy drops. Topical cyclosporine eye drops or tacrolimus 0.03% ointment may also be helpful [38–40]. In recalcitrant cases, carbon dioxide laser or cryoablation of the giant papillae can be attempted. Rarely, a prosthesis made of a different material (e.g., glass) may be considered.

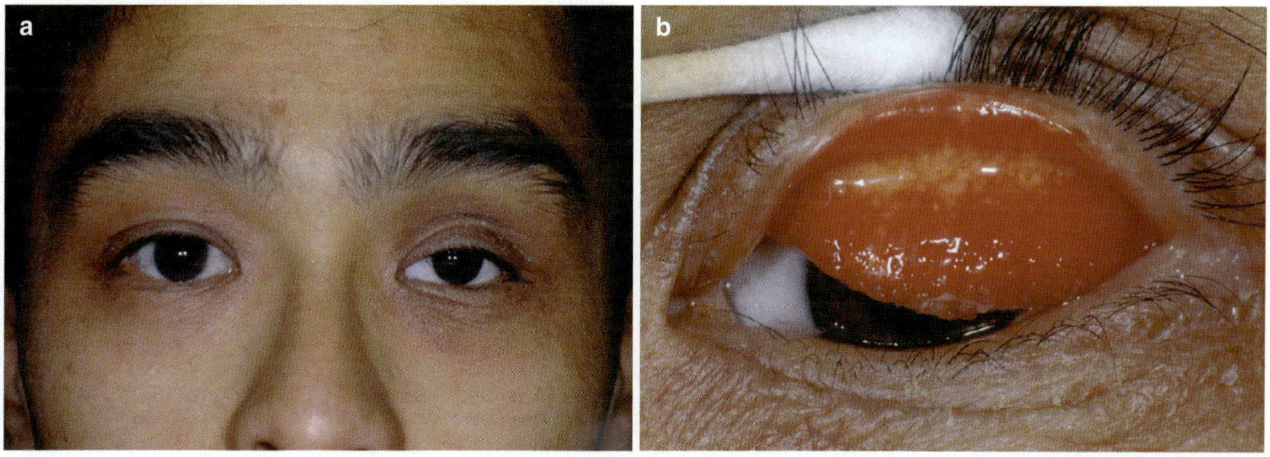

Fig. 60.2 (**a**) A 30-year-old male with a 5-year history of wearing an artificial eye presented with recurrent discharge and droopy left upper lid. (**b**) When the eyelid was everted, giant cobblestones typical of giant papillary conjunctivitis were seen along the tarsal plate

Lagophthalmos with Exposure of the Prosthesis Surface

Some individuals with nocturnal lagophthalmos may develop unsightly dried matter on the anterior surface of the prosthesis that results in the eyelid margin and/or lashes adhering to the anterior surface of the prosthesis. As the eyelid attempts to open upon awakening, it is pulled away from the prosthesis surface causing discomfort and irritation and contributing to conjunctival inflammation. Sometimes the debris can be cleaned without removing the prosthesis by rinsing the surface of the prosthetic eye with a soft contact lens irrigating solution or several drops of an artificial tear drop. If this is not successful, the artificial eye can be removed from the socket, and the debris wiped off the artificial eye surface under cool tap water using a wet paper towel [19–21]. Light mineral oil or a lubricating eye ointment (e.g., Lacri-lube) can be used at bedtime on the anterior surface of the prosthesis if debris buildup and eyelid sticking are a chronic problem.

Socket Pain

Pain and discomfort in the anophthalmic socket are uncommon but may range from mild to severe with resulting effects on daily life [37, 41–48]. A wide variety of problems can cause socket pain and discomfort, most of which can be diagnosed through a careful history and clinical examination of the prosthesis and eye socket (Table 60.1). Prosthetic care and handling should be assessed as well as the fit of the artificial eye. The socket implant should be evaluated for signs of migration and the conjunctiva for signs of inflammation, infection, or implant exposure. Migration of the implant may alter the fit of the prosthesis creating pressure on the tissue between the implant and prosthesis. Trochlear inflammation and pain (radiating along the superior orbital rim or into eye socket) secondary to the prosthetic edge hitting the trochlear area on a recurrent basis is also a consideration [42]. Palpation of the trochlea recreates the discomfort experienced by the patient. Triamcinolone injection (0.3–0.4 ml of 40 mg/ml vial) into the peritrochlear area may be very effective in resolving this type of discomfort. If an evisceration was performed, recurrent scleritis or postherpetic neuralgia is an uncommon cause of recurrent socket pain to consider. Patients with healthy-appearing sockets may be more challenging and rare etiologies (e.g., phantom eye pain, drug-seeking behavior, secondary gain, factitious) should be considered [2, 36, 48]. Persistent socket pain warrants neuroimaging (computerized tomography, magnetic resonance imaging) of the orbit, paranasal sinus, and brainstem to rule out an amputation neuroma, sinus infection or mass, or an intraorbital or central nervous system abnormality [2].

Table 60.1 Causes of socket pain

Eyelid malpositions
Entropion, ectropion, incomplete eyelid closure,
Conjunctival problems
Pyogenic granulomas, conjunctival inclusion cysts, giant papillary conjunctivitis, neoplasia (squamous cell),
Prosthesis issues
Poor fit, prosthetic surface breakdown, nicks, scratches, deposits, allergic reaction to the ocular prosthesis,
Implant problems
Infection, inflammation, migration, exposure,
Socket problems
Recurrent or new malignancy, amputation neuroma, trochleitis, scleritis (post-evisceration cases), socket contraction,
Lacrimal gland
Dry socket,
Referred pain from adjacent areas
Skull base/sinus/sphenoid wing tumors, postherpetic neuralgia,
Other
Complex regional pain syndrome, phantom eye pain, drug-seeking behavior, factitious.

Anterior Orbital Cysts

The development of a subconjunctival/anterior orbital cyst is occasionally seen and may be responsible for socket discomfort (aching, pressure sensation) as well as problems with the fit of a patient's prosthetic eye (Fig. 60.3) [49, 50]. These cysts arise from buried conjunctival epithelium that becomes incarcerated during wound closure. Management options include complete surgical excision of the cyst, marsupialization, absolute alcohol injection, and more recently trichloroacetic acid (TCA) injection [51–56]. Simple aspiration is not an adequate treatment on its own as recurrent cyst formation often occurs shortly after evacuation (days).

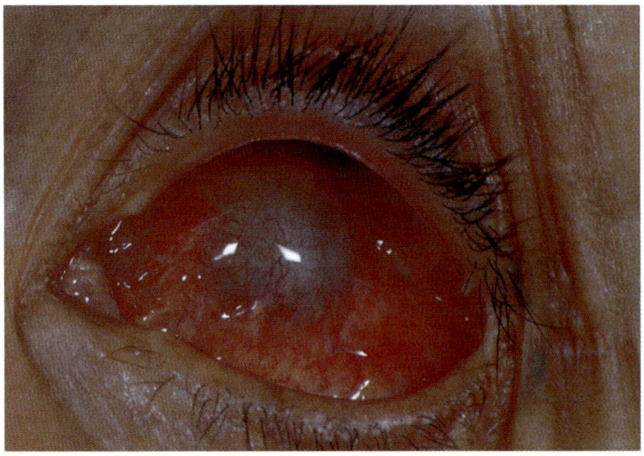

Fig. 60.3 A 60-year-old female presented with a pressure sensation in the left eye socket. Removal of the prosthesis revealed a prominent subconjunctival cyst centrally

Eyelid Malpositions

Lower eyelid laxity is a common problem that occurs with time in many artificial eye patients and results from the aging eyelid supporting the weight of the prosthesis as well as alterations of soft tissue support associated with removal of the eye (anophthalmic socket syndrome) (Fig. 60.1a–d) [10–12]. Lower eyelid laxity can be corrected with a tarsal strip-type procedure [57–59]. Horizontal lid tightening will help maintain the natural contour of the lower eyelid and lateral canthus and provide improved support for the prosthesis without sacrificing conjunctival tissue or inferior fornix volume. Some patients will also develop an inadequate inferior fornix secondary to anterior migration of inferior orbital fat and thinning or disruption of the suspensory ligament of the inferior fornix, resulting in anterior rotation of the lower edge of the prosthesis (Fig. 60.1b) [60–62]. The conjunctiva is not deficient but requires repositioning with suture fixation of the conjunctiva to the orbital rim periosteum to recreate the fornix [62–64].

With significant lid laxity, ectropion of the lower eyelid may develop. This may initially present as an aesthetic issue but eventually leads to difficulties with prosthesis retention. A tarsal strip-type procedure and in some a posterior lamellar spacer graft (e.g., auricular cartilage) may be required [57–60]. Occasionally there is a deficiency of anterior lamella (i.e., the skin) as well, requiring a myocutaneous transposition pedicle flap from the upper eyelid to the lower eyelid. If inadequate adjacent tissue is present for a transposition flap, a full-thickness skin graft may be indicated.

Eyelid margin entropion and vertically directed lashes are common in the anophthalmic patient in both the upper and lower eyelids, often resulting from contracture of the inferior or superior fornix. Fornix contracture as a result of surgery to remove the eye, alkali–/acid-induced scarring, or other trauma to the forniceal tissues and natural contracture of the forniceal conjunctiva over time (especially in those sockets with chronic inflammation or infection) are potential causes of eyelid margin entropion and vertical lashes. Eyelid rotational sutures or a marginal tarsotomy-type procedure can be very effective to rotate the misdirected lashes (Fig. 60.4a, b) [63–67]. More advanced cases may require posterior lamellar lengthening with a spacer graft (e.g., mucous membrane, auricular or nasal cartilage, hard palate mucosa, acellular dermis) (Figs. 60.5a–d and 60.6a–d) [60–62].

Upper eyelid ptosis may result from inadequate implant size, migration of the orbital implant, a poorly fit prosthesis, laxity of the fibrous connective tissue framework in the superior orbit (including Whitnall's ligament) with rotation of the orbital tissues posteriorly and inferiorly (post-enucleation socket syndrome), and trauma from the original injury/surgery or senile dehiscence of the levator aponeurosis [68–70]. The mechanisms producing anophthalmic ptosis are multifactorial and should be assessed carefully before surgical repair to achieve optimal functional and aesthetic results. Ocular prosthesis augmentation (artificial eye with a superior extension or flange) is a conservative nonsurgical method to correct mild anophthalmic upper eyelid ptosis. Levator-Mueller's muscle involutional changes may be corrected with either an anterior or posterior approach (Figs. 60.7a, b, 60.8a, b, and 60.9a, b) [70]. A superior conjunctivoplasty-Mullerectomy has been beneficial in those with an exceptionally deep superior fornix, ptosis, and chronic discharge (giant fornix syndrome) [33, 34].

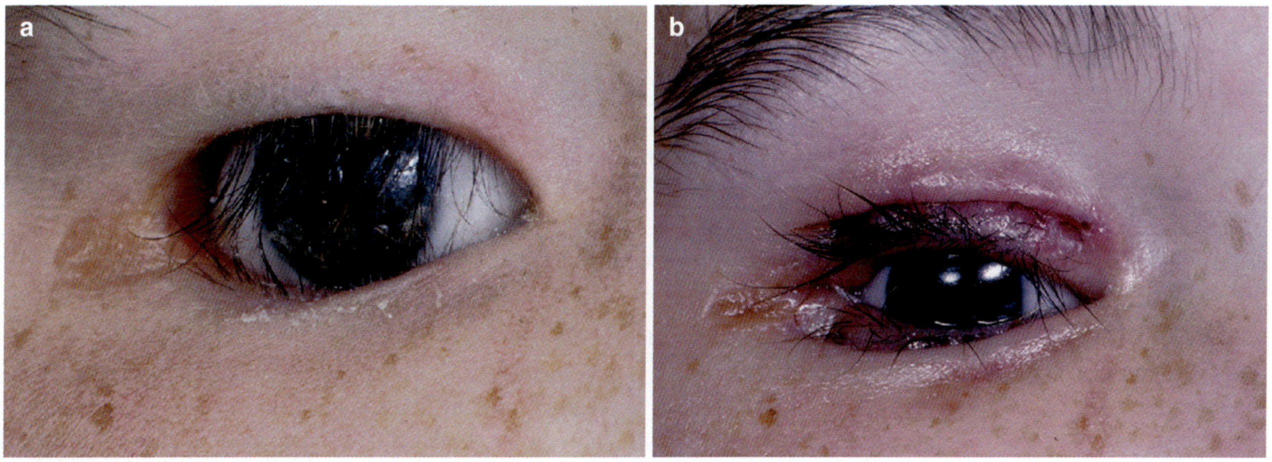

Fig. 60.4 (**a**) Vertically directed upper and lower eyelashes. (**b**) Three weeks post tarsal fracture surgery with lid margin rotation. The eyelashes are in a more normal position

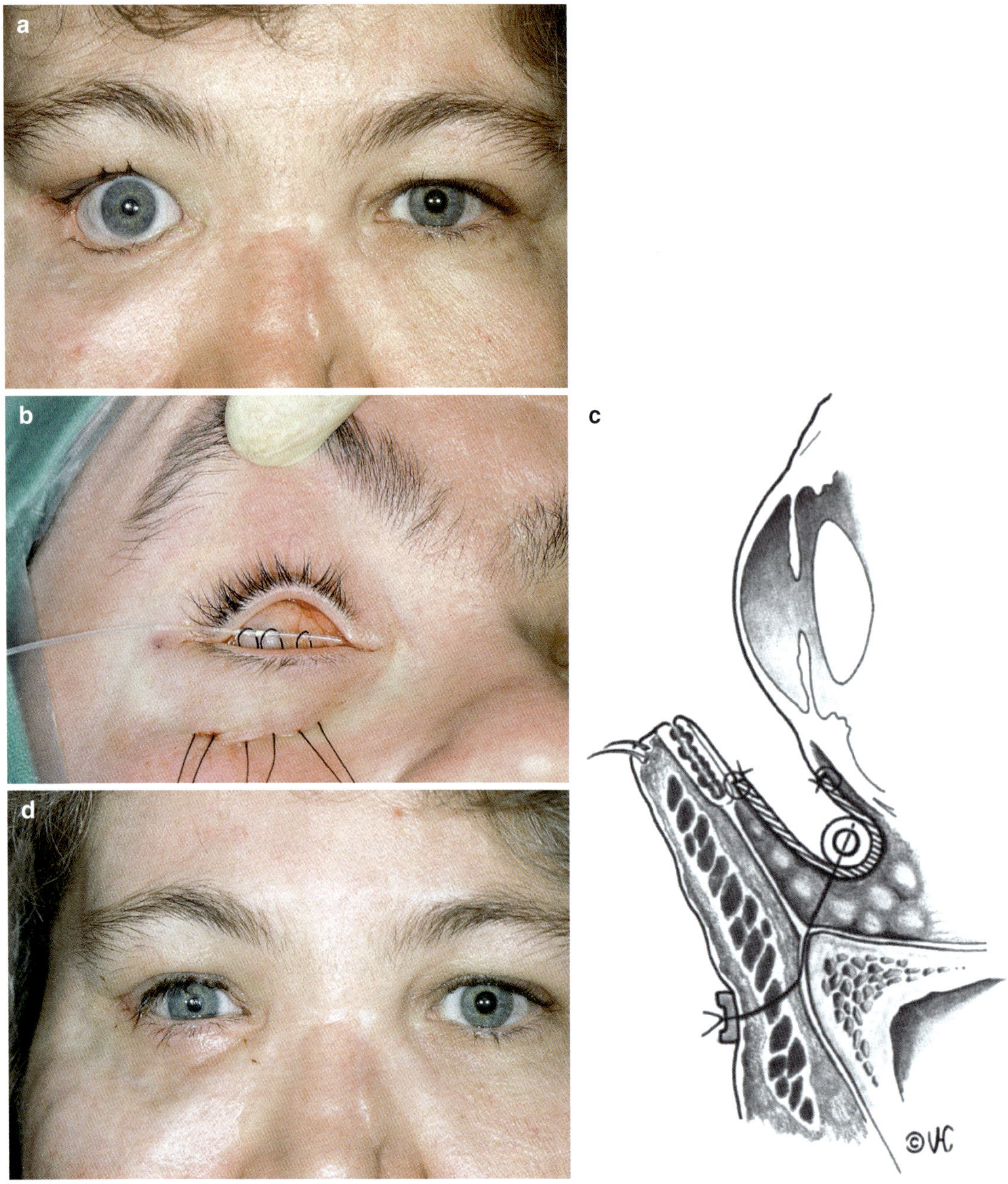

Fig. 60.5 (**a**) A 42-year-old female was seen with inability to retain her prosthetic eye due to a shortened inferior fornix. A mucous membrane graft was harvested from the lower lip with a Castroviejo handheld mucotome seen in Fig. 60.19. (**b**, **c**) The mucous membrane graft was sutured along the inferior tarsal border and remaining forniceal conjunctival edges toward the ball implant. The fornix was reformed with the aid of 4–0 slik sutures tied through a silicone band that was left in place for 4 weeks. (**d**) Three months postoperatively, the patient was able to retain her prosthesis without difficulty. The lower eyelid was in a normal position

Deep Superior Sulcus and Enophthalmos

The socket soft tissue and volume changes that occur following enucleation or evisceration surgery causing upper eyelid ptosis and lower eyelid malposition also contribute to deepening of the superior sulcus [10, 11]. Initially, following enucleation surgery and to a lesser degree after evisceration surgery, there may be an excellent cosmetic result that becomes less satisfactory over time. The implant may shift posteriorly and inferiorly due to the weight of the implant and progressive laxity of the orbital connective tissue framework. Combined with some rotary displacement of the orbital soft tissue from the superior to the posterior and from the posterior to the inferior orbit, the sulcus deepens, and the eye socket appears sunken (enophthalmic) [10, 11]. Inadequate volume replacement (too small an implant or no implant) at the time of the

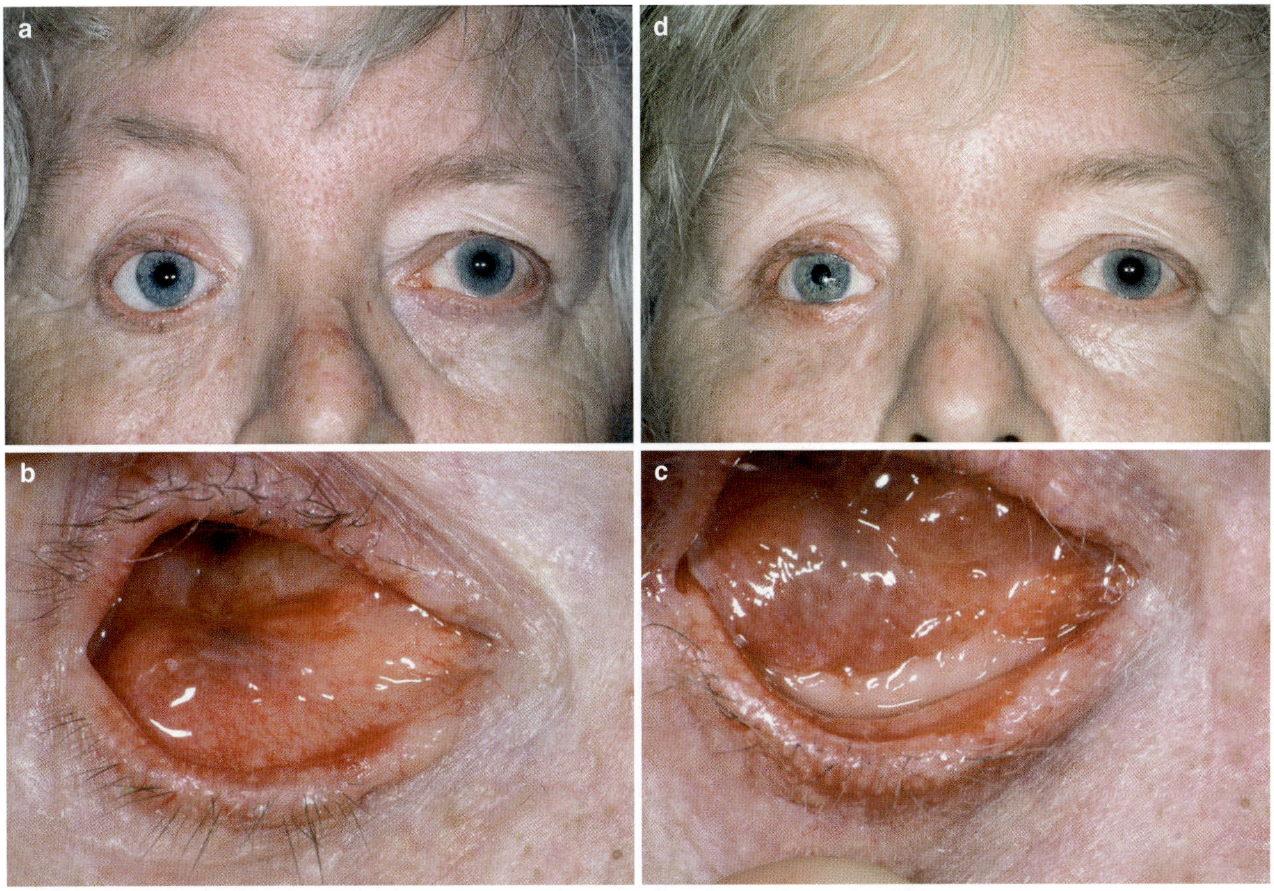

Fig. 60.6 (**a**, **b**) A 64-year-old female was seen with a retracted right lower eyelid as a result of inferior fornix shortening. (**c**) A hard palate graft was placed along the lower edge of tarsus and sutured in place. (**d**) Three months post-surgery, the right lower eyelid is in a much more normal position

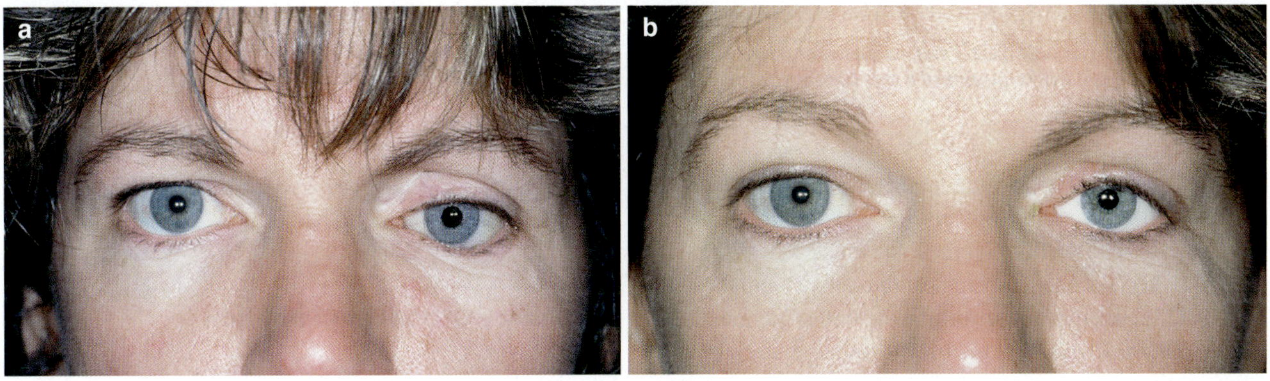

Fig. 60.7 (**a**) A 40-year-old female was seen with ptosis and enophthalmos of the left socket. Since her orbital implant was put in as a child and was rather small, it was elected to put in a larger implant as a first step to restore socket volume followed by an anterior approach levator advancement ptosis correction 3 months later. (**b**) Six months post-surgery, there was much more symmetry present between the two sides

enucleation or evisceration procedure and postsurgical orbital fat atrophy are other important factors in the development of a deep superior sulcus [10, 11, 13–16].

Conservative management of a superior sulcus deformity includes camouflage with lightly tinted spectacles or a weak plus lens (+1 to +2) that adds some magnification and helps make a narrow palpebral fissure appear larger. Alterations in the prosthesis can provide additional eyelid support and volume and help improve eyelid position and fullness. Surgical options include correcting bone defects from old orbital fractures, socket volume restoration (e.g., orbital floor wedge implant), and superior sulcus tissue

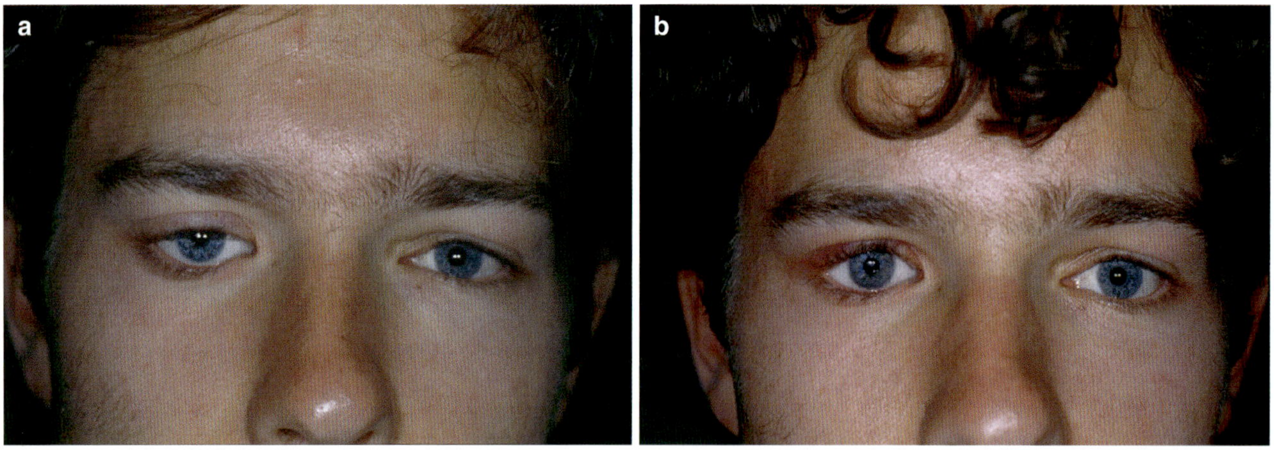

Fig. 60.8 (a) A 20-year-old male is seen with a right upper eyelid ptosis. The socket volume was fine (b). Three months following an anterior approach levator advancement procedure, there is much more symmetry

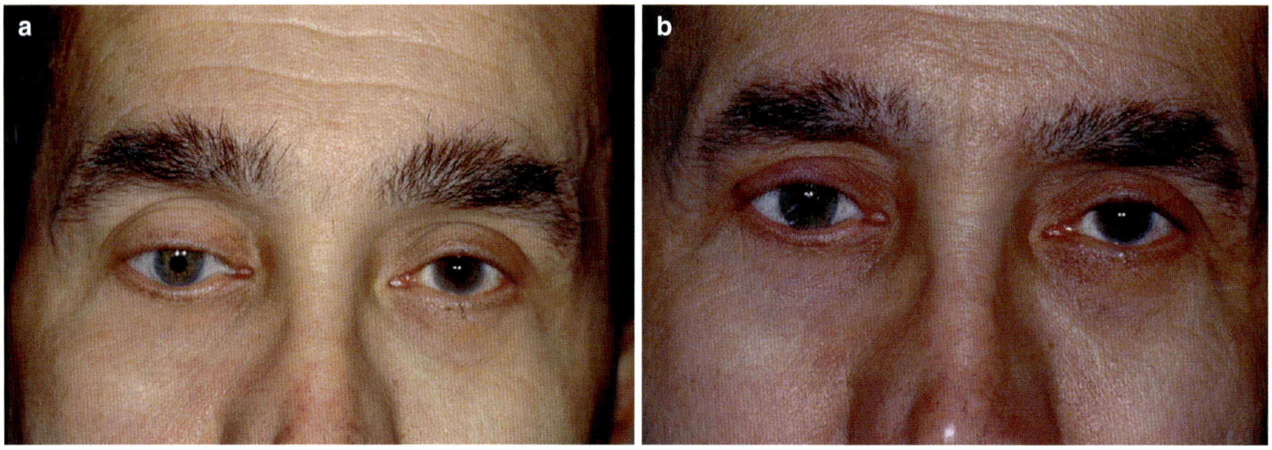

Fig. 60.9 (a) A 55-year-old male is seen with a right upper lid ptosis. The socket volume was fine. (b) Three months post anterior approach levator advancement surgery and fabrication of a new prosthetic eye, there is much more symmetry

grafting (dermis fat grafting or acellular human dermis graft – AlloDerm® – Lifecell Inc., Woodlands, Texas, USA, or DermaMatrix – Synthes, West Chester, PA, USA) [71–73]. Acrylic floor implants (polymethyl methacrylate) are usually adequate for orbital volume augmentation (Figs. 60.10a–c and 60.11a, b), but other materials have been utilized including bone grafts, silicone beads, hydroxyapatite, silicone, teflon, supramid sheets, and dermis fat as well as a variety of injectable products such as autogenous fat, injectable hydroxylapatite (Radiesse), cross-linked collagen, silicone oil, self-inflating hydrogel pellet expanders, and hard tissue replacement polymer [74–79]. Soft tissue fillers (e.g., hyaluronic acid-derived products) are a recent alternative to correct superior sulcus volume loss in the anophthalmic socket [29]. Some anophthalmic patients with deep superior sulci, enophthalmos, as well as various eyelid malpositions will require more than one surgical procedure to restore acceptable symmetry (Figs. 60.12a, b, 60.13a–d, and 60.14a–g).

Secondary Orbital Implantation

Enophthalmos may occur from fat atrophy secondary to orbital soft tissue changes following enucleation or evisceration, inadequate implant volume replacement, or implant extrusion. Insertion of a secondary intraconal orbital implant is a consideration to correct the enophthalmos and superior sulcus depression (Fig. 60.7a, b). Secondary orbital implantation may also be indicated to improve prosthesis motility or when implant exposure or migration has resulted in prosthetic fitting difficulties [80–85].

Secondary orbital implant surgery is often more complicated than enucleation or evisceration principally due to the

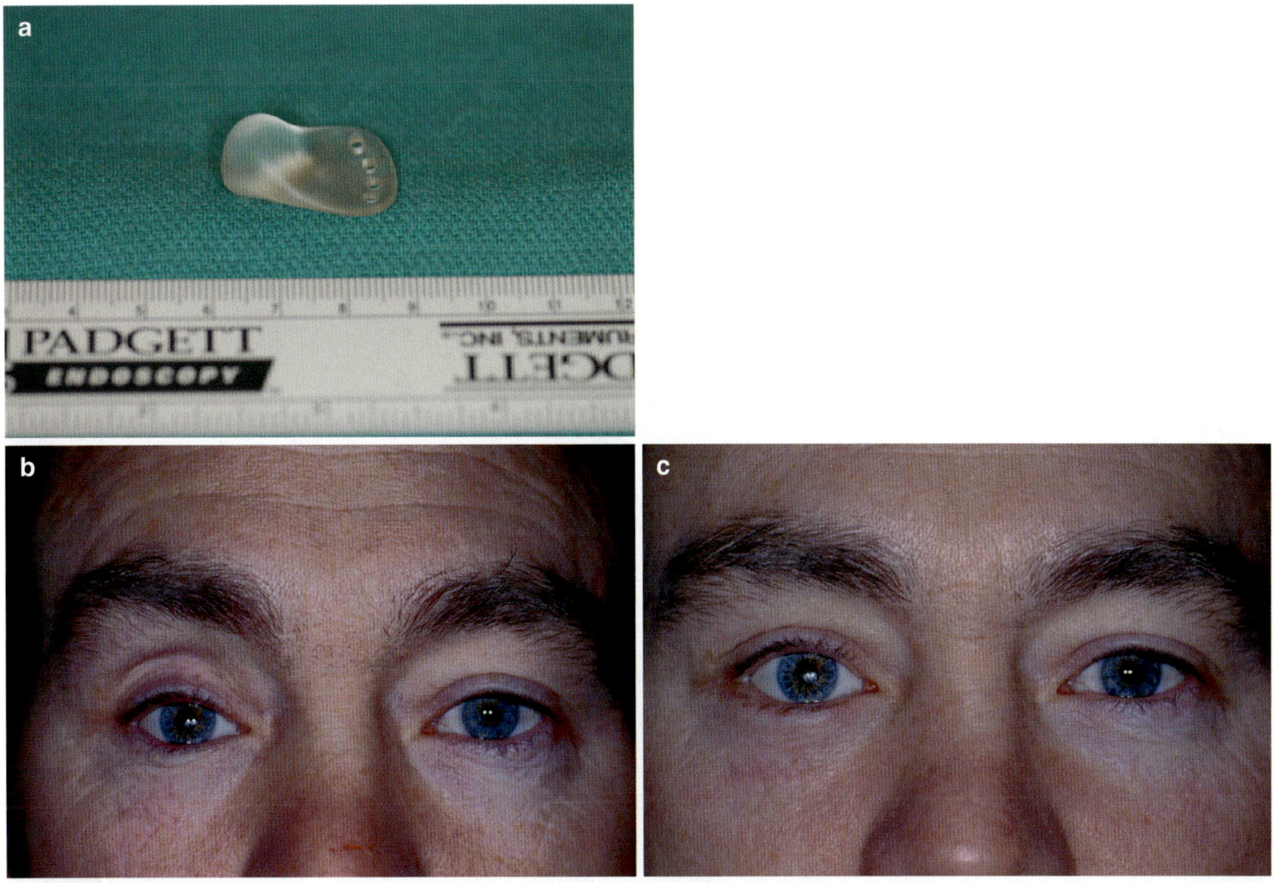

Fig. 60.10 (**a**) A subperiosteal floor implant ("Coderre implant," Oculo-Plastik, Inc., Montreal, Quebec). (**b**) A 35-year-old male presented 1-year post evisceration with a deep superior sulcus on the right side. (**c**) Three months post orbital floor implant, there was excellent symmetry

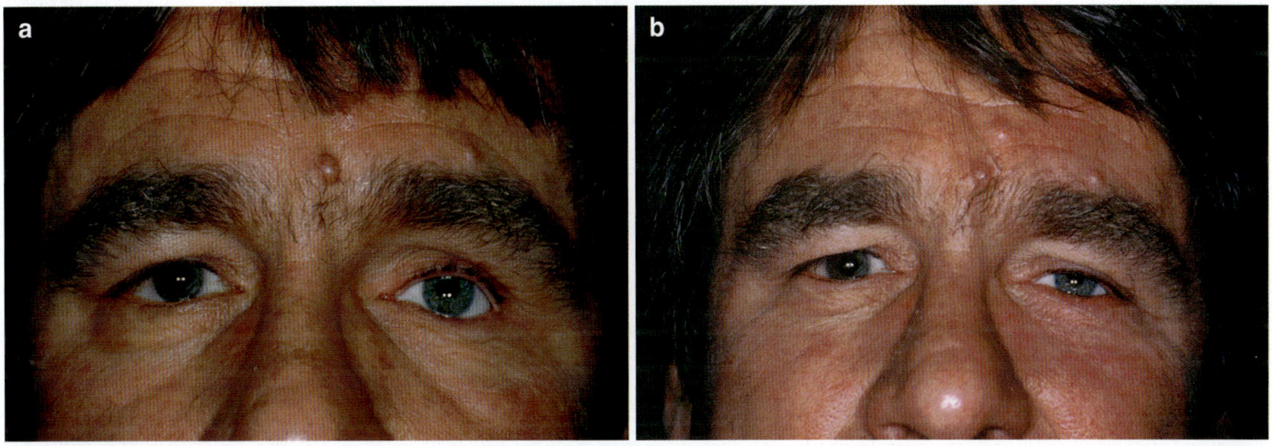

Fig. 60.11 (**a**) A 49-year-old male presented 3 years postenucleation with a deep superior sulcus. (**b**) Three months post orbital floor implant, there was excellent symmetry

disruption of anatomic planes with disorganization of the orbital tissues. In addition, varying degrees of fibrosis are often present throughout the orbital tissue as a result of the initial trauma or primary anophthalmic socket procedure. A variety of techniques for secondary orbital implantation have been described [80–84]. While secondary orbital implantation can be carried out without attempting to identify the rectus muscles, localization of the rectus muscles will typically help reposition the implant in a more anatomically correct position and improve socket motility [84].

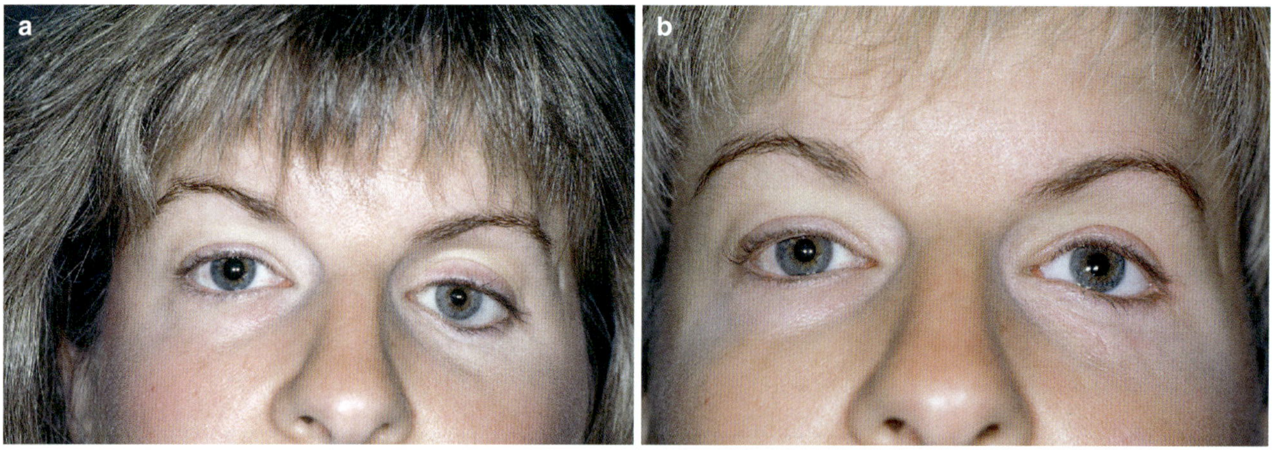

Fig. 60.12 Socket volume restoration, ptosis surgery, and lower lid retraction surgery. (**a**) A 35-year-old female was seen for assessment of enophthalmos, left lower lid retraction, and left upper eyelid ptosis. (**b**) An orbital floor implant was put in place first (Fig. 60.10a) followed in 3 months by a hard palate graft to the left inferior fornix, followed in 23 months by an anterior approach levator advancement procedure. (**b**) Four months following her last surgery and an adjustment to her artificial eye was happy with the symmetry between the two sides

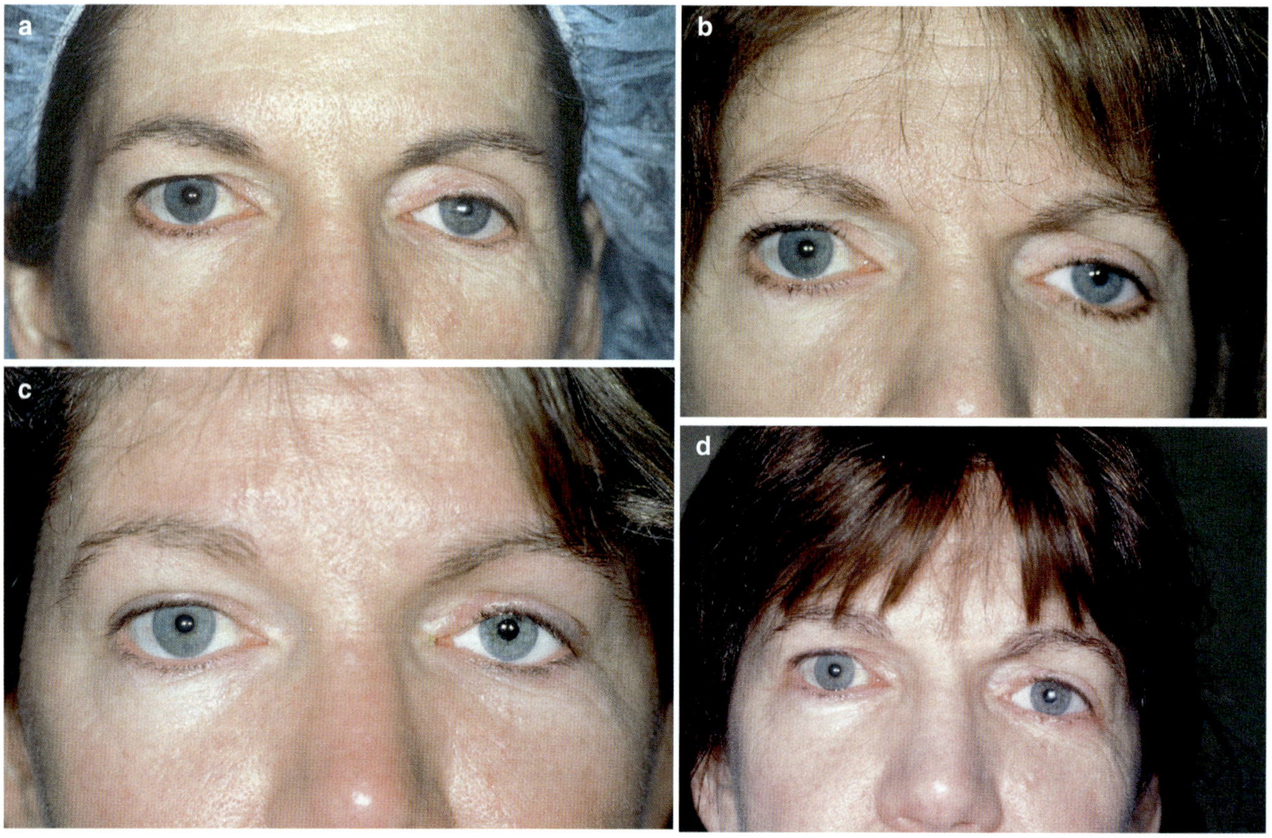

Fig. 60.13 (**a**) Same patient as Fig. 60.7 presented 7 years later with additional enophthalmos. An orbital floor implant (Fig. 60.10a) was suggested to augment the socket volume. (**b**) The patient is seen 3 months following the floor implant with further improvement to the sulcus and symmetry. The lower eyelid was also slightly down, but the patient did not want to correct it. (**c**) She returned 5 years later to have the left lower eyelid raised. An ear cartilage graft was placed in the lower lid. (**d**) Three months following the last surgery as well as a new prosthesis, the left lower eyelid was higher, and there was much more symmetry to the two sides

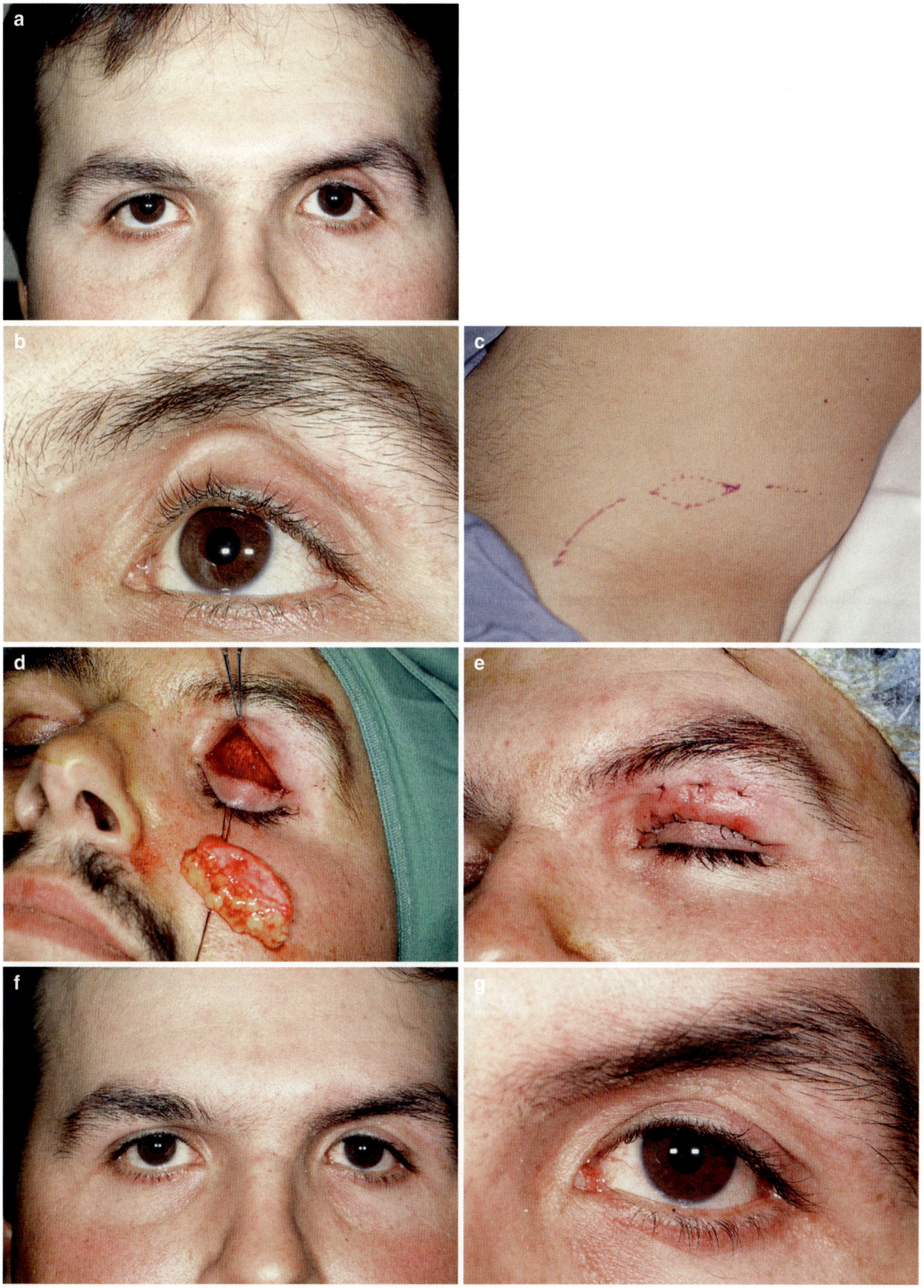

Fig. 60.14 (**a**, **b**) A 40-year-old male was seen with a very deep superior sulcus. A subperiosteal floor implant was considered, but the patient elected to have a dermis fat graft. (**c**, **d**) The dermis fat graft was harvested from the inside of his upper arm. The epithelium was removed, and the graft was placed just anterior to orbital septum and posterior to orbicularis. (**e**) Immediately after the procedure, the fullness to the sulcus is evident. The graft is being held in position with three bolster sutures coming through the skin. (**f**, **g**) Six months postsurgery, the superior sulcus is filled out nicely

Implant Migration

Implant migration may occur with long-standing orbital implants as a result of the progressive orbital soft tissue changes that occur with time in the anophthalmic socket [10, 11]. An early enucleation technique by Frost-Lange involved imbricating the extraocular muscles over unwrapped polymethyl methacrylate (PMMA) or silicone spheres [63]. Muscle imbrication over the anterior surface of a nonporous, non-wrapped alloplastic implant (e.g., polymethyl methacrylate, silicone) was a common practice many years ago and a frequent predisposing factor to "up and out" or "down and in" implant migration over time [85]. It is now well established that this technique leads to implant migration so it has largely been abandoned. Attaching the rectus muscles in their normal anatomic position to nonporous, wrapped spheres (e.g., PMMA, silicone) results in a very low migration rate with implants that are stable over many years. Nonporous alloplastic implants should not simply be placed within the orbit without some type of muscle fixation to stabilize their position.

Porous orbital implants were initially thought to decrease the chance of implant migration, but they also can migrate up and out or down and in. If one also considers anterior implant migration, the rate of implant migration with porous implants may be higher than nonporous implants as this type of migration manifests as implant exposure. These cases are then often grouped with other cases of implant exposure due to a variety of other factors (see below). Anterior migration is most often secondary to improper seating of the porous implant. Porous implants have a rough surface and drag tissue inward as they are placed into the orbit. The overlying tissue may be closed successfully over the implant, but with time, the tissues dragged inward may try to return to their original relaxed position. As this occurs, a gradual migration of the implant anteriorly with progressive conjunctival thinning and eventual tissue breakdown over the anterior implant surface (exposure) occurs. An implant inserter, tissue glide, and/or implant wrap may help avoid the posterior drag of anterior tissue.

A migrated implant may lead to poor motility and an uncomfortable, poorly positioned prosthesis. In mild cases, refitting the prosthesis may help socket motility and comfort. Alternatively, the migrated implant may have to be removed, and a secondary implant centrally positioned within the muscle cone with reattachment of the rectus muscles may be required [80–84].

Implant Exposure and Extrusion

Implant exposure may occur with any type of implant days to years following anophthalmic surgery and may lead to implant infection, extrusion, or explantation (Fig. 60.15a–c). It was anticipated that porous orbital implants would have a lower incidence of implant exposure than traditional nonporous implants because of their associated fibrovascular ingrowth. However, complications gradually became apparent with their widespread use over the past 30 years, and implant exposure is the most concerning problem with reported implant exposure rates ranging from 0% to 50%, causing some surgeons to avoid the use of porous implants [41, 42, 46, 86–113].

Factors predisposing to implant exposure include closing the wound under tension, poor wound closure techniques, infection, mechanical or inflammatory irritation from the spiculated surface of the porous implant, and delayed ingrowth of fibrovascular tissue with subsequent tissue breakdown [109]. Appropriate implant sizing and placement along with proper tissue closure are of primary importance in helping to prevent porous implant exposure [48, 98, 109, 113–115].

A variety of techniques are available to manage implant exposure. For nonporous implants, implant removal and secondary implantation are usually required [84]. For porous implants, management may include wound reclosure early on post-surgery (first few weeks) with or without a patch graft (e.g., sclera, temporalis fascia), vaulting of the prosthesis, and watchful waiting [115]. Persistent and or large implant exposures may require additional surgery. A variety of graft and flap techniques have been advocated to repair implant exposure including Tenon's flaps, bipedicle conjunctival flaps, tarsoconjunctival pedicle flaps, scleral patch grafts, temporalis fascia or fascia lata grafts, hard palate mucosa, or dermis fat grafts as well as other techniques [116–121].

Implant Infection

Infection of porous implants is a rare complication that may be difficult to treat without implant removal [36, 122–126]. Factors predisposing to infection include early conjunctival dehiscence with implant exposure, poor or delayed vascular ingrowth secondary to chronic illness (e.g., diabetes, immunosuppression, vasculopathy), chemotherapy, radiation therapy, prior socket reconstruction, or delayed fibrovascular ingrowth within a host scleral shell with no portals for vascular ingrowth [36]. Initial symptoms and signs are not always indicative of implant infection. Recurrent discharge, for example, may indicate implant infection but is also a common problem for some artificial eye patients without an infectious process. The constellation of socket findings including persistent mucopurulent discharge despite antibiotic coverage, recurrent pyogenic granuloma (indicative of implant exposure), and socket discomfort (aggravated by touching the implant) should raise suspicion for an implant infection (Fig. 60.16a, b) [122, 123]. Recurrent pyogenic

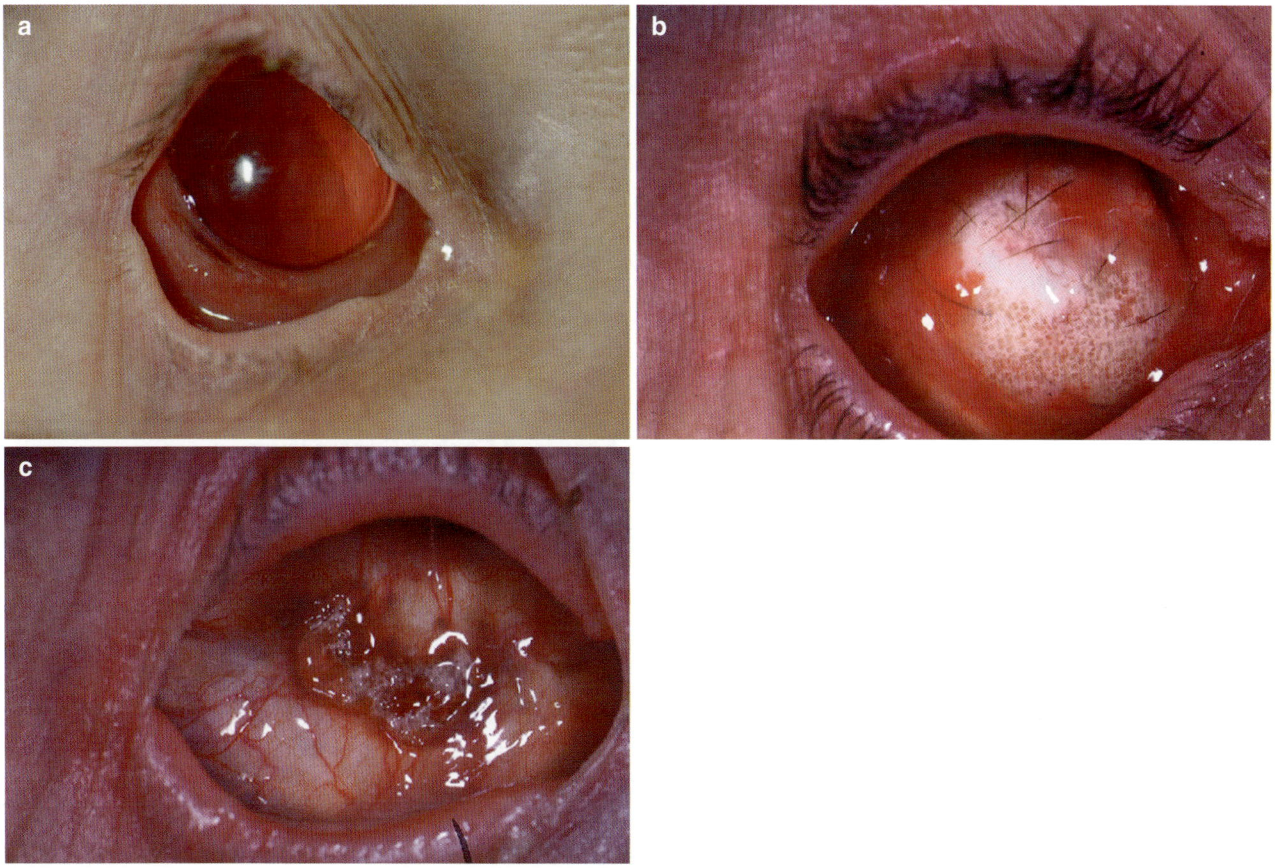

Fig. 60.15 (**a**) Exposed polymethyl methacrylate implant. (**b**) Exposed aluminum oxide orbital implant with multiple hairs on the implant surface. (**c**) Exposed aluminum oxide orbital implant 5 years post evisceration surgery

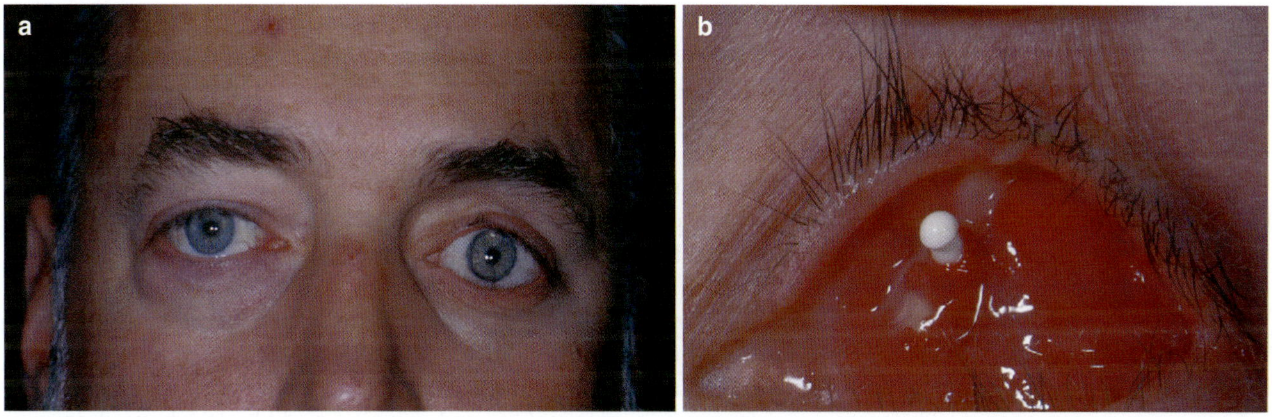

Fig. 60.16 (**a**) A 40-year-old male was seen in consultation 17 years following placement of a hydroxyapatite implant with eye socket discomfort, recurrent purulent/bloody discharge, and pyogenic granulomas. The prosthesis was difficult to retain. A peg had been in position for 15 years. (**b**) The socket revealed the presence of a polycarbonate peg with sleeve, gross inflammation of the entire conjunctiva, as well as a pyogenic granuloma around the peg. In addition, there was almost no superior fornix, and the superior tarsal plate was folded on itself. Implant infection was suspected. Implant removal and placement of dermis fat graft were suggested to help expand the conjunctival space

granulomas are often an indicator of small conjunctival dehiscences with underlying porous implant exposure [36]. These areas of tissue breakdown may allow entry of the causative bacteria before complete implant vascularization occurs (i.e., within the first 6 months following surgery). Alternatively, bacterial colonization of the implant may occur during initial surgical implantation. The eyelid margin is the most likely source of surgical infection, despite air fluid exchange of the implant in an antibiotic solution (e.g., bacitracin 500 units per ml) prior to implant placement. As the bacteria within the implant multiply and migrate to the surface, a conjunctival dehiscence occurs as well as a pyogenic granuloma. Once the infection becomes loculated, the pyogenic granulomas are the likely sites where bacteria migrate from within the implant to the conjunctival surface, explaining the persistent conjunctival inflammatory reaction, despite the topical application of numerous types of antimicrobial drops [36].

Small areas of porous implant exposures should be treated at any time with topical antibiotics and observed closely for signs of implant infection if spontaneous conjunctival wound closure does not occur. Implant infection typically requires implant explantation with the risk of rectus or levator muscle damage or oculomotor nerve injury as well as other socket tissue disruption that may limit subsequent reconstructive options [122–126]. Implant removal is unfortunate as it can be very destructive to the socket tissues, and it eliminates the primary advantage of the porous orbital implant, i.e., the potential for improved implant and prosthesis motility when the prosthesis is coupled to the orbital implant through a peg coupling subsystem.

Complications of Implant Pegging

One of the main advantages of porous orbital implants (e.g., hydroxyapatite, aluminum oxide, porous polyethylene) is the ability to directly integrate them with an overlying artificial eye through a pegging system (Fig. 60.17a). By coupling the orbital implant to the artificial eye via a peg, a wider range of prosthetic eye movements (as well as the fine darting eye movements seen during conversational speech) is possible. More dynamic artificial eye movement imparts a more lifelike quality to the prosthetic eye. Infrared oculography has demonstrated objective and significant improvement in horizontal gaze after motility peg placement [127]. Despite the improved motility, many surgeons and patients elect to avoid peg placement due to the satisfactory results without pegging and the risk of post-pegging complications [128–138].

Potential problems and complications associated with pegging include increased discharge, recurrent pyogenic granulomas, implant exposure around the peg, implant infection, tissue overgrowth, peg dislocation, clicking noises, and various fitting problems (Fig. 60.17b–d) [128–138]. Refitting the prosthesis, scleral patch grafting, peg removal, and at times implant removal may be required [128].

Although pegging has declined dramatically over the past 10 years or more, a precise and meticulous technique under local anesthesia with or without intravenous sedation in the appropriately selected patient can be a successful outpatient procedure [136, 137]. It is important to be selective in deciding which patients are candidates for a peg system. Proper care of the artificial eye and regular follow-up visits with the ocularist and ophthalmic plastic surgeon are important to help ensure minimal problems with the peg system. If the patient is unlikely, unable, or unwilling to maintain the postoperative visits required, then pegging should be avoided. Children under 15 years of age, the elderly (those over approximately 75 years of age), or individuals of any age with a chronic illness or vasculopathy (e.g., a collagen vascular disease, sarcoidosis, diabetes mellitus, immunosuppressive therapy, prior orbital radiation therapy, etc.) should not be considered for pegging in the author's opinion [135].

Acquired Socket Contracture

Acquired socket contracture results from shrinkage and shortening of part or all of the orbital tissues in the anophthalmic orbit, resulting in conjunctival fornices that are inadequate to allow retention of a prosthesis [139, 134]. Socket contracture may occur as a result of several processes including scar tissue associated with the initial injury, poor surgical techniques during previous surgeries (e.g., excessive destruction of conjunctiva, traumatic dissection/cauterization within the socket), multiple socket operations (poor vascular supply), prior ischemic ocular disease, alkali/acid burns, cicatrizing conjunctival diseases, radiation therapy (plaque or external beam), chronic socket inflammation, infection, not wearing a conformer or prosthesis, and a poorly fitting prosthesis.

Prevention is always an important consideration, so during enucleation, evisceration, and orbital trauma surgeries, it is essential to preserve tissue (e.g., conjunctiva), minimize dissection into the fornices, limit cauterization, restore tissues to their anatomic position, and utilize a conformer in the postoperative healing period. It is also important to recognize that each successive surgical procedure may cause further tissue trauma to the socket, with disruption of the already compromised vasculature, resulting in further potential contracture of the socket.

The goal of treatment in socket contracture is to identify and correct the underlying cause(s) (when possible), allow the patient to comfortably wear a prosthesis, and achieve the best motility and cosmesis possible. In advanced cases of socket contracture, success may be limited to the ability of the patient to wear a prosthesis, with motility of the prosthesis and symmetry to the contralateral side secondary considerations. No single surgical technique exists for the treatment of the contracted socket, particularly in advanced cases. The management of each case must be individualized to correct the specific problem of the affected socket. While classification of socket contracture has historically been somewhat complex, it can be simplified by dividing cases into mild, moderate, and severe contracture [139, 140].

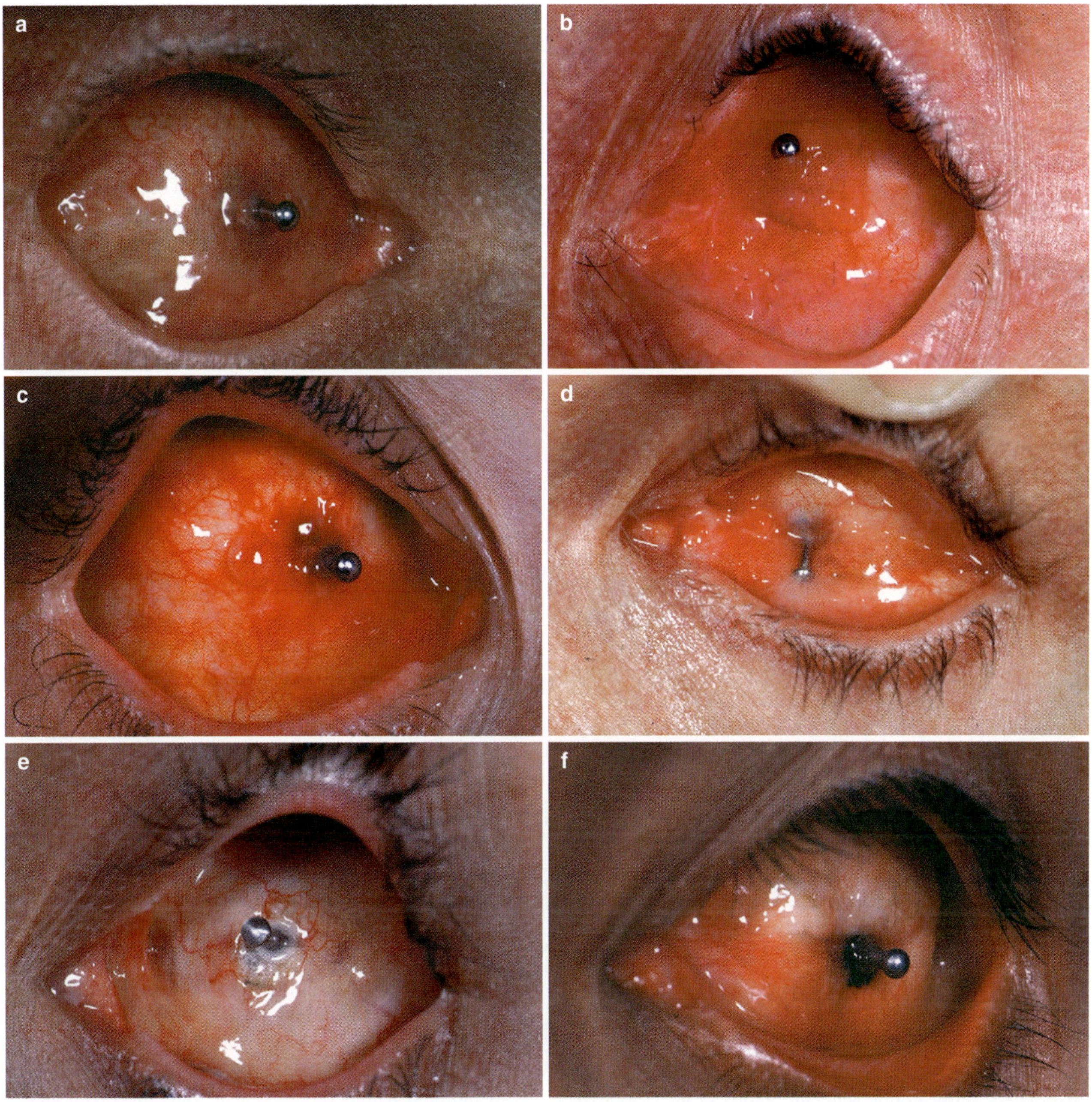

Fig. 60.17 (**a**) A nice looking titanium peg sitting within an aluminum oxide orbital implant. The conjunctiva is well opposed to the peg shaft without any sign of inflammation. (**b**) A large pyogenic granuloma surrounds a titanium peg. (**c**) A smaller pyogenic granuloma sitting just off the temporal side of a titanium peg. (**d**) The severe angulation of this peg makes the coupling with the prosthesis difficult. (**e**) Exposure of the peg sleeve and adjacent aluminum oxide orbital implant. (**f**) Accumulation of a black deposit leached away from the titanium peg is seen in the conjunctiva surrounding the peg

Mild Socket Contracture

Mild socket contracture involves shortening of the posterior lamella (tarsus, conjunctiva) of the upper and/or lower eyelids. It results in vertical lash orientation and marginal eyelid entropion and is generally not associated with significant loss of the fornices. Retaining a prosthesis is not usually a problem. A transverse tarsal incision (tarsotomy) with marginal rotation is the initial treatment of choice as discussed earlier (Fig. 60.6a, b) [65, 66]. If significant horizontal eyelid laxity coexists, the marginal lid rotation (tarsotomy) may be combined with horizontal lid shortening [67]. If these procedures do not correct the marginal lid entropion and vertical lashes, a spacer graft (e.g., hard palate, ear cartilage) may be required to lengthen the posterior lamella of the eyelid (Figs. 60.12b and 60.13c) [60–62].

In some sockets, there may be a decrease or loss of the inferior fornix space while maintaining an adequate amount of conjunctival tissue. This occurs secondary to anterior migration of the inferior orbital fat or thinning/disruption of the suspensory ligament of the inferior fornix [12–16, 60, 62, 67, 141]. The loss of the inferior conjunctival fornix fixation leads to a shallow inferior fornix causing prolapse of the inferior edge of the prosthesis, especially on upgaze, when the soft tissues of the socket shift anteriorly. Often these patients will also have an increase in the horizontal lid laxity of the lower eyelid. A lateral tarsal strip-type procedure combined with fornix reformation/reconstruction using large caliber sutures (2-0, 3-0 polyglactin) passed into the fornix, through the orbital rim periosteum onto the lower eyelid skin where they are either tied directly or over a bolster for 1–3 weeks may help restore adequate volume depth [57, 58, 59, 62, 67, 141].

In those patients with inferior eyelid retraction associated with lower fornix contraction, posterior lamellar lengthening by spacer graft insertion may be required. Homologous, synthetic, and autogenous materials have been advocated as spacers to lengthen the posterior lamella and deepen the inferior fornix [71–73, 142–172]. Homologous materials (e.g., donor sclera) have been used historically but potentially risk infectious disease transmission [165–167]. Although synthetic eyelid implants (e.g., porous polyethylene) initially looked promising, they are associated with a high risk of exposure, extrusion, and infection [144–149]. Many autogenous materials have been suggested such as spacer grafts including the fascia lata, buccal mucosa (Fig. 60.4a–d), nasal cartilage, hard palate (Fig. 60.5a–d), upper eyelid tarsus, and auricular cartilage (Figs. 60.12a, b and 60.13c, d). The fascia lata and buccal mucosa lengthen the posterior lamella but offer little support to the lower eyelid [150–152]. The nasal cartilage and hard palate harvesting prolong surgery time and may be associated with donor site problems [154, 156, 167]. Although upper eyelid tarsus may be useful in correcting retraction of the lower eyelid, the amount of donor tissue is limited and may be insufficient in treating patients with severe fornix contraction. Furthermore, the use of upper eyelid tarsus requires harvesting from the upper eyelid on the affected side or from a healthy eyelid on the contralateral side, potentially resulting in secondary upper eyelid malposition, tarsal kinking, and/or postoperative lagophthalmos [157, 158]. The use of auricular cartilage has several advantages over other autogenous grafts [60, 159–163, 168]. It is an ideal material for lifting the anophthalmic lower lid as it elevates the retracted lower eyelid, lengthens the shortened inferior conjunctival fornix, provides support for the prosthesis, and helps prevent forward migration of the artificial eye (barrier effect) (Fig. 60.13c, d) [60]. Auricular cartilage can be harvested anteriorly from the scaphoid fossa or posteriorly in the area of the helix. Donor site complications may include hemorrhage into the donor space, tenderness/pain secondary to inflammation of the transected cartilage, and occasionally a notch along the helix or a full-thickness auricular defect secondary to tissue necrosis. Unlike the cartilage obtained from the scaphoid fossa area, the cartilage obtained from the helix has a flatter surface in most patients. In either case, it is often necessary to trim the cartilage and score it with partial-thickness incisions (perpendicular to the direction of desired contour) in order to obtain an appropriately contoured piece that will fit. If an excessively ridged or curved piece is placed into the eyelid, it may be unacceptably visible and/or palpable. Two millimeters of cartilage graft for each millimeter of eyelid retraction is generally adequate for correction of the lower eyelid malposition.

Moderate Socket Contracture

Moderate socket contracture involves a more significant contracture and loss of tissue in the inferior and/or superior conjunctival fornix. Inferior fornix contracture is more common than superior fornix contracture. Superior fornix reconstruction techniques are similar to those in inferior fornix reconstruction; however, great care should be taken while dissecting superiorly to avoid injury to the levator complex. The superior fornix may undergo more contraction than the inferior fornix before a significant cosmetic deformity and prosthetic retention issue is produced. A shallow superior fornix will still retain a prosthesis in position; however, eyelid excursions and eyelid closure may be limited by the depth of the superior fornix. With moderate loss of inferior fornix depth, posterior rotation of the superior edge of the prosthetic eye with anterior rotation of the inferior edge allows the prosthesis to easily extrude, even with minimal eyelid movement or touching of the eyelid (Fig. 60.1a–d).

The goal of treatment in the moderately contracted eye socket is to enable the patient to comfortably wear a prosthesis with reasonably good cosmetic appearance. Prosthetic eye motility is often limited even with good operative results. The patient should be counseled regarding reasonable expectations, and that additional surgical procedures may be required. Significant contracture and loss of conjunctival surface area usually require a tissue grafting procedure. Amniotic membrane when tissue loss is mild or mucous membrane grafting (MMG) when more significant amounts of tissue are required are the most common tissues used for moderately contracted fornices [151, 152, 173–178]. Other suggested tissues have included dermis fat grafts [179–181], skin grafts [182, 183], and forearm free flaps [184–190]. Skin grafts are not ideal as they lack moisture, have a rough surface, and contain eccrine/apocrine/sebaceous glands and a keratinized epithelial surface that continues to turnover and slough; all contributing to a foul odor with increased socket discharge. In addition, shrinkage of the skin grafts may require repeated surgical intervention over time to maintain adequate forniceal volume needed for prosthetic retention [191].

In moderate socket contraction, mucous membrane transplantation remains the gold standard [152, 174–178]. Oral mucosa from the buccal area or the mucous membrane part of the lower lip is preferred and may be obtained either freehand or with a mucotome (e.g., Castroviejo dermatome) (Fig. 60.18a–c). Partial-thickness mucous membrane grafts are preferable as they are thinner and a closer match to the lost conjunctival tissue. The ideal thickness is 0.4–0.6 mm. Care is required to avoid the lip margin, gums, and opening of the parotid duct (Stenson's duct) adjacent to the second molar tooth. The fat and muscle layers of the oral mucosa should not be violated. Any submucosal tissue is removed from the graft. Grafts should be about 40–50% larger than the anticipated host defect to allow for anticipated graft contracture following implantation. Mucosal grafts are secured to the recipient conjunctiva with absorbable sutures at the graft edges followed by placement of a large conformer to secure the graft against the underlying vascularized socket tissue. Quilting sutures applied to the center of the graft will ensure better apposition with the recipient bed [192–194]. The donor area on the inside of the cheek is closed with a 4–0 chromic suture, while any mucosa harvested from inside the lip is left to heal by secondary intention. Once the mucous membrane graft is sutured in place and a conformer has been inserted, it is essential to place the tissue within the socket on stretch. Two or three temporary horizontal mattress tarsorrhaphy sutures (i.e., 4–0 silk) are placed across the upper and lower eyelids using a red rubber catheter or cotton bolster to limit skin erosion. The tarsorrhaphy sutures should be left in place for 4–5 weeks or as long as they maintain adequate tension. In a socket that has undergone prior irradiation, chemical or thermal injury, or extensive trauma, the tarsorrhaphy is left in place longer than 4 weeks. If the sutures loosen or erode through the eyelid, the tarsorrhaphy may need to be replaced to ensure adequate eyelid closure and

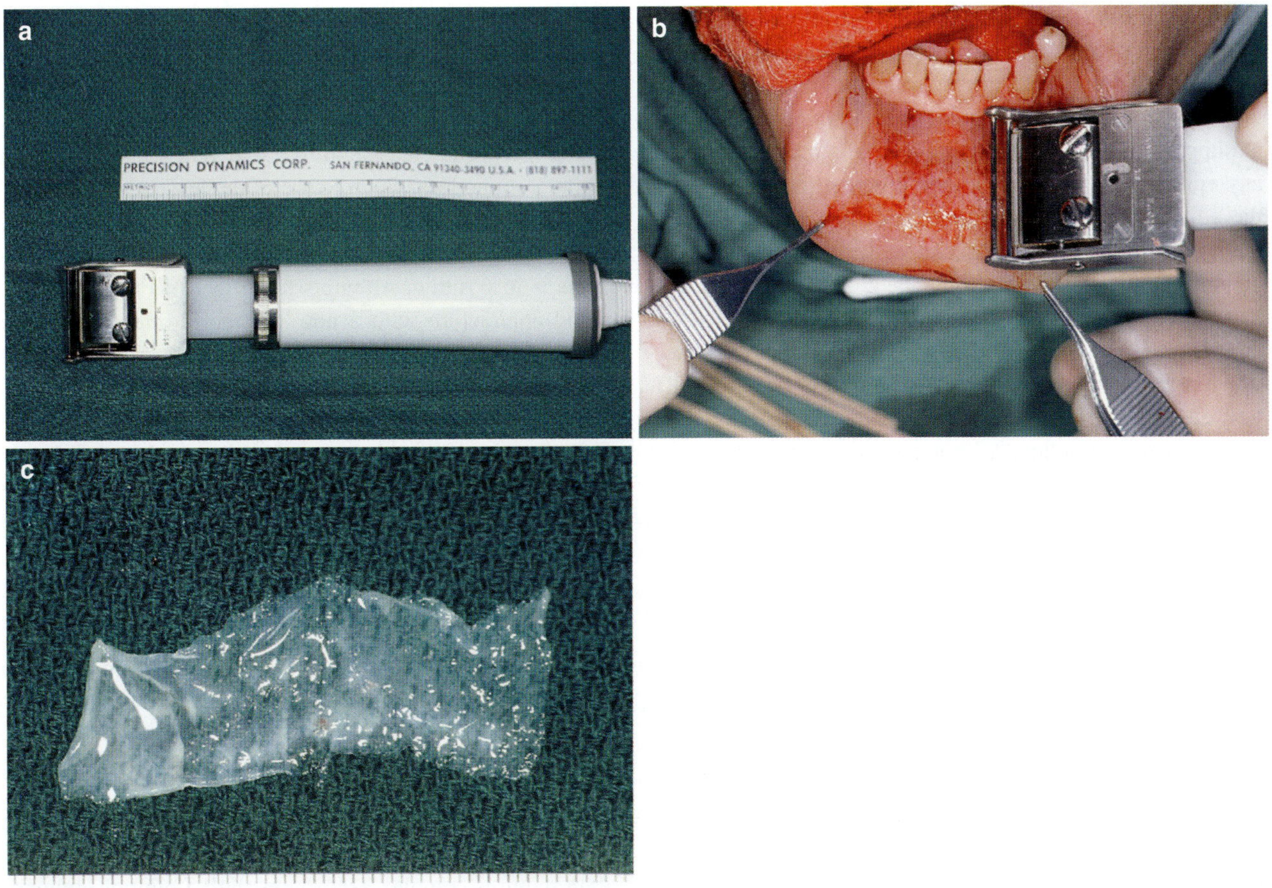

Fig. 60.18 (**a**) Castroviejo mucotome for harvesting mucous membrane grafts. (**b**) The inside of the lower lip is a good donor source of mucous membrane. (**c**) A thin piece of mucous membrane is ready for implantation

tension. With placement of large mucous membrane grafts, a silastic stent (e.g., 240 retinal band) can be positioned in the sulcus of the inferior fornix and anchored to the adjacent periosteum, with both arms of a double-armed suture passed in horizontal mattress fashion through the stent, the deepest part of the fornix, the periosteum of the inferior orbital rim, and finally through the full thickness of the eyelid (Fig. 60.4a–d). Cotton, silicone, or red rubber bolsters are used when the sutures are tied on the skin surface, anchoring the stent securely in the inferior fornix. These sutures may be removed in several weeks after adequate fibrosis has occurred between the inferior fornix and periosteum. A conformer must be in place until a prosthesis is custom fitted. The only downside to full-thickness mucous membrane grafting is that it may be thick and bulky and the produce mucous may create an annoying film over the prosthetic eye.

Amniotic membrane tissue (AMT) has been used as a graft in various conjunctival and orbital reconstructive procedures including those due to chemical burns, pterygium excision, symblepharon release (e.g., cicatricial pemphigoid, Stevens-Johnson syndrome), conjunctival fornix reformation, and in the repair of exposed orbital implants [195–199]. Amniotic membrane is a "substrate graft" in contrast to oral mucosa which is considered a "substitute graft." [191] Substrate grafts require healthy conjunctival epithelial cells to differentiate and multiply over the amniotic membrane surface. Substitute grafts are replacement grafts and provide the epithelial cells. They require an underlying vascular bed to supply them. Amniotic membrane grafts do not provide any epithelial cells. Instead, they promote the migration of the adjacent conjunctival epithelial cells over the amniotic membrane graft surface by secreting various growth factors and providing a basement membrane [200]. In addition, they have an antifibrotic and anti-inflammatory effect, as well as antimicrobial activity [191, 200–203]. Immunologic rejection has not been reported after AMT grafting [201]. AMT is best suited for those anophthalmic sockets with mild to moderate socket contraction. Advantages include its availability, lack of donor site morbidity, and antifibroblastic activity [202]. Comparable and favorable outcomes have been shown with either mucous membrane graft or amniotic membrane grafts [201, 202]. Further study is needed to determine the exact amount of recipient conjunctiva that is adequate for a successful outcome.

Dermis fat grafts may also be an option in patients with moderate socket contraction as well as socket volume deficiency (enophthalmos, deep superior sulcus) [179, 204, 205]. A dermis fat graft can improve orbital volume, as well as increase the conjunctival surface area [179, 204, 205]. As with amniotic membrane grafts, some normal recipient conjunctiva is required for a successful outcome. A healthy, vascularized socket is also required as the dermis fat graft is a free graft and its viability depends upon host fibrovascular ingrowth. Following placement of a dermis fat graft, the largest conformer that can be retained and permit eyelid approximation with a temporary tarsorrhaphy (4-0 silk horizontal mattress sutures over red rubber catheter or cotton bolster) should be inserted to limit postoperative tissue contracture. The tarsorrhaphy will help keep the eyelids and socket conjunctiva on traction for at least 3–4 weeks. Conjunctival epithelium will migrate over the anterior surface of the dermis fat graft during this time and expand the conjunctival surface area. Without the tarsorrhaphy sutures, progressive tissue contraction may occur (Figs. 60.19a–j and 60.20a–k).

Dermis fat grafts should be used with caution in those with a previous history of socket irradiation or in patients with severe or recurrent socket scarring as insufficient orbital vascularity will compromise success [206]. An unpredictable absorption rate is a disadvantage of the dermis fat graft in socket reconstruction.

Severe Socket Contracture

In the severely contracted socket, the conjunctival fornices are nearly absent or may be obliterated making it difficult to hold even a small prosthetic eye (Fig. 60.21a–d). In those that can still wear a prosthesis, enophthalmos with posterior displacement of the prosthesis may be evident along with poor or no prosthesis motility due to the contracted fornices. Retraction of the upper eyelid skin along the orbital roof with loss of the eyelid crease and fold may develop secondary to orbital volume loss. Contracture of the levator-superior rectus muscle complex may also contribute to the upper lid being retracted into an elevated position, even when no prosthesis is in position. Attempts to correct this type of upper eyelid contracture with a new prosthesis often result in a "staring" appearance (Fig. 60.21a, b). In addition to the discomfort and unsightly appearance of a poorly fit prosthesis, these patients often experience discharge and irritation.

Reconstruction of the severely contracted eye socket is often challenging. Patients should be counseled regarding the substantial challenges to achieve an acceptable outcome and the likelihood of several staged procedures being required. The primary goal in the treatment of severe socket contracture should be to enable the patient to retain a prosthesis with reasonable comfort and acceptable cosmetic appearance given their limited socket soft tissue. However, repair of severe socket contracture may also end in disappointment in the patient as well as the surgeon if too much surgery is attempted at once.

Complete socket reconstruction for severe contracture (loss of conjunctival fornices and orbital volume deficiency) often requires complex procedures with a multidisciplinary approach involving a craniofacial plastic or head and neck surgeon as well as an oculoplastic specialist (Fig. 60.21a–q).

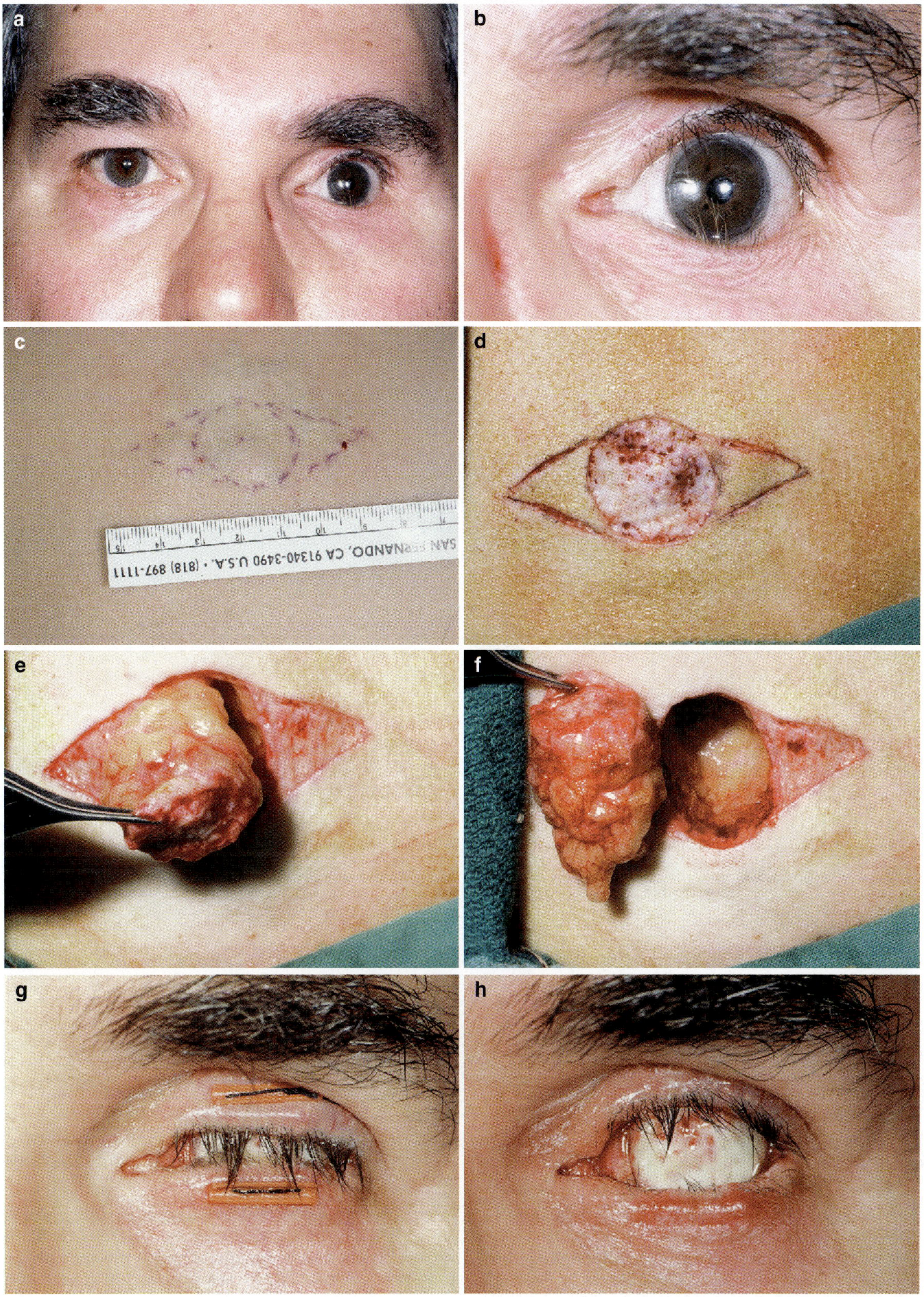

Fig. 60.19 Figure 60.11 – (**a**, **b**) – A 60-year-old man was seen in consultation for enophthalmos and inability to retain his prosthesis. On examination, there was enophthalmos and shortened fornices superiorly and inferiorly. It was elected to carry out a dermis fat graft. (**c**, **d**) The donor site was marked out over the upper outer quadrant of the buttock. The epithelium was removed leaving underlying dermis. (**e**, **f**) The dermis fat graft was harvested. (**g**) The graft was placed into the socket with a ring-shaped conformer to maintain the fornices. External red rubber bolsters were used to suture the lid margins together. (**h**) The bolsters have been removed, and the dermis fat graft is visualized. (**i**) In 2–4 weeks, epithelium grows over the dermis fat graft. (**j**) The enophthalmos has improved. He was happy with the results and the residual superior sulcus defect

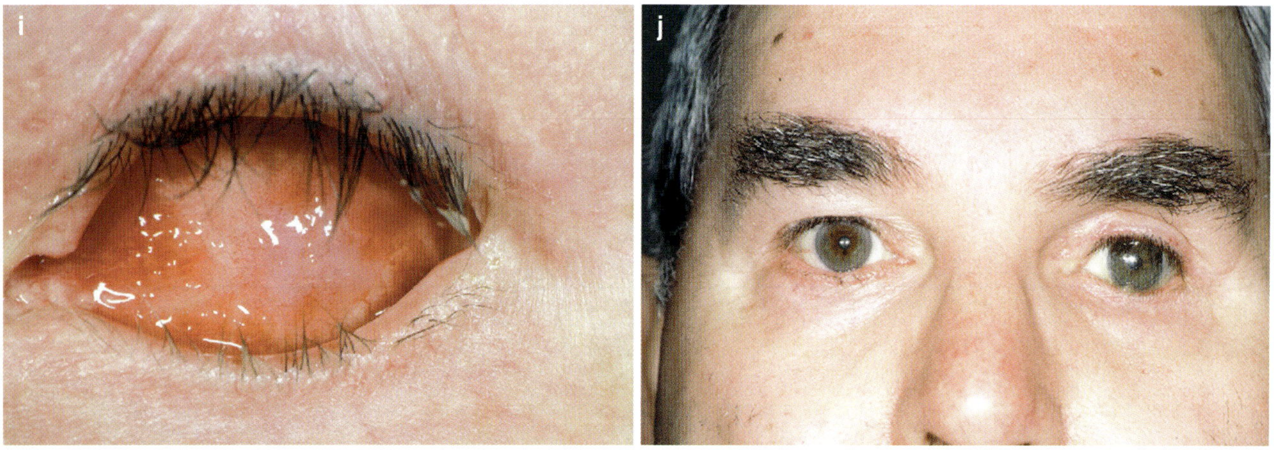

Fig. 60.19 (continued)

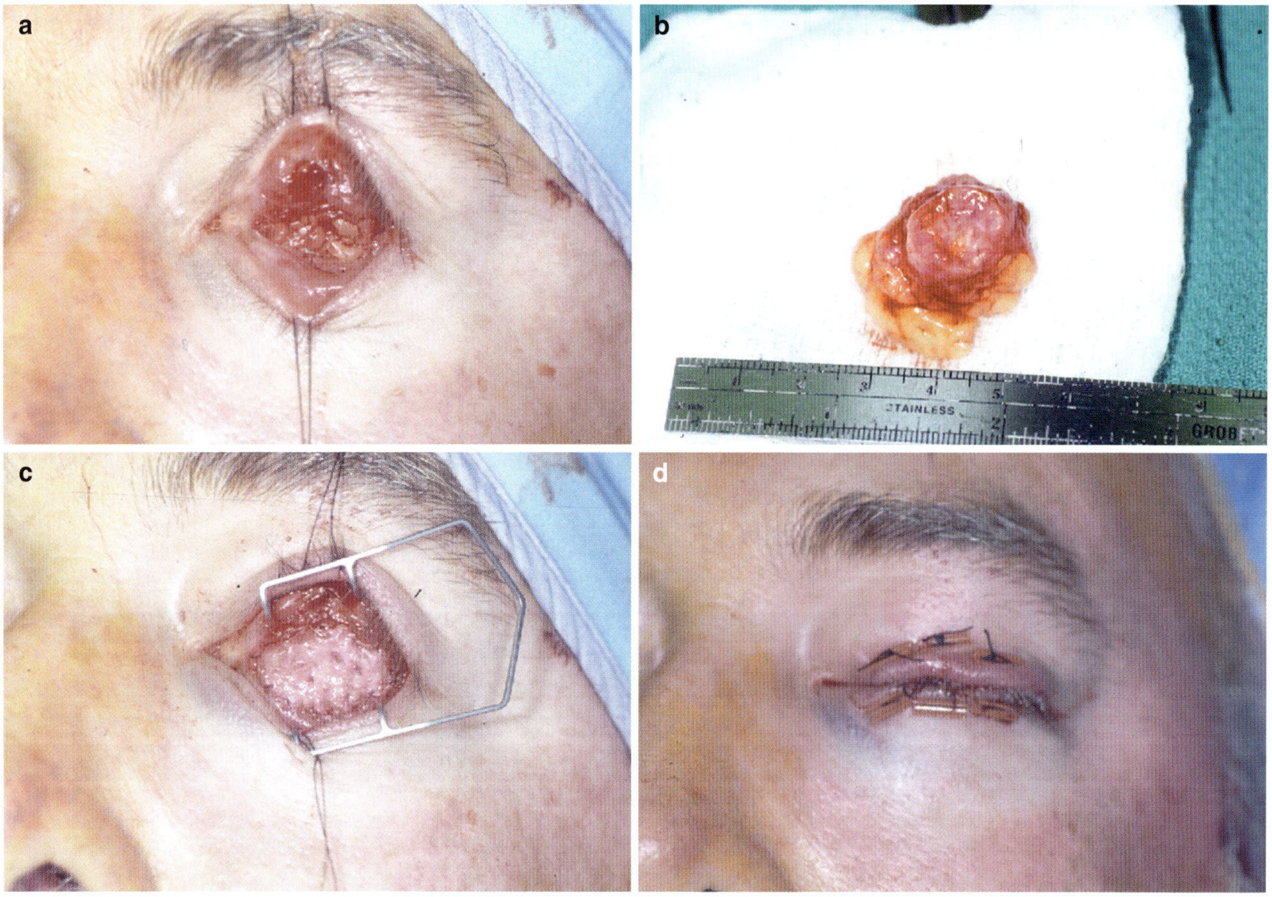

Fig. 60.20 Continuation of patient seen in Fig. 60.16 with suspected infected HA orbital implant. The first step was to remove the implant followed by implantation of a dermis fat graft. (**a**) A horizontal incision was used to remove the orbital implant and make space for the dermis fat graft. (**b**, **c**) The dermis fat graft was harvested and sutured into the socket followed by placement of a conformer. (**d**) The eyelids were sutured together over red rubber bolsters for 5 weeks and then removed. (**e**) The dermis fat graft appears healthy and is still being epithelialized. (**f**) The conjunctival epithelium has grown over the central aspect of the dermis fat graft by 8 weeks. (**g**) The patient is fit with a new prosthesis and has some residual ptosis. (**h**) The tarsal plate is no longer folded, but the superior fornix remains very deficient, and the eyelid was ptotic. An amniotic membrane graft was suggested to expand the superior fornix area. (**i**) The amniotic membrane graft is virtually transparent and ready to be implanted. (**j**) After dissecting into the superior fornix with a number 15 scalpel blade and Westcott scissors to create a fornix, the graft is sutured into the superior fornix with 7–0 chromic sutures followed by placement of a conformer. The lids are again sutured together over red rubber bolsters for 4–5 weeks at which time the prosthesis is adjusted. (**k**) 12 weeks post amniotic membrane graft, the superior fornix has been deepened

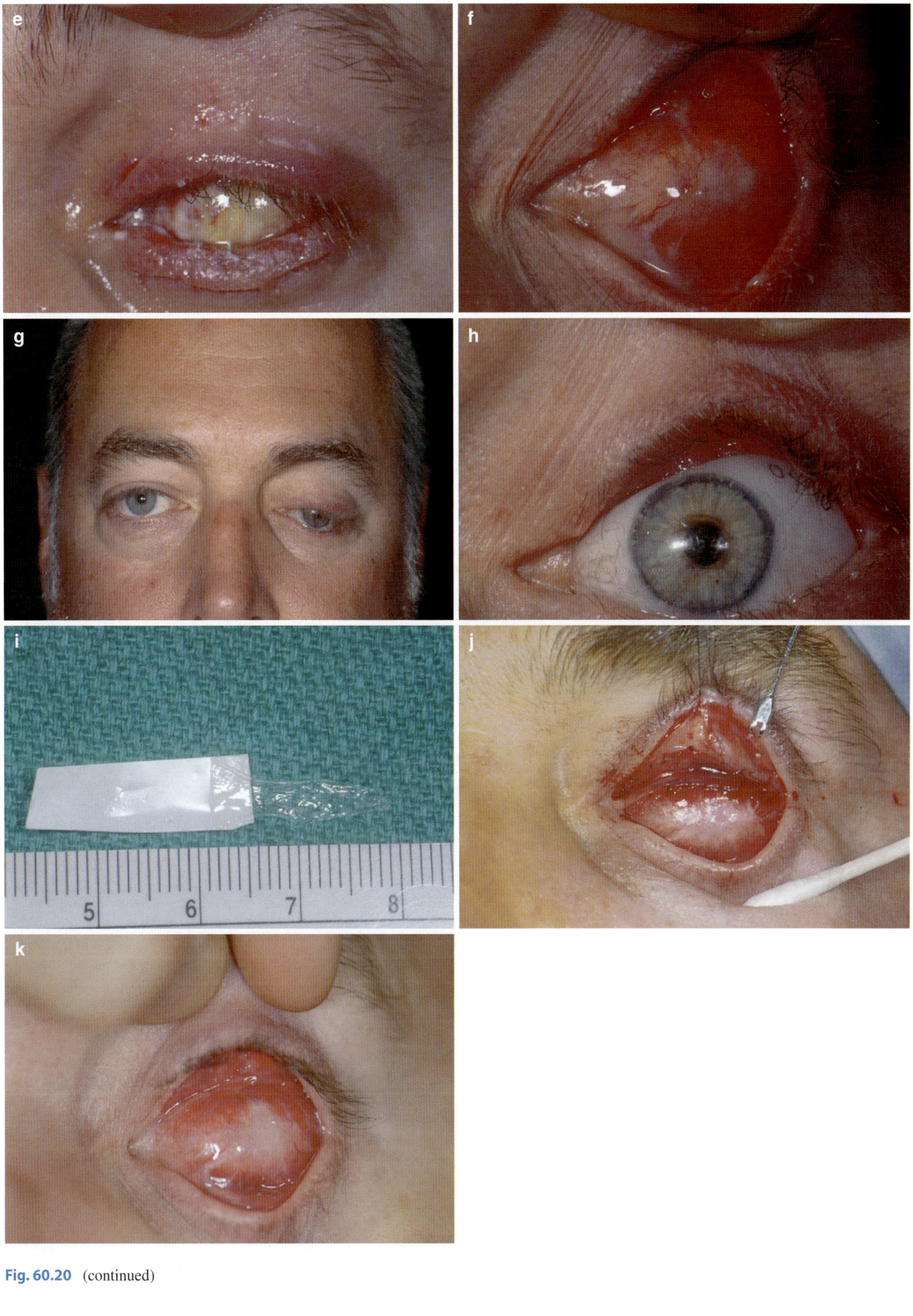

Fig. 60.20 (continued)

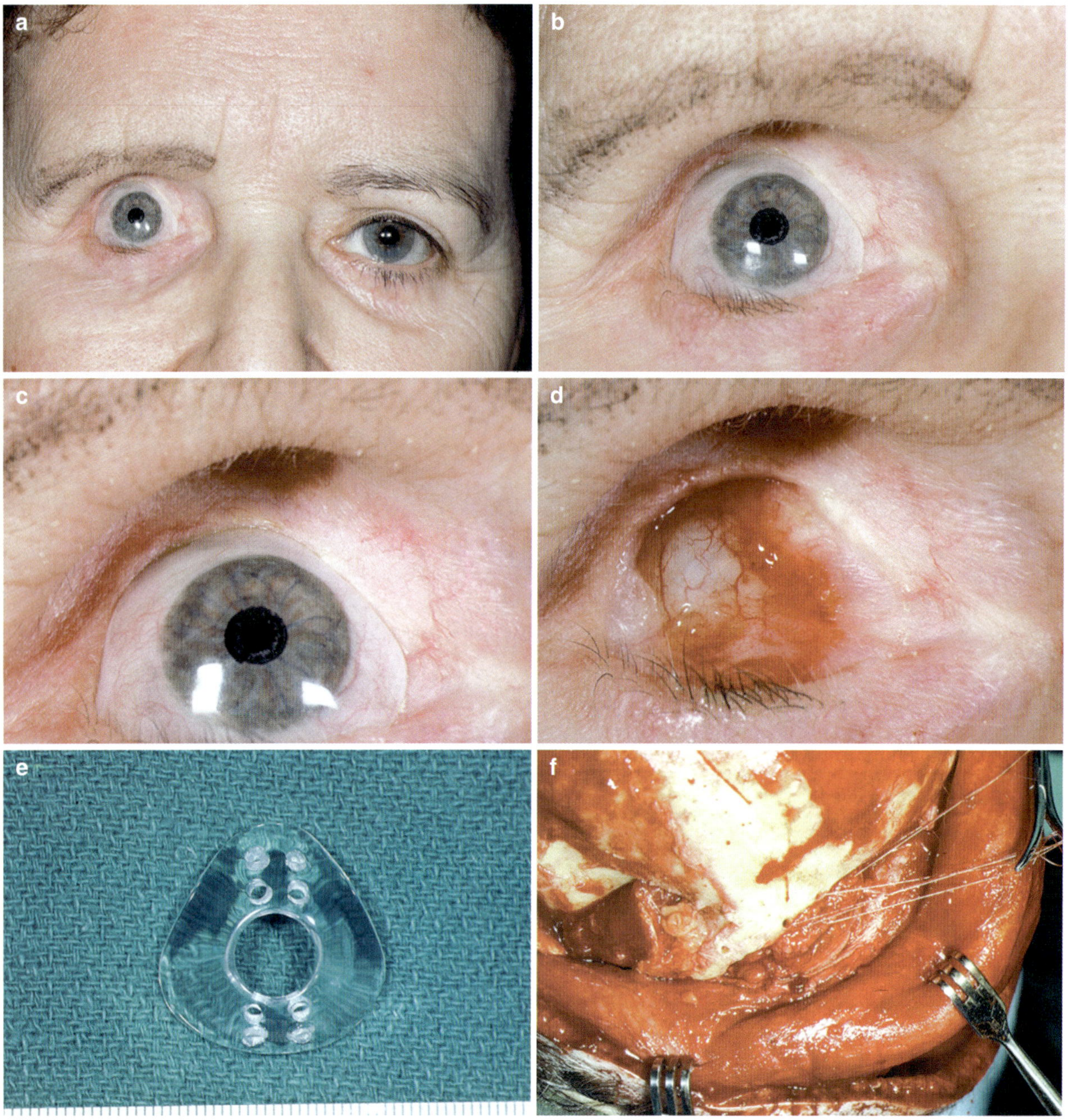

Fig. 60.21 (**a**) A 66-year-old female was seen in consultation for inability to wear her prosthesis. The eye had been removed following severe corneal exposure with corneal perforation as a result of an upper eyelid resection for basal cell carcinoma. Postoperative irradiation had been used following the lid surgery explaining the atrophic appearance of the upper eyelid tissue. (**a**, **b**) Severe enophthalmos is present, with loss of the right upper eyelid margin. (**c**, **d**) Loss of most of the upper eyelid and severe deficiency of the conjunctival space. (**e**) Example of a custom conformer that can be wired to the superior and inferior orbital rim. (**f**, **g**) a temporalis muscle transfer was performed with temporalis muscle placed into the eye socket through a tunnel in the lateral wall. (**h**, **i**) A custom conformer with a partial-thickness mucous membrane graft from the buccal mucosa was prepared and placed into the eye socket. It was not wired to the superior/inferior orbital rim. (**j**) The eyelids were sutured closed with 4–0 silk on red rubber catheter material. (**k**) A custom conformer with a champagne stem was placed in the fornices immediately following removal of the bolsters to try and maintain the fornices before an artificial eye was made. An eyepatch and tape were applied over the protruding stem. This applied pressure to the conformer sitting within the newly created fornices. (**l**, **m**) Following fabrication of the artificial eye, the right upper eyelid had a deficiency of the skin, and there was a retracted appearance to the upper eyelid. (**n**) A skin graft (supraclavicular) was put in place and held there with a sponge bolster. (**o**) Immediately following the bolster removal, the graft was healing well. (**p**, **q**) The patient is seen 12 weeks post skin graft placement and had a much more natural and symmetrical appearance. She was able to keep her prosthesis in place

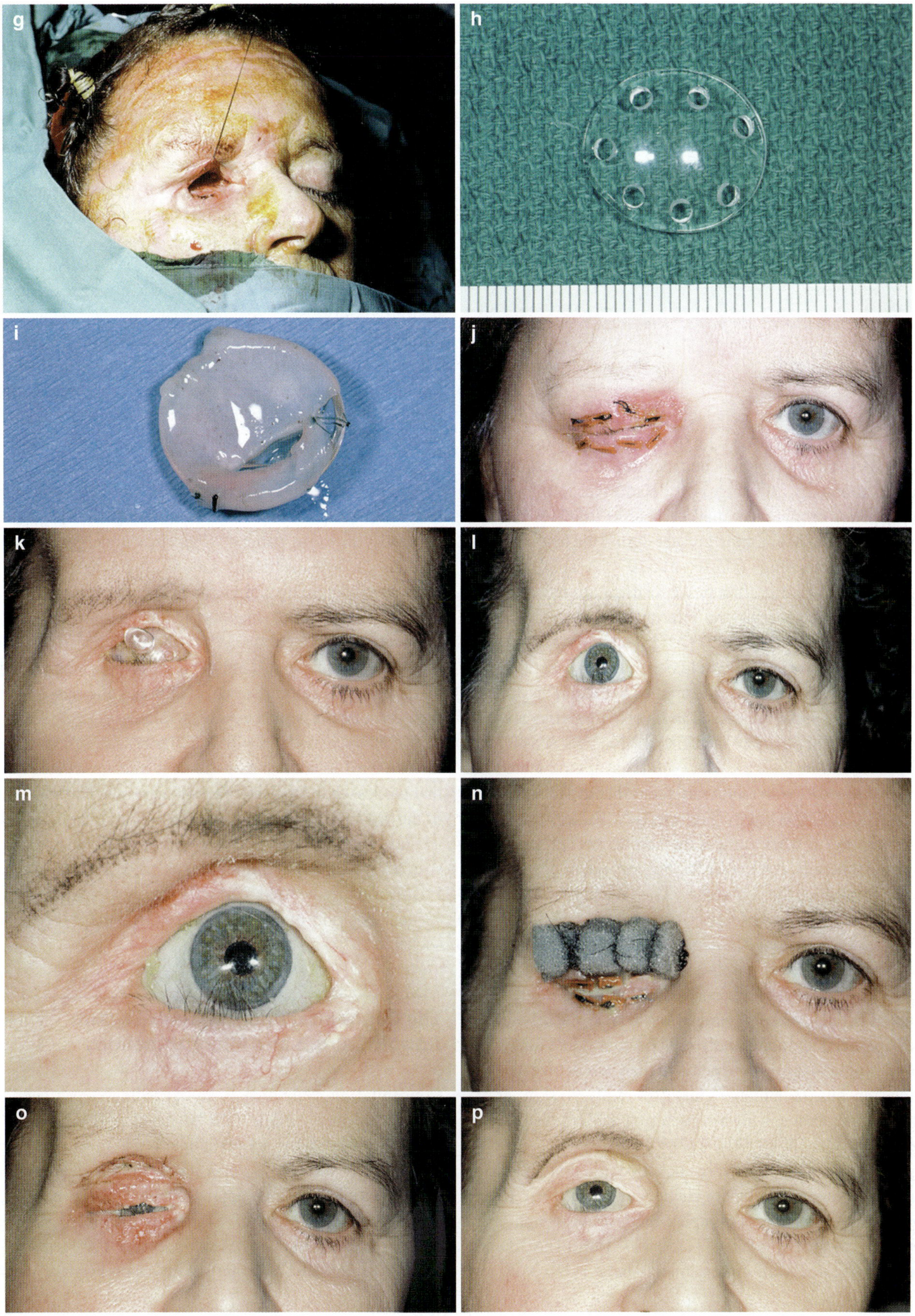

Fig. 60.21 (continued)

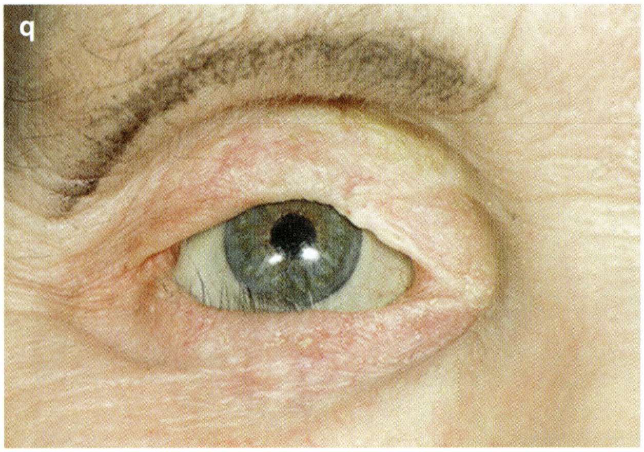

Fig. 60.21 (continued)

If volume deficiency is not an issue, buccal mucosal donor grafts are used but may not be of sufficient size to cover the entire socket. If enough mucous membrane can be obtained, wire fixation (e.g., 30 gauge) of a conformer to the inferior and superior orbital rims may be helpful to offset the contractive forces that are often present during the healing phase in these sockets (Fig. 60.21e, h) [207]. A split-thickness mucous membrane graft sutured to itself around a custom conformer with superior and inferior holes in it is our preferred technique (Fig. 60.21i) [207]. The wires are threaded through the conformer holes and bone tunnels superiorly and inferiorly, and gentle tension is applied to them. The skin and subcutaneous tissue are closed in layers. The wires are then twisted together on top of the skin incision over silastic, cotton, or red rubber bolsters. The eyelids are approximated and also tied together with temporary tarsorrhaphy sutures on red rubber or cotton bolsters (Fig. 60.21j). These bolsters are removed in 3–6 weeks unless they erode through the eyelid sooner. Generally, the longer the bolsters are in position, the more favorable the outcome. The wired conformer is removed when the new socket tissue appears quiet (typically 6–8 weeks). A custom conformer is then placed followed by a custom-made prosthesis 1–2 weeks later.

In poorly vascularized, contracted, and volume-deficient (enophthalmic) sockets, temporalis muscle flaps based on the superficial temporal artery may be considered to bring in blood supply to the orbit which will then vascularize an overlying mucous membrane graft (or rarely a skin graft). Mucous membrane is always preferred for reasons outlined earlier (Fig. 60.21f–q) [208–212].

Those patients with severe socket contraction and previous irradiation are extremely challenging [185, 186]. Radial forearm free flaps are a complex reconstructive option for severely contracted sockets [185, 187–190]. The forearm flap is harvested with dimensions as large as 10 × 20 cm, making it ideally suited for fornix reconstruction. Its vasculature is anatomically consistent during dissection and robust in caliber, and the diameter of the radial artery is comparable with the diameter of the anastomosing vessels in the maxillofacial region [189]. The vascular pedicle is flexible, and its length can be altered to accommodate varying facial anatomy as needed. Because of its multiple perforating feeding vessels, the entire flap can be folded while maintaining adequate perfusion [189]. In contrast to earlier methods where a bone window was used to tunnel a vascular pedicle, the radial forearm pedicle can be tunneled subcutaneously [185, 187]. Anastomosis is made with the facial artery or superior thyroid artery and the external jugular vein [189]. Alternatively, the superficial temporal artery may be used. The disadvantages of this technique include a cosmetically unfavorable forearm donor site, forearm numbness, and a decreased arterial flow to the forearm [189, 190]. Other techniques described to revascularize severely contracted sockets with volume deficiency include a short pedicled thoracodorsal artery trilobed adiposal flap, a retroauricular island flap, and a retroauricular fasciocutaneous flap [213–215].

Lastly, in those patients who have undergone multiple procedures with persistent failures, total excision of the residual socket lining with permanent closure of the lids (lid-sparing exenteration) may be indicated as a last resort. Fabrication of an oculofacial prosthesis, matched to the fellow side, in some cases, although immobile, may provide a better cosmetic result than any additional attempts at socket reconstruction in some cases (Fig. 60.22a–i) [216, 217].

Tinted eyeglass lenses in a full frame pair of glasses may also be used to add camouflage over a reconstructed socket that has less than the desired aesthetic result. The appearance of the prosthesis and eyelids may also be modified by adding a "plus or minus" spectacle lenses to magnify a small reconstructed socket or to minimize an enlarged appearing socket. Prisms can also be used to modify the apparent horizontal or vertical position of a malpositioned prosthetic eye or eye socket.

The Congenital Anophthalmic Socket: Anophthalmos and Microphthalmos

Congenital anophthalmia is an exceedingly rare condition where the optic vesicle fails to develop (Fig. 60.23a–c). Along with cyclopia, anophthalmia is the most severe malformation of the eye. Studies report the incidence of congenital anophthalmia as approximately 0.2–0.6 per 10,000 births [215, 218]. Many cases initially diagnosed as anophthalmos contain remnants of an underdeveloped eye, or vestigial eye tissue, and are more appropriately termed

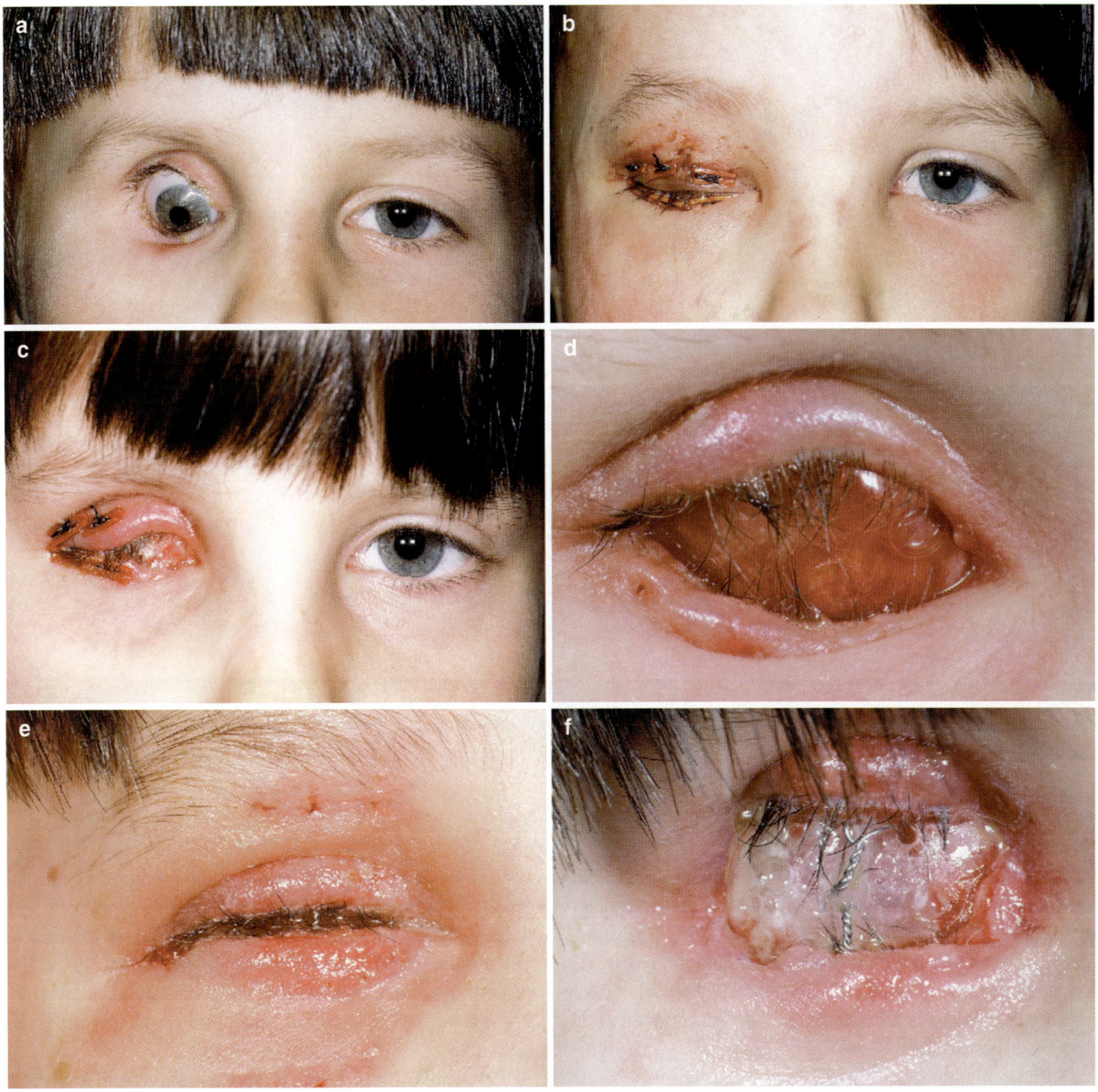

Fig. 60.22 (**a**) An 8-year-old female presented with an inability to retain her prosthesis and enophthalmos. The right eye had been removed due to retinoblastoma at age 1. There had been radiation therapy to the eye socket postoperatively. The child had difficulty retaining the prosthesis and a very retracted upper eyelid giving her a disfigured staring appearance. The superior and inferior fornices were shortened, and the socket was enophthalmic. The child underwent a dermis fat graft procedure to augment the socket volume and improve the fornices. (**b**) At 1 week, the eyelids were well opposed with temporary bolster tarsorrhaphy sutures. (**c**) By 3 weeks, one tarsorrhaphy suture had spontaneously released. (**d**) At 4 weeks, the other bolster sutures were removed; the fornices appeared to be contracting. At 7 weeks, it was elected to carry out socket reconstruction with a custom-made conformer that could be wired to the orbital rim (Fig. 60.21e), in addition to a buccal mucosal graft from the mouth. (**e**) At 2 weeks post socket reconstruction and 9 weeks post dermis fat grafting, the eyelids were in good position, and the fornices were well formed. (**f**) Six weeks following the socket reconstruction, the child had a volleyball hit her in the right periocular region. Within a week, socket contraction began. The eyelids are seen retracting superiorly and shrinking in size. (**g**) Four weeks later, the eyelids reveal further atrophy. The custom-made conformer was removed the following week. (**h**) Seven months following the volleyball blow, severe socket contraction has occurred with loss of the conjunctival fornices and atrophy of most of the upper and lower eyelids. (**i**) An oculofacial prosthesis, often used following exenteration, was used to cover the socket

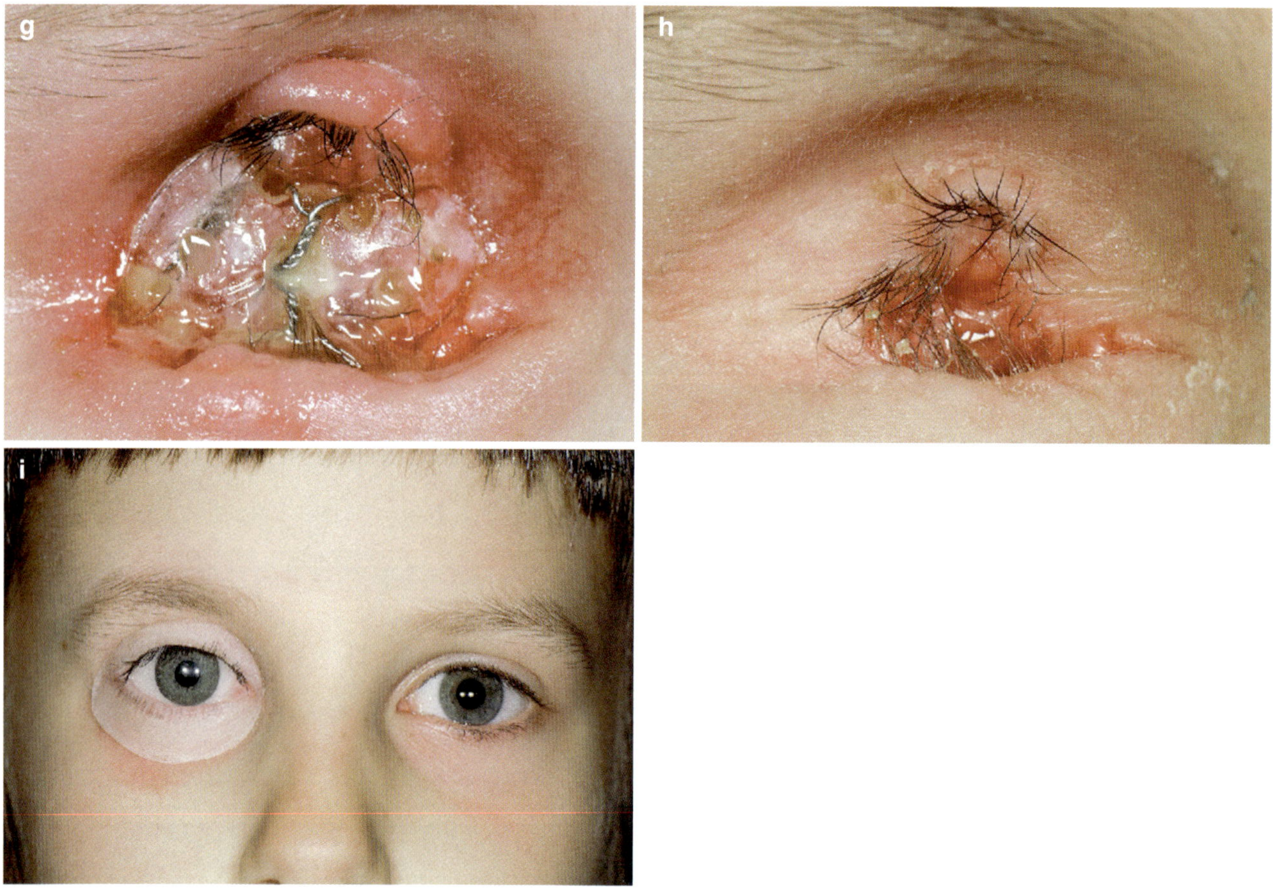

Fig. 60.22 (continued)

microphthalmos. Congenital microphthalmos is more common than congenital anophthalmos and has an incidence of between 1.2 and 1.8 per 10,000 births [219]. Ultrasound, computerized tomography, or more preferably magnetic resonance imaging (to avoid radiation) may be helpful in determining the presence of these remnants as well as documenting any other bone deformities (Fig. 60.23c).

Microphthalmos is a variable condition that is separated into "simple" or "complex" types according to the appearance of the globe. *Simple* or pure microphthalmos is defined as an eye that is essentially normal except for its decreased axial length. The microphthalmic eye has a diameter at birth of less than 15 mm (normal range, 15–19 mm) [220]. In most cases, the size of the anterior segment is within normal limits, whereas the posterior segment length is significantly decreased. In *complex* microphthalmos, the anterior and posterior segments of the globe are severely malformed, and the appearance of the globe varies considerably (Fig. 60.24). There may also be an associated coloboma or cystic component (Fig. 60.25a–j) [220–223].

Congenital deformations of the eye and orbit such as anophthalmos and microphthalmos vary in severity, and there is a spectrum of disease that exists between these two conditions. Both anophthalmia and microphthalmia may be unilateral or bilateral, and over 50% may be associated with other systemic abnormalities [218, 223–226]. In the case of unilateral anophthalmia or microphthalmia, there may also be developmental anomalies of the contralateral eye, including coloboma, lens, retina, and optic nerve abnormalities [226–228].

Practically, the clinical picture is often similar in both anophthalmos and microphthalmos. The eyelids are minified with deficient palpebral and bulbar conjunctiva and an underdeveloped orbital bone skeleton (Figs. 60.23, 60.24, and 60.26) [220]. The absence of a globe not only retards growth of the socket and eyelids but retards the development of the entire hemiface, impacting the growth of the maxilla, maxillary sinus, and mandible [229–234]. The eyelids are usually short both vertically and horizontally (phimosis). The levator muscle may also be absent causing blepharoptosis, and the conjunctival fornices are extremely shortened making placement and wearing of a prosthesis difficult. Without treatment, these patients may develop a significant decrease in the dimensions of the orbital entrance and deficient orbital volume (up to 60%). Orbital soft tissue volume is an indicator of orbital bone growth, and adequate volume replacement

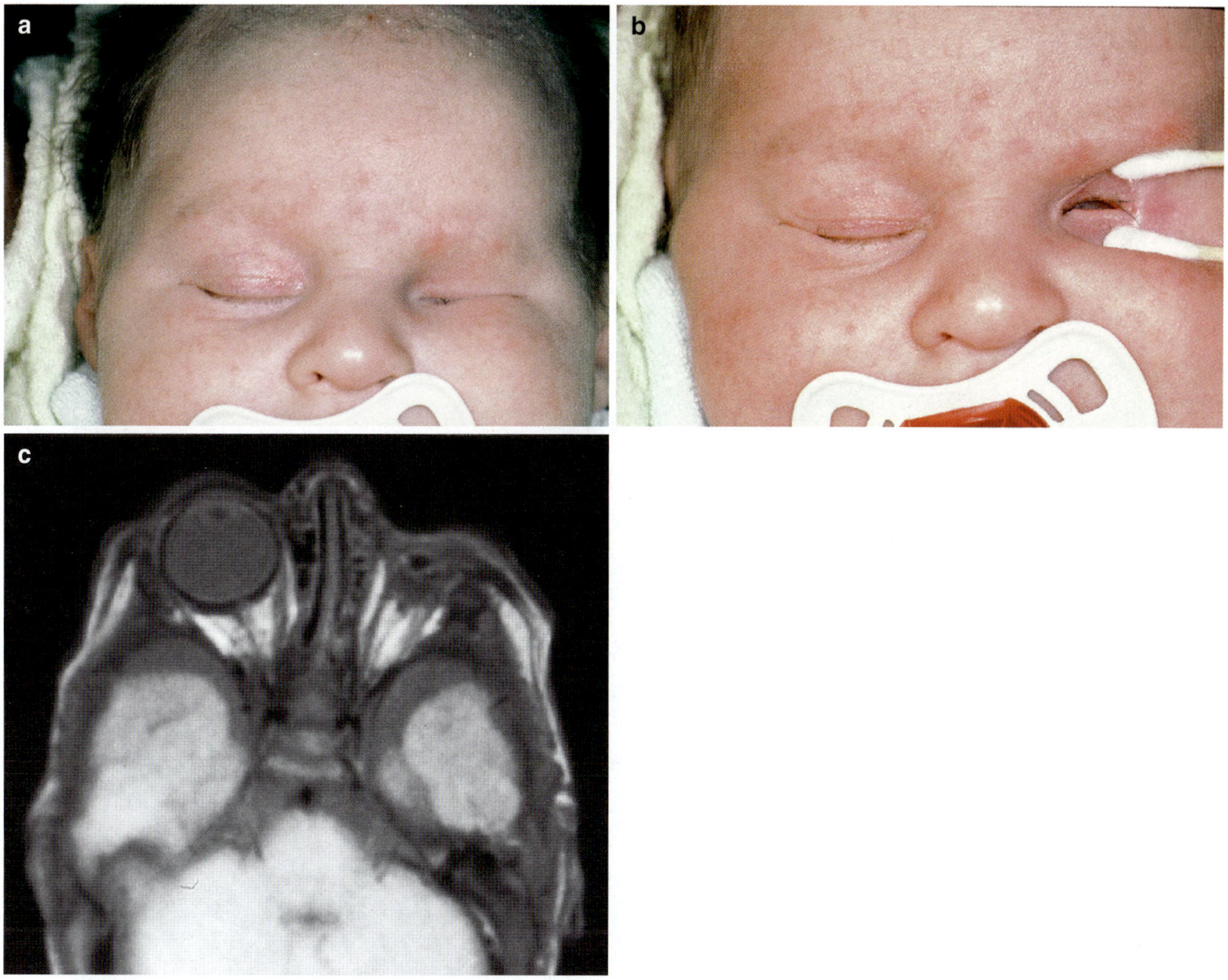

Fig. 60.23 (**a**) A 1-week-old child is seen with a microphthalmic vs anophthalmic socket. (**b**) Cotton-tipped applicators are used to open the tiny underdeveloped eyelids. A poorly formed conjunctival fornix was seen superiorly and inferiorly. A small custom-made conformer was placed in the socket. (**c**) An MRI scan done at 4 weeks of life revealed the underdeveloped left socket, no identifiable ocular remnant, and the presence of the custom conformer. The lack of an ocular remnant confirmed congenital anophthalmos rather than microphthalmos. The size of the bony orbit is already quite a bit smaller than the opposite side

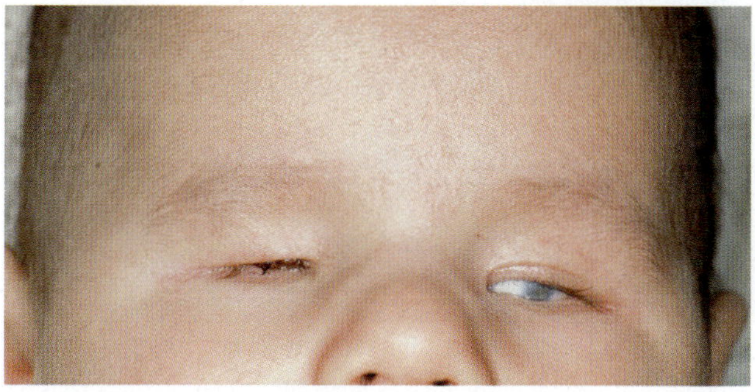

Fig. 60.24 A 2-month-old male is seen with anophthalmos on the right and a microphthalmos on the left. Vision was light perception on the left eye. The palpebral fissures are both underdeveloped (R > L). The bony orbits are also underdeveloped (R > L)

is a critical factor in continued orbital growth as well as adjacent facial growth [235–241].

The management of a child with suspected anophthalmia or microphthalmia often involves a number of health-care professionals including a pediatric ophthalmologist, pediatrician, social worker, oculoplastic/orbital specialist, geneticist, and an ocularist [224, 226, 241, 242]. A pediatric ophthalmologist and pediatrician usually carry out the initial assessment in the neonatal period. Early examination by a pediatric ophthalmologist will include both a diagnostic and visual assessment. It is important both eyes are examined as unilateral anophthalmia/microphthalmia eye patients may have other subtler abnormalities such as coloboma, optic nerve hypoplasia, retinal dystrophic changes, or cataract in the fellow eye. An ultrasound of the

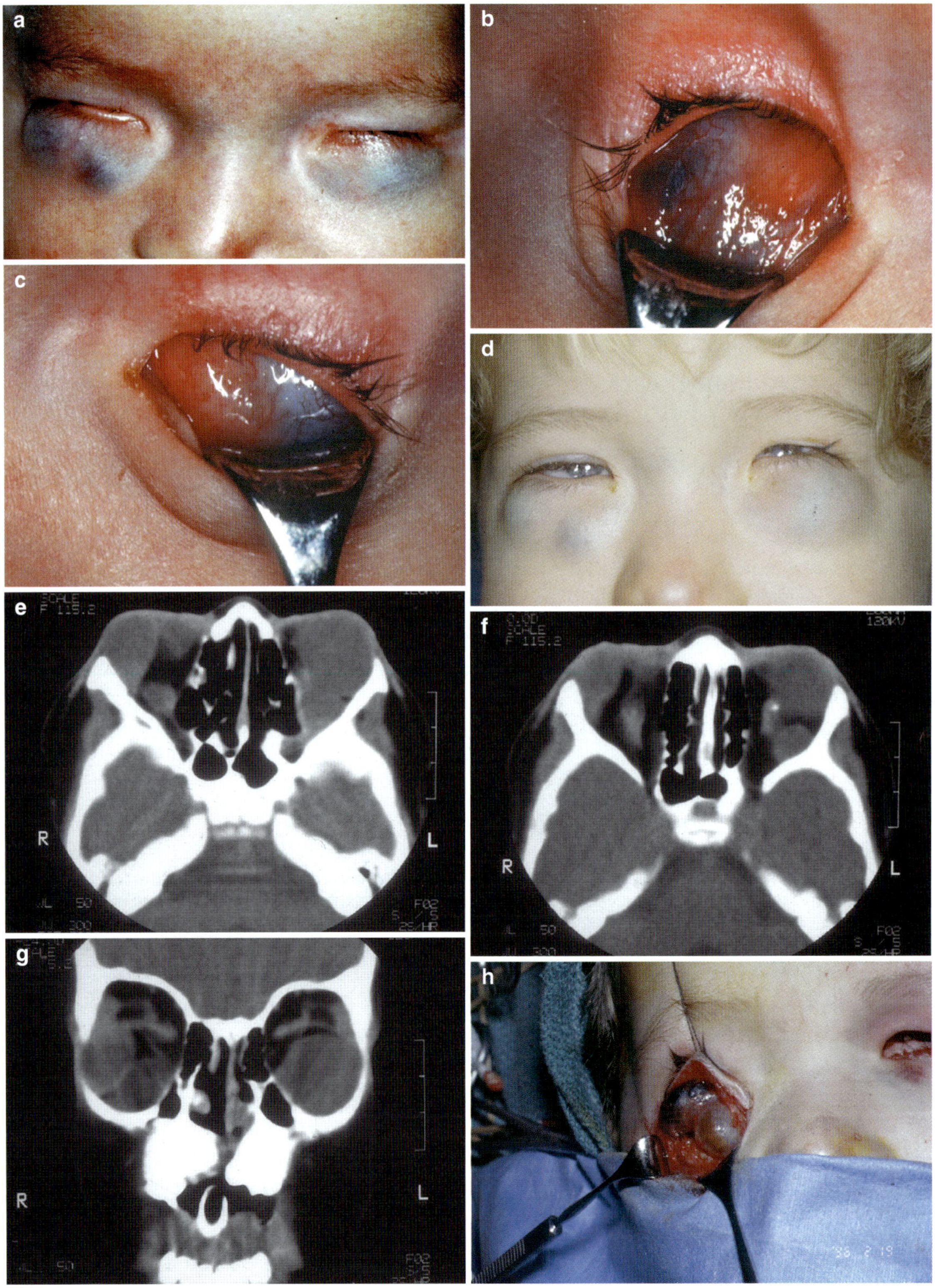

Fig. 60.25 (**a**) A 4-month-old male born with microphthalmos and cyst formation bilaterally as well as bilateral cleft lip and palate. (**b**, **c**) Large subconjunctival blue cystic masses seen bilaterally. (**d**) By 3 years of age, the eyelids and fornices were increasing in size. The prosthetic eyes were pushed superiorly by the inferior located cysts. The blue cystic masses were also helping to expand the bony orbit but gave the child a "battered" appearance, which was extremely troubling for their parents. (**e**, **f**) Axial CT view of cystic masses bilaterally, in (**f**), small ocular remnants were seen centrally; some calcification was present in the left remnant and to a smaller degree in the right remnant. (**g**) Coronal CT view of cystic masses bilaterally, the ocular remnants are also present centrally on each side. (**h–j**) The cystic masses were removed at age 3, H, right side, I, left side, J, cysts removed. (**k**) 2 months post cyst removal, the lids appear near normal. (**l**) At 3.5 years, the ocular remnants were removed, and 16 mm polymethyl methacrylate implants were put in place. (**m**) The child's prosthetic eyes fit much better, and he had a near-normal appearance (mild ptosis on the left). (**n**) By age 10, the child was doing well; the lid fissures and orbital volumes were symmetrical. He had a small degree of ptosis on the left

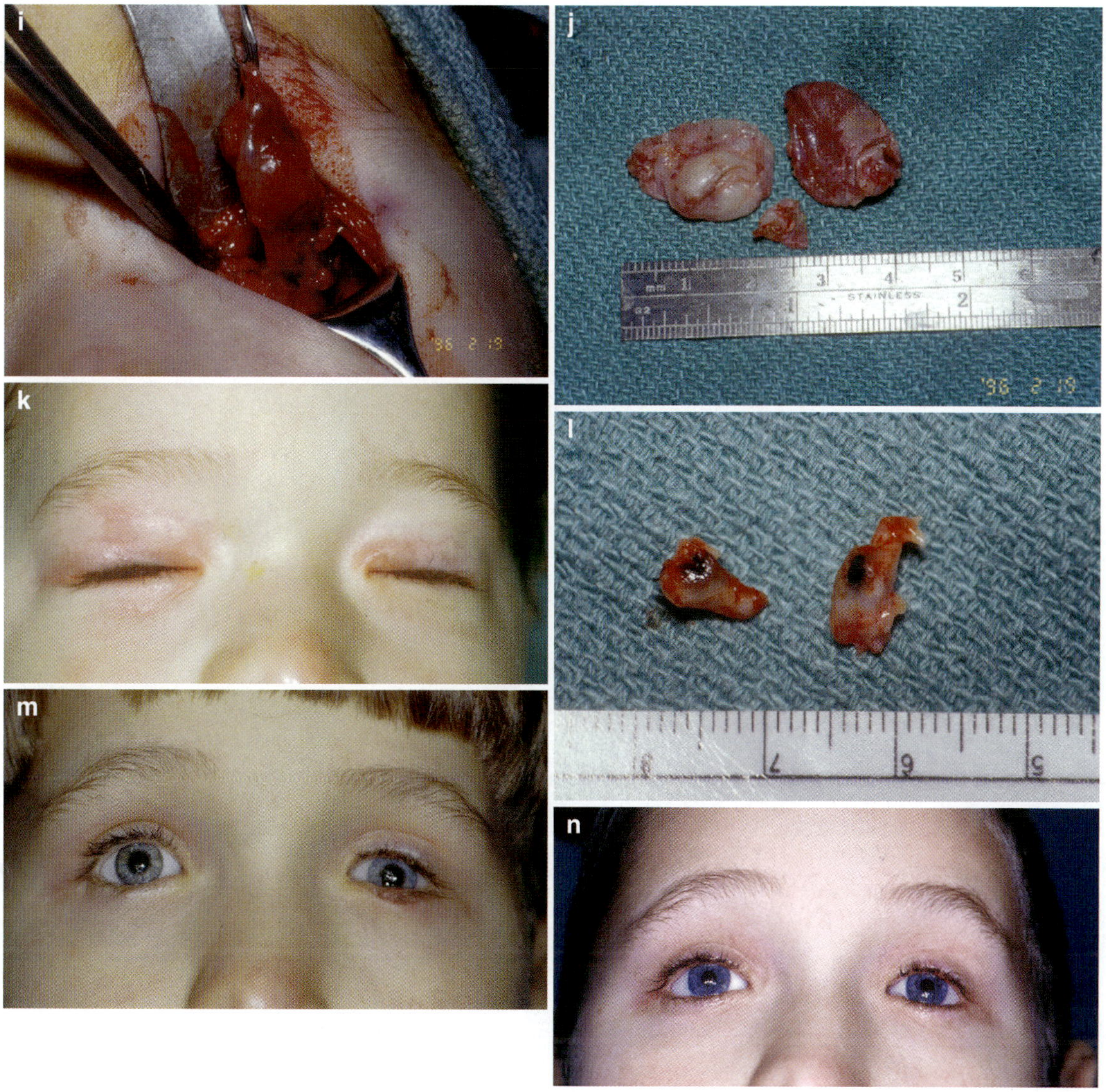

Fig. 60.25 (continued)

eye and orbit can be useful to assess the intraocular structures and the presence of an ocular remnant or cyst (Fig. 60.25) and to determine axial length in cases of microphthalmia. Vision is assessed using pediatric vision tests and electrodiagnostic testing if necessary. A flash visual-evoked potential (VEP) will establish if any visual function remains in cases of apparent anophthalmia or severe microphthalmia; a pattern VEP will help establish both a level of visual acuity and detect any optic nerve dysfunction, and an electroretinogram will identify if there is retinal dysfunction [223]. Even children with severe microphthalmia may have some vision, and it is important to establish this as early as possible, especially in bilateral cases, as it will guide the approach to socket expansion [223].

Early assessment by a pediatrician involves a complete history and physical examination searching for clues to the etiology and any associated systemic anomalies. The history should try to establish any relevant gestational factors or family history of other ocular or systemic abnormalities. The child may already be known to have other significant medical problems requiring active management. In the physical exam, particular attention is also focused upon the face, including the ear and palate, the cardiac system, genitalia, feeding difficulties which may indicate esophageal anomalies, and metabolic disturbances which may be due to pituitary underaction. A management plan is then made depending upon any systemic abnormalities identified [223]. Since many conditions that affect ocular development also affect brain growth, imaging of the brain with attention to the midline structures is commonly performed. Magnetic resonance imaging (MRI) is preferable to computerized tomography (CT) since there is higher resolution of soft tissue structures and no radiation exposure. Other testing will depend on the pediatrician's systemic assessment. Referral to a specialist in genetic counseling is beneficial but done at a later date once the family has adjusted to the situation and the management of the eye socket and other anomalies is

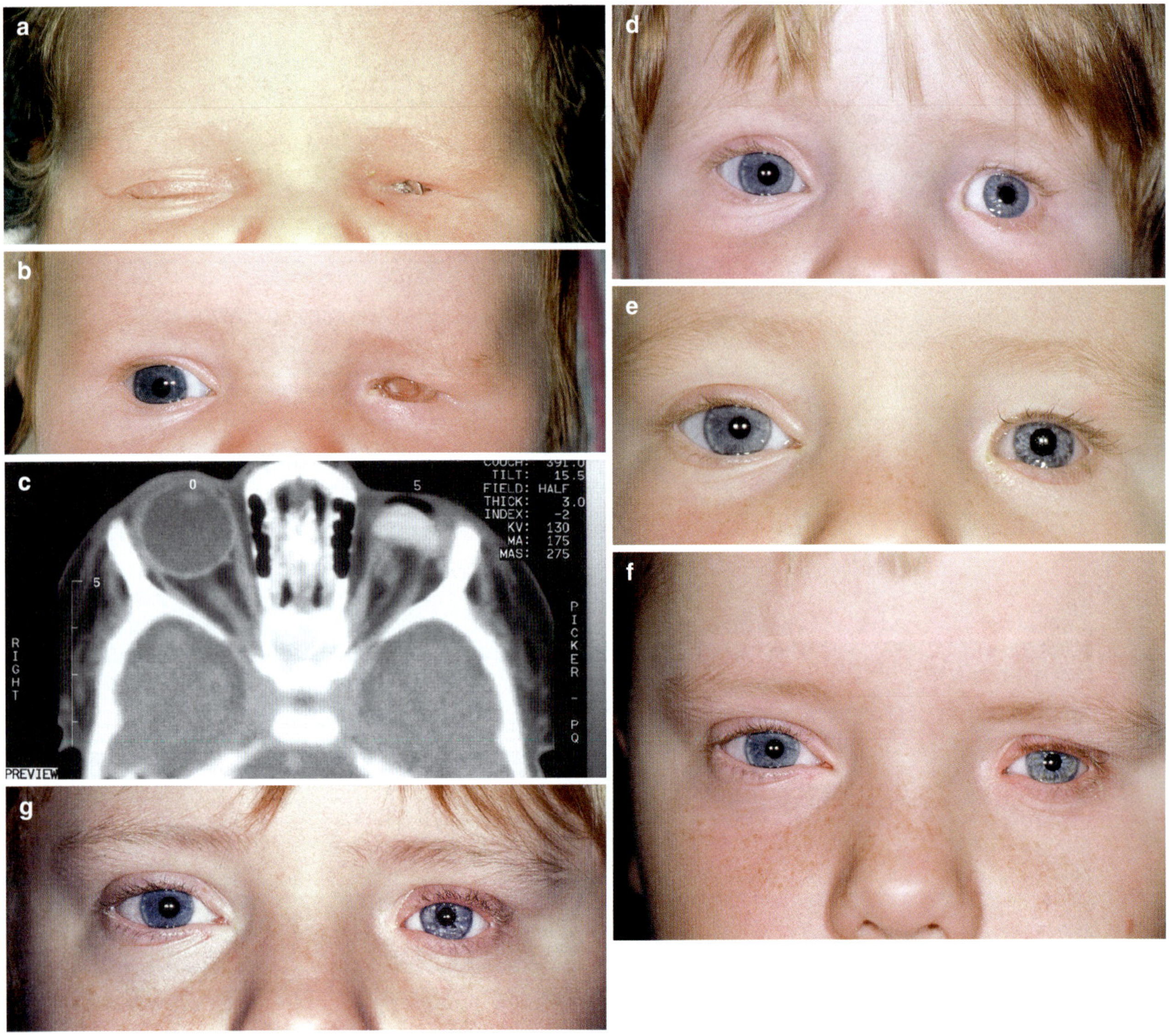

Fig. 60.26 (**a**) A 3-week-old male child is seen with a severly contracted eye socket. (**b**) By 6 weeks of age, the eyelids and conjunctival space have more than doubled in size with expanding conformers. (**c**) Computerized tomography reveals an ophthalmic remnant confirming severe microphthalmos. The orbital bones lag behind in their growth compared to the normal side. (**d**) By 24 months of age, the eyelids and conjunctival space have increased to about 75% of the normal side. (**e**) By 48 months of age, further development of the eyelids is present. A 16 mm polymethyl methacrylate implant was put in place shortly after this photo. (**f**) By 11 years of age, the eyelid fissures have continued to enlarge. (**g**) By 13 years of age, the eyelid fissures are approximately 80–85% of the normal side

under way. The development of the eye is highly complex. It is determined by a sequential and coordinated expression of eye development genes within the developing tissues. Although some individuals with anophthalmia or microphthalmia have relatives with other eye malformations, the frequent lack of clear Mendelian inheritance in these conditions has made identifying the genes for eye development challenging [223, 244].

Once the diagnosis of anophthalmos or microphthalmos (+/−cyst) has been established, it is important to discuss the diagnosis and complexity of the management with the parents. The pediatrician reviews the systemic malformations; the pediatric ophthalmologist discusses the ocular anomalies identified and the visual potential, while an oculoplastic/orbital specialist discusses the eyelid and eye socket problems. The initial meeting with the parents is often difficult. Not uncommonly, the parents have seen many individuals by the time they reach the oculoplastic/orbital specialist and have numerous concerns. Visual potential will be addressed by the pediatric ophthalmologist. Parents are also understandably interested in what can be done to improve their child's appearance. It is important to explain the complexity of management and guarded prognosis yet remain positive and encouraging. Parents should understand that any poten-

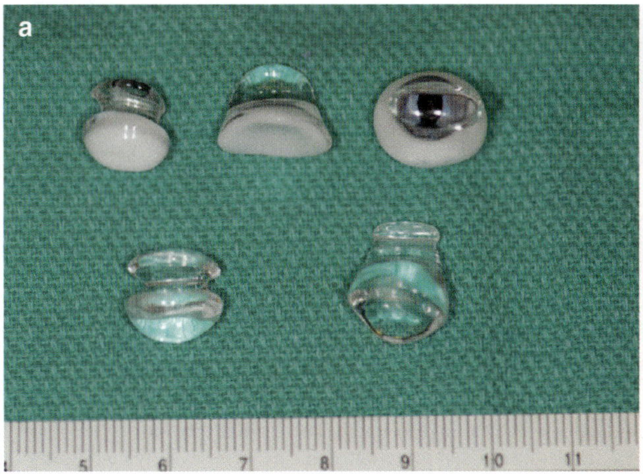

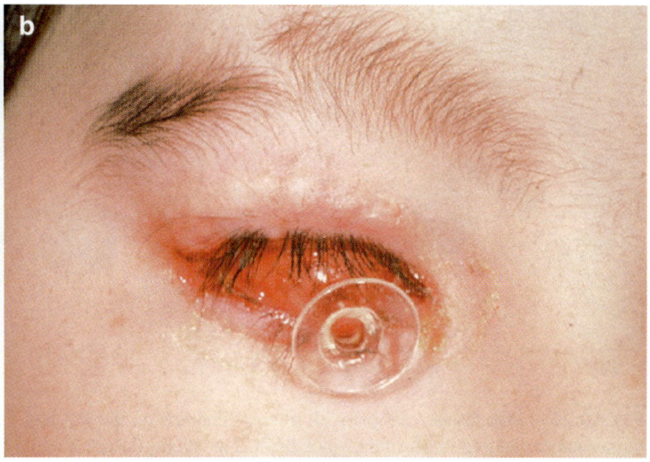

Fig. 60.27 (**a**) Examples of custom conformers of various sizes are used to progressively expand a congenital anophthalmic/microphthalmic socket. These are custom fit every 6–8 weeks and can be fashioned to resemble an eye when there is enough space to retain them (top row). (**b**) Champagne glass configuration-type conformer. Additional pressure to the fornices can sometimes be obtained by applying an eyepatch and tape over the protruding stem. The limiting factor is whether the child will tolerate the taped eye socket

tial aesthetic improvement with anophthalmos or microphthalmos relates to early socket expansion utilizing progressively larger-sized conformers (Fig. 60.27). This is followed by an ocular prosthesis and possibly an orbital implant which can provide acceptable results. Eyelid surgery and orbital cysts if present may be required but are usually deferred until the socket is more developed (e.g., 4–5 years of age).

The ideal management of anophthalmia and microphthalmia remains controversial, and no uniform strategy exists [223, 232, 242, 244]. Treatment of both the soft tissue hypoplasia (eyelids/conjunctival fornices) and bony hypoplasia is important to consider. Patients with phimotic lids and shortened conjunctival fornices all require early tissue expansion. Treatment of the orbital bone deficit may consist of observation only (e.g., microphthalmos with cyst – Fig. 60.25) or in severe cases may involve removal of a vestigial eye followed by placement of an orbital implant (expandable vs nonexpendable) [223, 232, 242, 243].

Treatment of these poorly developed eyelids and sockets should commence as early as possible (i.e., often within the first few weeks of life) and as previously mentioned requires the close collaboration of the ophthalmologist, ocularist, and most importantly the emotionally impacted parents [223, 224, 242, 243]. The eye and orbit develop most rapidly during the first year of life [249]. Seventy percent of the increase of the globe's volume occurs by 4 years of age and 90% by age 7 and is completed by early adolescence (around age 14) [246, 247]. With respect to orbital volume, 80% of adult orbital volume is reached by 5 years of age in normal pediatric individuals [237]. Orbital growth is completed by 11 years in females and approximately 15 years in males [236, 248]. By contrast, the face even by 3 months is only 40% of adult face size, but by 2 years, it is 70%, and by 5–6 years, 90% of adult size is achieved [249]. Both normal facial and orbital development are affected by a reduction in ocular volume. In anophthalmia and severe microphthalmia, there is underdevelopment of the bony orbit, the eyelids, the conjunctival fornices, as well as the side of the face [229, 230, 232–234, 241]. Without intervention, the socket remains underdeveloped, and the ability to wear a prosthesis is compromised. The under development and facial asymmetry become more pronounced as the child grows. The cosmetic deformity that results without intervention can lead to severe difficulties with social interaction. With appropriate treatment, orbital and facial disfigurement can be minimized. The earlier that treatment is initiated, the greater the effect on influencing the growth of the orbit, the orbital soft tissues, and the ipsilateral facial development.

Reconstruction efforts in anophthalmia or microphthalmia are designed to simultaneously expand the affected tissues in several dimensions:

1. Expansion of the eyelids both horizontally and vertically.
2. Expansion of the conjunctival space and forniceal depth.
3. Expansion of the orbital bone volume [250].

Treatment should begin promptly after birth (within weeks) and requires a commitment of time, energy, and resources by the parents, the physician team, and the ocularist [241, 243, 251–254]. Initial efforts are directed at expansion of the lid fissure as the severe phimosis prevents access to the orbital tissue. Traditionally, the lids and conjunctiva are expanded with a series of progressively enlarging acrylic conformers.

Ocular prosthesis management is critical to minimizing orbital growth retardation and preventing periorbital asymmetries [245, 251, 253, 254]. The ocularist may use a variety

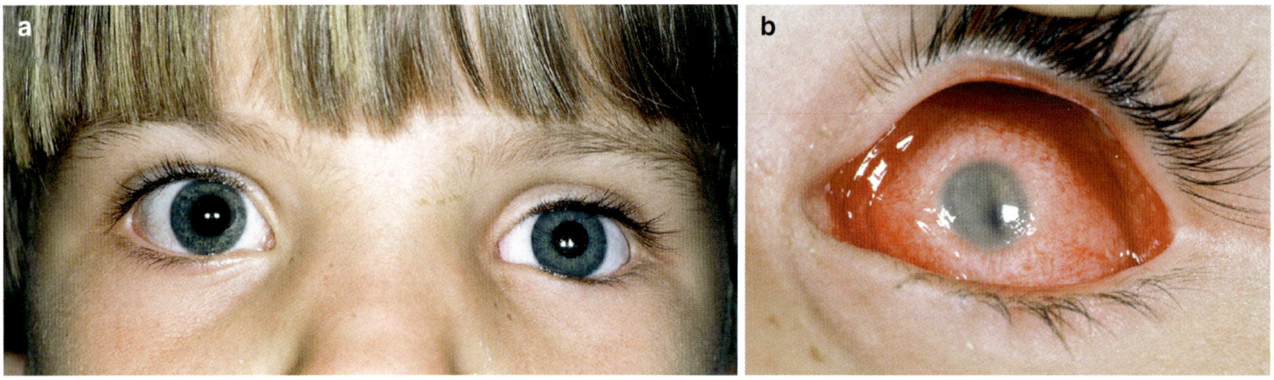

Fig. 60.28 (**a**) A 5-year-old girl with microphthalmos on the left had numerous expanding conformers since birth. The eyelid fissure height and horizontal length are very symmetrical to the normal side. (**b**) The microphthalmic left eye is approximately half the size of the normal eye. Both anterior and posterior segments were severely malformed

of conformers to expand the tissue including "dumbbell"-shaped conformers or "champagne glass configuration" conformer that help transmit pressure to the socket by application of tape over the external component of the conformer (Fig. 60.27a, b). The ocularist may enlarge the conformers weekly for the first few months of life and then every 6–8 weeks thereafter depending on the degree of tissue growth. These progressively enlarging conformers help expand the conjunctival fornices, eyelids, and periocular soft tissues and stimulate orbital bone development [245, 251, 253]. As the conformers get large enough, they can be painted and prepared to resemble an artificial eye to improve the cosmetic appearance (Figs. 60.26 and 60.28).

In recent years, another option to expand the eyelids and conjunctival fornices has involved hydrophilic expanders [223, 255–257]. Hydrophilic expanders are available in several sizes and can be placed into the conjunctival fornices or sutured into the underlying socket tissue. The eyelids are then closed over the expander with a temporary tarsorrhaphy, secured with sutures or Histoacryl glue [223, 256]. Approximately 2 months later, this is exchanged for an acrylic conformer, and socket expansion is considered [256].

In the case of mild to moderate microphthalmic eyes where there might be visual potential management, options vary. When the axial length is less than 16 mm, the eye is unlikely to promote normal orbital growth alone, and it is necessary to increase the socket volume early on to prevent asymmetry from becoming more pronounced as the child grows. In this situation, a custom-made cosmetic shell can be fit over the microphthalmic eye to promote orbital growth. Transparent shells should be fitted initially in the case of eyes with a positive VEP or with a near-normal size eye and cornea. Once the child grows and the vision has been established as useful or non-useful, consideration can be given to eye removal or placement of a more permanent custom-made prosthetic eye. The microphthalmic eye generally should only be removed if there are pathologic changes or symptoms that necessitate its removal. It is usually best to leave the eye in position and fit a prosthesis over it since this helps stimulate bone growth as the eye develops. A microphthalmic eye is a good template for an overlying prosthetic eye and usually has excellent motility, some of which may be transferred to a custom-made prosthesis (Fig. 60.28a, b). The question of when to change a clear prosthesis over a unilateral microphthalmic eye with some vision (e.g., light perception) for a custom-made painted prosthesis is difficult. A clear prosthesis allows maximal visual potential of the microphthalmic eye to be reached and the health of the underlying eye to be monitored. Eventually, once a stable visual development is achieved, it is unlikely to be significantly affected if the microphthalmic eye is covered with a custom prosthesis used to provide better cosmesis [223, 258]. A Gundersen conjunctival flap can also be used if the cornea shows intolerance to an acrylic shell or prosthesis. Removal of the microphthalmic eye is a consideration with some reconstructive socket procedures. Some surgeons advocate removal of a non-seeing microphthalmic eye and using a spherical implant, inflatable orbital tissue expander, or dermis fat graft at an early stage (see below). Our current preference is to try and preserve the microphthalmic eye even if there is no visual potential. The advantages of this approach are that the microphthalmic eye is likely to provide some stimulus to palpebral aperture and socket growth, particularly when the microphthalmos is mild or associated with an orbital cyst. Delay in intervention also avoids early invasive surgery with the potential risks associated with orbital implant placement (e.g., infection, migration, extrusion, ischemia).

For patients with anophthalmia or microphthalmia and an orbital cyst, gradual socket enlargement is usually achieved using increasing sized conformers for the fornices in conjunction with the natural expansion produced by the cyst (Fig. 60.25) [248]. The parents may need gentle reassurance that this is the best approach as initially the appearance may be unsatisfactory. The cysts may have a blue appearance subcutaneously which may appear to be ecchymosis and occasionally raise suspicion of child abuse (Fig. 60.28d). By the age of 3–5 years (before entering formal school education), the sockets in many of these cases have developed sufficiently for the orbital cyst to be removed [259, 260]. Once the cyst(s) is removed +/− an ocular remnant, an orbital implant is required to replace the volume deficit remaining. Alternatively, if the microphthalmic eye is left in place, a free fat graft can be placed into the socket to replace the volume loss [261, 262].

Once the eyelids of the anophthalmic or severely microphthalmic eye socket have been opened adequately and the fornices have been expanded, consideration of orbital volume augmentation and the bony skeleton is considered. This is ideally initiated within the first 2 years of life but may vary depending on the child's eyelid and orbital growth/development as well as family considerations and willingness. Since orbital growth does not cease until around 11–15 years of age, there is still some benefit if orbital expansion begins after infancy. A variety of orbital expanders are available to clinicians to treat the congenital orbital volume deficit including solid spherical implants, inflatable soft tissue expanders, dermis fat grafts, hydrogel expanders, and integrated orbital tissue expanders [263–265].

Solid orbital spheres have historically been the primary implant choice; however, inadequate orbital bone growth severely limits the size of the implants that can be placed. While small implants yield marginal results, larger implants risk extrusion [266]. Repeated implant exchanges require numerous anesthetics and surgical trauma to the conjunctiva and socket until skull maturation has occurred [267]. Despite the arduous process of serial replacements, volume disparity often remains apparent, and additional expansion may be required [259]. The inability to keep pace with the bony growth of the contralateral normal orbit also results in delayed development of the ipsilateral hemiface [229, 230]. Porous orbital implants are not recommended in this group of children as it may be difficult to get a large-sized implant in without risking exposure. Porous implants are also not readily replaced without a great deal of trauma to the socket. The real advantage of a porous implant is enhanced motility when they are coupled to a peg. Children are generally not peg candidates as most are unable or unwilling to adequately care for their socket. Polymethyl methacrylate implants are recommended with reassessment of the socket volume and motility at 16–20 years old at which time implant exchange with a larger porous implant may be considered.

Inflatable soft tissue (balloon) expanders are another option to increase the orbital dimensions in children with severe microphthalmos or anophthalmos. They are implanted through a bicoronal flap or temporoparietal scalp approach in conjunction with an orbitotomy [218, 220, 251, 255, 268]. Previous animal studies have shown that the placement of a solid sphere in an orbit results in partial expansion of the bony socket and that a fully inflated serially expanded silicone implant results in growth equal to the normal side [269–271]. There are several techniques available, with varying results [218, 220, 251, 255, 268]. Problems with extrusion and lack of control over the direction of expansion have been experienced [218, 271–275]. Frequently, uncontrolled forward protrusion of the expander during inflation will displace the conformer or result in premature extrusion [246, 267, 276]. Evisceration of the microphthalmic eye and using the scleral shell as a barrier may offer improved results [220]. The balloon expanders ideally are placed within the first year of life, but good results have been obtained even at 4–6 years old [220]. The balloon is inflated on a regular basis with saline via an externalized injection/inflation port placed distally from the orbit. The age of the subject at the time of implantation was not the sole determinant of the degree of eyelid and orbital growth in one series [220]. Similarly, severity of the deformity was not a dominant factor. The variable that seemed to most influence the degree of tissue growth was the time required to complete inflation of the expander [220]. A target inflation period of 20–36 weeks, initiated 3 months after expander placement, was associated with a low risk of extrusion [220]. The volume of saline required to reach an expander diameter of 22 mm ideally is divided equally into monthly injections over this period [220]. Advantages of this technique include predictable growth of the orbit, adjacent facial skeleton, eyelids, and conjunctiva. Only two surgical procedures are needed, and the technique does not produce significant conjunctival scarring [220]. However, disadvantages may include the lack of wide availability of the expanders, the need for multiple injections over a fairly rigid time sequence to obtain good results, and the inflation pressures that can sometimes reach 150–200 mmHg which can be uncomfortable for the patient and the parents [255, 275, 277]. To minimize inflation pressure spikes, a pulsatile orbital expander that transmitted steady carotid pulsations to the orbit was suggested but did not gain wide acceptance [278]. Additional risks associated with various expandable implant devices include tissue ischemia, infection, and extrusion [255].

Mazzoli et al. have suggested that an ideal orbital expander should have several characteristics including straightforward placement through a small incision, enlargement over a relatively short time, long-term soft tissue tolerance, avoidance of uncomfortable inflation spikes, resistance to infection, low likelihood of extrusion or inflator malfunction and minimal follow-up, intervention, manipulation, or revision [266].

Dermis fat grafts may also serve as orbital expanders in children [205, 241, 250, 279]. As dermis fat grafts are vascularized structures that grow with the child, they can potentially exert enough orbital pressure and volume to expand both the lids and socket [241, 250]. Dermis fat grafts have traditionally been used most frequently after extrusion of an orbital implant or removal of a migrated implant in adults where there is some loss of conjunctival tissues and shortened fornices. Conjunctival epithelium will migrate over the anterior surface of the dermis fat graft and potentially expand the conjunctival surface area. When used in the anophthalmic or microphthalmic socket, the growth of the fat may be so exuberant in some cases that debulking is required to avoid overexpansion. Placement of dermis fat grafts before the age of 3 years is associated with higher success [241, 250]. Because of the familiarity of the procedure and low risks of complications, this technique is popular and always combined with the serial expansion of conjunctival conformers both before and after the dermis fat graft is placed. Disadvantages of dermis fat grafts include an unpredictable rate of absorption with a resulting superior sulcus deformity and orbital volume deficiency. In addition, there is little or no transfer of eye socket movement to the overlying prosthesis resulting in an artificial eye with little natural motility.

After several years of use in Europe, a self-expanding hydrogel orbital expander has become another option in the anophthalmic/microphthalmic socket [223, 256, 268, 280]. Hydrogels are highly hydrophilic polymers that expand by osmotically imbibing water or tissue fluid [266]. These implantable spheres can absorb up to 2000% of their weight in water and can increase up to 30 times their original volume [245, 255]. The amount and rate of expansion can be engineered and precisely controlled. These characteristics combined with the ability to mold any desired shape and size make it an attractive material to consider in reconstructing congenital anophthalmic fornices and orbits [256, 280–282]. Three ophthalmic appliances have become available: a hemispherical-designed self-expanding conformer for conjunctival fornix expansion, an orbital sphere intended to help expand orbital bone volume (when a microphthalmic eye or remnant is not present), and self-inflating pellet expanders for those orbits that have a microphthalmic eye [255, 256, 283, 284]. Each is inserted in the dry, shrunken, and anhydrous state and gradually expand, nearly ten times, over several weeks. The conjunctival hemispherical conformer is placed into the conjunctival fornices, similar to a regular conformer and held in place with temporary suture tarsorrhaphy bolsters and/or tissue glue along the eyelid margins [223]. Normal tear secretion gradually swells the conformer to a maximum size within a few weeks, as it exerts a constant hydrostatic pressure of 20–30 mmHg [255]. Maximum expansion is achieved within 3–4 weeks, although the conformer can be retained for 2–3 months. Once maximum forniceal expansion is reached, a conventional prosthesis can be placed [223, 255, 256]. The orbital expanders are either spherical or pellet shaped. The selection depends upon whether a reasonably sized microphthalmic eye is present or an eye or eye remnant is absent [283, 284]. They come in various sizes and can be placed intraorbitally through a small lateral soft tissue incision, a central conjunctival incision (e.g., post enucleation), or in the case of the pellets, via an intraorbital injection using a customized trocar [223, 255, 256]. Because the hydrogel implants are self-inflating, there is no need for subfascial tracts and remote injection ports so there is less risk of inflator-related complications [255]. The orbital expanders like the conjuctival expanders exert a constant pressure of 20–25 mm Hg. As the hydrogel implant reaches its equilibrium of water content, the expansion forces are reduced substantially, and bone stimulation ceases [245]. The spherical orbital expander may require replacement to a larger size expander if orbital expansion is inadequate with the initially placed expander [256]. Although the hydrogel expander is an appealing alternative to the conventional implant options, the enthusiasm has been tempered by concern about the biomaterial's long-term fragility and ability to maintain sustained pressure on the orbit [266]. The requisite periodic exchanges to a larger diameter hydrogel sphere to maintain pressure holds little advantage over the conventional method of serial replacement with hard spheres of known geometry [255, 265]. In addition, although the use of spherical orbital expanders and conjunctival forniceal expanders has been described as "safe, simple and almost harmless," potential complications do exist [256, 266, 285]. The best methods for implantation as well as the intraorbital characteristics and side effect profile have yet to be clearly delineated [285]. In the largest series to date, the authors reported 14 failures with conjunctival socket expanders and 21 failures with orbital expanders out of a total of 127 expanders placed [256]. Unfortunately, the authors did not fully define failure [256]. They did however state that all complications could be corrected with another operation, and there had not yet been an irreparable failure [256]. These implants are foreign materials subject to infection and extrusion and their expansion and may potentially cause tissue ischemia [255]. Migration within the orbit and inadequate support of a conformer or ocular prosthesis are other possible problems [285, 286]. As with any new material or technique, there is always a potential for unintended or unexpected consequences that are not well-known until one use has been analyzed [255]. One unexpected and delayed (10 + years) complication reported with previous hydrogel appliances in the orbit (retinal buckling elements made of MIRAgel – MIRA,Waltham, MA) was a delayed breakdown of the hydrogel product attributed to uncontrolled swelling of the material beyond its initial size [255]. There are several reports of buckle extrusions, intraocular erosion and migration, intraorbital fibrosis, pain, foreign body granuloma formation, and inflammatory orbital pseudotumor as a result [287–292]. Although the current hydrogel polymers are reportedly more stable than the MIRAgel implants, it remains unknown how well tolerated this new material will be over the course of a child's life expectancy [255, 283].

In recent years, Tse et al. developed an integrated orbital tissue expander (OTE), (distributed by Marshfield Hills, MA) to address limitations of the conventional orbital expansion options that can be implanted using standard oculoplastic surgical procedures [263–265]. The OTE differs from earlier injectable orbital expanders as it consists of a flexible "balloon/expander" held in place by a titanium fixation plate that is anchored to the lateral orbital walls by screws (Fig. 60.29a–c). The direction of expansion and maintenance of expander fixation within the orbit are controlled allowing sustained omnidirectional expansion pressure. A 30-gauge needle connected to a 1 cc syringe is inserted into the OTE through an injection port. The injection track seals upon the removal of the needle, and increased pressure can then be applied to the orbit. Multiple surgeries are not required to maintain the OTE, and they can be easily inflated or deflated without surgery. To date, Tse et al. have used this device in nine patients ranging in age from 9 to 108 months [265]. Six of the nine received one subsequent inflation within 6 months of the initial implantation, and none have had more than one subsequent injection [265]. Using orbital CT-determined volumetric change as the primary outcome measure, all patients had an increase in the orbital volume after expander implantation (Fig. 60.29d–g). The orbital tissue expander also induced the growth of the adjacent frontal, maxillary, and zygomatic bones, leading to external improvements of the eyebrow position, cheek fullness, forward projection of the lateral canthal angle, and horizontal eyelid plane alignment [265]. These results validate the principle that the application of sustained biomechanical force to the craniofacial skeleton can achieve bone growth [265]. Three complications were encountered in the group of nine patients [265]. The first was associated with locating the injection port under the conjunctiva during the second inflation. The silicone globe of the orbital tissue expander of the first two patients inadvertently was punctured by the needle when palpation of the rounded tip of the T-plate was misinterpreted as the metal edge of the injection port. The ruptured expander had to be replaced immediately through a transconjunctival approach. The second complication involved the tip of the T-plate which protruded forward in a hypoplastic orbit, requiring conjunctival incision, temporary deflation, and repositioning of the plate. The third complication involved spontaneous deflation of the expander. The implant was removed and replaced. Examination of the expander revealed a small tear in the silicone rubber neck in the area where it was attached to the titanium injection valve [265].

Stimulation of orbital bone growth in congenital anophthalmos carries a significant biomedical and clinical burden. Management of the hypoplastic orbit requires simultaneous treatment of both the soft tissue hypoplasia and asymmetric bone growth [236]. The integrated orbital tissue expander described by Tse et al. appeared to fulfill all the essential criteria of an ideal orbital tissue expander (as described by Mazzoli and associates [266]) with the following added advantages: (1) small skin incision for implant placement, (2) ease of insertion, eliminating a lengthy implantation process, (3) collapsibility of the expander, facilitating insertion through a small opening, (4) no unpredictable implant movement or displacement, [5] sustained and uniform pressure delivered to constituent bones of the orbit without the need for serial implant exchanges, (6) reduced trauma by serial transconjunctival orbital tissue expander inflation with a needle rather than incising the conjunctiva, (7) well-tolerated long-term outcomes, (8) an implantation procedure that is familiar to orbital surgeons who routinely perform enucleation, and (9) a reduced number of procedures needed for effective orbital bone stimulation [265]. Overall, the integrated orbital tissue expander appeared safe and effective in stimulating anophthalmic socket bone growth. Validation of long-term effectiveness will require additional clinical studies with standardized protocol, pooling of data from participating clinical centers, and careful monitoring of adverse events [265]. Unfortunately, technical difficulties in the manufacturing process have yet to worked out, and it is presently unavailable for general use.

Long-Term Management of the Anophthalmic and Microphthalmic Socket

After the initial socket expansion over the first 5 years of life, the prosthesis and the socket require yearly examination. The microphthalmic eyes will also require follow-up with their pediatric ophthalmologist. Microphthalmic eyes may develop angle closure glaucoma, which may cause loss of what vision does exist and can also cause pain [291]. Children with chorioretinal coloboma and their parents should be aware of the increased risk of retinal detachment [293]. Glasses are prescribed for refractive error in the normal eye, for protection, and sometimes for providing lenses to minimize cosmetic defects (e.g., plus lenses to increase the size of a microphthalmic eye or prisms to equalize a height discrepancy).

The parents may wish to receive genetic counseling at some point regarding the risks of another child being affected. This may include chromosomal analysis and testing of particular genes [223]. Associated systemic abnormalities may have major implications for the child and often require considerable input from various pediatric specialties. It is important to reach a comprehensive diagnostic picture at some point as this helps direct future management. The parents are usually anxious to understand the nature of the condition, and coordinated counseling and management

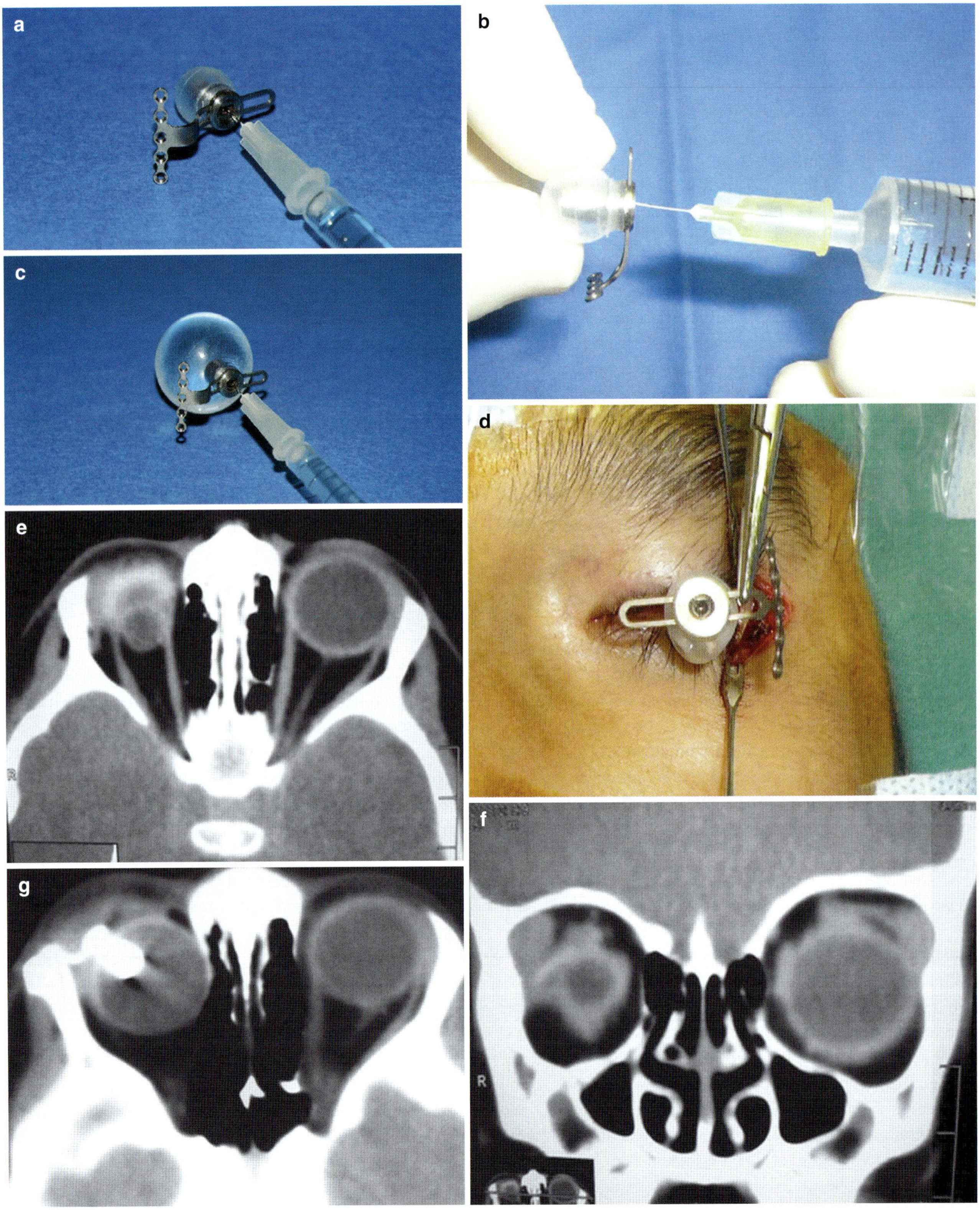

Fig. 60.29 (**a**) Deflated OTE orbital expander with needle tip sitting within the injection port. (Photos with permission of Dr. D. Tse and FCI Opthalmics, Marshfield Hills, MA). (**b**) Side view of OTE with needle in injection port. (**c**) OTE being inflated with saline. (**d**) Deflated OTE ready for insertion into the orbit of a 3-year-old male. (**e**) Preop axial Ct view of orbit before expansion. (**f**) Preop coronal CT view of orbit before expansion. (**g**) 24 months post placement of OTE, the axial CT scan shows orbital expansion. (**h**) 24 months post placement of OTE, the coronal CT scan shows orbital expansion

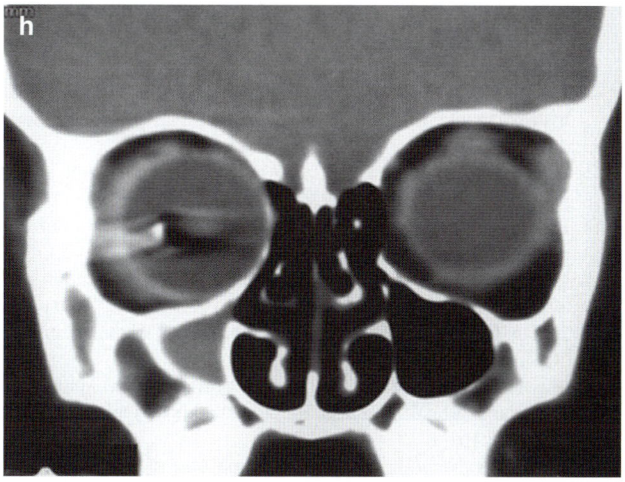

Fig. 60.29 (continued)

from pediatrics, ophthalmology, and genetics will help achieve this.

For those children with bilateral involvement, it is very important that they also receive assistance at an early age from low vision specialists. A social service worker should be involved from the early stages of those children bilaterally affected with anophthalmia/microphthalmia as they can help the family make connections with the various organizations for the visually impaired that will help them to obtain critical communication and survival skills. Early intervention undoubtedly makes a huge difference to the overall development of the child and the emotional well-being of the family [223].

Summary

Anophthalmic surgery is no longer simply about replacing a diseased eye with an orbital implant. There are multiple problems and complications that can occur with time. Ophthalmic surgeons working closely with ocularists must be focused on restoring a natural appearance to the patient's prosthesis with comfort, some motility, appropriate orbital volume, and eyelids that look symmetrical so they can integrate into the society with a near-normal appearance as possible. A variety of surgical techniques exist for correcting the different problems seen with the anophthalmic socket. Reconstruction of the contracted socket can be quite challenging as tissue loss and socket ischemia are difficult problems to overcome. Surgical techniques continue to evolve in the oculoplastic, craniofacial, and maxillofacial literature. Reconstructing congenitally anophthalmic/microphthalmic sockets poses particularly difficult social and surgical challenges that may result in frustration and disappointment for all concerned. Management of the hypoplastic orbit requires simultaneous treatment of both the soft tissue component (eyelids/conjunctiva) and the adjacent bone. Serial implant exchanges have significant limitations as they require numerous surgeries and have no dynamic component to stimulate bone growth. Although dermis fat grafts have a dynamic component and are popular among ophthalmologists, inflatable tissue expanders have the potential for controlled, gentle expansion of the eyelids, conjunctiva, and orbit. Until recently, the direction of expansion and maintenance of expander fixation within the orbit have been a problem, and migration/extrusion is not uncommon. Although a study by Tse et al. was small, their results with a new integrated orbital tissue expander (OTE) appear to be a breakthrough in the management of the congenital anophthalmic socket [265]. Their integrated orbital tissue expander appears to be safe, stable, and highly effective in stimulating anophthalmic orbital bone growth. Unfortunately, it is not yet available for general use.

References

1. Coday MP, Warner MA, Jarling KU, Rubin PA. Acquired monocular vision, functional consequences form the patients perspective. Ophthal Plast Reconstr Surg. 2002;18:55–63.
2. Bohman E, Roed Rassmussen ML, Dafgard Kopp E. Pain and discomfort in the anophthalmic socket. Curr Opin Ophthalmol. 2014;25:455–60.
3. Rasmussen ML, Ekholm O, Prause JU, Toft PB. Quality of life of eye amputated patients. Acta Ophthalmol. 2012;90:435–40.
4. Ahn JM, Lee SY, Yoon JS. Health related quality of life and emotional status of anophthalmic patients in Korea. Am J Ophthalmo. 2010;149:1005–11.
5. Masdottir S, Sahlin S. Patient satisfaction and results after evisceration with a split-sclera technique. Orbit. 2007;26:241–7.
6. McBain HB, Ezra DG, Rose GE, Newman SP. The psychological impact of living with an ocular prosthesis. Orbit. 2014;33:33–9.
7. Lost eye, coping with monocular vision after enucleation or eye loss from cancer, accident, or disease. Adkisson JD, editor. iUniverse, New York, 2006, Mental and Emotional Issues, chapter 22. p. 317–44.
8. Gougelmann HP. The evolution of the ocular motility implant. Int Ophthalmol Clin. 1970;10(4):689–711.
9. Jordan DR, Klapper SR, Mawn LA. The anophthalmic socket and complications. In Fay A, Dolman P, editors. Diseases and disorders of the orbit and ocular adnexa. Edinburgh London New York Oxfored Philedelphia St Louis Sydney Toronto: Elsevier. 2017, chapter 36. p. 657–75.
10. Smit TJ, Koornneef L, Zonnereld FW, Groet E, Otto AJ. Computed tomography in the assessment of the postenucleation socket syndrome. Ophthalmology. 1990;97:137–40.
11. Smit TJ, Koornneef L, Zonnereld FW, Groet E, Otto AJ. Primary and secondary implants in the anophthalmic orbit:preoperative and postoperative computed tomographic appearance. Ophthalmology. 1991a;98(1):106–10.
12. Soll DB. The anophthalmic socket. Ophthalmology. 1982;89:407–23.
13. Kaltreider SA. The ideal ocular prostheses. Analysis of prosthetic volume. Ophthal Plast Reconstr Surg. 2000;16(5):388–92.
14. Kaltreider SA, Lucarelli MJ. A simple algorithm for selection of implant size for enucleation and evisceration. Ophthal Plast Reconstr Surg. 2002;18:336–41.

15. Custer PL, Trinkaus KM. Volumetric determination of enucleation implant size. Am J Ophthalmol. 1999;128:489–94.
16. Thaller VT. Enucleation volume measurement. Ophthal Plast Reconstr Surg. 1997;13:18–20.
17. Allen L. Modified impression fitting. Int Ophthalmol Clin. 1970;10:747–62.
18. Parr GR, Goldman BM, Rahn AO. Post insertion care of the ocular prosthesis. J Pros Dentistry. 1983;49(2):220–4.
19. Pine KR, Sloan BH, Jacobs RJ. A proposed model of the response of the anophthalmic socket to prosthetic eye wear and its application to the management of mucoid discharge. Med Hypothesis. 2013a;81:300–5.
20. Pine KR, Sloan B, Stewart J, Jacobs RJ. The response of the anophthalmic socket to prosthetic eye wear. Clin Exp Optom. 2013b;96:338–93.
21. Pine KR, Sloan B, Jacobs RJ. Deposit build up on prosthetic eyes and implications for conjunctival inflammation and mucoid discharge. Clin Ophthalmol. 2012a;12(6):1755–62.
22. Pine KR, Sloan B, Stewart J, Jacobs RJ. A surgery of prosthetic eye wearers to investigate mucoid discharge. Clin Ophthal. 2012b;1(6):707–13.
23. Pine KR, Sloan B, Jacobs RJ. The development of measurement tools for prosthetic eye research. Clin Exp Optom. 2013c;96:32–8.
24. Osborn KL, Hottler D. A survey of recommendations on the care of ocular prostheses. Optometry. 2010;81:142–5.
25. Trawnik WR. Care of the ocular prostheses. Adv Ophthal Plas Reconstr Surg. 1990;8:146–8.
26. Fett DR, Scott R, Putterman AM. Evaluation of lubricants for prosthetic eye wearers. Ophthal Plast Reconstr Surg. 1986;2(1):29–31.
27. LeGrand JA. Chronic exudate: an unnecessary evil. J Ophthal Prosthetics. 1999;4(1):757–9.
28. Jones CA, Collin JRO. A classification and review of the causes of discharging sockets. Trans Ophthalmol UK. 1983;103:351–3.
29. Larned DC. Lacrimal mechanics in the enucleated state. Ophthal Plast Reconstr Surg. 1992;8:202–7.
30. Allen L, Kolder HE, Bulgarelli EM, Bulgarelli DM. Artificial eyes and tear measurements. Ophthalmology. 1980;87:155–7.
31. Kim SE, Yoon JS, Lee SY. Tear measurements in prosthetic eye users with Fourier-Domain optical coherence tomography. Am J Ophthal. 2010;149:602–7.
32. Vasquez RJ, Linberg JV. The anophthalmic socket and prosthetic eye: a clinical and bacteriologic study. Ophthal Plast Reconstr Surg. 1989;5:277–80.
33. Rose GE. The giant fornix syndrome: an unrecognized cause of chronic, relapsing, grossly purulent conjunctivitis. Ophthalmology. 2004;111:1539–45.
34. Jones DF, Lyle CE, Fleming JC. Superior conjunctivoplasty-Mullerectomy for correction of chronic discharge and concurrent ptosis in anophthalmic socket with enlarged superior fornix. Ophthal Plast Reconstr Surg. 2010;26:172–5.
35. Jordan DR, Brownstein S, Lee-Wing M, Ashenhurst M. Pyogenic granulomas following oculoplastic procedures: an imbalance in angiogenesis regulation. Can J Ophthalmol. 2001;36(5):260–8.
36. Jordan DR, Brownstein S, Faraji H. Clinicopathologic analysis of 15 explanted hydroxyapatite implants. Ophthal Plast Reconstr Surg. 2004a;20(4):285–90.
37. Chang WJ, Tse DT, Rosa RH, Huang A, et al. Conjunctival cytologic features of giant papillary conjunctivitis associated with ocular prostheses. Ophthal Plast Reconstr Surg. 2005;21(1):39–45.
38. Scrinivasan OD, Jakobiec FA, Iwamoto T, DeVoe G. Giant papillary conjunctivitis with ocular prostheses. Arch Ophthalmol. 1979;97:892–5.
39. Kymionis GD, Goldman D, Ide T, Yoo SH. Tacrolimus ointment 0.03% in the eye for treatment of giant papillary conjunctivitis. Cornea. 2008;27:228–9.
40. Attas-Fox L, Barkena Y, Iskhakov V, Rayvich S. Topical tacrolimus 0.03% ointment for intractable allergic conjunctivitis:an open-label pilot study. Curr Eye Res. 2008;33:545–9.
41. Remulla HD, Rubin PAD, Shore JW, Sutula FC, Townsend DJ, Woog JJ, Jahrling KV. Complications of porous spherical orbital implants. Ophthalmology. 1995;102:586–93.
42. Jordan DR, Bawazeer A. Experience with 120 synthetic hydroxyapatite implants ($FCI_{3)}$. Ophthal Plast Reconstr Surg. 2001;17:184–90.
43. Glaft HJ, Googe PB, Powers T, Apple DJ. Anophthalmic socket pain. Am J Ophthalmol. 1993;116:357–62.
44. Rasmussen ML, Prause JU, Toft PB. Phantom pain after eye amputation. Acta Ophthalmol. 2011;89:10–6.
45. Gerding H, Vo O, , Husstedt IW, Evers S, Soros P. Phantom pain after enucleation. Ophthalmology 2003;100:943–949.
46. Jordan DR. Anophthalmic orbital implants. Ophthal Clin NA. 2000;13(4):587–608.
47. Massary GC, Holds JB. Coralline hydroxyapatite spheres as secondary orbital implants in anophthalmos. Ophthalmology. 1995;102:161–6.
48. Jordan DR, Nerad J, Tse DT. An unusual case of orbital cellulitis. Can J Ophthal. 1990;25(4):210–2.
49. McCarthy RW, Beyer CK, Dallow RL, Burke JF, Lessell S. Conjunctival cysts of the orbit following enucleation. Ophthalmology. 1981;88(1):30–5.
50. Owji N, Aslani A. Conjunctival cysts of the orbit after enucleation: the use of trichloroacetic acid. Ophthal Plast Reconstr Surg. 2005;21(4):264–6.
51. Sanchez EM, Formento NA, Peres-Lopez M, Jimenez AA. Role of trichloroacetic acid in treating posterior conjunctival csyt in anophthalmic socket. Orbit. 2009;28:101–3.
52. Hornblass A, Bosniak S. Orbital cyst following enucleation: the use of absolute alcohol. Ophthal Surg. 1981;12:123–6.
53. Smit TJ, Koorneef L, Zonneveld FW. Conjunctival cysts in anophthalmic orbits. Br J Ophthalmol. 1991b;75:342–3.
54. Goldstein MH, Soparkar CNS, Kersten RC, Orcutt JC, Patrinely JR, Holds J. Conjunctival cysts of the orbit. Ophthalmology. 1998;105(11):2056–60.
55. Hanig CJ, Hornblass A. Treatment of post enucleation orbital cysts. Ann Ophthalmol. 1986;18:191–3.
56. Juneman A, Holbach LM. Epithelial giant inclusion cyst 50 years after enucleation without orbital implant. Klin Monatsbl Augenheilkd. 1998;212:127–8.
57. Anderson RL. The tarsal strip procedure for correction of eyelid laxity and canthal malposition in the anophthalmic socket. Ophthalmology. 1981;88:895–903.
58. Anderson RL, Gordy DD. The Tarsal strip procedure. Arch Ophthalmol. 1979;97(11):2192–6.
59. Jordan DR, Anderson RL. The lateral tarsal strip revisited: the enhanced Tarsal strip. Arch Ophthalmol. 1989;107(4):604–6.
60. Smith RJ, Malet T. Auricular cartilage grafting to correct lower conjunctival fornix retraction and eyelid malposition in anophthalmic patients. Ophthal Plast Reconstr Surg. 2008;24(1):13–8.
61. Ma'luf RN. Correction of the inadequate lower fornix in the anophthalmic socket. Br J Ophthalmol. 1999;83:881–2.
62. Neuhaus RW, Hawes MJ. Inadequate inferior cul-de-sac in the anophthalmic socket. Ophthalmology. 1992;99:153–7.
63. Rougraff PM, Tse DT, Johnson TE, Feuer W. Involutional entropion repair with fornix sutures and lateral tarsal strip. Ophthal Plast Reconstr Surg. 2001;17(4):281–7.
64. Ho SF, Pherwani A, Elsssherbiny SM, Reuser T. Lateral tarsal strip and Quickert Sutures for lower eyelid entropion. Ophthal Plast Reconstr Surg. 2005;21(5):345–8.
65. Kersten RC, Kleiner FP, Kulwin DR. Tarsotomy for the treatment of cicatricial entropion with trichiasis. Arch Ophthalmol. 1992;110:714–7.
66. Weis FA. Surgical treatment of entropion. J Int Coll Surg. 1954;21:758–60.

67. Allen LH. Four-snip procedure for involutional lower lid entropion: modification of Quickert and Jones procedures. Can J Ophthalmol. 1991;26(3):139–43.
68. Kaltreider S, Shields MD, Heipperd SC, Patrie J. Anopthalmic ptosis: investigation of the mechanisms and statistical analysis. Ophthal Plast Reconstr Surg. 2003;19(6):421–8.
69. Vistnes LM. Mechanism of upper eyelid ptosis in the anophthalmic orbit. Plast Reconstr Surg. 1976;58:539–45.
70. Karesh JW, Putterman AM, Fett DR. Conjunctival-Muellers muscle excision to correct anophthalmic ptosis. Ophthalmology. 1986;93:1068–71.
71. Lee EW, Berbos Z, Zaldivar RA, Lee MS, Harrison AR. Use of a Dermatrix graft in oculoplastic surgery. Opthal Plast Reconstr Surg. 2010a;26(3):153–4.
72. Rubin PA, Fay AM, Remulla HD, Maus M. Ophthalmic plastic applications of acellular dermal allografts. Ophthalmology. 1999;106:2091–7.
73. Shorr N, Perry JD, Glodberg RA, et al. The safety and applications of acellular human dermal allograft in ophthalmic plastic and reconstructive surgery. Opthal Plast Reconstr Surg. 2000;16:223–30.
74. Vagefi MR, McMullan TFW, Burroughs JR, White GW, McCann JD, Anderson RL. Injectable Calcium Hydroxylapatite for orbital volume augmentation. Arch Facial Plast Surg. 2007;9(6):439–42.
75. Cahill KV, Burns JA. Volume augmentation of the anophthalmic orbit with cross-linked collagen (Zyplast). Arch Ophthalmol. 1989;107(11):1684–6.
76. Hunter PD, Baker SS. The treatment of enophthalmos by orbital injection of fat autograft. Arch Otolaryngol Head Neck Surg. 1994;120(8):835–9.
77. Huang ZL, Ma L. Restoration of enophthalmos in anophthalmic socket by HTR polymer. Ophthal Plast Reconstr Surg. 2005;21(4):318–21.
78. Tenag MA, Madura T, Yano K, Hosokawa K. Use of calcium phosphate cement paste in orbital volume augmentation. Plast Reconstr Surg. 2006;117(4):1186–93.
79. Morley AMS, Mehryar T, Malhorta R, Goldberg R. Use of hyaluronic acid gel for upper eyelid filling and contouring. Opthal Plast Reconstr Surg. 2009;25:440–4.
80. Smit TJ, Koornneef L, Mourits MP, et al. Primary versus secondary intraorbital implants. Ophthal Plast Reconstr Surg. 1991c;6:115–8.
81. Georgiadis NS, Tezidou CD, Dimitriadis AS. Restoration of the anophthalmic socket with secondary implantation of a coralline hydroxyapatite sphere. Ophthal Surg Lasers. 1998;29:808–14.
82. Frueh BR, Kelker GV. Baseball implant, a method of secondary insertion of an intraorbital implant. Arch Ophthalmol. 1976;94:429–30.
83. Massry GG, Holds JB. Corralline hydroxyapatite spheres as secondary orbital implants in anophthalmos. Ophthalmology. 1995;102:161–6.
84. Jordan DR. Localization of extraocular muscles during secondary orbital implantation surgery. The tunnel technique: experience with 100 patients. Ophthalmology. 2004a;111:1048–54.
85. Allen L. The argument against imbrication the rectus muscles over spherical orbital implants after enucleation. Ophthalmology. 1983;90:1116–20.
86. Perry AC. Advances in enucleation. Ophthalmic Plast Reconstr Surg. 1991;4:173–82.
87. Dutton JJ. Coralline hydroxyapatite as an ocular implant. Ophthalmology. 1991;98:370–7.
88. Sheilds CL, Sheilds JA, De Potter P, et al. Lack of complications of the hydroxyapatite orbital implant in 250 consecutive cases. Trans Am Ophthal Soc. 1993;91:177–89.
89. Sheilds CL, Sheilds JA, De Potter P, et al. Problems with the hydroxyapatite orbital implant: experience with 250 consecutive cases. Br J Ophthalmol. 1994;78:702–6.
90. Nunery WR, Heinz GW, Bonnin JM, Martin RT, Cepela MA. Exposure rate of hydroxyapatite spheres in the anophthalmic socket: histopathologic correlation and comparison with silicone sphere implants. Ophthal Plast Reconstr Surg. 1993;9:96–104.
91. Goldberg RA, Holds JB, Ebrahimpour J. Exposed hydroxyapatite orbital implants: report of six cases. Ophthalmology. 1992;99:831–6.
92. Kim YD, Goldberg RA, Shorr N, Steinsapir KD. Management of exposed hydroxyapatite orbital implants. Ophthalmology. 1994;101:1709–15.
93. Oestreicher JH, Liu E, Berkowitz M. Complications of hydroxyapatite orbital implants: a review of 100 consecutive cases and a comparison of Dexon mesh (polyglycolic acid) with scleral wrapping. Ophthalmology. 1997;104:324–9.
94. Jordan DR, Brownstein S, Jolly SS. Abscessed hydroxyapatite orbital implants: a report of two cases. Ophthalmology. 1996a;103:1784–7.
95. Yoon JS, Lew H, Kim SJ, et al. Exposure rate of hydroxyapatite orbital implants. Ophthalmology. 2008;115:566–72.
96. Shoamanesh A, Pang N, Oestreicher JH. Complications of orbital implants; a review of 542 patients who have undergone orbital implantation and 275 subsequent peg placements. Orbit. 2007;25:173–82.
97. Custer PL, Trinkaus KM. Porous implant exposure: incidence, management, and morbidity. Ophthal Plast Reconstr Surg. 2007;23:1–7.
98. Jordan DR, Klapper SR, Gilberg SM. The use of vicryl mesh in 200 porous orbital implants. Ophthal Plast Reconstr Surg. 2003a;19:53–61.
99. Wang JK, Liao SL, Lai PC, et al. Prevention of exposure of porous orbital implants following enucleation. Am J Ophthalmol. 2007;143:61–7.
100. Blaydon SM, Shepler TR, Neuhaus RW, White WL, Shore JW. The porous polyethylene (Medpor) spherical orbital implant: a retrospective study of 136 cases. Ophthal Plast Reconstr Surg. 2003;19:364–74.
101. Karesh JW, Dresner SC. High density porous polyethylene (Medpor) as a successful anophthalmic implant. Ophthalmology. 1994;101:1688–96.
102. Ma Y, Schou KR, Maloney-Schou M, Harwin FM, NG J. The porous polyethylene/bioglass spherical orbital implant: a retrospective study of 170 cases. Ophthal Plast Reconstr Surg. 2011;27:21–7.
103. Mahoney NR, Grant MP, Illiff NT, Merbs SL. Exposure rate of smooth surface tunnel porous polyethylene implants after enucleation. Ophthal Plast Reconstr Surg. 2014;30:492–8.
104. Jordan DR, Munro SM, Brownstein S, Gilberg SM, Grahovac SZ. A synthetic hydroxyapatite implant: the so-called counterfeit implant. Ophthalmic Plast Reconstr Surg. 1998a;14(4):244–9.
105. Jordan DR, Mawn L, Brownstein S, McEachren TM, Gilberg SM, Hill V, Grahovac SZ, Adenis JP. The bioceramic orbital implant: a new generation of porous implants. Ophthalmic Plast Reconstr Surg. 2000;16:347–55.
106. Jordan DR, Gilberg S, Mawn LA. The bioceramic orbital implant: experience with 107 implants. Ophthalmic Plast Reconstr Surg. 2003b;19:128–35.
107. Alwitry A, West S, King J, Foss AJ, Abercrombie LC. Long term follow-up of porous polyethylene spherical implants after enucleation and evisceration. Ophthal Plast Reconstr Surg. 2007;23:11–5.
108. Ahmed Sadiq S, Mengher LS, Downes R. Integrated orbital implants – a comparison of hydroxyapatite and porous polyethylene implants. Orbit. 2008;27:37–40.
109. Jordan DR, Klapper SK, Gilberg SM, Dutton JJ, Wong A, Mawn L. The bioceraamic implant: evaluation of implant exposures in 419 implants ophthalmic. Plast Reconstr Surg. 2010;26:80–2.

110. Wang JK, Lai PC, Liao SL. Late exposure of the bioceramic orbital implant. Am J Ophthalmology. 2009;147:162–70.
111. Karslioglu SK, Buttanri IB, Fazil K, Serin D, Akbaba M. Long-term outcomes of pegged and unpegged bioceramic orbital implants. Ophthalmic Plast Reconstr Surg. 2012;28:264–7.
112. Jordan DR, Gilberg SM, Bawazeer A. The coralline hydroxyapatite orbital implant (Bio-Eye™): experience with 170 patients. Ophthal Plast Reconstr Surg. 2004b;20(1):69–71.
113. Jordan DR, Klapper SR. Anophthalmic orbital implants: current concepts and controverseys. Compre Ophthalmol. 2005;6(6):287–96.
114. Jordan DR. Problems after evisceration surgery with porous orbital implants: experience with 86 patients. Ophthal Plast Reconstr Surg. 2004b;20(5):374–80.
115. Pelletier C, Gilberg D, Jordan DR. Use of temporalis fascia for management of exposed hydroxyapatite implants. Ophthal Plast Reconstr Surg. 1998;14(3):198–203.
116. Buettner H, Bartley GB. Tissue breakdown and exposure associated with orbital hydroxyapatite implants. Am J Ophthalmol. 1992;113:669–73.
117. El-Sharhed FS, Sherief MM, Ali AT. Management of tissue breakdown and exposure associated with orbital hydroxyapatite implants. Ophthal Plast Recon Surg. 1995;11:91–4.
118. Neuhaus RW, Shorr N. Use of temporalis fascia and muscle as an auto graft. Arch Ophthalmol. 1983;101:262–4.
119. Oestreicher JH. Treatment of exposed coral implants after failed scleral patch graft. Ophthal Plast Reconstr Surg. 1994;10(2):110–3.
120. Wiggs EO, Becker BB. Extrusion of enucleation implants: treatment with secondary implants and autogenous temporalis fascia or fascia lata patch grafts. Ophthal Surg. 1992;23:472–6.
121. Soporkar CNS, Patrinely JR. Tarsal patch flap for orbital implant exposure. Ophthal Plast Reconstr Surg. 1998;6:391–7.
122. Jordan DR, Brownstein S, Joly SS. Abscessed hydroxyapatite orbital implants: a report of 2 cases. Ophthalmology. 1996b;103:1784–7.
123. Jordan DR, Klapper SR, Mawn L, et al. Abscess formation within a synthetic hydroxyapatite implant. Can J Opthalmol. 1998b;33:329–32.
124. Ainbinder DJ, Haik BG, Tallado M. Hydroxyapatite orbital implants abscess:histopathologic consideration of an infected implant following evisceration. Ophthal Plast Reconstr Surg. 1994;10:267–70.
125. Jordan DR, Brownstein S, Rawlings N, Robinson J. An infected porous polyethylene orbital implant. Ophthal Plast Reconstr Surg. 2007;23(5):413–5.
126. Jordan DR, Brownstein S, Robinson J. An infected aluminum oxide orbital implant. Ophthal Plast Reconstr Surg. 2006;22(1):66–7.
127. Guillinta P, Vasani SN, Granet DB, Kikkawa DO. Prosthetic motility in pegged versus unpegged integrated porous orbital implants. Ophthal Plast Reconstr Surg. 2003;19:119–22.
128. Jordan DR, Chan S, Mawn L, Gilberg S, Dean T, Brownstein S, Hill VE. Complications associated with pegging hydroxyapatite orbital implants. Ophthalmology. 1999a;106:505–12.
129. Fahim DK, Frueh BR, Musch DC, Nelson CC. Complications of pegged and non-pegged hydroxyapatite orbital implants. Ophthal Plast Reconstr Surg. 2007;23:206–10.
130. Jordan DR, Chan S, Mawn L, Gilberg SM, Brownstein S, Hill V. Complications associated with pegging hydroxyapatite orbital implants. Ophthalmology. 1999b;106:505–12.
131. Edelstein C, Shields CL, DePotter P, Shields JA. Complications of motility peg placement for the hydroxyapatite orbital implant. Ophthalmology. 1997;104:1616–21.
132. Lin CJ, Lio SL, Jou JR, Kao SC, Hou PK, Chen MS. Complications of motility peg placement for porous hydroxyapatite orbital implants. Br J Ophthalmol. 2002;86:394–6.
133. Jordan DR. Spontaneous loosening of hydroxyapatite peg sleeves. Ophthalmology. 2001;108:2041–4.
134. Cheng MS, Lio SL, Lin L. Late porous polyethylene implant exposure after motility coupling post placement. Am J Ophthalmol. 2004;138:420–4.
135. Lee SY, Jang JW, Lew H, Kim SJ, Kim HY. Complications in motility peg placement for hydroxyapatite orbital implants in anophthalmic socket. Jpn J Ophthalmol. 2002a;46:103–7.
136. Jordan DR, Klapper SR. A new titanium peg system for hydroxyapatite orbital implants. Ophthalmic Plast Reconstr Surg. 2000;16:380–7.
137. Johnson RLC, Ramstead CL, Nathoo N. Pegging the porous implant. Ophthalmic Plast Reconstr Surg. 2011;27:74–5.
138. Yazici B, Akova B, Sanli O. Complications of primary placement of motility post in porous polyethylene implants during enucleation. Am J Ophthalmol. 2007;143:828–4.
139. Krishna G. Contracted sockets (etiology and types). Indian J Ophthalmol. 1980;28:117–20.
140. Tawfik HA, Raslan AO, Talib N. Surgical management of acquired socket contracture. Curr Opin Ophthalmol. 2009;20:406–11.
141. Irahiem MF, Abdelaziz ST. Shallow inferior fornix in contracted socket and anophthalmic socket syndrome: a novel technique to deepen the fornix using fascia lata strips. J Ophthalmol. 2016;38:575–9.
142. Doxanas MT, Dryden RM. The use of sclera in the treatment of dysthyroid eyelid retraction. Ophthalmology. 1981;88:887–94.
143. Mourits MP, Koornneef L. Lid lengthening by sclera interposition for eyelid retraction in graves ophthalmopathy. Br J Ophthalmol. 1991;75:344–7.
144. Downes RN, Jordan K. The surgical management of dysthyroid related eyelid retraction using mersilelne mesh. Eye. 1989;3:385–90.
145. Fenton S, Kemp EG. A review of the outcome of upper lid lowering for eyelid retraction and complications of spacers at a single unit over 5 years. Orbit. 2002;21:289–94.
146. Wong JF, Soparkar CN, Patrinely JR. Correction of lower eyelid retraction with high density porous polyethylene: the medpor lower eyelid spacer. Orbit. 2001;20:217–25.
147. Tan J, Olver J, Wright M, et al. The use of porous polyethylene (medpor) lower eyelid spacers in lid heightening and stabilization. Br J Ophthalmol. 2004;88:1197–200.
148. Karesh JW, Fabrega MA, Rodriques MM, Glaros DS. Polytetrafluoroethylene as an interpositional graft material for the corrction of lower eyelid retraction. Ophthalmology. 1989;96:419–23.
149. Lee YJ, Khwarg SI. Polytetrafluoroethylene as a spacer graft for the correction of lower eyelid retraction. Korean J Ophthalmol. 2005;19:247–51.
150. Flanagan JC, Campbell CB. The use of autogenous fascia lata to correct lid and orbital deformities. Trans Am Ophthalmol Soc. 1981;79:227–42.
151. Klein M, Manneking H, Bier J. Reconstruction of the contracted ocular socket with free full-thickness mucosa graft. Int J Oral Maxillofac Surg. 1993;29:96–8.
152. Molgat YM, Hurwitz JJ, Webb MC. Buccal mucous membrane-fat graft in the management of the contracted socket. Ophthal Plast Reconstr Surg. 1993;9:267–72.
153. Darsonval V, Berthet V, Hubault P, et al. Treatment of the sequelae of enucleation by septal chondro-mucosal composite graft. Report of 21 cases. Ann Chir Plast Esthet. 1997;42:594–602.
154. Wearne MJ, Sandy C, Rose GE, et al. Autogenous hard palate mucosa; the ideal lower lid spacer? Br J Ophthalmol. 2004;137:1021–5.
155. Cohen MS, Shorr N. Eyelid reconstruction with hard palate mucosa grafts. Ophthal Plast Reconstr Surg. 1992;8:183–95.
156. Pang NK, Bartley GB, Bite U, Bradley EA. Hard palate mucosal grafts in oculoplastic surgery: donor site lessons. Am J Ophthalmol. 2004;137:1021–5.

157. Massry GG, Hornblass A, Rubin P, Holds JB. Tarsal switch procedure for the surgical rehabilitation of the eyelid and socket deficiencies of the anophthalmic socket. Ophthal Plast Reconstr Surg. 1999;15:333–40.
158. Ferri M, Oestreicher JH. Treatment of post-blepharoplasty lower lid retraction by free tarsoconjunctival grafting. Orbit. 2002;21:281–8.
159. Millard DR. Eyelid repairs with a chondromucosal graft. Plast Reconstr Surg. 1962;30:267–72.
160. Zybylski JR, LaRossa DD, Rich JD. Correction of lower eyelid ptosis in the anophthalmic orbit with an autogenous ear cartilage graft. Plast Reconstr Surg. 1978;61:220–4.
161. Bayliss HI, Rosen N, Neuhaus RW. Obtaining auricular cartilage for reconstructive surgery. Am J Ophthalmol. 1982;93:709–12.
162. Bayliss H, Perman KI, Feff DR, et al. Autogenous auricular cartilage grafting for the lower eyelid retraction. Ophthal Plast Reconstr Surg. 1985;1:23–7.
163. Marks MW, Argenta LC, Friedman RJ, Hall JD. Conchal cartilage and composite grafts for correction of lower lid retraction. Plast Reconstr Surg. 1989;83:629–35.
164. Jackson IT, Dubin B, Harris J. Use of contoured and stabilized Conchal cartilage grafts for lower eyelid support: a preliminary report. Plast Reconstr Surg. 1989;83:636–40.
165. Tullo AB, Buckley RJ, Kelly T, et al. Transplantation of ocular tissue from a donor with sporadic Creutzfeldt-Jacob disease. Clin Exp Ophthalmol. 2006;34:645–9.
166. Seiff SR, Chang JS, Hurt M, et al. Polymerase chain reaction identification of human immunodeficiency virus-1 in preserved human sclera. Am J Ophthalmol. 1994;118:528–30.
167. Mehta JS, Franks WA. The sclera, the prion, and the ophthalmologist. Br J Ophthalmol. 2002;86:587–92.
168. Kim JW, Kikkawa DO, Lemke BN. Donor site complications of hard palate mucosal grafting. Ophthalmol Reconstr Surg. 1997;13:36–9.
169. Moon JW, Choung HK, Khwerg SI. Correction of lower lid retraction combined with entropion using ear cartilage graft in the anophthalmic socket. Korean J Ophthalmol. 2005;19:161–7.
170. Chang M, Ahn SE, Baek S. The effect and applications of acellular dermal allograft (Alloderm) in ophthalmic plastic surgery. J Craniomaxillfac Surg. 2014;42(5):695–9.
171. Lee EW, Berbos Z, Zaldivar RA, Lee MS, Harrison AR. Use of Dermatrix graft in oculoplastic surgery. Ophthal Plast Reconstr Surg. 2010b;26(3):153–4.
172. Bee YS, Alonzo B, Ng JD. Review of Alloderm acellular human dermis regenerative tissue matrix in multiple types of oculofacial surgery. Ophthal Plast Reconstr Surg. 2015;31(5):348–57.
173. Kim CY, Woo YJ, Lee SY, Yoon JS. Postoperative outcomes of anophthalmic socket reconstruction using autologous buccal mucosa graft. J Craniofac Surg. 2014;25(4):1171–4.
174. Holck DE, Foster JA, Dutton JJ, Dillon HD. Hard palate mucosal grafts in the treatment of the contracted socket. Ophthal Plast Reconstr Surg. 1999;15:202–9.
175. Lee AC, Fedorovich I, Heinz GW, Kikkawa DO. Socket reconstruction with combined mucous membrane and hard palate mucous grafts. Ophthal Surg Lasers. 2002b;33:463–8.
176. Bowen Jones EJ, Nunes E. The outcome of oral mucosal grafts to the orbit: a three- and half-year study. Br J Plast Surg. 2002;55:100–4.
177. Karesh JW, Putterman AM. Reconstruction of the partially contracted ocular socket or fornix. Arch Ophthalmol. 1988;106:552–6.
178. Klein M, Menneking H, Bier J. Reconstruction of the contracted ocular socket with free full thickness mucous membrane graft. Int J Oral Maxillofac Surg. 2000;29:96–8.
179. Betharia SM, Patil ND. Dermis fat grafting in contracted sockets. Ind J Ophthalmol. 1988;36:110–2.
180. Bhattacharjee K, Kuri G, Bhattacharjee H, Kumar Das J. Comparative analysis of the use of porous orbital implant with mucous membrane graft versus dermis fat graft as a primary procedure in reconstruction of severely contracted socket (abstract). In: 67th All India Ophthalmological Congress Annual Meeting; 5–8 Feb2008; Banglore, India, 2008.
181. Guberina C, Hornblass A, Meltzer MA, et al. Autogenous dermis fat orbital implantation. Arch Ophthalmol. 1983;101:1586–9.
182. Betharia SM, Kanthamani, Prakash H, Kumar S. Skin grafting in severly contracted socket with the use of Compo. In J Ophthalmol. 1990;38:88–91.
183. Lee YH, Kim HC, Lee JS, et al. Surgical reconstruction of the contracted prbit. Plast Reconstr Surg. 1999a;4:1129–36.
184. Suh IS, Yang YM, Oh SJ. Conjunctival cul-de-sac reconstruction with radial forarm free flap in anophthalmic orbit syndrome. Plast Reconstr Surg. 2001;107:914–9.
185. Aihara M, Sakai S, Matsuzaki K, Ishida H. Eye socket reconstruction with free flaps in patients who have had postoperative radiotherapy. J Craniomaxillofac Surg. 1998;26:301–5.
186. Anita NH, Arora S. Malignant contracture of the eye socket. Plast Reconstr Surg. 1984;74:292–4.
187. Tahara S, Susuki T. Eye socket reconstruction with free radial forearm flap. Ann Plast Surg. 1989;23:112–6.
188. Sterker I, Frerich B. Secondary reconstruction of the eye socket with a free radial forarm flap. Ophthalmologe. 2007;104:978–82.
189. Li D, Jie Y, Liu H, et al. Reconstruction of anophthalmic orbits and contracted eye sockets with microvascular radial forearm free flaps. Ophthal Plast Reconstr Surg. 2008;24:94–7.
190. Soutar DS, Scheker LR, Tanner NS. The radial forarm flap: a versatile method for intr-oral reconstruction. Br J Plast Surg. 1983;36:1–8.
191. Bajaj MS, Pushker N, Kumar KS, Chandra M, Ghose S. Evaluation of amniotic membrane grafting in the reconstruction of contracted socket. Ophthalmic Plast Reconstr Surg. 2006;22(2):116–20.
192. Naugle TC, Lee WW, Couvillion S. Use of quilting sutures in ophthalmic plastic surgery. Ophthal Plast Reconstr Surg. 2004;20:237–9.
193. Davenport M, Daly J, Harvey I, et al. The bolus tie-over 'pressure' dressing in the management of full thickness skin grafts: is it necessary? Br J Plast Surg. 1988;41:28–32.
194. Solomon A, Pires RT, Tseng SC. Amniotic membrane transplantation after extensive removal of primary and recurrent pterygia. Ophthalmology. 2001;108:449–60.
195. Tsubota K, Satake Y, Ohyama M, et al. Surgical reconstruction of the ocular surface in advanced ocular cicatricial pemphigoid and Stevens-Johnson syndrome. Am J Ophthalmol. 1996;122:38–52.
196. Stewart JM, David S, Seiff SR. Amniotic membrane graft in the surgical management of cryptophthalmos. Ophthal Plast Reconstr Surg. 2002;110:93–100.
197. Solomon A, Espana EM, Tseng SC. Amniotic membrane transplantation for reconstruction of the conjunctival fornices. Ophthalmology. 2003;110:93–100.
198. Lee-Wing MW. Amniotic membrane for repair of exposed hydroxyapatite orbital implants. Ophthal Plast Reconstr Surg. 2003;19:401–2.
199. Koizumi NJ, Inatomi TJ, Sotozona CJ, et al. Growth factor mRNA and protein in preserved human amniotic membrane. Curr Eye Res. 2000;20:173–7.
200. Kumar S, Sugandhi P, Arora R, Pandey PK. Amniotic membrane transplantation versus mucous membrane grafting in the anophthalmic socket. Orbit. 2006;25:195–203.
201. Poonyathalang A, Preechawat P, Pomsathit J, Mahaisaviriya P. Reconstruction of contracted eye socket with amniotic membrane graft. Ophthal Plast Reconstr Surg. 2005;21:359–62.

202. Shimazaki J, Hao-Yung Y, Tsubota K. Amniotic membrane transplantation for ocular surface reconstruction in patients with chemical and thermal burns. Ophthalmology. 1997;104:2068–76.
203. Nunery WR, Hetzler KJ. Dermal-fat graft as a primary enucleation technique. Ophthalmology. 1985;92:1256–61.
204. Migliori ME, Putterman AM. The domed dermis-fat graft orbital implant. Ophthal Plast Reconstr Surg. 1991;7:23–30.
205. Raizada K, Shome D, Honavar I, et al. Management of an irradiated anophthalmic socket following dermis fat graft rejection: a case report. Indian J Ophthalmol. 2008;56:147–8.
206. Putterman AM, Karesh JW. A surgical technique for the successful and stable reconstruction of the totally contracted ocular socket. Ophthal Surg. 1988;19(3):193–201.
207. Mu X, Dong J, Chang T, et al. Correction of the contracted eye socket and orbitozygomatic hypoplasia using postauricular skin flap and temporalis fascial flap. J Craniofac Surg. 1999;1:11–7.
208. Tessier P, Krastinova D. Transplantation of the temporalis muscle into an anophthalmic orbit. Ann Chir Plast. 1982;27:211–20.
209. El-Khatib HA. Prefabricated temporalis fascia pedicled flap for previously skin grafted contracted eye socket. Plast Reconstr Surg. 2000;106:571–6.
210. Altintas M, Aydin Y, Yucei A. Eye socket reconstruction with the prefabricated temporal island flap. Plast Reconst Surg. 1998;102:980–7.
211. Lee YH, Kim HC, Lee JS, Park WJ. Surgical reconstruction of the contracted orbit. Plast Reconstr Surg. 1999b;103:1129–36.
212. Koshima I, Narushima M, Mihara M, et al. Short pedicle thoracodorsal artery perforator (TAP) adiposal flap for three dimensional reconstruction of contracted orbital cavity. J Plast Reconstr Aesthetic Surg. 2008;61:e13–7.
213. Lopez-Arcas JM, Martin M, Gomez E, et al. The Guyuron retroauricular island fklap for eyelid and eye socket reconstruction in children. Int J Oral Maxillofac Surg. 2009;38:744–50.
214. Krastinova D, Mihaylova M, Martin B. Surgical management of the anophthalmic orbit, part 2: post-tumoral. Plast Reconstr Surg. 2001;108:827–36.
215. Rycroft BW. An operation for treatment of severe contraction of the eye socket. Br J Ophthalmol. 1962;46:21–6.
216. Bardakjian TM, Steinberg L, Schneider A. The genetics of anophthalmia/microphthalmia. J Ophthal Prosthetics. 1997;2:15–22.
217. Tucker S, Jones D, Collin R. Systemic anomalies in 77 patients with congenital anophthalmos or microphthalmos. Eye. 1996;10:310–4.
218. Stoll C, Alembik Y, Dott B, et al. Epidemiology of congenital eye malformations in 131,760 consecutive births. Ophthal Pediatr Genet. 1992;13:179–86.
219. Gossman M, Mohay J, Roberts DM. Expansion of the human microphthalmic orbit. Ophthalmology. 1999;106:2005–9.
220. Weiss AH, Kousseff BG, Ross EA, Longbottom J. Simple Microphthalmos. Arch Ophthalmol. 1989;107:1625–30.
221. Warburg M. Classification of microphthalmos and coloboma. J Med Genet. 1993;30:664–9.
222. Ragge NK, Subak-Sharpe ID, Collin JRO. A practical guide to the management of anophthalmia and microphthalmia. Eye. 2007;21:1290–300.
223. Verma AS, Fitzpatrick DR. Anophthalmia and Micropthalmia. Orphanet J Rare Dis. 2007;2:47.
224. Plaisance J, Calvas P, Chassaing N. Genetic advances in microphthalmia. J Pediatr Genetics. 2016;5(4):184–8.
225. Skalicky E, White AJR, Grigg JR, et al. Microphthalmia, anophthalmia and coloboma and associated ocular and systemic features: understanding the spectrum. JAMA Ophthalmol. 2013;131(12):1517–24.
226. Gregory-Evans CY, Williams MJ, Halford S, Gregory-Evans K. Ocular coloboma: a reassessment in the age of molecular neuroscience. J Med Genetics. 2004;41:881–91.
227. Chang L, Blain D, Bertuzzi S, Broks BP. Uveal coloboma and basic science update. Curr Opin Ophthalmol. 2006;17:447–70.
228. Kennedy RE. The effect of early enucleation on the orbit in animals and humans. Trans Am Ophthal Soc. 1964;15(5):449–510.
229. Kennedy RE. The effect of early enucleation on the orbit in animals and humans. Adv Ophthal Plast Reconstr Surg. 1992;9:1–39.
230. Howard GM, Kinder RS, MacMillan AS. Orbital growth after unilateral enucleation in childhood. Arch Ophthlamol. 1965;73:80–3.
231. Kennedy RE. Growth retardation and volume determinations of the anophthalmic orbit. Trans Am Ophthalmol Soc. 1972;70:277–97.
232. Kastinova D, Kelly MBH, Mihaylora M. Surgical management of the anophthalmic orbit. Part I: congenital. Plast Reconstr Surg. 2001a;108(4):817–26.
233. Chen D, Heher K. Management of the anophthalmic socket in pediatric patients. Curr Opin Ophthalmol. 2004;15(5):449–53.
234. Kennedy RE. Bone changes in the adult anophthalmic orbit influencing oculoplastic reconstructive consideration. Trans Am Ophthalmol Soc. 1976;74:237–50.
235. Yago K, Furuta M. Orbital growth after unilateral enucleation in infancy without an orbital implant. Jpn J Ophthalmol. 2001;45(6):648–52.
236. Bentley RP, Sgouros S, Natarajan K, et al. Normal changes in orbital volume during childhood. J Neurosurg. 2002;96:742–6.
237. Cepela MA, Nunery WR, Martin RT. Stimulation of orbital growth by the use of expandable implants in the anophthalmic cat orbit. Ophthal Plast Reconstr Surg. 1992a;8:157–67.
238. Kaste SC, Chen G, Fontanesi J, et al. Orbital development in long-term survivors of retinoblastoma. J Clin Oncol. 1997;15:1183–9.
239. Fountain TR, Goldberger S, Murphree AL. Orbital development after enucleation in early childhood. Ophthal Plast Reconstr Surg. 1999;15:32–6.
240. Heher KL, Katowitz JA, Low JE. Unilateral dermis-fat graft implantation in the pediatric orbit. Ophthal Plast Reconstr Surg. 1998;14:81–8.
241. Clauser L, Sarti E, Dallera V, Galie M. Integrated reconstructive strategies for treating the anophthalmic orbit. J Craniomaxillofac Surg. 2004;32(5):279–90.
242. Kastinova D, Kelley MB, Mihaylova M. Surgical Management of the anophthalmic orbit, part I: congenital. Plast Reconstr Surg. 2001b;108(4):817–26.
243. Bar-Ysef U, Abuslaish I, Harel T, Hendler N, Ofir R, Birk OPS. CHX10 mutations cause non-syndromic microphthalmia/anophthalmia in Arab and Jewish Kindreds. Hum Genet. 2004;115(4):302–9.
244. Gundlach KKH, Gutoff RF, Hingst VHM, et al. Expansion of the socket and orbit for congenital clinical anophthalmia. Plast Reconstr Surg. 2005a;116:1214–22.
245. Dunaway DJ, David DJ. Intraorbital tissue expansion in the management of congenital anophthalmos. Br J Plast Surg. 1996;49:529–35.
246. Sinclair D, Dangerfiled P. Nervous system. In D Sinclair and P. Dangerfield (eds), Human growth after birth, Oxford: Oxford University Press, 1998, pg 87.
247. Furuta M. Measurement of orbital volume by computed tomography: especially on the growth of the orbit. J Jpn Ophthalmol. 2001;45(6):600–6.
248. Farkas LG, Posnick JC, Hrecko TM. Growth patterns in the orbital region: a morphometric study. Cleft Palate-Craniofac J. 1992;29:315–8.
249. Katowitz JA, Heher K, Handler L. Use of dermis fat graft as an orbital implant in congenital microphthalmia. J Ophthal Prosthetics. 1997;2:23–9.
250. Merritt JH, Trawnik WR. Prosthetic and surgical management of congenital anophthalmia. J Ophthal Prosthet. 1997;2:1–14.
251. Weingarten CT. Anophthalmia; psychological implications of an infants first visit to the ocularist. J Ophthal Prosth. 1997;2:31–7.

252. Kiskadden WS, McDowell AJ, Keiser T. Results of early treatment of congenital micropthalmia. J Ophthal Prosthes. 1997;2(1):1–14.
253. Price E, Simon JW, Calhoun JH. Prosthetic treatment of severe microphthalmia in infancy. J Pediatr Ophthalmol Stabismus. 1986;23(1):22–4.
254. Weise KG, Vogel M, Guthoff R, Gundlach K. Treatment of congenital anophthalmos with self-inflating polymer expands: a new method. J Craniomaxillofac Surg. 1999;27:72–6.
255. Gundlach KKH, Guthoff RF, Hingst VHM, Schittkowski MP, Bier UC. Expansion of the socket and orbit for congenital clinical anophthalmia. Plast Reconstr Surg. 2005b;116:1214–9.
256. Hou Z, Xian J, Chang Q, Wei W, Li D. Digital evaluation of orbital development after self-inflating hydrogel expansion in Chinese children with congenital microphthalmia. J Plast Reconstr Aesthet Surg. 2016;69(5):706–14.
257. Shawkat FS, Harris CM, Taylor DS, Thompson DA, Russell-Eggit I, Kriss A. The optokinetic response differences between congenital profound and nonprofound inilateral vision deprivation. Ophthalmology. 1995;102(11):1615–22.
258. Mclean CJ, Ragge NK, Jones RB, Collin JRO. The management of cysts associated with congenital microphthalmos and anophthalmos. Br J Ophthalmol. 2003;87(7):860–3.
259. Chaudry IA, Arat YO, Shamsi FA, et al. Congenital microphthalmos with orbital cysts; distinct diagnostic features and management. Ophthal Plast Reconstr Surg. 2004;20:452–7.
260. Wiwatwongwana D, Rootman J. Bilatral microphthalmos with cyst with free fat graft. Ophthal Plast Reconstr Surg. 2009;25(3):241–3.
261. Agrawal PK, Kumar H. Micropthalmos with cyst: a clinical study. Indian J Ophthalmol. 1993;41:177–9.
262. Tse DT, inventor; University of Miami (Miami, Fl) assignee. Integrated rigid fixation orbital expander. US patent 6,582,465 B2, June 2003.
263. Tse DT, Pinchuk L, Davis S, et al. Evaluation of an integrated orbital tissue expander in an anophthalmic feline model. Am J Ophthalmol. 2007;143(2):317–27.
264. Tse DT, Abdulhafez M, Orozco MA, Tse JD, Osma Azab A, Pinchuk L. Evaluation of an integrated orbital tissue expander in congenital anophthalmos: report of preliminary clinical experience. Am J Ophthalmol. 2011;151(3):470–82.
265. Mazzoli R, Raymond WR, Ainbinder DJ, Hansen EA. Use of self expanding, hydrophilic expanders (hydrogel) in the reconstruction of congenital clinical anophthalmos. Curr Opin Ophthalmol. 2004;15:426–31.
266. Tucker SM, Sapp N, Collin R. Orbital expansion of the congenitally anophthalmic socket. Br J Ophthalmol. 1995;79:667–71.
267. Bacskulin A, Vogel M, Weisse KG, et al. New osmotically active hydrogel expander for enlargement of the contracted anophthalmic socket. Graefes Arch Clin Exp Ophthalmol. 1995;238:24027.
268. Lo AK, Colcleugh RDG, Allen L, Van-Wyck L, Bite U. The role of tissue expanders in an anophthalmic animal model. Plast Reconstr Surg. 1990;86:399–408.
269. Epply BL, Holley S, Sadove AM. Experimental effects of intraorbital tissue expansion on orbitomaxillary growth in anophthalmos. Ann Plast Surg. 1993;31:19–27.
270. Cepela MA, Nunery WR, Martin RT. Stimulation of orbital growth by the use of expandable implants in the anophthalmic cat orbit. Ophthal Plast Reconst Surg. 1992b;8:157–67.
271. Berry FD. A modified tissue expander for socket enlargement in clinical anophthalmos. Ophthal Plast Reconstr Surg. 1991;7:41–7.
272. O'Keefe M, Webb M, Pasby RC, Wagman RD. Clinical anophthalmos. Br J Ophthalmol. 1987;71:635–8.
273. Downes R, Lavin M, Collin R. Hydrophilic expanders for the congenital anophthalmic socket. Adv Ophthal Plast Recconstr Surg. 1992;9:57–61.
274. Drennan M. Balloon expansion therapy in clinical anophthalmos. J Ophthal Prosth. 2002;5:9–15.
275. Anderson RL, Commentary on Cepala MA, Nunery MA, Martin RT. Stimulation of orbital growth by the use of expandable implants in the anophthalmic cat orbit. Ophthal Plast Reconstr Surg. 1992;8(3):168–9.
276. Brett J. Treating bilateral congenital anophthalmos. J Ophthal Prosth. 2002;7:17–21.
277. Waagner A, Schneider C, Lagogiannis G, et al. Pulsatile expansion therapy for orbital enlargement. Int J Oral Maxillofac Surg. 2000;29:91–5.
278. Mitchell KT, Hollsten DA, White WL, et al. The autogenous dermis-fat orbital implant in children. J AAPOS. 2001;5:367–9.
279. Ronert MA, Hofheinz H, Manassa E, Asgarouladi H, Olbrish RR. The beginning of a new era in tissue expansion: self-filling osmotic tissue expander- four-year clinical experience. Plast Reconstr Surg. 2004;114:1025–1031,2004.
280. Weise KG. Osmotically induced tissue expansion with hydrogels: a new dimension in tissue expansion? A preliminary report. J Craniomaxillofac Surg. 1993;21:309–13.
281. Wiese KG, Heineman DEH, Ostermeier D, et al. Biomaterial properties and biocompatibility in cell culture of a novel self-inflating hydrogel tissue expander. J Biomed Mater Res. 2001;54:179–88.
282. Schittkowski MP, Guthoff RF. Injectable self inflating hydrogel pellet expanders for the treatment of orbital volume deficiency in congenital microphthalmos; preliminary results with a new therapeutic approach. Br J Ophthalmol. 2006;90:1173–7.
283. Li TG, McCann JD, Goldberg RA. Orbital volume augmentation in anophthalmic patients using injectable hydrogel implants. ASOPRS Abstracts. 2003;91
284. Tao JP, LeBoyer RM, Hetzler K, Ng JD, Nunery WR. Inferolateral migration of hydrogel orbital implants in Microphthalmia. Ophthal Plast Reconstr Surg. 2010;26:14–7.
285. Manufacturer website for Osmed implant. Available at: http://iopinc.com/surgeons_and_medical_professional/osmed.
286. Marin JF, Tolentino FI, Refojo MF, et al. Long-term complications of the MAI hydrogel intrascleral buckling implant. Arch Ophthalmol. 1992;110:86–8.
287. Brown SL, Bloom SM. Spontaneous expulsion of a radial MIRAgel scleral buckle. Retina. 2004;24:306–7.
288. Le Rouic JF, Bejjani RA, Azan F, et al. Cryoextraction of episcleral Miragel buckle elements: a new technique to reduce fragmentation. Ophthal Surg Lasers. 2002;33:237–9.
289. Braunstein RA, Winnick M. Complications of Miragel: pseudotumor. Arch Ophthalmol. 2002;120:228–9.
290. Kawano T, Doi M, Miyamura M, et al. Extrusion and fragmentation of hydrogel exoplant 11 years after scleral buckling surgery. Ophthal Surg Lasers. 2002;33:240–2.
291. Roldan-Pallares M, del Castillo Sanz JL, Awad-El Susi S, et al. Long-term complications of silicone and hydrogel explants in retinal reattachment surgery. Arch Ophthalmol. 1999;117:197–201.
292. Daufenbach DR, Ruttum MS, Pulido JS, Keech RV. Chorioretinal colobomas in a pediatric population. Ophthalmology. 1998;1105(8):1455–8.
293. Dimirci H, Singh AD, Shileds JA, Sheilds CL, Eagale RC. Bilateral micropthalmos and orbital cyst. Eye. 2003;17:273–6.

Part X

Pediatric Considerations

Ann P. Murchison

Considerations in Pediatric Oculoplastic Examination

61

Christopher B. Chambers, William Rocamora Katowitz, and James A. Katowitz

Introduction

The oculoplastic examination of a child can be challenging and intimidating. Necessary measurements that are easily obtained in adults such as lid position, levator function, and globe position can be difficult to gather from a shy, scared, or active child. This chapter provides tips to help develop rapport with young children in the exam room that will help foster needed trust and cooperation. Tools and tricks will be explained to help the clinician complete the needed exam details. Important examination findings in children will be discussed, and pathology germane to the pediatric oculoplastic surgeon will be highlighted. The chapter will cover pediatric ptosis, eyelid tumors, tearing, orbital tumors, and trauma salient to the pediatric patient.

General Rapport

After spending any extended time in a pediatric office or hospital, you will, without fail, hear the quote "Children are not just small adults." Though this may seem cliché, it is very important to take this to heart. The more common oculoplastic and orbital conditions found in adults are often different in children. Even common diagnoses in an oculoplastic office such as ptosis often have different etiologies and must be evaluated and treated differently in children.

The examination of a child is also much different than the examination of an adult and can, at times, be intimidating. Setting up your office properly for a child can be extremely helpful in making the visit and examination go smoothly. Creating a special pediatric corner in a waiting room with toys, books, and small chairs can help the child feel at ease (Fig. 61.1). Avoiding long waits for kids will also increase the opportunity for a fruitful examination. Hungry and tired kids past naptime can be much more difficult to examine once in the chair.

Once in the examination lane, having colorful fixation targets, toys of gender specific interest (Fig. 61.2), and, if possible, cartoons playing in the exam room will aid in getting the attention of young children. The white coat can intimidate some children, so removing it before entering the room can help establish rapport.

The examination of a child can start before they are in the chair, and it may be helpful to observe the child playing in the waiting area. When entering an examination room, careful immediate observation will be of benefit. This may be the only chance you get to evaluate children before they begin crying or attempt to bury their heads in the shoulder of their parent. Carrying a camera into the room and snapping a quick photograph immediately can be helpful, as this image can be used to evaluate lid position, the adnexae, and ocular alignment.

Observation of the parents and siblings can also help aid diagnosis as many diseases such as blepharophimosis can be hereditary. Also, allowing the patient to sit in the parent's lap oftentimes will make the child feel more secure and comfortable.

Being outgoing, playful, and honest will allow the physician to gain the confidence of the child and parent, which can allow for a more accurate and shorter examination. Commenting on the child's clothes such as their flashing shoes or "cool" t-shirt will go a long way in building rapport.

C. B. Chambers (✉)
Division of Oculoplastic and Orbital Surgery, Department of Ophthalmology, University of Washington Harborview Medical Center, Seattle, WA, USA
e-mail: Cbc108@uw.edu

W. R. Katowitz
Perelman School of Medicine, The University of Pennsylvania, The Children's Hospital of Philadelphia and The Scheie Eye Institute, Division of Ophthalmology, Philadelphia, PA, USA

J. A. Katowitz
The Children's Hospital of Philadelphia and The Edwin and Fannie Gray Hall Center for Appearance, The University of Pennsylvania Perelman School of Medicine, Department of Ophthalmology, Philadelphia, PA, USA

J. J. Servat et al. (eds.), *Smith and Nesi's Ophthalmic Plastic and Reconstructive Surgery*,
https://doi.org/10.1007/978-3-030-41720-8_61

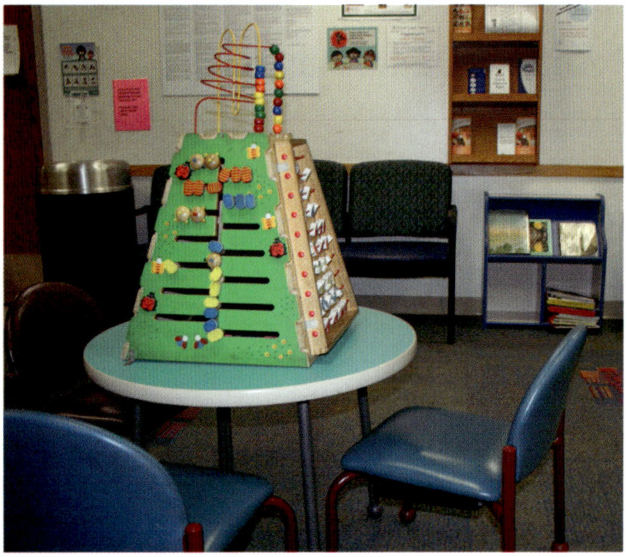

Fig. 61.1 Pediatric corner

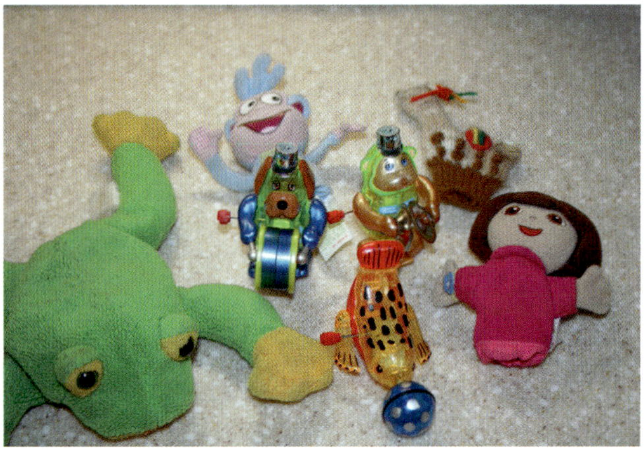

Fig. 61.2 Fixation targets and toys

Verbally engaging the child with easy questions will aid in examination. Kids want to be adults so referring to them as "big" or overestimating their age can make them feel at ease.

Making each step of the examination a game will aid in the examination as well. Describing the slit lamp as a motorcycle and telling them to hold on to the handlebars tight so that they won't fall off will get them excited and comfortable with an otherwise intimidating piece of equipment. Also, touching the muscle light with your finger and explaining how "cool" it is that this light can make your finger glow pink will gain their interest. After allowing them to light their finger up, directing the light to their eyes will be received with much more comfort (Fig. 61.3).

Using a smartphone with preloaded cartoons and pictures is an invaluable tool to stopping crying, squeezing, and getting the patient's head out from their parent's chest. The digital camera can be equally valuable. In an adult examination,

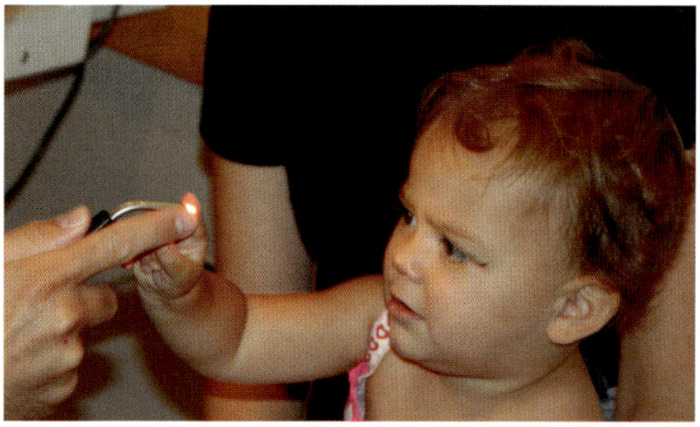

Fig. 61.3 Playing with examination tools can help children gain comfort

cooperation with using a ruler to evaluate lid height and levator function is much easier. Using a camera to snap a photograph of a child with a ruler placed near the eye will provide a frozen image to evaluate lid height, lid function, or intercanthal distance without struggling with an uncooperative patient.

When drops are needed for evaluation of tearing, to evaluate the response to phenylephrine, or for dilation, it can be helpful to have a technician place the drops in the child's eyes. This will help the physician avoid being the "bad guy" when it is time for the exam. For children under 6 months of age, 2.5% phenylephrine ophthalmic and 1% tropicamide can be used. If cycloplegia is necessary, 0.5% cyclopentolate should be considered. For children over 6 months of age, dilation with cycloplegia can be achieved with 1% tropicamide and 1% cyclopentolate.

Motility and Visual Examination

Examination of the sensory and motor systems in children with lid and orbital abnormalities is important for accurate diagnosis and appropriate treatment. Any ophthalmologist examining a pediatric patient with an oculoplastic or orbital disease must take great care to ensure amblyopia is not an issue. The prevalence of amblyopia in North America is between 2 and 4%, and it is the leading cause of childhood onset unilateral reduced vision. Amblyopia is caused by an abnormal visual experience early in life secondary to visual deprivation, strabismus, anisometropia, or isometropia. Most amblyopia is preventable through early detection and appropriate treatment [1].

A child with ptosis that presents to clinic must be evaluated for amblyopia. If the ptosis is severe enough to cover the visual axis, deprivation amblyopia can occur. Deprivation amblyopia takes less time to develop than strabismic or anisometropic amblyopia, and, in addition, the critical period occurs earlier in life [1]. Unilateral deprivation amblyopia is usually deeper than amblyopia produced by bilateral deprivation. If unilateral deprivation amblyopia is discovered, patching should be started, and urgent surgical repair of the ptosis is indicated. If the ptosis is so severe that the visual axis is not cleared by head position and maximal brow and levator effort, patching will not be effective as the visual axis will remain occluded. Patching of the healthy eye is particularly important in patients who will undergo a frontalis suspension sling to establish better vision and therefore provide motivation to lift the brow to clear the visual axis after surgery.

Though deprivation amblyopia must be a concern in a patient with ptosis, anisometropic amblyopia occurs more often than deprivation amblyopia in these patients. A good cycloplegic refraction should be performed on ptotic patients to rule out induced astigmatism from the low eyelid position [2]. As little as 1–2 diopters of astigmatism can induce mild amblyopia [1]. Other oculoplastic and orbital diseases, such as capillary hemangiomas or dermoid cysts, can also cause anisometropic amblyopia. Schwartz and colleagues explained that capillary hemangiomas of the lid and orbit larger than 1 cm in diameter have been shown to provide amblyogenic factors requiring treatment in up to half the patients studied [2]. The preventable nature of amblyopia if identified early reinforces the need for a thorough ocular examination.

Oculomotor abnormalities can often be associated with disorders of the lids and orbit [3, 4]. Extraocular dysfunction is due to either supranuclear abnormalities (disease above the oculomotor nuclei) or infranuclear abnormalities (disease below the oculomotor nuclei). Most forms of primary childhood strabismus, such as congenital esotropia, are secondary to supranuclear abnormalities of the oculomotor system. In contrast, most forms of strabismus associated with lid and orbital disease, which is separated into categories of restrictive and paralytic, are due to infranuclear disease. Understanding the type and classification of an associated extraocular muscle dysfunction can assist with diagnosis of the lid or orbital disorder. For example, paralytic strabismus associated with ptosis suggests cranial nerve dysfunction, whereas restrictive disease associated with lid retraction and proptosis can suggest thyroid ophthalmopathy [5].

Developing a good relationship with a strabismologist to help co-manage these patients is paramount. Typically, it is best to perform orbital surgery before strabismus surgery as ocular alignment can change after orbital surgery. Similarly, strabismus should be preformed before lid surgery, as changes in ocular alignment can cause a shift in lid position. Clearing the visual axis may take precedence over other surgeries in any patient developing amblyopia.

Epiphora

Epiphora is a common symptom affecting up to 20% of newborns; however, 90% of these obstructions resolve spontaneously within 1 year of age. It is can be helpful to understand the diagnostic pearls of epiphora in children, as most kids will not be as cooperative for an office probing and irrigation as an adult may be. Evaluation of epiphora is discussed in other sections of this text and therefore will not be discussed in detail here. Epiphora and the presence of an increased tear lake signify an imbalance between tear production and drainage. Though these symptoms may be secondary to a nasolacrimal duct obstruction, they may be also be secondary to non-obstructive functional abnormalities. In a moving child, abnormalities that affect the normal nasolacrimal pump mechanism such as entropion, ectropion, telecanthus, or coloboma may be overlooked. Irritation from infection, allergy, dry eyes, misdirected lashes secondary to epiblepharon, or incomplete blink due to Bell's palsy must also be ruled out. Finally, the child should be evaluated for the possible presence of a periocular mass at the medial canthal area, as this can suggest a nasolacrimal duct obstruction or may represent a periocular tumor such as a capillary hemangioma, encephalocele, mucocele, or dermoid cyst.

Diagnostic studies such as CT scan or MRI to rule out the presence of a periocular tumor or an encephalocele can be helpful. However, these studies may not be necessary with careful physical examination. Other studies such as the Jones dye test, basal tear secretion test, Schirmer test, and irrigation of the nasolacrimal system can be performed, but these studies are often not tolerated by children. The dye disappearance test is often well tolerated and can yield enough information for diagnosis combined with careful history and examination. In this test, fluorescein dye is placed in the cul-de-sac of each eye. After 5 minutes, the tear lake is observed with a blue light. A normal system will have cleared the dye, while an abnormal system will have dye left in the tear lake or will have dripped down the cheek. Remember, this test only identifies functional blockage, and other causes for epiphora as described above must be ruled out. Additionally this test may be difficult to evaluate if bilateral disease is present.

Eyelid

Ptosis

The management of pediatric ptosis can be one of the greatest challenges for an ophthalmologist. As explained previously, the risk of developing amblyopia is an important concern. The common etiologies of pediatric ptosis and modalities for surgical repair vary from those in the adult population. Getting as much information from a possibly challenging pediatric examination, using the techniques described above, can aid in the diagnosis and treatment to ensure the best possible visual and cosmetic outcome.

Correctly identifying the etiology of ptosis in each pediatric patient is essential to ensure proper management. Separating ptosis into four groups, myogenic, aponeurotic, neurogenic, and mechanical, can be helpful. Identifying cases of pseudoptosis secondary to conditions such as microphthalmos is important as well.

The evaluation for ptosis should include a thorough history beginning with the onset of ptosis in order to determine if it was present at birth or if it was acquired. Getting a birth history such as the method for delivery can be important in identifying if birth trauma could be a cause for ptosis. Detailed surgical history including craniofacial procedures or other ophthalmic procedures that have been performed should be gathered. Family history will also be beneficial to aid diagnosis as it may elicit an inherited reason for ptosis such as blepharophimosis syndrome.

Parents will often be able to fill in holes left by the physical examination. Evidence of synkinetic mechanisms or daily fluctuations can help identify causes such as jaw wink or myasthenia gravis. Also asking the parents to describe the degree of ptosis can be helpful to determine if the ptosis appears to interfere with daily vision and if the patient has adopted a chin up head posture that will indicate surgical treatment.

As discussed previously, visual function must be tested to identify amblyopia. Using HOTV, Teller, Allen cards, or even the 10-prism diopter test can be useful. The presence or absence of a Bell's phenomenon and adopted chin posture should be recorded. Again, cycloplegic refraction is indicated as the weight of the ptotic lid on the globe can cause a significant astigmatism [6)] Pupillary examination is also important to identify Horner syndrome or third nerve palsy causing the ptosis that will direct further testing. Placing a pacifier or bottle in a baby's mouth during examination may not only help with cooperation but may unmask synkinetic movement of the lid upon sucking or chewing (Fig. 61.4a, b).

Slit lamp examination should be conducted to evaluate the cornea for signs of exposure and to assess tear film quality. In an uncooperative child, slit lamp examination may not be practical, so a modified examination by placing fluorescein in the eye and observation of the cornea and tear film from a distance with a cobalt blue filter may be used to check for staining and evaluate tear breakup time. Normal tear breakup time is greater than 10 seconds.

Lid and adnexal examination should be performed as best permitted. Using a digital camera to photograph the lid is extremely helpful in children. The photographs can be used to supplement the medical record and with zoom features combined with a ruler placed near the face during the photograph can yield accurate lid measurements in an uncooperative child (Fig. 61.5a, b). A marginal reflex distance 1 (MRD1), distance from the corneal reflex to the upper eyelid in millimeters, of 1 mm or less can be categorized as severe. A MRD1 of 2 mm and 3 mm can be categorized as moderate and mild, respectively. Isolating the frontalis muscle during measurements or documenting the effect of brow use on the lid position should also be noted. Upon frontalis muscle engagement to lift the more ptotic lid can cause the other lid to appear "normal" while it too may be ptotic. Similarly, by Hering's law, overstimulation of a more ptotic lid can make the other lid appear in good position, while it may, in fact, be ptotic as well. This may be easily identified on an adult examination; however, it can be missed even by an experienced clinician during a difficult pediatric examination. Discussion with the parents about this principle is important

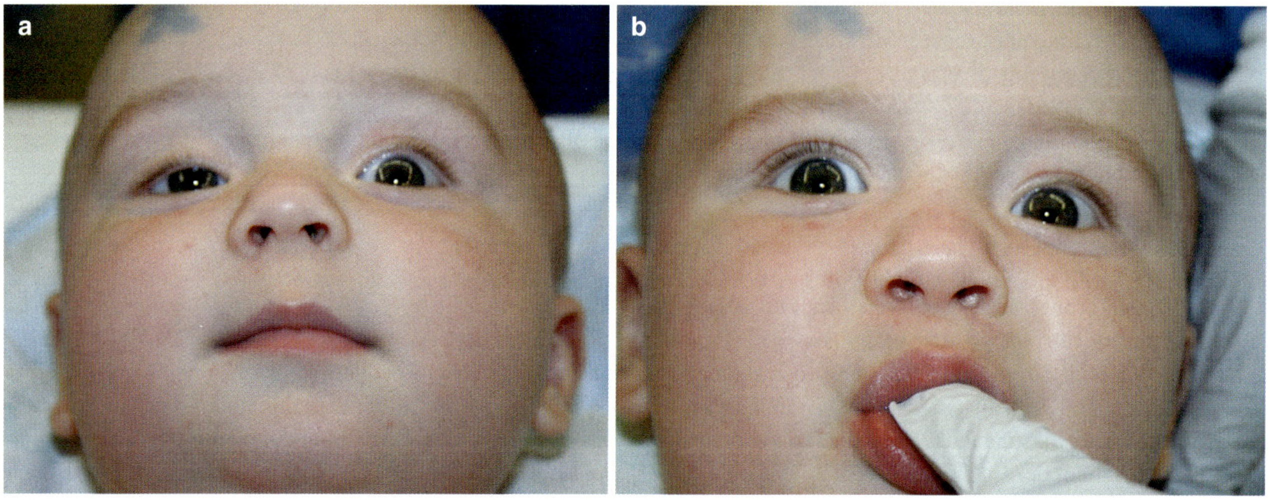

Fig. 61.4 (**a**, **b**) Marcus Gunn jaw wink unmasked by sucking on a gloved hand

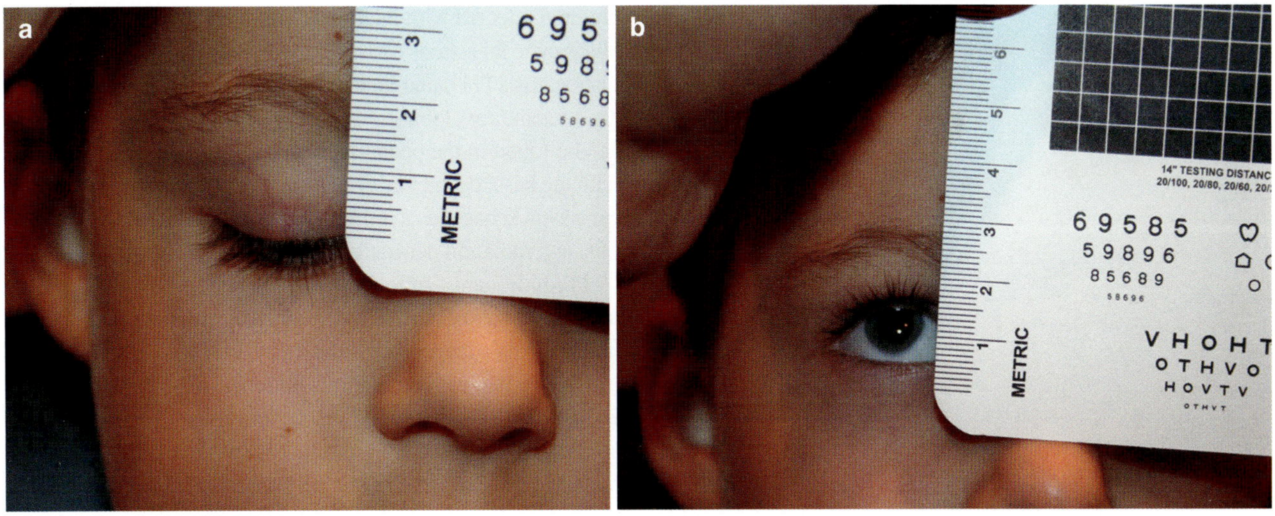

Fig. 61.5 (**a**, **b**) Using a digital camera with ruler can help with measurements in an uncooperative child. Shown in downgaze (**a**) and upgaze (**b**)

Table 61.1 Classification of levator function

Levator function	Eyelid excursion
Excellent	≥13 mm
Good	8–12 mm
Fair	5–7 mm
Poor	≤4 mm

Table 61.2 Graded response to 2.5% phenylephrine [8]

Response to phenylephrine	MRD1
Good	4–5
Moderate	3
Poor	≤2

so that they do not think ptosis of the other lid was caused by surgical intervention. Upper lid crease position should be observed especially in cases of unilateral ptosis, so that the lid crease can be matched to the fellow eye helping achieve symmetry postoperatively.

Observing lid position in upgaze and downgaze as well as identifying any lagophthalmos can be extremely important in determining the etiology of ptosis. If the amount of ptosis is less in downgaze than upgaze, this may indicate myogenic congenital ptosis. The characteristic lag in downgaze can be attributed to fibrotic levator muscle in this condition.

Likely the most important measurement in determining the type of surgical intervention in a pediatric patient is the levator function. The frontalis muscle should be immobilized if possible while moving a bright toy from inferior to superior in the child's view after obtaining the child's interest. The amount of levator function can then be classified as poor if the lid moves 4 mm or less. Lid movement of 5–7 mm should be documented as fair, good if 8–12 mm, and excellent if more than 13 mm (Table 61.1). Surgical selection for ptosis repair will be based on these measurements. Beard outlined the surgical treatment based on levator function stating that patients with excellent levator function should undergo aponeurotic advancement. Those with good levator function should have aponeurotic advancement or moderate levator resection of 14–17 mm. Patients with fair levator function should have 18–22 mm of levator resection, while those with poor levator function should undergo a frontalis suspension sling [7]. Details on these surgical techniques are addressed elsewhere in this text.

Finally, response of ptotic lids to 2.5% phenylephrine should be documented. This measurement may ultimately direct appropriate surgical correction. The lid position should be measured before and 5 minutes after instillation of a drop of 2.5% phenylephrine. Observation of the opposite lid should also be noted. As discussed earlier, the "normal" lid may become ptotic once the drive to lift the other lid is removed by instillation of phenylephrine due to Hering's law. The response to phenylephrine can be categorized as good if the MRD1 changes to 4–5 mm after instillation of the drop. If the MRD1 changes to 3 mm, the response can be noted as moderate and poor if the MRD1 is equal to or less than 2 mm (Table 61.2). If the ptotic eyelid demonstrates a good response to phenylephrine (Fig. 61.6a, b) and places the lid in good position, shortening the Muller's muscle by Putterman müllerectomy or by Fasanella-Servat müllerectomy with tarsectomy can be performed. If the response is moderate, a graded Fasanella-Servat or Werb procedure can be used. Finally, if the response is poor, levator surgery or frontalis suspension sling is likely appropriate based on the levator function described previously [8].

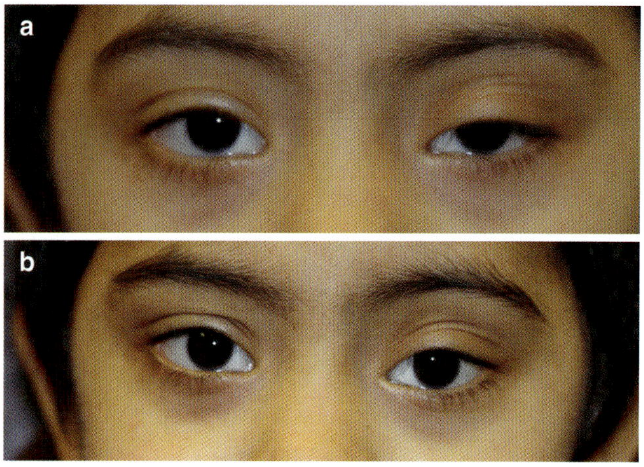

Fig. 61.6 (**a**) Lid position before application of 2.5% phenylephrine. (b) Lid position after application of 2.5% phenylephrine

Eyelid Tumors

Lid tumors can found in adult populations can also be identified in children, but the incidence and underlying etiology can be considerably different. Though one does not usually think of malignant tumors in a pediatric population, both malignant and benign tumors must be considered. Discussing each type of lid tumor is out of the scope of this chapter and is discussed in detail in other parts of this text, so only a limited differential and small description will be discussed here.

Benign Eyelid Tumors

Benign tumors of the eyelid found in the pediatric population include capillary hemangiomas, lymphangiomas, dermoid cysts, plexiform neurofibromas, nevi, pilomatrixomas, juvenile xanthogranuloma, and chalazions.

Malignant Eyelid Tumors

Malignant lid tumors are rare in the pediatric population and are not well documented in the literature. The Wilmer Institute pathology department published a review of 393 histopathologic specimens and found 3 malignant lesions: 1 basal cell carcinoma, 1 squamous cell carcinoma, and 1 metastatic embryonal cell carcinoma [9]. Though not common in the pediatric population, malignant lid lesions in children should be approached differently than in adults.

In contrast to adults where skin malignancies may be an isolated finding, pediatric skin malignancies may more often manifest from a systemic condition. Kaposi sarcoma can manifest in children infected with the human immunodeficiency virus [10]. Histiocytic lid lesions can be found in kids with Langerhans cell histiocytosis [11], and leukemic lid infiltrations can be secondary to acute myeloblastic leukemia [12]. Basal cell carcinoma can be found in the pediatric population and may be associated with the basal cell nevus syndrome, xeroderma pigmentosa, linear nevus sebaceous syndrome, epidermodysplasia verruciformis, and radiation dermatitis [13, 14].

Premalignant syndromes that can be identified in children include nevus of Ota [15], xeroderma pigmentosa, and the linear nevus sebaceous syndrome.

Sebaceous cell carcinoma which arises from the sebaceous glands of the eyelid, brow, and caruncle can be found as well as squamous cell carcinoma that is much more common in fair skin individuals on sun-exposed areas. Unusual malignant eyelid lesions may be found in children such as Merkel cell tumors originating from touch mechanoreceptors, mucinous carcinomas, and rhabdomyosarcoma that may present as a lid mass [14].

Orbit

Examination of a child with an orbital disease can be difficult, especially if the child is uncomfortable. Many of the examination tools and techniques can be intimidating to a child and should be deferred until later in the visit to yield the most information possible. Beginning with a detailed history obtained from the parent can give the child time to become comfortable with the surroundings and can provide valuable diagnostic information. The time of onset can be particularly helpful as acquired neoplasias typically do not occur in the first 6 months and usually are identified after the first year [16]. Congenital lesions are present at birth. However, it is important to keep in mind that in cases of an enlarging mass, a congenital tumor may not be noted until later in life. Reviewing photographs of the child provided by the family can help give the clinician a cross-sectional view of the progression. Birth history and eliciting any traumatic injury can be important as granulomas can be found in response to blood after an orbital hemorrhage. Progression of the lesion can help direct diagnosis, as slow-growing lesions are more likely benign while those with an intermediate growth pattern may be benign or malignant [16]. Rapid growth can indicate malignancies such as rhabdomyosarcoma; alternatively it may represent a benign process such as a ruptured dermoid cyst or cellulitis. Surgical history can be important to suggest a possible granuloma formation following strabismus surgery. Family history suggesting inherited disease such as neurofibromatosis can help with diagnosis as

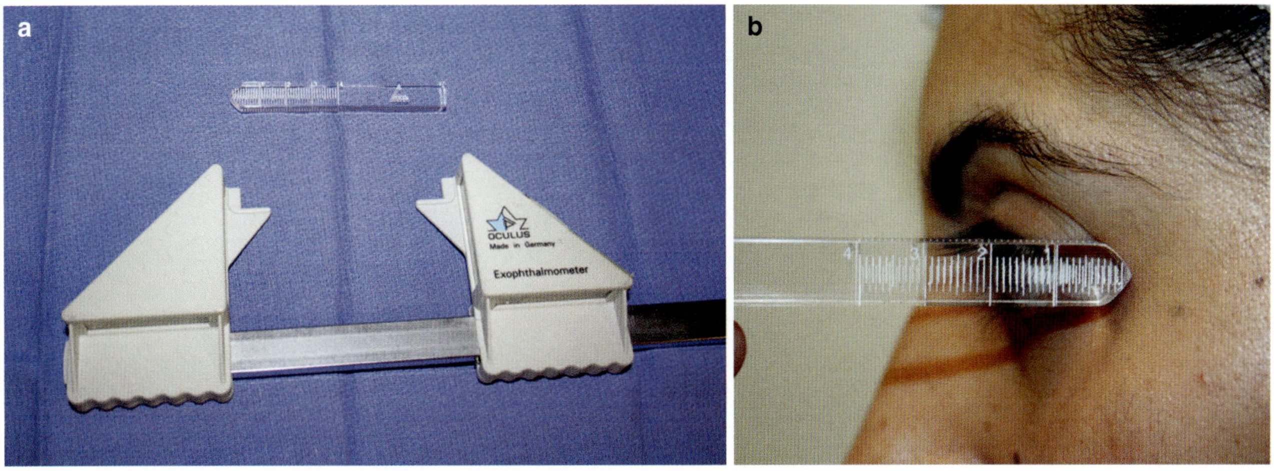

Fig. 61.7 (**a**) Hertel and Luedde exophthalmometers. (**b**) Luedde exophthalmometer in use

well. Developmental milestones and growth charts can identify systemic abnormalities.

Physical examination can be challenging; however, digital photography can help freeze a good view for a more thorough investigation. Using a ruler in the photograph can help identify lid position, extra-axial displacement, as well as vertical fissure height and intercanthal distances. Getting axial measurements using a Hertel exophthalmometer can be difficult, and using a Luedde exophthalmometer may be of benefit (Fig. 61.7a, b).

A detailed ocular examination noting vision, pupillary response, color vision, and refraction is important. Extraocular movement exam can identify restriction or may suggest a cranial nerve abnormality. Testing facial sensation can localize a process affecting the nerves.

Eyelid and adnexal examination should be conducted noting warmth that could suggest infection or color changes that may suggest lymphangioma, neuroblastoma, or capillary hemangioma. Notation of an S-shaped lid deformity or pulsatile movement of the lids that could indicate a plexiform neurofibroma or absence of the sphenoid wing found in some patients with neurofibromatosis.

A fundus examination can identify a retrobulbar mass causing choroidal folds or diagnose vascular abnormalities or flame hemorrhages suggesting a systemic association. Metastasis may also be identified in the retina or choroid. Optic nerve pallor may indicate mechanical stress or ischemic damage secondary to a mass.

Visual field measurements can help localize a lesion; however, it may be difficult or impossible to obtain in young children. Confrontational visual fields can be assessed using interesting toys that are presented in the periphery while maintaining a child's interest forward.

Imaging using ultrasound, MRI, or CT can be helpful in the diagnosis of an orbital examination and are discussed in other chapters of this text. It is important to consider the radiation exposure to a child with thin orbital cuts as well as the risk of sedation that may be necessary to obtain a quality film.

The incidence of pediatric orbital tumors differs from those in adults, and many reviews have attempted to provide an overview of these tumors. There is great variability in the literature, likely secondary to patient population and referral bias at different institutions. Reviews published from tertiary care centers will likely indicate a higher incidence of rare and complicated tumors, while reviews from a community ophthalmologist will show a higher incidence of such lesions as dermoid cysts or hemangiomas. The table included is modified from Katowitz's text, Pediatric Oculoplastic Surgery, and it compiles six large series of pediatric orbital tumors [16–22]. This table can be useful for the clinician to get a more balanced understanding of the most common pediatric orbital tumors that may be encountered (Table 61.3).

Hopefully some techniques explained in this chapter will aid in examination and provide some direction for diagnosis in the pediatric oculoplastic patient. With time, clinicians will gain their own style with children, develop their own examination "tricks," and become excellent pediatric oculoplastic physicians.

Table 61.3 Compilation of six large series of pediatric orbital lesions

	Iliff and Green Wilmer 1978 *N* = 174 [17]	Crawford Toronto 1983 *N* = 572 [18]	Shields et al. Wills 1986 *N* = 250 [19]	Rootman Univ of B.C. 1988 *N* = 241 [20]	Kodsi Mayo Clinic 1994 *N* = 340 [21]	Katowitz CHOP 1996 *N* = 243 [22]
Benign tumors						
Cystic lesions						
Dermoid	52	6	115	27	65	71
Lipodermoid	0	0	0	7	0	4
Microphthalmia w/ cyst	5	0	3	3	2	1
Sweat gland cyst	0	0	0	1	0	2
Mucocele	0	5	1	2	4	0
Implantation cyst	0	0	0	2	0	0
Simple epithelial cyst	1	0	12	1	5	6
Cephalocele	1	2	0	0	3	0
Lacrimal duct cyst	2	0	0	0	1	0
Infectious/inflammatory lesions						
Orbital cellulitis or abscess	0	226	0	17	0	2
Dacryoadenitis	0	1	5	0	0	0
Reactive lymphoid hyperplasia	0	0	5	0	0	0
Idiopathic orbital inflammation	9	5	41	14	20	13
Thyroid orbitopathy	0	107	0	24	0	0
Scleritis	0	0	0	1	0	0
Foreign body granuloma	0	0	0	0	7	0
Noninflammatory lacrimal abnormality	5	0	0	0	0	0
Neurogenic lesions						
Optic nerve glioma	9	17	5	13	47	2
Meningioma	5	0	1	2	9	3
Plexiform neurofibroma	11	14	2	9	16	33
Teratoma	3	1	0	0	2	3
Neurilemmoma	0	0	1	0	1	0
Paraganglioma	0	0	0	0	1	0
Vascular lesions						
Capillary hemangioma	14	0	10	23	40	14
Lymphangioma	10	4	4	14	12	7
Cavernous hemangioma	0	13	2	0	1	0
Varix	0	0	0	12	0	1
AV shunt	3	3	1	5	4	0
Vascular malformation	0	3	0	0	1	0
Angiofibroma	0	3	0	0	1	0
Hemangiopericytoma	0	0	0	0	1	0
Secondary hemorrhage	1	5	0	0	1	0
Trauma						
Fracture	0	0	0	16	0	0
Foreign body	0	0	0	2	0	5
Orbital hemorrhage	0	25	0	0	0	0
Degenerative						
Post-RT atrophy	0	0	0	5	0	0
Fat prolapse	1	0	0	1	0	0
Amyloidosis	1	0	0	0	0	0
Histiocytic lesions						
Langerhans histiocytosis	1	2	1	0	8	3
Juvenile xanthogranuloma	0	0	0	0	0	2
Fibrous histiocytosis	0	0	0	2	0	0
Bony lesions						
Fibrous dysplasia	2	4	0	7	13	5
Aneurysmal bone cyst	0	0	0	2	1	0
Osteoma	0	1	0	2	2	0

Table 61.3 (continued)

	Iliff and Green Wilmer 1978 $N = 174$ [17]	Crawford Toronto 1983 $N = 572$ [18]	Shields et al. Wills 1986 $N = 250$ [19]	Rootman Univ of B.C. 1988 $N = 241$ [20]	Kodsi Mayo Clinic 1994 $N = 340$ [21]	Katowitz CHOP 1996 $N = 243$ [22]
Orbital asymmetry	0	48	0	8	0	0
Ossifying granuloma	2	0	2	1	1	2
Osteoporosis	0	1	0	0	0	0
Hyperostosis	0	1	0	0	0	0
Fat-containing lesions	4	0	16	0	4	19
Pseudoproptosis	0	0	0	1	0	0
Malignant tumors						
Rhabdomyosarcoma	15	14	10	5	26	27
Leukemia/lymphoma	2	23	1	1	5	5
Soft tissue sarcomas	6	9	2	5	9	5
Secondary retinoblastoma	6	1	9	0	14	1
Histiocytosis X	0	18	0	3	4	3
Neuroblastoma	1	9	0	1	3	0
Adenoid cystic carcinoma of lacrimal gland	0	0	1	2	0	0
Malignant teratoma	1	0	0	0	1	0
Nasopharyngeal carcinoma	0	1	0	1	0	0
Esthesioneuroblastoma	0	0	0	0	1	1
Malignant schwannoma	0	0	0	0	0	1
Orbital melanoma	0	0	0	0	1	0
Medulloblastoma metastatic to optic nerve	0	0	0	1	0	0
Metastatic astrocytoma	1	0	0	0	0	0

References

1. Simon JW, Aaby AA, Drack AV, et al. Amblyopia. In: Cantor LB, editor. Basic and clinical science course section 6. American Academy of Opthalmology. San Francisco; 2006. p. 67–75.
2. Oral Y, Ozgur OR, Akcay L, Ozbas M, Dogan OK. Congenital ptosis and amblyopia. Pediatr Ophthalmol Strabismus. 2010;47(2): 101–4.
3. Miller MT. Ocular abnormalities in craniofacial malformation. Int Ophthalmol Clin. 1984;24:143.
4. Whitaker LA, Katowitz JA, Jacobs WE. Ocular adnexal problems in craniofacial deformities. J Maxillofac Surg. 1979;7:55.
5. Hertel RW, Quinn GE, Schaffer DB. Pediatric extraocular muscle surgery and oculoplastic disorders. In: Katowitz JA, editor. Pediatric oculoplastic surgery. New York: Springer-Verlag; 2002. p. 145–57.
6. Harrad RA, Graham CM, Collin JRO. Amblyopia and strabismus in congenital ptosis. Eye. 1988;2:625–7.
7. Beard C. Newer ptosis procedures. In: Ptosis. 2nd ed. St. Louis: Mosby; 1997. p. 189–212.
8. Heher KL, Katowitz JA. Pediatric ptosis. In: Katowitz JA, editor. Pediatric oculoplastic surgery. New York: Springer-Verlag; 2002. p. 253–88.
9. Doxanas MT, Green W, Arentsen JJ, Elsas FJ. Lid lesions of childhood: a histopathologic survey at the Wilmer Institute (1923-1974). J Pediatr Ophthalmol. 1976;13:7–13.
10. Stefan DC. Incidence of skin lesions of Kaposi sarcoma in HIV-positive children. Pediatr Blood Cancer. 2010;55(2):392.
11. Favara BE, Jaffe R. Pathology of Langerhans cell histiocytosis. Hematol Oncol Clin North Am. 1987;1:75–92.
12. Sandoval C, Davis A, Jayabose S. Eyelid mass as the presenting finding in a child with Down syndrome and acute megakaryoblastic leukemia. Pediatrics. 2005 Mar;115(3):810–1.
13. Anderson DE, Taylor WB, Falls HG, Davidson RT. The nevoid basal cell syndrome. Am J Hum Genet. 1967;19:12–22.
14. Fries P. Malignant pediatric eyelid tumors. In: Katowitz JA, editor. Pediatric oculoplastic surgery. New York: Springer-Verlag; 2002. p. 245–51.
15. Patterson CR, Acland K, Khooshabeh R. Cutaneous malignant melanoma arising in an acquired naevus of Ota. Australas J Dermatol. 2009 Nov;50(4):294–6.
16. Kazim M, Fries PD, Katowitz JA. Classification and evaluation of orbital disorders in children. In: Katowitz JA, editor. Pediatric oculoplastic surgery. New York: Springer-Verlag; 2002. p. 359–64.
17. Iliff WJ, Green WR. Orbital tumors in children. In: Jakobiec FA, editor. Ocular and adnexal tumors. Birmingham: Aesculapius Publishing Company; 1978. p. 669–84.
18. Crawford JS. Diseases of the orbit. In: Crawford JS, Morin JD, editors. The eye in childhood. New York: Grune & Stratton; 1983. p. 361–94.
19. Shields JA, Bakewell B, Ausburger JJ, et al. Space occupying orbital masses in children: a review of 250 consecutive biopsies. Ophthalmology. 1986;93:397–84.
20. Rootman J. Frequency and differential diagnosis of orbital disease. In: Rootman J, editor. Diseases of the orbit. Philadelphia: J.B. Lippencott Co.; 1988. p. 124.
21. Kodst SR, Sheltar KJ, Campbell RJ, et al. A review of 340 orbital tumors in children during a 60-year period. Am J Ophthalmol. 1994;117:177–82.
22. Katowitz JA. Unpublished data from the Children's Hospital of Philadelphia, 1996.

Child Abuse Concerns in Oculoplastics

62

Brian John Forbes

Childhood physical abuse is an important cause of pediatric morbidity and mortality and is associated with major physical and mental health problems that can extend into adulthood. Non-accidental trauma is a leading cause of childhood traumatic injury and death in the United States. It is estimated that some 1400 children die annually from maltreatment in the United States, and abusive head trauma accounts for approximately 80% of these deaths.

While it is unlikely that the oculoplastic surgeon will encounter such cases of child abuse, it is true that any form of trauma to the eye or adnexa can be due to abuse and should be considered in the differential diagnosis [1]. All physicians who work with children, even if the primary nature of their practice is the care of adults, are legally obligated to report the *suspicion* of child abuse. Each state has a system to receive and respond to reports of possible child abuse and neglect. Professionals and concerned citizens can call statewide hotlines, local child protective services, or law enforcement agencies to share their concerns in the United States as well as in virtually every developed nation. As such, oculoplastic surgeons must have a sufficient index of suspicion to prevent missing a case of abuse. It has been estimated that approximately 4–6% of physically abused children first present to the ophthalmologist [2]. Failure to recognize abuse will leave the child vulnerable to further injury or even death [3]. Ocular manifestations of non-accidental trauma include periorbital hematoma, eyelid laceration or burns, subconjunctival hemorrhage, subluxed or dislocated lens, cataracts, glaucoma, anterior chamber angle regression, iridodialysis, retinal dialysis or detachment, intraocular hemorrhage, optic atrophy, and papilledema though most commonly retinal hemorrhages which are often multilayered and occur in 60–85% of non-accidental head injuries [4].

B. J. Forbes (✉)
University of Pennsylvania, Department of Opthalmology, Philadelphia, PA, USA
e-mail: forbesb@email.chop.edu

Abusive burns to the face may involve the ocular adnexa, and a high percentage of childhood burns are due to abuse. The two kinds of burns most often seen in abused children are scald burns (from contact with hot liquids) and thermal burns (contact with hot objects) [5]. Additionally, periorbital ecchymosis is a cardinal sign of trauma and may certainly occur from abuse. Bilateral periorbital ecchymosis is more concerning for a non-accidental etiology although this finding can certainly also be seen following a variety of craniofacial surgeries, blunt trauma to the forehead with blood which can track down around both eyes, and medical conditions such as neuroblastoma or other coagulopathies. Orbital fracture and lid lacerations are common manifestations of accidental trauma, but can also be manifestations of child abuse [1]. More serious injuries such as a ruptured globe are infrequent though possible complications of child abuse and can certainly occur as the result of abuse, and the oculoplastic surgeon should maintain a healthy index of suspicion in such cases.

Several considerations may assist the oculoplastic surgeon in differentiating accidental versus non-accidental injury. In cases of abuse, the history may change frequently, be inconsistent with the observed injuries, or be inconsistent with the developmental level of the child [1]. For example, the story of a 10-month-old child running in the living room, tripping on the carpet, and striking their eyelid on a coffee table resulting in a laceration would be inconsistent with the developmental level at that age. Unusual presentation times or delays in seeking treatment should also prompt suspicion of abuse. A child who comes to see the oculoplastic surgeon for a lid laceration at 3:00 in the afternoon, accompanied by their parent and the school principal, with a history of the child having fallen off a slide in the school playground would not raise as much suspicion as the presentation of a 2-year-old child in the emergency room with a lid laceration allegedly sustained while playing at 3:00 in the morning. It is important to recognize that child abuse occurs without regard to race, religion, socioeconomic status, or other factors [6,

J. J. Servat et al. (eds.), *Smith and Nesi's Ophthalmic Plastic and Reconstructive Surgery*,
https://doi.org/10.1007/978-3-030-41720-8_62

7]. There are well-documented trends of over-reporting of visible minorities from lower socioeconomic groups and under-reporting of Caucasians from higher socioeconomic groups [7, 8].

The overwhelming majority of child abuse occurs as an act of frustration and loss of control rather than a preconceived intent to inflict a particular type of harm to a child, and the majority of perpetrators are remorseful [9]. Factors that are intrinsic to the perpetrator of abuse include relationship to the child and whether the perpetrator had been abused as a child. Perpetrators are likely to be young parents and female; however, males are more likely to be responsible for episodes of non-accidental trauma resulting in death [9]. Reporting is a means of intervening not only to protect the child but also to cease the cycle of events that lead to abuse through social intervention and medical care. The reporting ophthalmologist need not prove that abuse has occurred. If the medical scenario raises reasonable *suspicion* of possible abuse, then a prompt report to the appropriate child protective agency is warranted. Some physicians fear "getting involved" but should recognize that less than 1% of reporting ophthalmologists will end up testifying in court.

The oculoplastic surgeon may have to call upon their ability to examine the rest of the child. If the cause of an injury remains suspicious or unknown, undressing the child to look for other signs of injury, such as pattern marks on the body left by a beating with a belt, multiple bruises of apparently different ages, and bruising of areas not usually bruised in normal play (e.g., trunk, thorax, upper legs or arms, buttocks), will certainly raise the index of suspicion for abuse. Dating of bruising should not be attempted with regard to periorbital ecchymosis as the loose skin of the eyelids allow for a dramatic accumulation of blood that darkens the bruise and makes it often look older than it really is. Injuries should be documented by photography when possible. Parents should be informed that a report to child protective services will be taking place. It may be helpful to tell the parent simply that you are concerned that "someone may have injured your child." The physician should place no blame and clearly indicate to the family that no blame is being placed. Rather, the physician can develop a partnering alliance with the parents saying that "we do not want this to happen to your child again." The physician must put aside their fears that the parent may be unhappy with the report, get angry, or discourage other patients from seeing the physician. The primary mandate remains to protect a child who may have been injured. If the physician has access to a multidisciplinary child abuse team, as usually found in an academic medical center, reporting to child protective services can instead be triaged to evaluation by the multidisciplinary team who can in turn make the report on behalf of the ophthalmologist if indicated.

All physicians who treat children, regardless of their specific discipline, play an important role in the management of non-accidental trauma by early recognition of potentially suspicious injuries. It is essential for all physicians to maintain a high index of suspicion for non-accidental trauma in the management of pediatric patients and appropriately report cases of possible child abuse and neglect.

References

1. Levin A, Morad Y. Ocular manifestations of child abuse. In: Reece R, Christian C, editors. Child abuse: medical diagnosis and management. 3rd ed. Elk Grove Village: American Academy of Pediatrics; 2009. p. 211–25.
2. Friendly D. Ocular manifestations of physical child abuse. Trans Am Acad Ophthalmol Otolaryngol. 1971;75:318–32.
3. Jenny C, Hymel KP, Ritzen A, Reinert SE, Hay TC. Analysis of missed cases of abusive head trauma. JAMA. 1999;281(7):621–6.
4. Green MA, Lieberman G, Milroy CM, Parsons MA. Ocular and cerebral trauma in non-accidental injury in infancy: underlying mechanisms and implications for paediatric practice. Br J Ophthalmol. 1996;80(4):282–7.
5. Hobbs CJ. When are burns not accidental? Arch Dis Child. 1986;61(4):357–61.
6. Dashti SR, Decker DD, Razzaq A, et al. Current patterns of inflicted head injury in children. Pediatr Neurosurg. 1999;31:302–6.
7. Huang MI, O'Riordan MA, Fitzenrider E, et al. Increased incidence of nonaccidental head trauma in infants associated with the economic recession. J Neurosurg Pediatr. 2011;8:171–6.
8. Hampton R, Newberger E. Child abuse and reporting by hospitals: significance of severity, class, and race. Am J Public Health. 1985;75:56–60.
9. Mulpuri K, Slobogean BL, Tredwell SJ. The epidemiology of nonaccidental trauma in children. Clin Orthop Relat Res. 2011;469(3):759–67.

Genetics in Oculoplastics

63

Karthikeyan Arcot Sadagopan

Introduction

Genetic etiology is implicated in almost 50% of childhood blindness [1]. Several orbital and adnexal disorders have a genetic basis. An understanding of fundamental genetics and its clinical implications not only makes it possible to provide a comprehensive diagnosis and treatment but also helps to identify surveillance strategies for associated ocular and systemic findings, clarify prognosis, and provide families with genetic counseling and a disease-specific support. Knowledge of development of the orbit, eye, ocular adnexa, and face further supplements the oculoplastic surgeon's skills and enhances efficient decision-making especially in the management of congenital and other genetic oculoplastic disorders.

The Human Genome

Human DNA is comprised of approximately 30,000 genes. Each nucleated human cell except the ovum and sperm contains 23 pairs of chromosomes for a total of 46 chromosomes. The sperm and the ovum have only 23 chromosomes, and the 46 number of chromosomes is restored in the zygote after fertilization of the ovum by the sperm. The chromosomes are labeled 1 through 22, plus two X chromosomes in females and one X and one Y chromosome in males. The first 22 chromosomes are known as autosomes, while the X and Y chromosomes are known as the sex chromosomes. Each pair of genes is made up of one from the patient's mother and one from the patient's father. The term allele refers to one chromosome in a pair. Each allele contains the same genes as the fellow allele, but the sequences may be different. Every tissue in the body contains the same chromosomes and genes, but only certain genes are activated (turned on) or inactivated (turned off) in a specific given cell type. Genes code for proteins. Some proteins affect structure (e.g., fibrillin, collagen) and others, function (e.g., enzymes). Other genes, the transcription factors, code for proteins which regulate the expression other genes.

Gene Structure

Genes are made up protein coding sequences, called exons, and non-coding sequences, called introns. Introns are located between exons and are involved with appropriate linking of the protein components generated by transcribed exons to form the complete protein product of the gene.

The process by which DNA is copied to RNA is called transcription, and that by which RNA is used to produce proteins is called translation. This is the central dogma of molecular biology and involves DNA to RNA and RNA to protein.

Mutation and Polymorphism

Changes in the sequence of the nucleotides within a gene can occur in either an exon or intron causing changes in the intended protein product. When a sequence change results in an abnormal phenotype, it is referred to as a mutation. Sequence variations more often result in subtle protein variability that is not disease causing but rather responsible for normal human variability. These sequence variations are referred to as *benign polymorphisms*. Mutations may cause the substitution of one amino acid for another (missense mutation), premature truncation of the protein via and early stop in the reading of the DNA (nonsense), or a shift in the transcription leading to a jumbled protein and eventual stop

K. Arcot Sadagopan (✉)
CMER (SHENZHEN) Dennis Lam Eye Hospital, Department of Pediatric Ophthalmology & Ocular Genetics, Futian District, Shenzhen, China

J. J. Servat et al. (eds.), *Smith and Nesi's Ophthalmic Plastic and Reconstructive Surgery*,
https://doi.org/10.1007/978-3-030-41720-8_63

(frame shift). Mutations in an exon-intron boundary (splice sites) or within the intron may result in a failure to assemble the exon products correctly. Mutations can be inherited from one or both parents or occur as a new event. New spontaneous changes are referred to as de novo or sporadic mutations. A novel mutation is one that has not been reported previously in the literature. Previously reported mutations are often stored in web-based disease or gene-specific universal genome databases accessible globally. This aids the physician in distinguishing between a benign polymorphism and disease-causing mutation. Newly observed sequence variation must be evaluated for pathogenicity by assessing predicted biologic effect and ascertaining if the variation segregates within a family such that it is found only in those who have the disease.

Patterns of Inheritance

Mendelian Inheritance

Mendelian disorders are caused by mutations in single genes and follow the principles of inheritance as initially described by Sir Gregor Mendel in 1866.

Autosomal Dominant Inheritance

Autosomal dominant disorders manifest when only one autosomal gene copy is mutated. Transmission occurs regardless of sex and both sexes are equally affected. The risk of transmission to the next generation is 50% for each pregnancy. Different members of the family inheriting the mutation may manifest different levels of severity (variable expressivity). This is due to phenotype modification by other genes or by environmental factors. For example, in craniosynostoses, some members may have only very subtle findings that might be missed, but other members may have more obvious abnormalities of head shape. Hence examining family members may identify previously unrecognized affected individuals. When an individual has gene mutation but shows no clinical signs of the disease, the individual is said to be non-penetrant.

Autosomal Recessive Inheritance

Autosomal recessive disorders occur when both copies of a gene are mutated. The carrier parents of an affected individual are presumed to each harbor one abnormal gene copy which when simultaneously passed to the child result in disease. The risk to have an affected offspring is 25% at each pregnancy. When mutations in both copies of the gene are identical, the individual is said to be homozygous, and if the mutation on each copy of the gene is different, the individual is said to be compound heterozygous. Both sexes are affected equally and transmission is independent of sex. Autosomal recessive disorders are more common in consanguineous marriages and in constricted gene pools as it is more likely that each parent carries the same mutation in a given gene. Individuals with autosomal recessive disease would have to marry a carrier to have an affected child.

X-Linked Recessive Inheritance

X-linked disease occurs when the mutated gene lies on the X chromosome. In these disorders, males have the mutation on their single X chromosome (hemizygous) and thus manifest the disease, whereas females are carriers. There is no male-to-male transmission as an affected male must use his Y chromosome to create a son. In every cell, females only use one X chromosome with inactivation of the other X (lyonization). Rarely, a female may show signs of the disorder if she is adversely lyonized with more cells than expected using the mutated X. Females may also be affected as a result of obtaining a mutation on both copies of the X-linked gene. This can occur in disorders with a high frequency in the population such as red-green color vision deficiency where an affected daughter may be the product of a carrier mother and affected father. Turner syndrome is another clinical situation, where a female can be affected with an X-linked recessive disorder as she has only one X chromosome.

X-Linked Dominant Inheritance

In X-linked dominantly inherited disorders, only one copy of the X chromosome gene needs to be abnormal for disease to occur. Males who are hemizygous for the mutation usually have very severe disease or die, as they do not have another copy of the gene. Females who have heterozygous mutations are affected. Pedigrees often may show multiple miscarriages of male fetuses and exclusively female affliction. There is no male-to-male transmission. The risk of having an affected son/daughter with each conception for an affected female is 50%.

Non-Mendelian Inheritance

Mitochondrial Inheritance

Mitochondria have their own DNA (mtDNA) which is distinct from nuclear DNA. All mitochondria of an individual are inherited from the mother. All children born to affected females have the mutated mitochondrial DNA. Severity of disease in each child depends upon the proportion of abnormal mitochondria in affected tissues. Coexistence of normal and mutant mtDNA is called heteroplasmy [2]. When the percentage of mutant mtDNA reaches a certain threshold that may vary by tissue, manifestations of disease may be seen. Females and males are usually affected equally. Mitochondrial dysfunction may also occur as a result of mutations in nuclear genes whose protein products are used in the mitochondria. In these instances, inheritance is determined by Mendelian genetics as described above.

Chromosomal Aberrations

Whole chromosomes or part of chromosomes may be deleted or duplicated or otherwise altered in structure (e.g., translocation, inversion). Since such aberrations almost always involve more than one gene, patients often tend to have multisystem involvement with some developmental delay.

Genetic Testing

If a single gene disorder is suspected, mutation analysis of that gene may be available from a clinical laboratory. Interpretation of the results requires an understanding of the test methodology and the implications of a sequence change. Not all sequence changes are disease-causing mutations. Genetic testing may also involve assessment of chromosome structure (karyotype), tests for small deletions or duplications (chromosomal microarray), simultaneous sequencing of multiple genes that may be responsible for similar or the same disorder (panel testing), or even a simultaneous assessment of all coding genes (whole exome sequencing) or the entire genome (whole genome sequencing). Each test has an appropriate indication. The selection of the appropriate test is best conducted by consultation with a clinical or ocular geneticist who can also provide the required pre- and posttest counseling along with proper test result interpretation. Congenital Anomalies of the Orbit and Ocular Adnexa

MAC Spectrum: Anophthalmia, Microphthalmia, and Coloboma

Anophthalmia refers to the complete absence of ocular tissue in the orbit and is the most severe structural eye malformation. There is also absence of the optic nerve. The ocular adnexal structures are usually present but reduced in size. The term microphthalmia is used for an eye with an axial length of <19 mm in a 1-year-old child or <21 mm in an adult (2 SD below normal; Weiss et al. 1989a, b) [3]. Microphthalmia may be so severe that there is no visible globe on clinical examination, but remnants of the globe may be visualized only by orbital ultrasound, neuroimaging, or histologic examination (clinical anophthalmia). Nanophthalmos is a specific form of microphthalmia in which the eye is usually <18 mm in axial length and there is associated thickening of the sclera, shallowing of the anterior chamber, and a predisposition to peripheral subretinal effusion.

Simple microphthalmia refers to a small eye that is otherwise structurally normal. When microphthalmia is associated with other ocular malformations, it is designated as complex microphthalmia. Ocular coloboma is the most common major eye malformation and is due to an optic fissure closure defect (OFCD) during development. In most individuals with an OFCD, the genetic basis of the malformation is not known. The estimated prevalence of the MAC spectrum is 2–6 in 50,000 live births [4]. Prenatal ultrasound performed can detect anophthalmia or microphthalmia as early as 13–14 weeks. Risk factors for anophthalmia and microphthalmia include gestational-acquired infections (e.g., rubella), maternal vitamin A deficiency, and exposure to radiation and thalidomide [3, 5]. Warfarin and alcohol (fetal alcohol syndrome) transplacental transmission of gestational-acquired infections, with rubella, toxoplasmosis, varicella, and cytomegalovirus, has been shown to cause MAC spectrum.

Nanophthalmos

The term neonatal mean axial length is 17 mm [6]. Normal axial length at adulthood is 24 mm. The majority of this increase occurs during the first 3 years of life. Normal axial length at adulthood measures 24 mm. Nanophthalmos is derived from the Greek word meaning "dwarf eye." Nanophthalmos may be inherited either in an autosomal dominant or in a recessive pattern. All forms are characterized by a high hyperopia due to short axial length less than 18 mm, high lens/eye volume ratio, and a high incidence of angle closure glaucoma and uveal effusion. Thick sclera and uveal effusion are sine qua non of nanophthalmos. Clinically the eyes appear as a small hyperopic eye with narrow palpebral fissures placed in a deep set orbit. Strabismus, both accommodative and non-accommodative esotropia, occur. Amblyopia is common due to hyperopia and strabismus.

The loci for the genes causing nanophthalmos 1 (NNO1) and nanophthalmos 3 (NNO3) have been mapped to 11p and 2q11–q14, respectively. Autosomal recessive nanophthalmos (NNO2) is caused by homozygous or compound heterozygous mutations in the MFRP gene at 11q23, which encodes a Frizzled-related transmembrane protein that is selectively expressed in the retinal pigment epithelium (RPE) and ciliary body. Nanophthalmos 4 (NNO4) is a dominantly inherited disorder caused by heterozygous mutations in the Transmembrane Protein 98 (TMEM98) gene on chromosome 17q11 [7].

Nanophthalmos may be associated with autosomal dominant vitreo-choroidopathy (ADVIRC) when mutations involve the BEST1/VMD2 gene. ADVIRC is a rare condition characterized by a peripheral circumferential hyperpigmented band with punctate white opacities in the retina, chorioretinal atrophy, and fibrillary condensations in vitreous. Nanophthalmos in association with retinitis pigmentosa especially those with coats like picture has been reported with mutations in Crumbs Homologue 1 Gene (CRB1), a gene that is involved in several other retinal dystrophies including Leber congenital amaurosis.

Isolated and Syndromic Anophthalmia/Microphthalmos

Both anophthalmia and microphthalmia can occur unilaterally or more often bilaterally. They may occur in isolation or as part of a systemic syndrome. Unilateral microphthalmia is more common when it presents as isolated microphthalmia. Approximately one-third of microphthalmia have coloboma [4]. One-third to one-half of anophthalmia and microphthalmia cases occurs as part of a syndrome [4]. Neurological anomalies are the most common findings in patients with anophthalmia. Genitourinary anomalies are most common findings in colobomatous microphthalmia as in CHARGE syndrome (Fig. 63.1). Chromosome aberrations are found in 25–30% of individuals [8].

A/M spectrum is seen in several systemic syndromes. More than 200 syndromes with A/M have been listed in the London Dysmorphology Database. Inheritance patterns may be autosomal recessive, autosomal dominant, or X-linked [9]. The molecular basis of each syndrome is different.

Some of the common syndromes are shown in Table 63.1.

The "SOX2 Anophthalmia Syndrome"

The SOX2 anophthalmia syndrome has a well-recognizable pleiotropic phenotype. It is the commonest syndrome associated with anophthalmia and microphthalmos caused by het-

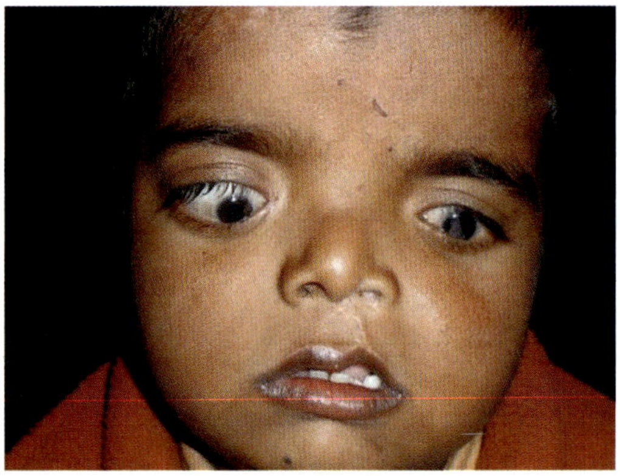

Fig. 63.1 CHARGE syndrome: This child with CHARGE syndrome has a broad rectangular forehead, bilateral iris coloboma, and repaired cleft lip and palate. The white reflex in the left pupil is caused by retinal detachment

Table 63.1 Important microphthalmia syndromes

Syndrome	Gene	Locus	Phenotype	Inheritance
SOX2 anophthalmia	SOX2 SRY (sex determining region Y)-box 2	3q26.33	Bilateral anophthalmia or severe microphthalmia, sclerocornea, cataracts, persistent hyperplastic primary vitreous and optic disc dysplasia	**AD**
Lenz microphthalmia syndrome	NAA10 BCOR	Xq28 Xp11.4	Clinical anophthalmia with malformations of the ears, teeth, fingers, skeleton, and/or genitourinary system, Colobomatous microphthalmos	X LR
Oculo-facio-cardiodental syndrome	BCOR	Xp11.4	Micro−/anophthalmia, congenital cataracts, radiculomegaly, cardiac defects, skeletal/digital anomalies, facial dysmorphia	X LR
Goltz syndrome (focal dermal hypoplasia)	PORCN	Xq28	Microphthalmia, coloboma, sclerocornea, linear skin lesions, digital anomalies, mental retardation	X L D
Midas syndrome MLS	HCCS COX7B NDUFB11	Xp22.2 Xq21 Xp11.3	Microphthalmia, linear skin pigmentation defects Linear skin defects with multiple anomalies	XLR
Nance-Horan syndrome	NHS	Xp22.13	Microcornea, cataract, dental anomalies, and intellectual disability	XLR
Norrie disease	NDP	Xp11.4	Bilateral severe microphthalmia, intellectual disability, sensorineural deafness	XLR
Waardenburg anophthalmia syndrome	SMOC1	14q24.2	Bilateral anophthalmia, with postaxial oligosyndactyly	AR
BRESHECK syndrome	MBTPS2	Xp22.12	Microphthalmia, CNS anomalies, skeletal anomalies, intellectual disability, renal hypoplasia	XLR
Renpenning syndrome	PQBP1 gene	Xp11.23	Developmental delay, microcephaly, short stature, and distinctive facial features. Intellectual disability. Cardiac defects, muscular atrophy, cleft palate, ocular colobomas	XLR

AD Autosomal dominant, *AR* Autosomal recessive, *XLR* X linked recessive, *XL D* X linked dominant erozygous mutations of the SOX2 gene. The phenotype is characterized by bilateral anophthalmia or severe microphthalmia. Other ocular findings include sclerocornea, cataracts, persistent hyperplastic primary vitreous, and optic disc dysplasia. Non-ocular features may include mild dysmorphic facial features, seizures, intellectual disability, neurological abnormalities, brain anomalies, esophageal pathology, male genital anomalies, and short stature. Developmental delay is common with delayed motor milestones, and children often have an unsteady ataxic gait. SOX2 mutations account for almost 10–15% of individuals with anophthalmia or microphthalmia [10]. De novo mutations account for most of these cases. Several reports of familial recurrence, even with a clinically unaffected parent, indicate the possibility of germline mosaicism in parents (usually the mother) [10].

Waardenburg Anophthalmia Syndrome

Ophthalmoacromelic syndrome (OAS), also known as Waardenburg anophthalmia syndrome, is characterized by the combination of eye malformations, most commonly bilateral anophthalmia, with postaxial oligosyndactyly [11].

X-Linked Microphthalmia Syndromes

The X-linked microphthalmia syndromes comprise a clinically and molecularly diverse group of disorders, a number of which overlap with X-linked mental retardation syndromes. A complete description of all syndromes is beyond the scope of this chapter. However, some of the more common and important syndromes are briefly discussed below.

Lenz Microphthalmia Syndrome

Lenz microphthalmia syndrome (LMS) is an X-linked disorder characterized by unilateral or bilateral microphthalmia and/or clinical anophthalmia with malformations of the ears, teeth, fingers, skeleton, and/or genitourinary system. Coloboma occurs in almost 60% of patients [12, 13]. LMS is caused by mutations of either NAA10 (MCOPS1 locus) or BCL-6 corepressor gene BCOR (MCOPS2 locus).

Oculo-Facio-Cardiodental (OFCD) Syndrome

It is another X-linked disorder which is an allelic disorder involving the BCOR gene and is characterized by ocular abnormalities (congenital cataracts, microphthalmia), facial anomalies, congenital cardiac defects, dental irregularities, and skeletal anomalies. Mutations in BCOR may be responsible for apparently isolated ocular anomalies. OFCD and Lenz microphthalmia syndromes are allelic disorders caused by mutation of the BCOR gene [14]. OFCD is lethal in males. Cataract may be the only ocular finding in females.

Microphthalmia, Dermal Aplasia, and Sclerocornea

MIDAS syndrome or microphthalmia with linear skin defects (MLS) syndrome is an X-linked dominantly inherited disorder with in utero lethality for affected males caused by mutations in *COX7B, HCCS,* or *NDUFB11* [15]. These skin lesions are present at birth, usually involve the face and neck and heal with age, leaving minimal residual scarring [15]. Systemic abnormalities include central nervous system involvement, developmental delay, heart defects, short stature, diaphragmatic hernia, nail dystrophy, preauricular pits and hearing loss, and genitourinary malformations. Corneal opacification and sclerocornea are common ocular manifestations in a microphthalmic eye. Retinal manifestations have also been reported [16].

Goltz syndrome Focal dermal hypoplasia is an extremely rare X-linked dominantly inherited multisystem disorder caused by mutations in the PORCN gene [17]. 95% of females with focal dermal hypoplasia have a de novo pathogenic variant, and 5% have inherited the pathogenic variant from a parent [18]. Ocular findings include colobomatous microphthalmos, cataracts, strabismus, and nystagmus. Cutaneous findings include congenital patchy skin aplasia along the lines of Blaschko. Lines of Blaschko correspond to cell migration pathways evident during embryonic and fetal skin development. These are similar to dermatomes in that the lines of Blaschko are linear on the limbs and circumferential on the trunk. However, unlike dermatomes, the lines of Blaschko do not correspond to innervation patterns. Congenital skin hypo- or hyperpigmentation that often follow Blaschko lines; congenital nodular fat herniation evidenced by soft nodules on the skin on the trunk and extremities; congenital ridged, dysplastic, or hypoplastic nails; and cutaneous telangiectasia are other cutaneous findings. Skeletal abnormalities include characteristic limb malformations that include syndactyly, ectrodactyly, oligodactyly, transverse limb defects, and long bone reduction defect (Fig. 63.2).

Other X-linked MAC spectrum includes Nance-Horan syndrome (Fig. 63.3), Norries disease, micro−/anophthalmia, ankyloblepharon, mental retardation, microphthalmia, microcornea and congenital cataract, and BRESHECK syndrome.

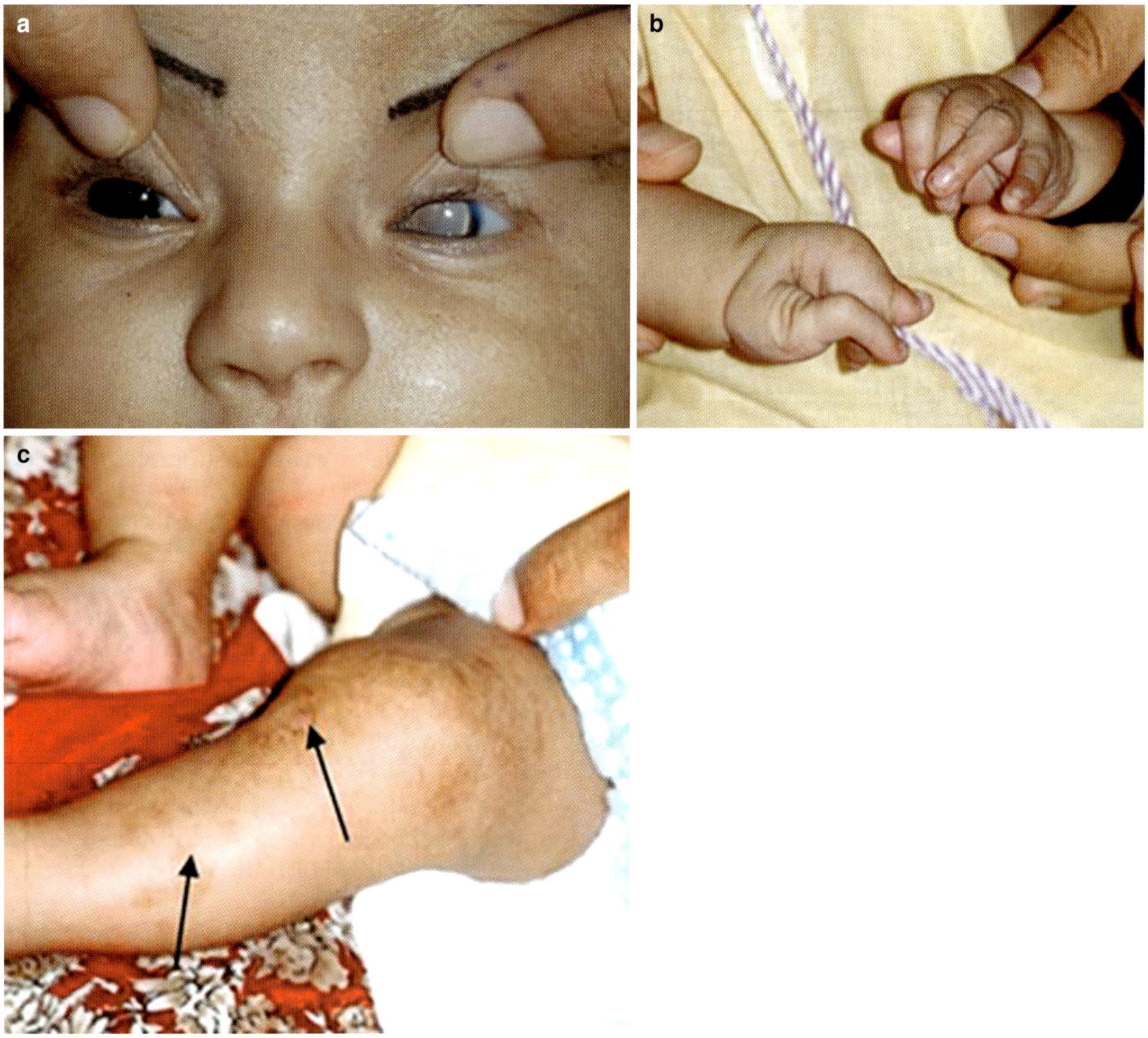

Fig. 63.2 Goltz syndrome (**a**) Leukocoria caused by coloboma in the left eye. (**b**) Upper limb anomaly ectrodactyly. (**c**) Fat herniation seen as soft nodules on the skin (black arrows). (Photo courtesy: Dr. Vijayalakshmi, Aravind Eye Care System, Madurai)

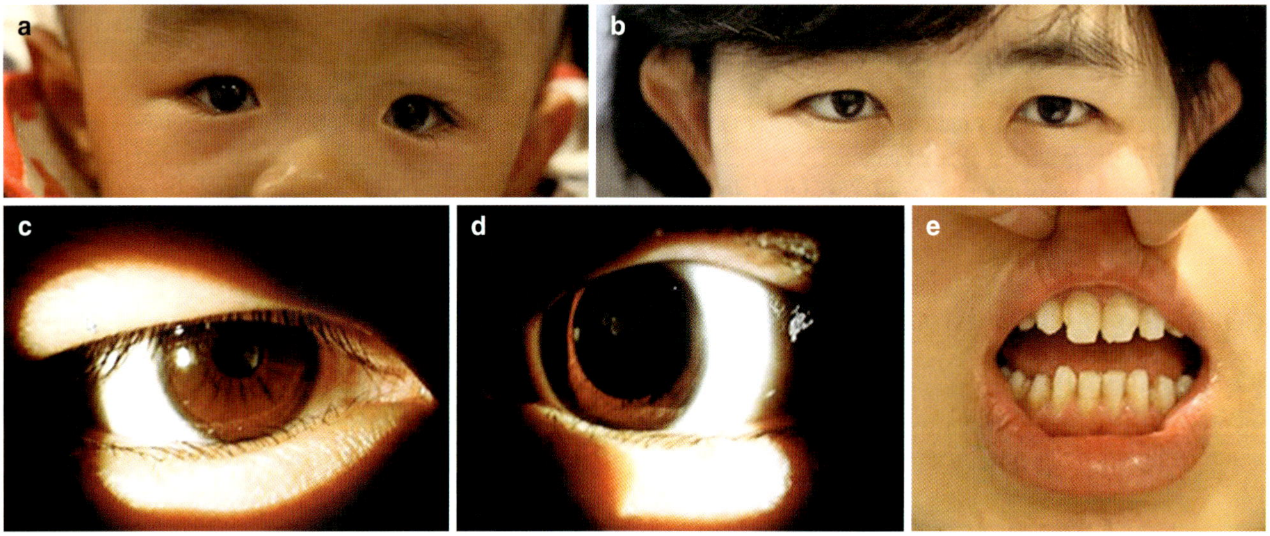

Fig. 63.3 Nance-Horan syndrome: (**a**) Child with microcornea and aphakia following cataract surgery. (**b**) Mother of child with slightly smaller corneas and prominent pinnae. (**c**, **d**) Cataract in carrier mother. (**e**) Dental anomalies in carrier mother

Genetic Testing and Counseling

Before genetic counseling or testing, when a patient has microphthalmia/anophthalmia, one must first determine if there is any evidence of a globe or optic stalk by imaging. The ophthalmologist must take a complete pedigree looking for other ocular disorders that may be associated (e.g., congenital cataract) and perform a full systemic examination of the patient in an attempt to identify a syndrome either of which may yield the correct inheritance pattern or pathway for genetic testing. Examination of the patient's parents is also useful. For example, a carrier parent may have subtle microphthalmia or an asymptomatic chorioretinal coloboma, which the parents were never aware they had (variable expression). The clinician should also carefully seek for non-genetic causes of the A/M spectrum. A specific pattern of associated features can provide a clinical diagnosis in approximately 25% of cases and help plan an appropriate genetic testing. The genetic cause is now identifiable in more than 50% of patients with a severe bilateral eye phenotype and in around 30% of all A/M patients taken together [19].

Several chromosomal anomalies have been reported to be associated with A/M including trisomy 13 (Patau syndrome) and mosaic trisomy 9. Genes known to cause isolated ocular involvement include CHX0, SHH, OTX2, PAX6, FOXE3, GDF6, and SIX6. Heterozygous mutations in SOX2, GDF6, OTX2, VSX2, CRYBA4, PAX2, PAX6, SIX3, and BMP4 genes and both homozygous and heterozygous mutations in FOXE3 gene can cause A/M spectrum. Additional genes associated with isolated or syndromic A/M include ALDH1A3, BCOR, BMP4, BMP7, COX7B (MLS), CRYBA4, FOXE3, GDF6, HCCS (MLS), MITF, NAA10, NDUFB11(MLS), PAX6, PRSS56, RAX, SALL1 (Townes-Brocks syndrome), SHH, SIX6, STRA6, TENM3, and VSX2 (CHX10). Holoprosencephaly and polydactyly may be seen along with anophthalmia in mutations of GLI2 gene [20]. Mutations of the STRA6 gene cause syndromic anophthalmia with associated findings that include congenital heart defects, pulmonary abnormalities, diaphragmatic hernia, and learning difficulties.

If no obvious syndrome is evident in infancy, further follow-up examinations may reveal the syndrome as many syndromes become more apparent by 3–4 years of age. Hence, it may require ongoing clinical genetics evaluation with monitoring of changes in growth and development overtime to make a syndromic diagnosis. However, if genetic testing is done and the results are contributory, an earlier syndromic diagnosis and an appropriate surveillance plan can be placed for the child and the family.

Presence of an intact globe is critical for the normal development of the orbit and the periocular tissues. A microphthalmic eye may result in orbital asymmetry and in severe cases may also result in facial asymmetry. Mild cases of microphthalmia may have normal or near-normal visual functions. When microphthalmia is severe with minimal or no potential for vision, scleral shells to promote periocular tissue growth are considered. Orbital implants of progressively enlarging size, such as an intraorbital balloon, may also be used in more severe cases [6]. Orbital volume-enhancing procedures like enucleation with dermal fat grafts and craniofacial surgery may rarely be indicated.

Cryptophthalmos

Cryptophthalmos (Greek, kryptos [hidden] + ophthalmos [eye]) was first described by Zehender and Manz in 1872 [21]. It is a rare congenital malformation that refers to the complete or incomplete failure of eyelid development. It is less common than microphthalmos/anophthalmia. However, it may be associated with M/A. The underlying globe is usually intact but may have severe compromise of the cornea.

Francois described three types of cryptophthalmos [22]. In typical or complete cryptophthalmos, there is complete absence of the eyelids, and the skin of the forehead extends onto the cheek passing over the orbit. The eyebrows are poorly developed, and all adnexal structures including lacrimal glands are absent. Incision of the skin in such patients often results in directly opening into the eye. Rudimentary eyelid structures may be seen in partial cryptophthalmos. In the third or the abortive form of cryptophthalmos, the upper eyelid partially fuses with the cornea. The rest of the cornea is often keratinized or vascularized or may be opaque.

Though cryptophthalmos can rarely occur as an isolated finding, it is usually a cardinal clinical manifestation of Fraser syndrome. Fraser syndrome is caused by homozygous mutations in FRAS1, FREM2, and GRIP1 [23]. There is usually no clear distinction between the upper and the lower eyelid. A tongue-shaped hair extends from the scalp to the periocular area (Fig. 63.4). Cryptophthalmos may coexist with eyelid coloboma. Grading system of congenital coloboma of the upper eyelid and cryptophthalmos with facial abnormalities is shown in Table 63.2. Systemic features include syndactyly, abnormal genitalia, and congenital anomalies of the ear, nose, and larynx. Bilateral renal agenesis when present often results in mortality. Intellectual disability may occur. Skeletal defects and umbilical hernia are other associated findings.

Manitoba-oculo-tricho-anal (MOTA) syndrome and bifid nose, renal agenesis, and anorectal malformations (BNAR) syndrome also are associated with mutations of the FREM1 gene [24].

MOTA syndrome is clinically characterized by a variable spectrum of eyelid malformations, including ocular hypertelorism, coloboma of the upper eyelid and corneopalpebral synechiae, absent eyebrow, aberrant hairline, bifid or broad

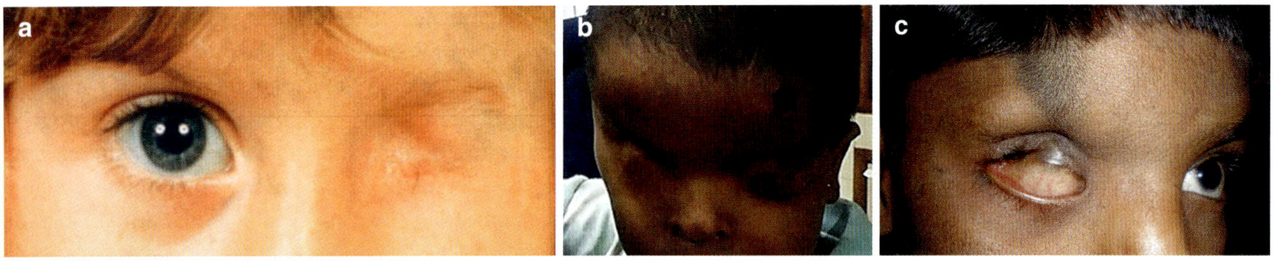

Fig. 63.4 (**a**) Fraser Syndrome: Cryptophthalmia with incomplete failure of lid development. (**b**) Bilateral Cryptophthalmos in Fraser syndrome. (**c**) Another child with unilateral Cryptophthalmia with pigmented skin extending from the brow to the forehead. (Photo Courtesy: Dr. Alex Levin (**a**, **b**), Dr. Vijayalakshmi (Aravind Eye Care system)-**c**)

Table 63.2 Grading system of congenital coloboma of the upper eyelid and cryptophthalmos with facial abnormalities

Grade	Cryptophthalmos	Skin
1	Coloboma without cryptophthalmos	No symblepharon
2	Coloboma with abortive cryptophthalmos	Forehead skin extends to the cornea in area of the coloboma
3	Coloboma with complete cryptophthalmos	Forehead skin extends over the cornea and merges with skin of the lower eyelid
4	Classic cryptophthalmos	Absence of all eyelid structures. Skin completely covers the eye
5	Severe cryptophthalmos	Grade 4 with severe deformity of the nose and ectropion of the upper lip

Adapted from [30]

nasal tip, and gastrointestinal anomalies that include anal stenosis and umbilical hernia. However, MOTA syndrome does not have syndactyly, ambiguous genitalia, cognitive impairment, ear anomalies, or limb anomalies that are often seen in Fraser syndrome.

The pathogenesis of cryptophthalmos is unclear. However, an understanding of the development of the eyelid will help in better understanding the spectrum of clinical findings seen in cryptophthalmos. Development of the lid is a complex process that includes interactions between the surface ectoderm and mesenchymal tissues. Five distinct phases, namely, eyelid formation, fusion, development, separation, and maturation of eyelid structures, have been recognized [25]. During development, the eyelids initially fuse and later separate. This initial fusion is critical before commencement of renal function (70 mm stage of the embryo), as when the kidneys begin to function, the urea, uric acid, and creatinine content of amniotic fluid increases significantly and this will have adverse effect on the ocular surface. Recent evidence also suggests that the fusion of the eyelids is necessary for subsequent differentiation of eyelid appendages. Hence morphogenesis of the eyelid involves very subtle yet strictly regulated morphogenetic episodes of tissue folding, proliferation, contraction, and migration. Many genes and molecular signaling pathways may play a role in this process. The cells involved in the development of the eyelids (periderm cells) are also concomitantly involved in temporary fusion of the digits [26, 27]. This could possibly explain why patients with Fraser syndrome may have syndactyly along with eyelid fusion anomalies [28]. Periderm cells are also precursors for the development of the tarsal conjunctiva and also play a role in corneal morphogenesis accounting for the corneopalpebral adhesions.

Orbit and eyelid reconstruction procedures form the mainstay of treatment, but the visual prognosis is guarded. The surgeon should anticipate a thinned or even absent cornea. Keratoplasty often has a very poor prognosis in such patients due to absence of a conjunctival sac and abnormal ocular surface [29]. In congenital symblepharon variant, there are an aborted cryptophthalmos with the upper lids partially fused with the globe and lagophthalmos resulting also in exposure keratopathy. Amniotic membrane grafts and mucous membrane grafts may be required in such patients in addition to lid procedures.

Congenital Coloboma of the Lids

Congenital coloboma of the lids may occur either as an isolated finding or more commonly as part of a systemic syndrome. Eyelid colobomas can be unilateral or bilateral and can be symmetrical or asymmetrical. It may or may not be associated with other ocular or facial deformities. It most commonly involves the upper eyelid. Congenital colobomas involving the upper eyelid, in particular, may threaten vision at a very early age and requires prompt management (Fig. 63.5) [28]. They may be associated with corneopalpebral adhesions. In contrast, children with lower lid colobomas often have a sufficient Bell phenomenon to protect the cornea from exposure, particularly in the early years [29]. This allows for surgical delay, and many children will not require surgical intervention for many years. Immediate attention at an early age through corneal protection, surgical repair of the eyelid defect, and monitoring of the visual development are essential.

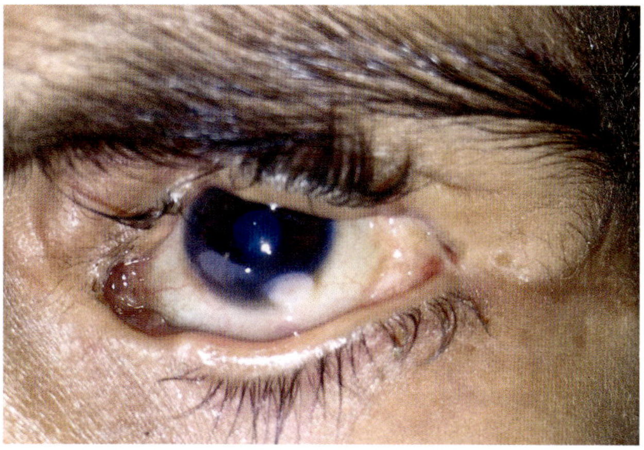

Fig. 63.5 Upper lid coloboma OS in a patient with Goldenhar syndrome. One can observe that the patient also has a limbal dermoid and an orbital dermoid. (Photo courtesy: Dr. Manju Meena. MS. Senior Consultant & International faculty, Oculoplasty & Ocular Oncology, CMER (Shenzhen) Dennis Lam Eye Hospital, Shenzhen, China)

Mustarde classified upper lid colobomas as three types, isolated coloboma, those associated with epibulbar tumors, and those associated with facial abnormalities [30]. Isolated colobomas lack corneopalpebral adhesions, are usually quadrangular in shape, demonstrate an intact eyelid margin medial to the coloboma, and almost always involve the upper lid. Conversely, colobomas associated with facial abnormalities may have corneopalpebral adhesions, are more triangular in shape, lack an intact eyelid margin medial to the coloboma, usually involve the lower lid, and often involve the proximal nasolacrimal system [30].

A new grading system has been suggested to classify cryptophthalmos and facial deformities with coloboma of the upper eyelid as one congenital anomaly (Table 63.1) [30]. Upper lid colobomas are often associated with eyelid adhesions to the conjunctiva or cornea, and this finding has led some to suggest an overlap with cryptophthalmia. These adhesions are similar to symblepharon but not acquired. Microphthalmos is often associated with these adhesions. Corneal surgery may be needed to obtain visual rehabilitation, but the dysplastic cornea may not be amenable to repair.

Systemic Syndromes with Lid Colobomas

The network and spectrum of genetic mutations responsible for upper eyelid colobomas remain largely unknown, and several possible environmental factors or mechanical events during pregnancy may contribute to the development. Fraser syndrome that has been discussed under cryptophthalmos may be associated with upper lid coloboma along with corneopalpebral adhesions.

Upper lid colobomas may be seen in oculoauriculovertebral spectrum (OAVS), including the subtype known as Goldenhar syndrome (Fig. 63.5). OAVS is due to abnormal development of the first and second branchial arches. Multiple loci and one gene, SALL1 (16q12.1), have been associated with autosomal dominant inheritance [31]. Ocular manifestations of OAVS also include limbal dermoid, lipodermoid, Duane syndrome, and less commonly microphthalmia or anterior segment dysgenesis. Patients can have bilateral OAVS with unilateral lid coloboma [32]. Other findings include mandibular hypoplasia, cleft lip/palate, microtia, preauricular skin tags, middle and inner ear malformations, macrostomia, and developmental delay. The presence of upper lid coloboma helps in differentiating OAVS from other similar syndromes such as Townes-Brocks, epibulbar dermoid with preauricular appendages and polythelia, oculoectodermal syndrome, and oculofaciocardiodental syndrome.

Other syndromes associated with lid colobomas include frontonasal dysplasia; manitoba-oculo-tricho-anal syndrome; ablepharon-macrostomia syndrome; nasopalpebral lipoma-coloboma syndrome; amniotic band sequence; oculoectodermal syndrome; CHARGE syndrome; several neurocutaneous syndromes like encephalo-cranio-cutaneous lipomatosis, Delleman syndrome, or oculo-cerebro-cutaneous syndrome; and linear nevus sebaceous syndrome.

Lower lid colobomas are most commonly associated with Treacher Collins-Franceschetti syndrome (Fig. 63.6) and are seen in almost 75% of these patients. The coloboma typically involves the junction of the medial 2/3 and outer one-third of the eyelid as a sharply demarcated defect, which has a more acute angle of upslant at its temporal edge. There are usually no lashes in the defect, and the proximal nasolacrimal drainage system may be absent. This condition is autosomal dominant and associated with mutations in the TCOF1 (5q32), POLR1D (13q12.2), or POLR1C genes (6p21.1). Hearing

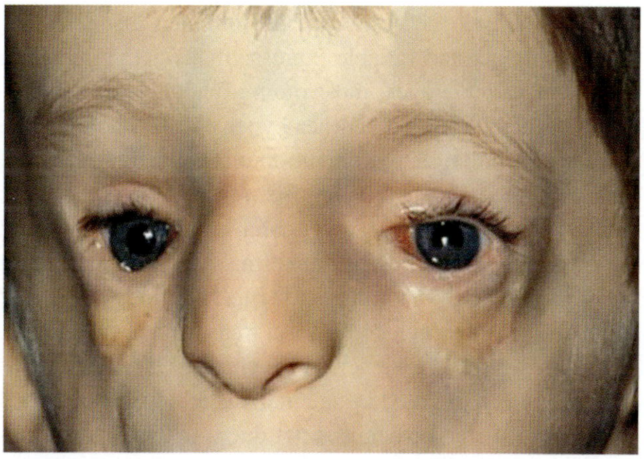

Fig. 63.6 Treacher Collins syndrome: Clinical photograph illustrating short horizontal lid fissures, downward slanting palpebral fissures, lower eyelid coloboma, and mid-face maxillary hypoplasia. Patient has had infraorbital plastic surgery. Note inferior corneal exposure left eye. (Photo courtesy: Dr. Alex Levin)

impairment is seen in almost 50% of the patients. It is inherited as an autosomal dominant condition.

Defects measuring less than one-quarter the eyelid margin can be closed directly. Full-thickness defects greater than one-third of the eyelid margin may require eyelid sharing techniques, such as Tenzel semicircular rotation flap, Hughes procedure, or lower eyelid rotation flap. Note that use of eyelid-sharing techniques may lead to iatrogenic amblyopia due to long periods of visual occlusion [33]. Eyelid colobomas especially those involving the upper eyelid are a potential threat to vision at an early age, requiring a multidisciplinary team, and involve close monitoring of the visual development of patients.

Distichiasis Syndromes

Distichiasis is the presence of an aberrant single eyelash or row of eyelashes originating from meibomian gland openings or from an ectopic location. This results when primary epithelial cells develop into a complete pilosebaceous unit rather than a specialized sebaceous gland of the tarsus [34]. It may lead to trichiasis, foreign body sensation, epiphora, and photophobia [34]. Congenital distichiasis was first reported by Becker in 1867. It may occur in isolation or as part of a congenital syndrome, such as lymphedema-distichiasis (LD) syndrome (also known as distichiasis-lymphedema-cleft palate syndrome) [35]. A coexistence of an atypically low level of serum cholinesterase was noted in a family with congenital distichiasis [36]. Low levels of serum cholinesterase can lead to prolonged apnea when given low doses of succinylcholine. Distichiasis has also been reported in one family as an autosomal dominant disorder associated with congenital heart and peripheral vascular abnormalities.

LD syndrome is an autosomal dominant disorder with high penetrance and variable expressivity [37]. Lymphedema begins at variable ages, most often after puberty. LD syndrome is associated with cornea hypoesthesia, photophobia, ptosis, congenital ectropion/entropion, congenital cataract, microphthalmia, blepharophimosis (see below), cleft palate, and webbing of the neck, vertebral anomalies, extradural cysts, varicose veins, renal abnormalities, and congenital heart disease. LD syndrome is due to mutations in *FOXC2* gene (16q24.3), which codes for a transcription factor [37]. Rare cases have been reported in which *FOXC2* mutations were found in isolated congenital distichiasis. Autosomal dominant isolated distichiasis not due to *FOXC2* mutations is also reported [37].

Removal of the eye lashes by electrolysis is done if only limited area of the lid is affected. Use of spacer grafts or eyelid splitting surgery may be considered when larger areas of the lid have trichiasis.

Congenital Ectropion

Congenital ectropion is a rare clinical condition caused by a vertical deficiency or shortening of the anterior lamella of the eyelids (blepharophimosis syndrome, ichthyosis, atrophic skin hypertrichosis syndrome, blepharo-cheilo-dontic syndrome) or by vertical elongation of the posterior lamella of the eyelid. Other possible pathophysiologic factors suggested include hypotonia of the orbicularis oculi (Down syndrome, congenital cutis laxa, Moebius syndrome with facial nerve paresis), birth trauma, and failure of the orbital septum to fuse with the levator aponeurosis.

It is commonly seen in ichthyosis (collodion baby) (Fig. 63.7). Congenital ichthyosis is a heterogeneous group of disorders of keratinization characterized primarily by abnormal skin scaling all over the body. Congenital ichthyosis is autosomal recessive and genetically heterogeneous. Harlequin ichthyosis (HI) is the most severe form of congenital ichthyosis and may be fatal. Collodion babies have a very taut, shiny, translucent, or opaque membrane that encases the entire body and lasts for few days to weeks. HI is an autosomal recessive disorder due to mutations of adenosine triphosphate-binding cassette A12 (ABCA12), a keratinocyte lipid transporter [38]. This mutation causes a disturbance of the epidermal lamellar granule lipid secretion and results in epidermal hyperkeratinization and defective desquamation. Neonates are prone to developing sepsis, dehydration, and impaired thermoregulation. Mutations in the ABCA12 gene can also cause another form of ichthyosis (autosomal recessive congenital ichthyosis) [39]. Children with HI develop thick hyperkeratotic plate-like scales with deep dermal fissures, severe congenital ectropion, alopecia,

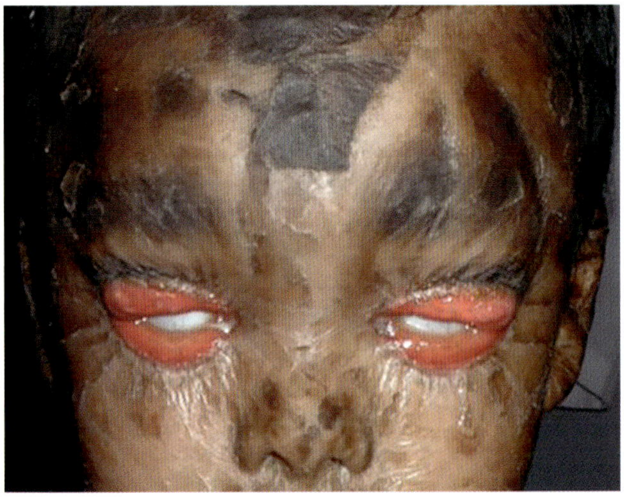

Fig. 63.7 Congenital ectropion: Ichthyosis causing bilateral congenital ectropion affecting both upper and lower eyelids. (Photo courtesy: Dr. Vijayalakshmi, Aravind Eye Care System, Madurai)

digital contractures, and growth delays. Mutations in the TGM1 (14q12) gene cause lamellar ichthyosis [40].

The conjunctiva often protrudes and is strangulated at its base by the lid margin obstructing venous return. This results in increased swelling and eversion of the eyelid as the palpebral portion of the orbicularis oculi contracts around the tarsal plate maintaining the lid in the everted position. Ectropion can also lead to lagophthalmos and exposure keratopathy.

Congenital Entropion

It is rarer than congenital ectropion and has been very rarely reported in the literature. Primary congenital upper eyelid entropion has been reported with Duane retraction syndrome [41]. It does not spontaneously improve. This condition may result in keratitis, corneal abrasion, or ulceration and opacification. Infants may develop corneal ulceration following trauma. Epiblepharon is frequently an associated finding especially in Asian ethnicity.

Euryblepharon

Euryblepharon is a congenital condition with increased length and width of the palpebral apertures and decreased vertical eyelid skin such that the lower lid appears to "hang away" from the globe laterally. The lateral contour of the globe is visible in primary position. Euryblepharon is usually bilateral and symmetric (Fig. 63.8). Lagophthalmos is common and patients tend to have lower blink rate.

The cause of euryeblepharon is unknown. Some of the theories postulated suggest tension of the skin, pull of the platysma, defective separation of the lids, and localized displacement of the lateral canthi as possible causes of euryeblepharon [42]. Euryblepharon may be seen in conjunction with lateral displacement of the proximal lacrimal drainage system, distichiasis, telecanthus, and strabismus.

It may be an isolated finding or occur as part of a syndrome. It is seen in Niikawa-Kuroki (formerly Kabuki make-up) syndrome and blepharo-cheilo-dontic syndrome. Kabuki syndrome is characterized by a peculiar facies which includes long palpebral fissures with eversion of the lateral third of the lower eyelids (reminiscent of the make-up of actors of Kabuki, a Japanese traditional theatrical form). Broad and depressed nasal tip, large prominent earlobes, a cleft, or high-arched palate are other facial features. Intellectual disability is a consistent finding. Other features include postnatal growth reduction; scoliosis; short fifth finger; presence of persistent finger pads; radiographic abnormalities of the vertebrae, hands, and hip joints; and recurrent otitis media in infancy. Kabuki syndrome-1 (KABUK1) is caused by heterozygous mutation in the MLL2 gene (KMT2D; 602,113) on chromosome 12q13 [43]. Kabuki syndrome-2 (300867) is caused by mutation in the KDM6A gene (300128) on chromosome Xp11.3 [43, 44].

Blepharocheilodontic syndrome-1 (BCDS1) is caused by heterozygous mutation in the CDH1 gene (192090) on chromosome 16q22. It is characterized by lower eyelid ectropion, upper eyelid distichiasis, euryeblepharon, lagophthalmos, ectropion, distichiasis, and hypertelorism. Systemic features include bilateral cleft lip and palate and conical teeth. Imperforate anus might be seen. Surgery for euryeblepharon involves horizontal eyelid shortening combined with repositioning of the lateral canthus.

Epicanthus

Epicanthus represents a nasal crescentic fold of skin directed downward with the concavity directed toward the medial canthus. Epicanthus is often a common and normal facial finding but is also a non-specific malformation associated

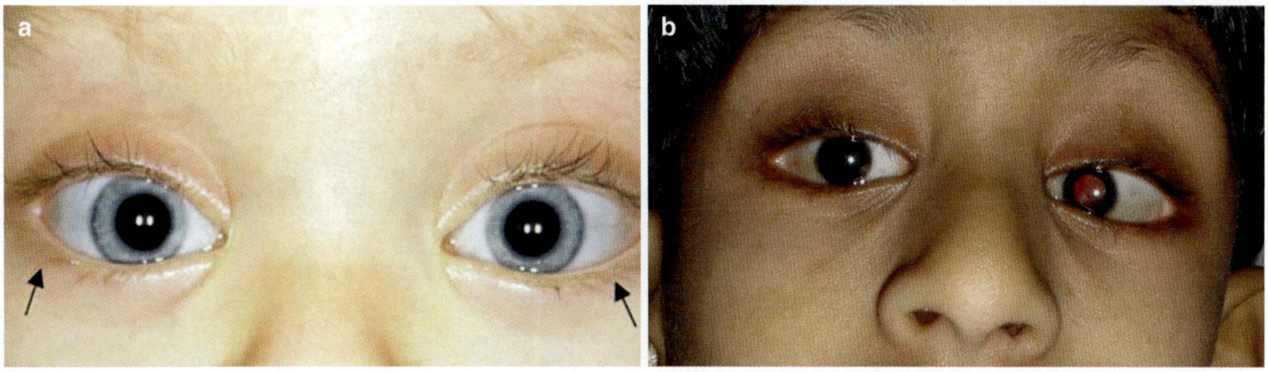

Fig. 63.8 (**a**) Euryblepharon (arrows). The lateral lower lids appear to "hang away" from the globe. (**b**) More prominent. (Photo courtesy: Dr. Alex Levin. Dr. Vijayalakshmi (Aravind Eye Care system)-**b**)

with many genetic syndromes. Epicanthic folds often become less prominent with facial development. There are four types of epicanthus depending upon the origin and amount of contribution of the upper and lower lid folds to the epicanthus. They are epicanthus supraciliaris, epicanthus tarsalis, epicanthus palpebralis, and epicanthus inversus.

In epicanthus supraciliaris, the fold of skin arises from close to the eyebrow and extends toward the lacrimal area. In epicanthus tarsalis, the major contribution is from the upper lid, and the fold of skin arises from the upper lid tarsus. Epicanthus tarsalis is often seen in those of East Asian decent as a fold of skin arising from the upper lid tarsus. Epicanthus palpebralis describes a redundant fold of skin arising from the upper lid above the tarsus and extending toward the lower margin of the orbit. The contributions from the upper and lower lids are equal. Epicanthus inversus is characterized by a redundant fold of skin arising mainly from the lower lid. It is one of the defining features of blepharophimosis syndrome [45].

The presence of epicanthic folds may impede favorable outcomes of ptosis repair, and consideration should be given to correcting both entities simultaneously [46]. The surgical technique to correct epiblepharon also needs to be modified in the presence of epicanthic folds as conventional techniques for epiblepharon repair in such situations may lead to higher risk of recurrence [47]. Surgical techniques include Y to V plasty, Mustarde 4 flap (jumping man), Roveda, and DelCampo.

Telecanthus

The Inter-pupillary distance (IPD) refers to the distance between the two pupils. The inner canthal distance (ICD) is the distance between the medial canthi. Mustarde ratio refers to the ratio of ICD and IPD (ICD/IPD).

Telecanthus is described by a Mustarde ratio (ICD/IPD) greater than 0.55 or increased distance between the medial canthal insertions. Telecanthus should be suspected in a patient in whom the lower lid puncta is located lateral to the medial limbus.

Hypertelorism

The interorbital distance (IOD) is the distance between the medial walls of the orbits. Hypertelorism describes an increase in the IOD. The interpupillary distance (IPD) is the distance between the two pupils. The inner canthal distance (ICD) is the distance between the medial canthi. The outer canthal distance (OCD) is the distance between the lateral canthi. The average IOD is 28 mm and 25 mm in men and women, respectively. Telecanthus may or may not be associated with hypertelorism. Telecanthus may be seen as a normal variant, particularly in those of East Asian decent with epicanthus. Patients with telecanthus may have pseudoesotropia. Telecanthus can be inherited as an autosomal dominant isolated anomaly or in association with cleft lip/palate, dental anomalies, or developmental delay. It is also a feature of many genetic syndromes. One of the classic examples is Waardenburg syndrome (Fig. 63.9).

Choristomas

A choristoma is an abnormal rest of normal tissues in an abnormal location. Ocular choristomas are typically located in the epibulbar region, ocular adnexa, and choroid. Four main histopathologic groups exist: dermoid, lipodermoids, single-tissue choristoma, and complex choristoma. Other histopathologic types of choristomas not included in the four main groups include dermoid cysts, epidermoid cysts, tera-

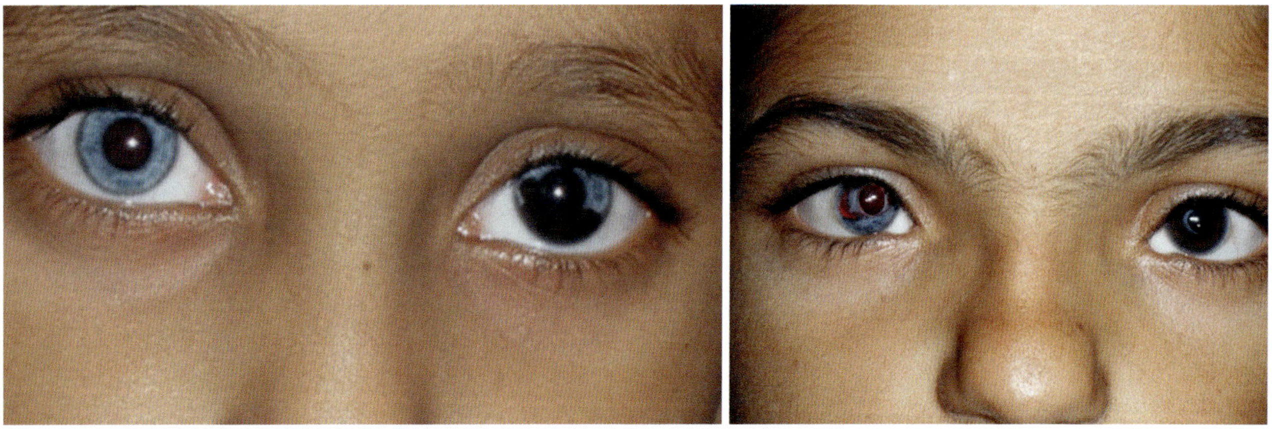

Fig. 63.9 (**a**) child with Waardenburg syndrome and heterochromia iris. (**b**) Child with Waardenburg syndrome with hypertelorism more prominent than in patient A. (Photo courtesy: **a** Dr. P. Vijayalakshmi, Aravind Eye care system; **b** Lumbini Eye Institute)

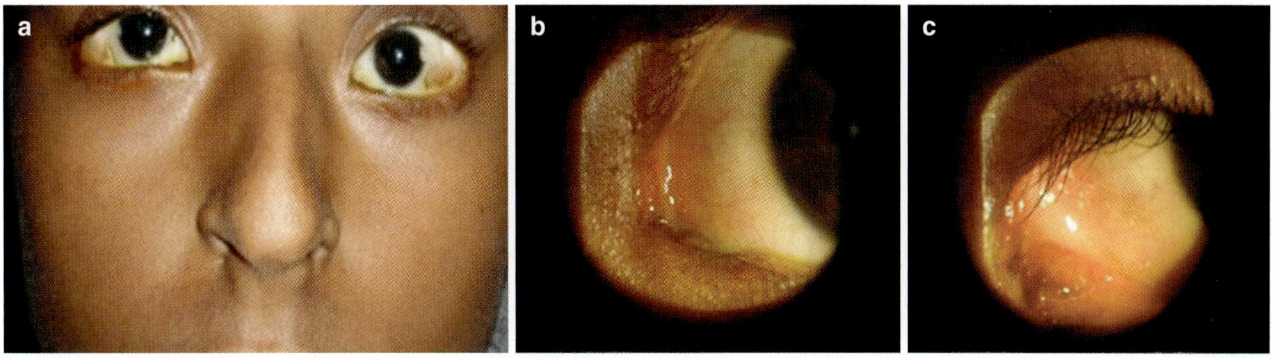

Fig. 63.10 Goldenhar syndrome: Oculo-auriculo-vertebral spectrum: (**a**) Dysmorphic facial features with bilateral lipodermoid. (**b**) Absence of caruncle at the left medial canthus. (**c**) Ectopic caruncular tissue on the medial aspect of the left lower lid. (Photo courtesy: Dr. Vijayalakshmi, Aravind Eye Care System, Madurai)

toma (tissues derived from three germinal layers), and teratoid tumors (tissues derived from two germinal layers).

The incidence of epibulbar choristomas is 1–3/10,000 live births, and this lesion constitutes 36% of epibulbar lesions presenting in the first decade of life [48]. Isolated choristomas may exhibit autosomal dominant, X-linked recessive, and possible autosomal recessive inheritance. About 10% of epibulbar choristomas are associated with Goldenhar syndrome or epidermal nevus syndrome [48]. Goldenhar syndrome (Figs. 63.5 and 63.10) is part of OAVS discussed earlier and can be associated with other epibulbar choristomas (limbal, subconjunctival, corneal), lacrimal abnormalities, eyelid coloboma, microtia, hemi facial asymmetry, vertebral anomalies, Duane syndrome, and preauricular skin tags. Goldenhar is inherited as an autosomal dominant disorder and has been associated with one gene, SALL1 (16.12.1) and multiple chromosomal loci. It should be differentiated from its allelic disorder, Townes-Brocks syndrome, which includes anal and renal malformations, cataract, and ocular coloboma.

Epidermal nevus syndrome (ENS) is characterized by skeletal abnormalities (kyphoscoliosis, lordosis, and cystic lesions of the long bones), neurologic abnormalities (seizures, intellectual disability, hemiparesis, cranial nerve palsies), vascular anomalies (cardiac malformations, arteriovenous malformations), and dermatologic disorders (linear epidermal nevi) [48]. Epidermal nevi follow the lines of Blaschko, S- or V-shaped linear patterns thought to represent the dorsoventral migratory pathways of the neuroectoderm during embryogenesis. The incidence of ENS is 1–3/1000 live births. Subsets of ENS include nevus sebaceous syndrome, Proteus syndrome, nevus comedonicus syndrome, Becker nevus associated with extracutaneous involvement syndrome, and phakomatosis pigmentokeratotica. Sebaceous nevus syndrome is characterized primarily by cutaneous sebaceous nevus, seizures, and epibulbar choristomas (Fig. 63.11).

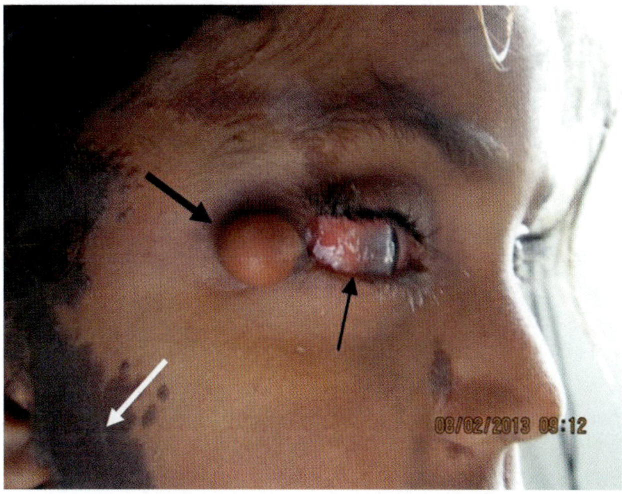

Fig. 63.11 Organoid nevus syndrome epibulbar choristomas (black arrows) and organoid or sebaceous nevus (white arrow). (Photo courtesy: Dr. Vijayalakshmi, Aravind Eye Care System, Madurai)

Encephalo-cranio-cutaneous lipomatosis (ECCL) is a rare sporadically occurring neurocutaneous disorder characterized by skin lesions, ocular and CNS anomalies. It was described by Haberland and Perou in 1970 [49]. Its genetic basis is unknown. Dermatologic findings include non-scarring alopecia, subcutaneous fatty masses, nevus psiloliparus, and nodular skin tags on eyelids, which histologically represent fibromas, lipomas, or fibrolipomas (Fig. 63.12) [50]. Ocular anomalies include epibulbar or limbal dermoid and lipodermoids. Intracranial findings consist of lipomas, most often located in the cerebellopontine angle, spinal lipomas, arachnoid cysts, porencephalic cysts, and hydrocephalus and leptomeningeal angiomatosis. Patients may also present with skeletal anomalies (e.g., jaw tumors) and congenital heart defects (e.g., coarctation of the aorta).

Ocular ectodermal syndrome is a congenital syndrome characterized by aplasia cutis congenita, epibulbar dermoids, umbilical hernia, eyelid papilloma, bladder exstro-

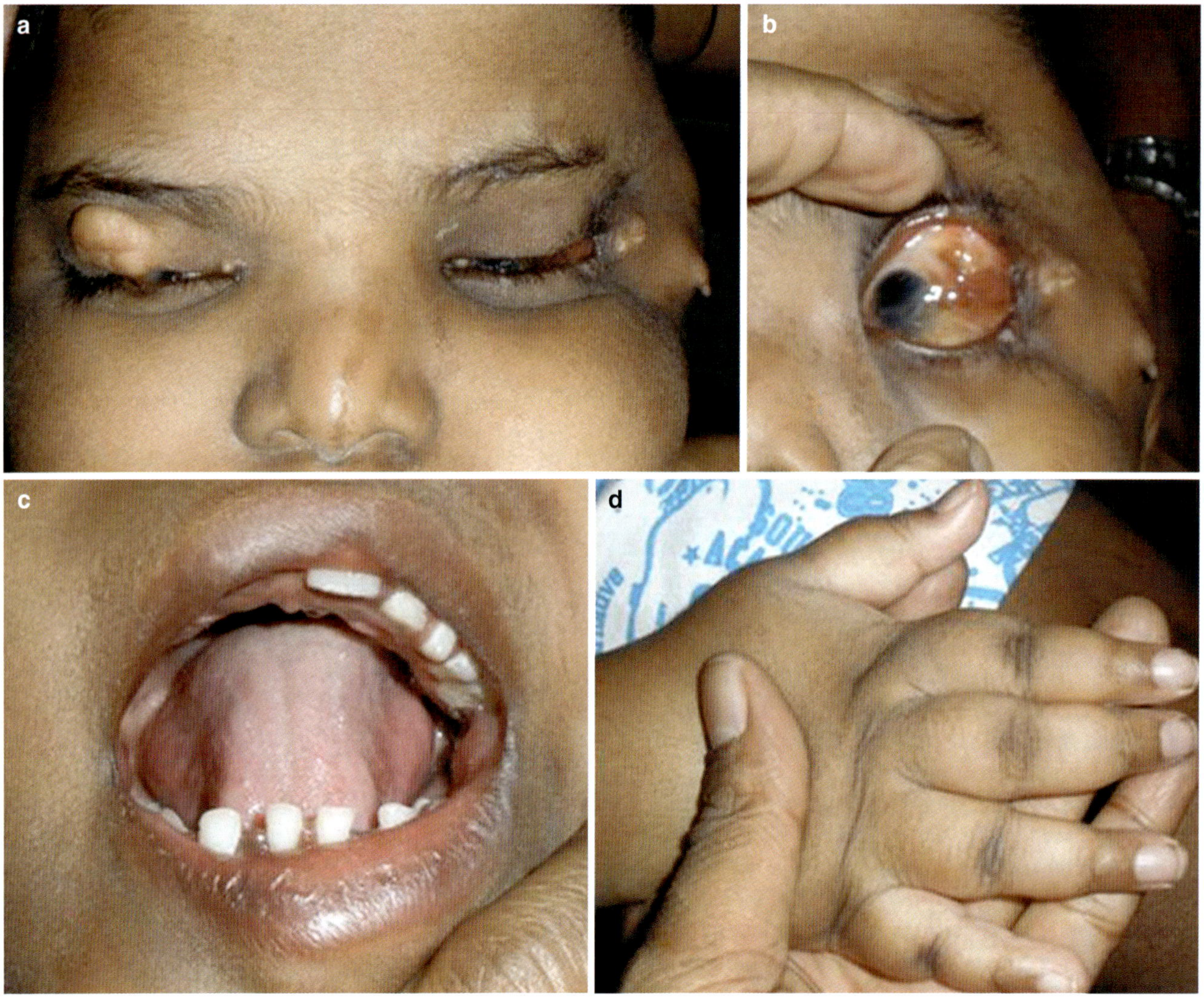

Fig. 63.12 Encephalo-cranio cutaneous lipomatosis. (**a**) Nodular skin tags on eyelid. (**b**) Lipodermoid. (**c**) Dental anomalies. (**d**) Anomaly of the digits. (Photo courtesy: Dr. Vijayalakshmi, Aravind Eye Care System, Madurai)

phy, epispadias, and cardiac anomalies [51]. Aplasia cutis congenita is the hallmark of ocular ectodermal syndrome describing absence of skin presenting as an ulcerated, eroded area of alopecia typically located on the scalp [52].

Hamartomas

Hamartomas are abnormal overgrowths of normal tissues that can occur throughout the body. Multiple hamartoma syndromes (MHS) include Cowden disease, Proteus syndrome, Bannayan-Riley-Ruvalcaba syndrome, and Lhermitte-Duclos disease. These are allelic disorders involving germline or somatic (Proteus) mutations in the PTEN gene (10q23.31) that encode for a tumor suppressor and are so currently also referred to as PTEN hamartoma tumor syndrome (PHTS).

Cowden disease or Cowden syndrome (CS) is a rare, autosomal dominant dermatologic disorder characterized by multiple facial papules (e.g., trichilemmomas), acral keratoses, oral papillomas and palmo-plantar keratoses, and mucocutaneous lesions of the gastrointestinal tract (GIT), thyroid, breast, and central nervous system [53]. Germline promoter methylation of KLLN; germline variations involving SDHB, SDHC, or SDHD; and germline mutations in AKT1 and PIK3CA have been observed in patients with Cowden syndrome and Cowden syndrome-like phenotypes that do not have PTEN involvement [54].

Proteus syndrome is a rare, highly variable, severe disorder of asymmetric and disproportionate overgrowth of body parts involving the skin, bone, muscle, and fatty tissue. It is characterized by macrocephaly, connective tissue nevi, epidermal nevi, dysregulated adipose tissue, and vascular malformations. Ocular findings include eyelid hamartomas, eyelid ptosis, hyperostosis, epidermal nevi, strabismus, nystagmus, high myopia, retinal pigmentary abnormalities, retinal coloboma, glaucoma, and posterior segment hamartomas [55].

Oculo-cerebro-cutaneous syndrome, also known as Delleman syndrome, consists of hamartomatous orbital cysts, microphthalmia, CNS malformations (e.g., intracranial cysts, agenesis of the corpus callosum, cerebellar hypoplasia, hydrocephalus, and seizures), focal aplasia cutis, and multiple skin appendages of the orbit and ear [56]. Oculo-cerebro-cutaneous syndrome may be associated with undescended testes and skeletal abnormalities (i.e., rib dysplasia). All cases have been sporadic and the genetic basis is unknown.

Craniofacial Disorders

Encephaloceles

An encephalocele is a sac-like protrusion containing brain and surrounding membranes extending out from the cranial vault through openings in the skull. If the protrusion contains only cerebrospinal fluid (CSF) and dura matter, the protrusion is called a meningocele. If the protrusion contains brain tissue, the protrusion is called an encephalomeningocele. Isolated encephalomeningocele is common in Southeast Asia, primarily Malaysia, Thailand, and Burma, with a reported incidence of 1:5000 [57].

The incidence of anterior meningoencephaloceles in North America is 1 in 10,000 to 15,000 live births [58]. Encephaloceles are classified as sincipital, occipital, parietal, and basal. Sincipital encephaloceles present in the front of the skull and are visible externally. They may be further subclassified into fronto-ethmoidal (naso-frontal, naso-ethmoidal, naso-orbital), inter-frontal, and craniofacial clefts (Fig. 63.13) [59]. Most sincipital encephaloceles are not genetic or syndromic but may be caused by exposure to an environmental agent in utero. Increased paternal age may be a risk factor.

Approximately 70–80% of encephaloceles occurs in the occipital region and is beyond the scope of this chapter [60]. Encephaloceles may be associated with intracranial abnormalities (i.e., agenesis of the corpus callosum, Dandy-Walker malformation, hydrocephalus, and holoprosencephaly), hypertelorism, telecanthus, and craniosynostosis (i.e., Apert syndrome, Goldenhar syndrome) [61]. The differential diagnosis of encephaloceles includes nasal glioma, dermoid cyst, hemangioma, lymphangioma, neurofibroma, and foreign body [62].

Frontonasal Dysplasia (FND)

Defects of the craniofacial midline result in a diverse spectrum of phenotypes and clinical entities that can be broadly defined as front nasal dysplasias (FNDs) (Fig. 63.14). Other names include frontonasal malformation, median cleft face syndrome, and frontal nasal syndrome. It is defined as two or more of the following: (1) true ocular hypertelorism, (2) broadening of nasal root, (3) median facial cleft affecting the nose and/or upper lip and palate, (4) unilateral or bilateral clefting of the alae nasi, (5) lack of formation of the nasal tip, (6) anterior cranium bifidum occultum, and (7) V-shaped or widow's peak frontal hairline [62]. FND is further classified as Sedano type A (hypertelorism, broad nasal root, absent nasal tip without median facial clefting), type B (hypertelorism, broad nasal root with medial facial groove or true cleft affecting the nose and/or upper lip and/or palate), type C (hypertelorism, broad nasal root and unilateral or bilateral notching of the alae nasi), or type D (types B and C with midline facial cleft and notching of the alae nasi). Frontal encephalocele is a common feature of FND and is in part responsible for the orbital hypertelorism. FND is part of many syndromes, well beyond the scope of this chapter.

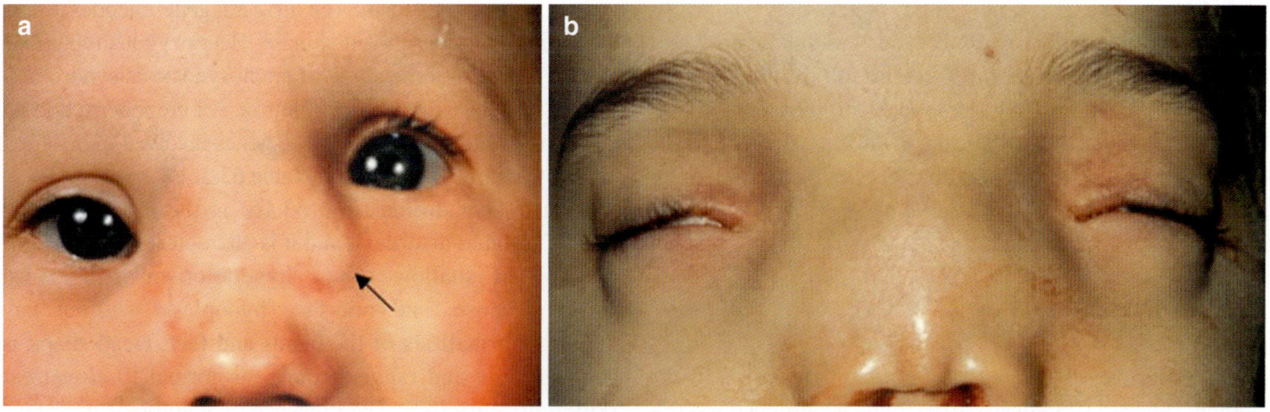

Fig. 63.13 (**a**) Naso-frontal encephalocele causing elevation of the left orbit. Arrow indicates subcutaneous encephalocele. (**b**) Frontonasal dysplasia causing hypertelorism, broad nasal root, and bifid nasal tip. The patient also has microphthalmos. (Photo courtesy: Dr. Alex Levin)

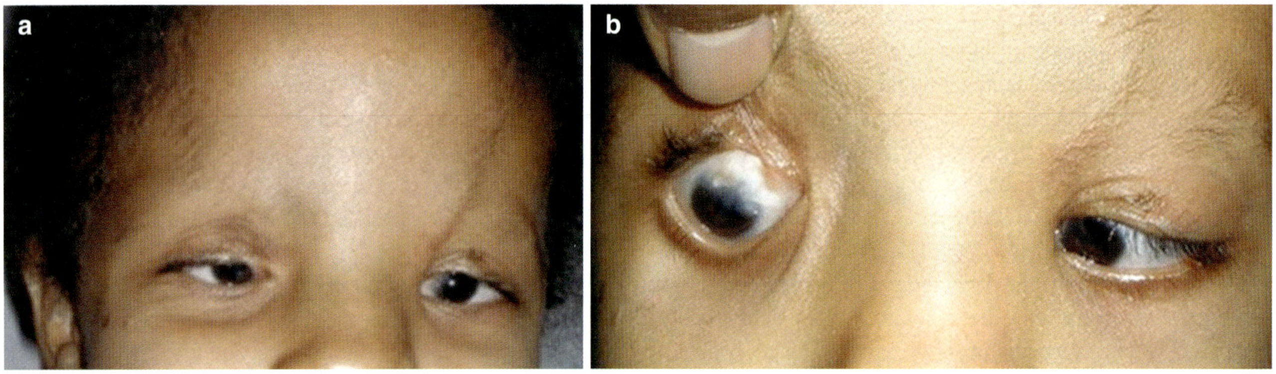

Fig. 63.14 Frontonasal dysplasia: (**a**) Another patient with FND. (**b**) Corneopalpebral adhesions. (Photo courtesy: Dr. Vijayalakshmi, Aravind Eye Care System, Madurai)

The syndromes within the FND spectrum are genetically very heterogeneous. There are currently six known genes associated with FND spectrum disorders that account for only a small fraction of cases with the majority of affected individuals still yet to attain a molecular diagnosis. Autosomal dominant, autosomal recessive, and X-linked FND syndromes have been reported.

Classic FND is an autosomal recessive disorder divided into frontorhiny, FND1 caused by mutations in the airstaless-like homeobox-3 (ALX3) gene (1p13.3), FND2 (ALX4, 11p11.2), and FND3 (ALX1, 12q21.3-q22). FND4 is due to deletion in SIX2 gene. CFNS or craniofrontonasal syndrome is characterized by severe hypertelorism, a bifid or hypoplastic nasal tip, coronal craniosynostosis, malformation of the clavicle, longitudinally grooved or split nails, and thick, wiry hair. The clinical findings are more distinct in females. One example of a syndromic form of anterior encephalocele is acro-fronto-facio-nasal dysostosis (AFFND) which is comprised of frontonasal dysplasia, facial and genital midline defects, and skeletal limb anomalies including polydactyly, tibial hypoplasia, and talipes equinovarus [63]. AFFND type I exhibits autosomal recessive inheritance and is characterized by short stature, hypertelorism, broad notched nasal tip, cleft lip or palate, postaxial campto-brachy polysyndactyly, and mental retardation. AFFND type II is similar to type I without mental retardation. One must be cautious against intranasal procedures (e.g., dacryocystorhinoscopy or silicone tube intubation) as the encephalocele extends into the nasal cavity [64]. Other ophthalmic features include microphthalmia, coloboma, and optic nerve hypoplasia.

Craniosynostosis

Craniosynostosis is defined as the premature fusion of the cranial sutures. Craniosynostosis may be grouped as primary, secondary, syndromic, or non-syndromic. Synostosis may involve a single suture causing typical skull deformities as growth continues to occur parallel to the closed suture. Multiple suture synostosis is less common than single suture and accounts for 15% of cases. Single suture synostosis most commonly affects the sagittal suture, followed by the coronal, metopic, and lambdoid sutures. Premature differentiation is considered the most probable factor leading to craniosynostosis. Other factors may include enhancement of proliferation, differentiation, and apoptosis of osteoblasts bordering the cranial suture mesenchyme [65].

Syndromic craniosynostosis accounts for approximately 15 percent of the craniosynostosis and demonstrates classic Mendelian patterns of inheritance with well-established genetic causes [66]. Non-syndromic craniosynostoses, which account for approximately 85 percent of cases, are genetically heterogeneous. The ocular features of most syndromic craniosynostosis overlap significantly. However, the systemic features may show specific features that is significantly different in each syndrome, and hence, it is easier to arrive at a clinical diagnosis by carefully observing the systemic features. Subtle skull and facial assmetry can be recognized by examining the patient from above and from below (Fig. 63.15). Examining the hands and feet provides critical clues to the type of craniosynostosis. The *FGFR2* gene encodes transmembrane receptor tyrosine kinase. Heterozygous mutations of FGFR2 cause three classical craniosynostosis syndromes, those of Apert, Crouzon, and Pfeiffer. All are inherited in an autosomal dominant manner. The genes involved in different craniosynostoses are shown in Table 63.3.

Crouzon syndrome (Fig. 63.16) is the mildest of the FGFR2-related disorders, and it is characterized by a combination of shallow orbits, hypertelorism, strabismus, abnormal nose, and mid-face hypoplasia without any major abnormalities of the hands and feet. Head shape is very variable and ranges from near-normal to cloverleaf skull deformity [67]. The presence of acanthosis nigricans in a patient with Crouzon indicates mutations in the

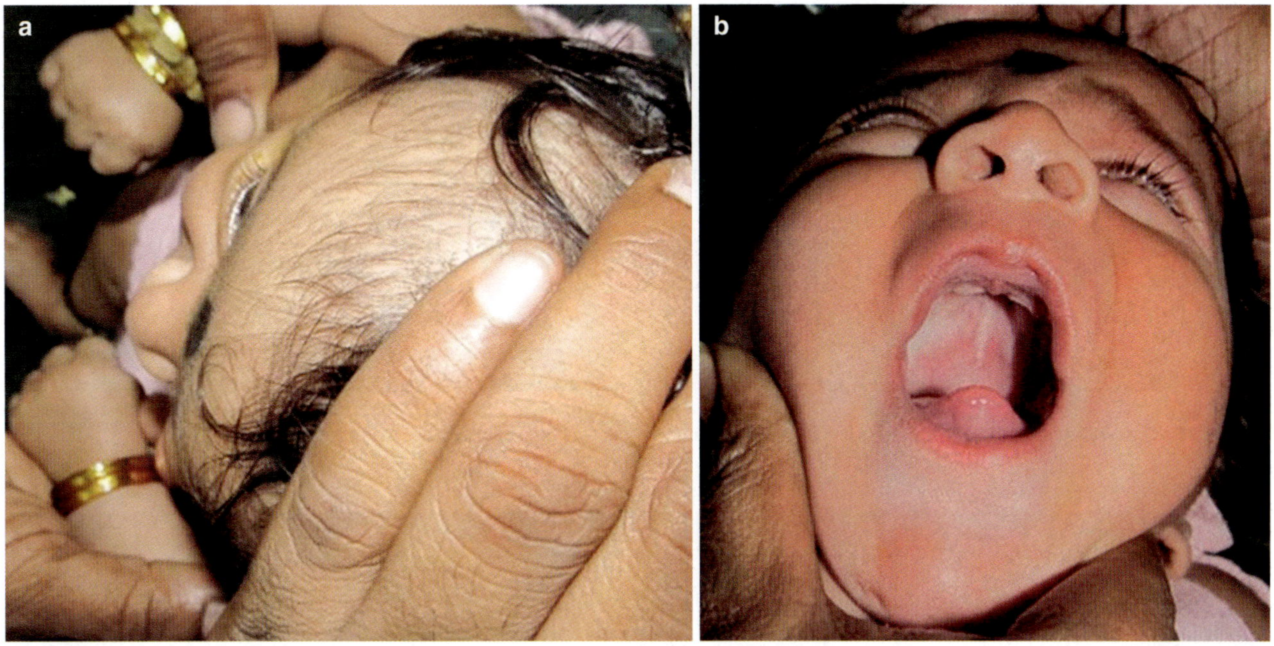

Fig. 63.15 Examining from above (**a**) and from below (**b**) will help in picking up even subtle facial asymmetry. (Photo courtesy: Dr. Vijayalakshmi, Aravind Eye Care System, Madurai)

Table 63.3 Craniosynostosis syndromes, genes, loci, and inheritance patterns

GENE	Loci	Syndrome	Inheritance
FGFR1	8p11.2 p11.1	Pfeiffer syndrome	AD
		Jackson-Weiss syndrome	
FGFR2	10q26.13	Crouzon	AD
		Apert syndrome	
		Jackson-Weiss	
		Saethre-Chotzen	
		Cutis gyrata	
		Isolated coronal craniosynostosis	
		Antley-Bixler syndrome	
FGFR3	4p16.3	Muenke syndrome	AD
		Achondroplasia	
		Crouzon with acanthosis nigricans (CAN)	
TWIST1	7p21	Saethre-Chotzen with or without eyelid anomalies	AD
RAB23	6p12.1-p11.2	Carpenter syndrome	AR
EFNB1	Xq13.1	Craniofrontonasal syndrome	XLR
MSX2	5p35.2	Craniosynostosis, Boston type	AD
POR	7q11.23	Antley-Bixler syndrome with genital anomalies	AR
ESCO2	8p21.1	Robert syndrome	AR
RECQL4	8p24.3	Baller-Gerold syndrome	AR
GLI3	7p14.1	Greig syndrome	AD

AD Autosomal dominant; *AR* Autosomal recessive; *XLR* X linked recessive

FGFR3 gene and not *FGFR2* (Crouzonodermoskeletal syndrome) [68]. Mutations in *FGFR3* can also cause Muenke syndrome.

Ocular findings include characteristic strabismus (often a V pattern with hypertropia of the adducting eye in side gazes) which may be due to anomalous extraocular eye muscle anatomy or excyclorotation of the orbits. Missing muscles and abnormal location of muscle insertion are common. Patients may have or develop exposure keratitis, luxation of globe, optic atrophy, and papilledema. These require emergency management. Other rare associations that have been reported include aniridia, anisocoria, blue sclera, cataract, corectopia, ectopia lentis, glaucoma, iris coloboma, microcornea, nystagmus, and optic nerve hypoplasia [69].

Apert syndrome (Fig. 63.17) is usually more severe than Crouzon though both disorders are allelic. It shares many of the skull vault, facial abnormalities, and ocular findings of Crouzon syndrome. Apert syndrome is however characterized by severe symmetric syndactyly of the hands and feet which is absent in Crouzon. Almost all Apert syndrome mutations are de novo and have been shown to be paternal in origin (originate exclusively from the father). Increased paternal age is a risk factor. Pfeiffer syndrome is usually characterized by broad, radially deviated thumbs and/or big toes sometimes with mild cutaneous syndactyly (Fig. 63.18). It can be caused either by mutations in *FGFR1* and FGFR2.

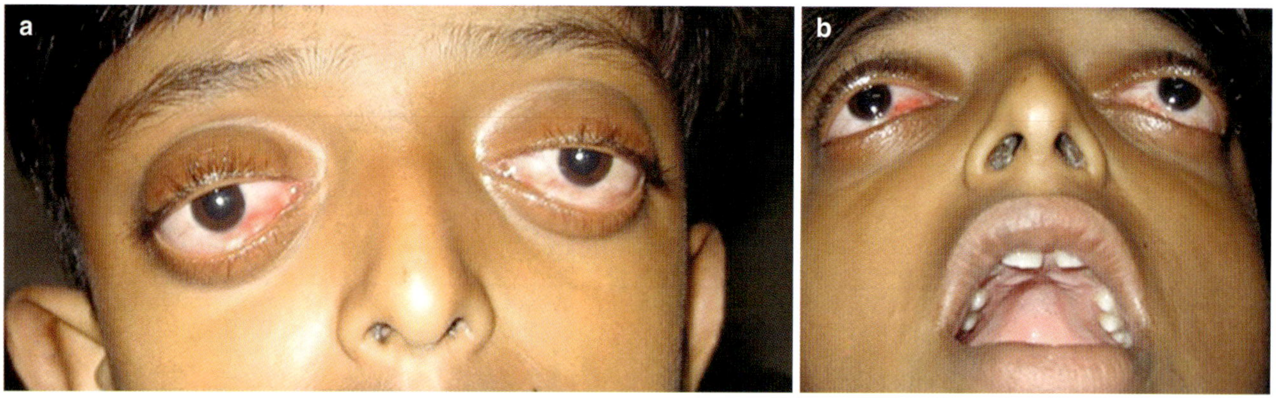

Fig. 63.16 Crouzon syndrome: (**a**) Shallow orbits and (**b**) high-arched palate (Photo courtesy Dr. Arjun Mallah Bhari)

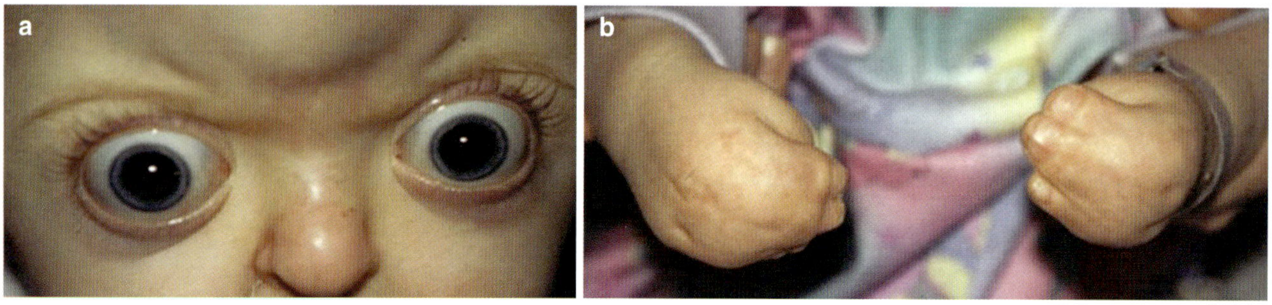

Fig. 63.17 (**a**) Clinical photograph depicting exorbitism, bullous or beaked nose, and mid-face hypoplasia. It may be seen in severe forms of Apert or Crouzon syndrome. (**b**) Syndactyly typically found in Apert syndrome. (Photo courtesy: Dr. Alex Levin)

Most genetically determined craniosynostoses are characterized by autosomal dominant inheritance; new mutations account for almost half of cases. Mutations in *FGFR2*, *FGFR3*, *TWIST1*, and *EFNB1* account for approximately 25% of craniosynostosis. Much rarer mutations in FGFR1 (mild Pfeiffer syndrome), POR (Antley-Bixler syndrome), RAB23 (Carpenter syndrome), *EFNA4* (non-syndromic coronal synostosis), *ESCO2* (Roberts syndrome), *GLI3* (Greig syndrome), *JAG1* (Alagille syndrome), *KRAS* (Noonan syndrome), *RECQL4* (Baller-Gerold syndrome), *TGFBR1* or *TGFBR2* (Loeys-Dietz syndrome) have been associated with craniosynostoses).

Examples of other syndromic craniosynostoses are Antley-Bixler, Saethre-Chotzen, Carpenter, and Muenke syndromes. Ptosis is common in Saethre-Chotzen syndrome. It occurs due to mutations in the *TWIST1* gene. Mutations in MSX2 gene (muscle segment homebox 2) have been reported in Boston-type craniosynostosis. FGFR3 p.Pro250Arg mutation is the most commonly found mutation in all cases of craniosynostosis, and genetic testing should be offered for all patients presenting with coronal or multisuture synostosis [70].

The main concerns for the oculoplastic surgeon are the corneal exposure due to exophthalmos, strabismus, and ptosis. Although the management of the ptosis is surgically not unique, the major issue is the worsened corneal exposure. Craniofacial surgery to advance the orbits may be needed if the corneal disease is significant.

Craniofacial Clefts

The most clinically useful and widely accepted classification is the Tessier system in which each major cranial, orbital, maximally, and mandibular cleft is assigned a number from 0 to 14 beginning with 0 in the lower facial midline. The Tessier system assigns clefts according to an architectural description rather than a true description of clinical syndromes. Several theories have been proposed hypothesizing the etiology of craniofacial clefts. These include fusional failures of normal embryonic clefts or facial processes, failure of neural crest cell migration, and degeneration of cells prior to migration [69].

Treacher Collins syndrome (TCS), also known as mandibulofacial dysostosis, is an autosomal dominant, but not always inherited (e.g., spontaneous mutation), disorder with variable penetrance involving congenital malformations of the first and second branchial arches (Fig. 63.7). TCS is caused by mutations in the TCOF1 gene (5Q32–33.1), which encodes for a nuclear phosphoprotein, Treacle [71]. TCS is

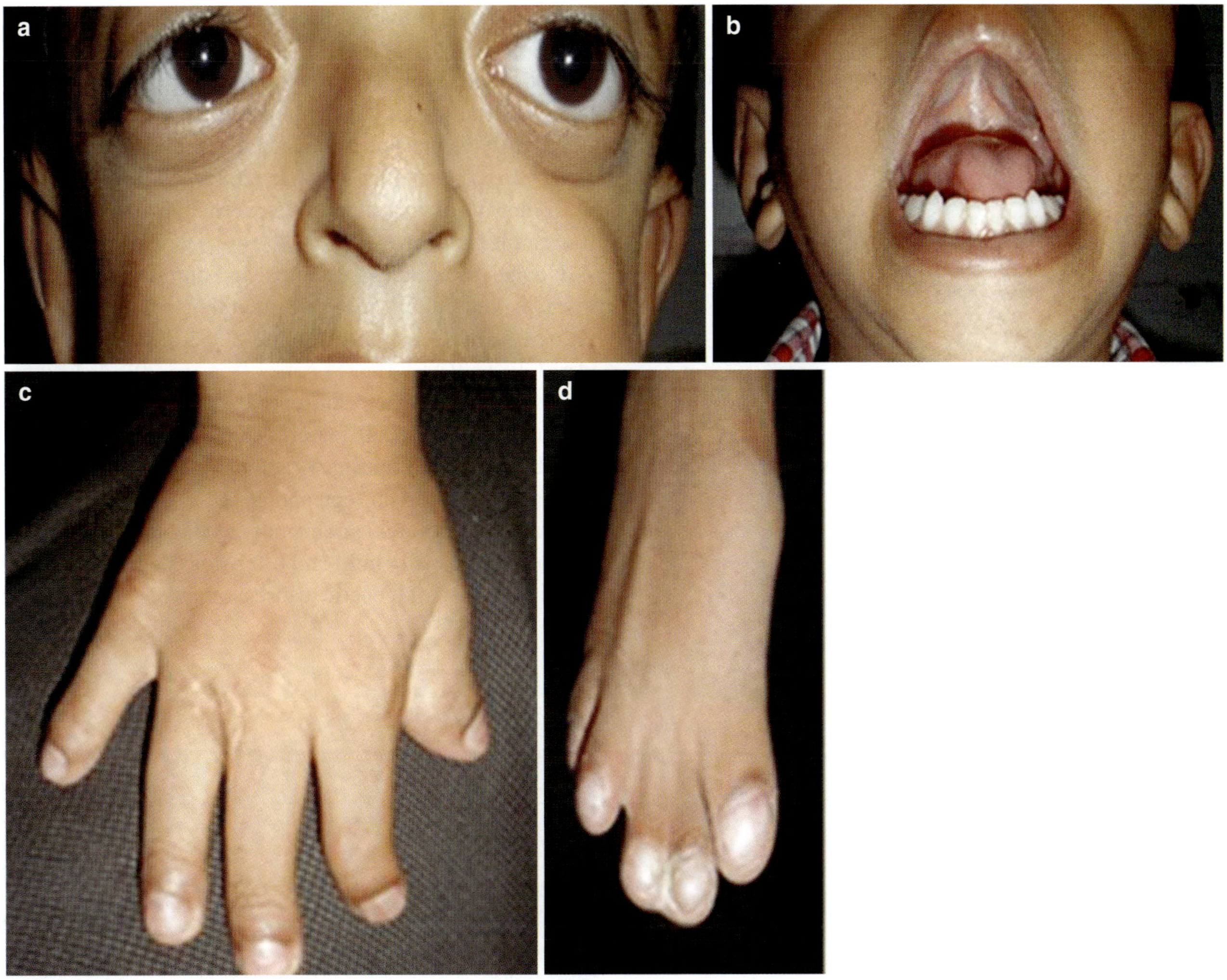

Fig. 63.18 Pfeiffer syndrome. (**a**) Maxillary hypoplasia, shallow orbits (**b**) high-arched palate (**c**) large and radially deviated thumb and great toe (**d**) Syndactyly of the toes. (Photo courtesy: Dr. Vijayalakshmi, Aravind Eye Care System, Madurai)

characterized by a steep downward slanting of the palpebral fissures, mandibular hypoplasia, notching (pseudo-coloboma) of the lower eyelids, paucity of lid lashes medial to defect, auditory malformations (e.g., auricular pinna malformation, altered position of the ears, irregular or absent auditory ossicles, deafness), and abnormal dentition. TCS has also been associated with microphthalmos, orbital hypoplasia, cataract, lacrimal duct atresia, corneal exposure (more in older children), proximal nasolacrimal system malformation, pupillary ectopia, astigmatism, ptosis, strabismus, and sinus abnormalities including airway obstruction and obstructive sleep apnea [71].

Genetic Forms of Ptosis

Isolated congenital ptosis is usually not heritable, but familial ptosis has been reported and linked to 1p32.1–34.1 (autosomal dominant) and Xq24–27.1. Congenital ptosis is also a common finding in a multitude of genetic syndromes such as trisomy 13, Turner syndrome, Saethre-Chotzen syndrome, Cornelia de Lange syndrome, Noonan syndrome, Smith-Lemli-Opitz syndrome, and many others (Table 63.4).

Some of the reports suggest the possibility of dominant inheritance and linkage to 1p34.1-p32 or Xq24-q27.1 [72]. The ZFH4 gene (8q21.1) may be a candidate gene [73].

The discussion of each syndrome is beyond the scope of this chapter, but two are described below as examples multi-system syndromic disorder.

Cornelia de Lange syndrome (CdLS) is an autosomal dominant or X-linked disorder caused by mutations in the NIPBL (5p13), SMC3 (10q25), or SMC1A (Xq11.2) genes (Fig. 63.19), all of which are involved with the chromosome cohesin complex. CdLS is characterized by dysmorphic facial features, hirsutism, limb reduction abnormalities, growth retardation, congenital heart disease, and varying degrees of developmental delay [73]. Ocular manifestations

Table 63.4 Syndromes with congenital ptosis

Arima syndrome
Blepharophimosis, ptosis, and epicanthus inversus syndrome
Cardiofaciocutaneous syndrome
Coach syndrome
Coffin-Siris syndrome
Congenital fibrosis of the extraocular muscles
Cornelia de Lange syndrome
Costello syndrome
Dandy-Walker syndrome
DiGeorge syndrome
Duane-radial ray syndrome
Duane retraction syndrome
Dubowitz syndrome
Kabuki syndrome
Kearns-Sayre syndrome
Jacobsen syndrome
Leopard syndrome 1
Loeys-Dietz syndrome
McDonough syndrome
Miller-Dieker lissencephaly syndrome
Moebius syndrome
Muenke syndrome
Myasthenic syndrome
Neurofibromatosis type 1
Noonan syndrome
Pallister-hall syndrome
Peters plus syndrome
Pierson syndrome
Potocki-Shaffer syndrome
Rubinstein-Taybi syndrome
Saethre-Chotzen syndrome
Shprintzen-Goldberg craniosynostosis
Smith-Lemli-Opitz syndrome
Smith-Magenis syndrome
Stiff person syndrome
Waardenburg syndrome
Warburg syndrome
Wolf-Hirschhorn syndrome

include synophrys that extends in a V pattern onto the bridge of the nose, long arcuate eyelashes, myopia, nasolacrimal duct obstruction (NLDO), blepharitis, microcornea, and nystagmus [74]. Ptosis is not an obligate feature but seen in 44% [75]. It may be unilateral or bilateral, usually without a good levator crease, and often accompanied by a brow lift. Severe ptosis may result in a chin lift severe enough that ambulation is even further delayed.

Noonan syndrome is an autosomal dominant congenital disorder caused by missense mutations in the PTPN11 (12q24.1), KRAS (12q12.1), or SOS1 (2p22.1), NRAS (1p13.2), or RAF1 (3p25) genes (Fig. 63.20). Autosomal recessive NS has also been reported [76]. NS is described by characteristic facial features, cardiopulmonary abnormalities, and genitourinary anomalies. Ocular findings include hypertelorism, epicanthal folds, downward slanting palpebral fissures, strabismus, nystagmus, and ptosis. The ptosis is usually mild and often does not require intervention. A list of genetic causes of ptosis is shown in Table 63.5.

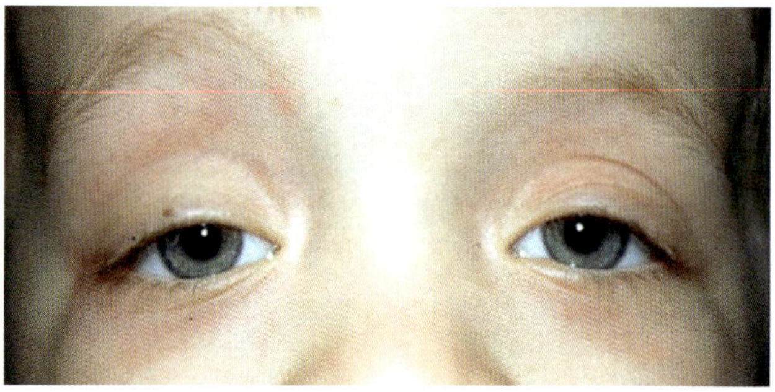

Fig. 63.20 Noonan syndrome. Clinical photograph demonstrating ptosis, hypertelorism, and downward slanting palpebral fissures. (Photo courtesy: Dr. Alex Levin)

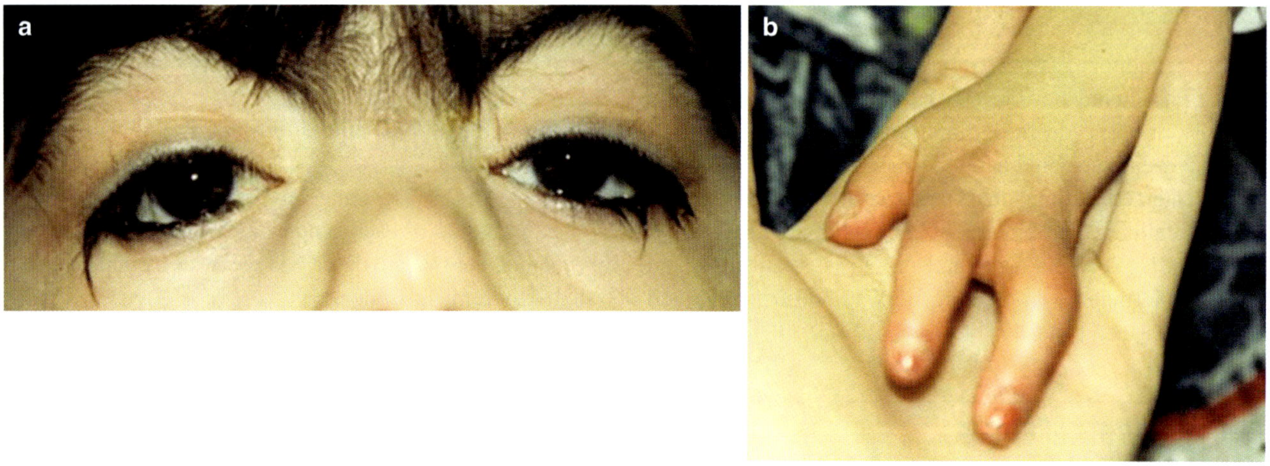

Fig. 63.19 (**a**) Cornelia de Lange syndrome (CdLS) with ptosis, hypertrichosis, and synophrys. (**b**) Hand anomaly in patient with CdLS. (Photo courtesy: Dr. Alex Levin)

Table 63.5 Ptosis of genetic etiology

Ocular phenotype	Gene	Loci	Inheritance pattern
Congenital ptosis			
Congenital simple ptosis	Not cloned	1p34.1-p32	AD
	Not cloned	Xq24-q27. 1	AD
	ZFH4	8q21.1	AD
Blepharophimosis			
Blepharophimosis-epicanthus inversus syndrome (BPES)	FOXL2	3q22.3	AD
Blepharophimosis-ptosis-intellectual disability syndrome (BPIDS)	UBE3B	12q23	AD
Congenital fibrosis of the extraocular muscles (CFEOM)			
CFEOM1	KIF21A	12q12	AD
CFEOM2	PHOX2A	11q13	AR
CFEOM3	TUBB3/KIF21A	16q24.3/12q12	AD
Tukel syndrome	TUBB3	16q24.3	AD
Marcus Gunn jaw winking ptosis	TUBB3/KIF21A	16q24.3/12q12	AD
Acquired ptosis			
Chronic progressive external ophthalmoplegia (CPEO)	POLG	15q25	AR
	ANT1	4q34	AR
Kearns-Sayre syndrome (KSS)	C10orf2	10q24	AR
Oculopharyngeal dystrophy	PABPN1	14q11.2	AD
Neurofibromatosis (NF1)	NF1	17q11.2	AD

AD Autosomal dominant; *AR* Autosomal recessive.
Adapted from [72]

BPES (Blepharophimosis Syndrome)

Blepharophimosis describes reduction of both the horizontal and vertical dimensions of the palpebral fissure as an isolated finding or part of a congenital syndrome. Blepharophimosis, ptosis, and epicanthus inversus syndrome (BPES) is an autosomal dominant disorder characterized by the presence of four adnexal features: shortened horizontal palpebral fissure length, ptosis, epicanthus inversus, and telecanthus (Fig. 63.21). Ptosis is usually severe due to dysplasia of the levator aponeurosis leading to poor levator function and absent upper lid crease. There are two subtypes. Type I is characterized by the additional finding of primary ovarian failure in affected females. Secondary sexual characteristics in BPES1 are normal. Type 2 does not have ovarian failure. Mutations in the fork head transcription factor gene FOXL2 have been found to be responsible for BPES. There has been only one report of autosomal recessive [77] transmission. Penetrance appears to be 100% in BPES1 and 96.5% in BPES2. In BPES1, there is transmission by males only as females are infertile. In BPES2, transmission occurs through both sexes. *FOXL2* is the only gene currently known to be associated with BPES. It has also been shown in mice that the Foxl2 gene is expressed in the mesenchyme of developing mouse eyelids and adult ovarian follicles.

Intellectual disability in patients with BPES may be due to larger deletions involving 3q22.3 or part of the blepharophimosis-ptosis-intellectual disability syndrome (BPIDS) caused by heterozygous mutations in the UBE3B gene (12q23) [78]. A patient with BPES and genital malformations was reported to have a deletion del (7) (q34) [79]. Waardenburg suggested that the ocular defects seen in this syndrome possibly occurred during the third month of intrauterine life as this timing coincides with the critical period in the development of the ovary and the beginning of formation of the uterus [80].

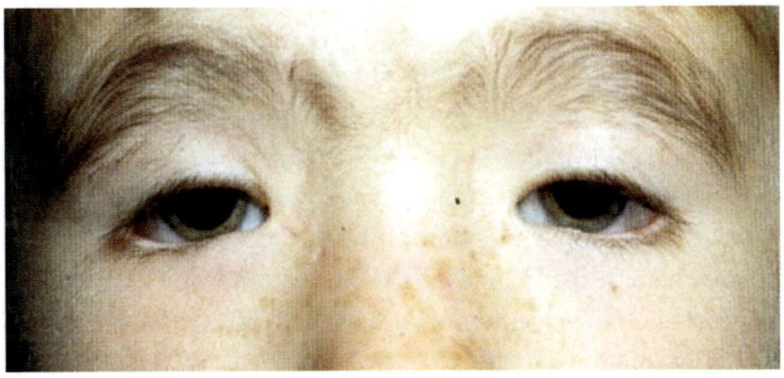

Fig. 63.21 Blepharophimosis syndrome: congenital ptosis, telecanthus, shortened horizontal palpebral fissure, and epicanthus inversus. (Photo courtesy: Dr. Alex Levin)

Hypoplastic supraorbital rims, bushy eyebrows, low set ears, and broad nasal bridge are other reported findings particularly in patients with deletions. Congenital nasolacrimal duct obstruction and strabismus also occur at a higher rate in BPES. There is often lateral displacement of the upper and lower lacrimal puncta, more than what would be expected from the lateral displacement of the inner canthi alone.

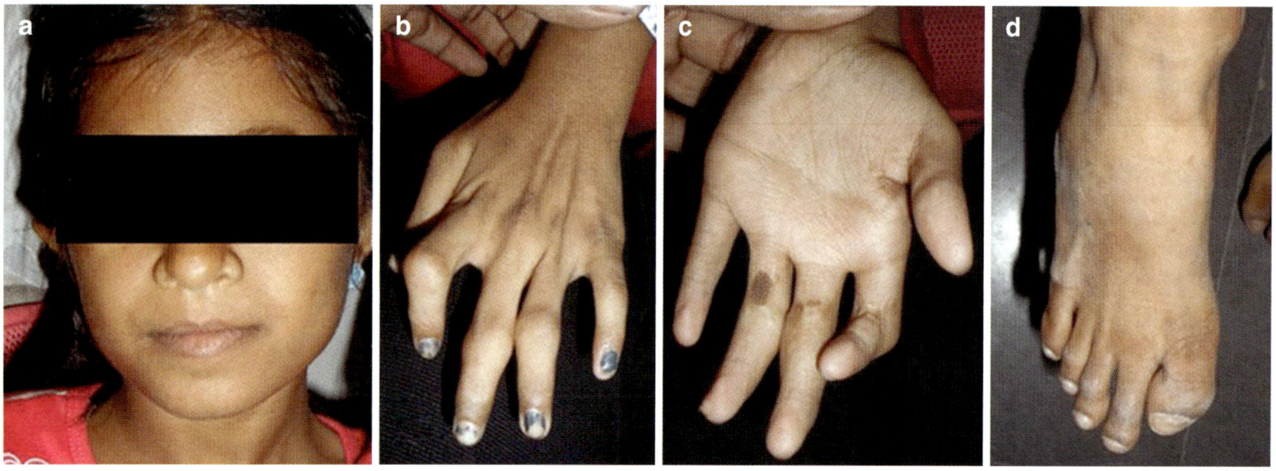

Fig. 63.22 Freeman-Sheldon syndrome. (**a**) Whistling face in Freeman-Sheldon syndrome. (**b**) Ulnar deviation of fingers. (**c**) Pigmentation at the flexural creases. (**d**) Deviation of the great toe. Photo courtesy: Dr. Vijayalakshmi, Aravind Eye Care System, Madurai

FOXL2 gene has a single exon and the encoded protein has an alanine-rich domain. Mutations predicted to result in proteins truncated before the polyalanine tract preferentially lead to BPES1. Polyalanine expansions preferentially lead to BPES2. Positive correlation between the size of the polyalanine expansion and the penetrance of the BPES phenotype has been reported [77].

Blepharophimosis as a feature may be seen in few other syndromes including Freeman-Sheldon syndrome (Fig. 63.22) (whistling face syndrome), Ohdo syndrome, and Say-Barber syndrome. Ohdo syndrome is an X-linked recessive disorder with blepharophimosis, developmental delay, and a characteristic facies. Say-Barber syndrome has blepharophimosis, developmental delay, thyroid dysfunction, and dental anomalies.

Congenital Fibrosis of the Extraocular Muscles

CFEOM is a congenital, non-progressive disorder characterized by restrictive ophthalmoplegia, misalignment of the eyes, and typically congenital ptosis. It is one of the congenital cranial dysinnervation disorders (CCDD). The motility limitation is most severe in vertical gaze (usually up gaze), and there is a variable limitation of horizontal gaze. Refractive errors and amblyopia are common.

Three subtypes have been identified based on the observation of specific eye findings and associated findings – CFEOM1, CFEOM2, and CFEOM3. CFEOM1 is an autosomal dominant inherited disorder caused by heterozygous mutations in KIF21A. CFEOM3 is caused by heterozygous mutations in *TUBB3* or *TUBB2B*. CFEOM2 is an autosomal recessive disorder caused by homozygous mutations in the transcription factor PHOX2A.

CFEOM type 1 is an autosomal dominant disorder demonstrating bilateral severe congenital ptosis, large angle exotropia, eyes fixed in down gaze, and the patient using a large chin lift to view straight ahead. Elevation of the eyes by inferior rectus recession will leave the eyes even more severely obstructed by the lids, and therefore upper lid sling procedures are often done prior to or in combination with the eye muscle surgery. CFEOM1 has two further subtypes. CFEOM1A is due to mutations in the KIF21A gene, which codes for a kinesin motor protein involved in the development of oculomotor axons by affecting the pathways involved in axonal guidance [81]. It is bilateral and usually symmetrical. The patient presents with ptosis and the eyes fixed in down gaze. It is not associated with any other additional neurologic abnormalities. MRI findings suggest a neurogenic etiology instead of a myopathic etiology. CFEOM1B is due to mutations in TUBB3.

CFEOM2

CFEOM2 is caused by homozygous mutations in the ARIX/PHOX2A (11q13). It clinically differs from other types in that the pupil is involved and the pupil reaction is often sluggish [81]. Retinal dysfunction also has been reported [82].

CFEOM3

It is caused by heterozygous mutations in the *TUBB3*. It has a more variable phenotype than other CFEOM. It may be unilateral or have asymmetric involvement. Ptosis may be absent. Unlike CFEOM1, other additional neurological abnormalities may be observed. Thinning or absence of the facial nerves, brainstem hypoplasia, and additional brain malformations have been reported. Patients with CFEOM3 may also have facial dysmorphism, cognitive impairment, thin corpus callosum, or digital anomalies [81]. Missense mutations in *TUBB3* have been reported to cause malformations of cortical development (MCD) without causing CFEOM. Individuals with these *TUBB3*-MCD variants have been found to have significant intellectual disability and motor developmental delays. Other associated abnormalities include Kallmann syndrome, cyclic vomiting, spasticity, progressive sensorimotor axonal polyneuropathy, and vocal cord paralysis.

Tukel Syndrome

Tukel syndrome refers to patients with CFEOM3 and post-axial oligodactyly/oligosyndactyly of the hands.

Marcus Gunn Jaw Winking Ptosis

Marcus Gunn jaw winking ptosis is being considered as one of the CCDD. The jaw winking phenomena has been reported to occur with mutations in TUBB3 and KIF21. CFEOM associated with polymicrogyria are due to pathogenic variant (c.1261G > A, p.Glu421Lys) in *TUBB2B* [81].

Congenital Myasthenic Syndromes

These are genetic disorders affecting the neuromuscular junction. Ocular findings include ptosis which typically shows variability and fatigability and ophthalmoplegia with a motility pattern not fitting in to any specific cranial nerve palsy. The pupil reactions are normal. Systemic findings include easy fatigability, and facial, neck, and limb weakness, or respiratory insufficiency. Genes encoding proteins involved in presynaptic, synaptic, or postsynaptic neuromuscular transmission are involved. RAPSN gene (11p11.2-p11.1) plays an active role in the clustering of acetylcholine receptors at the endplate, and the muscle-specific protein kinase (MUSK, 9q31.3-q32) gene is critical for synaptic differentiation [82]. Mutations in these genes are known to cause myasthenic syndromes.

Acquired Ptosis

It is imperative to understand that genetic disorders causing mitochondrial dysfunction may arise either due to mutations in the nuclear DNA or due to mutations in the mitochondrial DNA. In the former, they follow Mendelian pattern of inheritance. In the latter the inheritance is based on mitochondrial genetics. Mitochondrial DNA (mtDNA) deletion syndromes include progressive external ophthalmoplegia (PEO), Kearns-Sayre syndrome, and Pearson syndrome. Variants in mtDNA either can arise de novo or may be maternally inherited. Point mutations are usually inherited and large deletions usually are de novo. The mitochondrial mutations are confined only to the skeletal muscles in CPEO but involve all body tissues in KSS and Pearson syndrome.

Chronic Progressive External Ophthalmoplegia

Chronic progressive external ophthalmoplegia (CPEO) is a heterogeneous group of disorders characterized by chronic, progressive, bilateral, and mostly symmetric ocular motility deficit associated with ptosis and proximal limb weakness. CPEO may be autosomal recessive (e.g., POLG gene at 15q25) or dominant (e.g., twinkle helicase gene at 10q24, ANT1 at 4q35), but it is more often caused by mitochondrial DNA (mtDNA) mutations or deletions, most commonly mtDNA deletion of 4.9 kb position 8470 to 13,460. CPEO is a clinical diagnosis. The differential diagnosis for CPEO consists of myasthenia gravis, botulism, Eaton-Lambert syndrome, inflammatory disease (thyroid eye disease, idiopathic orbital myositis), neoplasm, infiltrative disease (sarcoid, amyloid), metabolic disease (primary cytochrome c oxidase deficiency, vitamin E deficiency), and neurologic disease (progressive supranuclear palsy, hereditary ataxias) [83]. The presence of ragged red fibers on muscle biopsy stained with Gomori trichrome as well as abnormal mitochondria and paracrystalline inclusions on electron microscopy is diagnostic.

Kearns-Sayre Syndrome

Kearns-Sayre syndrome is characterized by the triad of pigmentary retinopathy, CPEO, and onset before 20 years of age, with an additional finding of at least one of the following: cardiac conduction block, cerebellar ataxia, and increased CSF protein (greater than 100 mg/dL).

Other findings include endocrine abnormalities (diabetes mellitus, hypoparathyroidism, hyperaldosteronism, adrenal insufficiency, and hypogonadism and thyroid abnormalities).

Ptosis and ophthalmoplegia may occur early. However, diplopia is usually not a feature due to the progressive and symmetric involvement. Sensory neural hearing impairment is the commonest non-triad clinical finding. Intellectual impairment is common.

Large deletions associated with KSS and CPEO may be detected sometimes in skeletal muscle, and hence the role of muscle biopsy if blood testing does not show any mutations. Muscle biopsy also reveals the characteristic "ragged red fibers" on trichrome stain and hyperactive fibers with succinate dehydrogenase stain. Treatment with coenzyme Q10 has been shown to improve cardiac function and exercise tolerance; however, it does not appear to affect ophthalmoplegia, ptosis, or retinopathy.

Myotonic Dystrophy

It is an autosomal dominant inherited disorder caused by heterozygous mutations in the dystrophia myotonica protein kinase (*DMPK*) gene located at 19q13.32 resulting in trinucleotide repeat expansion (CTG)n units [84]. A repeat length exceeding 50 CTG units results in disease. The severity of the disease depends upon the number of repeats.

Ocular findings include ptosis, ophthalmoplegia, orbicularis weakness, posterior subcapsular cataract, and light-near dissociation, low intraocular pressure, and pigmentary retinopathy. Systemic features include myotonia, muscular dystrophy, hypogonadism, frontal balding, and cardiac and ECG abnormalities. Myotonic dystrophy differs from other muscular dystrophies in that it initially involves the distal muscles of the extremities and only later affects the proximal musculature. Atrophy of masseters, sternocleidomastoids, and the temporalis muscle results in a classic Hatchet facial appearance. During a handshake, the patient may have difficulty with release due to exaggerated myotonia. Since the trinucleotide repeat expansions tend to increase in subsequent generations, subsequent generations tend to be affected with more severity and at a younger age of onset. This is referred to as genetic anticipation [85].

Oculopharyngeal Muscular Dystrophy

Oculopharyngeal muscular dystrophy (OPMD) is characterized by ptosis and swallowing difficulties due to selective involvement of the muscles of the eyelid and pharynx, respectively.

Confirmatory diagnosis depends on detection of an expansion of a GCN trinucleotide repeat in the first exon of *PABPN1* [86]. Oculopharyngeal muscular dystrophy typically exhibits autosomal dominant inheritance with complete penetrance though autosomal recessive inheritance has been reported. The autosomal recessive forms have a later age of onset.

Syndromes with Lacrimal System Abnormalities

Congenital Secretory Anomalies

Congenital Alacrima

Congenital alacrima may be caused by an aplastic or hypoplastic lacrimal gland with or without abnormal innervations to the lacrimal system. Aplasia of the lacrimal glands is characterized by dry eyes. It may be with or without aplasia of the salivary glands resulting in dry mouth (xerostomia). Parents often present with the complains of child not able to produce tears when crying.

Isolated lacrimal gland aplasia is inherited as an autosomal dominant disorder caused by mutations involving the FGF10. Lacrimo-auriculo-dento-digital syndrome (LADD), also known as Levy-Hollister syndrome, is an allelic disorder with a more severe phenotype [87]. Besides alacrima and xerostomia, it is characterized by malformation of the external ears, teeth (unerupted and dysplastic teeth), kidneys (renal agenesis, nephrosclerosis), and auditory system (malformation of the auricles, auricular dysplasia, congenital hearing loss). Other syndromes associated with alacrima include Allgrove syndrome, Pierre-Robin sequence, BPES, and Hay-Wells syndrome (acro- dermato-ungal-lacrimal-tooth [ADULT] syndrome, Rapp-Hodgkin syndrome, and limb-mammary syndrome [LMS]), each of which mentioned has distinctive features and mostly involves the lacrimal drainage system. Clinical features of ADULT syndrome include ectrodactyly, onychodysplasia, excess freckling, lacrimal duct obstructions, and early loss of permanent teeth.

Allgrove syndrome (AS) is an autosomal recessive congenital disease, caused by mutations in the *AAAS* gene at 12q13, and is characterized by the triad of Addison's disease, achalasia, and alacrima [88]. It is also called as the Triple-A syndrome. A glycosylation disorder caused by mutations in GMPPA gene which shares features of Allgrove syndrome except Addison's disease has been reported [89]. Intellectual disability and autonomic dysfunction may occur in both. Signs of autonomic dysfunction include pupillary abnormalities, abnormal reaction to intradermal histamine, abnormal sweating, and orthostatic hypotension.

Riley-Day syndrome (RDS) which is an autosomal recessive disorder caused by mutations in the *IKBKAP* gene (9q31) is characterized by absent tears, corneal hypoesthesia, and autonomic dysfunction [90]. RDS is characterized by signs of autonomic dysfunction which include copious drooling, hypotonia, gastroesophageal reflux, decreased sensitivity to pain and temperature perception, hypoactive corneal and tendon reflexes, diminished taste (due to absence of lingual fungiform papillae), alacrima, dysautonomic crises, postural hypotension, and labile hypertension [91].

Alacrima has also been reported with blepharophimosis syndrome [92].

Nasolacrimal System Anomalies

Congenital nasolacrimal duct obstruction is a common disorder that is usually not strictly heritable although there are many instances where it seems to "run in families" or even portray an autosomal dominant pattern. This may be the coincidental effect of its very high rate of incidence. Congenital nasolacrimal system obstruction and other congenital abnormalities of the drainage system, including absent puncta or nasolacrimal fistula, may be part of multiple systemic syndromes. Although it may be difficult to distinguish between coincidental occurrence and true malformation association, some syndromes clearly have lacrimal drainage system anomalies. For example, nasolacrimal fistula is associated with trisomy 21 (Down syndrome), and these patients often have epiphora that may be due to floppy lids, nasolacrimal duct obstruction, blepharitis, or hypotonic lacrimal system pumping. A few other examples are offered below.

Johanson-Blizzard syndrome (JBS) is an autosomal recessive disorder caused by mutations in E3 ubiquitin ligase (UBR1) gene on chromosome 15q13–21.1.53 [93]. JBS is characterized by microcephaly, mid-face hypoplasia, severely hypoplastic nasal alae, cutis aplasia of the scalp, deafness, hypothyroidism, absent permanent teeth, pancreatic malabsorption, failure to thrive, nasolacrimal system malformations (lacrimal-cutaneous fistula, absent superior puncta, nasolacrimal duct obstruction), upslanting palpebral fissures, eyelid coloboma, strabismus, ptosis, and epicanthal folds.

Dyskeratosis congenita, which may be autosomal dominant, autosomal recessive, or X-linked recessive, often has proximal nasolacrimal system drainage anomalies in association with bone marrow failure, abnormal skin pigmentation, leukoplakia, and nail dystrophy. The phenotype is quite variable. Other features may include pulmonary fibrosis, ataxia, and teeth and bone abnormalities.

Phakomatoses with Oculoplastic Manifestations

Neurofibromatosis 1 (NF1)

NF1 is an autosomal dominant disorder caused primarily by mutations in the gene neurofibromin, which manufactures the GTPase activating enzyme neurofibromin (17q11.2) [94]. NF1 has an incidence of one in 3000 live births and is diagnosed by fulfilling any two of the following criteria: two or more neurofibromas on the skin or one plexiform neurofibroma, freckling of the groin or axilla, six or more café au lait spots measuring 5 mm in maximal diameter (>1.5 mm after puberty), skeletal abnormalities (e.g., sphenoid wing dysplasia, thinning of cortex of long bones), > 2 iris Lisch nodules (Fig. 63.23a, b), plexiform neurofibroma (Fig. 63.23c), glioma of the visual pathway (Fig. 63.23d), and affected first-degree relative. Oculoplastic manifestations include plexiform neurofibroma of the upper lid or orbit, facial subcutaneous neurofibromas, and proptosis. A pseudo-pulsatile proptosis occurs due to the transmitted pulsations caused by sphenoid wing dysplasia. The disorder can cause severe progressive orbital and facial malformation.

Tuberous Sclerosis (TS)

TS, also known as Bourneville disease, is an autosomal dominant disorder with incomplete penetrance and variable expressivity caused by mutations in the tuberous sclerosis complex (TSC) genes on chromosomes 9q34 (TSC1) and 16p13.3 (TSC2). Diagnostic criteria for TS include major criteria: facial angiofibromas, ungula fibromas, cortical tuber, subependymal hamartomas, multiple retinal hamartomas, and fibrous plaque on the forehead (Fig. 63.24). Minor

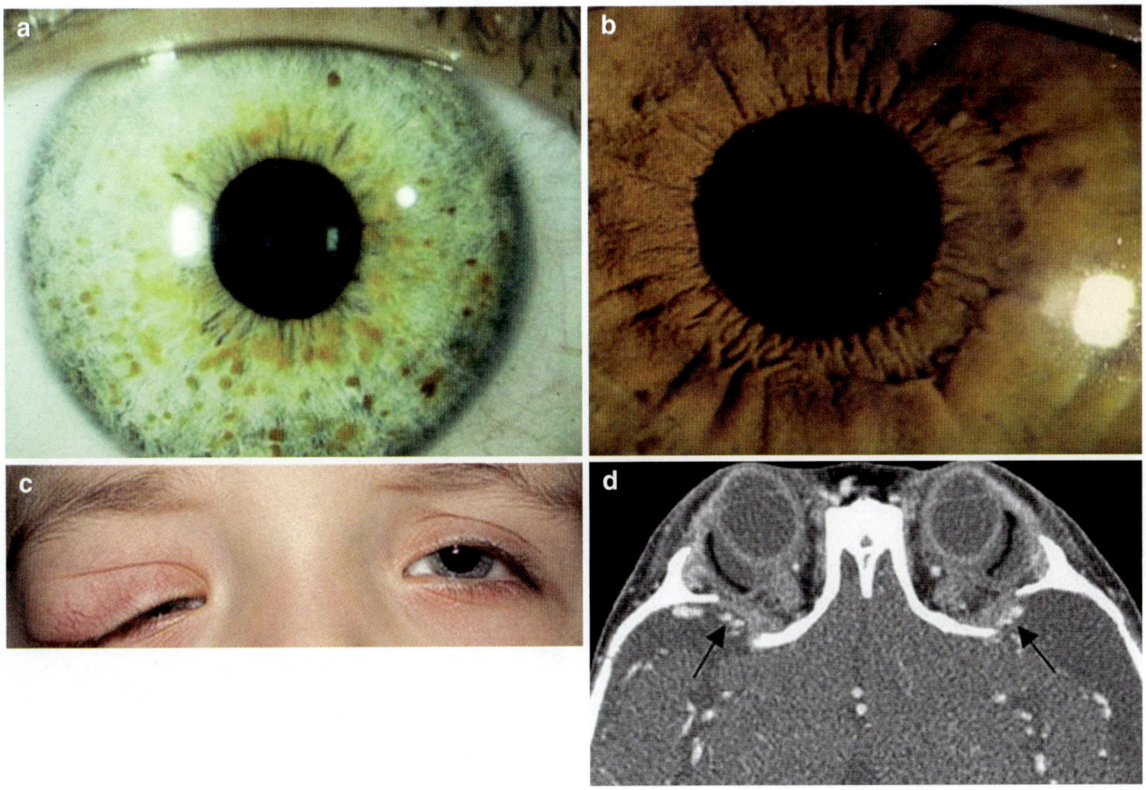

Fig. 63.23 Neurofibromatosis type 1. Common findings in NF1 include Lisch nodules (**a**, **b**), plexiform neurofibroma (**c**), and sphenoid wing dysplasia (**d**, arrows). (Photo courtesy: Dr. Alex Levin)

criteria consist of infantile spasms, hypopigmented macules, shagreen patch, single retinal hamartoma, bilateral renal angiomyolipomas or cysts, cardiac rhabdomyoma, and a first-degree relative with primary diagnosis of TS [95]. Other findings include seizures, mental retardation, and hamartomas in the brain, kidney, heart, skin, and retina [95].

Sturge-Weber Syndrome (SWS)

SWS, also known as leptomeningeal angiomatosis, are generally considered secondary to a somatic mutation and are not heritable (Fig. 63.25). SWS are characterized by port-wine mark, dermal vascular malformations, seizures, neuro-

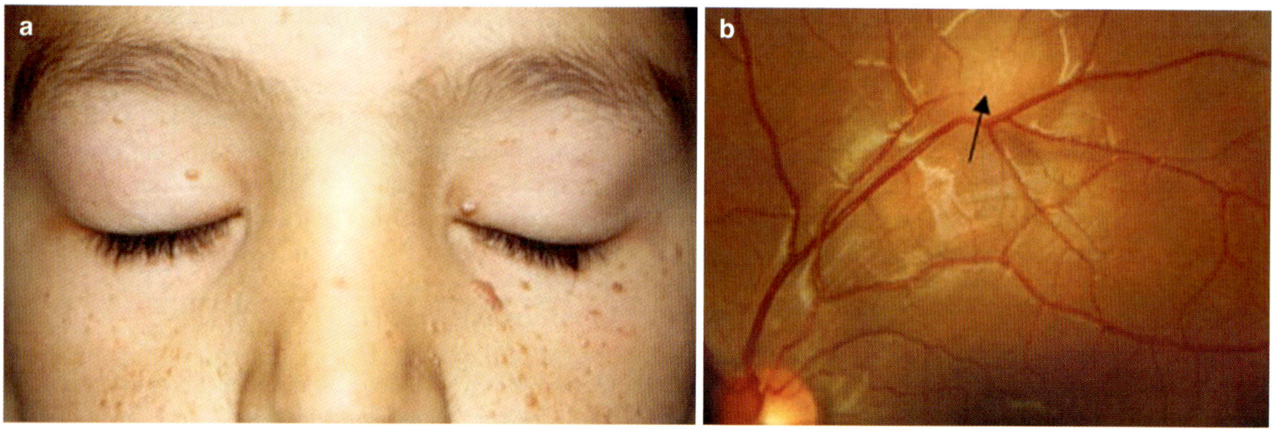

Fig. 63.24 (**a**) Facial angiofibromas of tuberous sclerosis. (**b**) Retinal astrocytic hamartoma (arrow). (Photo courtesy: Dr. Alex Levin)

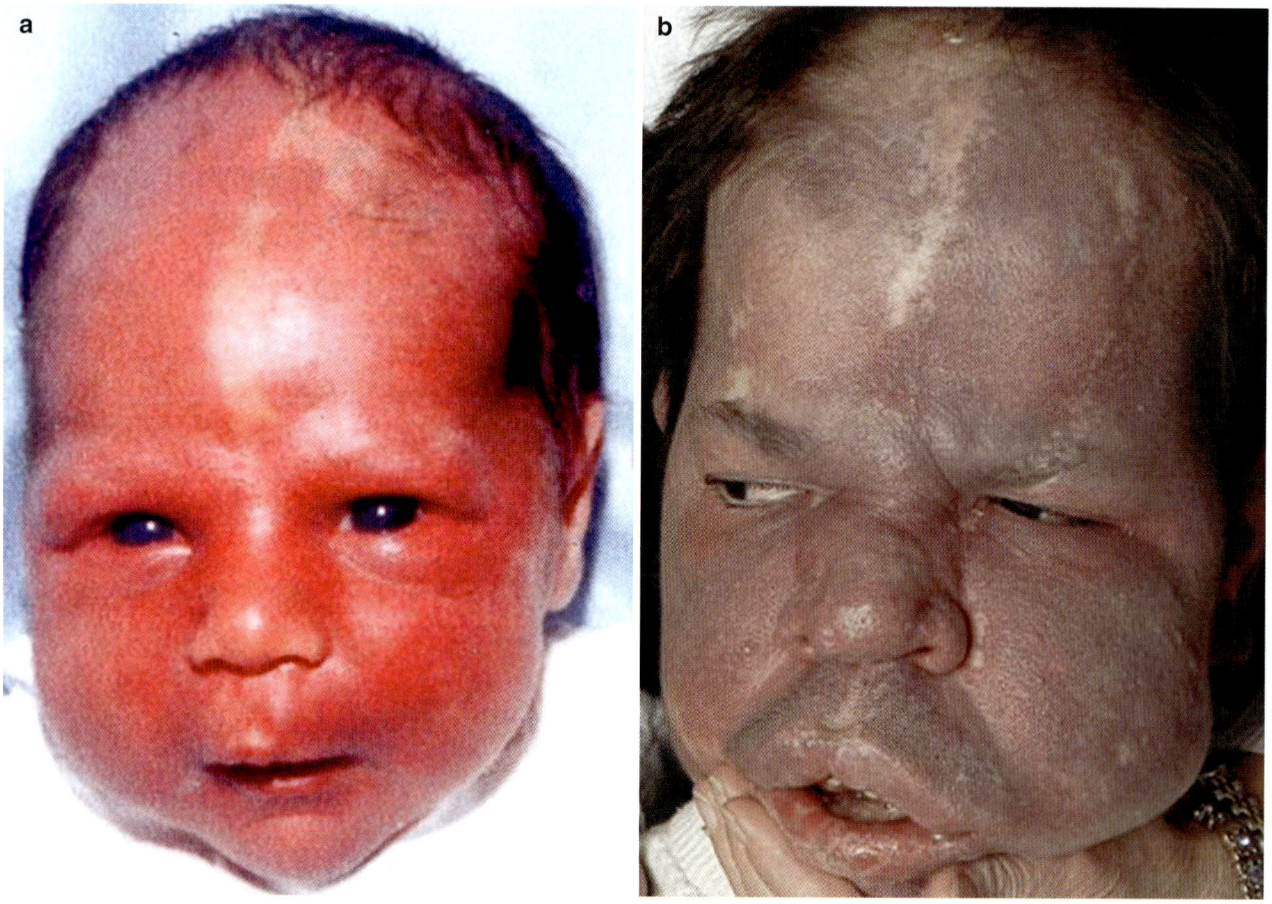

Fig. 63.25 Sturge-Weber syndrome. (**a**) Early port-wine mark. (**b**) Later evolution of port-wine mark, in another patient, with deep purple color and hypertrophy

logic deficits, choroidal hemangiomas, and glaucoma. MRI findings include cortical atrophy, abnormal meningeal vasculature, and tram track calcification. Pulse dye laser is a very effective treatment for the port-wine mark if started early in life. In the second and third decades, the marks begin to get a deeper purple in color and hypertrophy.

Acknowledgments This chapter is essentially written based on the initial framework of the chapter of its earlier edition with some modifications and new additional photographs. I sincerely acknowledge the enormous contributions of the authors (Dr. Alex V Levin and Dr. Kristina Pao) of this chapter of the earlier edition who were so generous and asked me to be the sole author for this edition. I thank Dr. Alex. V. Levin, my mentor in ocular Genetics for his enormous support and carrier guidance and for contributing some photographs to this chapter. I also thank Dr. P. Vijayalakshmi, my first mentor in pediatric ophthalmology for her career guidance and for granting permission to use photographs taken by me during my tenure at Aravind Eye Care system, Madurai. I also thank Dr. Manju Meena and Dr. Arjun Mallah Bhari for contributing of photographs for my Chapter.

References

1. Wygnanski-Jaffe T, Levin AV. Introductory genetics for the ophthalmologist. Focal Points. 2005;23:1–11.
2. Sadagopan KA, Capasso J, Levin AV. Genetics for the ophthalmologist. Oman J Ophthalmol. 2012;5(3):144–9.
3. Weiss AH, Kousseff BG, Ross EA, Longbottom J. Simple microphthalmos. Arch Ophthalmol. 1989;107:1625–30.
4. Deml B, Reis L, Lemyre E, Clark RD, Kariminejad A, Semina EV. Novel mutations in PAX6, OTX2 and NDP in anophthalmia, microphthalmia and coloboma. Eur J Hum Genet. 2016;24:535–41.
5. Smets KJ, Barlow T, Vanhaesebrouck P. Maternal vitamin a deficiency and neonatal microphthalmia: complications of biliopancreatic diversion? Eur J Pediatr. 2006;165(7):502–4. Epub 2006 Apr 29.
6. Levin AV. Congenital eye anomalies. Pediatr Clin N Am. 2003;50:55–76.
7. Khorram D, Choi M, Roos BR, Stone EM, Kopel T, Allen R, et al. Novel TMEM98 mutations in pedigrees with autosomal dominant nanophthalmos. Molec Vision. 2015;21:1017–23.
8. Verma AS, FitzPatrick DR. Anophthalmia and microphthalmia. Orphanet J Rare Dis. 2007;2:47.
9. Slavotinek AM. Eye development genes and known syndromes. Mol Genet Metab. 2011;104:448–56.
10. Schneider A, Bardakjian TM, Zhou J, Hughes N, Keep RB, Dorsainville D, et al. Familial recurrence of SOX2 anophthalmia syndrome: phenotypically normal mother with two affected daughters. Am J Med Genet A. 2008;146A(21):2794–8. https://doi.org/10.1002/ajmg.a.32384.
11. Rainger J, van Beusekom E, Ramsay JK, McKie L, Al-Gazali L, et al. Loss of the BMP antagonist, SMOC-1, causes Ophthalmo-Acromelic (Waardenburg Anophthalmia) syndrome in humans and mice. PLoS Genet. 2011;7(7):e1002114. https://doi.org/10.1371/journal.pgen.1002114.
12. Ng D, Hadley DW, Tifft CJ, Biesecker LG. Genetic heterogeneity of syndromic X-linked recessive microphthalmia-anophthalmia: is Lenz microphthalmia a single disorder? Am J Med Genet. 2002;110:308–14.
13. Ng D. Lenz microphthalmia syndrome. 2002 Jun 4 [updated 2014 Oct 2]. In: Adam MP, Ardinger HH, Pagon RA, et al., editors. GeneReviews® [internet]. Seattle: University of Washington; 1993–2019. Available from: https://www.ncbi.nlm.nih.gov/books/NBK1521/.
14. Hilton E, Johnston J, Whalen S, et al. BCOR analysis in patients with OFCD and Lenz microphthalmia syndromes, mental retardation with ocular anomalies, and cardiac laterality defects. Eur J Hum Genet. 2009;17(10):1325–35. https://doi.org/10.1038/ejhg.2009.52.
15. Van Rahden VA, Fernandez-Vizarra E, Alawi M, Brand K, Fellmann F, Horn D, et al. Mutations in NDUFB11, encoding a complex I component of the mitochondrial respiratory chain, cause microphthalmia with linear skin defects syndrome. Am J Hum Genet. 2015;96(4):640–50. https://doi.org/10.1016/j.ajhg.2015.02.002. Epub 2015 Mar 12
16. Vergult S, Leroy B, Claerhout I, Menten B. Familial cases of a submicroscopic Xp22.2 deletion: genotype-phenotype correlation in microphthalmia with linear skin defects syndrome. Mol Vis. 2013;19:311–8.
17. Stevenson DA, Chirpich M, Contreras Y, Hanson H, Dent K. Goltz syndrome and PORCN mosaicism. Int J Dermatol. 2014;53(12):1481–4. https://doi.org/10.1111/ijd.12605.
18. Bostwick B, Van den Veyver IB, Sutton VR. Focal dermal hypoplasia. 2008 May 15 [updated 2016 Jul 21]. In: Adam MP, Ardinger HH, Pagon RA, et al., editors. GeneReviews® [internet]. Seattle: University of Washington; 1993–2019. Available from: https://www.ncbi.nlm.nih.gov/books/NBK1543/.
19. Plaisancie J, Calvas P, Chassaing N. Genetic advances in microphthalmia. J Pediatr Genet. 2016;5(4):184–8. https://doi.org/10.1055/s-0036-1592350.
20. Bertolacini CD, Ribeiro-Bicudo LA, Petrin A, Richieri-Costa A, Murray JC. Clinical findings in patients with GLI2 mutations–phenotypic variability. Clin Genet. 2012;81(1):70–5. https://doi.org/10.1111/j.1399-0004.2010.01606.
21. Brazier DJ, Hardman-Lea SJ, Collin JR. Cryptophthalmos: surgical treatment of the congenital symblepharon variant. Br J Ophthalmol. 1986;70(5):391–5.
22. François J. Syndrome malformatif avec cryptophtalmie. Acta Genet Med Gemellol. 1969;18(1):18–50.
23. Fraser GR. Fraser syndrome: two millennia of cryptophthalmos from Pliny the elder to FRAS, FREM and GRIP: a historical perspective. Open J Genet. 2013;3:1–7.
24. Slavotinek AM, Baranzini SE, Schanze D, Labelle-Dumais C, Short KM, Chao R, et al. Manitoba-oculo-tricho-anal (MOTA) syndrome is caused by mutations in FREM1. J Med Genet. 2011;48(6):375–82. https://doi.org/10.1136/jmg.2011.089631. Epub 2011 Apr 20
25. Tawfik HA, Abdulhafez MH, Fouad YA, Dutton JJ. Embryologic and fetal development of the human eyelid. Ophthalmic Plast Reconstr Surg. 2016;32(6):407–14. https://doi.org/10.1097/IOP.0000000000000702.
26. Ohuchi H. Wakayama symposium: epithelial-mesenchymal interactions in eyelid development. Ocul Surf. 2012;10:212–6.
27. Maconnachie E. A study of digit fusion in the mouse embryo. J Embryol Exp Morphol. 1979;49:259–76.
28. Van Haelst MM, Scambler PJ, Hennekam RC, Fraser Syndrome Collaboration Group. Fraser syndrome: a clinical study of 59 cases and evaluation of diagnostic criteria. Am J Med Genet A. 2007;143A:3194–203.
29. Morax S, Hurbli T. The management of congenital malpositions of eyelids, eyes and orbits. Eye. 1988;2:207–19.
30. Nouby G. Congenital upper eyelid coloboma and cryptophthalmos. Ophthal Plast Reconstr Surg. 2002;18:373–7.
31. Vendramini-Pittoli S, Kokitsu-Nakata NM. Oculoauriculovertebral spectrum: report of nine familial cases with evidence of autosomal dominant inheritance and review of the literature. Clin Dysmorphol. 2009;18:67–77.

32. Grover AK, Chaudhuri Z, Malik S, et al. Congenital eyelid colobomas in 51 patients. J Pediatr Ophthalmol Strabismus. 2009;46:151–9.
33. Seah LL, Choo CT, Fong KS. Congenital upper lid colobomas management and visual outcome. Ophthal Plast Reconstr Surg. 2002;18:190–5.
34. Patil BB, Bell R, Brice G, et al. Distichiasis without lymphedema? Eye. 2004;18:1270–8.
35. Hoover RE, Kelley JS. Distichiasis and lymphedema; a hereditary syndrome with possible multiple defects: a report of a family. Tr Am Ophth Soc. 1971;69:293–306.
36. Shammas HF, Tabbara DK, Der Kaloustian VM. Atypical serum cholinesterase in a family with congenital distichiasis. J Med Genet. 1976;13:514–5.
37. Brooks BP, Dagenais SL, Nelson CC, et al. Mutation of FOXC2 gene in familial distichiasis. J AAPOS. 2003;7:354–7.
38. Young RJ. Congenital ectropion of the upper lids. Arch Dis Child. 1954;29:97–100.
39. Kelsell DP, Norgett EE, Unsworth H, et al. Mutations in ABCA12 underlie the severe congenital skin disease harlequin ichthyosis. Am J Hum Genet. 2005;76(5):794–803. https://doi.org/10.1086/429844.
40. Alallasi SR, Kokandi AA, Banagnapali B, et al. Exome analysis identifies a novel compound heterozygous alteration in TGM1 gene leading to lamellar ichthyosis in a child from Saudi Arabia: case presentation. Front Pediatr. 2019;7:44. https://doi.org/10.3389/fped.2019.00044.. Published 2019 Feb 21.
41. Patton N, Leatherbarrow B. Primary congenital upper eyelid entropion in association with Duane's retraction syndrome. Eye. 2000;14:385–7.
42. Keipert JA. Euryblepharon. Br J Ophthalmol. 1975;59:57–8.
43. Adam MP, Hudgins L, Hannibal M. Kabuki syndrome. 2011 Sep 1 [updated 2019 Feb 28]. In: Adam MP, Ardinger HH, Pagon RA, et al., editors. GeneReviews® [internet]. Seattle: University of Washington; 1993–2019. Available from: https://www.ncbi.nlm.nih.gov/books/NBK62111/.
44. Cheon CK, Ko JM. Kabuki syndrome: clinical and molecular characteristics. Korean J Pediatr. 2015;58(9):317–24. https://doi.org/10.3345/kjp.2015.58.9.317.
45. Guercio JR, Martyn LJ. Congenital malformations of the eye and orbit. Otolaryngol Clin N Am. 2007;40:113–40.
46. Jordan DR, Anderson RL. Epicanthal folds: a deep tissue approach. Arch Ophthalmol. 1989;107:1532–5.
47. Woo KB, Yi K, Kim YD. Surgical correction for lower lid epiblepharon in Asians. Br J Ophthalmol. 2001;84:1407–10.
48. Mansour AM, Barber JC, Reinecke RD, Wang FM. Ocular choristomas. Surv Ophthalmol. 1989;33:339–58.
49. Haberland C, Perou M. Encephalocraniocutaneous lipomatosis: a new example of ectomesodermal dysgenesis. Arch Neurol. 1970;22:144–55. [PubMed: 4902772] [Full Text].
50. Özdoğan S, Saymaz C, Yaltırık CK, et al. Encephalocraniocutaneous Lipomatosis: Haberland Syndrome. Am J Case Rep. 2017;18:1271–5. https://doi.org/10.12659/ajcr.907685. Published 2017 Dec 1.
51. Lees M, Taylor D, Atherton D, Reardon W. Oculo-ectodermal syndrome: report of two further cases. Am J Med Genet. 2000;91:391–5.
52. Gunduz K, Shields CL, Doych Y, Schnall B, Shields JA. Ocular ectodermal syndrome of epibulbar dermoid and cutaneous myxocapsular hamartoma. Br J Ophthalmol. 2000;84:669–70.
53. Bardenstein DS, McLean IW, Nerney J, Boatwright RS. Cowden's disease. Ophthalmology. 1988;95:1038–41.
54. Marsh DJ, Coulon V, Lunetta KL, Rocca-Serra P, Dahia PL, Zheng Z, et al. Mutation spectrum and genotype-phenotype analyses in Cowden disease and Bannayan-Zonana syndrome, two hamartoma syndromes with germline PTEN mutation. Hum Mol Genet. 1998;7:507–15.
55. De Becker I, Gajda DJ, Gilbert-Barness E, Cohen MM Jr. Ocular manifestations in proteus syndrome. Am J Med Genet. 2000;92:350–2.
56. Cambiaghi S, Levet PS, Guala G, et al. Delleman syndrome: report of a case with a mild phenotype. Eur J Dermatol. 2000;10:623–6.
57. Padmanabhan R. Etiology, pathogenesis and prevention of neural tube defects. Congenit Anom. 2006;46:55–67.
58. Bersani TA, Cecchi LM. Resection of anterior orbital meningoencephalocele in a newborn infant. Ophthal Plast Reconstr Surg. 2006;22:391–3.
59. David DJ, Sheffield L, Simpson D, White J. Fronto-ethmoidal meningoencephaloceles: morphology and treatment. Br J Plast Surg. 1984;37:271–84.
60. Agthong S, Wiwanitkit V. Encephalomeningocele cases over 10 years in Thailand: a case series. BMC Neurol. 2002;2:3–7.
61. Songur E, Mutluer S, Gurler T, et al. Management of frontoethmoidal (sincipital) encephalocele. J Craniofac Surg. 1999;10:135–9.
62. Wu E, Vargevik K, Slovetinek AM. Subtypes of frontonasal dysplasia are useful in determining clinical prognosis. Am J Med Genet. 2007;Part A 143A:3069–78.
63. Chaabouni M, Maazoul F, Hamida AB, et al. Autosomal recessive acro-fronto-facio-nasal dysostosis associated with genitourinary anomalies: a third case report. Am J Med Genet A. 2008;146A:1825–7.
64. Agthong S, Wiwanitkit V. Encephalomeningocele cases over ten years in Thailand: a case series. BMC Neurol. 2002;2:3–7.
65. Hwang SK, Park KS, Park SH, Hwang SK. Update of diagnostic evaluation of craniosynostosis with a focus on pediatric systematic evaluation and genetic studies. J Korean Neurosurg Soc. 2016;59(3):214–8. https://doi.org/10.3340/jkns.2016.59.3.214.
66. Derderian C, Seaward J. Syndromic craniosynostosis. Semin Plast Surg. 2012;26(2):64–75. https://doi.org/10.1055/s-0032-1320064.
67. Gray TL, Casey T, Selva D, Anderson PJ, David DJ. Ophthalmic sequelae of Crouzon syndrome. Ophthalmol. 2005;12:1129–34.
68. Mir A, Wu T, Orlow SJ. Cutaneous features of Crouzon syndrome with acanthosis Nigricans. JAMA Dermatol. 2013;149(6):737–41. https://doi.org/10.1001/jamadermatol.2013.3019.
69. Fries PD, Katowitz JA. Congenital craniofacial anomalies of ophthalmic importance. Surv Ophthalmol. 1990;25:87–119.
70. Johnson D, Wilkie AO. Craniosynostosis. Eur J Hum Genet. 2011;19(4):369–76. https://doi.org/10.1038/ejhg.2010.235.
71. Trainor PA, Dixon J, Dixon MJ. Treacher Collins syndrome: etiology, pathogenesis and prevention. Eur J Hum Genet. 2009;17:275–83.
72. Ganesh A, Al-Mujaini A, Levin AV. The genetic basis of oculoplastic disorders. Rev Ophthalmol. 2014. https://www.reviewofophthalmology.com/article/the-genetic-basis-of-oculoplastic-disorders.
73. Nallasamy S, Kherani F, Yaeger D, et al. Ophthalmologic findings in Cornelia de Lange syndrome: a genotype-phenotype correlation study. Arch Ophthalmol. 2006;124:552–7.
74. Levin AV, Seidman DJ, Nelson LB, Jackson LG. Ophthalmologic findings in the Cornelia de Lange syndrome. J Pediatr Ophthalmol Strabismus. 1990;27:94–102.
75. Wygnanski-Jaffe T, Shin J, Perruzza E, Abdolell M, Jackson LG, Levin AV. Ophthalmologic findings in the Cornelia de Lange syndrome. J AAPOS. 2005;9(5):407–15.
76. Van der Burgt I. Noonan syndrome. Orphanet J Rare Dis. 2007;2:4–9.
77. Nallathambi J, Moumne L, De Baere E, Beysen D, Usha K, Sundaresan P, et al. A novel polyalanine expansion in FOXL2: the first evidence for a recessive form of the blepharophimosis syndrome (BPES) associated with ovarian dysfunction. Hum Genet. 2007;121:107–12.

78. Basel-Vanagaite L, Dallapiccola B, Ramirez-Solis R, Segref A, Thiele H, Edwards A, Arends MJ, Miro X, White JK, Desir J, Abramowicz M, Dentici ML, and 24 others. Deficiency for the ubiquitin ligase UBE3B in a blepharophimosis-ptosis-intellectual-disability syndrome. Am J Hum Genet. 2012;91:998–1010 . [PubMed: 23200864.
79. Warburg M, Bugge M, Brøndum-Nielsen K. Cytogenetic findings indicate heterogeneity in patients with blepharophimosis, epicanthus inversus, and developmental delay. J Med Genet. 1995;32(1):19–24.
80. Karthikeyan Arcot S, Sneider A. Chapter 21: Ocular manifestations of systemic syndromes. In: Levin AV, Enzenauer RW, editors. The eye in pediatric systemic disease. Cham, Switzerland: Springer; 2017. p. 705–72.
81. Whitman MC, Engle CE. Ocular congenital cranial dysinnervation disorders (CCDDs): insights into axon growth and guidance. Hum Mol Genet. 2017;26(R1):R37–44.
82. Khan AO, Almutlaq M, Oystreck DT, Engle EC, Abu-Amero K, Bosley T. Retinal dysfunction in patients with congenital fibrosis of the extraocular muscles type 2. Ophthalmic Genet. 2016;37(2):130–6. https://doi.org/10.3109/13816810.2014.926942. Epub 2014 Jun 18.
83. Lee AG, Brazis PW. Chronic progressive external ophthalmoplegia. Curr Neurol Neurosci Rep. 2002;2:413–7.
84. Musova Z, Mazanec R, Krepelova A, Ehler E, et al. Highly unstable sequence interruptions of the CTG repeat in the myotonic dystrophy gene. Am J Med Genet. 2009;149A:1365–74.
85. Ashizawa T, Dunna PW. Anticipation in myotonic dystrophy. II Complex relationships between clinical findings and structure of the GCT repeat. Neurology. 1992;42(10):1877.
86. Brais B, Bouchard JP, Xie YG, Rochefort DL, Chretien N, Tome FM, et al. Short GCG expansions in the PABP2 gene cause oculopharyngeal muscular dystrophy. Nat Genet. 1998;18:164–7.
87. Rohmann E, Brunner HG, Kayserili H, Uyguner O, et al. Mutations in different components of FGF signaling in LADD syndrome. Nat Genet. 2006;38(4):414–7. Epub 2006 Feb 26
88. Li W, Gong C, Qi Z, Wu D, Cao B. Identification of AAAS gene mutation in Allgrove syndrome: a report of three cases. Exp Ther Med. 2015;10:1277–82.
89. Kohler K, et al. A novel TRAPPC11 mutation in two Turkish families associated with cerebral atrophy, global retardation, scoliosis, achalasia and alacrima. Am J Hum Genet. 2013;93:727–34.
90. Blumenfeld A, Slaugenhaupt SA, Liebert CB, Temper V, et al. Precise genetic mapping and haplotype analysis of the familial dysautonomia gene on human chromosome 9q31. Am J Hum Genet. 1999;64:1110–8.
91. Liebman SD. Riley-Day syndrome: long-term ophthalmologic observations. Tr Am OphthSoc. 1968;66:95–116.
92. Athappilly GK, Braverman RS. Congenital alacrima in a patient with blepharophimosis syndrome. Ophthalmic Genet. 2009;30(1):37–9. https://doi.org/10.1080/13816810802452176.
93. Cheung JC, Thomson H, Buncic JR, Heon E, Levin AV. Ocular manifestations of the Johanson-Blizzard syndrome. J AAPOS. 2009;13:512–4.
94. MacDonald IM, Bech-Hansen T, Britton WA, et al. The phakomatoses: recent advances in genetics. Can J Ophthalmol. 1997;32:4–11.
95. Leroy BP, Carton D, De Laey JJ. Ophthalmological signs of tuberous sclerosis. Societe Belge Dophtalmologie. 1996;262:115–21.

Congenital Soft Tissue Deformities

64

Antonio Augusto Velasco e Cruz and John C. Mustarde

Major Eyelid Deformities

Cryptophthalmos (Online Mendelian Inheritance in Man (OMIM)# 123570)

Cryptophthalmos, from the Greek "Krypto" (hidden), literally means hidden eye. In this condition the lids are not formed and the skin passes without interruption from the forehead over the orbit to the cheek. Although Zehender and Manz are cited as the first to have reported a child with cryptophthalmos [1] in 1872, this rare anomaly may have been recorded since the first century of the Common Era [2–4].

The authors of classic textbooks of ophthalmology, including Duke-Elder, knew that most patients with cryptophthalmos usually presented with a variety of other facial and systemic anomalies [5, 6]. In the 1960s Jules François wrote a preliminary note in French [7], which was later extended to a long article [8], pointing out that some subjects with unilateral cryptophthalmos presented less severe malformations in the fellow eye including upper eyelid colobomas with vestigial tissue fused to the bulbar conjunctiva. He also stressed that the ocular malformation was often part of a syndrome. Since then, cryptophthalmos has been classified as syndromic or isolated with complete and incomplete or partial forms [9, 10]. As discussed by Tawfik, there is some imprecision in this classification because incomplete forms of cryptophthalmos have been designated by several names including corneopalpebral adhesions, corneopalpebral synechiae, abortive cryptophthalmos, and congenital symblepharon [11]. Although we are not in a position to state if all these different upper eyelid anomalies share the same molecular basis, it is clear that they have a better surgical prognosis than that of the complete form of cryptophthalmos. Their surgical management will be discussed in the coloboma section.

Cryptophthalmos is an important diagnostic criterion of the Fraser syndrome (OMIM # 219000), being present in 88% of the affected individuals [3]. As discussed by Comstock [4], the syndrome was well described 90 years before 1962 when Fraser, acting as a consultant of the World Health Organization, presented a long paper on the mutational load of the human population to the IX session of the United Nations Scientific Committee on the Effects of Atomic Radiation in Geneva. In this communication, he described unpublished data of two sisters with cryptophthalmos, syndactyly, and many other malformations. Since then the association between cryptophthalmos, syndactyly, and a variety of systemic malformations has been known as Fraser syndrome (Fig. 64.1a, b). The incidence of this autosomal recessive condition is estimated to be 0.43 per 100,000 liveborn infants.

Complete or partial cryptophthalmos is also an important feature of the Manitoba-oculo-tricho-anal (MOTA) syndrome (OMIM # 248450), a rare recessive autosomal disorder described by Marles in 1992 in Indians of the Island Lake region of Northern Manitoba [12]. The affected subjects present with a variable combination of unilateral partial or complete cryptophthalmos, aberrant anterolateral scalp hairline, and nasal and anal anomalies. The nose of the patients is typically broad with a notch or groove on its tip (Fig. 64.2). It is interesting to note that the association of upper eyelid coloboma and wedge-shaped anterior hairline extension has already been interpreted as a Tessier cleft # 10 [13]. The overlap between MOTA and Fraser syndromes is evident. However, the patients with MOTA syndrome are less affected, and their prognosis is favorable because they have normal growth and no severe cognitive impairment. They usually have no internal organ abnormalities or syndactyly [14].

Modern molecular genetic research has shown that Fraser and MOTA syndromes, as well as isolated cryptophthalmos,

John C. Mustarde deceased at the time of publication.

A. A. V. e Cruz (✉)
Hospital das Clínicas- FMRP-USP, Department of Ophthalmology, Ribeirao Preto, SP, Brazil

J. J. Servat et al. (eds.), *Smith and Nesi's Ophthalmic Plastic and Reconstructive Surgery*,
https://doi.org/10.1007/978-3-030-41720-8_64

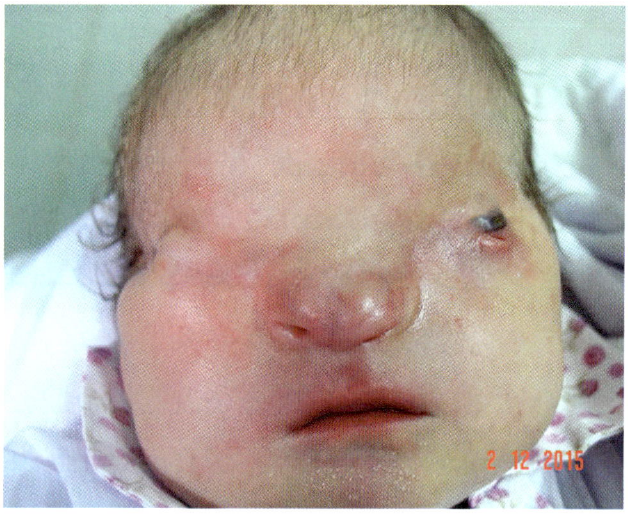

Fig. 64.1 Cryptophthalmos in Fraser syndrome. patient with complete cryptophthalmos on the right side and partial on the left

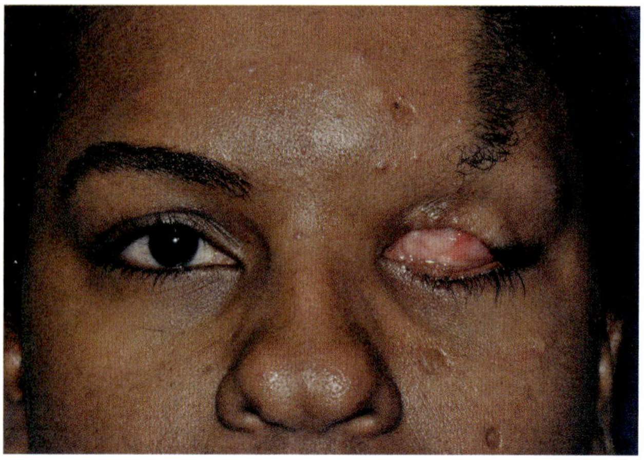

Fig. 64.2 Typical MOTA syndrome phenotype. Tongue-hair line extending to the orbital rim, absence of brow, bifid nose, and a partial cryptophthalmos that was surgically repaired

are caused by defects on the embryonic basement membrane proteins of the FRAS/FREM complex (FRAS1, FREM1, and FREM2). Fraser syndrome is caused by mutations in the FRAS1 and FREM2 genes or in GRIP1, a FRAS1-interacting protein [15, 16]. MOTA syndrome results from loss of function mutations in the FREM1 gene [17, 18], and isolated cryptophthalmos is also caused by mutations in the FREM2 gene [19].

The indication of surgical repair of cases of bilateral complete cryptophthalmos is a topic open to debate. In most cases, the malformed globe behind the skin has no potential for vision, and the purpose of the multiple procedures required to create a proper socket needs to be explained in detail to the family of patients with cognitive impairment [20]. First, a horizontal incision is performed to separate the skin from the globe. If a disorganized cystic eye is found, evisceration with an implant may be necessary if the size of the remnants is not sufficient to stimulate the normal bony growth of the orbit [10]. Multiple skin and mucous grafts [20, 21] are usually necessary to obtain a proper socket. Additional ear cartilage and hard palatal grafts may be necessary to provide a more rigid structure for the lid and to increase the posterior lamella [20].

Ablepharon Macrostomy Syndrome (OMIN # 200110) and Barber-Say (OMIM # 209885) Syndromes

The so-called ablepharon macrostomia syndrome (AMS) is an extremely rare condition first described in 1977 by McCarty [22]. The condition is caused by dominant mutations in the TWIST2 gene. A single lysine substitution in residue 75 of this gene results in a constellation of anomalies including macrostomia, redundant and lax skin, camptodactyly, and ambiguous genitalia. The clinical picture is dominated by the changes in the periocular area. The affected patients are born with severe shortening of all four lids and bilateral central corneal ulceration. To date, only 13 articles reporting 15 patients with AMS have been published [22–33]. In most of these articles, the lids of the patients were described as absent [22, 24, 29, 31, 32]. Our experience with this syndrome [26, 28] does not concur with this interpretation. Figure 64.3a shows a typical case of AMS who was operated in 2000. It is quite clear that the lids are only shortened and not absent. The palpebral conjunctiva is chemotic and redundant. Intraoperative lid dissection through an anterior approach allowed us to identify an intact orbital septum, levator muscle aponeurosis, pre-aponeurotic fat, and, of course, the palpebral conjunctiva. Tarsal plates are not formed. Figure 64.3b displays the same patient appearing in Fig. 64.3a 10 years after the placement of a simple skin graft over the inner surface of the Müller muscle/palpebral conjunctiva plane. The eyes are white, with no signs of active exposure. The amount of lagophthalmos with gentle occlusion is small.

In summary, the term ablepharon is a misnomer that should be avoided. The patients with this syndrome have rudimentary shortened eyelids (microblepharon). Their small lids can be lengthened with skin grafts if a proper dissection is performed. We do not recommend the use of lid-sharing procedures or masquerade flaps [34] in this syndrome.

In 1982 by two pediatricians Nancy Barber and Burhan Say described a 3.5-year-old girl who was born with several congenital anomalies including hypertrichosis, atrophic skin, and macrostomia [35, 36]. The condition was named as Barber-Say syndrome (BSS) by Martinez-Santana et al. who reported a third case in 1993 [37]. Several authors have noticed BBS and AMS share many clinical features [38]. Recent molecular genetic analyses have confirmed this rela-

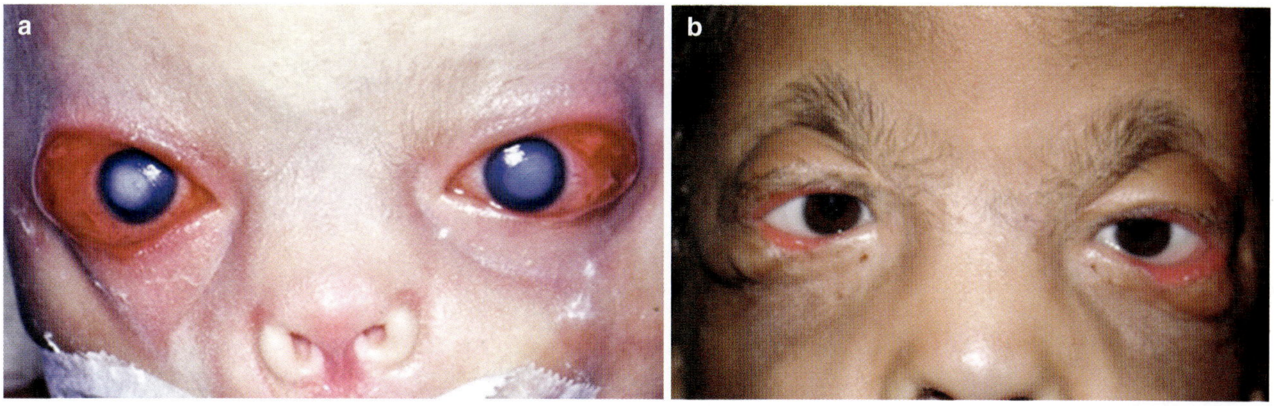

Fig. 64.3 (**a**) Neonate with ablepharon macrostomy syndrome. (**b**) Same patient after 10 years of lid repair with skin grafts placed over the Müller's muscle

tion but have shown that the two conditions are not the same at the molecular level. BSS is also caused by a dominant mutation in the TWIST2 gene. However, BSS results from a glutamine substitution rather than a lysine substitution at the same codon [23].

Despite many clinical similarities, the palpebral fissure changes in BSS are less severe than those observed in AMS. Ectropion was the term used to describe the eyelid condition in the first BSS case [35]. In a recent literature review of 22 BSS cases, ectropion and telecanthus were described in 19 patients and microblepharon in only 4 [39].

A more detailed clinical picture emerges from the rare descriptions of eyelid surgery of patients with BSS. A patient operated by Ng and Rajguru did not have ectropion but presented with lagophthalmos, weakness of the orbicularis oculi muscles, lower eyelid retraction, and euryblepharon. His lower eyelids were floppy with lateral canthal laxity and rounding [40]. A recent patient reported by Barreiro-Gonzalez [41] did have bilateral lower lid ectropion that was associated with an impressive canthal laxity and rounding. Euryblepharon was evident as well as shortening of the upper lid anterior lamella. The same pattern of euryblepharon, lax eyelids, and anterior lamella shortening was evident in the patient illustrated in Fig. 64.4 reported by Zuazo et al. [42]. It is important to notice that none of these patients developed significant corneal exposure of loss of vision. They were all described as having moderate inferior superficial keratopathy.

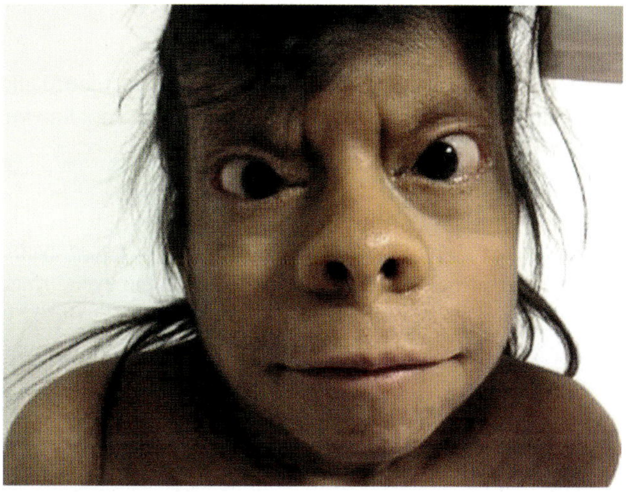

Fig. 64.4 Barber-Say syndrome. (Courtesy of Dr. Jose-Luis Tovilla-Canales). Notice the absence of ectropion, shortening of the upper eyelid anterior lamella laterally, euryblepharon, and lateral canthus rounding

Upper Eyelid Colobomas

Coloboma, from the Greek *koloboma* (Κολόβωμα), means a gap or defect in a tissue. Eyelid colobomas may be unilateral or bilateral with their base located always at the lid margin. There is a full-thickness missing segment of different sizes and shapes that is usually triangular or quadrilateral. Upper eyelid colobomas may be isolated, express partial forms of cryptophthalmos, and be associated with Tessier's facial cleft numbers 11, 10, and 9 or with other conditions such as the Goldenhar and other rare syndromes.

Isolated Colobomas

This type of coloboma is frequently unilateral, situated in the center of the middle third of the lid and, despite the presence of an eventual important corneal gap exposure, may be minimal or even absent. The size is quite variable and the shape is usually quadrangular (Fig. 64.5). By definition, these patients do not have any systemic or other ocular abnormalities. There is no skin or conjunctiva adhesion, there are no tags and no epibulbar lesions, and the brows and frontal region are normal [43, 44]. From a surgical point of view, these isolated cases have the best prognosis because the upper fornix

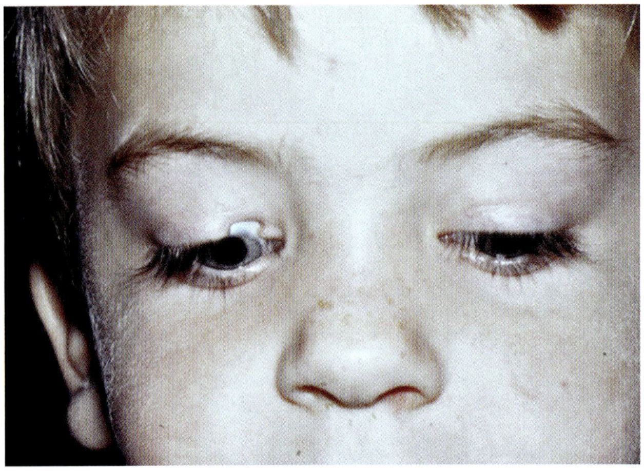

Fig. 64.5 Isolated coloboma of the upper lid without any signs of keratopathy

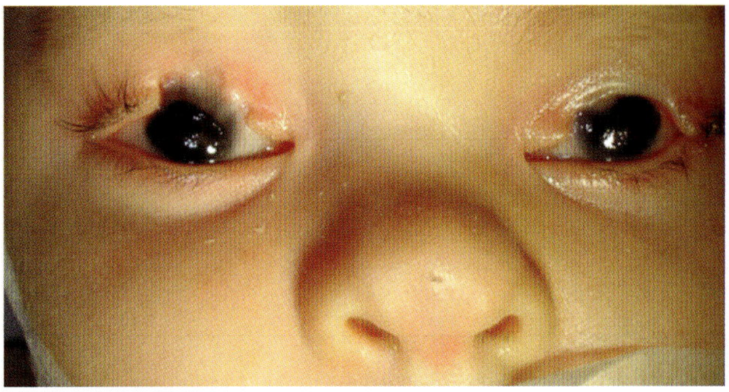

Fig. 64.6 Bilateral upper eyelid coloboma with corneopalpebral adhesions. (Courtesy of Dr. Fernando Procianoy, Porto Alegre, Brazil)

is deep with an intact bulbar conjunctiva. The incidence and molecular basis of this type of isolated defect are not known.

Colobomas with Corneopalpebral or Conjunctival Adhesions

Although there is a wide phenotypic variety of upper eyelid defects that present with adhesions between the eye surface and conjunctival or skin remnants of the upper eyelid [21, 45], these types of coloboma are likely to represent partial forms of cryptophthalmos and thus are probably caused by mutations of the FRAS/FREM complex [19]. As shown in Fig. 64.6, they can be bilateral.

The relation between these complex lid-eye defects and cryptophthalmos was noticed long before the advent of molecular biology. As mentioned before, François in 1969 had already pointed out that many cases of "superior symblepharon" were in fact associated with other contralateral or systemic anomalies typical of the mutations of the FRAX/FREM genes [8].

Craniofacial Cleft Numbers 11, 10, and 9

For several years after 1976, when Tessier published his landmark article on the classification of cranial clefting [46], there was a tendency to consider any type of upper eyelid coloboma as an expression of a Tessier cleft 11, 10, or 9. This position is no longer accepted. Tessier's system is purely morphologic, and the clinical features of some of his clefts involving the upper lid are similar to other conditions with a known molecular genetic basis.

According to the original Tessier's description, cleft # 11 is a coloboma of the medial third of the lid sometimes extending through the eyebrow. Since the patient he displayed to illustrate this cleft had no brow anomalies, the defect shown is indistinguishable from a simple coloboma.

Cleft # 10 is an upper "central" orbital defect occurring in the middle third of the supraorbital rim, lateral to the supraorbital nerve. The cleft may extend to the orbital roof and frontal bone (encephalocele). The coloboma is located in the middle third of the lid, sometimes amounting to total ablepharia. The eyebrow is divided into two portions, the lateral one vertically angulated joining the hairline of the scalp, while the medial portion is virtually absent. The patient displayed by Tessier had a huge bony defect involving the frontal area.

If these criteria are not strictly followed and the bone defect is ruled out, what is left is a central coloboma associated with a brow defect. In a large series of patients described as Tessier's cleft 10, none had bone defects, and their condition was closely similar to partial cryptophthalmos [47]. Figure 64.7 displays a child who was born with a large left lid coloboma. His brow was almost absent and his left frontal bone was thinned. The case was considered to be a facial cleft # 10, and immediate repair was advised due to severe keratopathy. One year after surgery, the abnormalities on the left frontal region were more evident.

Cleft # 9 is extremely rare and even Tessier had never seen one. We have seen a patient who had a classic combination of clefts 5 and 9 [48]. The upper lid was distorted upward by a lateral cicatricial coloboma, and severe keratopathy was present (Fig. 64.8a). After eyelid repair her cornea healed well. However, as she aged, the bony component of cleft 9 became prominent, and a combination of high refractive error and eye motility restriction induced a deep amblyopia (Fig. 64.8b).

Oculoauriculovertebral Spectrum (Goldenhar) and Other Rare Syndromes

Goldenhar syndrome (OMIM 164210), also called oculoauriculovertebral spectrum or first and second branchial arch syndrome, is a clinically and genetically heterogeneous disease mainly characterized by malformations of the ear, mouth, and mandible [49]. Most cases are sporadic, but there are families with autosomal dominant inheritance.

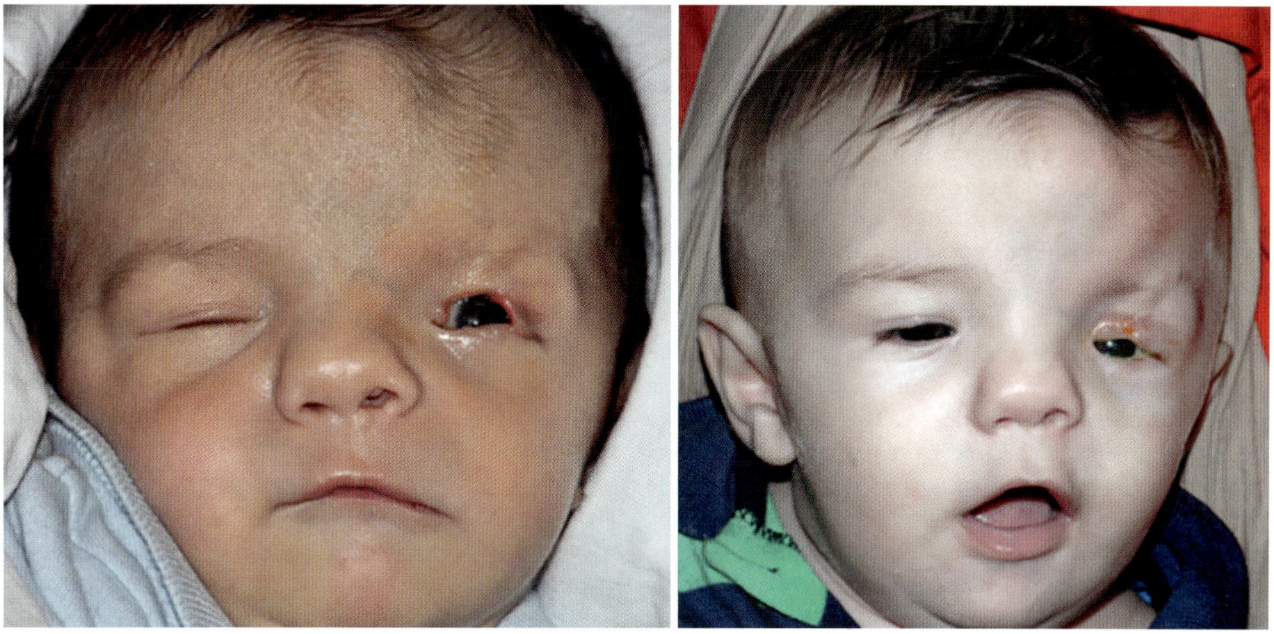

Fig. 64.7 Large upper eyelid coloboma associate with cleft 10. The defect was repaired with a sliding tarsal flap + skin graft

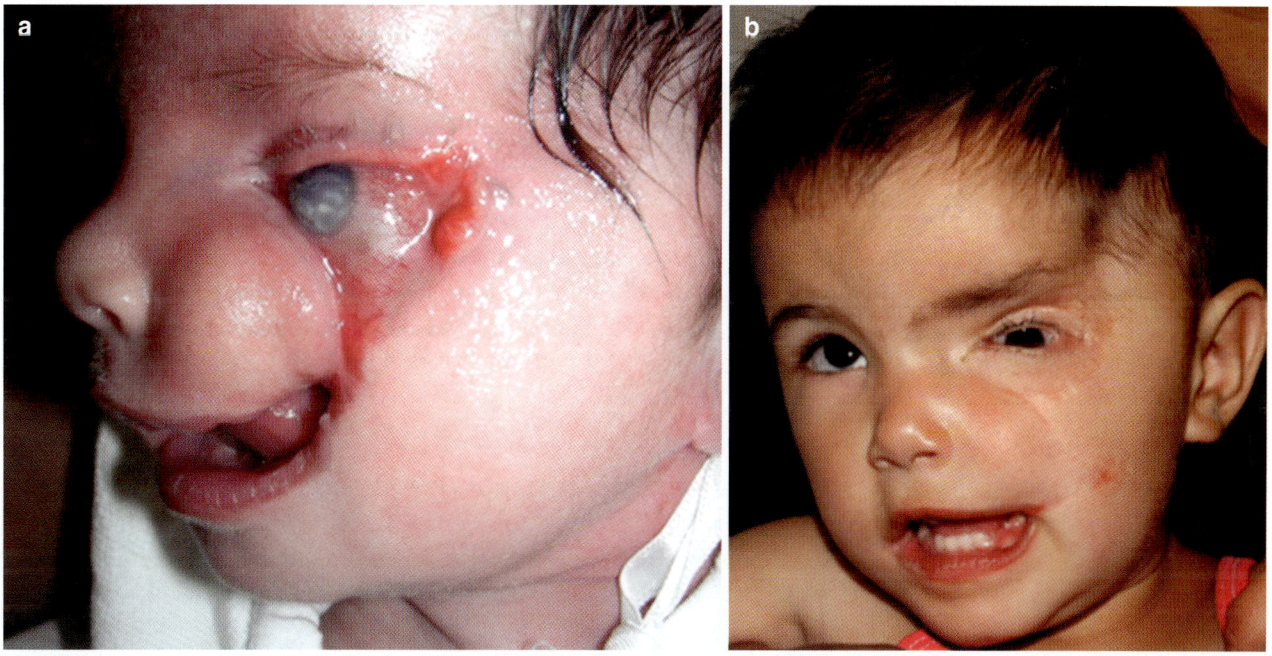

Fig. 64.8 A rare upper lid lateral coloboma due to a cleft 5/9. (**a**) Aspect of the infant, (**b**) lid fissure 7 years after surgical repair. The bony component of cleft 9 is now prominent

Epibulbar choristomas rather than upper eyelid colobomas are the most common ocular anomaly of the syndrome. Eyelid defects are seen in only 8 [50] to 11% [51] of affected patients.

Eyelid coloboma is also an exceptional finding in the CHARGE association [52] (Coloboma, Heart disease, Atresia of choanae, Retardation of growth and development, Genitourinary malformation, and Ear anomalies). Although letter C (coloboma) is the first in the acronym that names the condition, these defects are ocular, and in the most recent case series, not a single eyelid coloboma was found [53, 54]. Small cicatricial colobomas can also be found in rare neurocutaneous syndromes such as encephalocraniocutaneous lipomatosis [55].

Surgical Repair

The technique and time chosen to close an upper eyelid coloboma will vary according to a series of factors including size of the defect, degree of corneal exposure, possibility to use contralateral tarso-conjunctival flaps, and presence of corneal or conjunctival adhesions.

Isolated colobomas tend to induce minimal or no keratopathy, and thus, depending on the anxiety of the parents, surgery can be delayed. In such cases, the surgeon may decide intraoperatively which technique he will use. After removing the epithelial edges of the defect, both tarsal ends of the coloboma are pulled together. The surgeon can then judge if the defect can be repaired or not by direct closure. This is a critical choice because the defect should be closed without any tension, avoiding the risks of dehiscence or a tethered ptosis [45]. In order to increase the mobility of the lateral edge of the defect, canthotomy and cantholysis are performed. For larger defects, other options include different combinations of anterior and posterior lamella mobilization such as a semicircular Tenzel flap [56] (Fig. 64.9) with tarsal advancement techniques [57–59]) or free tarsal conjunctival grafts [60]. If there is a large bilateral defect, palatal mucosal grafts can be used together with anterior lamella rotational flaps. Finally, lid-sharing procedures such as Cutler-Beard or Mustarde flaps can also be used in selected cases.

Lower Eyelid Involvement in Craniofacial Clefting

Lower eyelid colobomas differ substantially from those of the upper lid because they are usually complex defects associated with cleft numbers 3, 4, and 5, which are collectively known as oblique clefts. Since these clefts involve other structures such as the nose, lacrimal system, orbit, and globe, surgical repair is a multistage individualized procedure requiring a multidisciplinary approach.

Cleft # 3, also known as oro-naso-ocular cleft, starts at cupid's bow, passes through the base of the nasal ala, and progresses cranially, provoking a medial lower eyelid coloboma. The lacrimal canaliculus and the nasal lacrimal duct are absent, and if the sac is present, it becomes a source of chronic dacryocystitis. The bony deformity may involve the pyriform aperture of the nasal cavity and the frontal process of the maxilla, shortening the vertical distance between the alar base and the medial canthus (Fig. 64.10). In complete forms, the nose, maxillary sinus, and orbit form a single cavity [61].

Cleft # 4, or oro-ocular cleft, passes laterally to the alar base and progresses cranially onto the cheek causing a central lid coloboma. The medial canthus is usually spared. The pyriform aperture is not involved and the nasal ala is only distorted. On the other hand, the orbital floor is widely opened into the maxillary sinus (Fig. 64.11).

Cleft # 5 is more rare than clefts 3 and 4. It decreases the distance between the angle of the mouth and the lower eyelid where it causes a lateral coloboma. It also causes a lateral defect on the orbital floor (Fig. 64.12).

As mentioned earlier, the surgical repair of clefts impacting the lower lid is challenging. The globe is often affected, and, in addition, rehabilitation of the lid coloboma socket is necessary. In a series of 21 patients with cleft #3, microphthalmia or anophthalmia was present in 5 patients (24%) [62]. Usually soft tissue surgery is performed early within the first year of life. Different variations of local flaps are employed to close the defects. Bony grafting is deferred at least until 5–6 years of age [63].

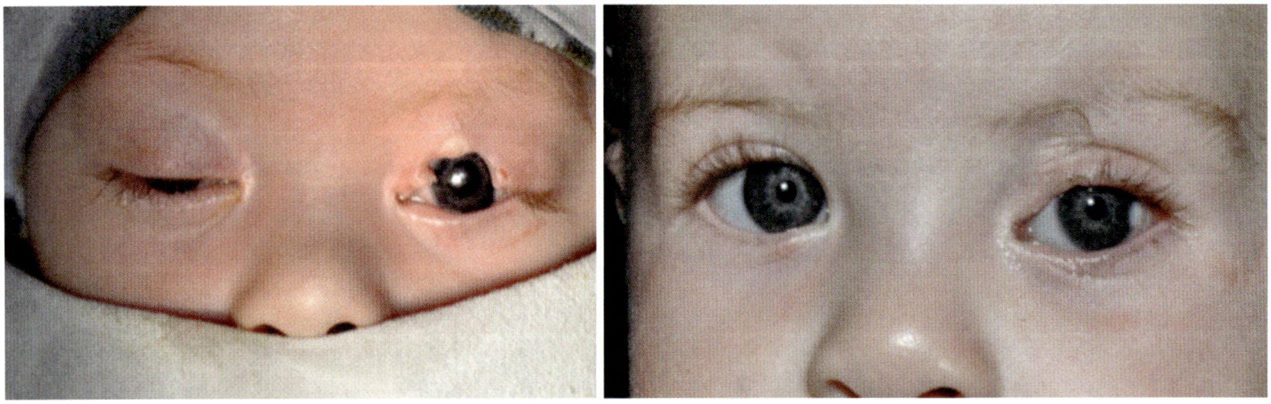

Fig. 64.9 Medium-size upper eyelid coloboma repaired with a semicircular Tenzel flap + direct closure

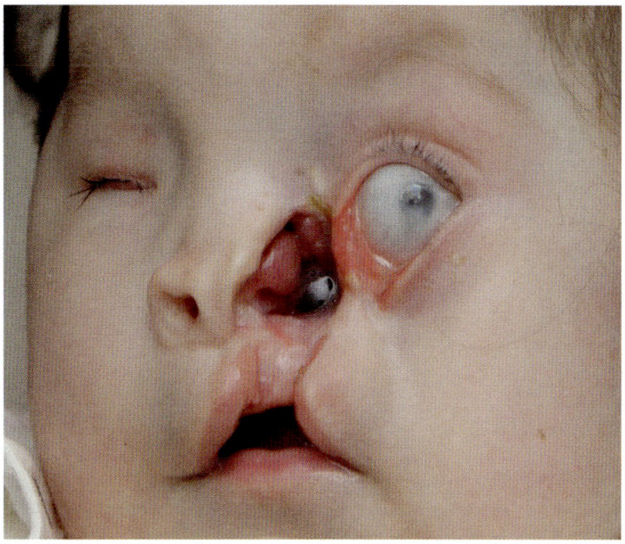

Fig. 64.10 Tessier's cleft # 3

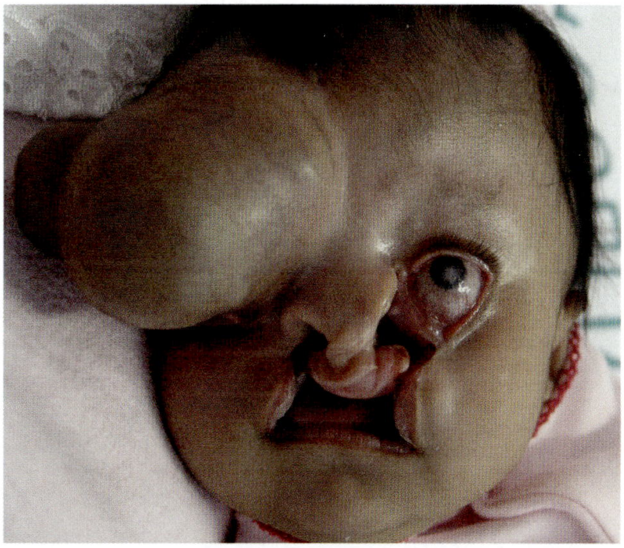

Fig. 64.11 Gigantic right orbital encephalocele and left Tessier's cleft # 4

Congenital Accessory Palpebral Fissure

An ectopic or accessory eyelid fissure is an extremely rare anomaly. To the best of our knowledge, only three cases have been reported [64–66], with the anomaly being unilateral in all of them. The patients presented with multiple malformations. The accessory fissure was above the upper lid margin and consisted of a short fissure with malformed tarsal plates and eyelashes. The second patient reported was diagnosed with oculocerebrocutaneous syndrome [65] (OMIM 164180).

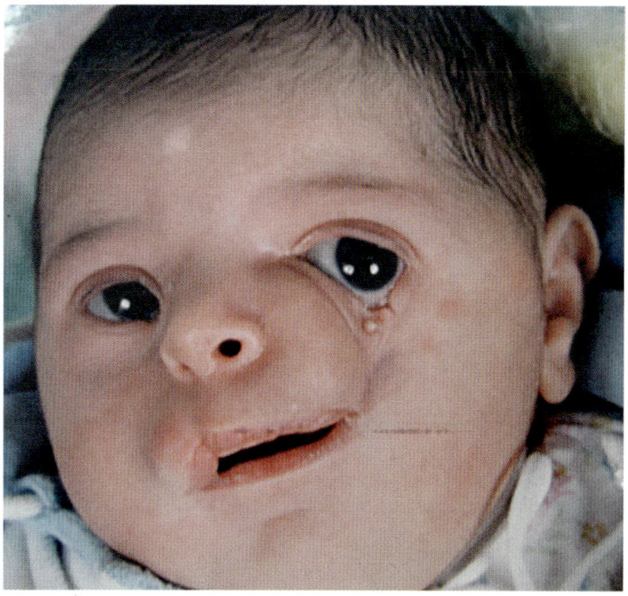

Fig. 64.12 Left Tessier's cleft # 5

Canthal Abnormalities

Medial Canthus

Epicanthal folds and telecanthus are the main congenital abnormalities of the inner canthus. Epicanthus may be defined as a vertical curved fold of skin overlying the medial canthus. Epicanthus is a normal finding in children of all ethnic backgrounds. In adults it is a normal characteristic of the Asian fissure. Von Ammon is quoted [67] as the first to have distinguished three types of epicanthus according to shape and area where the fold arises (brow = supraciliaris, upper lid = palpebralis, and lid crease = tarsalis). A fourth type of epicanthus arising from the lower eyelid and named epicanthus inversus was distinguished later [68, 69]. As discussed by Mustarde [70], this purely morphologic classification of the epicanthal folds is not relevant but is still mentioned in the modern literature [71].

Telecanthus was the term coined by Mustarde to design the lateral displacement of both inner canthi that he was diagnosing in many patients with ptosis [70, 72]. Implicit in the concept of telecanthus is a normal interorbital medial distance that differentiates telecanthus from hypertelorism. The displacement of the canthus results from an abnormal elongation of the medial canthal tendon.

Telecanthus can be associated with epicanthus or appear as an isolated abnormality. A typical example is Waardenburg syndrome type 1 (OMIN # 193500), an autosomal dominant condition caused by mutations in the PAX3 gene. In this syndrome telecanthus is a major diagnostic criterion found in 99% of the affected individuals (Fig. 64.13). In the genetic

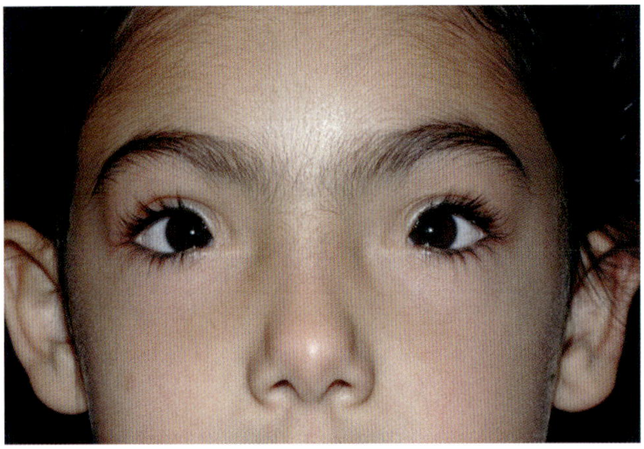

Fig. 64.13 Typical telecanthus of the Waardenburg syndrome type 1. The medial scleral triangle is not seen, and the lower puncta are close to the midpupil line

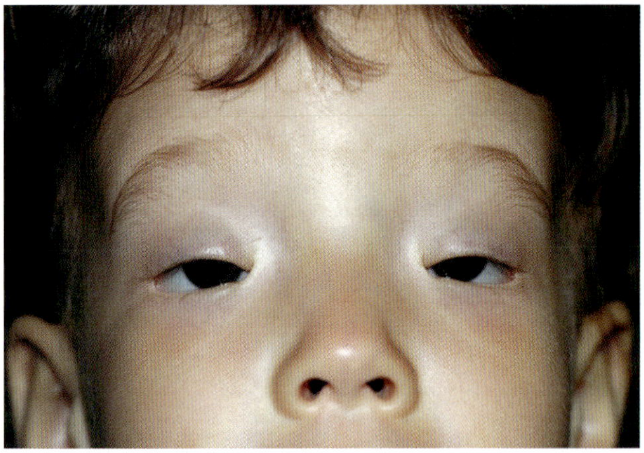

Fig. 64.14 Patient with BPES. Note the epicanthus inversus, severe ptosis with frontalis muscle recruitment (arched brows) and lateral lower lid retraction

literature, the telecanthus of the Waardenburg syndrome is referred to as *dystopia canthorum* [73, 74].

Blepharophimosis, Ptosis, and Epicanthus Inversus Syndrome (BPES) (OMIN #110100)

Epicanthus inversus and telecanthus are major findings in BPES (Fig. 64.14). This autosomal dominant syndrome was first described by Vignes in 1889 [75], and in 2001 it was demonstrated that the disease was associated with mutations on the forkhead box L2 (FOXL2) gene on chromosome 3q23 [76]. Since this gene is expressed not only in the developing eyelid mesenchyme but also in and fetal and adult ovaries, there is a subtype of patient (type I) with premature ovarian failure [77]. Type II patients have normal ovarian function [78].

The clinical characteristics of the syndrome have been well studied. Besides the three major findings (severe ptosis, epicanthus inversus, and telecanthus), the patients may display many other abnormalities including lower eyelid lateral ectropion, strabismus, high refractive errors, amblyopia, lacrimal abnormalities, and agenesis of the lacrimal gland [79–87].

The surgical repair of epicanthus and telecanthus involves shortening of the anterior crus of the medial canthal tendon and some skin manipulation to correct the two dog-ear folds formed when the medial canthus is advanced. While the discussion of how to shorten the medial canthal tendon mainly concerns whether or not to perform trans-nasal wiring, epicanthus management is a theme still open to debate. In Asia, where there is a high demand for cosmetic epicanthoplasty, a plethora of technical variants have been used [71, 88–97]. Huang analyzed 48 articles on different types of epicanthoplasties. Although Z-plasties were the most used procedures, the skin redraping technique became the most cited surgery after 2007 [98]. The skin redraping method was published by Oh as an option to reduce the scars induced by the classic Z-plasties and Y-V advancement flaps [99]. In 2012 the same technique was used for the first time in patients with BPES [100]. As shown in Fig. 64.15, we are very pleased with the skin redraping technique. The medial canthal tendon is easily exposed, and the scar is camouflaged in the lower lid infra-lash incision (Fig. 64.15).

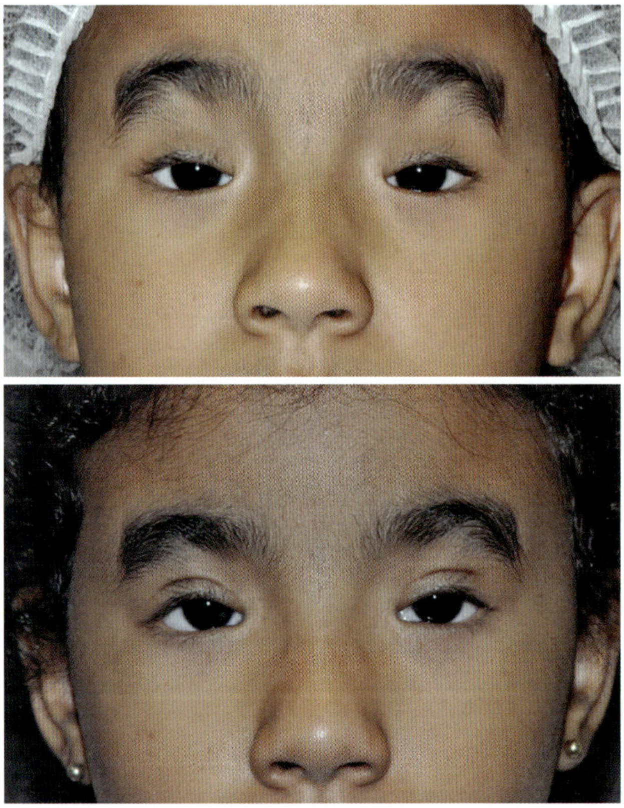

Fig. 64.15 Epicanthus inversus management with the skin redraping technique. The inconspicuous scars are under the lash line of the lower eyelids

Lateral Canthus

Treacher Collins/Franceschetti Syndrome

The Treacher Collins syndrome (TCS), also known as mandibulofacial dysostosis or Franceschetti syndrome, is a heterogeneous genetic disease transmitted by autosomal dominance (TCS1 and TCS2) or recessive inheritance (TCS3) [101].

The clinical features of this syndrome might have been known since the time of pre-Columbian civilizations [102]. According to Duke-Elder [103], the first mention in the English literature was by Berry, who reported in 1889 a mother and her son with antimongoloid palpebral fissure obliquity, lower eyelid colobomas, and micrognathia. Collins, a British ophthalmologist, reported several cases in 1990, adding to Berry's description hypoplasia of the malar bones. Franceschetti and Klein in 1944 and 1949 published several atypical cases and demonstrated the genetic background of the syndrome. They also coined the term mandibulofacial dysostosis, which is widely used in the modern literature [103].

TCS 1 (OMIM 154500) is the most frequent type caused by heterozygous mutations in the TCFO1 gene on chromosome 5q32. TCS 2 (OMIM 613717) has been diagnosed in a small subset of patients who display mutations in the POLR1D gene on chromosome 13q12, and TCS 3 (OMIM 248390) is the rarest form caused by compound heterozygous mutation in the POLR1C gene. A large series of patients with TCS showed high clinical variability and no phenotype-genotype correlation. In 4% of patients, the molecular defect was not identified [101].

Patients with TCS display a variety of bilateral anomalies in the craniofacial tissues derived from the first and second branchial arcs. Major findings include negative (antimongoloid) obliquity of the palpebral fissures, malar and mandibular hypoplasia, and conductive hearing loss. Microtia and small partial lateral lower lid colobomas are also frequent [101]. The palpebral fissure changes are typical. Besides the downward slant of the fissure, the eyelashes are often absent medially to the lid defect, and the lower lacrimal punctum and canaliculum are not formed [104]. The tarsal plates are also reduced or even absent [105].

The lateral canthus malformation is the main fissure abnormality. Hypoplasia of the frontal process of the zygomatic bone [105] with absence of the lateral canthal tendon [106] induces a marked canthal dystopia. The lateral canthus is rounded, and the horizontal diameter of the fissure is reduced. Three-dimensional reconstruction of the CT scans of the orbits of patients with TCS has confirmed that the main skeletal orbital deficiency is inferolateral [107].

Figure 64.16 illustrates the palpebral fissure anomalies in TCS.

Although the lateral canthal dystopia in TCS is well understood, its surgical correction is still a matter of discussion. Several surgical strategies have been proposed including bone grafting [108], musculocutaneous upper eyelid flaps [109, 110], Z-plasties [111], microvascular free flaps [112], fat grafting [110, 113], and subperiosteal lifting of the midface [113]. However, despite the usefulness of these techniques, the presence of residual scars and contour deformities affects the satisfaction of the patients with surgery. In a study of the long-term effect of facial reconstruction in TCS, 67% of the operated patients wished further correction of the periocular area [114].

Tessier's Cleft Number 8

This defect was not well defined by Tessier. According to his original drawings, cleft number 8 begins at the lateral canthus and extends horizontally over the temporal fossa [46, 61]. However, as mentioned by Kawamoto [61], this type of anomaly is rarely seen as an isolated cleft (Fig. 64.17), and Tessier stated that it belonged to Goldenhar and Treacher Collins syndromes [46]. Subsequent authors have shared the same concept that the lateral canthal anomaly, usually a

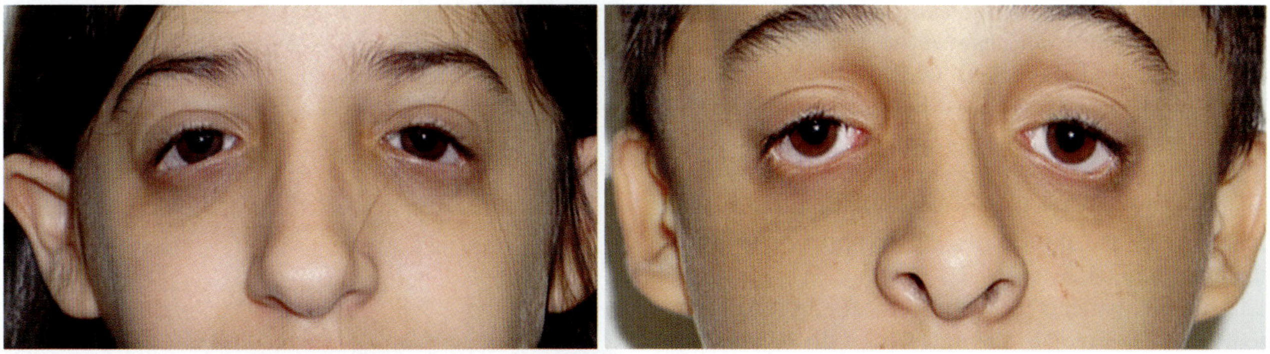

Fig. 64.16 Two siblings (dizygotic twins) with characteristic fissure findings of the Treacher Collins syndrome. A lateral notch on the lateral aspect of the lower eyelid, absence of lashes medial to the defect, absence of lower lacrimal punctum, and downward slant of the palpebral fissure

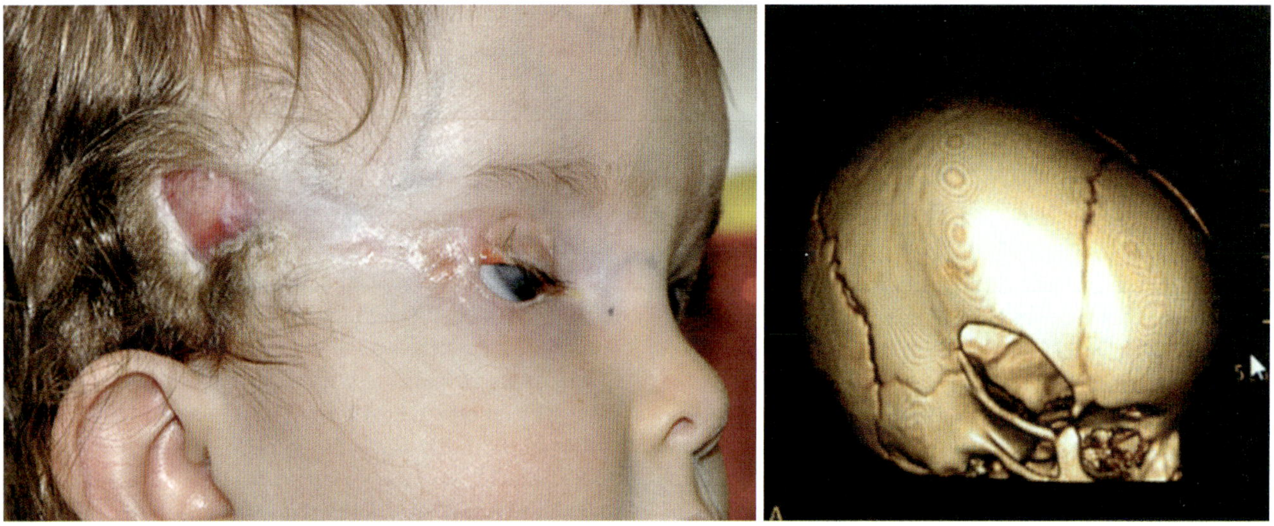

Fig. 64.17 Left: Clinical aspect of a lateral cleft extending from the lateral canthus to the temporal fossa. Right: Osseous defect of the cleft involving the lateral orbital rim and temporal and parietal bones

notch associated with an epibulbar choristoma on the lateral canthus, is a feature either of the Goldenhar or Treacher Collins syndrome [115, 116]. In a publication on cleft 8, all six cases described were examples of Goldenhar syndromes. The defects were characterized by dermolipomas on the lateral canthus adhered to the bulbar conjunctiva [117]. This type of defect can also be seen in rare neurocutaneous syndromes (Fig. 64.18).

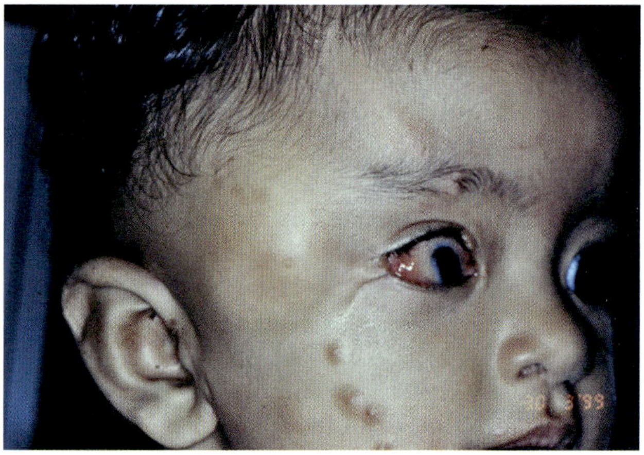

Fig. 64.18 Lateral canthal defect in a child with encephalocraniocutaneous lipomatosis. The lesion on the temporal fossa is a lipoma

Euryblepharon and Blepharocheilodontic Syndrome

Euryblepharon is a term used to describe a congenital bilateral and symmetrical enlargement of the palpebral fissure, especially laterally (Fig. 64.19). Most cases described are sporadic and of different etiology including Down syndrome [118]. In these patients with Down syndrome of the fissure is enlarged not only in the horizontal dimension but also vertically due to shortening of the anterior lamella of the upper lids. A variable degree of lower eyelid ectropion is often present [119–121].

Euryblepharon is an important feature of the blepharocheilodontic syndrome (BCD, OMIM 119580), an autosomal dominant condition caused by heterozygous mutations in two genes of the cadherin-catenin complex: CDH1 and CTNND1 [122]. The syndrome is characterized by abnormality in the lips (cleft lip/palate) and teeth (oligodontia, microdontia) and distichiasis, euryblepharon, and lagophthalmos (Figs. 64.20 and 64.21).

Although patients with the clinical signs and symptoms of BCD have been reported since the middle of the last century, the syndrome was recognized as a distinct condition by Korula in 1995 [123] and named by Gorlin in 1996 [124].

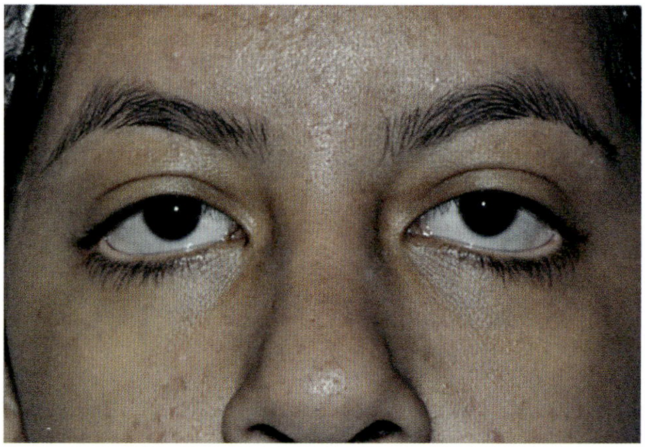

Fig. 64.19 Isolated euryblepharon. Notice the lateral lower lid ectropion and the increment on the width of the palpebral fissure

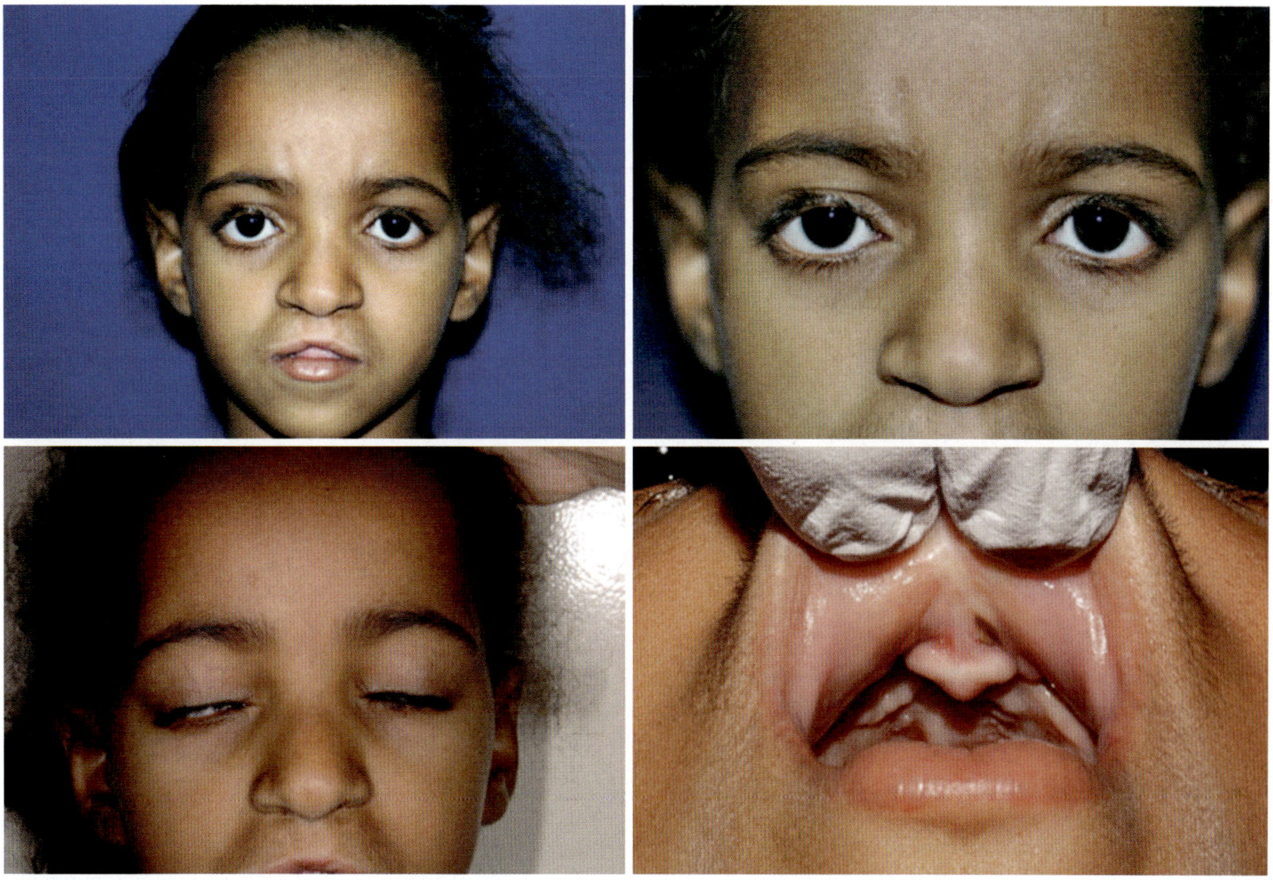

Fig. 64.20 Blepharocheilodontic syndrome: Top left, lip cleft and euryblepharon; right, segmental distichiasis; bottom left, mild lagophthalmos; right, hypodontia

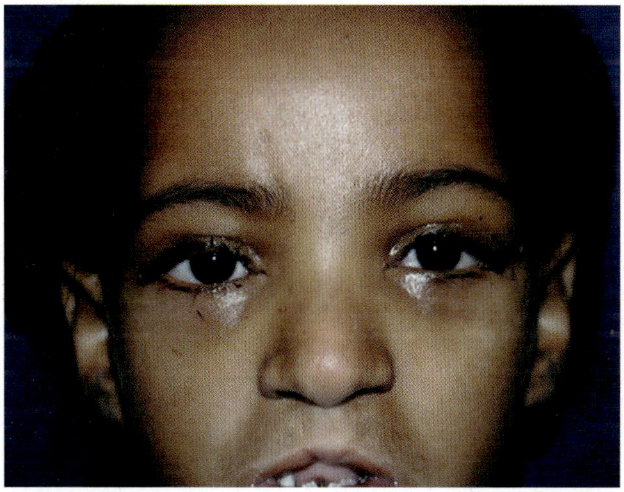

Fig. 64.21 Postoperative picture of the patient illustrated in Fig. 64.20

The ophthalmic literature on BCD syndrome is quite sparse. We are aware of just one article describing the correction of the fissure anomalies with lower eyelid retractor disinsertion, upper and lower lateral tarsal strips, myocutaneous advancement of the cheeks and eyelids, and lateral tarsorrhaphy [125]. The patient displayed in Fig. 64.17 was managed with a similar procedure (lower eyelid retractor and levator aponeurosis recession + midface lift).

Congenital Eyelid Malpositions

Upper Eyelid Eversion Associated with Lid Laxity

Congenital eversion of the upper eyelids is a relatively uncommon condition known since the nineteenth century [126]. Although the exact mechanism of this particular type of ectropion is not well established, the affected patients have lax upper lids which are everted with severe chemosis since birth. The lid eversion frequently occurs in both eyes [127–133], but the condition can be unilateral [128, 134]. Most cases are benign and successfully managed with conservative measures such as eyelid taping/patching, subconjunctival hyaluronidase injection, temporary lid sutures, and topical hypertonic saline instillation [128, 129, 135–138] (Fig. 64.22). Surgical treatment such as temporary tarsorrhaphy and excision of the redundant conjunctiva is rarely performed.

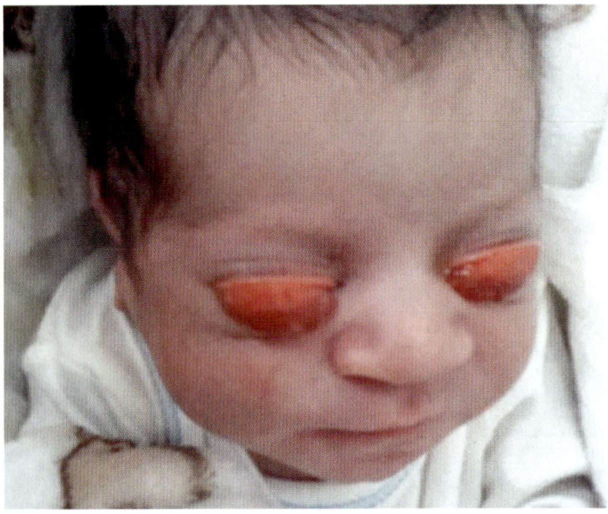

Fig. 64.22 Bilateral congenital eversion successfully corrected with patching. (Courtesy of Dr. Pedro Victorino Neto, Paraná, Brazil)

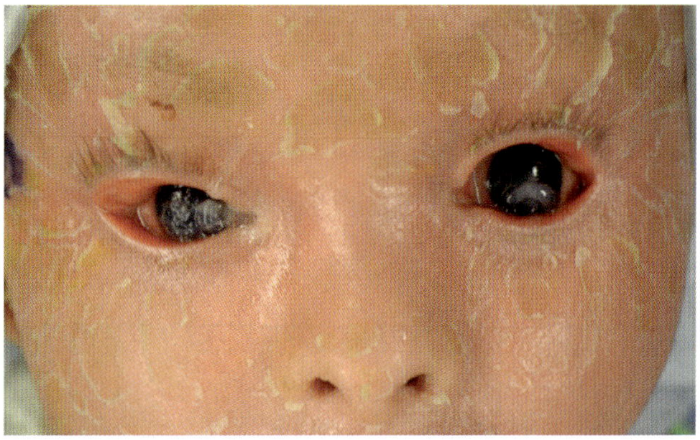

Fig. 64.23 Child with lamellar ichthyosis. The right eye was perforated before an upper eyelid lengthening could be performed

Eyelid Ectropion Associated with Anterior Lamella Shortening

The occurrence of congenital ectropion in Down syndrome is clearly caused by anterior lamella shortening, and skin grafts are required to reestablish a normal lid position [139, 140]. If harvesting a skin graft is not a problem in Down syndrome, in autosomal recessive congenital ichthyoses (ARCI), this task is not simple. ARCI is a heterogeneous group of non-syndromic disorders associated with mutations in at least 12 genes linked to lipid transportation to keratinocytes and lamellar granule formation [141]. This system is essential for the formation of the stratum corneum and the maintenance of skin barrier function [142]. Lamellar (LI) and especially Harlequin (HI) phenotypes are the most severe cases of ARCI. Harlequin patients are born encased in a dense colloidal membrane with extreme degrees of ectropion and eclabium causing a typical fishmouth appearance [143, 144]. They are at high risk for sepsis, respiratory failure, electrolyte imbalance, and temperature dysregulation. The availability of an intensive care unit is essential to avoid neonatal death [143].

The clinical picture is less severe in LI, but in both types, surgical lengthening of the upper eyelid anterior lamella may be necessary early in life (Fig. 64.23). Due to the generalized involvement of the disease, autogenous skin grafts may be difficult to harvest. Ectropion relief can be obtained with other types of tissues such as oral mucous membrane [145], engineered human skin [146], and a maternal skin allograft [147]. In our experience, whatever material is employed, graft contraction is a normal feature, and the patients need lifelong surveillance. Multiple procedures may be necessary to maintain adequate eye protection (Fig. 64.24).

Upper Eyelid Entropion

Congenital entropion of the upper eyelids is a rare condition reported in the literature as case reports or small case series. The affected children usually present with bilateral lid margin inversion, lacrimation, and keratitis due to continuous eyelash contact with the eye surface (Fig. 64.25). The condition is sporadically diagnosed in syndromic patients [148–153] or as a tarsal kink deformity in otherwise healthy children [154–160].

The mechanism responsible for the congenital horizontal deformation of the tarsal plate is not understood. Several hypotheses have been proposed to explain tarsal kinking [160] such as overaction of the orbicularis muscle, a primary tarsal defect, and direct mechanical pressure on the tarsus in utero with [155] or without disinsertion of the levator aponeurosis [159].

Probably due to the tarsal elasticity of the tarsal plate during childhood, congenital entropion has been successfully managed with different procedures [161] including anterior lamella reposition and lid crease reformation [159, 162], margin rotational operations [154, 157, 158], everting sutures [150, 151, 160], levator reinsertion + lid crease fixation [155], and temporary tarsorrhaphies [156, 163].

Eyelid Retraction

Primary congenital eyelid retraction is a diagnosis of exclusion. Only after a comprehensive examination, including measurement of thyroid-stimulating hormone receptor antibodies, orbital imaging and neuroimaging, and screening for congenital cranial dysinnervation disorders [164], can an upper or lower eyelid retraction be considered as an isolated primary anomaly. Prior to the widespread use of magnetic resonance imaging, scattered published cases of congenital upper eyelid retraction

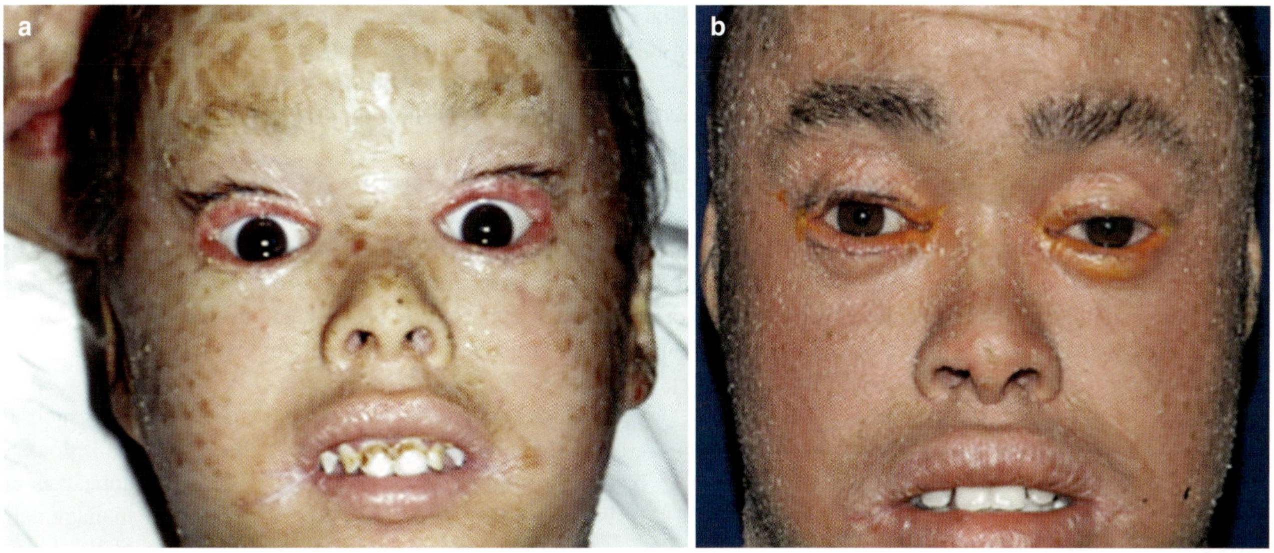

Fig. 64.24 (**a**) A child with marked upper eyelid ectropion. (**b**) Patient 12 years after two procedures performed in order to lengthen the upper lids

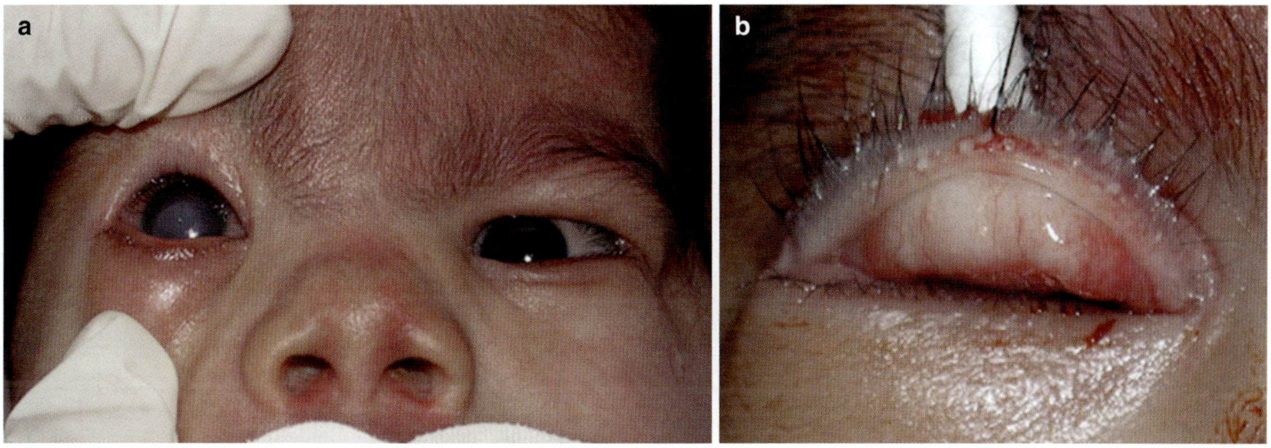

Fig. 64.25 (**a**) Bilateral tarsal kinking syndrome. Notice right corneal opacity. (**b**) The tarsal plate shows a groove parallel to the lid margin

were considered to be idiopathic [165–168]. More recent anatomical and clinical investigations have pointed out that some of these puzzling cases may be associated with abnormal orbital structures.

In 1990 Collins et al. published the largest series of congenital eyelid retraction [169]. In 19 patients the retraction affected the upper eyelid in 19 patients and the lower lid in 4. Surgical correction by an anterior or posterior approach was performed in 16 of the 19 patients with upper retraction and in all 4 patients with lower lid retraction. Since only 20% of the sample had symptoms or eye exposure and no systemic abnormalities were found in any patient, it was concluded that the condition was benign and did not require extensive investigation. No orbital imaging was performed in this series, and since three patients had strabismus with motility limitation, it is possible that some patients had congenital cranial dysinnervation disorders. More recently, Spierer and Bourla described four children with congenital upper lid retraction. No ocular or systemic anomalies could be detected, even when orbital imaging studies were performed [170].

The role of anatomic variations of the levator muscle in the pathogenesis of upper eyelid retraction has yet to be determined. Several anatomical studies have shown that in many orbits, there is a supernumerary muscle located medially to the medial border of the levator which inserts into the region of the trochlea. This muscle, also known as levator-trochlear, tensor levator-trochlear [171], gracillimus orbitis [172], accessory levator muscle of the upper eyelid [173], trochlea-levator tendon [174], and accessory levator muscle slips [175], is a vestigial structure found in 70% of the human fetuses [176]. The presence of the supernumerary levator muscle was well documented in at least one child with a congenital levator retraction. The patient reported by Wylen et al. [177] had unilateral lid retraction with a clear medial contour anomaly similar to that of the patient illustrated in Fig. 64.26.

Congenital eyelid retraction in downgaze in patients with full eye motility, lids normally positioned with normal contour and normal orbital imaging, is probably an atypical form of congenital dysinnervation disorder (Fig. 64.27).

Isolated congenital lower eyelid retraction is less frequent than retraction of the upper eyelid. Some case reports describing paradoxical lower eyelid retraction on upgaze have been described [178–180], and in one case, an abnormal muscle was identified as the cause of retraction [181].

Minor Deformities

Ankyloblepharon

It is well-known that during the fetal period, the lids are fused. The process of lid separation starts anteriorly and medially at 20 weeks and is completed at 32 weeks [182]. Extremely premature infants, at gestational ages between 19 and 28 weeks, are frequently born with fused eyelids, which spontaneously open within an average of 5.5 days of life [183].

Ankyloblepharon is a rare benign congenital anomaly characterized by adhesions between the upper and lower eyelids. When these adhesions are formed by fine bands of fibrovascular tissue, the condition is termed ankyloblepharon filiforme adnatum. According to Duke-Elder, this term was coined by Hasner in 1882 [184] (Fig. 64.28).

Ankyloblepharon may be part of a syndrome such as ankyloblepharon-ectodermal defects-cleft lip/palate (AEC) syndrome (OMIM 106260) [185] or appear as an isolated anomaly. In any case, its surgical management consists of only incision and cauterization of the tissue bands.

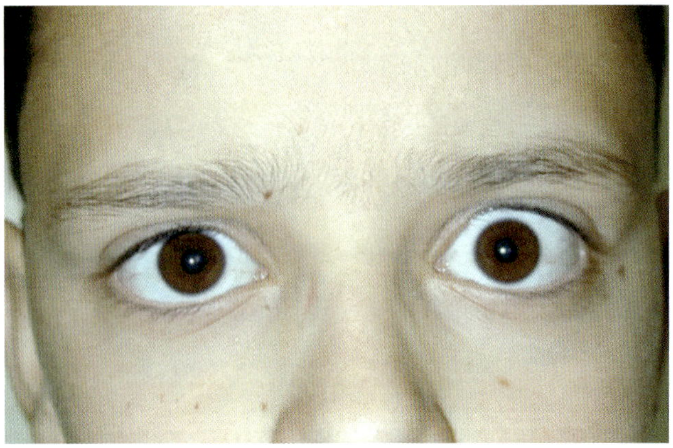

Fig. 64.26 Bilateral upper eyelid retraction more pronounced on the left eye. Notice the left medial contour abnormality

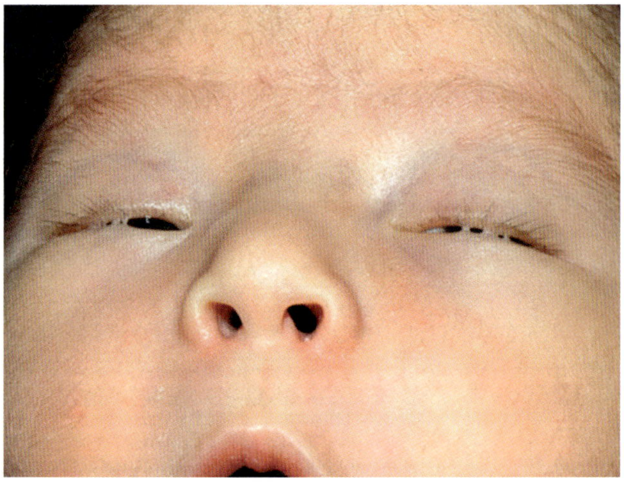

Fig. 64.28 Bilateral ankyloblepharon filiforme adnatum

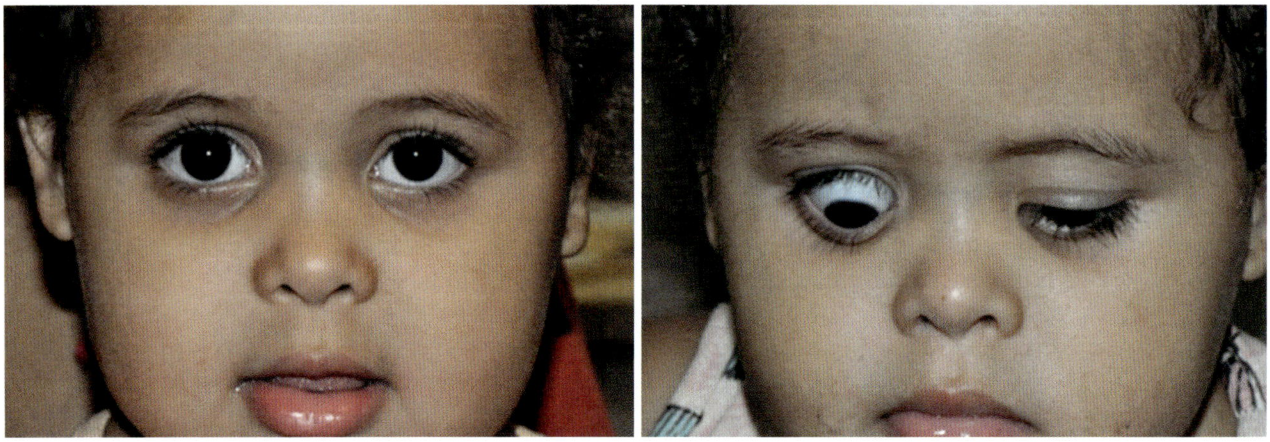

Fig. 64.27 Congenital upper eyelid retraction on downgaze

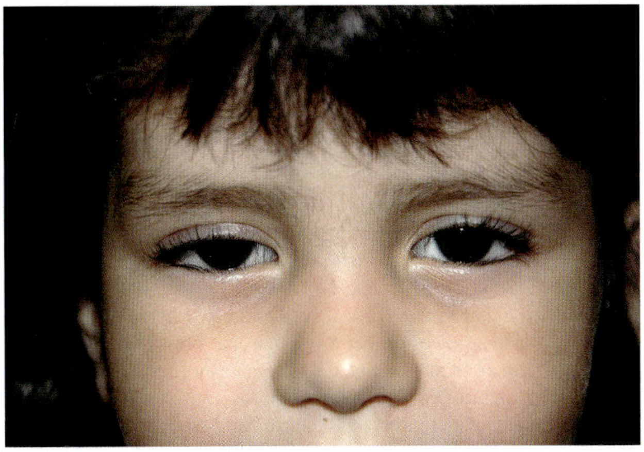

Fig. 64.29 Bilateral lower lid epiblepharon

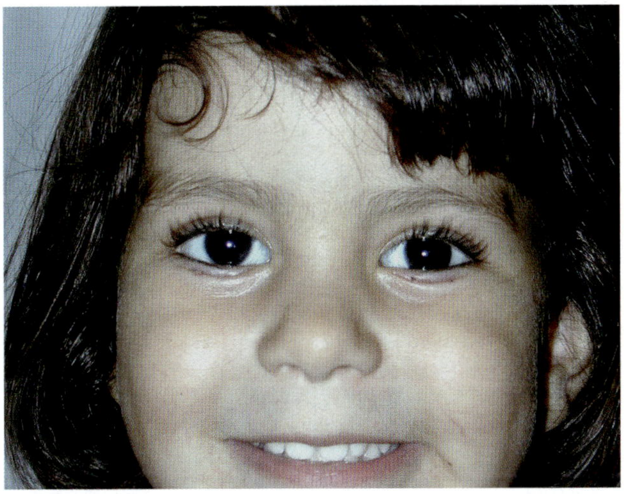

Fig. 64.30 Lower lid epiblepharon corrected with the Hotz procedure

Epiblepharon

Epiblepharon is a congenital upper or lower lid anomaly characterized by a horizontal fold of the anterior lamella running across the lid. The muscular-skin fold tends to overlap the lid margin inverting the lashes to the cornea. Epiblepharon should be differentiated from entropion. In the latter condition the whole margin is inverted, whereas in epiblepharon the position of the lid margin is normal (Fig. 64.29). Lower eyelid epiblepharon is a common feature of children of Asian descent. A Japanese study found a 46% prevalence of epiblepharon in infants [186].

The indication of surgical repair of epiblepharon should be individualized because not all affected children have complaints associated with keratopathy such as tearing, photophobia, discharge, ocular pain, and blurred vision, and the condition tends to spontaneously disappear with age [186]. Another important point is racial background and its standard concept of beauty. In Asians the creation of a lid crease with a skin-muscle resection (Hotz procedure) is not desirable [187], and a variety of techniques with minimal skin resection have been designed to simultaneously correct the epiblepharon and the epicanthal fold [188–190]. Non-incisional methods with everting sutures [191] and fillers [192] have also been advocated to correct mild degrees of epiblepharon.

If the creation of a crease on the lower eyelid might be problem in Asian children, in the Western population, a lower eyelid crease is totally acceptable and desirable because it is a normal feature of non-Asian children [193]. The old Hotz procedure is still a valid operation for Western patients (Fig. 64.30).

Acknowledgments We would like to thank Fernando Procianoy, Pedro Victorino Neto, and Jose-Luis Tovilla Canales for providing clinical documentation of their patients.

References

1. Thomas IT, Frias JL, Felix V, Sanchez de Leon L, Hernandez RA, Jones MC. Isolated and syndromic cryptophthalmos. Am J Med Genet. 1986;25(1):85–98.
2. Gattuso J, Patton MA, Baraitser M. The clinical spectrum of the Fraser syndrome: report of three new cases and review. J Med Genet. 1987;24(9):549–55.
3. Slavotinek AM, Tifft CJ. Fraser syndrome and cryptophthalmos: review of the diagnostic criteria and evidence for phenotypic modules in complex malformation syndromes. J Med Genet. 2002;39(9):623–33.
4. Comstock JM, Putnam AR, Opitz JM, Pysher TJ, Szakacs J. Prenatal death in Fraser syndrome. Fetal Pediatr Pathol. 2005;24(4–5):223–38.
5. Duke-Elder S. Cryptophthalmos. In: Duke-Elder S, editor. Textbook of ophthalmology the ocular Adnexa. V. London: Henry Kimpton; 1952. p. 4644–7.
6. Zinn S. Cryptophthalmia. Am J Ophthalmol. 1955;40(2):219–23.
7. Francois J. [Malformation syndrome with cryptophthalmos. (Preliminary report)]. Ophthalmologica. 1965;150(3):215–8.
8. Francois J. [Malformative syndrome with cryptophthalmos]. Acta Genet Med Gemellol (Roma). 1969;18(1):18–50.
9. Ding J, Hou Z, Li Y, Lu N, Li D. Eyelid and fornix reconstruction in abortive cryptophthalmos: a single-center experience over 12 years. Eye (Lond). 2017;31(11):1576–81.
10. Subramaniam N, Udhay P, Mahesh L. Prepucial skin graft for forniceal and socket reconstruction in complete cryptophthalmos with congenital cystic eye. Ophthalmic Plast Reconstr Surg. 2008;24(3):227–9.
11. Tawfik HA. Re: "Cryptophthalmos: reconstructive techniques–expanded classification of congenital symblepharon variant". Ophthalmic Plast Reconstr Surg. 2013;29(6):505–6.
12. Marles SL, Greenberg CR, Persaud TV, Shuckett EP, Chudley AE. New familial syndrome of unilateral upper eyelid coloboma, aberrant anterior hairline pattern, and anal anomalies in Manitoba Indians. Am J Med Genet. 1992;42(6):793–9.
13. Lee HM, Noh TK, Yoo HW, Kim SB, Won CH, Chang SE, et al. A wedge-shaped anterior hairline extension associated with a tessier number 10 cleft. Ann Dermatol. 2012;24(4):464–7.
14. Li C, Marles SL, Greenberg CR, Chodirker BN, van de Kamp J, Slavotinek A, et al. Manitoba Oculotrichoanal (MOTA) syndrome: report of eight new cases. Am J Med Genet A. 2007;143A(8):853–7.

15. van Haelst MM, Maiburg M, Baujat G, Jadeja S, Monti E, Bland E, et al. Molecular study of 33 families with Fraser syndrome new data and mutation review. Am J Med Genet A. 2008;146A(17):2252–7.
16. Nathanson J, Swarr DT, Singer A, Liu M, Chinn A, Jones W, et al. Novel FREM1 mutations expand the phenotypic spectrum associated with Manitoba-oculo-tricho-anal (MOTA) syndrome and bifid nose renal agenesis anorectal malformations (BNAR) syndrome. Am J Med Genet A. 2013;161A(3):473–8.
17. Mateo RK, Johnson R, Lehmann OJ. Evidence for additional FREM1 heterogeneity in Manitoba oculotrichoanal syndrome. Mol Vis. 2012;18:1301–11.
18. Slavotinek AM, Baranzini SE, Schanze D, Labelle-Dumais C, Short KM, Chao R, et al. Manitoba-oculo-tricho-anal (MOTA) syndrome is caused by mutations in FREM1. J Med Genet. 2011;48(6):375–82.
19. Yu Q, Lin B, Xie S, Gao S, Li W, Liu Y, et al. A homozygous mutation p.Arg2167Trp in FREM2 causes isolated cryptophthalmos. Hum Mol Genet. 2018;27(13):2357–66.
20. Saleh GM, Hussain B, Verity DH, Collin JR. A surgical strategy for the correction of Fraser syndrome cryptophthalmos. Ophthalmology. 2009;116(9):1707–12 e1.
21. Subramanian N, Iyer G, Srinivasan B. Cryptophthalmos: reconstructive techniques–expanded classification of congenital symblepharon variant. Ophthalmic Plast Reconstr Surg. 2013;29(4):243–8.
22. Mccarthy GT, West CM. Ablepharon macrostomia syndrome. Dev Med Child Neurol. 1977;19(5):659–63.
23. Marchegiani S, Davis T, Tessadori F, van Haaften G, Brancati F, Hoischen A, et al. Recurrent mutations in the basic domain of TWIST2 cause ablepharon macrostomia and Barber-Say syndromes. Am J Hum Genet. 2015;97(1):99–110.
24. Hornblass A, Reifler DM. Ablepharon macrostomia syndrome. Am J Ophthalmol. 1985;99(5):552–6.
25. Cesarino EJ, Pinheiro M, Freiremaia N, Meirasilva MC. Lid agenesis-macrostomia-psychomotor retardation forehead hypertrichosis – a new syndrome. Am J Med Genet. 1988;31(2):299–304.
26. Price NJ, Pugh RE, Farndon PA, Willshaw HE. Ablepharon macrostomia syndrome. Br J Ophthalmol. 1991;75(5):317–9.
27. Cruz AAV, Guimaraes FC, Obeid HN, Ferraz VEF, Noce TR, Martinez FE. Congenital shortening of the anterior lamella of all eyelids: the so-called ablepharon macrostomia syndrome. Ophthalmic Plast Rec. 1995;11(4):284–7.
28. Pellegrino JE, Schnur RE, BoghosianSell L, Strathdee G, Overhauser J, Spinner NB, et al. Ablepharon macrostomia syndrome with associated cutis laxa: possible localization to 18q. Hum Genet. 1996;97(4):532–6.
29. Cruz AAV, Souza CA, Ferraz VEF, Monteiro CAC, Martins FA. Familial occurrence of ablepharon macrostomia syndrome: eyelid structure and surgical considerations. Arch Ophthalmol Chic. 2000;118(3):428–30.
30. Stevens CA, Sargent LA. Ablepharon-macrostomia syndrome. Am J Med Genet. 2002;107(1):30–7.
31. Brancati F, Mingarelli R, Sarkozy A, Dallapiccola B. Ablepharon-macrostomia syndrome in a 46-year-old woman. Am J Med Genet A. 2004;127A(1):96–8.
32. Rohena L, Kuehn D, Marchegiani S, Higginson JD. Evidence for autosomal dominant inheritance of ablepharon-macrostomia syndrome. Am J Med Genet A. 2011;155A(4):850–4.
33. Feinstein E, Traish AS, Aakalu V, Kassem IS. A case report of ablepharon-macrostomia syndrome with amniotic membrane grafting. Case Rep Ophthalmol. 2015;6(3):366–72.
34. Hollanders K, Casteels I, Vandelanotte S, Reyniers R, Segers K, Nevens T, et al. Use of the masquerade flap in ablepharon-macrostomia syndrome: a case report. Cornea. 2018;37(7):929–32.
35. Barber N, Say B, Bell R, Merveille O. Macrostomia, ectropion, atrophic skin, hypertrichosis, and growth retardation. Syndr Ident. 1982;8(1):6–9.
36. De Maria B, Mazzanti L, Roche N, Hennekam RC. Barber-Say syndrome and ablepharon-macrostomia syndrome: an overview. Am J Med Genet A. 2016;170(8):1989–2001.
37. Martinez Santana S, Perez Alvarez F, Frias JL, Martinez-Frias ML. Hypertrichosis, atrophic skin, ectropion, and macrostomia (Barber-Say syndrome): report of a new case. Am J Med Genet. 1993;47(1):20–3.
38. Haensel J, Kohlschmidt N, Pitz S, Keilmann A, Zenker M, Ullmann R, et al. Case report supporting that the Barber-Say and ablepharon macrostomia syndromes could represent one disorder. Am J Med Genet A. 2009;149A(10):2236–40.
39. Singh A, Schanze D, Agarwal N, Prasad R, Mishra OP, Singh R, et al. Transmission of Barber-Say syndrome from a mosaic father to his child in an Indian family. Clin Dysmorphol. 2016;25(4):181–5.
40. Ng JD, Rajguru DS. Oculoplastic approach to treating Barber-Say syndrome. Ophthalmic Plast Reconstr Surg. 2006;22(3):232–4.
41. Barreiro-Gonzalez A, Barranco-Gonzalez H, Avino-Martinez J, Lopez Blanco E, Gutierrez Ontalvilla P, Evole-Buselli M. Multidisciplinary eyelid reconstruction in Barber-Say syndrome: a case report. Arch Soc Esp Oftalmol. 2019;94(4):196–9.
42. Zuazo F, Astiazaran MC, Rodriguez-Cabrera L, Garcia-Regil P, Chacon-Camacho O, Tovilla-Canales JL, et al. Clinical description, molecular analysis of TWIST2 gene, and surgical treatment in a patient with Barber-Say syndrome. Ophthalmic Plast Reconstr Surg. 2018;34(2):e61–e3.
43. Collin JR. Congenital upper lid coloboma. Aust N Z J Ophthalmol. 1986;14(4):313–7.
44. Nouby G. Congenital upper eyelid coloboma and cryptophthalmos. Ophthalmic Plast Reconstr Surg. 2002;18(5):373–7.
45. Tawfik HA, Abdulhafez MH, Fouad YA. Congenital upper eyelid coloboma: embryologic, nomenclatorial, nosologic, etiologic, pathogenetic, epidemiologic, clinical, and management perspectives. Ophthalmic Plast Reconstr Surg. 2015;31(1):1–12.
46. Tessier P. Anatomical classification facial, cranio-facial and latero-facial clefts. J Maxillofac Surg. 1976;4(2):69–92.
47. Fan X, Shao C, Fu Y, Zhou H, Lin M, Zhu H. Surgical management and outcome of tessier number 10 clefts. Ophthalmology. 2008;115(12):2290–4 e3.
48. Pereira FJ, Milbratz GH, Cruz AA, Vasconcelos JJ. Ophthalmic considerations in the management of Tessier cleft 5/9. Ophthalmic Plast Reconstr Surg. 2010;26(6):450–3.
49. Beleza-Meireles A, Clayton-Smith J, Saraiva JM, Tassabehji M. Oculo-auriculo-vertebral spectrum: a review of the literature and genetic update. J Med Genet. 2014;51(10):635–45.
50. Tasse C, Bohringer S, Fischer S, Ludecke HJ, Albrecht B, Horn D, et al. Oculo-auriculo-vertebral spectrum (OAVS): clinical evaluation and severity scoring of 53 patients and proposal for a new classification. Eur J Med Genet. 2005;48(4):397–411.
51. Rooryck C, Souakri N, Cailley D, Bouron J, Goizet C, Delrue MA, et al. Array-CGH analysis of a cohort of 86 patients with oculoauriculovertebral spectrum. Am J Med Genet A. 2010;152A(8):1984–9.
52. Russell-Eggitt IM, Blake KD, Taylor DS, Wyse RK. The eye in the CHARGE association. Br J Ophthalmol. 1990;74(7):421–6.
53. McMain K, Blake K, Smith I, Johnson J, Wood E, Tremblay F, et al. Ocular features of CHARGE syndrome. J AAPOS. 2008;12(5):460–5.
54. Nishina S, Kosaki R, Yagihashi T, Azuma N, Okamoto N, Hatsukawa Y, et al. Ophthalmic features of CHARGE syndrome with CHD7 mutations. Am J Med Genet A. 2012;158A(3):514–8.
55. Cruz AA, Schirmbeck T, Pina-Neto JM, Funayama CA. Cicatricial upper eyelid retraction in encephalocraniocutaneous lipomatosis: a report of two cases and review of literature. Ophthalmic Plast Reconstr Surg. 2002;18(2):151–5.
56. Kidwell ED, Tenzel RR. Repair of congenital colobomas of the lids. Arch Ophthalmol. 1979;97(10):1931–2.
57. Alexandridis E. A surgical technique for reconstruction of the upper and lower eyelid. Orbit. 1984;3:51–4.

58. Hashish A, Awara AM. One-stage reconstruction technique for large congenital eyelid coloboma. Orbit. 2011;30(4):177–9.
59. Malik A, Shah-Desai S. Sliding tarsal advancement flap for upper eyelid reconstruction. Orbit. 2014;33(2):124–6.
60. Toft PB. Reconstruction of large upper eyelid defects with a free tarsal plate graft and a myocutaneous pedicle flap plus a free skin graft. Orbit. 2016;35(1):1–5.
61. Kawamoto HK Jr. The kaleidoscopic world of rare craniofacial clefts: order out of chaos (Tessier classification). Clin Plast Surg. 1976;3(4):529–72.
62. da Silva FR, Alonso N, Busato L, Ueda WK, Hota T, Medeiros SH, et al. Oral-nasal-ocular cleft: the greatest challenge among the rare clefts. J Craniofac Surg. 2010;21(2):390–5.
63. Alonso N, Freitas Rda S, de Oliveira e Cruz GA, Goldenberg D, Dalloglio Tolazzi AR. Tessier no. 4 facial cleft: evolution of surgical treatment in a large series of patients. Plast Reconstr Surg. 2008;122(5):1505–13.
64. Prasanna M. Congenital accessory ectopic eyelid: case report. Br J Plast Surg. 1985;38(3):429–31.
65. Manudhane A, Arora R, Kapoor S, Rastogi A, Goyal JL. Congenital accessory palpebral aperture–an addition to the spectrum of Delleman syndrome. Ophthalmic Genet. 2013;34(1–2):109–11.
66. Bokman CL, Lo CC, Eichhorn K, Goldberg RA. Congenital accessory palpebral fissure and eyelid in a newborn: a case report. Ophthalmic Plast Reconstr Surg. 2018;34(4):e119–e21.
67. Duke-Elder S. Epicanthus. In: Duke-Elder S, editor. Text-book of ophthalmology the ocular adnexa. v. London: Henry Kimpton; 1952. p. 4653–61.
68. Johnson CC. Epicanthus and epiblepharon. Arch Ophthalmol. 1978;96(6):1030–3.
69. Johnson CC. Developmental abnormalities of the eyelids. The 1985 Wendell Hughes lecture. Ophthalmic Plast Reconstr Surg. 1986;2(4):219–32.
70. Mustarde JC. Epicanthus and telecanthus. Br J Plast Surg. 1963;16:346–56.
71. Saonanon P. The new focus on epicanthoplasty for Asian eyelids. Curr Opin Ophthalmol. 2016;27(5):457–64.
72. Mustarde J. Epicanthal folds and the problem of telecanthus. Trans Ophthalmol Soc U K. 1963;83:397–411.
73. Pingault V, Ente D, Dastot-Le Moal F, Goossens M, Marlin S, Bondurand N. Review and update of mutations causing Waardenburg syndrome. Hum Mutat. 2010;31(4):391–406.
74. Read AP, Newton VE. Waardenburg syndrome. J Med Genet. 1997;34(8):656–65.
75. Vignes M. Epicanthus héréditaire. Recueil d'Ophthalmologie. 1889:422–5.
76. Crisponi L, Deiana M, Loi A, Chiappe F, Uda M, Amati P, et al. The putative forkhead transcription factor FOXL2 is mutated in blepharophimosis/ptosis/epicanthus inversus syndrome. Nat Genet. 2001;27(2):159–66.
77. Heude E, Bellessort B, Fontaine A, Hamazaki M, Treier AC, Treier M, et al. Etiology of craniofacial malformations in mouse models of blepharophimosis, ptosis and epicanthus inversus syndrome. Hum Mol Genet. 2015;24(6):1670–81.
78. Zlotogora J, Sagi M, Cohen T. The blepharophimosis, ptosis, and epicanthus inversus syndrome: delineation of two types. Am J Hum Genet. 1983;35(5):1020–7.
79. Allen CE, Rubin PA. Blepharophimosis-ptosis-epicanthus inversus syndrome (BPES): clinical manifestation and treatment. Int Ophthalmol Clin. 2008;48(2):15–23.
80. Athappilly GK, Braverman RS. Congenital alacrima in a patient with blepharophimosis syndrome. Ophthalmic Genet. 2009;30(1):37–9.
81. Chawla B, Bhadange Y, Dada R, Kumar M, Sharma S, Bajaj MS, et al. Clinical, radiologic, and genetic features in blepharophimosis, ptosis, and epicanthus inversus syndrome in the Indian population. Invest Ophthalmol Vis Sci. 2013;54(4):2985–91.
82. Choi KH, Kyung S, Oh SY. The factors influencing visual development in blepharophimosis-ptosis-epicanthus inversus syndrome. J Pediatr Ophthalmol Strabismus. 2006;43(5):285–8.
83. Dawson EL, Hardy TG, Collin JR, Lee JP. The incidence of strabismus and refractive error in patients with blepharophimosis, ptosis and epicanthus inversus syndrome (BPES). Strabismus. 2003;11(3):173–7.
84. Garden JW. Blepharophimosis, ptosis, epicanthus inversus and lacrimal stenosis. Am J Ophthalmol. 1969;67(1):153–4.
85. Kohn R, Romano PE. Blepharoptosis, blepharophimosis, epicanthus inversus, and telecanthus–a syndrome with no name. Am J Ophthalmol. 1971;72(3):625–32.
86. Ng JK, Stout AU, Aaby AA, Ng JD. Blepharophimosis syndrome with absent tear production. Ophthal Plast Reconstr Surg. 2015;31(3):e62.
87. Duarte AF, Akaishi PM, de Molfetta GA, Chodraui-Filho S, Cintra M, Toscano A, et al. Lacrimal gland involvement in blepharophimosis-ptosis-epicanthus inversus syndrome. Ophthalmology. 2017;124(3):399–406.
88. Cho BC, Lee KY. Medial epicanthoplasty combined with plication of the medial canthal tendon in Asian eyelids. Plast Reconstr Surg. 2002;110(1):293–300; discussion 1.
89. Kao YS, Lin CH, Fang RH. Epicanthoplasty with modified Y-V advancement procedure. Plast Reconstr Surg. 1998;102(6):1835–41.
90. Lee Y, Lee E, Park WJ. Anchor epicanthoplasty combined with out-fold type double eyelid plasty for Asians: do we have to make an additional scar to correct the Asian epicanthal fold? Plast Reconstr Surg. 2000;105(5):1872–80.
91. Lee YJ, Baek RM, Song YT, Chung WJ, Lee JH. Periciliary Y-V epicanthoplasty. Ann Plast Surg. 2006;56(3):274–8.
92. Park JI. Modified Z-epicanthoplasty in the Asian eyelid. Arch Facial Plast Surg. 2000;2(1):43–7.
93. Wang G, Zhang S, Ma J, Li D, Xue H. Cosmetic and structural outcomes of two different techniques of medial epicanthoplasty according to epicanthal fold classification and severity: a cohort study. J Plast Reconstr Aesthet Surg. 2018;71(10):1453–61.
94. Yoo WM, Park SH, Kwag DR. Root z-epicanthoplasty in asian eyelids. Plast Reconstr Surg. 2002;109(6):2067–71; discussion 72–3.
95. Zan T, Jin R, Li H, Herrler T, Meng X, Huang X, et al. A novel U-flap epicanthoplasty for Asian patients. Aesthet Plast Surg. 2016;40(4):458–65.
96. Zhang H, Zhuang H, Yu H, Feng Y, Wang T, Hu S, et al. A new Z-epicanthoplasty and a concomitant double eyelidplasty in Chinese eyelids. Plast Reconstr Surg. 2006;118(4):900–7.
97. Zhang S, Xue HY. Adjustable V-flap epicanthoplasty based on desired eyelid morphology. Aesthet Plast Surg. 2018;42(6):1571–5.
98. Hwang K, Kim H. Historical vignettes of epicanthoplasty. J Craniofac Surg. 2016;27(4):1080–3.
99. Oh YW, Seul CH, Yoo WM. Medial epicanthoplasty using the skin redraping method. Plast Reconstr Surg. 2007;119(2):703–10.
100. Sa HS, Lee JH, Woo KI, Kim YD. A new method of medial epicanthoplasty for patients with blepharophimosis-ptosis-epicanthus inversus syndrome. Ophthalmology. 2012;119(11):2402–7.
101. Vincent M, Genevieve D, Ostertag A, Marlin S, Lacombe D, Martin-Coignard D, et al. Treacher Collins syndrome: a clinical and molecular study based on a large series of patients. Genet Med. 2016;18(1):49–56.
102. Poswillo D. The pathogenesis of the Treacher Collins syndrome (mandibulofacial dysostosis). Br J Oral Surg. 1975;13(1):1–26.
103. Duke-Elder S. Mandibulo-facial dysostosis. In: Duke-Elder S, editor. Text book of ophthalmology. The ocular adnexa. London: Henry Kimptom; 1952. p. 4720–7.
104. Bartley GB. Lacrimal drainage anomalies in mandibulofacial dysostosis. Am J Ophthalmol. 1990;109(5):571–4.

105. Wang FM, Millman AL, Sidoti PA, Goldberg RB. Ocular findings in Treacher Collins syndrome. Am J Ophthalmol. 1990;110(3):280–6.
106. Bachelor EP, Kaplan EN. Absence of the lateral canthal tendon in the Treacher-Collins syndrome. Br J Plast Surg. 1981;34(2):162–4.
107. Levasseur J, Nysjo J, Sandy R, Britto JA, Garcelon N, Haber S, et al. Orbital volume and shape in Treacher Collins syndrome. J Craniomaxillofac Surg. 2018;46(2):305–11.
108. Posnick JC, Ruiz RL. Treacher Collins syndrome: current evaluation, treatment, and future directions. Cleft Palate Craniofac J. 2000;37(5):434.
109. Jackson IT. Reconstruction of the lower eyelid defect in Treacher Collins syndrome. Plast Reconstr Surg. 1981;67(3):365–8.
110. Mitsukawa N, Saiga A, Satoh K. Changing the facial features of patients with Treacher Collins syndrome: protocol for 3-stage treatment of hard and soft tissue hypoplasia in the upper half of the face. Ann Plast Surg. 2014;73(1):39–42.
111. Kobus K, Wojcicki P. Surgical treatment of Treacher Collins syndrome. Ann Plast Surg. 2006;56(5):549–54.
112. Saadeh P, Reavey PL, Siebert JW. A soft-tissue approach to midfacial hypoplasia associated with Treacher Collins syndrome. Ann Plast Surg. 2006;56(5):522–5.
113. Franchi G, Kadlub N, Diner PA, Bandini M, Vazquez MP, Picard A. Orbital soft tissue surgery for patients with Treacher-Collins or Nager syndrome. A new surgical approach with early correction of soft tissue: prospective study. Br J Oral Maxillofac Surg. 2015;53(5):421–5.
114. Plomp RG, Versnel SL, van Lieshout MJ, Poublon RM, Mathijssen IM. Long-term assessment of facial features and functions needing more attention in treatment of Treacher Collins syndrome. J Plast Reconstr Aesthet Surg. 2013;66(8):e217–26.
115. David DJ, Moore MH, Cooter RD. Tessier clefts revisited with a third dimension. Cleft Palate J. 1989;26(3):163–84; discussion 84–5.
116. Fries PD, Katowitz JA. Congenital craniofacial anomalies of ophthalmic importance. Surv Ophthalmol. 1990;35(2):87–119.
117. Lessa S, Sebastia R, Pontello J. Lateral canthal clefts of the eyelid. Ophthalmic Plast Reconstr Surg. 2019;35(5):491–4.
118. Markowitz GD, Handler LF, Katowitz JA. Congenital euryblepharon and nasolacrimal anomalies in a patient with Down syndrome. J Pediatr Ophthalmol Strabismus. 1994;31(5):330–1.
119. Betharia SM, Dayal Y, Nayar RC. Euryblepharon. Indian J Ophthalmol. 1984;32(1):41–3.
120. D'Esposito M, Magli A, Del Prete A. Genetic study and surgical correction of euryblepharon. Ophthalmologica. 1979;178(6):396–403.
121. Gupta JS, Kumar K. Euryblepharon with ectropion. Am J Ophthalmol. 1968;66(3):554–5.
122. Kievit A, Tessadori F, Douben H, Jordens I, Maurice M, Hoogeboom J, et al. Variants in members of the cadherin-catenin complex, CDH1 and CTNND1, cause blepharocheilodontic syndrome. Eur J Hum Genet. 2018;26(2):210–9.
123. Korula S, Wilson L, Salomonson J. Distinct craniofacial syndrome of lagophthalmia and bilateral cleft lip and palate. Am J Med Genet. 1995;59(2):229–33.
124. Gorlin RJ, Zellweger H, Curtis MW, Wiedemann HR, Warburg M, Majewski F, et al. Blepharo-cheilo-dontic (BCD) syndrome. Am J Med Genet. 1996;65(2):109–12.
125. Yen MT, Lucci LM, Anderson RL. Management of eyelid anomalies associated with Blepharo-cheilo-dontic syndrome. Am J Ophthalmol. 2001;132(2):279–80.
126. Adams A. A case of double congenital ectropion. Med Fortnightly. 1896;9:137–8.
127. Young R. Congenital Ectropion of the upper lids. Arch Dis Child. 1954;29:97–100.
128. Bentsi-Enchill KO. Congenital total eversion of the upper eyelids. Br J Ophthalmol. 1981;65(3):209–13.
129. Fasina O. Management of bilateral congenital upper eyelid eversion with severe chemosis. J Ophthalmic Vis Res. 2013;8(2):175–8.
130. Cingu AK, Sahin A, Yuksel H, Ozkok A, Ari S, Caca I. Congenital bilateral upper eyelid eversion: report of a case. Semin Ophthalmol. 2014;29(1):36–8.
131. Ibraheem WA. Bilateral congenital upper eyelid eversion: the clinical course and outcome of conservative management. Pan Afr Med J. 2014;17:215.
132. Chinmayee J, Nagaraju G, Samhitha H, Kailash PC. Congenital eyelid eversion- a case report with review of literature. J Evid Based Med. 2015;2:1534–9.
133. Kirkpatrick A, Ledlow D, Dixon E, Philips JB. Congenital bilateral eyelid eversion and chemosis: a case study. Neonatal Netw. 2018;37(3):137–40.
134. Shinder R, Langer PD. Unilateral congenital eyelid eversion causing marked chemosis in a newborn. J Pediatr Ophthalmol Strabismus. 2011;48 Online:e1–2.
135. Stern EN, Campbell CH, Faulkner HW. Conservative management of congenital eversion of the eyelids. Am J Ophthalmol. 1973;75(2):319–20.
136. Watts MT, Dapling RB. Congenital eversion of the upper eyelid: a case report. Ophthalmic Plast Reconstr Surg. 1995;11(4):293–5.
137. Isawumi MA, Adeoti CO, Umar IO, Oluwatimilehin IO, Raji RA. Congenital bilateral eversion of the eyelids. J Pediatr Ophthalmol Strabismus. 2008;45(6):371–3.
138. Adeoti CO, Ashaye AO, Isawumi MA, Raji RA. Non-surgical management of congenital eversion of the eyelids. J Ophthalmic Vis Res. 2010;5(3):188–92.
139. Al-Hussain H, Al-Rajhi AA, Al-Qahtani S, Meyer D. Congenital upper eyelid eversion complicated by corneal perforation. Br J Ophthalmol. 2005;89(6):771.
140. Alvarez EV, Wakakura M, Alvarez EI. Surgical management of persistent congenital eversion of the upper eyelids. Ann Ophthalmol. 1988;20(9):353–4, 7.
141. Akiyama M. Pathomechanisms of harlequin ichthyosis and ABCA transporters in human diseases. Arch Dermatol. 2006;142(7):914–8.
142. Lima Cunha D, Alakloby OM, Gruber R, Kakar N, Ahmad J, Alawbathani S, et al. Unknown mutations and genotype/phenotype correlations of autosomal recessive congenital ichthyosis in patients from Saudi Arabia and Pakistan. Mol Genet Genomic Med. 2019;7(3):e539.
143. Glick JB, Craiglow BG, Choate KA, Kato H, Fleming RE, Siegfried E, et al. Improved management of harlequin ichthyosis with advances in neonatal intensive care. Pediatrics. 2017;139(1)
144. Chua CN, Ainsworth J. Ocular management of harlequin syndrome. Arch Ophthalmol. 2001;119(3):454–5.
145. Nayak S, Rath S, Kar BR. Mucous membrane graft for cicatricial ectropion in lamellar ichthyosis: an approach revisited. Ophthalmic Plast Reconstr Surg. 2011;27(6):e155–6.
146. Culican SM, Custer PL. Repair of cicatricial ectropion in an infant with harlequin ichthyosis using engineered human skin. Am J Ophthalmol. 2002;134(3):442–3.
147. Das S, Honavar SG, Dhepe N, Naik MN. Maternal skin allograft for cicatricial ectropion in congenital ichthyosis. Ophthalmic Plast Reconstr Surg. 2010;26(1):42–3.
148. Al-Faky YH, Salih MA, Mubarak M, Al-Rikabi AC. Bilateral congenital entropion with cutis laxa. Pediatr Dermatol. 2014;31(3):e82–4.
149. Amacher AG 3rd, Mazzoli RA, Gilbert BN, Hansen EA, Parmley VC, Ainbinder DJ, et al. Dominant familial congenital entropion with tarsal hypoplasia and atrichosis. Ophthalmic Plast Reconstr Surg. 2002;18(5):381–4.

150. Lucci LM, Fukumoto WK, Alvarenga LS. Trisomy 13: a rare case of congenital tarsal kink. Ophthalmic Plast Reconstr Surg. 2003;19(5):408–10.
151. Warner NJ, Wasserman BN, Lai YH. Bedside repair of congenital upper eyelid entropion: a variation of the Quickert suture technique. Am J Ophthalmol Case Rep. 2016;4:57–9.
152. Yazici B. Another case of neonatal progeroid syndrome and bilateral congenital upper eyelid entropion. Ophthalmic Plast Reconstr Surg. 2014;30(4):356–7.
153. Yazici B, Toka F, Comez AT. Anatomical characteristics and surgical treatment of bilateral congenital upper eyelid entropion in an infant with neonatal progeroid syndrome. Ophthalmic Plast Reconstr Surg. 2014;30(6):e164–6.
154. Biglan AW, Buerger GF Jr. Congenital horizontal tarsal kink. Am J Ophthalmol. 1980;89(4):522–4.
155. Dailey RA, Harrison AR, Hildebrand PL, Wobig JL. Levator aponeurosis disinsertion in congenital entropion of the upper eyelid. Ophthalmic Plast Reconstr Surg. 1999;15(5):360–2.
156. Demirel S, Firat C, Firat PG. Modified temporary eyelid margin suture for correction of congenital horizontal tarsal kink: a novel surgical technique. Ophthalmic Plast Reconstr Surg. 2012;28(4):300–2.
157. Firat T, Ozkan S. Bilateral congenital entropion of the upper eyelids. Br J Ophthalmol. 1973;57(10):753–4.
158. Naik MN, Honavar SG, Bhaduri A, Linberg JV. Congenital horizontal tarsal kink: a single-center experience with 6 cases. Ophthalmology. 2007;114(8):1564–8.
159. Unal M, Tunc M, Konuk O. Severe congenital horizontal tarsal kink without levator aponeurosis disinsertion. Ophthalmic Plast Reconstr Surg. 2003;19(1):79–81.
160. Vahdani K, Konstantinidis A, Thaller VT. A simple new technique for treatment of tarsal kink syndrome. Ophthalmic Plast Reconstr Surg. 2017;33(3S Suppl 1):S77–S9.
161. Sires BS. Congenital horizontal tarsal kink: clinical characteristics from a large series. Ophthalmic Plast Reconstr Surg. 1999;15(5):355–9.
162. Price NC, Collin JR. Congenital horizontal tarsal kink: a simple surgical correction. Br J Ophthalmol. 1987;71(3):204–6.
163. Pushker N, Meel R, Kaushal S, Bajaj MS, Mehta M, Lohia P. Congenital horizontal tarsal kink with microphthalmos corrected by intermarginal suture tarsorrhaphy. J Pediatr Ophthalmol Strabismus. 2010;47(1):51–3.
164. Stout AU, Borchert M. Etiology of eyelid retraction in children: a retrospective study. J Pediatr Ophthalmol Strabismus. 1993;30(2):96–9.
165. Leone CR Jr, Lewis R. Congenital upper eyelid retraction. J Pediatr Ophthalmol. 1976;13(6):350–2.
166. Ballen PH, Rochkopf L. Congenital retraction of the upper lid. Ophthalmic Surg. 1987;18(9):689–90.
167. Rovit AJ, Deupree DM, Zang YF, Biglan AW. Treatment of congenital unilateral upper eyelid retraction with a marginal myotomy procedure. Ophthalmic Surg. 1988;19(12):872–5.
168. Senyuva C, Yucel A, Yildirim I. Congenital upper eyelid retraction treated with gold weight implantation. Plast Reconstr Surg. 1997;99(7):2099–100.
169. Collin JR, Allen L, Castronuovo S. Congenital eyelid retraction. Br J Ophthalmol. 1990;74(9):542–4.
170. Spierer A, Bourla N. Primary congenital upper eyelid retraction in infants and children. Ophthalmic Plast Reconstr Surg. 2004;20(3):246–8.
171. Sacks JG. The levator-trochlear muscle. A supernumerary orbital structure. Arch Ophthalmol. 1985;103(4):540–1.
172. Jordan DR, Stoica B. The gracillimus orbitis muscle. Ophthalmic Plast Reconstr Surg. 2017;33(5):e120–e2.
173. Amonoo-Kuofi HS, Darwish HH. Accessory levator muscle of the upper eyelid: case report and review of the literature. Clin Anat. 1998;11(6):410–6.
174. Bartley GB. An anomalous trochlea-levator "tendon" observed during congenital blepharoptosis surgery. Ophthalmic Plast Reconstr Surg. 1989;5(4):288–90.
175. Yamaguchi K, Imai K, Fujimoto T, Takahashi M, Maruyama Y. Cosmetic comparison between the modified uchida method and the mustarde method for blepharophimosis-ptosis-epicanthus inversus syndrome. Ann Plast Surg. 2015;75(5):518–21.
176. Plock J, Contaldo C, von Ludinghausen M. Levator palpebrae superioris muscle in human fetuses: anatomical findings and their clinical relevance. Clin Anat. 2005;18(7):473–80.
177. Wylen EL, Brown MS, Rich LS, Hesse RJ. Supernumerary orbital muscle in congenital eyelid retraction. Ophthalmic Plast Reconstr Surg. 2001;17(2):120–2.
178. Yee RD, Odeh-Nasrala N. Congenital, paradoxical retraction of the lower eyelid. Am J Ophthalmol. 1974;78(6):1027–9.
179. Klapper SR, Jordan DR. Congenital, paradoxical lower eyelid retraction on upgaze. Ophthalmic Plast Reconstr Surg. 1999;15(2):100–5.
180. Mee JJ, McNab AA. Congenital retraction of the lower eyelid: two case reports. Ophthalmic Plast Reconstr Surg. 2002;18(1):75–8.
181. Richardson DR, Gadzala LA, Bonsall DJ, Hogg JP, Williams HJ, Nguyen J. Congenital paradoxical lower eyelid retraction with upgaze due to an anomalous extraocular muscle. Ophthalmic Plast Reconstr Surg. 2017;33(4):e101–e2.
182. Tawfik HA, Abdulhafez MH, Fouad YA, Dutton JJ. Embryologic and fetal development of the human eyelid. Ophthalmic Plast Reconstr Surg. 2016;32(6):407–14.
183. Duerksen K, Barlow WE, Stasior OG. Fused eyelids in premature infants. Ophthalmic Plast Reconstr Surg. 1994;10(4):234–40.
184. Duke-Elder S. Ankyloblepharon. In: Duke-Elder S, editor. Textbook of ophthalmology the ocular Adnexa. V. London: Henry Kimpton; 1952. p. 4664–466.
185. Guo S, Chen R, Xu Y, Mu Y, Chen L. Ankyloblepharon-ectodermal defects-cleft lip/palate syndrome. J Craniofac Surg. 2017;28(4):e349–e51.
186. Noda S, Hayasaka S, Setogawa T. Epiblepharon with inverted eyelashes in Japanese children. I. Incidence and symptoms. Br J Ophthalmol. 1989;73(2):126–7.
187. Woo KI, Kim YD. Management of epiblepharon: state of the art. Curr Opin Ophthalmol. 2016;27(5):433–8.
188. Ni J, Shao C, Wang K, Chen X, Zhou S, Lin H. Modified Hotz procedure combined with modified Z-epicanthoplasty versus modified hotz procedure alone for epiblepharon repair. Ophthalmic Plast Reconstr Surg. 2017;33(2):120–3.
189. Sung Y, Lew H. Epiblepharon correction in Korean children based on the epicanthal pathology. Graefes Arch Clin Exp Ophthalmol. 2019;257(4):821–6.
190. Jung JH, Kim HK, Choi HY. Epiblepharon correction combined with skin redraping epicanthoplasty in children. J Craniofac Surg. 2011;22(3):1024–6.
191. Seo JW, Kang S, Ahn C, Esmaeli B, Sa HS. Non-incisional eyelid everting suture technique for treating lower lid epiblepharon. Br J Ophthalmol. 2018;102(11):1504–9.
192. Naik MN, Pujari A, Ali MJ, Kaliki S, Dave TV. Nonsurgical correction of epiblepharon using hyaluronic acid gel. J AAPOS. 2018;22(3):179–82 e1.
193. Paiva RS, Minare-Filho AM, Cruz AA. Palpebral fissures changes in early childhood. J Pediatr Ophthalmol Strabismus. 2001;38(4):219–23.

Specific Issues in Pediatric Periocular Trauma

65

Ann P. Murchison and Jurij R. Bilyk

Introduction

Ocular and periocular injuries can cause significant morbidity. Periocular injuries occur in 5% of all serious injuries, according to the United States Eye Injury Registry, and the majority of these involve the canaliculus (81%) and/or eyelid (70%) [1]. Not surprisingly, many of these injuries occur in young children (23% in 0–9 years old) and older children/teenagers (18% in 10–19 years old). The management of periocular and orbital trauma is covered in detail elsewhere in this tome. The goal of this chapter is to address four issues of trauma that affect children in unique ways:

1. Periocular canine injuries.
2. Pediatric orbital fractures, especially white-eyed blowout fractures.
3. The use of computed tomography (CT) in children.
4. Orbital foreign bodies and their management.

Pediatric Periocular Dog Bite Injuries

Over one million Americans are bitten by dogs each year, leading to more than 330,000 emergency room visits, 13,000 hospitalizations, and 10 to 20 deaths, mostly among children [2]. These attacks are very costly and result in over $100 million in medical bills and approximately $400 million in associated insurance claims each year (www.iii.org/media/hottopics/insurance/dogbite) [3]. At least half of all dog bite injuries occur on the dog owner's property (www.iii.org/media/hottopics/insurance/dogbite).

Estimates show that over 50% of all children have been bitten by a dog at some point in their lives and that the majority of dog bite victims are young children (50–70%) [4, 5]. This can be attributed to many factors, including the unpredictable behavior of children, the close proximity of critical body parts to the animal, reduced ability to defend when attacked, and the breed and size of the dog [6, 7]. One large study of ophthalmic injuries secondary to dog bites found that pit bulls were the most common breed (25% overall and in 63% of attacks by strangers' dogs) and the most likely to cause complex periocular injury, and the dog involved was most commonly the patient's or neighbor's pet (90–93%) [7, 8]. Two large studies found that 97–99% of patients with ocular/periocular dog bite injuries had eyelid lacerations, with a 20–40% incidence of canalicular involvement; only 0–2% suffered a ruptured globe [7, 8]. Facial fractures are distinctly uncommon following dog bites, occurring in only 1.4–5.7% in two large studies, but are more common with injuries involving larger dogs, eyelid lacerations, severe soft tissue injury, and younger children [7–11].

The incidence rates of dog attacks are highest among children 9 years of age and younger, and over 70% of the injuries involve the face, head, and neck, with one in six involving the ocular adnexa [2, 7, 12]. Commonly associated with these areas of injury is trauma to the periocular area, leading to lacerations of the eyelid with potential for orbital fractures in 1.4% patients and more commonly damage to the canalicular system (Fig. 65.1) [11]. In one study, dog bites accounted for 40% of all canalicular laceration in children [12]. The canalicular system is particularly susceptible to injury [13] secondary to a dog bite for two reasons. First, the animal instinctively attempts to grab its victim by the snout, and the dog's incisors directly lacerate the medial canthus and canaliculus, often bilaterally. This is type of direct

A. P. Murchison (✉)
Associate Professor of Ophthalmology, Oculoplastic and Orbital Surgery Service and Director of Eye Emergency Room, Wills Eye Hospital and Thomas Jefferson University Hospital, Philadelphia, PA, USA
e-mail: amuchison@willseye.org

J. R. Bilyk
Attending Surgeon and Professor of Ophthalmology, Oculoplastic and Orbital Surgery Service, Wills Eye Hospital and Thomas Jefferson University Hospital, Philadelphia, PA, USA

J. J. Servat et al. (eds.), *Smith and Nesi's Ophthalmic Plastic and Reconstructive Surgery*,
https://doi.org/10.1007/978-3-030-41720-8_65

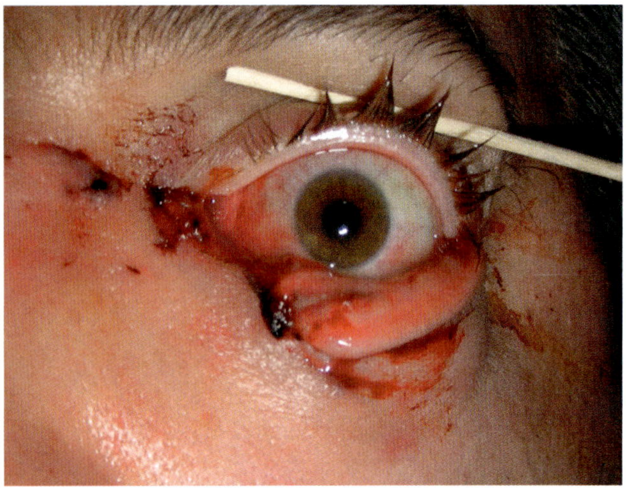

Fig. 65.1 Canalicular laceration and medial canthal avulsion for a dog bite. Note that the laceration from the dog's teeth extends anteriorly along the nose

canalicular injury is the most commonly encountered with dog bites, occurring in 92% of cases [14]. Second, cadaver studies have shown that the medial canthus is vulnerable to shearing forces applied to the lateral lid; presumably, the interdigitations of the lacrimal drainage system within the complex medial canthal anatomy act to weaken the tendinous insertions, resulting in canthal avulsion and secondary canalicular laceration [15–17]. Therefore, even a more lateral cheek bite may result in enough shearing force to avulse the medial canthus and lacerate the canaliculus, although this occurs in only a minority (8%) of dog bites that result in canalicular laceration [14]. Interestingly, in the aforementioned study by Wulc and Arterberry, 84% of *all* (not just dog bite) canalicular lacerations were due to an indirect, shearing injury, although a more recent study found an indirect cause in only 46% [14, 15].

When patients present after a dog bite attack to the face, head, or neck, it is important to evaluate and exclude injury to the eye and periocular structures; this may be difficult in uncooperative children (see Chap. 61). The identification and appropriate management of damage to the canalicular system are critical to prevent posttraumatic epiphora [18]. It is important to repair both upper and lower canalicular injuries, as both are vital in tear drainage: [19, 20] several studies have shown that both the upper and lower canaliculi contribute significantly to tear drainage [19, 20]. Furthermore, children have not yet developed age-related deficiencies in tear production and may experience long-term epiphora without intact upper and lower canaliculi.

Infection should be a main concern with all dog bite injuries, especially to the face [7]. The valveless venous supply to the face communicates with the venous system of the skull base and allows for direct access to intracranial structures of potentially life-threatening pathogens carried in the canine oral flora or the victim's skin [21]. Once a dog bite wound is identified, it should be cleaned and debrided of any foreign material. Punctures and lacerations should be carefully irrigated with copious amounts of saline [22]. Despite the concern for trapping these organisms in the repair site, primary wound closure of canalicular lacerations should be achieved within 1 week of the initial trauma. Delaying closure beyond 1 week has not been shown to reduce rates of infection and may lead to difficulty in finding the lacerated ends of the canaliculus [7, 8, 22].

The canine oral cavity contains a multitude of aerobic and anaerobic organisms that can become life-threatening pathogens once introduced into the body. More than 64 species of bacteria have been identified from the canine mouth [23–25]. The most commonly isolated organisms are *Staphylococci, Pasteurella, Streptococci, Moraxella, Neisseria, and Corynebacterium* species. Dog bite wounds typically harbor more than one organism, with one study demonstrating an average of five species per wound [24]. Two microorganisms are especially concerning in dog bite wounds – *Pasteurella multocida* and *Capnocytophaga canimorsus* – because of their aggressive pathogenicity and potential antibiotic resistance [4, 5].

Pasteurella multocida is a gram-negative coccobacillus associated with dog and cat bite wounds. Patients with wound infections from this organism can present with a variety of findings, including cellulitis, abscess formation, osteomyelitis, and even sepsis. Fortunately, the organism is highly susceptible to penicillin and several other antibiotics, including second- and third-generation cephalosporins, doxycycline, azithromycin, clarithromycin, trimethoprim-sulfamethoxazole, and fluoroquinolones [24].

Capnocytophaga canimorsus (formerly known as group DF-2) is a gram-negative, fermentative bacterium. It grows very slowly and is difficult to incubate on culture media. DF-2 has been associated with rapid-onset, severe infections leading to meningitis, sepsis, and even death in some patients after dog bite injury [26, 27]. Patients most susceptible to these severe complications include immunosuppressed and splenectomized patients. This population is at risk for fatal septicemia, making inquiry into immune and spleen status vital in all patients following canine injury. A necrotizing eschar at the wound site may be the only sign that this organism is present. DF-2 is susceptible to penicillins, cephalosporins, macrolides, and chloramphenicol.

Empiric antibiotic therapy of dog bite wounds should include coverage for skin flora, *P. multocida*, *C. canimorsus*, and anaerobes. Recommended therapy is listed in Table 65.1 [24]. In a recent, large study of periocular dog bite injuries, the most common antibiotic regimen was intravenous ampicillin/sulbactam followed by an oral course of amoxicillin/clavulanic acid, resulting in only a 2% incidence of postinjury infection [8]. However, another large study found a higher infection incidence of

10% overall, and *infection occurred in all patients that were not treated with prophylactic antibiotics* [7]. That said, a meta-analysis of antibiotic prophylaxis found the number needed to treat was 14 and recommend treatment only in high-risk patients [28].

Table 65.1 Recommended empiric antibiotic therapy for dog bite-related wounds

β-Lactam antibiotic plus β-lactamase inhibitor
Or
Second-generation cephalosporin with adequate activity against anaerobes
Or
Penicillin plus first-generation cephalosporin
For penicillin allergic patients
Clindamycin plus trimethoprim-sulfamethoxazole
Or
Clindamycin plus fluoroquinolone (fluoroquinolones should not be used in pediatric patients due to the increased risk of musculoskeletal complications)

Other infections can also be transmitted by dog bites, such as tetanus and rabies; the patient's tetanus status and health of the animal are therefore critical in management [7, 8]. Tetanus toxoid should be administered when necessary. Prophylaxis against rabies should be administered if there is any suspicion of infection, as it is almost universally fatal. Guidelines are available from the CDC and public health departments.

Surgical Technique

Canalicular laceration mandates primary repair. If not clearly evident, a canalicular laceration should be confirmed by probing and irrigation (P&I) of the lacrimal system (Fig. 65.2). A visible probe within the soft tissue laceration confirms the presence of canalicular injury (Fig. 65.3a, b). If probing cannot be performed definitively because of poor cooperation, then exploration in the operating room under anesthesia is necessary. The timing of the canalicular repair

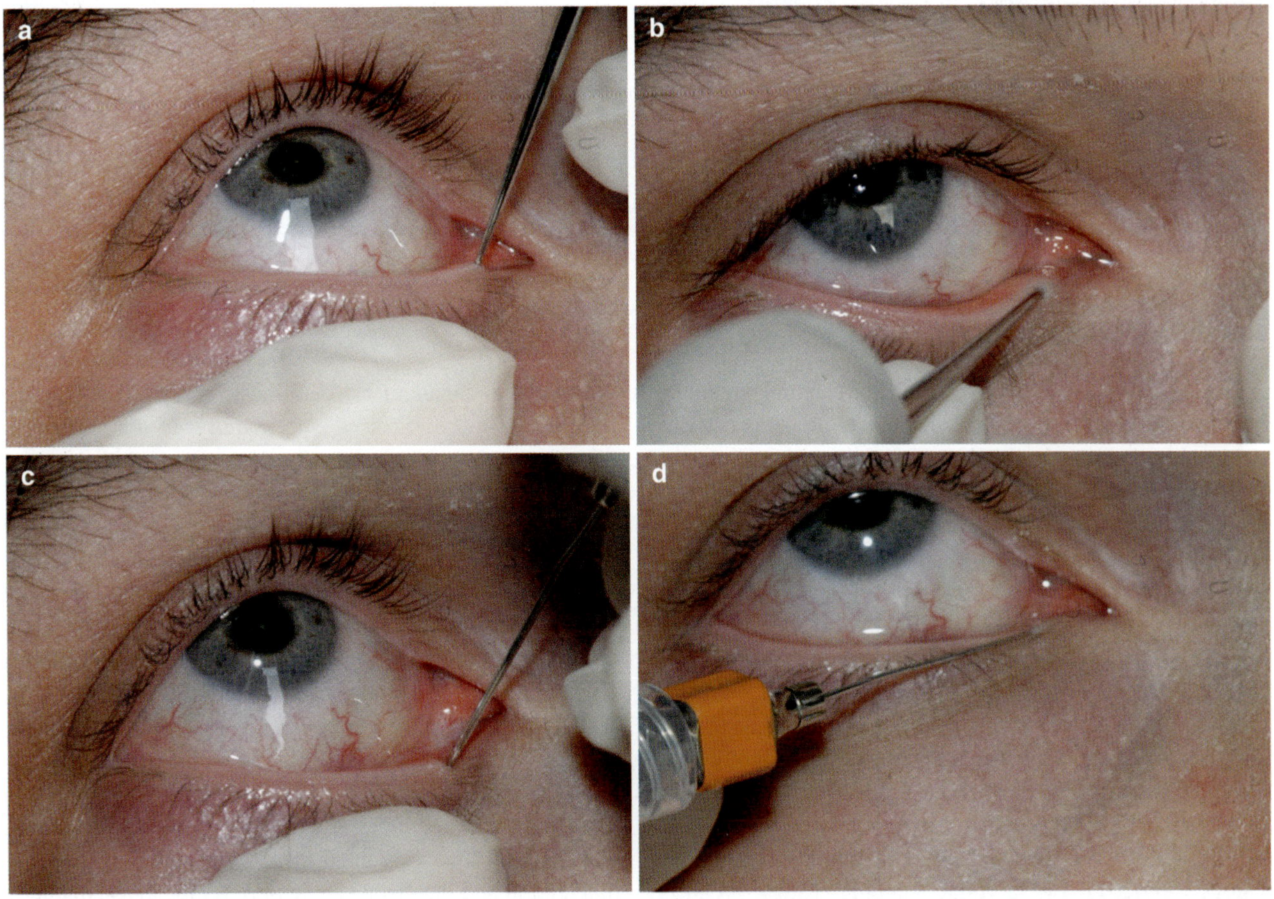

Fig. 65.2 Probing and irrigation. (**a**) After application of topical anesthesia, a pediatric punctum dilator is inserted into the punctum vertically with a gentle rotating motion, while lateral traction is applied to the lower eyelid. (**b**) The dilator is then turned horizontally and gently advanced, further dilating the punctum and proximal canaliculus. The dilator is then removed. (**c**) Next, either a #00 Bowman probe or, as shown here, a straight lacrimal cannula attached to a syringe, is passed into the canaliculus, first vertically and then horizontally. Once again, it is critical to maintain lateral traction on the lid to prevent bunching of soft tissue. The probe/cannula is advanced along the length of the horizontal canaliculus until bone (a "hard stop") is palpated. (**d**) The cannula is then pulled back slightly, and irrigation is performed to confirm intact nasolacrimal drainage. If at any point the tip of the probe or cannula is identified, a canalicular laceration is present

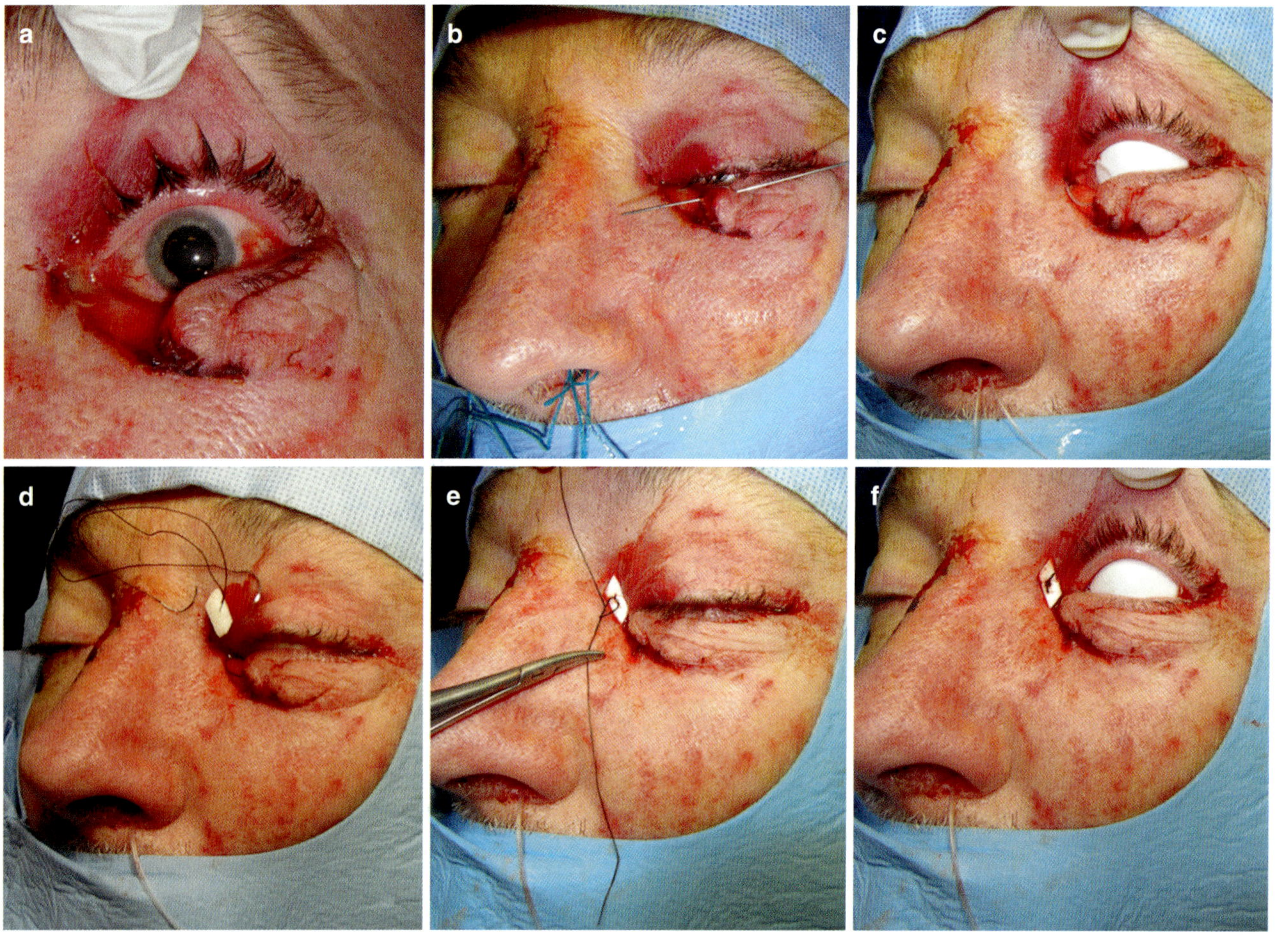

Fig. 65.3 Repair of medial canthal avulsion and canalicular laceration. a. Initial appearance with avulsion of the MCT evident. b. Confirmation of the canalicular laceration with a Bowman probe. c. Crawford bicanalicular tube in palce. d-f. See text for details.

is no longer guided by the historic recommendation of 6 hours; successful repair 5–7 days after injury is certainly achievable, but repair should proceed in a timely manner [29]. We recommend repair within 72 hours with utilization of optimal anesthesia and operating room staff.

The probing procedure should begin with topical ocular anesthetic (proparacaine, tetracaine, or viscous lidocaine) and use of a cotton-tipped applicator soaked in the same anesthetic and applied to the involved punctum for several minutes. The application of viscous lidocaine (lidocaine gel) may also be effective, although there is no good data to show the use of topical anesthetics decreases the discomfort of P&I; the patient should always be forewarned. The punctum is then dilated with a pediatric punctum dilator (Storz, #4366 or #E4340), followed by probing with a #00 Bowman probe (Storz; #E4201) or lacrimal cannula (Storz #E4404) (Fig. 65.2). The probe is first passed vertically for 2–4 mm and then rotated horizontally toward the nose. Gentle lateral traction on the eyelid facilitates advancement of the probe. If the canaliculus is intact, irrigation with tap water through a lacrimal cannula can be performed to document patency of the deeper lacrimal drainage system.

Although canalicular lacerations very proximal to the punctum can be repaired successfully in the office or minor procedure room under local anesthesia with a monocanalicular stent, the authors recommend that more distal injuries be repaired in the operating room under general anesthesia. Furthermore, while monocanalicular tubes are quite effective for proximal canalicular repair, they are more difficult to use for distal injury (i.e., injury closer to the common canaliculus and lacrimal sac) because distal injuries also usually involve some form of medial canthal avulsion. That said, a recent review of the available literature concluded that monocanalicular stenting is efficacious in canalicular laceration repair based on level III evidence [30]. In our experience, dog bit injuries involving the canaliculus are notorious for involving the deeper layers of the medial canthal tendon and the distal canaliculus. As the avulsed tendon is reapproximated, the monocanalicular tube tends to "accordion" in the soft tissue, precluding adequate reapproximation of the cut edges of the canaliculus. In such cases, some form of bicanalicular intubation (FCI Ophthalmics; Pembroke, MA. Crawford bicanaliculus intubation #S1.1270u) or a monocanalicular tube with an attached metal stent that can be passed down the nasolacrimal duct (FCI Ophthalmics; Pembroke, MA. Crawford monocanalicular intubation #S1.1901u or Ritleng monocanaliculus Intubation #S1.1451u) is preferable; these stents are passed down the nasolacrimal duct and externalized from beneath the inferior meatus. Thus, as the medial canthal tendon is reapproximated, tension can be placed on the exteriorized stent(s) and tube(s), minimizing any bunching of the silicone tube. If nasolacrimal duct stenting is to be used, general anesthesia is preferred because of potential pain during stent extraction from the nose. The inferior turbinate is packed with ½" by 3″ neurosurgical cottonoids soaked in oxymetazoline for vasoconstriction and easier access to the inferior meatus.

Exploration of an injured canaliculus is often frustrating, especially when the injury occurs deep within the medial canthal complex close to the lacrimal sac. During exploration, many of the canthal tendon fibers convincingly mimic the cut edge of the canalicular mucosa. Several surgical maneuvers increase the likelihood of finding the distal canaliculus and minimizing false passages that cause further injury to the soft tissue. First, the surgeon should avoid using an excess amount of local anesthetic infiltration, as this distorts the anatomy and may induce bleeding of the orbicularis oculi muscle. This is one reason why the authors have a low threshold for canalicular repair under general anesthesia, in which case no local anesthetic infiltration is used. Second, any exploration of the deeper soft tissue injury should be carried out exclusively with cotton-tipped applicators. The use of rake retractors and toothed forceps should be limited to skin retraction alone. The use of forceps during deeper soft tissue exploration results in further splaying and distortion of the medial canthal complex. Finally, the surgeon must resist the temptation of passing a Bowman probe in an impatient and haphazard fashion into soft tissue that "looks like it might be the canaliculus." A gentle exploration, although more time consuming initially, will increase the likelihood of successful identification of the distal canaliculus.

Once the distal canaliculus is identified, a #00 Bowman probe is passed medially into the canaliculus and lacrimal sac. Successful passage will result in a "hard stop" as the probe reaches the bony lacrimal sac fossa abutting the medial wall of the lacrimal sac. A "soft stop" typically indicates that a false passage has been made; the Bowman probe should be removed and additional exploration ensues. If a successful "hard stop" is palpated, the Bowman probe is then rotated almost 90 degrees along the superior orbital rim while maintaining gentle medial pressure with the tip of the probe against the lacrimal sac. As the probe rotates over the superior orbital rim, it should be held against the rim with a finger from the contralateral hand. Gentle pressure is applied inferiorly with the probe as it passes the 45-degree mark, palpating for the nasolacrimal duct with the tip. The nasolacrimal duct is usually accessible to the Bowman probe somewhere between the 45- and 90-degree rotation of the probe. Vigorous force must be avoided to prevent false passage into the nose. Once the probe enters the nasolacrimal duct, it is advanced just until it hits the floor of the nasopharynx. Additional pressure will simply force the probe more posteriorly in the nasopharynx.

At this juncture, the nasal packing is removed. A second, larger Bowman probe is then passed through the ipsilateral naris beneath the inferior turbinate into the inferior meatus. This can either be done using direct visualization with a nasal speculum or endoscope or, alternatively, simply by feel – the authors' preferred method. It is important to remember that the nasolacrimal duct exit in the inferior meatus is located "low and lateral" within the nasal cavity (Fig. 65.4). A tendency to look for the tip of the probe too superiorly and medially is common and should be avoided. A "metal on metal" scraping of one probe against the other indicates successful passage into the nasolacrimal duct.

If bicanalicular stents are used, then one end of the tube/stent is passed through the punctum of the involved eyelid and is pulled out through the proximal cut end of the canaliculus. While appropriate soft tissue retraction is performed by the assistant, the Bowman probe is gently backed out of the distal canaliculus and replaced with the stented tube, which is then passed into the lacrimal sac and down the nasolacrimal duct as just described. The stent and tube are then externalized from beneath the inferior meatus and naris by a variety of methods, depending on the specific type of tube and surgeon preference. For example, the Crawford tube system utilizes stents with bulbous ends, which can be retrieved by passing a Crawford hook (FCI Ophthalmics; Pembroke, MA. Crawford hook #S1.1275) into the nose to engage the stent (Fig. 65.4). The second stent is then passed through the uninvolved canaliculus and also exteriorized after being passed into the nasolacrimal duct (Fig. 65.3c).

With the canalicular system identified and intubated, further soft tissue repair ensues. Some surgeons will proceed with meticulous and admittedly frustrating reapproximation of the canalicular mucosa with fine suture, despite little evidence in the literature that this improves outcomes. One study by Chu et al. found a statistically significant improvement in anatomic patency in patients who had direct canalicular mucosal closure versus pericanalicular closure, but there was no difference in postoperative epiphora symptomatology [31]. The authors follow the recommendation of Kersten and Kulwin, who advocate repair of the pericanalicular orbicularis oculi muscle, anticipating that the stented canalicular mucosa will heal adequately once reapproximated [32]. Others have described good outcomes with similar techniques [12, 33–36].

In general, we prefer to repair the pericanalicular mucosa and medial canthal avulsion with one double-armed silk suture (Ethicon Inc., Bridgewater NJ, #735G, C-3 needles) that is exteriorized before tying for several reasons. First, silk is a relatively strong suture material and will provide enough

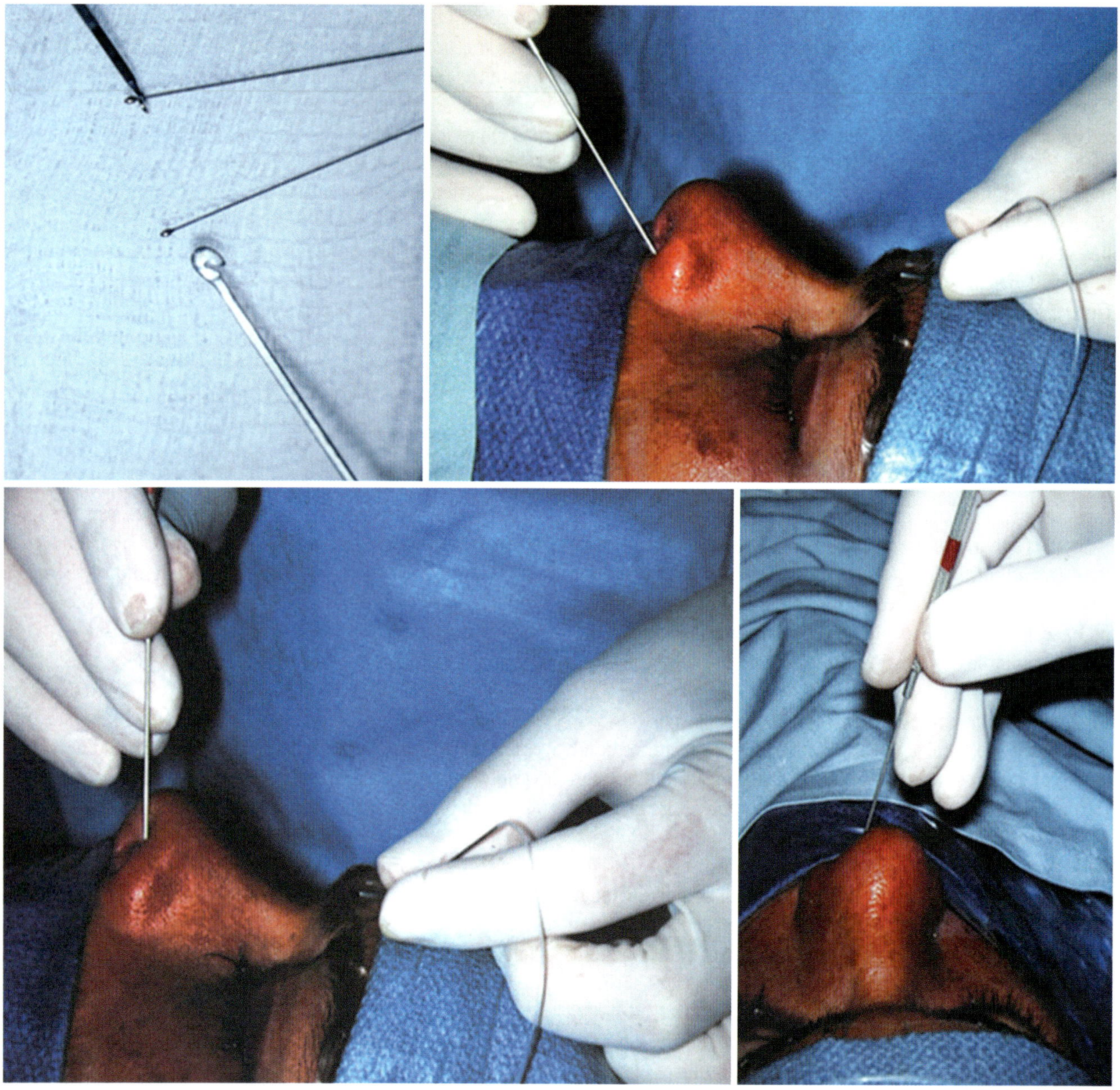

Fig. 65.4 Correct retrieval of a nasolacrimal stent. Top left, the bulbous end of the Crawford stents is engaged with a Crawford hook. Top right, *incorrect* positioning of the hook in the nose. Note the hook is being angled superiorly, toward the middle turbinate. Bottom, *correct* angulation of the Crawford hook, staying "low and lateral" to pass the hook beneath the inferior turbinate into the inferior meatus

medial tension to the lid without breaking. Second, silk incites an inflammatory reaction which presumably allows for more rapid healing of the lacerated MCT while the canaliculus is protected from complete contracture by the presence of the silicone tube. Finally, the large C-3 needles on the double-armed suture can be passed through the medial end of the lacerated canthal tendon in a posterior direction (to reproduce the correct vector of the MCT) through adequate soft tissue medially and still have enough needle length and curve to exteriorize the suture. This maneuver allows the surgeon to tie the suture over bolster material (the foam packing that comes with the suture is excellent), providing adequate medial and posterior vectors for the MCT, while avoiding the ofttimes difficult task of tying a deep suture under tension in a limited space. Of course, the use of nonabsorbable suture material necessitates timely patient follow-up and removal (7–10 days postoperatively); if there is any suspicion of noncomplaint follow-up at time of initial repair, then absorbable suture material should be considered.

The double-armed 4–0 silk suture is first passed above and below the proximal canaliculus through the orbicularis. Each needle is then passed individually above and below the distal canaliculus and gently rotated medially in a posterior to anterior direction. It is imperative not to force the needle, which will result in bending and eventually breakage. Instead, as the needle is passed, gentle posterior blunt force is applied with forceps on the skin overlying the lateral nasal bone, decreasing the soft tissue distance and facilitating exteriorization of the needles. Both needles are then passed through the foam bolster (Fig. 65.3d). The 4–0 silk suture is tied over the bolster, while gentle tension is applied to the stented tube(s) at the naris. As the silk suture is tied anteriorly, the eyelid will reappose against the globe as the medial canthus is pulled medially and posteriorly by the suture (Fig. 65.3d). Once the suture is tied, the MCT avulsion is essentially repaired (Fig. 65.3e, f). Skin sutures can be placed as needed. Typically, eyelid margin sutures are unnecessary. The scleral shell, placed over the eye at the start of the procedure, is removed before tying the tube to prevent tube migration. The final step is to place a hemostat at the level of the naris with gentle tension on the tube, cut the stents off of the tube, and tie the tube with one square knot, essentially forming a loop. The hemostat is gently released, and the tube retracts into the nasal cavity. The silk suture and bolster are removed in 7–10 days. The silicone stubs are left in place for 3–6 months if tolerated and removed in the office.

Overall success rate for canalicular laceration repair from all etiologies ranges between 37% and 95%, but this is dependent on the definition of success, which varies between studies [12, 32, 35, 37–52]. One study noted a significant difference in success depending on venue of repair (minor procedure room (37%) vs operating room (86%) and training level of the primary surgeon (resident (25%), oculoplastic fellow (44%), comprehensive ophthalmologist (29%), oculoplastic attending surgeon (84%)) [35], with a similar trend reported in a second cohort [36]. Counterintuitively, one study found a higher success rate in distal (>6 mm from punctum) canalicular laceration repair than proximal ones, but this was dependent on definition of success (complete or partial presence of epiphora) [51]. Of note, Bratton et al. reported a higher incidence of posttraumatic epiphora (19%) in their large cohort of dog bite-induced canalicular laceration, suggesting that repair of these injuries may have a lower success rate than those not related to dogs [7].

Pediatric Orbital Fractures

The epidemiology of pediatric orbital fractures is difficult to ascertain with any accuracy from the existing literature. Hatton and colleagues reported on a series of 96 patients (17 years or younger) who presented to a large academic institution (both as inpatients and outpatients) over an 8-year period [53]. The mean age was 12.5 years, with a majority of fractures (81.3%) occurring in males. The leading etiology for fracture was sports, regardless of gender, followed by assaults in boys and motor vehicle accidents in girls. Accompanying ocular injuries occurred in 50% of patients, ranging from mild to severe, emphasizing the importance of a detailed ocular exam in all pediatric orbital fractures. Overall, the most common wall involved in pediatric orbital fractures was the floor (67%), followed by combined floor and medial wall (14%), and isolated medial wall (8%). Isolated orbital roof fractures occurred in 6% and were distinctly more likely to occur in children younger than 10 years. Of note, a separate analysis of isolated orbital fractures across the entire pediatric age group revealed that orbital roof (30%) and medial wall fractures (28%) more common than floor fractures (24%), unlike Hatton's findings. Similar to Hatton, roof fractures were more common in patients younger than 8 years [54]. Overall, pediatric orbital fractures are less frequently associated with ocular injuries than their adult counterparts [54, 55].

The Pediatric Orbit and Orbital Roof Fractures

The pediatric facial skeleton differs significantly from its adult counterpart in several respects. First, the cranial to maxillofacial ratio in infants is very high (8:1) and progressively decreases to 2.5:1 in adulthood [53, 54, 56, 57]. Put another way, while the cranium undergoes a four-fold growth from birth to adulthood, the face grows by 12-fold [55]. Younger children also lack pneumatized frontal sinuses, which act to distribute forces applied to the forehead [54]. It is therefore not surprising to note a higher incidence of skull fractures in Hatton et al.'s series in children younger than 10 years and in Hink et al.'s review in children with an average age of 5.5 years [54]., in whom a larger cranium and at best rudimentary frontal sinuses predispose to this type of injury (Fig. 65.5) [53]. These findings are confirmed by an earlier study by Koltai and colleagues, who noted an average age of 4.7 ± 3.3 years in patients with orbital roof fractures, compared to 12.0 ± 4.2 years (p <0.01) in patients with other orbital fractures. The authors concluded that orbital roof fractures occur at a much higher frequency in children younger than 7 years [58]. A retrospective review of CT findings in 338 patients 18 years or younger found that an astounding 47–57% of all facial fractures occurring in patients younger than 9 years involved the orbital roof and were the most common facial fracture seen in the entire cohort [59]. Of note, only a minority of pediatric orbital roof fractures necessitated surgical intervention [53, 54, 58]. However, Chapman and colleagues note in their CT review that a significant number of orbital roof fractures were associated with subperiosteal orbital hematomas, with 61% of patients with orbital roof fractures also demonstrating exophthalmos on CT [59]. In addition, orbital roof fractures were

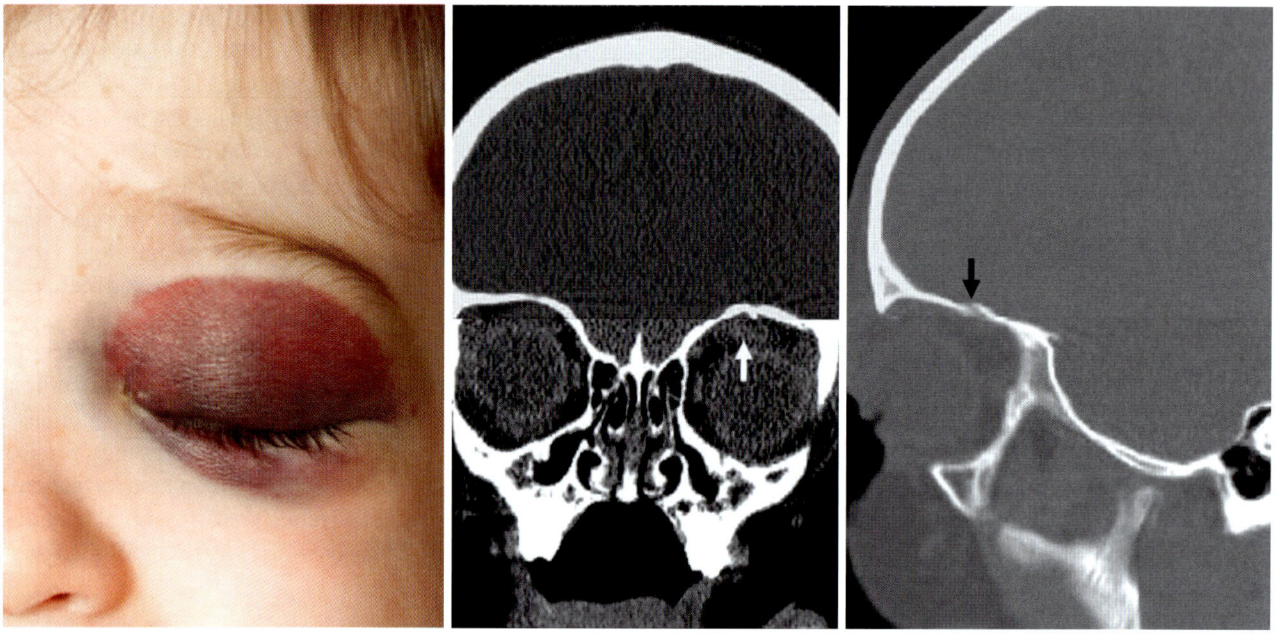

Fig. 65.5 Orbital roof fracture. Left. Clinical photograph of a 2-year-old girl who tripped and hit her forehead against concrete. Note the extensive periocular ecchymosis suggesting deeper injury and possible orbital hemorrhage. Coronal (center) and parasagittal (right) recombined images of the orbital and head CT showing a subperiosteal hematoma (white arrow) and orbital roof fracture (black arrow). No repair was needed

also associated with other skull fractures [59]. Therefore, while most children with orbital roof fractures will not require surgical repair, they should evaluated and followed for possible orbital compartment syndrome; neurosurgical consultation may also be warranted [60]. A large study of 312 patients by Hink and colleagues noted that in the pediatric age group, orbital fractures presented frequently (62%) with other craniofacial fractures, and that associated *neurologic* injury (23%) occurred as frequently as ophthalmic injury (20%); 4 patients died of their neurologic injury, with another 11% suffering from prolonged traumatic brain injury [54]. Not surprisingly, associated neurologic injury was more common with orbital roof fractures than with orbital floor fractures (31% vs 16%, p = 0.0024). Furthermore, younger age and more extensive craniofacial fractures (as opposed to isolated orbital fractures) had a significantly higher frequency of neurologic injury [55].

Concomitant to the expansion of the midface in relation to the cranium and to the pneumatization of the paranasal sinuses, the relatively flat face of the infant and toddler begins to "unfold" forward from beneath the protection of the overhanging cranium as the child grows [58]. Interestingly, this younger pediatric craniofacial anatomy appears to be protective against maxillofacial fractures: in a series of 1500 facial fractures, fewer than 5% occurred in children younger than 12 years [59, 61]. With increasing age, the midface expands faster than the cranium and paranasal sinuses become widely aerated, shifting the frequency of orbital fractures from the roof to the floor and toward a more adult fracture pattern (Fig. 65.6) [56].

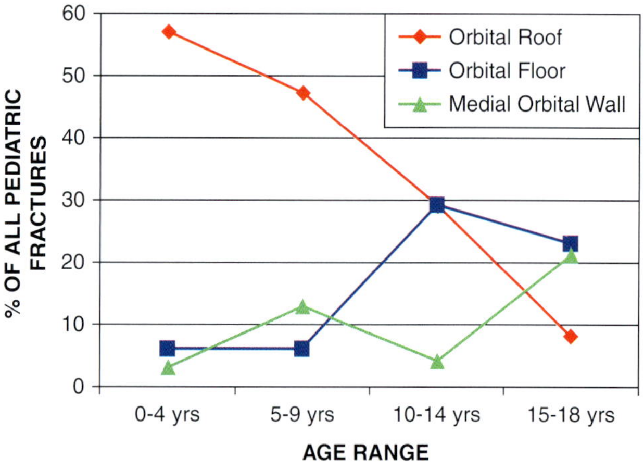

Fig. 65.6 Graphic representation of specific fracture incidence as a percentage of all pediatric orbital and midfacial fractures across multiple age groups. (Data compiled from Ref. 21)

The White-Eyed Blowout Fracture

The type of orbital wall fracture also differs in children and adults. Not only are the bones of children more flexible because of a thin cortex and relatively thicker cancellous component, but the paranasal sinuses in general are more rudimentary, changing the mechanics of the facial buttresses [56, 62]. In particular, the maxillary sinuses of children are not fully pneumatized, with a thicker overlying orbital floor [58]. It is therefore not surprising that significant differences exist in the clinical presentation of pediatric and adult orbital floor fractures. The more flexible bones in children result in the greenstick fractures common in this age group [63]. In addition, in many cases the more flexible facial buttresses may simply bend and not break [63].

Jordon and colleagues coined the term "white-eyed blowout fracture" (WEBOF) in a landmark 1998 publication, describing the clinical presentation of severe restrictive strabismus and diplopia coupled with a notable paucity of external signs of periocular injury (hence the term "white-eyed") and minimal, easily missed radiographic findings on CT [64]. The pathophysiology has been theorized to consist of a posterior buckling of the orbital rim from an applied force, which then leads to an inferior bending and cracking of the flexible orbital floor, resulting in a medially hinged trapdoor fracture. In addition to the buckling mechanism, a hydraulic force may be present simultaneously, effectively causing a momentary increase in soft tissue pressure within the orbit [65–69]. As the trapdoor opens, soft tissue is forced through the defect and is effectively incarcerated within the liner fracture as the trapdoor snaps shut. In addition to entrapped orbital fat, the inferior rectus muscle is often also caught within the bony confines of the fracture, resulting in typical clinical manifestations of WEBOF and possible ischemic injury to the muscle. Conversely, adult bone is more brittle, and the well-aerated and developed maxillary sinuses result in a thinner, wider-spanning orbital floor. A similar traumatic mechanism in an adult typically results in a more capacious orbital floor defect without a snapping trapdoor mechanism, minimizing the chance of muscle incarceration and ischemia.

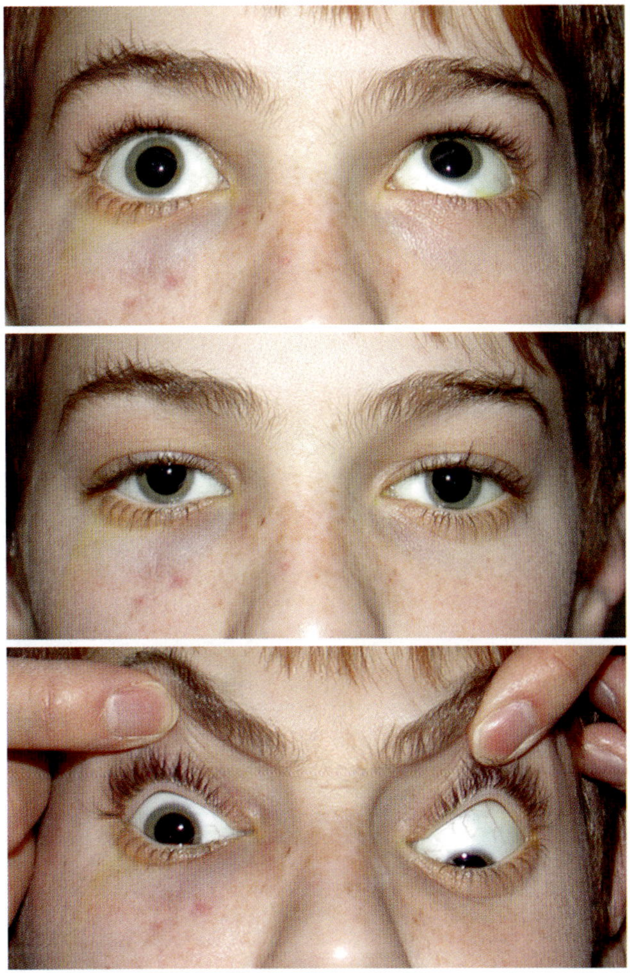

Fig. 65.7 Inferior wall WEBOF. A 12-year-old boy with severe nausea and vomiting after being struck in the right orbit with a baseball. He had been admitted for observation for 48 hours to an outside hospital with a diagnosis of concussion. After discharge, the patient did not tolerate oral intake because of persistent nausea and vomiting and was brought to Wills Eye Hospital by his parents for a second opinion. Note the minimal external signs of right periorbital injury coupled with severe vertical external ophthalmoplegia

WEBOF can occur at any age, including adulthood, but is overwhelmingly seen in the pediatric age group, with an average age of 10–12 years old [54, 63, 70, 71]. The classic presentation is that of an unimpressive external appearance after injury, with minimal bruising, edema, and ocular injury (ergo "white-eyed), but a marked external ophthalmoplegia (Fig. 65.7). Most WEBOF involve the orbital floor (71%) with a resultant vertical strabismus [70], but on occasion, the medial orbital wall is cracked, and an abduction deficit mimicking an abducens nerve palsy or a "pseudo-Duane syndrome" is present (Fig. 65.8) [72–74]. The child often complains of pain, especially in affected gazes, which in turn limits clinical evaluation. In addition, attempted ocular duction toward or away from the entrapped muscle stimulates the oculocardiac reflex, manifesting as nausea and vomiting [54]. Bradycardia and, rarely, cardiac arrhythmia/asystole may also be present [54, 75]. In an emergency room or pediatrician's office setting, a predictable cascade of understandable misdiagnosis ensues, with the leading concern being concussion or intracranial injury [76]. This then leads to axial CT of the brain rather than dedicated coronal imaging of the orbital bones, and not infrequently admission to the hospital for neurologic monitoring rather than complete ophthalmologic evaluation [76]. The potential for misdiagnosis is further increased by the fact that WEBOF in general has subtle radiographic findings even on appropriate coronal CT images and is easily missed radiographically (Fig. 65.9) [64].

Timely diagnosis of WEBOF is important, not only to reverse the oculocardiac reflex and its attendant symptomatology (nausea, vomiting, bradycardia) but also to minimize the possibility of permanent ischemic injury and contracture of the involved extraocular muscle, which could lead to long-term strabismus and diplopia [63, 64, 77].

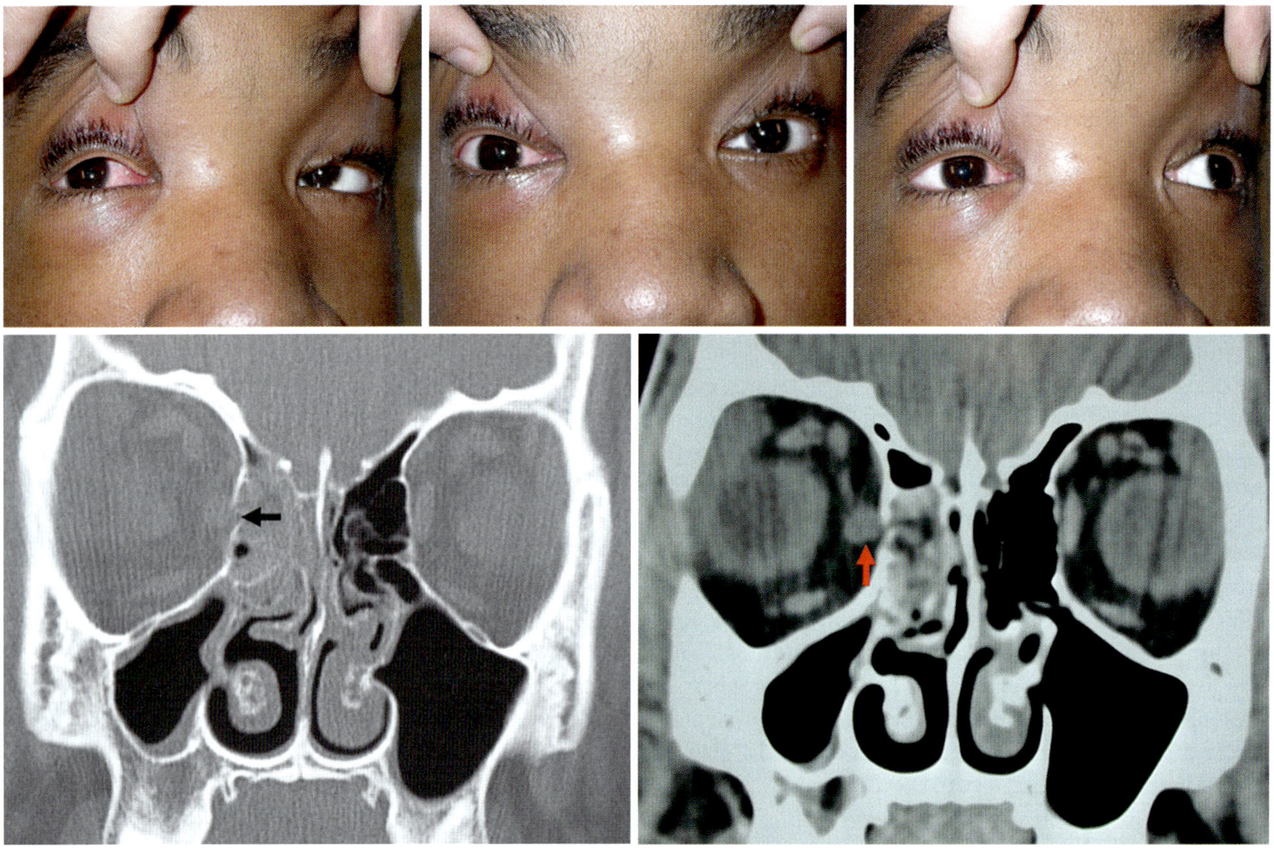

Fig. 65.8 Medial wall WEBOF. Top, clinical photographs demonstrating a pseudo-Duane syndrome from a medial wall fracture. Bottom, coronal CT images. Left, bone window shows the narrow fracture (black arrow). Right, soft tissue window demonstrating a markedly distorted medial rectus muscle (red arrow)

In the majority of cases, the diagnosis of WEBOF follows predictable patterns and should be considered a clinical diagnosis. While coronal CT imaging may be confirmatory, a negative CT should by no means rule out the presence of a subtle fracture. In fact, the authors suspect that most orbital specialists with experience in managing WEBOF would proceed with orbital exploration and fracture repair based on clinical findings, despite "normal" imaging, raising the question of whether WEBOF can be managed without any preoperative imaging at all. This last point is highly debatable, and the authors continue to recommend preoperative coronal CT, albeit utilizing pediatric imaging protocols with decreased radiation exposure (see next section).

Clinically, a patient with suspected WEBOF will have minimal or no external signs of injury, minimal or no exophthalmos, and yet exhibit a marked restrictive strabismus, usually greatest away from the action of the incarcerated muscle, with a lesser or no restriction toward the action of the muscle [64]. Thus, attempted upgaze in a WEBOF involving the inferior rectus will typically result in severe pain and a varying degree of nausea and vomiting, often limiting the clinical exam [78]. Nausea and vomiting are important symptoms, having a positive predictive value of 71%–83% in identifying patients with WEBOF [70, 76, 79]. On occasion, the child will also develop a chin-up position or tend to keep both eyes closed to minimize diplopia. Infraorbital hypesthesia with WEBOF of the orbital floor may be present in varying degrees; normal infraorbital nerve function does not effectively rule out WEBOF.

On imaging, WEBOF is often seen as a narrow crack in the orbital floor just medial to the infraorbital canal (Fig. 65.9). The fracture is classically linear and runs nearly parallel to the canal for a variable length. The medial hinge is often normal in appearance. A knuckle of soft tissue is usually present within the maxillary sinus abutting the fracture but may be misdiagnosed as "mucosal thickening" or "sinus polyp." [64, 71] The incarcerated muscle is often not noted within the fracture or sinus, but the portion remaining within the orbit may be significantly distorted when compared to the contralateral side, transitioning to a normal appearance anterior or posterior to the fracture. A very helpful finding is the "missing muscle sign": in the area of the fracture, the involved muscle seems to disappear (Fig. 65.10)

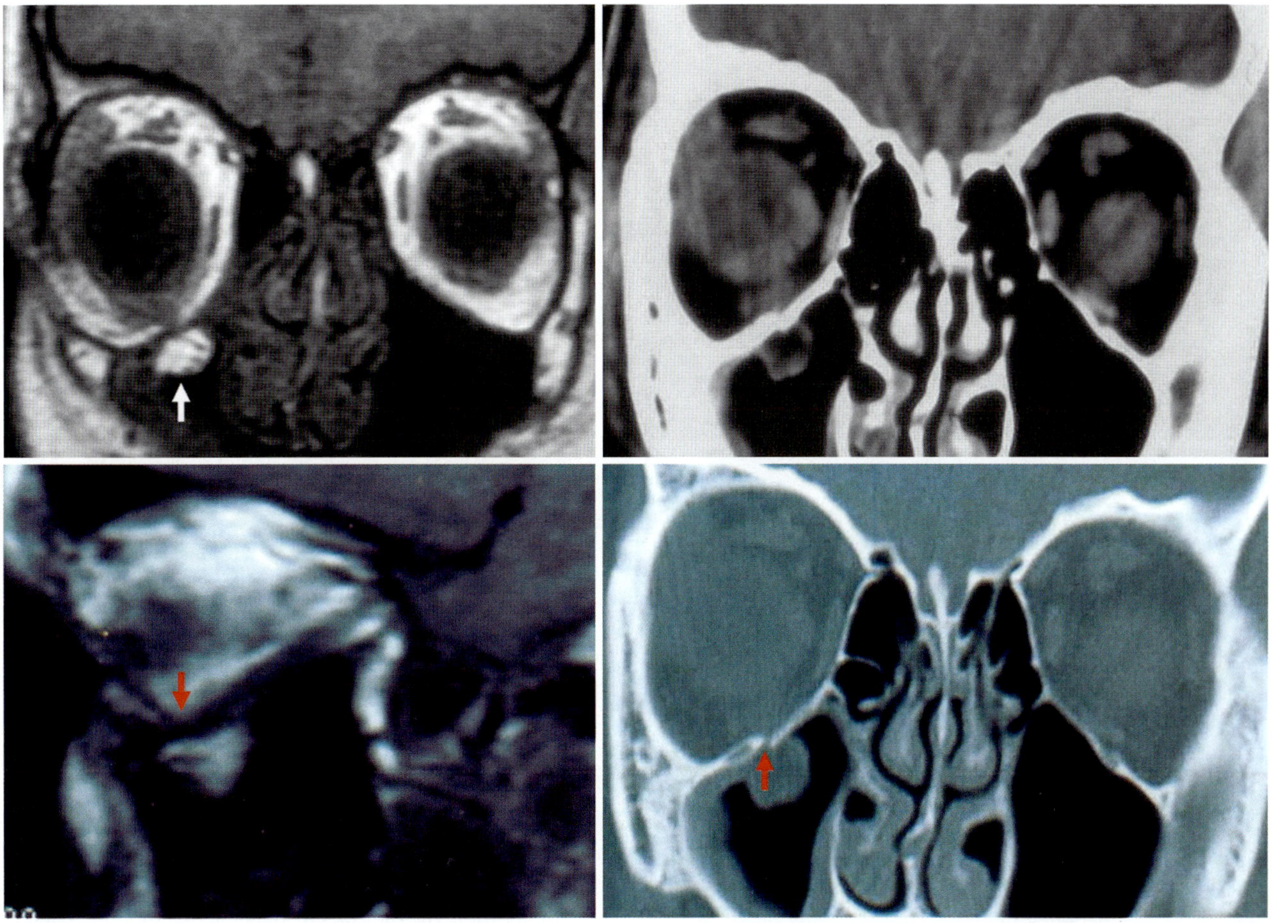

Fig. 65.9 Imaging of an inferior wall WEBOF. A 13-year-old girl was elbowed in the right eye with resultant diplopia with nausea and vomiting. Suspecting intracranial injury, her family doctor ordered an MRI of the head, which was read as normal. The report noted a right maxillary sinus polyp (white arrow) but no fracture on T1-weighted coronal orbital images (top left). On subsequent CT, a slight irregularity of the right orbital floor is noted on coronal soft tissue windows (top right), but the fracture (red arrow) is best demonstrated on coronal bone windows (bottom right), just medial to the infraorbital canal. An obvious acute angle distortion (red arrow) is present on parasagittal T1-weighted MRI (bottom left), consistent with inferior rectus incarceration. The "sinus polyp" is prolapsed orbital fat

[80]. This indicates that the entire belly of the muscle is incarcerated below the fracture within the maxillary sinus; it is usually not distinguishable from the incarcerated, edematous, and hemorrhagic fat. Careful review of coronal CT images is critical, and despite this, the fracture may be easily missed [54, 64, 70, 71]. It is therefore important to remember that muscle entrapment in WEBOF is a *clinical* rather than radiographic diagnosis [71].

Most studies of WEBOF have concluded that the entrapped tissue should be freed as soon as possible, ideally within 24–48 hours of the injury [63, 64, 81, 82]. This may be untenable for a variety of reasons, not least of which is delay in referral [76]. In addition to a full ophthalmic exam, other preoperative assessment is important. Patients with WEBOF may have suffered from nausea, vomiting, and poor oral intake for several days following initial injury and may be severely dehydrated. Intravenous rehydration and monitoring of electrolytes may be necessary before general anesthesia. If a severe oculocardiac reflex with bradycardia or arrhythmia is present, cardiac monitoring may be needed [83]. Forced duction testing to confirm entrapment is usually not necessary and is difficult to perform in an uncooperative patient.

Surgical Technique

All WEBOFs are repaired under general anesthesia. The authors prefer full endotracheal intubation in any orbital fracture repair because of possible bleeding from the paranasal sinuses into the nasopharynx and potential resultant laryngospasm or aspiration. Surgical draping includes both eyes in the sterile field, and this allows comparison between the eyes if needed. After anesthesia induction, forced ductions are performed as an initial baseline.

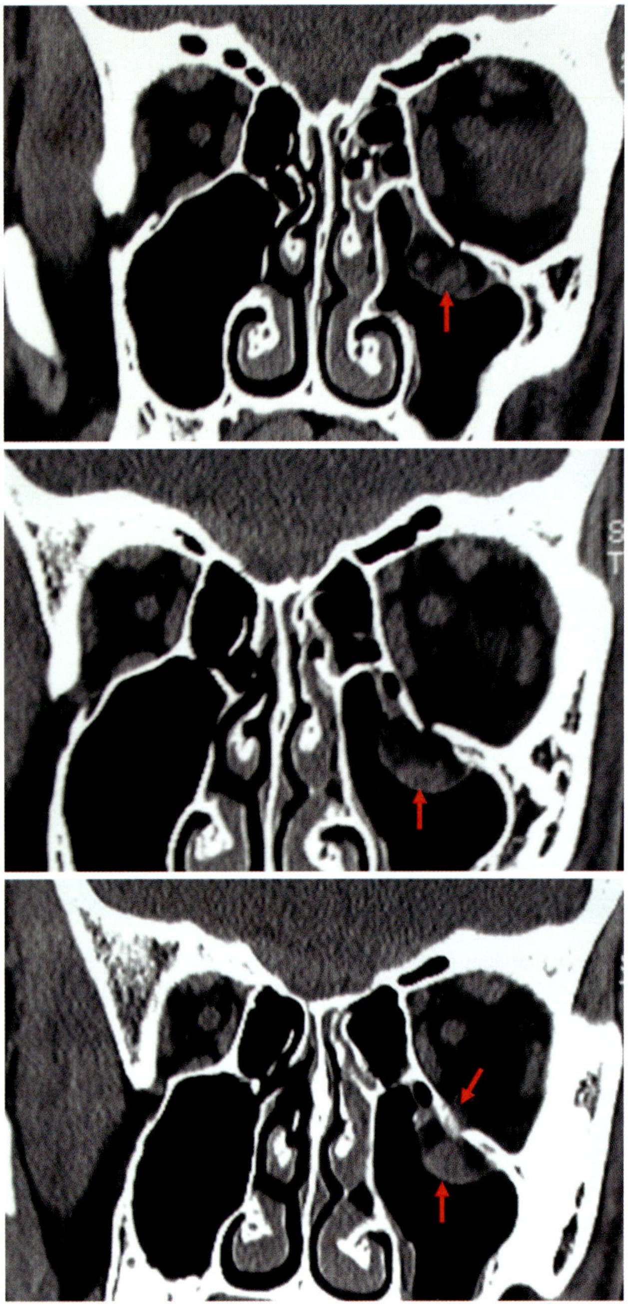

Fig. 65.10 The "missing muscle" sign. Coronal CT images (soft tissue window) of an inferior wall WEBOF. In the top two images, the left inferior rectus muscle appears to be missing within the orbit but is present within the knuckle of soft tissue herniated into the maxillary sinus (arrows). The muscle often is not clearly seen if the surrounding herniated fat is hemorrhagic. In the most posterior image (bottom), the muscle is still herniated, but a portion is reappearing within the orbit (arrows)

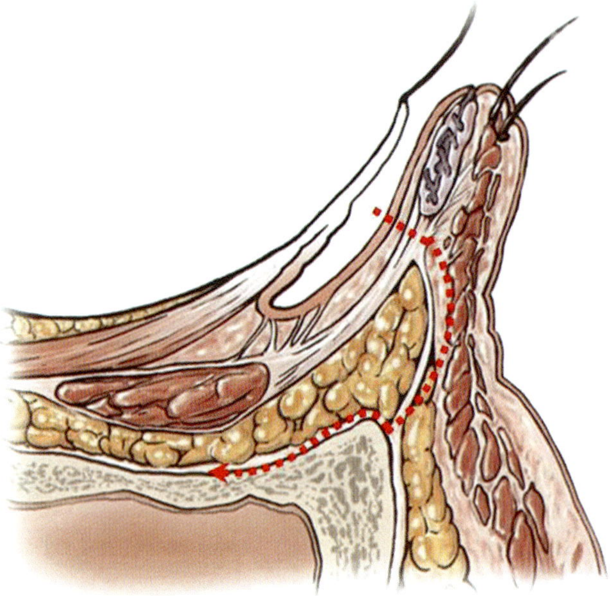

Fig. 65.11 Transconjunctival, preseptal dissection plane for WEBOF repair is shown as the dotted red arrow

A transconjunctival approach to the orbital floor is used. Lateral canthotomy and inferior cantholysis are rarely necessary for exposure in WEBOF repair. Several techniques have been described [84]; the discussion here will be limited to the authors' technique [85]. The dissection planes are shown in Fig. 65.11. After placement of a scleral shell and injection of the inferior cul-de-sac with local anesthetic containing epinephrine, a 4–0 silk suture is passed through the eyelid margin, and the eyelid is everted on a Desmarres retractor (Fig. 65.12a). Conjunctiva is cauterized 1 mm below the inferior border of the tarsal plate with bipolar cautery (Fig. 65.12b) and incised with scissors (Fig. 65.12c). A conjunctival/lower lid retractor flap is then elevated with Westcott scissors, through which an additional traction suture is placed (Fig. 65.12d). The dissection plane is carried preseptally toward the inferior orbital rim in a blunt fashion. Soft tissue overlying the inferior orbital rim is incised with Bovie cautery while protecting the globe and intraorbital contents with a malleable retractor (Fig. 65.12e). (NB: To avoid thermal injury to orbital soft tissue, a coated malleable retractor is preferred to the uncoated metal retractor shown in the figure.)

The periosteum is elevated around the arcus marginalis and orbital floor using a Freer elevator and malleable retractor in a hand-over-hand technique (Fig. 65.12f). Prolapsed and entrapped tissue is encountered a variable distance from the arcus marginalis. The surgeon should avoid the tendency of simply elevating soft tissue out of the maxillary sinus, which is a common and acceptable maneuver when repairing the wider orbital floor fractures seen in adults. In WEBOF, such traction on the entrapped tissue may cause further damage to the incarcerated muscle. Instead, the surgeon should gently push the hinged fracture into the maxillary sinus with the Freer elevator, effectively reopening the trapdoor and facilitating the elevation of prolapsed soft tissue back into the orbit. Typically, this maneuver is characterized by a

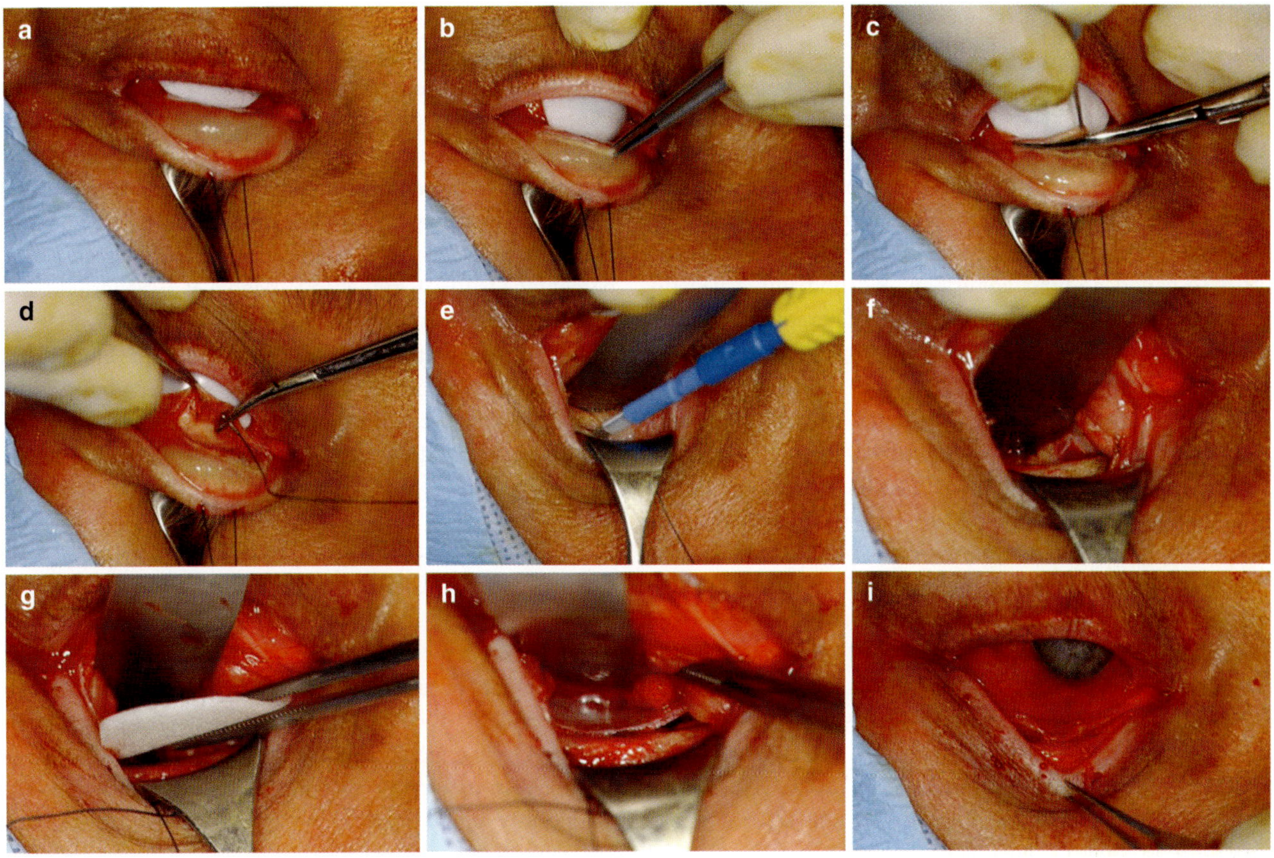

Fig. 65.12 Surgical technique for WEBOF repair. See text for details

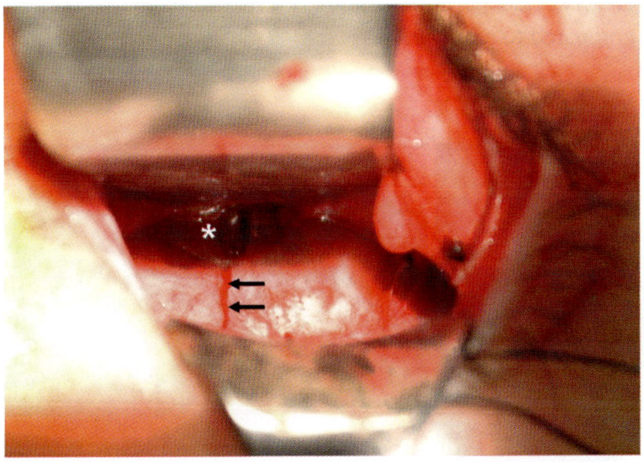

Fig. 65.13 Intraoperative findings in WEBOF. Note the linear trapdoor fracture (arrows) with incarceration of a dusky and edematous inferior rectus muscle (asterisk)

"push and sweep" motion with the elevator. The fracture and trapped tissue are followed posteriorly into the orbit until all tissue is freed and repositioned into the orbital space. The surgeon will often encounter an edematous and dusky rectus muscle, consistent with direct contusion and ischemic injury (Fig. 65.13). Forced duction are again performed, but on occasion may still be positive even with complete release of entrapped soft tissue because of edema or early fibrosis, especially if there is a significant delay in surgical repair.

Frequently, the fractured bone will realign with little or no defect noted. In such cases, some surgeons will opt against placement of any implant, while others will use absorbable materials, and still others will proceed with placement of a permanent alloplast such as porous polyethylene (Fig. 65.12g, h). Regardless of the alloplast, correct implant sizing and placement are critical to minimize iatrogenic entrapment and implant extrusion. In a properly sized and placed implant, there should be no soft tissue herniation around the implant (in other words, the inferior surface of the implant should abut bone only), and the anterior border should remain in the natural depression just behind the arcus marginalis. The position of the implant should be rechecked after forced ductions are performed. Any migration anterior to the arcus marginalis indicates incorrect positioning or an oversized implant. With proper sizing and placement, no additional implant fixation is needed. The authors also prefer to minimize closure of soft tissues and avoid layered closure of eyelid tissue, especially the orbital septum. Although many surgeons will close the conjunctiva, the authors typically avoid suturing altogether, and simply realign the conjunctival edges (Fig. 65.12i), followed by placement of a small amount of antibiotic ointment [85].

Postoperatively, the patient's vision and pupillary reactivity are checked in the postanesthesia care unit once awake to assure that there is no evidence of orbital compartment syndrome or optic neuropathy. Although there is an understandable trend toward outpatient orbital fracture repair in an ambulatory care setting, we still observe patients overnight as a so-called 23-hour admission. We find this especially important in children, who may be uncooperative postoperatively and not allow for adequate postoperative assessment of vision at home by the parents.

Postoperatively, nausea, vomiting, and pain with ductions should resolve almost immediately. Diplopia may linger for weeks and may paradoxically worsen in the immediate postoperative phase (Fig. 65.14). This is an important point to discuss with the patient and parents before surgery. It is not uncommon for the freed muscle to remain paretic for days to weeks, resulting in a marked hypertropia of the eye in the case of inferior wall WEBOF and exotropia with a medial WEBOF. As the injured rectus heals and recovers function, the strabismus improves and hopefully resolves completely (Fig. 65.14). On occasion, a small residual diplopia may persist in extreme gaze. If significant strabismus and diplopia is present several weeks after repair and an adequate reduction was performed intraoperatively, intramuscular fibrosis is likely present. Rarely, re-entrapment of the muscle may occur in the first week postoperatively and typically follows an activity that resulted in a Valsalva maneuver in patients where no orbital floor implant was placed. Very young patients (<4 years old) with postoperative diplopia or strabismus should be followed for the development of amblyopia. Otherwise, serial strabismus measurements should be performed to document improvement or stability. Hink and colleagues found complete resolution of restrictive external ophthalmoplegia in 63% of their WEBOF cohort, although long-term follow-up was limited and the actual percentage is likely higher [54]. Mehta et al. reported complete resolution of restrictive strabismus in 77–91% of patients, with a trend toward better outcome and faster recovery if the WEBOF was repaired within 24 hours from time of injury [82]. Strabismus surgery, when necessary, should be delayed for at least 6 months following initial repair.

CT Imaging in Children

A significant amount of data has been published since 2001 on the subject of radiation exposure from computed tomography (CT) [86–89], resulting in a broad spectrum of interpretation by the media and in the literature [90, 91] This, in turn, has led to appropriate concern among patients and the parents of young patients as to the potential cancer risk from CT. This section reviews the available data and summarizes the conclusions and recommendation of our radiology colleagues. Of note, most of the concerns regarding radiation effects of CT pertain to children (especially young children) compared to adults [91].

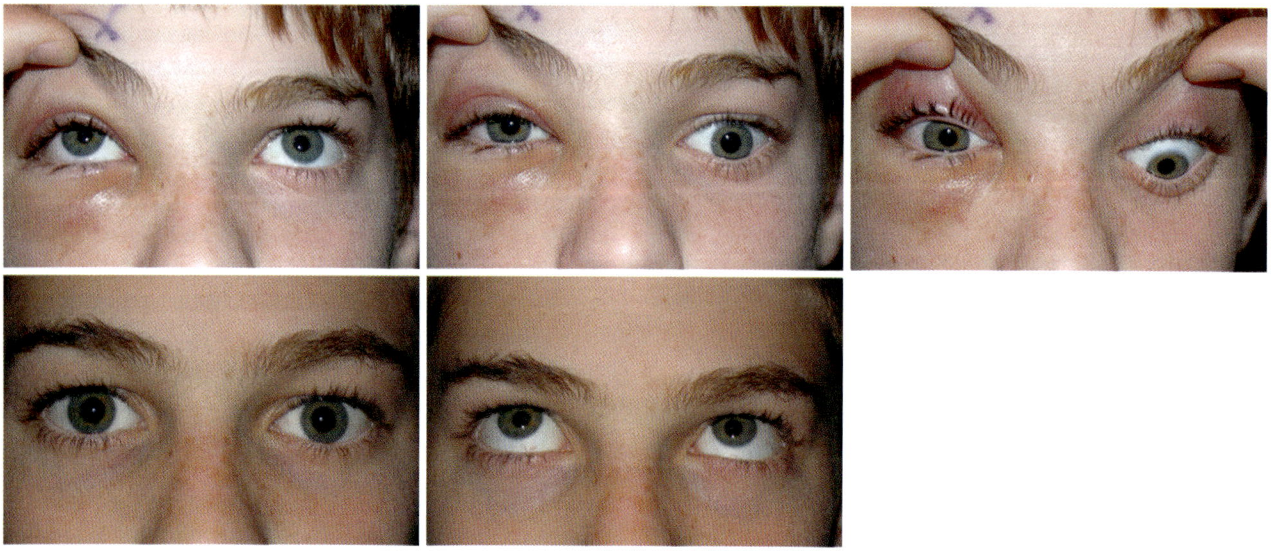

Fig. 65.14 Postoperative appearance of patient shown in Fig. 65.7. Top, 1 week after right WEBOF repair, the patient's vertical strabismus has worsened, with an obvious left hypotropia while fixating with the right eye (center). This is secondary to posttraumatic inferior rectus paresis (right) but is also consistent with a successful release of the entrapped right inferior rectus muscle and good supraduction (left). Bottom, 6 weeks after WEBOF repair, inferior rectus muscle function has recovered, and diplopia has resolved in all gazes

First, it is critical to remember that CT is an extremely powerful diagnostic tool that is readily available and is appropriate to use when clinically justified, even in children [92]. As a blanket statement, the risk of potential future cancer from a single CT is far less than the diagnostic benefit, especially in emergency situations [93, 94]. CT requires the use of a certain amount of ionizing radiation – there is simply no way around the basic physics of the technology. However, the radiation dosage of a diagnostic CT can be adjusted to lower levels without compromising diagnostic quality – the ALARA (As Low As Reasonably Achievable) concept.

Until recently, the actual risk of future cancer from low-level radiation exposure was not definitively quantified by any large study [93]. The majority of published conclusions relied on extrapolation from atomic bomb victims where there was whole-body exposure or from mathematical models [91, 95] However, since 2012 two major studies have been published which quantify CT radiation risk and reach some sobering conclusions [96, 97].

The study of ionizing radiation effects on the body is complex and beyond the scope of this chapter. Briefly, radiation affects specific tissues in different ways. As an example, studies on atomic bomb survivors concluded that the lung is more sensitive to the carcinogenic effects of radiation exposure than the liver, skeletal muscle, or skin [86, 94]. Furthermore, the dose of radiation from a CT study that strikes the body ("entrance dose") is not equivalent to the absorbed radiation by the body [96]. It is difficult to accurately quantify the risk of future malignancy from low-dose radiation exposure because low-dose radiation is a weak carcinogen [93, 96]. However, it is important to note that three expert panels, including the National Academy of Sciences, have concluded that there is a potential cancer risk even with low-level exposure and that this risk rises with increasing exposure [94]. In addition, the concept of "radiation effect" is critical in understanding the radiation risk from CT. Put simply, two types of radiation effects exist [91]. Deterministic effects are well-known to the orbitologist and are typified by high-dose radiation to the orbit (or any anatomic structure) over a short period of time, usually for the treatment of malignancy, resulting in myriad side effects (e.g., keratopathy, retinopathy, optic neuropathy, etc.). Stochastic effects are secondary to low doses of ionizing radiation absorbed over a long period of time, as seen in serial imaging, be it CT, mammography, etc. Although the side effects from such stochastic radiation are not immediately obvious, they do accumulate over time and are definitely more of an issue in the pediatric, rather than an adult, population.

The risk of radiation exposure is significantly different in children than in adults for multiple reasons [94]. First, children are more sensitive to the effects of radiation exposure than adults because of active tissue growth and development, with an estimated tenfold overall increased neoplastic potential [87]. Second, because of their age and statistically longer life span, children have more time in the ensuing decades to manifest any ill effects of radiation exposure; put simply, it is far more likely to see a radiation effect that takes 40 years to manifest in someone who is 10 years old than in someone who is 50 years old although, until recently, the magnitude of this risk from low-level exposure was difficult to accurately quantify. Third, unless the baseline radiation exposure parameters are adjusted for children, an equivalent dose has a higher effect on the smaller cross-sectional anatomic area of a child than of an adult; even with such adjustment, the final radiation dose to a child may be up to 50% higher than in an adult [98, 99]. Fourth and perhaps the most pertinent to the reader, the pediatric brain is especially sensitive to radiation effects [96], and at least a portion of the brain is unavoidably imaged during an orbital study. Finally, the ubiquity of CT in medicine and expanding indications for CT have led to ever-increasing utilization.

The use of diagnostic CT in the United States has risen by more than 20-fold, from two million studies annually in 1980 to almost 80 million in 2009 [88, 89]. Seven million CT studies are performed on children annually in the United States, and this number increases an average of 10% per year. Of note, the majority of brain CTs performed in children are for head trauma [87, 97, 100–102]. CT also accounts for a disproportionately high amount of total radiation exposure in medicine. A study from one academic radiology department published by Mettler and colleagues in 2000 concluded that although CT accounted for only 11% of procedures using ionizing radiation, 67% of all ionizing radiation was attributable to this modality [102].

Perhaps most importantly, CT of one organ system can be performed using a variety of techniques with a wide range of radiation exposure. This concept is extremely important to keep in mind for pediatric CT. As noted in a review by Brody and Frush, increasing the dose of radiation in an effort to improve image (and presumably diagnostic) quality has its limits, and after a certain threshold, additional radiation simply has no effect on improved diagnostic accuracy [94]. Therefore, lower doses of ionizing radiation in pediatric CT are preferable and do not necessarily compromise the quality of the study. The ALARA concept has markedly reduced radiation exposure in children from CT studies by 50–90% since about 2001, and these techniques continue to undergo refinement [87, 94, 97, 103].

The results of two recent large studies on radiation exposure from CT in children are worth summarizing in detail. Pearce and colleagues analyzed a National Health Care database in the United Kingdom and identified just over 175,000 pediatric patients that met the inclusion criteria of the study [96]. Of note, of 283,919 CT scans performed, the majority (64%) were of the head, an area of particular importance to the reader. The authors of the study estimated that the aver-

Table 65.2 Estimated radiation doses from one brain CT utilizing estimated standard CT dosages after 2001

	Males		Females	
Age at brain CT (years)	Brain dose (mGy)	Red bone marrow dose (mGy)	Brain dose (mGy)	Red bone marrow dose (mGy)
0	28	8	28	8
5	28	9	28	9
10	35	6	35	6
15	43	4	44	6
20	35	2	42	2

Reprinted in part from Pearce et al. [129]

age total dose from one brain CT in a child ranged between 28 and 44 mGy depending on age and gender (Table 65.2) [96]. The rates of leukemia and brain tumors (benign and malignant) in patients undergoing CT were analyzed based on dose. A significantly increased risk of both maladies was found in patients who received certain threshold cumulative radiation doses. Specifically, the relative risk (RR) of leukemia in patients with a cumulative dose of at least 30 mGy (mean 51.13 mGy) was 3.18 compared to those children who received less than 5 mGy. With regard to brain tumors, the RR was 3.32 in patients with a cumulative dose of 50 mGy (mean 104.16 mGy). The authors estimated that for children younger than 15 years, these threshold cumulative doses amounted to 5–10 head CTs for a 50 mGy bone marrow dose and 2–3 head CTs for a 60 mGy brain dose. Put another way, the authors concluded that one head CT before the age of 10 years would result in one excess case of leukemia and one excess brain tumor per 10,000 patients. Of note, multiple studies have concluded that younger children, especially those <5 years of age, are particularly sensitive to ionizing radiation [96, 97]. Admirably, Pearce et al. also pointed out that first, pediatric leukemia and brain tumors are relatively rare events and that tripling this risk from CT radiation exposure still makes these entities rare events; and second, the increased lifetime cancer risk from CT is "very small" compared with the natural occurrence of malignancy in the general population and with the benefits of CT "providing it is clinically justified." Herein lies the crux of the discussion: CT is a powerful and lifesaving technology with a now-proven underlying cancer risk and therefore should be used appropriately and judiciously.

In the second large study, Mathews and colleagues compared 680,211 pediatric patients who underwent CT with 10,939,680 who did not [97]. Mathews et al.'s study echoed the findings of Pearce et al. regarding subsequent leukemia development, providing independent confirmation of the previous study's findings; a cumulative dose of 30 mGy resulted in a relative risk of 3.18. Brain CT was associated with an excess incidence rate for brain cancer of 2.97/100,000 person-years. Put another way, the authors estimated 1 excess brain malignancy per 4000 brain CTs. As already noted, the authors also confirmed that children <5 years of age had the highest relative risk. However, even older children and adolescents showed an increased cancer risk following CT. Serial CT also increased the risk, presumably due to increased cumulative radiation dosages. Of particular interest to the reader, facial CT was associated with only a borderline increased RR of subsequent malignancy (IRR = 1.14). Since an orbital study is essentially a subseries of a standard maxillofacial protocol, it is reasonable to extrapolate this facial CT finding for orbital scans. In other words, based on the findings of Mathews et al., an orbital series should have a lower risk for subsequent brain or hematopoietic tumor development than a standard brain CT. However, this statement must be tempered by the varying protocols used at different healthcare facilities, some of which may extend a standard orbital series more cephalad, thereby exposing more of the brain to radiation, as well as the fact that in many (if not most) orbital injury cases, the brain is scanned along with the orbits as a precaution.

Mathews and colleagues also brought up some important limitations to their study (which do not change the prevailing opinion among radiologists that even low-dose radiation exposure increases cancer risk, albeit by a very small amount). First, as already noted, the authors point out that CT dosing protocols, especially for pediatric scans, have undergone a profound change since 2001 and that the current cancer risk from CT radiation may be smaller than calculated from older data. Second, the possibility of reverse causation may explain some of the increased brain tumor risk seen from head CT. In other words, symptomatology may have prompted initial brain imaging, which failed to diagnose an early, small lesion that went on to grow until diagnosis was made several years later; thus, the undiagnosed tumor prompted the initial CT, and therefore the CT did not cause the tumor. Of note, the authors still found an increased solid and hematopoietic cancer risk following CT exposure even when all brain tumors were excluded from analysis.

What, then, is the role of CT in pediatric orbital disease? First, as already stated, it is important to recognize that CT remains a valid and powerful tool in the pediatric population. In cases of head and orbital trauma, CT remains the imaging modality of choice because of its ready availability, rapid acquisition time, excellent resolution of bony and soft tissue orbital anatomy, and reasonable resolution of brain anatomy, especially in cases of acute intracranial hemorrhage. That said, it is also important to remember that a pediatric brain CT carries an increased risk of brain malignancy when compared to facial (i.e., orbital) CT based on the results of Mathews et al.'s study, and a brain CT should not be a knee-jerk response to every pediatric orbital trauma.

The authors recommend the following guidelines for the judicious and appropriate use of orbital CT, many of them gleaned from the recommendations of the American College of Radiology:

1. *The right scan for the right pathology*: In general, CT is excellent for imaging bone, and therefore is useful in the evaluation of trauma and orbital infection (which is often secondary to adjacent paranasal sinus disease). CT is also helpful in the diagnosis of metallic and wooden foreign bodies [104]. Unless indicated, avoid including a brain CT with the orbital study. Consider MRI in non-urgent orbital pathology.
2. *Avoid plain X-rays*: There are few indications for "screening" plain films of the face (see Table 65.3). On occasion, a plain X-ray is necessary to rule out occult metal prior to MRI. Otherwise, plain films should be avoided; they simply do not provide adequate detail of orbital or periocular pathology, but still expose the patient to radiation.
3. *Order the right scan the first time*: An axial imaging study of the brain is NOT equivalent to a dedicated orbital and facial study with axial and coronal views. Sometimes both the central nervous system and the orbit require imaging, but very often, imaging of the orbit suffices. In one study, the estimated effective dose from a head CT in a 5-year old child was 4mSV, equal to about 200 chest X-rays [94]. On occasion, the clinical findings may obviate the need for CT. As an already mentioned but also an admittedly controversial example, one could argue that routine CT imaging in a pediatric WEBOF is of little use because of the pathognomonic clinical features and predictable intraoperative findings; that said, at present pre-operative CT imaging of a suspected WEBOF remains the standard of care.
4. *Communicate*: Discuss with the radiologist or emergency room physician the *specific* area of concern, stressing the need for views limited to the orbit, unless brain imaging is indicated.
5. *Insist on seeing the actual scan* (and not simply the report) if the patient is being referred from another institution. In more routine cases, a delay of several days while the mislaid compact disc of the scan is being mailed is of little consequence. However, in an urgent situation (WEBOF, orbital abscess, etc.), absence of the actual images may force the physician to repeat the study, resulting in more radiation exposure for the child. If possible, make every attempt to obtain a digital copy of the original scan in a timely fashion to avoid reimaging.
6. *Make sure that your imaging facility has specific pediatric protocols* with decreased radiation exposure using the ALARA concept. All facilities accredited by the American College of Radiology must have pediatric protocols in place [94].
7. When possible, maximize diagnostic accuracy by having *the study interpreted by a pediatric radiologist or neuroradiologist*. Discuss any specific clinical suspicions (WEBOF, occult wooden foreign body, etc.) with the radiologist *prior* to the study to maximize CT technique.
8. *When possible, use single-pass technology with coronal reconstruction*. Newer multidetector CTs are extremely useful in certain clinical situations (CTA, etc.), but are usually unnecessary in typical trauma or infection cases [103]. Note that single-pass reconstruction does suffer from image degradation and may miss subtle abnormalities in WEBOF.
9. *Consider other imaging modalities* (MRI, ultrasound), especially if serial imaging is needed. When possible, use MR angiography rather than CT angiography in children. Note that MRI is typically avoided as the initial

Table 65.3 Comparison of radiologic procedures for an infant or child presenting with orbital asymmetry, proptosis, and visual loss

Radiologic procedure	Rating	Comments	RRL
MRI head and/or orbit without and with contrast	8		None
MRI head and/or orbit without contrast	7		None
CT head and/or orbit with contrast	6		3
CT head and or orbit without contrast	5		3
MRA head and neck	4	In selected cases when vascular disease is suspected	None
CTA head and neck	2	If vascular disease is suspected	4
X-ray orbit	1		1
Rating scale: 1–3, usually not appropriate; 4–6, may be appropriate; 7–9, usually appropriate			

In the rating column, higher numbers are safer. Note that CTA has a higher radiation dose than CT; when possible, MRA should be considered for suspected pediatric vascular disease. Also note that, despite having a low RRL, orbital X-ray has the lowest rating, mainly because it has such poor diagnostic value in orbital disease and yet exposes the child to radiation. Note that MRI/MRA is more time consuming than CT/CTA and may require general anesthesia or intravenous sedation; anesthesia risks are not included in rating scale. Modified from the American Academy of Radiology. For more details on imaging recommendation for specific orbital processes, see *"ACR Appropriateness Criteria. Orbits, Vision and Visual Loss,"* published by American College of Radiology. Available at https://acsearch.acr.org/docs/69486/Narrative/

CTA computed tomographic angiography, *MRA* magnetic resonance angiography, *RRL* relative radiation level.

imaging modality in trauma because of poor bone resolution, limited access to MRI compared to CT, length of study compared to CT, and possibility of an occult, posttraumatic metallic foreign body that may shift in the magnetic field of the MRI.

10. *Discuss with the patient's parents the rationale for the use of CT* in their particular clinical situation, the necessity of ionizing radiation in CT, and the fact that radiation dosages will be age- and size-adjusted. In one study, a majority of parents were unaware that CT exposed their child to ionizing radiation [105]. As importantly, this study also found that providing information about radiation exposure in CT did not change the parents' decision to proceed with imaging.

Periocular and Orbital Foreign Bodies

Orbital foreign bodies occur in about one of every six cases of penetrating orbital injury [107, 108]. The makeup of the foreign body (FB) varies widely and includes organic (wooden) and inorganic (metal, glass, etc.) materials [109]. Most intraorbital FBs are inorganic [109]. Multiple studies have shown that the diagnosis and management of periocular and orbital FBs is fraught with pitfalls for multiple reasons, which may be further compounded in the pediatric age group [104, 110, 111].

As a general rule, metallic FBs are easier to diagnose than nonmetallic substances, simply because metal is much more easily visualized on CT. By far the most difficult substance to diagnose and manage is wood [104].

Somewhat counterintuitively, history and examination may not be helpful in making the diagnosis of retained foreign body, especially in children. Multiple studies have shown that even in an acute trauma situation, the patient does not realize that the injury involved a penetrating foreign body [104, 110, 111]. In some cases, the initial trauma occurred months or even years previously, and no association is made by the patient and physician between the initial, distant trauma, and subsequent long-term sequelae [109]. In children, the history of the injury is notoriously inaccurate, either because the child does not recall the specifics of the incident or is afraid to admit them in front of the parents [109]. Clinical examination may also be misleading [112]. In one study of wooden intraorbital FBs, the authors found that in 53% of cases, no eyelid laceration was found because the entry wound occurred in the conjunctiva [104]. If there is a significant lag in initial presentation, the clinician may follow the wrong path of diagnosis: smoldering infection or inflammation from a retained FB may be misdiagnosed as idiopathic orbital inflammation (inflammatory orbital pseudotumor), allergy, leaking dermoid cyst, chronic conjunctivitis, and so forth.

Several rules regarding possible periocular and orbital FBs should be stressed. First, always suspect a retained foreign body in all cases of penetrating periocular trauma, regardless of the history (Fig. 65.15). Second, have a low index for imaging all patients with penetrating periocular injury, with several caveats to follow. Third, be suspicious of recurrent episodes of inflammation in children; retained FBs may respond temporarily to systemic antibiotics or corticosteroids. Finally, never attempt removal of a periocular foreign body without detailed imaging: the FB may have penetrated the globe, the frontal lobe of the brain, or the cavernous sinus and carotid siphon (Fig. 65.16) [109–113]. Orbital roof penetration by a transorbital FB appears to occur more frequently in children than in adults [111].

With regard to imaging, in general the initial modality is CT [104]. While plain X-rays may indeed show metallic FBs, they will miss organic materials and will not give the clinician enough anatomic detail if extirpation is planned (Fig. 65.17) [104, 114, 115]. Furthermore, as already mentioned in the previous section, plain X-rays will unnecessarily expose the patient to additional radiation. CT will reveal metallic FBs without difficulty in most cases, provided that the image width is adequate (Fig. 65.18). Here again the physician is faced with a clinical conundrum: decreased image width means more CT slices through a given volume and more radiation exposure; conversely, increased image width requires less radiation but may miss the foreign body. The final decision on image width is usually left up to the clinician and radiologist, but a determintion should be made prior to the initial study to decrease the need for additional imaging and radiation exposure. Although metal is usually easily imaged on CT, it also results in a significant amount of artifact, making visualization of surrounding bony and soft tissue anatomy difficult (Fig. 65.17). There is little that can be done about this metallic artifact, and in most cases, CT will still provide adequate anatomic information as to the tissue involved. Glass FBs are variably visualized on CT, depending largely on the amount of heavy metal contained within the glass (Fig. 65.19). Wooden FBs are notoriously difficult to image and are often either not seen at all or misdiagnosed initially as orbital emphysema (Fig. 65.20) [104, 116, 117]. Although MRI may be helpful in the diagnosis of wooden FBs [109], in general CT is still the imaging modality of choice. On occasion, CT and MRI play complimentary roles, especially with wooden FBs [113, 116, 118, 119].

Several principles regarding CT and intraorbital wooden FBs should be remembered. First, squared-off edges or a staghorn appearance are highly unlikely findings in true

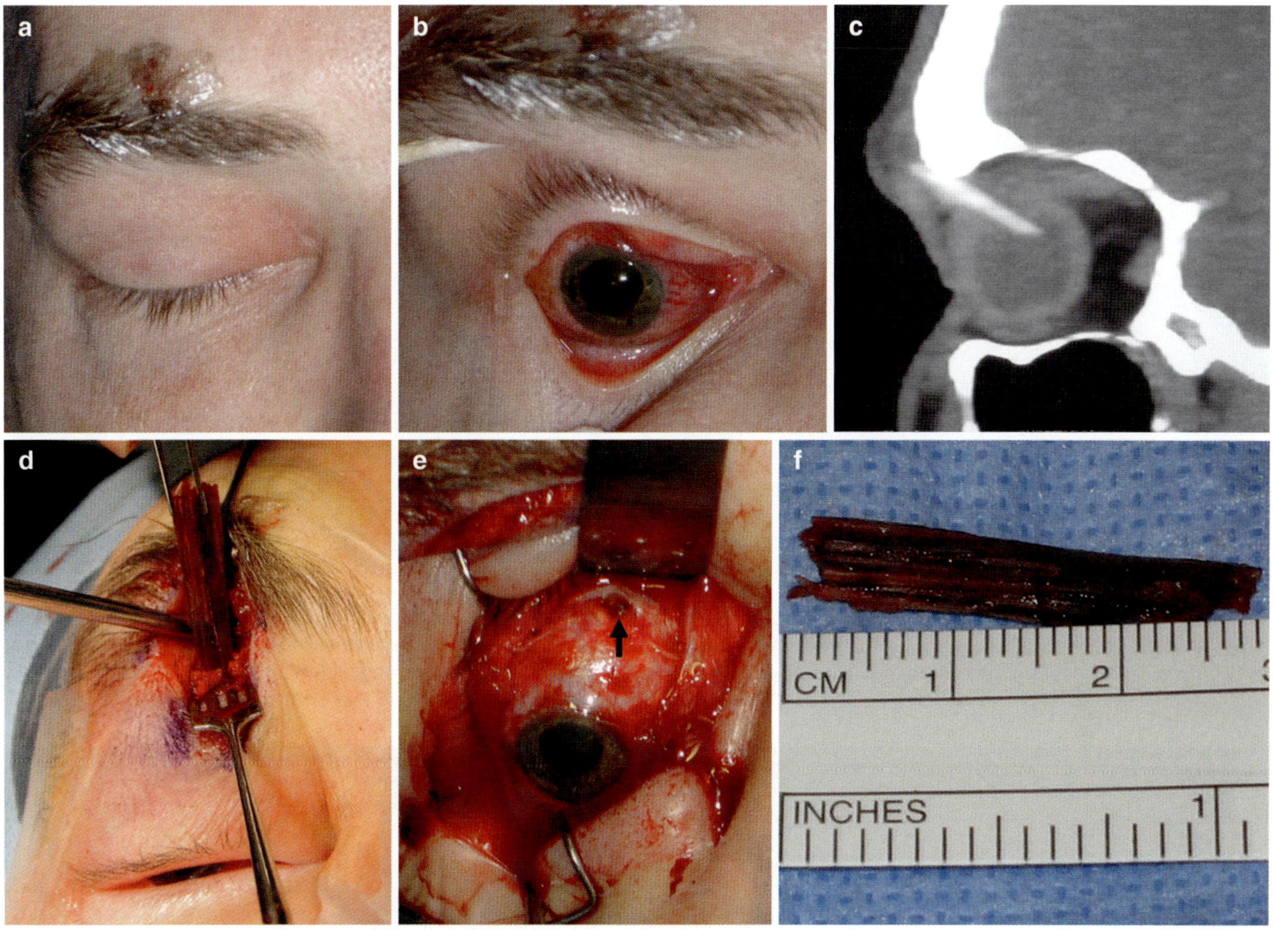

Fig. 65.15 Unsuspected orbital FB with globe rupture. (**a**) Clinical photograph of a patient who presented to a local emergency room after being struck in the right brow with a piece of pressure-treated lumber while using a power saw. (**a**) Superficial wood was removed and the brow laceration was glued. No imaging was performed. (**b**) A corneal abrasion and dense vitreous hemorrhage was noted on ophthalmic exam 2 days later. He had complete ptosis and could not elevate his globe. The patient was followed for 5 days before referral to the Wills Eye Hospital . (**c**) CT imaging revealed an orbital FB penetrating the globe. The wood appears opaque because of pressure treatment with chemicals. (**d**) During surgical exploration, the wood was backed out through the original brow laceration. (**e**) The globe rupture site (arrow) was repaired. (**f**) The wooden FB. The patient underwent subsequent vitrectomy and lensectomy with recovery of vision to 20/50. He never developed endophthalmitis

intraorbital emphysema (Fig. 65.20) [104]. In addition, unless the emphysema is significant and under pressure (described as a "tension pneumo-orbit"), air will not cause significant distortion of the globe and orbital soft tissue. Second, although to the human eye the density of wood may be identical to that of air, CT software often finds a significant disparity, regardless of the hydration and type of wood [104]. If a wooden FB is suspected, the clinician should ask the radiologist to obtain quantitative density measurements of known air (e.g., in the paranasal sinuses) and compare these to the lucency within the orbit (Fig. 65.21). If orbital emphysema is indeed present, the density measurements will correlate; if, on the other hand, wood is present, a significant disparity will be picked up by the CT's computer. If quantitative density measurements are not available, then the CT window settings can be optimized for identification of wooden FBs. One simple rule to remember is that standard bone windows are usually more sensitive than soft tissue windows for wooden FBs [104, 116, 120].

Management of periocular and orbital FBs also follows some general tenets [112, 113, 121, 122]. As already noted, extirpation should never be performed without adequate imaging. Because of the proximity of the orbit to other critical skull base structures, care must be taken in evaluating the orbital roof and cavernous sinus for signs of involvement. If skull base involvement is suspected, neurosurgical consultation may be prudent. This is especially important with suspected cavernous sinus involvement, since the carotid siphon

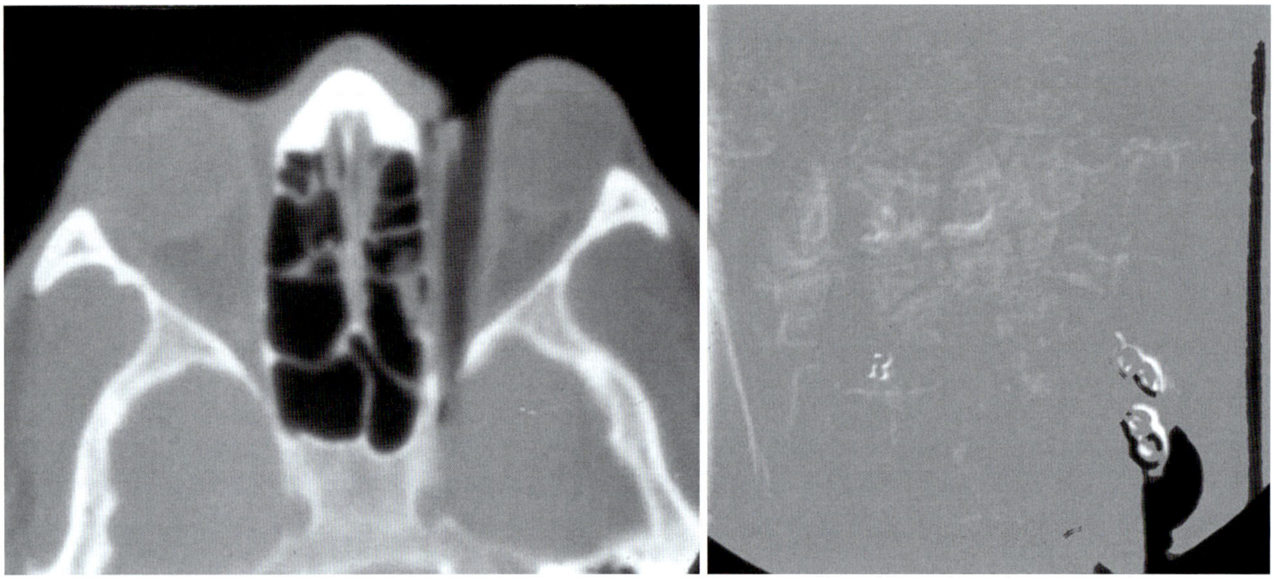

Fig. 65.16 Orbital FB penetrating the cavernous sinus through the superior orbital fissure. Left, axial CT demonstrates a radiolucent segment of wood with the tip in the cavernous sinus. Angiography was performed prior to removal and demonstrated penetration of the carotid siphon. Right, after adequate collateral flow via the circle of Willis was confirmed, the internal carotid artery was occluded with coils and the FB removed

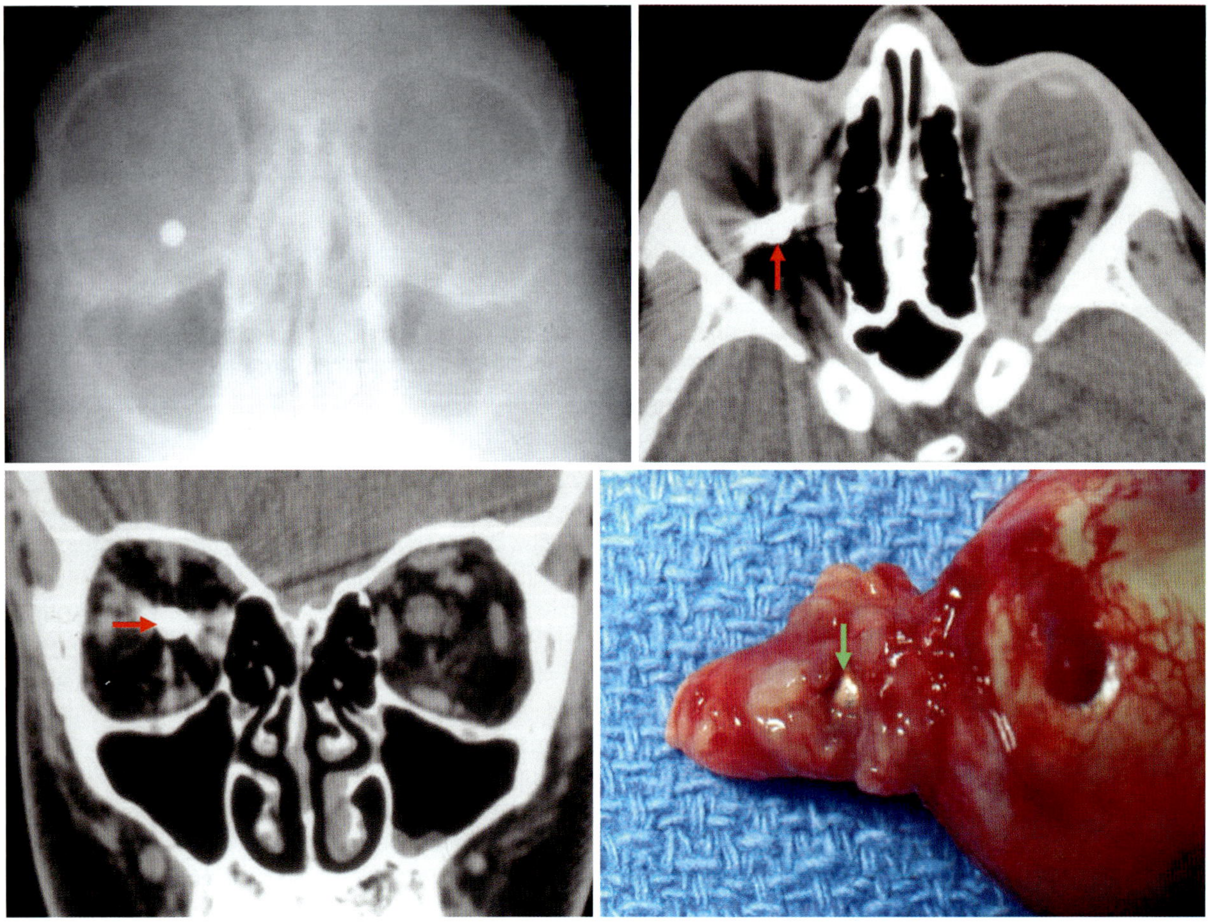

Fig. 65.17 Metallic orbital FB. Top left, a plain X-ray of an unfortunate 12-year-old boy shot in the left eye by a BB pellet. Although the pellet is clearly seen within the right orbit on the image, no additional anatomic detail is available. On axial (top right) and coronal (bottom left) soft tissue CT images, the BB is noted behind the globe in the area of the optic nerve. Note the distortion of the image by the metallic artifact. Bottom right, on subsequent enucleation, the BB was found imbedded in the optic nerve after penetrating the posterior sclera

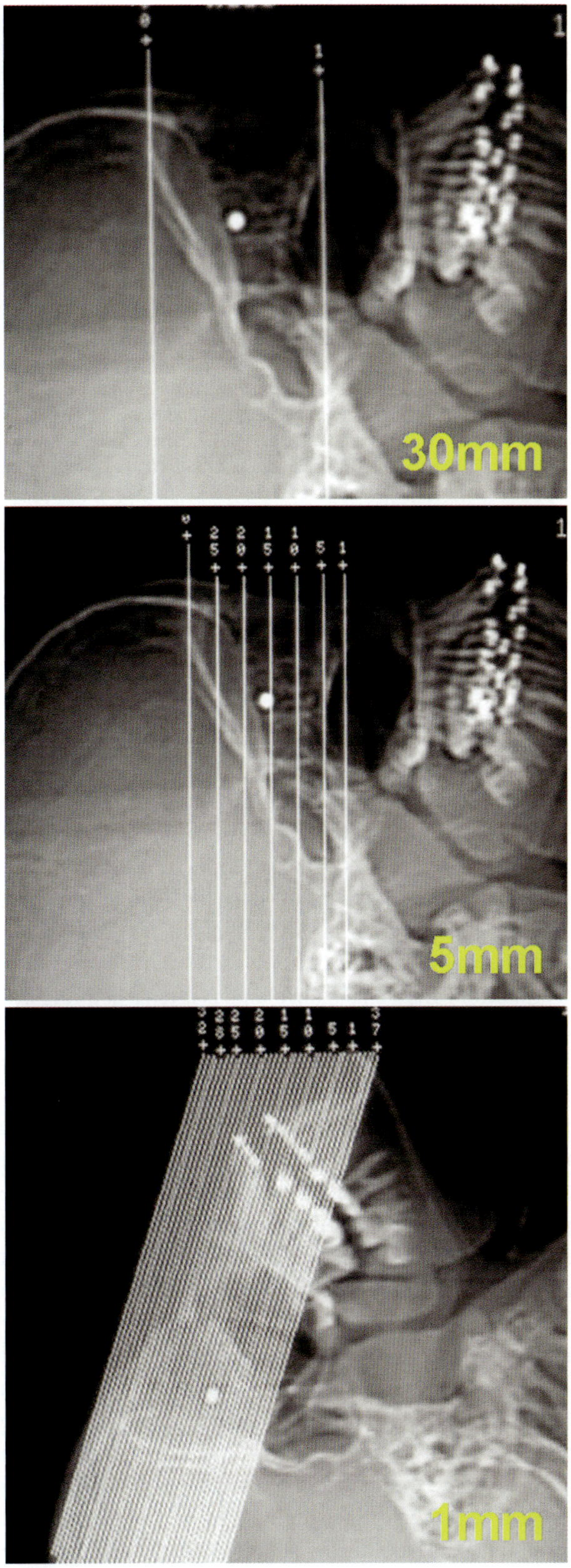

Fig. 65.18 Image width and FB localization. On scout films prior to coronal CT, various proposed CT widths are demonstrated. Top, a 30 mm width would miss the entire orbit. Middle, 5 mm cuts might also miss the FB, although scatter artifact from the metal would probably be noted. Bottom, 1 mm cuts would definitively demonstrate the FB but at a cost of higher radiation exposure

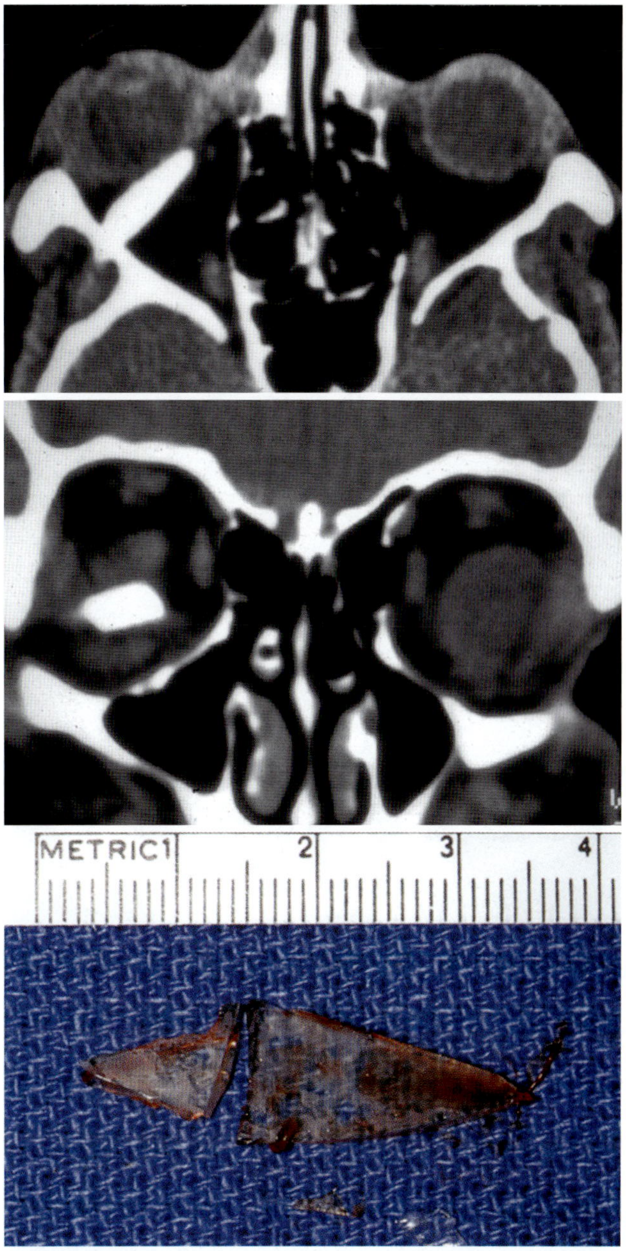

Fig. 65.19 Glass FB. An opaque FB is obvious on axial (top) and coronal (middle) soft tissue CT images. Bottom, the glass FBs after surgical removal

may be lacerated [123, 124]. Interventional arteriography with temporary or permanent carotid occlusion may be necessary before FB removal (Fig. 65.16) [125]. Extensive involvement of the paranasal sinuses may warrant otolaryngologic consultation for a combined FB extirpation.

In general, three broad findings will influence the decision of FB removal: FB makeup, intraorbital location, and extent of injury [113, 121]. Most metallic foreign bodies are inert and, unless they are directly causing optic neuropathy or other cranial neuropathy/external ophthalmoplegia, may be

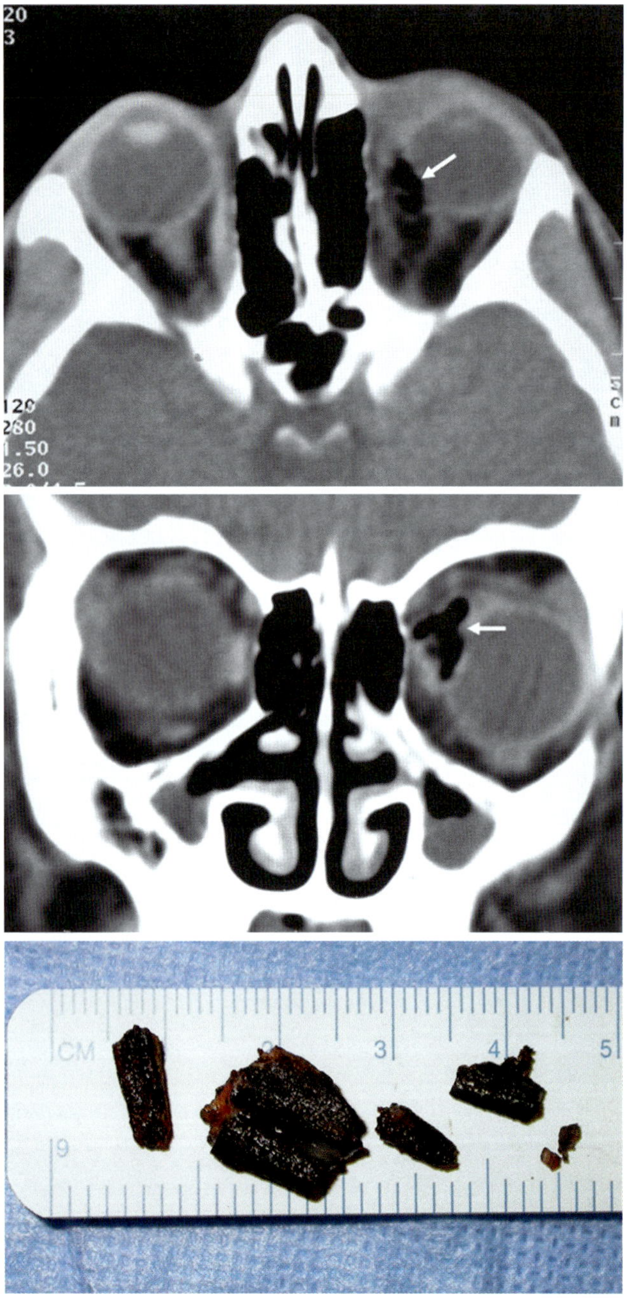

Fig. 65.20 Wooden FB. A child referred for possible laceration of the medial rectus muscle and orbital emphysema after falling while playing outside. Note the staghorn appearance of the intraorbital "air" and the distortion of the sclera (arrows). Surgical exploration revealed multiple wood splinters

left in place with little long-term consequence [121]. Three important exceptions to this rule should be considered: (1) copper results in a significant inflammatory response and, when possible, should be removed; (2) lead may cause systemic toxicity, although this is highly unlikely from a small intraorbital FB and to date has not been reported in the literature; and (3) intraorbital iron may theoretically result in siderosis bulbi and sequential electroretinography may be

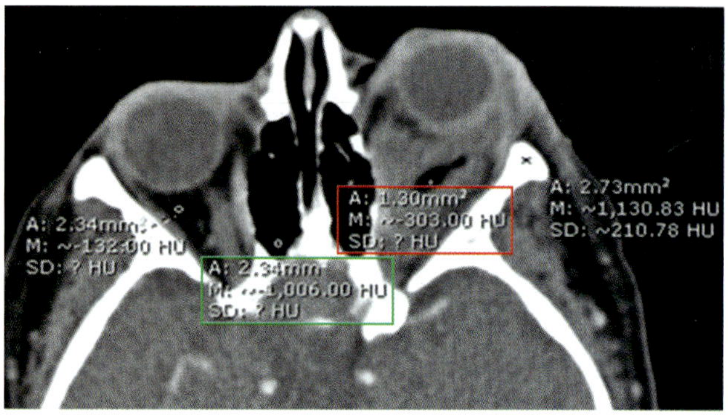

Fig. 65.21 Quantitative CT measurements. An axial view of a possible wooden FB initially read as emphysema. On quantitative analysis, note that known air has a different value (-1006HU, green box) when compared to the suspected FB (-303HU, red box). Surgical exploration confirmed the presence of a wooden FB. *HU*, Hounsfield unit. (Courtesy of Peter A. D. Rubin, MD)

warranted if the FB is left in place [113, 121, 126]. All patients with retained periocular or intraorbital metallic FBs should be warned to avoid MRI. Glass can also be left in place if no clinical deficits are noted and the FB is inaccessible. Wood, on the other hand, presents a problem, since infection is a common sequela (Fig. 65.22). Location within the orbit is also of paramount importance. An anteriorly located FB within the lids and orbit may be removed safely, regardless of makeup [121]. That said, surgical exploration for a FB is notoriously difficult, since the FB may move or be retracted during surgery [121]. If at all possible, the FB should be stabilized early during exploration. For eyelid or very anterior FBs, a chalazion clamp is often a helpful instrument (Peter A. D. Rubin, MD, personal communication). Unless organic, orbital apical FBs are usually left in place, since exploration in this area carries a significant risk of optic and other cranial neuropathy [113, 121]. If direct optic neuropathy is present, a difficult decision must be made by the patient: the possibility of successful FB removal with reversal of the optic neuropathy must be tempered by the risk of iatrogenically induced progression of optic neuropathy during surgical exploration (Fig. 65.23) [127]. Of note, most visual loss from inorganic FBs occurs at the time of initial trauma [113]. Conversely, because retained organic FBs may result in infection and incite a significant inflammatory reaction over time, the patient may develop a progressive optic neuropathy weeks to years following the initial trauma.

Removal of wooden foreign bodies in the acute phase may also be difficult, since multiple splintered pieces may be present [128]. The clinician should always warn the patient and family that complete removal of the wooden FB may not be tenable and that additional surgery may be needed in the future. Furthermore, there is a significant risk for infection from retained intraorbital wood, and the patient will need to be followed over the long term. Paradoxically, subsequent

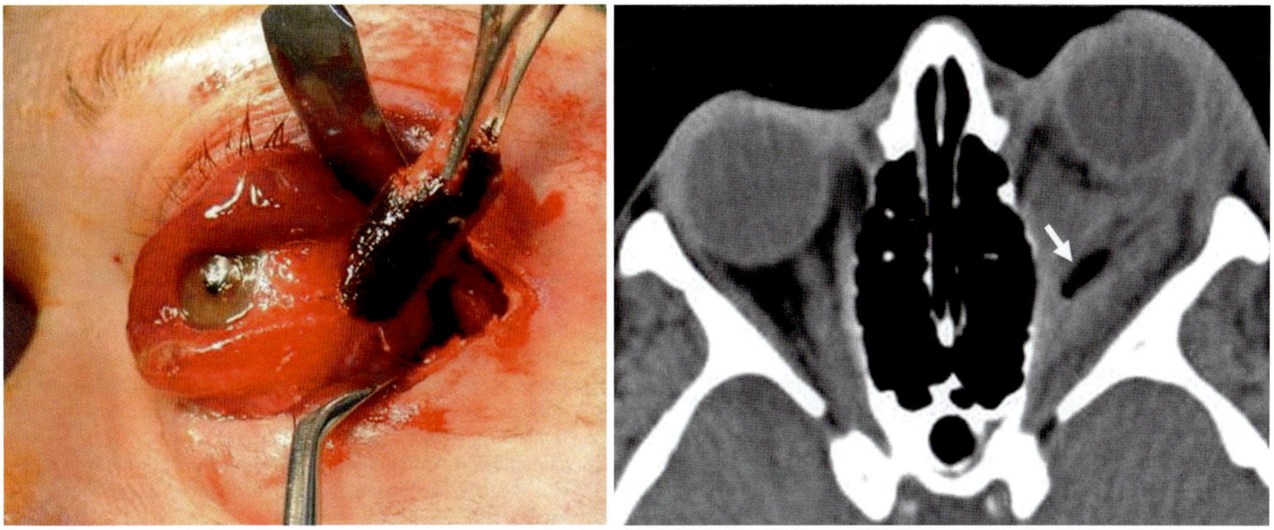

Fig. 65.22 Infection from a retained wooden orbital FB. The patient was admitted after trauma with initial CT imaging read as orbital emphysema (right). She was placed on intravenous corticosteroids for orbital edema that progressed over several days. Consultation with an orbital specialist was obtained after the patient lost vision. Quantitative CT measurements were performed (see Fig. 65.21), and urgent orbital exploration revealed a wooden FB surrounded by purulence. The patient did not regain significant vision postoperatively. (Courtesy of Peter A. D. Rubin, MD)

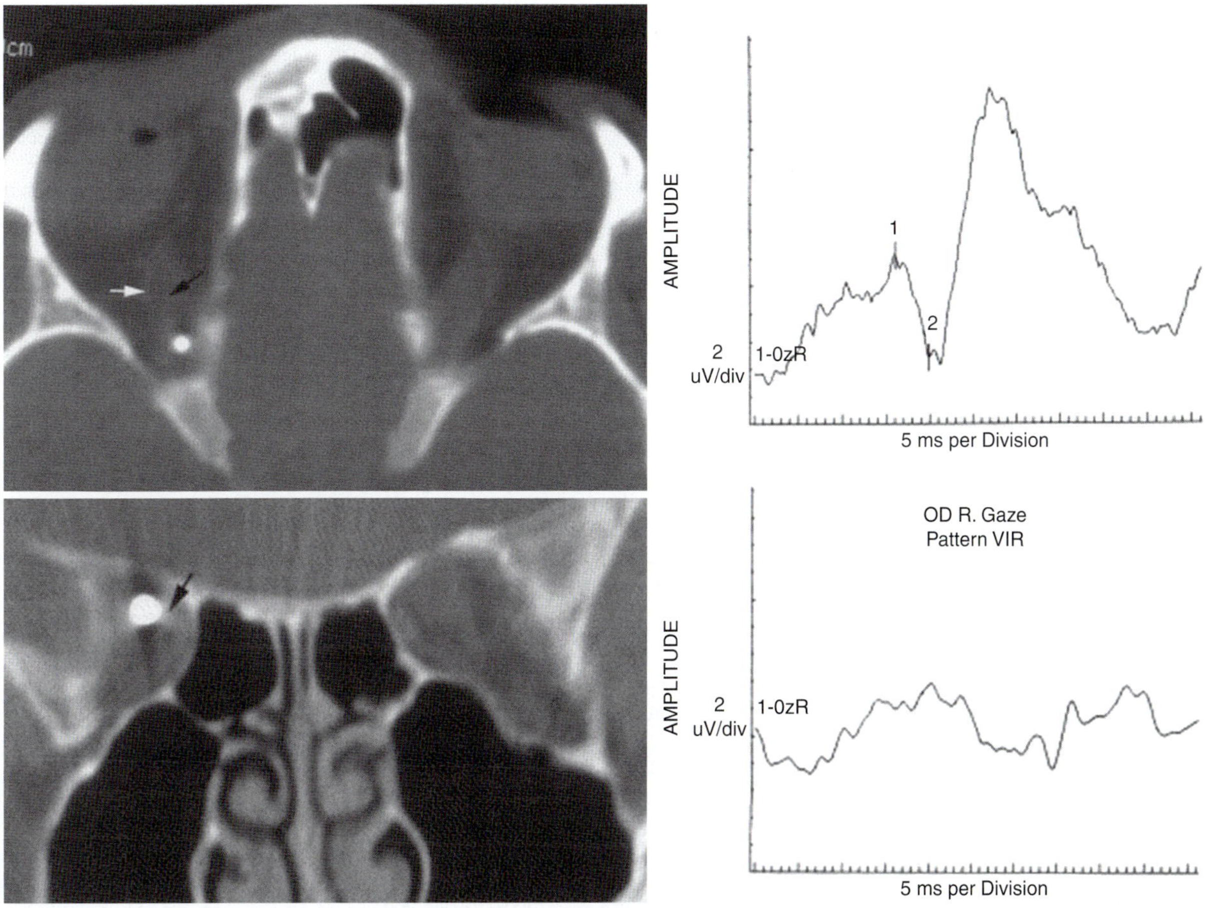

Fig. 65.23 Gaze-evoked amaurosis from an orbital apical FB. Left, axial (top) and coronal (bottom) CT of an apical birdshot causing gaze-evoked amaurosis in the right eye. The pellet is located beneath the superior rectus/levator complex (top black arrow) and superior ophthalmic vein (white arrow) and distorts the optic nerve medially (bottom black arrow). Right, visually evoked potential OD is normal in primary gaze (top) but markedly extinguishes in right gaze (bottom). A peripheral visual field defect was also present. Removal via craniotomy resulted in resolution of the amaurosis and optic neuropathy but caused diplopia requiring strabismus surgery

infection may be helpful in surgical location of the FB: the surgeon can often follow the purulent fistulous tract to the retained wood.

All patients with periocular or intraorbital FBs should receive a course of systemic antibiotics (especially if the FB is organic) although the specific agents and duration of therapy vary widely [104, 110, 111, 113].

References

1. Long JA, Tann T. Eyelid and lacrimal trauma. In: Kuhn F, Pieramici D, editors. Ocular trauma. New York: Thieme; 2002.
2. Weiss HB, Friedman DI, Coben JH. Incidence of dog bite injuries treated in emergency departments. JAMA. 1998;279:51–3.
3. Cornwell JM. Dog bite prevention: responsible pet ownership and animal safety. J Am Vet Med Assoc. 1997;210:1147–8.
4. Beck AM, Jones BA. Unreported dog bites in children. Public Health Rep. 1985;100:315–21.
5. Burroughs JR, Soparkar CN, Patrinely JR, Williams PD, Holck DE. Periocular dog bite injuries and responsible care. Ophthal Plast Reconstr Surg. 2002;18:416–9; discussion 9–20
6. Sacks JJ, Lockwood R, Hornreich J, Sattin RW. Fatal dog attacks, 1989–1994. Pediatrics. 1996;97:891–5.
7. Bratton EM, Golas L, Wei LA, Davies BW, Durairaj VD. Ophthalmic manifestations of facial dog bites in children. Ophthalmic Plast Reconstr Surg. 2018;34:106–9.
8. Prendes MA, Jian-Amadi A, Chang SH, Shaftel SS. Ocular trauma from dog bites: characterization, associations, and treatment patterns at a regional level I trauma center over 11 years. Ophthalmic Plast Reconstr Surg. 2016;32:279–83.
9. Gonnering RS. Ocular adnexal injury and complications in orbital dog bites. Ophthalmic Plast Reconstr Surg. 1987;3:231–5.
10. Tu AH, Girotto JA, Singh N, et al. Facial fractures from dog bite injuries. Plast Reconstr Surg. 2002;109:1259–65.
11. Wei LA, Chen HH, Hink EM, Durairaj VD. Pediatric facial fractures from dog bites. Ophthalmic Plast Reconstr Surg. 2013;29:179–82.
12. Murchison AP, Bilyk JR. Pediatric canalicular lacerations: epidemiology and variables affecting repair success. J Pediatr Ophthalmol Strabismus. 2014;51:242–8.
13. Wladis EJ, Dewan MA. Periorbital trauma from pit bull terrier attacks. Orbit. 2012;31:200–2.
14. Jordan DR, Ziai S, Gilberg SM, Mawn LA. Pathogenesis of canalicular lacerations. Ophthalmic Plast Reconstr Surg. 2008;24:394–8.
15. Wulc AE, Arterberry JF. The pathogenesis of canalicular laceration. Ophthalmology. 1991;98:1243–9.
16. Botek AA, Goldberg SH. Management of eyelid dog bites. J Craniomaxillofac Trauma. 1995;1:18–24.
17. Kersten RC. Re: "Pathogenesis of canalicular lacerations". Ophthalmic Plast Reconstr Surg. 2009;25:420–1; author reply 1
18. Jordan DR, Ziai S, Gilberg SM, Mawn LA. Pathogenesis of canalicular lacerations. Ophthal Plast Reconstr Surg. 2008;24:394–8.
19. White WL, Glover AT, Buckner AB, Hartshorne MF. Relative canalicular tear flow as assessed by dacryoscintigraphy. Ophthalmology. 1989;96:167–9.
20. Murgatroyd H, Craig JP, Sloan B. Determination of relative contribution of the superior and inferior canaliculi to the lacrimal drainage system in health using the drop test. Clin Exp Ophthalmol. 2004;32:404–10.
21. Barahimi B, Murchison AP, Bilyk JR. Forget me not. Surv Ophthalmol. 2010;55:467–80.
22. Slonim CB. Dog bite-induced canalicular lacerations: a review of 17 cases. Ophthal Plast Reconstr Surg. 1996;12:218–22.
23. Bailie WE, Stowe EC, Schmitt AM. Aerobic bacterial flora of oral and nasal fluids of canines with reference to bacteria associated with bites. J Clin Microbiol. 1978;7:223–31.
24. Talan DA, Citron DM, Abrahamian FM, Moran GJ, Goldstein EJ. Bacteriologic analysis of infected dog and cat bites. Emergency Medicine Animal Bite Infection Study Group. N Engl J Med. 1999;340:85–92.
25. Abrahamian FM, Goldstein EJ. Microbiology of animal bite wound infections. Clin Microbiol Rev. 2011;24:231–46.
26. Savar A, Kirszrot J, Rubin PA. Canalicular involvement in dog bite related eyelid lacerations. Ophthal Plast Reconstr Surg. 2008;24:296–8.
27. Lion C, Escande F, Burdin JC. Capnocytophaga canimorsus infections in human: review of the literature and cases report. Eur J Epidemiol. 1996;12:521–33.
28. Cummings P. Antibiotics to prevent infection in patients with dog bite wounds: a meta-analysis of randomized trials. Ann Emerg Med. 1994;23:535–40.
29. Hawes MJ, Segrest DR. Effectiveness of bicanalicular silicone intubation in the repair of canalicular lacerations. Ophthal Plast Reconstr Surg. 1985;1:185–90.
30. Wladis EJ, Aakalu VK, Tao JP, et al. Monocanalicular stents in eyelid lacerations: a report by the American Academy of Ophthalmology. Ophthalmology. 2019;126:1324.
31. Chu YC, Ma L, Wu SY, Tsai YJ. Comparing pericanalicular sutures with direct canalicular wall sutures for canalicular laceration. Ophthalmic Plast Reconstr Surg. 2011;27:422–5.
32. Kersten RC, Kulwin DR. "One-stitch" canalicular repair. A simplified approach for repair of canalicular laceration. Ophthalmology. 1996;103:785–9.
33. Della Rocca DA, Ahmad SM, Della Rocca RC. Direct repair of canalicular lacerations. Facial Plast Surg. 2007;23:149–55.
34. Loff HJ, Wobig JL, Dailey RA. The bubble test: an atraumatic method for canalicular laceration repair. Ophthalmic Plast Reconstr Surg. 1996;12:61–4.
35. Murchison AP, Bilyk JR. Canalicular laceration repair: an analysis of variables affecting success. Ophthalmic Plast Reconstr Surg. 2014;30:410–4.
36. Singh S, Ganguly A, Hardas A, Tripathy D, Rath S. Canalicular lacerations: factors predicting outcome at a tertiary eye care centre. Orbit. 2017;36:13–8.
37. Reifler DM. Management of canalicular laceration. Surv Ophthalmol. 1991;36:113–32.
38. Hawes MJ, Segrest DR. Effectiveness of bicanalicular silicone intubation in the repair of canalicular lacerations. Ophthalmic Plast Reconstr Surg. 1985;1:185–90.
39. Dortzbach RK, Angrist RA. Silicone intubation for lacerated lacrimal canaliculi. Ophthalmic Surg. 1985;16:639–42.
40. Jordan DR, Nerad JA, Tse DT. The pigtail probe, revisited. Ophthalmology. 1990;97:512–9.
41. Kennedy RH, May J, Dailey J, Flanagan JC. Canalicular laceration. An 11-year epidemiologic and clinical study. Ophthalmic Plast Reconstr Surg. 1990;6:46–53.
42. Naik MN, Kelapure A, Rath S, Honavar SG. Management of canalicular lacerations: epidemiological aspects and experience with Mini-Monoka monocanalicular stent. Am J Ophthalmol. 2008;145:375–80.
43. Anastas CN, Potts MJ, Raiter J. Mini Monoka silicone monocanalicular lacrimal stents: subjective and objective outcomes. Orbit. 2001;20:189–200.
44. Lee H, Chi M, Park M, Baek S. Effectiveness of canalicular laceration repair using monocanalicular intubation with Monoka tubes. Acta Ophthalmol. 2009;87:793–6.

45. Leibovitch I, Kakizaki H, Prabhakaran V, Selva D. Canalicular lacerations: repair with the Mini-Monoka(R) monocanalicular intubation stent. Ophthalmic Surg Lasers Imaging. 2010;41:472–7.
46. Eo S, Park J, Cho S, Azari KK. Microsurgical reconstruction for canalicular laceration using Monostent and Mini-Monoka. Ann Plast Surg. 2010;64:421–7.
47. Wu SY, Ma L, Chen RJ, Tsai YJ, Chu YC. Analysis of bicanalicular nasal intubation in the repair of canalicular lacerations. Jpn J Ophthalmol. 2010;54:24–31.
48. Nam SM. Microscope-assisted reconstruction of canalicular laceration using Mini-Monoka. J Craniofac Surg. 2013;24:2056–8.
49. Liang X, Lin Y, Wang Z, et al. A modified bicanalicular intubation procedure to repair canalicular lacerations using silicone tubes. Eye (Lond). 2012;26:1542–7.
50. Mauriello JA Jr, Abdelsalam A. Use of a modified monocanalicular silicone stent in 33 eyelids. Ophthalmic Surg Lasers. 1996;27:929–34.
51. Singh M, Gautam N, Ahir N, Kaur M. Is the distance from punctum a factor in the anatomical and functional success of canalicular laceration repairs? Indian J Ophthalmol. 2017;65:1114–9.
52. Tavakoli M, Karimi S, Behdad B, Dizani S, Salour H. Traumatic canalicular laceration repair with a new monocanalicular silicone tube. Ophthalmic Plast Reconstr Surg. 2017;33:27–30.
53. Hatton MP, Watkins LM, Rubin PA. Orbital fractures in children. Ophthal Plast Reconstr Surg. 2001;17:174–9.
54. Hink EM, Wei LA, Durairaj VD. Clinical features and treatment of pediatric orbit fractures. Ophthalmic Plast Reconstr Surg. 2014;30:124–31.
55. Alcala-Galiano A, Arribas-Garcia IJ, Martin-Perez MA, Romance A, Montalvo-Moreno JJ, Juncos JM. Pediatric facial fractures: children are not just small adults. Radiographics. 2008;28:441–61; quiz 618
56. McGraw BL, Cole RR. Pediatric maxillofacial trauma. Age-related variations in injury. Arch Otolaryngol Head Neck Surg. 1990;116:41–5.
57. Maisel H. Postnatal growth and anatomy of the face. In: Mathog RH, editor. Maxillofacial trauma. Baltimore: Willimas & Wilkins; 1984.
58. Koltai PJ, Amjad I, Meyer D, Feustel PJ. Orbital fractures in children. Arch Otolaryngol Head Neck Surg. 1995;121:1375–9.
59. Chapman VM, Fenton LZ, Gao D, Strain JD. Facial fractures in children: unique patterns of injury observed by computed tomography. J Comput Assist Tomogr. 2009;33:70–2.
60. Fulcher TP, Sullivan TJ. Orbital roof fractures: management of ophthalmic complications. Ophthal Plast Reconstr Surg. 2003;19:359–63.
61. Rowe NL. Fractures of the facial skeleton in children. J Oral Surg. 1968;26:505–15.
62. Khosla M, Boren W. Mandibular fractures in children and their management. J Oral Surg. 1971;29:116–21.
63. Grant JH 3rd, Patrinely JR, Weiss AH, Kierney PC, Gruss JS. Trapdoor fracture of the orbit in a pediatric population. Plast Reconstr Surg. 2002;109:482–9; discussion 90–5
64. Jordan DR, Allen LH, White J, Harvey J, Pashby R, Esmaeli B. Intervention within days for some orbital floor fractures: the white-eyed blowout. Ophthal Plast Reconstr Surg. 1998;14:379–90.
65. Kulwin DR, Leadbetter MG. Orbital rim trauma causing a blowout fracture. Plast Reconstr Surg. 1984;73:969–71.
66. Raflo GT. Blow-in and blow-out fractures of the orbit: clinical correlations and proposed mechanisms. Ophthalmic Surg. 1984;15:114–9.
67. Smith B, Regan WF Jr. Blow-out fracture of the orbit; mechanism and correction of internal orbital fracture. Am J Ophthalmol. 1957;44:733–9.
68. Fujino T, Makino K. Entrapment mechanism and ocular injury in orbital blowout fracture. Plast Reconstr Surg. 1980;65:571–6.
69. Anderson RL, Panje WR, Gross CE. Optic nerve blindness following blunt forehead trauma. Ophthalmology. 1982;89:445–55.
70. Bansagi ZC, Meyer DR. Internal orbital fractures in the pediatric age group: characterization and management. Ophthalmology. 2000;107:829–36.
71. Parbhu KC, Galler KE, Li C, Mawn LA. Underestimation of soft tissue entrapment by computed tomography in orbital floor fractures in the pediatric population. Ophthalmology. 2008;115:1620–5.
72. McInnes AW, Burnstine MA. White-eyed medial wall orbital blowout fracture. Ophthal Plast Reconstr Surg. 2010;26:44–6.
73. Tse R, Allen L, Matic D. The white-eyed medial blowout fracture. Plast Reconstr Surg. 2007;119:277–86.
74. Brannan PA, Kersten RC, Kulwin DR. Isolated medial orbital wall fractures with medial rectus muscle incarceration. Ophthal Plast Reconstr Surg. 2006;22:178–83.
75. Wartak SA, Mehendale RA, Lotfi A. A unique case of asystole secondary to facial injury. Case Rep Med. 2012;2012:382605.
76. Lane K, Penne RB, Bilyk JR. Evaluation and management of pediatric orbital fractures in a primary care setting. Orbit. 2007;26:183–91.
77. Smith B, Lisman RD, Simonton J, Della RR. Volkmann's contracture of the extraocular muscles following blowout fracture. Plast Reconstr Surg. 1984;74:200–16.
78. Egbert JE, May K, Kersten RC, Kulwin DR. Pediatric orbital floor fracture: direct extraocular muscle involvement. Ophthalmology. 2000;107:1875–9.
79. Cohen SM, Garrett CG. Pediatric orbital floor fractures: nausea/vomiting as signs of entrapment. Otolaryngol Head Neck Surg. 2003;129:43–7.
80. Wachler BS, Holds JB. The missing muscle syndrome in blowout fractures: an indication for urgent surgery. Ophthal Plast Reconstr Surg. 1998;14:17–8.
81. Burnstine MA. Clinical recommendations for repair of isolated orbital floor fractures: an evidence-based analysis. Ophthalmology. 2002;109:1207–10; discussion 10–1; quiz 12–3.
82. Mehta VJ, Chelnis JG, Chen Q, Mawn LA. Effect of time to operative intervention on motility outcomes following orbital floor fracture repair in children. Ophthalmic Plast Reconstr Surg. 2018;34:351–4.
83. Sires BS, Stanley RB Jr, Levine LM. Oculocardiac reflex caused by orbital floor trapdoor fracture: an indication for urgent repair. Arch Ophthalmol. 1998;116:955–6.
84. Bernardini FP, Nerad J, Fay A, Zambelli A, Cruz AA. The revised direct transconjunctival approach to the orbital floor. Ophthalmic Plast Reconstr Surg. 2017;33:93–100.
85. Lane KA, Bilyk JR, Taub D, Pribitkin EA. "Sutureless" repair of orbital floor and rim fractures. Ophthalmology. 2009;116:135–8. e2.
86. Brenner DJ, Hall EJ. Computed tomography–an increasing source of radiation exposure. N Engl J Med. 2007;357:2277–84.
87. Shah NB, Platt SL. ALARA: is there a cause for alarm? Reducing radiation risks from computed tomography scanning in children. Curr Opin Pediatr. 2008;20:243–7.
88. Brenner DJ, Hricak H. Radiation exposure from medical imaging: time to regulate? JAMA. 2010;304:208–9.
89. Hall EJ, Brenner DJ. Cancer risks from diagnostic radiology. Br J Radiol. 2008;81:362–78.
90. Tubiana M, Feinendegen LE, Yang C, Kaminski JM. The linear no-threshold relationship is inconsistent with radiation biologic and experimental data. Radiology. 2009;251:13–22.
91. Chen JX, Kachniarz B, Gilani S, Shin JJ. Risk of malignancy associated with head and neck CT in children: a systematic review. Otolaryngol Head Neck Surg. 2014;151:554–66.

92. Pearce MS. Patterns in paediatric CT use: an international and epidemiological perspective. J Med Imaging Radiat Oncol. 2011;55:107–9.
93. Amis ES Jr, Butler PF, Applegate KE, et al. American College of Radiology white paper on radiation dose in medicine. J Am Coll Radiol. 2007;4:272–84.
94. Brody AS, Frush DP, Huda W, Brent RL. Radiation risk to children from computed tomography. Pediatrics. 2007;120:677–82.
95. Brenner D, Elliston C, Hall E, Berdon W. Estimated risks of radiation-induced fatal cancer from pediatric CT. AJR Am J Roentgenol. 2001;176:289–96.
96. Pearce MS, Salotti JA, Little MP, et al. Radiation exposure from CT scans in childhood and subsequent risk of leukaemia and brain tumours: a retrospective cohort study. Lancet. 2012;380:499–505.
97. Mathews JD, Forsythe AV, Brady Z, et al. Cancer risk in 680,000 people exposed to computed tomography scans in childhood or adolescence: data linkage study of 11 million Australians. BMJ. 2013;346:f2360.
98. Meulepas JM, Ronckers CM, Smets AM, et al. Leukemia and brain tumors among children after radiation exposure from CT scans: design and methodological opportunities of the Dutch Pediatric CT Study. Eur J Epidemiol. 2014;29:293–301.
99. Ware DE, Huda W, Mergo PJ, Litwiller AL. Radiation effective doses to patients undergoing abdominal CT examinations. Radiology. 1999;210:645–50.
100. Frush DP, Applegate K. Computed tomography and radiation: understanding the issues. J Am Coll Radiol. 2004;1:113–9.
101. Linton OW, Mettler FA Jr. National conference on dose reduction in CT, with an emphasis on pediatric patients. AJR Am J Roentgenol. 2003;181:321–9.
102. Mettler FA Jr, Wiest PW, Locken JA, Kelsey CA. CT scanning: patterns of use and dose. J Radiol Prot. 2000;20:353–9.
103. Frush DP. Pediatric dose reduction in computed tomography. Health Phys. 2008;95:518–27.
104. Shelsta HN, Bilyk JR, Rubin PA, Penne RB, Carrasco JR. Wooden intraorbital foreign body injuries: clinical characteristics and outcomes of 23 patients. Ophthal Plast Reconstr Surg. 2010;26:238–44.
105. Larson DB, Rader SB, Forman HP, Fenton LZ. Informing parents about CT radiation exposure in children: it's OK to tell them. AJR Am J Roentgenol. 2007;189:271–5.
106. ACR Appropriateness Criteria. Orbits, Vision and Visual Loss. 2012. Accessed Sept 2016, at https://acsearch.acr.org/docs/69486/Narrative.
107. Boncoeur-Martel MP, Adenis JP, Rulfi JY, Robert PY, Dupuy JP, Maubon A. CT appearances of chronically retained wooden intraorbital foreign bodies. Neuroradiology. 2001;43:165–8.
108. Macrae JA. Diagnosis and management of a wooden orbital foreign body: case report. Br J Ophthalmol. 1979;63:848–51.
109. Nasr AM, Haik BG, Fleming JC, Al-Hussain HM, Karcioglu ZA. Penetrating orbital injury with organic foreign bodies. Ophthalmology. 1999;106:523–32.
110. Miller CF, Brodkey JS, Colombi BJ. The danger of intracranial wood. Surg Neurol. 1977;7:95–103.
111. Nishio Y, Hayashi N, Hamada H, Hirashima Y, Endo S. A case of delayed brain abscess due to a retained intracranial wooden foreign body: a case report and review of the last 20 years. Acta Neurochir. 2004;146:847–50.
112. Michon J, Liu D. Intraorbital foreign bodies. Semin Ophthalmol. 1994;9:193–9.
113. Fulcher TP, McNab AA, Sullivan TJ. Clinical features and management of intraorbital foreign bodies. Ophthalmology. 2002;109:494–500.
114. Ho VT, McGuckin JF Jr, Smergel EM. Intraorbital wooden foreign body: CT and MR appearance. AJNR Am J Neuroradiol. 1996;17:134–6.
115. Lagalla R, Manfre L, Caronia A, Bencivinni F, Duranti C, Ponte F. Plain film, CT and MRI sensibility in the evaluation of intraorbital foreign bodies in an in vitro model of the orbit and in pig eyes. Eur Radiol. 2000;10:1338–41.
116. Glatt HJ, Custer PL, Barrett L, Sartor K. Magnetic resonance imaging and computed tomography in a model of wooden foreign bodies in the orbit. Ophthal Plast Reconstr Surg. 1990;6:108–14.
117. Woolfson JM, Wesley RE. Magnetic resonance imaging and computed tomographic scanning of fresh (green) wood foreign bodies in dog orbits. Ophthal Plast Reconstr Surg. 1990;6:237–40.
118. Smely C, Orszagh M. Intracranial transorbital injury by a wooden foreign body: re-evaluation of CT and MRI findings. Br J Neurosurg. 1999;13:206–11.
119. McGuckin JF Jr, Akhtar N, Ho VT, Smergel EM, Kubacki EJ, Villafana T. CT and MR evaluation of a wooden foreign body in an in vitro model of the orbit. AJNR Am J Neuroradiol. 1996;17:129–33.
120. Dalley RW. Intraorbital wood foreign bodies on CT: use of wide bone window settings to distinguish wood from air. AJR Am J Roentgenol. 1995;164:434–5.
121. Finkelstein M, Legmann A, Rubin PA. Projectile metallic foreign bodies in the orbit: a retrospective study of epidemiologic factors, management, and outcomes. Ophthalmology. 1997;104:96–103.
122. Holt GR, Holt JE. Management of orbital trauma and foreign bodies. Otolaryngol Clin N Am. 1988;21:35–52.
123. Braun J, Gdal-On M, Goldsher D, Borovich B, Guilburd JN. Traumatic carotid aneurysm secondary to cavernous sinus penetration by wood: CT features. J Comput Assist Tomogr. 1987;11:525–8.
124. Doucet TW, Harper DW, Rogers J. Penetrating orbital foreign body with intracranial involvement. Ann Ophthalmol. 1983;15:325–7.
125. Cunningham EJ, Albani B, Masaryk TJ, Rasmussen PA. Temporary balloon occlusion of the cavernous carotid artery for removal of an orbital and intracranial foreign body: case report. Neurosurgery. 2004;55:1225.
126. Jacobs NA, Morgan LH. On the management of retained airgun pellets: a survey of 11 orbital cases. Br J Ophthalmol. 1988;72:97–100.
127. Danesh-Meyer HV, Savino PJ, Bilyk JR, Sergott RC, Kubis K. Gaze-evoked amaurosis produced by intraorbital buckshot pellet. Ophthalmology. 2001;108:201–6.
128. Mutlukan E, Fleck BW, Cullen JF, Whittle IR. Case of penetrating orbitocranial injury caused by wood. Br J Ophthalmol. 1991;75:374–6.
129. Cole TS, Jones LK, McGrogan P, et al. Emotional and behavioural difficulties in chronic granulomatous disease. Arch Dis Child. 2012;97:87.

Anesthesia and the Pediatric Oculoplastics Patient

66

Carlo Rob Bernardino

Introduction

Advances in the understanding of topical, local, and regional anesthetics have allowed ophthalmologists to transition rapidly from hospital-based surgery to ambulatory and office-based procedures. These advances, although often applicable in the pediatric population, are not easily generalized because "children are not small adults." When deciding whether to perform an office procedure, one needs to remember that efficacy and side effect profile of anesthetics and analgesics drastically change in the pediatric versus the adult population. Furthermore, the ability to perform procedures on a child will be limited by their mental capacity and acceptance of their caretakers or parents.

Role for Sedation

Whether performing an ocular examination or intervention, patient cooperation is key to obtain valuable information or to successfully perform the procedure. This is especially true in children. In dealing with children, one must determine if cooperation is essential, or if a child's lack of cooperation can be worked around to get a successful outcome.

In the office, an ophthalmologist might need to probe a small child to resolve a congenital nasolacrimal duct obstruction. One option is to papoose a child or have a staff member hold the child down. One study has recently shown that probing the lacrimal system in the office, under topical anesthesia, is efficacious in children under 6 months of age [1]. Depending on the age and size of the child, this could be easy or stressful and dangerous. The other option is to use sedation or general anesthesia to overcome the patient's lack of cooperation. However, the potential risks of sedation versus the outcome one might achieve from correcting the problem must be considered.

Another common scenario is evaluating a child with an eyelid laceration. Whether in the office or the emergency room, there are two components to the encounter: performing an adequate examination to determine the extent of the injury and repairing the eyelid in the same setting if possible. A thorough examination is key; the presence of a canthal avulsion or lacrimal system damage may necessitate special equipment or general anesthesia.

In the first scenario, since the probing takes only a few minutes, papoosing a child is reasonable. In the second case, examination and then surgical intervention can take an hour or longer. Therefore younger children, with poor understanding may be unable to cooperate, where an older child may be able to cooperate completely. Therefore, it is essential to develop a rapport with the child before injecting them with a needle. As a clinician considering a surgical intervention for a child, one should ask: "What is the mental capacity of the child?" "Can the parents and/or staff control the child with soothing words and hand holding?" "What is the emotional state of the child and/or the patient's family?" If there is any doubt of the child being able to cooperate, then sedation may be necessary.

Nonmedical Prevention of Anxiety

All patients will benefit from techniques (medical and nonmedical) to prevent anxiety during surgery; this is particularly true for pediatric patients and their families. Nonmedical techniques are the easiest and should become a part of the standard operating procedure. The most important is probably the attitude of the surgeon and staff. If the surgeon exudes confidence and talks with a calm and friendly voice before, during, and after the procedure, this will help keep a patient calm and relaxed during surgery.

C. R. Bernardino (✉)
Oculoplastics and Aesthetic Surgery, Vantage Eye Center, Monterey, CA, USA
e-mail: rbernardino@vantageeye.com

J. J. Servat et al. (eds.), *Smith and Nesi's Ophthalmic Plastic and Reconstructive Surgery*,
https://doi.org/10.1007/978-3-030-41720-8_66

Likewise, if the environment of the office and staff is calm and relaxing, the patient will be more at ease. A distracting office environment and a hyperkinetic staff can add to patient anxiety. The surgical suite, whether an examination lane or dedicated procedure room, should be comfortable. The surgical suite should be a kid-friendly environment, away from noise or adult patients. For children, it is important to allow them to get comfortable with the environment. Allowing them to "play" on the surgical table or with equipment, if they show interest, can be helpful to reduce anxiety. A familiar toy and blanket can also be comforting.

When examining children under anesthesia or performing procedures on children, a decision must be made as to whether a parent should be present. Certainly, a parent can help calm a child during the sedation process or even during a procedure. However, parents can also be a liability, either not being able to calm the child or becoming emotional and distraught, which in turn will make the child's cooperation worsen. In the worst-case scenario, a parent may get in the way of treating the child appropriately or may pass out becoming a "second patient." A frank discussion with the parents is a must if you want their help and cooperation. In some cases, hospital policy prohibits their participation, but a willing parent can be an ally during a difficult examination or procedure.

Distraction

Averting a child's attention away from the task at hand is also helpful in some situation. Distraction may involve allowing a child to listen to their favorite music or watch a video of choice. With the proliferation of smartphones, parents typically have a favorite app or program on their phone for their child to use.

If you are planning a procedure, working with the parents in this regard is helpful. Asking them to bring earphones and a music source, or having an iPod and earphones in the procedure suite, is an easy step. Having an iPad with preloaded videos can also be used. However, in ophthalmology, distraction by video is limited because periocular procedures typically preclude a patient from watching a video.

Talking at the Child's Level

All children should be reassured that someone will be with them at all times. Furthermore, speaking in terms which may be more accepting to them is appropriate; using terms like "sore" instead of "pain," or "make an opening" instead of "cut," can make a procedure more acceptable to a child. Children should be encouraged to ask questions.

Young children (aged 3–7) will have a limited capacity to understand, and their main concerns will be that of separation from their parents. Explaining things on their terms and that someone will always be with them is helpful. Honesty however is key. Trying to hide the fact that they need surgery can foster distrust and fear.

Elementary school children have more comprehension and therefore require more direct and honest explanation. Simple terms are appropriate, and explaining that the problem they have will not get better on its own without surgery is reasonable.

Adolescents have understanding similar to adults. Explanations can be fairly detailed and these children often have sophisticated concepts such as pain, disfigurement, and death. Children of this age will often not ask these questions due to fear; it is important to anticipate these questions and address them in a non-confrontational manner.

Working Without Sedation

At times it is neither convenient nor safe to employ sedation when examining or performing a procedure on a child. However, if a child is able to be reasoned with, particularly in the presence of a parent, medical and surgical procedures can be performed safely and efficiently. In these instances, it is key to constantly talk to the child in a calm, nonthreatening manner. Furthermore, it is useful to always give the child an out; if he or she suddenly becomes afraid or uncomfortable, it is reasonable to stop and try a different approach. If the proposed procedure cannot be stopped midway, though, then the procedure should be performed under sedation. Finally, if a procedure is performed on the cooperative child, the surgeon must be ready to react to a sudden change in disposition; a child can suddenly jerk or move when startled and therefore the surgeon needs to be prepared to pull sharp instruments from a child's face at a moment's notice.

Other times, sedation cannot be used but a child is not cooperative. In these cases, it is often essential to restrain or control a noncooperative child. The first step to restraining or papoosing a child is to ask permission from the parent or guardian. It is important to explain why restraining a distraught child is necessary and to obtain permission to proceed. Depending on the size and strength of a child, simple holding or hugging a child will suffice whereas in other cases papoosing is appropriate. When placing drops in child's eye or performing a quick examination, manual restraining of a child is safe and efficient. Usually this can be performed either with a parent or staff member. For small children, a child's head can be cradled with the head resting in the arm pit of a willing parent or assistant who is seated, and the free hand is used to hold the limbs down. Then the ophthalmologist can manipulate the face and eyes as needed.

Table 66.1 Levels of sedation

	Minimal sedation (anxiolysis)	Moderate sedation/analgesia (conscious sedation)	Deep sedation/analgesia	General anesthesia
Responsiveness	Normal response to verbal stimulation	Purposeful response to verbal or tactile stimulation	Purposeful response to repeated or painful stimulation	Unarousable, even to painful stimuli
Airway	Unaffected	No intervention required	Intervention may be required	Intervention often required
Spontaneous ventilation	Unaffected	Adequate	May be inadequate	Frequently inadequate
Cardiovascular function	Unaffected	Usually maintained	Usually maintained	May be impaired

In the case of a larger child, the child can sit on the lap of the parent or assistant, with legs wrapped around the waist. The ophthalmologist then sits in front of the parent or assistant, and the child is leaned back until the head/torso rests on their lap. The assistant can use both hands to restrain the child while the ophthalmologist can work.

In situations where more stable control of a child is needed, particularly for procedures, papoosing is necessary. Papoosing can be performed with a papoose board which is essentially a back board with usually Velcro panels to secure a child, his or her limbs, and to stabilize the head. When such devices are not available, using multiple towels or blankets wrapped around a child to keep the arms and legs against the body is effective. Whether using a papoose or the towel technique, make sure to have assistants help out and make sure to practice use of such devices before they are necessary. When deciding to papoose a child, though, offer to allow the parent to leave the room if they are uncomfortable seeing their child restrained. An emotional parent can make the procedure more difficult and dangerous. One study demonstrated that parents were accepting of the use of a papoose for dental procedure [2].

Levels of Sedation

Once you have determined that sedation is necessary, you will need to decide how deep the sedation is needed for the task. In some cases, such as a minor procedure in an older child, anxiolysis is all that's required, whereas in other cases, such as reconstructive surgery, general anesthesia is required. The surgeon must be mindful that sedation is independent of anesthesia. Sedation addresses anxiety and consciousness whereas anesthesia (local, region, or general) addresses tactile and pain stimulation. With proper patient selection and anesthesia use, sedation use and side effects can be minimized.

Surgery performed with minimal sedation is where oral medications are frequently used for anxiolysis. At this level of sedation, patients have normal responsiveness, and their breathing and cardiac function are unaffected. At moderate levels of sedation, often called conscious sedation, responsiveness is further depressed. Whether intramuscular, intravenous, or inhaled medications are used, patients can still respond to purposeful verbal or tactile stimulus. Respiratory and cardiac function remains unaffected. At deep levels of sedation, only painful or repeated stimulation causes a purposeful reaction from the patient. The patient's airway as well as spontaneous respiration can be affected, but cardiac function is intact. General anesthesia, the deepest level of sedation, involves complete loss of patient responsiveness, even to painful stimuli. Respiratory and cardiac function can be compromised without direct intervention. The levels of sedation (which were defined by the American Society of Anesthesiologists) are summarized in Table 66.1.

Table 66.2 Equipment necessary for sedation

1. Electronic/cycling BP monitor
2. Sphygmomanometer (manual or automated) with pediatric cuff
3. Oxygen tank and nasal cannula/mask/delivery system
4. Oxygen saturation monitor
5. EKG
6. Crash cart

Oral sedation, when used on adults, can be offered by the ophthalmologist for surgical procedures in the office safely. However, sedative use for the pediatric patient is more complicated, since children have specific dosing based on weight. Furthermore, children can often have paradoxical responses to sedation. If the pediatric patient is to be placed under conscious sedation, it is necessary to have appropriate monitoring devices on hand (Table 66.2). For these reasons, it is reasonable to offer sedation in the emergency room setting or in conjunction with an anesthesiologist, but not unmonitored in the office setting.

One also should evaluate the child for history of (or family history of) anesthesia intolerance and ability to obtain IV access. Without IV access, the anesthetic armamentarium is more limited.

Contraindications to Sedation

In general, children are excellent candidates for sedation for procedures. Most children are healthy and, if their vitals are normal, require no specific work-up. However, two important issues for the ophthalmologist to determine are fasting (NPO) status and if they had a recent upper respiratory tract infection (URI).

NPO status is important because although the risk of frank aspiration is less than in children, children are at risk for bronchospasm or pneumonia. Typically, surgery should be delayed at least 2 h if the patient had clear liquids, 4 h for breast milk, and 6 h for solids.

Like NPO status, a recent history of URI can lead to increased risk of laryngospasm, bronchospasm, and oxygen desaturation. Therefore, for elective surgery, a period of at least 4–6 weeks after URI is recommended.

Malignant hyperthermia (MH) is also a concern, usually raised by the family because of history in a family member. MH is diagnosed on clinical grounds; currently there are no good laboratory tests to determine predisposition to, or diagnosis of MH [3]. The incidence has been reported to be between 1:4500 and 1:60,000 procedures involving general anesthesia. Susceptibility to MH is often inherited as an autosomal dominant disorder.

Compounds most commonly implicated are inhalational anesthetics (sevoflurane, desflurane, isoflurane, halothane, enflurane, methoxyflurane) and succinylcholine – a depolarizing muscle relaxant. Other anesthetic drugs are considered safe. Local anesthetics such as lidocaine and bupivacaine, opiates, ketamine, propofol, etomidate, and benzodiazepines are unlikely to trigger MH.

The earliest signs of MH are tachycardia, a rise in end-tidal carbon dioxide concentration (despite increased minute ventilation), and muscle rigidity. Despite the name malignant hyperthermia, elevation of body temperature is often a late sign. Other signs may include acidosis, tachypnea (in a spontaneously breathing patient), and hyperkalemia. The criteria for diagnosing MH are summarized on Table 66.3 [4]. Treatment includes cooling blankets to reduce fever and medications like dantrolene, lidocaine, or beta-blockers to address cardiac arrhythmias.

Table 66.3 Criteria for diagnosing malignant hyperthermia

1. Respiratory acidosis (end-tidal CO_2 above 55 mmHg/7.32 kPa or arterial pCO_2 above 60 mmHg/7.98 kPa)
2. Heart involvement (unexplained sinus tachycardia, ventricular tachycardia, or ventricular fibrillation)
3. Metabolic acidosis (base excess lower than −8, pH < 7.25)
4. Muscle rigidity (generalized rigidity including severe masseter muscle rigidity) and muscle breakdown (CK > 20,000/L units, cola-colored urine or excess myoglobin in urine or serum, potassium above 6 mmol/L)
5. Temperature increase (rapidly increasing temperature, T > 38.8 °C)
6. Other (rapid reversal of MH signs with dantrolene, elevated resting serum CK levels)
7. Family history (autosomal dominant pattern)

Children with significant medical issues are beyond the scope of this chapter. However, in children with conditions which may affect the condition of their airway including juvenile rheumatoid arthritis, cervical spine injury, obesity, or prematurity, preoperative planning with anesthesiology is essential [5].

Finally, a discussion about the safety of exposure to anesthetics to the developing child is important to address. In 2016 and later clarified in April 2017, the FDA declared via a safety announcement that exposure to sedation or general anesthesia has been shown to cause nerve cell loss in the developing brain, particularly when a procedure is longer than 3 h, in the setting when a child has multiple exposures to anesthesia before the age of 3 [6].

However, there have been many studies refuting these findings. The GAS trial, published in 2015, looked at cognitive development in 2 years after patients were randomized to either have spinal anesthesia versus general anesthesia for hernia repair [7]. The study found no difference in cognitive testing at age 5; however, the mean exposure to general anesthesia was only 54 min.

The PANDA study was a retrospective study which looked at children who received one exposure to general anesthesia before the age of 36 months for hernia repair and compared their cognitive development to a sibling who did not have exposure to anesthesia during their first 36 months of life [8]. In the anesthesia cohort, the mean anesthesia exposure time was 80 min. Both groups were evaluated between ages 8 and 15 to determine cognitive development. The study found that there was no difference between the two groups in terms of cognitive development.

The MASK (Mayo Anesthesia Safety in Kids) study looked at two sets of children: single exposure and multiple anesthesia exposure before age of 3 and non-exposure children for neuropsychological testing at ages 8–12 or 15–20 years [9]. IQ which was a primary measure of the study was not different between the two exposure groups compared to the control, unexposed group. However, in secondary measures such as processing speed and fine motor skills, the multiple exposure group had decreased scores whereas the single exposure group was unaffected. Parents of the multiple exposure group also reported difficulty with behavior, executive function, and reading.

Given these studies and the FDA advisory, it is important to discuss risk of exposure to general anesthesia if your proposed procedure requires its use. For most ophthalmologic or periocular procedures, the exposure is brief (less than an hour), and therefore the risk for affecting cognitive development is unlikely. However, if you anticipate multiple exposures to anesthesia, such as serial retina examinations for retinopathy of prematurity, then it is important to discuss this risk with the parents of the patient.

Choice of Sedation

In the pediatric population, there are a number of choices of sedation route including: topical, intranasal, oral, rectal, inhalation, intramuscular, and intravenous. Compared to adults, children have rapid onset via mucous membranes by topical and inhalation routes. For longer procedures, intravenous is still the best because it can be titrated by an anesthesiologist.

In general, when performing a procedure in the hospital setting, young children are premedicated, where the child will drink the flavored pre-procedural sedative from a cup or syringe; this is often referred to in terms acceptable by the child such as, "this is Spider-man power juice." Children to bring a security object (blanket or stuffed animal) into the operating room (with a label). For children under 10, inhalation induction is preferred. Most will "help blow up the balloon" in the OR during sedation; toys on the anesthesia circuit can distract them. Once the child is sedated, IV access can be placed. An older patient may accept an IV more readily than mask anesthesia and premedication; topical EMLA cream at the IV site can aid the process.

For brief procedures in the emergency room, it is good to be familiar with some of the more commonly used systemic medications (Table 66.4). Midazolam, a benzodiazepine, is a short-acting sedative with some amnestic effect. This can be used by several routes. Midazolam syrup can be given orally (2 mg/mL) in a dose of 0.5 mg/kg up to about 20 mg. For the uncooperative child, intranasal, intramuscular, or rectal delivery is helpful [10].

Ketamine is an excellent product for sedation because of its many routes of administration. Ketamine rapidly crosses the blood-brain barrier [11]. It may also have a lower incidence of agitation with emergence from anesthesia.

Propofol is useful for brief procedures outside the traditional operating room. It is short-acting and has a rapid offset. It does, however, have a greater potential for respiratory depression compared with ketamine. Routine use of oxygen and monitoring of end-tidal CO2 might decrease the likelihood of that complication [12].

Each sedative has specific characteristics that may be helpful or harmful to the ophthalmic surgeon. Therefore, discussing proposed use of sedation with an anesthesiologist may aid in anesthetic choice. For example, Mizrak et al. found that ketamine was superior to propofol for strabismus surgery anesthesia [13]. However, propofol can decrease the need for antiemetics and the incidence of the oculocardiac reflex [14]. Ketamine and succinylcholine are thought to increase intraocular pressure and therefore may be contraindicated in ruptured globe repairs.

Anesthesia for Surgery

The goals of perioperative anesthesia include minimizing pain and sensation during a procedure, facilitating hemostasis via epinephrine injection (if desired), and preventing postoperative pain. Anesthetics for ocular and periocular surgery come in three varieties – topical, local injection, and regional block.

Topical Anesthetics

Topical ophthalmic anesthetics have many advantages over injectables (Table 66.5). These include fast onset, eliminating risk of globe injury/perforation from needles, and unaffected ocular motility and pupillary function. However, topical agents do not cause vasoconstriction; topical phenylephrine can be given concurrently if vasoconstriction is desired. Some topical medications (gel/viscous preparations) can block the bactericidal effects of povidone-iodine

Table 66.4 Commonly used systemic anesthetics

Systemic anesthetic	Onset	Length of action	Risks	Benefits	Routes of administration
Propofol	Brief	Short	Greater respiratory depression compared with ketamine	Rapid offset of effects	Sedation 25–100 mcg/kg/min Induction 1–2.5 mg/kg Maintenance 50–200 mcg/kg/min
Ketamine	Rapid (roughly 60 s)	Short	Higher incidence of postoperative nausea and vomiting and hallucinations	Dissociative	Intranasal (5.0 mg/kg) Oral (5–10 mg/kg in elixir) Rectal (5.0 mg/kg) Intravenous (1.0–2.0 mg/kg) Intramuscular (3.0 mg/kg)

Table 66.5 Common topical anesthetics used in ophthalmology

Name	Trade name	Strength	Notes
Cocaine topical solution		1–4%	Controlled substance
Lidocaine topical solution		4%	
Proparacaine	Alcaine [1]	0.5%	
Tetracaine		0.5%	More painful initially than proparacaine
Benoxinate/fluorescein	Fluress [2]	0.4%/0.25% sol	
Fluorescein/proparacaine	Fluoracaine [2]	0.25%/0.5% sol	
Lidocaine viscous gel	Akten [2]	3.5%	Povidone-iodine must be used first in surgery

(Betadine, Purdue Pharma LP, Stamford, CT); therefore betadine should be placed prior to the anesthetic.

Typically, topical anesthetics have an onset of 1 min and duration of 20–30 min. These topical anesthetics work only on mucous membranes, such as the ocular surface.

Ice and EMLA, or Eutectic Mixture of Local Anesthetic (APP Pharmaceuticals, LLC, Schaumburg, IL), are two effective topical anesthetics for skin use. Underutilized, ice can work as a quick anesthetic, particularly for small excisional biopsies or to dampen the pain from injections. It is quite helpful before other injections such as with botulinum toxin or fillers.

EMLA is a 5% mixture of topical prilocaine and lidocaine, which is thought to not have local ocular toxicity. It is commonly used prior to IV insertion but is useful before injections and laser skin surgery as well. However, its onset is up to 90 min and requires an occlusive dressing to facilitate skin absorption, which is more difficult in the periocular area. Common side effects from these topical anesthetics can include lightheadedness, local erythema, edema, and allergic reactions, while serious reactions including arrhythmias and seizures have been reported. Other topical anesthetics exist including topical lidocaine 3% in a lotion or cream (LidaMantle, PharmaDerm, Melville, NY), lidocaine 3.5% ophthalmic gel (Akten, Akorn, Inc., Lakeforest IL) as well as a generic 4% solution or 5% ointment; these all have similar efficacy.

A novel topical anesthesia is vibration distraction or vibration anesthesia. By using a vibrating instrument, such as a handheld massage unit adjacent to the injection site, the pain from injection is decreased [15]. The gate control theory of pain suggests that vibration nerve fibers transmit the sense of vibration while inhibiting the transmission of pain sensation. Therefore, using a massage device or directed vibration device such as Blaine Labs Vibration Anesthesia Device (Blaine Labs, Santa Fe Springs, CA) next to the injection site, the injection is better tolerated.

Injectable Anesthetics

Injectable anesthetics (Table 66.6) can be used locally around the surgical site and regionally via a nerve block. Local injections work well because the anesthetic is placed directly at the surgical site. If vasoconstriction is desired, epinephrine should be added to the anesthetic. Disadvantages of local anesthetic injections include tissue distortion and muscle paresis, both of which may be problematic particularly during external levator resection surgery, in which intraoperative titration of eyelid height and contour is critical for the optimal result. In such cases, the minimum amount of local anesthetic injection necessary should be used, i.e., less than 1 cc per upper eyelid.

Table 66.6 Common injectable anesthetics

Name	Maximum dose	Onset	Duration
Bupivacaine 0.25–0.75% (Marcaine1)	2 mg/kg or 175 mg/dose, 400 mg/24 h	2–10 min	3–6 h
Chloroprocaine 1–3% (Nesacaine2)	11 mg/kg or 800 mg/dose	6–12 min	0.5–1 h
Lidocaine 1–2% (Xylocaine2)	4 mg/kg or 280 mg/dose	4–6 min	0.75–1.5 h
Mepivacaine 1–2% (Carbocaine1)	4 mg/kg or 400 mg/dose	3–5 min	0.75–1.5 h
Procaine 1–4% (Novocain1)	10 mg/kg or 1000 mg/dose	2–5 min	0.5 h
Ropivacaine 0.25–1% (Naropin3)	2.5 mg/kg or 300 mg/dose	1–15 min	2–6 h

When choosing an injectable anesthetic, time of onset and duration are factors to consider. Typically, fast acting anesthetics have a shorter duration whereas longer lasting anesthetics have a longer time of onset, and therefore the surgeon has to plan appropriately. In order to take advantage of fast onset of one medication and longer duration of another, anesthetics can be mixed.

Regional blocks work by delivering anesthetic to a nerve supplying the surgical site. Examples include frontal, supraorbital, lacrimal, and infraorbital nerve blocks. The quantity of local anesthetic necessary is typically reduced with a regional block. Excellent intraoperative and postoperative pain control can be achieved, particularly if a long-acting anesthetic is used. However, the advantage of local vasoconstriction with epinephrine is lost, unless one combines a regional and local block.

There are no specific toxicity studies of these anesthetics in children, so side effects and dosing are derived from the adult literature. In normal healthy adults, the maximum recommended dose of lidocaine injection with epinephrine for local anesthesia other than spinal should not exceed 7 mg/kg, and the maximum total dose should not exceed

500 mg. The maximum recommended dose of lidocaine injection without epinephrine should not exceed 4.5 mg/Kg, and the maximum total dose should not exceed 300 mg. The maximum dose of lidocaine, once given, should not be repeated for 2 h [16]. Bupivacaine has a maximum recommended dosing of 2.5 mg/kg when used with epinephrine or 3 mg/kg when used without.

Injectables may be modified with the addition of epinephrine for vasoconstriction. All anesthetics cause vasodilatation, except cocaine, and can exacerbate bleeding. Therefore, epinephrine is compounded into many local anesthetics to improve hemostasis, prolong the anesthetic effect, and decrease systemic toxicity. Epinephrine should be avoided if pupil dilation is not desired.

Anesthetics are acidic by nature, and therefore buffering an anesthetic with sodium bicarbonate can reduce the pain associated with injection; sodium bicarbonate 8.4% is usually added to a local anesthetic in a 1:5 ratio.

Postoperative Nausea and Vomiting

Postoperative nausea and vomiting (PONV) can turn a surgical experience into a miserable one. Besides retching and vomiting, a patient may experience the unpleasant sensation of nausea. More worrisome to the surgeon, PONV can cause wound dehiscence, hematoma, orbital hemorrhage, and aspiration.

Thirty percent of all procedures are associated with PONV. Without prophylaxis, the rate of PONV after strabismus surgery varied from 37–90% [17]. The major risk factors for postoperative vomiting include age > 3 XE "Anesthesia and pediatric oculoplastics patient:postoperative nausea and vomiting (PONV)" years, duration of anesthesia >30 min, and a personal or family history of PONV or motion sickness.

Although there are many medications to prevent and/or treat PONV, many nonmedical interventions also work well. The first is preoperative fasting at least 6 h for solid meals and 2 h for liquids. Furthermore, reducing anxiety during the surgery may help prevent PONV. Controlling pain during and after surgery is important, although opioids may also contribute to PONV. Limiting position changes during surgery, i.e., sitting the patient up and down, can help prevent PONV.

If PONV needs to be treated, many medications are available and are quite effective (Table 66.7). All except ondansetron (Zofran, GlaxoSmithKline, London, UK) have the risk of extrapyramidal symptoms, in which patients develop involuntary muscle contractions. A history of this side effect may preclude use of these drugs.

Additionally, specific drugs may have additional side effects or benefits. Dimenhydrinate can be sedating and lead delay to discharge after surgery. Droperidol is very effective at stopping a single episode of vomiting, but in 2001, the FDA issued a black box warning because high doses of droperidol can cause QT prolongation. Dexamethasone (a corticosteroid) has excellent PONV prevention properties and has a synergistic effect when used with ondansetron [18].

Table 66.7 Treatment for postoperative nausea and vomiting

Medication	Dose
Dimenhydrinate	0.5 mg/kg
Metoclopramide	0.15 mg/kg, 0.25 mg/kg
Droperidol	0.075 mg/kg
Dexamethasone	0.15 mg/kg
Ondansetron	0.05–0.2 mg/kg

Table 66.8 Non-opioid pain medications

Drug	Dosing (mg/kg/day)	Number of doses/day
Acetaminophen	50–75	4
Diclofenac	1–3	2–3
Ibuprofen	15–40	2–4
Naproxen	10–15	2
Indomethacin	1–4	2–4
Piroxicam	0.2–0.3	1

Postoperative Pain Control

Proper intraoperative prevention of pain with appropriate anesthesia will help reduce postoperative pain. Nonetheless most patients will experience some discomfort after surgery. Educating the patient, and in this case the parents, to anticipate some degree of discomfort and appropriate dosing of analgesia can minimize postoperative pain and anxiety. Patients who are informed about the possibility of postoperative pain and the amount of discomfort they might experience are more accepting of it and are able to deal with it better, with potentially less anxiety about the pain. Therefore, telling the patient that there will be no discomfort after surgery is doing them a disservice and may reduce pain tolerance. Anticipating the amount of pain a patient may experience after a procedure is essential. This is no different whether the patient is an adult or a child. Discussions with the parents in front of the child about expected pain after a procedure is important. Also using language that the child will understand is important.

Treating postoperative pain should be performed in a staged approach. The first level of analgesics is NSAIDs or acetaminophen. These are effective for mild postoperative discomfort. However, NSAIDs and aspirin may increase the risk for postoperative hemorrhage or hematoma. The drugs used for mild pain relief are listed in Table 66.8.

Acetaminophen is an antipyretic with weak analgesic effects. The initial dose is 45 mg/kg administered rectally before waking. Additional doses can be given orally (10–15 mg/kg) or rectally (20 mg/kg) every 4–6 h for pain control. If they are given around the clock, rather than as needed, the medication can maintain an adequate blood level of

Table 66.9 Combination pain medications

Trade	Generic	Dose
Tylenol #3	30 mg codeine/300 mg APAP	1–2 every 4 h maximum 12 tabs in 24 h
Tylenol #3 elixir	120 mg acetaminophen/12 mg codeine per 5 mL elixir	3–7 years: 5 mL 3–4 times/day 7–12 years: 10 mL 3–4 times/day
Lortab elixir	2.5 mg hydrocodone/167 mg acetaminophen per 5 mL	0.27 mL/kg per dose every 4–6 h
Roxicet	5 mg oxycodone/325 mg acetaminophen per 5 mL	0.05–0.15 mg/kg of oxycodone every 4–6 h

10–20 micrograms/ml. The total dose should not exceed 100 mg/kg for children, 75 mg/kg for infants, and 60 mg/kg for term and preterm neonates. Combining non-opioids is also effective; ibuprofen and acetaminophen reduced the need for early analgesia by 50% following tonsillectomy when compared to acetaminophen alone [19].

Diclofenac provides effective analgesia after minor procedures in children. The dose is 1 mg/kg every 8 h rectally, orally, or intravenously. Ketorolac has been shown to be effective if given soon after induction in general anesthesia, since the onset of pain relief is 20–30 min. IV dosing of 0.5 mg/kg is the only available form in the USA.

Non-opioid analgesics can be used preoperatively, intraoperatively, and postoperatively. Some non-opioid analgesics can be administered shortly before the planned end of a procedure. In a study of ambulatory patients, administration of 1 g of paracetamol (aka acetaminophen) 30 min before the end of the procedure decreased postoperative pain by 86%.

For patients with moderate pain, adding a narcotic to a NSAID or acetaminophen is appropriate. For convenience, many combination drugs are available. Table 66.9 lists the most common combination analgesics. The use of opioids should be minimized by administering NSAIDs. Opioid medications, used in combination with NSAIDS or local anesthetics, provided improved analgesia or a reduction in the opioid consumption. Adjunctive therapy, or combination of multiple analgesic medications, can work in tandem to lower the total dose of anesthetic overall. Dexamethasone, when used in conjunction with administration of oxycodone, reduces postoperative pain [20].

For pain that is not well controlled by oral medications, it is worthwhile to admit a child to the hospital for intravenous pain management in conjunction with a pediatric service.

Conclusion

Pediatric patients can often be challenging to exam and to perform surgical procedures in part due to their lack of comprehension and cooperation. With a systematic approach of determining which children require sedation, choosing the appropriate anesthesia, working as a team with the parents and anesthesiologists, and preventing PONV and pain, an ophthalmologist can comfortably evaluate and treat children.

References

1. Shrestha JB, et al. Outcome of probing under topical anesthesia in children below 18 months of age with congenital nasolacrimal duct obstruction. Nepal Med Coll J. 2009;11(1):46–9.
2. Frankel RI. The Papoose Board and mothers' attitudes following its use. Pediatr Dent. 1991;13(5):284–8.
3. Litman R, Rosenberg H. Malignant hyperthermia: update on susceptibility testing. JAMA. 2005;293(23):2918–24.
4. Larach MG, Localio AR, Allen GC, et al. A clinical grading scale to predict malignant hyperthermia susceptibility. Anesthesiology. 1994;8(4):771–9.
5. Baker S, Parico L. Pathologic paediatric conditions associated with a compromised airway. Int J Paediatr Dent. 2010;20(2):102–11.
6. Federal Drug Administration. FDA Drug Safety Communication: FDA review results in new warnings about using general anesthetics and sedation drugs in young children and pregnant women. 2017. https://www.fda.gov/Drugs/DrugSafety/ucm554634.htm.
7. Davidson AJ, Disma N, de Graaf JC, et al. Neurodevelopmental outcome at 2 years of age after general anaesthesia and awake-regional anaesthesia in infancy (GAS): an international multicentre, randomised controlled trial. Lancet. 2016;387(10015):239–50.
8. Sun LS, Li G, Miller TLK, et al. Association between a single general anesthesia exposure before age 36 months and neurocognitive outcomes in later childhood. JAMA. 2016;315(21):2312–20.
9. Warner DO, Zaccariello MJ, Schroeder DR, et al. Neuropsychological and behavioral outcomes after exposure of young children to procedures requiring general anesthesia: the Mayo Anesthesia Safety in Kids (MASK) Study. Anesthesiology. 2018;129(1):89–105.
10. Gobeaux D, et al. Intranasal midazolam in pediatric ophthalmology. Can Anesthesiol. 1991;39(1):34–6.
11. Bergman SA. Ketamine: review of its pharmacology and its use in pediatric anesthesia. Anesthesia Prog. 1999;46:10–20.
12. Mahfouz AK, Khalaf MA. Comparative study of 2 anesthesia techniques for pediatric refractive surgery. J Cataract Refract Surg. 2005;31:2345–9.
13. Mizrak A, et al. Ketamine versus propofol for strabismus surgery in children. Clini Ophthalmol. 2010;4:673–9.
14. Choi SR, et al. Effect of different anesthetic agents on oculocardiac reflex in pediatric strabismus surgery. J Anesth. 2009;23:489–93.
15. Smith KC, Comite SL, Balasubramanian S, et al. Vibration anesthesia: a noninvasive method of reducing discomfort prior to dermatologic procedures. Dermatol Online J. 2004;10(2):1.
16. Murhammer J, Ross M, Bebout K. Lidocaine – maximum dosing recommendations. Rx Update. 2004;12. http://www.healthcare.uiowa.edu/pharmacy/RxUpdate/2004/12rxu.html.
17. Rodgers A, Cox RG. Anesthetic management for pediatric strabismus surgery: continuing professional development. Can J Anesth. 2010;57:602–17.
18. Schug SA, Chong C. Pain management after ambulatory surgery. Curr Opin Anesthesiol. 2009;22:738–43.
19. Elvir-Lazo OL, White PF. Postoperative pain management after ambulatory surgery: role of multimodal analgesia. Anesthesiol Clin. 2010;28:217–24.
20. Verghese ST, Hannallah RS. Acute pain management in children. J Pain Res. 2010;3:105–23.

Part XI

Eyelid and Orbital Trauma

Christopher J. Calvano and J. Javier Servat

Management of Ocular Adnexal Trauma

67

Jackson F. Lever, Anne Barmettler, and Mark R. Levine

Introduction

The evaluation and management of patients who have sustained ocular adnexal trauma can be challenging. Often these patients have multiple injuries and are being cared for by many different subspecialties. Evaluation of such patients may seem daunting secondary to substantial bleeding and edema. In addition, the emotional state of the patient and family members often makes history taking and examination especially difficult and time consuming. Despite these challenges, the examination and treatment of trauma patients can be straightforward and efficient if undertaken in a systematic fashion.

Before discussing the treatment of periocular trauma, a brief review of wound healing has been provided to improve surgical outcomes.

Principles of Wound Healing

Epithelial wound healing is a complex cascade that begins with tissue injury and ends with a goal of restoration of architectural integrity. The repair process is regulated and orchestrated by a myriad of cells, cytokines (signaling factors), and growth factors.

Overall, the cascade of cutaneous repair is best described as three overlapping stages known as inflammation, proliferation, and remodeling. The initial inflammatory phase is seen as hemostasis and inflammatory cellular infiltration. The proliferative phase is characterized by granulation, fibroplasia, contraction, and epithelialization. The final phase of remodeling allows for collagen synthesis and degradation to improve and strengthen the repair process.

Wound healing can be delayed for a number of reasons, including age, infection, smoking, and other underlying medical conditions, such as malnutrition, diabetes, and exogenous corticosteroid administration.

Phases of Wound Healing

Inflammation (Wounding Through Day 5)

Upon wounding, a series of hemostatic events begins the cascade that eventually leads to reestablishment of epithelial integrity. Chemical mediators are released by injured blood vessels activating the intrinsic portion of the coagulation cascade. This includes integrin receptors, such as GPIIb/IIIa, which mediates platelet adhesiveness and leads to vasoconstriction, platelet aggregation, and degranulation around damaged endothelium. A clot forms, which is initially made of collagen, platelets, thrombin, and fibronectin forms. This, in turn, releases additional cytokines and growth factors, serving as a chemo-modulator and scaffold of the wound healing response [1].

Chemotaxis and Activation

The formation of a stabilizing clot results in cellular signaling that attracts neutrophils, the initial cells in the wound healing cascade. Further accumulation of inflammatory mediators leads to rising prostaglandin levels, which leads to local vasodilation and loss of endothelial cell-cell adhesion. This allows for increased cellular traffic as neutrophils are attracted to the injured zone by interleukin-1 (IL-1), tumor

J. F. Lever (✉)
Country Hills Eye Center, Ogden, UT, USA

A. Barmettler
Albert Einstein College of Medicine, Montefiore Medical Center, Department of Ophthalmology, Bronx, NY, USA
e-mail: abarmett@montefiore.org

M. R. Levine
University Hospitals of Cleveland, Department of Ophthalmology, Cleveland, OH, USA
e-mail: mlevine@eye-lids.com

J. J. Servat et al. (eds.), *Smith and Nesi's Ophthalmic Plastic and Reconstructive Surgery*,
https://doi.org/10.1007/978-3-030-41720-8_67

necrosis factor-alpha (TNF-α), transforming growth factor-beta (TGF-β), PF4, and bacterial products. Neutrophils are responsible for clearing out invading bacteria and cellular debris by releasing caustic proteolytic enzymes. These proteases are categorized into serine proteases, which have broad specificity, and metalloproteinases (which contain zinc ions), which specifically digest collagen. Regardless of the protease, only the extracellular matrix of wounded tissue will be destroyed because of protease inhibitors, which protect unwounded tissue. Neutrophils also generate reactive oxygen free radicals (through a myeloperoxidase pathway) that combine with chlorine to help sterilize the wound from bacteria. To aid in bacterial killing, activated complement fragments promote opsonization and thus phagocytosis. These steps can be delayed in chronic wounds, where the protection of healthy tissue by protease inhibitors is overwhelmed and healthy tissue destroyed due to massive release or prolonged protease concentration. Another cause of delay in healing seen in chronic wounds is the prolonged or increased concentrations of oxygen free radicals.

The second cells attracted to the zone of injury and probably the most important in orchestrating wound healing are the macrophages. Around 48–96 hours post-wounding, monocytes are attracted to the area and transformed into macrophages. Activated macrophages are responsible for transitioning from the inflammatory to the proliferative phase of wound healing. This is accomplished by mediating angiogenesis through synthesis of vascular endothelial growth factor (VEGF), fibroblast growth factor (FGF), and tumor necrosis factor-alpha (TNF-α) and fibroplasia by transforming growth factor-beta (TGF-β), epidermal growth factor (EGF), platelet-derived growth factor (PDGF), IL-1 (interleukin-1), and TNF-α [2]. Further, nitric oxide (NO) is released by an inducible nitric oxide synthase activated IL-1 and TNF-α. Macrophages also play a role in pathogen killing and clearing of debris by synthesizing large quantities of NO. TNF and IL-1 stimulate macrophage iNOS to produce NO which will react with peroxide ion oxygen radicals to yield an even more toxic peroxynitrite and hydroxyl radicals. Debris clearing is accomplished by phagocytosis of devitalized material, bacteria, and apoptotic neutrophils. Further damaged extracellular matrix is cleared by matrix metalloproteinases (MMP), which are expressed by keratinocytes, fibroblasts, monocytes, and macrophages in response to TNF-α. This also enhances migration of cells through extracellular matrix [3].

Proliferation (Day 4–14)

This phase is characterized by epithelialization, angiogenesis, and provisional matrix formation. Epidermal growth factor (EGF) and tumor growth factor-alpha (TGF-α) are secreted by platelets and macrophages. This is the stimulus for epithelial cells at the wounded edge to send out projections to try and reestablish a protective barrier against further fluid loss and bacterial invasion. Reepithelialization begins shortly after wounding and is stimulated by inflammatory cytokines IL-1 and TNF-α. Further, fibroblasts synthesize keratinocyte growth factors to stimulate epidermal thickening and marginal basal cells to migrate into the wound, proliferate, and differentiate into epidermis. When these epithelial cells begin migrating, they do not divide until epidermal continuity is restored. These cells flatten and migrate as a sheet (a movement called epiboly) over the wound matrix. Cell adhesion proteins glycoproteins, such as tenascin and fibronectin, provide the "railroad" tracks to facilitate epithelial migration. After reestablishing the epithelial layer, keratinocytes and fibroblasts secrete collagen type IV to form the basement membrane. At this point the cells become more columnar and divide to form the normal layers of epidermis.

Circulating bone marrow-derived cells are signaled to migrate into the wound and develop into fibroblasts. Both fibroblasts and endothelial cells are the predominant activated cell types during this phase. Platelet-derived growth factor (PDGF) and epidermal growth factor (EGF) derived from macrophages and platelets stimulate fibroblasts to proliferate and to synthesize collagen. Further differentiation takes place among fibroblasts already present in the wound. Stimulation by macrophage-secreted transforming growth factor-beta-1 (TGF-β1) induces transformation into myofibroblasts for wound contraction. Transforming growth factor-beta (TGF-β) is important in orchestrating many processes during this phase. It peaks around day 7–14, which amplifies extracellular matrix (ECM) production and decreases its degradation. It also induces fibroblasts to begin synthesizing collagen type I, increases production of cell adhesion proteins, decreases production of matrix metalloproteinases (MMP), and increases production of metalloproteinase inhibitors [4]. TGF-β also plays a large role in wounds allowed to heal by secondary intention in which it stimulates larger quantities of myofibroblasts for wound contracture.

Vascular endothelial growth factor (VEGF) secreted mainly by keratinocytes at wound edges, but also macrophages, fibroblasts, platelets, and other endothelial cells, stimulates endothelial cells at venule edges to begin formation of new capillaries. VEGF production and release is also stimulated in response to hypoxia from nitric oxide (NO) released from endothelial cells [5]. This helps protect tissue from ischemia and reperfusion injury and causes endothelium to vasodilate.

After activation and proliferation, extracellular matrix (ECM) is laid down by fibroblasts. The initial matrix is provisional and is composed of fibrin, glycosaminoglycan (GAG), and hyaluronic acid (HA). Fibroblasts utilize hyaluronidase to digest the provisional hyaluronic acid-rich matrix, which allows for larger sulfated glycosaminoglycans to be deposited. Integrin receptors on cell surfaces bind to matrix glycosaminoglycans and glycoproteins. Adhesion glycoproteins, mainly fibronectin, laminin, and tenascin, are present in the early matrix to facilitate cell attachment and migration [6].

Concomitantly, while ECM is being laid down, disorganized collagens are also being synthesized and secreted by fibroblasts onto the fibronectin and GAG scaffold. Major fibrillar ECM collagens are types I and III in both wounded and normal skin. The ratio of collagen type I/III is 4:1 in the skin and healed mature scars. On the other hand, immature, wounded skin has a ratio closer to 2:1 with types I and III, where type I collagen is always the predominant type.

Dermal collagen is a right-handed triple helix synthesized and secreted by fibroblasts into the ECM. Here the N- and C-terminal pro-peptides are cleaved and tropocollagen molecules are formed. These molecules laterally aggregate and are covalently cross-linked by the enzyme lysyl oxidase to form collagen fibrils. These fibrils interact and aggregate into fibers.

In the proliferation stage, healing by secondary intention and open wounds are characterized by granulation tissue. Healthy granulation tissue has a typical beefy red appearance due to its dense population of blood vessels, macrophages, and fibroblasts embedded in a loose provisional matrix of fibronectin, hyaluronic acid, and collagen. Neo-angiogenesis induced by VEGF is directed at vascular endothelial progenitor cells to migrate and proliferate. This allows for the formation of the rich bed of new capillary networks seen in these healing wounds. Presence of granulation tissue is used as a clinical indicator of the health and overall ability of a wound to heal.

Healing by secondary intention is also characterized by wound contracture. Myofibroblasts are fibroblast-like cells that also contain α-smooth muscle actin and microfilaments, which confer the ability to generate contractile forces. Clinically, wound contraction allows for a smaller wound surface area, which then decreases time to heal and limits the amount of insensate scar that ensues. The amount of contraction is related to the size and location with areas such as the trunk and perineum allowing for the greatest contracture. Allowing wounds to heal by secondary intention can result in deformation and functional limitations on typically mobile areas. This is seen over joints and on the eyelids.

Remodeling Phase (14 Days to 1 Year)

This phase is characterized clinically by scar maturation. Overall, in the previous phases, the wound was internally debrided to sterile environment, and a structural extracellular matrix (ECM) was deposited haphazardly to facilitate wound closure and reestablishment of the internal milieu. A complex balance of ECM degradation, synthesis, and deposition of the initially disorganized repair characterizes the remodeling phase. This process also adds strength to wounded tissue and is seen clinically as a raised, red scar becoming flatter and more flesh-colored as the initially formed dense capillary network regresses. This phase clinically is very important due to the fact that wound strength and character are determined during this time. A weaker wound may result if patients have matrix deposition problems from diet or disease or may develop hypertrophic or keloid scars if the balance between collagen synthesis and degradation isn't regulated well.

Initially, the ECM is composed mainly of fibrin and fibronectin from the coagulation cascade of hemostasis and macrophages. Fibroblasts begin to secrete proteins such as glycosaminoglycans and proteoglycans as a preliminary and disorganized framework for the matrix made of primarily type III collagen, which is replaced by a stronger and more organized collagen matrix made of collagen type I. Initial deposition of type III collagen, which does not significantly contribute to wound strength, is not fully understood. It does however coincide with the presence of fibronectin, which has been thought to facilitate phagocytosis of denatured collagen by coating it.

Despite the complex wound healing process ultimately resulting in a scar, healed skin morphologically has a lack of connective tissue organization compared to pre-wounded skin. Collagen fibers are secreted by fibroblasts as early as 3 days into the wound healing cascade. Net collagen synthesis continues for up to 6 weeks partly from an increase in the number of fibroblasts and upregulated collagen synthesis per cell. Initially laid collagen is thinner and oriented parallel to the skin in a densely packed matrix. Granulation tissue collagen has a greater hydroxylation and glycosylation of lysine residues, which corresponds to thinner fibers [7]. The remodeling process degrades the initial collagen and replaces it with thicker fibers that are oriented along stress lines. Overall, this remains different than reticular pattern seen histologically in normal dermis. Increased tensile strength is positively correlated collagen thickness and orientation.

Most scars tend to be hypopigmented compared to the surrounding skin but can be hyperpigmented especially in darker skin types. Regardless, maturing scars should be kept out of the sun, and protective measures should be taken especially in sun-exposed areas such as the head, neck, and extremities.

Wound tensile strength rapidly increases from weeks 1 to 8. This initially is due to the increased content of collagen deposited. Further strengthening is accomplished by reorganization and cross-linking of collagen. Wound strength never returns to full strength. At week 1, it has 3% of final strength, at 3 weeks 30%, and at full maturity, the wound will achieve only 80% of pre-wounding strength [8]. This process utilizes lysyl oxidase as the major intermolecular collagen cross-linking enzyme. At the same time, matrix metalloproteinases (MMP) such as collagenases, gelatinases, and stromelysins degrade ECM components. The balance of collagen deposition and degradation is in part determined by regulation of MMP activity. Changing concentrations of cytokines such as TGF-β, PDGF, IL-1, and EGF influences activation. It is also further suppressed by tissue inhibitors of metalloproteinase (TIMP), secreted by fibroblasts, and upregulated by TGF-β and IL-6.

The final result of the wound healing cascade is a scar. Even in its final matured state, it will be more fragile and inelastic than the normal skin, in addition to missing skin appendages, such as hair follicles and sweat glands.

Clinical Factors Affecting Wound Healing

There are a number of factors that slow wound healing, including infection. Bacteria trigger acute and chronic inflammatory infiltrates, which inhibit the wound healing cascade by impairing fibroblast proliferation, resulting in decreasing ECM synthesis and deposition. More than 10^5 organisms/g of tissue constitute clinical infection and will delay wound healing.

Another important part of the anabolic wound healing process is nutrition. An adequate protein intake is necessary for many internal processes but is imperative for ECM deposition. Chronic protein depletion can result in poorly healed wounds and, in severe cases, dehiscence.

Other nutrients that are pivotal in the healing cascade are vitamins and minerals. Vitamin C (ascorbic acid) is necessary for hydroxylation of proline and lysine residues. Hydroxyproline allows for newly synthesized collagen to be transported out of cells. Hydroxylysine facilitates collagen cross-linking. Vitamin A (retinoic acid) is involved in many aspects of repair such as fibroplasia, collagen synthesis, and cross-linking as well as epithelialization.

Vitamin A requirements are increased following injury, and supplementation may be required to maintain normal serum levels. It has also been shown to reverse the impaired healing that occurs with chronic corticosteroid treatment. Being a fat-soluble vitamin, overdoses can occur, and the typical oral dose is important to note (25,000 IU every other day).

Vitamin B_6 (pyridoxine) is utilized for collagen cross-linking, and low levels of vitamin B_1 (riboflavin) are associated with poor wound healing. Minerals, such as zinc and copper, have been implicated in poor wound healing due to the fact that their divalent cations are cofactors in many important enzymatic reactions. Zinc deficiency has been associated with poor epithelialization and poor wound healing. This can be easily corrected as a patient only needs to supplement zinc for 10 days to improve the situation.

Systemic factors are a known impediment to healing. For example, a patient with arterial occlusions below the knee is unlikely to heal a posterior heel ulcer without revascularization. Similarly, diabetes mellitus is known to cause multiple cellular changes which delay healing. Growth factor and cytokine deficiencies have been found in both diabetic mouse and diabetic human wounds. Specifically, there are deficiencies in PDGF, VEGF, IGF-1, IGF-II, TGF-β, aFGF, and IL-6. Diabetics also have decreased angiogenesis, endothelial dysfunction, abnormalities in fibroblast function, extracellular matrix, and decreased cellular infiltrate [9]. These factors, in combination with the neuropathic changes and arterial occlusive disease that occur with diabetes over time, lead to very poor healing ability. Wound healing in diabetics proceeds far more effectively when tight glycemic control is maintained. One good indicator of diabetic blood glucose control in the prior 3 months is the hemoglobin A1C level. Any discrepancies or problems maintaining normal blood glucose levels should be referred to an endocrinologist.

Another outside factor on healing is smoking. Smoking has been shown to have deleterious effects on wound healing with one cigarette decreasing local blood supply by up to 30% for 2–4 h after each cigarette. Smoking cessation during the wound healing period can play a crucial role in the outcome.

The last important factor in healing is vascular supply. It is well established that wounds cannot heal without adequate blood flow, so a careful assessment of perfusion should be done for all wounds, particularly those on the distal extremities. Any patient with non-palpable, distal pulses should be referred for noninvasive testing or evaluation by a vascular surgeon. In addition, in patients, who have previously undergone revascularization procedures, reocclusion of the affected artery should be considered and evaluated in the setting of wound deterioration without other factors, such as infection, being present.

Excessive Healing

The normal wound healing cascade is characterized by numerous up- and downregulations of target cells, occurring at different times. When signals are ineffective or absent, the synthesis of ECM, especially collagen, may continue and result in excessive repair. The reasoning for this is not well understood, but certain aspects, such as overexpression of profibrotic cytokines, a lack of programmed cell death (apoptosis), and continued presence of ECM secreting activated fibroblasts, have been implicated.

One cause of excessive scarring can be attributed to the location of the wound, whether iatrogenic or traumatic, in unfavorable locations. Tension along the wound edge may cause separation and widening as well as some healing by secondary intention. To achieve the smallest and most cosmetically acceptable scar, placement of incisions should be made to create the least amount of tension on a wound. These areas are classically described as being within or parallel to natural skin creases (Langer's lines).

When excessive scarring occurs, this can be defined as hypertrophic and keloid. Hypertrophic scars are defined as raised scars that have not overgrown the boundaries of the original scar. They typically form as the result of tension on wound edges and are common across flexion surfaces of extremities, breasts, sternum, and neck. They are usually self-limited and will fade over time.

Keloid scars are characterized by overgrowth beyond the original boundaries and behave like a benign skin tumor. They are more commonly seen in darker-skinned patients with African Americans having an incidence between 6% and 16%. They have an autosomal dominant genetic predisposition. However, simple primary excision and closure usually results in recurrence. This may be due to excessive wound healing stimuli and/or inappropriate stopgap signals resulting in continued and unchecked repair. They are relatively acellular and are composed mainly of collagen. An appropriate number of fibroblasts at the wound edge seem to overproduce collagen and disturb the balance between synthesis and degradation. TGF-β causes a greater degree of collagen gene expression, and there is a greater degree of profibrotic growth factor expression in keloid compared to normal fibroblasts. Further studies have also found that keloid keratinocytes are phenotypically different and induce a greater proliferation and collagen expression in fibroblasts.

Eyelid Trauma

Systemic Considerations

Patients with ocular adnexal trauma may have other significant injuries. This is especially true in patients injured by motor vehicle accidents or falls. In general, the emergency medical staff will have already addressed the life-threatening medical conditions prior to obtaining an ophthalmic consultation. Nonetheless, it is important to use an appropriate treatment protocol for assessing patients with acute trauma that is systematic in nature. This includes assuring the basic ABCs of emergency care: establishing an adequate airway, controlling excessive bleeding, and stabilization of the patient's circulatory status [10]. The facial region is highly vascularized, and significant blood loss can rapidly occur. Control of bleeding can usually be achieved by a combination of pressure and ligation of large bleeding vessels. Significant blood loss should be treated with volume replacement. Ophthalmic evaluation and treatment should be delayed until life-threatening systemic problems have been addressed.

Because injuries to the lids may be associated with trauma to the head and neck region, it is mandatory to rule out a cervical spinal injury. Until an appropriate evaluation can be performed, the patient's neck should be immobilized in a cervical collar. The neurologic status should be evaluated, especially for signs of a closed head injury. If there is a possibility of an intracranial injury, obtain a head computed tomography (CT) scan and consultation with a neurosurgeon. Thorough full body exam should be done in conjunction with emergency medicine staff, ruling out diagnoses, such as occult chest and abdominal trauma.

General Principles

Once attention can be safely directed to the ocular adnexal region, priority should be first given to the preservation of vision. This entails evaluating the patient for any evidence of ocular or optic nerve injuries (Fig. 67.1). This may be difficult if the patient is uncooperative or unconscious. Furthermore, a proper examination may be difficult secondary to swelling of the eyelids or pain on opening of the lids. Bleeding may also hamper attempts to evaluate the globe. Light pressure to the lids usually controls generalized oozing; however, care should be taken to avoid pressure on the globe, especially if there is a risk of globe rupture. Treatment of eyelid injuries should be delayed until the globe is determined to be intact in order to prevent extrusion of intraocular contents. If a ruptured eye is suspected, further examination and treatment should be performed in an operating room setting [11].

If the adnexal injury is significant or there has been contamination, intravenous antibiotics should be administered and tetanus immunization status determined. Tetanus toxoid, 0.5 mL, should be administered if the patient has not had a tetanus immunization within 5 years. If the patient has never had a tetanus immunization, 250 units of human tetanus immune globulin should be given [12].

Pain can be severe in traumatized patients, and pain relief can facilitate the evaluation and treatment of injuries. However, care should be used in regard to the type and dosage of pain medication given, especially with regard to those with possible head injury and/or intoxication.

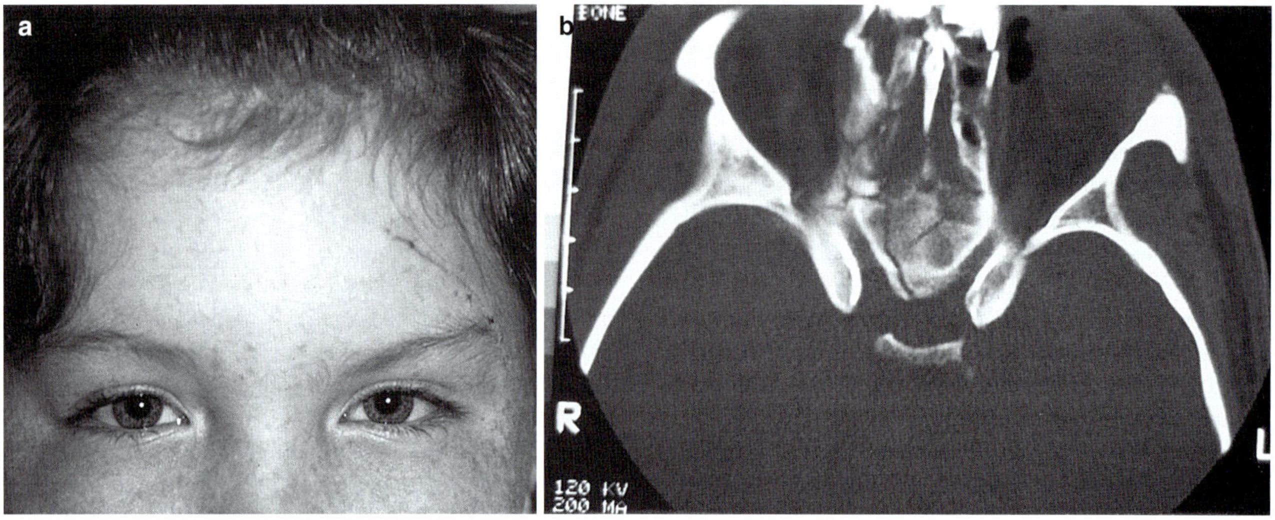

Fig. 67.1 (**a**) Soft tissue injury to the eyelid. (**b**) CT scan of the same patient with evidence of associated optic nerve injury

History

A carefully gathered history about the circumstances causing an injury can be of great help in determining the type and extent of the trauma, as well as for medicolegal documentation. The mechanism of injury can indicate the depth of a wound and if there may be a foreign body present. A history of sharp trauma with a pencil or knife should elicit suspicion of injury to deeper orbital structures like the levator muscle, optic nerve, or extraocular muscles. The object should be inspected, if possible, to ensure that its entirety has been removed. Likewise, a history of blunt injury to the periorbital tissues may raise suspicion of an underlying orbital fracture or canthal avulsion. Bite and claw injuries are notorious for causing canalicular lacerations.

In addition to asking about mechanism, documentation of the location where the injury took place (e.g., if at work) is also important. If the injury occurred at work, it is important to note time of injury and if goggles or other protective eyewear were being donned.

A patient's specific reports of symptoms can also suggest the type and extent of injury to be found. Decreased vision suggests an injury to the optic nerve or globe. Diplopia, hypesthesia, and pain on eye movement are indicative of an orbital fracture. Pain with jaw movement or chewing may indicate a zygomaticomaxillary complex fracture. Inquiry should be made about loss of consciousness and neck or trunk pain. If an animal bite is involved, it should be determined if the animal is up-to-date on its rabies immunizations and if the animal has been quarantined (for 10 days) [13–16]. A history of previous ocular abnormality as well as other medical problems should be elicited. Known allergies should be documented, and a compilation of medications should be noted. The most recent food or liquid ingestion should be documented. There is a delay in gastric emptying after significant trauma; so, if reasonable, surgery should be delayed for at least 8 h if general anesthesia is required [17].

Patient Evaluation

The examination should be divided into four basic parts: (1) the ocular examination, followed by (2) a periocular soft tissue examination, (3) orbital evaluation, and (4) examination of the face. Throughout the exam, excellent documentation and photographs should be taken for both medical and legal reasons.

First, an ocular examination must be performed first to rule out an injury of the globe. In the conscious patient, visual acuity, pupillary response, intraocular pressure, slit lamp examination, and a dilated fundus examination should be performed. Even in the unconscious patient, a complete ocular examination is usually possible. For some cases an evaluation under anesthesia is necessary because trying to manipulate the lids can cause further injury to the globe.

The second portion of the exam, periocular soft tissue examination, should delineate the extent and depth of lacerations. The eyelid margin should be examined carefully first. A notch or abnormality in the marginal contour should elicit suspicion for more extensive, full-thickness injury. Any laceration medial to the punctum should be inspected carefully for a canalicular laceration. Bite or claw injuries should raise suspicion for occult canalicular injury. Another sign of canalicular injury includes lateral punctal displacement. The punctal position can be compared with the contralateral punctum and the ipsilateral opposing punctum. If there is any possibility of a canalicular laceration, the involved canaliculus should be probed. A drop of tetracaine placed in the eye before probing will make this procedure more comfortable. Orbital fat prolapse through the eyelid indicates penetration through the orbital septum and potential deep orbital trauma and/or damage to the levator muscle. Lid position and levator function should be assessed. Displacement or rounding of the canthal angles should be noted.

The third portion of the exam, orbital evaluation, begins with testing of extraocular muscle function including range of motion and diplopia in all fields of gaze. Test for hypesthesia of the cheek, side of the nose, and upper lip and gum region as this may be seen in orbital floor fractures. Palpation of the bony orbital rims should be performed to evaluate for bony step-offs. Significant tightness of the orbit on palpation should raise suspicion of orbital compartment syndrome and possible compression of the optic nerve. Proptosis or enophthalmos is best assessed by bird's eye and worm's eye view and is optimally confirmed with a Hertel exophthalmometer. If a fracture or foreign body is suspected, a CT scan without contrast of the orbits and/or face is indicated. The CT scan is usually the study of choice in an acute trauma setting for several reasons; acquisition time is shorter, and there is better visualization of bony orbit and foreign bodies. Objects, such as wood and plastic, are better seen with CT or ultrasound, as they may not be seen on MRI. Direct axial and coronal views with thin cuts (less than or equal to 2 mm) should be obtained. A magnetic resonance image (MRI) scan of the orbits and/or face may be useful in identifying optic nerve injury.

Finally, because ocular adnexal injury is often associated with facial injuries, thorough examination of the head and neck should be performed. It is wise to involve other specialists as needed.

Surgical Management

The goals of surgical repair of adnexal trauma are to preserve the eye and vision, maintain function, and restore cosmesis [18]. The best way to accomplish these goals is through a well-executed primary repair.

At surgery, the first priority is to establish the extent of injury. If the globe is ruptured, it should be repaired and sealed to prevent loss of contents prior to any periocular or orbital exploration. A thorough exploration of all wounds should be performed, looking for deep orbital penetration, foreign bodies, or occult injury to the globe (Fig. 67.2). Debride only tissue that is clearly devitalized and avoid removal of tissue when possible. Gentle manipulation of the wound edges will minimize further trauma during the repair.

Care should be taken to remove foreign bodies, as retained foreign bodies can lead to chronic infection or abscesses, especially if the foreign body is organic. Even with extensive exploration and removal of foreign bodies, some small fragments, especially glass, may spontaneously extrude for months after the initial injury. Preoperative radiographic mapping of foreign bodies can be extremely helpful at the time of operation. In the case of inert, asymptomatic foreign bodies, especially in the posterior orbit, patients can be observed due to the risk of surgical risks of removal.

In cases with possible wound contamination, irrigation should be carried out initially to remove debris from the site of injury and reduce its bacterial load. Sterile saline solution can be used. Use of a large syringe fitted with an 18- to 19-gauge catheter creates a continuous stream under pressure, which can reduce bacterial counts by up to 1.5 log units and thus wound infection by 90% [19].

Once the wounds have been completely explored and decontaminated, the goal of surgical treatment is to restore the integrity of the five basic components of the eyelids: (1) anterior lamellae, skin and orbicularis muscle; (2) posterior lamellae, tarsus and conjunctiva; (3) canthal tendons; (4) upper and lower canaliculi; and (5) levator complex. If involved, the canthal tendons, lacrimal excretory system, and levator complex should be repaired first, and then attention can be directed to the eyelid margin and skin. Often it appears that there is loss of tissue when it merely is retraction of the wound margins secondary to normal elasticity of the eyelid structures or the thin tissue of the lids folding under itself. In closing a wound, first

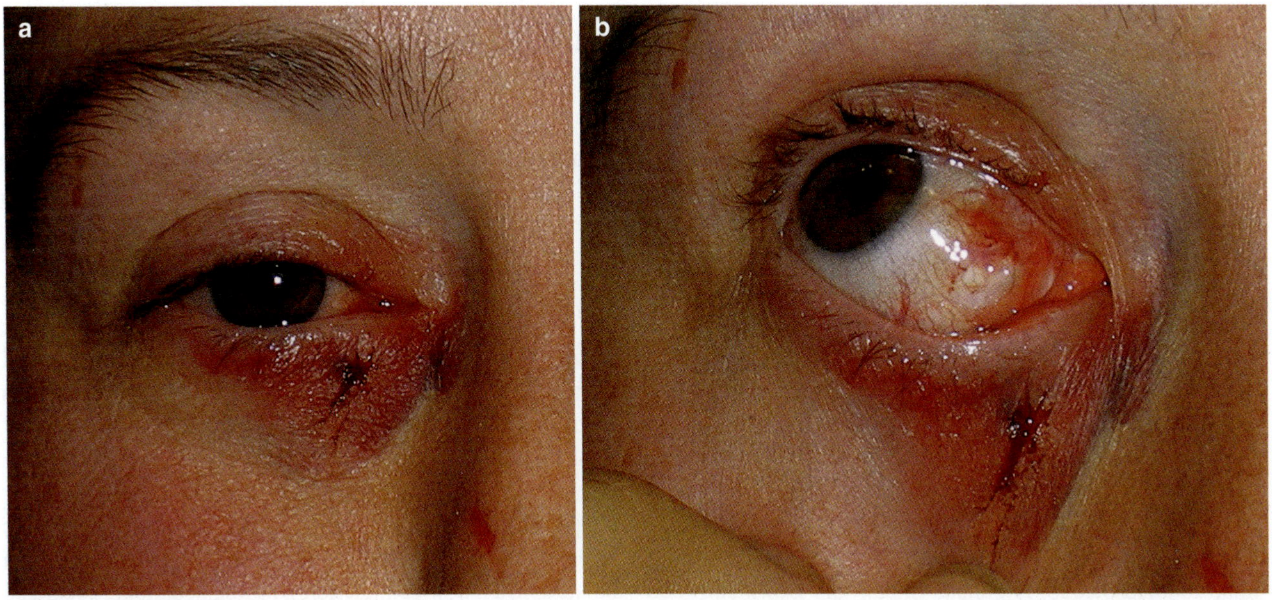

Fig. 67.2 43-year-old woman with unintentional self-inflected knife wound. (**a**) External photo shows what appears to be superficial laceration of the right lower lid. (**b**) Further examination reveals occult injury of the globe by full-thickness penetration through the right lower lid

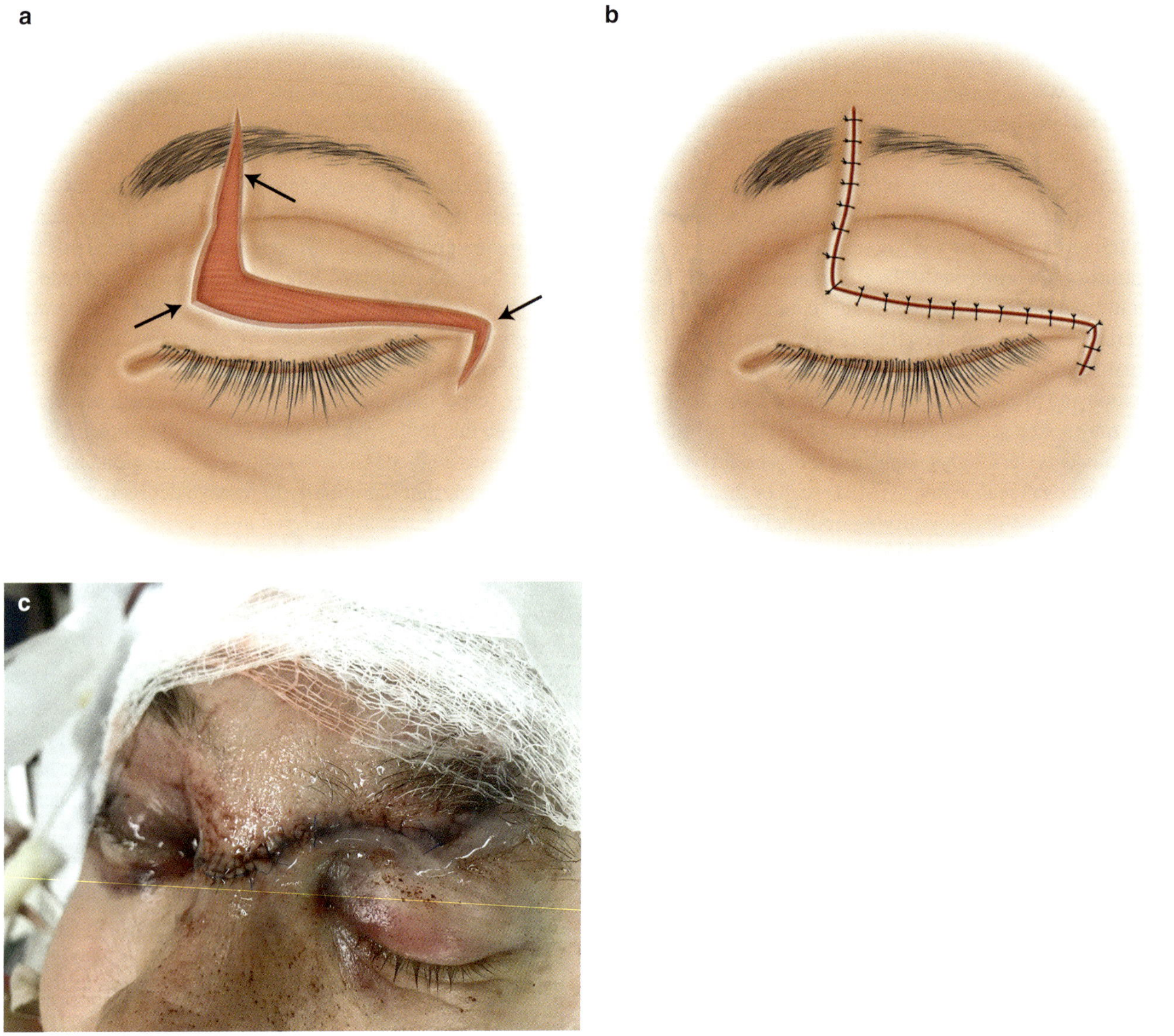

Fig. 67.3 54-year-old pedestrian struck by semi-truck presenting after initial closure by rural ED with poor approximation of key landmarks. (**a**) Key landmarks (arrows) include angles and apices, as well as the brow hair. (**b**) Appearance of laceration with proper approximation of key landmarks. (**c**) Immediate postoperative photograph demonstrating outcome of wound exploration with proper reapproximation of landmarks

pick identifying landmarks to reapproximate. These include points of acute angulation, hairline of the brow, and the apices of traumatic flaps (Fig. 67.3). The septum should not be incorporated in any repair of the traumatized lids, as this leads to marked lid retraction and lagophthalmos.

Operative Considerations

Most minor lacerations can be repaired bedside in the emergency room or intensive care unit. A small, specialized tray of instruments simplifies these repairs. This tray should include a Castroviejo needle holder, blunt Westcott scissors, and a small-toothed pickup. A punctal dilator and Bowman probe should be included (Fig. 67.4). Useful sutures for such minor repairs include 5-0 Prolene on TF needle, Vicryl with a S-14 needle, and plain gut with a G-1 needle. Local anesthesia can be obtained with a 1:1 ratio of 1% lidocaine with epinephrine 1:100,000 with 0.5% bupivacaine with epinephrine 1:200,000. The mix of short- and long-acting anesthesia provides anesthesia both during and after the cause for improved postoperative comfort. The epinephrine decreases bleeding.

In the operating room setting, most adnexal injuries can be repaired with local anesthesia and monitored sedation. General anesthesia should be used if there is a possibility of an open globe, but no depolarizing agent should be given at the time of induction. General anesthesia should also be used for extensive or complex injuries, canalicular lacerations, and in poorly cooperative individuals. Local anesthesia consisting of the same lidocaine and bupivacaine mixture described above can be administered in conjunction with the sedation. A regional nerve block can be used to augment the local infiltration [14].

The entire face is prepped with a dilute solution of 10% povidone-iodine (Betadine) paint. Contaminated wounds

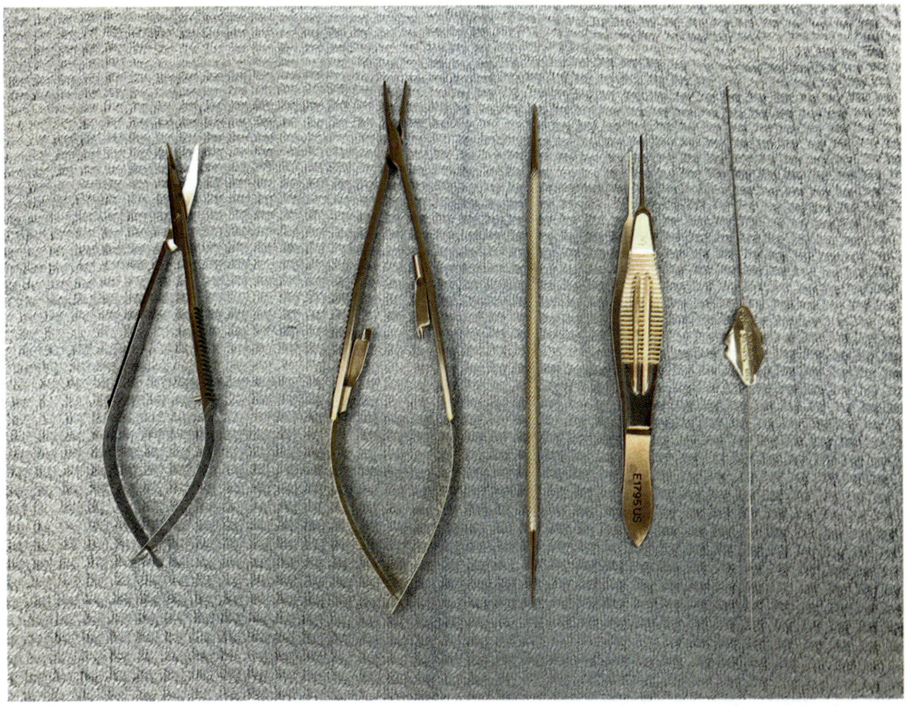

Fig. 67.4 Small ophthalmic plastic laceration tray consisting of blunt curved Shepard-Westcott scissors, Castroviejo locking needle holder, punctal dilator, Castroviejo fixation forceps 0.5 mm, and Bowman probe

should be thoroughly irrigated. At the end of surgery, an antibiotic ointment can be applied over the wounds. Patches should be used with caution in patients at risk for orbital compartment syndrome as this may delay diagnosis and thus management for this potentially vision-threatening condition.

Management of Blunt Trauma

Blunt trauma typically results in irregularly shaped lacerations and avulsion injuries. This type of injury is commonly seen in fist-related trauma or motor vehicle accidents when the face comes into contact with the dashboard.

Medial Canthal Injuries

Medial canthal tendon injuries are often associated with canalicular injuries, and intubation of the canaliculus should be performed before tendon repair. It is important to determine whether the posterior as well as the anterior horn of the medial canthal tendon has been injured. If the posterior horn has been transected, its repair is critical to proper lid apposition to the globe.

If both ends of the injured tendon can be found, it may be repaired using nonabsorbable suture. The 4-0 double-armed Polydek on a P-2 needle works well in this situation. Its small semicircular needle is invaluable in reattaching the canthal tendon in a posterior position. A horizontal mattress suture is placed through the distal avulsed end of the tendon, and the two needles are then brought from posterior to anterior through the proximal portion of the tendon. If the proximal portion of the tendon cannot be identified but there is intact periorbita, the needles can be passed through this in the region of the posterior lacrimal crest (Fig. 67.5). With complete avulsion of soft tissue from the bone, a microplate or miniature suture anchor can be used to fixate the medial canthal tendon into its normal position [20]. The microplate is attached to the thicker bone of the anterior lacrimal crest, and the posterior portion of the T-shaped plate is used to anchor the avulsed medial canthal tendon (Fig. 67.6). If using a miniature suture anchor, such as the Micro Quickanchor with 4-0 absorbable suture (DePuy Synthes, Indiana), the drill bit that comes with the anchor is used to drill the medial wall at the desired site. It is important to create a clear view of the bone (retracting periosteum) and to place the site about 2 mm superior than the normal anatomic position (which can be determined by comparing to the contralateral, non-involved medial canthus). Once placed, the sutures can be passed through the avulsed posterior medial canthal tendon or, if this is not available, the inferomedial tarsus and tied to the appropriate tension. Before repairing the medial canthal tendon, this region must be evaluated for evidence of bony fractures. Fractures must be stabilized before repair of the tendon. If the bone cannot be stabilized, then transnasal wiring of the medial canthal tendons should be used. The key point to remember in repairing the medial canthal tendon is that the repair must provide a superior and posterior pull to keep the lid well apposed to the globe and the lacrimal pump functioning normally.

Lateral Canthal Injuries

When both sides of the transected lateral canthal tendon can be identified, a 4-0 Polydek suture can be passed in a hori-

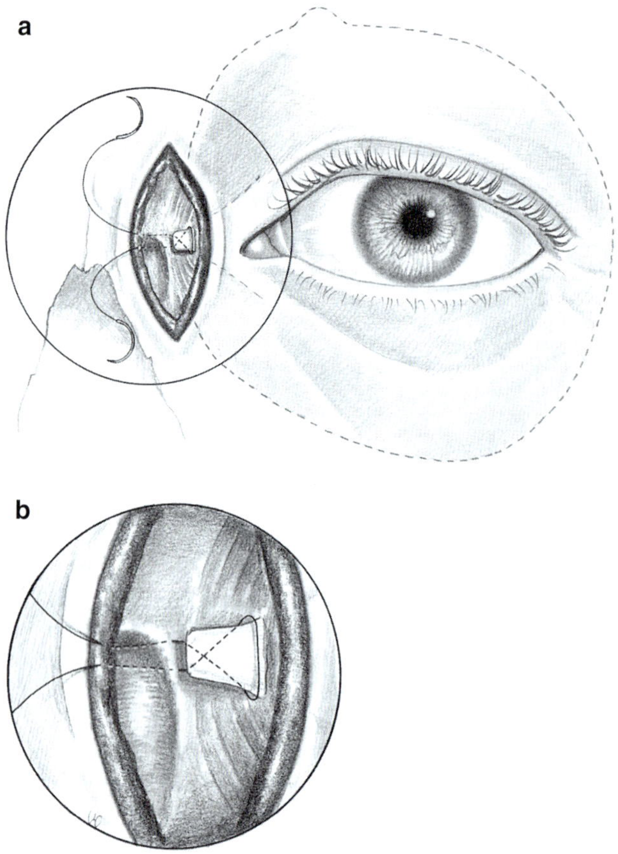

Fig. 67.5 Repair of an avulsion of the medial canthal tendon. (**a**) Medial canthal tendon has been avulsed from the periorbita, but the periorbita is intact. (**b**) A 4-0 Polydek suture is passed in a crisscross fashion through the cut end of the medial canthal tendon and then brought through the periorbita in the area of the posterior lacrimal crest in a posterior to anterior direction

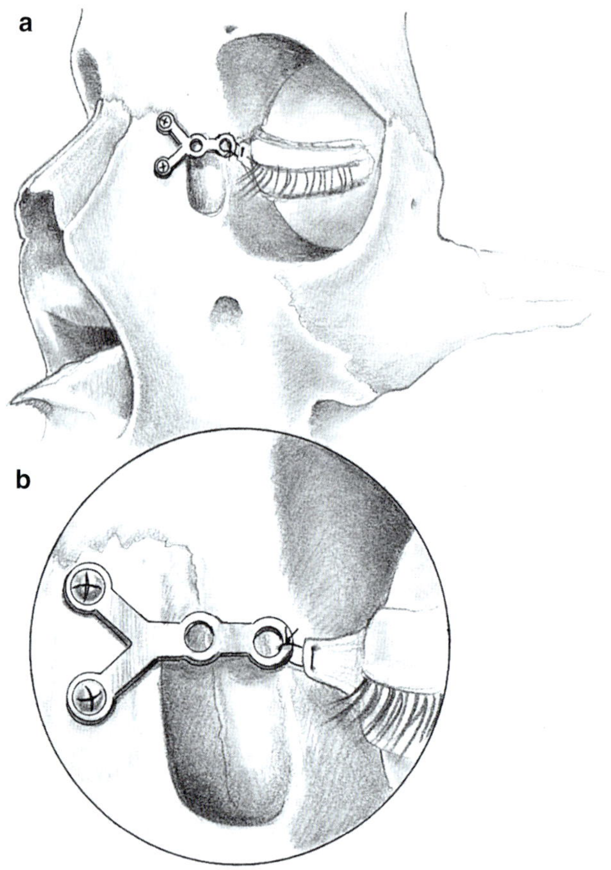

Fig. 67.6 When no periorbita remains, following a medial canthal tendon avulsion, a T-shaped microplate can be used to fixate the medial canthal tendon in its normal anatomic position

zontal mattress fashion across the cut ends of the tendon or to the periorbita if needed. With periosteal fixation, the transected tendon should be placed just above its normal anatomic position because wound contracture will tend to pull the canthal angle inferiorly [21]. If the periosteum at the desired area has been avulsed from the underlying lateral rim bone, small drill holes can be made through the lateral orbital rim, just above the lateral orbital tubercle and suture passed through these holes and tied. Just as in medial canthal tendon repairs, the lateral tendon should retain its superior and posterior pull to keep the lid in proper apposition with the globe.

Management of Sharp Trauma

Extramarginal Lacerations

Simple Lacerations

Simple lacerations are defined by involvement of only skin and underlying muscle with little tissue loss. It is important to examine the full extent of the wounds. What may at first appear to be a relatively superficial wound or small puncture may have significant underlying trauma.

The wound margins should be trimmed only if there is devitalized tissue. Slight undermining facilitates a good closure with eversion of the wound margin. Care should be taken so as not to have any significant tension on the wound. Lacerations, where the skin edges don't easily approximate, should be closed deeply with 6-0 Vicryl sutures. The eyelid skin is usually closed with 6-0 plain gut sutures. Interrupted sutures should be used for a curvilinear wound. Straight portions of the wound can be closed with a running suture. Cutaneous lacerations that extend past the eyelids should be closed with a 6-0 nonabsorbable suture; these sutures should be removed in 5–7 days. A 6-0 or 7-0 nonabsorbable suture, such as Prolene, can also be used to close eyelid skin but may pose issues should the patient have difficulty following up.

Complex Lacerations

Complex lacerations are defined as those with significant loss of tissue or injury to submuscular structures and include stellate lacerations. These wounds should be irrigated with

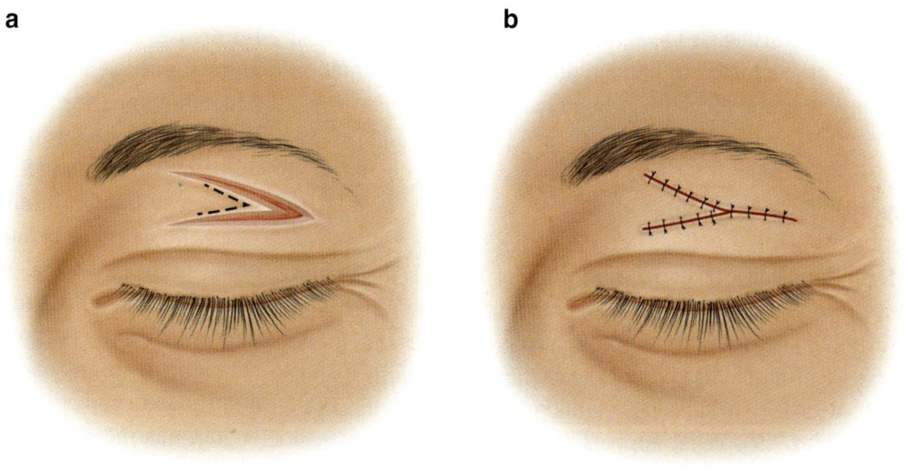

Fig. 67.7 (a) Complex laceration of the upper lid in a V-type configuration with devitalized apex. (b) Wound closure after devitalized tissue and wound edges are debrided with flap advanced

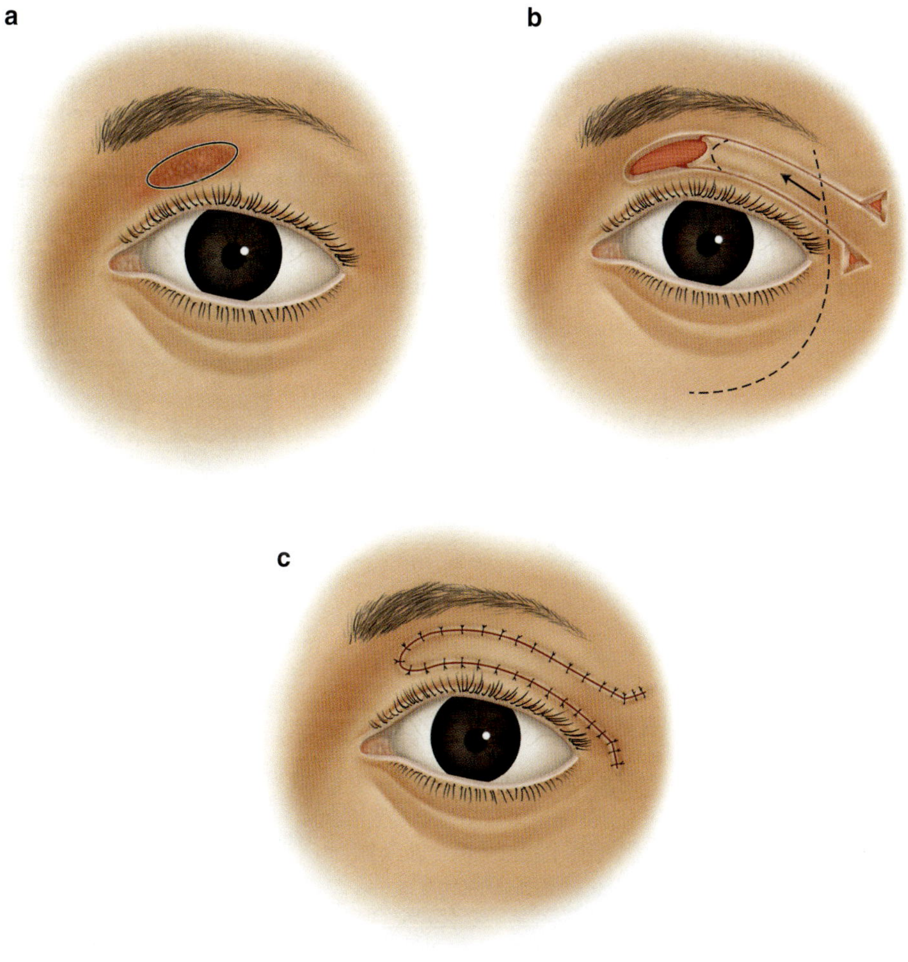

Fig. 67.8 (a) Injury to the upper lid involving avulsion of central portion of the anterior lamella. (b) Wound is debrided and margins freshened. A temporally based advancement flap is developed. (c) A sliding flap is then advanced and sutured into place with absorbable suture

normal saline and devitalized tissue debrided. Closure of these wounds is individualized and depends on the location and extent of injury. Lacerations of a V-type configuration in which the apex is devitalized can be transformed into a Y configuration after the devitalized tissue is removed (Fig. 67.7). Care must be taken not to shorten the anterior lamella enough to cause lid retraction. Wide undermining often facilitates wound closure. A valuable technique for tissue loss is the use of laterally or medially based advancement flaps (Fig. 67.8) [22]. Flaps advanced from the medial or lateral area (as opposed to from inferiorly) will help avoid creating eyelid retraction.

In general, it is advisable to minimize tissue rearrangement and grafting at the time of initial closure. Frost-type sutures may be used to prevent anterior lamella contraction during the initial phases of wound healing.

Eyelid Margin Lacerations

Meticulous closure of lacerations that involve the eyelid margin is crucial to achieve a correct anatomic repair and minimize postoperative complications. Failure to achieve these goals can lead to notching of the eyelid margin, poor contour of the lid, and lagophthalmos with corneal exposure (Fig. 67.9). What appears to be a small anterior eyelid laceration may have a more extensive posterior lamellar component (Fig. 67.10). A laceration that appears to be only a few millimeters in length anteriorly can completely disrupt the tarsal plate posteriorly. If possible, larger lacerations of the tarsal plate should be reapproximated with partial thickness, buried sutures in these cases to prevent eyelid contour abnormalities. In injuries with a small partial loss of tarsus, attempting primary closure without wound edge modification may lead to wound dehiscence or notching [23]. In these cases, the entire vertical portion of the tarsus needs to be removed corresponding to the width of the defect. Care must be taken to be sure that the tarsal excision is perpendicular to the margin. Vertical skin removal should not cross the upper eyelid crease, because incisions more superior can result in an unsightly scar with contracture and lagophthalmos. If needed, a superior lid crease incision can be made, anterior lamellae undermined, and advanced in a line parallel with the lid crease (Fig. 67.11). This gives a good cosmetic result and minimizes vertical contracture.

Eyelid margin lacerations can be closed in two ways. The older, more traditional method uses nonabsorbable suture, which must be removed postoperatively (Fig. 67.12). A 6-0 double-arm silk is passed through the tarsal plate as a vertical mattress suture, entering and exiting through the meibomian gland orifices 1.5–2 mm from the wound edges in a far-far, near-near fashion. This suture can be left long and used as a traction suture during the repair of the tarsus. The tarsal plate can be closed using 6-0 Vicryl sutures placed through an anterior approach at 90% depth, anterior to the conjunctiva, so as not to rub on the cornea [7]. Additional sutures can be placed at the anterior and posterior lash lines. Multiple sutures may be placed in the upper tarsus and one to two in the lower tarsus. The long arms of the marginal sutures are secured within the knot of an additional single interrupted suture to keep them from abrading the cornea. The remainder of the skin can be closed using 6-0 plain gut sutures. The margin sutures should be removed in 10–14 days. Earlier removal can lead to separation of the wound and notching.

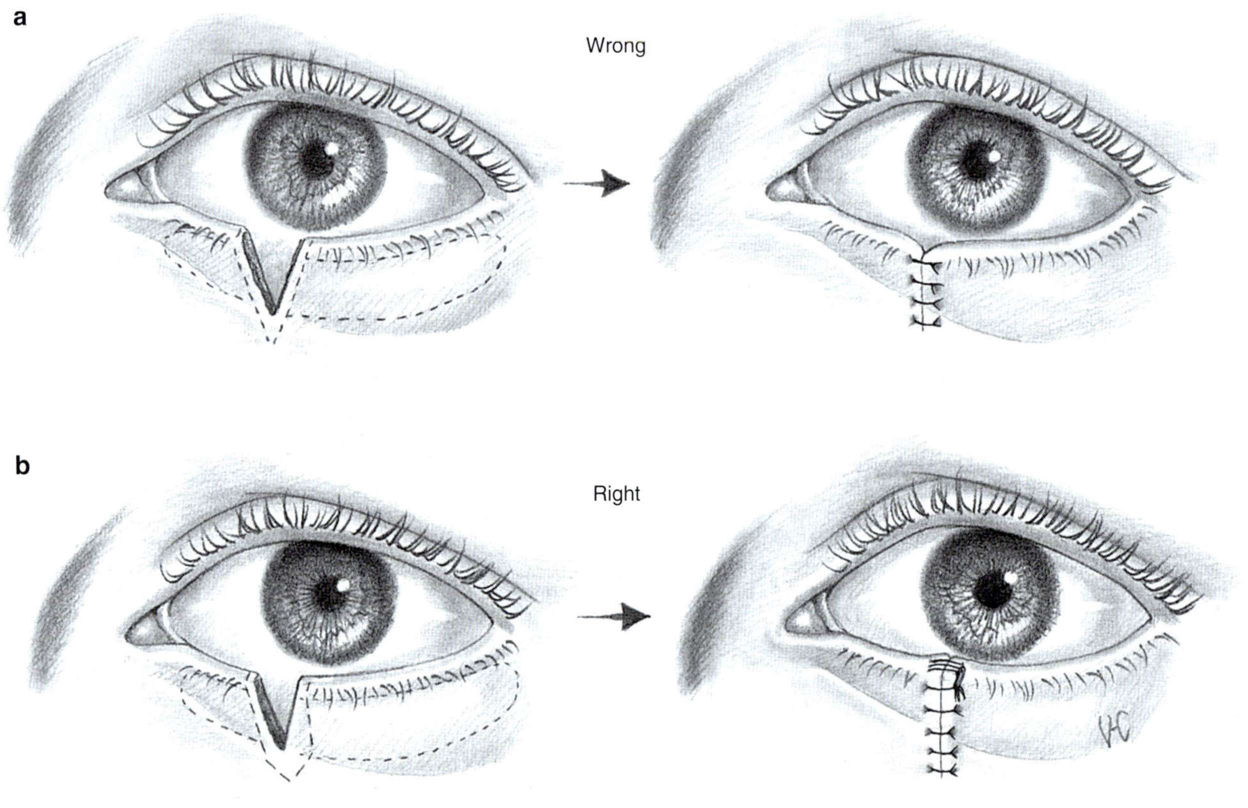

Fig. 67.9 (**a**) Debridement of a lid wound in a V-type configuration can lead to notching and poor lid contour after wound closure. (**b**) Debriding the wound in a line perpendicular to the lid margin gives a smooth lid margin without notching

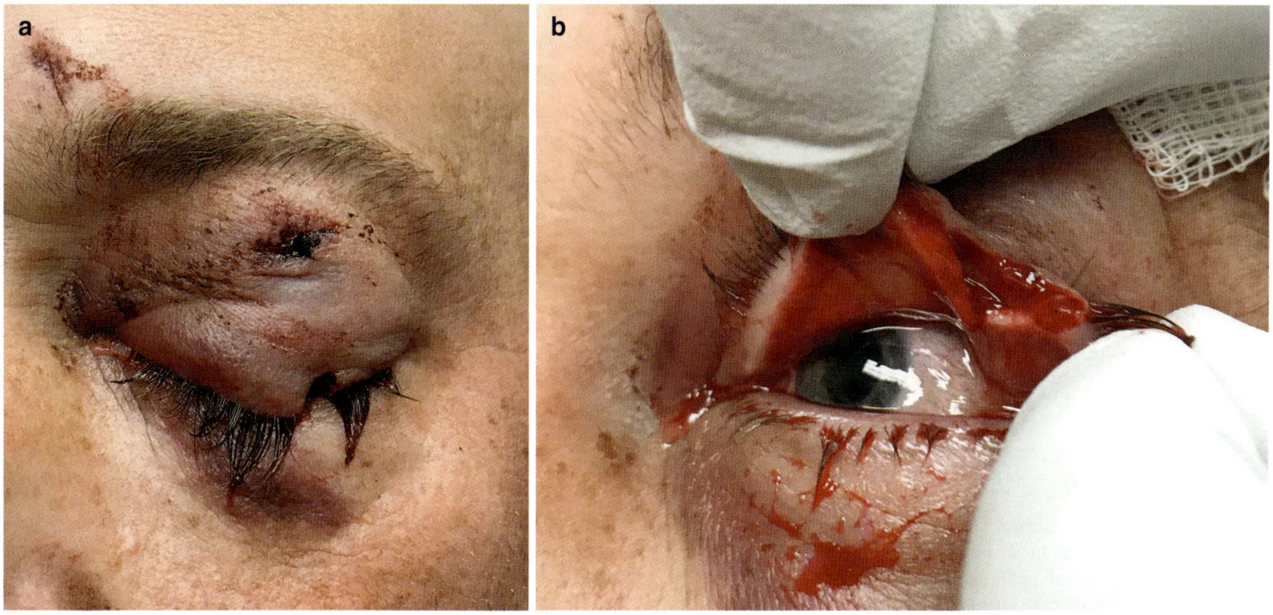

Fig. 67.10 (**a**) *Left upper* lid laceration involving the margin. (**b**) Everted lacerated eyelid showing involvement of the entire upper lid tarsal plate

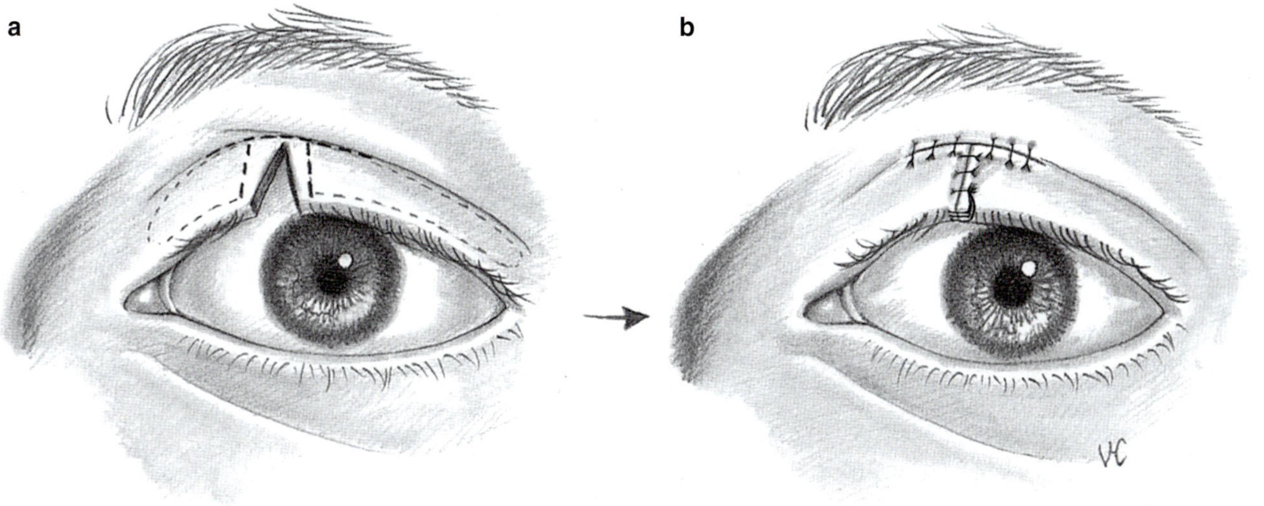

Fig. 67.11 Freshening an upper eyelid injury with excision of the tarsal plant perpendicular to the lid margin allows for improved aesthetic and functional outcomes. (**a**) The anterior and posterior lamella dissection and freshening is stopped at the superior lid crease and superior border of the tarsus, respectively. (**b**) The tarsus is then reapproximated directly. If necessary, horizontal skin flaps can be created by skin incisions in the lid crease to minimize vertical tension and contracture

The alternative way to close an eyelid margin laceration is to use a buried, absorbable suture at the eyelid margin. This avoids the need for postoperative suture removal, which can be difficult in even the most cooperative adult patient, let alone in children, the mentally disabled, or patients with questionable follow-up. For this method, the procedure remains the same except that the 6-0 double-arm silk passed through the tarsal plate is replaced by a 6-0 Vicryl passed through the tarsal plate at the eyelid margin as a buried, vertical mattress suture, entering and exiting through the meibomian gland orifices 1.5–2 mm from the wound edges.

Complex Eyelid Margin Lacerations

In cases of complex eyelid margin lacerations, where there is great tissue loss, undue tension should not be placed on the laceration at the margin as this leads to wound dehiscence and notching. When tissue loss is too great to primarily close the wound, horizontal relaxation of the lid is needed before wound closure. This can be achieved by means of a lateral canthotomy and graded cantholysis of the superior or inferior crux of the lateral canthal tendon (Fig. 67.13). The degree of cantholysis can be fashioned to

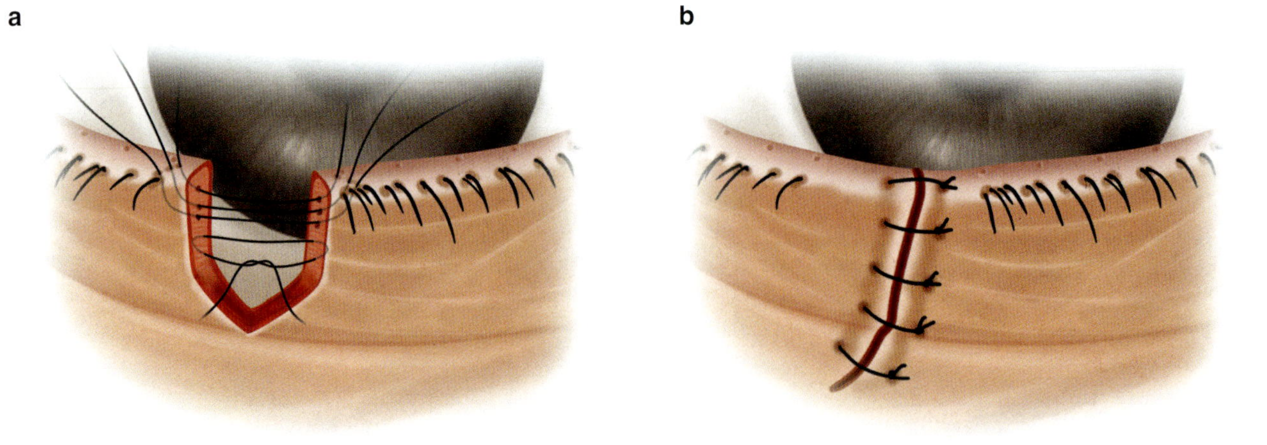

Fig. 67.12 (**a**) Eyelid margin laceration has been freshened in a pentagonal wedge configuration. First, silk suture is passed through the tarsal plate and exits the meibomian gland orifices (A). This suture is then tied, and the remaining tarsal plate is closed using partial-thickness 6-0 Vicryl sutures. Two more 6-0 silk sutures are placed behind the lash line (B) and in front of the lash line (C). (**b**) These marginal silk sutures are left long and incorporated into the first skin suture, and the remaining skin is closed using 6-0 mild chromic sutures. The inferior portion of the wound has been modified in a hockey stick configuration to reduce tissue puckering

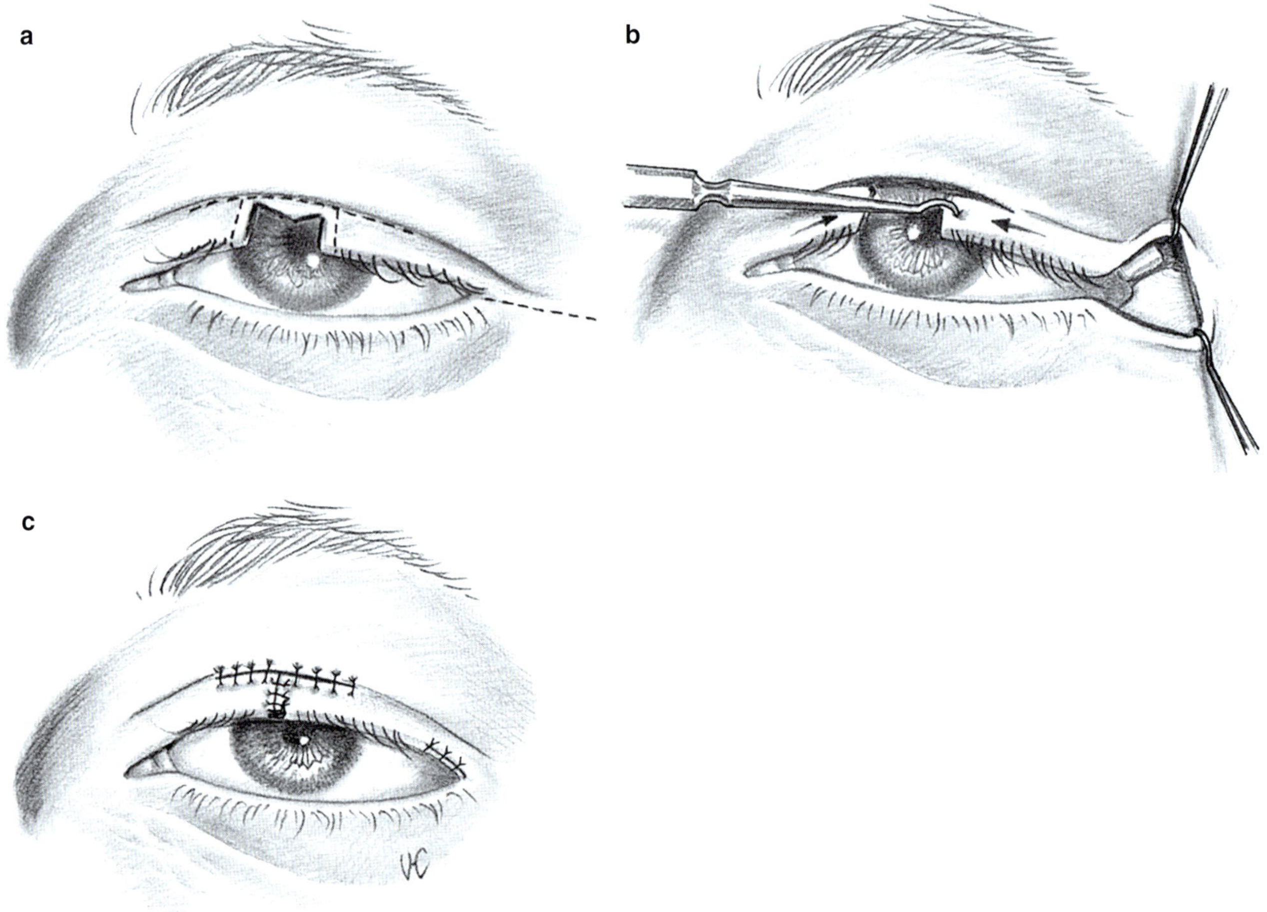

Fig. 67.13 Full-thickness eyelid laceration with moderate loss of tissue. (**a**) Wound is debrided and a lateral canthotomy performed. (**b**) Further relaxation of the upper lid is achieved by a superior cantholysis. (**c**) Wound is primarily closed, and the lateral canthotomy is closed with 5-0 Vicryl suture

the need of the defect. The lateral canthal site is closed with 6-0 plain gut or chromic sutures. A 5-0 Vicryl can be used to fixate orbicularis to lateral rim periosteum and to support the lateral canthal angle. If further anterior lamellar tissue is needed for proper closure of the wound, a modified Tenzel-type curvilinear flap can be raised as an extension of the canthotomy (Fig. 67.14). For upper lid defects, the arc of the circle should be below the lateral canthus, and for lower lid defects, above the canthus [24, 25]. Additionally, when repairing lid defects in this manner, a periosteal flap can be raised from the lateral orbital rim and sutured to the severed end of the lateral canthal tendon (Figure 67.14b) to minimize the development of late retraction and ectropion [13]. When lateral canthal supportive procedures are used, the lateral canthal angle should be placed 2–3 mm higher than its normal anatomic position because gravity and wound contracture will bring the angle into proper anatomic position in a few months. For those defects that have even greater tissue loss, Mustarde-type flaps or lid-sharing procedures can be used [26–28]. These techniques are covered in the chapters dedicated to eyelid reconstruction.

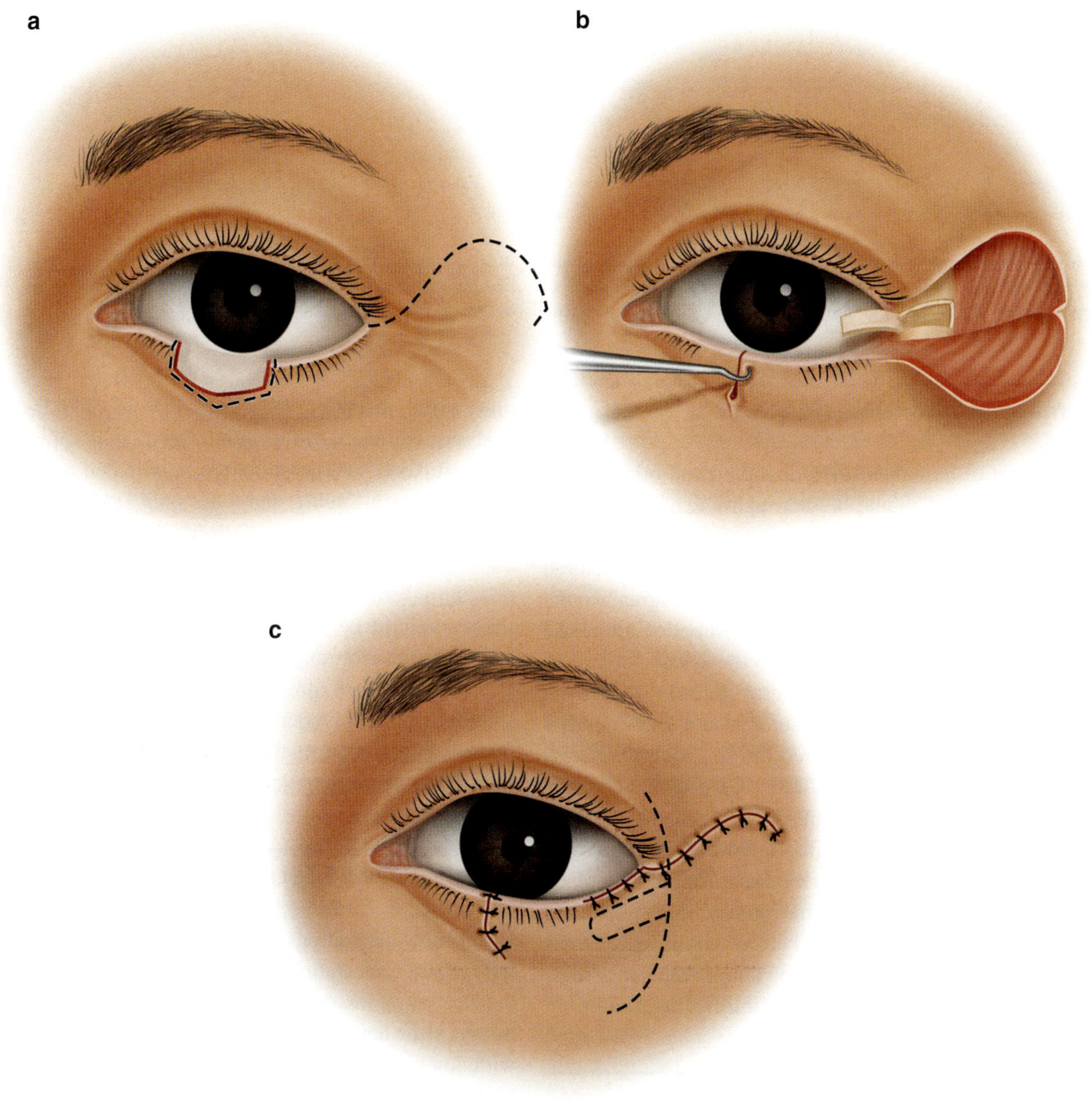

Fig. 67.14 Repair of lower eyelid defect with significant loss of tissue. (**a**) Outline of Tenzel rotational flap needed for closure. (**b**) Tenzel flap is elevated, and cantholysis is performed. Dotted line shows position of periosteal flap to be elevated. (**c**) Periosteal flap is sutured to lateral border of tarsal plate after the wound has been closed. Tenzel flap is rotated into position and closed

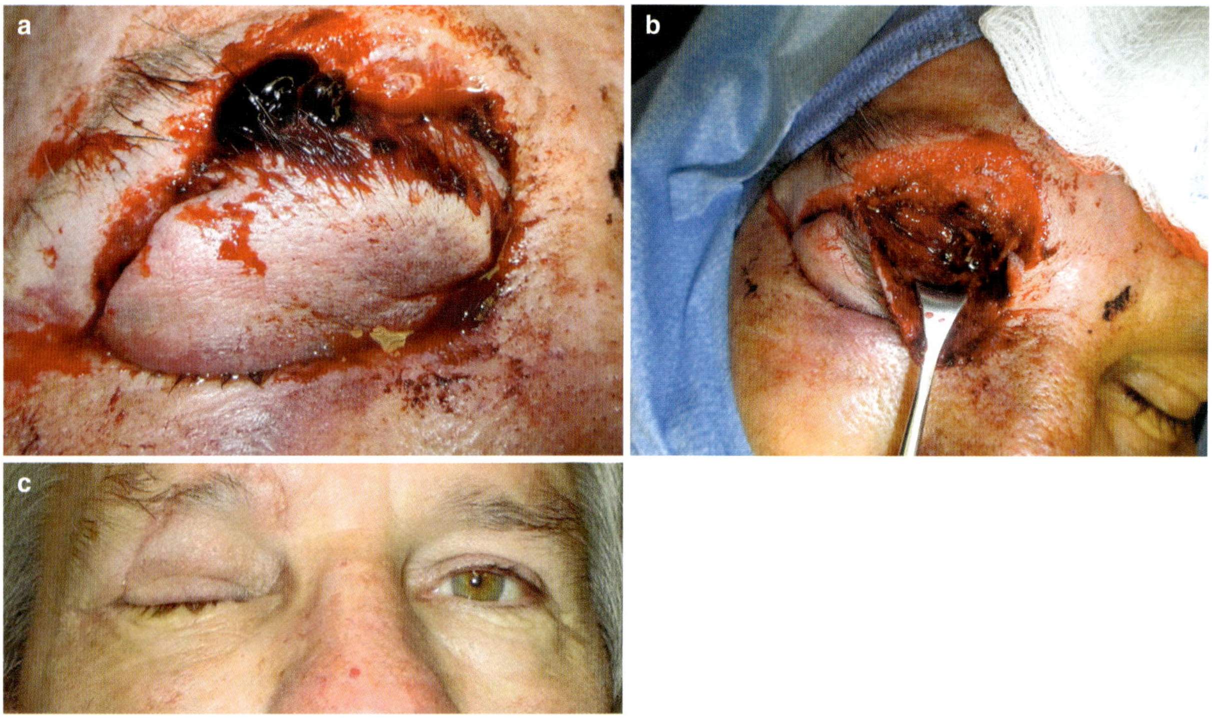

Fig. 67.15 (**a**) Patient suffered a laceration to the right upper lid and brow with complete ptosis. Due to the depth, the patient was taken to the operating room for exploration (**b**), showing a degloving injury with involvement of the levator aponeurosis. (**c**) Postoperatively, the patient had traumatic ptosis of the right upper lid. (Photos courtesy of Javier Servat, M.D.)

Traumatic Levator Dehiscence

If the septum of the upper lid is disrupted and orbital fat is exposed, the wound should be thoroughly explored and the levator complex identified to rule out damage (Fig. 67.15a). Injury to the levator aponeurosis or muscle should be repaired at the time of the primary wound closure. The original wound may need to be extended or a separate superior lid crease incision made to adequately explore the levator complex. Traumatic dehiscence of the levator muscle should be repaired with 5-0 nonabsorbable sutures such as Prolene. A detached levator should be sutured to the tarsal plate at its normal attachment level (Fig. 67.15b). Care should be taken not to extend these sutures in a full-thickness manner through the conjunctiva to avoid rubbing against the cornea. The levator muscle may also be dehisced in cases of blunt trauma. Patients with traumatic ptosis after blunt trauma should be observed for at least 6 months before definitive repair is attempted (Fig. 67.15c). Spontaneous improvement in levator function and lid height may occur during that time.

Secondary Repair

A wound should be closed as soon as possible. However, a delay in wound closure may be appropriate for a number of reasons. If the patient has life-threatening injuries or is otherwise unstable, these should be addressed first. Likewise, an open globe should be treated before soft tissue is repaired. If the patient is intoxicated or uncooperative, treatment delay may be indicated. If immediate wound repair cannot be performed, one can safely wait 24–48 h without an increase in the complication rate or a poor long-term outcome. Until surgery can be performed, tissues should be repositioned into as near their normal anatomic position as possible, topical antibiotic ointment applied, and a light dressing placed. Use of oral antibiotics should also be considered. At the time of surgery, debriding early granulation tissue from wound edges prior to repair will decrease risk of dehiscence.

Canalicular and Lacrimal System Trauma

Canalicular lacerations are a commonly missed adnexal injury. These lacerations may be caused by direct trauma to the canthal region or indirectly by avulsive forces caused by trauma elsewhere in the orbit (Fig. 67.16). They are common with dog bites to the midface. The diagnosis of a canalicular laceration is made by either direct visualization of the cut canaliculus or by probing of the canaliculus.

In the past, it was controversial as to whether monocanalicular lacerations should be repaired as some authors believe that upper canalicular obstruction seldom leads to epiphora.

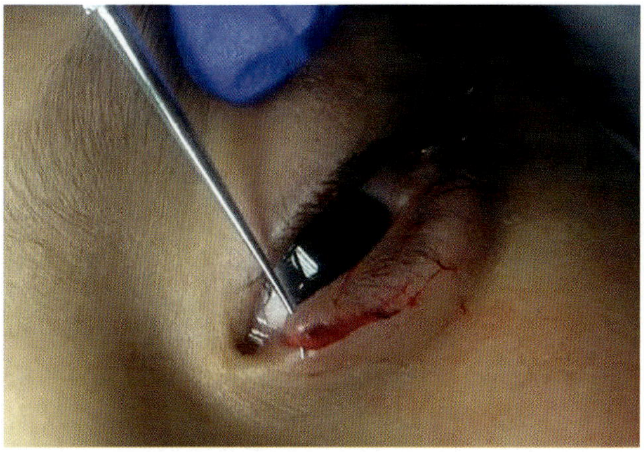

Fig. 67.16 Canalicular involving full-thickness laceration of the left lower lid. Note the punctal dilator exposing the laceration within the transverse canaliculus. (Photo courtesy of Dr. Anne Barmettler)

However, early, primary repair of canalicular trauma is significantly easier and has better outcomes than late repair. Primary repair of any canalicular laceration is thus recommended, ideally occurring within 48 to 72 hours, but achievable within 5 to 7 days.

The most important part of the canalicular repair is placement of a stent across the transected portion of severed canaliculus [29–31]. After the stent has been placed, two 7-0 Vicryl sutures are placed anteriorly and posteriorly through the adventitia of the severed canaliculus. These 7-0 sutures should be tagged and not tied until the first lid margin suture is placed (Fig. 67.17). If the canthal tendon has been severed, it should be repaired before the canalicular sutures are tied. The type of stent to be used will decide the type of anesthesia. For example, if planning to use a self-securing monocanalicular stent, like the Mini Monoka (FCI Ophthalmics, Pembroke, MA), this can be done under local anesthesia in the cooperative patient (Fig. 67.18) [32–34]. If planning on using a bicanalicular stent, such as the Crawford tube (FCI Ophthalmics, Pembroke, MA), general anesthesia will be ideal to allow for retrieval of the tube within the nose. In this case, prior to prepping and draping, the nostril can be packed with oxymetazoline-soaked cotton pledgets to decrease intranasal swelling and bleeding. After the wound has been approximated, the Silastic stent is tied with a simple square knot in the nose. There should be no tension at the puncta.

The stent is left in place for 3–6 months. If the lid laceration involves the punctum, the canaliculus can merely be marsupialized or a monocanalicular, self-retaining silicone stent can be placed to prevent stenosis. Occasionally it is difficult to locate the transected medial edge of the lacerated canaliculus. Fluorescein-dyed normal saline or viscoelastic material can be injected into the intact canaliculus with egress from the previously hidden canalicular opening. Methylene blue should be avoided because it stains all the

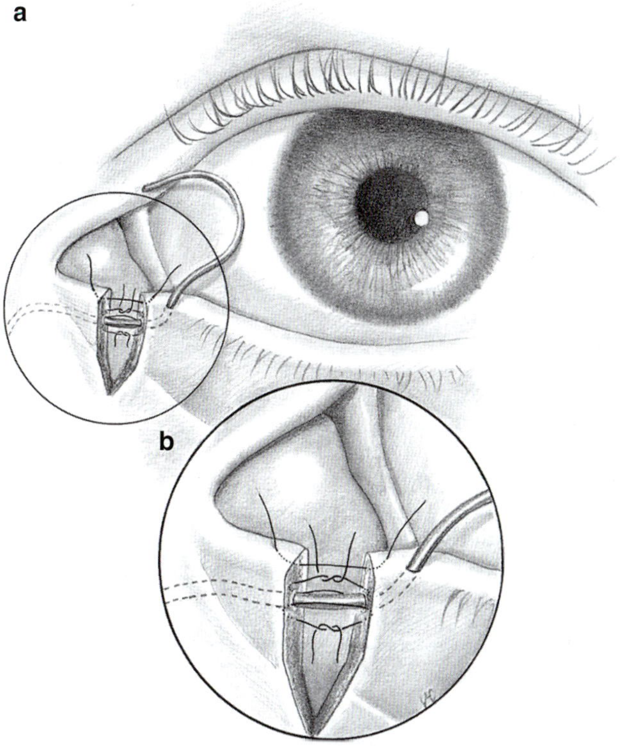

Fig. 67.17 Repair of transected canaliculus. The canaliculus is intubated with a silastic stent. Vicryl sutures (7-0) are placed both anteriorly and posteriorly and tied after the first lid margin suture has been placed and tied

tissue and makes identification of the canaliculus difficult. Another method to locate the hidden transected end of a canaliculus is to pool normal saline in the medial canthal area and then inject air through the intact canaliculus. Pigtail probes can be used but with caution and proper technique to avoid iatrogenic trauma to the canalicular system [35].

Management of Dog and Human Bites

There are greater than one million reported animal and human bites per year in the United States [36]. Animal bites and human bites account for approximately 1% of all emergency room visits; dog bites account for 80–90% of these cases. Children are particularly prone to dog bites because they tend to be on the same level as the animal and can inadvertently provoke the animal. Dog bites in children tend to be more severe as the injury occurs most commonly on the head, face, and neck (Fig. 67.19) [37, 38].

As with any other injury, it is important to elicit a complete history regarding the attack including the type of animal involved, vaccination history of the animal (specifically rabies), the mechanism of the injury, and whether or not the attack was provoked. It is especially important to document the patient's tetanus immunization status, drug allergies, and

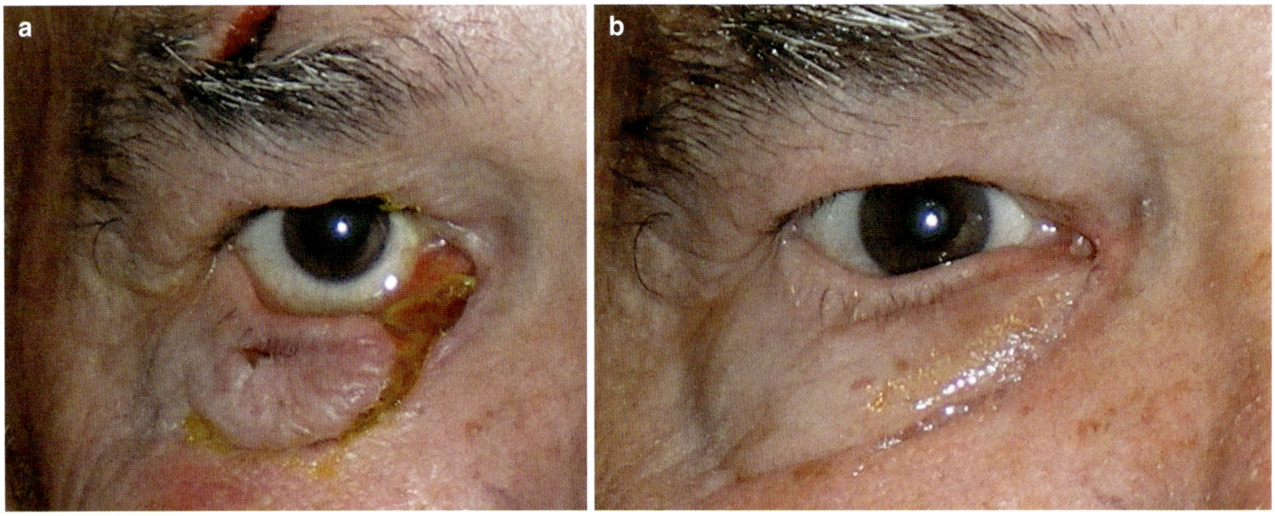

Fig. 67.18 (**a**) Right lower lid full-thickness laceration involving transverse canaliculus, (**b**) postoperative photo of reconstructed right lower lid with direct closure and plastic repair of canaliculus with monocanalicular Silastic intubation

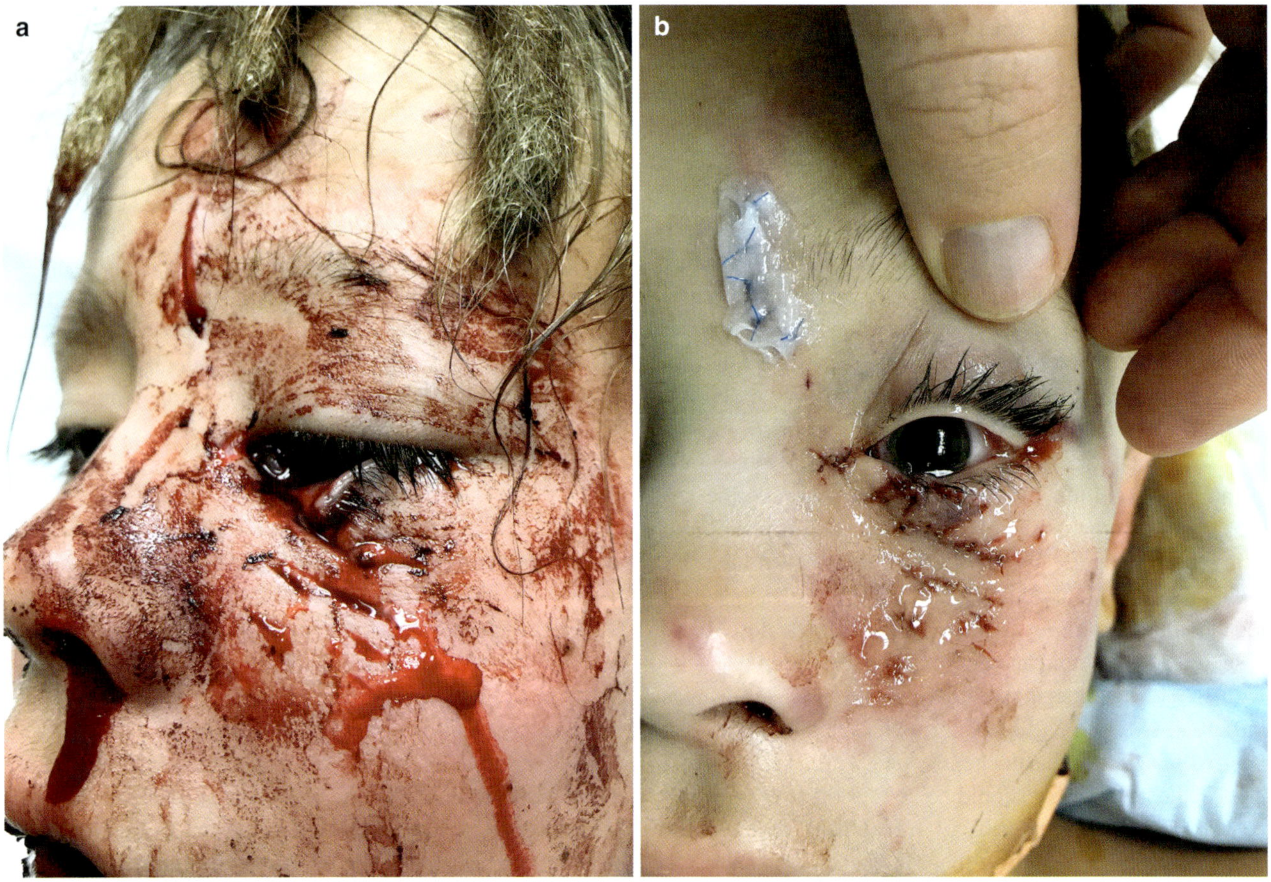

Fig. 67.19 (**a**) 8-year-old boy with non-canalicular full-thickness laceration of the left lower lid due to dog bite. (**b**) Immediate postoperative reconstruction of left lower lid full-thickness laceration and complex facial lacerations

any history of immunosuppression, splenectomy, or chronic disease [36].

The first priority on examination is to assess systemic stability and then the health of the eye. It is important to assess the visual acuity and rule out a ruptured globe or other serious injury to the eye. Once it is established that the eye is healthy and unharmed, the wound should be explored for depth as well as injury to other structures like the canalicular system, levator muscle, and canthal tendons [36]. As discussed previously, occult injury to the canalicular system is common in animal bites and scratches. It is important to inspect the defect and determine if there is missing tissue or if the tissue has just been avulsed and distorted secondary to the trauma and edema. Inspect the depth of the wound carefully for occult foreign bodies [36]. If the patient is in significant discomfort during the exploration, sometimes a mixture of lidocaine with epinephrine and tetracaine gel (LET) can be helpful if applied prior to the examination. Once foreign bodies have been removed or ruled out, it is prudent to irrigate the wound copiously with at least 150 mL of sterile saline through a 19-gauge catheter [39].

There is controversy regarding whether or not to close bite wounds primarily or secondarily due to risk of infection. However, in the face, primary repair of lacerations is almost universally recommended. This gives a better cosmetic result, and the excellent blood supply of the face is thought to decrease the incidence of infection here [37]. Care should be taken to preserve as much tissue as possible and minimize debridement [40].

That being said, the most common complication of bites is infection [32]. Two to five percent of dog bite wounds become infected [36]. Risk factors for bite infection include location on the face or scalp of an infant, puncture wounds, crush injury, treatment delay greater than 12 h, patient age greater than 50 years, immunosuppression, diabetes mellitus, chronic alcoholism, and vascular insufficiency [38].

Infections related to bite wounds are typically polymicrobial in nature, reflecting the abundant oral flora (aerobic and anaerobic) of the biter as well as skin flora of the victim [36]. The most common organisms cultured from infected dog bite wounds include *Pasteurella multocida*, *Pasteurella canis*, *Streptococci* sp., *Staphylococci* sp., and anaerobic gram-negative rods [38, 41]. The most common isolates from human bite wounds are *Staphylococcus aureus*, group A beta-hemolytic *Streptococcus*, and *Eikenella corrodens* [36].

The treatment of choice for all patients with a bite injury is amoxicillin-clavulanate, 500 mg po q 8 h. It has excellent coverage of skin flora as well as *Pasteurella* sp. [38]. In patients who are penicillin allergic, a combination of clindamycin and fluoroquinolone is recommended [41]. Indications for admission and IV antibiotics include fever, severe cellulitis, immunocompromise, and patients who have failed outpatient therapy [38].

Rarely, life-threatening sepsis may occur following dog bites contaminated with *Capnocytophaga canimorsus*. Eighty percent of patients who develop this serious infection have a predisposing risk factor, most commonly, asplenia. It is important to think about this potentially fatal pathogen in immunocompromised patients and those with asplenia. The treatment for *C. canimorsus* is IV penicillin G.

There are a few special circumstances for which additional treatment is necessary. Rabies is responsible for 20,000 deaths/year worldwide. There is approximately one case per year in the United States. An untreated person has a 20% chance of contracting the virus. When rabies is suspected, the wound should be irrigated with povidone-iodine as this is associated with a decreased transmission rate. In addition, the patient must receive passive immunization with the human rabies immune globulin (HRIG) as well as active immunization with the human diploid cell vaccine (HDCV) or rabies vaccine adsorbed (RVA). HRIG is administered on day 0 as a single 20 IU/kg dose, half of which is injected intramuscularly and the other half is injected around the site of the exposure. One milliliter of the HDCV/RVA is injected intramuscularly on days 0, 3, 7, 14, and 28. It is important that the intramuscular injection be in the deltoid of adults or the anterolateral thigh of infants. Injection in the gluteal region has been associated with failure [38].

Human immunodeficiency virus (HIV) and hepatitis B are of concern in cases of human bites wounds. The HIV status of the biter should be obtained if possible. If HIV is suspected, the wound should be irrigated with a virucidal agent like 1% povidone-iodine. A baseline HIV test should be obtained for the victim at the time of the injury with a follow-up test 6 months later [38]. In general, HIV prophylaxis is not recommended. Hepatitis B titers should be obtained from the victim as well. If the victim does not have hepatitis B antibodies, it is recommended to administer both the hepatitis B immunoglobulin and the HBV vaccination [36].

Gunshot Wounds of the Orbit

A firearm is now estimated to exist in a third of all US households [42]. Two-thirds of these weapons are loaded and stored within reach of children. This results in 150,000–500,000 missile injuries and 40,000–50,000 deaths annually [43]; this is a public safety concern.

Understanding the type of firearm and missile allows for velocity of the missile to be estimated, which guides diagnostic and management decisions. Damage from a gunshot wound is from the kinetic energy (KE) or energy due to a motion of a bullet penetrating tissue and/or bone. The kinetic energy of a moving object is a function of its mass and its velocity: $KE = 1/2\ mv^2$. Looking at the formula, it can be seen that increasing a mass only results in a linear increase in energy; however, increasing the velocity results in an increase in energy to the second power. Thus, higher missile velocities increase the rate of kinetic energy dissipation at impact, causing greater damage. On impact, these high-velocity bullets dissipate their kinetic energy into other forms of energy, i.e., high, vibration, and mechanic and vacuum forces, all of which can damage tissue. At very high velocities, the bullet is more likely to fragment, leading to greater tissue destruction (Table 67.1) to [44–46].

There are two types of firearm categories, non-powdered (BB and pellet) guns and powdered guns (0.38 Special and 0.357 Magnum). Non-powdered guns, like BB and pellet guns, use compressed air or gas to propel steel balls, lead, or plastic pellets. BBs are made of steel with copper or zinc plating, measuring 4.5 mm in diameter. Pellets can be made of lead or steel-tipped plastic and are generally 4.5 mm in diameter. Although most BB and pellet guns fire low-velocity missiles (muzzle velocity of less than 1000 ft./s), they are still fast enough to penetrate the cranium, abdomen, thorax, and paranasal sinuses (Fig. 67.20). Approximately 80% of these weapons have muzzle velocities greater than 350 ft./s, and 50% have velocities of 500–930 ft./s. A pellet velocity of only 150 ft./s is necessary to penetrate human skin and 200 ft./s to penetrate bone [47].

The other category of firearm is the powdered guns. Powdered bullet wounds can also be classified as either low-velocity or high-velocity wounds with 2000 ft./s being the cutoff in the American literature. It takes a speed of about 125–230 ft./s to penetrate skin and bone [48].

Missile velocities translate to differences in both amount and type of wounding. Entrance wounds are typically oval to circular in shape and have a punched-out, cleaned appearance with a surrounding zone of reddish damaged skin. Exit wounds can appear stellate, slit-like, crescentic, circular, or

Table 67.1 Mass and velocity of some common missiles

Velocity		
Weapon	Mass/grains	Meters/feet/second
12 Gauge	Variable	412.7/1354
0.22	49	323.1/1150
0.38 Special	158	257.6/755
0.38 Sp.H.V.	110	345.6/1020
0.357 Magnum	158	395.6/1235
0.45	225	259.1/900
M-16	55	990.6/3250
0.308 Winchester	150	859.5/2820
Daisy air rifles		
Spring	5.4 gr steel	76.2–91.4/250–300
Pneumatic	5.4 gr steel	91.4–228.6/300–750
CO_2 gun	7.7 gr lead	121.9/400

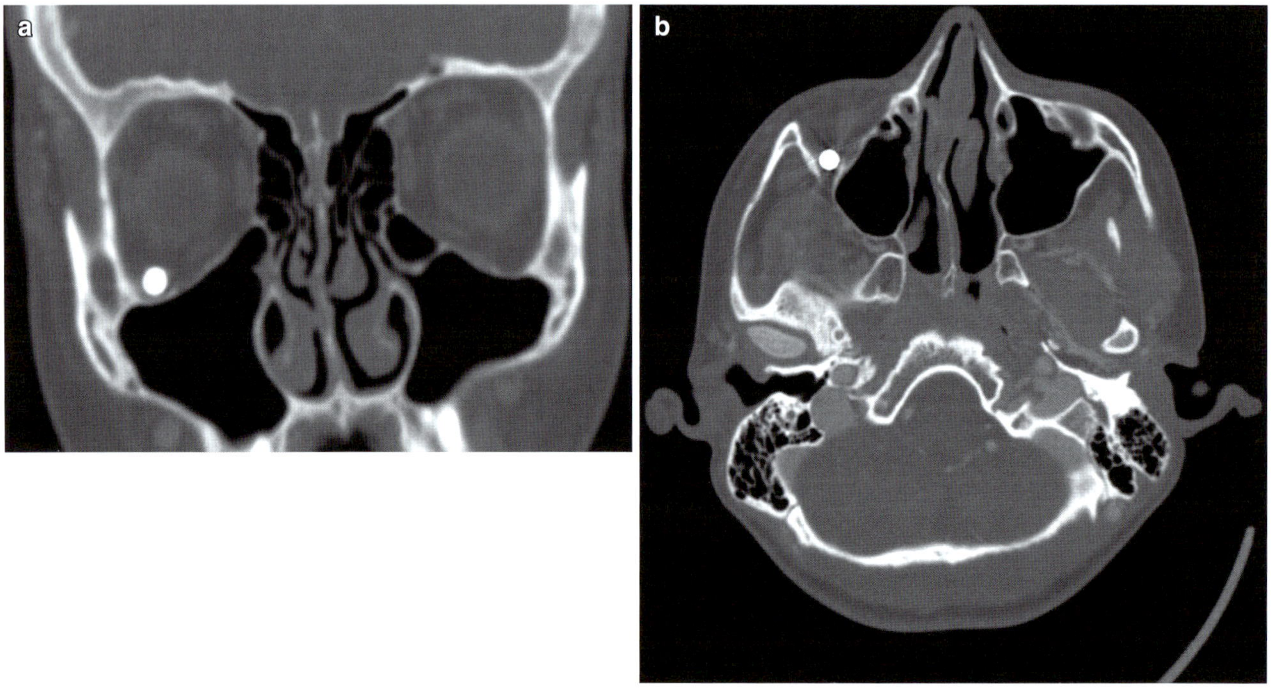

Fig. 67.20 14-year-old boy following BB penetrating of right lower lid skin; (**a**) coronal CT of the orbit with metallic foreign body in inferior temporal orbit; (**b**) axial CT of the same patient

completely irregular. With greater velocities, bullet deformation and tumbling within the body can result in exit wounds becoming larger and more irregular than entrance wounds.

In general, ocular gunshot injuries can be classified as either contusive or penetrating-perforating injuries. Contusive injuries result from the cavitation effect, where rapid changes in pressure lead to the formation of small vapor-filled cavities, which collapse when subjected to higher pressures. This causes shock waves and injuries like hemorrhage (hyphema, choroidal, vitreous, retina, and retrobulbar hemorrhage), angle recession iridocyclodialysis, concussive cataracts, lens dislocation, retinitis sclopetaria, retinal edema, retinal detachment, and nerve avulsion. Penetrating injuries can occur anywhere within the globe [49].

Late effects from severe orbitocranial trauma secondary to gunshot wounds consist of orbital hematomas, orbital cellulitis and abscess, meningitis, brain abscess, meningoencephaloceles, carotid cavernous fistula, cerebrospinal fluid rhinorrhea, proptosis, endophthalmitis, diplopia, and blindness [49].

The management of gunshot wounds to the orbit requires an interdisciplinary approach. As usual, airway and cardiopulmonary status is of prime consideration. Hemorrhage and shock should be controlled, and complete neurologic examination to rule out intracranial and spinal cord injuries should precede the ophthalmic examination. Every attempt should be made to obtain an accurate history with emphasis on type and mechanism of injury.

A complete orbital eyelid and ophthalmic examination is essential. In general, blunt or penetrating injuries associated with adnexal trauma presenting with decreased visual acuity, the presence of a relative afferent pupillary defect, absence of a red reflex, and presence of a retinal detachment are associated with a significantly higher rate of very poor vision and possible evisceration or enucleation. The examination is complemented by orbital ultrasound and CT and MRI scans of the head and orbit. Ultrasound can aid in detecting posterior ocular lesions such as a foreign body and retinal detachment that may have been obscured by anterior segment disruption and hyphema. Axial and coronal CT scanning is crucial in evaluating gunshot wounds. It provides visualization of soft tissue, bone structures, and foreign bodies. A CT angiogram is valuable for suspected vascular injuries such as carotid cavernous fistula or dural arteriovenous malformations.

In the initial assessment of trauma, CT should be the imagining modality of choice over MRI. Acquisition time for CT is dramatically shorter and shows excellent definition of bone and location of most foreign bodies. MRI requires significantly longer acquisition time and has poor bone definition. MRI may also cause movement of retained magnetic foreign bodies, potentially causing damage to the adjacent brain and intraocular structures. MRI does, however, provide better resolution for detecting optic nerve lacerations and avulsions. If wood is suspected, ultrasound is the best modality with the foreign body appearing hyperechoic with posterior shadowing [50].

Operative management depends on the type of injury and its mechanism. Contrary to popular belief, bullets are not sterilized on discharge. Furthermore, shotgun wadding (placement of a disc of material to seal gas or powder behind a projectile) has been associated with a high degree of wound contamination [43]. In addition, with high-velocity wounds, a vacuum is formed which may pull foreign material into the wound causing further wound contamination. Most low-velocity gunshot wounds may be safely treated nonoperatively on an outpatient basis with simple local wound care, consisting of superficial irrigation and careful cleaning followed by a dressing with or without systemic antibiotics. Higher-velocity gunshot wounds may be managed by debridement of the entrance and exit wound followed by copious irrigation with antibiotics as well as intravenous and systemic antibiotics with primary closure. Tetanus prophylaxis or a reinforcing booster shot should be administered as needed. Should the globe be ruptured, repair can occur once the patient is neurologically stable. Intravitreal antibiotics with vitrectomy can be considered to maximize an involved, but functioning globe. Careful follow-up for potential complications such as endophthalmitis, recurrence of hyphema, ocular siderosis, and sympathetic ophthalmia is most important.

If the patient is neurologically unstable, delayed primary closure is anticipated. The added delay may help the surgeon, patient, and family decide, depending on the remaining visual prognosis, whether to repair a globe perforation site surgically or to primarily eviscerate or enucleate the globe. Evisceration is preferred over enucleation because it leaves the orbital anatomy less disturbed. Sympathetic ophthalmia, although an ever-present threat, is uncommon. If sympathetic ophthalmia is a concern, enucleation should be considered and performed within 2 weeks of injury. Primary evisceration or enucleations should be avoided if possible.

References

1. Kurkinen MV. Sequential appearance of fibronectin and collagen in experimental granulation tissue. Lab Investig. 1980;43:7.
2. Gk G. Wound healing. Facial Plast Surg Clin North Am. 2002;10(2):119–27.
3. Abraham DS. Tumor necrosis factor alpha suppresses the induction of connective tissue growth factor by transforming growth factor-beta in normal and scleroderma fibroblasts. J Biol Chem. 2000;275:15220.
4. Goldman R. Growth factors and chronic wound healing: past, present and future. Adv Skin Wound Care. 2004;17:24.

5. Dulakk J, JĂłzkowicz A. Vascular endothelial growth factor synthesis in vascular smooth muscle cells is enhanced by 7-ketocholesterol and lysophosphatidylcholine independently of their effect on nitric oxide generation. Atherosclerosis. 2001;159:325–32.
6. Pierce GM. Role of platelet-derived growth factor in wound healing. J Cell Biochem. 1991;45:319–27.
7. Forrest L. Current concepts in soft connective tissue wound healing. Br J Surg. 1983;70:133.
8. Sabiston D. Textbook of surgery: the biological basis of modern surgical practice. 15th ed. St. Louis: Saunders; 1997.
9. Brem H. Surg Technol Int. 2003;11:23–31.
10. Committee on Trauma of the American College of Surgeons. Advanced trauma life support course. Chicago: American College of Surgeons; 1984.
11. Goldberg MF, Tessler HH. Occult intraocular perforations from brow and lid lacerations. Arch Ophthalmol. 1971;86:145.
12. Committee on Trauma of the American College of Surgeons: a guide to prophylaxis against tetanus in wound management, 1979 revision. Reprinted from the Bulletin of the American College of Surgeons; 1979.
13. Gonnering RS. Ocular adnexal injury and complications in orbital dog bites. Ophthal Plast Reconstr Surg. 1987;3:231.
14. Herman DC, Bartley GB, Walker RC. The treatment of animal bite injuries of the eye and ocular adnexa. Ophthal Plast Reconstr Surg. 1987;3:237.
15. Schultz RC, McMaster WD. The treatment of dog bite injuries, especially those of the face. Plast Reconstr Surg. 1972;49:494.
16. Shannon GM. The treatment of dog bite injuries of the eyelids and adnexa. Ophthalmic Surg. 1975;6:41.
17. Morris RE, Miller GW. Preoperative management of the patient with a full stomach. In: Giesecke AM, editor. Clinical anesthesia: anesthesia for the surgery of trauma. Philadelphia: FA Davis; 1976.
18. Garber PF, MacDonald D, Beyer-Machule CK. Management of trauma to the eyelids. In: Della Roca RC, Nesi FA, Lisman RD, editors. Ophthalmic plastic and reconstructive surgery, vol. I. St. Louis: CV Mosby; 1987.
19. Hildreth HR, Silver B. Sensory block of the upper eyelid. Arch Ophthalmol. 1967;77:230.
20. Shore JW, Rubin PA, Bilyk JR. Repair of telecanthus by anterior fixation of cantilevered miniplates. Ophthalmology. 1992;99:1133.
21. Leone CR. Lateral canthal reconstruction. Ophthalmology. 1987;94:238.
22. Ramecki JM, Nesi FA, Spoor TC. Management of injuries to the ocular adnexa. In: Spoor TC, Nesi FA, editors. Management of ocular, orbital, and adnexal trauma. New York: Raven; 1988.
23. Divine RD, Anderson RL. Techniques in eyelid wound closure. Ophthalmic Surg. 1982;13:283.
24. Tenzel RR. Reconstruction of the central one-half of an eyelid. Arch Ophthalmol. 1975;93:125.
25. Tenzel RR, Stewart WB. Eyelid reconstruction by the semicircle flap technique. Ophthalmology. 1978;85:1164.
26. Hughes WL. New method for rebuilding lower lid. Arch Ophthalmol. 1937;17:1008.
27. Hughes WL. Reconstructive surgery of the eyelids. 2nd ed. CV Mosby: St. Louis; 1954.
28. Mustarde JC. Repair and reconstruction in the orbital region. Edinburgh: Churchill Livingstone; 1971, chaps. 7–8.
29. Hawes MJ, Segrest DR. Effectiveness of bicanalicular silicone intubation in the repair of canalicular lacerations. Ophthal Plast Reconstr Surg. 1985;1:85.
30. Crawford JS. Intubation of obstructions in the lacrimal system. Can J Ophthalmol. 1977;12:289.
31. Crawford JS. Lacrimal intubation set with suture in the lumen. Ophthal Plast Reconstr Surg. 1988;4:249.
32. Gonnering RS. Simplified monocanalicular silicone intubation. Arch Ophthalmol. 1987;105:1024.
33. Long JA. A method of monocanalicular silicone intubation. Ophthalmic Surg. 1988;19:204.
34. Patrinely JR, Anderson RL. Monocanalicular silicone intubation. Arch Ophthalmol. 1988;106:579.
35. Saunders PH, Shannon CM, Flanagan J. The effectiveness of pigtail probe method of repairing canalicular lacerations. Ophthalmic Surg. 1978;9:33.
36. Brook I. Management of human and animal bite wound infection: an overview. Curr Infect Dis Rep. 2009;11:389–95.
37. Javaid M, Feldberg L, Gipson M. Primary repair of dog bites to the face: 40 cases. J R Soc Med. 1998;91:414–8.
38. Griego RD, Rosen T, Orengo IF, Wolf JE. Dog, cat, and human bites: a review. J Am Acad Dermatol. 1995;33:1019–29.
39. Graham WP III, Calabretta AM, Miller SH. Dog bites. Am Fam Physician. 1977;15:132–7.
40. Nerad JA. Techniques in ophthalmic plastic surgery. 1st ed. Philadelphia: Saunders Elsevier; 2010.
41. Talan DA, Citron DM, Abrahamian FM, Moran GJ, Goldstein EJ. Bacteriologic analysis of infected dog and cat bites. N Engl J Med. 1999;340(2):85–92.
42. Parker K, Horowitz JM, Igielnik R, Oliphant JB, Brown A. The demographics of gun ownership. https://pewsocialtrends.org/2017/06/22/the-demographics-of-gun-ownership/. Accessed 26 Apr 2019.
43. Bartlett CS, Helfet DL, et al. Ballistics and gunshot wounds: effects on musculoskeletal tissues. J Am Acad Orthop Surg. 2000;8(1):21–36.
44. Scott RF, editor. The shooter's bible. South Hackensack: Stoeger; 1983. p. 479–500.
45. Air Gun, From Wikipedia, https://en.wikipedia.org/wiki/Air_gun.
46. Great Lakes sports fishing council. www.great-lakes.org/reviews/review-09-04–06.html.
47. Chu A, Levine MR. Gunshot wounds of the eye and orbit. Ophthalmic Surg. 1989;20(10):729.
48. DiMaio VJ. Penetration and perforation of skin by bullets and missiles. A review of the literature. Am J Forensic Med Pathol. 1981;6(2):107–10.
49. Bower GW, Rossiter ND. Management of gunshot wounds of the limbs. Br Edit Soc Bone Joint Surg. 1997;79B(6):1031–6.
50. Jarraya M, Hayashi D, de Villiers RV, Roemer FW. Multimodality imaging of foreign bodies of the musculoskeletal system. Musculoskeletal Imaging. 2013;203(1):W92–W102.

Adnexal Burns

68

Wesley Lawrence Brundridge

Introduction

Ocular burns can be divided into those caused by thermal, chemical, or electrical current tissue injury. Thermal burns are typically a result of flame injuries and cause deeper burns that result in ocular sequelae [1]. Chemical burns are an ophthalmic emergency and require prompt management. Chemical burns can be categorized as alkali or acidic. Chemical burns may result in extensive long-term damage to the ocular surface and limbal stem cells. Limbal stem cell deficiency may lead to severely dry eyes, corneal neovascularization, corneal opacity, and conjunctivalization of the cornea [2]. Acidic chemical burns will precipitate proteins, thus creating a barrier to prevent deeper penetration. Alkali burns, however, can rapidly penetrate the cornea, reacting with cellular lipids to form soaps. The alkaline agents essentially dissolve the cell membranes [3]. The immediate phase begins the moment the chemical agent comes into contact with the surface. Prompt irrigation and removal of any particulate matter is the most important intervention for chemical burns [2]. The acute, intermediate, and chronic management of ocular chemical burns is extensive and beyond the scope of this chapter. Burns caused by an electrical current are unique because the underlying tissue destructions may be much more extensive than how superficial skin injury appears. Thus, a high suspicion for deep injury is required on all electrical burns [3].

Most ocular burns are thermal due to flame injuries. Ocular involvement in facial burns is not uncommon, with rates ranging from 7.5 to 36% in those admitted with burn injuries [4]. The loss of an eye primarily from a thermal injury is rare due to the protective mechanisms of the eye which include the blink reflex, Bell's phenomenon, and protective movements of the head and arms to avoid the source of a burn. Acute globe injury may result due to an absence of these protective reflexes in an obtunded patient or when reflexes are consciously suppressed [5]. In patients admitted to burn units, ocular injuries such as conjunctival burns, corneal abrasions, corneal burns, corneal perforations, and cataracts are far less common than eyelid burns. Thermal burn injury results in the release of multiple inflammatory mediators that result in vasodilation, pain, and edema. The exudation and edema from the wound are greatest in the first 24 hours, but the edema can take many days to resolve [1, 3]. The extent and depth of the burn depends on the intensity and duration of the heat exposure. Work by Moritz and Henrique [6] on time-temperature exposure relationship to depth of injury showed that as exposure temperature increases, time to produce a burn decreases. At temperatures below 44 C, a burn is unlikely to occur, even if there is exposure for several hours. However, an exposure for more than one second at 60 C (140 F) will cause epidermal sloughing (partial-thickness burn). A temperature greater than 70 C (158) will cause dermal protein denaturation which will produce full-thickness burns [1, 5].

Ocular burn patterns are rarely uniform and depend on the time exposure and temperature of exposure. The burn is dynamic as demonstrated by Jackson's burn wound model [7]. The center of the injury is referred to as the "zone of coagulation," where tissue is destroyed and no longer viable. This gives a characteristic white, leathery appearance due to coagulation necrosis with no blood flow. The area just peripheral to the center is the "zone of stasis," which temporarily has decreased vascularization but can recover barring further injury to insults such as infection, ischemia, or drying of the wound. This zone can be further divided into the superficial zone and a deeper zone. The superficial zone shows early stasis due to greater injury and becomes ischemic within 2 hours due to vasoconstriction and platelet aggregation. The deeper zone shows delayed stasis with ischemia beginning 4–24 hours after the injury. The third and outermost "zone of hyperemia" is the site of minimal cell involvement and undergoes early spontaneous recovery.

W. L. Brundridge (✉)
Aesthetic, Facial and Oculoplastic Surgery, San Antonio, TX, USA

J. J. Servat et al. (eds.), *Smith and Nesi's Ophthalmic Plastic and Reconstructive Surgery*,
https://doi.org/10.1007/978-3-030-41720-8_68

The vascular structures remain intact, and the area blanches with pressure. In this zone, there is no cell death due to prominent vasodilation which brings nutrients needed to support the zone of stasis and continue the inflammation process. The necrotic tissue from a burn is known as an eschar and is a good substrate for microorganisms. If the eschar is left untreated, it can become colonized, contaminated, and eventually infected [1, 3].

Classification of Thermal Eyelid Burns

Eyelid burns are classified like other burn injuries as first, second, or third. In 1994, however, to better describe their pathology, eyelid burns were classified as superficial, partial-thickness, and full-thickness [8]. In recent years, this has been further classified as epidermal, superficial partial-thickness, deep partial-thickness, full-thickness, and deep burns. Epidermal burns (first-degree) involve the epidermis only, and blistering is not common. Pain is due to local vasodilator prostaglandins, and healing is usually complete in 1 week. These are typically caused by sunburn, ultraviolet ray exposure, and flash burns [1, 3].

Partial-thickness burns (second degree) involve the dermis and epidermis and are typically caused by immersion scalds or flame injury. This area corresponds to the zone of stasis in Jackson's model. The skin often shrinks and blisters in partial-thickness burns. These burns are typically divided into superficial partial-thickness and deep partial-thickness. Superficial partial-thickness burns expose the superficial nerves of the dermis which make them painful. These burns will take approximately 2 weeks to regenerate the epidermis from keratinocytes within sweat glands and hair follicles. Thus, the rate of regeneration is partially dependent on the density of these structures. The eyelid skin is hairless. Thus, will take longer to heal than typical thicker or hairy skin. Deep partial-thickness burns typically have a pale white or mottled base beneath the blisters. There are few viable skin adnexa for regeneration at this depth, and healing will be slower. The blisters often break open, causing weeping and crusting of serous fluid which often causes contracture and scarring. In the eyelid region, early surgery for contracture and eyelid retraction is often necessary for deep partial-thickness burns [1, 3].

Third-degree burns (full-thickness) are the most serious. These burns involve the entire dermis and part or all of the subcutaneous tissue which destroy all the regenerative elements of Jackson's burn wound model. These burns are typically a result of chemical, electrical, and thermal significant exposure scaled injuries. The result is a dry, leathery skin due to heat coagulation of dermal blood vessels. The burn is typically avascular and white and is painless due to damage to sensory nerves. Healing will only occur from the edges and is associated with significant contracture. Figure 68.1 shows an example of full-thickness burns that caused significant contracture to the lower eyelids. Early excision of the affected tissue with skin grafting is almost always required for these burns. When full-thickness burns are deep enough to destroy underlying muscle, bone, and other vital structures, the result is severe contracture and prolonged disability [1, 3, 5].

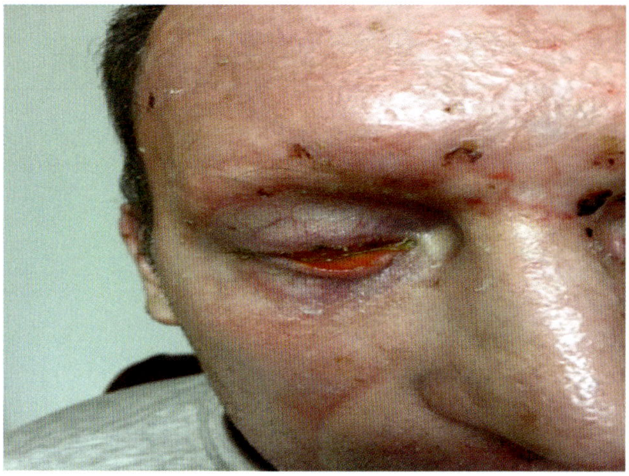

Fig. 68.1 Full-thickness burn with cicatricial ectropion

Evaluation and Acute Treatment

Patients with eyelid burns often have concomitant facial, neck, and upper torso burns. Airway compromise should always be considered. The priority should be to establish and maintain an adequate airway. In addition, these burns are often associated with life-threatening injuries, and immediate evaluation and treatment should follow ATLS and ACLS protocols [3].

Once the patient is stable, it is vital for an ophthalmologist to make an evaluation as soon as possible to assess the extent of the burns and to exclude further damage such as open globe injury and intraocular foreign body. If there is any doubt to the presence of a foreign body, a CT scan should be considered. It is important to evaluate the globe as early as possible because there is often massive swelling of the eyelids due to inflammation, edema, and aggressive fluid resuscitation. One of the most important assessments for an ophthalmologist is the integrity of the corneal surface. Epithelial defects should be evaluated and treated with antibiotics ointment due to risk of secondary bacterial infection [9]. Any damage to the globe or lagophthalmos should be documented [1, 3].

Immediate treatment should start with copious irrigation and debridement of foreign material such as dirt and debris. If the burn is chemical, thorough irrigation should be

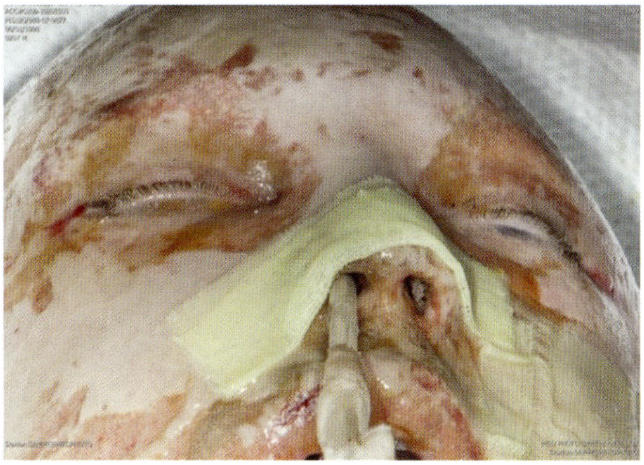

Fig. 68.2 Patient with significant eyelash singing and full-thickness eyelid burns

continued until the pH is near physiologic. Sloughing skin can also be removed gently, and the lids should then be covered with cool, moist bandages. Antibiotic ointment such as bacitracin or erythromycin can be used with bandaging. The depth and extent of burns in the eyelid and facial area should be assessed and photographed when possible. The presence of eyebrow hair and eyelashes should be documented as loss is associated with deep partial-thickness or full-thickness burns (Fig. 68.2). A complete and thorough exam that includes a portable slit lamp is essential as well to examine the conjunctiva, cornea, anterior segment structures, lens, and retina. Partial-thickness burns are associated with contracture and will produce progressive lagophthalmos within the first 2 weeks. Thus, corneal exposure is likely, and the presence or absence of a Bell's phenomenon should be documented. The Bell's phenomenon may be temporarily absent or diminished in a heavily sedated or paralyzed patient. A poor Bell's phenomenon can result in significant corneal exposure. It is important to examine the patient every day or every other day during the first 2 weeks [1, 3, 9].

Patients with significant burns will typically undergo aggressive fluid resuscitation in the first 24 hours after a massive burn. There is increased vascular permeability that leads to migration of water into the interstitium which will decrease the intravascular fluid volume. This necessitates significant replacement or there will be organ-specific hypoperfusion. The larger the burn, the larger the person, the more fluid needed to resuscitate. A popular formula used is the Parkland formula which estimates 4 mL/kg/% burn for the first 24 hours [10]. During this time, there is significant risk or orbital compartment syndrome and elevated IOP. Sullivan et al. [11] reported the occurrence of orbital compartment syndrome with IOP increasing greater than 30 mm Hg and requiring lateral canthotomy and cantholysis to reduce IOP in 5 out of 13 patients with burns greater than 25% TBSA. Thus, it's recommended to obtain IOP readings every 12–24 hours in patients undergoing aggressive fluid resuscitation.

Prophylactic ocular lubrication is a mainstay in all burn patients with a minimum of three applications a day since burn patients typically have reduced tear production, blink reflex, and eyelid mobility. At a minimum, carboxymethyl cellulose sodium 1.0% should be used four times daily with a white petroleum ointment before bedtime. Artificial tears are less effective than ointment, and typically an ointment such as bacitracin or Lacri-Lube is used. For more severe burns, the lubricating ointment may be needed every two hours [1]. In addition, moisture chamber goggles are often used to keep the moisture from evaporating from the surface of the eye. If the moisture chamber is ineffective or the patient is unable to tolerate it, a suture tarsorrhaphy can be placed [3, 5].

It is important to thoroughly assess the lacrimal system. Injuries that involve the medial one third of the lids can lead to both canalicular and punctal stricture. If the lacrimal system is involved, early stenting of the canalicular system is recommended with silicone tubing to prevent cicatrization and future obstruction and epiphora. The tubing is left in place for 3–9 months, until the cicatrizing changes have stopped or until the patient is unable to tolerate the tubes once healing has occurred. Monocanalicular intubation may be more beneficial than a bicanalicular tube since bicanalicular systems may cause cheese wiring of the canaliculi [3, 11, 12] (Figs. 68.3 and 68.4).

Tarsorrhaphy

In the acute setting, marked lid swelling can act as an auto tarsorrhaphy and can help protect the globe. As the swelling decreases, lagophthalmos may develop, with resultant exposure of the cornea. A temporary tarsorrhaphy suture can be placed to decrease lagophthalmos. This is created by passing a double-armed 5-0 suture through a bolster (small piece of foam, rubber, or plastic) and through the lower lid just inferior to the lashes. The needles are passed out through the lower lid gray line and into the upper lid line. The sutures are then passed out the upper lid skin above the lashes and through another bolster before the sutures are tied (Figs. 68.5 and 68.6). These sutures can then be tied into a slipknot to facilitate periodic examinations of the ocular surface. The bolsters are important to reduce the incidence of cheese wiring. It is important to note that temporary tarsorrhaphy will not prevent cicatricial changes. This type of tarsorrhaphy lasts approximately 2 weeks [1, 3, 13]. A newer modified forehead hitch technique was described recently by Lymperopoulos et al. [14]. This technique involves a lateral tarsorrhaphy with a horizontal mattress stitch being placed in each eyelid between and including the anterior lamella of the

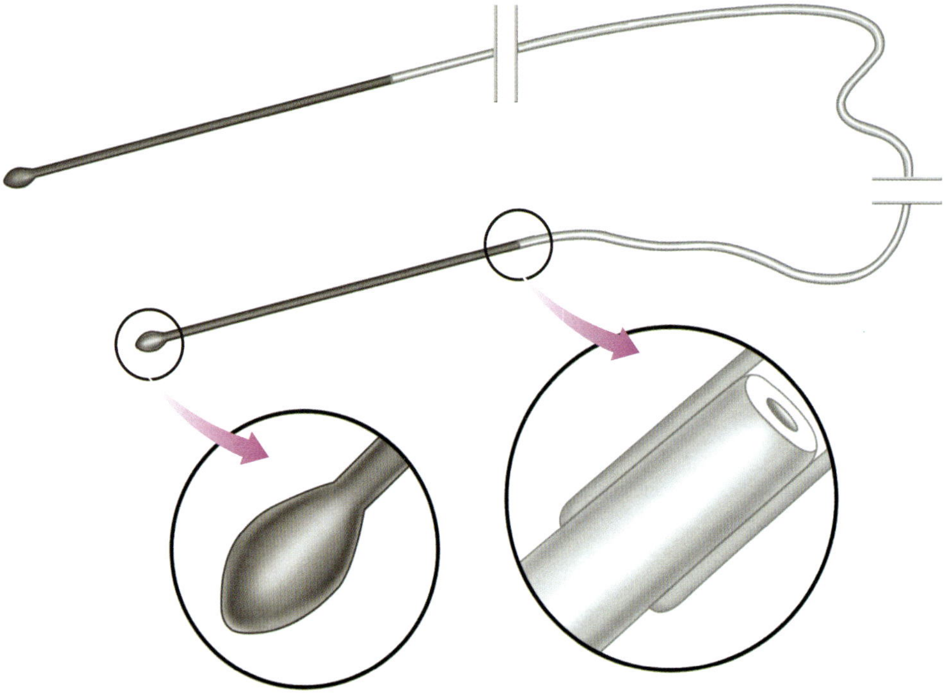

Fig. 68.3 Crawford stents [11]

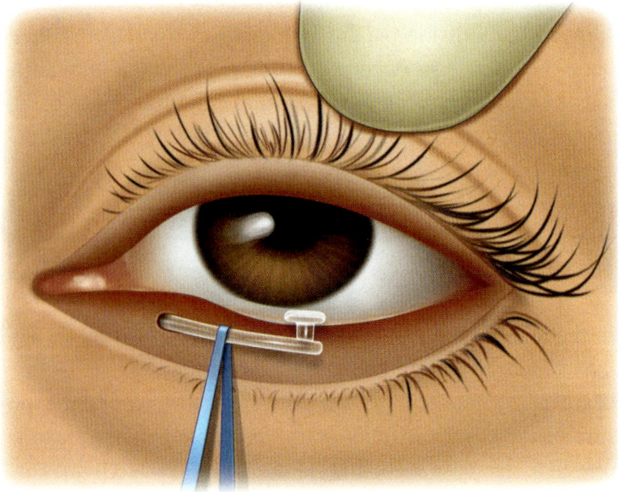

Fig. 68.4 Mini Monoka stent

tarsal plate. The suture is then hitched with a big bite to the skin of the supra-brow area using nonabsorbable suture material. This helps to counter the scar and gravity-related ectropic effect on the lower eyelids and protect the cornea.

Another technique was recently described by Yesiloglu et al. [15] to treat lagophthalmos and help possibly prevent cicatricial ectropion and contracture. The technique is based on V-Y advancement of the contracted eyelid or if necessary both upper and lower eyelids (Fig. 68.8). The V flap is harvested in musculocutaneous fashion by including eyelid skin and the orbicularis muscle to the flap and leaving the orbital septum intact for a tension-free closure. This technique has some limitations. First, it's not suitable for acute burns, and it's recommended to wait approximately 7–10 days after the initial injury. In the 7–10 days, a temporary tarsorrhaphy can be used to protect the globe. Second, the technique is not applicable in cases with severe burns with severe tissue deficiency [15].

A surgical tarsorrhaphy would theoretically seem ideal after 2 weeks. However, the use of a surgical tarsorrhaphy is very controversial. Some surgeons believe that tarsorrhaphies should not be used for several reasons. Early tarsorrhaphy does not appear to prevent or decrease wound contracture when cicatricial ectropion is present, and many surgeons feel that tissue replacement is the treatment of choice. Some surgeons perform a tarsorrhaphy at the time of skin grafting and leave it in place until the facial scars have matured. It is uncertain whether tarsorrhaphy at the time of skin grafting may prevent recurrent ectropion [1].

Masquerade Procedure

In severely damaged eyelids where most of the eyelid is absent, a masquerade procedure may be necessary to protect the globe. In this procedure, the remaining palpebral and bulbar conjunctivas from the upper and lower lid are mobilized and sutured together to cover the cornea. Then a split-thickness graft is placed on top of the conjunctiva and sutured to the skin edges. After 3 months, the flap can be divided to create two new eyelids [1, 3].

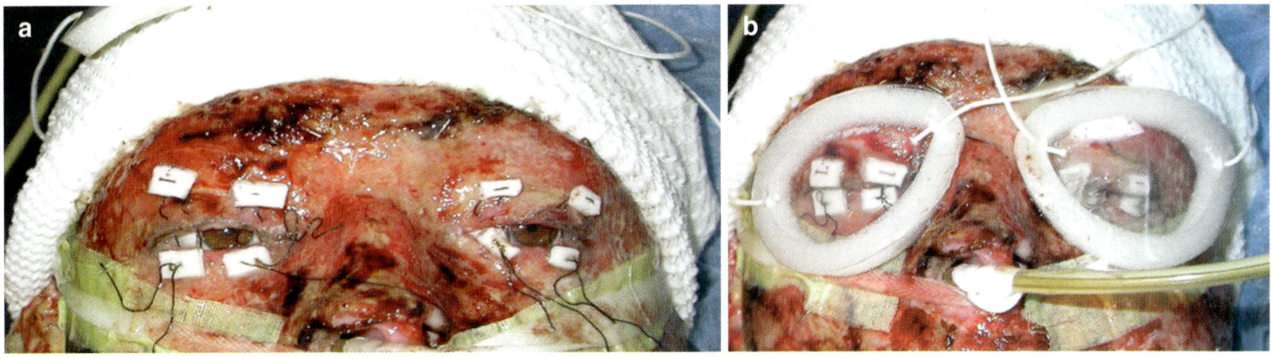

Fig. 68.5 (**a**) Patient with temporary tarsorrhaphy suture open. (**b**) Patient with temporary tarsorrhaphy suture closed

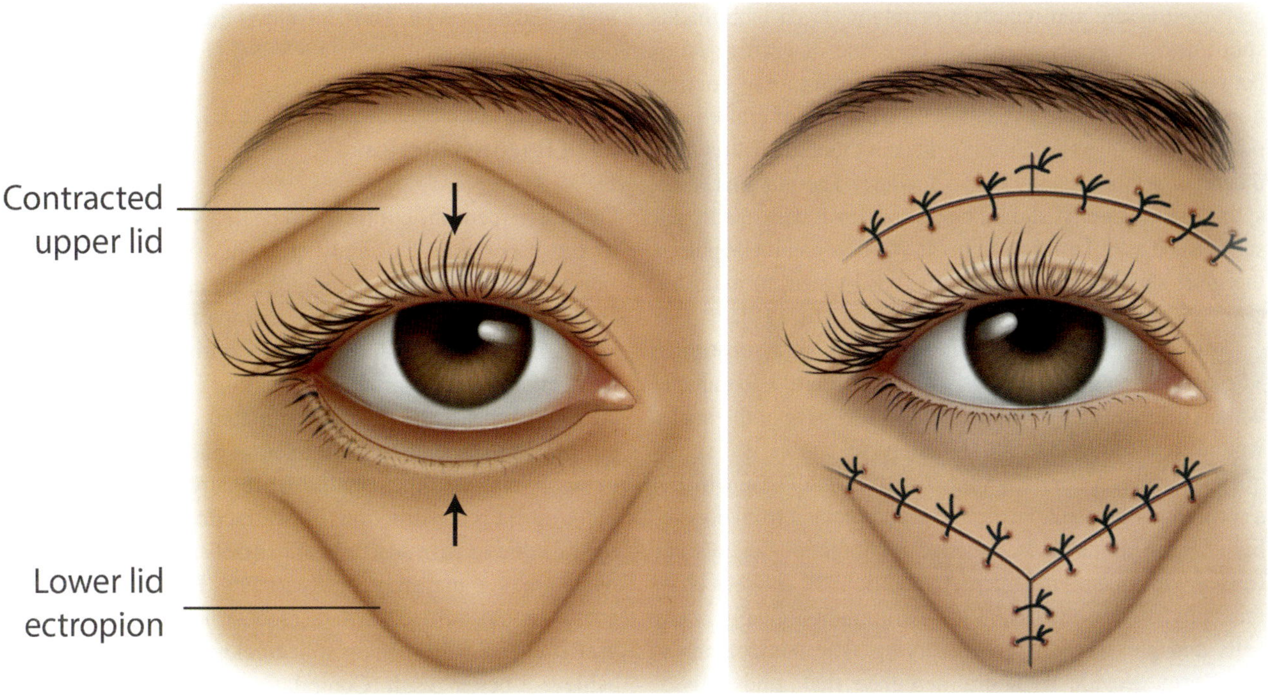

Fig. 68.6 Example of V-Y advancement [15]

Intermediate Care

It is generally agreed that progressive contracture and recurrent cicatricial ectropion is the norm in eyelid burns. This necessitates early and possibly repeated eyelid grafting during the early stages to both protect the cornea and help relieve eyelid retraction. This is considered one of the most important steps in the rehabilitation of eyelid burns. The timing of deep eyelid burn debridement is controversial. Often, clinical priorities necessitate that burns elsewhere on the body be treated and there may often be very little available skin graft. In addition, good blood supply and viable skin within the deep eyelid burn may help avoid contracture in the first 2 weeks [1, 3]. The judicious use of allograft could also be of benefit. The optimal time to perform a skin graft is also still controversial, as is whether the graft should be split or full thickness. The timing of grafting is often done at 2–3 weeks post injury and dictated by the emergence of eyelid contracture or lagophthalmos [1, 14]. However, a recent case report reported an optimal waiting time of 5 days for graft placement following debridement allowing healthy granulation tissue and bleeding observation [16].

Most burn injuries are limited to the skin and leave the underlying orbicularis muscle intact, which provides a rich vascular supply for the graft recipient bed. The release in the upper lid should be along the superior lid crease, approximately 10 mm from the lid margin, and extend appropriately medially and laterally. It is important to maximize the amount of normal skin that is left inferior to the crease over the tarsus. The lower lid release incision should be infraciliary. For both upper and lower eyelids, the dissection should be "canthus-to-canthus" and extend up to 2 cm beyond the lateral canthus. The upper lid is more important than the lower lid in protecting the globe, so grafting of the upper lid should be performed before the lower lids are treated. In addition, it is often thought best to perform grafting in separate sessions [1, 17].

In the early stages of healing, or if grafting sites are limited, split-thickness skin grafts can be used. Split-thickness grafts can be harvested from either the inner arm or thigh. These grafts should be relatively thick, in the range of 0.014–0.018 in. Using thinner grafts can lead to unacceptably high graft contracture and recurrent ectropion. Even with thicker split-thickness grafts, there can be a rate of graft rejection between 30% and 70%. Owing to this high rate of contraction, it is important to overcorrect the amount of grafted skin placed. This is best achieved by keeping the lid on stretch by means of a tarsorrhaphy or frost suture. The margins of the split-thickness grafts should be tacked down with absorbable suture such as 6-0 mild chromic. If a bolster cannot be placed, the graft should be covered with broad-spectrum antibiotic ointment and moist compresses for 5 days [1, 3, 17].

Another technique that can be used is skin substitutes. These are often used when donor skin is limited, to enhance wound healing, increase the dermal component of the healed wound, and reduce the inflammatory responses and subsequent scarring. A common matrix used is AlloDerm which is a commercially available dermal graft obtained from donated human skin tissue. It is screened for infectious agents and treated with an antiviral agent. In addition, the tissue is enzymatically processed to remove all immunologically active cells and preserved by freeze drying. The components of AlloDerm provide a natural template that guides tissue regeneration and can be used in patients whom large full-thickness periorbital skin grafts or flaps are either inappropriate or extremely difficult to perform [18, 19] (Fig. 68.7).

Whether to use a FTSG or STSG continues to be a debated subject. Traditionally, STSG was recommended for upper eyelids and FTSG for lower eyelids. This was thought to be that FTSG are too bulky for the upper eyelid and will give poor mobility and a poor cosmetic result. However, there have been multiple papers that have described using FTSG for both upper and lower eyelid burns with good results. Lille et al. [20] recently showed that FTSG to both upper and lower eyelids reduce the incidence of ectropion in comparison to STSG; FTSG are typically harvested from pre- or postauricular areas whenever possible. Otherwise, supraclavicular or if necessary inner arm or groin skin can be used. Ultimately, the capacity of a skin graft to inhibit wound contraction is directly proportional to the amount of intact dermal collagen present. Thus, it follows that a FTSG with more dermis will contract less than a STSG [1, 17].

Late Reconstruction

Definitive reconstruction should be delayed for 3 months to a year, if possible. This allows the phase of wound contraction to pass before determining the amount of graft needed to definitively correct cicatricial ectropion. It is important to ascertain if the lid malposition is due to contraction of the lid itself or is secondary to a scar pulling from the forehead, cheek, or neck (Fig. 68.8). Significant distal scarring can pull on the lids and cause retraction and ectropion. These extrinsic abnormalities should be repaired before proceeding with lid reconstruction. For retraction and ectropion of the lids due to burn scarring, skin grafts and adjacent tissue flaps are the mainstay of treatment. Full-thickness skin grafts should be used in late reconstruction because such grafts contrast less than split-thickness skin grafts and achieve a better result. Contralateral upper lid skin is best for repairing upper lid defects. The retroauricular area provides the best grafting site for lower lid defects or the upper lid, if contralateral skin is not available. Other possible sites

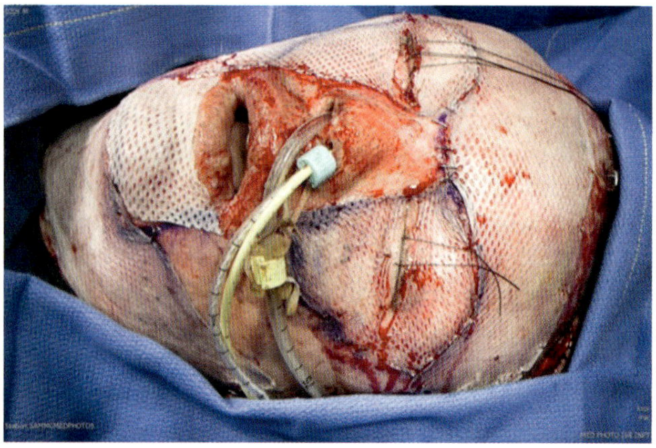

Fig. 68.7 Patient with AlloDerm placed at day 12 prior to skin grafting

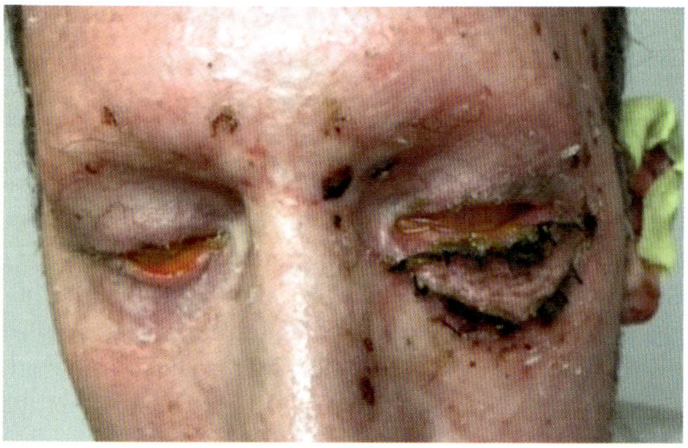

Fig. 68.8 Cicatricial contracture and ectropion of the lids with placement of FTSG to left lower eyelid

include the supraclavicular region, inner arms, and inner thighs. Although full-thickness skin grafts contract less than split-thickness skin grafts, up to 50% contraction can still occur.

It is uncommon that adjacent tissue skin or myocutaneous flaps are available in burn injuries. But if so, such flaps are useful because they contract less than grafts. They also have an intrinsic blood supply for better survival rates and usually are a good tissue match.

The technique used for full-thickness grafts is similar to that used in split-thickness grafts. Lid incision lines should extend beyond the lateral canthus and angle slightly superiorly. Regardless of where the graft is harvested, all subcutaneous tissue should be removed. The lid should be placed on stretch, and the graft sutured into the recipient bed with 6–0 mild chromic sutures. Antibiotic ointment is applied, and the graft is covered by a dressing of Telfa overlaid with molded dental wax. A light pressure dressing is then placed. The dressing is removed in 5–7 days (Fig. 68.9). Even after full-thickness grafts have been placed, there can be continued wound contraction necessitating the need to repeat these procedures [1, 3, 17].

When burns involve the posterior lamella and lid margin, reconstructive procedures described in the other sections of this book may be used. Such severe eyelid burns are typically associated with a very grave prognosis for survival.

Medial Canthal Reconstruction

Burns affecting the medial canthus and glabella can lead to webbing of the canthus contraction over the nasal bridge can pull the lids and puncta away from the globe. Multiple Z-plasties or Y-V plasties may be useful in correcting linear contractions if the wounds are relatively soft and not densely scarred. If eyelid tissue is in short supply, glabellar flaps can also be used. Otherwise, better results have been reported by excising the scar web, releasing the canthus,

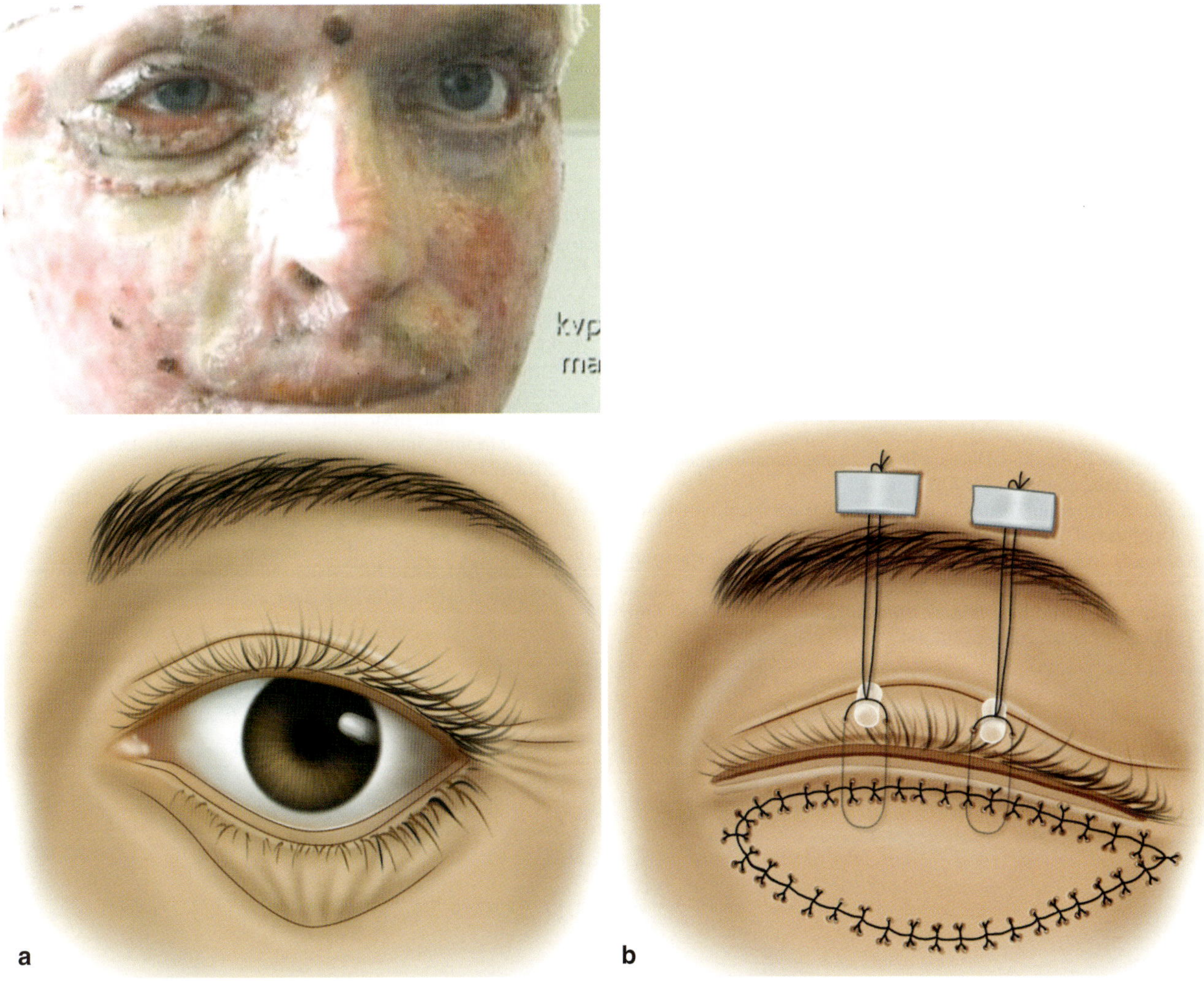

Fig. 68.9 Full-thickness skin graft for cicatricial ectropion to right lower eyelid. A full-thickness skin graft is harvested, thinned, and placed in the recipient bed. Frost sutures are placed to keep the lid on stretch postoperatively

and replacing the defect with a FTSG. In addition, local transposition flaps can be used to correct scan bands at the lateral canthus [1, 3, 21].

Tear Drainage System Abnormalities

In burn patients, the most common abnormalities of the lacrimal system involve the puncta, canaliculi, and tear sac either from the burn itself or scarring. Punctal stenosis is common and can typically be addressed with sequential punctal dilation with or without stents. If the stenosis is refractory to dilation or stenting, then the punctum can be opened with the two-snip procedure. Canalicular stenosis can be addressed dilation and stenting as well. If the canalicular obstruction persists despite dilation and stenting, a DCR can be performed [1, 3].

Summary

Eyelid involvement is common in facial burns and can be devastating to the patient both from a functional and psychological standpoint. Acute and subacute management focuses on protecting the eye and its visual potential and limiting the extent of the damage that has occurred to the eyelids and surrounding tissue. Long-term evaluation and management are critical to help minimize the complications and preserve the eyelid in terms of its functional components. As with other injuries to the adnexa, treatment is directed to preserving the eye and sight, maintaining function, and the restoration of cosmesis.

References

1. Malhotra R, Sheikh I, Dheansa B. The management of eyelid burns. Surv Ophthalmol. 2009;54(3):356–71.
2. Sharma N, et al. Treatment of acute ocular chemical burns. Surv Ophthalmol. 2018;63:214–35.
3. John D NG, Holck DEE. Management of eyelid burns. Ch 19. In: Ophthalmic care of the combat casualty: Office of the Surgeon General at TMM Publications, Borden Institute, Walter Reed Army Medical Center; 2003. p. 307–34.
4. Cabalag MS, et al. Early and late complications of ocular burn injuries. J Plast Reconstr Aesth Surg. 2015;68:356–61.
5. Fitzgerald O'Connor E, et al. Periorbital burns – a 6 year review of management and outcome. Burns. 2015;41:616–23.
6. Moritz AR, Henrique FC. Studies of thermal injury: II. The relative importance of time and surface temperature in the causation of cutaneous burns. Am J Pathol. 1947;23:695–720.
7. Jackson PM. The diagnosis of the depth of the burning. Br J Surg. 1953;40:558–96.
8. Johnson C. Pathologic manifestation of burn injury. Chap 3. In: Richard RL, Staly MJ, editors. Burn care and rehabilitation: principles and practice. Philadelphia: FA Davis Co; 1994.
9. Mauriellao JA Jr, Hollsten DA. Cicatricial ectropion due to thermal burns of the eyelids. Chap 9. In: Mauriella JA, editor. Unfavourable results of eyelid and lacrimal surgery, prevention and management. Boston: Butterworth-Heinemann; 2000. p. 219–26.
10. Gillenwater J, Garner W. Acute fluid management of large burns. Clin Plast Surg. 2017;44(3):495–503.
11. Meyer DR, Kersten RC, Kulwin DR. Management of canalicular injury associated with eyelid burns. Arch Ophthalmol. 1995;113(7):900.
12. Ricca AM, et al. Nasolacrimal stents: an introductory guide. Eyerounds.org. posted January 29, 2018. https://webeye.ophth.uiowa.edu/eyeforum/tutorials/Stents/index.htm. Accessed March 16, 2019.
13. Hollsten DA, White WL. Management of periorbital burns. Semin Ophthalmol. 1994;9:152–64.
14. Lymperopoulos NS, et al. A lateral tarsorraphy with forehead hitch to pre-empt and treat burns ectropion with a contextual review of burns ectropion management. Scars Burns Heal. 2016;2:1–11.
15. Yesiloglu N, et al. A simple method for the treatment of cicatricial ectropion and eyelid contraction in patients with Periocular burn: vertical V-Y advancement of the eyelid. Burns. 2014 Dec;40(8):1820–1.
16. Joethy J, Tan BK. A multi-staged approach to the reconstruction of burnt Asian face. Indian J Plast Surg. 2011;44(1):142–6.
17. Jovanovic N, et al. Case report of Wolfe grafting for the management of bilateral cicatricial eyelid ectropion following severe burn injuries. Annals of Medicine and Surgery. 2018;34:58–61.
18. Levin F, Tubin RE, Langer PD. Acellular human dermal matrix as a skin substitute for reconstruction of large periocular cutaneous defects. Ophthalmic Plast Reconstr Surg. 2011;27(1):44–7.
19. Wang Y, et al. Burn injury: challenges and advances in burn wound healing, infection, pain, and scarring. Adv Drug Deliv Rev. 2018;123:3–17.
20. Lille ST, Engrave LH, Caps MT, et al. Full-thickness grafting of acute eyelid burns should not be considered taboo. Plast Reconstr Surg. 1999;104(3):637–45.
21. Achauer BM, Adair SR. Acute and reconstructive management of the burned eyelid. Clin Plast Surg. 2000;7:87–95.

General Principles of Management of Orbital Fractures

69

Peter Timoney, Kevin Tomasko, William R. Nunery, and Hui Bae Harold Lee

Introduction

Orbital fractures are common forms of injury that occur with trauma to the midface. The severity can range from small, localized, non-displaced fractures to large fractures completely disrupting the orbit [1]. Typically, orbital fractures are defined by involvement of surrounding structures and location such as orbital floor, orbital roof, medial orbital wall, or lateral orbital wall. Assessment of patients with orbital fractures must be careful and meticulous, with visual function being of utmost importance. A thorough history and detailed examination including mechanism of injury, visual acuity, relative afferent pupillary defect, status of the globe, and presence or absence of extraocular muscle entrapment are crucial in evaluating all orbital trauma. Non-contrast computed tomography (CT) remains the gold standard imaging study for evaluating the extent of orbital trauma [2, 3]. Definitive management depends on a wide array of factors, which will be reviewed in the coming chapters.

Orbital Anatomy

The bony orbit develops from the mesenchyme that encircles the optic vesicle starting at the 6-week embryonic stage [4]. In the adult, the cone-shaped bony orbit encloses a volume of 30 cm [5]. The anterior entrance dimensions measure on average approximately 45 mm wide by 35 mm vertically. The orbit's widest dimension is situated approximately one cm posterior to the anterior bony rim. The angle between the lateral walls of each orbit is approximately 90°, whereas the angle between the lateral and medial walls is approximately 45°.

P. Timoney (✉)
University of Kentucky, Department of Ophthalmology, Lexington, KY, USA

K. Tomasko · W. R. Nunery
University of Louisville, Department of Ophthalmology & Visual Sciences, Louisville, KY, USA

H. B. H. Lee
St. Vincent Hospital, Department of Ophthalmology, Indianapolis, IN, USA

Orbital Roof

The orbital roof comprises the orbital plate of the frontal bone and the lesser wing of the sphenoid at the apex (Fig. 69.1). The roof is a thin plate with frequent dehiscences. It houses the lacrimal gland within the lacrimal gland fossa anterolaterally and the trochlea within the trochlear fossa anteromedially. The orbital roof separates the orbit from the frontal sinus anteriorly and the anterior cranial fossa posteriorly.

Medial Orbital Wall

The medial walls of the orbit are parallel to each other. They measure 45–50 mm in length from the orbital rim to the orbital apex. The medial wall is the thinnest of the orbital walls with the lamina papyracea measuring 0.2–0.4 mm in thickness. The medial wall is formed by the frontal process of the maxillary, ethmoid, lacrimal, and sphenoid bones (Fig. 69.1). The lamina papyracea of the ethmoid bone largely composes the medial wall with the body of the sphenoid, completing the medial wall posterior to the ethmoid bone. The lacrimal fossa is formed by the union of the lacrimal bone posteriorly and the frontal process of the maxilla anteriorly. The ethmoid bone joins the orbital roof at the frontoethmoid suture line, which marks the floor of the anterior cranial fossa at the level of the cribriform plate. Within the frontoethmoid suture line are the anterior and posterior ethmoidal foramina, which transmit branches of the nasociliary nerve as well as the

J. J. Servat et al. (eds.), *Smith and Nesi's Ophthalmic Plastic and Reconstructive Surgery*,
https://doi.org/10.1007/978-3-030-41720-8_69

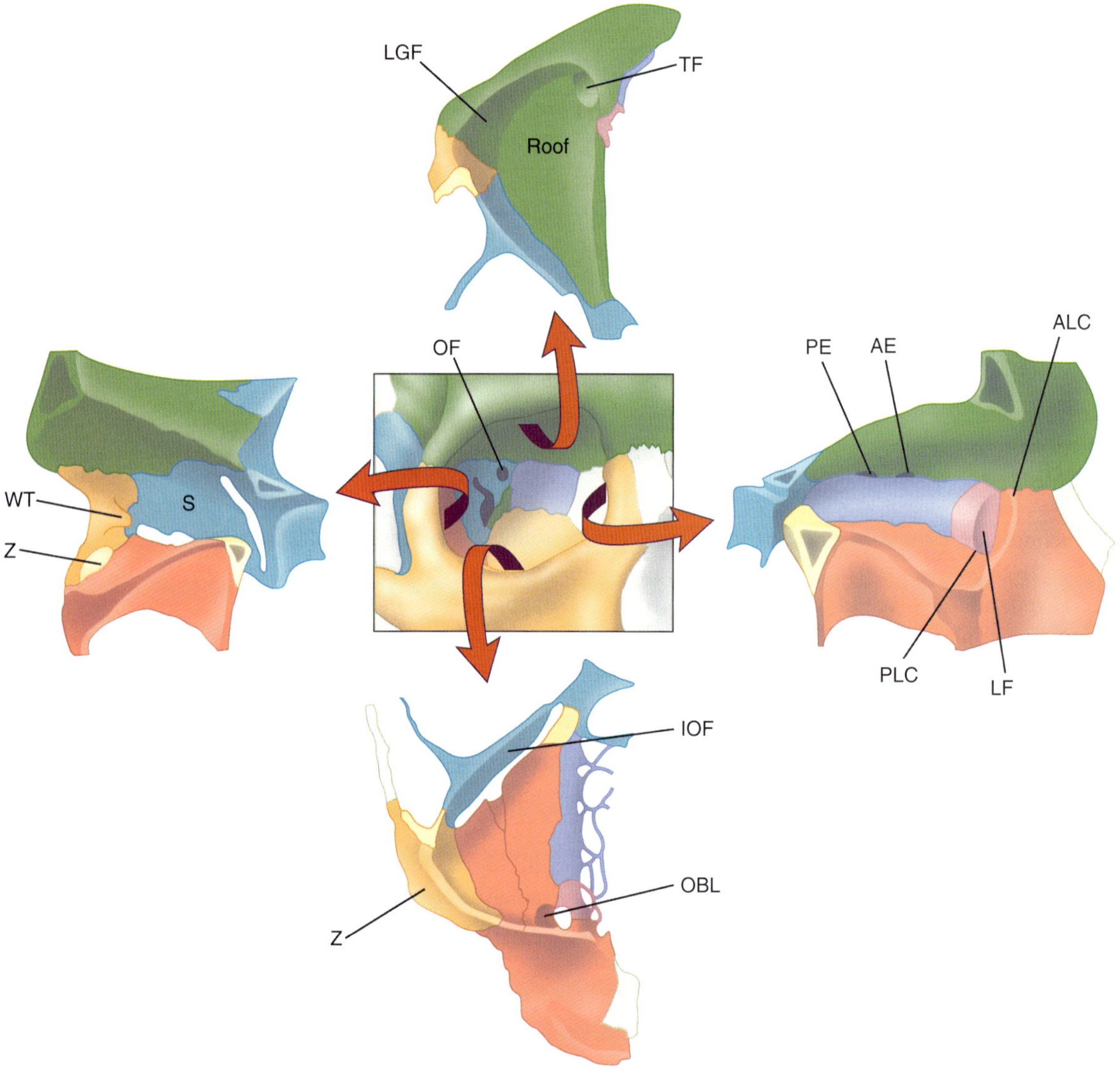

Fig. 69.1 Orbital walls. *The roof*: This wall is composed of the orbital plate of the frontal bone and a minor contribution from the lesser wing of the sphenoid bone. The anterolateral portion of the roof houses the lacrimal gland fossa (*LGF*) and the trochlear fossa (*TF*). The roof narrows posteriorly toward the orbital apex, where the optic foramen (*OF*) is located. *The lateral wall*: This wall is composed primarily of the zygomatic bone (*Z*) and the greater wing of the sphenoid bone (*S*). Whitnall's tubercle (*WT*), a small bony promontory located just within the lateral rim 11 mm below the frontozygomatic suture, is the attachment of several structures. There exists a groove that forms a canal that conducts both the zygomaticofacial and zygomaticotemporal neurovascular bundles. *The floor*: This wall is composed of the orbital plate of the maxilla, the zygomatic bone anterolaterally, and the orbital process of the palatine bone posteriorly. The inferior orbital fissure (*IOF*) separates the greater wing of the sphenoid bone from the floor. This fissure communicates with the pterygopalatine and the infratemporal fossae. This fissure transmits the maxillary division of the trigeminal nerve and its branches, branches of the inferior ophthalmic vein to the pterygoid plexus, the infraorbital artery, and branches of the sphenopalatine ganglion. The anteromedial area of the floor houses the origin of the inferior oblique muscle (*OBL*). *The medial wall*: This wall is composed of the ethmoid (lamina papyracea) and lacrimal bones centrally, the frontal bone superoanteriorly, and the sphenoid bone posteriorly. The lacrimal fossa (*LF*) lies between the anterior lacrimal crest (*ALC*), which is formed by the frontal process of the maxilla, and the posterior lacrimal crest (*PLC*), which is formed by the lacrimal bone. The anterior ethmoidal (*AE*) foramen transmits the anterior ethmoidal neurovascular bundle, and the posterior ethmoidal (*PE*) foramen transmits the posterior ethmoidal artery and occasionally a branch of the nasociliary nerve

anterior and posterior ethmoidal arteries, the latter being branches of the ophthalmic artery. The anterior ethmoidal neurovascular bundle is approximately 20–25 mm posterior to the anterior lacrimal crest. Approximately 12 mm separates the anterior and posterior neurovascular bundles. The posterior ethmoidal foramen lies approximately 4–8 mm anterior to the optic canal. These foramina are clinically important landmarks for the surgeon, as they define the level of the cribriform plate and point toward the optic canal position.

Orbital Floor

The triangular orbital floor is comprised of mostly the maxillary bone, with contributions from the zygomatic bone anterolaterally and the palatine bone posteriorly (Fig. 69.1). It is the shortest of the orbital walls, measuring 35–40 mm from the orbital rim. The floor does not extend to the orbital apex but rather ends at the posterior limit of the maxillary sinus. It is thinnest medial to the infraorbital canal; this is the most common site for blowout fractures. The inferior orbital fissure, which separates the floor from the lateral wall, transmits the maxillary division of the trigeminal nerve from the foramen rotundum, the maxillary artery, inferior ophthalmic vein branches, and postganglionic parasympathetic fibers which pass to the lacrimal gland. The inferior oblique muscle originates from the medial orbital floor just lateral to the nasolacrimal canal.

Lateral Orbital Wall

The lateral orbital wall is formed by the greater wing of the sphenoid posteriorly and by the zygomatic process of the frontal bone and the orbital process of the zygomatic bone anteriorly (Fig. 69.1). It is the most robust and strongest of the orbital walls. The thinnest portion of the lateral wall is at the zygomaticosphenoid suture. The alignment of the zygomaticosphenoid suture is crucial in reduction of a lateral wall fracture to achieve normal facial contour and symmetry.

At the junction of the lateral wall and the orbital roof is the superior orbital fissure, lying between the greater and lesser wings of the sphenoid. The lateral wall is separated from the orbital floor by the inferior orbital fissure. The lateral orbital (Whitnall's) tubercle is located within the lateral wall approximately 11 mm inferior to the frontozygomatic suture. This serves as the attachment site for several orbital structures such as the lateral canthal tendon, Lockwood's ligament, lateral horn of the levator aponeurosis and check ligament of the lateral rectus. The zygomaticofacial and zygomaticotemporal neurovascular bundles perforate the lateral wall near the anterior end of the inferior orbital fissure.

Evaluation

In conjunction with a comprehensive system review and examination, a complete ophthalmic examination should be undertaken in patients with suspected periorbital, orbital, and/or facial trauma. In addition to the general patient history, a focused patient history that details the mechanism of injury, presence of symptoms, and ophthalmic history (e.g., previous ocular surgery, eye medications, pre-injury visual acuity) should be obtained. The time of last ingestion of food and liquid should be determined along with the patient's tetanus status.

Assessment of the globes and the integrity of the optic nerves are of paramount importance. Penetrating globe injury should be identified, and a CT scan should be performed in cases of a suspected intraorbital foreign body, orbital fractures, or a ruptured globe. When attainable, the visual acuity, pupil response, and extraocular motility are essential elements of the initial examination.

Given the prognostic importance of visual acuity, each eye should be tested separately. Plus lenses may be necessary to obtain best near vision in patients with presbyopia. The swinging flashlight test elucidates the presence of a relative afferent papillary defect and may provide the only evidence of optic nerve injury in the neurologically incapacitated patient.

Limitation of extraocular motility may be seen in a variety of specific injuries. Edema or hemorrhage involving an extraocular muscle leads to diffuse reduction of motility, while entrapment of muscle or perimuscular tissue in the fracture site causes a "double diplopia" pattern of diplopia in the field of action of the involved extraocular muscle as well as the field of action of the antagonist muscle. Restriction due to a fracture is often accompanied by pain and guarding in attempted action of the involved extraocular muscle or its antagonist. Restriction of an extraocular muscle may also be detected by an increase in intraocular pressure greater than 4 mm when attempting to look in the field of diplopia.

Paralytic diplopia (i.e., cranial nerve III, IV, or VI) may also occur after head or orbit trauma but can usually be differentiated from restrictive diplopia by lack of intraocular pressure elevation in the diplopia field, lack of pain on eye movement, and presence of the typical cranial nerve pattern of diplopia.

Ocular motility is also important in the diagnosis of acute retrobulbar hematoma which is arguably the most urgent of all ocular emergencies. A "frozen globe" with limitation of motility in all positions of gaze when combined with proptosis, elevated intraocular pressure, tight and possibly ptotic eyelids, and retinal artery pulsations indicate sight-threatening compartment syndrome. This requires immediate canthotomy and cantholysis of both the superior and inferior rami of the lateral canthal tendon in order to reduce orbital pressure in hopes of limiting compression forces on the optic nerve.

Thorough examination of the retina and posterior segment should be performed in all neurologically stable patients but especially in those with suspected traumatic optic neuropathy to rule out intraocular sequela of acute trauma.

The ocular adnexa should be carefully evaluated for lacerations, possible lacrimal system trauma in medial canthal and/or midface trauma, upper eyelid ptosis, bone movement and/or discontinuities, palpable step-offs, telecanthus in midface trauma, pulsatile proptosis in cases with orbital roof fractures, orbital foreign bodies, and cranial nerve VII paresis.

Radiological Examination

Radiological evaluation following orbit trauma is an essential factor in complete patient evaluation. Radiological evaluation assists in identifying orbital foreign bodies, assessing the craniofacial bony structure, determining the integrity of the globes and optic nerves, and diagnosing retrobulbar hemorrhage or a subperiosteal abscess. Computed tomography (CT) is the primary imaging modality utilized in the initial evaluation of orbital trauma.

Even though CT imaging provides excellent bone detail and good orbital soft tissue resolution, it may underestimate the presence and extent of an orbital fracture. A standard orbital CT scan protocol includes helical CT scanning of 1–3 mm cuts in axial and coronal planes with soft tissue and bone windows. The usual windows include the cavernous sinus intracranially as well as the periorbital sinuses. Bone window exposures are best for detecting orbital fractures as soft tissue settings overexpose the bone and may obscure subtle fractures. This is particularly important in evaluating the pediatric population.

Orbital inflammation or infection can be evaluated with CT scans performed after IV contrast administration assuming normal renal function studies. If the patient presents with very poor vision and no definite globe abnormality and a compartment syndrome has been ruled out, then a detailed examination of orbital apex injuries and optic canal fractures should be evaluated using 1 mm intervals on CT scan images.

Generally, orbital fractures are evaluated on two-dimensional axial and coronal images (Fig. 69.2). Three-dimensional imaging techniques may demonstrate facial fracture displacement but increase the cost of the scans and may misinterpret thin bone (e.g., lamina papyracea and cribriform plate) as missing bone.

Magnetic resonance imaging (MRI) of the orbit has select indications in the assessment of orbital trauma patients. The MRI study cannot be used as the initial imaging modality until an orbital metallic foreign body is excluded via a plain film or CT scan evaluation. MRI provides poor bony detail, but it may be a useful adjunct in assessing injury to the optic nerve, extraocular muscles, orbital apex, cavernous sinus, and associated brain injury. A MRI protocol for orbital imaging includes T1- and T2-weighted images with gadolinium and fat suppression.

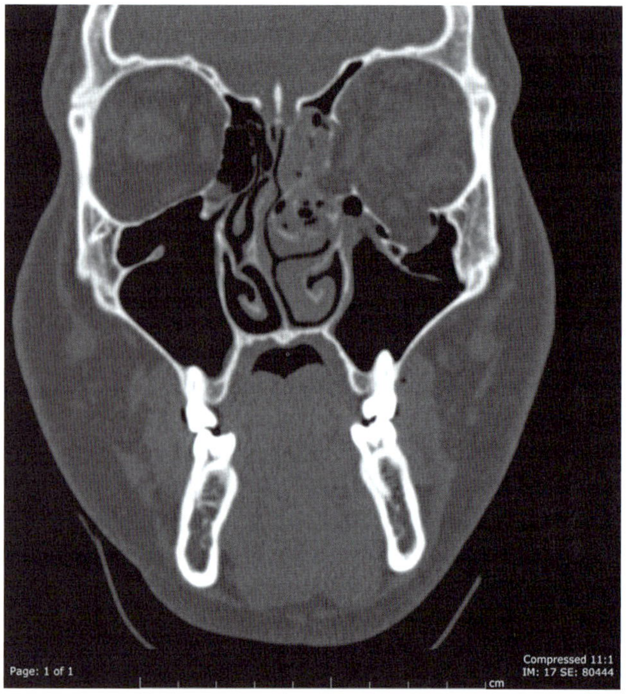

Fig. 69.2 Left orbital floor and medial wall fractures

General Management Principles of Orbital Fractures

Orbital fractures that are larger than 50% of the orbit floor and/or medial wall that demonstrate motility restriction or include both the medial wall and orbital floor require repair [6]. In these cases, orbital implants are necessary to prevent tissue incarceration and to restore normal anatomical relationships.

The optimal timing of surgical repair of most fractures is between 5 and 10 days following the injury. This allows resolution of orbital edema, provides adequate time for surgical decision-making, and allows surgical dissection before tissue healing creates fibrosis of the tissue planes. Fractures in the pediatric population require more urgent repair as fibrosis of extraocular motility with permanent diplopia occurs much more quickly in children than adults. Also, small fractures that incarcerate extraocular muscle tissue require immediate repair to prevent muscle necrosis. White-eyed blowout fractures are orbital floor fractures that occur in pediatric patients and display little or no soft tissue injury. Patients typically display upgaze restriction in the setting of an otherwise normal external exam. They may have symptoms of nausea, vomiting, or bradycardia secondary to inferior rectus muscle entrapment. Careful examination and urgent repair are required in these patients in order to prevent permanent damage to the inferior rectus [7]. In some cases, delayed fracture repair (2 weeks or longer after the injury) may be required in the setting of traumatic optic neuropathy or globe injury.

A variety of implant choices are available for repair of orbital wall fractures. These include materials such as nonadherent, nonporous alloplastic materials such as nylon foil sheets, silastic sheets, and silicone. Also, reabsorbable alloplastic materials such as LactoSorb may be used in some cases [8].

Preformed porous or titanium implants can provide structural support for the injured orbit but may also stimulate fibrosis to orbital tissue including orbital fat or extraocular muscles. This secondary fibrosis is responsible for post-repair orbital adherence syndrome with restrictive diplopia [9]. Our choice for repair of most orbital fractures is a nonporous implant, namely, a 0.4 mm nylon foil sheet that can be cut to fit the fracture size and dimensions. This provides excellent support without adherence to orbital tissue and can be wrapped from the medial wall to the floor to cover large fractures [10].

Autogenous bone grafts have largely been abandoned for orbital reconstruction due to donor site morbidity, increased surgery time, unpredictable reabsorption, and difficulty fashioning bone to exact orbital dimensions.

References

1. Bord SP, Linden J. Trauma to the globe and orbit. Emerg Med Clin North Am. 2008;26(1):97–123, vi–vii.
2. Vicinanzo MG, McGwin G Jr, Allamneni C, Long JA. Interreader variability of computed tomography for orbital floor fracture. JAMA Ophthalmol. 2015;133(12):1393–7.
3. Kubal WS. Imaging of orbital trauma. Radiographics. 2008;28(6):1729–39.
4. De Haan AB, Willekens BL. Embryology of the orbital wall. Mod Probl Ophthalmol. 1975;14:57.
5. Russel MD. The supraorbital torus: a most remarkable peculiarity. Curr Anthropol. 1985;26:337.
6. Hawes MJ, Dortzbach RK. Surgery on orbital floor fractures. Influence of time of repair and fracture size. Ophthalmology. 1983;90(9):1066–70.
7. Hammond D, et al. The white-eyed blowout fracture in the child: beware of distractions. J Surg Case Rep. 2013;2013(7):rjt054. https://doi.org/10.1093/jscr/rjt054.
8. Hollier LH, Rogers N, Nrezin E, et al. Resorbable mesh in the treatment of orbital floor fractures. J Craniofac Surg. 2001;12(3):242–6.
9. Lee HB, Nunery WR. Orbital adherence syndrome secondary to titanium implant material. Ophthal Plast Reconstr Surg. 2009;25(1):33–6.
10. Nunery WR, Tao JP, Johl S. Nylon foil "wraparound" repair of com bined orbital floor and medial wall fractures. Ophthal Plast Reconstr Surg. 2008;24(4):271–5.

Blowout Fractures of the Orbit

70

David R. Jordan, Louise Mawn, and Stephen R. Klapper

Introduction

An orbital floor fracture or "blowout fracture" is most often associated with midfacial trauma ranging from mild and seemingly insignificant to severe and debilitating. Initial assessment and management are guided by the severity and nature of the patient's injuries. Stabilization of the airway and cardiopulmonary system is of utmost importance, particularly in the polytrauma patient. A comprehensive ophthalmologic examination should be performed by an ophthalmologist. Once life- and sight-threatening injuries have been addressed and the patient is medically stable, the oculoplastic surgical assessment should include a thorough medical and surgical history. Determination of the mechanism of injury helps guide suspicion for injuries to the globe, eyelids, optic nerve, and adjacent ocular adnexal structures. It is useful to know the size and shape of the object, as well as the force and velocity at which the object struck the eye. With a small accelerating object such as a bungee cord or hockey puck, there is often more direct globe trauma than with larger objects like a fist or soccer ball where some of the force is absorbed by the orbital rim and periorbital area. Knowing the "mechanism of injury" gives you an idea of how serious the associated injuries may be.

The authors of this study do not have a commercial or proprietary interest in any of the products reviewed in this manuscript.

D. R. Jordan (✉)
Ottawa Hospital – General Campus, Eye Institute, Ottawa, ON, Canada

L. Mawn
Vanderbilt University Medical Center, Department of Ophthalmology, Nashville, TN, USA

S. R. Klapper
Ophthalmology/Oculoplastic Surgery, Klapper Eyelid and Facial Plastic Surgery, Carmel, IN, USA

Clinical Examination

Periocular injuries resulting in a floor and/or medial wall fracture generally occur following blunt trauma with a high velocity object larger than the orbital bone opening (e.g., baseball, fist, elbow), motor vehicle accidents, sports injuries, or a fall. If the object is smaller than the orbital bone aperture (e.g., squash or tennis ball), the impact is primarily on the lids and globe (Fig. 70.1). In these cases, the globe is retropulsed, and, while cushioned to some degree by the adjacent fat, significant globe injury including rupture may occur. It is essential to document the visual acuity, optic nerve function, corneal integrity, presence of anterior chamber hemorrhage or angle recession, and any retinal damage. With blunt injuries, there is often considerable soft tissue edema and ecchymosis which may make proper visual assessment and ocular examination quite difficult. Orbital emphysema may be present from air entering the periorbital soft tissues from the paranasal sinuses resulting in crepitus on palpation of the eyelids (Fig. 70.2a, b). Nose blowing will cause or exacerbate orbital emphysema so patients are advised to avoid nose blowing for the first 2 weeks post injury (or post surgical repair). A Desmarres lid retractor or a carefully folded paper clip are useful to retract the lids for a more accurate assessment of visual acuity and ocular motility (Fig. 70.3a, b). The cornea, anterior chamber, and pupil can also be evaluated with a bright, handheld light. Fundus examination is possible but may be only a partial view dependent upon patient cooperation. The more complete the ocular examination, the better, but patient cooperation may limit some elements of the examination.

A blowout fracture of the orbital floor or medial orbital wall may result in diplopia. Floor fractures are often associated with double vision in primary gaze that may increase on up or down gaze or be associated with worsening pain on vertical ductions. If the medial orbital wall is involved, diplopia and pain may be exacerbated by horizontal ductions. The motility restrictions may be secondary to edema or hemorrhage of the orbital tissues; fracture entrapment of the fat or orbital connective tissue framework adjacent to the

J. J. Servat et al. (eds.), *Smith and Nesi's Ophthalmic Plastic and Reconstructive Surgery*,
https://doi.org/10.1007/978-3-030-41720-8_70

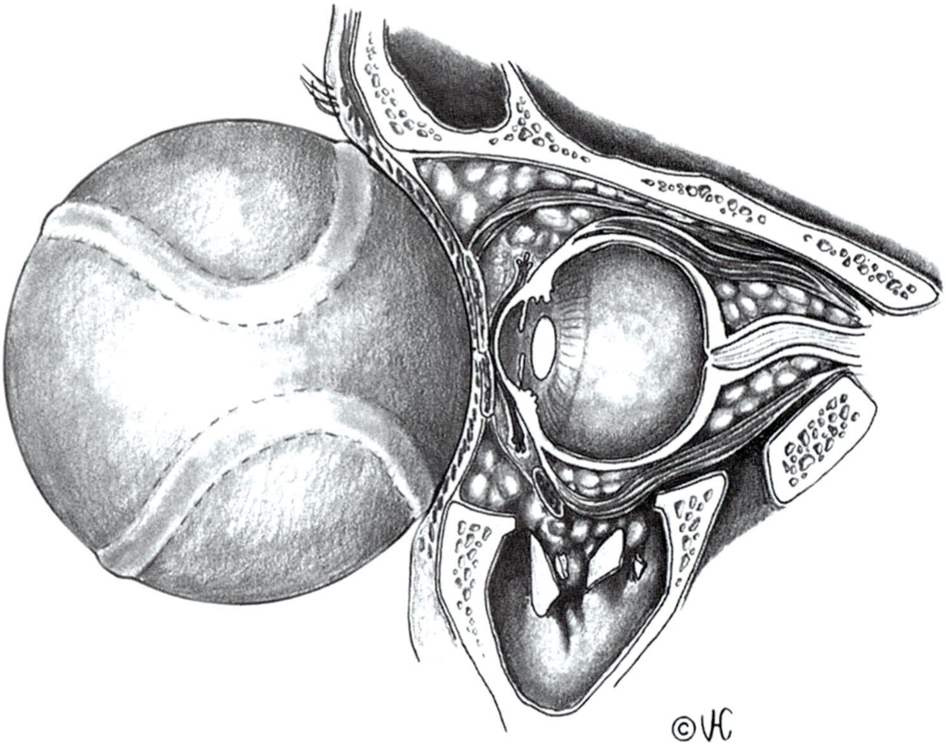

Fig. 70.1 Tennis ball striking eyelids and globe, retropulsing orbital contents, raising intraorbital pressure producing a blowout fracture

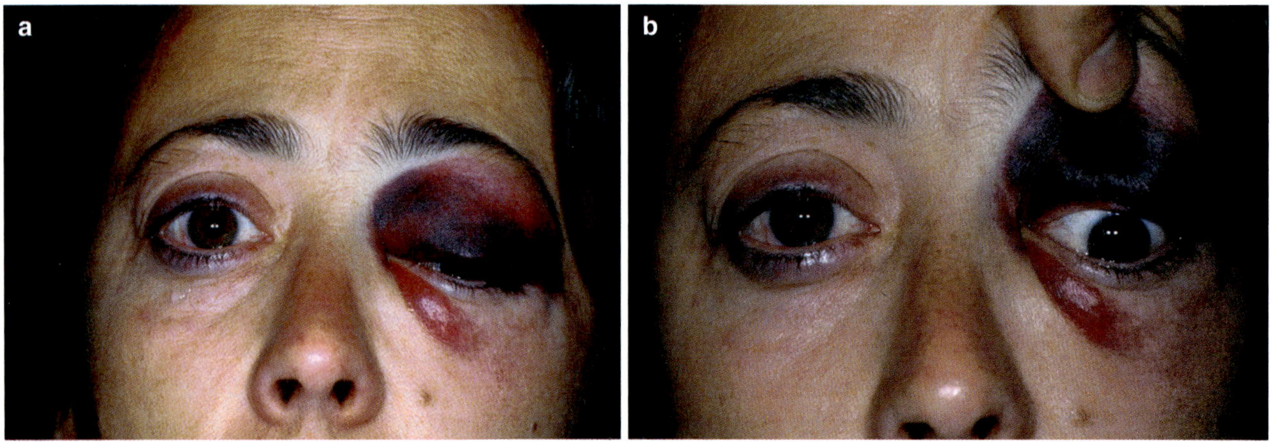

Fig. 70.2 (**a**) A 48-year-old lady with an orbital floor and medial wall fracture (left) is seen a few hours after she blew her nose. The left upper lid was very swollen and air was felt within the skin (crepitus). (**b**) The globe was shifted downward as a result of air that accumulated along the superior roof following a nose blow. The air resolved spontaneously over the next day

inferior rectus, medial rectus, and/or inferior oblique muscles; or incarceration of one or more of these muscles within the fracture site. Paresis of these muscles may also occur or a combination of any of these factors. Infraorbital hypesthesia including the lower eyelid, cheek, side of nose, and upper teeth is indicative of infraorbital injury and frequently associated with an orbital floor fracture. Proptosis may result from zygomaticotemporal complex fractures with displacement of the orbital bones into the orbit or more commonly from intraorbital edema or hemorrhage. Enophthalmos, typically associated with large orbital floor fractures or combined orbital floor-medial orbital wall fractures, may not be manifest until the orbital and periorbital edema resolves.

Orbital Imaging

Orbital imaging studies are invaluable in determining the radiologic severity of trauma and in guiding the surgical approach to fracture repair. The primary imaging modality to evaluate for orbital and facial bone trauma is high-resolution computed tomography (CT) in the axial and coronal planes

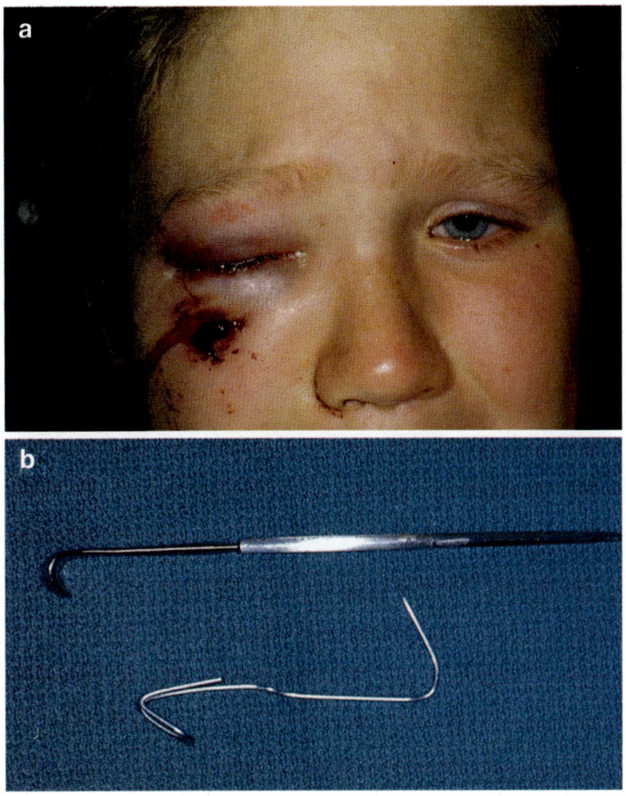

Fig. 70.3 (**a**) A 14-year-old male was hit in the right periocular area with a hockey stick and had upper and lower lid edema preventing the eyelids from opening. (**b**) A carefully folded paperclip was crafted to take the place of a Desmarres lid retractor. Topical anesthetic should be placed on the cornea before using either instrument. A hyphema was identified once the eyelids were opened. Computerized tomography revealed a floor fracture (see Fig. 70.4b)

[1]. While CT scans are excellent at imaging bones and identifying most fractures, small linear fractures may not be visualized, and the degree of soft tissue herniation into bone defects may be difficult to assess [2–4].

The fractured orbital floor (Fig. 70.4a) may appear as an inferiorly displaced plate of bone with one or more fragments The fractured bone may also appear depressed into the maxillary sinus but hinged medially with soft tissue herniation inferiorly (open trapdoor, Fig. 70.4b) or as a linear fracture line, with or without soft tissue herniation into the maxillary sinus (closed trapdoor, Fig. 70.4c) [5, 6]. An analogous clinical and imaging picture may occur with medial orbital wall fractures associated with pain and/or diplopia on horizontal gaze. The linear fracture presentation may occasionally be missed by the radiologist and the CT scan reported as normal [7]. This closed trapdoor picture is particularly dangerous in the pediatric group as muscle entrapment with a compartment syndrome and potentially ischemic contracture of the inferior (or medial) rectus may occur if the tissues are not released quickly (within 1–3 days) [2, 7–15]. The CT scan appearance should be assessed taking into consideration the patient's clinical presentation. In some cases the radiologist's CT scan interpretation may not correlate with the clinical situation (e.g., a fractured orbital floor that has swung back into position and does not appear fractured – a closed trapdoor) [4, 9–11, 15]. In a recent study, more than 50% of children had entrapment of orbital soft tissue that was not appreciated by the radiologist on the CT scan [4, 15]. Entrapment is therefore more of a clinical diagnosis than a radiological one [4]. Orbital CT imaging may reveal clues consistent with an occult fracture such as adjacent opacification from hemorrhage in the sinus. Subtle tenting of the inferior (or medial) rectus muscle or soft tissues incarceration within the fracture site may not be easily recognized, or depending on the degree of imaging resolution may not be detectable.

Parbhu et al. found that there was good correlation between imaging evidence of entrapment as noted by the radiologist and the intraoperative findings of entrapment in the adult group (concordance 87%) but less so with the pediatric group (concordance rate 50%) [4]. In the latter, the importance of noting soft tissue entrapment is especially relevant given the consequences of the closed trapdoor-type fracture that often occurs in this population [2, 8–10, 13, 15, 16]. This highlights the importance of a good clinical examination, to detect any limitation of motility suggesting the presence of entrapment and possible need for urgent surgical intervention [2, 7, 10].

The absence or minimal findings of entrapment by CT in patients with small fractures have been observed by other authors as well [2, 3, 7, 10, 11, 15]. The value of magnetic resonance imaging (MRI) was reported in a prospective study by Freund et al. [3]. Thirty consecutive patients with isolated orbital trauma underwent MRI and CT scanning. The authors noted that MRI had a similar sensitivity as CT in demonstrating orbital floor fractures but was superior to CT in showing soft tissue herniations [3].

In summary, although CT scanning is the modality of choice in the trauma setting, it is important to recognize its limitations in detecting entrapment of soft tissue, including the rectus muscles, in trapdoor fractures [4, 15]. It is important for the evaluating clinician to identify examination findings consistent with a clinically significant orbital fracture (diplopia or pain worsened on vertical or horizontal ductions) and to personally review the orbital CT images for evidence of an occult fracture [4, 10].

Buckling Theory Versus Hydraulic Theory

When an eye is struck forcibly by a large blunt object such as a fist or ball of greater dimension than the orbital aperture, the risk of globe rupture is less than with smaller objects. When the force of the injury is transmitted more widely to the periorbital structures, the thin bones of the orbital floor and/or medial wall are at risk for blowout fracture. The most

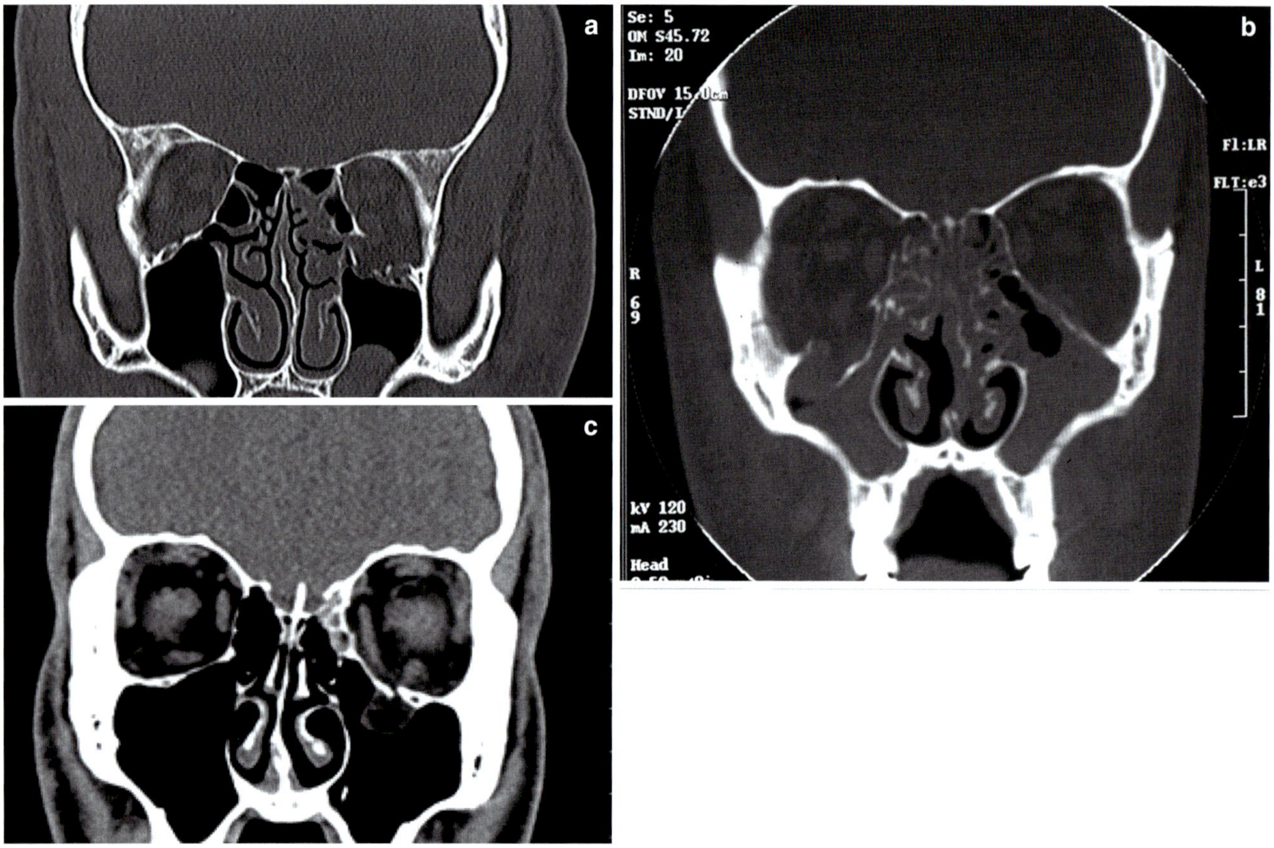

Fig. 70.4 (**a**) Fractured orbital floor may appear as an inferiorly displaced plate of bone with one or more fragments. (**b**) Fractured orbital floor, hinged medially with soft tissue herniation into sinus – open trapdoor. (**c**) Fractured orbital floor appears as a linear fracture line, with soft tissue herniation into sinus – closed trapdoor

commonly fractured wall of the orbit is the floor [1]. There is controversy as to the mechanism of these fractures [4, 9, 15, 17, 18]. According to the "buckling" theory, there is a blow to the orbital rim with sufficient force transmitted to the orbital floor which then fractures [17, 18]. In the "hydraulic" theory, it is believed that the force transmitted to the orbital floor occurs secondarily from the globe and orbital soft tissues [17, 18]. With this theory, a blowout fracture acts like a pressure release valve. The force of the blow to the eye raises the intraorbital pressure which is transmitted by the elastic ligaments, connective tissues, and fat of the orbit to the surrounding orbital bones. This pressure release valve mechanism is thought to provide some protection of globe integrity during orbital trauma, accidents, and altercations. It is likely that components of each of the above described mechanisms may contribute to the development of orbital floor and medial wall fractures. Orbital fat, connective tissue, extraocular muscle (inferior rectus/inferior oblique/medial rectus), or any combination of these structures may become herniated or entrapped within a fracture site.

Management

Fractures of the orbit are common in the facial trauma patient, and several surgical specialties may be involved in the management of these injured individuals. These fractures may be isolated to the orbital floor or medial orbital wall or may have associated orbital rim or adjacent bone (zygoma, maxilla, nasal, frontal) involvement. The varied spectrum of orbital fracture presentations, the involvement of numerous surgical specialties each with its own literature, and some disagreements within respective specialties have contributed to inconsistencies in the management of orbital fractures, particularly those involving the orbital floor [7, 8, 10, 19–31]. Over the past seven decades, recommendations have ranged from surgical repair of all fractures within 2 weeks to observation of all fractures for 4–6 months prior to intervention [19, 20, 24, 26]. Current controversies in the management of orbital floor fractures began following the presentation by Converse of his techniques in 1944 [32]. Two schools of thought evolved: one suggesting early surgical management (within 2 weeks) to restore normal orbital volume and anatomic relationships [26–29] and another favoring a more conservative, wait-and-watch management (4–6 months) [32–34]. Widely accepted indications for early surgery (within the first 2 weeks) include symptomatic diplopia (with positive forced ductions) and CT evidence of muscle entrapment without clinical improvement over 1–2 weeks; early enophthalmos of 2 mm or more; significant hypoglobus; a large orbital wall defect (more than 50% of the floor, substantial medial orbital wall involvement, or a combined floor and medial orbital wall defect) likely to result in late enophthalmos; or associated orbital rim or facial fractures with significant displacement [19, 20, 35, 36]. The indications for conservative observation without treatment include minimal diplopia with good motility with evidence of clinical improvement over several weeks, and without clear CT evidence of muscle entrapment; absence of significant enophthalmos or hypoglobus; and a small- to moderate-sized bone defect not likely to result in late enophthalmos [20, 36]. The two schools of thought have differed primarily in the determination of fracture severity that requires repair, in the importance of always releasing nonmuscular soft tissue incarceration and in the importance of restoring the orbital bone to near normal volume and contour [20]. While a dichotomy of approach remains, surgical intervention within 2 weeks for most cases with the aforementioned indications is well accepted and widely practiced [19–25].

With the exception of pediatric trapdoor fractures with muscle entrapment (the "white-eyed blowout" – discussed later) [2, 7–10], initial observation is recommended in each of the two management strategies (early vs late), to allow for improvement of orbital/periorbital edema, ecchymosis, and hemorrhage which may conceal motility deficits and signs of tissue entrapment, hypoglobus, and orbital volume deficits that may not otherwise be evident [20]. In the early management philosophy, if no improvement is seen within the first 2 weeks, surgical repair of the orbital floor or medial wall defect is felt to be important to restore normal orbital volume relationships [19, 20]. The herniated tissue (fat, muscle, connective tissue) is returned to its orbital position, and it is anticipated that ocular motility will improve (Fig. 70.5a–c). In the late management approach, Putterman and others suggest that in the majority of patients with orbital floor fractures, the orbital fat is entrapped rather than the inferior rectus muscle [26, 28, 29, 36]. They postulate that motility improves with time after an untreated blowout fracture as a result of resolution of edema and hemorrhage and stretching of the fat and connective tissue [36]. The patients who do not have resolution of their diplopia may either have their inferior rectus muscle entrapped within the maxillary sinus or possible injury to the rectus muscle or motor nerves [34]. Residual diplopia and enophthalmos is managed after 4–6 months if these symptoms are of concern to the patient (Fig. 70.6a–d) [20, 34–36].

In an editorial discussing the orbital fracture management, Kersten et al. [30] reviewed the two primary issues driving the ongoing debate, namely, the indications for surgical repair and the timing of intervention. Although there are no prospective, randomized clinical trials to help guide decision-making, review of the natural history of untreated orbital blowout fractures [26, 28–31, 37–44], surgeon experience [30, 31], and radiological studies showing a decrease in fracture size with time [45, 46] have influenced some to reconsider the indications for orbital fracture repair and suggest another paradigm shift to a more conservative approach for many of the adult blowout fractures [30, 47]. Kersten et al. emphasized that good results can be obtained when operating on fractures with persistent diplopia or enophthalmos, even when surgery is delayed well beyond the 2-week window [10, 30, 31, 38–43, 47]. Kasee et al. [44] recently found in 72 patients with blowout fractures followed without surgery that diplopia resolved in all but 1 patient by 6 months after injury, confirming what Putterman described over 40 years ago [26, 29, 36]. Nishida et al. [48] also found diplopia resolved in all unoperated patients by an average of 7 weeks after injury with a range of 19–143 days. In addition, multiple authors have found late enophthalmos is rare (even in the case of large fractures >50%), and it is difficult to predict from imaging studies in which patients it will develop [10, 30, 49–52]. In a recent study by Young et al. [45, 46], the authors observed that the size of an unoperated fracture on imaging often decreases over time as the initial traumatic edema resorbs and bone remodels [45]. Silverman et al. [52] have also reported on a prospective multicenter trial in which large fractures were observed for up to 6 months after injury. Of 46 patients enrolled, 37 patients did not demonstrate enophthalmos of 2 mm or more. Of the nine patients who did demonstrate significant enophthalmos, only 50% were sufficiently concerned with their appearance to consider surgical repair [30, 52]. With respect to orbital floor fracture patients with persistent double vision at 2 weeks post injury and beyond; some studies have found that delayed surgery may have a lower chance of curing symptomatic diplopia [53–55], but other studies (from several surgical disciplines) have found similar rates of resolution of double vision in early versus delayed intervention [30, 38–43]. With these observations in mind as well as clinical experience over several years, Kersten et al. believe it is time to reconsider the old paradigm of performing surgical repair of large fractures (>50%) or those associated with persistent diplopia within 2 weeks of injury [30, 47]. It has been their practice for several years to divide orbital floor fracture patients into two groups: the smaller group of patients (typically less than 25 years old) with trapdoor fractures and marked limitation of ductions (i.e., the white-eyed blowout fracture – discussed later) and the vast majority of other orbital fractures. In this latter group, they prefer a more prolonged observation

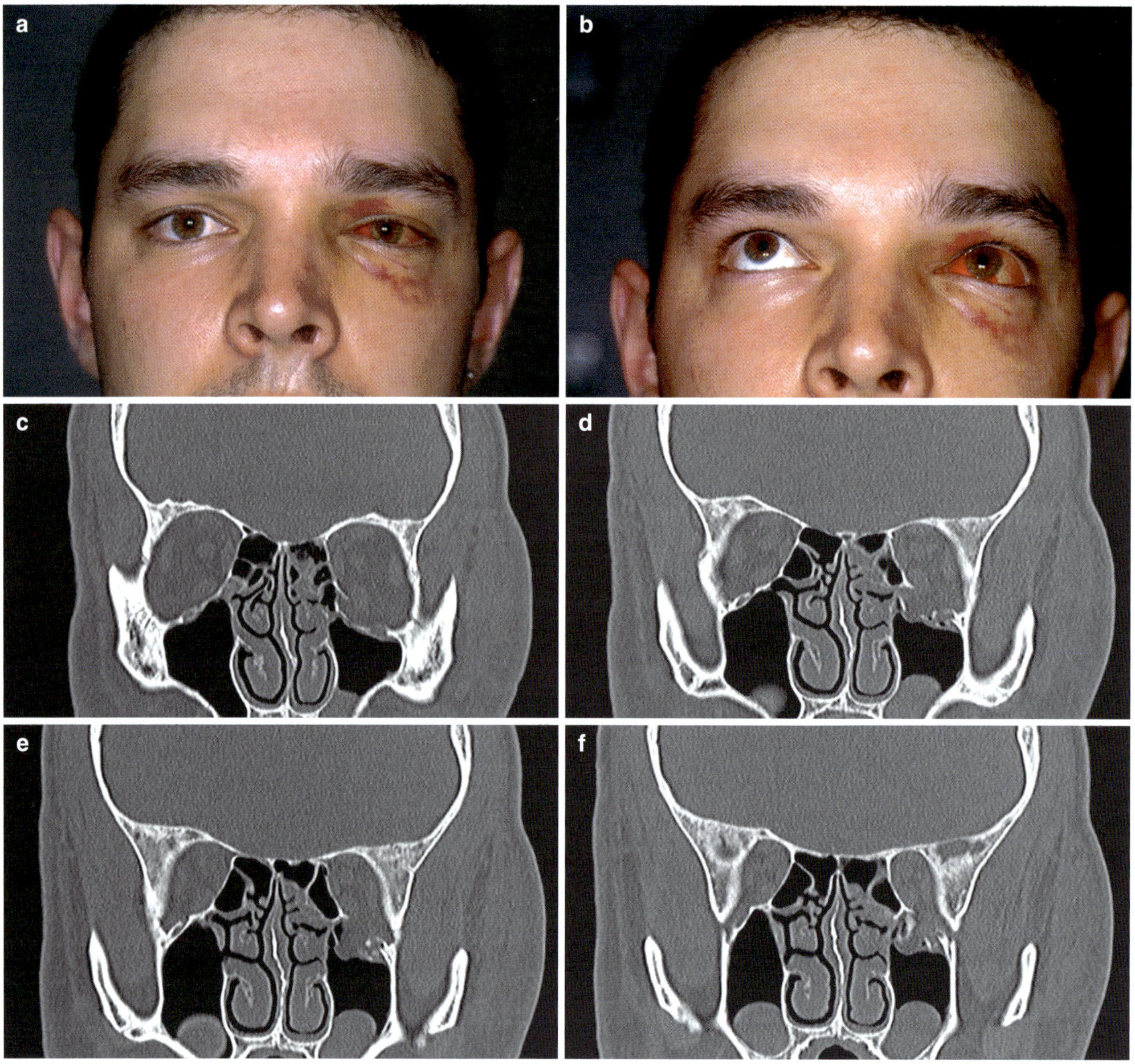

Fig. 70.5 (a, b) A 27-year-old male was seen 8 days following a blow (fist) to the left periocular area. Motility revealed −1 in upgaze and −2 in downgaze and was associated with enophthalmos (2 mm) and a large floor fracture (> than 50% of floor). Surgery was performed at day 12, postoperatively; he did well with full recovery

(6–8 weeks) to allow resolution of diplopia or development of significant enophthalmos [30, 47]. In those patients with diplopia, but without frank muscle entrapment, they reassure patients that their diplopia will typically resolve without surgical intervention, but should it persist, delayed surgery is still likely to achieve restoration of functional motility [30, 47]. Patients with large fractures can be reassured that the development of late enophthalmos is uncommon; however, if it occurs and late repair is needed, it can generally be accomplished without substantially increasing the risks of surgical complications [10, 30, 47].

A distinct and important subset of orbital floor fracture that requires earlier intervention than the guidelines discussed above is the so-called "white-eyed" blowout or small trapdoor fractures that typically occur in children and young adults (generally less than the age of 18–25 years) [2, 7–15]. With few clinical signs of soft tissue injury (i.e., the "white eye"), the potential severity of the clinical problem may not be appreciated leading to a delay in treatment. These patients often benefit from surgical release of the incarcerated orbital tissue within 1–3 days of injury, so prompt recognition is critical [7–10]. The history and clinical picture is quite distinct [2, 7–15]. The patients are young (generally less than 18–25 years of age) and have a significant trauma history but little clinical sign of soft tissue injury (little or no ecchymosis, little or no edema). Extraocular motility, however, is severely restricted (graded −3 or −4) in vertical gaze for fractures involving the orbital

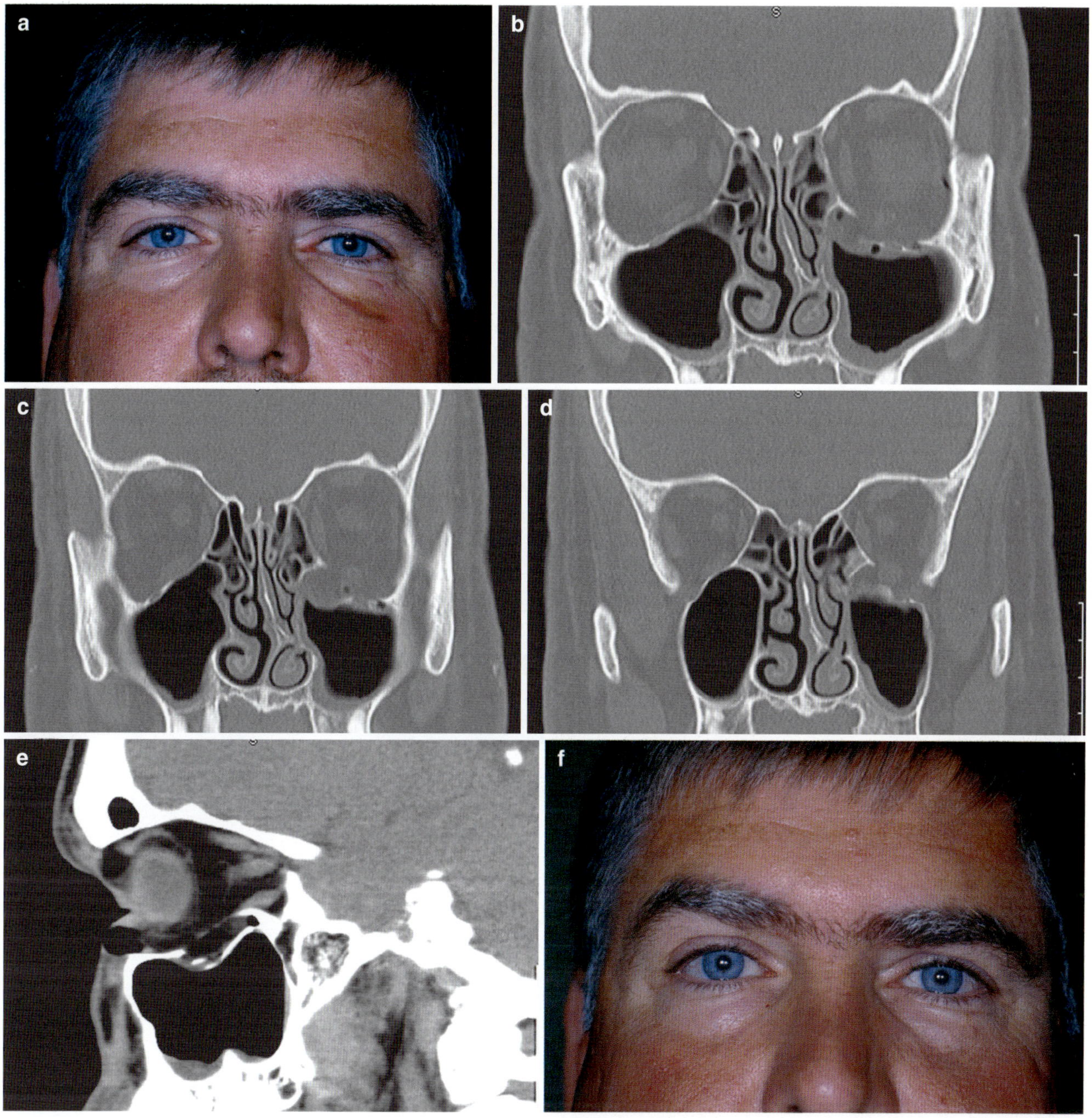

Fig. 70.6 (**a**) A 46-year-old male was seen 8 days following a tree branch blow to the left periocular area. Clinically there was some restriction in upgaze (−2) and downgaze (−2), 2 mm of enophthalmos, and no globe ptosis. The patient was happy to wait and observe. (**b–e**) Computerized tomography scan reveals a large floor fracture (50% of floor) with soft tissue herniation (fat) into the maxillary sinus. (**f**) At 3 months post injury, the patient had 3 mm of enophthalmos, full motility and was not bothered by the enophthalmos which was also difficult to detect clinically

floor and in horizontal gaze for medial orbital wall fractures resulting in marked diplopia. Substantial pain is often elicited in the affected field of gaze [7–9]. Vagal nerve stimulation may result in nausea and vomiting, and the oculocardiac reflex may be stimulated causing cardiac arrhythmias (e.g., bradycardia) [10, 56–59]. The patient's nausea (if present), rather than being taken as a sign of entrapment, may occasionally be attributed to the emotional reaction associated with the injury and of having to go to the emergency department [56].

Computed tomography scanning in this subset of patients reveals a small crack or trapdoor along the orbital floor or medial orbital wall with little or no bone displacement (closed trapdoor) often with a "teardrop" of tissue herniation into the adjacent maxillary (Figs. 70.4c and 70.7) or ethmoid sinus [4, 7, 10, 15] Occasionally, the inferior rectus muscle

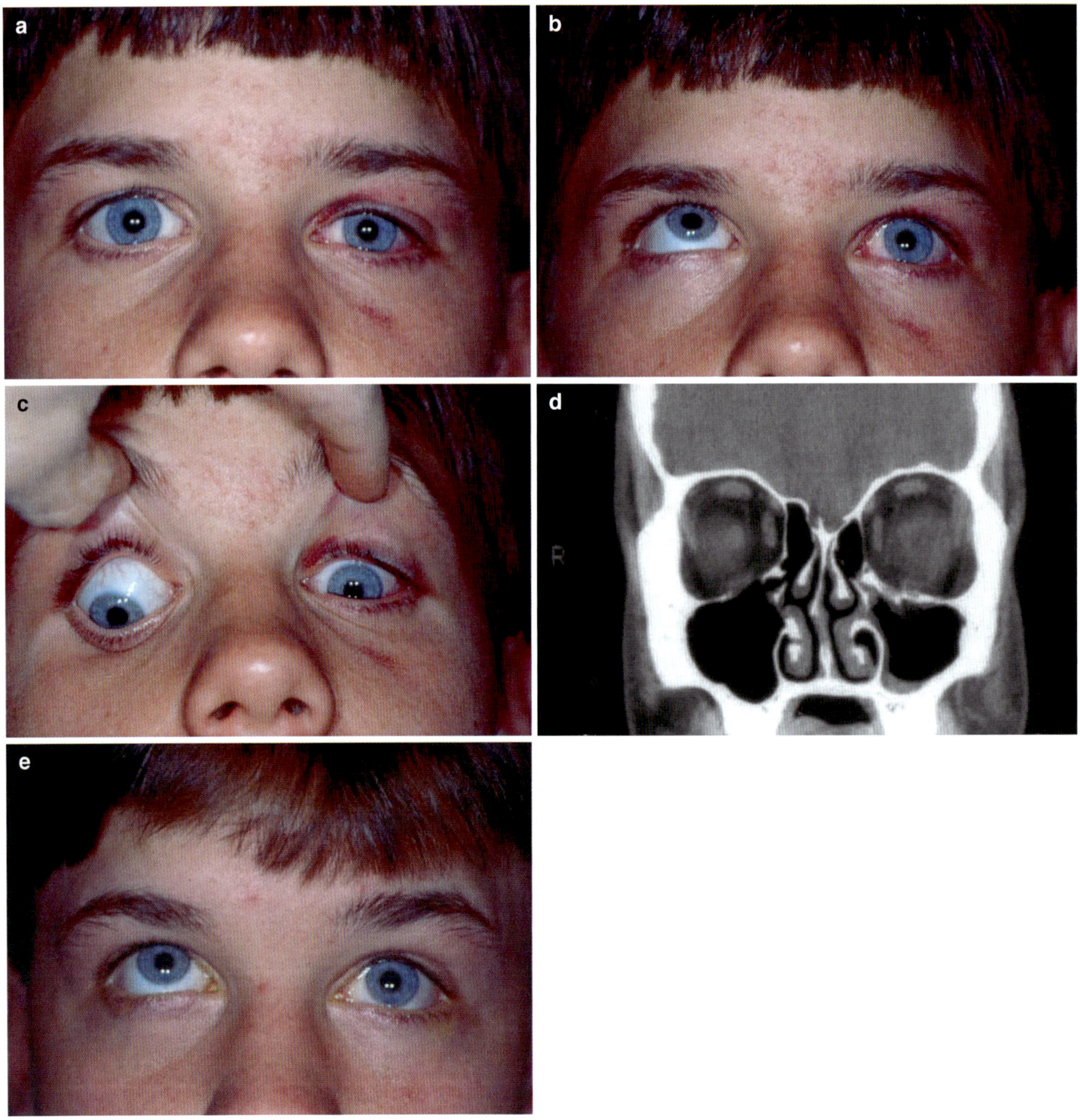

Fig. 70.7 (**a**–**c**) A 14-year-old male was seen 24 h following a blow to the left periocular area (fist). Clinically there was little sign of soft tissue edema and only mild ecchymosis but severe restriction of upgaze and downgaze (−4). (**d**) Computerized tomography scan revealed a linear crack on the orbital floor with minimal tissue herniation into the sinus. He was followed for 14 days and then taken to the operating room as the white-eyed blowout fracture had not been appreciated. (**e**) No improvement occurred following primary floor fracture repair or after re-exploration that was carried out 3 weeks post-op. He was left with permanent diplopia and muscle restriction

may not be visible within the orbit on the CT scan as it is buried within the tissue through herniating through the orbital floor (Figs. 70.8 and 70.9) [2, 4, 15].

Children have more flexible bones, and blunt trauma to the periocular region is more prone to result in a "greenstick-like" fracture into the adjacent sinus and a flexible "trapdoor" [7, 10, 11, 16]. The orbital floor or medial wall may spring back to a near normal position (closed trapdoor) entrapping tissue (muscle, connective tissue, fat or a combination of these soft tissue structures). Entrapment of the extraocular muscle and/or associated connective tissue may result in a compartment syndrome analogous to that described by Volkmann producing muscle ischemia, fibrosis, and restricted motility [60, 61]. Volkmann's theory of ischemic contraction

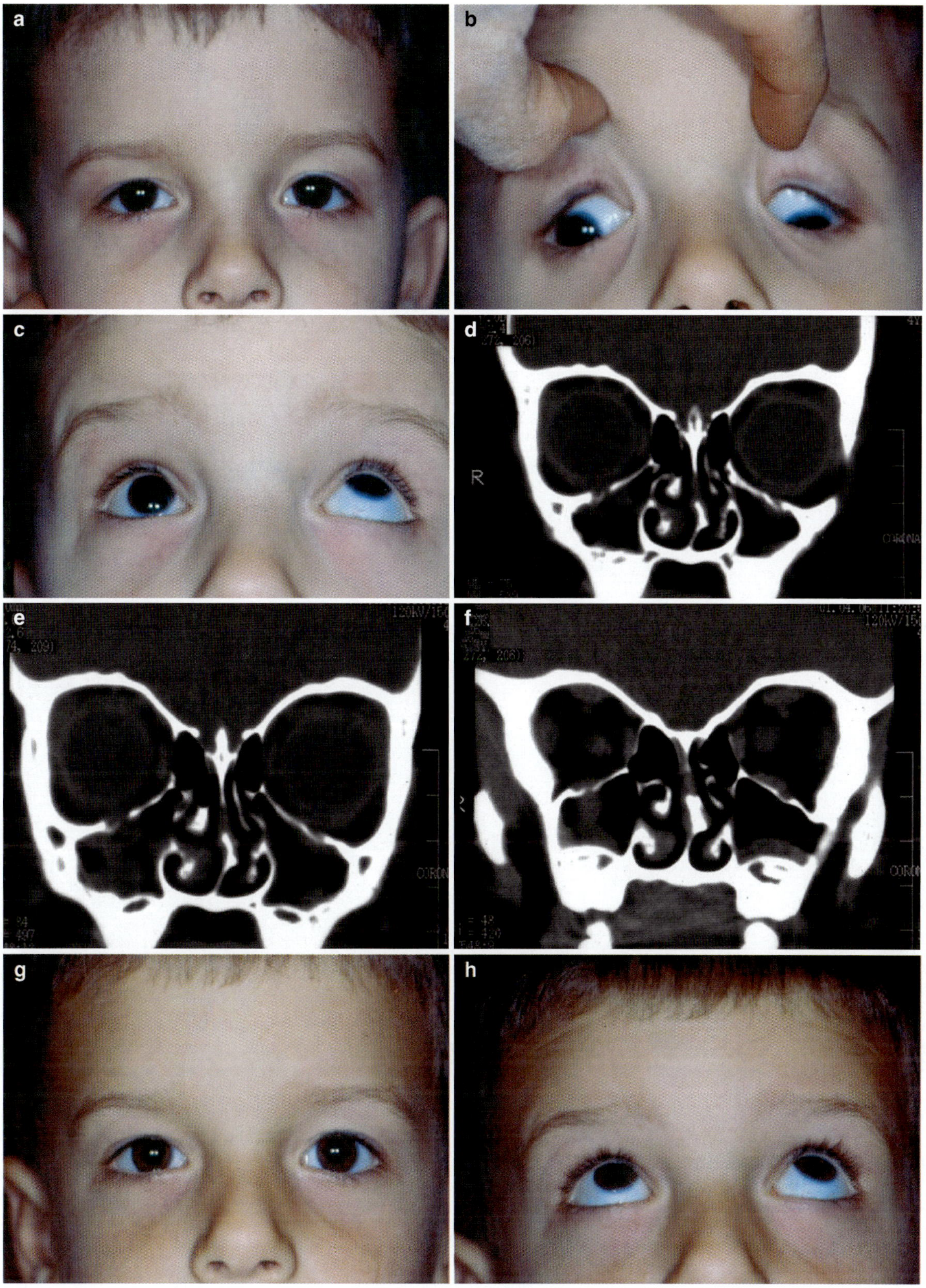

Fig. 70.8 (**a–c**) A 4-year-old male was seen 24 h following a blow to his right periocular area (knee) while jumping on the bed. He had some nausea and underactivity in upgaze (−3) and downgaze (−2). (**d**, **e**) Computerized tomography scan revealed an orbital floor that appeared to be intact (closed trapdoor) with a small teardrop of tissue within the sinus. (**f**) The inferior rectus is almost nonexistent in the orbit on this cut when compared to the opposite normal side. Urgent surgery (within 24 h of presentation) was carried out to repair the white-eyed blowout floor fracture and relieve the vagal symptoms of nausea and vomiting. (**g**, **h**) Postoperatively the child made a full recovery with motility back to normal within 4 weeks

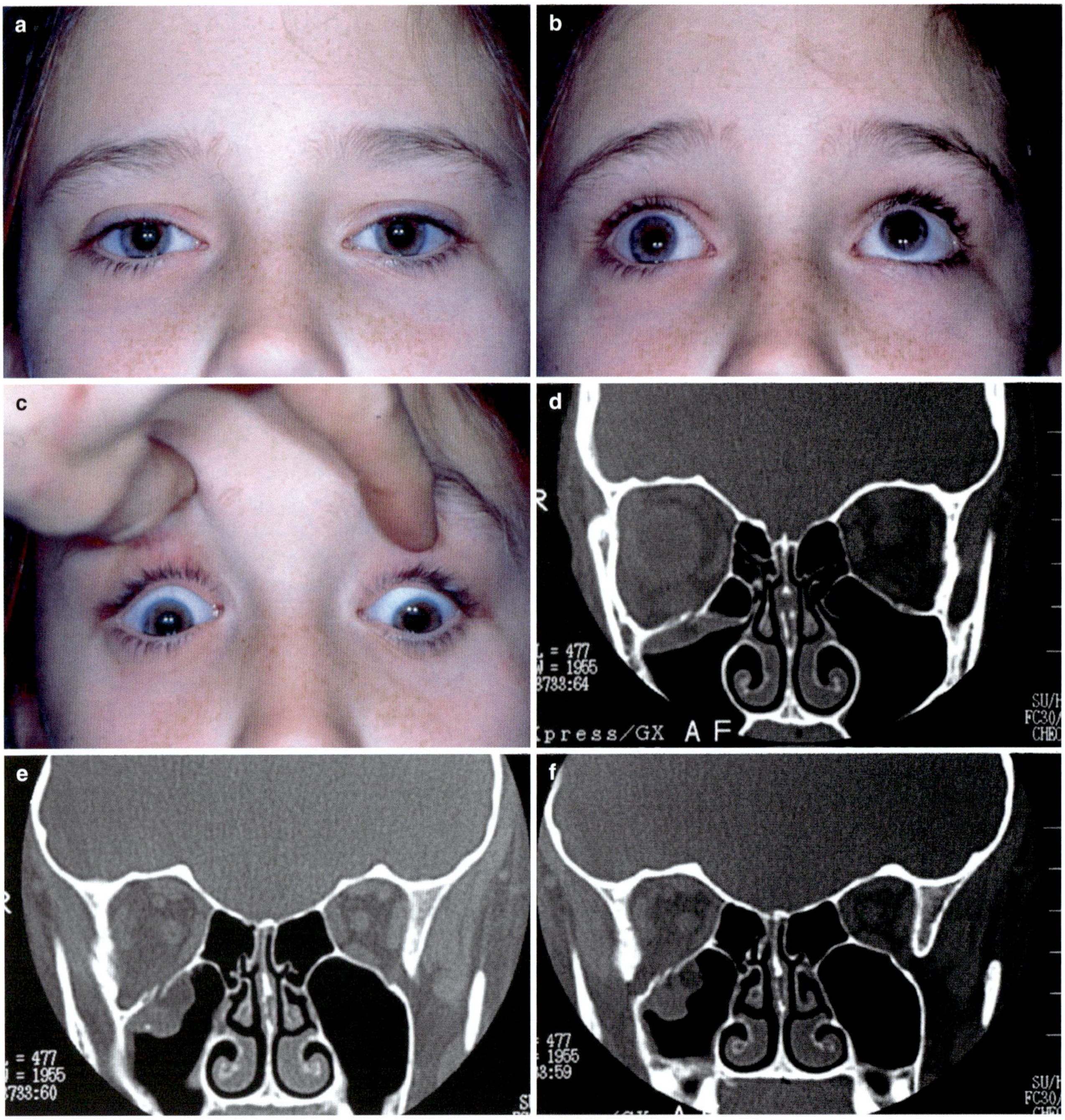

Fig. 70.9 (**a**) A 12-year-old female was seen 5 days after a sledding injury in which her knee hit the Rt periocular area. She was initially seen in Emergency and had vomiting and pain when moving her eyes. Over the subsequent 2 days, double vision was noticed, and she was referred to Ophthalmology. (**b**, **c**) Clinically, there was underactivity in upgaze (−3) and downgaze (−3). (**d**) Computerized tomography scan revealed a small crack (closed trapdoor) on the floor and herniated tissue within the sinus. The inferior rectus was initially present (**d**) and then absent on several cuts of the Ct (**e**, **f**) and then showed up toward the orbital apex (9**g**). The patient was taken to the operating room later that day (day 5 post injury) and had the floor fracture repaired. At the time of surgery, the floor was simply depressed downward while the orbital contents were repositioned. The floor came back to its normal position, and no implant was used. Postoperatively she improved dramatically. (**h**–**j**) At 6 months she had −1 in upgaze on the right that resolved by 1 year

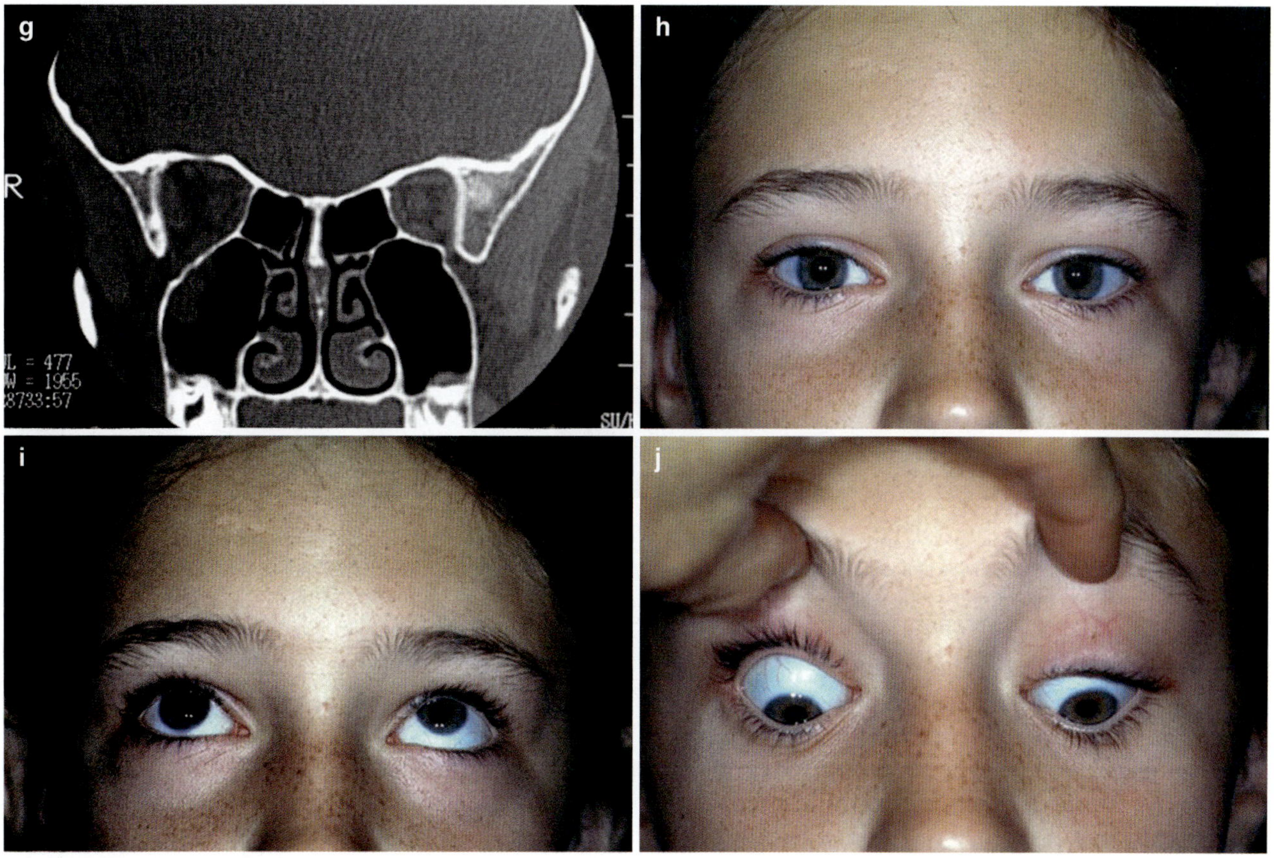

Fig. 70.9 (continued)

is dependent on the formation of a compartment around a muscle group. Such a compartment around the extraocular muscles has been demonstrated by the orbital dissection work of Koorneef [62].

There is a potential space around each extraocular muscle with a delicate network of fibrous and connective tissue septa. Attempts to measure pressure within this potential space both before and during surgery in normal muscle repeatedly indicate that no significant increase in pressure usually exists [60]. When the same technique is used to measure compartmental pressures during the period immediately after floor fractures of the orbit, some but not all of the patients exhibit high compartment pressures around the inferior rectus. Smith et al. suggest that small fractures are more likely to develop high inferior rectus compartment pressures [60]. If this Volkmann-type compartment syndrome is not relieved surgically, diplopia may be persistent. Furthermore, patients with compartment syndrome may be more likely to develop muscle paresis as demonstrated by saccadic velocities [60]. Smith et al. were able to demonstrate a definite cause-and-effect relationship between high compartment pressure (paresis-induced diplopia) and persistent motility abnormalities [60]. Those patients who required surgery in the face of a high compartment pressure and diplopia developed persistent diplopia. These muscles were later found to be fibrotic at extraocular muscle surgery.

When promptly recognized, release of the incarcerated rectus muscle within the first few days of the injury increases the likelihood of muscle recovery and eventual resolution of diplopia (Figs. 70.7a–e, 70.8a–h, and 70.9a–j) [2, 7–15]. If there is an associated arrhythmia as a result of the oculocardiac reflex being stimulated, surgery should be performed as soon as possible and the patient closely monitored until any arrhythmias have resolved [10, 56–59]. Urgent repair of white-eyed blowout fractures is important due to progressive tissue ischemia and potentially resultant muscle fibrosis (with permanent motility restriction) that occurs when the incarcerated tissue (rectus muscle, connective tissue, fat, or a combination) is entrapped for a prolonged period of time [7, 10, 11].

This management is in contrast to the adult with mature bone structure (typically >25 years old) where the bones are more mature, more brittle, and less flexible. Blunt periorbital trauma in these patients commonly produces a "blowout" of involved bone fragments toward the maxillary antrum (in orbital floor fractures) rather than remaining hinged medially and springing back in trapdoor fashion as previously discussed. An inferiorly displaced plate of bone with one or

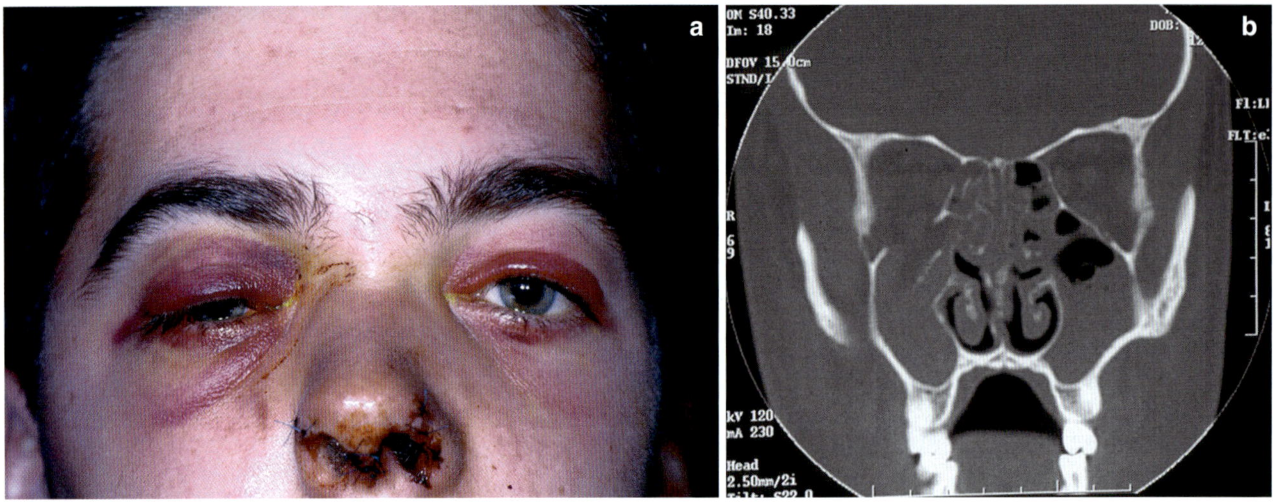

Fig. 70.10 (**a**) A 25-year-old male sustained a blow to the face when the air bags of his car deployed during a motor vehicle accident. He was seen 16 h post injury and had restriction in upgaze (−2) and downgaze (−2), infraorbital anesthesia and 2 mm of globe ptosis. (**b**) Computerized tomography showed a large floor fracture (>50%) with a depressed plate of bone sitting within the maxillary sinus. The patient underwent successful repair of the fracture 9 days post injury with resolution of the double vision

more associated fragments is commonly seen in the maxillary antrum (Figs. 70.5c–f, 70.6d, e, and 70.10b). Orbital soft tissue potentially including one or more extraocular muscles may herniate into the adjacent sinus cavity often resulting in motility restriction. A trapdoor fracture and associated compartment syndrome affecting an involved extraocular muscle occasionally occur in adult patients (Fig. 70.11b–e), and timely diagnosis and treatment might lead to a more favorable prognosis [37, 63]. White-eyed medial wall orbital blowout fractures with soft tissue herniation into the ethmoid sinus or those associated with an oculocardiac reflex (and potential arrhythmias) also benefit from early surgical intervention [64–66]. The oculocardiac reflex (and potential arrhythmias) may also be seen in adults with large, non-trapdoor-type orbital fractures without obvious extraocular muscle entrapment [67–69]. If present, emergent surgical intervention may be required. The white-eyed type blowout fracture of the floor or medial wall as well any fracture patient experiencing an arrhythmia secondary to the oculocardiac reflex are important to be aware of as the management is quite different than the guidelines for blowout fracture repair described earlier in the "early versus late" management controversy. Inappropriate timing of the fracture repair in these situations may have permanent consequences (e.g., irreversible muscle fibrosis) or potentially fatal (e.g., death secondary to a fatal arrhythmia associated with the oculocardiac reflex) [56–59, 67, 68]. With little clinical sign of soft tissue injury (white eye), the potential severity of the child's clinical problem may not be appreciated initially, and they may simply be observed. The patient's nausea (if present), rather than being taken as a sign of entrapment, may be attributed to the accident and emotion associated with the trauma and having to go to the hospital [56]. The patient (especially the child) may not be cooperative enough to examine properly. If the CT scan simply shows a crack, with little or no tissue herniation, the child is not uncommonly sent home. When it is obvious that no clinical improvement is occurring, they are reexamined. However, the longer the herniated tissue stays within the fracture, the greater the likelihood of ischemic damage to the tissue with some degree of persistent diplopia [7, 9–11]. Similarly, if an oculocardiac reflex is present, the longer it persists, the greater the likelihood of a problem as a result of the potential arrhythmias that may occur [56–59, 67, 68].

In addition to the closed trapdoor fracture scenario described above, where the orbital floor springs back into position, entrapping tissue and creating a compartment syndrome, some younger patients may have a trapdoor type of fracture that does not snap back and remains displaced into the sinus (open trapdoor – Fig. 70.4b) or may present with a segment of bone displaced into the sinus with tissue herniation (Fig. 70.4a) as commonly seen in the adult patient [10]. In either instance, minimal external signs of trauma may be visible, and the need for surgery may be seen as less urgent [10]. However, if orbital soft tissue incarceration is causing significant motility restriction, earlier surgical intervention (within days of the injury vs waiting 2 weeks) may be of benefit even if the orbital fracture is an open trapdoor or displaced bone fragment(s) (Figs. 70.12a–e) [63].

Some authors have suggested that blowout fractures be considered a soft tissue injury, and the degree of soft tissue disruption and displacement should be taken into account when thinking about the timing of surgery [23]. Those blowouts with soft tissue injury are more vulnerable to permanent

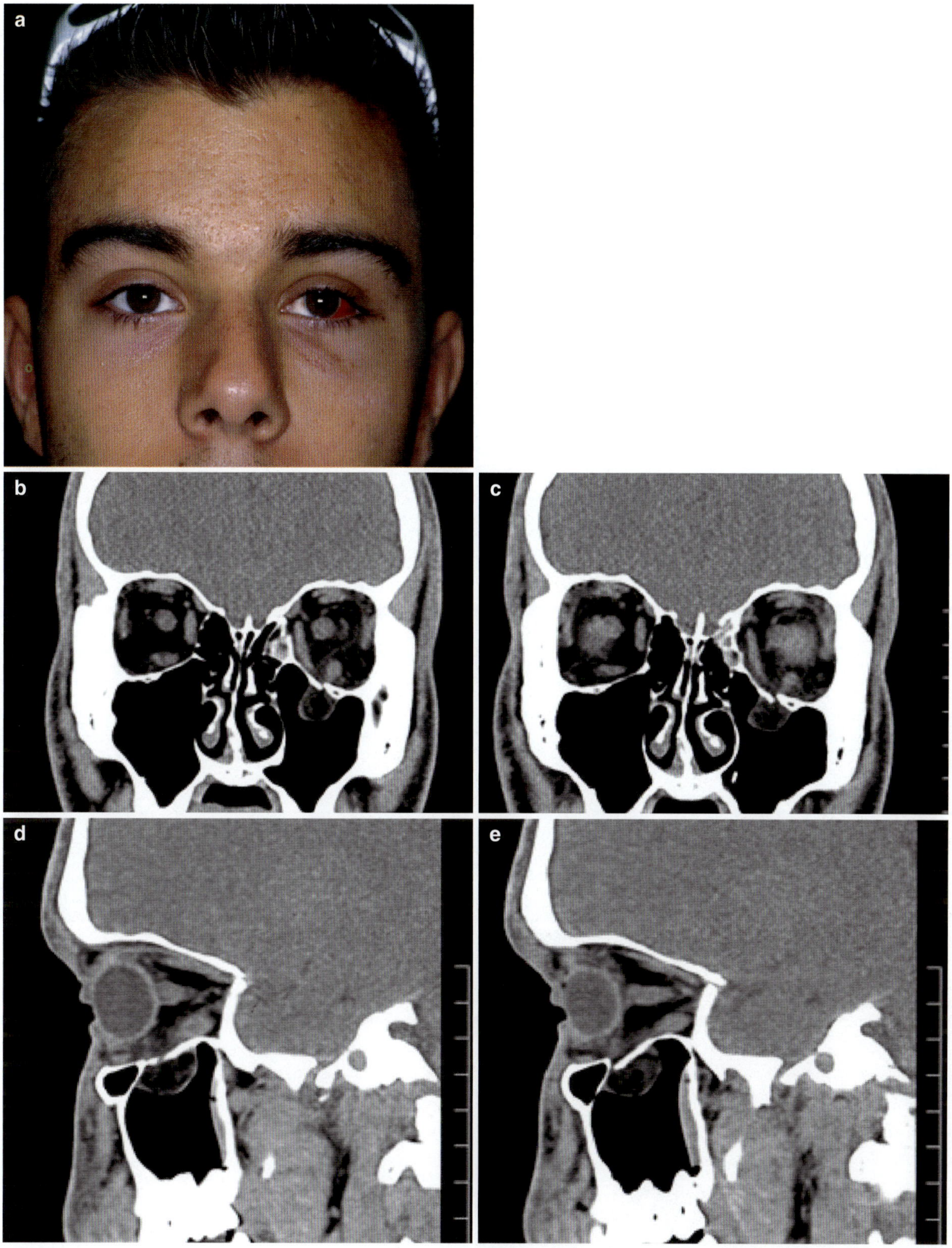

Fig. 70.11 (**a**) A 25-year-old male seen 2 days following a blow (fist) to the periocular area, complaining nausea and double vision in upgaze and downgaze. There was a subconjunctival hemorrhage but little in the way of eyelid edema or ecchymosis. The patient had restriction in upgaze (−2) and downgaze (−2), and the nausea was felt to be a vagal reaction. (**b**, **c**) Coronal CT scanning revealed a closed-type trapdoor with a great deal of tissue herniation and no enophthalmos. (**d**, **e**) Sagittal CT scan also revealed a closed trapdoor defect with tissue herniation into the sinus. The patient was taken to the operating room the following day. At the time of surgery, the floor was depressed, the contents were replaced, and the bone was simply placed back into position. No implant was required. His double vision resolved over the following 3 weeks

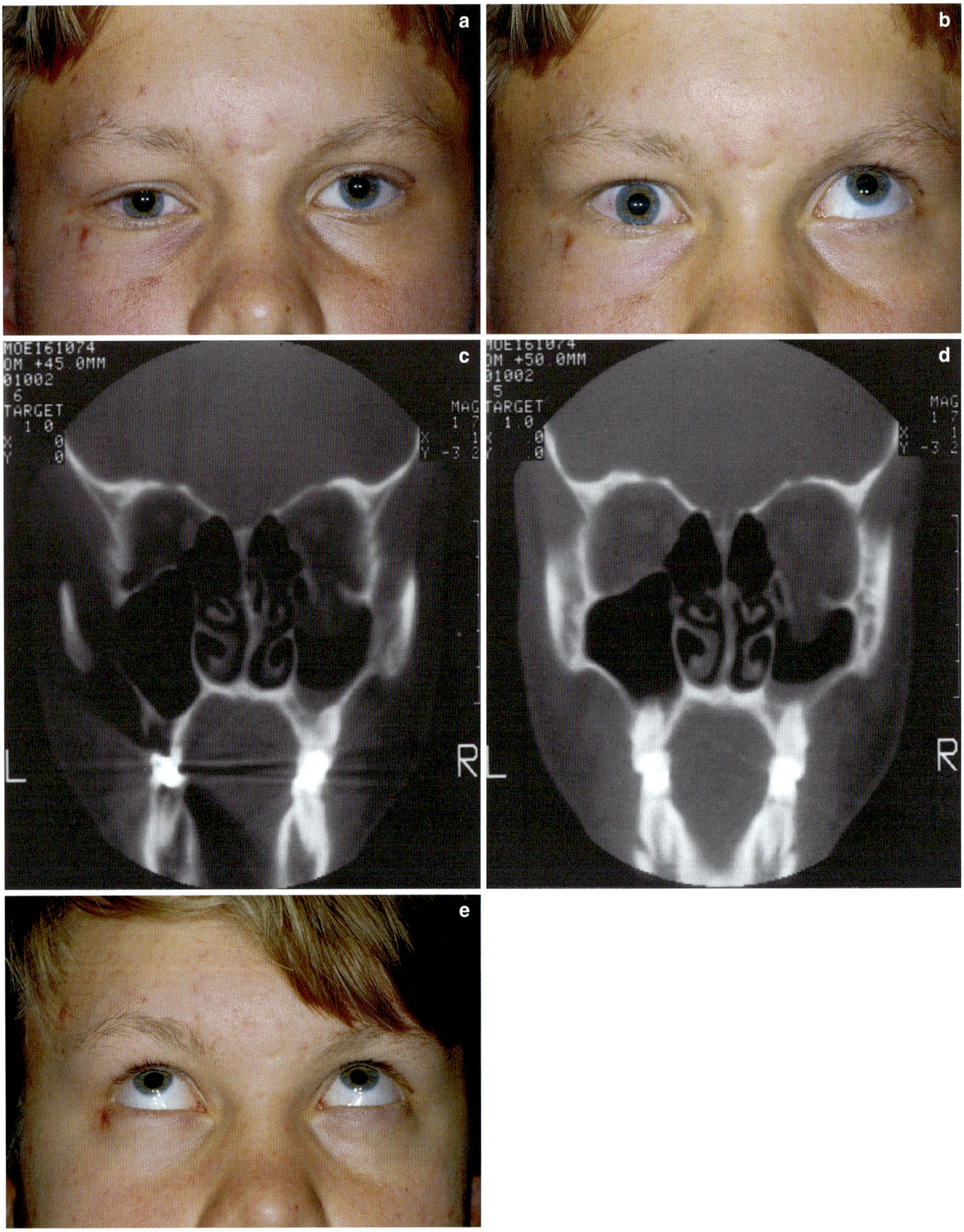

Fig. 70.12 (**a**, **b**) A 12-year-old male was seen 24 h following a blow to the right face (trampoline injury) with double vision and severe underactivity in upgaze (−4) due to soft tissue entrapment. (**c**, **d**) Computerized tomography scan revealed a floor fracture (open trap-door) with tissue herniation. The patient was taken to the operating room 4 days following the injury and had repositioning of the herniated tissue and an alloplastic floor implant. (**e**) Patient is seen 2 weeks post surgery and had full recovery of his motility

loss of function at any age. Greater degrees of soft tissue incarceration or prolapse with presumably greater intrinsic damage and subsequent fibrosis result in poorer motility outcomes despite complete release of the involved soft tissue [23]. Earlier intervention (less than 2 weeks) for such injuries might improve outcomes. The initial contusion, shearing, and laceration cannot be undone; early reversal of ongoing tissue crush or severe stretch might limit late fibrosis [23]. With this approach repairing a blowout fracture with significant tissue incarceration and motility restriction within a few days of injury (rather than waiting 2 weeks or more) may result in an improved recovery (assuming the periocular edema has cleared enough to allow an accurate clinical assessment) [63]. Orbital wall fractures with little or no soft tissue injury will often do better and many of these patients can be managed without intervention.

In summary, the management of orbital blowout fractures has been controversial for several decades and remains an area of significant ongoing debate [30, 31]. With a variety of orbital floor fracture presentations, it is important to guide the management approach based on the particular clinical and radiologic features associated with the injury. Isolated orbital floor and medial wall fractures not involving the orbital rim are often triaged differently than those involving the orbital rim, zygomaticotemporal, or nasoethmoidal structures [31]. The isolated floor fracture may be of the closed trapdoor variety with potential tissue incarceration, severe motility restriction, and substantial risk of muscle ischemia (the white-eyed blowout-type fracture more commonly occurring in children and young adults <18–25 years of age) (Figs. 70.4c, 70.7a–e, 70.8a–h, 70.9a–j, and 70.11a–e). Alternatively, an open trapdoor may be present with localized soft tissue herniation through the bone defect with potential enophthalmos, hypoglobus, and tissue entrapment without muscle strangulation resulting in functional diplopia (Figs. 70.3a, 70.4b, and 70.12a–e) [31]. Other patients may present with a displaced floor/medial wall fragment that may appear "punched out" with a free-floating segment of orbital wall bone evident in the adjacent sinus cavity with or without concomitant enophthalmos and/or motility deficit (Figs. 70.5a–f, 70.6a–f, and 70.10a, b).

With increasing awareness of the white-eyed blowout fracture clinical scenario [7, 10, 11, 36, 64, 65], the potential for the oculocardiac reflex to occur (and possible cardiac arrhythmias) in any fracture [56–59, 67, 68], as well as consideration of the degree of soft tissue injury [17], "current guidelines" for orbital fracture repair may be summarized as follows [2, 7–15, 23, 24, 26, 30, 31, 37, 56–59, 63, 67–72]:

1. Emergent surgery for those rare patients with globe luxation into the maxillary antrum [69–72].
2. Emergent surgery in the presence of a cardiac arrhythmia secondary to the oculocardiac reflex. Increased vagal tone may result in bradycardia, heart block, nausea, vomiting, hypotension or syncope, and potentially severe consequences (death) [10, 56–59, 67–69].
3. Surgery within the first few days (or as soon as can be coordinated) following the injury for those younger patients (generally children and young adults <18–25 years) with "white-eyed" blowout fractures of the orbital floor or medial wall and significant motility restriction and who have tissue entrapment (closed trapdoor configuration) on CT scan (Figs. 70.7, 70.8, 70.9, and 70.11) [2, 7–15, 64, 65]. If findings of the oculocardiac reflex are evident, more urgent release of the incarcerated tissue may be indicated as in #2 above [10, 56–59, 67–69].
4. Observation of 6–8 weeks for patients with mild/moderate diplopia, absence of significant motility restriction or clear signs of entrapment, and evidence of clinical improvement over the first few weeks following the injury (Fig. 70.6) [10, 30, 31]. The fractured orbital floor may appear as an inferiorly displaced plate of bone (Fig. 70.4a), hinged medially or laterally (open trapdoor configuration) with soft tissue herniation (Fig. 70.4b), or a linear fracture line with or without soft tissue herniation (closed trapdoor configuration) (Fig. 70.4c). These patients are reassessed once maximal symptomatic improvement is achieved. While historically the size of the floor or medial wall fracture (i.e., greater than 50%) or the presence of enophthalmos/hypoglobus (>2 mm) was considered an indication for surgery within 2 weeks of the injury (Figs. 70.5, 70.6, 70.10, and 70.13), these clinical and radiologic signs are no longer felt to be strong indications for earlier fracture repair.
5. Surgical consideration within 2–3 weeks following the injury for those cases with persistent, disabling diplopia, significant motility restriction, and no clinical sign of improvement. In some of these patients, the primary complaint and indication for surgery may be substantial pain on horizontal or vertical ductions consistent with soft tissue entrapment. There is generally CT evidence of rectus muscle entrapment and/or tissue herniation within the orbital wall defect (open trapdoor configuration on CT) (Fig. 70.12a–e). Early release of the incarcerated soft tissue may permit quicker resolution of debilitating symptoms than intervention months later [30, 38–43, 53–55]. In this group with clinically significant diplopia (± pain), repositioning of prolapsed tissue may also be technically less challenging with less intraoperative risk than surgical intervention 6–8 weeks or more after the initial insult. The risks and potential benefits of a longer wait and watch period are also discussed. The decision is not always clear and straightforward. Patient age, compliance, comorbidities, medications, occupation, and caregiver support are some of the additional considerations when discussing

surgical intervention versus continued observation. As in #4 above, we no longer use large fractures (>50% of the floor) or enophthalmos/hypoglobus (>2 mm) as an indication for surgery (Figs. 70.5 and 70.10) [10, 30, 31, 40]. If disfiguring enophthalmos/hypoglobus develops over time, surgical correction can be considered weeks or months later (Fig. 70.13a–i) [10, 30, 31, 40].

6. Observation is also recommended for another rare group of individuals; those patients with the unusual and sometimes difficult diagnosis to establish of inferior rectus muscle paresis – also benefit from close observation during the first several weeks following periorbital blunt trauma. An orbital fracture may or may not be evident on CT imaging. A positive forced generation test (limited duction in the direction of the involved rectus muscle) with a negative forced duction test.

Although late repair of orbital floor fractures (>2 months after trauma) has been shown to be less effective than repair performed before 2 months [53, 73], outcomes data are lacking for repairs performed 2–6 weeks after trauma. Recently, Dal Canto and Linberg [39] performed a retrospective review of orbital floor and/or medial wall fracture repairs and compared the results of patients undergoing early repair (less than 2 weeks) to those undergoing more delayed repair between 15 and 29 days (i.e., 3–4 weeks). They considered surgery beyond this time as "late" repair [39]. The author's results support delayed orbital floor and/or medial wall fracture repair (15–29 days after trauma) being as effective as early repair (less than 2 weeks) in regard to postoperative motility improvement and resolution of diplopia. This report has furthered the debate regarding the necessity of "early" orbital blowout fracture repair (Fig. 70.13a–i) [39]. Their study does not have implications for the "white-eyed" blowout fractures or complex midfacial fractures, zygomatico-temporal (tripod) factures, nasoethmoidal fractures, orbital roof fractures, or other orbital fractures not solely isolated to the orbital floor and/or medial wall [39]. The authors also emphasized that while delayed repair (15–29 days) was effective, surgery in this time frame is more technically challenging. They conclude that patients who present earlier and will predictably require surgery because of significant motility restriction should be considered for surgical repair within 1–2 weeks of the injury [39].

Surgical Technique for Orbital Floor Fracture Repair

After general anesthesia, forced duction studies may be done to confirm the degree of restriction and to help assess intraoperative tissue release. This may be done by directly grasping the inferior rectus muscle or passing a 4-0 silk suture through the inferior rectus insertion to recheck the forced ductions following repositing of the herniated orbital soft tissue and placement of an orbital floor implant. Surgeons should be aware of the possibility of intramuscular hemorrhage or localized hematoma formation following passage of the traction suture.

The lower eyelid and lateral canthal areas are injected with local anesthetic (50:50 mixture of lidocaine 2% with epinephrine 1:100,000 and bupivacaine 0.5% with epinephrine 1:200,000). The orbital floor may be approached through a subciliary incision or more commonly by the transconjunctival approach. A lateral canthotomy is accomplished with a full thickness cut through the lateral canthus to the lateral orbital rim (Fig. 70.14a). The inferior crus of the lateral canthal tendon is transected to initiate the swinging eyelid approach (Fig. 70.14b). Westcott scissors are utilized to incise the conjunctiva and lower eyelid retractors at the inferior tarsal edge from the lateral eyelid to the area just below the lower eyelid puncta (Fig. 70.14c). A 4-0 silk suture is placed centrally through the cut edge of the conjunctiva and lower eyelid retractors and placed on traction by attaching the silk to the forehead drape with a small clamp. Alternatively, the silk can be passed through the central gray line of the central upper lid and then clamped to the drape sheet above (Fig. 70.14d). The traction sutures should be released periodically during surgery to ensure adequate ocular perfusion and permit intraoperative examination of pupillary size and reactivity.

Sharp tissue dissection with a blunt-tipped Westcott or Stevens' tenotomy scissors as well as blunt dissection with cottontipped applicators is carried out in a sub-orbicularis muscle plane with orbital septum kept intact until the arcus marginalis is visualized. A Desmarres eyelid retractor is helpful during eyelid dissection and with providing exposure of the inferior orbital rim. An incision through the inferior orbital rim periosteum is made with a number 15 Bard Parker scalpel blade (Fig. 70.14e). The sharp edge of the periosteal elevator is used to reflect periosteum from its tight adherence to the inferior orbital rim and then from areas overlying intact bone medial and lateral to the orbital floor defect as far posterior as can be safely performed (generally at least to the mid-orbit). If the periosteal elevator is used further, the blunt end is utilized. A hand-over-hand soft tissue dissection technique using malleable orbit or brain retractors is performed to gently tease out the tissue herniating through the fracture site until all of the involved tissue is reposited. Cotton-tipped applicators may be helpful during this blunt dissection.

Once the entire orbital floor defect has been visualized, a floor implant (e.g., Suprafoil™, Teflon, Silastic, porous polyethylene, or other [74, 75]). Is placed over the fracture site to prevent prolapse of the orbital contents back into the maxillary sinus. The thickness of the floor implants ranges from 0.2mm to 0.75mm. The implant is trimmed down to a

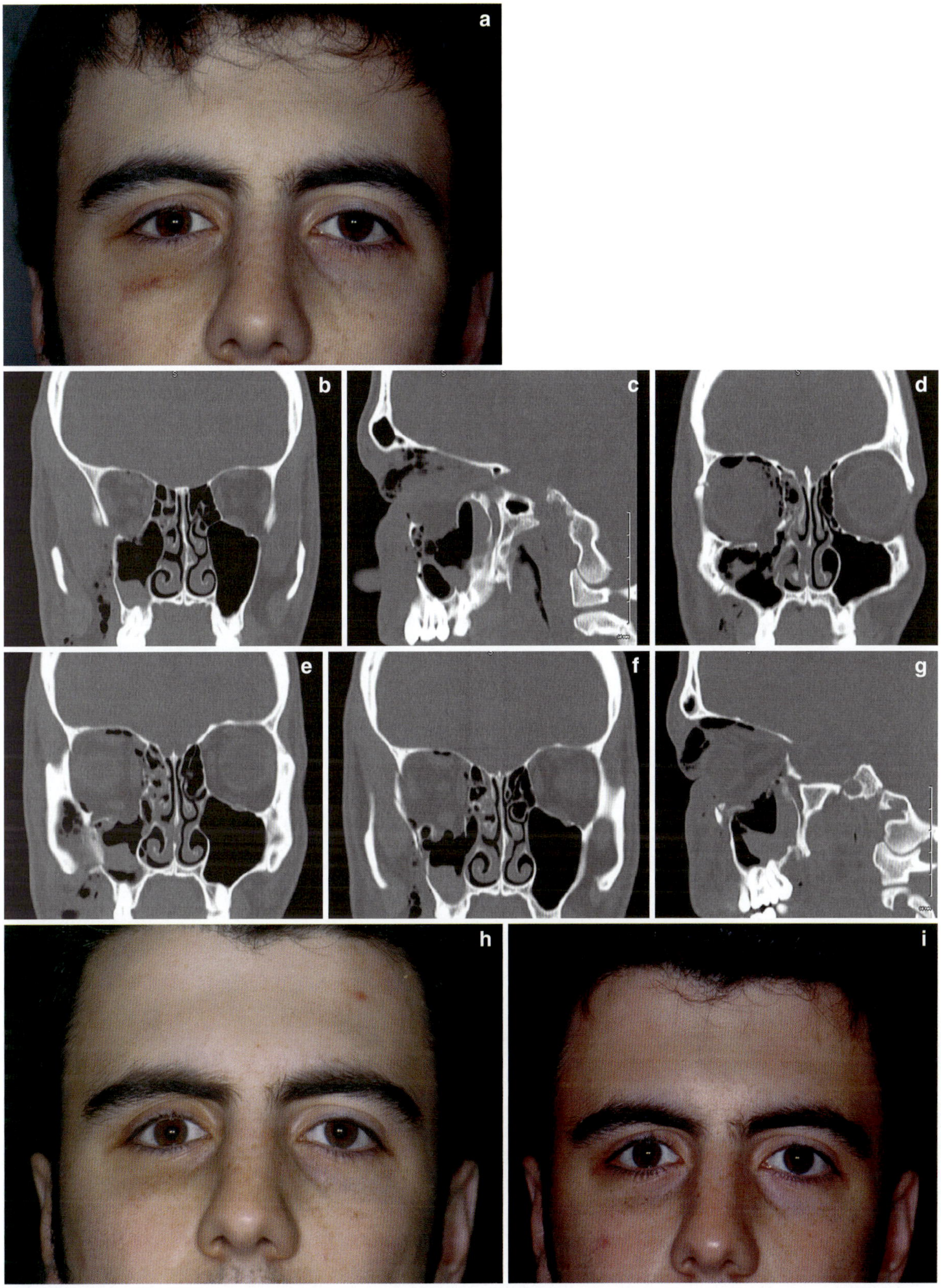

Fig. 70.13 (**a**) A 22-year-old male was seen 11 days following a blow to the right area. Clinically, there was minor underaction in upgaze (−1), the right globe was 1 mm ptotic and no enophthalmos was detected. (**b–g**) Computerized tomography scan revealed a large orbital floor fracture (>75%). The patient wanted to leave things be. (**h**) He was seen again at 20 days post injury with a deep superior sulcus, enophthalmos (2 mm), 2 mm of globe ptosis and full motility. He was bothered by the sunken appearance and decided to have surgery. Floor fracture surgery was carried out at 28 days post injury. (**i**) Postoperatively, he did well with full recovery

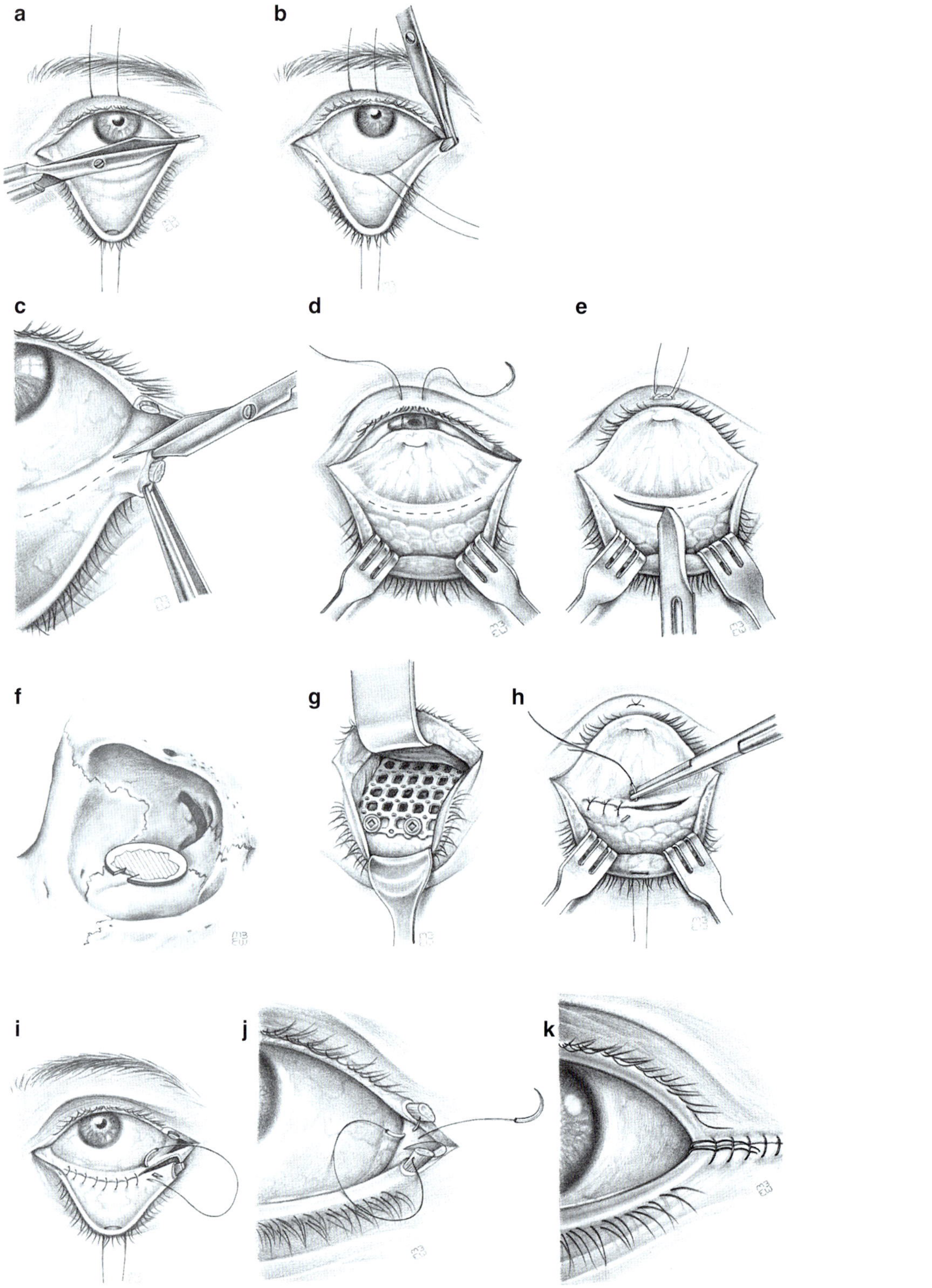

Fig. 70.14 (**a**) Lateral canthotomy. (**b**) Inferior lateral cantholysis. (**c**) Severing the eyelid conjunctiva and lower eyelid retractors from the inferior edge of tarsal plate. (**d**) A 4-0 silk, double-arm suture is passed through the lower eyelid conjunctiva and retractors and then to the forehead (some pass it through the upper eyelid and then to the forehead). (**e**) Periosteum over the inferior orbital rim is incised. A periosteal elevator is used to elevate periorbita away from the floor. Malleable retractors are used in a hand-over-hand technique to expose the orbital floor fracture and lift the orbital contents back into the orbit. (**f**) An alloplastic implant is placed over the floor fracture. A small tongue of tissue has been fashioned to slip inside the fracture and help secure it. (**g**) Titanium orbital floor implant as an alternative. (**h**) Periosteum is closed with absorbable sutures. (**i**) The conjunctiva is generally sutured to the inferior edge of tarsal border with a few 6-0 or 7-0 plane sutures. A sutureless closure is another possibility. (**j**) The lower eyelid tarsal plate is reanastomosed with the remaining superior crus of the lateral canthal tendon. (**k**). Skin is closed laterally with 1–3 sutures using a fine absorbable suture

size that will just cover the bone defect, often resulting in an implant shaped-like guitar pic. Fixation of the implant may or may not be necessary as the overlying soft tissue and underlying intact bone provide good fixation of an appropriately sized implant. If additional fixation is warranted, then two small cuts (4 mm depth and 2 mm apart) are made centrally in the anterior aspect of the implant [76]. The implant is placed over the fracture and the parts of the implant between the cuts (the tongue) are pushed downward into the sinus (Fig. 70.14f) to potentially minimize the risk of implant anterior migration. Cyanoacrylate glue can also be used to help keep the implant in position [77]. A variety of titanium plating systems are available but generally reserved for more extensive floor and medial wall fractures where there is inadequate bone support for a Suprafoil™ or porous polyethylene implant [78]. The implant may be secured directly to the orbital rim or via small microplate extensions (Fig. 70.14g) [78]. A historical and less optimal surgical technique used to repair orbital floor fractures is the Caldwell-Luc approach, in which the prolapsed orbital contents are elevated and then the maxillary sinus is packed with gauze. This approach is still performed by some otolaryngologists and oral maxillofacial surgeons.

After the implant is in place and forced duction studies have been satisfactorily repeated, the periosteum may be sutured over the orbital rim with interrupted, 4-0 polyglactin sutures (Fig. 70.14h). The importance of periosteal wound closure is not established, and many surgeons do not reapproximate the cut periosteum. Conjunctival wound closure is completed with a 6-0 plain or fast-absorbing gut suture or a 7-0 chromic suture using either a running or a simple, interrupted buried suture technique (Fig. 70.14i). Leaving the conjunctival wound unsutured is also an option [79]. The lateral canthal tissues are reapproximated with a 4-0 polyglactin suture passed through the lateral tarsal border and the superior crus of the lateral canthal tendon (Fig. 70.14j). Care is taken to not over tighten the lower eyelid in order to accommodate postoperative orbital edema and conjunctival chemosis. Skin wound closure is carried out with a few 6-0 plain gut sutures passed in interrupted fashion (Fig. 70.14k). If there is substantial risk of lower eyelid retraction (subciliary incision approach, additional lower eyelid trauma, or lacerations), then a 4-0 silk traction suture may be passed over a red rubber bolster and through the subciliary skin of the central lower eyelid exiting the meibomian gland orifices and then secured (taped) to the forehead. The patient and their caregivers should be aware of the importance of periodic release of the traction suture and regular visual acuity assessments following surgery.

The following surgical implant considerations are worth emphasizing [80]:

- Visualize the entire fracture margin prior to implant placement.
- Implants should be placed subperiosteally.
- The implant should cover the boundaries of the fracture without any residual tissue orbital tissue herniation.
- The implant should rest at least 3–4 mm posterior to the anterior orbital rim.
- The implant should not protrude into an adjacent sinus or about the nasolacrimal duct area.
- The edges of the implant should be smooth following customization.
- If forced duction testing repeated after implant placement appears to reveal continued restriction, the implant should be removed and resized or repositioned.
- Alloplastic implant complications, including those that may present years later, should be reviewed preoperatively with the patient and family (see below for further discussion).

Complications

Significant complications of orbital fracture repair have been reported in the literature including blindness, postoperative mydriasis, epiphora, worsening diplopia, cicatricial lower lid retraction, as well as problems with the implanted material (e.g., infection, extrusion, cicatricial eyelid changes) [19, 81–97]. Blindness is the most concerning complication with an estimated incidence of 1.0% [84]. The patient and their family should be made aware of this risk during the preoperative informed consent process [85, 86]. Blindness associated with orbital fracture repair has been attributed to retrobulbar hemorrhage (occurring within hours or up to several days following repair), malpositioned implant, optic nerve ischemia, or direct optic nerve injury [82–85]. Optic nerve ischemia and injury may result from vessel traction, compression, surgical sacrifice of vascular structures, thermal injury, mechanical/vibrating insults from drills/rongeurs, hypotension during anesthesia (or immediately postoperative), elevated intraorbital pressure resulting from bleeding or edema (compartment syndrome), or any combination thereof have also been implicated [85]. Those patients with multiple facial fractures undergoing surgical repair are at a higher risk of blindness (6.45%) [84]. Several factors may contribute to this increased risk, especially in severely traumatized orbit and midfacial injuries [85]. Traumatic optic neuropathy is more common in this group from the blow itself. The initial injury may then render the optic nerve more vulnerable to subsequent surgical or postsurgical insults [85]. Traumatic edema may be compounded by postoperative surgical edema and hemorrhage resulting intraorbital pressures that exceed optic nerve or retinal perfusion pressures [85]. Patients with cardiac or vascular disease (such as diabetes, hypertension) and a history of stroke or tobacco use may be at greater risk of sight-threatening perfusion-related complications.

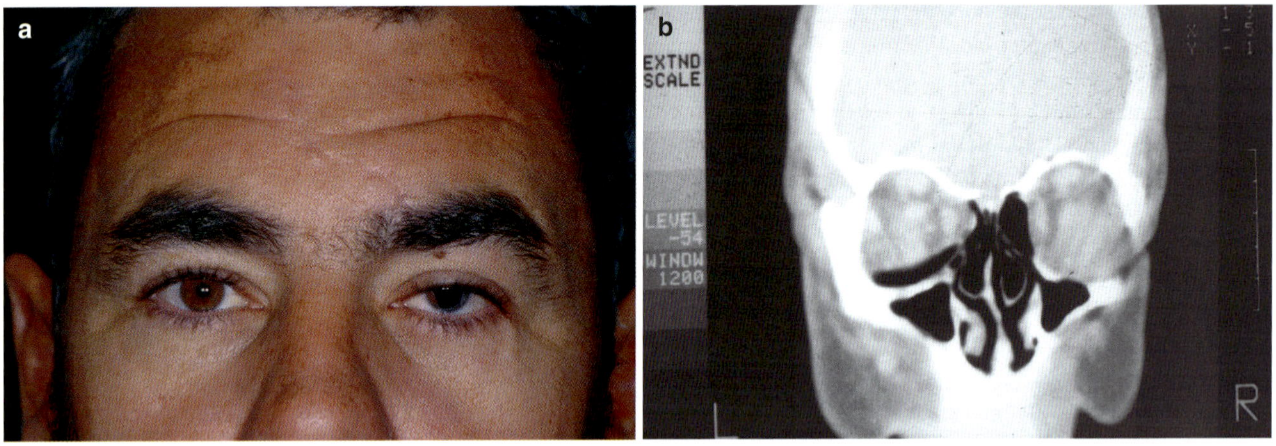

Fig. 70.15 (**a**) Eleven months post-orbital fracture repair, the patient presented with a pressure sensation in the socket during valsalva maneuvers while scuba diving. (**b**) Computerized tomography scan shows air along the orbital floor

There are certain precautions that should be followed to minimize the risk of vision loss following orbital fracture repair. Patients with coagulopathies or on anticoagulant medications should be co-managed with their treating physicians and counseled accordingly regarding the operative risks associated with surgery performed while taking medications that may impact clotting as well as the potential vascular risks of cessation of these medications (e.g., aspirin, anti-inflammatories, anticoagulants) [82, 85].

Intraoperatively, gentle manipulation of the orbital tissue, avoidance of undue pressure or traction on the globe and orbit, meticulous hemostasis, and headlight aided direct visualization can minimize the risk of injury to the optic nerve, retrobulbar hemorrhage, and orbital edema [85]. Properly sized, shaped, and positioned implants inserted under direct visualization also diminish these risks [82]. Avoidance of implant placement posterior to the posterior wall of the maxillary antrum is a wise surgical dictum as the orbital apex narrows substantially in this region placing the optic nerve and / or ophthalmic artery at risk of compromise. Postoperatively, vision monitoring in the post-anesthesia care unit, leaving the eye unpatched, and applying cold compresses on a frequent basis are recommended. All surgeons and nursing staff involved in orbital fracture procedures should be comfortable performing postoperative vision and pupillary examinations [86, 87]. Patient, caregivers, and/or family members should understand how to monitor for vision changes, be aware of the potential of postoperative hemorrhage during the first week, and immediately report any sudden visual loss or evidence of hematoma formation [85]. Carefully instructing the patient regarding the importance of rest, avoiding strenuous activity or exercise, and maintaining control of pain and nausea are important postoperative considerations. Although hemorrhage can occur in anyone, it is more likely to occur in those that are more active than they should be.

Complications associated with alloplastic implants are infrequent and usually reported as isolated case reports [80, 92]. Nylon foil (Suprafoil®) and porous polyethylene (Medpor®) are the most widely used and accepted orbital floor implant materials, but other alloplastic materials such as titanium, Teflon, silicone, Silastic sheeting, and hydroxyapatite may be well tolerated [74, 75, 78, 80, 98–101]. Orbital floor implants cover the orbital floor defect and prevent globe luxation into the fracture site as well as prevent scarring between the orbital contents and fracture site and sinus mucosa. The ideal orbital implant should provide good structural support over the defect and be nonreactive and well tolerated by the surrounding tissue, easily positioned, affordable, and readily available. Complications may occur soon after implant placement or years later [80, 92–113]. Reported complications include orbital infection, fistula formation, implant migration, extraocular muscle entrapment, double vision, dacryocystitis, globe malposition, intracapsular hemorrhage, cyst formation, and vision loss [80, 92–113].

Orbital infection may be secondary to the presence of a foreign body (implant), bacterial colonization in the adjacent sinus, or associated with an initial penetrating injury [102–104]. A cutaneous fistula or opening into one of the adjacent sinuses may develop (Fig. 70.15a, b) [80, 105–108]. Anterior implant migration may occur through the skin (Fig. 70.16a–c), or the implants may dislocate into the maxillary or ethmoid sinuses (Fig. 70.17a–c) [80, 103]. Persistent diplopia following orbital fracture repair may result from irreparable neuromuscular trauma, incomplete release of entrapped tissue, implant impingement on the inferior rectus or perimuscular connective tissue, or adherence of the implant material and orbital tissue [75, 109]. Hyperglobus may result from implant stacking, using too thick or too large an implant or placing an implant in an

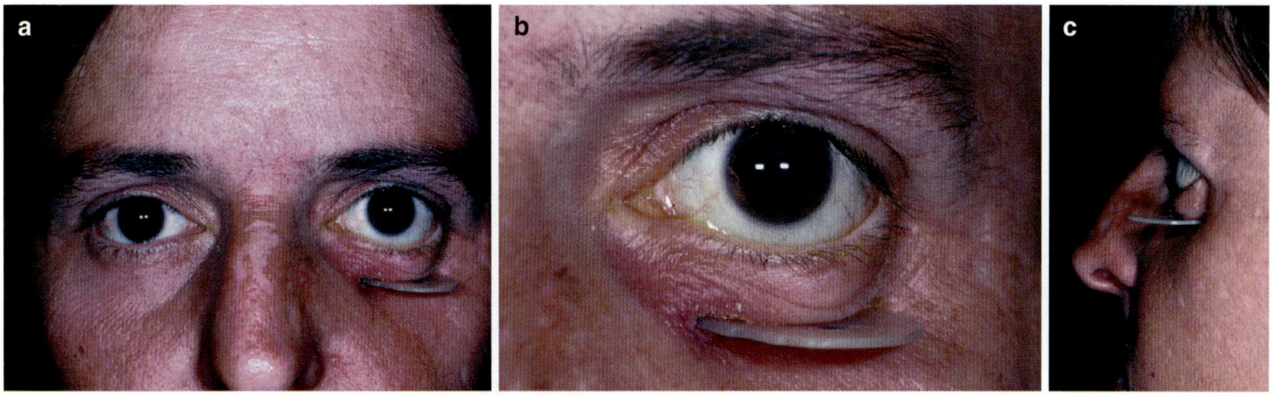

Fig. 70.16 (**a**–**c**) Five years post orbital floor fracture repair, the patient presented with implant extrusion

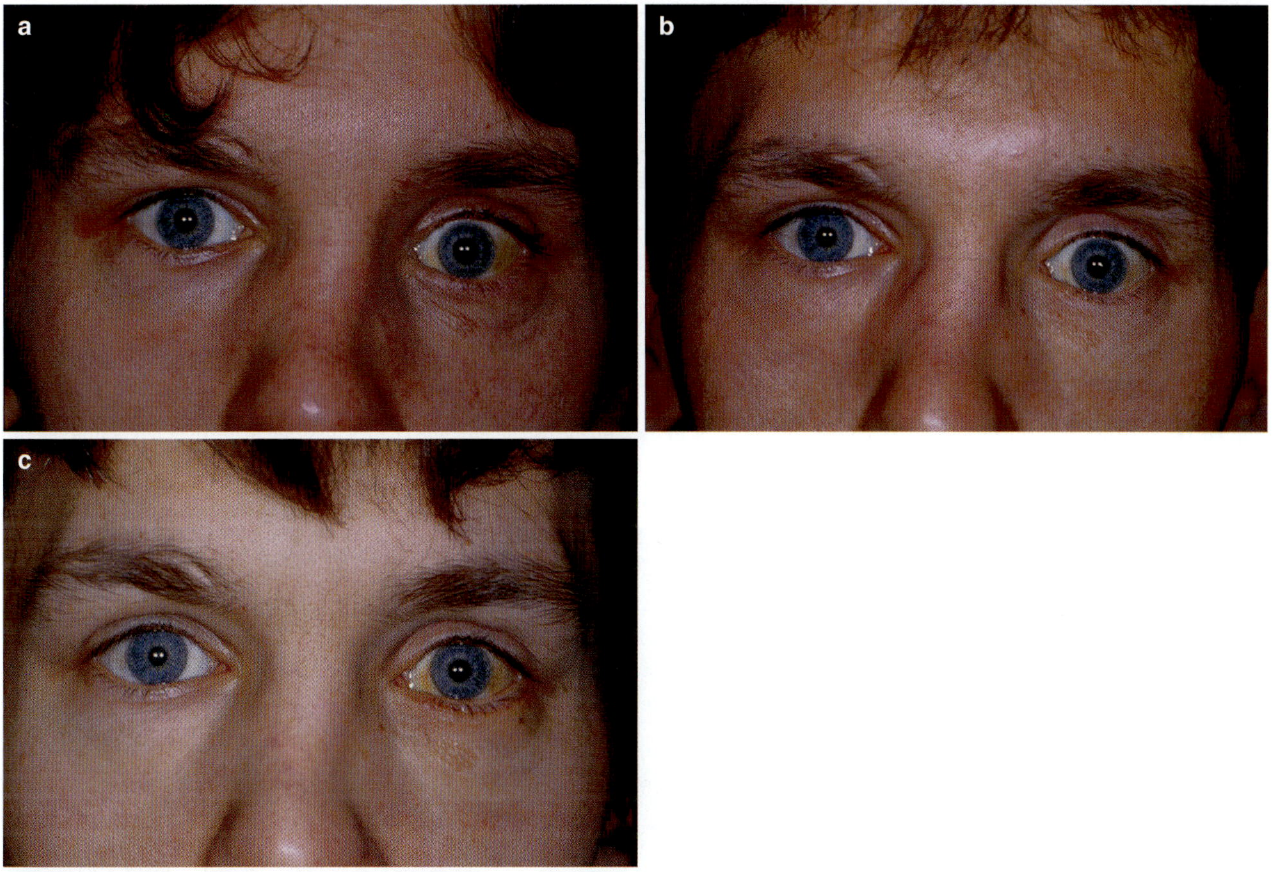

Fig. 70.17 (**a**) Patient is seen presurgical repair of his floor fracture with lid retraction and a deep sulcus, slight globe ptosis. The lid retraction and deep sulcus resolved following floor fracture repair. (**b**) Six months later the patient returned with a recurrence of the deep superior sulcus and lid retraction. The implant had migrated and could be felt along the inferior lateral orbital rim. He was taken back to surgery and had the implant repositioned and more securely placed over the floor fracture using a small titanium plate fastened to the implant and the orbital rim. (**c**) Post surgery, the lid retraction and superior sulcus disappeared again

unnatural position [98]. Cyst formation may occur with any of the absorbable implants as they are resorbed (Fig. 70.18a–c) [80, 101]. Sudden proptosis secondary to hemorrhage within the pseudocapsule around the floor implant is alarming for the patient but may resolve with conservative measures such as warm compresses (Fig. 70.19a, b), but surgical evacuation may be indicated in some cases [80].

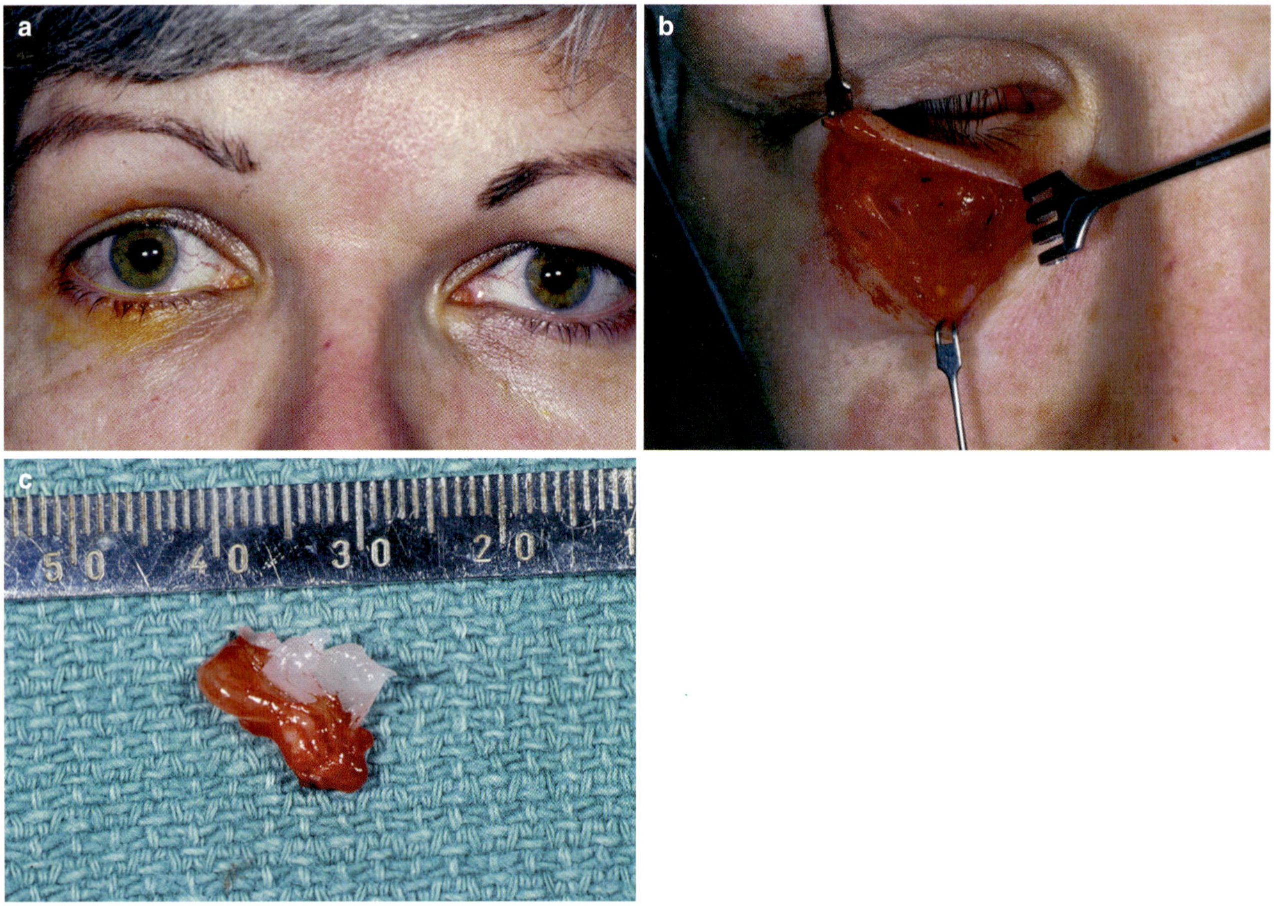

Fig. 70.18 (**a**) Two years after receiving a Gelfim implant for fracture repair, the patient presented with a mass along the right inferior orbital rim and some globe elevation. (**b**), (**c**) A cystic structure is transected and a gelatinous material came out

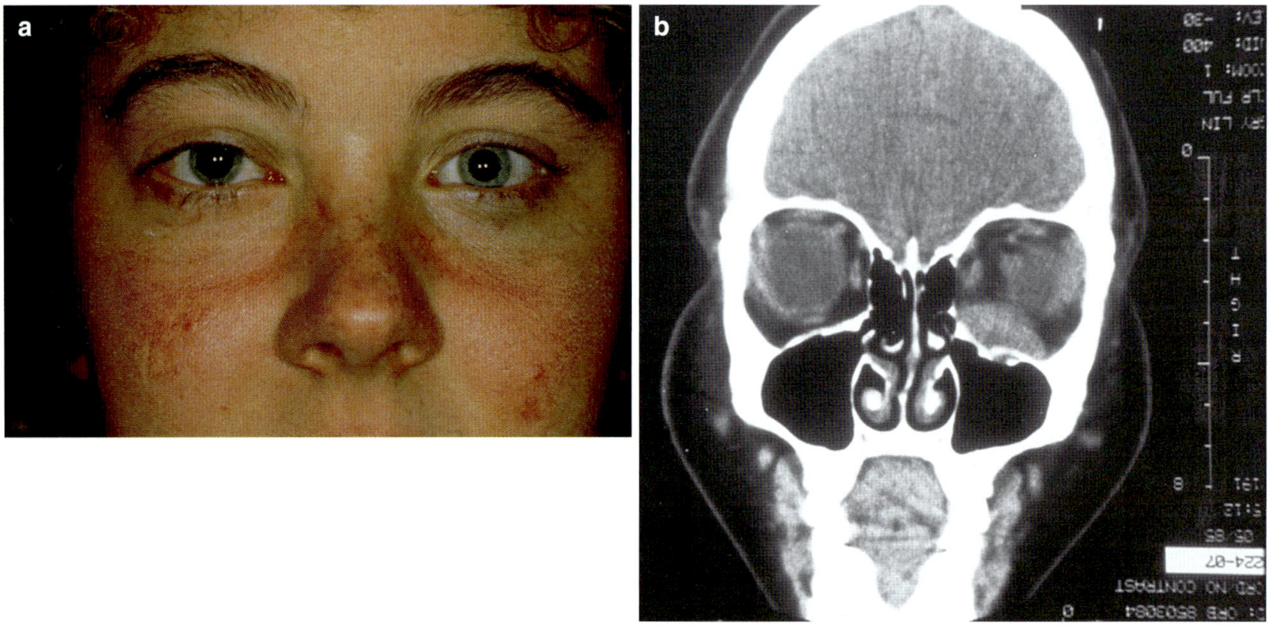

Fig. 70.19 (**a**) Patient presented 3 months after fracture repair with sudden onset of right-sided orbital fullness. (**b**) Mass sitting along right orbital floor consistent with a hematoma (CT scan, ultrasound) in the area of the floor implant. A conservative management plan was initiated, and the patient's symptoms and signs resolved

Summary

The orbital surgeon as a member of the facial trauma team should first attend to any life-threatening head or airway injuries. Determination of the nature and mechanism of injury is important to guide suspicion for globe and related site-threatening injuries. Following a comprehensive ophthalmologic assessment, a determination should be made regarding the presence of an orbital fracture. In those cases (generally children and young adults <18–25 yrs. of age) with significant extraocular muscle entrapment yet little clinical sign of trauma (i.e., the white-eyed blowout), surgical intervention is warranted within a few days of the periorbital trauma and sooner in any fracture patient (white-eyed or non-white-eyed blowout) if a new onset cardiac arrhythmia is detected [2, 7–15]. Both entrapment and arrhythmia (secondary to the oculocardiac reflex) need to be looked for clinically as these important findings may be overlooked and are significant in determining the timing of surgery [56–59, 67–69].

Management of adult orbital floor fractures with herniated tissue accompanied by mild/moderate double vision, absence of significant motility restriction, enophthalmos, and/or hypoglobus remains somewhat controversial [7, 8, 19, 47]. With progressive resolution of the double vision, periodic reassessment over 6–8 weeks is appropriate. There is also a trend toward less emphasis on fracture size and the presence of enophthalmos/hypoglobus in deciding whether to operate within the first 2 weeks following the injury [10, 30, 47, 49–52]. Successful improvement in asymmetries resulting from large orbital fractures can potentially be achieved, if necessary, several months or years after the initial trauma [30]. For those patients with clinically significant diplopia, signs of marked restriction, and/or disabling pain with ocular ductions and little evidence of improvement, surgical repair is often recommended within the first 2–3 weeks following the injury although discussing the risks and benefits of a wait-and-watch period of 6–8 weeks is also carried out [30, 38–43, 53–55]. Patient age, compliance, comorbidities, medications, occupation, and caregiver support are among some of the additional considerations when discussing surgical intervention versus continued observation. The decision is not always clear and straightforward. It is our goal to try and tailor the recommendation for repair to each individual, the particular fracture, and the degree of disability created by the fracture.

The management of orbital fractures requires a complete patient assessment, comprehensive discussion of the risks associated with surgical intervention, and adherence to meticulous surgical techniques if intervention is indicated.

References

1. Lee HJ, Jiliani M, Frohman L, Baker S. Ct of orbital trauma. Emerg Radiol. 2004;10:168–72.
2. Wachler BSB, Holds JB. The missing muscle syndrome in blowout fractures: an indication for urgent surgery. Ophthal Plast Reconstr Surg. 1998;14:17–8.
3. Freund M, Hahnel S, Sartor K. The value of magnetic resonance imaging in the diagnosis of orbital floor fractures. Eur Radiol. 2003;12:1127–33.
4. Parbhu KC, Galler KE, Li C, Mawn LA. Underestimation of soft tissue entrapment by computed tomography in orbital floor fractures in pediatric population. Ophthalmology. 2008;115:1620–5.
5. Soll DB, Poley BJ. Trapdoor variety of blowout fracture of theorbital floor. Am J Ophthalmology. 1965;60:269–72.
6. Soll SM. Trapdoor orbital fractures (letter to editor). Ophthal Plast Reconstr Surg. 2000;16(4):306–7.
7. Jordan DR, Allen LH, White J, et al. Intervention within days for some orbital floor fractures: the white-eyed blowout. Ophthal Plast Reconstr Surg. 1998;14:379–90.
8. Hatton MP, Watkins LM, Rubin PA. Orbital fractures in children. Ophthal Plast Reconstr Surg. 2002;109:482–9.
9. Grant JH III, Patrinely JR, Weiss AH, et al. Trapdoor fracture of the orbit in a pediatric population. Plast Reconstr Surg. 2002;109:482–9.
10. Chung SY, Langer PD. Pediatric orbital blowout fractures. Curr Opin Ophthalmol. 2017;28:470–6.
11. Mehta VJ, Chelnis JG, Chen Q, Mawn L. Effect of time to operative intervention on motility outcomes following orbital flor fracture repair in children. Ophthal Plast Reconatr Surg. 2018;34(34):351–4.
12. Wei LA, Durairaj VD. Pediatric orbital floor fractures. JAAPOS. 2011;15:173–80.
13. Lane K, Penne RB, Bilyk JR. Evaluation and management of pediatric orbital fractures in a primary care setting. Orbit. 2007;26:183–91.
14. Hink EM, Wei LA, Durairaj VD. Clinical features and treatment of pediatric orbital fractures. Ophthal Plast Reconstr Surg. 2014;30:124–31.
15. Criden MR, Ellis FJ. Linear nondisplaced orbital fractures with muscle entrapment. JAAPOS. 2007;11:142–7.
16. Kwon JH, Moon JH, Kwon MS, et al. The differences of blowout fracture of the inferior orbital wall between children and adults. Arch Otolaryngol Head and Neck Surg. 2005;131:723–7.
17. Warwar RE, Bullock JD, Ballal DR, Ballal RD. Mechanisms of orbital floor fractures: a clinical, experimental and theoretical study. Ophthal Plast Reconstr Surg. 2000;16:188–200.
18. Waterhouse N, Lyne J, Urdng M, Garey L. An investigation into the mechanism of orbital blowout fractures. Br J Plast Surg. 1999;52:607–12.
19. Burnstine MA. Clinical recommendations for repair of isolated orbital fractures: an eveidence-based analysis. Ophthalmology. 2002;109:1207–10.
20. Dutton JJ. Management of blow-out fractures of the orbital floor. Surv Ophthalmol. 1991;35:279–80.
21. Matteini C, Renzi G, Becelli R, et al. Surgical timing in orbital fracture treatment: experience with 108 consecutive cases. J Craniofac Surg. 2004;15:145–50.
22. Chang EW, Manolidis S. Orbital floor fracture management. Facial Plastic Surg. 2005;21:207–13.
23. Harris GJ. Orbital blow-out fractures: surgical timing and technique. Eye. 2006;20:1207–12.

24. Hartstein ME, Roper-all G. Update on orbital floor fractures: indications and timing for repair. Facial Plast Surg. 2000;16:95–106.
25. Cole P, Boyd V, Banerji S, et al. Comprhensive management of orbital fractures. Plast Reconstr Surg. 2007;120:57S–63S.
26. Putterman AM, Stevens T, Urist MJ. Non surgical management of blow-out fractures of the orbital floor. Am J Ophthalmol. 1974;767:232–9.
27. Smith B, Converse JM. Early treatment of orbital floor fractures. Trans Am Acad Opthalmol Otolaryngol. 1957;61:602–9.
28. Emery JM, Van Noorden GK, Sclernitzauer DA. Orbital floor fractures; long term follow-up of cases without surgical repair. Trans Am Acad Opthalmol Otolaryngol. 1971;75:802–12.
29. Putterman A. Interview: "Dr Allan M. Putterman on the subject of blow-out fractures of the orbital floor". Ophthal Plast Reconstr Surg. 1985;1:73–4.
30. Kersten RC, Vagefi MR, Bartley GB. Orbital "blowout" fractures: time for a new paradigm. Ophthalmology. 2018;125(6):796–7.
31. Beigi B, Khandwala M, Gupta D. Management of pure orbital fractures: a proposed protocol to prevent unnecessary or early surgery. Orbit. 2014;33:336–42.
32. Converse JM. Two plastic operatons for repair of the orbit following severe trauma and extensive comminuted fracture. Arch Ophthalmol. 1944;31:323–9.
33. Tajima S, Sugimoto C, Taniro R, et al. Surgical treatment of malunited fractures of zygoma with diplopia and with comments on blow-out fractures. J Maxillofacial Surg. 1974;2:201–10.
34. Wilkins R, Havins W. Current treatment of blow-out fracturee. Ophthalmology. 1982;89:464–6.
35. Manson PN, Iliff N. Management of blow-out fractures of the orbital floor. II: early repair of selected injuries. Surv Ophthamol. 1991;35:279–98.
36. Putterman AM. Management of blow-out fractures of the orbital floor. III: a conservative approach. Surv Ophthalmol. 1991;35:279–98.
37. Kum C, McCulley TJ, Yoon MK, Hwang TN. Adult orbital trapdoor fracture. Ophthal Plast Reconstr Surg. 2009;25(6):486–7.
38. Roncevic R, Stajcic Z. Surgical treatment of posttraumatic enophthalmos:a study of 72 patients. Ann Plast Surg. 1994;32:288–94.
39. Dal Canto AJ, Linberg JV. Comparison of orbital fracture repair perfomed within 14 days versus 15 to 29 days after trauma. Opthal Plast Reconstr Surg. 2008;24(6):437–43.
40. Simon GJ, Syed HM, McCann JD, Goldberg RA. Early versus late repair of orbital blowout fractures. Ophthalmic Surg Lasers Imaging. 2009;40:141–8.
41. Amrith S, Almousa R, Wong WL, Sundar G. Blowout fractures: surgical outcomes in relation to age, time of intervention, and other preoperative risk factors. Craniomaxillofac Trauma Reconstr. 2010;3:131–6.
42. Shin KH, Baek SH, Chi M. Comparison of the outcomes of non-trapdoor-type blowout fracture repair according to the time of surgery. J Craniofac Surg. 2011;22:1426–9.
43. Scawn RL, Lim LH, Whipple KM, et al. Outcomes of orbital blow-out fracture repair performed beyond 6 weeks after injury. Ophthal Plast Reconstr Surg. 2016;32:296–301.
44. Kasee A, Mirmohammadsadeghi A, Kaazemnezhad, et al. The predictive factors of diplopia and extraocular movement limitationsin isolated pure blow-out fracture. J Curr Ophthalmol. 2016;29:54–8.
45. Young SM, Kim YD, Kim SW, et al. Conservatively treated orbital blowout fractures: spontaneous radiological improvement. Ophthalmology. 2018;125:938–44.
46. Kocak ED, Kam JK, Hall AJ. Re: Young et al: Conservatively treated orbital blowout fractures: spontaneous radiologic improvement. Ophthalmology. 2018;125(12):e86–7.
47. Pfeiffer ML, Bergman NY, Merritt HA, et al. Re; Kersten et al: Orbital "blowout" fractures: time for a new paradigm. Ophthalmology. 2018;125(12):e87–8.
48. Nishida Y, Hayashi O, Miyake T. Quantitative evaluation of ocular motility in blow-out fractures for selection nonsurgically managed cases. Am J Ophthalmol. 2004;137:777–9.
49. Vicinanzo MG, McGwin G Jr, Allamneni C, Long JA. Interreader variability of computed tomography for orbital floor fracture. JAMA Ophthalmol. 2015;133:1393–7.
50. Goggin J, Jupiter DC, Czerwinski M. Simple computed tomography-based calculations of orbital floor fracture defect size are not sufficiently accurate for clinical use. J Oral Maxillofac Surg. 2015;73:112–6.
51. Gilbard SM, Mafee MF, Lagouros PA, Langer BG. Orbital blow-out fractures. The prognostic significance of computed tomography. Ophthalmology. 1985;92:1523–8.
52. Silverman N, Nakra T, Schinder R. Large orbital floor fracture – indication for surgery or not? In: 46th Annual Fall Scientific Symposium of the American Society of Ophthalmic Plastic and Reconstructive Surgery. Las Vegas; 2015 Nov 12–13.
53. Hawes MJ, Dortzbach RK. Surgery on orbital floor fractures. Influence of time or repair and fracture size. Ophthalmology. 2002;109:1207–10.
54. Harris GJ, Garcia GH, Logani SC, Murphy ML. Correlation of preoperative ocular motility in orbital blowout fractures. Ophthal Plast Reconstr Surg. 2000;16:179–87.
55. Liu SR, Song XF, Li ZK, et al. Postoperative improvement of diplopia and extraocular muscle movement in patients with reconstructive surgeries for orbital fractures. J Craniofac Surg. 2016;27:2043–9.
56. Sires BS, Stanley RB Jr, Levine LM. Oculocardiac reflex caused by orbital floor trapdoor fracture: an indication for urgent repair. Arch Ophthalmol. 1998;16:955–6.
57. Cohen SM, Garrett CG. Pediatric orbital floor fractures: nausea/vomiting as signs of entrapment. Otolaryngol Head Neck Surg. 2003;129:43–7.
58. Kim J, Lee H, Chi M, et al. Endoscopic-assisted repair of pediatric trapdoor fractures of the orbital floor: characterization and management. J Craniofac Surg. 2010;21:101–5.
59. Cobb A, Murthy R, Manisali M, et al. Oculovagal reflex in pediatric orbital floor fractures mimicking head injury. Emerg Med J. 2009;26:351–3.
60. Smith B, Lisman RD, Simontan J, et al. Volkman's contracture of the extarocular muscles following blow-out fracture. Plast Reconstr Surg. 1984;74:200–5.
61. Volkman R. Die ischemischen Muskella hmongen und fracturen. Centralbl Chir. 1881;8:801–5.
62. Koorneef L. Current concepts on the management of orbital blow-out fractures. Ann Plast Surg. 1982;9:185–200.
63. Carroll SC, Ng SG. Outcomes of orbital blowout fracture surgery in children and adolescents. Br J Opthamol. 2010;94:736–9.
64. McInnes AW, Burnstine MA. White-eyed medial wall orbital blowout fracture. Ophthal Plast Reconstr Surg. 2010;26(1):44–6.
65. Brannan PA, Kersten RC, Kulwin DR. Isolated medial wall fractures with medial rectus incarceration. Ophthal Plast Reconstr Surg. 2006;22:178–83.
66. Yenice O, Ogut MS, Onal S, Ozcan E. Conservative treatment of isolated medial wall fractures. Ophthal Surg Lasers Imaging. 2006;37:497–501.
67. Joseph JM, Rosenberg C, Zoulman CI, Zoulman RA, White M, Lisman RD. Oculocardiac reflex associated with a large orbital floor fracture. Ophthal Plast Reconstr Surg. 2009;25(6):496–8.
68. Mendelblatt FI, Firsch RE, Lemberg L. A study comparing methods of preventing the oculocardiac reflex. Am J Ophthalmol. 1962;53:506–12.

69. Pham CM, Couch SM. Oculocardiac reflex elicited by orbital floor fracture and inferior globe displacement. Am J Ophthalmol. 2017;3(6):4–6.
70. Amaral MB, Nery AC. Traumatic globe dislocation into the paranasal sinuses: literature review and treatment guideline. J Craniofac Surg. 2016;44:642–7.
71. Berkowitz RA, Putterman AM, Patel DB. Prolapse of the globe into the maxillary sinus after orbital floor fracture. Am J Ophthalmol. 1981;91:253–7.
72. Stasior OG, Roen JL. Traumatic enophthalmos. Ophthalmol. 1982;89:1267–73.
73. Converse JM, Smith B, Obear MF, Wood-Smith D. Orbital blowout fractures: a ten year survey. Plast Reconstr Surg. 1967;39:20–36.
74. Rinna C, Ungari C, Salteral A, et al. Orbital floor restoration. J Craniofacial Surg. 2005;16:968–72.
75. Nunery WR, Tao JP, Johl S. Nylon foil "wraparound" repair of combined orbital floor and medial wall fractures. Ophthal Plast Reconstr Surg. 2008;24:271–5.
76. Smith BC, Putterman AM. Fixation of orbital floor implants. Description of a simple technique. Arch Ophthalmol. 1970;83:598.
77. Tse DT. Cyanoacrylate tissue in securing orbital implants. Ophthal Surg. 1986;17:577–80.
78. Chang SH, Custer PL, Mohadjer Y, Scot E. Use of Lorenz titanium implants in orbital fracture repair. Ophthal Plast Reconstr Surg. 2009;25:119–22.
79. Lane KA, Bilyk JR, Taub D, Pribitkin EA. Sutureless repair of orbital floor and rim fractures. Ophthalmol. 2009;116:135–8.
80. Jordan DR, Onge S, Anderson RL, et al. Complications associated with alloplastic implants used in orbital fracture repair. Ophthalmology. 1992;99:160–8.
81. Greenwald HS, Keeney AH, Shannon GM. A review of 128 patients with orbital fractures. Am J Ophthalmol. 1974;78:655–64.
82. Liu D. Blindness after blow-out fracture repair. Ophthal Plast Reconstr Surg. 1994;10:206–10.
83. Girotto JA, Gamble WB, Robertson B, et al. Blindness after reduction of facial fractures. Plast Reconstr Surg. 1998;102:1821–34.
84. Gosaa M, Schoneich M, Drarnert FG, et al. Retrospective analysis of orbital floor fractures – complications, outcome and review of literature. Clin Oral Invest. 2011;15:305–13.
85. Jacobs SM, McInnis CP, Kapeles M, Chang SH. Incidence, risk factors and management of blindness after orbital surgery. Ophthalmology. 2018;125:1100–8.
86. Svider PF, Kovalerchik O, Mauro AC, et al. Legal liability in iatrogenic orbital injury. Laryngoscope. 2013;123:2099–103.
87. Peacock ZS, Boulos T, Miller JB, et al. Orbital fractures and ocu-locardiac injury; is a post-operative ophthalmology examination necessary? J Oral Maxillofacial Surg. 2014;72:111533–40.
88. Bodker FS, Cytryn AS, Putterman AM, Marschall MA. Postoperative mydriasis after repair of orbital floor fracture repair. Am J Ophthalmol. 1993;115:372–5.
89. Okinaka Y, Hara J, Takahashi M. Orbital blow-out fracture with persistent mobility deficit due to fibrosis of the inferior rectus muscle and perimuscular tissue. Ann Otol Rhinol Laryngol. 1999;108:1174–6.
90. Appling WD, Patrinely JR, Salzer TA. Transconjunctival approach vs subcilary skin-muscle flap approaches for orbital fracture repair. Arch Otolaryngol Head Neck Surg. 1993;19:1000–7.
91. Patel PC, Sobota BT, Patel NM, et al. Comparison of Transconjunctival versus subciliary approaches for orbital fracture; a review of 60 cases. J Craniomaxillofac Trauma. 1998;4:17–21.
92. Folketad L, Westin T. Long-term sequelae after surgery for orbital floor fractures. Otolaryngol Head and Neck Surg. 1999;120:914–21.
93. Lee HBH, Nunery WR. Orbital adherence syndrome secondary to titanium implant material. Ophthal Plast Reconstr Surg. 2009;25:33–6.
94. Custer PL, Lind A, Trinkaus KM. Complications of Supramid orbital implants. Ophthl Plast Reconstr Surg. 2003;19:62–7.
95. Morrison AD, Sanderson RC, Moos KF. The use of Silastic as an orbital implant for reconstruction of orbital wall defects: review of 311 cases treated over 20 years. J Oral Maxillofac Surg. 1995;53:412–7.
96. Polley JW, Ringer SL. The use of Teflon in orbital floor reconstruction following blunt facial trauma: a 20-year experience. Plast Reconstr Surg. 1987;79:39–43.
97. Oxturk S, Sengezer M, Isik S, et al. Long-term outcomes of ultrothin porous polyethylene implants used for reconstruction of orbital floor defects. J Craniofac Surg. 2005;16:973–7.
98. Taban M, Nakra T, Mancini R, Douglas RS, Goldberg RA. Orbital wall fracture repair using seprafilm. Ophthal Plast Reconstr Surg. 2009;25:211–4.
99. Buchel P, Raahal A, Seto I, iizuka T. Reconstruction of orital floor fracture woth polglactin 910/polydioxanon patch (Ethisorb):a retrospective study. J Oral Maxillofac Surg. 2002;31:367–73.
100. Bauman A, Burggasser G, Gauss N, Ewers R. Orbital floor reconstruction with an allolastic resobable polydioxanne sheet. Int J Oral Maxillofac Surg. 2002;31:367–73.
101. Loftfield K, Jordan DR, Fowler J, Anderson RL. Orbital cyst formation associated with gelfilm use. Ophthal Plast Reconstr Surg. 1988;3:187–91.
102. Browning CW. Alloplastic material in orbital repair. Am J Ophthalmol. 1967;63:955–62.
103. Weintraub B, Cucin RL, Jacobs M. Extrusion of an infected orbital-floor prosthesis after 15 years. Plast Reconstr Surg. 1981;68:586–7.
104. Mauriello JA Jr, Fiore PM, Kotch M. Dacryocystitis: late complication of orbital floor fracture repair with implant. Ophthalmology. 1987;94:248–50.
105. Goldman RJ, Hessburg PC. Appraisal of surgical correction in 130 cases of orbital floor fracture. Am J Ophthalmol. 1973;76:152–5.
106. Alpar JJ. Unuusual complication of orbital floor blowout fracture repair. Ann Ophthalmol. 1977;9:1173–6.
107. Aronwitz JA, Freeman BS, Spira M. Long-term stability of Teflon orbital implants. Plast Reconstr Surg. 1896;78:166–73.
108. Wolfe SA. Correction of lower eyelid deformity caused by multiple extrusions of alloplastic orbital floor implants. Plast Reconstr Surg. 1981;68:429–32.
109. Mauriello JA Jr. Inferior rectus muscle entrapped by Teflon implant after orbital floor fracture repair. Ophthal Plast Reconstr. 1990;6:218–20.
110. Kohn R, Romano PE, Puklin JE. Lacrimal obstruction after migration of orbital floor implant. Am J Ophthalmol. 1976;82(6):934–6.
111. Mauriello JA Jr, Flanagan JC, Peyster RG. An unusual late complication of orbital fracture repair. Ophthalmology. 1984;91:102–6.
112. Nicholson DH, Guzak S Jr. Visual loss complicating repair of floor fractures. Arch Ophthalmol. 1971;86:369–75.
113. Lederman IR. Loss of vision associated with surgical treatment of zygomatic-orbital floor fracture. Plast Reconstr Surg. 1981;68:94–8.

Zygomaticomaxillary Complex Fractures

71

Geoffrey M. Kwitko

Introduction

The zygomaticomaxillary complex (ZMC) is an essential anatomic and functional element of the aesthetic facial skeleton. It plays a key role in the structure, function, and aesthetic appearance of the facial skeleton. It provides normal cheek contour and separates the orbital contents from the temporal fossa and the maxillary sinus. Zygomaticomaxillary complex provides a key structural support to the orbit. Disruption in the anatomic location may result in a change in globe position resulting in enophthalmos, globe dystopia, as well as diplopia. The zygoma is the origin for the masseter and therefore affecting mastication. The bones of the ZMC create the inferior and lateral orbital socket thus potentially affecting the correct position of the globe and mobility of the extraocular muscles. The infraorbital nerve passes just inferior to the orbital rim, and damage to the infraorbital nerve can cause decreased sensation to the upper cheek, skin, lateral nose, lip, and gums. The zygoma makes up the anterolateral wall and inferotemporal floor of the orbit and the lateral aspect of the inferior orbital rim. It articulates with the zygomatic process of the temporal bone posterior laterally which forms the zygomatic arch. The arch is what provides contour to the lateral cheek and protects the temporalis muscle and coronoid process of the mandible. The zygoma articulates with the maxilla to make up the medial aspect of the inferior orbital rim and floor the orbit. The frontozygomatic suture is where the zygomatic process of the frontal bone articulates with the frontal process of the zygoma forming the lateral wall of the orbit. Needless to say, trauma to the ZMC not only causes cosmetic orbital and facial deformities but functional as well.

Frequency

The prominent convex shape of the zygoma makes it very susceptible to traumatic injury and typically results from a blow to the cheek. ZMC fractures are second only to nasal bone fractures in frequency which is the most common type of facial fracture. Even minimally displaced ZMC fractures can result in functional and cosmetic deformities (Fig. 71.1). As with any other fractures, successful repair of ZMC fractures requires accurate diagnosis via physical examination and appropriate imaging studies as well as appropriate surgical exposure and repair to reconstitute the complex three-dimensional anatomy. The incidence of ZMC fractures is higher in adult males who are between the ages of 20 and 30. Eighty percent of ZMC fractures occur in this group. Alcohol is involved in one third of these patients, and 65% of ZMC fractures are due to assault followed by motor vehicle accidents, falls, sports injuries, and work accidents. When females present with ZMC fractures and/or orbital fractures, it is imperative to investigate for domestic assault, and a careful history, examination, and photographic documentation should be obtained.

Evaluation

Patients will always present with a history of trauma and will complain of periorbital and cheek pain. They may complain of pain with mastication due to a fractured and displaced zygomatic arch impinging the temporalis muscle against the coronoid process. Facial asymmetry may or may not be evident due to swelling. Patients may complain of numbness on the cheek or gum on the ipsilateral side of the injury as well as double vision. However, if the edema is sufficient to cause the eye to be closed, double vision may not be evident. A complete dilated eye exam is imperative to make sure that there is no damage to the globe as well as a traumatic optic neuropathy. Due to orbital swelling, enophthalmos may not

G. M. Kwitko (✉)
University of South Florida, Department of Ophthalmology, Tampa, FL, USA

J. J. Servat et al. (eds.), *Smith and Nesi's Ophthalmic Plastic and Reconstructive Surgery*, https://doi.org/10.1007/978-3-030-41720-8_71

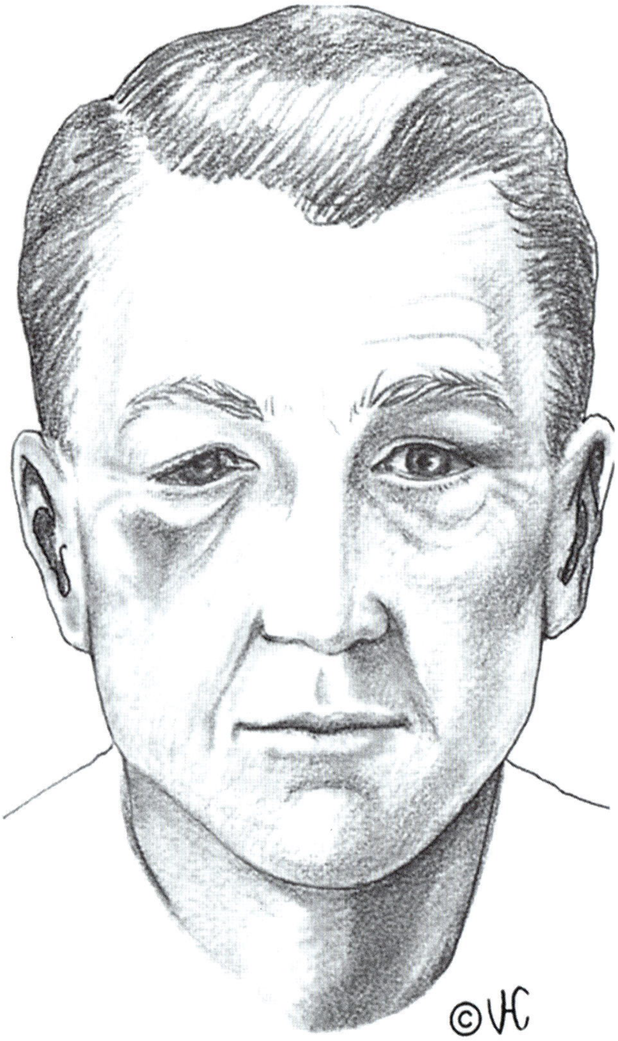

Fig. 71.1 Left zygomaticomaxillary complex fracture resulting in lateral canthal dystopia and visible malar flattening

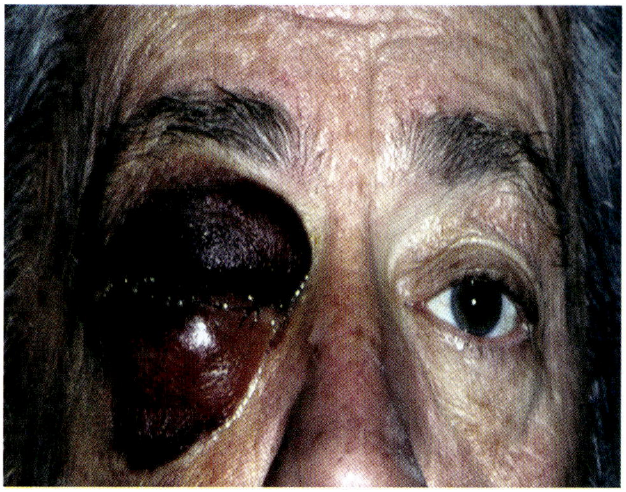

Fig. 71.2 Orbital hemorrhage

be initially evident, and double vision can be variable while the amount of swelling is changing. It is imperative to evaluate intraocular pressure as well as pupillary response to ensure that an orbital hemorrhage is not present to the degree that would cause a compressive optic neuropathy (Fig. 71.2). If this is the case, immediate canthotomy and canthal lysis (Figs. 71.3 and 71.4) should be performed to alleviate any pressure on the globe and optic nerve which is potentially vision saving. The inferior orbital rim should be palpated as well as the lateral orbital rim feeling for step-off deformity (Fig. 71.5). Extraocular movement should be evaluated; however this may be difficult with significant orbital and periorbital edema. Forced duction should be done if the exam shows limited extraocular movements and the patient is complaining of double vision. In a study published in 1987, there was a 14–40% incidence of significant intraocular injury in patients with ZMC fractures that involve the orbital floor. Extraocular muscle damage or entrapment may result in double vision usually resulting in decreased upward gaze and double vision present mostly in upward gaze due to entrapment of the inferior rectus muscle and the soft tissue surrounding it; however any of the extraocular muscles could be involved (Fig. 71.6). It is imperative to ensure that globe rupture has not occurred and repair of any globe rupture takes priority over repairing any fracture of the orbit or ZMC. Repairing ZMC or orbital floor fractures in the presence of an undiagnosed ruptured globe has the potential for causing additional intraocular damage.

Imaging

Non-contrast CT scans are essential for proper facial bone imaging (Fig. 71.7). These are easily obtained upon the patient's arrival. Axial, coronal, and sagittal cuts should be obtained to evaluate for ZMC fractures as well as orbital floor, medial wall, and orbital roof fractures. Additionally, it is important to evaluate for orbital hemorrhage especially in the setting of decreased vision and elevated intraocular pressure.

Indications for Surgery

Visual compromise and globe integrity take priority over repair of any fractures. Ruptured globes need to be repaired, and if visual potential is nil, then consideration for enucleation needs to be evaluated to avoid the small but real risk of sympathetic ophthalmia in the contralateral eye. Orbital hemorrhages that cause increased intraocular or intraorbital pressure to the point where compressive optic neuropathy is occurring need to be dealt with on an emergent basis with a lateral canthotomy canthal lysis to decrease pressure on the optic nerve.

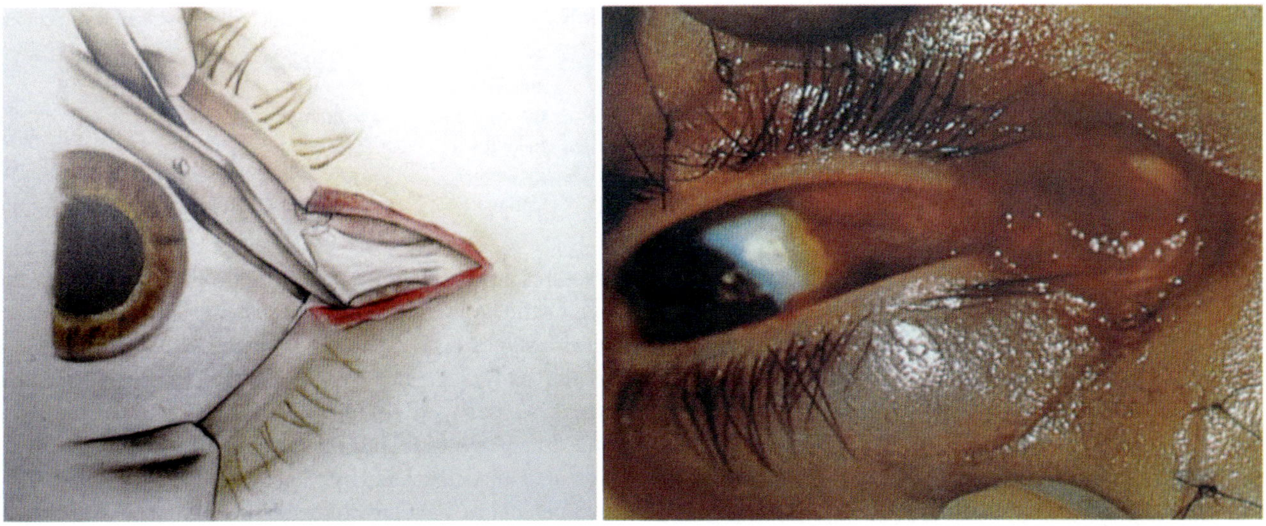

Figs. 71.3 and 71.4 Lateral canthotomy and cantholysis.

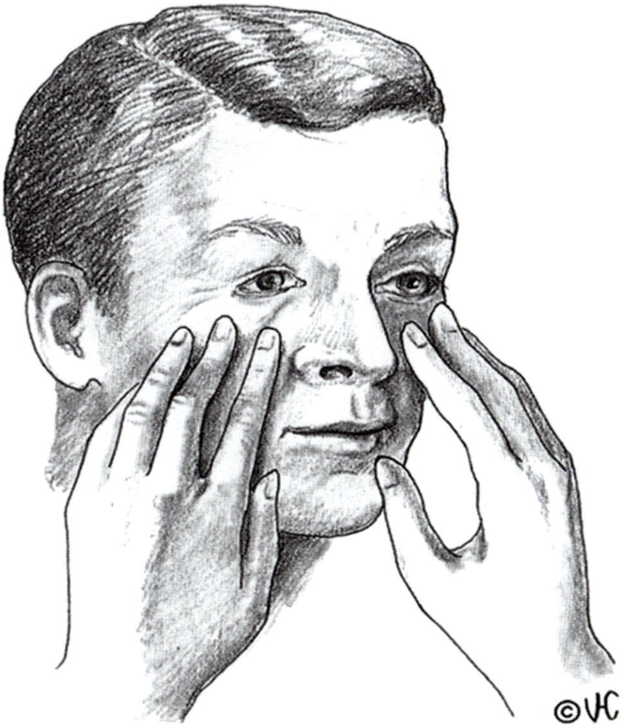

Fig. 71.5 Palpation over infraorbital and zygomaticofrontal areas may reveal step or gap deformities

Extraocular muscle dysfunction either by muscle contusion, local tissue edema, or extraocular muscle entrapment and strangulation can cause double vision via extraocular muscle dysfunction. While edema and contusions were usually resolved without any long-term effect, muscle entrapment does not resolve. If the muscle entrapment is not released, muscle necrosis with long-term double vision can occur.

Large orbital floor fractures (Fig. 71.8) can result in long-term enophthalmos and hypoglobus. Injuries involving 25–50% of the orbital floor pose a higher risk of long-term enophthalmos. In these patients as well as patients with entrapment of extraocular muscles, orbital floor exploration and repair should be considered.

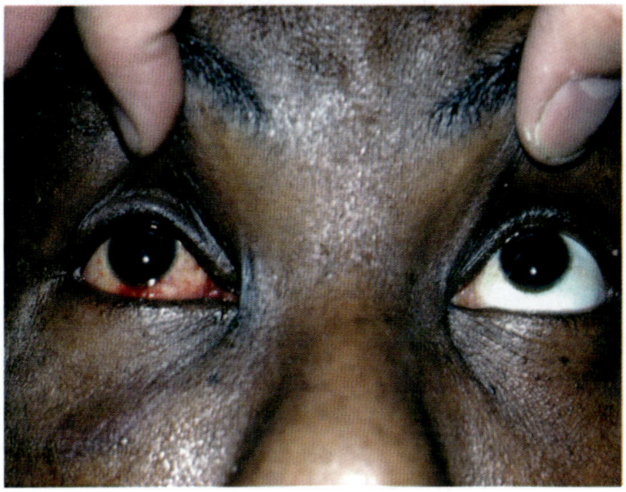

Fig. 71.6 Restricted upgaze associated with entrapment of the inferior rectus muscle

Displaced or comminuted fractures result in cosmetic deformity and as well require surgical repair.

Contraindications to Surgery

Medical instability and globe injuries. Additionally, if the orbit involved is the only seeing eye, it may be wise to defer orbital reconstruction to avoid risk to the patient's only seeing eye. Orbital exploration and reconstruction in the presence of a hyphema ruptured globe certainly runs the risk of making the injury worse and decreasing vision potential.

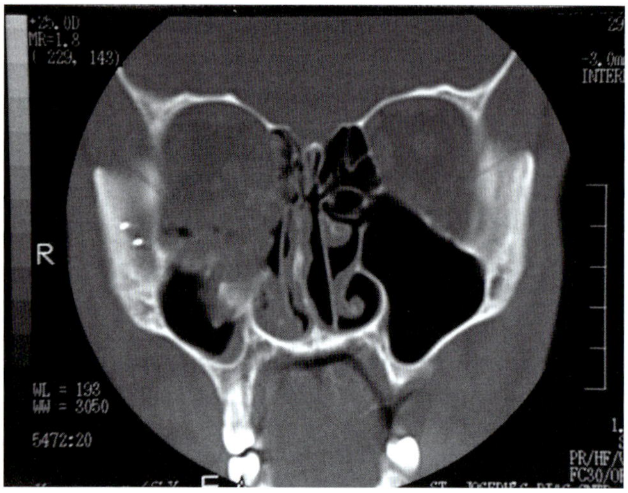

Fig. 71.7 Orbital floor fracture with total loss of the orbital floor

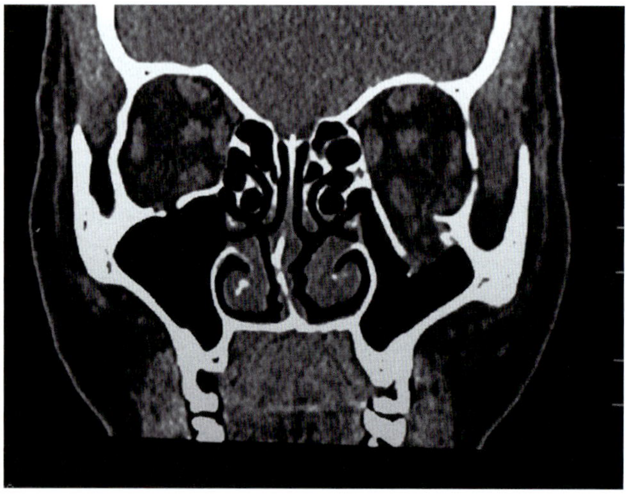

Fig. 71.8 Orbital floor fracture

Classification

ZMC fractures involve fractures where the zygoma meets the frontal bone, maxillary bone, and the sphenoid suture. These fractures are referred to as a tripod fracture or a tetrapod fracture because the inferior orbital floor or anterior wall of the maxillary sinus is also often fractured as well.

There are many classifications or ZMC fractures which are mostly of little clinical significance however are helpful in research and for physician communication. Zingg (1992) classified these injuries as to either A, B, or C. Type A fractures involved only one component of the tripod including the zygomatic arch which is a type AI, the lateral orbital wall which is a type A2, and the inferior orbital rim which is a type A3. Type B fractures involve all four buttresses. Type C fractures are complex fractures with comminution of the zygomatic bone itself. A second system classifies these fractures as types I–IV according to the degree of displacement of the bony segment. Type I fractures are nondisplaced, whereas type IV are completely displaced with no remaining attachment. Types II and III are classified based on the direction of displacement and rotation of the bony fragment. Sixty two percent of ZMC fractures or type B and C with type A fractures being relatively uncommon. Type B and C fractures occur at the zygomaticomaxillary and zygomaticotemporal buttresses. Significant disruption at this site usually implies a high-velocity injury with comminution in other areas. Type A3, B, and C injuries usually result in orbital floor disruption which puts the orbital contents at risk (Table 71.1).

Table 71.1 Classification of zygomaticomaxillary complex fractures

Type	Type of displacement	Direction of displacement
I	None	None
II	Incomplete	Inferior and lateral
IIIA	Incomplete	Inferior and lateral
IIIB	Incomplete	Superior and posterior
IV	Complete	Inferior with internal rotation at the rim

Type I usually result from low-velocity blunt trauma to the malar eminence. Non-contrast CT scanning shows a non-displaced fracture fragment plus or minus air-fluid levels in the maxillary sinus.

Type II usually result from blunt trauma with lateral trajectory to the inferior orbital rim. There is lateral displacement of the bony fragment, inferior orbital rim, and orbital floor (Fig. 71.8). There may be a palpable step-off of the inferior orbital rim plus or minus enophthalmos. Lateral canthal dystopia may be present. Non-contrast CT scan demonstrates separation of the zygomaticomaxillary suture, inferior orbital rim fracture, and possibly a separation of the arch.

Type III result from blunt trauma from above to the lateral orbital rim. These can present with lateral canthal dystopia and are classified as a type III a. The zygomaticomaxillary suture remains intact and attached, so no inferior orbital rim step-off is usually present. Imaging may show separation of the frontozygomatic suture and downward displacement of the bony zygoma fragment, and a gap may be palpable at the frontozygomatic suture (Fig. 71.9). Type IIIB fractures result from a blow to the lateral orbital wall from below which may cause telescoping of the frontozygomatic suture and displacement of the lateral orbital rim and zygoma superiorly (Fig. 71.10). Because the zygomaticomaxillary suture remains intact, there is usually no palpable step-off at the inferior orbital rim; however these patients may present with flat malar eminences and a deformity at the frontozygomatic suture. Non-contrast CT scan will show telescoping of the frontozygomatic suture displaced superiorly and posteriorly, and there may or may not be an orbital floor fracture.

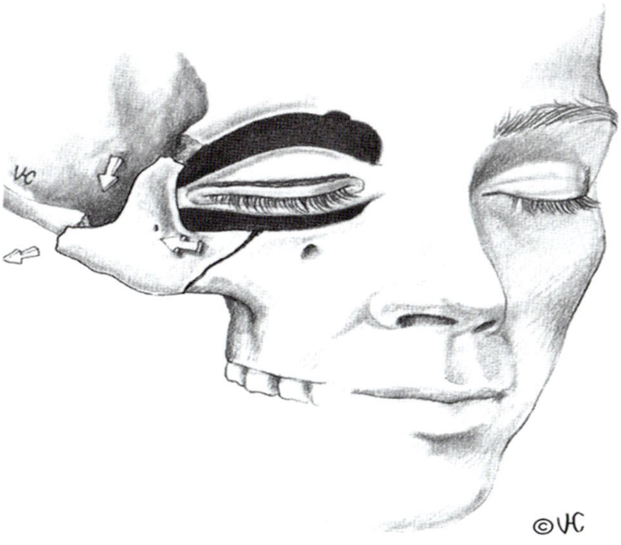

Fig. 71.9 ZMC fracture IIIa. Zygomatic bone is hinged at the zygomaticomaxillary suture. Lateral orbital tubercle is displaced downward. With inferior displacement of the lateral canthal angle

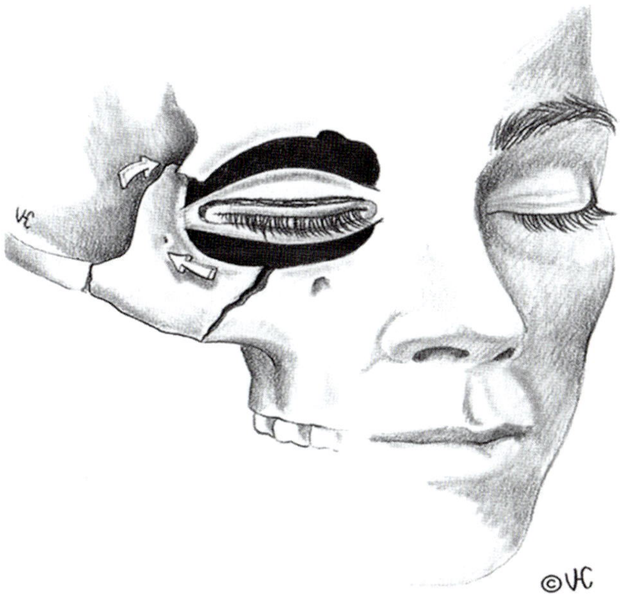

Fig. 71.10 ZMC fracture IIIb lateral orbital rim is displaced upwardly and posteriorly. This causes malar flattening associated with a bulge in the lateral orbital rim created by telescoping of the fracture fragments

Type IV result from high velocity blows to the zygoma or lateral wall involving a fist or motor vehicle accidents involving the dashboard or windshield. These patients present with flat malar eminences and prominent lateral canthal dystopia additionally complain of trismus and diplopia. Additionally, they complain of hypoesthesia to the cheek and gum. These fractures are significantly displaced at all suture lines and a rotated downward and inward. There is usually a palpable step-off along the inferior orbital rim as well as orbital floor fracture and a fracture of the zygomatic arch (Fig. 71.11).

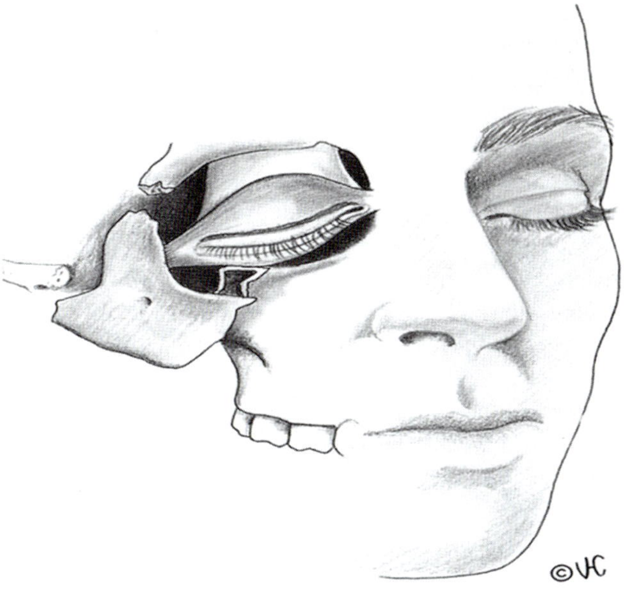

Fig. 71.11 ZMC fracture IV. Zygomatic bone is completely detached. There is downward and internal rotation of the inferior orbital and lateral orbital margins

Treatment

All patient should be started on broad-spectrum antibiotic therapy for 2 weeks as well as limiting activity and nose blowing for 2 weeks following trauma. A complete eye exam should be performed upon presentation ruling out ruptured globe, retrobulbar hemorrhage with possible compressive optic neuropathy. Additionally, a dilated funduscopic exam needs to be performed to rule out retinal detachment retinal or vitreous hemorrhage. If any of the above is present, they need to be addressed immediately before any attempt at bony repair is performed. If the eye is intact and there is no threat of compressive optic neuropathy, observation for a week or 2 is quite reasonable to allow for periorbital and orbital hemorrhage to resolve. CT scan should be done immediately, and if an obvious deformity is present in the malar eminence, the patient should be offered surgical intervention. If there is minimal displacement of the bony fragment without aesthetic, deformity observation without surgical intervention is appropriate.

Most (77–94%) of zygomaticomaxillary complex fractures require surgical intervention; however type I fractures usually do not require repair due to lack of flattening of the malar eminence without any aesthetic deformity. Type II fractures may require repair, and type III and IV fractures usually require repair again due to significant malar flattening and deformity.

Fractures causing flattening of the zygomatic arch can be repaired using a Gillies approach in type II and IIIa fractures. An incision 2–3 cm posterior to the hairline is made with the dissection going between the temporalis fascia and the temporalis muscle. The elevator is passed in this plane underneath the zygomatic arch, and the arch is lifted in an anterior and superior direction. Type IIIa fractures usually involve a Gillies approach as well as a subciliary approach for exploration of the orbital floor as well as the anterior wall of the maxillary sinus and lateral orbital rim. Appropriate plating can be performed after the zygomatic arch fracture is reduced. The surgical approach should be decided based on examination and CT scan findings to allow access to all fracture sites and permit ease of rigid fixation to minimize late complications of inward and downward rotation of the zygoma. The zygomaticomaxillary buttress can be approached through an intraoral transverse buccal sulcus incision where the incision is made 1 cm above the junction between the loose gingival mucosa and fixed mucosa. Mucosa is incised with a blade or Bovie and extends from the midline to the second maxillary molar. The fracture site is exposed with an elevator superiorly in the subperiosteal space care is taken not to violate the neurovascular bundle exiting from the infraorbital foramen. The frontozygomatic suture can be exposed to a brow incision or through a lateral canthotomy approach. This will allow evaluation of the lateral orbital wall and evaluation of the rotation of the zygomaticomaxillary complex. The inferior orbital rim is approached through a subciliary incision with dissection carried to the inferior orbital rim. Once the fracture is exposed, the periosteum is elevated with a freer elevator, and this also allows access to the anterior maxillary wall as well as the lateral orbital rim by simply extending the incision laterally. Once adequate exposure is achieved and all fractures are identified, the zygoma should be mobilized and the fracture reduced using clamps or appropriate hooks, and the zygomatic arch should be repositioned using a direct approach or through a Gillies approach. It may be necessary to do a Caldwell-Luc approach in order to further reduce the fracture and allow proper alignment and three-dimensional reconstruction of the zygoma and malar projection.

Once all fractures are reduced and aligned and 3D reconstruction achieved, rigid fixation is performed with microplates and screws. The zygomaticomaxillary buttress can be repaired using an L-shaped microplate. The inferior orbital rim is usually plated with a low-profile curved microplate. The plates are bent into position and fixated, and two screws are placed on each side of the fracture site. Remove all soft tissue from the fracture site, and any intervening fragmented bone should be preserved and secured into place with an additional screw with possible. Rigid fixation of the zygomatic arch is usually not necessary if other zygomatic fractures are secured with rigid fixation. Repair of the orbital floor is indicated in patients with significant enophthalamus of 2 mm or more, a large fracture involving 25–50% of the orbital floor, as well as entrapment of the inferior rectus muscle.

At the completion of the reduction, the malar projection should be evaluated; additionally forced ductions should be performed if there was evidence of preoperative entrapment of the inferior rectus muscle confirming that the entrapment was indeed released.

The patient is observed carefully postoperatively in the PACU looking for signs of orbital hemorrhage, and the vision is checked upon waking to ensure that vision has been preserved. Oral and topical antibiotics for prophylaxis are given for 2 weeks, and follow-up is the next day again to reevaluate vision and then 6–8 weeks following surgery.

Complications

Complications of ZMC fracture repair are relatively rare; however blindness due to compressive optic neuropathy from either for orbital hemorrhage or bony displacement is the most feared complication. Waiting a week or 2 from the time of injury to allow for orbital hemorrhage to subside as well as meticulous hemostasis at the time of surgery and careful manipulation of the bones will alleviate most of the risk. Additionally, the eye and vision should be checked immediately in the postoperative suite upon the patient waking to evaluate for loss of vision or orbital hemorrhage and if present should be dealt with immediately (Fig. 71.12).

Postoperative diplopia not present before surgery is relatively uncommon and can occur due to entrapment of orbital tissues following reduction of the zygoma. It's important to do intraoperative forced duction testing to ensure that entrapment has not occurred after all fractures are reduced and secured.

Lower lid retraction can additionally occur but can be reduced if a transconjunctival approach allows adequate exposure of the fracture site. Lid retraction can be repaired using spacers and tendon plication.

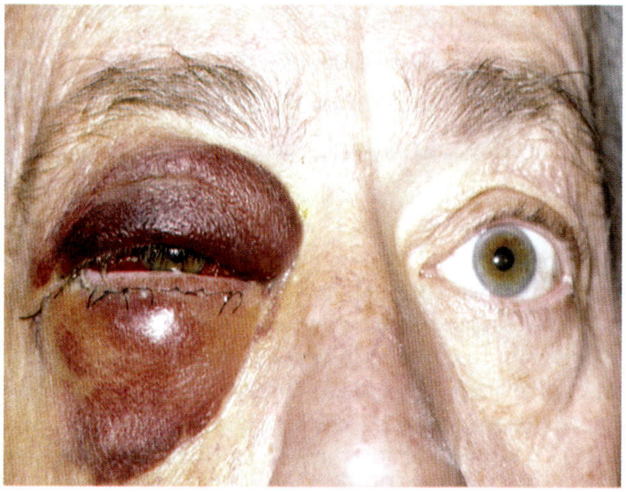

Fig. 71.12 Immediate postoperative orbital hemorrhage

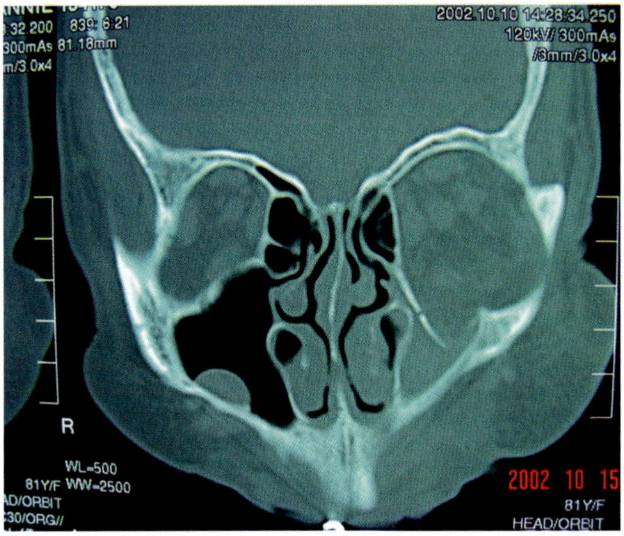

Fig. 71.13 Large floor fracture in a patient with infraorbital nerve damage

Infraorbital nerve damage causing numbness on the cheek and gums on the involved side should be assessed preoperatively and documented if present. Injury to the infraorbital nerve can occur intraoperatively, and the incidence ranges from 22% to 65% (Fig. 71.13). Visualization during surgery and taking care not to damage the infraorbital nerve will help to reduce the incidence of damage. Additionally, this should be discussed with the patient preoperatively, informing them that resolution or partial resolution may take 6–12 months following surgery.

Plate exposure is rare and may occur with a postop infection. If this occurs, the plate should be removed in the infection treated followed by reconstruction as needed. Resorbable plates should be used in children to prevent plate exposure due to growing bones.

Facial asymmetry requiring further surgical intervention is also rare. Mild facial asymmetry may be observed; however if significant facial asymmetry occurs, surgical intervention including implants or fat graft injection may be necessary. If trismus remains, removal of the coronoid process may be required for persistent trismus following reduction.

Suggested Readings

1. Nerad J. Techniques in ophthalmic plastics and reconstructive surgery: a personal tutorial. Saunders/Elsevier Printed in China; 2010.
2. Bogusiak K, Arkuszwski P. Characteristics and epidemiology of zygomaticomaxillary complex fractures. J Craniofac Surg. 2010;21(4):1018–23.
3. Arosarena OA, Fritsch TA, Hsueh Y, Aynehchi B, Haug R. Maxillofacial injuries and violence against women. Arch Facial Plast Surg. 2009;11(1):48–52.
4. Ellis E III, el-Attar A, Moos KF. An analysis of 2,067 cases of zygomatico-orbital fracture. J Oral Maxillofac Surg. 1985;43(6):417–28.
5. Fujii N, Yamashiro M. Classification of malar complex fractures using computed tomography. J Oral Maxillofac Surg. 1983;41(9):562–7.
6. Yanagisawa E. Symposium on maxillo-facial trauma. 3. Pitfalls in the management of zygomatic fractures. Laryngoscope. 1973;83(4):527–46.
7. Knight JS, North JF. The classification of malar fractures: an analysis of displacement as a guide to treatment. Br J Plast Surg. 1961;13:325–39.
8. Gillies HD, Kilner JP, Stone D. Fractures of the malar-zygomatic compound with a description of a new x-ray position. Br J Surg. 1927;14:651.
9. Shumrick KA, Kersten RC, Kulwin DR, Smith CP. Criteria for selective management of the orbital rim and floor in zygomatic complex and midface fractures. Arch Otolaryngol Head Neck Surg. 1997;23(4):378–84.
10. Lederman IR. Loss of vision associated with surgical treatment of zygomatic-orbital floor fracture. Plast Reconstr Surg. 1981;68(1):94–9.
11. Karlan MS, Cassisi NJ. Fractures of the zygoma. A geometric, biomechanical, and surgical analysis. Arch Otolaryngol. 1979;105(6):320–7.
12. Chuong R, Kaban LB. Fractures of the zygomatic complex. J Oral Maxillofac Surg. 1986;44(4):283–8.
13. Appling WD, Patrinely JR, Salzer TA. Transconjunctival approach vs subciliary skin-muscle flap approach for orbital fracture repair. Arch Otolaryngol Head Neck Surg. 1993;119(9):1000–7.
14. Wray RC, Holtmann B, Ribaudo JM, Keiter J, Weeks PM. A comparison of conjunctival and subciliary incisions for orbital fractures. Br J Plast Surg. 1977;30(2):142–5.
15. Zingg M, Laedrach K, Chen J, et al. Classification and treatment of zygomatic fractures: a review of 1,025 cases. J Oral Maxillofac Surg. 1992;50(8):778–90.
16. Stanley RB Jr. The zygomatic arch as a guide to reconstruction of comminuted malar fractures. Arch Otolaryngol Head Neck Surg. 1989;115(12):1459–62.

Le Fort Fractures

72

Gina M. Rogers-Hoffman and Richard C. Allen

History of Le Fort Fractures

In 1901, René Le Fort published his experimental findings of facial fracture patterns. His studies involved subjecting cadaver skulls to various forces of impact and analyzing the fractures that resulted. He described that fractures tended to occur in characteristic locations, which he noted corresponded to relatively weak areas of the facial skeleton [1]. With these findings, he introduced the term "pillars of resistance," which represent the strongest areas of the facial skeleton, and the fracture patterns he found occurred between these pillars. His report outlined three patterns of fractures with each bearing his name followed by a number, I, II, or III, depending on their location.

In clinical practice, facial and maxillary fractures often are not encountered in the isolated and complete patterns as described by Le Fort. Frequently, the force delivered is uneven between each side of the face, and the impact occurs at varying angles. In addition, penetrating injuries do not usually follow the patterns described by Le Fort. Fracture lines often diverge from the described pathways and may result in mixed-type fractures, unilateral fractures, or other atypical fractures. The resulting fractures may be asymmetric from one side of the face to the other (Le Fort II on right and III on the left), combined with other fractures creating a more complex pattern (Le Fort II and zygomaticomaxillary complex (ZMC) fracture), or in the setting of panfacial fractures. In addition, many midface fractures have some degree of comminution and are complicated by additional fractures not addressed in the Le Fort system. These additional fractures include palate, medial maxillary arch, dentoalveolar, and anterior maxillary fractures. Many feel the patterns described by Le Fort may be an oversimplified classification of fractures encountered today. However, knowledge of the patterns is not only important as historical background, but his classification schemes are still used widely although the pattern may not be isolated or exactly as those encountered in his studies. Osteotomies are created in similar formations in some instances of craniofacial reconstruction.

G. M. Rogers-Hoffman
Eye Physicians and Surgeons of Chicago, Chicago, IL, USA

R. C. Allen (✉)
Cullen Eye Institute, Baylor College of Medicine, Department of Ophthalmology, Houston, TX, USA

Relevant Anatomy

The maxilla represents the bridge between the cranial base superiorly and the dental occlusal plane inferiorly. The intimate relationship of the maxilla to the oral cavity, nasal cavity, and orbits, as well as the many structures contained within and adjacent to it, makes it a functionally and cosmetically important structure of the facial skeleton (Fig. 72.1).

Special mention of the pillars of support should be made as they provide the major support of the midface, and their understanding is crucial not only to recognizing Le Fort fracture patterns but also in understanding the physiology of the facial bones in the normal anatomic state. As Le Fort described that there are zones of weakness in the maxilla and associated bones of the midface, there are also zones of strength. These described *pillars of support* are commonly referred to as *buttresses* and consist of stronger bone [2]. The framework of the midface can be thought of as an arrangement of these vertical and horizontal buttresses. Again, the conceptualization of the facial buttresses is important in understanding the stronger planes of the facial skeleton, and their repair is an integral part of facial reconstruction [3].

Vertical Buttresses

There are three paired vertical buttresses and one unpaired vertical buttress. The three paired vertical buttresses are the (1) nasomaxillary buttress (medial), (2) zygomaticomaxillary

J. J. Servat et al. (eds.), *Smith and Nesi's Ophthalmic Plastic and Reconstructive Surgery*,
https://doi.org/10.1007/978-3-030-41720-8_72

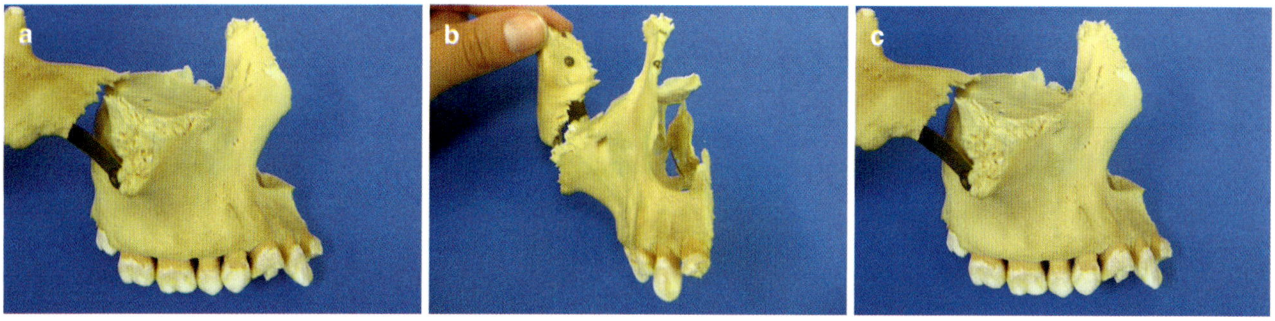

Fig. 72.1 The maxilla is formed by the fusion of the two maxillary bones at midline. It forms the roof of the oral cavity and holds the upper teeth, forms the floor of and contributes to the lateral wall and roof of the nasal cavity, houses the maxillary sinus, and contributes to the inferior rim and floor of the orbit. (**a**) Lateral view. (**b**) Anterior view. (**c**) Medial view

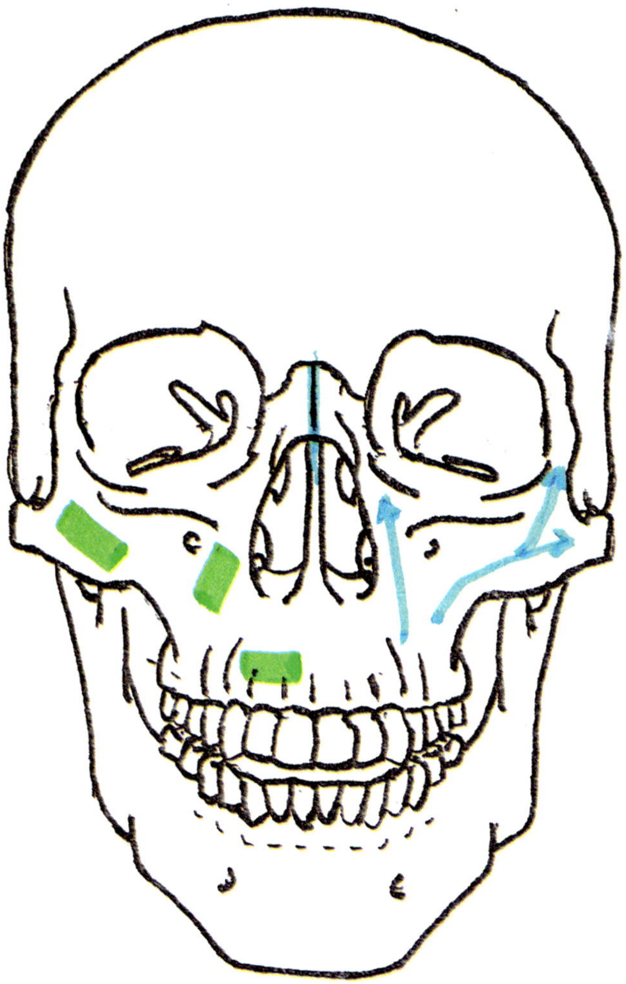

Fig. 72.2 Schematic drawing the pillars of resistance (*green*) and the vertical buttresses (*blue*). Of note, the pterygomaxillary (posterior) buttress is not depicted

buttress (lateral), and (3) pterygomaxillary buttress (posterior). The unpaired buttress is the midline frontoethmoidal-vomerine buttress. Collectively, the vertical pillars of support serve to diffuse the vertical forces of mastication over the cranial base and as shock absorbers to vertically oriented impact to the face (Fig. 72.2).

The nasomaxillary buttress is formed by the lower maxilla, the frontal process of the maxilla, the lacrimal bone, and the nasal process of the frontal bone. The nasomaxillary buttress transmits forces from the maxillary canine area through the lateral pyriform rim and frontal process of the maxilla and to the superior orbital rim. The zygomaticomaxillary buttress is formed from the lateral portion of the maxilla, zygoma, and lateral portion of the frontal bone. The zygomaticomaxillary buttress conducts forces from lateral alveolus above the anterior molars toward the zygomatic process of the frontal superiorly and the zygomatic arch laterally. The pterygomaxillary buttress extends from the maxillary tuberosity along the pterygoid plates to the skull base. The pterygomaxillary buttress transmits force through the palatine bone to the pterygoid plates and sphenoid base. Typically, no reconstruction is required for the posterior buttresses [4]. The frontoethmoidal-vomerine buttress is comprised of the median process of the frontal bone, the crista galli, the lamina perpendicularis of the ethmoid, and the nasal septum.

Horizontal Buttresses

The horizontal buttresses interconnect and provide support for the vertical buttresses. They include (1) frontal bar, (2) infraorbital rim and nasal bones, and (3) the hard palate and maxillary alveolus. These structures provide some protection against horizontal forces but can withstand much less force than the vertical buttresses (Fig. 72.3).

Classification of Le Fort Fractures

The categorization of the fracture patterns as described by Le Fort is felt to occur at relatively weak points in the facial skeleton. The common feature to Le Fort fractures is that the fractures extend through the pterygoid plates. By fracturing the pterygoid plates, a portion of the facial skeleton is separated from the skull base (Figs. 72.4 and 72.5).

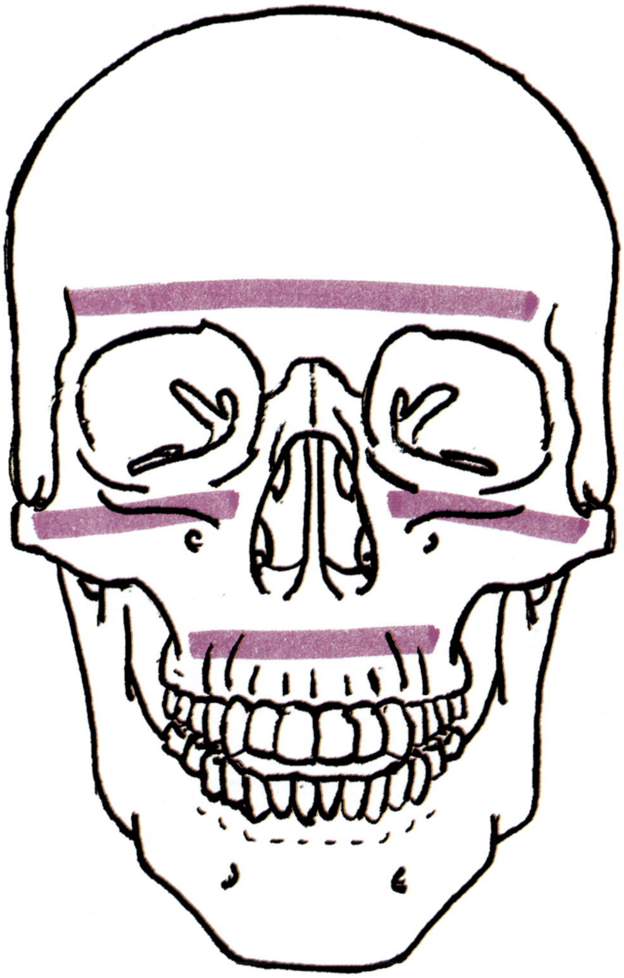

Fig. 72.3 Schematic drawing of the horizontal buttresses

Type I Le Fort Fracture

Le Fort I fractures (horizontal) classically result from a force of injury directed low on the maxillary alveolar rim in a downward direction. The fracture extends from the nasal septum to the lateral pyriform rims, travels horizontally above the dental apices, crosses below the zygomaticomaxillary junction, and traverses the pterygomaxillary junction to interrupt the pterygoid plates. There is no involvement of the orbital bones in this fracture pattern (Fig. 72.6).

Type II Le Fort Fracture

Le Fort II fractures (pyramidal) may result from impact directed at the lower or mid maxilla. The fracture extends from the nasal bridge at or below the nasofrontal suture through the frontal processes of the maxilla, inferolaterally through the lacrimal bones and inferior orbital floor and rim through or near the inferior orbital foramen, and inferiorly through the anterior wall of the maxillary sinus; it then travels under the zygoma, across the pterygomaxillary fissure, and through the pterygoid plates. The fracture fragment assumes a pyramidal shape and is separate from the upper craniofacial skeleton (Fig. 72.7).

Type III Le Fort Fracture

Le Fort III fractures (transverse), also termed *craniofacial dysjunction*, may follow impact to the nasal bridge or upper maxilla. These fractures start at the nasofrontal and

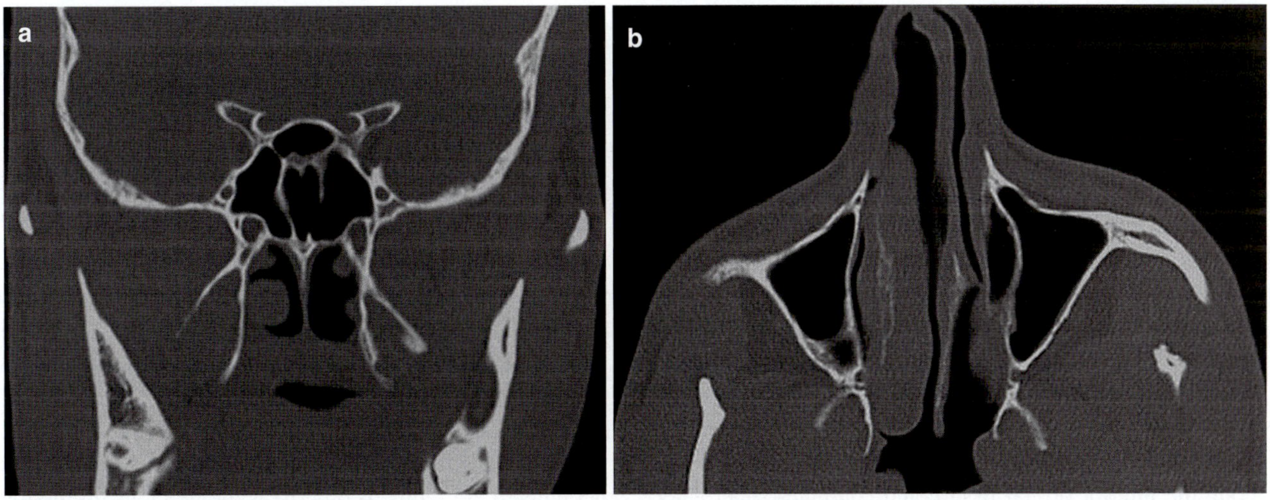

Fig. 72.4 Radiographic images of intact pterygoid plates. Pterygoid is Greek for “winglike”. (**a**) Coronal view. (**b**) Axial view

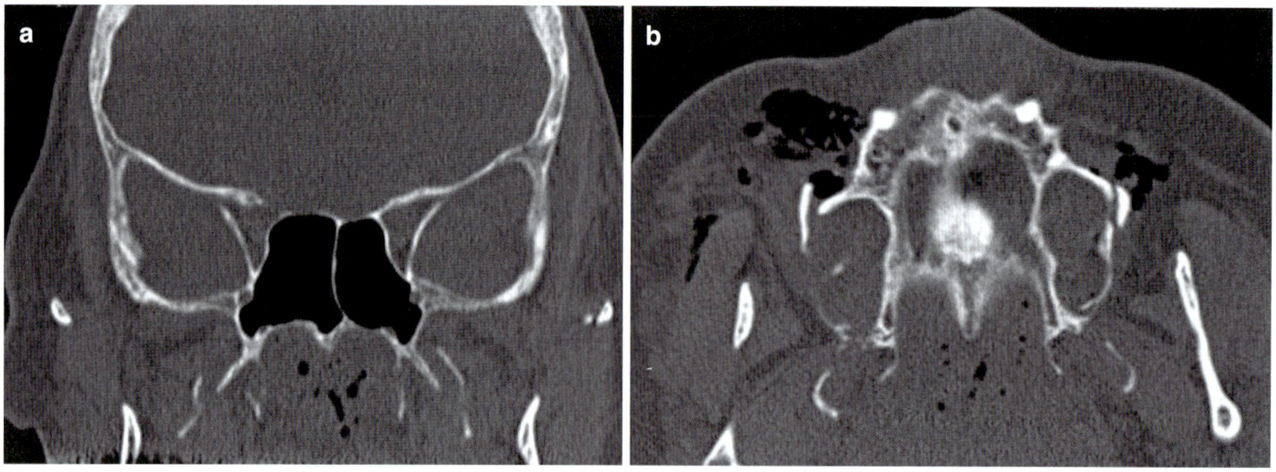

Fig. 72.5 Radiographic images of fractured pterygoid plates. (**a**) Coronal view. (**b**) Axial view

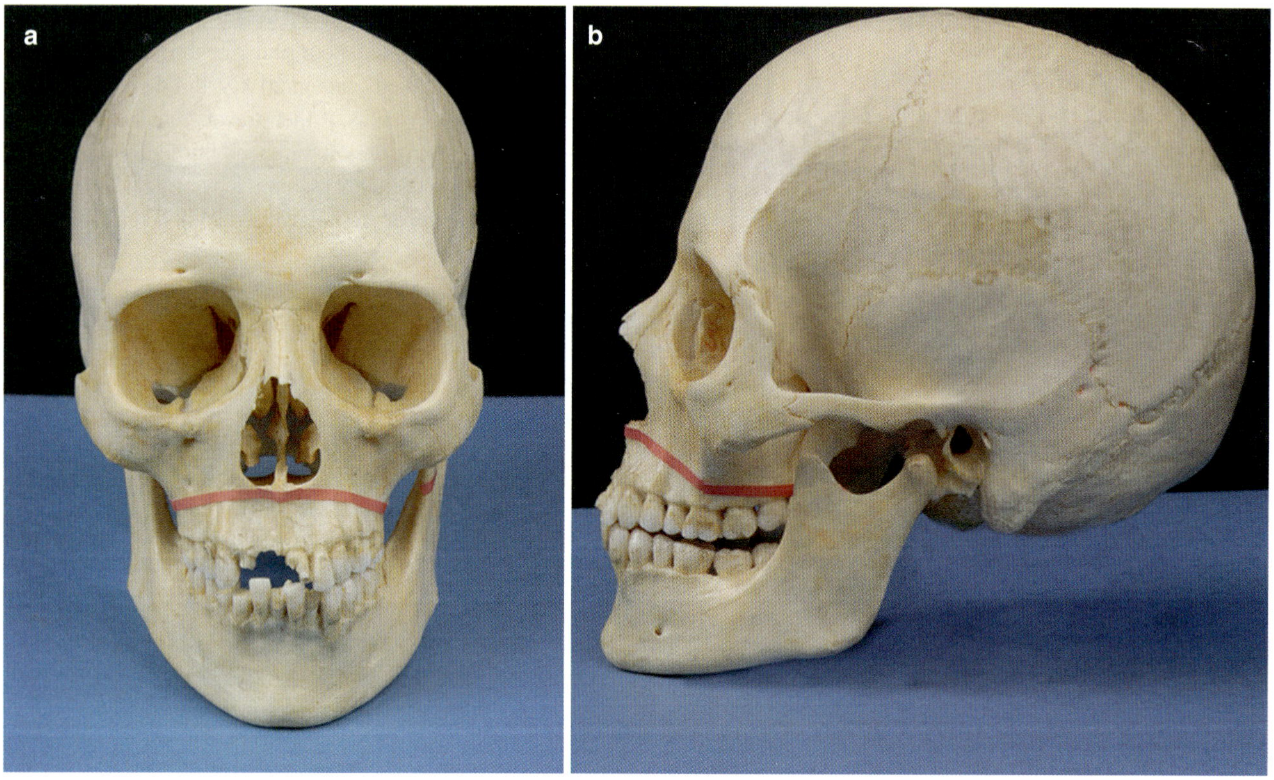

Fig. 72.6 Le Fort I. (**a**) Anterior view. (**b**) Lateral view

frontomaxillary sutures and extend posteriorly along the medial wall of the orbit through the nasolacrimal groove and ethmoid bones. The thicker sphenoid bone posteriorly usually prevents continuation of the fracture into the optic canal. Instead, the fracture continues along the floor of the orbit along the inferior orbital fissure and continues superolaterally through the lateral orbital wall, through the zygomaticofrontal junction and the zygomatic arch. Intranasally, a branch of the fracture extends through the base of the perpendicular plate of the ethmoid, through the vomer, and through the interface of the pterygoid plates to the base of the sphenoid. Generally, this is the least common of the fracture types, but when it occurs, it leads to a complete separation of the facial skeleton from the skull base (Fig. 72.8).

In clinical practice, the patterns of maxillary fractures encountered are rarely as orderly as the previous discussion suggests. The etiology of facial fractures may vary depending on the region of the country that one practices. For example, in urban settings, a much higher percentage of facial fractures occur secondary to assault, whereas in rural regions,

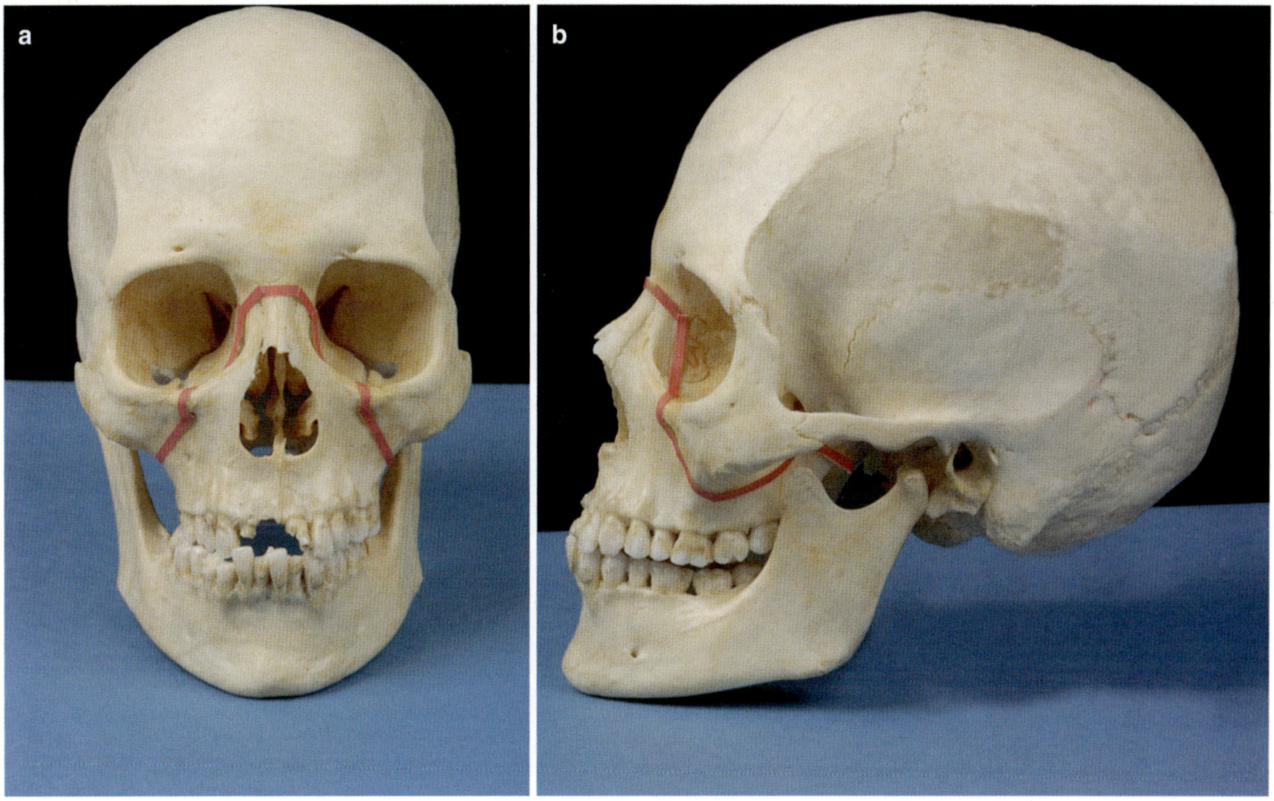

Fig. 72.7 Le Fort II. (**a**) Anterior view. (**b**) Lateral view

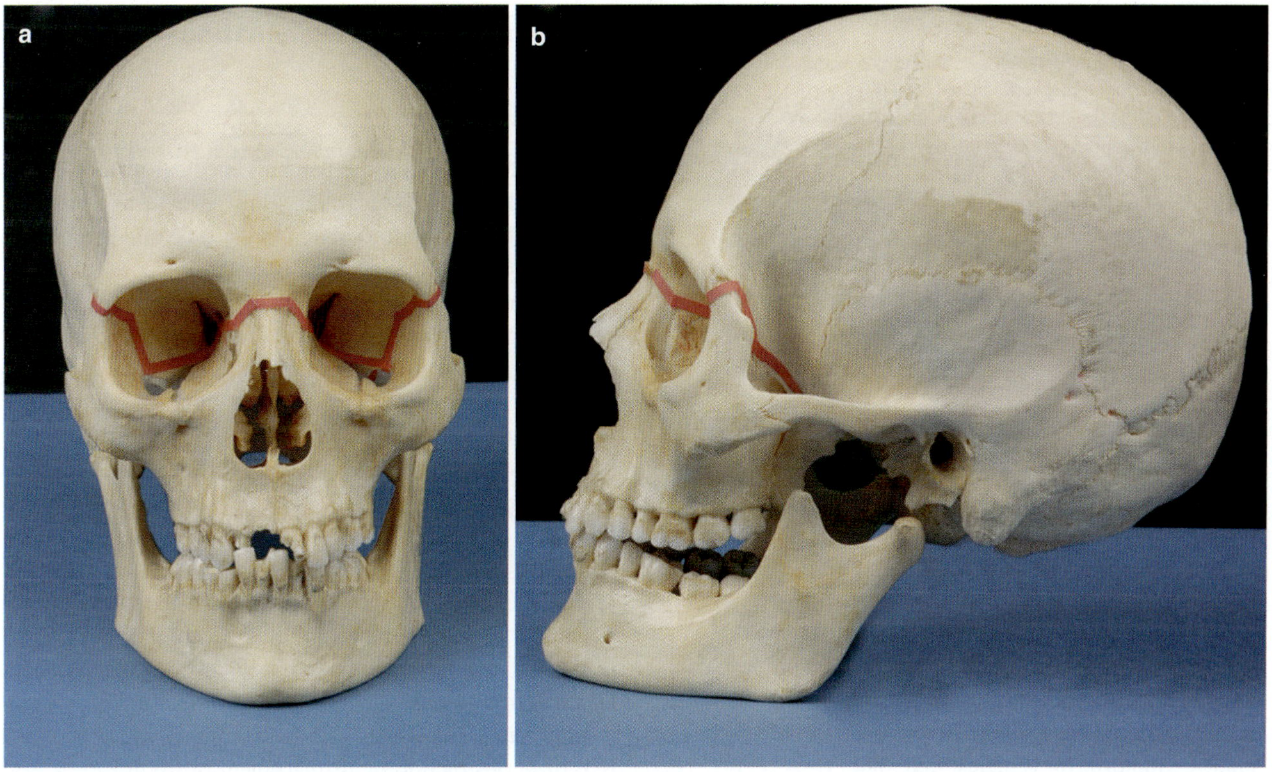

Fig. 72.8 Le Fort III. (**a**) Anterior view. (**b**) Lateral view

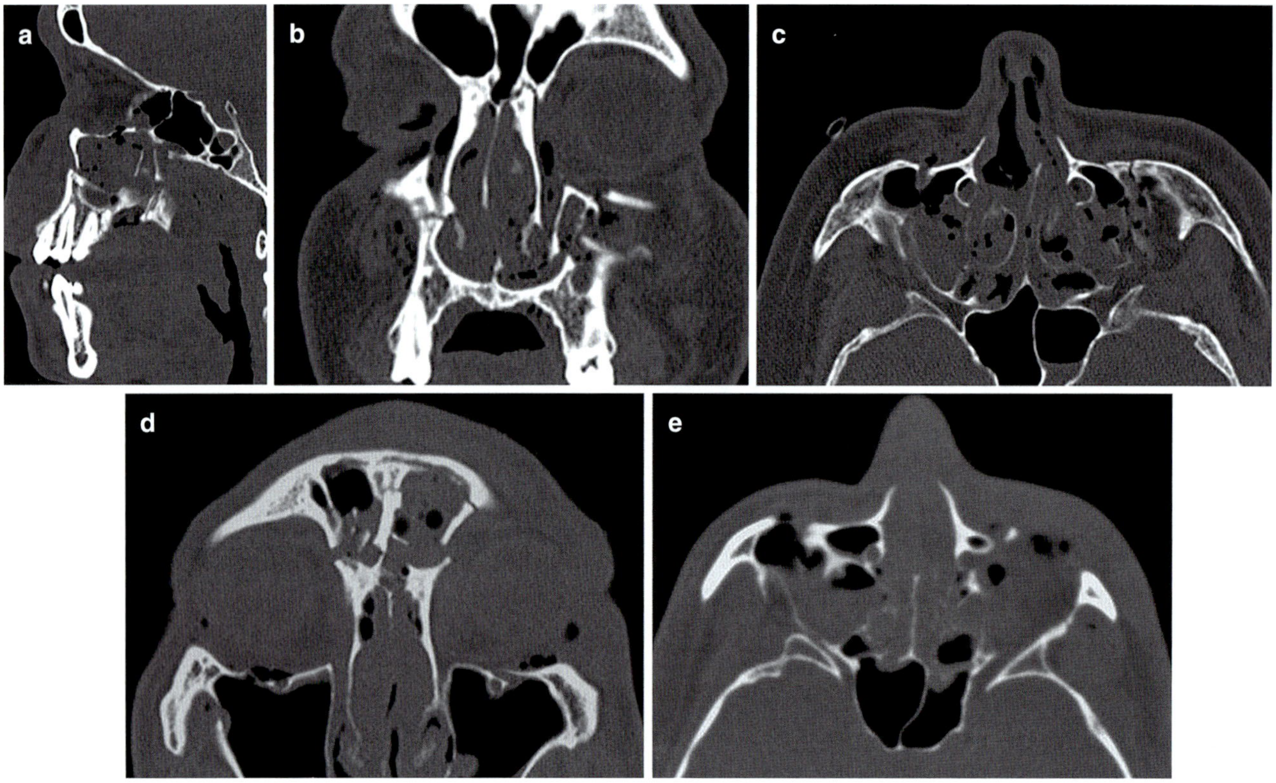

Fig. 72.9 (**a**). Sagittal view of Le Fort I. (**b**) Coronal view of Le Fort II. (**c**) Axial view of Le Fort II (same patient as **b**). (**d**) Coronal view of Le Fort III. (**e**) Coronal view of Le Fort III (same patient as **d**)

Table 72.1 Summary table

By definition, all Le Fort fractures extend posteriorly and involve fracture through the pterygoid plates. It is this fracture that allows for separation of the fracture segment from the skull base
Le Fort I (horizontal)
Separates the lower maxilla from remainder of midface
No orbital involvement
Le Fort II (pyramidal)
Separates midface from skull base
Violates the inferior orbital rim
Manipulation will produce mobility at the nasofrontal junction and medial aspect of the infraorbital rims
Le Fort III (transverse)
Also referred to as craniofacial dysjunction
Entire midface is separated from skull base
Creates posterior orbital fractures
Manipulation will produce mobility at the nasofrontal junction and zygomaticofrontal sutures

they are often the result of accidental trauma. The majority of injuries today are secondary to high-speed motor vehicle accidents. These high-velocity injuries often produce panfacial fractures that are extensive and not in the patterns as cleanly outlined by Le Fort. Remember in the time of his studies, motorized vehicles did not exist (Fig. 72.9; Table 72.1).

History and Physical Examination

History

It is prudent to obtain the patient's medical history and as much information regarding the event as possible. Specifically important to obtain is the time and mechanism of injury, and if possible, details of the impact such as the location, magnitude, and direction may be helpful. High-velocity trauma should raise concern of other possible concomitant injuries. A history of mental status changes or loss of consciousness warrants investigation for intracranial injury. The patient should be asked of any functional deficiencies, such as breathing, vision, hearing, or occlusion, as these symptoms may provide clues to fracture or injury location. The use of alcohol or illicit substances should be queried.

Initial evaluation should focus on evaluating for any potential life-threatening injuries according to ATLS (advanced trauma life support) protocol [5]. Special attention should be directed to the airway, cervical spine, and neurologic status. In patients with facial trauma, the airway is at risk from obstruction by displacement of the fractures, soft tissue edema, or from uncontrolled bleeding into the airway.

Early endotracheal intubation must be considered for these reasons. Once the patient is stable, a detailed maxillofacial and ophthalmic evaluation should be conducted.

In general, patients with facial fractures have sustained significant trauma, and their bony architecture may be obscured by soft tissue swelling, ecchymoses, gross blood, or hematomas. Examination should be performed in as complete a manner as possible. The face and cranium should be palpated to detect for bony irregularities, step-offs, crepitus, and point tenderness. Cranial nerves should be assessed for motor as well sensory function. Mobility of the midface may be tested by grasping the anterior alveolar arch and pulling forward while stabilizing the patient's forehead with the other hand. The authors suggest relying on diagnosis by reviewing imaging, rather than manipulating the fractures as this could cause additional injury. The size and location of the mobile segment may identify which type of Le Fort fracture is present. Palpation of the suture lines anticipated to be affected in a given fracture pattern can be done while mobilizing the midface. A global posterior retrusion of the midface creates a flattened appearance of the face and can be a sign of either a Le Fort II or Le Fort III fracture [6].

Any injury that causes periocular trauma or orbital fractures necessitates complete ophthalmic evaluation. This should begin with assessment of visual acuity, pupillary responses, extraocular motility, and evaluation of the globe with dilated fundus examination. Depending on the circumstance, additional examination of the periorbita including measurements of exophthalmometry, assessment of lid, medial, and lateral canthal tendon integrity, levator function, and intercanthal measurements. Concern of impaired motility should be assessed with forced duction testing to determine the presence of entrapment.

Dental occlusion must be assessed, and the patient should have an intraoral examination. Dentition should be noted and the gingiva examined. The alveolar ridge should be palpated and evaluated for integrity or additional fractures. The soft tissue and oral mucosa should be examined making note of any lacerations. Intranasal examination should be done paying particular attention to the identification of uncontrolled bleeding, sepal hematoma, and CSF rhinorrhea. Nasal fractures should be noted and addressed.

Remember to be prepared for assessment of the patient and have available the proper equipment that will be needed for a successful examination.

Special Considerations for Examination

Patients with Le Fort I fractures might not exhibit many signs of external trauma. The Le Fort I fracture pattern separates the lower maxilla from the remainder of the midface and cranium. The most common symptom in these patients is malocclusion. Displacement of the fractured segment posteriorly and inferiorly causes an anterior open bite with molars making contact prematurely. Intraorally, the palatal mucosa should be inspected for lacerations or bruising. There may be concomitant palatal fractures, which if they occur, typically do so at or adjacent to the midline longitudinally, dividing the palate (note Fig. 72.10). Palatal fractures can widen the palate and also lead to malocclusion. The teeth and gingiva should be inspected for the presence of laceration, fracture, or deformity. Dentoalveolar fractures are commonly displaced causing an asymmetric malocclusion and separate mobile segments.

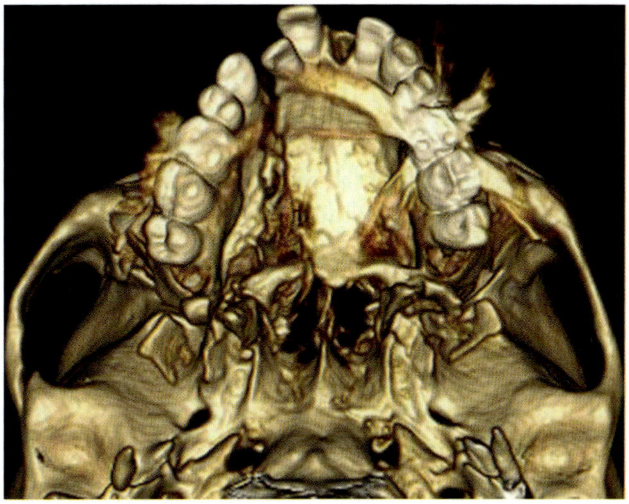

Fig. 72.10 Image of three-dimensional reconstruction demonstrating bilaterally fractured pterygoid plates and a right palatal-alveolar fracture

Le Fort II and III fractures exhibit more obvious external signs as they involve the orbits and nose. These patients may present with gross facial deformities, nasal deformities, epistaxis, periorbital edema and ecchymoses, and subconjunctival hemorrhages. Le Fort II fractures also can present with symptoms of malocclusion similar to Le Fort I fractures, but manipulating the fractured segment produces a larger mobile segment with mobility at the nasofrontal junction and medial aspect of the infraorbital rims. Given the involvement of the inferior orbital rim and possibly other orbital walls, globe trauma, motility problems, and infraorbital paresthesia may be encountered. Cerebrospinal fluid rhinorrhea may be detected and would indicate a likely fracture of the cribriform plate. Remember, Le Fort fractures allow the upper teeth to be moved freely away from the skull.

A Le Fort III fracture allows the entire midface (maxilla and zygoma) to move away from the skull; hence, why this fracture pattern is also referred to as *craniofacial dysjunction*. Le Fort III fracture patients again typically exhibit apparent external signs. Recalling the pattern of this fracture, the pterygoids, zygomaticofrontal sutures, inner orbits, and nasofrontal sutures are involved, and as such, many significant clinical findings may be encountered. The orbital rims may be intact. Dural tears in the area of the cribriform plate or the roof of the auditory canal may lead to CSF rhinorrhea or otorrhea, respectively. Bleeding and extravasation of blood along the path of the posterior auricular artery from basal skull fractures can lead to mastoid ecchymosis or the *Battles sign*. Globe, optic nerve, and periorbital trauma may be evident. Depending on the disarticulation of the fracture, significant displacement of orbital tissue can occur which could lead to entrapment or enophthalmos. Fractures of the medial orbital wall may produce telecanthus. Manipulation of the maxilla will exhibit mobility of the midface and can be felt at the nasofrontal junction and zygomaticofrontal sutures.

Imaging

Plain roentgenogram examination of facial fractures is inadequate. The imaging modality of choice is computed tomography (CT). Facial CT imaging should be ordered in both axial and coronal planes, and additional sagittal projections could be of utility as well. In the setting of orbital involvement, it is useful to obtain "fine cuts" which are obtained at 1 mm intervals through the orbit. CT is very useful in the setting of trauma as images through the various anatomical sites potentially involved in the injury can be obtained quickly. With the introduction of helical CT, which acquires data in a continuous fashion, computer-reformatted images can be produced, either coronal or sagittal, from the standard axial images. Three-dimensional reconstructions can be obtained from two-dimensional images but are usually not necessary for determining facial fractures. The reconstructions should not be used for primary diagnosis of fractures as some detail is lost in the digital reconstruction process. The 3D images do produce dramatic images of the injury and are easily recognizable to someone unfamiliar with reading conventional CT. Panorex images are especially useful in demonstrating the orthognathic relationship and occlusion and aid in evaluating mandibular fractures. Magnetic resonance imaging (MRI) is not particularly useful in the setting of routine fractures, as bony deformities are not visualized well.

Management and Surgical Treatment

In the setting of an emergency situation, such as airway compromise, uncontrollable bleeding, or vision-threatening injuries, immediate surgical intervention may be necessary. If the patient has multiple injuries, adequate consultations and examinations must be completed prior to surgical intervention. Generally, these patients are best treated in a trauma center where the appropriate specialists and equipment are available. Often in the setting of facial fractures only, surgical intervention can be carried out when facial swelling has diminished, often 5–7 days after initial injury. Ideally intervention should be undertaken within 14 days of the injury as permanent bone and soft tissue alterations may occur by this time. However, any concomitant globe injury should be addressed prior to periorbital manipulation, and fracture repair may need to be delayed on the side of the globe injury until it is deemed safe by the ophthalmologist.

Expectations of surgery have increased over the years, and patients expect not only good functional results but also good aesthetic results. With modern surgical technology and improved surgical technique, the oculofacial surgeon of this millennium can achieve successful outcomes in both respects. It is good practice to obtain photos at the time of injury, preoperatively, and postoperatively to aid in documentation of the extent of preoperative injury in comparison to the postoperative state.

Prior to surgery, informed consent should be obtained explaining the planned operative procedure, potential complications, and expected recovery. Especially important to address are the limitations and duration of maxillomandibular fixation (MMF) [synonyms: mandibulomaxillary fixation or intermaxillary fixation (IMF)] and any implants that will be used. Additionally, there are a host of potential complications that should be addressed. These include, but are not limited to, vision loss, diplopia, temporary or permanent paresthesia, cerebrospinal fluid leak, meningitis, anosmia, malocclusion, malunion, external deformity and scarring, plate exposure, tooth injury, infection, bleeding, death, and the possible need for additional surgery.

Extraskeletal fixation (any type of appliance applied outside of the facial tissues, to hold alignment, similar in principle to a halo for cervical fractures) is not usually necessary for Le Fort fractures. In patients with more extensive panfacial fractures, external fixation may be the only means of stabilization. This method alone typically leads to unsatisfactory functional outcomes. External fixation can also place excessive or misdirected force onto the fracture segments and cause shortening or further deformity of the midface.

Prior to any surgical intervention, good preoperative planning and preparation should be undertaken. Conventional computerized tomography (CT) images or 3D-reconstructed images available in the operating room are of great benefit for intraoperative guidance. The surgical team and equipment should be prepared as well as a complete maxillofacial plating set be available.

Intubation

Surgical management will need to address and correct the occlusion, often by means of maxillomandibular fixation (MMF). With this in mind, endotracheal intubation should not interfere with the placement of maxillomandibular fixation. Various means of endotracheal intubation are available and depend upon the clinical circumstance. Nasal intubation is adequate for Le Fort I fractures with or without mandibular fracture or when the nasal bones are not significantly displaced or comminuted. For Le Fort II and III fractures, nasal-orbital-ethmoid (NOE) fractures, and panfacial fractures, the establishment of an airway is not as simple. Surgical airways by means of tracheostomy may need to be established and are especially useful in the presence of panfacial or nasal fractures that will be repaired via a coronal approach. Oral airways may be acceptable in patients that are edentulous or partially dentate, where the tube can be placed through the space. Alternatively, it is often possible to successfully place an armored tube behind the mandibular molars. This tube is fixed with a wire to the posterior dentition, still allowing for MMF fixation to be applied. Another approach would be fiber-optic guided nasal intubation with fixation of maxillary, mandibular, and zygomatic fractures and then switching to oral intubation to address fractures of the frontal sinus and NOE complex [7]. Studies have suggested that even with involvement of the cribriform plate and CSF rhinorrhea, fiber-optic guided nasal intubation did not increase the incidence of complications or meningitis [8, 9].

Plating Systems

Years ago, facial fractures were reset in a closed manner which often resulted in unsatisfactory function and cosmesis. The repair of facial fractures has advanced greatly in the last century. The standard of repair today is by open reduction and internal fixation (ORIF). Plate and screw fixation systems via an open approach were first used widely in orthopedics and then later modified for use in the face. The advent and continued improvement of these plating systems now allows for fixation strong enough to prevent mobility of bony fragments during active use. The ability to achieve this secure fixation may allow for successful facial fracture repair without supplemental maxillomandibular or skeletal fixation. Titanium has surpassed other materials and is the most common material used in plating systems. Titanium is malleable enough to mold to fit the contours of the facial skeleton but is also strong enough to provide powerful fixation. It is advantageous to other metals because it minimizes artifact production on subsequent imaging and is safe for MRI. Bioresorbable materials such as polydioxanone, polyglycolic acid, polylactic acid, and their copolymers are being used but have not gained widespread acceptance at the time of this text [10, 11].

Whenever possible, separate plates are used to repair both the medial and lateral maxillary buttresses. Plating should be secured adequately into thick bone. Accurate contouring of the malleable plates is important for precise reduction and fixation. Monocortical, self-tapping, and self-drilling screws are ideal. Generally, at least two screws are necessary on both sides of the fracture. Care must be taken to avoid tooth roots when placing screws in maxilla. In these cases, it may be advantageous to use L-shaped, X-shaped, or Y-shaped plates for achieving stability [12].

Studies suggest that plating can bridge gaps up to 5 mm in the midface. Since the zygoma and maxilla are subjected to greater forces of stress, plating of gaps of any size in these bones becomes less successful in achieving good function. In general, gaps greater than 5 mm in dimension should be repaired with bone grafts or alloplastic material in addition to bridging plates and screws.

Maxillomandibular Fixation

Rigid fixation techniques are employed to stabilize the occlusion between the mandible and the maxilla. The goal in the repair of the fracture is to restore premorbid occlusion and allow the patient to resume mastication. There are several techniques to provide mandibulomaxillary fixation [13]. The majority of surgeons consider arch bars to be the gold standard of treatment; however, the fixation technique will depend on the clinical scenario. The common means of mandibulomaxillary fixation include arch bars, Ernst ligatures, Ivy loops, Gilmer wiring, Stout wiring, Kazanjian button, and intermaxillary fixation with screws, hanger plates, and interarch miniplates [14].

Surgical Approaches to Le Fort Fractures

The choice of incision(s) is directed by the extent of injury. Generally, these approaches are used in combination and typically result in hidden or acceptable scarring. Besides the surgical advances that have been made, antibiotics play a large role in the ability to repair these fractures combining intraoral and facial approaches.

Intraorally via Sublabial (Oral Vestibular) or Supramarginal Incision

These approaches allow for visualization of the lower half of the midface by making an incision through the oral mucosa. To perform a sublabial incision, the upper lip is retracted upward, and incision is placed in the oral vestibule just below the line of the gingival-mucosal junction taking care to preserve the mucosa for closure. The incision extends from approximately the frenulum to the canine tooth or molars and can be extended medially or laterally as necessary.

The supramarginal incision is made along the gingival margin in the dentulous patient. The extent of the incision is the same as that of the sublabial incision. This incision is useful in patients that have scarring of the gingival-mucosal junction. If one or more teeth are missing, the incision can be carried into the edentulous space. Once either incision is made, continue dissection to alveolar bone and elevate the periosteum superiorly to expose the buttresses, fracture lines, and other desired anatomical structures. Take caution not to injure the infraorbital neurovascular bundle. These approaches are generally tolerated very well but can have complications of infection, dehiscence, tooth damage, and scarring.

Periocular via the Subciliary (Lower Lid Transcutaneous), Lower Lid Transconjunctival, Combined Transconjunctival and Lateral Canthotomy, or Upper Eyelid Incision

Access to the inferior orbital rim, orbital floor, and portions of the medial orbital wall can be attained through a subciliary or transconjunctival incision. In the subciliary incision, an incision is made approximately 2–3 mm inferior to the lashes of the lower eyelid. The incision is extended from the level of the punctum medially to the lateral canthus laterally. The incision is made through the skin and orbicularis muscle and extended inferiorly between the orbicularis muscle and the orbital septum to the inferior orbital rim. The disadvantage of the subciliary incision is the external scar; however, in general, these incisions heal very well. An advantage of the subciliary incision is that an inferior cantholysis is not needed to gain easy access to the entire inferior orbital rim and orbital floor.

The transconjunctival incision is made through the conjunctiva, just inferior to the inferior border of the tarsus. This incision is often performed with a lateral canthotomy and inferior cantholysis to create a "swinging eyelid." The transconjunctival lateral canthotomy incision allows access to the entire lateral orbital wall, lateral portion of the orbital floor and roof, and the lateral orbital rim to the level of the frontozygomatic suture. The incision is extended from the level of the punctum medially to the lateral canthotomy incision laterally. Dissection is carried out through the conjunctiva, lower lid retractors, and orbital septum. Dissection is then continued in the same plane as noted above with the subciliary incision between the orbicularis muscle and the orbital septum to the inferior orbital rim. The advantage of the incision is the lack of an external incision. A disadvantage of the incision is manipulation of the lateral canthus which, if not placed in an appropriately overcorrected position superiorly and posteriorly at the end of surgery, could result in lateral canthal dystopia. The canthotomy incision heals very well with minimal scar. An additional disadvantage of the procedure is the proximity of the incision to the globe which some surgeons may not feel comfortable with, and also there can be some difficulty in finding the correct anatomical plane early in the adaption of this technique.

An upper lid incision approach provides excellent access to the frontozygomatic suture while allowing for good postoperative cosmesis. The incision is made in the upper lid skin crease from mid-pupil to the lateral orbital rim. Dissection is continued between the orbicularis muscle and the orbital septum and is extended toward the frontozygomatic suture and through the periosteum. Majority of the incisions will heal well and be hidden in the lid crease, but lid retraction and scarring are potential complications.

Brow Incision

The brow incision has a low incidence of complication but does leave a visible scar. The incision lies at the superior border of the lateral brow (overlying the region of the frontozygomatic suture). The incision is made first through the skin parallel to the hair shafts of the brow. The frontalis muscle is bluntly dissected down to the periosteum, which is then incised and freed from the underlying bone. As mentioned before, scarring and alopecia are associated with this approach. Extreme caution should be exercised to avoid severing the supraorbital nerve if working near the head of the brow to prevent permanent numbness of the forehead and scalp. Commonly, some degree of hypoesthesia in the area is present.

Coronal

This incision provides excellent exposure of the cranium and upper craniofacial skeleton. Think of this approach as providing exposure similar to a degloving injury of the upper face. The standard coronal incision runs from helical crus to helical crus approximately 2–3 cm posterior to the hairline. The incision is made through the scalp to the loose layer of scalp between the galea and pericardium. The incision must be designed cautiously to avoid injury to the frontal branch of the facial nerve. Dissection continues in the layer over the pericranium down to the supraorbital rim. The pericranium is incised, and the dissection of periosteum just above the supraorbital rim is completed [15]. This incision may be extended laterally to provide exposure to the zygomatic arches. Dissect just superficial to the temporalis fascia, and incise the temporalis fascia above the zygomatic arch. Develop a plane deep to the fascia down to the zygomatic arch [16]. Potential complications are scarring (especially visible in one with a receding hairline), alopecia, paresthesias posterior to the incision, weakness of the facial or temporal branch of the facial nerve, hematoma, or infection.

Existing Lacerations

Lacerations which involve any of the above dissection planes can be adapted as access points for fracture repair. The advantage of using these access points is the preexistence of an incision. However, if the laceration would need to be extended, or if the laceration does not involve the particular dissection plane needed to access the fracture, then it is probably wiser to close the laceration in the standard fashion than incorporate it into the repair.

General Principles for Repairing Panfacial Trauma

Reconstruct the load-bearing structures of the facial skeleton in a logical manner. Reconstruct the framework of the face, and position the fractured pieces into position, generally securing fractured elements to stable bone [17–19].

1. Reconstruct the projection of the face (anteroposterior dimension):
   (a) Affix zygomatic arches to stable temporal bone.
2. Reconstruct the width of the face (horizontal diameter):
   (a) Affix zygomas to the arches and to the frontal bone.
3. Reconstruct the area between the zygomas (NOE):
   (a) Orbital floor
   (b) Medial canthal tendon area
   (c) Nasal bridge
4. Reconstruct the posterior vertical height of the face:
   (a) Repair condylar fractures.
5. Perform mandibulomaxillary fixation and mandibular reconstruction.
6. Position the maxillary fragment to best approximate natural occlusion:
   (a) Complete reconstruction of the maxilla.

Specifics of Repair Depending on Fracture Pattern

Le Fort I Fractures

Minimally displaced Le Fort I fractures often can be reduced and stabilized sufficiently with MMF. When there is displacement or mobility of the maxilla, an open approach and additional means of fixation are required. The fracture is disimpacted. A sublabial incision is made and dissection continued until the fractures are exposed. The nasomaxillary and zygomaticomaxillary buttresses are plated orienting the plate along the load-bearing pathways. Occasionally, plating over either buttress on each side of the fracture will provide adequate, stable fixation. The occlusion is set via the desired technique of maxillomandibular fixation (see above section on MMF). The duration of MMF is directed by the degree of fracture and the stability obtained with repair. Careful follow-up is necessary to ensure that proper occlusion is maintained postoperatively and, if not, identified and corrected early.

Alternatively, suspension wiring may be used to secure the fracture. In this method, a 25- or 26-gauge wire is looped around the temporal aspect of the zygomatic arch, retrieved intraorally, and tightened to an intermediate wire loop connected to the arch bar.

Le Fort II Fractures

Nearly all Le Fort II fractures will require open reduction and internal fixation for adequate repair. Just as for Le Fort I fractures, a sublabial incision is made, and exposure of maxilla and fracture lines is performed. Additional exposure of the orbital rim is often necessary and can be achieved via either a subciliary or the more preferred, transconjunctival incision. First, the fracture is disimpacted and then the occlusion optimized. Next, the pyramidal-shaped fracture segment is positioned into place. The zygomaticomaxillary buttresses are secured by fixation with plating that spans the fracture lines. If the superior portion of the fracture remains unstable, then plate fixation of the inferior orbital rim and the nasomaxillary buttresses should be completed.

Alternatively, but much less commonly used today is fixation with interosseous wiring. To achieve this, small holes are placed into the appropriate bony segments on either side of the fracture line. Then, 28-gauge wire is passed through the holes and tightened together. If this method is used, a longer duration of MMF will be needed compared to plating.

Le Fort III Fractures

The force of impact to cause a Le fort III injury is significant. It is extremely rare that there would be such minimal displacement that occlusal fixation and plating of the buttresses through minimal incisions would be sufficient. The goal is to stabilize the mobile segments of bone to the stable mandible below and cranium above. Depending on the extent of the fracture, soft tissue incisions may be made in the same locations as for Le Fort II fractures (sublabial and periorbital, usually transconjunctival). If the zygomaticofrontal suture, zygomatic arch, or nasofrontal projections are not adequately visualized, then a more extensive incision such as a coronal incision or use of other additional incisions should be performed. Again, the initial step is to disimpact the maxilla, followed by establishment of occlusion and implementation of MMF. If there are concurrent cranial or mandibular fractures, they should be addressed prior to fixating the midface. For true Le Fort III fractures, bilateral zygomaticofrontal fixation may suffice. However, more commonly additional fixation at other locations such as the zygomatic arch, nasofrontal, and nasomaxillary is required.

Interosseous wiring and suspension wiring have been described for Le Fort III fractures and performed in the same manner, as discussed in the prior section. This method of repair is less reliable than plate fixation and is not an ideal means of repair of these fractures (Figs. 72.11 and 72.12).

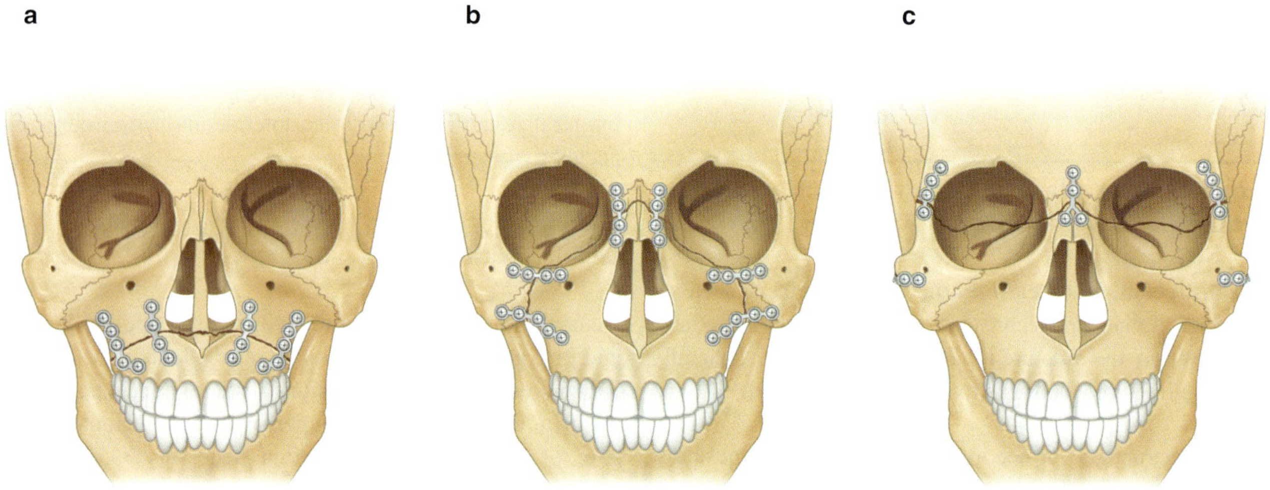

Fig. 72.11 Schematic examples of repaired fractures with plates. Ideally at least two screws are secured on each side of the fracture. Of note, there is normally a portion of the plate that crosses the fracture where no screw is placed. This was omitted to show the fracture lines. (**a**) Type I. (**b**) Type II. (**c**) Type III

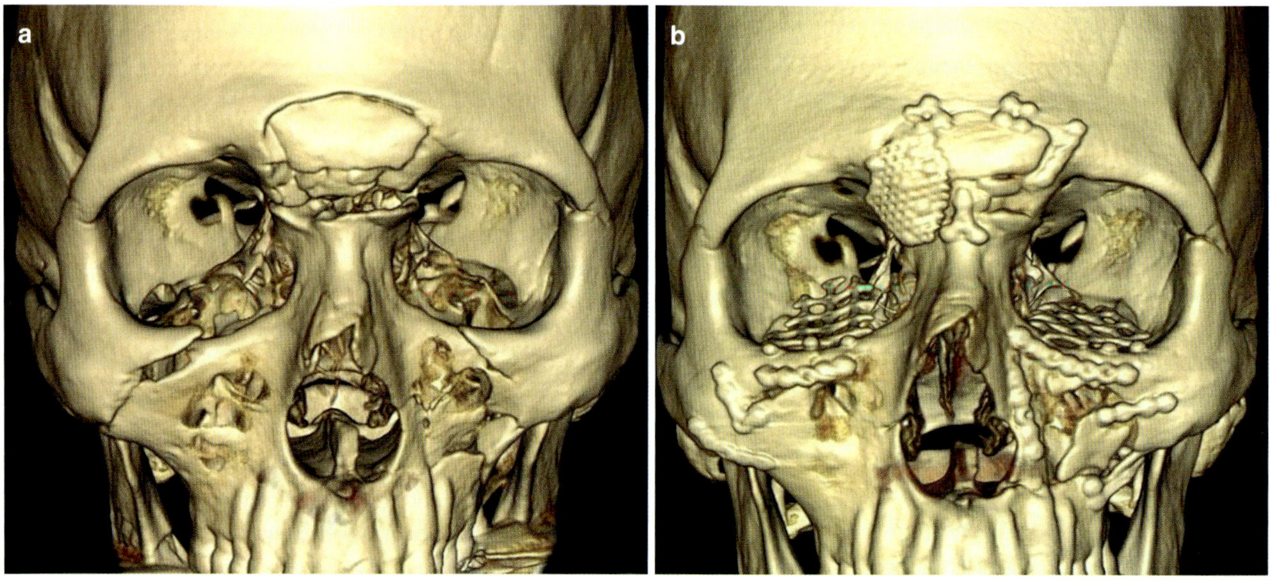

Fig. 72.12 Three-dimensional reconstructed images of a patient with Le Fort II, bilateral orbital floor, and frontal bone fractures pre- and post repair. (**a**) Preoperative image. (**b**) Postoperative image

Pediatric Le Fort Fractures

Pediatric facial fractures are often best managed via a conservative approach. There is significant potential for bone remodeling in the pediatric patient, and even some displaced bones can heal into a fairly normal position. Extensive periosteal stripping and plate fixation can disrupt facial and dental growth centers. Plate fixation is generally reserved for cases with considerable comminution. If it is determined that operative repair will be necessary, it should be done within 7–10 days before malunion and bony deformity from rapid healing occurs [20].

Postoperative Management

Patients with maxillary fractures should be treated with broad-spectrum antibiotics that cover both oral and sinus pathogens. Typically, antibiotics are started preoperatively and should continue for 5–10 postoperatively, depending on surgeon preference. Additionally, oral hygiene must be addressed. Chlorhexidine oral rinses three times daily should be used to control oral flora. MMF can be cleaned using pulsed irrigation or with a soft tipped bristle brush. Patients should be monitored closely for malunion, infection, or bleeding. The globe and vision should be checked and observed in any orbital involving injuries or procedures. Follow-up is determined by the procedure performed and if MMF was implemented.

Complications of Le Fort Fractures

One of the most challenging aspects of repair of these fractures is the restoration of normal function. Malunion is always a potential complication as is impaired mastication. Nerve function can be compromised from the initial insult or secondary to surgical repair. The bony facial structure may not be exact after injury and repair. There is a tendency for patients with these fractures to develop horizontal widening and midfacial depression. Because of this tendency, attention must be paid during fixation to not leave gaps in the horizontal dimension and to ensure that the fractured segment is properly repositioned in the anterior-posterior dimension. Orbital fractures and repair could lead to globe malposition leading to both a functional disability such as diplopia or extraocular motility impairment and cosmetic compromise via enophthalmos or hypoglobus.

Infection in the perioperative period may occur from a contaminated injury or from sinus, oral, or skin flora. Later in the postoperative course, the hardware may become infected and may need to be removed if antibiotic treatment fails. One must also consider the possibility of the development of osteomyelitis in refractory cases, which would require removal of the hardware and debridement of the bone. The hardware may also migrate and become visible through the skin. Injury to the tooth root can occur from misplaced plates and lead to nonviable teeth.

If meticulous closure is not conducted, soft tissue deformity or scarring may result [21]. We suggest closure be done in a two-layer fashion, first with re-approximation of the deeper soft tissue plane with absorbable suture (to allow soft tissue reconstruction as well as to remove tension from the skin layer) followed by skin closure in a manner that will slightly evert the skin edges. Eyelid malposition, most commonly upper or lower eyelid retraction or lower lid ectropion, can be encountered if dissection and closure are not executed properly.

References

1. Le Fort R. Ètude expérimentale sur les fractures de la mâchoire supériure. Rev chir paris 1901;23:208, 227, 360, 379, 479–507. Reprint translated by Tessier P. Plast Reconstr Surg. 1972;50:600–7.
2. Sicher H, Tandler J. Anatomie fur Zahnarazte. Vienna: Springer; 1928.
3. Donat TL, Endress C, Mathog RH. Facial fracture classification according to skeletal support mechanisms. Arch Otolaryngol Head Neck Surg. 1998;124:1306–14.
4. Rudderman RH, Mullen RL. Biomechanics of the facial skeleton. Clin Plast Surg. 1999;19(1):105–13.
5. American College of Surgeons. Advanced trauma life support. www.facs.org/dept/trauma/atls/index.html.
6. Derdyn C, Persing JA, Broaddus W, et al. Craniofacial trauma: an assessment of risk related to the timing of surgery. Plast Reconstr Surg. 1992;50:1264–8.
7. Smoot EC, Jernigan JR, Kinsley E, et al. A survey of operative airway management practices for midface fractures. J Craniofac Surg. 1997;8(3):157–242.
8. Bahr W, Stoll P. Nasal intubation in the presence of frontobasal fractures: a retrospective study. J Oral Maxillofac Surg. 1992;50:445–7.
9. Rhee KJ, Muntz CB, Donald PJ, et al. Does nasotracheal intubation increase complications in patients with skull base fractures? Ann Emerg Med. 1993;22:1145–7.
10. Yerit KC, Enislidis G, Schooper C, et al. Fixation of mandibular fractures with biodegradable plates and screws. Oral Surg Oral Med Oral Pathol Oral Radiol Endod. 2002;94(3):294–300.
11. Bell RB, Kindsfater CS. The use of biodegradable plates and screws to stabilize facial fractures. J Oral Maxillofac Surg. 2006;64(1):31–9.
12. Evans GR, Clark N, Manson PN, Leipziger LS. Role of mini- and microplate fixation in fractures of the midface and mandible. Ann Plast Surg. 1995;34(5):453–6.
13. Haug RH, Adama JM, Jordan RB. Comparison of the morbidity associated with maxillary fractures treated by maxillomandibular and rigid internal fixation. Oral Surg Oral Med Oral Pathol Oral Radiol Endod. 1995;80:629–37.
14. Arbeitsgemeinschaft für osteosynthesefragen/Association for the Study of Internal Fixation. www.aofoundation.org. Aug 2010.
15. Shaw RC, Parsons RW. Exposure through a coronal incision for initial treatment of facial fractures. Plast Reconstr Surg. 1975;56(3):254–9.

16. Frodel JL, Marentette LJ. The coronal approach anatomic and technical considerations and morbidity. Arch Otolaryngol Head Neck Surg. 1993;119:201–7.
17. Markowitz BL, Manson PN. Panfacial fractures: organization of treatment. Clin Plast Surg. 1989;16(1):105–14.
18. Marciani RD. Management of middle third facial fractures. J Oral Maxillofac Surg. 1993;51(5):535–42.
19. Gruss JS, Bubak PJ, Egbert MA. Craniofacial fractures: an algorithm to optimize results. Clin Plast Surg. 1992;19(1):195–206.
20. Haug RH, Foss J. Maxillofacial injuries in the pediatric patient. Oral Surg Oral Med Oral Pathol Oral Radiol Endod. 2000;90:126–34.
21. Frodel JL, Rudderman R. Facial soft tissue resuspension following upper facial skeletal reconstruction. J Craniomaxillofac Trauma. 1996;2:24–30.

Post-traumatic Enophthalmos and Three-Dimensional Imaging

73

Michael K. Yoon and Robert C. Kersten

Introduction

Enophthalmos following trauma can be a challenging condition to repair. Soon after the trauma, enophthalmos occurs secondary to an increase in orbital volume [1]. With late enophthalmos, there is evidence that traumatic atrophy of soft tissue plays a role [2]. When enophthalmos occurs, patients may report abnormalities in blink, ocular discomfort, visible deformity, or diplopia. Globe projection asymmetry of 2 mm or greater is typically cosmetically noticeable [3, 4]. In this chapter, we review the relevant anatomy of the orbit, the pathophysiology of enophthalmos, mechanisms of injury, evaluation, and management. Other masqueraders of traumatic enophthalmos will be discussed. The use of modern three-dimensional imaging techniques and custom-made patient-specific implants in reconstruction will also be examined.

Enophthalmos following trauma occurs secondary to an increase in orbital volume although traumatic atrophy of soft tissue may play a role [1, 2]. Whether presenting in the acute or chronic phase, such cases can be challenging to evaluate and manage. Patients may report abnormalities in blink, ocular discomfort, visible deformity, or diplopia. Globe projection asymmetry of 2 mm or greater is typically cosmetically noticeable [3, 4]. In this chapter, we review the relevant anatomy of the orbit, the pathophysiology of enophthalmos, mechanisms of injury, evaluation, and management. Other masqueraders of traumatic enophthalmos will be discussed. The use of modern three-dimensional imaging techniques and its role in reconstruction will also be examined.

M. K. Yoon (✉)
Mass Eye and Ear, Department of Ophthalmology, Harvard Medical School, Boston, MA, USA
e-mail: Michael_yoon@meei.harvard.edu

R. C. Kersten
University of California – San Francisco, Department of Ophthalmology, San Francisco, CA, USA

Anatomy and Pathophysiology

The orbit is a quadrilateral pyramidal-shaped bony cavity with the base oriented anteriorly. The position of the globe within this cavity is dependent on the relative volumes of orbital fat, extraocular muscles, nerves, blood vessels, and other adnexal structures. The anterior limit of the orbit is the orbital septum.

With trauma, injury to the orbital walls with subsequent bone displacement is responsible for an increase in bony orbital volume. However, disruption of the periorbita as well as suspensory ligaments of the globe is also necessary for globe displacement [1, 5]. This concept is also encountered with orbital decompression where incision of the periorbita is performed after bony removal for the soft tissue to shift. Finally, orbital fat atrophy can result in further net increase in the orbital volume, contributing approximately 1/3 of the effect [2]. In response to these factors, the globe is shifted in a direction corresponding to the location of fracture, e.g., posteriorly and occasionally inferiorly with orbital floor fracture, giving rise to enophthalmos and globe dystopia (Fig. 73.1a–c).

Diplopia associated with enophthalmos is uncommon (outside the acute setting). When it does occur, it is usually due to entrapment of soft tissue or cranial nerve palsy. Entrapment of the extraocular muscles within the fracture is the most common cause of restrictive strabismus in patients with post-traumatic enophthalmos. Trauma may result in cranial nerve palsy affecting the oculomotor (III), trochlear (IV), or abducens (VI) nerves which may or may not recover following injury [6]. The location of the nerve injury may be within the orbit or from intracranial injury associated with the original trauma. Furthermore, following restrictive strabismus repair with tissue release, latent muscle paresis may be unmasked [7]. Severe enophthalmos may result in slack extraocular muscles with resultant limitation of extraocular excursions and diplopia [8].

J. J. Servat et al. (eds.), *Smith and Nesi's Ophthalmic Plastic and Reconstructive Surgery*,
https://doi.org/10.1007/978-3-030-41720-8_73

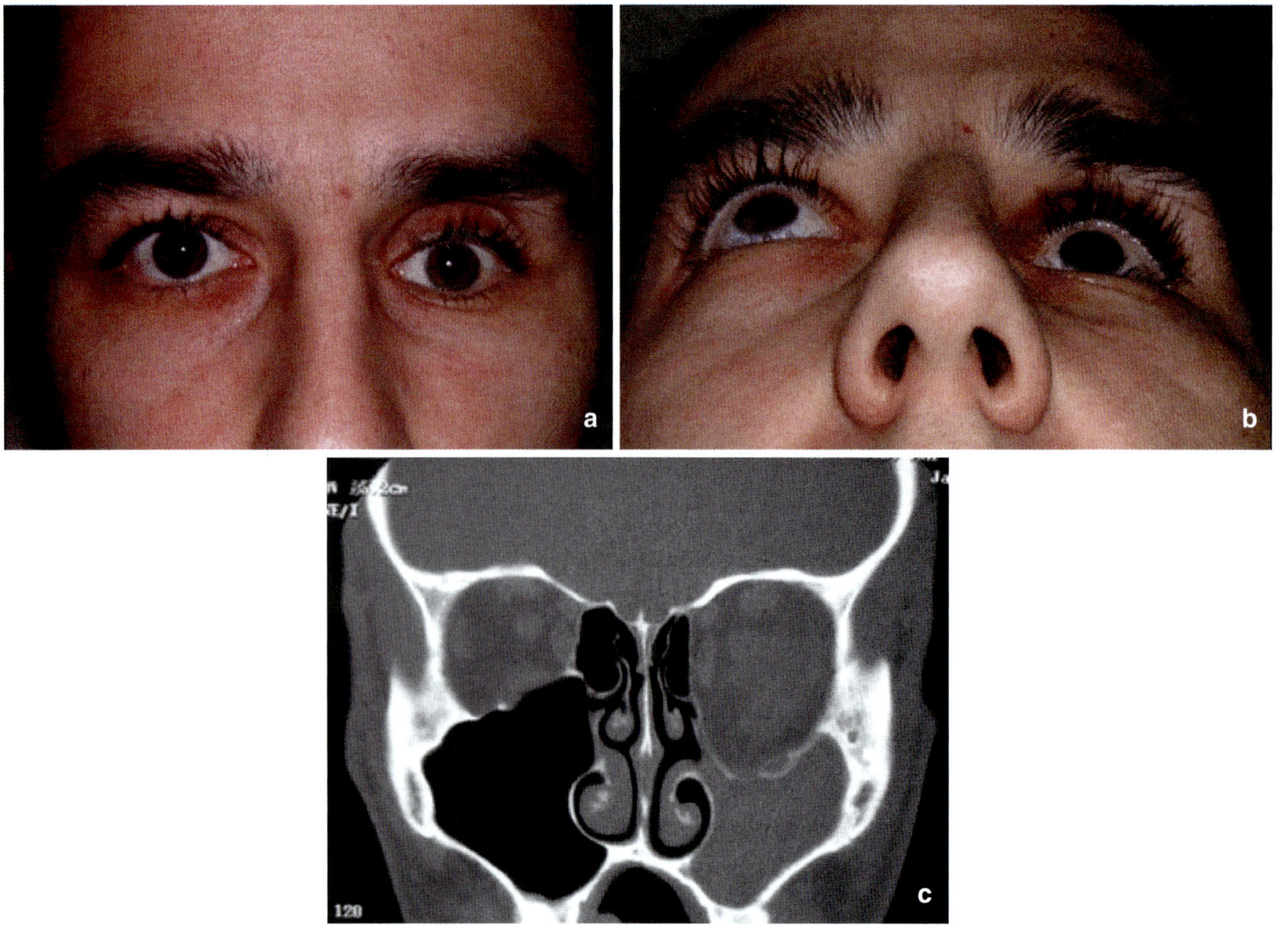

Fig. 73.1 A man with history of trauma, demonstrating enophthalmos. (**a**) Demonstrates enophthalmos of the left eye with hypoglobus. (**b**) Worm's-eye view accentuates the enophthalmos. Note the flattening of the maxillary prominence. (**c**) Coronal CT scan showing a large left orbital floor fracture with opacification of the adjacent maxillary sinus

Mechanisms of Traumatic Orbital Wall Displacement

Periocular trauma, whether directly to the soft tissues of the globe and orbit or to the orbital rims, transfers kinetic energy to the orbital walls, which can result in a fracture. Injuries to multiple walls are not uncommon. When occurring in conjunction with other facial and systemic injuries, these fractures have a higher rate of late enophthalmos [9].

Floor

The orbital floor is the most common location for orbital fracture. These fractures are considered "internal" or "blow-out" when they involve the floor without an associated fracture affecting the orbital rim. More complex fractures with multiple wall involvement may occur and may further contribute to development of enophthalmos. With the maxillary sinus inferior to the floor, orbital tissue may herniate through the floor and into this space. Isolated orbital floor fractures typically are found medial to the infraorbital canal, involving the maxillary bone.

Medial Wall

The medial orbital wall is the thinnest bony wall of the orbit (approximately 0.5 mm in thickness) and is often referred to as the lamina papyracea. Despite being half the thickness of the orbital floor, it is less commonly fractured. Although isolated medial wall fractures may occur, more often they occur in association with other orbital walls, especially the orbital floor [10].

Lateral Wall

The lateral wall is the thickest of the orbital bones, requiring high-energy forces to fracture the zygomatic and sphenoid

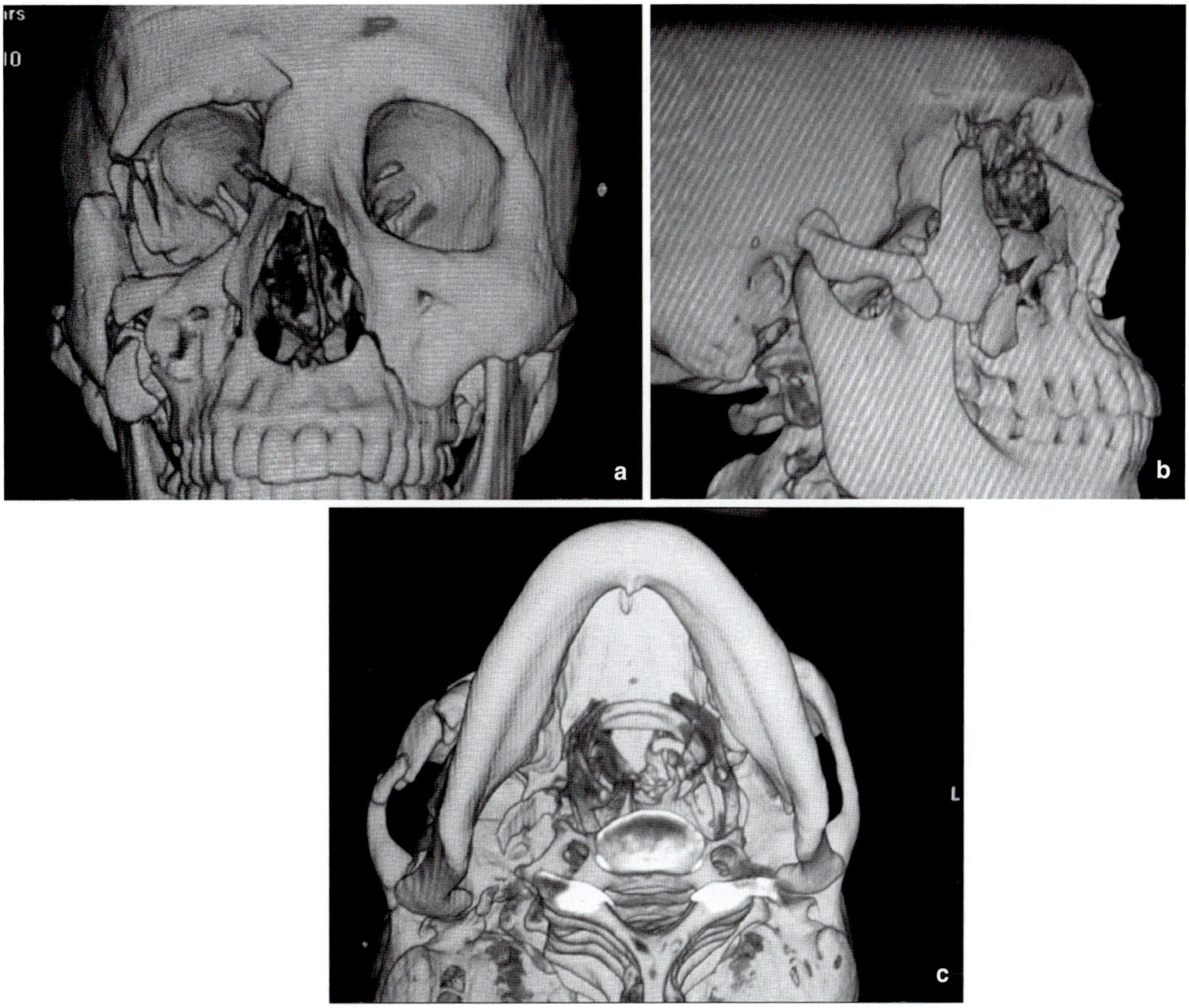

Fig. 73.2 Three-dimensional reconstruction of a CT scan demonstrating a right zygomaticomaxillary complex fracture. (**a**) The fracture involves the medial orbital wall at the frontal process of the maxillary bone, the inferior orbital rim with a comminuted maxillary bone, and the lateral orbital rim at the fronto-zygomatic suture. (**b**) Lateral view of the reconstruction illustrates the depressed maxillary sinus. (**c**) Inferior view illustrates the fracture of the right zygomatic arch

bones. Fractures in this region are almost universally found in conjunction with zygomaticomaxillary complex (ZMC) fractures. Here, a large block of bone is displaced, typically with a rotational or telescoping component. ZMC fractures are a common cause of enophthalmos, even after initial repair [11, 12] (Fig. 73.2a–c).

Roof

Fractures to the orbital roof are uncommon in adults. This is believed to be secondary to the pneumatized frontal sinus which serves as a "crumple zone" preventing severe roof injury. When these fractures do occur, they typically involve high-energy injuries, such as motor vehicle accidents. However, in children, roof fractures are more commonly encountered if the sinuses have not yet developed [13].

Dislocations of bone are typically minimal, with the relatively durable dura mater and brain preventing large superior displacements, and gravity preventing superior globe dystopia. "Blow-in" fractures, with downward displacement of bone into the orbit, generally require impact to the supraorbital rim with an abrupt elevation in intracranial pressure [14]. These may cause proptosis due to the net decrease in the bony orbital volume. Roof fractures generally do not cause enophthalmos. These injuries should be managed in consultation with neurosurgery.

Evaluation

Whether in the acute or chronic presentation, all patients with enophthalmos require complete ophthalmic examination to rule out globe injury, since even days or weeks after the initial injury, patients may not have had a full evaluation. Associated facial injuries should be assessed in conjunction with other facial surgeons as needed.

Clear discussion with the patient regarding their subjective complaints is essential for planning any intervention. Both functional and aesthetic concerns are usually present and should be adequately addressed.

Physical evaluation begins with the external examination of the face and eyelids. Hollowing of the superior palpebral sulcus is often found as an associated sign of enophthalmos. The location and shape of the lateral canthus may suggest a zygomaticomaxillary complex fracture as inferior rotation of the complex may result in an anti-mongoloid slant. The medial canthus may be altered with naso-orbito-ethmoidal fractures [15] producing telecanthus and enophthalmos with an abnormal nasal bridge. Epiphora or other evidence of associated nasolacrimal duct injury should be assessed.

Extraocular motility including ductions (uniocular) and versions (binocular) should be carefully assessed to evaluate for extraocular muscle entrapment. Enophthalmos in the presence of a chronically entrapped muscle may occur. Exophthalmometry should be performed to evaluate for exophthalmos or enophthalmos. If the lateral orbital wall is also fractured and posteriorly displaced, enophthalmos may not be detected by Hertel exophthalmometry, as that instrument relies on the lateral orbital rim as its reference point. It is useful to view the globe projection from below with the patient's chin tipped upward (worm's-eye view) to detect gross enophthalmos in this setting. Furthermore, depression of the maxilla may be more obvious with this perspective. Superior or inferior globe dystopia may suggest an inferior blow-in fracture or blowout fracture.

Assessment of the orbital bones should be specifically performed to address all orbital walls. Careful palpation of the orbital rims and zygomatic arch may reveal gross step-off displacement or tenderness, suggesting underlying fracture. Cutaneous sensation of the cheek should be evaluated, with hypesthesia of the infraorbital nerve suggestive of an orbital floor fracture [16]. Finally, the presence of trismus or malocclusion may be present with a zygomaticomaxillary complex fracture.

Preoperative photography should be carried out in the office to document the preoperative status of the patient.

Imaging

Computed tomography (CT) imaging is the best method to evaluate the orbital anatomy and bony structures of the face. Fine cuts (0.625–1.25 mm) of the orbits in the axial, coronal, and sagittal planes are recommended. With modern helical CT scanners, rapid scans (from 104 to 18 s) with lower radiation dose [17], and software multiplanar reconstruction have increased safety and image quality.

In almost all cases, recent imaging (less than 3 months) is necessary to completely evaluate the injury. If the patient has had previous surgery, new imaging should be obtained to reveal the location of existing implants or other hardware as their location is critical to planning subsequent intervention.

Timing of Intervention

Absolute indications for early surgery to address acute enophthalmos from orbital fracture are rare. Subluxation of the globe into the maxillary sinus usually requires urgent surgical reduction [18, 19]. It is very rare to encounter enophthalmos in association with a trapdoor fracture (where there is entrapment and incarceration of an extraocular muscle), since there is rarely any significant bone displacement. However, if frank entrapment is present, early release of this muscle, especially within 24 h, is associated with greater return of function [20, 21]. Trapdoor fractures are typically seen in children (who have more elastic, thicker orbital bone), although they have been described in patients up to 37 years of age [22]. Trapdoor fractures of the medial orbital may also occur [23, 24]. If there are associated severe fractures of the skull base or facial skeleton, they must be addressed in conjunction with appropriate consulting services.

Floor and Medial Wall Fractures

It is rare to encounter enophthalmos immediately following bony trauma as it usually takes several days to weeks for initial soft tissue swelling to subside. Even in the presence of multiple wall fractures with significant displacement, early enophthalmos is uncommon. Although historically it was felt that operating on fractures within 2 weeks of injury resulted in better outcomes, more recent literature has shown no difference in postoperative outcomes whether fractures were operated within this early time window, or if surgery was delayed until ultimate enophthalmos could be better evaluated [25, 26]. In fact, in relation to orbital blowout fractures (both floor and medial wall), early surgical repair may actually result in less satisfactory correction of ultimate enophthalmos [27]. For the large majority of patients, surgical repair to correct enophthalmos may be scheduled in a nonurgent manner and should be delayed until confounding edema and ecchymosis have resolved.

Lateral Wall Fractures

Lateral orbital wall fractures are commonly found in association with zygomaticomaxillary complex (ZMC) fractures. Symptoms include trismus and malocclusion from interference of the fracture with the adjacent temporalis and masseter muscles that may warrant more expedient treatment. However, timing of surgery is controversial, and it is generally accepted that midfacial fractures involving the orbital rims should be repaired earlier than pure blowout fractures since soft tissue contracture may result in more significant displacement of the orbital rims and midfacial bones. Late revision of ZMC fractures may require osteotomy for mobilization of the displaced fragments, which add complexity and risk to the procedure.

Predictors of Enophthalmos

In the acute setting, most patients do not have visible enophthalmos, owing to orbital edema and hemorrhage from the trauma, as well as difficulty in assessment from facial swelling. Late enophthalmos may occur in 10–76% [28–31] of patients who do not meet indications for immediate repair. In order to predict which patients that might develop late enophthalmos, several groups have attempted CT-based analysis of orbital volume. Results by various studies have shown in inconsistent results due to the variations in methodology. Similarly, our experience has been that enophthalmos correlates poorly with the volume displacement. Therefore, our preference is to allow soft tissue swelling to resolve and to then look for functionally or cosmetically significant enophthalmos before deciding on surgical repair (Fig. 73.3a–d).

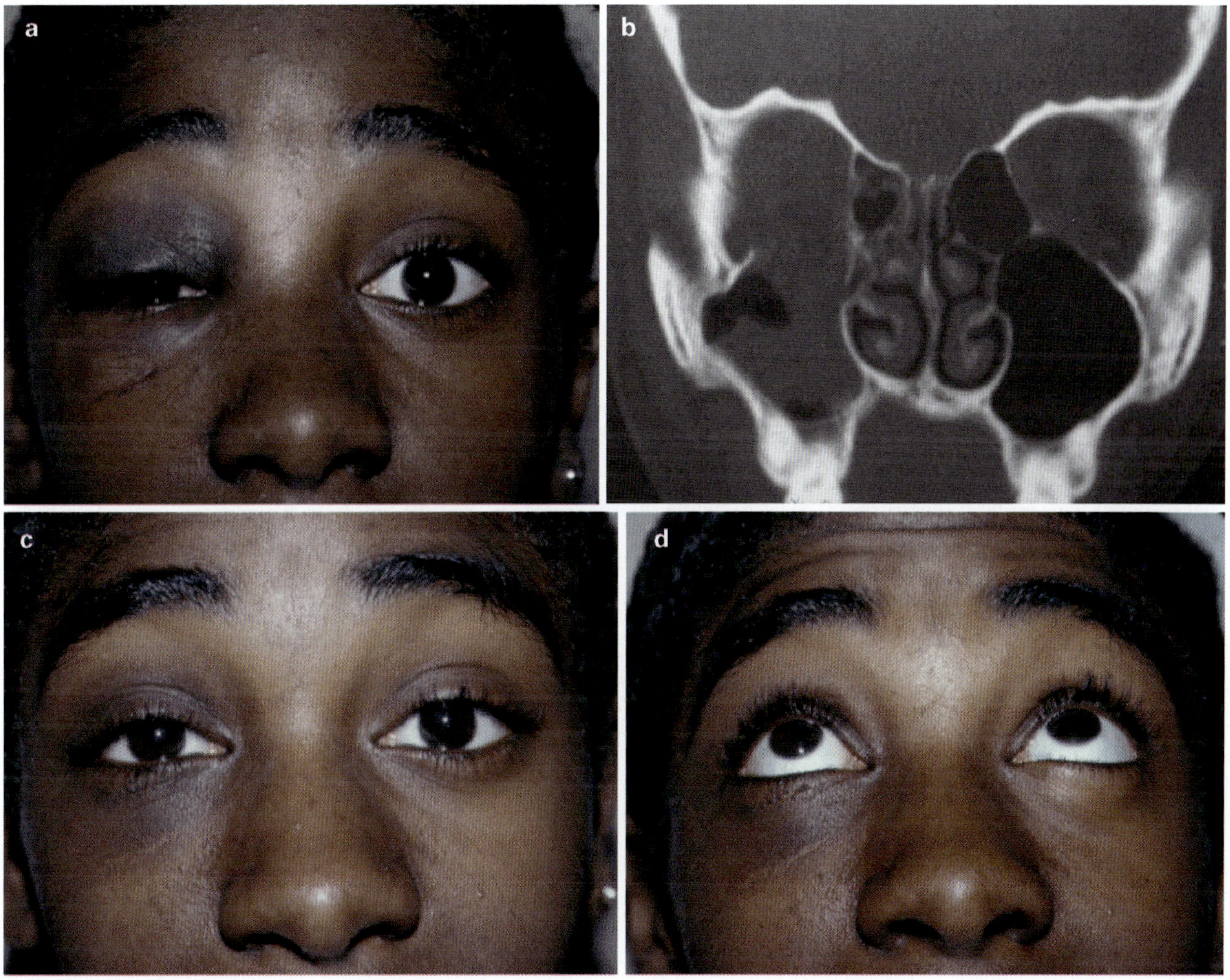

Fig. 73.3 Enophthalmos is difficult to predict based on CT imaging. (**a**) Girl immediately following trauma to the right eye. (**b**) Coronal CT scan shows a large right orbital floor fracture and medial wall fracture. (**c**) Six weeks later without any surgical intervention. Edema has largely improved. (**d**) No enophthalmos developed and extraocular motility was full

However, there are those who do believe there is a role for image-based volumetric analysis in determining patients who are at risk for late enophthalmos. Whitehouse et al. analyzed CT images of a mixed population of fractures (13 orbital floor, 3 medial wall, and 21 combined medial and floor) calculating that with 1 cm^3 in orbital volume resulted in 0.8 mm of enophthalmos [32]. Fan et al. found nearly identical results in a similar study [33]. Ahn et al. correlated 1 cm^3 of increased orbital volume with 0.84 mm of enophthalmos [34].

Orbital floor fractures were investigated with CT-based volumetric analysis of orbital volume. An increase in over 13% of orbital volume (compared to the non-traumatized side) resulted in a significant risk of late enophthalmos (in 92% of patients) [35].

Isolated medial orbital wall fractures have been examined. By inference calculations from CT scans, regression analysis determined that 0.9 cm^3 of herniated orbital tissue or 1.9 cm^2 of fracture area correlated with 2 mm enophthalmos, while 2.1 cm^3 or 3.2 cm^2 correlated with 3 mm enophthalmos [36]. Lee et al. calculated an estimated defect area of 0.55 cm^2 correlated with 1 mm enophthalmos [31]. Here too, calculations were based on CT scan measurements with the assumption that the bony defects were elliptical in nature, making them estimates at best.

The most convincing data for the mechanism and quantification of post-traumatic enophthalmos was presented by Cohen et al. [2]. This group quantified the bony orbital volume as well as the orbital fat volume in 13 orbits with unilateral orbital fracture that did not undergo repair. The volumes were quantified using CT scans at least 3 months after injury comparing the traumatized orbit as well as the uninjured control orbit. The mean increase in bony volume (due to displaced bone) was 2.1 cc (range 0.7–2.7, SD 1.3), while the decrease in fat volume was 0.9 cc (range 0.1–2.1, SD 0.6). This was the first group to quantify that fat atrophy does occur in patients with late post-traumatic enophthalmos.

Non-volumetric studies have also been performed. Matic et al. investigated rounding of the inferior rectus muscle on coronal CT scan as a predictor of late enophthalmos [28]. In an evaluation of 18 isolated floor fractures that were managed nonsurgically for 6 months or greater, late enophthalmos in 2 patients was significantly correlated to rounding of the inferior rectus muscle (defined as height-to-width ratio of 1 or greater). Similarly, looking at the medial rectus in isolated medial orbital wall fractures, rounding of the medial rectus in the coronal plane correlated significantly with the development of late enophthalmos [37]. It has been our experience that rounding of the adjacent rectus muscle is extremely common after orbital wall fractures, the majority of whom do not develop clinically significant enophthalmos.

Surgical Techniques

Planning surgery requires complete evaluation of the patient clinically as well as appropriate imaging to correlate exam findings. Functional and cosmetic concerns should be completely evaluated and discussed in detail to enter surgery with appropriate goals and expectations.

Materials

In repairing orbital fractures, numerous implantable materials have been utilized and reported. Historically, autologous bone grafts, most commonly from iliac crest or calvarium, were harvested from the patient for restoration of bony volume and contour [38–40]. Similarly, sliced or diced autologous cartilage has been historically used to replace volume with reasonable success [41–44]. With the development of synthetic alloplastic materials, the use of autologous materials declined significantly over the past several decades. The shorter operating time with these packaged materials and the elimination of morbidity from a surgical harvest site have made them the new gold standard in industrialized nations.

When selecting from the myriad of materials, the primary consideration is how the implant will integrate with orbital tissues or "bio-integrate." Porous materials have channels allowing for fibrovascular ingrowth, which contribute to stabilization of the implant and minimization of long-term migration. In addition, complete vascularization of the material may help to resist infection. Porous polyethylene is one such material that has been used for orbital reconstructions following fracture [45]. Specific advantages include ease of handling, the ability to shape and contour the material intraoperatively, and the ability to fixate it to surrounding bone. Variations of this material exist, including Supor (Poriferous, Newnan, GA, USA) and Medpor (Stryker, Kalamazoo, MI, USA), each with different pore density, thicknesses, and handling characteristics. Medpor™ Titan (Stryker, Kalamazoo, MI, USA) is porous polyethylene with an impregnated titanium mesh. Each face of the implant is either porous or nonporous, which can affect handling and ingrowth. The addition of the titanium allows for increased strength as well as presence of a radiopaque medium to visualize the implant on postimplantation CT scans [46]. These materials offer an advantage over bare titanium mesh, which can be difficult to pass through incisions due to rough edges which may become hung up on adjacent soft tissue. Additional complications include orbital adherence syndrome, where an "intense fibrotic adherence" between the titanium implant and orbital soft tissues occurs [47, 48], and displacement leading to diplopia [49] and orbital emphysema [50].

Although nonporous materials may have a role in fracture repair, the inability to radiographically visualize the implant after surgery and the generally lower maximum load they can sustain make them less popular for this indication [51]. Furthermore, dozens of reports of cystic implant encapsulation and hemorrhage due to late migration of a nonporous implant have been published [52, 53]. Perhaps related to this, porous implants are most commonly used by oculofacial plastic surgeons (53%) compared to nonporous nylon and silicone (39%) [54].

Fixation of the implant to the surrounding skeleton is not always necessary. When there is concern for implant migration, or to ensure proper apposition of the implant to bone, implantable titanium screws may be used (Fig. 73.4).

To help facilitate the speed and accuracy of orbital fracture repair, preformed implants have been developed. These are implants that have been developed by a manufacturer based on templates derived from averaged orbital datasets. Often the manufacturer will make different sizes as well as specific right- and left-sided implants. Although these preformed implants are not custom-made for each patient, they can have benefits over flat two-dimensional implants such as sheets [55]. Various manufacturers make implants for the orbit and are available in the United States including Stryker (Kalamazoo, MI), Synthes (West Chester, PA), KLS Martin (Jacksonville), and Biomet (Parsippany, NJ). Although the authors do not believe these to be needed commonly, they may be useful in certain cases with large, displaced fractures where typical landmarks (e.g., orbital strut) are missing.

Over the past several years, the use of patient-specific implants for orbital reconstruction has increased. These implants are custom-made for each patient and developed prior to surgery. Numerous implant materials are available including titanium mesh [56], porous polyethylene, polyether ether ketone (PEEK) [57], and polymethyl methacrylate (PMMA) [58] among others. Although there are several methods of their design, most patient-specific implants are created based on a 3D mirror image of the non-traumatized orbit. The mirror image and the injured orbit are overlaid in imaging software, and an implant is manufactured to fill the difference between the two. Some implants are thin and are only the thickness of titanium mesh [56], while others have substantial thickness of several millimeters (Fig. 73.5). These implants have been used in both primary fracture repair, revision fracture repair, post-traumatic enophthalmos, and post-oncologic reconstruction. Habib and colleagues presented their work using PEEK and porous polyethylene implants for silent sinus syndrome, revision orbital fracture repair, and post-oncologic reconstruction with success [59]. They have found that these implants are most useful for complex reconstruction or revision surgery, as opposed to more common orbital floor or single-wall fractures. One hurdle for using this technology is the relatively high cost compared to standard sheet implants (over 10× more expensive) and the need to plan for this reconstruction. However, as this technology becomes further adopted, the cost will likely reduce.

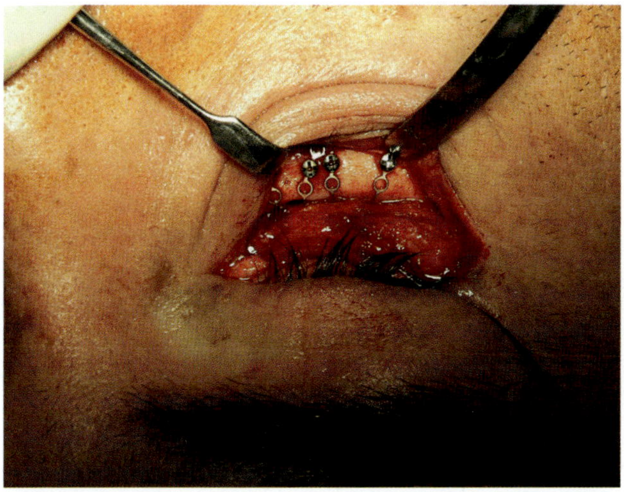

Fig. 73.4 Surgeon's view of the right eye. Using a conjunctival incision, the inferior orbital rim is exposed. Titanium screws are used to affix the implant (not visible) to the rim with the assistance of titanium mini-plates

Principles

Historically, the correction of post-traumatic enophthalmos was believed to require substantial dissection and mobilization – complete subperiosteal dissection of the orbit 360° from the rim anteriorly to 1 cm from the apex posteriorly, release of the periorbita from the bony fragments, osteotomies to mobilize and reposition the orbital framework, and reconstruction of the walls with bone grafts [60]. The extensive dissection required added to additional morbidity and is no longer routinely performed unless all orbital walls are being treated.

However, general principles in performing orbital fracture repair should be followed. Mobilization of the involved soft tissues (and periorbita) around the fracture is critical. A subperiosteal dissection plane is key to identify the edges of the fracture and to expose the bare stable bone upon which the implant will sit. Failure to place the implant in this plane will impinge on the extraocular muscles and may induce atrophy of soft tissue (orbital fat) that is trapped between the bone and implant. Complete reduction of the herniated soft tissue restores the orbital soft tissue volume. Restriction of extraocular motility may result from soft tissue displacement, as there are fine septae between the orbital fat and extraocular muscles. Fractures involving the orbital rim should be repositioned into their anatomic location allowing for proper contour. Although no consensus exists for removal of displaced fine orbital bone fragments (e.g., lamina papyracea

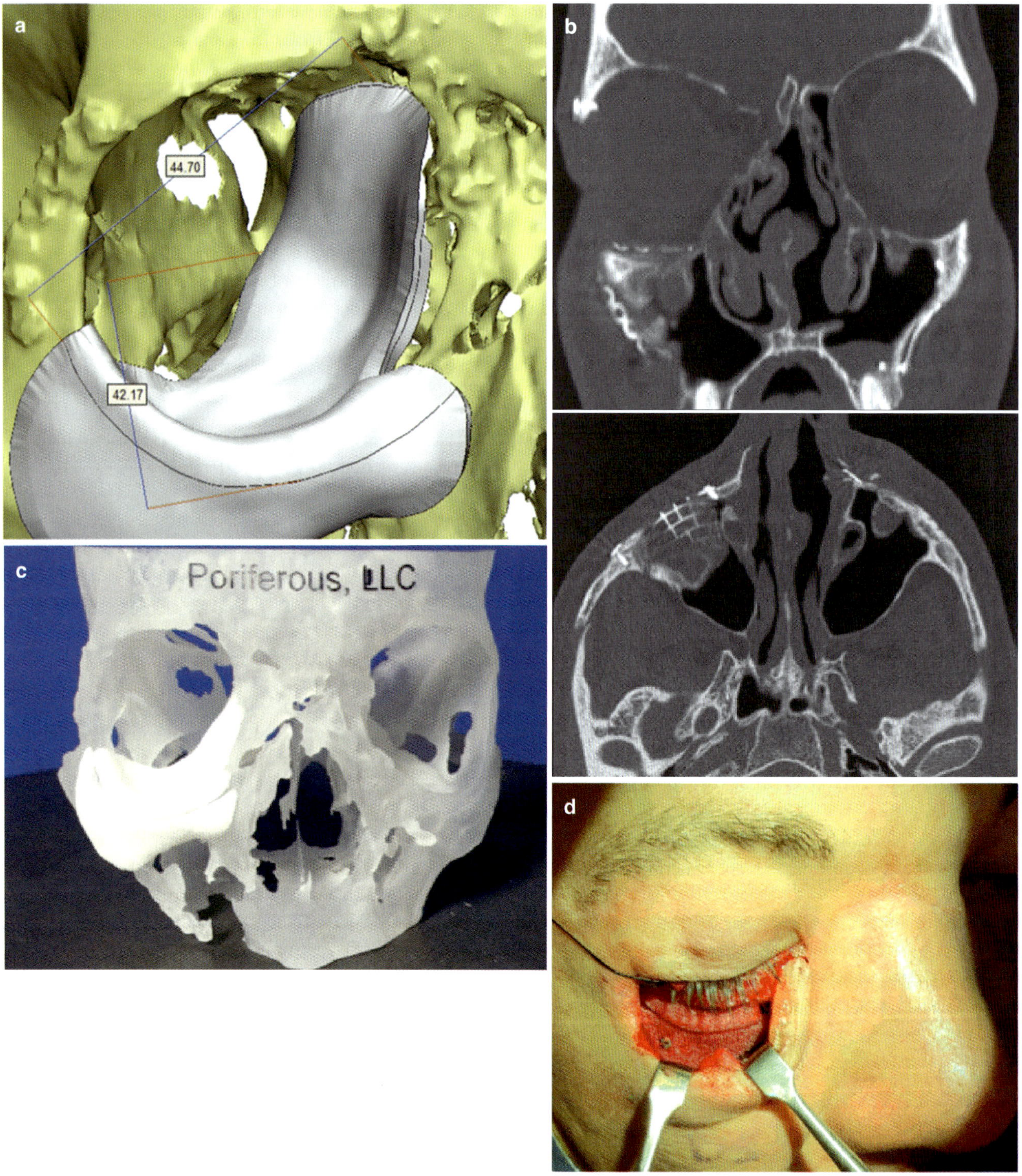

Fig. 73.5 Example of a case using a patient-specific implant. (**a**) The manufacturer's design of a patient-specific implant. The proposed implant, shown in white, spans a combined right inferior rim, inferior wall, and medial orbital wall fractures. The dimensions of the implant in millimeters are shown. (**b**) The preoperative CT scan showing previously placed titanium mesh implants that are improperly positioned. The medial wall fracture has not been reduced. (**c**) Model of the fracture with the implants placed overlying the defect. (**d**) Intraoperative photograph of the implants placed in the orbit and on the rim

within the ethmoid sinus), there is evidence that bony fragments may resorb [61] or partially reduce itself [62]. Finally, reattaching the eyelids to the bone at the proper medial and lateral canthal locations will allow for proper structure and function of the eyelids and adnexa [63].

Orbital Floor

Correlation of the clinical findings to imaging is crucial to properly address orbital volume restoration. Proper identification of the site of fracture and resultant orbital volume increase will direct the surgical approach. In orbital floor fractures, if the primary cause of enophthalmos is the floor defect, then this should be primarily addressed. Although medial wall fractures commonly occur concurrently, if small, they do not always require repair (Fig. 73.6a, b).

Even after previous surgery for repair of orbital floor fractures, enophthalmos may persist in 14–27% of patients [29, 64]. It usually occurs due to one of three causes. Often there is an unrecognized or untreated medial wall fracture. This is especially true when imaging is acquired weeks after the injury with resolution of ethmoid sinus hemorrhage and opacification on imaging. A second cause is failure to place the implant over the posterior ledge of the fracture (the "posterior ledge" formed by the nondisplaced portion of the posterior orbital floor/maxillary sinus roof). The orbital floor slopes in a posterior and superior direction from the inferior orbital rim. If the implant is not resting on the posterior ledge, then it will simply "fall" into the maxillary sinus. Inadequate posterior dissection during surgery from fear of injuring orbital apex structures may prevent visualization of this bony ledge. The surgeon may be reassured by remembering that the anterior-posterior length of the orbital floor is 35–40 mm. Intraoperative measurements and review of the imaging may properly identify the posterior extent of the fracture. Rarely with extensive fractures, a posterior ledge is not present, and a cantilevered implant with hardware fixation may be necessary. Third, migration of the previously placed implant may occur. This is an uncommon occurrence with proper placement (extending to and resting over the posterior ledge) as well as use of a bio-integratable implant.

When addressing orbital floor fractures, the use of a transconjunctival incision should always be employed, even in the presence of a cutaneous laceration over the orbital rim. The development of inflammation, full-thickness cicatrix formation, and/or adhesion of eyelid soft tissue to the implant can result in ectropion or eyelid retraction when using a transcutaneous approach. This can occur in up to 28% percent of patients, compared to about 3% of patients using the transconjunctival incision [65].

Medial Orbital Wall

The presence of large floor and medial orbital wall fractures requires addressing both components. The medial wall is commonly injured as part of facial and periorbital injuries [30]. This can result in medial dystopia of the globe with an apparent hypotelorism (Fig. 73.7a–e). If volume is restored only in one location (e.g., the lateral wall) without repairing the medial wall, the globe may be improperly positioned either due to lack of medial support (causing persistent medial globe dystopia) or overcompensation with implant volume in the incorrect location (causing medial or other globe displacement) [66] (Fig. 73.8a–h). Therefore, it is critical to assess the patient clinically as well as carefully examine the orbital imaging to plan the proper approach. If patients have had surgical repair by another surgeon, then secondary repair may be successfully performed by removing the inappropriate implants and adding volume in the correct location (Fig. 73.9a–g).

At the time of surgery, it is recommended to slightly overcorrect the amount of volume deficit. Through the authors'

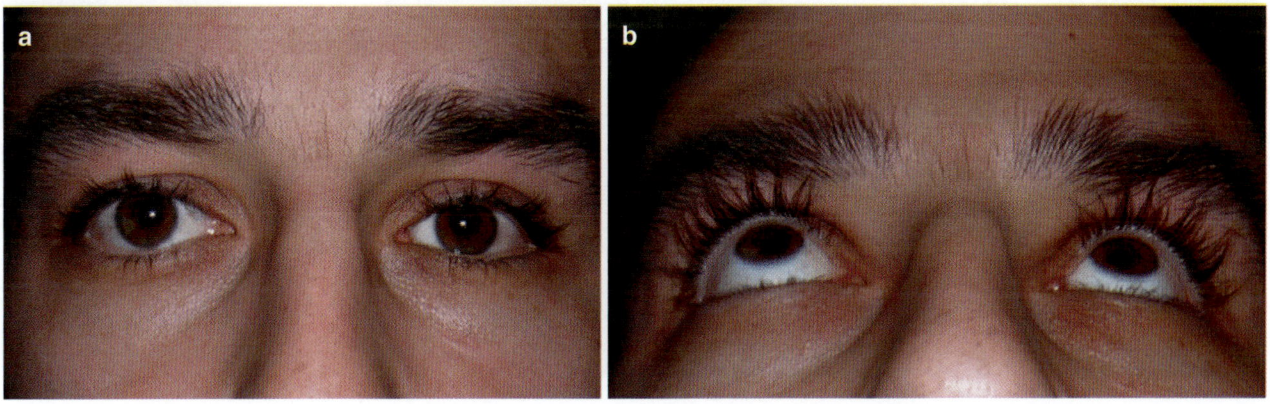

Fig. 73.6 The same patient is from Fig. 73.1 following repair of the left orbital floor fracture. (**a**) Hypoglobus has improved with a more symmetric appearance of the eyelids. (**b**) Significantly improved enophthalmos is demonstrated compared to Fig. 73.1b

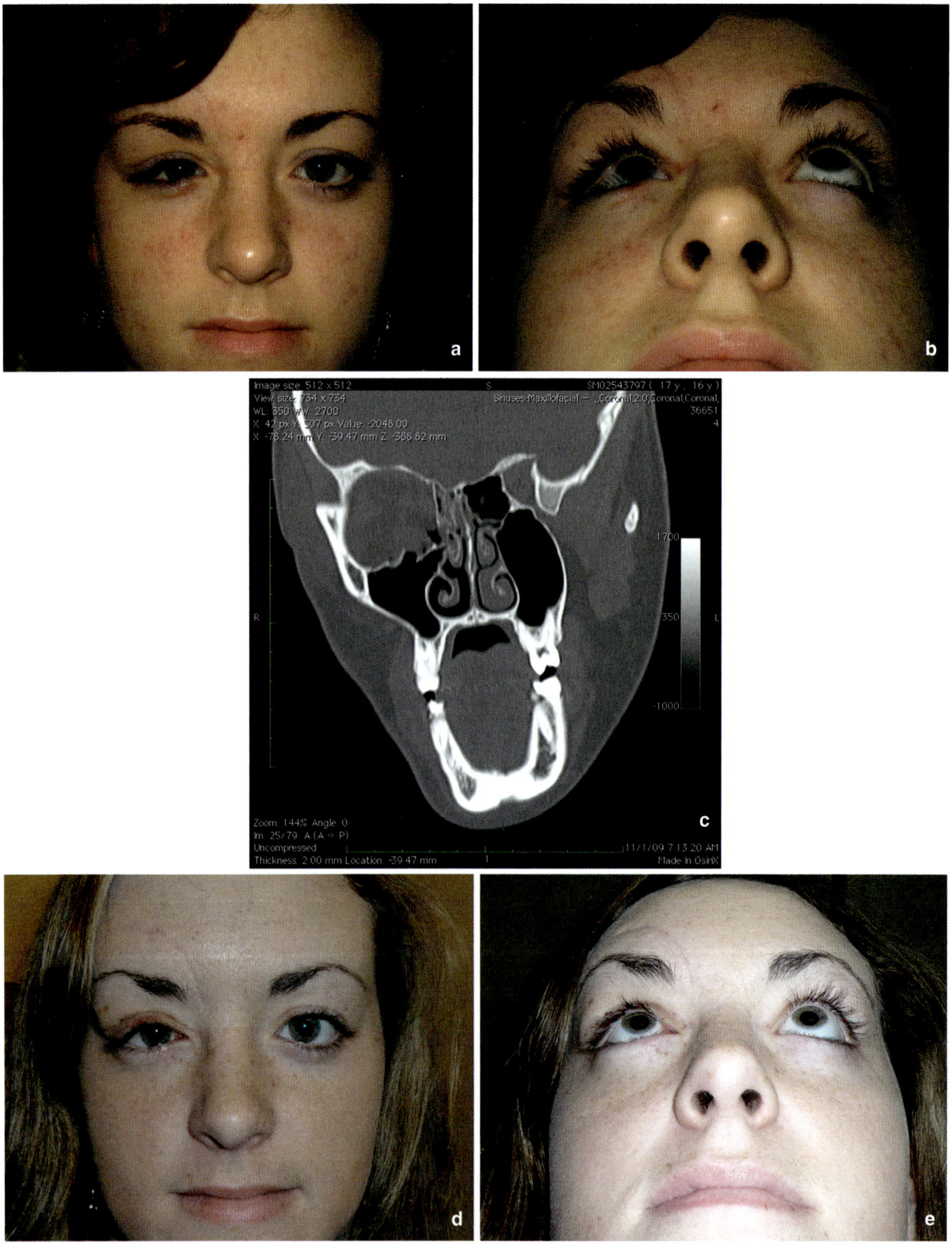

Fig. 73.7 A 16-year-old girl 4 months after a motor vehicle accident. No previous surgery had been performed. (**a**) Right enophthalmos is evident. In addition, the right globe appears to be shifted medially. (**b**) Worm's-eye view of the patient demonstrates 4 mm of right enophthalmos. (**c**) CT scan demonstrates a right orbital floor and medial wall fracture. (**d**) Following porous polyethylene implants to the medial and lateral walls, there is marked improvement in the position of the globe. (**e**) Enophthalmos has greatly improved

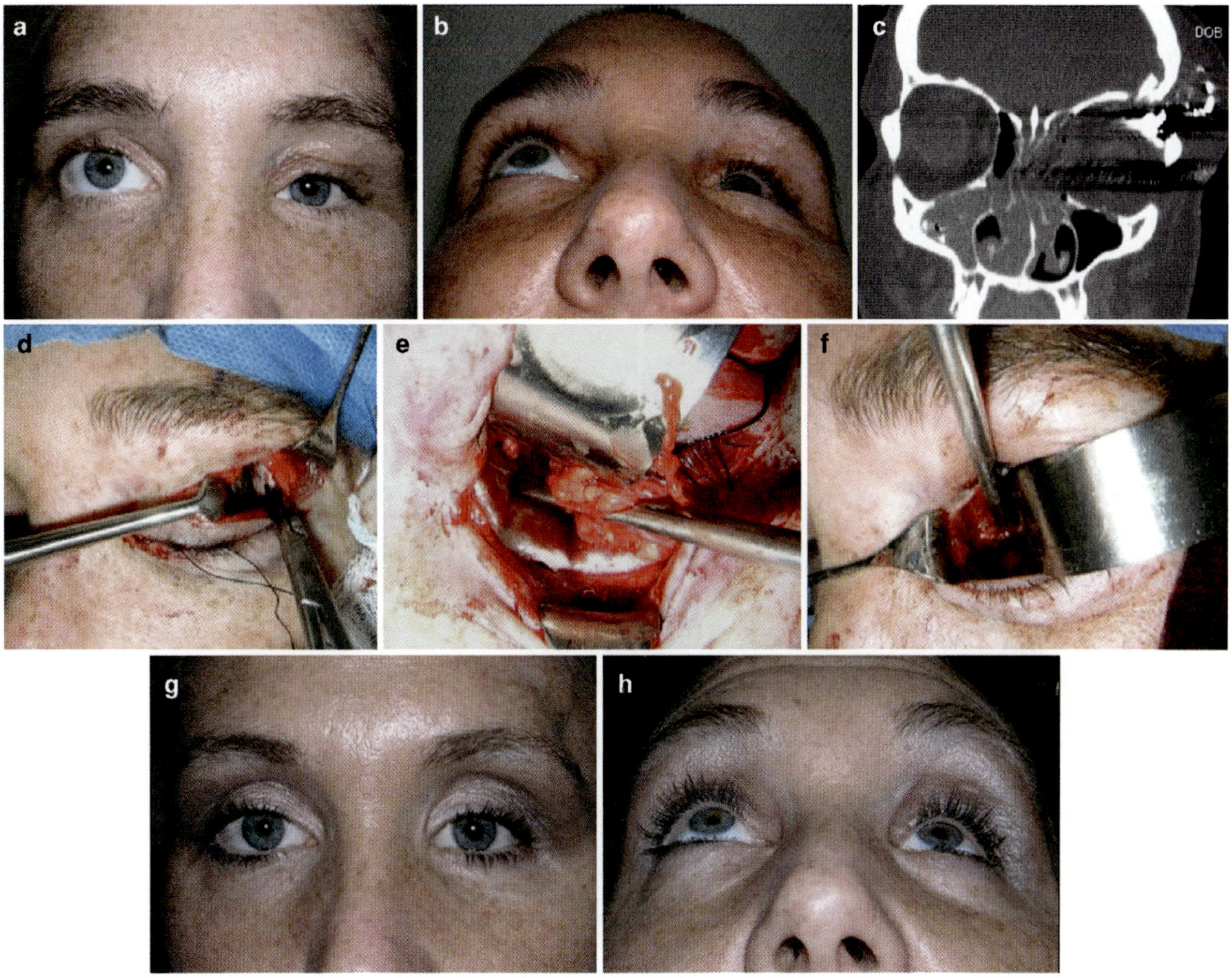

Fig. 73.8 Woman who suffered a gunshot injury to the left face. She had not had orbital surgery. The patient has no light perception on the left due to the injury. (**a**) Marked enophthalmos of the left globe. (**b**) Enophthalmos measured 7 mm on the left. (**c**) Coronal CT scan shows fractures involving the medial wall, floor, lateral wall, and roof of the left orbit. Imaging artifacts are from metallic foreign bodies related to the gunshot. (**d**) Repair was addressed by placing porous polyethylene sheets into the superolateral orbit via a lid crease incision. (**e**) The floor and medial wall were repaired through an inferior fornix and transcaruncular incision. A porous polyethylene sheet is shaped to reform the injured walls. (**f**) Through a transconjunctival incision, the medial wall may be well visualized and accessed. (**g**) Postoperative appearance with marked improvement in enophthalmos and hypoglobus. (**h**) Slight residual enophthalmos following surgery

experience, when patients appear to have equal globe prominence immediately at completion of surgery, they often have a small recurrence of enophthalmos several months after surgery (perhaps due to resolution of intraoperative edema and hemorrhage). Aiming for approximately 1 mm of exophthalmos generally results in eventual equivalent prominence.

Three-Dimensional (3D) Imaging

Over the past few decades, advances in imaging techniques have vastly improved visualization of orbital fractures [67]. Higher resolution of both bony defects and soft tissues has allowed for precise evaluation of complicated fractures and pathologies. Historically, image analysis has generally been limited to qualitative analysis of injuries, but with newer modalities, it is now possible to measure orbital defects quantitatively using imaging software. This allows the surgeon to preoperatively assess the size of the fracture and approximate the degree of orbital volume replacement. 3D simulation and modeling techniques for surgery involve registering data from fine-cut CT scans into various computer software programs to create a three-dimensional computer model. From this stage, there are three general uses for these models: to create a physical model to preoperatively plan surgery, to create a template on which to preoperatively bend or fashion a flat alloplastic implant, or to manufacture a custom implant.

The first type of model can be used to perform simulated surgery with the computer program to plan the location of

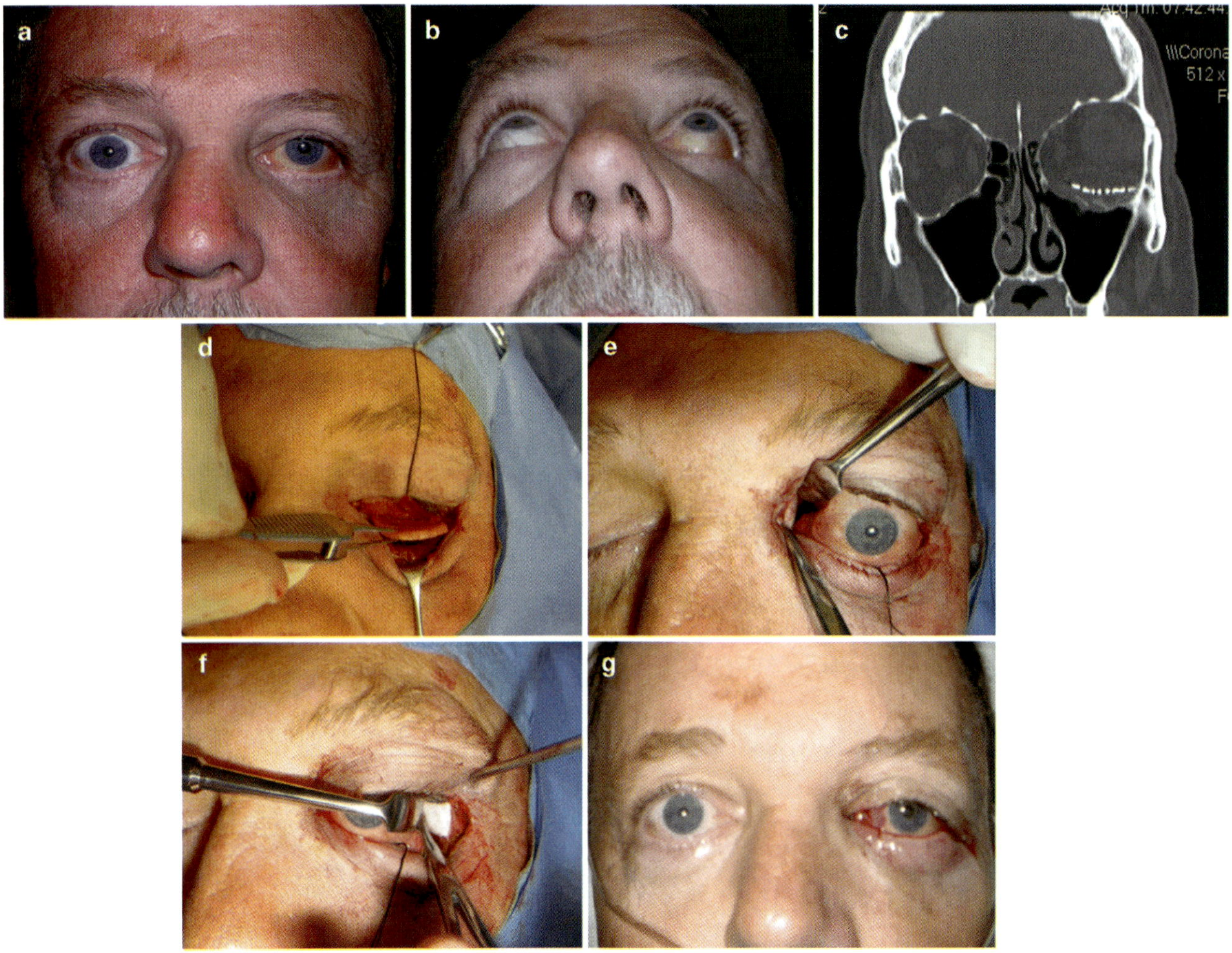

Fig. 73.9 Patient who had a large left medial wall and floor fracture. He reported double vision following surgical repair at an outside institution. (**a**) Note left hyperglobus. (**b**) Although there is no enophthalmos, the globe remains dystopic. (**c**) Coronal CT scan following the first surgery illustrates the floor implant. However, the medial wall fracture is not addressed. The globe was simply pushed superiorly. (**d**) The previous implant was removed and replaced with a porous polyethylene implant. (**e**) A second implant was placed along the medial wall via a transconjunctival incision. (**f**) A third implant was placed along the lateral wall via a lateral canthotomy incision to restore volume without malposition of the globe. (**g**) Immediate postoperative appearance with resolution of diplopia and hyperglobus

osteotomies and predict movement, reposition, and fixation of bones [68]. Additionally, skull or orbital models may be fabricated to more directly visualize the reconstructed orbital fracture and associated injuries. This can be particularly useful in complex trauma affecting multiple areas where mobilization of a bone may affect many articulations simultaneously.

The second application allows for a template to be fashioned. Numerous reports of titanium mesh shaped onto the model manually by the surgeon to later be implanted into the patient have been published [69–71]. This can be useful to reduce time intraoperatively, since the implant has been prebent. However, the implant must be sterilized after molding, which cannot be done for all materials. Additionally, this sterilization process can take some time to complete. Another similar application has been to fashion a mold to be used intraoperatively. This mold can then sterilized and used during surgery to bend and trim an unaltered implant [72].

Individual custom-fabricated implants have also been utilized based on fracture location [73] as well as pre-drilled screw fixation holes based on surrounding bone thickness [74] using bioceramic and titanium, respectively. Porous polyethylene and polyether ether ketone (PEEK) have also been used effectively in the periorbital region [59]. Finally, preformed implants have gained popularity in some centers. These implants, available from multiple suppliers, are manufactured based on anatomic norms calculated from hundreds of normal scans. While they are not custom, but rather "off-the-shelf," these preformed implants are particularly useful for large orbital floor fractures with few remaining stable, nondisplaced areas to support a hand-carved implant. Mahoney and colleagues [55] further used 3D digital fracture assessment to compare the best fit of the various available preformed implants to reduce surgical time and anatomic fit.

Success has been generally good using the implants with improvement in enophthalmos in almost all cases. There are several advantages to using these techniques. Improved visualization of the fracture allows the surgeon to better plan the surgical approach, which may be more useful in complicated cases involving extensive injuries to the craniofacial skeleton. Operative time is decreased since shaping the implant is not necessary. Primary disadvantages include the relatively high cost of fabricating a model and the time required for production. This technology remains promising for fast and efficient repair of post-traumatic enophthalmos.

Masqueraders

Rarely there are other causes of enophthalmos that may apparently be secondary to orbital wall fracture. Careful history and examination of the scalp will reveal whether patients have undergone orbitozygomatic-pterional craniotomy for neurosurgery. In this approach, the lateral wall and roof of the orbit are removed, and incomplete orbital wall reconstruction may result in enophthalmos. Silent sinus syndrome [75] is an implosion of the maxillary sinus and secondary expansion of the orbit due to an occluded osteomeatal complex from sinus disease with presumed chronic negative pressure within the sinus. This may be a preexisting condition only noted after the patient more carefully inspects their facial anatomy following minor trauma [76]. Notably, post-traumatic silent sinus syndrome has been reported with the trauma as the cause of osteomeatal occlusion [77–79].

Complications

There are numerous potential complications of orbital surgery, although most are uncommon. Retrobulbar hemorrhage is rare following orbital surgery. Careful postoperative observation and rapid decompression in case of hemorrhage may prevent severe visual loss. Nosocomial infections of implanted materials may be minimized with pre- and postoperative antibiotics and sterile technique, although if they occur, explantation is often necessary. Persistent enophthalmos may occur with inadequate volume restoration at the time of surgery, failure to recognize concomitant fractures, or implant dislocation or migration. Postoperative ptosis and cranial neuropathies typically resolve without intervention. Fortunately, most complications may be avoided with proper preoperative planning and meticulous technique.

Conclusions

Post-traumatic enophthalmos can result in ocular signs and symptoms as well as unacceptable appearance. Following complete ophthalmic and facial examination, thorough inspection of radiographic scans will reveal the size and location of any orbital wall fractures and defects. Prediction of late enophthalmos is difficult based on early examination and imaging findings. There are rare indications for immediate repair, and the vast majority of orbital fractures may be successfully repaired in a delayed fashion. Operating on a "large" fracture in a patient who does not yet have clinically visible enophthalmos is strongly discouraged. Many of these patients will not go on to develop enophthalmos (see Fig. 73.3). Surgical intervention should be carried out only after thorough discussion with the patient to identify goals and expectations of surgery. Restoration of volume should be directed toward the affected walls to successfully address the areas of need. Generally alloplastic, bio-integratable implants are favored for their ease of use and potentially fewer long-term complications. Three-dimensional imaging can improve visualization of the injury and preoperative shaping of an implant, although is not necessary. With proper surgical planning, traumatic enophthalmos may be successfully managed.

References

1. Manson PN, Grivas A, Rosenbuam A, Vannier M, Zinreich J, Iliff N. Studies on enophthalmos: II. The measurement of orbital injuries and their treatment by quantitative computed tomography. Plast Reconstr Surg. 1986;77(2):203–14.
2. Cohen LM, Habib LA, Yoon MK. Quantified orbital fat atrophy in late post-traumatic enophthalmos: volumetric analysis of unoperated orbital fractures. Presented at the 49th annual fall symposium of the American Society of Ophthalmic Plastic and Reconstructive Surgery, Chicago. October 2018.
3. Dulley B, Fells P. Long-term follow up of orbital blowout fracture with or without surgery. Mod Probl Ophthalmol. 1970;19:467.
4. Osguthorpe JD. Orbital wall fractures: evaluation and management. Otolaryngol Head Neck Surg. 1991;105:702.
5. Mustarde JC. The role of Lockwood's suspensory ligament in preventing downward displacement of the eye. Br J Plast Surg. 1968;21:73.
6. Memon MY, Paine KW. Direct injury of the oculomotor nerve in craniocerebral trauma. J Neurosurg. 1971;35:461–4.
7. Mauriello JA, Antonacci R, Mostafavi R, Narain K, Caputo AR, Wagner RS, Palydowicz S. Paresis and restriction of the extraocular muscles after orbital fracture: a study of 16 patients. Ophthal Plast Reconstr Surg. 1996;12(3):206–10.
8. Yoon MK, Economides J, Horton JC. Slack extraocular muscles cause diplopia on eccentric gaze in enophthalmos. North American Neuro-Ophthalmological Society: Vancouver; 2011.
9. Seider N, Gilboa M, Miller B, Hadar RS, Beiran I. Orbital fractures complicated by late enophthalmos: higher prevalence in patients with multiple trauma. Ophthal Plast Reconstr Surg. 2007;23(2):115–8.

10. Jank S, Schuchter B, Emshoff R, Strobl H, Koehler J, Nicasi A, Norer B, Baldissera I. Clinical signs of orbital wall fractures as a function of anatomic function. Oral Surg Oral Med Oral Pathol. 2003;96(2):149–53.
11. Ellis E III, El-Attar A, Moos KF. An analysis of 2067 cases of zygomatico-orbital fracture. J Oral Maxillofac Surg. 1985;43:417–28.
12. Gassner R, Tarkan T, Hachl O, et al. Cranio-maxillofacial trauma: a 10 year review of 9543 cases with 21067 injuries. J Craniomaxillofac Surg. 2003;31:51–61.
13. Hink EM, Wei LA, Durairaj VD. Clinical features and treatment of pediatric orbit fractures. Ophthalmic Plast Reconstr Surg. 2014;30(2):124–31.
14. Sullivan WG. Displaced orbital roof fractures: presentation and treatment. Plast Reconstr Surg. 1991;87(4):657–61.
15. Baril SE, Yoon MK. Naso-orbito-ethmoidal (NOE) fractures: a review. Int Ophthalmol Clin. 2013;53(4):149–55.
16. Homer N, Glass LR, Lee NG, et al. Assessment of infraorbital hypesthesia following orbital floor and zygomaticomaxillary fractures using a novel sensory grading system. Ophthalmic Plast Reconstr Surg. 2019;35(1):53–5.
17. Lakits A, Prokesch R, Scholda C, Nowotny R, Kaider A, Bankier A. Helical and conventional CT in the imaging of metallic foreign bodies in the orbit. Acta Ophthalmol Scand. 2000;78:79–83.
18. Berkowitz RA, Putterman AM, Patel DB. Prolapse of the globe into the maxillary sinus after orbital floor fracture. Am J Ophthalmol. 1981;91(2):253–7.
19. Abrishami M, Aletaha M, Bagheri A, Salour SH, Yazdani S. Traumatic subluxation of the globe into the maxillary sinus. Ophthal Plast Reconstr Surg. 2007;23(2):156–8.
20. Bansagi ZC, Meyer DR. Internal orbital fractures in the pediatric age group: characterization and management. Ophthalmology. 2000;107(5):829–36.
21. Jimenez-Perez JC, Yoon MK. Posterior orbital floor fracture. Presented at the spring Symposium of the American Society of Ophthalmic Plastic and Reconstructive Surgery, Vancouver. June 2017.
22. Kum C, McCulley TJ, Yoon MK, Hwang TN. Adult orbital trapdoor fracture. Ophthal Plast Reconstr Surg. 2009;25(6):486–7.
23. McCulley TJ, Yip CC, Kersten RC, Kulwin DR. Medial rectus muscle incarceration in pediatric medial orbital wall trapdoor fractures. Eur J Ophthalmol. 2004;14(4):330–3.
24. Brannan PA, Kersten RC, Kulwin DR. Isolated medial wall fractures with medial rectus muscle incarceration. Ophthal Plast Reconstr Surg. 2006;22(3):178–83.
25. Dal Canto AJ, Linberg JV. Comparison of orbital fracture repair performed within 14 days versus 15 to 29 days after trauma. Ophthal Plast Reconstr Surg. 2008;24(6):437–43.
26. Simon GJ, Syed HM, McCann JD, Goldberg RA. Early versus late repair of orbital blowout fractures. Ophthalmic Surg Lasers Imaging. 2009;40(2):141–8.
27. Scawn RL, Lim LH, Whipple KM, et al. Outcomes of orbital blow-out fracture repair performed beyond 6 weeks after injury. Ophthalmic Plast Reconstr Surg. 2016;32(4):296–01.
28. Matic DB, Tse R, Banerjee A, Moore CC. Rounding of the inferior rectus muscle as a predictor of enophthalmos in orbital floor fractures. J Craniofac Surg. 2007;18(1):127–32.
29. Roncevic R, Stajcic Z. Surgical treatment of post-traumatic enophthalmos: a study of 72 patients. Ann Plast Surg. 1992;32:288.
30. Burm JS, Chung CH, Oh SJ. Pure orbital blowout fracture: new concepts and importance of medial orbital blowout fracture. Plast Reconstr Surg. 1999;103:1839–49.
31. Lee WT, Kim HK, Chung SM. Relationship between small-size medial orbital wall fracture and late enophthalmos. J Craniofac Surg. 2009;20(1):75–80.
32. Whitehouse RW, Batterbury M, Jackson A, Noble JL. Prediction of enophthalmos by computed tomography after "blow out" orbital fracture. Br J Ophthalmol. 1994;78:618–20.
33. Fan X, Li J, Zhu J, Li H, Zhang D. Computer-assisted orbital volume measurement in the surgical correction of late enophthalmos caused by blowout fractures. Ophthal Plast Recontr Surg. 2003;19(3):207–11.
34. Ahn HB, Ryu WU, Yoo KW, Park WC, Rho SH, Lee JH, Choi SS. Prediction of enophthalmos by computer-based volume measurement of orbital fractures in a Korean population. Ophthal Plast Reconstr Surg. 2008;24(1):36–9.
35. Raskin EM, Millman AL, Lubkin V, Della Rocca RC, Lisman RD, Maher EA. Prediction of late enophthalmos by volumetric analysis of orbital fractures. Ophthal Plast Reconstr Surg. 1998;14(1):19–26.
36. Jin HR, Shin SO, Choo MJ, Choi YS. Relationship between the extent of fracture and the degree of enophthalmos in isolated blowout fractures of the medial orbital wall. J Oral Maxillofac Surg. 2000;58:617–20.
37. Kim YK, Park CS, Kim HK, Lew DH, Tark KC. Correlation between changes of the medial rectus muscle section and enophthalmos in patients with medial orbital wall fracture. J Plast Reconstr Aesthet Surg. 2009;62:1379–83.
38. Converse JM, Cole G, Smith B. Late treatment of blowout fractures of the orbit. Plast Reconstr Surg. 1961;64:676–88.
39. Pearl RN. Surgical management of volumetric changes in the boy orbit. Ann Plast Surg. 1987;19:349–58.
40. McDermott MW, Durity FA, Rootman J, Woodhurst WB. Combined frontotemporal-orbitozygomatic approach for tumors of the sphenoid wing and orbit. Neurosurgery. 1990;26(1):107–16.
41. Matsuo K, Hirose T, Furuta S, Hayashi M, Watanabe T. Semiquantitative correction of posttraumatic enophthalmos with sliced cartilage grafts. Plast Reconstr Surg. 1989;83(3):429–37.
42. Lee JW. Preplanned correction of enophthalmos using diced cartilage grafts. Br J Plast Surg. 2000;53:17–23.
43. Nishi Y, Kiyokawa K, Watanabe K, Rikimaru H, Yamauchi T. A surgical treatment of severe late posttraumatic enophthalmos using sliced costal cartilage chip grafts. J Craniofac Surg. 2006;17(4):673–9.
44. Lee JW. Treatment of enophthalmos using corrective osteotomy with concomitant cartilage-graft implantation. J Plast Reconstr Aesthet Surg. 2010;63:42–53.
45. Rubin PA, Bilyk JR, Shore JW. Orbital reconstruction using porous polyethylene sheets. Ophthalmology. 1994;10(10):1697–708.
46. Garibaldi DC, Iliff NT, Grant MP, Merbs SL. Use of porous polyethylene with embedded titanium in orbital reconstruction: a review of 106 patients. Ophthal Plast Reconstr Surg. 2007;23(6):439–44.
47. Lee HB, Nunery WB. Orbital adherence syndrome secondary to titanium implant material. Ophthalmic Plast Reconstr Surg. 2009;25(1):33–6.
48. Lee GH, Ho SY. Orbital adherence syndrome following the use of titanium precontoured orbital mesh for the reconstruction of posttraumatic orbital floor defects. Craniomaxillofac Trauma Reconstr. 2017;10(1):77–83.
49. Costa PJC, de Guaw JH, Costa Filho JZ, et al. Late complication associated with the treatment of orbital floor fracture with titanium mesh. J Craniofac Surg. 2019;29(6):e623–4.
50. Roelofs KA, Starks V, Yoon MK. Orbital emphysema: a case report and comprehensive review of the literature. Ophthalmic Plast Reconstr Surg. 2019;35(1):1–6.
51. Haug RH, Nuveen E, Bredbenner T. An evaluation of the support provided by common internal orbital reconstruction materials. J Oral Maxillofac Surg. 1999;57:564–70.
52. Rosen CE. Late migration of an orbital implant causing orbital hemorrhage with sudden proptosis and diplopia. Ophthal Plast Reconstr Surg. 1996;12(4):260–2.

53. Custer PL, Lind A, Trinkaus KM. Complications of supramid orbital implants. Ophthal Plast Reconstr Surg. 2003;19(1):62–7.
54. Cohen LM, Shaye D, Yoon MK. Isolated orbital floor fracture management: a survey and comparison of American oculofacial and facial plastic surgeon preferences. Craniomaxillofac Trauma Reconstr. 2019;12:112. https://doi.org/10.1055/s-0038-1639350.
55. Mahoney NR, Peng MY, Merbs SL, et al. Virtual fitting, selection, and cutting of preformed anatomic orbital implants. Ophthalmic Plast Reconstr Surg. 2017;33:196–201.
56. Gander T, Essig H, Meltzer P, et al. Patient specific implants (PSI) in reconstruction of orbital floor and wall fractures. J Craniomaxillofac Surg. 2015;43(1):126–30.
57. Jalbert F, Boetto S, Nadon F, et al. One-step primary reconstruction for complex craniofacial resection with PEEK custom-made implants. J Craniomaxillofac Surg. 2014;42(2):141–8.
58. Dave TV, Tiple S, Vempati S, et al. Low-cost three-dimensional printed orbital template-assisted patient-specific implants for the correction of spherical orbital implant migration. Indian J Ophthalmol. 2018;66(11):1600–7.
59. Habib LA, Cohen LM, Yoon MK. Patient specific implants for orbital reconstruction. Presented at the 49th annual fall symposium of the American Society of Ophthalmic Plastic and Reconstructive Surgery, Chicago. October 2018.
60. Tessier P, Rougier J, Hervouet F, et al. Sequelae of orbital trauma. Plastic surgery of the orbit and eyelids [transl by Wolfe SA]. New York: Masson Publishing USA; 1981. p. 99.
61. Campbell AA, Cunnane ME, Dunn GP, et al. Spontaneous resorption of a penetrating orbital bone fracture fragment. Ophthalmic Plast Reconstr Surg. 2015;31(5):e123–5.
62. Young SM, Kim YD, Kim SW, et al. Conservatively treated orbital blowout fractures: spontaneous radiologic improvement. Ophthalmology. 2018;125(6):938–44.
63. Grant MP, Iliff NT, Manson PN. Strategies for the treatment of enophthalmos. Clin Plast Surg. 1997;24:539–50.
64. Yeatts RP. Measurement of the globe position in complex orbital fractures: II. Patient evaluation utilizing a modified exophthalmometer. Ophthal Plast Reconstr Surg. 1992;8:119.
65. Appling WD, Patrinely JR, Salzer TA. Transconjunctival approach vs subciliary skin-muscle flap approach for orbital fracture repair. Arch Otolaryngol Head Neck Surg. 1993;119(9):1000–7.
66. McNichols CH, Hatef DA, Thornton JF, et al. A paradigm shift in correcting medial orbital fracture-related enophthalmos: volumetric augmentation through a lateral approach. J Craniofac Surg. 2012;23(3):762–6.
67. Bite U, Jackson IT, Forbes GS, Gehring DG. Orbital volume measurements in enophthalmos using three-dimensional CT imaging. Plast Reconstr Surg. 1985;75(4):502–8.
68. Fan X, Zhou H, Lin M, Fu Y, Li J. Late reconstruction of the complex orbital fractures with computer-aided design and computer-aided manufacturing technique. J Craniofac Surg. 2007;18(3):665–73.
69. Schon R, Metzger MC, Zizelmann C, Weyer N, Schmelzelsen R. Individually preformed titanium mesh implants for a true-to-original repair of orbital fractures. Int J Oral Maxillofac Surg. 2006;35:990–5.
70. Guo L, Tian W, Feng F, Long J, Li P, Tang W. Reconstruction of orbital floor fractures: comparison of individual prefabricated titanium implants and calvarial bone grafts. Ann Plast Surg. 2009;63(6):624–31.
71. Tang W, Guo L, Long J, Wang H, Lin Y, Liu L, Tian W. Individual design and rapid prototyping in reconstruction of orbital wall defects. J Oral Maxillofac Surg. 2010;68:562–70.
72. Kang S, Kwon J, Ahn CJ, et al. Generation of customized orbital implant templates using 3-dimensional printing for orbital wall reconstruction. Eye (Lond). 2018;32(12):1864–70.
73. Klein M, Glatzer C. Individual CAD/CAM fabricated glass-bioceramic implants in reconstructive surgery of the bony orbital floor. Plast Reconstr Surg. 2006;117:565–70.
74. Lieger O, Richards R, Liu M, Lloyd R. Computer-assisted design and manufacture of implants in the late reconstruction of extensive orbital fractures. Arch Facial Plast Surg. 2010;12(3):186–91.
75. Soparkar CN, Patrinely JR, Cuaycong MJ, et al. The silent sinus syndrome: a cause of spontaneous enophthalmos. Ophthalmology. 1994;101:772–8.
76. Lin GC, Sedaghat AR, Bleier BS, et al. Volumetric analysis of chronic maxillary atelectasis. Am J Rhinol Allergy. 2015;29(3):166–9.
77. Gagnon MR, Yeatts RP, Williams Z, et al. Delayed enophthalmos following a minimally displaced orbital floor fracture. Ophthal Plast Reconstr Surg. 2004;20:241–3.
78. Ross JJ, Kersten RC. Late enophthalmos mimicking silent sinus syndrome secondary to orbital trauma. J Craniofac Surg. 2005;16:840–3.
79. Montezuma SR, Gopal H, Savar A, Turalba A, Cestari DM, Torun N. Silent sinus syndrome presenting as enophthalmos long after orbital trauma. J Neuroophthalmol. 2008;28:107–10.

Orbital Foreign Bodies and Penetrating Orbital Injuries

74

Alan A. McNab and Khami Satchi

Introduction

Penetrating orbital injuries with or without retained intraorbital foreign bodies (IOrbFBs) are uncommon but often dramatic injuries. In legend and history, there have been some notable examples of this type of trauma. Homer related how Odysseus, on his wanderings, visited the cave of the Cyclops, was imprisoned by one of them, Polyphemus, and was only able to escape by spearing the monster's single eye, blinding him, and then escaping among the sheep and goats in the morning when the cave was opened to let them out. The blinded Polyphemus felt along the backs of the animals as they passed in an attempt to detect any escapees, but Odysseus evaded detection by slinging himself under the belly of the leading ram. At the Battle of Hastings in 1066, England's King Harold famously sustained a penetrating orbital injury with an arrow but probably died of other injuries sustained on the battlefield.

The sport of jousting was derived from the battlefield and became popular among the nobility and kings of Europe. The best documented royal orbital injury was that of Henry the second of France [1]. Henry had married Catherine de' Medici in one of the great unions of Europe's royal families. Their youngest daughter, Elisabeth, was betrothed at the age of 14 to Philip the second of Spain, a diplomatic union between two royal families. To celebrate the betrothal of Phillip and Elisabeth, Henry organized a jousting tournament to be held at the Place des Vosges in Paris. He rode twice and on the second ride suffered a heavy blow and was probably concussed. He wanted to ride a third time, and no one could argue with the king. Henry climbed back in the saddle, somewhat dazed, and forgot to fasten the visor of his helmet. He charged toward his opponent, Gabriel de Montgomery, whose lance struck the king on the shoulder, shattered, and continued up under the king's visor and into his right orbit. Courtiers rushed to the king's aid, the visible wooden splinters were removed, but others were left behind.

The king was taken to his palace and put in his sick bed. Montgomery, his opponent, despite being pardoned by the king, made a tactical retreat to Brittany. The two most famous doctors of the day were summoned, one French and the other Flemish. The Frenchman Ambroise Parè is now regarded as the father of trauma surgery, and Vesalius had already published his famous anatomy text. They decided to let any residual foreign bodies "exfoliate," the term for allowing foreign bodies to float out on a sea of pus. Experiments were conducted on the severed heads of criminals with jousting lances, and it was concluded that the lance had not penetrated the cranial cavity. Despite that, both doctors felt the king was doomed from the complications of infection. Henry duly died 9 days after the injury. A postmortem confirmed the injury was confined to the orbit but revealed suppuration in the orbit had spread to the meninges and brain along the orbital veins. Catherine de' Medici, who had always hated jousting, turned the Place des Vosges into a garden, as it remains today.

Henry's orbital injury and retained wooden foreign bodies highlight some of the dangers of this type of injury. Apart from the initial trauma to the eye and orbital contents, there is the almost inevitable risk of infection, which, untreated, can have fatal consequences. Indeed, the risk of death with this type of injury was very high in the pre-antibiotic era.

Prevention

As in all areas of medicine, the best means of treatment is prevention. With penetrating orbital injuries and retained IOrbFBs, avoidance of risky behaviors particularly in children can minimize risk. Parents routinely and wisely advise

A. A. McNab (✉)
Royal Victorian Eye and Ear Hospital, Orbital Plastic and Lacrimal Clinic, East Melbourne, VIC, Australia

K. Satchi
Orbital Plastic and Lacrimal Clinic, Royal Victorian Eye and Ear Hospital, Melbourne, VIC, Australia

J. J. Servat et al. (eds.), *Smith and Nesi's Ophthalmic Plastic and Reconstructive Surgery*,
https://doi.org/10.1007/978-3-030-41720-8_74

their offspring to avoid running or playing with sticks. In the industrial setting, appropriate protective eye wear can reduce but will not eliminate risk [2].

Perhaps the commonest area where penetrating orbital injuries with or without retained IOrbFBs occur is the battlefield. Recent conflicts have been no exception, and in the Iraqi insurgency of 2004, 82% of severe ocular and orbital injuries were from blast fragmentation, often from improvised explosive devices [3]. It has been shown that appropriate eye protection can reduce the severity and frequency of eye and orbital injuries [4] which remain often very severe in comparison to the types of injury encountered in civilian practice.

Classification

There are several factors in penetrating orbital injuries and IOrbFBs that can be classified, and while such a classification is not particularly helpful in managing the individual patient, it gives a good framework on which to consider different types of injury and to compare management and outcomes.

With respect to the penetrating injury itself, the following factors may be considered:

1. Speed of foreign body – high speed versus low speed.
2. Point of entry – via the eyelid, conjunctiva, or globe itself or from outside the orbit, for example, via the temporal fossa, the face and paranasal sinuses, the nasal cavity, or the cranial cavity.
3. Direction of penetration – this is an important consideration when injuries penetrate beyond the orbit. Foreign bodies entering via the orbit may exit through the superior orbital fissure, the orbital roof, and posterolateral orbital wall into the cranial cavity; they may exit via the inferior orbital fissure into the skull base area, or via the paranasal sinuses and nasal cavity and beyond, and inferiorly even into the oral cavity, upper aerodigestive tract, or neck (see Fig. 74.1).
4. The nature of the penetration – entry only (such as with a retained wooden foreign body or stick), entry and removal via the same wound (as in a stabbing injury), or through and through injuries where the foreign body enters perhaps via the orbit and then exits the body at some distant point.

With respect to a retained IOrbFB itself, the following factors may be considered:

1. Visible or occult – some larger IOrbFBs may be only partly within the orbit or beyond, with the remainder visible externally. Some will be completely buried and not visible.
2. Nature of the IOrbFB – organic (wood, plant material, animal matter), metallic (and the type of metal), or other inorganic materials (plastic, etc.) or combinations of these (for instance, with a pencil or pen).
3. Duration that the IOrbFB has been present – most patients present acutely soon after their injury, but occasionally, they may present days, months, or years after the initial injury, sometimes unable to recall the original injury and sometimes with little morbidity associated with a long-retained IOrbFB.

Clinical Assessment

The most important aspect of the management of a patient with an apparent or suspected penetrating orbital injury and IOrbFB is the history and examination. Because of the often major morbidity associated with penetrating orbital injuries and retained IOrbFBs, a high index of suspicion is important to minimize the risk of perhaps missing a retained IOrbFB or a penetrating wound that may extend into the cranial cavity or skull base. A careful history of the nature of the injury will often point to the possibility of deeper penetration or a retained IOrbFB. Falls in gardens or wooded areas with often small wounds in the lid or conjunctiva should always raise suspicions of the possibility of deeper penetration or retained wooden IOrbFBs.

Preverbal or older children are at particular risk of having a significant injury or retained IOrbFB overlooked. Children may be unable or unwilling to tell the doctor the details of their injury, and a high index of suspicion should always be maintained. Such children may present some days or weeks after an apparently trivial injury with infective complications that then lead to the discovery of retained IOrbFBs (see Fig. 74.2). Unconscious patients, often with multiple injuries, present another group where occult injuries and IOrbFBs may be more easily missed.

It goes without saying that a careful and thorough examination is critical in patients with these types of injuries. Entry wounds may be very small or hidden in the conjunctival fornices. A complete ocular and adnexal examination and assessment of the upper cranial nerves may reveal evidence of deeper penetration, and assessment and monitoring of the neurological status is important where there is the possibility of penetration of the cranial cavity. If there is any possibility of orbital penetration or penetration beyond the orbit, with or without IOrbFBs, appropriate imaging should be obtained.

Imaging Penetrating Orbital Injuries and IOrbFBs

The first-line investigation in a patient with a possible penetrating orbital injury and IOrbFB is computed tomography (CT). The cranial cavity, not just the orbit, should be imaged.

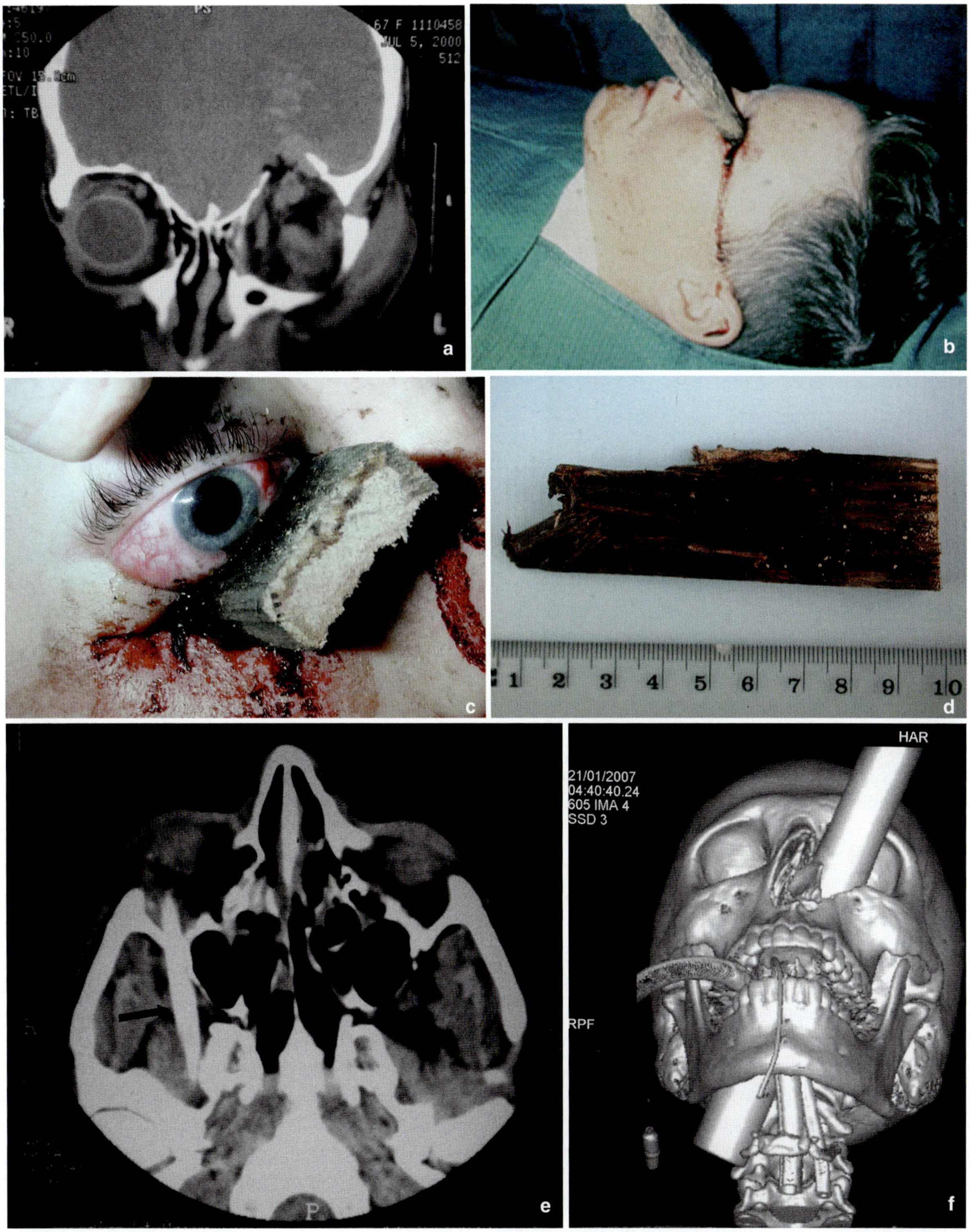

Fig. 74.1 (**a**) A coronal CT scan of a woman who bent over in the garden and stabbed herself through the upper eyelid with a garden stake that penetrated the orbital roof and frontal lobe of the brain. (**b**) A young boy fell from a tree onto a large garden stake that penetrated his left orbit and orbital roof, crossing the midline with the tip of the foreign body finishing up in the right temporal lobe. (**c**) A young boy was speared in the right orbit by a large piece of wood that was sawn off before presenting to hospital. The wood passed through the orbital floor and inferior orbital fissure into the infratemporal fossa. (**d**) The wooden FB removed from the boy in Fig. 74.1c. (**e**) An axial CT scan of a surfer who suffered a penetrating orbital injury by a needle fish. The fish's jaw (*arrow*) penetrated via the inferior orbital fissure into the skull base area, with its tip coming to rest only a few millimeters from the internal carotid artery. (**f**) A 3-D reformatted CT image of a young man assaulted with an aluminum chair leg. The leg of the chair penetrated the left orbit and orbital floor medially, passing through the nasal cavity, the palate, and the oropharynx and came to rest in the right side of the neck

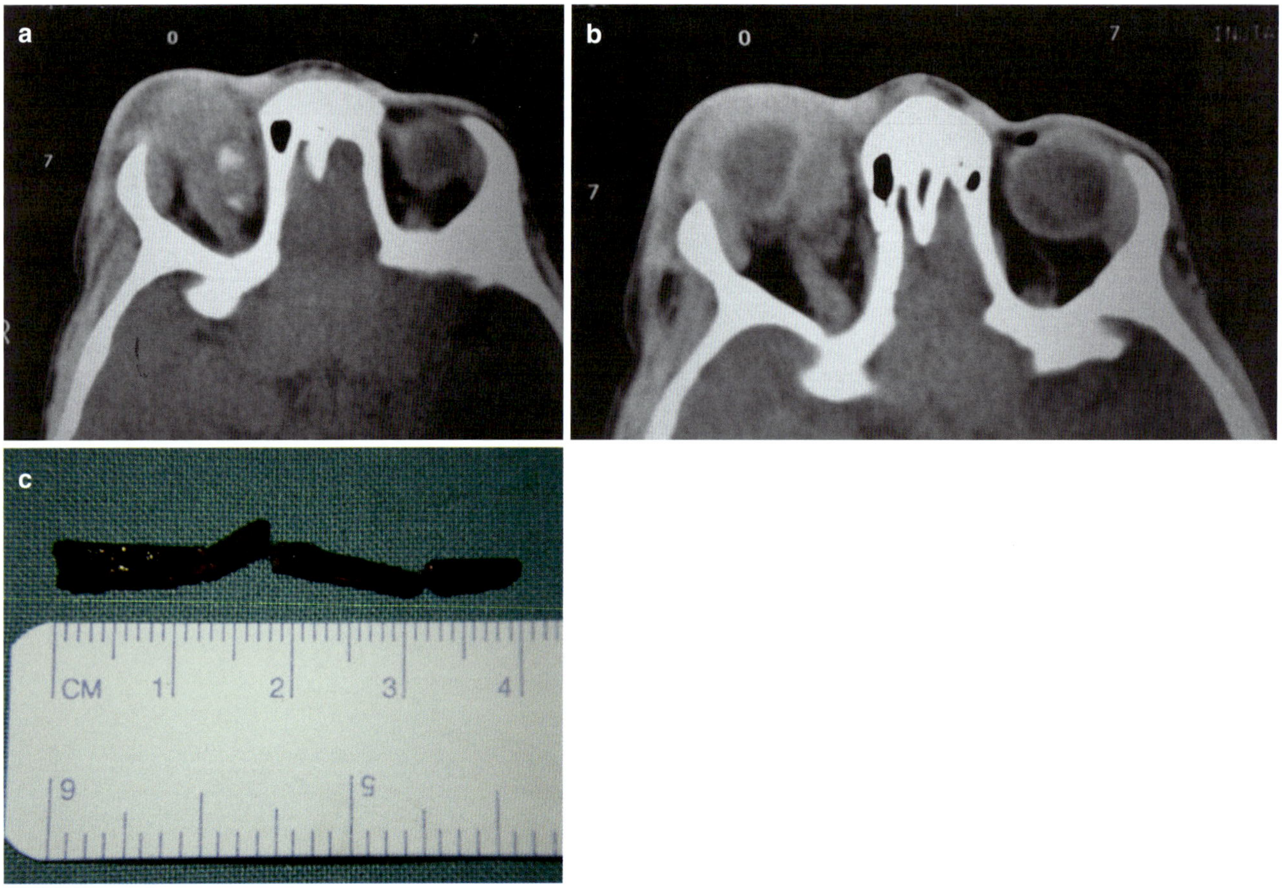

Fig. 74.2 (**a**) A 4-year-old child presented 5 days after an innocuous injury to the upper eyelid that was not witnessed by her parents. She developed a large intraorbital abscess with several higher density objects within it. (**b**) The abscess compressed the globe significantly. (**c**) At surgery, several pieces of a stick were removed from the center of the orbital abscess

Clues to penetrating injuries include the presence of air bubbles along the course of the penetration (see Fig. 74.3), the presence of hemorrhage, and when the penetration extends beyond the orbit, the presence of small, often apparently insignificant fractures in the orbital walls (see Fig. 74.4). CT is also safe when there is the possibility of a ferromagnetic foreign body.

Wooden foreign bodies have presented some particular difficulties when trying to detect them with imaging. In some reported cases, CT has missed wooden foreign bodies [5]. Wood, especially dry wood, can be isodense with air or orbital fat (see Fig. 74.5), making them difficult to detect on CT [6]. The wooden foreign body may be hypodense compared to the surrounding fat, especially when that fat has blood or inflammatory cells within it (see Fig. 74.6) [7]. However, with appropriate window settings on CT, experimental models of wooden IOrbFBs have found CT to be superior to MRI [8]. Glatt et al. have shown that the optimal window setting for detection of intraorbital wood by CT is a window width of 1000 Hounsfield units. They also found that all types of wood were hypointense to orbital fat on MRI, and small pieces of wood were surrounded by an MRI truncation artifact, making their detection easier [8]. Others have confirmed the superiority of CT over MRI in the detection of wooden FBs in experimental models [9]. Similarly, in larger clinical series, CT has been shown to be superior to MRI in detecting wooden IOrbFBs [10].

If a foreign body is suspected and it is not detected by CT, even with appropriate window settings, then obtaining MR images would seem prudent.

MRI and Suspected Metallic IOrbFBs

One group of patients worth special consideration is the group where an MRI is planned, but in whom there is the possibility of a retained ferromagnetic metallic IOrbFB. If a patient with a retained metallic IOrbFB (or intraocular FB) has an MRI, there is the potential for serious injury, although such injuries are extremely uncommon. The metallic FB may shift or more likely become heated during the MRI and may cause mechanical or thermal injury. Based on large surveys,

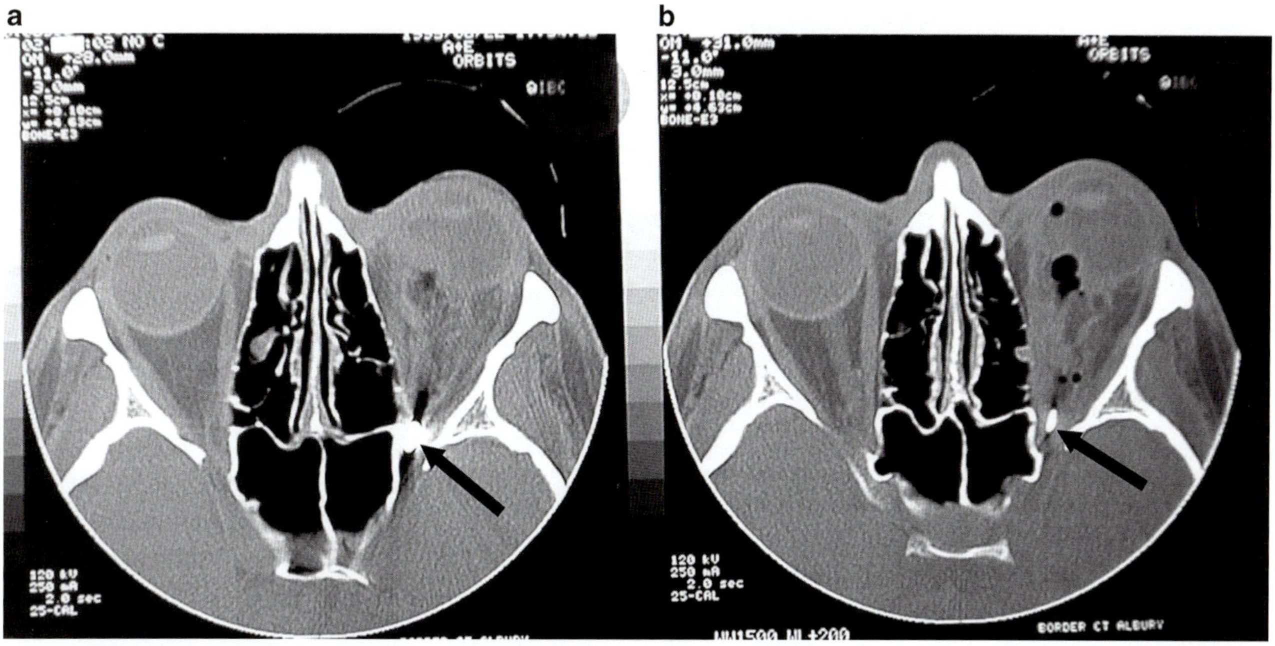

Fig. 74.3 Axial CT scans ((a) soft tissue windows and (b) bone windows to better show the foreign body) of a metal worker who suffered a through and through globe injury from a metallic FB (*black arrow*) that came to rest at the orbital apex just anterior to the superior orbital fissure. Note the air bubbles scattered along the course of the FB

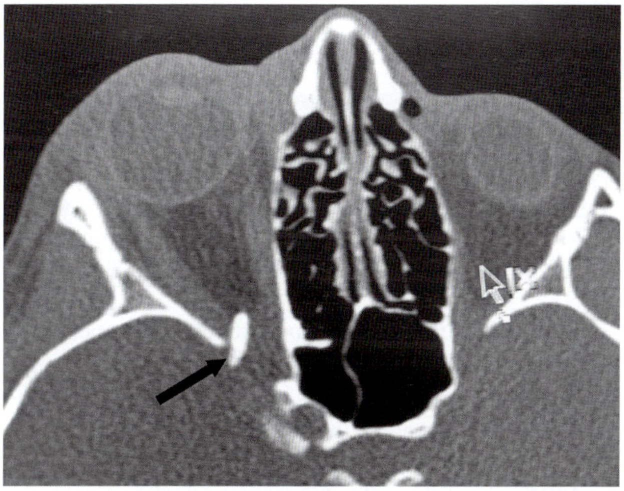

Fig. 74.4 An axial CT scan of the boy illustrated in Fig. 74.7. Note the small bone fragment (*black arrow*) that has been presumably pulled back into the orbit when a long stick was pulled out from the orbit and cranial cavity by his friend

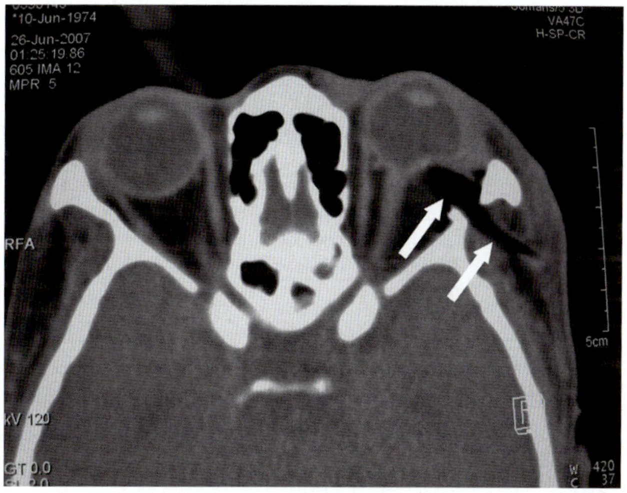

Fig. 74.5 An axial CT scan of a patient who was speared in the temporal fossa with a long piece of wood that broke off after penetrating the lateral orbital wall. The wood (two *white arrows*) is similar density to air and slightly hypodense compared to orbital fat

it has been shown that the prevalence of metallic IOrbFBs in the population of patients having MRI is low at 0.27% [11]. This same study found a higher prevalence of 2.5% in patients identified as being at risk of IOrbFBs. Examining the number of MRIs performed annually in the USA, and establishing that 5% of departments did not perform any screening examinations, these authors estimated that more than 2400 patients had undergone MRI from 1986 to 1993 with an unsuspected metallic IOrbFB present, but none had a reported injury from the presence of the FB. They inferred from this that the risk of eye or ocular adnexal injury from MRI in the presence of a ferromagnetic IOrbFB was extremely low and argued that radiographic screening was probably unnecessary prior to MRI [11]. Despite this, most radiology departments will screen patients undergoing MRI by asking appropriately directed questions about previous trauma that may have led to a possible IOrbFB and will also ask about occupational or recreational risk factors for IOrbFBs such as welding, grinding, or metal work [12]. Most will perform plain radiographs (85%), many will

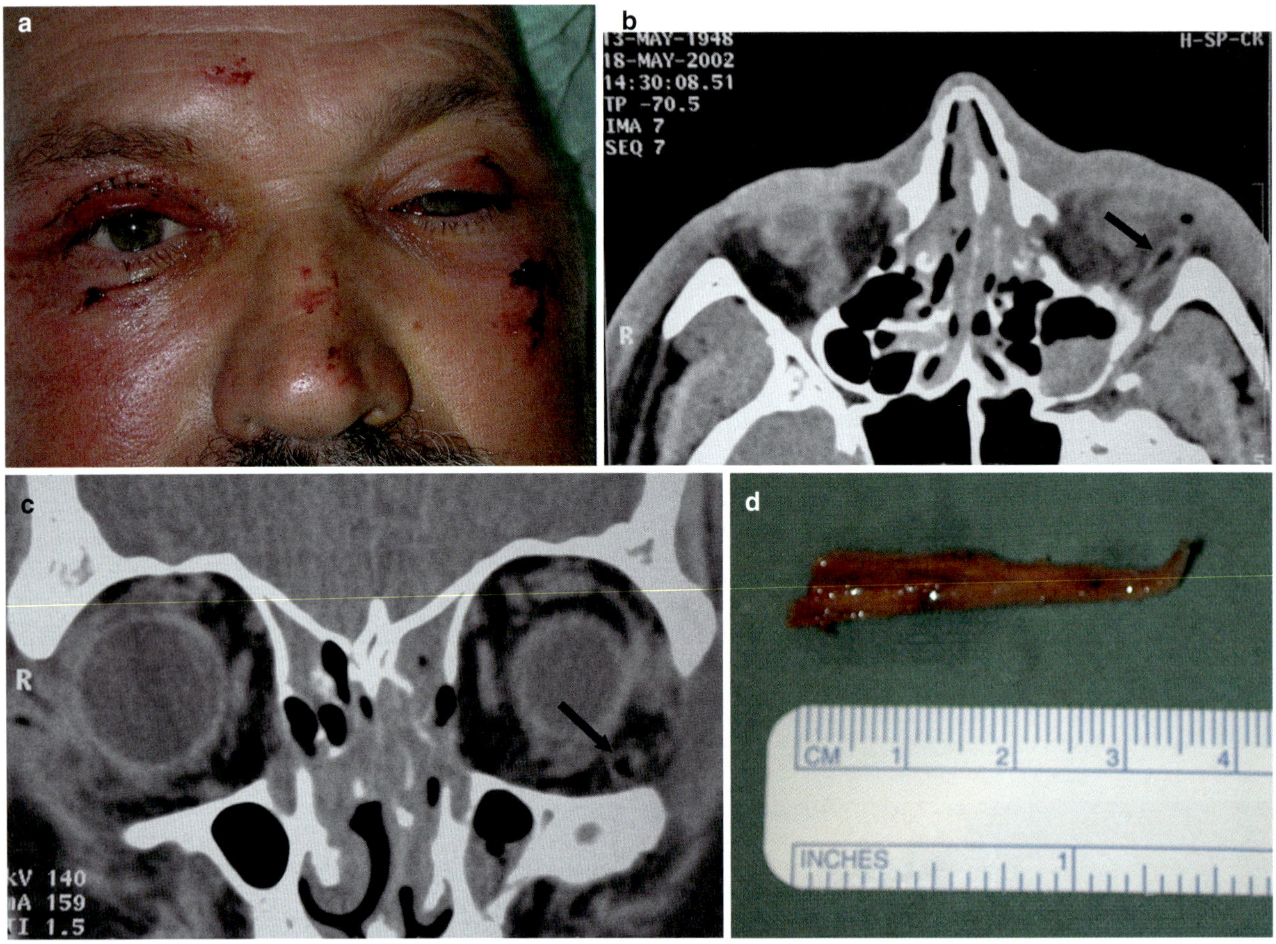

Fig. 74.6 (**a**) A man fell into a woody shrub and sustained several small lacerations on his eyelids and face. (**b**) An axial CT of the patient in (**a**) shows a low density linear object in the infero-lateral orbit, made more obvious by surrounding orbital tissue which is of greater than normal density. (**c**) A coronal CT of the same patient in (**a**). The object in the infero-lateral orbit (*arrow*) is of similar density to the orbital fat but is highlighted by the tissue reaction around it. (**d**) The patient in (**a**) was surgically explored and a 4 cm piece of wood was removed

screen with CT for selected indications (45%), and a small number use metal detectors or magnetometers (12%) [12].

Appropriate questionnaires will pick up most patients with metallic IOrbFBs. One study reported the results of plain x-rays in screening 2626 patients undergoing MRI. In this group, 17 (0.65%) were found to have metallic IOrbFBs, and of these, 16 gave a history of known injury or had knowledge of likely orbital metallic FBs. The remaining patient had an occupational history with a higher risk (a welder) [13]. Another study has looked at the cost utility of radiographic screening for IOrbFBs prior to MRI and has shown that clinical screening (asking the patient if they had a history of IOrbFB and if it was completely removed by their doctor) increases the cost-effectiveness of foreign body screening by an order of magnitude [14].

If on screening, a metallic IOrbFB is found, the question arises as to whether it should then be removed. This will depend on the present and future need for MRI examinations and whether alternative imaging techniques will be adequate and safe. If it is deemed to be important for the patient to be able to undergo MRI, then removal of the FB would seem prudent, although the risk of its removal has to be taken into account also. There are reports of patients successfully undergoing removal of IOrbFBs specifically to allow ongoing MRI examinations [15, 16].

Complications of Retained IOrbFBs

Most of the morbidity of penetrating orbital injuries and IOrbFBs is from the original injury [17]. However, some IOrbFBs may cause delayed complications. These include the following:

1. Infection and abscess formation
2. Discharging sinus
3. Noninfectious inflammation and fibrosis
4. Migration and spontaneous extrusion
5. Gaze-evoked amaurosis

Retained IOrbFBs may be tolerated for many years and never require intervention. This applies particularly to inert metallic and nonorganic FBs [17]. However, the commonest complication of a retained IOrbFB is infection, and this is commoner with organic or wooden FBs [10, 17]. Infection may not become apparent for some days, and less commonly, a delay of weeks or months may occur before infection becomes manifest. This presumably depends on the load of infective organisms introduced with the FB and the host response to them.

Another factor which may lead to delay in presentation is the use of antibiotics. Prolonged broad-spectrum antibiotics may mask or delay the development of infection when a foreign body is present. An illustrative case is shown in Fig. 74.7. This young boy fell off his bicycle into a hedge. He emerged with a long stick protruding from his orbit which was pulled out by his friend. He presented to hospital where he was found to have a sixth nerve palsy and signs on imaging of penetration through the orbit and superior orbital fissure into the posterior cranial fossa and cerebellum almost to

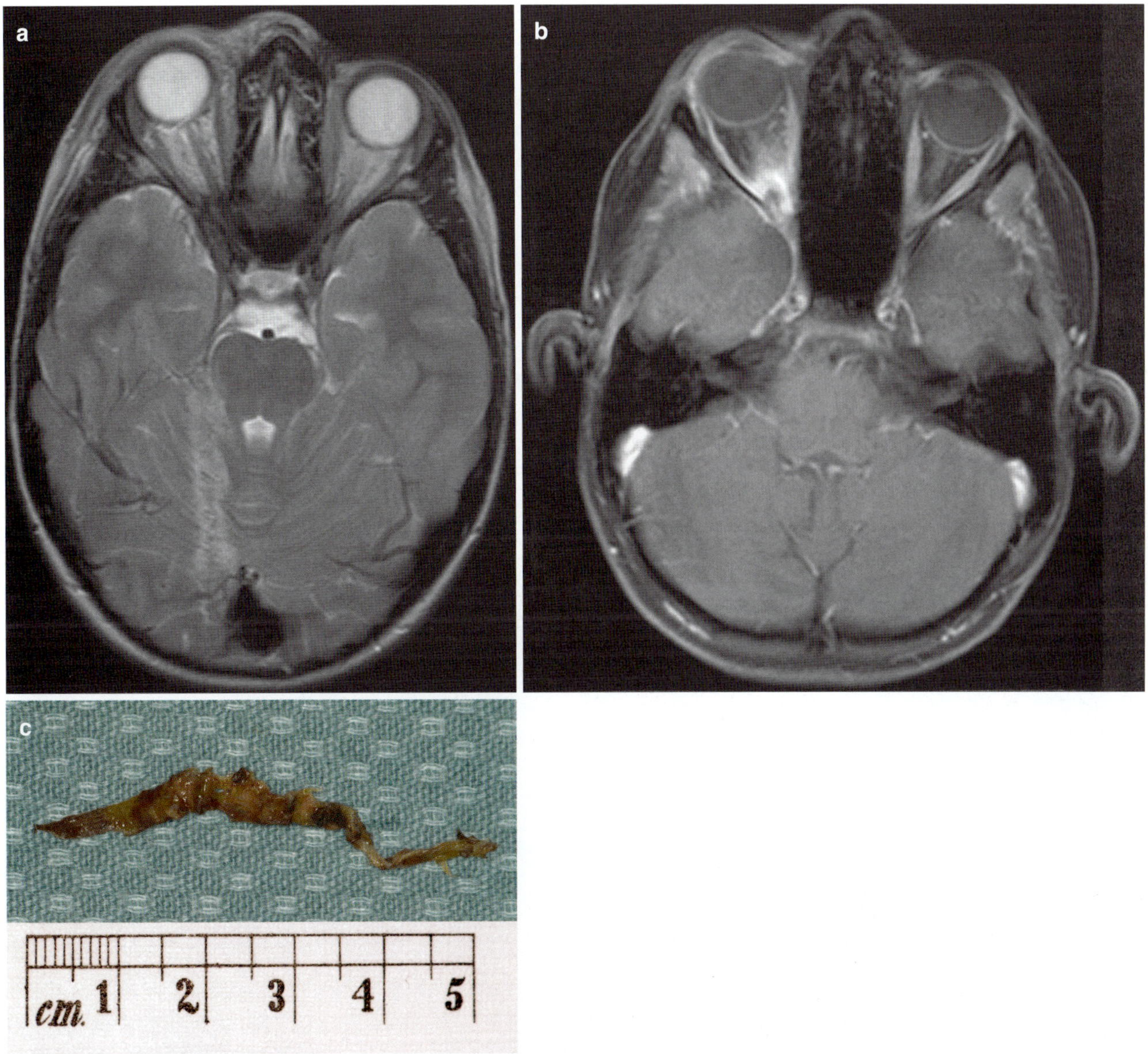

Fig. 74.7 (**a**) A T2-weighted axial MRI of a 7-year-old boy who fell from his bike into a bush. A long stick penetrated his right orbit, passed through the superior orbital fissure, skirted the internal carotid artery and the cerebral peduncle, and penetrated the cerebellum almost as far as the occiput. Apart from a right sixth nerve palsy and some mild cerebellar signs, he was otherwise intact. He was treated with broad-spectrum antibiotics for several weeks. (**b**) An axial T1-weighted MRI with contrast of the boy in (**a**) taken 4 weeks after his injury shows an enhancing mass at the orbital apex with a lower density area in its center. He had developed an optic neuropathy. (**c**) The orbital apex was explored via a subperiosteal lateral orbital approach. In the center of the small abscess cavity, a long piece of curled up bark was found and removed. His optic nerve function returned to normal

the occiput (see Fig. 74.7a). There was no evidence of retained foreign body. He was treated with high-dose parenteral and then prolonged oral broad-spectrum antibiotics to prevent intracranial infection. His vision was initially normal, but 4 weeks after the injury, he presented with optic neuropath; reimaging suggested a collection at the orbital apex adjacent to a small fracture in the region of the superior orbital fissure (see Fig. 74.7b). The area was explored, and a large curled up piece of bark was extracted from an abscess cavity in the superior orbital fissure (see Fig. 74.7c). His vision fully recovered.

One complication of IOrbFB with infection is the production of a "fistula," where there is a chronically or intermittently discharging wound in the eyelid or conjunctiva, with a retained FB at the base of the discharging orifice (see Fig. 74.8). Strictly, this is not a fistula as the discharge is not from an epithelially lined structure, but more correctly should be called a sinus. A common cause of presentation with a "fistula" or sinus is a retained FB [18], although other causes such as an incompletely removed dermoid cyst, osteomyelitis, and chronic paranasal sinus infection with discharge and lacrimal fistula should be considered [19].

Some retained IOrbFBs may induce a significant inflammatory response with dense fibrosis (see Fig. 74.9). This response may lead to complications such as restrictive strabismus and optic neuropathy. One such patient is illustrated in Fig. 74.9. The patient had sustained an injury 2 years earlier when she was inebriated and fell in the garden. A wooden FB had been removed at the time, but she returned with restrictive strabismus and optic neuropathy. There was a dense fibrotic infiltrate in the posterior orbit extending into the superior orbital fissure. The MRI suggested the possible presence of small wooden foreign bodies within the mass of fibrotic tissue (see Fig. 74.9f). At surgery, a dense mass of fibrous tissue was found with several small splinters of wood in its center. The fibrous mass persisted after removal of the

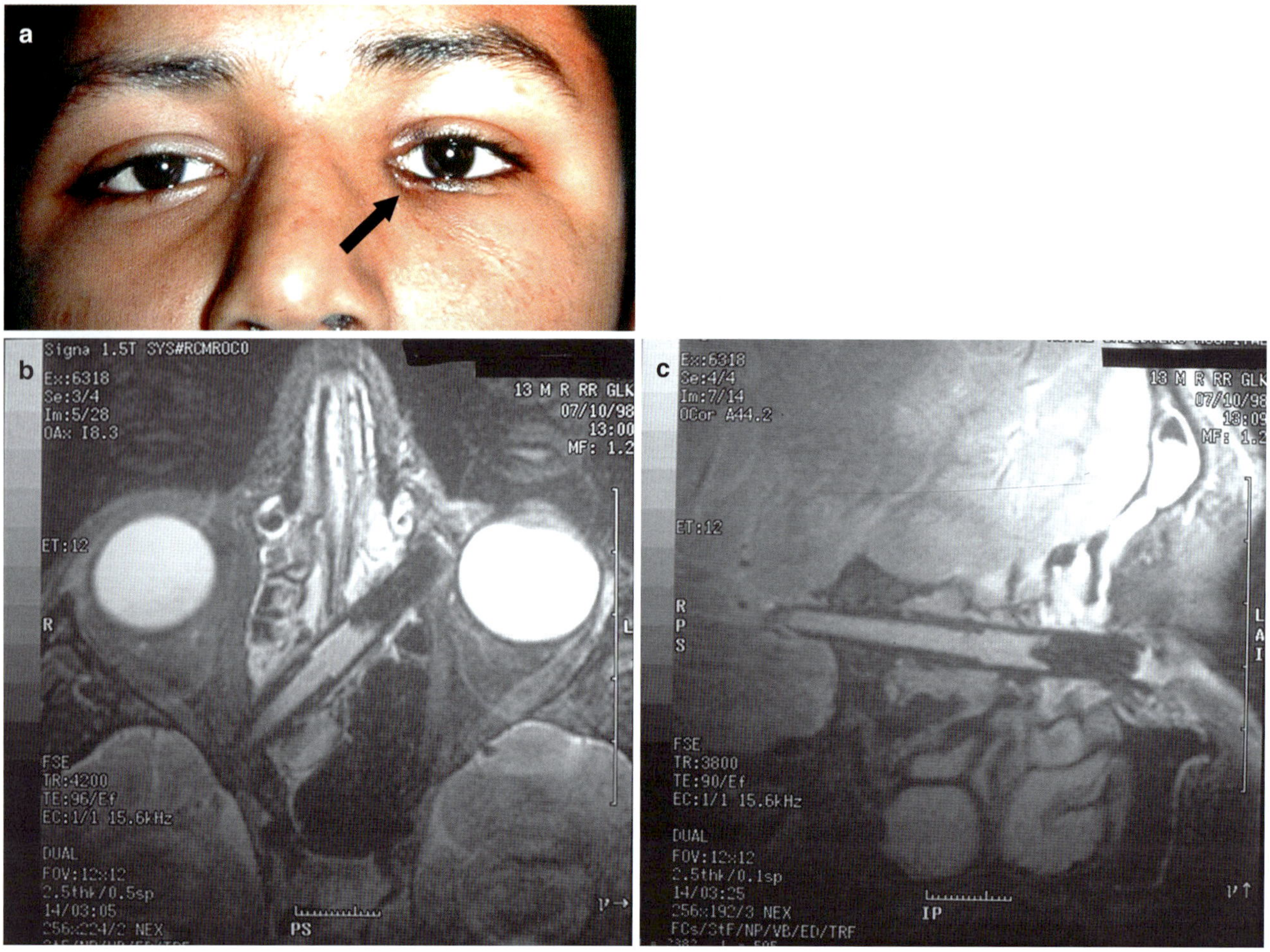

Fig. 74.8 (**a**) A 14-year-old boy presented 2 years after being stabbed with a pen at school with a small discharging sinus below his medial canthus (*arrow*) and no other symptoms. (**b**) An axial MRI shows a pen passing from near the left medial canthus across the nasal cavity and paranasal sinuses. (**c**) A sagittal MRI shows the tip of the pen just penetrating the opposite temporal lobe. It was removed via a craniotomy without any complications

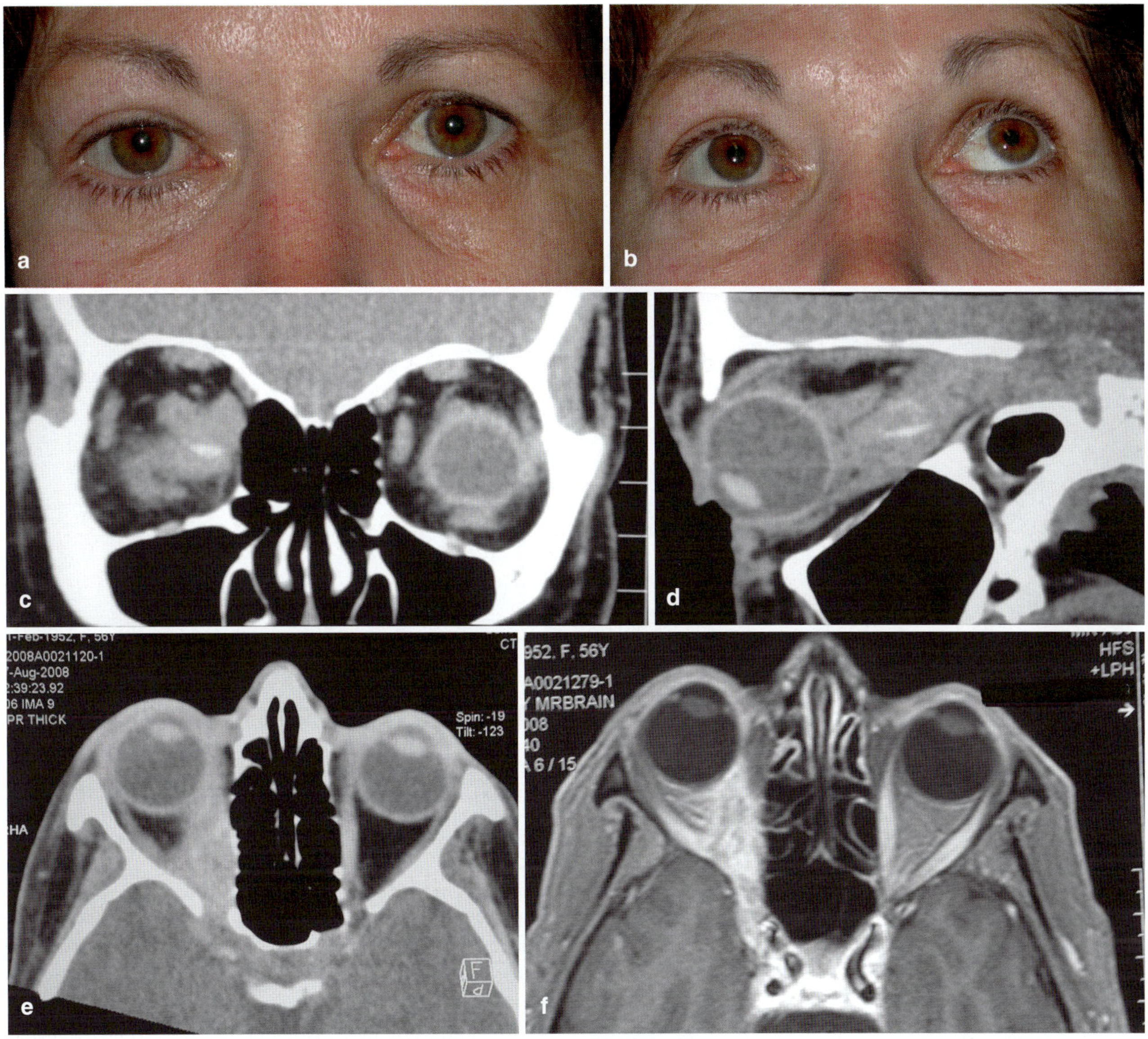

Fig. 74.9 (**a**) A woman presented some months after a fall in the garden with diplopia on upgaze. (**b**) She had limited elevation of the right eye. (**c**) A coronal CT scan shows a dense intraconal mass in the right orbit with a higher density area within it. (**d**) A sagittal CT scan shows the higher density area within the mass to be linear. It was removed at surgery and found to be a small wooden foreign body. (**e**) An axial CT scan of the same patient as in (**a**) who presented 2 years later with worsening diplopia and optic neuropathy. There was a larger mass within the central and posterior orbit extending through the superior orbital fissure where the normal fat space was obliterated. (**f**) An axial T1-weighted MRI shows some linear areas within the mass of lower signal. The dense fibrotic mass was explored and several very small splinters of wood were removed. The mass has persisted

residual FBs. Histopathological examination of the fibrotic mass did not show any organisms or fungal elements.

Retained IOrbFBs may migrate over time. There is a tendency for them to migrate toward the surface, particularly with subcutaneous FBs, which may extrude spontaneously sometimes years after the original injury. Larger and deeper FBs may also spontaneously extrude years later, either to the surface or into some other cavity such as the paranasal sinuses, nasal cavity, or mouth. Occasionally, IOrbFBs may migrate from a position where there was no associated morbidity to another place where symptoms may occur. I have seen a patient with a deep metallic IOrbFB (a small piece of shrapnel from a war injury) migrate years later to a position between the globe and the medial rectus where it began to cause pain on eye movement 40 years after the original injury (see Fig. 74.10). Removing the FB abolished the symptoms.

Very rarely, an intraorbital FB may produce gaze-evoked amaurosis. This unusual symptom can occur with any intraconal orbital mass and also with optic nerve

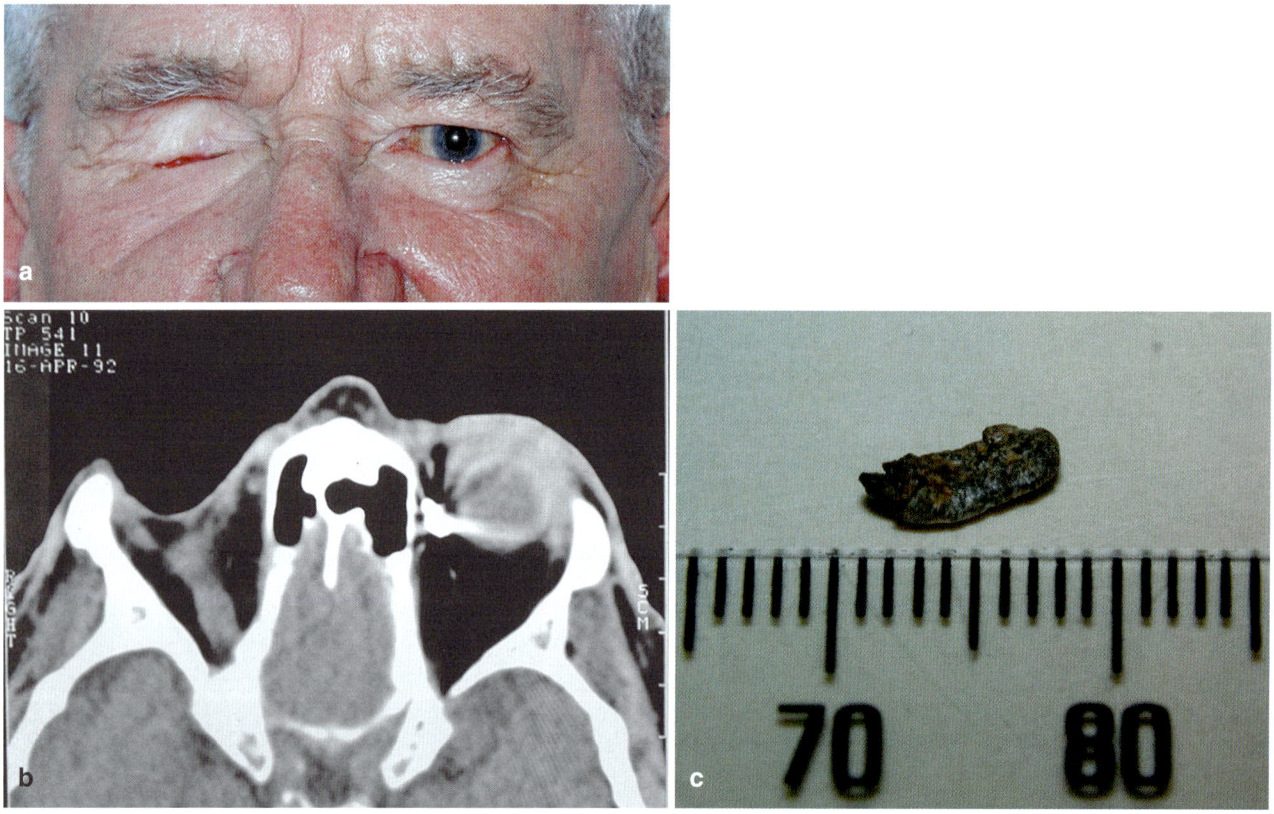

Fig. 74.10 (**a**) An elderly man had been injured as a tail gunner in a bomber during World War II. His right eye was injured and removed and several pieces of shrapnel had penetrated his body. Forty-five years later, he developed pain on eye movement. (**b**) An axial CT scan shows a metallic foreign body lying adjacent to the globe near the medial rectus muscle. It had presumably migrated to a position where it began to produce symptoms. (**c**) The piece of shrapnel was removed from the left orbit and the symptoms were abolished

sheath meningiomas. The patient presents with loss if vision in one direction of gaze, with associated pupil changes in that direction of gaze [20].

Treatment of Penetrating Orbital Injuries and IOrbFBs

In general, all penetrating orbital injuries with or without retained foreign bodies should be treated with broad-spectrum antibiotics. If material is available to culture, it should be taken before instituting antibiotic therapy. If the patient is taken to the operating theater, the foreign body may be sent for culture, and the wound may also be swabbed. In general, broad coverage of aerobic and anaerobic organisms should be provided. There is usually no indication for antifungal agents, and infection with fungi after penetrating injuries of the orbit and IOrbFBs is very rare. The patient should also have appropriate tetanus immunization if required.

The specific treatment of penetrating orbital injuries with or without retained FBs will depend on a number of factors. Each patient will need a careful and thorough clinical assessment and appropriate imaging. The main decision to make in the presence of a foreign body will be whether it needs to be removed or whether the FB can be safely left. In making this decision, the nature of the foreign body, its size, and position will need to be taken into account.

Larger protruding FBs (see Fig. 74.1b, c, f) clearly have to be removed. Careful surgical planning may be required when a large foreign body lies within the orbit but extends into other body cavities. For example, the foreign body may lie close to or penetrate large blood vessels, and plans should be made to deal with potential catastrophic hemorrhage.

Foreign bodies that penetrate the cranial cavity will need the assistance of neurosurgeons, and a decision will need to be made about the possible need for a craniotomy either for access to the FB or to deal with intracranial complications such as hematoma, abscess, tissue necrosis, or dural injury and cerebrospinal fluid leak (see Fig. 74.8). Careful preoperative imaging will help in planning the safe removal of orbito-cranial foreign bodies [21].

Deeply buried IOrbFBs may not need to be removed. This applies particularly to smaller metallic foreign bodies which may be tolerated indefinitely [17, 22, 23]. The risk of removing such a deep foreign body will usually outweigh the risk of leaving it in situ (see Fig. 74.3).

Organic IOrbFBs should, in general, be removed because of the much higher risk of infection [10, 17, 18]. Most organic foreign bodies are wood or plant related and carry with them a range of organisms that can cause infection.

The surgical approach to a retained IOrbFB will be dictated by several factors. Chief among these is whether the foreign body lies entirely within the orbit or whether it also extends into the cranial cavity or adjacent tissue spaces such as the paranasal sinuses or skull base area. In such cases, help should be sought from appropriate surgical colleagues [24].

The surgical approach will also be determined by the location of the FB within the orbit and the time since the injury. If a patient presents acutely, soon after their injury, the wound made by the penetrating foreign body is the best route to take to reach a more deeply placed foreign body. Not only does this approach minimize tissue damage, it also generally leads directly to the foreign body. Similarly, if there is a discharging abscess or sinus, then the sinus track should be followed in order to reach the FB. Often, thin malleable retractors can be placed into the wound, and the orbit can be explored often into its depths to locate and remove an FB. If necessary, the wound can be enlarged to facilitate deeper exposure.

If an IOrbFB has been present within the orbit for a long time, it will often become "walled off" by inflammatory and fibrous tissue. Entering this inflammatory mass with sharp dissection to reach its center will often locate an abscess cavity with the FB in its center.

Once an FB is located, especially a wooden FB, careful inspection and exploration should proceed until the surgeon is happy there are no more FBs present. Wood is often in multiple fragments or splinters, and care needs to be taken to remove all of them. Irrigating the wound thoroughly with antiseptic solutions is also helpful. Finally, a passive drain should be inserted to the point where the FB was and left for 24–48 hours to allow infective material and blood to drain. Broad-spectrum antibiotics should be continued for at least 5 days or longer, depending on the nature of the FB, and the severity and site of the infection.

Smaller FBs may be difficult to locate within the orbital soft tissues. Orbital tissues move with surgical manipulation and dissection, and what seems to be a simple surgical procedure can turn into a prolonged search for an FB within shifting orbital tissues. Some authors have advocated the use of intraoperative fluoroscopy to help in the location and removal of radiopaque IOrbFBs [16, 25], and this can certainly be helpful in such cases.

Generally, loss of visual function and other morbidity associated with penetrating orbital injuries and IOrbFBs are the result of the original injury, and the removal of an IOrbFB is much less likely to cause visual loss or other complications [17]. Despite that, caution should always be exercised when considering the removal of a deeply placed foreign body, particularly one that is inorganic, metallic, and inert, when leaving the FB in situ may be less dangerous than trying to remove it.

Summary

A high index of suspicion and a careful history and examination are critical in assessing patients with definite or possible penetrating orbital injuries with or without retained IOrbFBs, whether they present acutely or in a delayed fashion. The possibility of deeper penetration, especially of the cranial cavity, should always be kept in mind. Appropriate imaging should be obtained, and the first-line examination is CT. MRI may be helpful when CT is equivocal in the detection of possible wooden FBs. Antibiotics should always be given after obtaining material for microbiological examination (if available). The decision to operate and remove an FB must be individualized, but in general, all organic FBs should be removed. Larger and more anteriorly placed inorganic IOrbFBs can be removed, but smaller and deeply placed inorganic IOrbFBs can often be left without any significant subsequent morbidity.

References

1. Martin G. The death of Henry II of France: a sporting death and post-mortem. Aust N Z J Surg. 2001;71:318–20.
2. Al Hashmi A, Cheng A, Nikolarakos D, Goss A. Penetrating injuries to the orbit despite safety equipment. Br J Oral Maxillofac Surg. 2009;47:71–2.
3. Mader TH, Carroll RD, Slade CS, George RK, Ritchey JP, Neville SP. Ocular war injuries in the Iraqi insurgency, January – September 2004. Ophthalmology. 2006;113:97–104.
4. Andreotti G, Lange JL, Brundage JF. The nature, incidence, and impact of eye injuries among US military personnel: implications for prevention. Arch Ophthalmol. 2001;119:1693–7.
5. Green BF, Kraft SP, Carter KD, Buncic JR, Nerad JA, Armstrong D. Intraorbital wood. Detection by magnetic resonance imaging. Ophthalmology. 1990;97:608–11.
6. Specht CS, Varga JH, Jalali MM, Edelstein JP. Orbitocranial wooden foreign body diagnosed by magnetic resonance imaging. Dry wood can be isodense with air and orbital fat by computed tomography. Surv Ophthalmol. 1992;36:341–4.
7. Adesanya OO, Dawkins DM. Intraorbital wooden foreign body (IOFB): mimicking air on CT. Emerg Radiol. 2007;14:45–9.
8. Glatt HJ, Custer PL, Barrett L, Sartor K. Magnetic resonance imaging and computed tomography in a model of wooden foreign bodies in the orbit. Ophthal Plast Reconstr Surg. 1990;6:108–14.
9. McGuckin JF Jr, Akhtar N, Ho VT, Smergel EM, Kubacki EJ, Villafana T. CT and MR evaluation of a wooden foreign body in an in vitro model of an orbit. Am J Neuroradiol. 1996;17:129–33.
10. Shelsta HN, Bilyk JR, Rubin PA, Penne RB, Carrasco JR. Wooden intraorbital foreign body injuries: clinical characteristics and outcomes in 23 patients. Ophthal Plast Reconstr Surg. 2010;26:238–44.
11. Williamson MR, Espinosa MC, Boutin RD, Orrison WW Jr, Hart BL, Kelsey CA. Metallic foreign bodies in the orbits of patients

undergoing MR imaging: prevalence and value of radiography and CT before MR. Am J Roentgenol. 1994;162:985–6.
12. Boutin RD, Briggs JE, Williamson MR. Injuries associated with MR imaging: survey of safety records and methods used to screen patients for metallic foreign bodies before imaging. Am J Roentgenol. 1994;162:189–94.
13. Murphy KJ, Brunberg JA. Orbital plain films as a prerequisite for MR imaging: is a known history of injury a sufficient screening criterion? Am J Roentgenol. 1996;167:1053–5.
14. Seidenwurm DJ, McDonnell CH III, Raghavan N, Breslau J. Cost utility of radiographic screening for an orbital foreign body before MR imaging. Am J Neuroradiol. 2000;21:245–7.
15. Deen HG, Miller DA, Kostick DA, Jaeckle A. Removal of an orbital metallic foreign body to facilitate magnetic resonance imaging: technical case report. Neurosurgery. 2006;58:E999; discussion E999.
16. Cho RI, Kahana A, Patel B, Sivak-Callcott J, et al. Intraoperative fluoroscopy-guided removal of orbital foreign bodies. Ophthal Plast Reconstr Surg. 2009;25:215–8.
17. Fulcher TP, McNab AA, Sullivan TJ. Clinical features and management of intraorbital foreign bodies. Ophthalmology. 2002;109:494–500.
18. Nasr AM, Haik BG, Fleming JC, Al-Hussain HM, Karcioglu ZA. Penetrating orbital injury with organic foreign bodies. Ophthalmology. 1999;106:523–32.
19. Wang WJ, Li CX, Sebag J, Ni C. Orbital fistula. Causes and treatment of 20 cases. Arch Ophthalmol. 1983;101:1721–3.
20. Danesh-Meyer HV, Savino PJ, Bilyk JR, Sergott RC, Kubis K. Gaze-evoked amaurosis produced by intraorbital buckshot pellet. Ophthalmology. 2001;108:201–6.
21. Fezza J, Wesley R. The importance of CT scans in planning the removal of orbital-frontal lobe foreign bodies. Ophthal Plast Reconstr Surg. 1999;15:366–8.
22. Finkelstein M, Legmann A, Rubin PAD. Projectile metallic foreign bodies in the orbit. A retrospective study of epidemiologic factors, management, and outcomes. Ophthalmology. 1997;104:96–103.
23. Gönül E, Akbörü M, Izci Y, Timrkaynak E. Orbital foreign bodies after penetrating gunshot wounds: retrospective analysis of 22 cases and clinical review. Minim Invasive Neurosurg. 1999;42:207–11.
24. Liu D, Shail EA. Retained orbital wooden foreign body. A surgical technique and rationale. Ophthalmology. 2002;109:393–9.
25. Yoganathan P, Conti SM, Kavalec C. The use of intraoperative fluoroscopy as an aid for removal of radiopaque intraorbital foreign bodies. Ophthalmic Surg Lasers Imaging. 2008;39:436–7.

Combat Casualty Ophthalmic Care for the Oculoplastic and Orbital Surgeon

75

Donovan S. Reed, Brett W. Davies, and Christopher J. Calvano

Introduction

Since the onset of battle, military physicians have been faced with the management of complex oculofacial injuries in unfamiliar environments with limited resources. Prior to the establishment of sub-specialized medical care, military physicians without formalized ophthalmic training were responsible for the management of injuries involving the eye and orbit. With advanced warfare tactics and weaponry, particularly following World War II, the US military recognized the necessity for maintaining physicians with formal training in the field of ophthalmology, specifically focused on providing ophthalmic care in a combat environment. With advances in medical equipment and surgical technique, in addition to improved medical evacuation systems, the prognosis for oculofacial and orbital injuries in combat has greatly improved. Nevertheless, warfare is constantly evolving, requiring the combat ophthalmologist to continue to innovate and adapt to provide the best care possible. Unfortunately, with the increasing frequency of terrorist acts targeting civilians, mass shootings with advanced weaponry, and domestic bombings, these challenges are no longer unique to the military ophthalmologist and facial surgeon. The ability to manage complex oculofacial and orbital trauma, triage casualties, and appropriately evacuate injured patients is paramount to the oculofacial and orbital surgeon [1].

D. S. Reed
Brooke Army Medical Center, Department of Ophthalmology, Fort Sam Houston, TX, USA

B. W. Davies (✉)
Ophthalmic Plastic and Reconstructive Surgery, Brooke Army Medical Center/Wilford Hall Eye Center, Department of Ophthalmology, Lackland, TX, USA

C. J. Calvano
San Antonio Military Medical Center/Wilford Hall Ambulatory Surgery Center, Department of Ophthalmology and Oculoplastic Surgery, San Antonio, TX, USA

Casualty Care Goals

Oculofacial and orbital injuries faced in a combat environment are unique (see Fig. 75.1). Often, these patients have suffered significant life-threatening trauma involving multiple organ systems. Not infrequently the status of the eye and orbit are secondary to lifesaving casualty care. Rarely is there an isolated ocular or orbital injury. As such, it is critical for the ophthalmic and facial surgeon to identify those injuries requiring urgent evaluation and address those injuries promptly. Seamless coordination with other subspecialties is key to the appropriate management of combat trauma casualties.

Despite advances in modern armor, ocular and facial injuries were present in approximately 20% of combat casualties

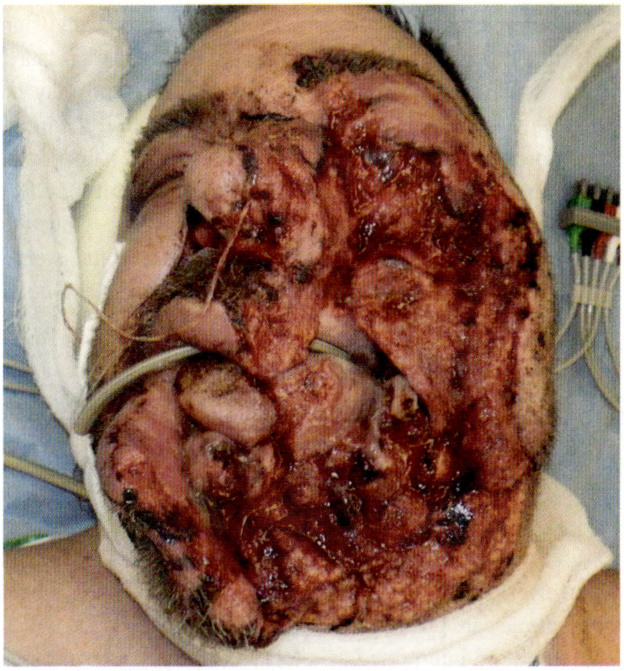

Fig. 75.1 Facial gunshot wound with associated polytrauma

J. J. Servat et al. (eds.), *Smith and Nesi's Ophthalmic Plastic and Reconstructive Surgery*,
https://doi.org/10.1007/978-3-030-41720-8_75

during Operations Iraqi and Enduring Freedom [1]. As such, it is crucial to maintain a high suspicion for ocular injury in combat multi-trauma victims. Still, the evaluation and treatment of vision-threatening ocular and orbital injuries in a combat environment remains challenging, particularly if evacuation of causalities is delayed secondary to the austere nature of the environment or the presence of a mass casualty situation. Small metallic foreign bodies are able to penetrate the eye leaving the clinical appearance of a relatively intact globe, and blunt trauma with occult posterior rupture remains incredibly difficult to appreciate during rapid clinical assessment. Additionally, it is not uncommon for combat trauma patients to be unconscious and, therefore, unable to report changes in vision or pain. Particular focus to the mechanism of injury suggesting possible penetrating/perforating or blunt ocular trauma is therefore critical [2, 3].

Assessment

Visual acuity immediately following the trauma is the most important prognostic indicator for future visual outcome and is therefore paramount to assess if possible. Assessment of visual function for both the injured and non-injured eye can be effectively estimated with the patient's ability to read letters or labels of medical supplies, count fingers, detect hand motions, or appreciate a bright light. Utilizing any bright light source, assessment of a relative afferent pupillary defect offers a quick indication of retina and optic nerve function and remains essential in conditions such as orbital compartment syndrome secondary to retrobulbar hemorrhage. Presence of a relative afferent pupillary defect is also an important prognostic sign for future potential vision. Assessment of intraocular pressure, if no obvious or suspected globe injury is present, may be effectively estimated with the two-finger method. If the intraocular pressure is elevated, the globe feels firm to palpation in comparison to the contralateral globe, and the orbit may feel tense in the presence of a retrobulbar hemorrhage. Once the patient is stabilized, a more detailed ocular and orbital examination will provide further information regarding the complexity of ocular and orbital injury [4].

Pain Management and Prevention of Further Damage

Pain control is an essential component of tactical combat casualty care, including ocular and orbital injuries, though often overlooked in the acute management by the combat ophthalmic care provider. Even in the absence of pain, which should not be interpreted as a lack of injury, ocular injuries often cause significant anxiety. As this may impede appropriate care, an anxiolytic such as a benzodiazepine may be administered to facilitate evaluation and treatment. As the traumatized eye remains highly susceptible to further damage, appropriate administration of eye protection is critical, particularly during patient transport. If no fox shield is readily available, anything appropriately sized to cover the globe and orbit such as a small taped cup may be utilized. Further, administration of antiemetic medications remains essential to prevent retching, which may elevate the pressure to a level resulting in further damage [3, 4].

Evacuation

As the determination of the full extent of ophthalmic injuries associated with combat trauma remains challenging in a hostile environment with limited resources, evacuation remains a high priority of the ocular combat casualty provider in an austere environment. Determination of the threat of permanent vision loss is crucial, as prompt evacuation of all casualties may not be possible in every situation. The ultimate goal is definitive management of all potential vision-threatening injuries within 24 hours of the initial trauma. As such, the establishment of contact with subspecialty care surgeons in preparation for casualty arrival is key to the successful transition of ophthalmic casualty care [4].

Ocular Injuries

A brief description of combat ocular and orbital injuries is provided. Full-length discussion of the medical and surgical management of each condition is beyond the scope of this chapter.

Open Globe Injury

Open globe injuries result from penetrating and perforating trauma or from globe rupture secondary to compressive forces following blunt trauma. Corneoscleral lacerations with prolapsed ocular contents are obvious exam findings (see Fig. 75.2) but may not be present with all injuries. Other findings which should raise suspicion for an open globe injury include penetrating periocular trauma, peaked pupil, and abnormal anterior chamber depth. The goals in a combat environment include the prevention of further damage to the eye, prophylaxis for endophthalmitis, and prompt evacuation for definitive management. With any suspicion of possible open globe injury, a rigid eye shield without gauze or bandaging under the shield should be placed. Endophthalmitis prophylaxis with moxifloxacin 400 mg PO and antiemetic therapy with ondansetron 4 mg oral dissolving tablet or intravenously should also be administered promptly. The

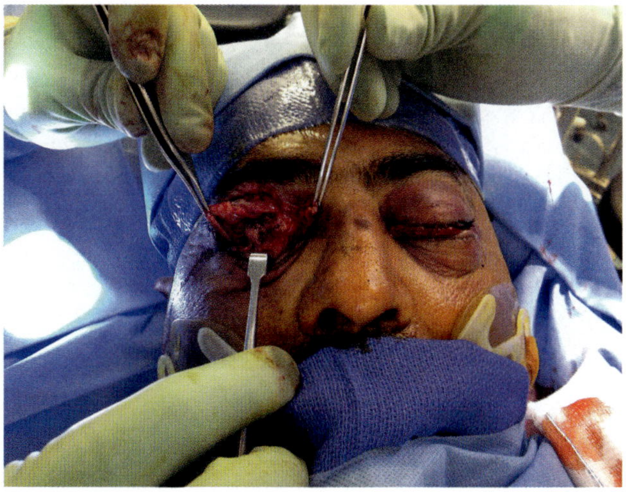

Fig. 75.2 Open globe injury, right eye

head of the patient should be kept elevated to approximately 30–45 degrees. Patient movements should be minimized, and pain control addressed. Evaluation should be repeated with any reported change in vision or pain, and evacuation and coordination of definitive surgical repair should be initiated. Description of the repair of complex corneoscleral lacerations is beyond the scope of this chapter [5].

Blunt Trauma

Closed globe injury may result in severe vision loss and is often overlooked in the management of complex multi-system trauma at the point of injury. As these injuries are typically not as obvious to non-ophthalmic providers and identification may require advanced ophthalmic assessment including dilated posterior examination, suspicion of injury secondary to mechanism is key to appropriate combat care management. Anterior segment blunt injury may result in traumatic hyphema, which may lead to increased intraocular pressure causing optic neuropathy and corneal blood staining. The risk of intraocular pressure elevation and further damage increases with the grade of hyphema and with rebleeding. Upon the identification of hyphema in a combat environment, a rigid shield should be placed and the head elevated. Antiemetics should be administered, and nonsteroidal anti-inflammatory medications should be avoided due to the risk of worsened intraocular hemorrhage. Topical corticosteroid drops, prednisolone acetate 1%, four times daily, and cycloplegic agents should be administered. The eye should be monitored for rebleeding or increasing intraocular pressure which results in vision changes and increasing size of the hyphema. If elevated intraocular pressure is present, ocular hypotensive medications should be initiated. Administration of acetazolamide is contraindicated in patients with sickle cell disease or trait [6].

Injury to the posterior segment as a result of blunt injury often damages the retina and optic nerve, leading to vision loss. Decreased visual acuity, loss of the red reflex, a positive relative afferent pupillary defect, and visual field defect may signify vitreous hemorrhage or retinal detachment. Initiation of supplemental oxygen therapy prior to and during transport may improve visual outcomes with retinal detachment [7]. Prompt consultation with a retina specialist is crucial to achieving the best possible outcomes during transition of care. It is important to remember ophthalmic ultrasound, which may allow for diagnosis of posterior segment trauma and is contraindicated if there remains the possibility of open globe injury. Ultimately, there are no altitude evacuation restrictions required for blunt closed globe injury [2].

Chemical Injury

Chemical injuries can cause significant ocular damage leading to permanent visual loss. As such, chemical injury to the eye should be considered an ophthalmic emergency. Alkali chemical burns have more potential for damage due to lipid peroxidation and subsequent penetration into deeper structures within the eye. Acid injuries typically cause coagulative necrosis, limiting further penetration of ocular structures. Assessment of the initial pH and degree of injury, particularly the presence and extent of limbal ischemia, is key to determining the prognosis. Regardless of the cause or extent of injury, immediate and aggressive irrigation is crucial in the early period following the initial burn. Utilization of a Morgan Lens © or other device for irrigation at the point of injury, with continuation throughout the evacuation process, is key to the ultimate visual outcome and future eye salvage. The ultimate goal at the point of injury is to initiate irrigation with at least two liters of sterile/clean water or IV fluids as rapidly as possible to reduce further damage. Utilization of ocular anesthetics as needed may help facilitate irrigation. However, these should be avoided for pain control as continued use may impair corneal epithelial healing. Additionally, the eye should be examined, with particular attention to the fornices, for retained particulate matter, which should be removed if present. Copious irrigation should be continued throughout the evacuation process until it can be definitively determined the eye has returned to a physiologic pH [8].

Once the patient has reached definitive care, treatment will be based on the extent of ocular injury. The modified Hughes classification may be utilized as a guide for further ophthalmic care. Grade I injuries should be treated with a topical antibiotic ointment 3–4 times daily, with cycloplegia for photophobia. Preservative-free artificial tears should be utilized liberally between antibiotic ointment applications. Grade II–IV injuries require topical moxifloxacin 0.5% antibiotic drops four times daily, in addition to topical corticosteroids. Additionally, oral doxycycline and oral vitamin C may be utilized for its anti-inflammatory and anti-collagenase properties, respectively [8].

Soft Tissue Trauma

Eyelid Laceration

Lid lacerations as demonstrated in Fig. 75.3 result from both penetrating and blunt periorbital trauma. Ultimately, the primary concern when lid lacerations are present remains assessment of the integrity of the underlying globe. Consideration of the possibility of ocular or orbital foreign body should be maintained in all penetrating soft tissue trauma. Ultimately, meticulous closure should be undertaken, ideally within 24 hours of injury. Fortunately, given the extensive blood supply to the lid and face, eyelid lacerations have a relatively low incidence of infection. This is not true if the mechanism of injury is an animal or human bite wound. The possible need for rabies vaccination should always be considered when an animal bite has occurred. Tetanus prophylaxis should also be administered if appropriate. Presence of fat within the laceration is indicative of orbital septum violation. As a barrier to the spread of infection, if the orbital septum has been violated, antibiotic coverage and expedient evacuation for surgical exploration and repair should be undertaken. Additionally, attempts to maintain any avulsed tissue should be undertaken, and such tissue should be preserved in chilled saline and transported with the patient to definitive care. There should be no attempt to debride, excise, or suture exposed orbital tissue in a combat environment, as uncontrolled orbital bleeding may occur. Gentle wound irrigation may be attempted with sterile saline or clean water, and temporary closure with steri strips prior to definitive surgical repair is appropriate [9].

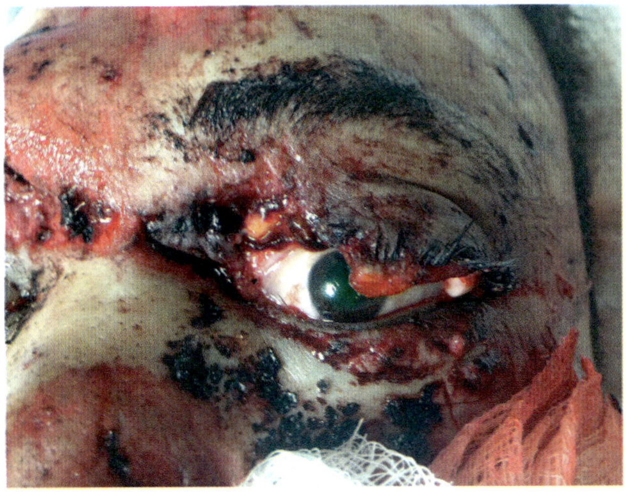

Fig. 75.3 Complex margin-involving left upper eyelid laceration and associated periorbital facial burn secondary to an improvised explosive device blast injury

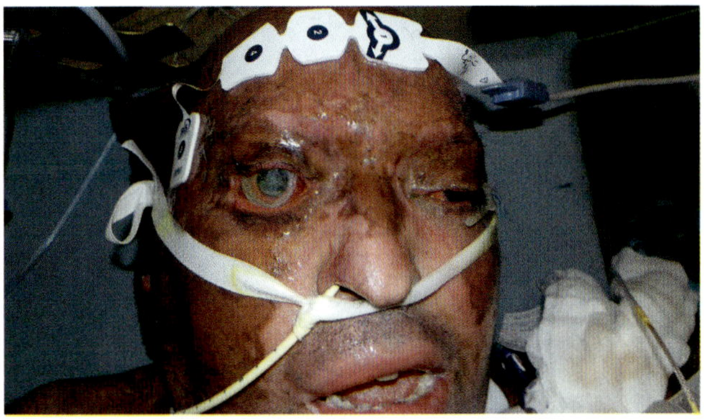

Fig. 75.4 Periorbital thermal facial burn with significant lagophthalmos and inferior lid ectropion of the right eye

Thermal Burn

Periorbital facial burns result in high risk for exposure keratopathy secondary to the loss of the normal blink reflex, impaired tear production and tear film dynamics, entropion, lid retraction, and lagophthalmos (see Fig. 75.4) [10]. Furthermore, patients with facial thermal burns are often intubated due to concern of inhalation injury and therefore are unable to vocalize complaints of worsening vision or eye pain. Early ocular surface protection with lubricating drops and ointments should be initiated [11]. Additionally, ophthalmic safe antibiotic ointments should be applied every 2 to 4 hours for all periorbital and facial thermal burns. Gentle tape tarsorrhaphy may be utilized during evacuation and transport prior to definitive management. If available, coverage of the eyes from the brow to the maxilla with food-grade polyethylene film to prevent drying can be considered. If periorbital thermal burns are present, consideration for early lateral canthotomy and cantholysis should be considered, as fluid resuscitation requirements may be extensive [2].

Orbital Trauma

Orbital Compartment Syndrome

The most common cause of orbital compartment syndrome, particularly in the combat environment, is retrobulbar hemorrhage. Usually associated with blunt orbital trauma, bleeding into the confined orbital space results in increased ocular pressure leading to ischemia of critical structures, ultimately leading rapidly to irreversible vision loss if not promptly addressed. Other causes of orbital compartment syndrome in a combat environment include orbital congestion secondary to aggressive fluid resuscitation in burn victims and orbital emphysema following extensive orbital fractures (see below). As orbital compartment syndrome may have a delayed onset, continued surveillance for its development, particularly in the evacuation period, is crucial to prompt management and prevention of vision loss. Exam findings include proptosis, increased orbital pressure, loss of visual acuity, and presence of a relative afferent pupillary defect. If these findings are present in association with a history of trauma, prompt lateral canthotomy and cantholysis should be performed without delay. If the orbital compartment syndrome persists despite appropriate superior and inferior lateral cantholysis, blepharotomies and ultimately orbital floor decompression may be required. Following this, ice packs may be applied, and compressive dressings should be avoided. Monitoring for recurrence of elevated intraocular pressure should be continued throughout the evacuation period until definitive management is reached. Initiation of acetazolamide and hypertonic saline IV or IV mannitol may be considered to further lower intraocular pressure, in addition to one dose of 1 g IV methylprednisolone to decrease inflammation. Of note, the presence of orbital compartment syndrome does not result in altitude restrictions for evacuation management of casualties [12–14].

Orbital Wall Fracture

When an object larger than the width of the orbit strikes the orbit, expansion of orbital contents and mechanical buckling forces may fracture the orbital bones. Resultant herniation of contents into the surrounding sinuses and extraocular muscle entrapment within the fracture site may occur. Exam findings concerning for orbital wall fracture include diplopia, a palpable and painful orbital rim step-off, enophthalmos, extraocular motility restriction, and infraorbital hypoesthesia. Complex facial fractures involving the orbital bones such as zygomaticomaxillary complex fractures may result in trismus and malocclusion. Fortunately, orbital wall fractures are not typically considered ophthalmic emergencies. Still, the presence of a restriction of extraocular motility and concern for an orbital fracture in pediatric trauma (white-eyed trapdoor blowout fracture) and the presence of an oculocardiac reflex are concerning, requiring urgent evaluation and evacuation for definitive surgical care. It is important to note the "white-eyed" blowout fracture is not exclusive to the pediatric population, and has been described in the young adult population. If there is concern for an orbital wall fracture in a combat environment, the patient should be instructed in sinus precautions such as no nose blowing, and initiation of nasal decongestants such as oxymetazoline nasal spray should be considered. Appropriate antibiotic coverage with amoxicillin/clavulanic acid 875 mg/125 mg by mouth every 12 hours or ertapenem 1 g intravenously daily should be initiated to prevent the spread of sinus pathogens into the orbital tissues. Ice packs for 20 minutes every 1 to 2 hours for the first 48 hours should be utilized to reduce swelling. During evacuation, there should be continued monitoring for the delayed development of orbital compartment syndrome given the possibility of concurrent retrobulbar hematoma [12].

Mass Casualty

A mass casualty event is present when the number of casualties is greater than the amount of immediately available medical capabilities, which includes personnel, supplies, and/or equipment. Unfortunately, this scenario is becoming more and more common in not only the combat environment but also in the civilian sector of medicine. Effective response relies on the principle of triage, which is the structure of sorting and prioritizing casualties based on the situation and available resources, as demonstrated in Figs. 75.5 and 75.6. The ultimate goal is to provide the greatest number of good outcomes within the limitations of the available capabilities present at the given time. Triage is constantly in evolution, and should be performed at all levels of care, from point of injury to definitive care facilities [13, 15].

Within the triage paradigm, ocular injuries fall into one or multiple traditional categories, being immediate, delayed, minimal, and expectant. Immediate injuries are those requiring attention within minutes to 2 hours upon arrival to avoid death or major disability. Immediate oculofacial injuries include chemical burns and those injuries leading to orbital compartment syndrome such as a retrobulbar hematoma. Delayed injuries are those ultimately requiring surgery, but treatment may be delayed without unjustifiably endangering life or eyesight. Delayed oculofacial injuries include open globe trauma and facial fractures without compromise of the airway. Additionally, periorbital facial burns without airway compromise can be considered delayed. Minimal injuries are those minor injuries in which the individual may care for themselves or require only minimal medical care. Those with minimal injuries may often be utilized for additional resources or manpower, potentially assisting with the movement, evacuation, and care of others injured. Casualties with injuries overwhelming available medical capabilities at the cost of treating potentially salvageable patients fall into the expectant category, such as transcranial gunshot wounds with coma and burns without reasonable chance for survival and/or recovery. A few situations require special consideration. Wounded victims contaminated by a biological or chemical attack must be decontaminated prior to evacuation to a treatment facility; however, appropriate prehospital care

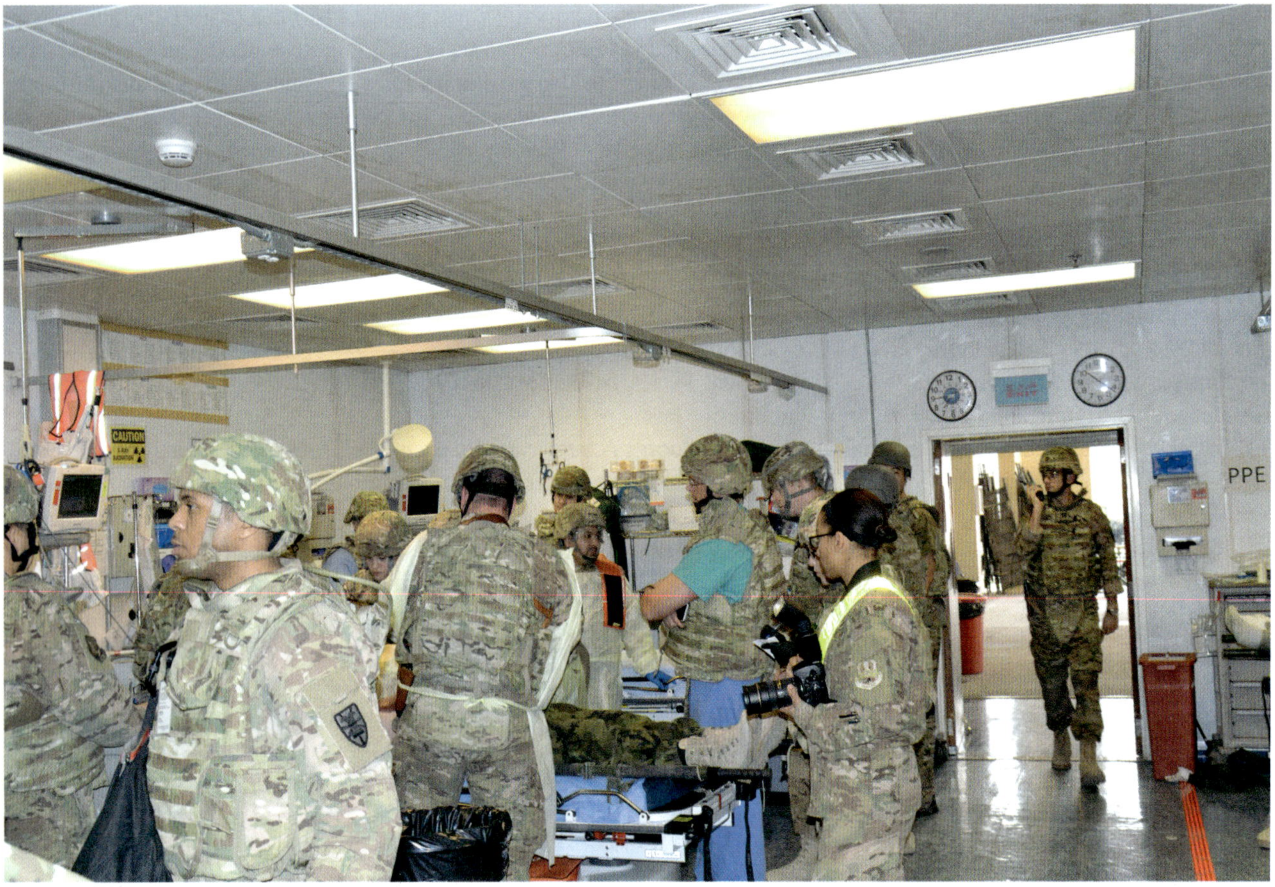

Fig. 75.5 Mass casualty trauma bay in a deployed combat environment

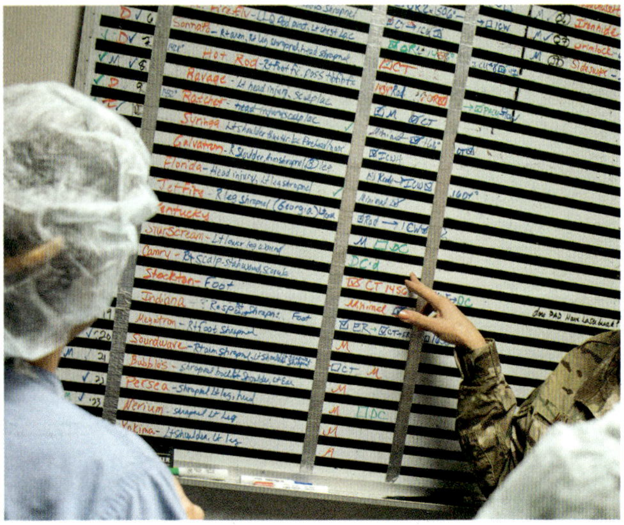

Fig. 75.6 Mass casualty board in a deployed combat environment

may still be provided by appropriately protected medical personnel. Further, patients with retained unexploded ordnance require immediate segregation and should be treated last to decrease the chance of causing further injury to medical care personnel or other casualties [13].

It is important to continually reassess casualties as the triage status may change with care, worsening of the clinical condition, or a change in the availability of resources and medical capabilities. Triage remains fluid at all levels, as situations alter and resources become available. Additionally, attempts to decrease further damage to the eye and orbit, such as placement of a rigid eye shield, should be utilized throughout the triage and evacuation efforts [2]. Ultimately, appropriate and prompt evacuation to the appropriate level of care improves overall prognosis and chances of vision salvage for multi-trauma and mass casualty patients.

Packing and Planning Considerations

Well-thought planning and preparation for the combat environment or mass casualty situation improves overall prognosis and visual outcomes for oculofacial casualties. In a combat environment, the minimum required equipment includes rigid eye shields, bright light source, visual acuity estimate reference, and lateral canthotomy/cantholysis instrument sets. Additionally, teleconsultation capability should be immediately available. Furthermore, pH test strips, ice packs, polyethylene film, and steri strips may prove beneficial. Ultimately, the ability to have a portable slit lamp or direct ophthalmoscope with portable ultrasound would be ideal; however, this may or may not be feasible in a combat environment or at the point of injury. Recommended medications include moxifloxacin 400 mg oral tablets, clindamycin 300 mg oral tablets, ondansetron intravenous or oral dissolving tablets, tetracaine eye drops, fluid for ocular irrigation, and fluorescein ophthalmic stain. Additionally, oxymetazoline nasal spray, ophthalmic antibiotic ointments, and cycloplegic eye drops improve capabilities in an austere environment. Additional medications to consider if available include intravenous mannitol, acetazolamide 250 mg oral tablets, intravenous corticosteroids or corticosteroid eye drops, artificial tears, vitamin C, and the tetanus and rabies vaccines. Ultimately, the specific environment and medical personnel capabilities will dictate the appropriate medical equipment and instruments to have available [2].

References

1. Pan A, Davies B. History of military ophthalmology in Calvano. In: Ophthalmology in military and civilian casualty care. New York, NY: Springer; 2018. p. 1–4.
2. Reynolds M, et al. Ocular injuries and vision-threatening conditions in prolonged field care (CPG ID:66). Joint Trauma Sys Clin Practe Guidel. 2017:1–20.
3. Joint Trauma System clinical practice guideline. Initial care of ocular and adnexal injuries by non-ophthalmologists at role 1, role 2, and nonophthalmic role 3 facilities. 24 Nov 2014. http://www.usaisr.amedd.army.mil/cpgs/Initial_Care_of_Ocular_and_Adnexal_Injuries_24Nov2014.pdf. Accessed 1 Nov 2017.
4. Committee on Tactical Combat Casualty Care. Tactical Combat Casualty Care guidelines for medical personnel. http://www.usaisr.amedd.army.mil/pdfs/TCCCGuidelinesforMedicalPersonnel170131Final.pdf. Accessed 1 Nov 2017.
5. Bhagat N, Nagori S, Zarbin M. Post-traumatic infectious endophthalmitis. Surv Ophthalmol. 2011;56:214–51.
6. Walton W, Von Hagen S, Grigorian R, et al. Management of traumatic hyphema. Surv Ophthalmol. 2002;47:297–334.
7. Mervin K, Valter K, Maslin J, et al. Limiting photoreceptor death and deconstruction during experimental retinal detachment: the value of oxygen supplementation. Am J Ophthalmol. 1999;128:155–64.
8. Colby K. Chemical injuries of the cornea. In: Focal points: clinical modules for ophthalmologists. San Francisco, CA: American Academy of Ophthalmology; 2010, module 1.
9. Rapp J, Plackett TP, Crane J, et al. Acute traumatic wound management in the prolonged field care setting. J Spec Oper Med. 2017;17(2):132–49.
10. Peterson K, Colyer MH, Hayes DK, et al. Prevention of infections associated with combat-related eye, maxillofacial, and neck injuries. J Trauma. 2011;71:S264–9.
11. Saritas TB, Bozkurt B, Simsek B, et al. Ocular surface disorders in intensive care unit patients. ScientificWorldJournal. 2013;2013:182038.
12. Long J, Tann T. Orbital trauma. Ophthalmol Clin N Am. 2002;15:249–53.
13. Ord RA. Postoperative retrobulbar haemorrhage and blindness complicating trauma surgery. Br J Oral Surg. 1981;19:202–7.
14. Lima V, Burt B, Leibovitch I, et al. Orbital compartment syndrome: the ophthalmic surgical emergency. Surv Ophthalmol. 2009;54:441–9.
15. Banks D. Mass casualty and triage. In: Cubano M, editor. Emergency war surgery. 5th ed. Fort Sam Houston: Borden Institute; 2018. p. 29–45.

Index

A

Abaxial proptosis, 884
Abducens nerve, 680
Aberrant oculomotor nerve regeneration (AONR), 257
Ablepharon macrostomy syndrome (AMS), 1146, 1147
Abnormal globe, 622
Abscess formation, 377
Accessory canalicular channels, 516
Accessory canaliculi, 513, 516
Accessory lacrimal glands, 506
Accreditation Council for Graduate Medical Education (ACGME), 100
Acellular dermis, 1019, 1020
Acetaminophen, 1197
Acidic chemical burns, 1223
Acidosis, 683
Acinic cell carcinoma, 735, 736
Acoustic neuromas, 578
Acquired ptosis, 1137
  anatomy and physiology, 295, 296
  anesthesia, 307, 308
  anterior approach, 308
  aponeurotic ptosis, 296
  clinical presentation, 296
  eyelid measurements, 302, 303
  Fasanella Servat operation, 318–320
  frontalis suspension surgery, 310–313
  Guillain–Barré syndrome, 300
  levator aponeurosis surgery, 313–316, 318
  Marcus Gunn jaw-winking phenomenon, 300
  mechanical ptosis, 301
  Müller's muscle–conjunctival resection, 320, 321
  multiple sclerosis, 300
  myogenic ptosis
    CPEO, 296, 298
    myasthenia gravis, 296, 297
    myotonic dystrophy, 298
  neurogenic ptosis, 298
  nonsurgical management, 308, 309
  ocular sympathetic paresis, 299, 300
  ophthalmoplegic migraine, 300
  patient history, 302
  photographic documentation, 303, 304
  physical examination, 302
  posterior approach, 308
  pseudoptosis, 301, 302
  psychological aspects, 304
  ptosis correction, 308
  third cranial nerve palsy, 299
  traumatic ptosis, 301
  visual fields, 304
Acquired socket contracture, 1070
Acro-fronto-facio-nasal dysostosis (AFFND), 1130
Actinic keratoses, 401, 402
Actinomyces israelii, 532
Actinomyces meyeri, 533
Actinomycin D, 932
Acute dacryocystitis, 21, 531, 549, 640
Acute hemorrhagic cysts, 901
Acute myelogenous leukemia, 653
Acute orbital dacryoadenitis, 722
Acute vision loss, 937
Acyclovir, 685
AdatoSil, 376
Adenocarcinoma, 498
  clinical pearls, 944, 945
  clinical presentation, 945
  computed tomography, 945
  histopathology, 945
  magnetic resonance imaging, 945
  prognosis, 945
  treatment, 945
Adenoid cystic carcinoma (ACC), 498, 672, 690, 731, 733, 734, 847, 946
  Adie's pupil, 731
  clinical pearls, 945, 946
  clinical presentation, 946
  computed tomography, 946
  diagnosis, 731
  drug delivery, 733
  extraperiosteal approach, 731
  histopathologic appearance, 731
  histopathology, 946, 947
  IACC protocol, 733, 734
  imaging, 730
  inflammatory pseudotumor, 731
  initial presentation, 731
  intra-arterial cytoreductive chemotherapy, 733
  lacrimal gland, 650
  local tumor clearance, 732
  loss of heterozygosity, 734
  magnetic resonance imaging, 946
  microdissection genotyping, 734
  MOPP therapy, 733
  optimal local therapy, 731
  prevalence, 730
  prognosis, 947
  proliferative phase, 731
  recurrence rate, 732
  survival outcome, 732
  symptoms, 730
  treatment, 733, 947
  tumor suppressor gene loss, 734

J. J. Servat et al. (eds.), *Smith and Nesi's Ophthalmic Plastic and Reconstructive Surgery*,
https://doi.org/10.1007/978-3-030-41720-8

Adjunctive radiotherapy, 903, 937, 940, 947
Adjuvant chemotherapy, 861, 904, 906, 922, 925
Adriamycin, 937
Adult orbital xanthogranulomatous diseases, 761
Agenesis, canalicular atresia and, 516
AIDS-related lymphoma (ARL), 788, 789
Ali ibn Isa's method, 92
Alkali burns, 1223
Allergic conjunctivitis, 535
Allgrove syndrome (AS), 1138
AlloDerm, 1228
Alloplastic material, 1021
Alm retractor, 567
Alopecia, facelift, 394, 395
Aluminum oxide (Al_2O_3), 1034
Aluminum oxide orbital implant, 1071
Alveolar rhabdomyosarcomas, 931
Amblyopia, 1104
Amelanotic malignant melanoma, 626, 954
American Society of Ophthalmic Plastic and Reconstructive Surgery (ASOPRS), 99, 100
Aminoquinolones, 361
Amniotic bands, 518
Amniotic membrane grafts, 1074
Amniotic membrane tissue, 1074
Amniotic membrane transplantation (AMT), 237
Amniotocele, 516
Amoxicillin, 1166
Amphotericin B, 683, 684
Ampulla, 524, 527
Amyloidosis, 737
Analytical reasoning, 121
Anatomic obstruction, 545
Ancillary chemotherapy, 903
Anesthesia and pediatric oculoplastics patient
  at child's level, 1192
  distraction, 1192
  injectable anesthetics, 1196, 1197
  non-medical prevention of anxiety, 1191, 1192
  post-operative nausea and vomiting, 1197
  post-operative pain control, 1197, 1198
  sedation
    choice of, 1195
    contraindications to, 1193, 1194
    equipment necessary for, 1193
    levels of, 1193
    role of, 1191
    working without, 1192, 1193
  for surgery, 1195
  topical anesthetics, 1195, 1196
Aneurysmal bone cyst, 934
  clinical pearls, 933
  clinical presentation, 933
  computed tomography, 934
  histopathology, 934
  magnetic resonance imaging, 934
  prognosis, 934
  treatment, 934
Aneurysm rupture, 677
Angiocath, 579
Angiolymphoid hyperplasia with eosinophilia (ALHE), 761, 762
Angiosarcomas, 903
  clinical pearls, 902
  clinical presentation, 902
  CT scan, 902
  histopathology, 903
  magnetic resonance imaging, 903
  prognosis, 903
  treatment, 903
Anisocoria, 258
Anisometropia, 1104
Anisometropic amblyopia, 1105
Ankyloblepharon, 1158
Anophthalmic socket, 1029, 1031, 1032, 1037, 1056
  acquired socket contracture, 1070
  changes associated with, 1056, 1057
  charactersitics of, 1055
  congenital anophthalmic socket, 1080, 1082–1091
  implant exposure and extrusion, 1068, 1069
  implant infection, 1068–1070
  implant migration, 1068
  implant pegging, complications of, 1070
  long-term management of, 1091, 1093
  mild socket contracture, 1071, 1072
  moderate socket contracture, 1072–1076
  problems, management of
    anterior orbital cysts, 1060
    deep superior sulcus, 1062–1064, 1066, 1067
    discharge and irritation, 1058, 1059
    enophthalmos, 1062–1064, 1066, 1067
    eyelid malpositions, 1061–1064
    lagophthalmos with exposure of prosthesis surface, 1060
    socket dryness, 1058
    socket pain, 1060
  secondary orbital implant surgery, 1064, 1065
  severe socket contracture, 1074, 1078, 1080, 1081
  surgery, 1034, 1055
Anophthalmos/anophthalmia, 1080, 1082–1091, 1117, 1118, 1121
Anterior migration, 1035, 1068
Anterior orbital cysts, 1060
Anterior scleral wound, 1046
Antibiotics, DES, 511
Antibody therapy, 991, 992
Anticholinergic class drugs, 222
Anticoagulation, 681
Antiestrogen tamoxifen, 951
Anti-neutrophil cytoplasmic antibody (ANCA) test, 641
Anxiety, non-medical prevention of, 1191, 1192
Apert syndrome, 1132
Aponeurotic ptosis, 243, 296
Apraclonidine, 300
Apraxia of eyelid opening (AEO), 221, 249, 250
Aqueous tear deficiency (ATD), 507
Arginine vasopressin (AVP), 670
Arnica montana gel, 371
ArteFill, 375
Arteriovenous malformation (AVM), 660, 661, 817–819
Artificial eye, fabrication, care, and maintenance of, 1056–1058
Artificial tears, 509, 1225
Artist's conception, 1030, 1032
As Low As Reasonably Achievable (ALARA) concept, 1179, 1181
Aseptic cavernous sinus thrombosis
  clinical presentation, 678
  pathogenesis, 677, 678
Asian blepharoplasty
  anatomy, 343–345
  complications, 348, 349
  postoperative care, 348
  preoperative evaluation, 345
  surgical techniques, 345–348
  upper eyelid blepharoplasty, 343

Aspergillosis, 684
Aspergillus, 684
Atelectasis, 880
Atypia, 432, 541, 738, 804, 917, 920, 921, 926, 940, 958
Atypical lymphoid hyperplasia, 770
Auricular cartilage, 1072
Autoantigens in TED, 986, 987
Autoenucleation, 163
Autogenous bone grafts, 1235
Autoimmune disorders, sarcoidosis, 751, 752
Autoimmune orbital granulomatous disease, 751
Autoimmune processes, 593
Autoimmune thyroiditis, 773
Autologen, 372
Autologous auricular cartilage, 1015–1017
Autosomal dominant inheritance, 1116
Autosomal recessive congenital ichthyoses (ARCI), 1156
Autosomal recessive inheritance, 1116
Autosomes, 1115
Avitene®, 597
Axial displacement, orbital evaluation, 606
Axial proptosis, 606, 884
Azathioprine, 991
Azithromycin, 1166

B

Bacitracin, 1225
Bacterial orbital cellulitis, 832, 833
  clinical features, 744
  complications, 747–749
  diagnosis, 744, 745
  differential diagnosis, 746, 747
  orbital nocardiosis, 749
  treatment, 747
Bacterial organisms, 635
Bacterial preseptal cellulitis, 832
Baker–Gordon formula, 117
Balanced decompression, 1011
Balanced salt solution (BSS)., 587
Balloon at valve of Hasner, 588
Balloon catheter system, 587
Balloon dacryoplasty, 114, 587, 588
Balloon dilatation, failed dacryocystorhinostomy, 596
Banked sclera, 1022
Barber-Say syndrome (BSS), 1146, 1147
Barrow's angiographic subtypes, 673
Basal cell adenocarcinoma
  clinical pearls, 954
  clinical presentation, 954
  computed tomography, 955
  histopathology, 955
  magnetic resonance imaging, 955
  prognosis, 955
  treatment, 955
Basal cell carcinoma (BCC), 423, 455, 459, 956, 1108
  clinical pearls, 955, 956
  clinical presentation, 424, 425, 956
  histopathology, 956, 957
  magnetic resonance imaging, 956
  management, 425
  MMS, 465, 468
  pathologic features, 423, 424
  prognosis, 957
  treatment, 957
Battles sign, 1278
Bayes theorem/regression analysis, 121
B-cell lymphoma, 771
Bell's palsy, 208, 251, 578
Bell's phenomenon, 137, 1106, 1223, 1225
Bell's phenomenon, anesthesia, and dryness (BAD), 208
Belotero balance, 373
Benign cartilaginous tumors
  clinical pearls, 926
  clinical presentation, 926
  computed tomography, 926
  histopathology, 926
  magnetic resonance imaging, 926
  prognosis, 927
  treatment, 926
Benign essential blepharospasm (BEB), 247, 249, 250
Benign Essential Blepharospasm Research Foundation (BEBRF), 225
Benign eyelid tumors, 1108
Benign fibrous histiocytomas, 921
Benign mixed tumor, *see* Pleomorphic adenoma
Benign orbital tumors, 860
Benign polymorphisms, 1115
Beta-blockers, 1194
Betamethasone, 598
Bicanalicular intubation, 561
Bicanalicular stent, 561, 562
Bicoronal flap, 1089
Bilateral ankyloblepharon filiforme adnatum, 1158
Bilateral complete cryptophthalmos, 1146
Bilateral congenital eversion, 1156
Bilateral dacryocystogram, 524
Bilateral follicular lymphoma, 652
Bilateral lower lid epiblepharon, 1159
Bilateral MALT lymphoma, 651
Bilateral optic glioma, 637
Bilateral orbital varices, 661
Bilateral periorbital ecchymosis, 1113
Bilateral postoperative lagophthalmos, 411
Bilateral scirrhous breast metastasis, 655
Bilateral tarsal kinking syndrome, 1157
Bilateral upper eyelid coloboma, 1148
Bilateral upper eyelid retraction, 1158
Bilobed flap, 457
Binocular diplopia, 608
Bio-alcamid, 376
Bioceramic implants, 1034, 1038
Bio-Eye™ hydroxyapatite implant, 1032
Biofilm formation, 375, 377
Biopsy
  excisional, 707
  fine-needle aspiration biopsy, 706, 707
  incisional, 707
Biosynthetic polymers, 374–376
Blaine Labs vibration anesthesia device, 1196
Bleeding, 597
Bleomycin, 961
Blepharochalasis repair, 90
Blepharocheilodontic syndrome, 1125, 1154, 1155
Blepharocheilodontic syndrome-1 (BCDS1), 1125
Blepharophimosis-ptosis-epicanthus-inversus syndrome (BPES), 280, 1126, 1135, 1136, 1138, 1152
Blepharophimosis-ptosis-intellectual disability syndrome (BPIDS), 1135

Blepharoplasty, 409, 1014
canthal webbing, 410, 411
complications, 412
fire and facial burns, 412
hemorrhage, 412
ocular injury, 412
dry eye and exposure keratopathy, 411
lacrimal gland injury, 412
lagophthalmos, 411, 412
lid/crease asymmetry, 410
lower lid retraction after, 415
operative complications, 410, 414
fire/facial burns, 416
hemorrhage, 416
ocular injuries, 416
postoperative complications, 410, 413, 414
blindness, 414, 418
canalicular laceration and epiphora, 417
conjunctival chemosis, 417
diplopia, 414, 417
incision irregularities, 413
infection, 413, 414, 417
inflammation, 418
lower lid blepharoplasty, complications of, 414
nonaesthetic incision and incision irregularities, 416, 417
numbness, 414
wound dehiscence, 413
preoperative planning/surgical judgement, complications, 410
ectropion and eyelid retraction, 414, 415
overcorrected/undercorrected herniated orbital fat, 416
overcorrected/undercorrected redundant skin, 415, 416
preoperative planning/surgical judgement, errors in, 410, 414
ptosis, 412
residual left lower lid skin, 415
superior sulcus deformity, 411
undercorrected redundant skin/fat, 410
upper lid blepharoplasty, 409, 410
Blepharoptosis, 364
Blepharospasm
botulinum toxin therapy, 222, 223
causes, 219
classification, 219, 220
clinical presentation, 220, 221
etiologic factors, 221
functional and cosmetic deformities, 219
myectomy surgery, 223–225
oral drug therapy, 222
patient support, 225
periocular injections, 222
supportive therapies, 221, 222
therapeutic protocol, 225
treatment, 219
Blindness, blepharoplasty, 414
Blind, painful eyes, non-surgical management of, 1042
Blowout fracture
buckling theory vs. hydraulic theory, 1239, 1240
clinical examination, 1237–1239
complications, 1255–1258
computed tomography imaging, 1238, 1239
fractured orbital floor, 1239, 1240
magnetic resonance imaging, 1239
mechanism of injury, 1237
treatment
alloplastic floor implant, 1250, 1254, 1255
blunt periorbital trauma, 1247
computed tomography, 1243
conjunctival wound closure, 1254, 1255
conservative observation, 1241
double arm suture, 1254
floor fracture surgery, 1253
guidelines, 1251, 1252
inferior lateral cantholysis, 1252, 1254
lateral canthotomy, 1252, 1254
lower eyelid tarsal, 1254
periosteal elevator, 1254
periosteum closure, 1254, 1255
skin wound closure, 1254, 1255
surgical implant, 1255
titanium orbital floor implant, 1254
"white-eyed" blowout or small trapdoor fractures, 1242
Blunt trauma, 630, 1209
B mode ultrasound, orbital evaluation, 610
Body harvest site, fat transfer, 379, 380
Bone loss, 359
Bone remodeling, 926
Bone, tumors of, 888
Bony anatomy, 861
Bony nasolacrimal canal, 518
Bony orbit, 618, 619
Bony reconstruction, 865, 866
Bortezomib, 489
Bothersome epiphora, 486
Botulinum neurotoxin type A (BoNTA), 359
adjuvant use, 367
complications, 367, 368
history, 360, 361
injection technique for, 362
lower face, 366, 367
mid face, 365, 366
pathophysiology, 359, 360
technique, 361, 362
treatment, 362, 363
upper face, 363–365
Botulism, 270, 271
Bourneville disease, *see* Tuberous sclerosis (TS)
Bovine spongiform encephalopathy (BSE), 1038
Bowen's disease, 469
Bowman lacrimal probe, 568, 573, 597, 1169
Brain abscess, 681
Brainlab's Kick and Curve, 873
Brainstem ocular motility disorders, 124
Breakdown phase, 1057
Breast carcinoma, 950, 951
clinical pearls, 950
clinical presentation, 950
computed tomography, 950
histopathology, 951
magnetic resonance imaging, 951
prognosis, 951
treatment, 951
Bromelain, 370
Bronchogenic carcinoma
clinical pearls, 951
clinical presentation, 951
computed tomography, 951, 952
histopathology, 952
magnetic resonance imaging, 952
prognosis, 952
treatment, 952
Brow ptosis, 364
Brueghel syndrome, 219, 220
Buckling theory, 1239, 1240

Bulbar conjunctiva, 485
Bullous pemphigoid, 231
Bunny lines, 365
Buphthalmos, 622
Bupivacaine, 1197
Burkitt lymphoma (BL), 785, 786, 847
Butanediol diglycidyl ether (BDDE), 372

C

Calcium hydroxylapatite, 374
Caldwell–Luc decompression, 99
Canalicular atresia, 516
Canalicular cyst, 528
Canalicular lacerations, 417, 560, 561, 1166–1168, 1171, 1206, 1208, 1216, 1217
Canalicular stenosis, 486, 489, 1230
Canalicular stents, 563
Canaliculi, 513, 521, 522, 528, 537, 554
  abducens nerve (VI), 48
  ciliary ganglion and parasympathetic nerves, 49, 50
  conjunctiva, 34
  extraocular muscles, 44–46
  eyebrow, 22, 23
  eyelid, 34, 35
    anatomy, 22
    development, 39, 40
    margin, 26, 27
    nerves, 36–39
    vessels, 35–37
  globe topography, 46, 47
  lacrimal excretory development, 21, 22
  lacrimal excretory system, 19, 20
  levator palpebrae superioris, 30–33
  lower eyelid retractors, 32, 33
  lymphatic system, 52, 53
  medial and lateral canthal ligaments, 28–30
  meibomian glands, 34
  Müller's muscle, 33
  nasolacrimal sac and duct, 21
  orbicularis oculi muscle, 27, 28
  orbit, 40
  orbital arteries nerves, 50–52
  orbital fascia, 40–43
  orbital fat, 43, 44
  orbital nerves, 47
    nerves (II), 47
    nerves (III), 47, 48
  orbital septum, 30, 31
  orbital veins, 52
  periorbita, 40
  superficial eyelid anatomy, 25, 26
  superficial musculoaponeurotic system, 23, 24
  sympathetic nerve, 49
  tarsal plates, 33, 34
  trigeminal nerve (V), 48, 49
  trochlear nerve (IV), 48
Canaliculitis, 559
  bicanalicular repair, 561, 562
  dog bites, 560
  examination, 560
  intracanalicular plugs, 560
  lacrimal system obstructions, 532, 533
  lacrimal trauma, 560
  monocanalicular stent, 562
  pigtail probe, 562, 563
  punctal ectropion, 563, 564
  repair, 561
  stent, choice of, 561
  stent removal, 563
Canalization, 513
Cancer therapy
  oculoplastic complications
    chalazia, 489
    chemotherapy, 488
    epiphora, canalicular stenosis, and nasolacrimal duct blockage, 488, 489
    head and neck cancer, ablative surgery in, 490, 491
    orbital and periorbital edema, 490
    radiation therapy, 483, 484
    trichomegaly, 489
  orbital bone, 486, 487
  secondary neoplasms, 487, 488
  tissue damage
    eyelid, 485, 486
    lacrimal system, 486
    skin and conjunctiva, 484, 485
  wound healing, 487
Canthal dystopia, 491
Canthal webbing, 410, 411
Cantholysis, 1264, 1265
Capillary hemangiomas, 653–655, 841, 897, 898
  clinical pearls, 896, 897
  clinical presentation, 897
  CT scan, 897
  histopathology, 897
  MRI, 897
  prognosis, 898
  treatment, 897, 898
Capillary vascular malformations (CVM), 398
Capnocytophaga canimorsus, 1166, 1219
Capsulopalpebral fascia (CPF), 620
Carbon dioxide lasers, 401
Carcinoids
  clinical pearls, 903, 904
  clinical presentation, 904
  CT scan, 904
  histopathology, 904
  magnetic resonance imaging, 904
  prognosis, 904
  treatment, 904
Carcinosarcoma, 736
Carotid-cavernous fistulas(CCF), 661, 674, 827, 828
  classification, 673
  clinical presentation, 674
  evaluation, 674
  observation, 675
  outcomes and prognosis, 674, 675
  pathogenesis, 673
  surgical options, 675–677
  venous drainage, 673, 674
Cartesian coordinate system, 871
Catastrophic onset, 885
Catheter cerebral angiography (CCA), 258
Caudal elevator, 572
Cautery, 539
Cavernous hemangiomas, 655, 659, 738, 823, 825, 884, 886, 899
  clinical pearls, 898
  clinical presentation, 898
  CT scan, 898
  histopathology, 899
  MRI, 898, 899
  prognosis, 899
  treatment, 899

Cavernous ICA aneurysms
clinical presentation, 677
prognosis, 677
Cavernous malformations, 655, 657
Cavernous sinus, 667–670
Cavernous sinus thrombosis (CST), 667, 677
Cavernous vascular malformation, *see* Cavernous hemangioma
Celecoxib, 377
Central implant fibrovascularization, 1033
Central medial canthal defect, 456
Central nervous system neurosarcoidosis, 635
Cephalosporins, 1166
Cerebral dural venous plexus, 669
Cerebrospinal fluid rhinorrhea, 1277
Chalazia, 190, 489
CHARGE syndrome, 1118
Chemical burns, 1223
Chemical peeling, 116
Chemiluminescence, lacrimal system obstruction, 554
Chemodenervation, 364–366
Chemotaxis, 1201, 1202
Chemotherapy, 488, 908, 919, 920, 925, 945, 954
Chiasmal injury, 146, 163, 164
Child abuse in oculoplastics, 1113, 1114
pediatric morbidity and mortality, 1113
scald burns, 1113
thermal burns, 1113
Chinese characters, 938
Chlamydia trachomatis, 532
Chloramphenicol, 1166
Cholesterol granuloma, 935
clinical pearls, 934, 935
clinical presentation, 935
computed tomography, 935
histopathology, 935
magnetic resonance imaging, 935
prognosis, 936
treatment, 935
Chondromas, 926
Chondromesenchymal hamartomas, 926
Choristomas, 837, 838, 1126–1128
Choroidal detachments, 623
Choroidal hemangiomas, 628
Choroidal melanoma, 627, 762, 953
Chromosomal aberrations, 1117
Chronic blepharitis, 190
Chronic canaliculitis, 533
Chronic maxillary sinus atelectasis, 879, 880
Chronic progressive external ophthalmoplegia (CPEO), 134, 135, 254, 255, 296, 298, 1137
Chronic socket discharge, 1050
Churg-Strauss syndrome (CSS), 753, 754
Cicatricial ectropion, 1224, 1226–1229
Cicatricial entropion, 186, 190
causes, 182
treatment, 183, 185
Cicatricial nasolacrimal duct drainage obstruction, 529
Cilia incarnata, 189
Cisplatin, 908, 951, 961
Clarithromycin, 1166
Clavulanic acid, 1166
C-Line CIS, 586
Clinical activity score (CAS), 987
Clinical congenital anophthalmia, 113
Closed trapdoor fracture, 1239, 1244–1246, 1248
Cluster headache (CH), 271, 272
Coats' disease, 624, 625
Cobalt, 542
Cold compresses, 569
Collagen, 372
Collared punctal plugs, 538
Collarless intracanalicular plugs, 538–539
Coloboma, 622, 1119
Colobomas with corneopalpebral/conjunctival adhesions, 1148
Colobomatous cysts, 896
clinical pearls, 895, 896
clinical presentation, 896
CT scan, 896
histopathology, 896
MRI, 896
prognosis, 896
treatment, 896
Combat casualty ophthalmic care
blunt trauma, 1315
chemical injuries, 1315, 1316
evacuation, 1314
eyelid laceration, 1316
facial gunshot wound, 1313
goals, 1313, 1314
lid lacerations, 1316
mass casualty, 1317, 1318
open globe injuries, 1314, 1315
orbital trauma
orbital compartment syndrome, 1316, 1317
orbital wall fracture, 1317
packing and planning, 1318, 1319
pain management and prevention, 1314
periorbital thermal facial burn, 1316
soft-tissue trauma
eyelid laceration, 1316
thermal burn, 1316
visual function assessment, 1314
Combination pain medications, 1198
Combined chemotherapy, 961
Combined radiotherapy, 961
Compartment syndrome, 1011, 1012
Complete/partial cryptophthalmos, 1145
Complex eyelid margin lacerations, 1213, 1215
Complex microphthalmia/microphthalmos, 1082, 1117
Composite rhytidectomy, 393
Compressive optic neuropathy (CON), 911, 1001, 1003
Computed tomography (CT), 886
adenocarcinoma, 945
adenoid cystic carcinoma, 946
aneurysmal bone cyst, 934
angiosarcomas, 902
basal cell adenocarcinoma, 955
basal cell carcinoma, 956
benign cartilaginous tumors, 926
breast carcinoma, 950
bronchogenic carcinoma, 951, 952
carcinoids, 904
cavernous hemangiomas, 898
in children, 1178–1182
avoid plain X-rays, 1181
communicate, 1181
imaging modalities, 1181
ionizing radiation effects, 1179
in pediatric orbital disease, 1180
radiation exposure, risk of, 1179
right scan for right pathology, 1181
single-pass technology with coronal reconstruction, 1181

cholesterol granuloma, 935
Ewing sarcoma, 936
fibrosarcoma, 920
fibrous dysplasia, 938
fibrous histiocytoma, 921
giant cell reparative granulomas, 939
inverted papillomas, 957
juvenile xanthogranuloma, 922
lacrimal system obstruction, 551, 552
leiomyosarcomas, 924
lipoblastomas, 925
lipodermoids, 927
lipomas, 928
liposarcomas, 929
lymphangiomas, 900
malignant melanoma, 953
meningocele, 907
MPNST, 905
mucoepidermoid carcinomas, 948
neuroblastoma, 908
ONSM, 911, 912
optic pathway glioma, 909, 910
orbital evaluation, 610
orbital radiology, 615
ossifying fibromas, 940, 941
osteoblastomas, 942
osteomas, 942, 943
osteosarcoma, 944
pleomorphic adenomas, 949
plexiform neurofibromas, 913
rhabdomyosarcoma, 931
schwannomas, 915
sinonasal carcinoma, 959
solitary fibrous tumor, 932
solitary neurofibromas, 917
sphenoid wing meningioma, 918
squamous cell carcinomas, 960
varices, 901, 902
Cone-beam computed tomography, 552
Congenital accessory palpebral fissure, 1151
Congenital alacrimia, 1138
Congenital anophthalmic socket, 1080, 1082–1091
Congenital coloboma, 1121–1123
Congenital dermoid cysts, 736, 737
Congenital distichiasis, 1124
Congenital ectropion, 1124, 1125
Congenital entropion, 1125
epiblepharon, 181
surgical repair, 181
Congenital fibrosis of the extraocular muscles (CFEOM), 252, 1136
Congenital fibrosis of the extraocular muscles 2 (CFEOM2), 1136
Congenital fibrosis of the extraocular muscles 3 (CFEOM3), 1136, 1137
Congenital ichthyosis, 1124
Congenital lacrimal amniocele, 516
Congenital myasthenic syndromes, 1137
Congenital nasolacrimal duct obstructions, 583, 587
Congenital ptosis, 1107, 1133
Congenital punctal agenesis, 516
Congenital punctal atresia, 515, 516
Congenital secretory anomalies
congenital alacrimia, 1138
nasolacrimal system anomalies, 1138, 1139
Congenital soft tissue deformities
canthal abnormalities
lateral canthus, 1153–1155
medial canthus, 1151, 1152
congenital eyelid malpositions
eyelid ectropion associated with anterior lamella shortening, 1156
eyelid retraction, 1156–1158
upper eyelid entropion, 1156
upper eyelid eversion associated with lid laxity, 1155
major eyelid deformities
ablepharon macrostomy syndrome, 1146, 1147
congenital accessory palpebral fissure, 1151
cryptophthalmos, 1145, 1146
lower eyelid involvement in craniofacial clefting, 1150
upper eyelid colobomas, 1147–1150
minor deformities
ankyloblepharon, 1158
epiblepharon, 1159
Congenital upper eyelid retraction, 1158
Conjunctiva, 563
cancer therapy, 484, 485
chemosis, blepharoplasty, 417
dermoid cyst of, 891
melanoma, 433, 478, 863
melanocytic tumors, 432
clinical presentation, 433
management, 433
pathologic features, 432
SLNB, 478
squamous cell carcinoma, 434
squamous neoplasia, 433
clinical presentation, 433, 434
management, 434
pathologic features, 433
Conjunctivochalasis, 527, 546
Conjunctivodacryocystorhinostomy (cDCR), 443
Contralateral upper eyelid retraction, 244, 245
Contrast dacryocystography, 550, 551
Controlled tissue necrosis, 90
Corneal scarring, 237
Corneal sensitivity, 523
Cornelia de Lange syndrome (CdLS), 1133, 1134
Corrugator supercilii, 363
Corticosteroids, 679, 897, 989–992, 1003
Cosmetic oculoplastic surgery, 100, 101
Cottonoids, 587
Cotton-tipped applicator (CTA), 1007, 1049
Covered stents, 676
Cowden disease, 1128
C psittaci-positive marginal-zone B-cell lymphoma, 727
Cranial neuropathy, 667, 674, 680
Craniofacial clefts, 1132, 1133
lower eyelid involvement in, 1150
numbers 11, 10 and 9, 1148
Craniofacial deformities, 518
Craniofacial dysjunction, 1273, 1277
Craniofacial osteosarcomas, 944
Craniosynostosis, 1131, 1132
Crawford hook, 561, 585
Crawford lacrimal intubation, 584, 585
Crawford silicone tube, 569
Crawford stents, 585, 1226
C-reactive protein, 609
Crigler massage, 583
Crohn's disease (CD), 836
Cross-hatching, 371
Cross linking technology, 372
Crouzon syndrome, 1131, 1132
Crow's feet, 364

Crumbs homologue 1 gene (CRB1), 1118
Cryoprobe, 890
Cryptophthalmos, 1121, 1122, 1145, 1146
Cupid's bow, 370
Curvilinear incision, 566
Cutaneous fistula, 1256
Cutaneous neuroendocrine carcinoma, 431
Cutler-Beard bridge flap technique, 440, 451, 452
Cyclophosphamide, 236, 908, 932, 937, 951
Cyclosporine, 991
Cystic lesions, 887
  colobomatous cysts
    clinical pearls, 895, 896
    clinical presentation, 896
    CT scan, 896
    histopathology, 896
    MRI, 896
    prognosis, 896
    treatment, 896
  dermoid cyst
    clinical pearls, 889
    clinical presentation, 889
    computed tomography, 889, 890
    of conjunctival origin, 890, 891
    histopathology, 890
    magnetic resonance imaging, 890
    prognosis, 890
    treatment, 890
  epithelial cysts
    clinical pearls, 892
    clinical presentation, 892
    computed tomography, 892
    histopathology, 893
    magnetic resonance imaging, 892
    prognosis, 893
    treatment, 893
  mucocele and mucopyocele
    clinical pearls, 894
    clinical presentation, 894
    computed tomography, 895
    histopathology, 895
    MRI, 895
    prognosis, 895
    treatment, 895
  respiratory epithelial cyst
    clinical pearls, 893
    clinical presentation, 893
    computed tomography, 893, 894
    histopathology, 894
    magnetic resonance imaging, 894
    prognosis, 894
    treatment, 894
Cytogenetics, periocular tissues, 700
Cytologic techniques, periocular tissues, 699

D

Dacarbazine, 908
Dacryoadenitis, 641, 722, 758, 887
Dacryocystectomy, 501
Dacryocystitis, 516, 517, 530, 532, 535, 593, 606, 640
Dacryocystoceles, 534
Dacryocystography, 524, 551, 556, 595
Dacryocystorhinostomy (DCR), 95, 114, 443, 489, 551, 571
Dacryoliths, 533, 534, 539, 540
Dacryops, 736
Dacryoscintigraphy/dacryoscintillography, 553, 595
Dacryostenosis, 516, 538, 539
Dantrolene, 1194
Dark circles, 335
Deep superior sulcus, 1062–1064, 1066, 1067
Deferoxamine, 682
Delayed tear clearance, 523
Delleman syndrome, *see* Oculo-Cerebro-cutaneous syndrome
Demyelinating disease, 630, 631
de novo/sporadic mutations, 1116
Dental occlusion, 1277
Dentoalveolar fractures, 1277
Depressor anguli oris, 366
Deprivation amblyopia, 1104
Dermal collagen, 1203
Dermal fillers, 369
  biosynthetic polymers, 374–376
  collagen, 372
  complications, 376, 377
  history, 368
  hyaluronic acid, 372–374
  products, 371
  technique, 370, 371
  treatment areas
    lower face, 370
    midface, 369, 370
    upper face, 368, 369
Dermatitis, 485
Dermatochalasis, 189, 244
Dermis fat grafts (DFG), 1015, 1050, 1074, 1089, 1090
Dermoid cysts, 885, 889–891
  clinical pearls, 889
  clinical presentation, 889
  computed tomography, 889, 890
  of conjunctival origin
    clinical pearls, 890, 891
    clinical presentation, 891
    computed tomography, 891
    histopathology, 891
    magnetic resonance imaging, 891
    prognosis, 891
    treatment, 891
  histopathology, 890
  magnetic resonance imaging, 890
  prognosis, 890
  treatment, 890
Dermolipoma, 838, 888, 927, 928
  See also Lipodermoids
Desmarres lid retractor, 67, 1176, 1239
Dexamethasone, 1198
Diabetic ketoacidosis (DKA), 683
Diclofenac, 1198
Diffuse canalicular occlusion, 596
Diffuse large B-cell lymphoma (DLBCL), 773, 781, 783
Digital subtraction contrast dacryocystogram, 550
Dilated tortuous episcleral vessels, 885
Dimenhydrinate, 1197
Diplopia, 414, 417, 884, 894, 905, 929, 1233, 1235, 1263, 1267, 1268, 1285
Direct external ethmoidectomy, 1002
Distichiasis-lymphedema-cleft palate syndrome, *see* Lymphedema-distichiasis (LD) syndrome
Distichiasis syndromes, 189, 540, 1124
Diverticuli, 549
Divinyl sulfone (DVS), 372
DNA-binding fluorescent dyes, 700

Docetaxel, 488, 541, 951
Dog and human bites, 1217, 1219
Dorsal midbrain syndrome, 125
Double diplopia, 1233
Double elevator palsy, 280
Down syndrome, 522, 1138, 1154
Doxorubicin, 908, 937, 951, 961
Doxycycline, 1166
Draping, 105
Droperidol, 1197
Dry eye syndrome (DES), 486, 505–507
  blepharoplasty, 411
  good history taking, 507
  oculoplastic approach, 511
  patient medical and dietary history, 507
  patient medication list, 507
  physical examination, 507, 508
  treatment, 508–511
Duane retraction syndrome (DRS), 250, 1123, 1125
Dye disappearance test (DDT), 514, 515, 547, 1105
Dynamic vascular imaging, 618
Dyskeratosis congenita, 1139
Dysplasia, 907
Dysport, 360, 362
Dystopia canthorum, 1152

E

Earlobe deformity, 395
Eaton-Lambert Syndrome, 361
EBV-associated lymphoproliferative disease, 774
Ecchymosis, 417
Ectropion, 414, 415, 1125
Edrophonium (Tensilon) testing, 264
Eisler's pocket, 30
Electromagnetic (EM) based stereotaxy, 872, 873
Electromagnetic navigated surgery, 871
Electron microscopy, periocular tissues, 699
Embryonal rhabdomyosarcoma, 932
Embryonal tumors, 931
Empiric antibiotic therapy, 1166, 1167
Encephalocele, 1129
Encephalocraniocutaneous lipomatosis (ECCL), 1127, 1128, 1154
Endocanalicular laser dacryocystorhinostomy (ELADCR), 589
Endonasal endoscopic orbital decompression (medial wall and floor), 1011, 1012
Endonasal surgery, 1002
Endophytic lesions, 889
Endoscopic-assisted endonasal approaches, 598
Endoscopic conjunctivodacryocystorhinostomy
  advantages of, 578
  complications, postoperative evaluation and management of, 581, 582
  Gladstone–Putterman Modified Jones Tube, 577
  indications, 578
  postoperative care, 580, 581
  preoperative evaluation, 577
  surgical technique, 578–580
Endoscopic orbital surgery, 713
Endotine™ forehead fixation device, 356
Enophthalmos, 245, 246, 491, 607, 1062–1064, 1066, 1067, 1263, 1265
  anatomy, 1285
  clinical evaluation, 1288
  computed tomography imaging, 1288
  floor, 1288
  fronto-zygomatic suture, 1287
  intervention timing, 1288
  lateral orbital wall fractures, 1286, 1287, 1289
  medial orbital wall fractures, 1286, 1288
  orbital floor, 1286
  orbital roof, 1287
  pathophysiology, 1285, 1286
  predictors of, 1289, 1290
  surgical technique
    complications, 1297
    conjunctival incision, 1291
    masqueraders, 1297
    medial orbital wall, 1293, 1295, 1296
    non-porous materials, 1291
    orbital floor, 1293
    patient-specific implant, 1292
    porous materials, 1290
    pre-formed implants, 1291
    principles, 1291, 1293
    3D imaging, 1295–1297
  traumatic orbital wall displacement, 1286
Enucleation, 1029, 1065
  vs. evisceration, 1042
  historical perspective, 1029–1032
  indications for, 1041
  postoperative care, 1048–1050
  preoperative preparation for, 1040, 1041
  socket volume considerations, 1037, 1038
  surgical technique, 1042–1045
Enzyme immunohistochemistry, 700
Eosinophilic granuloma, 645
Ephelides, 399
Epiblepharon, 181, 182, 189, 1125, 1159
Epibulbar choristomas, 1127, 1149
Epicanthus inversus, 1126
Epicanthus palpebralis, 1126
Epicanthus supraciliaris, 1126
Epicanthus tarsalis, 1126
Epidermal growth factor (EGF), 1202, 1204
Epidermal nevus syndrome (ENS), 1127
Epidermoid, 645
Epinephrine, 541, 1197
Epiphora, 488, 489, 514, 521, 535, 536, 555, 1105
Epirubicin, 951
Epithelial cysts, 892–894
  clinical pearls, 892
  clinical presentation, 892
  computed tomography, 892
  histopathology, 893
  magnetic resonance imaging, 892
  prognosis, 893
  treatment, 893
Epithelial membrane antigen (EMA), 919
Epithelial suture tunnels, 413
Epithelial tumors, 498, 499
Epstein-Barr virus (EBV), 958, 959
Equilibrium phase, 1056
Erythrocyte sedimentation rate, 609
Erythromycin, 511
Eschar, 682
Ethmoidectomy, 568
Ethmoid sinuses, 8, 9, 12
Etoposide, 937
European Group on Graves' Orbitopathy (EUGOGO) classification, 987
Euryblepharon, 1125, 1147, 1154, 1155

Eutetic Mixture of Local Anesthetic (EMLA), 370, 1196
Evisceration, 1029, 1039, 1046
vs. enucleation, 1042
historical perspective, 1029–1032
indications for, 1041, 1042
with keratectomy, 1046
with porous orbital implant, 1030
postoperative care, 1048–1050
preoperative preparation for, 1040, 1041
socket volume considerations, 1037, 1038
surgical technique (with keratectomy), 1044–1047
Evolence, 372
Ewing sarcoma (ES), 845, 846, 936, 937
clinical pearls, 936
clinical presentation, 936
computed tomography, 936
histopathology, 936, 937
magnetic resonance imaging, 936
prognosis, 937
treatment, 937
Excisional biopsy, periocular tissues, 689, 690, 707
Exophthalmometry, 302, 607, 1288
Exposure keratopathy, blepharoplasty, 411
External beam radiotherapy, 944
Extranodal marginal zone B-cell lymphoma (EMZL), 779, 780
Extraocular dysfunction, 1105
Extraocular motility, 608
Extraocular muscle, 619, 620, 1285, 1288, 1291
metastasis, 654
surgery, 1012
Eyelid adnexal reconstruction, 439
eyelid defects, 440, 441
frozen-section histopathologic examination/Mohs surgery, 439
lateral canthal defects, 454
lower eyelid defects, 443–445
medial canthal defects, 454, 455, 457, 458
moderate defects, 443
principles, 439, 440
small defects, 441–443
upper eyelid margin
large defects involving, 449, 450, 452, 454
moderate defects involving, 445, 447, 449
small defects, 445
Eyelid ectropion
anterior lamellar shortening, 196, 197, 1156
clinical presentation, 195
distraction test, 196
etiology, 195
eyelid margin, 196
eyelid puncta, 196
lateral canthus evaluation, 197
medial canthus evaluation, 197
orbicularis oculi muscle tone, 197
physical examination, 196
posterior eyelid inspection, 197
snap back test, 196
treatment, 198
anterior lamellar skin graft, 202, 203
cicatricial ectropion, 202
congenital ectropion, 202
involutional ectropion, 197
lateral tarsal strip, 197–199
lazy-T procedure, 200, 201
mechanical ectropion, 202
medial spindle with rotational suture, 198–200
mixed mechanism ectropion, 203
paralytic ectropion, 202
retractor advancement, 200
skin flaps, 202
upper eyelid ectropion, 203
Eyelid laceration, 1316
Eyelid malpositions, 1061–1064
Eyelid margin lacerations, 446, 1212, 1213
Eyelid neoplasms
BCC, 423
clinical presentation, 424
management, 425
pathologic features, 423, 424
clinical presentation, 425
lymphoma, 432
malignant melanoma, 429
clinical presentation, 429, 430
management, 430, 431
pathologic features, 429
Merkel cell carcinoma, 431
metastatic lesions, 432
pathologic features, 424
SCC, 425
clinical presentation, 426
management, 426, 427
pathologic features, 425, 426
sebaceous carcinoma, 427
clinical presentation, 428
management, 428, 429
pathologic features, 427, 428
vascular tumors, 431
Eyelid repair and reconstruction, 87–91
Eyelid retraction, 414, 415, 605, 1001, 1156–1158
Eyelid-sparing exenteration, 862, 863
Eyelid surgery
etiology of eyelid changes in TED, 1013, 1014
lower eyelid retraction repair, 1014, 1015
post-operative considerations, 1022, 1023
spacer graft materials, 1015, 1022
acellular dermis, 1019, 1020
alloplastic material, 1021
autologous auricular cartilage, 1015–1017
banked sclera, 1022
free tarsal grafts, 1021
hard palate mucosa, 1016, 1019, 1020
upper eyelid recession, 1014
anterior approach (full thickness blepharotomy), 1014
posterior approach, 1014
Eyelid swelling, 417
Eyelid tumors, 1108
benign eyelid tumors, 1108
malignant eyelid tumors, 1108
SLNB, 478

F

Facelift, 391
anatomy
facial nerve, 392
greater auricular nerve, 392
platysma, 391, 392
SMAS, 391
complications
alopecia, 394, 395
earlobe deformity, 395
hematoma, 394
infection, 394

midface, rejuvenation of, 395
nerve injury, 394
scars, 394
patient evaluation, 392
surgical techniques
skin excision, 392
sub-SMAS rhytidectomy, 392–394
Facial aging, 359, 378
Facial angiofibromas of tuberous sclerosis, 1140
Facial burns, 412
Facial buttress, 4
Facial clefts, nasolacrimal duct obstruction, 518
Facial fractures, 1165
Facial gunshot wound, 1313
Facial infections, 680
Facial muscles, 361
Facial palsy
aberrant regeneration, 214, 215
anatomy, 205–207
Bell's palsy, 208
browlift, 213
clinical presentation, 208
clinical syndromes, 205, 208
corneal neurotization, 216
ectropion repair, 210–212
facial suspension, 213–215
gold weight implantation, 212, 213
medical therapy, 209, 210
nerve grafting, 214
physical examination, 208
rehabilitation, 205
tarsorrhaphy, 210
lateral, 210, 211
medial, 210, 211
Facial rejuvenation, 359
Facial rhytids, 359
Failed dacryocystorhinostomy
balloon dilatation, 596
causes of, 593
clinical evaluation and diagnostic testing, 594, 595
computed tomography, 595
endoscopic-assisted endonasal and transcanalicular approaches, 598
external approach via skin incision, 597, 598
management, 595, 596
medical conditions, 594
mitomycin C, 598
MRI, 595
prolonged postoperative silicone stent placement, 594
repeat dacryocystorhinostomy, 596
silicone intubation, 599
surgical success in, 593
tearing, cause of, 594
Farnsworth D-15 panel test, 609
Farnsworth–Munsell 100-hue test, 609
Fasanella Servat operation (FSO), 93, 318–320, 1107
Fat harvesting technique, 379
Fat isolation techniques, 381
Fat transfer, 378, 380, 382, 383
complications, 383, 385
history and rationale, 378
post-operative evaluations, 383
pre-operative exam, 379
procedural technique, 379, 380
FCI aluminum oxide (Bioceramic) implant, 1034
FCI synthetic hydroxyapatite implant, 1033
Fetal alcohol syndrome, 1117
Fibroblastic meningioma, 912
Fibro-osseous lesions, 643, 645
Fibrosarcoma
clinical pearls, 919
clinical presentation, 920
computed tomography, 920
histopathology, 920
magnetic resonance imaging, 920
prognosis, 920
treatment, 920
Fibrous dysplasia (FD), 844, 845, 938
clinical pearls, 937
clinical presentation, 937, 938
computed tomography, 938
histopathology, 938
magnetic resonance imaging, 938
prognosis, 939
treatment, 939
Fibrous histiocytoma
clinical pearls, 920
clinical presentation, 920, 921
computed tomography, 921
histopathology, 921
magnetic resonance imaging, 921
prognosis, 922
treatment, 922
Filtering, 380
Fine-needle aspiration, 699, 706, 707
Fire/facial burns, 412, 416
Fistula, 1308
Fitzpatrick phototype scale, 333
5-fluorouracil, 488, 541, 961
Floppy eyelid syndrome (FES), 251, 252
Flow cytometry, periocular tissues, 700
Fluorescein appearance test, 548
Fluorouracil, 951
Foam rubber bolster, 455
Focal dermal hypoplasia, *see* Goltz syndrome
Focal dystonias, 247
Focal trichiasis, 189
Follicular lymphoma (FL), 780
Forearm flap, 1080
Forehead flaps, 453
Forehead/brow ptosis
anatomic considerations, 352
clinical evaluation, 351, 352
coronal forehead lift, 354
direct and temporal direct brow lift, 353
endoscopic forehead lift, 354, 356, 357
medical management, 352, 353
midforehead lift, 353
pretrichial forehead lift, 354
surgical management, 353
transblepharoplasty brow lift, 354
FOXL2 gene, 1136
Fractional lasers, 401
Fractured orbital floor, 1239
Frame-based stereotaxy, 871
Franceschetti syndrome, *see* Treacher Collins syndrome (TCS)
Fraser syndrome, 1122, 1123, 1145, 1146
Freeman Sheldon syndrome, 1136
Freer elevator, 572
Free tarsal grafts, 1021
Freign bodies, 540
French-Canadian ancestry, 298

Frey's syndrome, 360
Frontal bone, 618
Frontal branch, 620
Frontalis muscle, 363
Frontalis sling surgery, 113
Frontalis suspension surgery, 310–312
Frontal sinus, 12
Frontoethmoidal-vomerine buttress, 1272
Frontoethmoid suture line, 1231
Frontonasal dysplasias (FNDs), 1129–1131
Frontozygomatic craniotomy, 717
Frontozygomatic suture, 1232, 1233, 1263, 1266, 1268, 1280
Frozen sections, periocular tissues, 691, 692
Full thickness blepharotomy, 1014
Full thickness burn, 1224
Fungal granulomas, 684
Fungal orbital cellulitis, 749
  aspergillosis, 749, 750
  mucormycosis, 750
Fusiform schwannoma, 915

G
Gadolinium, 886, 890, 906, 931, 933, 938, 946
Gastrointestinal mucormycosis, 682
Gaze-evoked amaurosis, 1309
Gelfim implant, 1258
Gelfoam®, 597
Gene structure, 1115
Genetic anticipation, 1138
Genetic testing, 1117
Gene translocations, 700
Gentian violet mark, 1049
Genzyme, 373
Giant cell reparative granulomas, 939
  clinical pearls, 939
  clinical presentation, 939
  computed tomography, 939
  histopathology, 940
  magnetic resonance imaging, 940
  prognosis, 940
  treatment, 940
Giant papillary conjunctivitis (GPC), 1059
Gillies approach, 1267, 1268
Glabella, 363, 377
Gladstone–Putterman modified Jones tube, 577
Glasgow Coma Score (GCS), 165
Glial fibrillary acidic protein (GFAP), 910
Glioma, 909
Globe ptosis, 42
Glogau photoaging classification, 333
Glycosaminoglycans (GAGs), 985
Goldenhar syndrome, 1123, 1127, 1148, 1149
Goldmann kinetic perimetry, 609
Goldmann's equation, 675
Goltz syndrome, 1119
Gomori trichrome, 1137
Gonioscopy, 675
Gorlin-Goltz syndrome, 1120
Gradenigo's syndrome, 56, 120
Granulation tissue, 1203, 1216
Granuloma annulare, 755
Granuloma formation, 377
Granulomatosis with polyangiitis (GPA), 835
Granulomatous diseases, 534
Graves' disease (GD), 636, 645–647, 834, 884, 886, 984, 985, 987–990
  radioactive iodine, 988, 989
  surgical thyroidectomy, 989, 990
  thioamide drugs, 988
Graves' ophthalmopathy, 486
Graves' orbitopathy, 725, 885
Greater auricular nerve, 392
Gross lacrimal function, 545
Guibor and Jackson stents, 586
Guillain–Barré syndrome (GBS), 208, 255, 300
Gummy smile, 366
Gunshot wounds, 1219–1221
Gustatory tearing, 208

H
Hair loss, 394
Hamartomas, 837, 1128, 1129
Handheld mirror, 409
Hard palate mucosa, 1016, 1019, 1020
Hard palate mucosal grafting, 1018, 1019
Harlequin ichthyosis (HI), 1124
Hasner's membrane, 545
Hasner's valves, 556
Hay-Wells syndrome, 1138
Headache, 368
Head and neck cancer, ablative surgery in, 490, 491
Hemangioma, 884
Hemangiopericytoma (HPC), 738, 825, 827, 887
Hemifacial spasm (HFS), 250
  clinical presentation, 226
  diagnosis, 226
  etiologic factors, 226
  incidence rate, 226
  medical therapy, 227
  surgical treatment, 227
Hemorrhage, blepharoplasty, 412, 416, 630
Hemosiderin-laden macrophages, 935
Hering's law, 245, 246
Herniated orbital fat, 738
Herpes zoster virus (HZV), 377, 684
Herrick plugs, 539
Herring's law effects, 303
Hertel exophthalmometers, 919, 1109, 1288
Heteroplasmy, 1117
Histiocytic tumors, 846, 847
Histiocytosis, 645, 649
Horizontal buttresses, 1272
Horizontal forehead rhytids, 363
Horner–Duverney lacrimal muscle, 13, 21
Horner syndrome (HS), 127, 266–272, 299, 300, 620, 907, 1106
Hotz's procedure, 1159
House–Brackmann scale, 208, 209
Hughes tarsoconjunctival flap, 440, 485
Human diploid cell vaccine (HDCV), 1219
Human genome, 1115
Human immunodeficiency virus (HIV), 1219
Human rabies immune globulin (HRIG), 1219
Hyaluronic acid fillers, 368, 369, 372–374
Hyaluronidase, 374
Hybridization techniques, 700
Hydraulic theory, 1239, 1240
Hydrogels, 1090
Hydrophilic expanders, 1088
Hydroxyapatite implants, 1032, 1033

Hydroxyproline, 1204
Hylacross technology, 373
Hylaform, 373
Hyperbaric oxygen, 684
Hyperglobus, 1256
Hyperlacrimation, 594
Hyperostotic meningioma, 938
Hypersecretion syndrome, 556
Hypertelorism, 1126
Hyperthyroidism, 883
Hypertrophic scars, 1205
Hypoglobus, 491
Hypointense melanoma, 953
Hypophysitis, parasellar syndromes, 679
Hypothetico-deductive model, 121
Hypoxia, 986
Hypoxia-inducible factor-1 (HIF-1)-dependent pathways, 986

I

Iatrogenic obstruction, 538, 539
Iatrogenic ptosis, 363
Ibuprofen, 1198
Ichthyosis (collodion baby), 1124
Idiopathic canalicular inflammatory disease (ICID), 533
Idiopathic inflammatory pseudotumor, *see* Idiopathic orbital inflammation (IOI)
Idiopathic optic neuritis, 633
Idiopathic orbital inflammatory disease (IOID), 636, 644, 723, 724, 770
- clinical features, 755, 756
- treatment, 756, 757

Idiopathic orbital myositis, 644
Idiopathic perineuritis, 636
Idiopathic posterior scleritis, 759
Ifosfamide, 937
IgG4 disease, 610
Image guided orbital surgery, 871, 874
- stereotactic surgery, 873, 874
  - basic technique, 874
  - EM-based stereotaxy, 873
  - history of, 872
  - Kick EM navigation system, 873
- stereotaxy
  - benefits of, 874, 876
  - in orbital surgery, 872, 873
  - science of, 871, 872

Imatinib mesylate, 490
Immunosuppressants, DES, 510
Impaired tear outflow, 522
Implants
- classification and terminology, 1036
- exposure and extrusion, 1068, 1069
- infection, 1068–1070
- migration, 1068
- pegging, complications of, 1070
- sampling of, 1031
- selection in adults and children, 1036, 1037

Impression-fitted custom prosthesis, 1050
Incisional biopsy, 707
Incisional microabscesses, 413
Infantile and juvenile fibrosarcomas, 920
Infantile hemangiomas (IH)/infantile capillary hemangioma, 658, 659, 825–827
Infectious orbital disease, 832
Inferior left globe displacement, 608
Inferior oblique muscle, 417, 620, 642
Inferior petrosal sinuses, 668, 674, 676
Inferior punctal atresia, 516
Inferior rectus, 642
Inferior turbinate, 514, 584
Infiltrative (morpheaform) basal cell carcinoma, 424
Inflammatory bowel disease (IBD), 836
Inflammatory lesions, 887
Infliximab, 991
Infraorbital dark circles, 402
Infraorbital hollow, 369
Injectable anesthetics, 1196, 1197
Inner canthal distance (ICD), 1126
Inorganic IOrbFBs, 1311
Insulin-like growth factor-1 receptor (IGF-1R), 985
Intense pulsed light, 398, 399, 403
Intergroup Rhabdomyosarcoma Study (IGRS), 932
Interleukin-1 (IL-1), 1201, 1202, 1204
Intermittent proptosis, 885
Internal carotid artery (ICA), 667, 670, 673
Internal punctum, 521
International Consensus Statement on Mucous Membrane Pemphigoid, 231
International prognostic index (IPI), 807
Internuclear ophthalmoplegia (INO), 124, 125
Interorbital distance (IOD), 1126
Interpupillary distance (IPD), 1126
Intra-arterial cytoreductive chemotherapy (IACC), 733
Intracanalicular plugs, 538, 539, 560
Intracranial abscesses, 635
Intracranial orbital relationships
- carotid and intracranial ophthalmic arteries, 56, 57
- cavernous sinus, 53–55
- cranial nerves, 55–57
- dura matter, 53
- optic chiasm, 57
- pertinent intracranial osteology, 53, 54

Intralesional sclerosing therapy, 901
Intraocular masses
- choroidal hemangiomas, 628
- ocular calcification, 629
- ocular inflammation, 629, 630
- ocular melanoma, 626, 628
- retinal angiomas, 628
- retinoblastoma, 626
- trauma, 630

Intraocular pressure, 609
Intraocular tumor–related orbital inflammation, 762
Intraorbital antifungal therapy, 859
Intraorbital foreign bodies (IOrbFBs) and penetrating orbital injuries, 852
- classification, 1302
- clinical assessment, 1302, 1304
- computed tomography imaging, 1302, 1304–1306
- history, 1301
- prevention, 1301, 1302
- retained IOrbFBs, 1306–1309
- suspected metallic IOrbFBs, 1304–1306
- treatment, 1310, 1311

Intraorbital steroid injections, 991
Intravascular thrombosis, 899
Intravenous immunoglobulin therapy (IVIg), 236
Intrinsic canalicular tumors, 528

Intrinsic inflammation
infectious lesions
bacterial, 722
fungal, 722
viral, 722
noninfectious lesions
Graves' orbitopathy, 725
idiopathic orbital inflammatory disease, 723, 724
sarcoidosis, 725
Sjogren's syndrome, 724
systemic lupus erythematosus, 725
Wegener's granulomatosis, 725
Intubation, 1278, 1279
Invasive squamous cell carcinoma, 469, 484
Inverted papillomas, 528, 537, 957
clinical pearls, 957
clinical presentation, 957
computed tomography, 957
histopathology, 958
magnetic resonance imaging, 958
prognosis, 958
treatment, 958
Involutional entropion, 182
causes, 181
lower eyelid laxity, 181
therapeutic procedure, 182
treatment, 182, 183
Iridium brachytherapy, 542
Ischemic optic neuropathy, 150
Isolated coloboma, 1147, 1148, 1150
Isolated congenital lower eyelid retraction, 1158
Isolated congenital ptosis, 1133
Isolated euryblepharon, 1154
Ivory osteoma, 943

J
Jackson's burn wound model, 1223, 1224
Johanson-Blizzard syndrome (JBS), 1139
Jones dilator, 573
Juvederm Ultra Plus, 373
Juvenile xanthogranuloma (JXG), 922
clinical pearls, 922
clinical presentation, 922
computed tomography, 922
histopathology, 923
magnetic resonance imaging, 922, 923
prognosis, 923
treatment, 923

K
Kabuki syndrome, 1125
Kabuki syndrome-1 (KABUK1), 1125
Kaposi sarcoma, 431, 1108
Kearns-Sayre syndrome (KSS), 135, 136, 255, 1137
Keloid keratinocytes, 1205
Keloid scars, 1205
Keratoacanthoma, 469
Keratoconjunctivitis sicca, 724
Keratome, 572
Keratoplasty, 1122
Kerrison bone rongeur, 567, 573, 579, 597
Ketamine, 1195
Kimura's disease (KD), 737, 761, 762
Kollner–Hughes procedure, 89
Kronlein lateral orbitotomy approach, 99
Kuhnt-Szymanowski procedure, 200

L
LacriCath® STENTube, 596
Lacrilube, 1225
Lacrimal bone, 567, 568
Lacrimal drainage apparatus, 486, 545
Lacrimal drainage-associated lymphoid tissue (LDALT), 773
Lacrimal endoscopes, 522
Lacrimal excretory osteology, 12–17
Lacrimal excretory outflow system, 522
Lacrimal fossa, 567
Lacrimal gland disease
acute presentation, 721
amyloidosis, 737
benign and malignant lymphoid lesions, 726
benign tumors
myoepithelioma, 730
oncocytoma, 730
pleomorphic adenoma, 727–730
blepharoplasty, 412
cavernous hemangiomas, 738
chronic presentation, 722
congenital dermoid cysts, 736, 737
dacryops, 736
hemangiopericytoma, 738
herniated orbital fat, 738
intrinsic inflammation (*see* Intrinsic inflammation)
Kimura's disease, 737
lymphoproliferative disorders
anatomic and immunologic studies, 725–726
atypical lymphoid hyperplasia, 726
C psittaci-positive marginal-zone B-cell lymphoma, 727
complete systemic evaluation, 727
management of, 727
mucosal-associated lymphoid tissue, 727
ocular adnexal MALT lymphoma, 727
orbital lymphoid tumors, 726
primary intraocular lymphomas, 726
primary ocular adnexal lymphoma, 726
radiation therapy, 727
rituximab, 727
systemic lymphoma, 727
malignant tumors
acinic cell carcinoma, 735, 736
adenoid cystic carcinoma, 730–734
carcinosarcoma, 736
malignant myoepithelial carcinoma, 736
mucoepidermoid carcinoma, 735
pleomorphic adenocarcinoma, 735
primary adenocarcinoma, 734, 735
squamous cell carcinoma, 736
management protocols, 722
neoplastic and inflammatory diseases, 721
solitary fibrous tumors, 737, 738
subacute presentation, 721
Warthin's tumor, 737
Lacrimal gland lesions, 888
Lacrimal gland neoplasms, 646
Lacrimal gland tumors, 847, 884
adenocarcinoma
clinical pearls, 944, 945
clinical presentation, 945
computed tomography, 945
histopathology, 945
magnetic resonance imaging, 945
prognosis, 945
treatment, 945

adenoid cystic carcinoma, 847
clinical pearls, 945, 946
clinical presentation, 946
computed tomography, 946
histopathology, 946, 947
magnetic resonance imaging, 946
prognosis, 947
treatment, 947
mucoepidermoid carcinomas
clinical pearls, 947
clinical presentation, 947, 948
computed tomography, 948
histopathology, 948
magnetic resonance imaging, 948
prognosis, 948
treatment, 948
pleomorphic adenomas
clinical pearls, 948, 949
clinical presentation, 949
computed tomography, 949
histopathology, 949
magnetic resonance imaging, 949
prognosis, 950
treatment, 949, 950
Lacrimal irrigation, 594
Lacrimal pump, 29, 523
Lacrimal pump failure, 578
Lacrimal sac, 528, 529, 554
flaps, 574
incision of, 574
tenting of, 573
Lacrimal sac tumors, 497
classification of, 499
clinical features, 497
diagnostic evaluation, 498
management, 500
pathology, 498, 500
prognosis, 502
Lacrimal secretors, 14, 16, 18, 19
Lacrimal surgery, 95, 96
Lacrimal system, 1225, 1230
cancer therapy, 486
congenital secretory anomalies
congenital alacrimia, 1138
nasolacrimal system anomalies, 1138, 1139
NF1, 1139
Sturge-Weber syndrome, 1140, 1141
tuberous sclerosis, 1139, 1140
orbital radiology, 621
Lacrimal system obstructions, 521, 545
canaliculus, 528
chemiluminescence, 554
clinical diagnosis, 545
clinical history, 545, 546
congenital etiology of, 515
dacryoliths, 539, 540
diagnostic imaging techniques
computed tomography, 551, 552
contrast dacryocystography, 550, 551
diagnostic ultrasonography, 549, 550
magnetic resonance dacryocystography, 552
radionuclide dacryoscintigraphy, 552, 553
diagnostic tests, 554–556
duct, 529, 530
dye disappearance test, 547
etiological causes
canaliculitis, 532, 533
dacryoliths, 533, 534
endogenous origin, 534, 535
exogenous factors, 535
fractures, 537, 538
iatrogenic obstruction, 538, 539
infectious, 531, 532
inflammation, 534
traumatic injury, 537
tumors (neoplastic), 535–537
examination, 522, 523, 546
history, 521, 522
imaging studies, 524
lacrimal pump, 523
lacrimal sac, 528, 529
mechanical compression, 539
medications, 540, 541
nasolacrimal duct, nasal portion obstruction, 530
nasolacrimal endoscopy, 554
percutaneous contrast dacryocystography, 553, 554
primary jones dye test, 547, 548
probing, 548
radiation, 541, 542
Rose Bengal staining, 547
Schirmer tests, 546, 547
secondary jones dye test, 548
stenosis/occlusion, location of, 524, 527
tear break-up time, 547
thermography, 554
Lacrimal trauma, 560
Lacrimo-auriculo-dento-digital syndrome (LADD), 1138
Lacripen, 508
Lactate dehydrogenase (LDH), 804, 806, 807
LactoSorb, 1235
Lagophthalmos, 411, 412, 1125, 1226
Lambert–Eaton myasthenic syndrome (LEMS), 133
Lamellar ichthyosis, 1125, 1156
Lamina papyracea, 1231, 1232, 1234
Lamina propria, 528
Langerhans' cell histiocytosis (LCH), 760, 761, 1108
Large defects, upper eyelid margin, 449, 450, 452, 454
Large upper eyelid coloboma, 1149
Laser fiber optic probe, 589
Laser probe, intranasal visualization of, 590
Lasers
definition, 397
developement, 397
electromagnetic spectrum, 397
infraorbital dark circles, 402
periorbital skin
adnexal structures, 403, 404
CVM, 398
defective venous morphogenesis, 398
hemangiomas, 398
periorbital photodamage and rejuvenation, 401, 402
pigmented concerns, 399–401
pulsed dye laser, 398
purpura, 399
safety and complications, 404, 405
selective photothermolysis, 397
skin resurfacing, 117
spontaneous emission, 397
thermal relaxation time, 398
xanthelasma, 402, 403

Lashes, nasolacrimal duct obstruction, 515
Lash ptosis, 189
Lateral canthal injuries, 1209, 1210
Lateral canthal rhytids, 364, 367
Lateral canthal tendon, 442
Lateral canthotomy, 1264, 1265, 1268, 1280
Lateral canthus
  blepharocheilodontic syndrome, 1154, 1155
  euryblepharon, 1154, 1155
  Tessier's cleft number 8, 1153, 1154
  Treacher Collins syndrome, 1153
Laterality, 885
Lateral nasal mucosa, 572
Lateral nasal wall, 590
Lateral orbital decompression, 1006
Lateral orbital wall, 1233
Lateral orbitotomy, 711–713, 899
Lateral periocular defect, 440
Lateral tarsorrhaphy, 210, 211
Lateral wall decompression, 1005–1009
Lateral wall fractures, 851, 852
Lazy-T procedure, 200, 564
Le Fort fractures
  anatomy, 1271
  complications, 1283
  computed tomography, 1278
  craniofacial dysjunction, 1277
  extraskeletal fixation, 1278
  fractured pterygoid plates, 1272, 1274
  history, 1271
  horizontal buttresses, 1272, 1273
  intact pterygoid plates, 1272, 1273
  intubation, 1278, 1279
  magnetic resonance imaging, 1278
  malocclusion, 1277, 1278
  maxillomandibular fixation, 1278, 1279
  panfacial trauma, 1281
  patient's history, 1276, 1277
  plating systems, 1279
  postoperative management, 1283
  surgical treatment, 1278
    brow incision, 1280
    coronal incision, 1280, 1281
    sublabial incision, 1279–1281
    supramarginal incision, 1280
    transconjunctival incision, 1280
    upper lid incision approach, 1280
  type I, 1273, 1274, 1281
  type II, 1273, 1275, 1281
  type III, 1273–1276, 1281, 1282
  vertical buttresses, 1271, 1272
Leber congenital amaurosis, 1118
Left orbital lipoma, 928
Left Tessier's cleft # 5, 1151
Leiomyosarcomas, 924
  clinical pearls, 923
  clinical presentation, 923
  computed tomography, 924
  histopathology, 924
  magnetic resonance imaging, 924
  prognosis, 925
  treatment, 924, 925
Lentigines, 399
Lentigo maligna of lower eyelid, 430
Lenz microphthalmia syndrome (LMS), 1119
Leptomeningeal angiomatosis, *see* Sturge-Weber Syndrome (SWS)
Leudde exophthalmometer, 1109
Leukemia, orbital, 647
Leukemic neoplasia, 848, 849
Leukocoria, orbital radiology, 623
Levator aponeurosis surgery, 313–316, 318
Levator muscle aponeurosis, 1146
Levy-Hollister syndrome, *see* Lacrimo-auriculo-dento-digital syndrome (LADD)
Lichen planus, 535
Lid/crease asymmetry, 410
Lid hygiene, 509
Lid lacerations, 1316
Lid malpositions
  ectropion, 94
  entropion, 94–95
  full-thickness eyelid incision, 94
  lateral canthal suspension, 94
  surgical approaches, 92
Lid retractor system, 620
Lidocaine, 361, 565, 1194, 1196
Light cautery, 597
Limbal stem cell deficiency, 1223
Linear threading technique, 371
Lipiflow, 509
Lipoblastomas
  clinical pearls, 925
  clinical presentation, 925
  computed tomography, 925
  histopathology, 926
  magnetic resonance imaging, 925
  prognosis, 926
  treatment, 926
Lipodermoids
  clinical pearls, 927
  clinical presentation, 927
  computed tomography, 927
  histopathology, 927, 928
  of lacrimal gland, 648
  magnetic resonance imaging, 927
  prognosis, 928
  treatment, 928
Lipomas, 645
  clinical pearls, 928
  clinical presentation, 928
  computed tomography, 928
  histopathology, 929
  magnetic resonance imaging, 928, 929
  prognosis, 929
  treatment, 929
Liposarcomas
  clinical pearls, 929
  clinical presentation, 929
  computed tomography, 929
  histopathology, 930
  magnetic resonance imaging, 930
  prognosis, 930
  treatment, 930
Lipstick lines, 366
Liquid silicone, 376
Local tarsoconjunctival flap, 1048
Localized orbital melanomas, 954
Locally aggressive tumors, 922
Lockwood's ligament, 42, 1233
Loeys-Dietz syndrome, 1132
Lower eyelid blepharoplasty
  aftercare and recovery, 340
  aging, 333
  anesthesia, 336

canthoplasty/canthopexy, 339
complications of, 414
description, 333
eyelid skin resurfacing, 339
fat grafting, 339, 340
Frank ectropion, 415
injectable fillers, 340
lower eyelid aging, 334
lower eyelid fat modification, 336–338
orbicularis suspension, 338, 339
physical examination, 333, 335, 336
skin excision, 338
Lower eyelid colobomas, 1123, 1150
Lower eyelid defects, 443–445
Lower eyelid laxity, 1061
Lower eyelid, nodular melanoma of, 430
Lower eyelid retractors, 563
Lower lid ectropion, 535
Lower lid epiblepharon, 1159
Lower system obstructions
amniotocele and dacryocystitis, 516
anatomical variation causing, 516, 517
dacryostenosis, 516
Lung cancer, 951
Lymphangiomas, 659, 662, 887, 900
clinical pearls, 899
clinical presentation, 899, 900
CT scan, 900
histopathology, 900, 901
magnetic resonance imaging, 900
prognosis, 901
treatment, 901
Lymphatic malformations, 659, 660
Lymphedema-distichiasis (LD) syndrome, 1124
Lymphoid hyperplasia, 770
Lymphoma, 432, 593, 672, 770
Lymphoproliferative diseases, 536, 646
Lymphoproliferative lesions, 888, 889
Lymphoproliferative tumors, 847
Lympho-venous malformation (LVM), 821–824
Lymph node examination, 606
Lysyl oxidase, 1203, 1204

M

Macrolides, 1166
Madibulocutaneous ligaments, 393
Magnetic resonance dacryocystography, lacrimal system obstruction, 552
Magnetic resonance imaging (MRI), 886
adenocarcinoma, 945
adenoid cystic carcinoma, 946
aneurysmal bone cyst, 934
angiosarcomas, 903
basal cell adenocarcinoma, 955
basal cell carcinoma, 956
benign cartilaginous tumors, 926
breast carcinoma, 951
bronchogenic carcinoma, 952
carcinoids, 904
cavernous hemangiomas, 898, 899
cholesterol granuloma, 935
Ewing sarcoma, 936
fibrosarcoma, 920
fibrous dysplasia, 938
fibrous histiocytoma, 921
giant cell reparative granulomas, 940
inverted papillomas, 958
juvenile xanthogranuloma, 922, 923
leiomyosarcomas, 924
lipoblastomas, 925
lipodermoids, 927
lipomas, 928, 929
liposarcomas, 930
lymphangiomas, 900
malignant melanoma, 953
meningocele, 907
MPNST, 905
mucoepidermoid carcinomas, 948
neuroblastoma, 908
ONSM, 912
optic pathway glioma, 910
orbital radiology, 615, 618
ossifying fibromas, 941
osteoblastomas, 942
osteomas, 943
osteosarcoma, 944
pleomorphic adenomas, 949
plexiform neurofibromas, 913, 914
rhabdomyosarcoma, 931
schwannomas, 915
sinonasal carcinoma, 959
solitary fibrous tumor, 933
solitary neurofibromas, 917
sphenoid wing meningioma, 918, 919
squamous cell carcinomas, 960, 961
varices, 902
Magnevist®, 140
Major eyelid deformities
ablepharon macrostomy syndrome, 1146, 1147
cryptophthalmos, 1145, 1146
upper eyelid colobomas, 1147
colobomas with corneopalpebral/conjunctival adhesions, 1148
craniofacial clefts numbers 11, 10 and 9, 1148
isolated colobomas, 1147, 1148
oculoauriculovertebral spectrum, 1148, 1149
surgical repair, 1150
Malformations of cortical development (MCD), 1137
Malignant eyelid tumors, 1108
Malignant hyperthermia (MH), 1194
Malignant melanoma (MM), 429, 953
clinical pearls, 952
clinical presentation, 429, 430, 952, 953
computed tomography, 953
histopathology, 953
magnetic resonance imaging, 953
management, 430, 431
pathologic features, 429
prognosis, 954
treatment, 953, 954
Malignant mixed tumor, *see* Pleomorphic adenocarcinoma
Malignant myoepithelial carcinoma, 736
Malignant peripheral nerve sheath tumor (MPNST), 905, 906
clinical pearls, 905
clinical presentation, 905
computed tomography, 905
histopathology, 906
magnetic resonance imaging, 905
prognosis, 906
treatment, 906
Malignant pleomorphic adenomas, 949
Mandibulofacial dysostosis, *see* Treacher Collins syndrome (TCS)
Manitoba-oculo-tricho-anal (MOTA) syndrome, 1121, 1145
Mantle cell lymphoma (MCL), 785

Manual compression, 675
Mapped serial excision, 473
Marcus Gunn jaw winking ptosis, 261, 262, 300, 1137
Marginal reflex distance 1 (MRD1), 409, 1106
Marionette lines, 366, 370
Masquerade procedure, 1226
Mass casualty, 1317, 1318
Masseter muscle hypertrophy, 366
Masson trichrome stain, 931
Mastisol, 383
Matrix metalloproteinases (MMP), 1202, 1204
Maxillary sinus, 7, 11, 12
Maxillomandibular fixation (MMF), 1278, 1279
Mayo Anesthesia Safety in Kids (MASK) study, 1194
McCune-Albright's syndrome, 937
Mechanical compression, 539
Mechanical ptosis, 301
Medial canthus, 457, 1151, 1152
  blepharophimosis, ptosis and epicanthus inversus syndrome, 1152
  defects, 454, 455, 457, 458
  tendon injuries, 1209
Medial orbital decompression, 1011
Medial orbital wall, 657, 1231, 1232
Medial rectus, 1049
Medial tarsorrhaphy, 210, 211
Medial transconjunctival approach to orbit, 1008–1011
Medial transconjunctival wall decompression, 1010
Medical parsimony/Occam's razor, 120
Medicamentosa, 541
MEDPOR® implant, 1033, 1040
Medtronic StealthStation™, 873
Meibography, 508, 509
Meibomian glands, 486, 505, 621
  dysfunction, 505, 508, 511, 535
  with turbid secretions, 508, 509
Meige syndrome, 219, 220
Melanocytic tumors, 432
Melanoma in situ and invasive malignant melanoma, 472–474
Mendelian inheritance, 1116
Meningocele, 1129
  clinical pearls, 906
  clinical presentaion, 906, 907
  CT scan, 907
  histopathology, 907
  magnetic resonance imaging, 907
  prognosis, 907
  treatment, 907
Meningoencephalocele, *see* Meningocele
Mentalis, 366
Merkel cell carcinoma (MC), 431, 471
Mesenchymal tumors, 887, 888
  aneurysmal bone cyst
    clinical pearls, 933
    clinical presentation, 933
    computed tomography, 934
    histopathology, 934
    magnetic resonance imaging, 934
    prognosis, 934
    treatment, 934
  benign cartilaginous tumors
    clinical pearls, 926
    clinical presentation, 926
    computed tomography, 926
    histopathology, 926
    magnetic resonance imaging, 926
    prognosis, 927
    treatment, 926
  cholesterol granuloma
    clinical pearls, 934, 935
    clinical presentation, 935
    computed tomography, 935
    histopathology, 935
    magnetic resonance imaging, 935
    prognosis, 936
    treatment, 935
  Ewing sarcoma
    clinical pearls, 936
    clinical presentation, 936
    computed tomography, 936
    histopathology, 936, 937
    magnetic resonance imaging, 936
    prognosis, 937
    treatment, 937
  fibrosarcoma
    clinical pearls, 919
    clinical presentation, 920
    computed tomography, 920
    histopathology, 920
    magnetic resonance imaging, 920
    prognosis, 920
    treatment, 920
  fibrous dysplasia
    clinical pearls, 937
    clinical presentation, 937, 938
    computed tomography, 938
    histopathology, 938
    magnetic resonance imaging, 938
    prognosis, 939
    treatment, 939
  fibrous histiocytoma
    clinical pearls, 920
    clinical presentation, 920, 921
    computed tomography, 921
    histopathology, 921
    magnetic resonance imaging, 921
    prognosis, 922
    treatment, 922
  giant cell reparative granulomas
    clinical pearls, 939
    clinical presentation, 939
    computed tomography, 939
    histopathology, 940
    magnetic resonance imaging, 940
    prognosis, 940
    treatment, 940
  juvenile xanthogranuloma
    clinical pearls, 922
    clinical presentation, 922
    computed tomography, 922
    histopathology, 923
    magnetic resonance imaging, 922, 923
    prognosis, 923
    treatment, 923
  leiomyosarcomas
    clinical pearls, 923
    clinical presentation, 923
    computed tomography, 924
    histopathology, 924
    magnetic resonance imaging, 924
    prognosis, 925
    treatment, 924, 925
  lipoblastomas
    clinical pearls, 925
    clinical presentation, 925
    computed tomography, 925
    histopathology, 926

magnetic resonance imaging, 925
prognosis, 926
treatment, 926
lipodermoids
clinical presentation, 927
computed tomography, 927
histopathology, 927, 928
magnetic resonance imaging, 927
prognosis, 927, 928
treatment, 928
lipomas
clinical pearls, 928
clinical presentation, 928
computed tomography, 928
histopathology, 929
magnetic resonance imaging, 928, 929
prognosis, 929
treatment, 929
liposarcomas
clinical pearls, 929
clinical presentation, 929
computed tomography, 929
histopathology, 930
magnetic resonance imaging, 930
prognosis, 930
treatment, 930
ossifying fibromas
clinical pearls, 940
clinical presentation, 940
computed tomography, 940, 941
histopathology, 941
magnetic resonance imaging, 941
prognosis, 941
treatment, 941
osteoblastomas
clinical pearls, 941, 942
clinical presentation, 942
computed tomography, 942
histopathology, 942
magnetic resonance imaging, 942
prognosis, 942
treatment, 942
osteomas
clinical pearls, 942
clinical presentation, 942
computed tomography, 942, 943
histopathology, 943
magnetic resonance imaging, 943
prognosis, 943
treatment, 943
osteosarcoma
clinical pearls, 943, 944
clinical presentation, 944
computed tomography, 944
histopathology, 944
magnetic resonance imaging, 944
prognosis, 944
treatment, 944
rhabdomyosarcoma
clinical pearls, 930, 931
clinical presentation, 931
computed tomography, 931
histopathology, 931
magnetic resonance imaging, 931
prognosis, 932
treatment, 932
solitary fibrous tumor
clinical pearls, 932
clinical presentation, 932
computed tomography, 932
histopathology, 933
magnetic resonance imaging, 933
prognosis, 933
treatment, 933
Metallic IOrbFBs, 1184, 1306
Metastases
orbital radiology, 649
parasellar syndromes, 672
Metastatic disease, 537
Metastatic lesions, 432
Metastatic tumors, 884, 888
breast carcinoma
clinical pearls, 950
clinical presentation, 950
computed tomography, 950
histopathology, 951
magnetic resonance imaging, 951
prognosis, 951
treatment, 951
bronchogenic carcinoma
clinical pearls, 951
clinical presentation, 951
computed tomography, 951, 952
histopathology, 952
magnetic resonance imaging, 952
prognosis, 952
treatment, 952
leukemic neoplasia, 848, 849
malignant melanoma
clinical pearls, 952
clinical presentation, 952, 953
computed tomography, 953
histopathology, 953
magnetic resonance imaging, 953
prognosis, 954
treatment, 953, 954
midfacial or maxillofacial fractures, 849
neuroblastomas, 848
pediatric facial trauma, 849
Methicillin-resistant *Staphylococcus aureus* (MRSA), 532
Methimazole, 988
Methotrexate (MTX), 951, 961, 991
Meticulous surgical technique, 926
Micophthalmos, 1080, 1082–1091
Microcystic adnexal carcinoma (MAC), 471, 472
Microdebrider, 573
Microdermabrasion, 117
Microphthalmia, 1117, 1118, 1121
Microphthalmia, dermal aplasia and sclerocornea (MIDAS) syndrome, 1119
Microphthalmia with linear skin defects (MLS) syndrome, 1119
Microphthalmic socket, 1090, 1091, 1093
Microphthalmos, 624, 837, 896, 1080, 1082–1084, 1086–1089, 1118, 1119, 1123, 1129, 1132
Microporous expanded polytetrafluoroethylene (e-PTFE), 1038
Microspheres, 375
Microvascular free flaps, 865
Midazolam, 1195
Middle aqueous layer, 505
Middle turbinate, 565, 572, 590, 598
Mid-face hypoplasia, 1132
Midface lifts, 391
complications
midface, rejuvenation of, 395
nerve injury, 394
midface anatomy, 395
Midfacial/maxillofacial fractures, 849
Migrated polymethylmethacrylate orbital implant, 1049

Mild amblyopia, 1105
Mild microphthalmos, 896
Mild socket contracture, 1071, 1072
Milia, 413
Mini-lift, 394
Mini Monoka stent, 1226
Minocycline, 377
MIRAgel implants, 1090
Missiles, 1220
Missing muscle sign, 1174, 1176
Mitek™, 356
Mitochondrial inheritance, 1116, 1117
Mitochondrial myopathies, 134, 135, 137
Mitomycin C, 433, 541, 598
Moderate socket contracture, 1072–1076
Modified Hughes procedure, 444
Modified impression technique, 1056
Moebius syndrome, 1124
Mohs micrographic surgery (MMS), periorbital area, 425, 459, 461, 462, 691
 basal cell carcinoma, 465, 467, 468
 clinical features, 462, 463
 histologic features, 463
 history, 459, 460
 indications, 462
 MAC, 471, 472
 margin control, 460
 melanoma in situ and invasive malignant melanoma, 472–474
 Merkel cell carcinoma, 471
 patient considerations, 463
 periorbital considerations, 463
 relative contraindications, 463
 SCC and squamous cell carcinoma in situ, 468, 469
 sebaceous carcinoma, 469–471
 technique, 463–466
 training, 462
 treatment, 459
 WLE, 460, 461
Monocanalicular intubation, 1225
Monocanalicular stent, 561, 562
Monoclonal B-cell proliferations, 769
MOTA syndromes, 1145, 1146
Motor nerves injury
 abducens nerve (CN-VI) injury, 166, 170–174
 diagnosis, 166, 167
 loss of consciousness, 165
 management, 173
 oculomotor nerve (CN-III) injury, 166–170, 173, 174
 trochlear nerve (CN-IV) injury, 168, 169, 171, 174
Moyamoya disease, 1007
MUC7, 523
Mucins, 528
Mucocele, 895
 clinical pearls, 894
 clinical presentation, 894
 computed tomography, 895
 histopathology, 895
 MRI, 895
 prognosis, 895
 treatment, 895
Mucocutaneous junction of upper lid, 509
Mucoepidermoid carcinomas, 497, 735, 947, 948
 clinical pearls, 947
 clinical presentation, 947, 948
 computed tomography, 948
 histopathology, 948
 magnetic resonance imaging, 948
 prognosis, 948
 treatment, 948
Mucopurolent discharge, nasolacrimal duct obstruction, 515
Mucopyocele, 672
 clinical pearls, 894
 clinical presentation, 894
 computed tomography, 895
 histopathology, 895
 MRI, 895
 prognosis, 895
 treatment, 895
Mucosal-associated lymphoid tissue (MALT), 646, 727, 773, 779, 780
Mucous membrane grafts (MMG), 1062, 1072, 1073
Mucous membrane pemphigoid (MMP), 231
 causes, 231
 clinical presentation, 231, 232
 corneal scarring, 237
 diagnosis, 233, 234
 differential diagnosis, 234, 235
 first line therapy, 235
 grading systems, 232, 233
 pathophysiology, 233
 second line therapy, 236
 surgical therapies, 237
 third line therapy, 236, 237
 treatment, 235
Muenke syndrome, 1131
Muir–Torre syndrome, 470
Mullerectomy, 114
Müller's muscle, 33, 320, 321, 620
Multiagent chemotherapy, 944
Multidiode™ fiber optic, 590
Multi-factorial tearing process, 593
MultiHance®, 140
Multiple hamartoma syndromes (MHS), 1128
Multiple orbital foreign bodies, 631
Multiple sclerosis (MS), 300, 630
Muscular fascia, 41
Mustarde cheek rotational flap, 445, 1124
Mustarde ratio, 1126
Myasthenia gravis (MG), 132, 133, 261–266
Mycophenolate mofetil (MMF), 235, 991
Mycosis fungoides (MF), 432, 791
Mycotic orbital cellulitis, 833, 834
Myocutaneous flaps, 865
Myoepithelioma, 730
Myogenic ptosis
 CFEOM, 252, 253
 chronic progressive external ophthalmoplegia, 254, 255, 296, 298
 Guillain-Barré syndrome, 255
 myasthenia gravis, 296
 myotonic dystrophy, 253, 298
 oculopharyngeal muscular dystrophy, 253–255
Myositis, 757, 758
Myotonic dystrophy (MD), 137, 253, 298, 1138
Myxoid fibrous histiocytomas, 921
Myxoid fibrous stroma, 949

N

Nance Horan syndrome, 1119, 1120
Nanophthalmos, 1117, 1118
Nasal and paranasal sinuses, 11
Nasal endoscopy, 577, 594
Nasal intubation, 1279
Nasalis muscle, 365
Nasal mucosal flap, 572
Nasal-orbital-ethmoid (NOE) fractures, 1279
Nasal packing, 575
Nasal passageway, 572

Nasal septum, 598
Nasoantral window procedures, 539
Nasociliary artery, 620
Nasofrontal encephalocele, 1129
Nasojugal groove, 383
Nasolabial folds, 365, 369, 383
Nasolacrimal drainage system, 536
Nasolacrimal duct, 514, 521, 522, 862, 867
Nasolacrimal duct intubation
in adults, 583, 584
cancer therapy, 488, 489
in children, 583
C-Line CIS, 586
complications, 586
Crawford, 584, 585
Guibor and Jackson stents, 586
Ritleng, 585, 586
tube removal, 587
Nasolacrimal duct obstruction (NLDO), 505, 530, 534, 546, 548, 551, 552, 565, 593, 594, 942
amniotic bands, 518
anatomy and embryology, 513, 514
canalicular abnormalities
accessory canaliculi and accessory canalicular channels, 516
canalicular atresia and agenesis, 516
congenital punctal agenesis, 516
congenital punctal atresia, 515, 516
diagnostic studies, 515
facial clefts, 518
lacrimal system obstructions, congenital etiology of, 515
lower system obstructions
amniotocele and dacryocystitis, 516
anatomical variation causing, 516, 517
dacryostenosis, 516
punctal abnormalities, 515
supernumerary (anlage) ducts, 517
symptoms
epiphora, 514
lashes and mucopurolent discharge, mattering of, 515
periocular mass, 515
tumors and mass effect, 518
upper system obstructions, 515
Nasolacrimal endoscopy, 554
Nasolacrimal sac, 514
Nasolacrimal system, 513, 549, 606
Nasolacrimal system anomalies, 1138, 1139
Nasomaxillary buttress, 1272
Nasopharyngeal carcinomas, 671, 958, 959
Naso-sinus tumor, 959
National Acute Spinal Cord Injury Studies (NASCIS), 159
National Institutes of Health (NIH), 279
Natural killer/T-cell Lymphoma (NKTL), 789, 790
Necrobiotic xanthogranuloma, 792
Nerve injury, facelift, 394
Neural integrated arm, 506
Neural tumors, 649, 651, 887
carcinoid
clinical pearls, 903, 904
clinical presentation, 904
CT scan, 904
histopathology, 904
magnetic resonance imaging, 904
prognosis, 904
treatment, 904
malignant peripheral nerve sheath tumor
clinical pearls, 905
clinical presentation, 905
computed tomography, 905
histopathology, 906
magnetic resonance imaging, 905
prognosis, 906
treatment, 906
meningocele
clinical pearls, 906
clinical presentaion, 906, 907
CT scan, 907
histopathology, 907
MRI, 907
prognosis, 907
treatment, 907
neuroblastoma
clinical pearls, 907
clinical presentation, 907
CT scan, 908
histopathology, 908
magnetic resonance imaging, 908
prognosis, 908, 909
treatment, 908
optic nerve sheath meningioma
clinical pearls, 910, 911
clinical presentation, 911
computed tomography, 911, 912
histopathology, 912
magnetic resonance imaging, 912
prognosis, 912, 913
treatment, 912
optic pathway glioma
clinical pearls, 909
clinical presentation, 909
computed tomography, 909, 910
histopathology, 910
MRI, 910
prognosis, 910
treatment, 910
plexiform neurofibromas
clinical pearls, 913
clinical presentation, 913
computed tomography, 913
histopathology, 914
MRI, 913, 914
prognosis, 914
treatment, 914
schwannomas
clinical pearls, 914, 915
clinical presentation, 915
computed tomography, 915
histopathology, 915, 916
magnetic resonance imaging, 915
prognosis, 916
treatment, 916
solitary neurofibroma
clinical pearls, 916
clinical presentation, 916, 917
computed tomography, 917
histopathology, 917
magnetic resonance imaging, 917
prognosis, 917
treatment, 917
sphenoid wing meningioma
clinical pearls, 918
clinical presentation, 918
computed tomography, 918
histopathology, 919
magnetic resonance imaging, 918, 919
prognosis, 919
treatment, 919

Neurilemoma, *see* Schwannomas
Neuroblastoma, 848, 908
  clinical pearls, 907
  clinical presentation, 907
  CT scan, 908
  histopathology, 908
  magnetic resonance imaging, 908
  prognosis, 908, 909
  treatment, 908
Neurofibromas, 651, 917
Neurofibromatosis 1 (NF1), 637, 905, 1139
Neurogenic ptosis, 243, 298
  aberrant oculomotor nerve regeneration, 257–259
  botulism, 270, 271
  catheter cerebral angiography, 258
  cluster headache, 271, 272
  computed tomographic arteriography, 258
  congenital oculomotor palsies, 258
  Horner syndrome (oculosympathetic paresis), 266–272
  isolated pupillary dilation, 258
  magnetic resonance arteriography, 260, 261
  Marcus Gunn Jaw-Winking synkinesis, 261
  myasthenia gravis, 261–266
  oculomotor nerve dysfunction, 256, 257
  recurrent ophthalmoplegic cranial neuropathy, 271
Neuro-ophthalmology approach
  abducens (sixth) nerve
    anatomy, 128
    monocular esotropia, 128
    pathology, 128
  basal ganglia diseases, 123, 124
  botulism, 134
  brainstem ocular motility disorders, 124
  carotid-cavernous fistula, 130, 131
  cavernous sinus
    anatomy, 128, 129
    pathology, 129
    Tolosa–Hunt syndrome, 130
  cerebral gaze deviation, 122, 123
  cerebral ptosis, 123
  clinical localization, 119, 120
  common anatomy, 120
  CT angiography, 139
  CT scans, 138
  differential diagnosis, 121
  dorsal midbrain syndrome, 125
  eye movement disorders localization, 122
  Gadolinium, 140
  internuclear ophthalmoplegia, 124, 125
  Lambert–Eaton myasthenic syndrome, 133
  mitochondrial myopathies, 134, 135, 137
  MR angiography, 139, 140
  MRI, 138, 139
  myasthenia gravis, 132, 133
  myotonic dystrophy, 137
  nephrogenic systemic fibrosis, 140
  neuroophthalmic imaging techniques, 138
  oculomotor (third) nerve
    anatomy, 126
    paralysis, 126
    pathology, 126, 127
  oculopharyngeal dystrophy, 137, 138
  in oculoplastics, 122
  orbital apex syndrome, 131, 132
  Parkinson's disease, 123
  progressive supranuclear palsy, 124
  rare myopathies, 138
  skew deviation, 125
  trochlear (fourth) nerve
    anatomy, 127
    hypertropia, 127
    pathology, 128
Neuropathic ophthalmoplegia, 884
Neurosurgical approaches, 714
Neutrophils, 1201, 1202
Nevoid basal cell carcinoma syndrome, 465
Newer Methods of Ophthalmic Plastic Surgery, 88
Niikawa-Kuroki (formerly Kabuki make-up) syndrome, 1125
Nodular basal cell carcinoma (BCC), 423, 424
Nodular melanoma, 430
Non-accidental trauma, 1113
Nonaxial displacement, orbital evaluation, 606, 608
Nonepithelial lesions, 528
Nonepithelial tumors, 499, 500
Non-medical prevention of anxiety, 1191, 1192
Nonmobile subcutaneous mass, 499
Non-opioid analgesics, 1198
Non-opioid pain medications, 1197
Nonporous implants, 1034, 1035, 1037, 1068
Nonspecific orbital inflammation (NSOI), *see* Idiopathic orbital inflammation (IOI)
Nonsteroidal anti-inflammatory drugs (NSAIDs), 758, 1197, 1198
Non-syndromic craniosynostoses, 1131
Noonan syndrome, 1134
Nuclear factor kappa-light-chain-enhancer of B cells (NF-κB) pathway, 771
Numbness, 414

O

Oblique muscles, 619
Obstructive sleep apnea (OSA), 251
Ocular adnexa, 1113, 1234
Ocular adnexal lymphoproliferative disease (OALD)
  classification, 777
    Burkitt and Hodgkin lymphoma, 778
    diffuse large B-cell lymphoma, 781, 783
    follicular lymphoma, 780
    initial Rappaport classification, 777
    MALT lymphoma, 779, 780
    mantle cell lymphoma, 785
    REAL classification, 777, 778
    T-cell lymphoma, 778
  clinical presentation, 794, 795
  cytogenetic aberrations, 793, 794
  definitions, 769, 770
  epidemiology, 770, 771
  imaging, 798, 800–803
  immunohistochemistry, 793
  lymphoid hyperplasia, 770
  lymphoma, 770
  management
    staging, 807
    tissue diagnosis, 807
    treatment, 808, 809
  pathogenesis
    adaptive immune response, 771
    B-cell lymphoma, 771
    chronic antigenic stimulation, 773
    chronic immune stimulation, 771
    chronic immunosuppression, 771, 774
    class-switch recombination, 772

infectious organisms/chronic antigenic stimulation, 775, 776
innate immune response, 771
mucosa-associated lymphoid tissue, 773
NF-κB, 771
normal B-cell immune response, 771
normal somatic hypermutation, 771
ocular adnexal, 773
ophthalmic lymphoma, 773
post-transplant lymphoproliferative disorder, 774, 775
somatic hypermutation, 772
pathognomonic aberrations, 794
prognostic indicators, 804
international prognostic index, 807
lactate dehydrogenase, 804, 806, 807
Rappaport classification, 769
REAL classification, 769
uncommon and unusual ocular adnexal lymphomas
AIDS-related lymphoma, 788, 789
Burkitt lymphoma, 785, 786
high-grade lymphoma, 786, 787
multiple myeloma, 792
natural killer/T-cell Lymphoma, 789–791
WHO reclassification, 769
Ocular adnexal MALT lymphoma (OAML), 727
Ocular adnexal reconstruction, 439
eyelid defects, 440, 441
frozen-section histopathologic examination/Mohs surgery, 439
lateral canthal defects, 454
lower eyelid defects, 443–445
medial canthal defects, 454, 455, 457, 458
moderate defects, 443
principles, 439, 440
small defects, 441–443
upper eyelid margin
large defects involving, 449, 450, 452, 454
moderate defects involving, 445, 447, 449
small defects, 445
Ocular adnexal trauma
dog and human bites management, 1217–1219
evaluation, 1201
eyelid trauma
ABCs of emergency care, 1205
adnexal injury, 1205
blunt trauma, 1209
lateral canthal tendon, 1209, 1210
local anesthesia, 1208
medial canthal tendon injuries, 1209, 1210
nerve injuries, 1205, 1206
neurologic evaluation, 1205
ocular examination, 1206
ophthalmic plastic laceration tray, 1209
orbital evaluation, 1206, 1207
patient history, 1206
periocular soft tissue examination, 1206
surgical repair, 1207, 1208
gunshot wounds of the orbit, 1219–1221
sharp trauma
canalicular laceration, 1216–1218
eyelid margin lacerations, 1210–1215
secondary repair, 1216
simple lacerations, 1210
traumatic levator dehiscence, 1216
wound healing
chemotaxis and activation, 1201, 1202
clinical factors, 1204
excessive healing, 1204, 1205
inflammation, 1201
principles, 1201
proliferation phase, 1202, 1203
remodeling phase, 1203, 1204
smoking, 1204
vascular supply, 1204
vitamin A (retinoic acid), 1204
vitamin B6 (pyridoxidine), 1204
vitamin C (ascorbic acid), 1204
Ocular and periocular injuries, 1165
Ocular burns
alkali burns, 1223
chemical burns, 1223
clinical evaluation, 1224
intermediate care, 1227, 1228
FTSG or STSG, 1228
skin substitutes, 1228
split-thickness skin grafts, 1228
late reconstruction, 1228, 1229
masquerade procedure, 1226
medial canthal reconstruction, 1229, 1230
tarsorrhaphy, 1225–1227
tear drainage system abnormalities, 1230
thermal eyelid burns, 1223, 1224
treatment, 1224, 1225
Ocular calcification, 629
Ocular cicatricial pemphigoid
causes, 231
definition, 231
Ocular coloboma, 1117
Ocular detachments, 622, 623
Ocular ectodermal syndrome, 1127
Ocular injuries, blepharoplasty, 412, 416
Ocularist, 1050
Ocular melanoma, 626
Ocular metastasis, 626–628
Ocular motility, 884, 1233
Ocular nerve, 622
Ocular rosacea, 507
Ocular surface health, 505, 506, 510
Ocular sympathetic paresis, 299, 300
Oculoauriculovertebral spectrum (OAVS), 1123, 1148, 1149
Oculocardiac reflex, 1243, 1247, 1248, 1251, 1259
Oculo-cerebro-cutaneous syndrome, 1123, 1129
Oculofaciocardiodental (OFCD) syndrome, 1119, 1123
Oculomotor nucleus, 669
Oculopharyngeal muscular dystrophy (OPMD), 137, 138, 253, 298, 1138
Oculophotodynia, 222
Oculoplastics, child abuse in, 1113, 1114
pediatric morbidity and mortality, 1113
scald burns, 1113
thermal burns, 1113
Oculoplastics, genetics in
chromosomal aberrations, 1117
gene structure, 1115
genetic testing & counseling, 1117, 1121
human genome, 1115
lacrimal system abnormalities, syndromes with (*see* Lacrimal system abnormalities, syndromes with)
mutation and polymorphism, 1115, 1116
orbit and ocular adenexa, congenital anomalies of
acquired ptosis, 1137
anophthalmia, 1117, 1118
blepharophimosis syndrome, 1135, 1136
CFEOM, 1136

Oculoplastics, genetics in (*cont.*)
choristomas, 1126–1128
complex microphthalmia, 1117
congenital coloboma, 1122, 1123
congenital ectropion, 1124, 1125
congenital entropion, 1125
congenital fibrosis of the extraocular muscles 2, 1136
congenital fibrosis of the extraocular muscles 3, 1136, 1137
congenital myasthenic syndromes, 1137
CPEO, 1137
craniofacial clefts, 1132, 1133
craniosynostosis, 1131, 1132
cryptophthalmos, 1121, 1122
distichiasis syndromes, 1124
encephalocele, 1129
epicanthus, 1125, 1126
euryblepharon, 1125
frontonasal dysplasias, 1129–1131
Goltz syndrome, 1119
hamartomas, 1128, 1129
hypertelorism, 1126
Kearns-Sayre syndrome, 1137
Lenz microphthalmia syndrome, 1119
Marcus Gunn jaw winking ptosis, 1137
microphthalmia, 1117, 1118
MIDAS syndrome, 1119
myotonic dystrophy, 1138
nanophthalmos, 1117, 1118
OFCD syndrome, 1119
OPMD, 1138
ptosis, genetic forms of, 1133, 1134
simple microphthalmia, 1117
SOX2 anophthalmia syndrome, 1118, 1119
systemic syndromes with lid colobomas, 1123, 1124
telecanthus, 1126
Tukel syndrome, 1137
Waardenburg anophthalmia syndrome, 1119
X-linked microphthalmia syndromes, 1119
patterns of inheritance
autosomal dominant inheritance, 1116
autosomal recessive inheritance, 1116
Mendelian inheritance, 1116
mitochondrial inheritance, 1116, 1117
X-linked dominant inheritance, 1116
X-linked recessive inheritance, 1116
Oculoplastic surgery, 87, 511
Oculosympathetic paresis, *see* Horner syndrome (HS)
Odansetron, 1197
Oedipism, 163
Ollier/Maffucci syndromes, 926
Omega-3 fatty acids, 510
OnabotulinumtoxinA, 368
Oncocytoma, 730
Online Mendelian Inheritance in Man (OMIM), 1145, 1146
Open globe injury, 1315
Open reduction and internal fixation (ORIF), 1279
Ophthalmic and plastic reconstructive surgery (OPRS), 290
Ophthalmic artery, 620
Ophthalmic lymphomas, 726
Ophthalmic nerve schwannoma, 655
Ophthalmic plastic surgery
adjuvant agents, 68, 69
balloon dacryoplasty, 114, 115
bipolar cautery, 68
bone and cartilage, 111, 112
canalicular laceration repair, 114
canalicular stents, 114
carbon dioxide laser, 68
chemical peeling, 116
dog ears, 74, 75
draping, 105
dry eye evaluation, 111
electroepilation, 106
endoscopic brow lifting, 115
endoscopic DCR, 115, 116
endoscopic surgery, 114, 115
eyelid reconstruction, 81–85
facial skin rejuvenation, 116
fat grafting, 116
flaps, 74–78
frontalis sling surgery, 113, 114
hemostasis technology, 67, 109, 110
high-frequency electrocautery, 68
hot-wire cautery, 68
hydroxyapatite, 113
incisions, 66, 67, 106, 107
integrated (porous) implants, 113
intraoperative hemostasis, 67
laser skin resurfacing, 117
microdermabrasion, 117
nonintegrated (nonporous) implants, 113
orbital spherical implants, 113
orbital tissue expanders, 113
patient preparation, 65, 66
pegged implants, 113
perioperative antibiotics, 66
perioperative hemostasis, 67
perioperative planning, 67
photography, 105
porous polyethylene (Medpor), 113
postoperative care, 69
preoperative bleeding studies, 67
primary closure, 72–75
repair of orbital fractures, 112
retraction and exposure, 67
silicone (polyorganosiloxane) injection, 116
skin defects, 72
skin markings and local anesthesia, 66
soft tissue grafts, 110, 111
surgeon position, 106
surgical field exposure, 107, 109
surgical marking, 105
suture materials, 71, 73
suture needles, 69, 70
suture placement, 69–73
tissue dissection, 106–109
traction and exposure, 110, 111
wound closure, 69
wrapping materials, 113
Z-plasty, 76–83
Ophthalmoacromelic syndrome (OAS), *see* Waardenburg anophthalmia syndrome
Ophthalmoplegia, 901
Ophthalmoplegic migraine, 300
Opioid medications, 1198
Optic disk abnormalities, 622
Optic fissure closure defect (OFCD), 1117
Optic nerve, 619, 622, 630
anatomy, 146
avulsion, 163
compression, 817
gliomas, 632, 909, 910

Optic nerve head drusen, 629
Optic nerve sheath meningioma (ONSM), 911, 912
clinical pearls, 910, 911
clinical presentation, 911
computed tomography, 911, 912
histopathology, 912
magnetic resonance imaging, 912
prognosis, 912, 913
treatment, 912
Optic neuritis, 630, 631
Optic pathway glioma (OPGs), 838, 839
clinical pearls, 909
clinical presentation, 909
computed tomography, 909, 910
histopathology, 910
magnetic resonance imaging, 910
prognosis, 910
treatment, 910
Optic perineuritis, 632, 758
Optic sheath meningioma, 632, 638, 639
OptiMark®, 140
Orbicularis oculi, 1124
Orbicularis oris, 366, 370
Orbit and ocular adenexa, congenital anomalies of, 1108, 1109
acquired ptosis, 1137
anatomy of, 618
anophthalmia, 1117, 1118
blepharophimosis syndrome, 1135, 1136
choristomas, 1126–1128
chronic progressive external ophthalmoplegia, 1137
complex microphthalmia, 1117
congenital coloboma, 1122, 1123
congenital ectropion, 1124, 1125
congenital entropion, 1125
congenital fibrosis of the extraocular muscles, 1136, 1137
congenital myasthenic syndromes, 1137
craniofacial clefts, 1132, 1133
craniosynostosis, 1131, 1132
cryptophthalmos, 1121, 1122
distichiasis syndromes, 1124
encephalocele, 1129
epicanthus, 1125, 1126
euryblepharon, 1125
frontonasal dysplasias, 1129–1131
genetic testing & counseling, 1121
Goltz syndrome, 1119
hamartomas, 1128–1129
hypertelorism, 1126
infection, 632–636
Kearns-Sayre syndrome, 1137
Lenz microphthalmia syndrome, 1119
Marcus Gunn jaw winking ptosis, 1137
microphthalmia, 1117, 1118
MIDAS syndrome, 1119
myotonic dystrophy, 1138
nanophthalmos, 1117, 1118
OFCD syndrome, 1119
OPMD, 1138
ptosis, genetic forms of, 1133, 1134
simple microphthalmia, 1117
SOX2 anophthalmia syndrome, 1118, 1119
systemic syndromes with lid colobomas, 1123, 1124
telecanthus, 1126
Tukel syndrome, 1137
vascular masses of, 653
vascular supply of, 620, 621
Waardenburg anophthalmia syndrome, 1119
X-linked microphthalmia syndromes, 1119
Orbital apex, 9–11, 131, 132, 618, 667, 668
Orbital aspergillosis, 749, 750, 859
Orbital bone, cancer therapy, 486, 487
Orbital cellulitis, 414
Orbital compartment syndrome (OCS), 852, 853, 1316, 1317
Orbital decompression, 871–874, 876
history, 1002
indications for, 1004
post-operative considerations, 1012
pre-operative planning, 1003, 1004
surgical techniques, 1001, 1005
endonasal endoscopic orbital decompression (medial wall and floor), 1011, 1012
lateral wall decompression, 1005–1009
medial transconjunctival approach to orbit, 1008–1011
orbital fat decompression, 1005
orbital floor decompression, 1011
surgical timing, 1003
Orbital dermoid cysts, 837
Orbital edema, 490
Orbital emphysema, 1237
Orbital epithelial cysts, 837
Orbital evaluation
B mode ultrasound, 610
CT imaging, 610
examination
accessory tests, 609
axial displacement, 606
external, 605, 606
extraocular motility, 608
eye, anterior segment, 608, 609
eye, posterior segment, 609
lacrimal gland, 606
lymph node, 606
nasolacrimal system, 606
nonaxial displacement, 606, 608
pupils, 604, 605
visual acuity, 604
family history, 603
imaging, 610
laboratory evaluation, 609, 610
MRI, 610
patient history, 603
patient management, 610, 611
social history, 604
Orbital exenteration, 859
bony reconstruction, 865, 866
complications of, 866, 867
definition of, 859
extended exenteration with bone removal and/or additional resection, 863
eyelid-sparing exenteration, 862, 863
indications for, 859, 860
orbital prostheses, 867, 868
preoperative evaluation and planning, 860, 861
primary reconstruction of, 863, 864
rehabilitation of exenterated socket, 867
skin grafting, 864
soft tissue reconstruction, 864, 865
special clinical considerations, 866
spontaneous granulation, 863, 864
subtotal exenteration, 863
total exenteration, 861, 862

Orbital fat, 621, 1005
Orbital fibroblasts, 985, 986
Orbital floor, 657, 849, 850, 862, 866, 867, 1233, 1234, 1266
decompression, 1011
and medial wall fractures, 1234
See also Blowout fracture
Orbital fractures, 1113
computed tomography, 1234
definition, 1231
evaluation
extraocular motility, 1233
ocular adnexa, 1234
ocular motility, 1233
paralytic diplopia, 1233
penetrating globe injury, 1233
swinging flashlight test, 1233
history, 1231
intraorbital foreign bodies, 852
lateral orbital wall, 851, 852, 1233
magnetic resonance imaging, 1234
management, 1234, 1235
medial orbital wall, 1231, 1232
non-contrast computed tomography, 1231
orbital anatomy, 1231
orbital floor and medial wall fractures, 849, 850, 1233, 1234
orbital hemorrhage, 852, 853
orbital roof fractures, 850, 851, 1231, 1232
traumatic optic neuropathy, 853
zygomaticomaxillary complex fractures, 852
Orbital hemorrhage, 412, 852, 853, 1264
arterial occlusion, 150
blunt-tipped Westcott or curved Stevens scissors, 155
castroviejo or Bishop Harmon forceps, 155
causes, 149
clinical evaluation, 152
clinical presentation, 150, 151
external ophthalmoplegia, 150
gentle examination techniques, 150, 151
globe tenting, 153
inferior cantholysis, 153, 154
inferior septolysis, 154
intraocular pressure measurement, 150, 152
intraorbital pressure, 150
intravenous corticosteroids, 153
ischemic optic neuropathy, 150
lateral canthotomy, 153
medical therapy, 153
orbital compartment syndrome, 152
CT imaging, 152
surgical treatment, 154, 155
topical antiglaucoma medications, 153
tear-drop sign, 153
transnasal endoscopic decompression, 154
visual loss, 150
Orbital hypoplasia, 486
Orbital implant wrapping, 1038, 1039
Orbital inflammation, 985, 991
adult orbital xanthogranulomatous diseases, 761
angiolymphoid hyperplasia with eosinophilia, 761, 762
autoimmune disorders
Churg-Strauss syndrome, 753, 754
granuloma annulare, 755
sarcoidosis, 751, 752
Sjögren's syndrome, 754
Wegener's granulomatosis, 752, 753
autoimmune orbital granulomatous disease, 751
bacterial orbital cellulitis
clinical features, 744
complications, 747–749
diagnosis, 744, 745
differential diagnosis, 746, 747
orbital nocardiosis, 749
treatment, 747
clinical evaluation, 743, 744
dacryoadenitis, 758
fungal orbital cellulitis, 749
aspergillosis, 749, 750
mucormycosis, 750
idiopathic orbital inflammation
clinical features, 755, 756
treatment, 756, 757
idiopathic posterior scleritis, 759
infection, 744
intraocular tumors, 762
Kimura disease, 761, 762
Langerhans' cell histiocytosis, 760, 761
myositis, 757, 758
optic perineuritis, 758
Tolosa-Hunt syndrome, 760
trochleitis, 758
Orbital inflammatory syndrome (OIS), *see* Idiopathic orbital inflammation (IOI)
Orbital invasion, 490
Orbital lymphangiomas, 842, 843
Orbital lymphoma, 646, 885
Orbital margin, 4
Orbital medial wall fractures, 850
Orbital meningiomas, 840, 841
Orbital mucormycosis, 643, 750, 859
Orbital neural cysts, 837
Orbital neurofibromas, 839, 840
Orbital neurofibromatosis, 885
Orbital nocardiosis, 749
Orbital pain, 884, 946
Orbital radiology, 615
abnormal globe and optic disk abnormalities, 622
arteriovenous malformation, 660, 661
bony orbit, 618, 619
buphthalmos, 622
capillary hemangioma, 653–655
carotid cavernous fistula, 661
cavernous malformations, 655, 657
Coats' disease, 624, 625
coloboma, 622
CT imaging, 615
dermoid, epidermoid and lipoma, 645
dynamic vascular and positional imaging, 618
extraocular muscles, 619, 620
fibro-osseous lesions, 643, 645
globe and optic nerve, 619
histiocytosis, 645
intraocular masses
choroidal hemangiomas, 628
ocular calcification, 629
ocular inflammation, 629, 630
ocular melanoma, 626, 628
retinal angiomas, 628
retinoblastoma, 626
trauma, 630
IOID, 636
lacrimal gland neoplasms, 646

lacrimal system, 621
leukemia, 647
leukocoria, 623
lid retractor system, 620
lymphatic and venolymphatic malformations, 659, 660
metastases, 649
MR imaging, 615, 618
neural structures, 621
neural tumors, 649, 651
ocular detachments, 622, 623
ocular, optic nerve, and orbital pathology, 622, 630
optic nerve gliomas, 632
optic neuritis and demyelinating disease, 630, 631
optic perineuritis, 632
optic sheath meningioma, 632
orbit
anatomy of, 618
infection, 632–636
lymphoma, 646
varix, 658
vascular masses of, 653
vascular supply of, 620, 621
papilledema, 622
PHPV, 623, 624
retinoblastoma, 623
rhabdomyosarcoma, 647, 649
ROP, 625
sarcoidosis, 638, 640
Sjögren's syndrome, 641, 643
staphyloma, 622
surgical change, 630
thyroid orbitopathy, 636, 638
Toxocara canis infection, 625
trauma, 652
tumors and tumorlike lesions, 643
Wegener's granulomatosis, 641
Orbital radiotherapy, 992
Orbital roof fracture, 850, 851, 861, 863, 865–867, 1171, 1172, 1231, 1234
Orbital schwannomas, 841
Orbital shape and development, 3–5
Orbital soft tissues sarcomas, 845
Orbital surgery
acrylic prostheses, 97
age, 703
anticoagulants, 703–704
Bartisch's method, 96
biopsy
excisional biopsy, 707
fine-needle aspiration biopsy, 706, 707
incisional biopsy, 707
Caldwell–Luc decompression, 99
cryoprobe, 706
endoscopic orbital surgery, 706, 713
enucleation implants, 97
hollow-ball implant, 97
hydroxyapatite orbital implant, 97
image guidance procedures, 706
imaging, 704
infra orbital lesions
transconjunctival approach, 708, 709
transcutaneous approach, 708
instruments
bloodless field, 706
cotton applicators, 706
drills, 706
microdissecting instruments, 706
peanut sponges, 706
periosteal elevators, 706
retractors, 704
integrated orbital implant, 97
intraoperative complications, 714
Kronlein lateral orbitotomy approach, 99
lateral orbitotomy, 711–713
local/general anesthesia, 704
Lynch transcutaneous incision, 99
medial lid crease approach, 713
medial orbital lesions
transcaruncular approach, 711
transconjunctival approach, 709
transcutaneous approach, 709
neurosurgical approaches, 714
ocular prosthesis, 97
orbital decompression, 99
perioperative antibiotics, 703
postoperative complications
emergent, 714, 715
non-emergent, 715
revolutionalized orbital surgery, 97
Ruedmann implant, 97
superior orbital lesions
transconjunctival approach, 708
transcutaneous approach, 707
transconjunctival incision, 97
Troutman's implant, 97, 98
universal implant, 97
vertical full-thickness lid split approach, 97
Orbital tissue expander (OTE), 1091, 1092
Orbital tissues, 984–986
Orbital trauma
orbital compartment syndrome, 1316, 1317
orbital wall fracture, 1317
Orbital tumors, 540
age at onset, 885
ancillary imaging techniques, 886
bone, tumors of, 888
clinical evaluation, 883
computerized tomography, 886
cystic lesions, 887
colobomatous cysts, 895, 896
dermoid cyst, 889–891
epithelial cysts, 892, 893
mucoceles, 894, 895
mucopyocele, 894, 895
respiratory epithelial cyst, 893, 894
differential diagnosis, 883
incidence of, 886, 887
inflammatory lesions, 887
lacrimal gland lesions, 888
lacrimal gland tumors
adenocarcinoma, 944, 945
adenoid cystic carcinoma, 945–947
mucoepidermoid carcinomas, 947, 948
pleomorphic adenomas, 948–950
lymphoproliferative lesions, 888, 889
mesenchymal tumors, 887, 888
aneurysmal bone cyst, 933, 934
benign cartilaginous tumors, 926, 927
cholesterol granuloma, 934–936
Ewing sarcoma, 936, 937
fibrosarcoma, 919, 920
fibrous dysplasia, 937–939

Orbital tumors (*cont.*)
fibrous histiocytoma, 920–922
giant cell reparative granulomas, 939, 940
juvenile xanthogranuloma, 922, 923
leiomyosarcomas, 923–925
lipoblastomas, 925, 926
lipodermoids, 927, 928
lipomas, 928, 929
liposarcomas, 929, 930
ossifying fibromas, 940, 941
osteoblastomas, 941, 942
osteomas, 942, 943
osteosarcoma, 943, 944
rhabdomyosarcoma, 930–932
solitary fibrous tumor, 932, 933
metastatic tumors, 888
breast carcinoma, 950, 951
bronchogenic carcinoma, 951, 952
malignant melanoma, 952–954
MRI, 886
nature of onset, 885
neural tumors, 887
carcinoid, 903, 904
malignant peripheral nerve sheath tumor, 905, 906
meningocele, 906, 907
neuroblastoma, 907–909
optic nerve sheath meningioma, 910–913
optic pathway glioma, 909, 910
plexiform neurofibromas, 913, 914
schwannomas, 914–916
solitary neurofibromas, 916, 917
sphenoid wing meningioma, 918, 919
ophthalmic and medical history, 883
ophthalmic examination, 883, 884
secondary tumors, 889
basal cell adenocarcinoma, 954, 955
basal cell carcinoma, 955–957
inverted papillomas, 957, 958
sinonasal carcinoma, 958, 959
squamous cell carcinomas, 960, 961
signs and symptoms of
laterality, 885
ocular motility, 884
orbital pain, 884
periorbital inflammation, 885
proptosis, 884
visual loss, 884
temporal onset of, 885
unusual features, 885, 886
vascular lesions, 887
angiosarcomas, 902, 903
capillary hemangiomas, 896–898
cavernous hemangiomas, 898, 899
lymphangiomas, 899–901
varices, 901, 902
Orbital varix, 658
Orbital walls, 1231–1233
congenital dehiscences, 9
epidermoid, 649
frontoethmoidal and maxilloethmoidal sutures, 8, 9
infraorbital groove, 8
lateral nasal wall, 7
medial wall, 8
menin-golacrimal foramen, 6
nasal anatomy, 6
nasal development, 6
orbital apex, 6
orbital floor, 8
orbital plate, 8
orbital rim and nasal cavity, 8
superior and inferior orbital fissures, 7
triangular orbital roof, 6
zygomaticotemporal and zygomaticofacial foramina, 8
zygomatic process, 7
Organic IOrbFBs, 1311
Organoid nevus syndrome epibulbar choristomas, 1127
Original polycarbonate peg, 1040
Oro-naso-ocular cleft, 1150
Osseointegration, 720
Ossifying fibromas, 941
clinical pearls, 940
clinical presentation, 940
computed tomography, 940, 941
histopathology, 941
magnetic resonance imaging, 941
prognosis, 941
treatment, 941
Osteitis fibrosa generalisata, 844
Osteoblastomas
clinical pearls, 941, 942
clinical presentation, 942
computed tomography, 942
histopathology, 942
magnetic resonance imaging, 942
prognosis, 942
treatment, 942
Osteochondromas, 926
Osteoclasts, 486
Osteoconduction, 720
Osteoinduction, 720
Osteomas, 943
clinical pearls, 942
clinical presentation, 942
computed tomography, 942, 943
histopathology, 943
magnetic resonance imaging, 943
prognosis, 943
treatment, 943
Osteoradionecrosis, 486
Osteosarcoma
clinical pearls, 943, 944
clinical presentation, 944
computed tomography, 944
histopathology, 944
magnetic resonance imaging, 944
prognosis, 944
treatment, 944
Osteotomy, 567, 568, 597
Outer canthal distance (OCD), 1126
Oxycodone, 1198
Oxymetazoline HCl, 572

P

Paclitaxel, 951
Pagetoid spread, 427
Palatal fractures, 1277
Palpebral conjunctiva, 485
Palpebral fissure asymmetry, 365
Panfacial trauma, 1281
Papilledema, 622, 623
Papillomas, 536, 957

Papoosing, 1191–1193
Paracetamol, 1198
Paralytic diplopia, 1233
Paralytic strabismus, 1105
Paranasal sinuses, 537, 670, 744
Parasellar syndromes, 667, 668
  anatomy, 667
  aseptic cavernous sinus thrombosis, 677
    clinical presentation, 678
    pathogenesis, 677, 678
  aspergillosis, 684
  carotid-cavernous fistulas, 673
    classification, 673
    clinical presentation, 674
    evaluation, 674
    observation, 675
    outcomes and prognosis, 674, 675
    pathogenesis, 673
    surgical options, 675–677
    venous drainage, 673, 674
  cavernous ICA aneurysms, 677
    clinical presentation, 677
    prognosis, 677
  cavernous sinuses, 668–670
  differential diagnosis, 670, 671
  hypophysitis, 679
  infection, 679, 680
  inflammation, 678
  lymphoma, 672
  meningiomas, 672
  metastases, 672
  nasopharyngeal carcinomas, 671
  orbital apex, 667, 668
  outcomes and prognosis, 675
  paranasal sinuses, 670
  pituitary adenoma, 672
  pituitary gland, 670
  rhino-cerebral-orbital mucormycosis, 682
    clinical presentation, 682
    diagnosis, 683
    risk factors, 682, 683
    treatment, 683, 684
  septic CST, 680
    clinical presentation, 680
    neuroimaging, 680
    outcomes and prognosis, 680, 681
    treatment, 681, 682
  Tolosa Hunt syndrome, 678
    clinical presentation, 678, 679
    neuroimaging, 679
    treatment, 679
  trauma, 671
  treatment, 675, 677
  tumors, 671
  vascular, 673
  zoster neuropathy, 684, 685
Parasitic obstruction, 532
Paredrine, 300
Paresis, 1238, 1247
Parinaud syndrome, 251
Parkinson's disease (PD), 123
Parkland formula, 1225
Partial thickness burns (second degree), 1224
Pasteurella multocida, 1166
Patau syndrome, 1121
Paton's folds, 609
Patternless pattern, 933
Patterns of inheritance
  autosomal dominant inheritance, 1116
  autosomal recessive inheritance, 1116
  Mendelian inheritance, 1116
  mitochondrial inheritance, 1116, 1117
  X-linked dominant inheritance, 1116
  X-linked recessive inheritance, 1116
Pearly gray borders, 424
Pearson syndrome, 1137
Pediatric corner, 1104
Pediatric facial trauma, 849
Pediatric oculoplastic examination, 1103
  epiphora, 1105
  eyelid, ptosis, 1105–1108
  eyelid tumors, 1108
    benign eyelid tumors, 1108
    malignant eyelid tumors, 1108
  general rapport, 1103, 1104
  motility and visual examination, 1104, 1105
  orbit, 1108, 1109
Pediatric orbital disease
  bacterial orbital cellulitis, 832, 833
  bacterial preseptal cellulitis, 832
  congenital orbital tumors and cysts
    choristomas, 837, 838
    hamartoma, 837
  Crohn's disease, 836
  development and anatomy, 831
  granulomatosis with polyangiitis, 835
  idiopathic orbital inflammation, 834
  infectious, 832
  inflammatory disease, 834
  lacrimal gland tumors, 847
  mesenchymal tumors
    Burkitt lymphoma, 847
    Ewing sarcomas, 845, 846
    fibrous dysplasia, 844, 845
    histiocytic tumors, 846, 847
    lymphoproliferative tumors, 847
    orbital soft tissues sarcomas, 845
    rhabdomyosarcoma, 843, 844
  metastatic tumors
    facial trauma, 849
    leukemic neoplasia, 848, 849
    midfacial/maxillofacial fractures, 849
    neuroblastomas, 848
  mycotic orbital cellulitis, 833, 834
  neural tumors
    optic pathway gliomas, 838, 839
    orbital meningiomas, 840, 841
    orbital neurofibromas, 839, 840
    orbital schwannomas, 841
  orbital fractures
    intraorbital foreign bodies, 852
    lateral wall fractures, 851, 852
    orbital floor fractures, 849, 850
    orbital hemorrhage, 852, 853
    orbital medial wall fractures, 850
    orbital roof fractures, 850, 851
    traumatic optic neuropathy, 853
    zygomaticomaxillary complex fractures, 852
  periarteritis nodosa/polyarteritis nodosa, 835, 836
  sarcoidosis, 836
  Sjogren's syndrome, 837
  systemic lupus erythematosus, 835
  thyroid eye disease, 834, 835
  vascular tumors
    infantile hemangiomas, 841, 842
    orbital lymphangiomas, 842, 843

Pediatric orbital fractures, 1171
and orbital roof fractures, 1171, 1172
surgical technique, 1175–1178
white-eyed blowout fracture, 1172–1175
Pediatric orbital mesenchymal tumors
Burkitt lymphoma, 847
Ewing sarcomas, 845, 846
fibrous dysplasia, 844, 845
histiocytic tumors, 846, 847
lymphoproliferative tumors, 847
orbital soft tissues sarcomas, 845
rhabdomyosarcoma, 843, 844
Pediatric orbital neural tumors
optic pathway gliomas, 838, 839
orbital meningiomas, 840, 841
orbital neurofibromas, 839, 840
orbital schwannomas, 841
Pediatric orbital vascular tumors
infantile hemangiomas, 841, 842
orbital lymphangiomas, 842, 843
Pediatric periocular dog bite injuries, 1165–1167
Capnocytophaga canimorsus, 1166
incidence rate, 1165
Pasteurella multocida, 1166
surgical technique, 1167–1171
Pediatric periocular trauma, specific issues of
CT imaging in children, 1178–1182
avoid plain X-rays, 1181
communicate, 1181
imaging modalities, 1181
ionizing radiation effects, 1179
in pediatric orbital disease, 1180
radiation exposure, risk of, 1179
right scan for right pathology, 1181
right scan the first time, 1181
single-pass technology with coronal reconstruction, 1181
pediatric orbital fractures, 1171
and orbital roof fractures, 1171, 1172
surgical technique, 1175–1178
white-eyed blowout fracture, 1172–1175
pediatric periocular dog bite injuries, 1165–1167
Capnocytophaga canimorsus, 1166
incidence rate, 1165
Pasteurella multocida, 1166
surgical technique, 1167–1171
periocular and orbital foreign bodies, 1182–1188
Pediatric thyroid eye disease (TED), 834, 835
Pegging porous orbital implants, 1039, 1040
Pemphigus vulgaris, 231
Penetrating orbital injuries and IOrbFBs
classification, 1302
clinical assessment, 1302
computed tomography imaging, 1302, 1304, 1305
history, 1301
metallic IOrbFBs, 1305
MRI, 1304
prevention, 1301, 1302
retained IOrbFBs complications, 1306–1310
suspected metallic IOrbFBs, 1305, 1306
treatment, 1310, 1311
Penicillin, 1166
Peplomycin, 961
Percutaneous contrast dacryocystography, 553, 554
Periarteritis nodosa/polyarteritis nodosa (PAN), 835, 836
Pericanalicular orbicularis muscle, 561
Pericranial flap, 720
Perineural invasion, 426, 955
Perineuritis, 632
Periocular BCC, 424
Periocular infantile hemangiomas, 841, 842
Periocular mass, 515
Periocular necrotizing fasciitis, 860
Periocular tissues
cytogenetics, 700
cytologic techniques, 699
electron microscopy, 699
enzyme immunohistochemistry, 700
flow cytometry, 700
frozen sections, 691, 692
histologic stains, 696
immunohistochemistry, 696–699
molecular techniques, 700
ophthalmic pathology, pitfall prevention, 701
pathologic diagnosis, rendering
histologic diagnosis, limitations of, 695
histopathologic diagnosis, 694, 695
issuing pathology reports, 695
pathologic specimens, medicolegal considerations of, 695, 696
previous pathologic material, 694
pathologic specimens, processing
dissection, 693, 694
gross examination, 692
mishandling, 694
surgical margins, identification of, 694
pathologic specimens, resection and handling
classification, 689, 690
method, 690, 691
pathology request form, pathologic specimens and completing, 692
radiographic study, 700
surgical pathology, special techniques in, 696
tissue fixation, 692
Perioral rhytids, 366
Periorbital area, MMS, 459, 461, 462
basal cell carcinoma, 465, 467, 468
clinical features, 462, 463
histologic features, 463
history, 459, 460
indications, 462
MAC, 471, 472
margin control, 460
melanoma in situ and invasive malignant melanoma, 472–474
Merkel cell carcinoma, 471
patient considerations, 463
periorbital considerations, 463
relative contraindications, 463
SCC and squamous cell carcinoma in situ, 468, 469
sebaceous carcinoma, 469–471
technique, 463–466
training, 462
treatment, 459
WLE, 460, 461
Periorbital ecchymosis, 1113
Periorbital edema, 490
Periorbital hematoma, 1113
Periorbital inflammation, 885
Periorbital thermal facial burn, 1316
Periosteal elevator, 567, 568, 1252, 1254
Periosteum, 567
Peripheral T-cell lymphoma (PTCL), 792
Persistent hyperplastic primary vitreous (PHPV), 623, 624
Pfeiffer syndrome, 1133
PHACES syndrome, 825

Phakomatoses with oculoplastic manifestations
 neurofibromatosis 1, 1139
 Sturge-Weber Syndrome, 1140, 1141
 tuberous sclerosis, 1139, 1140
Phased array coils, 615
Photography, 105
Phthisis bulbi, 629
Physiological dysfunction, 547, 549, 555, 556
Pillars of resistance, 1271, 1272
Pilosebaceous units, 928
Pituitary adenoma, 672
Pituitary apoplexy, 672
Plasmacytoma, 792
Plastic embedding, 700
Platelet-derived growth factor (PDGF), 1202
Platysma, 391, 392
Pleomorphic adenomas, 650, 727–730, 735, 949, 950
 clinical pearls, 948, 949
 clinical presentation, 949
 computed tomography, 949
 histopathology, 949
 magnetic resonance imaging, 949
 prognosis, 950
 treatment, 949, 950
Pleomorphic rhabdomyosarcoma, 931
Pleuripotential mesenchymal cells, 920
Plexiform neurofibromas, 914
 clinical pearls, 913
 clinical presentation, 913
 computed tomography, 913
 histopathology, 914
 MRI, 913, 914
 prognosis, 914
 treatment, 914
Pneumatic retinopexy, 632
Polyalanine, 1136
Polycarbonate safety lenses, 1058
Polyglactin, 1044
Poly-L-lactic acid (PLLA), 375
Polymethylmethacrylate (PMMA), 1031, 1033, 1035, 1037, 1068, 1291
Polymorphism, 1115, 1116
Porous orbital implants, 1032, 1037, 1068, 1089
 bioceramic implants, 1034
 hydroxyapatite implants, 1032, 1033
 vs. nonporous implants, 1034, 1035
 pegging, 1039, 1040
 porous polyethylene implants, 1033
 synthetic hydroxyapatite implants, 1033, 1034
Porous polyethylene implants, 1033
Porous polyethylene, polyetheretherketone (PEEK), 1291
Porous stents, 676
PosiSep®, 574, 575
Post-dacryocystorhinostomy, 550
Post enucleation socket syndrome, 1056
Posterior indirect TON (PITON), 145
 asymmetric PITON, 158
 bilateral PITON, 158
 CT imaging, 158, 159
 diagnosis, 158, 159
 head and neck injuries, 158
 management, 158
 MRI, 159
 nonimpinging fractures, 159
 optic nerve assessment, 159
 prognosis, 162, 163
 shearing injury, 158
 treatment
  experimental modalities, 161, 162
  megadose intravenous corticosteroid therapy, 159, 160
  optic canal decompression, 160, 161
 visual acuity, 158
Posterior lacrimal sac flap, 574
Posterior scleritis, 630
Posterior sclerotomy technique, 1046, 1047
Post-operative nausea and vomiting (PONV), 1197
Postoperative radiotherapy, 950, 961
Postseptal cellulitis, 633
Post-transplant lymphoproliferative disorder (PTLD), 774, 775
Post-viral optic neuritis, 634
Potassium titanyl phosphate (KTP), 589
Preauricular/retroauricular grafts, 441
Preseptal orbital cellulitis, 414, 640
Primary acquired dacryostenosis, 523
Primary acquired melanosis (PAM), 432, 952
Primary acquired nasolacrimal duct obstruction (PANDO), 524
Primary adenocarcinoma, 734, 735, 944, 945
Primary cutaneous anaplastic large cell lymphoma (ALCL), 792
Primary ductal adenocarcinomas, 945
Primary endoscopic dacryocystorhinostomy
 complications, 575, 576
 patient selection, 571
 postoperative care, 575
 process, 572–575
 surgical equipment, 572
Primary external dacryocystorhinostomy
 anesthesia, 565
 postoperative care, 569, 570
 procedure, 565, 567–569
 surgical principles, 565
Primary intraocular lymphomas (PIOL), 726
Primary jones dye test, 547, 548
Primary ocular adnexal lymphoma (OAL), 726
Primary orbital melanomas, 952, 953
Primary/solitary extramedullary plasmacytoma, 792
Primary uveal or conjunctival melanomas, 952
Probing, 1167, 1168
 in adults, 583, 584
 in children, 583
 complications, 586
 lacrimal system obstruction, 548
 technique, 584
 tube removal, 587
Probing and irrigation (P&I), 1167
Profill, 376
Progressive external ophthalmoplegia (PEO), 1137
Progressive supranuclear palsy (PSP), 124
Prolonged hypothyroidism, 988
Prophylactic ocular lubrication, 1225
Propofol, 1195
Proptosis, 605, 681, 884, 896, 898, 900, 915, 936, 937, 939, 1004
 abaxial, 884
 axial, 884
 definition of, 884
Propylthiouracil (PTU), 988
Prostaglandin-endoperoxide H synthase-2 (PGHS-2), 985
Prosthetic eye, living with, 1058
Proteus syndrome, 1128
Psammomatoid ossifying fibroma, 941
Pseudoenophthalmos, 299
Pseudolymphoma, 770
Pseudopemphigoid, 235

Pseudoptosis, 296, 301, 302
aberrant facial nerve regeneration, 251
causes, 244
contralateral upper eyelid retraction, 244, 245
dermatochalasis, 244, 245
Duane retraction syndrome, 250, 251
enophthalmos, 245–247
FES, 251
globe asymmetry, 246
margin-to-reflex distance, 244
ocular misalignment, 246–249
Parinaud syndrome, 251
pathology, 244
spastic disorders, 247, 250
PTEN hamartoma tumor syndrome (PHTS)., 1128
Pterygomaxillary buttress, 1272
Ptosis, 1104–1108, 1137
anatomy, 280
anesthesia, 282
anterior cutaneous approach, 90
aponeurotic ptosis, 243
bilateral congenital ptosis, 290, 292
blepharochalasis repair, 90, 92
blepharoplasty, 412
blepharoptosis correction, 243
Bowman's posterior approach, 90, 92
BPES, 280
clinical documentation, 243
clinical evaluation, 280, 281
definition, 279
degree of ptosis, 282
double elevator palsy, 280
etiology, 279
eyebrow suspension, 283, 291
frontalis sling procedure, 285, 289, 290
genetic associations, 279, 280
genetic forms of, 1133, 1134
informed consent process, 281, 282
levator function, 283
levator resection, 283–286, 288–289
myogenic ptosis (*see* Myogenic ptosis)
neurogenic etiologies, 243
neurogenic ptosis (*see* Neurogenic ptosis)
neurologic ptosis, 243
pathology, 279
physical examination, 243
physiologic anisocoria, 244
preoperative examination, 282
Putterman's procedure, 92
relaxed eyelid treatment, 90
retrieval of autogenous fascia lata, 290, 291
skin excision limitations, 90
surgery, 90
suspensions, 92
tarsectomy/mullerectomy, 90–93
Punctal abnormalities, 515
Punctal ectropion, 563, 564
Punctal occlusion, 509, 538
Punctal plugs, 528
Punctal stenosis, 489, 527, 546, 559, 1230
Punctoplasty, 538, 559
Punctual stenosis, 540
Punctum, 524, 527, 548
bicanalicular repair, 561, 562
monocanalicular stent, 562
pigtail probe, 562, 563
punctal ectropion, 563, 564
stent removal, 563
Pupils, orbital evaluation, 604, 605
Putterman müllerectomy, 1107
Putterman's procedure, 92
Pyoceles, 672
Pyogenic granuloma, 528, 539, 1059
Pyridostigmine, 367

Q

Quasi-integrated (or indirectly integrated) implants, 1036, 1037

R

Rabies vaccine adsorbed (RVA), 1219
Radial sclerotomies, 1046
Radiation effect, 1179
Radiation therapy, 425, 427, 431, 483, 484
Radiesse, 370, 374
Radioactive iodine (RAI), 988–990
Radioiodine ablation, 542
Radioiodine uptake testing (RAIU), 989
Radionuclide dacryoscintigraphy, 552, 553, 556
Radiotherapy, 904, 910, 912, 923, 932, 934, 939, 945, 951, 952, 955, 958
Ragged red fibers, 1137
Rare eyelid neoplasms, 431
Recombinant interferon alpha-2, 897–898
Rectus muscles, 619, 1235
Recurrent ophthalmoplegic cranial neuropathy, 271
Redraping technique, 338
Regulatory T cells (Treg), 986
Relative risk (RR), 1180
Residual fluorescein, 548
Resorption atelectasis, 880
Respiratory epithelial cyst
clinical pearls, 893
clinical presentation, 893
computed tomography, 893, 894
histopathology, 894
magnetic resonance imaging, 894
prognosis, 894
treatment, 894
Restasis, 510
Restylane products, 372, 373
Retinal angiomas, 628
Retinal detachment, 622
Retinoblastoma, 623, 624, 626, 762
Retinoid acid receptor-alpha (RARα), 985
Retinopathy of prematurity (ROP), 625
Retrobulbar hematoma, 657
Retrobulbar hemorrhage, 1297
Retrobulbar rhabdomyosarcoma, 931
Retrocaruncular, 1008
Retro-orbicularis oculi fat (ROOF), 326
Retro-orbital pathology, 667
Retroscope, 336
Revised European-American lymphoma (REAL), 769
Rhabdomyosarcoma (RMS), 647, 649, 843, 844, 888, 930, 931, 1108
clinical pearls, 930, 931
clinical presentation, 931
computed tomography, 931
histopathology, 931
magnetic resonance imaging, 931
prognosis, 932
treatment, 932
Rheology, 373
Rhino-cerebral-orbital mucormycosis (RCOM), 682
clinical presentation, 682
diagnosis, 683

risk factors, 682, 683
treatment, 683, 684
Rhomboid flaps, 440
Right frontoethmoid mucocele, 895
Right inferior globe displacement, 607
Riley day syndrome (RDS), 1138
Rim-sparing orbital decompression, 1005
Ritleng hook, 586
Ritleng NLD intubation system, 585, 586
Ritleng stent, 585
Rituximab, 991
Rongeur, 568
Rose Bengal staining, 547
Rosenmuller's valves, 556
Ruedmann implant, 97

S
Saethre-Chotzen syndrome, 1132
Sarcoidosis, 638, 640, 725, 836, 883, 887
Sarcomas, 488
Say-Barber syndrome, 1136
Scald burns, 1113
Scars, facelift, 394
Schirmer testing, 507, 546, 547
Schlemm's canal, 675
Schwannomas, 884, 915, 916
clinical pearls, 914, 915
clinical presentation, 915
computed tomography, 915
histopathology, 915, 916
magnetic resonance imaging, 915
prognosis, 916
treatment, 916
Sculptra, 375
Sebaceous carcinoma (SC), 427
clinical presentation, 428
lower eyelid, 428
management, 428, 429
MMS, 469–471
pathologic features, 427, 428
Sebaceous cell carcinoma, 863, 1108
Seborrheic keratoses, 190
Secondary acquired lacrimal drainage obstruction (SALDO), 524
Secondary acquired nasolacrimal duct obstruction, 525–527
Secondary glaucoma, 675
Secondary jones dye test, 548
Secondary neoplasms, cancer therapy, 487, 488
Secondary orbital implants, 1048, 1064, 1065
clinical scenarios, 1047
placement surgical technique, 1048, 1049
postoperative care, 1048–1050
Secondary tumors, orbital, 889
basal cell adenocarcinoma
clinical pearls, 954
clinical presentation, 954
computed tomography, 955
histopathology, 955
magnetic resonance imaging, 955
prognosis, 955
treatment, 955
basal cell carcinoma
clinical pearls, 955, 956
clinical presentation, 956
computed tomography, 956
histopathology, 956, 957
magnetic resonance imaging, 956
prognosis, 957
treatment, 957
inverted papillomas
clinical pearls, 957
clinical presentation, 957
computed tomography, 957
histopathology, 958
magnetic resonance imaging, 958
prognosis, 958
treatment, 958
sinonasal carcinoma
clinical pearls, 958
clinical presentation, 958, 959
computed tomography, 959
histopathology, 959
magnetic resonance imaging, 959
prognosis, 959
treatment, 959
squamous cell carcinomas
clinical pearls, 960
clinical presentation, 960
computed tomography, 960
histopathology, 961
magnetic resonance imaging, 960, 961
prognosis, 961
treatment, 961
Sedation
choice of, 1195
contraindications to, 1193, 1194
equipment necessary for, 1193
levels of, 1193
role of, 1191
working without, 1192, 1193
Selective photothermolysis, 397
Sentinel lymph node (SLN), 477, 478
Sentinel lymph node biopsy (SLNB), 477, 478
for conjunctival and eyelid tumors, 478
evaluation, 480
feasibility, safety, and false-negative rate, 478
indications, 480, 481
risks, 480
SPECT/CT scan, 479
technique, 478–480
Septic CST, 680
clinical presentation, 680
neuroimaging, 680
outcomes and prognosis, 680, 681
treatment, 681, 682
Severe socket contracture, 1074, 1078, 1080, 1081
Sex chromosomes, 1115
Short scar lift, 394
Shotgun wadding, 1221
Sickle blade, 572
Sight-threatening disease, 983
Signal-to-noise ratio (SNR), 615
Silent sinus syndrome (SSS), 248, 879
diagnosis, 880
differential diagnosis, 881
epidemiology, 879
imaging, 881
pathophysiology, 879, 880
presentation, 880
treatment, 881, 882
Silicone, 375
Silicone intubation, 486

Silicone stents, 574, 575
Silicone tubes, 488, 489, 569, 574, 590, 597
Simple lacerations, 1210
Simple/pure microphthalmos, 1082, 1117
Sincipital encephalocele, 1129
Sinonasal carcinoma
  clinical pearls, 958
  clinical presentation, 958, 959
  computed tomography, 959
  histopathology, 959
  magnetic resonance imaging, 959
  prognosis, 959
  treatment, 959
Sinonasal fibrosarcomas, 920
Sinus cranialization, 720
Sinus histiocytosis, 534
Sinus obliteration, 720
Sinus of Maier, 513
Sinus tumors, 537
Sjogren's syndrome, 641, 643, 724, 754, 837
Skin, cancer therapy, 484, 485
Skin grafting, 864
Skin marking, 105
Skin redraping technique, 1152
Skin substitutes, 1228
Sliding tarsal flap, 448
Slowly progressive proptosis, 942
Smoker's lines, 366
Smoking, 1204
Socket dryness, 1058
Socket pain, 1060
Soft tissue augmentation, 367, 369, 374, 376
Soft tissue fillers, 1064
Soft tissue reconstruction, 864, 865
Soft-tissue trauma
  lid lacerations, 1316
  thermal burn, 1316
Solid orbital spheres, 1089
Solid tumors, 488
Solitary fibrous tumor (SFT), 737, 738, 827, 932, 933
  clinical pearls, 932
  clinical presentation, 932
  computed tomography, 932
  histopathology, 933
  magnetic resonance imaging, 933
  prognosis, 933
  treatment, 933
Solitary neurofibroma, 916, 917
  clinical pearls, 916
  clinical presentation, 916, 917
  computed tomography, 917
  histopathology, 917
  magnetic resonance imaging, 917
  prognosis, 917
  treatment, 917
Sonidegib, 425
SOX2 anophthalmia syndrome, 1118, 1119
Spastic disorders, 247
Spastic paretic hemifacial contracture (SPHC), 250
Sphenoid sinus, 10, 12, 667, 669, 677, 682, 684
Sphenoid wing meningioma, 918
  clinical pearls, 918
  clinical presentation, 918
  computed tomography, 918
  histopathology, 919
  magnetic resonance imaging, 918, 919
  prognosis, 919
  treatment, 919
Split-thickness skin grafts, 864, 865, 1228
Spontaneous emission, 397
Spontaneous granulation, 458
Squamous cell carcinoma (SCC), 425, 426, 459, 485, 497, 672, 736, 952, 959–961
  clinical pearls, 960
  clinical presentation, 426, 960
  computed tomography, 960
  histopathology, 961
  magnetic resonance imaging, 960, 961
  management, 426, 427
  MMS, 468, 469
  pathologic features, 425, 426
  prognosis, 961
  treatment, 961
Squamous cell carcinoma in situ, 468, 469
Squamous neoplasia, 433
  clinical presentation, 433, 434
  management, 434
  pathologic features, 433
Stable tear film, 505
Staphylococcus aureus, 681
Staphyloma, 622
Static rhytids, 359
Stem cell transplantation, 237
Stent, choice of, 561
Stereotactic fractionated radiotherapy, 912
Stereotactic surgery, 871, 873, 874
  basic technique, 874
  EM-based stereotaxy, 873
  history of, 872
  Kick EM navigation system, 873
Stereotaxy, 871
  benefits of, 874, 876
  in orbital surgery, 872, 873
  science of, 871, 872
Steroids, 510, 682
Stevens-Johnson syndrome, 233
Strabismus surgery, 1001, 1012, 1013, 1104, 1105, 1108
Stryker navigation system III, 873
Sturge-Weber Syndrome (SWS), 1140, 1141
Suborbicularis orbital fat (SOOF), 28, 395, 415
Subperiosteal and orbital abscesses, 642
Subperiosteal floor implant, 1065
Subperiosteal orbital abscess, 641
Sub-SMAS rhytidectomy, 392–394
Substrate graft, 1074
Subtotal exenteration, 863
Sump syndrome, 593, 598
Superficial injection, 364
Superficial musculoaponeurotic system (SMAS), 23, 24, 352, 367, 391, 393
Superior conjunctivoplasty-Mullerectomy procedure, 1059, 1061
Superior fornix reconstruction techniques, 1072
Superior oblique muscle, 621
Superior orbital fissure, 619
Superior sulcus deformity, 411, 1063
Superior symblepharon, 1148
Supernumerary (anlage) ducts, 517, 518
Superomedial orbital varix enlarging with valsalva, 901
Superotemporal migration, 1035
Surface coils, 615
Surgical thyroidectomy, 989, 990
Suscle-specific antigen (SMA), 924

Suspected metallic IOrbFBs, 1304–1306
Sweat gland tumors, 431
Swinging flashlight test, 1233
Sympathetic fibers, 621
Symptomatic diplopia, 1241
Symptomatic orbital vascular anomalies, 817
Symptomatic tearing, 593
Syndromic craniosynostosis, 1131
Synostosis, 1131
Synthetic hydroxyapatite implants, 1033, 1034
Syphilis, 679
Systemic anesthetics, 1195
Systemic corticosteroids, 923
Systemic lipoblastomas, 925
Systemic lupus erythematosus (SLE), 725, 835, 991
Systemic propranolol, 898
Systemic syndromes with lid colobomas, 1123, 1124

T

T cell lymphoma, 790, 791
Target Guided Surgery™ (TGS) navigation system, 873
Targeted immunotherapies, 991
Tarsoconjunctival flaps, 443, 444
Tarsorrhaphy, 1225–1227
Tear break-up time, 547
Tear drainage system abnormalities, 1230
Tear film, 505, 523
Tear production testing, 593
Tear pump function, 593
Tearing, 521
Telangiectasia, 424, 508
Telecanthus, 1126, 1151, 1152
Temporal forehead transposition flap, 454
Temporoparietal scalp approach, 1089
Teniposide, 908
Tenon's capsule, 41, 619
Tenon's flaps, 1068
Tenon's tissue, 1044
Tension pneumo-orbit, 1183
Tenzel semicircular rotation flap, 447, 1124
Teprotumumab, 992
Teratomas/teratomatous cyst, 838
Tessier's cleft # 3, 1151
Tessier's cleft # 4, 1151
Tessier's cleft number 8, 1153, 1154
Tessier's system, 1132
Tetanus prophylaxis, 1316
Tetanus toxoid, 1167, 1205
Tetracyclines, 510
Therapy-induced carcinogenesis, 487
Thermal eyelid burns, 1113, 1224
Thermal relaxation time (TRT), 398
Thermographic camera, 554
Thermography, 554
Thioamide drugs, 988
Thioamides, 988
Third cranial nerve palsy, 299
Third degree burns (full-thickness), 1224
Three-snip punctoplasty, 559
Thyroid carcinoma, 489
Thyroid eye disease (TED), 871, 874, 983, 984
  clinical features of, 983
  clinical monitoring and classification systems, 987, 988
  diagnosis and autoantigens in, 986, 987
  endocrine management of systemic Graves' disease
    radioactive iodine, 988, 989
    surgical thyroidectomy, 989, 990
    thioamide drugs, 988
  immunology, 984, 985
  lymphocytes, role of, 986
  medical management of
    antibody therapy, 991, 992
    conservative measures, 990
    corticosteroids, 990, 991
    targeted immunotherapies, 991
  orbital fibroblasts, 985, 986
  orbital radiotherapy, 992
  pathogenesis of, 984
  surgical management of, 1001, 1002
    eyelid surgery (*see* Eyelid surgery)
    orbital decompression (*see* Orbital decompression)
    strabismus surgery, 1012, 1013
  thyroid dysfunction in, 983
Thyroid function tests (TFTs), 987
Thyroid orbitopathy, 636, 638
Thyroid stimulating hormone (TSH), 609
Thyroid-stimulating immunoglobulin, 984
Tissue fixation, periocular tissues, 692
Tissue inhibitors of metalloproteinase (TIMP), 1204
Tissue motion stabilization, 383
Titanium, 1279
Tocilizumab, 992
Tolosa Hunt syndrome (THS), 129, 130, 678, 760
  clinical presentation, 678, 679
  neuroimaging, 679
  treatment, 679
Topical anesthetics, 1195, 1196
Topical phenylephrine, 1195
Total exenteration, 861, 862
Total thyroidectomy, 990
Tourette's syndrome, 124
Town-Brocks syndrome, 1127
Toxocara canis infection, 625
Tram-tracking, 911
Transcanalicular approaches, 598
Transcanalicular laser-assisted dacryocystorhinostomy
  outcomes, 590, 591
  patient selection, 589
  postopertative care, 590
  procedure, 589, 590
Transconjunctival approach, 1176
Transconjunctival entropion repair, 183, 184
Transcranial orbitotomy approach
  craniofacial preoperative prepping and draping, 717, 718
  frontozygomatic craniotomy, 717
  indication, 717
  inner table calvarial grafts, 719
  ophthalmic plastic surgeon, 717, 720
  orbital exposure and dissection, 717, 718
  reconstruction and closure, 719
  tumor debulking and orbital decompression, 717
Transforming growth factor-beta (TGF-β), 1202, 1204, 1205
Transient chemosis, 417
Transitional cell carcinoma, 502
Transitional meningioma, 912
Transmembrane protein 98 (TMEM98) gene, 1118
Transvenous access, 676
Transvenous embolization, 676
Trauma
  ocular, 630
  orbital radiology, 652
  parasellar syndromes, 671

Traumatic cranial neuropathies, 145
Traumatic globe rupture, 630
Traumatic injury, 537
Traumatic levator dehiscence, 1216
Traumatic optic neuropathy (TON), 853
  anterior and posterior form, 145
  anticoagulants management, 155–158
  chiasmal injury, 146
  direct TON, 145, 147–150
  incidence rate, 145
  indirect injury, 145–148
  Miller's classification, 145
  PITON (*see* Posterior indirect TON (PITON))
Traumatic orbital wall displacement, 1286
Traumatic ptosis, 301
Treacher-Collins-Franceschetti syndrome, 1123
Treacher Collins syndrome (TCS), 1123, 1132, 1153
Triamcinalone injection, 1060
Trichiasis, 540
  accidental or surgical lid margin trauma, 190
  causes, 189
  chronic blepharitis, 190
  cicatricial entropion, 190
  cilia incarnata, 189
  cryotherapy technique, 191, 192
  definition, 189
  electrolysis, 190, 191
  entropion and ectropion, 190
  focal trichiasis, 189
  laser technique, 192
  lash ptosis, 189
  lid splitting technique, 192, 193
  ocular irritation, 189
  pentagonal wedge excision and repair, 190
  seborrheic keratoses, 190
  surgical repair, 190
  treatment, 189
  upper lid lash ptosis, 190, 191
Trichomegaly, 489
Trigeminal nerve, 670
Trigeminal neuropathy, 724
Trimethoprim-sulfamethoxazole, 1166
Tripod fracture, 1266
Trisomy 13, 1121
Trisomy 21, 1138
Trochleitis, 758
Troutman's implant, 97
True tear, 510
Tuberous sclerosis (TS), 1139, 1140
Tuberous sclerosis complex (TSC) genes, 1139
Tukel syndrome, 1137
Tumorlike lesions, 643
Turbid secretions, meibomian glands with, 508, 509
Turkey gobbler, 391
Two-snip procedure, 1230
Tyndall effect, 368, 369, 374

U
Ultratine™ forehead fixation device, 356
Uncinate process, 578, 579
Undifferentiated carcinoma (UC), 959
Unilateral deprivation amblyopia, 1105
Unilateral tearing, 522
Upper eyelid blepharoplasty, 343, 409, 410, 413
  anesthesia, 327
  beauty evolution, 325
  central fat pad, 329
  crease fixation, 329, 330
  incision closure, 329
  incision marking, 327
  lid crease height in men, 327
  medial fat pad exposure, 329
  musculocutaneous flap removal, 328
  patient-centered approach, 325
  post-operative management, 329, 330
  pre-operative and post-operative brow lift, 326
  skin marking, 328
  surgical planning, 325–329
Upper eyelid colobomas, 1123, 1145, 1147, 1149, 1150
  with corneopalpebral/conjunctival adhesions, 1148
  craniofacial clefts numbers 11, 10 and 9, 1148
  isolated colobomas, 1147, 1148
  oculoauriculovertebral spectrum, 1148, 1149
  surgical repair, 1150
Upper eyelid defects, 441, 445
Upper eyelid ectropion, 1157
Upper eyelid entropion, 1156
Upper eyelid eversion associated with lid laxity, 1155
Upper eyelid margin
  large defects involving, 449, 450, 452, 454
  moderate defects involving, 445, 447, 449
  small defects, 445
Upper lid lash ptosis, 190
Upper respiratory tract infection (URI), 1194
Upper system obstructions, 515
Uveal melanoma, 762

V
V flap, 1226
Valsalva maneuver, 901
Valve of Hasner, 583, 588
Valve of Rosenmüller, 513, 529
Vancomycin, 681
Varices, 901, 902
  clinical pearls, 901
  clinical presentation, 901
  CT scan, 901, 902
  histopathology, 902
  magnetic resonance imaging, 902
  prognosis, 902
  treatment, 902
Vascular anomalies
  arteriovenous malformation, 817–819
  carotid-cavernous fistula, 827, 828
  cavernous hemangioma, 823, 825
  digital subtraction angiography, 817
  dynamic non-invasive imaging, 817
  hemangiopericytomas, 827
  infantile hemangiomas, 825–827
  lympho-venous malformation, 821–824
  MRI technology, 817
  optic nerve compression, 817
  solitary fibrous tumor, 827
  venous malformations, 819–822
Vascular endothelial growth factor (VEGF), 1202–1204
Vascularized osseocutaneous flaps, 865
Vascularized pedicle flaps, 88
Vascular lesions, 887
  angiosarcomas
    clinical pearls, 902
    clinical presentation, 902
    CT scan, 902
    histopathology, 903
    magnetic resonance imaging, 903

prognosis, 903
treatment, 903
capillary hemangiomas
clinical pearls, 896, 897
clinical presentation, 897
CT scan, 897
histopathology, 897
MRI, 897
prognosis, 898
treatment, 897, 898
cavernous hemangiomas
clinical pearls, 898
clinical presentation, 898
CT scan, 898
histopathology, 899
MRI, 898, 899
prognosis, 899
treatment, 899
lymphangiomas
clinical pearls, 899
clinical presentation, 899, 900
CT scan, 900
histopathology, 900, 901
magnetic resonance imaging, 900
prognosis, 901
treatment, 901
varices
clinical pearls, 901
clinical presentation, 901
CT scan, 901, 902
histopathology, 902
magnetic resonance imaging, 902
prognosis, 902
treatment, 902
Vascular parasellar syndromes, 673
Vascular tumors, 431
Velcro®, 1035
Venetian method, 1032
Venolymphatic malformations, 659, 660
Venous drainage, 673, 674
Venous malformations, 819–822
Verruca vulgaris, 532
Vertical buttresses, 1271, 1272
Vertical diplopia, 880
Vertical lip lines, 366
Vertical platysmal bands, 367
Vincristine, 908, 932, 937
Vision, inflammation, strabismus, and appearance/exposure (VISA) system, 988
Vision loss, 377
Vismodegib, 425
Visual deprivation, 1104
Visual evoked potential (VEP), 1085
Visual field testing, 304, 609
Visual loss, 884
Vitamin A (retinoic acid), 1204
Vitamin B1 (riboflavin), 1204
Vitamin B6 (pyridoxidine), 1204
Vitamin C (ascorbic acid), 1204
Vitamin K cream, 371
Volkmann's theory of ischemic contraction, 1244

W
Waardenburg anophthalmia syndrome, 1119, 1126, 1151, 1152
Warthin's tumor, 737
Wegener's granulomatosis (WG), 534, 594, 641, 648, 725, 752, 753, 887
See also Granulomatosis with polyangiitis (GPA)
Weil-Blakesley forceps, 572, 573
Westcott scissors, 559
White-eyed blowout fracture (WEBOF), 1172–1178, 1242
Whitnall's ligament, 42
Whitnall's tubercle, 1232
Whole genome sequencing, 1117
Wide local excision (WLE), 460, 461
Wound dehiscence, 413
Wound healing, 487
Wound tensile strength, 1203

X
Xanthelasma, 402, 403
Xeomin, 360, 362
Xeroderma pigmentosa, 1108
Xerophthalmia, 542
Xiidra, 511
X-linked dominant inheritance, 1116
X-linked microphthalmia syndromes, 1119
X-linked recessive inheritance, 1116

Z
Zinc chloride, 460
Zinc deficiency, 1204
Zone of coagulation, 1223
Zone of hyperemia, 1223
Zone of stasis, 1223, 1224
Zoster neuropathy, 684, 685
Zoster ophthalmoplegia, 685
Z-plasties and Y-V advancement flaps, 440, 1152
Zyderm, 372
Zygomaticofacial and zygomaticotemporal neurovascular bundles, 1233
Zygomaticomaxillary buttress, 1268, 1272
Zygomaticomaxillary complex (ZMC), 852
cantholysis, 1264, 1265
classifications, 1266
type I, 1266
type II, 1266
type III, 1266, 1267
type IV, 1267
complications, 1268, 1269
contraindications to surgery, 1265
floor fracture with infraorbital nerve damage, 1269
frequency, 1263
inferior orbital rim, 1264, 1265
inferior rectus muscle, 1264, 1265
lateral canthal dystopia, 1264
lateral canthotomy, 1264, 1265
malar flattening, 1264
non-contrast CT scans, 1264
orbital hemorrhage, 1264
post-operative orbital hemorrhage, 1268
role, 1263
surgery indications, 1264, 1265
treatment, 1267, 1268
Zygomatico-temporal complex fractures, 1238
Zygomaticus muscles, 365
Zygomaticus smile, 365
Zyplast, 372